GOODMAN and GILMAN's
The Pharmacological Basis
of Therapeutics

EDITORS

Alfred Goodman Gilman
M.D., Ph.D.

Professor and Chairman, Department of Pharmacology,
Southwestern Medical School, University of Texas
Health Science Center at Dallas, Dallas, Texas

Louis S. Goodman
M.A., M.D., D.Sc.(Hon.)

Distinguished Professor of Pharmacology,
University of Utah College of Medicine,
Salt Lake City, Utah

Theodore W. Rall
Ph.D., D.Med.(Hon.)

Professor of Pharmacology,
University of Virginia School of Medicine,
Charlottesville, Virginia

Ferid Murad
M.D., Ph.D.

Chief of Medicine, Veterans Administration
Medical Center, Palo Alto, California; Professor of
Medicine and Pharmacology, and Associate Chairman,
Department of Medicine, Stanford University School
of Medicine, Stanford, California

GOODMAN and GILMAN's
The Pharmacological Basis of Therapeutics

SEVENTH EDITION

MACMILLAN PUBLISHING COMPANY

New York

COLLIER MACMILLAN CANADA, INC.

Toronto

COLLIER MACMILLAN PUBLISHERS

London

In this textbook, reference to proprietary names of drugs is ordinarily made only in chapter sections dealing with preparations. Such names are given in SMALL-CAP TYPE, usually immediately following the official or nonproprietary titles. Proprietary names of drugs also appear in the Index.

PREFACE TO THE SEVENTH EDITION

T H E first edition of this textbook, published nearly 45 years ago, was written when basic pharmacology was not fully accepted as a meaningful or relevant biomedical discipline. The appearance of that book did much to change the picture. An eminent pharmacologist, commenting on the first edition many years after its publication, stated that it provided a renaissance or perhaps more properly the *naissance* of the teaching and practice of pharmacology. The second edition, published in the mid-1950s, reflected the immense impact of the post–World War II burgeoning of biomedical research. Subsequent editions have been written as multiauthored works—a reflection of the enormous change in the content, stature, and function of pharmacology; its role in the biomedical sciences; and its impact on the clinical sciences and rational therapeutics. The Preface to the First Edition is reprinted herein, because it clearly states the three primary objectives that have guided the writing of all subsequent editions. Adherence to these objectives has encouraged widespread and successful use of *Goodman and Gilman's The Pharmacological Basis of Therapeutics* by students and practitioners of medicine and other health professions, both in the United States and abroad.

Those familiar with previous editions of this textbook will immediately recognize the organization of the present volume, which remains largely intact from the sixth edition. Nevertheless, the revision of the text has been extensive. This is a reflection not only of the dozens of new therapeutic agents that have become available to the clinician during the past 5 years but also of tremendous advances in both basic pharmacology and the application of that knowledge to medical practice. It is increasingly necessary for the pharmacologist to be a complete biologist, versed in biochemistry, physiology, biophysics, cell biology, and molecular genetics. Technics developed by molecular biologists are now having a profound impact in pharmacology. Molecular cloning of DNA and biosynthesis of the encoded products permit large-scale production of agents such as human insulin and growth hormone. Of even greater significance, detailed information on the primary structure of important macromolecules has become available as a result. These proteins include receptors for acetylcholine and insulin, the voltage-sensitive sodium channel, the receptor for low-density lipoprotein, and many others. While this could not have been anticipated a decade ago, the next few years will see an explosion of such information. To follow will be the capability to predict the tertiary structure of such proteins and, ultimately, to design drugs to alter their functions selectively and predictably. Coupled with these advances have been similarly impressive strides in such areas as mechanisms of receptor function, transmembrane signaling events, regulation of second-messenger synthesis, and so forth. Discussion of such topics appears throughout the textbook. Increased knowledge of pharmacokinetics and its practical application have kept pace with advances in pharmacodynamics. One indication of this growth is the near doubling of the drugs for which detailed pharmacokinetic data are presented in Appendix II. These are just a few of the major trends that are emphasized in the seventh edition.

Most of the contributors to the sixth edition were able and anxious to participate in the current undertaking, and we are pleased with this loyalty. We also welcome several outstanding new authors. Two of us are delighted with the efforts of the two new editors of this volume, Theodore W. Rall and Ferid Murad.

In addition to paying tribute to our collaborators, we gratefully acknowledge the advice and help received from scores of individuals, too numerous to mention by name. However, special note is made of certain extraordinary efforts. Michele Ferguson reviewed all sections of the text on pharmaceutical preparations and dosage with skill and exceptional diligence. Dr. Murray Smigel catalyzed the passage of untold megabytes of text past the guardians of several computers. Our editorial assistants—Wendy Deaner, Jane Rall, and Kathryn Gilman—spent literally thousands of hours in the performance of countless tasks, almost all with outstanding good humor. The importance of their efforts cannot be overstated. We also note the special relationship between this textbook and Joan Carolyn Zulch, Publisher and Editor-in-Chief, Medical/Nursing/Health Sciences Department, Macmillan Publishing Company. Miss Zulch has edited this textbook for six editions over a period of more than 30 years.

Finally, we would like to record some of our feelings about Alfred Gilman, who wrote the first two editions of this textbook in collaboration with Louis S. Goodman and who served as an editor until his death in 1984. He was a gentle and unpretentious man; a kind and thoughtful colleague, friend, father. Alfred Gilman's major contributions to biology and medicine have been chronicled in detail by others; they spanned supervision of the first clinical trial of nitrogen mustard to the global review of drug efficacy undertaken by the National Academy of Sciences/National Research Council. He was committed to the integration of basic science and clinical medicine, particularly as a teacher, author, and editor. On the occasion of his receipt of an honorary degree in 1979, Dartmouth University President John Kemeny stated: "Far more than an isolated exercise in pharmacology, your book has provided for generations of students and practitioners the essential, but difficult, bridge between the basic medical sciences and the practice of medicine. Indeed, it could be said that long before the concept of an integrated curriculum became a popular educational philosophy in medical schools, it was a reality in the form of your textbook." We reaffirm this principle and dedicate this volume to the memory of Alfred Gilman.

ALFRED GOODMAN GILMAN
LOUIS S. GOODMAN
THEODORE W. RALL
FERID MURAD

PREFACE TO THE FIRST EDITION

T H R E E objectives have guided the writing of this book—the correlation of pharmacology with related medical sciences, the reinterpretation of the actions and uses of drugs from the viewpoint of important advances in medicine, and the placing of emphasis on the applications of pharmacodynamics to therapeutics.

Although pharmacology is a basic medical science in its own right, it borrows freely from and contributes generously to the subject matter and technics of many medical disciplines, clinical as well as preclinical. Therefore, the correlation of strictly pharmacological information with medicine as a whole is essential for a proper presentation of pharmacology to students and physicians. Furthermore, the reinterpretation of the actions and uses of well-established therapeutic agents in the light of recent advances in the medical sciences is as important a function of a modern textbook of pharmacology as is the description of new drugs. In many instances these new interpretations necessitate radical departures from accepted but outworn concepts of the actions of drugs. Lastly, the emphasis throughout the book, as indicated in its title, has been clinical. This is mandatory because medical students must be taught pharmacology from the standpoint of the actions and uses of drugs in the prevention and treatment of disease. To the student, pharmacological data per se are valueless unless he is able to apply his information in the practice of medicine. This book has also been written for the practicing physician, to whom it offers an opportunity to keep abreast of recent advances in therapeutics and to acquire the basic principles necessary for the rational use of drugs in his daily practice.

The criteria for the selection of bibliographic references require comment. It is obviously unwise, if not impossible, to document every fact included in the text. Preference has therefore been given to articles of a review nature, to the literature on new drugs, and to original contributions in controversial fields. In most instances, only the more recent investigations have been cited. In order to encourage free use of the bibliography, references are chiefly to the available literature in the English language.

The authors are greatly indebted to their many colleagues at the Yale University School of Medicine for their generous help and criticism. In particular they are deeply grateful to Professor Henry Gray Barbour, whose constant encouragement and advice have been invaluable.

Louis S. Goodman
Alfred Gilman

New Haven, Connecticut
November 20, 1940

CONTRIBUTORS

Baldessarini, Ross J., M.D. Professor of Psychiatry and in Neuroscience, Harvard Medical School; Interim Director, Mailman Laboratories for Psychiatric Research, McLean Hospital, Belmont, Massachusetts

Benet, Leslie Z., Ph.D. Professor and Chairman, Department of Pharmacy, School of Pharmacy, University of California, San Francisco, California

Bianchine, Joseph R., M.D., Ph.D. Clinical Professor, Department of Medicine, Ohio State University School of Medicine, Columbus, Ohio; Department of Clinical Research and Development, Hoffmann-LaRoche, Inc., Nutley, New Jersey

Bigger, J. Thomas, Jr., M.D. Professor of Medicine and Pharmacology, and Director of Cardiology, Columbia University College of Physicians and Surgeons, New York, New York

Blaschke, Terrence F., M.D. Associate Professor of Medicine and Pharmacology, and Chief, Division of Clinical Pharmacology, Stanford University School of Medicine, Stanford, California

Bloom, Floyd E., M.D. Member, Research Institute of Scripps Clinic, La Jolla, California

Brown, Michael S., M.D., D.Sc.(Hon.). Paul J. Thomas Professor of Genetics and Medicine, Southwestern Medical School, University of Texas Health Science Center at Dallas, Dallas, Texas

Brunton, Laurence L., Ph.D. Assistant Professor of Medicine, Division of Pharmacology, University of California, San Diego, School of Medicine, La Jolla, California

Calabresi, Paul, M.D. Professor and Chairman, Department of Medicine, Brown University; Physician-in-Chief, Roger Williams General Hospital, Providence, Rhode Island

Cohn, Victor H., Ph.D. Professor of Pharmacology, George Washington University Medical Center, Washington, D.C.

Corr, Peter B., Ph.D. Associate Professor of Pharmacology and Medicine, Washington University School of Medicine, St. Louis, Missouri

Coulston, Ann M., M.S., R.D. Research Dietitian, Stanford University Hospital; Lecturer, Department of Medicine, Stanford University School of Medicine, Stanford, California

Douglas, William W., M.D., Ch.B., F.R.S. Professor of Pharmacology, Yale University School of Medicine, New Haven, Connecticut

Finch, Clement A., M.D. Professor of Medicine, University of Washington School of Medicine, Seattle, Washington

Flower, Roderick J., D.Sc., Ph.D. Professor and Chairman, Department of Pharmacology, School of Pharmacy and Pharmacology, The University of Bath, Claverton Down, Bath, United Kingdom

Franz, Donald N., M.S., Ph.D. Professor of Pharmacology, University of Utah College of Medicine, Salt Lake City, Utah

Gilman, Alfred Goodman, M.D., Ph.D. Professor and Chairman, Department of Pharmacology, Southwestern Medical School, University of Texas Health Science Center at Dallas, Dallas, Texas

Goldstein, Joseph L., M.D., D.Sc.(Hon.). Paul J. Thomas Professor and Chairman, Department of Molecular Genetics, Southwestern Medical School, University of Texas Health Science Center at Dallas, Dallas, Texas

Greene, Nicholas M., M.D. Professor of Anesthesiology, Yale University School of Medicine, New Haven, Connecticut

Gross, Jeffrey B., M.D. Assistant Professor of Anesthesiology, University of Pennsylvania School of Medicine, Philadelphia, Pennsylvania

Harvey, Stewart C., Ph.D. Professor of Pharmacology, University of Utah College of Medicine, Salt Lake City, Utah

Haynes, Robert C., Jr., M.D., Ph.D. Professor of Pharmacology, University of Virginia School of Medicine, Charlottesville, Virginia

Hays, Richard M., M.D. Professor of Medicine and Director, Division of Nephrology, Albert Einstein College of Medicine of Yeshiva University, Bronx, New York

Hillman, Robert S., M.D. Professor of Medicine, University of Vermont College of Medicine, Burlington, Vermont; Chief of Medicine, Maine Medical Center, Portland, Maine

Hoffman, Brian F., M.D. David Hosack Professor of Pharmacology, Columbia University College of Physicians and Surgeons, New York, New York

Jaffe, Jerome H., M.D. Director, Addiction Research Center, National Institute on Drug Abuse; Alcohol, Drug Abuse, and Mental Health Administration, Baltimore, Maryland

Johnson, Eugene M., Jr., Ph.D. Professor of Pharmacology, Washington University School of Medicine, St. Louis, Missouri

Klaassen, Curtis D., Ph.D. Professor of Pharmacology and Toxicology, University of Kansas Medical Center, Kansas City, Kansas

Larner, Joseph, M.D., Ph.D., D.Sc.(Hon.). Alumni Professor and Chairman, Department of Pharmacology, University of Virginia School of Medicine, Charlottesville, Virginia

Mamelok, Richard D., M.D. Assistant Professor of Medicine and Pharmacology, Stanford University School of Medicine, Stanford, California

Mandel, H. George, Ph.D. Professor and Chairman, Department of Pharmacology, George Washington University Medical Center, Washington, D.C.

Mandell, Gerald L., M.D. Professor of Medicine, and Head, Division of Infectious Diseases, and Owen R. Cheatham Professor of the Sciences, University of Virginia School of Medicine, Charlottesville, Virginia

Marcus, Robert, M.D. Director, Aging Study Unit, Geriatrics Research, Education and Clinical Center, Veterans Administration Medical Center, Palo Alto, California; Associate Professor of Medicine, Stanford University School of Medicine, Stanford, California

Marshall, Bryan E., M.D., F.R.C.P. Horatio C. Wood Professor of Anesthesia, University of Pennsylvania School of Medicine, Philadelphia, Pennsylvania

Martin, William R., M.D. Professor and Chairman, Department of Pharmacology, University of Kentucky College of Medicine, Lexington, Kentucky

Moncada, Salvador, M.D., Ph.D., D.Sc. Director of the Therapeutic Research Division, The Wellcome Research Laboratories, Beckenham, Kent, United Kingdom

Mudge, Gilbert H., M.D. Emeritus Professor of Pharmacology and Medicine, Dartmouth Medical School, Hanover, New Hampshire

Murad, Ferid, M.D., Ph.D. Chief of Medicine, Veterans Administration Medical Center, Palo Alto, California; Professor of Medicine and Pharmacology, and Associate Chairman, Department of Medicine, Stanford University School of Medicine, Stanford, California

Needleman, Philip, Ph.D. Professor and Head, Department of Pharmacology, Washington University School of Medicine, St. Louis, Missouri

Nies, Alan S., M.D. Professor of Medicine and Pharmacology, and Head, Division of Clinical Pharmacology, University of Colorado School of Medicine, Denver, Colorado

O'Reilly, Robert A., M.D., F.A.C.P. Chairman, Department of Medicine, Santa Clara Valley Medical Center, San Jose, California; Professor of Medicine, Stanford University, Stanford, California; Clinical Professor of Medicine, University of California, San Francisco, California

Parks, Robert E., Jr., M.D., Ph.D. Professor of Medical Science, Brown University, Providence, Rhode Island

Pathak, Madhu A., B.Sc.(Hon.), M.B., M.Sc. (Tech), Ph.D. Senior Associate in Dermatology, Harvard Medical School and Massachusetts General Hospital, Boston, Massachusetts

Rall, Theodore W., Ph.D., D.Med.(Hon.). Professor of Pharmacology, University of Virginia School of Medicine, Charlottesville, Virginia

Ritchie, J. Murdoch, Ph.D., D.Sc., F.R.S. Eugene Higgins Professor of Pharmacology, Yale University School of Medicine, New Haven, Connecticut

Ross, Elliott M., Ph.D. Associate Professor of Pharmacology, Southwestern Medical School, University of Texas Health Science Center at Dallas, Dallas, Texas

Rudd, Peter, M.D. Associate Professor of Medicine (Clinical), Division of General Internal Medicine, Stanford University School of Medicine, Stanford, California

Sande, Merle A., M.D. Professor and Vice-Chairman, Department of Medicine, University of California School of Medicine, San Francisco; Chief, Medical Services, San Francisco General Hospital, San Francisco, California

Schleifer, Leonard S., M.D., Ph.D. Assistant Professor of Neurology, Cornell University Medical College; Assistant Attending Neurologist, New York Hospital, New York, New York

Sheiner, Lewis B., M.D. Professor of Laboratory Medicine and Medicine, University of California School of Medicine, San Francisco, California

Smith, Theodore Craig, M.D. Professor of Anesthesiology and Pharmacology, Stritch School of Medicine, Loyola University of Chicago, Maywood, Illinois

Swinyard, Ewart A., M.S., Ph.D., D.Sc. (Hon.). Professor Emeritus of Pharmacology and Former Dean, College of Pharmacy, and Professor Emeritus of Pharmacology, University of Utah College of Medicine, Salt Lake City, Utah

Taylor, Palmer, Ph.D. Professor and Head, Division of Pharmacology, Department of Medicine, University of California, San Diego, School of Medicine, La Jolla, California

Vane, John R., D.Sc., F.R.S. Group Research and Development Director, The Wellcome Foundation, Ltd., Beckenham, Kent, United Kingdom

Webster, Leslie T., Jr., M.D., Sc.D.(Hon.). John H. Hord Professor and Chairman, Department of Pharmacology, and Professor of Medicine, Case Western Reserve University School of Medicine, Cleveland, Ohio

Weiner, Irwin M., M.D. Professor of Pharmacology, State University of New York, Upstate Medical Center, Syracuse, New York

Weiner, Norman, M.D. Professor and Chairman, Department of Pharmacology, University of Colorado School of Medicine, Denver, Colorado

Wollman, Harry, M.D. Robert Dunning Dripps Professor and Chairman, Department of Anesthesia, and Professor of Pharmacology, University of Pennsylvania School of Medicine, Philadelphia, Pennsylvania

CONTENTS

SECTION
XIII

Chemotherapy of Neoplastic Diseases

SECTION
XIV

Drugs Acting on the Blood and the Blood-Forming Organs

SECTION
XV

Hormones and Hormone Antagonists

SECTION
XVI

The Vitamins

SECTION
XVII

Toxicology

GOODMAN and GILMAN's
The Pharmacological Basis
of Therapeutics

General Principles

INTRODUCTION

Leslie Z. Benet and Lewis B. Sheiner

In its entirety, *pharmacology* embraces the knowledge of the history, source, physical and chemical properties, compounding, biochemical and physiological effects, mechanisms of action, absorption, distribution, biotransformation and excretion, and therapeutic and other uses of drugs. Since a *drug* is broadly defined as any chemical agent that affects living processes, the subject of pharmacology is obviously quite extensive.

For the clinician and the student of health sciences, however, the scope of pharmacology is less expansive than indicated by the above definitions. The clinician is interested primarily in drugs that are useful in the prevention, diagnosis, and treatment of human disease. Study of the pharmacology of these drugs can be reasonably limited to those aspects that provide the basis for their rational clinical use. Secondarily, the clinician is also concerned with chemical agents that are not used in therapy but are commonly responsible for household and industrial poisoning as well as environmental pollution. Study of these substances is justifiably restricted to the general principles of prevention, recognition, and treatment of such toxicity or pollution. Finally, all health professionals share in the responsibility to help resolve the continuing sociological problem of the abuse of drugs.

The basic pharmacological concepts summarized in this section apply to the characterization, evaluation, and comparison of all drugs. A clear understanding of these principles is essential for the subsequent study of the individual drugs. The relationship between the dose of a drug given to a patient and the utility of that drug in treating the patient's disease is described by two basic areas of pharmacology: *pharmacokinetics* and *pharmacodynamics*. Operationally, these terms may be defined as what the body does to the drug (pharmacokinetics) and what the drug does to the body (pharmacodynamics).

Pharmacokinetics (Chapter 1) deals with the *absorption, distribution, biotransformation,* and *excretion* of drugs. These factors, coupled with dosage, determine the concentration of a drug at its sites of action and, hence, the intensity of its effects as a function of time. Many basic principles of biochemistry and enzymology and the physical and chemical principles that govern the active and passive transfer and the distribution of substances across biological membranes are readily applied to the understanding of this important aspect of pharmacology.

The study of the biochemical and physiological *effects* of drugs and their *mechanisms of action* is termed *pharmacodynamics* (Chapter 2). As a border science, pharmacodynamics borrows freely from both the subject matter and the experimental technics of physiology, biochemistry, cellular and molecular biology, microbiology, immunology, genetics, and pathology. It is unique mainly in that attention is focused on the characteristics of drugs. As the name implies, the subject is a dynamic one. The student who attempts merely to memorize the pharmacodynamic properties of drugs is foregoing one of the best opportunities for correlating the entire field of preclinical medicine. For example, the actions and effects of the saluretic agents can be fully understood only in terms of the basic principles of renal physiology and of the pathogenesis of edema. Conversely, great insight into normal and abnormal renal physiology can be gained by the study of the pharmacokinetics and pharmacodynamics of the saluretic agents.

The clinician is understandably interested mainly in the effects of drugs in man. This emphasis on *clinical pharmacology* is justified, since the effects of drugs are often characterized by significant interspecies variation, and since they may be further modified by disease. In addition, some drug effects, such as those on mood and behavior, can be adequately studied only in man. However, technical, legal, and ethical considerations limit pharmacological evaluation in man, and the choice of drugs must be based in part on their pharmacological evaluation in animals. Consequently, some knowledge of *animal pharmacology* and *comparative pharmacology* is helpful in deciding the extent to which claims for a drug based upon studies in animals can be reasonably extrapolated to man.

Pharmacotherapeutics (Chapter 3) deals with the use of drugs in the prevention and treatment of disease. Many drugs stimulate or depress biochemical or physiological function in man in a sufficiently reproducible manner to provide relief of symptoms or, ideally, to alter favorably the course of disease. Conversely, chemotherapeutic agents are useful in therapy because they have only minimal effects on man but can destroy or eliminate pathogenic cells or organisms.

Whether a drug is useful for therapy is crucially dependent upon its ability to produce its desired effects with only tolerable undesired effects. Thus, from the standpoint of the clinician interested in the therapeutic uses of a drug, the *selectivity* of its effects is one of its most important characteristics. Drug therapy is rationally based upon the correlation of the actions and effects of drugs with the physiological, biochemical, microbiological, immunological, and behavioral aspects of disease. In addition, disease may modify the pharmacokinetic properties of a drug by alteration of its absorption into the systemic circulation and/or its disposition.

Toxicology (Section XVII) is that aspect of pharmacology that deals with the adverse effects of drugs. It is concerned not only with drugs used in therapy but also with the many other chemicals that may be responsible for household, environmental, or industrial intoxication. The adverse effects of the pharmacological agents employed in therapy are properly considered an integral part of their total pharmacology. The toxic effects of other chemicals is such an extensive subject that the clinician must usually confine his attention to the general principles applicable to the prevention, recognition, and treatment of drug poisonings of any cause.

1 PHARMACOKINETICS: THE DYNAMICS OF DRUG ABSORPTION, DISTRIBUTION, AND ELIMINATION

Leslie Z. Benet and Lewis B. Sheiner

To produce its characteristic effects, a drug must be present in appropriate concentrations at its sites of action. Although obviously a function of the amount of drug administered, the concentrations attained also depend upon the extent and rate of its absorption, distribution, binding or localization in tissues, biotransformation, and excretion. These factors are depicted in Figure 1–1.

PHYSICOCHEMICAL FACTORS IN TRANSFER OF DRUGS ACROSS MEMBRANES

The absorption, distribution, biotransformation, and excretion of a drug all involve its passage across cell membranes. It is essential, therefore, to consider the mecha-nisms by which drugs cross membranes and the physicochemical properties of molecules and membranes that influence this transfer. Important characteristics of a drug are its molecular size and shape, solubility at the site of its absorption, degree of ionization, and relative lipid solubility of its ionized and nonionized forms.

When a drug permeates a cell, it must obviously traverse the cellular plasma membrane. Other barriers to drug movement may be a single layer of cells (intestinal epithelium) or several layers of cells (skin). Despite these structural differences, the diffusion and transport of drugs across these various boundaries have many common characteristics, since drugs in general pass through cells rather than between them. The plasma membrane thus represents the common barrier.

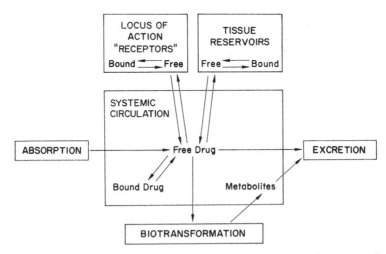

Figure 1–1. *Schematic representation of the interrelationship of the absorption, distribution, binding, biotransformation, and excretion of a drug and its concentration at its locus of action.*

Possible distribution and binding of metabolites are not depicted.

Cell Membranes. Initially, cell membranes were hypothesized to consist of a thin layer of lipid-like material interspersed with minute water-filled channels. Subsequent studies suggested that the plasma membrane consisted of a bilayer of amphipathic lipids, with their hydrocarbon chains oriented inward to form a continuous hydrophobic phase and their hydrophilic heads oriented outward. This hypothesis has been broadened to a more dynamic fluid-mosaic model, where globular protein molecules penetrate into either side of or entirely through a fluid phospholipid bilayer (Singer and Nicolson, 1972). Individual lipid molecules in the bilayer can move laterally, endowing the membrane with fluidity, flexibility, high electrical resistance, and relative impermeability to highly polar molecules. However, it is also appreciated that complexes of intrinsic membrane proteins and lipids can form either hydrophilic or hydrophobic channels that allow transport of molecules with different characteristics.

Passive Processes. Drugs cross membranes either by passive processes or by mechanisms involving the active participation of components of the membrane. In the former, the drug molecule usually penetrates by *passive diffusion* along a concentration gradient by virtue of its solubility in the lipid bilayer. Such transfer is directly proportional to the magnitude of the concentration gradient across the membrane and the lipid:water partition coefficient of the drug. The greater the partition coefficient, the higher is the concentration of drug in the membrane and the faster is its diffusion. After a steady state is attained, the concentration of the free drug is the same on both sides of the membrane, if the drug is a nonelectrolyte. For ionic compounds, the steady-state concentrations will be dependent on differences in pH across the membrane, which may influence the state of ionization of the molecule on each side of the membrane, and on the electrochemical gradient for the ion. Most biological membranes are relatively permeable to water, either by diffusion or by flow that results from hydrostatic or osmotic differences across the membrane. Such bulk flow of water can carry with it small, water-soluble substances. Most cell membranes permit passage only of water, urea, and other small, water-soluble molecules by this mechanism. Such substances generally do not pass through cell membranes if their molecular weights are greater than 100 to 200.

While most inorganic ions would seem to be sufficiently small to penetrate the membrane, their hydrated ionic radius is relatively large. The concentration gradient of many inorganic ions is largely determined by active transport (*e.g.,* sodium and potassium ions). The transmembrane potential determines the distribution of other ions (*e.g.,* chloride) across the membrane. Channels with selectivity for individual ions are often controlled to allow regulation of specific ionic fluxes. Such mechanisms are of obvious importance in the generation of action potentials in nerve and muscle (*see* Chapter 4) and in transmembrane signaling events (*see* Chapter 2).

Weak Electrolytes and Influence of pH. Most drugs are weak acids or bases that are present in solution as both the nonionized and ionized species, and they must pass membrane barriers by diffusion through the bilayer. The nonionized molecules are usually lipid soluble and can diffuse across the cell membrane. In contrast, the ionized fraction is usually unable to penetrate the lipid membrane because of its low lipid solubility.

The distribution of a weak electrolyte is usually determined by its pK_a and the pH gradient across the membrane. To illustrate the effect of pH on distribution of drugs, the partitioning of a weak acid ($pK_a = 4.4$) between plasma (pH = 7.4) and gastric juice (pH = 1.4) is depicted in Figure 1–2. It is assumed that the gastric mucosal membrane behaves as a simple lipid barrier that is permeable only to the lipid-soluble, nonionized form of the acid. The ratio of nonionized to ionized drug at each pH can be calculated from the Henderson-Hasselbalch equation. Thus, in plasma, the ratio of nonionized to ionized drug is 1:1000; in gastric juice, the ratio is 1:0.001. The total concentration ratio between the plasma and the gastric juice would therefore be

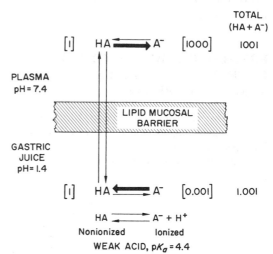

Figure 1–2. *Influence of pH on the distribution of a weak acid between plasma and gastric juice, separated by a lipid barrier.*

Only the nonionized moiety can readily penetrate the membrane; hence, it diffuses along its concentration gradient until, at steady state, its concentration is the same in both compartments. The degree of dissociation of the acid on each side depends on the pH of the plasma and gastric juice. The total concentration difference between the two sides is a direct function of the pH gradient across the membrane.

The values in brackets represent relative concentrations of the ionized and nonionized forms on each side of the membrane. The thick horizontal arrows point in the direction of the predominant form of the weak acid at the indicated pH.

1000:1 if such a system came to a steady state. For a weak base with a pK_a of 4.4 ($BH^+ \rightleftharpoons B + H^+$), the ratio would be reversed. These considerations have obvious implications for the absorption and excretion of drugs, as will be discussed more specifically below. The establishment of concentration gradients of weak electrolytes across membranes with a pH gradient is a purely physical process and does not require an active transport system. All that is necessary is a membrane preferentially permeable to one form of the weak electrolyte and a pH gradient across the membrane. The establishment of the pH gradient is, however, an active process.

Bulk flow through *intercellular pores* is the major mechanism of passage of drugs across most capillary endothelial membranes, with the important exception of the central nervous system (CNS) (*see* below). These intercellular gaps are sufficiently large that diffusion across most capillaries is limited by blood flow and not by the lipid solubility of drugs or pH gradients. This is an important factor in absorption of drugs after parenteral administration and in filtration across glomerular membranes in the kidney (*see* below). *Tight junctions* are characteristic of capillaries of the CNS and a variety of epithelia. Intercellular diffusion is consequently limited. *Pinocytosis,* the formation and movement of vesicles across cell membranes, has been implicated in drug absorption. However, the quantitative significance of pinocytosis is questionable.

Carrier-Mediated Membrane Transport. While passive diffusion through the bilayer is dominant in the absorption and distribution of most drugs, more active and selective mechanisms can play important roles. *Active transport* of some drugs occurs across neuronal membranes, the choroid plexus, renal tubular cells, and hepatocytes. The characteristics of active transport—selectivity, competitive inhibition by congeners, a requirement for energy, saturability, and movement against an electrochemical gradient—may be important in the mechanism of action of drugs that are subject to active transport or that interfere with the active transport of natural metabolites or neurotransmitters. The term *facilitated diffusion* describes a carrier-mediated transport process to which there is no input of energy, and movement of the substance in question thus cannot occur against an electrochemical gradient. Such mechanisms, which may also be highly selective for specific conformational structures of drugs, are necessary for the transport of endogenous compounds whose rate of movement across biological membranes by simple diffusion would otherwise be too slow.

DRUG ABSORPTION, BIOAVAILABILITY, AND ROUTES OF ADMINISTRATION

Absorption may be described as the rate at which a drug leaves its site of administration and the extent to which this occurs.

However, the clinician is primarily concerned with a parameter designated as *bioavailability,* rather than absorption. Bioavailability is a term used to indicate the extent to which a drug reaches its site of action *or* a biological fluid from which the drug has access to its site of action. For example, a drug that is absorbed from the stomach and intestine must first pass through the liver before it reaches the systemic circulation. If the drug is metabolized in the liver or excreted in the bile, some of the active drug will be inactivated before it can reach the general circulation and be distributed to its sites of action. If the metabolic or excretory capacity of the liver for the agent in question is great, bioavailability will be substantially decreased (the so-called first-pass effect). This decrease in availability is a function of the anatomical site from which absorption takes place; other anatomical, physiological, and pathological factors can influence bioavailability (*see* below), and the choice of the route of drug administration must be based on an understanding of these conditions. Moreover, factors that modify the absorption of a drug can change its bioavailability.

Factors That Modify Absorption. Many variables, in addition to the physicochemical factors that affect transport across membranes, influence the absorption of drugs. Absorption, regardless of the site, is dependent upon drug *solubility.* Drugs given in aqueous solution are more rapidly absorbed than those given in oily solution, suspension, or solid form because they mix more readily with the aqueous phase at the absorptive site. For those given in solid form, the rate of *dissolution* may be the limiting factor in their absorption. Local conditions at the site of absorption alter solubility, particularly in the gastrointestinal tract. Aspirin, which is relatively insoluble in acidic gastric contents, is a common example of such a drug. The *concentration* of a drug influences its rate of absorption. Drugs ingested or injected in solutions of high concentration are absorbed more rapidly than are drugs in solutions of low concentration. The *circulation to the site of absorption* also affects drug absorption. Increased blood flow, brought about by massage or local application of heat, enhances absorption of a drug; decreased blood flow, produced by vasoconstrictor agents, shock, or other disease factors, can slow absorption. The area of the *absorbing surface* to which a drug is exposed is one of the more important determinants of the rate of drug absorption. Drugs are absorbed very rapidly from large surface areas such as the pulmonary alveolar epithelium, the intestinal mucosa, or, in a few cases after extensive application, the skin. The absorbing surface is determined largely by the *route of administration*. Each of these factors separately or in conjunction with one another may have profound effects on the efficacy and toxicity of a drug.

Enteral (Oral) vs. Parenteral Administration. Often there is a choice of the route by which a therapeutic agent may be given, and a knowledge of the advantages and disadvantages of the different routes of administration is then of primary importance. Some characteristics of the major routes employed for systemic drug effect are compared in Table 1–1.

Oral ingestion is the most common method of drug administration. It is also the safest, most convenient, and most economical. Disadvantages to the oral route include emesis as a result of irritation to the gastrointestinal mucosa, destruction of some drugs by digestive enzymes or low gastric pH, irregularities in absorption or propulsion in the presence of food or other drugs, and necessity for cooperation on the part of the patient. In addition, drugs in the gastrointestinal tract may be metabolized by the enzymes of the mucosa, the intestinal flora, or the liver before they gain access to the general circulation.

The parenteral injection of drugs has certain distinct advantages over oral administration. In some instances, parenteral administration is essential for the drug to be absorbed in active form. Absorption is usually more rapid and more predictable than when a drug is given by mouth. The effective dose can therefore be more accurately selected. In emergency therapy, parenteral administration is particularly serviceable. If a patient is unconscious, uncooperative, or unable to retain anything given by mouth, parenteral therapy may become a necessity. The injection of drugs also has its disadvantages. Asepsis must be maintained to avoid infection, an intravascular injection

Table 1–1. SOME CHARACTERISTICS OF COMMON ROUTES OF DRUG ADMINISTRATION *

ROUTE	ABSORPTION PATTERN	SPECIAL UTILITY	LIMITATIONS AND PRECAUTIONS
Intravenous	Absorption circumvented Potentially immediate effects	Valuable for emergency use Permits titration of dosage Suitable for large volumes and for irritating substances, when diluted	Increased risk of adverse effects Must inject solutions *slowly*, as a rule Not suitable for oily solutions or insoluble substances
Subcutaneous	Prompt, from aqueous solution Slow and sustained, from repository preparations	Suitable for some insoluble suspensions and for implantation of solid pellets	Not suitable for large volumes Possible pain or necrosis from irritating substances
Intramuscular	Prompt, from aqueous solution Slow and sustained, from repository preparations	Suitable for moderate volumes, oily vehicles, and some irritating substances	Precluded during anticoagulant medication May interfere with interpretation of certain diagnostic tests (*e.g.,* creatine phosphokinase)
Oral ingestion	Variable; depends upon many factors (*see* text)	Most convenient and economical; usually more safe	Requires patient cooperation Availability potentially erratic and incomplete for drugs that are poorly soluble, slowly absorbed, unstable, or extensively metabolized by the liver

* *See* text for more complete discussion and for other routes.

may occur when it is not intended, pain may accompany the injection, and it is sometimes difficult for a patient to perform the injection himself if self-medication is a necessary procedure. Expense is another consideration.

Oral Ingestion. Absorption from the gastrointestinal tract is governed by factors that are generally applicable, such as surface area for absorption, blood flow to the site of absorption, the physical state of the drug, and its concentration at the site of absorption. Since most drug absorption from the gastrointestinal tract occurs via passive processes, absorption is favored when the drug is in the nonionized and more lipophilic form. Thus, one might expect the absorption of weak acids to be optimal in the acidic environment of the stomach, whereas absorption of bases might be favored in the relatively alkaline small intestine. However, it is an oversimplification to extrapolate the pH-partition concept presented in Figure 1–2 to a comparison of two different biological membranes, such as the epithelia of the stomach and the intestine. The stomach is lined by a thick, mucus-covered membrane with small surface area and high electrical resistance. The primary function of the stomach is digestive. In contrast, the epithelium of the intestine has an extremely large surface area; it is thin, it has low electrical resistance, and it serves the primary function of facilitating the absorption of nutrients. Thus, any factor that accelerates gastric emptying will be likely to increase the rate of drug absorption, while any factor that delays gastric emptying will probably have the opposite effect. The experimental data available from the classical work of Brodie (1964) and more recent studies (Prescott and Nimmo, 1981) are all consistent with the following conclusion: the nonionized form of a drug will be absorbed more rapidly than the ionized form at any particular site in the gastrointestinal tract. However, the rate of absorption of a drug from the intestine will be greater than that from the stomach even if the drug is predominantly ionized in the intestine and largely nonionized in the stomach.

Drugs that are destroyed by gastric juice or that cause gastric irritation are sometimes administered in dosage forms with a coating that prevents dissolution in the acidic gastric contents. However, some *enteric-coated* preparations of a drug also may resist dissolution in the intestine, and very little of the drug may be absorbed.

Controlled-Release Preparations. The rate of absorption of a drug administered as a tablet or other solid oral-dosage form is partly dependent upon its rate of dissolution in the gastrointestinal fluids. This factor is the basis for the so-called *controlled-release, timed-release, sustained-release,* or *prolonged-action* pharmaceutical preparations that are designed to produce slow, uniform absorption of the drug for 8 hours or longer. Potential advantages of such preparations are reduction in the frequency of administration of the drug as compared with conventional dosage forms, possibly with improved compliance by the patient, maintenance of a therapeutic effect overnight, and decreased incidence of undesired effects by elimination of the peaks in drug concentration that often occur after administration of other dosage forms.

Some controlled-release preparations fulfill these theoretical expectations. Unfortunately, not all marketed preparations are reliable. The dissolution rate of some preparations in gastrointestinal fluid may be quite irregular because of technical problems associated with their manufacture or because of variations in gastrointestinal pH, gastric emptying, intestinal motility, and other physiological factors that influence drug absorption. Moreover, slow absorption from the gastrointestinal tract is often incomplete and erratic. In addition, each drug must be evaluated separately for its suitability as a controlled-release preparation. Drugs given for a brief therapeutic effect should not be in the controlled-release form. Conversely, controlled-release preparations are not needed for drugs with an inherent long duration of effect. Also, controlled-release preparations of some drugs might not be safe. Since the total dose of drug ingested at one time may be several times the dose of the conventional form of the drug, faulty release of the entire amount at once could lead to toxicity. Finally, failure of adequate release may compromise the therapeutic effect. It is thus incumbent on the clinician who uses preparations of this type to establish a need for a controlled-release preparation and also to assure himself of its uniformity, reliability, and safety. This is especially necessary since the controlled-release formulations of different manufacturers may vary considerably from each other.

Sublingual Administration. Absorption from the oral mucosa has special significance for certain drugs, despite the fact that the surface area available is small. For example, nitroglycerin is effective when retained sublingually because it is nonionic and has a very high lipid solubility. The drug is also very *potent;* relatively few molecules need to be absorbed to produce the therapeutic effect.

Since venous drainage from the mouth is to the superior vena cava, the drug is also protected from rapid first-pass metabolism by the liver. Hepatic first-pass metabolism is sufficient to *prevent* the appearance of any active nitroglycerin in the systemic circulation if the conventional tablet is swallowed.

Rectal Administration. The rectal route is often useful when oral ingestion is precluded by vomiting or when the patient is unconscious. Approximately 50% of the drug that is absorbed from the rectum will pass through the liver before entry into the systemic circulation; the potential for hepatic first-pass metabolism is thus less than that for an oral dose. However, rectal absorption is often irregular and incomplete, and many drugs cause irritation of the rectal mucosa.

Parenteral Injection. The major routes of parenteral administration are intravenous, subcutaneous, and intramuscular. Absorption from subcutaneous and intramuscular sites occurs by simple diffusion along the gradient from drug depot to plasma. The rate is limited by the area of the absorbing capillary membranes and by the solubility of the substance in the interstitial fluid. Relatively large aqueous channels in the endothelial membrane account for the indiscriminate diffusion of molecules regardless of their lipid solubility. Larger molecules, such as proteins, slowly gain access to the circulation by way of lymphatic channels.

Drugs administered into the systemic circulation by any route, excluding the intra-arterial, are subject to possible first-pass elimination in the lung prior to distribution to the rest of the body. The lungs serve as a temporary clearing site for a number of agents, especially basic compounds, apparently by their partition into lipid. The lungs also serve as a filter for particulate matter that may be given intravenously, and, of course, they provide a route of elimination for volatile substances.

Intravenous. The factors concerned in absorption are circumvented by intravenous injection of drugs in aqueous solution, and the desired concentration of a drug in blood is obtained with an *accuracy* and *immediacy* not possible by any other procedure. In some instances, as in the induction of surgical anesthesia by a barbiturate, the dose of a drug is not predetermined but is adjusted to the response of the patient.

Also, certain irritating solutions can be given only in this manner, for the blood vessel walls are relatively insensitive and the drug, if injected slowly, is greatly diluted by the blood.

As there are assets to the use of this route of administration, so are there liabilities. Unfavorable reactions are prone to occur, since high concentrations of drug may be attained rapidly in both plasma and tissues. Once the drug is injected there is no retreat. Repeated intravenous injections are dependent upon the ability to maintain a patent vein. Drugs in an oily vehicle or those that precipitate blood constituents or hemolyze erythrocytes should not be given by this route. *Intravenous injection must usually be performed slowly and with constant monitoring of the responses of the patient.*

Subcutaneous. Injection into a subcutaneous site is often utilized for the administration of drugs. It can be used only for drugs that are not irritating to tissue; otherwise, severe pain, necrosis, and slough may occur. The rate of absorption following subcutaneous injection of a drug is often sufficiently constant and slow to provide a sustained effect. Moreover, it may be varied intentionally. For example, the rate of absorption of a suspension of insoluble insulin is slow compared with that of a soluble preparation of the hormone. The incorporation of a vasoconstrictor agent in a solution of a drug to be injected subcutaneously also retards absorption. Absorption of drugs implanted under the skin in a solid pellet form occurs slowly over a period of weeks or months; some hormones are effectively administered in this manner.

Intramuscular. Drugs in aqueous solution are absorbed quite rapidly after intramuscular injection, depending upon the rate of blood flow to the injection site. Joggers who inject insulin into their thigh may experience a precipitous drop in blood sugar that is not seen following injection into the arm or abdominal wall, since running markedly increases blood flow to the leg. Generally the rate of absorption following injection of an aqueous preparation into the deltoid or vastus lateralis is faster than when the injection is made into the gluteus maximus. The rate is particularly slower for females after injection into the gluteus maximus. This has been attributed to the different distribution of subcutaneous fat in males and females, since fat is relatively poorly perfused. Very obese or emaciated patients may exhibit unusual patterns of absorption following intramuscular or subcutaneous injection. Very slow, constant absorption from the intramuscular site results if the drug is injected in solution in oil or suspended in various other repository vehicles. Penicillin is often administered in this manner. Substances too irritating to be injected subcutaneously may sometimes be given intramuscularly.

Intra-arterial. Occasionally a drug is injected directly into an artery to localize its effect in a particular tissue or organ. However, this practice usually has dubious therapeutic value. Diagnostic agents are sometimes administered by this route. Intra-arterial injection requires great care and should be reserved for experts. The first-pass and cleansing effects of the lung are not available when drugs are given by this route.

Intrathecal. The blood-brain barrier and the blood–cerebrospinal fluid barrier often preclude or slow the entrance of drugs into the CNS. Therefore, when local and rapid effects of drugs on the meninges or cerebrospinal axis are desired, as in spinal anesthesia or acute CNS infections, drugs are sometimes injected directly into the spinal subarachnoid space.

Intraperitoneal. The peritoneal cavity offers a large absorbing surface from which drugs enter the circulation rapidly, but primarily by way of the portal vein; first-pass hepatic losses are thus possible. Intraperitoneal injection is a common laboratory procedure, but it is seldom employed clinically. The dangers of infection and adhesions are too great to warrant the routine use of this route in man.

Pulmonary Absorption. Gaseous and volatile drugs may be inhaled and absorbed through the pulmonary epithelium and mucous membranes of the respiratory tract. Access to the circulation is rapid by this route, because the surface area is large. The principles governing absorption and excretion of the anesthetic gases and vapors are discussed in Chapter 13.

In addition, solutions of drugs can be atomized and the fine droplets in air (aerosol) inhaled. Advantages are the almost instantaneous absorption of a drug into the blood, avoidance of hepatic first-pass loss, and, in the case of pulmonary disease, local application of the drug at the desired site of action. For example, epinephrine can be given in this manner for the treatment of bronchial asthma. The main disadvantages are poor ability to regulate the dose, cumbersomeness of the methods of administration, and the fact that many gaseous and volatile drugs produce irritation of the pulmonary epithelium.

Pulmonary absorption is an important route of entry of toxic environmental substances of varied composition and physical states (*see* Section XVII). Both local and systemic reactions to allergens may occur subsequent to inhalation; the lung is thus the target of action of numerous pharmacological agents.

Topical Application. *Mucous Membranes.* Drugs are applied to the mucous membranes of the conjunctiva, nasopharynx, oropharynx, vagina, colon, urethra, and urinary bladder primarily for their local effects. Occasionally, as in the application of antidiuretic hormone to the nasal mucosa, systemic absorption is the goal. Absorption through mucous membranes occurs readily. In fact, local anesthetics applied for local effect may sometimes be absorbed so rapidly that they produce systemic toxicity.

Skin. Few drugs readily penetrate the intact skin. Absorption of those that do is proportional to the surface area over which they are applied and to their lipid solubility, since the epidermis behaves as a lipid barrier. The dermis, however, is freely permeable to many solutes; consequently, systemic absorption of drugs occurs much more readily through abraded, burned, or denuded skin. Inflammation and other conditions that increase cutaneous blood flow also enhance absorption. Toxic effects are sometimes produced by absorption through the skin of highly lipid-soluble substances (*e.g.,* a lipid-soluble insecticide in an organic solvent). Absorption through the skin can be enhanced by suspending the drug in an oily vehicle and rubbing the resulting preparation into the skin. This method of administration is known as *inunction.* Because hydrated skin is more permeable than dry skin, the dosage form may be modified or an occlusive dressing may be used to facilitate absorption. Controlled-release topical patches are recent innovations. A patch containing scopolamine, placed behind the ear where body temperature and blood flow enhance absorption, releases sufficient drug to the systemic circulation to protect the wearer from motion sickness. Patches containing nitroglycerin are utilized to provide sustained delivery of a drug that is subject to extensive first-pass metabolism after oral administration (*see* Wester and Maibach, 1983).

Eye. Topically applied ophthalmic drugs are used primarily for their local effects. Systemic absorption that results from drainage through the nasolacrimal canal is usually undesirable. In addition, drug that is absorbed after such drainage is not subject to first-pass hepatic elimination. Systemic toxicity may occur for this reason when β-adrenergic antagonists are administered as ophthalmic drops. Local effects usually require absorption of the drug through the cornea; corneal infection or trauma may thus result in more rapid absorption. Ophthalmic delivery systems that provide prolonged duration of action (*e.g.,* suspensions and ointments) are useful additions to ophthalmic therapy. Ocular inserts, developed more recently, have been very successful. They provide continuous delivery of low amounts of drug. Very little is lost through drainage and, hence, systemic side effects are minimized.

Bioequivalence. Pharmaceutical formulations of a drug are termed *chemically equivalent* if they meet the chemical and physical standards established by governmental or other regulatory agencies. They are said to be *biologically equivalent* if they yield similar concentrations of drug in blood and tissues, and they are designated *therapeutically equivalent* if they provide equal therapeutic benefit in clinical trial. Pharmaceutical preparations that are chemically equivalent but not biologically or therapeutically equivalent are said to differ in their *bioavailability*. Dosage forms of a drug from different manufacturers and even different lots of preparations from a single manufacturer sometimes differ in their bioavailability. Such differences are seen primarily among oral dosage forms of poorly soluble, slowly absorbed drugs. They result from differences in crystal form, particle size, or other physical characteristics of the drug that are not rigidly controlled in formulation and manufacture of the preparations. These factors affect disintegration of the dosage form and dissolution of the drug and, hence, rate and extent of drug absorption.

Biological nonequivalence of different drug preparations is a particularly acute problem because bioavailability of a preparation in man does not always correlate with laboratory tests of tablet dissolution or with tests of bioavailability in animals. Biological nonequivalence of practical importance has been detected among the preparations of a number of important drugs, including the cardiac glycoside digoxin and several antibiotics. Responsible drug manufacturers, interested medical and pharmaceutical scientists, and governmental agencies are cooperating to speed resolution of the problem by establishing tests for bioavailability of pharmaceutical preparations in man and by devising *in-vitro* tests for drug dissolution that have satisfactory predictive value. The significance of possible nonequivalence of drug preparations is further discussed in connection with drug nomenclature and the choice of drug name in prescription order writing (*see* Appendix I; Berliner *et al.*, 1974; American Pharmaceutical Association, 1978).

DISTRIBUTION OF DRUGS

After a drug is absorbed or injected into the bloodstream, it may be distributed into interstitial and cellular fluids. Patterns of drug distribution reflect certain physiological factors and physicochemical properties of drugs. An initial phase of distribution may be distinguished that reflects cardiac output and regional blood flow. Heart, liver, kidney, brain, and other highly perfused organs receive most of the drug during the first few minutes after absorption. Delivery of drug to muscle, most viscera, skin, and fat is slower, and these tissues may require several minutes to several hours before equilibration is attained. A second phase of drug distribution may therefore be distinguished; this is also limited by blood flow, and it involves a far larger fraction of the body mass than does the first phase. Superimposed on patterns of distribution of blood flow are factors that determine the rate at which drugs diffuse into tissues. Diffusion into the interstitial compartment occurs rapidly, because of the highly permeable nature of capillary endothelial membranes (except in brain). Lipid-insoluble drugs that permeate membranes poorly are restricted in their distribution and, hence, in their potential sites of action. Distribution may also be limited by drug binding to plasma proteins, particularly albumin for acidic drugs and α_1-acid glycoprotein for basic drugs. An agent that is totally and strongly bound has no access to cellular sites of action, nor can it be metabolized and eliminated. Drugs may accumulate in tissues in higher concentrations than would be expected from diffusion equilibrium as a result of pH gradients, binding to intracellular constituents, or partitioning into lipid.

Drug that has accumulated in a given tissue may serve as a reservoir that prolongs drug action in that same tissue or at a distant site reached through the circulation. An example that illustrates many of these factors is the use of the intravenous anesthetic thiopental, a very lipid-soluble drug. Because blood flow to the brain is so high, the drug reaches its maximal concentration in brain within a minute after it is injected intravenously. After injection is concluded, the plasma concentration falls as thiopental diffuses into other tissues such as muscle. The concentration of the drug in brain follows that of the plasma, because there is little binding of the drug to brain constituents. Thus, onset of anesthesia is rapid, but so is its termination. Both are directly related to the concentration of the drug in brain. A third phase of distribution for this drug is due to the slow, blood flow–limited uptake by fat. With administration of successive doses of thiopental, accumulation of drug takes place in fat and other tissues that can store large amounts of the compound. These can become reservoirs for the maintenance of the plasma concentration, and, therefore, the brain concentration at or above the threshold required for anesthesia. Thus, a drug that is short acting because of rapid *redistribution* to sites at which the agent has no pharmacological action can become long acting when these storage sites are "filled" and termination of the drug's action becomes dependent on biotransformation and excretion (*see* Benet, 1978).

Since the pH difference between intracellular and extracellular fluids is small (7.0 vs. 7.4), this factor can result in only a relatively small concentration gradient of drug across the plasma membrane. Weak bases are concentrated slightly inside of cells, while the concentration of weak acids is slightly lower in the cells than in extracellular fluids. Lowering the pH of extracellular fluid increases the intracellular concentration of weak acids and decreases that of weak bases, provided that the intracellular pH does not also change and that the pH change does not simultaneously affect the binding, biotransformation, or excretion of the drug. Elevating the pH produces the opposite effects (*see* Figure 1–2).

Central Nervous System and Cerebrospinal Fluid. The distribution of drugs to the CNS from the blood stream is unique, mainly in that entry of drugs into the CNS extracellular space and cerebrospinal fluid is restricted. The restriction is similar to that across the gastrointestinal epithelium. Endothelial cells of the brain capillaries differ from their counterparts in most tissues by the absence of intercellular pores and pinocytotic vesicles. Tight junctions predominate, and aqueous bulk flow is thus severely restricted. This is not unique to the CNS capillaries (tight junctions appear in many muscle capillaries as well). It is likely that the unique arrangement of pericapillary glial cells also contributes to the slow diffusion of organic acids and bases into the CNS. The drug molecules probably must traverse not only endothelial but also perivascular cell membranes before reaching neurons or other drug target cells in the CNS. Cerebral blood flow is the only limitation to permeation of the CNS by highly lipid-soluble drugs. With increasing polarity the rate of diffusion of drugs into the CNS is proportional to the lipid solubility of the nonionized species (*see* Rall in the volume edited by La Du *et al.*, 1971). Strongly ionized agents such as quaternary amines or the penicillins are normally unable to enter the CNS from the circulation.

In addition, organic ions are extruded from the cerebrospinal fluid into blood at the choroid plexus by transport processes similar to those in the renal tubule. Lipid-soluble substances leave the brain by diffusion through the capillaries and the blood–choroid plexus boundary. Drugs and endogenous metabolites, regardless of lipid solubility and molecular size, also exit with bulk flow of the cerebrospinal fluid through the arachnoid villi.

The blood-brain barrier is adaptive in that exclusion of drugs and other foreign agents such as penicillin or *d*-tubocurarine protects the CNS against severely toxic effects. However, the barrier is neither absolute nor invariable. Very large doses of penicillin may produce seizures; meningeal or encephalic inflammation increases the local permeability. Maneuvers to increase permeability of the blood-brain barrier are potentially important to enhance the efficacy of chemotherapeutic agents that are used to treat infections or tumors localized in the brain.

Drug Reservoirs. As mentioned, the body compartments in which a drug accumulates are potential reservoirs for the drug. If stored drug is in equilibrium with that in plasma and is released as the plasma concentration declines, a concentration of the drug in plasma and at its locus of action is sustained, and pharmacological effects of the drug are prolonged. However, if the reservoir for the drug has a large capacity and fills rapidly, it so alters the distribution of the drug that larger quantities of the drug are required initially to provide a therapeutically effective concentration in the target organ.

Plasma Proteins. Many drugs are bound to plasma proteins, mostly to plasma albumin for acidic drugs and to α_1-acid glycoprotein for basic drugs; binding to other plasma proteins generally occurs to a much smaller extent. The binding is usually reversible; covalent binding of reactive drugs such as alkylating agents occurs occasionally.

The fraction of total drug in plasma that is bound is determined by the drug concentration, its affinity for the binding sites, and the number of binding sites. Simple mass-action equations are used to describe the free and bound concentrations. At low concentrations of drug (less than the plasma protein–binding dissociation constant), the fraction bound is a function of the concentration of binding sites and the dissociation constant. At high drug concentrations (greater than the dissociation constant), the fraction bound is a function of the number of binding sites and the drug concentration. Therefore, statements that a given drug is bound to a specified extent only apply over a limited range of concentrations. The percentage values listed in Appendix II refer only to the therapeutic range of concentrations for each drug.

Binding of a drug to plasma proteins limits its concentration in tissues and at its locus of action, since only unbound drug is in equilibrium across membranes. Binding also limits glomerular filtration of the drug, since this process does not immediately change the concentration of free drug in the plasma (water is also filtered). However, plasma protein binding does *not* generally limit renal tubular secretion or biotransformation, since these processes lower the free drug concentration, and this is rapidly followed by dissociation of the drug-protein complex. If a drug is avidly transported or metabolized and its clearance, calculated on the basis of unbound drug, exceeds organ plasma flow, binding of the drug to plasma protein may be viewed as a transport mechanism that fosters drug elimination by delivering drug to sites for elimination.

Since binding of drugs to plasma proteins is rather nonselective, many drugs with similar physicochemical characteristics compete with each other and with endogenous substances for these binding sites. For example, displacement of unconjugated bilirubin from binding to albumin by the sulfonamides and other organic anions is known to increase the risk of bilirubin encephalopathy in the newborn, and drug toxicity has sometimes been attributed to similar competition between drugs for binding sites. Such interactions are often more complex than generally stated. Since drug displaced from plasma protein will redistribute into its full potential volume of distribution, the concentration of free drug in plasma and tissues after redistribution may be increased only slightly. The interaction may also involve altered elimination of the drug. Risk of adverse effect is greatest if the displaced drug has a limited volume of distribution, if the competition extends to the drug bound in tissues, if elimination of the drug is also reduced, or if the displacing drug is administered in high dosage by rapid intravenous injection. Competition of drugs for plasma protein binding sites may also cause misinterpretation of measured concentrations of drugs in serum.

Cellular Reservoirs. Many drugs accumulate in muscle and other cells in higher concentrations than in the extracellular fluids. If the intracellular concentration is high and if the binding is reversible, the tissue involved may represent a sizable drug reservoir, particularly if the tissue represents a large fraction of body mass. For example, during chronic administration of the antimalarial agent quinacrine, the concentration of the drug in liver may be several thousand times that in plasma. Accumulation in cells may be the result of active transport or, more commonly, binding. Tissue binding of drugs usually occurs with proteins, phospholipids, or nucleoproteins and is generally reversible.

Fat as a Reservoir. Many lipid-soluble drugs are stored by physical solution in the neutral fat. In obese persons, the fat content of the body may be as high as 50%, and even in starvation it constitutes 10% of body weight; hence, fat can serve as an important reservoir for lipid-soluble drugs. For example, as much as 70% of the highly lipid-soluble barbiturate thiopental may be present in body fat 3 hours after administration. However, fat is a rather stable reservoir because it has a relatively low blood flow.

Bone. The tetracycline antibiotics (and other divalent-metal-ion chelating agents) and heavy metals may accumulate in bone by adsorption onto the bone-crystal surface and eventual incorporation into the crystal lattice. Bone can become a reservoir for the slow release of toxic agents such as lead or radium into the blood. Their effects can thus persist long after exposure has ceased. Local destruction of the bone medulla may also lead to reduced blood flow and prolongation of the reservoir effect, since the toxic agent becomes sealed off from the circulation; this may further enhance the direct local damage to the bone. A vicious cycle results whereby the greater the exposure to the toxic agent the slower is its rate of elimination.

Transcellular Reservoirs. Drugs also cross epithelial cells and may accumulate in the transcellular fluids. The major transcellular reservoir is the gastrointestinal tract. Weak bases are passively concentrated in the stomach from the blood, because of the large pH differential between the two fluids, and some drugs are secreted in the bile in an active form or as a conjugate that can be hydrolyzed in the intestine. In these cases and when an orally administered drug is slowly absorbed, the gastrointestinal tract serves as a drug reservoir.

Other transcellular fluids, including *cerebrospinal fluid, aqueous humor, endolymph,* and *joint fluids,* do not generally accumulate significant total amounts of drugs.

Redistribution. Termination of drug effect is usually by biotransformation and excretion, but it may also result from redistribution of the drug from its site of action into other tissues or sites. Redistribution is a factor in terminating drug effect primarily when a highly lipid-soluble drug that acts on the brain or cardiovascular system is administered rapidly by intravenous injection or by inhalation. The factors involved in redistribution of drugs have been discussed above.

Placental Transfer of Drugs. The potential transfer of drugs across the placenta is important, since drugs may cause congenital anomalies. Administered immediately prior to delivery, they may also have adverse effects upon the neonate. Drugs cross the placenta primarily by simple diffusion. Lipid-soluble, nonionized drugs readily enter the fetal blood from the maternal circulation. Penetration is least with drugs possessing a high degree of dissociation or low lipid solubility. The view that the placenta is a barrier to drugs is inaccurate. A more appropriate approximation is that the fetus is to at least some extent exposed to essentially all drugs taken by the mother (*see* Merkin and Singh, 1973).

BIOTRANSFORMATION OF DRUGS

Many drugs are lipid-soluble, weak organic acids or bases that are not readily eliminated from the body. For example, after filtration at the renal glomerulus they are readily reabsorbed by diffusion through the renal tubular cells. Drug metabolites usually are more polar and less lipid soluble than the parent molecule, and this enhances their excretion and reduces their volume of distribution. Biotransformation not only fosters drug elimination but also often results in inactivation of the compound. However, many drug metabolites have pharmacological activity. They may exert effects that are similar to or different from those of the parent molecule, and they may be responsible for important toxic effects that follow drug administration. Furthermore, advantage may sometimes be taken of drug-metabolizing enzymes by administration of an agent in an inactive form as a *prodrug*. This is necessary, for example, for purine or pyrimidine analogs used for cancer chemotherapy; in these cases the active chemical species, the nucleotide, is too polar to penetrate to intracellular sites of action, and drug is administered in the form of the purine or pyrimidine base or the corresponding nucleoside. If drug metabolites are active, termination of action takes place by further biotransformation or by excretion of the active metabolite in the urine. (For excellent summaries of drug biotransformation, *see* La Du *et al.,* 1971; Goldstein *et al.,* 1974; Lee *et al.,* 1977; Jenner and Testa, 1981; Mitchell and Horning, 1984.)

Patterns of Biotransformation. The chemical reactions concerned in the biotransformation of drugs are classified as phase-I and phase-II reactions. *Phase-I reactions* usually convert the parent drug to a more polar metabolite by oxidation, reduction, or hydrolysis. The resulting metabolite may be more active than the parent molecule (which then may be designated as a prodrug), less active, or inactive. *Phase-II reactions*, which are also called synthetic or conjugation reactions, involve coupling between the drug or its metabolite and an endogenous substrate, such as glucuronic acid, sulfuric acid, acetic acid, or an amino acid.

Although many details of drug biotransformation are necessarily based upon observations in animals, the mechanisms in man are often similar. However, rates of the reactions in the various species are often quite different, and the patterns of biotransformation may be qualitatively different.

Various patterns of biotransformation, involving phase-I and phase-II reactions and representing both activation and inactivation of drugs, are illustrated in Table 1–2. These reactions also emphasize that most drugs are converted concurrently or con-

secutively to multiple metabolites. The hepatic microsomal enzyme systems are responsible for the biotransformation of the majority of drugs. Other tissues, including plasma, kidney, lung, and the gastrointestinal tract, also contribute to drug biotransformation.

The first reaction in Table 1–2, involving morphine, illustrates the common process of inactivation by glucuronide formation. The second series of reactions depicts the inactivation of the antiepileptic agent phenobarbital by oxidation. Subsequent conjugations of two types further facilitate excretion of the metabolite. The third reaction, oxidation of the antiepileptic agent trimethadione to the active metabolite dimethadione (DMO), demonstrates that oxidation need not inactivate a drug and that biotransformation does not always proceed to conjugation. DMO is not further metabolized but is slowly excreted in the urine. Oxidation may also result in conversion of an inactive drug to an active metabolite or the formation of a metabolite with qualitatively different activity than that of the parent drug, for example, the biotransformation of the antipyretic-analgesic phenacetin to a metab-

Table 1–2. REPRESENTATIVE PATTERNS OF DRUG BIOTRANSFORMATION

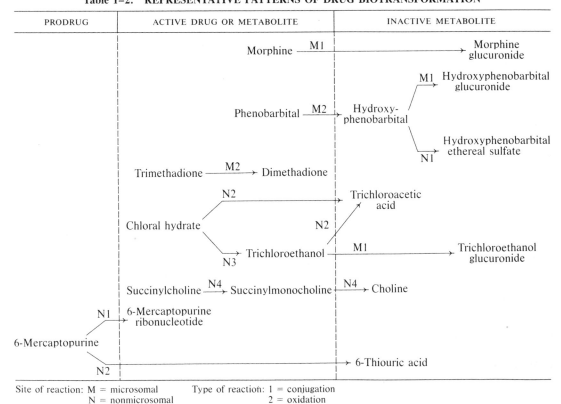

Site of reaction: M = microsomal   Type of reaction: 1 = conjugation
                  N = nonmicrosomal   2 = oxidation
                                                       3 = reduction
                                                       4 = hydrolysis

olite that causes methemoglobin formation. The fourth reaction sequence illustrates that a drug may be converted concurrently to active and inactive metabolites. The sedative-hypnotic chloral hydrate is both oxidized to inactive trichloroacetic acid and reduced to the active metabolite trichloroethanol, which is subsequently inactivated by conjugation. The time course of drug effect after administration of chloral hydrate thus depends upon the relative rates of the three reactions. The fifth series of reactions involves the third general type of phase-I reaction, hydrolysis. The neuromuscular blocking agent succinylcholine is hydrolyzed to succinyl-monocholine, and this metabolite with weak activity is then further hydrolyzed to inactive choline. The final reaction sequence illustrates that conjugation, in this case resulting in the conversion of 6-mercaptopurine to its ribonucleotide, occasionally results in activation of a drug.

Hepatic Microsomal Drug-Metabolizing Systems. The enzyme systems concerned in the biotransformation of many drugs are primarily located in the hepatic smooth endoplasmic reticulum. Fragments of this network are isolated by centrifugation of liver homogenates in the fraction generally called *microsomes*. These enzymes are present in other organs such as the kidney and gastrointestinal epithelium. Drugs absorbed from the intestine may thus be subject to the *first-pass effect*. This represents the combined action of gastrointestinal epithelial and hepatic drug-metabolizing enzymes, which may prevent the appearance of significant amounts of a drug in the circulation after oral administration, as discussed above.

The endoplasmic reticulum resembles a canal system within the cell, and it also functions in intracellular transport. The reticulum consists of a membrane that bears small ribonucleoprotein particles, *ribosomes*, which cause the reticulum to have a rough surface. The rough-surfaced reticulum is the site of protein synthesis, including the synthesis of the smooth-surfaced reticulum that contains the enzymes that metabolize drugs.

The microsomal enzymes catalyze glucuronide conjugations and most of the oxidations of drugs (*see* Table 1–3). Reduction and hydrolysis of drugs are catalyzed by both microsomal and nonmicrosomal enzymes. Lipid solubility is an important, but not the only, requirement for a drug to be metabolized by the hepatic microsomes since this property favors the penetration of a drug into the endoplasmic reticulum and

its binding with cytochrome P-450, a primary component of the oxidative enzyme system (Figure 1–3). Most endogenous metabolic intermediates are polar compounds and are not substrates. However, the microsomal enzymes do contribute to the biotransformation of fatty acids and steroid hormones and also conjugate bilirubin.

The hepatic microsomal enzyme systems are notable; not only do they participate in the biotransformation of many drugs but also the activity of these enzymes can be induced by many drugs and by chemicals encountered in the environment (*see* below). Both normal individual differences in microsomal enzyme activity and susceptibility to induction are genetically determined. Rates of biotransformation of drugs among individuals may vary sixfold or more.

The evolutionary development of drug-metabolizing systems is probably related to exposure of both vertebrates and invertebrates to toxic alkaloids in plants on which they have fed. Thus, drug metabolism has evolved as a means of protection against environmental toxins. However, the notion that biotransformation is equivalent to detoxication is incorrect, particularly with regard to drugs and man-made pollutants.

Oxidation. The hepatic endoplasmic reticulum contains an important group of oxidative enzymes called *mixed-function oxidases* or *monooxygenases* that require both a reducing agent, nicotinamide adenine dinucleotide phosphate (NADPH), and molecular oxygen. These enzymes are involved in the biotransformation of many drugs. Epoxide intermediates in these reactions are capable of covalent binding with macromolecules and may be responsible for tissue necrosis, carcinogenicity, and other toxic effects of drugs. The toxicity of several drugs (*e.g.,* acetaminophen, isoniazid, furosemide, methyldopa) appears to be due, at least in part, to the formation of such reactive electrophils (*see* below and Figure 1–4).

The reactions catalyzed by the microsomal mixed-function oxidases include N- and O-dealkylation, aromatic ring and side chain hydroxylation, sulfoxide formation, N-oxidation, N-hydroxylation, deamination of primary and secondary amines, and

Table 1–3.   DRUG BIOTRANSFORMATION REACTIONS

I. *Oxidative Reactions* (Microsomal)

(1) N- and O-Dealkylation

$$RNHCH_2CH_3 \xrightarrow{[O]} RNH_2 + CH_3CHO$$

$$ROCH_3 \xrightarrow{[O]} ROH + CH_2O$$

(2) Side Chain (Aliphatic) and Aromatic Hydroxylation

$$RCH_2CH_3 \xrightarrow{[O]} R\overset{\overset{\displaystyle OH}{|}}{C}HCH_3$$

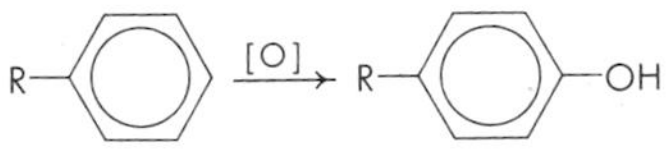

(3) N-Oxidation and N-Hydroxylation

$$(R)_3N \xrightarrow{[O]} R_3N{=}O$$

$$RNHR' \xrightarrow{[O]} R\overset{\overset{\displaystyle OH}{|}}{N}R'$$

(4) Sulfoxide Formation

$$RSR' \xrightarrow{[O]} R\overset{\overset{\displaystyle O}{\|}}{S}R'$$

(5) Deamination of Amines

$$RCH_2NH_2 \xrightarrow{[O]} RCHO + NH_3$$

(6) Desulfuration

$$RSH \xrightarrow{[O]} ROH$$

II. *Glucuronide Synthesis* (Microsomal)

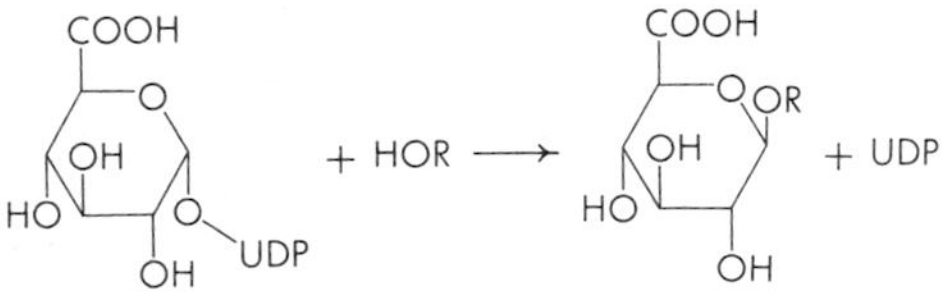

UDP–Glucuronic Acid

the replacement of a sulfur by an oxygen atom (desulfuration). These reactions are depicted in Table 1–3.

The electron transport scheme involved in microsomal drug oxidation is illustrated in Figure 1–3. The terminal oxidase in the pathway is one of a large group of related hemoproteins designated cytochromes P-450, so named because they absorb light at 450 nm when exposed to carbon monoxide. This property is also the basis for their analytical determination. Furthermore, carbon monoxide blocks the metabolism of many drugs by the system. The primary electron donor is NADPH; the electron transfer involves a flavoprotein, cyto-

chrome P-450 reductase. Phospholipid is essential for activity of the reconstituted system.

A drug substrate binds with oxidized cytochrome P-450 ($[Fe^{3+}]$ in Figure 1–3). The resulting drug-cytochrome complex is reduced by the reductase, and the reduced complex then combines with molecular oxygen. A second electron and two hydrogen ions are acquired from the donor system, and the subsequent products are oxidized metabolite and water, with regeneration of the oxidized cytochrome P-450.

Interactions of substrates and inhibitors with oxidized cytochrome P-450 produce characteristic changes in the absorbance spectrum of the microsomes. These originally provided the basis for the designation of two types of drug binding sites or at

Table 1–3. DRUG BIOTRANSFORMATION REACTIONS (Continued)

III. *Other Conjugation Reactions*

(1) Acetylation

$$RNH_2 + CH_3\overset{\displaystyle O}{\overset{\|}{C}}SCoA \longrightarrow RNH\overset{\displaystyle O}{\overset{\|}{C}}CH_3 + CoA—SH$$
Acetyl CoA

(2) Conjugation with Glycine

$$RCOOH \longrightarrow R\overset{\displaystyle O}{\overset{\|}{C}}SCoA + NH_2CH_2COOH \longrightarrow R\overset{\displaystyle O}{\overset{\|}{C}}NHCH_2COOH + CoA—SH$$

(3) Conjugation with Sulfate

$$ROH + 3'\text{-phosphoadenosine } 5'\text{-phosphosulfate} \longrightarrow RO\overset{\displaystyle O}{\underset{\underset{\displaystyle O}{\|}}{\overset{\|}{S}}}OH + 3'\text{-phosphoadenosine } 5'\text{-phosphate}$$

(4) O-, S-, and N-Methylation

$$R—XH + S\text{-adenosylmethionine} \longrightarrow R—X—CH_3 + S\text{-adenosylhomocysteine}$$
(X = O, S, N)

IV. *Hydrolysis of Esters and Amides*

$$R\overset{\displaystyle O}{\overset{\|}{C}}OR' \longrightarrow RCOOH + R'OH$$

$$R\overset{\displaystyle O}{\overset{\|}{C}}NR' \longrightarrow RCOOH + R'NH_2$$

V. *Reduction*

(1) Azo Reduction

$$RN{=\!\!=}NR' \longrightarrow RNH_2 + R'NH_2$$

(2) Nitro Reduction

$$RNO_2 \longrightarrow RNH_2$$

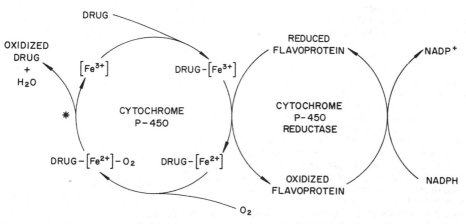

* Denotes contribution of a second electron and two hydrogen ions from NADH–flavoprotein–cytochrome b_5 or from NADPH–flavoprotein.

Figure 1–3. *Major components of the hepatic microsomal drug-metabolizing enzyme system.*

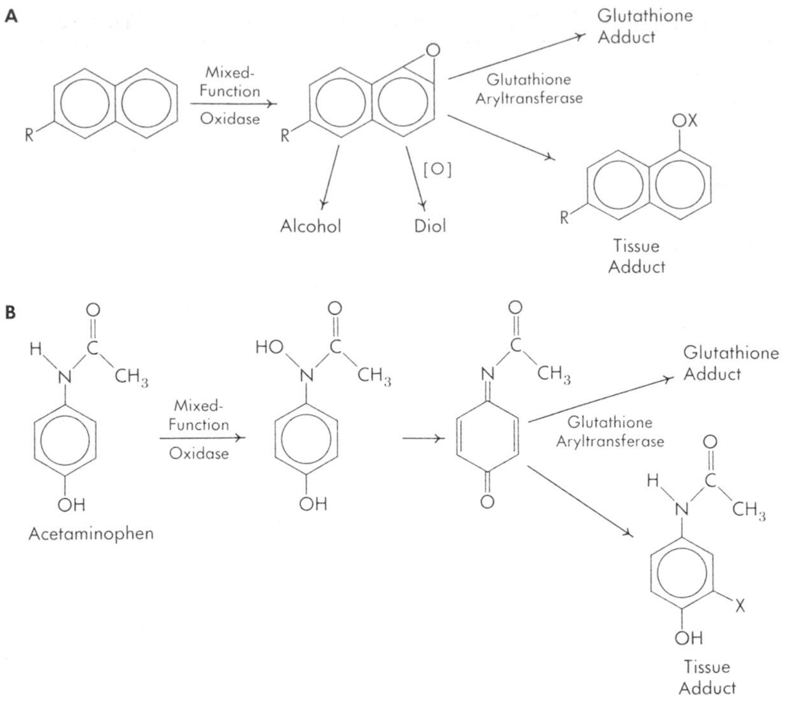

Figure 1–4. *Formation of reactive intermediates during the metabolism of environmental substances and drugs.*

A. A compound with an aromatic ring susceptible to hydroxylation may be metabolized to an arene oxide (epoxide) that can be converted spontaneously to the monoalcohol. The epoxide also can be converted enzymatically to a "diol" or can react with glutathione. The latter compound is eventually excreted as a mercapturic acid derivative. When concentrations of compounds such as glutathione are limiting, reaction can occur with macromolecular constituents of tissues.

B. Acetaminophen may be converted to a quinone type of reactive intermediate that is rapidly transformed to a mercapturate when the concentration of glutathione is not limiting. (The major route of acetaminophen metabolism is to an O-glucuronide.) X represents a tissue site of covalent reaction.

least two types of cytochrome P-450 molecules. Technics of protein purification and molecular cloning by recombinant DNA technology have now led to the view that there are many cytochromes P-450, each encoded by a specific gene. These various proteins differ in their substrate specificity and in their inducibility by drugs and other xenobiotics. Clarification of the relationships between these proteins is an area of active research.

The rate of drug biotransformation by the mixed-function oxidase system is determined by the concentration of cytochrome P-450, the proportions of the various forms of cytochrome P-450 and their affinities for the substrate, the concentration of cytochrome P-450 reductase, and the rate of reduction of the drug–cytochrome P-450 complex. Rate of biotransformation may also be influenced by competing endogenous and exogenous substrates. These many factors are responsible for the sometimes marked species, strain, and individual variations in drug metabolism by the microsomal system.

Glucuronide Synthesis. Glucuronides constitute the major proportion of metabolites of many phenols, alcohols, and carboxylic acids. Glucuronides are generally inactive and are rapidly secreted into the urine and bile by the transport mechanisms for anions. However, concentrations of some glucuronide conjugates in plasma may approach those of the parent compound. Glucuronides eliminated in the bile may be subsequently hydrolyzed by intestinal or bacterial β-glucuronidase, and the liberated drug may be reabsorbed. This enterohepatic cycling may prolong the action of the drug.

Glucuronide formation is catalyzed by various microsomal glucuronyltransferases, with uridine diphosphate–glucuronic acid as the donor of glucuronic acid (Table 1–3). It is generated from glucose by enzymes in the cytosol. Glucuronide conjugation also occurs in the kidney and other tissues to a lesser extent.

Inhibition of Microsomal Drug Metabolism. Competitive inhibition between the many substrates for the microsomal enzymes is readily demonstrated *in vitro.* Such interactions are not usually of practical significance *in vivo.* This is not unexpected, since the inactivation of most drugs *in vivo* exhibits exponential (first-order) rather than linear (zero-order) kinetics; that is, the activity of drug-metabolizing enzymes is usually not rate limiting. Drug concentrations are commonly well below those necessary to saturate metabolizing enzymes, and competition between substrates is minimized under these conditions. An important corollary, however, is that significant mutual inhibition of drug metabolism is to be expected for drugs that normally exhibit saturable inactivation kinetics. For example, dicumarol inhibits the metabolism of phenytoin and can increase the incidence and severity of side effects of phenytoin, such as ataxia and drowsiness. Concurrent administration of allopurinol and 6-mercaptopurine results in elevated concentrations of the latter chemotherapeutic agent due to competitive inhibition of xanthine oxidase by allopurinol.

Reduction in the rate of drug metabolism may also occur when biotransformation is so rapid that hepatic blood flow is the rate-limiting factor. Hepatic blood flow may decrease acutely after β-adrenergic blockade, and this can affect the rate of metabolism of drugs that are cleared from the plasma at very high rates (*e.g.,* lidocaine). Microsomal drug metabolism is inhibited by carbon monoxide and by hepatotoxic agents that destroy cytochrome P-450, interfere with hepatic metabolism, or chronically decrease hepatic blood flow. Certain drugs can inhibit the activity of cytochrome P-450 irreversibly because of covalent interaction with a reactive intermediate generated by the enzyme. Identification of drugs in this category is growing rapidly.

Induction of Microsomal Enzyme Activity. The activity of the microsomal enzymes can be increased by administration of certain drugs and by exposure to various chemicals in the environment; these inducers need not be substrates for the enzymes

that are affected. The capacity of foreign compounds to induce microsomal drug metabolism is important for drug therapy and the transformation of environmental substances into highly toxic agents. That a drug can increase its own metabolism and that of other substrates has wide implications for chronic toxicity tests, crossover drug studies in animals and man, chronic drug therapy with single or multiple drugs, and the development of tolerance to drugs. (Chapter 3 and chapters on specific classes of drugs provide more information about the pharmacological and therapeutic aspects of induction of microsomal enzymes.)

In animals, the several hundred compounds known to stimulate the microsomal enzyme systems are loosely classified into two types, namely, those that resemble phenobarbital and those that are similar to the carcinogenic polycyclic hydrocarbons. Stimulation of the microsomal system by phenobarbital results in altered biotransformation of a wide variety of substrates. The increase in enzyme activity is attributed to induced synthesis of cytochromes P-450, cytochrome P-450 reductase, and other enzymes involved in drug metabolism. Indeed, induction caused by phenobarbital, but not all other inducers, is associated with proliferation of the endoplasmic reticulum and increases in liver weight, hepatic blood flow, bile flow, and other hepatic proteins, including those thought to be important in the uptake of organic anions into the hepatocyte. Stimulation of the microsomal enzyme system by the polycyclic hydrocarbons is also attributed to induced protein synthesis, but the increase in drug metabolism is limited to relatively few substrates, does not result in an increase in cytochrome P-450 reductase, and is associated with the appearance of a qualitatively different terminal oxidase. Different receptors and different genes are thus probably involved in induction by these two classes of compounds. A widely used defoliant, trichlorophenoxyacetic acid (2,4,5-T), contains an inducer of this type as a contaminant, tetrachlorodibenzo-*p*-dioxin. This compound can produce permanent induction of microsomal enzymes when submicrogram doses are given to experimental animals. This class of inducer can also accelerate the formation of reactive intermediates during metabolism of other drugs or of environmental chemicals.

Enzyme induction also occurs to a limited extent in kidney, gastrointestinal tract, adrenal, lung, placenta, skin, and pancreas. Upon removal of most inducing agents, the effects wane over a period of days or weeks, depending in part upon the time course for accumulation or elimination of the inducing agent.

Since chronic administration of a drug may stimulate its own metabolism and that of other agents, interactions may occur between drugs that are simultaneously administered. The concomitant administration of phenobarbital and warfarin results in lower plasma concentrations of warfarin and less anticoagulant effect than when the anticoagulant is administered alone. The desired therapeutic effect can be attained if dosage of the anticoagulant is increased. However, if the phenobarbital medication is stopped after the dosage of the anticoagulant has been adjusted, the plasma concentration and effect of warfarin increase, and severe bleeding may occur. Thus, during multiple-drug therapy involving an agent that stimulates drug metabolism, the effects of the other drugs must be carefully monitored, both when medication with the inducing agent is initiated and when it is discontinued.

Relationship of Drug Metabolism to Drug Toxicity. Reference has been made above to the formation of toxic metabolites as the result of microsomal oxidation of drugs. Microsomal oxidation can cause the formation of highly reactive compounds that normally have such a transient existence that they exert no biological action. Two examples of formation and inactivation of such substances are shown in Figure 1–4. As long as the terminal hydroxylation or conjugation keeps pace, accumulation of reactive intermediates does not occur. However, when induction occurs or when very large amounts of drug are present, oxidation by cytochrome P-450 is accelerated. Since glutathione is in limited supply in liver and kidney and can be depleted, the drug epoxide or quinone may reach a sufficient concentration to react with nucleophilic cell constituents. Hepatic or renal necrosis results. The discovery that the availability of glutathione determines the threshold for the toxic response has led to attempts to use thiols, for example, N-acetylcysteine, to treat poisoning by drugs such as acetaminophen.

Polycyclic hydrocarbons are potent inducers of microsomal metabolism and cause the accumulation of relatively small amounts of reactive intermediates that presumably intercalate into the DNA helix and initiate carcinogenesis. The experimental basis of this concept is well established; its clinical significance is not clear.

Drug Metabolism in the Fetus and Neonate. Activity of the hepatic microsomal enzyme systems is low in the neonate, particularly premature babies. Reduced conjugating activity contributes to the hyperbilirubinemia of the neonate and the risk of bilirubin encephalopathy. It is also the basis of the increased toxicity in the neonate of drugs such as chloramphenicol or certain opioid analgesics that are inactivated by glucuronide formation. Activity of nonmicrosomal enzymes involved in drug biotransformation is also reduced. The combination of a poorly developed blood-brain barrier, weak drug-metabolizing activity, and immature mechanisms for excre-

tion combine to make the fetus and neonate very sensitive to toxic effects of drugs. Biotransformation capacity increases during the early months of postnatal life, although the pattern for different enzymes is variable.

Nonmicrosomal Drug Biotransformation. All conjugations other than glucuronide formation and some oxidation, reduction, and hydrolysis of drugs are catalyzed by nonmicrosomal enzymes. Such reactions contribute to the biotransformation of a number of common drugs, including aspirin and the sulfonamides. In addition, drugs that are only slowly metabolized may compete effectively with endogenous substrates. In certain such cases, as illustrated by the inhibition of xanthine oxidase by allopurinol, drug action and biotransformation are intimately related.

Nonmicrosomal biotransformation of drugs occurs primarily in the liver but also in plasma and other tissues. Although drug metabolism by the gastrointestinal tract and intestinal flora is usually minor relative to total drug elimination, biotransformation in the gastrointestinal tract sometimes contributes to what is superficially interpreted as poor oral absorption of a drug. Minor metabolites from the intestinal metabolism of a drug may contribute to drug toxicity. Intestinal hydrolysis of glucuronides secreted in the bile is an integral link in the enterohepatic cycling of drugs.

Individual variation in rates of drug biotransformation is about the same for the nonmicrosomal enzymes as for the microsomal enzymes, namely, sixfold or greater. None of the nonmicrosomal enzymes involved in drug biotransformation is known to be inducible. Several, including butyrylcholinesterase and the acetylating enzymes, exhibit genetic polymorphism. (*See* La Du *et al.,* 1971, for an excellent discussion of genetic modification of drug biotransformation.)

Conjugations. Inactivation of aromatic primary amines and hydrazines by conjugation with *acetic acid,* with acetyl coenzyme A as the acetyl donor, involves several N-acetyl transferases. These enzymes appear to represent the products of multiple genes, since genetic polymorphism (slow or fast acetylation by different individuals) is exhibited only to some substrates, including isoniazid, hydralazine, and many sulfonamides.

Aromatic carboxylic acids, such as salicylic acid, are often inactivated by conjugation with *glycine*. This reaction may exhibit saturable kinetics when drug concentrations are high and first-order kinetics when they are lower. The kinetics of elimination of drugs metabolized by glycine conjugation thus appears to be highly variable, and adjustment of dosage may be very difficult.

Conjugation with *glutathione*, with subsequent formation of a mercapturate derivative, is not a quantitatively important route of biotransformation, but it contributes to inactivation of toxic epoxide intermediates produced by hydroxylation reactions (*see* discussion above and Figure 1–4).

Still other nonmicrosomal conjugations include *sulfate* conjugation of phenolic compounds, including steroids; *O-, S-,* and *N-methylation* of amines and phenols, including epinephrine and norepinephrine; and *ribonucleoside* and *ribonucleotide* formation, usually of analogs of the purines and pyrimidines to form active antimetabolites (*see* Figure 1–3).

Hydrolysis. Esters, such as procaine, are hydrolyzed by a variety of nonspecific esterases in liver, plasma, gastrointestinal tract, and other tissues. Hydrolysis of amides, such as lidocaine, occurs primarily in the liver. Peptidases in plasma, erythrocytes, and many other tissues are involved in the biotransformation of the biologically active polypeptides.

Oxidation. Some drugs are oxidized by a variety of flavoprotein enzymes in mitochondria and cytosol of the liver and other tissues. Examples include the oxidation of alcohols and aldehydes by *alcohol and aldehyde dehydrogenases,* the purine antimetabolite 6-mercaptopurine by *xanthine oxidase,* and drugs related to the catecholamines by *tyrosine hydroxylase* and *monoamine oxidase*.

Reduction. Microsomal and nonmicrosomal enzymes in the liver and other tissues can catalyze the reduction of nitro groups and the cleavage and reduction of the azo linkage. Examples include the nitro reduction of chloramphenicol and the azo reduction of PRONTOSIL. Reduction of nitro and azo compounds *in vivo* is often catalyzed by the intestinal flora in the anaerobic environment of the gut (Scheline, 1973).

EXCRETION OF DRUGS

Drugs are eliminated from the body either unchanged or as metabolites. Excretory organs, the lung excluded, eliminate polar compounds more efficiently than substances with high lipid solubility. Lipid-soluble drugs are thus not readily eliminated until they are metabolized to more polar compounds.

The kidney is the most important organ for elimination of drugs and their metabolites. Substances excreted in the feces are mainly unabsorbed orally ingested drugs or metabolites excreted in the bile and not reabsorbed from the intestinal tract. Excretion of drugs in milk is important not because of the amounts eliminated but because the excreted drugs are potential sources of unwanted pharmacological effects in the nursing infant. Pulmonary excretion is important mainly for the elimination of anesthetic gases and vapors (*see* Chapter 13); occasionally, small quantities of other drugs or metabolites are excreted by this route.

Renal Excretion. Excretion of drugs and metabolites in the urine involves three processes: glomerular filtration, active tubular secretion, and passive tubular reabsorption.

The amount of drug entering the tubular lumen by *filtration* is dependent on its fractional plasma protein binding and glomerular filtration rate. In the proximal renal tubule, certain organic anions and cations are added to the glomerular filtrate by active, carrier-mediated tubular *secretion*. Many organic acids, such as penicillin, and metabolites, such as glucuronides, are transported by the system that secretes naturally occurring substances such as uric acid; organic bases, such as tetraethylammonium, are transported by a separate system that secretes choline, histamine, and other endogenous bases.

Both carrier systems are relatively nonselective, and organic ions of similar charge compete for transport. Both transport systems can also be bidirectional, and at least some drugs are both secreted and actively reabsorbed. However, transport of most exogenous ions is predominantly secretory. The outstanding example of the bidirectional tubular transport of an endogenous organic acid is uric acid. The characteristics of tubular transport systems for organic compounds are described in detail in Chapter 38.

In the proximal and distal tubules, the nonionized forms of weak acids and bases undergo net passive *reabsorption*. The concentration gradient for back diffusion is created by the reabsorption of water with sodium and other inorganic ions. Since the tubular cells are less permeable to the ionized forms of weak electrolytes, passive reabsorption of these substances is pH dependent. When the tubular urine is made more alkaline, weak acids are excreted more rapidly, primarily because they are more ionized and passive reabsorption is decreased. When the tubular urine is made more acid, the excretion of weak acids is reduced. Alkalinization and acidification of the urine have the opposite effects on the excretion of weak bases. In the treatment of drug poisoning, the excretion of some drugs can be hastened by appropriate alkalinization or acidification of the urine. Whether alteration of urine pH results in significant change in drug elimination depends upon the extent and persistence of the pH change and the contribution of pH-dependent passive reabsorption to total drug elimination. The effect is greatest for weak acids and bases with pK_a values in the range of urinary pH (5 to 8). However, alkalinization of urine can produce a fourfold to sixfold increase in excretion of a relatively strong acid such as salicylate when urinary pH is changed from 6.4 to 8.0. The fraction of nonionized drug would decrease from 1% to 0.04%.

Biliary and Fecal Excretion. Many metabolites of drugs formed in the liver are excreted into the intestinal tract in the *bile*. These metabolites may be excreted in the feces; more commonly, they are reabsorbed into the blood and ultimately excreted in the urine. Both organic anions, including glucuronides, and organic cations are actively transported into bile by carrier systems similar to those that transport these substances across the renal tubule. Both transport systems are nonselective, and ions of like charge may compete for transport. Steroids and related substances are transported into bile by a third carrier system. The effectiveness of the liver as an excretory organ for glucuronide conjugates is very much limited by their enzymatic hydrolysis after the bile is mixed with the contents of the small intestine.

Excretion by Other Routes. Excretion of drugs into *sweat, saliva,* and *tears* is quantitatively unimportant. Elimination by these routes is dependent mainly upon diffusion of the nonionized, lipid-soluble form of drugs through the epithelial cells of the glands and is pH dependent. Reabsorption of the nonionized drug from the primary secretion probably also occurs in the ducts of the glands, and active secretion of drugs across the ducts of the gland may also occur. Drugs excreted in the saliva enter the mouth, where they are usually swallowed. Their fate thereafter is the same as that of drugs taken orally. The concentration of some drugs in saliva parallels that in plasma. Saliva may therefore be a useful biological fluid in which to determine drug concentrations when it is difficult or inconvenient to obtain blood.

The same principles apply to excretion of drugs in *milk*. Since milk is more acidic than plasma, basic compounds may be slightly concentrated in this fluid, and the concentration of acidic compounds in milk is lower than in plasma. Nonelectrolytes, such as ethanol and urea, readily enter milk and reach the same concentration as in plasma, independent of the pH of the milk. (*See* summary of Plaa, in La Du *et al.,* 1971.)

Although excretion into *hair* and *skin* is also quantitatively unimportant, sensitive methods of detection of toxic metals in these tissues have forensic significance. Arsenic in hair, detected 150 years after administration, has raised interesting questions about how Napoleon died, and by whose hand. Mozart's manic behavior during the preparation of his last major work, the *Requiem,* may have been due to mercury poisoning; traces of the metal have been found in his hair.

CLINICAL PHARMACOKINETICS

A fundamental hypothesis of clinical pharmacokinetics is that a relationship exists between the pharmacological or toxic response to a drug and the concentration of the drug in a readily accessible site in the body (*e.g.,* blood). This hypothesis has been documented for many drugs (*see* Appendix II), although it is apparent for some drugs that no clear or simple relationship has been found between pharmacological effect and concentration in plasma. In most cases, as depicted in Figure 1–1, the concentration of drug in the systemic circulation will be related to the concentration of drug at its sites of action. The pharmacological effect that results may be the clinical effect desired, a toxic effect, or, in some cases, an effect unrelated to efficacy or toxicity. Clinical pharmacokinetics plays its role in the dose-efficacy scheme by attempting to provide a more quantitative relationship between dose and efficacy and by providing the framework with which to interpret measurements of concentrations of drugs in biological fluids. The importance of pharmacokinetics in patient care rests on the improvement in efficacy that can be attained by attention to its principles when dosage regimens are chosen and modified.

The various physiological and pathophysiological variables that dictate adjustment of dosage in individual patients often do so as a result of modification of pharmacokinetic parameters. The three most important parameters are *bioavailability,* the fraction of drug absorbed as such into the systemic circulation; *clearance,* a measure of the body's ability to eliminate drug; and *volume of distribution,* a measure of the apparent space in the body available to contain the drug. Of lesser importance are the *rates* of availability and distribution of the agent.

CLEARANCE

Clearance is the most important concept to be considered when a rational regimen for drug administration is to be designed. The clinician usually wants to maintain steady-state concentrations of a drug within a known therapeutic range (*see* Appendix II). Assuming complete bioavailability, the steady state will be achieved when the rate of drug elimination equals the rate of drug administration:

$$\text{Dosing rate} = CL \cdot C_{ss} \qquad (1)$$

where CL is clearance and C_{ss} is the steady-state concentration of drug. Thus, if the desired steady-state concentration of drug in plasma or blood is known, the rate of clearance of drug by the patient will dictate the rate at which the drug should be administered.

The concept of clearance is extremely useful in clinical pharmacokinetics because clearance of a given drug is usually constant over the range of concentrations encountered clinically. This is true because systems for elimination of drugs are not usually saturated and, thus, the *absolute* rate of elimination of the drug is essentially a linear function of its concentration in plasma. A synonymous statement is that the elimination of most drugs follows first-

order kinetics—a constant *fraction* of drug is eliminated per unit time. If mechanisms for elimination of a given drug become saturated, the kinetics become zero order—a constant *amount* of drug is eliminated per unit time. Under such a circumstance, clearance becomes variable. Principles of drug clearance are similar to those of renal physiology, where, for example, creatinine clearance is defined as the rate of elimination of creatinine in the urine relative to its concentration in plasma. At the simplest level, clearance of a drug is the rate of elimination by all routes normalized to the concentration of drug, C, in some biological fluid:

$$CL = \text{Rate of elimination}/C \qquad (2)$$

It is important to note that clearance does not indicate how much drug is being removed but, rather, the volume of biological fluid such as blood or plasma that would have to be completely freed of drug to account for the elimination. Clearance is expressed as a volume per unit of time. Clearance is usually further defined as blood clearance (CL_b), plasma clearance (CL_p), or clearance based on the concentration of unbound or free drug (CL_u), depending on the concentration measured (C_b, C_p, or C_u). (For additional discussion of clearance concepts, *see* Benet *et al.,* 1984.)

Clearance by means of various organs of elimination is additive. Elimination of drug may occur as a result of processes that occur in the kidney, liver, and other organs. Division of the rate of elimination by each organ by a concentration of drug (*e.g.,* plasma concentration) will yield the respective clearance by that organ. Added together, these separate clearances will equal total systemic clearance:

$$CL_{renal} + CL_{hepatic} + CL_{other} = CL_{systemic} \qquad (3)$$

Other routes of elimination could include that in saliva or sweat, partition into the gut, and metabolism at other sites.

Total systemic clearance may be determined at steady state by using equation 1. For a *single* dose of a drug with complete bioavailability and first-order (linear) kinetics of elimination, total systemic clearance may be determined from mass balance and the integration of equation 2 over time.

$$CL = \text{Dose}/AUC \qquad (4)$$

where AUC is the total area under the curve that describes the concentration of drug in the systemic circulation as a function of time (from zero to infinity).

Examples. In Appendix II, the plasma clearance for cephalexin is reported as 4.3 ml · min^{-1} · kg^{-1}, with 91% of the drug excreted unchanged in the urine. For a 70-kg man, the total body clearance from plasma would be 300 ml/min, with renal clearance accounting for 91% of this elimination. In other words, the kidney is able to excrete cephalexin at a rate such that approximately 273 ml of plasma would be freed of drug per minute. Because *clearance* is usually assumed to remain constant in a stable patient, the total rate of *elimination* of cephalexin will depend on the concentration of drug in the plasma (equation 2). Propranolol is cleared at a rate of 12 ml · min^{-1} · kg^{-1} (or 840 ml/min in a 70-kg man), almost exclusively by the liver. Thus, the liver is able to remove the amount of drug contained in 840 ml of plasma per minute. Of the drugs listed in Appendix II, one of the highest values of plasma clearance is that for imipramine—1050 ml/min; this value exceeds the rate of plasma flow to the liver, the dominant organ for elimination of this drug. However, because imipramine partitions readily into red blood cells ($C_{rbc}/C_p = 2.7$), the amount of drug delivered to the excretory organ is considerably higher than suspected from measurement of its concentration in plasma. The relationship between plasma and blood clearance at steady state is given by:

$$\frac{CL_p}{CL_b} = \frac{C_b}{C_p} = 1 + H\left(\frac{C_{rbc}}{C_p} - 1\right) \qquad (5)$$

One may solve for imipramine clearance from blood by substituting the red blood cell to plasma concentration ratio and the average value for the hematocrit ($H = 0.45$). Clearance of imipramine, when measured in terms of its concentration in blood, is actually 595 ml/min, a more reasonable value. Thus the plasma clearance may assume values that are not "physiological." A drug with an extremely low concentration in plasma that is concentrated in erythrocytes (*e.g.*, mecamylamine) can show a plasma clearance of tens of liters per minute. However, if the concentration in blood is used to define clearance, the maximal clearance possible is equal to the sum of blood flows to the various organs of elimination.

As mentioned, clearance of most drugs is constant over the range of concentration in plasma or blood that is encountered in clinical settings. This means that elimination is not saturated and the rate of elimination of drug is directly proportional to its concentration (equation 2). For drugs that exhibit saturable or dose-dependent elimination (nonlinear clearance), clearance will vary with the concentration of drug:

$$\text{Total plasma clearance} = V_m/(K_m + C_p) \qquad (6)$$

where K_m represents the plasma concentration at which half of the maximal rate of elimination is reached (in units of mass/volume) and V_m is equal to the maximal rate of elimination (in units of mass/time). This equation is entirely analogous to the Michaelis-Menten equation for enzyme kinetics. Design of dosage regimens for such drugs is more complex (*see* below).

A further definition of clearance is useful for understanding the effects of pathological and physiological variables on drug elimination, particularly with respect to an individual organ. The rate of elimination of a drug by an individual organ can be defined in terms of the blood flow to the organ and the concentration of drug in the blood. The rate of presentation of drug to the organ is the product of blood flow (Q) and the arterial drug concentration (C_A), and the rate of exit of drug from the organ is the product of blood flow and the venous drug concentration (C_V). The difference between these rates at steady state is the rate of drug elimination.

$$\text{Rate of elimination} = Q \cdot C_A - Q \cdot C_V$$
$$= Q(C_A - C_V) \qquad (7)$$

Division of equation 7 by the concentration of drug that enters the organ of elimination, C_A, yields an expression for clearance of the drug by the organ in question:

$$CL_{organ} = Q\left(\frac{C_A - C_V}{C_A}\right) = Q \cdot E \qquad (8)$$

The expression $(C_A - C_V)/C_A$ in equation 8 can be referred to as the extraction ratio for the drug (E).

Hepatic Clearance. The concepts developed in equation 8 have important implications for drugs that are eliminated by the liver. Consider a drug that is efficiently removed from the blood by hepatic processes—biotransformation and/or excretion of unchanged drug into the bile. In this instance, the concentration of drug in the blood leaving the liver will be low, the extraction ratio will approach unity, and the clearance of the drug from blood will become limited by hepatic blood flow. Drugs that are cleared efficiently by the liver (*e.g.*, drugs in Appendix II with clearances greater than $6 \, ml \cdot min^{-1} \cdot kg^{-1}$, such as chlorpromazine, diltiazem, imipramine, lidocaine, morphine, and propranolol) are restricted in their rate of elimination not by intrahepatic processes but by the rate at which they can be transported in the blood to hepatic sites of elimination.

Additional complexities have also been considered. For example, the equations presented above do not account for drug binding to components of blood and tissues, nor do they permit an estimation of the intrinsic ability of the liver or kidney to eliminate a drug in the absence of limitations imposed by blood flow. Extensions of the relationships of equation 8 to include expressions for protein binding and intrinsic clearance have been provided by Roland and colleagues (1973) and by Wilkinson and Shand (1975). These models indicate that, when the capacity of the eliminating organ to metabolize the drug is large in comparison with the rate of presentation of drug, the clearance will approximate the organ blood flow. In contrast, when the metabolic capability is small in comparison to the rate of drug presentation, the clearance will be proportional to the unbound fraction of drug in blood and the intrinsic clearance. Appreciation of these concepts allows one to understand a number of possibly puzzling experimental results. For example, enzyme induction or hepatic disease may change the rate of drug metabolism in an isolated hepatic microsomal enzyme system but not change clearance in the whole animal. For a drug with a high extraction ratio, clearance is limited by blood flow, and changes in the intrinsic clearance due to enzyme induction or hepatic disease should have no effect. Similarly, for drugs with high extraction ratios, changes in protein binding due to disease or competitive binding interactions should have no effect on clearance. In contrast, changes in intrinsic clearance and protein binding will affect the clearance of drugs with low extraction ratios but changes in blood flow should have little effect.

Renal Clearance. Renal clearance of a drug results in its appearance as such in the urine; changes in the pharmacokinetic properties of drugs due to renal disease may also be explained in terms of clearance concepts. However, the complications that relate to filtration, active secretion, and reabsorption must be considered. The rate of filtration of a drug depends on the volume of fluid that is filtered in the glomerulus and the unbound concentration of drug in plasma, since drug bound to protein is not filtered. The rate of secretion of drug by the kidney will depend on the binding of drug to the proteins involved in active transport relative to that bound to plasma proteins, the degree of saturation of these carriers, the rate of transfer of the drug across the tubular membrane, and the rate of delivery of the drug to the secretory site. The influences of changes in protein binding, blood flow, and the number of functional nephrons are analogous to the examples given above for hepatic elimination.

DISTRIBUTION

Volume of Distribution. Volume is a second fundamental parameter that is useful in discussing processes of drug disposition. The volume of distribution (V) relates the amount of drug in the body to the concentration of drug (C) in the blood or plasma, depending upon the fluid measured. This volume does not necessarily refer to an identifiable physiological volume, but merely to the fluid volume that would be required to account for all the drug in the body:

$$V = \text{Amount of drug in body}/C \qquad (9)$$

The plasma volume of a normal 70-kg man is 3 liters, blood volume is about 5.5 liters, extracellular fluid volume outside the plasma is 12 liters, and the volume of total body water is approximately 42 liters. However, many drugs exhibit volumes of distribution far in excess of these known fluid volumes. For example, if 500 μg of digoxin were in the body of a 70-kg subject, plasma concentration of approximately 0.7 ng/ml would be observed. Dividing the amount of drug in the body by the plasma concentration yields a volume of distribution for digoxin of about 700 liters, or a value ten times greater than the total body volume of a 70-kg man. In fact, digoxin, which is relatively hydrophobic, distributes preferentially into muscle and adipose tissue, leaving a very small amount of drug in the plasma. For drugs that are extensively bound to plasma proteins but that are not bound to tissue components, the volume of distribution will approach that of the plasma volume. In contrast, certain drugs have high volumes of distribution even though most of the drug in the circulation is bound to albumin because these drugs are also sequestered elsewhere.

The volume of distribution may vary widely depending on the pK_a of the drug, the degree of binding to plasma proteins, the partition coefficient of the drug in fat, the degree of binding to other tissues, differences in regional blood flow, and so forth. As might be expected, the volume of distribution for a given drug can change as a function of the patient's age, gender, disease, and body composition.

Several volume terms are commonly used, and they have been derived in a number of ways. The volume of distribution defined in equation 9 considers the body as a single homogeneous compartment (Figure 1–1). In this one-compartment model, all drug administration occurs directly into the central compartment and distribution of drug is instantaneous throughout volume (V). Clearance of drug from this compartment occurs in a first-order fashion, as defined in equation 2; that is, the amount of drug eliminated per unit time depends on the amount (concentration) of drug in the body compartment. Figure 1–5 and equation 10 describe the decline of plasma concentration with time for a drug introduced into this compartment.

$$C = (\text{Dose}/V) \cdot exp(-kt) \qquad (10)$$

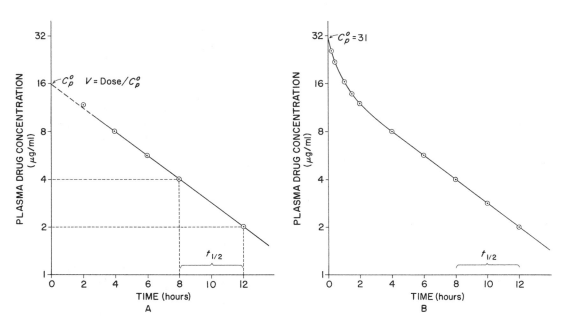

Figure 1–5. *Plasma concentration-time curves following intravenous administration of a drug (500 mg) to a 70-kg man.*

A. In this example, drug concentrations are measured in plasma 2 hours after the dose is administered. The semilogarithmic plot of plasma concentration versus time appears to indicate that the drug is eliminated from a single compartment by a first-order process (equation 10) with a half-life of 4 hours ($k = 0.693/t_{1/2} = 0.173$ hr^{-1}). The volume of distribution (V) may be determined from the value of C_p obtained by extrapolation to $t = 0$ ($C_p^o = 16$ μg/ml). Volume of distribution (equation 9) for the one-compartment model is 31.3 liters or 0.45 liter/kg ($V = $ dose/C_p^o). The clearance for this drug is 92 ml/min; for a one-compartment model, $CL = k \cdot V$.

B. Sampling before 2 hours indicates that, in fact, the drug follows multiexponential kinetics. The terminal disposition half-life is 4 hours, clearance is 103 ml/min (equation 4), V_{area} is 28 liters (equation 11), and V_{ss} is 25.4 liters (equation 12). The initial or "central" distribution volume for the drug ($V_1 = $ dose/C_p^o) is 16.1 liters. The example chosen indicates that multicompartment kinetics may be overlooked when sampling at early times is neglected. In this particular case, there is only a 10% error in the estimate of clearance when the multicompartment characteristics are ignored. However, for many drugs multicompartment kinetics may be observed for significant periods of time, and failure to consider the distribution phase can lead to significant errors in estimates of clearance and in predictions of the appropriate dosage.

where k is the rate constant for elimination of the drug from the compartment. This rate constant is inversely related to the half-life of the drug ($k = 0.693/t_{1/2}$).

For most drugs the idealized one-compartment model discussed above does not describe the entire time course of the plasma concentration. That is, certain tissue reservoirs can be distinguished from the central compartment, and the drug concentration appears to decay in a manner that can be described by multiple exponential terms (*see* Figure 1–5, *B*).

Rate of Drug Distribution. The multiple exponential decay observed for a drug that is eliminated from the body with first-order (linear) kinetics results from differences in the rates at which the drug equilibrates with tissue reservoirs. The rate of equilibration will depend upon the ratio of the perfusion of the tissue to the partition of drug into the tissue. In many cases, groups of tissues with similar perfusion/partition ratios all equilibrate at essentially the same rate, such that only one apparent phase of distribution (rapid initial fall of concentration, as in Figure 1–5, *B*) is seen. It is as though the drug starts in a "central" volume, which consists of plasma and tissue reservoirs that are in rapid equilibrium with it, and distributes to a "final" volume, at which point concentrations in plasma decrease in a log-linear fashion at rate k (*see* Figure 1–5, *B*).

If the pattern or ratio of blood flows to various tissues changes within an individual or differs between individuals, rates of drug distribution to tissues will also change. However, changes in blood flow may also cause some tissues that were originally in the "central" volume to equilibrate sufficiently more slowly so as to appear only in the "final" volume. This means that central volumes will appear to vary with disease states that cause altered regional blood flow. After an intravenous bolus dose, drug concentrations in plasma may be higher in individuals with poor perfusion (*e.g.*, shock) than they would be if perfusion were better. Thus, the effect of a drug at various sites of action can be variable, depending on perfusion of these sites.

Multicompartment Volume Terms. Two different terms have been used to describe the volume of distribution for drugs that follow multiple exponential decay. The first, designated V_{area}, is calculated as the ratio of clearance to the rate of decline of concentration during the elimination (final) phase of the logarithmic concentration versus time curve.

$$V_{area} = \frac{CL}{k} = \frac{\text{Dose}}{k \cdot AUC} \qquad (11)$$

The calculation of this parameter is straightforward, and the volume term may be determined after administration of drug by intravenous or enteral routes (where the dose used must be corrected for bioavailability). However, another multicompartment volume of distribution may be more useful, especially when the effect of disease states on pharmacokinetics is to be determined. The volume of distribution at steady state (V_{ss}) represents the volume in which a drug would appear to be distributed during steady state if the drug existed throughout that volume at the same concentration as that in the measured fluid (plasma or blood). This volume can be determined by the use of areas, as described by Benet and Galeazzi (1979).

$$V_{ss} = (\text{Dose}_{iv})(AUMC)/AUC_2 \qquad (12)$$

where $AUMC$ is the area under the first moment of the curve that describes the time course of the plasma or blood concentration, that is, the area under the curve of the product of time, t, and plasma or blood concentration, C, over the time span zero to infinity.

Although V_{area} is a convenient and easily calculated parameter, it varies when the rate constant for drug elimination changes, even when there has been no change in the distribution space. This is because the terminal rate of decline of the concentration of drug in blood or plasma depends not only on clearance but also on the rates of distribution of drug between the central and final volumes. V_{ss} does not suffer from this disadvantage (*see* Benet *et al.*, 1984).

HALF-LIFE

The half-life ($t_{1/2}$) is the time it takes for the plasma concentration or the amount of drug in the body to be reduced by 50%. For the simplest case, the one-compartment model (Figure 1–5, *A*), half-life may be determined readily and utilized to make decisions about drug dosage. However, as indicated in Figure 1–5, *B*, drug concentrations in plasma often follow a multiexponential pattern of decline; two or more half-life terms may thus be calculated. The half-life that is usually reported is that which corresponds to the terminal log-linear rate of elimination.

Early studies of pharmacokinetic properties of drugs in disease were compromised by their reliance on half-life as the sole measure of alterations of drug disposition. Only recently has it been appreciated that half-life is a derived parameter that changes as a function of both clearance and volume of distribution. A useful approximate relationship between the terminal log-linear half-life, clearance, and volume of distribution is given by:

$$t_{1/2} \cong 0.693 \cdot V/CL \qquad (13)$$

Clearance is the measure of the body's ability to eliminate a drug. However, the organs of elimination can only clear drug from the blood or plasma with which they are in direct contact. As clearance decreases due, for example, to a disease process, half-life would be expected to increase. However, this reciprocal relationship is exact only when the disease does not change the volume of distribution. For example, the half-life of diazepam increases with increasing age; however, it is not clearance that changes as a function of age, but the volume of distribution (Klotz *et al.*, 1975). Similarly, changes in protein binding of the drug may affect its clearance as well as its volume of distribution, leading to unpredictable changes in half-life as a function of disease. The half-life of tolbutamide, for example, decreases in patients with acute viral hepatitis, exactly the opposite from what one might expect. The disease appears to modify protein binding in both plasma and tissues, causing no change in volume of distribution but an *increase* in total clearance because higher concentrations of free drug are present (Williams *et al.*, 1977).

Although it can be a poor index of drug elimination, half-life does provide a good indication of the time required to reach steady state after a dosage regimen is initiated (*i.e.*, four half-lives to reach approximately 94% of a new steady state), the time for a drug to be removed from the body, and a means to estimate the appropriate dosing interval (*see* below).

Steady State. Equation 1 indicates that a steady-state concentration will eventually be achieved when a drug is administered at a constant rate. At this point, drug elimination (the product of clearance and concentration; equation 2) will equal the rate of drug availability. This concept also extends to intermittent dosage (*e.g.*, 250 mg of drug every 8 hours). During each interdose interval, the concentration of drug rises and falls. At steady state, the entire cycle is repeated identically in each interval. Equation 1 still applies for intermittent dosing, but it now describes the average drug concentration during an interdose interval.

Steady-state dosing is illustrated in Figure 1–6.

EXTENT AND RATE OF AVAILABILITY

Bioavailability. It is important to distinguish between the rate and extent of drug absorption and the amount that ultimately reaches the systemic circulation, as discussed above. The amount of the drug that reaches the systemic circulation can be expressed as a fraction of the dose, *F*, which is often called bioavailability. Reasons for incomplete absorption have been discussed above. Also, as noted previously, if the drug is metabolized in the liver or excreted in bile, some of the active drug absorbed from the gastrointestinal tract will be inactivated by the liver before it can reach the general circulation and be distributed to its sites of action.

When drugs are administered by a route that is subject to first-pass loss, the equations presented previously that contain the terms dose or dosing rate (equations 1, 4, 10, and 11) must also include the bioavailability term, *F*, such that the available dose or dosing rate is utilized. For example, equation 1 is modified to:

$$F \cdot \text{Dosing rate} = CL \cdot C_{ss} \qquad (14)$$

Rate of Absorption. Although the rate of drug absorption does not, in general, influence the average steady-state concentration of the drug in plasma, it may still influence drug therapy. If a drug is absorbed very rapidly (*e.g.*, a dose given as an intravenous bolus) and has a small central volume, the concentration of drug will be high initially. It will then fall as the drug is distributed to its final (larger) volume (*see* Figure 1–5, *B*). If the same drug is absorbed more slowly (*e.g.*, by slow infusion), it will be distributed while it is being given, and peak concentrations will be lower and will occur later. A given drug may act to produce both desirable and undesirable effects at several sites in the body, and the rates of distribution of drug to these sites may not be the same. The relative intensities of these different effects of a drug may thus vary transiently when its rate of administration is changed.

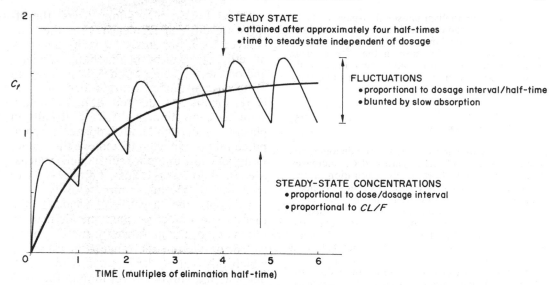

Figure 1–6. *Fundamental pharmacokinetic relationships for repeated administration of drugs.*

Light line is the pattern of drug accumulation during repeated administration of a drug at intervals equal to its elimination half-time, when drug absorption is ten times as rapid as elimination. As the relative rate of absorption increases, the concentration maxima approach 2 and the minima approach 1 during the steady state. Heavy line depicts the pattern during administration of equivalent dosage by continuous intravenous infusion. Curves are based upon the one-compartment model.

Average concentration ($\overline{C}_{ss}$) when the steady state is attained during intermittent drug administration:

$$\overline{C}_{ss} = \frac{F \cdot \text{dose}}{CL \cdot T}$$

where F = fractional bioavailability of the dose and T = dosage interval (time). By substitution of infusion rate for $F \cdot \text{dose}/T$, the formula is equivalent to equation 1 and provides the concentration maintained at steady state during continuous intravenous infusion.

NONLINEAR PHARMACOKINETICS

Nonlinearity in pharmacokinetics (*i.e.*, changes in such parameters as clearance, volume of distribution, and half-life as a function of dose or concentration of drug) is usually due to saturation of protein binding, hepatic metabolism, or active renal transport of the drug.

Saturable Protein Binding. As the molar concentration of drug increases, the unbound fraction must eventually also increase (as all binding sites become saturated). This usually occurs only when drug concentrations in plasma are in the range of tens to hundreds of micrograms per milliliter. For a drug that is metabolized by the liver with a low ratio of extraction, saturation of plasma protein binding will cause both V and clearance to increase as drug concentrations increase; half-life may thus remain constant (*see* equation 13). For such a drug, C_{ss} will not increase linearly as the rate of drug administration is increased. For drugs that are cleared with high extraction ratios, C_{ss} can remain

linearly proportional to the rate of drug administration. In this case, hepatic clearance would not change, and the increase in V would increase the half-time of disappearance by reducing the fraction of the total drug in the body that is delivered to the liver per unit time. Most drugs fall between these two extremes, and the effects of nonlinear protein binding may be difficult to predict.

Saturable Metabolism. In this situation, the Michaelis-Menten equation (equation 6) usually describes the nonlinearity. All active processes are undoubtedly saturable, but they will appear to be linear if values of drug concentrations encountered in practice are much less than K_m. When they exceed K_m, nonlinear kinetics is observed. The major consequences of saturation of metabolism are the opposite of those for saturation of protein binding. When both conditions are present simultaneously, they may virtually cancel each others' effects, and surprisingly linear kinetics may result; this occurs over a certain range of concentrations for salicylic acid.

Saturable metabolism causes first-pass metabolism to be less than expected (higher F), and there is a greater fractional increase in C_{ss} than the corresponding fractional increase in the rate of drug administration. The latter can be seen most easily by substituting equation 6 into equation 1 and solving for the steady-state concentration.

$$C_{ss} = \frac{\text{Dosing rate} \cdot K_m}{V_m - \text{Dosing rate}} \qquad (15)$$

As the dosing rate approaches V_m, the denominator of equation 15 approaches zero and C_{ss} increases disproportionately. Fortunately, saturation of metabolism should have no effect on V; thus, as clearance decreases, the apparent half-life for elimination increases and the approach to the (disproportionate) new steady state is slow. However, the concept of "four half-lives to steady state" is not applicable for drugs with nonlinear metabolism in the usual range of clinical concentrations.

Phenytoin provides an example of a drug for which metabolism becomes saturated in the therapeutic range of concentration (*see* Appendix II). K_m is typically near the lower end of the therapeutic range ($K_m = 5$ to 10 mg/liter). For some individuals, especially children, K_m may be as low as 1 mg/liter. If, for such an individual, the target concentration is 15 mg/liter and this is attained at a dosing rate of 300 mg per day, then, from equation 15, V_m equals 320 mg per day. For such a patient, a dose 10% less than optimal (*i.e.*, 270 mg per day) will produce a C_{ss} of 5 mg/liter, well below the desired value. In contrast, a dose 10% greater than optimal (330 mg per day) will exceed metabolic capacity (by 10 mg per day) and cause a long and slow but unending climb of concentration until toxicity occurs. Dosage cannot be controlled so precisely (less than 10% error); for those patients in whom the target concentration for phenytoin is more than tenfold greater than the K_m, alternating inefficacious therapy and toxicity is almost unavoidable.

DESIGN AND OPTIMIZATION OF DOSAGE REGIMENS

When chronic therapy is initiated, a pharmacodynamic question must be asked: what degree of drug effect is desired and achievable? If some effect of the drug is easily measured (*e.g.*, blood pressure), it can be used to guide dosage, and a trial-and-error approach to optimal dosage is both practical and sensible. Even in this ideal case, certain quantitative issues arise, such as how often to change dosage and by how much. These can usually be settled with simple rules of thumb based on the principles discussed (*e.g.*, change dosage by no more than 50% and no more often than every three to four half-lives).

Target Level. For some drugs, the effects are difficult to measure (or the drug is given for prophylaxis), toxicity and lack of efficacy are both potential dangers, and/or the therapeutic index is narrow. In these circumstances a target-level strategy is reasonable. A desired (target) steady-state concentration of the drug (usually in plasma) is chosen, and a dosage is computed that is expected to achieve this value. Drug concentrations are subsequently measured, and dosage is adjusted if necessary to approximate the target more closely.

To apply the target-level strategy, the therapeutic objective must be defined in terms of a desirable range for the C_{ss}, often called the therapeutic range. For drugs for which this can be done, such as theophylline and digoxin, the lower limit of the therapeutic range appears to be approximately equal to the drug concentration that produces about half of the greatest possible therapeutic effect. The upper limit of the therapeutic range is fixed by toxicity, not by efficacy. It can be essentially unbounded for a very nontoxic drug. In general, however, the upper limit of the therapeutic range is such that no more than 5 to 10% of patients will experience a toxic effect. For many drugs, this may mean that the upper limit of the range is no more than twice the lower limit. Of course, these figures can be highly variable, and some patients may benefit greatly from drug concentrations that exceed the therapeutic range while others may suffer significant toxicity at much lower values. Barring more specific information, however, the target is usually chosen as the center of the therapeutic range.

Maintenance Dose. In most clinical situations, drugs are administered in a series of repetitive doses or as a continuous infusion in order to maintain a steady-state concentration of drug in plasma within a given therapeutic range. Thus, calculation of the appropriate maintenance dosage is a primary goal. To maintain the chosen steady-state or target concentration, the rate of drug administration is adjusted such that the rate of input equals the rate of loss. This relationship was defined previously in equations 1 and 14 and is expressed here in terms of the desired target concentration:

Dosing rate = Target · CL/F (16)

If the clinician chooses the desired concentration of drug in plasma and knows the clearance and availability for that drug in a particular patient, the appropriate dose and dosing interval can be calculated.

Example. A steady-state plasma concentration of theophylline of 15 mg/liter is desired to relieve acute bronchial asthma in a 68-kg patient. If the patient does not smoke and is otherwise normal except for the asthmatic condition, one can use the mean clearance given in Appendix II, that is, 0.65 ml · min^{-1} · kg^{-1}. Because the drug is to be given as an intravenous infusion, $F = 1$.

Dosing rate = Target · CL/F
= 15 μg/ml · 0.65 ml · min^{-1} · kg^{-1}
= 9.75 μg · min^{-1} · kg^{-1}
= 40 mg/hr for a 68-kg patient

Since almost all intravenous preparations of theophylline are available as the ethylenediamine salt (aminophylline), which contains 85% theophylline, the infusion rate will be 47 mg/hr of aminophylline [(40 mg/hr)/(0.85)].

Dosing Interval for Intermittent Dosage. In general, marked fluctuations in drug concentrations between doses are not beneficial. If absorption and distribution were instantaneous, fluctuation of drug concentrations between doses would be governed entirely by the drug's elimination half-life. If the dosing interval (T) was chosen to be equal to the half-life, then the total fluctuation would be twofold; this is usually a tolerable variation.

Pharmacodynamic considerations modify this. If a drug is relatively nontoxic, such that concentrations many times that necessary for therapy can easily be tolerated, doses can be large and the dosing interval can be much longer than the elimination half-life (for convenience). The half-life of penicillin G is less than 1 hour, but it is often given in very large doses every 6 or 12 hours.

For some drugs with a narrow therapeutic range, it may be important to estimate the maximal and minimal concentrations that will occur for a particular dosing interval. If the dosing interval chosen corresponds to a time during the log-linear phase of drug disposition (Figure 1–5, *B*), then the minimal steady-state concentration, $C_{ss,min}$, may be reasonably determined by the use of equation 17.

$$C_{ss},min = \frac{F \cdot \text{dose}/V_{ss}}{1 - exp(-kT)} \cdot exp(-kT) \qquad (17)$$

where k is the terminal rate constant for elimination (*see* Figure 1–5, *B*) and T is the dosing interval. The term $exp(-kT)$ is, in fact, the fraction of the last dose (corrected for bioavailability) that remains in the body at the end of a dosing interval.

For drugs that follow multiexponential kinetics and that are administered orally, the estimation of the maximal steady-state concentration, $C_{ss,max}$, involves a complicated set of exponential constants for distribution and absorption. If these terms are ignored for multiple oral dosing, one may easily predict a maximal steady-state concentration by omitting the $exp(-kT)$ term in the numerator of equation 17 (*see* equation 18, below). Because of the approximation, the predicted maximal concentration from equation 18 will be greater than that actually observed.

Example. When the acute asthmatic attack in the patient discussed above is relieved, the clinician might want to maintain the plasma concentration of theophylline at 15 mg/liter, with oral dosage at intervals of 6, 8, or 12 hours. The correct rate of drug administration, independent of consideration of the dosing interval, is 40 mg/hr for this patient, as calculated above, since the availability of theophylline from an oral dose is 100%. Thus, the appropriate intermittent doses would be 240 mg every 6 hours, 320 mg every 8 hours, or 480 mg every 12 hours. All of these regimens would yield the same average concentration, 15 mg/liter, but different maximal and minimal concentrations would pertain. For a 12-hour dosing interval, the following maximal and minimal concentrations would be predicted:

$$\begin{aligned} C_{ss,max} &= \frac{F \cdot \text{dose}/V_{ss}}{1 - exp(-kT)} \\ &= \frac{480 \text{ mg}/34 \text{ liters}}{0.65} = 22 \text{ mg/liter} \end{aligned} \qquad (18)$$

$$\begin{aligned} C_{ss,min} &= C_{ss,max} \cdot exp(-kT) \\ &= (21.7 \text{ mg/liter}) \cdot (0.35) = 7.6 \text{ mg/liter} \end{aligned} \qquad (19)$$

The calculations in equations 18 and 19 were performed assuming oral doses of 480 mg every 12 hours of a drug with a half-life of 8 hours ($k = 0.693/8$ hr $= 0.0866$ hr^{-1}), a volume of distribution of 0.5 liter/kg ($V_{ss} = 34$ liters for a 68-kg patient), and an oral availability of 1. Since the predicted minimal concentration, 7.6 mg/liter, falls below the suggested effective concentration and the predicted maximal concentration is above that suggested to avoid toxicity (*see* Appendix II), the choice of a 12-hour dosing interval is probably inappropriate. A more appropriate choice would be 320 mg every 8 hours or 240 mg every 6 hours; for $T = 6$ hr, $C_{ss,max} = 17$ mg/liter; $C_{ss,min} = 10$ mg/liter. The clinician must of course balance the problem of compliance with regimens that involve frequent dosage against the problem of periods when the patient may be subjected to concentrations of the drug that could be too high or too low.

Loading Dose. The "loading dose" is one or a series of doses that may be given at the onset of therapy with the aim of achieving the target concentration rapidly. The appropriate magnitude for the loading dose is:

$$\text{Loading dose} = \text{Target } C_p \cdot V_{ss}/F \qquad (20)$$

A loading dose may be desirable if the time required to attain steady state by the administration of drug at a constant rate (four elimination half-lives) is long relative to the temporal demands of the condition being treated. For example, the half-life of lidocaine is usually more than 1 hour. Arrhythmias encountered after myocardial infarction may obviously be life threatening, and one cannot wait for 4 to 6 hours to achieve a therapeutic concentration of lidocaine by infusion of the drug at the rate required to *maintain* this concentration. Hence, use of a loading dose of lidocaine in the coronary care unit is standard.

The use of a loading dose also has significant disadvantages. First, the particularly sensitive individual may be exposed abruptly to a toxic concentration of a drug. Moreover, if the drug involved has a long half-life, it will take a long time for the concentration to fall if the level achieved was excessive. Loading doses tend to be large, and they are often given parenterally and rapidly; this can be particularly dangerous if toxic effects occur as a result of actions of the drug at sites that are in rapid equilibrium with plasma.

Individualizing Dosage. To design a rational dosage regimen, the clinician must know F, CL, V_{ss}, and $t_{1/2}$, and have some knowledge about rates of absorption and distribution of the drug. Moreover, one must judge what variations in these parameters might be expected in a particular patient. Usual values for the important parameters and appropriate adjustments that may be necessitated by disease or other factors are presented in Appendix II. There

is, however, unpredictable variation between normal individuals; for many drugs, one standard deviation in the values observed for F, CL, and V_{ss} is about 20%, 50%, and 30%, respectively. This means that 95% of the time the C_{ss} that is achieved will be between 35% and 270% of the target; this is an unacceptably wide range for a drug with a low therapeutic index. If values of C_p are measured, one can estimate values of F, CL, and V_{ss} directly, and this permits more precise adjustment of a dosage regimen. Such measurement and adjustment are appropriate for many drugs with low therapeutic indices (*e.g.*, cardiac glycosides, antiarrhythmic agents, anticonvulsants, theophylline, and others).

THERAPEUTIC DRUG MONITORING

The major use of measured concentrations of drugs (at steady state) is to refine the estimate of CL/F for the patient being treated (using equation 14 as rearranged below):

$$CL/F \text{ (patient)} = \text{Dosing rate}/C_{ss} \text{ (measured)} \qquad (21)$$

The new estimate of CL/F can be used in equation 16 to adjust the maintenance dose to achieve the desired target concentration.

Certain practical details and pitfalls related to therapeutic drug monitoring should be kept in mind. The first of these concerns the time of sampling for measurement of the drug concentration. If intermittent dosing is utilized, when, during a dosing interval, should samples be taken? It is necessary to distinguish between two possible uses of measured drug concentrations in order to understand the possible answers. A concentration of drug measured in a sample taken at virtually any time during the dosing interval will provide information that may aid in the assessment of drug toxicity. This is one type of therapeutic drug monitoring. It should be stressed, however, that such use of a measured concentration of drug is fraught with difficulties caused by interindividual variability in sensitivity to the drug. When there is a question of toxicity, the drug concentration can be no more than just one of many items that serve to inform the clinician.

Changes in the effects of drugs may be delayed relative to changes in plasma concentration because of a slow rate of distribution or pharmacodynamic factors. Concentrations of digoxin, for example, regularly exceed 2 ng/ml (a potentially toxic value) shortly after an oral dose, yet these peak concentrations do not cause toxicity; indeed, they occur well before peak effects. Thus, concentrations of drugs in samples obtained shortly after administration can be uninformative or even misleading.

When concentrations of drugs are used for purposes of adjusting dosage regimens, samples obtained shortly after administration of a dose are almost invariably misleading. The point of sampling during supposed steady state is to modify one's estimate of CL/F and thus one's choice of dosage. Early postabsorptive concentrations do not reflect clearance; they are determined primarily by the rate of absorption, the central (rather than the steady-state) volume of distribution, and the rate of distribution, all of which are pharmacokinetic features of virtually no relevance to long-term, steady-state dosage. When the goal of measurement is adjustment of dosage, the sample should be taken well after the previous dose—as a rule of thumb just before the next planned dose, when the concentration is at its minimum. There is an exception to this approach. Some drugs are nearly completely eliminated between doses and act only during the initial portion of each dosing interval. If, for such drugs, it is questionable whether efficacious concentrations are being achieved, a sample taken shortly after a dose may be helpful. Yet, if another concern is that low clearance (as in renal failure) may cause accumulation of drug, concentrations measured just before the next dose will reveal such accumulation and are considerably more useful for this purpose than is knowledge of the maximal concentration. For such drugs, determination of both maximal and minimal concentrations is thus recommended.

A second important aspect of the timing of sampling is its relationship to the beginning of the maintenance dosage regimen. When constant dosage is given, steady state is reached only after four half-lives have passed. If a sample is obtained too soon after dosage is begun, it will not accurately reflect clearance. Yet, for toxic drugs, if one waits until steady state is assured, the damage may have been done. Some simple guidelines can be offered. When it is important to maintain careful control of concentrations, one may take the first sample after two half-lives (as calculated and expected for the patient), assuming no loading dose has been given. If the concentration already exceeds 90% of the eventual expected mean steady-state concentration, the dosage rate should be halved, another sample obtained in another two (supposed) half-lives, and the dosage halved again if this sample exceeds the target. If the first concentration is not too high, one proceeds with the initial rate of dosage; even if the concentration is lower than expected, one can usually await the attainment of steady state in another two estimated half-lives and then proceed to adjust dosage as described above.

If dosage is intermittent, there is a third concern with the time at which samples are obtained for determination of drug concentrations. If the sample has been obtained just prior to the next dose, as recommended, concentration will be a minimal value, not the mean. However, as discussed above, the estimated mean concentration may be calculated by using equation 17 if the dosing interval chosen corresponds to a time during the log-linear phase of drug disposition (*i.e.*, the rates of drug absorption and distribution are fast relative to the rate of drug elimination). Since $C_{ss,min}$ is directly related to dose, the ratio between the measured and desired concentrations can be used to adjust the dose.

$$\frac{C_{ss,min}(\text{measured})}{C_{ss,min}(\text{desired})} = \frac{\text{Dose(initial)}}{\text{Dose(new)}} \quad (22)$$

When absorption is known to be slow or when the interval between doses is less than 50% of the half-life, then the criteria for calculation of $C_{ss,min}$ with equation 17 are not met. Under these conditions, the concentration measured at the end of a dosing interval may be assumed to approximate the mean or steady-state concentration and equation 14 can be used to adjust dosage.

Other difficulties of interpretation of drug concentrations arise from problems with specificity of assays. Some assays for drugs measure not only the active compound but other substances or metabolites as well. When this is so, the usual relationship of concentration to effect may appear to change over time (*e.g.*, as metabolites that are devoid of pharmacological activity accumulate). This may be especially noticeable in patients with renal failure. The opposite results from accumulation of active metabolites that are not measured by a specific assay. As specific and sensitive assays for drugs and metabolites are developed, such problems should decrease.

General References

Goldstein, A.; Aronow, L.; and Kalman, S. M. *Principles of Drug Action: The Basis of Pharmacology,* 2nd ed. John Wiley & Sons, Inc., New York, **1974.**

Levine, R. R. *Pharmacology: Drug Actions and Reactions,* 3rd ed. Little, Brown & Co., Boston, **1983.**

Melmon, K. L., and Morrelli, H. F. (eds.). *Clinical Pharmacology: Basic Principles in Therapeutics,* 2nd ed. Macmillan Publishing Co., New York, **1978.**

Historical Background

Holmstedt, B., and Liljestrand, G. (eds.). *Readings in Pharmacology.* Pergamon Press, Ltd., Oxford, **1963.**

Shuster, L. (ed.). *Readings in Pharmacology.* Little, Brown & Co., Boston, **1962.**

Absorption, Distribution, Biotransformation, and Excretion

American Pharmaceutical Association. *The Bioavailability of Drug Products,* cumulative ed. The Association, Washington, D. C., **1978.**

Berliner, R. W.; Clubb, L. E.; Doluisio, J. T.; Melmon, K. L.; Nados, A. S.; Oates, J. A.; Reigelmen, S.; Shideman, F. E.; Zelin, M.; and Robbins, F. C. *Drug Bioequivalence.* Office of Technological Assessment, U.S. Government Printing Office, Washington, D. C., **1974.**

Brodie, B. B. Physicochemical factors in drug absorption. In, *Absorption and Distribution of Drugs.* (Binns, T. B., ed.) The Williams & Wilkins Co., Baltimore, **1964,** pp. 16–48.

Green, T. P.; O'Dea, R. F.; and Mirkin, B. L. Determinants of drug disposition and effect in the fetus. *Annu. Rev. Pharmacol. Toxicol.,* **1979,** *19,* 285–322.

Jenner, P., and Testa, B. (eds.). *Concepts in Drug Metabolism. Drugs and the Pharmaceutical Sciences Series,* Vol. 10, Pt. B. Marcel Dekker, Inc., New York, **1981.**

La Du, B. N.; Mandel, H. G.; and Way, E. L. (eds.). *Fundamentals of Drug Metabolism and Drug Disposition.* The Williams & Wilkins Co., Baltimore, **1971.**

Lee, D. H. K.; Falk, H. L.; Murphy, S. D.; and Geiger, S. R. (eds.). *Reactions to Environmental Agents. Handbook of Physiology,* Sect. 9. American Physiological Society, Bethesda, **1977.** (*See* especially Chapters 12 to 34 for absorption, distribution, and excretion of foreign agents.)

Merkin, B. L., and Singh, S. Placental transfer of pharmacologically active molecules. In, *Perinatal Pharmacology and Therapeutics.* (Mirkin, B. L., ed.) Academic Press, Inc., New York, **1973,** pp. 1–69.

Mitchell, J. R., and Horning, M. G. (eds.). *Drug Metabolism and Drug Toxicity.* Raven Press, New York, **1984.**

Prescott, L. F., and Nimmo, W. S. (eds.). *Drug Absorption.* Adis Press, New York, **1981.**

Reidenberg, M. M. *Renal Function and Drug Action.* W. B. Saunders Co., Philadelphia, **1971.**

Routledge, P. A., and Shand, D. G. Presystemic drug elimination. *Annu. Rev. Pharmacol. Toxicol.,* **1979,** *19,* 447–468.

Scheline, R. R. Metabolism of foreign compounds by gastrointestinal microorganisms. *Pharmacol. Rev.,* **1973,** *25,* 451–523.

Singer, S. J., and Nicolson, G. L. The fluid-mosaic model of the structure of membranes. *Science,* **1972,** *175,* 720–731.

Symposium. (Various authors.) Pharmacogenetics. (Vesell, E. S., ed.) *Fed. Proc.,* **1972,** *31,* 1253–1330.

Symposium. (Various authors.) Clinical implications of drug-protein binding. (Levy, R., and Shand, D., eds.) *Clin. Pharmacokinet.,* **1984,** *9,* Suppl. 1, 1–104.

Wester, R. C., and Maibach, H. E. Cutaneous pharmacokinetics: 10 steps to percutaneous absorption. *Drug Metab. Rev.,* **1983,** *14,* 169–205.

Pharmacokinetic Principles

Atkinson, A. J., Jr., and Kushner, W. Clinical pharmacokinetics. *Annu. Rev. Pharmacol. Toxicol.,* **1979,** *19,* 105–128.

Benet, L. Z. Effect of route of administration and distribution on drug action. *J. Pharmacokinet. Biopharm.,* **1978,** *6,* 559–585.

Benet, L. Z., and Galeazzi, R. L. Noncompartmental determination of the steady-state volume of distribution. *J. Pharm. Sci.,* **1979,** *68,* 1071–1074.

Benet, L. Z.; Massoud, N.; and Gambertoglio, J. G. (eds.). *Pharmacokinetic Basis for Drug Treatment.* Raven Press, New York, **1984.**

Gibaldi, M., and Perrier, D. *Pharmacokinetics,* 2nd ed. Marcel Dekker, Inc., New York, **1982.**

Klotz, U.; Avant, G. R.; Hoyumpa, A.; Schenker, S.; and Wilkinson, G. R. The effects of age and liver disease on the disposition and elimination of diazepam in adult man. *J. Clin. Invest.,* **1975,** *55,* 347–359.

Nies, A. S.; Shand, D. G.; and Wilkinson, G. R. Altered hepatic blood flow and drug disposition. *Clin. Pharmacokinet.,* **1976,** *1,* 135–155.

Rowland, M.; Benet, L. Z.; and Graham, G. G. Clearance concepts in pharmacokinetics. *J. Pharmacokinet. Biopharm.,* **1973,** *1,* 123–136.

Wagner, J. G. *Biopharmaceutics and Relevant Pharmacokinetics.* Drug Intelligence, Hamilton, Ill., **1971.**

Wilkinson, G. R., and Shand, D. G. A physiologic approach to hepatic drug clearance. *Clin. Pharmacol. Ther.,* **1975,** *18,* 377–390.

Williams, R. L.; Blaschke, T. F.; Meffin, P. J.; Melmon, K. L.; and Rowland, M. Influence of acute viral hepatitis on disposition and plasma binding of tolbutamide. *Clin. Pharmacol. Ther.,* **1977,** *21,* 301–309.

CHAPTER

2 PHARMACODYNAMICS: MECHANISMS OF DRUG ACTION AND THE RELATIONSHIP BETWEEN DRUG CONCENTRATION AND EFFECT

Elliott M. Ross and Alfred G. Gilman

Pharmacodynamics may be defined as the study of the biochemical and physiological effects of drugs and their mechanisms of action. The latter aspect of the subject is perhaps the most fundamental challenge to the investigator in pharmacology, and information derived from such study is of basic utility to the clinician. The objectives of the analysis of drug action are identification of the primary action (as distinguished from description of resultant effects), delineation of the details of the chemical interaction between drug and cell, and characterization of the full sequence of actions and effects. Such a complete analysis provides a truly satisfactory basis for the rational therapeutic use of a drug on the one hand and for the design of new and superior chemical agents on the other.

MECHANISMS OF DRUG ACTION

While there are several types of exceptions, the effects of most drugs result from their interaction with functional macromolecular components of the organism. Such interaction alters the function of the pertinent cellular component and thereby initiates the series of biochemical and physiological changes that are characteristic of the response to the drug. This concept—now almost obvious—had its origins in the experimental work of Ehrlich and Langley during the late nineteenth and early twentieth centuries. Ehrlich was struck by the high degree of chemical specificity for the antiparasitic and toxic effects of a variety of synthetic organic agents. Langley noted the ability of the South American arrow poison, curare, to inhibit the contraction of skeletal muscles caused by nicotine; however, the tissue remained responsive to di-

rect electrical stimulation. The terms *receptive substance* and, more simply, *receptor* were coined to denote the component of the organism with which the chemical agent was presumed to interact. There are fundamental corollaries to the statement that the receptor for a drug can be any functional macromolecular component of the organism. One is that a drug is potentially capable of altering the rate at which *any* bodily function proceeds; a second is that, by virtue of interactions with such receptors, drugs do not *create* effects but merely modulate ongoing function. A simple pharmacological dictum thus states that a drug cannot impart a new function to a cell. While modern technics of molecular genetics may challenge this principle, it remains valid for the immediate future (*see*, for example, Mishina *et al.*, 1985).

Whereas any functional macromolecular component of the organism may serve as a drug receptor, we will make special mention below of a group of cellular proteins that *normally* serve as receptors for endogenous regulatory ligands (*e.g.*, hormones, neurotransmitters). Many drugs mimic at least some of the effects of such endogenous compounds by interaction with the appropriate physiological receptor; such agents are termed *agonists*. In this context it is most important to note that other compounds may have no intrinsic regulatory activity at a given receptor but may still be able to bind to the macromolecule; a result of such binding may be interference with the effect of an agonist. Compounds that are themselves devoid of intrinsic pharmacological activity but cause effects by inhibition of the action of a specific agonist (*e.g.*, by competition for agonist binding sites) are designated as *antagonists*.

DRUG RECEPTORS

Chemical Properties. At least from a numerical standpoint, the proteins of the cell form the most important class of drug receptors. Obvious examples are the enzymes of crucial metabolic or regulatory pathways (*e.g.,* dihydrofolate reductase, acetylcholinesterase), but of equal interest are proteins involved in transport processes (*e.g.,* Na^+,K^+-ATPase) or those that serve structural roles (*e.g.,* tubulin). Specific binding properties of other cellular constituents can also be exploited. Thus, nucleic acids are important drug receptors, particularly for chemotherapeutic approaches to the control of malignancy; plant lectins show remarkably specific recognition of carbohydrate moieties in glycoproteins (use of this property may be forthcoming in the synthesis of lectin-drug hybrids that are targeted to specific cells); drugs such as general anesthetics interact with and alter the structure and function of the lipids of cellular membranes.

The binding of drugs to receptors, in various cases, involves all known types of interactions—ionic, hydrogen, hydrophobic, van der Waals, and covalent. If binding is covalent, the duration of drug action is frequently, but not necessarily, prolonged. Noncovalent interactions of high affinity may also appear to be essentially irreversible. In most interactions between drugs and receptors it is likely that bonds of multiple types are important (*see* Goldstein *et al.,* 1974).

Structure-Activity Relationship. The affinity of a drug for a specific macromolecular component of the cell and its intrinsic activity are intimately related to its chemical structure. The relationship is frequently quite stringent, and relatively minor modifications in the drug molecule, particularly including such subtle changes as stereoisomerism, may result in major changes in pharmacological properties. Exploitation of structure-activity relationships has on many occasions led to the synthesis of valuable therapeutic agents. Since changes in molecular configuration need not alter all actions and effects of a drug equally, it is sometimes possible to develop a *congener*

with a more favorable ratio of therapeutic to toxic effects, enhanced selectivity among different cells or tissues, or more acceptable secondary characteristics than those of the parent drug. In addition, effective therapeutic agents have been fashioned by developing structurally related competitive antagonists of other drugs or of endogenous substances known to be important in biochemical or physiological function. Minor modifications of structure can also have profound effects on the pharmacokinetic properties of drugs.

Cellular Sites of Drug Action. The general and major determinants of the primary site of drug action must be the localization and functional capacity of the specific receptors with which the drug interacts and the concentration of drug to which the receptor is exposed. Localization of drug action is not necessarily dependent upon selective distribution of the drug. If a drug acts by interaction with a receptor that serves functions common to most cells, its effects will be widespread. If this is a vital function, the drug will be particularly dangerous to use. Nevertheless, such a drug may be clinically important. Digitalis glycosides, important in the treatment of heart failure, are potent inhibitors of an ion transport process that is vital to most cells. As such, they can cause widespread toxicity, and their margin of safety is dangerously low. Other examples could be cited, particularly in the area of cancer chemotherapy. Attempts have been made to restrict or direct the distribution of drugs by their attachment to soluble or insoluble carriers or by their encapsulation in liposomes. Another approach is the design of prodrugs that can be preferentially converted to the active species in only certain types of cells. These are areas of active investigation.

If a drug interacts with specialized receptors unique to specific types of differentiated cells, its effects are more specific. The hypothetical ideal drug would cause its therapeutic effect by virtue of such types of action. Side effects would be minimized, but toxicity might not be. If the differentiated function is a vital one, this type of drug could also be very dangerous. Some of the most lethal chemical agents known (*e.g.,* botulinus toxin) show such specificity and toxicity. Note also that even if the *action* of a drug is localized, the effects of the drug may be widespread and disseminated by a variety of secondary forces, chemical and physical.

RECEPTORS FOR PHYSIOLOGICAL REGULATORY MOLECULES

In the discussion above, the term *receptor* has been used operationally to denote any cellular macromolecule to which a drug binds to initiate its effects. The functional properties of the receptors that have been used as examples are evident. In addition, however, there exist groups of cellular proteins whose *normal function* is to act as receptors for endogenous regulatory ligands—particularly hormones, neurotransmitters, and autacoids (*see* Kleinzeller and Martin, 1983). The function of such physiological receptors, many of which are components of the plasma membrane, consists of binding the appropriate ligand and propagating its regulatory signal in the target cell, either by virtue of a direct intracellular effect or by promoting the synthesis or release of another intracellular regulatory molecule, a *second messenger*. The two functions of a receptor, ligand binding and message propagation, have led to speculation on the existence of functional domains within the receptor: a *ligand-binding domain* and an *effector domain*. The evolution of different receptors for diverse ligands that act by similar biochemical mechanisms on the one hand and of multiple receptors for a single ligand that act by unrelated mechanisms on the other is consistent with such a concept. In some cases, an individual receptor molecule may interact with closely associated cellular proteins in order to generate its effect; this constitutes a *receptor-effector system*. An example of such is the hormone-sensitive adenylate cyclase system. Here, receptors regulate the activity of the enzyme adenylate cyclase, the effector that synthesizes the second messenger adenosine $3',5'$-monophosphate (cyclic AMP). This system is complex, in that two separate guanine nucleotide-binding regulatory proteins act as intermediaries between receptors and the enzyme. One serves to transduce stimulatory signals, while the other is involved with inhibitory events (Gilman, 1984).

Receptors (and their associated effector and coupling proteins) also act as *integrators* of extracellular information as they coordinate signals from multiple ligands with each other and with the metabolic activities of the cell (*see* below). This integrative function is particularly evident when one considers that the different receptors for scores of chemically unrelated ligands utilize relatively few biochemical mechanisms to exert their regulatory functions, and that even these few pathways may share common elements (*see* Figure 2–1).

Intracellular receptors for steroids, thyroid hormone, and some other hormonal lipids (*e.g.,* vitamins A and D) *induce the synthesis of specific proteins* by binding to nuclear chromatin and thereby enhancing the transcription of the appropriate genes (*see* R1, Figure 2–1). Receptors for several neurotransmitters (*e.g.,* acetylcholine, gamma-aminobutyric acid, glycine) are themselves *ion channels* (or are associated with ion channels) in the plasma membranes of target cells. They open in response to agonists and thus control the cell's membrane potential and influence its ionic composition (Conti-Tronconi and Raftery, 1982; *see* R2, Figure 2–1). Numerous receptors ($R3_s$, $R3_i$, Figure 2–1) act to either stimulate or inhibit adenylate cyclase, cumulatively leading to an increase or decrease in the intracellular concentration of *cyclic AMP* (Smigel et al., 1984). These receptors act by way of distinct guanosine triphosphate (GTP)–binding regulatory proteins (G_s and G_i, respectively). G_s is activated to a form that can stimulate adenylate cyclase (A.C.) by binding GTP, and such binding is accelerated by the appropriate agonist-receptor ($R3_s$) complex. Deactivation occurs by the hydrolysis of GTP to guanosine diphosphate (GDP). G_i can be similarly activated to a form that can inhibit the activation of G_s and, probably indirectly, inhibit adenylate cyclase. Cyclic AMP (cAMP), in turn, acts within the cell to stimulate cyclic AMP–dependent protein kinases (cA-Dep. Kinase), which catalyze the phosphorylation of numerous enzymes and other proteins on seryl residues. Ca^{2+} entry into the cell is controlled by distinct receptors (R4). *Cytoplasmic Ca^{2+}* regulates some functions directly and regulates others only when it is bound to the intracellular Ca^{2+}-dependent regulatory protein calmodulin (CaM). The CaM-Ca^{2+} complex controls the functions of some proteins directly and others by activating a distinct group of protein kinases, of which myosin light-chain kinase (MLCK) is an important example.

Receptors for many hormones and neurotransmitters (R5, Figure 2–1) appear to cause the accumulation of multiple intracellular second messengers. For example, a fundamental event in some

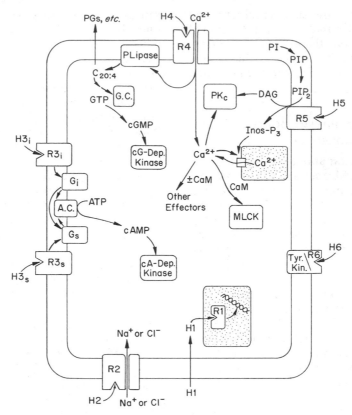

Figure 2–1. *Receptor-mediated regulatory mechanisms.*

    Classes of receptors (R1, R2, *etc.*) are shown with the understanding that several different types of receptors within a class may coexist in a single cell. *See* text for further discussion. Abbreviations not defined in the text are as follows: H = hormone, neurotransmitter, autacoid, *etc.*; PI = phosphatidylinositol; PIP = phosphatidylinositol-4-phosphate. Proteins are designated within solid lines; cellular organelles are stippled. Major sites of intracellular storage of Ca^{2+} include mitochondria and, particularly in muscle, sarcoplasmic reticulum.

systems appears to be the receptor-stimulated formation of *inositol-1,4,5-triphosphate* (Inos-P$_3$) and *diacylglycerol* (DAG) as the result of hydrolysis of a membrane phospholipid, phosphatidylinositol-4,5-biphosphate (PIP$_2$). The formation of inositol triphosphate is tightly (and perhaps causally) linked to the release of Ca^{2+} from intracellular stores. In addition to its general functions mentioned above, Ca^{2+} in the presence of diacylglycerol also activates a distinct protein kinase, denoted protein kinase C (PK$_c$) (*see* Berridge, 1984). Other secondary events that appear to occur in such a cascade involve the hydrolysis of arachidonic acid (C$_{20:4}$) from membrane phospholipids by Ca^{2+}-activated phospholipases (PLipase), with subsequent generation of *prostaglandins* (PGs), *prostacyclin, leukotrienes*, and related compounds (eicosanoids). These oxidative events lead further to the activation of guanylate cyclase (G.C.), with resultant elevation of the intracellular concentration of guanosine 3′,5′-monophosphate (cyclic GMP; cGMP). This cyclic nucleotide is the activator of yet a fourth class of protein kinases (cG-Dep. Kinase).

Receptors for insulin and several polypeptide growth factors (R6) are themselves agonist-stimulated, plasma membrane–bound *protein kinases* (Tyr. Kin.). Physiological substrates for these kinases are just being identified, but their phosphorylation is distinctive in that it is localized to tyrosyl rather than seryl or threonyl residues (Cobb and Rosen, 1984). Given this profusion of protein kinases, it should be noted that a given protein may be a substrate for several kinases that phosphorylate the same or different amino acid residues with varied consequences.

    If a cell has several receptors that utilize a single effector mechanism, multiple extracellular signals may be integrated to yield a cumulative intracellular signal. For example, individual submaximal stimulation of two receptors that activate adenylate cyclase and of one receptor that inhibits the enzyme will be expressed as a unique rate of synthesis of cyclic AMP. Receptors that act by different primary mechanisms can be coordinated at other levels. Thus, release of intracellular calcium and the activation of adenylate cyclase can lead to the phosphorylation and activation (or deactivation) of the same metabolic enzymes or of distinct enzymes with opposing or synergistic functions. Alternatively, signal integration can be built into the receptor-effector complex; hormonal inhibition of adenylate cyclase may reflect the competition between the stimulatory and inhibitory coupling proteins for a shared, common subunit (Gilman, 1984).

Regulation of Receptors. It is important to recognize that receptors not only are the determinants of acute regulation of physiological and biochemical function but also are themselves subject to regulatory and homeostatic control. For example, continued stimulation of cells with agonists generally results in a state of *desensitization* (also referred to as *refractoriness* or *down regulation*), such that the effect that follows subsequent exposure to the same concentration of drug is diminished (Harden, 1983). This can become very important in therapeutic situations; an example is the repeated use of β-adrenergic bronchodilators such as isoproterenol for the treatment of asthma (*see* Chapter 8). Multiple mechanisms exist that account for desensitization of different types. In some cases the signal from only a specific receptor becomes interrupted. This may involve alteration of the receptor or, in some cases, the actual destruction of the receptor or its relocalization within the cell. In other situations, receptors for different hormones that, for example, may all stimulate the adenylate cyclase of a single cell become less effective; this type of regulation presumably is directed at some common point in the effector pathway distal to the receptor itself. Conversely, *hyperreactivity* or *supersensitivity* to receptor agonists is also frequently observed to follow reduction in the chronic level of receptor stimulation. Situations of this type can result from the long-term administration of antagonists such as propranolol (*see* Chapter 9). In at least some cases supersensitivity may result from the synthesis of additional receptors.

Detection of Receptors by Ligand-Binding Assays. As suggested by the discussion above, there has been notable recent progress in the identification, purification, and characterization of receptors. Receptors can no longer be considered as metaphysical constructs. Much of this success reflects the development of radioactive ligands with great affinity and specificity for individual receptors; this allows the direct study of the drug-binding properties of receptors and reduces the need for reliance on the measurement of distal physiological responses. There are significant benefits to this approach. Physiological and pathological alterations that influence the number or binding properties of individual receptors may be analyzed without the need to infer their change from an alteration in the response that is observed. This is necessary, since the response may be many steps removed from the receptor, and may be influenced by change at any site in the pathway leading from receptor to ultimate effector. Research of this type has led to understanding of mechanisms of pathophysiology and therapeutic effects. For example,

we now appreciate the neuromuscular disorder myasthenia gravis as an autoimmune disease wherein antibodies are directed toward the nicotinic cholinergic receptor (*see* Chapters 6 and 11). Ligand-binding studies with preparations from the central nervous system can localize receptors and, by inference, specific synapses. This facilitates the mapping of pathways of neurotransmission. Furthermore, ligand-binding assays for many individual receptors are requisite for their purification and molecular characterization. Again, one may not be able to rely on the response that is characteristic of the drug-receptor complex for assay during receptor purification, since other components of the system necessary for the response may be lost. The ultimate goal of this type of research is to analyze the molecular events that are responsible for the interactions between the essential components of the system. Studies of this kind will allow a detailed definition of the differences between subtypes of receptors (*e.g.*, nicotinic and muscarinic receptors for acetylcholine) and an understanding of how receptors function and are regulated.

Classification of Receptors and Drug Effects. Drug receptors have traditionally been identified and classified primarily on the basis of the effect or lack thereof of selective antagonists and by the relative potencies of representative agonists—the structure-activity relationship. For example, the effects of acetylcholine that are mimicked by the alkaloid muscarine and that are selectively antagonized by atropine are termed *muscarinic effects*. Other effects of acetylcholine that are mimicked by nicotine and that are not readily antagonized by atropine but are selectively blocked by other agents (*e.g.*, *d*-tubocurarine) are described as *nicotinic effects*. By *extension*, these two types of cholinergic effects are said to be mediated by muscarinic or nicotinic receptors. Such classification of receptors results in an internally consistent scheme that gives support to the view that two types of receptor are involved. Although it frequently contributes little to delineation of mechanism of drug action, such categorization does provide a convenient basis for summarizing drug effects. If the effects and receptors in the various tissues have been classified, a statement that a drug activates a specified type of receptor is a succinct summary of its spectrum of effects and of the agents that will antagonize it. Similarly, a statement that a drug blocks a certain type of receptor specifies the agents that it will antagonize and at what sites.

Significance of Receptor Subtypes. As the diversity and selectivity of drugs have increased, it has become clear that multiple subtypes of receptors exist within many previously defined classes of receptors. In the case of the nicotinic cholinergic receptor, referred to above, there are distinct differences in the ligand-binding and functional properties between the receptors that are found in the ganglia of the autonomic nervous system and those at the somatic neuromuscular junction. This difference is exploited for therapeutic benefit. Thus, antagonists that act preferentially at the nicotinic receptors in ganglia can be used to control blood pressure; they do not, happily, paralyze skeletal muscle. *d*-Tubocurarine and related agents constitute the converse example, and their ability to antagonize the action of acetylcholine is relatively well confined to the receptor sites at the neuromuscular junction. These subtypes of the nicotinic receptor or, for example, the subtypes of the β-adrenergic receptor for catecholamines (*e.g.*, β_1 in the heart, β_2 in the bronchi) are conceptually analogous to tissue-specific isozymes of an enzyme; the mechanisms of action of these subtypes are largely identical. However, subtypes of some classes of receptors (*e.g.*, α_1- and α_2-adrenergic) also display fundamental differences in the biochemical regulatory activities of the different receptor proteins. Regardless of their mechanistic meaning (or lack thereof), these schemes of classification have facilitated the recent development of a number of therapeutic agents that have selectivity for specific types or subtypes of receptors. This has allowed the clinician to utilize more fully the therapeutic efficacy of these compounds, while limiting the frequency or intensity of unwanted effects.

ACTIONS OF DRUGS NOT MEDIATED BY RECEPTORS

If one restricts the definition of receptors to *macro*molecules, then several drugs may be said not to act by virtue of combination with receptors. Certain drugs may interact specifically with small molecules or ions that are normally or abnormally found in the body. The chelating agents, capable of forming strong bonds with a variety of metal cations, are an excellent example, and chelators are available that show a remarkable degree of preference for specific ionic species—even among divalent cations. Thus, the affinity of ethylenediaminetetraacetate is ten orders of magnitude greater for Pb^{2+} than it is for Ba^{2+}, Sr^{2+}, or Mg^{2+}. A rather less specific but nonetheless often gratifying example is the therapeutic neutralization of gastric acid by a base (antacid).

Certain drugs that are structural analogs of normal biological constituents may be incorporated into cellular components and thereby alter their function. This has been termed a "counterfeit incorporation mechanism" (*see* Goldstein *et al.*, 1974), and has been particularly explored with analogs of pyrimidines and purines that can be incorporated into nucleic acids and that have clinical utility in cancer chemotherapy (*see* Chapter 55).

Additionally, there is a group of agents that act more by virtue of their colligative effects than by more classical chemical mechanisms. A hint of this type of mechanism is provided by a lack of requirement for highly specific chemical structure. Stereoisomers of such drugs would not be expected to differ in their potency or efficacy. For example, certain relatively benign compounds, such as mannitol, can be administered in quantities sufficient to increase the osmolarity of various body fluids, and thereby cause appropriate changes in the distribution of water. Depending on the agent and route of administration, this effect can be exploited to promote diuresis, catharsis, expansion of circulating volume in the vascular compartment, or reduction of cerebral edema. The volatile general anesthetic agents interact with membranes to depress excitability. They appear to act colligatively as solutes in the lipid bilayer of the membrane. Their diversity of structure is consistent with such a mechanism; their individual potencies correlate best with their oil:water partition coefficients.

QUANTITATION OF DRUG-RECEPTOR INTERACTIONS

As early as 1878, even before he coined the term *receptive substance,* Langley suggested that drug-cell combinations, and hence the actions and effects of drugs, were probably governed by the law of mass action. This view was extensively developed by A. J. Clark in the 1920s, and it remains the keystone of most theories of drug action. Thus, the quantitative analysis of drug action borrows freely from theory developed for ligand-binding reactions and for enzyme-substrate interaction, and there is obvious coalescence when the effect of a drug results from a direct interaction with an enzyme.

When one attempts to extend analysis of drug-receptor interactions beyond the initial reaction—the binding of drug to receptor—important questions arise as to the relationship between the concentration of drug-receptor complex and the magnitude of the effect that is observed. In the classical receptor theory developed by Clark, it was assumed that the effect of a drug is proportional to the fraction of receptors occupied by drug, and that maximal effect results when all receptors are occupied. While these assumptions are probably true in some cases, exceptions are common, particularly when the pathway leading from receptor to effect is complex (*e.g.,* drug-receptor interaction → → alteration of cardiac contractility). However, the simplifying assumption serves as a useful point of departure.

Quantitative Descriptions of Drug Action. If one assumes that an agonist drug interacts reversibly with its receptor and that the resultant effect is proportional to the number of receptors occupied, the following reaction equation can be written:

$$\text{Drug } (D) + \text{Receptor } (R) \underset{k_2}{\overset{k_1}{\rightleftharpoons}} DR \longrightarrow \text{Effect} \tag{1}$$

This reaction sequence is analogous to the interaction of substrate with enzyme, and the magnitude of effect can be analyzed in a manner similar to that for enzymatic product formation.

The applicable equation is identical in form with the Michaelis-Menten equation:

$$\text{Effect} = \frac{\text{Maximal Effect } [D]}{K_D + [D]} \tag{2}$$

where $[D]$ is the concentration of free drug and K_D (equal to k_2/k_1) is the dissociation constant for the drug-receptor complex. This equation describes a simple rectangular hyperbola. There is no effect at $[D] = 0$; the effect is half-maximal when $[D] = K_D$,

that is, when half of the receptors are occupied; the maximal effect is approached asymptotically as $[D]$ increases above K_D (Figure 2–2, *A*). It is frequently convenient to plot the magnitude of effect versus log $[D]$, since a wide range of drug concentrations is easily displayed and a portion of the curve is more linear. In this case, the result is the familiar sigmoidal log dose-effect curve (Figure 2–2, *B*).

Data analysis can be further facilitated if a linear form of the equation is written. This may be obtained by taking the reciprocal of both sides of the expression and constructing the equivalent of the Lineweaver-Burk plot:

$$\frac{1}{\text{Effect}} = \frac{K_D}{\text{Max. Effect } [D]} + \frac{1}{\text{Max. Effect}} \tag{3}$$

A plot of 1/Effect versus 1/$[D]$ yields a straight line that intersects the Y-axis at 1/(Max. Effect) and that has a slope equal to K_D/(Max. Effect). Extrapolation of this line to the X-axis yields the value of the intercept, easily shown to be $-1/K_D$ (Figure 2–2, *C*). Thus, values for K_D and for the maximal effect can be readily calculated from such a plot. This representation is particularly useful for the analysis of drug antagonism. Additional numerical and graphic analytical methods are discussed by Segel (1984). Numerous software systems designed specifically to analyze pharmacodynamic data are also available (*see,* for example, Munson and Rodbard, 1980).

As stated above, certain drugs, termed antagonists, interact with the receptor or with other components of the effector mechanism to inhibit the action of an agonist, while initiating no effect themselves. If the inhibition can be overcome by increasing the concentration of the agonist, ultimately achieving the same maximal effect, the antagonist is said to be *surmountable* or *competitive.* This type of inhibition is commonly observed with antagonists that bind reversibly at the receptor site. A somewhat similar situation would also result from reversible or irreversible interaction of the antagonist at other sites so that the affinity of the receptor for the agonist is decreased. This is, however, more appropriately referred to as negative cooperativity between the two drugs than as competitive antagonism. Since the maximal effect can still be achieved if sufficient agonist is used, the double reciprocal plots of agonist alone versus agonist plus competitive antagonist *must* meet at the 1/Effect axis, where the concentration of agonist is infinite. The lines diverge at lower agonist concentrations; the apparent affinity of agonist for receptor is lowered (Figure 2–2, *D*). In the presence of a competitive antagonist, the log dose-effect curve for the agonist is shifted to the right (Figure 2–2, *E*). The maximal effect is unaltered, but the agonist appears to be less potent.

A noncompetitive antagonist *prevents* the agonist from producing any effect at a given receptor site. This could result from irreversible interaction of the antagonist at any site to prevent binding of agonist. It could also follow reversible or irreversible interaction with any component of the system so as to decrease the effect of the binding of agonist. Intuitively, these results may be conceptual-

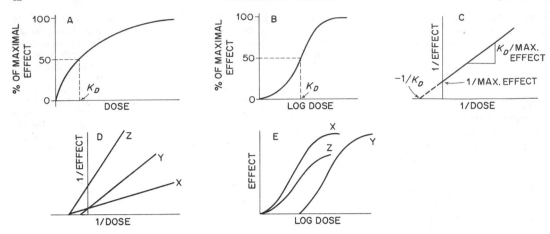

Figure 2–2. *Different representations of dose-effect curves.*

　　A. The ideal relationship between the concentration (dose) of a drug and the magnitude of response to it. When plotted on a linear scale of dose, a typical hyperbolic curve results.
　　B. A sigmoidal dose-effect curve results when the magnitude of effect observed is plotted versus the logarithm of the drug dose.
　　C. A double-reciprocal plot of the concentration dependence of drug effect (*see* text for explanation).
　　D and E. Representative double-reciprocal plots (*D*) and log dose-effect curves (*E*).
　　Curves X and Y. Two agonists with similar efficacy but differing in potency (X more potent than Y) *or* an agonist in the absence (X) and presence (Y) of a competitive antagonist.
　　Curves X and Z. Two agonists with similar potency but differing in efficacy (full agonist, X, and partial agonist, Z) *or* an agonist in the absence (X) and presence (Z) of a noncompetitive antagonist.

ized as *removal* of receptor or response potential from the system. The maximal effect possible is reduced, but agonist can act normally at receptor-effector units not so influenced. The affinity of the agonist for the receptor and its potency are thus unaltered. The double reciprocal plot shows intersection of agonist and antagonist plus agonist lines on the 1/[D] axis at $-1/K_D$ (the affinity is unaltered). The maximal effect is different (Figure 2–2, *D*). Similarly, the log dose-effect curves show unaltered potency and reduced efficacy (Figure 2–2, *E*).

　　Antagonists may thus be classified as acting reversibly or irreversibly. If the antagonist binds at the active site for the agonist, reversible antagonists will be competitive and irreversible antagonists will be noncompetitive. If binding is elsewhere, however, these simple rules do not hold, and any combination is possible.

　　If two drugs bind to the same receptor at the same site, why can one be an agonist and the other produce no effect—acting as an antagonist because of its presence? This question lies at the heart of the biophysics of protein structure and protein-ligand interactions. Its answer is still incompletely known. However, the following *model* may help to conceptualize a working answer to this question.

　　Consider a receptor that can exist in two conformations: active (*a*) or inactive (*i*). These might correspond to the open and closed states of an ion channel or the active and inactive forms of a protein kinase. If these states are in equilibrium and the inactive state predominates when no ligand for

the receptor is present, then an agonist will cause activation of the receptor if it binds preferentially to (has greater affinity for) the active conformation.

$$R_i \rightleftharpoons R_a$$
$$\Big\updownarrow \qquad\qquad \Big\updownarrow$$
$$D \cdot R_i \rightleftharpoons D \cdot R_a$$

The *extent* to which the equilibrium $R_i \rightleftharpoons R_a$ is perturbed, and thus the magnitude of effect, is determined by the *relative* affinity of the drug for the two conformations (Figure 2–3). Thus, if a different but perhaps structurally analogous compound binds to the same site on R but with only slightly greater affinity for R_a than for R_i, the magnitude of effect observed may be less, despite the presence of maximally effective concentrations of the agent. A drug that displays such intermediate effectiveness is referred to as a *partial agonist*. (Partial agonists are not hypothetical; they are quite common.) It then follows that an agent that has equal affinity for R_i and R_a will not alter the preexisting equilibrium; this compound will have no activity as an agonist but, when bound, will act as an antagonist because it impairs the ability of an agonist to alter the equilibrium and produce a response. (A drug with preferential affinity for R_i will actually inhibit the system, although if the *preexisting* equilibrium lies far in the direction of R_i this may be difficult to observe and the agent will be difficult to distinguish from the simple antagonist just described.) Finally, a partial agonist, when it binds to receptors but fails

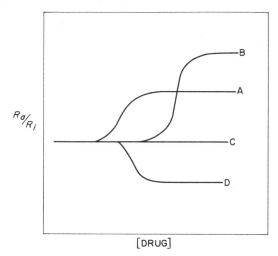

Figure 2–3. *Effects of drugs on the relative concentrations of two hypothetical forms of a receptor, R_a and R_i, that are in equilibrium* $(R_i \rightleftharpoons R_a)$.

Drugs A–D all bind to both forms of the receptor but with differing absolute and relative affinities. For drug A, affinity (K) for $R_a > R_i$ and binding affinity is relatively high; for drug B, K for $R_a \ggg R_i$, but binding affinity is relatively poor; for drug C, K for $R_a = R_i$ (or K for $R_a = R_i = 0$); for drug D, K for $R_a < R_i$. *(See text for additional explanation.)*

to produce a maximal response, can also act as an antagonist. A greater concentration of a full agonist will be required to produce a maximal effect because of the competitive effect of either a partial agonist or, of course, an antagonist.

It is obvious that something different from a simple receptor-occupancy theory has now been invoked, in that antagonists and partial agonists occupy receptors fully but do not produce maximal effects. It is thus useful to develop the concept of *intrinsic activity* or *efficacy* of drugs that act at the same receptor site but fail to produce equal effects. Quantitatively, the idea of efficacy can be used to modify the occupancy theory presented above. If the efficacy of an agonist is taken to be 1, that of an antagonist is 0, and that of a partial agonist is between 0 and 1, the effect will be equal to the product of fractional occupancy of the receptor and the fractional efficacy.

It should be noted at this point that the use of the word *efficacy* can, at times, be confusing. While an antagonist has no efficacy in this sense as an initiator of an action-effects sequence, it may have great therapeutic efficacy when used as an antagonist.

Even if the molecular *action* of an agonist at a receptor site is proportional to its efficacy and to the number of receptor sites occupied, additional complications frequently make difficult the quantitative interpretation of the dose dependence of effect. This is particularly true when the drug-receptor interaction is but one event in a complex

sequence of reactions that ultimately result in an observable effect. For example, while occupancy of a certain number of receptors by agonist may initially lead to response, a later step in the pathway may become limiting at this stimulated level of function. Further receptor occupancy can then produce no additional effect. Analysis of situations of this type has led to the concept of *spare receptors,* wherein a maximal effect can be achieved when a relatively small fraction of receptors is occupied; in at least some such situations a certain number of receptors can be lost (*e.g.,* with an irreversible antagonist) without diminution of the maximal observable response. Conversely, if a drug is acting to inhibit a step in a reaction sequence, the ultimate consequences of receptor occupation will be visible only when the step inhibited is or becomes the limiting step. It may be necessary to occupy the majority of the receptors before any change in function is observed. In both this situation and in the case of "spare receptors," it should be apparent that the concentration of drug producing a half-maximal effect bears a complex relationship to the dissociation constant for the drug-receptor complex. When there are spare receptors, the concentration of drug required for a half-maximal effect is less than K_D, whereas the opposite holds when occupation of the initial fraction of receptors fails to cause a change in the function of interest (Figure 2–4).

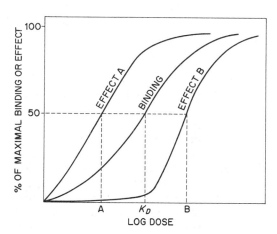

Figure 2–4. *Anomalous relationships between receptor occupation and response to a drug.*

The central curve, labeled *binding,* depicts the occupation of receptor by increasing concentrations of drug. Hypothetical dose-effect curve (*A*) is seen if maximal response results from less than maximal receptor occupation (spare receptors). Dose-effect curve (*B*) is seen if a significant fraction of receptors must be occupied before noticeable response to the drug occurs. The concentration of drug required to produce a half-maximal effect (*A* or *B*) thus bears a complex relationship to the dissociation constant of the drug-receptor complex (K_D).

Still other situations have required consideration of the possibilities that certain receptors may have multiple active sites or other drug binding (allosteric) sites. These sites may not act independently, and drug attachment at one point may alter the affinity for binding or reaction characteristics of agonists or antagonists at other locations. It should be pointed out that different receptor theories may be required when there are fundamental differences in the mechanism of drug action or in the structural and functional complexity of the responding system. These theories need not be mutually exclusive, and each may be true for individual situations. Further analysis of these models of receptor function may be found in the textbook by Goldstein and associates (1974); *see also* Colquhoun (1979).

RELATIONSHIP BETWEEN DOSE OF DRUG AND RESPONSE IN THE PATIENT

As discussed above, the relationship between the concentration of a drug and the magnitude of the response that is observed may be complicated by numerous considerations, even where proximate responses to the agent are examined in simplified systems *in vitro*. However, under most such circumstances, dose-effect curves of the type shown in Figure 2–2 can be observed. When drugs are administered *in vivo*, however, there is no single characteristic relationship between intensity of drug effect and drug dosage. A dose-effect curve may be linear, concave upward, concave downward, or sigmoid. Moreover, if the observed effect is the composite of several effects of the drug, such as the change in blood pressure produced by a combination of cardiac, vascular, and reflex effects, the dose-effect curve need not be monotonic. However, such a composite dose-effect curve can frequently be resolved into simple curves for each of its components. These simplified dose-effect curves, whatever their precise shape, can be viewed as having four characteristic variables: potency, slope, maximal efficacy, and individual variation. These are illustrated in Figure 2–5 for the common sigmoid log dose-effect curve. As mentioned, the logarithmic transformation of dosage is often employed for the dose-effect relationship because it permits display of a wide range of doses on a single graph and because it facilitates visual comparisons between dose-effect curves

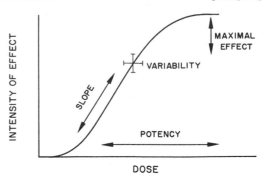

Figure 2–5. *The log dose-effect relationship.*

Representative log dose-effect curve, illustrating its four characterizing variables (*see* text for explanation).

for different drugs or for different responses to a single drug.

Potency. The location of its dose-effect curve along the *dose axis* is an expression of the potency of a drug. Potency *in vivo* is influenced by the absorption, distribution, biotransformation, and excretion of a drug, as well as being determined by its inherent ability to combine with its receptors and the functional relationship between the receptor and the effector system. While knowledge of a drug's potency is obviously of paramount importance for decisions regarding drug dosage, potency *per se* is a relatively unimportant characteristic of a drug for clinical purposes. Thus, it makes little difference whether the effective dose of a drug is 1 μg or 100 mg, as long as the drug can be administered conveniently. Potency is not necessarily correlated with any other characteristic of a drug, and there is no justification for the view that the more potent of two drugs is clinically superior. Low potency is a disadvantage only if the effective dose is so large that it is awkward to administer. Extremely potent drugs, particularly if they are volatile or are absorbed through the skin, may be hazardous and may require special handling.

For therapeutic applications, the potency of a drug is necessarily stated in *absolute* dosage units (25 μg, 10 mg/kg, *etc.*); for comparison of drugs, *relative potency* (i.e., the ratios of equieffective doses) is a more convenient expression.

Maximal Efficacy. The maximal effect produced by a drug is referred to as its *maximal efficacy* or, simply, *efficacy*. Maximal efficacy of a drug may be determined by its inherent properties or those of the receptor-effector system and be reflected as a plateau in the dose-effect curve. However, maximal efficacy may also be imposed by other factors. If the undesired effects of a drug limit its dosage, its efficacy will be correspondingly limited, even though it is inherently capable of producing a greater effect. Maximal efficacy of a drug is clearly one of its major characteristics. One of many important differences between morphine and aspirin is the difference in their maximal efficacy. The opioid provides relief of pain of nearly all intensities, whereas the salicylate is effective only against mild-to-moderate pain.

Efficacy and potency of a drug are not necessarily correlated, and these two characteristics of a drug should not be confused.

Slope. The slope of the dose-effect curve reflects the mechanism of action of a drug as well as the shape of the curve that describes its binding to the receptor. For example, if a drug must bind to most of the receptor molecules before a response is detected, the slope of the dose-effect curve will be increased considerably (*see* Figure 2–4). While such phenomena are usually of little more than theoretical importance, they can have therapeutic significance. For example, a steep dose-effect curve for a CNS depressant implies that there is a small ratio between the dose that produces coma and that which causes mild sedation, and that excessive or inadequate effect may occur if the dose of the drug is not carefully adjusted. Nevertheless, many factors influence the margin of safety of a drug and the variability of its effects, and these characteristics of a drug are properly expressed by methods that summarize the contributions of all factors (*see* below).

Biological Variation. For our purposes, variation or *variance* can be defined as the appearance of differences in the magnitude of response among individuals in the same population given the same dose of drug.

The more important factors that modify drug effect are discussed in Chapter 3. However, even when all known sources of variation are controlled or taken into account, drug effects are never identical in all patients, or even in a given patient on different occasions. A dose-effect curve applies only to a single individual at one time or to the average individual. The intersecting brackets in Figure 2–5 indicate that biological variation of the dose-effect relationship can be visualized in either of two ways. The vertical bracket expresses the fact that a range of effects will be produced if a given dose of a drug is administered to a group of individuals; alternatively, the horizontal bracket expresses the fact that a range of doses is required to produce a specified intensity of effect in all individuals.

Dose-Percent Curve. The dose of a drug required to produce a specified effect in an individual is termed the *individual effective dose*. As defined simply, this is a *quantal* rather than a *graded* response, since the specified effect is either present or absent. Individual effective doses of most drugs are lognormally distributed, which means that the familiar *normal curve* of variation is obtained if the logarithms of the individual effective doses for a group of patients are expressed as a frequency distribution (Figure 2–6, *A*). A cumulative frequency distribution of individual effective doses, that is, the percentage of individuals that exhibit the effect plotted as a function of logarithm of dose, is known as a dose-percent curve or a quantal dose-effect curve. This is the integrated form of the normal frequency distribution. Although also a sigmoid curve, the dose-percent curve is an expression of individual variability for a single effect and has a slightly different meaning from the graded dose-effect curve discussed above. However, the graded dose-effect curve can be viewed similarly as representing the integral (summation) of a large number of quantal (molecular) responses.

The dose of a drug required to produce a specified intensity of effect in 50% of individuals is known as the *median effective dose* and is abbreviated ED50 (Figure 2–6, *B*). If death is the end point, the me-

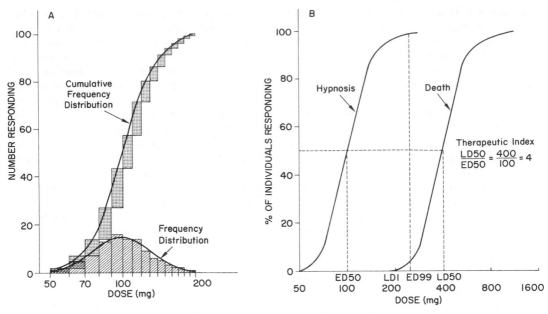

Figure 2–6. *Frequency distribution curves and quantal dose-effect curves.*

    A. An experiment was performed on 100 subjects and the effective dose to produce a quantal response was determined for each individual. The number of subjects who required each dose is plotted, giving a lognormal frequency distribution (bars with diagonal lines). The stippled bars demonstrate that the normal frequency distribution, when summated, yields the cumulative frequency distribution—a sigmoidal curve that is a quantal dose-effect curve.

    B. *Quantal Dose-Effect Curves.* Animals were injected with varying doses of a sedative-hypnotic, and the responses determined and plotted (*see* text for additional explanation).

dian effective dose is termed the *median lethal dose* (LD50). The doses required to produce the stated effect in other percentages of the population are similarly expressed (ED20, LD90, *etc.*). Variation in the population and the diverse shapes of observed dose-response curves require consideration of the significance of ED99 and LD1. If variation is marked, these doses may overlap even though the ED50 and LD50 differ by a wide margin (*see* below).

Terminology. Specific terms are used to refer to individuals who are unusually sensitive or unusually resistant to a drug, and to describe those in whom a drug produces an unusual effect.

If a drug produces its usual effect at unexpectedly low dosage, the individual is said to be *hyperreactive* or *hypersensitive.* The latter term may, however, be confused with the pattern of effects associated with drug allergy. Hyperreactivity to a drug is usually termed *supersensitivity* only if the increased sensitivity is the result of denervation. Supersensitivity may also result from continued administration of a receptor antagonist, the pharmacological equivalent of denervation. If a drug produces its usual effect only at unusually large dosage, the individual is said to be *hyporeactive.* Decreased sensitivity is also described as *tolerance,* but this term has the connotation of hyporeactivity acquired as the result of prior exposure to the drug. Tolerance that develops rapidly after administration of only a few doses of a drug is termed *tachyphylaxis.* Reduced sensitivity should be described as *immunity* only if the acquired tolerance is the result of antibody formation.

An *unusual effect* of a drug, of whatever intensity and irrespective of dosage, that occurs in only a small percentage of individuals is often termed *idiosyncrasy.* However, this term is frequently considered a synonym for drug allergy and has so many other connotations that it perhaps should be abandoned. Unusual effects of drugs should simply be described as such or, when possible, by terms that refer to the underlying mechanism; they are often types of drug allergy or a consequence of genetic differences.

Selectivity. A drug is usually described by its most prominent effect or by the action thought to be the basis of that effect. However, such descriptions should not obscure the fact that *no drug produces only a single effect*. Morphine is correctly described as an analgesic, but it also suppresses cough and causes sedation, respiratory depression, constipation, bronchiolar constriction, release of histamine, antidiuresis, and a variety of other effects. A drug is adequately characterized only in terms of its full *spectrum of effects*. The relationship between the doses of a drug required to produce undesired and desired effects is termed its *therapeutic index, margin of safety,* or *selectivity*. Rarely is a drug sufficiently selective to be described as being *specific*. For therapeutic applications, selectivity of a drug is clearly one of its more important characteristics.

Furthermore, a drug does not have a single therapeutic index, but many. The margin of safety of aspirin for relief of headache is greater than its margin of safety for relief of arthritic pain, since the latter use requires larger dosage. Similarly, several therapeutic indices can be calculated for each desired effect. A synthetic opioid may cause less constipation than morphine and yet afford no advantage over the parent compound with regard to respiratory depression or sedation. Moreover, a drug may be selective within one context yet still be nonselective within another. The antihistamines are correctly described as selective antagonists of histamine, yet none of these drugs produces this selective peripheral effect without also causing significant central sedation. Finally, a drug may be correctly described as having an adequate margin of safety in most patients, but this description is meaningless for the patient who exhibits an unusual response to the drug. Penicillin is essentially nontoxic in the great majority of patients, yet it can cause death in those who have become allergic to it.

In clinical studies, drug selectivity is often expressed indirectly by summarizing the pattern and incidence of adverse effects produced by therapeutic doses of the drug and by indicating the proportion of patients who were forced to decrease drug dosage or discontinue medication because of adverse effects. These indirect procedures are often adequate, but comparison of dose-effect curves for desired and undesired effects is more consistently meaningful and is preferred whenever feasible (Figure 2–6, *B*).

In laboratory studies, therapeutic index is usually defined as the ratio between the median toxic dose and the median effective dose (TD50/ED50) or the median lethal dose and median effective dose (LD50/ED50). Because the ideal drug produces its desired effect in all patients without causing toxic effects in any, and because dose-percent curves need not be parallel, it can be logically argued that therapeutic index should be defined as the ratio between the minimal toxic dose and the maximal effective dose. However, minimal and maximal toxic and effective doses cannot be estimated with precision, particularly in the variable human population with which medical practice is concerned.

Ariëns, E. J., and Beld, A. J. The receptor concept in evolution. *Biochem. Pharmacol.*, **1977**, *26*, 913–918.

Baxter, J. D., and Funder, J. W. Hormone receptors. *N. Engl. J. Med.*, **1979**, *301*, 1149–1161.

Berridge, M. J. Inositol triphosphate and diacylglycerol as second messengers. *Biochem. J.*, **1984**, *220*, 345–360.

Clark, A. J. *The Mode of Action of Drugs on Cells.* E. Arnold & Co., London, **1933**.

Cobb, M. H., and Rosen, O. M. The insulin receptor and tyrosine protein kinase activity. *Biochim. Biophys. Acta*, **1984**, *734*, 1–8.

Colquhoun, D. The link between drug binding and response: theories and observations. In, *The Receptors: A Comprehensive Treatise*, Vol. 1. (O'Brien, R. D., ed.) Plenum Press, New York, **1979**, pp. 93–142.

Conti-Tronconi, B. M., and Raftery, M. A. The nicotinic cholinergic receptor: correlation of molecular structure with functional properties. *Annu. Rev. Biochem.*, **1982**, *51*, 491–530.

Featherstone, R. M. (ed.). *A Guide to Molecular Pharmacology-Toxicology*, Pts. I–II. Marcel Dekker, Inc., New York, **1973**.

Gilman, A. G. Guanine nucleotide-binding regulatory proteins and dual control of adenylate cyclase. *J. Clin. Invest.*, **1984**, *73*, 1–4.

Goldstein, A.; Aronow, L.; and Kalman, S. M. *Principles of Drug Action: The Basis of Pharmacology*, 2nd ed. John Wiley & Sons, Inc., New York, **1974**.

Harden, T. K. Agonist-induced desensitization of the β-adrenergic receptor–linked adenylate cyclase. *Pharmacol. Rev.*, **1983**, *35*, 5–32.

Kleinzeller, A., and Martin, B. R. (eds.). *Membrane Receptors. Current Topics in Membranes and Transport,* Vol. 18. Academic Press, Inc., New York, **1983.**

Klinge, E. (ed.). *Receptors and Cellular Pharmacology. Proceedings of the Sixth International Congress of Pharmacology,* Vol. 1. Pergamon Press, Ltd., Oxford, **1976.**

Korolkovas, A. *Essentials of Molecular Pharmacology.* John Wiley & Sons, Inc., New York, **1970.**

Mishina, M.; Tobimatsu, T.; Imoto, K.; Tanaka, K.; Fujita, Y.; Fukuda, K.; Kurasaki, M.; Takahashi, H.; Morimoto, Y.; Hirose, T.; Inayama, S.; Takahashi, T.; Kuno, M.; and Numa, S. Location of functional regions of acetylcholine receptor α-subunit by site-directed mutagenesis. *Nature,* **1985,** *313,* 364–369.

Munson, P. J., and Rodbard, D. LIGAND: a versatile computerized approach for characterization of ligand-binding systems. *Anal. Biochem.,* **1980,** *107,* 220–239.

Rang, H. P. Receptor mechanisms: Fourth Gaddum Memorial Lecture, School of Pharmacy, University of London, January 1973. *Br. J. Pharmacol.,* **1973,** *48,* 475–495.

Segel, I. H. *Enzyme Kinetics,* 2nd ed. John Wiley & Sons, Inc., New York, **1984.**

Smigel, M. D.; Ross, E. M.; and Gilman, A. G. Role of the β-adrenergic receptor in the regulation of adenylate cyclase. In, *Cell Membranes: Methods and Reviews,* Vol. 2. (Elson, E. L.; Frazer, W. A.; and Glaser, L.; eds.) Plenum Press, New York, **1984,** pp. 247–294.

Smythies, J. R., and Bradley, R. J. (eds.). *Receptors in Pharmacology.* Marcel Dekker, Inc., New York, **1978.**

3 PRINCIPLES OF THERAPEUTICS

Terrence F. Blaschke, Alan S. Nies, and Richard D. Mamelok

THERAPY AS A SCIENCE

Over a century ago Claude Bernard formalized criteria for gathering valid information in experimental medicine, but application of these criteria to therapeutics and to the process of making decisions about therapeutics has, until recently, been slow and inconsistent. At a time when the diagnostic aspects of medicine had become scientifically sophisticated, therapeutic decisions were often made on the basis of impressions and traditions. Historically, the absence of accurate data on the effects of drugs in man was in large part due to ethical standards of human experimentation. "Experimentation" in human beings was precluded, and it was not generally conceded that *every* treatment by any physician should be designed and in some sense recorded as an experiment.

Although there must always be ethical concern about experimentation in man, principles have been defined, and there are no longer ethical restraints on the gathering of either experimental or observational data on the efficacy and toxicity of drugs in *adults*. Furthermore, it should now be considered absolutely unethical to utilize the *art* as opposed to the *science* of therapeutics on any patient who directly (the adult or child) or indirectly (the fetus) receives drugs for therapeutic purposes. Observational (nonexperimental) technics that can greatly add to our knowledge of the effects of drugs can be applied to all populations. The fact that such observational technics have largely been applied in a nonsystematic fashion has led us to rely on a relative paucity of information about many drugs. Therapeutics must now be dominated by objective evaluation of an adequate base of factual knowledge.

Conceptual Barriers to Therapeutics as a Science. The most important barrier that inhibited the development of therapeutics as a science seems to have been the belief that multiple variables in diseases and in the effects of drugs are uncontrollable. If this were true, the scientific method would not be applicable to the study of pharmacotherapy. In fact, therapeutics is the aspect of patient care that is most amenable to the acquisition of useful data, since it involves an intervention and provides an opportunity to observe a response. It is now appreciated that clinical phenomena can be defined, described, and quantified with some precision. Analysis of measurements has become mathematically sound; experiments can be designed to yield valid conclusions about the pharmacological effects of drugs used for the treatment of patients. The approach to complex clinical data has been artfully discussed by Feinstein (1983).

Another barrier to the realization of therapeutics as a science was overreliance on traditional *diagnostic labels* for disease. This encouraged the physician to think of a disease as a static rather than a dynamic entity, to view patients with the same "label" as a homogeneous rather than a heterogeneous population, and to consider a disease as an entity even when information about pathogenesis was not available. If diseases are not considered to be dynamic, "standard" therapies in "standard" doses will be the order of the day; decisions will be reflexive. Needed instead is an attitude that makes the physician responsible for recognition of and compensation for changes that occur in pathophysiology as the underlying process evolves. For example, the term *myocardial infarction* refers to localized destruction of myocardial cells caused by the interruption of the blood supply; however, decisions about therapy must take into account a variety of autonomic, hemodynamic, and electrophysiological variables that change as a function of time, as well as with the size of the infarction and its location. Furthermore, one often must focus on the presence of other diseases that could contribute to the infarction and that may require primary care separate from hemodynamic support (*e.g.,* management of the metabolic status of a patient with diabetes who has sustained a myocardial infarction). Failure to take all such variables into account while planning a therapeutic maneuver may result in ineffective therapy or avoidable toxicity. Differences in these variables among patients who are receiving the same therapy can account for different outcomes; conversely, if heterogeneous groups of patients receive alternative treatments, true differences in efficacy or toxicity between therapies may go unrecognized. A diagnosis or label of a disease or syndrome usually indicates a spectrum of possible causes and outcomes. Therapeutic experiments that fail to match groups for the known variables that affect prognosis yield uninterpretable data.

A third conceptual barrier was the incorrect notion that data derived empirically are useless because they are not generated by application of the scientific method. Empiricism is often defined as the practice of medicine founded on mere experience, without the aid of science or a knowledge of principles. The connotations of this definition are misleading; empirical observations need not be scientifically unsound. In fact, concepts of therapeutics have been greatly advanced by the astute clinical observer who makes careful and controlled observations on the outcome of a therapeutic intervention. The results, even when the mechanisms of disease and their interactions with the effects of drugs are not understood, are nevertheless often crucial to appropriate therapeutic decisions. Often the initial suggestion that a drug may be efficacious in one condition arises from careful, empirical observations that are made while the drug is being used for another purpose. Recent examples of valid empirical observations that have resulted in new uses of drugs

include the use of penicillamine to treat arthritis, lidocaine to treat cardiac arrhythmias, and propranolol and clonidine to treat hypertension. Conversely, empiricism, when not coupled with appropriate observational methods and statistical technics, often results in findings that are inadequate or invalid.

Clinical Trials. Application of the scientific method to experimental therapeutics is exemplified by a well-designed and well-executed clinical trial. Clinical trials form the basis for therapeutic decisions by all physicians, and it is therefore essential that they be able to evaluate the results and conclusions of such trials critically. To maximize the likelihood that useful information will result from the experiment, the objectives of the study must be defined, homogeneous populations of patients must be selected, appropriate control groups must be found, meaningful and sensitive indices of drug effects must be chosen for observation, and the observations must be converted into data and then into valid conclusions (Feinstein, 1977b). A number of excellent, critical summaries of the scientific requirements for clinical trials have been published (Hill, 1960, 1962). The *sine qua non* of any clinical trial is its controls. Many different types of controls may be used, and the term *controlled study* is not synonymous with *randomized double-blind technic*. Selection of a proper control group is as critical to the eventual utility of an experiment as the selection of the experimental group (*see* Feinstein, 1977a). Although the randomized, double-blind controlled trial is the most effective design for distributing bias and unknown variables between the "treatment" and the "control" groups, it is not necessarily the optimal or applicable design for all studies. It may be impossible to use this design to study disorders that occur rarely, disorders in populations of patients that cannot, by regulation or ethics or both, be studied (*e.g.,* children, women of child-bearing age, the fetus, or some patients with psychiatric diseases), or the treatment of patients with a uniformly fatal disorder (*e.g.,* patients with rabies, where historical controls can be used).

There are several requirements in the design of clinical trials to test the relative effects of *alternative* therapies. (1) *Specific outcomes* of therapy that are clinically relevant and quantifiable must be measured. (2) The *accuracy of diagnosis* and the *severity of the disease* must be comparable in the groups being contrasted; otherwise, false-positive and false-negative errors may occur. (3) The *dosages* of the drugs must be chosen and individualized in a manner that allows relative efficacy to be compared at equivalent toxicities or allows relative toxicities to be compared at equivalent efficacies (Meffin *et al.,* 1977). (4) *Placebo effects,* which occur in a large percentage of patients, can confound many studies—particularly those that involve subjective responses; controls must take this into account (Beecher, 1959). Special designs, such as the "preference technic" (Jick *et al.,* 1966), may be required to evaluate the efficacy of drugs used for the relief of symptoms. In fact, subjective assessments that relate to the quality of life can be generated by the experimental subject and can be objectively tabulated and incorporated into evaluation of a therapy (Sheiner, 1979). (5) *Compliance* to the experimental regimens should be assessed *before* subjects are assigned to experimental or control groups. The drug-taking behavior of the subjects should be reassessed during the course of the trial. Noncompliance, even if randomly distributed between both groups, may cause falsely low estimates of the true potential benefits or toxicity of a particular treatment. (6) *Sample size* should be estimated prior to beginning a clinical trial and must be taken into account in interpreting the results of the trial. Depending upon such factors as the overall prognosis of the disease and the anticipated improvement in outcome or toxicity from the new treatment, very large numbers of subjects may be needed; otherwise, the possibility of a false-negative result is high (*i.e.,* no statistically significant differences between the two treatments will be found, even though differences actually exist) (Freiman *et al.,* 1978). (7) *Ethical considerations* may be major determinants of the types of controls that can be used and must be evaluated explicitly (Curran, 1979). For example, in therapeutic trials that involve life-threatening diseases, the use of a placebo is unethical, and new treatments must be compared with "standard" therapies.

The results of clinical trials of new therapeutic agents or of old agents for new indications may have severe limitations in terms of what can be expected of drugs when they are used in an office practice. The selection of the patients for experimental trials usually eliminates those with coexisting diseases, and such trials usually assess the effect of only one or two drugs, not the many that might be given to or taken by the same patient under the care of a physician. Clinical trials are usually performed with relatively small numbers of patients for periods of time that may be shorter than are necessary in practice, and compliance may be better controlled than it can be in practice. All these factors, plus those that are described below (*see* section on Drug Development), lead to several inescapable conclusions:

1. Even if the result of a valid clinical trial of a drug is thoroughly understood, the physician can only develop a hypothesis about what the drug might do to a particular patient, and there can be no assurance that what occurred in other patients will be seen. In effect, the physician uses the results of a clinical trial to establish an experiment in each patient (Ingelfinger *et al.,* 1983). The detection of anticipated and unanticipated effects and the determination of whether or not they are due to the drug(s) being used are important responsibilities of the physician during the supervision of a therapeutic regimen. If an effect of a drug is not seen in a clinical trial, it may still be revealed in the setting of clinical practice. About one half or more of both useful and adverse effects of drugs that were not recognized in the initial formal trials were subsequently discovered and reported by practicing physicians.

2. If an anticipated effect of a drug has *not* occurred in a patient, this does not mean that the effect cannot occur in that patient or in others. *Many factors in the individual patient may contribute to lack of efficacy of a drug.* They include, for example, misdiagnosis, poor compliance by the patient to the regimen, poor choice of dosage or dosage intervals, coincidental development of an undiagnosed separate illness that influences the outcome, the use of other agents that interact with primary drugs to nullify or alter their effects, undetected genetic or environmental variables that modify the disease or the pharmacological actions of the drug, or unknown therapy by another physician who is caring for the same patient. Such factors must be considered when a regimen is failing. Of equal importance, even when a regimen appears to be efficacious and innocuous, a physician should not uncritically attribute all improvement to the therapeutic regimen chosen, nor should a physician assume that

a deteriorating condition reflects only the natural course of the disease. Similarly, if an anticipated untoward or toxic effect is not seen in a particular patient, it can still occur in others. Physicians who use *only* their own experience with a drug to make decisions about its use unduly expose their patients to unjustifiable risk or unrealized efficacy. For example, simply because a doctor has not seen a case of chloramphenicol-induced aplastic anemia in his own practice does not mean that such a disaster may not occur; the drug should still be used for the proper indications.

3. Rational therapy is therapy based on the use of observations that have been evaluated critically. It is no less crucial to have a scientific approach to the treatment of an individual patient than to use this approach when investigating drugs in a research setting. In both instances, it is the patient who benefits.

INDIVIDUALIZATION OF DRUG THERAPY

As has been implied above, therapy as a science does not apply simply to the evaluation and testing of new, investigational drugs in animals and man. It applies with equal importance to the treatment of each patient as an individual. Therapists of every type have long recognized and acknowledged that individual patients show wide variability in response to the same drug or treatment modality. Progress has been made in identifying the sources of variability (Vesell, 1979). Important factors are presented in Figure 3–1; the basic principles that underlie these sources of variability have been presented in Chapters 1 and 2. The following discussion relates to the strategies that have been developed to minimize variability in the clinical setting. (*See also* Appendixes I to III; Sheiner *et al.,* 1975; Sheiner and Tozer, 1978.)

VARIATION IN DISPOSITION OF A DRUG

Interpatient and intrapatient variation in disposition of a drug must be taken into account in choosing a drug regimen. For a given drug, there may be wide variation

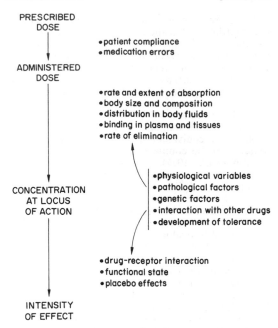

Figure 3–1. *Factors that determine the relationship between prescribed drug dosage and drug effect.* (Modified from Koch-Weser, 1972.)

among individuals in its pharmacokinetic properties. For some drugs, this variability may account for one half or more of the total variation in eventual response. The relative importance of the many factors that contribute to these differences depends in part on the drug itself and on its usual route of elimination. Drugs that are excreted primarily unchanged by the kidney tend to have smaller differences in disposition than do drugs that are inactivated by metabolism. Of drugs that are extensively metabolized, those with slower biotransformation tend to have the largest variation in such rates between individuals. Studies in identical and nonidentical twins have revealed that genotype is a most important determinant of differences in the rates of metabolism (Penno and Vesell, 1983; Vesell, 1983). For many drugs, physiological and pathological variations in organ function are major determinants of their rate of disposition. For example, the clearance of digoxin and gentamicin is related to the rate of glomerular filtration, whereas that of lidocaine and propranolol is primarily dependent on the rate of hepatic blood flow. The effect of disease states, especially those that involve the kidneys or liver, is to impair elimination and to increase the variability in the disposition of drugs. In such settings, measurements of concentrations of drugs in biological fluids can be used to assist in the individualization of drug therapy (Koch-Weser, 1972). Since renal or hepatic diseases may also affect the responsiveness of target tissues (*e.g.*, the brain), the physician should be alert to the possibility of a shift in the range of therapeutic concentrations.

A test should not be performed simply because an assay is available. More assays of drugs are available than are generally useful. Determinations of concentrations of drug in blood, serum, or plasma are particularly useful when well-defined criteria are fulfilled. (1) There must be a demonstrated relationship between the concentration of the drug in plasma and the eventual therapeutic effect that is desired. (2) There should be substantial *interpatient* variability in disposition of the drug (and small *intrapatient* variation). Otherwise, concentrations of drug in plasma could be predicted from dose alone. (3) It should be difficult to monitor intended or unintended effects of the drug. Whenever clinical effects or minor toxicity are easily measured (*e.g.*, the effect of a drug on blood pressure), such effects should be preferred in the decision to make any necessary adjustment of dosage of the drug. However, the effects of drugs in certain settings are not easily monitored. For example, the hemodynamic changes caused by digitalis glycosides may be delayed and difficult to measure. For some drugs, the *initial* manifestation of toxicity may be serious (*e.g.*, hypoglycemia or hemorrhage). The same concepts apply to a number of agents used for cancer chemotherapy. Other drugs (*e.g.*, antiarrhythmic agents) produce toxic effects that mimic symptoms or signs of the disease being treated. Many drugs are used for *prophylaxis* of an uncommon or dangerous event; examples include anticonvulsants and antiarrhythmic agents. In each of these situations, titration of drug dosage may be aided by measurements of concentrations of the drug in blood. (4) The therapeutic index of the drug should be low, and its toxic effects should have the potential to increase morbidity. If this criterion is not met, patients could simply be given the largest dose known to be necessary to treat a disorder, as is commonly done with penicillin. However, if there is an overlap in the concentration-response relationship for desirable and undesirable effects of the drug, as is true for theophylline, determinations of concentration of drug in plasma may allow the dose to be optimized. All four of the above-described criteria should be met if the measurement of drug concentrations is to be of significant value in the adjustment of dosage. Knowledge of concentrations of drugs in plasma or urine is also particularly useful for detection of therapeutic failures that are due to lack of patient compliance with a medical regimen or for identification of patients with unexpected extremes in the rate of drug disposition.

Assay of drugs to assist the physician in achieving a desired concentration of drug in blood or plasma (*i.e.*, "targeting" the dose) is an example of the use of an *intermediate end point of therapy*. An intermediate end point is defined as a specific goal of treatment that is used in place of the ultimate clinical goal, which may be difficult to assess. The concept of intermediate end points, including concentrations of drugs, as a guide to individualization of therapy can also be applied in other ways; one is to provide an indication for a change in the choice of drug therapy. Measurements of concentrations of drugs in plasma or preferably measurements of one or more pharmacological effects of the drug can provide an indication of probable lack of efficacy. Other issues of importance with regard to the measurement and interpretation of drug concentrations are discussed in Chapter 1 and Appendix II.

PHARMACODYNAMIC VARIABILITY

The availability of precise information about the pharmacokinetic properties of many drugs has contributed to understanding of the importance of differences in the responsiveness of target tissues to pharmacological agents. It is clear that considerable residual variation in response remains after the concentration of drug has been adjusted to the desired value; for some drugs this accounts for most of the total variation in the responsiveness of the individual. These observations have led to an increased interest in attempts to define and measure "sensitivity" to drugs in a clinical setting. Important progress has been made in understanding some of the determinants of sensitivity to drugs that act at specific receptors. For example, the number of receptors for insulin may be altered in diabetes (Flier *et al.*, 1979); responsiveness to adrenergic agonists (*e.g.*, isoproterenol or norepinephrine) may change because of disease (thyrotoxicosis) or because of the prior administration of either adrenergic agonists or antagonists (Lefkowitz *et al.*, 1984); resistance to the antineoplastic agent methotrexate may occur because of gene amplification and subsequent synthesis of large quantities of the receptor for the cytotoxic action of this drug, dihydrofolate reductase (Brown *et al.*, 1983). Receptors for drugs are not static components of the cell (*see* Chapter 2). They are in a dynamic state and are modulated by a variety of exogenous and endogenous factors that play a major role in the response to treatment.

OTHER FACTORS THAT AFFECT THERAPEUTIC OUTCOME

The variation in pharmacokinetic and pharmacodynamic parameters that accounts for much of the need to individualize therapy has been discussed. Other factors, listed in Figure 3–1, also should be considered as potential determinants of success or failure of therapy. The following presentation serves as an introduction to these subjects, certain of which are also discussed elsewhere in this textbook.

Drug-Drug Interactions. The concomitant use of drugs is often essential to obtain a desired therapeutic objective. Examples abound, and the choice of drugs to be employed concurrently can be based on sound pharmacological principles. In the treatment of hypertension, a single drug is effective in only a modest percentage of patients. In the treatment of heart failure, the concurrent use of a cardiac glycoside and a

diuretic is often essential to achieve an adequate cardiac output and to maintain the patient in an edema-free state. Multiple-drug therapy is usual in cancer chemotherapy and for the treatment of certain infectious diseases. The goals in these cases are usually to improve efficacy and to delay the emergence of malignant cells or of microorganisms that are resistant to the effects of available drugs. When the physician uses several drugs concurrently, he must face at least two difficult problems related to their interactions. One is the acquisition of a perspective on the rapidly expanding body of information in this area. The other problem is to know whether a specific combination in a given patient has the potential to result in an interaction, and, if so, how to take advantage of the interaction if it leads to improvement in efficacy or how to avoid the consequences of an interaction if they are adverse.

A *potential drug interaction* refers to the possibility that one member of a class of drugs may alter the intensity of pharmacological effects of another drug given concurrently. The net result may be enhanced or diminished effects of one or both of the drugs. Interactions may be either pharmacokinetic (alteration of the absorption, distribution, or disposition of one drug by another) or pharmacodynamic (*e.g.*, interactions between agonists and antagonists at drug receptors). Mechanisms are detailed in Appendix III.

Beneficial Drug-Drug Interactions. Interactions between drugs may be employed for the treatment of drug toxicity. This is most effective if a specific receptor blocking agent is available to counter the effects of a given agonist (*e.g.*, naloxone to treat opioid overdosage). Alteration of the pharmacokinetic parameters of one drug by the administration of another may also be used for benefit. A familiar example is the administration of probenecid to inhibit the secretion of penicillin by the proximal tubule of the kidney. Drugs may be utilized to alter the pharmacokinetic profile of a toxicant (*see* Chapter 68).

Adverse Drug-Drug Interactions. Interactions that are classified as adverse either compromise therapeutic efficacy, enhance toxicity, or both. These are also numerous, and the frequency of adverse interactions, as would be expected, increases with the number of drugs that a patient receives (Steel *et al.*, 1981). The major mechanisms that lead to adverse interactions between drugs involve changes in the pharmacokinetic profile. Thus, one drug may interact with another to retard absorption, compete for binding sites on plasma proteins, alter metabolism by enzyme induction or inhibition, or change the rate of renal excretion. Adverse pharmacodynamic interactions can also occur.

Adverse drug interactions may frequently be avoided by appropriate modifications of dose, time, or route of administration, or by careful monitoring of the patient who is concurrently receiving drugs that may interact. Many drugs that have the potential to interact adversely must nevertheless be used in combination for optimal patient care (*e.g.*, digitalis and diuretics, even though K^+ loss due to diuretics may increase the toxicity of cardiac glycosides).

The frequency of significant beneficial or adverse drug interactions is unknown. Surveys that include data obtained *in vitro*, in animals, and in case reports tend to predict a frequency of interactions that is higher than actually occurs. While such reports have contributed to skepticism about the overall importance of drug interactions (Aronson and Grahame-Smith, 1981), the physician must be alert for their occurrence. Recognition of beneficial effects and recognition and prevention of adverse drug interactions require a thorough knowledge of the intended and possible effects of drugs that are prescribed, a mental set to attribute unusual events to drugs rather than to disease, and adequate observation of the patient. Automated monitoring of prescription orders in the hospital or outpatient pharmacy may decrease the physician's need to memorize potential interactions. Nevertheless, knowledge of likely mechanisms of drug interactions is the only way the clinician can be prepared to analyze new findings systematically. It is incumbent upon the physician to be familiar with the basic principles of drug-drug interactions in planning a therapeutic regimen. Such reactions are discussed for individual drugs throughout this text and are summarized in Appendix III. (*See also* Hansten, 1985; Mangini, 1985.)

The concomitant use of two or more drugs adds to the complexity of individualization of drug therapy. The dose of each drug should be adjusted to achieve optimal benefit. Thus, patient compliance is essential yet more difficult to achieve. To obviate the latter problem many fixed-dose drug combinations are marketed. The use of such combinations is advantageous only if the ratio of the fixed doses corresponds to the needs of the individual patient.

In the United States, a fixed-dose combination of drugs must be approved by the Food and Drug Administration (FDA) before it can be marketed, even though the individual drugs are available for concurrent use. To be approved, certain conditions must be met. The two drugs must act as synergists to achieve a better therapeutic response than either drug alone (*e.g.*, many antihypertensive drug combinations); or one drug must act to reduce the incidence of adverse effects caused by the other (*e.g.*, a diuretic that promotes the urinary excretion of potassium combined with a potassium-sparing diuretic).

Placebo Effects.   The net effect of drug therapy is the sum of the pharmacological effects of the drug and the nonspecific placebo effects associated with the therapeutic effort. Although identified specifically with administration of an inert substance in the guise of medication, *placebo effects are associated with the taking of any drug, active as well as inert.*

Placebo effects result from the physician-patient relationship, the significance of the therapeutic effort to the patient, and the mental "set" imparted by the therapeutic setting and by the physician. They vary significantly in different individuals and in any one patient at different times. Placebo effects are commonly manifest as alterations of mood, other subjective effects, and objective effects that are under autonomic or voluntary control. They may be favorable or unfavorable relative to the therapeutic objectives. Exploited to advantage, placebo effects can significantly supplement pharmacological effects and can represent the difference between success and failure of therapy. (*See* Bourne, 1978; Benson and McCallie, 1979.)

A placebo (in this context, better termed *dummy medication*) is an indispensable element of the controlled clinical trial. In contrast, a placebo has only a limited role in the routine practice of medicine. Although the inert medication may be an effective vehicle for a placebo effect, the physician-patient relationship is generally preferable. Relief or lack of relief of symptoms upon administration of a placebo is *not* a reliable basis for determining whether the symptoms have a "psychogenic" or "somatic" origin.

Tolerance. Tolerance may be acquired to the effects of many drugs, especially the opioids, barbiturates, and other CNS depressants. When this occurs, *cross-tolerance* may develop to the effects of pharmacologically related drugs, particularly those acting at the same receptor site, and drug dosage must be increased to maintain a given therapeutic effect. Since tolerance does not usually develop equally to all effects of a drug, the therapeutic index may decrease. However, there are also examples of the development of tolerance to the undesired effects of a drug and a resultant increase in its therapeutic index (*e.g.,* tolerance to sedation and respiratory depression produced by phenobarbital when used as an anticonvulsant).

The mechanisms involved in the development of tolerance are only partially understood. In animals, tolerance often occurs as the result of induced synthesis of the hepatic microsomal enzymes concerned in drug biotransformation; the possible significance of this *drug-disposition* or *pharmacokinetic tolerance* during chronic medication in man is an area of continuing investigation. The most important factor in the development of tolerance to the opioids, barbiturates, and ethanol is some type of neuronal adaptation vaguely referred to as *cellular* or *pharmacodynamic tolerance.* Tachyphylaxis, such as that to histamine-releasing agents and to the sympathomimetic amines that act indirectly by releasing norepinephrine, has been attributed to depletion of available mediator, but other mechanisms may also contribute. The subject of tolerance is discussed in more detail in Chapter 23.

Genetic Factors. Genetic factors are the major determinants of the normal variability of drug effects and are responsible for a number of striking quantitative and qualitative differences in pharmacological activity (Vesell, 1983). Many of these differences are polygenic, but some, such as the prolonged apnea in some patients after administration of usual doses of the neuromuscular blocking agent succinylcholine, have been traced to monogenic influences on the enzymes involved in *drug biotransformation.* Other variations in drug effect, such as the greater incidence of drug-induced hemolytic anemia in non-Caucasians than in Caucasians, have been found to be related to genetic differences that modify the actions of drugs.

The objectives of *pharmacogenetics* include not only identification of differences in drug effects that have a genetic basis but also development of simple methods by which susceptible individuals can be recognized *before* the drug is administered.

APPROACH TO INDIVIDUALIZATION

After it has been determined that pharmacotherapy is necessary to modify the symptoms or outcome of a disease, the therapist is faced with two types of decisions: the first is qualitative (the initial choice of a specific drug) and the second quantitative (the initial dosage regimen). Optimal treatment will result only when the physician is aware of the sources of variation in response to drugs and when the dosage regimen is designed on the basis of the best-available data about the diagnosis, severity and stage of the disease, presence of concurrent diseases or drug treatment, and *predefined goals* of acceptable efficacy and limits of acceptable toxicity. If objectively assessable expectations of drug therapy are not set before therapy is initiated, the patient is likely to be treated until he *obviously* responds in a grossly positive or grossly negative way before reconsideration of therapy will be likely.

In most clinical settings, the decision about the choice of drug is substantially influenced by the confidence the physician has in the accuracy of his diagnosis and estimates of the extent and severity of disease. Based on the best-available information, the physician must decide on an initial drug from a group of reasonable alternatives. The extent of this evaluation is itself dependent on many factors, including a cost-benefit analysis of diagnostic tests (Ingelfinger *et al.,* 1983), and this must be based on the availability and specificity of alternative therapies (*e.g., see* Finnerty, 1975; Melby, 1975). The initial dosage regimen is determined by estimation, if possible, of the pharmacokinetic properties of the drug in the individual patient. The estimate must be based on an appreciation of the variables that are most likely to affect the disposition of the particular drug. These variables have been discussed above (*see* Figure 3–1; Appendix II). Subsequent adjustments should be based on whether the regimen is efficacious, either without adverse effects or at an acceptable level of toxicity.

It has been stated above that every therapeutic plan is and should be treated as an experiment. As such, most of the considerations that were specified in the discussion of clinical trials must be applied to individual patients. Of utmost importance is the definition of specific goals of treatment and the means to assess whether these goals are being achieved successfully. Whenever possible, the objective end point should be related as closely as possible to the clinical goals of therapy (*e.g.*, suppression of an arrhythmia, shrinkage of a tumor, eradication of an infection). Many clinical goals are, however, difficult to assess (*e.g.*, the prevention of cardiovascular complications associated with hypertension and diabetes). In such cases it is necessary to set intermediate end points to therapy, such as a reduction in blood pressure or the concentration of glucose in plasma. These intermediate end points are based on demonstrated *or assumed* correlations with the ultimate clinical benefit. In many cases, such as normalization of the concentration of plasma glucose or reduction of the concentration of cholesterol in plasma by drugs, the link between the intermediate goal and the ultimate goal is controversial.

Certain general considerations apply to the individualization of a drug regimen and the concept of intermediate end points. The value or utility of the regimen obviously needs to be assessed at intervals during the course of therapy. The utility of a regimen can be defined as the benefit it produces plus the dangers of not treating the disease minus the sum of the adverse effects of therapy. Another common expression of the usefulness of a regimen is its ratio of risks to benefits (representing a balance between the efficacious and toxic effects of the drug). A definitive evaluation of the utility of a drug is not easy; nevertheless, some sense of value of a regimen must be established in the minds of the physician and the patient. Knowledge of the usefulness of a given regimen may be a critical determinant of protracted compliance by the patient to a chronic regimen or logical discontinuation by the physician of a marginally efficacious and risky therapy.

DRUG REGULATION AND DEVELOPMENT

DRUG REGULATION

The history of drug regulation in the United States reflects the growing involvement by governments of most countries to assure some degree of efficacy and safety in marketed medicinal agents. The first act, the Federal Pure Food and Drug Act of 1906, was concerned only with the purity of drugs. There were no restrictions on sale nor obligations to establish efficacy and safety. However, few new drugs were marketed between 1908 and the advent of the sulfonamides in the mid 1930s, an era of therapeutic nihilism. The federal act was amended in 1938, following an epidemic of deaths that resulted from the marketing of a solution of sulfanilamide in diethylene glycol, an excellent but highly toxic solvent. The amended act, the enforcement of which was entrusted to the Food and Drug Administration (FDA), was primarily concerned with the labeling and safety of drugs. Toxicity studies were required, as well as approval of a new drug application (NDA), before a drug could be promoted and distributed. However, no proof of efficacy was required, and extravagant claims for therapeutic indications were commonly made. Drugs could go from the laboratory to clinical testing without approval by the FDA.

In this relatively relaxed atmosphere, research in basic and clinical pharmacology burgeoned in both industrial and academic laboratories. The result was a flow of new and effective drugs, called "wonder drugs" by the lay press, for the treatment of both infectious and organic disease. The risk-to-benefit ratio was seldom mentioned, but it emerged in dramatic fashion early in the 1960s. At that time thalidomide, a hypnotic with no obvious advantage over other drugs in its class, was introduced in the European market. After an appropriate period, it became apparent that the incidence of a relatively rare birth defect, phocomelia, was increasing. It soon reached epidemic proportion, and retrospective epidemiological research firmly established the causative agent to be thalidomide, taken early in the course of pregnancy. The reaction to the dramatic demonstration of the teratogenicity of a needless drug was worldwide. In the United States it resulted, in 1962, in the Harris-Kefauver Amendment to the Federal Pure Food and Drug Act.

The Harris-Kefauver Amendment is sound legislation. It requires extensive pharmacological and toxicological research before a drug can be tested in man. The data from such studies must be submitted in the form of an application for an investigational new drug (IND) and approved by the FDA before clinical studies can begin. Three extensive phases of clinical testing (*see* below) must be completed before a new drug application (NDA) can be submitted. For drugs introduced after 1962, proof of efficacy is required, as is documentation of relative safety in terms of the risk-to-benefit ratio for the disease entity to be treated. The amendment also required proof of efficacy, retroactively, for all drugs marketed between 1938 and 1962.

The provisions of the amendment have greatly increased the time and the cost required to market a new drug. Moreover, although the law requires action on the part of the FDA within a period of 6 months, an NDA may be repeatedly returned to the applicant at 6-month intervals for additional basic or clinical research. The result has been a barrage of criticism from both the pharmaceutical industry and organized medicine, not of the law but of the rigid regulations imposed by the FDA in its enforcement. On the other hand, some consumer groups, with little appreciation of risk-to-benefit ratio, demand the recall of drugs that may play an important role in the therapeutic regimen of appropriately selected patients. In this climate, further amendments to the Federal Pure Food and Drug Act are being considered to speed the process of approval of an NDA without weakening, and hopefully even strengthening, requirements for safety and efficacy.

A seemingly contradictory directive to the FDA is also contained in the Federal Pure Food and Drug Act—that is, the FDA cannot interfere with the practice of medicine. Thus, once the efficacy of a new agent has been proven in the context of acceptable toxicity, the drug can be marketed. The physician is allowed to determine its most appropriate use. It is expected that physicians will discover true rates of anticipated effects and the severity and rates of unanticipated effects in the actual clinical setting. This expectation may be invalid and it has not been realized, because most physicians rely heavily on unrealistic guarantees from the tests performed prior to marketing of a new drug. Physicians must realize that new drugs are inherently more "risky" because of the relatively small amount of data about their effects. Yet there is no practical way to increase knowledge about a drug before it is marketed. A systematic method for postmarketing surveillance would appear to be an indispensable requirement for early optimization of drug use.

Before a drug can be marketed, an acceptable package insert must be prepared. This is a cooperative effort between the FDA and the pharmaceutical company. The insert usually contains basic pharmacological information, as well as essential clinical information in regard to approved indications, contraindications, precautions, warnings, adverse reactions, usual dosage, and available preparations. Advertising material cannot deviate from information contained in the insert.

DRUG DEVELOPMENT

Except for concern about the so-called drug lag (Kennedy, 1978) and governmental interference with the practice of medicine, the average physician has not considered it to be important to understand the process of drug development. Yet an appreciation of this process is necessary if the therapist wishes to have the ability to estimate the risk-to-benefit ratio of a drug and to realize just when regulations can and cannot be relied upon for

guarantees of efficacy and safety of a marketed product.

By the time an IND has been approved and a drug reaches the stage of testing in man, extensive evaluation of its pharmacokinetic, pharmacodynamic, and toxic properties have been performed in several species of animals and *in vitro*. As indicated above, the FDA issues regulations and guidelines that govern the type and extent of preclinical testing. Although the value of many requirements for preclinical testing is self-evident, such as those that screen for direct toxicity to organs and characterize dose-related effects, the value of others is controversial, particularly because of the well-known interspecies variation in the effects of drugs. Interestingly, although many of the preclinical tests have not been convincingly shown to predict effects that are eventually observed in man, the risk of cautious testing of a new drug in a normal person is surprisingly low.

Trials of drugs in man in the United States are generally conducted in phases, three of which must be completed before an NDA can be approved; these are outlined in Figure 3–2. Although assessment of risk is a major objective of such testing, this is far more difficult than is the determination of whether a drug is efficacious for a selected clinical condition (Temple *et al.*, 1979). Usually about 500 to 3000 carefully selected patients receive a new drug during phase-3 clinical trials. At most, only a few hundred are treated for more than 3 to 6 months, regardless of the likely duration of therapy that will be required in practice. Thus, the most profound and overt risks that occur almost immediately after the drug is given can be detected in a phase-3 study, if these occur more often than once per 100 administrations. Risks that are medically important but delayed or less frequent than 1 in 1000 administrations will not be revealed (Idanpaan-Heikkilä, 1983). However, to withhold a drug with important and proven efficacy until all of its untoward effects or unanticipated beneficial actions have been demonstrated is unreasonable. For instance, to detect an effect of a drug that occurs with a frequency of 1 in 50,000 administrations at a relative risk of 2 (*i.e.*, the treated population would develop the event twice as frequently as it would appear spontaneously) within 1 year of giving the drug, requires the study of more than 1.5 million patients (Strom and Melmon, 1979). It is thus obvious that a number of unanticipated adverse and beneficial effects of drugs are only detectable after the drug is approved for distribution. The same can be more convincingly stated about most of the effects of drugs on children or the fetus, where premarketing experimental studies are restricted. It is for these reasons that many countries are considering the establishment of systematic methods for the surveillance of the effects of drugs after they have been approved for distribution (*see* Slone *et al.*, 1979; Venning, 1983).

The problem of recognizing adverse effects during clinical trials is due not only to the limited number of studies but also to the selection of patients who are included. After marketing, the drug is used

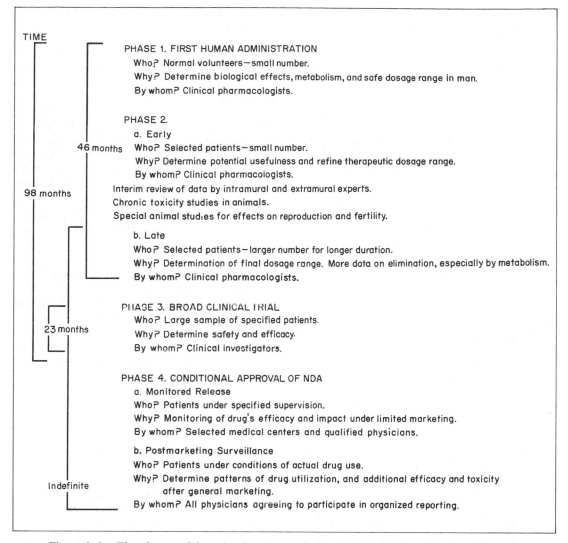

Figure 3–2. *The phases of drug development in the United States.* (Modified from Melmon and Morrelli, 1978.)

in patients with greater variations in their rates of absorption and elimination of drugs, in patients who have coexisting diseases, and so forth. Adverse reactions that may occur rarely or never in a carefully selected patient population, no matter how large, may be relatively frequent in the general population of patients (*e.g., see* Naranjo *et al.,* 1979). Thus, while most physicians realize that it is medically and morally impractical to delay the release of a drug while awaiting the "definitive" information on all possible adverse effects, the limitations of available data at the time of release place an additional burden on the physician to be observant and critical in his use of new drugs and to consider the possibility of iatrogenic illness when undesirable reactions occur (Venning, 1983).

ADVERSE DRUG REACTIONS AND DRUG TOXICITY

Very few physicians believe that any drug, no matter how trivial its actions, is free of toxic effects. The use of the term *safe* in the 1938 amendments to the Federal Pure Food and Drug Act has led to unnecessary misunderstandings between the regulatory agencies, the medical profession, and consumers of drugs. Patients, to a much greater extent than physicians, do not understand the limitations of premarketing evaluation of risks, and the difficulties faced by the FDA in gathering systematically useful information on the effects caused by drugs. Although resistance seems to be waning, the agency has had only limited success in cajoling the pharmaceutical industry into limited *postmarketing* studies. Generally, the public has had unwarranted confidence and expectations about the safety of drugs. More recently, the public has been told that thousands of patients are dying needlessly because of adverse effects of drugs. As is most often the case, the true situation lies somewhere between these two extremes, but precisely or even approximately where is unknown. For a review of the problems of defining, recognizing, classifying, and measuring the economic and human costs of adverse drug reactions, *see* Adverse Drug Reactions in the United States (1974) and Karch and Lasagna (1975).

As with drug interactions, classification of adverse effects of drugs according to information about their causes provides a framework for the transfer of principles to the clinical setting. Such classification appears in Chapter 68. In addition, the clinician obviously also needs to know the frequencies and types of untoward effects caused by each individual drug he prescribes; such information is presented throughout this textbook.

There is a danger that overemphasis of adverse drug reactions may cause physicians to lose sight of a most important aspect of therapy—the ratio of risks to benefits. Without consideration of this ratio it is impossible to establish the value of a drug. Procedures to estimate risk-to-benefit ratios for individuals (Pauker and Kassirer, 1975) and for populations (Schoenbaum, 1978) have been tried but are not proven. A generally applicable method for the quantitation of utility will remain elusive until the rates of anticipated efficacy of a drug can be determined and until quantitative values can be placed on the state of health and on the probability of anticipated and unanticipated decreases in longevity, quality of life, and function. It must also be remembered that the physician and the patient may have very disparate opinions of these values.

GUIDE TO THE "THERAPEUTIC JUNGLE"

The flood of new drugs in recent years has provided many dramatic improvements in therapy, but it has also created a number of problems of equal magnitude. Not the least of these is the "therapeutic jungle," the term used to refer to the combination of the overwhelming number of drugs, the confusion over nomenclature, and the associated uncertainty of the status of many of these drugs. A reduction in the marketing of close congeners and drug mixtures and an improvement in the quality of advertising are important ingredients in the remedy for the "therapeutic jungle." However, the physician can also contribute to the remedy by employing nonproprietary rather than proprietary names whenever appropriate, by using prototypes both as an instructional device and in clinical practice, by adopting a properly critical attitude toward new drugs, and by knowing and making use of reliable sources of pharmacological information. Most important, he should develop a "way of thinking about drugs" based upon pharmacological principles.

Drug Nomenclature. The existence of many names for each drug, even when reduced to a minimum, has led to a lamentable and confusing situation in drug nomenclature. In addition to its formal *chemical* name, a new drug is usually assigned a *code* name by the pharmaceutical manufacturer. If the drug appears promising, and the manufacturer wishes to place it on the market, a *United States Adopted Name* (USAN) is selected by the USAN Council, which is jointly sponsored by the American Medical Association, the American Pharmaceutical Association, and the United States Pharmacopeial Convention, Inc. This *nonproprietary* name is often referred to as the *generic* name. This term has become entrenched, but by definition it should be more properly reserved to designate a chemical or pharmacological class of drugs, such as sulfonamides or sympathomimetics. If the drug is eventually admitted to *The United States Pharmacopeia* (*see* below), the USAN becomes the *official* name. However, the nonproprietary name and the official name of an older drug may differ. Subsequently, the drug will also be assigned a *proprietary* name or *trademark* by the manufacturer. If the drug is marketed by more than one company, it may have several proprietary names. If mixtures of the drug with other agents are marketed, each such mixture may also have a separate proprietary name.

There is increasing worldwide adoption of the same name for each therapeutic substance. For newer drugs, the USAN is usually adopted for the nonproprietary name in other countries, but this is not true for older drugs. International agreement on drug names is mediated through the World Health Organization and the pertinent health agencies of the cooperating countries.

The nonproprietary or official name of a drug should be used whenever possible, and such a practice has been adopted in this textbook. The use of the nonproprietary name is clearly less confusing when the drug is available under multiple proprietary names, and when the nonproprietary name more readily identifies the drug with its pharmacological class. The best argument for the proprietary name is that it is frequently more easily pronounced and remembered as a result of advertising. For purposes of identification, representative proprietary names, designated by SMALL-CAP TYPE, appear throughout the text in chapter sections dealing with preparations as well as in the Index. This list is far from complete, since the number for a single drug may be large and since proprietary names differ from country to country.

When the physician prescribes drugs, the question arises as to whether the nonproprietary name or a proprietary name should be employed. In practically all states with generic drug laws, a pharmacist may substitute a preparation that is presumably equivalent *unless* the physician indicates "no substitution" on the prescription. Likewise, if the nonproprietary name of a drug is employed, the physician has the privilege of indicating its source. In view of the discussion above on the individualization of drug therapy, it is understandable why a physician who has carefully adjusted the

dose of a drug to a patient's individual requirements for chronic therapy may be reluctant to surrender control over the source of the drug that the patient receives.

Based on a number of considerations, such as the frequency of use of a drug that is only available from a single manufacturer, the cost of filling a prescription, and the markup of the pharmacist, it appears as though the *overall savings* to society of prescribing the least expensive nonproprietary preparation is about 5% (*see* Trout and Lee, 1981). Of course, savings in individual situations can be very much greater. On the other hand, prescribing by nonproprietary name could result in the patient receiving a preparation of inferior quality or of uncertain bioavailability, and therapeutic failures due to decreased bioavailability do occur. On the urging of the Senate Subcommittee on Health, the FDA has been attempting to establish standards for bioavailability and to compile information about the interchangeability of drug products (*see* Drug Bioequivalence: A Report of the Office of Technology Assessment, Drug Bioequivalence Study Panel, 1974). Unfortunately, at present there is still no single, comprehensive source of data on the bioequivalency of different products. In spite of this limitation, potential cost savings to the individual patient and simplification of the "therapeutic jungle" dictate that nonproprietary names be used when prescribing, except for those drugs with known differences in bioavailability among marketed products (Koch-Weser, 1974; Bioavailability of Drug Products, 1978).

Use of Prototypes. It is obviously crucial for the physician to be thoroughly familiar with the pharmacological properties of a drug before it is administered. It follows that the patient will benefit if the physician avoids the temptation to choose from many different drugs for the patient's regimen. A physician's needs for therapeutic agents can usually be satisfied by thorough knowledge of one or two drugs in each therapeutic category. Inevitably, a small number of drugs can be used more effectively. When the clinical setting calls for a drug that the physician uses infrequently, he should feel obligated to learn about its effects, to use great caution in its administration, and to apply appropriate procedures in monitoring its effects.

For teaching purposes in this textbook, the confusion created by the welter of similar drugs is reduced by restricting major attention to prototypes in each pharmacological class. Focusing on the representative drugs results in better characterization of a class as a whole, and thereby permits sharper recognition of the occasional member that possesses unique properties. A teaching prototype is often the agent most likely to be employed in clinical use, but this is not always true. A particular drug may be retained as the prototype, even though a new congener is clinically superior, either because more is known about the older drug or because it is more illustrative for the entire class of agents.

Attitude toward New Drugs. A reasonable attitude toward new drugs is summarized by the adage that advises the physician to be "neither the first to use a new drug nor the last to discard the old." Only a minor fraction of the new drugs represents a significant therapeutic advance. The limitation of information about toxicity and efficacy at the time of release of a drug has been emphasized above, and this is particularly pertinent to comparisons with older agents in the same therapeutic class. Nevertheless, the important advances in therapeutics in the last 40 years emphasize the obligation to keep abreast of significant advances in pharmacotherapy.

SOURCES OF DRUG INFORMATION

The physician's need for objective, concise, and well-organized information on drugs is obvious. Among the available sources are textbooks of pharmacology and therapeutics, leading medical journals, drug compendia, professional seminars and meetings, and advertising. Despite this cornucopia of information, responsible medical spokesmen insist that most practicing physicians are unable to extract the objective and unbiased data required for the practice of rational therapeutics (*see* Task Force, 1969).

Depending on their aim and scope, *pharmacology textbooks* provide (in varying proportions) basic pharmacological principles, critical appraisal of useful categories of therapeutic agents, and detailed descriptions of individual drugs or prototypes that serve as standards of reference for assessing new drugs. In addition, pharmacodynamics and pathological physiology are correlated. Therapeutics is considered in virtually all textbooks of medicine, but often superficially. For obvious reasons, textbooks cannot contain information on the most recently introduced drugs.

The source of information described as most often used by physicians in an industry survey is the *Physicians' Desk Reference* (PDR). The brand-name manufacturers whose products appear support this book. No comparative data on efficacy, safety, or cost are included. The information is nearly identical to that contained in drug package inserts, which are largely based on the results of phase-3 testing; its primary value is thus in learning what indications for use of a drug have been approved by the FDA.

There are, however, several inexpensive, unbiased sources of information on the clinical uses of drugs that are preferable to the industry-supported PDR. All recognize that the physician's legitimate use of a drug in a particular patient is not limited by FDA-approved labeling in the package insert. *The United States Pharmacopeia Dispensing Information* (USPDI), first published in 1980, comes in two volumes. One, *Drug Information for the Health Care Provider,* consists of drug monographs that contain practical, clinically significant information aimed at minimizing the risks and enhancing the benefits of drugs. Monographs are developed by USP staff and are reviewed by advisory panels and other reviewers. The *Advice for the Patient* volume is intended to reinforce, in lay language, the oral consultation provided by the therapist, and this may be provided to the patient in written form. It is planned that the volumes will be published frequently. The *American Hospital Formulary Service* (AHFS), published by the American Society of Hospital

Pharmacists, is a collection of monographs that are kept current by periodic supplements. The monographs are written on a single drug; there are also general discussions of drugs that are included in a defined class. *AMA Drug Evaluations*, compiled by the American Medical Association Department of Drugs in cooperation with the American Society for Clinical Pharmacology and Therapeutics, includes general information on the use of drugs in special settings (*e.g.*, pediatrics, geriatrics, renal insufficiency, *etc.*) and reflects the consensus of a panel on the effective clinical use of therapeutic agents. *Facts and Comparisons*, published by a division of J. B. Lippincott Company, is also organized by pharmacological classes and is updated monthly. Information in monographs is presented in a standard format and incorporates FDA approved information, which is supplemented with current data obtained from the biomedical literature. A useful feature is the comprehensive list of preparations with a "Cost Index," an index of the average wholesale price for equivalent quantities of similar or identical drugs.

Industry promotion, in the form of direct-mail brochures, journal advertising, displays, professional courtesies, or the detail man, is intended to be persuasive rather than educational. The pharmaceutical industry cannot, should not, and indeed does not purport to be responsible for the education of physicians in the use of drugs.

Over 1500 medical journals are published regularly in the United States. However, of the two to three dozen medical publications with circulations in excess of 70,000 copies, the great majority are sent to physicians free of charge and paid for by the industry. Objective journals, which are not supported by drug manufacturers, include *Clinical Pharmacology and Therapeutics*, which is devoted primarily to the evaluation of the actions and effects of drugs in man. The *New England Journal of Medicine, Annals of Internal Medicine, Archives of Internal Medicine, British Medical Journal, Lancet*, and *Postgraduate Medicine* offer timely therapeutic reports and reviews. Three publications deserve special emphasis here because they exemplify effective attempts to provide objective drug information in easily assimilable form. These are *The Medical Letter, Clin-Alert*, and *Rational Drug Therapy. The Medical Letter* provides summaries of scientific reports and consultants' evaluations of the safety, efficacy, and rationale for use of a drug. *Clin-Alert* consists mainly of abstracts from the literature on drugs. *Rational Drug Therapy* presents a monthly review article on groups of drugs or on the management of specific conditions.

The United States Pharmacopeia (USP) and *The National Formulary* (NF) were recognized as "official compendia" by the Federal Pure Food and Drug Act of 1906. The approved therapeutic agents used in medical practice in the United States are described and defined with respect to source, chemistry, physical properties, tests for identity and purity, assay, and storage. The two official compendia are now published in a single volume.

Benson, H., and McCallie, D. P. Angina pectoris and the placebo effect. *N. Engl. J. Med.*, **1979**, *300*, 1424–1425.

Bristow, M. R.; Ginsburg, R.; Minobe, W.; Cubicciotti, R. S.; Sageman, W. S.; Lurie, K.; Billingham, M. E.; Harrison, D. C.; and Stinson, E. B. Decreased catecholamine sensitivity and β-adrenergic-receptor density in failing human hearts. *N. Engl. J. Med.*, **1982**, *307*, 205–211.

Curran, W. J. Reasonableness and randomization in clinical trials: fundamental law and governmental regulation. *N. Engl. J. Med.*, **1979**, *300*, 1273–1275.

Feinstein, A. R. Clinical biostatistics. XLI. Hard science, soft data and the challenges of choosing clinical variables in research. *Clin. Pharmacol. Ther.*, **1977a**, *22*, 485–498.

———. An additional basic science for clinical medicine. *Ann. Intern. Med.*, **1983**, *99*, 393–397, 544–550, 705–712, 843–848.

Freiman, J. A.; Chalmers, T. C.; Smith, H.; and Kuebler, R. R. The importance of beta, the type II error and sample size in the design and interpretation of the randomized control trial. *N. Engl. J. Med.*, **1978**, *299*, 690–694.

Jick, H.; Slone, D.; Dinan, B.; and Muench, H. Evaluation of drug efficacy by a preference technique. *N. Engl. J. Med.*, **1966**, *275*, 1399–1403.

Kennedy, D. A calm look at "drug lag." *J.A.M.A.*, **1978**, *239*, 423–426.

Lefkowitz, R. J.; Caron, M. G.; and Stiles, G. L. Mechanisms of membrane-receptor regulation. Biochemical, physiological, and clinical insights derived from studies of the adrenergic receptors. *N. Engl. J. Med.*, **1984**, *310*, 1570–1579.

Meffin, P. J.; Winkle, R. A.; Blaschke, T. F.; Fitzgerald, J.; and Harrison, D. C. Response optimization of drug dosage: antiarrhythmic studies with tocainide. *Clin. Pharmacol. Ther.*, **1977**, *22*, 42–57.

Naranjo, C. A.; Pontigo, E.; Valdenegro, C.; Gonzalez, G.; Ruiz, I.; and Bustio, U. Furosemide-induced adverse reactions in cirrhosis of the liver. *Clin. Pharmacol. Ther.*, **1979**, *25*, 154–160.

Pauker, S. G., and Kassirer, J. P. Therapeutic decision making: a cost-benefit analysis. *N. Engl. J. Med.*, **1975**, *293*, 229–234.

Penno, M. B., and Vesell, E. S. Monogenic control of variations in antipyrine metabolite formation. *J. Clin. Invest.*, **1983**, *71*, 1698–1709.

Schoenbaum, S. C. Vaccination for influenza—any alternatives? *N. Engl. J. Med.*, **1978**, *298*, 621–622.

Sheiner, L. B.; Halkin, H.; Peck, C.; Rosenberg, B.; and Melmon, K. L. Improved computer-assisted digoxin therapy: a method using feedback of measured serum digoxin concentrations. *Ann. Intern. Med.*, **1975**, *82*, 619–627.

Slone, D.; Shapiro, S.; Miettinen, O. S.; Finkle, W. D.; and Stolley, P. D. Drug evaluation after marketing. *Ann. Intern. Med.*, **1979**, *90*, 257–261.

Steel, K.; Gertman, P. M.; Cresienze, C.; and Anderson, J. Iatrogenic illness on a general medical service at a university hospital. *N. Engl. J. Med.*, **1981**, *304*, 638–642.

Temple, R. J.; Jones, J. K.; and Crout, J. R. Adverse effects of newly marketed drugs. *N. Engl. J. Med.*, **1979**, *300*, 1046–1047.

Monographs and Reviews

Adverse Drug Reactions in the United States: An Analysis of the Scope of the Problem and Recommendations for Future Approaches. Medicine in the Public Interest, Inc., Washington, D. C., **1974**.

AMA Drug Evaluations, 5th ed. American Medical Association, Chicago, **1983**.

American Hospital Formulary Service. American Society of Hospital Pharmacists, Bethesda, Md., **1985**.

Aronson, J. K., and Grahame-Smith, D. C. Adverse drug interactions. *Br. Med. J. [Clin. Res.],* **1981**, *282*, 288–291.

Beecher, H. K. *Measurement of Subjective Responses: Quantitative Effects of Drugs.* Oxford University Press, New York, **1959**.

Bioavailability of Drug Products, cumulative ed. American Pharmaceutical Association, Washington, D. C., **1978**.

Bourne, H. R. Rational use of placebo. In, *Clinical Pharmacology: Basic Principles in Therapeutics,* 2nd ed. (Melmon, K. L., and Morrelli, H. F., eds.) Macmillan Publishing Co., New York, **1978**, pp. 1052–1062.

Boyd, J. R. (ed.). *Facts and Comparisons.* Facts and Comparisons, Div. of J. B. Lippincott Co., St. Louis, **1985**.

Brown, P. C.; Johnston, R. N.; and Schimke, R. T. Approaches to the study of mechanisms of selective gene amplification in cultured mammalian cells. In, *Gene Studies in Regulation and Development.* Alan R. Liss, Inc., New York, **1983**, pp. 197–212.

Drug Bioequivalence: A Report of the Office of Technology Assessment, Drug Bioequivalence Study Panel. U.S. Government Printing Office, Washington, D. C., **1974**.

Feinstein, A. R. *Clinical Biostatistics.* C. V. Mosby Co., St. Louis, **1977b**.

Finnerty, F. A. Extensive hypertensive work-up: con. *J.A.M.A.*, **1975**, *231*, 402–403.

Flier, J. S.; Kahn, C. R.; and Roth, J. Receptors, antireceptor antibodies and mechanisms of insulin resistance. *N. Engl. J. Med.*, **1979**, *300*, 413–419.

Hansten, P. D. *Drug Interactions,* 5th ed. Lea & Febiger, Philadelphia, **1985**.

Hill, A. B. *Controlled Clinical Trials: Conference of Council for International Organizations of Medical Sciences.* Blackwell Scientific Publications, Ltd., Oxford, **1960**.

———. *Statistical Methods in Clinical and Preventive Medicine.* Oxford University Press, New York, **1962**.

Idanpaan-Heikkilä, J. *A Review of Safety Information Obtained from Phase I–II and Phase III Clinical Investigations of Sixteen Selected Drugs.* U.S. Department of Health and Human Services, Food and Drug Administration Office of New Drug Evaluation, Washington, D. C., **1983**.

Ingelfinger, J. A.; Mosteller, F.; Thibodeau, L. A.; and Ware, J. H. *Biostatistics in Clinical Medicine.* Macmillan Publishing Co., New York, **1983**.

Karch, F. E., and Lasagna, L. Adverse drug reactions: a critical review. *J.A.M.A.*, **1975**, *234*, 1236–1241.

Koch-Weser, J. Serum drug concentrations as therapeutic guides. *N. Engl. J. Med.*, **1972**, *287*, 227–231.

———. Bioavailability of drugs. *N. Engl. J. Med.*, **1974**, *291*, 233.

Mangini, R. J. (ed.). *Drug Interaction Facts.* Facts and Comparisons, Div. of J. B. Lippincott Co., St. Louis, **1985**.

Melby, J. C. Extensive hypertensive work-up: pro. *J.A.M.A.*, **1975**, *231*, 399–401.

Melmon, K. L. Preventable drug reactions—causes and cures. *N. Engl. J. Med.*, **1971**, *284*, 1361–1368.

Melmon, K. L., and Morrelli, H. F. Drug reactions. In, *Clinical Pharmacology: Basic Principles in Therapeutics,* 2nd ed. (Melmon, K. L., and Morrelli, H. F., eds.) Macmillan Publishing Co., New York, **1978**, pp. 951–981.

Morrelli, H. F., and Melmon, K. L. Drug interactions. In, *Clinical Pharmacology: Basic Principles in Therapeutics,* 2nd ed. (Melmon, K. L., and Morrelli, H. F., eds.) Macmillan Publishing Co., New York, **1978**, pp. 982–1007.

Peck, C. C. Qualitative aspects of therapeutic decision making. In, *Clinical Pharmacology: Basic Principles in Therapeutics,* 2nd ed. (Melmon, K. L., and Morrelli, H. F., eds.) Macmillan Publishing Co., New York, **1978**, pp. 1063–1083.

Sheiner, L. B. Clinical trials and the illusion of objectivity. In, *Drug Therapeutics: Concepts for Physicians.* (Melmon, K. L., *et al.*, eds.) Elsevier North-Holland, Inc., New York, **1979**, pp. 167–182.

Sheiner, L. B., and Melmon, K. L. The utility function of antihypertensive therapy. In, *Mild Hypertension: To Treat or Not to Treat.* (Perry, H. M., Jr., and Smith, W. M., eds.) *Ann. N.Y. Acad. Sci.*, **1978**, *304*, 112–122.

Sheiner, L. B., and Tozer, T. N. Clinical pharmacokinetics: the use of plasma concentrations of drugs. In, *Clinical Pharmacology: Basic Principles in Therapeutics,* 2nd ed. (Melmon, K. L., and Morrelli, H. F., eds.) Macmillan Publishing Co., New York, **1978**, pp. 71–109.

Smith, W. M. Drug choice in disease states. In, *Clinical Pharmacology: Basic Principles in Therapeutics,* 2nd ed. (Melmon, K. L., and Morrelli, H. F., eds.) Macmillan Publishing Co., New York, **1978**, pp. 3–24.

Strom, B. L., and Melmon, K. L. Can post-marketing surveillance help to effect optimal drug therapy? *J.A.M.A.*, **1979**, *242*, 2420–2423.

———. Major challenges to effective post-marketing surveillance. In, *Drug-Induced Sufferings: Medical, Pharmaceutical and Legal Aspects.* (Soda, T., ed.) International Congress Series, No. 513. Excerpta-Medica, Amsterdam, **1980**, pp. 184–194.

Task Force on Prescription Drugs. *Final Report.* Department of Health, Education and Welfare, U.S. Government Printing Office, Washington, D. C., **1969**.

Trout, M. E., and Lee, A. M. Generic substitution: a boon or a bane to the physician and the consumer? In, *Drug Therapeutics: Concepts for Physicians.* (Melmon, K. L., ed.) Elsevier North-Holland, Inc., New York, **1981**.

The United States Pharmacopeia, 21st rev., and *The National Formulary,* 16th ed. The United States Pharmacopeial Convention, Inc. Mack Printing Co., Easton, Pa., **1985**.

The United States Pharmacopeia Dispensing Information. The United States Pharmacopeial Convention, Inc. Mack Printing Co., Easton, Pa., **1985**.

Venning, G. R. Identification of adverse reactions to new drugs. *Br. Med. J. [Clin. Res.]*, **1983**, *286*, 199–202, 289–292, 365–368, 458–460, 544–547.

Vesell, E. S. Pharmacogenetics—multiple interactions between genes and environment as determinants of drug response. *Am. J. Med.*, **1979**, *66*, 183–187.

————. Assessment of methods to identify sources of interindividual pharmacokinetic variations. *Clin. Pharmacokinet.*, **1983**, *8*, 378–409.

Drugs Acting at Synaptic and Neuroeffector Junctional Sites

CHAPTER

4 NEUROHUMORAL TRANSMISSION: THE AUTONOMIC AND SOMATIC MOTOR NERVOUS SYSTEMS

Norman Weiner and Palmer Taylor

The theory of *neurohumoral transmission* received direct experimental validation over 80 years ago (Euler, 1981), and extensive investigation during the ensuing years has led to its general acceptance. Nerves transmit their impulses across most synapses and neuroeffector junctions by means of specific chemical agents known as *neurohumoral transmitters*. The actions of the so-called autonomic drugs that affect smooth muscle, cardiac muscle, and gland cells can be understood and classified in terms of their mimicking or modifying the actions of the neurohumoral transmitters released by the autonomic fibers at either ganglia or effector cells.

Most of the general principles concerning the *physiology* and *pharmacology* of the peripheral autonomic nervous system and its effector organs apply with certain modifications to the neuromuscular junctions of skeletal muscle also, and in a more limited sense to the central nervous system (CNS). In fact, the study of neurotransmission in the CNS has benefited greatly from the delineation of this process in the periphery (*see* Chapter 12).

A clear understanding of the anatomy and physiology of the autonomic nervous system is essential to a study of the pharmacology of the *autonomic drugs*. The actions of an autonomic agent on various organs of the body can often be predicted if the responses to nerve impulses that reach the organs are known.

ANATOMY AND GENERAL FUNCTIONS OF THE AUTONOMIC NERVOUS SYSTEM

The autonomic nervous system is also called the visceral, vegetative, or involuntary nervous system. In the periphery, its representation consists of nerves, ganglia, and plexuses that provide the innervation to the heart, blood vessels, glands, other visceral organs, and smooth muscles. It is therefore widely distributed throughout the body and regulates autonomic functions, which occur without conscious control.

Differences between Autonomic and Somatic Nerves. The efferent nerves of the involuntary system supply all innervated structures of the body except skeletal muscle, which is served by somatic nerves. The most distal synaptic junctions in the autonomic reflex arc occur in ganglia that are entirely outside of the cerebrospinal axis; somatic nerves contain no peripheral ganglia, and the synapses are located entirely within the CNS. Many autonomic nerves form extensive peripheral plexuses, whereas such networks are absent from the somatic system. While motor nerves to skeletal muscles are myelinated, postganglionic autonomic nerves are generally nonmyelinated. When the cerebrospinal nerves are interrupted, the skeletal muscles that they innervate are completely paralyzed and undergo atrophy, whereas smooth muscles and glands generally show some level of spontaneous activity independent of intact innervation.

Visceral Afferent Fibers. The *afferent* fibers from visceral structures are the first link in the *reflex arcs of the autonomic system*. With certain exceptions, such as local axon reflexes, most visceral reflexes are mediated through the CNS. The afferent fibers are, for the most part, nonmyelinated fibers and are carried into the cerebrospinal axis by the vagus, pelvic, splanchnic, and other autonomic nerves. For example, about four fifths of the vagal nerve fibers are sensory. Other autonomic afferents from blood vessels in skeletal muscles and from certain integumental structures are carried in the somatic nerves. The cell bodies of visceral afferent fibers lie in the dorsal root ganglia of the spinal nerves and in the corresponding sensory ganglia of certain cranial nerves, such as the nodose ganglion of the vagus. The *efferent* link of the autonomic reflex arc is discussed in the sections that follow.

The autonomic afferent fibers are concerned with the mediation of visceral sensation (including pain and referred pain); with vasomotor, respiratory, and viscerosomatic reflexes; and with the regulation of interrelated visceral activities. An example of an autonomic afferent system is that arising from the pressoreceptive endings in the carotid sinus and the aortic arch, and from the chemoreceptor cells in the carotid and aortic bodies; this system is important in the reflex control of blood pressure, heart rate, and respiration, and its afferent fibers pass in the glossopharyngeal and vagus nerves to the medulla.

The neurohumoral agents that mediate transmission from sensory fibers have not been established unequivocally. However, substance P is present in afferent sensory fibers, in the dorsal root ganglia, and in the dorsal horn of the spinal cord, and this peptide is a leading candidate for the neurotransmitter that functions in the passage of nociceptive stimuli from the periphery to the spinal cord and higher structures (Jessell, 1983; Pernow, 1983). Other neuroactive peptides, including somatostatin, vasoactive intestinal polypeptide (VIP), and cholecystokinin, have also been found in sensory neurons (Hökfelt *et al.*, 1980), and one or more such peptides may play a role in the transmission of afferent impulses from autonomic structures. Enkephalins, present in interneurons in the dorsal spinal cord, have antinociceptive effects that may

be brought about by a presynaptic action to inhibit the release of substance P or other peptides (Duggan and North, 1983).

Central Autonomic Connections. There are probably no purely autonomic or somatic centers of integration, and extensive overlap occurs. Somatic responses are always accompanied by visceral responses and *vice versa*. Autonomic reflexes can be elicited at the level of the *spinal cord*. They are clearly demonstrable in the spinal animal, including man, and are manifested in sweating, blood pressure alterations, vasomotor responses to temperature changes, and reflex emptying of the urinary bladder, rectum, and seminal vesicles. Extensive central ramifications of the autonomic nervous system exist above the level of the spinal cord. For example, the integration of the control of blood pressure and respiration in the *medulla oblongata* is well known. The *hypothalamus* is generally regarded as the principal locus of integration of the entire autonomic system and is concerned in the regulation of body temperature, water balance, carbohydrate and fat metabolism, blood pressure, emotions, sleep, and sexual reflexes, although higher centers, including the cerebral cortex, also contribute crucially to these processes. Stimulation of the hypothalamus activates highly organized neuronal systems that induce a variety of integrated functions in the organism, including autonomic responses; these involve the cortex, the limbic system, and other structures in the brain (Hess, 1957; Morgane, 1981). Much information concerning central integration of autonomic functions has come not only from physiological experimentation but also from clinical investigation of such syndromes as diabetes insipidus, dystrophia adiposogenitalis, narcolepsy, hypothermia, hyperthermia, and diencephalic autonomic epilepsy (*see* Appenzeller, 1982; Bannister, 1983). The hypothalamic nuclei that lie posteriorly and laterally are sympathetic in their main connections, and their stimulation results in massive discharge of the sympathoadrenal system. Parasympathetic functions are evidently integrated by the midline nuclei in the region of the tuber cinereum and by nuclei lying anteriorly. The baroreceptor reflex is mediated via neural connections in the posteromedial hypothalamus, which originate in an ascending polysynaptic pathway from the nucleus of the solitary tract (Mancia and Zanchetti, 1981). Lesion of this nucleus is associated with the production of profound hypertension; a similar effect is elicited by lesions in the anterior hypothalamus (Reis *et al.*, 1976). The supraoptic nuclei are involved in water metabolism through their connections with the posterior lobe of the hypophysis. This hypothalamiconeurohypophyseal system represents a centrally located autonomic mechanism that exerts its peripheral effects on the kidney by means of the antidiuretic hormone (ADH). The neostriatum is probably concerned in the regulation of certain vegetative functions, as indicated clinically by the autonomic disturbances accompanying lesions in this region. The *cortex* provides another suprasegmental level of integration for sympathetic and parasympathetic functions. It is also a locus for correlation between somatic and vegetative functions, both sensory and motor. The activities of the cardiovascular, gastrointestinal, and many other systems are partially regulated at this highest level. The *limbic* system, which includes the olfactory lobe, hippocampal formation, and the pyriform lobe, is also important in the integration of emotional state with motor and visceral activities.

The actions of autonomic drugs on CNS transmission, although not fully understood, are often prominent and may overshadow the peripheral effects (*e.g.,* scopolamine, dextroamphetamine, diisopropyl phosphorofluoridate, *etc.*). Likewise, many centrally acting drugs may exert important visceral effects (*e.g.,* phenothiazines, barbiturates, morphine, *etc.*) (*see* Chapter 12).

Divisions of the Peripheral Autonomic System.

On the efferent or motor side, the autonomic nervous system consists of two large divisions: (1) the *sympathetic* or *thoracolumbar* outflow and (2) the *parasympathetic* or *craniosacral* outflow. Only the briefest outline of those anatomical features necessary for an understanding of the actions of autonomic drugs will be given here.

The arrangement of the principal parts of the peripheral autonomic nervous system is presented schematically in Figure 4–1. As will be discussed subsequently, the neurohumoral transmitter of all preganglionic autonomic fibers, all postganglionic parasympathetic fibers, and a few postganglionic sympathetic fibers is *acetylcholine* (ACh); these so-called *cholinergic fibers* are depicted in *blue.* The *adrenergic fibers,* shown in *red,* comprise the majority of the postganglionic sympathetic fibers; here the transmitter is *norepinephrine (noradrenaline, levarterenol).* As mentioned, the transmitter(s) of the *primary afferent fibers,* shown in *green,* has not been identified conclusively. Substance P and perhaps glutamate are prime candidates, since both are present in high concentrations in the dorsal regions of the spinal cord. The terms *cholinergic* and *adrenergic* were proposed originally by Dale to describe neurons that liberate ACh and norepinephrine, respectively. Subsequently, Dale (1954) suggested the terms *cholinoceptive* and *adrenoceptive* to denote postjunctional sites that are acted upon by the respective transmitters, but the terms *cholinergic receptor* and *adrenergic receptor* have been adopted more generally.

Sympathetic Nervous System. The cells that give rise to the *preganglionic fibers* of this division lie mainly in the intermediolateral columns of the spinal cord and extend from the first thoracic to the second or third lumbar segment. The axons from these cells are carried in the anterior nerve roots and synapse with neurons lying in sympathetic ganglia outside the cerebrospinal axis. The sympathetic ganglia are found in three locations: paravertebral, prevertebral, and terminal.

The *paravertebral sympathetic ganglia* consist of 22 pairs that lie on either side of the vertebral column to form the lateral chains. The ganglia are connected to each other by nerve trunks and to the spinal nerves by rami communicantes. The *white rami* are restricted to the segments of the thoracolumbar outflow; they carry the preganglionic myelinated fibers that exit from the spinal cord by way of the anterior spinal roots. The *gray rami* arise from the ganglia and carry postganglionic fibers back to the spinal nerves for distribution to sweat glands and pilomotor muscles, and to blood vessels of skeletal muscle and skin. The *prevertebral ganglia* lie in the abdomen and the pelvis near the ventral surface of the bony vertebral column, and consist mainly of the celiac (solar), superior mesenteric, aorticorenal, and inferior mesenteric ganglia. The *terminal ganglia* are few in number, lie near the organs that they innervate, and consist especially of those connected with the urinary bladder and rectum. In addition to the above ganglionic system, there are small *intermediate ganglia,* especially in the thoracolumbar region, that lie outside the conventional vertebral chain. They are variable in number and location, but are usually in close proximity to the communicating rami and to the anterior spinal nerve roots. Since they are not readily accessible to surgical resection, their continued presence after conventional types of sympathectomy may explain the incomplete denervation and the consequent return of autonomic function after surgery.

Preganglionic fibers issuing from the spinal cord may synapse with the neurons of more than one sympathetic ganglion. Their principal ganglia of termination need not correspond to the original level from which the preganglionic fiber exits the spinal cord. Many of the preganglionic fibers from the fifth to the last thoracic segment pass through the paravertebral ganglia and form the *splanchnic nerves.* Most of the splanchnic nerve fibers do not synapse until they reach the celiac ganglion; others directly innervate the adrenal medulla (*see* below).

Postganglionic fibers arising from sympathetic ganglia innervate the visceral structures of the thorax, abdomen, head, and neck. The trunk and the limbs are supplied by means of sympathetic fibers in spinal nerves, as previously described. The prevertebral ganglia contain cell bodies, the axons of which innervate the glands and the smooth muscles of the abdominal and the pelvic viscera. Many of the upper thoracic sympathetic fibers from the vertebral ganglia form *terminal plexuses,* such as the cardiac, esophageal, and pulmonary. The sympathetic distribution to the head and the neck (vasomotor, pupillodilator, secretory, and pilomotor) is by way of the cervical sympathetic chain and its three ganglia. All postganglionic fibers in this chain arise from cell bodies located in these three ganglia; all preganglionic fibers arise from the upper thoracic segments of the spinal cord, there being no sympathetic fibers that leave the CNS above the first thoracic level.

The *adrenal medulla* and other chromaffin tissue are embryologically and anatomically homologous to sympathetic ganglia; all are derived from the neural crest. The adrenal medulla differs from sympathetic ganglia in that the principal catecholamine that is released in man and many other species is *epinephrine (adrenaline)*. The chromaffin cells in the adrenal medulla are innervated by typical preganglionic fibers.

Parasympathetic Nervous System. This system consists of preganglionic fibers that originate in three areas of the CNS and their postganglionic connections. The regions of central origin are the midbrain, the medulla oblongata, and the sacral part of the spinal cord. The *midbrain* or tectal outflow consists of fibers arising from the Edinger-Westphal nucleus of the *third* cranial nerve and going to the ciliary ganglion in the orbit. The *medullary* outflow comprises the parasympathetic components of the seventh, ninth, and tenth cranial nerves. The fibers in the seventh cranial, or *facial*, nerve form the chorda tympani, which innervates the ganglia lying on the submaxillary and sublingual glands. They also form the greater superficial petrosal nerve, which innervates the sphenopalatine ganglion. The ninth cranial, or *glossopharyngeal*, autonomic components innervate the otic ganglion. Postganglionic parasympathetic fibers from these ganglia supply the sphincter of the iris, the ciliary muscle, the salivary and lacrimal glands, and the mucous glands of the nose, mouth, and pharynx. These fibers also include vasodilator nerves to the organs mentioned. The tenth cranial, or *vagus*, nerve arises in the medulla and contains preganglionic fibers, most of which do not synapse until they reach the many small ganglia lying directly on or in the viscera of the thorax and abdomen. In the intestinal wall, the vagal fibers terminate around ganglion cells in the plexuses of Auerbach and Meissner. The preganglionic fibers are thus very long and the postganglionic fibers quite short. The vagus nerve in addition carries a far greater number of afferent fibers (but apparently not pain fibers) from the viscera into the medulla; the cell bodies of these fibers lie mainly in the nodose ganglion. The *sacral* outflow consists of axons that arise from cells in the second, third, and fourth segments of the sacral cord and proceed as preganglionic fibers to form the pelvic nerves (nervi erigentes). They synapse in terminal ganglia lying near or within the bladder, rectum, and sexual organs. The vagal and sacral outflows provide motor and secretory fibers to thoracic, abdominal, and pelvic organs, as indicated in Figure 4–1. The functions of these nerves are subsequently described.

Differences between Sympathetic and Parasympathetic Nerves.

The *sympathetic system* is distributed to effectors throughout the body whereas the parasympathetic distribution is much more limited. Furthermore, the *sympathetic fibers* ramify to a much greater extent. A preganglionic sympathetic fiber may traverse a considerable distance of the sympathetic chain and pass through several ganglia before it finally synapses with a postganglionic neuron; also, its terminals make contact with a large number of postganglionic neurons. In some ganglia, the ratio of preganglionic axons to ganglion cells may be 1:20 or more. In this manner, a diffuse discharge of the sympathetic system is possible. In addition, there is an overlapping of synaptic innervation so that one ganglion cell may be supplied by several preganglionic fibers.

The *parasympathetic system,* by contrast, has its terminal ganglia very near to or within the organs innervated and thus can be more circumscribed in its influences. While in some organs a 1:1 relationship between the number of preganglionic and postganglionic fibers has been suggested, the ratio of preganglionic vagal fibers to ganglion cells in Auerbach's plexus has been estimated as 1:8000. Hence, this distinction between the two systems does not apply to all sites.

Details of Innervation. The axon of each *somatic motoneuron* divides into many branches, each of which innervates a single muscle fiber, so that more than 100 muscle fibers may be supplied by one motoneuron to form a *motor unit.* At each neuromuscular junction, or *motor end-plate,* the axonal terminal loses its myelin sheath and forms a terminal arborization that lies in apposition to a specialized surface of the muscle membrane. Mitochondria and a collection of synaptic vesicles are concentrated at the nerve terminal.

The terminations of the *postganglionic autonomic fibers* at smooth muscle and gland cells differ from the foregoing pattern. In most autonomic effector organs, the innervation forms a rich plexus or terminal reticulum. The terminal reticulum is a triad and consists of the final ramifications of the postganglionic sympathetic (adrenergic), parasympathetic (cholinergic), and visceral afferent fibers, all of which are enclosed within a frequently interrupted sheath of satellite or Schwann cells (*see* Hillarp, 1959). At these interruptions, varicosities packed with vesicles are seen in the efferent fibers. Such varicosities occur repeatedly along the course of the ramifications of the axon. There is apparently wide variation in the distance between the nerve varicosities and smooth muscle fibers, ranging from 200 Å in the vas deferens to 10,000 Å in certain blood vessels (Gabella, 1981).

"Protoplasmic bridges" occur between the smooth muscle fibers themselves at points of contact between their plasma membranes. They are believed to permit the conduction of impulses from cell to cell without the intervention of nervous elements. These structures have been variously termed nexuses, caveolae, or tight junctions. Through these structures the direct actions of neurohumoral transmitters or drugs on a limited portion of the total cell population could be extended indirectly to large numbers of effector cells.

Sympathetic ganglia have been shown to be extremely complex, both anatomically (Elfvin, 1963a, 1963b) and pharmacologically (Chapter 10). The preganglionic fibers lose their myelin sheaths, and divide repeatedly into a vast number of end fibers with diameters ranging from 0.1 to 0.3 μm; except at points of synaptic contact, they retain their satellite-cell sheaths. The vast majority of synapses are axodendritic. Apparently, a given axonal terminal may synapse with one or more dendritic processes at several points. Additional elements of yet-unknown physiological significance that are present in varying numbers in sympathetic ganglia are small, catecholamine-containing cells (termed small, intensely fluorescent [SIF] cells). Some of these appear to make synaptic contact with ganglion cells. Others are clustered predominantly around blood vessels (Eränkö *et al.*, 1980).

Responses of Effector Organs to Autonomic Nerve Impulses. A clear understanding of the response of the various effector organs to autonomic nerve impulses makes it possible to anticipate the actions of drugs that mimic or inhibit the actions of these nerves. In most instances, the sympathetic and parasympathetic systems can be viewed as physiological antagonists. If one system inhibits a certain function, the other usually augments that function. Most viscera are innervated by both divisions of the autonomic nervous system, and the level of activity at any one moment represents the integration of influences of the two components. The action of one system is most easily demonstrated by surgical removal or drug-induced paralysis of the opposing system. However, despite the conventional concept of antagonism between the two portions of the autonomic nervous system, their activities on specific structures may be either different and independent or integrated and interdependent. For example, the effects of sympathetic and parasympathetic stimulation of the heart and the iris follow a highly integrated pattern of antagonism. Their actions on male sexual organs are complementary and are integrated to promote sexual function. The control of blood pressure is probably almost entirely due to sympathetic control of arteriolar resistance. The effects of stimulating the sympathetic (adrenergic) and parasympathetic (cholinergic) nerves to various organs, visceral structures, and effector cells are summarized in Table 4–1.

General Functions of the Autonomic Nervous System. The integrating action of the autonomic nervous system is of vital importance for the well-being of the organism. In general, the autonomic nervous system regulates the activities of structures that are not under voluntary control and that, as a rule, function below the level of consciousness. Thus, respiration, circulation, digestion, body temperature, metabolism, sweating, and the secretions of certain endocrine glands are regulated, in part or entirely, by the autonomic nervous system. As Claude Bernard (1878–1879) and Cannon (1929, 1932) have emphasized, the constancy of the internal environment of the organism is to a large extent controlled by the vegetative, or autonomic, nervous system.

The sympathetic and parasympathetic systems have contrasting functions in regulating the internal environment. The *sympathetic system* and its associated adrenal medulla are not essential to life, and animals completely deprived of the sympathoadrenal system can survive within the sheltered confines of the laboratory. Under circumstances of stress, however, the lack of the sympathoadrenal functions becomes evident. Body temperature cannot be regulated when environmental temperature varies; the concentration of glucose in blood does not rise in response to urgent need; compensatory vascular responses to hemorrhage, oxygen want, excitement, and work are lacking; resistance to fatigue is lessened; sympathetic components of instinctive reactions to fright and danger are lost; pilomotor responses are absent; and other serious deficiencies in the protective forces of the body are discernible.

The *sympathetic system* is normally active at all times, the degree of activity varying from moment to moment and from organ to organ; in this manner, adjustments to a constantly changing environment are accomplished. The *sympathoadrenal system* can also discharge as a unit. This occurs especially during rage and fright, under which circumstances sympathetically innervated structures over the entire body are affected simultaneously. The heart rate is accelerated; the blood pressure rises; red blood cells are poured into the circulation from the spleen (in certain species); blood flow is shifted from the skin and splanchnic region to the skeletal muscles; blood glucose rises; the bronchioles and pupils dilate; and, on the whole, the organism is better prepared for "fight or flight." Many of these effects result primarily from, or are reinforced by, the actions of epinephrine, secreted by the adrenal medulla (*see* below).

The *parasympathetic system* is organized mainly for discrete and localized discharge and is concerned primarily with the functions of conservation of energy and maintenance of organ function during periods of minimal activity. It slows the heart rate, lowers the blood pressure, stimulates the gastrointestinal movements and secretions, aids absorption of nutrients, protects the retina from excessive light, and empties the urinary bladder and rectum. No useful purpose would be served in the body if the parasympathetic nerves all discharged at once.

NEUROHUMORAL TRANSMISSION

Nerve impulses elicit responses in smooth, cardiac, and skeletal muscles, exocrine glands, and postsynaptic neurons through liberation of specific chemical substances. The steps involved and the evidence for them will be outlined in some detail because the concept of chemical mediation of nerve impulses profoundly affects our knowledge of the mechanism of action of drugs at these sites.

HISTORICAL ASPECTS

The earliest concrete proposal of a neurohumoral mechanism was made shortly after the turn of the present century. Lewandowsky (1898) and Langley (1901) noted independently the similarity between the effects of injection of extracts of the adrenal gland and stimulation of sympathetic nerves. A few years later, in 1905, T. R. Elliott, while a student at Cambridge, England, extended these observations and postulated that sympathetic nerve impulses release minute amounts of an epinephrine-like substance in immediate contact with effector cells. He considered this substance to be the chemical step in the process of transmission. He also noted that long after sympathetic nerves had degenerated, the effector organs still responded characteristically to the hormone of the adrenal medulla. In 1905, Langley suggested that effector cells have excitatory and inhibitory "receptive substances," and that the response to epinephrine depended on which type of substance was present. In 1907, Dixon was so impressed by the correspondence between the effects of the alkaloid muscarine and the responses to vagal stimulation that he advanced the important idea that the vagus nerve liberated a muscarine-like substance that acted as a chemical transmitter of its impulses. In the same year, Reid Hunt described the actions of acetylcholine (ACh) and other choline esters. In 1914, Dale thoroughly reinvestigated the pharmacological properties of ACh. He was so intrigued with the remarkable fidelity with which this drug reproduced the responses to stimulation of parasympathetic nerves that he introduced the term *parasympathomimetic* to characterize its effects. Dale also noted the brief duration of the action of this chemical and proposed that an esterase in the tissues rapidly splits ACh to acetic acid and choline, thereby terminating its action.

The brilliant researches of Otto Loewi, begun in 1921, provided the first proof of the chemical mediation of nerve impulses by the release of specific chemical agents. He stimulated the vagus nerve of a perfused (donor) frog heart and allowed the perfusion fluid to come in contact with a second (recipient) frog heart used as a test object. It was thus evident that a substance was liberated from the first organ that slowed the rate of the second. Loewi referred to this chemical substance as *Vagusstoff* ("vagus-substance"; parasympathin); subsequently, Loewi and Navratil (1926) presented evidence for its identification as ACh. Loewi also discovered that an accelerator substance similar to epinephrine was liberated into the perfusion fluid in summer, when the action of the sympathetic fibers in the frog's vagus, a mixed nerve, predominated over that of the inhibitory fibers. Loewi's discoveries were eventually confirmed and are now universally accepted.

Evidence that the cardiac vagus-substance is also ACh in mammals was obtained in 1933 by Feldberg and Krayer. Many other investigations established quite conclusively that a chemical mediator, ACh, is instrumental in the transmission of parasympathetic impulses in mammals to other structures, including the iris, salivary glands, stomach, and small intestine.

In addition to the role of ACh as the transmitter of all postganglionic parasympathetic fibers and of a few postganglionic sympathetic fibers, such as those to the sweat glands and the sympathetic vasodilator fibers, this substance has been shown to have transmitter function in three additional classes of nerves: (1) preganglionic fibers of both the sympathetic and the parasympathetic systems, (2) motor nerves to skeletal muscle, and (3) certain neurons within the CNS.

Mention has already been made of Loewi's discovery of an accelerator substance released from frog hearts under certain conditions. In the same year, Cannon and Uridil (1921) reported that stimulation of the sympathetic hepatic nerves resulted in the release of an epinephrine-like substance that increased the blood pressure and the heart rate. Subsequent experiments, mainly by Cannon and coworkers, firmly established that this substance is the chemical mediator liberated by sympathetic nerve impulses at neuroeffector junctions. The mediator was originally called "sympathin" by Cannon.

In many of its pharmacological and chemical properties, Cannon's "sympathin" closely resembled epinephrine, but the two substances differed in certain important respects. When epinephrine is injected into the body, it elicits both excitatory and inhibitory effects. Thus, it accelerates the rate of the heart but simultaneously dilates certain vascular beds while constricting others. In contrast, the excitatory effects of "sympathin" could be elicited

Table 4–1. RESPONSES OF EFFECTOR ORGANS TO AUTONOMIC NERVE IMPULSES

EFFECTOR ORGANS	Receptor Type [2]	ADRENERGIC IMPULSES [1] Responses [3]	CHOLINERGIC IMPULSES [1] Responses [3]
Eye			
Radial muscle, iris	α_1	Contraction (mydriasis) ++	
Sphincter muscle, iris			Contraction (miosis) +++
Ciliary muscle	β	Relaxation for far vision +	Contraction for near vision +++
Heart			
S-A node	β_1	Increase in heart rate ++	Decrease in heart rate; vagal arrest +++
Atria	β_1	Increase in contractility and conduction velocity ++	Decrease in contractility, and shortened action-potential duration ++
A-V node	β_1	Increase in automaticity and conduction velocity ++	Decrease in conduction velocity; A-V block +++
His-Purkinje system	β_1	Increase in automaticity and conduction velocity +++	Little effect
Ventricles	β_1	Increase in contractility, conduction velocity, automaticity, and rate of idioventricular pacemakers +++	Slight decrease in contractility claimed by some
Arterioles			
Coronary	$\alpha; \beta_2$	Constriction +; dilatation [4] ++	Dilatation ±
Skin and mucosa	α	Constriction +++	Dilatation [5]
Skeletal muscle	$\alpha; \beta_2$	Constriction ++; dilatation [4,6] ++	Dilatation [7] +
Cerebral	α	Constriction (slight)	Dilatation [5]
Pulmonary	$\alpha; \beta_2$	Constriction +; dilatation [4]	Dilatation [5]
Abdominal viscera	$\alpha; \beta_2$	Constriction +++; dilatation [6] +	
Salivary glands	α	Constriction +++	Dilatation ++
Renal	$\alpha_1; \beta_1, \beta_2$	Constriction +++; dilatation [6] +	
Veins (Systemic)	$\alpha_1; \beta_2$	Constriction ++; dilatation ++	
Lung			
Tracheal and bronchial muscle	β_2	Relaxation +	Contraction ++
Bronchial glands	$\alpha_1; \beta_2$	Decreased secretion; increased secretion	Stimulation +++
Stomach			
Motility and tone	$\alpha_2; \beta_2$	Decrease (usually) [8] +	Increase +++
Sphincters	α	Contraction (usually) +	Relaxation (usually) +
Secretion		Inhibition (?)	Stimulation +++
Intestine			
Motility and tone	$\alpha_1; \beta_1, \beta_2$	Decrease [8] +	Increase +++
Sphincters	α	Contraction (usually) +	Relaxation (usually) +
Secretion		Inhibition (?)	Stimulation ++
Gallbladder and Ducts	β_2	Relaxation +	Contraction +
Kidney	β_1	Renin secretion ++	
Urinary Bladder			
Detrusor	β	Relaxation (usually) +	Contraction +++
Trigone and sphincter	α	Contraction ++	Relaxation ++
Ureter			
Motility and tone	α	Increase	Increase (?)
Uterus	$\alpha; \beta_2$	Pregnant: contraction (α); relaxation (β_2). Nonpregnant: relaxation (β_2)	Variable [9]
Sex Organs, Male	α	Ejaculation +++	Erection +++
Skin			
Pilomotor muscles	α	Contraction ++	
Sweat glands	α	Localized secretion [10] +	Generalized secretion +++
Spleen Capsule	$\alpha; \beta_2$	Contraction +++; relaxation +	

Table 4–1. RESPONSES OF EFFECTOR ORGANS TO AUTONOMIC NERVE IMPULSES (Continued)

EFFECTOR ORGANS	ADRENERGIC IMPULSES [1]		CHOLINERGIC IMPULSES [1]
	Receptor Type [2]	*Responses* [3]	*Responses* [3]
Adrenal Medulla		———	Secretion of epinephrine and norepinephrine (nicotinic effect)
Skeletal Muscle	β_2	Increased contractility; glycogenolysis; K^+ uptake	———
Liver	α; β_2	Glycogenolysis and gluconeogenesis [11] +++	Glycogen synthesis +
Pancreas Acini Islets (β cells)	 α α_2 β_2	 Decreased secretion + Decreased secretion +++ Increased secretion +	 Secretion ++ ——— ———
Fat Cells	α; β_1	Lipolysis [11] +++	———
Salivary Glands	α_1 β	Potassium and water secretion + Amylase secretion +	Potassium and water secretion +++
Lacrimal Glands		———	Secretion +++
Nasopharyngeal Glands		———	Secretion ++
Pineal Gland	β	Melatonin synthesis	———
Posterior Pituitary	β_1	Antidiuretic hormone secretion	———

[1] The anatomical classes of adrenergic and cholinergic nerve fibers are described on page 68 and depicted in Figure 4–1 in red and blue, respectively. A long dash signifies no known functional innervation.

[2] Where a designation of subtype is not provided, the nature of the subtype has not been determined unequivocally.

[3] Responses are designated 1+ to 3+ to provide an approximate indication of the importance of adrenergic and cholinergic nerve activity in the control of the various organs and functions listed.

[4] Dilatation predominates *in situ* due to metabolic autoregulatory phenomena.

[5] Cholinergic vasodilatation at these sites is of questionable physiological significance.

[6] Over the usual concentration range of physiologically released, circulating epinephrine, β-receptor response (vasodilatation) predominates in blood vessels of skeletal muscle and liver; α-receptor response (vasoconstriction), in blood vessels of other abdominal viscera. The renal and mesenteric vessels also contain specific dopaminergic receptors, activation of which causes dilatation (*see* review by Goldberg *et al.*, 1978).

[7] Sympathetic cholinergic system causes vasodilatation in skeletal muscle, but this is not involved in most physiological responses.

[8] It has been proposed that adrenergic fibers terminate at inhibitory β receptors on smooth muscle fibers, and at inhibitory α receptors on parasympathetic cholinergic (excitatory) ganglion cells of Auerbach's plexus.

[9] Depends on stage of menstrual cycle, amount of circulating estrogen and progesterone, and other factors.

[10] Palms of hands and some other sites ("adrenergic sweating").

[11] There is significant variation among species in the type of receptor that mediates certain metabolic responses; α and β responses have not been determined in man.

in the absence of dilatation of some vascular beds, with more marked increases in total peripheral resistance and diastolic blood pressure. As early as 1910, Barger and Dale noted that the effects of sympathetic nerve stimulation were more closely reproduced by the injection of sympathomimetic primary amines than by that of epinephrine or other secondary amines. The possibility that demethylated epinephrine (*norepinephrine, levarterenol, noradrenaline*) might be "sympathin" had been repeatedly advanced by Z. M. Bacq and others, but definitive evidence for its role as the sympathetic nerve mediator was not obtained until specific chemical and biological assay methods were developed for the quantitative determination of

small amounts of sympathomimetic amines in extracts of tissues and body fluids. Euler in 1946 found that the sympathomimetic substance in highly purified extracts of sympathetic nerves and effector organs resembled norepinephrine by all criteria used. He proposed that the sympathetic transmitter is norepinephrine. Numerous workers have confirmed and extended these observations; *norepinephrine* is the predominant sympathomimetic substance in the postganglionic sympathetic nerves of mammals and is the adrenergic mediator liberated by their stimulation. (*See* Euler, 1972.) Norepinephrine, its immediate precursor, dopamine, and epinephrine are also neurohumoral transmitters in the CNS (*see* Chapter 12).

EVIDENCE FOR NEUROHUMORAL TRANSMISSION

The concept of neurohumoral transmission was first developed primarily to explain observations relating to the transmission of impulses from postganglionic autonomic fibers to effector cells. The general lines of evidence in its support have included: (1) demonstration of the presence of a physiologically active compound, and of the enzymes necessary for its synthesis, at appropriate sites; (2) recovery of the compound from the perfusate of an innervated structure during periods of nerve stimulation, but not (or in greatly reduced amounts) in the absence of stimulation; (3) demonstration that the compound, when administered appropriately, is capable of producing responses identical with those to nerve stimulation; and (4) demonstration that the responses to nerve stimulation and to the administered compound are modified in the same manner by various drugs.

General acceptance of neurohumoral, rather than electrogenic, transmission at autonomic ganglia and the neuromuscular junction of skeletal muscle was withheld for a considerable period, chiefly for two reasons: (1) the extremely rapid time factors involved, in contrast to those at autonomic effector sites; and (2) discrepancies between the amount of the putative transmitter, ACh, recovered during nerve stimulation and that required to produce characteristic responses. Both objections have, for the most part, been answered by the development of modern technics of intracellular recording and microiontophoretic application of drugs.

One important feature of junctional transmission that supports the concept of a neurohumoral mechanism is the irreducible latent period between the arrival of an impulse at the axonal terminal and the appearance of the postjunctional potential. Physiologists had long recognized a synaptic delay, sometimes as brief as a fraction of a millisecond, that could not be accounted for in terms of known conduction velocities in the presynaptic or postsynaptic neurons. However, there remained the possible explanation that conduction might be considerably slowed in the fine preterminal axonal branches. This limitation was overcome in an investigation of the giant synapse of the squid. Bullock and Hagiwara (1957) inserted fine-recording micropipettes into the presynaptic and postsynaptic fibers and simultaneously recorded from both following presynaptic stimulation. There was invariably a delay of 0.5 to 2.0 milliseconds, depending upon the temperature, between the arrival of the impulse at the presynaptic electrode and the recording of postsynaptic activity; furthermore, depolarization or hyperpolarization of either the presynaptic or the postsynaptic element induced no detectable change in the potential of the other (Hagiwara and Tasaki, 1958). These findings are consistent with the chemical mediation of synaptic transmission and not with the direct spread of electrical current across the synapse.

There are instances where synaptic transmission undoubtedly does occur by the direct spread of current across the junction. Such electrotonic transmission of information across "gap junctions" occurs in the CNS (Schmitt et al., 1976), and it might also have effects on synchronous firing of peripheral autonomic neurons.

Neurohumoral transmission in the peripheral and central nervous systems was once believed to conform to the hypothesis that each neuron contains only one transmitter substance. However, enkephalins, substance P, somatostatin, and other peptides have been found in nervous tissue, and these peptides can depolarize or hyperpolarize nerve terminals or postsynaptic cells (see Barker, 1983). Furthermore, histochemical, immunocytochemical, and autoradiographic studies have demonstrated that one or more of these peptides is present in the same neurons that contain one of the classical biogenic amine neurotransmitters (Gilbert and Emson, 1983). For example, enkephalins are found in postganglionic sympathetic neurons, preganglionic cholinergic neurons, and adrenal medullary chromaffin cells. There is considerable evidence to suggest that VIP is localized in peripheral cholinergic neurons that innervate exocrine glands. The VIP may be responsible for the vasodilatation that accompanies secretion following nerve stimulation (Lundberg et al., 1981). Livett and associates (1983) have reported that preganglionic stimulation of cholinergic nerves to the adrenal medulla is associated with the release of both substance P and ACh. Substance P may prevent desensitization of the nicotinic receptor for ACh that is present on the chromaffin cells. These observations suggest that in many instances synaptic transmission may be mediated by the release of more than one neurohumoral agent. (For further discussion of neuropeptides, see Iversen et al., 1983.)

STEPS INVOLVED IN NEUROHUMORAL TRANSMISSION

The sequence of events involved in neurohumoral transmission is of particular importance pharmacologically, since the actions of a great number of drugs can be related directly to the individual steps. The term *conduction* is reserved for the passage of an impulse along an axon or muscle fiber; *transmission* refers to the passage of an impulse across a synaptic or neuroeffector junction. With the exception of the local anesthetics, which are infiltrated in high concentrations in the immediate vicinity of nerve trunks, very few drugs modify axonal conduction in the doses employed therapeutically. Hence, this process will be described only briefly in order to introduce its role in triggering the first step in transmission.

Axonal Conduction. The current model that describes axonal conduction stems largely from the investigative work of Hodgkin and Huxley (1952).

At rest, the interior of the typical mammalian axon is approximately 70 mV negative to the exterior. The *resting potential* is essentially a *diffusion potential*, based chiefly on the 30- to 50-fold higher concentration of potassium ion in the axoplasm as compared with the extracellular fluid, and the relatively high permeability of the resting axonal membrane to potassium ions. Sodium and chloride ions are present in higher concentrations in the extracellular fluid than in the axoplasm, but their concentration gradients across the membrane are somewhat lower than that of potassium, and the axonal membrane at rest is considerably less permeable to these ions; hence their contribution to the resting potential is relatively minor. These ionic gradients are maintained by an energy-dependent active-transport or pump mechanism, which involves an adenosine triphosphatase (ATPase) activated by sodium at the inner and by potassium at the outer surface of the membrane (*see* Armstrong, 1974; Grundfest, 1975). In some excitable tissues an electrogenic sodium pump may also contribute to the net resting potential (Fleming, 1980).

In response to a stimulus above the threshold level, a nerve *action potential* (AP) or nerve impulse is initiated at a local region of the membrane. This is detectable first by a rapid deflection of the internal resting potential from its negative value toward zero, and continuing uninterruptedly to a positive overshoot. This local depolarization is due to a sudden, selective increase in the permeability of the membrane to *sodium* ions, which flow rapidly inward in the direction of their concentration gradient. Repolarization of the membrane follows immediately and results from the rapid replacement of this change by one of increased permeability to *potassium*. Separate channels appear to be involved. The transmembrane ionic currents produce local circuit currents around the axon. As a result of such localized changes in membrane potential, adjacent inactive channels in the axon are activated, and excitation of the next excitable portion of the axonal membrane occurs. This brings about the propagation of the AP without decrement along the axon. The region that has undergone depolarization remains momentarily in a refractory state. In myelinated fibers, permeability changes occur only at the nodes of Ranvier, thus causing a rapidly progressing type of jumping, or saltatory, conduction. The puffer fish poison, *tetrodotoxin*, and a close congener found in some shellfish, *saxitoxin*, selectively block axonal conduction; they do so by preventing the increase in permeability to sodium ion associated with the rising phase of the AP (Kao, 1966). In contrast, *batrachotoxin*, an extremely potent steroidal alkaloid secreted by a South American frog, produces paralysis through a selective increase in sodium permeability, which induces a persistent depolarization (Albuquerque *et al.*,

1973). Scorpion toxins are peptides that also cause persistent depolarization, but they do this by inhibiting the inactivation process. The pharmacological aspects of axonal conduction have been reviewed in detail by Narahashi (1975) and Catterall (1980).

Junctional Transmission. The arrival of the action potential (AP) at the axonal terminals initiates a series of events that effect the neurohumoral transmission of an excitatory or inhibitory impulse across the synapse or neuroeffector junction (*see* reviews by Katz, 1966; Eccles, 1973; Krnjević, 1974). These events, diagramed in Figure 4–2, are as follows:

1. *Release of the Transmitter.* The neurohumoral transmitters are probably synthesized in the region of the axonal terminals and stored there within the synaptic vesicles (*see* below). During the resting state, there is a continual, slow release of isolated quanta of the transmitter, ordinarily insufficient to cause initiation of a propagated impulse at the postjunctional site. However, this release of small amounts of transmitter produces electrical responses at the postjunctional membrane (miniature end-plate potentials, mepps) that are associated with the maintenance of physiological responsiveness of the effector organ (*see* Katz, 1969; Changeux, 1981). The AP causes the synchronous release of several hundred quanta. The depolarization of the axonal terminal triggers this process; however, the intermediate steps are uncertain. One step is the influx of calcium ion, which enters the axonal cytoplasm and is believed to promote fusion of those vesicles in close proximity to the axoplasmic membrane with the axoplasmic membrane. The contents of the vesicles are then discharged to the exterior by a process termed *exocytosis*. Other components of the vesicle, including enzymes and other proteins, are also discharged. Measurement of these components may provide useful information about the intensity and duration of prejunctional activity (*see* Weiner, 1979a).

A variety of chemical substances can inhibit the neurally mediated release of either norepinephrine or ACh by interaction with putative presynaptic receptors on the appropriate nerve terminals. Norepinephrine is able to interact with a presynaptic α_2-adrenergic receptor (termed an *autoreceptor*)

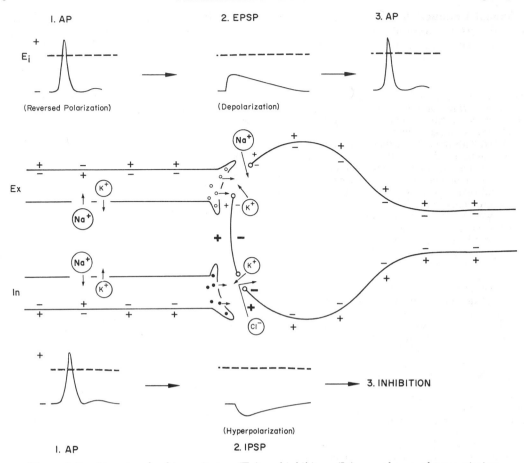

Figure 4–2. *Steps involved in excitatory* (Ex) *and inhibitory* (In) *neurohumoral transmission.*

1. The nerve action potential (AP), consisting in a self-propagated *reversal* of negativity (the internal potential, E_i, goes from a negative value, through zero potential, indicated by the broken line, to a positive value) of the axonal membrane, arrives at the presynaptic terminal and causes release of the excitatory (○) or inhibitory (●) transmitter.

2. Combination of the excitatory transmitter with postsynaptic receptors produces a localized depolarization, the excitatory postsynaptic potential (EPSP), through an increase in permeability to cations, most notably Na^+. The inhibitory transmitter causes a selective increase in permeability to the smaller ions (K^+ and Cl^-), resulting in a localized hyperpolarization, the inhibitory postsynaptic potential (IPSP).

3. The EPSP initiates a conducted AP in the postsynaptic neuron; this can, however, be prevented by the hyperpolarization induced by a concurrent IPSP.

The transmitter is dissipated by enzymatic destruction, by re-uptake into the presynaptic terminal or adjacent glial cells, or by diffusion. (Modified from Eccles, 1964, 1973; Katz, 1966; others.)

and inhibit neurally mediated release of norepinephrine. Administration of nonselective or selective α_2-adrenergic antagonists causes a marked increase in the release of norepinephrine per nerve impulse. In an analogous fashion, neurally mediated release of ACh from cholinergic neurons is inhibited by α_2-adrenergic agonists. Conversely, stimulation of presynaptic β_2-adrenergic receptors is associated with a modest enhancement of norepinephrine release. Adenosine, methacholine, dopamine, prostaglandins, and enkephalins all inhibit

neurally mediated release of norepinephrine by means of interactions with specific presynaptic receptors (*see* Langer, 1980; Starke, 1981). There is evidence that adenosine 3′,5′-monophosphate (cyclic AMP) facilitates the release of neurotransmitters and that agents that modulate the process may act via receptor-coupled stimulation (enhanced release) or inhibition (reduced release) of adenylate cyclase (*see* Weiner, 1979a).

In cholinergic neurons, presynaptic muscarinic receptors have been detected at those synapses where there are postjunctional muscarinic receptors. They are found in parasympathetic nerves that innervate the heart and eye and in the ganglia of the myenteric plexus. These receptors mediate inhibition of the evoked release of acetylcholine, and the output of acetylcholine is thus decreased with repetitive stimulation. The evoked release of ACh is also blocked by inhibitors of acetylcholinesterase (AChE), and it is enhanced by muscarinic antagonists (Kilbinger, 1984). Presynaptic muscarinic receptors have not been detected in sympathetic ganglia or somatic motor nerves (*see* Bowman, 1980; Chapter 11).

2. Combination of the Transmitter with Postjunctional Receptors and Production of the Postjunctional Potential. The transmitter diffuses across the synaptic or junctional cleft and combines with specialized macromolecular receptors on the postjunctional membrane; this results generally in a localized, nonpropagated increase in the ionic permeability, or conductance, of the membrane. With certain exceptions, noted below, either of two types of permeability change can occur: (1) a generalized increase in permeability of the channel to cations (notably Na^+), resulting in a localized depolarization of the membrane, that is, an *excitatory postsynaptic potential* (EPSP); or (2) a selective increase in channel permeability to only the smaller ions (*e.g.*, potassium and chloride), resulting in stabilization or actual hyperpolarization of the membrane, which constitutes an *inhibitory postsynaptic potential* (IPSP).

It should be emphasized that the potential changes associated with the EPSP and IPSP at most sites are the results of passive fluxes of extracellular and intracellular ions down their concentration gradients. The changes in channel permeability that cause these potential changes are specifically regulated by the specialized postjunctional receptors for the neurotransmitter that initiates the response (*see* Chapter 2 and the remainder of this section). Under normal conditions, these receptors may be highly localized on the effector-cell surface, as seen at the neuromuscular junctions of skeletal muscle, or distributed in a more uniform fashion, as observed in smooth muscle.

3. Initiation of Postjunctional Activity. If an EPSP exceeds a certain threshold value, it initiates a propagated AP in a post-synaptic neuron or a muscle AP in most skeletal muscles or in cardiac muscle. In smooth muscle, in which propagated impulses are minimal, an EPSP may initiate a localized contractile response; in gland cells, it initiates secretion. An IPSP will tend to oppose excitatory potentials initiated by other neuronal sources at the same time and site; whether a propagated impulse or other response ensues will depend on the algebraic sum of all these effects. In the CNS, and possibly at other sites, inhibition can also result from an action of a transmitter on presynaptic terminals, which brings about a reduction in the amount of transmitter released by selective alteration of the permeability of ion channels such that impulse-induced depolarization of nerve terminals is reduced (Eccles, 1964). This phenomenon of *presynaptic inhibition* has provided a tentative explanation of the mechanism of action of some centrally acting drugs and neuromodulators.

4. Destruction or Dissipation of the Transmitter. When impulses can be transmitted across junctions at frequencies ranging from a few up to several hundred per second, it is obvious that there must be an efficient means of disposing of the transmitter following each impulse. At most cholinergic junctions, a highly specialized enzyme, *acetylcholinesterase* (AChE), is available for this function. Upon inhibition of AChE, removal of the transmitter is accomplished principally by diffusion. Under these circumstances, the effects of released ACh are potentiated and prolonged.

It is unlikely that any particular enzyme is directly involved in terminating the action of the adrenergic transmitter at the immediate receptor site in most organs; this is probably effected by a combination of simple diffusion and re-uptake of most of the released norepinephrine by the axonal terminals (*see* Iversen, 1967, 1975). Peptide neurotransmitters are hydrolyzed by various peptidases and dissipated by diffusion; specific uptake mechanisms have not been demonstrated for these substances.

5. Nonelectrogenic Functions. The continual, quantal release of neurotransmitters in amounts not sufficient to elicit a postjunctional response is probably important in the transjunctional control of neurotransmitter action. Both the activity and synthesis of enzymes involved in the synthesis and inactivation of neurotransmitters and the density of presynaptic and postsynaptic receptors are probably controlled by *trophic* actions of neurotransmitters or other substances released by the neuron or the target cells (Thesleff, 1973; Fambrough, 1979). For example, nerve growth factor (NGF) is apparently produced by target cells and taken up by adrenergic nerve terminals. It is then transported in a retrograde fashion to the perikaryon, where it exerts its trophic effect on various neuronal functions (Iversen *et al.*, 1975).

CHOLINERGIC TRANSMISSION

In close association with the neurotransmitter, ACh, are two enzymes, *choline acetyltransferase* and *acetylcholinesterase* (*AChE*), which are involved in its synthesis and hydrolysis, respectively.

Choline Acetyltransferase. Choline acetyltransferase catalyzes the final step in the synthesis of ACh—the acetylation of choline with acetyl coenzyme A (CoA) (*see* Hebb, 1972; Rossier, 1977). This enzyme, which has only recently been purified and characterized, has a molecular weight of approximately 68,000 (Tucek, 1982).

Acetyl CoA for this reaction is derived from pyruvate via the multistep pyruvate dehydrogenase reaction or is synthesized by acetate thiokinase, which catalyzes the reaction of acetate with adenosine triphosphate (ATP) to form an enzyme-bound acyladenylate (acetyl AMP). In the presence of CoA, transacetylation and synthesis of acetyl CoA proceed.

Tremendous variations in choline acetyltransferase activity occur in mammalian nerve tissue. In general, high concentrations have been reported for peripheral cholinergic nerves (*e.g.*, ventral spinal roots, superior cervical ganglion) and thousandfold lower values are detected in afferent nerves (*e.g.*, dorsal spinal roots, optic nerve). Similar differences have been found by ultramicrodetermination and immunocytochemical studies of choline acetyltransferase in single cholinergic and noncholinergic neurons of autonomic ganglia and in the CNS.

Choline acetyltransferase, like other protein constituents of the neuron, is synthesized within the perikaryon and is then transported along the length of the axon to its terminal. The synaptic vesicles appear to be formed at the terminal, and the axonal terminals contain a large number of mitochondria,

where acetyl CoA is synthesized. Choline is taken up from the extracellular fluid into the axoplasm by active transport. The final step in the synthesis occurs within the cytoplasm, following which most of the ACh is sequestered within the synaptic vesicles. Moderately potent, selective inhibitors of choline acetyltransferase are available (Cavallito *et al.*, 1969), but they have not proven to be effective in therapy, presumably because they are relatively weak inhibitors of the enzyme *in vivo* and because the uptake of choline appears to be the rate-limiting step in the biosynthesis of ACh.

The transport of choline into neuronal tissues is accomplished by distinct high- and low-affinity systems. The high-affinity system is unique to cholinergic neurons, is inhibited by hemicholinium, and is believed to be responsible for the delivery of choline to the cholinergic nerve endings. The transport system is dependent on Na^+ and may be in part regulated by intracellular concentrations of Na^+ and K^+ (*see* Jope, 1979).

Acetylcholinesterase. For ACh to serve as the neurohumoral agent in peripheral junctional transmission, the ester must be removed or inactivated within the time limits imposed by the response characteristics of visceral neuroeffector junctions, motor end-plates, and various types of neurons. At the neuromuscular junction, the mediator must be destroyed almost immediately—with "flashlike suddenness," as Dale has expressed it. Modern biophysical methods have revealed that the time required for this process is less than a millisecond. Body fluids and tissues contain enzymes, first called *cholinesterase,* that rapidly hydrolyze ACh to choline and acetic acid. The choline produced possesses only 10^{-5} the vasodepressor potency of ACh. The general characteristics and distribution of acetylcholinesterases are discussed below; a more complete account of their molecular structure, catalytic properties, and the effect of various inhibitors is presented in Chapter 6.

Acetylcholinesterase (AChE; also known as specific or true ChE) is found in neurons, at the neuromuscular junction, and in certain other tissues (*see* below); it is responsible for the hydrolysis of ACh released from cholinergic nerve terminals. Hydrolysis occurs in the immediate vicinity of the nerve ending. *Butyrylcholinesterase* (BuChE; also known as cholinesterase, ChE, serum esterase, or pseudoChE) is present in various types of glial or satellite cells but only to a limited extent in neuronal elements of the central and peripheral nervous systems. It is also present in the plasma, liver, and other organs; its physiological function is unknown. Although both types of enzyme can hydrolyze ACh and certain other aliphatic and aromatic esters and as a group are inhibited selectively by physostigmine, they can be distinguished by the use of selective inhibitors. Almost all the pharmacological effects of the anti-ChE agents (Chapter 6) are due to the inhibition of AChE, with the consequent accumulation of endogenous ACh.

AChE hydrolyzes ACh at a greater velocity than choline esters with acyl groups larger than acetate. The enzyme also hydrolyzes methacholine, and it is inhibited selectively by low concentrations of several *bis*-quaternary ammonium compounds and by other agents. BuChE, on the other hand, exhibits a maximal velocity of hydrolysis with butyrylcholine as a substrate; it does not hydrolyze methacholine; and it is more sensitive than AChE to inhibition by certain organophosphorus agents and quaternary ammonium compounds (*see* Chapter 6).

It is possible to visualize, by histochemical technics, the sites of enzyme activity in relation to the various structural components of tissues and cells (*see* review by Koelle, 1975). Such studies have shown that neurons that give rise to the three categories of peripheral cholinergic fibers (postganglionic parasympathetic, preganglionic autonomic, somatic motor) contain relatively high concentrations of AChE throughout their entire length (dendrites, perikarya, axons). The concentrations in noncholinergic peripheral neurons (adrenergic, primary afferent) are, in general, considerably lower. A small percentage of sympathetic ganglion cells in most species contains concentrations of AChE equivalent to those of their respective parasympathetic ganglion cells; evidence has been obtained that in the cat the former cells give rise to the cholinergic sympathetic fibers that innervate the sweat glands (Sjöqvist, 1963).

At the motor end-plates of skeletal muscle, most of the AChE is localized at the surface and infoldings of the postjunctional membrane. Accordingly, it is situated strategically for the rapid hydrolysis of ACh following the production of the end-plate potential (EPP). Several distinct molecular forms of the enzyme exist, and activity appears to be localized in both the postsynaptic membrane and the outer basal lamina in the neuromuscular junction of skeletal muscle. Both nerve and muscle have the capacity to synthesize AChE, and the enzyme present at the end-plate probably derives from both tissues.

Storage and Release of Acetylcholine. Fatt and Katz (1952) recorded at the motor end-plate of skeletal muscle and observed the random occurrence of small (approximately 0.1 to 3.0 mV), spontaneous depolarizations at a frequency of approximately one per second. The magnitude of these miniature end-plate potentials (mepps) is considerably below the threshold required to fire a muscle AP; that they are due to the release of ACh is indicated by their enhancement by neostigmine and their blockade by *d*-tubocurarine. This was the first evidence that ACh is released from motor-nerve endings in constant amounts or *quanta*. A likely morphological counterpart of this phenomenon was discovered shortly thereafter, in the form of synaptic vesicles noted in electron micrographs of nerve terminals by De Robertis and Bennett (1955). The storage and release of ACh have been investigated most extensively at motor end-plates; nevertheless, most of the principles discovered at this locus probably apply to other sites of cholinergic transmission as well, and in many respects to noncholinergic transmission (*see* reviews by Hubbard, 1973; Krnjević, 1974; Reichardt and Kelly, 1983).

When an AP arrives at the motor-nerve terminal, there is an explosive release of 100 or more quanta (or vesicles) of ACh, following a latent period of approximately 0.75 millisecond (Katz and Miledi, 1965). The intermediate steps appear to be as follows: the depolarization of the terminal permits the influx of calcium ions, which hypothetically then bind to sites bearing negative charges on the internal surface of the terminal axoplasmic membrane (active zones). This could facilitate fusion of axonal and vesicular membranes, resulting in the extrusion of the contents of the vesicles. Calcium ionophores, which allow extracellular calcium to permeate the nerve ending, stimulate vesicular release of ACh. Release can be inhibited by excess magnesium.

While there is general agreement regarding certain steps involved in the storage and release of ACh, many of the details are still unknown. Estimates of the ACh content of the synaptic vesicles range from 1000 to over 50,000 molecules per vesicle, and it has been calculated that a single motor-nerve terminal contains 300,000 or more vesicles. In addition, an uncertain but significant amount of ACh is present in the extravesicular cytoplasm. Recording of the electrical events associated with the opening of single channels at the motor end-plate during continuous application of ACh has permitted estimation of the potential change induced by a single molecule of ACh (3×10^{-7} V); from such calculations, it is evident that even the lower estimate of the ACh content per vesicle (1000 molecules) is sufficient to account for the magnitude of the mepps (Katz and Miledi, 1972). Although it is clear that ACh is stored in vesicles and that release is quantal, exocytotic release has been questioned as the sole mechanism (*see* Ceccarelli and Hurlbut, 1980; Cooper and Meyer, 1984).

The superior cervical ganglion is able to support a remarkably high rate of ACh synthesis and release. When it is stimulated supramaximally at a frequency of 20 cycles per second, the ACh output during 1 hour is approximately six times the original content (Birks and MacIntosh, 1961).

The release of ACh by exocytosis through the prejunctional membrane is inhibited by toxin produced by *Clostridium botulinum*, one of the most potent toxins known. A small number of molecules of this toxin binds irreversibly to their sites of action, producing an essentially irreversible blockade of all cholinergic junctions (*see* Kao *et al.,* 1976; Simpson, 1981). Death results from respiratory failure. Black widow spider toxin has a site of action similar to that of botulinus toxin, but with the opposite effect. Clumping of vesicles at the prejunctional membrane is associated with the release of excessive amounts of ACh (Pumplin and Reese, 1977; Howard and Gunderson, 1980).

Characteristics of Cholinergic Transmission at Various Sites.

From the comparisons noted above, it is obvious that there are marked differences between various sites of cholinergic transmission with respect to general-architectural and fine-structural arrangements, the distributions of AChE, and the temporal factors involved in normal functioning. For example, in skeletal muscle the junctional sites occupy a small, discrete portion of the surface of the individual fibers and are relatively isolated from those of adjacent fibers; in the superior cervical ganglion, in contrast, approximately 100,000 ganglion cells are packed within a volume of a few cubic millimeters, and both the presynaptic and postsynaptic neuronal processes form complex networks. It is therefore to be expected that the specific features of cholinergic transmission will vary markedly at different sites.

1. *Skeletal Muscle.* Stimulation of a motor nerve results in the release of ACh from perfused muscle; close intra-arterial injection of ACh produces muscular contraction similar to that elicited by stimulation of the motor nerve. The amount of ACh (10^{-17} mole) required to elicit an EPP following its microiontophoretic application to the motor end-plate of a rat diaphragm muscle fiber is equivalent to that recovered from each fiber following stimulation of the phrenic nerve (Krnjević and Mitchell, 1961).

The combination of ACh with the receptors at the external surface of the postjunctional membrane induces an immediate, marked increase in permeability to Na^+ and K^+. Upon activation by ACh, the channel of each receptor molecule opens for about 1 millisecond; during this interval about 50,000 cations traverse the channel (Katz and Miledi, 1972). This is the basis for the localized depolarizing EPP, which triggers the muscle AP. The latter in turn leads to contraction. Further details concerning these events and their modification by neuromuscular blocking agents are presented in Chapter 11.

Following section and degeneration of the motor nerve to skeletal muscle or of the postganglionic fibers to autonomic effectors, there is a marked reduction in the threshold doses of the transmitters and of certain other drugs required to elicit a response, that is, *denervation supersensitivity* (Cannon and Rosenblueth, 1949). In skeletal muscle this change is accompanied by a spread of the cholinoceptive sites from the end-plate region to the adjacent portions of the sarcoplasmic membrane, which eventually involves the entire muscle surface (Axelsson and Thesleff, 1959). Embryonic muscle also exhibits this uniform sensitivity to ACh prior to innervation (Fambrough, 1979).

The most important sources of material for study of both molecular and biochemical properties of the nicotinic cholinergic receptor have been the electric organs of the eel (*Electrophorus* species) and the electric elasmobranchs (*Torpedo, Raia* species) (Changeux, 1981). A more detailed discussion is given in Chapter 11.

2. *Autonomic Effectors.* In contrast to other cholinergically innervated cells (*i.e.*, skeletal muscle and neurons), smooth muscle and the cardiac conduction system (S-A node, atrium, A-V node, and the His-Purkinje system) normally exhibit intrinsic activity, both electrical and mechanical, that is modified but not initiated by nerve impulses. In the basal condition, smooth muscle and the cardiac conduction system exhibit spikes, or waves of increased membrane conduction, that are propagated from cell to cell at rates considerably slower than the AP of axons or skeletal muscle. The spikes are apparently initiated by rhythmic fluctuations in the membrane resting potential; in intestinal smooth muscle, the site of the pacemaker activity continually shifts, whereas in the heart it normally arises from the S-A node but can under certain circumstances arise from any part of the conduction system (*see* Chapter 31).

The addition of ACh (10^{-7} to 10^{-6} M) to isolated intestinal muscle causes a fall in the resting potential (*i.e.*, the membrane potential becomes less negative) and an increase in the frequency of spike production, accompanied by a rise in tension. The primary action of ACh in initiating these effects is probably the partial depolarization of the cell membrane, brought about by an increase in sodium and, in some instances, calcium conductances (Bolton, 1979). ACh can also produce contraction of some smooth muscles when the membrane has been completely depolarized by high concentrations of potassium, provided calcium is present. Although the physiological significance of this observation is uncertain, there is increasing evidence that calcium ion fluxes across the muscle plasma membrane and mobilization of calcium from intracellular sites are affected by ACh and are directly involved in contraction.

In the cardiac conduction system, particularly from the S-A to the A-V node, stimulation of the cholinergic innervation (of which the preganglionic fibers are in the vagus nerve) or the direct application of ACh causes inhibition, associated with hyperpolarization of the fiber membrane and a marked decrease in the rate of depolarization. These effects are due, at least in part, to a selective increase in permeability to potassium (Trautwein *et al.*, 1956).

It is likely that, in those smooth muscle fibers where cholinergic impulses are inhibitory, ACh produces inhibition by hyperpolarization, with resultant decrease in the frequency of spike production. The hyperpolarization in most cases appears to be mediated by increased permeability to potassium. In this case, the potassium channels may be activated by increases in the intracellular concentration of calcium.

3. *Autonomic Ganglia.* The evidence for cholinergic transmission in autonomic ganglia is similar to that obtained at the neuromuscular junction of skeletal muscle. For example, when the perfusate from the isolated cat superior cervical ganglion is tested, ACh appears in the perfusion fluid after preganglionic but not after antidromic stimulation; it is not liberated spontaneously in significant amounts. The ganglion cells can be discharged by injecting very small amounts of ACh into the ganglion (Feldberg and Gaddum, 1934).

Ganglionic transmission is a highly complex process, and several secondary transmitters or modulators are involved. These either enhance or diminish the sensitivity of the postganglionic cell to ACh. This sensitivity appears to be related to the membrane potential of the postsynaptic nerve cell body or its dendritic branches. Ganglionic transmission is discussed in more detail in Chapter 10.

Actions of Acetylcholine at Prejunctional Sites. Considerable attention has been focused on the possible involvement of *prejunctional cholinoceptive sites* in both cholinergic and noncholinergic transmission and in the actions of various drugs. The intra-arterial injection of ACh or an anti-ChE agent (physostigmine or neostigmine) produces both fasciculations (synchronous contractions of the skeletal muscle fibers of *entire motor units*) and antidromic APs that are conducted from the terminals of the motor nerves to the ventral spinal roots. Both effects are blocked by curare. These and related observations suggest that the compounds act at the prejunctional axonal terminals as well as at the postjunctional cholinoceptive sites (Riker *et al.*, 1957; Riker and Okamoto, 1969; Bowman, 1980; *see also* Chapter 11). ACh can also cause the release of norepinephrine by an action of nicotinic receptors on cardiac and other sympathetic nerve endings (*see* Higgins *et al.*, 1973; Westfall, 1977).

While cholinergic innervation of blood vessels is limited, prejunctional cholinergic muscarinic receptors appear to be present on sympathetic vasoconstrictor nerves (Steinsland *et al.*, 1973). The physiological role of these receptors is unclear, but their activation causes inhibition of neurally mediated release of norepinephrine (*see* Weiner, 1979a). Because ACh is so rapidly hydrolyzed by local and circulating esterases, it is very unlikely that it plays a role as a circulating hormone analogous to that of epinephrine.

Dilatation of blood vessels in response to administered choline esters could involve several sites of action, including prejunctional inhibitory synapses on sympathetic fibers and inhibitory cholinergic receptors in the vasculature that are not innervated. The vasodilator effect of ACh on isolated blood vessels requires an intact endothelium. Activation of muscarinic receptors apparently results in the liberation of a vasodilator substance (endothelium-dependent relaxing factor) that diffuses to the smooth muscle and causes relaxation (Furchgott, 1984).

ADRENERGIC TRANSMISSION

Under this general heading are included *norepinephrine*, the transmitter of most sympathetic postganglionic fibers and of certain tracts in the CNS, and *dopamine*, the predominant transmitter of the mammalian extrapyramidal system and of several mesocortical and mesolimbic neuronal pathways, as well as *epinephrine*, the major hormone of the adrenal medulla.

A tremendous amount of information about catecholamines and related compounds has accumulated during recent years, motivated in part by the importance of interactions between the endogenous catecholamines and many of the drugs used in the treatment of hypertension, mental disorders, and a variety of other conditions. The details of these interactions and of the pharmacology of the sympathomimetic amines themselves will be found in subsequent chapters. The basic physiological, biochemical, and pharmacological features are presented briefly here.

Synthesis, Storage, and Release of Catecholamines. The *synthesis* of epinephrine from tyrosine, by the steps shown in Figure 4–3, was proposed by Blaschko in 1939. The enzymes involved have been identified and characterized. Three of these enzymes (tyrosine hydroxylase, dopamine β-hydroxylase, and phenylethanolamine-N-methyltransferase) appear to have regions of amino acid sequence homology and may be under common genetic control (Joh *et al.*, 1984). It is important to note

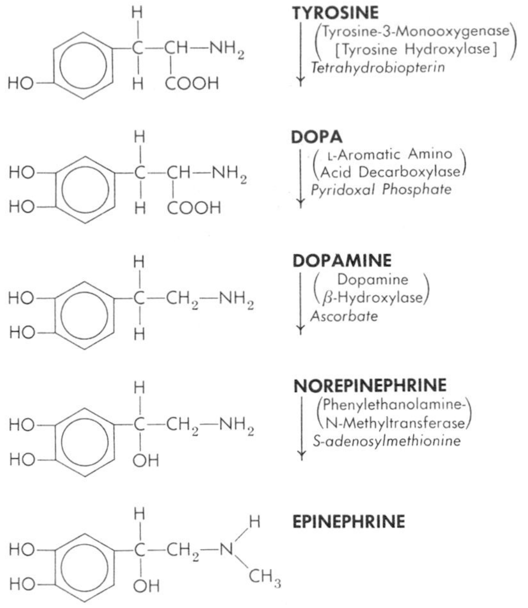

Figure 4–3. *Steps in enzymatic synthesis of dopamine, norepinephrine, and epinephrine.*

The enzymes involved are shown in parentheses; essential cofactors, in italics. The final step occurs only in the adrenal medulla and in a few epinephrine-containing neuronal pathways in the brain stem.

that none of these enzymes is highly specific; consequently, many other endogenous substances as well as certain drugs are similarly acted upon at the various steps. For example, 5-hydroxytryptamine (5-HT, serotonin) can be produced by L-aromatic amino acid decarboxylase (or dopa decarboxylase) from 5-hydroxy-L-tryptophan. Dopa decarboxylase can also convert the drug methyldopa to α-methyldopamine, which, in turn, is converted by dopamine β-hydroxylase to the "false transmitter," α-methylnorepinephrine. Tyramine can be hydroxylated to octopamine, the phenol analog of norepinephrine, by dopamine β-hydroxylase; while octopamine is present only in small amounts in mammals, it is probably the major adrenergic transmitter in certain invertebrates (Barker *et al.*, 1972).

The hydroxylation of tyrosine is generally regarded as the rate-limiting step in the biosynthesis of catecholamines (Weiner, 1979b), and tyrosine hydroxylase is activated following stimulation of adrenergic nerves or the adrenal medulla. The en-

zyme is a substrate for cyclic AMP–dependent protein kinase (Weiner *et al.*, 1984), and kinase-catalyzed phosphorylation is associated with increased hydroxylase activity (Vulliet *et al.*, 1980). The enzyme is also a substrate for Ca^{2+}-activated protein kinases (Yamauchi *et al.*, 1981). In addition, tyrosine hydroxylase is inhibited by catechol compounds in a manner that is competitive with its pterin cofactor, tetrahydrobiopterin. It is thus subject to end-product feedback inhibition (Weiner *et al.*, 1972).

Current knowledge concerning the *cellular sites and mechanisms of synthesis, storage, and release* of catecholamines has been derived from studies of both adrenergically innervated organs and adrenal medullary tissue. Nearly all the *norepinephrine* content of the former is confined to the postganglionic sympathetic fibers; it disappears within a few days after section of the nerves.

Understanding of the localization and function of adrenergic nerves has advanced rapidly because of the development of formaldehyde vapor histofluorescence procedures and immunocytochemical technics. The former has allowed visualization of a dense network of catecholamine-containing nerve fibers in smooth and cardiac muscle, blood vessels, and certain exocrine glands. Much of the catecholamine is present in frequently occurring minute swellings (varicosities) that are in close apposition to the muscle and gland cells and that probably represent sites of release of the transmitter (Carlsson *et al.*, 1962).

Other approaches that are of considerable value for investigating the functions of adrenergic innervation are the production of *immunosympathectomy* and *chemosympathectomy*. The former arose from observations that a protein, *nerve-growth factor*, causes a marked hypertrophy of sympathetic ganglia, both in tissue culture and in newborn animals. When an *antiserum* to the nerve-growth factor is injected into newborn animals under proper conditions, the development of the peripheral sympathetic system is suppressed (Levi-Montalcini and Angeletti, 1968). The same result can be obtained more simply in both newborn and adult animals by the administration of the chemosympathectomizing agent 6-hydroxydopamine. This compound is taken up selectively by adrenergic fibers and results in their destruction, presumably as a result of the formation of reactive intermediates that damage the structures of the nerve terminal (Thoenen, 1972; Jonsson *et al.*, 1975; Chapter 9).

The main features of the mechanisms of synthesis, storage, and release of catecholamines and their modifications by drugs are summarized in Figure 4–4. Electron-dense

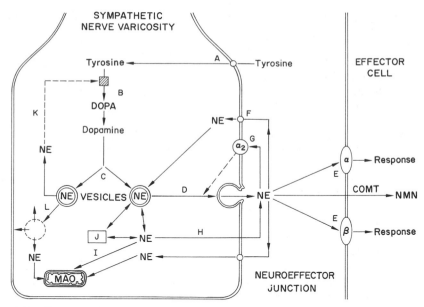

Figure 4–4. *Proposed sites of action of drugs on the synthesis, action, and fate of norepineph-rine at sympathetic neuroeffector junctions.*

The events proposed to occur in this model of a sympathetic neuroeffector junction are as follows. Tyrosine is transported actively into the axoplasm (*A*) and is converted to dopa and then to dopamine by cytoplasmic enzymes (*B*). Dopamine is transported into the vesicles of the varicosity, where the synthesis and the storage of norepinephrine (NE) take place (*C*). An action potential causes an influx of Ca^{2+} into the nerve terminal (not shown), with subsequent fusion of the vesicle with the plasma membrane and exocytosis of NE (*D*). The transmitter then activates α and β receptors in the membrane of the postsynaptic cell (*E*). NE that penetrates into these cells (uptake-2) is probably rapidly inactivated by catechol-O-methyltransferase (COMT) to normetanephrine (NMN). The most important mechanism for termination of the action of NE in the junctional space is by active re-uptake into the nerve (uptake-1) and the storage vesicles (*F*). Norepinephrine in the synaptic cleft can also activate presynaptic (α_2) receptors (*G*), the result of which is to inhibit further exocytotic release of norepinephrine (dashed line).

NE can also be displaced from storage vesicles by sympathomimetic amines such as tyramine, which gain access to the nerve terminal by active uptake as in *F*. A portion of this NE diffuses out of the nerve (*H*) to interact with receptors. Another portion of the NE released in this manner, or by spontaneous diffusion, is deaminated by mitochondrial monoamine oxidase (MAO) (*I*). Observations suggest that only a fraction of the total NE content is available for release by either nerve stimulation or tyramine, and indicate that there may be pools of the transmitter that are held in reserve (*J*). These may be vesicles that reside deep within the nerve terminals.

The most important mechanism of regulation of NE synthesis involves the rate-limiting step, the hydroxylation of tyrosine. This regulation is complex but in part involves feedback inhibition by NE (*K*) and activation of the enzyme by cyclic AMP–dependent protein kinase and, perhaps, by Ca^{2+}-dependent protein kinases.

Sites of drug action in this scheme include:

1. Inhibition of MAO (*e.g.*, by pargyline) or COMT (no pharmacologically significant example of inhibitor).

2. Inhibition of plasma membrane uptake mechanism for NE (*F*) by tricyclic antidepressants or cocaine, making more NE available for binding to receptors.

3. Inhibition of vesicular storage of NE by reserpine and, in part, by guanethidine (*L*). The NE thereby released is normally inactivated by MAO. Guanethidine and bretylium also block coupling of the action potential to the release of NE.

4. Displacement of NE by indirectly acting sympathomimetic amines (*H*). Exocytosis of vesicular contents does not occur.

5. Direct interaction with adrenergic receptors by agonists and antagonists (*E, G*).

Anatomical elements are not drawn to scale. Mitochondria are about 0.25 μm in diameter and 0.75 μm long; vesicles, 0.05 μm; a nerve varicosity, 2 to 10 μm; the junctional space, 0.1 μm or more.

vesicles, 0.05 to 0.2 μm in diameter, have been noted in electron micrographs of adrenergically innervated tissues (Bloom, 1973; Cooper *et al.*, 1982). These vesicles or granules contain extremely high concentrations of catecholamines (approximately 21% dry weight) and ATP, in a molecular ratio of 4:1, as well as specific proteins or *chromogranins,* the enzyme dopamine β-hydroxylase (DBH), ascorbic acid, and peptides (*e.g.,* enkephalin precursors). In the course of synthesis (Figure 4–3), the hydroxylation of tyrosine to dopa and the decarboxylation of dopa to dopamine take place in the cytoplasm. Dopamine then enters the granules, where it is converted to norepinephrine by DBH. In the adrenal medulla, there are two distinct catecholamine-containing cell types: those with norepinephrine and those with primarily epinephrine (Goldstein *et al.*, 1972). The latter cell population contains the enzyme phenylethanolamine-N-methyltransferase. In these cells, the norepinephrine formed in the granules leaves these structures, presumably by diffusion, and is methylated in the cytoplasm to epinephrine. Epinephrine then re-enters the chromaffin granules, where it is stored until released. In the human adult, epinephrine accounts for approximately 80% of the catecholamines of the adrenal medulla, with norepinephrine making up most of the remainder. (*See* reviews by Axelrod, 1963; Euler, 1972; Stjärne, 1972; Rubin, 1982.)

The enzymes that participate in the formation of norepinephrine are synthesized in the cell bodies of the adrenergic neurons and are then transported along the axons to their terminals. This can occur either slowly (1 to 3 mm per day) by bulk flow through axoplasm, as appears to be the case for tyrosine hydroxylase, or much more rapidly (1 to 10 mm per hour), as with DBH. The microtubular system may participate in such rapid axonal transport and also in the formation and extrusion of the granules in which catecholamines are stored (*see* review by Kopin and Silberstein, 1972).

A major factor that controls the rate of synthesis of *epinephrine,* and hence the size of the store available for release from the adrenal medulla, is the level of glucocorticoids secreted by the adrenal cortex. The latter hormones are carried in high concentration, by the intra-adrenal portal vascular system, directly to the adrenal medullary chromaffin cells, where they induce the synthesis of phenylethanolamine-N-methyltransferase (Figure 4–3). The activities of both tyrosine hydroxylase and

DBH are also increased in the adrenal medulla when the secretion of glucocorticoids is stimulated (*see* Weiner, 1975). Thus, any stress that persists sufficiently to invoke an enhanced secretion of corticotropin mobilizes the appropriate hormones of both the adrenal cortex (predominantly cortisol) and medulla (epinephrine) (*see* review by Wurtman *et al.,* 1972).

This remarkable relationship is present only in certain mammals, including man, where the adrenal chromaffin cells are enveloped entirely by steroid-secreting cortical cells. In the dogfish, for example, where the chromaffin cells and steroid-secreting cells are located in independent, noncontiguous glands, no epinephrine is formed (*see* review by Coupland, 1972).

In addition to its synthesis *de novo,* outlined above, there is a second major mechanism for replenishment of the norepinephrine of the terminal portions of the adrenergic fibers, namely, recapture by active transport of norepinephrine previously released to the extracellular fluid (Iversen, 1967). This process is responsible for the termination of the effects of adrenergic impulses in most organs; the blood vessels apparently constitute an exception, where the immediate disposition of released norepinephrine is accomplished largely by a combination of extraneuronal uptake (*see* below) and enzymatic breakdown and diffusion (Spector *et al.*, 1972). In order to effect the re-uptake of norepinephrine into adrenergic nerve terminals and to maintain the concentration gradient of norepinephrine within the granules, at least two carrier-mediated transport systems are involved: one, across the axoplasmic membrane from the extracellular fluid to the cytoplasm; and the other, from the cytoplasm into the storage granules.

The capacity of the adrenergic nerve terminal to store the neurotransmitter is exceptionally high. The carrier-mediated transport system in the membrane of the nerve ending and the transport of catecholamines into granules or vesicles may result in a 10,000-fold concentration of norepinephrine.

Due to the relative ease of isolating pure preparations of granules, especially from the adrenal medulla, the transport system of the storage granule has been well characterized. It can concentrate catecholamines against a 200-fold gradient across the granular membrane. The intragranular free norepinephrine is in equilibrium with a catecholamine-ATP-protein complex. This transport system requires ATP and magnesium ion, and it is blocked by very low concentrations (40 nM) of reserpine (Kirshner, 1962; Carlsson *et al.*, 1963). Uptake of catecholamine and ATP into isolated chromaffin granules appears to be driven by pH and potential gradients that are established by an ATP-dependent proton translocase (Winkler *et al.*, 1981). The amine transport system across the axoplasmic membrane is Na$^+$ dependent and is blocked selectively by a number of drugs, including *cocaine* and the *tricyclic antidepressants,* such as imipramine.

Certain sympathomimetic drugs (*e.g., ephedrine, tyramine*) produce most of their effects indirectly, chiefly by displacing norepinephrine from the nerve-ending binding sites to the extracellular fluid, where the released endogenous transmitter then acts at the receptor sites of the effector cells. This action of so-called indirectly acting sympathomimetic amines is associated with the phenomenon of *tachyphylaxis.* For example, repeated administration of tyramine results in rapidly decreasing effectiveness, whereas the effect of repeated administration of norepinephrine is not reduced and, in fact, reverses the tachyphylaxis to tyramine. One possible explanation of tachyphylaxis to tyramine and similarly acting sympathomimetic agents is that the pool of neurotransmitter available for displacement by these drugs is quite small relative to the total amount stored in the sympathetic nerve ending. This pool is presumed to reside in close proximity to the plasma membrane, and the norepinephrine of such vesicles may be replaced by the less potent amine following repeated administration of the latter substance. Neurotransmitter release by displacement is not associated with the release of DBH and is thus presumed not to involve exocytosis.

The adrenergic neuronal uptake system for catecholamines and other phenylethylamines is characterized by a high affinity for norepinephrine and a somewhat lower affinity for epinephrine; the synthetic β-adrenergic agonist isoproterenol is not a substrate for this system. The neuronal uptake process has been termed uptake-1 (Iversen, 1975). There is also an extraneuronal amine transport system, termed uptake-2, which exhibits a low affinity for norepinephrine, a somewhat higher affinity for epinephrine, and a still higher affinity for isoproterenol. This uptake process is quite ubiquitous and is present in glial, hepatic, myocardial, and other cells. Uptake-2 is inhibited by metanephrine and corticosteroids, but it is not affected by imipramine or cocaine. It is probably of relatively little physiological importance unless the neuronal uptake mechanism is blocked or is otherwise not functional (Iversen, 1975; Trendelenburg, 1980). It may be of greater importance in the disposition of circulating catecholamines than in the removal of amines that have been released from adrenergic nerve terminals.

The full sequence of steps by which the nerve impulse effects the release of norepinephrine from adrenergic fibers is not known. In the adrenal medulla, the triggering event is the liberation of ACh by the preganglionic fibers and its interaction with nicotinic receptors on the chromaffin cells to produce a localized depolarization; a succeeding step is the entrance of calcium ions into these cells, which results in the extrusion by exocytosis of the granular contents, including epinephrine, ATP, some neuroactive peptides or their precursors (Gilbert and Emson, 1983; Viveros and Wilson, 1983; Costa *et al.*, 1984), chromogranins, and DBH (Kirshner, 1974; Weiner, 1979a; Winkler *et al.*, 1981). Calcium likewise appears to play an essential role in coupling the nerve impulse with the release of norepinephrine at adrenergic nerve terminals (Burn and Gibbons, 1965), as has been demonstrated also at cholinergic terminals. Enhanced activity of the sympathetic nervous system is accompanied by an increased concentration of both DBH and chromogranins in the circulation, supporting the notion that the process of release following adrenergic nerve stimulation also involves exocytosis.

A number of cytoplasmic and cytoskeletal proteins have been implicated in the process of exocytosis, including tubulin, calmodulin, neurin (actin-like), and stenin (myosin-like) (*see* Weiner, 1979a). Another cytoplasmic protein, synexin, can induce the fusion of chromaffin granules *in vitro* in the presence of low concentrations of calcium when certain unsaturated fatty acids (*e.g.,* arachidonic acid) are also present. This protein may play an important role in the fusion of secretory granules with the plasma membrane that precedes exocytosis (Creutz, 1981; Pollard *et al.*, 1981; Creutz *et al.*, 1983).

Adrenergic fibers can sustain the output of norepinephrine during prolonged periods of stimulation without exhausting their reserve supply, provided synthesis and uptake of the transmitter are unimpaired. To meet increased needs for norepinephrine, acute regulatory mechanisms come into play that involve activation of tyrosine hydroxylase (*see* above). However, the physiological response to prolonged or intense nerve stimulation may diminish before the stores of transmitter are exhausted. This may be due to a failure of conduction of nerve impulses into the axon terminals, a failure of stimulus-secretion coupling, or the exhaustion of stores of transmitter in vesicles present at critical subsynaptic sites adjacent to the plasma membrane. Postsynaptic sensitivity to the transmitter may also be regulated, either by alteration of the state or number of receptors or by changes in their ability to influence the activity of other components of the response system (Harden, 1983).

Termination of the Actions of Catecholamines. The actions of norepinephrine and epinephrine are terminated by (1) re-uptake into nerve terminals; (2) dilution by diffusion out of the junctional cleft and uptake at extraneuronal sites; and (3) metabolic transformation. Two enzymes are important in the initial steps of metabolic transformation of catecholamines—monoamine oxidase (MAO) and catechol-O-methyltransferase (COMT) (*see* Axelrod, 1966; Kopin, 1972). It was evident that a powerful enzymatic mechanism, such as that provided by AChE, was absent from the adrenergic nervous system. Axelrod and colleagues then demonstrated the significance of re-uptake of norepinephrine into the sympathetic nerve ending (*see* reviews by Axelrod, 1966, 1973). Consistent with this are the observations that inhibitors of norepinephrine uptake by the nerve terminal (*e.g.*, cocaine, imipramine) potentiate the effects of the neurotransmitter; inhibitors of MAO and COMT have little effect. However, transmitter that is released *within* the nerve terminal is metabolized by

MAO; COMT, particularly in the liver, plays a major role in the metabolism of endogenous circulating and administered catecholamines.

Both MAO and COMT are widely distributed throughout the body, including the brain; the highest concentrations of each are in the liver and the kidney. However, there are distinct differences in their cytological locations; whereas MAO is associated chiefly with the outer surface of mitochondria, including those within the terminals of adrenergic fibers, COMT is located largely in the cytoplasm and, to a smaller degree, in membranes. COMT apparently has no selective association with adrenergic nerves. These factors are of importance both in determining the primary metabolic pathways followed by catecholamines in various circumstances and in explaining the effects of certain drugs. There are two different isozymes of MAO that are found in widely varying proportions in different cells in the CNS and in peripheral tissues. Selective inhibitors of these two isozymes are available (*see* Chapters 19 and 21).

Most of the epinephrine and norepinephrine that enters the circulation, from the adrenal medulla or following administration, or that is released by exocytosis from adrenergic fibers is first methylated by COMT to metanephrine or normetanephrine, respectively (Figure 4–5). Norepinephrine that is released intraneuronally by drugs such as reserpine is initially deaminated by MAO to 3,4-dihydroxyphenylglycolaldehyde (DOPGAL) (Figure 4–5). The aldehyde is reduced by aldehyde reductase to the glycol, 3,4-dihydroxyphenylethylene glycol (DOPEG) within the neuron. If the amine is deaminated at extraneuronal sites, such as the intestine or liver, the aldehyde is largely oxidized by aldehyde dehydrogenase to 3,4-dihydroxymandelic acid (DOMA). Circulating catecholamines are preferentially oxidized to the acid, while catecholamines in the CNS are preferentially reduced to the glycol. In either case, most of the metabolites formed by either MAO or COMT are then converted by the other enzyme to the common product, either 3-methoxy-4-hydroxyphenylethylene glycol (MOPEG or MHPG) or 3-methoxy-4-hydroxymandelic acid, generally but incorrectly called "vanillylmandelic acid" (VMA). These substances constitute the major metabolites of catecholamines excreted in the urine. The corresponding product of the metabolic degradation of dopamine, which contains no hydroxyl group in the side chain, is homovanillic acid (HVA). Other metabolic reactions are described in Figure 4–5. Normally in man the 24-hour urinary excretion of metabolites of endogenous norepinephrine and epinephrine includes 2 to 4 mg of VMA, 1.2 to 1.8 mg of MOPEG (about 20 to 30% of this metabolite is believed to be formed in the CNS), 100 to 300 μg of normetanephrine, and 100 to 200 μg of metanephrine. In addition, 25 to 50 μg of norepinephrine and 2 to 5 μg of epinephrine appear in the urine.

Inhibitors of MAO (*e.g., pargyline, nialamide*)

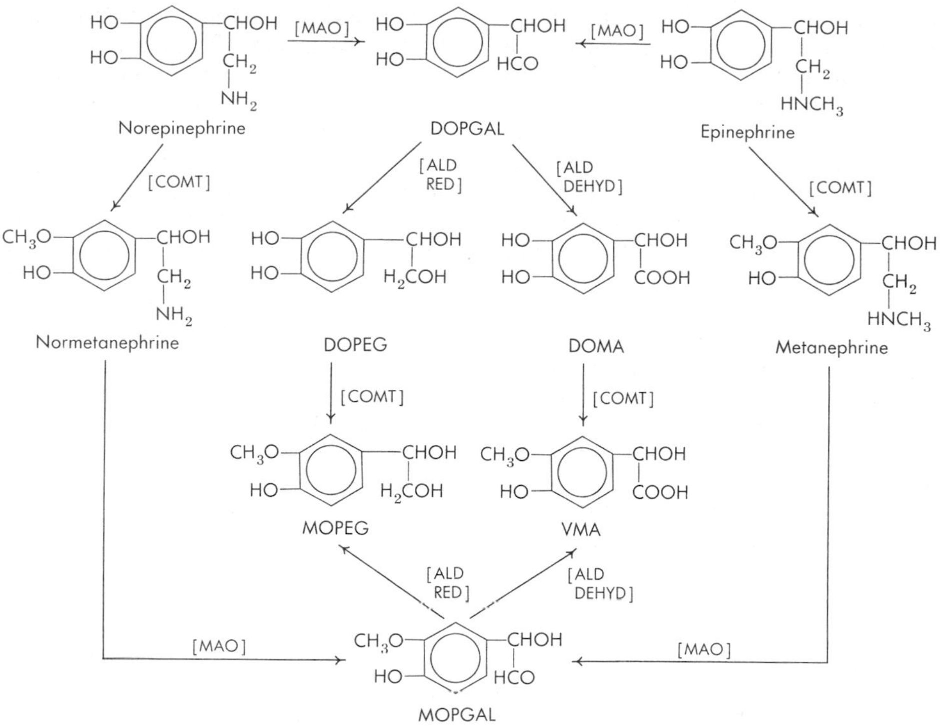

Figure 4–5. *Steps in the metabolic disposition of catecholamines.*

Both norepinephrine and epinephrine are first oxidatively deaminated by monoamine oxidase (MAO) to 3,4-dihydroxyphenylglycolaldehyde (DOPGAL) and then either reduced to 3,4-dihydroxyphenylethylene glycol (DOPEG) or oxidized to 3,4-dihydroxymandelic acid (DOMA). Alternatively, they can initially be methylated by catechol-O-methyltransferase (COMT) to normetanephrine and metanephrine, respectively. Most of the products of either type of reaction are then metabolized by the other enzyme to form the major excretory products, 3-methoxy-4-hydroxyphenylethylene glycol (MOPEG or MHPG) and 3-methoxy-4-hydroxymandelic acid (VMA). The glycol and, to some extent, the O-methylated amines and the catecholamines may be conjugated to the corresponding sulfates or glucuronides. (MOPGAL = 3-methoxy-4-hydroxyphenylglycolaldehyde; ALD RED = aldehyde reductase; ALD DEHYD = aldehyde dehydrogenase.) (Modified from Axelrod, 1966; others.)

can cause an increase in the level of norepinephrine, dopamine, and 5-HT in the brain and other tissues accompanied by a variety of pharmacological effects. No striking pharmacological action can be attributed to the inhibition of COMT.

General Actions of Adrenergic Transmitters. The effects of norepinephrine released by adrenergic nerve impulses at various effector organs are listed in Table 4–1, and the actions of the catecholamines and other sympathomimetic agents are presented in detail in Chapter 8. Hence, it is necessary here to mention only the general principles relating to the role of the catecholamines as neurohumoral transmitters. Norepinephrine, epinephrine, and other

catecholamines can cause either excitation or inhibition of *smooth muscle contraction,* depending on the site, the dose, and the catecholamine chosen. Norepinephrine is a potent excitatory catecholamine and has correspondingly low activity as an inhibitor; *isoproterenol* exhibits the reverse pattern of activity. Epinephrine is potent both as an excitor and as an inhibitor of smooth muscle contraction. On the basis of such observations, Ahlquist (1948) proposed the terms α and β *receptors* for sites on smooth muscles where catecholamines produce excitatory and inhibitory responses, respectively. The gut is generally relaxed by catecholamines, but here the inhibitory response is mediated by both α and β receptors. Cardiac pacemakers and muscle respond to catecholamines and adrenergic impulses with an increase in rate and force of contraction (positive chronotropic and inotropic effects), but these have the pharmacological properties of β-adrenergic responses. Isoproterenol is thus the most potent agent in producing these effects. This classification of receptors has been corroborated by the findings that certain drugs (*e.g.*, *phenoxybenzamine*) produce selective blockade of the effects of adrenergic nerve impulses and sympathomimetic agents at α-receptor sites, whereas others (*e.g.*, *propranolol*) produce β-adrenergic blockade.

β Receptors can be subdivided into β_1 receptors (chiefly at cardiac sites) and β_2 receptors (elsewhere) on the basis of the relative selectivity of effects of both agonists and antagonists (Lands *et al.*, 1967; Molinoff *et al.*, 1981b). The continuing development of highly selective drugs in these categories offers distinct therapeutic advantages (*see* Chapters 8 and 9).

There are also two subtypes of α-adrenergic receptors (*see* Chapter 8). α_1 Receptors probably have a predominant postjunctional location and thus are responsible for the initiation of excitatory postsynaptic events. α_2 Receptors are in part located on presynaptic nerve terminals; activation of these receptors results in inhibition of the release of transmitter. Thus, α_2 receptors on adrenergic nerve terminals appear to mediate feedback inhibition of norepinephrine release (Figure 4–4), while such receptors on the cholinergic nerve terminals in the gastrointestinal tract are probably responsible for inhibitory effects of α-adrenergic agonists at this site. In addition, postjunctional α_2 receptors also appear to be present at extrasynaptic sites in blood vessels and in the CNS. Stimulation of the latter receptors is associated with reduced sympathetic outflow from the CNS. Selective agonists and antagonists for α_1 and α_2 receptors are available, and some have important clinical uses (*see* Chapters 8 and 9).

In the smooth muscle of the guinea pig *vas deferens*, where adrenergic nerve impulses cause contraction by activation of α receptors, Burnstock and Holman (1961) have shown that effects at the muscle fiber membrane are quite similar to the excitatory effect of ACh. Each adrenergic nerve impulse causes localized, partial depolarization as a result of increased Na^+ conductance. When the summation of successive responses attains a critical level of depolarization, a spike potential is induced; this is conducted over the adjacent muscle fibers and is accompanied by contraction.

In contrast, in the guinea pig *taenia coli* and other gastrointestinal smooth muscle, where the spontaneous rhythmic activity is inhibited by adrenergic nerve impulses through activation of both α and β receptors, the opposite effects are produced: suppression of spike discharges, abolition of conducted responses to electrical stimulation, and hyperpolarization. The basis for these effects is considerably more complex. A site of α-adrenergic action is most likely on the stimulatory cholinergic neurons that innervate the muscle, and the effect is to hyperpolarize the neuron and decrease its rate of firing by a presynaptic mechanism. In addition, α-receptor stimulation of the smooth muscle itself causes hyperpolarization by activation of calcium-dependent potassium channels (*see* Bolton, 1979). The β-receptor inhibitory component is exerted on the smooth muscle cell but is apparently not associated with any significant change in conductance. The effects that result from the occupation of β-adrenergic receptors on smooth muscle cells are perhaps mediated by an increase in intracellular cyclic AMP, as discussed below (Bolton, 1979; Bülbring *et al.*, 1981).

In addition to the foregoing pharmacodynamic effects, epinephrine and its congeners produce an important group of *metabolic effects,* the manifestations of which include hyperglycemia, hyperlactacidemia, hyperlipemia, increased oxygen consumption, and hyperkalemia (*see* review by Stull and Mayer, 1979). The key compound that is involved in the mediation of these effects, as well as those of a great number of other hormones, is *cyclic AMP,* as was demonstrated in investigations initiated by Sutherland, Rall, and their associates (*see* Robison *et al.*, 1971; Rall, 1972). Epinephrine enhances the accumulation of cyclic

AMP by activating (via β receptors) a membrane-bound enzyme, adenylate cyclase, which catalyzes the conversion of ATP to cyclic AMP. Cyclic AMP then initiates a series of intracellular events that result in the characteristic metabolic effects of the catecholamines (Figure 4–6). Cyclic AMP also appears to mediate or modify the other actions of catecholamines that are exerted by means of β-adrenergic receptors.

β-Adrenergic receptors are located in the plasma membranes, with their catecholamine-binding sites oriented externally; the interaction of the receptor with adenylate cyclase requires a guanine nucleotide–binding regulatory protein (G_s) that is responsible for the activation of the catalytic component of adenylate cyclase (*see* Figure 4–6; Gilman, 1984; Smigel *et al.*, 1984). β-Adrenergic receptors have

been quantified and characterized in many tissues by ligand-binding technics (*see* Molinoff *et al.*, 1981a; Lefkowitz *et al.*, 1983; Abramson and Molinoff, 1984). The receptor protein has now been purified to homogeneity from several sources, and its interactions with G_s are being studied in detail (Ross *et al.*, 1983). Such work indicates that the receptor and G_s interact in the membrane bilayer, and that the crucial function of the agonist-receptor complex is to catalyze the binding of guanosine triphosphate (GTP) to G_s and the activation of the regulatory protein.

Hyperglycemia induced by catecholamines and by glucagon is attributable in part to activation, via cyclic AMP, of hepatic *glycogen phosphorylase*. This enzyme converts glycogen to glucose-1-phosphate, the rate-limiting step in *glycogenolysis*. In addition, the action of cyclic AMP results in the inactivation of *glycogen synthase*, the enzyme that catalyzes the transfer of glycosyl units from UDP-glucose to glycogen. These two effects of cyclic

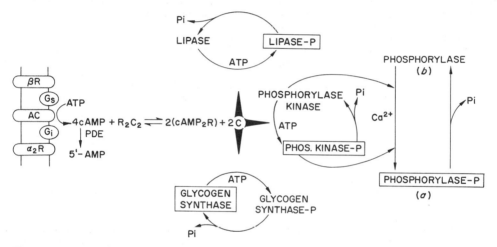

Figure 4–6. *Regulation of metabolism through β-adrenergic receptors.*

Adenosine 3′,5′-monophosphate (cyclic AMP, *cAMP*) is synthesized by adenylate cyclase (*AC*) at the cytoplasmic face of the plasma membrane consequent to activation of β-adrenergic receptors (*βR*) by epinephrine or other β-adrenergic agonists. To accomplish the activation of adenylate cyclase, the receptor interacts with a stimulatory guanine nucleotide–binding regulatory protein (G_s). G_s then binds GTP, and GTP · G_s interacts with and activates the actual catalyst of the enzyme complex. The regulatory protein possesses GTPase activity, and the hydrolysis of bound GTP results in reversal of this process. A closely related regulatory protein (G_i) also binds GTP in response to interaction with appropriate inhibitory receptors (*e.g.*, $α_2$-adrenergic receptors; $α_2R$). The interaction of G_i · GTP with the components of the system cause inhibition of adenylate cyclase. The intracellular receptor for cyclic AMP is a protein kinase (R_2C_2) that exists as a tetramer consisting of two regulatory (R) and two catalytic (C) subunits. Reaction with cyclic AMP causes dissociation and activation of the enzyme. The dissociated catalytic subunit phosphorylates a variety of proteins. The reactions shown in the figure are those that are the most important ones for the regulation of glycogenolysis and lipolysis by the autonomic nervous system. Phosphorylation of triglyceride lipase and phosphorylase kinase increases enzyme activity. Phosphorylation of glycogen synthase, however, deactivates this enzyme. (The activated form of each enzyme is shown enclosed in a box.) Stimulation of glycogenolysis is thus the consequence of the concerted phosphorylation of two enzymes that have opposing actions. Removal of the hormonal stimulus is followed by rapid dephosphorylation of all the proteins by phosphoprotein phosphatases. *PDE* = cyclic nucleotide phosphodiesterase.

AMP thus summate to increase the output of glucose from the liver.

The mechanism of action of cyclic AMP to produce these enzymatic changes is complex and is the result of the initiation of a cascading series of protein phosphorylation reactions (Figure 4–6). Cyclic AMP interacts with its intracellular receptor, a *cyclic AMP–dependent protein kinase,* and causes the dissociation of this enzyme into activated catalytic subunits and regulatory subunits (the cyclic AMP–binding component). The activated protein kinase can phosphorylate a variety of proteins, ATP being used as a substrate. Thus, protein kinase phosphorylates glycogen synthase, and the result is *inactivation* of the enzyme. Concurrently, the activated protein kinase phosphorylates and *activates* the enzyme *phosphorylase kinase.* Phosphorylase kinase is in fact another protein kinase, and it catalyzes the phosphorylation and *activation* of phosphorylase. This sequence of successive phosphorylation steps allows for considerable amplification of the initial signal. Stimulation of a small number of receptors can activate a large number of phosphorylase molecules in a very brief span of time. The hyperglycemia that ensues derives largely from the liberation of glucose from liver into the blood. Since muscle does not contain glucose-6-phosphatase, an end product of glycogenolysis in muscle is lactate, and *hyperlactacidemia* results.

Similar types of reactions result in the activation of triglyceride lipase in adipose tissue, with resultant hyperlipemia (Figure 4–6). Through this mechanism catecholamines provide an increased supply of substrate for oxidative metabolism.

Hyperglycemia is also promoted by other catecholamine-induced mechanisms. *Gluconeogenesis* from lactate and amino acids is stimulated, via cyclic AMP, by catecholamines and glucagon. The mechanism of this action is less precisely understood. The critical reactions occur in mitochondria and appear to involve the enhanced formation of phosphoenolpyruvate. The latter is then converted to glucose by the action of several cytoplasmic enzymes. This is also an important action of glucocorticoids (*see* Chapter 63), by mechanisms not directly involving cyclic AMP.

Catecholamines have both an inhibitory effect on the secretion of insulin by the β cells of the pancreatic islets, via α receptors, and a cyclic AMP–mediated stimulatory effect, by means of β receptors. The inhibitory effect predominates strongly *in vivo*. Since insulin antagonizes many of the metabolic effects of catecholamines and glucagon, this inhibitory effect on the secretion of insulin reinforces the metabolic actions described above.

The important question of a causal relationship between the accumulation of cyclic AMP induced by catecholamines and the actions of these agents at autonomic effectors remains a subject of extensive investigation. Most if not all the actions of catecholamines at β-*receptor* sites appear to be linked to activation of adenylate cyclase and the consequent increase in the intracellular concentrations of cyclic AMP. This applies to inhibitory effects on smooth muscle, excitatory effects on the myocardium, secretory responses of exocrine glands, and quite possibly the action of norepinephrine as a neurotransmitter in the CNS (Cohen, 1982; Drummond, 1983). However, only in the case of the metabolic changes produced by catecholamines is the pathway between cyclic AMP accumulation and the response well delineated.

Protein kinases that are not dependent on cyclic AMP also modulate intracellular events and are coupled directly or indirectly to membrane-bound receptors. Such enzymes include protein kinase C (Nishizuka, 1984) and a group of calmodulin-dependent protein kinases (Kakiuchi *et al.,* 1982). The activities of these enzymes are regulated in part by intracellular concentrations of calcium. Several such kinases are probably involved in the regulation of contractile processes; they also may be responsible for the enhanced glycogenolysis and gluconeogenesis produced by stimulation of α receptors in the liver of some animal species. In the heart, stimulation of β-adrenergic receptors leads to an increased inotropic response. Increased intracellular concentrations of cyclic AMP and enhanced phosphorylation of proteins such as troponin and phospholamban are detected after β-adrenergic stimulation. Although these phosphorylation events appear to influence both the action and the disposition of cellular Ca^{2+}, other events may also contribute to the inotropic response (England *et al.,* 1984). Receptor-induced contraction of smooth muscle is in general mediated by an increase in the concentration of free intracellular Ca^{2+}. Ca^{2+} activates the calmodulin-dependent myosin light-chain kinase, and phosphorylation of myosin is, in turn, associated with the development of tension (Murphy *et al.,* 1983; Kamm and Stull, 1985). Stimulation of β-adrenergic receptors usually results in an increase in cyclic AMP concentrations and relaxation of smooth muscle. While a cyclic AMP–dependent phosphorylation event is probably involved, the precise nature of this pathway remains unknown (*see* Kamm and Stull, 1985).

In several systems, α_2-adrenergic stimulation inhibits adenylate cyclase. This effect appears to involve an inhibitory, GTP-binding regulatory protein (G_i) in the cell membrane (*see* Figure 4–6). G_s and G_i are structurally related and have opposing effects on adenylate cyclase activity in many cells (Gilman, 1984).

RELATIONSHIP BETWEEN THE NERVOUS AND THE ENDOCRINE SYSTEMS

The concept that "humors" are secreted at certain sites to act elsewhere in the body can be traced back to Aristotle. In modern terms, the theory of neurohumoral transmission by its very designation implies at least a superficial resemblance between the nervous and the endocrine systems. Yet it should now be clear that the similarities extend considerably deeper, particularly with respect to the autonomic nervous system. In the regulation of homeostasis, the autonomic nervous system is responsible for rapid adjustments to changes in the total environment, which it effects at both its ganglionic relays and postganglionic terminals by the liberation of chemical agents that act transiently at their immediate sites of release. The endocrine system, in contrast, regulates slower, more generalized adaptations by releasing its hormonal agents into the systemic circulation to act at distant, widespread sites over periods of hours or days. Both systems have major central representations in the hypothalamus, where they are integrated with each other and with subcortical, cortical, and spinal influences. The neurohumoral theory may thus be said to provide a unitary concept of the functioning of the nervous and the endocrine systems, in which the differences are essentially only quantitative.

PHARMACOLOGICAL CONSIDERATIONS

In the foregoing sections, there are numerous references to the actions of drugs considered primarily as tools for the dissection and elucidation of physiological mechanisms. Here will be presented a classification of drugs that act upon the peripheral nervous system and its effector organs at some stage of neurohumoral transmission. In the immediately succeeding chapters, as well as elsewhere in the text, the systematic pharmacology of the important members of each of these classes is described.

Before proceeding with any classification of drugs, it is essential to emphasize an important general principle. The "first adage" of pharmacology is: "No drug has a single effect." Thus, a drug may be classified as an "anti-ChE agent," but this does not preclude its having direct effects at postsynaptic cholinoceptive sites or elsewhere. Drugs are placed in a given class on the basis of what appears to be their primary or predominant action, but the decision is often an arbitrary one. Additional effects or side effects constitute the major limitation to the usefulness of drugs as tools in the analysis of physiological and pharma-

cological mechanisms and in drug therapy. For example, there are serious limitations to the use of ganglionic blocking agents in the treatment of hypertension because of their lack of *selectivity* between sympathetic and parasympathetic ganglia. Nonselective β-adrenergic antagonists, used in the treatment of various cardiovascular conditions, produce unwanted effects because they block hepatic and bronchial smooth-muscle β receptors. For these reasons both the pharmacologist and the clinician are constantly seeking drugs that have more selective effects, with respect to both mechanism and site.

Each step involved in neurohumoral transmission (Figure 4–2) represents a potential point of drug attack. This is depicted in the diagram of the adrenergic terminal and its postjunctional site, in Figure 4–4. Drugs that affect processes concerned in each step of transmission at both cholinergic and adrenergic junctions are summarized in Table 4–2, which lists representative agents that act by the mechanisms described below.

Interference with the Synthesis or Release of the Transmitter. *Cholinergic. Hemicholinium* (HC-3), a synthetic compound, blocks the transport system by which choline accumulates in the terminals of cholinergic fibers and thus it limits the synthesis of the ACh store available for release (Birks and MacIntosh, 1957). *Botulinus toxin* has been shown to prevent the release of ACh by all types of cholinergic fibers studied; death results from peripheral respiratory paralysis. Apparently, the toxin blocks release of vesicular ACh at the preterminal portion of the axon, but why this effect is confined to cholinergic fibers is not known (Simpson, 1981).

Adrenergic. α-*Methyltyrosine (metyrosine)* blocks the synthesis of norepinephrine by inhibiting tyrosine hydroxylase, the enzyme that catalyzes the rate-limiting step. On the other hand, *methyldopa,* an inhibitor of aromatic L-amino acid decarboxylase, is, like dopa itself, successively decarboxylated and hydroxylated in its side chain to form the putative "false neurotransmitter," α-*methylnorepinephrine. Bretylium* and *guanethidine* act by prevent-

Table 4–2.   TYPES OF ACTION OF REPRESENTATIVE AGENTS AT PERIPHERAL CHOLINERGIC AND ADRENERGIC SYNAPSES AND NEUROEFFECTOR JUNCTIONS

MECHANISM OF ACTION	SYSTEM	AGENTS	EFFECT
1. Interference with synthesis of transmitter	Cholinergic	Hemicholinium	Block of choline uptake with consequent depletion of ACh
	Adrenergic	α-Methyltyrosine	Depletion of norepinephrine
2. Metabolic transformation by same pathway as precursor of transmitter	Adrenergic	Methyldopa	Displacement of norepinephrine by false transmitter (α-methylnorepinephrine)
3. Blockade of transport system of membrane of nerve terminal	Adrenergic	Cocaine, imipramine	Accumulation of norepinephrine at receptors
4. Blockade of transport system of storage granule membrane	Adrenergic	Reserpine	Destruction of norepinephrine by mitochondrial MAO, and depletion from adrenergic terminals
5. Displacement of transmitter from axonal terminal	Cholinergic	Black widow spider venom	Cholinomimetic followed by anticholinergic
	Adrenergic	Amphetamine, tyramine	Sympathomimetic
6. Prevention of release of transmitter	Cholinergic	Botulinus toxin	Anticholinergic
	Adrenergic	Bretylium, guanethidine	Antiadrenergic
7. Mimicry of transmitter at postsynaptic receptor	Cholinergic Muscarinic Nicotinic	Methacholine Nicotine	Cholinomimetic Cholinomimetic
	Adrenergic $Alpha_1$ $Alpha_2$	Phenylephrine Clonidine	Sympathomimetic Sympathomimetic (periphery) Reduced sympathetic outflow (CNS)
	$Beta_{1,2}$ $Beta_1$ $Beta_2$	Isoproterenol Dobutamine Terbutaline	Nonselective β-adrenomimetic Selective cardiac stimulation Selective inhibition of smooth muscle contraction
8. Blockade of endogenous transmitter at postsynaptic receptor	Cholinergic Muscarinic Nicotinic	Atropine d-Tubocurarine, hexamethonium	Cholinergic blockade Cholinergic blockade
	Adrenergic Alpha $Beta_{1,2}$ $Beta_1$	Phenoxybenzamine Propranolol Metoprolol	α-Adrenergic blockade β-Adrenergic blockade Selective adrenergic blockade (cardiac)
9. Inhibition of enzymatic breakdown of transmitter	Cholinergic	Anti-ChE agents (physostigmine, di*iso*propyl phosphorofluoridate [DFP])	Cholinomimetic
	Adrenergic	MAO inhibitors (pargyline, nialamide, tranylcypromine)	Little direct effect on norepinephrine or sympathetic responses; potentiation of tyramine

ing the release of norepinephrine by the nerve impulse. However, both guanethidine and bretylium can transiently stimulate the release of norepinephrine, as a result of their ability to displace the amine from storage sites. Guanethidine can also partially deplete tissue stores of catecholamines by inhibition of the vesicular transport system for such amines.

Promotion of the Release of the Transmitter. *Cholinergic.* The ability of cholinergic agents to promote the release of ACh is limited, presumably because ACh and other cholinomimetic agents are quaternary ammonium compounds and do not readily cross the axonal membrane into the nerve ending. Black widow spider venom is known to cause a transient release of ACh before a permanent block is elicited (Howard and Gunderson, 1980).

Adrenergic. Several drugs that promote the release of the adrenergic mediator have already been discussed. On the basis of the *rate* and the *duration* of the drug-induced release of norepinephrine from adrenergic terminals, one of two opposite effects can predominate. Thus, *tyramine, ephedrine, amphetamine,* and related drugs cause a relatively rapid, brief liberation of the transmitter and hence produce a sympathomimetic effect. On the other hand, *reserpine,* by causing blockade of vesicular uptake of amines, produces a slow, prolonged release of the adrenergic transmitter within the nerve terminal, where it is largely metabolized by intraneuronal MAO. The resultant depletion of transmitter produces the equivalent of adrenergic blockade. Reserpine also causes the depletion of 5-HT, dopamine, and possibly other, unidentified amines from central and peripheral sites, and many of its major effects may be consequent to the depletion of transmitters other than norepinephrine.

Combination with Postjunctional Receptor Sites. *Cholinergic.* The majority of therapeutically useful agents that affect the peripheral cholinergic systems are in this category, and much research on drug development is directed to discovery of agents that interact with specific subtypes of cholinergic receptors. Since ACh is the neuro-

humoral transmitter at various peripheral junctions, the postjunctional cholinergic receptors presumably share certain common features. However, it has long been known that individual drugs vary in potency, relative to ACh, at different cholinoceptive sites. The various receptors must therefore have certain distinctive features, in addition to their common ones, based either on intrinsic differences in the structure of the binding site or differences induced by proteins that interact with the receptor. This constitutes the major basis of selectivity of drug action (*see* Figure 4–7). When a drug combines with a cholinergic receptor, it may produce a response resembling that of ACh (*i.e., cholinomimetic*). Alternatively, such a drug may cause no direct effect but, by occupation of the ACh binding site or a site that results in noncompetitive interference with the binding of ACh to its receptor, it may block the action of endogenous ACh (*i.e., cholinergic blockade*). Some substances, such as nicotine, produce both effects in sequence.

Before many congeners of ACh were synthesized, the effects of the alkaloids *muscarine* and *nicotine* on cholinergic junctions provided the basis for Dale's classical differentiation of receptor types, which is still accurate for both the peripheral and central nervous systems. By convention, the cholinomimetic effects of drugs and of ACh at *autonomic effector cells* are referred to as *muscarinic effects,* since the alkaloid activates these receptors. From the early work of Langley it is known that nicotine in low doses stimulates, and in higher doses paralyzes, autonomic ganglia; the same sequence was later shown to occur at the motor end-plates of certain types of skeletal muscle. The stimulation and then blockade of *autonomic ganglia* and the *end-plates of skeletal muscle,* as exhibited by ACh and various other drugs, are thus termed *nicotinic effects.* It must be emphasized that these effects by no means describe the full pharmacological spectra of muscarine and nicotine, which also have marked effects on the CNS and, at least in the case of nicotine, on some afferent nerve endings.

The "nicotinic" receptors of autonomic ganglia and skeletal muscle are not identical

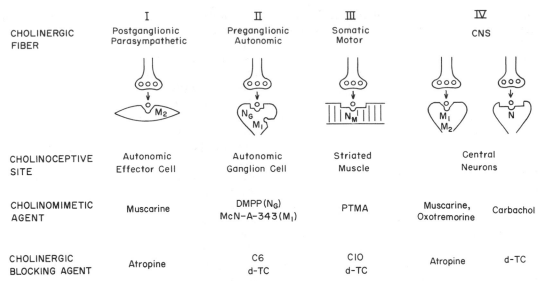

Figure 4–7. *Relative specificity of action of cholinomimetic and cholinergic blocking agents.*

Acetylcholine (ACh; depicted above as ○), released by the nerve action potential from the four classes of cholinergic fibers (*I–IV*) or introduced from an exogenous source, can combine with the cholinoceptive sites of the corresponding postjunctional cells (*I–IV*) to produce its characteristic transmitter effects. The receptors of autonomic effector cells (*I*) are classified as *muscarinic* (M), those of autonomic ganglion cells (*II*) are muscarinic and nicotinic (N), and those of striated muscle (*III*) are classified as *nicotinic*. Although certain drugs act at nicotinic receptors on both *II* and *III* (*e.g., d*-tubocurarine, *d*-TC), others are more selective for *II* (*e.g.,* hexamethonium, C6) or *III* (*e.g.,* decamethonium, C10); hence the receptors are designated here as N_G and N_M, respectively. Cholinoceptive neurons of the CNS have predominantly either nicotinic (spinal cord and optic tectum) or muscarinic (midbrain, cerebral cortex) receptors.

Examples of drugs that act selectively to produce cholinomimetic effects at the foregoing cholinoceptive sites are muscarine (*I*), dimethylphenylpiperazinium (DMPP) (*II-N*), McN-A-343 (*II-M*), phenyltrimethylammonium (PTMA) (*III*), muscarine or oxotremorine (*IV-M*), and carbachol (*IV-N*). All muscarinic receptors do not show identical specificities, hence the classification M_1 and M_2. M_1 receptors are found preferentially in ganglia, and McN-A-343 is a relatively specific agonist for M_1 receptors; pirenzepine is a corresponding M_1 antagonist. Cholinergic blocking agents also combine relatively selectively at such sites but have no important effects directly; their effects are due to blockade of the approach of endogenous ACh or exogenous cholinomimetic agents. Examples of drugs acting in this manner are atropine (*I*), hexamethonium (C6) (*II*), decamethonium (C10) (*III*), atropine (*IV-M*), and *d*-tubocurarine (*IV-N*).

since they respond differently to certain stimulating and blocking agents, as can be seen in Figure 4–7. *Dimethylphenylpiperazinium* (DMPP) and *phenyltrimethylammonium* (PTMA) are highly selective stimulants of autonomic ganglion cells and end-plates of skeletal muscle, respectively. *Tetraethylammonium* and *hexamethonium* are likewise selective ganglionic blocking agents. While d-*tubocurarine* effectively blocks transmission at both motor end-plates and autonomic ganglia, its action at the former site predominates, whereas *decamethonium*, a depolarizing agent, pro-

duces selective neuromuscular blockade. The snake toxins, which cause neuromuscular paralysis, also exhibit selectivity for the nicotinic cholinergic receptor at the neuromuscular junction. Transmission at autonomic ganglia is further complicated by the presence of muscarinic receptors, in addition to the principal nicotinic receptors (*see* Chapter 10).

Muscarinic receptors can be divided into two subclasses, M_1 and M_2, based upon the selectivity of certain agonists and antagonists (*see* Chapters 5 and 7). *Atropine* blocks all the muscarinic responses to injected ACh and related cholinomimetic drugs, whether they are excitatory, as in the intestine, or inhibitory, as in the heart. However, it is less effective in blocking responses to stimulation of certain postganglionic parasympathetic fibers. For example, although small doses of atropine prevent cardiac slowing or salivary secretion after nerve stimulation, even large doses will not abolish fully the responses of the smooth muscle of the intestine and urinary bladder to nerve impulses. A partial explanation is that such impulses are mediated in fact by purinergic, or ATP-releasing, fibers. Most muscarinic antagonists are approximately equipotent at both subtypes of muscarinic receptors. An exception is pirenzepine, a recently discovered muscarinic antagonist. This compound may provide new insights into achieving additional therapeutic specificity for this class of drugs (*see* Chapter 7).

Adrenergic. A vast number of synthetic compounds that bear structural resemblance to the naturally occurring catecholamines can combine at α- or β-adrenoceptive sites, or both, and produce sympathomimetic effects (*see* Chapter 8). *Phenylephrine* acts selectively at α_1-receptor sites, while *clonidine* is a selective α_2 agonist. *Isoproterenol* exhibits agonist activity at both β_1- and β_2-adrenergic receptors. Preferential stimulation of cardiac β_1 receptors follows the administration of *dobutamine*. *Terbutaline* is an example of a drug with relatively selective action on β_2 receptors; that is, it produces effective bronchodilatation with minimal effects on the heart. The main features of adrenergic blockade, including the selectivity of various blocking agents for α and β receptors, have been discussed. Here too, partial dissociation of effects at β_1- and β_2-adrenergic receptors has been achieved, as exemplified by the β_1-blocking agent *metoprolol*, which blocks the cardiac actions of catecholamines without causing an equivalent degree of antagonism at bronchioles. Several important drugs that promote the release of norepinephrine or deplete the transmitter resemble, in their effects, activators or blockers of postjunctional receptors (*e.g., tyramine* and *reserpine,* respectively) (*see* Chapters 8 and 9).

Interference with the Destruction of the Transmitter. *Cholinergic.* The *anti-ChE agents* (Chapter 6) constitute a large group of compounds, the primary action of which is inhibition of AChE, with the consequent accumulation and action of endogenous ACh at sites of cholinergic transmission.

Adrenergic. The re-uptake of norepinephrine by the adrenergic nerve terminals is probably the major mechanism for terminating its transmitter action. Interference with this process has been proposed as the basis of the potentiating effect of *cocaine* on responses to adrenergic impulses and injected catecholamines. It has also been suggested that the antidepressant actions and some of the side effects of *imipramine* and related drugs are due to a similar action at adrenergic synapses in the CNS (*see* Chapter 19). Inhibitors of COMT, such as pyrogallol and tropolone, produce only slight enhancement of the actions of catecholamines, whereas MAO inhibitors, such as *tranylcypromine,* potentiate the effects of tyramine but not of catecholamines.

OTHER AUTONOMIC NEUROTRANSMITTERS

It has become evident that the concept of an autonomic nervous system whose neurons contain only ACh or norepinephrine as transmitters and whose effects are mediated only by release of these two transmitters is a considerable simplification. A host of other agents, such as purines, prostaglandins, peptides, other biogenic amines, and amino acids, clearly modulate or mediate the responses that follow stimulation of autonomic nerves; a major question is whether these agents meet the criteria necessary to designate them as neurotransmitters.

The purines (ATP and adenosine) exert predominantly inhibitory effects in the gastrointestinal tract and appear to be involved with inhibition of peristalsis and relaxation of sphincters. Extensive studies by Burnstock and colleagues have marshalled substantial evidence for purinergic autonomic nerves in the gastrointestinal and genitourinary tracts (Burnstock, 1981). ATP is stored in postganglionic neurons; it is released and subsequently degraded following nerve stimulation. Two types of purinergic receptors, designated P_1 and P_2, have been proposed. P_1 receptors are most sensitive to adenosine and are blocked by the methylxanthines, while P_2 receptors respond to ATP (Su, 1983). Purinergic nerves likely exist in other visceral organs, but their function is less well defined. 5-HT (serotonin) is also a candidate as an excitatory transmitter in enteric smooth muscle, although its precise neuronal location is unclear (*see* Chapter 26).

Several peptides, including the opioids, substance P, vasoactive intestinal polypeptide (VIP), neurotensin, bombesin, and cholecystokinin, have been localized by immunohistochemical methods to autonomic nerves in the gastrointestinal tract. However, current studies have not clearly established their function as autonomic transmitters; some may serve as sensory transmitters or neuromodulators. Many of these agents are also likely neurotransmitters in autonomic ganglia and in the CNS (*see* above; *see also* Chapters 10 and 12).

Ahlquist, R. P. A study of the adrenotropic receptors. *Am. J. Physiol.*, **1948**, *153*, 586–600.

Albuquerque, E. X.; Seyama, I.; and Narahashi, T. Characterization of batrachotoxin-induced depolarization of the squid giant axons. *J. Pharmacol. Exp. Ther.*, **1973**, *184*, 308–314.

Axelsson, J., and Thesleff, S. A study of supersensitivity in denervated mammalian skeletal muscle. *J. Physiol. (Lond.)*, **1959**, *147*, 178–193.

Barger, G., and Dale, H. H. Chemical structure and sympathomimetic action of amines. *J. Physiol. (Lond.)*, **1910**, *41*, 19–59.

Barker, D. L.; Molinoff, P. B.; and Kravitz, E. A. Octopamine in the lobster nervous system. *Nature [New Biol.]*, **1972**, *236*, 61–63.

Birks, R. I., and MacIntosh, F. C. Acetylcholine metabolism of a sympathetic ganglion. *Can. J. Biochem. Physiol.*, **1961**, *39*, 787–827.

Blaschko, H. The specific action of L-dopa decarboxylase. *J. Physiol. (Lond.)*, **1939**, *96*, 50P–51P.

Bullock, T. H., and Hagiwara, S. Intracellular recording from the giant synapse of the squid. *J. Gen. Physiol.*, **1957**, *40*, 565–577.

Burn, J. H., and Gibbons, W. R. The release of noradrenaline from sympathetic fibres in relation to calcium concentrations. *J. Physiol. (Lond.)*, **1965**, *181*, 214–223.

Burnstock, G., and Holman, M. E. The transmission of excitation from autonomic nerve to smooth muscle. *J. Physiol. (Lond.)*, **1961**, *155*, 115–133.

Cannon, W. B., and Uridil, J. E. Studies on the conditions of activity in endocrine glands. VIII. Some effects on the denervated heart of stimulating the nerves of the liver. *Am. J. Physiol.*, **1921**, *58*, 353–354.

Carlsson, A.; Falck, B.; and Hillarp, N.-Å. Cellular localization of brain monoamines. *Acta Physiol. Scand.*, **1962**, *56*, Suppl. 196, 1–27.

Carlsson, A.; Hillarp, N.-Å.; and Waldeck, B. Analysis of the Mg^{++}-ATP dependent storage mechanism in the amine granules of the adrenal medulla. *Acta Physiol. Scand.*, **1963**, *59*, Suppl. 215, 1–38.

Cavallito, C. J.; Yun, H. S.; Smith, J. C.; and Foldes, F. F. Choline acetyltransferase inhibitors. Configurational and electronic features of styrylpyridine analogs. *J. Med. Chem.*, **1969**, *12*, 134–138.

Creutz, C. E. *Cis*-unsaturated fatty acids induce the fusion of chromaffin granules aggregated by synexin. *J. Cell Biol.*, **1981**, *91*, 247–256.

Creutz, C. E.; Dowling, L. G.; Sando, J. J.; Villar-Palasi, C.; Whipple, J. H.; and Zaks, W. J. Characterization of the chromobindins: soluble proteins that bind to the chromaffin granule membrane in the presence of Ca^{2+}. *J. Biol. Chem.*, **1983**, *258*, 14664–14674.

Dale, H. H. The action of certain esters and ethers of choline, and their relation to muscarine. *J. Pharmacol. Exp. Ther.*, **1914**, *6*, 147–190.

De Robertis, E., and Bennett, H. S. Some features of the submicroscopic morphology of synapses in frog and earthworm. *J. Biophys. Biochem. Cytol.*, **1955**, *1*, 47–58.

Dixon, W. E. On the mode of action of drugs. *Med. Mag. (Lond.)*, **1907**, *16*, 454–457.

Elfvin, L.-G. The ultrastructure of the superior cervical sympathetic ganglion of the cat. I. The structure of the ganglion cell processes as studied by serial sections. *J. Ultrastruct. Res.*, **1963a**, *8*, 403–440. II. The structure of the preganglionic end fibers and the synapses as studied by serial sections. *Ibid.*, **1963b**, *8*, 441–476.

Elliot, T. R. The action of adrenalin. *J. Physiol. (Lond.)*, **1905**, *32*, 401–467.

Fatt, P., and Katz, B. Spontaneous subthreshold activity at motor nerve endings. *J. Physiol. (Lond.)*, **1952**, *117*, 109–128.

Feldberg, W., and Gaddum, J. H. The chemical transmitter at synapses in a sympathetic ganglion. *J. Physiol. (Lond.)*, **1934**, *81*, 305–319.

Feldberg, W., and Krayer, O. Das Auftreten eines azetylcholinartigen Stoffes in Herzvenenblut von Warmblütern bei Beizung der Nervi vagi. *Naunyn Schmiedebergs Arch. Exp. Pathol. Pharmakol.*, **1933**, *172*, 170–193.

Hagiwara, S., and Tasaki, I. A study of the mechanism of impulse transmission across the giant synapse of the squid. *J. Physiol. (Lond.)*, **1958**, *143*, 114–137.

Hodgkin, A. L., and Huxley, A. F. A quantitative description of membrane current and its application to conduction and excitation in nerve. *J. Physiol. (Lond.)*, **1952**, *117*, 500–544.

Hökfelt, T.; Lundberg, J. M.; Schultzberg, M.; Johansson, O.; Skirboll, L.; Änggård, A.; Fredholm, B.; Hamberger, B.; Pernow, B.; Rehfeld, J.; and Goldstein, M. Cellular localization of peptides in neural structures. *Proc. R. Soc. Lond. [Biol.]*, **1980**, *210*, 63–77.

Iversen, L. L.; Stöckel, K.; and Thoenen, H. Autoradiographic studies of the retrograde axonal transport of nerve growth factor in mouse sympathetic neurones. *Brain Res.*, **1975**, *88*, 37–43.

Kao, I.; Drachman, D. B.; and Price, D. L. Botulinum toxin: mechanism of presynaptic action. *Science*, **1976**, *193*, 1256–1258.

Katz, B., and Miledi, R. The measurement of synaptic delay, and the time course of acetylcholine release at the neuromuscular junction. *Proc. R. Soc. Lond. [Biol.]*, **1965**, *161*, 483–495.

———. The statistical nature of the acetylcholine potential and its molecular components. *J. Physiol. (Lond.)*, **1972**, *224*, 665–699.

Kirshner, N. Uptake of catecholamines by a particulate fraction of the adrenal medulla. *J. Biol. Chem.*, **1962**, *237*, 2311–2317.

Krnjević, K., and Mitchell, J. F. The release of acetylcholine in the isolated rat diaphragm. *J. Physiol. (Lond.)*, **1961**, *155*, 246–262.

Lands, A. M.; Arnold, A.; McAuliff, J. P.; Luduena, F. P.; and Brown, R. G., Jr. Differentiation of receptor systems activated by sympathomimetic amines. *Nature*, **1967**, *214*, 597–598.

Langley, J. N. Observations on the physiological action of extracts of the supra-renal bodies. *J. Physiol. (Lond.)*, **1901**, *27*, 237–256.

Lewandowsky, M. Ueber eine Wirkung des Nebennieren-extractes auf das Auge. *Zentralbl. Physiol.*, **1898**, *12*, 599–600.

Livett, B. G.; Boksa, P.; Dean, D. M.; Mizobe, F.; and Lindenbaum, M. H. Use of isolated chromaffin cells to study basic release mechanisms. *J. Auton. Nerv. Syst.*, **1983**, *7*, 59–86.

Loewi, O. Über humorale Übertragbarkeit der Herznervenwirkung. *Pflügers Arch. Gesamte Physiol.*, **1921**, *189*, 239–242.

Loewi, O., and Navratil, E. Über humorale Übertragbarkeit der Herznervenwirkung. X. Mitteilung. Über das Schicksal des Vagusstoff. *Pflügers Arch. Gesamte Physiol.*, **1926**, *214*, 678–688.

Lundberg, J. M.; Änggård, A.; and Fahrenkrug, J. Complementary role of vasoactive intestinal polypeptide (VIP) and acetylcholine for cat submandibular gland blood flow and secretion. I. VIP release. *Acta Physiol. Scand.*, **1981**, *113*, 317–327.

Pumplin, D. W., and Reese, T. S. Action of brown widow spider venom and botulinum toxin on the frog neuromuscular junction examined with the freeze fracture technique. *J. Physiol. (Lond.)*, **1977**, *273*, 444–457.

Riker, W. F.; Roberts, J.; Standaert, F. G.; and Fujimoru, H. The motor nerve terminal as the primary focus for drug-induced facilitation of neuromuscular transmission. *J. Pharmacol. Exp. Ther.*, **1957**, *121*, 286–312.

Sjöqvist, F. Pharmacological analysis of acetylcholinesterase-rich ganglion cells in the lumbo-sacral sympathetic system of the cat. *Acta Physiol. Scand.*, **1963**, *157*, 352–362.

Spector, S.; Tarver, J.; and Berkowitz, B. Effects of drugs and physiological factors in the disposition of catecholamines in blood vessels. *Pharmacol. Rev.*, **1972**, *24*, 191–202.

Steinsland, O. S.; Furchgott, R. F.; and Kirpekar, F. M. Inhibition of adrenergic neurotransmission by parasympathomimetics in the rabbit ear artery. *J. Pharmacol. Exp. Ther.*, **1973**, *184*, 346–356.

Thesleff, S. Functional properties of receptors in striated muscle. In, *Drug Receptors*. (Rang, H. P., ed.) University Park Press, Baltimore, **1973**, pp. 121–133.

Trautwein, W.; Kuffler, S. W.; and Edwards, C. Changes in membrane characteristics of heart muscle during inhibition. *J. Gen. Physiol.*, **1956**, *40*, 135–145.

Viveros, O. H., and Wilson, S. P. The adrenal chromaffin cell as a model to study cosecretion of enkephalins and catecholamines. *J. Auton. Nerv. Syst.*, **1983**, *7*, 41–58.

Vulliet, P. R.; Langan, T. A.; and Weiner, N. Tyrosine hydroxylase: a substrate of cAMP-dependent protein kinase. *Proc. Natl. Acad. Sci. U.S.A.*, **1980**, *77*, 92–96.

Yamauchi, T.; Nakata, H.; and Fujisawa, H. A new activator protein that activates tryptophan-5-monooxygenase and tyrosine-3-monooxygenase in the presence of Ca^{++}-calmodulin dependent protein kinase. *J. Biol. Chem.*, **1981**, *256*, 5404–5409.

Monographs and Reviews

Abramson, S. N., and Molinoff, P. B. In vitro interactions of agonists and antagonists with β-adrenergic receptors. *Biochem. Pharmacol.*, **1984**, *33*, 869–875.

Appenzeller, O. *The Autonomic Nervous System*. Elsevier Publishing Co., Amsterdam, **1982**.

Armstrong, C. M. Ionic pores, gates and gating currents. *Q. Rev. Biophys.*, **1974**, *7*, 179–209.

Axelrod, J. The formation, metabolism, uptake and re-

lease of noradrenaline and adrenaline. In, *The Clinical Chemistry of Monoamines*. (Varley, H., and Gowenlock, A. H., eds.) Elsevier Publishing Co., Amsterdam, **1963**, pp. 5–18.

——. Methylation reactions in the formation and metabolism of catecholamines and other biogenic amines: the enzymatic conversion of norepinephrine (NE) to epinephrine (E). *Pharmacol. Rev.*, **1966**, *18*, 95–113.

——. The fate of noradrenaline in the sympathetic neurone. *Harvey Lect.*, **1973**, *67*, 175–197.

Bannister, R. (ed.). *Autonomic Failure: A Textbook of Clinical Disorders of the Autonomic Nervous System*. Oxford University Press, Oxford, **1983**.

Barker, J. L. Peptide effects on the excitability of single nerve cells. In, *Neuropeptides*. (Iversen, L. L.; Iversen, S. D.; and Snyder, S. H.; eds.) *Handbook of Psychopharmacology*, Vol. 16. Plenum Press, New York, **1983**, pp. 489–517.

Bernard, C. *Leçons sur les phénomènes de la vie communs aux animaux et aux végétaux*. Baillière, Paris, **1878–1879**. (Two volumes.)

Birks, R. I., and MacIntosh, F. C. Acetylcholine metabolism at nerve-endings. *Br. Med. Bull.*, **1957**, *13*, 157–161.

Bloom, F. E. Ultrastructural identification of catecholamine-containing central synaptic terminals. *J. Histochem. Cytochem.*, **1973**, *21*, 333–348.

Bolton, T. B. Mechanisms of action of transmitters and other substances on smooth muscle. *Physiol. Rev.*, **1979**, *59*, 606–718.

Bowman, W. C. Prejunctional and postjunctional cholinoceptors at the neuromuscular junction. *Anesth. Analg.*, **1980**, *59*, 935–943.

Bülbring, E.; Ohashi, H.; and Tomita, T. Adrenergic mechanisms. In, *Smooth Muscle: An Assessment of Current Knowledge*. (Bülbring, E.; Brading, A. F.; Jones, A. W.; and Tomita, T.; eds.) University of Texas Press, Austin, **1981**, pp. 219–248.

Burnstock, G. Neurotransmitters and trophic factors in the autonomic nervous system. *J. Physiol. (Lond.)*, **1981**, *313*, 1–35.

Cannon, W. B. Organization for physiological homeostasis. *Physiol. Rev.*, **1929**, *9*, 399–431.

——. *The Wisdom of the Body*. W. W. Norton & Co., Inc., New York, **1932**.

Cannon, W. B., and Rosenblueth, A. *The Supersensitivity of Denervated Structures: A Law of Denervation*. The Macmillan Co., New York, **1949**.

Catterall, W. A. Neurotoxins that act on voltage-sensitive sodium channels in excitable membranes. *Annu. Rev. Pharmacol. Toxicol.*, **1980**, *20*, 15–43.

Ceccarelli, B., and Hurlbut, W. P. Vesicle hypothesis of the release of quanta of acetylcholine. *Physiol. Rev.*, **1980**, *60*, 396–441.

Changeux, J.-P. The acetylcholine receptor: an "allosteric" membrane protein. *Harvey Lect.*, **1981**, *75*, 85–254.

Cohen, P. P. The role of protein phosphorylation in neural and hormonal control of cellular activity. *Nature*, **1982**, *296*, 613–620.

Cooper, J. R.; Bloom, F. E.; and Roth, R. H. *The Biochemical Basis of Neuropharmacology*, 4th ed. Oxford University Press, New York, **1982**.

Cooper, J. R., and Meyer, E. M. Possible mechanisms involved in the release and modulation of release of neuroactive agents. *Neurochem. Int.*, **1984**, *6*, 419–433.

Costa, E.; Guidotti, A.; Hanbauer, I.; Kageyama, H.; Kataoka, Y.; Panula, P.; Quach, T. T.; and Schwartz, J. P. Adrenal medulla: regulation of biosynthesis and secretion of catecholamines and enkephalins. In, *Neurology and Neurobiology*. (Usdin, E.; Carlsson, A.; Dahlström, A.; and Engel, J.; eds.) *Catecholamines: Basic and Peripheral Mechanisms*, Vol. 8A. Alan R. Liss, Inc., New York, **1984**, pp. 153–161.

Coupland, R. E. The chromaffin system. In, *Catechol-*

amines. (Blaschko, H., and Muscholl, E., eds.) *Handbuch der Experimentellen Pharmakologie,* Vol. 33. Springer-Verlag, Berlin, **1972,** pp. 16–45.

Dale, H. H. The beginnings and the prospects of neurohumoral transmission. *Pharmacol. Rev.,* **1954,** *6,* 7–13.

Drummond, G. I. Cyclic nucleotides in the nervous system. *Adv. Cyclic Nucleotide Res.,* **1983,** *15,* 373–494.

Duggan, A. W., and North, R. A. Electrophysiology of opioids. *Pharmacol. Rev.,* **1983,** *35,* 219–281.

Eccles, J. C. *The Physiology of Synapses.* Springer-Verlag, Berlin; Academic Press, Inc., New York, **1964.**

——. *The Understanding of the Brain.* McGraw-Hill Book Co., New York, **1973.**

England, P. J.; Pask, H. T.; and Mills, D. Cyclic AMP–dependent phosphorylation of cardiac contractile proteins. *Adv. Cyclic Nucleotide Protein Phosphorylation Res.,* **1984,** *17,* 383–390.

Eränkö, O.; Sonila, S.; and Paiverinta, M. *Histochemistry and Cell Biology of Autonomic Neurons, SIF Cells and Paraneurons.* Academic Press, Inc., New York, **1980.**

Euler, U. S. von. Synthesis, uptake and storage of catecholamines in adrenergic nerves. The effects of drugs. In, *Catecholamines.* (Blaschko, H., and Muscholl, E., eds.) *Handbuch der Experimentellen Pharmakologie,* Vol. 33. Springer-Verlag, Berlin, **1972,** pp. 186–230.

——. Historical perspective: growth and impact of the concept of chemical neurotransmission. In, *Chemical Neurotransmission—75 Years.* (Stjärne, L.; Hedqvist, P.; Lagercrantz, H.; and Wennmalm, Å.; eds.) Academic Press, Ltd., London, **1981,** pp. 3–12.

Fambrough, D. M. Control of acetylcholine receptors in skeletal muscle. *Physiol. Rev.,* **1979,** *59,* 165–227.

Fleming, W. W. The electrogenic Na^+,K^+-pump in smooth muscle: physiologic and pharmacologic significance. *Annu. Rev. Pharmacol. Toxicol.,* **1980,** *20,* 129–149.

Furchgott, R. F. The role of endothelium in the responses of vascular smooth muscle to drugs. *Annu. Rev. Pharmacol. Toxicol.,* **1984,** *24,* 175–197.

Gabella, G. Structure of smooth muscles. In, *Smooth Muscle: An Assessment of Current Knowledge.* (Bülbring, E.; Brading, A. F.; Jones, A. W.; and Tomita, T.; eds.) University of Texas Press, Austin, **1981,** pp. 1–46.

Gilbert, R. F. T., and Emson, P. C. Neuronal coexistence of peptides with other putative transmitters. In, *Neuropeptides.* (Iversen, L. L.; Iversen, S. D.; and Snyder, S. H.; eds.) *Handbook of Psychopharmacology,* Vol. 16. Plenum Press, New York, **1983,** pp. 519–556.

Gilman, A. G. Guanine nucleotide-binding regulatory proteins and dual control of adenylate cyclase. *J. Clin. Invest.,* **1984,** *73,* 1–4.

Goldberg, L. I.; Volkman, P. H.; and Kohli, J. D. A comparison of the vascular dopamine receptor with other dopamine receptors. *Annu. Rev. Pharmacol. Toxicol.,* **1978,** *18,* 57–80.

Goldstein, M.; Fuxe, K.; and Hökfelt, T. Characterization and tissue localization of catecholamine synthesizing enzymes. *Pharmacol. Rev.,* **1972,** *24,* 293–309.

Grundfest, H. Physiology of electrogenic excitable membranes. In, *The Nervous System,* Vol. 1. (Tower, D. B., ed.) Raven Press, New York, **1975,** pp. 153–164.

Harden, T. K. Agonist-induced desensitization of the β-adrenergic receptor-linked adenylate cyclase. *Pharmacol. Rev.,* **1983,** *35,* 5–32.

Hebb, C. O. Biosynthesis of acetylcholine in nervous tissue. *Physiol. Rev.,* **1972,** *52,* 918–957.

Hess, W. R. *The Functional Organization of the Diencephalon.* Grune & Stratton, Inc., New York, **1957.**

Higgins, C. B.; Vatner, S. F.; and Braunwald, E. Parasympathetic control of the heart. *Pharmacol. Rev.,* **1973,** *19,* 119–155.

Hillarp, N.-Å. The construction and functional organiza-

tion of the autonomic innervation apparatus. *Acta Physiol. Scand.,* **1959,** *46,* Suppl. 157, 1–39.

Howard, B. D., and Gunderson, C. B., Jr. Effects and mechanisms of polypeptide neurotoxins that act presynaptically. *Annu. Rev. Pharmacol. Toxicol.,* **1980,** *20,* 307–336.

Hubbard, J. I. Microphysiology of vertebrate neuromuscular transmission. *Physiol. Rev.,* **1973,** *53,* 674–723.

Iversen, L. L. *The Uptake and Storage of Noradrenaline in Sympathetic Nerves.* Cambridge University Press, London, **1967.**

——. Uptake processes for biogenic amines. In, *Handbook of Psychopharmacology,* Vol. 3. (Iversen, L. L.; Iversen, S. D.; and Snyder, S. H.; eds.) Plenum Press, New York, **1975,** pp. 381–442.

Iversen, L. L.; Iversen, S. D.; and Snyder, S. H. (eds.). *Neuropeptides. Handbook of Psychopharmacology,* Vol. 16. Plenum Press, New York, **1983.**

Jessell, T. M. Substance P in the nervous system. In, *Neuropeptides.* (Iversen, L. L.; Iversen, S. D.; and Snyder, S. H.; eds.) *Handbook of Psychopharmacology,* Vol. 16. Plenum Press, New York, **1983,** pp. 1–105.

Joh, T. H.; Baetge, E. E.; Ross, M. E.; and Reis, D. J. Similar gene coding regions for catecholamine biosynthetic enzymes: possible existence of ancestral precursor gene. In, *Neurology and Neurobiology.* (Usdin, E.; Carlsson, A.; Dahlström, A.; and Engel, J.; eds.) *Catecholamines: Basic and Peripheral Mechanisms,* Vol. 8A. Alan R. Liss, Inc., New York, **1984,** pp. 203–221.

Jonsson, G.; Malmfors, T.; and Sachs, C. (eds.). *6-Hydroxydopamine as a Denervation Tool in Catecholamine Research. Chemical Tools in Catecholamine Research,* Vol. I. American Elsevier Publishing Co., Inc., New York, **1975,** pp. 3–372.

Jope, R. S. High-affinity choline transport and acetyl CoA production in brain and their roles in the regulation of acetylcholine synthesis. *Brain Res. Rev.,* **1979,** *1,* 313–344.

Kakiuchi, S.; Hidaka, H.; and Means, A. R. (eds.). *Calmodulin and Intracellular Calcium Receptors.* Plenum Press, New York, **1982.**

Kamm, K. E., and Stull, J. T. Function of myosin and myosin light chain kinase in smooth muscle. *Annu. Rev. Pharmacol. Toxicol.,* **1985,** *25,* 593–620.

Kao, C. Y. Tetrodotoxin, saxitoxin and their significance in the study of excitation phenomena. *Pharmacol. Rev.,* **1966,** *18,* 997–1049.

Katz, B. *Nerve, Muscle, and Synapse.* McGraw-Hill Book Co., New York, **1966.**

——. *The Release of Neural Transmitter Substances.* Charles C Thomas, Publisher, Springfield, Ill., **1969.**

Kilbinger, H. Presynaptic muscarine receptors modulating acetylcholine release. *Trends Pharmacol. Sci.,* **1984,** *5,* 103–105.

Kirshner, N. Function and organization of chromaffin vesicles. *Life Sci.,* **1974,** *14,* 1153–1167.

Koelle, G. B. Microanatomy and pharmacology of cholinergic synapses. In, *The Nervous System,* Vol. 1. (Tower, D. B., ed.) Raven Press, New York, **1975,** pp. 363–371.

Kopin, I. J. Metabolic degradation of catecholamines. The relative importance of different pathways under physiological conditions and after administration of drugs. In, *Catecholamines.* (Blaschko, H., and Muscholl, E., eds.) *Handbuch der Experimentellen Pharmakologie,* Vol. 33. Springer-Verlag, Berlin, **1972,** pp. 271–282.

Kopin, I. J., and Silberstein, S. D. Axons of sympathetic neurons: transport of enzymes *in vivo* and properties of axonal sprouts *in vitro. Pharmacol. Rev.,* **1972,** *24,* 245–254.

Krnjević, K. Chemical nature of synaptic transmission in vertebrates. *Physiol. Rev.,* **1974,** *54,* 418–540.

Langer, S. Z. Presynaptic regulation of the release of catecholamines. *Pharmacol. Rev.,* **1980,** *32,* 337–362.

Lefkowitz, R. J.; Stadel, J. M.; and Caron, M. G. Adenylate cyclase-coupled beta-adrenergic receptors: structure and mechanisms of activation and desensitization. *Annu. Rev. Biochem.*, **1983**, *52*, 159–186.

Levi-Montalcini, R., and Angeletti, P. U. Nerve growth factor. *Physiol. Rev.*, **1968**, *48*, 534–569.

Lewis, R. V., and Stern, A. S. Biosynthesis of the enkephalins and enkephalin-containing polypeptides. *Annu. Rev. Pharmacol. Toxicol.*, **1983**, *23*, 353–372.

Limbird, L. Activation and attenuation of adenylate cyclase. *Biochem. J.*, **1981**, *195*, 1–13.

Mancia, G., and Zanchetti, A. Hypothalamic control of autonomic function. In, *Handbook of the Hypothalamus*, Vol. 3, Pt. B. *Behavioral Studies of the Hypothalamus.* (Morgane, P. J., and Panksepp, J., eds.) Marcel Dekker, Inc., New York, **1981**, pp. 147–202.

Molinoff, P. B.; Weiland, G. A.; Heidenreich, K. A.; Pittman, R. N.; and Minneman, K. P. Interactions of agonists and antagonists with β-adrenergic receptors. *Adv. Cyclic Nucleotide Res.*, **1981a**, *14*, pp. 51–67.

Molinoff, P. B.; Wolfe, B. B.; and Weiland, G. A. Quantitative analysis of drug-receptor interactions. II. Determination of the properties of receptor subtypes. *Life Sci.*, **1981b**, *29*, 427–443.

Morgane, P. J. Historical and modern concepts of hypothalamic organization and function. In, *Anatomy of the Hypothalamus.* (Morgane, P. J., and Panksepp, J., eds.) *Handbook of the Hypothalamus*, Vol. 1. Marcel Dekker, Inc., New York, **1981**, pp. 1–64.

Murphy, R. A.; Aksoy, M. O.; Dillon, P. F.; Gerthoffer, W. T.; and Kamm, K. E. The role of myosin light chain phosphorylation in regulation of the cross-bridge cycle. *Fed. Proc.*, **1983**, *42*, 51–56.

Narahashi, T. Neurotoxins: pharmacological dissection of ionic channels of nerve membranes. In, *The Nervous System*, Vol. 2. (Tower, D. B., ed.) Raven Press, New York, **1975**, pp. 101–110.

Nishizuka, Y. The role of protein kinase C in cell surface signal transduction and tumour promotion. *Nature*, **1984**, *308*, 693–698.

Pernow, B. Substance P. *Pharmacol. Rev.*, **1983**, *35*, 85–141.

Pollard, H. B.; Pazoles, C. J.; and Creutz, C. E. Mechanism of calcium action and release of vesicle-bound hormones during exocytosis. *Recent Prog. Horm. Res.*, **1981**, *37*, 299–332.

Rall, T. W. Role of adenosine 3′,5′-monophosphate (cyclic AMP) in actions of catecholamines. *Pharmacol. Rev.*, **1972**, *24*, 399–410.

Reichardt, L. F., and Kelly, R. B. A molecular description of nerve terminal function. *Annu. Rev. Biochem.*, **1983**, *52*, 871–926.

Reis, D. J.; Nathan, M. A.; Doba, N.; and Amer, M. S. Two models of arterial hypertension in rat produced by lesions of inhibitory areas of brain. In, *The Nervous System in Arterial Hypertension.* (Julius, S., and Esler, M. D., eds.) Charles C Thomas, Publisher, Springfield, Ill., **1976**, pp. 119–143.

Riker, W. F., Jr., and Okamoto, M. Pharmacology of motor nerve terminals. *Annu. Rev. Pharmacol.*, **1969**, *9*, 173–208.

Robison, G. A.; Butcher, R. W.; and Sutherland, E. W. *Cyclic AMP.* Academic Press, Inc., New York, **1971**.

Ross, E. M.; Pedersen, S. E.; and Florio, V. A. Hormone-sensitive adenylate cyclase: identity, function and regulation of the protein components. In, *Current Topics in Membranes and Transport*, Vol. 18. (Kleinzeller, A., and Martin, B. R., eds.) Academic Press, Inc., New York, **1983**, pp. 109–142.

Rossier, J. Choline acetyltransferase: a review with special reference to its cellular and subcellular localization. *Int. Rev. Neurobiol.*, **1977**, *20*, 283–337.

Rubin, R. P. *Calcium and Cellular Secretion.* Plenum Press, New York, **1982**.

Schmitt, F. O.; Dev, P.; and Smith, B. H. Electrotonic processing of information by brain cells. *Science*, **1976**, *193*, 114–120.

Simpson, L. L. The origin, structure and pharmacological activity of botulinum toxin. *Pharmacol. Rev.*, **1981**, *33*, 155–188.

Smigel, M. D.; Ross, E. M.; and Gilman, A. G. Role of the β-adrenergic receptor in the regulation of adenylate cyclase. In, *Cell Membranes: Methods and Reviews*, Vol. 2. (Elson, E. L.; Frazier, W. A.; and Glaser, L.; eds.) Plenum Press, New York, **1984**, pp. 247–294.

Starke, K. Presynaptic receptors. *Annu. Rev. Pharmacol. Toxicol.*, **1981**, *21*, 7–30.

Stjärne, L. The synthesis, uptake and storage of catecholamines in the adrenal medulla. The effects of drugs. In, *Catecholamines.* (Blaschko, H., and Muscholl, E., eds.) *Handbuch der Experimentellen Pharmakologie*, Vol. 33. Springer-Verlag, Berlin, **1972**, pp. 231–269.

Stull, J. T., and Mayer, S. E. Adrenergic and cholinergic mechanisms of modulation of myocardial contractility. In, *Heart*, Vol. 1. Sect. 2, *The Cardiovascular System. Handbook of Physiology.* (Berne, R. M., ed.) American Physiological Society, Bethesda, **1979**, pp. 741–774.

Su, C. Purinergic neurotransmission and neuromodulation. *Annu. Rev. Pharmacol. Toxicol.*, **1983**, *23*, 397–411.

Thoenen, H. Surgical, immunological, and chemical sympathectomy. In, *Catecholamines.* (Blaschko, H., and Muscholl, E., eds.) *Handbuch der Experimentellen Pharmakologie*, Vol. 33. Springer-Verlag, Berlin, **1972**, pp. 813–844.

Trendelenburg, U. A kinetic analysis of the extraneuronal uptake and metabolism of catecholamines. *Rev. Physiol. Biochem. Pharmacol.*, **1980**, *87*, 33–115.

Tucek, S. The synthesis of acetylcholine. In, *Handbook of Neurochemistry*, 2nd ed., Vol. 4. (Lajtha, A., ed.) Plenum Press, New York, **1982**, pp. 219–249.

Weiner, N. Control of the biosynthesis of adrenal catecholamines by the adrenal medulla. In, *Adrenal Gland*, Vol. 6. Sect. 7, *Endocrinology. Handbook of Physiology.* (Blaschko, H.; Sayers, G.; and Smith, A. D.; eds.) American Physiological Society, Washington, D.C., **1975**, pp. 357–366.

————. Multiple factors regulating the release of norepinephrine consequent to nerve stimulation. *Fed. Proc.*, **1979a**, *38*, 2193–2202.

————. Tyrosine-3-monooxygenase (tyrosine hydroxylase). In, *Aromatic Amino Acid Hydroxylases: Biochemical and Physiological Aspects.* (Youdim, M. B. H., ed.) John Wiley & Sons, Inc., New York, **1979b**, pp. 141–190.

Weiner, N.; Cloutier, G.; Bjur, R.; and Pfeffer, R. I. Modification of norepinephrine synthesis in intact tissue by drugs and during short-term adrenergic nerve stimulation. *Pharmacol. Rev.*, **1972**, *24*, 203–232.

Weiner, N.; Yanagihara, N.; Tank, A. W.; Baizer, L.; and Langan, T. A. Studies of the mechanism of activation of tyrosine hydroxylase *in situ* in PC 12 cells. In, *Neurology and Neurobiology.* (Usdin, E.; Carlsson, A.; Dahlström, A.; and Engel, J.; eds.) *Catecholamines: Basic and Peripheral Mechanisms*, Vol. 8A. Alan R. Liss, Inc., New York, **1984**, pp. 173–181.

Westfall, T. C. Local regulation of adrenergic neurotransmission. *Physiol. Rev.*, **1977**, *57*, 659–728.

Winkler, H.; Fischer-Colbrie, F.; and Weber, A. Molecular organization of vesicles storing transmitter: chromaffin vesicles as a model. In, *Chemical Neurotransmission—75 Years.* (Stjärne, L.; Hedqvist, P.; Lagercrantz, H.; and Wennmalm, Å.; eds.) Academic Press, Ltd., London, **1981**, pp. 57–68.

Wurtman, R. J.; Pohorecky, L. A.; and Baliga, B. S. Adrenocortical control of the biosynthesis of epinephrine and proteins in the adrenal medulla. *Pharmacol. Rev.*, **1972**, *24*, 411–426.

CHAPTER
5 CHOLINERGIC AGONISTS

Palmer Taylor

Cholinergic agonists have as their primary action the excitation or inhibition of autonomic effector cells that are innervated by postganglionic parasympathetic nerves. When acting in this capacity, they may be referred to as *parasympathomimetic agents*. Additional actions are exerted on ganglia, on the neuromuscular junction, and on cells that do not receive extensive parasympathetic innervation but nevertheless possess cholinergic receptors. These drugs may be divided into two groups: (1) acetylcholine (ACh) and several synthetic choline esters and (2) the naturally occurring cholinomimetic alkaloids (particularly pilocarpine, muscarine, and arecoline) and their synthetic congeners. In addition, the anticholinesterase (anti-ChE) agents (Chapter 6) and the ganglionic stimulants (Chapter 10) have parasympathomimetic actions, but they also produce prominent effects at locations other than the postganglionic cholinergic effector site.

CHOLINE ESTERS

Acetylcholine (ACh) has had virtually no therapeutic applications because of its diffuseness of action and its rapid hydrolysis by both acetylcholinesterase (AChE) and plasma butyrylcholinesterase. Consequently, numerous derivatives have been synthesized in attempts to obtain drugs with more selective and prolonged actions. Only the latter objective has met with much success.

History. ACh was first synthesized by Baeyer in 1867. Investigations culminating in its identification as a neurohumoral transmitter are described in Chapter 4.

Of several hundred synthetic choline derivatives investigated, only methacholine, carbachol, and bethanechol have had clinical application. The structures of these compounds are shown in Table 5–1. Although *methacholine*, the β-methyl analog of ACh, was studied by Hunt and Taveau as early as 1911, it was not until the systematic investigations of this compound by Simonart (1932) and Starr and associates (1933) that the drug received adequate therapeutic trial. *Carbachol*, the carbamyl ester of choline, and *bethanechol*, its β-methyl analog, were synthesized in the early 1930s; their pharmacological actions were investigated by Molitor (1936) and others.

Mechanism of Action. The mechanisms of action of endogenous ACh at the postjunctional membranes of the effector cells and neurons that correspond to the four classes of cholinergic synapses are discussed in Chapter 4. By way of recapitulation, these are (1) autonomic effector sites, innervated by postganglionic parasympathetic fibers; (2) sympathetic and parasympathetic ganglion cells and the adrenal medulla, innervated by preganglionic autonomic fibers; (3) motor end-plates on skeletal muscle, innervated by somatic motor nerves; and (4) certain synapses within the central nervous system (CNS). When ACh is administered systemically, it has the potential to act at all of these sites; however, as a quaternary ammonium compound its penetration into the CNS is limited, and butyrylcholinesterase reduces the concentrations of ACh that reach areas in the periphery with low blood flow.

Since muscarine was characterized originally as acting relatively selectively at *autonomic effector cells* to produce qualitatively the same effects as ACh, actions of ACh and related drugs at these sites are referred to as *muscarinic*. Accordingly, the *muscarinic*, or *parasympathomimetic*, actions of the drugs considered in this chapter are practically equivalent to the effects of postganglionic parasympathetic nerve impulses listed in Table 4–1 (page 72); the differences between the actions of the classical muscarinic agonists are largely quantitative, with limited selectivity for one organ system or another. It is now known that *muscarinic* receptors are also present

Table 5–1. STRUCTURAL FORMULAS OF CHOLINE, ACETYLCHOLINE, AND CHOLINE ESTERS EMPLOYED CLINICALLY

Choline chloride	$(CH_3)_3\overset{+}{N}CH_2CH_2OH$	Cl^-
Acetylcholine chloride	$(CH_3)_3\overset{+}{N}CH_2CH_2O\overset{\overset{\displaystyle O}{\|\|}}{C}CH_3$	Cl^-
Methacholine chloride	$(CH_3)_3\overset{+}{N}CH_2\underset{\underset{\displaystyle CH_3}{\|}}{C}HO\overset{\overset{\displaystyle O}{\|\|}}{C}CH_3$	Cl^-
Carbachol chloride	$(CH_3)_3\overset{+}{N}CH_2CH_2O\overset{\overset{\displaystyle O}{\|\|}}{C}NH_2$	Cl^-
Bethanechol chloride	$(CH_3)_3\overset{+}{N}CH_2\underset{\underset{\displaystyle CH_3}{\|}}{C}HO\overset{\overset{\displaystyle O}{\|\|}}{C}NH_2$	Cl^-

to a variable degree on autonomic ganglion cells and on certain cortical and subcortical neurons; although these muscarinic receptors appear to differ in chemical selectivity from those found on postganglionic effector sites in smooth muscle, cardiac tissue, and secretory organs, the drugs of this class may have secondary effects at these sites. All the actions of ACh and its congeners at muscarinic receptors can be blocked by *atropine* (*see* Chapter 7). The *nicotinic* actions of cholinergic agonists refer to their initial stimulation, and in high doses to subsequent blockade, of autonomic ganglion cells and the neuromuscular junction, actions comparable to those of nicotine.

Properties of Muscarinic Receptors. The muscarinic receptor has been quantified and characterized in various tissues in the periphery and in the CNS by analysis of binding of antagonists that interact with the putative receptor (Snyder *et al.*, 1974; Birdsall *et al.*, 1978). Specificity of ligand binding to the receptor has been examined by study of competition by agonists, saturability, and stereospecificity of interaction. Specific binding is found in tissues where muscarinic receptors are demonstrable pharmacologically. Understanding of the events associated with activation of the receptor remains relatively meager. Stimulation of muscarinic receptors in the various tissues can lead to hyperpolarization or depolarization (Krnjević, 1974), and the responses are sufficiently slow to suggest that intracellular events could mediate the changes in membrane potential. Accumulation of

guanosine 3′,5′-monophosphate (cyclic GMP) (George *et al.*, 1970), enhanced permeability to monovalent cations (Burgen and Spero, 1968), hydrolysis of phosphoinositides (Jafferji and Michell, 1976), mobilization of or increases in the concentration of intracellular Ca^{2+} (Putney, 1978; Bolton, 1981), and inhibition of adenylate cyclase (Murad *et al.*, 1962; Watanabe, 1983) have all been correlated with muscarinic stimulation. It seems likely that a multiplicity of intracellular events are linked to stimulation of muscarinic receptors, and the particular result or sequence of intermediary steps depends on the tissue and perhaps on the type of muscarinic receptor.

Structure-Activity Relationship. The structure-activity relationship of cholinergic agonists has been described in detail (Bebbington and Brimblecombe, 1965; Kosterlitz, 1967; Rand and Stafford, 1967). Attention is accorded here only to those drugs that are of therapeutic interest.

Acetyl-β-methylcholine (methacholine) differs from ACh chiefly in its greater duration and selectivity of action. Its action is more prolonged because it is hydrolyzed by AChE at a considerably slower rate than ACh and is almost totally resistant to hydrolysis by nonspecific cholinesterase or butyrylcholinesterase. Its selectivity is manifested by slight nicotinic and a predominance of muscarinic actions, the latter being most marked on the cardiovascular system (Table 5–2).

Carbachol and *bethanechol*, which are unsubstituted carbamyl esters, are totally resistant to hydrolysis by either AChE or nonspecific cholinesterases; their half-lives are thus sufficiently long that they are distributed to areas of low blood flow. Bethanechol has mainly muscarinic actions, but both drugs act with some selectivity on the smooth muscle of the gastrointestinal tract and urinary bladder. Carbachol retains substantial nicotinic activity, particularly on autonomic ganglia. It is likely that both its peripheral and its ganglionic actions are due, in part, to the release of endogenous ACh from the terminals of cholinergic fibers.

PHARMACOLOGICAL PROPERTIES

Cardiovascular System. ACh has three primary effects upon the cardiovascular system: *vasodilatation,* a decrease in cardiac rate (the *negative chronotropic* effect), and a decrease in the force of cardiac contraction (the *negative inotropic* effect). The last-named effect is of lesser significance in ventricular than in atrial muscle. Certain of the above effects can be obscured by the release by ACh of catecholamines from both cardiac and extracardiac tissues and the dampening of the direct effects of ACh by baroreceptor and other reflexes.

Although ACh is rarely given systemically as a drug, its cardiac actions are of

Table 5–2. SOME PHARMACOLOGICAL PROPERTIES OF CHOLINE ESTERS

CHOLINE ESTER	SUSCEPTIBILITY TO CHOLINESTERASES	PHARMACOLOGICAL ACTIONS Muscarinic					Nicotinic
		Cardiovascular	Gastrointestinal	Urinary Bladder	Eye (Topical)	Antagonism by Atropine	
Acetylcholine	+++	++	++	++	+	+++	++
Methacholine	+	+++	++	++	+	+++	+
Carbachol	−	+	+++	+++	++	+	+++
Bethanechol	−	±	+++	+++	++	+++	−

importance because of the involvement of cholinergic vagal impulses in the actions of the cardiac glycosides, antiarrhythmic agents, and many other drugs. The intravenous injection of a small (1 to 5 μg/kg) dose of ACh in an anesthetized animal produces an evanescent fall in blood pressure due to generalized vasodilatation, accompanied usually by reflex tachycardia. A considerably larger dose is required to elicit bradycardia or block of A-V nodal conduction from the direct action of ACh on the heart. If large doses of ACh are injected after the administration of atropine, an increase in blood pressure is observed due to stimulation of release of catecholamines from the adrenal medulla and activation of sympathetic ganglia. In *man,* intravenous infusions of ACh (20 to 60 mg per minute) produce little change other than vasodilatation and a slight fall in blood pressure, because of the rapid enzymatic hydrolysis of ACh and the efficient compensatory cardiovascular reflexes mediated through the caroticoaortic baroreceptors. When large doses (90 to 140 mg per minute) are administered intravenously, the complete pattern of bradycardia, hypotension, and the expected responses of other autonomic effectors is obtained.

ACh, when injected, produces *dilatation* of essentially *all vascular beds,* including the pulmonary (Aviado, 1965) and coronary (Levy and Martin, 1979). Coronary vasodilatation may be elicited by cardiovascular reflexes or by direct electrical stimulation of the vagus (Feigl, 1975). However, it is unlikely that either parasympathetic vaso-

dilator or sympathetic vasoconstrictor tone plays a major role in the regulation of coronary blood flow, in comparison with the effects of local oxygen tension and autoregulatory metabolic factors such as adenosine (Berne and Rubio, 1979).

The dilatation of vascular beds by choline esters is due to the presence of muscarinic receptors, despite the lack of apparent cholinergic innervation of most blood vessels. The muscarinic receptors responsible for relaxation actually appear to be in the endothelial cells of the vasculature; when these cells are stimulated, they release an unidentified mediator (endothelium-dependent relaxing factor) that diffuses to the smooth muscle and causes it to relax (Furchgott and Zawadzki, 1980).

ACh has important actions on all types of specialized cardiac cells; the same is qualitatively true of vagal impulses, since cholinergic parasympathetic fibers are distributed extensively to the S-A and A-V nodes and the atrial muscle. Cholinergic innervation of the ventricular myocardium is sparse, and the parasympathetic fibers terminate predominantly on specialized conduction tissue such as the Purkinje fibers (Kent *et al.,* 1974; Priola *et al.,* 1977).

In the *S-A node,* each normal cardiac impulse is initiated by the spontaneous depolarization of the pacemaker cells (*see* Chapter 31). At a critical level, the threshold potential, this depolarization initiates an action potential (AP). The AP is conducted over the course of the atrial muscle fibers to the A-V node and thence through the Purkinje system to the ventricular muscle. ACh slows the heart rate by hyperpolarization and by decreasing the rate of spontaneous diastolic depolarization at the S-A node; this delays the attainment of the threshold potential and the succeeding events in the cardiac cycle.

In *atrial muscle,* ACh decreases the strength of contraction. It also slows the rate of conduction of the AP and shortens the durations of the AP and the effective refractory period. The combination of these factors is the basis for the perpetuation or exacerbation by vagal impulses of atrial flutter or fibrillation arising at an ectopic focus. In contrast, primarily in the *A-V node* and to a much lesser extent in the *Purkinje conducting system,* ACh slows conduction but increases the refractory period. The decrement in A-V nodal conduction is usually responsible for the complete heart block that may be observed when large quantities of cholinergic agonists are administered systemically. With an increase in vagal tone, such as is produced by the digitalis glycosides, the increased refractory period can contribute to the reduction in the frequency with which aberrant atrial impulses are transmitted to the ventricle, and thus decrease the ventricular rate during atrial flutter or fibrillation.

In the *ventricle,* ACh, whether released by vagal stimulation or applied directly, also has a negative inotropic effect, although it is much smaller than that observed in the atrium. The effect is more obvious when contractility is enhanced by adrenergic stimulation (*see* Higgins *et al.,* 1973; Levy and Martin, 1979). Automaticity of Purkinje fibers is suppressed, and the threshold for ventricular fibrillation is increased (Kent *et al.,* 1974; Kent and Epstein, 1976). Sympathetic and vagal nerve terminals lie in close proximity, and muscarinic receptors are believed to exist at presynaptic as well as postsynaptic sites (*see* Watanabe, 1983). Inhibition of adrenergic stimulation of the heart arises from the capacity of ACh to modulate or depress the myocardium's response to catecholamines as well as from a capacity to inhibit the release of norepinephrine from sympathetic nerve endings. These effects can be explained in part by the inhibitory effect of muscarinic agonists on adenylate cyclase activity (*see* Chapter 4) and by their ability to interfere with the intracellular actions of adenosine 3',5'-monophosphate (cyclic AMP) (Watanabe, 1983; Symposium, 1984). At excessive concentrations, ACh may cause a positive inotropic effect, mainly through the local release of catecholamine (Buccino *et al.,* 1966).

The effects produced in man by constant *intravenous* infusion of *methacholine* are identical with those obtained with ACh, but the effective dose is only about 0.5% as large. After a *subcutaneous* dose of 20 mg, a transient fall in blood pressure and a compensatory tachycardia occur.

In contrast to ACh and methacholine, the cardiovascular effects of *carbachol* and *bethanechol* ordinarily are less conspicuous following usual subcutaneous or oral doses that affect the gastrointestinal and urinary tracts; these generally consist only in a slight, transient fall in diastolic pressure accompanied by a mild reflex tachycardia.

Gastrointestinal System. All the compounds of this class are capable of producing increases in tone, amplitude of contractions, and peristaltic activity of the stomach and intestines, as well as enhanced secretory activity of the gastrointestinal tract. The enhanced motility may be accompanied by nausea, belching, vomiting, intestinal cramps, and defecation.

Urinary Tract. *Carbachol* and *bethanechol,* in contrast to ACh and methacholine, stimulate rather selectively the urinary tract as well as the gastrointestinal tract. The choline esters increase ureteral peristalsis, contract the detrusor muscle of the urinary bladder, increase the maximal voluntary voiding pressure, and decrease the capacity of the bladder. In addition, the trigone and external sphincter are relaxed. In animals with experimental lesions of the spinal cord or sacral roots, these drugs bring about satisfactory evacuation of the neurogenic bladder.

Miscellaneous Effects. ACh and its analogs stimulate secretion by all *glands* that receive parasympathetic innervation, including the lacrimal, tracheobronchial, salivary, digestive, and exocrine sweat glands. The effects on the *respiratory system,* in addition to increased tracheobronchial secretion, include bronchoconstriction and stimulation of the chemoreceptors of the carotid and aortic bodies. When instilled into the eye, they produce *miosis;* however, the resultant fall in the intraocular tension may be preceded by a temporary elevation due to an increase in the permeability of the blood–aqueous humor barrier and vasodilatation of small vessels.

The effects of ACh on *autonomic ganglia* and at the *neuromuscular junction* of skeletal muscle are described in Chapters 10 and 11, respectively. While the cholinergic agonists considered here can produce similar effects in isolated preparations, these are not significant with the doses employed clinically, with the exception of carbachol. Muscarinic receptors are also found at *presynaptic sites* and, when stimulated, they inhibit the release of norepinephrine or ACh (*see* Chapter 4). These sites at the nerve ending do not differ in chemical specificity from postjunctional muscarinic receptors (Fuder *et al.,* 1982).

Synergisms and Antagonisms. ACh and methacholine are hydrolyzed by AChE, and their effects are markedly enhanced by the prior administration of anti-ChE agents. The latter drugs produce only additive effects with the stable analogs, carbachol and bethanechol.

The *muscarinic* actions of all the drugs of this class are blocked selectively by atropine, through competitive occupation of cholinergic receptor sites on the autonomic effector cells and on the secondary muscarinic receptors of autonomic ganglion cells. Epinephrine and other sympathomimetic amines antagonize many muscarinic effects by actions at sites where adrenergic and cholinergic impulses produce opposing responses (Table 4–1).

The *nicotinic* actions of ACh and its derivatives at autonomic ganglia are blocked by hexamethonium and related drugs; their actions at the neuromuscular junction of skeletal muscle are antagonized by *d*-tubocurarine and other competitive blocking agents.

Preparations, Routes of Administration, and Dosage. *Acetylcholine chloride* is used practically exclusively as an intraocular solution (MIOCHOL INTRAOCULAR). It is available in vials for the extemporaneous preparation of a 1% solution in 3% mannitol.

Methacholine chloride (acetyl-β-methylcholine chloride) is rarely used clinically.

Bethanechol chloride (*carbamylmethylcholine chloride;* URECHOLINE, others) is available in tablets containing 5, 10, 25, or 50 mg and as an injection (5 mg/ml). It is used to stimulate contraction of the urinary bladder and gastrointestinal tract. The

oral dose for adults varies from 10 to 50 mg; the *subcutaneous* dose is 2.5 to 5.0 mg. The single dose may be given two to four times daily. *The drug should not be administered by the intramuscular or intravenous route.*

Carbachol (carbamylcholine chloride) is used as an ophthalmic solution (CARBACEL, ISOPTO CARBACHOL) in concentrations of 0.75, 1.5, 2.25, and 3.0%. It is also available as *carbachol intraocular solution* (MIOSTAT INTRAOCULAR), a 0.01% solution that is used to produce miosis during ocular surgery. The solution (0.5 ml) is instilled into the anterior chamber.

Precautions, Toxicity, and Contraindications. Drugs of this class should be administered only by the *oral* or *subcutaneous* route for systemic effects; they are also used locally in the eye. If they are given intravenously or intramuscularly, their relative selectivity of action no longer holds, and the incidence and severity of toxic side effects are greatly increased. In order to *counteract* serious toxic reactions to these drugs, *atropine sulfate* (0.5 to 1.0 mg) should be given intramuscularly or intravenously, and should be readily available. *Epinephrine* (0.1 to 1.0 mg, subcutaneously) is also of value in overcoming severe cardiovascular or bronchoconstrictor responses.

Among the major *contraindications* to the use of the choline esters are *asthma, hyperthyroidism, coronary insufficiency,* and *peptic ulcer.* As noted previously, their bronchoconstrictor action is liable to precipitate an asthmatic attack, and hyperthyroid patients may develop atrial fibrillation. Hypotension induced by these agents can severely reduce coronary blood flow, especially if it is already compromised. The gastric acid secretion produced by the choline esters can aggravate the symptoms of peptic ulcer.

After administration of *bethanechol,* untoward effects related to the cardiovascular system are less liable to occur. Undesirable effects may include flushing, sweating, asthma attacks, hypotension, epigastric distress, abdominal cramps, belching, a sensation of tightness in the urinary bladder, difficulty in visual accommodation, headache, and salivation.

THERAPEUTIC USES

Bethanechol is used as a stimulant of the smooth muscle of the gastrointestinal tract and, particularly, the urinary bladder; *car-*

bachol is less desirable for these purposes because of its relatively larger component of nicotinic action at autonomic ganglia. The unpredictability of the intensity of response has virtually eliminated the use of *methacholine* as a vasodilator and cardiac vagomimetic agent.

Gastrointestinal Disorders. Bethanechol is of value in certain cases of *postoperative abdominal distention* and *gastric atony* or *gastroparesis.* The oral route is preferred; the usual dose is 10 to 20 mg, three or four times daily. It may be necessary to insert a rectal tube to facilitate passage of flatus. The drug has likewise been used to advantage in certain patients with adynamic ileus secondary to toxic states. *Gastric atony and retention following bilateral vagotomy* for peptic ulcer are often satisfactorily relieved by bethanechol; in this condition, neostigmine is ineffective. Bethanechol is given by mouth with each main meal in cases without complete retention; when gastric retention is complete and nothing passes into the duodenum, the subcutaneous route is necessary because the drug is not adequately absorbed from the stomach. Bethanechol increases the volume and the acidity of secretion of the vagotomized stomach and hence should be given only with meals. Bethanechol is also of value in selected cases of *congenital megacolon.* Bethanechol has been shown in some studies to be of benefit in the treatment of esophageal reflux (Saco *et al.,* 1982; Thanik *et al.,* 1982). Lower esophageal sphincter pressure and esophageal motility are increased, and acid reflux into the esophagus is decreased; however, symptomatic improvement does not necessarily correlate with these parameters.

Urinary Bladder Disorders. *Bethanechol* may be useful in combating *urinary retention* and *inadequate emptying of the bladder when organic obstruction is absent,* as in postoperative and postpartum urinary retention and in certain cases of *chronic hypotonic, myogenic,* or *neurogenic bladder* (Khanna, 1976; Finkbeiner and Bissada, 1980). α-Adrenergic antagonists have been reported to be a useful adjunct in reducing outlet resistance of the internal sphincter. Bethanechol may enhance contractions of the detrusor muscle after spinal injury if the vesical reflex is intact, and some benefit has been noted in partial sensory or motor paralysis of the bladder. Catheterization, with its attendant risk of urinary tract infection, can thus be avoided. For *acute retention,* the drug is injected subcutaneously in the usual dose of 5 mg, which can be repeated after 15 to 30 minutes if necessary. The stomach should be empty at the time the drug is injected. In *chronic cases,* 50 mg of the drug may be given orally, three times daily, until voluntary or automatic voiding begins and then its administration is slowly withdrawn. Too large a dose will result in detrusor-sphincter dyssynergia. Bethanechol has also been reported to be effective in the treatment of *malacoplakia* of the bladder (Zornow *et al.,* 1979).

Ophthalmological Uses. *Acetylcholine,* 1%, or *carbachol,* 0.01%, is used in cataract extractions and certain other surgical procedures on the anterior segment when it is desired to produce miosis rapidly; the action of acetylcholine is brief. For the chronic therapy of noncongestive, wide-angle glaucoma, *carbachol* (0.75 to 3.0%) has been employed. Carbachol will often reduce intraocular pressure in patients who have become resistant to pilocarpine or physostigmine.

Diagnostic Uses. If a patient is suspected of having poisoning due to atropine or other belladonna alkaloids, 10 to 30 mg of *methacholine* may be injected subcutaneously. The failure of appearance of the characteristic flush, sweating, lacrimation, rhinorrhea, salivation, and enhanced peristalsis is pathognomonic of *belladonna intoxication.* The specific antidote for this condition is *physostigmine* (*see* Chapter 6).

Methacholine and *bethanechol* have also been employed diagnostically in place of secretin as a test for *pancreatic enzymatic function;* by simultaneously stimulating secretion and constricting the ampullary mechanism, the drugs should normally cause an increase in the plasma amylase level. *Acetylcholine* has been employed as a transient vasodilator to improve visualization of hypovascular renal neoplasms.

CHOLINOMIMETIC NATURAL ALKALOIDS AND SYNTHETIC ANALOGS

The three major natural alkaloids in this group—*pilocarpine, muscarine,* and *arecoline*—have the same principal sites of action as the choline esters discussed above. Muscarine acts almost exclusively at *muscarinic* receptor sites, their classification as such being derived from this fact. Arecoline acts in addition at *nicotinic* receptors. Pilocarpine has a dominant muscarinic action, but it causes anomalous cardiovascular responses and the sweat glands are particularly sensitive to the drug. Although these naturally occurring alkaloids are of great value as pharmacological tools, present clinical use is largely restricted to the employment of pilocarpine as a miotic agent. Since evidence is beginning to accumulate that there are distinct subtypes of muscarinic receptors, there has been a renewed interest in synthetic analogs that may enhance the tissue selectivity of muscarinic agonists (*see* below).

History and Sources. *Pilocarpine* is the chief alkaloid obtained from the leaflets of South American shrubs of the genus *Pilocarpus.* Although it was long known by the natives that the chewing of leaves of *Pilocarpus* plants caused salivation, the first experiments were apparently performed in 1874 by a Brazilian physician named Coutinhou. The alkaloid was isolated in 1875, and shortly thereafter the actions of pilocarpine on the pupil as well as on the sweat and salivary glands were described by Weber.

The poisonous effects of certain species of mushrooms have been known since ancient times, but it was not until Schmiedeberg isolated the alkaloid *muscarine* from *Amanita muscaria* that the properties of the drug could be systematically investigated. Schmiedeberg and Koppe published the first careful pharmacological study of muscarine in 1869. The role played by muscarine in the development of the neurohumoral theory has been recounted in Chapter 4.

Arecoline is the chief alkaloid of areca or betel nuts, the seeds of *Areca catechu*. The *betel nut* has been consumed as a euphoretic by the natives of the East Indies from early times in a masticatory mixture known as *betel* and composed of the nut, shell lime, and leaves of *Piper betle*, a climbing species of pepper.

Structure-Activity Relationship. The muscarinic alkaloids show marked differences as well as interesting relationships in structure (Table 5–3). *Arecoline* and *pilocarpine* are tertiary amines, but the former is pharmacologically active chiefly in the protonated form. *Muscarine*, a quaternary ammonium compound, has three asymmetrical carbon atoms; all four pairs of enantiomorphs have been synthesized (Eugster *et al.*, 1958), including the naturally occurring L(+) form. *Oxotremorine* is a

synthetic compound that is used as an investigative tool. In the periphery, it acts as a potent muscarinic agonist. Its parkinsonism-like central effects include tremor, ataxia, and spasticity, which result apparently from activation of muscarinic receptors in the basal ganglia and elsewhere (Cho *et al.*, 1962). The chemistry and pharmacology of many natural and synthetic muscarinic compounds have been reviewed by Bebbington and Brimblecombe (1965).

Certain muscarinic antagonists, such as *pirenzepine,* show selectivity for receptors in specific tissues. Although it is not entirely clear whether sensitivity to pirenzepine is a consequence of structurally distinct subtypes of muscarinic receptors, the receptors that possess high and low affinities for pirenzepine have been termed M_1 and M_2 receptors, respectively (*see* Chapters 4 and 7). Some synthetic agonists also exhibit selectivity among sites for activation; among them is McN-A-343 (Table 5–3), which selectively stimulates M_1 receptors. Upon systemic injection of McN-A-343, there is a rise in blood pressure and an increase in peripheral vascular resistance that are consequences of stimulation of sympathetic ganglia in the absence of stimulation of cardiac and vascular postganglionic muscarinic receptors (*see* Roszkowski, 1961; Hammer and Giachetti, 1982). Muscarinic receptors with M_1 sensitivity are found in ganglia and the CNS, whereas M_2 sites exist at the postganglionic effector organs.

PHARMACOLOGICAL PROPERTIES

Smooth Muscle. Pilocarpine, when applied locally to the *eye,* causes pupillary constriction,

Table 5–3. STRUCTURAL FORMULAS OF CHOLINOMIMETIC NATURAL ALKALOIDS AND SYNTHETIC ANALOGS

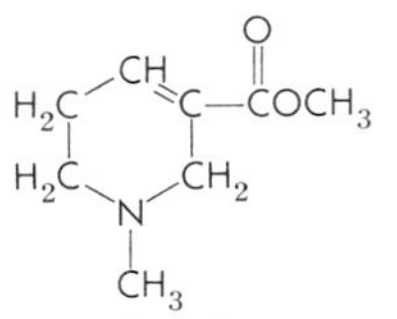

Arecoline

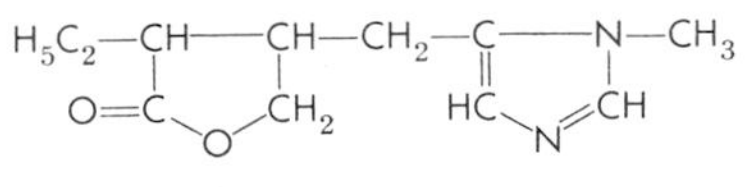

Pilocarpine

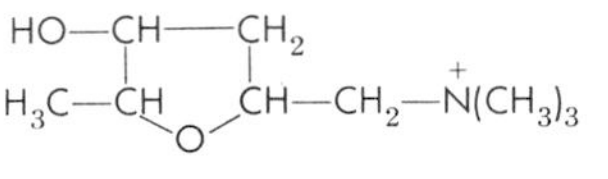

Muscarine

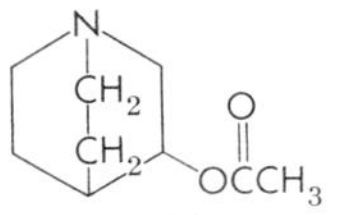

Aceclidine

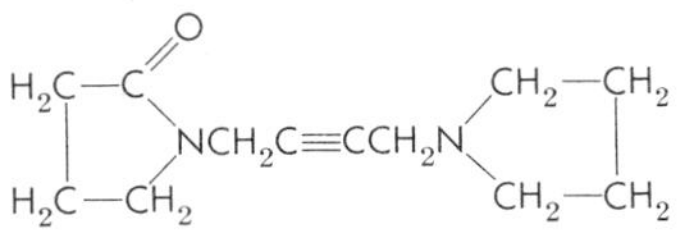

Oxotremorine

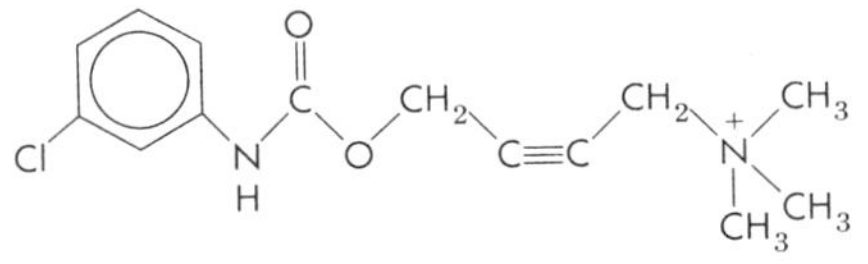

McN-A-343

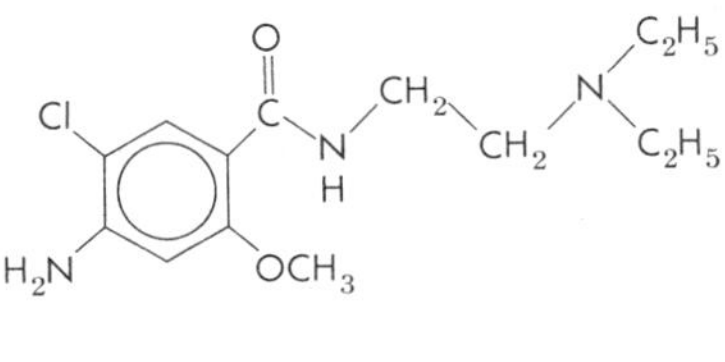

Metoclopramide

spasm of accommodation, and a transitory rise in intraocular pressure, followed by a more persistent fall. Miosis lasts from several hours to a day, but the effect on accommodation disappears in about 2 hours. The muscarinic alkaloids stimulate the smooth muscles of the *intestinal tract,* thereby increasing tone and motility; large doses cause marked spasm and tenesmus. The *bronchial musculature* is also stimulated; asthmatic patients uniformly respond to pilocarpine with a reduction in vital capacity, and a typical asthmatic attack may be precipitated. The tone and motility of the *ureters, urinary bladder, gallbladder,* and *biliary ducts* are also enhanced by pilocarpine and muscarine.

Exocrine Glands. Pilocarpine (10 to 15 mg, subcutaneously) causes marked diaphoresis in man; 2 to 3 liters of sweat may be secreted. Accompanying side effects may include hiccough, salivation, nausea, vomiting, weakness, and occasionally collapse. Muscarine and arecoline are also potent diaphoretic agents. The intradermal injection of a solution of pilocarpine or ACh in normally innervated skin causes local sweating and vasodilatation, which can be blocked by atropine. The salivary, lacrimal, gastric, pancreatic, and intestinal glands, and the mucous cells of the respiratory tract are also stimulated by these alkaloids. Normal saliva is hypotonic and is also unique in containing a larger amount of potassium than does the extracellular fluid from which it is derived; after pilocarpine, the composition of the saliva tends to approach that of an ultrafiltrate of the plasma. The *gastric glands* are stimulated to secrete a juice rich in acid but especially abundant in pepsin and mucin, resembling that resulting from vagal stimulation.

Cardiovascular System. The most prominent cardiovascular effects following the intravenous injection of extremely small doses (0.01 to 0.03 μg/kg) of *muscarine* in various species are a marked fall in the blood pressure and a slowing or temporary cessation of the heart. The actions of *pilocarpine* on the cardiovascular system defy satisfactory explanation. An intravenous injection of 0.1 mg/kg of pilocarpine produces a brief fall in blood pressure. However, if this is preceded by an appropriate dose of a nicotinic blocking agent, pilocarpine produces a marked rise in pressure. Both the vasodepressor and pressor responses are prevented by atropine; the latter effect is also abolished by α-adrenergic blocking agents (Levy and Ahlquist, 1962).

Central Nervous System. Pilocarpine, muscarine, and arecoline evoke a characteristic cortical arousal or activation response in cats following the intravenous injection of relatively small doses, similar to that produced by the injection of ACh or anti-ChE agents, or by electrical stimulation of the brain stem reticular formation. The arousal response to all these drugs is reduced or blocked by atropine and related agents. The spectrum of the known central actions of this group of drugs, ranging from those on individual neurons to the modification of complex behavioral processes, has been reviewed by Krnjević (1974).

Toxicology. Poisoning from pilocarpine, muscarine, or arecoline is characterized chiefly by exaggeration of their various parasympathomimetic effects, and resembles that produced by consumption of mushrooms of the genus *Inocybe* (*see* below). *Treatment* consists in the parenteral administration of atropine, and adequate measures to support the respiration and the circulation and to counteract pulmonary edema.

Preparations and Dosage. Preparations of pilocarpine include ophthalmic solutions of both *pilocarpine hydrochloride* and *pilocarpine nitrate.* Pilocarpine hydrochloride solutions include methylcellulose or a similar polymer and are available under a variety of trade names in concentrations ranging from 0.25 to 10%, while the concentrations of pilocarpine nitrate solutions range from 0.5 to 6%. Combinations of pilocarpine with epinephrine or physostigmine are also available.

A drug-delivery system (OCUSERT PILO-20 or 40) is available for achieving the sustained release of pilocarpine; it is placed in the cul-de-sac of the eyes. This is an elliptically shaped unit consisting of a pilocarpine-containing reservoir bounded by two layers of copolymer that control delivery of the drug. A relatively constant release of pilocarpine (20 or 40 μg per hour, corresponding to 1% and 2% pilocarpine solutions) is maintained for 7 days. However, variation in duration of action between individuals is substantial. Intraocular pressure may be effectively controlled without the stinging sensation and the myopia experienced immediately after the application of pilocarpine solution. Diurnal control of intraocular pressure may also be improved. Some patients find the foreign body uncomfortable and have difficulty with insertion of the device.

THERAPEUTIC USES

Pilocarpine is used in the treatment of *glaucoma,* where it is generally administered as a 0.5 to 4.0% aqueous solution. It is usually better tolerated than are the anticholinesterases, and pilocarpine is the standard cholinergic agent for initial treatment of open-angle glaucoma. Reduction of intraocular pressure occurs within a few minutes and lasts for 4 to 8 hours. The initial irritation and miosis can be bothersome, and care should be used when patients at risk for retinal detachment are treated (Beasley and Fraunfelder, 1979). The miotic action of pilocarpine is useful in overcoming the mydriasis produced by atropine; alternated with mydriatics, pilocarpine is employed to break adhesions between the iris and the lens.

Aceclidine (GLAUCOSTAT) is a synthetic compound that resembles arecoline (Table 5–3). In concentrations of 0.5 to 4.0%, it is approximately as effective as pilocarpine in reducing intraocular pressure in glaucoma, and it is a useful alternative for patients in whom the latter drug is unsatisfactory (Romano, 1970). The drug is employed in Europe but is not currently available in the United States.

Metoclopramide (REGLAN) acts peripherally to enhance the action of ACh at muscarinic synapses and in the CNS to antagonize dopamine. The latter action is responsible for its effectiveness as an antiemetic agent in cancer chemotherapy. It has found some use in radiological examination of the gastrointestinal tract, the treatment of esophageal reflux, and the control of gastroparesis in diabetics (Schulze-Delrieu, 1981; Snape *et al.*, 1982). An increase in both esophageal sphincter pressure and gastric emptying should be facilitated by cholinergic stimulation; however, the symptomatic improvement in gastroparesis may relate more closely to the antiemetic effect of the drug than to that on gastric emptying. Adverse dystonic or extrapyramidal effects, while infrequent, can limit the use of this agent.

MUSHROOM POISONING (MYCETISM)

Mushroom poisoning has been known for centuries. The Greek poet Euripides (fifth century B.C.) is said to have lost his wife and three children from this cause. In recent years the number of cases of mushroom poisoning has been increasing as the result of the current popularity of the consumption of wild mushrooms (*see* Medical Letter, 1984).

Although *Amanita muscaria* is the source from which *muscarine* has generally been isolated, its content of the alkaloid is so low (approximately 0.003%) that muscarine cannot be responsible for the major toxic effects. Much higher concentrations of muscarine are present in various species of *Inocybe* and *Clitocybe*. The symptoms of intoxication attributable to muscarine develop within 30 to 60 minutes of ingestion; they include salivation, lacrimation, nausea, vomiting, headache, visual disturbances, abdominal colic, diarrhea, bronchospasm, bradycardia, hypotension, and shock. Treatment with atropine (2 mg, parenterally) effectively blocks these effects.

Intoxication produced by *A. muscaria* and related species arises from the anticholinergic and hallucinogenic properties of a variety of isoxazole derivatives. Symptoms include irritability, restlessness, ataxia, hallucinations, and delirium. Treatment is mainly supportive; atropine is contraindicated, and sedatives are of questionable value (Becker *et al.*, 1976).

The most serious form of mycetism is produced by *Galerina* species, *A. verna*, *A. virosa*, *A. ocreata*, and *A. phalloides*, which are fairly common in both North America and Europe. These species account for over 90% of all fatal cases. The principal toxins are the *amatoxins* (α and β amanitin), a group of cyclic octapeptides that inhibit RNA polymerase II and hence block the synthesis of mRNA. This causes cell death, particularly in the gastrointestinal mucosa, liver, and kidneys. Initial symptoms, which are slow in onset, include diarrhea and abdominal cramps. Death occurs in 4 to 7 days from renal and hepatic failure (Becker *et al.*, 1976; Wieland and Faulstich, 1978). Treatment is largely supportive (Mitchel, 1980); thioctic acid

may be an effective antidote in the treatment of this type of mushroom poisoning, but the evidence for this is largely based on anecdotal studies (Mitchel, 1980).

Beasley, H., and Fraunfelder, F. T. Retinal detachments and topical ocular miotics. *Ophthalmology (Rochester)*, **1979**, *85*, 95–98.

Becker, C. E.; Tong, T. G.; Boerner, U.; Roe, R. L.; Scott, R. A. T.; MacQuarrie, M. B.; and Bartter, F. Diagnosis and treatment of *Amanita phalloides*–type mushroom poisoning. *West. J. Med.*, **1976**, *125*, 100–109.

Birdsall, N. J. M.; Burgen, A. S. V.; and Hulme, E. C. The binding of agonists to brain muscarinic receptors. *Mol. Pharmacol.*, **1978**, *14*, 737.

Buccino, R. A.; Sonnenblick, E. H.; Cooper, T.; and Braunwald, E. Direct positive inotropic effect of acetylcholine on myocardium. Evidence for multiple cholinergic receptors in the heart. *Circ. Res.*, **1966**, *11*, 1097–1108.

Burgen, A. S. V., and Spero, L. The action of acetylcholine and other drugs on the efflux of potassium and rubidium from smooth muscle of guinea pig intestine. *Br. J. Pharmacol.*, **1968**, *34*, 99–115.

Cho, A. K.; Haslett, W. L.; and Jenden, D. J. The peripheral actions of oxotremorine, a metabolite of tremorine. *J. Pharmacol. Exp. Ther.*, **1962**, *138*, 249–257.

Eugster, C. H.; Häfliger, F.; Denss, R.; and Girod, E. Die Spaltung von *d,l*-Muscarin in die optischen Antipoden. *Helv. Chim. Acta*, **1958**, *41*, 886–888.

Feigl, E. O. Reflex parasympathetic coronary vasodilatation elicited from cardiac receptors in the dog. *Circ. Res.*, **1975**, *37*, 175–182.

Fuder, H.; Rink, D.; and Muscholl, E. Sympathetic nerve stimulation on the perfused rat heart. *Naunyn Schmiedebergs Arch. Pharmacol.*, **1982**, *318*, 210–219.

Furchgott, R. F., and Zawadzki, J. V. The obligatory role of endothelial cells in relaxation of arterial smooth muscle by acetylcholine. *Nature*, **1980**, *288*, 373–376.

George, W. J.; Polson, J. B.; O'Toole, A. G.; and Goldberg, N. D. Elevation of guanosine 3′,5′ cyclic phosphate in rat heart after perfusion with acetylcholine. *Proc. Natl. Acad. Sci. U.S.A.*, **1970**, *66*, 398–403.

Hammer, R., and Giachetti, A. Muscarinic receptor subtypes: biochemical and functional characterization. *Life Sci.*, **1982**, *31*, 2991–2998.

Jafferji, S. S., and Michell, R. H. Muscarinic cholinergic stimulation of phosphoinositol turnover in longitudinal smooth muscle of guinea-pig ileum. *Biochem. J.*, **1976**, *154*, 63–67.

Kent, K. M., and Epstein, S. E. Neural basis for the genesis and control of arrhythmias associated with myocardial infarction. *Cardiology*, **1976**, *61*, 61–74.

Kent, K. M.; Epstein, S. E.; Cooper, T.; and Jacobowitz, D. M. Cholinergic innervation of the canine and human ventricular conducting system. *Circulation*, **1974**, *50*, 948–955.

Khanna, O. P. Disorders of micturition: neuropharmacologic basis and results of drug therapy. *Urology*, **1976**, *8*, 316–327.

Levy, B., and Ahlquist, R. P. A study of sympathetic ganglionic stimulants. *J. Pharmacol. Exp. Ther.*, **1962**, *137*, 219–228.

Medical Letter. Mushroom poisoning. **1984**, *26*, 67–70.

Molitor, H. A comparative study of the effects of five choline compounds used in therapeutics: acetylcholine chloride, acetyl-beta-methycholine chloride, carbaminoyl choline, ethyl ether beta-methylcholine chloride, carbaminoyl beta-methylcholine chloride. *J. Pharmacol. Exp. Ther.*, **1936**, *58*, 337–360.

Murad, F.; Chi, Y.-M.; Rall, T. W.; and Sutherland, E. W. Adenyl cyclase: the effect of catecholamines and choline esters on the formation of adenosine 3',5'-phosphate by preparations from cardiac muscle and liver. *J. Biol. Chem.*, **1962**, *237*, 1233–1238.

Priola, D. V.; Spurgeon, M. A.; and Geis, W. P. The intrinsic innervation of the canine heart: a functional study. *Circ. Res.*, **1977**, *40*, 5056.

Romano, J. H. Double-blind cross-over comparison of aceclidine and pilocarpine in open-angle glaucoma. *Br. J. Ophthalmol.*, **1970**, *54*, 510–521.

Roszkowski, A. P. An unusual type of ganglionic stimulant. *J. Pharmacol. Exp. Ther.*, **1961**, *132*, 156–170.

Saco, L. S.; Orlando, R. C.; Levinson, S. L.; Buzymki, K. M.; Jones, J. D.; and Frakes, J. T. Double-blind controlled trial of bethanechol and antacid versus placebo and antacid in the treatment of erosive esophagitis. *Gastroenterology*, **1982**, *82*, 1369–1373.

Schulze-Delrieu, K. Metoclopramide. *N. Engl. J. Med.*, **1981**, *305*, 28–33.

Simonart, A. On the action of certain derivatives of choline. *J. Pharmacol. Exp. Ther.*, **1932**, *46*, 157–193.

Snape, W. J.; Battle, W. M.; Schwartz, S. S.; Braunstein, S. N.; Goldstein, H. A.; and Alavi, A. Metoclopramide treatment of gastroparesis due to diabetes mellitus. *Ann. Intern. Med.*, **1982**, *96*, 444–446.

Starr, I., Jr.; Elsom, K. A.; Reisinger, J. A.; and Richards, A. N. Acetyl-β-methylcholin: action on normal persons with note on action of ethyl ether of β-methylcholin. *Am. J. Med. Sci.*, **1933**, *186*, 313–323.

Thanik, K.; Chey, W. K.; Shak, A.; Hamilton, D.; and Nadelson, N. Bethanechol or cimetidine in the treatment of symptomatic reflex esophagitis. *Arch. Intern. Med.*, **1982**, *142*, 1479–1481.

Zornow, D. H.; Landes, R. R.; Morganstern, S. L.; and Fried, F. A. Malacoplakia of the bladder: efficacy of bethanechol chloride therapy. *J. Urol.*, **1979**, *122*, 703–704.

Monographs and Reviews

Aviado, D. M. Acetylcholine and other parasympathomimetics. In, *The Lung Circulation*. Vol. 1, *Physiology and Pharmacology*. Pergamon Press, Ltd., Oxford, **1965**, pp. 329–341.

Bebbington, A., and Brimblecombe, R. W. Muscarinic receptors in the peripheral and central nervous systems. *Adv. Drug Res.*, **1965**, *2*, 143–172.

Berne, R. M., and Rubio, R. Coronary circulation. In, *The Cardiovascular System*, Vol. 1. (Berne, R. M., ed.) *Handbook of Physiology*, Sect. II. American Physiological Society, Bethesda, **1979**, pp. 873–952.

Bolton, T. B. Action of acetylcholine on the smooth muscle membrane. In, *Smooth Muscle*. (Bulbring, C.; Brading, A. F.; Jones, A. W.; and Tomita, T.; eds.) University of Texas Press, Austin, **1981**, pp. 199–217.

Finkbeiner, A. E., and Bissada, N. K. Drug therapy for lower urinary tract dysfunction. *Urol. Clin. North Am.*, **1980**, *7*, 3–16.

Higgins, C. B.; Vatner, S. F.; and Braunwald, E. Parasympathetic control of the heart. *Pharmacol. Rev.*, **1973**, *25*, 119–155.

Kosterlitz, H. W. Effects of choline esters on smooth muscle and secretions. In, *Physiological Pharmacology*. Vol. 3, *The Nervous System—Part C: Autonomic Nervous System Drugs*. (Root, W. S., and Hofmann, F. G., eds.) Academic Press, Inc., New York, **1967**, pp. 97–161.

Krnjević, K. Chemical nature of synaptic transmission in vertebrates. *Physiol. Rev.*, **1974**, *54*, 418–540.

Levy, M. N., and Martin, P. J. Neural control of the heart. In, *The Cardiovascular System*, Vol. 1. (Berne, R. M., ed.) *Handbook of Physiology*, Sect. II. American Physiological Society, Bethesda, **1979**, pp. 581–620.

Mitchel, D. H. *Amanita* mushroom poisoning. *Annu. Rev. Med.*, **1980**, *31*, 51–57.

Putney, J. W. Stimulus-permeability coupling: role of calcium in the receptor regulation of membrane permeability. *Pharmacol. Rev.*, **1978**, *30*, 209–245.

Rand, M. J., and Stafford, A. Cardiovascular effects of choline esters. In, *Physiological Pharmacology*. Vol. 3, *The Nervous System—Part C: Autonomic Nervous System Drugs*. (Root, W. S., and Hofmann, F. G., eds.) Academic Press, Inc., New York, **1967**, pp. 1–95.

Schmiedeberg, O., and Koppe, R. *Das Muscarin, das giftige Alkaloid des Fliegenpilzes*. F. C. W. Vogel, Leipzig, **1869**.

Snyder, S. H.; Chang, K. J.; Kuhar, M. J.; and Yamamura, H. I. Biochemical identification of the mammalian muscarinic cholinergic receptor. *Fed. Proc.*, **1974**, *34*, 1915–1921.

Symposium. (Various authors.) Parasympathetic neuroeffector mechanisms in the heart. *Fed. Proc.*, **1984**, *43*, 2597–2623.

Watanabe, A. M. Cholinergic agonists and antagonists. In, *Cardiac Therapy*. (Rosen, M. R., and Hoffman, B. F., eds.) Martinus Nijhoff Publishing, Hingham, Mass., **1983**, pp. 95–144.

Wieland, T., and Faulstich, H. Amatoxins, phallotoxins, phallolysin and antamanide: the biologically active components of poisonous *Amanita* mushrooms. *CRC Crit. Revbiochem.*, **1978**, *5*, 185–260.

6 ANTICHOLINESTERASE AGENTS

Palmer Taylor

The function of acetylcholinesterase (AChE) in terminating the action of acetylcholine (ACh) at the junctions of the various cholinergic nerve endings with their effector organs or postsynaptic sites is considered in Chapter 4. Drugs that inhibit AChE are called *anticholinesterase* (anti-ChE) agents. They cause ACh to accumulate at cholinergic receptor sites and thus are potentially capable of producing effects equivalent to excessive stimulation of cholinergic receptors throughout the central and peripheral nervous systems. In view of the widespread distribution of cholinergic neurons, it is not surprising that the anti-ChE agents as a group have received more extensive application as toxic agents, in the form of agricultural insecticides and potential chemical-warfare "nerve gases," than as therapeutic agents. Nevertheless, several members of this class of compounds are clinically useful.

Prior to World War II, only the "reversible" anti-ChE agents were generally known, of which *physostigmine (eserine)* is the outstanding example. Shortly before and during World War II, a comparatively new class of highly toxic chemicals, the *organophosphates,* was developed chiefly by Schrader, of I.G. Farbenindustrie, first as agricultural insecticides and later as potential chemical-warfare agents. The extreme toxicity of these compounds was found to be due to their "irreversible" inactivation of AChE, thereby exerting long-lasting inhibitory activity. Since the pharmacological actions of both classes of anti-ChE agents are qualitatively similar, they will be discussed as a group. Certain effects of anti-ChE agents and their interactions with other drugs at autonomic ganglia and the neuromuscular junction are described in Chapters 10 and 11.

History. *Physostigmine,* also called *eserine,* is an alkaloid obtained from the Calabar or ordeal bean, the dried ripe seed of *Physostigma*

venenosum Balfour, a perennial plant in tropical West Africa. The Calabar bean, also called Esére nut, chop nut, or bean of Etu Esére, was once used by native tribes of West Africa as an "ordeal poison" in trials for witchcraft.

The Calabar bean was brought to England in 1840 by Daniell, a British medical officer stationed in Calabar, and early investigations of its pharmacological properties were conducted by Christioson (1855), Fraser (1863), and Argyll-Robertson (1863). A pure alkaloid was isolated by Jobst and Hesse in 1864 and named *physostigmine;* the following year, Vee and Leven obtained the same alkaloid, which they named *eserine.* The first therapeutic use of the drug was in 1877 by Laqueur, in the treatment of glaucoma, one of its few clinical uses today. M. and M. Polonovski, Stedman, and Barger elucidated the chemical structure of physostigmine in the 1920s. Interesting accounts of the history of physostigmine have been presented by Karczmar (1970) and Holmstedt (1972).

As a result of the basic research of Stedman (1929a, 1929b) and associates in elucidating the chemical basis of the activity of physostigmine, others began systematic investigations of a series of substituted phenyl esters of alkyl carbamic acids. *Neostigmine,* a most promising member of this series, was introduced into therapeutics in 1931 for its stimulant action on the intestinal tract. It was subsequently reported to be effective in the symptomatic therapy of myasthenia gravis.

It is remarkable that the first account of the synthesis of a highly potent compound of the *organophosphorus anti-ChE* series, *tetraethyl pyrophosphate* (TEPP), was published by Clermont in 1854, 10 years prior to the isolation of physostigmine. More remarkable still, as Holmstedt (1963) has pointed out, is the fact that the investigator survived to report on the compound's taste; a few drops of the pure compound placed on the tongue would be expected to prove rapidly fatal. Modern investigations of the organophosphorus compounds date from the 1932 publication of Lange and Krueger on the synthesis of dimethyl and diethyl phosphorofluoridates. The authors' statement that inhalation of these compounds caused a persistent choking sensation and blurred vision apparently was instrumental in leading Schrader to explore this class for insecticidal activity.

During the synthesis of approximately 2000 compounds, Schrader (1952) defined the structural requirements for insecticidal (and, as learned subsequently, for anti-ChE) activity (*see* below). One compound in this early series, *parathion,* later became the most widely employed insecticide of this class. Prior to and during World War II, the efforts of Schrader's group were directed toward the development of chemical-warfare agents. The synthesis of several compounds of much greater toxicity than parathion, such as *sarin, soman,* and *tabun,* was kept secret by the German government. Investigators in the Allied countries also followed Lange and Krueger's lead in the search for potentially toxic compounds; di*iso*propyl phosphorofluoridate (DFP), synthesized by McCombie and Saunders (1946), was the organophosphorus compound studied most extensively by British and American scientists.

In the 1950s, a series of heterocyclic, aromatic, and naphthyl *carbamates* was synthesized and found to have a high degree of selective toxicity against insects and to be potent anti-ChE agents (Gysin, 1954). Among those currently employed as insecticides are 1-naphthyl N-methylcarbamate (carbaril or carbaryl; SEVIN) and 2-isopropoxyphenyl N-methylcarbamate (BAYGON) (*see* Fukuto, 1972; Hayes, 1982; Murphy, 1985).

Structure of Acetylcholinesterase. AChE exists in two classes of molecular forms: simple oligomers (*i.e.,* monomers, dimers, and tetramers) of a 70,000-dalton catalytic subunit, and elongated forms of complex molecular structures (Massoulié and Bon, 1982). The simple oligomers often contain a hydrophobic surface and are found in association with the plasma membrane. The elongated forms consist of tetramers of the catalytic subunit, but the tetramers in turn are linked in groups of three by disulfide bonds to a filamentous structure (50 × 2 nm). The molecular weights of these forms approach 10^6, and their structure is analogous to balloons attached to a branching stalk (Cartaud *et al.,* 1975). The filamentous subunits are collagen-like in composition (Lwebuga-Mukasa *et al.,* 1976; Rosenberry and Richardson, 1977) and serve only a structural role. The composition of the elongated forms, their susceptibility to dissolution from the synapse by collagenases, and their retention in synaptic areas after degeneration of the nerve and muscle plasma membranes all indicate that these forms are localized in the outer basal lamina (basement membrane) of the synapse, rather than in the plasma membrane of the nerve ending or muscle end-plate. Deposition of the elongated forms occurs during synaptogenesis, and these forms are primarily found in junctional areas of skeletal muscle (Hall, 1973; Massoulié and Bon, 1982).

The active center of AChE consists of a negative subsite, which attracts the quaternary group of choline through both coulombic and hydrophobic forces, and an esteratic subsite, where nucleophilic attack occurs on the acyl carbon of the substrate (Figure 6–1, *I*). The catalytic mechanism resembles that of other serine esterases, where a serine hydroxyl group is rendered highly nucleophilic through a charge-relay system involving the close apposition of an imidazole group and, presumably, a carboxyl group on the enzyme. During enzymatic attack on the ester, a tetrahedral intermediate between enzyme and ester is formed that collapses to an acetyl enzyme conjugate with the concomitant release of choline. The acetyl enzyme is labile to

hydrolysis, which results in the formation of acetate and active enzyme (*see* Froede and Wilson, 1971; Rosenberry, 1975). AChE is one of the most efficient enzymes known and has the capacity to hydrolyze 3×10^5 ACh molecules per molecule of enzyme per minute; this is equivalent to a turnover time of 150 microseconds.

Mechanism of Action of AChE Inhibitors. The mechanisms of action of compounds that typify the three classes of anti-ChE agents are also shown in Figure 6–1 (*II, III, IV*).

Quaternary compounds inhibit the enzyme reversibly by combining either at the active center or at a site spatially removed from the active center called the peripheral anionic site (Mooser and Sigman, 1974; Taylor and Lappi, 1975). The potent reversible inhibitor, *edrophonium,* binds selectively to the active center. The complex is stabilized by interaction of the quaternary nitrogen at the anionic subsite and by hydrogen bonding (Wilson and Quan, 1958) (Figure 6–1, *II*). Edrophonium has a brief duration of action owing to the reversibility of its binding to AChE and rapid renal elimination following systemic administration.

Drugs such as *physostigmine* and *neostigmine* that have a carbamyl ester linkage are hydrolyzed by AChE, but much more slowly than is ACh (Wilson *et al.,* 1960). Both the quaternary amine, neostigmine, and the tertiary amine, physostigmine, exist as cations at physiological pH; this contributes to their association with the active center. By serving as alternate substrates (Figure 6–1, *III*), the alcohol moiety is cleaved, giving rise to the carbamylated enzyme. In contrast to the acetyl enzyme, methylcarbamyl AChE or dimethylcarbamyl AChE is far more stable ($t_{1/2}$ for hydrolysis of the dimethylcarbamyl enzyme is 15 to 30 minutes) (Wilson and Harrison, 1961). Sequestration of the enzyme in its carbamylated form thus precludes the enzyme-catalyzed hydrolysis of ACh for extended periods of time. *In vivo,* the duration of inhibition by the carbamylating agents is 3 to 4 hours.

The *organophosphorus inhibitors,* such as DFP, serve as true hemisubstrates, since the resultant phosphorylated or phosphonylated enzyme is extremely stable (Figure 6–1, *IV*). Reaction occurs at the esteratic subsite and is enhanced by the geometry of the tetrahedral phosphates, which resemble the transition state for acetyl ester hydrolysis. Certain quaternary organophosphorus compounds (*e.g.,* echothiophate) interact with both the esteratic and anionic subsites in the active center to produce a stable complex; this contributes to the high potency of these agents (*see* Holmstedt, 1963). If the alkyl groups in the phosphorylated enzyme are ethyl or methyl, spontaneous regeneration of active enzyme requires several hours. Secondary (as in DFP) or tertiary alkyl groups further enhance the stability of the phosphorylated enzyme, and significant regeneration of active enzyme is not observed. Hence, the return of AChE activity depends on

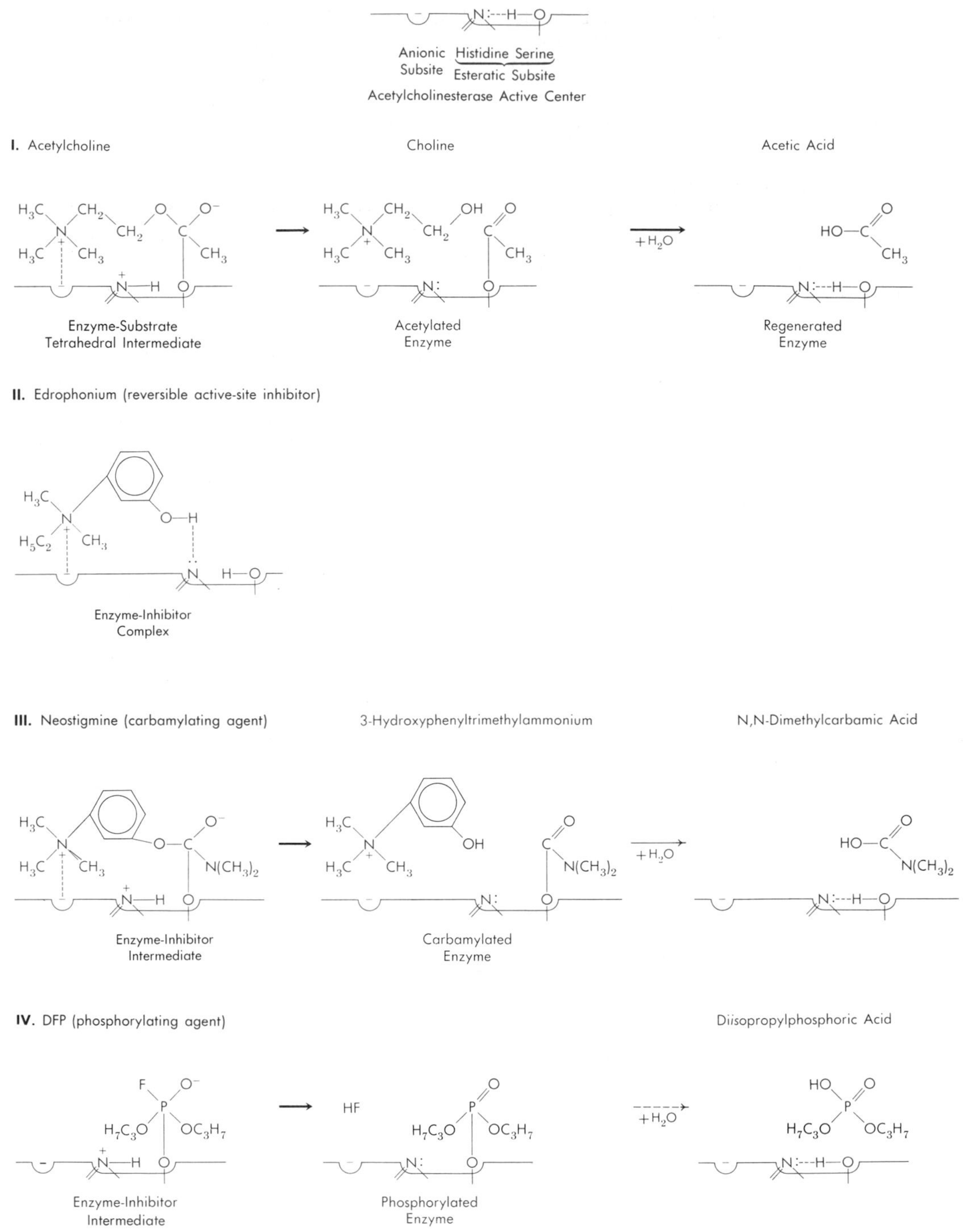

Figure 6–1. *Steps involved in the hydrolysis of acetylcholine (ACh) by acetylcholinesterase (AChE)* (I), *and in the inhibition of AChE by reversible* (II), *carbamyl ester* (III), *and organophosphorus* (IV) *agents.*

Heavy, light, and dashed arrows represent extremely rapid, intermediate, and extremely slow or insignificant reaction velocities, respectively. *See* text and references for description. Structures of the inhibitors appear in Tables 6–1 and 6–2.

synthesis of new enzyme. The stability of the phosphorylated enzyme is also enhanced through "aging," which results from the loss of one of the alkyl groups (*see* Figure 6–2; Aldridge, 1976; Hobbiger, 1976).

From the foregoing account, it is apparent that the terms "reversible" and "irreversible," as applied to the carbamyl ester and organophosphorus anti-ChE agents, respectively, reflect only quantitative differences in rates of deacylation, and that both classes of drugs react covalently with the enzyme in essentially the same manner as does ACh.

Action at Effector Organs. The characteristic pharmacological effects of the anti-ChE agents are due primarily to the prevention of hydrolysis of ACh by AChE at sites of cholinergic transmission. Transmitter thus accumulates, and the action of ACh that is liberated by cholinergic impulses or that spontaneously leaks from the nerve ending is enhanced. With most of the organophosphorus agents, such as DFP, virtually all the acute effects of moderate doses are attributable to this action. For example, the characteristic miosis that follows local application of DFP to the eye is not observed after chronic postganglionic denervation of the eye because there is no source from which to release endogenous ACh. The consequences of enhanced concentrations of ACh at motor end-plates are unique to these sites and are discussed below.

Among the classical anti-ChE agents, physostigmine, a tertiary amine, exerts a minimum of effects that are not related to inhibition of AChE. The quaternary ammonium anti-ChE compounds all have additional direct actions at some cholinergic receptor sites, either as agonists or antagonists. For example, the effects of neostigmine on the spinal cord and neuromuscular junction are based on a combination of its anti-ChE activity and direct cholinergic stimulation.

Chemistry and Structure-Activity Relationship. The structure-activity relationship of anti-ChE drugs has been reviewed extensively for the "reversible" inhibitors (Long, 1963), the organophosphorus agents (Holmstedt, 1963), and both classes of compounds (Karczmar, 1967; Usdin, 1970). Only those agents that are of general therapeutic or toxicological interest will be considered here.

"Reversible" Carbamate Inhibitors. Drugs of this class that are of therapeutic interest are shown in Table 6–1. From Stedman's early studies (1929a,

Table 6–1. REPRESENTATIVE "REVERSIBLE" ANTICHOLINESTERASE AGENTS EMPLOYED CLINICALLY

Physostigmine

Neostigmine

Edrophonium

Pyridostigmine

Demecarium

Ambenonium

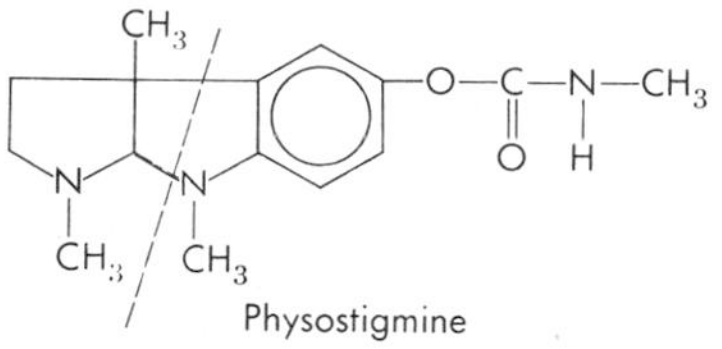

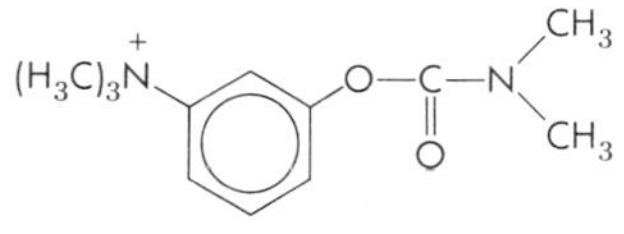

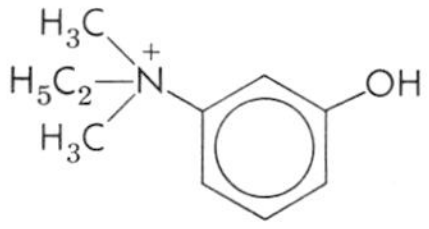

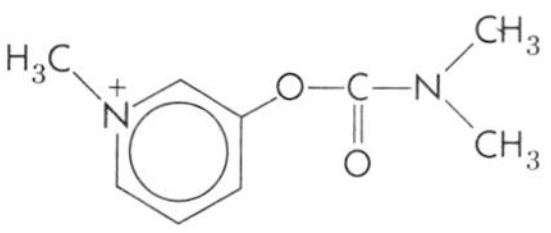

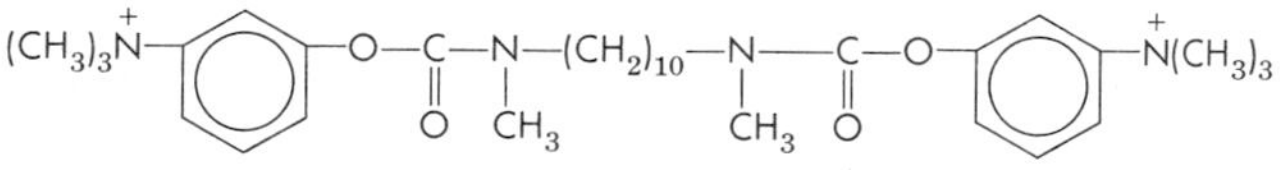

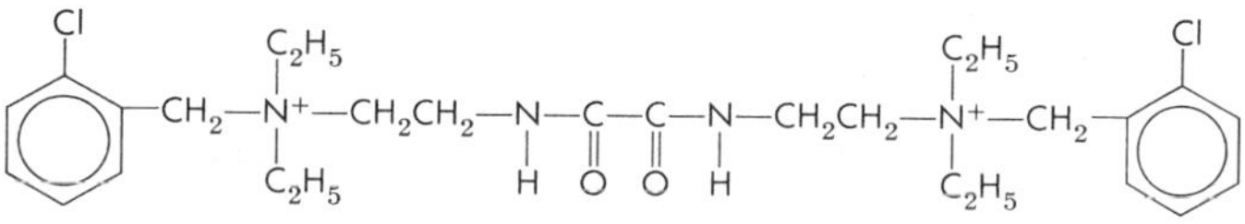

1929b), it was concluded that the essential moiety of the physostigmine molecule was the methyl carbamate of a basically substituted simple phenol (right of the dash line in Table 6–1). The quaternary ammonium derivative, *neostigmine*, is a compound of greater stability and equal or greater potency. *Pyridostigmine* is a close congener that is also employed in the treatment of myasthenia gravis. Analogs of neostigmine that lack the carbamyl group, such as *edrophonium*, are less potent and shorter-acting anti-ChE agents.

An increase in anti-ChE potency and duration of action can result from the linking of two quaternary ammonium nuclei by a chain of appropriate structure and length. One such example is the miotic agent *demecarium*, which consists of two neostigmine molecules connected at their carbamate nitrogens by a series of ten methylene groups. The second quaternary group confers additional stability to the interaction on the enzyme surface since negative subsites peripheral to the active center have been identified on AChE. Another class of *bis*-quaternary compounds is represented by *ambenonium*, used in the treatment of myasthenia gravis. Ambenonium does not react covalently with AChE but binds reversibly with a high affinity. This drug has additional actions at both prejunctional and postjunctional sites of the skeletal muscle motor end-plate (Hobbiger, 1976).

The insecticide *carbaril* (*carbaryl*), which is extensively used in garden products, inhibits ChE in a fashion identical to other carbamylating inhibitors. The signs and symptoms of poisoning closely resemble those of the organophosphates (Murphy, 1985). Carbaril has a particularly low toxicity from dermal absorption. It is used for control of head lice in some countries. Its structure is as follows:

Carbaril

Several analogs of carbaril are employed as agricultural and garden insecticides and have similar inhibitory properties (*see* Hayes, 1982). However, not all carbamates found in garden formulations are cholinesterase inhibitors; the dithiocarbamates are fungicidal.

Organophosphorus Inhibitors. The general formula for this class of cholinesterase inhibitors is presented in Table 6–2. A great variety of substituents is possible: R_1 and R_2 may be alkyl, alkoxy, aryloxy, amido, mercaptan, or other groups, and X, the leaving group, may represent a halide, cyanide, thiocyanate, phenoxy, thiophenoxy, phosphate, or carboxylate group. A useful chemical classification of the compounds that are of particular pharmacological or toxicological interest has been developed by Holmstedt (1963), upon which the listing in Table 6–2 is based. Compilations of the organophosphorus compounds and their toxic-

ity may be found in the publications of Gaines (1969) and Hayes (1982).

Diisopropyl phosphorofluoridate (DFP) is perhaps the best-known and most extensively studied compound of this general class as the result of its toxicological evaluation during World War II. It produces virtually irreversible inactivation of AChE and other esterases by alkylphosphorylation. Its lipid solubility, low molecular weight, and volatility facilitate inhalation and transdermal absorption. DFP also readily penetrates the central nervous system (CNS).

The "nerve gases," *tabun, sarin,* and *soman,* are among the most potent synthetic toxic agents known; they are lethal to laboratory animals in submilligram doses.

Parathion was synthesized by Schrader in 1944. Because of its low volatility and stability in aqueous solution, it became widely used as an insecticide. It continues to be used extensively in agriculture, but less hazardous compounds have become popular for home and garden use. Early studies demonstrated that parathion, purified from its contaminants, was inactive in inhibiting AChE *in vitro* and that *paraoxon* was the active metabolite. The sulfur-for-oxygen substitution is carried out predominantly in liver by the mixed-function oxygenases in the endoplasmic reticulum. Other tissues also have some capacity for such conversion. Parathion has probably been responsible for more cases of accidental poisoning and death than any other organophosphorus compound. The trade names that have been employed to designate the compound include NIRAN, ETILON, and FOLIDOL. Other insecticides possessing the phosphorothiolate structure are widely employed for home, garden, and agricultural use. These include *dimpylate* (DIAZINON), *fenthion,* and *chlorpyrifos.*

Malathion (CHEMATHION, MALA-SPRAY) also requires replacement of a sulfur atom with oxygen *in vivo.* This insecticide can be detoxified by hydrolysis of the carboxyl ester linkage by plasma carboxylesterases. The detoxication reaction is much more rapid in mammals and birds than in insects, giving rise to an additional degree of selective toxicity (*see* Murphy, 1985). In recent years, *malathion* has been employed in aerial spraying of relatively populous areas for control of fruit flies and mosquitos. Little evidence for acute toxicity has been reported. The lethal dose in mammals is about 1 g/kg. Exposure to the skin results in a small fraction (<10%) of systemic absorption.

Among the quaternary ammonium organophosphorus compounds (group E, Table 6–2), only *echothiophate* is useful clinically. It is relatively resistant to spontaneous hydrolysis and can thus be stored for several weeks in aqueous solution.

PHARMACOLOGICAL PROPERTIES

Generally the pharmacological properties of anti-ChE agents can be predicted merely by knowing those loci where ACh is released physiologically by nerve impulses

Table 6–2. CHEMICAL CLASSIFICATION OF REPRESENTATIVE ORGANOPHOSPHORUS COMPOUNDS OF PARTICULAR PHARMACOLOGICAL OR TOXICOLOGICAL INTEREST *

General formula (Schrader, 1952):

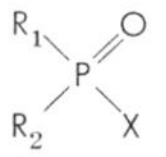

$$\begin{array}{c} R_1 \\ \diagdown \\ P = O \\ \diagup \ \diagdown \\ R_2 \quad\ X \end{array}$$

Group A, X = halogen, cyanide, or thiocyanate; group B, X = alkylthio, arylthio, alkoxy, or aryloxy; group C, thiol- or thionophosphorus compounds; group D, pyrophosphates and similar compounds; group E, quaternary ammonium compounds

GROUP	STRUCTURAL FORMULA	COMMON, CHEMICAL, AND OTHER NAMES	COMMENTS
A	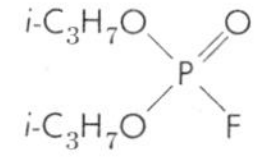 $i\text{-}C_3H_7O$, O, $i\text{-}C_3H_7O$, F (P center)	DFP Diisopropyl phosphorofluoridate	Potent, irreversible inactivator
	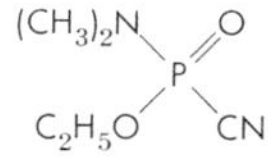 $(CH_3)_2N$, O, C_2H_5O, CN (P center)	Tabun Ethyl N-dimethylphosphoramido-cyanidate	Extremely toxic "nerve gas"
	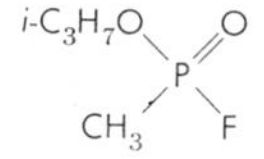 $i\text{-}C_3H_7O$, O, CH_3, F (P center)	Sarin (GB) Isopropyl methylphosphonofluoridate	Extremely toxic "nerve gas"
	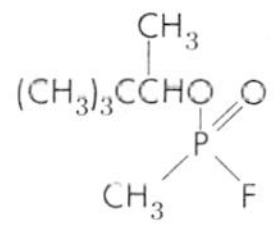 CH_3 / $(CH_3)_3CCHO$, O, CH_3, F (P center)	Soman Pinacolyl methylphosphonofluoridate	Extremely toxic "nerve gas"
B	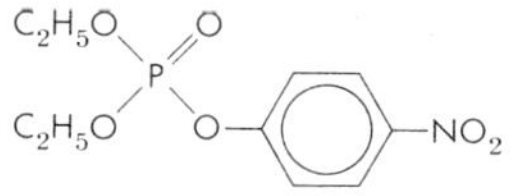 C_2H_5O, O, C_2H_5O, $O\text{--}C_6H_4\text{--}NO_2$ (P center)	Paraoxon, Mintacol, E 600 O,O-Diethyl O-(4-nitrophenyl)-phosphate	Active metabolite of parathion
C	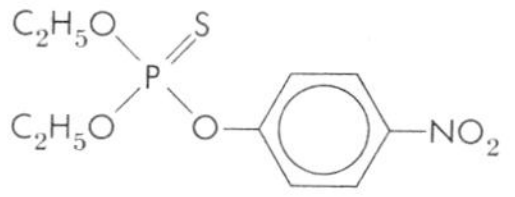 C_2H_5O, S, C_2H_5O, $O\text{--}C_6H_4\text{--}NO_2$ (P center)	Parathion (see trade names in text) O,O-Diethyl O-(4-nitrophenyl)-phosphorothioate	Employed as agricultural insecticide, resulting in numerous cases of accidental poisoning
	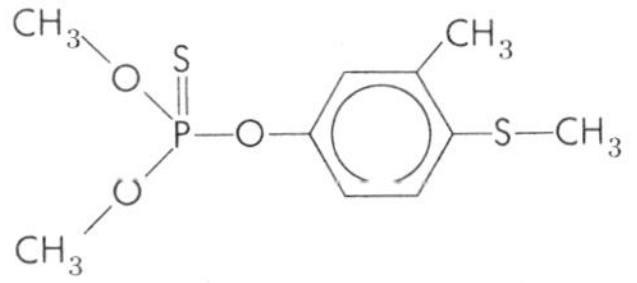 CH_3O, S, CH_3O, O–(4-methylthio-m-tolyl) (P center)	Fenthion O,O-Dimethyl O-4-methylthio-m-tolyl phosphorothioate	Insecticide with high lipid solubility; agricultural use
	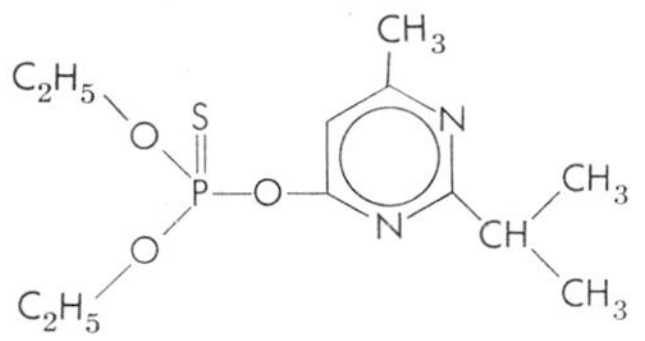 C_2H_5O, S, C_2H_5O, O–(2-isopropyl-6-methyl-4-pyrimidinyl) (P center)	Dimpylate (DIAZINON) O,O-Diethyl 2-isopropyl-6-methyl-4-pyrimidinyl phosphorothioate	Insecticide in wide use for gardening and agriculture
	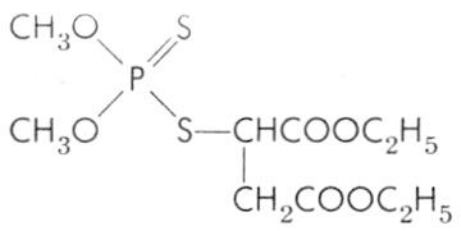 CH_3O, S, CH_3O, $S\text{--}CHCOOC_2H_5$ / $CH_2COOC_2H_5$ (P center)	Malathion (see trade names in text) O,O-Dimethyl S-(1,2-dicarbethoxyethyl) phosphorodithioate	Widely employed insecticide of greater safety than parathion or other agents because of rapid detoxication by higher organisms
D	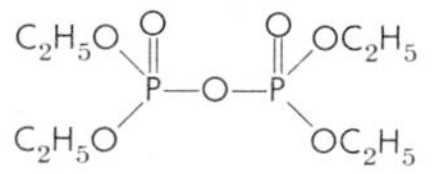 C_2H_5O, O, O, OC_2H_5 / C_2H_5O–P–O–P–OC_2H_5	TEPP Tetraethyl pyrophosphate	Early insecticide
E	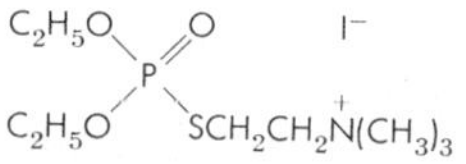 C_2H_5O, O, I^-, C_2H_5O, $SCH_2CH_2\overset{+}{N}(CH_3)_3$ (P center)	Echothiophate, Phospholine, 217MI Diethoxyphosphinylthiocholine iodide	Extremely potent choline derivative; employed in treatment of glaucoma; relatively stable in aqueous solution

* After Holmstedt, 1963. See also Hobbiger, 1976; Hayes, 1982.

115

and the responses of the corresponding effector organs to ACh (*see* Chapter 4). While this is true in the main, the diverse locations of cholinergic synapses increase the complexity of the response. Potentially, the anti-ChE agents can produce all the following effects: (1) stimulation of muscarinic receptor responses at autonomic effector organs; (2) stimulation, followed by depression or paralysis, of all autonomic ganglia and skeletal muscle (nicotinic actions); and (3) stimulation, with occasional subsequent depression, of cholinergic receptor sites (primarily muscarinic) in the CNS. Following toxic or lethal doses of anti-ChE agents, most of these effects can actually be noted (*see* below). However, with smaller doses, particularly those employed therapeutically, several modifying factors are significant. The response of effector organs also depends on whether they receive cholinergic nerve impulses continuously or phasically. Compounds such as parathion become more toxic when distributed systemically, owing to conversion to the active form, paraoxon. In general, compounds containing a quaternary ammonium group do not penetrate cell membranes readily; hence, anti-ChE agents in this category are absorbed poorly from the gastrointestinal tract and are excluded by the blood-brain barrier from exerting significant action on the CNS after moderate doses. On the other hand, such compounds act relatively selectively at the neuromuscular junctions of skeletal muscle, exerting their action both as anti-ChE agents and as direct agonists. They have comparatively less effect at autonomic effector sites; their ganglionic actions are generally intermediate. In contrast, the more lipid-soluble agents, which are uncharged at physiological pH, are well absorbed after oral administration and have ubiquitous effects at both peripheral and central cholinergic receptor sites. The lipid-soluble organophosphates are also well absorbed through the skin, and the volatile agents are readily transferred across the alveolar membrane.

The actions of anti-ChE agents on autonomic effector cells and on cortical and subcortical sites in the CNS, where the receptors are largely of the muscarinic type, are blocked by *atropine*. Likewise, atropine blocks some of the excitatory actions of anti-ChE agents on autonomic ganglia, since such agents also activate muscarinic receptors of the ganglion cells, in addition to nicotinic receptors primarily involved in ganglionic synaptic transmission (*see* Chapter 10).

The main actions of anti-ChE agents that are of therapeutic importance are concerned with the *eye*, the *intestine,* and the *skeletal neuromuscular junction;* most of the other actions are of toxicological interest.

Eye. When applied locally to the conjunctiva, anti-ChE agents cause conjunctival hyperemia and constriction of the sphincter pupillae muscle around the pupillary border of the iris (miosis) and the ciliary muscle (block of accommodation reflex and focusing to near vision). Miosis is apparent in a few minutes, becomes maximal in 0.5 hour, and lasts for several hours to days. Although the pupil may be "pinpoint" in size, it generally contracts further when exposed to light. The block of accommodation is more transient and generally disappears before termination of the miosis. Intraocular pressure usually falls concomitantly, as the result of facilitation of outflow of the aqueous humor; the reduction in tension is likely to be particularly marked in eyes in which the pressure is elevated. However, in some cases anti-ChE agents may cause a transient increase in intraocular pressure due to dilatation and engorgement of the finer blood vessels and to increased permeability of the vascular–aqueous humor barrier. (A more complete account is given below in the discussion of glaucoma.)

Gastrointestinal Tract. While the actions of various anti-ChE agents on the gastrointestinal tract are nearly identical, *neostigmine* has been studied most extensively in this regard. In man, neostigmine enhances *gastric* contractions and increases the secretion of gastric acid from the parietal cells. The drug tends to counteract the inhibition of gastric tone and motility induced by atropine, and enhances the stimulatory effect of morphine. After bilateral vagotomy, the effects of neostigmine on gastric motility are greatly reduced. The lower portion of the *esophagus* is stimulated by neostigmine; in patients with marked achalasia and dilatation of the esophagus, the drug can cause a salutary increase in tone and peristalsis.

Neostigmine augments the motor activity of the *small and large bowel;* the colon is particularly stimulated. Atony may be overcome or prevented, propulsive waves are increased in amplitude and frequency, and transport is thus promoted. The total effect of anti-ChE agents on intestinal motility probably represents a combination of actions at the ganglion cells of Auerbach's plexus and at the muscle fibers, as a result of the preservation of ACh released by the cholinergic preganglionic and postganglionic fibers, respectively.

Skeletal Neuromuscular Junction. Most of the effects of potent anti-ChE drugs on muscle fibers can be adequately explained on the basis of their inhibition of AChE at neuromuscular junctions. However, there is good evidence for an accessory component of *direct action* of neostigmine and other quaternary ammonium anti-ChE agents on skeletal muscle. For example, the intra-arterial injection of neostigmine into chronically denervated muscle, or into normally innervated muscle in which essentially all the AChE has been inactivated by prior administration of DFP, evokes an immediate contraction, whereas physostigmine does not.

Normally, a single nerve impulse in a terminal motor-axon branch liberates enough ACh to produce a localized depolarization (end-plate potential) of sufficient magnitude to initiate a propagated muscle action potential. The ACh released is rapidly hydrolyzed by AChE, such that the lifetime of free ACh within the synapse (~200 microseconds) is shorter than the decay of the end-plate potential or the refractory period of the muscle (Colquhoun, 1979). Therefore, each nerve impulse gives rise to a single wave of depolarization. After inhibition of AChE the residence time of ACh in the synapse increases, allowing for rebinding of transmitter to multiple receptors. A prolongation of the decay of the end-plate potential is observed (about threefold) due to

successive stimulation at neighboring receptors. Quanta released by individual nerve impulses are no longer isolated. This destroys the synchrony between end-plate depolarization and the development of the action potential. Consequently, asynchronous excitation and fibrillation of muscle fibers are observed. When ACh persists in the synapse, it may also depolarize the axon terminal, resulting in antidromic firing of the motoneuron; this contributes to fasciculations, which involve the entire motor unit. The effect may result from a direct action on prejunctional sites or involve release of potassium into the synapse. With sufficient inhibition of AChE, depolarization of the end-plate predominates and blockade due to depolarization ensues (*see* Chapter 11). Thus, a small dose of physostigmine or neostigmine may increase the skeletal muscle contraction produced by a single maximal nerve stimulus, but larger doses or repetitive nerve stimulation at a rapid rate results in depression or block of neuromuscular transmission.

The anti-ChE agents act as "decurarizing" drugs and will reverse the antagonism of competitive neuromuscular blocking agents. Neostigmine is not usually effective against the skeletal muscle paralysis caused by decamethonium or succinylcholine, since these agents also produce neuromuscular blockade by depolarization. However, partial reversal can often be achieved if the duration of action of succinylcholine is prolonged and phase-II block is evident (Futter *et al.*, 1983; *see* Chapter 11).

Actions at Other Sites. *Secretory glands* that are innervated by postganglionic cholinergic fibers include the bronchial, lacrimal, sweat, salivary, gastric (antral G cells and parietal cells), intestinal, and acinar pancreatic glands; low doses of anti-ChE agents cause, in general, augmentation of their secretory responses to nerve stimulation, and higher doses produce an increase in the resting rate of secretion.

Smooth muscle fibers of the bronchioles and ureters are contracted by these drugs, and the ureters may show increased peristaltic activity.

The *cardiovascular actions* of anti-ChE agents are extremely complex, since they reflect both ganglionic and postganglionic effects of accumulated ACh on the heart and blood vessels. The predominant effect on the *heart* from the peripheral action of accumulated ACh is bradycardia, resulting in a fall in cardiac output. Blood pressure is usually affected by higher doses; this is often a consequence of effects of anti-ChE agents in the CNS.

The effective refractory period of cardiac muscle fibers is shortened, and the refractory period and conduction time of the conducting tissue are increased. The *blood vessels* are in general dilated, although the coronary and pulmonary circulation may show the opposite response. The sum of the foregoing effects should result in hypotension, but at the ganglionic level ACh has first an excitatory and at higher concentrations an inhibitory action. Hence, the excitatory action on the parasympathetic ganglion cells would tend to reinforce the diminished cardiac output, whereas the opposite sequence would result from the action of ACh on sympathetic ganglion cells. Excitation followed by inhibition is also produced by ACh at the medullary vasomotor and cardiac centers. All these effects are complicated further by the hypoxemia resulting from the bronchoconstrictor and other actions of accumulated ACh on the respiratory system; this would reinforce both sympathetic tone and ACh-induced discharge of epinephrine from the adrenal medulla. Hence, it is not surprising that a wide variety of hemodynamic effects has been reported following anti-ChE agents, depending on the drug, dose, route of administration, species, and other factors.

At *autonomic ganglia,* as indicated above, low concentrations of ACh or of anti-ChE agents cause spontaneous firing of the ganglion cells in response to submaximal preganglionic stimulation. This effect results primarily from the activation of *muscarinic* receptors. The ganglionic blockade from higher concentrations of anti-ChE drugs apparently results from persistent depolarization of the cell membrane induced at the *nicotinic* receptors, which masks the preceding excitatory effect (Dolivo and Koelle, 1970; *see also* Chapter 10).

The effects of anti-ChE drugs on the CNS are likewise characterized by stimulation or facilitation at various sites, succeeded by inhibition or paralysis at higher concentrations. In the EEG, for example, the initial characteristic change noted is desynchronization, or the appearance of waves of low voltage and high frequency, probably reflecting stimulation of the ascending reticular activating system. The respiratory and other subcortical centers likewise show stimulation after low doses and depression with higher or toxic doses. Hypoxemia is probably a major factor in CNS depression that appears after large doses of anti-ChE agents. The stimulant effects are antagonized by atropine, although not as completely as are the muscarinic effects at peripheral autonomic effector sites.

Absorption, Fate, and Excretion. *Physostigmine* is readily absorbed from the gastrointestinal tract, subcutaneous tissues, and mucous membranes. The conjunctival instillation of solutions of the drug may result in systemic effects if measures (*e.g.,* pressure on inner canthus) are not taken to prevent absorption from the nasal mucosa. The alkaloid is largely destroyed in the body, mainly by hydrolytic cleavage at the ester linkage by plasma esterases; renal excretion plays only a minor role in its disposal. In man, a 1-mg dose of physostigmine injected subcutaneously is largely destroyed in 2 hours.

Neostigmine and related quaternary ammonium drugs are absorbed poorly after oral administration, such that much larger doses are needed than by the parenteral route. Whereas the effective parenteral dose of neostigmine in man is 0.5 to 2.0 mg, the equivalent oral dose may be 15 to 30 mg or more. Large oral doses may prove toxic if intestinal absorption is enhanced for any reason. Neostigmine is destroyed by plasma esterases, and the quaternary alcohol and parent compound are excreted in the urine. Pyridostigmine and its quaternary alcohol are also the predominant entities found in urine after administration of this drug to man (Somani *et al.,* 1972; Cohan *et al.,* 1976; Appendix II).

The commonly encountered *organophosphorus anti-ChE agents* are, with certain exceptions (*e.g.,* echothiophate), highly lipid-soluble liquids; many have high vapor pressures at ordinary temperatures. The less volatile agents that are commonly employed as agricultural insecticides (*e.g.,* parathion, malathion) are generally dispersed as aerosols or as dusts consisting of the organophosphorus compound adsorbed to an inert, finely particulate material. Consequently, the compounds are rapidly and effectively *absorbed* by practically all routes, including the gastrointestinal tract, as well as through the skin and mucous membranes following contact with moisture, and by the lungs after inhalation of the vapors, dusts, or aerosols.

Following their absorption, most organophosphorus compounds are *excreted* almost entirely as hydrolysis products in the urine. Plasma and tissue enzymes are responsible for hydrolysis to the corresponding phosphoric and phosphonic acids. However, *oxidative enzymes* are also involved in the metabolism of some organophosphorus compounds.

The organophosphorus anti-ChE agents are hydrolyzed in the body by a group of enzymes known as *A-esterases* or *paroxonase*. The enzymes are found in plasma and in the hepatic endoplasmic reticulum and can hydrolyze a large number of organophosphorus compounds (*e.g.,* DFP, tabun, sarin, paraoxon, TEPP) by splitting the anhydride, P—F, P—CN, or ester bond. The enzymes are not inhibited by organophosphorus compounds, presumably because the phosphorylated active site reacts rapidly with water to regenerate the free form, in contrast to its high stability in the case of the cholinesterases. Acquired resistance of insects to certain insecticides of this class results from the adaptive elaboration of such enzymes. Malathion and other organophosphorus compounds containing carboxylesters undergo hydrolysis at these ester linkages. This reaction is catalyzed by plasma esterases that can be inhibited by organophosphorus compounds. Thus, the activity and toxicity from exposure to two organophosphorus insecticides may be supra-additive (Su *et al.,* 1971; Murphy, 1985).

TOXICOLOGY

The toxicological aspects of the anti-ChE agents are of practical importance to the physician. In addition to numerous cases of accidental intoxication from the use and manufacture of organophosphorus compounds as agricultural insecticides, these agents have been employed frequently for homicidal and suicidal purposes, largely because of their accessibility. Occupational exposure is most common by the dermal and pulmonary routes, while oral ingestion is most common in cases of nonoccupational poisoning. In addition, chronic exposure to several organophosphorus com-

pounds, in particular triarylphosphates, can produce a delayed neuropathy characterized by demyelination and axonal degeneration; these effects are apparently not due to inhibition of cholinesterases but rather to inhibition of a separate enzyme, termed the *neurotoxic esterase*. It is common practice to screen for this toxicity in the evaluation of the safety of new insecticides.

Acute Intoxication. The effects of acute intoxication by anti-ChE agents are manifested by muscarinic and nicotinic signs and symptoms and, except for compounds of extremely low lipid solubility, by signs referable to the CNS. Effects may be *localized* or *generalized*. Local effects are due to the action of vapors or aerosols at their site of contact with the eyes or respiratory tract, or to the local absorption after liquid contamination of the skin or mucous membranes, including those of the gastrointestinal tract. General effects rapidly follow systemic absorption by any route; they appear most rapidly after inhalation of vapors or aerosols, where severe effects are present within a few minutes. In contrast, after gastrointestinal and percutaneous absorption, the onset of symptoms is delayed. The *duration* of effects is determined largely by the properties of the compound: its lipid solubility, whether it must be activated, the stability of the organophosphorus-AChE bond, and whether "aging" of the phosphorylated enzyme has occurred.

After *local exposure* to vapors or aerosols or after their *inhalation*, ocular and respiratory effects generally appear first. Ocular effects include marked miosis, ocular pain, conjunctival congestion, diminished vision, ciliary spasm, and brow ache. With acute systemic absorption, miosis may not be evident due to sympathetic discharge in response to the hypotension. In addition to rhinorrhea and hyperemia of the upper respiratory tract, respiratory effects consist in "tightness" in the chest and wheezing respiration, due to the combination of bronchoconstriction and increased bronchial secretion. Gastrointestinal symptoms occur earliest after *ingestion*, and include anorexia, nausea and vomiting, abdominal cramps, and diarrhea. With *percutaneous absorption* of liquid, localized sweating and muscular fasciculation in the immediate vicinity are generally the earliest manifestations.

Additional *muscarinic* effects after systemic absorption include those discussed under pharmacological properties; severe intoxication is manifested by extreme salivation, involuntary defecation and urination, sweating, lacrimation, bradycardia, and hypotension.

Nicotinic actions at the *neuromuscular junctions* of skeletal muscle usually consist in fatigability and generalized weakness, involuntary twitchings, scattered fasciculations, and eventually severe weakness and paralysis; a central component of action may contribute to some of these effects. The most serious consequence of the neuromuscular actions is paralysis of the respiratory muscles.

The broad spectrum of effects on the CNS include confusion, ataxia, slurred speech, loss of reflexes, Cheyne-Stokes respiration, generalized convulsions, coma, and central respiratory paralysis. Actions on the vasomotor and other cardiovascular centers in the medulla oblongata further complicate the hemodynamic pattern and lead to hypotension.

The *time of death* after a single acute exposure may range from less than 5 minutes to nearly 24 hours, depending upon the dose, route, agent, and other factors. The *cause of death* is primarily *respiratory failure*, usually accompanied by a secondary *cardiovascular* component. Muscarinic, nicotinic, and central actions all contribute to respiratory embarrassment; they include laryngospasm, bronchoconstriction, increased tracheobronchial and salivary secretion, compromised voluntary control of the diaphragm and intercostal muscles, and central respiratory depression. Although the blood pressure may fall to alarmingly low levels and cardiac irregularities intervene, these effects probably result as much from hypoxemia as from the specific actions mentioned, since they are often reversed by the establishment of adequate pulmonary ventilation.

Diagnosis and Treatment. The *diagnosis* of severe, acute anti-ChE intoxication is readily made from the history of exposure and the characteristic signs and symptoms. In suspected cases of milder acute or chronic intoxication, determination of the ChE activities in erythrocytes and plasma will generally establish the diagnosis. Although these values vary considerably in the normal population, they will usually be depressed well below the normal range before any symptoms due to systemic anti-ChE intoxication are evident. Such figures do not reflect with any accuracy the activities of the corresponding enzymes in the tissues, the depression of which is the basis of the toxic effects.

Treatment is both specific and highly effective. *Atropine* in sufficient dosage (*see* below) effectively antagonizes the actions at muscarinic receptor sites, including the increased tracheobronchial and salivary secretion, the bronchoconstriction, the peripheral ganglionic stimulation, and to a moderate extent the central actions. Larger doses are required to get appreciable concentrations of atropine into the CNS. Atropine is virtually without effect against the peripheral neuromuscular activation and subsequent paralysis. The last-mentioned action of the anti-ChE agents as well as all other peripheral effects can be reversed by *pralidoxime,* a cholinesterase reactivator that is discussed in detail below.

In moderate or severe anti-ChE intoxication, the recommended adult dose of pralidoxime is 1 to 2 g, infused intravenously within not less than 5 minutes. If weakness is not relieved or if it recurs after 20 minutes, the dose may be repeated. Early treatment is very important to assure that the oxime reaches the phosphorylated AChE while the latter can still be reactivated. Many of the alkylphosphates are extremely lipid soluble, and, if there has been extensive partitioning into body fat, the onset of toxicity may be delayed and symptoms may recur after initial treatment. It has been necessary to continue treatment with atropine and pralidoxime for several weeks in some cases.

In addition, certain general supportive measures may be necessary. These include (1) termination of exposure, by removal of the patient or application of a gas mask if the atmosphere is contaminated, copious washing of contaminated skin or mucous membranes with water, or gastric lavage; (2) maintenance of a patent airway, including endobronchial aspiration; (3) artificial respiration, if required; (4) administration of oxygen; (5) alleviation of persistent convulsions with diazepam (5 to 10 mg, intravenously) or sodium thiopental (2.5% solution, intravenously); and (6) treatment of shock (*see* Wills, 1970).

Atropine should be given in very large doses. Following an initial injection of 2 to 4 mg, given intravenously if possible, otherwise intramuscularly, the 2-mg dose should be repeated every 5 to 10 minutes until muscarinic symptoms disappear, and also if they reappear. As much as 50 mg may be required the first day. A mild degree of atropine block should then be maintained, by the oral administration of 1 or 2 mg at intervals of several hours, as long as symptoms are in evidence. Whereas the AChE *reactivators* can be of great benefit in the therapy of anti-ChE intoxication (*see* below), their use must be supplemented by the administration of atropine as described.

Cholinesterase Reactivators. While the phosphorylated esteratic site of AChE undergoes hydrolytic regeneration at a slow or negligible rate (Figure 6–2, upper reaction), Wilson (1951) found that nucleophilic agents, such as hydroxylamine (H_2NOH), hydroxamic acids (RCONHOH), and oximes (RCH=NOH), reactivate the enzyme more rapidly than does spontaneous hydrolysis. He reasoned that selective reactivation could be achieved by a site-directed nucleophil, wherein interaction of a quaternary nitrogen with the negative subsite of the active center would place the nucleophil in close apposition to the phosphorus. This goal was achieved to a remarkable degree by Wilson and Ginsburg (1955) with pyridine-2-aldoxime methyl chloride (2-PAM, 2-formyl-1-methyl-

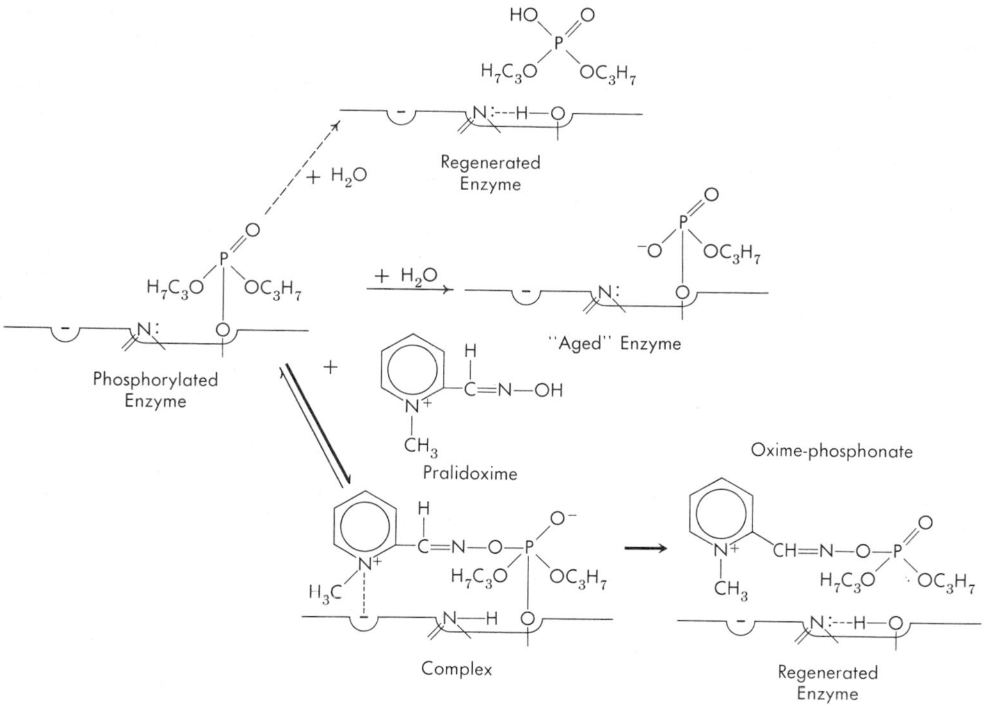

Figure 6–2. *Reactivation of alkylphosphorylated acetylcholinesterase (AChE).*

Following alkylphosphorylation of AChE by DFP (at left), spontaneous hydrolytic reactivation occurs at a slow rate (upper reaction), as indicated by the dashed arrow. "Aging" is the loss of one of the isopropoxy residues; the product is very resistant to hydrolysis and regeneration by pralidoxime. Pralidoxime (in lower reaction) combines with the anionic site by electrostatic attraction of its quaternary N atom, which orients the nucleophilic oxime group to react with the electrophilic P atom; the oxime-phosphonate is split off, leaving the regenerated enzyme. (Modified from Wilson, 1959; Froede and Wilson, 1971; Aldridge, 1976.)

pyridinium chloride oxime, *pralidoxime;* Figure 6–2); reactivation with this compound occurs at a million times the rate of that with hydroxylamine. The oxime is oriented proximally to exert a nucleophilic attack on the phosphorus; the oxime-phosphonate is then split off, leaving the regenerated enzyme (Figure 6–2, lower reaction) (Wilson, 1959).

A number of *bis*-quaternary oximes were subsequently shown to be even more potent as reactivators; an example is *obidoxime chloride* (Hobbiger and Vojvodić, 1966), the structure of which follows:

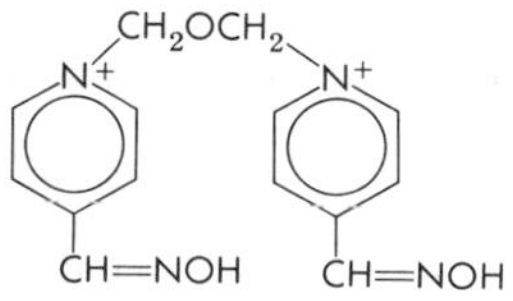

Obidoxime

Several such compounds appear to be more effective than pralidoxime as antidotes for nerve gas poisoning (*see* below; Ellin, 1982).

The velocity of reactivation of phosphorylated AChE by pralidoxime varies with the nature of the phosphoryl group, and in general follows the same sequence as the order for spontaneous hydrolytic reactivation, that is, dimethylphosphoryl-AChE > diethylphosphoryl-AChE > di*iso*propyl-phosphoryl-AChE, and so forth. Furthermore, phosphorylated AChE can undergo a fairly rapid process of "aging," so that within the course of minutes or hours it becomes completely resistant to the reactivators. The "aging" is probably due to the loss of one alkyl or alkoxy group, leaving a much more stable monoalkyl- or monoalkoxy-phosphoryl-AChE (Fleisher and Harris, 1965) (*see* Figure 6–2). Phosphonates containing tertiary alkoxy groups are more prone to "aging" than are the secondary or primary congeners (Aldridge, 1976). The oximes are not effective in antagonizing the toxicity of the carbamyl ester inhibitors, and, since pralidoxime itself has weak anti-ChE activity, *they are contraindicated in the treatment of overdosage with neostigmine or physostigmine or poisoning with carbaril* (Hayes, 1982; Murphy, 1985).

Pharmacology, Toxicology, and Disposition. The reactivating action of oximes and hydroxamic acids *in vivo* is most marked at the skeletal neuromuscular junction. Following a dose of an organophosphorus compound that produces total blockade of transmission, the intravenous injection of an oxime can restore the response to stimulation of the motor nerve within a few minutes. Antidotal effects are less striking at autonomic effector sites and insignificant in the CNS.

High doses of pralidoxime and related compounds can in themselves cause neuromuscular blockade and other effects, including inhibition of AChE; such actions are minimal at the doses recommended for clinical use, 1 to 2 g intravenously. If pralidoxime is injected intravenously at a rate more rapid than 500 mg per minute, it can cause mild weakness, blurred vision, diplopia, dizziness, headache, nausea, and tachycardia.

The oximes as a group are largely metabolized by the liver, and the breakdown products are excreted by the kidney.

Chronic Neurotoxicity of Organophosphorus Compounds. Certain fluorine-containing alkylorganophosphorus anti-ChE agents (*e.g.,* DFP, mipafox) have in common with the triarylphosphates, of which triorthocresylphosphate (TOCP) is the classical example, the property of inducing delayed neurotoxicity. This syndrome first received widespread attention following the demonstration that TOCP, an adulterant of Jamaica ginger, was responsible for an outbreak of thousands of cases of paralysis that occurred in the United States during prohibition.

The *clinical picture* is that of a severe polyneuritis that begins several days after exposure to a sufficient single or cumulative amount of the toxic compound. It is manifested initially by mild sensory disturbances, ataxia, weakness, and ready fatigability of the legs, accompanied by reduced tendon reflexes and the presence of muscle twitching, fasciculation, and tenderness to palpation. In severe cases, the weakness may progress eventually to complete flaccid paralysis that, over the course of weeks or months, is often succeeded by a spastic paralysis with a concomitant exaggeration of reflexes. During these phases, the muscles show marked wasting. Recovery may require 2 or more years.

Certain triarylphosphates and fluorine-containing alkylphosphates have the greatest propensity to produce the characteristic neurotoxic pattern, clinically and experimentally. Accordingly, it does not seem to be dependent upon inhibition of AChE or other cholinesterases. The *pathological lesion*, studied most thoroughly in the chicken, is characterized by *axonal* swelling, segmentation, and eventual breakdown into granular debris; the marked *demyelination* is probably secondary to the aforementioned axonal changes. Increasing evidence points to inhibition of a different esterase, termed a neurotoxic esterase, as being linked to the lesions (Abou-Donia, 1981; Johnson, 1982). Aging of the esterase-alkylphosphate conjugate in a manner similar to that described for AChE may be required for the genesis of the disease. No specific therapy is known. Experimental myopathies that result in generalized necrotic lesions and changes in end-plate cytostructure are also found after chronic treatment with organophosphates (Laskowski and Dettbarn, 1977).

PREPARATIONS

The compounds described here are those commonly used as anti-ChE drugs and cholinesterase reactivators in the United States. *Conventional dosages* and *routes of administration* are given in the discussion of therapeutic applications of these agents (*see* below).

Physostigmine salicylate (ANTILIRIUM) injection contains 1-mg amounts in 1-ml syringes. *Physostigmine sulfate ophthalmic ointment* (0.25%) and *physostigmine salicylate ophthalmic solution* (0.25% and 0.5%) are also available.

Neostigmine bromide (PROSTIGMIN) is available for *oral* use in 15-mg tablets. *Neostigmine methylsulfate* (PROSTIGMIN) is marketed for *parenteral* injection in sterile solution in ampuls and vials containing 0.25, 0.5, or 1.0 mg/ml.

Ambenonium chloride (MYTELASE) is available for *oral* use in 10-mg tablets.

Pyridostigmine bromide (MESTINON) is available for *oral* use in 60-mg tablets, in 180-mg sustained-release tablets, and in a syrup that contains 12 mg/ml, as well as in an *injectable* form that contains 5 mg/ml in 2-ml ampuls.

Edrophonium chloride (TENSILON) is marketed for *parenteral* injection in ampuls and vials containing 10 mg/ml.

Demecarium bromide ophthalmic solution (HUMORSOL) is available in concentrations of 0.125 and 0.25%.

Echothiophate iodide for ophthalmic solution (PHOSPHOLINE IODIDE) is marketed as a powder in 1.5-, 3.0-, 6.25-, and 12.5-mg amounts. Solutions of appropriate strength must be freshly prepared in a diluent supplied by the manufacturer. Once prepared, the solution is stable for about 6 months if kept refrigerated. The powder must not be applied to the eye.

Isoflurophate ophthalmic ointment (FLOROPRYL) contains 0.025% isoflurophate (di*iso*propyl phosphorofluoridate, DFP) in an anhydrous vehicle.

Malathion lotion (PRIODERM LOTION) contains 0.5% *malathion* in isopropyl alcohol for treatment of head lice. It is pediculicidal and ovicidal. A single treatment is usually sufficient to eradicate the infestation.

Pralidoxime chloride (PROTOPAM CHLORIDE) is the only AChE reactivator currently available for general use in the United States. It is dispensed in vials in sterile, 1-g amounts for extemporaneous solution in 20 ml of sterile water. It is also marketed in 500-mg tablets.

Other reactivators of AChE not currently available in the United States include *obidoxime chloride* (TOXOGENIN), its analog *trimedoxime bromide* (TMB-4), and *diacetyl monoxime* (*see* Ellin, 1982). *Obidoxime* is more potent than pralidoxime; the recommended dose is 3 to 6 mg/kg, injected intravenously over 5 to 10 minutes. The dose of *diacetyl monoxime* is 1 g, injected intravenously at a rate of 200 mg per minute; unlike pralidoxime or obidoxime, it penetrates the blood-brain barrier and reactivates AChE in the CNS. Both drugs can also be repeated in the same doses after 20 minutes.

THERAPEUTIC USES

Although anti-ChE agents have been recommended for the treatment of a wide variety of conditions, their superiority to other drugs and widespread acceptability have been established mainly in four areas: *atony of the smooth muscle of the intestinal tract and urinary bladder, glaucoma, myasthenia gravis,* and *termination of the effects of competitive neuromuscular blocking drugs.* In these conditions, certain anti-ChE agents can be recommended as the drugs of choice; other classes of drugs may sometimes be indicated as adjuncts or in preference to the anti-ChE agents. *Physostigmine* is also useful in the treatment of *atropine intoxication* (*see* below) and of poisoning with *phenothiazines* and *tricyclic antidepressants* (Chapter 19). *Edrophonium* can be used for terminating attacks of *paroxysmal supraventricular tachycardia.*

Paralytic Ileus and Atony of the Urinary Bladder. In the treatment of both these conditions, *neostigmine* is generally the most satisfactory of the anti-ChE agents. The direct parasympathomimetic agents, discussed in Chapter 5, are employed for the same purposes.

Neostigmine is used for the relief of *abdominal distention* from a variety of medical and surgical causes. The usual subcutaneous dose of neostigmine methylsulfate for postoperative paralytic ileus is 0.5 to 1.0 mg. Peristaltic activity commences in 10 to 30 minutes after parenteral administration, whereas 2 to 4 hours is required after oral administration of neostigmine bromide (15 mg). A rectal tube should be inserted to facilitate expulsion of gas, and it may be necessary to assist evacuation with a small low enema. The drug should not be used when there is mechanical obstruction of the intestine or urinary bladder, when peritonitis is present, or when the viability of the bowel is doubtful. Other supportive measures include intubation and suction as well as appropriate therapy with fluids and electrolytes. Indeed, neostigmine and other drugs are to be viewed mainly as adjuvant agents in the treatment of distention. The drug is not likely to be helpful in relieving atony of the stomach or upper gastrointestinal tract after vagotomy.

When neostigmine is employed for the treatment of atony of the detrusor muscle of the *urinary bladder,* postoperative dysuria is relieved and the time interval between operation and spontaneous urination is shortened. The drug is used in the same dose and manner as in the management of paralytic ileus.

Glaucoma. Glaucoma is a disease complex characterized chiefly by an increase in intraocular pressure that, if sufficiently high and persistent, leads to damage to the optic disc at the juncture of the optic nerve and the retina; this can cause irreversible blindness. Of the three types—primary, secondary, and congenital—anti-ChE agents are of great value in the management of the primary as well as of certain categories of the secondary type (*e.g.,* aphakic glaucoma, following cataract extraction); the congenital type rarely responds to therapy other than surgical treatment. Primary glaucoma is subdivided into narrow-angle (acute congestive) and wide-angle (chronic simple) types, based on the configuration of the angle of the anterior chamber where reabsorption of the aqueous humor occurs. Anti-ChE agents produce a fall in intraocular pressure in both types of primary glaucoma, chiefly by lowering the resistance to outflow of the aqueous humor. Effects on the volumes of the various intraocular vascular beds (*e.g.,* those of the iris, ciliary body, *etc.*) and on the rate of secretion of the aqueous humor into the posterior chamber may contribute secondarily to the lowering of pressure, or conversely may produce a rise in pressure preceding the fall. In narrow-angle glaucoma, the aqueous outflow is facilitated by the freeing of the entrance to the trabecular space at the canal of Schlemm from blockade by the iris, as the result of the drug-induced contraction of the sphincter muscle of the iris.

In wide-angle, or chronic simple, glaucoma, there is no physical obstruction to the entry to the trabeculae; rather, the trabeculae, which are a meshwork of pores of small diameter, lose their patency. In this circumstance, contraction of the sphincter muscle of the iris and the ciliary muscle enhances tone and alignment of the trabecular network to improve resorption and outflow of aqueous humor through the network to the canal of Schlemm (*see* reviews by Watson, 1972; Schwartz, 1978; Kaufman *et al.,* 1984).

The foregoing distinctions are of great importance for therapy, since the roles of miotic drugs, including the anti-ChE agents, are quite different in the management of the two types of primary glaucoma. Acute congestive (narrow-angle) glaucoma is nearly always a medical emergency in which the drugs are essential in controlling the acute attack, but the long-range management is usually based predominantly on surgery (*e.g.*, peripheral or complete iridectomy). Chronic simple (wide-angle) glaucoma, on the other hand, has a gradual, insidious onset and is not generally amenable to surgical improvement; in this type, control of intraocular pressure is usually dependent upon drug therapy on a permanent basis.

Acute congestive glaucoma may be precipitated by the injudicious use of a mydriatic agent in patients over 40, or by a variety of factors that can cause pupillary dilatation or engorgement of intraocular vessels. The cardinal signs and symptoms include marked ocular inflammation, a semidilated pupil, severe pain, and nausea. Every effort must be made to reduce the intraocular pressure to the normal level and maintain it there for the duration of the attack. In general, an anti-ChE agent is instilled in the conjunctival sac in combination with a parasympathomimetic agent for greatest effectiveness. One such combination that is frequently employed is a solution of *physostigmine salicylate*, 0.5%, plus *pilocarpine nitrate*, 4%. This combination should be instilled six times at 10-minute intervals, then three times at 30-minute intervals, and thereafter as required. *Adjunctive therapy* should include the intravenous administration of a carbonic anhydrase inhibitor, such as *acetazolamide*, to reduce the secretion of aqueous humor, or of an osmotic agent, such as *mannitol* or *glycerin*, to induce intraocular dehydration. The long-acting organophosphorus compounds are not indicated in narrow-angle glaucoma because of vascular engorgement and an increase in the angle block.

Chronic simple glaucoma and *secondary glaucoma* require careful consideration of the needs of the individual patient in selecting the drug or combination of drugs to be employed. The choices available include (1) parasympathomimetic agents (*e.g., pilocarpine nitrate*, 0.5 to 6%; *see* Chapter 5); (2) anti-ChE agents that are short acting (*e.g., physostigmine salicylate*, 0.25 and 0.5%) or long acting (*demecarium bromide*, 0.125 to 0.25%; *echothiophate iodide*, 0.03 to 0.25%; *isoflurophate*, 0.025%); (3) β-adrenergic antagonists such as *timolol maleate* (*see* Chapter 9), a long-acting agent that is administered at 12-hour intervals, does not directly affect pupillary aperture but reduces production of aqueous humor (Boger *et al.*, 1978; Lotti *et al.*, 1984), and avoids the partial block of accommodation and the untoward effects of the long-acting anti-ChE agents; and paradoxically (4) sympathomimetic agents (*e.g., epinephrine*, 0.25 to 2%; *phenylephrine*, 10%; *see* Chapter 8). Drugs of the last-mentioned class are often most effective when used in combination with AChE inhibitors or cholinergic agonists. They reduce intraocular pressure by decreasing secretion of aqueous humor, and they prevent engorgement of small blood vessels.

Since the cholinergic agonists and cholinesterase inhibitors block accommodation, these agents produce transient blurring of far vision. The block of accommodation usually occurs after administration of relatively high doses and is of shorter duration. With long-term administration of the cholinergic agonists and anti-ChE agents, the response diminishes; this, in part, is a consequence of a diminished number of receptors for ACh.

Despite the convenience of less frequent administration and the high potency of long-acting anti-ChE agents, their use entails a greater risk of development of lenticular opacities and untoward autonomic effects (*see* below). Of the organophosphorus agents, *DFP* has the longest duration of action and is extremely potent when applied locally; solutions in peanut or sesame oil require instillation from once daily to once weekly, and may control intraocular pressure in severe cases that are resistant to other drugs. The oily vehicle is unpleasant to most patients. Consequently, DFP has largely been replaced by echothiophate.

Anti-ChE agents have been employed locally in the treatment of a variety of other ophthalmological conditions, including accommodative esotropia and myasthenia gravis confined to the extraocular and eyelid muscles. *Adie* (or tonic pupil) *syndrome* results from dysfunction of the ciliary body, perhaps because of local nerve degeneration. Low concentrations of physostigmine are reported to decrease the blurred vision and pain associated with this condition (Wirtschafter and Herman, 1980). In alternation with a mydriatic drug such as atropine, short-acting anti-ChE agents have proven useful for the breaking of adhesions between the iris and the lens or cornea. (For a complete account of the use of anti-ChE agents in ocular therapy, *see* Havener, 1983; Kaufman *et al.*, 1984.)

Untoward Effects. Treatment of glaucoma with potent, long-acting anti-ChE agents (including demecarium, echothiophate, and isoflurophate) for 6 months or longer carries a high risk of the development of a specific type of *cataract*, which begins as anterior subcapsular vacuoles (Axelsson and Holmberg, 1966; de Roetth, 1966; Shaffer and Hetherington, 1966). Although formation of spontaneous cataracts is quite common within comparable age groups, the incidence of lenticular opacities under such circumstances can be as high as 50%; the hazard is apparently increased in proportion to the strength of the solution, frequency of instillation, duration of therapy, and age of the patient. The underlying mechanism remains elusive (*see* Laties, 1969; Kaufman *et al.*, 1984).

Most of the studies that have implicated the long-acting anti-ChE agents in the formation of cataracts have been retrospective and uncontrolled. The reported incidence of cataracts attributable to such drugs may thus be distorted by selection of patients with more severe glaucoma; nevertheless, cataractogenesis should be considered when therapeutic decisions are made. Long-acting anti-ChE agents are, of course, not indicated when glaucoma can be controlled by timolol, parasympathomimetic drugs, physostigmine, or other agents. Since glaucoma leads to irreversible blindness if not adequately controlled, the long-acting cholinesterase inhibitors retain their therapeutic importance in situations where other agents are inadequate.

Treatment with *pilocarpine* (4%), alone or in combination with *physostigmine* (0.2%), one to five times daily, was found to entail no higher incidence of the development of lenticular opacities than appeared spontaneously in untreated patients in comparable age groups (Axelsson, 1969). At present, it seems clear that pilocarpine and other shorter-acting miotic drugs should be employed as long as they provide adequate control of intraocular tension. If they fail to do so, the hazards of cataract development must be balanced against those of increased intraocular pressure before resorting to the use of the potent, long-acting anti-ChE agents. When such drugs are used, patients should be examined for the appearance of lenticular opacities at intervals of 6 months or less.

Miscellaneous ocular side effects that may occur following local instillation of anti-ChE agents are headache, brow pain, blurred vision, phacodinesis, pericorneal injection, congestive iritis, various allergic reactions, and, rarely, retinal detachment. When anti-ChE drugs are instilled intraconjunctivally at frequent intervals, sufficient absorption may occur to produce various systemic effects, which result from inhibition of AChE and butyryl-ChE. Hence, cholinergic autonomic function will be augmented, the duration of action of local anesthetics with an ester linkage will be prolonged (*see* Chapter 15), and the neuromuscular blockade produced by succinylcholine will be enhanced and prolonged (*see* Chapter 11). Individuals with vagotonia and allergies are at particular risk. Systemic absorption of the drug can be minimized by digital compression of the inner canthus of the eye during and for a short period following its instillation.

Myasthenia Gravis. Myasthenia gravis is a neuromuscular disease characterized by weakness and marked fatigability of skeletal muscle (*see* Drachman, 1978; Grob, 1981); exacerbations and partial remissions occur frequently. Its clinical manifestations were described before the turn of the century (Jolly, 1895; Campbell and Bramwell, 1900). Jolly noted the similarity between the symptoms of myasthenia gravis and curare poisoning in animals and suggested that *physostigmine*, an agent then known to antagonize curare, might be of therapeutic value. Forty years elapsed before his suggestion was given systematic trial (Walker, 1934). Remen (1932) and Walker (1935) independently showed *neostigmine* to be useful in the management of the disease, and, although *pyridostigmine* is also frequently employed today, neostigmine remains a standard for comparison of new agents.

The defect in myasthenia gravis is in synaptic transmission at the neuromuscular junction. When a motor nerve of a normal subject is stimulated at 25 Hz, electrical and mechanical responses are well sustained. A suitable margin of safety exists for maintenance of neuromuscular transmission. Initial responses in the myasthenic patient may be normal, but they diminish rapidly, which explains the difficulty experienced by the patient in maintaining voluntary muscle activity for more than brief periods. When the patient is given an appropriate dose of neostigmine, the response to tetanic stimulation is improved, along with symptomatic improvement in muscle strength. The same dose of neostigmine in control subjects leads to a *reduced* response to tetanic stimulation, accompanied by fasciculations, local weakness, and repetitive action potentials in response to a single stimulus. Elmqvist and coworkers (1964) observed that the amplitude of miniature end-plate potentials was reduced in patients with myasthenia gravis and, since they were unable to demonstrate a reduction of receptor sensitivity, postulated that the change was due to a reduction in the number of ACh molecules per quantum. However, Simpson had proposed in 1960 that the disease was a consequence of an autoimmune response to the nicotinic receptor for ACh. The relative importance of prejunctional and postjunctional defects was a matter of considerable debate until Patrick and Lindstrom (1973) found that rabbits immunized with the nicotinic receptor purified from electric eels slowly developed muscular weakness and respiratory difficulties that resembled the symptoms of myasthenia gravis. The rabbits also exhibited decremental responses following repetitive nerve stimulation, enhanced sensitivity to curare, and symptomatic and electrophysiological improvement of neuromuscular transmission following administration of anti-ChE agents. Although this *experimental allergic myasthenia gravis* and the naturally occurring disease differ somewhat, particularly in the marked acute phase of the experimental condition, this critical development of an animal model prompted intense investigation into whether the natural disease represented an autoimmune response directed toward the ACh receptor. Antireceptor antibody was soon identified in patients with myasthenia gravis (Almon *et al.*, 1974). Receptor-binding antibody has been detected in sera of 80 to 90% of patients with myasthenia gravis, although the clinical status of the patients does not correlate precisely with the antibody titer (Lindstrom *et al.*, 1976; Drachman *et al.*, 1982). Passive transfer of antibody, by use of an immunoglobulin fraction prepared from myasthenic patients, produces the myasthenic syndrome in recipient animals (Toyka *et al.*, 1975). By use of the snake α-neurotoxins that bind with high affinity to the nicotinic receptor (*see* Chapter 11), Fambrough and associates (1973) were able to detect a 70 to 90% reduction in the number of receptors per end-plate in myasthenic patients. This finding provided crucial support for the hypothesis that a decrease in receptors in the postsynaptic membrane accounts for the defects of the disease.

The picture that emerges is that myasthenia gravis is caused by an autoimmune response to the ACh receptor at the postjunctional end-plate. Antibodies, which are also present in plasma, reduce the number of receptors detectable either by toxin-binding assays or by electrophysiological measurements of ACh sensitivity (Drachman, 1978). The autoimmune reaction enhances receptor degradation (Drachman *et al.*, 1982). Immune complexes have been detected at the postsynaptic membrane, along with marked ultrastructural abnormalities in the synaptic cleft (Engel *et al.*, 1977). The latter appear to be a consequence of complement-mediated lysis of junctional folds in the end-plate.

Diagnosis. Although the diagnosis can usually be made from the history, signs, and symptoms, its differentiation from certain neurasthenic, infectious, endocrine, neoplastic, and degenerative neuromuscular diseases may be difficult. However, myasthenia gravis is the only condition in which the aforementioned deficiencies can be improved dramatically by anti-ChE medication. The *edrophonium test* is performed by injecting intravenously 2 mg of edrophonium chloride, followed 45 seconds later by an additional 8 mg if the first dose is without effect; a positive response consists of brief improvement in strength, unaccompanied by lingual fasciculation (which generally occurs in nonmyasthenic patients).

An excessive dose of an anti-ChE drug results in a *cholinergic crisis*. The condition is characterized by weakness resulting from generalized depolarization of the motor end-plate; other features result from overstimulation of muscarinic receptors. The weakness resulting from depolarization block may closely resemble *myasthenic weakness*, which is due to insufficient anti-ChE medication. The distinction is of obvious practical importance, since the former is treated by withholding, and the latter by administering, the anti-ChE agent. When the edrophonium test is performed cautiously, limiting the dose to 1 or 2 mg, and with facilities for respiratory resuscitation immediately available, a further decrease in strength indicates cholinergic crisis, while improvement signifies myasthenic weakness. *Atropine sulfate,* 0.6 mg or more intravenously, should be given immediately if a severe muscarinic reaction ensues (for complete details, *see* Osserman and Genkins, 1966; Osserman *et al.*, 1972).

Although a provocative test with 0.1 to 0.5 mg of *d*-tubocurarine to elicit muscular weakness has been used to confirm the diagnosis, it is potentially hazardous. The quantitation of antireceptor antibodies in muscle biopsies or plasma is now widely employed.

Treatment. Neostigmine, pyridostigmine, and *ambenonium* are the standard anti-ChE drugs used in the symptomatic treatment of myasthenia gravis. All can increase the response of myasthenic muscle to repetitive nerve impulses, primarily by the preservation of endogenous ACh; receptors over a greater cross-sectional area of the end-plate are then presumably exposed to concentrations of ACh that are sufficient for stimulation.

When the diagnosis of myasthenia gravis has been established, the optimal single oral dose of an anti-ChE agent can be determined by either of two empirical methods involving oral or intravenous titration.

In the oral test, baseline recordings are made of grip strength, vital capacity, and a number of signs and symptoms that reflect the strength of various muscle groups. The patient is then given an oral dose of neostigmine (7.5 mg), pyridostigmine (30 mg), or ambenonium (2.5 mg). The improvement in muscle strength and changes in other signs and symptoms are noted at frequent intervals until there is a return to the basal state. After an hour or longer in the basal state, the drug is given again with the dose increased to one and one-half times the initial amount, and the same observations are repeated. This sequence is continued, with increasing increments of one half the initial dose, until the optimal response is obtained. The result can be confirmed by the *edrophonium test.* If the dose of the longer-acting anti-ChE agent was insufficient, a further improvement in muscle strength will result. If the dose was adequate or excessive, no further change or a reduction in muscle strength will be evident. The optimal single oral dose may range from the initial doses given above to more than ten times these amounts.

Alternatively, dosage can be optimized by recording the above parameters before and following the intravenous injection of successive, small increments of neostigmine (0.125 mg) or pyridostigmine (0.5 mg), at intervals of a few minutes (Osserman *et al.*, 1972). Prior to injection of the anti-ChE agent, the patient is given an intravenous injection of 0.4 to 0.6 mg of atropine to prevent muscarinic side effects. When the optimal total intravenous dose has been established, and confirmed by the edrophonium test, the optimal single oral dose is estimated as approximately 30 times that amount.

The duration of action of these drugs is such that the interval between oral doses required to maintain a reasonably even level of strength is usually 2 to 4 hours for neostigmine and 3 to 6 hours for pyridostigmine or ambenonium. However, the amount required may vary from day to day, and physical or emotional stress, intercurrent infections, and menstruation usually necessitate an increase in the frequency or size of the dose. In addition, unpredictable exacerbations and remissions of the myasthenic state may require adjustment of the dosage upward or downward. Although all patients with myasthenia gravis should be seen by a physician at regular intervals, most can be taught to modify their dosage regimens according to their changing requirements. *Pyridostigmine* is available in sustained-release tablets containing a total of 180 mg, of which 60 mg is released immediately and 120 mg over several hours; this preparation should be limited to use at bedtime and is of value in maintaining patients for 6- to 8-hour periods. Muscarinic cardiovascular and gastrointestinal side effects of anti-ChE agents can generally be controlled by atropine or other anticholinergic drugs (Chapter 7). However, it should be recognized that anticholinergics mask the side effects of an excessive dose of anticholinesterase. Many patients learn to titrate dosage by symptomatic improvement of muscle function and development of side effects. In most patients, tolerance is developed eventually to the muscarinic effects, so that anticholinergic medication is not necessary. A number of drugs, including curariform agents and certain antibiotics and general anesthetics, interfere with neuromuscular transmission (*see* Chapter 11); their administration to patients with myasthenia gravis is hazardous without proper adjustment of anti-ChE dosage and other appropriate precautions. Parenteral administration of the standard anti-ChE agents is sometimes required in desperately ill myasthenic patients who do not respond adequately to oral medication.

In cases where administration of anti-ChE agents at optimal doses is not sufficient to enable near-normal motor activity, other therapeutic measures must be considered. Controlled studies reveal that *corticosteroids* promote clinical improvement in a high percentage of patients (Engel, 1976; Howard *et al.*, 1976). However, when treatment with steroids is continued over a prolonged period, a high incidence of undesirable side effects may result (*see* Chapter 63). Gradual lowering of maintenance doses and alternate-day regimens of short-acting steroids are used as means for minimizing side effects (Howard *et al.*, 1976). In addition, initiation of steroid treatment augments muscle weakness; however, as the patient improves with continued administration of steroids, doses of anti-ChE drugs can be reduced (Drachman, 1978). The immunosuppressive activity of corticosteroids is likely of primary importance, since antireceptor activity is diminished in circulating lymphocytes following such treatment (Abramsky *et al.*, 1975).

Thymectomy should be considered in myasthenia associated with a thymoma or when the disease is not adequately controlled by anti-ChE agents and steroids. An improved prognosis following thymectomy is likely, and apparent remissions have been observed in some cases (Buckingham *et al.*, 1976). However, the relative risks and benefits of the surgical procedure versus anti-ChE and corticosteroid treatment requires careful assessment in each case (McQuillen and Leone, 1977; Rowland, 1980; Grob, 1981). Since the thymus contains myoid cells and a predominance of patients have thymic abnormalities, it has been suggested that the disease arises in this tissue (*see* Drachman, 1978); however, the thymus is not required for perpetuation of the condition.

In keeping with the presumed autoimmune etiology of myasthenia gravis, *plasmapheresis* has been performed with beneficial results in patients who have remained disabled despite thymectomy and treatment with steroids and anti-ChE agents (Dau, 1981). The treatment seems most effective when coupled with steroids or other immunosuppressive agents. Improvement in muscle strength correlates with the reduction of the titer of antibody directed against the cholinergic nicotinic receptor.

Intoxication by Anticholinergic Drugs. Many of the peripheral and central effects of poisoning by atropine and related antimuscarinic drugs (Chapter 7) can be reversed by intravenous injection of physostigmine. Many other drugs, such as the phenothiazines, antihistamines, tricyclic antidepressants, and benzquinamide, have central, as well as peripheral, anticholinergic activity, and *physostigmine salicylate* may be useful in reversing the central anticholinergic syndrome and the cardiac arrhythmias produced by overdosage or an unusual reaction to these drugs (Aquilonius, 1977; Nilsson, 1982). The effectiveness of physostigmine as an antidote for those agents that have anticholinergic activity has been clearly documented. An initial intravenous dose of 0.5 to 2 mg of physostigmine is indicated, with additional increments given as necessary. Physostigmine, a tertiary amine, crosses the blood-brain barrier in contrast to the quaternary anti-AChE drugs. The use of anti-ChE agents to reverse the effects of competitive neuromuscular blocking agents is discussed in Chapter 11.

Alzheimer's Disease. A deficiency of functional cholinergic neurons has been observed by several groups in patients with progressive dementia of the Alzheimer type. Physostigmine has been employed in the earlier stages of the disease to improve memory. Results have been variable, although some investigators have employed dosage schedules that appear to cause transient improvement (*see* Thai *et al.*, 1983). More extensive analyses over longer periods will be necessary to establish the efficacy of such regimens.

Abramsky, O.; Aharonov, A.; Teitelbaum, D.; and Fuchs, S. Myasthenia gravis and the acetylcholine receptor: effect of steroids in the clinical course and cellular immune response to acetylcholine receptor. *Arch. Neurol.*, **1975**, *32*, 684–687.

Almon, R. R.; Andrew, C. G.; and Appel, S. H. Serum globulin in myasthenia gravis: inhibition of α-bungarotoxin binding to acetylcholine receptors. *Science*, **1974**, *186*, 55–57.

Argyll-Robertson, D. The Calabar bean as a new agent in ophthalmic practice. *Edinb. Med. J.*, **1863**, *8*, 815–820.

Axelsson, U. Glaucoma miotic therapy and cataract. *Acta Ophthalmol. (Kbh.)*, **1969**, Suppl. 102, 1–37.

Axelsson, U., and Holmberg, A. The frequency of cataract after miotic therapy. *Acta Ophthalmol. (Kbh.)*, **1966**, *44*, 421–429.

Boger, W.; Steinert, R.; Puliafito, C.; and Pavah-Langston, D. Clinical trial comparing timolol ophthalmic solution in patients with open angle glaucoma. *Am. J. Ophthalmol.*, **1978**, *86*, 8–18.

Buckingham, J. M.; Howard, F. M.; Bernatz, P. E.; Payne, W. S.; Harrison, E. G.; O'Brien, P. C.; and Weiland, L. H. The value of thymectomy in myasthenia gravis. *Ann. Surg.*, **1976**, *184*, 543–548.

Campbell, H., and Bramwell, E. Myasthenia gravis. *Brain*, **1900**, *23*, 277–336.

Cartaud, J.; Reiger, F.; Bon, S.; and Massoulié, J. Fine structure of electric eel acetylcholinesterase. *Brain Res.*, **1975**, *88*, 127–130.

Christioson, R. On the properties of the ordeal bean of Old Calabar. *Mon. J. Med. (Lond.)*, **1855**, *20*, 193–204.

Cohan, S. L.; Pohlmann, J. L. W.; Mikszewki, J.; and O'Doherty, D. S. The pharmacokinetics of pyridostigmine. *Neurology (Minneap.)*, **1976**, *26*, 536–539.

Dau, P. C. Response to plasmapheresis and immunosuppressive drug therapy in sixty myasthenia gravis patients. *Ann. N.Y. Acad. Sci.*, **1981**, *377*, 700–708.

de Roeth, A., Jr. Lenticular opacities in glaucoma patients receiving echothiophate iodide therapy. *J.A.M.A.*, **1966**, *195*, 664–666.

Dolivo, M., and Koelle, G. B. Properties of nicotinic and muscarinic receptors in isolated rat ganglia. *Experientia*, **1970**, *26*, 679.

Drachman, D. B.; Adams, R. N.; Josifek, L. F.; and Self, S. G. Functional activities of autoantibodies to acetylcholine receptors and the clinical severity of myasthenia gravis. *N. Engl. J. Med.*, **1982**, *307*, 769–775.

Elmqvist, D.; Hoffman, W. W.; Kugelberg, J.; and Quastel, D. M. J. An electrophysiological investigation of neuromuscular transmission in myasthenia gravis. *J. Physiol. (Lond.)*, **1964**, *174*, 417–434.

Engel, A. G.; Lambert, E. H.; and Howard, F. M., Jr. Immune complexes (IgG and C3) at the motor endplate in myasthenia gravis. *Mayo Clin. Proc.*, **1977**, *52*, 267–280.

Engel, W. K. Myasthenia gravis: corticosteroids and anticholinesterases. *Ann. N.Y. Acad. Sci.*, **1976**, *274*, 623–630.

Fambrough, D. M.; Drachman, D. B.; and Satyamurti, S. Neuromuscular junction in myasthenia gravis; decreased acetylcholine receptors. *Science*, **1973**, *182*, 293–295.

Fleisher, J. H., and Harris, L. W. Dealkylation as a mechanism for aging of cholinesterase after poisoning with pinacolyl methylphosphonofluoridate. *Biochem. Pharmacol.*, **1965**, *14*, 641–650.

Fraser, T. R. On the characters, actions and therapeutical uses of the ordeal bean of Calabar (*Physostigma venenosum*, Balfour). *Edinb. Med. J.*, **1863**, *9*, 36–56, 123–132, 235–248.

Futter, M. E.; Donati, F.; Sodikor, A. S.; and Bevan, D. R. Neostigmine antagonism of succinylcholine phase II block: a comparison with pancuronium. *Can. Anaesth. Soc. J.*, **1983**, *30*, 575–580.

Gaines, T. B. Acute toxicity of pesticides. *Toxicol. Appl. Pharmacol.*, **1969**, *14*, 515–534.

Gysin, H. Über einige neue Insektizide. *Chimia*, **1954**, *8*, 205–210, 221–228.

Hall, Z. W. Multiple forms of acetylcholinesterase and their distribution in endplate and non-endplate regions of rat diaphragm muscle. *J. Neurobiol.*, **1973**, *4*, 343–361.

Hobbiger, F., and Vojvodić, V. The reactivating and antidotal actions of N,N'-trimethylenebis(pyridinium-4-aldoxime) (TMB-4) and N,N'-oxydimethylenebis-(pyridinium-4-aldoxime) (toxogenin) with particular reference to their effect on phosphorylated acetylcholinesterase in brain. *Biochem. Pharmacol.*, **1966**, *15*, 1677–1690.

Howard, F. M., Jr.; Duane, D. D.; Lambert, E. H.; and Daube, J. R. Alternate-day prednisolone: preliminary report of a double-blind controlled study. *Ann. N.Y. Acad. Sci.*, **1976**, *274*, 596–607.

Jolly, F. Pseudoparalysis myasthenica. *Neurol. Zentralbl.*, **1895**, *14*, 34.

Laties, A. M. Localization in cornea and lens of topically-applied irreversible cholinesterase inhibitors. *Am. J. Ophthalmol.*, **1969**, *68*, 848–857.

Lindstrom, J. M.; Seybold, M. E.; Lennon, V. A.; Whittingham, S.; and Duane, D. D. Antibody to acetylcholine receptor in myasthenia gravis: prevalence, clinical correlates and diagnostic value. *Neurology (Minneap.)*, **1976**, *26*, 1054–1059.

Lwebuga-Mukasa, J. S.; Lappi, S.; and Taylor, P. Molecular forms of acetylcholinesterase from *Torpedo californica*: their relationship to synaptic membranes. *Biochemistry*, **1976**, *15*, 1425–1434.

McCombie, H., and Saunders, B. C. Alkyl fluorophosphonates: preparation and physiological properties. *Nature*, **1946**, *157*, 287–289.

McQuillen, M. P., and Leone, M. G. A treatment carol: thymectomy revisited in the corticosteroid era. *Neurology (Minneap.)*, **1977**, *27*, 1103–1106.

Mooser, G., and Sigman, D. S. Ligand binding properties of acetylcholinesterase determined with fluorescent probes. *Biochemistry*, **1974**, *13*, 2299–2307.

Nilsson, E. Physostigmine treatment in various drug-induced intoxications. *Ann. Clin. Res.*, **1982**, *14*, 165–172.

Osserman, K. E., and Genkins, G. Critical reappraisal of the use of edrophonium (tensilon) chloride tests in myasthenia gravis and significance of clinical classification. *Ann. N.Y. Acad. Sci.*, **1966**, *135*, 312–326.

Patrick, J. L., and Lindstrom, J. Autoimmune response to acetylcholine receptor. *Science*, **1973**, *180*, 871–872.

Remen, L. Zur Pathogenese und Therapie der Myasthenia gravis pseudoparalytic. *Dtsch. Z. NervHeilk.*, **1932**, *128*, 66–78.

Rosenberry, T. L., and Richardson, J. M. Structure of 18S and 14S acetylcholinesterase. Identification of collagen-like subunits that are linked by disulfide bonds to catalytic subunits. *Biochemistry*, **1977**, *16*, 3550–3558.

Shaffer, R. N., and Hetherington, J., Jr. Anticholinesterase drugs and cataracts. *Am. J. Ophthalmol.*, **1966**, *62*, 613–618.

Somani, S. M.; Roberts, J. B.; and Wilson, A. Pyridostigmine metabolism in man. *Clin. Pharmacol. Ther.*, **1972**, *13*, 393–399.

Stedman, E. III. Studies on the relationship between chemical constitution and physiological action. Part II. The miotic activity of urethanes derived from the isomeric hydroxybenzyldimethylamines. *Biochem. J.*, **1929a**, *23*, 17–24.

———. Chemical constitution and miotic action. *Am. J. Physiol.*, **1929b**, *90*, 528–529.

Su, M.; Kinoshita, F. K.; Frawley, F. P.; and DuBois, K. P. Comparative inhibition of aliesterases and cholinesterases in rats fed eighteen organophosphorus insecticides. *Toxicol. Appl. Pharmacol.*, **1971**, *20*, 241–249.

Taylor, P., and Lappi, S. Interaction of fluorescent probes with acetylcholinesterase. The site and specificity of propidium binding. *Biochemistry*, **1975**, *14*, 1989–1997.

Thai, L. J.; Fuld, P. A.; Masur, D. M.; and Sharpless, N. S. Oral physostigmine and lecithin improve memory in Alzheimer's disease. *Ann. Neurol.*, **1983**, *13*, 491–496.

Toyka, K. V.; Drachman, D. B.; Pestronk, A.; and Kao, I. Myasthenia gravis: passive transfer from man to mouse. *Science*, **1975**, *190*, 397–399.

Walker, M. B. Treatment of myasthenia gravis with physostigmine. *Lancet*, **1934**, *1*, 1200–1201.

———. Case showing effect of prostigmine on myasthenia gravis. *Proc. R. Soc. Med.*, **1935**, *28*, 759–761.

Wilson, I. B. Acetylcholinesterase. XI. Reversibility of tetraethyl pyrophosphate inhibition. *J. Biol. Chem.*, **1951**, *190*, 111–117.

Wilson, I. B., and Ginsburg, S. A powerful reactivator of alkyl phosphate–inhibited acetylcholinesterase. *Biochim. Biophys. Acta*, **1955**, *18*, 168–170.

Wilson, I. B., and Harrison, M. A. Turnover number of acetylcholinesterase. *J. Biol. Chem.*, **1961**, *236*, 2292–2295.

Wilson, I. B.; Hatch, M. A.; and Ginsburg, S. Carbamylation of acetylcholinesterase. *J. Biol. Chem.*, **1960**, *235*, 2312–2315.

Wilson, I. B., and Quan, C. Acetylcholinesterase: studies on molecular complementariness. *Arch. Biochem. Biophys.*, **1958**, *73*, 131–143.

Wirtschafter, J. D., and Herman, W. K. Low concentration eserine therapy for the tonic pupil (Adie) syndrome. *Ophthalmology (Rochester)*, **1980**, *87*, 1037–1043.

Monographs and Reviews

Abou-Donia, M. B. Organophosphorus ester-induced delayed neurotoxicity. *Annu. Rev. Pharmacol. Toxicol.*, **1981**, *21*, 511–548.

Aldridge, W. N. Survey of major points of interest about reactions of cholinesterases. *Croat. Chem. Acta*, **1976**, *47*, 225–233.

Aquilonius, S.-M. Physostigmine in the treatment of drug overdose. In, *Cholinergic Mechanisms and Psychopharmacology*, Vol. 24. (Jenden, D. J., ed.) Plenum Press, New York, **1977**, pp. 817–825.

Colquhoun, D. The link between drug binding and response: theories and observations. In, *The Receptors: A Comprehensive Treatise*, Vol. I. (O'Brien, R. D., ed.) Plenum Press, New York, **1979**, pp. 93–142.

Drachman, D. H. Myasthenia gravis. *N. Engl. J. Med.,* **1978**, *298,* 136–142, 186–193.

Ellin, R. I. Anomalies in theories and therapy of intoxication by potent organophosphorus anticholinesterase compounds. *Gen. Pharmacol.,* **1982**, *13,* 457–466.

Froede, H. C., and Wilson, I. B. Acetylcholinesterase. In, *The Enzymes*, Vol. 5. (Boyer, P. D., ed.) Academic Press, Inc., New York, **1971**, pp. 87–114.

Fukuto, T. R. Metabolism of carbamate insecticides. *Drug Metab. Rev.,* **1972**, *1,* 117–151.

Gosselin, R. E.; Hodge, H. C.; Smith, R. P.; and Gleason, M. N. *Clinical Toxicology of Commercial Products,* 5th ed. The Williams & Wilkins Co., Baltimore, **1984**.

Grob, D. Myasthenia gravis: pathophysiology and management. *Ann. N.Y. Acad. Sci.,* **1981**, *377,* 1–902.

Havener, W. H. *Ocular Pharmacology,* 5th ed. C. V. Mosby Co., St. Louis, **1983**.

Hayes, W. J., Jr. *Pesticide Studies in Man,* 2nd ed. The Williams & Wilkins Co., Baltimore, **1982**, pp. 284–435, 436–467.

Hobbiger, F. Reactivation of phosphorylated acetylcholinesterase. In, *Cholinesterases and Anticholinesterase Agents*. (Koelle, G. B., ed.) *Handbuch der Experimentellen Pharmakologie*, Vol. 15. Springer-Verlag, Berlin, **1963**, pp. 921–988.

———. Pharmacology of anticholinesterase drugs. In, *Neuromuscular Junction*. (Zaimis, E., ed.) *Handbuch der Experimentellen Pharmakologie*, Vol. 42. Springer-Verlag, Berlin, **1976**, pp. 487–581.

Holmstedt, B. Structure-activity relationships of the organophosphorus anticholinesterase agents. In, *Cholinesterases and Anticholinesterase Agents*. (Koelle, G. B., ed.) *Handbuch der Experimentellen Pharmakologie*, Vol. 15. Springer-Verlag, Berlin, **1963**, pp. 428–485.

———. The ordeal bean of Old Calabar: the pageant of *Physostigma venenosum* in medicine. In, *Plants in the Development of Modern Medicine*. (Swain, T., ed.) Harvard University Press, Cambridge, **1972**, pp. 303–360.

Johnson, M. K. The target for initiation of delayed neurotoxicity by organophosphorus esters. In, *Reviews in Biochemical Toxicology*, Vol. 4. (Hodgson, E.; Band, E.; and Philpot, R. M.; eds.) Elsevier Publishing Co., New York, **1982**, pp. 141–272.

Karczmar, A. G. Pharmacologic, toxicologic, and therapeutic properties of anticholinesterase agents. In, *Physiological Pharmacology*. Vol. 3, *The Nervous System— Part C: Autonomic Nervous System Drugs*. (Root, W. S., and Hofmann, F. G., eds.) Academic Press, Inc., New York, **1967**, pp. 163–322.

———. History of the research with anticholinesterase agents. In, *Anticholinesterase Agents*, Vol. 1. *International Encyclopedia of Pharmacology and Therapeutics*, Sect. 13. (Karczmar, A. G., ed.) Pergamon Press, Ltd., Oxford, **1970**, pp. 1–44.

Kaufman, P. L.; Weidman, T.; and Robinson, J. R. Cholinergics. In, *Pharmacology of the Eye*. (Sears, M. L., ed.) *Handbook of Experimental Pharmacology*, Vol. 69. Springer-Verlag, Berlin, **1984**, pp. 149–192.

Laskowski, M. B., and Dettbarn, W. D. The pharmacology of experimental myopathies. *Annu. Rev. Pharmacol. Toxicol.,* **1977**, *17,* 387–409.

Lindstrom, J., and Engel, A. Myasthenia gravis and the nicotinic cholinergic receptor. In, *Receptors and Recognition*, Vol. 13. (Cuatrecasas, P., and Greaves, M., eds.) Chapman & Hall, London, **1981**, pp. 161–214.

Long, J. P. Structure-activity relationships of the reversible anticholinesterase agents. In, *Cholinesterases and Anticholinesterase Agents*. (Koelle, G. B., ed.) *Handbuch der Experimentellen Pharmakologie*, Vol. 15. Springer-Verlag, Berlin, **1963**, pp. 374–427.

Lotti, V. J.; Le Douarec, S. C.; and Stone, C. A. Autonomic nervous system: adrenergic antagonists. In, *Pharmacology of the Eye*. (Sears, M. L., ed.) *Handbook of Experimental Pharmacology*, Vol. 69. Springer-Verlag, Berlin, **1984**, pp. 249–278.

Massoulié, J., and Bon, S. The molecular forms of cholinesterase and acetylcholinesterase in vertebrates. *Annu. Rev. Neurosci.,* **1982**, *5,* 106.

Mounter, L. A. Metabolism of organophosphorus anticholinesterase agents. In, *Cholinesterases and Anticholinesterase Agents*. (Koelle, G. B., ed.) *Handbuch der Experimentellen Pharmakologie*, Vol. 15. Springer-Verlag, Berlin, **1963**, pp. 486–504.

Murphy, S. D. Pesticides. In, *Casarett and Doull's Toxicology: The Basic Science of Poisons*, 3rd ed. (Klaassen, C. D.; Amdur, M. O.; and Doull, J.; eds.) Macmillan Publishing Co., New York, **1985**.

Osserman, K. E.; Foldes, F. F.; and Genkins, G. Myasthenia gravis. In, *Neuromuscular Blocking and Stimulating Agents*, Vol. 11. *International Encyclopedia of Pharmacology and Therapeutics*, Sect. 14. (Cheymol, J., ed.) Pergamon Press, Ltd., Oxford, **1972**, pp. 561–618.

Rosenberry, T. L. Acetylcholinesterase. *Adv. Enzymol.,* **1975**, *43,* 103–213.

Rowland, L. P. Controversies about treatment of myasthenia gravis. *J. Neurol. Neurosurg. Psychiatry,* **1980**, *43,* 644–659.

Schrader, G. *Die Entwicklung neuer Insektizide auf Grundlage von Organischen Fluor- und Phosphorverbindungen*. Monographie No. 62, Verlag Chemie, Weinheim, **1952**.

Schwartz, B. The glaucomas. *N. Engl. J. Med.,* **1978**, *290,* 182–186.

Usdin, E. Reactions of cholinesterases with substrates inhibitors and reactivators. In, *Anticholinesterase Agents*, Vol. 1. *International Encyclopedia of Pharmacology and Therapeutics*, Sect. 13. (Karczmar, A. G., ed.) Pergamon Press, Ltd., Oxford, **1970**, pp. 47–354.

Watson, P. G. (ed.). Glaucoma. *Br. J. Ophthalmol.,* **1972**, *56,* 145–318.

Wills, J. H. Toxicity of anticholinesterases and treatment of poisoning. In, *Anticholinesterase Agents*, Vol. 1. *International Encyclopedia of Pharmacology and Therapeutics*, Sect. 13. (Karczmar, A. G., ed.) Pergamon Press, Ltd., Oxford, **1970**, pp. 355–471.

Wilson, I. B. Molecular complementarity and antidotes for alkyl phosphate poisoning. *Fed. Proc.,* **1959**, *18,* 752–758.

7 ATROPINE, SCOPOLAMINE, AND RELATED ANTIMUSCARINIC DRUGS

Norman Weiner

The drugs described in this chapter inhibit the actions of acetylcholine (ACh) on autonomic effectors innervated by postganglionic cholinergic nerves as well as on smooth muscles that lack cholinergic innervation. Since they antagonize the muscarinic actions of ACh, they are known as *antimuscarinic* or *muscarinic cholinergic blocking* agents. Because the main actions of all members of this class of drugs are qualitatively similar to those of the best-known member, atropine, the terms *atropinic* and *atropine-like* are also appropriately used.

In general, antimuscarinic agents have little effect on the actions of ACh at nicotinic receptor sites. Thus, at autonomic ganglia, where transmission primarily involves an action of ACh on nicotinic receptors, atropine produces partial block only at relatively high doses. At the neuromuscular junction, where the receptors are principally or exclusively nicotinic, extremely high doses of atropine or related drugs are required to cause any degree of blockade. However, quaternary ammonium analogs of atropine and related drugs generally exhibit varying degrees of nicotinic blocking activity and, consequently, are likely to interfere with ganglionic or neuromuscular transmission in doses that more closely approximate those that produce muscarinic block. In the central nervous system (CNS), cholinergic transmission appears to be predominantly nicotinic in the spinal cord and both muscarinic and nicotinic at subcortical and cortical levels in the brain (Brimblecombe, 1974). Many or most of the CNS effects of atropine-like drugs at ordinary doses are probably attributable to their central antimuscarinic actions. At high or toxic doses, the central effects of atropine and related drugs consist, in general, of stimulation followed by depression.

There is an increased release and turnover of ACh in the CNS associated with the administration of antimuscarinic drugs; this may result in the activation of nicotinic receptors in the brain and contribute to the central effects of this class of drugs (Weiner, 1974). Since quaternary compounds penetrate the blood-brain barrier poorly, antimuscarinic drugs of this type show little in the way of central effects.

Parasympathetic neuroeffector junctions in different organs are not equally sensitive to the antimuscarinic agents. However, the relative sensitivity of various parasympathetically innervated organs to blockade by atropinic agents varies little among the drugs currently available. Small doses depress salivary and bronchial secretion and sweating. With larger doses, the pupil dilates, accommodation of the eye is inhibited, and vagal effects on the heart are blocked so that the heart rate is increased. Larger doses inhibit the parasympathetic control of the urinary bladder and gastrointestinal tract, thus inhibiting micturition and decreasing the tone and motility of the gut. Still larger doses are required to inhibit gastric secretion and motility. Since only the primary phase of gastric secretion is controlled by the vagus, the remaining hormonally controlled secretion remains unaffected. Thus, doses of atropine and related antimuscarinic drugs that reduce the tone and motility of the stomach and the duodenum and depress gastric secretion also invariably affect salivary secretion, ocular accommodation, and micturition. The drugs produce the functional equivalent of resection or paralysis of postganglionic cholinergic nerves.

The actions and effects of the antimuscarinic agents usually differ only quantitatively from those of atropine, which is considered in detail as the prototype of the group. The properties of other antimuscarinic drugs are discussed in terms of their differences from those of atropine.

Recent evidence suggests that subclasses of muscarinic receptors are present in both the CNS and peripheral organs (*see* Chapter 4; Hammer *et al.*, 1980; Symposium, 1980, 1984). These receptor subtypes exhibit differing affinities for certain muscarinic agonists and antagonists. This raises the possibility that antimuscarinic agents may be developed that will have selective actions on gastric secretion, heart rate, or gastrointestinal or other smooth muscle. For example, pirenzepine, a muscarinic antagonist, appears to interact rather selectively with cholinergic receptors that mediate gastric secretion, and it is less potent at muscarinic receptors in the atria, salivary glands, and gastrointestinal smooth muscle.

History. The naturally occurring antimuscarinic drugs are the alkaloids of the belladonna plants. The most important of these are *atropine* and *scopolamine*. Preparations of belladonna were known to the ancient Hindus and have been used by physicians for many centuries. During the time of the Roman Empire and in the Middle Ages the deadly nightshade plant was frequently used to produce obscure and often prolonged poisoning. This prompted Linné to name the shrub *Atropa belladonna,* after Atropos, the oldest of the Three Fates, who cuts the thread of life.

Accurate study of the actions of belladonna dates from the isolation of atropine in pure form by Mein in 1831. In 1867, Bezold and Bloebaum showed that atropine blocks the cardiac effects of vagal stimulation, and 5 years later Heidenhain found that it prevents salivary secretion due to stimulation of the chorda tympani. Many semisynthetic congeners of the belladonna alkaloids, usually quaternary ammonium derivatives, and a large number of synthetic antimuscarinic compounds have been prepared, primarily with the objective of depressing gastric secretion without undesired antimuscarinic

effects on other organs. The drugs that are currently available have few advantages over the naturally occurring alkaloids and their derivatives, but more selective agents may yet be developed.

ATROPINE, SCOPOLAMINE, AND RELATED BELLADONNA ALKALOIDS

Sources and Members. The belladonna drugs are widely distributed in nature, especially in the Solanaceae plants. *Atropa belladonna,* the deadly nightshade, yields mainly the alkaloid *atropine* (*dl-hyoscyamine*). The same alkaloid is found in *Datura stramonium,* known as Jamestown or Jimson weed, stinkweed, thorn-apple, and devil's apple. The alkaloid *scopolamine* (*hyoscine*) is found chiefly in the shrub *Hyoscyamus niger* (henbane) and *Scopolia carniolica.* Preparations of belladonna act chiefly by virtue of their content of atropine.

Chemistry. These alkaloids are organic esters formed by combination of an aromatic acid, *tropic acid,* and complex organic bases, either *tropine* (tropanol) or *scopine.* Scopine differs from tropine only in having an oxygen bridge between the carbon atoms designated as 6 and 7 in the structural formulas in Table 7–1. Homatropine is a semisynthetic compound produced by combining the base tropine with mandelic acid. *Methylatropine nitrate, methscopolamine bromide,* and *homatropine methylbromide* are the corresponding quaternary ammonium derivatives, modified by the addition of a second methyl group to the nitrogen.

Structure-Activity Relationship. The intact ester of tropine and tropic acid is essential for the antimuscarinic action of atropine, since neither the free acid nor the base exhibits significant antimuscarinic activity. The presence of a free OH group in the acid portion of the ester is also important. Substitution of other aromatic acids for tropic acid modifies but does not necessarily abolish the antimuscarinic activity. When given parenterally, quaternary ammonium derivatives of atropine and scopolamine are, in general, more potent than their

Table 7–1.   **STRUCTURAL FORMULAS OF ATROPINE, SCOPOLAMINE, AND HOMATROPINE**

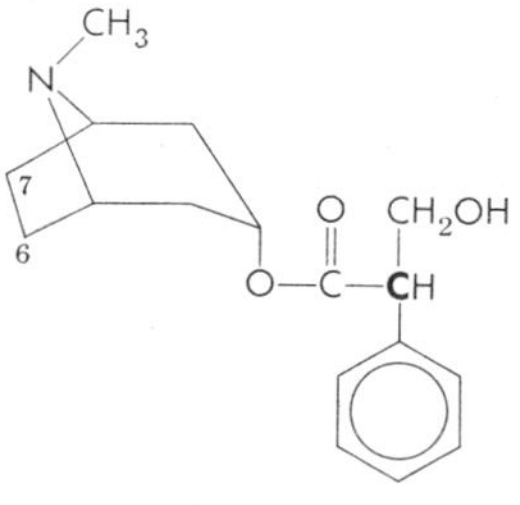

Atropine 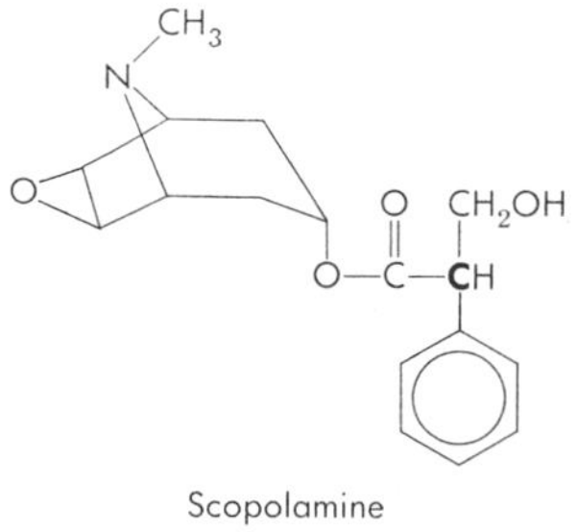   Scopolamine 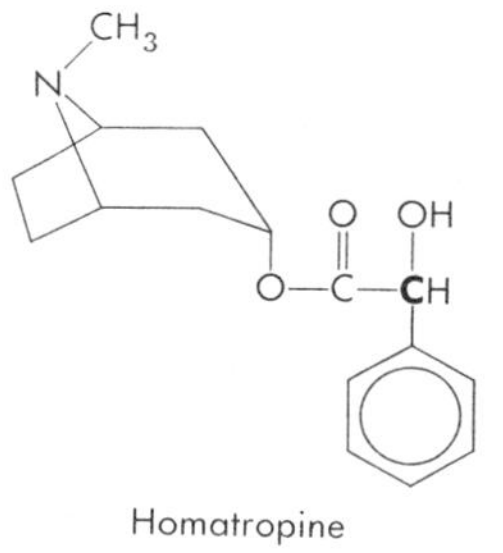   Homatropine parent compounds in both antimuscarinic and ganglionic blocking activity, and lack CNS activity because of poor penetration into the brain. Given orally, they are poorly and unreliably absorbed, as are other quaternary ammonium compounds.

There is an asymmetrical carbon atom in tropic and mandelic acids (boldface **C** in the formulas in Table 7–1). Scopolamine is *l*-hyoscine and is much more active than *d*-hyoscine. Atropine is racemized during extraction and consists of a mixture of equal parts of *d*- and *l*-hyoscyamine, but the antimuscarinic activity is almost wholly due to the naturally occurring *l* form.

Mechanism of Action. Antimuscarinic agents are *competitive* antagonists of the actions of ACh and other muscarinic agonists. The antagonism can therefore be overcome by increasing sufficiently the concentration of ACh at receptor sites of the effector organ. The receptors affected are those of peripheral structures that are either stimulated or inhibited by muscarine, that is, exocrine glands and smooth and cardiac muscle. Responses to postganglionic cholinergic nerve stimulation are also inhibited by antimuscarinic drugs, but less readily than are responses to injected choline esters. The difference may be due to release of ACh by cholinergic nerve terminals so close to receptors that very high concentrations of the neurotransmitter gain access to the receptors in the synaptic cleft. In addition, diffusion and other factors may limit the concentration of antagonist that can be attained at these receptor sites.

Interaction of Atropine and Related Drugs with Muscarinic Receptors. Much evidence supports the notion that atropine and related compounds compete with muscarinic agonists for identical binding sites on muscarinic receptors (Brimblecombe, 1974; Yamamura and Snyder, 1974; Hulme et al., 1978).

While pharmacological observations made more than 25 years ago suggested that muscarinic receptors in the heart had different properties than those in the gastrointestinal tract, it was not until 1978 that substantial evidence for the existence of subtypes of muscarinic receptors began to accumulate. Pertinent pharmacological observations came from the study of cholinergic regulation of the lower esophageal sphincter (see Rattan and Goyal, in Symposium, 1984). Vagal stimulation causes relaxation of this structure. However, while some muscarinic agonists (*e.g.,* McN-A-343) also cause relaxation, others (*e.g.,* bethanechol) produce contraction. The effects of both bethanechol and McN-A-343 are readily antagonized by atropine, but effective blockade of vagally induced relaxa-

tion requires the use of both atropine and a ganglionic blocking agent. These observations, together with the capacity of McN-A-343 to cause *contraction* of the sphincter in the presence of tetrodotoxin, suggested that vagal fibers innervate intrinsic neurons. These neurons are believed to elaborate an inhibitory substance that is primarily responsible for the relaxation in response to vagal stimulation. The interneurons can apparently be activated by either muscarinic or nicotinic cholinergic receptors. Moreover, the muscarinic receptors on these neurons (termed M_1) appear to be different from those on the smooth muscle cells (termed M_2). The M_1 receptors can be preferentially stimulated by McN-A-343. This results in relaxation of the esophageal sphincter. Bethanechol acts preferentially on M_2 receptors. Similar complexities may underlie muscarinic regulation of gastric acid secretion (see Pagani et al., in Symposium, 1984).

At the same time, detailed examination of the ligand-binding properties of cerebral cortical membranes indicated that there were two major populations of binding sites with differing affinities for muscarinic agonists (Birdsall et al., 1978). In contrast, only one type of binding site for muscarinic antagonists could be demonstrated in these preparations (Hulme et al., 1978). However, the recent availability of the selective muscarinic antagonist pirenzepine and the use of the tritiated compound as a radioligand have provided additional evidence in support of the existence of at least two subtypes of muscarinic receptors (see Watson et al., in Symposium, 1984). Relatively large amounts of binding sites with a high affinity for pirenzepine (M_1 receptors) are present in corpus striatum, cerebral cortex, hippocampus, and, presumably, autonomic ganglia. The low-affinity receptor (M_2) appears to be predominant in heart, cerebellum, and ileum. Moreover, pirenzepine preferentially antagonizes the effects of McN-A-343 on the lower esophageal sphincter (see Rattan and Goyal, in Symposium, 1984). Thus, the nomenclature that arose independently from studies of intact smooth muscle and from examination of ligand-binding properties has been brought into register (see MacIntosh, in Symposium, 1984).

It is hypothesized that the M_2 receptor is linked to adenylate cyclase, and its activation is associated with inhibition of this enzyme. The M_2 receptor may also exist on cholinergic and adrenergic nerve terminals, and its activation may result in inhibition of the release of neurotransmitter. Its interaction with a guanine nucleotide–binding regulatory protein (see Chapter 2) is inferred from the pronounced effect of guanosine triphosphate (GTP) on the binding of agonists in analogy with other receptors that are coupled to adenylate cyclase (see Birdsall et al. and Watson et al., in Symposium, 1984). The M_1-receptor type may be involved in the regulation of Ca^{2+} fluxes and the generation of phosphorylated derivatives of inositol.

Selectivity of Antagonism. Although atropine does not discriminate between M_1 and M_2 receptors, it is a highly selective antagonist of muscarinic agents at the corresponding receptors of smooth and cardiac muscle and exocrine gland cells. This antagonism is so selective that atropine blockade of the actions of a noncholinomimetic drug has been taken as evidence that the drug acts indirectly either through release of ACh or by some other cholinergic mechanism. For example, the stimulant action of 5-hydroxytryptamine (5-HT) on guinea pig ileum has been attributed to activation of intramural cholinergic neurons because it is blocked by atropine. However, atropine and other antimuscarinic agents are no exceptions to the general rule that selectivity of antagonism is rarely absolute and is usually lost when high doses are used. Under appropriate experimental conditions and usually in higher doses than are needed to antagonize ACh, atropine may block or reduce responses to histamine, 5-HT, and norepinephrine. Atropine is moderately active in relieving histamine-induced bronchoconstriction in man and experimental animals. It also antagonizes the action of 5-HT on rat uterus, the respiratory tract smooth muscle of guinea pig and cat, guinea pig atria, and the aneural smooth muscle of chick amnion, where 5-HT is presumed to act directly.

PHARMACOLOGICAL PROPERTIES

Atropine and scopolamine differ quantitatively in antimuscarinic actions. Scopolamine has a more potent action on the iris, ciliary body, and certain secretory (salivary, bronchial, and sweat) glands, but atropine is the more potent on heart, intestine, and bronchial muscle, and has a more prolonged action. Atropine does not depress the CNS in doses that are used clinically and, therefore, is given in preference to scopolamine for most purposes. When some central depressant effect is no disadvantage or is desired, as in preanesthetic medication, scopolamine is frequently administered.

Central Nervous System. *Atropine* stimulates the medulla and higher cerebral centers. In doses used clinically (0.5 to 1.0 mg), this effect is usually confined to mild vagal excitation. The rate and occasionally the depth of breathing are increased, but this effect is probably the result of bronchiolar dilatation and the subsequent increase in physiological "dead space." With toxic doses of atropine, central excitation becomes more prominent, leading to restlessness, irritability, disorientation, hallucinations, or delirium (*see* discussion of atropine poisoning). With still larger doses, stimulation is followed by depression, coma ensues, and medullary paralysis causes death. Even moderate doses of atropine may depress certain central motor mechanisms controlling muscle tone and movement, as seen in the salutary effect on the tremor and rigidity of parkinsonism (*see* Chapter 21 and Therapeutic Uses, below).

Scopolamine in therapeutic doses normally causes drowsiness, euphoria, amnesia, fatigue, and dreamless sleep with a reduction in rapid-eye-movement (REM) sleep. These effects are sometimes sought when scopolamine is used as an adjunct to anesthetic agents or for preanesthetic medication. However, the same doses of scopolamine occasionally cause excitement, restlessness, hallucinations, or delirium, especially in the presence of severe pain. These excitatory effects, which resemble the central effects of toxic doses of atropine, occur regularly after large doses of scopolamine.

Central Antimuscarinic Action. Doses of atropine required to inhibit peripheral responses to choline esters or anticholinesterase (anti-ChE) agents produce almost no detectable central effects; large doses are required. This may reflect difficulty of penetration of the drug into the CNS. Physostigmine is able to reverse the atropine-induced depression of the hypothalamus and reticular activating system in animals and the central effects of atropine poisoning in man. In animals, atropine antagonizes the action of ACh applied locally to the cerebral cortex and spinal cord. However, atropine also depresses the effects of noncholinergic stimuli, indicating that the drug has central actions other than blocking cholinergic synapses. (*See* Krnjević, 1969, 1974.)

EEG. Atropine promptly restores to normal the increased EEG activity due to isoflurophate (di*iso*propyl phosphorofluoridate, DFP). Given alone, it reduces the voltage and frequency of the *alpha* rhythm and consistently shifts the EEG rhythm to slow activity, a pattern typical of the EEG in drowsiness. Both atropine and scopolamine also depress the EEG arousal response to photostimulation. In experimental animals, atropine and particularly scopolamine antagonize EEG activation by hypothalamic or reticular formation stimulation and by several drugs, including sympathomimetic agents. Atropine or scopolamine disrupts several behavioral responses in experimental animals at the same time as the EEG is altered. In many cases physostigmine promptly and simultaneously restores both to normal (*see* Longo, 1966).

Antitremor Activity. The belladonna alkaloids and related antimuscarinic agents have long been used in parkinsonism. A central antimuscarinic mechanism is likely, since physostigmine reverses the beneficial effects of atropinic drugs and aggravates the symptoms in untreated patients. The salutary effect of levodopa in parkinsonism has led to considerable insight into the relations between cholinergic and dopaminergic mechanisms in this disease (*see* Chapter 21).

Vestibular Function. Scopolamine is effective in preventing motion sickness. This action is probably either on the cortex or more peripherally on the vestibular apparatus.

Eye. The atropinic drugs block the responses of the sphincter muscle of the iris and the ciliary muscle of the lens to cholinergic stimulation (Table 7–3, page 139). Thus, they dilate the pupil (*mydriasis*) and paralyze accommodation (*cycloplegia*). The wide pupillary dilatation results in photophobia; the lens is fixed for far vision, near objects are blurred, and sometimes micropsia occurs. The normal pupillary reflex constriction to light or upon convergence of the eyes is abolished. These effects can occur after either local or systemic administration of the alkaloids. However, conventional systemic doses of atropine (0.6 mg) have little ocular effect, in contrast to equal doses of scopolamine, which cause definite mydriasis and loss of accommodation. Locally applied atropine or scopolamine produces ocular effects of considerable duration; accommodation and pupillary reflexes may not fully recover for 7 to 12 days. The atropinic mydriatics differ from the sympathomimetic agents in that the latter cause pupillary dilatation without loss of accommodation. Pilocarpine, choline esters, physostigmine, and DFP in sufficient concentrations can reverse the ocular effects of atropinic drugs at least partially.

Atropinic drugs when administered systemically have little effect on *intraocular pressure* except in patients with narrow-angle glaucoma, where the pressure may occasionally rise dangerously. This effect is because the iris, crowded back into the angle of the anterior chamber of the eye, interferes with drainage of aqueous humor. The drugs may precipitate a first attack in unrecognized cases of this rare condition. In patients with wide-angle glaucoma, a significant rise in pressure is unusual. Atropinic drugs can generally be used safely in this latter condition, particularly if the patient is also adequately treated with an appropriate miotic agent.

Cardiovascular System. *Heart.* The main effect of atropine on the heart is to alter *rate*. With average clinical doses (0.4 to 0.6 mg), the rate often decreases transiently, possibly due to central vagal stimulation, which may occur prior to the onset of peripheral muscarinic cholinergic blockade. A similar effect may be seen with low doses of atropine that do not produce peripheral antimuscarinic effects. The slowing is rarely marked, about 4 to 8 beats per minute, and is usually absent after rapid intravenous injection. There are no accompanying changes in blood pressure or cardiac output. Larger doses cause progressively increasing tachycardia by blocking vagal effects on the S-A nodal pacemaker. The resting heart rate is increased by about 35 to 40 beats per minute in young men given 2 mg intramuscularly; the maximal heart rate (*e.g.*, in response to exercise) is not altered by atropine. The influence of atropine is most noticeable in healthy young adults, in whom vagal tone is considerable. In infancy and old age, even large doses of atropine may fail to accelerate the heart. Atropine often causes cardiac arrhythmias, but without significant cardiovascular symptoms. Atrial arrhythmias and atrioventricular dissociation occur, the former most commonly in children given small doses that slow the heart, the latter usually in adults after small or large doses (Dauchot and Gravenstein, 1971; Hayes *et al.*, 1971).

With low doses of scopolamine (0.1 or 0.2 mg) the cardiac slowing is greater than with atropine. With higher doses, cardioacceleration occurs initially, but it is short lived and is followed within 30 minutes either by a return to the normal rate or by bradycardia. Thus, after a short initial period, doses of scopolamine that produce ocular effects do not accelerate cardiac rate. With atropine, ocular effects are accompanied by tachycardia.

Adequate doses of atropine can abolish many types of reflex vagal cardiac slowing or asystole, for example, from inhalation of irritant vapors, stimulation of the carotid sinus, pressure on the eyeballs, peritoneal stimulation, central stimulation of vagal nuclei, or the normal afferent impulses causing respiratory arrhythmia. It also prevents or abruptly abolishes bradycardia or asystole caused by choline esters, anti-ChE agents, or other parasympathomimetic drugs, as well as cardiac arrest from electrical stimulation of the vagus.

The removal of vagal influence on the heart by atropine may also cause changes in *conduction*. A-V conduction time is decreased, even when heart rate is kept constant by atrial pacing, and the P-R interval is shortened. In certain cases of partial heart block, in which vagal activity is an etiological factor, atropine may lessen the degree of block. In some patients with complete heart block, the idioventricular rate may be accelerated by atropine; in others it is stabilized. Atropine may improve the clinical condition of patients with early myocardial infarction by relieving severe sinus or nodal bradycardia or A-V block (*see* Adgey *et al.,* 1968; and below). In contrast, toxic doses and, occasionally, a large therapeutic dose of atropine may cause A-V block and nodal rhythm.

Circulation. Atropine, in clinical doses, completely counteracts the peripheral vasodilatation and sharp fall in blood pressure caused by choline esters. In contrast, when given alone, its effect on blood vessels and blood pressure is neither striking nor constant. This is expected, because most vascular beds probably lack significant cholinergic innervation and the cholinergic sympathetic vasodilator fibers to vessels supplying skeletal muscle do not appear to be involved to any important extent in the normal regulation of tone.

Toxic amounts of atropine usually, and therapeutic doses occasionally, dilate cutaneous blood vessels, especially those in the blush area (*atropine flush*). The mechanism of this anomalous vascular response is unknown. It may be a compensatory reaction permitting the radiation of heat to offset the atropine-induced rise in temperature. On the other hand, it may represent a direct vasodilator action unrelated to cholinergic blockade. The scarlet appearance of the flushed skin, coupled with fever, has caused atropine intoxication to be mistakenly diagnosed as scarlet fever.

Gastrointestinal Tract. Interest in the actions of antimuscarinic drugs on the stomach and intestine has led to their use as antispasmodic agents for gastrointestinal disorders and in the treatment of peptic ulcer. Although atropine can completely abolish the effects of ACh (and other parasympathomimetic drugs) on the gastrointestinal tract, it inhibits only incompletely the effects of vagal impulses. This difference is particularly striking in the effects of atropine on motility of the gut. The cause is not known; it appears likely that it may be due to the involvement of gastrointestinal hormones or neurohumoral transmitters other than ACh and norepinephrine.

Secretion. *Salivary secretion* is particularly sensitive to inhibition by antimuscarinic agents, which can completely abolish the copious, watery, parasympathetically induced secretion. The mouth becomes dry, and swallowing and talking become difficult.

Gastric secretion is reduced in volume and total acid content. However, this reduction is notable only when relatively large doses are given to experimental animals. Gastric secretion in *man* is not greatly altered by conventional doses of the belladonna drugs; to be effective, doses must usually be given (1 mg or more) that invariably cause dry mouth, increase in heart rate, ocular disturbances, and other side effects. Secretion during both psychic and gastric phases is reduced but not abolished. Volume is usually reduced, but the concentration of acid is not necessarily lowered. The intestinal phase of gastric secretion may be somewhat inhibited. Full doses of atropine diminish and may completely abolish the interdigestive (fasting) secretion of acid; this action is less prominent in patients with peptic ulcers. The duration of the effect of atropine on gastric secretion is brief when compared with that on salivary glands. Secretion induced by histamine, alcohol, or caffeine is reduced but not abolished by the doses of atropine tested in man.

The gastric cells that secrete mucin and enzymes are more directly under vagal influence than are the acid-secreting cells, and full doses of atropine may decrease the concentration of these organic constituents. Atropine completely blocks the copious secretion of gastric juice, rich in both acid and proteolytic enzymes, elicited by injection of choline esters (methacholine and carbachol) or pilocarpine.

Atropine reduces the loss of plasma proteins from the everted gastric mucosal pouch of vagally denervated dogs. The increased shedding of plasma proteins across the gastric mucosa produced by either histamine or ACh is also substantially inhibited by atropine, whereas that produced by ethanol is not affected (Davenport and Kauffman, 1975; Kauffman and Davenport, 1975). These results are of interest, since it has been reported that prolonged oral administration of antimuscarinic agents such as propantheline or atropine is efficacious in the management of Menétrièr's disease, which is associated with giant hypertrophy of the gastric mucosa, peripheral edema, and excessive loss of protein from the stomach (Smith and Powell, 1978).

Atropine has little effect on secretion by the pancreas, intestine, or liver; these processes are largely under hormonal rather than vagal control.

Motility. The belladonna alkaloids have marked effects on motility of the gastrointestinal tract, since the parasympathetic nerves almost exclusively supply the extrinsic nervous motor control of the gut; sympathetic nerve impulses play a relatively small part in the physiological regulation of tone and motility. The parasympathetic nerves enhance both tone and motility, and relax sphincters, thereby favoring the passage of chyme through the gut. However, the intestine has a complex system of intramural nerve plexuses that are mainly responsible for motility, and impulses from the CNS only modify the effects of the intrinsic reflexes. The terminal neurons of the intramural plexuses are cholinergic, and the effects of their activity can be blocked by atropine. However, atropine-resistant alterations in the tone and movements of the gut are also demonstrable.

Both in normal subjects and in patients with gastrointestinal disease, full therapeutic doses of atropine produce definite and prolonged inhibitory effects on the motor activity of the stomach, duodenum, jejunum, ileum, and colon, characterized by a decrease in tone and in amplitude and frequency of peristaltic contractions. It should be noted that the doses needed to produce inhibition are more than enough to depress salivary secretion and usually produce ocular and cardiac effects.

Atropine abolishes or prevents the excess motor activity of the gastrointestinal tract induced by parasympathomimetic drugs and anti-ChE agents. In moderate doses, the alkaloids do not block responses to other directly acting stimulants, such as histamine and vasopressin, that do not act on ACh receptors. However, responses to drugs acting through the intramural plexuses, such as nicotine, morphine, and 5-HT, are inhibited.

Respiratory Tract. The belladonna alkaloids inhibit secretions of the nose, mouth, pharynx, and bronchi, and thus dry the mucous membranes of the respiratory tract. This action is especially marked if there is excessive secretion, and is the basis for the use of atropine and scopolamine in preanesthetic medication. The smooth muscles of bronchi and bronchioles are relaxed, with a resulting slight widening of the airway, which decreases airway resistance but increases the volume of residual air. The increase in "dead space" due to bronchiolar dilatation may be the basis of the respiratory stimulation produced by atropine. Atropine is more potent than scopolamine as a bronchodilator. It is particularly effective against bronchoconstriction produced by parasympathomimetic drugs such as methacholine and anti-ChE agents, but it is also moderately active in histamine-induced experimental asthma in both animals and man. However, atropine is less effective than epinephrine or isoproterenol as a bronchial relaxant, even against bronchoconstriction from electrical stimulation of the vagus. The role of cholinergic factors in the causation of bronchial asthmatic attacks remains to be elucidated.

Atropine and scopolamine reduce the occurrence of laryngospasm during general anesthesia. This appears to be due to depression of respiratory tract secretions that can precipitate reflex laryngospasm. The contraction of the laryngeal skeletal muscle is not directly blocked by atropine.

Other Smooth Muscle. *Urinary Tract.* Intravenous urographic studies in man indicate that atropine (1.2 mg, intravenously) dilates the pelves, calyces, ureters, and bladder, and increases the visibility of the kidneys. Atropine decreases the normal tone and amplitude of contractions of the *ureter* and *bladder,* and often eliminates drug-induced enhancement of ureteral tone.

Biliary Tract. Atropine exerts a mild antispasmodic action on the gallbladder and bile ducts in man. However, this is not sufficient to overcome or prevent the marked spasm and increase in biliary duct pressure induced by opioids. Both nitrites and theophylline are more effective than atropine in this respect. Atropine has no consistent effect on the choledochal sphincter mechanism in man. Emptying of the human gallbladder in response to a fat meal is delayed by prior administration of atropine. There is little basis for the use of atropine alone as a biliary antispasmodic.

Uterus. Atropine and scopolamine have negligible effects on the human uterus. Although the drugs cross the placental barrier, the fetus is apparently not adversely affected and the respiration of the newborn is not depressed.

Sweat Glands and Temperature. Small doses of atropine or scopolamine inhibit the activity of *sweat glands,* despite the vasodilatation the drugs may cause in some skin areas. The skin becomes hot and dry; sweating may be depressed enough to raise the body temperature, but only notably so after toxic doses. Atropine more readily blocks sweating induced by injected muscarinic agents than it does thermoregulatory sweating. The anhidrotic action of atropine and stimulation of sweating by muscarinic agents appeared for many years to be a pharmacological anomaly, as the sweat glands are supplied only by nerves that are anatomically sympathetic. However, these fibers are, in fact, mainly cholinergic.

The rise in body temperature due to the belladonna alkaloids is usually significant only after large doses. Nevertheless, in infants and small children moderate doses induce "atropine fever." In atropine poisoning in infants, the temperature may reach 43° C or higher. Suppression of sweating is doubtless a considerable factor in the production of the fever, especially when the environmental temperature is high, but other mechanisms may be important when large doses are taken. Atropine may exert a central effect on temperature regulation; however, animals that do not sweat, such as the dog, do not exhibit fever after atropine.

Absorption, Fate, and Excretion. The belladonna alkaloids are absorbed rapidly from the gastrointestinal tract. They also enter the circulation when applied locally to the mucosal surfaces of the body. Only limited absorption occurs from the intact skin. The total absorption of quaternary ammonium derivatives of the alkaloids after an oral dose is only about 10 to 25% (Jonkman et al., 1977); nevertheless, some of these compounds, applied locally to the eye, can cause mydriasis and cycloplegia. Atropine has a half-life of about 2.5 hours, and most of the drug is excreted in the urine within the first 12 hours, in part unchanged. Only about 1% of an oral dose of scopolamine is eliminated as such in the urine. Traces of atropine are found in various secretions, including milk.

Poisoning by Belladonna Alkaloids. The deliberate or accidental ingestion of belladonna alkaloids or other classes of drugs with atropinic properties is a major cause of poisonings. Many H_1-histaminergic blocking agents, phenothiazines, and tricyclic antidepressants have antimuscarinic activity and, in sufficient dosage, may produce syndromes that include features of atropine intoxication. Infants and young children are especially susceptible to the toxic effects of atropinic drugs (Rumack, 1973). Indeed, many cases of intoxication in children have resulted from conjunctival instillation of atropinic drugs, systemic absorption occurring either from the nasal mucosa after the drug has traversed the nasolacrimal duct or from the intestinal tract if it is swallowed. Delirium or toxic psychoses, without undue peripheral manifestations, have been reported in adults after instillation of atropine eyedrops. Poisoning also occurs from overdoses of the many "over-the-counter" sleeping medicines containing scopolamine, and from purposeful ingestion, for hallucinatory effects, of nonprescription remedies for asthma that contain belladonna. Serious intoxication may occur in children who ingest berries or seeds containing belladonna alkaloids. Reports of stramonium poisoning due to tea made from Jimson weed seeds date as far back as 1676 in the United States and are described in *earlier editions* of this textbook.

Shein and Smith (1978) have quantified the antimuscarinic activity of a series of tricyclic antidepressants. Agents such as imipramine, nortriptyline, protriptyline, and amitriptyline are approximately 1/20 to 1/80 as potent as atropine in inhibiting the effects of ACh on the guinea pig ileum. However, since these drugs are administered in therapeutic doses considerably higher than the effective dose of atropine, antimuscarinic effects are often observed clinically (*see* Chapter 19). Treatment of intoxication by tricyclic antidepressants may thus require the administration of physostigmine (*see* below; Rumack, 1973; Aquilonius, 1978).

Fatalities from intoxication with atropine and scopolamine are rare, but they sometimes occur in children, in whom 10 mg or less may be lethal. Idiosyncratic reactions are more common with scopolamine than with atropine, and ordinary therapeutic doses sometimes cause alarming effects. Homatropine methylbromide is well tolerated in doses much larger than those used for therapy and is only about 1/50 as toxic as atropine. Table 7–2 shows the doses of atropine giving undesirable responses or symptoms of overdosage. In cases of full-blown poisoning with atropine, the syndrome may last for 48 hours or longer. In addition to the effects described in Table 7–2, convulsions may occur. Depression and circulatory collapse are evident only in cases of severe intoxication; the blood pressure declines, respiration becomes inadequate, and death due to respiratory failure may follow after a period of paralysis and coma (*see* Shader and Greenblatt, 1972).

The *diagnosis* of atropine poisoning is suggested by the widespread paralysis of organs innervated by parasympathetic nerves. Subcutaneous injection of 1 mg of the anti-ChE agent physostigmine may be used for confirmation. If the typical salivation, sweating, and intestinal hyperactivity do not

Table 7–2. EFFECTS OF ATROPINE IN RELATION TO DOSAGE

DOSE	EFFECTS
0.5 mg	Slight cardiac slowing; some dryness of mouth; inhibition of sweating
1.0 mg	Definite dryness of mouth; thirst; acceleration of heart, sometimes preceded by slowing; mild dilatation of pupil
2.0 mg	Rapid heart rate; palpitation; marked dryness of mouth; dilated pupils; some blurring of near vision
5.0 mg	All the above symptoms marked; speech disturbed; difficulty in swallowing; restlessness and fatigue; headache; dry, hot skin; difficulty in micturition; reduced intestinal peristalsis
10.0 mg and more	Above symptoms more marked; pulse rapid and weak; iris practically obliterated; vision very blurred; skin flushed, hot, dry, and scarlet; ataxia, restlessness, and excitement; hallucinations and delirium; coma

occur, intoxication with atropine or a related agent is almost certain.

Measures to limit intestinal absorption should be initiated without delay if the poison has been taken orally. *Physostigmine* is the rational therapy. For example, the slow intravenous injection of 1 to 4 mg of physostigmine (0.5 mg in children) rapidly abolishes the delirium and coma caused by large doses of atropine. Since physostigmine is metabolized rapidly, the patient may again lapse into coma within 1 to 2 hours, and repeated doses may be needed (*see* Ketchum *et al.*, 1973; Rumack, 1973). If marked excitement is present and more specific treatment is not available, diazepam is most suitable for sedation and for control of convulsions. Large doses should be avoided because the central depressant action may coincide with the depression occurring late in atropinic poisoning. Phenothiazines should not be used because their antimuscarinic action is likely to intensify toxicity. Artificial respiration may be necessary. Ice bags and alcohol sponges help to reduce fever, especially in children.

Preparations, Dosage, and Routes of Administration. *Belladonna tincture* is a preparation that consists of an aqueous-alcoholic extract of belladonna leaf. The adult dose is 0.6 to 1.0 ml, which contains approximately 0.2 to 0.3 mg, respectively, of the alkaloids of the leaf (mainly atropine). *Belladonna extract* may be given in tablets; the dose is 15 mg, equivalent to approximately 0.2 mg of atropine. *Atropine* is the main alkaloid of belladonna as the free base. The readily soluble salt, *atropine sulfate,* is available in tablet form, as an injectable solution, as an ophthalmic solution and ointment, and as a solution to be given by nebulization. The average oral or parenteral dose of atropine sulfate for adults is 0.5 mg. *Scopolamine* (*l*-hyoscine) is marketed as the readily soluble salt, *scopolamine hydrobromide;* the adult oral or parenteral dose is 0.6 mg. Scopolamine is also available in an ophthalmic solution and in transdermal patches (*see* below).

SYNTHETIC AND SEMISYNTHETIC SUBSTITUTES FOR BELLADONNA ALKALOIDS

The lack of selectivity of the belladonna alkaloids for those parasympathetic functions that might profitably be blocked in various diseases, particularly of the gastrointestinal tract, has led to intensive efforts to discover antimuscarinic drugs with more selective effects. Success has been limited, and the available agents are not wholly satisfactory. Although there are minor variations, the sequence of block in various organ systems is very similar for all antimuscarinic drugs now used clinically.

The main differences in pharmacological properties are seen with those compounds having a quaternary ammonium structure. These drugs are poorly and unreliably absorbed after oral administration, and valid comparisons of their potencies with those of the belladonna alkaloids can be made only after parenteral administration (Jonkman *et al.*, 1977). Penetration of the conjunctiva is also poor, so that most quaternary ammonium compounds are of little value in ophthalmology. Central effects are generally lacking, because these agents do not readily pass the blood-brain barrier. The quaternary ammonium compounds usually have a somewhat more prolonged action; little is known of the fate and excretion of most of these agents. The ratio of ganglionic blocking to antimuscarinic activity is greater for compounds with the quaternary ammonium structure because of their greater potency at nicotinic receptors; some of the side effects seen after high doses are due to ganglionic blockade. Thus, impotence and postural hypotension can occur in patients who are given these drugs. Poisoning with quaternary ammonium compounds may also cause a curariform neuromuscular block, leading to respiratory paralysis. Thus, toxic doses of these agents produce the usual manifestations of antimuscarinic poisoning with additional effects of ganglionic and, rarely, neuromuscular block, but usually without significant CNS involvement.

There is a clinical impression that the quaternary ammonium compounds have a relatively greater effect on gastrointestinal activity and that the doses necessary to treat gastrointestinal disorders are, consequently, somewhat more readily tolerated; this has been attributed to the additional element of ganglionic block. These drugs, like atropine, do not produce adequate control of gastric secretion or gastrointestinal motility at doses that are devoid of significant side effects due to muscarinic blockade at other sites (Ivey, 1975a). However, there is a suggestion that propantheline, taken orally, significantly reduces secretion of gastric acid stimulated by food to the same extent at low doses (15 mg per day) as when larger amounts are given (45 mg per day); only the higher dose caused pronounced side effects (Feldman *et al.*, 1977).

The pharmacological properties of the drugs discussed below differ little from those of other agents in the same general category and range between those of atropine and those of oxyphenonium and methantheline, the quaternary ammonium compounds with the greatest ratio of ganglionic blocking to antimuscarinic activity.

Homatropine.   This drug (Table 7–1) has about one tenth the potency of atropine. It is used almost exclusively as a topical *mydriatic* and *cycloplegic* in the form of 2 and 5% *homatropine hydrobromide ophthalmic solution,* for which purposes it is preferable to atropine in many cases because of its rapid onset and shorter duration of action (Table 7–3). Accommodation is usually normal within 24 hours, but a briefer cycloplegia can be obtained by use of a 1% solution. Homatropine does not usually cause complete cycloplegia in children. Some conjunctival vasodilatation occurs after instillation of the drug.

QUATERNARY AMMONIUM DERIVATIVES OF BELLADONNA ALKALOIDS

Methscopolamine Bromide.   *Methscopolamine bromide* (PAMINE) lacks the central actions of scopolamine. It is less potent than atropine and is poorly absorbed; however, its action is more prolonged, the usual oral dose (2.5 mg) acting for 6 to 8 hours. Its limited use has been chiefly in gastrointestinal diseases. The drug is available in 2.5-mg tablets.

Homatropine Methylbromide.   *Homatropine methylbromide* is less potent than atropine in antimuscarinic activity, but it is four times more potent as a ganglionic blocking agent. It is available in some combination products intended for relief of gastrointestinal spasm.

REPRESENTATIVE SYNTHETIC QUATERNARY AMMONIUM COMPOUNDS

Methantheline.   *Methantheline bromide* (BANTHINE) is a quaternary ammonium compound that differs from atropine in having a particularly high ratio of ganglionic blocking to antimuscarinic activity. Its structural formula is as follows:

Methantheline

Table 7–3.   MYDRIATIC AND CYCLOPLEGIC PROPERTIES OF ANTIMUSCARINIC AGENTS

DRUG	STRENGTH OF SOLUTION * (percent)	MYDRIASIS		PARALYSIS OF ACCOMMODATION	
		Maximal (minutes)	*Recovery † (days)*	*Maximal (hours)*	*Recovery ‡ (days)*
Atropine sulfate	1.0	30–40	7–10	1–3	7–12
Scopolamine hydrobromide	0.5	20–30	3–7	½–1	5–7
Homatropine hydrobromide	1.0 §	40–60	1–3	½–1	1–3
Cyclopentolate hydrochloride	0.5–1.0	30–60	1	½–1	1
Tropicamide	0.5–1.0 ‖	20–40	¼	½	<¼

* One instillation of 1 drop of solution. Preparations of ophthalmic solutions currently available in the United States include atropine sulfate, 0.5–3%; scopolamine hydrobromide, 0.25%; homatropine hydrobromide, 2 and 5%; cyclopentolate hydrochloride, 0.5–2%; and tropicamide, 0.5 and 1%.

† To within 1 mm of original pupillary diameter.

‡ To within 2 diopters of original accommodative power; ability to read fine print is possible by the third day after instillation of atropine or scopolamine and by 6 hours after homatropine.

§ Full mydriasis and loss of accommodation require instillation of a 5% solution.

‖ Adequate loss of accommodation lasting about 30 minutes requires instillation of a 1% solution.

High doses may cause impotence, an effect rarely produced by purely antimuscarinic drugs and indicative of ganglionic block. Toxic doses may paralyze respiration by neuromuscular block. CNS manifestations of restlessness, euphoria, fatigue, or, very rarely, acute psychotic episodes may appear in occasional patients. Gastrointestinal effects of methantheline appear to be relatively greater than those of atropine, and many clinicians have the impression that the doses of methantheline used in the treatment of gastrointestinal disorders cause fewer antimuscarinic side effects than does atropine. The action is somewhat more prolonged than that of atropine, the effects of a therapeutic dose (50 to 100 mg) lasting 6 hours. An additional toxic manifestation unrelated to the blocking actions is the occasional appearance of skin rashes, including exfoliative dermatitis.

Propantheline. *Propantheline bromide* (PRO-BANTHINE) resembles methantheline chemically (isopropyl groups replace the ethyl substituents on the quaternary N atom). Its pharmacological properties are also similar to those of methantheline, but it is two to five times more potent. It is one of the more widely used of the synthetic antimuscarinic drugs. Very high doses block the skeletal neuromuscular junction. The usual clinical dose (15 mg) acts for about 6 hours. Propantheline bromide, administered orally, slows gastric emptying in man (Hurwitz *et al.*, 1977). The significance of this pharmacological action of propantheline and other atropine-like compounds in the management of peptic ulcer has not been clarified.

Other Compounds. Other drugs in this category include *anisotropine methylbromide* (VALPIN), *clidinium bromide* (QUARZAN; also in combination with chlordiazepoxide as LIBRAX and others), *glycopyrrolate* (ROBINUL; also used parenterally in conjunction with anesthesia), *hexocyclium methylsulfate* (TRAL), *isopropamide iodide* (DARBID), *mepenzolate bromide* (CANTIL), *oxyphenonium bromide* (ANTRENYL BROMIDE), and *tridihexethyl chloride* (PATHILON). Their structural formulas appear in *earlier editions* of this textbook. Many of these drugs, as well as the belladonna alkaloids, are found in a large number of combination products that include sedatives and, in some cases, other agents.

SYNTHETIC TERTIARY-AMINE ANTIMUSCARINIC COMPOUNDS

Certain of these agents are particularly useful in ophthalmology; included in this category are *cyclopentolate hydrochloride* (CYCLOGYL) and *tropicamide* (MYDRIACYL). Their structural formulas are as follows:

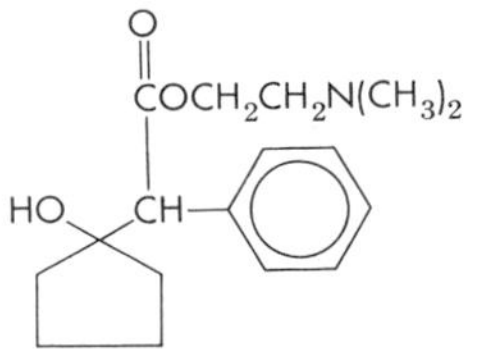

Cyclopentolate

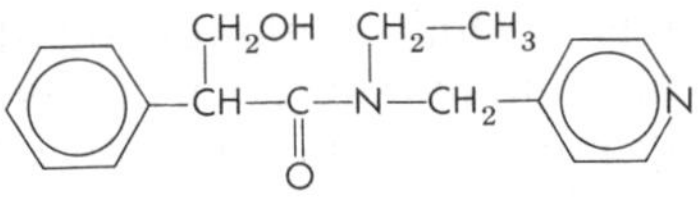

Tropicamide

Ophthalmological properties and preparations of these two drugs are listed in Table 7–3.

TERTIARY AMINES WITH ANTISPASMODIC PROPERTIES

Dicyclomine hydrochloride (BENTYL, others), *oxyphencyclimine hydrochloride* (DARICON), and *thiphenamil hydrochloride* decrease spasm of the gastrointestinal tract, biliary tract, ureter, and uterus without producing characteristic atropinic effects on the salivary, sweat, or gastrointestinal glands, the eye, or the cardiovascular system, except in large doses. The structural formula of dicyclomine is as follows:

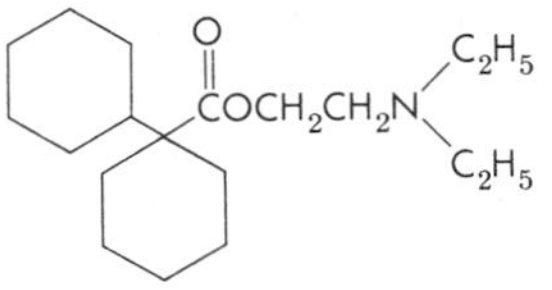

Dicyclomine

The major action of these agents is purported to be a nonspecific direct relaxant action on smooth muscle rather than a competitive antagonism of ACh. Thiphenamil is chemically related to the local anesthetics and has local anesthetic activity. Clinical use of these drugs has been disappointing.

THERAPEUTIC USES OF ANTIMUSCARINIC DRUGS

The belladonna alkaloids have been employed in a wide variety of clinical conditions, predominantly to inhibit effects of parasympathetic nervous system activity. However, the lack of selectivity of the antimuscarinic agents makes it difficult to obtain desired therapeutic responses without concomitant side effects. The latter usually are not serious but are sufficiently disturbing to the patient to limit sharply the dosage tolerated and therefore the usefulness of these agents, particularly for chronic administration. In addition, the efficacy of atropine-like drugs for several gastrointestinal disorders, their major use, is marginal. Fortunately, H_2-receptor blockers are now available as an alternative for the treatment of ulcer disease.

Certain of the synthetic belladonna substitutes are used much more extensively than are the natural alkaloids in a number of clinical conditions. However, there are few situations in which this preference is supported by evidence. With the discovery of subclasses of muscarinic receptors, it is possible that more selective antimuscarinic agents may be developed. Pirenzepine shows promise as a selective inhibitor of gastric secretion and may be of value in the management of peptic ulcer. However, its place in clinical practice is yet to be defined.

Gastrointestinal Tract. Antimuscarinic agents have been widely employed in the management of peptic ulcer. Although these drugs can reduce the secretion of gastric acid and gastric motility, the doses required to produce these effects are usually associated with pronounced side effects, such as dryness of the mouth, loss of visual accommodation, photophobia, and difficulty in urination. As a consequence, patient compliance in the long-term management of symptoms of peptic ulcer with these drugs is poor. Although Feldman and co-workers (1977) reported that propantheline can inhibit the secretion of gastric acid (stimulated by food) in doses that produce minimal side effects, most investigators have concluded that antimuscarinic agents that are currently available, even when administered in relatively high doses, are not unequivocally efficacious in the management of patients with peptic ulcer (Ivey, 1975a).

If an antimuscarinic drug is to be used, belladonna tincture is the most economical and is readily titrated to what can be considered the patient's optimal dose. A relatively high dose is less troublesome if taken at bedtime, so that peak side effects as well as inhibition of gastric secretion occur during sleep. The use of H_2-receptor blocking agents has resulted in marked improvement in the treatment of peptic ulcer (see Chapter 26). Most patients with this disease will also respond well to appropriate doses of antacids, which may be given alone or in conjunction with an H_2 blocker if necessary. It is thus difficult to describe a useful role for antimuscarinic agents in the treatment of peptic ulcer.

The belladonna alkaloids and their synthetic substitutes have been employed and recommended in a wide variety of conditions known or supposed to involve increased tone ("spasticity") or motility of the gastrointestinal tract. These agents can reduce tone and motility when administered in maximal tolerated doses, and they might be expected to have a real effect if the condition in question is in fact due to excessive smooth muscle contraction, a point that is often in doubt. Although antimuscarinic agents are commonly used in the management of irritable colon syndrome, there is no convincing evidence that these drugs are effective in this condition. A difficulty in evaluation of the efficacy of any treatment for the management of irritable colon syndrome is the observation that placebo medication has been found to be effective in over 35% of patients with this condition (Ivey, 1975b).

The intestinal hypermotility and increased frequency of stools associated with administration of two antihypertensive agents, guanethidine and reserpine, are frequently well controlled by atropine-like drugs. Similarly, diarrhea sometimes associated with irritative conditions of the lower bowel, such as mild dysenteries and diverticulitis, may respond to such therapy. In these conditions, both the frequency of bowel movements and the associated abdominal cramps may be reduced or fully controlled. However, more severe conditions such as salmonella dysenteries, ulcerative colitis, and regional enteritis respond poorly.

The belladonna alkaloids and synthetic substitutes are very effective in reducing excessive salivation, such as that associated with heavy-metal poisoning or parkinsonism; indeed, the dosage must be adjusted carefully to avoid reducing secretion to the point where dry mouth is troublesome. Although these agents are rarely effective alone in relieving biliary colic, they are commonly administered with morphine or another opioid. Antimuscarinic agents can reduce the volume and tryptic activity of pancreatic secretion, perhaps largely secondary to retarded entry of acid gastric contents into the duodenum and thus delayed release of secretin. Several agents, particularly methantheline and propantheline, have been tried in the treatment of acute pancreatitis; however, evidence for their efficacy in this condition remains entirely unconvincing.

Uses in Ophthalmology. Effects limited to the eye are obtained by local administration of an antimuscarinic drug to produce mydriasis and cycloplegia. Cycloplegia is not attainable without mydriasis and requires higher concentrations or more prolonged application of a given agent. Mydriasis is often necessary for thorough examination of the retina and optic disc and in the therapy of acute iritis, iridocyclitis, and keratitis. The belladonna mydriatics may be alternated with miotics for breaking or preventing the development of adhesions between the iris and the lens. Complete cycloplegia may be necessary in the treatment of iridocyclitis and choroiditis, following cataract surgery, and for accurate measurement of refractive errors. In instances where complete cycloplegia is required, agents such as atropine or scopolamine, which are more effective, are preferred to drugs such as cyclopentolate and tropicamide. Details of the drugs commonly used and the duration of action of the usual solutions are given in Table 7–3. One or 2 drops of an aqueous solution, often containing a surface-active agent to facilitate penetration, is instilled into the conjunctival sac and repeated as necessary to produce the desired intensity and duration of effect. The values given vary with the frequency and duration of contact with the solution and with individual susceptibility. Although the effect of a single drop of a solution of atropine on healthy eyes is very prolonged, in acute inflammation two or three instillations a day may be required to maintain a full effect. Atropine occasionally causes local irritation of the eye, and in susceptible persons it may produce swelling of the eyelids and conjunctivitis. With continued use, the conjunctivitis may become chronic. Therapy with antihistaminic agents may control the atropine conjunctivitis, or therapy may be continued with another agent (*e.g.,* scopolamine).

Shorter-acting substitutes for atropine or scopolamine are used when prolonged mydriasis and cycloplegia are not required or may pose a hazard to the patient. The standard agents for this purpose are homatropine, cyclopentolate, and tropicamide. Of these, homatropine has the longest action but may not provide adequate cycloplegia even with 5% solutions. Where mydriasis alone is desired, the weaker solutions of cyclopentolate or tropicamide may be used, if necessary in combination with a sympathomimetic drug such as phenylephrine. Psychotic reactions, behavioral disturbances, and convulsions have appeared after ophthalmic use of cyclopentolate.

It is of great importance to recognize patients who are predisposed to narrow-angle glaucoma. The ophthalmic use of any of the antimuscarinic drugs may increase intraocular pressure in eyes with a narrow angle between iris and cornea, precipitating an attack of *acute glaucoma* with the potential hazard of ensuing blindness, particularly if mydriasis is prolonged. Atropine and scopolamine are therefore particularly dangerous. Systemic use of the antimuscarinic agents can also precipitate glaucoma in such predisposed patients. In wide-angle glaucoma the drugs generally do not cause dangerous elevation of intraocular pressure, particularly if the patient is treated soon afterward with locally applied miotics. Although narrow-angle glaucoma is a very rare condition, the use of drugs with antimuscarinic properties is not; careful ophthalmological evaluation, including examination with tonometer and gonioscope, should be undertaken to detect the possible presence of a narrow-angle anterior chamber before starting therapy with these agents, particularly if therapy is to be intensive or prolonged. Mydriasis due to the shorter-acting agents may be counteracted by local application of pilocarpine (1 to 4%); mydriasis from atropine and scopolamine is usually only partly counteracted, even by physostigmine (0.25%) or isoflurophate (0.025%).

The photophobia associated with mydriasis may require that the patient wear dark glasses. Although absorption into the blood stream from the conjunctival sac is minimal, systemic toxicity can occur from an antimuscarinic agent that reaches more absorptive mucosal surfaces by way of the nasolacrimal duct. This danger should be minimized by pressure on the inner canthus of the eye for a few minutes after each instillation. This precaution is particularly important in small children, who are highly susceptible to the toxic effects of belladonna alkaloids.

Respiratory Tract. Atropine and other belladonna alkaloids and substitutes reduce secretion in both the upper and the lower respiratory tract. This effect in the nasopharynx may provide some symptomatic relief of *acute rhinitis* associated with *coryza* or *hay fever,* but such therapy does not affect the natural course of the condition. It is probable that the contribution of antihistamines employed in "cold" mixtures is primarily due to their antimuscarinic properties, except in conditions with an allergic basis.

The belladonna alkaloids can induce bronchial dilatation and were formerly in common use as a remedy for bronchial asthma. They appear to have beneficial effects when there is obstruction of the airway associated with chronic bronchitis. *Ipratropium bromide,* a congener of methylatropine that is currently available only for experimental use in the United States, is an effective bronchodilator when administered by inhalation in doses of 40 to 80 μg (Poppius and Salorinne, 1973). In this dose, ipratropium appears to be as effective as the β_2-adrenergic agonist albuterol (200 μg, by inhalation) in relieving airway obstruction in patients with chronic bronchitis. In contrast, albuterol is much more effective in cases of bronchial asthma (Petrie and Palmer, 1975). Ipratropium, administered by aerosol, produces a significant increase in forced expiratory volume (FEV_1) without significantly affecting the viscosity or volume of sputum. It appears to cause fewer systemic side effects than do β-adrenergic agonists used in the treatment of obstructive pulmonary disease and may become a useful agent for the management of selected patients with such afflictions (Symposium, 1975; May and Palmer, 1977). The concurrent use of ipratropium and a β-adrenergic agonist such as fenoterol or albuterol produces additive effects on FEV_1 and functional ventilation capacity when administered by aerosol (Jenkins *et al.,* 1982). The duration of action of ipratropium when given by this route is approximately 6 hours.

When administered systemically, antimuscarinic agents may reduce the volume of bronchial secretion, which can result in decreased fluidity and subsequent inspissation of the residual secretion. This viscid material is difficult to remove from the respiratory tree, and its presence can dangerously obstruct airflow and predispose to infection. Because of the effect on bronchial secretion, repeated administration of any antimuscarinic drug to a patient with chronic lung disease is considered by some authorities to be potentially hazardous.

Cardiovascular System. Aside from inhibition of certain reflexes during anesthesia and surgery, the cardiovascular effects of the belladonna alkaloids have limited clinical application, and the synthetic substitutes are little used in this field. Atropine is a specific antidote for the cardiovascular collapse that may result from the injudicious administration of a choline ester.

Atropine may be of value in the *initial* treatment of carefully selected patients with *acute myocardial infarction* in whom excessive vagal tone causes sinus or nodal bradycardia accompanied by a falling blood pressure and a low cardiac output, or a high-grade A-V block resulting in ectopic ventricular tachyarrhythmia (*see* Thomas and Woodgate, 1966; Adgey *et al.,* 1968). Administered intravenously, small doses of atropine (0.2 to 0.4 mg) may restore a normal heart rate and increase the blood pressure to an adequate level within a few minutes. However, there are very substantial risks in this therapeutic maneuver. If the drug accelerates heart rate without improving coronary perfusion, myocardial ischemia will be even more pronounced. Uncontrollable tachyarrhythmias, including ventricular tachycardia and fibrillation, may result (*see* Richman, 1974). Repeated doses of atropine must therefore be avoided. Bradycardia, if persistent, should be controlled by the insertion of a pacemaker as soon as possible.

Atropine is occasionally useful in reducing the severe bradycardia and syncope associated with a *hyperactive carotid sinus reflex*. It has little effect on most ventricular rhythms. In some patients atropine may eliminate ventricular premature contractions associated with a very slow atrial rate. It may also reduce the degree of A-V block when increased vagal tone is a major factor in the conduction defect. Atropine is occasionally useful in the diagnosis of *anomalous A-V conduction* (Wolff-Parkinson-White syndrome) by restoring the QRS complex to normal duration.

Central Nervous System. For many years the belladonna alkaloids and subsequently the tertiary-amine synthetic substitutes were the only agents helpful in the treatment of *parkinsonism*. Levodopa is now the treatment of choice, but concurrent therapy with the synthetic antimuscarinic agents may be required (*see* Chapter 21). Synthetic agents such as benztropine are also useful in the treatment of parkinsonism-like symptoms induced by phenothiazines or butyrophenones (*see* Chapter 19).

The belladonna alkaloids were among the first drugs to be used in the prevention of *motion sickness*. Scopolamine is the most effective prophylactic agent for short (4- to 6-hour) exposures to severe motion, and probably for periods up to several days. Oral doses of 0.1 mg protect 75% of susceptible persons, and do not affect vision and rarely cause dryness of the mouth. Intramuscular injection of 0.2 mg controls symptoms of most seasick individuals; sedation is the major disadvantage. (*See* Brand and Whittingham, 1970.) The superiority of scopolamine is more apparent the more susceptible the subject and the more severe the stress. The drug is not recommended for nausea and vomiting due to most other causes. All agents used to combat motion sickness should be given *prophylactically;* they are much less effective after severe nausea or vomiting has developed. A preparation for the transdermal administration of scopolamine (TRANSDERM SCŌP) has been shown to be highly effective for the prevention of motion sickness (Price *et al.*, 1981). The drug is incorporated into an adhesive unit that is applied behind the ear. For optimal effects, the application should be made at least 4 hours before the antiemetic effect is required. The duration of action of the preparation is about 72 hours, during which time approximately 0.5 mg of scopolamine is delivered. Although anticholinergic side effects are generally not pronounced, dry mouth, blurred vision, and drowsiness have been associated with use of this preparation. (For further discussion of motion sickness, *see* Chapter 26.)

The sedation, tranquilization, and amnesia produced by scopolamine are useful in a variety of circumstances, including *labor*. In this situation it is almost always combined with agents that produce analgesia or sedation. Given alone in the presence of pain or severe anxiety, scopolamine may induce outbursts of uncontrolled behavior.

Uses in Anesthesia. The belladonna alkaloids were often used prior to the administration of a general anesthetic agent, mainly to inhibit excessive salivation and secretions of the respiratory tract; their concomitant bronchodilator action is also of value. The increasing use of relatively nonirritating anesthetics lessens the importance of antimuscarinic agents for this purpose. Scopolamine may contribute to tranquilization and amnesia (*see* Chapter 13). Atropine is commonly given with neostigmine to counteract its parasympathomimetic effects when the latter agent is used to end curarization after surgery. Serious cardiac arrhythmias have occasionally occurred, perhaps due to the combination of initial central vagal stimulation by atropine and the cholinomimetic effect of neostigmine.

Genitourinary Tract. Atropine has often been given with an opioid in the treatment of *renal colic* in the hope that it will relax the ureteral smooth muscle; however, as in biliary colic, it probably does not make a major contribution to the relief of pain. The belladonna alkaloids and several synthetic substitutes can lower intravesicular pressure, increase capacity, and reduce the frequency of urinary bladder contractions by antagonizing the parasympathetic control of this organ. The block is less complete than in many other organs, but it has been taken as a basis for the use of such agents in *enuresis* in children, particularly when a progressive increase in bladder capacity is the objective, to reduce urinary frequency in spastic paraplegia, and to increase the capacity of the bladder in conditions in which irritation has led to hypertonicity. However, it has not been established that antimuscarinic drugs make a major contribution to the treatment of any of these conditions. Tricyclic antidepressants are used to manage enuresis; it is possible that at least a component of the efficacy of this approach is due to the atropine-like properties of this class of drugs.

Anticholinesterase and Mushroom Poisoning. The use of atropine in large doses for the treatment of poisoning by anti-ChE organophosphorus insecticides is discussed in detail in Chapter 6. Atropine may also be used to antagonize the parasympathomimetic effects of neostigmine or other anti-ChE agents administered in the treatment of myasthenia gravis. It does not interfere with the salutary effects at the skeletal neuromuscular junction, and is particularly useful early in therapy, before tolerance to muscarinic side effects has developed.

Atropine is a specific antidote for the so-called *rapid type* of *mushroom poisoning* due to the cholinomimetic alkaloid muscarine, found in *Amanita muscaria* and a few other fungi. Atropine is of no value in the *delayed type* of mushroom poisoning due to the toxins of *A. phalloides* and certain other species of the same genus. (*See* Chapter 5.)

Adgey, A. A. J.; Geddes, J. S.; Mulholland, H. C.; Keegan, D. A. J.; and Pantridge, J. F. Incidence, significance, and management of early bradyarrhythmia complicating acute myocardial infarction. *Lancet,* **1968,** *2,* 1097–1101.

Aquilonius, S.-M. Physostigmine in the treatment of drug overdose. In, *Cholinergic Mechanisms and Psychopharmacology,* Vol. 24. (Jenden, D. J., ed.) Plenum Press, New York, **1978,** pp. 817–825.

Birdsall, N. J. M.; Burgen, A. S. V.; and Hulme, E. C. The binding of agonists to brain muscarinic receptors. *Mol. Pharmacol.,* **1978,** *14,* 723–736.

Brand, J. J., and Whittingham, P. Intramuscular hyoscine in control of motion sickness. *Lancet,* **1970,** *2,* 232–234.

Dauchot, P., and Gravenstein, J. S. Effects of atropine on the electrocardiogram in different age groups. *Clin. Pharmacol. Ther.,* **1971,** *12,* 274–280.

Davenport, H. W., and Kauffman, G. L. Plasma shedding by the canine oxyntic and pyloric glandular mucosa induced by topical action of acetylcholine. *Gastroenterology,* **1975,** *69,* 190–197.

Feldman, M.; Richardson, C. T.; Peterson, W. L.; Walsh, J. H.; and Fordtran, J. S. Effect of low-dose propantheline on food-stimulated gastric acid secretion. *N. Engl. J. Med.,* **1977,** *297,* 1427–1430.

Hammer, R.; Berrie, C. P.; Birdsall, N. J. M.; Burgen, A. S. V.; and Hulme, E. C. Pirenzepine distinguishes between different subclasses of muscarinic receptors. *Nature,* **1980,** *283,* 90–92.

Hayes, A. H., Jr.; Copelan, H. W.; and Ketchum, J. S. Effects of large intramuscular doses of atropine on cardiac rhythm. *Clin. Pharmacol. Ther.,* **1971,** *12,* 482–486.

Hulme, E. C.; Birdsall, N. J. M.; Burgen, A. S. V.; and Mehta, P. The binding of antagonists to brain muscarinic receptors. *Mol. Pharmacol.,* **1978,** *14,* 737–750.

Hurwitz, A.; Robinson, R. G.; and Herrin, W. F. Prolongation of gastric emptying by oral propantheline. *Clin. Pharmacol. Ther.,* **1977,** *22,* 206–210.

Ivey, K. J. Anticholinergics: do they work in peptic ulcer? *Gastroenterology,* **1975a,** *68,* 154–166.

———. Are anticholinergics of use in the irritable colon syndrome? *Ibid.,* **1975b,** *68,* 1300–1307.

Jenkins, C. R.; Chow, C. M.; Fisher, B. L.; and Marlin, G. E. Ipratropium bromide and fenoterol by aerosolized solution. *Br. J. Clin. Pharmacol.,* **1982,** *14,* 113–115.

Jonkman, J. H. G.; Van Bork, L. E.; Wijsbeek, J.; De Zeeuw, R. A.; and Orie, N. G. M. Variations in the bioavailability of thiazinamium methylsulfate. *Clin. Pharmacol. Ther.,* **1977,** *21,* 457–463.

Kauffman, G. L., and Davenport, H. W. Effect of atropine in reducing plasma protein shedding by the canine oxyntic glandular mucosa induced by topical irrigation with histamine or cobra venom. *Gastroenterology,* **1975,** *69,* 198–199.

Ketchum, J. S.; Sidell, F. R.; Crowell, E. B., Jr.; Aghajanian, G. K.; and Hayes, A. H., Jr. Atropine, scopolamine, and ditran: comparative pharmacology and antagonists in man. *Psychopharmacologia,* **1973,** *28,* 121–145.

May, C. S., and Palmer, K. N. V. Effect of aerosol ipratropium bromide (Sch 1000) on sputum viscosity and volume in chronic bronchitis. *Br. J. Clin. Pharmacol.,* **1977,** *4,* 491–492.

Petrie, G. R., and Palmer, K. N. V. Comparison of aerosol ipratropium bromide and salbutamol in chronic bronchitis and asthma. *Br. Med. J.,* **1975,** *1,* 430–432.

Poppius, H., and Salorinne, Y. Comparative trial of a new anticholinergic bronchodilator, Sch 1000, and salbutamol in chronic bronchitis. *Br. Med. J.,* **1973,** *4,* 134–136.

Price, N. M.; Schmitt, L. G.; McGuire, J.; Shaw, J. E.; and Trobough, G. Transdermal scopolamine in the prevention of motion sickness at sea. *Clin. Pharmacol. Ther.,* **1981,** *29,* 414–419.

Richman, S. Adverse effect of atropine during myocardial infarction. Enhancement of ischemia following intravenously administered atropine. *J.A.M.A.,* **1974,** *228,* 1414–1416.

Rumack, B. H. Anticholinergic poisoning: treatment with physostigmine. *Pediatrics,* **1973,** *52,* 449–451.

Shein, K., and Smith, S. E. Structure-activity relationships for the anticholinoceptor action of tricyclic antidepressants. *Br. J. Pharmacol.,* **1978,** *62,* 567–571.

Smith, R. L., and Powell, D. W. Prolonged treatment of Ménétrièr's disease with an oral anticholinergic drug. *Gastroenterology,* **1978,** *74,* 903–906.

Thomas, M., and Woodgate, D. Effect of atropine on bradycardia and hypotension in acute myocardial infarction. *Br. Heart J.,* **1966,** *28,* 409–413.

Yamamura, H. I., and Snyder, S. H. Muscarinic cholinergic receptor binding in the longitudinal muscle of the guinea pig ileum with (^{3}H) quinuclidinyl benzilate. *Mol. Pharmacol.,* **1974,** *10,* 861–867.

Monographs and Reviews

Brimblecombe, R. W. *Drug Actions on Cholinergic Systems.* University Park Press, Baltimore, **1974.**

de Wied, D., and de Jong, W. Drug effects and hypothalamic–anterior pituitary function. *Annu. Rev. Pharmacol.,* **1974,** *14,* 389–412.

Goldstein, A.; Aronow, L.; and Kalman, S. M. *Principles of Drug Action: The Basis of Pharmacology,* 2nd ed. John Wiley & Sons, Inc., New York, **1974,** p. 111.

Krnjević, K. Central cholinergic pathways. *Fed. Proc.,* **1969,** *28,* 113–120.

———. Chemical nature of synaptic transmission in vertebrates. *Physiol. Rev.,* **1974,** *54,* 418–540.

Longo, V. G. Behavioral and electroencephalographic effects of atropine and related compounds. *Pharmacol. Rev.,* **1966,** *18,* 965–996.

Shader, R. I., and Greenblatt, D. J. Belladonna alkaloids and synthetic anticholinergics: uses and toxicity. In, *Psychiatric Complications of Medical Drugs.* (Shader, R. I., ed.) Raven Press, New York, **1972,** pp. 103–147.

Symposium. (Various authors.) The place of parasympatholytic drugs in the management of chronic obstructive airways disease. (Hoffbrand, B. I., ed.) *Postgrad. Med. J.,* **1975,** *51,* Suppl. 7, pp. 1–161.

Symposium. (Various authors.) Proceedings of the second international symposium on pirenzepine. Advances in basic and clinical pharmacology of pirenzepine. (Baron, J. H., and Londong, W., eds.) *Scand. J. Gastroenterol.,* **1980,** *15,* Suppl. 66, pp. 1–114.

Symposium. (Various authors.) Subtypes of muscarinic receptors. (Hirschowitz, B. I.; Hammer, R.; Giachetti, A.; Keirns, J. J.; and Levine, R. R.; eds.) *Trends Pharmacol. Sci.,* **1984,** Suppl., 1–103.

Toman, J. E. P., and Davis, J. P. The effects of drugs upon the electrical activity of the brain. *Pharmacol. Rev.,* **1949,** *1,* 425–492.

Weiner, N. Neurotransmitter systems in the central nervous system. In, *Drugs and the Developing Brain.* (Vernadakis, A., and Weiner, N., eds.) Plenum Press, New York, **1974,** pp. 105–131.

CHAPTER

8 NOREPINEPHRINE, EPINEPHRINE, AND THE SYMPATHOMIMETIC AMINES

Norman Weiner

The sympathetic nervous system is vitally involved in the homeostatic regulation of a wide variety of functions, among which are heart rate, force of cardiac contraction, vasomotor tone, blood pressure, bronchial airway tone, and carbohydrate and fatty acid metabolism. Stimulation of the sympathetic nervous system normally occurs in response to physical activity, psychological stress, generalized allergic reactions, and other situations in which the organism is provoked. Because of the diverse functions that are mediated or modified by the sympathetic nervous system, agents that mimic or alter its activity are useful in the treatment of several clinical disorders, including hypertension, shock, cardiac failure and arrhythmias, asthma, allergy, and anaphylaxis.

The host of physiological and metabolic responses that follows stimulation of sympathetic nerves in mammals is usually mediated by the neurotransmitter, norepinephrine. As part of the response to stress, the adrenal medulla is also stimulated, resulting in elevation of the concentrations of epinephrine and norepinephrine in the circulation. The actions of these two catecholamines are very similar at some sites but differ significantly at others. For example, both compounds stimulate the myocardium; however, epinephrine dilates blood vessels to skeletal muscle, whereas norepinephrine has a minimal constricting effect on them. Dopamine is a third, naturally occurring catecholamine. While it is found predominantly in the basal ganglia of the central nervous system (CNS), dopaminergic nerve endings and specific receptors for this catecholamine have been identified elsewhere in the CNS and in the periphery. The role of the catecholamines in the CNS is detailed in Chapter 12 and elsewhere. As might be expected, sympathomimetic amines—naturally occurring catecholamines and drugs that mimic their actions—comprise one of the more extensively studied groups of pharmacological agents.

Most of the actions of such compounds can be classified into six broad types: (1) a *peripheral excitatory action* on certain types of smooth muscle, such as those in blood vessels supplying skin and mucous membranes, and on gland cells, such as those in salivary and sweat glands; (2) a *peripheral inhibitory action* on certain other types of smooth muscle, such as those in the wall of the gut, in the bronchial tree, and in blood vessels supplying skeletal muscle; (3) a *cardiac excitatory action*, responsible for an increase in heart rate and force of contraction; (4) *metabolic actions*, such as an increase in rate of glycogenolysis in liver and muscle, and liberation of free fatty acids from adipose tissue; (5) *endocrine actions*, such as modulation of the secretion of insulin, renin, and pituitary hormones; and (6) *CNS actions*, such as respiratory stimulation and, with some of the drugs, an increase in wakefulness, psychomotor activity, and a reduction in appetite. All sympathomimetic drugs do not show each of the above types of action to the same degree. However, many of the differences in their effects are only quantitative, and description of the effects of each compound would be unnecessarily repetitive. Therefore, the pharmacological properties of these drugs as a class are described in detail for the prototypical agent, *epinephrine*.

History. The pressor effect of suprarenal extracts was first shown by Oliver and Schäfer in 1895. The active principle was named epinephrine by Abel in 1899 and synthesized independently by Stolz and Dakin (*see* Hartung, 1931). The development of our knowledge of epinephrine and norepinephrine as neurohumoral transmitters is outlined in Chapter 4. Barger and Dale (1910) studied the pharmacological activity of a large series of synthetic amines related to epinephrine and termed their action *sympathomimetic*. This important study determined the basic structural requirements for activity. When it was later found that cocaine or chronic denervation of effector organs reduced the responses to ephedrine and tyramine but enhanced the effects of epinephrine, it became clear that the differences between sympathomimetic amines were not simply quantitative. It was suggested that epinephrine acted directly on the effector cell while ephedrine and tyramine had an indirect effect by acting on the nerve endings. The discovery that reserpine depletes tissues of norepinephrine (Bertler *et al.*, 1956) was followed by evidence that tyramine and certain other sympathomimetic amines do not act on tissues from animals that have been treated with reserpine; this too indicated that they act by releasing endogenous norepinephrine (Burn and Rand, 1958).

Sites and Mechanism of Action. *α- and β-Adrenergic Receptors, or Adrenoceptors.* In his classical studies, Ahlquist (1948) examined the effects of epinephrine, norepinephrine, and isoproterenol on a variety of target tissues and concluded that differences in the actions of these catecholamines could be explained by the presence of two distinct types of receptors for the catecholamines, denoted as α and β. Subsequently, the development of more selective agonists and antagonists that act at adrenergic receptors has allowed their subclassification. Lands and coworkers (1967a, 1967b) categorized β receptors as either β_1 or β_2; β_1-adrenergic receptors predominate in cardiac tissues, while β_2 receptors are present primarily in smooth muscle and gland cells. However, different tissues may possess both β_1 and β_2 receptors in varying proportions (*see* Minneman *et al.*, 1979). α Receptors also appear to be heterogeneous. Those designated α_1 predominate at postsynaptic effector sites of smooth muscle and gland cells; α_2 receptors, which are proposed to exist on nerve terminals, are believed to mediate the presynaptic feedback inhibition of neural release of norepinephrine and, perhaps, acetylcholine. Activation of such α_2 receptors on cholinergic nerve terminals may contribute to the inhibition of intestinal activity caused by α-adrenergic agonists. α_2 Receptors are also present at postjunctional sites in several tissues, including the brain, uterus, parotid gland, and certain regions of vascular smooth muscle. Many of the adrenergic receptors in the CNS have not been definitively classified at the present time.

The relative sensitivities of these adrenergic receptors to epinephrine, norepinephrine, and isoproterenol are as follows: (1) at α_1 receptors, epinephrine is equal to or more potent than norepinephrine, which in turn is much more potent than isoproterenol; (2) at α_2 receptors, epinephrine is either more or less potent than norepinephrine, depending on the tissue, and isoproterenol is ineffective; (3) at β_1 receptors, isoproterenol is more potent than epinephrine, which is equipotent with norepinephrine; (4) at β_2 receptors, isoproterenol is equal to or more potent than epinephrine, which is much more potent than norepinephrine. Drugs that activate or block these receptors more selectively are detailed in this and the next chapter. Particularly notable has been the development of β_1- and β_2-adrenergic agonists and of β_1 antagonists. The distributions of these receptors and the responses that occur when they are activated are detailed in Table 4–1 (page 72).

In general, the effect of activation of α_1 receptors in smooth muscle is excitatory while that of β_2 receptors at such sites is inhibitory, although this is not an absolute rule. In other tissues, β-adrenergic receptors can mediate stimulatory effects (*see* Table 4–1). Thus, activation of β_2 receptors results in stimulation of various secretions (*e.g.*, that of insulin), and the stimulatory effects of catecholamines on the heart are mediated by β_1 receptors.

Catecholamines inhibit propulsive contractions and reduce the tone of most intestinal smooth muscle; these effects appear to be mediated by both α- and β-adrenergic receptors. Activation of β receptors located on smooth muscle cells results in their relaxation. α Receptors appear to inhibit gastrointestinal motility primarily by a presynaptic action. Thus, activation of α_2 receptors on cholinergic nerve terminals within the intestinal wall is associated with inhibition of the release of acetylcholine. For this reason the presence of both an α- and a β-blocking agent is required to prevent completely the inhibitory effect of epinephrine on the intestine.

An important factor in the response of an organ to sympathomimetic amines is the proportion and density of α and β receptors in the tissue. Norepinephrine has little effect on bronchial air flow because the receptors in bronchial smooth muscle appear to be largely of the β_2 type. In contrast, isoproterenol and epinephrine are potent bronchodilators. Cutaneous blood vessels possess α receptors almost exclusively; thus, norepinephrine and epinephrine cause marked constriction of such vessels, while isoproterenol has little effect. The smooth muscle of blood vessels supplying skeletal muscles has both β_2 receptors, the activation of which by low concentrations of epinephrine causes vasodilatation, and α receptors that allow epinephrine to constrict these vessels. In this tissue the threshold concentration of epinephrine for activation of β_2 receptors is lower, but when both types of receptors are activated the response to α receptors predominates.

Release of Stored Norepinephrine. Many sympathomimetic drugs, such as *amphetamine* and *ephedrine*, exert a large fraction of their effects by releasing norepinephrine from storage sites in the sympathetic nerves to the effector organ. Such agents are termed *indirectly acting sympathomimetic amines.* The responses they elicit are therefore similar to those of norepinephrine but are slower in onset and generally longer lasting than those of a single equipressor dose of norepinephrine. They also exhibit tachyphylaxis; that is, repeated injections or continuous infusions of these indirectly acting drugs become less effective. The tachyphylaxis is often said to result from depletion of the "releasable stores" of norepinephrine. However, there seems to be some circularity in this assertion, since the nerve endings still contain the catecholamine and responses to nerve stimulation remain intact. Many sympathomimetic drugs owe only part of their effect to norepinephrine release and also act directly on adrenergic receptors. These agents are generally called *mixed-acting sympathomimetic amines* (*see* below).

Role of Sympathomimetic Amines in the Modulation of Neural Release of Norepinephrine. α-Adrenergic agonists are able to inhibit profoundly the release of norepinephrine by neurons (Haggendahl, 1970; Starke, 1971; Enero *et al.,* 1972; Cubeddu and Weiner, 1975). Conversely, when the sympathetic nerve to a tissue is stimulated in the presence of a nonselective α-adrenergic antagonist, there is a marked increase in the amount of norepinephrine released per nerve impulse (Brown and Gillespie, 1957; DePotter *et al.,* 1971). The inhibitory effect of norepinephrine on its release from noradrenergic nerve terminals appears to be mediated by α receptors that are pharmacologically distinct from the classical α_1 postsynaptic receptor. As mentioned, these receptors have been designated α_2 and are presumed to be located on presynaptic nerve terminals (Starke, 1972). Certain drugs, such as nordefrin (α-methylnorepinephrine) and clonidine, are more potent agonists at α_2 than at α_1 receptors, and, at appropriate concentrations, they preferentially inhibit the release of norepinephrine. A major component of the antihypertensive effect of these agents may rely on this action, predominantly at central sites (*see* Chapter 32). Phenylephrine and methoxamine, in contrast, activate postsynaptic α_1 receptors at much lower concentrations than are required to inhibit the release of transmitter (*see* Langer, 1977; Starke, 1977). While β-adrenergic agonists appear to enhance the release of norepinephrine from neurons, these effects are modest and may not be significant under normal circumstances *in vivo* (Dixon *et al.,* 1979).

Reflex Effects. The ultimate response of a target organ to sympathomimetic amines is determined not only by the direct effects of the agent but also by the reflex homeostatic adjustments of the organism. One of the most striking effects of many sympathomimetic amines is a rise in arterial blood pressure due to stimulation of α receptors in vascular beds. This elicits compensatory reflexes through the caroticoaortic baroreceptor system, resulting in a diminution of overall sympathetic tone and an increase in vagal tone; both responses act to slow the heart. This compensatory mechanism is of special importance for drugs having little β-receptor activity and, therefore, little direct cardioaccelerator action. For example, one such drug, phenylephrine, can be used to treat paroxysmal atrial or nodal tachycardia because it raises blood pressure and thereby reflexly lessens sympathetic cardioaccelerator tone and increases parasympathetic cardiodecelerator tone, the combined effects of which may be enough to terminate the episode of tachycardia.

Mechanism of Direct Action on Sympathetic Effectors. Catecholamines act directly on sympathetic effector cells by binding to receptors located in cellular plasma membranes. It is now generally accepted that the effects of stimulation of β_1- and β_2-adrenergic receptors are at least largely mediated by the activation of adenylate cyclase and the resultant accumulation and action of adenosine 3′,5′-monophosphate (cyclic AMP). The immediate consequences of stimulation of α receptors are less well understood; they appear to involve, in part, the mobilization of Ca^{2+} and/or the formation of inositol triphosphate (α_1 receptors) and the inhibition of adenylate cyclase (α_2 receptors). This subject is discussed in Chapters 2 and 4.

The relationships of electrical phenomena, ion fluxes, and changes of tension in smooth muscle are complex and differ between smooth muscles. Visceral smooth muscle contractions are generally associated with slow waves of partial depolarization, in some muscles with superimposed action potentials that travel for some distance along adjacent cells. Contractions due to α-receptor stimulation are accompanied in some muscles by graded depolarization only; in others, there is a concomitant appearance or increased frequency of superimposed action potentials. The ionic mechanisms associated with these changes are also discussed in Chapter 4. In muscles inhibited by β-receptor stimulation the membrane may become hyperpolarized and action potentials may disappear or become less frequent. It is generally believed that such inhibition is caused by reduction of the cytosolic concentration of free Ca^{2+}. This may be mediated by cyclic AMP, but the mechanism is unknown; both enhanced sequestration and efflux of Ca^{2+} may be involved. Relaxation of intestinal smooth muscle in some species is also associated with activation of α-adrenergic receptors. This may be caused, at least in part, by hyperpolarization of the cell membrane as a consequence of increased permeability to K^+ and Cl^- (Tomita and Watanabe, 1973). As mentioned, inhibition of smooth muscle tone by α-adrenergic agonists can also be mediated by inhibition of acetylcholine (ACh) release from cholinergic neurons. Contraction of intestinal sphincter muscle (and other smooth muscles) by α-adrenergic agonists appears to result from a more generalized increase in ion permeability (to Na^+,

K^+, Cl^-, and perhaps Ca^{2+}), and this is associated with a decreased membrane potential.

Localization of Adrenergic Receptors. There is increasing evidence to support the notion that α_1- and β_1-adrenergic receptors are located in the immediate vicinity of adrenergic nerve terminals in peripheral target organs, strategically placed for activation during stimulation of adrenergic nerves. In addition to those located on nerve terminals, both α_2- and β_2-adrenergic receptors also appear to be situated in postjunctional regions that are relatively remote from sites of release of norepinephrine. It is hypothesized that the latter receptors are preferentially stimulated by circulating catecholamines. In some instances, the physiological role of these and other adrenergic receptors (*e.g.,* those on leukocytes and platelets) is not well understood.

Refractoriness to Catecholamines. Chronic exposure of catecholamine-sensitive cells and tissues to adrenergic agonists causes a diminution in their capacity to respond to such agents. This phenomenon is variously termed refractoriness, desensitization, down regulation, or tachyphylaxis. While descriptions of such adaptive changes are common in a variety of experimental and clinical situations, mechanisms are only partially understood. They have been studied extensively in cells that synthesize cyclic AMP in response to β-adrenergic agonists. Following the constant application of isoproterenol or similar agents to such cells, the capacity to synthesize cyclic AMP may be markedly reduced within a few hours. There is evidence for multiple points of regulation. Under some circumstances β-adrenergic receptors become phosphorylated and apparently inactivated. This is presumably a feedback regulatory mechanism that is mediated by cyclic AMP. Under other circumstances the interaction between the receptor and adenylate cyclase is impaired by processes that are not yet understood. In addition, the number of receptors detectable by radioactive ligand-binding assays may be reduced (apparently because of their internalization), triggered in some way by the agonist (*see* Harden, 1983; Lefkowitz *et al.,* 1984). Regulation of this type is not unique to adrenergic receptors; rather, it is the rule in most neural and endocrine systems.

Chemistry and Structure-Activity Relationship of Sympathomimetic Amines. β-Phenylethylamine (Table 8–1) can be viewed as the parent compound of the sympathomimetic amines, consisting of a benzene ring and an ethylamine side chain. The structure permits substitutions to be made on the aromatic ring, the α- and β-carbon atoms, and the terminal amino group, to yield a great variety of compounds with sympathomimetic activity. Norepinephrine, epinephrine, dopamine, and isoproterenol have OH groups substituted in the 3 and 4 positions of the benzene ring. Since *o*-dihydroxybenzene is also known as *catechol,* sympathomimetic amines with these OH substitutions in the aromatic ring are termed *catecholamines.*

Most directly acting sympathomimetic drugs influence both α and β receptors, but the ratio of the α and β activity varies tremendously between

Table 8–1. CHEMICAL STRUCTURES AND MAIN CLINICAL USES OF IMPORTANT SYMPATHOMIMETIC DRUGS †

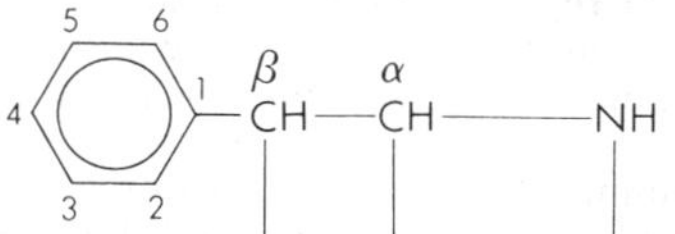

Prototypical formula: benzene ring (positions 5, 6, 4, 1, 3, 2) attached to β CH — α CH — NH

Drug	Ring substituent	β	α	N	α Receptor A N P V	β Receptor B C U	CNS,0
Phenylethylamine		H	H	H			
Epinephrine	3-OH,4-OH	OH	H	CH$_3$	A, P,V	B,C	
Norepinephrine	3-OH,4-OH	OH	H	H	P		
Dopamine	3-OH,4-OH	H	H	H	P		
Dobutamine	3-OH,4-OH	H	H	1 *		C	
Ethylnorepinephrine	3-OH,4-OH	OH	CH$_2$CH$_3$	H		B	
Isoproterenol	3-OH,4-OH	OH	H	CH(CH$_3$)$_2$		B,C	
Isoetharine	3-OH,4-OH	OH	CH$_2$CH$_3$	CH(CH$_3$)$_2$		B	
Metaproterenol	3-OH,5-OH	OH	H	CH(CH$_3$)$_2$		B	
Terbutaline	3-OH,5-OH	OH	H	C(CH$_3$)$_3$		B, U	
Metaraminol	3-OH	OH	CH$_3$	H	P		
Phenylephrine	3-OH	OH	H	CH$_3$	N,P		
Tyramine	4-OH	H	H	H			
Hydroxyamphetamine	4-OH	H	CH$_3$	H			
Ritodrine	4-OH	OH	CH$_3$	2 *		U	
Prenalterol	4-OH	OH ‡	H	-CH(CH$_3$)$_2$		C	
Methoxamine	2-OCH$_3$,5-OCH$_3$	OH	CH$_3$	H	P		
Albuterol	3-CH$_2$OH,4-OH	OH	H	C(CH$_3$)$_3$		B, U	
Amphetamine		H	CH$_3$	H			CNS,0
Methamphetamine		H	CH$_3$	CH$_3$			CNS,0
Benzphetamine		H	CH$_3$	3 *			0
Ephedrine		OH	CH$_3$	CH$_3$	N,P	B,C	
Phenylpropanolamine		OH	CH$_3$	H	N		0
Mephentermine		H	4 *	CH$_3$	N,P		
Phentermine		H	4 *	H			0
Fenfluramine	3-CF$_3$	H	CH$_3$	C$_2$H$_5$			0
Propylhexedrine	5 *	H	CH$_3$	CH$_3$	N		
Diethylpropion			6 *				0
Phenmetrazine			7 *				0
Phendimetrazine			8 *				0

Substituent structures:

1. —CH(CH$_3$)—(CH$_2$)$_2$—[ring]—OH
2. —CH$_2$—CH$_2$—[ring]—OH
3. —N(CH$_3$)—CH$_2$—[ring]
4. —C(CH$_3$)$_3$
5. cyclohexane ring
6. —C(O)—CH(CH$_3$)—N(C$_2$H$_5$)(C$_2$H$_5$)
7. —CH(O—CH$_2$)(CH$_2$)—CH—NH—CH$_3$ (morpholine ring)
8. —CH(O—CH$_2$)(CH$_2$)—CH—N(CH$_3$)(CH$_3$) (morpholine ring)

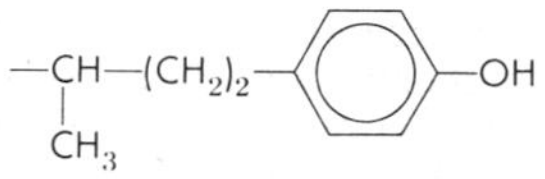

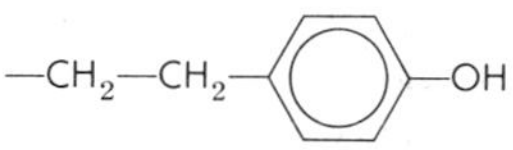

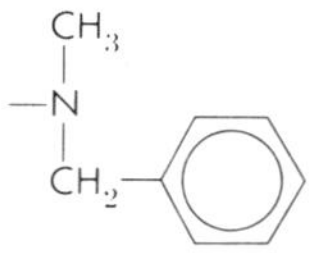

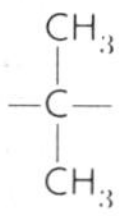

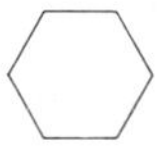

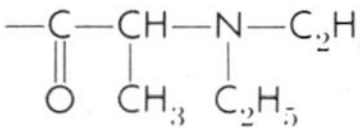

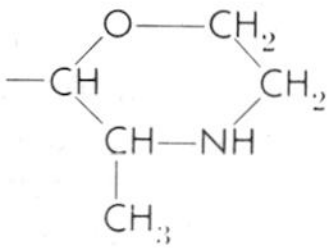

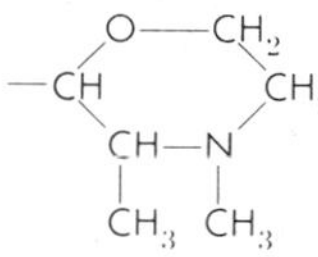

α Activity
A = Allergic reactions (includes β action)
N = Nasal decongestion
P = Pressor (may include β action)
V = Other local vasoconstriction
   (e.g., in local anesthesia)

β Activity
B = Bronchodilator
C = Cardiac
U = Uterus

CNS = Central nervous system
0 = Anorectic

* Numbers bearing an asterisk refer to the substituents numbered in the bottom rows of the table; substituent 3 replaces the N atom, substituent 5 replaces the phenyl ring, and 6, 7, and 8 are attached directly to the phenyl ring, replacing the ethylamine side chain.

† The α and β in the prototypical formula refer to positions of the C atoms in the ethylamine side chain.

‡ Prenalterol has —OCH$_2$— between the aromatic ring and the carbon atom designated as β in the prototypical formula.

drugs, in a continuous spectrum from an almost pure α activity (phenylephrine) to an almost pure β activity (isoproterenol). The structure-activity relationship of directly acting agents is best studied in isolated systems, where indirect and reflex effects will not confuse interpretation. Despite the multiplicity of the sites of action of sympathomimetic amines, several generalizations can be made, as presented below.

Separation of Aromatic Ring and Amino Group. By far the greatest sympathomimetic activity occurs when two carbon atoms separate the ring from the amino group. This rule applies with few exceptions to all types of action.

Substitution on the Amino Group. The effects of amino substitution are most readily seen in the actions of catecholamines on α and β receptors. Increase in the size of the alkyl substituent increases β-receptor activity (*e.g.*, isoproterenol). Norepinephrine has, in general, rather feeble β_2 activity; this is greatly increased in epinephrine with the addition of a methyl group. A notable exception is phenylephrine, which has a N-methyl substituent but is almost a pure α agonist. Selective β_2-receptor stimulants require a large amino substituent, but depend on other substitutions for their selectivity for β_2 rather than for β_1 receptors. In general, the less the substitution on the amino group the greater is the selectivity for α activity, although N-methylation increases the potency of primary amines. Thus, α activity is maximal in epinephrine, less in norepinephrine, and almost absent in isoproterenol.

Substitution on the Aromatic Nucleus. Maximal α and β activity depends on the presence of OH groups in the 3 and 4 positions. When one or both of these groups are absent, without other aromatic substitution, the overall potency is reduced. Phenylephrine is thus less potent than epinephrine on both α and β receptors, with β activity almost completely absent. Hydroxy groups in the 3 and 5 positions confer β_2-receptor selectivity on compounds with large amino substituents. Thus, metaproterenol, terbutaline, and other similar compounds relax the bronchial musculature in patients with asthma without causing significant direct cardiac stimulation. The response to noncatecholamines is in part determined by their capacity to release norepinephrine from sites of storage. These agents thus cause mostly effects that are mediated by α and β_1 receptors, since norepinephrine is a weak β_2 agonist. Phenylethylamines that lack both hydroxyl groups on the ring and the β-hydroxyl group on the side chain act almost exclusively by causing the release of norepinephrine from adrenergic nerve terminals.

Since substitution of polar groups on the phenylethylamine structure makes the resultant compounds less lipophilic, unsubstituted or alkyl-substituted compounds cross the blood-brain barrier more readily and have more central activity. Thus, ephedrine, amphetamine, and methamphetamine exhibit considerable CNS activity. In addition, as mentioned, the absence of polar hydroxyl groups results in a loss of direct peripheral sympathomimetic activity.

Catecholamines have only a brief duration of action and are ineffective after oral administration because they are rapidly inactivated in the intestinal mucosa and in the liver before reaching the systemic circulation (*see* Chapter 4). Compounds without one or both OH substituents, particularly the 3-OH group, are not acted upon by catechol-O-methyltransferase (COMT), and their oral effectiveness and duration of action are enhanced.

Groups other than OH have been substituted on the aromatic ring. In general, potency on α receptors is reduced and β-receptor activity is minimal; the compounds may even block β receptors. For example, methoxamine, with methoxy substituents on positions 2 and 5, has highly selective α-stimulating activity and in large doses blocks β receptors. Albuterol, a selective β_2-receptor stimulant, has a CH_2OH substituent on position 3 and is an important exception to the general rule of low β activity.

Substitution on the α-Carbon Atom. This substitution blocks oxidation by monoamine oxidase (MAO), thus greatly prolonging the duration of action of noncatecholamines, the detoxication of which depends largely on breakdown by MAO. The duration of action of drugs such as ephedrine or amphetamine is thus measured in hours rather than in minutes. Since intraneuronal MAO is an important enzyme for degradation of phenylethylamines that lack an α-methyl substituent, compounds with such a group persist in the nerve terminal and are more likely to release norepinephrine from sites of storage. Agents such as metaraminol thus exhibit a greater degree of indirect sympathomimetic activity.

Substitution on the β-Carbon Atom. Substitution of an OH group on the β carbon generally decreases central stimulant action, largely because of the lower lipid solubility of such compounds. However, such substitution greatly enhances agonistic activity, both at α and β receptors. Thus, ephedrine is less potent than methamphetamine as a central stimulant, but it is more powerful in dilating bronchioles and increasing blood pressure and heart rate.

Absence of the Benzene Ring. CNS stimulant activity is reduced without a corresponding decrease in α and β activity when the benzene ring is replaced by a saturated ring (*e.g.*, cyclopentamine, propylhexedrine), or by a different unsaturated ring (*e.g.*, naphazoline; Table 8–2). Naphazoline, in fact, is a powerful α-receptor stimulant, but it differs from most other sympathomimetic amines in that it depresses instead of stimulates the CNS, presumably because it, like clonidine and oxymetazoline, exhibits preferential effects on α_2 receptors (*see* Chapters 9 and 32).

The proportion of α to β activity varies with the compound; however, in general the amines that do not possess a benzene ring have rather more marked α than β activity. Consequently, many of them are used primarily as nasal decongestants because of their vasoconstrictor properties.

Optical Isomerism. Substitution on either α or β carbon yields optical isomers. Levorotatory substitution on the β carbon confers the greater peripheral activity, so that the naturally occurring *l*-epi-

Table 8–2.   CHEMICAL STRUCTURES OF IMIDAZOLINE DERIVATIVES

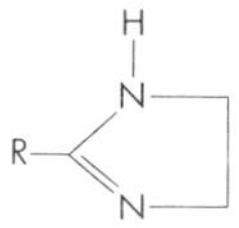

| R = | Naphazoline | Tetrahydrozoline | Oxymetazoline | Xylometazoline |

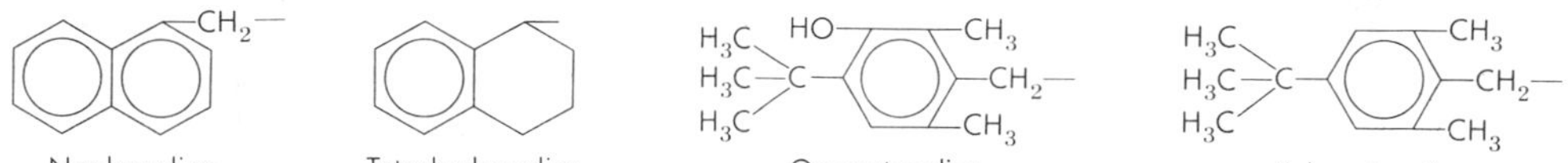

nephrine and *l*-norepinephrine are ten or more times as potent as their unnatural *d* isomers. Dextrorotatory substitution on the α carbon generally provides a more potent compound than the *l* isomer in central stimulant activity. *d*-Amphetamine is more potent than *l*-amphetamine in central but not peripheral activity.

I. Catecholamines

EPINEPHRINE

PHARMACOLOGICAL PROPERTIES

Epinephrine is a potent stimulator of both α- and β-adrenergic receptors, and its effects on target organs are thus complex. Most of the responses listed in Table 4–1 (page 72) are seen after injection of epinephrine in man, although the occurrence of sweating, piloerection, and mydriasis depends on the physiological state of the subject. Particularly prominent are the actions on the heart and the vascular and other smooth muscle. So enormous is the literature on almost every aspect of the many changes in bodily function caused by epinephrine that this discussion is limited largely to the actions of the drug in man and refers to the more abundant results in animals when studies in man are limited.

Blood Pressure. Epinephrine is one of the most potent vasopressor drugs known. Given rapidly *intravenously* it evokes a characteristic effect on blood pressure, which rises rapidly to a peak that is proportional to the dose. The increase in systolic pressure is greater than the rise in diastolic pressure, so that the pulse pressure increases. As the response wanes, the mean pressure falls below normal before return-

ing to the control level. Repeated doses of epinephrine continue to have the same pressor effect, in sharp contrast to amines that owe a major part of their effect to release of norepinephrine.

The mechanism of the rise in blood pressure due to epinephrine is threefold: a direct myocardial stimulation that increases the strength of ventricular contraction (positive inotropic action); an increased heart rate (positive chronotropic action); and, most important, vasoconstriction in many vascular beds, especially in the precapillary resistance vessels of skin, mucosa, and kidney, along with marked constriction of the veins. The pulse rate, at first accelerated, may be slowed markedly at the height of the rise of blood pressure by compensatory vagal discharge. This bradycardia is absent if the effects of vagal discharge are blocked by atropine. Minute doses of epinephrine (0.1 μg/kg) may cause the blood pressure to fall. The depressor effect of small doses and the biphasic response to larger doses are due to greater sensitivity to epinephrine of vasodilator β_2 receptors than of constrictor α receptors.

The effects are somewhat different when the drug is given by slow *intravenous infusion* or by *subcutaneous injection*. Absorption of epinephrine after subcutaneous injection is slow due to the drug's local vasoconstrictor action; the effects of doses as large as 0.5 to 1.5 mg can be duplicated by intravenous infusion at a rate of 10 to 30 μg per minute. There is a moderate increase in systolic pressure due to increased cardiac contractile force and a rise in cardiac output (Figure 8–1). Peripheral resistance decreases, due to the dominant action on β_2 receptors of vessels in skeletal mus-

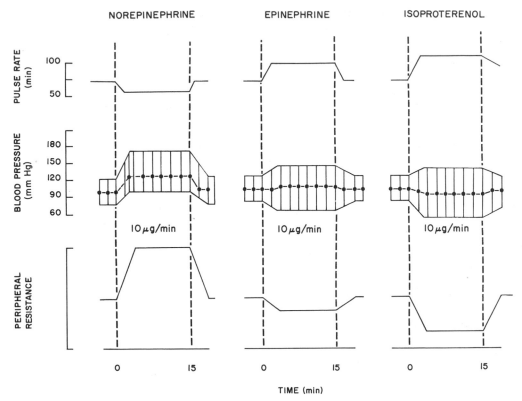

Figure 8–1. *The effects of intravenous infusion of norepinephrine, epinephrine, and isoproterenol in man.* (After Allwood, Cobbold, and Ginsburg, 1963. Courtesy of the *British Medical Bulletin.*)

cle, where blood flow is enhanced; as a consequence, diastolic pressure usually falls. Since the mean blood pressure is not, as a rule, greatly elevated, compensatory reflexes do not antagonize appreciably the direct cardiac actions. There may be no change or even a slight rise in peripheral resistance and diastolic pressure, depending upon the dose administered and the resultant ratio of α to β responses in the various vascular beds. Heart rate, cardiac output, stroke volume, and left ventricular work per beat are increased due to direct cardiac stimulation and to increased venous return to the heart, which is reflected by an increase in right atrial pressure. The details of the effects of intravenous infusion of epinephrine, norepinephrine, and isoproterenol in man are compared in Table 8–3 and Figure 8–1.

Vascular Effects. The chief vascular action of epinephrine is exerted on the smaller arterioles and precapillary sphincters, although veins and large arteries also respond to the drug. Various vascular beds react differently (*see* Table 4–1, page 72).

Injected epinephrine markedly reduces *cutaneous blood flow,* constricting precapillary vessels and subpapillary venules. However, skin pallor due to cutaneous vasoconstriction during "flight-or-fight" reactions is mainly due to increased sympathetic discharge rather than to released epinephrine. Cutaneous vasoconstriction accounts for a marked decrease in blood flow in the hands and feet. The "aftercongestion" of mucosae following the vasoconstriction from locally applied epinephrine is probably due to changes in vascular reactivity as a result of tissue hypoxia rather than to β-receptor activity of the drug on mucosal vessels.

Blood flow to *skeletal muscles* is increased by therapeutic doses in man. Epinephrine infused intravenously in man at

Table 8–3. COMPARISON OF THE EFFECTS OF INTRAVENOUS INFUSION OF EPINEPHRINE AND NOREPINEPHRINE IN MAN *

	EPINEPH-RINE	NOREPINEPH-RINE
Cardiac		
Heart rate	+	− †
Stroke volume	+ +	+ +
Cardiac output	+ + +	0,−
Arrhythmias	+ + + +	+ + + +
Coronary blood flow	+ +	+ +
Blood Pressure		
Systolic arterial	+ + +	+ + +
Mean arterial	+	+ +
Diastolic arterial	+,0,−	+ +
Mean pulmonary	+ +	+ +
Peripheral Circulation		
Total peripheral resistance	−	+ +
Cerebral blood flow	+	0,−
Muscle blood flow	+ + +	0,−
Cutaneous blood flow	− −	− −
Renal blood flow	−	−
Splanchnic blood flow	+ + +	0,+
Metabolic Effects		
Oxygen consumption	+ +	0,+
Blood glucose	+ + +	0,+
Blood lactic acid	+ + +	0,+
Eosinopenic response	+	0
Central Nervous System		
Respiration	+	+
Subjective sensations	+	+

* 0.1 to 0.4 μg/kg/min

+ = increase; 0 = no change; − = decrease; † = after atropine, +

(After Goldenberg, Aranow, Smith, and Faber, 1950. Courtesy of *Archives of Internal Medicine*.)

the rate of 30 μg per minute causes a very large but transient increase in blood flow, followed by a fall to about double the resting flow. This is due in part to a powerful β_2-receptor vasodilator action that is partially counterbalanced by a vasoconstrictor action on the α receptors that are also present in the vascular bed. These vascular effects are independent of cardiac or central reflex effects and occur also in sympathectomized limbs. If an α-adrenergic blocking agent is given, the pronounced vasodilatation in muscle due to epinephrine is sustained, the total peripheral resistance is decreased, and the mean blood pressure falls (epinephrine reversal). After the administration of a nonselective β-adrenergic antagonist, only vasoconstriction occurs, and the administration of epinephrine is associated with a considerable pressor effect. This marked rise in blood pressure is not elicited by epinephrine in the presence of a selective β_1 antagonist (Houben *et al.*, 1982).

The effect of epinephrine on *cerebral circulation* is related to systemic blood pressure. In usual therapeutic doses the drug has no significant constrictor action on cerebral arterioles; cerebral blood flow increases, and there is no change in cerebrovascular resistance. However, autoregulatory mechanisms tend to limit the increase in cerebral blood flow due to increased blood pressure.

Intravenous infusion of 0.1 μg/kg per minute in man markedly increases *hepatic blood flow* and decreases *splanchnic vascular resistance,* concomitantly with a large increase in hepatic glucose output and in the consumption of oxygen as measured in the splanchnic vascular bed (*see* Greenway and Stark, 1971).

Doses of epinephrine that have little effect on mean arterial pressure consistently increase *renal vascular resistance* and reduce *renal blood flow* by as much as 40%. All segments of the renal vascular bed contribute to the increased resistance. Since the glomerular filtration rate is only slightly and variably altered, the filtration fraction is consistently increased. Excretion of sodium, potassium, and chloride is decreased; urine volume may be increased, decreased, or unchanged. Maximal tubular reabsorptive and excretory capacities are unchanged. The secretion of renin is increased as a consequence of a direct action of epinephrine on β_1 receptors in the juxtaglomerular apparatus.

Arterial and venous *pulmonary pressures* are raised. Although direct pulmonary vasoconstriction can be shown under suitable conditions, redistribution of blood from the systemic to the pulmonary circulation, due to constriction of the more powerful musculature in the systemic great veins, doubtless plays an important part in the increase in pulmonary pressure. Overdosage of epinephrine may cause death by pulmonary edema precipitated by elevated pulmonary capillary filtration pressure.

Coronary blood flow is enhanced by epinephrine or by cardiac sympathetic stimulation in man as well as in animals. The increased flow occurs even with doses that do not increase the aortic blood pressure and is the net result of three factors. The first is the increased duration of diastole (*see* below); this is partially offset by decreased blood flow during systole due to more forceful contraction of the surrounding myocardium and an increase in mechanical compression of the coronary vessels. The increased flow during diastole is further enhanced if aortic blood pressure is elevated by epinephrine, and, as a consequence, there may be an increase in total coronary flow because of this effect. The second factor is the direct action of the drug on coronary vessels, which have both α and β receptors; in man this is predominantly constrictor via α receptors (Anderson *et al.*, 1972). This direct action normally is of little importance compared to the overriding influence of the third factor, a metabolic dilator effect consequent upon the increased strength of contraction and myocardial oxygen consumption. This vasodilatation is mediated in large part by adenosine that is released from the cardiac myocytes (*see* Dempsey and Cooper, 1972; Berne *et al.*, 1983).

Cardiac Effects. Epinephrine is a powerful cardiac stimulant. It acts directly on β_1 receptors of the myocardium and of the cells of the pacemaker and conducting tissues. This stimulation is independent of alterations in cardiac function secondary to increased venous return and other peripheral vascular effects. The heart rate increases and the rhythm is often altered. Cardiac systole is shorter and more powerful, cardiac output is enhanced, and the work of the heart and its oxygen consumption are markedly increased. Cardiac efficiency (work done relative to oxygen consumption) is lessened. The direct actions of epinephrine uncomplicated by secondary effects can be most readily observed in isolated cardiac preparations from animals. Responses include increases in contractile force, accelerated rate of rise of isometric tension, enhanced rate of relaxation, decreased time to peak tension, increased excitability, enhanced oxygen consumption, acceleration of the rate of spontane-

ous beating, and induction of automaticity in quiescent muscle.

In accelerating the heart within the physiological range, epinephrine shortens systole more than diastole so that the duration of diastole per minute is increased. Epinephrine speeds the heart by accelerating the slow depolarization of S-A cells that takes place during diastole, that is, during phase 4 of the action potential. Thus, the transmembrane potential of the pacemaker cells falls more rapidly to the threshold level at which the action potential is initiated. The amplitude of the action potential and the maximal rate of depolarization (phase 0) are also increased. A shift in the location of the pacemaker in the S-A node often occurs, indicating the activation of latent pacemaker cells. In Purkinje fibers, epinephrine accelerates diastolic depolarization and further facilitates activation of latent pacemaker cells. These changes do not occur in atrial and ventricular muscle fibers, where epinephrine has little effect on the stable, phase-4 membrane potential after repolarization. Some effects of epinephrine on cardiac tissues are largely secondary to the increase in heart rate, and are small or inconsistent in preparations where the heart rate is kept constant. For example, the effect of epinephrine on repolarization of atrium, Purkinje fibers, or ventricle is small if the heart rate is unchanged. When the heart rate is increased, the duration of the action potential is consistently shortened, and the refractory period is correspondingly decreased. Similarly, acceleration of the heart rate plays an important part in increasing the conduction velocity in the bundle of His, Purkinje fibers, and ventricle. Thus, the drug shortens the refractory period of atrial and ventricular muscle. It also decreases the grade of A-V block occurring as a result of disease, drugs, or vagal stimulation.

Conduction through the Purkinje system depends on the level of membrane potential at the time of excitation. Excessive reduction of this potential results in conduction disturbances, ranging from slowed conduction to complete inexcitability. Epinephrine increases the membrane potential and improves conduction in canine Purkinje fibers that have been excessively depolarized. Since circumstances favoring such excessive depolarization are common in diseased hearts, this mechanism may play some role in the salutary effects of epinephrine in various human arrhythmias—as, for example, in patients with complete heart block until more definitive measures can be instituted (Singer *et al.*, 1967). If large doses of epinephrine are given, premature ventricular systoles occur and may herald more serious ventricular arrhythmias. This is rarely seen with conventional doses in man, but ventricular extrasystoles, tachycardia, or even fibrillation may be precipitated by release of endogenous epinephrine when the heart has been sensitized to this action of epinephrine by certain anesthetics or in cases of myocardial infarction. The mechanism of induction of these cardiac arrhythmias is not clear. However, α-adrenergic blocking agents such as phenoxybenzamine protect against epinephrine-induced cardiac irregularities during anesthesia; protection is due in part to prevention of the rise in blood pressure (which sensitizes the myocardium to epinephrine-induced ectopic rhythms).

The refractory period of the human A-V node is normally shortened by epinephrine, but may be prolonged indirectly by doses that slow the heart through reflex vagal discharge, an effect reversed by atropine. Supraventricular arrhythmias are apt to occur from the combination of epinephrine and cholinergic stimulation. Depression of sinus rate and A-V conduction by vagal discharge probably plays a part in epinephrine-induced ventricular arrhythmias, since various drugs that block the vagal effect confer some protection. The cardiac arrest occasionally caused by vagal discharge due to pressure on the eyeball or carotid sinus can be abolished by epinephrine, which induces or accelerates impulse formation in the ventricles. The action of epinephrine in enhancing cardiac automaticity and its action in causing arrhythmias are effectively antagonized by β-blocking agents such as propranolol. However, there do appear to be α receptors in at least some regions of the heart, since the α-receptor stimulant phenylephrine and, during β-receptor block, epinephrine prolong the refractory period and strengthen contractions of isolated atria; these effects are antagonized by α-blocking agents (Benfey and Varma, 1967; Schumann *et al.*, 1978).

Cardiac arrhythmias have been recorded in man after accidental intravenous administration of conventional subcutaneous doses of epinephrine. Systolic and diastolic pressures rise alarmingly, sometimes as high as 400/300 mm Hg for a short time; cerebrovascular hemorrhage has occurred from this error. Venous pressure rises, hyperventilation occurs (occasionally preceded by a brief period of apnea), pallor and palpitation are prominent, and heart rate is accelerated after a transient bradycardia. Ventricular premature systoles usually appear within the first minute after injection, frequently followed by multifocal ventricular tachycardia (prefibrillation rhythm). As the effects on the ventricle subside 1 or 2 minutes after their appearance, a marked atrial tachycardia ensues, occasionally associated with A-V block.

With respect to the electrocardiogram (ECG), epinephrine decreases the amplitude of the T wave in all leads in normal persons. In animals given relatively larger doses, additional effects are seen on the T wave and S-T segment. After being decreased in amplitude, the T wave may become biphasic and the S-T segment deviates either above or below the isoelectric line before abnormal ventricular deflections appear. Such S-T segment changes are similar to the downward deviation found in patients with *angina pectoris* during spontaneous or epinephrine-induced attacks of pain. These electrical changes have therefore been attributed to myocardial hypoxia.

Effects on Smooth Muscles. The effects of epinephrine on the smooth muscles of different organs and systems depend upon the type of adrenergic receptor in the muscle (Table 4–1, page 72). Gastrointestinal smooth muscle is, in general, relaxed by epinephrine. Intestinal tone and the frequency and amplitude of spontaneous contractions are reduced. The stomach is usually relaxed and the pyloric and ileocecal sphincters are contracted, but these effects depend upon the preexisting tone of the muscle. If tone is already high, epinephrine causes relaxation; if low, contraction. Epinephrine contracts the *splenic capsule* and reduces the size of the spleen in some species but not in man.

The responses of *uterine muscle* to epinephrine vary with species, phase of the sexual cycle, state of gestation, and the dose given. Epinephrine contracts strips of pregnant or nonpregnant human uterus *in vitro* in any effective concentration by interaction with α receptors. The effects of epinephrine on the human uterus *in situ*, however, differ. During the last month of pregnancy and at parturition, epinephrine inhibits uterine tone and contractions; this effect is of no clinical value because it is brief and accompanied by cardiovascular effects. However, other more selective β_2-receptor stimulants, such as ritodrine or terbutaline, have been used successfully to delay premature labor. (*See* Caritis, 1983; Chapter 39.)

Epinephrine relaxes the detrusor muscle of the *bladder* as a result of activation of β receptors and contracts the trigone and sphincter muscles due to its α-agonistic activity. This can result in hesitancy in urination and may contribute to retention of urine in the bladder.

Respiratory Effects. Epinephrine stimulates respiration, but this effect is brief and has no clinical value. Given intravenously to animals or man, epinephrine may cause a brief period of apnea before stimulation is seen. The apnea is probably due in part to a transient reflex inhibition of the respiratory center through the baroreceptor mechanism and in part to direct inhibition of the center.

Epinephrine can affect respiration more significantly by its peripheral actions, particularly by relaxing bronchial muscle. It has a powerful bronchodilator action, most evident when bronchial muscle is contracted due to disease, as in bronchial asthma, or in response to drugs or various autacoids. In such situations, epinephrine has a striking therapeutic effect as a physiological antagonist to the constrictor influences since it is not limited to specific competitive antagonism such as occurs with antihistaminic drugs against histamine-induced bronchoconstriction. Epinephrine also alters respiration by its α-receptor action in both normal and asthmatic persons; it increases vital capacity by relieving congestion of the bronchial mucosa and, when its action is limited as much as possible to the pulmonary vascular bed by administration as an aerosol, by constricting pulmonary vessels. Its effect in asthma may be due in part to inhibition of antigen-induced release of histamine; this action is shared by selective β_2-receptor stimulants (*see* Chapter 26).

Epinephrine increases respiratory rate and tidal volume, and thereby reduces alveolar carbon dioxide content in normal subjects. However, inordinately large doses in man may cause death by interference with gaseous exchange due to development of pulmonary edema. Administration of a rapidly acting α-blocking agent or intermittent positive-pressure respiration (to increase intra-alveolar pressure) may be lifesaving.

Effects on Central Nervous System. Epinephrine in conventional therapeutic doses is not a powerful CNS stimulant. This is largely due to the inability of this rather polar compound to enter the CNS. While the drug may cause restlessness, apprehension, headache, and tremor in many persons, these effects may in part be secondary to the profound cardiorespiratory and peripheral metabolic effects of the catecholamine.

In animals, small intravenous doses cause arousal from natural sleep and large doses cause stupor, emesis, exaggerated knee jerks, spasticity, and even convulsions. In patients with Parkinson's disease, epinephrine increases rigidity and tremor, but the locus and mechanism of action are unclear.

Metabolic Effects. Epinephrine has a number of important influences on metabolic processes. Epinephrine elevates the concentrations of *glucose* and *lactate* in blood by mechanisms described in Chapter 4. *Insulin secretion* is inhibited via α receptors and is enhanced by activation of β_2 receptors; the predominant effect seen with epinephrine is inhibition. Glucagon secretion is enhanced by an action on the β receptors of the α cells of pancreatic islets. Epinephrine also decreases the uptake of glucose by peripheral tissues, at least in part because of its effects on the secretion of insulin. Glycosuria rarely occurs. The effect of epinephrine to stimulate glycogenolysis in most tissues and in most species involves β receptors (*see* Chapter 4).

Epinephrine raises the concentration of *free fatty acids* in blood by activation of triglyceride lipase, which accelerates the breakdown of triglycerides to form free fatty acids and glycerol. Fat is deposited in muscle and liver, probably due to the increased amount of free fatty acid in the blood. This lipolytic action also appears to be mediated by cyclic AMP via β_1-adrenergic receptors. Infusions of epinephrine generally increase plasma cholesterol, phospholipid, and low-density lipoproteins. The *calorigenic action* of epinephrine (increase in metabolism) is reflected in man by an increase of 20 to 30% in oxygen consumption after conventional doses. Studies in animals have shown that this effect, although composite, is mainly due to enhanced breakdown of triglycerides in brown adipose tissue, providing an increase in oxidizable substrate. (*See* Himms-Hagen, 1972; Ellis, 1980; Chapter 4.)

Miscellaneous Effects. Epinephrine reduces circulating *plasma volume* by loss of protein-free fluid to the extracellular space, thereby increasing *erythrocyte* and *plasma protein concentrations*. However, conventional doses of epinephrine in man do not significantly alter plasma volume or packed red-cell volume under normal conditions, although such doses are reported to have variable effects in shock, hemorrhage, hypotension, and anesthesia. Epinephrine increases *total leukocyte count* but causes *eosinopenia*. Epinephrine has long been known to accelerate blood coagulation in animals and man, an effect probably due to increased activity of factor V (Forwell and Ingram, 1957).

The effects of epinephrine on *secretory glands* are not marked; in most glands secretion is usually inhibited, partly due to reduced blood flow caused by vasoconstriction. Epinephrine stimulates *lacrimation* and a scanty mucous secretion from salivary glands. *Sweating* and *pilomotor activity* are not seen after systemic administration of epinephrine, but occur after intradermal injection of very dilute solutions of either epinephrine or norepinephrine. Such effects are inhibited by α-blocking agents.

Mydriasis is readily seen during physiological sympathetic stimulation but not when epinephrine is instilled into the conjunctival sac of normal eyes. However, epinephrine usually lowers *intraocular pressure* from normal levels and in wide-angle glaucoma; the mechanism is not clear, but both reduced production of aqueous humor due to vasoconstriction and enhanced outflow probably occur (*see* Grant, 1969). Paradoxically, timolol, a β-receptor antagonist, also reduces intraocular pressure and is useful in the treatment of glaucoma (*see* Chapter 9).

Although epinephrine does not directly excite *skeletal muscle,* it facilitates neuromuscular transmission, particularly that following prolonged rapid stimulation of the motor nerve. This effect appears to involve both α- and β-adrenergic receptors. Stimulation of the latter may increase cyclic AMP presynaptically, thereby facilitating the release of neurotransmitter (Weiner, 1980). In apparent contrast to the effects of α-receptor activation at presynaptic nerve terminals in the autonomic nervous system, stimulation of α-adrenergic receptors causes a more rapid increase in transmitter release from the somatic motoneuron, perhaps as a result of enhanced influx of Ca^{2+} (*see* Bowman, 1981; Snider and Gerald, 1982). These actions may explain in part the ability of epinephrine (given intraarterially) to cause a brief increase in motor power of the injected limb of patients with myasthenia gravis. Given orally, ephedrine and amphetamine have this same effect; although these two drugs have been used clinically in this condition, the improvement in muscle strength does not approach that seen after neostigmine. Epinephrine also acts directly on white, fast-contracting muscle fibers to prolong the active state, thereby increasing peak tension. Of greater physiological and clinical importance is the capacity of epinephrine and selective β_2-adrenergic agonists to shorten the active state of red, slow-contracting mammalian muscle, apparently by accelerating the sequestration of cytosolic Ca^{2+}; this causes incomplete fusion of contractile events at physiological rates of nerve stimulation and a reduction in developed tension. These effects, together with a β-receptor-mediated enhancement of discharge of muscle spindles, are thought to be important in the production of the tremor that sometimes accompanies the use of adrenergic bronchodilators (*see* Bowman, 1981). Skeletal muscles of hypocalcemic patients are hypersensitive to epinephrine, which causes immediate local tetany upon intra-arterial injection; the mechanism of this action is not known.

Epinephrine produces a transient rise in the concentration of *potassium* in plasma, mainly due to release of the ion from the liver. This hyperkalemia is followed by a more prolonged fall in plasma potassium. During these changes hepatic potassium rapidly enters the blood and is taken up by muscle. Subsequently the pool of potassium in muscle falls during the period of hypokalemia and is transferred

to the liver. β_2-Adrenergic agonists, such as albuterol, have been used in the management of hyperkalemic familial periodic paralysis, which is characterized by episodic flaccid paralysis, hyperkalemia, and depolarization of skeletal muscle. Albuterol is apparently able to correct the impairment in the ability of the muscle to accumulate and retain potassium, presumably by stimulating the Na^+,K^+-ATPase (*see* Bowman, 1981).

Large or repeated doses of epinephrine or other sympathomimetic amines given to experimental animals lead to *damage to arterial walls and myocardium,* so severe as to cause the appearance of necrotic areas, indistinguishable in the heart from myocardial infarcts. The mechanism of this injury is not yet clear, but verapamil (which inhibits entry of calcium into the myocardial cell), propranolol, phentolamine, dipyridamole, indomethacin, or aspirin gives substantial protection against the damage. Similar lesions occur in many patients with pheochromocytoma or after prolonged infusions of norepinephrine (*see* Vliet *et al.,* 1966).

Absorption, Fate, and Excretion. *Absorption.* Epinephrine does not reach pharmacologically active concentrations in the body after oral administration because it is rapidly conjugated and oxidized in the gastrointestinal mucosa and liver. Absorption from subcutaneous tissues occurs slowly because of local vasoconstriction; heat and massage hasten the rate. Absorption is more rapid after intramuscular than after subcutaneous injection. When relatively concentrated solutions (1%) are nebulized and inhaled, the actions of the drug are largely restricted to the respiratory tract; however, systemic reactions such as arrhythmias may occur, particularly if larger amounts are used.

Fate and Excretion. Epinephrine is rapidly inactivated in the body despite its stability in the blood. The liver, which is rich in both of the enzymes responsible for destruction of circulating epinephrine, is an important, although not essential, tissue in the degradation process. While only small amounts appear in the urine of normal persons, the urine of patients with pheochromocytoma contains large amounts of epinephrine, norepinephrine, and their metabolites.

The greater part of a dose of epinephrine injected into man is excreted as metabolites in the urine. Most of the injected drug is first metabolized by COMT and MAO, as already described (*see* Figure 4–5, page 87). Congeners of epinephrine are metabolized by the same enzyme systems; amines lacking the 3-OH group are unaffected by COMT, and their disposal depends upon MAO or other enzymes, mostly in the liver. Destruction of these amines is generally slower than that of epinephrine, and inhibition of MAO by a variety of drugs may prolong their action in the body. (*See* Sharman, 1973.) Amines with an α-methyl substituent are resistant to deamination by MAO.

Preparations, Dosage, and Routes of Administration. Many preparations of epinephrine are available. Epinephrine is the official USP term; adrenaline, the BP term.

Epinephrine is the *l* isomer of β-(3,4-dihydroxyphenyl)-α-methylaminoethanol (*see* Table 8–1). It is only very slightly soluble in water but forms water-soluble salts with acids. It is unstable in alkaline solution and on exposure to air or light, turning pink from oxidation to adrenochrome and then brown from formation of polymers. Epinephrine may be given by injection, usually subcutaneously, inhaled as an aerosol, or applied locally to mucous membranes or abraded surfaces as an aqueous solution.

Epinephrine injection is a 1:1000 or a 1:10,000 sterile solution of epinephrine hydrochloride in water. The usual adult dose given *subcutaneously* ranges from 0.2 to 1 mg. The *intravenous* route is used cautiously if an immediate and reliable effect is mandatory. If the solution is given by vein, it must be adequately diluted and injected *very slowly*. The dose is seldom as much as 0.25 mg, except for cardiac arrest, when 0.5 mg can be given every 5 minutes. *Intracardiac* injection is occasionally used for attempted resuscitation in emergencies (0.3 to 0.5 mg). An aqueous 1:200 suspension of crystalline epinephrine (SUS-PHRINE) has a prolonged duration of action because of its low solubility. Injected subcutaneously the initial adult dose is 0.1 ml, and the maximum is 0.3 ml, repeated no sooner than after 6 hours. *Epinephrine suspensions must never be injected intravenously.*

Epinephrine inhalation is a nonsterile 1% aqueous solution of epinephrine hydrochloride for oral (not nasal) inhalation, either from a nebulizer or from an intermittent positive-pressure breathing apparatus. It is used to relieve bronchial constriction. *Every precaution must be taken not to confuse this 1:100 solution with the 1:1000 solution designed for parenteral administration.* Injection of the 1:100 solution has caused death.

Epinephrine nasal solution is a 1:1000 preparation of epinephrine hydrochloride identical with *epinephrine injection* except that it is not sterile. It is generally used in preparing more dilute solutions (1:50,000 to 1:2000) for sprays to constrict vessels of mucosa or abraded skin. *Epinephrine bitartrate* is available as a 2% *ophthalmic* solution and as a pressurized *aerosol* (MEDIHALER-EPI) delivering measured doses of 0.3 mg (0.16 mg of epinephrine base) for oral inhalation.

Epinephrine hydrochloride (0.1 to 2%) and *epinephrine borate* (0.5 to 2%) are also available for topical ophthalmic use.

Toxicity, Side Effects, and Contraindications. Epinephrine may cause disturbing reactions, such as *fear, anxiety, tenseness, restlessness, throbbing headache, tremor, weakness, dizziness, pallor, respiratory difficulty,* and *palpitation*. The effects rapidly subside with rest, quiet, recumbency, and reassurance, but the patient is often alarmed. Hyperthyroid and hypertensive individuals are particularly susceptible to the untoward and pressor responses to epinephrine. In psychoneurotic individuals, existing symptoms are often markedly aggravated by the administration of epinephrine.

More serious reactions include *cerebral hemorrhage* and *cardiac arrhythmias*. The use of large doses or the accidental rapid *intravenous* injection of epinephrine may result in cerebral hemorrhage from the sharp rise in blood pressure. Subarachnoid hemorrhage and hemiplegia have occurred even after a subcutaneous dose of 0.5 ml of the 1:1000 solution. Rapidly acting vasodilators such as the nitrites or sodium nitroprusside can counteract the marked pressor effects of large doses of epinephrine; α-blocking agents may also be of use.

Ventricular arrhythmias may follow the administration of epinephrine. If ventricular fibrillation develops, it is usually fatal unless immediate remedial measures are employed; fibrillation is particularly likely to occur if the drug is used unwisely during anesthesia, especially with halogenated hydrocarbon anesthetics, or in individuals with organic heart disease. Patients with long-standing bronchial asthma and a significant degree of emphysema, who have reached the age at which degenerative heart disease is prevalent, must be given epinephrine only with considerable caution. In patients suffering from shock, the drug may accentuate the underlying disorder. Anginal pain is readily induced by epinephrine in patients with angina pectoris.

Therapeutic Uses. Epinephrine has a wide variety of clinical uses in medicine and surgery. In general, these are based on the actions of the drug on blood vessels, heart, and bronchial muscle. The most common uses of epinephrine are to relieve respiratory distress due to *bronchospasm,* to provide rapid relief of *hypersensitivity reactions* to drugs and other allergens, and to *prolong the action of infiltration anesthetics.* Its cardiac effects may be of use in restoring cardiac rhythm in patients with *cardiac arrest* due to various causes. It is also used as a *topical hemostatic* on bleeding surfaces. The therapeutic uses of epinephrine are further discussed later in this chapter, together with those of other sympathomimetic drugs.

NOREPINEPHRINE (LEVARTERENOL)

Norepinephrine (levarterenol, *l*-noradrenaline, *l*-β-[3,4-dihydroxyphenyl]-α-aminoethanol) is the chemical mediator liberated by mammalian postganglionic adrenergic nerves. It differs from epinephrine only by lacking the methyl substitution in the amino group (*see* Table 8–1). Norepinephrine constitutes 10 to 20% of the catecholamine content of human adrenal medulla and as much as 97% in some pheochromocytomas. The history of its discovery and its role as a neurohumoral mediator are discussed in Chapter 4.

Pharmacological Actions. The pharmacological actions of norepinephrine and epinephrine have been extensively compared *in vivo* and *in vitro* (*see* Table 8–3). Both drugs are direct agonists on effector cells, and their actions differ mainly in the ratio of their effectiveness in stimulating α and β_2 receptors. Both are approximately equipotent in stimulating β_1 (cardiac) receptors. Norepinephrine is a potent agonist at α receptors and has little action on β_2 receptors; however, it is somewhat less potent than epinephrine on the α receptors of most organs.

Cardiovascular Effects. The cardiovascular effects of intravenous infusion of 10 μg of norepinephrine per minute in man are shown in Figure 8–1. Systolic and diastolic pressures and usually pulse pressure are increased. Cardiac output is unchanged or decreased, and the total peripheral resistance is raised. Compensatory vagal reflex activity slows the heart, overcoming the direct cardioaccelerator action, and the stroke volume is thus increased. The peripheral vascular resistance increases in most vascular beds, and the blood flow is

reduced through kidney, liver, and usually skeletal muscle. A marked venoconstriction contributes to the increased resistance. Glomerular filtration rate is maintained unless the decrease in renal blood flow is quite marked. Norepinephrine constricts mesenteric vessels and reduces splanchnic and hepatic blood flow in man. Coronary flow is substantially increased, probably due to both indirectly induced coronary dilatation, as with epinephrine, and elevated blood pressure. However, patients with Prinzmetal's variant angina apparently are supersensitive to the α-adrenergic vasoconstrictor effects of norepinephrine, epinephrine, and sympathetic nerve discharge. In such patients, endogenous or exogenous norepinephrine will reduce coronary blood flow. They can experience angina at rest even though their vascular bed may be relatively free of atherosclerotic lesions, and the decrease in coronary blood flow may be sufficiently great and prolonged to cause myocardial infarction (*see* Chapter 33).

Unlike epinephrine, small doses of norepinephrine do not cause vasodilatation or lower blood pressure, since the blood vessels of skeletal muscle are constricted instead of dilated; α-blocking agents therefore abolish the pressor effects but do not cause significant reversal. The circulating blood volume is reduced by loss of protein-free fluid to the extracellular space, probably due to postcapillary vasoconstriction. The usual ECG change is sinus bradycardia due to a reflex increase in vagal tone, with or without prolongation of the P-R interval. Nodal rhythm, A-V dissociation, bigeminal rhythm, ventricular tachycardia, and fibrillation have also been observed.

Other Effects. Other responses to norepinephrine are not prominent in man. The drug causes hyperglycemia and other metabolic effects similar to those produced by epinephrine, but these are observed only when larger doses are given. Respiratory minute volume is slightly increased. Effects on the CNS are somewhat less prominent than those of epinephrine. Intradermal injection of suitable doses in man causes sweating that is not blocked by atropine. Increased frequency of contraction of the pregnant human uterus has been observed, but the effects on the other smooth muscles are slight.

Absorption, Fate, and Excretion. Norepinephrine, like epinephrine, is ineffective when given orally and is absorbed poorly from sites of subcutaneous injection. It is rapidly inactivated in the body by the same enzymes that methylate and oxidatively deaminate epinephrine (*see* above). Negligible amounts are normally found in the urine, but as much as 15 mg per day may be excreted by persons with pheochromocytoma.

Preparations, Dosage, and Route of Administration. *Norepinephrine bitartrate* (LEVOPHED BITARTRATE) is the water-soluble, crystalline monohydrate salt. Like epinephrine, it is readily oxidized. *Norepinephrine bitartrate injection* is a 0.2% sterile solution of the bitartrate, equivalent to 0.1% of norepinephrine base. It is usually given by *intravenous infusion*, as a solution containing 4 μg/ml of norepinephrine base. After the cardiovascular response to a test dose of 0.1 to 0.2 μg/kg of body weight is observed, the infusion is adjusted to obtain the desired pressor response. Normally the infusion of 2 to 4 μg of base per minute (0.5 to 1.0 ml per minute) is adequate. The pressor response to the drug can be readily controlled since it disappears within 1 or 2 minutes after the infusion is stopped. In patients in whom intravenous infusion of large volumes of fluid is undesirable, less dilute solutions may be used cautiously.

Toxicity, Side Effects, and Precautions. The untoward effects of norepinephrine are similar to those of epinephrine, but they are usually less pronounced and less frequent. Anxiety, respiratory difficulty, awareness of the slow, forceful heart beat, and transient headache are the most common effects. Overdoses or conventional doses in hypersensitive persons (*e.g.*, hyperthyroid patients) cause severe hypertension with violent headache, photophobia, stabbing retrosternal pain, pallor, intense sweating, and vomiting. The risk of cardiac arrhythmias contraindicates the use of the drug during anesthesia with agents that sensitize the automatic tissue of the heart.

Care must be taken that *necrosis* and *sloughing* do not occur at the site of intravenous injection, due to extravasation of the drug. The infusion should be made high in the limb, preferably through a long plastic cannula extending centrally, and the site of infusion should be changed at least every 12 hours. Impaired circulation at injection sites, with or without extravasation of norepinephrine, may be relieved by hot packs and infiltration of the area with phentolamine or a local anesthetic. Norepinephrine infusions should never be left unattended. Blood pressure must be determined at least every 15 minutes during the infusion and more frequently during initial adjustment of the rate. Blood pressure should not be raised to more than normotensive levels. Reduced blood flow to vital areas is a constant danger in the use of norepinephrine. The drug should not be used in pregnant women because of its contractile action on the pregnant uterus.

Therapeutic Uses and Status. Norepinephrine has only limited therapeutic value. The therapeutic use of norepinephrine and of other sympathomimetic amines in hypotension due to shock is discussed later in this chapter.

ISOPROTERENOL

Isoproterenol (isopropylarterenol, isopropylnorepinephrine, isoprenaline, isopropylnoradrenaline, *dl*-β-[3,4-dihydroxyphenyl]-α-isopropylaminoethanol) (Table 8–1) is the most potent of the sympathomimetic amines that act almost exclusively on β receptors.

Pharmacological Actions. Isoproterenol has a powerful action on all β receptors and almost no action on α receptors. Its main actions, therefore, are on the heart, the smooth muscle of bronchi, skeletal muscle vasculature, and the alimentary tract. In addition, it exerts prominent metabolic effects in adipose tissue, skeletal muscle, and, in some species, liver. The major cardiovascular effects of isoproterenol, epinephrine, and norepinephrine in man are compared in Figure 8–1.

Cardiovascular System. Intravenous infusion of isoproterenol in man lowers peripheral vascular resistance, mainly in skeletal muscle but also in renal and mesenteric vascular beds, and diastolic pressure falls. Cardiac output is raised because of the positive inotropic and chronotropic actions of the drug. With usual doses of isoproterenol in man, the increase in cardiac output is generally enough to maintain or raise the systolic pressure, although the mean pressure is reduced. Renal blood flow is decreased in normotensive subjects but is markedly increased in patients in cardiogenic or septicemic shock. Pulmonary arterial pressure is unchanged. Larger doses cause a striking fall in mean blood pressure.

Smooth Muscle. Isoproterenol relaxes almost all varieties of smooth muscle when the tone is high, but this action is most pronounced on bronchial and gastrointestinal smooth muscle. It prevents or relieves bronchoconstriction due to drugs and bronchial asthma in man, but tolerance to this effect develops with overuse of the drug. Its effect in asthma may be due in part to an additional action to inhibit antigen-induced release of histamine; this action is shared by selective β_2-receptor stimulants. The drug decreases the tone and motility of intestinal musculature and inhibits uterine motility even when epinephrine causes contraction.

Metabolic and Central Nervous System Actions. In man, isoproterenol causes less hyperglycemia than does epinephrine, in part because insulin secretion is stimulated by direct β-adrenergic activation of pancreatic islet cells. However, the drug is as effective as epinephrine in releasing *free fatty acids,* and the *calorigenic* actions of the two agents are similar. Like epinephrine, isoproterenol can cause central excitation, but this is not significant with doses used clinically.

Absorption, Fate, and Excretion. Isoproterenol is readily absorbed when given parenterally or as an aerosol. It is metabolized primarily in the liver and other tissues by COMT. Isoproterenol is a relatively poor substrate for MAO and is not taken up by sympathetic neurons to the same extent as are epinephrine and norepinephrine. The duration of action of isoproterenol may therefore be longer than that of epinephrine, but it is still brief.

Preparations, Dosage, and Routes of Administration. *Isoproterenol hydrochloride* (ISUPREL HCL) is a white, water-soluble powder; it is oxidized on exposure to air or alkali. *Isoproterenol hydrochloride inhalation* is available as a 0.25% aerosol (ISUPREL MISTOMETER, NORISODRINE AEROTROL) and as solutions (0.25 to 1%) for nebulization. A usual dose to relieve bronchoconstriction in asthma is 0.5 ml of the 0.5% solution. This is diluted to approximately 2.5 ml with water or isotonic saline solution and is given as a mist over 10 to 20 minutes. The drug is also available as *isoproterenol hydrochloride injection,* containing 200 μg/ml. *Isoproterenol sulfate* is available as a powder for use with an inhaler. Sublingual and oral preparations of isoproterenol are unreliable, and their use is not recommended.

Toxicity and Side Effects. The acute toxicity of isoproterenol is much less than that of epinephrine. Palpitation, tachycardia, headache, and flushing of the skin are common; anginal pain, nausea, tremor, dizziness, weakness, and sweating are less frequent. Cardiac arrhythmias can occur readily, although they are not usually serious. Large or repeated doses in animals may lead to myocardial necrosis, as with epinephrine, or to cardiac arrest when the heart is subjected to an increased work load (Lockett, 1965).

Overdosage of isoproterenol administered by inhalation can be fatal, presumably as a result of the induction of ventricular arrhythmias. Approximately 15 years ago, an isoproterenol nebulizer containing five times the usual concentration of the drug was introduced for use in England and Wales for the management of intractable asthma. This nebulizer provided approximately 0.4 mg of isoproterenol per inhalation. During the time when this preparation was popular in the United Kingdom, there was a considerable increase in mortality among asthmatics. A similar increase was not seen in other countries where such preparations were not available. This unfortunate experience serves to illustrate dramatically the hazards of excessive doses of β-adrenergic agonists (Stolley, 1972).

Therapeutic Uses. Isoproterenol is employed clinically only as a *bronchodilator* in respiratory disorders and as a *cardiac stimulant* in heart block, cardiogenic shock after myocardial infarction, and septicemic shock. Its use in these conditions and its value in relation to other sympathomimetic agents are discussed later in this chapter.

ETHYLNOREPINEPHRINE

Ethylnorepinephrine hydrochloride (BRONKEPHRINE) is primarily a β-adrenergic agonist, despite the fact that it is a primary amine (Table 8–1). Its use is as a bronchodilator. The drug also has α-adrenergic agonist activity; this may cause local vasoconstriction and thereby reduce bronchial congestion. Ethylnorepinephrine is administered intramuscularly or subcutaneously. Bronchodilatation is achieved within 5 to 10 minutes and lasts about 1 to 2 hours. The drug is available in a solution for injection that contains 2 mg/ml, and the usual dose is 1 to 2 mg.

DOPAMINE

Dopamine (3,4-dihydroxyphenylethylamine) (Table 8–1) is the immediate metabolic precursor of norepinephrine and epinephrine; it is a central neurotransmitter (Chapters 12, 19, and 21) and possesses important intrinsic pharmacological properties. Dopamine is a substrate for both MAO and COMT and thus is ineffective when administered orally.

Cardiovascular Effects. Dopamine exerts a positive inotropic effect on the myocardium, acting as an agonist at β_1 receptors. In addition, it has the capacity to release norepinephrine from nerve terminals, and this also contributes to its effects on the heart. Tachycardia is less prominent during infusions of dopamine than of isoproterenol. Dopamine appears to increase systolic and pulse pressure and has either no effect on or slightly increases diastolic blood pressure. Total peripheral resistance is usually unchanged when low or intermediate therapeutic doses are given. This is probably due to the ability of dopamine to reduce regional arterial resistance in the mesentery and the kidney, while producing minor increases in other vascular beds. The effect of dopamine on the renal vasculature appears to be mediated by a specific dopaminergic receptor. In relatively low doses, infusion of dopamine is associated with an increase in glomerular filtration rate, renal blood flow, and sodium excretion. As a consequence, dopamine is especially useful in the management of cardiogenic, traumatic, or hypovolemic shock, where major increases in sympathetic activity may particularly compromise renal function. Since dopamine is a potent sympathomimetic agent, its use in life-threatening states of shock must be carefully monitored, and particular attention must be paid to avoidance of elevated blood pressure or reduction in renal function as a consequence of renal vasoconstriction. This may occur during administration of high doses of dopamine as a consequence of its direct and indirect stimulatory effects at α receptors. Many aspects of the pharmacology of dopamine have been reviewed by Goldberg (1972).

Other Effects. Although there are specific dopaminergic receptors in the CNS, injected dopamine usually has no central effects because it does not readily cross the blood-brain barrier (*see* Chapters 12, 19, and 21).

Preparations, Dosage, and Route of Administration. *Dopamine hydrochloride* (INTROPIN, DOPASTAT) is a water-soluble, light-sensitive, white crystalline powder, marketed in solutions for injection that contain 40, 80, and 160 mg/ml. It is used only by the intravenous route. The drug is usually diluted to a concentration of 0.8 to 1.6 mg/ml and is administered at a rate of 2 to 5 μg/kg per minute initially; this rate may be increased gradually up to 20 to 50 μg/kg per minute as the clinical situation dictates. During the infusion, all patients require intermittent evaluation of blood volume and fre-

quent assessment of myocardial function, perfusion of vital organs, and the production of urine. Most patients should receive intensive care, with monitoring of arterial and venous pressures and the ECG. Reduction in urine flow, tachycardia, and the development of arrhythmias may be indications to slow or terminate the infusion. The duration of action of dopamine is quite brief, and hence the rate of administration can be used to control the intensity of effect.

Precautions, Adverse Reactions, and Contraindications. Before dopamine is administered to patients in shock, hypovolemia should be corrected by transfusion of whole blood, plasma, or appropriate fluids. The patient must be monitored as indicated above. Untoward effects due to overdosage are generally attributable to excessive sympathomimetic activity (although this may also be the response to worsening shock). Nausea, vomiting, tachycardia, anginal pain, arrhythmias, headache, hypertension, and vasoconstriction may be encountered during infusion of dopamine. Since the drug has an extremely short half-life in plasma, these effects usually disappear quickly if the infusion is slowed or interrupted. Rarely, the use of a short-acting α-blocking agent such as phentolamine may be required. Extravasation of large amounts of dopamine during infusion may cause ischemic necrosis and sloughing. Rarely, gangrene of the fingers or toes has followed the prolonged infusion of the drug. If this is threatened, local infiltration of the region with phentolamine should be instituted.

Dopamine should be avoided or used at a much reduced dosage (one tenth or less) if the patient has received an inhibitor of MAO. Careful adjustment of dosage is also necessary for the patient who is taking tricyclic antidepressants.

Therapeutic Uses. Dopamine is useful in the treatment of some types of shock. It is particularly beneficial for patients with oliguria and with low or normal peripheral vascular resistance. The drug is also of value in the treatment of cardiogenic and bacteremic shock, as well as profound hypotension following removal of pheochromocytoma (from patients who were inadequately treated with adrenergic blocking agents prior to surgery). In all such situations the prognosis is more favorable when therapy is instituted early and especially before the rate of urine flow is seriously decreased (below 0.3 ml per minute). The management of shock is more fully discussed later in this chapter. Dopamine may also be of value in the treatment of *chronic refractory congestive heart failure* (*see* Goldberg, 1974).

DOBUTAMINE

Dobutamine resembles dopamine chemically but possesses a bulky aromatic substituent on the amino group (Table 8–1). Despite the absence of a β-OH group, dobutamine is a directly acting agent with selectivity for β_1 receptors; its indirect actions are slight (Sonnenblick *et al.*, 1979).

Cardiovascular Effects. Dobutamine appears to be relatively more effective in enhancing the contractile force of the heart than in increasing heart rate (Tuttle and Mills, 1975; Tuttle *et al.*, 1976). The drug acts directly on β_1 receptors to produce its inotropic effect. While dobutamine enhances the automaticity of the sinus node in man, this action is not as prominent as that produced by isoproterenol. Dobutamine does not appear to affect atrial conduction velocity in man, although it does augment conduction velocity through the A-V node. There is little or no effect on ventricular impulse conduction. In contrast to dopamine, dobutamine does not have an effect on the dopaminergic receptors in the renal vasculature and, therefore, does not produce renal vasodilatation (Goldberg *et al.*, 1977).

In animals, dobutamine, administered at a rate of 2.5 to 15 μg/kg per minute, increases cardiac contractility and cardiac output. Total peripheral resistance is not much affected. The heart rate increases only modestly when the rate of administration of dobutamine is maintained at less than 20 μg/kg per minute. After administration of β-blocking agents, infusion of dobutamine fails to increase cardiac output, but total peripheral resistance increases, suggesting that dobutamine does have modest direct effects on α receptors in the vasculature. Reflex tachycardia associated with isoproterenol-induced hypotension cannot explain the greater chronotropic effect of isoproterenol as compared with dobutamine, since neither vagotomy nor agents that interfere with the function of sympathetic neurons eliminate the difference in the chronotropic effects of the two drugs.

Route of Administration, Dosage, and Preparations. Dobutamine is not effective when given orally, and, since its half-life in plasma is approximately 2 minutes, it must be administered by continuous intravenous infusion. The usual dose is 2.5 to 10 μg/kg per minute. The drug is rapidly metabolized in the liver to inactive conjugates with glucuronic acid and to 3-O-methyldobutamine.

Dobutamine hydrochloride (DOBUTREX) is supplied in 20-ml vials that contain 250 mg of the drug. The compound is dissolved in 10 ml of sterile water or 5% dextrose solution, and this solution is then further diluted to at least 50 ml for use.

Toxicity and Precautions. Since the electrophysiological effects caused by dobutamine are not markedly different from those of isoproterenol or dopamine, serious arrhythmias may be expected; however, it appears that the incidence is lower (Sonnenblick *et al.*, 1979). Nevertheless, because dobutamine enhances A-V conduction, the drug should be used with considerable caution or avoided in individuals with atrial fibrillation. In approximately 5 to 10% of patients, dobutamine may produce a marked increase in heart rate or systolic pressure. These effects can be rapidly reversed by reduction in the rate of administration of the drug. Less frequent side effects include nausea, headache, palpitations, shortness of breath, and anginal pain. Infusions of the drug have been performed for as long as 3 days.

Therapeutic Uses. Dobutamine causes a dose-related improvement in cardiac output in patients with congestive heart failure. Infusions at rates ranging from 2.5 to 15 μg/kg per minute produce progressive increases in cardiac output and decreases in pulmonary wedge pressure, indicative of a reduction in diastolic filling pressure in the left ventricle. Urine output and sodium excretion are increased, presumably secondarily to the improvement in cardiovascular status. Dobutamine appears to be particularly useful in patients who have undergone procedures involving cardiopulmonary bypass. Even greater beneficial effects are obtained under these circumstances when sodium nitroprusside is administered concomitantly with dobutamine.

Dobutamine appears to have advantages over other catecholamines for the improvement of myocardial function in heart failure. Since the effects of dobutamine on heart rate and systolic pressure are minimal in comparison to the other catecholamines, the oxygen demands of the myocardium are increased to a lesser degree. Increased contractility and reduction in left ventricular filling pressure in the failing heart should augment the gradient for diastolic coronary blood flow. The reduction in heart size also reduces wall tension at any given level of systolic pressure, and this tends to reduce oxygen demand. These favorable effects on myocardial perfusion are less likely to occur in the absence of cardiac failure. As a consequence, the use of dobutamine has been recommended for patients with acute myocardial infarction when congestive heart failure is superimposed (particularly if peripheral vascular resistance and heart rate are high) (*see* Goldstein *et al.,* 1980). If cardiogenic shock and severe hypotension are also present, coronary perfusion may be compromised and, under these circumstances, a vasopressor or expansion of plasma volume may also be required. Such procedures should be instituted only if pulmonary arterial and pulmonary wedge pressures can be monitored. Dobutamine, as well as other inotropic agents, is contraindicated in patients with marked obstruction to cardiac ejection, such as in idiopathic hypertrophic subaortic stenosis.

II. Noncatecholamines

For many years it was presumed that all sympathomimetic amines produced their effects by acting directly on adrenergic receptors. However, this notion was challenged by the findings that the effects of tyramine and many other noncatecholamines were reduced or abolished following chronic postganglionic adrenergic denervation or treatment with cocaine or reserpine. Under these circumstances, the effects of epinephrine and especially norepinephrine were often enhanced. These observations led to the proposal that tyramine and related amines acted indirectly, following uptake into the adrenergic nerve terminal, by stoichiometric displacement of norepinephrine from storage sites in the synaptic vesicles or from extravesicular binding sites (Burn and Rand, 1958). Norepinephrine could then exit from the adrenergic nerve terminal and interact with receptors to produce the sympathomimetic effects. The depletion of tissue stores of catecholamines that follows treatment with reserpine or degeneration of adrenergic nerve terminals would explain the lack of effect of tyramine under these conditions. In the presence of cocaine, the high-affinity neuronal transport system for catecholamines and certain congeners is inhibited,

and tyramine and related amines are unable to enter the adrenergic nerve terminal. In this manner cocaine inhibits the actions of indirectly acting sympathomimetic amines, while potentiating the effects of directly acting agents that are normally removed from the synaptic cleft by this transport system (*see* Chapter 4).

In assessing the proportion of direct and indirect actions of a sympathomimetic amine, the most common experimental procedure is to compare the dose-response curve for the agent on a particular target tissue before and after treatment with reserpine (Trendelenburg, 1972). Those drugs whose actions are essentially unaltered after treatment with reserpine are classified as directly acting sympathomimetic amines (*e.g.,* norepinephrine, phenylephrine), while those whose actions are abolished are termed indirectly acting (*e.g.,* tyramine). Most agents exhibit some degree of residual sympathomimetic activity after the administration of reserpine, but higher doses of these amines are required to produce comparable effects. These are classified as mixed-acting sympathomimetic amines; that is, they have both direct and indirect actions. The proportion of direct and indirect actions can vary considerably between different tissues and species. The general structural features that appear to govern the pattern of responses obtained have been described above.

Since the actions of norepinephrine are more marked on α and β_1 receptors than on β_2 receptors, many noncatecholamines that release norepinephrine have predominantly α-receptor-mediated and cardiac effects. However, many noncatecholamines with both direct and indirect effects on adrenergic receptors show powerful β_2-agonistic activity and are widely used clinically for the effects that result. Thus, ephedrine, although dependent upon norepinephrine release for some of its effects, relieves bronchospasm by its action on β_2 receptors in bronchial muscle, an effect virtually absent with norepinephrine. It must also be recalled that some noncatecholamines, for example, phenylephrine, act primarily and directly on effector cells. It is therefore impossible to predict precisely the characteristic effects of noncatecholamines simply on the basis that they all provoke the release of at least some norepinephrine.

With few exceptions the actions and effects of noncatecholamines, except those on the CNS, fit within the framework of α- and β-receptor activity as listed in Table 4–1 (page 72), and, therefore, only the main differences in their properties will be presented. The additional CNS effects, most prominent with sympathomimetic amines lacking substituents on the benzene ring, have been most extensively studied with amphetamine and, consequently, are discussed in detail in relation to the properties and clinical uses of that drug.

False-Transmitter Concept. As indicated above, indirectly acting amines are taken up into adrenergic nerve terminals and storage vesicles, where they presumably replace norepinephrine in the storage complex. Phenylethylamines that lack a β-hydroxyl group are retained there poorly, but β-hydroxylated phenylethylamines and compounds that subsequently become hydroxylated in the synaptic vesicle by dopamine β-hydroxylase are retained in the synaptic vesicle for relatively long periods of time (Musacchio *et al.*, 1965; Kopin, 1968). Such substances can produce a persistent diminution in the content of norepinephrine at functionally critical sites in the adrenergic nerve terminal. When the nerve is stimulated, the content of a relatively constant number of synaptic vesicles is presumably released by exocytosis. If these vesicles contain a considerable proportion of phenylethylamines that are much less potent than norepinephrine, activation of postsynaptic adrenergic receptors will be diminished.

This hypothesis, known as the *false-transmitter concept,* is a possible explanation for the hypotensive effect that results from the administration of inhibitors of MAO. Phenylethylamines are normally synthesized in the gastrointestinal tract as a result of the action of bacterial tyrosine decarboxylase. The tyramine that is formed in this fashion is usually oxidatively deaminated in the gastrointestinal tract and the liver, and the amine does not reach the systemic circulation in significant concentrations. However, when an MAO inhibitor is administered, tyramine may be absorbed systemically. It is transported into the adrenergic nerve terminal, where its catabolism is again prevented because of the inhibition of MAO at this site; it is

then β-hydroxylated to octopamine and stored in the vesicles in this form. As a consequence, there is gradual displacement of norepinephrine, and stimulation results in the release of a relatively small amount of norepinephrine along with a fraction of octopamine. The latter amine has relatively little ability to activate either α- or β-adrenergic receptors. There is thus a functional impairment of sympathetic nerve transmission following chronic administration of MAO inhibitors.

Despite such functional impairment, patients who have received MAO inhibitors may experience severe hypertensive crises if they ingest cheese, beer, or red wine. These and related foods, which are produced by a fermentation process, contain a large quantity of tyramine and, to a lesser degree, other phenylethylamines. When gastrointestinal and hepatic MAO is inhibited, the large quantity of tyramine that is ingested is absorbed rapidly and reaches the systemic circulation in high concentration. A massive and precipitous release of norepinephrine can result, with consequent hypertension that can be sufficiently severe to cause myocardial infarction or a cerebrovascular accident (*see* Chapter 19).

The false-transmitter concept can also be invoked to explain the hypotension that often follows infusions of metaraminol. Metaraminol possesses both direct and indirect sympathomimetic actions and has been infused for many hours for the maintenance of blood pressure in individuals who are severely hypotensive. When the infusion is terminated, patients may relapse into a severe hypotensive state, despite correction of the factors responsible for their shock. Presumably, the maintenance of adequate blood pressure at this time is largely dependent upon intrinsic sympathomimetic activity. However, a considerable fraction of the norepinephrine in the nerve terminal may have been replaced by metaraminol, and the release of this less potent sympathomimetic amine, along with norepinephrine, is apparently insufficient to produce adequate vasoconstriction. To manage this problem, patients can be given an infusion of norepinephrine for a period of time sufficient to allow replenishment of the stores of the neurotransmitter.

Absorption, Distribution, and Fate of Noncatecholamines. In contrast to the catecholamines, most of the noncatecholamines that are used clinically are effective when given orally and many act for long periods. These properties are due in part to resistance to the inactivating enzymes of liver and other tissues and in part to the fact that relatively large amounts are given. Phenylisopropylamines, the most commonly used noncatecholamines, are widely distributed in tissues, and, in contrast to catecholamines, they cross the blood-brain barrier. This accounts in part for their relatively powerful CNS activity.

Although several pathways, including *p*-hydroxylation, N-demethylation, deamination, and conjugation in the liver, take part in their disposal, a substantial fraction of these drugs is excreted in the urine unchanged. Urinary excretion of amphetamine and many other noncatecholamines is greatly influenced by urinary pH. For example, the pK_a of amphetamine is 9.9, and at pH 8.0 only 2 to 3% is excreted. If the urine is acidic, urinary excretion may be as much as 80%. Thus, acidification of the urine by the administration of ammonium chloride is a logical procedure in the treatment of amphetamine poisoning. Since a large number of noncatecholamines have pK_a values between 9.0 and 10.3, similar striking effects of urinary pH can be expected.

Patients treated with MAO inhibitors should not take noncatecholamines or ingest foods that contain tyramine (*see* above). Even sympathomimetic drugs that are resistant to MAO (*e.g.*, amphetamine and ephedrine) should not be administered to such individuals, since these drugs provoke the release of norepinephrine, and the actions of the neurotransmitter can be potentiated by MAO inhibitors in this circumstance (Smith, 1966).

AMPHETAMINE

Amphetamine, racemic β-phenylisopropylamine (Table 8–1), has powerful CNS stimulant actions in addition to the peripheral α and β actions common to indirectly acting sympathomimetic drugs. Unlike epinephrine, it is effective after oral administration and its effects last for several hours.

PHARMACOLOGICAL PROPERTIES

Cardiovascular Responses. In man and animals, amphetamine given orally raises both systolic and diastolic blood pressures. Heart rate is often reflexly slowed; with large doses, cardiac arrhythmias may occur. Cardiac output is not enhanced by therapeutic doses, and cerebral blood flow is little changed. The *l* isomer is slightly more potent than the *d* isomer in its cardiovascular actions.

Other Smooth Muscles. In general, smooth muscles respond to amphetamine as they do to other sympathomimetics. The contractile effect on the urinary bladder sphincter is particularly marked, and has been used in treating enuresis and incontinence. Pain and difficulty in micturition occasionally occur. The gastrointestinal effects of amphetamine are unpredictable. If enteric activity is pronounced, amphetamine may cause relaxation and delay the movement of intestinal contents; if the gut is already relaxed, the opposite effect may be seen. The response of the human uterus varies, but usually there is an increase in tone.

Central Nervous System. Amphetamine is one of the most potent sympathomimetic amines with respect to stimulation of the CNS. It stimulates the medullary respiratory center, lessens the degree of central depression caused by various drugs, and produces other signs of stimulation of the CNS. These effects are thought to be due to cortical stimulation and possibly to stimulation of the reticular activating system. In contrast, the drug can obtund the maximal electroshock seizure discharge and prolong the ensuing period of depression. In elicitation of CNS excitatory effects, the *d* isomer (dextroamphetamine) is three to four times as potent as the *l* isomer.

In man, the *psychic* effects depend on the dose and the mental state and personality of the individual. The main results of an oral dose of 10 to 30 mg are as follows: wakefulness, alertness, and a decreased sense of fatigue; elevation of mood, with increased initiative, self-confidence, and ability to concentrate; often elation and euphoria; increase in motor and speech activity. Performance of only simple mental tasks is improved; and, although more work may be accomplished, the number of errors is not necessarily decreased. Physical performance, for example, in athletes, is improved, and the drug is abused for this purpose. These effects are not invariable, and may be reversed by overdosage or repeated usage. Prolonged use or large doses are nearly always followed by mental depression and fatigue. Many individuals given amphetamine experience headache, palpitation, dizziness, vasomotor disturbances, agitation, confusion, dysphoria, apprehension, delirium, or fatigue. (*See* Chapter 23.)

Fatigue and Sleep. Prevention and reversal of fatigue by amphetamine have been studied extensively in the laboratory, in military field studies, and in athletics. In general, the duration of adequate performance is prolonged before fatigue appears and the effects of fatigue are at least partly reversed. The most striking improvement due to amphetamine appears to occur when performance has been reduced by fatigue and lack of sleep. Such improvement may be partly due to alteration of unfavorable attitudes toward the task. However, amphetamine reduces the frequency of attention lapses that impair performance after prolonged sleep deprivation, and thus improves execution of tasks requiring sustained attention. The need for sleep may be postponed, but it obviously cannot be indefinitely avoided. When the drug is discontinued after long use, the pattern of sleep may take as long as 2 months to return to normal. (*See* reviews by Weiss and Laties, 1962; Oswald, 1968.)

Analgesia. Amphetamine and some other sympathomimetic amines have a small analgesic effect in man and experimental animals; this is not sufficiently pronounced to be useful therapeutically. However, amphetamine can enhance the analgesia produced by morphine-like drugs (*see* Chapter 22).

EEG. In general, amphetamine accelerates and desynchronizes the EEG. It causes a shift of the resting EEG toward the higher frequencies in man, but to a smaller degree than that occurring during attention. It reduces the amplitude and the duration of the large delta waves that are present during sleep after prolonged insomnia and in narcolepsy. In children with behavioral disorders and abnormal EEG (6-cycle-per-second rhythm), amphetamine may improve behavior with or without altering the EEG.

Spinal Cord, Reticular Formation, and Respiratory Center. Amphetamine facilitates monosynaptic and polysynaptic transmission in the spinal cord. In common with ephedrine, it enhances excitatory activity, promotes righting movements and postural activity, and speeds the recovery of responses in spinal, decerebrate, and decorticate animals.

The *respiratory center* is stimulated by amphetamine in animals, and the rate and depth of respiration are increased. In normal man, usual doses of the drug do not appreciably increase respiratory rate or minute volume. Nevertheless, when respiration is depressed by centrally acting drugs, amphetamine may stimulate respiration.

Depression of Appetite. Amphetamine and similar drugs have been widely used in the treatment of obesity, although the wisdom of this use is at best questionable. Weight loss in obese humans treated with amphetamine is almost entirely due to reduced food intake and only in small measure to increased metabolism. The site of action is probably in the lateral hypothalamic feeding center; injection of amphetamine into this area, but not into the ventromedial satiety center, suppresses food intake (*see* Blundell and Leshem, 1973). In man, some drug-induced loss of acuity of smell and taste has been described, and increased physical activity may also contribute to the loss of weight. In dogs, the effect is powerful and may lead to complete starvation if amphetamine is given each day 1 hour before the daily meal. The effect is much less in man, and tolerance to acceptable doses develops rapidly. The effect is insufficient to reduce weight continuously in obese individuals without dietary restriction. Amphetamine has little effect in reducing food intake in those persons whose overeating is impelled by psychological factors.

Mechanisms of Action in the CNS. Amphetamine appears to exert most or all of its effects in the CNS by releasing biogenic amines from their storage sites in the nerve terminals. The alerting effect of amphetamine, its anorectic effect, and at least a component of its locomotor-stimulating action are presumably mediated by release of norepinephrine from central noradrenergic neurons. These effects can be prevented by treatment of the animal with α-methyltyrosine, an inhibitor of tyrosine hydroxylase and, therefore, of catecholamine synthesis. Some aspects of locomotor activity and the stereotyped behavior induced by amphetamine are probably a consequence of the release of dopamine from dopaminergic nerve terminals, particularly in the neostriatum. Higher doses are required to produce these behavioral effects, and this is correlated with the need for higher concentrations of amphetamine to release dopamine from brain slices or synaptosomes *in vitro*. With still higher doses of amphetamine, disturbances of perception and overt psychotic behavior occur. These effects may be due to release of 5-hydroxytryptamine (5-HT) from tryptaminergic neurons and of dopamine in the mesolimbic system. In addition, amphetamine may exert direct agonistic effects on central receptors for 5-HT (*see* Weiner, 1972).

Metabolic Effects. Although large doses of amphetamine markedly increase oxygen consumption in animals, conventional therapeutic doses cause either no change, a small fall, or a modest rise (10 to 15%) in the metabolic rate in man. Some patients show a slight increase in body temperature. The apparent calorigenic action may be due to restlessness caused by the drug.

Preparations and Route of Administration. *Amphetamine sulfate* is a white, water-soluble powder, available in 5- and 10-mg tablets. The *d* isomer is available as *dextroamphetamine sulfate* (DEXEDRINE, others) in 5- and 10-mg tablets, in an elixir (1 mg/ml), and in 5-, 10-, and 15-mg slow-release capsules. Dosage is discussed under specific therapeutic applications (*see* below). The amphetamines are schedule-II drugs under federal regulations (*see* Appendix I).

Toxicity and Side Effects. The *acute toxic effects* of amphetamine are usually extensions of its therapeutic actions and, as a rule, result from overdosage. The *central effects* commonly include restlessness, dizziness, tremor, hyperactive reflexes, talkativeness, tenseness, irritability, weakness, insomnia, fever, and sometimes euphoria. Confusion, assaultiveness, increased libido, anxiety, delirium, paranoid hallucinations, panic states, and suicidal or homicidal tendencies occur, especially in mentally ill patients. However, these psychotic effects can be elicited in any individual if sufficient quantities of amphetamine are ingested for a prolonged period. Fatigue and depression usually follow the central stimulation. *Cardiovascular effects* are common and include headache, chilliness, pallor or flushing, palpitation, cardiac arrhythmias, anginal pain, hypertension or hypotension, and circulatory collapse. Excessive sweating occurs. Symptoms referable to the *gastrointestinal system* include dry mouth, metallic taste, anorexia, nausea, vomiting, diarrhea, and abdominal cramps. Fatal poisoning usually terminates in convulsions and coma, and cerebral hemorrhages are the main pathological finding.

The *toxic dose* of amphetamine varies widely. Toxic manifestations occasionally occur as an idiosyncrasy after as little as 2 mg, but are rare with doses of less than 15 mg. Severe reactions have occurred with 30 mg, yet doses of 400 to 500 mg are not uniformly fatal. Larger doses can be tolerated after chronic use of the drug.

Treatment of acute amphetamine intoxication should include acidification of the urine by administration of ammonium chloride; excretion of amphetamine is vastly increased in acidic urine. Chlorpromazine is effective treatment for the CNS symptoms, and additionally its α-receptor blocking action reduces the elevated blood pressure. A nitrite, sodium nitroprusside, or a rapidly acting α-receptor blocking agent (*e.g.*, phentolamine) may also be required if hypertension is marked.

Chronic intoxication with amphetamine causes symptoms similar to those of acute overdosage, but abnormal mental conditions are more common. Weight loss may be marked. A psychotic reaction with vivid hallucinations and paranoid delusions, often mistaken for schizophrenia, is the most common serious effect. Recovery is usually rapid after withdrawal of the drug, but occasionally the condition becomes chronic. In these persons amphetamine may act as a precipitating factor hastening the onset of an incipient schizophrenia (*see* Angrist and Gershon, 1972).

Precautions and Contraindications. The abuse of amphetamine by the laity as a means of overcoming sleepiness and of increasing energy and alertness should be discouraged. The drug should be used only under medical supervision. The additional *contraindications* and *precautions* in the use of amphetamine are generally similar to those described above for epinephrine. Its use is inadvisable in patients with anorexia, insomnia, asthenia, psychopathic personality, or a history of homicidal or suicidal tendencies.

Dependence and Tolerance. Psychological dependence often occurs when amphetamine or dextroamphetamine is used chronically, as discussed in Chapter 23. *Tolerance* almost invariably develops to the anorexigenic effect of amphetamines, and is often seen also in the need for increasing doses to maintain improvement of mood in psychiatric patients. Tolerance is striking in individuals who are dependent on the drug, and a daily intake of 1700 mg without apparent ill effects has been reported. Development of tolerance is not invariable, and cases of narcolepsy have been treated for years without requiring an increase in the initially effective dose.

Therapeutic Uses. Amphetamine and dextroamphetamine are used chiefly for their CNS effects. Dextroamphetamine, with greater CNS action and less peripheral action, is generally preferred to amphetamine; it is used in obesity, narcolepsy, and *attention-deficit disorder* in children. These uses are discussed later in this chapter.

METHAMPHETAMINE

Methamphetamine is closely related chemically to amphetamine and ephedrine (Table 8–1). Small doses have prominent central stimulant effects without significant peripheral actions; somewhat larger doses produce a sustained rise in systolic and diastolic blood pressures, due in man mainly to cardiac stimulation. Cardiac output is increased, although the heart rate may be reflexly slowed. Venous constriction causes peripheral venous pressure to increase. These factors tend to increase the venous return and, therefore, the cardiac output. Pulmonary arterial pressure is raised, probably secondary to increased cardiac output. Renal blood flow is also enhanced. Although moderate doses stimulate cardiac contraction, excessive doses depress the myocardium. (*See* Aviado, 1970.)

Preparations, Route of Administration, and Dosage. *Methamphetamine hydrochloride* (DESOXYN, METHAMPEX) is the *d* isomer. It is available in tablets containing 5 and 10 mg and in sustained-release tablets containing 5, 10, or 15 mg. The usual oral dose for central effects varies from 5 to 25 mg daily in single or divided doses, depending on the formulation used. Methamphetamine is a schedule-II drug under federal regulations (*see* Appendix I).

Therapeutic Uses. Methamphetamine is principally used for its *central effects,* which are more pronounced than those of amphetamine and are accompanied by less prominent peripheral actions. These uses are discussed below in the section of this chapter on therapeutic uses.

EPHEDRINE

Ephedrine occurs naturally in various plants. It was used in China for at least 2000 years before being introduced into Western medicine in 1924 (*see* Chen and Schmidt, 1930). Its central actions are less pronounced than those of the amphetamines. Ephedrine stimulates both α and β receptors and has clinical uses related to both types of action. The drug owes part of its peripheral action to release of norepinephrine, but it also has direct effects on receptors and exhibits substantial effects in reserpine-treated animals and man. Tachyphylaxis develops to its peripheral actions, and rapidly repeated doses become less effective.

Since ephedrine contains two asymmetrical carbon atoms, four compounds are possible. Only *l*-ephedrine and racemic ephedrine are commonly used clinically; their pharmacological properties and uses are essentially similar. The structure of ephedrine is depicted in Table 8–1.

Pharmacological Actions. Ephedrine differs from epinephrine mainly in its efficacy after oral administration, its much longer duration of action, its more pronounced central actions, and its much lower potency. *Cardiovascular effects* of ephedrine are in many ways similar to those of epinephrine, but they persist about ten times as long. The drug elevates the systolic and usually also the diastolic pressure in man, and pulse pressure increases. Pressor responses are due partly to vasoconstriction but mainly to cardiac stimulation. The heart rate may not be altered, but it increases if vagal reflexes are blocked. The force of myocardial contraction is enhanced by the drug, and cardiac output is augmented, provided venous return is adequate. The renal and splanchnic blood flows are decreased whereas the coronary, cerebral, and muscle blood flows are increased.

Bronchial muscle relaxation is less prominent but more sustained with ephedrine than with epinephrine. Consequently, ephedrine is of value only in milder cases of acute asthma and in chronic cases that need continued medication. *Mydriasis* occurs after local application of the drug to the eye. Reflexes to light are not abolished, accommodation is unaffected, and intraocular pressure is unchanged. Ephedrine and other sympathomimetics are of little use as mydriatics in the presence of inflammation. The drug is less effective in individuals who have heavily pigmented irides than in those in whom the iris is light colored. Other smooth muscles are generally affected by ephedrine in the same manner as by epinephrine. However, the activity of the human *uterus* is usually reduced by ephedrine, regardless of the effect of epinephrine. Ephedrine is less effective than epinephrine in elevating the concentration of *glucose* in the *blood*. The *CNS effects* of ephedrine are similar to those of amphetamine but are considerably less marked.

Preparations, Routes of Administration, and Dosage. *Ephedrine sulfate* is the *l* isomer. It is available in 25- and 50-mg capsules and in syrups; the oral dose varies from 15 to 50 mg. For continued medication, small doses are given at 3- to 4-hour intervals. Sterile solutions (25 and 50 mg/ml) are available; 25 to 50 mg may be given subcutaneously, intramuscularly, or intravenously. Solutions and a jelly are available for nasal mucosal decongestion. Ephedrine is also available in combination with other agents for use in asthma, as a nasal decongestant, and for topical application to the eye.

Toxic Reactions. These are similar to the untoward reactions observed after epinephrine, with additional reactions referable to the CNS effects of ephedrine. Insomnia is common with continued medication, but it is readily counteracted by sedatives if necessary. *Precautions* in the use of ephedrine are similar to those outlined for epinephrine and the amphetamines.

Therapeutic Uses. The main clinical applications of ephedrine are in *bronchospasm*, in *Stokes-Adams syndrome*, as a *nasal decongestant*, and in certain *allergic disorders*. The drug has also been employed as a *pressor* agent, particularly during spinal anesthesia, and for its central stimulant action in *narcolepsy*. These uses are discussed below in the section of this chapter on therapeutic uses.

MEPHENTERMINE

Mephentermine is N-methyl-ω-phenyl-*tertiary*-butylamine (Table 8–1). It is one of several pressor agents that can be used in various hypotensive conditions. Its duration of action is prolonged, and pressor effects last for up to 4 hours after intramuscular doses. Mephentermine acts both directly and by release of endogenous norepinephrine. Cardiac contraction is enhanced, and cardiac output and systolic and diastolic pressures are usually increased. The change in heart rate is variable, depending on the degree of vagal tone; large doses can depress the heart. The pressor response involves both increased cardiac output and peripheral vasoconstriction. In some cases the net vascular effect may be vasodilatation, which appears not to involve β receptors (Caldwell and Goldberg, 1970). Coronary blood flow is increased, forearm blood flow is reduced, and venous tone is increased. Marked mucosal vasoconstriction can be produced by local application of the drug. CNS effects are usually modest with the recommended doses of mephentermine, but they become more prominent with larger doses. These include drowsiness, weeping, incoherence, and convulsions, and rapidly disappear on withdrawal of the drug.

Preparations, Routes of Administration, and Dosage. *Mephentermine sulfate* (WYAMINE SULFATE) is available in sterile solution (15 and 30 mg/ml) for parenteral injection. Given *intramuscularly* the dose is usually 15 to 45 mg. Slow *intravenous infusions* are also given, the rate being varied to produce the desired pressor effect.

Therapeutic Uses. Mephentermine is mainly used as a pressor agent in various *hypotensive states*, as discussed below.

HYDROXYAMPHETAMINE

The chemical structure of hydroxyamphetamine differs from that of amphetamine only by the addition of a 4-OH group (*see* Table 8–1). The actions of hydroxyamphetamine resemble those of ephedrine, with the exception that the drug almost entirely lacks CNS stimulant activity. While the drug has been employed for the treatment of hypotensive states and to maintain an adequate ventricular rate in the Stokes-Adams syndrome, the only current use of hydroxyamphetamine in the United States is as a mydriatic. *Hydroxyamphetamine hydrobromide* (PAREDRINE) is available as a 1% ophthalmic solution.

METARAMINOL

Metaraminol, 3-hydroxyphenylisopropanolamine (Table 8–1), is used almost exclusively for the treatment of hypotensive states. It has both direct and indirect actions and its overall effects are similar to those of norepinephrine, but it is much less potent and has a more prolonged action. It lacks CNS stimulant effects. Metaraminol is absorbed after oral administration; however, for equal effects, oral doses must be five or six times greater than doses given intramuscularly or intravenously. The pressor effect of an intramuscular dose of 5 mg lasts for about 1.5 hours.

Cardiovascular Actions. The cardiovascular actions in man are reflected in a sustained rise in systolic and diastolic pressures, almost entirely due to vasoconstriction and usually accompanied by a marked reflex bradycardia. In normotensive subjects, cardiac output is unchanged or may decrease slightly, but the force of myocardial contraction is enhanced. Cardiac output increases strikingly when slowing of the heart is prevented by atropine. Increased cardiac output may play a larger role in patients with hypotension and shock. Metaraminol increases venous tone and decreases renal and cerebral blood flows, the latter even when blood pressure is raised as much as 40%. Pulmonary vasoconstriction occurs, and the pulmonary blood pressure is elevated by the drug even when cardiac output is reduced.

Preparations, Routes of Administration, and Dosage. *Metaraminol bitartrate* (ARAMINE) is available as a sterile solution (10 mg/ml) for intramuscular injection, usually in a dose of 2 to 10 mg, or, after suitable dilution, for intravenous infusion. The rate of administration is regulated according to the individual's response to the drug.

Therapeutic Uses. The principal use of metaraminol is as a pressor agent in certain *hypotensive states*, the treatment of which is discussed below in the section of this chapter on therapeutic uses.

PHENYLEPHRINE

Phenylephrine differs chemically from epinephrine only in lacking an OH in the 4 position on the benzene ring (Table 8–1).

Phenylephrine is a powerful α_1-receptor stimulant with little effect on the β receptors of the heart. A direct action on receptors accounts for the greater part of its effects, only a small part being due to its ability to release norepinephrine. Central stimulant action is minimal.

Cardiovascular Actions. The predominant actions of phenylephrine are on peripheral arterioles. Intravenous, subcutaneous, or oral administration causes a rise in systolic and diastolic pressures. Responses persist for 20 minutes after intravenous and as long as 50 minutes after subcutaneous injection. Accompanying the pressor response to phenylephrine is a marked reflex bradycardia that can be blocked by atropine; after atropine, large doses of the drug increase the heart rate only slightly. In man, cardiac output is slightly decreased and peripheral resistance is considerably increased. Circulation time is slightly prolonged, and venous pressure is slightly increased; venous constriction is not marked. Most vascular beds are constricted, and renal, splanchnic, cutaneous, and limb blood flows are reduced but coronary blood flow is increased. Pulmonary vessels are constricted, and pulmonary arterial pressure is raised. Cardiac irregularities are seen only very rarely even with large doses, and the reflex slowing is sufficient to permit use of the drug to end attacks of paroxysmal atrial tachycardia.

Preparations, Routes of Administration, and Dosage. *Phenylephrine hydrochloride* (NEO-SYNEPHRINE, others) is the *l* isomer. It is available as a sterile solution (10 mg/ml) for parenteral use and in various nasal and ophthalmic solutions, as a nasal jelly, and as a viscous ophthalmic solution. Phenylephrine is also present in a large number of combination products, primarily for use as a decongestant. Absorption after oral administration is unreliable. For treatment of hypotension during spinal anesthesia, the usual dose is 2 to 3 mg, administered subcutaneously or intramuscularly. The rate of intravenous infusion in hypotensive states should be regulated according to the patient's response.

Therapeutic Uses. Phenylephrine is used mainly as a *nasal decongestant*, a pressor agent in *hypotensive states*, a *mydriatic*, and a local vasoconstrictor (0.005%) in solutions of local anesthetics, as well as in the relief of *paroxysmal atrial tachycardia*. These uses are discussed below in the section of this chapter on therapeutic uses.

METHOXAMINE

Methoxamine is β-hydroxy-β-(2,5-dimethoxyphenyl) isopropylamine (Table 8–1). Its pharmacological properties are almost exclusively those characteristic of α-receptor stimulation, and it acts directly at these sites. Its pharmacological actions are thus similar to those of phenylephrine. The outstanding effect is an increase in blood pressure, due entirely to vasoconstriction. The drug has virtually no stimulant action on the heart and lacks β-receptor action on smooth muscle. It causes little or no CNS stimulation.

Cardiovascular Actions. Methoxamine, given intravenously or intramuscularly in man, causes a rise in systolic and diastolic blood pressures that persists for 60 to 90 minutes. Cardiac output is decreased or unchanged. Renal blood flow is reduced in man to a greater extent than after equipressor doses of norepinephrine or metaraminol. Cerebral, splanchnic, and limb blood flows are reduced in dogs, and coronary blood flow is unchanged; whether the effects are similar in man is not known. In man, the venous pressure increases, but the constrictor action on forearm veins is feeble. Methoxamine does not increase the ventricular rate in patients with heart block. Reflex bradycardia is prominent, and, therefore, the drug is used clinically to relieve attacks of paroxysmal atrial tachycardia. When the vagal effects are blocked by atropine, methoxamine often slows the heart slightly. This is probably due to a direct action on α receptors. Injection of the drug into the artery leading to the sinus node slows the heart, an effect blocked by phentolamine (James *et al.*, 1968). Methoxamine does not appear to precipitate cardiac arrhythmias. In contrast to epinephrine, methoxamine prolongs ventricular muscle action potentials and refractory period and slows A-V conduction.

In man, pressor doses of methoxamine cause pilomotor stimulation and often a desire to micturate. Occasionally tingling of the extremities and a feeling of coldness follow intravenous injection of the drug.

Preparations, Routes of Administration, and Dosage. *Methoxamine hydrochloride* (VASOXYL) is available as a solution (20 mg/ml) for intramuscular injection. The dose varies from 5 to 20 mg. Intravenous injections of 3 to 5 mg may also be given with the precautions properly accorded to intravenous injections of sympathomimetic amines.

Therapeutic Uses. Methoxamine is almost solely used as a pressor agent in *hypotensive states* and to end attacks of *paroxysmal atrial tachycardia*. These conditions are discussed below in the section of this chapter on therapeutic uses.

SELECTIVE β_2-ADRENERGIC STIMULANTS

The considerable incidence and intensity of untoward effects of isoproterenol, when administered either parenterally or by inhalation for the treatment of bronchoconstrictive disease, have caused investigators to conduct an intensive search for more specific β_2-adrenergic agonists. *Metaproterenol, terbutaline, isoetharine, albuterol*, and *ritodrine* have already been introduced into therapy in the United States. Other β_2 agonists include *carbuterol, fenoterol, quinterenol, rimiterol, salmefamol, soterenol*, and *tretoquinol* (Webb-Johnson and Andrews, 1977). The structures of the agents available in the United States are shown in Table 8–1. Because of their relative specificity for β_2 receptors, these drugs relax smooth muscle of the bronchi, uterus, and vascular supply to skeletal muscle, but generally have much less stimulant action on the heart than does isoproterenol. Thus, in asthmatic patients cardiac stimulation can be sufficiently limited to give these drugs appreciable therapeutic advantage over isoproterenol.

METAPROTERENOL

Metaproterenol is quite similar to isoproterenol chemically, except that the two hydroxyl groups are attached at the meta positions on the benzene ring rather than at the meta and para positions. As a consequence, metaproterenol is resistant to methylation by COMT. It is effective when administered orally and has a somewhat longer duration of action than does isoproterenol.

Pharmacological Properties. Metaproterenol is primarily a β_2-adrenergic agonist. When administered by inhalation, it has relatively little effect on the β_1 receptors of the heart. Following either oral administration or inhalation of metaproterenol, there is an increase in 1-second forced expiratory volume (FEV_1) and in the maximal rate of forced expiratory flow (FEF), and a decrease in airway resistance. With a single oral dose of 20 mg of the drug, significant improvement in airway function is demonstrable for up to 4 hours. After administration of the drug by inhalation, improved respiratory function is apparent for a more variable period of time, but usually for 3 to 4 hours. There is some suggestion that tolerance develops after repeated administration of metaproterenol. This is manifested primarily as a shortened duration of action of the drug. A similar phenomenon is seen with ephedrine.

Approximately 40% of metaproterenol is absorbed after oral administration. The drug is excreted in the urine primarily as conjugates with glucuronic acid.

Preparations, Routes of Administration, and Dosage. *Metaproterenol sulfate* (ALUPENT, METAPREL) is available for oral inhalation as a micronized powder. The metered-dose inhaler contains 225 mg of the drug, and approximately 0.65 mg is nebulized per dose. Administration is generally performed by 2 or 3 deep inhalations, and this may be repeated at 3- to 4-hour intervals; the total daily dose should not exceed 12 inhalations. An oral inhalant solution can also be utilized. For oral administration, metaproterenol is supplied as 10- and 20-mg tablets. The usual adult dose is 20 mg, taken three or four times a day. A syrup (10 mg/5 ml) is suitable for use in children. The usual dose in children who are 6 to 9 years of age or who weigh less than 27 kg is 5 ml, given three or four times a day. Children over 9 years of age or who weigh over 27 kg may receive 10 ml three or four times a day.

Toxicity and Precautions. Adverse reactions are generally those expected from sympathomimetic stimulation and include tachycardia, hypertension, nervousness, tremor, palpitations, nausea, and vomiting. The drug should be used with special caution in patients with hypertension, coronary artery disease, congestive heart failure, hyperthyroidism, or diabetes.

Therapeutic Uses. Metaproterenol is useful as a *bronchodilator* in the treatment of bronchial asthma and for reversible bronchospasm associated with bronchitis or emphysema. When administered by inhalation, it is approximately as effective as isoproterenol and its duration of action is considerably longer. When administered orally, it is at least as effective as ephedrine.

TERBUTALINE

Terbutaline sulfate is a synthetic sympathomimetic agent that is administered orally, subcutaneously, and by inhalation for the treatment of reversible obstruction of the airway. It is a relatively selective β_2 agonist. Like metaproterenol, terbutaline is not a catechol and is not methylated by COMT.

Pharmacological Properties. Terbutaline, given orally in a dose of 5 mg to patients with asthma, produces bronchodilatation after about 1 hour that lasts for approximately 7 hours. There is a significant increase in pulmonary function, as demonstrated by an increase of 15% or more in FEV_1 and FEF. When the drug is administered subcutaneously, the improvement in pulmonary function occurs in approximately 5 minutes and persists for up to 4 hours. However, the selectivity of this agent for β_2 receptors is much less apparent when the drug is administered by this route, and cardiovascular effects similar to those caused by isoproterenol may be expected.

Side effects associated with the administration of terbutaline are generally those produced by other sympathomimetic agents. Nervousness and muscle tremors are common; other effects include headache, tachycardia, palpitations, drowsiness, nausea, vomiting, and sweating. These reactions are usually mild, and their frequency appears to diminish with continued therapy. The precautions to be observed are the same as those for other sympathomimetic drugs.

Preparations, Routes of Administration, and Dosage. *Terbutaline sulfate* (BRETHAIRE, BRETHINE, BRICANYL) may be administered subcutaneously, orally, or by inhalation. Its use in children under 12 years of age is not recommended. The usual subcutaneous dose is 0.25 mg. If significant clinical improvement does not occur in 15 to 30 minutes, a second dose may be administered. A total dose of 0.5 mg should not be exceeded within a 4-hour period. The usual oral dose of terbutaline is 5 mg, administered at intervals of approximately 6 hours three times a day. If side effects are notable, the dose may be reduced to 2.5 mg three times daily. The inhalational dose is 2 sprays every 4 to 6 hours. Terbutaline is available in tablets containing either 2.5 or 5 mg of the drug, as an injection containing 1 mg/ml, and as an aerosol containing 0.2 mg per spray.

Therapeutic Uses. Terbutaline is an effective *bronchodilator* when administered orally and is useful in the management of asthma and other bronchospastic diseases. Like metaproterenol and other relatively selective β_2 agonists, terbutaline

appears to possess modest therapeutic advantages over less selective bronchodilators such as ephedrine.

ALBUTEROL

Albuterol is a selective β_2-adrenergic agonist with pharmacological properties and therapeutic indications similar to those of terbutaline. It is administered either by inhalation or orally for the symptomatic relief of bronchospasm associated with chronic or acute asthma, bronchitis, or other obstructive pulmonary diseases. When administered by inhalation, it produces significant bronchodilatation within 15 minutes and effects are demonstrable for 3 to 4 hours. The cardiovascular effects of albuterol are considerably less than those of isoproterenol when doses that produce comparable bronchodilatation are administered by inhalation (Ahrens and Smith, 1984).

Preparations, Routes of Administration, and Dosage. *Albuterol* (PROVENTIL, VENTOLIN) (*salbutamol* in Canada and Europe) is marketed in 2- and 4-mg tablets (as the sulfate) for oral administration and as an aerosol. Each inhalation delivers approximately 90 μg of the drug; no more than 2 inhalations every 4 to 6 hours is recommended. The initial oral dose is 2 to 4 mg, given three to four times daily; a total daily dose of 32 mg should not be exceeded. The safety and efficacy of albuterol in children under 12 years of age has not been established.

RITODRINE

Ritodrine is a selective β_2-adrenergic agonist that was developed specifically for use as a uterine relaxant. Nevertheless, its pharmacological properties closely resemble those of the other agents in this group. Ritodrine is the only β_2-adrenergic agonist that is currently approved in the United States for use to delay or prevent premature parturition; other drugs, such as terbutaline and fenoterol, have been used extensively for this purpose in Europe and elsewhere (*see* Caritis, 1983).

Ritodrine is rapidly but incompletely (30%) absorbed following oral administration, and 90% of the drug is excreted in the urine as inactive conjugates; about 50% of ritodrine is excreted unchanged after intravenous administration. The pharmacokinetic properties of ritodrine are complex and incompletely defined (*see* Caritis, 1983).

Therapeutic Uses. Ritodrine is administered intravenously to selected patients in order to arrest premature labor; if successful, oral therapy is then instituted. The preparations, dosage, indications, and contraindications for the use of ritodrine are presented in Chapter 39.

OTHER SELECTIVE β AGONISTS

Isoetharine is available for the treatment of bronchospastic disease as a solution for nebulization (BRONKOSOL) or in a metered-dose, pressurized inhaler as the mesylate (BRONKOMETER). It is purported to produce fewer cardiac side effects than does either epinephrine or isoproterenol, but isoetharine appears to be less selective for β_2-adrenergic receptors than is albuterol or metaproterenol.

Prenalterol is a selective β_1-adrenergic agonist that is under investigation for use as a cardiac stimulant in the management of chronic congestive heart failure. Intravenous or oral administration of prenalterol is associated with small increases in heart rate and mean arterial pressure and a positive inotropic effect; total peripheral resistance is not significantly altered (Jennings *et al.*, 1983). Muscle tremors are not apparent during the administration of prenalterol, in keeping with the notion that it is selective for β_1 receptors. Its therapeutic value in the treatment of heart failure remains to be established.

MISCELLANEOUS SYMPATHO-MIMETIC DRUGS

Several sympathomimetic drugs are used primarily as vasoconstrictors for local application to the nasal mucous membrane or the eye. Their structures are depicted in Tables 8–1 and 8–2. Their nonproprietary and trade names as well as representative preparations are as follows: *propylhexedrine* (BENZEDREX), nasal inhaler (250 mg); *naphazoline hydrochloride* (PRIVINE), 0.05% nasal spray or solution and 0.012 to 0.1% ophthalmic solution; *tetrahydrozoline hydrochloride*, 0.05 and 0.1% nasal solutions (TYZINE) and 0.05% ophthalmic solution (VISINE, others); *oxymetazoline hydrochloride* (AFRIN, others), 0.025 and 0.05% nasal solution (spray or drops); *xylometazoline hydrochloride* (OTRIVIN, others), 0.05 and 0.1% nasal solutions (spray or drops).

Phenylephrine (*see* above), pseudoephedrine (a stereoisomer of ephedrine), and phenylpropanolamine are the sympathomimetic drugs most commonly used in oral preparations for the relief of nasal congestion. *Pseudoephedrine hydrochloride* (SUDAFED, others) is available in 30- and 60-mg tablets, 120-mg timed-release capsules, and a liquid (6 mg/ml). The usual dose is 60 mg every 6 hours (or one timed-release capsule every 12 hours) for adults, 15 mg for children aged 2 to 5 years, and 30 mg for children aged 6 to 12 years. The dosing interval in all cases is not less than 6 hours. *Phenylpropanolamine hydrochloride* (PROPAGEST, others) shares the pharmacological properties of ephedrine and is approximately equal in potency except that it causes less CNS stimulation. The drug is available in 25- and 50-mg tablets, 75-mg timed-release capsules, and a syrup (12.5 mg/5 ml). Numerous proprietary mixtures marketed for the oral treatment of nasal and sinus congestion contain one of these sympathomimetic amines, usually in combination with an H_1-antihistaminic drug.

THERAPEUTIC USES OF SYM-PATHOMIMETIC DRUGS

The success that has attended efforts to develop therapeutic agents that can influence adrenergic receptors selectively and the variety of vital functions that are regulated by the sympathetic nervous system have resulted in a class of drugs that have a large number of important therapeutic uses.

Use of Vascular Effects. *Control of Hemorrhage.* The vasoconstrictor action of epinephrine may control superficial hemorrhage from skin and mucous membranes when the drug is applied topically as a spray or on cotton or gauze pledgets. It is effective only against bleeding from arterioles and capillaries and does not control venous oozing or hemorrhage from larger vessels.

Decongestion of Mucous Membranes. Sympathomimetic amines with α-receptor action cause marked vasoconstriction and blanching when applied to nasal and pharyngeal mucosal surfaces. They are therefore useful in the treatment of mucosal congestion accompanying *hay fever, allergic rhinitis, acute coryza, sinusitis,* and other respiratory conditions. Some of the sympathomimetic amines more widely used topically for nasal decongestion are indicated as *N* in Table 8–1. All have the disadvantage that their use may be followed by "aftercongestion" and that prolonged use often results in chronic rhinitis. Some (*e.g.,* naphazoline) also irritate the nasal mucosa, causing a brief but sharp stinging sensation when first applied. Sufficient absorption of any of the imidazoline derivatives (Table 8–2) may cause CNS depression, leading to coma and marked reduction in body temperature, especially in infants. These drugs should not be used in young children.

Epinephrine is used in many surgical procedures on the nose, throat, and larynx, to shrink the mucosa and improve visualization by limiting hemorrhage. Since epinephrine is relatively nonirritating, it is especially suitable for use in treatment of congestion of the conjunctiva.

The efficacy of locally applied sympathomimetic vasoconstrictors in shrinking the nasal mucosa has led to the use of amines that may have this effect when given orally. Since the vessels of the nasal mucosa have not been shown to be more sensitive than most other vessels to sympathomimetic drugs, doses of orally administered sympathomimetics large enough to afford relief from nasal congestion will be expected to constrict other vascular beds. Phenylephrine, phenylpropanolamine, and pseudoephedrine have been given orally as nasal decongestants; their effects on nasal congestion due to colds are not of much consequence, but *allergic rhinitis* often responds well. Several oral preparations promoted for the relief of colds and other upper respiratory conditions contain a sympathomimetic amine in combination with a variety of other agents (*e.g.,* antihistamines, antimuscarinic drugs, antipyretic-analgesics, caffeine, antitussives). There is no convincing evidence that such concoctions provide other than the symptomatic relief that is likely due to the presence of the aspirin-like drug.

Use with Local Anesthetics. Epinephrine is widely used to retard the absorption of local anesthetics. Other sympathomimetic amines are of value in preventing the fall in blood pressure that may accompany spinal anesthesia (*see* Chapter 15).

Hypotension. Sympathomimetic amines with predominant α-receptor activity can be used to relieve hypotension in various conditions, such as that associated with spinal anesthesia or due to overdosage of an antihypertensive agent. However, hypotension *per se* is not a sufficient reason to use pressor agents. There should be evidence that the hypotension is the cause of inadequate perfusion of vital organs before treatment with such drugs is initiated, and other maneuvers may be safer and more effective. For example, hypotension during spinal anesthesia may be managed by attention to fluid volumes and tilting of the patient. Sympathomimetic amines must be used very cautiously in patients under general anesthesia, since halogenated hydrocarbons sensitize the heart to the arrhythmic action of catecholamines and related drugs.

Administration of sympathomimetic agents for their pressor effect may be a useful *emergency measure* until other therapy can be instituted in certain hypotensive states (*e.g.,* in acute hemorrhage). Sympathomimetics may be used to raise the blood pressure and sustain the coronary and cerebral circulation until measures can be taken to restore an adequate circulating blood volume. However, this therapy must be regarded as only a temporary expedient that can obscure the extent of blood-volume replacement required and can in itself cause loss of fluid from the vascular compartment. Vasopressor therapy can thus increase the risk of further circulatory deterioration.

The release of large amounts of catecholamines during operation on patients with *pheochromocytoma* can lead to a considerable decrease in the circulating blood volume, and the blood pressure may drop precipitously as soon as the tumor has been removed. Infusion of norepinephrine has been used to sustain the blood pressure postoperatively, but adequate fluid-volume replacement appears to be more rational therapy. Alternatively, the loss of circulating volume can be largely prevented and the postoperative fall in pressure much reduced or

eliminated by inhibiting the vasoconstriction due to released catecholamines with an α-adrenergic blocking agent, both prior to and during surgery (*see* Chapter 9).

The blood pressure of patients with *orthostatic hypotension* due to various factors, including neurological diseases such as syringomyelia and tabes dorsalis, may be supported by treatment orally with ephedrine or other long-acting pressor sympathomimetic agents. However, responses are highly variable and control of the blood pressure in these conditions remains a very difficult problem.

Shock. Shock is a clinical state in which there is inadequate perfusion of tissues. The management of shock and the prognosis are determined by the pathogenesis of the syndrome. For example, hypovolemic shock due to the loss of fluid from either the vascular or extravascular compartment is treated by replacement of blood, plasma, or water and electrolytes, as appropriate. Adequate delivery of oxygen and the restoration of circulating blood volume, in addition to correction of the factors that resulted in hypovolemia, are generally sufficient to treat hypovolemic shock. Although these maneuvers are not likely to be adequate for other forms of shock, they are no less important in the treatment of the syndrome no matter what the cause.

Cardiogenic shock as a consequence of myocardial infarction is a vexing problem; there is no standard, accepted treatment, and the prognosis is poor no matter what the therapy. Replacement of fluid to restore circulatory volume is essential, but judicious administration is mandatory and the consequences must be monitored by measurement of either central venous pressure or pulmonary arterial pressure. Blood pressure must be adequate to restore perfusion of vital organs, including the heart, but the pressure should not be so high as to place undue demands for oxygen on an already severely compromised myocardium; the output of urine must be assessed as an index of renal perfusion, especially if α-adrenergic agonists are employed to restore blood pressure. Dopamine appears to be particularly appropriate for this purpose, because of its ability to produce vasoconstriction while maintaining flow through the renal and mesenteric vascular beds. Dobutamine has been recommended because of its positive inotropic effects that are accompanied by modest peripheral vasoconstriction. Isoproterenol has also been employed. Prenalterol may also prove to be useful in the management of cardiogenic shock, but this has yet to be demonstrated. Improvement of cardiac performance and cardiac output can lead to a rise in blood pressure and improved perfusion of tissues. Unfortunately there are no convincing data that support the use of one drug in preference to another in this condition.

Under exceptional circumstances peripheral vasoconstrictors may be required to maintain an adequate blood pressure. Infusions of norepinephrine, metaraminol, and mephentermine, as well as epinephrine, have been employed for this purpose. As was discussed above, care must be taken to avoid an excessive increase in blood pressure, since the advantages of improving coronary perfusion may be more than offset by the increased demands placed on the myocardium; circulation to the kidneys and other vital organs may also be compromised. It is well to remember that, except in neurogenic shock and shock associated with spinal anesthesia, reflex vasoconstriction mediated by the sympathetic nervous system is probably already intense, and vasoconstrictors may only further compromise blood flow.

Because of the intense vasoconstriction associated with most forms of shock, several investigators have recommended the use of either α-adrenergic antagonists or vasodilators in the management of this condition. Such agents are likely to improve blood flow to tissues if a minimally effective blood pressure can be maintained. In addition, the reduction of afterload and preload on the heart reduces cardiac work and the myocardial requirement for oxygen at any given cardiac output. Rapidly acting vasodilator agents such as sodium nitroprusside appear to be superior to α-blocking agents in this circumstance, in part because of the ease of moment-to-moment control of the action of the drug (*see* Chapters 32 and 33).

The hemodynamic abnormalities of septic shock are treated in a manner similar to that for cardiogenic shock, at least insofar as one can apply the same principles of adequate oxygenation, tissue perfusion, and circulating volume, as well as maintenance of a respectable, but not excessive, blood pressure and correction of electrolyte or acid-base imbalance. Administration of appropriate antibiotics is of course indicated. Claims have also been made for the value of administration of large doses of adrenocorticosteroids and other agents that may reduce the elaboration of the vasoactive substances that are mediators of this syndrome. There is no convincing evidence of the efficacy of such treatment.

Use of Reflex Cardiac Effects of Pressor Drugs. Attacks of *paroxysmal atrial* or *nodal tachycardia* may be ended by reflex vagal discharge caused by pressor responses to phenylephrine or methoxamine, drugs without significant cardiac excitatory action. The dose, given slowly intravenously, should not raise the blood pressure above 160 mm Hg; for phenylephrine, the dose may be 0.15 to 0.8 mg; for methoxamine, 3 to 5 mg. A short-acting anticholinesterase agent such as edrophonium may be safer for this purpose (*see* Chapter 6).

Use of Cardiac Effects. *Cardiac Arrest and Heart Block with Syncopal Seizures.* Syncope in *Stokes-Adams syndrome,* generally occurring at the transition from partial to complete A-V block, may be due to ventricular standstill or to prefibrillatory rhythm leading to ventricular fibrillation. Epinephrine and isoproterenol are of value in prophylaxis and symptomatic treatment of the attacks, but physical measures should be applied first in the acute attack. Circulation may sometimes be restored by a precordial blow followed by external cardiac compression or, if readily at hand, by an electrical pacemaker or defibrillator. Next, cardiac puncture with or without intracardiac injection of epinephrine may be effective and, as a last resort,

thoracotomy and manual cardiac massage may rarely be required. To restore the intrinsic cardiac rhythm once some circulation has been established, intravenous infusion of epinephrine or isoproterenol may be necessary. These catecholamines are likely to precipitate ventricular fibrillation if injudiciously used in patients with prefibrillatory rhythm, and, therefore, extreme care should be taken in their *intravenous* administration. When the indications are less urgent, repeated subcutaneous injections of epinephrine or intramuscular injections of epinephrine in oil may give the desired results. Epinephrine has been used to maintain an adequate ventricular rate (30 to 40 beats or more per minute) for as long as a week, but other sympathomimetic amines are more suitable for prolonged and prophylactic treatment. Ephedrine is both orally effective and longer acting. *However, drug therapy is a temporary measure only to be used until an electrical pacemaker can be fitted to supply optimal and reliable ventricular regulation.*

The problem of reviving patients apparently dead from *drowning, electrocution,* or *anesthetic accidents* is not substantially different from that of the syncope in Stokes-Adams syndrome, and the same principles apply. In all cases of cardiac arrest, adequate artificial ventilation is crucial. Anesthetic cardiac accidents may be due either to asystole or to ventricular fibrillation. Since the heart is sensitized to the arrhythmic action of epinephrine by many anesthetics, the drug may convert asystole to ventricular fibrillation. Physical measures, especially the use of an electrical pacemaker, are obviously more appropriate. Electrical countershock is indicated in ventricular fibrillation. Although the use of epinephrine in anesthetic accidents is theoretically inadvisable in cardiac arrest or after defibrillation, many patients have recovered when the drug has been administered. It is impossible to decide whether recovery is due to the drug, to mechanical stimulation of the myocardium by the needle prick, or to other procedures simultaneously applied. In patients who do not respond to other measures, it is not unreasonable to resort to the cardiac excitatory action of epinephrine. (*See* Bellet, 1960; Zoll and Linenthal, 1963.)

Uses in Allergic Disorders. *Bronchial Asthma.* Epinephrine, isoproterenol, and the newer selective β_2-receptor stimulants are the mainstay of the symptomatic treatment of respiratory distress due to bronchospasm. Relief is due to the β_2-receptor action that relaxes smooth muscle; with epinephrine, a contributory factor may be an α-receptor action that constricts bronchial mucosal vessels, thereby reducing congestion and edema. Acute asthmatic attacks are usually relieved within 3 to 5 minutes after subcutaneous injection of 0.2 to 0.5 mg of epinephrine or after oral inhalation of a 1% solution of epinephrine, a 0.5 to 1% solution of isoproterenol, or 0.65 mg of metaproterenol from a metered-dose inhaler. The decrease in vital capacity and the increase in residual air characteristic of these attacks are rapidly corrected, and maximal breathing capacity and velocity of expiration increase.

Whatever the drug or route of administration, the smallest dose affording relief should be used. Inhalations of isoproterenol or epinephrine may have to be repeated at intervals of 2 or 3 minutes, and subcutaneous injections of epinephrine at 15- to 20-minute intervals until relief of acute attacks is obtained. If symptoms recur, massage of the site of injection may give relief by enhancing absorption of the drug. With the longer-acting β_2-receptor stimulants such as albuterol, 1 or 2 inhalations are often sufficient and repetition is unnecessary for 4 hours.

Complete refractoriness to epinephrine and isoproterenol is not uncommon after protracted therapy in severe cases and in status asthmaticus, especially when bronchospasm is associated with the presence of viscid mucus plugs in the bronchi. Epinephrine reduces bronchial secretion and may make these plugs more viscid and difficult to dislodge. Measures to facilitate removal of mucus plugs are important in these cases and include expectorants and increased hydration of the patient to liquefy the plugs, and mechanical removal of retained secretion by bronchoscopic suction. Suitable chemotherapy is used to combat respiratory infection when this common precipitating cause is present.

In cases of *refractory asthma,* intravenous administration of aminophylline is sometimes useful, but administration of adrenocorticosteroids is often required to interrupt the severe asthmatic cycle. Because of the serious side effects of prolonged use of such steroids (*see* Chapter 63), their administration should be discontinued as early as practicable; fortunately, such discontinuation is possible in most cases. Susceptibility to small doses of epinephrine and other sympathomimetic amines is usually restored once repeated and progressive bronchial relaxation has been achieved. For prolonged relief from bronchospasm, usually in chronic asthma, metaproterenol (20 mg) or terbutaline (5 mg), administered orally every 6 hours, is useful. Ephedrine (20 to 50 mg), given at 4-hour intervals, is also an effective prophylactic. The use of methylxanthines such as aminophylline in asthma is discussed in Chapter 25.

Miscellaneous Allergic Disorders. Epinephrine is the drug of choice to relieve the symptoms of acute hypersensitivity reactions to drugs (*e.g.,* penicillin) and of other acute allergic reactions. A subcutaneous injection of epinephrine rapidly relieves itching, urticaria, and swelling of lips, eyelids, and tongue, and the drug may be lifesaving when edema of the glottis threatens suffocation. Only epinephrine is administered to relieve these acute reactions since it acts particularly rapidly; however, ephedrine, having a more prolonged action, can be used for the continued treatment of allergic disorders, such as hay fever. When skin tests are performed for hypersensitivity to various foods, drugs, pollens, or other allergens, epinephrine should always be at hand to control acute untoward reactions. If chronic medication with ephedrine is being used for allergic conditions, the drug should not be given for at least 12 hours before sensitivity tests are made; otherwise, positive reactions may be prevented. When conjunctival tests for serum or drug hypersensitivity are made, epinephrine solution instilled into the eye readily controls the local discomfort of positive reactions.

Ophthalmic Uses. Local application of various sympathomimetic amines to the conjunctiva is used to dilate the pupil, mainly to permit adequate examination of the fundus. The mydriatic effect of these drugs, notably ephedrine (0.1%), hydroxyamphetamine (1%), and phenylephrine (1 to 2.5%), lasts for only a few hours. The sympathomimetics have the additional advantage that they do not cause cycloplegia and usually do not increase intraocular pressure. Sympathomimetic mydriatics are also used to reduce the incidence of posterior synechiae in uveitis, and epinephrine (0.25 to 2%) or phenylephrine (2.5 to 10%) is used to treat wide-angle glaucoma, reducing the intraocular pressure by their local vasoconstrictor action, which decreases production of aqueous humor.

Use of Central Effects. Apart from a series of drugs used only as anorectics (*see* below), the main sympathomimetics used for central effects are ephedrine, amphetamine, dextroamphetamine, methamphetamine, and mephentermine. Of these, dextroamphetamine and methamphetamine are most widely employed. The peripheral actions of ephedrine, mephentermine, and, to a lesser extent, amphetamine are disproportionately great, and central effects cannot be obtained without side effects from the peripheral actions.

Narcolepsy. Ephedrine, amphetamine, methamphetamine, and dextroamphetamine have been used to treat narcoleptic patients. The amphetamines largely prevent attacks of sleep in nearly all patients, and cataplexy is often much improved. The usual dose of dextroamphetamine varies from 5 to 60 mg daily, in divided portions, the last dose being taken not later than 4 P.M. so that the nocturnal sleep is not prevented. Tolerance does not appear to develop to these agents in the treatment of narcolepsy.

Parkinsonism. Dextroamphetamine partially alleviates various symptoms of parkinsonism, but it has been superseded by levodopa and other antiparkinsonism drugs. If levodopa cannot be tolerated, dextroamphetamine can be given as an adjuvant to the other drugs. It has little effect on tremor, but decreases rigidity in many patients and frequently relieves oculogyric crises. The drug brings about a better sleep cycle, a subjective improvement in muscle strength and rigidity, and elevates the mood, a most important objective in the treatment of the patients. The total daily dose varies from 10 to 50 mg or more. In certain other diseases of the extrapyramidal system, such as *spasmodic torticollis* and spasmodic movements of a limb, dextroamphetamine may relieve symptoms.

Obesity and Weight Reduction. Whatever the etiology of obesity, a factor common to all cases is necessarily an intake of amounts of food that supply more energy than the body uses. Of the two possible measures to correct this imbalance, attempts to reduce food intake have been more popular in Western civilization. Persistent dietary restraint has proven both essential and difficult to achieve, and various sympathomimetic and related drugs that depress appetite have been used to make a low-calorie diet more tolerable. These appetite depressants are of no value without an accompanying stringent dietary regimen, and it has been regularly demonstrated that, without consistent supervision, no prescribed regimen of drug or diet is predictably successful. Several factors have a part in determining this unsatisfactory situation. In many patients the etiology of obesity is psychological, and compulsive overeating is difficult to eradicate even with psychiatric help. The central-stimulant and appetite-suppressant effects of most of these drugs have proven inseparable. This compromises their use in the latter part of the day; given after 4 P.M., they interfere with sleep at night. Since much of the overeating takes place in the evening, their value is obviously limited. In addition, tolerance develops within a few weeks and increased dosage is limited both by the peripheral actions that these drugs exert and by such symptoms of central stimulation as nervousness and irritability. Even during the early period of administration, peripheral effects, although seldom pronounced, are rarely completely absent.

None of the drugs used in obesity has proven superior to dextroamphetamine or methamphetamine, either in effectiveness or in lack of peripheral side effects. However, certain other agents have not so far presented a significant problem of drug abuse and, therefore, are preferable. *Phenylpropanolamine* (*see* above) is available in a wide variety of "over-the-counter" anorexiants in tablets or capsules or in combination with other drugs, such as caffeine or various mixtures of vitamins. The daily dosage should not exceed 75 mg. A number of authorities suggest that the daily dosage should be no more than 50 mg in order to avoid alarming elevations in blood pressure and other side effects; continuation of this agent as an "over-the-counter" drug is a matter of controversy.

Among those agents appearing in schedule IV of the Controlled Substances Act are *fenfluramine, diethylpropion, mazindol,* and *phentermine*. *Fenfluramine hydrochloride* (PONDIMIN), in contrast to other phenylethylamines, is a CNS depressant and causes drowsiness. It is therefore the preferred drug in individuals who are anxious and in whom CNS stimulant effects should be avoided. It should not be administered in conjunction with other CNS depressants and should not be used in individuals with a history of depression. Although sympathomimetic effects are not observed in usual doses, such effects can be elicited when excessive doses are administered. Fenfluramine is available in 20-mg tablets, and the usual dosage is 20 to 40 mg three times a day. *Diethylpropion hydrochloride* (TENUATE, others) possesses pharmacological properties similar to those of amphetamine, although CNS side effects appear to be less severe and cardiovascular effects are minimal. Diethylpropion is therefore regarded as the preferred anorexiant in individuals with hypertension or cardiovascular disease. It is available in 25-mg tablets and 75-mg sustained-release tablets. The usual dose is 25 mg three times a day or one sustained-release tablet daily. *Mazindol* (MAZANOR,

SANOREX), an imidazoline derivative, appears to resemble the tricyclic antidepressants in that it is able to block the neuronal uptake of norepinephrine and dopamine; the effects of catecholamines can thus be potentiated by this agent. Mazindol is a weaker CNS stimulant than amphetamine and related drugs, but modest cardiovascular stimulation is associated with the use of this agent. Mazindol is available in 1- and 2-mg tablets; the usual adult dose is 1 or 2 mg once daily or 1 mg given three times daily with meals. *Phentermine hydrochloride* (PHENTROL, others) is available in tablets and capsules that contain from 8 to 37.5 mg of the drug. The usual adult dose is 8 mg three times daily or 15 to 37.5 mg taken once daily.

Included in schedule III of the Controlled Substances Act are *benzphetamine* and *phendimetrazine*. *Benzphetamine hydrochloride* (DIDREX) suppresses appetite in doses that produce fewer cardiovascular and CNS effects than does amphetamine. It is available in 25- and 50-mg tablets; the usual adult dose is 25 to 50 mg, given one to three times daily. *Phendimetrazine tartrate* (ANOREX, others) is available in tablets or capsules containing 35 mg of the drug and in 105-mg sustained-release capsules. The dosage is 35 mg, taken two to three times daily (or one sustained-release capsule, taken once daily).

Phenmetrazine hydrochloride (PRELUDIN) is included in schedule II of the Controlled Substances Act, along with dextroamphetamine and methamphetamine. Phenmetrazine is available in 25-mg tablets and in sustained-release tablets containing 50 or 75 mg of the drug.

Attention-Deficit Disorder (Hyperkinetic Syndrome). The amphetamines have a dramatic effect in calming a high proportion of abnormally hyperactive children. Restlessness, distractibility, and impulsive behavior are reduced; attention span is lengthened; and behavior becomes more tolerable to parents and teachers. Concomitant psychotherapy and parent counseling are necessary. Long-term drug therapy is essential; withdrawal leads to deterioration of performance. However, since the demands of school aggravate the condition, the drug can often be stopped during vacations. The usual dose of dextroamphetamine is 5 to 10 mg three times daily. Tolerance to this effect does not appear to develop. Side effects include insomnia, headache, irritability, depression, periods of excessive crying, and gastrointestinal cramps, but these do not often require discontinuation of the drug. Continued use of dextroamphetamine depresses growth in these children by reducing appetite; a rebound weight gain occurs when the drug is stopped. Methylphenidate, which is equally effective, may cause less inhibition of growth. There is evidence that the long-term use of these stimulant drugs does not lead to subsequent abuse of the drug. It is alarming that the number of so-called hyperkinetic children is estimated at 5%. A careful assessment of the condition must be made before therapy is begun. (*See* Sroufe and Stewart, 1973; Chapters 19 and 24.)

The mechanism of action of amphetamine in children with this syndrome is probably related to the effect of the drug on CNS neurotransmitters (*see*

Weiner, 1972; Snyder, 1973). It is not difficult to correlate the alerting and attention-span effects of the drug with its central actions, but the calming effect seems paradoxical.

Miscellaneous Uses. Ephedrine and amphetamine have been reported to prevent *syncopal reactions* of the vagal or vasodepressor type due to abnormal sensitivity of the carotid sinuses. Ephedrine, amphetamine, and other sympathomimetics have been used with variable success to treat *urinary incontinence* and *nocturnal enuresis*. The benefit may be due partly to central effects of the drugs and partly to contraction of the vesical sphincter. The use of ritodrine and other selective β_2 agonists to delay delivery in *premature labor* is discussed in Chapter 39.

Ahlquist, R. P. A study of adrenotropic receptors. *Am. J. Physiol.*, **1948**, *153*, 586–600.

Ahrens, R. C., and Smith, G. D. Albuterol: an adrenergic agent for use in the treatment of asthma. Pharmacology, pharmacokinetics and clinical use. *Pharmacotherapy*, **1984**, *4*, 105–120.

Anderson, R.; Holmberg, S.; Svedmyr, N.; and Åberg, G. Adrenergic α- and β-receptors in coronary vessels in man: an *in vitro* study. *Acta Med. Scand.*, **1972**, *191*, 241–244.

Barger, G., and Dale, H. H. Chemical structure and sympathomimetic action of amines. *J. Physiol. (Lond.)*, **1910**, *41*, 19–59.

Benfey, B. G., and Varma, D. R. Interactions of sympathomimetic drugs, propranolol and phentolamine, on atrial refractory period and contractility. *Br. J. Pharmacol. Chemother.*, **1967**, *30*, 603–611.

Bertler, A.; Carlsson, A.; and Rosengren, E. Release by reserpine of catecholamines from rabbit hearts. *Naturwissenschaften*, **1956**, *43*, 521.

Blundell, J. E., and Leshem, M. B. Dissociation of the anorexic effects of fenfluramine and amphetamine following intrahypothalamic injection. *Br. J. Pharmacol.*, **1973**, *47*, 183–185.

Brown, G. L., and Gillespie, J. S. The output of sympathetic transmitter from the spleen of the cat. *J. Physiol. (Lond.)*, **1957**, *138*, 81–102.

Burn, J. H., and Rand, M. J. The action of sympathomimetic amines in animals treated with reserpine. *J. Physiol. (Lond.)*, **1958**, *144*, 314–336.

Caldwell, R. W., and Goldberg, L. I. An evaluation of the vasodilation produced by mephentermine and certain other sympathomimetic amines. *J. Pharmacol. Exp. Ther.*, **1970**, *172*, 297–309.

Cubeddu, L. X., and Weiner, N. Release of norepinephrine and dopamine-β-hydroxylase by nerve stimulation. III. Effects of norepinephrine depletion on the alpha presynaptic regulation of release. *J. Pharmacol. Exp. Ther.*, **1975**, *192*, 1–14.

DePotter, W. P.; Chubb, I. W.; Put, A.; and De Schaepdryver, A. F. Facilitation of the release of noradrenaline and dopamine-β-hydroxylase at low stimulation frequencies by α-blocking agents. *Arch. Int. Pharmacodyn. Ther.*, **1971**, *193*, 191–197.

Dixon, W. R.; Mosimann, W. F.; and Weiner, N. The role of presynaptic feedback mechanisms in regulation of norepinephrine release by nerve stimulation. *J. Pharmacol. Exp. Ther.*, **1979**, *209*, 196–204.

Enero, M. A.; Langer, S. Z.; Rothlin, R. P.; and Stefano, F. J. E. Role of the alpha-adrenergic receptor in regulating noradrenaline overflow by nerve stimulation. *Br. J. Pharmacol.*, **1972**, *44*, 672–688.

Forwell, G. D., and Ingram, G. I. C. The effect of adren-

aline infusion on human blood coagulation. *J. Physiol. (Lond.)*, **1957**, *135*, 371–383.

Goldberg, L. I. Dopamine—clinical uses of an endogenous catecholamine. *N. Engl. J. Med.*, **1974**, *291*, 707–710.

Goldenberg, M.; Aranow, H., Jr.; Smith, A. A.; and Faber, M. Pheochromocytoma and essential hypertensive vascular disease. *Arch. Intern. Med.*, **1950**, *86*, 823–836.

Goldstein, R. A.; Passamani, E. R.; and Roberts, R. A comparison of digoxin and dobutamine in patients with acute infarction and cardiac failure. *N. Engl. J. Med.*, **1980**, *303*, 846–850.

Haggendahl, J. Some further aspects on the release of the adrenergic transmitter. In, *Bayer Symposium II. New Aspects of Storage and Release Mechanisms of Catecholamines.* (Schumann, H. J., and Kroneberg, G., eds.) Springer-Verlag, Berlin, **1970**, pp. 100–109.

Harden, T. K. Agonist-induced desensitization of the β-adrenergic receptor-linked adenylate cyclase. *Pharmacol. Rev.*, **1983**, *35*, 5–32.

Hartung, W. H. Epinephrine and related compounds: influence of structure on physiologic activity. *Chem. Rev.*, **1931**, *9*, 389–465.

Houben, H.; Thien, T.; and van 't Laar, A. Effect of low-dose epinephrine infusion on hemodynamics after selective and nonselective beta-blockade in hypertension. *Clin. Pharmacol. Ther.*, **1982**, *31*, 685–690.

James, T. N.; Bear, E. S.; Lang, K. F.; and Green, E. W. Evidence for adrenergic alpha receptor depressant activity in the heart. *Am. J. Physiol.*, **1968**, *215*, 1366–1375.

Jennings, G.; Bobik, A.; Oddie, C.; Hargreaves, M.; and Korner, P. Cardioselectivity of prenalterol and isoproterenol. *Clin. Pharmacol. Ther.*, **1983**, *34*, 749–757.

Lands, A. M.; Arnold, A.; McAuliff, J. P.; Luduena, F. P.; and Brown, T. G., Jr. Differentiation of receptor systems activated by sympathomimetic amines. *Nature*, **1967a**, *214*, 597–598.

Lands, A. M.; Luduena, F. P.; and Buzzo, H. J. Differentiation of receptors responsive to isoproterenol. *Life Sci.*, **1967b**, *6*, 2241–2249.

Lockett, M. Dangerous effects of isoprenaline in myocardial failure. *Lancet*, **1965**, *2*, 104–106.

Minneman, K. P.; Hegstrand, L. R.; and Molinoff, P. B. Simultaneous determination of beta-1 and beta-2 adrenergic receptors in tissues containing both receptor subtypes. *Mol. Pharmacol.*, **1979**, *15*, 286–298.

Musacchio, J. M.; Kopin, I. J.; and Weise, V. K. Subcellular distribution of some sympathomimetic amines and their β-hydroxylated derivatives in the rat heart. *J. Pharmacol. Exp. Ther.*, **1965**, *148*, 22–28.

Oliver, G., and Schäfer, E. A. The physiological effects of extracts from the suprarenal capsules. *J. Physiol. (Lond.)*, **1895**, *18*, 230–276.

Schumann, H. J.; Wagner, J.; Knorr, A.; Reidemeister, J. C.; Sadony, V.; and Schramm, G. Demonstration in human atrial preparations of alpha-adrenoceptors mediating positive inotropic effects. *Naunyn Schmiedebergs Arch. Pharmacol.*, **1978**, *302*, 333–336.

Singer, D. H.; Lazzara, R.; and Hoffman, B. F. Interrelationships between automaticity and conduction in Purkinje fibers. *Circ. Res.*, **1967**, *21*, 537–558.

Smith, C. B. The role of monoaminoxidase in the intraneuronal metabolism of norepinephrine released by indirectly-acting sympathomimetic amines or by adrenergic nerve stimulation. *J. Pharmacol. Exp. Ther.*, **1966**, *151*, 207–220.

Smythe, C. McC.; Nickel, J. F.; and Bradley, S. E. The effect of epinephrine (USP), *l*-epinephrine and *l*-norepinephrine on glomerular filtration rate, renal plasma flow and the urinary excretion of sodium, potassium and water in normal man. *J. Clin. Invest.*, **1952**, *31*, 499–506.

Snider, R. M., and Gerald, M. C. Studies on the mechanism of (+)-amphetamine enhancement of neuromuscular transmission: muscle contraction, electrophysiological and biochemical results. *J. Pharmacol. Exp. Ther.*, **1982**, *221*, 14–21.

Snyder, S. H. How amphetamine acts in minimal brain dysfunction. *Ann. N.Y. Acad. Sci.*, **1973**, *205*, 310–320.

Sonnenblick, E. H.; Frishman, W. H.; and LeJemtel, T. H. Dobutamine: a new synthetic cardioactive sympathetic amine. *N. Engl. J. Med.*, **1979**, *300*, 17–22.

Starke, K. Influence of alpha receptor stimulants on noradrenaline release. *Naturwissenschaften*, **1971**, *58*, 420.

————. Alpha-sympathomimetic inhibition of adrenergic and cholinergic transmission in the rabbit heart. *Naunyn Schmiedebergs Arch. Pharmakol.*, **1972**, *274*, 18–45.

Stolley, P. D. Asthma mortality—why the United States was spared an epidemic of deaths due to asthma. *Am. Rev. Respir. Dis.*, **1972**, *105*, 883–890.

Tomita, T., and Watanabe, H. A comparison of the effects of adenosine triphosphate with noradrenaline and with the inhibitory potential of the guinea-pig taenia coli. *J. Physiol. (Lond.)*, **1973**, *231*, 167–177.

Trendelenburg, U.; Muskus, A.; Fleming, W. W.; and de la Sierra, B. G. A. Modification by reserpine of the action of sympathomimetic amines in spinal cats: a classification of sympathomimetic amines. *J. Pharmacol. Exp. Ther.*, **1962**, *138*, 170–180.

Tuttle, R. R.; Hillman, C. C.; and Toomey, R. E. Differential β adrenergic sensitivity of atrial and ventricular tissue assessed by chronotropic, inotropic, and cyclic AMP responses to isoprenaline and dobutamine. *Cardiovasc. Res.*, **1976**, *10*, 452–458.

Tuttle, R. R., and Mills, J. Dobutamine: development of a new catecholamine to selectively increase cardiac contractility. *Circ. Res.*, **1975**, *36*, 185–196.

Vliet, P. D. V.; Burchell, H. B.; and Titus, J. L. Focal myocarditis associated with pheochromocytoma. *N. Engl. J. Med.*, **1966**, *274*, 1102–1108.

Webb-Johnson, D. C., and Andrews, J. L. Bronchodilator therapy. *N. Engl. J. Med.*, **1977**, *297*, 476–482.

Wolfe, J. D.; Tashkin, D. P.; Calvarese, B.; and Simmons, M. Bronchodilator effects of terbutaline and aminophylline alone and in combination in asthmatic patients. *N. Engl. J. Med.*, **1978**, *298*, 363–367.

Yamaguchi, N.; DeChamplain, J.; and Nadeau, R. A. Regulation of norepinephrine release from cardiac sympathetic fibers in the dog by presynaptic alpha and beta receptors. *Circ. Res.*, **1977**, *41*, 108–117.

Monographs and Reviews

Allwood, M. J.; Cobbold, A. F.; and Ginsburg, J. Peripheral vascular effects of noradrenaline, isopropylnoradrenaline and dopamine. *Br. Med. Bull.*, **1963**, *19*, 132–136.

Angrist, B. M., and Gershon, S. Psychiatric sequelae of amphetamine use. In, *Psychiatric Complications of Medical Drugs.* (Shader, R. I., ed.) Raven Press, New York, **1972**, pp. 175–199.

Aviado, D. M., Jr. *Sympathomimetic Drugs.* Charles C Thomas, Publisher, Springfield, Ill., **1970**.

Bellet, S. Mechanism and treatment of A-V heart block and Adams-Stokes syndrome. *Prog. Cardiovasc. Dis.*, **1960**, *2*, 691–705.

Berne, R. M.; Winn, H. R.; Knabb, R. M.; Ely, S. W.; and Rubio, R. Blood flow regulation by adenosine in heart, brain, and skeletal muscle. In, *Regulatory Function of Adenosine.* (Berne, R. M.; Rall, T. W.; and Rubio, R.; eds.) Martinus Nijhoff, Boston, **1983**, pp. 293–317.

Bowman, W. C. Effects of adrenergic activators and inhibitors on the skeletal muscles. In, *Adrenergic Activators and Inhibitors.* (Szekeres, L., ed.) *Handbook of Experimental Pharmacology*, Vol. 54, Pt. II. Springer-Verlag, Berlin, **1981**, pp. 47–128.

Caritis, S. N. Treatment of preterm labour. A review of therapeutic options. *Drugs*, **1983**, *26*, 243–261.

Chen, K. K., and Schmidt, C. F. Ephedrine and related substances. *Medicine (Baltimore)*, **1930**, *9*, 1–117.

Dempsey, P. J., and Cooper, T. Pharmacology of the coronary circulation. *Annu. Rev. Pharmacol.*, **1972**, *12*, 99–110.

Ellis, S. Effects on the metabolism. In, *Adrenergic Activators and Inhibitors.* (Szekeres, L., ed.) *Handbook of Experimental Pharmacology*, Vol. 54, Pt. I. Springer-Verlag, Berlin, **1980**, pp. 319–349.

Goldberg, L. I. Cardiovascular and renal actions of dopamine: potential clinical applications. *Pharmacol. Rev.*, **1972**, *24*, 1–29.

Goldberg, L. I.; Hsieh, Y.-Y.; and Resnekov, L. Newer catecholamines for treatment of heart failure and shock; an update on dopamine and a first look at dobutamine. *Prog. Cardiovasc. Dis.*, **1977**, *19*, 327–340.

Grant, W. M. Action of drugs on movement of ocular fluids. *Annu. Rev. Pharmacol.*, **1969**, *9*, 85–94.

Greenway, C. V., and Stark, R. D. Hepatic vascular bed. *Physiol. Rev.*, **1971**, *51*, 23–65.

Himms-Hagen, J. Effects of catecholamines on metabolism. In, *Catecholamines.* (Blaschko, H., and Muscholl, E., eds.) *Handbuch der Experimentellen Pharmakologie*, Vol. 33. Springer-Verlag, Berlin, **1972**, pp. 363–462.

Kopin, I. J. False adrenergic transmitters. *Annu. Rev. Pharmacol.*, **1968**, *8*, 377–394.

Langer, S. Z. Presynaptic receptors and their role in the regulation of transmitter release. *Br. J. Pharmacol.*, **1977**, *60*, 481–497.

Lefkowitz, R. J.; Caron, M. G.; and Stiles, G. L. Mechanisms of membrane receptor regulation. Biochemical, physiological and clinical insights derived from studies of the adrenergic receptors. *N. Engl. J. Med.*, **1984**, *310*, 1570–1579.

Oswald, I. Drugs and sleep. *Pharmacol. Rev.*, **1968**, *20*, 273–303.

Sharman, D. F. The catabolism of catecholamines: recent studies. *Br. Med. Bull.*, **1973**, *29*, 110–115.

Sroufe, L. A., and Stewart, M. A. Treating problem children with stimulant drugs. *N. Engl. J. Med.*, **1973**, *289*, 407–413.

Starke, K. Regulation of noradrenaline release by presynaptic receptor systems. *Rev. Physiol. Biochem. Pharmacol.*, **1977**, *77*, 1–124.

Trendelenburg, U. Factors influencing the concentration of catecholamines at the receptors. In, *Catecholamines.* (Blaschko, H., and Muscholl, E., eds.) *Handbuch der Experimentellen Pharmakologie*, Vol. 33. Springer-Verlag, Berlin, **1972**, pp. 726–761.

Weiner, N. Regulation of norepinephrine synthesis. *Annu. Rev. Pharmacol.*, **1970**, *10*, 273–290.

————. Pharmacology of central nervous system stimulants. In, *Drug Abuse: Proceedings of the International Conference.* (Zarafonetis, C. J. D., ed.) Lea & Febiger, Philadelphia, **1972**, pp. 243–251.

————. The role of cyclic nucleotides in the regulation of neurotransmitter release from adrenergic neurons by neuromodulators. In, *Essays in Neurochemistry and Neuropharmacology*, Vol. 4. (Youdim, M. B. H.; Lovenberg, W.; Sharman, D. F.; and Lagnado, J. R.; eds.) John Wiley & Sons, Inc., New York, **1980**, pp. 69–124.

Weiss, B., and Laties, V. G. Enhancement of human performance by caffeine and the amphetamines. *Pharmacol. Rev.*, **1962**, *14*, 1–36.

Zaimis, E. Vasopressor drugs and catecholamines. *Anesthesiology*, **1968**, *29*, 732–762.

Zoll, P. M., and Linenthal, A. J. A program for Stokes-Adams disease and cardiac arrest. *Circulation*, **1963**, *27*, 1–4.

9 DRUGS THAT INHIBIT ADRENERGIC NERVES AND BLOCK ADRENERGIC RECEPTORS

Norman Weiner

Many substances of diverse structure and mechanism of action interfere with the function of the sympathetic nervous system. Several such drugs are extremely valuable in clinical medicine, particularly for the control of hypertension and cardiac disorders.

Certain drugs, termed *adrenergic neuron blocking agents,* interfere with the release of norepinephrine consequent to nerve stimulation. They may produce this effect by inhibition of the synthesis, storage, or release of the neurotransmitter. Irrespective of the precise mechanism, the consequence of these effects is a reduction in the amount of norepinephrine released by each nerve impulse. Such agents do not interfere significantly with the actions of circulating or exogenous catecholamines or other sympathomimetic amines that act directly on postsynaptic adrenergic receptors. Since the physiology and pharmacology of peripheral adrenergic neurons that innervate different organs are quite similar, drugs that interfere with adrenergic neuronal function affect all peripheral adrenergic neurons in a similar manner. A subgroup of this class of agents, of which clonidine and methyldopa are members, inhibits sympathetic nervous activity by reducing impulse traffic from sympathetic centers in the brain that modulate the activity of peripheral sympathetic neurons.

Other drugs, *adrenergic receptor blocking agents,* inhibit the ability of the neurotransmitter or other sympathomimetic amines to interact effectively with their receptors. Since the pharmacological sensitivities of adrenergic receptors vary considerably, these agents may interfere selectively with the different responses that are normally mediated by the sympathetic nervous system. For example, selective blockers of β_1-adrenergic receptors antagonize the actions of epinephrine and norepinephrine on the heart, have less effect on β_2-adrenergic receptors in bronchial smooth muscle, and do not block vasoconstrictor responses mediated by α receptors.

A knowledge of autonomic physiology and the sites of action of drugs that interfere with sympathetic function is essential for understanding the pharmacology and clinical uses of these important classes of drugs. The appropriate background is presented in Chapters 4 and 8.

Side Effects Common to Agents That Interfere with the Function of Sympathetic Neurons. The sympathetic nervous system is intimately involved in the modulation of a host of homeostatic mechanisms. Interference with its functions impairs the capacity of the organism to generate appropriate physiological responses that are required to react to adverse or provocative environmental inputs. As a consequence, a number of effects that are associated with the administration of such blocking agents are predictable. Since many of the side effects caused by these drugs are common to all agents that interfere with sympathetic function, they can be discussed collectively. Exceptions will be mentioned at this point and explained in more detail in the discussion of the individual drugs.

Postural Hypotension. Hypotension, and particularly postural hypotension, is a common effect of agents that interfere with sympathetic function. The sympathetic nervous system is critically involved in the regulation of blood pressure, particularly by modulation of vasomotor tone and cardiac rate and contractility. Venous tone is under the control of the sympathetic nervous system, and, if this regulation is impaired, blood pools in the capacitance vessels when the erect position is assumed.

Thus, postural hypotension is particularly troublesome in individuals with minimal sympathetic nervous system function. Postural hypotension is especially common with adrenergic neuron blocking agents such as guanethidine and methyldopa and with α-adrenergic blocking agents.

Sedation or Depression. Agents that interfere with adrenergic function in the central nervous system (CNS) frequently cause sedation or depression. Locomotor activity, alertness, and affect appear to be importantly regulated by central noradrenergic neurons (*see* Chapter 12). Agents that interfere with peripheral adrenergic function and that are sufficiently lipophilic to enter the CNS may therefore be expected to produce behavioral effects. Drugs of this type include reserpine, methyldopa, phenoxybenzamine, and clonidine. The effects of guanethidine on the CNS are minimal, since this very polar compound does not gain access to central adrenergic neurons to any significant degree.

Monoamine oxidase (MAO) inhibitors, which interfere with peripheral sympathetic nervous system function, enhance affect and stimulate psychomotor activity by a central mechanism; several factors appear to contribute. The rates of synthesis and release of catecholamines appear to be considerably greater in the CNS than in the periphery. It is likely that inhibition of the metabolism of catecholamines is more significant when their rate of turnover is more rapid. Furthermore, interference with peripheral adrenergic activity by MAO inhibitors is hypothesized to be due, in part, to the accumulation of false neurotransmitters derived from dietary amines such as tyramine (*see* Chapter 8); penetration of tyramine into the CNS is not nearly as rapid as it is into peripheral adrenergic neurons.

Increased Gastrointestinal Motility and Diarrhea. Sympathomimetic agents inhibit gastrointestinal function by two mechanisms. β-Adrenergic agonists cause relaxation of intestinal smooth muscle directly; α agonists may exert a direct relaxant effect on the smooth muscle and also act presynaptically to inhibit the release of neurotransmitter from cholinergic neurons in the intestinal wall (Chapter 8; Furness and Burnstock, 1975). Thus, it is to be expected that agents that interfere with sympathetic function would increase gastrointestinal motility and cause diarrhea. These side effects are seen particularly with drugs such as reserpine, methyldopa, and guanethidine.

Impaired Ability to Ejaculate. Contraction of the vas deferens and other accessory reproductive organs is mediated by the sympathetic nervous system, and agents that interfere with sympathetic function will thus inhibit ejaculation. This problem is most frequent when the more powerful adrenergic neuron blocking agents, such as guanethidine and methyldopa, are administered.

Increased Blood Volume and Sodium Retention. Hypotension can cause a reduction of renal blood flow. If the rate of glomerular filtration is reduced, more complete reabsorption of sodium and water can occur, and there will be an increase in the volume of blood and extracellular fluid. These effects tend to negate the reduction in blood pressure and may account for the tolerance to the hypotensive effect that may accompany the use of certain antihypertensive agents. Retention of sodium is particularly prominent with the more powerful hypotensive agents, such as guanethidine and methyldopa. This side effect accounts for one of the attributes of the concomitant use of a diuretic agent in the treatment of hypertension (*see* Chapters 32 and 36).

Nasal Stuffiness. This is an annoying side effect that is common to agents that block either adrenergic neurons or α receptors. It is due to vasodilatation in the mucous membranes of the nasopharynx.

Extrapyramidal Symptoms. Symptoms of akinesia, rigidity, and tremor, characteristic of Parkinson's disease, are commonly caused by agents that enter the CNS and interfere with sympathetic nervous function by a presynaptic mechanism. These alterations are presumably due to interference with the function of dopaminergic neurons. Reserpine and methyldopa commonly produce such side effects.

Side Effects Limited to α-Adrenergic Blocking Agents. Agents that interfere with sympathetic function by blockade of α receptors cause most of the side effects listed above, with the exception of extrapyramidal symptoms. In addition, reflex tachycardia is an important side effect of such drugs. Postural hypotension with reflex stimulation of the sympathetic nervous system results in tachycardia and increased myocardial contractility, effects mediated by β receptors and not blocked by α-adrenergic antagonists. In addition, many α blocking agents that act at postsynaptic (α_1) receptors also inhibit presynaptic (α_2) receptors; this results in enhanced output of norepinephrine per nerve impulse and presumably intensifies the effects of reflex sympathetic stimulation on the heart. Phentolamine and phenoxybenzamine produce this presynaptic effect, whereas prazosin is relatively ineffective in blocking presynaptic α_2 receptors. Prazosin is thus less likely to cause reflex tachycardia.

Side Effects Limited to β-Adrenergic Blocking Agents. The side effects common to β-adrenergic blocking agents are largely restricted to the cardiovascular and respiratory systems and to alterations of metabolism. Bradycardia and reduced cardiac output are important changes, particularly when the contractility of the myocardium is already impaired; congestive heart failure may be precipitated. Sensitivity to insulin and oral hypoglycemic drugs is also associated with the administration of β blockers, since glycogenolysis in muscle and, in some species, in liver is mediated by β receptors. Bronchoconstriction is a common side effect of β_2-blocking drugs and nonselective β-adrenergic antagonists, particularly in patients with pulmonary disease.

Epinephrine, which is secreted by the adrenal medulla, is an important physiological bronchodilator. The release of catecholamines from the adrenal medulla is not greatly affected by the usual doses of adrenergic neuron blocking agents. Thus, drugs that interfere with the function of the sympathetic nervous system by a presynaptic mechanism but do not affect secretion of epinephrine by the adrenal medulla do not interfere to any significant extent with the compensatory mechanisms that are evoked by bronchoconstriction or hypoglycemia.

I. α-Adrenergic Blocking Agents

α-Adrenergic blocking agents bind selectively to the α class of adrenergic receptors and thereby interfere with the capacity of sympathomimetic amines to initiate actions at these sites. Phenoxybenzamine (and its congener dibenamine) binds covalently to the α receptor and produces an irreversible and insurmountable type of blockade. Phentolamine, tolazoline, and prazosin bind reversibly and antagonize the actions of sympathomimetic amines competitively.

There are prominent differences in the relative abilities of α-adrenergic blocking agents to antagonize the effects of sympathomimetic amines at the two subtypes of α receptors. Prazosin is much more potent in blocking α_1 (postsynaptic) receptors than α_2 receptors that, among other effects, modulate neural release of transmitter (presumed presynaptic receptors). Phenoxybenzamine is a moderately selective α_1-blocking agent, while phentolamine is

only three to five times more potent in inhibiting α_1- than α_2-adrenergic receptors. In contrast, yohimbine is a selective α_2 blocker and has been shown to prevent the antihypertensive effects of clonidine, an α_2 agonist (Starke *et al.*, 1975; Langer, 1977).

PHENOXYBENZAMINE AND RELATED HALOALKYLAMINES

Phenoxybenzamine and *dibenamine* are haloalkylamines with a relatively specific capability to interact with and block α-adrenergic receptors; they have no α-adrenergic agonistic activity (Nickerson and Goodman, 1947). Phenoxybenzamine is the only member of this series of compounds that has been studied extensively in man.

Chemistry. The structural formula of phenoxybenzamine is as follows:

Phenoxybenzamine

Dibenamine is N,N-dibenzyl-β-chloroethylamine and differs from phenoxybenzamine only in the replacement of the phenoxyisopropyl moiety with a benzyl group.

The haloalkylamine adrenergic blocking agents are closely related chemically to the nitrogen mustards; like the latter, the tertiary amine cyclizes to form a reactive ethylenimonium intermediate (Chapter 55). The molecular configuration directly responsible for blockade is probably a highly reactive carbonium ion formed when the three-membered ring breaks. The relatively slow onset of action, even after intravenous administration, is probably due to the time required for the formation of these reactive intermediates, which can then alkylate various biological materials. It is presumed that the arylalkyl amine moiety of the molecule is responsible for the relative specificity of action of these agents, since the reactive intermediate can presumably react with sulfhydryl, amino, and hydroxy groups on many macromolecules.

Locus and Mechanism of Action. α-Adrenergic blockade is due to a direct action of these drugs on α receptors. β-Adrenergic receptors are not affected by conventional doses of these blocking agents.

The presence of a catecholamine or an α-adrenergic blocking agent of the competitive type during development of blockade by a haloalkylamine can decrease the degree of block attained. This appears to involve a competition for the same population of receptors. However, after blockade by a haloalkylamine has fully developed, it is unaffected by exposure to another drug capable of interacting with the same receptors. This stage is referred to as *irreversible* or *nonequilibrium blockade* and is the result of formation of a stable covalent bond between the antagonist and the receptor (Nickerson, 1957).

While it was anticipated that a radioactive haloalkylamine could be used to label the α-adrenergic receptor selectively to facilitate its identification and purification, this has not been possible because of reaction of such compounds with many other macromolecules. However, more selective (although noncovalently binding) radioactive ligands such as (^{3}H)dihydroergocryptine and (^{3}H)prazosin have been used successfully to quantify and characterize α-adrenergic receptors in various tissues (Lefkowitz *et al.*, 1984).

In addition to producing postsynaptic α-adrenergic blockade, the haloalkylamines, and to varying degrees other classes of α-blocking agents, exert important effects on the metabolism of catecholamines. Phenoxybenzamine increases the rate of turnover of norepinephrine in the periphery, which is associated with increased tyrosine hydroxylase activity. In intact animals, these effects are probably predominantly due to increased sympathetic nerve activity, a reflex response to α-adrenergic blockade, since the effect can be inhibited by ganglionic blocking agents (Mueller *et al.*, 1970). Phenoxybenzamine and other α-blocking agents also increase the amount of neurotransmitter released by each nerve impulse. This appears to be due to blockade of presynaptic α_2 receptors, which mediate a negative feedback mechanism that inhibits the release of norepinephrine (Langer, 1977; Starke, 1977; Weiner, 1980). There is a parallel increase in the output of both norepinephrine and dopamine β-hydroxylase, implicating the facilitation of exocytosis in the mechanism. Phenoxybenzamine and many congeners inhibit the uptake of catecholamines into both adrenergic nerve terminals and extraneuronal tissues (Cubeddu *et al.*, 1974).

PHARMACOLOGICAL PROPERTIES

Phenoxybenzamine effectively inhibits responses that are mediated by α-adrenergic agonists. Thus, α-receptor-mediated excitatory responses of smooth muscle and exocrine glands are antagonized (Table 4–1, page 72). While the *actions* of all sympathomimetic agents that stimulate α receptors are inhibited essentially to the same extent, the *net effects* of different sympathomimetic amines on a complex parameter such as blood pressure may be antagonized to very different degrees because of different effects of these agonists on other receptors. For example, a dose of phenoxybenzamine that completely eliminates the pressor response to epinephrine or converts it to a depressor response may produce only a partial inhibition of the pressor response to norepinephrine. Epinephrine produces both vasoconstriction and vasodilatation, and moderate inhibition of the former may allow the latter to predominate; norepinephrine, on the other hand, has very little vasodilator action, and all of the residual constriction is manifested in the pressor response. Even when high doses of α-adrenergic antagonists are given, norepinephrine can exert a small pressor effect because of its cardiac stimulant actions. It should also be noted that the effects of any blocking agent are highly dependent on the level of activity of the system on which it acts. Thus, the vasodilatation induced by phenoxybenzamine may vary markedly in different vascular beds, depending on their degree of adrenergic vasomotor tone, and may vary over a wide range in a single vascular bed, depending on its physiological state.

Blockade by most haloalkylamines develops relatively slowly, and the peak effect is usually not attained in less than an hour after intravenous administration. The blockade produced by a single dose of phenoxybenzamine disappears with a half-life of roughly 24 hours in intact laboratory animals and man. Demonstrable effects persist for at least 3 or 4 days, and the effects of daily administration are cumulative for nearly a week.

Many tissues appear to contain receptors in excess of the number required for a full response to most agonists ("spare receptors"), and a considerable proportion can be inactivated irreversibly before the tissue is incapable of a maximal response (*see* Chapter 2). With increasing doses of the blocking agent, the dose-response curve for an agonist is shifted progressively to the right as the number of available receptors is reduced. When the number of functional receptors is reduced to the degree that the original maximal response is no longer attainable with a full agonist, the dose-response curve does not shift further to the right; additional receptor blockade now causes a depression of the maximal response. The reduction in maximal response then is proportional to the further irreversible blockade of the remaining receptors. Many aspects of the general pharmacology of the haloalkylamines are reviewed by Nickerson and Hollenberg (1967) and Furchgott (1972).

In addition to the blockade of α-adrenergic receptors, the haloalkylamines can inhibit responses to 5-hydroxytryptamine (5-HT, serotonin), histamine, and acetylcholine (ACh). Somewhat higher doses are usually required to inhibit the actions of these substances; this is especially apparent for ACh.

Cardiovascular System. *Blood Pressure.* The usual blocking dose of phenoxybenzamine (1.0 mg/kg in man) infused slowly intravenously into recumbent, normovolemic subjects causes little change in systemic blood pressure, although the diastolic pressure tends to fall somewhat. However, a sharp drop may occur in any situation involving compensatory sympathetic vasoconstriction, such as upright posture or hypovolemia. Thus, a prominent effect of the blockade is *postural hypotension*. In addition, impairment of compensatory vasoconstriction sensitizes to the hypotensive effects of a variety of agents and conditions that tend to produce vasodilatation, including hypercapnia, anesthetic agents, and analgesics such as morphine and meperidine. Rapid injection of a haloalkylamine can cause a precipitous fall in blood pressure, which probably involves factors other than α-adrenergic blockade.

Blood Flows. Phenoxybenzamine produces a prominent and progressive increase in cardiac output and decrease in total peripheral resistance in normal recumbent subjects. However, the changes in blood flow and resistance induced in specific vascular beds vary widely with the conditions under which the blocking agent is administered. In general, the greater the degree of adrenergic vasomotor tone in a vascular bed, the more pronounced is the relaxant effect of the haloalkylamines. Cerebral and coronary resistances are not significantly altered by α-adrenergic blockade *per se*. Cerebral flow is little affected unless the blood pressure is greatly reduced, and coronary flow increases in parallel with reflex cardiac stimulation. Phenoxybenzamine increases resting blood flow in muscle and, in a cool environment, enhances cutaneous blood flow. However, sympathetic vasoconstriction exerts little restraint on muscle blood flow during exercise or on cutaneous blood flow in a warm environment, and under these conditions α blockade produces little change. Splanchnic and renal blood flows are not altered remarkably in the normovolemic subject at rest; however, in the presence of the increased adrenergic vasoconstrictor tone induced by circumstances such as hypovolemia, phenoxybenzamine increases flow to a major degree in both these areas. In the kidney, perfusion of the outer cortex is most markedly affected. Pulmonary arteries and veins are also relaxed; however, because of a greater systemic vasodilatation, blood volume in the pulmonary circuit is usually decreased.

Phenoxybenzamine and other agents that inhibit sympathetic vasoconstriction cause a shift of fluid from the interstitial to the vascular compartment, the result of differential effects on precapillary and postcapillary resistance vessels (Hollenberg and Nickerson, 1970).

Responses to Adrenergic Stimuli. Pressor responses to epinephrine and other sympathomimetic amines are blocked or reversed by phenoxybenzamine (Figure 9–1). A reduction in the pressor response without reversal is usually seen when the capacity for adrenergic vasodilatation is limited by any factor, for example, the sympathomimetic amine used (norepinephrine, phenylephrine, or other agents with minimal β_2-adrenergic agonistic activity).

Cardiac Effects. The chronotropic and inotropic effects of epinephrine, norepinephrine, and direct or reflex sympathetic nerve stimulation on the mammalian myocardium are not inhibited by the haloalkylamines or by other α-adrenergic blocking agents. Indeed, the reflex tachycardia in intact animals is usually exaggerated because the pressor response is prevented and reflex vagal stimulation is minimized. The reflex tachycardia is further accentuated by enhanced release of norepinephrine and decreased inactivation of the amine due to inhibition of neuronal and extraneuronal uptake mechanisms.

In both laboratory animals and man, haloalkylamines effectively inhibit cardiac arrhythmias that involve catecholamines in their genesis, with or without specific sensitization of the myocardium by drugs such

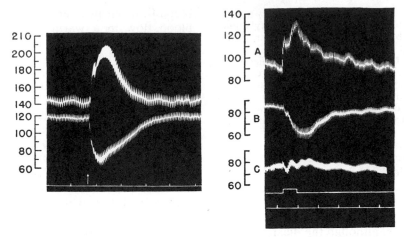

Figure 9–1. *Effect of dibenamine on blood pressure responses of anesthetized cat.*

Left. Responses to a small dose of epinephrine. Upper record before and lower record after intravenous administration of dibenamine (15 mg/kg). The arrow indicates intravenous injections of epinephrine (2.5 µg/kg). The pressor response is converted to depressor by selective blockade of the vasoconstrictor (α-receptor) action of epinephrine, which allows expression of the concurrent vasodilator (β₂-receptor) action. Ordinate, blood pressure in mm Hg; abscissa, time in minutes.

Right. Responses to splanchnic nerve stimulation. *A* before and *B* after dibenamine; *C* after dibenamine and removal of adrenal glands. Ordinate, blood pressure in mm Hg; abscissa, time in minutes. Period of stimulation is indicated by upward deflection of signal line. The initial sharp component of the pressor response in tracing A is due to the local effect of norepinephrine released from sympathetic nerve endings in splanchnic vessels. The subsequent slower component of the rise is predominantly due to catecholamines released from the adrenal medulla. In tracing B each of the two components of the original pressor response is reversed. The initial rapid fall is small. The second, slower component of the reversal represents the vasodilator response to circulating catecholamines, predominantly the effect of epinephrine. After removal of the adrenal glands, only the local (splanchnic) component of the response remains. (After Nickerson and Goodman, 1947. Courtesy of the *Journal of Pharmacology and Experimental Therapeutics.*)

as halogenated anesthetics. Both inhibition of the adrenergic pressor response and a direct blocking effect on the heart are involved, but it is not known if the latter is related to the small component of α-adrenergic receptors that is present in the myocardium. However, arrhythmias following acute coronary artery occlusion or precipitated by hypothermia are not inhibited.

Metabolic Effects. The receptors involved in metabolic responses to catecholamines are predominantly β, but important α-adrenergic actions also participate. For example, agents such as epinephrine stimulate hepatic glycogenolysis (β, in some species) and inhibit insulin secretion (α). However, there is also a weaker β-adrenergic stimulatory effect on insulin secretion. In the presence of phenoxybenzamine, the inhibitory action of epinephrine on insulin secretion is blocked, and the response to β-receptor stimulation and the direct

effect of glucose are revealed. The subsequent rise in insulin concentration may facilitate glucose uptake to the extent that hyperglycemia (from glycogenolysis) is obscured. The result is an *apparent* block of the glycogenolytic effect of epinephrine by phenoxybenzamine when, in fact, this is not the case. Phenoxybenzamine does not specifically antagonize the effects of catecholamines on glycogenolysis in muscle, nor does it inhibit catecholamine-augmented lipolysis. In some species, however (*e.g.*, rat), phenoxybenzamine can block the effect of catecholamines on hepatic glycogenolysis.

Central Nervous System. Phenoxybenzamine can stimulate the CNS to cause nausea, vomiting, hyperventilation, motor excitability, and even convulsions, particularly when a relatively large dose is rapidly injected intravenously. These effects develop and terminate much more rapidly than does the blockade, and hydrolysis products of the active agents, which do not block α receptors, are also effective CNS stimulants. More typically, mild-to-moderate sedation commonly results from the slow intravenous infusion of the usual blocking dose of phenoxybenzamine in man, and fatigue and lethargy may accompany oral medication.

Other Effects. Phenoxybenzamine effectively antagonizes the wide variety of responses to endogenous and exogenous sympathomimetic amines that are mediated by α-adrenergic receptors. Stimulation of the radial fibers of the iris is readily blocked, and miosis is a prominent component of the response to phenoxybenzamine in man, but accommodation is not significantly affected. Contractions of the nictitating membrane, retractor penis, arrector pili, and the uterus of several species are inhibited. Motility of the nonpregnant human uterus *in situ* is reduced, and stimulation by norepinephrine is prevented. Estrogen-induced tubal block of ovum transport is inhibited in rabbits, and it is of interest that the circular fibers of the human tubal isthmus have a particularly dense adrenergic innervation (Owman *et al.*, 1967).

Inasmuch as the predominantly inhibitory effects of sympathomimetic agents on the gastrointestinal tract are mediated by α as well as by β receptors, combined α- and β-adrenergic blockade is usually required to inhibit completely relaxation by epinephrine or norepinephrine. Phenoxybenzamine alone does not appreciably alter transit time through the human gastrointestinal tract.

Absorption, Fate, and Excretion. Phenoxybenzamine is effective when administered by all routes, but injection should be only intravenously because of its irritant properties. Absorption from the gastrointestinal tract is incomplete and somewhat capricious; 20 to 30% of orally administered phenoxybenzamine appears to be absorbed in active form.

Phenoxybenzamine has a high lipid solubility at body pH, and accumulation in fat may occur after large doses. The metabolic fate of these highly unstable agents is poorly understood. Over 50% of the radioactivity of intravenously administered phenoxybenzamine is excreted in 12 hours and over 80% in 24 hours, but small amounts remain in various tissues for considerably longer.

Preparations, Routes of Administration, and Dosage. *Phenoxybenzamine hydrochloride* (DIBENZYLINE) is available for *oral* use in 10-mg capsules. The oral dose usually varies between 20 and 60 mg per day, and full dosage should be approached incrementally.

Toxicity, Side Effects, and Precautions. Untoward effects of phenoxybenzamine are largely due to the blockade of α-adrenergic receptors. Loss of vasomotor control can result in postural hypotension and reflex tachycardia in ambulatory patients, or a sharp fall in blood pressure in those who are hypovolemic. The postural hypotension and palpitation may disappear despite continued blockade, but can reappear under conditions that promote vasodilatation, such as exercise, eating a large meal, or consuming alcohol. Inhibition of compensatory vasoconstriction also exaggerates the effects of vasodilators. Other results of α-receptor blockade include miosis, nasal stuffiness, and inhibition of ejaculation. Effects not clearly related to blockade are local tissue irritation, sedation, and a generalized feeling of weakness and tiredness. Local irritation is probably involved in the nausea and occasional vomiting that may follow large oral doses, particularly if administered on an empty stomach.

Therapeutic Uses. The clinical uses of phenoxybenzamine are discussed below, along with those of other α-adrenergic blocking agents.

PHENTOLAMINE AND TOLAZOLINE

Tolazoline (2-benzyl-2-imidazoline) was first reported in the pharmacological literature as a vasodepressor agent with effects similar to those of histamine. Its α-adrenergic blocking action was noted only during subsequent investigations. *Phentolamine* was introduced later, with particular attention to its α-adrenergic blocking activity.

Chemistry. The 2-substituted imidazolines have a wide range of pharmacological actions, including adrenergic blocking, sympathomimetic, antihypertensive, antihistaminic, histamine-like, and cholinomimetic; slight changes in structure may make one or another of these properties dominant. The structural formulas of *phentolamine* and *tolazoline* are as follows:

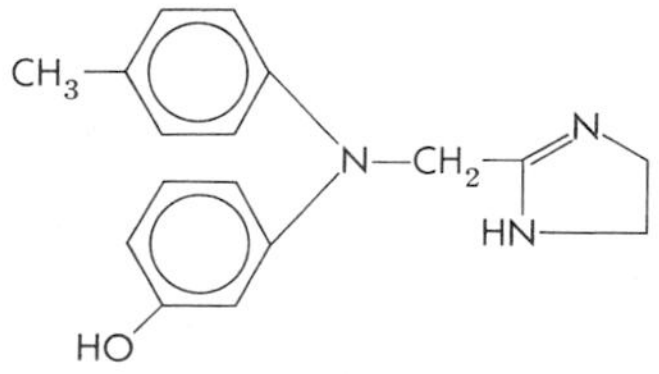

Phentolamine

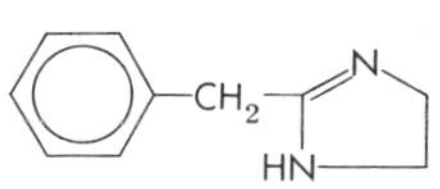

Tolazoline

PHARMACOLOGICAL PROPERTIES

Phentolamine and *tolazoline* produce a moderately effective competitive *α*-adrenergic blockade that is relatively transient. Responses to 5-HT are also inhibited. These substances have other important actions on cardiac and smooth muscle that include cardiac stimulation, stimulation of the gastrointestinal tract that is blocked by atropine, stimulation of gastric secretion, and peripheral vasodilatation. Phentolamine is a considerably more potent *α*-adrenergic blocking agent than is tolazoline, and its other effects are somewhat less prominent.

Tolazoline or phentolamine given intravenously produces vasodilatation and cardiac stimulation; the blood pressure response varies with the relative contributions of the two effects. Phentolamine usually causes a fall in pressure, but the net effect of tolazoline commonly is pressor. Both agents can decrease peripheral resistance and increase venous capacity. The dilatation is predominantly due to a *direct action on vascular smooth muscle* in the dose range now usually employed in man. Pulmonary arterial pressure and vascular resistance are usually reduced by tolazoline or phentolamine.

Therapeutic doses of phentolamine and tolazoline cause cardiac stimulation that is more than just a reflex response to peripheral vasodilatation, and this can be associated with cardiac arrhythmias in both laboratory animals and man (Das and Parratt, 1971). Enhanced neural release of norepinephrine due to presynaptic α_2 blockade may contribute to these effects.

Phentolamine and tolazoline can block many responses that involve *α*-adrenergic receptors. However, the intrinsic eye muscles are relatively resistant, and tolazoline may cause mydriasis rather than miosis. The imidazoline blocking agents stimulate salivary, lacrimal, respiratory tract, and pancreatic secretion, and tolazoline can cause profuse sweating in man. This may be due to a direct action of the drug on muscarinic cholinergic receptors. Phentolamine and tolazoline produce hyperperistalsis and diarrhea, effects that are blocked by atropine. Abdominal discomfort is a very common side effect of phentolamine administration. Phentolamine and tolazoline stimulate gastric secretion of both acid and pepsin.

Absorption, Fate, and Excretion. *Tolazoline* is well absorbed after both parenteral and oral administration. However, it is considerably less effective when given orally because rapid renal excretion prevents accumulation of adequate concentrations during the slow absorption from the gastrointestinal tract. It is largely excreted unchanged by the organic-base transport system of the renal tubules. Little is known about the fate of *phentolamine* in the body. It is not more than 20% as active after oral as after parenteral administration, and only 10% of an injected dose is recovered in the urine in active form.

Toxicity, Side Effects, and Precautions. The most disturbing clinical side effects of phentolamine and tolazoline are attributable to cardiac and gastrointestinal stimulation. Both drugs can cause alarming tachycardia, cardiac arrhythmias, and anginal pain, most frequently after parenteral administration. Tolazoline has been implicated as a precipitating factor in myocardial infarction. Gastrointestinal stimulation may result in abdominal pain, nausea, vomiting, diarrhea, and exacerbation of peptic ulcer. Effective doses of tolazoline quite frequently produce piloerection, chilliness, and apprehension. The imidazoline blocking agents should be used with caution in patients with gastritis, peptic ulcer, or coronary artery disease.

Preparations, Routes of Administration, and Dosage. *Phentolamine mesylate* (REGITINE) is marketed for parenteral use in sterile vials containing 5 mg. The standard dose that has been employed in the diagnosis of pheochromocytoma in adults is 5 mg, given intravenously or intramuscularly. However, it is more prudent to initiate testing with lower doses, particularly if suspicion is high that the patient does indeed have a pheochromocytoma.

Tolazoline hydrochloride (PRISCOLINE HCL) is marketed for injection in 10-ml multiple-dose vials (25 mg/ml). A full parenteral dose is 10 to 50 mg four times daily, given intravenously, intramuscularly, or subcutaneously. Tolazoline is infrequently administered except for investigational purposes.

Therapeutic Uses. Clinical applications of the adrenergic blocking and vasodilating actions of phentolamine and tolazoline are discussed with those of other *α*-adrenergic blocking agents later in this chapter.

PRAZOSIN

Prazosin is an antihypertensive agent that appears to exert its vasodilator action through blockade of postsynaptic α_1 receptors. Administration of prazosin causes reversal of pressor responses to epinephrine, and it blocks pressor responses to norepinephrine. Prazosin appears to be a rather selective α_1-blocking agent, and it has little effect on α_2 receptors; it thus does not cause enhanced neural release of norepinephrine. This may explain the relatively modest degree of tachycardia associated with the administration of this *α*-adrenergic antagonist. Prazosin reduces vascular tone in both resistance and capacitance vessels. This is associated with a reduction in venous return and cardiac output. The hemodynamic effects associated with prazosin, namely, decreased arterial pressure, reduction in arterial and venous tone, and relatively little change in cardiac output, heart rate, or right atrial pressure, are similar to the hemodynamic consequences of directly acting vasodilators, such as sodium nitroprusside (Graham and Pettinger, 1979). Additional information about prazosin is presented in Chapter 32.

TRIMAZOSIN

Trimazosin is chemically related to prazosin and appears to exhibit similar pharmacological properties. However, it is a less potent inhibitor of α_1-adrenergic receptors and has been reported to possess direct arteriolar vasodilator activity. It is rapidly absorbed when administered orally and has a half-life of approximately 2 hours. It is extensively metabolized in the liver. Trimazosin has been effective in the treatment of hypertension, usually when a diuretic is administered concurrently (Chrysant et al., 1981; Weber et al., 1982). The usual dose of trimazosin in adults is 25 to 300 mg two or three times daily. It is not currently approved for general use in the United States.

ERGOT ALKALOIDS

The ergot alkaloids were the first adrenergic blocking agents to be discovered, and most aspects of their general pharmacology were disclosed by the classical studies of Dale (1906).

Ergot alkaloids exhibit a complex variety of pharmacological properties. To varying degrees, these agents act as partial agonists or antagonists at α-adrenergic, tryptaminergic, and dopaminergic receptors (Berde and Stürmer, 1978; see Table 39–2).

Chemistry. Details of the chemistry of the ergot alkaloids are presented in Chapter 39. In general, compounds of the ergonovine type, which lack a polypeptide side chain, have no adrenergic blocking activity. Of the natural ergot preparations, "ergotoxine" has the greatest α-adrenergic blocking potency. It is a mixture of three alkaloids— ergocornine, ergocristine, and ergocryptine; fortunately, these have very similar pharmacological properties. Dihydrogenation of the lysergic acid nucleus increases α-adrenergic blocking activity and decreases, but does not eliminate, the ability to stimulate smooth muscle by an action on tryptaminergic receptors.

PHARMACOLOGICAL PROPERTIES

Both the natural and the dihydrogenated peptide alkaloids produce α-adrenergic blockade. This is relatively persistent for a competitive antagonist, but it is of much shorter duration than that produced by phenoxybenzamine. These drugs also are effective antagonists of 5-HT. Although the hydrogenated ergot alkaloids are among the most potent α-adrenergic blocking agents known, side effects prevent the administration of doses that could produce more than minimal blockade in man.

The most important effects of all the ergot alkaloids are due to actions on the CNS and direct stimulation of smooth muscle. The latter occurs in many different organs (see Chapter 39), and even dihydroergotoxine has been observed to produce spastic contractions of the intestine in man.

The peptide ergot alkaloids can reverse the pressor response to epinephrine to depressor. However, all the natural ergot alkaloids cause a significant rise in blood pressure as a result of peripheral vasoconstriction, which is more pronounced in postcapillary than in precapillary vessels. Although hydrogenation reduces this action, dihydroergotamine is still an effective vasoconstrictor, and a residual constrictor action of dihydroergotoxine is also demonstrable. Ergotamine, ergonovine, and other ergot alkaloids can produce coronary vasoconstriction, often with associated ischemic changes in the ECG and anginal pain in patients with coronary artery disease. The ergot alkaloids usually induce bradycardia even when the blood pressure is not increased. This is predominantly due to increased vagal activity, but a central reduction in sympathetic tone and direct myocardial depression may also be involved.

Several aspects of the pharmacology of the ergot alkaloids are discussed in more detail by Nickerson and Hollenberg (1967) and in a volume edited by Berde and Schild (1978).

Toxicity and Side Effects. The dose of dihydroergotoxine in man is strictly limited by the production of nausea and vomiting. Prolonged or excessive administration of any of the natural peptide ergot alkaloids can cause vascular insufficiency and gangrene of the extremities. This is particularly likely to occur in the presence of preexisting vascular pathology or infection. In severe cases, prompt vasodilatation is essential. There have been no comparative studies on the treatment of this sporadic condition, but a direct-acting drug such as nitroprusside appears to be most effective (Carliner et al., 1974). Toxic effects of the ergot alkaloids are described in more detail in Chapter 39.

Therapeutic Uses and Preparations. The primary uses of ergot alkaloids are to stimulate contraction of the uterus post partum and to relieve the pain of migraine. These and other applications are described in Chapter 39; the effect of bromocriptine on the secretion of prolactin, of which advantage is taken clinically, is described in Chapter 59. The various preparations of ergot alkaloids are listed in Chapter 39.

OTHER α-ADRENERGIC BLOCKING AGENTS

Natural and synthetic compounds of several other chemical classes exhibit α-adrenergic blocking activity. Chlorpromazine, haloperidol, and many other neuroleptic drugs produce significant α blockade in both laboratory animals and man. Chlorpromazine has also been reported to prolong and, under appropriate conditions, enhance the pressor response to norepinephrine, possibly as a result of the capability of this compound to block neuronal re-uptake of the neurotransmitter. Haloperidol also inhibits dopamine-induced renal vaso-dilatation, which is not affected by the common α- or β-adrenergic blocking agents.

Yohimbine. Yohimbine is an indolealkylamine alkaloid with a chemical similarity to reserpine. Yohimbine and a diastereoisomer, *corynanthine,* and a derivative, *ethyl yohimbine,* produce competitive α-adrenergic blockade of limited duration. Yohimbine also blocks peripheral 5-HT receptors. It has little direct effect on smooth muscle, but readily penetrates the CNS and produces a complex pattern of responses in doses lower than those required to produce peripheral α-adrenergic blockade. These include antidiuresis, due to release of antidiuretic hormone (ADH), and a general picture of central excitation, including elevations of blood pressure and heart rate, increased motor activity, irritability, and tremor in both unanesthetized laboratory animals and man. Yohimbine is known to block central α_2 receptors, and these effects are generally opposite to those of clonidine, an α_2 agonist. Sweating, nausea, and vomiting are also common after parenteral administration in man. Since yohimbine is a relatively selective inhibitor of α_2-adrenergic receptors, it can enhance neural release of norepinephrine at concentrations less than those required to block postsynaptic α_1 receptors. This may account for some of the effects of this drug, which resemble those of sympathomimetic agents (Starke, 1977).

THERAPEUTIC USES OF α-ADRENERGIC BLOCKING AGENTS

α-Adrenergic blockade has been employed or suggested as therapy in a wide variety of conditions, but it has few well-established uses. Quite possibly the clinical application of these drugs will always be severely limited by the fact that efferent sympathetic pathways operating through α-adrenergic receptors are critical to the cardiovascular reflexes that allow man to function as a biped, and it is often difficult to balance the therapeutic benefits of blockade against the disadvantages of disrupting this essential regulatory function.

Cardiovascular Uses. *Hypertension.* Several drugs currently used in the treatment of essential hypertension act by inhibiting sympathetic vasoconstrictor tone. However, with the exception of prazosin, results with α-adrenergic blocking agents in this condition have been disappointing. An important factor is that β receptors are unaffected, and reflex tachycardia and palpitation are added to the other side effects associated with inhibition of sympathetic vasoconstriction. The usefulness of

prazosin in hypertension may in part be due to its lack of potency in inhibiting presynaptic α_2 receptors. Small doses of phenoxybenzamine have been found useful in patients who have developed resistance to adrenergic neuron blocking drugs on the basis of vascular supersensitivity to catecholamines (Sandler *et al.,* 1968). Phenoxybenzamine and phentolamine have also been used successfully to control acute hypertensive episodes due to sympathomimetics, and to certain foods and drugs in the presence of MAO inhibition. The treatment of hypertension is discussed in Chapter 32.

Pheochromocytoma. Many pharmacological tests for the diagnosis of pheochromocytoma have been employed in the past, including provocative tests with histamine, methacholine, and glucagon, as well as blocking tests with phentolamine and other drugs. Determinations of the amounts of catecholamines and their metabolites, particularly vanillylmandelic acid, metanephrine, and nor-metanephrine in urine and catecholamines in plasma, are now generally accepted as the most reliable methods of diagnosis. While the pharmacological tests are now much less helpful, there are a few patients with symptoms and signs that are very suggestive of pheochromocytoma who will not have abnormal concentrations of catecholamines or their metabolites in plasma or urine, despite the presence of the tumor. The patient can be treated with phentolamine prior to the performance of a histamine challenge test. Protection is thus secured from hypertension or arrhythmias caused by catecholamines. However, high concentrations of catecholamines may be detected in plasma just after the histamine is administered or in urine collected for 2 hours after the test.

Adrenergic blocking agents are useful in the *pre-operative management* of patients with pheochromocytoma, for *prolonged treatment* if the tumor is malignant or otherwise not amenable to surgery, and to prevent paroxysmal hypertension during *operative manipulation* of the tumor. Oral phenoxybenzamine is the preferred drug in the first two of these situations. The stable, persistent blockade may allow improvement in the general cardiovascular status of the patient prior to operation, and it permits expansion of the blood volume, which may be severely reduced as a result of the excessive adrenergic vasoconstriction. Patients with inoperable tumors have been adequately controlled with phenoxybenzamine for many years (*see* Engelman and Sjoerdsma, 1964). A β-adrenergic antagonist is also frequently employed in these patients in order to block the effects of catecholamines on the heart. In the preoperative management of pheochromocytoma, phenoxybenzamine can be administered orally, starting with daily doses of 10 to 20 mg. If the patient has evidence of catecholamine-induced myocarditis or cardiomyopathy, such treatment can be continued for weeks. The drug is given for shorter periods if cardiovascular and metabolic abnormalities are corrected quickly. During the operation, 2 to 5 mg of phentolamine can also be given intravenously to block effects of large amounts of catecholamines that may be released suddenly. If preoperative treatment is effective, removal of the tumor should not precipitate a period of hypotension. The judicious use of small doses of propranolol or special anesthetic procedures may be necessary to prevent arrhythmias (*see* Ross *et al.*, 1967; Crout and Brown, 1969). Preoperative treatment with metyrosine, an inhibitor of catecholamine synthesis, may be preferred if the patient is sensitive to adrenergic blocking agents (*see* below).

Shock. Largely because of preoccupation with low blood pressure as a criterion of shock, vasopressor agents have been used extensively in its treatment. However, vasoconstriction is a prominent feature of shock *per se*, and there is little evidence that its accentuation by drugs is beneficial, as long as a minimally acceptable blood pressure can be maintained (*see* Chapter 8).

Many agents that induce vasodilatation by inhibiting sympathetic vasoconstriction or by directly relaxing vascular smooth muscle improve the survival rate of experimental animals subjected to various shock-inducing procedures. Protection can be attributed to at least three distinct cardiovascular effects: (1) increased cardiac output and total blood flow; (2) local redistribution of blood flow so that a larger percentage passes through channels that readily exchange metabolites with tissue cells, presumably true capillaries; and (3) reversal of the vasoconstriction-induced shift of fluid from the vascular to the interstitial compartment. Two other effects of α-blocking agents such as phentolamine can make important contributions to the practical clinical management of this condition: (1) The fall in blood pressure induced when it is administered in the presence of hypovolemia provides a quick and reliable indication of the adequacy of intravascular fluid–volume replacement, a point often difficult to determine even with careful monitoring of the central venous pressure. (2) The shift of blood from the pulmonary to the systemic vascular bed associated with blockade of sympathetic vasomotor tone allows administration of larger volumes of fluid more rapidly than would otherwise be possible, particularly in patients with some myocardial inadequacy. It should be emphasized that any drug therapy in shock is secondary to fully adequate replacement of intravascular fluid volume with blood or other appropriate fluids. *Phentolamine or phenoxybenzamine should not be given unless the central venous pressure has been elevated by fluid administration without an adequate circulatory response;* inhibition of vasoconstrictor reflexes makes the circulation highly vulnerable to hypovolemia. In addition, the blocking agent must be administered slowly and suitable fluids must be immediately available for use if a sharp drop in blood pressure indicates that replacement has in fact been inadequate. (*See* Nickerson, 1962; Hardaway, 1968.) Direct vasodilators are also being used to treat shock, particularly that associated with myocardial failure (*see* Chapter 33).

Peripheral Vascular Disease. Many α-adrenergic blocking drugs, direct-acting vasodilators (*see also* Chapter 33), and drugs with mixed actions are promoted for the treatment of inadequacies of blood flow, particularly to the skin and muscles of the extremities. Ischemia in these areas arises from a variety of pathological processes, but morphological changes that limit flow in relatively large vessels are commonly involved. In general, the results of drug therapy in this broad group of diseases have been disappointing, and vasoactive drugs should not be given precedence over conservative medical management or surgery, where the latter is indicated and possible. Although there are many reports of the efficacy of α-adrenergic blocking agents and of other vasodilators in *intermittent claudication*, there is no convincing evidence that any agent or procedure can increase skeletal muscle blood flow beyond the level produced by exercise to the limit of tolerance. Such exercise is also generally accepted as the most effective mechanism for improving the collateral circulation to ischemic muscle.

The most favorable clinical responses to α-adrenergic blockade are in conditions with a large component of adrenergic vasoconstriction, such as *Raynaud's phenomenon* and *acrocyanosis*. These are less common and threatening than occlusive arterial disease, but even here drug therapy is probably secondary to other measures. Phenoxybenzamine, prazosin, and tolazoline have been observed to relieve vasospasm and reduce sensitivity to cold in Raynaud's phenomenon. Satisfactory results are obtained in most cases with oral doses that produce only a relatively low level of adrenergic blockade (Gifford, 1971). Vasospasm induced by an exogenous sympathomimetic is readily antagonized, and local infiltration with 5 to 10 mg of phentolamine in 10 ml of 0.9% sodium chloride solution effectively prevents the severe local vasoconstriction and skin necrosis that can be associated with infusion of a vasoconstrictor such as norepinephrine, particularly if there is some extravasation.

Other Cardiovascular Uses. High spinal cord transection commonly leads to autonomic hyperreflexia with paroxysmal elevations in blood pressure from both cutaneous and visceral stimuli, particularly those from the urinary bladder. It has been reported that these pressor episodes and the associated signs and symptoms can be well controlled by relatively small oral doses of phenoxybenzamine (Sizemore and Winternitz, 1970).

Any inadequacy of cardiac output, particularly of relatively acute onset, can cause an increase in sympathetic vasomotor tone, which increases peripheral resistance and decreases venous compliance. Because the constriction is greater in the systemic bed, blood is shifted to the pulmonary circuit, and increased pulmonary blood volume and pressure can cause *pulmonary congestion* and *edema*. It has been repeatedly shown that block of sympathetic vasoconstriction can rapidly reverse these processes and decrease myocardial work and pulmonary congestion. α-Adrenergic blockade has been shown to be beneficial in heart failure with pulmonary edema (*see* Majid *et al.*, 1971) and in acute myocardial infarction where pain can accentuate the vasoconstriction (Kelly *et al.*, 1973). Other vasodilator drugs such as nitroprusside are also effective.

II. β-Adrenergic Blocking Agents

β-Adrenergic blocking agents have received major attention because of their utility in the management of cardiovascular disorders, including hypertension, angina pectoris, and cardiac arrhythmias (Prichard *et al.*, 1980).

The first drug shown to produce a selective blockade of β-adrenergic receptors was *dichloroisoproterenol* (DCI) (Powell and Slater, 1958). Studies with DCI made a substantial contribution to the understanding of effects mediated by β receptors, but it was not used in man, largely because it has a prominent β-receptor stimulant action; that is, it is a partial agonist. *Propranolol* was the first β-adrenergic antagonist to come into wide clinical use, and it remains the most important of these compounds. It is a highly potent, nonselective β-adrenergic blocking agent with no intrinsic sympathomimetic activity. However, because of its ability to block β receptors in bronchial smooth muscle and skeletal muscle, propranolol interferes with bronchodilatation produced by epinephrine and other sympathomimetic amines and with glycogenolysis, which ordinarily occurs during hypoglycemia. Thus, the drug is usually not used in individuals with bronchial asthma and must be used cautiously in diabetics who are receiving insulin or oral hypoglycemic agents. As a consequence, there has been a search for β-adrenergic blocking agents that are cardioselective (*see* Karow *et al.*, 1971), and a number of drugs have now been developed that exhibit some degree of specificity for β$_1$-adrenergic receptors. *Practolol* was the first such agent, and it was widely employed in Europe and elsewhere for the treatment of hypertension. However, disturbing toxicities that involved epithelial structures in particular were noted after long-term use of the drug.

Among the relatively *nonselective β-adrenergic blocking agents* that are either available in the United States or under clinical investigation are propranolol, alprenolol, bunolol, nadolol, oxprenolol, penbutolol, pindolol, sotalol, and timolol. Propranolol, timolol, nadolol, and pindolol are currently available for systemic use in the United States. *Selective β$_1$-adrenergic*

blocking agents that have either been introduced into therapy or are under investigation include *metoprolol, atenolol, acebutolol, bevantolol, pafenolol,* and *tolamolol. Metoprolol* and *atenolol* have been approved for use in the United States. It is important to remember that the selectivity of the β$_1$ blockers is not absolute; larger doses of these compounds will inhibit all β-adrenergic receptors (*see* Prichard, 1978). Propranolol and metoprolol will be discussed as prototypes of nonselective and cardioselective β$_1$-adrenergic blocking agents, respectively.

Butoxamine is a somewhat selective β$_2$-adrenergic antagonist. It blocks β$_2$-vasodilator and other smooth muscle inhibitory effects of isoproterenol, but relatively little antagonism of the cardiac effects is observed in anesthetized animals; in unanesthetized dogs, however, it blocks the chronotropic action (Levy, 1966; Burns *et al.*, 1967). This may be due to the presence of β$_2$ receptors in the atria.

Chemistry. The structural formulas of the β-adrenergic blocking agents that are available for general use in the United States are as follows:

Nonselective Antagonists

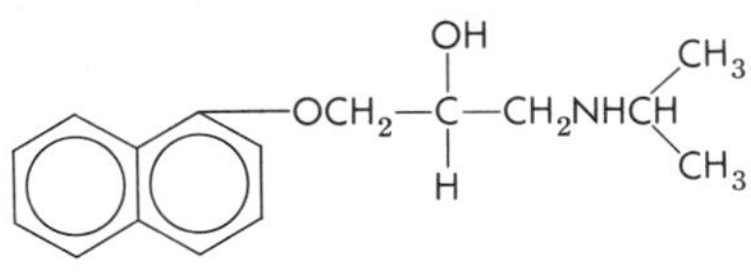

Propranolol

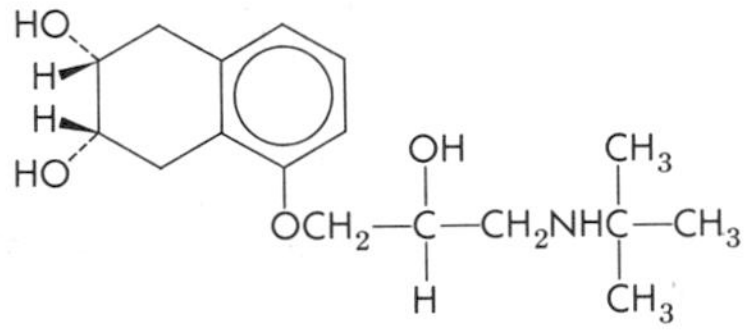

Nadolol

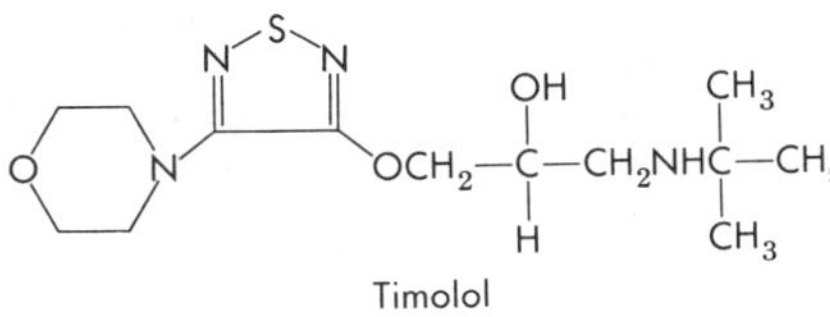

Timolol

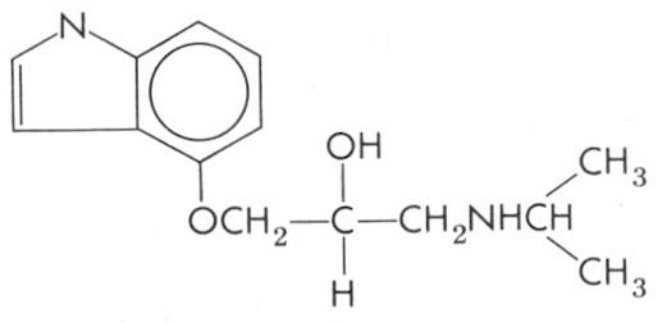

Pindolol

β_1-*Selective Antagonists*

Metoprolol

Atenolol

The structural similarity between β-receptor agonists and antagonists is closer than in the case of drugs acting at α receptors. The side chain with an isopropyl or bulkier substituent on the amine appears to favor interaction with β receptors. The nature of substituents on the aromatic ring determines whether the effect will be predominantly activation or blockade. These substituents also affect cardioselectivity. The aliphatic hydroxyl appears to be essential for activity. It confers on the molecule optical activity, and the levorotatory forms of both β-adrenergic agonists and antagonists are much more potent than the dextrorotatory forms. This difference is useful in distinguishing the effects of β-receptor blockade from those of other pharmacological actions of the molecule; for example, the *d* isomer of propranolol has less than 1% of the potency of the *l* isomer of propranolol in blocking β-adrenergic receptors, but the two are equipotent as local anesthetics.

PHARMACOLOGICAL PROPERTIES

As in the case of the α-adrenergic blocking agents, much of the pharmacology of β-adrenergic blockade can be deduced from a knowledge of the functions subserved by the involved receptors (Table 4–1, page 72) and the physiological or pathological conditions under which they are activated. Thus, β-receptor blockade has little effect on the normal heart with the subject at complete rest, but may have profound effects when sympathetic control of the heart is high, as during exercise. The overall response to a β-adrenergic blocking agent may also be modified by other properties of the drug in question. β-Receptor stimulation ("intrinsic sympathomimetic activity"; partial agonist activity) is an important pharmacological property of certain β-adrenergic antagonists, such as practolol, pindolol, acebutolol, alprenolol, and oxprenolol (Prichard, 1978). The clinical significance of this partial agonist activity is uncertain,

although agents with this activity do not elicit as pronounced a bradycardia or negative inotropic effect at rest (Prichard *et al.*, 1980; Symposium, 1982; McDevitt, 1983). Some of these drugs also have direct actions on cell membranes, which are commonly described as membrane stabilizing, local anesthetic, and quinidine-like. The local anesthetic potency of propranolol is about equal to that of lidocaine, while oxprenolol is about half as potent; other agents are almost devoid of this property (*see* Table 9–1).

In isolated atria, propranolol and oxprenolol decrease spontaneous frequency, maximal driving frequency, and contractility, and increase electrical threshold. They also increase A-V conduction time and decrease the spontaneous rate of depolarization of ectopic pacemakers in intact hearts. Resting membrane potential and repolarization are not greatly affected by propranolol, but the height and rate of rise of the action potential are reduced because the drug decreases the inward sodium current (Tarr *et al.*, 1973). These quinidine-like effects are associated with generalized depression of myocardial function, which can cause death with large doses. It has been suggested that β-adrenergic blocking agents without membrane-stabilizing activity are less likely than propranolol to precipitate heart failure. However, direct myocardial depression requires doses much higher than those necessary for β-adrenergic blockade, and it appears that block of sympathetic stimulation is by far the most important factor in the occasional precipitation of heart failure in a patient with an inadequate cardiac reserve. The quinidine-like effects of β-adrenergic blocking drugs appear to contribute little to their efficacy in the treatment of cardiac arrhythmias; effective concentrations of propranolol in blood are below those that cause much membrane stabilization, and β blockers without this property are also effective antiarrhythmic agents (*see* Black and Prichard, 1973; Shand, 1975).

Binding Studies with Labeled β-Adrenergic Antagonists. β-Adrenergic receptors have been identified and characterized in many tissues with the use of highly potent and selective β-adrenergic blocking agents that are labeled with a radioisotope of high specific activity. Such studies have allowed determination of the molecular properties of the receptor and have increased the knowledge about its mechanism of interaction with adenylate cyclase (*see* Smigel *et al.*, 1984). Furthermore, the affinities of various agents for β_1 and β_2 receptors can be determined with precision (Minneman *et al.*, 1979a). Thus, metoprolol and practolol exhibit the greatest (10- to 20-fold) degree of selectivity for β_1 receptors, while atenolol is about threefold more potent in binding to β_1- than to β_2-adrenergic receptors; propranolol, pindolol, sotalol, and timolol have equal affinity for both subtypes. The greater

Table 9–1. PHARMACOLOGICAL CHARACTERISTICS OF β-ADRENERGIC RECEPTOR BLOCKING AGENTS *

COMPOUND	POTENCY AS β BLOCKER (PROPRANOLOL = 1.0)	LOCAL ANESTHETIC ACTIVITY	INTRINSIC SYMPATHOMIMETIC ACTIVITY	HALF-LIFE IN PLASMA (HOURS) †
I. Nonselective (β$_1$ + β$_2$) Adrenergic Blocking Agents				
Alprenolol	0.3–1	+	+ +	2–3
Bunolol	50	0	0	6
Nadolol	0.5	0	0	14–18
Oxprenolol	0.5–1	+	+ +	1–2
Penbutolol	5–10	+	0	26 ‡
Pindolol	5–10	±	+ +	3–4
Propranolol	1	+ +	0	3–5
Sotalol	0.3	0	0	5–12
Timolol	5–10	0	±	4
II. Cardioselective (β$_1$) Adrenergic Blocking Agents				
Acebutolol	0.3	+	+	3
Atenolol	1	0	0	6–8
Metoprolol	0.5–2	±	0	3–4
Practolol	0.3	0	+ +	5–10
Tolamolol	0.3–1	±	0	3–6

* Based on data in Waal-Manning, 1976; Brogden *et al.*, 1977; McDevitt, 1977; Benson *et al.*, 1978; Prichard, 1978; Scriabine, 1979. *See also* Appendix II.

† The duration of effect, in general, is considerably longer than might be expected from the plasma $t_{1/2}$.

‡ Plasma $t_{1/2}$ of slow phase of disposition. A rapid phase ($t_{1/2}$, 1 to 2 hours) is also demonstrable.

selectivity of metoprolol for β$_1$ receptors (compared to atenolol) in binding studies is in contrast to clinical observations and other *in-vivo* studies, where atenolol appears to be more cardioselective. The reason for this discrepancy is not known. The relative proportions of β$_1$ and β$_2$ receptors in a tissue can also be determined by ligand-binding technics (Minneman *et al.*, 1979b). For example, in rat tissues, the proportion of β$_1$ to β$_2$ receptors is about 4:1 in heart and cerebral cortex and about 1:5 in lung and cerebellum.

β-Adrenergic receptors have been purified to homogeneity from various sources by affinity chromatographic technics (Shorr *et al.*, 1982). The receptor is a single glycosylated polypeptide, although its molecular weight varies among sources. It is possible to reconstitute purified receptor in phospholipid vesicles with purified guanine nucleotide–binding regulatory proteins (*see* Chapter 2) and the catalytic component of adenylate cyclase; the mechanisms of interactions between these proteins can thus be studied in detail (Brandt *et al.*, 1983).

NONSELECTIVE β-ADRENERGIC BLOCKING AGENTS: PROPRANOLOL

As mentioned, propranolol is a nonselective β-adrenergic blocking agent that is used widely for the treatment of hypertension, the prophylaxis of angina pectoris, and the control of certain types of cardiac arrhythmias. It blocks both β$_1$ and β$_2$ receptors competitively and does not exhibit any intrinsic agonistic properties.

Cardiovascular System. The most important effects of β-adrenergic blocking drugs are on the cardiovascular system, predominantly due to actions on the heart. Propranolol decreases heart rate and cardiac output, prolongs mechanical systole, and slightly decreases blood pressure in resting subjects (Robin *et al.*, 1967; Helfant *et al.*, 1971). The effects on cardiac output and heart rate are more dramatic during exercise. Peripheral resistance is increased as a result of compensatory sympathetic reflexes, and blood flow to all tissues except the brain is reduced (Nies *et al.*, 1973).

The cardiac effects of β-adrenergic blockade are often reflected in changes in sodium excretion. The normal diurnal pattern is reversed, as in patients with moderate myocardial inadequacy, and there is a slow adjustment to a new steady state with increased total body sodium and extracellular fluid volume. These effects are most obvious in patients with some preexisting myocardial inadequacy. In some patients with severe heart disease, β-adrenergic blockade can cause progressive accumulation of sodium and water, edema, and frank congestive heart failure. These effects on sodium excretion probably result from intrarenal hemodynamic changes that are part of the adjustment to the decreased cardiac output (Nies *et al.*, 1971). The magnitude of the effect appears to parallel the dependence of the heart on adrenergic stimulation to maintain adequate function. Occasionally a β-adrenergic blocking agent, particularly when given intravenously, can precipitate acute heart failure.

The effect of β-adrenergic blockade on the heart is more marked under conditions of increased demand and sympathetic tone. The cardiac response to fluid load is reduced, as is the tachycardia associated with exercise, nitrite hypotension, or the Valsalva maneuver (Black and Prichard, 1973). Ventricular dimensions and contractility are little affected in normal, supine, resting subjects, but the decreases in end-diastolic and end-systolic ventricular size and the increase in myocardial contractility associated with exercise are reduced. In patients with occlusive coronary artery disease, propranolol can cause significant increases in ventricular end-diastolic volumes and pressures, and in the tension-time index; it can also cause or increase ventricular asynergy. Maximal exercise tolerance is considerably decreased in normal individuals, but can be increased in patients with angina pectoris (Sowton *et al.*, 1971).

Total myocardial oxygen consumption and coronary blood flow are also decreased as a result of reductions of heart rate, ventricular systolic pressure, and contractility. The reduction is predominantly in subepicardial blood flow, which leads to a relative redistribution of flow (Gross and Winbury, 1973). A similar internal shunting after β-adrenergic blockade allows blood flow to ischemic areas of the heart to be altered less than that to other regions (Pitt and Craven, 1970). While prolongation of systolic ejection and dilatation of the ventricle caused by propranolol tend to increase oxygen requirements, the oxygen-sparing effects predominate (*see* Chapter 33).

Blood Pressure. Propranolol is an effective antihypertensive agent. Chronic treatment of hypertensive patients with a β-adrenergic blocking agent results in a slowly developing reduction in blood pressure. Propranolol is particularly useful clinically in combination with vasodilators that act directly on the vasculature. The reflex tachycardia that is a prominent feature of the response to the latter drugs is effectively blocked by the β-adrenergic antagonist (*see* Chapter 32).

Several mechanisms have been proposed for the efficacy of propranolol in the management of hypertension, and more than one mechanism may contribute to this effect. Reduction in cardiac output occurs rather promptly after administration of propranolol. However, the hypotensive effects of propranolol do not usually appear as rapidly. β-Adrenergic agonists are known to increase modestly the release of norepinephrine from adrenergic nerve terminals (Starke, 1977; Dixon *et al.*, 1979). Propranolol blocks this effect, and such impairment of the release of norepinephrine following sympathetic nerve stimulation might contribute to the antihypertensive effects of the drug.

The release of renin from the juxtaglomerular apparatus is stimulated by β-adrenergic agonists, and this effect is blocked by drugs such as propranolol (*see* Chapter 27). They also reduce, but do not completely block, the increase in plasma renin activity induced by sodium deprivation. Buhler and associates (1972) observed that the antihypertensive effect of propranolol, administered in relatively modest doses, is much more prominent in individuals with elevated plasma renin activity than in those in whom this value is relatively low. It has thus been proposed that propranolol may exert at least a portion of its antihypertensive effect by inhibiting the secretion of renin by the kidney. However, hypertensive patients who have low activity of renin in plasma do respond to propranolol if larger doses are employed (Oates *et al.*, 1977). Furthermore, some β-blocking agents reduce blood pressure but do not inhibit the secretion of renin significantly (*see* Stokes *et al.*, 1974; Weber *et al.*, 1974).

Esler and coworkers (1977) have suggested that hypertensive patients who respond to propranolol can be classified into two groups. Those who exhibit hypotensive responses when the concentration of propranolol in plasma is relatively low (3 to 30 ng/ml) tend to have high activity of renin in plasma and elevated concentrations of circulating catecholamines. Many of the remaining subjects respond when the concentration of propranolol in plasma is in the range of 30 to 100 ng/ml.

Effect on Vascular Responses to Drugs. Propranolol and other nonselective β-adrenergic blocking drugs inhibit the vasodepressor and vasodilator effects of isoproterenol, and augment the pressor effect of epinephrine. Pressor responses to norepinephrine may be slightly decreased because its cardiac actions are blocked, but those to phenylephrine are unchanged. These effects are entirely predictable from a knowledge of the relative activities of different sympathomimetics on vascular α and β receptors. Vasodilatation due to histamine, ACh, and nitroglycerin is unaffected. β-Adrenergic blockade does not inhibit renal vasodilatation induced by dopamine, although the limited responses to isoproterenol in this vascular bed and to dopamine in the femoral vasculature are eliminated.

Effects on Cardiac Rhythm and Automaticity.
Propranolol reduces sinus rate, decreases the spontaneous rate of depolarization of ectopic pacemakers, and slows conduction in the atria and in the A-V node. Large doses of propranolol appear to exert a quinidine-like effect on the myocardium, which might contribute to the antiarrhythmic effect of this drug. However, the β-adrenergic blocking activity of propranolol appears to be its major mechanism of action (Shand, 1975). The utility of propranolol in the management of cardiac arrhythmias is discussed in Chapter 31.

β-Adrenergic antagonists can reduce the incidence of reinfarction and death after myocardial infarction (*see* below). The mechanism of this important therapeutic effect of these drugs is not known.

Central Nervous System. Propranolol readily penetrates into the brain, but it has few, if any, effects that can be clearly attributed to blockade of β-adrenergic receptors in the CNS. While there has been speculation that central actions of propranolol might contribute to its antihypertensive effects, there is no convincing evidence.

Metabolic Effects. β-Adrenergic blocking agents can considerably modify carbohydrate and fat metabolism, although many species and tissue variations as well as composite effects confuse this complex field (*see* Ellis, 1980). Most of the effects of catecholamines on carbohydrate and fat metabolism are mediated by β receptors and changes in adenylate cyclase activity, with resultant production of adenosine 3',5'-monophosphate (cyclic AMP). Adrenergic blocking agents that inhibit metabolic responses act on this sequence of events. In man, propranolol inhibits the rise in plasma free fatty acids induced by sympathomimetic amines or by enhanced sympathetic nervous system activity. It also effectively and selectively inhibits the lipolytic action of catecholamines on isolated adipose tissue of several species. The actions of adrenergic blocking agents on carbohydrate metabolism are more complicated. The hyperglycemic response to epinephrine is reduced by β-adrenergic blocking drugs in most species and by α blockers in only a few. The effects of the latter agents also involve actions on insulin secretion (*see* above). Glycogenolysis in heart and skeletal muscle is inhibited by β- and not by α-adrenergic blocking drugs. The effects on hepatic glycogenolysis are dependent on the species (*see* Chapter 4). The release of insulin by isoproterenol is blocked by propranolol. Propranolol does not affect plasma glucose or insulin concentrations in normal individuals, or the rate or magnitude of the fall of plasma glucose after insulin, but it does slow the subsequent recovery of glucose concentration and prevents the usual rebound of plasma glycerol. These effects are presumably due to inhibition of the glycogenolytic and lipolytic actions of endogenous catecholamines released in response to hypoglycemia. Consequently, β-adrenergic blocking agents must be used with caution in patients prone to hypoglycemia and particularly in diabetics treated with insulin (*see* Chapter 64).

Other Effects. Propranolol blocks the action of sympathomimetic amines on β-adrenergic receptors in many structures. However, when administered in the absence of a specific agonist, the most important response to β blockade outside of the cardiovascular system is that of the bronchi and bronchioles. Adrenergic bronchodilatation is mediated by β_2 receptors, but the presence of significant intrinsic adrenergic bronchodilator activity was not demonstrated before the clinical availability of β-adrenergic blocking agents. Propranolol consistently increases airway resistance. This effect is small and of no clinical significance in normal individuals, but it can be marked and potentially dangerous in asthmatics. Because bronchodilatation is a β_2-adrenergic response, selective β_1 blockers such as metoprolol are much less likely than propranolol to induce bronchoconstriction, and they have been used in asthmatic patients with minimal effects on airway resistance.

β-Adrenergic blocking agents antagonize relaxation of the uterus by catecholamines, but they have no effect under conditions in which the response is excitatory. Propranolol increases the activity of the human uterus, more in the nonpregnant than in the pregnant state (Wansbrough *et al.,* 1968). β-Receptor blockade inhibits the action of epinephrine that prevents local edema formation in response to the injection of a variety of irritants in the rat paw (*see* Green, 1972), and blocks the "antianaphylactic" effect of catecholamines on antigen-induced histamine release from sensitized lung (Assem and Schild, 1971). Circulating eosinophils increase in man during the administration of propranolol, and the reduction characteristically induced by epinephrine is blocked (Koch-Weser, 1968).

The effects of β-adrenergic blocking agents on skeletal neuromuscular transmission are variable. Drugs that block β-adrenergic receptors antagonize epinephrine-induced tremor in man. However, propranolol is not consistently effective in controlling the tremor of parkinsonism, and its efficacy in the management of essential tremor is controversial (Gilligan *et al.,* 1972).

Absorption, Fate, and Excretion. Propranolol is almost completely absorbed following oral administration. However, much of the administered drug is metabolized by the liver during its first passage through the portal circulation, and only about one third reaches the systemic circulation. In addition, there is considerable interindividual variation in the degree of presystemic hepatic elimination of propranolol, and this contributes to the great variability (up to 20-fold) in plasma concentrations found after oral administration of comparable doses to patients. The degree of hepatic extraction of propranolol is less as the dose is increased, suggesting that a saturable mechanism is involved (Evans *et al.,* 1973b). Furthermore, somewhat less of the drug is removed during the first circulation through the liver after repeated administration than after the initial dose, which accounts for a gradual increase in the half-life of the drug after chronic oral administration (about 4 hours) compared with the half-life of the initial oral dose (about 3 hours) (Shand, 1975). The ingestion of food reduces the first-pass metabolism of propranolol and increases its bioavailability.

Propranolol is bound to plasma proteins to the extent of 90 to 95% (Evans *et al.,* 1973a). This may contribute to the relative unreliability of total plasma concentration as a guide to therapeutic efficacy.

Propranolol is virtually completely metabolized before excretion in the urine. One of the products of hepatic metabolism is 4-hydroxypropranolol, which appears to exhibit β-adrenergic blocking activity comparable to that of the parent compound. However, the half-life of 4-hydroxypropranolol is short, and it probably contributes relatively little to the therapeutic effect of the drug. Other metabolic products that have been identified in the urine include naphthoxylactic acid, isopropylamine, and propranolol glycol. A considerable fraction of the metabolites of propranolol is apparently glucuronide conjugates (Shand, 1975; Oates *et al.,* 1977).

Preparations, Routes of Administration, and Dosage. *Propranolol hydrochloride* (INDERAL) is available in tablets containing 10 to 90 mg for oral administration, and in 1-ml ampuls containing 1.0 mg for intravenous use. It is also available in sustained-release capsules (INDERAL LA).

In the management of hypertension, propranolol is administered orally. The initial dose is usually 40 mg, given twice daily, or 80 mg once daily (sustained-release capsule). The dose is increased gradually to a level of 120 to 240 mg per day (or up to 640 mg in some cases). When the doses are large, the drug can often be taken once daily. In the treatment of angina pectoris or for the control of arrhythmias, doses of 40 to 320 mg per day may be employed. As in the treatment of hypertension, the initial doses should be low and increased gradually until either therapeutic benefit or toxicity is noted. Propranolol may be administered intravenously for the management of life-threatening arrhythmias. Under these circumstances the usual dose is 1 to 3 mg, administered slowly and with careful and frequent measurement of blood pressure, ECG, and cardiac function. If an adequate response is not obtained, a second dose may be given after a few minutes. In the event of overdosage, atropine should be administered to counteract the bradycardia, and cardiac glycosides and diuretics should be given in the event of cardiac failure. Vasopressors may be required to counteract a profound fall in blood pressure. The recommended dose of propranolol after myocardial infarction is 180 to 240 mg per day in three or four divided portions.

Toxicity, Side Effects, and Precautions. The major dangers of therapy with propranolol or other β-adrenergic blocking drugs are related to the blockade *per se.* Serious cardiac depression is uncommon, but heart failure may develop suddenly or slowly, usually in patients whose hearts are severely compromised by disease or by other drugs (*e.g.,* anesthetics). Acute failure is rare with oral administration. Propranolol should be given with caution to any patient with inadequate myocardial function, but it may be beneficial if the patient has severe hypertension or a treatable arrhythmia or if excessive sinus rate contributes significantly to the inadequacy. The inotropic action of digitalis is not prevented by propranolol, but both drugs depress A-V conduction. Propranolol can cause A-V dissociation and cardiac arrest in patients with preexisting partial heart block due to digitalis or other factors.

Administration of propranolol, and presumably any β-adrenergic blocking agent that lacks partial agonist activity, renders patients susceptible to a withdrawal syndrome that may be due to supersensitivity of β-adrenergic receptors (due, hypothetically, to adaptive changes in receptor number). Some patients may experience a severe exacerbation of anginal attacks, and myocardial infarction has occurred. Patients being treated for hypertension may have a life-threatening rebound of blood pressure to levels that can exceed pretreatment values. Such problems appear within hours to 1 to 2 days after the drug is abruptly discontinued. Some patients develop premonitory signs and symptoms, such as nervousness, sweating, and tachycardia. If therapy is to be stopped, it should be done gradually. If the patient discontinues his own medication, treatment should be reinstituted promptly and, if there is evidence of difficulty, in the hospital. The withdrawal syndrome is claimed to be less severe in patients who have received a β-adrenergic antagonist with partial agonist activity (e.g., pindolol) (see below; see also Symposium, 1982; Frishman, 1983).

Another important danger from β-adrenergic blockade is an increase in airway resistance, which can be life threatening in asthmatics. Asthma is a contraindication to the use of propranolol. The effectiveness of epinephrine in the treatment of acute allergic reactions may be reduced in patients who receive propranolol chronically. Cardioselective (β_1) adrenergic antagonists should be utilized in asthmatics and other patients with a history of severe allergy. However, none of the compounds developed thus far is sufficiently selective to be considered safe in patients with obstructive airway disease. They should not be administered to such individuals unless the therapist is prepared to counter unwanted bronchoconstriction.

Propranolol augments the hypoglycemic action of insulin by reducing the compensatory effect of sympathoadrenal activation, and masks the tachycardia that is an important sign of developing hypoglycemia. Consequently, any patient susceptible to episodes of hypoglycemia who is also taking propranolol must be taught to respond to subtle signs of hypoglycemia. If possible, propranolol should not be given to diabetic patients who are being treated with insulin or oral hypoglycemic agents.

Side effects of propranolol that are not extensions of the desired pharmacological action are usually not serious and frequently disappear during continued drug administration. Nausea, vomiting, mild diarrhea, and constipation have been reported (see Jacob et al., 1983). CNS effects are not common, but a variety of reactions has been noted, including hallucinations, nightmares, insomnia, lassitude, dizziness, and depression (see Greenblatt and Shader, 1972). In double-blind studies, many of these CNS complaints occurred with equal frequency during administration of a placebo. Rash, fever, and purpura probably reflect an allergic response; they are infrequent but require discontinuation of the drug. Unwanted effects of propranolol have been reviewed by Greenblatt and Koch-Weser (1973).

Therapeutic Uses. Propranolol can be especially useful in the management of hypertension. In general, the drug is combined with a diuretic agent. It is also frequently used as an adjunct to treatment with a vasodilator in order to minimize reflex tachycardia and compensatory increases in cardiac output (see Holland and Kaplan, 1976; see also Chapter 32). Propranolol is indicated for the management of both supraventricular and ventricular arrhythmias. It seems to be especially valuable in the management of arrhythmias associated with digitalis intoxication (see Chapter 31). Propranolol has proven efficacious in the prophylaxis of angina pectoris; this subject is discussed in Chapter 33.

Recent studies with several β-adrenergic antagonists, including propranolol, metoprolol, timolol, and oxprenolol, have indicated their effectiveness in reducing the incidence of reinfarction and death after myocardial infarction. In some studies, treatment was initiated only after patients were clinically stable. In one such trial with timolol, the cumulative reinfarction rates after 33 months of treatment were 20% in the placebo group and 14% in the timolol group (Norwegian Multicenter Study Group, 1981). In those trials in which therapy was initiated early in the acute phase of the attack, the estimated size of the infarct was also reduced. The mechanism presumably involves reduced cardiac work and thus oxygen demands in the presence of β-adrenergic blockade. In the metoprolol trial, where therapy was initiated early, there were 40 deaths (of 698 patients) in the treated group during the initial 3 months after infarction, compared with 62 deaths (of 697 patients) in the control group. After this time all patients in the study received metoprolol (Symposium, 1984). Although such studies are difficult to evaluate from an epidemiological and statistical point of view (Hamptom, 1981), the preponderance of evidence indicates the efficacy of such therapy, and it has been approved and adopted widely. It is generally felt that treatment should be continued for at least 2 years. (*See also* NHLBI, 1982; Taylor *et al.,* 1982; Vedin and Wilhelmsson, 1983; International Collaborative Study Group, 1984.)

Propranolol is also used in *hypertrophic obstructive cardiomyopathies*. In these conditions forceful contraction of the myocardium along a ventricular outflow tract can greatly increase outflow resistance, particularly during exercise. β-Adrenergic blockade may have little effect when the patient is at rest, but it has been shown to improve hemodynamic parameters considerably during exercise, and relatively long-term treatment has been reported to be beneficial (*see* Shand *et al.,* 1971). Propranolol is sometimes useful in the management of tachycardia and arrhythmias in patients with *pheochromocytoma*. However, it is less important than α-adrenergic blockade in this condition and should not be given except in the presence of the latter. When used alone, β-adrenergic blocking drugs can cause a dangerous increase in blood pressure, presumably due to the blockade of vasodilatation in skeletal muscle. This should be less of a concern with selective β_1 antagonists. Similarly,

propranolol can accentuate vasospasm in conditions such as Raynaud's phenomenon.

β-Adrenergic blockade has been shown to have palliative value in a variety of conditions that involve adrenergic signs and symptoms. In *hyperthyroidism* propranolol decreases heart rate, cardiac output, and tremor; the drug provides rapid, dramatic improvement in thyroid crises (*see* Malcolm, 1972; Chapter 60). Propranolol has been claimed to reduce portal hypertension in patients with alcoholic cirrhosis. In a controlled clinical trial in patients with cirrhosis and a history of recurrent bleeding from esophageal varices, propranolol was reported to reduce the incidence of bleeding (Lebrec *et al.,* 1981). However, in a subsequent study in patients with varices from cirrhosis of unspecified cause, propranolol was not found to be efficacious (Burroughs *et al.,* 1983). Propranolol is effective in controlling *acute panic symptoms* in individuals who are required to perform in public or in other anxiety-provoking situations. Thus, public speakers and actors appear to be considerably calmed by the prophylactic administration of the drug, and the performance of musicians may be improved (Brantigan *et al.,* 1982). Tachycardia, palpitations, and other evidence of increased sympathetic activity are reduced. A central mechanism of action has been suggested to explain the beneficial effects of propranolol in various anxiety states, but peripheral block of symptoms such as palpitation and tremor, which tend to reinforce the anxiety, appears to be the most likely mechanism (*see* Bonn *et al.,* 1972). Propranolol is not effective in the management of chronic anxiety or in anxiety where somatic symptoms are not significant.

Well-controlled studies have demonstrated that propranolol is an effective agent for the *prophylaxis of migraine* (Weber and Reinmuth, 1972). The pathophysiology of migraine is complex and incompletely understood, and the mechanism of action of propranolol to prevent such headaches is unknown (*see* Chapter 39). Propranolol has *not* been demonstrated to be an effective agent for the management of the symptoms of an acute attack. The dose of propranolol for the prophylaxis of migraine must be determined for each patient. The usual procedure is to begin with 80 mg per day in single or divided doses. If no effect is observed, this is gradually increased to a maximal dose of 240 mg per day. If there is no benefit in 4 to 6 weeks, therapy with propranolol is gradually discontinued. Other β-adrenergic antagonists that lack partial agonist activity also have been reported to be effective in preventing migraine attacks. Agents that possess partial agonist activity are apparently less effective or ineffective, perhaps because they dilate cerebral blood vessels (Peatfield, 1983).

NADOLOL

Nadolol is a long-acting, nonselective β-adrenergic receptor blocking agent. It is not metabolized extensively and is excreted largely unchanged in the urine. It has a half-life of approximately 16 to 20 hours and therefore can be administered once daily for its antihypertensive activity. Dosage should be reduced in patients with impaired renal function.

In contrast to propranolol, nadolol does not possess membrane-stabilizing activity; it also lacks partial agonist activity. Because of its low solubility in lipid, nadolol does not readily pass the blood-brain barrier. The usefulness of agents such as atenolol and nadolol in hypertension, despite the fact that they do not readily enter the CNS, strongly suggests that the antihypertensive action of this class of agents is not mediated centrally (*see* Symposium, 1979). The major adverse reactions that follow the administration of nadolol appear to be the same as those described above for propranolol. The pharmacological properties of nadolol have been reviewed by Frishman (1981).

Nadolol (CORGARD) is available for oral administration in tablets (40 to 160 mg). The usual initial dose, either for angina pectoris or hypertension, is 40 mg once daily. Dosage is gradually adjusted upward in increments of 40 to 80 mg until optimal effects are obtained. A dose of 80 to 240 mg is usually required for treatment of angina. For hypertension, 80 to 320 mg is usually satisfactory, although 640 mg per day may be required.

TIMOLOL

Timolol is a nonselective β-adrenergic antagonist without demonstrable local anesthetic properties; it has minimal intrinsic sympathomimetic activity. Timolol is five to ten times more potent than propranolol as a β-adrenergic blocking agent (Scriabine *et al.*, 1973). Although timolol is well absorbed when given orally, it undergoes considerable first-pass hepatic metabolism. Timolol and its metabolites are excreted in the urine relatively rapidly, and the half-life in plasma is approximately 4 hours.

Timolol is effective in the management of hypertension and, like other β-adrenergic blocking agents, is probably useful in the management of patients with angina pectoris (*see* Frishman, 1982). In addition, timolol has been shown to be effective in reducing the incidence of reinfarction and death after myocardial infarction (*see* above).

Timolol maleate (BLOCADREN) is available in tablets that contain 5, 10, or 20 mg; the usual initial dose is 10 mg twice daily. Modification of dosage to achieve optimal antihypertensive effects should be instituted at intervals of at least 7 days. The usual maintenance dose is 20 to 40 mg per day. For long-term use to prevent recurrence of myocardial infarction, timolol is administered in a dose of 10 mg twice daily.

Timolol maleate is also available as an ophthalmic preparation (TIMOPTIC) for the treatment of chronic wide-angle glaucoma, aphakic glaucoma, and secondary glaucoma. β-Adrenergic blocking agents have been shown to lower intraocular pressure, presumably by reducing the production of aqueous humor; however, the exact mechanism of this effect is unclear. Timolol does not change the size of the pupil nor the tone of the ciliary body, and it does not interfere with vision. The drug is administered as eyedrops, and solutions of 0.25 and 0.5% are available. The recommended initial dosage is 1 drop of 0.25% timolol solution in the affected eye twice a day. The duration of the beneficial effect of timolol is in excess of 7 hours. Although mild ocular irritation is noted occasionally, the side effects with this agent are minimal; patients may rarely complain of blurred vision. Systemic absorption of the drug can occur, leading to slowing of the heart, and the drug should be used with caution in individuals with asthma, heart block, or heart failure.

In a comparative study of timolol and pilocarpine in the management of wide-angle glaucoma, Boger and associates (1978) demonstrated that these agents reduce intraocular pressure to an equal degree. Preparations of timolol were better accepted by the patients, since there was no evidence of miosis and spasm of accommodation. In this study, tolerance to the effect of timolol did not develop over a period of 10 weeks.

PINDOLOL

Pindolol is a nonselective β-adrenergic antagonist with considerable partial agonist activity; it lacks membrane-stabilizing activity in usual doses. In man, the intrinsic sympathomimetic activity of pindolol is evidenced by a smaller reduction in resting cardiac output and heart rate than is seen with agents that are not partial agonists. Thus, pindolol may be preferred in individuals with less cardiac reserve or who are liable to severe bradycardia. However, the increases in cardiac output and heart rate associated with exercise appear to be blocked by pindolol to a degree comparable to that seen with other β-adrenergic blocking agents.

Although pindolol is efficiently absorbed and undergoes relatively little first-pass metabolism in the liver, approximately 50% of the drug is eventually metabolized. The principal metabolites are hydroxylated derivatives, which are subsequently conjugated with either glucuronide or sulfate and excreted in the urine. The half-life of pindolol is relatively short, averaging 3 to 4 hours. However, the antihypertensive effect and other effects of pindolol persist for a considerably longer period.

The major current indication for pindolol is as an antihypertensive agent, although its potential is probably similar to that of other nonselective β-adrenergic blocking agents. Side effects are also similar to those seen with the other drugs in this class. Because of its intrinsic sympathomimetic activity, it has been argued that supersensitivity to catecholamines, exacerbation of angina, and increased likelihood of myocardial infarction and ventricular arrhythmias are less likely to occur following abrupt withdrawal of pindolol. Although there have been several reports of enhanced sensitivity to catecholamines following abrupt termination of pindolol, the effects appear to be less marked with this agent than with propranolol, metoprolol, or other agents that lack intrinsic sympathomimetic activity. Nevertheless, it seems prudent to reduce the dosage of pindolol gradually when therapy is discontinued (Rangno *et al.*, 1982; Symposium, 1982; Frishman, 1983; Schirger *et al.*, 1983).

Pindolol (VISKEN) is available in 5- and 10-mg tablets. The recommended initial dose is 10 mg twice daily or 5 mg three times a day. Dosage is generally increased at intervals of 2 to 3 weeks and in increments of 10 mg per day. The maximal recommended dose is approximately 60 mg per day.

CARDIOSELECTIVE (β_1) ADRENERGIC BLOCKING AGENTS: METOPROLOL

Metoprolol is a relatively selective β_1-adrenergic antagonist that is devoid of agonist activity. Metoprolol effectively inhibits the inotropic and chronotropic responses to isoproterenol; its potency in this regard is similar to that of propranolol. In contrast, to inhibit the vasodilator response to isoproterenol, the dose of metoprolol must be 50 to 100 times that of propranolol. This relative β_1 selectivity of metoprolol is the basis for its potential therapeutic advantage over less selective agents (Ablad *et al.*, 1973).

Metoprolol reduces plasma renin activity in hypertensive patients and in normal subjects and inhibits the rise in the plasma renin activity normally induced by cardiovascular stress, such as prolonged standing. These observations form part of the evidence for the classification of receptors in juxtaglomerular cells as β_1.

Absorption, Distribution, and Excretion. Metoprolol is efficiently and rapidly absorbed from the gastrointestinal tract. However, metoprolol, like propranolol, is subject to first-pass metabolism in the liver, and, in man, only about 40% of the drug reaches the systemic circulation. Peak concentrations in plasma are achieved after 90 minutes (*see* Brogden *et al.*, 1977). Metoprolol has a relatively short half-life in the plasma, averaging about 3 hours. The drug is extensively metabolized in the body, and 10% or less of the drug is excreted unchanged. The metabolites of metoprolol, which include hydroxylated and O-demethylated compounds, appear to lack significant pharmacological activity. There is genetic polymorphism in the hydroxylation of metoprolol; slow hydroxylators may have markedly higher concentrations of the active drug in plasma (Lennard *et al.*, 1982).

Toxicity, Side Effects, and Precautions. Metoprolol causes some reduction in forced expiratory volume (FEV_1) in asthmatic patients, but the effect is less than that produced by propranolol when the drugs are administered in doses that cause equal degrees of β_1-adrenergic blockade. In contrast to propranolol, metoprolol does not significantly inhibit the bronchodilatation induced by isoproterenol. However, exacerbation of respiratory symptoms has occurred in asthmatic patients who have received relatively high doses of metoprolol. Such individuals should probably not be treated with metoprolol unless bronchoconstriction is controlled simultaneously with a β_2-adrenergic agonist or other antiasthmatic drug (Brogden *et al.*, 1977).

There is some evidence that metoprolol may impair glucose tolerance in diabetic patients and perhaps in normal individuals, implying that the β-receptor-mediated release of insulin is to some degree inhibited by this drug. Should hypoglycemia occur in a diabetic patient, metoprolol, like propranolol, can mask some of the signs because of inhibition of the associated reflex tachycardia.

The most common side effects associated with the administration of metoprolol are fatigue, headache, dizziness, and insomnia. These effects are generally not sufficiently severe to require cessation of treatment.

As with all β-adrenergic antagonists, metoprolol should not be used if there is a risk of congestive heart failure unless the patient is monitored closely; the administration of digitalis may be necessary. Similarly, the drug must be used with caution in individuals with disturbances of cardiac conduction.

Preparations, Routes of Administration, and Dosage. *Metoprolol tartrate* (LOPRESSOR) is available for oral use in 50- and 100-mg tablets. The initial dosage is 100 mg daily in single or divided doses, and this may be gradually increased to a maximum of 450 mg per day, depending upon the response.

Metoprolol is also available in injectable form (5 mg/5 ml) for use in the early phase of suspected or definite acute myocardial infarction. Three bolus injections of 5 mg each are given at 2-minute intervals as soon as the patient's hemodynamic condition has stabilized. Blood pressure, heart rate, and ECG should be monitored. If the patient tolerates the full intravenous dose, oral dosage (50 mg every 6 hours) is started 15 minutes later. Maintenance dosage of 100 mg twice daily is initiated after 2 days. Patients who do not tolerate intravenous metoprolol or who have contraindications to early treatment may be started on maintenance doses as soon as their condition allows. Contraindications include bradycardia (heart rate < 45 beats/min), heart block greater than first degree, systolic blood pressure less than 100 mm Hg, or moderate-to-severe cardiac failure.

Therapeutic Uses. Metoprolol is an effective antihypertensive agent, and its efficacy appears to be comparable to that of propranolol in the management of mild or moderate disease (*see* Koch-Weser, 1979). Metoprolol is frequently administered in combination with other antihypertensive drugs (*see* Chapter 32). Metoprolol is also effective in the control of anginal attacks. As described above, metoprolol reduces the incidence of recurrent myocardial infarctions and mortality in patients who receive the drug after an infarction. It also reduces the apparent size of the infarct and the incidence of fatal arrhythmias.

ATENOLOL

Atenolol is a selective β_1-adrenergic receptor blocking agent with insignificant partial agonist activity and weak membrane-stabilizing properties (*see* Robertson *et al.*, 1983). The drug is incompletely absorbed when administered orally and is excreted largely unchanged in the urine. Atenolol has a half-life in plasma of approximately 6 to 8 hours, but its antihypertensive effect appears to last for a considerably longer period. It can thus be administered once a day for the treatment of hypertension. The dosage interval should be increased if renal impairment is significant. Like nadolol, atenolol does not appear to enter the CNS to a significant degree; however, fatigue and depression are not uncommon. Other side effects and precautions are similar to those observed with metoprolol. Unlike nonselective β blocking agents, atenolol does not appear to potentiate insulin-induced hypoglycemia. This agent can thus be used with caution in diabetics and in patients with bronchoconstrictive disease whose hypertension is not controlled by other antihypertensive medication.

Comparisons of atenolol and metoprolol with nonselective β blockers in hypertensive patients reveal that each agent reduces systolic blood pressure to a comparable degree in usual therapeutic doses. However, during infusion of epinephrine and presumably during stress, patients treated with atenolol or metoprolol experience a much smaller elevation of systolic and diastolic blood pressures than do subjects who have received a nonselective antagonist (Houben *et al.*, 1982; McGibney *et al.*, 1983). This might be expected, since epinephrine-mediated vascular dilatation, which involves β_2 receptors, is not blocked by the β_1-selective agents.

Atenolol (TENORMIN) is available in 50- and 100-mg tablets for oral use. Initial dosage is generally 50 mg once a day. If optimal response is not obtained in 1 to 2 weeks, the dose may be increased to 100 mg per day.

OTHER β-ADRENERGIC BLOCKING AGENTS

Many β-adrenergic blocking agents have been synthesized since the introduction of propranolol and the realization that this class of agents has a diverse number of therapeutic applications. In addition to those described above, several agents are still under investigation and have not been approved for general use in the United States. Their properties are summarized in Table 9–1.

LABETALOL

Labetalol is an antihypertensive agent with unique and complex pharmacological properties; it exhibits both selective α_1- and nonselective β-adrenergic blocking activity (Brittain and Levy, 1976; Richards and Prichard, 1978). It is also able to inhibit the re-uptake of norepinephrine into nerve terminals. The structural formula of labetalol is as follows:

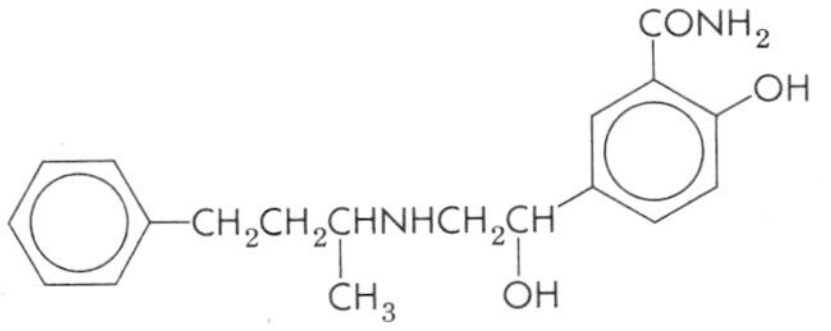

Labetalol has two asymmetrical centers and is supplied as a mixture of four isomers. The relative ability to interact with α- and β-adrenergic receptors differs among them (Sybertz *et al.*, 1981).

Labetalol is approximately one tenth as potent as phentolamine in its ability to block α receptors, and it is approximately one third as potent as propranolol in blocking β receptors. In man, the ratio of α to β blockade has been estimated to be about 1:3 and 1:7 after oral or intravenous administration, respectively. After ganglionic blockade, labetalol has little effect on heart rate, but it produces vasodilatation that is blocked by propranolol (*see* Baum and Sybertz, 1983). Labetalol thus appears to possess intrinsic sympathomimetic activity that is largely confined to β_2-adrenergic receptors.

Labetalol is well absorbed when administered orally. Like propranolol, a considerable fraction of the drug is metabolized in the first circulation through the liver. Its half-life in plasma is approximately 5 hours, and about 5% of the drug is excreted in the urine unchanged.

Labetalol is a potent hypotensive agent (Prichard and Boakes, 1976). It has been used successfully to treat essential hypertension, the hypertension and other cardiovascular effects associated with pheochromocytoma, and the hypertensive response during abrupt withdrawal of clonidine (Rosei *et al.*,

1976). Heart rate and cardiac output are little changed, total peripheral resistance is reduced, and plasma renin activity may be reduced (*see* Bloomfield *et al.*, 1983; Lund-Johansen, 1983; Wallin *et al.*, 1983). Postural hypotension occurs in a small fraction of patients. Other side effects are those that might be expected from a combination of α- and β-receptor blockade. In addition, an increased titer of antinuclear antibodies has been noted in some patients treated with labetalol. Rashes are not uncommonly associated with its use.

Labetalol hydrochloride (NORMODYNE, TRANDATE) was introduced in 1984 for general clinical use in the United States. Its full therapeutic potential thus remains to be evaluated. It is available as 200- and 300-mg tablets. The initial dose is 100 mg twice daily; the usual maintenance dose is 200 to 400 mg twice daily.

III. Centrally Acting Agents That Interfere with Adrenergic Neuronal Function

The activity of the peripheral sympathetic nervous system is regulated by the CNS in a complex manner that remains incompletely understood. Psychic factors can profoundly affect sympathetic activity, suggesting that the cortex is involved in this process. Regions of the brain stem such as the hypothalamus and nucleus tractus solitarius also are critically involved in central sympathetic regulation of cardiovascular activity and blood pressure. Neurons in these regions of the brain stem that are *themselves* adrenergic are involved in regulation of peripheral sympathetic activity, but the nature and mechanism of this control are unclear (*see* below).

Clonidine (and related agents *guanabenz* and *guanfacine*) and *methyldopa* are useful antihypertensive agents that act by inhibiting the outflow of sympathetic neural traffic from the CNS. While their pharmacological properties are primarily presented in Chapter 32, brief descriptions of these drugs follow to facilitate comparison with other agents that interfere with the function of the sympathetic nervous system.

CLONIDINE

Clonidine is an antihypertensive agent that, paradoxically, possesses primarily α₂-adrenergic agonistic properties. However, clonidine owes its antihypertensive

effect to a predominant action on the CNS, where it apparently produces a decrease in the sympathetic outflow from the brain. Guanabenz and guanfacine are also α₂ agonists that appear to act primarily in the CNS. Their pharmacological properties are similar to those of clonidine (*see* Chapter 32).

The major pharmacological actions of clonidine appear to be related to its capacity to stimulate both central and peripheral α₂-adrenergic receptors. Shortly after the parenteral administration of clonidine, an elevation in blood pressure is observed. This appears to be the result of direct interaction of the drug with peripheral α₂ receptors that are thought to reside on the smooth muscle cells of blood vessels in areas that are somewhat remote from adrenergic nerve terminals. Within a short period of time, the hypotensive effect of clonidine becomes apparent, presumably as a result of a direct α₂-agonistic effect in the CNS.

The exact site at which clonidine exerts this central effect is not precisely known. It appears to inhibit central sympathetic outflow by acting upon α₂ receptors in the lower brain stem region, possibly in the nucleus tractus solitarius (Haeusler, 1973a, 1973b, 1974). This region of the brain is rich in cell bodies and nerve terminals that contain epinephrine or norepinephrine (Van der Gugten *et al.*, 1976). In some species, notably the rat, lesion of this region is associated with a fulminating hypertensive response (*see* Brody, 1981). Conversely, electrical stimulation of this region is associated with a reduction in blood pressure (De Jong *et al.*, 1975). However, the actions of clonidine on blood pressure may be mediated in the lower brain stem, in the spinal cord, or at several levels in the cerebrospinal axis.

The hypotensive effect of clonidine persists after depletion of catecholamines in the CNS with reserpine or after destruction of central adrenergic neurons with 6-hydroxydopamine. In addition, the effect of clonidine on blood pressure can be inhibited by yohimbine, which is primarily an α₂ antagonist (Starke and Altmann, 1973). It thus seems likely that the central actions of this drug involve stimulation of postsynaptic α₂-adrenergic receptors. Clonidine has also been shown to exhibit potent agonist activity on presynaptic α₂ receptors. As a consequence, neural release of norepinephrine is inhibited by the drug. This could lead to a reduction of central and peripheral sympathetic neuronal activity, which might contribute to the reduced peripheral sympathetic outflow. However, this effect seems to be less significant than the action of clonidine on postsynaptic α₂ receptors in the brain stem.

METHYLDOPA

It is now generally accepted that methyldopa exerts its antihypertensive effect by a central mechanism (Porter *et al.*, 1977; *see*

Chapter 32). The drug enters the CNS quite readily, and it is then decarboxylated to α-methyldopamine and β-hydroxylated to α-methylnorepinephrine in central adrenergic neurons. The α-methylnorepinephrine that is released from such neurons is a potent agonist at α_2 receptors in the CNS and, in some manner, perhaps analogous to that of clonidine, inhibits central sympathetic outflow. α-Methylnorepinephrine, like clonidine, is a more potent stimulator at α_2 receptors than at α_1 receptors (Starke, 1977).

IV. Adrenergic Neuron Blocking Agents

Interference with chemical mediation at postganglionic adrenergic nerve endings can occur by several mechanisms, including depletion of the stores of mediator and direct prevention of its release. However, many drugs in this class appear to act by more than one mechanism, and the contribution of each to a given effect is often unclear. It is particularly difficult to assess the contribution of reduced norepinephrine content to inhibition of the function of adrenergic neurons. In some cases block occurs only after extensive depletion; in others, with only minor changes in total content. In the latter instance the assumption has often been made that a crucial "pool" or "compartment" of transmitter has been depleted. However, it is equally likely in such cases that the blockade of the adrenergic neuron is unrelated to the depletion of norepinephrine.

GUANETHIDINE

Guanethidine may be considered representative of drugs that depress the function of postganglionic adrenergic nerves. Guanethidine and related compounds, such as bretylium (see below), have a strongly basic moiety such as the guanidine grouping or a quaternary nitrogen. The structural formula of guanethidine is as follows:

Guanethidine

Locus and Mechanism of Action. The major effect of guanethidine is inhibition of responses to stimulation of sympathetic nerves and to indirectly acting sympathomimetic amines (e.g., tyramine, amphetamine). The site of this inhibition is clearly presynaptic and, during chronic administration of guanethidine, it is due to impaired release of neurotransmitter from peripheral adrenergic neurons.

Guanethidine has considerable local anesthetic activity, but concentrations that prevent responses to adrenergic nerve stimulation do not block conduction along adrenergic axons. Essentially complete inhibition of responses to adrenergic nerve activity can develop very rapidly, and this change precedes any detectable alteration in tissue stores of catecholamines, which subsequently decline slowly. Chronic administration of guanethidine can, however, greatly reduce tissue concentrations of norepinephrine, and the depletion persists for several days after the drug has been discontinued.

Guanethidine is taken up by and stored in adrenergic nerves, and this accumulation is essential for its action. Uptake involves the same mechanism responsible for the nerve membrane transport of norepinephrine, and the uptake and subsequent action of guanethidine can thus be inhibited by sympathomimetic amines, phenoxybenzamine, cocaine, phenothiazines, and tricyclic antidepressants. Guanethidine apparently accumulates in and displaces norepinephrine from intraneuronal storage granules, and is itself released by nerve stimulation. Thus, it fits the definition of a "false transmitter," but this mechanism appears not to be responsible for its effects. Guanethidine can also be released by reserpine, amphetamine, and tyramine; release by the latter two drugs is associated with a decreased response. (See Boura and Green, 1965; Furst, 1967; Mitchell and Oates, 1970; Kirpekar and Furchgott, 1972; Shand et al., 1973.)

A considerable part of the norepinephrine released from adrenergic nerve terminals by guanethidine is first deaminated by intraneuronal MAO. However, sufficient amounts of unchanged norepinephrine are released initially to produce sympathomimetic effects, including hypertension, contraction of the nictitating membrane, piloerection, and cardiac stimulation. Guanethidine directly depresses the myocardium previously depleted of catecholamines.

Chronic administration of guanethidine produces a supersensitivity of effector cells that is very similar to that due to sympathetic postganglionic denervation. It reaches a maximum in 10 to 14 days, is greater for norepinephrine than for epinephrine, and can be explained by chronic absence of released mediator. Guanethidine can also cause an acute increase in the sensitivity of tissues to catecholamines. This could involve a "presynaptic" component due to competition for the amine transport mechanism at the nerve membrane.

PHARMACOLOGICAL PROPERTIES

The most important effects of guanethidine are attributable to reduction of responses to sympathetic nerve activation because of diminution in the release of transmitter. Thus, in contrast to adrenergic blocking agents, responses mediated by α- and β-adrenergic receptors are suppressed about equally. Guanethidine usually causes a roughly parallel shift to the right of frequency-response curves for stimulation of adrenergic nerves, but with some preferential block of responses to low frequencies. The concentration of catecholamines in the adrenal medulla is not lowered by guanethidine, and responses that involve the release of amines from this site may be unaffected or even augmented. Similarly, concentrations of catecholamines in the CNS are not altered by guanethidine, since this polar drug does not penetrate the blood-brain barrier in sufficient concentrations to exert prominent CNS effects.

Cardiovascular System. Rapid intravenous injection of guanethidine produces a characteristic triphasic response. There is an initial rapid fall in blood pressure associated with increased cardiac output and decreased peripheral resistance; the latter is probably due to a transient direct action of the drug on resistance vessels. The fall in blood pressure is followed by hypertension, which may persist for several hours and is much accentuated by prior ganglionic blockade or spinal cord section. Infusion of the doses employed in man causes a definite, but relatively small and transient increase in blood pressure.

In both laboratory animals and man, the initial changes are followed by a progressive fall in both systemic and pulmonary arterial pressures that may last for several days. This period of hypotension is usually associated with bradycardia, decreased pulse pressure, and decreased cardiac output. Systolic pressure in the erect position is most markedly reduced, and changes in supine blood pressure are often small. Peripheral resistance is not usually decreased, but in view of the reduced cardiac output, the absence of compensatory vasoconstriction is indicative of some impairment of sympathetic regulation of vascular tone. At least under resting conditions the distribution of blood flow is not greatly affected, although the hepatosplanchnic and renal beds may receive a smaller percentage of the cardiac output after guanethidine.

During chronic administration of guanethidine, the cardiac output may return toward or to normal, probably as a result of the sodium and water retention and increased blood volume induced by guanethidine. The heart rate is usually decreased for the duration of the antihypertensive response. The effect of guanethidine on plasma renin activity has received little attention, but it appears to cause a decrease, as do most other drugs and procedures that decrease stimulation at β_1-adrenergic receptors in the kidney.

Guanethidine inhibits cardiovascular reflexes such as those elicited by bilateral carotid artery occlusion in laboratory animals or by the Valsalva maneuver or cold pressor test in man. Blockade may be incomplete with the doses usually employed in man. However, a significant antihypertensive effect is always associated with some impairment of cardiovascular adjustments, and postural and exercise hypotension are common. (*See* review by Sannerstedt and Conway, 1970.)

Other Effects. Guanethidine has been studied primarily for its cardiovascular effects. However, it has been shown to produce a generalized depression of responses to sympathetic nerve stimulation and augmentation of responses to catecholamines in both *in-vivo* and *in-vitro* experiments on a large number of tissues and organs.

Guanethidine and most other adrenergic neuron blocking drugs increase *gastrointestinal motility* and can cause diarrhea. This is commonly attributed to parasympathetic predominance after blockade of adrenergic fibers, but it is not well correlated with such blockade; for example, reserpine causes relatively more and bethanidine relatively less diarrhea than does guanethidine.

Absorption, Fate, and Excretion. Under the usual conditions of chronic oral administration, absorption of guanethidine can vary from 3 to about 30%; it appears to be relatively constant in a given patient. However, differences in absorption account for only part of the wide variation in dose required for a satisfactory antihypertensive effect. Guanethidine is rapidly cleared by the kidney, but small amounts may remain in the body for as long as 14 days; retention probably involves both specific (adrenergic nerves) and nonspecific tissue uptake. Almost all the guanethidine that enters the circulation in man is accounted for by renal excretion of the parent compound and of two more polar and much less active metabolites. Metabolism appears to be by hepatic microsomal enzymes, and the percentage metabolized is considerably higher after oral than after parenteral administration. (*See* McMartin and Simpson, 1971.)

Preparations, Route of Administration, and Dosage. *Guanethidine monosulfate* (ISMELIN SULFATE) is available in 10- and 25-mg tablets for oral administration. The usual daily dose is 25 to 50 mg, but it varies widely; because of its long duration of action, a single daily dose is satisfactory. The starting dose for ambulatory patients is usually 10 mg, and this may be increased at intervals of about 1 week until the desired effects are obtained or unacceptable side effects supervene. Carefully supervised patients in the hospital may receive a somewhat higher initial dose, and it may be increased more rapidly.

Toxicity, Side Effects, and Precautions. The effects of guanethidine are cumulative over extended periods. Adverse effects can appear or progress for many days or even weeks after an increase in dosage, and may not subside for several days after complete cessation of therapy. The therapeutic effect of guanethidine can be antagonized by tricyclic antidepressants (Mitchell *et al.*, 1970), and a similar antagonism has been reported with chlorpromazine. If high doses of guanethidine are administered to overcome such antagonism, subsequent withdrawal of, for example, a tricyclic antidepressant can lead to profound hypotension and shock if the dose of guanethidine is not adjusted appropriately beforehand. Sensitization by guanethidine to some directly acting sympathomimetics found in "cold remedies" can result in hypertensive crises.

The most important complication of guanethidine therapy is *postural hypotension;* it is most prominent shortly after arising from sleep and may be accentuated by hot weather, alcohol, or exercise. Hypotensive episodes may be associated with symptoms of cerebral and myocardial ischemia. It is important that both standing and supine blood pressures be considered in adjusting dosage. A generalized subjective "weakness" is common; it is partially but not entirely attributable to postural hypotension. Fluid retention occurs and can lead to edema and resistance to the antihypertensive effect if a diuretic is not given concurrently. Guanethidine can also decrease myocardial competence by decreasing adrenergic nerve effects, and this plus fluid accumulation can lead to frank heart failure in patients with limited cardiac reserve. Some tendency to diarrhea is associated with guanethidine therapy in a high percentage of cases, but this can often be controlled by relatively small doses of an anticholinergic agent, an opioid, or a kaolin-pectin preparation. Guanethidine can cause severe hypertensive reactions in patients with pheochromocytoma.

Therapeutic Uses. The only major use of guanethidine is in the treatment of *hypertension*. This subject is discussed in Chapter 32. It also effectively controls the pressor episodes associated with the hyperreflexia of high spinal cord lesions.

GUANADREL

The pharmacological properties of guanadrel are similar to those of guanethidine. Its structural formula is as follows:

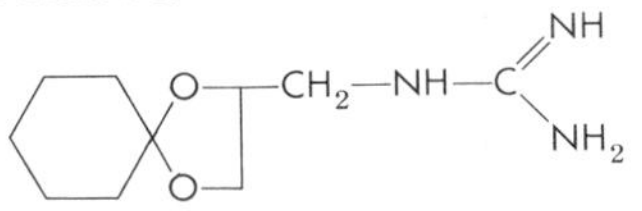

Guanadrel

Guanadrel appears to exert its antihypertensive action by blocking the release of norepinephrine from adrenergic nerve terminals. The antihypertensive effect is more pronounced in the standing position, and postural hypotension, dizziness, and weakness on standing are frequent side effects. Patients may exhibit increased sensitivity to circulating catecholamines.

Guanadrel is rapidly absorbed after oral administration. The half-life of the drug is approximately 10 hours, and a significant fraction of guanadrel is eliminated unchanged in the urine. The maximal hypotensive effect is achieved approximately 4 to 6 hours after oral administration. Guanadrel does not enter the CNS. As with guanethidine, tricyclic antidepressants and phenothiazines interfere with the action of guanadrel, and indirectly acting sympathomimetic amines can reverse the effect of the drug.

Preparations, Route of Administration, and Dosage. *Guanadrel sulfate* (HYLOREL) is available for oral administration in 10- and 25-mg tablets. The usual initial dose is 10 mg per day. This is adjusted at weekly or monthly intervals. The usual dosage range for control of hypertension is 20 to 75 mg per day, divided into two or more doses.

BRETYLIUM

Choline 2,6-xylyl ether (TM10) was the first of many strongly basic compounds shown to inhibit responses to adrenergic nerve stimulation without impairing responses to exogenous catecholamines; interest in this type of specific blockade of adrenergic nerves led to the study of many congeners, of which *bretylium* was the first to be used in man.

Discovered in the late 1950s, bretylium was first regarded as a potentially useful antihypertensive agent. Its development was greatly hampered, however, because of its poor and unpredictable absorption after oral administration. More recently, bretylium has been demonstrated to be an effective antiarrhythmic agent, and it is now available for use in the United States for that purpose. Only the effects of bretylium on the function of the adrenergic neuron will be discussed here; other pharmacological properties of this drug are described in Chapter 31.

Bretylium, like guanethidine, inhibits the release of norepinephrine from adrenergic nerve endings. Autoradiographic studies have shown that the drug is concentrated in adrenergic nerve terminals, and it appears to exert a selective local anesthetic effect at that site. As with many compounds that affect sympathetic neurons, bretylium exerts multiple effects on the metabolism of norepinephrine. Acute, parenteral administration of bretylium may be associated with sympathomimetic effects as a result of the capacity of this agent to release norepinephrine from nerve terminals. Subsequently, bretylium blocks the release of norepinephrine associated with nerve stimulation. Bretylium also inhibits the uptake of norepinephrine and epinephrine into adrenergic nerve endings. As a consequence, bretylium is able to potentiate the actions of circulating catecholamines.

Bretylium and guanethidine produce very similar early inhibition of responses to adrenergic nerve stimulation and to amphetamine and other indirectly acting sympathomimetics, although the action of bretylium is more readily antagonized by such drugs. Agents that block the amine transport mechanism at adrenergic nerve-terminal membranes, such as imipramine, inhibit the action of both guanethidine and bretylium. It is possible that this particular drug interaction can be used to advantage. Bretylium is a useful antiarrhythmic agent; however, postural hypotension is a major side effect. Since the antiarrhythmic action is not dependent on the uptake of bretylium into the adrenergic neuron, whereas hypotension due to neuronal blockade is, inhibition of bretylium uptake into the neuron would be expected to eliminate the side effect. Woosley and associates (1982) have shown that protriptyline is able to antagonize the hypotensive effect of bretylium without reducing the antiarrhythmic efficacy of the drug.

In contrast to guanethidine, a single blocking dose of bretylium produces little reduction of the concentrations of catecholamines in tissues. Only large, repeated doses produce depletion. Bretylium can cause an initial increase in tissue catecholamines, antagonize the depleting action of guanethidine, and delay the release of norepinephrine during nerve degeneration. The initial ''sympathomimetic'' effects of bretylium are less prominent and more transient than those of guanethidine. Like guanethidine, bretylium does not block release of catecholamines from the adrenal medulla, and responses of effector cells to circulating catecholamines may be much increased.

BETHANIDINE, DEBRISOQUIN

Two other compounds, *bethanidine* (1-benzyl-2,3-dimethylguanidine) and *debrisoquin* (3,4-dihydro-2[1H]-isoquinolinecarboxamidine), are effective antihypertensive drugs with hemodynamic effects that are essentially the same as those of guanethidine or bretylium. Compared to guanethidine, their durations of action are much shorter, they produce lesser sympathomimetic effects when injected intravenously, and they cause considerably less depletion of norepinephrine stores. In occasional patients the shorter duration of action of bethanidine and debrisoquin or the lesser tendency to produce diarrhea may be a significant advantage. These compounds are not available for general use in the United States.

RESERPINE

History. Descriptions of the use of extracts of plants resembling rauwolfia may be traced back to ancient Hindu ayurvedic writings. They were used in primitive Hindu medicine for a variety of diseases, including snakebite (because of the resemblance of the root to a snake), hypertension, insomnia, and insanity. *Rauwolfia serpentina* (Benth) is a climbing shrub of the Apocynaceae family, indigenous to India and neighboring countries. Therapeutic applications of the whole root for the treatment of psychoses and hypertension were described in an Indian medical journal in 1931 by Sen and Bose. Little attention was paid to this finding until 1955, when Vakil wrote the first report of its antihypertensive effect in a Western medical journal.

In 1954, Kline reported that rauwolfia or reserpine was helpful in the treatment of psychotic patients. Subsequent discovery of the ability of rauwolfia alkaloids and related compounds to deplete biogenic amines from storage sites in the body initiated a great number of investigations directed at elucidating the interactions between these amines and reserpine.

Chemistry. There are a number of rauwolfia alkaloids with complex structures. The structure of reserpine is as follows:

Reserpine

Locus and Mechanism of Action. Reserpine depletes stores of catecholamines and 5-HT in many organs, including the brain and adrenal medulla, and most of its pharmacological effects have been attributed to this action. Depletion is slower and less complete in the adrenal medulla than in other tissues.

Reduced concentrations of catecholamines can be measured within an hour after administration of reserpine, and depletion is maximal by 24 hours. Most of the catecholamine is deaminated intraneuronally, and pharmacological effects of the released mediator are minimal unless MAO has been inhibited. The doses used in most laboratory experiments reduce tissue catecholamines to negligible levels. Major impairment of adrenergic nerve function usually begins at levels below 30% of normal, and is roughly related to the degree of depletion below that value. Tissue catecholamines are restored slowly; consequently, repeated doses have a cumulative action when administered even at intervals of up to a week or longer. Chronic administration

of reserpine in doses of less than 1.0 mg per day produces a marked depletion of the norepinephrine content of the human myocardium.

Depletion of catecholamines by reserpine is at least partially dependent on nerve activity and can be reduced by spinal cord section or ganglionic blockade. Studies with labeled drug indicate that reserpine itself is not released by nerve activity even in the period up to 18 hours after administration when some of the drug is reversibly bound; all reserpine remaining in tissues after 24 to 30 hours is firmly bound and may persist for many days.

It is clear that reserpine interferes with intracellular storage of catecholamines, but the amounts of reserpine in tissues are much too small to assume a stoichiometric displacement. Reserpine antagonizes the uptake of norepinephrine by isolated chromaffin granules, apparently by inhibiting the $ATP\text{-}Mg^{2+}$–dependent uptake mechanism of the granule membrane. This may be irreversible, because it appears that restoration of normal intraneuronal stores of norepinephrine is dependent on transport of new storage vesicles down the axon. Inhibition of reserpine-induced depletion of catecholamines by MAO inhibitors has been attributed to an increased intracellular concentration of free amine. The decrease in norepinephrine synthesis induced by reserpine may be due to block of dopamine uptake into storage granules that contain the enzyme dopamine β-hydroxylase. Furthermore, the increased concentration of free catecholamine presumably feeds back to inhibit tyrosine hydroxylase, since norepinephrine competes with the pterin cofactor for the enzyme (Pfeffer *et al.*, 1975). On the other hand, the compensatory increased firing of adrenergic nerves after reserpine and other drugs that inhibit their effects causes an acute increase in tyrosine hydroxylase activity, and chronic administration of reserpine is associated with induction and increased levels of the enzyme and an increased turnover rate of norepinephrine. (*See* Weiner, 1970; Weiner *et al.*, 1978.)

Supersensitivity to catecholamines is observed following chronic administration of reserpine. The site of change is presumably postjunctional and may be due to alterations of the adrenergic receptors. Such adaptive change is usual following chronic deprivation of transmitter.

Pharmacological Properties. After a transient sympathomimetic effect, seen only after parenteral administration of relatively large doses, reserpine causes a slowly developing fall in blood pressure frequently associated with bradycardia. In recumbent subjects, the reduction in blood pressure may involve a decrease in peripheral resistance; this is most marked in the skin, and cutaneous blood flow may be increased. However, the antihypertensive effect of chronic administration of reserpine is usually associated with a reduced cardiac output (Cohen *et al.*, 1968). Pressor responses, such as those induced by carotid artery occlusion or stimulation of the central end of the cut vagus nerve, are effectively inhibited by the doses of reserpine commonly employed in experimental animals. Most observations in man indicate that cardiovascular reflexes are only partially inhibited, probably because of the small doses administered. However, reflex responses of veins can be comparably depressed by guanethidine and reserpine, and the two drugs appear to have a similar potential to decrease cardiac output and produce postural hypotension at equivalent levels of inhibition of efferent nerve function. (*See* reviews by Alper *et al.,* 1963; Sannerstedt and Conway, 1970.)

Reserpine acts centrally to produce characteristic sedation and a state of indifference to environmental stimuli. These central effects resemble those of the phenothiazines (Chapter 19), but they are not identical. It is assumed that these changes are due to depletion of stores of catecholamines and 5-HT in the brain. Following prolonged administration of high doses, extrapyramidal effects are noted.

Preparations, Route of Administration, and Dosage. The oral antihypertensive dose of reserpine ranges from 0.1 to 1.0 mg daily, usually taken in two divided doses. Higher doses are now rarely employed because of increased side effects. It requires up to 3 weeks for the full antihypertensive effect to develop. Reserpine is now used only rarely in psychiatric patients for its behavioral effects.

The rauwolfia fractions, alkaloids, and derivatives are available in a large variety of preparations. These include the whole root, *Rauwolfia serpentina,* and the purified alkaloid, *reserpine.* Rauwolfia serpentina (RAUDIXIN, others) is available in tablets containing 50 or 100 mg. Orally, 200 to 300 mg of powdered whole root is equivalent to 0.5 mg of reserpine. Reserpine (SANDRIL, SERPASIL, others) is available in tablets that contain 0.1, 0.25, or 1 mg or in capsules that contain 0.5 mg.

Toxicity, Side Effects, and Precautions. Untoward responses to reserpine are predominantly referable to the CNS and the gastrointestinal tract, and have resulted in a progressive reduction in the doses employed in the treatment of hypertension.

The mild sedative effect of small doses may be desirable in some apprehensive patients. However, even doses as small as 0.25 mg per day can produce a considerable incidence of nightmares and psychic depression, sometimes severe enough to require hospitalization or to end in suicide. *Reserpine should not be administered to patients with a history of depressive episodes,* and it should be discontinued if suggestive signs or symptoms develop. Extrapyramidal disturbances rarely occur with the usual antihypertensive dose. Reserpine commonly increases gastrointestinal tone and motility, with abdominal cramps and diarrhea. Single doses of 0.25 mg or more quite consistently increase gastric acid secretion. The secretory effects of chronic administration and their relation to reports of gastrointestinal ulceration and hemorrhage are less clear-cut, but reserpine probably should not be given to patients with a history of peptic ulcer and it should be discontinued if signs or symptoms of peptic ulceration appear. Reserpine quite commonly causes weight gain.

Hypotensive episodes are rare with doses of less than 1 mg of reserpine per day, but patients may be sensitized to this reaction following a cerebrovascular accident. Vascular side effects include flushing and nasal congestion; these are usually of minor importance, but the latter may occasionally cause serious respiratory problems in infants born of mothers receiving reserpine.

In a retrospective study in the United States, subsequently confirmed in the United Kingdom and Finland, it was found that the long-term administration of reserpine as an antihypertensive drug in women was associated with over a threefold increase in the incidence of *carcinoma of the breast* (*see* Boston Collaborative Drug Surveillance Program, 1974; Editorial, 1974). However, considerable controversy ensued over the statistical validity of this conclusion. It remains uncertain if the chronic administration of reserpine is associated with an increased incidence of any type of malignancy.

Therapeutic Uses. The only important application of the cardiovascular effects of reserpine is in the treatment of *hypertension;* this subject is discussed in Chapter 32. Because of the severity of the dose-related side effects of reserpine, the drug is administered in low doses and is used only in conjunction with other types of antihypertensive agents.

SPECIFIC INHIBITORS OF CATECHOLAMINE SYNTHESIS

Much of the work on adrenergic neuron blocking drugs has assumed a cause-and-effect relationship between depletion of norepinephrine stores and failure of nerve function. Consequently, it appeared that inhibition of norepinephrine synthesis would represent the ultimate mechanism of adrenergic neuron blockade. Inhibitors of each step of the biosynthesis have been studied, but major depletion occurs only with drugs that act on the rate-limiting step, the hydroxylation of tyrosine.

METYROSINE

Metyrosine (α-methyltyrosine) is a competitive inhibitor of tyrosine hydroxylase, the enzyme that catalyzes the synthesis of dihydroxyphenylalanine (DOPA) from tyrosine. Inhibition of tyrosine hydroxylase results in a reduction in the rate of synthesis of norepinephrine and dopamine in both the CNS and the periphery. Tissue concentrations of these catecholamines thus gradually decline at a rate that is correlated with the rate of turnover of catecholamines in the tissue. Because of the large stores of catecholamines in the adrenal medulla and the relatively low rate of their turnover in this tissue, depletion of the adrenal medulla or adrenal medullary tumors proceeds relatively slowly.

Metyrosine is well absorbed when administered orally, and a considerable fraction of the drug is excreted unchanged in the urine. A very small fraction of the administered drug is converted to α-methyl analogs of DOPA and other catecholamines.

The pharmacological effects of metyrosine are largely a consequence of inhibition of catecholamine synthesis and result from impaired peripheral and central sympathetic activity. The most common side effect is moderate-to-severe sedation. Extrapyramidal side effects, such as tremor and locomotor impairment, may also be seen. Diarrhea is a common complaint. Because the bulk of the drug is excreted in the urine and this amino acid is relatively insoluble in water, renal crystalluria is a potential hazard; water intake should be maintained at an adequate level.

Metyrosine is used in the management of patients with pheochromocytoma. It is administered preoperatively for at least 5 to 7 days. The drug may be employed for prolonged periods of time in the management of such patients when surgery is not indicated or when a malignant pheochromocytoma is not amenable to surgical resection.

Metyrosine (DEMSER), which is available in 250-mg capsules, is generally administered in an initial dose of 250 mg four times a day. Adequacy of treatment is monitored by measurement of urinary catecholamine metabolites or, if the patient is hypertensive, by monitoring blood pressure. To achieve the desired effect, it may be necessary to increase the dose to 500 mg to 1 g four times a day. Phenoxybenzamine is often employed concurrently (*see* above).

MONOAMINE OXIDASE INHIBITORS

Monoamine oxidase (MAO) inhibitors were introduced into therapy for the treatment of depression in 1957. Paradoxically, these agents, which inhibit the oxidative deamination of norepinephrine, were found to cause hypotension. However, because of their toxicity and the occurrence of dangerous interactions between MAO inhibitors and certain other drugs and foods, they are now used only occasionally as antidepressants (*see* Chapter 19); they currently have little or no place in the management of hypertension.

The effects of MAO inhibitors on blood pressure are attributed both to a central effect, where the protected norepinephrine appears to stimulate α_2 receptors (in analogy with the actions of methyldopa and clonidine), and to the accumulation of false transmitters (impotent phenylethylamines) in peripheral adrenergic neurons. The false-transmitter concept is discussed in Chapter 8.

There has been a resurgence of interest in MAO inhibitors as possible therapeutic agents following the discovery that there are isozymes of MAO and that these isozymes have different substrate specificities and can be inhibited selectively. This subject is discussed in Chapters 19 and 21.

DRUGS THAT DESTROY ADRENERGIC NERVE FIBERS

Interest in 6-hydroxydopamine (6-OHDA) was first aroused by the observation that it caused a prolonged decrease in the catecholamine content of the heart (Porter *et al.,* 1963). This effect was subsequently shown to be due to destruction of sympathetic nerve endings. Most peripheral sympathetic nerves are affected by adequate doses, but there are some quantitative differences in sensitivity. The adrenal medulla and peripheral cholinergic neurons are unaffected. 6-OHDA does not penetrate the CNS from the blood stream, but it can act on central neurons after local or intraventricular administration. 6-OHDA does not damage peripheral adrenergic nerve-cell bodies or proximal axons in adult animals, and regeneration of the terminal usually occurs completely. In newborn animals the entire adrenergic neuron may be destroyed and a permanent sympathectomy produced. This is usually more complete than that produced by antisera against the nerve-growth factor (immunosympathectomy) (*see* Levi-Montalcini and Angeletti, 1966). There is little regeneration of central neurons at any age.

The action of 6-OHDA on adrenergic nerves is dependent on its accumulation by the nerve-membrane amine pump and can be prevented by drugs such as desipramine that block this process. Although 6-OHDA is taken up by intraneuronal storage granules, this step appears not to be necessary for nerve damage because the drug is fully effective in animals pretreated with reserpine.

While 6-OHDA has been evaluated for the long-term therapy of glaucoma, repeated subconjunctival injections have been necessary and have caused inflammation and fibrosis. The pharmacology of 6-OHDA has been reviewed by Thoenen and Tranzer (1973) and Kostrzewa and Jacobowitz (1974).

Ablad, B.; Carlsson, B.; Carlsson, E.; Dahlof, C.; Ek, L.; and Hultberg, E. Cardiac effects of β-adrenergic antagonists. *Adv. Cardiol.*, **1974**, *12*, 290–302.

Ablad, B.; Carlsson, E.; and Ek, L. Pharmacological studies of two new cardioselective adrenergic beta-receptor antagonists. *Life Sci.*, **1973**, *12*, Pt. I, 107–119.

Assem, E. S. K., and Schild, H. O. Antagonism by β-adrenoceptor blocking agents of the antianaphylactic effect of isoprenaline. *Br. J. Pharmacol.*, **1971**, *42*, 620–630.

Benson, M. K.; Berrill, W. T.; Cruickshank, J. M.; and Sterling, G. S. A comparison of four β-adrenoceptor antagonists in patients with asthma. *Br. J. Clin. Pharmacol.*, **1978**, *5*, 415–419.

Boger, W. P., III; Steinert, R. F.; Puliafito, C. A.; and Pavan-Langston, D. Clinical trial comparing timolol ophthalmic solution to pilocarpine in open-angle glaucoma. *Am. J. Ophthalmol.*, **1978**, *86*, 8–18.

Bonn, J. A.; Turner, P.; and Hicks, D. C. Beta-adrenergic receptor blockade with practolol in treatment of anxiety. *Lancet*, **1972**, *1*, 814–815.

Boston Collaborative Drug Surveillance Program. Reserpine and breast cancer. *Lancet*, **1974**, *2*, 669–671.

Brandt, D. R.; Asano, T.; Pedersen, S. E.; and Ross, E. M. Reconstitution of catecholamine-stimulated GTPase activity. *Biochemistry*, **1983**, *22*, 4357–4362.

Brantigan, C. O.; Brantigan, T. A.; and Joseph, N. Effect of beta blockade and beta stimulation on stage fright. *Am. J. Med.*, **1982**, *72*, 88–94.

Brittain, R. T., and Levy, G. P. A review of the animal pharmacology of labetalol, a combined alpha and beta adrenoceptor blocking drug. *Br. J. Clin. Pharmacol.*, **1976**, *3*, 681–694.

Brogden, R. N.; Heel, R. C.; Speight, T. M.; and Avery, G. S. Metoprolol: a review of its pharmacological properties and therapeutic efficacy in hypertension. *Drugs*, **1977**, *14*, 321–348.

Buhler, F. R.; Laragh, J. H.; Baer, L.; Vaughn, D. E.; and Brunner, H. R. Propranolol inhibition of renin secretion. *N. Engl. J. Med.*, **1972**, *287*, 1209–1214.

Burns, J. J.; Salvador, R. A.; and Lemberger, L. Metabolic blockade by methoxamine and its analogs. *Ann. N.Y. Acad. Sci.*, **1967**, *139*, 833–840.

Burroughs, A. K.; Jenkins, W. J.; Sherlock, S.; Dunk, A.; Walt, R. P.; Osuafor, T. O. K.; Mackie, S.; and Dick, R. Controlled trial of propranolol for the prevention of recurrent variceal hemorrhage in patients with cirrhosis. *N. Engl. J. Med.*, **1983**, *309*, 1539–1542.

Carliner, N. H.; Denune, D. P.; Finch, C. S., Jr.; and Goldberg, L. I. Sodium nitroprusside treatment of ergotamine-induced peripheral ischemia. *J.A.M.A.*, **1974**, *227*, 308–309.

Chrysant, S. G.; Miller, R. F.; Brown, J. L.; and Danisa, K. Long-term hemodynamic and metabolic effects of trimazosin in essential hypertension. *Clin. Pharmacol. Ther.*, **1981**, *30*, 600–604.

Cohen, S. I.; Young, M. W.; Lau, S. H.; Haft, J. I.; and

Damato, A. N. Effects of reserpine therapy on cardiac output and atrioventricular conduction during rest and controlled heart rates in patients with essential hypertension. *Circulation*, **1968**, *37*, 738–746.

Crout, J. R., and Brown, B. R., Jr. Anesthetic management of pheochromocytoma: the value of phenoxybenzamine and methoxyflurane. *Anesthesiology*, **1969**, *30*, 29–36.

Cubeddu, L. X.; Barnes, E.; Langer, S. Z.; and Weiner, N. Release of norepinephrine and dopamine-β-hydroxylase by nerve stimulation. I. Role of neuronal and extraneuronal uptake and of alpha presynaptic receptors. *J. Pharmacol. Exp. Ther.*, **1974**, *190*, 431–450.

Das, P. K., and Parratt, J. R. Myocardial and haemodynamic effects of phentolamine. *Br. J. Pharmacol.*, **1971**, *41*, 437–444.

De Jong, W.; Zandberg, P.; and Bohus, P. Central inhibitory noradrenergic cardiovascular control. *Prog. Brain Res.*, **1975**, *42*, 285–298.

Dixon, W. R.; Mosimann, W. F.; and Weiner, N. The role of presynaptic feedback mechanisms in regulation of norepinephrine release by nerve stimulation. *J. Pharmacol. Exp. Ther.*, **1979**, *209*, 196–204.

Editorial. Rauwolfia derivatives and cancer. *Lancet*, **1974**, *2*, 701–702.

Engelman, K., and Sjoerdsma, A. Chronic medical therapy for pheochromocytoma: a report of four cases. *Ann. Intern. Med.*, **1964**, *61*, 229–241.

Esler, M.; Zweifler, A.; Randall, O.; and DeQuattro, V. Pathophysiologic and pharmacokinetic determinants of the antihypertensive response to propranolol. *Clin. Pharmacol. Ther.*, **1977**, *22*, 299–308.

Evans, G. H.; Nies, A. S.; and Shand, D. G. The disposition of propranolol. III. Decreased half-life and volume of distribution as a result of plasma binding in man, monkey, dog and rat. *J. Pharmacol. Exp. Ther.*, **1973a**, *186*, 114–122.

Evans, G. H.; Wilkinson, G. R.; and Shand, D. G. The disposition of propranolol. IV. A dominant role for tissue uptake in the dose-dependent extraction of propranolol by the perfused rat liver. *J. Pharmacol. Exp. Ther.*, **1973b**, *186*, 447–454.

Gay, A. J.; Salmon, M. L.; and Wolkstein, M. A. Topical sympatholytic therapy for pathologic lid retraction. *Arch. Ophthalmol.*, **1967**, *77*, 341–344.

Gifford, R. W., Jr. The arteriospastic diseases: clinical significance and management. *Cardiovasc. Clin.*, **1971**, *3*, No. 1, 128–139.

Gilligan, B. S.; Veale, J. L.; and Wodak, J. Propranolol in the treatment of tremor. *Med. J. Aust.*, **1972**, *1*, 320–322.

Graham, R. M., and Pettinger, W. A. Drug therapy: prazosin. *N. Engl. J. Med.*, **1979**, *300*, 232–236.

Green, K. L. The anti-inflammatory effect of catecholamines in the peritoneal cavity and hind paw of the mouse. *Br. J. Pharmacol.*, **1972**, *45*, 322–332.

Gross, G. J., and Winbury, M. M. *Beta* adrenergic blockade on intramyocardial distribution of coronary blood flow. *J. Pharmacol. Exp. Ther.*, **1973**, *187*, 451–464.

Haeusler, G. Activation of the central pathway of the baroreceptor reflex, a possible mechanism of the hypotensive action of clonidine. *Naunyn Schmiedebergs Arch. Pharmacol.*, **1973a**, *278*, 231–246.

———. Further similarities between the action of clonidine and a central activation of the depressor baroreceptor reflex. *Ibid.*, **1973b**, *285*, 1–14.

———. Clonidine-induced inhibition of sympathetic nerve activity: no indication for a central presynaptic or an indirect sympathomimetic mode of action. *Ibid.*, **1974**, *286*, 97–111.

Hampton, J. R. The use of beta blockers for the reduction of mortality after myocardial infarction. *Eur. Heart J.*, **1981**, *2*, 259–268.

Helfant, R. H.; Herman, M. V.; and Gorlin, R. Abnormalities of left ventricular contraction induced by beta adrenergic blockade. *Circulation*, **1971**, *43*, 641–647.

Hollenberg, N. K., and Nickerson, M. Changes in pre- and postcapillary resistance in pathogenesis of hemorrhagic shock. *Am. J. Physiol.*, **1970**, *219*, 1483–1489.

Houben, H.; Thien, T.; and van't Laar, A. Effect of low-dose epinephrine infusion on hemodynamics after selective and nonselective β blockade in hypertension. *Clin. Pharmacol. Ther.*, **1982**, *31*, 685–690.

International Collaborative Study Group. Reduction of infarct size with the early use of timolol in acute myocardial infarction. *N. Engl. J. Med.*, **1984**, *310*, 9–15.

Jacob, H.; Brandt, L. J.; Farkas, P.; and Frishman, W. Beta-adrenergic blockade and the gastrointestinal system. *Am. J. Med.*, **1983**, *74*, 1042–1050.

Kelly, D. T.; Delgado, C. E.; Taylor, D. R.; Pitt, B.; and Ross, R. S. Use of phentolamine in acute myocardial infarction associated with hypertension and left ventricular failure. *Circulation*, **1973**, *47*, 729–735.

Kirpekar, S. M., and Furchgott, R. F. Interaction of tyramine and guanethidine in the spleen of the cat. *J. Pharmacol. Exp. Ther.*, **1972**, *180*, 38–46.

Koch-Weser, J. Beta adrenergic blockade and circulating eosinophils. *Arch. Intern. Med.*, **1968**, *121*, 255–258.

Lebrec, D.; Poynard, T.; Hillon, P.; and Benhamou, J.-P. Propranolol for prevention of recurrent gastrointestinal bleeding in patients with cirrhosis: a controlled study. *N. Engl. J. Med.*, **1981**, *305*, 1371–1374.

Lennard, M. S.; Silas, J. H.; Freestone, S.; Ramsay, L. E.; Tucker, G. T.; and Woods, H. F. Oxidation phenotype—a major determinant of metoprolol metabolism and response. *N. Engl. J. Med.*, **1982**, *307*, 1558–1560.

Levy, B. The adrenergic blocking activity of N-*tert*-butylmethoxamine (butoxamine). *J. Pharmacol. Exp. Ther.*, **1966**, *151*, 413–422.

McDevitt, R. G. The assessment of β-adrenoceptor blocking drugs in man. *Br. J. Clin. Pharmacol.*, **1977**, *4*, 413–425.

McGibney, D.; Singleton, W.; Silke, B.; and Taylor, S. H. Observations on the mechanism underlying the differences in exercise and isoprenaline tachycardia after cardioselective and non-selective β-adrenoceptor antagonists. *Br. J. Clin. Pharmacol.*, **1983**, *15*, 15–19.

McMartin, C., and Simpson, P. The absorption and metabolism of guanethidine in hypertensive patients requiring different doses of the drug. *Clin. Pharmacol. Ther.*, **1971**, *12*, 73–77.

Majid, P. A.; Sharma, B.; and Taylor, S. H. Phentolamine for vasodilator treatment of severe heart-failure. *Lancet*, **1971**, *2*, 719–724.

Minneman, K. P.; Hegstrand, L. R.; and Molinoff, P. B. The pharmacological specificity of beta-1 and beta-2 adrenergic receptors in rat heart and lung *in vitro*. *Mol. Pharmacol.*, **1979a**, *15*, 21–33.

————. Simultaneous determination of beta-1 and beta-2 adrenergic receptors in tissues containing both receptor subtypes. *Ibid.*, **1979b**, *15*, 34–46.

Mitchell, J. R.; Cavanaugh, J. H.; Arias, L.; and Oates, J. A. Guanethidine and related agents. III. Antagonism by drugs which inhibit the norepinephrine pump in man. *J. Clin. Invest.*, **1970**, *49*, 1596–1604.

Mitchell, J. R., and Oates, J. A. Guanethidine and related agents. I. Mechanism of the selective blockade of adrenergic neurons and its antagonism by drugs. *J. Pharmacol. Exp. Ther.*, **1970**, *172*, 100–107.

Mueller, R. A.; Thoenen, H.; and Axelrod, J. Inhibition of neuronally induced tyrosine hydroxylase by nicotinic receptor blockade. *Eur. J. Pharmacol.*, **1970**, *10*, 51–56.

NHLBI β-Blocker Heart Attack Trial Research Group. A randomized trial of propranolol in patients with acute myocardial infarction. I. Mortality results. *J.A.M.A.*, **1982**, *247*, 1707–1714.

Nickerson, M., and Goodman, L. S. Pharmacological properties of a new adrenergic blocking agent:

N,N-dibenzyl-β-chloroethylamine (dibenamine). *J. Pharmacol. Exp. Ther.*, **1947**, *89*, 167–185.

Nies, A. S.; Evans, G. H.; and Shand, D. G. Regional hemodynamic effects of beta-adrenergic blockade with propranolol in the unanesthetized primate. *Am. Heart J.*, **1973**, *85*, 97–102.

Nies, A. S.; McNeil, J. S.; and Schrier, R. W. Mechanism of increased sodium reabsorption during propranolol administration. *Circulation*, **1971**, *44*, 596–604.

Norwegian Multicenter Study Group. Timolol-induced reduction in mortality and reinfarction in patients surviving acute myocardial infarction. *N. Engl. J. Med.*, **1981**, *304*, 801–807.

Owman, C.; Rosengren, E.; and Sjöberg, N.-O. Adrenergic innervation of the human female reproductive organs: a histochemical and chemical investigation. *Obstet. Gynecol.*, **1967**, *30*, 763–773.

Pfeffer, R. I.; Mosimann, W. F.; and Weiner, N. Time course of the effect of reserpine administration on tyrosine hydroxylase activity in adrenal glands and vasa deferentia. *J. Pharmacol. Exp. Ther.*, **1975**, *193*, 533–548.

Pitt, B., and Craven, P. Effect of propranolol on regional myocardial blood flow in acute ischaemia. *Cardiovasc. Res.*, **1970**, *4*, 176–179.

Porter, C. C.; Totaro, J. A.; and Stone, C. A. Effect of 6-hydroxydopamine and some other compounds on the concentration of norepinephrine in the hearts of mice. *J. Pharmacol. Exp. Ther.*, **1963**, *140*, 308–316.

Powell, C. E., and Slater, I. H. Blocking of inhibitory adrenergic receptors by a dichloro analog of isoproterenol. *J. Pharmacol. Exp. Ther.*, **1958**, *122*, 480–488.

Prichard, B. N. C., and Boakes, A. J. Labetalol in long term treatment of hypertension. *Br. J. Clin. Pharmacol.*, **1976**, *3*, 743–750.

Rabkin, R.; Stables, D. P.; Levin, N. W.; and Suzman, M. M. The prophylactic value of propranolol in angina pectoris. *Am. J. Cardiol.*, **1966**, *18*, 370–380.

Rangno, R. E.; Langlois, S.; and Stewart, J. Cardiac hyper- and hyporesponsiveness after pindolol withdrawal. *Clin. Pharmacol. Ther.*, **1982**, *31*, 564–571.

Richards, D. A., and Prichard, B. N. C. Concurrent antagonism of isoproterenol and norepinephrine after labetalol. *Clin. Pharmacol. Ther.*, **1978**, *23*, 253–258.

Robertson, J. I. S.; Kaplan, N. M.; Caldwell, A. D. S.; and Speight, T. M. (eds.). β-Blockade in the 1980s: focus on atenolol. *Drugs*, **1983**, *25*, Suppl. 2, 1–340.

Robin, E.; Cowan, C.; Puri, P.; Ganguly, S.; DeBoyrie, E.; Martinez, M.; Stock, T.; and Bing, R. J. A comparative study of nitroglycerin and propranolol. *Circulation*, **1967**, *36*, 175–186.

Rosei, E. A.; Brown, J. J.; Lever, A. F.; Robertson, A. S.; Robertson, J. I. S.; and Trust, P. M. Treatment of phaeochromocytoma and of clonidine withdrawal hypertension with labetalol. *Br. J. Clin. Pharmacol.*, **1976**, *3*, 809–815.

Ross, E. J.; Prichard, B. N. C.; Kaufman, L.; Robertson, A. I. G.; and Harries, B. J. Preoperative and operative management of patients with phaeochromocytoma. *Br. Med. J.*, **1967**, *1*, 191–198.

Roth, J. A. Guanethidine and adrenaline used in combination in chronic simple glaucoma. *Br. J. Ophthalmol.*, **1973**, *57*, 507–510.

Rydén, L., and others. A double-blind trial of metoprolol in acute myocardial infarction. *N. Engl. J. Med.*, **1983**, *308*, 614–618.

Sandler, G.; Leishman, A. W. D.; and Humberstone, P. M. Guanethidine-resistant hypertension. *Circulation*, **1968**, *38*, 542–551.

Schirger, A.; Sheps, S. G.; Spiekerman, R. E.; Harman, T. R.; and Kleven, M. K. Pindolol, a new β-adrenergic blocking agent with intrinsic sympathomimetic activity in the management of mild and moderate hypertension. *Mayo Clin. Proc.*, **1983**, *58*, 315–318.

Scriabine, A. β-Adrenoceptor blocking drugs in hypertension. *Annu. Rev. Pharmacol. Toxicol.*, **1979**, *19*, 269–284.

Scriabine, A.; Torchiana, M. L.; Stavorski, J. M.; Ludden, C. T.; Minsker, D. H.; and Stone, C. A. Some cardiovascular effects of timolol, a new beta adrenergic blocking agent. *Arch. Int. Pharmacodyn. Ther.*, **1973**, *205*, 76–93.

Sen, G., and Bose, K. C. *Rauwolfia serpentina*, a new Indian drug for insanity and high blood pressure. *Indian Med. World*, **1931**, *2*, 194–201.

Shand, D. G.; Morgan, D. H.; and Oates, J. A. The release of guanethidine and bethanidine by splenic nerve stimulation: a quantitative evaluation showing dissociation from adrenergic blockade. *J. Pharmacol. Exp. Ther.*, **1973**, *184*, 73–80.

Shand, D. G.; Sell, C. G.; and Oates, J. A. Hypertrophic obstructive cardiomyopathy in an infant—propranolol therapy for three years. *N. Engl. J. Med.*, **1971**, *285*, 843–844.

Shorr, R. G. L.; Heald, S. L.; Jeffs, P. W.; Lavin, T. N.; Strohsacker, M. W.; Lefkowitz, R. J.; and Caron, M. G. The β-adrenergic receptor: rapid purification and covalent labeling by photoaffinity cross-linking. *Proc. Natl. Acad. Sci. U.S.A.*, **1982**, *79*, 2778–2782.

Sizemore, G. W., and Winternitz, W. W. Autonomic hyper-reflexia—suppression with alpha-adrenergic blocking agents. *N. Engl. J. Med.*, **1970**, *282*, 795.

Sowton, E.; Smithen, C.; Leaver, D.; and Barr, I. Effect of practolol on exercise tolerance in patients with angina pectoris. *Am. J. Med.*, **1971**, *51*, 63–70.

Starke, K., and Altmann, K. P. Inhibition of adrenergic neurotransmission by clonidine: an action on prejunctional α-receptors. *Neuropharmacology*, **1973**, *12*, 339–347.

Starke, K.; Borowski, E.; and Endo, T. Preferential blockade of presynaptic alpha receptors by yohimbine. *Eur. J. Pharmacol.*, **1975**, *34*, 385–388.

Stokes, G. S.; Weber, M. A.; and Thornell, I. R. β-Blockers and plasma renin activity in hypertension. *Br. Med. J.*, **1974**, *1*, 60–62.

Sybertz, E. J.; Sabin, C. S.; Pula, K. K.; Vander Vliet, G.; Glennon, J.; Gold, E. H.; and Baum, T. Alpha and beta adrenoceptor blocking properties of labetalol and its R,R-isomer, SCH 19927. *J. Pharmacol. Exp. Ther.*, **1981**, *218*, 435–443.

Tarr, M.; Luckstead, E. F.; Jurewicz, P. A.; and Haas, H. G. Effect of propranolol on the fast inward sodium current in frog atrial muscle. *J. Pharmacol. Exp. Ther.*, **1973**, *184*, 599–610.

Taylor, S. H.; Silke, B.; Ebbutt, A.; Sutton, G. C.; Prout, B. J.; and Burley, D. M. A long-term prevention study with oxprenolol in coronary heart disease. *N. Engl. J. Med.*, **1982**, *307*, 1293–1301.

Van der Gugten, J.; Palkovits, M.; Wijnen, H. L. J. M.; and Versteeg, D. H. G. The regional distribution of adrenaline in the rat brain. *Brain Res.*, **1976**, *107*, 171–175.

Waal-Manning, H. J. Which beta-blocker? *Drugs*, **1976**, *12*, 412–441.

Wansbrough, H.; Nakanishi, H.; and Wood, C. The effect of adrenergic receptor blocking drugs on the human uterus. *J. Obstet. Gynaecol. Br. Commonw.*, **1968**, *75*, 189–198.

Weber, M. A.; Brewer, D. D.; Drayer, J. I. M.; Aronow, W. S.; Lipson, J. L.; and Ricci, B. A. A vasodilator that avoids renin stimulation and fluid retention: antihypertensive treatment with trimazosin. *Clin. Pharmacol. Ther.*, **1982**, *31*, 572–578.

Weber, M. A.; Stokes, G. S.; and Gain, J. M. Comparison of the effect of renin release of beta adrenergic antagonists with differing properties. *J. Clin. Invest.*, **1974**, *54*, 1413–1419.

Weber, R. G., and Reinmuth, O. M. The treatment of migraine with propranolol. *Neurology (Minneap.)*, **1972**, *22*, 366–369.

Weiner, N.; Lee, F.-L.; Dreyer, E.; and Barnes, E. The activation of tyrosine hydroxylase in noradrenergic neurons during acute nerve stimulation. *Life Sci.*, **1978**, *22*, 1197–1216.

Woosley, R. L.; Reele, S. B.; Roden, D. M.; Nies, A. S.; and Oates, J. A. Pharmacologic reversal of hypotensive effect complicating antiarrhythmic therapy with bretylium. *Clin. Pharmacol. Ther.*, **1982**, *32*, 313–321.

Monographs and Reviews

Alper, M. H.; Flacke, W.; and Krayer, O. Pharmacology of reserpine and its implications for anesthesia. *Anesthesiology*, **1963**, *24*, 524–542.

Baum, T., and Sybertz, E. J. Antihypertensive actions of an isomer of labetalol and other vasodilator-β-adrenoceptor blockers. *Fed. Proc.*, **1983**, *42*, 176–181.

Berde, B., and Schild, H. O. (eds.). *Ergot Alkaloids and Related Compounds*. Handbuch der Experimentellen Pharmakologie, Vol. 49. Springer-Verlag, Berlin, **1978**.

Berde, B., and Stürmer, E. Introduction to the pharmacology of ergot alkaloids and related compounds as a basis of their therapeutic application. In, *Ergot Alkaloids and Related Compounds*. (Berde, B., and Schild, H. O., eds.) *Handbuch der Experimentellen Pharmakologie*, Vol. 49. Springer-Verlag, Berlin, **1978**, pp. 1–28.

Black, J. W., and Prichard, B. N. C. Activation and blockade of β adrenoceptors in common cardiac disorders. *Br. Med. Bull.*, **1973**, *29*, 163–167.

Bloomfield, S. S.; Lucas, C. P.; Gantt, C. L.; Poland, B. A.; and Medakovic, M. Step II treatment with labetalol for essential hypertension. *Am. J. Med.*, October 17, **1983**, *75*, Suppl., 81–86.

Boura, A. L. A., and Green, A. F. Adrenergic neurone blocking agents. *Annu. Rev. Pharmacol.*, **1965**, *5*, 183–212.

Brody, M. J. New developments in our knowledge of blood pressure regulation. *Fed. Proc.*, **1981**, *40*, 2257–2261.

Dale, H. H. On some physiological actions of ergot. *J. Physiol. (Lond.)*, **1906**, *34*, 163–206.

Ellis, S. Effects on the metabolism. In, *Adrenergic Activators and Inhibitors*. (Szekeres, L., ed.) *Handbook of Experimental Pharmacology*, Vol. 54, Pt. I. Springer-Verlag, Berlin, **1980**, pp. 319–349.

Frishman, W. H. Nadolol: a new β-adrenoceptor antagonist. *N. Engl. J. Med.*, **1981**, *305*, 678–682.

———. Drug therapy: atenolol and timolol, two new systemic beta-adrenoceptor antagonists. *Ibid.*, **1982**, *306*, 1456–1462.

———. Pindolol: a new β-adrenoceptor antagonist with partial agonist activity. *Ibid.*, **1983**, *308*, 940–944.

Frishman, W. H.; Furberg, C. D.; and Friedewald, W. T. Beta-adrenergic blockade for survivors of acute myocardial infarction. *N. Engl. J. Med.*, **1984**, *310*, 830–837.

Furchgott, R. F. The classification of adrenoceptors (adrenergic receptors). An evaluation from the standpoint of receptor theory. In, *Catecholamines*. (Blaschko, H., and Muscholl, E., eds.) *Handbuch der Experimentellen Pharmakologie*, Vol. 33. Springer-Verlag, Berlin, **1972**, pp. 283–335.

Furness, J. B., and Burnstock, G. Role of circulating catecholamines in the gastrointestinal tract. In, *Adrenal Gland*, Vol. 6. Sect. 7, Endocrinology. Handbook of Physiology. (Blaschko, H.; Sayers, G.; and Smith, A. D.; eds.) American Physiological Society, Washington, D. C., **1975**, pp. 515–536.

Furst, C. I. The biochemistry of guanethidine. *Adv. Drug Res.*, **1967**, *4*, 133–161.

Ganong, W. F. Biogenic amines, sympathetic nerves, and renin secretion. *Fed. Proc.*, **1973**, *32*, 1782–1784.

Greenblatt, D. J., and Koch-Weser, J. Adverse reactions to propranolol in hospitalized medical patients: a report from the Boston Collaborative Drug Surveillance Program. *Am. Heart J.*, **1973**, *86*, 478–484.

Greenblatt, D. J., and Shader, R. I. On the psychopharmacology of beta adrenergic blockade. *Curr. Ther. Res.*, **1972**, *14*, 615–625.

Hardaway, R. M., III. *Clinical Management of Shock.* Charles C Thomas, Publisher, Springfield, Ill., **1968**.

Holland, O. G., and Kaplan, N. M. Propranolol in the treatment of hypertension. *N. Engl. J. Med.*, **1976**, *294*, 930–936.

Karow, A. M., Jr.; Riley, M. W.; and Ahlquist, R. P. Pharmacology of clinically useful beta-adrenergic blocking drugs. *Fortschr. Arzneimittforsch.*, **1971**, *15*, 103–122.

Koch-Weser, J. Metoprolol. *N. Engl. J. Med.*, **1979**, *301*, 698–703.

Kostrzewa, R. M., and Jacobowitz, D. M. Pharmacological actions of 6-hydroxydopamine. *Pharmacol. Rev.*, **1974**, *26*, 199–288.

Langer, S. Z. Presynaptic receptors and their role in the regulation of transmitter release. *Br. J. Pharmacol.*, **1977**, *60*, 481–497.

Lefkowitz, R. J.; Caron, M. G.; and Stiles, G. L. Mechanisms of membrane receptor regulation. Biochemical, physiological and clinical insights derived from studies of the adrenergic receptors. *N. Engl. J. Med.*, **1984**, *310*, 1570–1579.

Levi-Montalcini, R., and Angeletti, P. U. Immunosympathectomy. *Pharmacol. Rev.*, **1966**, *18*, 619–628.

Lund-Johansen, P. Short- and long-term (six-year) hemodynamic effects of labetalol in essential hypertension. *Am. J. Med.*, October 17, **1983**, *75*, Suppl., 24–31.

McDevitt, D. G. Beta-adrenergic blocking drugs and partial agonist activity: is it clinically relevant? *Drugs*, **1983**, *25*, 331–338.

Malcolm, J. Adrenergic beta receptor inhibition and hyperthyroidism. *Acta Cardiol.*, **1972**, Suppl. 15, 307–326.

Nickerson, M. Nonequilibrium drug antagonism. *Pharmacol. Rev.*, **1957**, *9*, 246–259.

———. Drug therapy of shock. In, *Shock: Pathogenesis and Therapy* (a Ciba Foundation symposium). (Bock, D. K., ed.) Springer-Verlag, Berlin, **1962**, pp. 356–370.

Nickerson, M., and Hollenberg, N. K. Blockade of α-adrenergic receptors. In, *Physiological Pharmacology.* Vol. 4, *The Nervous System—Part D: Autonomic Nervous System Drugs.* (Root, W. S., and Hofmann, F. G., eds.) Academic Press, Inc., New York, **1967**, pp. 243–305.

Oates, J. A.; Conolly, M. E.; Prichard, B. N. C.; Shand, D. G.; and Schapel, G. The clinical pharmacology of antihypertensive drugs. In, *Antihypertensive Agents.* (Gross, F., ed.) *Handbuch der Experimentellen Pharmakologie*, Vol. 39. Springer-Verlag, Berlin, **1977**, pp. 571–632.

Peatfield, R. Migraine. Current concepts of pathogenesis and treatment. *Drugs*, **1983**, *26*, 364–371.

Porter, C. C.; Torchiana, M. L.; and Stone, C. A. False transmitters as antihypertensive agents. In, *Antihypertensive Agents.* (Gross, F., ed.) *Handbuch der Experimentellen Pharmakologie*, Vol. 39. Springer-Verlag, Berlin, **1977**, pp. 263–297.

Prichard, B. N. C. β-Adrenergic receptor blockade in hypertension, past, present and future. *Br. J. Clin. Pharmacol.*, **1978**, *5*, 379–399.

Prichard, B. N. C.; Owens, C. W. I.; and Tuckman, J. Clinical features of adrenergic agonists and antagonists. In, *Adrenergic Activators and Inhibitors.* (Szekeres, L., ed.) *Handbook of Experimental Pharmacology*, Vol. 54, Pt. II. Springer-Verlag, Berlin, **1980**, pp. 559–697.

Sannerstedt, R., and Conway, J. Hemodynamic and vascular responses to antihypertensive treatment with adrenergic blocking agents: a review. *Am. Heart J.*, **1970**, *79*, 122–127.

Shand, D. G. Drug therapy: propranolol. *N. Engl. J. Med.*, **1975**, *293*, 280–284.

Smigel, M. D.; Ross, E. M.; and Gilman, A. G. Role of the β-adrenergic receptor in the regulation of adenylate cyclase. In, *Cell Membranes: Methods and Reviews*, Vol. 9. (Elson, E. L.; Frazier, W. A.; and Glaser, L.; eds.) Plenum Press, New York, **1984**, pp. 247–294.

Starke, K. Regulation of noradrenaline release by presynaptic receptor systems. *Rev. Physiol. Biochem. Pharmacol.*, **1977**, *77*, 1–124.

Symposium. (Various authors.) Interrelationship of angina pectoris and hypertension. *Br. J. Clin. Pharmacol.*, **1979**, *7*, Suppl. 2, 157S–267S.

Symposium. (Various authors.) Pindolol: the relevance of intrinsic sympathomimetic activity after 12 years of experience. (Aellig, W. H.; Hedges, A.; Turner, P.; and Waite, R.; eds.) *Br. J. Clin. Pharmacol.*, **1982**, *13*, Suppl. 2, 143S–450S.

Symposium. (Various authors.) Hypertension and hemodynamics: therapeutic implications. (Sonnenblick, E. H., ed.) *Am. J. Med.*, October 17, **1983**, *75*, Suppl., 1–114.

Symposium. (Various authors.) The Goteborg metoprolol trial in acute myocardial infarction. (Roberts, W. C., ed.) *Am. J. Cardiol.*, **1984**, *53*, 1D–50D.

Thoenen, H., and Tranzer, J. P. The pharmacology of 6-hydroxydopamine. *Annu. Rev. Pharmacol.*, **1973**, *13*, 169–180.

Vedin, J. A., and Wilhelmsson, C. E. Beta receptor blocking agents in the secondary prevention of coronary heart disease. *Annu. Rev. Pharmacol. Toxicol.*, **1983**, *23*, 29–44.

Wallin, J. D.; Wilson, D.; Winer, N.; Maronde, R. F.; Michelson, E. L.; Langford, H.; Maloy, J.; and Poland, M. Treatment of severe hypertension with labetalol compared with methyldopa and furosemide. Results of a long-term, double-blind, multicenter trial. *Am. J. Med.*, October 17, **1983**, *75*, Suppl., 87–94.

Weiner, N. Regulation of norepinephrine biosynthesis. *Annu. Rev. Pharmacol.*, **1970**, *10*, 273–290.

———. The role of cyclic nucleotides in the regulation of neurotransmitter release from adrenergic neurons by neuromodulators. In, *Essays in Neurochemistry and Neuropharmacology*, Vol. 4. (Youdim, M. B. H.; Lovenberg, W.; Sharman, D. F.; and Lagnado, J. R.; eds.) John Wiley & Sons, Inc., New York, **1980**, pp. 69–124.

CHAPTER

10 GANGLIONIC STIMULATING AND BLOCKING AGENTS

Palmer Taylor

The pharmacology of ganglionic transmission is based largely on modifications of the availability or action of the primary neurotransmitter, acetylcholine (ACh). Accordingly, the passage of impulses in autonomic ganglia can be influenced by drugs that (1) interfere with the storage or synthesis of the transmitter (*e.g.,* hemicholinium), (2) prevent the liberation of ACh from the preganglionic nerve endings (*e.g.,* botulinus toxin, local anesthetics), (3) inactivate ganglionic cholinesterases (*e.g.,* physostigmine, DFP), and (4) either mimic or prevent the actions of ACh at its receptor sites in ganglia.

Neurotransmission in autonomic ganglia has long been recognized to be a far more complex process than that described by a single neurotransmitter-receptor system, and intracellular recordings reveal at least four different changes in potential that can be elicited by stimulation of the preganglionic nerve (Eccles and Libet, 1961; Nishi and Koketsu, 1968; Weight *et al.,* 1979). The *primary event* involves the rapid depolarization of postsynaptic sites by ACh. The receptors are classified as nicotinic, and the pathway is sensitive to classical non-depolarizing blocking agents such as *hexamethonium.* Activation of this primary pathway gives rise to an initial *excitatory postsynaptic potential* (EPSP). This depolarization is primarily due to an inward Na^+ current. It is rapid, since there is a tightly coupled relationship between occupation of the receptor by ACh and activation of the channel to conduct current. The mechanism of generation of the initial EPSP parallels that seen at the neuromuscular junction (*see* Chapter 11). The secondary pathways are thought to amplify or suppress this signal.

An *action potential* is generated in the postganglionic neuron when the initial EPSP attains a critical amplitude. In mammalian sympathetic ganglia *in vivo,* it may be necessary for multiple synapses to be activated before transmission is effective.

Iontophoretic application of ACh to the ganglion results in a depolarization with a latency of less than 1 millisecond; this decays over a period of 10 to 50 milliseconds (Ascher *et al.,* 1979; MacDermott *et al.,* 1980). These kinetic characteristics also indicate that the channel associated with nicotinic receptors in ganglia is very similar to that found at the neuromuscular junction (*see* Chapter 11). The two channels show similar conductances when they are open. In some ganglia, two types of fast channels have been detected (Gray and Rang, 1983).

The *secondary events or pathways* are insensitive to hexamethonium or other nicotinic antagonists. They include the slow EPSP, the late, slow EPSP, and an inhibitory postsynaptic potential (IPSP). The slow EPSP is generated by agonists acting on muscarinic receptors, and it is blocked by atropine or antagonists that are selective for M_1 receptors (Libet, 1970). The slow EPSP has a longer latency and a duration of 30 to 60 seconds. In contrast, the late, slow EPSP lasts for several minutes and is initiated by the action of peptides that are found in specific ganglia (*see* below). The peptides and ACh are released from the same nerve ending, but the enhanced stability of the peptide in the ganglion extends its sphere of influence to postsynaptic sites beyond those in immediate proximity to the nerve ending (Jan *et al.,* 1983). The slow EPSPs result from a decreased K^+ conductance (Weight *et al.,* 1979). Depolarization activates a K^+ channel, and the muscarinic agonists or peptides suppress channel conductance. The K^+ conductance has been called an *M current,* and it regulates the sensitivity of the cell to repetitive fast-depolarizing events (Adams *et al.,* 1982).

Like the slow EPSP, the IPSP is unaffected by the classical ganglionic blocking agents but, in many systems, is sensitive to blockade by atropine. Substantial electrophysiological and morphological evidence has accumulated to suggest that catecholamines participate in the generation of the IPSP. Dopamine and norepinephrine cause hyperpolarization of ganglia, and both the IPSP and the catecholamine-induced hyperpolarization are blocked by α-adrenergic antagonists. Since the IPSP is sensitive in most systems to blockade by *both* atropine and α-adrenergic antagonists, ACh that is released at the preganglionic terminal may act on a catecholamine-containing interneuron to stimulate the release of dopamine or norepinephrine; the catecholamine, in turn, produces hyperpolarization (an IPSP) of the ganglion cell (Eccles and Libet, 1961; Libet, 1970). Morphological studies indicate that catecholamine-containing cells are present in ganglia. These include the dopamine- or norepinephrine-containing small, intensely fluorescent (SIF) cells and adrenergic nerve terminals. The precise role played by the SIF cells and the electrogenic mechanism of the IPSP remain to be resolved (Eranko *et al.*, 1980).

The relative importance of the secondary pathways and even the nature of the modulating transmitters appear to differ among individual ganglia and between parasympathetic and sympathetic ganglia. A variety of peptides, including *luteinizing hormone–releasing hormone* (LH-RH), *substance P, angiotensin*, and *enkephalins,* have been identified in ganglia by immunofluorescence, and they appear to be released upon preganglionic nerve stimulation (Sejnowski, 1982; Jan *et al.*, 1983). Precise details of their modulatory actions are not understood, but they appear to be most closely associated with the late, slow EPSP and inhibition of the M current in various ganglia. Other substances, such as *5-hydroxytryptamine* (Saum and de Groat, 1973; Wood and Mayer, 1979) and *gamma-aminobutyric acid,* are known to modify ganglionic transmission. It should be emphasized that the secondary synaptic events only modulate the initial EPSP. Conventional ganglionic blocking agents can inhibit ganglionic transmission completely; the same cannot be said for muscarinic antagonists or α-adrenergic agonists (*see* Weight *et al., 1979;* Volle, 1980).

Drugs that stimulate cholinergic receptor sites on autonomic ganglia can be grouped into two major categories. The first group consists of drugs with nicotinic specificity, including *nicotine* itself. Their excitatory effects on ganglia are rapid in onset, are blocked by non-depolarizing ganglionic blocking agents, and mimic *the initial EPSP.* The second group is composed of agents such as *muscarine, McN-A-343,* and *methacholine,* and, in part, the *anticholinesterase* (anti-ChE) *agents.* Their excitatory effects on ganglia are delayed in onset, blocked by atropine-like drugs, and mimic the *slow EPSP.*

Ganglionic blocking agents impair transmission by actions at the primary nicotinic receptor and also may be classified into two groups. The *first group* includes those drugs that initially stimulate the ganglia by an ACh-like action and then block because of a persistent depolarization (*e.g.,* nico-

tine); prolonged application of nicotine results in desensitization of the cholinergic receptor site and continued blockade. (*See* review by Volle, 1980.) The blockade of autonomic ganglia produced by the *second group* of blocking drugs, of which *hexamethonium* and *trimethaphan* can be regarded as prototypes, does not involve prior ganglionic stimulation or changes in the ganglionic potentials. These agents impair transmission either by competing with ACh for ganglionic cholinergic receptor sites or by blocking the channel when it is open. Trimethaphan acts by competition with ACh, analogous to the mechanism of action of curare at the neuromuscular junction. Blockade of the channel by hexamethonium appears to occur after the channel opens. This shortens the duration of current flow, since the open channel either becomes occluded or closes (Rang, 1982; Gurney and Rang, 1984). Irrespective of the mechanism, the initial EPSP is blocked and ganglionic transmission is inhibited. Compounds in this group have no effect on nerve conduction or on the release of transmitter substance from the nerve terminals. It is this class of conventional ganglionic blocking agents that is employed in therapy (*see* below).

GANGLIONIC STIMULATING DRUGS

History. Two natural alkaloids, nicotine and lobeline, owe much of their pharmacological activity to their actions at autonomic ganglia. *Nicotine* (Table 10–1) was first isolated from leaves of tobacco, *Nicotiana tabacum,* by Posselt and Reiman in 1828, and Orfila initiated the first pharmacological studies of the alkaloid in 1843. Langley and Dickinson (1889) painted the superior cervical ganglion of rabbits with nicotine and demonstrated that its site of action was the ganglion, rather than the preganglionic or postganglionic nerve fiber. *Lobelia* (Indian tobacco) is obtained from the dried leaves and tops of an herb, *Lobelia inflata. Lobeline* (α-lobeline) (Table 10–1) is the chief constituent of lobelia and was first obtained in crystalline form by Wieland in 1915. Lobeline has many of the same actions in the body as nicotine but is less potent.

A number of synthetic compounds also have prominent actions at ganglionic receptor sites. The actions of the *onium compounds,* of which *tetramethylammonium* (TMA) is the simplest prototype, were explored in considerable detail in the last half of the nineteenth century and in the early twentieth century. In 1951, Chen and coworkers described the ganglionic stimulating properties of

Table 10–1. GANGLIONIC STIMULANTS

Nicotine

Lobeline

Tetramethylammonium

1,1-Dimethyl-4-phenylpiperazinium

1,1-dimethyl-4-phenylpiperazinium (DMPP) iodide, a relatively specific ganglionic stimulant.

NICOTINE

Nicotine is of considerable medical significance because of its toxicity, presence in tobacco, and propensity for conferring a dependence on its users. The chronic effects of nicotine and the untoward effects of the chronic use of *tobacco* are considered in Chapter 23.

Chemistry. *Nicotine* is one of the few natural liquid alkaloids. It is a colorless, volatile base ($pK_a = 8.5$) that turns brown and acquires the odor of tobacco on exposure to air. The alkaloid is readily soluble in water and forms water-soluble salts.

Pharmacological Actions. The complex and often unpredictable changes that occur in the body after administration of nicotine are due not only to its actions on a variety of neuroeffector and chemosensitive sites but also to the fact that the alkaloid has both stimulant and depressant phases of action. The ultimate response of any one system represents the summation of the several different and opposing effects of nicotine. For example, the drug can increase the heart rate by excitation of sympathetic or paralysis of parasympathetic cardiac ganglia, and it can slow the heart rate by paralysis of sympathetic or stimulation of parasympathetic cardiac ganglia. In addition, the effects of the drug on the chemoreceptors of the carotid and aortic bodies and on medullary centers influence heart rate, as do also the cardiovascular compensatory reflexes resulting from changes in blood pressure caused by

nicotine. Finally, nicotine causes a discharge of epinephrine from the adrenal medulla, and this hormone accelerates cardiac rate and raises blood pressure.

Peripheral Nervous System. The major action of nicotine consists initially in transient stimulation and subsequently in a more persistent depression of all autonomic ganglia. Small doses of nicotine stimulate the ganglion cells directly and facilitate the transmission of impulses. When larger doses of the drug are applied, the initial stimulation is followed very quickly by a blockade of transmission. Whereas stimulation of the ganglion cells coincides with their depolarization, depression of transmission by adequate doses of nicotine occurs both during the depolarization and after it has subsided. Nicotine also possesses a biphasic action on the adrenal medulla; small doses evoke the discharge of catecholamines, and larger doses prevent their release in response to splanchnic nerve stimulation.

Nicotine also causes the release of catecholamines in a number of isolated organs. This action results in a sympathomimetic response to nicotine that is blocked by drugs known to prevent the effects of catecholamines.

The effects of nicotine on the neuromuscular junction are similar to those on ganglia. However, with the exception of avian and denervated mammalian muscle, the stimulant phase is largely obscured by the rapidly developing paralysis. In the latter stage, nicotine also produces neuromuscular blockade by receptor desensitization.

Nicotine, like ACh, is known to stimulate a number of sensory receptors. These include mechanoreceptors that respond to stretch or pressure of the skin, mesentery, tongue, lung, and stomach; chemoreceptors of the carotid body; thermal receptors of the skin and tongue; and pain receptors. Prior administration of hexamethonium prevents the stimulation of the sensory receptors by nicotine, but has little effect, if any, on the activation of the sensory receptors by physiological stimuli.

Central Nervous System. Nicotine markedly stimulates the central nervous system (CNS). Appropriate doses produce *tremors* in both man and laboratory animals; with somewhat larger doses, the tremor is followed by *convulsions*. The *excitation of respiration* is a prominent action of nicotine; although large doses act directly on the medulla oblongata, smaller doses augment respiration reflexly by excitation of the chemoreceptors of the carotid and aortic bodies. Stimulation of the CNS is followed by depression, and death results from failure of respiration due to both central paralysis and peripheral blockade of muscles of respiration.

Nicotine and lobeline cause *vomiting* by central and peripheral actions. The central component of the vomiting response is due to stimulation of the emetic chemoreceptor trigger zone in the area postrema of the medulla oblongata. In addition, nicotine activates vagal and spinal afferent nerves that form the sensory input of the reflex pathways involved in the act of vomiting.

Cardiovascular System. When administered intravenously to the dog, nicotine characteristically produces an increase in heart rate and blood pressure. The latter is usually a more sustained response. In general, the cardiovascular responses to nicotine are due to stimulation of sympathetic ganglia and the adrenal medulla, together with the discharge of catecholamines from sympathetic nerve endings. Also contributing to the sympathomimetic response to nicotine is the activation of chemoreceptors of the aortic and carotid bodies, which reflexly results in *vasoconstriction, tachycardia,* and *elevated blood pressure.*

Gastrointestinal Tract. In contrast to the cardiovascular actions of nicotine, the effects of the drug on the gastrointestinal tract are due largely to parasympathetic stimulation. The combined activation of parasympathetic ganglia and cholinergic nerve endings results in increased tone and motor activity of the bowel. Nausea, vomiting, and occasionally diarrhea are observed following systemic absorption of nicotine.

Exocrine Glands. Nicotine causes an initial stimulation of salivary and bronchial secretions that is followed by inhibition. Salivation caused by smoking is reflexly produced by the irritant smoke rather than by a systemic effect of nicotine.

Absorption, Fate, and Excretion. Nicotine is readily absorbed from the respiratory tract, buccal membranes, and skin. Severe poisoning has resulted from percutaneous absorption. Being a relatively strong base, its absorption from the stomach is limited unless intragastric pH is raised. Intestinal absorption is far more efficient.

Approximately 80 to 90% of nicotine is altered in the body, mainly in the liver but also in the kidney and lung. A significant fraction of inhaled nicotine is metabolized by the lung (Turner *et al.,* 1975). The major metabolites of nicotine are cotinine and nicotine-1'-N-oxide, which are formed respectively from oxidation of the α carbon and N-oxidation of the pyrrolidine ring. The half-life of nicotine following inhalation or parenteral administration is about 2 hours. Both nicotine and its metabolites are rapidly eliminated by the kidney (Russell and Feyerabend, 1978). The rate of urinary excretion of nicotine is dependent upon the pH of the urine; excretion diminishes when the urine is alkaline. Nicotine is also excreted in the *milk* of lactating women who smoke. The milk of heavy smokers may contain 0.5 mg per liter.

Acute Nicotine Poisoning. Poisoning from nicotine may occur from accidental ingestion of insecticide sprays in which nicotine is present as the effective agent or in children from ingestion of tobacco products. The acutely fatal dose of nicotine for an adult is probably about 60 mg of the base. Smoking tobacco usually contains 1 to 2% nicotine. Apparently the gastric absorption of nicotine from tobacco taken by mouth is delayed because of slowed gastric emptying, so that vomiting caused by the central effect of the initially absorbed fraction may remove much of the tobacco remaining in the gastrointestinal tract.

The onset of symptoms of acute, severe nicotine poisoning is rapid; they include nausea, salivation, abdominal pain, vomiting, diarrhea, cold sweat, headache, dizziness, disturbed hearing and vision, mental confusion, and marked weakness. Faintness and prostration ensue; the blood pressure falls; breathing is difficult; the pulse is weak, rapid, and irregular; and collapse may be followed by terminal convulsions. Death may result within a few minutes from respiratory failure.

Therapy. Vomiting should be induced with syrup of ipecac, or gastric lavage should be performed. Alkaline solutions should be avoided. A slurry of activated charcoal is then passed through the tube and left in the stomach. Respiratory assistance and treatment of shock may be necessary.

OTHER GANGLIONIC STIMULANTS

Stimulation of ganglia by TMA or DMPP differs from that produced by nicotine in that the initial stimulation is not followed by a dominant blocking action. Demonstration of ganglionic blockade caused by DMPP or TMA requires large intra-arterial doses or application of the drug *in vitro.* Their stimulatory action for the most part mimics the initial EPSP and is blocked by hexamethonium. DMPP is about three times more potent than nicotine. Parasympathomimetic drugs (muscarine, pilocarpine, and the synthetic choline esters) can also stimulate ganglia; however, their effects are usually obscured by stimulation of other neuroeffector sites.

GANGLIONIC BLOCKING DRUGS

The chemical diversity of compounds that block autonomic ganglia without causing prior stimulation is shown in Table 10–2. The structure-activity relationship of these compounds has been extensively analyzed (Paton and Zaimis, 1952; Ing, 1956).

HEXAMETHONIUM AND RELATED DRUGS

History and Structure-Activity Relationship. Although Marshall (1913) and Burn and Dale (1915) first described the "nicotine paralyzing" action of *tetraethylammonium* (TEA) on ganglia, TEA was largely overlooked until Acheson and Moe (1946) and Acheson and Pereira (1946) published their definitive analyses of the effects of the ion on the cardiovascular system and autonomic ganglia. They also proposed the use of TEA for the treatment of hypertension. The more potent *bis*-quaternary ammonium salts were developed and studied independently by Barlow and Ing (1948) and Paton and Zaimis (1949, 1952). The prototypical ganglionic blocking drug in this series, *hexamethonium* (C6), has a bridge of six methylene groups between the two quaternary nitrogen atoms (Table 10–2). C6 and its congener C5 have minimal neuromuscular and muscarinic blocking activity.

Subsequently, several series of *bis*-quaternary ammonium compounds were investigated for gan-

Table 10–2.   NON-DEPOLARIZING GANGLIONIC BLOCKING AGENTS

$$CH_3 \overset{\underset{\displaystyle CH_3}{|}}{\overset{\displaystyle CH_3}{\overset{|}{N^+}}}\!\!-\!(CH_2)_6\!-\!\overset{\underset{\displaystyle CH_3}{|}}{\overset{\displaystyle CH_3}{\overset{|}{N^+}}}\!\!-\!CH_3$$

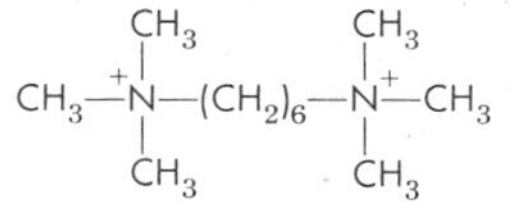

Hexamethonium (C6)

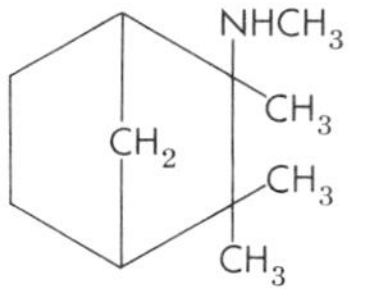

Mecamylamine

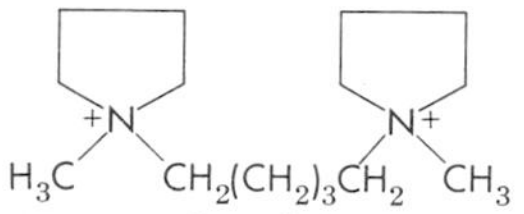

Pentolinium

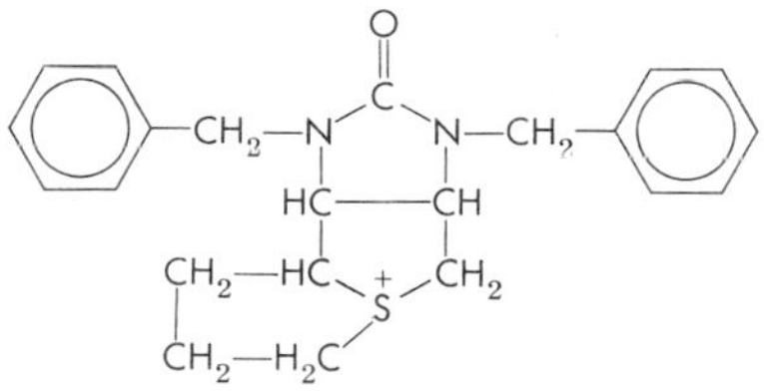

Trimethaphan

sented a departure in the chemistry of these agents. The pharmacological properties of *mecamylamine* (Table 10–2) were reported in the mid-1950s, and the drug was soon introduced into therapy. *Pempidine*, a tertiary amine with similar properties, was introduced shortly after mecamylamine.

Pharmacological Properties. Nearly all of the physiological alterations observed after the administration of hexamethonium and related drugs can be attributed to the blockade of transmission in autonomic ganglia by the mechanisms already considered. These alterations can be anticipated with reasonable accuracy by a careful inspection of Figure 4–1 (facing page 68) and by knowing which division of the autonomic nervous system exercises dominant control of various organs (Table 10–3). For example, blockade of sympathetic ganglia interrupts adrenergic control of arterioles and results in vasodilatation, improved peripheral blood flow in some vascular beds, and a fall in blood pressure.

Generalized ganglionic blockade may result also in atony of the bladder and gastrointestinal tract, cycloplegia, xerostomia, diminished perspiration, and, by abolishing circulatory reflex pathways, postural hypotension. These changes represent the generally undesirable features of ganglionic blockade, which limit the therapeutic efficacy of ganglionic blocking agents.

Cardiovascular System. The importance of existing sympathetic tone in determining the degree to which blood pressure is lowered by ganglionic blockade is illustrated by the fact that blood pressure may be decreased only minimally in recumbent normotensive subjects but may fall markedly in sitting or standing subjects. Postural hypotension is a major problem in ambulatory patients receiving ganglionic blocking drugs; it is relieved to some extent by muscular activity and completely by recumbency, and tends to become less prominent after continued medication. Sympathetically mediated vasomotor reflexes are inhibited, and the cold pressor response is reduced.

Changes in *cardiac rate* following ganglionic blockade depend largely on existing vagal tone. In man, mild tachycardia usually accompanies the hypotension, a sign that indicates fairly complete

glionic blocking activity, and some drugs so discovered, such as *pentolinium,* have been employed clinically. Pentolinium has a longer duration of action than hexamethonium and was widely used to produce controlled hypotension in anesthesia after Enderby's favorable report in 1954. Triethylsulfoniums, like the quaternary and *bis*-quaternary ammonium ions, possess ganglionic blocking actions. This knowledge led to the development of sulfonium ganglionic blocking agents such as *trimethaphan* (Table 10–2). The synthesis of secondary amines with ganglionic blocking activity repre-

Table 10–3.   USUAL PREDOMINANCE OF SYMPATHETIC (ADRENERGIC) OR PARASYMPATHETIC (CHOLINERGIC) TONE AT VARIOUS EFFECTOR SITES, WITH CONSEQUENT EFFECTS OF AUTONOMIC GANGLIONIC BLOCKADE

SITE	PREDOMINANT TONE	EFFECT OF GANGLIONIC BLOCKADE
Arterioles	Sympathetic (adrenergic)	Vasodilatation; increased peripheral flow; hypotension
Veins	Sympathetic (adrenergic)	Dilatation; pooling of blood; decreased venous return; decreased cardiac output
Heart	Parasympathetic (cholinergic)	Tachycardia
Iris	Parasympathetic (cholinergic)	Mydriasis
Ciliary muscle	Parasympathetic (cholinergic)	Cycloplegia
Gastrointestinal tract	Parasympathetic (cholinergic)	Reduced tone and motility; constipation
Urinary bladder	Parasympathetic (cholinergic)	Urinary retention
Salivary glands	Parasympathetic (cholinergic)	Xerostomia
Sweat glands	Sympathetic (cholinergic)	Anhidrosis

ganglionic blockade. However, a decrease may occur if the heart rate is initially high.

Cardiac output is often reduced by ganglionic blocking drugs in patients with normal cardiac function as a consequence of diminished venous return resulting from venous dilatation and peripheral pooling of blood. In patients with cardiac failure, ganglionic blockade frequently results in increased cardiac output due to a reduction in peripheral resistance. In hypertensive subjects, cardiac output, stroke volume, and left ventricular work are diminished.

Although *total systemic vascular resistance* is decreased in patients who receive ganglionic blocking agents, changes in *blood flow* and *vascular resistance* of individual vascular beds are variable. *Skin temperature* is elevated mostly in the hands and feet, and blood flow to the limbs may increase. Reduction of *cerebral blood flow* is small unless mean systemic blood pressure falls below 50 to 60 mm Hg (Miletick and Ivankovich, 1978). *Skeletal muscle blood flow* is unaltered, and *splanchnic and renal blood flow* decrease following ganglionic blockade. Renal vascular resistance increases, and the rate of glomerular filtration falls. Trimethaphan appears to cause some vasodilatation by a direct mechanism (Wang *et al.*, 1977).

Other Effects. Gastrointestinal secretions are generally decreased by ganglionic blocking agents, and the tone and motility of the gastrointestinal tract are reduced. Ganglionic blockade causes partial or total impairment of the voiding contractions of the *urinary bladder,* with a resultant increase in vesical capacity and incomplete voiding. This is due to blockade of parasympathetic ganglia along the efferent pathways of the spinal reflex concerned with micturition, so that bladder distention causes no urge to void. Penile erection and ejaculation are impaired. Ganglionic blockade causes incomplete *mydriasis* and partial loss of *accommodation* as a result of impaired transmission in the ciliary ganglion. *Sweating* is reduced.

Untoward Responses and Severe Reactions. Among the milder untoward responses observed are visual disturbances, dry mouth, conjunctival suffusion, urinary hesitancy, decreased potentia, subjective chilliness, moderate constipation, occasional diarrhea, abdominal discomfort, anorexia, heartburn, nausea, eructation and bitter taste, and the signs and symptoms of syncope caused by postural hypotension. These side effects tend to become less pronounced as administration of the drug is continued. More severe reactions include *marked hypotension, constipation, paralytic ileus, urinary retention,* and *cycloplegia.* Syncope may occur without warning. Unlike the quaternary ganglionic blocking agents, which do not readily reach the CNS, large doses of *mecamylamine* can produce *prominent central effects,* resulting in tremors, mental confusion, seizures, mania, or depression.

Absorption, Fate, and Excretion. The absorption of quaternary ammonium and sulfonium compounds from the enteric tract is incomplete and

unpredictable. This is due both to the limited ability of these ionized substances to penetrate cell membranes and to the depression of propulsive movements of the small intestine. Gastric emptying time may be so delayed that two or three doses may be retained in the stomach; the gastric contents may then suddenly enter the duodenum, and the absorption of the accumulated toxic amounts of drug can cause severe hypotension and collapse. Although the absorption of mecamylamine is less erratic, a danger exists of reduced bowel activity leading to frank paralytic ileus.

After absorption, the quaternary ammonium and sulfonium blocking agents are confined primarily to the extracellular space. Most of a parenteral dose is excreted unchanged by the kidney. Mecamylamine is not confined to the extracellular space; high concentrations accumulate in the liver and kidney. Mecamylamine is excreted slowly by the kidney in unchanged form and has a relatively long duration of action.

Preparations, Routes of Administration, and Dosage. Of the ganglionic blocking agents that have appeared on the therapeutic scene, only *mecamylamine* and *trimethaphan* are currently utilized in the United States. *Pempidine* and *pentolinium* are still used to a limited extent in Europe.

Mecamylamine hydrochloride (INVERSINE) is available for oral administration in tablets containing 2.5 mg of the drug. The usual initial dose is 2.5 mg, given twice daily.

Trimethaphan camsylate (ARFONAD) is available as an injection (50 mg/ml). It possesses a short duration of action and is administered by intravenous drip. When administered in this manner, a 0.1% solution in 5% dextrose is employed.

THERAPEUTIC USES

Historically the major therapeutic use of the ganglionic blocking agents was in the management of *hypertensive cardiovascular disease.* However, these drugs have been supplanted by superior agents for the treatment of *chronic hypertension.* Some physicians still use ganglionic blocking agents for the treatment of *hypertensive crises* and for the initial control of blood pressure in patients with *acute dissecting aortic aneurysm.* In such situations, trimethaphan is infused intravenously at a rate of 0.3 to 3 mg per minute with frequent monitoring of blood pressure. Abrupt reduction of blood pressure or reduction below the normal range is particularly dangerous in individuals with coronary or cerebrovascular insufficiency. Since trimethaphan can stimulate the release of histamine, it should be used with caution in patients with a history of allergy.

An additional therapeutic use of the ganglionic blocking agents is in the production of *controlled hypotension;* a reduction in blood pressure during surgery may be sought deliberately to minimize hemorrhage in the operative field, to reduce blood loss in various orthopedic procedures, and to facilitate surgery on blood vessels (Leigh, 1975; Salem, 1978). Trimethaphan may be used as an alternative to *sodium nitroprusside,* since some patients are resistant to the latter drug. Cardiac output and contractility are reduced to a greater extent with ganglionic blocking agents than with sodium nitroprusside (Wang *et al.,* 1977).

Trimethaphan can be employed in the management of *autonomic hyperreflexia.* This syndrome is typically seen in patients with injuries of the upper spinal cord and results from a massive sympathetic discharge. A common stimulus for such discharge is distention of the bladder; it is often associated with catheterization or irrigation of the bladder, cystoscopy, or transurethral resection. Since normal central inhibition of the reflex is lacking in such patients, the spinal reflex is dominant. It can be controlled successfully with ganglionic blocking agents (Basta *et al.,* 1977).

Acheson, G. H., and Moe, G. K. The action of tetraethylammonium ion on the mammalian circulation. *J. Pharmacol. Exp. Ther.,* 1946, *87,* 220–236.

Acheson, G. H., and Pereira, S. A. The blocking effect of tetraethylammonium ion on the superior cervical ganglion of the cat. *J. Pharmacol. Exp. Ther.,* 1946, *87,* 273–280.

Adams, P. R.; Brown, D. A.; and Constanti, A. Pharmacological inhibition of the M-current. *J. Physiol. (Lond.),* 1982, *332,* 223–262.

Ascher, P.; Large, W. A.; and Rang, H. P. Studies on the mechanism of action of acetylcholine antagonists on rat parasympathetic ganglion cells. *J. Physiol. (Lond.),* 1979, *295,* 139–170.

Barlow, R. B., and Ing, H. R. Curare-like action of polymethylene bis-quaternary ammonium salts. *Br. J. Pharmacol. Chemother.,* 1948, *3,* 298–304.

Basta, J. W.; Nlejadlik, K.; and Pallares, V. Autonomic hyperflexia: intraoperative control with pentolinium tartrate. *Br. J. Anaesth.,* 1977, *49,* 1087–1090.

Burn, J. H., and Dale, H. H. The action of certain quaternary ammonium bases. *J. Pharmacol. Exp. Ther.,* 1915, *6,* 417–438.

Eccles, R. M., and Libet, B. Origin and blockade of the synaptic responses of curarized sympathetic ganglia. *J. Physiol. (Lond.),* 1961, *157,* 484–503.

Gray, P. T. A., and Rang, H. P. Analysis of current noise evoked by nicotinic agonists in rat submandibular ganglion neurones. *Br. J. Pharmacol.,* 1983, *80,* 235–240.

Gurney, A. M., and Rang, H. P. The channel-blocking action of methonium compounds on rat submandibular ganglion cells. *Br. J. Pharmacol.,* 1984, *82,* 623–642.

Langley, J. N., and Dickinson, W. L. On the local paralysis of peripheral ganglia, and on the connexion of different classes of nerve fibers with them. *Proc. R. Soc. Lond. [Biol.],* 1889, *46,* 423–431.

MacDermott, A. B.; Connor, E. A.; Dionne, V. E.; and Parsons, R. L. Voltage clamp study of fast excitatory synaptic currents in bullfrog sympathetic ganglion cells. *J. Gen. Physiol.,* 1980, *75,* 39–60.

Marshall, C. R. Studies on the pharmaceutical action of tetra-alkyl-ammonium compounds. *Trans. R. Soc. Edinb.,* 1913, *1,* 17–40.

Nishi, S., and Koketsu, K. Early and late after-discharges of amphibian sympathetic ganglion cells. *J. Neurophysiol.,* 1968, *31,* 109–121.

Paton, W. D. M., and Zaimis, E. J. The pharmacological actions of polymethylene bistrimethylammonium salts. *Br. J. Pharmacol. Chemother.,* 1949, *4,* 381–400.

Rang, H. P. The action of ganglionic blocking drugs on the synaptic responses of submandibular ganglion cells. *Br. J. Pharmacol.,* 1982, *75,* 151–168.

Saum, W. P., and de Groat, W. C. The actions of 5-hydroxytryptamine on the urinary bladder and on vesical autonomic ganglia in the cat. *J. Pharmacol. Exp. Ther.,* 1973, *185,* 70–82.

Turner, D. M.; Armitage, A. K.; Briant, R. H.; and Dollery, C. T. Metabolism of nicotine by the isolated perfused dog lung. *Xenobiotica,* 1975, *5,* 539–551.

Wang, H. H.; Liu, L. M. P.; and Katz, R. L. A comparison of the cardiovascular effects of sodium nitroprusside and trimethaphan. *Anesthesiology,* 1977, *46,* 40–48.

Wood, J. D., and Mayer, C. J. Serotonergic activation of tonic-type enteric neurons in guinea pig small bowel. *J. Neurophysiol.,* 1979, *42,* 582–593.

Monographs and Reviews

Eranko, O.; Sonila, S.; and Paiverinta, H. *Histochemistry and Cell Biology of Autonomic Neurons, SIF Cells and Paraneurons.* Academic Press, Inc., New York, 1980.

Ing, H. R. Structure-action relationships of hypotensive drugs. In, *Hypotensive Drugs.* (Harrington, M., ed.) Pergamon Press, Ltd., Oxford, 1956, pp. 7–22.

Jan, Y. N.; Bowers, C. W.; Branton, D.; Evans, L.; and Jan, L. Y. Peptides in neuronal function: studies using frog autonomic ganglia. *Cold Spring Harbor Symp. Quant. Biol.,* 1983, *43,* 363–374.

Leigh, J. M. The history of controlled hypotension. *Br. J. Anaesth.,* 1975, *47,* 745–749.

Libet, B. Generation of slow inhibitory and excitatory postsynaptic potentials. *Fed. Proc.,* 1970, *29,* 1945–1956.

Miletick, D. J., and Ivankovich, A. D. Cardiovascular effects of ganglionic blocking drugs. *Int. Anesthesiol. Clin.,* 1978, *16,* 151–170.

Paton, W. D. M., and Zaimis, E. J. The methonium compounds. *Pharmacol. Rev.,* 1952, *4,* 219–253.

Russell, M. A. H., and Feyerabend, C. Cigarette smoking: a dependence on high nicotine level boli. *Drug Metab. Rev.,* 1978, *8,* 29–57.

Salem, M. R. Therapeutic uses of ganglionic blocking drugs. *Int. Anesthesiol. Clin.,* 1978, *16,* 171–200.

Sejnowski, T. J. Peptidergic synaptic transmission in sympathetic ganglia. *Fed. Proc.,* 1982, *41,* 2923–2928.

Volle, R. L. Nicotinic ganglion-stimulating agents. In, *Pharmacology of Ganglionic Transmission.* (Kharkevich, D. A., ed.) Springer-Verlag, Berlin, 1980, pp. 281–312.

Weight, F. F.; Schulman, J. A.; Smith, P. A.; and Busis, N. A. Long-lasting synaptic potentials and the modulation of synaptic transmission. *Fed. Proc.,* 1979, *38,* 2084–2094.

CHAPTER
11 NEUROMUSCULAR BLOCKING AGENTS

Palmer Taylor

Several drugs employed clinically have as their major action the interruption of transmission of the nerve impulse at the skeletal neuromuscular junction. On the basis of distinct electrophysiological differences in their mechanism of action, they are classified either as *competitive* (*stabilizing*) agents, of which curare is the classical example, or as *depolarizing* agents, such as succinylcholine.

History, Sources, and Chemistry. *Curare* is a generic term for various South American arrow poisons. The drug has a long and romantic history. It has been employed for centuries by the Indians along the Amazon and Orinoco Rivers and in other parts of the continent for killing wild animals used for food; death results from paralysis of skeletal muscles. The technic of preparation of curare was long shrouded in mystery and was entrusted only to tribal witch doctors. Soon after the discovery of the American continent, Sir Walter Raleigh and other early explorers and botanists became interested in curare, and late in the sixteenth century samples of the native preparations were brought to Europe for examination and investigation. Following the pioneering work of the scientist-explorer von Humboldt, in 1805, the *botanical sources* of curare quite early became the object of much field search. The curares from eastern Amazonia contain various species of *Strychnos* as their chief ingredient. It is noteworthy that most of the South American species of *Strychnos* examined contain chiefly quaternary, neuromuscular blocking alkaloids, whereas the Asiatic, African, and Australian species nearly all contain tertiary, strychnine-like alkaloids. Certain species of *Chondrodendron* also yield curare. Research on curare was greatly accelerated by the work of Gill (1940), who, after prolonged and intimate study of the native methods of preparing curare, brought to the United States a sufficient amount of the authentic drug prepared from *C. tomentosum* to permit chemical and pharmacological investigations.

The modern clinical use of curare probably dates from 1932, when West employed highly purified fractions in patients with tetanus and spastic disorders. In 1940, Bennett introduced the drug as an adjuvant in the pentylenetetrazol shock treatment of psychiatric disorders. The first trial of curare for promoting muscular relaxation in general anesthesia was reported by Griffith and Johnson (1942). The advantage of obtaining the desired degree of muscular relaxation without the use of dangerously high concentrations of anesthetic became recognized over the next decade. The achievement of muscle relaxation during abdominal surgery or tracheal intubation thus emerged as the chief therapeutic use of curare.

The fascinating history of curare, the reports of early travelers, and the complex problems of botanical source, nomenclature, and chemical identification of the curare alkaloids have been presented in extensive reviews (*see* Bovet, 1972; McIntyre, 1972; and *previous editions* of this textbook).

The essential structure of *d-tubocurarine* was established by King in 1935. One of the nitrogen atoms was later found to constitute a tertiary amine (Table 11–1). A synthetic derivative, *metocurine* (formerly called *dimethyl d-tubocurarine*), contains three additional methyl groups, one of which quaternizes the tertiary nitrogen; the other two form methyl ethers at the phenolic hydroxyl groups. This compound possesses about three times the potency of *d*-tubocurarine in man.

The most potent of all curare alkaloids are the *toxiferines,* obtained from *Strychnos toxifera.* A semisynthetic derivative, *alcuronium chloride* (*N,N'-diallylnortoxiferinium dichloride*), is employed clinically in Europe (Table 11–1). The seeds of the trees and shrubs of the genus *Erythrina,* widely distributed in tropical and subtropical areas, contain substances with curare-like activity. A hydrogenated derivative, *dihydro-β-erythroidine,* of the parent alkaloid, *erythroidine,* has been studied carefully and subjected to clinical trial.

Gallamine (Table 11–1) is one of a series of synthetic substitutes for curare described by Bovet and coworkers in 1949 (*see* review by Bovet, 1972). Exploration of the structure-activity relationship of the plant alkaloids led to the development of the *polymethylene bis-trimethylammonium series* (referred to herein by the generic term *methonium compounds*) simultaneously and independently by Barlow and Ing (1948) and Paton and Zaimis (1949 *et seq.*). The most potent agent was found when the chain contained ten carbon atoms (*decamethonium* [*C10*], Table 11–1). The member of the series containing six carbon atoms in the chain, *hexamethonium* (*C6*), was found to be particularly effective as a ganglionic blocking agent (*see* Chapter 10).

The use of curarized animals by Hunt and Taveau in 1906 in experiments on *succinylcholine* (Table 11–1) prevented them from observing the neuromuscular blocking activity of the drug, and this property went unrecognized for more than 40 years. In 1949, the curariform action of the compound was described independently by workers in Italy, Great Britain, and the United States, and its

Table 11–1. STRUCTURAL FORMULAS OF MAJOR NEUROMUSCULAR BLOCKING AGENTS

COMPETITIVE AGENTS

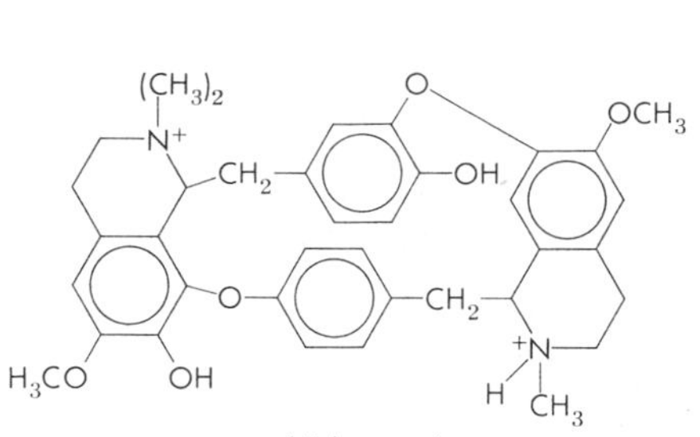

d-Tubocurarine

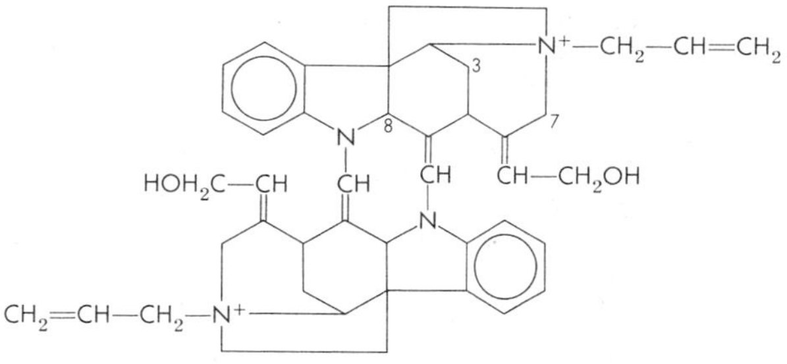

Alcuronium

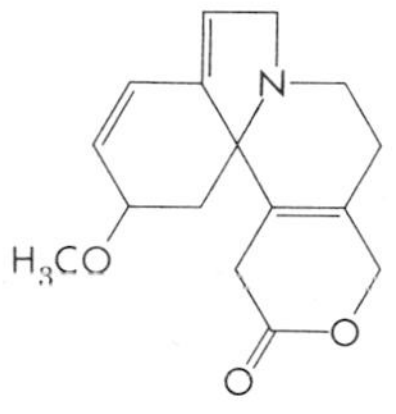

β-Erythroidine

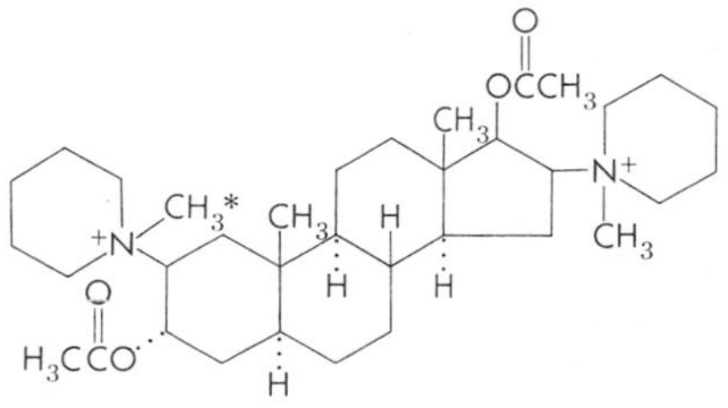

Pancuronium

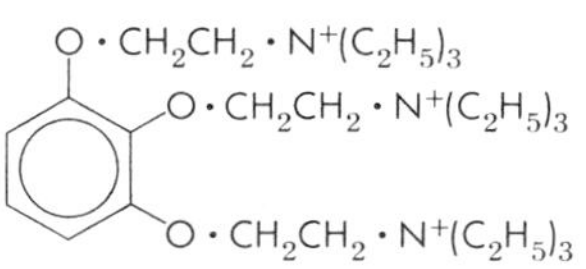

Gallamine

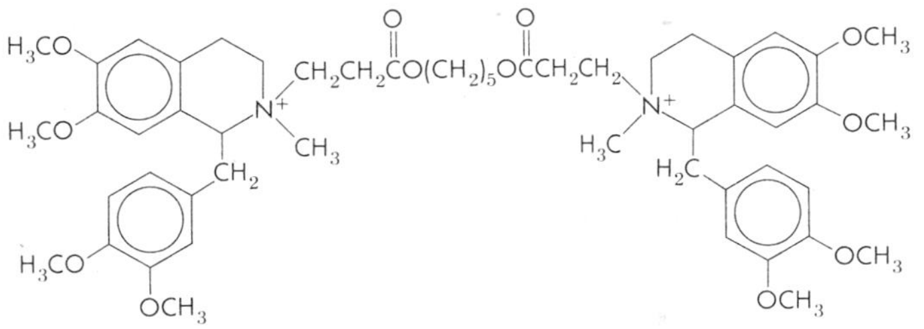

Atracurium

DEPOLARIZING AGENTS

$(CH_3)_3\overset{+}{N}—(CH_2)_{10}—\overset{+}{N}(CH_3)_3$

Decamethonium

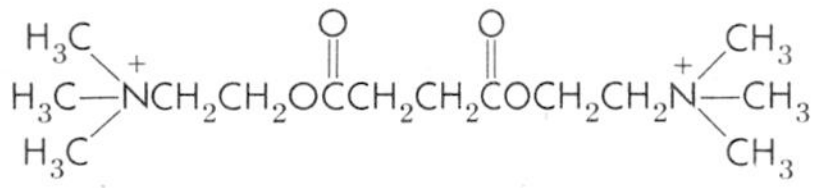

Succinylcholine

* The adjacent methyl group is absent in *vecuronium*.

clinical application soon followed (*see* Dorkins, 1982).

Pancuronium is a member of a series of *bis*-quaternary ammonium steroids that were synthesized in 1964. Extensive pharmacological and clinical studies have shown that it is approximately five times as potent as *d*-tubocurarine as a competitive neuromuscular blocking agent, with minimal cardiovascular and little histamine-releasing or hormonal actions (Buckett *et al.*, 1968; Speight and Avery, 1972). *Vecuronium* is a congener of pancuronium in which the 2β-methyl group has been removed. This small modification has been shown to reduce inhibition of plasma butyrylcholinesterase and minimize further the cardiovascular effects of

this agent. It has recently been released for general clinical use in the United States. Its potency is equivalent to or slightly greater than that of pancuronium (Agoston *et al.*, 1980). *Atracurium* is another new synthetic competitive blocking agent of intermediate duration of action. It undergoes both spontaneous and enzymatically catalyzed conversion to inactive metabolites and, hence, is less dependent on renal elimination for termination of its action (Hughes and Chapple, 1981). It is three to four times less potent than pancuronium. *Fazadinium* was developed in Great Britain as a competitive blocking agent. Its extensive metabolism by the liver (reduction of a diazo group) makes it unique among this class of drugs.

Structure-Activity Relationship. The first attempts to analyze the structure-activity relationship of drugs were made in the field of neuromuscular blocking agents by Crum Brown and Fraser in the 1860s, although neither the structure of the active ingredients of curare nor the role of acetylcholine (ACh) in neuromuscular transmission was then known.

For both theoretical and practical reasons, the structural features that distinguish *competitive* from *depolarizing* neuromuscular blocking agents have received particular attention. Although exceptions can be cited, a few useful generalizations can be made about the differences in structure between these two groups of agents. The *competitive* or *stabilizing* agents are for the most part relatively bulky, rigid molecules (*e.g.*, *d*-tubocurarine, the toxiferines, *β*-erythroidine, gallamine, pancuronium), whereas the *depolarizing* agents (*e.g.*, decamethonium, succinylcholine) generally have a more flexible structure that enables free bond rotation (*see* Table 11–1; Bovet, 1972; Cheymol and Bourillet, 1972). While the distance between quaternary groups in the flexible depolarizing agents can vary up to the limit of the maximal bond distance (1.45 nm for decamethonium), the distance for the rigid competitive blockers is usually 1.0 ± 0.1 nm. The *tris*-quaternary compound gallamine, the tertiary amine *β*-erythroidine, and fazadinium, in which the cationic charge is delocalized, represent exceptions to this generalization. The crystal structure of *d*-tubocurarine has been elucidated (Sobell *et al.*, 1972), and the internitrogen distance is 1.03 nm. Moreover, all the polar oxygen groups reside on the convex surface of this saucer-shaped molecule. *l*-Tubocurarine, which is 20- to 60-fold less potent than the *d* isomer, has an equivalent internitrogen distance but does not have its polar groups confined to one surface.

The functional relationship of curare to ACh focuses attention on the role of quaternary ammonium groups. Many well-known drugs (atropine, quinine, strychnine, *etc.*) show a marked increase in neuromuscular blocking potency when their nitrogen atom is quaternized. On the other hand, many nonquaternary ammonium compounds block the neuromuscular junction (quinine, nicotine, erythroidine derivatives, *etc.*). The neuromuscular blocking activity of *β*-erythroidine and dihydro-*β*-erythroidine is actually abolished by quaternization of the nitrogen. Other atoms can substitute for cationic quaternary nitrogen; thus, neuromuscular blocking activity has been reported for sulfonium, phosphonium, arsonium, stibonium, iodinium, platinum, and osmium compounds.

The *bis*-quaternary ammonium structure of most of the compounds in Table 11–1 suggests that electrostatic or coulombic association occurs between the two ionized cationic centers of the drug and certain anionic groups of the receptor site; for example, replacement of one quaternary moiety of decamethonium by a primary amine group results in a considerable loss of potency, which is likely a consequence of increased hydration of the cation. The quaternary moiety ensures that the cationic charge is maintained in a minimally hydrated environment.

Cholinergic Receptor Site. The concept of the nicotinic cholinergic receptor, with which ACh combines to initiate the end-plate potential (EPP), is introduced in Chapter 4. By taking advantage of specialized evolutionary events related to cholinergic neurotransmission, it has been possible in recent years to isolate and characterize the nicotinic receptor. These accomplishments represent landmarks in the development of molecular pharmacology. The electric organs from the aquatic species of *Electrophorus* and, especially, *Torpedo* provide rich sources of receptor. The electric organ is derived embryologically from myoid tissue; however, in contrast to skeletal muscle, a significant fraction of the surface of the membrane is excitable and contains cholinergic receptors. In vertebrate skeletal muscle, motor end-plates occupy 0.1% or less of the cell surface. The discovery of seemingly irreversible antagonism of neuromuscular transmission by an α toxin from venoms of the krait, *Bungarus multicinctus,* or varieties of the cobra, *Naja naja* (Chang and Lee, 1963), offered a suitable marker for identification of the receptor. The α toxins are peptides of about 8000 molecular weight that can be isolated and labeled with radioisotopes. The interaction of α toxins with the receptor was initially applied to an assay for identification of the isolated cholinergic receptor *in vitro* by Changeux and colleagues in 1970. The α toxins have extremely high affinities and slow rates of dissociation from the receptor, yet the interaction is noncovalent. *In situ* and *in vitro* their behavior resembles that expected for a high-affinity antagonist.

Parallel studies employing a site-directed, irreversible sulfhydryl-labeling reagent, *maleimidobenzyl trimethylammonium,* identified a 40,000-dalton peptide in the preparations containing receptor, the labeling of which is protected by agonists (Karlin, 1969). This peptide also predominates in preparations that were subsequently purified by use of the α-toxin assay (Karlin and Cowburn, 1973). Thus, two separate approaches, which rely on distinctly different aspects of receptor specificity, identified the same protein (or peptide therefrom) as the nicotinic cholinergic receptor. Further evidence that the isolated protein was the receptor came from immunological studies (Patrick and Lindstrom, 1973), since initial attempts at reconstitution of receptor function in isolated membranes met with marginal success. Immunization of experimental animals with purified receptor from electric fish results in the production of antibody that reacts with endogenous nicotinic receptors and a syndrome that in many ways resembles the human disease *myasthenia gravis* (*see* Chapter 6). Apart from the importance of the α toxins in isolation of the receptor, these peptides are also of value as markers for examination of the biosynthesis, location, and turnover of the receptor (Fambrough, 1979; Changeux, 1981).

Despite its relative paucity in muscle, the nicotinic receptor has also been isolated from mammalian skeletal muscle; it has virtually the same biochemical properties as does the receptor of electric fish (Dolly and Barnard, 1977). Subcellular fractions that bind α toxins have been extracted from brain and a cultured pheochromocytoma (Patrick and Stallcup, 1977). In the latter cells, the ACh receptor that mediates changes in ion permeability is distinct from the α-neurotoxin binding entity. This is not totally unexpected, since the nicotinic receptor of cells that originate from the neural crest (which gives rise to autonomic ganglia) has a different pharmacological specificity than does the receptor of the neuromuscular junction (*see* Chapter 10). Thus, α toxins may be specific markers only for nicotinic receptors whose embryonic origin is skeletal muscle.

The nicotinic receptor is a pentamer composed of four distinct subunits in the stoichiometric ratio of $\alpha_2\beta\gamma\delta$. The individual subunits show partial homology of their amino acid sequences, suggesting that they arise from a common primordial gene (Numa *et al.*, 1983). Only the α subunits carry the primary recognition sites for ACh, the reversible antagonists, and the snake α toxins. The binding of these ligands is mutually exclusive with each other. Each of the subunits has an extracellular and an intracellular exposure on the postsynaptic membrane, and they are arranged in such a manner as to circumscribe an internally located channel in a fashion similar to petals on a lily (Changeux, 1981; Kistler *et al.*, 1982; Figure 11–1). In each subunit there are at least three short sequences of hydrophobic amino acids, which are the likely domains that span the membrane. The receptor is an asymmetrical molecule (14 nm × 8 nm) of 250,000 daltons, and the bulk of the nonmembrane spanning domains is on the extracellular surface (Figure 11–1). Measurement of the number of receptors per unit area and the membrane conductance have demonstrated that rates of ion translocation are sufficiently rapid (5×10^7 ions per second) to require movement through an open channel, rather than by a rotating carrier of ions. Moreover, agonist-mediated changes in ion permeability (inward movement of sodium and outward movement of potassium) occur through a single class of channels (Dionne *et al.*, 1978). Thus, the agonist binding site appears to be intimately coupled with an ion channel; binding of two agonist molecules results in a rapid conformational change that opens the channel, which is internal to the five subunits in the pentameric receptor molecule.

In junctional areas the receptor is present in high densities ($10,000/\mu m^2$) (Cartaud *et al.*, 1978). On the extracellular surface, an internal cavity (presumably the channel) collects electron-dense stain. Thus, the view perpendicular to the membrane surface is of closely packed, rosette-like structures, 8 nm in diameter (*see* Kistler *et al.*, 1982).

PHARMACOLOGICAL PROPERTIES

Skeletal Muscle. The localization of the paralytic action of curare to the junction between nerve and muscle was first adequately described in the classical reports of

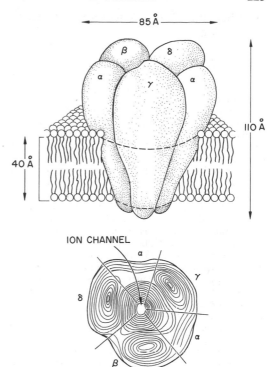

Figure 11–1. *Molecular structure of the cholinergic receptor at the neuromuscular junction.*

The structure of the receptor is described in the text. A side view of a model of the receptor is shown above, while a cross-section at the level of the dashed line in the side view is shown below. (Modified from Kistler *et al.*, 1982.)

Claude Bernard in the 1850s. The cellular locus and mechanism of action of *d-tubocurarine* and other *competitive* neuromuscular blocking agents have now been well defined by modern technics, including microiontophoretic application of drugs and intracellular recording. In brief, *d-tubocurarine* combines with the cholinergic receptor sites at the postjunctional membrane and thereby blocks competitively the transmitter action of ACh. When the drug is applied directly to the end-plate of a single isolated muscle fiber under microscopic control, the muscle cell becomes insensitive to motor-nerve impulses and to directly applied ACh; however, the end-plate region and the remainder of the muscle fiber membrane retain their normal sensitivity to the application of potassium ions, and the muscle fiber still responds to direct electrical stimulation.

To analyze the action of antagonists at the neuromuscular junction further, it is important to consider certain details of receptor activation. The steps involved in the release of ACh by the nerve action potential (AP), the development of miniature end-plate potentials (mepps), their summation to form a postjunctional end-plate potential (EPP), the triggering of the muscle AP, and contraction have been described in Chapter 4. In the past 15 years electrophysiological experimentation has revealed the electrical event associated with the opening and closing of the individual receptor channels associated with activation by agonist. This was achieved by statistical analysis of membrane potential or conductance fluctuations during continuous administration of agonist (Katz and Miledi, 1972; Anderson and Stevens, 1973) and by direct recording from single receptor channels with a suction or patch electrode on denervated skeletal muscle (Neher and Sakmann, 1976). The fundamental event elicited by agonist is an "all-or-none" opening and closing of channels, which gives rise to a square-wave pulse with an average open-channel conductance of ~30 picoSiemens and a duration that is exponentially distributed around a time of about 1 millisecond. The duration of channel opening is far more dependent on the nature of the agonist than is the value of the open-channel conductance (Colquhoun, 1979).

The influence of increasing concentrations of the competitive antagonist, d-tubocurarine, is progressively to diminish the amplitude of the EPP. The amplitude of the EPP may fall to below 70% of its initial value before it is insufficient to initiate the propagated muscle AP; this provides a safety factor in neuromuscular transmission. Analysis of the antagonism of d-tubocurarine on single-channel events shows that it reduces the frequency of channel-opening events but does not affect the conductance or duration of opening for a single channel (Katz and Miledi, 1973). This behavior is precisely that expected for a competitive antagonist. At higher concentrations, curare and other competitive antagonists will block the channel directly in a fashion that is noncompetitive with agonists. The magnitude of this inhibition is dependent on membrane potential (Colquhoun et al., 1979). The rates of onset and offset of antagonism by curare are slower than those of ACh because of the tendency of curare to rebind to successive receptors before exit from the synapse by diffusion (Armstrong and Lester, 1979).

The duration of the end-plate current (or EPP) parallels the lifetime for channel closing. Since the former event is a consequence of multiple quanta of ACh interacting with receptors during nerve stimulation, individual ACh molecules released presynaptically do not successively rebind to receptors to activate multiple channels before hydrolysis by acetylcholinesterase. The concentration of unbound ACh diminishes more rapidly than does the decay of the end-plate current.

If anticholinesterase (anti-ChE) drugs are present, the EPP (or end-plate current) is prolonged, which is indicative of rebinding of transmitter to neighboring receptors before removal from the synapse (Mageby and Terrar, 1975). It is then not surprising that anti-ChE agents and d-tubocurarine are competitive, since increasing the duration of action of ACh in the synapse should favor occupation of the receptor by transmitter relative to d-tubocurarine. d-Tubocurarine also partially prevents the prolongation of the EPP by the anti-ChE compounds (Mageby and Terrar, 1975). This is, in part, a consequence of longer diffusion distances between unoccupied receptors and a diminished probability of agonist rebinding to neighboring receptors when antagonist is present.

At the level of the individual receptor molecules, simultaneous binding by two agonist molecules (one on each α subunit) is required for activation. Activation shows positive cooperativity, and thus occurs over a narrow range of concentrations (Dionne et al., 1978; Sine and Taylor, 1980). Although two competitive antagonist or snake α-toxin molecules can bind to each receptor molecule, also on the α subunits, the binding of one molecule of antagonist to each receptor is sufficient to render it nonfunctional (Sine and Taylor, 1981; Taylor et al., 1983). The binding constants of antagonists for the two α subunits do not appear to be identical.

The *depolarizing agents*, such as *succinylcholine* and *decamethonium*, act by a different mechanism. Their initial action is to depolarize the membrane by opening channels in the same manner as ACh; however, since they persist at the neuromuscular junction, the depolarization is longer lasting. This results in a brief period of repetitive excitation, which may be manifested by transient muscular fasciculation. This phase is followed by block of neuromuscular transmission and flaccid paralysis. The details of the sequence of excitation and depression vary with different species and muscles in the same species, so that the dominance of repetitive excitation, contracture, or block will differ. In man, the sequence of repetitive excitation (fasciculations) followed by block of transmission and neuromuscular paralysis is observed; however, even this sequence is influenced by such factors as the anesthetic agent used concurrently, the type of muscle, and the interval between doses of drug. Depolarization blockade exhibits several distinct differences from that produced by d-tubocurarine and related drugs; these are listed in Table 11–2.

Table 11–2.   COMPARISON OF COMPETITIVE (*d*-TUBOCURARINE) AND DEPOLARIZING (DECAMETHONIUM) BLOCKING AGENTS *

	d-TUBOCURARINE	DECAMETHONIUM (C10)
Effect of *d*-tubocurarine chloride administered previously	Additive	Antagonistic
Effect of decamethonium administered previously	No effect, or antagonistic	Some tachyphylaxis; usually no cumulative effect
Effect of anti-ChE agents on block	Reversal of block	No antagonism
Effect on motor end-plate	Elevated threshold to ACh; no depolarization	Partial, persisting depolarization
Initial excitatory effect on striated muscle	None	Transient fasciculations
Character of muscle response to indirect tetanic stimulation during *partial* block	Poorly sustained contraction	Well-sustained contraction
Effect of KCl or of a tetanus on block	Transient reversal of the block	No antagonism
Effect of current applied to end-plate region:		
—cathodal	Lessens paralysis	Intensifies paralysis
—anodal	Intensifies paralysis	Lessens paralysis
Effect of lowering muscle temperature on block	Antagonism and shortening of effect	Amplification and prolongation of effect
Effect on denervated mammalian muscle	Transient fibrillation	Contracture

* Based on data in Paton and Zaimis, 1949, 1952; Zaimis, 1976; Zaimis and Head, 1976.

A partial explanation of these distinctive features of neuromuscular blockade by the depolarizing agents was provided by the discovery by Burns and Paton (1951) that, in contrast to the stabilizing action of *d*-tubocurarine on the motor end-plate, decamethonium produces an immediate and persistent depolarization of both the end-plate and the immediately adjacent area of the sarcoplasmic membrane in the gracilis muscle of the cat. Much the same result is obtained with high, paralyzing doses of ACh in the presence of an anti-ChE agent. Thus, it was assumed that neuromuscular blockade was due to the inability of the depolarized area just beyond the end-plate to initiate propagated muscle APs in response to the continued depolarization of the end-plate itself. However, this proposal did not fully explain several subsequent observations (*see* below).

Many of the characteristics of depolarizing blocking agents listed in Table 11–2 apply only to man and to the twitch ("white") muscles of the cat. In all muscles investigated in the monkey, dog, rabbit, and rat, and in the slowly contracting soleus muscle of the cat, decamethonium and succinylcholine produce a type of blockade that combines certain features of both the depolarizing and the competitive agents described above and that has some characteristics not associated with either; this type of action has been termed a "dual" mechanism by Zaimis (1976). In such cases, the depolarizing agents produce initially the characteristic fasciculations and potentiation of the maximal twitch, followed by the rapid onset of neuromuscular block; this block is potentiated by anti-ChE agents. However, following the onset of blockade, there is a poorly sustained response to tetanic stimulation of the motor nerve, intensification of the block by

d-tubocurarine, and usual reversal by anti-ChE agents.

The dual action of the depolarizing blocking agents is also seen in intracellular recordings of membrane potential; when agonist is applied continuously, the initial depolarization is followed by a gradual repolarization (Elmqvist and Thesleff, 1962). The second phase, repolarization, resembles receptor desensitization (Katz and Thesleff, 1957).

In man, most of the early evidence indicated that decamethonium and succinylcholine produced a depolarization blockade, wherein anti-ChE drugs potentiate depolarization. However, behavior characteristic of a dual type of blockade has also been frequently reported under clinical circumstances. Here, with increasing concentrations of succinylcholine and in time, the block converts slowly from a depolarizing to a non-depolarizing type, termed phase-I and phase-II block (Durant and Katz, 1982). Zaimis (1976) has observed that the pattern of neuromuscular blockade produced by depolarizing drugs in anesthetized patients has changed in recent years. Prolonged apnea and slow recovery are now observed more frequently, and the characteristics of depolarization blockade are less evident following prolonged administration of succinylcholine or decamethonium. Zaimis has suggested that the general anesthetic employed may be an important factor, with fluorinated hydrocarbons predisposing the system to non-depolarization blockade (*see also* Fogdall and Miller, 1975). Thus, the anesthetic may induce some change in the postsynaptic membrane so that different features of neuromuscular blockade are accentuated.

During the initial phase of application, depolarizing agents produce channel opening, which can be measured by the statistical analysis of fluctuation of EPPs. The probability of channel opening associated with the binding of drug to the receptor is less with decamethonium than with ACh or carbamylcholine (Katz and Miledi, 1973). The diminished probability of channel opening would serve to classify decamethonium as a partial agonist that acts on the postsynaptic membrane. Higher concentrations of decamethonium also interfere with ion translocation by blocking the channel directly (Adams and Sakmann, 1978).

Although the observed fasciculations may result from stimulation of the prejunctional motor-nerve terminal by the depolarizing agent, giving rise to stimulation of the motor unit in an antidromic fashion (Riker, 1975), the primary site of action of both competitive and depolarizing blocking agents is the postjunctional membrane (Katz and Miledi, 1965; Standaert and Adams, 1965; Auerbach and Betz, 1971). Presynaptic actions of the competitive agents may become significant upon repetitive, high-frequency stimulation, since prejunctional nicotinic receptors may be involved in the mobilization of ACh for release from the nerve terminal (Bowman, 1980).

Many ions, drugs, and toxins block neuromuscular transmission by other mechanisms, such as interference with the synthesis or release of ACh (*see* Chapter 4), but most of these agents are not employed clinically for this purpose. An exception is dantrolene, which has proven to be valuable in the treatment of malignant hyperthermia. Dantrolene blocks release of Ca^{2+} from the sarcoplasmic reticulum. The sites of action and interrelationship of several agents that serve as pharmacological tools are indicated in Figure 11–2.

Sequence and Characteristics of Paralysis. When an appropriate dose of *d*-tubocurarine is injected intravenously in man, the onset of effects is rapid. Motor weakness gives way to a total flaccid paralysis. Small, rapidly moving muscles such as those of the fingers and eyes are involved before those of the limbs, neck, and trunk. Ultimately the intercostal muscles and fi-

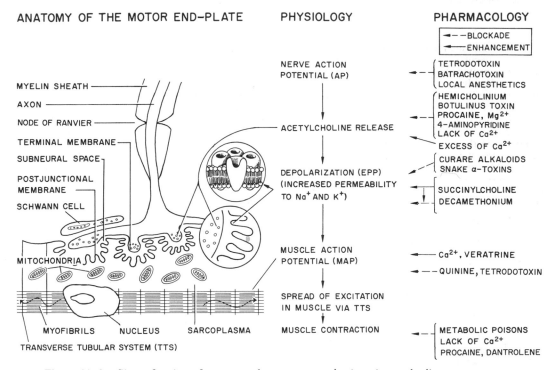

Figure 11–2. *Sites of action of agents at the neuromuscular junction and adjacent structures.*

The anatomy of the motor end-plate, shown at the left, and the sequence of events from liberation of acetylcholine (ACh) by the nerve action potential (AP) to contraction of the muscle fiber, indicated in the middle column, are described in some detail in Chapter 4. The modification of these processes by various agents is shown on the right; the dashed arrows indicate inhibition or block; the solid arrows, enhancement or activation. The circled inserts are an enlargement of the indicated structures. The highest magnification depicts the receptor in the bilayer of the postsynaptic membrane (Ross *et al.*, 1977). A more detailed view of the receptor is shown in Figure 11–1. (Modified from Waser, 1958.)

nally the diaphragm are paralyzed, and respiration then ceases. Recovery of muscles usually occurs in the reverse order to that of their paralysis, and thus the diaphragm is ordinarily the first to regain function.

Prior to causing paralysis, *depolarizing agents* such as succinylcholine evoke transient muscular fasciculations, observed especially over the chest and abdomen; however, these are less common in the anesthetized patient. As the paralytic effect progresses, the neck, arm, and leg muscles are involved at a time when there is only slight weakness of facial, masticatory, lingual, pharyngeal, and laryngeal muscles; at this stage, respiratory muscular weakness is not pronounced and vital capacity is reduced only 25%.

After a single intravenous dose of 10 to 30 mg of *succinylcholine,* muscular fasciculation ensues briefly; then relaxation occurs within 1 minute, becomes maximal within 2 minutes, and disappears as a rule within 5 minutes. Transient apnea usually occurs at the time of maximal effect. Muscular relaxation of longer duration can be achieved by repeated injections at appropriate intervals or by continuous intravenous infusion. Even after discontinuance of an infusion, the effects of the drug usually disappear rapidly because of its rapid hydrolysis by the butyrylcholinesterase of the plasma and liver. The degree of muscular relaxation can usually be altered within 30 to 60 seconds by a change in the rate of infusion. Muscle soreness may follow the administration of succinylcholine. Small doses of competitive blocking agents have been employed to minimize fasciculations and muscle pain caused by succinylcholine. However, this procedure is controversial, since it increases the requirement for the depolarizing drug.

During prolonged depolarization, muscle cells may lose significant quantities of K^+ and gain Na^+, Cl^-, and Ca^{2+}. In patients in whom there has been extensive injury to soft tissues, the efflux of K^+ following continued administration of succinylcholine can be life threatening. The change in the nature of the blockade produced by succinylcholine (from phase I to phase II) presents an additional complication with long-term infusion.

Central Nervous System.   *d*-Tubocurarine and other quaternary neuromuscular blocking agents are virtually devoid of central effects following the intravenous administration of ordinary clinical doses because of their inability to penetrate the blood-brain barrier.

The most decisive experiment performed to settle the problem whether curare significantly affects central functions in the dose range employed clinically is that of Smith and associates (1947). Smith (an anesthesiologist) permitted himself to receive intravenously two and one-half times the amount of *d*-tubocurarine necessary for paralysis of all skeletal muscles. Adequate respiratory exchange was maintained by artificial respiration with oxygen. At no time was there any evidence of lapse of consciousness, impairment of memory, clouding of sensorium, analgesia, disturbance of special senses, or alteration in the resting EEG or its response to pattern vision. No evidence of central respiratory or vasomotor stimulation was observed. Despite adequate artificially controlled respiration, "shortness of breath" was experienced, and the accumulation of unswallowed saliva in the pharynx caused the sensation of choking. The experience was definitely unpleasant. It was concluded that *d*-tubocurarine given intravenously even in large doses has no significant central stimulant, depressant, or analgesic effect in man, and that its sole action in anesthesia is the peripheral paralytic effect on skeletal muscle.

Autonomic Ganglia.   Although the nicotinic receptors of autonomic ganglion cells have certain features in common with those at the motor end-plate, the two types are not identical, as discussed above and in Chapter 4. Hence, neuromuscular blocking agents vary with respect to their relative potencies in producing ganglionic blockade. Just as at the motor end-plate, ganglionic blockade by *d*-tubocurarine and other stabilizing drugs is antagonized effectively by anti-ChE agents, such as neostigmine; however, in ganglia, the antagonism is reinforced by the additional action of endogenous ACh at the muscarinic receptors of the ganglion cells, as described in Chapters 6 and 10.

At the doses of *d*-tubocurarine employed clinically, some degree of blockade is probably produced, both at autonomic ganglia and at the adrenal medulla, which results in a fall in blood pressure and tachycardia. Gallamine in doses used clinically blocks selectively the cardiac vagus nerve, probably at the postganglionic muscarinic sites.

This action results in sinus tachycardia and occasionally in cardiac arrhythmias and hypertension. Pancuronium, metocurine, and alcuronium show less ganglionic blockade at common clinical doses. Atracurium and, particularly, vecuronium are even more selective (Son *et al.*, 1981; Basta *et al.*, 1982; Sutherland, *et al.*, 1983); the vagolytic and the hypotensive effects from blockade of autonomic ganglia appear to be minimal with these agents. The maintenance of cardiovascular reflex responses is usually desired during anesthesia.

Of the *depolarizing agents,* succinylcholine (or decamethonium) rarely causes effects attributable to ganglionic blockade; although instances of bradycardia, tachycardia, and even cardiac arrest have been reported, it is difficult to dissociate such occurrences from the actions of the anesthetic agent or other circumstances. Cardiovascular effects that are probably due to the successive stimulation of vagal ganglia (manifested by bradycardia) and of sympathetic ganglia (resulting in hypertension and tachycardia) are more frequently associated with the administration of succinylcholine. With extremely high doses, ganglionic blockade may ensue (*see* Foldes, 1966).

Histamine Release. *d*-Tubocurarine produces typical histamine-like wheals when injected intracutaneously or intra-arterially in man, and certain clinical responses to *d*-tubocurarine (bronchospasm, hypotension, excessive bronchial and salivary secretion) appear to be caused by the release of histamine. Metocurine, succinylcholine, and atracurium also cause histamine release, but to a lesser extent. Decamethonium, pancuronium, alcuronium, vecuronium, and gallamine have even less tendency to release histamine after intradermal or systemic injection (Bowman, 1982; Ertama, 1982).

Cardiovascular System. The rapid intravenous injection of large doses of *d*-tubocurarine in man may cause a rapid and severe fall in blood pressure. The major causes of the hypotension are peripheral vasodilatation from the release of histamine and sympathetic ganglionic blockade. Additional factors are diminished venous return due to loss of skeletal muscle tone, diminished respiratory excursion, and the consequences of intermittent positive pressure in the airway for the purpose of restoring the adequacy of respiration. Pancuronium is unique in that rapid injection can increase blood pressure, possibly because of ganglionic stimulation. Little change in blood pressure or heart rate is noted upon injection of atracurium or vecuronium.

Miscellaneous Actions. Ganglionic blockade is chiefly responsible for the decreased tone and motility of the gastrointestinal tract. Decamethonium and succinylcholine exhibit muscarinic actions, but only in extremely high doses; the latter drug may cause an increase in intraocular tension. The depolarizing agents can release potassium rapidly from intracellular sites; this may be a factor in the production of prolonged apnea that has been noted in patients who receive these drugs while in electrolyte imbalance (Dripps, 1976). Such alterations in the distribution of potassium may be particularly important in patients with congestive heart failure who are receiving digitalis or diuretics. Caution should be used or depolarizing blocking agents should be avoided in patients with extensive soft-tissue trauma or burns. A higher dose of a competitive blocking agent is often required in these patients. Neonates may have an enhanced sensitivity to competitive neuromuscular blocking agents and some resistance to depolarizing drugs (Smith, 1976).

Synergisms and Antagonisms. The interactions between the competitive and depolarizing neuromuscular blocking agents have already been considered. From a clinical viewpoint, the most important pharmacological interactions of these drugs are with certain *general anesthetics,* certain *antibiotics, calcium channel blockers,* and *anti-ChE compounds.*

Since the anti-ChE agents neostigmine, pyridostigmine, and edrophonium preserve endogenous ACh and also act directly on the neuromuscular junction, they can be employed in the treatment of overdosage with *d*-tubocurarine or other competitive blocking agents. Similarly, upon completion of the surgical procedure many anesthesiologists employ neostigmine or edrophonium to reverse and decrease the duration of competitive neuromuscular blockade (Dripps, 1976). A muscarinic antagonist (atropine or glycopyrrolate) is used concomitantly to prevent stimulation of muscarinic receptors. The anti-ChE agents, however, are synergistic with the depolarizing blocking agents, particularly in their initial phase of action. Thus, the distinction in the type of neuromuscular blocking agent must be clear.

Many inhalational anesthetics (*e.g.,* halothane, *methoxyflurane, isoflurane,* and *enflurane*) exert a stabilizing effect on the postjunctional membrane and, therefore, act synergistically with the *competitive blocking agents.* Consequently, when such blocking drugs are employed for muscular relaxation as adjuncts to these anesthetics, their doses should be reduced (*see* Fogdall and Miller, 1975).

Aminoglycoside antibiotics produce neuromuscular blockade by inhibition of ACh release from the preganglionic terminal (through competition with calcium ions) and to a lesser extent by stabilization of the postjunctional membrane. The blockade is antagonized by calcium salts, but only inconsistently by anti-ChE agents (*see* Chapter 51). The *tetracycline antibiotics* can also produce neuromuscular block, possibly by chelation of calcium ions; Ca^{2+} will also reverse their block. Additional antibiotics that have neuromuscular blocking action, through both presynaptic and postsynaptic actions, include the *peptides* (*polymyxins A* and *B, colistin*), *clindamycin*, and *lincomycin* (*see* Sokoll and Gergis, 1981). Accordingly, when neuromuscular blocking agents are to be administered to patients who are receiving any of these antibiotics, special consideration should be given to the dose and to the judicious use of a calcium salt as an antagonist if recovery of spontaneous respiration is delayed. *Calcium channel blockers* also enhance neuromuscular blockade produced by both competitive and depolarizing antagonists. It is not clear if this is a result of a diminution of calcium-dependent release of transmitter from the nerve ending or a postsynaptic action (Durant *et al.*, 1984).

Miscellaneous drugs that may have significant interactions with either competitive or depolarizing neuromuscular blocking agents include *trimethaphan, opioid analgesics, procaine, lidocaine, quinidine, phenelzine, propranolol, magnesium salts, corticosteroids, digitalis glycosides, chloroquine, catecholamines*, and *diuretics* (*see* Zaimis, 1976; Argov and Mastaglia, 1979).

Toxicology. The important untoward responses of the neuromuscular blocking agents are *prolonged apnea, cardiovascular collapse*, and those resulting from *histamine release*.

Failure of respiration to become adequate in the postoperative period may not always be due directly to the drug. An obstruction of the airway, decreased arterial carbon dioxide tension secondary to hyperventilation during the operative procedure, or the neuromuscular depressant effect of excessive amounts of neostigmine used to reverse the action of the competitive blocking drugs are also causes of the failure to resume adequate ventilation. Directly related factors may also include alterations in body temperature (an increased temperature potentiating the competitive drugs, and a decreased temperature exerting the same effect on the action of the depolarizing substances); electrolyte imbalance, particularly of potassium; decreased plasma cho-

linesterase (*e.g.*, congenital deficiency or liver disease, resulting in reduction in the rate of destruction of succinylcholine); the presence of latent myasthenia gravis or of malignant disease such as oat-cell carcinoma of the bronchus (myasthenic syndrome); reduced blood flow to skeletal muscles causing delayed removal of the blocking drugs; decreased elimination of the relaxants secondary to reduced renal function; and interactions with any of the drugs noted above. Great care should be taken when administering muscle relaxants to dehydrated or desperately ill patients.

A severe rapid rise in temperature has occurred occasionally in patients receiving *halothane* and *succinylcholine*, and more rarely with other combinations of general anesthetics and neuromuscular blocking agents. This condition, known as *malignant hyperthermia*, has a familial tendency and an estimated incidence between 1 in 15,000 and 1 in 50,000. The inducing agent causes widespread muscular rigidity and enhanced heat production by muscle. The hyperthermia may be fatal, and steps should be taken to dissipate heat quickly. Subsequent muscle damage is usually evident. Malignant hyperthermia should be treated by rapid cooling, inhalation of 100% oxygen, and control of the acidosis that is generally present. Dantrolene is administered intravenously. The drug blocks release of Ca^{2+} from the sarcoplasmic reticulum, which reduces muscle tone and heat production (Symposium, 1978; Denborough, 1980).

Treatment of respiratory paralysis should be by positive-pressure artificial respiration with oxygen and maintenance of a patent airway until the complete recovery of normal respiration is assured. With the competitive blocking agents, this may be hastened by the administration of neostigmine methylsulfate (1 to 3 mg, intravenously) or edrophonium (10 mg, intravenously, repeated as required). These agents are usually given together with atropine or glycopyrrolate to counteract the effects of excessive muscarinic stimulation.

Neostigmine antagonizes only the skeletal muscular blocking action of the competitive blocking agents effectively, and it may aggravate such side effects as hypotension or bronchospasm. In such circumstances, sympathomimetic amines may be given to support the blood pressure. The position of the patient should be such as to favor the return of venous blood from the flaccid musculature. Antihistamines are definitely beneficial to counteract the responses that follow the release of histamine, particularly if they are administered before the neuromuscular blocking agent.

Absorption, Fate, and Excretion. Quaternary ammonium neuromuscular blocking agents are very poorly and irregularly absorbed from the gastrointestinal tract. *d*-Tubocurarine is inactive after oral administration, unless huge doses are ingested; this fact was well known to the South American Indians, who ate with impunity the flesh of game killed with curare-poisoned arrows. Absorption is quite adequate from intramuscular sites.

When a single moderate dose of *d-tubocurarine* is injected intravenously, the action begins to wear off in about 20 minutes, yet some residual effect is still discernible after 2 to 4 hours or more. However, when a second dose is given as late as 24 hours after a first, less drug is needed for an equivalent degree of paralysis. The brief duration of paralysis following the initial dose is probably due to redistribution of the drug; when repeated doses are administered, the tissues become saturated and factors of degradation and excretion then directly influence intensity and duration of action. In man, up to two thirds of an administered dose of *d*-tubocurarine is excreted in the urine over a period of several hours, independent of dose and parenteral route of injection; smaller quantities appear in the bile, and a variable amount is metabolized (Crankshaw and Cohen, 1975). The slow redistribution is responsible for the decline of plasma concentrations after a single dose even in cases of renal failure (Maclagan, 1976). In patients with renal insufficiency, accumulation may occur following multiple doses (Gibaldi *et al.*, 1972). Insignificant amounts of *d*-tubocurarine cross the placenta late in pregnancy.

Distribution and elimination of *metocurine* are similar to those of *d*-tubocurarine, as is its duration of action (Savarese *et al.*, 1977). *Pancuronium* is partially hydroxyl-

ated in the liver but also has a similar duration of action (Agoston *et al.*, 1977). *Gallamine* and *decamethonium* are almost entirely excreted by the kidney, with no apparent metabolic degradation. *Atracurium* is converted to less active metabolites by plasma esterases and by spontaneous nonenzymatic rearrangement (Hughes and Chapple, 1981; Basta *et al.*, 1982). This accounts for its briefer duration of action, which is about one half that of pancuronium. *Vecuronium* is metabolized to an appreciable extent, and its duration of action is also about one half that of *pancuronium*. The drug shows little cumulation with multiple doses (Agoston *et al.*, 1980; Fahey *et al.*, 1981).

The extremely brief duration of action of *succinylcholine* is due largely to its rapid hydrolysis by the butyrylcholinesterase of liver and plasma. The initial metabolite, *succinylmonocholine*, has a much weaker, predominantly competitive type of neuromuscular blocking action. Among the occasional patients who exhibit prolonged apnea following the administration of succinylcholine, a considerable number have an atypical plasma cholinesterase or a deficiency of the enzyme, due to a genetic factor, hepatic disease, or a nutritional disturbance; however, in some the enzymatic activity in plasma is normal (Whittaker, 1980).

Preparations, Routes of Administration, and Dosage. Neuromuscular blocking agents are administered parenterally and nearly always *intravenously*. Detailed information on *dosage* can be found in anesthesiology textbooks (*see* Vickers *et al.*, 1978; Miller, 1981; Feldman, 1984). The neuromuscular blocking agents are potentially hazardous drugs. Consequently, they should be administered to patients only by anesthesiologists and other clinicians who have had extensive training in their use and in a setting where facilities for respiratory and cardiovascular resuscitation are immediately at hand.

Tubocurarine chloride (d-tubocurarine chloride) is marketed as a solution containing 3 mg/ml. The use of *d*-tubocurarine to produce muscular relaxation for surgical purposes may be cited as an example of one dose schedule employed. In conjunction with usual preanesthetic medication and light surgical anesthesia, 6 to 9 mg of the drug may be given as a single intravenous injection in adults. One half of this dose may be given after 3 to 5 minutes, if necessary, and small supplements employed later, as required. With certain general anesthetics, lower doses should be employed.

Metocurine iodide (dimethyl tubocurarine iodide; METUBINE IODIDE) is available as a solution containing 2 mg/ml. Since this drug is about two times as potent as *d*-tubocurarine in man, the doses employed are only one half those of the parent alkaloid.

Gallamine triethiodide (FLAXEDIL) is available as a solution containing 20 mg/ml. For muscular relaxation in conjunction with surgical anesthesia, gallamine triethiodide is usually injected intravenously in a dose of 1.0 mg/kg of body weight, and an additional amount (0.5 to 1.0 mg/kg) may be given after 40 to 50 minutes, if necessary.

Pancuronium bromide (PAVULON) is available in solutions containing 1 or 2 mg/ml. The usual intravenous dose is 0.04 to 0.10 mg/kg.

Vecuronium bromide (NORCURON) is available in vials containing 10 mg. Usual initial doses are 0.08 to 0.1 mg/kg, administered intravenously. Additional doses of 0.01 to 0.015 mg/kg are given as necessary.

Atracurium besylate (TRACRIUM) is marketed as a solution (10 mg/ml); it should be administered intravenously at doses of 0.4 to 0.5 mg/kg initially. Maintenance doses are usually one fifth of the initial doses.

Succinylcholine chloride (ANECTINE, others) is marketed as a sterile powder and as a solution containing 20, 50, or 100 mg/ml. For brief surgical procedures in adults, the usual intravenous dose is 20 mg, but the optimal dose varies considerably (10 to 30 mg or more). The drug is given by intravenous drip infusion for more prolonged procedures, in order to obtain sustained muscular relaxation; the dose varies widely from patient to patient (0.5 to 5.0 mg or more per minute), and must be highly individualized. Moment-to-moment control of relaxation can be obtained by careful attention to the rate of infusion and the response of the patient.

Hexafluorenium bromide (MYLAXEN; hexamethylenebis [9-fluorenyldimethylammonium]) is a selective inhibitor of plasma cholinesterase with mild competitive neuromuscular blocking potency. It is given to prolong the blocking action of *succinylcholine* and to minimize the fasciculations that occur prior to neuromuscular block with this agent. The drug is available as a solution (20 mg/ml). Following an intravenous dose of hexafluorenium of 0.4 mg/kg (not to exceed a total dose of 36 mg), the initial dose of succinylcholine is 0.2 mg/kg, intravenously (not to exceed a total dose of 18 mg), which causes muscular relaxation for 20 to 30 minutes.

Alcuronium chloride (ALLOFERIN) is provided in ampuls containing 5 mg/ml; the recommended intravenous dose is 0.2 to 0.3 mg/kg initially. The drug is not marketed in the United States.

Fazadinium bromide is employed in Europe as a rapidly acting competitive blocking agent. It is unique among the neuromuscular blocking agents in that the decline of plasma concentrations is primarily due to reduction of the diazo linkage in the liver (Brittain and Tyers, 1973). The agent may have advantages in short surgical or diagnostic procedures or in patients whose renal function is compromised. The agent has yet to be marketed or tested extensively in the United States.

Decamethonium bromide is no longer marketed in the United States.

Measurement of Neuromuscular Blockade in Man. Assessment of neuromuscular block is usually performed by stimulation of the ulnar nerve. Responses are monitored from compound action potentials or muscle tension developed in the adductor pollicis muscle. Responses to repetitive or tetanic stimuli are most useful for evaluation of blockade of transmission since individual measurements of twitch tension must be related to control values obtained prior to the administration of drugs. Thus, stimulus schedules such as the "train of four" or responses to tetanic stimulation are preferred procedures (Waud and Waud, 1972; Ali and Savarese, 1976).

THERAPEUTIC USES

The main clinical use of the neuromuscular blocking agents is as an *adjuvant in surgical anesthesia* to obtain relaxation of skeletal muscle, particularly of the abdominal wall, so that operative manipulations are facilitated. With muscular relaxation no longer dependent upon the depth of general anesthesia, a much lighter level of anesthesia suffices. This situation is of obvious advantage since the risk of respiratory and cardiovascular depression is minimized. Moreover, the postanesthetic recovery period is reduced. Muscle relaxation is also of value in various orthopedic procedures, such as the correction of dislocations and the alignment of fractures. Neuromuscular blocking agents of short duration are often employed to facilitate intubation with an endotracheal tube and have been used to facilitate laryngoscopy, bronchoscopy, and esophagoscopy in combination with a general anesthetic.

Use to Prevent Trauma in Electroshock Therapy. Electroconvulsive therapy of psychiatric disorders is occasionally complicated by trauma to the patient; the seizures induced may cause dislocations or fractures. Inasmuch as the muscular component of the convulsion is not essential for benefit from the procedure, neuromuscular blocking agents and thiopental are employed. The combination of the blocking drug, the anesthetic agent, and postictal depression usually results in respiratory depression or temporary apnea. An endotracheal tube and oxygen should always be available, and the previously described precautions must be rigidly observed. An oropharyngeal airway should be inserted as soon as the jaw muscles relax (after the seizure) and provision made to prevent aspiration of mucus and saliva. Succinylcholine is most often used because of the brevity of its effect. A cuff may be applied to one extremity to prevent the effects of the drug in that limb; evidence of an effective electroshock is provided by contraction of the group of protected muscles.

Diagnostic Uses. Curare can be employed diagnostically for the *detection of pain due to nerve-root compression* masked by painful spasm of muscles involved in protective splinting. The use of d-tubocurarine to assist in the *diagnosis of myasthenia gravis* and its potential hazards are presented in Chapter 6.

Adams, P. R., and Sakmann, B. Decamethonium both blocks and opens end plate channels. *Proc. Natl. Acad. Sci. U.S.A.*, **1978**, *75*, 2994–2998.

Agoston, S.; Crul, J. F.; Kersten, U. W.; and Scaf, A. H. J. Relationship of serum concentration of pancuronium to its neuromuscular activity in man. *Anesthesiology*, **1977**, *15*, 509–512.

Agoston, S.; Salt, P.; Newton, D.; Bencini, A.; Boomsma, P.; and Erdmann, W. The neuromuscular blocking action of Org NC 45, a new pancuronium derivative, in anaesthetized patients. *Br. J. Anaesth.*, **1980**, *52*, 53S–59S.

Ali, H. H., and Savarese, J. J. Monitoring of neuromuscular function. *Anesthesiology*, **1976**, *14*, 216–249.

Anderson, C. R., and Stevens, C. F. Voltage clamp analysis of acetylcholine produced current fluctuations at the frog neuromuscular junction. *J. Physiol. (Lond.)*, **1973**, *235*, 655–672.

Armstrong, D. L., and Lester, H. A. The kinetics of tubocurarine action and restricted diffusion within the synaptic cleft. *J. Physiol. (Lond.)*, **1979**, *294*, 365–386.

Auerbach, A., and Betz, W. Does curare affect transmitter release? *J. Physiol. (Lond.)*, **1971**, *213*, 691–705.

Barlow, R. B., and Ing, H. R. Curare-like action of polymethylene *bis*-quaternary ammonium salts. *Br. J. Pharmacol. Chemother.*, **1948**, *3*, 298–304.

Basta, S. J.; Ali, H. H.; Savarese, J. J.; Sander, N.; Gionfriddo, M.; Clouter, G.; Lineberry, G.; and Cato, A. E. Clinical pharmacology of atracurium besylate: a new non-depolarizing muscle relaxant. *Anesth. Analg.*, **1982**, *61*, 723–729.

Bennett, A. E. Preventing traumatic complications in convulsive shock therapy by curare. *J.A.M.A.*, **1940**, *114*, 322–324.

Brittain, R. T., and Tyers, M. B. The pharmacology of AH 8165: a rapid-acting, short-lasting competitive neuromuscular blocking drug. *Br. J. Anaesth.*, **1973**, *45*, 837–843.

Buckett, W. R.; Marjoribanks, C. E. B.; Marwick, F. A.; and Morton, M. B. The pharmacology of pancuronium bromide (Org.NA97), a new potent steroidal neuromuscular blocking agent. *Br. J. Pharmacol. Chemother.*, **1968**, *32*, 671–682.

Burns, B. D., and Paton, W. D. M. Depolarization of the motor end-plate by decamethonium and acetylcholine. *J. Physiol. (Lond.)*, **1951**, *115*, 41–73.

Cartaud, J.; Benedetti, E. C.; Sobel, A.; and Changeux, J.-P. A morphological study of the cholinergic receptor protein from *Torpedo marmorata* in its membrane environment and in its detergent extracted form. *J. Cell Sci.*, **1978**, *29*, 313–325.

Chang, C. C., and Lee, C. Y. Isolation of neurotoxins from the venom of *Bungarus multicinctus* and their modes of neuromuscular blocking action. *Arch. Int. Pharmacodyn. Ther.*, **1963**, *144*, 241–257.

Colquhoun, D.; Dreyer, F.; and Sheridan, R. E. The actions of tubocurarine at the frog neuromuscular junction. *J. Physiol. (Lond.)*, **1979**, *293*, 247–284.

Dionne, V. E.; Steinbach, J. H.; and Stevens, C. F. An analysis of the dose-response relationship at voltage-clamped frog neuromuscular junctions. *J. Physiol. (Lond.)*, **1978**, *281*, 421–444.

Dolly, J. O., and Barnard, E. A. Purification and characterization of an acetylcholine receptor from mammalian skeletal muscle. *Biochemistry*, **1977**, *16*, 5053–5060.

Durant, N. N.; Nguyen, N.; and Katz, R. L. Potentiation of neuromuscular blockade by verapamil. *Anesthesiology*, **1984**, *60*, 298–303.

Ertama, P. M. Histamine liberation in surgical patients following administration of neuromuscular blocking drugs. *Ann. Clin. Res.*, **1982**, *14*, 27–31.

Fahey, M. R.; Morris, R. B.; Miller, R. D.; Sohn, Y. J.; Cronnelly, R.; and Gencarelli, P. Clinical pharmacology of ORG NC45. *Anesthesiology*, **1981**, *55*, 6–11.

Fogdall, R. P., and Miller, R. D. Neuromuscular effects of enflurane, alone and combined with d-tubocurarine, pancuronium and succinylcholine in man. *Anesthesiology*, **1975**, *42*, 173–178.

Gibaldi, M.; Levy, G.; and Hayton, W. L. Tubocurarine and renal failure. *Br. J. Anaesth.*, **1972**, *44*, 163–165.

Griffith, H. R., and Johnson, G. E. The use of curare in general anesthesia. *Anesthesiology*, **1942**, *3*, 418–420.

Hughes, R., and Chapple, D. J. The pharmacology of atracurium: a new competitive neuromuscular blocking agent. *Br. J. Anaesth.*, **1981**, *53*, 31–44.

Karlin, A., and Cowburn, D. W. The affinity-labeling of partially purified acetylcholine receptor from electric tissue of *Electrophorus*. *Proc. Natl. Acad. Sci. U.S.A.*, **1973**, *70*, 3636–3640.

Katz, B., and Miledi, R. Propagation of electric activity in motor nerve terminals. *Proc. R. Soc. Lond. [Biol.]*, **1965**, *161*, 453–482.

———. The statistical nature of the acetylcholine potential and its molecular components. *J. Physiol. (Lond.)*, **1972**, *224*, 665–699.

———. The characteristics of "end plate noise" produced by different depolarizing drugs. *Ibid.*, **1973**, *231*, 549–574.

Katz, B., and Thesleff, S. A study of "desensitization" produced by acetylcholine at the motor end-plate. *J. Physiol. (Lond.)*, **1957**, *138*, 63–80.

Kistler, J.; Stroud, R. M.; Klymkowsky, M. W.; Lalaneethee, R. A.; and Fairclough, R. H. Structure and function of an acetylcholine receptor. *Biophys. J.*, **1982**, *37*, 371–383.

Mageby, K., and Terrar, D. A. Factors affecting the time course of decay of end-plate currents: a possible cooperative action of acetylcholine on receptors at the frog neuromuscular junction. *J. Physiol. (Lond.)*, **1975**, *244*, 467–482.

Neher, E., and Sakmann, B. Single channel currents recorded from the membrane of denervated frog muscle fibres. *Nature*, **1976**, *260*, 799–800.

Paton, W. D. M., and Zaimis, E. J. The pharmacological actions of polymethylene bistrimethylammonium salts. *Br. J. Pharmacol. Chemother.*, **1949**, *4*, 381–400.

Patrick, J., and Lindstrom, J. Auto-immune response to acetylcholine receptor. *Science*, **1973**, *180*, 871–872.

Patrick, J., and Stallcup, B. α-Bungarotoxin binding and cholinergic receptor function on a rat sympathetic nerve line. *J. Biol. Chem.*, **1977**, *252*, 8629–8633.

Ross, M. J.; Klymkowsky, M. W.; Agard, D. A.; and Stroud, R. M. Structural studies of a membrane-bound acetylcholine receptor from *Torpedo californica*. *J. Mol. Biol.*, **1977**, *116*, 635–659.

Savarese, J. J.; Ali, H. H.; and Antonio, R. P. The clinical pharmacology of metocurine. *Anesthesiology*, **1977**, *47*, 277–284.

Sine, S., and Taylor, P. Relationship between agonist occupation and the permeability response of the cholinergic receptor revealed by bound cobra toxin. *J. Biol. Chem.*, **1980**, *255*, 10144–10156.

———. Relationship between reversible antagonist occupancy and the functional capacity of the acetylcholine receptor. *Ibid.*, **1981**, *256*, 6692–6698.

Smith, S. M.; Brown, H. O.; Toman, J. E. P.; and Goodman, L. S. The lack of cerebral effects of *d*-tubocurarine. *Anesthesiology*, **1947**, *8*, 1–14.

Sobell, H. M.; Sokore, T. D.; Tavale, S. S.; Canepa, F. G.; Pauling, P.; and Petcher, T. J. Stereochemistry of a curare alkaloid: O,O′,N-trimethyl-*d*-tubocurarine. *Proc. Natl. Acad. Sci. U.S.A.*, **1972**, *69*, 2212–2215.

Son, S. L.; Waud, B. E.; and Waud, D. R. A comparison of the neuromuscular and vagolytic effects of ORG NC 45 and pancuronium. *Anesthesiology*, **1981**, *55*, 12–18.

Standaert, F. G., and Adams, J. E. The actions of succinylcholine on the mammalian motor nerve terminal. *J. Pharmacol. Exp. Ther.*, **1965**, *149*, 113–123.

Sutherland, G. A.; Squire, J. B.; Gibb, A. J.; and Marshall, I. G. Neuromuscular blocking and autonomic effects of vecuronium and atracurium in the anaesthetized cat. *Br. J. Anaesth.*, **1983**, *55*, 1119–1126.

Waser, P. Pharmakologie der Muskelendplatten. *Schweiz. Arch. Neurol. Psychiatr.*, **1958**, *82*, 298 319.

Waud, B. E., and Waud, D. R. The relation between the response to "train of four" stimulation and receptor occlusion during competitive neuromuscular block. *Anesthesiology*, **1972**, *37*, 413–416.

Zaimis, E. J. Motor end-plate differences as a determining factor in the mode of action of neuromuscular blocking substances. *J. Physiol. (Lond.)*, **1953**, *122*, 238–251.

Monographs and Reviews

Argov, Z., and Mastaglia, F. L. Disorders of neuromuscular transmission caused by drugs. *N. Engl. J. Med.*, **1979**, *301*, 409–413.

Bovet, D. Synthetic inhibitors of neuromuscular transmission, chemical structures and structure activity relationships. In, *Neuromuscular Blocking and Stimulating Agents*, Vol 1. *International Encyclopedia of Pharmacology and Therapeutics*, Sect. 14. (Cheymol, J., ed.) Pergamon Press, Ltd., Oxford, **1972**, pp. 243–294.

Bowman, W. C. Pre- and postjunctional cholinoreceptors at the neuromuscular junction. *Anesth. Analg.*, **1980**, *59*, 935–943.

———. Non-relaxant properties of neuromuscular blocking drugs. *Br. J. Anaesth.*, **1982**, *54*, 147–159.

Changeux, J.-P. The acetylcholine receptor: an allosteric membrane protein. *Harvey Lect.*, **1981**, *75*, 85–254.

Cheymol, J., and Bourillet, F. Inhibitors of post-synaptic receptors. In, *Neuromuscular Blocking and Stimulating Agents*, Vol. 1. *International Encyclopedia of Pharmacology and Therapeutics*, Sect. 14. (Cheymol, J., ed.) Pergamon Press, Ltd., Oxford, **1972**, pp. 297–356.

Colquhoun, D. The link between drug binding and response: theories and observations. In, *The Receptors: A Comprehensive Treatise*. (O'Brien, R. D., ed.) Plenum Press, New York, **1979**, pp. 93–142.

Crankshaw, D. P., and Cohen, E. N. Uptake, distribution and elimination of skeletal muscle relaxants. In, *Muscle Relaxants*. (Katz, R., ed.) Excerpta Medica, Amsterdam, **1975**, pp. 125–141.

Denborough, M. The pathopharmacology of malignant hyperpyrexia. *Pharmacol. Ther.*, **1980**, *9*, 357–365.

Dorkins, H. R. Saxamethonium—the development of a modern drug from 1906 to the present day. *Med. Hist.*, **1982**, *26*, 145–168.

Dripps, R. D. The clinician looks at neuromuscular blocking drugs. In, *Neuromuscular Junction*. (Zaimis, E., ed.) Springer-Verlag, Berlin, **1976**, pp. 583–592.

Durant, N. N., and Katz, R. L. Saxamethonium. *Br. J. Anaesth.*, **1982**, *54*, 195–208.

Elmqvist, D., and Thesleff, S. Ideas regarding receptor desensitization at the motor end plate. *Rev. Can. Biol.*, **1962**, *21*, 220–234.

Fambrough, D. Control of acetylcholine receptors in skeletal muscle. *Physiol. Rev.*, **1979**, *59*, 165–227.

Feldman, S. Neuromuscular blocking drugs. In, *A Practice of Anaesthesia*, 5th ed. (Churchill-Davidson, H. C., and Wylie, W. D., eds.) Year Book Medical Publishers, Inc., Chicago, **1984**, pp. 722–734.

Foldes, F. F. (ed.). *Muscle Relaxants*. F. A. Davis Co., Philadelphia, **1966**.

Gill, R. C. *White Waters and Black Magic*. Henry Holt & Co., New York, **1940**.

Karlin, A. Chemical modification of the active site of the acetylcholine receptor. *J. Gen. Physiol.*, **1969**, *54*, 245S–264S.

McIntyre, A. R. History of curare. In, *Neuromuscular Blocking and Stimulating Agents*, Vol. 1. *International Encyclopedia of Pharmacology and Therapeutics*, Sect. 14. (Cheymol, J., ed.) Pergamon Press, Ltd., Oxford, **1972**, pp. 187–203.

Maclagan, J. Competitive neuromuscular blocking drugs. In, *Neuromuscular Junction*. (Zaimis, E., ed.) Springer-Verlag, Berlin, **1976**, pp. 421–474.

Miller, R. D. (ed.). *Pharmacology of Muscle Relaxants, Their Agonists and the Monitoring of Neuromuscular Function*. Churchill Livingston, Inc., New York, **1981**, pp. 487–538.

Numa, S.; Noda, M.; Takahashi, H.; Tanabe, T.; Toyosato, M.; Furutani, Y.; and Kikyotani, S. Molecular structure of the nicotinic acetylcholine receptor. *Cold Spring Harbor Symp. Quant. Biol.*, **1983**, *48*, 57–70.

Paton, W. D. M., and Zaimis, E. J. The methonium compounds. *Pharmacol. Rev.*, **1952**, *4*, 219–253.

Riker, W. F. Prejunctional effects of neuromuscular blocking and facilitatory drugs. In, *Muscle Relaxants*. (Katz, R., ed.) Excerpta Medica, Amsterdam, **1975**, pp. 59–102.

Smith, S. C. Neuromuscular blocking drugs in man. In, *Neuromuscular Junction*. (Zaimis, E., ed.) Springer-Verlag, Berlin, **1976**, pp. 593–660.

Sokoll, M. D., and Gergis, S. D. Antibiotics and neuromuscular function. *Anesthesiology*, **1981**, *55*, 148–159.

Speight, T. M., and Avery, G. S. Pancuronium bromide: a review of its pharmacological properties and clinical application. *Drugs*, **1972**, *4*, 163–226.

Symposium. (Various authors.) *Second International Symposium on Malignant Hyperthermia*. (Aldrete, A., and Britt, B. A., eds.) Grune & Stratton, Inc., New York, **1978**, pp. 1–560.

Taylor, P.; Brown, R. D.; and Johnson, D. A. The linkage between ligand occupation and response of the nicotinic acetylcholine receptor. In, *Current Topics in Membranes and Transport*, Vol. 18. (Kleinzeller, A., and Martin, B. R., eds.) Academic Press, Inc., New York, **1983**, pp. 407–444.

Vickers, M. D.; Wood-Smith, F. G.; and Stewart, H. C. *Drugs in Anaesthetic Practice*. Butterworths, London, **1978**.

Whittaker, M. Plasma cholinesterase variants and the anaesthetist. *Anaesthesia*, **1980**, *35*, 174–197.

Zaimis, E. The neuromuscular junction: area of uncertainty. In, *Neuromuscular Junction*. (Zaimis, E., ed.) Springer-Verlag, Berlin, **1976**, pp. 1–18.

Zaimis, E., and Head, S. Depolarizing neuromuscular blocking drugs. In, *Neuromuscular Junction*. (Zaimis, E., ed.) Springer-Verlag, Berlin, **1976**, pp. 365–420.

Zaimis, E. J. Mechanisms of neuromuscular blockade. In, *Curare and Curare-like Agents*. (Bovet, D.; Bovet-Nitti, F.; and Marini-Bettòlo, G. B.; eds.) Elsevier Publishing Co., Amsterdam, **1959**, pp. 191–203.

III

Drugs Acting on the Central Nervous System

CHAPTER

12 NEUROHUMORAL TRANSMISSION AND THE CENTRAL NERVOUS SYSTEM

Floyd E. Bloom

Drugs that act upon the central nervous system (CNS) influence the lives of everyone, everyday. These agents are invaluable therapeutically because they can produce specific physiological and psychological effects. Without general anesthetics, modern surgery would be impossible. Drugs that affect the CNS may selectively relieve pain or fever, suppress disorders of movement, or prevent seizures. They may induce sleep or arousal, reduce the desire to eat, or allay the tendency to vomit. They may be used to treat anxiety, mania, depression, or schizophrenia without altering consciousness. The brain may also be affected by drugs that are used to treat diseases of peripheral organs.

The nonmedical, self-use of CNS drugs is widely practiced. Socially acceptable stimulants and antianxiety agents produce stability, relief, and even pleasure for many. However, the excessive use of these and other drugs can also adversely affect lives when their use leads to physical dependence on the drug or to toxic side effects that may include lethal overdosage.

The unique quality of drugs that affect the nervous system and behavior places investigators who study the CNS in the midst of an extraordinary scientific challenge—the attempt to understand the cellular and molecular basis for the enormously complex and varied functions of the human brain. In this effort, pharmacologists have two major goals: to use drugs to dissect the mechanisms that operate in the normal CNS and to develop appropriate drugs to correct pathophysiological events in the abnormal CNS.

Approaches to the elucidation of the sites and mechanisms of action of CNS drugs demand understanding of the cellular and molecular biology of the brain. Although knowledge of the anatomy, physiology, and chemistry of the nervous system is far from complete, the acceleration of interdisciplinary research on the CNS has led to remarkable progress. This chapter introduces guidelines and fundamental principles for the comprehensive analysis of drugs that affect the CNS. Specific therapeutic approaches to neurological and psychiatric disorders are discussed in the chapters that follow in this section.

ORGANIZATIONAL PRINCIPLES OF THE BRAIN

The brain is an assembly of interrelated neural systems that regulate their own and each other's activity in a dynamic, complex fashion. The large anatomical divisions provide a superficial classification of the distribution of brain functions.

MACROFUNCTIONS OF BRAIN REGIONS

Cerebral Cortex. The two cerebral hemispheres constitute the largest division of the brain. Regions of the cortex are classified in several ways: (1) by the modality of information processed (*e.g.*, sensory, including somatosensory, visual, auditory, and olfactory, as well as motor and associational); (2) by anatomical position (frontal, temporal, parietal, and occipital); and (3) by the geometrical relationship between cell types in the major cortical layers (so-called cytoarchitectonic classifications). Presently, emphasis on cortical structure is focused upon the rather regular columnar organization of cells within vertically oriented cylinders at right angles to the cortical surface. Each of these vertical arrays contains slightly more than 100 neurons. One such unit may constitute the elemental module for processing information in the cortex. Individual columns can be assembled into large ensembles of hundreds to thousands of neurons by functional association with adjacent vertical arrays or with functionally related units in other areas of the cortex. Mountcastle and Edelman (1978) view these ensembles as "interconnected . . . nested distributed systems" and suggest that the associations are rapidly modifiable as information is processed. The 50 billion neurons of the human cortex provide an astronomical number of possibilities for such processing. Cortical areas termed association areas receive and somehow process information that is relayed to the primary cortical sensory regions, producing the still-unexplained higher cortical functions such as abstract thought, memory, and consciousness.

The cerebral cortices also provide for supervisory integration of the autonomic nervous system, and they may integrate somatic and vegetative functions, including those of the cardiovascular and gastrointestinal systems. For example, the control of blood pressure and of gastric motility may be susceptible to conscious feedback control in human beings (Miller, 1978).

Limbic System. This region, which consists of the *hippocampus, amygdaloid complex, septum, hypothalamus, olfactory* and *pyriform lobes, basal ganglia,* and parts of the *thalamus,* is sometimes called the visceral brain. These structures lie beneath the cortical mantle and act in a complex manner to integrate emotional state with motor and visceral activities.

Parts of the limbic system also participate individually in functions that are capable of more precise definition. Thus, the basal ganglia or neostriatum (the *caudate nucleus, putamen, globus pallidus,* and *lentiform nucleus*) form an essential segment of the *extrapyramidal motor system.* This system complements the function of the pyramidal (or voluntary) motor system; damage to the extra-pyramidal system depresses the ability to initiate voluntary movements and causes disorders characterized by involuntary movements, such as the tremors and rigidity of Parkinson's disease or the uncontrollable limb movements of Huntington's chorea. Similarly, the hippocampus may be crucial to the formation of recent memory, since this function is lost in patients with extensive bilateral damage to the hippocampus.

The *thalamus* lies in the center of the brain, beneath the cortex and basal ganglia and above the hypothalamus. The neurons of the thalamus are arranged into distinct clusters, or nuclei, which are either paired or midline structures. These nuclei act as relays between the incoming sensory pathways and the cortex, between the discrete regions of the thalamus and hypothalamus, and between the basal ganglia and the association regions of the cerebral cortex. The thalamic nuclei and the basal ganglia also exert regulatory control over visceral functions; aphagia and adipsia, as well as general sensory neglect, follow damage to the corpus striatum.

The *hypothalamus* is the principal integrating region for the entire autonomic nervous system, and it regulates among other functions, body temperature, water balance, intermediary metabolism, blood pressure, sexual and circadian cycles, secretion of the adenohypophysis, sleep, and emotion. Recent advances in the cytophysiological and chemical dissection of the hypothalamus have clarified the connections and possible functions of individual hypothalamic nuclei (Guillemin, 1978).

Midbrain and Brain Stem. The *mesencephalon, pons,* and *medulla oblongata* connect the cerebral hemispheres and thalamus-hypothalamus to the spinal cord. These "bridge portions" of the CNS contain most of the nuclei of the cranial nerves, as well as the major inflow and outflow tracts from the cortices and spinal cord. It is within these regions that the *reticular activating system* is found, which is an important but incompletely characterized region of gray matter linking peripheral sensory and motor events with higher levels of nervous integration. The major monoamine-containing neurons of the brain are found within this zone. These regions together represent the points of central integration for coordination of essential reflexive acts such as swallowing and vomiting and those that involve the cardiovascular and respiratory systems; these areas also include the primary receptive regions for most visceral afferent sensory information. The reticular activating system is essential for the regulation of sleep, wakefulness, and level of arousal, as well as for coordination of eye movements. The fiber systems projecting from the reticular formation have been called "nonspecific" because the targets to which these fibers project are considerably more diffuse in distribution than are the connections from many other neurons (*e.g.*, specific thalamocortical projections). However, the reticular systems may innervate targets in a coherent, functional manner even though their targets are widely distributed (*see* Foote *et al.*, 1983).

Cerebellum. This small and highly organized cortical region arises from the posterior pons behind the cerebral hemispheres. Although it is also highly laminated and redundant in its detailed cytological organization, the lobules and folia of the cerebellum project onto specific deep cerebellar nuclei, which in turn make relatively selective projections to the motor cortex (by way of the thalamus) and to the brain stem nuclei concerned with vestibular (position-stabilization) function. The cerebellum is generally regarded as playing an important role in the maintenance of appropriate body posture in space. In addition to maintaining the proper tone of antigravity musculature and providing continuous feedback during volitional movements of the trunk and extremities, the cerebellum may also regulate heart rate, possibly to maintain blood flow despite changes in posture.

Spinal Cord. The cord extends from the caudal end of the medulla oblongata to the lower lumbar vertebrae. Within this mass of nerve cells and tracts, the sensory information from skin, muscles, joints, and viscera is locally coordinated with motoneurons and with primary sensory relay cells that project to and receive signals from higher levels. The spinal cord is divided into anatomical segments (cervical, thoracic, lumbar, and sacral) that correspond to divisions of the peripheral nerves and spinal column. Ascending and descending tracts of the spinal cord are located within the white matter at the perimeter of the cord, while intersegmental connections and synaptic contacts are concentrated within the H-shaped internal mass of gray matter. Within the H, sensory information flows into the dorsal portion, and motor outflow exits from the ventral portion. The preganglionic neurons of the autonomic nervous system are found in the intermediolateral columns of the gray matter, approximately at the external boundary of the middle of the H of the gray matter. Autonomic reflexes (*e.g.*, changes in skin vasculature with alteration of temperature) can easily be elicited within local segments of the cord, as shown by the maintenance of these reflexes after the cord is severed.

MICROANATOMY OF THE BRAIN

Cellular Organization of the Brain. Present understanding of the cellular organization of the CNS can be viewed simplistically according to three main patterns of neuronal connectivity. In the first, *long-hierarchical* neuronal organizations are typically found in the primary sensory and motor pathways. Here the transmission of information is highly sequential, and interconnected neurons are related to each other in a hierarchical fashion. Primary receptors (in the retina, inner ear, olfactory epithelium, tongue, or skin) transmit first to primary relay cells, then to secondary relay cells, and finally to the primary sensory fields of the cerebral cortex. For motor output systems, the reverse sequence holds, descending from the motor cortex to the final common output of the spinal motoneuron. The essential feature of the hierarchical scheme of CNS organization is that chains of neurons provide a precise flow of information, but such organization suffers the disadvantage that destruction of any link incapacitates the system. As yet, few specific neurotransmitters have been identified for any of the major links in the sensory or motor pathways. The final junction between motoneuron and muscle uses acetylcholine (ACh) as the transmitter. Substance P and other peptides may function in some sensory neurons (Nicoll *et al.*, 1980b; Krieger *et al.*, 1983).

The second pattern of organization involves neurons whose connections are mainly established within the immediate vicinity of their location. Such local-circuit neurons are frequently small and may have very few processes. They are thought to regulate the flow of information through their small spatial domain, and they may do this *without* the necessity for the generation of action potentials, which are essential for the long-distance transmission between hierarchically connected neurons. Local-circuit neurons appear to use many different transmitter substances, including the amino acids gamma-aminobutyrate (GABA), glycine, glutamate, and aspartate, as well as several families of peptides.

A third pattern of organization is utilized by certain neuronal systems of the hypothalamus, pons, and brain stem. These systems contain either a monoamine—norepinephrine (NE), dopamine (DA), or 5-hydroxytryptamine (5-HT)—or one of a number of peptides. These include vasopressin, oxytocin (Swanson and Sawchenko, 1983), beta-endorphin (*see* Bloom, 1983), corticotropin-releasing factor (Swanson *et al.*, 1983; Vale *et al.*, 1983), and growth hormone–releasing factor (Guillemin *et al.*, 1982; Spiess *et al.*, 1983). From a single anatomical location, these neurons extend multiple-branched and divergent connections to many target cells, almost all of which lie outside of the brain region in which the neurons are located. In no case do these cells appear to be sequential elements within any known hierarchical system; rather, they appear to be special local-circuit neurons whose spatial domains are one to two orders of magnitude larger than the classical intraregional interneurons. For example, NE-containing neurons of the locus ceruleus project from pons to cerebellum, spinal cord, thalamus, and several cortical zones, but the function of these target regions is not obviously disrupted when the adrenergic fibers are destroyed experimentally, indicating their divergent but nonhierarchical structure. These systems could mediate linkages between regions that may require temporary integration. Many other long projecting systems that arise from the midbrain could also fit into this organizational scheme, which is neither hierarchical nor strictly local circuit. The neurotransmitters are not yet known for most of these types of internuncial connections.

Cell Biology of Neurons. Morphological properties of central neurons have been very useful for the description of their functional characteristics. Neurons are classified in many different ways, including designation according to function (sensory, motor, or interneuron), the location, or the identity of the transmitter they synthesize and release. Microscopic analysis focuses on their general shape, and, in particular, the number of extensions from the cell body. Most neurons have one axon, which carries signals from the cell of origin to other cells. Other processes extend from the nerve cell to receive synaptic contacts from other neurons; these processes, called dendrites, may branch in extremely complex patterns. Neurons exhibit the cytological characteristics of highly active secretory cells: large nuclei; large amounts of smooth and rough endoplasmic reticulum; and frequent clusters of specialized smooth endoplasmic reticulum (Golgi apparatus), where secretory products of the cell are packaged into organelles bound with membrane for transport out of the cell (Figure 12–1). The synaptic vesicles that are characteristic of distal axons are not easily observed within the neuronal cell body; larger vesicles seen in the Golgi zone may thus form the synaptic vesicles after transport to the nerve terminals. Neurons and their cellular extensions are rich in microtubules—elongated tubules of approximately 24-nm diameter. Their functions may be to support the elongated axons and dendrites and to assist in the reciprocal transport of essential macromolecules and organelles between the cell body and the distant axon or dendrites.

Synaptic Relationships. Synaptic arrangements in the CNS fall into a wide variety of morphological and functional forms that are specific for the cells involved. Specific synaptic connections that have one origin will tend to form contacts upon particular surface zones of their target cells in a mosaic arrangement that may reflect the underlying distribution of chemical receptors. Electron microscopic observations of target neurons reveal two major structural details as characteristic of the site presumed to be the active zone of contact. The presynaptic structure is enriched in small vesicles; their shape, size, and chemical properties vary with the identity of the neurotransmitter. Each vesicle probably contains several thousand molecules of transmitter, a number that approaches the lower estimate of transmitter molecules in a "quantum," the elemental package responsible for miniature postsynaptic potentials (*see* Chapter 4). In addition, the presynaptic and postsynaptic membranes exhibit a specialized attachment site, termed the *synaptolemma* by Bodian (1972).

Many spatial arrangements are possible within synaptic relationships (Figure 12–1). The most common arrangement, typical of the hierarchical pathways, is the axodendritic or axosomatic arrangement in which the axons of the cell of origin make their functional contact with the dendrites or cell body of the target. In other cases, functional contacts may occur between the adjacent cell bodies (somasomatic) or between overlapping dendrites (dendrodendritic). The latter is typical of some of the monoaminergic neurons within their nuclei of origin. Many local-circuit neurons do not possess distinct axons and yet enter into synaptic relationships through modified dendrites, sometimes termed *telodendrites;* these modified dendrites can be either the presynaptic or the postsynaptic element. Another relatively frequent arrangement, particularly within the spinal cord, is the serial axoaxonic relationship in which the axon of an interneuron ends upon the terminal of a long-distance neuron as that terminal contacts a dendrite in the dorsal horn. Many presynaptic axons contain enlargements along their length that show collections of typical synaptic vesicles, often without a specialized synaptolemma. It is not yet clear if such sites also act as specific sites of release of transmitter; "nonspecialized" axonal enlargements (or *boutons en passage*) could also be sites of some other function. Neurons of the peripheral autonomic nervous system do not exhibit specialized synaptolemma at the point of their contact with glandular or smooth muscle cells, where transmitter is certainly released; they do, however, exhibit typical axodendritic, dendrodendritic, and somasomatic contacts within autonomic ganglia.

The bioelectric properties of neurons and junctions in the CNS generally follow the outlines and details already described for the peripheral autonomic nervous system (*see* Chapter 4), except that a much more varied range of intracellular mechanisms has been discerned in CNS. Although not yet fully clarified, some description of these various forms of presumptive exchange of information appears below.

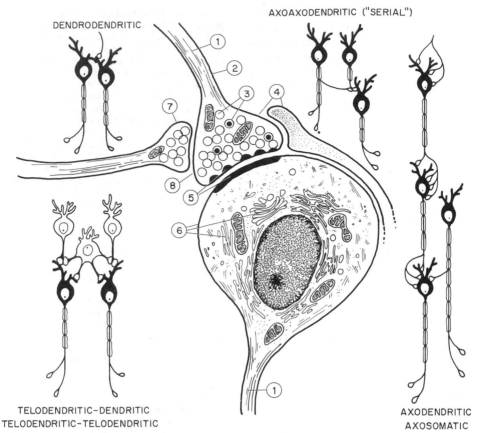

Figure 12–1.   *Drug-sensitive sites in synaptic transmission.*

Schematic view of the drug-sensitive sites in some prototypical synaptic complexes. In the center, a postsynaptic neuron receives a somatic synapse (shown greatly oversized) from an axonic terminal; an axoaxonic terminal is shown in contact with this presynaptic nerve terminal. Drug-sensitive sites include: (*1*) microtubules responsible for orthograde and retrograde transport of macromolecules between the neuronal cell body and distal processes; (*2*) electrically conductive membranes; (*3*) sites for the synthesis and storage of transmitters; (*4*) sites for the active uptake of some transmitters into nerve terminals or glia; (*5*) sites for the release of transmitter and sites (receptors) to generate responses; (*6*) cytoplasmic organelles and postsynaptic membranes for maintenance of synaptic activity and for long-term mediation of altered physiological states; and (*7*) presynaptic receptors on adjacent presynaptic processes and (*8*) on nerve terminals (autoreceptors). Around the central neuron are schematic illustrations of the more common synaptic relationships in the CNS. (Modified from Bodian, 1972, and Cooper *et al.,* 1983.)

IDENTIFICATION OF CENTRAL TRANSMITTERS

The rigorous scientific identification of the transmitter for a given central synaptic connection requires data to satisfy the same criteria that were utilized to demonstrate that ACh and NE were the predominant transmitters of the autonomic nervous system (*see* Chapter 4).

1. *The transmitter must be shown to be present in the presynaptic terminals of the synapse and in the neurons from which those presynaptic terminals arise.* Extensions of this criterion involve the demonstration that the presynaptic neuron synthesizes the transmitter substance, rather than simply storing it after accumulation from a nonneural source. Microscopic cytochemistry (*see* Cooper *et al.,* 1983) and subcellular fractionation and analysis of brain tissue are particularly useful to evaluate this criterion in the CNS. These technics are often combined with the production of surgical or

chemical lesions of presynaptic neurons or their tracts to demonstrate that the lesion causes the disappearance of the alleged transmitter from the target region.

2. *The transmitter must be released from the presynaptic nerve concomitantly with presynaptic nerve activity.* This criterion is generally evaluated by electrical stimulation of the nerve pathway *in vivo* and collection of the transmitter in an enriched extracellular fluid within the synaptic target area (Cheramy *et al.*, 1983). However, devices for collection such as push-pull cannulas are still hundreds of times larger than individual synapses, and the sensitivity of the methods for detection of transmitters requires that collection extend for periods that are thousands of times longer than most known synaptic potentials. Thus, this "release" criterion has not yet been rigorously satisfied for single synapses in the CNS. However, methods have recently been developed that may provide sufficient sensitivity to permit collection of substances *in situ* within the spatial and temporal bounds of transmission at a single synapse (Buda *et al.*, 1983; Ewing *et al.*, 1983). Release of transmitter can also be studied *in vitro* by ionic or electrical activation of thin brain slices or subcellular fractions that are enriched in nerve terminals. The release of all transmitter substances so far studied is voltage dependent and requires the influx of Ca^{2+} into the presynaptic terminal. However, transmitter release is relatively insensitive to extracellular Na^+ or to tetrodotoxin, which blocks transmembrane movement of Na^+.

3. *The effects of the alleged substance, when applied experimentally to the target cells, must be identical to the effects of stimulating the presynaptic pathway.* This criterion can be met loosely by qualitative comparisons (*e.g.*, both the substance and the pathway inhibit or excite the target cell). More convincing is the demonstration that the ionic conductances activated by the pathway are the same as those activated by the candidate transmitter. More specifically, the equilibrium value of the synaptic potential and that to which the cell is driven by the alleged transmitter should be identical. These tests require intracellular recording for long periods of time, and this is difficult to achieve *in vivo,* especially for smaller or deeply placed target neurons. The use of preparations of brain slices *in vitro* may overcome such problems (Lynch and Schubert, 1980). Alternatively, the criterion can be satisfied less rigorously by demonstration of pharmacological identity of receptors. In general, pharmacological antagonism of the pathway's actions and those of the candidate transmitter should be achieved by similar doses of the same drug. To be convincing, the antagonistic drug should not affect responses of the target neurons to other unrelated pathways or to chemically distinct transmitter candidates. Actions that are qualitatively identical to those that follow stimulation of the pathway should also be observed with synthetic agonists that mimic the transmitter. Pharmacological characterization of the actions of various agonists and antagonists will define various subsets of receptors for the presumed natural agonist (*e.g.*, muscarinic or nicotinic cholinergic receptors, β_1- or β_2-adrenergic receptors, *etc.*).

Recent studies, especially those that have implicated peptides as transmitters in the central and peripheral nervous systems, suggest that many synapses may contain more than one transmitter substance. Although rigorous proof is lacking, substances that coexist in a given synapse are presumed to be released together and to act jointly on the postsynaptic membrane. Clearly, if more than one substance transmits information, no single agonist or antagonist would necessarily provide faithful mimicry or total antagonism of activation of the presynaptic element.

Assessment of Receptor Properties. Central synaptic receptors may be characterized by examination of their ability to bind high-specific-activity radiolabeled agonists or antagonists or of the ability of other unlabeled compounds to compete for such binding sites (*see* Chapter 2). The specificity of such binding must be evaluated with care. Radioligand-binding assays can be used to quantify binding sites within a region, to follow their appearance throughout the phylogenetic scale and during brain development, and to determine how physiological or pharmacological manipulation regulates receptor number or affinity. Radioligand-binding assays helped characterize the central and peripheral opioid receptors and motivated the eventual detection of a previously unknown group of structurally related peptides, known generally as the *endorphins* (*see* below). Similar approaches are being pursued to determine if there are endogenous ligands to account for the existence of macromolecular binding sites for such drugs as phencyclidine or the benzodiazepines.

The properties of the cellular response to the transmitter can be studied electrophysiologically by the use of *microiontophoresis* (combination of recordings from single cells and highly localized drug administration). The *patch clamp technic* can be used to study the electrical properties of single ionic channels and their regulation by neurotransmitters. These direct electrophysiological tests of neuronal responsiveness can provide qualitative and quantitative information on the effects of a putative transmitter substance. In some cases, receptor properties can also be studied biochemically when the activated receptor is coupled to an enzymatic reaction, such as the synthesis of a cyclic nucleotide.

With limitations, these biochemical and electrophysiological methods can provide quantitative information on the adaptive self-regulation of receptors for a neurotransmitter that follows pharmacological or pathological perturbations (*e.g.*, denervation supersensitivity, drug-induced subsensitivity, *etc.*). Drug-receptor interactions should be considered to be constantly modifiable relationships. Postsynaptic receptivity on CNS neurons is continuously regulated in terms of the number of receptive sites and the threshold required for generation of a response. Receptor number is often dependent upon the concentration of agonist to which the target cell is exposed. Thus, chronic excess of agonist can lead to a reduced number of receptors (desensitization or down-regulation) and consequently to subsensitivity or tolerance to the transmitter. A deficit of transmitter can lead to increased numbers of receptors and supersensitivity of the system (*see* Symposium, 1983). These adaptive processes become especially important when drugs are used to treat chronic illness of the CNS. *With prolonged periods of exposure to drug, the actual mechanisms underlying the therapeutic effect may differ strikingly from those that operate when the agent is first introduced into the system.* Similar adaptive modifications of neuronal systems can also occur at presynaptic sites, such as those concerned with transmitter synthesis, storage, re-uptake, and release. These adaptive changes frustrate attempts to interpret the effects of behaviorally active drugs in terms of specific neurotransmitters (*see* Iversen and Iversen, 1979).

NEUROTRANSMITTERS, NEUROHORMONES, AND NEUROMODULATORS: CONTRASTING PRINCIPLES OF NEURONAL REGULATION

Neurotransmitters. The criteria for identification of synaptic transmitters rely heavily on the demonstrations that a substance contained in a neuron is secreted by that neuron to transmit information to its postsynaptic target. Given this level of functional description and a definite effect of neuron A on its target cell B, a substance found in neuron A, secreted from neuron A, and producing the effect of A on B would then operationally be the transmitter from A to B. Within this broad definition, substances may act to transmit their information in a variety of ways, many of which are only now beginning to be characterized as to mechanisms. In some cases, transmitters may produce minimal effects on bioelectric properties, yet activate or inactivate biochemical mechanisms necessary for responses to other circuits. Alternatively, the action of a transmitter may vary with the context of ongoing synaptic events—enhancing excitations or inhibitions, rather than operating to impose direct excitation or inhibition. Each chemical substance that fits within the broad definition of a transmitter may, therefore, require operational definition within the spatial and temporal domains in which a specific cell-cell circuit is defined. Those same properties may or may not be generalized to other cells that are contacted by the same presynaptic neurons, with the differences in operation related to differences in the postsynaptic receptor and the mechanisms by which the activated receptor produces its effect (Bloom, 1975).

Classically, electrophysiological signs of the action of a *bona fide* transmitter fall into two major categories: *excitation* (in which ion channels are opened to permit net influx of positively charged ions, leading to depolarization with a reduction in the electrical resistance of the membrane) and *inhibition* (in which selective ion movements lead to hyperpolarization, also with decreased membrane resistance). More recent work suggests there may be many "nonclassical" transmitter mechanisms operating in the CNS. In some cases, either depolarization or hyperpolarization is accompanied by a *decreased* ionic conductance (increased membrane resistance) as actions of the transmitter lead to the closure of ion channels (so-called leak channels) that are normally open in some resting neurons (Shepherd, 1983). For some transmitters, such as monoamines and some peptides, a "conditional" action may be involved.

That is, a transmitter substance may enhance or suppress the response of the target neuron to classical excitatory or inhibitory transmitters while producing little or no change in membrane potential or ionic conductance when applied alone. Such conditional responses have been termed *modulatory*, and specific categories of modulation have been hypothesized (*see* Foote *et al.,* 1983; Bloom, 1984; *see also* Nicoll *et al.,* 1980a; Madison and Nicoll, 1982; Waterhouse *et al.,* 1982). Regardless of the mechanisms that underlie such synaptic operations, their temporal and biophysical characteristics differ substantially from the rapid onset-offset type of effect previously thought to describe all synaptic events. These differences have thus raised the issue of whether substances that produce slow synaptic effects should be described with the same term—*neurotransmitter*. Some of the alternate terms deserve brief survey with regard to mechanisms of drug action.

Neurohormones. Peptide-secreting cells of the hypothalamicohypophyseal circuits were originally described as neurosecretory cells, a form of neuron that was both fish and fowl, receiving synaptic information from other central neurons yet secreting their transmitter in a hormone-like fashion into the circulation (Scharrer, 1969; *see* Chapter 59). The transmitter of such neurons was termed a *neurohormone,* that is, a substance secreted into the blood by a neuron. However, this term has lost most of its original meaning because these hypothalamic neurons may also form traditional synapses with many central neurons (Krieger *et al.,* 1983; Swanson and Sawchenko, 1983). Cytochemical evidence would indicate that transmission at these sites is also mediated by the same substance that is secreted as a hormone in the posterior pituitary (oxytocin, antidiuretic hormone). Thus, the designation of *hormone* relates to the site of release at the pituitary and does not necessarily describe all of the actions of the peptide.

Neuromodulators. Florey (1967) employed the term *modulator* to describe substances that can influence neuronal activity differently than do neurotransmitters. In the context of this definition, the distinctive feature of a modulator is that it originates from cellular and nonsynaptic sites, yet influences the excitability of nerve cells. Florey specifically designated substances such as CO_2 and ammonia, arising from active neurons or glia, as potential modulators through nonsynaptic actions. Similarly, circulating steroid hormones, locally released adenosine, and prostaglandins might all now be regarded as modulators.

Neuromediators. Substances that participate in the elicitation of the postsynaptic response to a transmitter fall under this heading. The clearest examples of such mediation are provided by the involvement of adenosine 3',5'-monophosphate (cyclic AMP), and perhaps of guanosine 3',5'-monophosphate (cyclic GMP), as second messengers at specific sites of synaptic transmission (Bloom, 1975; Greengard, 1978). However, it is technically difficult to demonstrate that a change in the concentration of cyclic nucleotides occurs prior to the generation of the synaptic potential and that this change in concentration is both necessary and sufficient for the generation of the synaptic potential. Possibly, the changes in the concentration of cyclic nucleotides that can be observed under certain conditions supplement and enhance the generation of the synaptic potentials. Activation of cyclic nucleotide–dependent protein phosphorylation reactions (*see* Chapter 4) can alter properties of membrane proteins that are known to be substrates in these reactions (Greengard, 1978; Nestler and Greengard, 1984). These possibilities are particularly pertinent to the action of the central catecholaminergic circuits described below.

ACTIONS OF DRUGS IN THE CNS

Specificity and Nonspecificity of CNS Drug Action. The effect of a drug is considered to be specific when it affects an identifiable molecular mechanism unique to target cells that bear receptors for the drug. Conversely, a drug is regarded as nonspecific when it produces effects on many different target cells and acts by diverse molecular mechanisms. This terminology thus distinguishes *broad* actions at many levels of the CNS through effects on specific molecular mechanisms (*e.g.*, atropine blockade of muscarinic receptors) from nonspecific actions. This separation is often a property of the dose-response relationship of the drug and the cell or mechanisms under scrutiny. Even a drug that is highly selective when tested at a low concentration may exhibit nonspecific actions at substantially higher doses. (For example, many specific antagonists of β-adrenergic receptors can also cause local anesthesia at high concentrations; similar nonspecific effects may be seen with tricyclic antidepressants at doses one to two orders of magnitude higher than those required to cause selective changes in rates of transmitter uptake or release.) Conversely, even generally acting drugs may not act equally on all levels of the CNS. For example, sedatives, hypnotics, or general anesthetics would have very limited utility if central neurons that control the respiratory and cardiovascular systems were not less sensitive to their actions. Drugs with specific actions may produce nonspecific effects when the dose and route of administration initially produce high tissue concentrations; their specificity of action becomes apparent only later, when the concentrations fall.

As the number of putative neurotransmitters has increased and as technics have evolved for the analysis of the actions of drugs upon specific target neurons, the list of drugs that have been regarded as having general actions has become considerably shorter. Thus, more and more drugs exhibit actions that can be related to specific mechanisms. For example, the effects of the broadly acting stimulants strychnine and picrotoxin can now be attributed to interference with inhibitory actions that are mediated at receptors for glycine and GABA, respectively (Curtis *et al.*, 1971); similarly, barbiturates have been found to have relatively selective effects on synaptic mechanisms (Macdonald and McLean, 1982).

Drugs whose mechanisms currently appear to be general or nonspecific are classed according to whether they produce behavioral depression or stimulation, while specifically acting CNS drugs can be classed more definitively according to their locus of action or specific therapeutic usefulness.

General (Nonspecific) CNS Depressants. This category includes the anesthetic gases and vapors, the aliphatic alcohols, and some hypnotic-sedative drugs. These agents share the ability to depress excitable tissue at all levels of the CNS by stabilization of neuronal membranes, leading to a decrease in amount of transmitter released by the nerve impulse, as well as to general depression of postsynaptic responsiveness and ion movement.

General (Nonspecific) CNS Stimulants. The drugs that remain in this category are pentylenetetrazol and related agents that are capable of powerful excitation of the CNS and the methylxanthines, which have a much weaker stimulant action. Stimulation may be accomplished by one of two general mechanisms: by blockade of inhibition or by direct neuronal excitation (which may involve increased transmitter release, more prolonged transmitter action, labilization of the postsynaptic membrane, or a decrease in synaptic recovery time).

Drugs That Selectively Modify CNS Function. The agents in this group *may* cause either depression or excitation. In some instances, a drug may produce both effects simultaneously on different systems. Some agents in this category have little effect upon the level of excitability in doses that are used therapeutically. The principal classes of these CNS drugs are the following: anticonvulsants, antiparkinsonism drugs, opioid and nonopioid analgesics, appetite suppressants, antiemetics, analgesic-antipyretics, certain stimulants, neuroleptics (antidepressants and antimanic and antipsychotic agents), tranquilizers, sedatives, and hypnotics.

Although selectivity of action may be remarkable, a drug usually affects several CNS functions to varying degrees. When only one constellation of effects is wanted in a therapeutic situation, the remaining effects of the drug are regarded as limitations in selectivity (*i.e.*, unwanted or side effects).

The specificity of a drug's action is frequently overestimated. This is partly due to the fact that the drug is identified with the effect that is implied by the class name. For example, levodopa, atropine and other muscarinic antagonists, and some antihistamines are all antiparkinsonism drugs, yet all have substantial additional effects that are therapeutically useful. However, since all centrally acting drugs are more or less selective, it will be profitable to consider some of the probable bases for their selectivity; such considerations are inseparable from discussion of the mechanisms of their action.

Factors That Affect the Intensity and Duration of the Effects of Drugs on the CNS. Apart from the exceptional instances in which drugs are introduced directly into the CNS, the concentration of the agent in the blood after oral or parenteral administration obviously has great bearing on the concentration in the CNS. However, this relationship is often not as simple as for peripheral structures.

Although not thoroughly defined anatomically, the *blood-brain barrier* represents an important boundary between the peripheral and central nervous systems in the form of a permeability barrier to the passive diffusion of substances from the blood stream into various regions of the CNS. Evidence of the barrier is provided by the greatly diminished rate of access of chemicals from plasma to the brain (*see* Chapter 1). This phenomenon is much less prominent in the hypothalamus and in several small specialized organs lining the third and fourth ventricles of the brain: the median eminence, area postrema, pineal gland, subfornical organ, and subcommissural organ. While severe limitations are imposed upon the diffusion of macromolecules, selective barriers to permeation also exist for small charged molecules such as neurotransmitters, their precursors and metabolites, and some drugs. These diffusional barriers are at present best conceived as a combination of the partition of solute across the vasculature (which governs passage by definable properties such as molecular weight, charge, and lipophilicity) and the presence or absence of energy-dependent transport systems. Active transport of certain agents

may occur across the barrier in either direction. The diffusional barriers retard the movement of substances from brain to blood as well as from blood to brain, but the brain clears metabolites of transmitters into the cerebrospinal fluid by excretion through the acid transport system of the choroid plexus (*see* Wood, 1979). Substances that can rarely gain access to the brain from the blood stream can often reach the brain after injection directly into the cerebrospinal fluid.

Other factors may also influence the *duration* of a drug's effect. Where the action of a drug is to reduce storage of a transmitter substance, the onset of the effect may be delayed; however, the drug may have a prolonged effect that persists after it has disappeared from the CNS. For example, reserpine reduces stores of catecholamines and 5-HT in the central and peripheral nervous systems. The full biochemical and behavioral effect of this drug appears only after many hours but is apparent for a considerable time after reserpine has been eliminated from the body; yet long-term therapy with reserpine may result in transmitter stores that are only slightly reduced. Covalent or high-affinity binding of a drug to a receptor can also, of course, produce a prolonged effect.

General Characteristics of CNS Drugs. Combinations of centrally acting drugs are frequently administered to therapeutic advantage (*e.g.*, an anticholinergic drug and levodopa for Parkinson's disease). However, other combinations of drugs may be detrimental because of potentially dangerous additive or mutually antagonistic effects.

The effect of a CNS drug is additive with the physiological state and with the effects of other depressant and stimulant drugs. For example, anesthetics are less effective in a hyperexcitable subject than in a normal patient; the converse is true with respect to the effects of stimulants. In general, depressant effects of drugs from all categories are additive (*e.g.*, the fatal combination of barbiturates or benzodiazepines with ethanol), as are the effects of stimulants. Therefore, respiration depressed by morphine is further impaired by depressant drugs, while stimulant drugs can augment the excitatory effects of morphine to produce vomiting and convulsions.

Antagonism between depressants and stimulants is variable. Some instances of true pharmacological antagonism among CNS drugs are known; for example, opioid antagonists are very selective in blocking the effects of opioid analgesics, and ethosuximide (an anticonvulsant) completely blocks the convulsions produced by pentylenetetrazol over a wide dosage range. However, the antagonism exhibited between two CNS drugs is usually physiological in nature. Thus, an individual who has received one drug cannot be returned entirely to normal by another.

The selective effects of drugs on specific neurotransmitter systems may be additive or competitive. This potential for drug interaction must be considered whenever such drugs are administered concurrently. The prolonged duration of action of certain agents may necessitate a drug-free period before therapy with other drugs can be started in order to avoid such interactions. An excitatory effect on some functions is commonly observed with low concentrations of some depressant drugs due either to depression of inhibitory systems or to a transient increase in the release of excitatory transmitters. Examples are the "stage of excitement" during induction of general anesthesia and the "stimulant" effects of alcohol. The excitatory phase occurs only with low concentrations of the depressant; uniform depression ensues with increasing drug concentration. The excitatory effects can be minimized, when appropriate, by pretreatment with a depressant drug that is devoid of such effects (*e.g.*, benzodiazepines in preanesthetic medication). Acute, excessive stimulation of the cerebrospinal axis is normally followed by depression (amphetamine, strychnine), which is in part the consequence of neuronal fatigue and exhaustion of metabolites and stores of transmitters. This postictal depression is additive with the effects of depressant drugs. Acute, drug-induced depression is not, as a rule, followed by stimulation. However, chronic drug-induced sedation or depression is followed by prolonged hyperexcitability upon abrupt withdrawal of medication (barbiturates, alcohol). This type of hyperexcitability can be effectively controlled by the same or another depressant drug (*see* Chapter 23).

Organization of CNS-Drug Interactions. The structural and functional properties of neurons provide a means to specify the possible sites at which drugs could interact specifically or generally in the CNS (Figure 12–1). In this scheme, drugs that affect neuronal energy metabolism, maintenance of membrane integrity, or transmembrane ionic equilibria would be generally acting compounds. Similarly general in action would be drugs that affect the two-way intracellular transport systems (*e.g.*, colchicine). These general effects can still exhibit different dose-response or time-response relationships among different neurons based, for example, on such neuronal properties as rate of firing, dependence of discharge on external stimuli or internal pacemaker, resting ionic fluxes, or axon length. In contrast, when drug actions can be related to specific aspects of the metabolism, release, or function of a neurotransmitter, the site, specificity, and mechanism of action of a drug can be defined by systematic studies of dose-response and time-response relationships. From such data the most sensitive, rapid, or persistent neuronal event can be identified.

Transmitter-dependent actions of drugs can be organized conveniently into *presynaptic* and *postsynaptic* categories. The presynaptic category includes all of the events in the perikaryon and nerve terminal that regulate transmitter synthesis (including the acquisition of adequate substrates and cofactors), storage, release, re-uptake, and catabolism. Transmitter concentrations can be lowered by blockade of synthesis or storage or both. The amount of transmitter released per impulse is generally stable but can also be regulated. For example, 5-HT produces a cyclic AMP–mediated phosphorylation of presynaptic membrane proteins in certain invertebrate neurons. This leads to increased influx of Ca^{2+} and release of transmitter at the affected synapse (Siegelbaum *et al.*, 1982). The effective concentration of transmitter may be increased by inhibition of re-uptake or by blockade of catabolic enzymes. The transmitter that is released at a synapse can also exert actions upon the terminal from which it was released by interaction with receptors at these sites (termed *autoreceptors*). Activation of presynaptic autoreceptors can slow the rate of discharge of transmitter and thereby provide a feedback mechanism that controls the concentration of transmitter in the synaptic cleft (*see* Carlsson, 1975; Chapters 4 and 8).

The postsynaptic category includes all of the events that follow release of the transmitter in the vicinity of the postsynaptic receptor—in particular, the molecular mechanisms by which occupation of the receptor by the transmitter produces changes in the properties of the membrane of the postsynaptic cell (shifts in membrane potential) as well as more enduring biochemical actions (changes in intracellular cyclic nucleotides, protein kinase activity, and related substrate proteins). Direct postsynaptic effects of drugs generally require relatively high affinity for the receptors or resistance to metabolic degradation. Each of these presynaptic or postsynaptic actions is potentially highly specific and can be envisioned as being restricted to a single, chemically defined subset of CNS cells.

CENTRAL NEUROTRANSMITTERS

In examining the effects of drugs on the CNS with reference to the neurotransmitters for specific circuits, attention should be devoted to the general organizational principles of neurons. The view that synapses represent drug-modifiable control points within neuronal networks thus requires the explicit delineation of the sites at which given neurotransmitters may operate and the degree of specificity or generality by which such sites may be affected. One principle that underlies the following summaries of individual transmitter substances is the chemical-specificity hypothesis of Dale (1935), which holds that a given neuron releases the same transmitter substance at every one of its synaptic terminals. In the face of growing indications that some neurons may contain more than one transmitter substance (Hokfelt *et al.,* 1980, 1983),

Dale's hypothesis has been modified to indicate that a given neuron will secrete the same set of transmitters from all its terminals. However, even this view may require revision. For example, it is not clear whether a neuron that secretes a given peptide will process the precursor peptide to the same end product at all of its synaptic terminals. This principle could also be taken to mean that a transmitter produces the same functional effect (hyperpolarization, depolarization) wherever it is released (functional specificity), but this latter corollary has *not* yet been established. Table 12–1 provides an overview of the pharmacological properties of those amino acid and monoamine transmitters that have been most fully studied in the CNS.

Amino Acids. The CNS contains uniquely high concentrations of certain amino acids, notably glutamate and gamma-aminobutyrate (GABA); these amino acids are extremely potent in their ability to alter neuronal discharge. However, many physiologists were extremely reluctant to accept these simple substances as central neurotransmitters. This reluctance was based in part on conceptual problems of how to discriminate amino acids acting as transmitters from the same compounds as precursors for protein synthesis. The ubiquitous distribution of amino acids within the brain also posed problems in relating release to activity of a single neuronal circuit. Other important arguments against amino acids as transmitters were that they produced prompt, powerful, and readily reversible but redundant effects on every neuron tested; the dicarboxylic amino acids produced excitation, and the monocarboxylic ω-amino acids (*e.g.*, GABA, glycine, β-alanine, taurine) produced qualitatively similar inhibitions (Kelly and Beart, 1975). This redundancy of effect was taken as further support of a nonspecific action on neuronal discharge, and this view was seemingly supported by the early observations that iontophoretic application of amino acids produced excitations or inhibitions that differed from those produced by activation of relevant synapses. Research was also hampered by the facts that selective antagonists of the amino acids were not

Table 12–1. OVERVIEW OF THE PHARMACOLOGY OF AMINO ACID AND MONOAMINE TRANSMITTERS IN THE CENTRAL NERVOUS SYSTEM

TRANSMITTER	ANATOMY-CYTOLOGY	PRESYNAPTIC PHARMACOLOGY			POSTSYNAPTIC PHARMACOLOGY			
		Synthesis	Storage	Re-uptake	Receptor Subtypes and Agonists	Antagonists	Receptor Mechanisms	Catabolism
GABA	Supraspinal interneurons	—	—	2-Hydroxy-GABA, guvacine, and nipecotic acid inhibit	A: Muscimol	Bicuculline, picrotoxin	Increases chloride conductance; hyperpolarizes	Blocked with aminooxyacetic acid
					B: Baclofen	—	—	
Glycine	Spinal interneurons	—	—	—	Taurine (?), β-alanine (?)	Strychnine	Increases Cl^- conductance; hyperpolarizes	—
Glutamate; aspartate	Interneurons at all levels	—	—	—	Quisqualate, ibotenate	Glutamate diethylester	Increases cation conductance; depolarizes	—
					N-Me-D-aspartate	α-Amino adipate, 2-amino-5-phosphonovalerate		
					Kainate	Lactonized kainate		
Acetylcholine	All levels; probable long and short connections	Hemicholinium blocks	—	Choline uptake can be enhanced with loading	M₁; Muscarine, McN-A-343 ‡	Quinuclidinyl benzoate, atropine, pirenzepine	Excitatory *	Cholinesterase inhibitors block
					M₂: Bethanechol	Atropine	Inhibitory *	
	Motoneuron–Renshaw cell				Nicotine	Dihydro-β-erythroidine	Excitatory	

248

Transmitter	Anatomical distribution	Synthesis	Storage and release	Reuptake	Receptor: agonist	Antagonist	Effect on adenylate cyclase	Monoamine oxidase inhibitors block
Dopamine	All levels; short, medium, and long connections	α-Methyltyrosine inhibits; levodopa enhances	Tetrabenazine, reserpine, α-methyl-*m*-tyrosine inhibit; amphetamine releases; γ-hydroxybutyrate inhibits release	Benztropine, amitriptyline inhibit; 6-hydroxydopamine accumulates and is toxic	D_1: —	Phenothiazines, thioxanthenes	Activates adenylate cyclase; inhibitory *	
					D_2: Apomorphine	Phenothiazines, thioxanthenes, butyrophenones	Unlinked to or inhibits adenylate cyclase; inhibitory *	
Norepinephrine	All levels; long axons from pons and brain stem	Same as for dopamine; FLA-63 † and diethyldithiocarbamate inhibit dopamine β-hydroxylase	Reserpine, tetrabenazine, α-methyl-*m*-tyrosine inhibit; amphetamine releases	Desipramine inhibits; 6-hydroxydopamine accumulates and is toxic	α_1: Phenylephrine	Prazosin	—	Same as for dopamine
					α_2: Clonidine	Rauwolscine, yohimbine	Inhibitory *	
					β_1: Dobutamine ‡	Metoprolol, practolol	Activates adenylate cyclase; inhibitory *	
					β_2: Terbutaline ‡	Butoxamine ‡		
Epinephrine	Midbrain and brain stem to diencephalon	Same as for norepinephrine	Probably same as for norepinephrine	—	Probably same as for norepinephrine	Probably same as for norepinephrine	—	Probably same as for dopamine
5-Hydroxytryptamine	Midbrain and pons to all levels	p-Chlorophenylalanine blocks; tryptophan may increase	Reserpine, tetrabenazine inhibit	Clomipramine and fluoxetine inhibit; 5,7-dihydroxytryptamine accumulates and is toxic	5-HT_1: LSD	Metergoline, methysergide	Inhibitory *	Same as for dopamine
					5-HT_2: LSD	Spiroperidol, pirenperone	—	

* Excitatory and inhibitory refer to the effects of agonists on the rates of firing of responsive neurons in the CNS.

† FLA-63 is *bis*-(1-methyl-4-homopiperazinyl-thiocarbonyl) disulfide.

‡ Predicted on the basis of peripheral actions.

available and there were no cytochemical methods that could visualize such junctions. In the last 20 years most of these conceptual arguments have proven to be unjustified, and the evidence is quite strong that certain amino acids, especially GABA and glycine, are central transmitters.

GABA was identified as a unique chemical constituent of brain in 1950, but its potency as a CNS depressant was not immediately recognized. In the crustacean stretch receptor, GABA mimicked the actions of stimulation of the inhibitory nerve, and picrotoxin antagonized both the effects of applied GABA and stimulation of the inhibitory nerve. In the crustacean, work by Kravitz and coworkers (1963) demonstrated that GABA was the only inhibitory amino acid found exclusively in the inhibitory nerve and that the inhibitory potency of extracts of this nerve were accounted for by their content of GABA. Release of GABA was then correlated with the frequency of nerve stimulation. Intracellular recordings from the muscle indicated that the inhibitory nerve and GABA produced identical increases of Cl⁻ conductance in the muscle. These observations thus fully satisfy the criteria for identification of a transmitter (*see* Otsuka, 1973).

These same physiological and pharmacological properties were later found to be useful models in tests of a role for GABA in the CNS. Evidence strongly supports the idea that GABA mediates the inhibitory actions of local interneurons in the brain and that GABA may also mediate presynaptic inhibition within the spinal cord. Presumptive GABA-ergic inhibitory synapses have been demonstrated most clearly between cerebellar Purkinje neurons and their targets in Deiter's nucleus; between small interneurons and the major output cells of cerebellar cortex, olfactory bulb, cuneate nucleus, hippocampus, and the lateral septal nucleus; and between the vestibular nucleus and the trochlear motoneurons. GABA may also mediate the effects of inhibitory neurons within the cerebral cortex (*see* Kelly and Beart, 1975). The existence of a GABA-ergic pathway from caudate nucleus to substantia nigra is supported by neurochemical and cytochemical evidence (Kelly and Beart, 1975). Presumptive GABA-ergic neurons and nerve terminals have been localized with immunocytochemical methods that visualize glutamic acid decarboxylase. The reaction catalyzed by this pyridoxal phosphate–requiring enzyme provides the major source of GABA. The most useful drugs for confirmation of GABA-ergic mediation have been *bicuculline* and *picrotoxin;* however, many convulsants whose actions were previously unexplained (including penicillin and pentylenetetrazol) may also act as selective antagonists of GABA (Macdonald and McLean, 1982). Useful therapeutic effects have not yet been obtained by the use of agents that mimic GABA (such as muscimol), that inhibit the active re-uptake of the transmitter (2,4-diaminobutyrate, nipecotic acid, and guvacine; *see* Johnston, 1978), or that alter the rate of synthesis or degradation of

GABA (such as aminooxyacetic acid; *see* Iversen, 1978). Picrotoxin and bicuculline appear to antagonize the actions of GABA. However, while bicuculline competes with GABA for putative receptor binding sites, picrotoxin cannot (Iversen, 1978). Benzodiazepines can potentiate responses to GABA, apparently by interacting with a drug receptor located within the GABA-ergic receptor complex (Olsen, 1982). Two types of receptors for GABA have been proposed: GABA-A receptors, where muscimol is a potent agonist, bicuculline is a competitive antagonist, and binding of GABA may be enhanced by benzodiazepines; and GABA-B sites, where baclofen is an agonist and GABA has a relatively low potency that is unaffected by benzodiazepines (Wojcik and Neff, 1984).

Glycine was found not to be a particularly potent agent when its inhibitory effects were first evaluated by the iontophoretic technic in spinal cord. However, Werman and associates (1968) have assembled neurochemical and electrophysiological evidence that strongly supports a role for glycine as the inhibitory transmitter between spinal interneurons and motoneurons.

Glycine is the most abundant amino acid with inhibitory activity found in the ventral-quadrant gray matter of the spinal cord, and concentrations of glycine drop in proportion to the degeneration of ventral-quadrant interneurons following transient ischemia of the cord. Glycine has also been localized to spinal interneurons by electron-microscopic autoradiography. It is concentrated in nerve terminals that can be discriminated from those that accumulate GABA (Iversen, 1978). The hyperpolarization of motoneurons produced by iontophoretic application of glycine is relatively transient but approaches the equilibrium potential for the indirectly activated inhibitory postsynaptic potential; however, tests with GABA also indicate similar electrophysiological effects and a similar increase in Cl⁻ conductance. The major evidence that favors glycine as the mediator of intraspinal postsynaptic inhibition is the selective antagonism of its effects by strychnine. Strychnine does not usually antagonize responses to GABA (*see* Ryall, 1975), but it is able to inhibit the hyperpolarizing responses to β-alanine, another naturally occurring amino acid (*see* Zieglgänsberger, 1982). Glycine also appears to be the most likely inhibitory transmitter in the reticular formation (excluding the cuneate nucleus). Except for experiments with strychnine, there has been little pharmacological manipulation of neurons that release glycine. Aspects of the synthesis or degradation of glycine that are unique to the CNS are not appreciated.

Glutamate and *aspartate* are found in very high concentrations in brain, and both of these amino acids have extremely powerful excitatory effects on neurons in virtually every region of the CNS. However, the widespread distribution of these two dicarboxylic acids in the CNS and their roles in intermediary metabolism have tended to obscure the action that they might have as transmitters.

While a strong circumstantial case can be built for glutamate as the transmitter at the neuromuscular junction of insect muscle (Usherwood and

Machili, 1968), efforts to support either glutamate or aspartate as excitatory transmitters in the mammalian CNS have been hampered by the unavailability of a convincingly selective receptor antagonist. Evidence for selective, high-affinity re-uptake systems for glutamate and aspartate favors a transmitter role, as does the correlation of the concentrations of glutamate and aspartate with microdissections of brain regions following selective lesions (Nadler *et al.,* 1978). Glutamic acid diethylester (GDEE) may selectively suppress effects of glutamate on thalamic neurons without suppressing responses to either ACh or aspartate (Krogsgaard-Larsen and Honore, 1983). Glutamate and a rigid analog, kainic acid, have been employed as neurotoxins to produce lesions in neuronal cell bodies while selectively sparing axons in the vicinity (Coyle *et al.,* 1977); these effects may depend upon the existence of postsynaptic receptors for glutamate, but all neurons are not equally susceptible to the toxic action.

Acetylcholine. After it was established that ACh is the transmitter at neuromuscular and parasympathetic neuroeffector junctions, as well as at the major synapse of autonomic ganglia (*see* Chapter 4), the amine began to receive considerable attention as a potential central neurotransmitter. Based on the finding of an irregular distribution within the regions of the CNS and the observation that peripheral cholinergic drugs could produce marked behavioral effects after central administration, many were willing to consider that ACh might be "the" central neurotransmitter. In the late 1950s Eccles and colleagues demonstrated the recurrent excitation of spinal Renshaw neurons to be sensitive to nicotinic cholinergic antagonists; these cells were also found to be cholinoceptive. Such observations were consistent with the chemical and functional specificity of Dale's hypothesis that all branches of a neuron released the same transmitter substance and, in this case, produced similar types of postsynaptic action (*see* Eccles, 1964). Although the ability of ACh to elicit neuronal discharge has subsequently been replicated on scores of CNS cells (*see* Shepherd, 1983), the spinal Renshaw cell remains the best if not the sole example of a central cholinergic nicotinic junction.

In most regions of the CNS, the effects of ACh, assessed either by iontophoresis or by radioligand receptor-displacement assays (Kuhar, 1978), would appear to be generated by interaction with a mixture of nicotinic and muscarinic receptors. Several sets of presumptive cholinergic pathways have been proposed in addition to that of the motoneuron-Renshaw cell. These include the following: medial septal nucleus to dentate gyrus and subiculum of hippocampus habenula to interpeduncular nucleus; cortical interneurons to cortical pyramidal neurons; and thalamus, putamen, and caudate to neurons in the caudate. More precise maps of presumptive cholinergic neural circuits have been made possible by immunocytochemical localization of choline acetyltransferase (Levey *et al.,* 1983). These maps emphasize prominent cholinergic circuits in cerebral, limbic, and thalamic regions, and they include both long-divergent and local-circuit connections. Many of the iontophoretic actions of ACh on a host of identified test cells are reversed by muscarinic antagonists, including those on the cerebrocortical and the hippocampal pyramidal neurons (Stone, 1972). Subsets of cholinergic muscarinic sites have also been described (Hirschowitz *et al.,* 1984).

Thus, while ACh has long been the subject of intense investigation as a CNS transmitter, compelling evidence has been accumulated for only a few sites. The present data are fully in keeping with the possibility that both interregional and intraregional circuits may have ACh as their transmitter. When administered to man and animals, both cholinergic and anticholinergic drugs cause marked behavioral effects (*see* Chapters 6 and 7; Iversen and Iversen, 1979).

Catecholamines. The brain contains separate neuronal systems that utilize three different catecholamines—*dopamine, norepinephrine,* and *epinephrine.* Each system is anatomically distinct and presumably serves separate functional roles. There has been extensive investigation of these systems with a variety of technics, and a wealth of descriptive details is thus available for each (*see* Moore and Bloom, 1978, 1979; Symposium, 1979).

Dopamine. Although originally regarded only as a precursor of norepinephrine, assays of distinct regions of the CNS eventually revealed that the distributions of dopamine and norepinephrine are markedly different. In fact, more than half of the CNS content of catecholamine is dopamine, and extremely high amounts are found in the basal ganglia (especially the caudate nucleus), the nucleus accumbens, the olfactory tubercle, the central nucleus of the amygdala, the median eminence, and restricted fields of the frontal cortex. Due to the availability of histochemical methods that can reveal all the catecholamines (formaldehyde- or glyoxylic acid–induced fluorescence; Dahlstrom and Fuxe, 1964) or immunohistochemical methods for enzymes that synthesize individual catecholamines (Hokfelt *et al.,* 1978), the anatomical connections of the dopamine-containing neurons are known with some precision, at least for the rodent brain.

These studies indicate that there are three major morphological classes of dopaminergic neurons: (1) ultrashort neurons within the amacrine cells of the retina and periglomerular cells of the olfactory bulb; (2) intermediate-length neurons within the tuberobasal ventral hypothalamus that innervate the median eminence and intermediate lobe of the pituitary, incertohypothalamic neurons that connect the dorsal and posterior hypothalamus with the lateral septal nuclei, and small series of neurons within the perimeter of the dorsal motor nucleus of the vagus, the nucleus of the solitary tract, and the periaqueductal gray matter; and (3) long projections between the major dopamine-containing nuclei in the substantia nigra and ventral tegmentum and their targets in the striatum, in the limbic zones of the cerebral cortex, and in other major regions of the limbic system except the hippocampus (see Moore and Bloom, 1978). At the cellular level, the nature of the actions of dopamine remains somewhat controversial. While most iontophoretic studies indicate that inhibition is the predominant action, studies of the effects of electrical stimulation on transmembrane properties of the target neurons in the striatum suggest that there are depolarizing effects (Siggins, 1978; Brown and Arbuthnott, 1983). Many, but not all, classes of antipsychotic drugs have been shown to antagonize the ability of dopamine to activate adenylate cyclase (see Chapter 19). However, most antipsychotic agents show greater affinity for a subset of receptors for dopamine (D_2) that do not activate adenylate cyclase. At concentrations higher than needed for binding to D_2-dopaminergic receptors, neuroleptic drugs may influence the rate of release and synthesis of dopamine. Some of these drugs will also inhibit cholinergic and adrenergic transmission, as well as interfere with the regulation of cyclic nucleotide phosphodiesterase by Ca^{2+}-calmodulin (Seeman, 1981; Creese et al., 1983). Acute treatment of experimental animals with antipsychotic agents can inhibit the effect of dopamine on its target neurons and produce an acute secondary increase in the synthesis of dopamine. Chronic treatment results either in loss of this antagonism or in greatly diminished rates of metabolism of dopamine. The molecular mechanism responsible for the therapeutic effect is therefore not known (Symposium, 1977).

Norepinephrine. Relatively large amounts of norepinephrine occur within the hypothalamus and in certain zones of the limbic system, such as the central nucleus of the amygdala and the dentate gyrus of the hippocampus, but this catecholamine is also present in significant but lower amounts in most brain regions. Detailed mapping studies indicate that most noradrenergic neurons arise either in the locus ceruleus of the pons or in neurons of the lateral tegmental portion of the reticular formation. From these neurons, multiple branched axons innervate specific target cells in a large number of cortical, subcortical, and spinomedullary fields (Foote et al., 1983).

Examination of the effects of iontophoretic application of norepinephrine and of stimulation of the locus ceruleus indicates that the predominant acute effect of norepinephrine on cortical structures is inhibitory. This is mediated by β-adrenergic receptors and results in hyperpolarization of the postsynaptic membrane, accompanied by an increase in the passive resistance of the membrane. These actions are relatively slower in onset and longer in duration than are effects of inhibitory amino acids (Siggins et al., 1971a, 1971b), and they can be simulated by iontophoretic application of cyclic AMP on cerebellar Purkinje cells, hippocampal pyramidal cells, and cerebrocortical pyramidal cells (see Bloom, 1975). These results support those of Rall and coworkers that demonstrate a β-adrenergic-sensitive adenylate cyclase system in cerebellar slices (see Rall, 1972). In some brain regions the effects of norepinephrine on adenylate cyclase may involve both α- and β-adrenergic receptors (see Bloom, 1975; Kebabian and Nathanson, 1982). In diencephalic and mesencephalic systems, α-adrenergic receptors produce excitatory effects that are qualitatively opposite to the effects of norepinephrine on β-adrenergic receptors elsewhere (Menkes et al., 1983).

As in the periphery, four subtypes of adrenergic receptors have been described in the CNS (i.e., α_1, α_2, β_1, and β_2). Even though the proportion varies from region to region, β_1-adrenergic receptors may be associated predominantly with neurons, while β_2-adrenergic receptors may be more characteristic of glial and vascular elements. Stimulation of β_1- and β_2-adrenergic receptors results in activation of adenylate cyclase. Stimulation of α_2-adrenergic receptors on noradrenergic neurons leads to marked inhibition of firing. Both α_1- and α_2-adrenergic receptors have been detected in regions of the CNS that are targets for noradrenergic neurons (see Bylund and U'Prichard, 1983; Menkes et al., 1983; Symposium, 1983).

Depending on the species and brain region examined, *adenosine* can markedly potentiate the effects of norepinephrine and other biogenic amines on the synthesis of cyclic AMP. While the methylxanthines potentiate the effects of norepinephrine, cyclic AMP, and stimulation of the locus ceruleus on cerebellar Purkinje cells, they *antagonize* the ability of adenosine to activate adenylate cyclase or to inhibit the discharge of cells that are targets for norepinephrine (see Chapter 25; Bloom, 1975). Antipsychotic drugs, especially phenothiazines, also have effects upon the norepinephrine-activated adenylate cyclase in certain cortical areas. Tricyclic antidepressants influence binding of α-receptor ligands as well as their better-known ability to inhibit the re-uptake of norepinephrine. Although the latter action potentiates the effects of norepinephrine acutely, chronic treatment with these drugs can result in desensitization of noradrenergic receptors (Symposium, 1983).

Examination of the effects of lesions of noradrenergic pathways and of parenterally injected drugs has suggested a long list of physiological events that are regulated by norepinephrine. These include feeding, sleeping, memory, learning, and attention. Because the neurophysiological bases of these functions are not well understood, details of the involvement of norepinephrine in the multiple circuits that underlie such behaviors remain to be elucidated (Foote *et al.*, 1983).

Epinephrine. Neurons in the CNS that contain epinephrine were recognized only relatively recently following the development of sensitive enzymatic assays for phenylethanolamine-N-methyltransferase (*see* Chapter 4) and immunocytochemical staining technics for the enzyme (Hokfelt *et al.*, 1974). Epinephrine-containing neurons are found in the medullary reticular formation and make restricted connections to a few pontine and diencephalic nuclei, eventually coursing as far rostrally as the paraventricular nucleus of the dorsal midline thalamus (Hokfelt *et al.*, 1974). The physiological properties of these connections have not been studied as yet.

5-Hydroxytryptamine. Following the chemical determination that a biogenic substance found both in serum ("serotonin") and in gut ("enteramine") was 5-HT, assays for this substance revealed its presence in brain (Brodie and Shore, 1957). Since that time, studies of 5-HT have had a pivotal role in the neuropharmacology of the CNS. Various cytochemical methods have been used to trace the central anatomy of 5-HT-containing neurons in several species (*see* Azmitia, 1978). Tryptaminergic neurons are localized to some nine nuclei lying in or adjacent to the midline (raphe) regions of the pons and upper brain stem, corresponding to well-defined nuclear ensembles (Dahlstrom and Fuxe, 1964).

More precise patterns of innervation emerge from the use of orthograde and retrograde tracing technics (Azmitia, 1978). The most rostral raphe nuclei appear to innervate forebrain regions, while the more caudal raphe nuclei project within the brain stem and spinal cord. The median raphe nucleus contributes a major portion of the tryptaminergic innervation of the limbic system, and the dorsal raphe nucleus contributes a major portion of similar innervation of cortical regions and the neostriatum.

In the mammalian CNS, cells receiving cytochemically demonstrable tryptaminergic input, such as the suprachiasmatic nucleus, ventrolateral geniculate body, and amygdala, exhibit a uniform and dense investment of reactive terminals. Recordings obtained from such neurons show uniform inhibition after stimulation of the raphe neurons, and this effect is mimicked by iontophoretic application of 5-HT (Aghajanian and Wang, 1978).

Of the many different drugs that antagonize 5-HT in autonomic ganglia or smooth muscle (*see* Chapter 26), none blocks 5-HT at any proven tryptaminergic synapse within the CNS (Aghajanian

and Wang, 1978). This result is remarkable since much speculation on the function of 5-HT in the CNS was predicted on knowledge of the hallucinogenic properties of lysergic acid diethylamide (LSD) and its ability to antagonize the actions of 5-HT on smooth muscle. Although LSD, in high concentration, does block the action of 5-HT at peripheral tryptaminergic receptors, it mimics 5-HT in the CNS, especially on 5-HT-containing neurons (Aghajanian and Wang, 1978). LSD and some of the other peripheral antagonists of 5-HT can inhibit responses to 5-HT applied by microiontophoresis to randomly encountered cells in various regions of the CNS. However, none of these cells has been proven to be a physiological target for a tryptaminergic neuron. As with other transmitters, there appear to be at least two subtypes of receptor for 5-HT (Janssen, 1983; Peroutka and Snyder, 1983); these differ in their affinity for 5-HT, for neuroleptics, and for LSD. Functional differences between these two sites are not yet clear (*see* Quach *et al.*, 1982).

It has been hypothesized that altered function of tryptaminergic pathways is a factor in various mental illnesses and CNS dysfunctions. Drug treatments of animals and correlations of 5-HT metabolism with experimental manipulations have provided some indications that 5-HT-containing neurons may also be involved in other, simpler functions, such as regulation of temperature, neuroendocrine control (regulation of release of hypophysiotropic hormones), and activity of the extrapyramidal system (*see* Symposium, 1974). These proposals of behavioral functions of such highly divergent and overlapping long-axon systems are subject to the limitations mentioned above for the catecholamines. Many different classes of centrally active drugs can affect physiological or biochemical parameters of various tryptaminergic neuronal systems by influencing direct responses to 5-HT or its uptake, synthesis, storage, release, or catabolism. The list includes hallucinogens such as LSD, N,N-dimethyltryptamine (DMT), and other tryptamine congeners, mescaline, reserpine, chlorpromazine, tricyclic antidepressants, monoamine oxidase inhibitors, amphetamines (particularly the chloroamphetamines), lithium, morphine, methylxanthines, and ethyl alcohol. These drugs have also been demonstrated to have effects on catecholamine-containing and other chemically defined neurons, making the functional importance of the effects on mechanisms that involve 5-HT difficult to interpret.

LSD is among the most interesting of the compounds that interact with 5-HT. It reduces turnover of 5-HT in the brain, and it inhibits the firing of raphe neurons (*see* Freedman and Halaris, 1978). In iontophoretic tests, LSD and 5-HT are both potent inhibitors of the firing of raphe (5-HT) neurons, but LSD and other hallucinogens are far less potent depressants than is 5-HT on neurons that receive innervation from the raphe. The inhibitory effect of LSD on raphe neurons offers a plausible explanation of the drug's hallucinogenic effects, namely, that they result from depression of activity in a system that tonically inhibits visual and other sensory inputs. However, typical LSD-induced behavior is still seen in animals with raphe nuclei destroyed or after blockade of the synthesis of 5-HT by *p*-chlorophenylalanine. Other evidence against this explanation of LSD-induced hallucinations is the potentiation of LSD by administration of the precursor of 5-HT, 5-hydroxytryptophan. In addition, at least one LSD-like behavioral response in rats (poor habituation to sensory stimulation) is replicated by electrical stimulation of raphe nuclei (*see* Freedman and Halaris, 1978).

Histamine.   For many years, histamine and antihistamines that are active in the periphery have been known to produce significant effects on animal behavior. Only relatively recently, however, has evidence accumulated to suggest that histamine might be a central neurotransmitter.

Efforts to document the presence of histamine within neurons are hampered by lack of an effective cytochemical method and by the presence of mast cells, which have rich stores of histamine, in the CNS. However, only about half of the brain content of histamine can be released by drugs such as compound 48/80 or polymyxin B, which are effective in liberating the amine from mast-cell granules; the histamine that remains can be localized by subcellular fractionation technics to fractions of brain homogenates rich in nerve terminals. The histamine content varies from one hypothalamic nucleus to another, which is suggestive of a neuron-specific distribution. Furthermore, lesions of the lateral hypothalamus result in a depletion of histidine decarboxylase activity on the side of the lesion. The time course of disappearance parallels that expected for postlesion nerve-fiber degeneration (Schwartz, 1975). Unlike the monoamines and amino acid transmitters, there does not appear to be an active re-uptake process for histamine to conserve transmitter after its release. In fact, no direct evidence has been obtained for histamine release *in vivo* or *in vitro* associated with neuronal activity.

Two classes of receptor for histamine are known: H_1 and H_2 (Chapter 26). Only the H_2 sites are directly linked to activation of adenylate cyclase in the CNS (*see* Ganellin and Parsons, 1982). The ability of histamine to enhance the accumulation of cyclic AMP is potentiated by adenosine; this involves both H_1 and H_2 receptors (*see* Kebabian and Nathanson, 1982). In brain regions with high contents of histamine, such as hypothalamus and reticular formation, the effects of iontophoretically applied histamine are inhibitory; in some cases, these effects can be simulated by application of cyclic AMP and potentiated by inhibitors of cyclic nucleotide phosphodiesterase (*see* Bloom, 1975). Cyclic AMP may serve as a second messenger to mediate the actions of histamine in the CNS. The functions of presumptive histaminergic neural systems remain uncertain.

Peptides.   The continuing discovery of novel peptides in the CNS that are capable of regulating one or another aspect of neural function has produced considerable excitement (*see* Guillemin, 1978; Krieger, 1983; Krieger *et al.*, 1983). Technics for rapid determination of the amino acid sequences of such peptides and for their synthesis in large quantities have greatly facilitated progress. The peptide's physiological effects can then be studied, and its localization can be probed by radioimmunoassay and by immunocytochemical procedures.

An imposing catalog of previously unknown neuropeptides has accumulated. In addition, certain peptides previously thought to be restricted to the gut or to endocrine glands have also been found in the CNS. Relatively detailed maps are now available for neurons that show immunoreactivity to peptide-specific antisera.

There are literally scores of peptides that may function in the CNS, either on their own or in combination with a coexisting transmitter. Some hypothalamic neurons may contain more than two possible transmitters (*see* Hokfelt *et al.*, 1983). At this time at least three schemes appear to have some utility in attempting to organize the peptidergic systems of neurons.

Organization by Peptide Families.   Based on the detection of significant homology in amino acid sequences, families of related molecules can be defined (Blundell and Humbel, 1980; Niall, 1982). These families may be *ancestral* or *concurrent*. The ancestral relationship is illustrated by peptides such as the substance-P or the vasotocin family, in which species differences can be correlated with modest variations in peptide structure. The concurrent relationship is best exemplified by the endorphins and by the glucagon-secretin family. In the "superfamily" endorphin, three major systems of endorphin peptides (pro-opiomelanocortin, proenkephalin, and prodynorphin) exist in independent neuronal circuits (*see* Bloom, 1983). These arise from independent, but homologous, genes. The peptides all share some actions at receptors once classed generally as "opioid" and now undergoing progressive refinement (*see* Chapters 22 and 59). In the glucagon family, multiple and somewhat homologous peptides are found simultaneously in different cells of the same organism but in separate organ systems: glucagon and vasoactive intestinal polypeptide (VIP) in pancreatic islets; secretin in duodenal mucosa; VIP and related peptides in enteric, autonomic, and central neurons (*see* Blundell and Humbel, 1980; Iversen, 1983); and growth hormone–releasing factor in central neurons only (Guillemin *et al.*, 1982). The general metabolic effects produced by this family can be viewed as leading to increased blood glucose (*see* Magistretti *et al.*, 1982). To some degree, ancestral and concurrent relationships are not mutually exclusive, since multiple members of the substance-P family have now been reported (Nawa *et al.*, 1983); this may account for the apparent existence of subsets of receptors for substance P (Iversen *et al.*, 1982). The mammalian terminus of the vasotocin family shows two concurrent products as well, vasopressin and oxytocin, each having evolved to perform separate effects that were once executed by single vasotocin-related peptides in lower phyla.

Organization by Anatomic Pattern. Some peptide systems follow rather consistent anatomical organizations. Thus, the hypothalamic peptides oxytocin, vasopressin, proopiomelanocortin, luteinizing hormone–releasing hormone, and growth hormone–releasing factor all tend to be made by single large clusters of neurons that give off multibranched axons to several distant targets. Others, such as systems that contain somatostatin, cholecystokinin, and enkephalin, can have many forms, with patterns varying from moderately long, hierarchical connections to short-axon, local-circuit neurons that are widely distributed throughout the brain (*see* Krieger *et al.*, 1983).

Organization by Function. Since almost all peptides were identified initially on the basis of bioassays, their names reflect these functions (*e.g.*, thyrotropin-releasing hormone, vasoactive intestinal polypeptide, *etc.*). These names become trivial if more ubiquitous distributions and additional functions are discovered. Although some general integrative role might be hypothesized for widely separated neurons (and other cells) that make the same peptide, a more parsimonious view would be that each peptide has unique messenger roles at the cellular level and that these are used again and again in functionally similar pathways within large systems that differ in their overall functions (*see* Bloom, 1984).

Comparison with Other Transmitters. Peptides differ in several important respects from the monoamine and amino acid transmitters considered earlier. Synthesis of a peptide is performed in the rough endoplasmic reticulum, where mRNA for the propeptide can be translated into an amino acid sequence. The propeptide is then cleaved (processed) to the form that is secreted as the secretory vesicles are transported from the perinuclear cytoplasm to the nerve terminals. Further, no active re-uptake mechanisms for peptides have been described; this increases the dependency of nerve terminals on distant sites of synthesis. Perhaps most importantly, linear chains of amino acids can assume many tertiary conformations at their receptors, making it difficult to detect the sequences and their steric relationships that are critical for activity. The lack of predictive capability has severely limited the development of agonists or antagonists that will interact with specific receptors for peptides. Nature has also had limited success in this regard, since only one plant alkaloid, morphine, has been found to act selectively at peptidergic synapses. Fortunately for pharmacologists, morphine was discovered before the endorphins, or there might not yet be any example of a rigid molecule that is capable of acting at receptors for a peptide.

PERSPECTIVES FOR FUTURE DEVELOPMENT

Concepts of the relationship between the actions of a drug and the functions of specific brain systems have progressed through three phases, particularly in the relatively brief history of psychopharmacology (Mandell, 1973). In the first phase, drug-induced changes in function were correlated directly with changes in the concentrations of neurotransmitters or their metabolites. An exemplary anomaly revealed at this stage was the relationship between the behavioral depression that follows administration of reserpine and the decreased storage of 5-HT (and also norepinephrine and dopamine) in the brain (Brodie and Shore, 1957). The time course of the change in behavior coincides initially with alterations in the content of biogenic amines; however, when the analysis is extended past the first 48 hours, it becomes clear that the concentrations of amines remain depressed while behavior returns toward normal.

A second phase of investigation began with demonstrations that many drugs with potent behavioral actions (*e.g.*, LSD, amphetamine, tricyclic antidepressants, antipsychotics) produced relatively minor changes in the concentrations of transmitter. Attempts were thus made to relate the effects of drugs to alterations in the dynamics of neuronal metabolism, from which it was hoped that information about changes in neuronal activity could be inferred. For example, estimates have been made of the turnover rates of neurotransmitters (*see* Costa and Meek, 1974), and single-unit electrophysiological recordings have also been employed as indices of the effects of drugs on the functional activity of chemically characterized neuronal systems. This approach suffers from at least two problems that are also shared by experiments that rely on assessment of concentrations of transmitters. (1) Neurochemical experiments proceed on a time scale of minutes to hours, while neuronal events occur in milliseconds or seconds; changes that are measured may therefore be quite removed from those that occur at the primary site of action. (2) Neurotransmitters that have not yet been identified obviously cannot be measured. Because of these and other limitations, it is entirely possible for changes to occur after a drug treatment that are correctly correlated, perhaps even selectively, with aspects of the metabolism or action of one or more transmitter substances, and yet the two effects—that on function and that on specific neuronal systems—may not be causally related.

Current efforts in CNS pharmacology are also in a third phase that focuses on the adaptive changes imposed on the nervous system by chronic treatment with drugs. Thus, for example, the therapeutic effects of lithium or of tricyclic antidepressants require periods of treatment of 1 to 2 weeks before therapeutic results are evident (*see* Chapter 19; Symposium, 1983). While the metabolic changes and functional effects that are observed during acute treatment were assumed to continue, it has become clear that they do not persist and are replaced by changes that may in fact be opposite to those seen acutely. For example, tricyclic antidepressants, when given acutely, potentiate the cellular and behavioral effects of norepinephrine by inhibition of its re-uptake. It has been inferred that depression results from a deficiency of catecholamine and that tricyclic antidepressants are effective by increasing the amounts of catecholamine at the postsynaptic receptor. However, in animals treated chronically with desmethylimipramine, sensitivity of β-adrenergic receptors is decreased, even though presynaptic re-uptake of norepinephrine remains fully inhibited (Symposium, 1983).

Future efforts to provide explanations for drug-induced neurological changes will undoubtedly continue to focus on synaptic transmitters and their mechanisms. Many more transmitter peptides probably remain to be discovered, if estimates of the complexity of brain-specific mRNA are any indication (Milner and Sutcliffe, 1983). Use of recombinant DNA technology has already lengthened the list of putative transmitter peptides considerably (Tatemoto and Mutt, 1980; Tatemoto, 1982; Itoh *et al.*, 1983;

Nawa *et al.*, 1983). As more transmitters are discovered and their neuronal systems are mapped, new target cells will become available for the study of unique or common mechanisms of action. In this regard it may be useful to consider three general properties by which neuronal circuits can be described and to employ them in efforts to correlate the molecular actions of drugs with the neurological and behavioral effects that result. A *spatial domain* describes those areas of the brain or of peripheral receptive fields that feed signals to a given cell and those areas to which that cell sends its signals. A *temporal domain* describes the duration of the effects of a cell on its targets. A *functional domain* describes the molecular mechanisms by which the cell influences its targets. Within these three domains, neurons can be defined in terms of their transmitters, receptors, and functional location, as well as in the more classical categories of sensory, motor, or interneuronal. All of these properties must be borne in mind simultaneously in the attempt to develop comprehensive explanations of the acute and chronic effects of drugs.

Brodie, B. B., and Shore, P. A. A concept for a role of serotonin and norepinephrine as chemical mediators in the brain. *Ann. N.Y. Acad. Sci.*, **1957**, *66*, 631–642.

Brown, J. R., and Arbuthnott, G. W. The electrophysiology of dopamine (D_2) receptors: a study of the actions of dopamine on corticostriatal transmission. *Neuroscience*, **1983**, *10*, 349–355.

Buda, M.; De Simoni, G.; Gonon, F.; and Pujol, J.-F. Catecholamine metabolism in rat locus coeruleus as studied by *in vivo* differential pulse voltammetry. I. Nature and origin of contributors to the oxidation current at +0.1V. *Brain Res.*, **1983**, *273*, 197–206.

Cheramy, A.; Chesselet, M. F.; Romo, R.; Leviel, V.; and Glowinski, J. Effects of unilateral electrical stimulation of various thalamic nuclei on the release of dopamine from dendrites and nerve terminals of neurons of the two nigrostriatal dopaminergic pathways. *Neuroscience*, **1983**, *8*, 767–780.

Coyle, J. T.; Schwarcz, R.; Bennet, J. P.; and Campochiaro, P. Clinical, neuropathologic and pharmacologic aspects of Huntington's disease: correlates with a new animal model. *Prog. Neuro-psychopharmacol.*, **1977**, *1*, 13–30.

Curtis, D. R.; Duggan, A. W.; Felix, D.; Johnston, G. A. R.; and McLennan, H. Antagonism between bicuculline and GABA in the cat brain. *Brain Res.*, **1971**, *33*, 57–73.

Dahlstrom, A., and Fuxe, K. Evidence for the existence of monoamine-containing neurons in the central nervous system. I. Demonstration of monoamines in the cell bodies of brain stem neurons. *Acta Physiol. Scand.*, **1964**, *232*, Suppl. 62, 1–55.

Ewing, A. G.; Bigelow, J. C.; and Wightman, R. M. Direct *in vivo* monitoring of dopamine released from two striatal compartments in the rat. *Science,* **1983,** *221,* 169–171.

Guillemin, R.; Brazeau, P.; Bohlen, P.; Esch, F.; Ling, N.; and Wehrenberg, W. B. Growth hormone–releasing factor from a human pancreatic tumor that caused acromegaly. *Science,* **1982,** *218,* 585–587.

Hokfelt, T.; Fahrenkrug, J.; Tatemoto, K.; Mutt, V.; Werner, S.; Hulting, A. L.; Terenius, L.; and Chang, K. J. The PHI-27/corticotropin releasing factor/enkephalin immunoreactive hypothalamic neuron: possible morphological basis for integrated control of prolactin, corticotropin, and growth hormone secretion. *Proc. Natl. Acad. Sci. U.S.A.,* **1983,** *80,* 895–898.

Hokfelt, T.; Fuxe, K.; Goldstein, M.; and Johansson, O. Immunohistochemical evidence for the existence of adrenaline neurons in the rat brain. *Brain Res.,* **1974,** *66,* 235–251.

Itoh, N.; Obata, K. I.; Yanaihara, N.; and Okamoto, H. Human preprovasoactive intestinal polypeptide contains a novel PHI-27-like peptide, PHM-27. *Nature,* **1983,** *304,* 547–549.

Iversen, L. L.; Hanley, M. R.; Sandberg, B. E.; Lee, C. M.; Pinnock, R. D.; and Watson, S. P. Substance P receptors in the nervous system and possible receptor subtypes. *Ciba Found. Symp.,* **1982,** *91,* 186–205.

Kravitz, E. A.; Kuffler, S. W.; and Potter, D. D. Gamma-aminobutyric acid and other blocking compounds in Crustacea. Their relative concentrations in separated motor and inhibitory axons. *J. Neurophysiol.,* **1963,** *26,* 739–751.

Levey, A. I.; Wainer, B. H.; Mufson, E. J.; and Mesulam, M. M. Co-localization of acetylcholinesterase and choline acetyltransferase in the rat cerebrum. *Neuroscience,* **1983,** *9,* 9–22.

Macdonald, R. L., and McLean, M. J. Cellular bases of barbiturate and phenytoin anticonvulsant drug action. *Epilepsia,* **1982,** *23,* Suppl. 1, S7–S18.

Madison, D. V., and Nicoll, R. A. Noradrenaline blocks accommodation of pyramidal cell discharge in the hippocampus. *Nature,* **1982,** *299,* 636–638.

Magistretti, P. J.; Morrison, J. H.; Shoemaker, W. J.; Sapin, V.; and Bloom, F. E. Vasoactive intestinal polypeptide induces glycogenolysis in mouse cortical slices: a possible regulatory mechanism for the local control of energy metabolism. *Proc. Natl. Acad. Sci. U.S.A.,* **1982,** *78,* 6535–6539.

Mandell, A. J. Redundant macromolecular mechanisms in central synaptic regulation. In, *New Concepts in Neurotransmitter Regulation.* (Mandell, A. J., ed.) Plenum Press, New York, **1973,** pp. 259–277.

Menkes, D. B.; Gallager, D. W.; Reinhard, J. F.; and Aghajanian, G. K. α_1-Adrenoceptor denervation supersensitivity in brain: physiological and receptor binding studies. *Brain Res.,* **1983,** *272,* 1–12.

Milner, R. J., and Sutcliffe, J. G. Gene expression in rat brain. *Nucleic Acids Res.,* **1983,** *11,* 5497–5520.

Morrison, J. H.; Magistretti, P. J.; Benoit, R.; and Bloom, F. E. The distribution and morphological characteristics of the intracortical VIP-positive cell: an immunocytochemical analysis. *Brain Res.,* **1984,** *292,* 269–282.

Nadler, J. V.; White, W. F.; Vaca, K. W.; Perry, B. W.; and Cotman, C. W. Biochemical correlates of transmission mediated by glutamate and aspartate. *J. Neurochem.,* **1978,** *31,* 147–155.

Nawa, H.; Hirose, T.; Takashima, H.; Inayama, S.; and Nakanishi, S. Nucleotide sequences of cloned cDNAs for two types of bovine brain substance P precursor. *Nature,* **1983,** *306,* 32–36.

Nicoll, R. A.; Alger, B. E.; and Jahr, C. E. Enkephalin blocks inhibitory pathways in the vertebrate CNS. *Nature,* **1980a,** *287,* 22–25.

Otsuka, M. Gamma aminobutyric acid and some other transmitter candidates in the nervous system. In, *Pharmacology and the Future of Man: Proceedings of the Fifth International Congress on Pharmacology,* Vol. 4. (Acheson, G. H., and Bloom, F. E., eds.) S. Karger, Basel, **1973,** pp. 186–201.

Quach, T. T.; Rose, C.; Duchemin, A. M.; and Schwartz, J. C. Glycogenolysis induced by serotonin in brain: identification of a new class of receptors. *Nature,* **1982,** *298,* 373–375.

Siegelbaum, S. A.; Camardo, J. S.; and Kandel, E. R. Serotonin and cyclic AMP close single K+ channels in *Aplysia* sensory neurones. *Nature,* **1982,** *299,* 413.

Siggins, G. R.; Hoffer, B. J.; Oliver, A. P.; and Bloom, F. E. Activation of a central noradrenergic projection to cerebellum. *Nature,* **1971a,** *233,* 481–483.

Siggins, G. R.; Oliver, A. P.; Hoffer, B. J.; and Bloom, F. E. Cyclic adenosine monophosphate and norepinephrine: effects on transmembrane properties of cerebellar Purkinje cells. *Science,* **1971b,** *171,* 192.

Spiess, J.; Rivier, J.; and Vale, W. Characterization of rat hypothalamic growth hormone releasing factor. *Nature,* **1983,** *303,* 532–535.

Stone, T. W. Cholinergic mechanisms in the rat somatosensory cerebral cortex. *J. Physiol. (Lond.),* **1972,** *225,* 485–499.

Swanson, L. W.; Sawchenko, P. E.; Rivier, J.; and Vale, W. W. Organization of ovine corticotropin releasing factor immunoreactive cells and fibers in the rat brain: an immunohistochemical study. *Neuroendocrinology,* **1983,** *36,* 165–186.

Tatemoto, K. Neuropeptide Y: complete amino acid sequence of the brain peptide. *Proc. Natl. Acad. Sci. U.S.A.,* **1982,** *79,* 5485–5489.

Tatemoto, K., and Mutt, V. Isolation of two novel candidate hormones using a chemical method for finding naturally occurring polypeptides. *Nature,* **1980,** *285,* 417–418.

Usherwood, P. N. R., and Machili, P. Pharmacological properties of excitatory neuromuscular synapses in the locust. *J. Exp. Biol.,* **1968,** *49,* 341–361.

Waterhouse, B. D.; Moises, H. C.; Yeh, H. H.; and Woodward, D. J. Norepinephrine enhancement of inhibitory synaptic mechanisms in cerebellum and cerebral cortex: mediation by β adrenergic receptors. *J. Pharmacol. Exp. Ther.,* **1982,** *221,* 495–506.

Werman, R.; Davidoff, R. A.; and Aprison, M. H. Inhibitory action of glycine on spinal neurons in the cat. *J. Neurophysiol.,* **1968,** *31,* 81–95.

Wojcik, W. J., and Neff, N. H. γ-Aminobutyric acid B receptors are negatively coupled to adenylate cyclase in brain and in the cerebellum these receptors may be associated with granule cells. *Mol. Pharmacol.,* **1984,** *25,* 24–28.

Monographs and Reviews

Aghajanian, G. K., and Wang, R. Y. Physiology and pharmacology of central serotonergic neurons. In, *Psychopharmacology—A Generation of Progress.* (Lipton, M. A.; DiMascio, A.; and Killam, K. F.; eds.) Raven Press, New York, **1978,** pp. 171–184.

Azmitia, E. C. The serotonin-producing neurons of the midbrain median and dorsal raphe nuclei. In, *Handbook of Psychopharmacology,* Sect. II, Vol. 9. (Iversen, L. L.; Iversen, S. D.; and Snyder, S. H.; eds.) Plenum Press, New York, **1978,** pp. 233–314.

Barker, J. L. Physiological roles of peptides in the nervous system. In, *Peptides in Neurobiology.* (Gainer, H., ed.) Plenum Press, New York, **1977,** pp. 295–344.

Bloom, F. E. The role of cyclic nucleotides in central synaptic function. *Rev. Physiol. Biochem. Pharmacol.,* **1975,** *74,* 1–103.

———. The endorphins: a growing family of pharmacologically pertinent peptides. *Annu. Rev. Pharmacol. Toxicol.,* **1983,** *23,* 344–351.

———. The functional significance of neurotransmitter

diversity. *Am. J. Physiol.*, **1984**, *246* (Cell Physiol. 15), C184–C194.

Blundell, T. L., and Humbel, R. E.   Hormone families: pancreatic hormones and homologous growth factors. *Nature*, **1980**, *287*, 781–786.

Bodian, D.   Neuron junctions: a revolutionary decade. *Anat. Rec.*, **1972**, *174*, 73–82.

Bylund, D. B., and U'Prichard, D. C.   Characterization of α_1 and α_2 adrenergic receptors. *Int. Rev. Neurobiol.*, **1983**, *24*, 343–427.

Carlsson, A.   Autoreceptors. In, *Pre- and Postsynaptic Receptors*. (Usdin, E., and Bunney, W. E., Jr., eds.) Marcel Dekker, Inc., New York, **1975**, pp. 49–65.

Cooper, J. R.; Bloom, F. E.; and Roth, R. H.   *The Biochemical Basis of Neuropharmacology*, 4th ed. Oxford University Press, New York, **1983**.

Costa, E., and Meek, J. L.   Regulation of biosynthesis of catecholamines and serotonin in the CNS. *Annu. Rev. Pharmacol.*, **1974**, *14*, 491–512.

Creese, I.; Sibley, D. R.; Hamblin, M. W.; and Leff, S. E.   The classification of dopamine receptors: relationship to radioligand binding. *Annu. Rev. Neurosci.*, **1983**, *6*, 43–72.

Dale, H. H.   Pharmacology and nerve endings. *Proc. R. Soc. Med.*, **1935**, *28*, 319–332.

Eccles, J. C.   *The Physiology of Synapses.* Academic Press, Inc., New York, **1964**.

Florey, E.   Neurotransmitters and modulators in the animal kingdom. *Fed. Proc.*, **1967**, *26*, 1164–1176.

Foote, S. L.; Bloom, F. E.; and Aston-Jones, G.   The nucleus locus coeruleus: new evidence of anatomical and physiological specificity. *Physiol. Rev.*, **1983**, *63*, 844–914.

Freedman, D. X., and Halaris, A.   Monoamines and the biochemical mode of action of LSD at synapses. In, *Psychopharmacology—A Generation of Progress.* (Lipton, M. A.; DiMascio, A.; and Killam, K. F.; eds.) Raven Press, New York, **1978**, pp. 347–360.

Ganellin, C. R., and Parsons, M. E. (eds.).   *Pharmacology of Histamine Receptors.* Wright PSG, Bristol, **1982**.

Greengard, P.   *Cyclic Nucleotides, Phosphorylated Proteins, and Neuronal Function: Distinguished Lecture Series of the Society of General Physiologists*, Vol. 1. Raven Press, New York, **1978**.

Guillemin, R.   Peptides in the brain: the new endocrinology of the neuron. *Science*, **1978**, *202*, 390–402.

Hirschowitz, B. I.; Hammer, R.; Giachetti, A.; Keirns, J. J.; and Levine, R. R. (eds.).   Subtypes of muscarinic receptors. *Trends Pharmacol. Sci.*, **1984**, Suppl. 1, 1–103.

Hokfelt, T.; Johansson, O.; Ljungdahl, A.; Lundberg, J. M.; and Schutzberg, M.   Peptidergic neurons. *Nature*, **1980**, *284*, 515–521.

Hokfelt, T., and others.   Aminergic and peptidergic pathways in the nervous system with special reference to the hypothalamus. In, *The Hypothalamus.* (Reichlin, S.; Baldessarini, R. J.; and Martin, J. B.; eds.) Raven Press, New York, **1978**, pp. 69–136.

Iversen, L. L.   Biochemical psychopharmacology of GABA. In, *Psychopharmacology—A Generation of Progress.* (Lipton, M. A.; DiMascio, A.; and Killam, K. F.; eds.) Raven Press, New York, **1978**, pp. 25–38.

———.   Nonopioid neuropeptides in mammalian CNS. *Annu. Rev. Pharmacol. Toxicol.*, **1983**, *23*, 1–27.

Iversen, S. D., and Iversen, L. L.   *Behavioral Pharmacology*, 2nd ed. Oxford University Press, New York, **1979**.

Iversen, L. L.; Nicoll, R. A.; and Vale, W. W.   Neurobiology of peptides. *Neurosci. Res. Program Bull.*, **1978**, *16*, 214–370.

Janssen, P. A. J.   5-HT$_2$ receptor blockade to study serotonin-induced pathology. *Trends Pharmacol. Sci.*, **1983**, *4*, 198–206.

Johnston, G. A. R.   Neuropharmacology of amino acid inhibitory transmitters. *Annu. Rev. Pharmacol. Toxicol.*, **1978**, *18*, 269–289.

Kebabian, J. W., and Nathanson, J. A. (eds.).   *Cyclic Nucleotides. Handbook of Experimental Pharmacology*, Vol. 58. Springer-Verlag, Berlin, **1982**.

Kelly, J. S., and Beart, P. M.   Amino acid receptors in CNS. II. GABA in supraspinal regions. In, *Handbook of Psychopharmacology*, Sect. I, Vol. 4. (Iversen, L. L.; Iversen, S. D.; and Snyder, S. H.; eds.) Plenum Press, New York, **1975**, pp. 129–209.

Krieger, D. T.   Brain peptides: what, where, and why? *Science*, **1983**, *222*, 975–985.

Krieger, D. T.; Brownstein, M. J.; and Martin, J. B. (eds.).   *Brain Peptides.* John Wiley & Sons, Inc., New York, **1983**.

Krogsgaard-Larsen, P., and Honore, T.   Glutamate receptors and new glutamate agonists. *Trends Pharmacol. Sci.*, **1983**, *4*, 31–33.

Kuhar, M. J.   Central cholinergic pathways: physiologic and pharmacologic aspects. In, *Psychopharmacology—A Generation of Progress.* (Lipton, M. A.; DiMascio, A.; and Killam, K. F.; eds.) Raven Press, New York, **1978**, pp. 199–204.

Lynch, G., and Schubert, P.   The use of *in vitro* brain slices for multidisciplinary studies of synaptic function. *Annu. Rev. Neurosci.*, **1980**, *3*, 1–22.

McIlwain, H.   Extended roles in the brain for second-messenger systems. *Neuroscience*, **1977**, *2*, 357–372.

Miller, N. E.   Biofeedback and visceral learning. *Annu. Rev. Psychol.*, **1978**, *29*, 237–250.

Moore, R. Y., and Bloom, F. E.   Central catecholamine neuron systems: anatomy and physiology of the dopamine systems. *Annu. Rev. Neurosci.*, **1978**, *1*, 129–169.

———.   Central catecholamine neuron systems: anatomy and physiology. *Ibid.*, **1979**, *2*, 113–168.

Mountcastle, V. B., and Edelman, G. M.   An organizing principle for cerebral function: the unit module and the distributed system. In, *The Mindful Brain.* (Edelman, G. M., and Mountcastle, V. B., eds.) The MIT Press, Cambridge, Mass., **1978**, pp. 7–50.

Nestler, E. J., and Greengard, P.   *Protein Phosphorylation in the Nervous System.* John Wiley & Sons, New York, **1984**.

Niall, H. D.   The evolution of peptide hormones. *Annu. Rev. Physiol.*, **1982**, *44*, 615–624.

Nicoll, R. A.; Schenker, C.; and Leeman, S. E.   Substance P as a transmitter candidate. *Annu. Rev. Neurosci.*, **1980b**, *3*, 227–268.

Olsen, R. W.   Drug interactions at the GABA receptor–ionophore complex. *Annu. Rev. Pharmacol. Toxicol.*, **1982**, *22*, 245–277.

Pardridge, W. M.   Neuropeptides and the blood-brain barrier. *Annu. Rev. Physiol.*, **1983**, *45*, 73–82.

Peroutka, S. J., and Snyder, S. H.   Multiple serotonin receptors and their physiological significance. *Fed. Proc.*, **1983**, *42*, 213–217.

Rall, T. W.   Role of adenosine 3'-5'-monophosphate (cyclic AMP) in actions of catecholamines. *Pharmacol. Rev.*, **1972**, *24*, 399–409.

Rothlin, E., and Berde, B.   The structural and functional principles of the autonomic nervous system. *Aerztl. Monatsschr.*, **1953**, *5*, 865–905.

Ryall, R. W.   Amino acid receptors in CNS. I. GABA and glycine in spinal cord. In, *Handbook of Psychopharmacology*, Sect. I, Vol. 4. (Iversen, L. L.; Iversen, S. D.; and Snyder, S. H.; eds.) Plenum Press, New York, **1975**, pp. 83–128.

Scharrer, B.   Neurohumors and neurohormones: definitions and terminology. *J. Neurovisc. Relat.*, **1969**, *9*, Suppl., 1–20.

Schwartz, J. C.   Histamine as a transmitter in brain. *Life Sci.*, **1975**, *17*, 503–513.

Seeman, P. Brain dopamine receptors. *Pharmacol. Rev.,* **1981,** *32,* 229–313.

Shepherd, G. M. *Neurobiology.* Oxford University Press, New York, **1983.**

Siggins, G. R. Electrophysiological role of dopamine in striatum: excitatory or inhibitory? In, *Psychopharmacology—A Generation of Progress.* (Lipton, M. A.; DiMascio, A.; and Killam, K. F.; eds.) Raven Press, New York, **1978,** pp. 143–158.

Snyder, S. H. Brain peptides as neurotransmitters. *Science,* **1980,** *290,* 976–983.

Swanson, L. W., and Sawchenko, P. E. Hypothalamic integration: organization of the paraventricular and supraoptic nuclei. *Annu. Rev. Neurosci.,* **1983,** *6,* 269–325.

Symposium. (Various authors.) Serotonin—new vistas: histochemistry and pharmacology. (Costa, E.; Gessa, G. L.; and Sandler, M.; eds.) *Adv. Biochem. Psychopharmacol.,* **1974,** *10,* 1–329.

Symposium. (Various authors.) Nonstriatal dopaminergic neurons. (Costa, E., and Gessa, G. L., eds.) *Adv. Biochem. Psychopharmacol.,* **1977,** *16,* 1–686.

Symposium. (Various authors.) *Catecholamines—Basic and Clinical Frontiers: Proceedings of the Fourth International Catecholamine Symposium.* (Usdin, E., ed.) Pergamon Press, Ltd., Oxford, **1979.**

Symposium. (Various authors.) Molecular mechanisms in the actions of drugs active in mania and depression. *Neuropharmacology,* **1983,** *22,* 359–446.

Vale, W.; Rivier, C.; Brown, M. R.; Spiess, J.; Koob, G.; Swanson, L.; Bilezikjian, L.; Bloom, F.; and Rivier, J. Chemical and biological characterization of corticotropin releasing factor. *Recent Prog. Horm. Res.,* **1983,** *39,* 245–270.

Weindl, A., and Sofroniew, M. V. Relation of neuropeptides to mammalian circumventricular organs. *Adv. Biochem. Psychopharmacol.,* **1981,** *28,* 303–320.

Werman, R. Amino acids as central transmitters. In, *Neurotransmitters: Proceedings of the Association for Research in Nervous and Mental Disease,* Vol. 50. (Kopin, I. J., ed.) The Williams & Wilkins Co., Baltimore, **1972,** pp. 147–180.

Wood, J. W. (ed.). *Neurobiology of the Cerebrospinal Fluid.* Plenum Press, New York, **1979.**

Zieglgänsberger, W. Actions of amino acids, amines and neuropeptides on target cells in the mammalian central nervous system. *Prog. Brain Res.,* **1982,** *55,* 297–320.

13 HISTORY AND PRINCIPLES OF ANESTHESIOLOGY

Theodore C. Smith and Harry Wollman

I. History of Surgical Anesthesia

Anesthesia before 1846. Surgical procedures were uncommon before 1846. Understanding of the pathophysiology of disease and of the rationale for its treatment by surgery was rudimentary. Aseptic technic and the prevention of wound infection were almost unknown. In addition, the lack of satisfactory anesthesia was a major deterrent. Because of all these factors few operations were attempted and mortality was frequent. Typically, surgery was of an emergency nature—for example, amputation of a limb for open fracture or drainage of an abscess. Fine dissection and careful technic were not possible in patients for whom relief of pain was inadequate.

Some means of attempting to relieve surgical pain were available and, in fact, had been used since ancient times (Davison, 1965). Drugs like alcohol, hashish, and opium derivatives, taken by mouth, provided some consolation. Physical methods for the production of analgesia, such as packing a limb in ice or making it ischemic with a tourniquet, were occasionally used. Unconsciousness induced by a blow to the head or by strangulation did provide relief from pain, although at a high cost. However, the most common method used to achieve a relatively quiet surgical field was simple restraint of the patient by force. It is no wonder that surgery was looked upon as a last resort.

Although the analgesic properties of both nitrous oxide and diethyl ether had been known to a few for years, the agents were not utilized for medical purposes (Keys, 1963). Nitrous oxide was synthesized by Priestley in 1776, and both he and Humphry Davy some 20 years later commented upon its anesthetic properties (Faulconer and Keys, 1965). Davy in fact suggested that ". . . it may probably be used with advantage during surgical operations in which no great effusion of blood takes place." Another 20 years passed before Michael Faraday wrote that the inhalation of diethyl ether produced effects similar to those of nitrous oxide. However, except for their inhalation in carnival exhibitions or to produce "highs" at "ether frolics," these drugs were not used in man until the mid-nineteenth century.

Greene (1971) has presented an analysis of the reasons for the introduction of anesthesia in the 1840s. The time was then right, since concern for the well-being of one's fellows, a humanitarian attitude, was more prevalent than it had been in the previous century. "So long as witches were being burned in Salem, anesthesia could not be discovered 20 miles away in Boston." While humanitarian concern extended to the relief of pain, chemistry and medicine had simultaneously advanced to such an extent that a chemically pure drug could be prepared and then used with some degree of safety. There was, too, growth of the inquisitive spirit—a search for improvement of man's lot.

Public Demonstration of Ether Anesthesia. Dentists were instrumental in the introduction of both diethyl ether and nitrous oxide. They, even more than physicians, came into daily contact with persons complaining of pain; often, as a by-product of their work, they produced pain. It was at a stage show that Horace Wells, a dentist, noted that one of the participants, while under the influence of nitrous oxide, injured himself yet felt no pain. The next day Wells, while breathing nitrous oxide, had one of his own teeth extracted, painlessly, by a colleague. Shortly thereafter, in 1845, Wells attempted to demonstrate his discovery at the Massachusetts General Hospital in Boston. Unfortunately the patient cried out during the operation, and the demonstration was deemed a failure.

William T. G. Morton, a Boston dentist (and medical student), was familiar with the use of nitrous oxide from a previous association with Horace Wells. Morton learned of ether's anesthetic effects, thought it more promising, and practiced with it on animals and then on himself. Finally, he asked permission to demonstrate the drug's use, publicly, as a surgical anesthetic.

The story of this classical demonstration in 1846 has been retold countless times. The operating room ("ether dome") at the Massachusetts General Hospital remains as a memorial to the first public demonstration of surgical anesthesia. In the gallery of this room skeptical spectators gathered, for the news had spread that a second-year medical student had developed a method for abolishing surgical pain. The patient, Gilbert Abbott, was brought in and Dr. Warren, the surgeon, waited in formal morning clothes. Operating gowns, masks, gloves, surgical asepsis, and the bacterial origin of infection were entirely unknown at that time. Everyone was ready and waiting, including the strong men to hold down the struggling patient, but Morton did not appear. Fifteen minutes passed, and the surgeon, becoming impatient, took his scalpel and turning to the gallery said, "As Dr. Morton has not arrived, I presume he is otherwise engaged." While the audience smiled and the patient cringed, the surgeon turned to make his incision. Just then Morton entered, his tardiness being due to the necessity for completing an apparatus with which to administer the ether. Warren stepped back, and pointing to the man strapped to the operating table said, "Well, sir, your patient is ready." Surrounded by a silent and unsympathetic audience, Morton went quietly to work. After a few minutes of ether inhalation, the patient was unconscious, whereupon Morton looked up and said, "Dr. Warren, *your* patient is ready." The operation was begun. The patient showed no sign of pain, yet he was alive and breathing. The strong men were not needed. When the operation was completed, Dr. Warren turned to the astonished audience and made the famous statement, "Gentlemen, this is no humbug." Dr. Henry J. Bigelow, an eminent surgeon attending the demonstration, remarked, "I have seen something today that will go around the world."

Following initial disbelief, news of the successful demonstration spread rapidly. Within a month, ether was in use in other cities of the United States and had been given in Great Britain as well. Its use was soon established as legitimate medical therapy.

The lives of those involved in the introduction of surgical anesthesia did not have so salubrious an outcome. Morton initially tried to patent the use of ether to produce anesthesia and, when this failed, patented instead his device for its administration. Considerable wrangling ensued as to who was the legitimate discoverer of anesthesia. Never receiving what he felt to be his due, Morton died an embittered man.

Charles Jackson, Morton's chemistry teacher at Harvard, also claimed priority in the discovery; it was he who had suggested that Morton use pure sulfuric ether. Jackson became insane, a fate that also befell Horace Wells, the man who had failed in the public demonstration of nitrous oxide anesthesia. Crawford Long, a physician in rural Georgia, had used ether anesthesia since 1842 but neglected to publish his experiences. He survived and prospered, but Morton rightfully receives credit for the introduction of surgical anesthesia. A monument erected by the citizens of Boston over the grave of Dr. Morton in Mt. Auburn Cemetery near Boston bears the following inscription written by Dr. Jacob Bigelow:

WILLIAM T. G. MORTON
Inventor and Revealer of Anaesthetic Inhalation.
Before Whom, in All Time, Surgery Was Agony.
By Whom Pain in Surgery Was Averted and Annulled.
Since Whom Science Has Control of Pain.

Anesthesia after 1846. Although it is rarely used today, ether was the ideal "first" anesthetic. Chemically, it is readily made in pure form. It is relatively easy to administer, since it is a liquid at room temperature but is readily vaporized. Ether is potent, unlike nitrous oxide, and thus a few volumes percent can produce anesthesia without diluting the oxygen in room air to hypoxic levels. It supports both respiration and circulation, crucial properties at a time when human physiology was not understood well enough for assisted respiration

and circulation to be possible. And ether is not toxic to vital organs.

The next anesthetic to receive wide use was chloroform. Introduced by the Scottish obstetrician James Simpson in 1847, it became quite popular, perhaps because of its more pleasant odor. Other than this and its nonflammability, there was little to recommend it (Sykes, 1960). The drug is a hepatotoxin and a severe cardiovascular depressant. Despite the relatively high incidence of intraoperative and postoperative death associated with the use of chloroform, it was championed, especially in Great Britain, for nearly 100 years (Duncum, 1947). Because of the danger and difficulty in administering chloroform, distinguished British physicians early became interested in anesthetics and their administration, a trend that was evident in the United States only 100 years later.

The course of anesthesiology in the United States, after the initial burst of enthusiasm, was one of slow change and limited progress (Vandam, 1973). Furthermore, despite the relative comfort that the surgical patient experienced, the amount and scope of surgery increased only slightly in the 1840s and 1850s (Greene, 1979). The incidence of mortality was little changed, for postoperative infection was still a serious problem. Only with the introduction of aseptic technics 20 years after the discovery of anesthesia did surgery come into its own.

Other Anesthetic Agents. Nitrous oxide fell into disuse after the apparent failure in Boston in 1845. It was reintroduced in 1863 into American dental and surgical practice, largely through the efforts of a showman, entrepreneur, and partially trained physician, Gardner Q. Colton. In 1868, the administration of nitrous oxide with oxygen was described by Edmond Andrews, a Chicago surgeon, and soon thereafter the two gases became available in steel cylinders, greatly increasing their practicality (Thomas, 1975). Nitrous oxide is still widely used today.

The anesthetic properties of cyclopropane were accidentally discovered in 1929 when chemists were analyzing impurities in an isomer, propylene (Lucas, 1961). After extensive clinical trial at the University of Wisconsin, the drug was introduced into practice; cyclopropane was perhaps the most widely used general anesthetic for the next 30 years. However, with the prominent risk of explosion in the operating room brought about by the increasing use of electronic equipment, the need for a safe, nonflammable anesthetic increased, and several groups pursued the search. Efforts by the British Research Council and by chemists at Imperial Chemical Industries were rewarded by the development of halothane, a nonflammable anesthetic. It was introduced into clinical practice in 1956, and it revolutionized inhalational anesthesia. Most of the newer agents, which are halogenated hydrocarbons and ethers, are modeled after halothane.

The skeletal muscle relaxants (neuromuscular blocking agents) were also discovered and their pharmacological properties demonstrated long before their introduction into clinical practice (McIntyre, 1959; Bennett, 1967). Curare, in crude form, had long been used by South American Indians as a poison on their arrow tips (*see* Chapter 11). Its first clinical use was in spastic disorders, where it could decrease muscle tone without embarrassing respiration excessively. It was then used to modify the violent muscle contractions associated with convulsive therapy of psychiatric disorders. Finally, in the 1940s, anesthesiologists used curare to provide the muscular relaxation that previously could be obtained only with deep levels of general anesthesia. Over the next half-dozen years several synthetic substitutes were made and used clinically. It is difficult to overemphasize the importance of muscle relaxants in anesthetic practice. Their use permits adequate conditions for surgery with light levels of general anesthesia; cardiovascular depression is thus minimized, and the patient awakens promptly when the anesthetic is discontinued.

Although the desirability of an intravenous anesthetic agent must have been apparent to physicians early in the twentieth century, the drugs at hand were few and unsatisfactory. The situation changed dramatically in 1935, when Lundy demonstrated the clinical usefulness of thiopental, a rapidly acting thiobarbiturate. It was originally considered useful as a sole anesthetic agent, but the heroic doses required resulted in serious depression of the circulatory, respiratory, and nervous systems. Thiopental has, however, been enthusiastically accepted as an agent for the rapid induction of general anesthesia.

Various combinations of intravenous drugs from several classes have been used recently as anesthetic agents, usually in combination with nitrous oxide. However convenient these agents may be, their utility has been limited to special situations because of their side effects and lack of rapid reversibility. The future will probably bring better drugs for intravenous use along with specific antagonists to these drugs, making intravenous anesthesia more feasible without supplementation with inhalational agents.

II. Principles of the Administration of General Anesthetics

UPTAKE AND DISTRIBUTION OF INHALATIONAL ANESTHETICS

A firm understanding of general anesthesia requires appreciation of the pharmacokinetics of drugs that are inhaled. During general anesthesia produced with an inhalational agent, the depth of anesthesia varies directly with the tension of anesthetic agent in the brain, and the rates of induction and recovery depend upon the rate of change of tension in this tissue. The terms *tension* and *partial pressure* are used interchangeably. The tension of anesthetic agent in the brain is always approaching the tension in arterial blood. The factors that determine the tension of anesthetic gas in the arterial blood and in the brain can be considered under four headings: (1) concentration of the anesthetic agent in inspired gas, (2) pulmonary ventilation delivering the anesthetic to the lungs, (3) transfer of the gas from the alveoli to the blood flowing through the lungs, and (4) loss of the agent from the arterial blood to all the tissues of the body.

CONCENTRATION OF THE ANESTHETIC AGENT IN INSPIRED GAS

The tension of an individual gas in a mixture of gases is proportional to its concentration, and one often refers to them interchangeably when speaking of the inspired gases.

When a constant tension of anesthetic gas is inhaled, the tension in arterial blood approaches that of the agent in the inspired mixture, in the manner shown in Figure 13–1 for several different anesthetics. (The tension of the inspired vapor or gas is called the "inspired tension.") For drugs such as nitrous oxide, the arterial tension reaches 90% of the inspired tension in about 20 minutes. When methoxyflurane is administered, the approach to a steady state is much slower, and 90% of the inspired tension would be reached in arterial blood only after many hours. This difference is determined by the physical properties of the two agents (*see* below).

In practice the inspired tension is rarely constant. An anesthetizing concentration of some agents may irritate the airway of an awake or lightly anesthetized patient, so that the inspired concentration must be increased slowly. In other cases, where the vapor is not irritating, the speed of induction may be increased by giving the inhalational anesthetics in concentrations greater than those ultimately desired. Anesthetic tensions are thus produced in blood and tissues sooner than would be possible if maintenance concentrations were used for induction. As anesthesia proceeds, the inspired concentration of anesthetic is re-

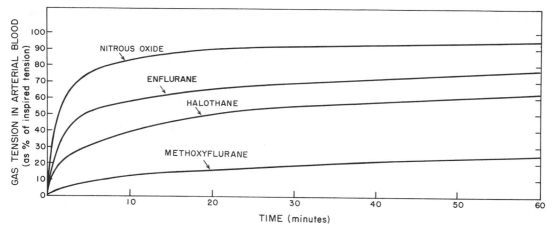

Figure 13–1. *The tensions of anesthetic gases in arterial blood.*

The curves demonstrate how arterial blood tension of the anesthetics increases toward the inspired tension. The increase in partial pressure is rapid for the relatively insoluble gases, and slower for those that are more soluble in blood. The course of events is illustrated here for an idealized situation, where the inhaled concentration remains constant, and pulmonary ventilation and cardiac output and its regional distribution remain constant at normal values. In fact, as anesthesia deepens, alveolar ventilation and cardiac output fall, and distribution of regional circulation and agent solubility are variably altered. These and other factors can result in up to 11% difference between predicted and actual concentration (Cowles *et al.*, 1972). Alinear analyses have been proposed that take these factors into consideration (Smith *et al.*, 1972; Munson *et al.*, 1973).

duced to a level suitable for the maintenance of anesthesia.

PULMONARY VENTILATION

Each inspiration delivers some anesthetic gas to the lung. If the respiratory minute ventilation is great, the tension of the anesthetic in alveoli increases quickly, as does its tension in arterial blood. Thus, the partial pressure of anesthetic gas in blood can be increased by overventilation during induction. Conversely, decreased ventilation (resulting, for instance, from respiratory depression by premedication or an anesthetic agent) can lead to a slower rate of change of alveolar and arterial gas tension.

The effects of the rate of respiration to slow or speed induction are transient for gases such as nitrous oxide that have low solubility in blood and tissues and thus equilibrate quickly. However, the volume of respiration exerts a more significant and prolonged effect on the rate of uptake of more soluble and slowly equilibrating drugs such as methoxyflurane. (For further discussion, *see* Eger, 1964.)

TRANSFER OF ANESTHETIC GASES FROM ALVEOLI TO BLOOD

The normal alveolar membrane poses no barrier to the transfer of anesthetic gases in both directions. Although the diffusion of anesthetic gases may be normal, certain situations can occur during clinical anesthesia that impede the efficient transfer of gases into blood flowing through the lung. One of these is maldistribution of alveolar ventilation such as may occur in pulmonary emphysema. There is then a lower tension of anesthetic gas in the poorly ventilated alveoli, and thus a lower anesthetic tension in the blood draining them. The contribution of this blood to the arterial pool results in slowing of the rate of change of tension of the anesthetic in arterial blood. Any mismatch of ventilation and perfusion in the lung that may occur as a result of a variety of pulmonary disorders produces a difference between alveolar and arterial tensions of anesthetic gases. This, too, results in slowing of the rate of induction of, or recovery from, anesthesia (*see* Eger and Severinghaus, 1964).

In the absence of ventilation-perfusion

disturbances, three factors determine how rapidly anesthetics pass from the inspired gases to blood. These are (1) the solubility of the agent in blood, (2) the rate of blood flow through the lung, and (3) the partial pressures of the agent in arterial and mixed venous blood.

Solubility of the Agent in Blood. This is usually expressed as the blood:gas partition coefficient, or λ, which represents the ratio of anesthetic concentration in blood to anesthetic concentration in a gas phase when the two are in equilibrium (*i.e.,* when the partial pressure is equal in both phases). The blood:gas partition coefficient is as high as 12 for very soluble agents such as methoxyflurane and as low as 0.47 for relatively insoluble anesthetics such as nitrous oxide. *The more soluble an anesthetic is in blood, the more of it must be dissolved in blood to raise its partial pressure there appreciably. Therefore, the blood tension of soluble agents rises slowly. The potential reservoir for relatively insoluble gases is small and can be filled more quickly. Therefore, their tension in blood can increase more rapidly.*

The blood:gas partition coefficients for the commonly used anesthetic agents are given in Table 14–1 (page 277). The feature of the curves in Figure 13–1 that is largely determined by the blood solubility of the agents is the height of the bend, or "knee," in the uptake curve. The more soluble the agent (*i.e.,* the higher the λ), the lower is the "knee" of the curve, and the slower is the approach of blood tension to that of the inhaled gases.

Rate of Pulmonary Blood Flow. The pulmonary blood flow (*i.e.,* the cardiac output) affects the rate at which anesthetics pass from the alveolar gases into the arterial blood. An increase in pulmonary blood flow slows the initial portion of the arterial tension curve; but the latter part of the curve tends to catch up, with the overall result that there is little change in the total time required for complete equilibration. (For the reasons why this should be so, *see* Eger, 1964.)

Partial Pressures in Arterial and Mixed Venous Blood. After taking up anesthetic gas in the lung, the blood circulates to the tissues, and anesthetic gas is transferred from the blood to all tissues of the body. Blood cannot approach equilibrium with inhaled gas tension until this process, which tends to decrease the blood tension, is nearly complete. The mixed venous blood returning to the lungs has more anesthetic gas in it with each passage through the body. After a few minutes of anesthesia the difference between arterial (or alveolar) and mixed venous gas tension decreases continuously. Since the rate of diffusion across the pulmonary membrane is proportional to the difference between alveolar and mixed venous gas tensions, the volume of gas transferred to arterial blood during each minute decreases as time passes. Thus, arterial tension rises more slowly in the final portion of the curves in Figure 13–1.

LOSS OF ANESTHETIC GASES FROM ARTERIAL BLOOD TO TISSUES

When the inhalational agents are delivered by arterial blood to the tissues, the tension rises in tissues to approach that in arterial blood. The rate at which a gas passes into tissues depends on (1) the solubility of the gas in the tissues, (2) the rate at which the gas is delivered to the tissues (*i.e.,* the blood flow to the various areas of the body), and (3) the partial pressures of the gas in arterial blood and tissues. Note that these three factors affecting transfer of the gas from blood to tissue are similar to the three that affect transfer of the anesthetic from lung to blood (*see* above).

Solubility of Gas in Tissues. This is expressed as a tissue:blood partition coefficient, a concept analogous to the blood:gas partition coefficient previously discussed. With most anesthetic agents, the tissue:blood partition is near unity for many of the body's lean tissues; that is, these agents are equally soluble in lean tissue and blood. An anesthetic concentration in blood or tissue is the product of partial pressure and solubility. Thus, the concentration of most anesthetics in lean tissues, such as the gray matter of brain, approaches that in blood as tissue tension builds up toward arterial blood tension. On the other hand, the tissue:blood coefficient for all anesthetics is large for fatty tissues. Their concentration in the fatty tissue is much greater than that in blood at the time of equilibrium (when tissue tension equals blood tension).

Tissue solubility is of importance in determining the slope of the final portion, or "tail," of the gas tension curves (Figure 13–1). High tissue solubility, especially high fat solubility, tends to depress the rate of rise of the "tail" of the curve.

Tissue Blood Flow. The higher the blood flow to a tissue, the faster is the delivery of the anesthetic agent, and the more rapidly will its tension and concentration rise in that area. Thus, the concentration of an inert gas in brain approaches that in arterial blood more rapidly when cerebral blood flow is high, and more slowly when cerebral blood flow decreases. It has been suggested that anesthetic induction and emergence can be speeded by allowing the patient to inhale some carbon dioxide. This agent, by increasing ventilation, accelerates the rise in the arterial tension curve (*see* above). In addition, by dilating cerebral vessels, carbon dioxide increases cerebral blood flow and thus hastens the rate at which brain tension of the anesthetic changes. Since brain tension of the anesthetic is the important factor for anesthesia, this procedure results in more rapid induction or emergence but *not* in more profound anesthesia.

Only tissues with high rates of blood flow will exhibit rapid rises in concentration of anesthetic, and only high-flow areas take up significant amounts of the agent during the early stages of anesthesia. Since blood flow to adipose tissue is very limited, anesthetic gases will be delivered to, and taken up by, fatty tissues so slowly that these tissues contain a significant amount of anesthetic agent only after a considerable time has elapsed.

Partial Pressures in Arterial Blood and Tissues. As the tissues take up anesthetic agent, the partial pressure of the gas in tissues increases toward that of the arterial blood. Since the rate at which gas diffuses from arterial blood to tissues varies with the partial-pressure difference between them, tissue concentration changes rapidly in the early minutes of anesthesia; however, as the tissue tension comes closer to the arterial tension, the tissue uptake of gas slows.

In *summary,* during the administration of an anesthetic, its tension in blood rises toward that in the inspired gas, at first rapidly, then more slowly. Tissue tensions increase concomitantly, approaching the arterial tension. The partial pressure increases most rapidly in tissues with high rates of blood flow, and lags considerably in areas where blood flow is lower.

ELIMINATION OF INHALATIONAL ANESTHETICS

The major factors that affect rate of elimination of the anesthetics are the same as those that are important in the uptake phase: pulmonary ventilation, blood flow, and solubility in blood and tissue. However, the administration of anesthesia is usually completed before arterial tension has reached inspired tension, and long before tissues of low blood flow or high gas solubility have reached inspired tension. As ventilation with anesthetic-free gas washes out the lungs, the arterial blood tension declines first, followed by that in the tissues. An example of tissue concentrations during 60 minutes of nitrous oxide inhalation and 45 minutes of washout is shown in Figure 13–2 (*see* Cowles *et al.,* 1968). Soon after elimination begins, the tension in lung and blood has fallen to very low (nonanesthetic) levels. Because of the high blood flow to brain, its tension of anesthetic gas decreases rapidly, accounting for the rapid awakening from anesthesia noted with relatively insoluble agents such as nitrous oxide. The agent persists for a longer time in tissues with lower blood flow such as muscle, and for yet longer times in fat where blood flow is very low, and from which the agent is therefore very slowly released.

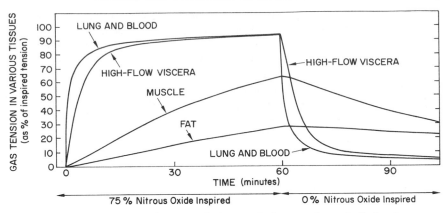

Figure 13–2. *Tissue tensions of an anesthetic gas during uptake and elimination.*

The curves demonstrate how tissue tensions of nitrous oxide approach the inspired tension during a 60-minute anesthetic uptake phase and a subsequent 45-minute elimination phase. The high-blood-flow viscera include brain, heart, and kidney. Liver and intestine have lower blood flows, and their tensions would lie between those of the high-blood-flow viscera and muscle. (Modified from Cowles, Borgstedt, and Gillies, 1968.)

OTHER ROUTES OF ELIMINATION
OF ANESTHETICS

The anesthetic gases are metabolized in the body to a variable extent. With most agents this is small. However, up to 15% of halothane and 70% of methoxyflurane are metabolized to various intermediate compounds, and in some cases to ionized halogens (*see* Chapter 14; Cohen, 1971). The bulk of metabolism of anesthetics occurs after clinical anesthesia has been discontinued, and is greatest for the more fat-soluble drugs (Berman *et al.*, 1973). The importance of the metabolism of anesthetic agents is not in the termination of their action; rather, metabolites of anesthetics may be responsible for certain of their toxic effects or aftereffects.

Additional small losses of anesthetic gases from the body occur by diffusion across skin and mucous membranes, and by means of urinary excretion of the agent or its breakdown products (Stoelting and Eger, 1969; Cohen, 1971).

MINOR EFFECTS

Minor pharmacokinetic effects distinguish the uptake, distribution, and elimination of gases such as nitrous oxide from those of relatively less solubility, such as nitrogen or helium.

Concentration Effect and Second-Gas Effect.
The *concentration effect* may be defined as follows: when higher concentrations of an anesthetic gas are inhaled, arterial tension increases at a slightly greater rate than it would have if a lesser concentration of the anesthetic had been inhaled (*see* Eger, 1963). Consider a patient who is inhaling 75% nitrous oxide and 25% oxygen. Although nitrous oxide is relatively insoluble, when the inhaled concentration is high, the rate of uptake of the gas by blood and tissues may be as great as 1 liter per minute during the early minutes of anesthesia. As

this volume of gas disappears from the lung, fresh gases are literally sucked into the lung from the breathing circuit to replace the volume taken up. The rate at which the inspired gas mixture is delivered to the lung is then 1 liter per minute greater than the minute ventilation would have provided without this effect. Therefore, the rate of rise of the arterial tension curve for nitrous oxide is increased during induction of anesthesia. However, if only 10% nitrous oxide is inhaled, the body's uptake of approximately 150 ml per minute results in no significant change in the rate of gas delivery to the lung, and there is little or no acceleration of the arterial tension.

The simultaneous presence of two anesthetic gases in the lung can introduce a closely related phenomenon known as the *second-gas effect.* An illustration may be taken in which 75% nitrous oxide and 1% halothane are administered together with 24% oxygen. The same disappearance of 1 liter per minute of nitrous oxide from the lung into the body takes place, and the rate at which 1% halothane is delivered to the alveoli becomes 1 liter per minute greater than the minute ventilation would otherwise have provided. As a result, the arterial tension of halothane rises a little more rapidly in the presence of nitrous oxide. (*See* Epstein *et al.*, 1964.)

Diffusion Hypoxia. The reverse of the concentration effect can occur after the anesthetic has been discontinued, and will be illustrated for nitrous oxide. The elimination of nitrous oxide from blood to lung may proceed at a rate as great as the uptake. The additional gas added to the alveoli dilutes the available oxygen, and reduces alveolar oxygen concentration. The phenomenon is known as *diffusion hypoxia* (*see* Fink, 1955). It is seen in the early minutes following the end of a nitrous oxide administration, if the patient is breathing air. The hypoxia is usually mild, and is rarely a clinical threat. It can be prevented by oxygen inhalation for a few minutes at the end of the anesthetic administration.

Although *diffusion hypoxia* can theoretically occur after the withdrawal of any anesthetic agent, its magnitude is insignificant unless high concentrations of a soluble agent such as nitrous oxide have been inhaled for some time. Under these circumstances a considerable volume of inert gas has been dissolved in the body (up to 30 liters), and much of it is eliminated through the lungs in the first few minutes after its administration is discontinued. When lower concentrations of an agent (*e.g.*, 2% halothane) are inhaled, even after a long time only a few liters will have been taken up in the body. When administration is discontinued, the elimination of 100 ml per minute or less of halothane is not sufficient to dilute the alveolar oxygen to hypoxic levels.

Intertissue Diffusion. During the approach to equilibrium, the gas being inhaled may be present at different partial pressures in adjacent tissues, the partial pressure being higher in the areas with greater flow and in those where the gas is less soluble. The anesthetic will diffuse into the areas where its tension is lower. The rates of diffusion are such that tissue tensions are not much affected in areas with high blood flow and areas where the gas is relatively insoluble. However, tissue concentrations can be significantly changed by diffusion in areas where flow rates are low and gas solubility is high, as in adipose tissue (*see* Eger, 1973).

ADMINISTRATION OF INHALATIONAL ANESTHETICS

ANESTHETIC MACHINES

With these devices, the anesthesiologist is able to deliver measured quantities of anesthetic gases and oxygen through accurate flowmeters, and with the use of special vaporizers it is possible to add the vapor of volatile anesthetic liquids to the gas stream. The mixture of oxygen and anesthetic agents is then delivered to a breathing circuit for administration to patients.

Vaporizers. Liquid anesthetic agents can be vaporized in several ways (*see* Hill, 1968). They may be slowly dripped into the gas stream. They may be vaporized by a gas stream that passes over the surface of the liquid, or past a wick saturated with the liquid. A gas may also be passed through the liquid, in "saturation-type" vaporizers. In these devices, gas bubbles pass through a liquid anesthetic in such a way that saturation of the gas bubbles with the liquid agent is complete. Equilibration occurs within the vaporizer, the amount of liquid volatilized by the gas depending only upon the vapor pressure, which, in turn, is determined by the particular liquid and its temperature. As the vapor pressures of many liquid anesthetics are several hundred millimeters Hg at room temperature (*see* Table 14–1, page 277), saturation vaporizers can deliver far more than is necessary or desirable. Therefore, the outflow of gases from the vaporizer is diluted with additional flows of oxygen or nitrous oxide to attain the desired anesthetic concentrations.

Most often liquid anesthetic agents are vaporized into a stream of oxygen and nitrous oxide by an agent-specific vaporizer, which has been designed and calibrated to deliver the chosen concentration of a particular anesthetic. The concentration is accurately maintained over a range of gas flows and ambient temperatures by a combination of the methods available for vaporization and dilution.

Breathing Circuits. The gases and vapors are delivered into a system of wide-bore tubes with valves, a distensible bag that provides a reservoir for the gases, and a method for elimination of expired carbon dioxide. Gases are administered to the patient by means of a face mask or endotracheal tube. Two types of gas delivery systems are illustrated in Figure 13–3.

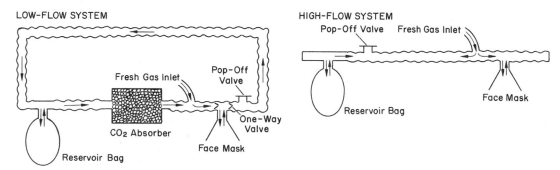

Figure 13–3. *Systems used for delivering inhalational anesthetics.*

Two breathing circuits are shown; they are made up of similar components arranged in slightly different ways. In the low-flow system, gas flow is unidirectional around the circle, and exhaled carbon dioxide is absorbed chemically. In the high-flow system, the movement of gases is bidirectional. As long as the inflow of fresh gas is approximately as great as the respiratory minute volume, carbon dioxide is diluted and washed out via the pop-off valve.

Low-Flow System (Circle System). Unidirectional valves near the connection of the circuit to the patient ensure that gases circulate in one direction around the circle. The exhaled carbon dioxide is absorbed chemically by a material such as soda lime. This system permits rebreathing of the exhaled gases, and only small amounts of fresh gas need be added through the flowmeters and vaporizer to replace the oxygen and the anesthetic gases taken up by the patient. If larger amounts of fresh gas are added, the excess is eliminated through the one-way pop-off valve. A distensible bag provides a reservoir of gas from which the patient can inhale. The bag partially empties during inhalation and refills during exhalation. The bag also provides a means for the assistance or control of respiration by the anesthesiologist, who can compress the bag and thus force gas into the patient's lungs. When pressure on the bag is released, the lungs empty and the bag refills.

High-Flow System. The fresh gas inflow in this system moves to and fro as the patient inhales gases from the bag and exhales. Since the rate of gas inflow exceeds the amount of oxygen utilized and anesthetic taken up, the excess gas escapes through the one-way pop-off valve, carrying the exhaled carbon dioxide with it.

Information on Exact Concentrations. If the anesthesiologist has accurate flowmeters for gases and a dependable vaporizer for liquids, he can determine what concentrations of anesthetics and oxygen are being delivered to the breathing circuit. However, rebreathing occurs in low-flow systems, and the gas mixture inhaled by the patient is not the same as that delivered to the breathing circuit. Denitrogenation of the patient dilutes the gases in the system; humidification of the gases in the system lowers their concentrations somewhat; oxygen is lost from the system as the patient utilizes it for metabolic requirements; and anesthetic gases are taken up by the patient at a changing rate. At the same time, small amounts of oxygen and anesthetic are added to the circuit. It is apparent that in a low-flow system, the inhaled gases are a mixture with a composition that is difficult to estimate. As the flow rates increase, the characteristics of the system change, and the inhaled gas concentrations approach the concentrations of fresh gases being delivered from the flowmeters and the vaporizer. Nitrous oxide is most frequently delivered in high-flow systems; the anesthesiologist is then assured of at least 20% inhaled oxygen and very nearly 80% inhaled concentration of this rather weak anesthetic gas.

Gas, Heat, and Water Exchange in Anesthesia Systems. Three liters of nitrogen may be eliminated from the lung and from tissues in the first hour of anesthesia if a nitrous oxide–oxygen mixture is inspired. This nitrogen must be exhausted from the breathing circuit if high concentrations of both oxygen and nitrous oxide are desired. Unlike carbon dioxide, it cannot be absorbed, but it can be eliminated by dilution and venting through a pop-off valve.

Water vapor and the heat to vaporize it are provided under normal conditions by the nasal turbinates. However, during anesthesia, the machine delivers dry gas and the patient inspires it through oropharyngeal or endotracheal tubes that bypass the nasal turbinates; cooling and drying of the tracheobronchial mucosa thus occur. While the heat and water loss may be tolerable in a normal patient for a short operation, the small, the elderly, and those who lose a great deal of heat and water when a large mass of tissue is exposed during long procedures benefit from the conservation of water and heat. This may be provided by the use of low-flow systems or by warming and humidifying inspired gases. Such measures are often undertaken in pediatric anesthesia.

DOSAGE AND POTENCY OF GENERAL ANESTHETICS

General anesthetics are among the most dangerous drugs approved for general use, in that the margin of safety in their use is small. Therapeutic indices range from about two to four. That is, the dose that produces circulatory failure may be only two to four times that which produces adequate anesthesia (Wolfson *et al.*, 1978). Thus, accurate methods are required for choosing the dose of an anesthetic and for evaluating the depth of anesthesia.

When a tablet is swallowed or a solution injected into a muscle, the dose is described in terms of the mass of drug that is administered. However, when a drug is inhaled as a gas or vapor, only a relatively small amount is actually absorbed; a very large fraction is exhaled within the next 1 or 2 seconds. Moreover, since it is the brain and not the lung that is the site of action of inhalational anesthetics, the agent must first partition between the alveolar gas and the blood and then again between the blood and the brain cells before exerting its action. It is difficult to specify the concentration in the brain of experimental animals and impossible to measure it in man. Yet the need to specify a dose to facilitate pharmacological and physiological studies and to permit the administration of general anesthesia is inescapable. Anesthesiologists have therefore accepted a measure of potency of inhalational agents known as MAC, which stands for *minimum alveolar concentration* of anesthetic at 1 atmosphere that produces immobility in 50% of patients or animals exposed to a noxious stimulus (Eger *et al.*, 1965). The rationale for using the concentration in the alveoli rather than that in the brain to measure a dose is based on the following considerations: concentration in the lung can be easily, frequently, and accurately measured; near equilibrium, the partial pressure of anesthetic in the lung and the partial pressure in the brain are almost equal; and relatively high blood flow to the brain causes rapid transport of blood-borne agents to the brain and thus rapid equilibration between blood and brain.

Among the characteristics of MAC that recommend it as a measure of anesthetic dose and potency are that MAC is invariant with a variety of noxious stimuli, from tail clamping to abdominal incision; that variability within individuals of a given species is small; that sex, height, weight, and duration of anesthesia do not alter MAC, although temperature and age do (Stevens *et al.*, 1975; Lerman *et al.*, 1983); and, finally, that doses of anesthetic agents appear to be additive (*i.e.*, one half of a MAC of one drug plus one half of a MAC of another drug will cause immobility following noxious stimulation in 50% of individuals tested) (Cullen *et al.*, 1969; Millar *et al.*, 1969).

The slopes of the dose-response curves for inhalational anesthetics are steep. Thus, although only 50% of individuals may fail to respond to stimulation at 1.0 MAC, 99% are unresponsive at a dose of 1.3 MAC (*see* de Jong and Eger, 1975). The latter concentration is, therefore, the surgically useful dose of each anesthetic if it is used without supplementation. Modern anesthesiologists tend to provide "light" anesthesia with concentrations of inhaled anesthetic of 0.8 to 1.2 MAC, in combination with judicious use of adjuvant drugs.

MAC represents only a single point on the dose-response curve for the production of anesthesia. Doubling the concentration of an anesthetic may produce more or less than a doubling of the intensity of another effect (*e.g.*, decrease in blood pressure), depending on the slope of the dose-response curve of that drug for that effect.

DEPTH OF ANESTHESIA

SIGNS AND STAGES OF ANESTHESIA

Between 1847 and 1858, John Snow described certain signs that helped him determine the depth of anesthesia in patients receiving chloroform or ether. These included the onset of rhythmic, auto-matic breathing and the loss of winking in response to touching the conjunctiva as surgical anesthesia was reached, and the gradual disappearance of intercostal muscle activity and cessation of eyeball movement as anesthesia was deepened. In 1920, Guedel, using these and other signs, outlined four stages of general anesthesia, dividing the third stage, that of surgical anesthesia, into four planes. Guedel's observations related primarily to ether, a substance with such great solubility in blood that the onset and progressive deepening of anesthesia were predictably slow. Opportunity was thus afforded the anesthesiologist to watch the unfolding of a series of changes involving respiration, muscle tone, and reflex activity. The somewhat arbitrary division is as follows: I—stage of analgesia; II—stage of delirium; III—stage of surgical anesthesia; IV—stage of medullary depression.

I. *Stage of Analgesia.* The first stage begins with the administration of the anesthetic and lasts until consciousness is lost. Certain major operations requiring minimal muscular relaxation can be completed during the analgesia characterizing this stage.

II. *Stage of Delirium.* This stage extends from the loss of consciousness to the beginning of surgical anesthesia. Excitement and involuntary activity may be minimal or marked. The jaw becomes set, skeletal muscular tone increases, and breathing is irregular. Incontinence of urine and feces may occur, as may retching or vomiting. The pupils may dilate. Hypertension and tachycardia may be marked. Anesthesiologists try to reduce the duration and the intensity of this stage to the minimum.

III. *Stage of Surgical Anesthesia.* The third stage extends from the end of the second stage until cessation of spontaneous respiration occurs. The transition to stage III occurs when the excitement and the respiratory irregularity of stage II disappear. The third stage can be divided into four planes, numbered from 1 to 4, in order of increasing depth of anesthesia. The major differences in physical signs in the various planes relate to the character of the *respiration,* the character of the *eyeball movements,* the presence or absence of certain *reflexes,* and the size of the *pupils.*

IV. *Stage of Medullary Depression.* This stage starts as soon as the weakened respiration of plane 4 ceases, and it ends with failure of the circulation.

These signs and stages are partly recognizable during administration of many other general anesthetics, although they are often obscured by modern anesthetic technics. For example, the use of neuromuscular blocking agents deprives the anesthesiologist of much information about depth of anesthesia, as does controlled ventilation. Complete muscular paralysis eliminates all the skeletal muscular indices of depth, such as eyeball movement, changes in respiration, tightness of the jaw, and ability to phonate, swallow, move, or close the glottis. Eye signs may be obscured by the intense pupillary constriction that accompanies administration of opioid analgesics. Other preanesthetic medications may obscure still other signs of the depth of anesthesia, and rapid induction of anesthesia with thiopental virtually eliminates the stage of excitement. Cullen and coworkers (1972) demonstrated that no single one of the major signs described by Guedel correlated satisfactorily with the measured alveolar concentrations of anesthetic during prolonged stable states.

A PRACTICAL APPROACH TO EVALUATING DEPTH OF ANESTHESIA

The following approach is useful for almost any general anesthetic. If the eyelids blink when the eyelashes are stroked, if the patient is swallowing, if respiration is irregular in rate and depth, and if one knows that not a great deal of anesthetic has been administered, surgical anesthesia is *not* present.

Loss of the eyelash reflex and the development of rhythmic respiration indicate the beginning of surgical anesthesia. If the skin incision is made at once, indications of "light" anesthesia may include an increase in respiratory rate or a rise in arterial blood pressure. Jaw muscles may become tight, and even if the mouth can be opened an oral airway may not be tolerated; an attempt to insert it may produce gagging, coughing, vomiting, or laryngospasm.

As anesthesia deepens, these responses are reduced in degree or abolished altogether. With most of the general anesthetics, an increase in depth brings progressive reduction in respiratory tidal volume. Tracheal tug may become evident as accessory muscles of respiration come into play. Diaphragmatic activity becomes jerky or snapping in character, and the lower chest is pulled in as the diaphragm descends. When the potent halogenated agents are used, arterial blood pressure tends to vary directly with the depth of anesthesia, and hypotension can be used as an index of dosage. Suggestions that anesthesia is becoming "lighter" are the formation of tears, apnea following peritoneal stimulation, increasing resistance to inflation of the lungs, and the return of those indices of light anesthesia listed above.

Severe respiratory depression or cessation of breathing (excluding breath-holding seen during early phases of anesthesia) and marked hypotension or asystole must be regarded as evidence of deep anesthesia unless other causes, for example, the effect of muscle relaxants, blood loss, and hyp-

oxia, or the influence of vagal reflexes, can explain these findings.

Thus, common sense and experience, combined with constant observation of the patient's responses to anesthetic drugs and to stimuli, permit the successful estimation of depth of anesthesia.

The Electroencephalogram as an Index of Depth of General Anesthesia. A number of workers have classified the EEG changes produced by the inhalational agents and barbiturates (*see* Faulconer and Bickford, 1960; Clark and Rosner, 1973; Rosner and Clark, 1973). However, use of the EEG as the sole index of anesthetic depth is unreliable, since many factors influence the activity of the central nervous system (CNS). Hypoxia, hypocarbia, hypoglycemia, hypothermia, and inadequate cerebral circulation can markedly alter the EEG at a time when anesthetic concentration remains constant. Furthermore, although EEG changes produced by a given agent may correlate with brain concentration, they also vary widely when different anesthetics are compared. (For a detailed examination of this subject, the reader should consult Clark and Rosner, 1973; Rosner and Clark, 1973; McDowall, 1976; Levy *et al.*, 1980.) Another approach is to use the evoked response to auditory, visual, or peripheral electrical stimulation. Averages of 100 or more of such stimulations yield a relatively reproducible, multiphasic wave response; the characteristics of this response vary with depth of anesthesia (*see* Grundy, 1983; Thornton *et al.*, 1983).

PREANESTHETIC MEDICATION

Preanesthetic medication should decrease anxiety without producing excessive drowsiness, provide amnesia for the perioperative period while maintaining cooperation prior to loss of consciousness, and relieve preoperative and postoperative pain if it is present. Secondary goals include minimization of undesirable side effects associated with some of the anesthetic agents, notably salivation, bradycardia, coughing, and postanesthetic vomiting. The accomplishment of these multiple purposes usually requires the concomitant use of two or three drugs. The most commonly employed classes include sedative-hypnotics, antianxiety agents, opioids, antiemetics, and anticholinergics. An informative, supportive preoperative visit by the anesthesiologist has long been known to be as effective as a traditional sedative-hypnotic drug (Egbert *et al.*, 1963). The wide variety of preanesthetic regimens in current use testifies to the lack of agreement on optimal combinations.

SEDATIVE-HYPNOTICS AND ANTIANXIETY AGENTS

While drowsiness does not imply loss of all anxiety, most drugs in use for preanesthetic medication have some of both effects.

Benzodiazepines. The members of this class of drugs are used extensively for preanesthetic medication. They provide amnesia in 60% of patients after doses that produce only mild sedation (Pandit *et al.,* 1976). Benzodiazepines can raise the threshold for CNS toxicity of local anesthetics (de Jong and Heavner, 1973). *Diazepam* has been most widely used in doses of 5 to 10 mg. It is active orally but is less predictable after intramuscular injection. It has little effect on respiration at usual doses, and does not potentiate respiratory depression produced by opioids (Aukburg *et al.,* 1976). *Lorazepam* is used extensively and may be given intramuscularly. It appears to produce amnesia frequently (Fragen and Caldwell, 1976). *Midazolam,* which is not yet available in the United States, acts more rapidly after any route of administration and is perhaps most likely to produce amnesia as well as tranquility (Fragen *et al.,* 1983). Lorazepam and midazolam are less likely to produce hangover or cumulative effects than is diazepam.

Barbiturates. Pentobarbital and *secobarbital* are the barbituric acid derivatives used most frequently to provide sedation and relieve apprehension before operation. They may be administered orally or intramuscularly to adults in doses of 100 to 200 mg, and to infants and children in doses of 3 to 5 mg/kg of body weight. These drugs have minimal depressant action on respiration and circulation and rarely produce nausea or vomiting. Tolerance to the usually administered doses of barbiturates is observed in patients who have been taking many kinds of drugs, including other barbiturates, alcohol, and even aspirin and some anticoagulants.

Antihistamines. Sedation is a variable side effect of this group of drugs. *Hydroxyzine,* 25 to 100 mg intramuscularly, has found wide usage. It exhibits many minor benefits, such as bronchodilatory, antisialogogic, antiemetic, antiarrhythmic, and ataractic effects. It produces minimal circulatory and respiratory depression and does not prolong anesthesia. *Diphenhydramine* (10 to 50 mg intravenously or intramuscularly) is a mild sedative as well as an H_1 blocker, and this combination of effects is desirable in certain patients. In others, it is desirable to reduce secretion of gastric acid with an H_2 antagonist.

Phenothiazines. Phenothiazines have sedative, antiarrhythmic, antihistaminic, and antiemetic properties. They are sometimes combined in reduced dosage with a barbiturate or an opioid. Prolongation of postanesthetic sleep and greater respiratory depression are probable, and decrease in blood pressure is possible. The value of phenothiazines in premedication must be carefully weighed against their side effects. Phenothiazines commonly used in premedication include *promethazine* and *propiomazine,* both in intramuscular dosage of 20 to 50 mg.

Butyrophenones. The usual dose for premedication is 2.5 to 10 mg of droperidol. Some antiemetic activity can be expected, and there is reasonable cardiovascular stability, despite slight α-adrenergic blocking activity. Both restlessness and extrapyramidal dyskinesia can occur, especially in chil-

dren; these effects may be countered by the administration of atropine.

OPIOIDS

Surgical pain is often severe, and even minor preoperative pain is deleterious to smooth induction of anesthesia. Opioids are thus frequently used for preanesthetic medication. The major difference among opioids that governs the choice for premedication is duration of activity (*see* Chapter 22).

Morphine. Morphine in doses of 8 to 12 mg intramuscularly is frequently used prior to operation. If pain is present before operation, morphine is one of the drugs of choice. It is the pain-relieving property that in all probability minimizes the incidence of restlessness or excitation during emergence from general anesthesia. The drug is useful also for depressing the cough reflex. Preanesthetic medication with an opioid reduces the amount of general anesthetic required by 10 to 20%.

Unfortunately, morphine may have undesirable side effects. It often prolongs the awakening from general anesthesia since its clinical effects persist for 4 to 6 hours. Its stimulant effect on smooth muscle may cause spasm of the bile duct or of the ureters; colicky pain, often relieved by atropine but always abolished by naloxone, may result from this effect on smooth muscle. Wheezing may develop in patients with asthma. Constipation and urinary retention may be annoying. Nausea and vomiting are not uncommon. A vagotonic effect may be evidenced by bradycardia. Hypotension can occur after the use of morphine or other opioid analgesics. The respiratory depressant action of morphine may increase intracranial pressure through retention of carbon dioxide and subsequent cerebral vasodilatation. While this can be undesirable in patients in whom intracranial pressure is already elevated, the effect can be abolished through adequate pulmonary ventilation.

Meperidine. This drug is utilized in doses of 50 to 100 mg intramuscularly. It shares all the disadvantages of morphine, including depression of blood pressure, cardiac output, and respiration. Tachycardia occasionally occurs, posing a problem in differential diagnosis. Respiratory depression lasts 2 to 3 hours.

Fentanyl. This synthetic opioid is useful in some cases because of its short duration of action, 1 to 2 hours. The usual dose is 0.05 to 0.10 mg intramuscularly.

ANTIEMETICS

Often the sequelae of prophylactic antiemetics (notably hypotension) are as disturbing and frequent as emetic episodes. However, if a drug is otherwise useful in a given instance, its antiemetic effect is an additional welcome benefit. *Droperidol* and *hydroxyzine* are sometimes useful for their antiemetic effects. *Benzquinamide* is a mild vasopressor and hence does not share some of the drawbacks of other antiemetics. *Other drugs* that provide an antiemetic effect following intramuscular administration include scopolamine, 0.4 to

0.6 mg; cyclizine, 50 mg; trimethobenzamide, 200 mg; and a variety of phenothiazines.

ANTICHOLINERGIC DRUGS

The excessive respiratory tract secretions seen during open-drop administration of ether suggested the use of an anticholinergic drug prior to anesthetization. With the advent of less irritating anesthetic agents, secretions have become less of a problem. The emphasis has now shifted to the desire to counteract the vagal effects that may frequently occur during anesthesia. Thus, atropine or a similar substance continues to be given by most anesthesiologists.

Atropine. Atropine produces oral dryness and blurred vision within 10 to 15 minutes after intramuscular injection of the standard 0.4- to 0.6-mg dose. The vagal blocking action of such an amount may not be sufficient to prevent parasympathetically induced cardiovascular effects such as hypotension and bradycardia that result from increase in ocular pressure, visceral traction, manipulation of the carotid sinus, or injection of multiple doses of succinylcholine. However, the intravenous injection of an additional dose of atropine often promptly restores the cardiac rate and the arterial pressure toward normal.

Atropine is not contraindicated in patients with glaucoma. Increased intraocular pressure does not result from the doses recommended. Some have advised that anticholinergic premedication be omitted in patients with asthma. However, inspissation of respiratory secretions has not proven to be a problem when the drugs are used in asthmatics. Their use in febrile patients may be unwise, since they depress the mechanism of heat loss by sweating.

Scopolamine. Scopolamine is usually given intramuscularly, in a dose of 0.4 to 0.6 mg. It is superior to atropine as an antisialogogue but is less effective in preventing reflex bradycardia during general anesthesia, particularly in children. The sedative effect of scopolamine is more marked than that of atropine; occasionally, however, patients become restless or disoriented after scopolamine, and the incidence of emergence excitement appears greater after its administration.

Glycopyrrolate. This longer-acting quaternary amine produces less sedation than scopolamine and is a more effective antisialogogue than atropine. It is less likely to cause significant tachycardia than atropine, while it simultaneously blocks bradyarrhythmias more effectively (Odura, 1975; Myer and Tomeldan, 1979). It is also more effective in blocking the secretion of gastric acid.

MOLECULAR MECHANISM OF ACTION OF GENERAL ANESTHETICS

A myriad of molecular species are capable of producing anesthesia, including inert gases (*e.g.,* xenon), simple inorganic and organic compounds (*e.g.,* nitrous oxide and chloroform), and more complex organic molecules (*e.g.,* halogenated alkanes and ethers). Yet there remains no satisfactory explanation as to *how* these drugs produce general anesthesia.

Most theories that attempt to explain how anesthetics exert their actions are based on the physicochemical characteristics of the anesthetic drugs. These proposals relate closely to the correlation between the potency of an anesthetic agent and the solubility of the drug in oil, first demonstrated by Meyer (1899, 1901) and Overton (1901). The precise nature of this correlation is demonstrated in Figure 13–4, where the MAC value for a number of anesthetics is plotted versus the olive oil:gas partition coefficient at 37° C. Interpretation of this fundamental result is thought to be crucial to the understanding of the action of anesthetics. It should be noted that other properties of molecules are also correlated with their potency as anesthetics. These include the ability to reduce surface tension (Traube, 1904; Clements and Wilson, 1962) and the ability to induce the formation of clathrates of water (ordered, crystal-like structures) (Miller, 1961; Pauling, 1961). However, such molecular properties are closely related to the fundamental physical forces that determine hydrophobicity.

The physical force that promotes the high relative solubility of molecules in oil compared to water is the so-called hydrophobic interaction. Molecules such as potent anesthetics that cannot form a significant number of hydrogen bonds and that are nonpolar distribute to sites in which they are removed from the aqueous environment. For this reason and because of the correlation of lipophilicity with anesthetic potency, it has been concluded that the primary site of action of anesthetics is either the lipid matrix of the biological membrane or hydrophobic regions of specific membrane-bound proteins. Anesthetics can bind to proteins, presumably to hydrophobic sites. However, the absence of a satisfactory structure-activity relationship for anesthetic agents suggests that they do not produce their effects by specific interaction with a receptor protein. Thus, the most attractive possibility is that the primary action of anesthetics is exerted on the lipid matrix of the biological membrane.

Anesthesia in experimental animals can be reversed by the application of moderate pressure (~100 atmospheres) (Miller *et al.,* 1973). One interpretation of this observation is that a large change of volume may be crucially associated with the fundamental action of anesthetics. Phospholipids in artificial (model) membranes undergo a change of state as temperature is increased—the so-called gel-liquid crystalline transition of the phospholipid matrix. The temperature at which this occurs is dependent on the identity of the phospholipid, and the change in state is associated with an increase in the molar volume of the lipid. If anesthetics are present, the transition from the gel to the liquid crystalline state of the phospholipids is more likely to happen; that is, it occurs at lower temperatures (Trudell *et al.,* 1973b). It is possible to rationalize the effect of pressure to reverse anesthesia based on such considerations. Furthermore, anesthetics broaden the melting curve for the gel-liquid crystal-

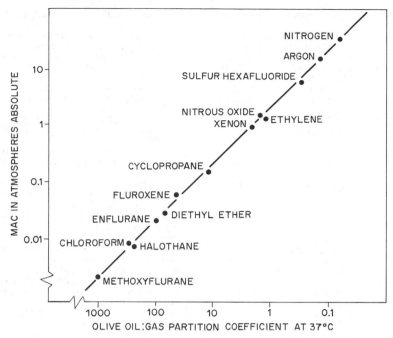

Figure 13–4. *The correlation of anesthetic potency with olive oil:gas partition coefficient.*

The correlation is shown for a number of general anesthetic agents and other inert gases not usually used for anesthesia. Note the log scales and the excellent correlation over a very wide range of fat solubilities and potencies (*see* Paton, 1974). (Modified from Eger, Lundgren, Miller, and Stevens, 1969; Miller, Paton, Smith, and Smith, 1972.)

line transition (as if water melted between 0° and 5° C), indicative of a reduction in the number of phospholipid molecules that interact cooperatively at any time. The application of physical technics, such as nuclear-magnetic resonance and electron-spin resonance, indicates that anesthetics cause a local disordering of the lipid matrix (Trudell *et al.,* 1973a; Trudell and Hubbell, 1976). Because anesthetics appear to decrease the number of molecules of phospholipid that alternate *simultaneously* between the gel and liquid crystalline states, these drugs reduce the magnitude of fluctuations of volume that probably occur in dynamic biological membranes (Mountcastle *et al.,* 1978). It is hypothesized that such fluctuations are sufficiently large to be important in the regulation of the structural state of membrane-bound proteins (*e.g.,* their state of aggregation) and, therefore, of their functional properties (*see* Halsey, 1974). As inhibitors of such fluctuations, anesthetics could readily influence the fluxes of ions, which are crucial determinants of neuronal excitability, or other functions of membranes that are determined by the proteins that function in the milieu of a dynamic lipid matrix.

Aukburg, S. J.; Miller, J.; and Smith, T. C. Interaction between meperidine and diazepam on the ventilatory response to carbon dioxide. *Clin. Res.,* **1976,** *24,* 506a.

Bennett, A. E. How "Indian arrow poison" curare became a useful drug. *Anesthesiology,* **1967,** *28,* 446–451.

Berman, M. L.; Lowe, H. J.; Bochantin, J.; and Hagler, K. Uptake and elimination of methoxyflurane as influenced by enzyme induction in the rat. *Anesthesiology,* **1973,** *38,* 352–357.

Clements, J. A., and Wilson, K. M. The affinity of narcotic agents for interfacial films. *Proc. Natl. Acad. Sci. U.S.A.,* **1962,** *48,* 1008–1014.

Cowles, A. L.; Borgstedt, H. H.; and Gillies, A. J. Uptake and distribution of inhalation anesthetic agents in clinical practice. *Anesth. Analg.,* **1968,** *47,* 404–414.

————. The uptake and distribution of four inhalation anesthetics in dogs. *Anesthesiology,* **1972,** *36,* 558–570.

Cullen, D. J., and others. Clinical signs of anesthesia. *Anesthesiology,* **1972,** *36,* 21–36.

Cullen, S. C.; Eger, E. I., II; Cullen, B. F.; and Gregory, P. Observations on the anesthetic effect and the combination of xenon and halothane. *Anesthesiology,* **1969,** *31,* 305–309.

de Jong, R. H., and Eger, E. I., II. MAC expanded: AD_{50} and AD_{95} values of common inhalation anesthetics in man. *Anesthesiology,* **1975,** *42,* 384–389.

de Jong, R. H., and Heavner, J. E. Diazepam and lidocaine-induced cardiovascular changes. *Anesthesiology,* **1973,** *39,* 633–638.

Egbert, L. D.; Battit, G. E.; Turndorf, H.; and Becker, H. K. The value of a preoperative visit by an anesthetist. *J.A.M.A.,* **1963,** *185,* 533–555.

Eger, E. I., II. Effect of inspired anesthetic concentration on the rate of rise of alveolar concentration. *Anesthesiology,* **1963,** *24,* 153–157.

————. Respiratory and circulatory factors in uptake and distribution of volatile anaesthetic agents. *Br. J. Anaesth.,* **1964,** *36,* 155–171.

————. Intertissue diffusion of anesthetics. *Anesthesiology*, **1973**, *38*, 201.

Eger, E. I., II; Lundgren, C.; Miller, S. F.; and Stevens, W. C. Anesthetic potencies of sulfur hexafluoride, carbon tetrafluoride, chloroform and ETHRANE in dogs: correlation with the hydrate and lipid theories of anesthetic action. *Anesthesiology*, **1969**, *30*, 129–135.

Eger, E. I., II; Saidman, L. J.; and Brandstater, B. Minimum alveolar anesthetic concentration, a standard of anesthetic potency. *Anesthesiology*, **1965**, *26*, 756–763.

Eger, E. I., II, and Severinghaus, J. W. Effect of uneven pulmonary distribution of blood and gas on induction with inhalation anesthetics. *Anesthesiology*, **1964**, *25*, 620–626.

Epstein, R. M.; Rackow, H.; Salanitre, E.; and Wolf, G. Influence of the concentration effect on the uptake of anesthetic mixtures: the second gas effect. *Anesthesiology*, **1964**, *25*, 364–371.

Fink, B. R. Diffusion anoxia. *Anesthesiology*, **1955**, *16*, 511–519.

Fragen, R. J., and Caldwell, N. Lorazepam premedication. *Anesth. Analg.*, **1976**, *55*, 792–796.

Fragen, R. J.; Funk, D. I.; Avram, M. J.; Costello, C.; and DeBruine, K. Midazolam versus hydroxyzine as intramuscular premedicant. *Can. Anaesth. Soc. J.*, **1983**, *30*, 136–141.

Greene, N. M. A consideration of factors in the discovery of anesthesia and their effects on its development. *Anesthesiology*, **1971**, *35*, 515–522.

————. Anesthesia and the development of surgery (1846–1896). *Anesth. Analg.*, **1979**, *58*, 5–12.

Halsey, M. J. Mechanisms of general anesthesia. In, *Anesthetic Uptake and Action*. (Eger, E. I., II, ed.) The Williams & Wilkins Co., Baltimore, **1974**, pp. 45–76.

Hill, D. W. The design and calibration of vaporizers for volatile anaesthetic agents. *Br. J. Anaesth.*, **1968**, *40*, 648–659.

Lerman, J.; Robinson, S.; Willis, M. M.; and Gregory, G. A. Anesthetic requirements for halothane in young children 0–1 month and 1–8 months of age. *Anesthesiology*, **1983**, *59*, 421–424.

Lucas, G. H. The discovery of cyclopropane. *Anesth. Analg.*, **1961**, *40*, 15–27.

McDowall, D. G. Monitoring the brain. *Anesthesiology*, **1976**, *45*, 117–134.

McIntyre, A. R. Historical background, early use and development of muscle relaxants. *Anesthesiology*, **1959**, *20*, 409–415.

Meyer, H. H. Zur Theorie de Alkoholnarkose. I. Mitt. Welche Eigenschaft der Anästhetika bedingt ihre narkotische Wirkung? *Arch. Exp. Pathol. Pharmakol.*, **1899**, *42*, 109.

————. Zur Theorie der Alkoholnarkose. III. Mitt. Der Einfluss wechselnder Temperatur auf Wirkungsstärke und Teilungskoefficient der Narkotika. *Ibid.*, **1901**, *46*, 338.

Millar, R. D.; Wahrenbrock, E. A.; Schroeder, C. F.; Knipstein, T. W.; Eger, E. I., II; and Buechel, D. R. Ethylene-halothane anesthesia: addition or synergism? *Anesthesiology*, **1969**, *31*, 301–304.

Miller, K. W.; Paton, W. D. M.; Smith, E. B.; and Smith, R. A. Physicochemical approaches to the mode of action of general anesthetics. *Anesthesiology*, **1972**, *36*, 339–351.

Miller, K. W.; Paton, W. D. M.; Smith, R. A.; and Smith, E. B. The pressure reversal of general anesthesia and the critical volume hypothesis. *Mol. Pharmacol.*, **1973**, *9*, 131–143.

Miller, S. L. A theory of gaseous anesthetics. *Proc. Natl. Acad. Sci. U.S.A.*, **1961**, *47*, 1515–1524.

Mountcastle, D. B.; Biltonen, R. L.; and Halsey, M. J. Effect of anesthetics and pressure on the thermotropic behavior of multilamellar dipalmitoylphosphatidyl cho-

line liposomes. *Proc. Natl. Acad. Sci. U.S.A.*, **1978**, *75*, 4906–4910.

Munson, E. S.; Eger, E. I., II; and Bowers, D. L. Effects of anesthetic-depressed ventilation and cardiac output on anesthetic uptake: a computer nonlinear simulation. *Anesthesiology*, **1973**, *38*, 251–259.

Myer, E. F., and Tomeldan, S. A. Glycopyrrolate compared with atropine in prevention of the oculocardiac reflex during eye-muscle surgery. *Anesthesiology*, **1979**, *51*, 350–352.

Odura, K. A. Glycopyrrolate methylbromide. Comparison with atropine sulfate. *Can. Anaesth. Soc. J.*, **1975**, *22*, 466–473.

Overton, E. *Studien über die Narkose zugleich ein Beitrag zur allgemeinen Pharmakologie.* G. Fischer, Jena, **1901**.

Pandit, S. K.; Heisterkamp, D. V.; and Cohen, P. J. Further studies of the anti-recall effect of lorazepam. *Anesthesiology*, **1976**, *45*, 495–500.

Pauling, L. A molecular theory of general anesthesia. *Science*, **1961**, *134*, 15–21.

Rosner, B. S., and Clark, D. L. Neurophysiologic effects of general anesthetics. II. Sequential regional actions in the brain. *Anesthesiology*, **1973**, *39*, 59–81.

Smith, N. T.; Zwart, A.; and Beneken, J. E. W. Interaction between the circulatory effects and the uptake and distribution of halothane: use of a multiple model. *Anesthesiology*, **1972**, *37*, 47–58.

Stevens, W. C.; Dolan, W. M.; Gibbons, R. T.; White, A.; Eger, E. I., II; Miller, R. D.; de Jong, R. H.; and Elashoff, R. M. Minimum alveolar concentrations (MAC) of isoflurane with and without nitrous oxide in patients of various ages. *Anesthesiology*, **1975**, *42*, 197–200.

Stoelting, R. K., and Eger, E. I., II. Percutaneous loss of nitrous oxide, cyclopropane, ether and halothane in man. *Anesthesiology*, **1969**, *30*, 278–289.

Thornton, C.; Catley, D. M.; Jordan, C.; Lehane, J. R.; Royston, D.; and Jones, J. G. Enflurane anaesthesia causes graded changes in the brainstem and early cortical auditory evoked response in man. *Br. J. Anaesth.*, **1983**, *55*, 479–486.

Traube, J. Theorie der Osmose und Narkose. *Arch. Ges. Physiol.*, **1904**, *105*, 541–559.

Trudell, J. R., and Hubbell, W. L. Localization of molecular halothane in phospholipid bilayer model nerve membranes. *Anesthesiology*, **1976**, *44*, 202.

Trudell, J. R.; Hubbell, W. L.; and Cohen, E. N. The effect of two inhalation anesthetics on the order of spin-labeled phospholipid vesicles. *Biochim. Biophys. Acta*, **1973a**, *291*, 321–327.

————. Pressure reversal of inhalation anesthetic-induced disorder in spin-labeled phospholipid vesicles. *Ibid.*, **1973b**, *291*, 328–334.

Vandam, L. D. Early American anesthetists—the origins of professionalism in anesthesia. *Anesthesiology*, **1973**, *38*, 264–274.

Wolfson, B.; Hetrick, W. D.; Kake, C. L.; and Siker, E. S. Anesthetic indices—further data. *Anesthesiology*, **1978**, *48*, 187–190.

Monographs and Reviews

Clark, D. L., and Rosner, B. S. Neurophysiologic effects of general anesthetics. I. The electroencephalogram and sensory evoked responses in man. *Anesthesiology*, **1973**, *38*, 564–582.

Cohen, E. N. Metabolism of the volatile anesthetics. *Anesthesiology*, **1971**, *35*, 193–202.

Davison, M. H. A. *The Evolution of Anesthesia.* The Williams & Wilkins Co., Baltimore, **1965**.

Duncum, B. M. *The Development of Inhalation Anesthesia.* Oxford University Press, New York, **1947**.

Faulconer, A., Jr., and Bickford, R. G. *Electroencephalography in Anesthesiology.* Charles C Thomas, Publisher, Springfield, Ill., **1960.**

Faulconer, A., and Keys, T. E. (eds.). *Foundations of Anesthesiology.* Charles C Thomas, Publisher, Springfield, Ill., **1965.**

Grundy, B. L. Intraoperative monitoring of sensory-evoked potentials. *Anesthesiology,* **1983,** *58,* 72–87.

Keys, T. E. *The History of Surgical Anesthesia.* Dover Publications, Inc., New York, **1963.**

Levy, W. J.; Shapiro, H. M.; Maruchak, G.; and Meathe, E. Automated EEG processing for intraoperative monitoring. *Anesthesiology,* **1980,** *53,* 223–236.

Paton, W. D. M. Unconventional unanaesthetic molecules. In, *Molecular Mechanisms in General Anaesthesia.* (Halsey, M. J.; Millar, R. A.; and Sutton, J. A.; eds.) Churchill-Livingstone, Ltd., London, **1974,** pp. 48–64.

Sykes, W. S. *Essays on the First Hundred Years of Anesthesia.* E. & S. Livingstone, Edinburgh, **1960.**

Thomas, K. B. *The Development of Anaesthetic Apparatus.* Blackwell Scientific Publications, Oxford, **1975.**

14 GENERAL ANESTHETICS

Bryan E. Marshall and Harry Wollman

The state of general anesthesia is a drug-induced absence of perception of all sensations. Depths of anesthesia appropriate for the conduct of surgical procedures can be achieved with a wide variety of drugs, either alone or, more often, in combinations. General anesthetics can be administered by a variety of routes, but intravenous or inhalational administration is preferred, because the effective dose and the time course of action are more predictable when these technics are used. In this chapter the inhalational general anesthetic agents are described in some detail. The intravenous agents, including the barbiturates, benzodiazepines, opioids, and neuroleptics, are discussed in detail elsewhere (see Index) and, therefore, only their use for anesthesia will be presented here.

I. Inhalational Anesthetics

An ideal inhalational general anesthetic agent would be characterized by: (1) rapid and pleasant induction of, and recovery from, anesthesia; (2) rapid changes in the depth of anesthesia; (3) adequate relaxation of skeletal muscles; (4) a wide margin of safety; and (5) the absence of toxic effects or other adverse properties in normal doses. However, the availability of ultrashort-acting intravenous agents, potent opioid analgesics with short durations of action, and specific muscle relaxants has reduced the necessity for the first three properties. The margin of safety of inhalational drugs has become less of an issue, since lower concentrations of the anesthetic can be administered in combination with useful intravenous supplements. The incidence of adverse effects is, therefore, the principal factor that now determines the acceptability of a general anesthetic agent.

The inhalational general anesthetic agents in wide use are nitrous oxide, halo-

thane, enflurane, and isoflurane; methoxyflurane is usually employed only for analgesia during obstetrical procedures. The inorganic compound nitrous oxide (N_2O) is a gas at normal ambient temperature and pressure, whereas the other four agents are volatile organic liquids (Table 14–1). Certain generalizations are appropriate concerning the relative potency and the properties that result from their physical and chemical characteristics (see also Chapter 13).

Potency. A standard of comparison for potency of general anesthetic agents was elusive, but the introduction of the concept of *minimum alveolar concentration* (MAC; see Chapter 13) by Eger and associates (1965) provided an important and practical definition. A dose of 1 MAC will prevent movement in response to surgical incision in 50% of subjects; doses that span the approximate range of 0.5 to 2 MAC are necessary for adequate anesthesia in individual patients. A dose of less than 1 MAC may also be effective when requirements are reduced by disease or the presence of other drugs. The values of MAC in Table 14–1 demonstrate both the wide range of relative potencies and the greater potencies of the volatile agents compared to nitrous oxide. Technics for vaporization and administration of volatile anesthetic agents are described in Chapter 13. The saturated vapor pressures for the volatile anesthetics are shown in Table 14–1; also listed are the maximum concentrations of anesthetic vapor that can be delivered by an efficient vaporizer.

Induction of Anesthesia. None of the agents listed in Table 14–1 is irritating to breathe, and their odors are not unpleasant. The depth of anesthesia that can be achieved depends on the potency relative to the maximum amount of agent that can

Table 14–1. PROPERTIES OF INHALATIONAL ANESTHETIC AGENTS

ANESTHETIC	MAC * (%)	VAPOR PRESSURE (mm Hg at 20° C)	MAXIMUM VAPOR CONCENTRATION (% at 20° C)	BLOOD:GAS PARTITION COEFFICIENT (at 37° C)	OIL:GAS PARTITION COEFFICIENT (at 37° C)
Methoxyflurane	0.16	22.5	3	12.0	970
Halothane	0.75	243	32	2.3	224
Enflurane	1.68	175	23	1.9	98
Isoflurane	1.15	250	33	1.4	99
Nitrous oxide	105 †	Gas	—	0.47	1.4

* MAC = minimum alveolar concentration (see text for further definition).
† A value of MAC greater than 100% means that hyperbaric conditions would be required to reach 1 MAC.

be vaporized. Table 14–1 illustrates the fact that concentrations far higher than usually necessary can be delivered when halothane, enflurane, and isoflurane are used. The speed with which induction of anesthesia can be accomplished is inversely related to the solubility of the agent in most body tissues (blood:gas partition coefficient), as described in Chapter 13. The greater the oil:gas partition coefficient (Table 14–1), the greater the capacity of fatty tissues to absorb the agent; this results in slower equilibration with fatty tissues and longer periods of elimination after discontinuation of the anesthetic following prolonged administration.

Most of what follows in this chapter concerns the pharmacological properties of anesthetic drugs. Their influences on the lungs, heart, and circulation, as well as the less apparent actions on other organ systems, are side effects that always accompany general anesthesia; accurate knowledge of these properties is required for safe management of the patient. Although inhalational anesthetics in current use are relatively inert and nontoxic, some are more prone than others to be metabolized. Certain metabolic products are now believed to determine the long-term toxic effects that may follow the use of these drugs.

HALOTHANE

Chemistry and Physical Properties. *Halothane* (FLUOTHANE) is 2-bromo-2-chloro-1,1,1-trifluoroethane (Table 14–2). Mixtures of halothane with air or oxygen are not flammable or explosive. Partition coefficients and the MAC value for halothane are listed in Table 14–1.

With the exception of chromium, nickel, and titanium, most metals are tarnished or corroded by

halothane. The compound interacts with rubber and some plastics, but not with polyethylene.

The solubility of halothane in rubber can theoretically slow the induction of and the emergence from anesthesia as a consequence of the uptake or release of the anesthetic from the rubber elements in the anesthesia circuit when low-flow technics are used.

PHARMACOLOGICAL PROPERTIES

General Characteristics. The general and special properties of halothane are discussed in greater detail than are those of the other volatile agents because halothane represents the first of the series of drugs now in common use, and it is the standard to which others are compared. Halothane is a potent anesthetic agent with properties that allow a smooth and rather rapid loss of consciousness that progresses to anesthesia with abolition of responses to painful stimulation. In practice, the rapidity, convenience, and pleasantness associated with the intravenous administration of thiopental

Table 14–2. STRUCTURES OF VOLATILE GENERAL ANESTHETIC AGENTS *

* Note the varying halogen substitutions and that all of the agents, except halothane, are ethers. While isoflurane and enflurane are isomers, there are some important differences in their pharmacological properties (see text).

are usually preferred for induction of anesthesia; halothane is then introduced for maintenance of anesthesia during the surgical procedure. The circumstances and requirements of the surgical procedure determine whether the trachea is intubated; whether the patient is allowed to breathe spontaneously or is ventilated manually or mechanically; and whether additional drugs, such as muscle relaxants or analgesics, are administered.

Following its introduction in 1956, the clinical popularity of halothane was based primarily on its lack of flammability, the ease with which depth of anesthesia can be changed, the rapid awakening (less than 1 hour) when its administration is stopped, and the relatively low incidence of toxic effects associated with its use. However, the margin of safety of halothane is not wide; circulatory depression with profound reduction of arterial blood pressure is readily produced (Eger, 1974).

The signs of depth of anesthesia with halothane that are of most practical value are the blood pressure, which is progressively depressed, and the response to surgical stimulation (*e.g.*, pulse rate, blood pressure, movement, or even awakening). The concentration of anesthetic agent that is necessary in the inspired gas mixture for induction of anesthesia must be appropriately reduced as the alveolar concentration increases during maintenance if progressive increase in depth of anesthesia and decrease in blood pressure are to be avoided.

Circulation. Administration of halothane is characterized by a dose-dependent reduction of arterial blood pressure (Eger *et al.*, 1970). Hypotension results from two main effects. First, there is a direct depression of the myocardium and decreased cardiac output; second, the normal baroreceptor-mediated tachycardia in response to hypotension is obtunded. With halothane and the other commonly used volatile agents, anesthesia is not associated with increased sympathoadrenal activity; concentrations of catecholamines in blood do not increase (Perry *et al.*, 1974), and cardiovascular depression is evident. However, at clinical depths of anesthesia, sympathoadrenal response to stimulation is not abolished by halothane. An appropriate stimulus, for example, increased carbon dioxide tension or surgical stimulation, may cause an active sympathetic response with increases of blood pressure, heart rate, and concentrations of catecholamines in plasma.

Heart. When anesthesia is induced by inspiration of halothane at concentrations commonly necessary for surgical anesthesia (0.8 to 1.2%), cardiac output is reduced by 20 to 50% from the level characteristic of the awake state (Marshall *et al.*, 1969). Both increased concentration of halothane and reduced arterial carbon dioxide tension (hyperventilation) accentuate the reduction (Prys-Roberts *et al.*, 1968).

The contractility of preparations of heart muscle *in vitro* is depressed in a dose-dependent fashion (Sugai *et al.*, 1968). There is also general agreement that myocardial contractility is reduced during halothane anesthesia in man (Sonntag *et al.*, 1978). However, after some 2 to 5 hours of constant halothane anesthesia, all of the cardiovascular changes (*i.e.*, hypotension, depressed cardiac output, and bradycardia) tend to return toward normal; this has been attributed to sympathetic activation with time (Eger *et al.*, 1970). Animal studies have established that autoregulation of coronary flow remains intact and that any reduction of flow that is observed reflects the reduced oxygen consumption and work of the heart. No deficiency in supply of metabolic substrates to the myocardium is detectable in the normal heart, and there is no evidence of anaerobic metabolism. Merin and associates (1977) have concluded that interference with myocardial metabolism does not account for changes in contractility. While the mechanism of this depression of contractility is thus unclear, it can be reversed experimentally by administration of Ca^{2+}. It is suggested that halothane may interfere with the availability of Ca^{2+} in the sarcoplasm (Lynch *et al.*, 1981). This hypothesis remains to be confirmed.

Cardiac Rhythm. The heart rate is slowed during anesthesia with halothane. This is, in part, reversible by atropine and is due to reduction of cardiac sympathetic activity with consequent vagal predominance. However, direct slowing of the S-A nodal discharge *in vitro* was observed by Reynolds and associates (1970), and atropine does not alter this effect. There appears to be both a reduction of the rate of phase-4 depolarization, which is normally responsible for the automaticity of pacemaker tissue, and an increased threshold for the generation of an action potential. During halothane anesthesia in man, vagal activity is further enhanced by manipulation of the airway. Sinus bradycardia, wandering pacemaker, or junctional rhythms are not uncommon at this time, but they are generally benign.

Tachyarrhythmias may also occur in the presence of halothane. Some of these may be of the reentrant type (*see* Chapter 31). Since halothane slows the conduction of impulses and also probably increases refractory periods in conducting tissue, it creates the conditions necessary for reentry, a unidirectional block with slow retrograde conduction (Atlee and Rusy, 1977).

Halothane may also increase the automaticity of the myocardium; this effect is exaggerated by adrenergic agonists and leads to propagated impulses from ectopic sites within the atria or ventricles (Zink *et al.,* 1975). Increased secretion of endogenous epinephrine may result from stimulation during surgery, if anesthesia is insufficient, or from increased arterial tension of carbon dioxide, if ventilation is inadequate. Alternatively, exogenously administered epinephrine may initiate the arrhythmia. Tachyarrhythmias are unlikely if, in the presence of halothane anesthesia, ventilation is adequate and the use of epinephrine for hemostasis is limited to concentrations of 1:100,000 or less and the dose in adults does not exceed 0.1 mg in 10 minutes or 0.3 mg in 1 hour (Katz *et al.,* 1962).

While all of the above-mentioned arrhythmias are generally benign in patients with a healthy myocardium, they may not be so in the presence of cardiac disease, hypoxia, acidosis, or electrolyte abnormalities.

Baroreceptor Control. Early work on this system demonstrated that halothane influenced the afferent discharge by "resetting" the baroreceptors to respond around a lower "set point," depressed the vasomotor response of the brain stem, and reduced the sympathetic outflow that results. However, the observed changes were small, and other investigations of the entire baroreceptor system led to the conclusion that the action of halothane on its central neural components accounted for only part of the depression of baroreceptor response (Wang *et al.,* 1968). In addition, there is little effect of halothane on the response of preganglionic sympathetic neurons to stimulation of baroreceptors (Skovsted *et al.,* 1969). It is concluded that the predominant actions of halothane are at the effector sites in the heart that control cardiac rate and/or contractility.

Organ Blood Flow. Halothane influences the blood flow to every organ. In the skin and cerebral circulation, flow may increase as the vessels dilate. However, the cerebrovascular bed, as well as the renal and splanchnic circulations, loses some of its ability to autoregulate flow, and perfusion of these tissues decreases if blood pressure falls excessively. The coronary circulation remains responsive to myocardial needs for oxygen; vasodilatation occurs in poorly ventilated areas of the lung because of inhibition of pulmonary vasoconstriction that normally occurs in response to hypoxia.

In an individual patient, blood flow to each of these organs can be influenced by pH and carbon dioxide tension, posture, temperature, age, disease, and the administration of other drugs. It is, therefore, not surprising that conflicting results have been reported. However, there is agreement that, despite the differences from organ to organ, the total peripheral vascular resistance changes very little when hypotension occurs with halothane (Eger *et al.,* 1970; Sonntag *et al.,* 1978). Dilatation in one organ bed is offset by reduced flow in another, and, thus, generalized peripheral vasodilatation is not the primary cause of hypotension.

Respiration. If the patient anesthetized with halothane is allowed to breathe spontaneously, an increased partial pressure of carbon dioxide in the arterial blood is common and is indicative of ventilatory depression; there is also an increased difference between the partial pressure of oxygen in the alveolar gas and in the arterial blood, indicating less efficient exchange of gas. Halothane thus influences both ventilatory control and the efficiency of oxygen transfer. To compensate for these effects, ventilation is frequently assisted or controlled by manual or mechanical means, and the concentration of inspired oxygen is increased.

Ventilatory Control. Characteristically, respirations are rapid and shallow during halothane anesthesia. Minute volume is reduced, and arterial carbon dioxide tension is increased from 40 mm Hg to approximately 50 mm Hg. Halothane causes a dose-related reduction in the ventilatory response to carbon dioxide (Knill and Gelb, 1978). While the precise effects of the anesthetic on the function of central and peripheral chemoreceptors are uncertain, the changes in the ventilatory response to carbon dioxide and the altered pattern of breathing caused by halothane are probably predominantly mediated at central sites of action.

In the awake state, the total ventilatory response to carbon dioxide is altered little by denervation of peripheral chemoreceptors. Therefore, despite evidence that halothane depresses the activity of the carbon dioxide–stimulated carotid body, it seems unlikely that this effect can be responsible for the ventilatory depression that is observed.

The increased ventilation in response to arterial hypoxemia, which is mediated by the carotid bodies, is abolished by denervation and by halothane (Knill and Gelb, 1978). It follows that adequacy of oxygenation during anesthesia cannot be assessed by observing ventilatory exchange. However, halothane depresses responsiveness to carbon dioxide even when the blood is hyperoxic.

The above considerations lead to the conclusion that depression of respiratory sensitivity to carbon dioxide by halothane results from a central action on the respiratory centers themselves. This view is further supported by investigations of factors that determine the rapid and shallow pattern of ventilation that accompanies halothane anesthesia. Some evidence of minor changes in sensitivity of pulmonary stretch receptors has been adduced by Coleridge and associates (1968), but, in general, the phasic activity of the vagal afferents is unchanged by halothane, and the essential sites of action are in the brain stem.

Pulmonary Oxygen Transfer. Efficient transfer of oxygen from the alveolar gas to hemoglobin in the alveolar capillary red blood cell depends on a proper balance between alveolar ventilation and perfusion. This balance is importantly controlled by the effects of gravity and various structural mechanical factors, and fine adjustments are provided by changes in the tone of the smooth muscle of bronchial airways and pulmonary vessels. All of these may be altered during halothane anesthesia. The influence of gravity obviously differs when the patient is in the horizontal position, particularly when ventilation is achieved by intermittent positive pressure. Halothane changes the relative movements of the rib cage and diaphragm (Tusiewicz *et al.,* 1977), alters lung volume (Laws, 1968), dilates constricted bronchial smooth muscle (a useful property in asthmatic patients) (Hirshman *et al.,* 1982), depresses mucociliary flow (Forbes, 1976), and inhibits pulmonary vascular constriction in the presence of hypoxia (Benumof and Wahrenbrock, 1975). The outcome is more or less impairment of oxygen exchange (Marshall and Wyche, 1972), with evidence of an increased fraction of blood to which no oxygen is added as it traverses the lungs (pulmonary shunt) and increased mismatching of ventilation and perfusion (Dueck *et al.,* 1980).

Nervous System. Electrical activity of the cerebral cortex recorded by a frontooccipital EEG shows progressive replacement of fast, low-voltage activity by slow waves of greater amplitude as halothane anesthesia is deepened. Surgical stimulation may reverse this pattern, and such arousal reactions may be associated with recall of intraoperative events by patients, as in a dream (Bimar and Bellville, 1977). This sequence resembles arousal of the brain by activation of the brain stem reticular formation, but reticular neuronal activity is depressed by halothane (Shimoji *et al.,* 1977).

Cerebral vessels dilate during halothane anesthesia, cerebral blood flow increases unless blood pressure falls excessively (Wollman *et al.,* 1964), autoregulation is impaired (Miletich *et al.,* 1976), and cerebrospinal fluid pressure increases (Lassen and Christensen, 1976). The cerebral metabolic consumption of oxygen is reduced and the delivery of oxygen and substrates to the brain appears to be adequate, despite decreased blood flow. There is no indication that halothane anesthesia interferes with energy metabolism in the brain unless excessive doses are employed (Smith and Wollman, 1972; Michenfelder and Theye, 1975).

Recovery of mental function after even brief anesthesia with halothane is not complete for several hours (Korttila *et al.*, 1977), but this phenomenon probably contributes little to the more prolonged impairment of psychological performance that has been reported after major surgery. Shivering during recovery is common and probably represents both a response to heat loss and an ill-defined expression of neurological recovery.

Muscle. Relaxation of skeletal muscle is desirable or necessary for many surgical procedures. Anesthesia with halothane causes some relaxation by central depression; in addition, the duration and magnitude of the muscular relaxation induced by non-depolarizing skeletal muscle relaxants such as *d*-tubocurarine or pancuronium are increased. The mechanism of this effect is not known but appears to be based on increased sensitivity of the end-plate to the action of the competitive neuromuscular blocking agents (Waud and Waud, 1979).

Rarely, induction of anesthesia with halothane or any of the other halogenated inhalational anesthetics triggers a peculiar, uncontrolled hypermetabolic reaction in skeletal muscle of susceptible patients. The resultant syndrome of *malignant hyperpyrexia* is characterized by a rapid rise in body temperature, a massive increase in oxygen consumption, and production of carbon dioxide; death may result. This peculiar syndrome may occur when calcium uptake by sarcoplasmic reticulum fails in genetically susceptible muscle (Gronert, 1980).

Uterine smooth muscle is relaxed by halothane. This effect is of sufficient magnitude to allow manipulation of the fetus (version) during the prenatal period. Inhibition of natural or induced uterine contractions by halothane during parturition may prolong the process of delivery, as well as increase blood loss. Thus, other agents or technics may be preferred for the relief of obstetrical pain.

Kidney. Anesthesia with halothane at a level of about 1 MAC causes dose-dependent reductions of renal blood flow and the rate of glomerular filtration to approximately 40% and 50% of normal, respectively (Mazze *et al.*, 1963). These effects can be attenuated by preoperative hydration (Barry *et al.*, 1964) and prevention of hypotension. Halothane does not interfere greatly with autoregulation of renal blood flow nor, in the normotensive state, with the distribution of flow between the renal cortex and medulla (Leighton and Bruce, 1975). Anesthesia is normally accompanied by the production of a small volume of concentrated urine. The changes in urine volume are probably secondary to circulatory responses and reduced glomerular filtration (Deutsch *et al.*, 1966). The renal effects of halothane anesthesia are rapidly reversed, and there is no evidence of postoperative renal impairment. In an occasional patient (usually elderly), retention of water postoperatively results in hyponatremia, reduced plasma osmolality, and mental confusion. There is no direct evidence that halothane anesthesia is responsible for this syndrome of inappropriate secretion of antidiuretic hormone.

Liver and Gastrointestinal Tract. Compared to older agents (*e.g.*, ether and cyclopropane), the incidence and duration of postoperative nausea and vomiting are much reduced with the inhalational anesthetics in current use. Factors such as age, sex, site and duration of surgery, disease state, and other medications have a greater influence than does the specific inhalational agent selected. However, the injectable anesthetic agents generally result in an even lower incidence of nausea and vomiting.

Splanchnic and, therefore, hepatic blood flow is reduced by halothane as a passive consequence of reduced perfusion pressure, but there is no evidence of overt ischemia (Epstein *et al.*, 1966). Hepatic cellular functions are, however, depressed, and the ability of the microsomal enzyme systems to metabolize drugs is reduced when halothane is administered. The extent of this depression is similar to that produced by other inhalational anesthetics, and it is rapidly reversed when administration of halothane is stopped.

Hepatitis. Hepatitis that occurs in the postoperative period is most often due to transmission of hepatitis virus (*e.g.*, in transfused blood), involvement of the liver by disease processes, or damage by known hepatotoxic drugs. However, a retrospective analysis of the records of more than 850,000 administrations of anesthetics suggested a small incidence of hepatic necrosis in which the above etiological factors did not appear to be present (Summary of the National Halothane Study, 1966).

Typically, some 2 to 5 days after anesthesia and surgery, a fever develops, accompanied by anorexia, nausea, and vomiting. Occasionally, a rash occurs and analysis of blood reveals eosinophilia and biochemical abnormalities characteristic of hepatitis. There may be a progression to hepatic failure, and death occurs in about 50% of these patients. The incidence of the syndrome is low, approximately 1 in 10,000 anesthetic administrations. Since it is seen most often after repeated administrations of halothane over a short period of time, the term *halothane hepatitis* is used.

A possible basis for the above-described syndrome has been provided by the observation that halothane and all other general anesthetic agents are metabolized, at least to some extent (*see* below). Chemically reactive or immunogenic products may result. An excess of a toxic product or of a metabolite capable of inducing an immune response may lead to hepatitis. Evidence that such reactions occur has been obtained in both animals and man, but this has been observed only in extraordinary circumstances (Sipes and Brown, 1976; Williams *et al.*, 1977). While the specificity of this effect has stimulated particular interest, it should be emphasized that other complications of general anesthesia occur with much greater frequency.

Biotransformation. Approximately 60 to 80% of absorbed halothane is eliminated unchanged in the exhaled gas in the first 24 hours after its administration, and smaller amounts continue to be exhaled for several days or even weeks. Of the fraction not exhaled, approximately 15% undergoes biotransformation, and the rest is eliminated unchanged by other routes.

The mixed-function oxidase or cytochrome P-450 system in the endoplasmic reticulum of the hepatocyte is responsible for this metabolism (Cohen, 1971). Chloride and bromide ions are removed from halothane but only a small amount of fluoride (the bond energy for C-F is nearly twice that for C-Br or C-Cl). It has been suggested that the concentrations of circulating bromide may be sufficient to cause changes in mood or intellectual function in the postoperative period (Johnstone *et al.*, 1975). The urine contains organic fluorine-containing compounds, mostly trifluoroacetic acid (Rehder *et al.*, 1967; Sakai and Takaori, 1978). Induction of microsomal enzymes may follow repeated exposure to various drugs, including halothane, and metabolic breakdown may thereby be increased (Sipes and Brown, 1976).

Several studies have suggested that occupational exposure to an environment containing halothane or other anesthetic agents for a prolonged period may result in an increased incidence of miscarriage of pregnancy (Vessey, 1978). While this has not yet been confirmed, effective steps to reduce environmental contamination are relatively simple and have already been instituted in most operating rooms; this seems prudent, indeed.

Evaluation. *Disadvantages and Limitations.* General anesthesia for surgery requires sleep, analgesia, suppression of visceral reflexes, and, to a variable extent, muscle relaxation; only the first is completely obtained with halothane. Analgesia must often be accomplished by the use of opioids or nitrous oxide, muscular relaxation is enhanced by specific relaxant drugs, and visceral reflexes are managed with other drugs as appropriate (*e.g.*, atropine for bradycardia or local anesthesia to obtund responses to visceral traction). Hypoxemia, hypotension, and transient arrhythmias may occur and sometimes require modification of the anesthetic technic; respiratory depression usually necessitates supplemental ventilation.

Advantages and Uses. Halothane has a moderately high potency and a moderately low blood:gas partition coefficient. Induction of and recovery from anesthesia are, therefore, not prolonged. Halothane is non-flammable. The larynx is not irritated, bronchospasm is uncommon, and, thus, induction is smooth. Nevertheless, thiopental is most commonly injected to induce sleep prior to the administration of halothane. Halothane is compatible with soda lime and may be used with oxygen to provide maximal oxygenation or combined with other gas mixtures such as nitrous oxide and oxygen. Its potential for inducing hypotension is sometimes utilized deliberately to reduce blood loss under carefully controlled conditions. Uterine relaxation can be valuable during version or extraction of a fetus.

Status. Halothane has enjoyed wide popularity for over 25 years, and it is utilized for the entire range of surgical procedures. Its administration is associated with an excellent safety record (Summary of the National Halothane Study, 1966). Appropriate equipment is available for precise administration of this agent in all situations. The introduction of enflurane and isoflurane, together with the availability of a variety of intravenous agents, has reduced the use of halothane, but it remains the standard for comparison.

ENFLURANE

Chemistry and Physical Properties. *Enflurane* (ETHRANE) is 2-chloro-1,1,2-trifluoroethyl difluoromethyl ether. It is a clear, colorless, non-flammable liquid with a mild, sweet odor. It is extremely stable chemically. It does not attack aluminum, tin, brass, iron, or copper. The partition coefficients and the MAC value for enflurane are listed in Table 14–1. Enflurane is soluble in rubber (partition coefficient = 74), and this may prolong induction and recovery somewhat, as described for halothane.

PHARMACOLOGICAL PROPERTIES

General Characteristics. The physical properties of enflurane assure that induction of and emergence from anesthesia and adjustment of anesthetic depth during maintenance can be smooth and moderately rapid. Technics of administration are very similar to those for halothane. Induction of anesthesia to depths appropriate for surgery may be achieved in less than 10 minutes when approximately 4% enflurane is inhaled. A short-acting barbiturate is usually infused intravenously to render the patient unconscious. As with any inhalational agent, the alveolar concentration approaches the inspired concentration with time, and the latter must be progressively reduced. Anesthesia is maintained with inspired concentrations of 1.5 to 3% enflurane.

There is mild stimulation of salivation and tracheobronchial secretions, but these are not usually troublesome. Laryngeal and pharyngeal reflexes are obtunded early, and excitement during induction is seldom observed.

The pupils remain small, and eye movements are not prominent; respiration is depressed, and ventilatory assistance is usually required; and, as with halothane, the most useful signs of depth of anesthesia are changes in arterial blood pressure, pulse rate, or movement in response to surgical stimulation.

Circulation. Arterial blood pressure decreases progressively as the depth of anesthesia increases with enflurane, to about the same degree as it does with halothane. Studies of the effects of the agent on the baroreceptor responses and preganglionic sympathetic activity are also similar (Skovsted and Price, 1972); there is evidence of reduced adrenergic activity, and there is no increase in the concentration of circulating catecholamines (Göthert and Wendt, 1977).

In-vitro preparations of myocardium show dose-dependent, reversible depression of contractility (Shimosato *et al.*, 1969), similar to that caused by halothane at equivalent doses. In the intact animal, Merin and associates (1976) have demonstrated that depression of myocardial work is paralleled by diminished consumption of oxygen by the heart. There is no evidence of myocardial hypoxia.

No major differences between the potent volatile anesthetic agents have been observed with regard to their effects on blood flow to vital organs. There are, however, small differences. Bradycardia does not usually occur during anesthesia with enflurane; the pulse rate remains constant. Cardiac output is not decreased as much as with halothane (Marshall *et al.*, 1971), at least at concentrations below 1.5 MAC, and the decreased blood pressure is due, in part, to greater peripheral vascular dilatation. In response to surgical stimulation or hypercarbia, cardiovascular depression may be reversed and blood pressure and cardiac output return toward preanesthetic levels. Administration of the β-adrenergic antagonist propranolol exaggerates hypotension induced by enflurane (Horan *et al.*, 1977); this is also observed with other anesthetic agents. Doses of general anesthetics are, therefore, often reduced for patients who are receiving such drugs, or the β-adrenergic antagonist is reduced in dosage or eliminated before anesthesia.

Cardiac Rhythm. In addition to the absence of bradycardia with enflurane, there is also a reduced tendency to arrhythmias. Enflurane does not interfere with impulse conduction in the heart to the same extent as does halothane (Atlee and Rusy, 1977), and the heart is not as sensitized to catecholamines (Johnston *et al.*, 1976). Hypercarbia or the use of epinephrine for hemostasis or prolongation of the action of local anesthetic agents seldom promotes cardiac arrhythmias in patients receiving enflurane. Thus, somewhat more epinephrine can be used with enflurane than with halothane.

Respiration. Enflurane causes increasing respiratory depression as its concentration is increased. At the level of 1 MAC, the arterial tension of carbon dioxide is greater than with other anesthetics, and depression of the responses to both hypoxia and hypercarbia are greater than with halothane (Hirshman *et al.*, 1977). Curiously, and in contrast to halothane, tachypnea is less common. Assisted or controlled ventilation is usually employed; nevertheless, in order to reduce the incidence of central nervous system (CNS) seizure activity (*see* below), hyperventilation should be avoided. As with all inhalational agents, pulmonary exchange of oxygen may become less efficient during anesthesia, and inspired oxygen concentrations of 35% or more are given to avoid hypoxemia, especially in the elderly. Enflurane causes bronchodilatation and usually inhibits bronchoconstriction.

Nervous System. The occurrence of tonic-clonic muscle activity in a small proportion of subjects was noted early in the clinical use of enflurane (Clark and Rosner, 1973). Subsequently it was demonstrated that a characteristic EEG pattern may emerge when higher concentrations of enflurane are used or when there is hypocarbia. A high-voltage, fast-frequency (14- to 18-Hz) pattern progresses to spike-dome complexes; these alternate with periods of electrical silence or frank seizure activity with motor movements. Jerking or twitching of the muscles of the jaw, face, neck, or limbs may be seen. The seizures are of short duration, are self-limited, and may be prevented by avoiding deep anesthesia and/or hyperventilation. This excitatory action of enflurane is not thought to be of special concern, but the drug should be avoided in patients with seizure foci.

The other effects of enflurane on the CNS are similar to those of halothane. Cerebral oxygen consumption is reduced. Cerebral blood flow is increased when perfusion pressure remains constant, since vasodilatation occurs, and intracranial pressure is also increased. As the blood pressure declines, cerebral blood flow is at first maintained and then decreases if low values of pressure are reached.

Muscle. Skeletal muscle relaxation increases with the depth of anesthesia and is greater than that produced by halothane (Fogdall and Miller, 1975). Relaxation may be sufficient for abdominal surgery. Competitive skeletal muscle relaxants are more effective in the presence of enflurane (Waud, 1977), and the administration of small doses of these agents allows the use of lighter stages of anesthesia. The muscle relaxant activity of enflurane is caused by actions in the CNS and at the postjunctional membrane of the neuromuscular junction; it is not reversed by neostigmine.

Uterine muscle is relaxed by enflurane, and increased blood loss may occur during parturition, cesarean section, or therapeutic abortion.

Kidney. Reductions of renal blood flow, glomerular filtration rate, and urine volume during anesthesia with enflurane are similar to those that occur with equivalent depths of anesthesia from halothane; they are reversed rapidly when the anesthetic is discontinued.

Fluoride is a metabolite of enflurane (Mazze *et al.,* 1977; Sakai and Takaori, 1978); however, despite circulating concentrations (up to 20 μM) that far exceed those derived from halothane, concentrations of fluoride do not usually reach the threshold for renal toxicity (>40 μM). Even when there is renal failure in animals, plasma concentrations of fluoride decline rapidly after enflurane is discontinued, probably due to entry of the anion into bone. It is probable that anesthesia with enflurane is safe in patients with renal disease as long as the depth and duration are not excessive.

Liver and Gastrointestinal Tract. No unusual effects on the gastrointestinal tract have been reported. Splanchnic blood flow is reduced in proportion to perfusion pressure, but delivery of oxygen is not compromised. Nausea and vomiting occur in the postoperative period in perhaps 3 to 15% of patients.

Evidence of hepatic impairment has been obtained during and after surgical anesthesia with enflurane. However, postanesthetic impairment is not apparent in volunteers and the hepatic effects of enflurane are rapidly reversed. Hepatic necrosis associated with repeated administration of enfluranc has bccn rcportcd, and another anesthetic agent should be selected if sensitivity is suspected from a previous administration of the drug (*see* above).

Biotransformation. About 80% of the enflurane that is administered can be recovered unchanged in the expired gas. Of the remainder, some 2 to 5% is metabolized in the liver. This quantity is small because the presence of fluorine and chlorine, the absence of bromine, and the incorporation of an ether bond in the molecule increase its stability. In addition, the oil:gas partition coefficient is less than that of other halogenated anesthetic agents. For this reason, enflurane leaves the fatty tissues more rapidly in the postoperative period and is available for degradation for a relatively brief time. Biotransformation may be increased if hepatic enzymes are induced. The metabolic products that have been identified include difluoromethoxydifluoroacetic acid and fluoride ion. The significance of circulating fluoride with regard to renal function is discussed above.

Evaluation. *Disadvantages and Limitations.* Deep anesthesia with enflurane is associated with respiratory and circulatory depression. Seizure activity may occur when concentrations of enflurane are relatively high, especially when there is hypocarbia. This agent should be avoided when patients have preexisting abnormalities in the EEG or history of a seizure disorder. Uterine relaxation caused by enflurane provides a relative contraindication to the use of deep levels of enflurane anesthesia during labor.

Advantages. Enflurane allows rapid, smooth adjustments of the depth of anesthesia with little change in pulse or respiratory rate. While arrhythmias, postoperative shivering, nausea, and vomiting occur, they do so to a lesser extent than with halothane or methoxyflurane. Relaxation of skeletal muscle is often adequate for surgery, and interactions with competitive muscle relaxants allow smaller doses of enflurane or of relaxants to be used. If epinephrine is used parenterally with the same precautions as are described for halothane, arrhythmias are even less likely to occur than with the latter agent.

Status. Enflurane was introduced into general clinical use in 1973. It was utilized initially mainly as a substitute to avoid repeated administration of halothane, but it is now employed quite widely whenever an inhalational anesthetic agent is desired.

ISOFLURANE

Chemistry and Physical Properties. *Isoflurane* (FORANE) is 1-chloro-2,2,2-trifluoroethyl difluoromethyl ether. The chemical and physical properties of isoflurane are similar to those of its isomer enflurane (Table 14–1). It is not flammable in air or oxygen. Its vapor pressure is high, and delivery of safe concentrations necessitates the use of a precision vaporizer.

PHARMACOLOGICAL PROPERTIES

General Characteristics. The properties of isoflurane are such that there is a smooth and rapid induction of, and emergence from, general anesthesia. Isoflurane has a lower blood:gas solubility coefficient than enflurane; a smaller volume of anesthetic vapor must therefore be transferred to achieve the same tension in blood (or brain), and changes in anesthetic depth can thus be achieved more rapidly with isoflurane than with enflurane. Induction of anesthesia can be achieved in less than 10 minutes with an inhaled concentration of 3% isoflurane in oxygen, and this concentration is subsequently reduced to 1.5 to 2.5% for maintenance of anesthesia. Induction is usually assisted by the injection of a rapidly acting barbiturate. The use of other adjuvant drugs, such as opioids, nitrous oxide, and/or muscle relaxants, reduces the dose of volatile anesthetic that is required to achieve the conditions optimal for surgery.

The clinical signs by which depth of anesthesia is judged include progressive decreases in blood pressure and in respiratory volume and rate, as well as an increase in heart rate. When ventilation is controlled, changes in not only blood pressure and heart rate but also responses to surgical stimulation are the most reliable indices. The pupils are small and responsive to light and are not a useful guide to depth of anesthesia with isoflurane.

Circulation. Systemic arterial blood pressure decreases progressively with increasing depth during anesthesia with isoflurane, as it does with halothane and enflurane. However, in contrast to the latter agents, cardiac output is well maintained with isoflurane, and the hypotension is due to decreased vascular resistance; vasodilatation occurs particularly in skin and muscle (Stevens *et al.,* 1971). While myocardial depression has been demonstrated *in vitro,* this action is not observed with normal concentrations of the anesthetic in intact animals or man. The maintenance of cardiac output and the absence of a negative inotropic effect, together with unaltered coronary blood flow and decreased myocardial oxygen consumption, suggest that isoflurane may have a wider margin of cardiovascular safety than is provided by halothane or enflurane. The cardiac and peripheral vascular effects of isoflurane are abolished by treatment with propranolol, and they are

therefore thought to result in part from stimulation of β-adrenergic receptors.

Cardiac Rhythm. Heart rate is increased with isoflurane, but arrhythmias are not precipitated. Isoflurane does not interfere with atrioventricular conduction and does not sensitize the heart to catecholamines. When epinephrine is utilized for local hemostasis, three times the dose that induces arrhythmias in the presence of halothane is well tolerated with isoflurane (Johnston *et al.,* 1976).

Respiration. Isoflurane depresses respiration progressively as the concentration increases. With a concentration of 1 MAC, the arterial carbon dioxide tension is increased to about the same level as with halothane ($\cong$50 mm Hg), but the ventilatory responses to excess carbon dioxide or to hypoxia are depressed somewhat more than with the other volatile agents (Hirshman *et al.,* 1977). With spontaneous respiration, depression of ventilation is characterized by a reduction in tidal volume with little change in respiratory rate. Respiratory depression is exacerbated by premedication with opioids; assisted or controlled ventilation is generally employed to avoid excessive hypercarbia.

Reductions of pulmonary compliance and functional residual capacity, as well as inhibition of hypoxic pulmonary vasoconstriction, also contribute to the inefficiency of gas exchange that occurs with all of the volatile agents. Isoflurane reduces the tone of constricted bronchi in a manner similar to that of halothane (Hirshman *et al.,* 1982). Until adequate levels of anesthesia are attained, isoflurane may stimulate airway reflexes, resulting in increased secretions, coughing, and laryngospasm. The incidence is greatly reduced by the use of adequate preanesthetic medication and by induction of anesthesia with thiopental or another intravenous agent prior to the administration of isoflurane.

Nervous System. Cerebral blood flow is increased during isoflurane anesthesia, while cerebral metabolism is reduced to an extent that is only slightly less than that with halothane. The cerebral circulation remains responsive to carbon dioxide. Intracranial pressure is increased as a result of cerebral vasodilatation, but this can be controlled by hyperventilation. The EEG reveals progressive changes with increasing depth of anesthesia (Clark and Rosner, 1973). At 1 MAC, slow waves with increased voltage predominate; this declines to burst suppression at 1.5 MAC and electrical silence at 2 MAC. Unlike its isomer, enflurane, convulsive activity is not observed with isoflurane.

Muscle. Isoflurane reduces the response of skeletal muscle to sustained nerve stimulation and enhances the neuromuscular blocking effects of both non-depolarizing and depolarizing muscle relaxants. It is more potent in this regard than halothane, and, for the same depth of anesthesia, only half as much tubocurarine may be required with isoflurane (or enflurane) to achieve satisfactory muscular relaxation. This effect is desirable, because it reduces the requirement for drugs and allows lighter levels of anesthesia. The muscle relaxant activity results from actions on the CNS and neuromuscular junction that are similar to those of enflurane; in addition, the increased muscle blood flow that accompanies anesthesia with isoflurane accelerates delivery and removal of neuromuscular blocking drugs. Uterine muscle is relaxed by isoflurane, as it is by halothane and enflurane, and these agents are not recommended for procedures that depend on adequate uterine contraction to limit blood loss.

Kidney. Depression of renal blood flow, the rate of glomerular filtration, and urinary flow accompanies anesthesia with isoflurane, as with all the volatile anesthetic agents. However, all changes in renal function observed during anesthesia are rapidly reversed during recovery. The quantity of fluoride released by metabolic degradation of isoflurane is small, and renal injury is not observed with single or repeated exposures. This agent is not contraindicated for patients with renal diseases.

Liver and Gastrointestinal Tract. The incidence of nausea and vomiting following isoflurane is similar to that for other haloge-

nated anesthetics and is dependent on other factors, discussed above for halothane.

Blood flow to the liver and gastrointestinal tract is reduced with increasing depth of anesthesia as the systemic arterial pressure decreases. Tests of hepatic function show minimal changes that are reversed with recovery from anesthesia. Hepatic failure has not been reported following the administration of isoflurane. Experience with this agent is still accumulating, but the limited extent to which isoflurane is metabolized encourages confidence that hepatotoxicity will occur less frequently than with halothane and enflurane.

Biotransformation. Only 0.2% of the isoflurane that enters the body is metabolized (Holaday *et al.,* 1975). This is approximately 1% of the amount of halothane that is metabolized and about 10% of the value for its isomer, enflurane. The small quantities of fluoride and trifluoroacetic acid that are generated as degradation products of isoflurane are insufficient to cause cell damage, and this accounts for the lack of renal or hepatic toxicity. Isoflurane does not appear to be a mutagen, teratogen, or carcinogen (Eger *et al.,* 1978).

Evaluation. *Disadvantages and Limitations.* Isoflurane has a more pungent odor than halothane; supplemental intravenous agents are used to overcome this drawback. Anesthesia with isoflurane is associated with progressive respiratory depression and hypotension. Uterine relaxation can be undesirable. At present, the cost of the agent is a principal factor restricting its use.

Advantages. The depth of anesthesia can be rapidly adjusted with isoflurane. Cardiac output is well sustained, and arrhythmias are uncommon; epinephrine can be used in greater amounts for hemostasis than with halothane. Isoflurane potentiates the action of muscle relaxants and reduces the dosage of such drugs that are required. Isoflurane is metabolized to a minimal extent; hepatic and renal toxicity have not been reported.

Status. Isoflurane was introduced in 1981 and has already become widely adopted for surgery requiring general anesthesia, for the reasons detailed above. It is expected that widespread adoption of iso-flurane will be limited only by economic considerations.

METHOXYFLURANE

Chemistry and Physical Properties. *Methoxyflurane* (PENTHRANE) is 2,2-dichloro-1,1-difluoro-ethyl methyl ether (Table 14–2). It is a clear, colorless liquid with a sweet, fruity odor. It is stable in the presence of soda lime and is nonflammable and nonexplosive in air or oxygen in anesthetic concentrations. Physical properties of methoxyflurane and its MAC value are listed in Table 14–1; it is very soluble in rubber (partition coefficient = 635).

PHARMACOLOGICAL PROPERTIES

General Characteristics. Methoxyflurane is the most potent of the inhalational agents. Because of its low vapor pressure at room temperature, the maximal inspired concentration that can be obtained is only 3%. Because of extreme solubility in rubber, as much as 30% of the administered drug may be absorbed by components of an anesthetic circuit, thus reducing the concentration available. Furthermore, the unusually large blood:gas partition coefficient reduces still further the alveolar and hence the arterial tension of the drug early in administration. Nevertheless, since the MAC is only 0.16%, induction of anesthesia with methoxyflurane can be accomplished with inhaled concentrations of 2 to 3%. Induction is slow, requires perhaps 20 to 30 minutes, and is often associated with a stage of excitement. Overdosage is obviously unusual at this stage. For these reasons and because it is desirable to minimize the total dose, methoxyflurane is usually administered after anesthesia has been induced by the intravenous administration of a rapidly acting barbiturate. The inspired concentration of methoxyflurane that is required for maintenance of anesthesia is between 0.2% and 0.8%, and muscle relaxants are used as required. As with all inhalational agents, the administered concentration must be reduced as time passes, to maintain a constant depth of anesthesia. This may be estimated by evaluation of the extent of respiratory and circulatory depression, particularly as reflected in response to surgical stimulation. The extraordinarily great solubility of methoxyflurane in lipid results in its accumulation in fatty tissue. Slow diffusion from these sites accounts for the prolonged and sometimes restless, albeit pain-free, recovery period.

Methoxyflurane is utilized effectively for analgesia during labor. It is administered by the patient to herself with a special inhaler that limits the total dose to 15 ml of liquid methoxyflurane. The inhaled concentration is between 0.1% and 0.6%, and the patient learns to time the intermittent inhalations to anticipate the period when analgesia is desired. The technic has proven to be safe and practical.

Circulation. Cardiovascular depression with methoxyflurane is generally similar to that pro-duced by halothane (Walker *et al.*, 1962). Systemic arterial blood pressure, pulse rate, and cardiac output are decreased progressively with increasing depth of anesthesia. Total peripheral vascular resistance is not changed, and, as with halothane, the primary effect appears to be decreased myocardial contractility (Shimosato and Etsten, 1969). Myocardial consumption of oxygen and coronary blood flow decrease, but there is no evidence of myocardial hypoxia.

Anesthesia with this agent is not accompanied by stimulation of the sympathetic nervous system, and concentrations of circulating catecholamines do not increase (Millar and Morris, 1961). Cardiac arrhythmias are not frequent, but sinus bradycardia is the most common; it is responsive to atropine (Reynolds *et al.*, 1970). If anesthesia is profound, A-V nodal rhythm may occur. If the sympathetic nervous system is activated by hypercarbia or by tracheal or surgical stimulation in the presence of an inadequate depth of anesthesia, ventricular arrhythmias may occasionally appear. The myocardium is sensitized to the action of injected epinephrine, but less so than with halothane. Arrhythmias can be avoided by observation of the same precautions.

Respiration. Ventilatory depression, as measured by the arterial tension of carbon dioxide, the response to increased carbon dioxide, or the response to hypoxia, is proportional to the depth of anesthesia and is similar to that observed with halothane (Larson *et al.*, 1969). When spontaneous respiration is allowed, changes in ventilatory minute volume can be useful as a sign of depth of anesthesia. Methoxyflurane is not irritating to the respiratory tract. Secretions are not stimulated (hence premedication with atropine is not necessary), and bronchoconstriction does not occur (Coon and Kampine, 1975).

Muscle. Relaxation of skeletal muscles can be marked at deeper levels of anesthesia with methoxyflurane. The action appears to be a combination of central and peripheral effects and is additive with the action of the competitive neuromuscular blocking agents (Waud and Waud, 1975). However, the latter drugs are usually used to achieve relaxation of skeletal muscle so that the dose of methoxyflurane can be minimized.

Methoxyflurane does not relax the uterus and in normal doses has little effect on uterine contractions during labor. Its use in obstetrical practice, particularly during the first stage of labor, is thus of value.

Nervous System. As anesthesia is established with methoxyflurane, the fast, low-amplitude pattern that is characteristic of the EEG of the awake subject is progressively replaced by slower waves of greater amplitude. Dilatation of cerebral vessels occurs and results in increased cerebral blood flow and increased intracranial pressure; cerebral consumption of oxygen is decreased (Lassen and Christensen, 1976).

Liver and Gastrointestinal Tract. Depression of hepatic function occurs as it does with other agents and is rapidly reversible. Postoperative hepatic necrosis, probably related to the effects of metabolic products, has been reported (*see* above).

Nausea or vomiting may occur in the postoperative period. The incidence is less than 20% and varies with the surgical procedure, premedication, and other factors.

Kidney. Renal blood flow, glomerular filtration rate, and urine flow are reduced, as they are with halothane. However, in the postoperative period, high-output renal failure may occur under certain circumstances. Crandell and associates (1966) first drew attention to this association, but 5 years passed before the cause-and-effect nature of the relationship was established by Mazze and coworkers (1971). All patients who receive methoxyflurane have concentrations of circulating fluoride as a result of biotransformation of the anesthetic. When the administration of methoxyflurane exceeds the *equivalent* of a dose of 1 MAC for more than 2 hours, the concentration of fluoride in plasma may exceed 40 μM, and direct damage to the renal tubules occurs. The toxic syndrome is characterized by an inability to concentrate the urine, even in response to vasopressin (Cousins and Mazze, 1973). The resulting polyuria may result in dehydration, hypernatremia, and azotemia. In those who survive, recovery of renal function is usual, but it may take a year; mortality rates in such patients have been reported to be as high as 20%.

It is this complication that has curtailed the use of methoxyflurane. To avoid renal toxicity, the dose and duration must be limited. Justification of its use for analgesia in labor is based on intermittent administration of the agent immediately preceding each uterine contraction.

Biotransformation. Methoxyflurane is metabolized to a greater extent than any other inhalational agent (Sakai and Takaori, 1978). As much as 50 to 70% of the absorbed dose is metabolized in the liver to free fluoride, oxalic acid, difluoromethoxy-acetic acid, and dichloroacetic acid. The first two substances, particularly fluoride, cause renal damage.

Two characteristics of methoxyflurane are responsible for this occurrence. The molecule, despite the ether bond, is more susceptible to metabolism than are the other halogenated methyl ethyl ethers. Probably of greater importance is the great propensity of methoxyflurane to diffuse into fatty tissues. The drug is released slowly from this reservoir and becomes available for biotransformation for many days. The peak concentration of free fluoride in the plasma is found on the second to fourth postanesthetic day. There is considerable variation in the concentration of fluoride that is achieved. It is greater in obese subjects, in the elderly, and after induction of hepatic microsomal enzymes by drugs such as phenobarbital.

Evaluation. *Disadvantages and Limitations.* The potential renal toxicity of this agent dictates that it should not be used to achieve profound anesthesia nor for prolonged periods of time. Contraindications to its use include the presence of renal disease or the concomitant administration of drugs that induce hepatic enzymes or that are nephrotoxic. Respiratory and circulatory depression can be profound. Induction, maintenance, and adjustment of the depth of anesthesia are slow compared to halothane or enflurane.

Advantages and Uses. This agent was quite widely used for all types of anesthesia following its introduction into clinical practice in 1960. It is nonflammable, and it provides profound analgesia and good relaxation of skeletal muscles. Uterine contractions are not inhibited. Postoperative nausea and vomiting are not troublesome.

Status. As a result of its renal toxicity, the use of methoxyflurane as a general anesthetic is limited. It is valued mainly for its analgesic potency during labor, where small doses administered discontinuously do not result in sufficient accumulation of methoxyflurane or its metabolites to produce observable renal toxicity.

NITROUS OXIDE

Chemistry and Physical Properties. *Nitrous oxide* (dinitrogen monoxide; N_2O) is a colorless gas without appreciable odor or taste. It is the only inorganic gas that is practical for clinical anesthesia. It is marketed in steel cylinders as a colorless liquid under pressure and in equilibrium with its gas phase. As it is released from the cylinder, some of the liquid nitrous oxide returns to the gaseous state; the pressure in the tank thus remains nearly constant until all the liquid has evaporated. The heat required for its vaporization is obtained from the walls of the cylinder and surrounding air, with the result that the tank becomes cold. Nitrous oxide is heavier than air. Although nitrous oxide is not flammable, it supports combustion as actively as does oxygen when it is present in proper concentration with a flammable anesthetic. Fatal explosions have occurred with ether–nitrous oxide mixtures.

Nitrous oxide has relatively low solubility in blood, the blood:gas partition ratio at 37° C being 0.47. Other properties are listed in Table 14–1.

PHARMACOLOGICAL PROPERTIES

General Characteristics. Since Colton administered nitrous oxide in 1844, it has passed through periods of greater or lesser popularity. It is currently used as an adjuvant during most procedures in which general anesthesia is employed.

Nitrous oxide can cause surgical anesthesia predictably only when administered under hyperbaric conditions. Paul Bert demonstrated this in 1879 by the use of 85% nitrous oxide in oxygen at 1.2 atmospheres in a pressure chamber. The MAC value is 105%, but there is considerable variability among individuals. Analgesia equivalent to that produced by morphine follows the inspiration of 20% nitrous oxide; some patients lose consciousness when breathing 30% nitrous oxide in oxygen, and most will become unconscious with 80%.

Nitrous oxide has been used as the sole anesthetic agent at inspired concentrations up to 80% and even beyond. In this situation the danger of hypoxia is obvious. The avoidance of hypoxic organ damage and the maintenance of satisfactory anesthesia for any but the briefest of procedures require maneuvering between very narrow limits, and this should no longer be attempted.

Another technic for the administration of nitrous oxide that has enjoyed considerable success includes induction of sleep by the intravenous administration of thiopental, accomplishment of skeletal muscle relaxation with neuromuscular blocking agents, and hyperventilation to reduce the arterial tension of carbon dioxide to approximately 25 mm Hg. It has been suggested that the total muscle paralysis and the absence of respiratory drive augment the analgesia provided by nitrous oxide. Conditions for surgery are excellent, organ functions are depressed minimally, and recovery is rapid. However, there have been several reports of recall by patients of events that occurred during this type of "anesthesia." The subjects are immobilized and unable to communicate and their unconsciousness cannot be assured without appropriate supplementation with potent inhalational agents or intravenous drugs such as morphine.

The value of nitrous oxide is as an adjuvant. In the presence of 70% nitrous oxide in oxygen, the concentration of potent inhalational agents can be reduced. Reductions of MAC values in these circumstances are from 0.75% to 0.29% for halothane, from 1.68% to 0.6% for enflurane, and from 1.15% to 0.5% for isoflurane. Smaller doses of the halogenated agents, combined with some nitrous oxide, result in less respiratory and circulatory depression and more rapid recovery.

The uptake and distribution of nitrous oxide are influenced in relatively unique ways by its physical properties (Eger, 1974). A normal adult breathing 70% nitrous oxide will achieve 90% equilibration in about 15 minutes. During this time, approximately 10 liters of nitrous oxide will have been absorbed from the alveolar gas into the body. This volume change is more than ten times that which occurs during the inhalation of 1% halothane. This large uptake of gas has two effects, called the second-gas effect and the concentration effect (see Chapter 13). As nitrous oxide is removed from the alveoli, some additional fresh gas must flow in from the airways; this augments the ventilatory volume and increases the delivery of all the gases to the alveoli. This is the second-gas effect. At the same time, the flow of nitrous oxide into the blood stream reduces somewhat the total gas volume, so that the remaining gases are concentrated; this is the concentration effect. Clinically, the second-gas and concentration effects are useful during induction of anesthesia, since they increase the rapidity of uptake of a potent inhalational agent and also increase the alveolar concentration of oxygen, thus minimizing hypoxia. The reverse process occurs when the administration of nitrous oxide is discontinued (see Chapter 13). If air is abruptly substituted, the exchange of nitrous oxide from tissue and blood to alveolar gas results in a transient substantial decrease in the alveolar tension and, hence, the arterial tension of oxygen. This has been labeled *diffusional hypoxia* and can be a cause of postoperative hypoxemia, particularly when there also is respiratory depression following prolonged hyperventilation. Diffusional hypoxia has a limited time span, and adverse effects can be avoided by the administration of supplemental oxygen during the early recovery period.

Nitrous oxide exchanges with nitrogen whenever a nitrous oxide–containing mixture of gases is administered to a patient who had previously been breathing air. Since the blood:gas partition coefficient for nitrous oxide is 34 times that for nitrogen, a great deal more nitrous oxide is available for exchange. As a result, when nitrous oxide is administered, pockets of trapped gas in the body will expand as nitrogen leaves and is replaced by larger amounts of nitrous oxide (see Chapter 13). Such pockets may be found in an occluded middle ear, a pneumothorax, loops of intestine, lung, or renal cysts. Even air within the skull following a pneumoencephalogram is subject to expansion. This can result in large increases in pressure and volume, and nitrous oxide is thus best avoided in these circumstances.

Circulation. Nitrous oxide is generally employed as only one of several agents for general anesthesia. The potent inhalational agents have such marked effects on the cardiovascular system that the subtle influence of nitrous oxide may be easily overlooked.

When nitrous oxide is added to halothane in combined concentrations that do not alter the depth of anesthesia, the pupils dilate and the concentration of circulating norepinephrine increases. Under these conditions, arterial blood pressure, total peripheral vascular resistance, and cardiac output all rise (Hornbein *et al.*, 1969; Smith *et al.*, 1970). Nitrous oxide depresses myocardial contractility *in vitro* but increases the responsiveness of vascular smooth muscle to epinephrine. The net effect of supplementation of halothane with nitrous oxide is a substantial reduction in the amount of halothane required to maintain anesthesia and, thus, less hypotension.

Supplementation of enflurane anesthesia with 70% nitrous oxide results in reduction of the concentration of enflurane that is required and in similar, but less marked, activation of the sympathetic nervous system (Smith *et al.*, 1978). Similarly, when nitrous oxide is administered with isoflurane, respiratory depression and systemic hypotension are less than with the same depth of anesthesia achieved with isoflurane alone. When combined with narcotics, nitrous oxide causes only further circulatory depression.

Respiration. The effects of nitrous oxide on ventilatory drive are generally small. Slight or no depression of the response to carbon dioxide has been reported with 50% nitrous oxide; however, when nitrous oxide is added to other anesthetic agents, further depression is unequivocal (Hornbein *et al.*, 1969). The response to hypoxia is reduced when 50% nitrous oxide is given alone (Yacoub *et al.*, 1976).

The relatively nonspecific changes in respiratory function that may result in an increased difference between alveolar and arterial oxygen tension during general anesthesia reemphasize the importance of augmentation of the tension of inspired oxygen. A concentration of not less than 30%

oxygen is wise, and, therefore, not more than 70% nitrous oxide should be employed.

Effects on Other Organs. Nitrous oxide does not exert toxic effects on the CNS. Cerebral blood flow remains responsive to carbon dioxide, and autoregulation continues as perfusion pressure changes in the presence of 70% nitrous oxide (Wollman *et al.*, 1965).

Skeletal muscle does not relax in the presence of 80% nitrous oxide, and blood flow to muscle does not change. Unlike the halogenated general anesthetics, nitrous oxide is most unlikely to contribute to the production of malignant hyperpyrexia.

The liver, kidneys, and gastrointestinal tract show no marked effects of nitrous oxide, and there is no evidence of toxicity. Nausea or vomiting occurs postoperatively in approximately 15% of patients.

Following very prolonged administration of nitrous oxide, there is evidence of interference with production of both leukocytes and red blood cells by bone marrow (Lassen *et al.*, 1956). These effects do not occur within the time frame of clinical surgery (Amess *et al.*, 1978). Nitrous oxide can oxidize the cobalt atom in vitamin B_{12} and thereby cause megaloblastic changes in the bone marrow and a neuropathy in experimental animals (*see* Chapter 57). While long-term inhalation of nitrous oxide has been utilized to treat pain and discomfort, its value is limited. Of more practical concern is the effect of long-term, low-dose exposure of operating room personnel to the gas. As with halothane, there is little definitive evidence of adverse effects, although mild CNS depression is detectable at a concentration of 500 ppm. However, with simple procedures to prevent contamination, the atmosphere of an operating room should not contain more than 50 ppm of nitrous oxide. A neuropathy similar to that of vitamin B_{12} deficiency has been observed in dentists who use nitrous oxide as an anesthetic (Layzer, 1978).

Biotransformation. Nitrous oxide is rapidly and predominantly eliminated as such in the expired gas, and a little diffuses out through the skin. Sufficiently precise methods have not been utilized to determine to what extent biotransformation may occur.

Evaluation. *Disadvantages.* Nitrous oxide is a weak agent with no muscle relaxant activity, and attempts to provide adequate anesthesia may be accompanied by hypoxia if it is used alone. Transient postanesthetic hypoxia may also occur as large volumes of nitrous oxide are exhaled. Air pockets in closed spaces may expand in the abdomen, chest, and skull.

Advantages. Nitrous oxide is a nonflammable, nonirritating, and powerful analgesic agent; there is very rapid onset of and recovery from its effects, and it causes little or no toxicity during ordinary clinical use. Its principal application is as a supplement to other specific and/or potent agents, and this results in the use of smaller doses of the latter, shorter recovery time, and reduced likelihood of complications.

Status. As a sole agent, nitrous oxide is used intermittently to provide analgesia for dental procedures and during the first stage of parturition. In combination with other drugs, nitrous oxide is given to the majority of patients who require general anesthesia.

OBSOLETE ANESTHETIC AGENTS

Diethyl ether (ether), *ethyl chloride, vinyl ether, fluroxene, cyclopropane,* and *ethylene* are chemically and physically dissimilar, but they have in common one property that renders them essentially obsolete. They are all flammable and/or explosive at concentrations necessary for anesthesia, particularly in oxygen-enriched mixtures. They have no advantages that offset this property and, in fact, have other disadvantages that also render them less desirable than the newer agents. Further information on these drugs can be found in the *fifth* and *previous editions* of this textbook. Trichloroethylene and chloroform are older and now less useful halogenated compounds. They were popular in the past but are no longer used. Chloroform is hepatotoxic and nephrotoxic.

II. Intravenous Anesthetics

The requirements for general anesthesia and surgery may necessitate the administration of several intravenous drugs with different actions to ensure hypnosis, analgesia, relaxation, and control of visceral reflex responses. The use of intravenous drugs thus adds flexibility and permits the administration of lower doses of inhalational agents. Intravenous drugs are also frequently used to induce anesthesia rapidly.

In this section the special properties of barbiturates, benzodiazepines, opioids, and other agents that have utility in surgical procedures will be discussed. More detailed discussions of each class of drug and their uses in other circumstances are presented elsewhere (*see* Index).

BARBITURATES

Barbiturates with a duration of action appropriate to the requirements of surgery became available with the introduction of thiopental by Lundy in 1935. Its use during general anesthesia continues greatly to exceed that of any other barbiturate.

Chemistry and Preparations. *Thiopental* is supplied for clinical use as the water-soluble sodium salt, *thiopental sodium for injection* (PENTOTHAL). When thiopental sodium is diluted in sterile water, a 3.4% solution is isotonic; concentrations less than 2% may cause hemolysis. Other ultrashort-acting barbiturates include *methohexital* (BREVITAL SODIUM) and *thiamylal* (SURITAL).

PHARMACOLOGICAL PROPERTIES

Pharmacokinetics. Following a single intravenous anesthetic dose of thiopental sodium, unconsciousness occurs after 10 to 20 seconds (the time required for the drug to circulate from the arm to the brain). The depth of anesthesia may increase for up to 40 seconds and then decreases progressively until consciousness returns in 20 to 30 minutes. This sequence reflects the changes in concentration of thiopental at its sites of action in the brain and is a consequence of the initial distribution of the drug to the brain, followed by its subsequent redistribution to other tissues (plasma half-life is 3 minutes). This is discussed fully in Chapters 1 and 17. At the time of awakening, the plasma concentration may be 10% of the peak value. When all tissues contain sufficient quantities of thiopental, redistribution does not result in such a precipitous drop of the concentrations in plasma, and the duration of action is prolonged. Thus, when too great a total quantity of thiopental is administered, recovery may require many hours (elimination half-time is 9 hours).

Thiopental is metabolized slowly in the liver, and this is not a very significant factor in limiting the duration of anesthesia except after excessive dosage. For methohexital, metabolic degradation may be of somewhat greater importance (Breimer, 1977). Other factors, such as the binding of thiopental by plasma proteins, change in the nonionized fraction of the drug following changes in blood pH, or changes in the distribution of blood flow, may also influence the depth of anesthesia, time of recovery, and duration of action.

General Anesthetic Action. The effects of barbiturates on the CNS are discussed in Chapter 17. The signs of anesthesia are not particularly characteristic; pupils are of small or normal size, eyeballs are fixed and usually central, eyelash and tendon reflexes are diminished, and respiration and circulation are somewhat depressed. However, thiopental and other barbiturates are poor analgesics and may even increase the sensitivity to pain when administered in inadequate amounts (Dundee, 1960). In these circumstances, evidence of sympathetic response becomes manifest with tachycardia, dilated pupils, tears, sweating, tachypnea, increased blood pressure, and movement or vocalization in response to surgery.

Respiration. Unlike some of the inhalational anesthetics, thiopental is not irritating to the respiratory tract, and yet coughing, laryngospasm, and even bronchospasm occur with some frequency. The basis of these reactions is unknown; they disappear as a deeper phase of anesthesia is established. The presence of saliva, the insertion of an airway, or partial obstruction by soft tissues may trigger one or all of these responses. Moderate doses of thiopental do not depress these airway reflexes.

Thiopental produces a dose-related depression of respiration that can be profound. Both the response to carbon dioxide and the response to hypoxia are reduced or even abolished (Hirshman *et al.*, 1975).

Following a dose of thiopental sufficient to cause sleep, tidal volume is decreased, and, despite a small increase of respiratory rate, the minute volume is reduced; the arterial tension of carbon dioxide rises slightly. Larger doses of thiopental cause more profound changes, and respiration is maintained only by movements of the diaphragm. Surgical manipulations provide a stimulus to respiration and, within limits, can offset the respiratory depression.

Circulation. *In vivo,* following the administration of an anesthetic dose of thiopental to a normal adult, the arterial blood pressure decreases only *transiently* and then returns essentially to normal. Cardiac output is usually decreased somewhat, but total peripheral vascular resistance is unchanged or increased. Blood flow to the skin and brain is decreased, but that to other organs remains essentially normal.

However, in the presence of hemorrhage or other form of hypovolemia, circulatory instability, sepsis, toxemia, or shock, the administration of a "normal" dose of thiopental may result in hypotension, circulatory collapse, and cardiac arrest. In such patients, thiopental or any other general anesthetic agent should be used very cautiously.

The baroreceptor system appears unaffected, but there is a reduction of sympathetic nerve activity. Concentrations of catecholamines in plasma are not increased, and the heart is not sensitized to epinephrine. Arrhythmias are uncommon except in the presence of hypercarbia or arterial hypoxemia.

Cerebral blood flow and cerebral metabolic rate are reduced with thiopental and other barbiturates. There is a marked reduction of intracranial pressure, and this effect is utilized clinically in anesthesia for neurosurgery or in other circumstances when elevated intracranial pressures are expected (Shapiro, 1975).

Other Organs. Relaxation of skeletal muscle is transient and occurs only at the onset of anesthesia. Thiopental has little effect on uterine contractions, but it does cross the placenta and depresses the fetus. The functions of liver and kidney are depressed only with large doses, and then only transiently.

Clinical Use. Thiopental sodium is administered intravenously. It may be injected either as a single bolus, intermittently, or as a continuous infusion. The use of a continuous infusion increases the likelihood of overdosage, with a subsequent prolonged recovery period. For single or intermittent injections of thiopental sodium, the concentration employed should not exceed 2.5% in aqueous solution. Injections are most safely made into the side port of a flowing intravenous infusion of saline solution or 5% dextrose in water.

If concentrations greater than 2.5% are injected extravascularly, the pain may be severe and tissue necrosis can occur. Of even greater concern are the results of inadvertent intra-arterial injection of concentrated solutions of thiopental. The arterial endothelium and deeper layers are immediately damaged and endarteritis follows, often with thrombosis exacerbated by arteriolar spasm as norepinephrine is released (Brown *et al.*, 1968). Vascular ischemia and even gangrene may result. Because damage to the arterial wall is instantaneous, the aim of treatment is to reduce the response and hence limit the lesion. If the infusion needle is still *in situ*, 5 to 10 ml of 1% procaine may serve to reduce the pain and the arteriospasm. Heparin may inhibit thrombosis, and a regional block of the sympathetic nerves may also induce arterial dilatation. Permanent and serious sequelae have not been reported to follow intra-arterial injection of 2.5% solutions of thiopental and do not occur with 1% solutions of methohexital.

For induction of anesthesia in an adult patient, the usual procedure is to inject a 50-mg test dose moderately rapidly, observe the response, and then inject an additional 100 to 200 mg over 20 seconds. In a muscular, robust individual, as much as 500 mg may occasionally be necessary to induce general anesthesia. If the dose is injected too slowly, a stage of excitement may be encountered. Such excitatory movements are more common with methohexital. Conversely, if too much drug is injected too rapidly, profound anesthesia may supervene with apnea and hypotension. The usual response after a correctly chosen dose is for the patient to experience a faint taste of garlic, followed by a suppressed yawn and then the smooth, rapid appearance of sleep. There is an initial and transient period of relaxation, which may be appropriate for very short procedures such as correction of a dislocation, and the airway may become impaired by the infolding of soft tissues around the tongue and pharynx.

After this point the drugs to be used for maintenance of anesthesia can be administered. Most commonly, these will be an inhalational agent with or without nitrous oxide, opioid analgesics, or muscle relaxants. For short procedures that are not especially painful, intermittent doses of thiopental combined with nitrous oxide are satisfactory, particularly if an analgesic was given preoperatively. A total dose of 1 g of thiopental should not generally be exceeded if prolonged recovery is to be avoided. The larger the initial dose of thiopental that is required, the larger the supplementary doses must be, even in patients of the same size. Patients who require a large initial dose of thiopental will awaken despite plasma concentrations that would normally cause sleep. This phenomenon is termed *acute tolerance,* and, while its nature is obscure, it is important in its effects on total drug dosage.

Recovery following thiopental should be characterized by smooth, rapid awakening to consciousness. However, if there is postoperative pain, restlessness may become evident and analgesics should be given (an antianalgesic effect of thiopental at low circulating concentrations may be partially responsible). There is often shivering postoperatively as heat is generated to restore body temperature that has decreased during anesthesia and surgery. Postural hypotension may be encountered, and patients should not be moved too hurriedly.

Evaluation. *Disadvantages.* Most of the complications associated with the use of thiopental are minor and can be avoided or minimized by judicious use of the drug. Extravenous or intra-arterial injection should be uncommon and, if concentrations no greater than 2.5% are used, are unlikely to cause serious damage. Cough, laryngospasm, and bronchospasm can be serious in certain patients, such as those with elevated intracranial pressure, pharyngeal infections, unstable aneurysms, or asthma. In each such case, adequate anesthesia should be ensured prior to stimulation of the airway.

Overdosage can occur if the specific requirements for each patient are not estimated correctly. There is no effective agent to antagonize the actions of the barbiturates. Hexobarbital and methohexital both cause a higher incidence of motor movements during induction of anesthesia.

The presence of *variegate porphyria* (South African) or *acute intermittent porphyria* constitutes an absolute contraindication to the use of barbiturates. In these two forms of porphyria, thiopental or other barbiturates may precipitate a widespread demyelination of peripheral and cranial nerves and disseminated lesions throughout the CNS, resulting in pain, weakness, and paralysis that may be life threatening (Dean, 1971). Other types of porphyria do not contraindicate the use of barbiturates; this has been a point of confusion.

Advantages. The outstanding advantages of thiopental are rapid, pleasant induction of anesthesia and fast recovery therefrom, with little postanesthetic excitement or vomiting. The use of methohexital is associated with even more rapid recovery of consciousness. These drugs may be given to induce anesthesia prior to administration of another agent, or they can be used alone to provide anesthesia for short procedures that are associated with little pain. They are useful to promote light sleep during regional local anesthesia and for quieting excitement or controlling convulsions.

Status. The ultrashort-acting barbiturates have an important place in the practice of anesthesiology. Thiopental sodium remains the standard for comparison. Thiamylal is very similar; methohexital is more potent and has a somewhat shorter duration of effect. General anesthesia is most often initiated by an injection of thiopental to induce sleep prior to administration of the agents that are necessary for the surgical procedure.

BENZODIAZEPINES

Benzodiazepines were first introduced for the treatment of anxiety, and a large number of these compounds with sedative, antianxiety, anticonvulsant, and muscle relaxant properties have now been synthesized (*see* Chapters 17, 19, 20, and 21). Hypnosis and unconsciousness may be produced with large doses of benzodiazepines, and *diazepam* and *lorazepam* have become widely used for preanesthetic medication and to supplement or to induce and maintain anesthesia. A new benzodiazepine, *midazolam,* may become employed even more frequently in the future.

Preparations. *Diazepam* (VALIUM) is insoluble in water and is supplied for injection in a solution of 5 mg of diazepam per milliliter of organic solvents; it should not be diluted. The solution is injected intravenously into the side port of a running intravenous infusion to minimize a burning sensation on injection and the possibility of venous thrombosis. *Lorazepam* (ATIVAN) is supplied at a concentration of 2 or 4 mg/ml of organic solvent for injection. Lorazepam is somewhat less irritating than diazepam, but the same precautions should be observed during injection. Its onset of action is slower, but lorazepam is about three times more potent than diazepam. Otherwise, their pharmacological properties are similar.

PHARMACOLOGICAL PROPERTIES

Diazepam is discussed as the prototype, and the properties of lorazepam and midazolam are compared where appropriate.

Pharmacokinetics. Following an intravenous injection of 0.1 to 1 mg/kg of diazepam, the drug is rapidly distributed to the brain but, unlike thiopental, there is a delay of up to several minutes before the onset of drowsiness. The concentration in plasma declines rapidly due to redistribution, with an initial half-time of 10 to 15 minutes; however, there is often a return of drowsiness with an increased concentration of diazepam in plasma after 6 to 8 hours. This is probably due to absorption from the gastrointestinal tract after excretion in the bile. The onset of drowsiness is slightly less rapid after administration of lorazepam and is slightly more rapid with midazolam. Additional information is given in Chapter 17 and Appendix II.

General Anesthetic Action. *Central Nervous System.* The effects of the benzodiazepines on the CNS are described in detail in Chapters 17, 19, 20, and 21. In the doses used to supplement or induce anesthesia, these drugs cause amnesia in 50% or more of patients. The amnesia may last for up to 6 hours and is characteristically antegrade, with little or no retrograde effect. CNS depression induced by benzodiazepines is partially antagonized by physostigmine (2 mg intravenously), probably due to inhibition of acetylcholinesterase. If physostigmine is used for this purpose, atropine (1 mg intravenously) should be given to prevent excessive salivation, abdominal cramps, nausea, and vomiting. If the dose of diazepam is very large, the CNS depression may return as physostigmine is eliminated. The intravenous administration of aminophylline (1 to 2 mg/kg) can also accelerate recovery from the CNS depressant effects of diazepam (Arvidsson *et al.,* 1982).

Circulation and Respiration. By themselves, the benzodiazepines cause only moderate depression of the circulation and respiration. Large doses may cause a 15 to 20% decline in systemic blood pressure and vascular resistance. Changes in heart rate vary from a mild decrease to a moderate increase. If tachycardia occurs, it may compensate for a small decrease in stroke volume and thus limit the modest tendency toward reduction in cardiac output. Stability of the cardiovascular system has encouraged the use of these drugs for anesthesia in patients with cardiac impairment (particularly for diagnostic procedures) (Samuelson *et al.,* 1981). Benzodiazepines are not analgesics, and it is necessary to combine several drugs to achieve surgical levels of anesthesia with a balance of sedation, analgesia, amnesia, relaxation, and freedom from reflex stimulation. When opioids are given concurrently with benzodiazepines, the combination may produce severe cardiovascular depression, probably as a result of a sympatholytic action. The same considerations apply to the respiratory effects of benzodiazepines, which are minimal by themselves but, in combination with opioids, may result in severe and prolonged depression of the respiratory response to hypoxia and to carbon dioxide (Forster *et al.*, 1980; Gross *et al.*, 1983). Transient apnea may follow the rapid injection of diazepam, and facilities for the support of respiration should always be available.

Other Organs. Diazepam neither causes emesis nor prevents it and has little effect on renal, hepatic, or reproductive functions. While the drug induces relaxation of spastic muscle, which is centrally mediated, it has no effect on the neuromuscular junction and does not enhance or antagonize the actions of specific muscle relaxants. Diazepam crosses the placenta readily and can depress the fetus.

Use in Anesthesia. Diazepam (5 to 10 mg) may be administered orally, intramuscularly, or intravenously for preanesthetic medication about an hour before the patient is transported to the operating area. Benzodiazepines are useful as the sole agent for procedures that do not require analgesia, such as bronchoscopy, cardioversion, cardiac catheterization, and a spectrum of radiodiagnostic procedures. For induction of anesthesia, the benzodiazepines are given intravenously. However, it is important that the injection be given slowly and that the rate of administration not be so rapid that an excessive dose is given during the period of delayed onset of action. A total dose of 0.6 mg/kg of diazepam administered to an adult will usually result in a sequence of drowsiness, amnesia, and, finally, unconsciousness. Induction with lorazepam is similar but requires approximately one half the dose necessary for diazepam. A special application for these drugs is the control and prevention of seizures induced by local anesthetics during regional technics. Benzodiazepines are also frequently employed as part of a technic of balanced anesthesia, combined with thiopental for rapid induction, muscle relaxants, analgesics, and, often, an inhalational anesthetic agent. Such a technic has the advantage of requiring a reduced dose of each drug while providing rapid and more precise control of side effects.

Status. The benzodiazepines have achieved a useful place for their contribution to preanesthetic medication and to induction and maintenance of anesthesia. *Midazolam* is a new benzodiazepine. It is soluble in water, and its injection is neither painful nor irritating. Furthermore, the onset of action of midazolam is shorter, its potency is greater, and its elimination is more rapid than the other drugs discussed above. Midazolam may thus be used extensively in the future.

ETOMIDATE

Etomidate is a potent hypnotic agent without analgesic properties. It has recently become available for use and is supplied for injection in a solution containing 2 mg/ml (AMIDATE).

An intravenous injection of 0.3 mg/kg of etomidate to an adult patient will induce sleep that lasts for approximately 5 minutes. Cardiovascular and respiratory depression do not usually occur, although hypotension and carbon dioxide retention can happen occasionally. Involuntary muscle movements are a frequent occurrence and necessitate the administration of other drugs, such as diazepam. The induction of anesthesia with etomidate is usually followed by the administration of analgesic and muscle relaxant drugs and/or potent inhalational anesthetic agents. Nausea and vomiting are common during the recovery period, particularly when opioids have been used. The use of etomidate to produce prolonged sedation can inhibit adrenal steroidogenesis in some patients; low concentrations of cortisol in plasma and increased mortality have been observed (Wagner *et al.*, 1984).

OPIOID ANALGESICS

The detailed pharmacology of the opioids is discussed in Chapter 22. Morphine, meperidine, fentanyl, or other analgesics are frequently employed as supplements during general anesthesia with inhalational or intravenous agents (Kitahata and Collins, 1982). For this purpose, intravenous doses of 1 to 2 mg of morphine, 10 to 25 mg of meperidine, and 0.05 to 0.1 mg of fentanyl are approximately equivalent and may provide analgesia for about 90, 45, and 30 minutes, respectively. Respiratory depression, mild decreases in blood pressure, some delay in awakening, and an appreciable incidence of postoperative nausea or vomiting accompany the use of these drugs.

In some situations, very large doses of morphine may be infused to obtain anesthesia. Morphine given slowly intravenously in doses of 1 to 3 mg/kg over 15 to 20 minutes induces analgesia and unconsciousness. Respiratory depression is severe, and ventilation must be mechanically controlled, often for extended periods of time. The addition of nitrous oxide adds further to the anesthesia, and administration of competitive skeletal muscle relaxants provides good conditions for surgery. It is perhaps unexpected that the cardiovascular system is not severely depressed with such large doses of morphine. Lowenstein and associates (1969) showed that patients with normal cardiac function experienced no significant changes, while an increase in cardiac output and stroke volume and a decrease in total peripheral resistance often occur in those with cardiac disease. Blood flow to organs is maintained. For example, autoregulation of the cerebral circulation is unimpaired even at the higher dose range (3 mg/kg); similarly, renal function is well maintained.

The morphine–nitrous oxide technic has been utilized quite widely for cardiac surgery. Despite the large doses of morphine, some patients are evidently not sufficiently anesthetized and may become hypertensive during surgery; postoperative recall of events as a terrifying dream or psychosis may also occur.

When large doses of fentanyl (50 to 100 μg/kg) are administered slowly intravenously, profound analgesia and unconsciousness are induced. While this state is similar to that caused by morphine, the incidence of incomplete amnesia, hypotension, and hypertension is less than that associated with morphine; the duration of respiratory depression is also shorter (Kitahata and Collins, 1982). For these reasons, fentanyl has largely replaced morphine for anesthesia, and it is utilized particularly during cardiac surgery, usually combined with muscle relaxants and nitrous oxide or small doses of other inhalational anesthetics. Rigidity of respiratory muscles may be prominent during induction of anesthesia with large doses of morphine or fentanyl, and administration of a muscle relaxant may be necessary to permit artificial ventilation.

Following intravenous administration of fentanyl, the onset of action is within one circulation time. The drug is rapidly redistributed, and the duration of action is approximately 30 minutes. However, accumulation of fentanyl occurs with repeated administration or following injection of large doses, leading to a prolonged duration of sedation and respiratory depression. Fentanyl is metabolized by the liver and is eliminated with a half-life of 3.5 hours.

Alfentanil and *sufentanil* are newer and more potent opioid analgesics. Alfentanil has approximately one fourth the potency of fentanyl, and its duration of action is shorter by two thirds. Sufentanil (SUFENTA) has a potency about ten times that of fentanyl, and its duration of action is about one half as long, even after administration of large doses. Both of these drugs can induce profound analgesia and, in sufficient doses, anesthesia; cardiovascular stability is impressive.

Status. Opioid analgesics are widely used to provide relief from pain during general anesthesia of all types. Judicious use of these agents intravenously can provide analgesia of rapid onset and appropriate duration; smaller doses of general anesthetics are then required. When large or repeated doses of opioids are administered for general anesthesia, sedation and respiratory depression can be prolonged and mechanical ventilation may be necessary. These effects can be reversed by the use of specific opioid antagonists (*see* Chapter 22). Small doses (increments of 0.02 to 0.05 mg) of naloxone may be repeated until the desired reversal is achieved; careful titration will prevent precipitous awakening and return of discomfort. The duration of action of naloxone is 60 to 90 minutes, and the patient must remain under close observation for recurrence of respiratory depression. Naltrexone and certain investigational opioid antagonists have a longer duration of action. Some practitioners prefer to employ the mixed opioid agonist-antagonists, nalbuphine or butorphanol, for anesthetic uses.

NEUROLEPTIC-OPIOID COMBINATIONS

Neuroleptic compounds, such as the butyrophenone derivative *droperidol* (INAPSINE), produce a state of quiescence with reduced motor activity, reduced anxiety, and indifference to the surroundings. Sleep is not necessarily induced, and patients are responsive to commands. In addition to inducing neurolepsis, droperidol has adrenergic blocking, antiemetic, antifibrillatory, and anticonvulsant actions, and it enhances the effects of other CNS depressants.

When a potent opioid analgesic such as fentanyl citrate is combined with droperidol, a state of neurolept analgesia is established, during which a variety of diagnostic or minor surgical procedures can be accomplished; these include bronchoscopy, radiological studies, burn dressings, cystoscopy, and the like. Neurolept analgesia can be converted to neurolept anesthesia by the concurrent administration of 65% nitrous oxide in oxygen.

Clinical Use. Droperidol and fentanyl citrate may be used alone or together, the dose of each being adjusted individually, but most often a precompounded mixture (INNOVAR) is used. Each milliliter of this preparation contains 0.05 mg of fentanyl citrate and 2.5 mg of droperidol.

A useful technic for adults is to mix a dose of 0.1 ml/kg of INNOVAR in 250 ml of 5% dextrose in water and to infuse this solution intravenously over a period of 5 to 10 minutes. If the rate of infusion is too slow, delirium and excitement may occur, sometimes with laryngospasm. If the rate is too rapid, spasm of the chest wall may supervene, and respiratory exchange can become impossible, even by artificial means. This untoward response is easily managed by the intravenous administration of a rapidly acting neuromuscular blocking agent, such as succinylcholine. Normally, after approximately 3 to 4 minutes, the recipient appears to fall asleep and may cease to breathe, except on command. Should an endotracheal tube be required to ensure adequate ventilation, a smaller dose of the combination will suffice if the larynx and trachea are anesthetized by the topical application of a local anesthetic.

Circulatory effects of neurolept anesthesia are not generally marked. Droperidol has a slight α-adrenergic blocking action that results in moderate hypotension. A parasympathomimetic effect of fentanyl accounts for bradycardia; administration of atropine will prevent this. Cerebral blood flow and cerebral metabolism are not altered in human subjects, and there may be reduction of elevated intracranial pressure, provided that the arterial tension of carbon dioxide does not increase when respiration is depressed. Care should be taken to avoid abrupt changes in posture, since severe hypotension may be precipitated. Other than bradycardia, cardiac arrhythmias are rare, and the heart is not sensitized to the effects of epinephrine.

In contrast to the circulatory effects, respiratory depression is marked (Dunbar *et al.*, 1967). Assisted or controlled ventilation is necessary, and respiration of an oxygen-enriched gas mixture is desirable.

Droperidol has a prolonged duration of action (3 to 6 hours), whereas fentanyl exerts its analgesic effect for only about 30 minutes. Following induction of neurolept anesthesia, supplementary doses of fentanyl alone (1 μg/kg) are injected at intervals of approximately 20 minutes. Indications for additional doses include evidence of sympathetic activity with increasing pulse rate and blood pressure, sweating, and limb movements.

Recovery. Consciousness is recovered rapidly after the administration of nitrous oxide is stopped, but patients remain free of pain and drowsy, although arousable. Nausea or vomiting occurs in 5 to 10% of patients; confusion and a depressed mental state may become apparent.

Respiratory depression may persist into the postoperative period and can last for 3 to 4 hours (Harper *et al.*, 1976). The opioid antagonist naloxone can reverse this respiratory depression (*see* above).

A side effect of droperidol is the occurrence of extrapyramidal muscle movements. Approximately 1% of patients receiving droperidol exhibit this side effect, which is sometimes delayed for 12 hours after the termination of anesthesia. The movements are self-limited and can be controlled with atropine or benztropine. Neurolept analgesia should not be used for patients with Parkinson's disease.

Status. Neurolept analgesia and neurolept anesthesia are safe and simple procedures, although induction of these states is slow. Circulatory changes are minimal unless the patient is hypovolemic or subjected to postural changes. Respiratory depression is severe but predictable. This is a useful technic in the elderly or the seriously ill or debilitated.

When neuromuscular blocking agents are also used, adequate conditions can be provided for all types of surgery, but the technic is generally not preferred over the use of potent inhalational agents for most types of major surgery. It has specialized uses for certain diagnostic procedures and for some types of peripheral operations.

DISSOCIATIVE ANESTHESIA

Some arylcycloalkylamines may induce a state of sedation, immobility, amnesia, and marked analgesia. The name *dissociative anesthesia* is derived from the strong feeling of dissociation from the environment that is experienced by the subject to whom such an agent is administered. This condition is similar to neurolept analgesia but results from the administration of a single drug (Winters *et al.*, 1972).

Phencyclidine was the first drug used for this purpose, but the frequent occurrence of unpleasant hallucinations and psychological problems soon led to its abandonment. These effects are much less frequent with *ketamine hydrochloride* (2-[*o*-chlorophenyl]-2-[methylamino] cyclohexanone hydrochloride; KETALAR).

Ketamine hydrochloride is supplied in solution for intravenous or intramuscular use in vials containing 10, 50, or 100 mg of ketamine base per milliliter.

Clinical Use. For the induction of dissociative anesthesia in an adult, ketamine hydrochloride is administered in a dose of 1 to 2 mg/kg over a period of about 1 minute. (A similar induction follows the intramuscular injection of 6 to 13 mg/kg.) A sensation of dissociation is noticed within 15 seconds, and unconsciousness becomes apparent within another 30 seconds. Intense analgesia and amnesia are established rapidly. Following a single dose, unconsciousness lasts for 10 to 15 minutes and analgesia persists for some 40 minutes; amnesia may be evident for a period of 1 to 2 hours following the initial injection. If anesthesia of longer duration is necessary, supplementary doses of about one third or one half of the initial amount may be administered.

Muscular relaxation is poor, muscle tone may be increased, purposeless movements sometimes occur, and occasionally violent and irrational responses to stimuli are observed. A soothing and quiet environment is necessary for success with this technic.

Hypoxic or hypercarbic stimulation of respiration is not seriously affected following usual doses of ketamine (Hirshman *et al.*, 1975). Pharyngeal and laryngeal reflexes are retained, and, while the cough reflex is depressed, airway obstruction does not normally occur. Airway resistance is in fact decreased, and bronchospasm may be abolished (Bovill *et al.*, 1971). Arterial blood pressure increases by as much as 25%, and cardiac output and rate increase. When myocardial tissue is exposed to ketamine *in vitro*, depression of contractility occurs. The stimulation observed *in vivo* is attributed to increased sympathetic activity. When ketamine is used to induce anesthesia in hypovolemic patients, hypotension may occur, but the incidence is less than when inhalational agents are used. Cerebral blood flow, metabolic rate, and intracranial pressure are augmented (Lassen and Christensen, 1976), as is intraocular pressure.

Recovery. Unlike the conventional intravenous agents, ketamine does not act primarily on the reticular activating system in the brain stem; rather, it acts on the cortex and the limbic system (Winters *et al.*, 1972). Perhaps this is the reason that recovery after ketamine has some unusual features. Awakening often requires several hours and is not infrequently characterized by disagreeable dreams and even hallucinations. Sometimes these unpleasant occurrences may recur days or weeks later. Almost half of adults over the age of 30 years exhibit delirium or excitement, or experience visual disturbances. The incidence of such adverse psychological experiences is greatly reduced in children and young adults. It is thought that the incidence of such unpleasant effects can be lowered by the prior administration of morphine and scopolamine and by the substitution of diazepam or thiopental for the last dose of ketamine.

Status. Ketamine hydrochloride is not indicated for patients with hypertension or psychiatric disorders. Intraocular pressure is increased with ketamine and, therefore, its use is not advisable for many types of eye surgery. It can be employed for induction of anesthesia, or, in combination with nitrous oxide, to produce adequate general anesthesia.

Ketamine is especially useful in children for the management of minor surgical or diagnostic procedures or for repeated procedures that require intense analgesia, such as changing burn dressings. When the burns involve the face and neck, the maintenance of an unobstructed airway with ketamine makes it a valuable agent.

Amess, J. A. L.; Burman, J. F.; Rees, G. M.; Nancekievill, D. G.; and Mollin, D. L. Megaloblastic hemopoiesis in patients receiving nitrous oxide. *Lancet,* **1978,** *2,* 339–341.

Arvidsson, S. B.; Ekstrom-Jodal, B.; Martinell, S. A. G.; and Niemand, D. Aminophylline antagonises diazepam sedation. *Lancet,* **1982,** 2, 1467.

Atlee, J. L., and Rusy, B. F. Atrioventricular conduction times and atrioventricular nodal conductivity during enflurane anesthesia in dogs. *Anesthesiology,* **1977,** *47,* 498–503.

Barry, K. G.; Mazze, R. I.; and Schwartz, F. D. Prevention of surgical oliguria and renal-hemodynamic suppression by sustained hydration. *N. Engl. J. Med.,* **1964,** *270,* 1371–1377.

Benumof, J., and Wahrenbrock, E. A. Local effects of anesthetic on regional hypoxic pulmonary vasoconstriction. *Anesthesiology,* **1975,** *43,* 525–532.

Bimar, J., and Bellville, J. W. Arousal reaction during anesthesia in man. *Anesthesiology,* **1977,** *47,* 449–454.

Bovill, J. G.; Clarke, R. S. J.; Davis, E. A.; and Dundee, J. W. Some cardiovascular effects of ketamine in man. *Br. J. Pharmacol.,* **1971,** *41,* 411P–412P.

Breimer, D. D. Clinical pharmacokinetics of hypnotics. *Clin. Pharmacokinet.,* **1977,** *2,* 93–109.

Brown, S. S.; Lyons, S. M.; and Dundee, J. W. Intraarterial barbiturates: a study of some factors leading to intravascular thrombosis. *Br. J. Anaesth.,* **1968,** *40,* 13–19.

Clark, D. L., and Rosner, B. D. Neurophysiologic effects of general anesthetics. 1. The electroencephalogram and sensory evoked responses in man. *Anesthesiology,* **1973,** *38,* 564–582.

Coleridge, H. M.; Coleridge, J. C. G.; Luck, J. C.; and Norman, J. The effect of four volatile anaesthetic agents in the impulse activity of two types of pulmonary receptor. *Br. J. Anaesth.,* **1968,** *40,* 484–492.

Coon, R. L., and Kampine, J. P. Hypocapnic bronchoconstriction and inhalation anesthetics. *Anesthesiology,* **1975,** *43,* 635–641.

Cousins, M. J., and Mazze, R. I. Methoxyflurane nephrotoxicity: a study of dose-response in man. *J.A.M.A.,* **1973,** *225,* 1611–1616.

Crandell, W. B.; Pappas, S. G.; and MacDonald, A. Nephrotoxicity associated with methoxyflurane anesthesia. *Anesthesiology,* **1966,** *27,* 591–607.

Deutsch, S.; Goldberg, M.; Stephens, G. M.; and Wu, W. H. Effects of halothane anesthesia on renal function in normal man. *Anesthesiology,* **1966,** *27,* 793–804.

Dueck, R.; Young, I.; Clauson, J.; and Wagner, P. D. Altered distribution of pulmonary ventilation and blood flow following induction of inhalational anesthesia. *Anesthesiology,* **1980,** *52,* 113–125.

Dunbar, B. S.; Ovassapian, A.; Dripps, R. D.; and Smith, T. C. The respiratory response to carbon dioxide during INNOVAR–nitrous oxide anaesthesia in man. *Br. J. Anaesth.,* **1967,** *39,* 861–866.

Dundee, J. W. Alterations in response to somatic pain associated with anaesthesia. II. The effect of thiopentone and pentobarbitone. *Br. J. Anaesth.,* **1960,** *32,* 407–414.

Eger, E. I., II; Saidman, L. J.; and Brandstater, B. Minimum alveolar anesthetic concentration: a standard of anesthetic potency. *Anesthesiology,* **1965,** *26,* 756–763.

Eger, E. I., II; Smith, N. T.; Stoelting, R. K.; Cullen, D. J.; Kadis, L. B.; and Whitcher, C. E. Cardiovascular effects of halothane in man. *Anesthesiology,* **1970,** *32,* 396–409.

Eger, E. I., II; White, A.; Brown, C.; Biava, C.; Corbett, T.; and Steven, W. A test of carcinogenicity of enflurane, isoflurane, halothane, methoxyflurane, and nitrous oxide in mice. *Anesth. Analg.,* **1978,** *57,* 678–694.

Epstein, R. M.; Deutsch, S.; Cooperman, L. H.; Clement, A. J.; and Price, H. L. Splanchnic circulation during halothane anesthesia and hypercapnia in normal man. *Anesthesiology,* **1966,** *27,* 654–661.

Fogdall, R. P., and Miller, R. D. Neuromuscular effects of enflurane alone and combined with *d*-tubocurarine, pancuronium, and succinylcholine in man. *Anesthesiology,* **1975,** *42,* 173–178.

Forbes, A. R. Halothane depresses mucociliary flow in the trachea. *Anesthesiology,* **1976,** *45,* 59–63.

Forster, A.; Gardaz, J. P.; Suter, P. M.; and Gemperle, M. Respiratory depression by midazolam and diazepam. *Anesthesiology,* **1980,** *53,* 494–497.

Göthert, M., and Wendt, J. Inhibition of adrenal medullary catecholamine secretion by enflurane. I. Investigations *in vivo. Anesthesiology,* **1977,** *46,* 400–403.

Gronert, G. A. Malignant hyperthermia. *Anesthesiology,* **1980,** *53,* 395–423.

Gross, J. B.; Zebrowski, M. E.; Carel, W. D.; Gardner, S.; and Smith, T. C. Time course of ventilatory depression after thiopental and midazolam in normal subjects and in patients with chronic obstructive pulmonary disease. *Anesthesiology,* **1983,** *59,* 46–50.

Harper, M. H.; Hickey, R. F.; Cromwell, T. H.; and Linwood, S. The magnitude and duration of respiratory depression produced by fentanyl and fentanyl plus droperidol in man. *J. Pharmacol. Exp. Ther.,* **1976,** *199,* 464–468.

Hirshman, C. A.; Edelstein, G.; Peetz, S.; Wayne, R.; and Downes, H. Mechanism of action of inhalational anesthesia on airways. *Anesthesiology,* **1982,** *56,* 107–111.

Hirshman, C. A.; McCullough, R. E.; Cohen, P. J.; and Weil, J. V. Hypoxic ventilatory drive in dogs during thiopental, ketamine or pentobarbital anesthesia. *Anesthesiology,* **1975,** *43,* 628–634.

———. Depression of hypoxic ventilatory response by halothane, enflurane and isoflurane in dogs. *Br. J. Anaesth.,* **1977,** *49,* 957–963.

Holaday, D. A.; Fiseroua-Bergerova, V.; Latto, I. P.; and Zumbiel, M. A. Resistance of isoflurane to biotransformation in man. *Anesthesiology,* **1975,** *43,* 325–332.

Horan, B. F.; Prys-Roberts, C.; Hamilton, W. K.; and Roberts, J. G. Haemodynamic responses to enflurane anaesthesia and hypovolaemia in the dog and their modification by propranolol. *Br. J. Anaesth.,* **1977,** *49,* 1189–1197.

Hornbein, T. F.; Martin, W. E.; Bonica, J. J.; Freund, F. G.; and Parmentier, P. Nitrous oxide effects on the circulatory and ventilatory responses to halothane. *Anesthesiology,* **1969,** *31,* 250–260.

Johnston, R. R.; Eger, E. I., II; and Wilson, C. A comparative interaction of epinephrine with enflurane, isoflurane and halothane in man. *Anesth. Analg.,* **1976,** *55,* 709–712.

Johnstone, R. E.; Kennell, E. M.; Behar, M. G.; Brummond, W.; Ebersole, R. C.; and Shaw, L. M. Increased serum bromide concentration after halothane anesthesia in man. *Anesthesiology,* **1975,** *42,* 598–601.

Katz, R. L.; Matteo, R. S.; and Papper, E. M. The injection of epinephrine during general anesthesia. II. Halothane. *Anesthesiology,* **1962,** *23,* 597–600.

Knill, R. L., and Gelb, A. W. Ventilatory responses to hypoxia and hypercapnia during halothane sedation and anesthesia in man. *Anesthesiology,* **1978,** *49,* 244–251.

Korttila, V.; Tammisto, T.; Ertama, P.; Pfaffli, P.;

Blomgren, E.; and Hakkinen, S. Recovery, psychomotor skills and simulated driving after brief inhalational anesthesia with halothane or enflurane combined with nitrous oxide and oxygen. *Anesthesiology*, **1977**, *46*, 20–27.

Larson, C. P.; Eger, E. I., II; Maullem, M.; Buechel, D. R.; Munson, E. S.; and Eisele, J. H. The effects of diethyl ether and methoxyflurane on ventilation. II. A comparative study in man. *Anesthesiology*, **1969**, *30*, 174–184.

Lassen, H. C. A.; Henriksen, E.; Neukirch, F.; and Kristensen, H. S. Treatment of tetanus: severe bone-marrow depression after prolonged nitrous-oxide anaesthesia. *Lancet*, **1956**, *1*, 527–530.

Lassen, N. A., and Christensen, M. S. Physiology of cerebral blood flow. *Br. J. Anaesth.*, **1976**, *48*, 719–734.

Laws, A. K. Effects of induction of anaesthesia and muscle paralysis on functional residual capacity of the lungs. *Can. Anaesth. Soc. J.*, **1968**, *15*, 325–331.

Layzer, R. B. Myeloneuropathy after prolonged exposure to nitrous oxide. *Lancet*, **1978**, *2*, 1227–1230.

Leighton, K., and Bruce, C. Distribution of kidney blood flow: a comparison of methoxyflurane and halothane effects as measured by heated thermocouple. *Can. Anaesth. Soc. J.*, **1975**, *22*, 125–137.

Lowenstein, E.; Hallowell, P.; Levine, F. H.; Daggett, W. M.; Austen, W. G.; and Laver, M. B. Cardiovascular response to large doses of intravenous morphine in man. *N. Engl. J. Med.*, **1969**, *281*, 1389–1393.

Lundy, J. S. Intravenous anesthesia: preliminary report of the use of two new thiobarbiturates. *Proc. Staff Meet. Mayo Clin.*, **1935**, *10*, 536–543.

Lynch, C.; Vogel, S.; and Sperelakis, N. Halothane depression of myocardial slow action potentials. *Anesthesiology*, **1981**, *55*, 360–368.

Marshall, B. E.; Cohen, P. J.; Klingenmaier, C. H.; and Aukburg, S. Pulmonary venous admixture before, during and after halothane:oxygen anesthesia in man. *J. Appl. Physiol.*, **1969**, *27*, 653–657.

Marshall, B. E.; Cohen, P. J.; Klingenmaier, C. H.; Neigh, J. L.; and Pender, J. W. Some pulmonary and cardiovascular effects of enflurane (ETHRANE) anaesthesia with varying $PaCO_2$ in man. *Br. J. Anaesth.*, **1971**, *43*, 996–1002.

Mazze, R. I.; Calverley, R. K.; and Smith, N. T. Inorganic fluoride nephrotoxicity: prolonged enflurane and halothane anesthesia in volunteers. *Anesthesiology*, **1977**, *46*, 265–271.

Mazze, R. I.; Schwartz, F. D.; Slocum, H. C.; and Barry, K. G. Renal function during anesthesia and surgery. I. The effects of halothane anesthesia. *Anesthesiology*, **1963**, *24*, 279–284.

Mazze, R. I.; Shue, G. L.; and Jackson, S. H. Renal dysfunction associated with methoxyflurane anesthesia. *J.A.M.A.*, **1971**, *216*, 278–288.

Merin, R. G.; Kumazawa, T.; and Luka, N. L. Enflurane depresses myocardial function, perfusion and metabolism in the dog. *Anesthesiology*, **1976**, *45*, 501–507.

Merin, R. G.; Verdouw, P. D.; and de Jong, J. W. Dose-dependent depression of cardiac function and metabolism by halothane in swine (*Sus scrofa*). *Anesthesiology*, **1977**, *46*, 417–423.

Michenfelder, J. D., and Theye, R. A. *In vivo* toxic effects of halothane on canine cerebral metabolic pathways. *Am. J. Physiol.*, **1975**, *229*, 1050–1055.

Miletich, D. J.; Ivankovich, A. D.; Albrecht, R. F.; Reimann, C. R.; Rosenberg, R.; and McKissic, E. D. Absence of autoregulation of cerebral blood flow during halothane and enflurane anesthesia. *Anesth. Analg.*, **1976**, *55*, 100–109.

Millar, R. A., and Morris, M. E. A study of methoxyflurane anesthesia. *Can. Anaesth. Soc. J.*, **1961**, *8*, 210–215.

Perry, L. B.; VanDyke, R. A.; and Theye, R. A. Sympathoadrenal and hemodynamic effects of isoflurane, halothane, and cyclopropane in dogs. *Anesthesiology*, **1974**, *40*, 465–470.

Prys-Roberts, C.; Kelman, G. R.; Greenbaum, R.; Kain, M. L.; and Bay, J. Hemodynamic and alveolar-arterial PO_2 differences at varying $PaCO_2$ in anesthetized man. *J. Appl. Physiol.*, **1968**, *25*, 80–87.

Rehder, K.; Forbes, J.; Alter, H.; Hessler, O.; and Stier, A. Halothane biotransformation in man: a quantitative study. *Anesthesiology*, **1967**, *28*, 711–715.

Reynolds, A. K.; Chiz, J. F.; and Pasquet, A. F. Halothane and methoxyflurane. A comparison of their effects on cardiac pacemaker fibers. *Anesthesiology*, **1970**, *33*, 602–610.

Sakai, T., and Takaori, M. Biodegradation of halothane, enflurane, and methoxyflurane. *Br. J. Anaesth.*, **1978**, *50*, 785–791.

Samuelson, P. M.; Reves, J. G.; Kouchoukos, N. T.; Smith, L. R.; and Dole, K. M. Hemodynamic responses to anesthetic induction with midazolam or diazepam in patients with ischemic heart disease. *Anesth. Analg.*, **1981**, *60*, 802–809.

Shapiro, H. M. Intracranial hypertension: therapeutic and anesthetic considerations. *Anesthesiology*, **1975**, *43*, 445–471.

Shimoji, K.; Matsuki, M.; Shimizu, H.; Maruyama, Y.; and Aida, S. Dishabituation of mesencephalic reticular neurons by anesthetics. *Anesthesiology*, **1977**, *47*, 349–352.

Shimosato, S., and Etsten, B. E. Effect of anesthetic drugs on the heart: a critical review of myocardial contractility and its relationship to hemodynamics. *Clin. Anesth.*, **1969**, *3*, 17–72.

Shimosato, S.; Sugai, N.; Iwatsuki, N.; and Etsten, B. E. The effect of ETHRANE on cardiac muscle mechanics. *Anesthesiology*, **1969**, *30*, 513–518.

Sipes, I. G., and Brown, B. R. An animal model of hepatotoxicity associated with halothane anesthesia. *Anesthesiology*, **1976**, *45*, 622–628.

Skovsted, P., and Price, H. L. The effects of ETHRANE on arterial pressure, preganglionic sympathetic activity and barostatic reflexes. *Anesthesiology*, **1972**, *36*, 257–262.

Skovsted, P.; Price, M. L.; and Price, H. L. The effects of halothane on arterial pressure, preganglionic sympathetic activity, and barostatic reflexes. *Anesthesiology*, **1969**, *31*, 507–514.

Smith, A. L., and Wollman, H. Cerebral blood flow and metabolism. Effect of anesthetic drugs and techniques. *Anesthesiology*, **1972**, *36*, 378–400.

Smith, N. T.; Calverley, R. K.; Prys-Roberts, C.; Eger, E. I., II; and Jones, C. W. Impact of nitrous oxide on the circulation during enflurane anesthesia in man. *Anesthesiology*, **1978**, *48*, 345–349.

Smith, N. T.; Eger, E. I., II; Stoelting, R. K.; Whayne, T. F.; Cullen, D.; and Kadis, L. B. The cardiovascular and sympathomimetic responses to the addition of nitrous oxide to halothane in man. *Anesthesiology*, **1970**, *32*, 410–421.

Sonntag, H.; Donath, U.; Hillebrand, W.; Merin, R. G.; and Radke, J. Left ventricular function in conscious man and during halothane anesthesia. *Anesthesiology*, **1978**, *48*, 320–324.

Stevens, W. C.; Cromwell, T. H.; Halsey, M. J.; Eger, E. I., II; Shakespeare, T. F.; and Bahlman, S. H. The cardiovascular effects of a new inhalation anesthetic, FORANE, in human volunteers at constant arterial carbon dioxide tension. *Anesthesiology*, **1971**, *35*, 8–16.

Sugai, N.; Shimosato, S.; and Etsten, B. E. Effect of halothane on force-velocity relations and dynamic stiffness of isolated heart muscle. *Anesthesiology*, **1968**, *29*, 267–274.

Summary of the National Halothane Study. *J.A.M.A.*, **1966,** *197,* 775–788.

Tusiewicz, K.; Bryan, A. C.; and Froese, A. B. Contributions of changing rib cage-diaphragm interactions to the ventilatory depression of halothane anesthesia. *Anesthesiology,* **1977,** *47,* 327–337.

Vessey, M. P. Epidemiological studies of the occupational hazards of anaesthesia—a review. *Anaesthesia,* **1978,** *33,* 430–438.

Wagner, R. L.; White, P. F.; Kan, P. B.; Rosenthal, M. H.; and Feldman, D. Inhibition of adrenal steroidogenesis by the anesthetic etomidate. *N. Engl. J. Med.,* **1984,** *310,* 1415–1421.

Walker, J. A.; Eggers, G. W. N.; and Allen, C. R. Cardiovascular effects of methoxyflurane anesthesia in man. *Anesthesiology,* **1962,** *23,* 639–642.

Wang, H.; Epstein, R. A.; Markee, S. J.; and Bartelstone, H. J. The effects of halothane on peripheral and central vasomotor control mechanisms of the dog. *Anesthesiology,* **1968,** *29,* 877–886.

Waud, B. E., and Waud, D. R. Comparison of the effects of general anesthetics on the end-plate of skeletal muscle. *Anesthesiology,* **1975,** *43,* 540–547.

———. Effects of volatile anesthetics on directly and indirectly stimulated skeletal muscle. *Ibid.,* **1979,** *50,* 103–110.

Williams, B. D.; White, N.; Amlot, P. L.; Slaney, J.; and Toseland, P. A. Circulating immune complexes after repeated halothane anaesthesia. *Br. Med. J.,* **1977,** *2,* 159–162.

Winters, W. D.; Ferrer-Allado, T.; and Guzman-Flores, C. The cataleptic state induced by ketamine: a review of the neuropharmacology of anesthesia. *Neuropharmacology,* **1972,** *11,* 303–315.

Wollman, H.; Alexander, S. C.; Cohen, P. J.; Chase, P. E.; Melman, E.; and Behar, M. G. Cerebral circulation of man during halothane anesthesia: effects of hypocarbia and *d*-tubocurarine. *Anesthesiology,* **1964,** *25,* 180–184.

Wollman, H.; Alexander, S. C.; Cohen, P. J.; Smith, T. C.; Chase, P. E.; and van der Molen, R. A. Cerebral circulation during general anesthesia and hyperventilation in man. Thiopental induction to nitrous oxide and *d*-tubocurarine. *Anesthesiology,* **1965,** *26,* 329–334.

Yacoub, O.; Doell, D.; Kryger, M. H.; and Anthonisen, N. R. Depression of hypoxic ventilatory response by nitrous oxide. *Anesthesiology,* **1976,** *45,* 385–389.

Zink, J.; Sasyniuk, B. I.; and Dresel, P. E. Halothane-epinephrine-induced cardiac arrhythmias and the role of heart rate. *Anesthesiology,* **1975,** *43,* 548–555.

Monographs and Reviews

Aldrete, J. A., and Britt, B. A. (eds.). *Malignant Hyperthermia.* Grune & Stratton, Inc., New York, **1978.**

Cohen, E. N. Metabolism of the volatile anesthetics. *Anesthesiology,* **1971,** *35,* 193–202.

Dean, G. *Porphyrias: A Story of Inheritance and Environment,* 2nd ed. Pitman, London, **1971.**

Eger, E. I., II. *Anesthetic Uptake and Action.* The Williams & Wilkins Co., Baltimore, **1974.**

———. Isoflurane: a review. *Anesthesiology,* **1981,** *55,* 559–576.

Kitahata, L. M., and Collins, J. G. *Narcotic Analgesics in Anesthesiology.* The Williams & Wilkins Co., Baltimore, **1982.**

Marshall, B. E., and Wyche, M. Q. Hypoxemia during and after anesthesia. *Anesthesiology,* **1972,** *37,* 178–209.

Waud, B. E. Neuromuscular blocking agents. In, *Current Problems in Anesthesia and Critical Care Medicine,* Vol. 4. (Brunner, E. A., ed.) Year Book Medical Publishers, Inc., Chicago, **1977,** pp. 5–47.

CHAPTER

15 LOCAL ANESTHETICS

J. Murdoch Ritchie and Nicholas M. Greene

GENERAL PHARMACOLOGY OF LOCAL ANESTHETICS

Local anesthetics are drugs that block nerve conduction when applied locally to nerve tissue in appropriate concentrations. They act on any part of the nervous system and on every type of nerve fiber. For example, when they are applied to the motor cortex impulse transmission from that area stops, and when they are injected into the skin they prevent the initiation and the transmission of sensory impulses. A local anesthetic in contact with a nerve trunk can cause both sensory and motor paralysis in the area innervated. Many kinds of compounds interfere with conduction, but they often permanently damage the nerve cells. The great practical advantage of the local anesthetics is that their action is reversible; their use is followed by complete recovery in nerve function with no evidence of structural damage to nerve fibers or cells.

History. The first local anesthetic to be discovered was cocaine, an alkaloid contained in large amounts (0.6 to 1.8%) in the leaves of *Erythroxylon coca,* a shrub growing in the Andes Mountains 1000 to 3000 m above sea level. Nearly 9 million kilograms of these leaves are consumed annually by about 2 million inhabitants of the highlands of Peru, who chew or suck the leaves for the sense of well-being it produces.

The pure alkaloid was first isolated by Niemann, who noted that it had a bitter taste and produced a peculiar effect on the tongue, making it numb and almost devoid of sensation. Von Anrep in 1880 observed that the skin became insensitive to the prick of a pin when cocaine was infiltrated subcutaneously. He recommended that the alkaloid be used clinically as a local anesthetic. His suggestion, however, was not acted upon. The clinical use of cocaine was in fact initiated by two young Viennese physicians, Sigmund Freud and Karl Koller. In 1884, Freud made a general study of the physiological effects of cocaine (*see* Byck, 1975). He was particularly impressed by the central actions of the drug and used it to wean one of his colleagues from morphine. He was successful in this attempt, but at the cost of producing one of the first-known cocaine addicts of modern times. Koller quickly appreciated that the anesthetizing properties of cocaine had great practical importance and soon introduced cocaine into ophthalmology as a local anesthetic. Within a short time, Hall in 1884 introduced local anesthesia into dentistry, and the next year Halsted, by demonstrating that cocaine could stop transmission in nerve trunks, laid the foundation for nerve block anesthesia in surgery. Corning in 1885 produced spinal anesthesia in dogs, but several years passed before his technic was employed in clinical surgery.

A chemical search for synthetic substitutes for cocaine started in 1892 with the work of Einhorn and his colleagues. This resulted in 1905 in the synthesis of procaine, which is still a prototype for local anesthetic drugs.

Properties Desirable in Local Anesthetics. A good local anesthetic should combine several properties. It should not be irritating to the tissue to which it is applied, nor should it cause any permanent damage to nerve structure; most local anesthetics in common use fulfill these requirements. Its systemic toxicity should be low because it is eventually absorbed from its site of application. The ideal local anesthetic must be effective regardless of whether it is injected into the tissue or whether it is applied locally to mucous membranes. It is usually important that the time required for the onset of anesthesia should be as short as possible. Furthermore, the action must last long enough to allow time for the contemplated surgery, yet not so long as to entail an extended period of recovery. Many agents satisfy this latter requirement. Occasionally, a local anesthetic action lasting for days or even weeks or months is desirable, for example, in the control of chronic pain. Unfortunately, the available compounds employed for anesthesia of such long duration have high local toxicity. Neurolysis with slough and necrosis of surrounding tissues occurs, and partial or complete transverse injury of the spinal cord with permanent paralysis may result if such a reaction occurs in the vicinity of the cord.

GENERAL PROPERTIES

The local anesthetics have many actions in common, and before discussing the pharmacology of the individual members these general properties will be considered. (For reviews, *see* de Jong, 1977; Fink, 1980; Strichartz, 1985.)

Chemistry and Structure-Activity Relationship. Table 15–1 shows that the structure of typical anesthetics contains hydrophilic and hydrophobic domains that are separated by an intermediate alkyl chain. The hydrophilic group is usually a tertiary amine, but it may also be a secondary amine; the hydrophobic domain is an aromatic residue. Linkage to the aromatic group is of either the ester or amide type, and the nature of this bond determines certain of the pharmacological properties of these agents. The ester link is important because this bond is readily hydrolyzed during metabolic degradation and inactivation in the body. Procaine, for example, can be divided into three main portions: the aromatic acid (para-aminobenzoic), the alcohol (ethanol), and the tertiary amino group (diethylamino). Changes in any part of the molecule alter the anesthetic potency and the toxicity of the compound. Increasing the length of the alcohol group leads to a greater anesthetic potency. It also leads to an increase in toxicity; compounds with an ethyl ester, such as procaine, exhibit the least toxicity. The length of the two terminal groups on the tertiary amino nitrogen is similarly important. The structure-activity relationship and the physicochemical properties of local anesthetics have been reviewed by Büchi and Perlia (1971).

Mechanism of Action. Local anesthetics prevent the generation and the conduction of the nerve impulse. Their main site of action is the cell membrane, and there is seemingly little direct action of physiological importance on the axoplasm in the concentrations used to produce local anesthesia. The work of Hodgkin, Huxley, and their colleagues has led to a better understanding of the nature of the nerve impulse, and it is now relatively easy to account for the action of local anesthetics within the framework of the ionic theory of nervous activity.

Local anesthetics and other classes of agents (*e.g.*, alcohols and barbiturates) block conduction by decreasing or preventing the large *transient* increase in the permeability of the membrane to sodium ions that is produced by a slight depolarization of the membrane (*see* Strichartz, 1981; Strichartz and Ritchie, 1985). As the anesthetic action progressively develops in a nerve, the threshold for electrical excitability gradually increases and the safety factor for conduction decreases; when this action is sufficiently well developed, block of conduction is produced.

Raising the calcium concentration in the medium bathing a nerve may either relieve or intensify conduction block produced by local anesthetics. Relief occurs because calcium alters the surface potential on the membrane, and hence the transmembrane electrical field. This, in turn, reduces the degree of inactivation of the sodium channels and the affinity of the latter for the local anesthetic molecules (*see* Hille, 1977). Calcium, however, may also intensify the degree of conduction block by altering the kinetics of opening of the sodium channel (Strichartz, 1980).

The local anesthetics also reduce the permeability of *resting* nerve to potassium as well as to sodium ions. Since changes in

Table 15–1.   STRUCTURAL FORMULAS OF SELECTED LOCAL ANESTHETICS

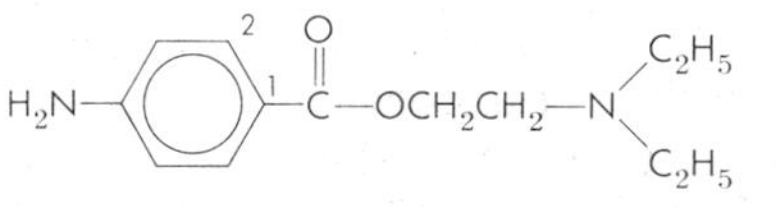

Procaine *

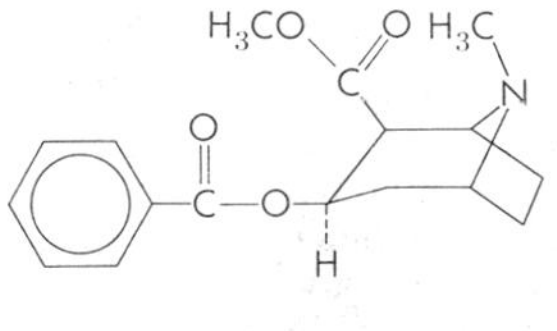

Cocaine

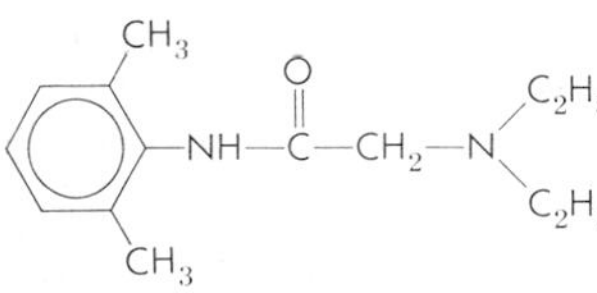

Lidocaine

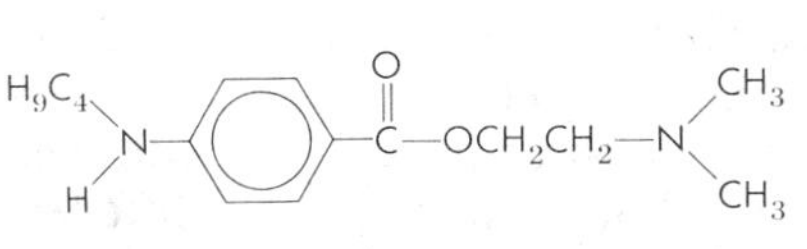

Tetracaine

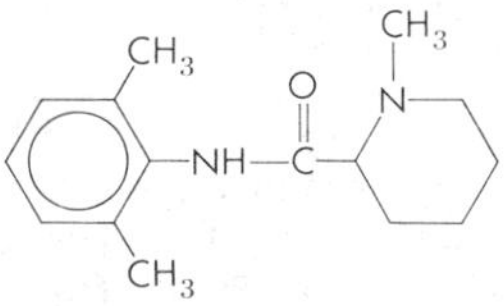

Mepivacaine †

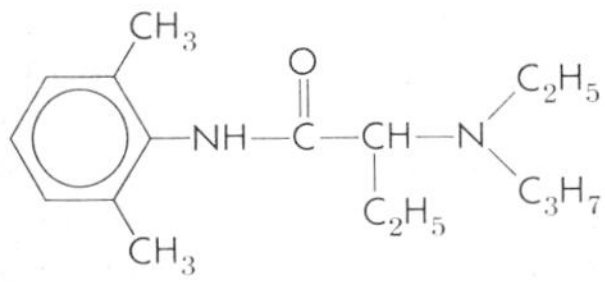

Etidocaine

* Chloroprocaine has a chlorine atom in position 2 of the aromatic moiety of procaine.
† Bupivacaine has a butyl group in place of the N-methyl substituent of mepivacaine.

permeability to potassium require higher concentrations of local anesthetic, blockade of conduction is not accompanied by any large or consistent change in the resting potential.

Quaternary analogs of local anesthetics block conduction when applied internally to perfused giant axons of squid, but they are relatively ineffective when applied externally. These observations, together with others on the effects of varying pH on the potency of related tertiary amines, suggest that the site at which local anesthetics act, at least in their charged form, is accessible only from the inner surface of the membrane (Narahashi and Frazier, 1971; Strichartz and Ritchie, 1985). Local anesthetics applied externally must therefore first cross the membrane, in the uncharged form, before they can exert a blocking action. Furthermore, several studies show that the binding of the charged form of the local anesthetic to its site of action is voltage dependent, in a way that suggests that the receptor is about halfway down the sodium channel (Strichartz, 1981).

The relative anesthetic potency of a series of compounds exactly parallels their effectiveness in increasing the surface pressure of monomolecular films of lipids (see Skou, 1961). On the basis of this work, Shanes (1958) suggested that local anesthetics achieve block by increasing the surface pressure of the lipid layer that constitutes the nerve membrane, thereby closing the pores through which ions move. This would cause a general decrease in the resting permeability and would also limit the increase in sodium permeability, the fundamental change necessary for the generation of the action potential. In contrast, Metcalfe and Burgen (1968) have suggested that local anesthetics affect permeability by increasing the degree of disorder of the membrane. The partial reversal of local anesthetic block by high external pressure (Kendig and Cohen, 1977) is consistent with this latter view. However, the major mechanism of action of local anesthetics involves their combination with a specific receptor site within the sodium channel, hence physically blocking it (see Ritchie, 1975; Hille, 1980; Strichartz and Ritchie, 1985).

The proteins that comprise the sodium channel have recently been purified extensively and reconstituted functionally; more complete understanding of the mechanism of action of local anesthetics can thus be anticipated in the near future (see Agnew, 1984; Catterall, 1984). The mammalian sodium channel appears to consist of three dissimilar subunits of glycosylated proteins with an aggregate molecular size in excess of 300,000 daltons. After incorporation of the purified polypeptides into phospholipid vesicles, sodium flux into the vesicles occurs in response to veratridine, a substance known to cause persistent activation of sodium channels. This transport can be blocked by the neurotoxins tetrodotoxin and saxitoxin (see below) and by local anesthetics (Tamkun et al., 1984). By use of a nonpermeant quaternary analog of lidocaine, it is possible to show that local anesthetics and tetrodotoxin interact at opposite ends of the sodium channel (Rosenberg et al., 1984).

Radioactive neurotoxins and antibodies to the purified channel proteins have permitted visualization of sodium channels in plasma membranes of electrically excitable cells (see Catterall, 1984); their distribution is nonuniform. For example, while few channels can be detected in the internodal regions of myelinated axons, sodium channels appear to occupy at least 15% of the membrane surface at the nodes of Ranvier. Thus, local anesthetics need have access only to the nodal regions in order to produce blockade of conduction.

Differential Sensitivity of Nerve Fibers to Local Anesthetics. As a general rule, small nerve fibers seem to be more susceptible to the action of local anesthetics than are large fibers. This was clearly established for the myelinated A fibers by Gasser and Erlanger (1929), who showed that when cocaine is applied to a cutaneous nerve the δ waves (from small cutaneous afferent fibers) are the first and the α waves (from large fibers) the last to disappear. The smallest mammalian nerve fibers are nonmyelinated and, on the whole, are blocked more readily than the myelinated fibers. However, the spectrum of sensitivity of the nonmyelinated fibers overlaps that of the myelinated fibers to some extent. Thus, some myelinated A δ fibers are blocked earlier, and with lower concentrations of anesthetic, than are most of the C fibers (Nathan and Sears, 1961). The sensitivity to local anesthetics is not determined by fiber size alone, therefore, but also by the anatomical fiber type. This is not surprising in view of the great difference between the physiological mode of conduction in the myelinated fibers, in which conduction is saltatory, and that of the nonmyelinated fibers, in which it is continuous. Still other factors may determine the susceptibility of a fiber to a local anesthetic. For example, in the rabbit vagus nerve the myelinated autonomic B fibers seem to have a greater safety factor for conduction than do the larger myelinated A fibers (Gissen et al., 1982); this would account for their lower sensitivity to local anesthetics (Gissen et al., 1980). Although there is general agreement on the differential rate of blockade produced by local anesthetics in fibers of different sizes, there is some question whether a similar differential effect obtains after sufficient time has been allowed for full equilibration of the local anesthetic with the tissue. Indeed, Franz and Perry (1974) found that *absolute* differential blockade occurred only when the length of nerve exposed to the anesthetic was limited to a few millimeters.

The sensitivity of a fiber to local anesthetics does not seem to depend on whether it is sensory or motor. Although application of local anesthetic to a muscle-nerve trunk leads to blockade of contractions elicited reflexly before those elicited by electrical stimulation of the nerve, both muscle proprioceptive afferent and muscle efferent fibers are equally sensitive. These two types of fibers have the same diameter, which is larger than the γ *motor* fibers that supply the muscle spindles. It is the more rapid blockade of these smaller motor fibers, rather than the sensory fibers, that leads to the preferential loss of the muscle reflexes.

Computer simulation suggests that the safety factor for conduction in a homologous population of myelinated fibers (*e.g.,* in a somatic nerve) should be largely independent of fiber diameter (Chiu and Ritchie, 1984). This agrees with the suggestion of Franz and Perry (1974) that differential block cannot result from differences in minimal concentrations necessary to block axons of different diameters. Rather, it results from differences in the critical lengths of axons that must be exposed to the anesthetic, smaller axons having shorter critical lengths because of their smaller internodal distances. In the early stages of development of anesthetic action, small discrete lengths of the most accessible portions of the nerve trunk are the first to be exposed to the anesthetic as it diffuses inward along various intrafascicular routes. Smaller fibers with their shorter critical lengths are thus blocked more quickly by anesthetic solutions than are larger fibers; the same reasoning accounts for their slower recovery when the process is reversed.

The differential sensitivity to block exhibited by fibers of varying sizes is of great practical importance and may explain why there is a definite order in which the sensory functions of a nerve are affected by local anesthetics. Fortunately for the patient, the sensation of pain is usually the first modality to disappear, and it is followed in turn by the sensations of cold, warmth, touch, and deep pressure, although there is great individual variation.

Effect of pH. The local anesthetics in the form of the unprotonated amine tend to be only slightly soluble. Therefore, they are generally marketed in the form of their water-soluble salts, usually the hydrochlorides. Inasmuch as the local anesthet-

ics are weak bases, these salt solutions are quite acidic, a condition that fortunately increases the stability of the local anesthetic and any accompanying vasoconstrictor substance. A small amount of unprotonated amine must, however, always be present, and it is in this form that the drug can penetrate the tissues.

Numerous investigations in which anesthetics were applied to isolated nerve trunks or to the cornea, where the buffering capacity of the tissue fluids is limited, have shown that the addition of base to local anesthetic solutions enhances activity. However, alkaline solutions of the drugs are not more effective clinically. The explanation probably is that, under conditions usually encountered in clinical use, the pH of the local anesthetic is rapidly brought to that of the extracellular fluids, regardless of the pH of the solution in which it is injected.

All the commonly used local anesthetics contain a tertiary (or secondary) nitrogen atom and, therefore, can exist either as the uncharged tertiary (or secondary) amine or as the positively charged substituted ammonium cation, depending on the dissociation constant (pK_a) of the compound and the pH of the solution. The ionization of a typical local anesthetic may be depicted as follows:

$$R_2\overset{\displaystyle R_1}{\underset{\displaystyle R_3}{-}}\overset{+}{N}H \rightleftharpoons R_2\overset{\displaystyle R_1}{\underset{\displaystyle R_3}{-}}N + H^+$$

The pK_a of a typical local anesthetic lies between 8.0 and 9.0, so that only 5 to 20% will be unprotonated at the pH of the tissues. This fraction, although small, is important because the drug usually has to diffuse through connective tissue and other cellular membranes to reach its site of action, and it is generally agreed that it can do so only in the form of the uncharged amine. Once the anesthetic has reached the nerve the form of the molecule active in nerve fibers seems to be the cation. This conclusion has been supported by the results of experiments on anesthetized mammalian nonmyelinated fibers (Ritchie and Greengard, 1966) in which conduction could be blocked or unblocked merely by setting the pH of the bathing medium at pH 7.2 or pH 9.6, respectively, without altering the amount of anesthetic present. When the pH is low and conduction is blocked, most of the anesthetic must be in its cationic form. This indicates that it is the cation that combines with some receptor in the membrane to prevent the generation of an action potential. Furthermore, the *major* role of the cation has been clearly demonstrated by Narahashi and colleagues using quaternary analogs of the amine local anesthetics (Narahashi and Frazier, 1971).

However, it is now evident that both molecular forms possess anesthetic activity; whether there is only a single receptor site for these two forms remains unsettled (Hille, 1977; Mrose and Ritchie, 1978; Ritchie, 1979; Strichartz and Ritchie, 1985).

Frequency Dependence and Use Dependence. The degree of block produced by a given concentration of local anesthetic depends markedly on how much and how recently the nerve has been stimulated. Thus, a resting nerve is much less sensitive to a local anesthetic than one that has been recently and repetitively stimulated: the higher the frequency of preceding stimulation, the greater is the degree of block obtained to a test shock. These frequency- and use-dependent effects of local anesthetics occur because the local anesthetic molecule in its quaternary form gains access to the receptor only when the "gates" at the inner face of the sodium channel are open and because the local anesthetic binds more tightly to and stabilizes the inactive state of the sodium channel (*see* Hille, 1980). Local anesthetics exhibit these properties to different extents, depending, for example, on their pK_a, lipid solubility, and molecular size (Courtney, 1980). An anesthetic that blocked high-frequency sensory discharge while permitting passage of low-frequency motor discharge would clearly be valuable clinically.

Prolongation of Action by Vasoconstrictors. The duration of action of a local anesthetic is proportional to the time during which it is in contact with nervous tissues. Consequently, procedures that keep the drug at the nerve prolong the period of anesthesia. Cocaine itself constricts blood vessels by potentiating the action of norepinephrine (*see* Chapters 4 and 8); therefore, it prevents its own absorption. Braun in 1903 demonstrated that the addition of epinephrine to local anesthetic solutions greatly prolongs and intensifies their action. In clinical practice, therefore, the solution of a local anesthetic usually also contains epinephrine (1 part in 200,000), norepinephrine (1 part in 100,000), or a suitable synthetic congener, for example, phenylephrine. In general, the concentration of such constrictor agents should be kept at the minimal effective level. The epi-

nephrine performs a dual service. By decreasing the rate of absorption, epinephrine not only localizes the anesthetic at the desired site but also allows the rate at which it is destroyed in the body to keep pace with the rate at which it is absorbed into the circulation. This reduces its systemic toxicity.

Some of the vasoconstrictor agent may be absorbed systemically, occasionally to an extent sufficient to cause untoward reactions, such as restlessness, an increase in heart rate, palpitation, and chest pain. In such circumstances, the use of α- or β-adrenergic antagonists should be considered to counter any prominent untoward manifestations of adrenergic stimulation. There may also be a delay in wound healing, tissue edema, or necrosis after local anesthesia. These effects seem to occur in part because sympathomimetic amines increase the oxygen consumption of the tissue, and this, together with the vasoconstriction, leads to hypoxia and local tissue damage. This is particularly serious when local anesthetics are used in surgery on the digits, hands, or feet. Prolonged constriction of major arteries in the presence of limited collateral circulation can produce irreversible hypoxic damage and gangrene. In addition, the local anesthetics themselves may interfere with the reparative processes of wound healing.

Pharmacological Actions. In addition to blocking conduction in nerve axons in the peripheral nervous system, local anesthetics interfere with the function of all organs in which conduction or transmission of impulses occurs. Thus, they have important effects on the central nervous system (CNS), the autonomic ganglia, the neuromuscular junction, and all forms of muscle fiber (for review, *see* de Jong, 1977). The danger of such adverse reactions is proportional to the concentration of local anesthetic that is achieved in the circulation. This is highly dependent on the agent administered, the dose employed, and the site and technic of use. These important issues are considered below in the section on Clinical Uses of Local Anesthetics.

Central Nervous System. Following absorption, all nitrogenous local anesthetics may cause stimulation of the CNS, producing restlessness and tremor that may proceed to clonic convulsions. In general, the more potent the anesthetic the more readily convulsions may be produced. Alterations of CNS activity are thus predictable from the local anesthetic agent in question and the blood concentration achieved. Unfortunately, EEG patterns give little or no consistent warning of impending convulsive activity (Covino, 1985). Central stimulation is followed by depression, and death is usually due to respiratory failure. It is possible to protect animals from several lethal doses of a local anesthetic by the use of artificial respiration.

The apparent stimulation and subsequent depression produced by applying local anesthetics to the CNS may both be due solely to *depression* of neuronal activity. Since local anesthetics produce only depression of monosynaptic and polysynaptic spinal reflexes or of directly evoked electrical responses in isolated slabs of cerebral cortex, a selective depression of inhibitory neurons may account for the excitatory phase *in vivo*. This would be consistent with the suppressive effects of local anesthetics against convulsions in both experimental animals and epileptic patients (*see* Covino, 1985).

Rapid systemic administration of local anesthetics, or large doses of the more toxic agents administered locally, may produce death with only transient or no signs of CNS stimulation. Under these conditions the concentration of the drug probably rises so rapidly that all neurons are depressed simultaneously. In addition, the function of critical centers that control respiration and vasomotor tone may be impaired quickly, depriving neurons that are involved in apparently stimulatory effects of local anesthetics of oxygen and glucose.

The support of respiration is the essential feature of treatment in the late stage of intoxication. While the barbiturates arrest convulsions resulting from toxic doses of local anesthetics, near-anesthetic doses are required. The usual sedative dose affords little protection. Diazepam administered intravenously is the drug of choice for both the prevention and the arrest of convulsions (*see* Chapter 20).

All the local anesthetics stimulate the CNS. For example, although drowsiness is the most frequent complaint, lidocaine may produce dysphoria or euphoria and muscle twitching at a blood concentration of 5 μg/ml. However, both lidocaine and procaine may produce loss of consciousness that is preceded only by symptoms of sedation (*see* Covino, 1985). While shared to some extent by other local anesthetics, cocaine has a particularly prominent effect on mood and behavior (*see* Van Dyke and Byck, 1982; Fishman *et al.*, 1983). These effects of cocaine and its potential for abuse are discussed in Chapter 23.

Neuromuscular Junction and Ganglionic Synapse. Local anesthetics also affect transmission at the neuromuscular junction. Close intra-arterial injection of 0.2 mg of procaine into the cat's tibialis anterior muscle reduces twitches and tetanic responses evoked by maximal motor-nerve volleys, and the response of the muscle to injected acetylcholine. The muscle, however, responds normally to direct electrical stimulation. Other work suggests that procaine also diminishes the release of acetylcholine by the motor-nerve endings (*see* de Jong, 1977). Similar effects are obtained when procaine is added to the fluid perfusing an autonomic ganglion. The effects of procaine and physostigmine are antagonistic, and those of procaine and curare additive. The postsynaptic action of procaine, however, differs from that of curare in that the end-plate current is much prolonged by local anesthetics and has a multicomponent time course of decay (*see* Ruff, 1977). Local anesthetics do not interfere with transmission by simply competing with acetylcholine for the receptor. Rather, it appears that a complex of transmitter, receptor, and local anesthetic is formed that seems to have negligible conductance (Ruff, 1977).

Cardiovascular System. Following systemic absorption, local anesthetics act on the cardiovascular system (*see* Feldman *et al.*, 1982; Covino, 1985). The primary site of action is the myocardium, where decreases in electrical excitability, conduction rate, and force of contraction occur. In addition, most local anesthetics cause arteriolar dilatation. The cardiovascular effects are usually seen only after high systemic concentrations are attained and effects on the CNS are produced (Scott, 1981). However, on rare occasion small amounts of anesthetic employed for simple infiltration anesthesia will cause cardiovascular collapse and death. The exact mechanism is unknown, but it probably results from cardiac arrest due to either an action on the pacemaker or the sudden onset of ventricular fibrillation. Such a reaction may follow inadvertent intravascular administration of the agent, particularly if epinephrine is present in the preparation. Both the ionized and the nonionized forms of the local anesthetic may be important for these effects.

Studies on isolated atrial and ventricular muscle reveal that procaine resembles quinidine in its cardiac action in that it increases the effective refractory period, raises the threshold for stimulation, and prolongs conduction time. These cardiac actions and the accompanying characteristic changes in the ECG would be of therapeutic interest were it not for the rapid metabolic destruction of procaine and its propensity to cause central stimulation. Studies of procaine congeners led to the introduction of *procainamide,* the cardiac actions of which are fully discussed in Chapter 31.

Smooth Muscle. The local anesthetics depress contractions in the intact bowel and in strips of isolated intestine (*see* Zipf and Dittmann, 1971). There is, however, little correlation between anesthetic potency and antispasmodic efficacy. They also relax vascular and bronchial smooth muscle, although low concentrations may initially produce contraction (*see* Covino, 1985).

Spinal and epidural anesthesia, as well as instillation of local anesthetics into the peritoneal cavity, cause sympathetic nervous system paralysis that can result in increased tone of gastrointestinal musculature. Most local anesthetics may increase the resting tone and decrease the contractions of isolated human uterine muscle; however, uterine contractions are seldom depressed during intrapartum regional anesthesia (de Jong, 1977).

Hypersensitivity to Local Anesthetics. Rare individuals are hypersensitive to local anesthetics. This may manifest itself as an allergic dermatitis, a typical asthmatic attack, or a fatal anaphylactic reaction (*see* de Jong, 1977). Hypersensitivity seems to occur most prominently with local anesthetics of the *ester type* and frequently extends to chemically related compounds. For example, individuals sensitive to procaine may also react to structurally similar compounds (*e.g.,* tetracaine). Although agents of the amide type are essentially free of this problem, solutions of such agents may contain preservatives that are not (Covino, 1985). Certain antihistamines are occasionally used as local anesthetics for individuals who have become hypersensitive to all the conventional agents. These antihistamines presumably have the general structural features necessary for local anesthetic activity without sharing the specific antigenic determinants of the conventional drugs.

Fate of Local Anesthetics. The metabolic fate of local anesthetics is of great practical importance because their toxicity depends largely on the balance between their rate of absorption and their rate of destruction. As noted above, the rate of absorption can be reduced considerably by the incorporation of a vasoconstrictor agent in the anesthetic solution. However, the rate of destruction of local anesthetics varies greatly, and this is a major factor in determining the safety of a particular agent. Binding of the anesthetic to tissues reduces the amount that appears in the systemic circulation and, consequently, reduces toxicity. For example, in intravenous regional anesthesia of an extremity, about half of the original anesthetic dose is still tissue bound 30 minutes after release of the tourniquet (de Jong, 1977).

Many of the common local anesthetics (*e.g.,* procaine and tetracaine) are esters, and their toxicity is usually lost as the result of hydrolysis. This is accomplished primarily by a plasma esterase, probably plasma cholinesterase; the liver also participates. Since spinal fluid contains little or no esterase, anesthesia produced by the intrathecal injection of an anesthetic agent will persist until the local anesthetic agent has been absorbed into the blood.

The amide-linked local anesthetics are, in general, degraded by the hepatic endoplasmic reticulum, the initial reactions involving N-dealkylation and subsequent hydrolysis (Arthur, 1985). However, with prilocaine the initial step is hydrolytic, forming *o*-toluidine metabolites that can cause methemoglobinemia. Animals with experimentally produced hepatic damage are much more susceptible to the toxic actions of local anesthetics; the extensive use of amide-linked local anesthetics in patients with severe hepatic damage should be avoided. The amide-linked local anesthetics are extensively (55 to 95%) bound to plasma proteins, particularly α_1-acid glycoprotein. Many factors increase (cancer, trauma, myocardial infarction, smoking, uremia) or decrease (oral contraceptive agents) the concentration of this protein in plasma. This results in changes in the amount of anesthetic delivered to the liver for metabolism, thus influencing systemic toxicity (*see* Arthur, 1985). Uptake by the lung may also play an important role in the distribution of amide-linked local anesthetics in the body (Rothstein *et al.*, 1983; Arthur, 1985).

COCAINE

Source. Cocaine occurs in the leaves of *Erythroxylon coca* and other species of *Erythroxylon*, trees indigenous to Peru and Bolivia, where the leaves have been used for centuries by the natives to increase endurance and promote a sense of well-being.

Chemistry. Cocaine is benzoylmethylecgonine. Ecgonine is an amino alcohol base closely related to tropine, the amino alcohol in atropine. Cocaine is thus an ester of benzoic acid and a nitrogen-containing base. It has the fundamental structure previously described for the synthetic local anesthetics (*see* Table 15–1).

Pharmacological Actions. The most important action of cocaine clinically is its ability to block the initiation or conduction of the nerve impulse following local application. Its most striking systemic effect is stimulation of the CNS. In addition, cocaine has numerous important side actions.

Central Nervous System. Cocaine stimulates the CNS generally. In man, this is manifested first in a feeling of well-being and euphoria; sometimes dysphoria may result. These effects may be accompanied by garrulousness, restlessness, and excitement. After small amounts of cocaine, motor activity is well coordinated; however, as the dose is increased, tremors and eventually clonic-tonic convulsions result. The vasomotor and vomiting centers may also share in the stimulation, and emesis may result. Central stimulation is soon followed by depression. Eventually the vital medullary centers are depressed, and death results from respiratory failure. The cerebral actions of cocaine and the subject of *cocaine abuse* are discussed in Chapter 23.

Cardiovascular System. Small doses of cocaine given systemically may slow the heart as a result of central vagal stimulation, but after moderate doses the heart rate is increased. The increased cardiac rate probably results from increased central sympathetic stimulation as well as from the peripheral effects of cocaine on the sympathetic nervous system, as discussed below. Although the blood pressure may finally fall, there is at first a prominent rise in blood pressure due to sympathetically mediated tachycardia and vasoconstriction. A large intravenous dose of cocaine may cause immediate death from cardiac failure due to a direct toxic action on the heart muscle.

Skeletal Muscle. There is no evidence that cocaine increases the intrinsic strength of muscular contraction. The relief of fatigue by cocaine seems to result from central stimulation, which masks the sensation of fatigue.

Body Temperature. Cocaine is markedly pyrogenic. The increased muscular activity attending stimulation by cocaine augments heat production; vasoconstriction decreases heat loss. Also, cocaine may have a direct action on the heat-regulating centers, for the onset of cocaine fever is often heralded by a chill, which indicates that the body is adjusting its temperature to a higher level. Cocaine pyrexia is often a striking feature of cocaine poisoning and can easily be elicited in animals by sublethal doses.

Sympathetic Nervous System. Cocaine potentiates the responses of sympathetically innervated organs to norepinephrine, sympathetic nerve stimulation, and, to a lesser degree, epinephrine. It is well established that cocaine blocks the uptake of catecholamines at adrenergic nerve endings; this uptake process is primarily responsible for terminating the actions of both adrenergic impulses and circulating catecholamines (*see* Chapter 4). Other local anesthetics do not share this capability to alter the uptake of norepinephrine, to produce sensitization to catecholamines, or to produce vasoconstriction and mydriasis. The peripheral component of the cardioacceleration produced by cocaine is probably of similar origin.

Local Anesthetic Actions. The most important local action of cocaine is its ability to block nerve conduction. Cocaine was once used extensively in ophthalmological procedures, but it causes sloughing of the corneal epithelium. Because of this, and because of its potential for abuse, cocaine is now restricted to topical use, especially in the upper respiratory passages. Even this use may be accompanied by severe toxicity.

Absorption, Fate, and Excretion. Cocaine is absorbed from all sites of application, including mucous membranes and the gastrointestinal mucosa. Absorption is enhanced in the presence of inflammation, and systemic effects of the drug may thereby be markedly increased. For example, such may occur if cocaine is used in cystoscopy when the urinary bladder is inflamed.

After absorption, cocaine is degraded by plasma esterases (Van Dyke *et al.*, 1976) and, at least in some animals, by hepatic enzymes (*see* de Jong, 1977). Small amounts are excreted unchanged in the urine. The half-life of cocaine in the plasma after oral or nasal administration is approximately 1 hour (Van Dyke *et al.*, 1978).

Tolerance, Abuse, and Acute Poisoning. As noted, cocaine is often abused for its effects on the CNS. The symptoms and treatment of poisoning and the misuse of cocaine are discussed in Chapter 23.

Preparations and Dosage. *Cocaine* and *cocaine hydrochloride* are the official preparations of the alkaloid. Cocaine is not prepared legitimately to be used internally or injected. Solutions employed clinically for surface anesthesia usually vary from 1 to 4%, depending on the mucosa being anesthetized. Epinephrine is sometimes incorporated in these solutions. Occasionally, dry cocaine powder is moistened with epinephrine solution to form so-called cocaine mud for use on the nasal mucosa. In view of the dangerous potentiative interaction between cocaine and catecholamines, this practice is to be condemned.

Cocaine is included among the drugs controlled by the federal drug-abuse regulations (*see* Appendix I).

LIDOCAINE

Lidocaine, introduced in 1948, is one of the most widely used local anesthetics. Its chemical structure is shown in Table 15–1.

Pharmacological Actions. The pharmacological actions that lidocaine shares with other local anesthetic drugs have been presented. Lidocaine produces more prompt, more intense, longer-lasting, and more extensive anesthesia than does an equal concentration of procaine. Unlike procaine it is an aminoethylamide. It is an agent of choice, therefore, in individuals sensitive to ester-type local anesthetics.

Absorption, Fate, and Excretion. Lidocaine is relatively quickly absorbed after parenteral administration and from the gastrointestinal tract (*see* Boyes *et al.*, 1971; Hansson, 1971; Keenaghan and Boyes, 1972). Although it is effective when used without any vasoconstrictor, in the presence of epinephrine the rate of absorption and the toxicity are thereby decreased and the duration of action is prolonged. Lidocaine is metabolized in the liver by mixed-function oxidases by dealkylation to monoethylglycine and xylidide. The latter compound retains significant local anesthetic and toxic activity. In man about 75% of xylidide is excreted in the urine as the further metabolite, 4-hydroxy-2,6-dimethylaniline (*see* Arthur, 1985).

Toxicity. In experimental animals, overdosage of lidocaine produces death from ventricular fibrillation or cardiac arrest; procaine, on the other hand, tends to depress respiration rather than the circulation (de Jong, 1977). A notable side effect of lidocaine is sleepiness. There is also a high incidence of dizziness, which may be caused by a metabolite rather than by lidocaine itself (Boyes *et al.*, 1971).

Preparations. *Lidocaine hydrochloride* (*lignocaine;* XYLOCAINE, others) is very soluble in water and alcohol. Preparations include injections and a cream, ointment, jelly, topical solution, and topical aerosol. Market preparations (0.5 to 5%), available in ampuls, vials, or prefilled syringes with and without epinephrine (1:50,000 to 1:200,000), are suitable for infiltration (0.5 to 1%), block (1 to 2%), and topical mucosal anesthesia (1 to 5%).

Clinical Uses. Lidocaine has a variety of clinical uses as a local anesthetic. In addition, lidocaine is employed intravenously as an antiarrhythmic agent, as described in Chapter 31.

PROCAINE

Procaine was synthesized by Einhorn in 1905 and introduced under the trade name NOVOCAIN. It is still a useful local anesthetic. The chemical structure is presented in Table 15–1.

Pharmacological Actions. The pharmacological actions that procaine shares with other local anesthetic drugs have been presented. Procaine and many other ester-type local anesthetics are hydrolyzed in the body to produce para-aminobenzoic acid, which inhibits the action of sulfonamides. This fact is occasionally of practical importance. Procaine and its congeners also interfere with the chemical determination of sulfonamide concentration in biological fluids.

Absorption, Fate, and Excretion. Procaine is readily absorbed following parenteral administration and thus does not long remain at the site of injection. In order to retard absorption, vasoconstrictor drugs may be added to procaine solutions. Following absorption, procaine, like the other ester-type drugs, is rapidly hydrolyzed by a plasma esterase.

Preparations. *Procaine hydrochloride* (NOVOCAIN) occurs as a white crystalline powder that is freely soluble in water. Market preparations include ampuls or vials of a 1, 2, or 10% solution without epinephrine; a vasoconstrictor may be added when the preparation is used. Solutions usually contain 0.25 to 0.5% procaine for infiltration anesthesia, 0.5 to 2% for peripheral nerve block, and 10% for spinal anesthesia.

Clinical Uses. Procaine has a variety of clinical uses as a local anesthetic, which are discussed below.

Procaine can form poorly soluble salts or conjugate with other drugs and prolong their action. This property is unrelated to the ability of procaine to produce local anesthesia. For example, after the intramuscular injection of procaine penicillin G, the antibiotic is absorbed very slowly so that detectable concentrations of penicillin exist in the blood and urine for prolonged periods, as discussed in more detail in Chapter 50. The possibility of allergy to procaine must be considered when hypersensitivity to such preparations occurs. The amount of procaine given with large intramuscular doses of procaine penicillin G can also cause CNS toxicity.

OTHER SYNTHETIC LOCAL ANESTHETICS

The number of synthetic local anesthetics is so large that it is impractical to consider all of them. Therefore, discussion will be limited mainly to those that are official in the USP.

Some local anesthetic agents are too toxic to be given by injection. Their use is restricted to topical application to the eye, the mucous membranes, or the skin. Many local anesthetics are suitable, however, for infiltration or injection to produce nerve block; some of them are also useful for topical application. The main categories of local anesthetics are given below; the agents are listed alphabetically.

LOCAL ANESTHETICS SUITABLE FOR INJECTION

Bupivacaine hydrochloride (MARCAINE) is an amide type of local anesthetic; its structure is identical to that of mepivacaine except that a butyl group replaces the methyl substituent on the amino nitrogen. It is a potent agent capable of producing prolonged anesthesia. Its mean duration of action is greater than that of tetracaine, while the toxicity of the two compounds is similar. Bupivacaine hydrochloride is available in solutions for injection (0.25, 0.5, and 0.75%) with or without epinephrine (1:200,000). The 0.75% solution should not be used for obstetrical anesthesia.

Chloroprocaine hydrochloride (NESACAINE) is a halogenated derivative of procaine, the pharmacological properties of which it shares almost completely. Its anesthetic potency is at least twice as great as that of procaine, and its toxicity is lower because of its more rapid metabolism. A question has recently been raised about the possibility of neurological toxicity from the use of chloroprocaine (Ravindran *et al.*, 1982; *see* Covino, 1985). Chloroprocaine hydrochloride is available in solutions for injection (1.0, 2.0, and 3.0%).

Dibucaine hydrochloride (cinchocaine; NUPERCAINE) is a quinoline derivative. It is one of the most potent, most toxic, and longest acting of the commonly employed local anesthetics. It is about 15 times as potent and as toxic as procaine, and its anesthetic action lasts about three times as long. Dibucaine hydrochloride is infrequently used by injection.

Etidocaine hydrochloride (DURANEST) is a long-acting derivative of lidocaine. The time required for induction of anesthesia with etidocaine is about the same as that for lidocaine, but its analgesic action lasts two to three times longer (*see* de Jong, 1977). It is not employed for spinal anesthesia, but is useful for epidural and for all types of infiltration and regional anesthesia. Etidocaine hydrochloride is marketed in solutions for injection (1.0%) with or without epinephrine (1:200,000) and in a 1.5% solution with epinephrine (1:200,000).

Mepivacaine hydrochloride (CARBOCAINE) is a local anesthetic of the amide type (*see* Table 15–1). Its pharmacological properties are similar to those of lidocaine, which it resembles chemically. Its action is more rapid in onset and somewhat more prolonged than that of lidocaine. It has been employed for all types of infiltration and regional nerve block anesthesia as well as for spinal anesthesia. Mepivacaine hydrochloride is marketed in solutions for injection (1.0, 1.5, 2.0, and 3.0% without, and 2% with, levonordefrin as a vasoconstrictor).

Prilocaine hydrochloride (CITANEST) is a local anesthetic of the amide type. Its pharmacological properties resemble those of lidocaine. Its onset and duration of action are longer than those of lidocaine. Like lidocaine, it may produce sleepiness. A unique toxic aftereffect is *methemoglobinemia*, and its use is declining for this reason. It has been employed for all types of infiltration and regional nerve block anesthesia as well as for spinal anesthesia. Prilocaine hydrochloride is marketed in solutions for injection (1.0, 2.0, and 3.0%).

Tetracaine hydrochloride (PONTOCAINE) is a derivative of para-aminobenzoic acid (*see* Table 15–1). It is about ten times more toxic and more active than procaine after intravenous injection. For topical anesthesia of the eye, a 0.5% solution or ointment is used; for the mucous membranes of the nose and throat, a 2.0% solution. For spinal anesthesia, a total dose of 5 to 20 mg is adequate. Tetracaine has been extensively employed for continuous caudal anesthesia, but its onset of action at this site is very slow. The usual initial dose is 30 ml of a 0.25% solution. The effects are longer lasting than those of procaine. Tetracaine hydrochloride is available in solutions and in ampuls containing the dry salt. An ophthalmic solution of tetracaine and an ophthalmic ointment of 0.5% tetracaine base in white petrolatum are also marketed.

LOCAL ANESTHETICS LARGELY RESTRICTED TO OPHTHALMOLOGICAL USE

While certain of the agents described above can be used in the eye, the following local anesthetic agents are largely restricted to the production of corneal anesthesia. Their main advantage over the prototype, cocaine, is that they produce little or no mydriasis or corneal injury.

Benoxinate hydrochloride is a benzoic acid ester related to procaine. A single instillation of 1 or 2 drops of a 0.4% solution produces within 60 seconds a sufficient degree of anesthesia to permit Schiötz tonometry. It is marketed as a 0.4% solution.

Proparacaine hydrochloride (ALCAINE, OPHTHAINE) is a benzoate ester, but it is chemically distinct from procaine, benoxinate, and tetracaine. This difference in chemical structure may explain the lack of cross-sensitization between proparacaine and other local anesthetic agents. It is about as potent as tetracaine. Unlike some topical anesthetics, proparacaine hydrochloride produces little or no initial irritation. It is available in a 0.5% ophthalmic solution for topical application.

LOCAL ANESTHETICS USED MAINLY TO ANESTHETIZE MUCOUS MEMBRANES AND THE SKIN

Some anesthetics are either too irritating or too ineffective to be applied to the eye. However, they are useful as topical anesthetic agents on the skin and mucous membranes. These preparations are effective in the symptomatic relief of anal and genital pruritus, ivy poisoning, and numerous other acute and chronic dermatoses.

Cyclomethycaine sulfate (SURFACAINE) acts on damaged or diseased skin and on the mucosa of the rectum and genitourinary system, but it is relatively ineffective on the mucous membranes of the mouth, nose, bronchi, and eye. The compound is marketed as a cream (0.5%), an ointment (1.0%), and a jelly for urethral application (0.75%).

Dyclonine hydrochloride (DYCLONE) has a rapid onset of action and a duration of effect comparable to that of procaine. It is absorbed through the skin and mucous membranes. The compound is used as a 0.5 to 1.0% solution for topical anesthesia in otolaryngology and for anogenital anesthesia.

Hexylcaine hydrochloride (CYCLAINE) was previously used for infiltration, spinal, topical, and nerve block anesthesia. It is about twice as potent as procaine. Hexylcaine hydrochloride is available for topical application as a 5% solution.

Pramoxine hydrochloride (TRONOTHANE) is a surface anesthetic agent that is not of the benzoate ester type. Its distinct chemical structure is likely to minimize the danger of cross-sensitivity reactions in patients allergic to other local anesthetics. Pramoxine produces satisfactory surface anesthesia and is reasonably well tolerated on the skin and mucous membranes. It is too irritating to be used on the eye or in the nose. Preparations are available for topical application as a 1% cream, jelly, or lotion.

ANESTHETICS OF LOW SOLUBILITY

Some local anesthetics are poorly soluble in water and, consequently, too slowly absorbed to be toxic. They can be applied directly to wounds and ulcerated surfaces, where they remain localized for long periods of time to produce a sustained anesthetic action. Chemically, they are esters of para-aminobenzoic acid that lack the terminal amino group possessed by the previously described local anesthetics. The most important members of the series are *benzocaine* (*ethyl aminobenzoate;* AMERICAINE ANESTHETIC) and *butamben picrate* (*butyl aminobenzoate;* BUTESIN PICRATE). Benzocaine is identical to procaine structurally, except that it lacks the terminal diethylamino group. They may be applied as dusting powders, undiluted or diluted with sterile talc. They are soluble in oil and may be incorporated in oily solutions, ointments, and suppositories.

Some salts of the tertiary amino group of local anesthetics are very insoluble. For example, the hydroiodide salt of tetracaine may produce anesthesia of 45-hours' duration when sprinkled in a surgical wound (Cherney, 1963).

TETRODOTOXIN AND SAXITOXIN

These toxins are two of the most potent poisons known, the minimal lethal dose of each in the mouse being about 8 μg/kg. Both toxins are responsible for outbreaks of fatal poisoning in man. Tetrodotoxin is found in the gonads and other tissues of some fish of the order Tetraodontiformes (to which the Japanese *fugu,* or puffer fish, belongs); it also occurs in the skin of some newts of the family Salamandridae and of the Costa Rican frog *Atelopus.* Saxitoxin, and possibly some related toxins, are elaborated by the dinoflagellates *Gonyaulax catenella* and *Gonyaulax tamerensis,* and are retained in the tissues of clams and other shellfish that eat these organisms. Given the right conditions of temperature and light the *Gonyaulax* may multiply so rapidly as to discolor the ocean— hence the term *red tide.* Shellfish feeding on *Gonyaulax* at this time become extremely toxic to man and are responsible for the periodic outbreaks of *paralytic shellfish poisoning* (*see* Kao, 1972; Ritchie, 1980).

Although the toxins are chemically different from each other, their *mechanism of action* seems identical (*see* Ritchie, 1980). Both toxins, in nanomolar concentrations, specifically block the sodium channels in the membranes of excitable cells. As a result, the sodium currents are inhibited and the action potential is blocked. Blockade of vasomotor nerves, together with a relaxation of vascular smooth muscle, seems to be responsible for the hypotension that is characteristic of tetrodotoxin poisoning (Kao, 1972). Both toxins cause death by paralysis of the respiratory muscles. The *treatment* of severe cases of poisoning therefore requires artificial ventilation. Early gastric lavage and therapy to support the blood pressure are also indicated. If the patient survives paralytic shellfish poisoning for 24 hours, the prognosis is good (*see* Ogura, 1971; Schantz, 1971).

Apart from toxicological considerations, there are two other reasons for current interest in these toxins. First, since the toxins are much more specific and potent than the local anesthetics described above, they might serve as prototypes for new chemical classes of local anesthetics. Indeed, in animal experiments a combination of saxitoxin and a local anesthetic produces nerve block of longer duration than does either agent alone (Adams *et al.,* 1976). Second, they are important in the analysis of the molecular basis of the action potential. Experiments with radioactively labeled toxins have been used to determine the density of sodium channels in a variety of nerves (*see* Ritchie, 1980).

CLINICAL USES OF LOCAL ANESTHETICS

Local anesthesia is the loss of sensation without the loss of consciousness, and central control of vital functions is not impaired. A major advantage, therefore, is that the physiological trespass associated with general anesthesia is avoided. Local anesthetics are not, however, devoid of the potential to produce deleterious side effects. The choice of a local anesthetic and the technic of its use are the determinants of such toxicity.

The following discussion concerns the pharmacological and physiological consequences of the use of local anesthetics; these are evaluated in terms of the potential advantages and disadvantages of local anesthetics under clinical conditions. Technics for the administration of local anesthetics are described in detail elsewhere (Moore, 1965; Bromage, 1978).

SURFACE ANESTHESIA

Anesthesia of mucous membranes of the nose, mouth, throat, tracheobronchial tree, esophagus, and genitourinary tract can be produced by direct application of aqueous solutions of salts of many local anesthetics. Tetracaine (2%), lidocaine (2 to 5%), and cocaine (4%) are most often used. Cocaine is used only in the nose, nasopharynx, mouth, and throat. Other local anesthetics are clinically unsatisfactory; they penetrate mucous membranes too poorly. Cocaine has the unique advantage of producing vasoconstriction as well as anesthesia. The shrinking of mucous membranes decreases operative bleeding while improving surgical visualization. Comparable vasoconstriction can be achieved with other local anesthetics by the addition of a low concentration of a vasoconstrictor such as phenylephrine (0.005%). Phenylephrine should not be added to solutions of cocaine. Epinephrine, topically applied, has no significant local effect and does not prolong the duration of action of local anesthetics applied to mucous membranes because it penetrates mucous membranes too poorly. Maximal safe total dosages for topical anesthesia in a healthy 70-kg adult are 750 mg for lidocaine and 50 mg for cocaine and tetracaine.

Peak anesthetic effect following topical application of cocaine or lidocaine occurs within 2 to 5 minutes (3 to 8 minutes with tetracaine), and anesthesia lasts for 30 to 45 minutes (30 to 60 minutes with tetracaine). Anesthesia is entirely superficial; it does not extend to submucosal structures. This technic does not alleviate pain or discomfort from pressure or distortion of adjacent structures.

Local anesthetics are rapidly absorbed into the circulation following topical application to mucous membranes. Such topical anesthesia thus always carries the risk of systemic toxic reactions. Absorption is particularly rapid when local anesthetics are applied to the tracheobronchial tree. Concentrations in blood after instillation of local anesthetics into the airway are nearly the same as those that follow intravenous injection. Blood concentrations are lower and peak values are reached more slowly when a given amount of topical anesthetic is applied over a longer period of time. When topical anesthetics are applied to the mouth, nose, or throat, the patient should be cautioned to expectorate the excess solution of the anesthetic to avoid excessive absorption. Surface anesthetics for the skin and cornea have been described above.

INFILTRATION ANESTHESIA

Infiltration anesthesia consists in injection of a solution of local anesthetic directly into the tissue to be incised or mechanically stimulated. Infiltration anesthesia can be so superficial as to include only the skin. It can also include deeper structures, including intra-abdominal organs when these, too, are infiltrated.

The duration of infiltration anesthesia can be approximately doubled by the addition of epinephrine (1:200,000; 5 μg/ml) to the solution. By decreasing the rate of absorption of drug into the blood stream, epinephrine also decreases peak concentrations of local anesthetics in blood and the rate at which these are achieved. The likelihood of adverse systemic reactions is thereby proportionately decreased. Epinephrine-containing solutions should not, however, be injected into tissues supplied by end arteries, for example, fingers and toes, ears, the nose, and the penis. To do so may result in gangrene. For the same reason, epinephrine should be avoided in solutions injected intracutaneously. Since epinephrine is also absorbed into the circulation, it should not be used in patients in whom adrenergic stimulation is undesirable, especially those with ventricular arrhythmias, hypertension, or hyperthyroidism.

The local anesthetics most frequently used for infiltration anesthesia are lidocaine (0.5 to 1.0%), procaine (0.5 to 1.0%), and bupivacaine (0.125 to 0.25%). When used without epinephrine, up to 4.5 mg/kg of lidocaine, 7 mg/kg of procaine, or 2.5 mg/kg of bupivacaine can be employed in adults. When epinephrine is added, these amounts can be increased by one third.

The advantage of infiltration anesthesia and other regional anesthetic technics is that it is possible to provide good anesthesia without disruption of normal bodily functions. The chief disadvantage of infiltration anesthesia is that relatively large amounts of drug must be used to anesthetize relatively small areas. This is no problem with minor surgery. When major surgery is performed, however, the amount of local anesthetic that is required may make systemic toxic reactions likely. Whereas intra-abdominal procedures are technically feasible under infiltration anesthesia, substantially better operating conditions are more readily and safely achieved with lesser amounts of local anesthetic administered by other regional technics or with general anesthesia.

FIELD BLOCK ANESTHESIA

Field block anesthesia is produced by subcutaneous injection of a solution of local anesthetic in such a manner as to interrupt nerve transmission proximal to the site to be anesthetized. For example, subcutaneous infiltration of the proximal portion of volar surface of the forearm results in an extensive area of cutaneous anesthesia that starts 2 to 3 cm distal to the site of injection. The same principle can be applied with particular benefit to the scalp, the anterior abdominal wall, and the lower extremity.

The drugs used and the concentrations and doses recommended are the same as for infiltration anesthesia. The advantage of field block anesthesia is that less drug can be used to provide a greater area of anesthesia than when infiltration anesthesia is used. Knowledge of the relevant neuroanatomy is obviously essential for successful field block anesthesia.

NERVE BLOCK ANESTHESIA

Injection of a solution of a local anesthetic into or about individual peripheral nerves or nerve plexuses produces even greater areas of anesthesia with a smaller amount of drug than do the technics described above. Blockade of mixed peripheral nerves and nerve plexuses also usually anesthetizes somatic motor nerves, a matter of importance in certain types of surgery. The areas of sensory and motor denervation usually start several centimeters distal to the site of injection. Particularly useful are blocks of the brachial plexus for procedures on the upper extremity distal to insertion of the deltoid, intercostal nerve blocks for anesthesia and relaxation of the anterior abdominal wall, cervical plexus block for surgery of the neck, sciatic and femoral nerve blocks for surgery distal to the knee, blocks of individual nerves at the wrist and at the ankle or blocks of individual nerves such as the median or ulnar at the elbow, and blocks of sensory cranial nerves.

The onset of sensory anesthesia following injection about a peripheral nerve depends on the pK_a of the anesthetic, that is, the amount that exists in the unprotonated form at a tissue pH of 7.4. The onset of action of lidocaine occurs in about 3 minutes; 35% of lidocaine is in the basic form at this pH. Onset of action of bupivacaine requires about 15 minutes; only 5 to 10% of bupivacaine is not protonated at pH 7.4. Latency is also determined by the need for diffusion of the agent from its site of injection to its site of action. Diffusion is more important in determining rapidity of onset when nerve plexuses are blocked than when single nerves are anesthetized. The latency of the anesthetic effect of lidocaine injected about the ulnar nerve is 3 minutes, but this value is nearly 15 minutes when the drug is injected about the brachial plexus. The latency of bupivacaine is over 20 minutes in brachial plexus block.

Duration of nerve block anesthesia depends upon the physical characteristics of the local anesthetic used. Especially important are lipid solubility and protein binding. In general, local anesthetics can be divided into three categories: those such as procaine with a short duration of action (20 to 45 minutes) following anesthetization of a mixed peripheral nerve; those with an intermediate duration of action (60 to 120 minutes), such as lidocaine, mepivacaine, and prilocaine; and those with a long duration of action (400 to 450 minutes), such as tetracaine, bupivacaine, and etidocaine. Duration of nerve block anesthesia can be extended by increasing the amount of drug injected. However, this is of relatively limited value because the possibility of systemic toxic reactions is increased more than is the duration of action of the drug. Increasing the volume of anesthetic injected also increases the likelihood of spread of the solution to nearby structures that one may not wish to affect. In an attempt to produce long-lasting anesthesia with rapid onset, combinations of agents such as lidocaine and bupivacaine have been employed. However, any theoretical advantages may be thwarted by practical issues, such as the pH of commercial solutions relative to the pK_a of the local anesthetics. Duration of action is more safely prolonged by the addition of epinephrine.

The types of nerve fibers that are blocked when a local anesthetic is injected about a mixed peripheral nerve depend upon the concentration of drug used, nerve-fiber size, internodal distance, and frequency and pattern of nerve-impulse transmission (*see* above). Anatomical factors are similarly important. A mixed peripheral nerve or nerve trunk consists of individual nerves surrounded by an investing epineurium. The vascular supply is usually centrally located. When a local anesthetic is deposited about a peripheral nerve, it diffuses from the outer surface toward the core along a concentration gradient (Winnie *et al.*, 1977). Consequently, nerves located in the outer mantle of the mixed nerve are blocked first. These fibers are usually distributed to more proximal anatomical structures than are those situated near the core of the mixed nerve. If the volume and concentration of local anesthetic solution deposited about the nerve are adequate, the local anesthetic will eventually diffuse inwardly in amounts adequate to block even the most centrally located fibers. Lesser amounts of drug will block only nerves in the mantle and smaller and more sensitive central fibers. Furthermore, since uptake of local anesthetics usually occurs primarily in the core of a mixed nerve or nerve trunk where the vascular supply is located, the duration of blockade of centrally located nerves is shorter than that of more peripherally situated fibers.

Which local anesthetic is to be used for a nerve block, as well as the amount and concentration to be used, depends upon which nerves or plexuses are to be blocked, the types of fibers to be blocked, the duration of anesthesia required, and the size and physical status of the patient. Procaine (0.5 to 2.0% solution) and lidocaine (1.0 to 2.0% solution) can be used in the amounts recommended above under Infiltration Anesthesia. Mepivacaine (up to 7 mg/kg of a 1.0 to 3.0% solution) provides anesthesia that lasts as long as that from lidocaine. Bupivacaine (0.25 to 0.75% solution) can be used when long duration of action is required. Chloroprocaine (1 to 2% solution) is especially useful when short duration of effect is desired; up to 20 mg/kg may be injected because chloroprocaine is so rapidly hydrolyzed by plasma cholinesterase. As with other regional anesthetic technics, addition of 1:200,000 epinephrine prolongs duration and allows the use of greater amounts of local anesthetic.

Peak concentrations of local anesthetics in blood and the potential for systemic reactions depend upon the amount injected, the physical characteristics of the local anesthetic, and whether epinephrine is used. They also are determined by the rate of blood flow to the site of injection. This is of particular importance in nerve block anesthesia. Peak concentrations of lidocaine in blood following injection of 400 mg for intercostal nerve blocks average 7 μg/ml; the same amount of lidocaine used for block of the brachial plexus results in peak concentrations in blood of approximately 3 μg/ml (Covino and Vassallo, 1976). The amounts of local anesthetic that can be safely injected as outlined in the preceding paragraph must, therefore, be adjusted according to the anatomical site of the nerve(s) to be blocked. Multiple nerve blocks (*e.g.*, intercostal block) require reduction in the amount of anesthetic that can be safely given because the surface area for absorption is increased. Nerve blocks in richly vascular areas must also be performed with less drug.

Successful nerve blocks depend upon thorough knowledge of neuroanatomy. Armed with such knowledge, however, the expert anesthesiologist can predictably block any nerve by using one of two technics. He can place the needle for injection in the same fascial compartment in which the nerve to be blocked lies and then inject a relatively large volume of anesthetic solution. Diffusion of the solution is restricted by anatomical boundaries, and an effective concentration can thus be delivered to the nerve. Alternatively, the anesthesiologist can assure himself that the tip of the needle lies immediately adjacent to the nerve to be blocked. Smaller amounts of local anesthetic need then be injected because of reliance on accurate placement of the drug. Assurance that the tip of the needle lies immediately adjacent to the nerve requires that a paresthesia be elicited, and the most accurate placement is ensured when a paresthesia is produced by injection of the anesthetic solution.

INTRAVENOUS REGIONAL ANESTHESIA

Intravenous regional anesthesia consists in the injection of local anesthetic solution into a vein of an extremity previously exsanguinated with an Esmarch bandage and kept exsanguinated by a pneumatic tourniquet placed on the upper part of the extremity and inflated above arterial pressure. Lidocaine (1.5 mg/kg of 0.5% solution) is frequently used for intravenous regional anesthesia of the upper extremity. Onset of anesthesia occurs in 2 to 3 minutes. At the end of surgery when the tourniquet is released, approximately 15 to 30% of the lidocaine injected into the isolated extremity enters the systemic circulation. Peak concentrations in blood, reached within 4 to 5 minutes, are less than those observed following brachial plexus or lumbar epidural block. Bupivacaine is not approved for use in intravenous regional anesthesia.

Intravenous regional anesthesia is not as effective in the lower as it is in the upper extremity. In the latter case it is used for operations at the level of or distal to the elbow. Intravenous regional anesthesia cannot be used when fractures or other tender lesions exist in the extremity because of pain produced by exsanguination with the Esmarch bandage. The safety of intravenous regional anesthesia depends upon maintenance of pressure in the tourniquet adequate to occlude arterial flow at all times.

SPINAL ANESTHESIA

Spinal anesthesia is produced by injection of a local anesthetic into the lumbar subarachnoid space below the termination of the cord (second lumbar vertebra). Spread of the agent within the subarachnoid space and, thus, the level of anesthesia are controlled by the injection of solutions that are heavier or lighter than cerebrospinal fluid; the patient is then placed in the head-up or head-down position. Addition of 10% glucose solution to that of the local anesthetic produces a solution that is heavier than cerebrospinal fluid (hyperbaric spinal anesthesia). With the patient in the head-down position the glucose–local anesthetic solution then ascends in the subarachnoid space. The height that it achieves is determined by the volume of solution injected and the degree of tilt of the patient. Hyperbaric solutions remain in the distal subarachnoid space when injected with the patient sitting or in the head-up position. Hypobaric spinal anesthesia is produced by addition of sterile distilled water to the solution of local anesthetic. These mixtures are used less frequently than are hyperbaric solutions.

The concentration of local anesthetic in cerebrospinal fluid decreases rapidly after injection as the drug is bound to tissue and absorbed into the vascular system. Furthermore, within 10 to 15 minutes a hyperbaric solution becomes isobaric. At this point changes in position of the patient no longer affect distribution of the local anesthetic within the subarachnoid space. The level of anesthesia becomes "fixed."

Local anesthetics within the subarachnoid space act on superficial layers of the spinal cord, but their primary site of anesthetic action is on nerve fibers. Because the concentration of local anesthetic in spinal fluid decreases as a function of distance from the site of injection and because different types of nerve fibers differ in their sensitivity to the effects of local anesthetics, zones of differential anesthesia develop. Since preganglionic sympathetic fibers are blocked by concentrations of local anesthetics that are inadequate to affect somatic sensory or motor fibers, the level of sympathetic denervation during hyperbaric spinal anesthesia extends an average of two spinal segments cephalad to the level that is unresponsive to painful stimuli. On the other hand, since somatic motor fibers are more resistant to the action of local anesthetics than are somatic sensory fibers, the level of motor blockade is an average of two spinal segments below the level made unresponsive to painful stimuli during hyperbaric spinal anesthesia.

The goal of spinal anesthesia is to block somatic sensory and motor fibers. The accompanying sympathetic denervation, however, alters physiological responses. Blood concentrations of local anesthetics during spinal anesthesia are relatively low and play no role in altering physiological responses. The amount of drug that is injected is too low, and the rate of absorption is too slow. The physiological effects of spinal anesthesia are those of sympathetic blockade, and the safe practice of spinal anesthesia requires comprehension of its consequences (Greene, 1983).

Cardiovascular Consequences of Sympathetic Blockade in Spinal Anesthesia. The most cephalad preganglionic sympathetic fibers arise from the spinal cord at the level of the first thoracic segment.

Because of the two-segment zone of differential sympathetic block, sympathetic denervation is complete when sensory anesthesia is obtained at the third thoracic segmental level. Since the physiological responses to spinal anesthesia depend upon the level of sympathetic denervation, the consequences of spinal anesthesia with sensory loss to midcervical levels are essentially the same as those associated with sensory effects that extend only to the third thoracic segmental level. Furthermore, sympathetic denervation by spinal anesthesia involves preganglionic fibers, and each preganglionic fiber ascends and descends in the paravertebral chain to synapse with up to 18 postganglionic fibers, which are then distributed peripherally in a nonsegmental manner. Thus, blockade of sympathetic fibers at, for example, the fourth thoracic segmental level is associated with diffuse peripheral responses that extend three or four segments above the peripheral sensory area that is innervated by fibers arising at the fourth thoracic segmental level.

Even low segmental levels of sensory spinal anesthesia are usually associated with some degree of sympathetic blockade. The most distal preganglionic sympathetic fibers arise from the spinal cord at the second lumbar segmental level. Spinal anesthetic solutions are usually injected between the third and fourth lumbar vertebrae. Turbulence associated with injection, together with subsequent diffusion of the local anesthetic in spinal fluid, almost invariably results in sympathetic blockade at the second lumbar segmental level, even when sensory denervation involves only low lumbar or sacral roots.

The most important consequence of the sympathetic blockade of spinal anesthesia is alteration of cardiovascular function. Arteries and arterioles dilate in sympathetically denervated areas; total peripheral vascular resistance and mean arterial blood pressure thus decrease. Reduction in blood pressure due to peripheral vasodilatation during spinal anesthesia is, however, not proportional to the extent of the sympathetic block. Compensatory vasoconstriction occurs in areas where sympathetic innervation is intact. This increases regional vascular resistance and tends to restore blood pressure. Compensatory vasoconstriction occurs mainly in the upper extremities. It does not involve the cerebral vasculature. However, even with total sympathetic blockade the decrease in total peripheral resistance averages no more than 12 to 14% in normal individuals. The change is relatively small because the smooth muscles of arteries and (especially) arterioles retain a certain degree of autonomous tone, and they do not dilate maximally. Because the decrease in total peripheral resistance is relatively minor in normal individuals, even with total sympathetic blockade during spinal anesthesia, severe arterial hypotension is not brought about by changes in the arterial side of the circulation.

The most important cardiovascular responses to spinal anesthesia are those that result from changes in the venous side of the circulation. Sympathetic tone to veins and venules is lost during spinal anesthesia to the same extent as is that to arteries and arterioles. Unlike arteries and arterioles, however, denervated veins and venules retain little autonomous tone. They can dilate maximally, and the extent to which they do is determined by intraluminal hydrostatic pressure. As they increase their capacity, they sequester within them a greater percentage of the blood volume, and venous return to the heart decreases. This can cause an appreciable fall in cardiac output and blood pressure.

The safety of spinal anesthesia thus depends upon maintenance of an adequate venous return to the heart. This is best accomplished by elevation of sympathetically blocked areas above the level of the right atrium. The slight (10° to 15°) head-down position is appropriate. In normal individuals in the slight head-down position, cardiac output remains normal even during total preganglionic sympathetic blockade. The head-up position, on the other hand, is associated with severe decreases in cardiac output and profound arterial hypotension. Cardiac arrest may occur. The head-up position should, of course, be used to restrict spread of hyperbaric anesthetic solutions in the subarachnoid space; however, if the level of anesthesia becomes unexpectedly high or if severe hypotension develops, the patient must unhesitatingly and immediately be placed in the head-down position. The resulting level of anesthesia may be embarrassingly high, but the patient will survive. Because adequate venous return is essential to the safe management of patients during spinal anesthesia, this form of anesthesia is contraindicated in the presence of hypovolemia from any cause.

Treatment of arterial hypotension during spinal anesthesia should, as a general rule, be initiated if systolic blood pressure falls by approximately 25% of normal *resting* levels. The patient is placed in the slight head-down position and oxygen is administered. Vasopressors are of some value but should not be relied upon exclusively. When used, vasopressors should be given intravenously in small doses. α-Adrenergic agonists, such as methoxamine and phenylephrine, are best avoided. The increase in peripheral vascular resistance produced by such agents may so increase afterload that the myocardium, already suffering from a decrease in preload, may fail acutely. Agents that increase blood pressure by increasing heart rate are also best avoided. Atropine, for example, increases blood pressure and thus improves coronary blood flow, but the increase in myocardial oxygen supply is offset by an even greater increase in oxygen demands associated with the tachycardia. Drugs that act solely by virtue of their positive inotropic effects are also of limited value in the absence of an adequate venous return. The most satisfactory vasopressors are those that decrease venous compliance. While no vasopressor acts solely on the venous circulation, agents such as mephentermine and ephedrine have desirable effects. They also have moderate positive inotropic effects, yet do not produce severe and undesirable increases in peripheral vascular resistance. Hypotension during spinal anesthesia may also be treated by the rapid intravenous infusion of balanced salt solutions, sometimes in amounts as great as 1.5 to 2 liters or more. While hypovolemia must be treated during spinal anesthesia (or any other type of anesthesia), the administration of large volumes of intravenous fluids to normovolemic patients rendered hypotensive by sympathetic blockade during spinal anesthesia may be questioned. Cardiac output is restored by rapid infusion of balanced salt solutions to the extent that venous return is increased, but the increase is accomplished by hemodilution, not by increasing the output of blood with a normal content of oxygen. Use of large volumes of intravenous fluids in this way also sharply increases the incidence of postoperative urinary retention and the need for catheterization.

Spinal anesthesia is, in the absence of parasympatholytic premedication, characterized by a decrease in pulse rate. The bradycardia is due to a combination of two factors: preganglionic blockade of cardiac accelerator fibers (first through fourth thoracic spinal segments), and responses of intrinsic stretch receptors in the right side of the heart that mediate chronotropic responses to changes in central venous and right atrial pressure. The role of intrinsic stretch receptors in regulation of heart rate during spinal anesthesia to midthoracic levels is illustrated by the effects of changes in posture on heart rate after the local anesthetic is fixed and changes in the level of anesthesia are no longer possible; lowering the patient's head increases pulse rate as venous return and right atrial pressure increase, while elevation of the head decreases pulse rate as venous return and right atrial pressure decrease.

Coronary blood flow decreases during spinal anesthesia in proportion to the decrease in mean aortic pressure. Myocardial work, however, also decreases. Myocardial oxygen requirements decrease because of the decrease in afterload, the decrease in preload, and the bradycardia. In normal individuals the decrease in the myocardial requirement for oxygen slightly exceeds the decrease in oxygen supply (coronary flow); the myocardium is thus relatively overperfused. It is not known if the same relationship holds true in patients with coronary artery disease.

Cerebrovascular autoregulatory mechanisms maintain cerebral circulation at normal levels even though arterial hypotension may develop during spinal anesthesia. Only when mean aortic pressure decreases to the range of 55 to 60 mm Hg does cerebral blood flow begin to diminish. The level of blood pressure at which cerebrovascular autoregulation is no longer able to compensate for decreases in arterial perfusion pressure is greater in hypertensive than in normotensive patients. Thus, hypotension should be treated sooner in hypertensive patients than in normal subjects.

Renovascular autoregulation also compensates for changes in arterial blood pressure over a wide range. When arterial hypotension is severe enough to diminish renal blood flow, glomerular filtration and urinary output decrease, but circulation usually remains adequate to maintain the viability of glomerular and tubular cells. The oliguria is then transient and disappears as the effects of the spinal anesthetic wear off and blood pressure returns to normal.

Respiratory Complications. Pulmonary ventilation is little affected by spinal anesthesia. Even levels of sensory denervation high enough to include lower cervical dermatomes are associated with normal tensions of carbon dioxide and oxygen in arterial blood. The phrenic nerves remain unaffected during such high levels of anesthesia because of the existence of the two-segment zone of differential motor blockade mentioned above. The diaphragm compensates for intercostal paralysis, particularly since relaxation of the anterior abdominal wall associated with intercostal paralysis decreases resistance to descent of the diaphragm during inhalation. Diaphragmatic excursions during high spinal anesthesia may be impaired, however, in obese patients, in patients with ascites, in pregnant women at term, or in other situations in which intra-abdominal pressure may be increased, including use of the extreme head-down or Trendelenburg position.

While respiratory tidal volume and maximal inspiratory capacity are unaffected by high spinal anesthesia, forced expiration is impaired because of paralysis of the abdominal musculature. Patients with high spinal anesthesia are unable to cough normally. High spinal anesthesia may therefore be hazardous in patients with excessive tracheobronchial secretions.

Respiratory arrest, while rare, can occur during spinal anesthesia. Its most frequent cause is ischemic paralysis of the medullary respiratory centers associated with profound decreases in cardiac output and arterial blood pressure. Only a small percentage of such incidents is due to phrenic nerve paralysis during lumbar spinal anesthesia. Apnea is also not due to ascent of the local anesthetic in cerebrospinal fluid with direct depression of chemotactic respiratory neurons in the brain stem. Concentrations of local anesthetic in cisternal spinal fluid during high spinal anesthesia are inadequate to produce pharmacological effects; they are even lower in ventricular cerebrospinal fluid and have no effect on either vasomotor or respiratory nuclei in the medulla.

The fundamental importance of inadequate cerebral perfusion as the primary cause of apnea during spinal anesthesia is demonstrated by the observation that respiratory arrest almost always immediately precedes or follows cardiac arrest. Furthermore, prompt restoration of cardiac output by appropriate means will result in immediate restoration of ventilation. This would not occur if the apnea were due to phrenic nerve paralysis or to direct depression of the respiratory centers.

The incidence, magnitude, and type of postoperative respiratory complications are the same after spinal anesthesia (or other forms of regional anesthesia) as after general anesthesia for the same operative procedure. Postoperative respiratory complications are related to age, sex, smoking habits, use of narcotics, quality of intraoperative and postoperative ventilatory care, preexisting pulmonary disease, and, above all, the anatomical site and nature of the surgery. When these factors are taken into consideration, postoperative respiratory complications are not related to the type of anesthesia. Regional anesthesia, including spinal anesthesia, provides no advantage for the avoidance of pulmonary complications in the postoperative period.

Hepatic Function. Hepatic function is largely unaffected by spinal anesthesia, even in the presence of hypotension. Postoperative hepatic function is principally determined by the type and nature of the surgery performed. Spinal and other forms of regional anesthesia confer no special benefits in patients with liver disease.

Neurological Complications. Residual neurological deficits associated with spinal anesthesia are so rare in modern practice that, if they do occur, aggressive and complete diagnostic tests must be undertaken immediately to assure that they are not due to other causes. When neurological deficits occur that are directly ascribable to spinal anesthesia, they may present themselves either immediately or they may develop days or a week or more after the procedure. Neurological complications with acute onset may be due to the injection of a local anesthetic with histotoxic properties or to the injection of an excessive concentration of a local anesthetic that normally does not cause histotoxicity. Tetracaine, procaine, and lidocaine are devoid of neurotoxicity. When neurological complications follow the use of these local anesthetics, they are, in the absence of chemical contamination of the solution, the result of injection in such a manner as to expose nerve roots and the spinal cord to excessive concentrations of the drug. They are not due to "allergic" responses to the agent.

Another cause of the immediate appearance of neurological deficits following spinal anesthesia is traumatic damage to a nerve root incurred during performance of the lumbar puncture. This characteristically involves a single nerve root. Nerve damage during lumbar puncture usually occurs when the needle is directed so far laterally that it impinges on a nerve root at its point of exit from the subarachnoid space through the dura—the point at which a nerve is sufficiently fixed to be susceptible to direct trauma. Such damage to a nerve root in the cauda equina is rare.

Neurological sequelae of spinal anesthesia that are delayed in onset are usually the result of chronic arachnoiditis; this is produced by the inadvertent injection of materials (lint, talc, *etc.*) or chemicals that initiate a chronic inflammatory response. Avoidance of this type of reaction depends upon meticulous attention to details of technic during administration of the drug and the use of equipment that is chemically uncontaminated as well as sterile.

Spinal anesthesia is commonly regarded as contraindicated in patients with preexisting disease of the spinal cord. No experimental evidence exists to support this hypothesis. It is, nonetheless, prudent to avoid spinal anesthesia in patients with progressive diseases of the spinal cord, since worsening of the disease may be blamed on the anesthetic agent or the procedure.

Headaches may follow any lumbar puncture, whether for diagnostic or anesthetic purpose. Characteristically postural in nature, these disappear when the patient is supine. The incidence of such headaches is related to the size of the needle used and to the age and sex of the patient. When 25-gauge needles are used, the incidence of headaches after spinal anesthesia is 1% or less (even in obstetrical patients, who constitute the most susceptible group). Spinal needles larger than 22-gauge should be avoided.

Dosage and Duration of Anesthesia. Dosages of local anesthetics used for spinal anesthesia vary according to the volume of the subarachnoid space (*i.e.*, the height of the patient), the segmental level of anesthesia desired, and the duration of anesthesia required. Although five local anesthetics are presently approved for use in spinal anesthesia in the United States (procaine, lidocaine, tetracaine, bupivacaine, and dibucaine), only two, lidocaine and tetracaine, enjoy widespread clinical use. The concentration of tetracaine injected for spinal anesthesia should not exceed 0.5%; the injected concentration of lidocaine should not exceed 5%. When high thoracic levels of anesthesia are sought, 16 mg of tetracaine or 100 mg of lidocaine may be used.

The duration of spinal anesthesia is governed by the rate at which the local anesthetic is absorbed from the subarachnoid space, the spinal cord, and, after diffusion through the dura, the epidural space. Duration thus decreases with increases in the absorptive surface to which the drug is exposed as it spreads within the subarachnoid space. Duration also depends upon lipophilicity of the local anesthetic. Tetracaine, which is highly lipid soluble, provides 2 to 3 hours of anesthesia, while that with the less lipid-soluble lidocaine lasts about an hour. Epinephrine (0.2 to 0.5 mg) prolongs the duration of spinal anesthesia with tetracaine by about 30%. For reasons that remain to be clarified, epinephrine fails to produce significant prolongation of lidocaine-induced spinal anesthesia (Greene, 1983).

Evaluation of Spinal Anesthesia. Modern spinal anesthesia is a safe and effective technic. Its value is greatest during surgery involving the lower abdomen, the extremities, or the perineum. It is often combined with intravenous medication to provide sedation and amnesia. With low spinal anesthesia the potential for physiological trespass is less than that associated with general anesthesia. The same does not apply for high spinal anesthesia. The sympathetic blockade that accompanies levels of spinal anesthesia adequate for mid or upper abdominal surgery is so extensive that equally satisfactory and safer operating conditions are usually achieved by the administration of a general anesthetic and a neuromuscular blocking agent. Low spinal anesthesia and high spinal anesthesia are, in physiological terms, totally different technics. One is frequently indicated, the other only rarely.

EPIDURAL ANESTHESIA

Injection of a solution of local anesthetic into the epidural space is a popular form of regional anesthesia. When injected into the lumbar, or less frequently, the thoracic area, the anesthetic acts in two places. It diffuses across the dura into the subarachnoid space, where it acts on nerve roots and the spinal cord much as it does when injected directly into the subarachnoid space during spinal anesthesia. The drug also diffuses into the paravertebral area through the intervertebral foramina, producing, in essence, multiple paravertebral nerve blocks. The former is the more important site of action. When local anesthetics are injected into the epidural space via the caudal canal (caudal anesthesia), the anesthetic acts less by diffusing across the dura and more by blocking nerves as they pass through the epidural space; diffusion through sacral foramina also plays an important role.

The choice of drugs to be used during epidural anesthesia is dictated primarily by the duration of anesthesia desired. Particularly popular are bupivacaine, when long duration is sought, and lidocaine, when intermediate duration is indicated. Chloroprocaine provides rapid onset and very short duration of action. However, its use in epidural anesthesia has been clouded by controversy regarding its potential to cause neurological complications if the drug is accidentally injected into the subarachnoid space. The duration of action of lidocaine is frequently prolonged (and its systemic toxicity decreased) by addition of epinephrine (1:200,000). Duration of anesthesia is also frequently extended by serial injections through a catheter placed in the epidural space.

The volumes of local anesthetic injected during epidural anesthesia are determined principally by the segmental level of anesthesia required. The larger the volume, the greater is the spread within the epidural space and the more extensive the area of anesthesia.

Concentrations of local anesthetic used are determined by the types of nerve fibers to be blocked. The lowest concentrations are used when only sympathetic fibers are to be blocked. The highest concentrations are used when sympathetic, somatic sensory, and somatic motor blockade are required. Intermediate concentrations allow somatic sensory anesthesia without muscle relaxation. The total amounts of drug that can be safely injected at one time are approximately the same as those mentioned above in the section on Nerve Block Anesthesia and the section on Infiltration Anesthesia. The technic of epidural anesthesia and the volumes, concentrations, and types of drugs used are described in detail by Bromage (1978).

A significant difference between epidural and spinal anesthesia is that drugs used with the epidural technic are injected in amounts sufficient to produce high concentrations in blood following absorption. Peak concentrations of lidocaine in blood following injection of 400 mg (without epinephrine) into the lumbar epidural space average 3 to 4 μg/ml. The same amount of lidocaine injected into the caudal epidural space results in slightly higher values. Addition of epinephrine (1:200,000) to the lidocaine decreases peak concentrations in blood by about 25%. Peak concentrations of bupivacaine in blood after the lumbar epidural injection of 150 mg average 1.0 μg/ml. These concentrations are a function of the total dose of drug rather than the concentration or volume of solution following epidural or other forms of regional anesthesia, except for spinal anesthesia (Covino and Vassallo, 1976).

Another difference between epidural and spinal anesthesia is that there is no zone of differential sympathetic blockade with epidural anesthesia, and the level of sympathetic denervation is thus the same as the level of sensory denervation. On the other hand, the zone of differential motor blockade is four to five spinal segments with epidural anesthesia, whereas it is only two segments with spinal anesthesia.

Because epidural anesthesia is not associated with the zone of differential sympathetic blockade that is observed during spinal anesthesia, cardiovascular responses to epidural anesthesia would be expected to be less prominent. In practice, this is not the case; this potential advantage of epidural anesthesia is offset by the cardiovascular responses to the high concentration of anesthetic in blood that is achieved during epidural anesthesia. This is most apparent when, as is often the case, epinephrine is added to the epidural injection. The resulting concentration of epinephrine in blood is sufficient to produce significant β-adrenergic stimulation. As a consequence, peripheral vasodilatation is so pronounced that blood pressure decreases, even though cardiac output increases due to the positive inotropic and chronotropic effects of epinephrine. The result is peripheral hyperperfusion and hypotension. Differences in cardiovascular responses to equal levels of spinal and epidural anesthesia are also observed when a local anesthetic such as lidocaine is used without epinephrine. The direct effects of the high concentration of lidocaine on peripheral smooth muscle and the effects of the agent on the heart may become significant. The magnitude of the differences in responses to equal sensory levels of spinal and epidural anesthesia varies, however, with the local anesthetic used for the epidural injection (assuming no epinephrine is used). Local anesthetics such as bupivacaine, which are highly lipid soluble, are distributed less into the circulation than are less lipid-soluble agents such as lidocaine.

High concentrations of local anesthetics in blood during epidural anesthesia are of special importance when this technic is used to control pain during labor and delivery. Local anesthetics cross the placenta, enter the fetal circulation, and may cause depression of the neonate (Scanlon et al., 1974). The extent to which they do so is determined by dosage, the level of protein binding in both maternal and fetal blood (Tucker, et al., 1970), placental blood flow, and solubility of the agent in fetal tissue. The persistence of abnormal neonatal neurobehavioral activity for 24 or even 48 hours after delivery may be related to placental transfer of local anesthetics during labor and delivery and to the relative inability of the neonate to metabolize the drugs, particularly those of the amide type. These potential hazards to the neonate can be offset to some extent by use of local anesthetics (e.g., bupivacaine) that are less distributed into the circulation. On the other hand, should high plasma concentrations of bupivacaine be achieved, the resulting systemic toxicity may be less readily reversed.

The greater zone of differential motor blockade that results with epidural anesthesia means that this procedure has less effect on pulmonary ventilation than does an equal sensory level of spinal anesthesia. This potential benefit is offset, however, during abdominal operations, because higher sensory levels of epidural anesthesia must be achieved to obtain the same degree of surgical relaxation of abdominal muscles that is produced by spinal anesthesia.

Epidural and Intrathecal Opioid Analgesia. Small amounts of opioids injected intrathecally or epidurally relieve postoperative and chronic pain (Kitahata *et al.*, 1974; Yaksh and Rudy, 1976). The resulting analgesia is localized to spinal cord segments at the site of injection. Sympathetic, sensory, and motor fibers remain functionally intact. Hypotension, sensory anesthesia, and motor paralysis are avoided. Compared with their systemic administration, the duration of analgesia (12 to 18 hours) is longer and there is less sedation and respiratory depression with intrathecal or, more commonly, epidural administration of opioids. Side effects of intrathecal or epidural opioids include pruritus and urinary retention; rarely, severe respiratory depression appears 6 to 8 hours after injection. The latter complication is apparently due to the rostral spread of opioids in the cerebrospinal fluid (Bromage *et al.*, 1982). Close monitoring of ventilatory function is essential whenever opioids are used in this manner.

Adams, H. J.; Blair, M. R.; and Takman, B. H. The local anesthetic activity of saxitoxin alone and with vasoconstrictor and local anesthetic agents. *Arch. Int. Pharmacodyn. Ther.*, **1976**, *224*, 275–282.

Boyes, R. N.; Scott, D. B.; Jebson, P. J.; Godman, M. J.; and Julian, D. G. Pharmacokinetics of lidocaine in man. *Clin. Pharmacol. Ther.*, **1971**, *12*, 105–116.

Bromage, P. R.; Camporesi, E. M.; Durant, P. A. C.; and Nielsen, C. H. Rostral spread of epidural morphine. *Anesthesiology*, **1982**, *56*, 431–436.

Cherney, L. S. Tetracaine hydroiodide: a long-lasting local anesthetic agent for the relief of pain. *Anesth. Analg.*, **1963**, *42*, 477–481.

Chiu, S. Y., and Ritchie, J. M. On the physiological role of potassium channels and the security of conduction in myelinated nerve fibres. *Proc. R. Soc. Lond. [Biol.]*, **1984**, *220*, 415–422.

Courtney, K. R. Structure-activity relations for frequency-dependent sodium channel block in nerve by local anesthetics. *J. Pharmacol. Exp. Ther.*, **1980**, *213*, 114–119.

Feldman, H. S.; Covino, B. M.; and Sage, D. J. Direct chronotropic and inotropic effects of local anesthetic agents in isolated guinea pig atria. *Reg. Anaesth.*, **1982**, *7*, 149–156.

Fishman, M. W.; Schuster, C. R.; and Rajfer, S. A comparison of the subjective and cardiovascular effects of procaine and cocaine in humans. *Pharmacol. Biochem. Behav.*, **1983**, *18*, 711–716.

Franz, D. N., and Perry, R. S. Mechanisms for differential block among single myelinated and non-myelinated axons by procaine. *J. Physiol. (Lond.)*, **1974**, *236*, 193–210.

Gasser, H. S., and Erlanger, J. The role of fiber size in the establishment of a nerve block by pressure or cocaine. *Am. J. Physiol.*, **1929**, *88*, 581–591.

Gissen, A. J.; Covino, B. G.; and Gregus, J. Differential sensitivities of mammalian nerve fibers to local anesthetic agents. *Anesthesiology*, **1980**, *53*, 467–474.

——. Differential sensitivity of fast and slow fibers in mammalian nerve. II. Margin of safety for nerve transmission. *Anesth. Analg.*, **1982**, *61*, 561–569.

Hille, B. Local anesthetics: hydrophilic and hydrophobic pathways for the drug-receptor reaction. *J. Gen. Physiol.*, **1977**, *69*, 497–515.

Keenaghan, J. B., and Boyes, R. N. The tissue distribution, metabolism and excretion of lidocaine in rats, guinea pigs, dogs and man. *J. Pharmacol. Exp. Ther.*, **1972**, *180*, 454–463.

Kendig, J., and Cohen, E. N. Pressure antagonism to nerve conduction block by anesthetic agents. *Anesthesiology*, **1977**, *47*, 6–10.

Kitahata, L. M.; Kosada, Y.; Taub, A.; Bonikos, K.; and Hoffer, M. Lamina-specific suppression of dorsal-horn unit activity by morphine sulfate. *Anesthesiology*, **1974**, *41*, 39–48.

Matthews, P. B. C., and Rushworth, G. The relative sensitivity of muscle nerve fibres to procaine. *J. Physiol. (Lond.)*, **1957**, *135*, 263–269.

Metcalfe, J. C., and Burgen, A. S. V. Relaxation of anaesthetics in the presence of cyto-membranes. *Nature*, **1968**, *220*, 587–588.

Mrose, H., and Ritchie, J. M. Local anesthetics: do benzocaine and lidocaine act at the same site? *J. Gen. Physiol.*, **1978**, *71*, 223–225.

Nathan, P. W., and Sears, T. A. Some factors concerned in differential nerve block by local anaesthetics. *J. Physiol. (Lond.)*, **1961**, *157*, 565–580.

Ravindran, R. S.; Turner, M. S.; and Muller, I. Neurological effects of subarachnoid administration of 2-chloroprocaine—CE, bupivacaine and low pH normal saline in dogs. *Anesth. Analg.*, **1982**, *61*, 279–283.

Rosenberg, R. L.; Tomiko, S. A.; and Agnew, W. S. Reconstitution of neurotoxin-modulated ion transport by the voltage-regulated sodium channel isolated from the electroplax of *Electrophorus electricus*. *Proc. Natl. Acad. Sci. U.S.A.*, **1984**, *81*, 1239–1243.

Rothstein, P.; Arthur, G. R.; Feldman, H. S.; and Covino, B. G. The lung modifies arterial concentrations of bupivacaine in humans. *Reg. Anaesth.*, **1983**, *8*, 44.

Ruff, R. L. A quantitative analysis of local anaesthetic alteration of miniature end-plate currents and end-plate current fluctuations. *J. Physiol. (Lond.)*, **1977**, *264*, 89–124.

Scanlon, J. W.; Brown, W. U., Jr.; Weiss, J. B.; and Alper, M. H. Neurobehavioral responses of newborn infants after maternal epidural anesthesia. *Anesthesiology*, **1974**, *40*, 121–128.

Scott, D. B. Toxicity caused by local anaesthetic drugs. *Br. J. Anaesth.*, **1981**, *53*, 553–554.

Skou, J. C. The effect of drugs on cell membranes with special reference to local anaesthetics. *J. Pharm. Pharmacol.*, **1961**, *13*, 204–217.

Strichartz, G. R. Use-dependent conduction block produced by volatile general anesthetic agents. *Acta Anaesthesiol. Scand.*, **1980**, *24*, 402–406.

Tamkun, M. M.; Talvenheimo, J. A.; and Catterall, W. A. The sodium channel from rat brain: reconstitution of neurotoxin-activated ion flux and scorpion toxin binding from purified components. *J. Biol. Chem.*, **1984**, *259*, 1676–1688.

Tucker, G. T.; Boyes, R. N.; Bridenbaugh, P. O.; and Moore, D. C. Binding of anilide-type local anesthetics in human plasma. II. Implications *in vivo*, with special reference to transplacental distribution. *Anesthesiology*, **1970**, *35*, 304–314.

Van Dyke, C.; Barash, P. G.; Jatlow, P.; and Byck, R.

Cocaine: plasma concentrations after intranasal application in man. *Science*, **1976**, *191*, 859–861.

Van Dyke, C.; Jatlow, P.; Ungerer, J.; Barash, P. G.; and Byck, R. Oral cocaine: plasma concentrations and central effects. *Science*, **1978**, *200*, 211–213.

Winnie, A. P.; Tay, C. H.; Patel, K. P.; Ramanmurthy, S.; and Durrani, Z. Pharmacokinetics of local anesthetics during plexus blocks. *Anesth. Analg.*, **1977**, *56*, 852–861.

Yaksh, T. L., and Rudy, T. A. Analgesia mediated by a direct spinal action of narcotics. *Science*, **1976**, *192*, 1357–1358.

Monographs and Reviews

Agnew, W. S. Voltage-regulated sodium channel molecules. *Annu. Rev. Physiol.*, **1984**, *46*, 517–530.

Arthur, G. R. Pharmacokinetics. In, *Local Anesthetics.* (Strichartz, G. R., ed.) *Handbook of Experimental Pharmacology.* Springer-Verlag, Berlin, **1985**, in press.

Bromage, P. R. *Epidural Analgesia.* W. B. Saunders Co., Philadelphia, **1978**.

Büchi, J., and Perlia, X. Structure-activity relations and physicochemical properties of local anesthetics. In, *Local Anesthetics*, Vol. 1. *International Encyclopedia of Pharmacology and Therapeutics*, Sect. 8. (Lechat, P., ed.) Pergamon Press, Ltd., Oxford, **1971**, pp. 39–130.

Byck, R. (ed.). *Cocaine Papers: Sigmund Freud.* Stonehill, New York, **1975**.

Catterall, W. A. The molecular basis of neuronal excitability. *Science*, **1984**, *223*, 653–661.

Covino, B. G. Toxicity and systemic effects of local anesthetic agents. In, *Local Anesthetics.* (Strichartz, G. R., ed.) *Handbook of Experimental Pharmacology.* Springer-Verlag, Berlin, **1985**, in press.

Covino, B. G., and Vassallo, H. G. *Local Anesthetics: Mechanisms of Action and Clinical Use.* Grune & Stratton, Inc., New York, **1976**.

de Jong, R. H. *Local Anesthetics.* Charles C Thomas, Publisher, Springfield, Ill., **1977**.

Fink, B. R. (ed.). *Molecular Mechanisms of Anesthesia.* Vol. 2, *Progress in Anesthesiology.* Raven Press, New York, **1980**.

Greene, N. M. *Physiology of Spinal Anesthesia.* 3rd ed. The Williams & Wilkins Co., Baltimore, **1981**.

————. Uptake and elimination of local anesthetics during spinal anesthesia. *Anesth. Analg.*, **1983**, *62*, 1013–1024.

Hansson, E. Absorption, distribution, metabolism and excretion of local anesthetics. In, *Local Anesthetics*, Vol. 1. *International Encyclopedia of Pharmacology and Therapeutics*, Sect. 8. (Lechat, P., ed.) Pergamon Press, Ltd., Oxford, **1971**, pp. 239–260.

Hille, B. Theories of anesthesia: general perturbations versus specific receptors. In, *Mechanisms of Anesthesia.* (Fink, B. R., ed.) Vol. 2, *Progress in Anesthesiology.* Raven Press, New York, **1980**, pp. 1–5.

Kao, C. Y. Pharmacology of tetrodotoxin and saxitoxin. *Fed. Proc.*, **1972**, *31*, 1117–1123.

Moore, D. C. *Regional Block.* Charles C Thomas, Publisher, Springfield, Ill., **1965**.

Narahashi, T., and Frazier, D. T. Site of action and active form of local anesthetics. *Neurosci. Res.*, **1971**, *4*, 65–99.

Ogura, Y. Fugu (puffer-fish) poisoning and the pharmacology of crystalline tetrodotoxin poisoning. In, *Neuropoisons: Their Pathophysiological Actions.* Vol. 1, *Poisons of Animal Origin.* (Simpson, L. L., ed.) Plenum Press, New York, **1971**, pp. 139–156.

Ritchie, J. M. Mechanism of action of local anesthetic agents and biotoxins. *Br. J. Anaesth.*, **1975**, *74*, 191–198.

————. A pharmacological approach to the structure of sodium channels in myelinated axons. *Annu. Rev. Neurosci.*, **1979**, *2*, 341–362.

————. Tetrodotoxin and saxitoxin and the sodium channels of excitable tissues. *Trends Pharmacol. Sci.*, **1980**, *1*, 275–279.

Ritchie, J. M., and Greengard, P. On the mode of action of local anesthetics. *Annu. Rev. Pharmacol.*, **1966**, *6*, 405–430.

Schantz, E. J. Paralytic shellfish poisoning and saxitoxin. In, *Neuropoisons: Their Pathophysiological Actions.* Vol. 1, *Poisons of Animal Origin.* (Simpson, L. L., ed.) Plenum Press, New York, **1971**, pp. 159–168.

Shanes, A. M. Electrochemical aspects of physiological and pharmacological action in excitable cells. *Pharmacol. Rev.*, **1958**, *10*, 59–273.

Strichartz, G. R. Current concepts of the mechanism of action of local anesthetics. *J. Dent. Res.*, **1981**, *60*, 1460–1467.

————. (ed.). *Local Anesthetics. Handbook of Experimental Pharmacology.* Springer-Verlag, Berlin, **1985**, in press.

Strichartz, G. R., and Ritchie, J. M. Action of local anesthetics on ion channels of excitable tissues. In, *Local Anesthetics.* (Strichartz, G. R., ed.) *Handbook of Experimental Pharmacology.* Springer-Verlag, Berlin, **1985**, in press.

Van Dyke, C., and Byck, R. Cocaine. *Sci. Am.*, **1982**, *246*, 128–141.

Zipf, H. F., and Dittmann, E. C. General pharmacological effects of local anesthetics. In, *Local Anesthetics*, Vol. 1. *International Encyclopedia of Pharmacology and Therapeutics*, Sect. 8. (Lechat, P., ed.) Pergamon Press, Ltd., Oxford, **1971**, pp. 191–238.

16 THE THERAPEUTIC GASES

Oxygen, Carbon Dioxide, Helium, and Water Vapor

Theodore C. Smith, Jeffrey B. Gross, and Harry Wollman

The therapeutic gases discussed in this chapter, most notably oxygen, are obviously not uniquely relevant to the central nervous system. They are placed in Section III primarily for proximity to the general anesthetic agents, many of which are also administered by inhalation.

OXYGEN

The importance of oxygen, water, and food to the animal organism is fundamental. Of these three basic essentials for the maintenance of life, the deprivation of oxygen leads to death most rapidly. Therapy with oxygen is useful or necessary for life in several diseases and intoxications that interfere with normal oxygenation of the blood or tissues. In addition, pure oxygen administered at ambient pressures greater than 1 atmosphere has both unique applications as a therapeutic agent and multiple toxic effects.

History. Soon after Priestley's discovery of oxygen in 1772 and Lavoisier's elucidation of its role in respiration, oxygen therapy was introduced in England by Beddoes. His publication in 1794, entitled "Considerations on the Medicinal Use and Production of Factitious Airs," can be considered the beginning of inhalational therapy. Beddoes, overcome with enthusiasm for his project, treated all kinds of diseases with oxygen. They included such diverse conditions as scrofula, leprosy, and paralysis. Such indiscriminate therapeutic applications naturally led to many failures, and Beddoes died a disconsolate man. It is interesting to note that Beddoes' collaborator was James Watt, engineer and inventor of the steam engine, and his assistant was Sir Humphry Davy. When Beddoes' experiments proved disappointing, Davy left the laboratory in order to pursue his own investigations on the properties of nitrous oxide. Davy's contribution to the history of anesthesia is mentioned in Chapter 13.

It was only following such pioneer investigations as those of Haldane, Hill, Barcroft, Krogh, L. J.

Henderson, and Y. Henderson that oxygen therapy was placed upon a sound physiological basis (*see* Sackner, 1974). Although Paul Bert had studied therapeutic aspects of hyperbaric oxygen in 1870, and identified oxygen toxicity (Bert, 1873), the extension of the "dose" of oxygen above 1 atmosphere for therapeutic purposes did not begin until the 1950s (*see* Lambertsen *et al.*, 1953; Boerema *et al.*, 1960).

NORMAL OXYGENATION

Oxygen Cascade. A cascade of alternating convective and diffusive steps carries oxygen from the air to the cells within the body. Since the inspired air contains 20.9% oxygen at normal barometric pressure (760 mm Hg), the partial pressure (or tension) of oxygen (P_{O_2}) in the inspired air is 159 mm Hg. The oxygen cascade starts with convective transport of oxygen when ambient air is inhaled and delivered to the alveoli of the lung. The P_{O_2} in the alveoli is about two thirds of that in inspired gas. This is due to humidification in the airway, which dilutes all the inspired gases; dilution with carbon dioxide, which is delivered to alveoli by blood returning from tissues; and loss of alveolar oxygen to blood flowing through the lung. The next step in the cascade is diffusion through the alveolar-capillary membrane into the blood. The arrangement of gas spaces and capillaries in the lung is an efficient one, and the P_{O_2} of arterial blood is thus normally close to the alveolar P_{O_2}.

The cascade continues with convective transport of oxygen via the arterial blood to tissue capillaries, where diffusion carries oxygen away from the blood through the capillary endothelium, extracellular fluid, and cell membranes to the intracellular space. As a result of this loss to the tissues, the P_{O_2} in venous blood (about 40 mm Hg) is considerably lower than that in the arterial blood. However, the P_{O_2} in the tissues is even lower than that in venous blood, due to the limited rate of diffusion and ongoing utilization of oxygen. In the mitochondria, where the rate of oxygen consumption is greatest, P_{O_2} is lowest.

Carriage of Oxygen in Blood. Oxygen is carried in the blood mainly in chemical combination with hemoglobin and to a small extent in physical solution. The amount of oxygen combined with hemoglobin depends on the P_{O_2} of blood, as illustrated by the sigmoid-shaped oxygen-hemoglobin dissocia-

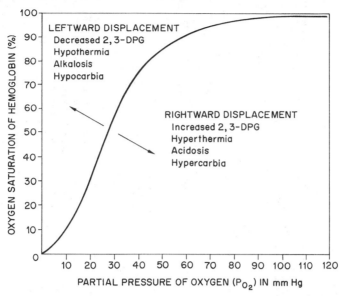

Figure 16–1. *The oxygen-hemoglobin dissociation curve.*

Saturation of normal hemoglobin with oxygen is determined by the partial pressure of oxygen (P_{O_2}) and is modified by a number of other factors. The most important of these are certain phosphate compounds, temperature, and pH. Molecular CO_2 has a small effect in the same direction as that of the hydrogen ions that result from hydration and dissociation of CO_2. A leftward shift of the curve limits the availability of oxygen, since a lower P_{O_2} is required to remove the same fraction of hemoglobin-bound oxygen. A rightward shift increases the supply of oxygen available to tissues. Different hemoglobins may have different dissociation curves. For example, the curve for fetal hemoglobin is above and to the left of normal. 2,3-DPG is 2,3-diphosphoglycerate. (*See* Samaja *et al.*, 1981.)

tion curve (Figure 16–1). When fully saturated with oxygen, each gram of hemoglobin binds 1.3 volumes % of oxygen. When air is breathed at sea level, arterial P_{O_2} is 97 mm Hg and hemoglobin is more than 98% saturated with oxygen. As arterial P_{O_2} increases (*e.g.*, during inhalation of oxygen), the carriage of additional oxygen depends almost entirely on its physical solution. At 37° C, the solubility of oxygen in blood is such that 0.003 volume % is dissolved per mm Hg of P_{O_2}. Under conditions of hyperbaric oxygenation (3 atmospheres of oxygen) more than 25% of the oxygen in blood is carried in solution. These relationships are illustrated in Table 16–1.

Also shown in Table 16–1 is the oxygen content and P_{O_2} of mixed venous blood. At normal cardiac output and metabolic rate, venous oxygen content is always about 5 volumes % less than arterial. When air is the inspired gas, the hemoglobin in venous blood is only about 74% saturated. Venous P_{O_2} is only slightly higher when 40% oxygen is inhaled. However, the inhalation of oxygen at a pressure of 3 atmospheres leads to a venous oxygen content of 20 volumes %; in this circumstance the hemoglobin in venous blood remains nearly 100% saturated.

When the oxygen content of arterial blood is very low, cyanosis of skin and mucous membranes may occur due to the darker color of deoxyhemo-

globin. Cyanosis appears when about 5 g/dl of deoxyhemoglobin is present in arterial blood. At normal concentrations of hemoglobin (15 g/dl), this value will occur at a saturation of 67%. Cyanosis is an insensitive sign of low arterial oxygen content. For example, at an altitude of 4.3 km (14,000 ft), arterial P_{O_2} is only 42 mm Hg, the oxygen saturation of hemoglobin in arterial blood is above 75%, and cyanosis would not be evident (Table 16–1). In addition, the clinical recognition of cyanosis is extremely variable (*see* Hudson and Pierson, 1981).

OXYGEN DEPRIVATION

Etiology of Hypoxia. *Hypoxia* is a broad term used to designate insufficient oxygenation of tissues. Since hypoxia can arise from a variety of causes, and because methods of treatment are closely allied to etiology, a classification of the causes of hypoxia is useful. Three categories can be delineated:

1. *Prepulmonary Causes of Hypoxia.* Hypoxia may be due to low inspired concentration of oxygen at normal ambient pressure, such as occurs when inert gases

Table 16–1. THE CARRIAGE AND TRANSFER OF OXYGEN IN BLOOD *

INSPIRED GAS	ARTERIAL OXYGEN TENSION (mm Hg)	ARTERIAL OXYGEN CONTENT (vol %)			MIXED VENOUS OXYGEN CONTENT (vol %)			MIXED VENOUS OXYGEN TENSION (mm Hg)
		Dissolved	*Bound to Hemoglobin*	*Total*	*Dissolved*	*Bound to Hemoglobin*	*Total*	
Air at 4.3 km (14,000 ft) above sea level	42	0.1	14.8	14.9	0.1	9.8	9.9	27
Air at sea level	97	0.3	19.3	19.6	0.1	14.5	14.6	41
Oxygen (40%) at sea level	210	0.6	19.5	20.1	0.1	15.0	15.1	43
Oxygen (100%) at sea level	600	1.8	19.6	21.4	0.1	16.3	16.4	49
Oxygen (100%) at 3 atmospheres	1800	5.4	19.6	25.0	0.5	19.5	20.0	150

* The table illustrates the carriage and transfer of oxygen in blood under a variety of circumstances. As arterial oxygen tension increases, so does the amount of dissolved oxygen, which is directly proportional to the P_{O_2}. As oxygen tension increases, oxygen bound to hemoglobin rises to, but does not exceed, 19.6 volumes % (100% saturation of hemoglobin at 15 g/dl). Increasing the oxygen tension by increasing inspired concentration, pressure, or both increases the amount of dissolved oxygen, which can be used by tissues. This is a small fraction of the total demand at normal oxygen tension, but at elevated ambient pressures (in hyperbaric facilities) dissolved oxygen may supply a large part or all of the requirement for oxygen.

The figures in this table are approximations based on the assumptions of 15 g/dl of hemoglobin, 5 volumes % of oxygen extraction by the whole body, constant cardiac output, and the ventilatory changes usually observed under the circumstances illustrated. When severe anemia is present, arterial oxygen tensions are little affected, but arterial content of oxygen is lower. Oxygen extraction continues, and, therefore, mixed venous blood has a considerably lower oxygen content and oxygen tension.

are present in greater-than-normal concentration. Alternatively, it may be caused by low ambient pressure, such as occurs at high altitude. Hypoxia may also occur when gas at normal P_{O_2} is available but is not delivered to the lungs in adequate amounts. This may be due to respiratory tract obstruction, to muscular weakness induced by disease (*e.g.,* myasthenia gravis) or by drugs (*e.g.,* neuromuscular blocking agents), or to lack of respiratory drive because of central nervous system (CNS) disease or the effect of central respiratory depressant drugs (*e.g.,* opioids, barbiturates, and general anesthetics).

2. *Pulmonary Causes of Hypoxia.* In the presence of a normal P_{O_2} in the inspired air and adequate ventilation, a defect in pulmonary function can prevent the normal oxygenation of blood. The defect in pulmonary function may be a diffusion block, due to thickening of the alveolar-capillary membrane. It may be caused by venous-arterial (right-to-left) shunts. It may also reflect a functional inequality of ventilation and perfusion in the lung, such as occurs in most acute and chronic pulmonary diseases.

3. *Postpulmonary Causes of Hypoxia.* Despite normal arterial P_{O_2}, the arterial blood may fail to deliver sufficient oxygen to the tissues. This can be caused by low cardiac output, as in shock, or by maldistribution of the cardiac output, such as occurs following thrombosis or vasospasm. Other causes include impaired oxygen-carrying capacity of the blood (*e.g.,* anemia, abnormal hemoglobins, and carbon monoxide poisoning) and impaired release of oxygen from hemoglobin due to hypocapnia or a deficiency of 2,3-diphosphoglycerate (2,3-DPG).

In other situations, the tissues may be unable to extract and utilize enough oxygen from the normally oxygenated blood that is delivered. This may be due to abnormally high metabolic demand (*e.g.,* thyrotoxicosis, hyperpyrexia) or to malfunctioning cellular enzyme systems (*e.g.,* cyanide poisoning, uncoupling of oxidative phosphorylation) (*see* Robin, 1977).

In prepulmonary and pulmonary hypoxia, there is hypoxemia, and both the *content* and *tension* of oxygen are low in arterial blood. The administration of oxygen alleviates the hypoxemia in most cases and thereby corrects the tissue hypoxia. In some cases of prepulmonary hypoxia, it may, of course, be necessary to relieve airway obstruction or to ventilate patients mechanically in order to deliver the supplemental oxygen to the lungs. The administration of oxygen may be minimally effective in correcting tissue hypoxia when oxygenation of blood is normal, and correction of the basic cause of poor delivery or extraction of oxygen is required (*see* Anthonisen, 1982). In those cases of postpulmonary hypoxia where the defect is impaired oxygen-carrying capacity of blood or abnormally high metabolic demand, administration of oxygen *is* useful.

Actually, a combination of several kinds of hypoxia may exist and the dangers are then far greater. For instance, an organ with low blood flow due to atherosclerotic changes can sustain serious damage if the P_{O_2} of its arterial supply should decrease only slightly.

Effects of Hypoxia. The signs and symptoms of hypoxia are varied and widespread. They are most clearly seen in the individual who is subjected to inadequate oxygenation of the blood acutely or subacutely, as with inhalation of low oxygen mixtures, respiratory depression, or respiratory obstruction. The changes produced by hypoxia include respiratory, cardiovascular, and CNS alterations, as well as effects on individual organs and tissues and on metabolism. These effects are discussed below.

Respiration. Hypoxia stimulates both rate and depth of respiration reflexly through the chemoreceptors of the carotid and aortic bodies. Although moderate reductions in oxygen saturation fail to increase the respiratory minute volume markedly, the inhalation of gas mixtures containing 7% or less of oxygen nearly doubles the pulmonary ventilation. Furthermore, interactions at the carotid chemoreceptors enhance the ventilatory response to carbon dioxide when the P_{O_2} of arterial blood is lowered (Lahiri *et al.,* 1981). It is important to realize that, as a result of the hyperpnea induced by hypoxia, there is a fall in arterial carbon dioxide tension (P_{CO_2}). Some of the physiological changes observed in hypoxic persons may be partly due to this mild hypocarbia. With decrease in the normal carbon dioxide central respiratory drive, the increase in ventilation due to hypoxia at the peripheral chemoreceptors is somewhat diminished.

Normal individuals breathing low concentrations of oxygen fail to experience dyspnea because hypoxia and dyspnea are not necessarily associated. Dyspnea occurs when the respiratory minute volume approaches the maximal breathing capacity. In the normal individual, with a maximal breathing capacity of 160 liters per minute, an extreme degree of hypoxia does not provide sufficient stimulus for the minute ventilation to reach levels associated with dyspnea. On the other hand, if the maximal breathing capacity is reduced to 15 to 30 liters per minute by pulmonary abnormalities, any slight respiratory stimulation might raise the minute volume sufficiently to cause dyspnea. There are many stimuli to respiration in addition to hypoxia, for example, acidosis, hypercarbia, and activation of stretch receptors originating in the lungs. Thus, the indication for oxygen therapy is not dyspnea but hypoxia or the threat of severe hypoxemia. When oxygen is given to a patient who has both hypoxia and dyspnea, therapy should not be stopped if oxygen fails to relieve the dyspnea.

Cardiovascular System. The cardiac output increases with hypoxia, largely due to an increase in heart rate and a decrease in peripheral vascular resistance. Tachycardia is probably initiated somewhere in the CNS, rather than by the carotid and aortic chemoreceptors (Krasney and Koehler, 1977), and it also reflects in part the release of catecholamines from the adrenal medulla (*see* Cohen *et al.*, 1967; Schwartz *et al.*, 1981). Hypoxia produces dilatation of the coronary, cerebral, and much of the peripheral vasculature, largely due to autoregulatory mechanisms. However, significant changes in blood pressure are not observed unless the hypoxia becomes severe, such as that produced in normal individuals breathing less than 10% oxygen; hypertension then ensues. Lesser degrees of hypoxia do cause pulmonary vasoconstriction and pulmonary hypertension. This response is an exaggeration of the pulmonary arterial vasomotion that matches regional perfusion to regional ventilation in the normal lung (*see* Glasser *et al.*, 1983).

In normal individuals exposed to reduced P_{O_2} in the inspired air, the increase in pulse rate varies with the oxygen saturation of arterial blood, reaching about a 30% increase at 70% saturation. Tachycardia is such a consistent response to hypoxia that a reduction in heart rate of 10 beats per minute within a few minutes after the initiation of oxygen therapy has been taken as presumptive evidence that acute hypoxia existed. Continuing severe hypoxia, however, can result in a decrease in heart rate toward normal values, and the prolonged inhalation of 4 to 5% oxygen can produce circulatory failure (Kafer and Sugioka, 1981).

Central Nervous System. Hypoxia affects both the function and morphology of the CNS. An acute reduction of the arterial oxygen saturation to 85% (P_{O_2}=50 mm Hg) decreases mental effectiveness, visual acuity, emotional stability, and finer muscular coordination. Further reduction to 75% saturation (P_{O_2}=40 mm Hg) leads to faulty judgment, analgesia, and considerable impairment of muscular coordination. If the arterial oxygen saturation is reduced below 65% (P_{O_2}=32 mm Hg), unconsciousness and a progressive, descending depression of the CNS supervene. Finally, circulatory failure occurs. Because hypoxia is so pernicious and reduces acuity of sensation and judgment, a person inhaling a low oxygen mixture may lose consciousness before realizing that any changes have taken place.

Under certain conditions the inhalation of carbon dioxide may offer some protection to the hypoxic brain, for three reasons. First, it counteracts the respiratory alkalosis produced when hypoxia induces hyperpnea, thus moving the oxygen dissociation curve to the right and making more oxygen available to tissues. Second, it increases the ventilation, resulting in more rapid delivery of oxygen to alveoli and therefore in a higher arterial P_{O_2}. Third, it tends to dilate cerebral vessels and increase blood flow to the brain (*see* Karl *et al.*, 1978).

The manifestations of cerebral hypoxia produced by acute arrest of the cerebral circulation are sudden and dramatic. Changes in the EEG include the appearance of high-voltage slow waves (δ waves), which occur within seconds, as does the loss of consciousness. The first histological changes occur in cortical gray matter and some thalamic and hippocampal cells after less than 5 minutes of circulatory occlusion. The cerebellum is more resistant to hypoxic damage, and the brain stem and cord are most resistant (Pulsinelli *et al.*, 1982). Full return of function cannot be expected if circulatory arrest exceeds 5 minutes, and irreversible damage and death may be expected if the cerebral circulation remains static for longer periods (*see* Safer *et al.*, 1978; Orlowski, 1983).

Individual Organs and Tissues. The brain is usually the first organ to manifest hypoxic damage; the myocardium is also highly susceptible. Hypoxic injury to other organs is slower in onset, but can occur as a result of generalized circulatory insufficiency. Cerebrovascular responses and compensatory vasomotor reflexes combine to deflect an inordinately large proportion of the cardiac output from visceral channels to organs such as the brain and heart (Koehler *et al.*, 1980). Under these circumstances, hypoxic damage to the liver and kidney as well as other organs can be demonstrated. The effect of oxygen lack on the eye is loss of visual acuity, which is manifested most noticeably by the abrupt development of a sensation of brightening following restoration of the normal supply of oxygen. Muscle is capable of sustaining an oxygen debt for periods of several hours by means of anaerobic metabolism.

Metabolism. Oxygen consumption and carbon dioxide production by the whole body and by various organs do not change measurably until extremes of hypoxia are reached. However, there are changes in carbohydrate metabolism associated with a shift from aerobic to anaerobic metabolic pathways. Those changes most frequently observed are hyperglycemia and increased production of lactic acid, with an increase in the lactate:pyruvate ratio in blood and metabolic acidosis. A summary of the metabolic effects of hypoxia has been provided by Astrup (1982).

Adaptation to Chronic Hypoxia. Individuals who have resided at high altitudes since birth (highlanders) display a number of physiological differences from those born near sea level (lowlanders) (*see* Cruz *et al.*, 1980). Highlanders display increased lung growth, more alveoli, more muscle myoglobin, a higher hemoglobin concentration in blood, and a decreased ventilatory response to hypoxia; the latter limits the respiratory alkalosis that results from hyperventilation induced by hypoxia. Lowlanders who travel to high altitudes (sojourners) can acclimatize within weeks toward the highlander's state. The mechanisms of adaptation are as yet obscure (*see* Houston, 1980). In cases where adaptation fails to occur, a syndrome known as *acute mountain sickness* appears (generally at altitudes greater than 2.5 km). The symptoms include headache, nausea, vomiting, disturbed sleep, difficulty in mentation, and dyspnea. The syndrome can progress to a stage in which pulmonary and cerebral edema occur; administration of oxygen and descent to lower altitude are required. Treatment with diuretics and anti-inflammatory steroids may be helpful (Johnson *et al.*, 1984). The syndrome may be avoided by slow ascent, permitting gradual acclimatization. Acclimatized individuals may lose tolerance and develop a syndrome known as *chronic mountain sickness,* characterized by severe polycythemia; this condition can end in heart failure unless the individual returns to lower altitudes. The greater resistance to hypoxia manifested by the newborn of most mammalian species might be regarded as an adaptation to the chronic mild hypoxia that exists *in utero* (*see* Newth, 1979).

EFFECTS OF OXYGEN INHALATION

The administration of oxygen to a hypoxic patient can often restore normal oxygen tensions in blood and tissues; if irreversible changes due to severe hypoxia have not occurred, normal function will be restored. In normal individuals, the inhalation of oxygen at 1 or more atmospheres raises the arterial P_{O_2} to many times its normal value (*see* Table 16–1) and increases the degree of oxygenation of tissues. These changes are followed by alterations in other blood gases and by physiological adjustments in the respiratory and cardiovascular systems. Under some circumstances, there is significant toxicity.

Effect on Other Blood Gases. *Carbon Dioxide.* One of the ways in which carbon dioxide is carried by blood is in the form of bicarbonate. This mechanism of carbon dioxide transfer operates more readily when a hydrogen ion acceptor is made available, as occurs in the capillaries when oxyhemoglobin is converted to deoxyhemoglobin, a stronger base and therefore a better hydrogen ion acceptor. When large amounts of oxygen are carried in simple solution (*e.g.*, during hyperbaric oxygenation), the amount of physically dissolved oxygen may be sufficient to satisfy the requirements of tissue (*see* Table 16–1). Little or no oxygen is then extracted from oxyhemoglobin, and deoxyhemoglobin is not formed. Carbon dioxide is then carried away from tissues less efficiently, and the P_{CO_2} of the tissues rises by several mm Hg (*see* Plewes and Farhi, 1983).

Nitrogen. Normally, the blood is in equilibrium with alveolar air, which contains close to 80% nitrogen. As a result, several liters of this inert gas are in solution in body fluids and are present in body cavities. When pure oxygen is inhaled, the partial pressure of nitrogen in the alveoli falls rapidly. Nitrogen diffuses from the tissues to be eliminated by the lungs. Most of the nitrogen of the body can be exhaled in this manner within a few hours. The effects of this absence of "inert gas" from the body are discussed in the section on Untoward Effects of Oxygen Inhalation, as well as under Therapeutic Uses.

Respiration. The immediate effect of the inhalation of 100% oxygen by normal subjects is a mild respiratory depression, presumably due to withdrawal of tonic impulses from the chemoreceptors. However, there is an increase in ventilation within a few minutes (Lambertsen, 1978). This is due to an increase in the P_{CO_2} in the CNS that results from its less efficient removal by the blood (*see* above).

Cardiovascular System. There is a slight decrease in the heart rate of normal subjects inhaling pure oxygen. Cardiac output is reduced by 8 to 20%, which may be caused in part by oxygen-induced myocardial depression. There is little change in blood pressure. The inhalation of oxygen also affects blood flow to some important vascular beds. Coronary blood flow in the dog is reduced by the administration of oxygen. Cerebral blood flow is decreased slightly. This is related in part to the mild hypocarbia attending oxygen inhalation (Fishman, 1961). There also seems to be cerebrovascular constriction due to increased sensitivity to adrenergic agonists under hyperoxic conditions (Nakajima *et al.*, 1983). In the pulmonary vascular bed, high tensions of oxygen cause dilatation and reduced pulmonary arterial pressure. Oxygen inhalation appears to relax the pulmonary vasculature in hypoxic animals and man, and in persons with pulmonary hypertension.

Metabolism. When 100% oxygen is inhaled by man, changes are not detectable in oxygen consumption, carbon dioxide production, respiratory quotient, or glucose utilization.

UNTOWARD EFFECTS OF OXYGEN INHALATION

The administration of oxygen, particularly at more than 1 atmosphere of pressure, can cause undesirable effects. However, none of these should interdict the use of high partial pressures of oxygen when they are indicated.

Respiratory Depression. In several situations the response of the respiratory centers to carbon dioxide may be so depressed that respiration is maintained largely by the activity of the carotid and aortic chemoreceptors. This phenomenon may attend cerebral injuries involving the respiratory centers, barbiturate intoxication, or long periods of exposure to hypercarbia or hypoxia (*e.g.*, chronic pulmonary disease). In these instances, the administration of oxygen may cause hypoventilation or apnea by the removal of the chemoreceptor drive to respiration (Aubier *et al.*, 1980). The occurrence of respiratory depression is not a contraindication to, but rather a convincing indication of the need for, the administration of oxygen. It is better to have the patient well oxygenated with controlled artificial respiration than to have him poorly oxygenated from breathing spontaneously, but inadequately, in response to a hypoxic drive from the chemoreceptor mechanism.

Fortunately, in many cases it is possible to administer carefully controlled concentrations of oxygen sufficient to increase arterial oxygenation, but not great enough to cause respiratory depression; the patient must be monitored constantly and the conditions controlled stringently.

Retrolental Fibroplasia. Retrolental fibroplasia occurs in some premature infants who are exposed to high concentrations of oxygen before 44 weeks of gestational age (Betts *et al.*, 1977). It is believed to result from oxygen-induced spasm and subsequent degeneration of immature retinal arterioles. Retinal changes become noticeable in 3 to 6 weeks. These may regress entirely or may progress through retinal detachment to blindness. The incidence of this disease has been greatly reduced in recent years by careful monitoring of arterial or transcutaneous oxygen tensions of infants receiving supplemental oxygen. The inspired P_{O_2} is limited to that required to maintain an arterial P_{O_2} of 60 to 70 mm Hg (Ashton, 1979). It is the *arterial* P_{O_2} and not the *inspired* P_{O_2} that is the crucial determinant of this disease. Retinal damage can also occur in adults following inhalation of 100% oxygen at greater-than-atmospheric pressures. This is particularly liable to occur in those patients whose retinal circulation has been previously compromised, for example, by retinal detachment (*see* Kushner *et al.*, 1977).

Oxygen Toxicity. In the course of evolution, the P_{O_2} in the earth's atmosphere increased, and mechanisms to protect cellular constituents from oxidative damage became necessary. These consist of enzymes (such as superoxide dismutases), reducing agents (such as glutathione and ascorbate), and compounds that scavenge free radicals. These normal defenses may become inadequate when high concentrations of oxygen are inhaled. At elevated oxygen tensions, highly reactive forms of oxygen are present in abnormal concentrations. These include free radicals (*e.g.*, superoxide and hydroxyl radical) and activated molecular oxygen in the form of hydrogen peroxide or singlet oxygen (*see* Gilbert, 1981; Phelps, 1982; Crapo *et al.*,

1983). Oxygen toxicity results particularly from the destruction of membrane lipids, nucleic acids, and thioamino acids. There is as yet no protective treatment of demonstrated value in man (*see* Barthelemy *et al.*, 1981).

Respiratory Tract. Pulmonary oxygen toxicity is the most common form of oxygen toxicity in man. The inhalation, at atmospheric pressure, of 80% oxygen for more than about 12 hours can cause a symptom complex that begins with irritation of the respiratory tract. Normal subjects exposed to these tensions of oxygen in the inspired air manifest a progressive decrease in vital capacity, coughing, nasal stuffiness, sore throat, and substernal distress. Continued exposure results in tracheobronchitis and later in the development of pulmonary congestion, transudation, exudation, and atelectasis (*see* Miller and Winter, 1981).

Pulmonary oxygen toxicity is not experienced by subjects breathing 50% oxygen, nor by those breathing 100% oxygen at ½ atmosphere for 24 hours or longer. Thus, it is clear that the important factor in the causation of this symptom complex is the P_{O_2} and *not* the concentration of oxygen in the inhaled gas. The onset and progression of signs and symptoms are more rapid at greater inspired P_{O_2}. When inspired P_{O_2} becomes greater than 2 atmospheres, CNS toxicity is the first symptom to appear (Lambertsen, 1965). Figure 16–2 shows a comparison of the times of onset of pulmonary and CNS symptoms of oxygen toxicity.

The mechanisms of pulmonary oxygen toxicity are complex (Deneke and Fanburg, 1982). Endothelial and type-I alveolar cells are most susceptible to injury, and the loss of integrity of the alveolar capillary membrane leads to an increase in interstitial fluid and protein. Breathing of oxygen also depresses the mucociliary transport mechanism of the respiratory tract, with subsequent inhibition of the tracheal flow of mucus. This effect can be demonstrated after several hours of inhalation of oxygen and is proportional to the inspired oxygen concentration. Inhibition of mucociliary transport impairs the host's pulmonary defenses (*see* Barnes *et al.*, 1983; Davis *et al.*, 1983).

Central Nervous System. When pure oxygen is inhaled at pressures greater than 2 atmospheres, a characteristic syndrome is

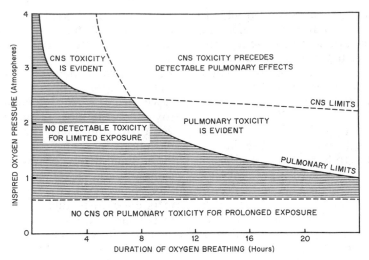

Figure 16–2. *Oxygen-toxicity limits in man.*

The two areas most affected are the CNS and the lungs. The occurrence of toxicity depends upon both the inspired oxygen pressure (P_{O_2}) and the duration of exposure. The safe duration of exposure becomes shorter as the inspired P_{O_2} increases. Below ½ atmosphere of inspired oxygen, indefinite exposure appears to be safe; between ½ and approximately 2 atmospheres, pulmonary toxicity occurs after prolonged exposures but CNS effects are not detectable; above 2 atmospheres, CNS toxicity appears before pulmonary effects are detectable. (Adapted from Lambertsen, 1978.)

observed. Signs and symptoms include mood changes, nausea, vertigo, muscular twitching, generalized convulsions, and loss of consciousness. The appearance of this syndrome is related both to the length of exposure and to the ambient P_{O_2}. The symptoms may appear in persons at rest in less than 2 hours at 3 atmospheres, in 0.5 hour at 4 atmospheres, and in a few minutes at 6 atmospheres of oxygen. However, wide individual variations are observed in the susceptibility to oxygen poisoning. The latent period before oxygen toxicity appears is decreased by physical exertion and by inhalation of carbon dioxide. CNS toxicity produced by high pressures of oxygen appears to be reversible with decrease in the inspired P_{O_2}. Following a period of postictal depression, recovery of normal function is complete and relatively rapid.

PREPARATIONS

Preparations of oxygen are of a specified purity. Oxygen is marketed in a compressed form in steel cylinders fitted with reducing valves for delivery of the gas. They are usually color coded (green in the United States), and those for use on anesthetic machines are pin indexed.

METHODS OF ADMINISTRATION

The various methods for the administration of oxygen will be discussed only briefly. They have been reviewed by Leigh (1974).

A simple device for the administration of oxygen is a soft rubber or plastic catheter, which is inserted into a nostril. Short, paired catheters that just extend into both nares are called nasal prongs. Humidified oxygen is passed through these tubes, and the rate of flow largely determines the concentration that enters the alveoli. It is rare that more than 50% oxygen can be introduced into the lungs by this means.

Another, more effective method for the administration of oxygen is a face mask. Such masks may be equipped with a system of valves to permit elimination of carbon dioxide and dilution of the inspired oxygen with ambient air, if this is desired. As long as the rate of oxygen inflow exceeds the minute ventilation, it is possible to administer nearly 100% oxygen with a tightly fitted face mask and reservoir bag. Masks are almost essential for use at high altitudes, in aviation, and in pressure chambers. Furthermore, they make possible the use of assisted or controlled ventilation, which can be of value in the treatment of pulmonary edema, asthma, and certain chronic pulmonary diseases.

Oxygen tents or hoods that fit over the patient's head in a fairly airtight manner are sometimes used for pediatric patients. They are comfortable for the patient and require minimal cooperation but restrict access of attendants. Oxygen must be delivered to them at relatively high flow rates. Administration of oxygen through an endotracheal tube or a tracheostomy in conjunction with mechanical ventilation is used for the seriously ill.

THERAPEUTIC USES

Haldane stated years ago that *hypoxia not only stops the machine but wrecks the machinery*. The treatment of hypoxia is obviously a medical emergency, and, therefore, all therapeutic measures for its relief should be marshaled. Since the causes of hypoxia are diverse, the administration of oxygen frequently does not correct the basic defect. Rather, oxygen is employed as a stopgap until more fundamental measures can be instituted or become effective, or occasionally because specific therapy for the underlying disease is unavailable. In this capacity the administration of oxygen can be lifesaving. The alert therapist does not wait until the signs and symptoms of severe hypoxia are evident but administers the gas in anticipation of its need.

The therapeutic uses of oxygen are conveniently considered under the headings used above to classify the etiology of hypoxia.

Prepulmonary Causes of Hypoxia. When there is a deficiency of oxygen in the atmosphere, for example, at high altitudes, the administration of supplemental oxygen will assure an adequate P_{O_2} in the alveoli. Above an altitude of 3.7 km (12,000 ft), where barometric pressure is below 500 mm Hg, it is necessary to administer supplemental oxygen; above 10.1 km (33,000 ft), even 100% oxygen will not maintain normal alveolar P_{O_2}.

Inadequate oxygenation of the normal lung does not always call for therapy with oxygen. Rather, the basic cause of the hypoxia should be addressed. For example, obstruction of the airway can often be corrected by mechanical means; insufficiency of the respiratory muscles or respiratory depression calls for artificial ventilation. However, there are circumstances under which oxygen therapy can be of great value. For instance, when obstruction to breathing is due to bronchoconstriction that proves difficult to overcome, hypoxia can be relieved when oxygen is administered by mask.

Pulmonary Causes of Hypoxia. These problems constitute the most frequent indications for oxygen therapy.

Diffusion Barriers. In certain situations there is a barrier to diffusion of oxygen through the alveolar-capillary membrane. This can occur when there are anatomical changes, as in pulmonary fibrosis, or when the membrane is temporarily thickened, as in pulmonary edema. In such situations, oxygen inhalation is of great value in overcoming the diffusion barrier, and adequate arterial oxygenation can usually be obtained with only a small increase in inspired oxygen concentration. Pure diffusion block is rare, and other pulmonary defects in association with it are usually of greater functional importance.

Ventilation-Perfusion Inequalities. When some alveoli are poorly ventilated, the oxygenation of blood flowing past them is decreased. This blood will mix with well-oxygenated blood coming from more normal areas of lung, and the resulting mixed arterial blood will be intermediate in its content of oxygen. If the ventilation-perfusion defect is serious enough to produce significant desaturation of the arterial blood, therapy with oxygen is indicated. This treatment increases the P_{O_2} of gas in alveoli that receive any ventilation, and some reversal of hypoxemia can be expected.

Venous-Arterial Shunts. A small amount of right-to-left shunting of blood is normal from Thebesian and pleural veins. Abnormal degrees of shunting may be due to congenital anatomical defects, or they may be acquired, as in patients with atelectasis or pneumonia. Since the shunted blood is never exposed to respiratory gases, administration of oxygen cannot increase its saturation. The increase in oxygen content of blood draining normal oxygen-containing alveoli is small, as it represents mostly dissolved oxygen (*see* Table 16–1). When this blood mixes with partially unsaturated blood, the resulting arterial pool may still be inadequately oxygenated. Thus, some improvement can be obtained by administering oxygen in the presence of right-to-left shunting; however, if the defect is great, arterial blood saturation may not be returned completely to normal.

Mixed Defects in Pulmonary Function. In most pulmonary disease states, more than one factor contributes to the production of hypoxemia. For example, in *pneumonia* there is a diffusion defect. Atelectasis is present in some areas of the lung, and there is also a ventilation-perfusion defect. Finally, tachypnea and shallow respiration result in less effective alveolar ventilation. In this disease, as in many others, oxygen administration compensates for some of the abnormalities better than for others. It may overcome the diffusion barrier completely and successfully treat the ventilation-perfusion defect, but may only partially compensate for the shunting of blood past atelectatic alveoli. The inefficient ventilatory pattern usually improves with relief of the hypoxia. Oxygen obviously does not remove the basic cause of the disease; improvement is symptomatic.

In the treatment of *pulmonary edema*, the administration of oxygen by mask or endotracheal tube with controlled or assisted ventilation can be of value. Particular benefit derives from the increased intrapulmonary pressure that is transmitted to the great veins, thereby retarding the flow of blood into the right heart.

Maintenance of positive airway pressure throughout the ventilatory cycle is frequently beneficial in patients with impaired pulmonary gas exchange. The resulting increase in functional residual capacity decreases the tendency of alveoli to collapse during part of the ventilatory cycle. The decrease in shunting and improved matching of ventilation to perfusion frequently allow adequate arterial oxygenation to be achieved without increasing inspired oxygen tensions to toxic levels (*see* Tyler, 1983).

Postpulmonary Causes of Hypoxia. Oxygen is useful in some types of postpulmonary hypoxia in which it provides a valuable adjunct to more fundamental therapy.

Hemoglobin Deficiency. The administration of oxygen is of importance in the treatment of *carbon monoxide poisoning,* because it accelerates the conversion of carboxyhemoglobin to oxyhemoglobin. In addition, the breathing of pure oxygen leads to increased transport of this gas in solution in the plasma, and in this manner tissue hypoxia is partially relieved (*see* Chapter 70). Similarly, oxygen inhalation can also be of value in anemia.

Circulatory Deficiency. Oxygen has been used effectively in certain instances of generalized circulatory deficiency, including cardiac decompensation and shock. In *cardiac decompensation* the oxygen saturation of the blood may be reduced due to pulmonary edema. In addition, there is tissue hypoxia associated with circulatory inadequacy. Oxygen therapy often results in the relief of cyanosis and a slowing of the pulse rate. Although treatment should be directed primarily toward improving cardiac function, oxygen affords temporary relief due to better oxygenation of the myocardium.

Oxygen administration is of limited value in the therapy of the tissue hypoxia present during *shock.* Nevertheless, oxygen is often administered to patients with peripheral circulatory failure for whatever benefit can be gained from the increase in blood P_{O_2} and the additional oxygen carried in solution.

Oxygen may also be of some value in cases of localized circulatory deficiency, such as occurs in *coronary occlusion.* The higher P_{O_2} and oxygen content of the circulating blood may aid in the delivery of oxygen to hypoxic areas of the myocardium. Improvement is frequently noted, with relief of pain and restlessness, improvement of circulation, and relief of cyanosis. Oxygen inhalation may also be of value in some instances of *cerebrovascular accidents,* permitting better oxygenation of marginally hypoxic areas of the brain. In situations of abnormally high metabolic demand, such as hyperthermia or thyrotoxicosis, inhalation of oxygen can also be helpful.

Miscellaneous Uses of Oxygen. A unique although uncommon use of oxygen is in the treatment of *abdominal distention.* In such conditions as intestinal obstruction, ileus, or postoperative distention, the gas accumulating in the bowel consists largely of nitrogen. Very little of this nitrogen will dissolve in blood, for it has already been exposed in the lungs to an atmosphere containing 80% nitrogen. If, however, 100% oxygen is breathed and the partial pressure of nitrogen in the alveoli falls, nitrogen diffuses out of the gas in the intestine and into the blood, and is eliminated through the lungs. For similar reasons, inhalation of 100% oxy-gen has also been suggested for treatment of *spontaneous pneumothorax* and *air embolism* (Chadha and Cohn, 1983).

Oxygen inhalation is also used by workers in *pressurized spaces,* to decrease the inhaled nitrogen concentration and thus to lessen the likelihood of *caisson disease,* or bends, to shorten the required decompression time, and to minimize nitrogen narcosis. Under these conditions one must be careful not to exceed the time and concentration limits for avoidance of oxygen toxicity.

Finally, in *anesthesia,* oxygen is a common diluent for the gaseous and volatile anesthetic agents. The anesthetized patient may inhale up to 98% oxygen when 2% halothane is being administered in a non-rebreathing system, or as little as 20% oxygen when 80% nitrous oxide is given.

HYPERBARIC OXYGEN THERAPY

Although most uses of oxygen do not require more than 1 atmosphere of the gas, there are some conditions where administration of greater tensions may be desirable.

Hyperbaric oxygenation is accomplished in pressure chambers. These range in size from those designed for a few small experimental animals, through those large enough for a man, up to chambers that accommodate an entire operating suite. Since it is neither practical nor economical to fill the larger chambers with oxygen, they may be brought to ambient pressures of more than 1 atmosphere with compressed air. The patients then inhale oxygen at these ambient pressures through a face mask or mouthpiece.

There are many practical difficulties associated with this type of treatment. The facilities and their proper maintenance and operation are expensive; there is a fire hazard in the enclosed space of the chamber; oxygen toxicity and nitrogen narcosis are distinct possibilities; and decompression sickness can occur in patients or attendants. However, many potential uses for this method of therapy have been explored. Presently its use is justified in a few situations (Vorosmarti, 1981; Davis, 1983).

Gas Emboli and Bubbles. Hyperbaric oxygenation can be useful in the treatment of decompression sickness. It can also provide immediate relief of symptoms in situations where gas emboli in the vascular tree can be compressed by high pressures, such as diving accidents and postcardiopulmonary-bypass gas emboli. During slow decompression these bubbles, which become filled with oxygen, are gradually absorbed.

Anaerobic Infections. Intermittent treatment with hyperbaric oxygen may be of value in the treatment of infections produced by *Clostridium perfringens,* the anaerobic bacillus causing *gas gangrene.* The increased tissue oxygen pressure achieved inhibits growth and production of toxin by these bacteria. Antibiotics and other supportive therapy are still necessary. Results are less satisfactory in the treatment of *tetanus* with hyperbaric oxygen, as the toxin may already be bound to neural tissue, and, although the microorganism is killed or prevented from multiplying, irreversible damage may have occurred.

Hyperbaric oxygen may prove to be useful in the treatment of other anaerobic infections, some mixed aerobic and anaerobic infections, certain refractory mycoses, and some cases of chronic, refractory osteomyelitis.

Carbon Monoxide Poisoning. The use of 2 atmospheres of oxygen will result in faster conversion of carboxyhemoglobin to oxyhemoglobin than will 100% oxygen at sea level. Little practical benefit is gained by increasing pressure much further. One treatment with 2 atmospheres of oxygen for 30 to 90 minutes is usually sufficient even for patients who are comatose. The greatest difficulty encountered in the use of this therapy is the problem of rapidly transporting the patient to a hyperbaric chamber. The use of 1 atmosphere of oxygen during transport is recommended and may make hyperbaric treatment unnecessary (*see* Chapter 70).

Circulatory Disturbances. With the hope of improving tissue oxygenation by raising the arterial blood P_{O_2}, hyperbaric oxygen has been used as a therapeutic measure in such *local circulatory disturbances* as stroke, peripheral arterial insufficiency, compromised skin grafts, radiation necrosis, and crush injuries. The possibility of oxygen toxicity makes continuous therapy dangerous, and, therefore, intermittent treatments are used. The efficacy of this method of therapy in these diseases depends on the presence of some circulation to the tissues, that is, only partial occlusion of vessels or the existence of collateral channels for those that are blocked. This application of hyperbaric oxygen has had minimal success.

CARBON DIOXIDE

It was not until the end of the eighteenth century that Priestley discovered this gas and Lavoisier described its role in respiration. A century later Miesher demonstrated its effects on the respiration of man. The gas is of paramount importance in the regulation of many vital functions, and small changes in P_{CO_2} in the body have marked physiological effects.

Transfer and Elimination of Carbon Dioxide

Approximately 200 ml per minute of carbon dioxide are produced by the body's metabolism at rest, and up to ten times that much during heavy exercise. The gas diffuses readily from the cells that produce it into the blood stream, where it is carried partly as bicarbonate ion, partly in chemical combination with hemoglobin and plasma proteins, and also in solution at a partial pressure of about 46 mm Hg in mixed venous blood. It is transported to the lung, where it is normally exhaled at the same rate at which it is produced, leaving a partial pressure of about 40 mm Hg in the alveoli and in the arterial blood.

When carbon dioxide is inhaled, or when alveolar ventilation is decreased, the P_{CO_2} in arterial blood rises and its pH falls. This decrease in pH is referred to as *respiratory acidosis*. When overventilation lowers the P_{CO_2} of blood, the pH rises and *respiratory alkalosis* is present. As carbon dioxide can freely diffuse into and out of cells, the changes in blood P_{CO_2} and pH are soon reflected by intracellular changes of P_{CO_2} and pH (*see* Chapter 35).

Effects of Carbon Dioxide

Alterations of P_{CO_2} and pH have widespread effects in the body. Here a description will be given of the important effects of carbon dioxide on respiration, circulation, and the CNS. (For a more complete discussion of these and other effects, *see* Nunn, 1977.)

Respiration. Carbon dioxide is a potent stimulus to respiration. The inhalation of 2% carbon dioxide produces a measurable increase in both rate and depth of ventilation. Ten percent carbon dioxide can produce respiratory volumes of 75 liters per minute in normal individuals. The inhalation of even higher concentrations produces little additional increase in ventilation. Respiratory stimulation begins in seconds following the inhalation of even low concentrations of carbon dioxide, and maximal stimulation by the inhaled carbon dioxide is usually attained in less than 5 minutes (*see* Lourenco, 1976). The respiratory effects of carbon dioxide inhalation disappear within a few minutes after its withdrawal.

There are at least two *sites* where carbon dioxide acts to stimulate respiration. Respiratory integration areas in the brain stem are acted upon by impulses from medullary chemoreceptors and from peripheral arterial chemoreceptors. The mechanism by which carbon dioxide acts on these receptors particularly involves the decrease in pH produced by the gas (*see* Neff and Talmage, 1978; Drysdale *et al.*, 1981). Elevated P_{CO_2} causes bronchodilatation, while hypocarbia causes constriction of airway smooth muscle; these responses may play a role in matching pulmonary ventilation and perfusion (Duane *et al.*, 1979).

Circulation. The circulatory effects of carbon dioxide are the result of its direct local effects and its centrally mediated effects on the autonomic nervous system. The direct effect of carbon dioxide on the *heart* results from pH changes and produces diminished contractile force and slowing of the rate of contraction (van den Bos *et al.*, 1979). The cardiac rhythm is usually not affected. The direct effect on systemic *blood vessels* results in vasodilatation.

The autonomic effects of carbon dioxide result in widespread activation of the *sympathetic nervous system,* resulting in an increase in concentration of epinephrine, norepinephrine, angiotensin, and other vasoactive peptides in plasma (Staszewska-Barczak and Dusting, 1981). The response is mediated by various subcortical centers in the hypothalamus, brain stem reticular formation, and medulla. These areas can be locally excited by carbon dioxide, but they also receive afferents from the carotid and aortic chemoreceptors that are sensitive to changes in carbon dioxide in the blood. The results of sympathetic nervous system activation are, in general, opposite to the local effects of carbon dioxide. The sympathetic effects consist in increase in the force and rate of cardiac contraction and constriction of many vascular beds.

The total circulatory response to carbon dioxide, therefore, is determined by the balance of the opposing effects on local tissues and the sympathetic nervous system effects. The overall effects of carbon dioxide inhalation in normal man are increase in cardiac output and heart rate, elevation of systolic and diastolic blood pressures, and increase in pulse pressure (Rasmussen *et al.*, 1978; Lin *et al.*, 1983). There is a *decrease* in total peripheral resistance when carbon dioxide is breathed. The local vasodilating effects of carbon dioxide appear to exert more of an influence than do the sympathetically mediated vasoconstrictor effects. In the heart, the marked increase in cardiac output reflects a predominance of the sympathetic over the local effects. The cerebral circulation, which does not have functionally important sympathetic innervation, undergoes significant dilatation when carbon dioxide is inhaled. Carbon dioxide is also a potent coronary vasodilator (Ely *et al.*, 1982). Renal and splanchnic blood flow are not significantly affected by increased P_{CO_2}.

In isolated cardiac preparations, carbon dioxide increases the threshold for catecholamine-induced arrhythmias (de Castuma *et al.*, 1977). In the intact organism, however, the amount of catecholamine released during hypercarbia may be sufficient to overwhelm this protective effect. Arrhythmias are especially likely to occur if the myocardium has been sensitized by such factors as inhalation of halogenated anesthetics.

The circulatory effects of lower-than-normal tensions of carbon dioxide consist in decreased blood pressure, vascular dilatation in muscle, and vasoconstriction in skin, intestine, brain, kidney, and heart. If the hypocarbia results from voluntary hyperventilation, cardiac output and heart rate increase because of increased venous return and increased metabolic demands of the respiratory muscles. In contrast, mechanical hyperventilation reduces heart rate and cardiac output. This effect is probably related to the increased intrathoracic pressure caused by mechanical ventilation.

Central Nervous System. The inhalation of low concentrations of carbon dioxide depresses the excitability of the cerebral cortex and increases the threshold for the production of seizures by drugs or electroshock. It also increases the cutaneous pain threshold through a central action. This central depression is of importance in the therapeutic application of the gas, for carbon dioxide can cause further depression of an already depressed brain. However, when high concentrations of carbon dioxide (25 to 30%) are breathed, subcortical areas that have cortical projections are activated. This activation overcomes the depressant effect of carbon dioxide on the cortex. The increased cortical excitability that results can progress to convulsions. The inhalation of even higher concentrations of carbon dioxide (about 50%) produces marked cortical and subcortical depression of a type similar to that produced by anesthetic agents. Acute decreases in P_{CO_2}, resulting from voluntary or mechanical hyperventilation, may cause symptoms of hypocalcemia, including carpopedal spasms (Argent, 1982).

Untoward Effects of Carbon Dioxide Inhalation. The normal subject inhaling concentrations of carbon dioxide up to 5 or 6% experiences the sensation of increased respiration, but rarely experiences dyspnea. Some notice an acidic taste, as carbon dioxide forms carbonic acid in the presence of water. The inhalation of higher concentrations, up to about 10%, produces dyspnea, headache, dizziness, sweating, restlessness, paresthesias, and a general feeling of discomfort. Higher concentrations result in pronounced discomfort. The CNS effects of very high concentrations of carbon dioxide are described above. As with oxygen poisoning, the CNS toxicity of carbon dioxide is a reversible phenomenon. Cardiovascular effects of hypercarbia include marked elevation of blood pressure, tachycardia, and arrhythmias. These effects are related to the sympathoadrenal activation that accompanies elevated carbon dioxide tensions.

Following the abrupt withdrawal of inhaled concentrations of carbon dioxide above 5%, a few subjects experience headache or dizziness. These symptoms can be avoided by slowly decreasing the inhaled concentration rather than withdrawing it suddenly.

CHEMISTRY, PREPARATIONS, AND
METHODS OF ADMINISTRATION

Carbon dioxide is approximately one and one-half times as dense as air. It is marketed in metal cylinders as carbon dioxide itself or mixed with oxygen. For medicinal purposes, carbon dioxide is usually administered by means of a face mask at a concentration of 5 to 10% in combination with oxygen. It is also possible to deliver 100% carbon dioxide from a cylinder through a tube held a few centimeters above the patient's face. Although this technic requires little equipment, it does not allow one to know the inhaled concentration of carbon dioxide. Another method of administration of carbon dioxide is by rebreathing, for example, from a paper bag. This obviously cannot be continued for longer than a few minutes.

THERAPEUTIC USES

Inhalation of carbon dioxide has been suggested as a means of therapy in many commonly encountered situations, but for most of these there are other treatments available that are more effective and offer fewer disadvantages.

Respiratory Depression, Asphyxia, and Coma. The usefulness of carbon dioxide in stimulating depressed respiration is very limited. When respiratory minute volume is reduced, the tension of this gas in blood and tissues rises. Thus, there is already an elevated P_{CO_2}. A further elevation of the tension by the administration of carbon dioxide may not increase ventilation and will only worsen the respiratory acidosis; it may also further depress the neurons of the respiratory centers.

Carbon Monoxide Poisoning. The inhalation of 5 to 7% carbon dioxide in oxygen has been used in the treatment of carbon monoxide poisoning, as carbon dioxide increases both the ventilatory exchange and the rate of dissociation of carbon monoxide from carboxyhemoglobin. A disadvantage is the production of serious acidosis when the respiratory acidosis produced by carbon dioxide is added to the metabolic acidosis already present in cases of severe carbon monoxide poisoning.

Uses in Anesthesia. Carbon dioxide inhalation can increase the speed of induction and emergence from anesthesia by increasing minute ventilation and cerebral blood flow (*see* Chapter 13). However, some degree of respiratory acidosis is inevitable. Hyperventilation with its attendant respiratory alkalosis has some uses in anesthesia. It increases the apparent depth of anesthesia. By constricting the cerebral vessels, it decreases brain size slightly and may facilitate the performance of neurosurgical operations.

Miscellaneous Uses. Inhalation of carbon dioxide is one of many suggested treatments for *hiccoughs,* and it has been successful in some cases. Sudden deafness has been treated successfully by inhalation of mixtures of carbon dioxide and oxygen, presumably because of increased cochlear circulation and delivery of oxygen (Fisch, 1983). Because it does not support combustion, carbon dioxide is often insufflated during endoscopic procedures when electrocauterization is used (Bigard *et al.,* 1979).

HELIUM

Helium is an inert gas. Its limited medical applications derive from its special physical properties. The low density of helium (specific gravity = 0.14) reduces resistance to turbulent gas flow and is the basis for its use when respiration is embarrassed by airway obstruction. However, helium's high kinematic viscosity (eight times that of air) acts in the opposite direction, and it decreases airflow in most obstructed airways below the major bronchi. The low aqueous solubility of helium (one half that of nitrogen) makes it useful for divers and others who work in environments with high ambient pressure to minimize inert gas narcosis, decompression time, and "the bends." Its high velocity of sound

transmission (four times that of air) causes voice distortion, and its high thermal conductivity (six times that of air) can cause excessive heat loss.

History and Preparation. Helium was identified spectroscopically in the sun's atmosphere in 1868, as α radiation from uranium ore in 1895, and as a component in natural gas in 1905. The sole commercial source of helium is recovery after liquefaction of natural gas from fields in the western United States. It is marketed in compressed form in steel cylinders.

Methods of Administration. The apparatus that is used to breathe helium is chosen largely on the basis of the specific application. In saturation diving applications, individuals are placed in a closed environment consisting largely of helium. In pulmonary function testing, one breath of helium may be inhaled or it may be breathed from closed spirometers by way of a mask or mouthpiece. For intermittent positive-pressure breathing, a non-rebreathing circuit is commonly employed with either a mask or endotracheal tube.

Applications. The clinical uses of helium have been summarized by Mathewson (1982). It has been employed in respiratory obstruction, in investigative and diagnostic testing, and in hyperbaric applications.

Respiratory Obstruction. During normal breathing, gas flow in the airways is mostly laminar and the energy required to produce flow is dependent on both the kinematic viscosity and the density of the gas. While the kinematic viscosity of helium is high, its density is sufficiently low that the work of breathing is decreased by about 25% in normal subjects breathing 78% helium (DeWeese *et al.,* 1983). However, when there is turbulent flow of gas in the airway, the energy required to produce flow is *inversely* related to the density of the gas. This may occur when there is laryngeal or tracheal obstruction, a high volume of ventilation, or very high ambient pressures. In this situation, mixtures of helium and oxygen may be respired more easily than air, resulting in greater washout of carbon dioxide (Brice and Welch, 1983). However, such mixtures are always less effective than is 100% oxygen in raising the P_{O_2} in blood. Beneficial results have not been conclusively documented from the use of mixtures of helium and oxygen in respiratory obstruction, but some patients may improve temporarily (Chan-Yeung *et al.,* 1976).

Diagnostic Uses. Helium is useful in pulmonary function testing because it is nearly as insoluble as hydrogen but is not flammable. When a patient breathes from a spirometer containing a mixture of helium, very little helium is dissolved in body tissues, and all the helium lost from the spirometer is diluted in the lungs. This permits calculation of diffusing capacity and functional residual capacity of the lungs.

Hyperbaric Applications. The production of oxygen toxicity at 2 atmospheres and of nitrogen narcosis at 6 atmospheres limits the barometric pressure at which man can function in either oxygen or air. Furthermore, under high pressure, significant amounts of nitrogen dissolve in blood and, particularly, in lipid. If decompression is rapid, nitrogen will effervesce from body stores and produce gas emboli in joints, the CNS, and blood; the results are excruciating pain, chronic disability, and even death. This decompression sickness, also known as "the bends" or caisson disease, can be avoided by slow decompression, which permits the dissolved nitrogen to diffuse gradually into the blood and be eliminated by the lungs. Because helium is markedly less soluble than nitrogen in both water and lipids and because it has little demonstrable narcotic effect up to 30 atmospheres (Brauer and Way, 1970), respiration of mixtures of helium and oxygen permits deeper diving and safer, quicker decompression. Furthermore, helium's low density reduces the work of breathing required at very high pressures. In some undersea missions, subjects have lived in a helium-oxygen atmosphere. Problems encountered included distorted speech, increased loss of body heat, and gas emboli at the junction of skin and subcutaneous fat or of body fat and blood vessels. The latter is due to the phenomenon of isobaric counterdiffusion of nitrogen and helium (Lambertsen and Idicula, 1975).

WATER VAPOR

Because of extensive hydrogen bonding, water is a liquid with a large heat of vaporization, a high specific heat, and considerable ability to dissolve or disperse a wide variety of other compounds. Inhalation and exhalation of water vapor normally take place with every breath, and inhalation of supplemental amounts of water vapor can be an important therapeutic procedure.

Inspired air is warmed to body temperature and humidified to saturation by the time it reaches the larynx or upper trachea. While deep, rapid breathing may move the boundary of saturation into the lung, the air-conditioning function of the nasal turbinates and upper airway still provides the bulk of humidification. Normal man can tolerate a temporary shift in the site of humidification to the tracheobronchial tree during endotracheal anesthesia (Knudsen et al., 1973) or the chronic shift that results from tracheostomy if no additional stress is placed on the airways. Since about 50 mg of water is needed for each liter of inspired dry gas to saturate it at body temperature, sedentary individuals require approximately 500 ml of water per day for this purpose.

Uses of Inspired Water. Water vapor is particularly therapeutic for patients whose airways are chronically intubated (as in respiratory care units); it decreases crusting of respiratory mucosa, liquefies thick secretions, promotes mucociliary clearance, limits the loss of body water, and tends to conserve body heat by limiting evaporation in the airway (Chalon et al., 1979). Inhalation of humidified gases warmed to slightly above body temperature can help to warm hypothermic patients (Caldwell et al., 1981).

Water aerosols may be used instead of water vapor. Either cool or warm aerosols may be soothing in laryngitis and croup. Aerosols also permit delivery of drugs such as bronchodilators, mucolytics, hydroscopics, steroids, and antibiotics to the respiratory tract (Pierce and Saltzman, 1974).

Methods of Administration. Inspired water may be provided as vapor from humidifiers or as vapor and particulate water from aerosol generators (nebulizers). Either may provide water warmed to body temperature or cooled below room temperature, as occasionally desired in laryngitis. The water used may be distilled water or dilute solutions of sodium chloride; isotonic saline is preferred for nebulizers (Shephard et al., 1983).

While the content of water vapor in inspired gas is limited to a maximum set by temperature, additional water may be administered with an aerosol generator. Control of the size of the aerosol particles permits some control over the site of deposition of the aerosol. Particles larger than 50 μm tend to settle rapidly or coalesce, forming the rain familiar in oxygen tents and hoods. Particles of 10 to 20 μm tend to impact on the walls of the upper airway and trachea. Particles of 5 to 10 μm are mainly deposited in medium-sized and small bronchi, while those of 1 to 5 μm may penetrate all the way to the alveolar ducts and alveoli. Most particles of less than 1 μm are completely exhaled in the subsequent breath. They are neither heavy enough to impact on the airways nor light enough to diffuse from alveolar ducts to alveoli during the course of one breath. Aerosol deposition tends to be increased at points of increased airway resistance and collections of secretions (Kim et al., 1983). Regardless of particle size, slow deep breaths favor more alveolar penetration of droplets while fast short breaths favor upper airway deposition (Stahlhofen et al., 1983).

Untoward Effects. Potential problems include thermal damage from overheated inspired gas, fluid overload from absorption of excess water, and coughing and bronchoconstriction from direct irritation of the bronchi by water droplets. Prior administration of lidocaine aerosol can inhibit coughing, and administration of isoproterenol, atropine, or cromolyn sodium can inhibit bronchoconstriction (Waltemath and Bergman, 1973; Shephard et al., 1983). Thermal damage is due not only to the temperature of the gas but also to the delivery of 580 cal for each gram of vapor that is condensed. Chronic inhalation of an aerosol mist can result in the net absorption of more than 500 ml of water a day by adult patients and disproportionately more (relative to weight) by children and infants. Humidification devices must be cleaned scrupulously to reduce the incidence of nosocomial infections (see Brain, 1980).

Anthonisen, N. R. Hypoxemia and O_2 therapy. *Am. Rev. Respir. Dis.*, **1982**, *126*, 729–733.
Argent, V. P. Treatment of severe tetany due to hyperventilation during labour with a mixture of nitrous

oxide, oxygen, and carbon dioxide. *Br. Med. J.*, **1982**, *285*, 117–118.

Ashton, N. The pathogenesis of retrolental fibroplasia. *Ophthalmology (Rochester)*, **1979**, *86*, 695–699.

Aubier, M.; Murciano, D.; Milic-Emili, J.; Touaty, E.; Daghfous, J.; Pariente, R.; and Derenne, J. P. Effects of the administration of O_2 on ventilation and blood gases in patients with chronic obstructive pulmonary disease during acute respiratory failure. *Am. Rev. Respir. Dis.*, **1980**, *122*, 747–754.

Barnes, S. D.; Agee, C. C.; Peace, R. J.; and Leffler, C. W. Effects of elevated P_{O_2} upon tracheal explants. *Respir. Physiol.*, **1983**, *53*, 285–293.

Barthelemy, L.; Belaud, A.; and Chastel, C. A comparative study of oxygen toxicity in vertebrates. *Respir. Physiol.*, **1981**, *44*, 261–268.

Bert, P. Experience sur l'empoisonment par l'oxygene. *Gaz. Méd. Paris*, **1873**, *28*, 387.

Betts, E. K.; Downes, J. J.; Schaffer, D. B.; and Johns, R. Retrolental fibroplasia and oxygen administration during general anesthesia. *Anesthesiology*, **1977**, *47*, 518–520.

Bigard, M.; Gaucher, P.; and Lassalle, C. Fatal colonic explosion during colonoscopic polypectomy. *Gastroenterology*, **1979**, *77*, 1307–1310.

Boerema, I.; Meyne, N. G.; Brummelkamp, W. K.; Bouma, S.; Mensch, M. H.; Kamermans, F.; Stern Hanf, M.; and Van Aalderen, W. Life without blood. *J. Cardiovasc. Surg. (Torino)*, **1960**, *1*, 133–146.

Brauer, R. W., and Way, R. O. Relative narcotic potencies of hydrogen, helium, nitrogen and their mixtures. *J. Appl. Physiol.*, **1970**, *29*, 23–31.

Brice, A. G., and Welch, H. G. Metabolic and cardiorespiratory responses to He-O_2 breathing during exercise. *J. Appl. Physiol.*, **1983**, *54*, 387–392.

Caldwell, C.; Crawford, R.; and Sinclair, I. Hypothermia after cardiopulmonary bypass in man. *Anesthesiology*, **1981**, *55*, 86–87.

Chadha, T. S., and Cohn, M. A. Noninvasive treatment of pneumothorax with oxygen inhalation. *Respiration*, **1983**, *44*, 147–152.

Chalon, J.; Patel, C.; Ali, M.; Ramanathan, S.; Capan, L.; Tang, C. K.; and Turndorf, H. Humidity and the anesthetized patient. *Anesthesiology*, **1979**, *50*, 195–198.

Chan-Yeung, M.; Abboud, R.; Ming, S. T.; and MacLean, L. Effect of helium on maximum expiratory flow in patients with asthma before and during induced bronchoconstriction. *Am. Rev. Respir. Dis.*, **1976**, *113*, 434–443.

Cohen, P. J.; Alexander, S. C.; Smith, T. C.; Reivich, M.; and Wollman, H. Effects of hypoxia and normocarbia on cerebral blood flow and metabolism in conscious man. *J. Appl. Physiol.*, **1967**, *23*, 183–189.

Crapo, J. D.; Freeman, B. A.; Barry, B. E.; Turrens, J. F.; and Young, S. L. Mechanisms of hyperoxic injury to the pulmonary microcirculation. *Physiologist*, **1983**, *26*, 170–176.

Cruz, J. C.; Reeves, J. T.; Grover, R. F.; Maher, J. T.; McCullough, R. E.; Cymerman, A.; and Denniston, J. C. Ventilatory acclimatization to high altitude is prevented by CO_2 breathing. *Respiration*, **1980**, *39*, 121–130.

Davis, W. B.; Rennard, S. I.; Bitterman, P. B.; and Crystal, R. G. Pulmonary oxygen toxicity: early reversible changes in human alveolar structures induced by hyperoxia. *N. Engl. J. Med.*, **1983**, *309*, 878–883.

de Castuma, E. S.; Mattiazzi, A. R.; and Cingolani, H. E. Effect of hypercapnic acidosis on induction of arrhythmias by catecholamines in cat papillary muscles. *Arch. Int. Physiol. Biochim.*, **1977**, *85*, 509–518.

DeWeese, E. L.; Sullivan, T. Y.; and Yu, P. L. Ventilatory and occlusion pressure responses to helium breathing. *J. Appl. Physiol.*, **1983**, *54*, 1525–1531.

Drysdale, D. B.; Jensen, J. I.; and Cunningham, D. J. C.

The short-latency respiratory response to sudden withdrawal of hypercapnia and hypoxia in man. *Q. J. Exp. Physiol.*, **1981**, *66*, 203–210.

Duane, S. F.; Weir, E. K.; Stewart, R. M.; and Niewoehner, D. E. Distal airway responses to changes in oxygen and carbon dioxide tensions. *Respir. Physiol.*, **1979**, *38*, 303–311.

Ely, S. W.; Sawyer, D. C.; and Scott, J. B. Local vasoactivity of oxygen and carbon dioxide in the right coronary circulation of the dog and pig. *J. Physiol. (Lond.)*, **1982**, *332*, 427–439.

Fisch, U. Management of sudden deafness. *Otolaryngol. Head Neck Surg.*, **1983**, *91*, 3–8.

Glasser, S. A.; Domino, K. B.; Lindgren, L.; Parcella, P.; Marshall, C.; and Marshall, B. E. Pulmonary blood pressure and flow during atelectasis in the dog. *Anesthesiology*, **1983**, *58*, 225–231.

Johnson, T. S.; Rock, P. B.; Fulco, C. S.; Trad, L. A.; Spark, R. F.; and Maher, J. T. Prevention of acute mountain sickness by dexamethasone. *N. Engl. J. Med.*, **1984**, *310*, 683–686.

Karl, A. A.; McMillan, G. R.; Ward, S. L.; Kissen, A. T.; and Souder, M. E. Effects of increased ambient CO_2 on brain tissue oxygenation and performance in the hypoxic rhesus. *Aviat. Space Environ. Med.*, **1978**, *49*, 984–989.

Kim, C. S.; Brown, L. K.; Lewars, G. G.; and Sacknet, M. A. Depression of aerosol particles and flow resistance in mathematical and experimental airway models. *J. Appl. Physiol.*, **1983**, *55*, 154–163.

Knudsen, J.; Lomholt, N.; and Wisborg, K. Postoperative pulmonary complications using dry and humidified anesthetic gases. *Br. J. Anaesth.*, **1973**, *45*, 363–368.

Koehler, R. C.; McDonald, B. W.; and Krasney, J. A. Influence of CO_2 on cardiovascular response to hypoxia in conscious dogs. *Am. J. Physiol.*, **1980**, *239*, H545–H558.

Krasney, J. A., and Koehler, R. C. Influence of arterial hypoxia on cardiac and coronary dynamics in the conscious sinoaortic-denervated dog. *J. Appl. Physiol.*, **1977**, *43*, 1012–1018.

Kushner, B. J.; Essner, D.; Cohen, I. J.; and Flynn, J. T. Retrolental fibroplasia. II. Pathologic correlation. *Arch. Ophthalmol.*, **1977**, *95*, 29–38.

Lahiri, S.; Mokashi, A.; Mulligan, E.; and Nishino, T. Comparison of aortic and carotid chemoreceptor responses to hypercapnia and hypoxia. *J. Appl. Physiol.*, **1981**, *51*, 55–61.

Lambertsen, C. J., and Idicula, J. A. A new gas lesion syndrome in man induced by "isobaric gas counter diffusion." *J. Appl. Physiol.*, **1975**, *39*, 434–443.

Lambertsen, C. J.; Kough, R. H.; Cooper, D. Y.; Emmel, G. L.; Loeschcke, H. H.; and Schmidt, C. F. Oxygen toxicity. Effects in man of oxygen inhalation at 1 and 3.5 atmospheres upon blood gas transport, cerebral circulation and cerebral metabolism. *J. Appl. Physiol.*, **1953**, *5*, 471–486.

Leigh, J. M. Evolution of oxygen therapy apparatus. *Anaesthesia*, **1974**, *29*, 462–485.

Lin, Y. C.; Shida, K. K.; and Hong, S. K. Effects of hypercapnia, hypoxia, and rebreathing on circulatory response to apnea. *J. Appl. Physiol.*, **1983**, *54*, 172–177.

Lourenco, R. V. Clinical methods for the study of regulation of ventilation. *Chest*, **1976**, *70*, 109–195.

Mathewson, H. S. Helium—who needs it? *Respir. Care*, **1982**, *27*, 1400–1401.

Nakajima, S.; Meyer, J. S.; Amano, T.; Shaw, T.; Okabe, T.; and Mortel, K. F. Cerebral vasomotor responsiveness during 100% oxygen inhalation in cerebral ischemia. *Arch. Neurol.*, **1983**, *40*, 271–276.

Neff, T. A., and Talmage, P. Neuromuscular and chemical control of breathing. *Chest*, **1978**, *73*, 247–308.

Orlowski, J. P. Pediatric cerebral resuscitation. *Cleve. Clin. Q.*, **1983**, *50*, 317–321.

Phelps, D. L. Neonatal oxygen toxicity—is it preventable? *Pediatr. Clin. North Am.*, **1982**, *29*, 1233–1239.

Plewes, J. L., and Farhi, L. E. Peripheral circulatory responses to acute hyperoxia. *Undersea Biomed. Res.*, **1983**, *10*, 123–129.

Pulsinelli, W. A.; Brierley, J. B.; and Plum, F. Temporal profile of neuronal damage in a model of transient forebrain ischemia. *Ann. Neurol.*, **1982**, *11*, 491–498.

Rasmussen, J. P.; Dauchot, P. J.; DePalma, R. G.; Sorensen, B.; Regula, G.; Anton, A. H.; and Gravenstein, J. S. Cardiac function and hypercarbia. *Arch. Surg.*, **1978**, *113*, 1196–1200.

Robin, E. D. Dysoxia—abnormal tissue oxygen utilization. *Arch. Intern. Med.*, **1977**, *137*, 905–910.

Sackner, M. A. A history of oxygen usage in chronic obstructive pulmonary disease. *Am. Rev. Respir. Dis.*, **1974**, *110*, Suppl., 25–34.

Safar, P.; Bleyaert, A.; Nemoto, E. M.; Moossy, J.; and Snyder, J. V. Resuscitation after global brain ischemia-anoxia. *Crit. Care Med.*, **1978**, *6*, 215–227.

Samaja, M.; Mosac, A.; Luzzana, M.; Rossi-Bernardi, L.; and Winslow, R. M. Equations and nomogram for the relationship of human blood p50 to 2,3-diphosphoglycerate, CO_2 and H^+. *Clin. Chem.*, **1981**, *27*, 1856–1861.

Schwartz, S.; Frantz, R. A.; and Shoemaker, W. C. Sequential hemodynamic and oxygen transport responses in hypovolemia, anemia, and hypoxia. *Am. J. Physiol.*, **1981**, *241*, H864–H871.

Shephard, D.; Rizk, N. W.; Boushey, H. A.; and Bethel, R. A. Mechanism of cough and bronchoconstriction induced by distilled water aerosol. *Am. Rev. Respir. Dis.*, **1983**, *127*, 691–694.

Stahlhofen, W.; Gibhart, J.; Hayder, J.; and Scheuck, G. Disposition pattern of droplets from medical nebulizers in the human respiratory tract. *Bull. Eur. Physiopath. Respir.*, **1983**, *19*, 459–463.

Staszewska-Barczak, J., and Dusting, G. J. Importance of circulating angiotensin II for elevation of arterial pressure during acute hypercapnia in anaesthetized dogs. *Clin. Exp. Pharmacol. Physiol.*, **1981**, *8*, 189–201.

Tyler, D. C. Positive end-expiratory pressure: a review. *Crit. Care Med.*, **1983**, *11*, 300–308.

van den Bos, G. C.; Drake, A. J.; and Noble, M. I. M. The effect of carbon dioxide upon myocardial contractile performance, blood flow, and oxygen consumption. *J. Physiol. (Lond.)*, **1979**, *287*, 149–161.

Vorosmarti, J. Hyperbaric oxygen therapy. *Am. Fam. Physician*, **1981**, *23*, 169–173.

Waltemath, C. L., and Bergman, N. A. Increased respiratory resistance provoked by endotracheal administration of aerosols. *Am. Rev. Respir. Dis.*, **1973**, *108*, 520–525.

Monographs and Reviews

Astrup, J. Energy-requiring cell functions in the ischemic brain. *J. Neurosurg.*, **1982**, *56*, 482–497.

Brain, J. Aerosol and humidity therapy. *Am. Rev. Respir. Dis.*, **1980**, *122*, 17–21.

Davis, J. C. *Hyperbaric Oxygen Therapy: A Committee Report.* Undersea Medical Society, Inc., Bethesda, Md., **1983**.

Deneke, S. M., and Fanburg, B. 1. Oxygen toxicity of the lung: an update. *Br. J. Anaesth.*, **1982**, *54*, 737–749.

Fishman, A. P. Respiratory gases in the regulation of the pulmonary circulation. *Physiol. Rev.*, **1961**, *41*, 214–280.

Gilbert, D. L. (ed.). *Oxygen and Living Processes: An Interdisciplinary Approach.* Springer-Verlag, New York, **1981**.

Houston, C. S. *Going High: The Story of Man and Altitude.* The American Alpine Club, New York, **1980**.

Hudson, L. D., and Pierson, D. J. Comprehensive respiratory care for patients with chronic obstructive pulmonary disease. *Med. Clin. North Am.*, **1981**, *65*, 629–645.

Kafer, E. R., and Sugioka, K. Respiratory and cardiovascular responses to hypoxemia and the effects of anesthesia. *Int. Anesthesiol. Clin.*, **1981**, *19*, 85–122.

Lambertsen, C. J. Effects of oxygen at high partial pressure. In, *Respiration*, Vol. 2. Sect. 3, *Handbook of Physiology.* (Fenn, W. O., and Rahn, H., eds.) American Physiological Society, Washington, D. C., **1965**, pp. 1027–1040.

————. Effects of hyperoxia on organs and their tissues. In, *Extrapulmonary Manifestations of Respiratory Disease.* (Robin, E. D., ed.) Vol. 8, *Lung Biology in Health and Disease.* (Lenfant, C., ed.) Marcel Dekker, Inc., New York, **1978**, pp. 239–303.

Miller, J. W., and Winter, P. M. Clinical manifestations of pulmonary oxygen toxicity. *Int. Anesthesiol. Clin.*, **1981**, *19*, 179–199.

Newth, C. J. L. Recognition and management of respiratory failure. *Pediatr. Clin. North Am.*, **1979**, *26*, 617–641.

Nunn, J. F. Carbon dioxide. In, *Applied Respiratory Physiology*, 2nd ed. Butterworths, London, **1977**, pp. 334–374.

Pierce, A. K., and Saltzman, H. A. The scientific basis of respiratory therapy (the Sugarloaf Conference). *Am. Rev. Respir. Dis.*, **1974**, *110*, Pt. 2, 1–204.

CHAPTER

17 HYPNOTICS AND SEDATIVES

Stewart C. Harvey

The principal use of sedative-hypnotic drugs is to produce drowsiness and promote sleep. The application of the term *sedative* to this group is somewhat misleading. It dates from the era when the sedative-hypnotic compounds were the only drugs (apart from alcohol, opioids, and belladonna) that could be used to calm anxious and disturbed patients. With the proliferation of psychopharmacological agents, the drugs traditionally described as "sedative-hypnotics" have come to play a lesser role in daytime sedation. This role will be discussed in connection with the pharmacotherapy of anxiety in Chapter 19. In the present chapter, the hypnotic properties and uses of these drugs are emphasized.

A *sedative* drug decreases activity, moderates excitement, and calms the recipient. A *hypnotic* drug produces drowsiness and facilitates the onset and maintenance of a state of sleep that resembles natural sleep in its electroencephalographic characteristics and from which the recipient may be easily aroused; the effect is sometimes called hypnosis, but the sleep induced by hypnotic drugs does not resemble that artificially induced passive state of suggestibility also called hypnosis. Sedation, pharmacological hypnosis, and general anesthesia are usually regarded as only increasing depths of a continuum of central nervous system (CNS) depression. Indeed, most sedative or hypnotic drugs, when used in high doses, can induce general anesthesia. One important exception, however, is the benzodiazepines.

Since sedative-hypnotic drugs usually have the capability of producing widespread depression of the CNS, it is not surprising to find that CNS functions, in addition to the state of wakefulness, are usually depressed by these drugs. Thus, various sedative-hypnotic drugs are employed as antiepileptic agents (Chapter 20), muscle relaxants (Chapter 21), and antianxiety drugs (Chapter 19); some may also be used to produce amnesia or general anesthesia (Chapter 14). It is not certain whether the effects of these drugs on wakefulness and anxiety are truly distinct, and their separation in this textbook may represent an artificial division.

History. Since antiquity, potions have been used to induce sleep. History and folklore have provided accounts of both sinister and romantic uses of laudanum, alcoholic beverages, and various herbals to produce stupor, during which intrigue, adultery, or magical transformation could take place. Potions were also used for sedation and hypnosis, but they were too unpredictable to bequeath to modern medicine. The first agent to be specifically introduced as a sedative and soon thereafter as a hypnotic was bromide (1853, 1864). Only four more sedative-hypnotic drugs (chloral hydrate, paraldehyde, urethan, and sulfonal) were in use before 1900. Barbital was introduced in 1903 and phenobarbital in 1912. Their success spawned the synthesis and testing of over 2500 barbiturates, of which approximately 50 were distributed commercially. The barbiturates held the stage so dominantly that less than a dozen other sedative-hypnotics were successfully marketed before 1960, and several popular old drugs slipped into oblivion.

The partial separation of sedative-hypnotic-anesthetic from anticonvulsant properties, embodied in phenobarbital, led to searches for agents with more selective effects on the functions of the CNS. As a result, relatively nonsedative anticonvulsants, notably phenytoin and trimethadione, were developed in the late 1930s and early 1940s (*see* Chapter 20). The advent of chlorpromazine and meprobamate in the early 1950s, with their taming effects in animals, and the development of increasingly sophisticated methods for evaluation of the behavioral effects of drugs set the stage in 1957 for the synthesis of chlordiazepoxide by Sternbach and the discovery of its unique pattern of actions by Randall (*see* Symposium, 1982). With its introduction into clinical medicine in 1961, chlordiazepoxide ushered in the era of benzodiazepines; more than 3000 have been synthesized, over 120 have been tested for biological activity, and 25 are in clinical use in various parts of the world.

Most of the benzodiazepines that have reached the marketplace were selected for high anxiolytic potential and low potency as general depressants of CNS function. Their extraordinary popularity in clinical medicine is largely due to their ability to relieve symptoms of anxiety with minimal interference with cognitive function or wakefulness. Nevertheless, the benzodiazepines all possess sedative-hypnotic properties to varying degrees; these are extensively exploited clinically, especially to facilitate sleep. Mainly because of their remarkably low capacity to produce fatal CNS depression, the benzodiazepines have largely displaced the barbiturates as sedative-hypnotic agents. Meanwhile, a few agents other than benzodiazepines continue to appear and command careful examination.

BENZODIAZEPINES

While the benzodiazepines in clinical use exert qualitatively similar effects, there are important quantitative differences in their pharmacodynamic spectra and pharmacokinetic properties that have led to varying patterns of therapeutic application. There is now reason to believe that a number of distinct mechanisms of action contribute in varying degrees to the sedative-hypnotic, muscle relaxant, anxiolytic, and anticonvulsant effects of the benzodiazepines; these mechanisms are currently under intense investigation. While only those benzodiazepines used primarily for hypnosis will be discussed in detail, this chapter will describe the general properties of the group and the important differences between individual agents (*see also* Chapters 19 and 20).

Chemistry. The structures of the benzodiazepines in use in the United States are shown in Table 17–1, as are those of a few related compounds to be discussed below.

The term *benzodiazepine* refers to the portion of the structure composed of a benzene ring (A) fused to a seven-membered diazepine ring (B). However, since all of the important benzodiazepines contain a 5-aryl substituent (ring C) and a 1,4-diazepine ring, the term has come to mean the 5-aryl-1,4-benzodiazepines. Various modifications in the structure of the ring systems have yielded compounds with similar activities. These include 1,5-benzodiazepines (*e.g.*, *clobazam*) and the replacement of the fused benzene ring (A) with heteroaromatic systems such as thieno or pyrazolo (*see* Fryer, in Symposium, 1983a). The 5-aryl substituent greatly enhances potency but can be replaced by a five-membered ring fused to positions 3 and 4 to form an anthramycin.

The chemical nature of substituents at positions 1 to 3 can vary widely and can include triazolo or imidazo rings fused at positions 1 and 2. Electron-withdrawing groups at position 7 markedly enhance activity; electron-releasing or large groups at this position or substituents elsewhere in ring A reduce activity. Electron-withdrawing groups at the 2' (or ortho) position in ring C enhance potency, while substituents elsewhere decrease activity (*see* Sternbach, in Symposium, 1973). Replacement of ring C with a keto function at position 5 and a methyl substituent at position 4 are important structural features of a specific benzodiazepine antagonist (Ro 15-1788) (*see* Haefely *et al.*, in Symposium, 1983a).

PHARMACOLOGICAL PROPERTIES

The effects of the benzodiazepines virtually all result from actions of these drugs on the CNS, even when lethal doses are taken. In man and other mammals, the most prominent of these effects are sedation, hypnosis, decreased anxiety, muscle relaxation, and anticonvulsant activity. One benzodiazepine, alprazolam, appears to have antidepressant activity in certain clinical settings. Only two effects of these drugs appear to result from actions on peripheral tissues: coronary vasodilatation, seen after intravenous administration of therapeutic doses of certain benzodiazepines, and neuromuscular blockade, seen only with very high doses.

Central Nervous System. While the benzodiazepines affect activity at all levels of the neuraxis, some structures are affected to a much greater extent than are others. In addition, some effects of the drugs are indirect. The benzodiazepines are not general neuronal depressants, as are the barbiturates. All of the benzodiazepines have the same pharmacological profile, except for the anticonvulsant and possibly analgesic effects of certain members. Nevertheless, there are wide differences in selectivity among the drugs, and the clinical usefulness of individual benzodiazepines thus varies considerably. While some of these differences are described below, detailed discussion may be found in the monographs and reviews listed in the bibliography.

The pharmacological profile for a given drug varies markedly from species to species. In some species, the subject may become alert before there is evidence of CNS depression. For example, the 7-nitrobenzodiazepines induce hyperactivity in mice, rats, and monkeys, but not in most other species; flurazepam causes convulsions only in cats. Interestingly, muscle relaxation in cats and anticonvulsant activity

Table 17–1. BENZODIAZEPINES: NAMES AND STRUCTURES *

BENZODIAZEPINE	R_1	R_2	R_3	R_7	$R_{2'}$
Alprazolam	[Fused triazolo ring] [b]		—H	—Cl	—H
Chlordiazepoxide [a]	(—)	—NHCH$_3$	—H	—Cl	—H
Clonazepam	—H	=O	—H	—NO$_2$	—Cl
Clorazepate	—H	=O	—COO$^-$	—Cl	—H
Demoxepam [a,1,2]	—H	=O	—H	—Cl	—H
Diazepam	—CH$_3$	=O	—H	—Cl	—H
Flurazepam	—CH$_2$CH$_2$N(C$_2$H$_5$)$_2$	=O	—H	—Cl	—F
Halazepam	—CH$_2$CF$_3$	=O	—H	—Cl	—H
Lorazepam	—H	=O	—OH	—Cl	—Cl
Midazolam [2]	[Fused imadazo ring] [c]		—H	—Cl	—F
Nitrazepam [2]	—H	=O	—H	—NO$_2$	—H
Nordazepam [2,3]	—H	=O	—H	—Cl	—H
Oxazepam	—H	=O	—OH	—Cl	—H
Prazepam	—CH$_2$—CH$\langle$CH$_2$ / CH$_2\rangle$	=O	—H	—Cl	—H
Temazepam	—CH$_3$	=O	—OH	—Cl	—H
Triazolam	[Fused triazolo ring] [b]		—H	—Cl	—Cl
Ro 15-1788 [a,2]	[Fused imidazo ring] [d]		—H	—F	[=O at C$_5$] [e]

* Alphabetical footnotes refer to alterations of the general formula; numerical footnotes are used for other comments.
  [a] No substituent at position 4, except for chlordiazepoxide and demoxepam, which are N-oxides; R$_4$ is —CH$_3$ in Ro 15-1788, in which there is no double bond between positions 4 and 5.

[e] No ring C.
[1] Major metabolite of chlordiazepoxide.
[2] Not available for clinical use in the United States.
[3] Major metabolite of diazepam and others; also referred to as nordiazepam and desmethyldiazepam.

against pentylenetetrazol in mice correlate better with the sedative, antianxiety, and hypnotic properties in man than do the actions to suppress motor activity, induce sleep, and release suppressed behavior in experimental animals.

In man, as the dose of a benzodiazepine is increased, sedation progresses to hypnosis and hypnosis to stupor, as expected of a general CNS depressant. The clinical literature often refers to the ''anesthetic'' effects and uses of certain benzodiazepines, but the drugs do not cause a true general anesthesia, since awareness usually persists and relaxation sufficient to allow surgery can-

not be achieved. However, anterograde amnesia may occur, which creates the illusion of previous anesthesia. For true surgical anesthesia, benzodiazepines must be combined with other CNS depressant drugs. Similarly in some experimental animals, righting reflexes or certain other CNS functions are not abolished until lethal or nearly lethal doses of benzodiazepines are given. In contrast, the barbiturates can cause anesthesia.

As with probably all sedative-hypnotic drugs, ''preanesthetic'' doses of benzodiazepines impair recent memory and interfere with the establishment of the memory trace. Hence they cause anterograde amnesia for events that occur subsequent to the administration of the drug.

The question whether the so-called antianxiety effects of benzodiazepines are the same as or different from the sedative and hypnotic effects has not been resolved. Contributing to this uncertainty are the difficulty in defining and measuring sedation in both man and experimental animals, the difficulty in assessing antianxiety effects in man (*see* Chapter 19), and the unproven validity of various models of anxiety in animals.

In experimental animals, most attention has been focused on the ability of benzodiazepines to increase locomotor, feeding, or drinking behavior that has been suppressed by novel or aversive stimuli. For example, animals have been tested in various ways in which behavior that had been previously rewarded by food or water is periodically punished by an electric shock. The time during which shocks are delivered is signaled by some auditory or visual cue, and untreated animals stop performing almost completely when the cue is perceived. The administration of a benzodiazepine can eliminate the difference in behavioral responses during the punished and unpunished periods, usually at doses that do not reduce the rate of unpunished responses or produce other signs of impaired motor function. Similarly, rats placed in an unfamiliar environment exhibit markedly reduced exploratory behavior ("neophobia"), while animals treated with benzodiazepines do not. Opioid analgesics and neuroleptic (antipsychotic) drugs do not increase suppressed behaviors, while phenobarbital and meprobamate usually do so only at doses that also reduce spontaneous or unpunished behaviors or produce ataxia. Descriptions of these and other experimental procedures, as well as discussions of their potential relationship to anxiety in man, can be found in the proceedings of several recent symposia (*see* Symposium, 1983a, 1983b, 1983c).

The ratio of the dose required to impair motor function to that necessary to increase punished behavior varies widely among the benzodiazepines and depends, not surprisingly, on the species and experimental protocol. For example, in the squirrel monkey this ratio ranges from about 1 for flurazepam to over 300 for clonazepam (*see* Randall and Kappell, in Symposium, 1973). While such data may have encouraged the marketing of flurazepam only as a sedative-hypnotic agent, they have not predicted with any accuracy the relative frequency or intensity of sedative effects among those benzodiazepines marketed as anxiolytic agents (*see* Linnoila, in Symposium, 1983a).

Studies on tolerance in animals are often cited to support the belief that disinhibitory effects of benzodiazepines are separate from their general depressant effects. For example, tolerance to the depressant effects on rewarded or neutral behavior occurs after several days of treatment with benzodiazepines, while the disinhibitory effects of the drugs on punished behavior appear to be augmented. Although tolerance to the impairment of certain aspects of psychomotor performance (*e.g.*, visual tracking) in man is not usually observed (*see* Linnoila, in Symposium, 1983a), most patients who ingest benzodiazepines chronically report that drowsiness wanes over a few days (*see* Lader and Petursson, in Symposium, 1983c). The development of tolerance to the anxiolytic effects of benzodiazepines has not been studied adequately. However, most patients maintain themselves on a fairly constant dose; increases or decreases in dosage appear to correspond to changes in problems or stresses. Nevertheless, some patients either do not reduce their dosage when stress is relieved or steadily escalate dosage without apparent reason (*see* Lader and Petursson, in Symposium, 1983c). Such behavior may be associated with the development of drug *dependence* (*see* below).

Some benzodiazepines induce muscle hypotonia without interfering with normal locomotion. They also decrease decerebrate rigidity in cats and rigidity in patients with cerebral palsy. They increase the patellar reflex. In cats, muscle relaxation is effected in doses that are two (flurazepam) to four (clonazepam) orders of magnitude less than those that abolish the righting reflex. Diazepam is ten times more selective than meprobamate. However, this remarkable degree of selectivity is not seen in man; clonazepam in nonsedative doses does cause muscle relaxation in man, but diazepam and most other benzodiazepines do not. Tolerance occurs to both the muscle relaxant and ataxic effects of these drugs.

Experimentally, benzodiazepines inhibit seizure activity induced by either pentylenetetrazol or picrotoxin, but strychnine- and maximal electroshock-induced seizures are suppressed only with doses that also severely impair locomotor activity. Flunitrazepam, triazolam, clonazepam, bromazepam, and nitrazepam are more selective anticonvulsants than are other benzodiazepines. Benzodiazepines also suppress photic seizures in baboons and ethanol-withdrawal seizures in man. The development of tolerance to the anticonvulsant effects has limited the usefulness of benzodiazepines in the treatment of seizure disorders in man (*see* Chapter 20).

Only diazepam is selectively analgesic in mice. In man, it causes a transient analgesia after intravenous administration. No analgesic effect in man has been reported for other benzodiazepines. Various interactions with the effects of different analgesics have been observed in experimental animals. Their clinical significance remains to be clarified. Unlike the barbiturates, benzodiazepines do not cause hyperalgesia.

Effects on EEG and Sleep Stages. The effects of benzodiazepines on the waking EEG resemble those of other sedative-hypnotic drugs. Alpha activity is decreased, and there is an increase in low-voltage, fast activity, especially beta activity. The shift in activity occurs more in the frontal and rolandic areas than elsewhere in the brain; unlike the effect of barbiturates, there is little or no posterior spread. The benzodiazepines reduce the amplitude of cortical somatosensory-evoked potentials in the human EEG; the latency of the early peak is shortened and that of the late peak prolonged. This effect and the shift to beta activity appear to correlate with the antianxiety effects. Benzodiazepines resemble barbiturates in that tolerance occurs to the effects on the EEG.

There continues to be much effort devoted to understanding the stages of sleep. Some characteristics of these stages are summarized in Table 17–2. The effects of benzodiazepines on the stages of sleep have been studied widely. An excellent compilation of findings and discussion of 66 studies may be found in the review by Kay and associates (1976) (*see also* Greenblatt and Shader, 1974; Mendelson *et al.,* 1977). It may be concluded that, with a few important exceptions, the benzodiazepines are all rather similar in their effects on the important sleep parameters. However, a few studies suggest that high doses of some benzodiazepines produce effects that are qualitatively different from those that are seen after low doses. Many studies have been on normal subjects. It appears that insomniacs and patients with various psychiatric disorders may respond differently than do normal individuals.

Most benzodiazepines decrease sleep latency, especially when first used, and diminish the number of awakenings and the time spent in stage 0 (a stage of wakefulness). They have been shown to increase the awakening threshold. Time in stage 1 (descending drowsiness) is usually decreased by flurazepam, lorazepam, nitrazepam, and temazepam, but it is increased by chlordiazepoxide, diazepam, and oxazepam. Time spent in stage 2 (which is the major fraction of non-rapid-eye-movement [REM] sleep) is increased by all benzodiazepines. Benzodiazepines (with the possible exception of temazepam) prominently decrease the time spent in slow-wave sleep (SWS; stages 3 and 4); usually both stages 3 and 4 are shortened, but in neurotic patients or those with endogenous depression temazepam has been found to prolong stage 3 and shorten stage 4. The shortening of stage-4 sleep does not decrease the total number of delta waves during a night because they are transferred to stage 2. The decrease in stage-4 sleep is accompanied by a reduction in night terrors and nightmares; however, if the decrease is marked, these phenomena may be shifted to the waking hours ("daymares").

Much attention has been paid to the effects on REM sleep. Most benzodiazepines increase REM latency (time from onset of spindle sleep to the first REM burst), except that flurazepam has been reported to shorten latency in some insomniac neurotic or psychotic individuals. The frequency of eyeball movement during REM sleep is decreased. The time spent in REM sleep is usually shortened. However, REM sleep may not be shortened when temazepam or lower doses of flurazepam, clobazam, or perhaps other benzodiazepines are used, even though substantial shortening of SWS and prolongation of stage-2 sleep may occur. Temazepam and triazolam diminish REM sleep in the early hours, but the lost time is made up later in the sleep time. Even with benzodiazepines that cause a substantial reduction in total time spent in REM sleep, the number of cycles of REM sleep is usually increased, mostly late in the sleep time. Various benzodiazepines may actually increase time in REM sleep and fast activity during REM sleep in depressed schizophrenics and other psychotics, patients with endogenous depression or neuroses, unspecified insomniacs, and persons who alternately work during the day or night. Nitrazepam often increases REM sleep.

Benzodiazepines do not appear to lessen the relaxation of neck muscles that occurs at the onset of REM sleep. They diminish the magnitude of the bursts of tachycardia that occur during REM sleep and the fluctuations in skin resistance that occur in both stage-2 and REM sleep. Tolerance rapidly develops to the effects on skin resistance. Flunitrazepam increases the sexual and aggressive content of dreams during REM sleep.

Despite the shortening of stage-4 and REM sleep, the net effect of administration of benzodiazepines is usually an increase in total sleep time. The effect is greatest in subjects with the shortest baseline total sleep time, for whom sleep time may triple, and least (or even insignificant) in those who normally enjoy a long sleep time. In addition, despite the increase in the number of REM cycles, the number of shifts to lighter sleep stages (1 and 0) and the amount of body movement are diminished. The nocturnal peaks in the concentration of growth hormone in plasma and the concentrations of prolactin and luteinizing hormone are not affected by flurazepam or nitrazepam.

Use of benzodiazepines imparts a sense of deep or refreshing sleep, but it is uncertain to which effect on sleep parameters this can be attributed. Some have ascribed it to the diminution in REM sleep, but this is not consistent with the high regard insomniacs have for triazolam and temazepam, which have little effect on total REM sleep time. Others attribute it to the suppression of SWS, but this is an inconsistent effect of temazepam.

During chronic nocturnal use of benzodiazepines the effects on the various stages of sleep usually

Table 17–2.   ELECTROENCEPHALOGRAPHIC AND OTHER CHARACTERISTICS
OF THE STAGES OF SLEEP

STAGE *	EEG WAVE ACTIVITY †	EYEBALL ACTIVITY	EFFECT OF DEPRIVATION	OTHER OBSERVATIONS
0 (Awake) Eyes open Eyes closed	Beta Alpha	Irregular, except slowly rolling when drowsy	—	Insomniacs have longer stages 0 and 1 than normal subjects
1 ("Descending" sleep; dozing)	Alpha Beta Theta	Slight, but bursts of rolling movement	Prevents all following sleep stages; no selective deprivation	
2 (Unequivocal sleep)	Theta Spindles K complexes	Slight rolling movements; occasional REM ‡	Prevents following stages	Subject easily aroused; sensory stimuli evoke K complexes
Slow-Wave Sleep (SWS, Deep Sleep, Delta Sleep) — *3* (Deep-sleep transition)	Theta Delta Spindles K complexes	Slight	Prevents stage 4	Subject hard to arouse; K complexes are hard to evoke
4 ("Cerebral" sleep)	Delta	Slight	Suicidal ideation and day terrors Rebound excessive; SWS begins on first night of restored sleep and may last for weeks	Subject very hard to arouse; K complexes cannot be evoked Night terrors and somnambulism occur in this stage Insomniacs have normal SWS
REM sleep ‡ (REMS)	Mixed frequency but no spindles or K complexes	Considerable; darting, irregular, in bursts (REM) ‡·§	Anxiety, overeating, behavioral disturbances, decreased concentration and learning, hypersexuality, decreased seizure threshold	Stage of recallable dreaming; 74% of dreams occur in REMS Dreams are more vivid, sexual, and bizarre than in non-REMS; nightmares usually occur during REMS In the male, REMS frequently begins with an erection

* Order of sleep stages is 0, 1, 2, 3, 4, REMS, 1, 2, 3, 4, REMS, *etc.;* stage 0 may also be repeated, especially in insomniacs. A complete cycle takes approximately 90 minutes. Narcoleptics may bypass any or all of stages 1 to 4. In young adults, the percentage of total sleep time spent in the various stages is as follows: stage 0, 1 to 2%; stage 1, 3 to 6%; stage 2, 40 to 52%; stage 3, 5 to 8%; stage 4, 10 to 19%; REMS, 23 to 34%.

† Alpha is high-amplitude, sinusoidal activity of 8 to 14 cycles per second (cps); beta is low amplitude, 15 to 35 cps; delta is high amplitude (>75 μvolt), 0.5 to 3 cps; theta is low amplitude, 4 to 7 cps; spindles are bursts (each, 0.5-second duration) of high amplitude, 12 to 15 cps; K complex is a high-amplitude negative wave followed by a positive wave, with spindles sometimes superimposed.

‡ REM stands for rapid eyeball movement.

§ REM activity is expressed as "density," *i.e.,* number of movements per epoch.

decline within a few nights but do not disappear. Tolerance is more pronounced to the effects on the REM-sleep than to the non-REM-sleep parameters. During chronic use the number of dreams may double, although dreams usually are less bizarre. If after 3 to 4 weeks of nightly use of a benzodiazepine the drug is discontinued, there may be a considerable rebound in the amount and density of REM sleep. Withdrawal from clorazepate, lorazepam, or nitrazepam causes a rebound decrease in REM-sleep latency and an increase in REM-sleep time that may last for a long period. With flurazepam, temazepam, and triazolam, the rebound in REM sleep appears to be slight or negligible, possibly due to their slight effect on total REM sleep time. During the period of such rebound the number of dreams per night is about the same as before the drug was taken, but their bizarre character may increase. There is also usually a rebound in SWS, which may exceed the rebound in REM sleep.

Withdrawal of flurazepam causes only a slight rebound, perhaps because of the extremely long half-life of the active metabolite, N-desalkylflurazepam. After flunitrazepam, SWS may remain depressed for several weeks, gradually returning to the baseline condition without rebound. In some studies a rebound increase in total wake time has been found; this was especially evident with triazolam and midazolam but negligible with flurazepam (*see* Kales *et al.*, 1983b). However, several other studies have failed to find significant rebound insomnia after triazolam.

Sites and Mechanisms of CNS Actions. Currently, there is general agreement that most, if not all, of the actions of benzodiazepines are a result of potentiation of the neural inhibition that is mediated by gamma-aminobutyric acid (GABA). This view is supported by behavioral and electrophysiological evidence that the effects of benzodiazepines are reduced or prevented by prior treatment with antagonists of GABA (*e.g.*, bicuculline) or inhibitors of the synthesis of the transmitter (*e.g.*, thiosemicarbazide). Although possible actions that lead to increased release of GABA cannot be excluded, most attention has been focused on the ability of benzodiazepines to potentiate the actions of GABA on neurons at all levels of the neuraxis. As a result of the detection and characterization of specific binding sites for benzodiazepines, a substantial body of biochemical evidence has accumulated that suggests a close molecular association between sites of action for GABA and the benzodiazepines. The various categories of evidence have been brought together by the recent discovery that certain congeners of the benzodiazepines are potent and selective inhibitors of both their biological effects and their binding to putative sites of action. One such antagonist (Ro 15-1788) is currently under investigation for possible use in the treatment of overdosage with benzodiazepines. The sites and mechanism of action of the benzodiazepines have been reviewed recently by Haefely and colleagues (1981), Mennini and Garrattini (1982), Olsen (1982), Skolnick and Paul (1982), and Dubnick and colleagues (1983), as well as in several symposia (Symposium, 1983a, 1983b, 1983c).

While the GABA-potentiation hypothesis does not yet provide detailed explanations for the therapeutic actions of the benzodiazepines, it does supply a versatile framework with which to connect diverse observations. For example, the remarkable safety of the benzodiazepines can be accounted for by the self-limited nature of neuronal depression that requires the release of an endogenous inhibitory neurotransmitter to be expressed. Although barbiturates have similar effects at low doses, they also inhibit the release of excitatory neurotransmitters and mimic the inhibitory actions of GABA at higher doses; thus, they can produce profound depression of the CNS (*see* below). Further, the ability of benzodiazepines to release suppressed behaviors as well as to produce sedation can be ascribed in part to potentiation of GABA-ergic pathways that serve to regulate the firing of neurons containing various monoamines (*see* Chapter 12); these neurons are known to promote behavioral arousal as well as to be important mediators of the inhibitory effects of fear and punishment on behavior. Finally, inhibitory effects on muscular hypertonia or the spread of seizure activity can be rationalized by potentiation of inhibitory GABA-ergic circuits at various levels of the neuraxis. However, there are problems that will require refinement of this hypothesis. For example, potentiation of the action of GABA to increase chloride ion conductance requires concentrations of benzodiazepines at least tenfold higher than those achieved in the cerebrospinal fluid (CSF) during therapy; at therapeutic concentrations, direct inhibitory effects on the excitability of some neurons are produced, which in part appear to involve changes in the conductances of ions other than chloride (MacDonald and Barker, 1982; Carlen *et al.*, 1983). There is also no adequate explanation for the large variation in the ratio of doses of different benzodiazepines required to produce release of inhibited behavior as opposed to sedative-ataxic effects in experimental animals. In any event, the benzodiazepine antagonists are equally potent in preventing both of these categories of effects and can also inhibit those electrophysiological effects of benzodiazepines that do not involve potentiation of GABA.

In the vast majority of studies conducted *in vivo* or *in situ,* the local or systemic administration of benzodiazepines reduces the spontaneous or evoked electrical activity of major (large) neurons in all regions of the brain and spinal cord; significant effects can usually be detected at doses that are consistent with those used in man. The activity of these neurons is regulated in part by small inhibitory interneurons (predominantly GABA-ergic) arranged in both feedback and feedforward types of circuits (see Chapter 12). In the former, axonal branches activate the interneurons, which in turn inhibit the large neuron by way of axosomatic and, sometimes, axodendritic synapses. In feedforward circuits, some or all of the excitatory inputs to the large neuron send collateral axons to inhibitory interneurons that make synaptic contact with the large neuron and/or with excitatory nerve terminals; the latter arrangement is termed presynaptic inhibition. The magnitude of the effects produced by benzodiazepines can vary widely and depends upon such factors as the types of inhibitory circuits that are operating, the sources and intensity of ongoing excitatory input, and the manner in which experimental manipulations are performed and assessed. For example, the inhibitory synapses on the neuronal soma, especially those near the axon hillock, are the most powerful and are usually supplied predominantly by recurrent pathways. The synaptic or exogenous application of GABA to this region can prevent neuronal discharge in response to either orthodromic or antidromic stimuli; this involves a GABA-induced increase in the conductance of chloride ions, thereby shunting electrical currents that would otherwise depolarize the membrane of the initial segment. Accordingly, benzodiazepines markedly prolong the period that follows brief activation of recurrent GABA-ergic pathways, during which neither spontaneous nor applied excitatory stimuli can evoke neuronal discharge; this effect is reversed by the administration of bicuculline.

Similar effects of the benzodiazepines have been observed with brain slices incubated in vitro. For example, as little as 50 nM diazepam facilitates recurrent inhibition of CA_1 pyramidal cells in hippocampal slices from the rat (see Haefely et al., in Symposium, 1983a). However, data indicate that this effect may not be due to potentiation of the actions of GABA per se. In studies that employed intracellular recording and the iontophoretic application of GABA to the soma of hippocampal CA_1 pyramidal cells, approximately 1 μM diazepam was required to observe augmentation of the actions of GABA (Alger and Nicoll, 1982). In similar studies, various benzodiazepines were found to reduce the excitability of resting pyramidal cells without either the addition of GABA or the participation of changes in chloride conductance. The concentration dependence of these effects was bell shaped, commencing at less than 1 nM and disappearing at 100 nM, a concentration that was not sufficient to produce augmentation of the actions of GABA (Carlen et al., 1983). Thus, while potentiation of inhibition mediated by GABA-ergic pathways (and, perhaps, effects unrelated to GABA) may be important at the usual clinical doses, it is possible that the ability of benzodiazepines to en-

hance the actions of GABA itself may participate in the CNS depression produced only at higher doses.

Specific binding sites for benzodiazepines have been detected in the CNS of various species, including man; the binding capacity is greatest in the cerebral cortex and least in the spinal cord. The affinity of these sites for the binding of benzodiazepines (but not of the antagonist, Ro 15-1788) is enhanced by both GABA and chloride ion. These effects also occur in preparations of binding sites after solubilization in detergent and extensive purification; this suggests a close association between sites of action for benzodiazepines and a macromolecular complex composed of GABA-ergic receptors and chloride channels.

The relative binding affinities correlate reasonably well with the relative potencies of benzodiazepines in producing release of inhibited behaviors and antagonism of pentylenetetrazol-induced seizures, especially when adjustment is made for the formation of active metabolites. Further, the magnitude of these effects has been correlated with estimates of the fractional occupancy of binding sites in vivo. Finally, certain imidazobenzodiazepines (e.g., Ro 15-1788) compete for binding sites with benzodiazepines in a strictly competitive fashion and antagonize their biological effects. Taken together, such data provide strong evidence that these sites mediate the actions of the benzodiazepines. Despite the fact that Ro 15-1788 has little effect in vivo in the absence of benzodiazepines, these data have also prompted investigation of the possible existence of endogenous substances that can exert physiological or pathophysiological actions by binding to these sites.

Experiments performed with other agents that can compete for binding sites for benzodiazepines suggest that there may be multiple populations of such sites. These compounds include triazolopyridazines, which are reported to produce anxiolytic effects with little sedation, and β-carbolines, which antagonize the effect of both benzodiazepines and sedative barbiturates. It is thus possible that the various actions of the benzodiazepines are mediated by interactions at different sites and that agents with a more limited spectrum of effects may be developed.

Respiration. The benzodiazepines have only slight effects on respiration; hypnotic doses are without effect in normal subjects. Preanesthetic doses of diazepam and flurazepam slightly depress alveolar ventilation and cause respiratory acidosis as the result of a decrease in hypoxic rather than hypercapnic drive. The rate of expiratory flow is depressed only under hypoxic conditions. In doses used for endoscopy, benzodiazepines decrease alveolar ventilation and P_{O_2}, increase P_{CO_2}, and may cause CO_2 narcosis in patients with chronic obstructive pulmonary disease (see Rao et al., 1973; Gross et al., 1983). Furthermore, diazepam can cause apnea during anesthesia and also when given with opioids. Despite the occasional adverse interaction with opioids, the benzodiazepines do not alter the effect of meperidine on the response to CO_2 (see Greenblatt and Shader, 1974). It is noteworthy that in scores of cases of intoxication involving benzodiazepines the only patients who required respiratory assistance were those who had also taken another CNS-depressant drug, especially alcohol (*see* Greenblatt *et al.*, 1977).

Cardiovascular System. The cardiovascular effects of benzodiazepines are minor, except in severe intoxication. In so-called anesthetic doses, all benzodiazepines decrease blood pressure and increase heart rate. With flunitrazepam and midazolam, the effects are secondary to a decrease in peripheral resistance (Seitz *et al.*, 1977), but with diazepam and lorazepam they are secondary to a decrease in left ventricular work and cardiac output (*see* Rao *et al.*, 1973; Al-Khudhairi *et al.*, 1982). Bromazepam and midazolam diminish systolic and diastolic pressures about equally. Diazepam increases coronary flow in man (Ikram *et al.*, 1973) and dogs, possibly by an action to increase interstitial concentrations of adenosine. In large doses, midazolam decreases considerably both cerebral blood flow and oxygen assimilation (Nugent *et al.*, 1982).

Gastrointestinal Tract. Antianxiety benzodiazepines are thought by some gastroenterologists to improve a variety of "anxiety-related" gastrointestinal disorders. There is a paucity of evidence for direct actions. Benzodiazepines partially protect against stress ulcers in rats, and diazepam markedly decreases nocturnal gastric secretion in humans.

Pharmacokinetics. The physicochemical and pharmacokinetic properties of the benzodiazepines greatly affect their clinical utility. They all have high lipid:water distribution coefficients in the nonionized form; nevertheless, lipophilicity varies more than 50-fold according to the polarity and electronegativity of various substituents.

All of the benzodiazepines are essentially completely absorbed, with the exception of clorazepate; this drug is rapidly decarboxylated in gastric juice to N-desmethyldiazepam (nordazepam), which is subsequently absorbed completely. Some benzodiazepines (*e.g.*, prazepam and flurazepam) reach the systemic circulation only in the form of active metabolites. After oral administration the time to peak concentration in plasma ranges from 0.5 to 8 hours for the various benzodiazepines. Among those commonly used for their hypnotic effects, peak concentrations of triazolam occur in plasma within 1 hour, while the absorption of temazepam is somewhat slower and more variable. Peak concentrations of active metabolites of flurazepam are attained in 1 to 3 hours. With the exception of lorazepam, the absorption of benzodiazepines tends to be erratic after intramuscular injection.

The benzodiazepines and their active metabolites bind to plasma proteins. The extent of binding correlates strongly with lipid solubility and ranges from about 70% for alprazolam to nearly 99% for diazepam. The concentration in the CSF is approximately equal to the concentration of free drug in plasma. While competition with other protein-bound drugs may occur, no clinically significant examples have been reported.

The plasma concentrations of most benzodiazepines exhibit patterns that are consistent with two-compartment models (*see* Chapter 1 and Appendix II), but three-compartment models appear to be more appropriate for the compounds with the highest lipid solubility. Accordingly, there is rapid uptake of benzodiazepines into the brain and other highly perfused organs after intravenous administration (or oral administration of a rapidly absorbed compound); this is followed by a phase of redistribution into tissues that are less well perfused, especially muscle and fat. Redistribution is most rapid for drugs with the highest lipid solubility. In the regimens used for nighttime sedation, the rate of redistribution can sometimes have a greater influence on the duration of CNS effects than the rate of biotransformation (*see* Dettli, in Symposium, 1983a). The kinetics of redistribution of diazepam and other lipophilic benzodiazepines is complicated by enterohepatic circulation. The volumes of distribution of the benzodiazepines are large (*see* Appendix II), and many are increased in elderly patients (*see* Swift and Stevenson, in Symposium, 1983a). These drugs cross the placental barrier and are secreted into milk.

The benzodiazepines are metabolized extensively, particularly by several different microsomal enzyme systems in the liver. Because active metabolites are generated that are biotransformed more slowly than the parent compound, the duration of action of many benzodiazepines bears little relationship to the half-time of elimination of the drug that has been administered. For example, the half-life of flurazepam in plasma is 2 to 3 hours, but that of a major active metabolite (N-desalkylflurazepam) is 50 hours or more. Conversely, the rate of biotransformation of those agents that are inactivated by the initial reaction is an important determinant of their duration of action; these include oxazepam, lorazepam, temazepam, and triazolam. Metabolism of the benzodiazepines occurs in three major stages. These and the relationships between the drugs and their metabolites are shown in Table 17–3.

For those benzodiazepines that bear a substituent at position 1 (or 2) of the diazepine ring, the initial and most rapid phase of metabolism involves modification and/or removal of the substituent. With the exception of triazolam and alprazolam, which contain a fused triazolo ring, the eventual products are N-desalkylated compounds; these are all biologically active. One such compound, nordazepam, is a major metabolite common to the biotransformation of diazepam, clorazepate, prazepam, and halazepam; it is also formed from demoxepam, an important metabolite of chlordiazepoxide. The second stage involves hydroxylation at position 3 and also usually yields an active derivative (*e.g.,* oxazepam from nordazepam). The rates of these reactions are usually very much slower than the first stage (half-times greater than 40 to 50 hours), such that appreciable accumulation of hy-

droxylated products with intact substituents at position 1 does not occur. The accumulation of small amounts of temazepam during the chronic administration of diazepam (not shown in Table 17–3) is an exception to this rule. The third major stage is the conjugation of the 3-hydroxyl compounds, principally with glucuronic acid; the half-times of these reactions are usually between 6 and 12 hours, and the products are invariably inactive. Conjugation is the only major route of metabolism available for oxazepam and lorazepam, and it is the preferred pathway for temazepam because of its slower conversion to oxazepam. Triazolam and alprazolam are metabolized principally by initial hydroxylation of the methyl group on the fused triazolo ring; the absence of a chlorine residue in ring C of alprazolam slows this reaction significantly (Table 17–3). The products, sometimes referred to as α-hydroxylated compounds, are quite active but are metabolized very rapidly, primarily by conjugation with glucuronic acid, such that there is no appreciable accumulation of active metabolites. These drugs are also metabolized to a significant extent by hydroxylation at position 3 of the benzodiazepine ring; the rate of this reaction appears to be unusually swift compared to that for compounds without the triazolo ring. These metabolites are rapidly conjugated or oxidized further to benzophenone derivatives and excreted.

The aromatic rings (A and C) of the benzodiazepines are hydroxylated to only a small extent. The only important metabolism at these sites is the reduction of the 7-nitro substituents of clonazepam, nitrazepam, and flunitrazepam; the half-times of

Table 17–3.   MAJOR METABOLIC RELATIONSHIPS BETWEEN SOME OF THE BENZODIAZEPINES *

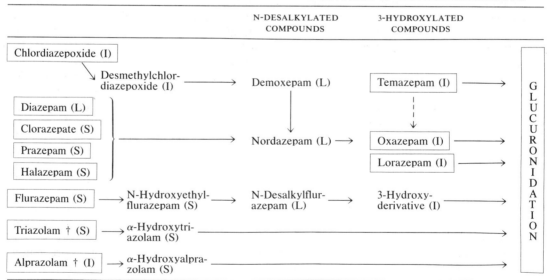

* Compounds enclosed in boxes are marketed in the United States. The approximate half-lives of the various compounds are denoted in parentheses: S = <6 hours; I = 6 to 20 hours; L = >20 hours. All compounds except clorazepate are biologically active; the activity of 3-hydroxydesalkylflurazepam has not been determined. Clonazepam (not shown) is a N-desalkyl compound, and it is metabolized primarily by reduction of the 7-NO$_2$ group to the corresponding amine (inactive), followed by acetylation; its half-life is 20 to 40 hours.

† *See* text for discussion of other pathways of metabolism.

these reactions are usually 20 to 40 hours. The resulting amines are inactive and are acetylated to varying degrees before excretion.

Since the benzodiazepines apparently do not induce the synthesis of hepatic microsomal enzymes significantly, their chronic administration usually does not result in the accelerated metabolism of other substances or of the benzodiazepines. Cimetidine and oral contraceptives inhibit N-dealkylation and 3-hydroxylation of benzodiazepines. Ethanol, isoniazid, and phenytoin are less effective in this regard. These reactions are usually reduced to a greater extent in the aged and in patients with chronic liver disease than are those involving conjugation. However, the half-life of temazepam is markedly longer in elderly women compared to young adults or to men of the same age (Smith et al., 1983).

Ideally, a useful hypnotic agent would have a rapid onset of action when taken at bedtime, a sufficiently sustained action to facilitate sleep throughout the night, and no residual action by the following morning. Among those benzodiazepines that are commonly used as hypnotic agents, triazolam theoretically fits this description most closely. Because of the slow rate of elimination of desalkylflurazepam, flurazepam might seem to be unsuitable for this purpose. However, in practice there appear to be some disadvantages to the use of agents that have a relatively rapid rate of disappearance; these are not well defined at present but include the phenomena of "rebound" daytime anxiety and early-morning insomnia that are experienced by some patients (see below). With careful selection of dosage, flurazepam and other benzodiazepines with slower rates of elimination than triazolam can be used effectively. The biotransformation and pharmacokinetic properties of the benzodiazepines have been reviewed by Breimer (1979), Bellantuono and associates (1980), Breimer and Jochemsen (in Symposium, 1981), Greenblatt and coworkers (1981, 1982, 1983a, 1983b, 1983c), van der Kleijn and colleagues (1981), and Schütz (1982), as well as in recent symposia (Symposium, 1983a, 1983b).

Untoward Effects. At the time of peak concentration in plasma, hypnotic doses of benzodiazepines can be expected to cause varying degrees of light-headedness, lassitude, increased reaction time, motor incoordination, ataxia, impairment of mental and psychomotor functions, disorganization of thought, confusion, dysarthria, anterograde amnesia, dry mouth, and a bitter taste. Cognition appears to be affected less than motor performance. All of these effects greatly impair driving and other psychomotor skills. When the drug is given before the intended time of sleep, they may not even be noticed, but the persistence of these effects during the waking hours is adverse. *Interaction with ethanol* may be especially serious. Significant residual effects have been observed after administration of hypnotic doses of a variety of benzodiazepines. For example, the incidence after flurazepam and temazepam is about 11 and 17%, respectively (see Rickels, 1983). While triazolam in a dose of 0.25 mg does not appear to cause significant residual effects, even in the elderly (Carskadon et al., 1982), higher doses may do so (Roth et al., 1981). The intensity and incidence of CNS toxicity generally increase with age; both pharmacokinetic and pharmacodynamic factors are involved (see Meyer, 1982; Swift et al., in Symposium, 1983a). The effects of benzodiazepines on performance have recently been reviewed by Bond and Lader (in Symposium, 1981) and by Linnoila (in Symposium, 1983a).

Other relatively common side effects of benzodiazepines are weakness, headache, blurred vision, vertigo, nausea and vomiting, epigastric distress, and diarrhea; joint pains, chest pains, and incontinence may occur in a few percent or less of recipients. Anticonvulsant benzodiazepines sometimes actually increase the frequency of seizures in patients with epilepsy.

The possible adverse effects of alterations in the sleep pattern will be discussed at the end of this chapter.

Adverse Psychological Effects. Benzodiazepines may cause paradoxical effects. Nitrazepam frequently and flurazepam occasionally increase the incidence of nightmares, especially during the first week of use. Flurazepam occasionally causes garrulousness, anxiety, irritability, tachycardia, and sweating. Euphoria, restlessness, hallucinations, and hypomanic behavior have been reported to occur during use of various benzodiazepines. Antianxiety benzodiazepines have been reported to release bizarre uninhibited behavior in some users with low levels of anxiety; hostility and rage may occur in others. Paranoia, depression, and suicidal ideation occasionally also accompany the use of these agents. However, the incidence of such paradoxical reactions is extremely small (*see* Hall and Zisook, 1981).

Although benzodiazepines have a reputation for causing only a low incidence of *abuse* and *dependence,* the possibility of this adverse complication of chronic use must not be overlooked. The overwhelming preponderance of reported cases involves benzodiazepines used to treat anxiety, often in combination with other abused drugs. High doses and prolonged periods of use appear to be necessary. The number of documented cases of dependence is small considering the large number of patients for whom these drugs are prescribed. Very few individuals increase dosage or manifest compulsive drug-seeking behavior after discontinuation of a benzodiazepine. Even among habitual drug abusers, benzodiazepines are seldom preferred to barbiturates or even ethanol (*see* O'Brien *et al.,* 1982).

Nevertheless, after discontinuation of a therapeutic regimen, withdrawal syndromes probably occur far more frequently than are recognized. The incidence may be as high as 45%, but the symptoms are usually quite moderate; their intensity is generally inversely proportional to the duration of action of the benzodiazepine that had been ingested. After use in the treatment of anxiety, the original symptoms may recur and may be exaggerated. Dysphoria, irritability, sweating, headache, sleep abnormalities and unpleasant dreams, tremors, anorexia, faintness, and dizziness may also occur. After a regimen of high or, occasionally, of conventional dosage, discontinuation may evoke more severe symptoms; these include agitation, depression, panic, paranoia, delirium, myalgia, muscle twitches, and even frank convulsions (Lader and Petursson, 1983). Habituation and dependence upon benzodiazepines have been reviewed by Marks (1978), Petursson and Lader (1981), MacKinnon and Parker (1982), Owen and Tyrer (1983), and Schöpf (1983), as well as in several symposia (Symposium, 1983b, 1983c).

Rebound insomnia is another type of withdrawal phenomenon (*see* Kales *et al.,* 1983a, 1983b). A decrease in the number of sleep spindles can sometimes be detected subsequent to a single dose of a benzodiazepine (Borbély *et al.,* 1983). A similar phenomenon may also be involved in the early-morning insomnia that is sometimes manifested during treatment at constant dosage. Rebound insomnia has been reported to be especially intense following the use of the short-acting benzodiazepines, such as midazolam and triazolam; daytime symptoms that resemble those of anxiety may also occur during continuous hypnotic use of these agents. However, these claims have been disputed; factors such as excessive dosage and the psychiatric profile of the patients that were studied may have contributed to the conflicting observations. These and related issues have been reviewed by Nicholson (1980, 1981), Carskadon and coworkers (1982), Wincor (1982), and Bliwise and colleagues (1983).

In spite of the adverse effects reviewed above, the benzodiazepines are relatively safe drugs. Even huge doses are rarely fatal unless other drugs are taken concomitantly. Ethanol is a common contributor to deaths involving benzodiazepines, and true coma is uncommon in the absence of another CNS depressant. While overdosage with a benzodiazepine rarely causes severe cardiovascular or respiratory depression, therapeutic doses can further compromise respiration in patients with chronic obstructive respiratory disease.

A wide variety of allergic, hepatotoxic, and hematologic reactions to the benzodiazepines may occur, but the incidence is quite low; these have been associated with the use of flurazepam and triazolam, but not with temazepam. The concern that diazepam may be teratogenic is not supported by recent evidence (Rosenberg *et al.,* 1983). Large doses taken just prior to or during labor may cause hypothermia, hypotonia, and mild respiratory depression in the neonate. Abuse by the pregnant mother can result in a withdrawal syndrome in the newborn infant.

Except for additive effects with other CNS-depressant drugs, most frequently ethanol and valproate, reports of clinically important, pharmacodynamic drug interactions between benzodiazepines and other drugs have been rare and unconfirmed. Ethanol increases both the absorption of benzodiazepines and the CNS depression. Valproate and benzodiazepines in combination may cause psychotic episodes. Pharmacokinetic interactions are mentioned above.

THERAPEUTIC USES

The use of the benzodiazepines as hypnotics is discussed at the end of this chapter; there is also some discussion of their employment as sedatives. (*See also* Mitler, 1981; McElnay *et al.*, 1982; Roth *et al.*, 1983.) Other uses of benzodiazepines are as antianxiety agents (Chapter 19), anticonvulsants (Chapter 20), muscle relaxants (Chapter 21), for preanesthetic medication (Chapter 13), and in anesthesia (Chapter 14).

Preparations and Dosage. The aqueous solubility of benzodiazepines ranges from less than 1/10,000 (chlordiazepoxide, lorazepam, oxazepam) to 1/2 (flurazepam hydrochloride). Solubilities in lipid are generally low; however, because of the generally low aqueous solubilities, lipid:water partition coefficients are usually high. The official names, trade names, preparations, and sedative and hypnotic doses of these agents are given in Table 17–4.

BARBITURATES

The barbiturates once enjoyed a long period of extensive use as sedative-hypnotic drugs; however, except for a few specialized uses, they have been largely replaced by the much safer benzodiazepines. A more detailed description of the barbiturates can be found in the *fifth edition* of this textbook.

Chemistry. Barbituric acid is 2,4,6-trioxohexahydropyrimidine. The compound lacks central-depressant activity, but the presence of alkyl or aryl groups at position 5 confers sedative-hypnotic and sometimes other activities. The general structural formula for the barbiturates and the structures of those compounds available in the United States are shown in Table 17–5.

The carbonyl group at position 2 takes on acidic character because of lactam ("keto")–lactim ("enol") tautomerization favored by its location between the two electronegative amido nitrogens. The lactim form is favored in alkaline solution, and salts result. The barbituric acid derivatives do not dissolve readily in water, although they are quite soluble in nonpolar solvents, a feature that they share with many other organic compounds that depress the CNS. The sodium salts of barbiturates dissolve in water, forming alkaline and often unstable solutions.

Barbiturates in which the oxygen at C2 is replaced by sulfur are called *thiobarbiturates*. Although only those compounds having a barbituric acid ring (oxygen at C2) are properly called *barbiturates*, it has become common practice to refer to both groups of compounds as barbiturates and to distinguish between them, when necessary, by using the terms *thiobarbiturates* and *oxybarbiturates*. Thiobarbiturates are more lipid soluble than the corresponding oxybarbiturates.

In general, structural changes that increase lipid solubility decrease duration of action, decrease latency to onset of activity, accelerate metabolic degradation, and often increase hypnotic potency. Thus, large aliphatic groups at C5 confer greater activity than do methyl groups, but the compounds have a shorter duration of action; however, groups larger than seven carbons tend to have convulsant activity. Introduction of polar groups, such as ether, keto, hydroxyl, amino, or carboxyl groups, into alkyl side chains decreases lipid solubility and abolishes hypnotic activity. Methylation of the 1-N atom increases lipid solubility and shortens duration of action, although demethylation to a longer-acting metabolite may occur. Lipid solubility also favors interaction with hydrophobic regions in proteins. It correlates roughly with binding to plasma protein and cytochrome P-450.

PHARMACOLOGICAL PROPERTIES

The barbiturates reversibly depress the activity of all excitable tissues. The CNS is exquisitely sensitive, and, when barbiturates are given in sedative or hypnotic doses, there is very little effect on skeletal, cardiac, or smooth muscle. Even in anesthetic concentrations, direct effects on peripheral excitable tissues are weak and do not create difficulties if the duration of anesthesia is not prolonged. However, if depression is extended, as in acute barbiturate intoxication, serious deficits in cardiovascular and other peripheral functions occur.

Central Nervous System. The barbiturates can produce all degrees of depression of the CNS, ranging from mild sedation to general anesthesia. The use of barbiturates for general anesthesia is discussed in Chapter 14. Certain barbiturates, particularly those containing a 5-phenyl substituent (phenobarbital, mephobarbital) have selective anticonvulsant activity (*see* Chapter 20). The barbiturates, especially phenobarbital, have been used for the treatment of anxiety. However, their antianxiety properties are not equivalent to those exerted by benzodiazepines, especially with respect to the degree of sedation that is produced. The barbiturates may have euphoriant effects, which, when maximal, are comparable to those of morphine.

Except for the anticonvulsant activities of phenobarbital and its congeners, the barbiturates possess a low degree of selectivity and therapeutic index. Thus, it is not possible to achieve a desired effect without evidences of general depression of the CNS. However, there is one function, namely, pain perception and reaction, that is relatively unimpaired until the moment of unconsciousness.

Table 17–4. HALF-LIVES, DOSAGE FORMS, AND ORAL DOSES OF SEDATIVE-HYPNOTIC DRUGS

DRUG CLASSES, NON PROPRIETARY NAMES, AND TRADE NAMES	HALF-LIFE (*hours*)	DOSAGE [1] FORMS	ADULT ORAL DOSE (*mg*) Sedative	ADULT ORAL DOSE (*mg*) Hypnotic
Benzodiazepines				
Clordiazepoxide (LIBRIUM)	5–15	C,T,I	10–100, 1–3xd [2,3]	50–100 [3]
Clorazepate (TRANXENE)	50–80 [4]	C,T	3.75–15, 2–4xd [3]	15–30 [3]
Diazepam (VALIUM)	30–60	T,ERC,I	5–10, 3–4xd [3]	5–10 [3]
Flurazepam (DALMANE)	50–100 [4]	C	—	15–30
Lorazepam (ATIVAN)	10–20	T,I	—	2–4
Oxazepam (SERAX)	5–10	C,T	15–30, 3–4xd [3]	15–30 [3]
Temazepam (RESTORIL)	10–17	C	—	15–30
Triazolam (HALCION)	1.5–3	T	—	0.25–0.5
Barbiturates				
Amobarbital (AMYTAL)	8–42	C,T,E,I	15–50, 2–3xd	65–200
Aprobarbital (ALURATE)	14–34	E	40, 3xd	40–160
Butabarbital (BUTISOL)	34–42	C,T,E	15–30, 3–4xd	50–100
Butalbital	—	M [5]	50–100, 3–4xd	100–200
Mephobarbital (MEBARAL)	11–67	T	32–100, 3–4xd	—
Pentobarbital (NEMBUTAL)	15–48	C,E,I,S	20, 3–4xd [6]	100
Phenobarbital (LUMINAL)	80–120	C,ERC,T E,L,D,I	15–40, 2–3xd	100–320
Secobarbital (SECONAL)	15–40	C,T,S,I	30–50, 3–4xd	100–200
Talbutal (LOTUSATE)	—	T	30–60, 2–3xd	120
Miscellaneous				
Chloral hydrate (NOTEC)	4–9.5 [4]	C,E,L,S	250, 3xd	500–1000
Ethchlorvynol (PLACIDYL)	10–25 [7]	C	100–200, 2–3xd	500–1000
Ethinamate (VALMID)	—	C	—	500–1000
Glutethimide (DORIDEN)	5–22	C,T	—	250–500
Meprobamate (MILTOWN)	6–17	ERC,T	400, 3–4xd	800
Methyprylon (NOLUDAR)	3–6	C,T	50–100, 3–4xd	200–400
Paraldehyde (PARAL)	—	L,I	2–5 ml, 2–4xd	10–30 ml
Triclofos (TRICLOS)	—	T,L	—	1500

[1] C = capsule; T = tablet; ERC = extended-release capsule; L = liquid; E = elixir; D = drops; I = injection; S = suppository.
[2] Dose, number per day.
[3] Approved as a sedative-hypnotic drug only for management of CNS-depressant drug withdrawal; dose in a nontolerant individual would be smaller.
[4] Half-life of the active metabolite, to which effects can be attributed.
[5] Marketed only in mixtures.
[6] Dose refers to the base.
[7] For acute use, half-life of distribution phase (1–3 hours) may be more appropriate.

Table 17–5. BARBITURATES AVAILABLE CURRENTLY IN THE UNITED STATES: NAMES AND STRUCTURES

GENERAL FORMULA:

BARBITURATE	R_{5a}	R_{5b}
Amobarbital	ethyl	isopentyl
Aprobarbital	allyl	isopropyl
Butabarbital	ethyl	sec-butyl
Butalbital	allyl	isobutyl
Mephobarbital *	ethyl	phenyl
Metharbital *	ethyl	ethyl
Methohexital *	allyl	1-methyl-2-pentynyl
Pentobarbital	ethyl	1-methylbutyl
Phenobarbital	ethyl	phenyl
Secobarbital	allyl	1-methylbutyl
Talbutal	allyl	sec-butyl
Thiamylal †	allyl	1-methylbutyl
Thiopental †	ethyl	1-methylbutyl

* R_3 = H, except in mephobarbital, metharbital, and methohexital, where it is replaced by CH_3.

† O, except in thiamylal and thiopental, where it is replaced by S.

Indeed, in small doses, the barbiturates are *hyperalgesic* and increase the reaction to painful stimuli. Hence they cannot be relied upon to produce sedation or sleep in the presence of even moderate pain.

In some individuals and in some circumstances, such as in the presence of pain, barbiturates cause overt excitement instead of sedation. The fact that such paradoxical excitement occurs with other CNS depressants suggests that it may result from depression of inhibitory centers. As with ethanol, the degree and quality of excitement are variable, depending on both personality and environment.

Effects on EEG. In small intravenous doses or after oral ingestion, barbiturates decrease low-frequency electrical activity determined by electroencephalography and increase the low-voltage, fast activity (15 to 35 Hz). Fast activity from the frontal cortex spreads to the parietal and occipital cortex and recedes in the reverse order as the effect of the drug wanes. The early high-frequency response resembles that from electrical arousal of the reticular formation, but true arousal does not occur.

Activation of the EEG is accompanied by clouding of consciousness and, occasionally, euphoria. As the dose is increased, large-amplitude, random slow waves (5 to 12 Hz) similar to those in sleep appear in spindle-shaped bursts. Consciousness is lost, although the patient may continue to respond to strong, painful stimuli. The EEG is very stable in this and subsequent stages.

A further increase in dose causes the wave frequency to decrease to 1 to 3 Hz. Limbic neuronal firing rates become depressed. Mild-to-moderate noxious stimuli now fail to evoke responses. With still higher doses the amplitudes of the waves diminish, and there are occasional brief periods of electrical silence, but EEG coherence among the limbic structures persists even during such burst suppression. Major surgical procedures can be undertaken at this time. The periods of electrical silence become longer as depression becomes more severe, and eventually all electrical activity disappears. The EEG patterns are grossly similar to those produced by gaseous and volatile anesthetic agents (Chapter 14); however, there are minor differences, particularly during induction.

Effects on Stages of Sleep. Hypnotic doses of barbiturates always alter the stages of sleep, and they do so in a dose-dependent manner. They decrease sleep latency, slightly increase delta bursts and fast-EEG activity during sleep, decrease the number of stage shifts to stages 0 and 1 (number of awakenings), and decrease body movement. Stages 3 and 4 (slow-wave sleep, SWS) are generally shortened considerably, except in some patients with anxiety and in barbiturate addicts. Furthermore, phenobarbital sometimes increases stage-4 sleep in healthy persons and may also increase total SWS in enuretic and somnambulistic persons. The latent period before REM sleep is prolonged, and total time spent in REM sleep, the number of REM cycles, and REM activity are diminished; with the short-acting barbiturates, these effects occur primarily during the first third of the night and are compensated for in the last third. It is of interest that administration of barbiturates during the day may decrease REM sleep at night (Feinberg *et al.*, 1974).

During repetitive nightly administration, some tolerance to the effects on sleep occurs within a few days, and the effect on total sleep time may be reduced by as much as 50% after 2 weeks of use. In all of nine studies reviewed by Kay and associates (1976), discontinuation led to rebound increases in all the parameters reported to be decreased by barbiturates. There may be an increase in REM sleep even if there was no reduction of this phenomenon during the time of drug administration. A rebound decrease in stage-2 sleep is said also to occur. However, effects on SWS and total sleep time may not occur after discontinuation of secobarbital, and rebound increases in REM sleep do not occur consistently (*see* Feinberg *et al.*, 1974).

The effects of barbiturates on sleep have been reviewed by Kay and associates (1976) and Mendelson and coworkers (1977).

Tolerance. Both pharmacodynamic (functional) and pharmacokinetic tolerance to barbiturates can occur. The former contributes more to the decreased effect than does the latter. Indeed, after a single dose of barbiturate, the concentration in plasma upon awakening may be higher than when sleep ensued and a higher concentration is required to reestablish sleep. Acute tolerance thus appears to occur substantially earlier than does induction of microsomal enzymes. With chronic administration of gradually increasing doses, pharmacodynamic tolerance continues to develop over a period of weeks to months, depending upon the dosage schedule, whereas pharmacokinetic tolerance reaches its peak in a few days. Tolerance to the effects on mood, sedation, and hypnosis occurs more readily and is greater than that to the anticonvulsant and lethal effects; thus, as tolerance increases, the therapeutic index decreases. When tolerance becomes maximal, the effective dose of a barbiturate may be increased by as much as six times; this is twofold to threefold greater than can be accounted for by enhanced metabolic disposition.

Supervised chronic sedation for weeks to months with therapeutic doses of secobarbital or pentobarbital causes a negligible degree of tolerance (*see* Wikler, 1976), and it might be concluded that once-a-day use of recommended hypnotic doses would be unlikely to cause tolerance. However, tolerance to the effects on sleep stages may occur or the chronic disruption of the normal sleep pattern may in itself make sleep less satisfying; the result is that the patient may increase his dosage in an attempt to improve his sleep and therein enhance the probability or degree of tolerance.

Tolerance to barbiturates confers tolerance to all general CNS-depressant drugs, including ethanol. There may even be cross-tolerance to the pharmacodynamically dissimilar opioids and phencyclidine, only a part of which is due to induction of hepatic enzymes. There is some evidence of cross-tolerance to the antianxiety and hypnotic effects of benzodiazepines, but not to the muscle relaxant effects.

Abuse and Dependence. Like other CNS-depressant drugs, barbiturates are abused, and some individuals develop a dependence upon them. These topics are discussed in Chapter 23.

Sites and Mechanisms of Action on the CNS. Barbiturates act throughout the CNS, although not with equal potency in all regions. Pertinent to their sedative-hypnotic effects is the fact that the mesencephalic reticular activating system is exquisitely sensitive to these drugs. In whatever region of the neuraxis, nonanesthetic doses preferentially suppress polysynaptic responses. Facilitation is diminished, and inhibition is usually enhanced. In neuronal cell cultures, low concentrations sometimes increase the frequency of spontaneous discharge and decrease it at slightly higher concentrations. The increase is possibly due to disinhibition by a depressant action on proximal inhibitory neurons. Effects to increase synaptic inhibition occur at the lowest concentrations. The synaptic site of inhibition is either *postsynaptic,* as at cortical and cerebellar pyramidal cells and in the cuneate nucleus, substantia nigra, and thalamic relay neurons, or *presynaptic,* as in the spinal cord. Furthermore, inhibition occurs only at synapses where physiological inhibition is GABA-ergic and not glycinergic or monoaminergic. The effect, however, may not be entirely mediated by GABA.

The barbiturates exert several distinct effects on excitatory and inhibitory synaptic transmission. For example, in cultures of spinal neurons, both hypnotic-anesthetic (*e.g.,* pentobarbital) and anticonvulsant barbiturates (*e.g.,* phenobarbital) po-

tentiate GABA-induced increases in chloride ion conductance and reduce glutamate-induced depolarization at about the same concentrations (50 to 75 μM). At higher concentrations, the barbiturates depress calcium-dependent action potentials, reduce the calcium-dependent release of neurotransmitters, and enhance chloride ion conductance in the absence of GABA (so-called GABA-mimetic action). However, pentobarbital is much more potent than phenobarbital in producing these effects. Thus, the more selective anticonvulsant properties of phenobarbital and its higher therapeutic index might be explained by its lower capacity to produce profound depression of neuronal function as compared with the anesthetic barbiturates (*see* Macdonald and McLean, 1982).

The capacity of the barbiturates to facilitate GABA-ergic inhibition resembles some of the actions of the benzodiazepines, discussed above. However, barbiturates do not displace benzodiazepines from their binding sites. Instead, they enhance such binding by increasing the affinity for benzodiazepines; they also enhance the binding of GABA and its agonist analogs to specific sites in neural membranes. These effects are almost completely dependent upon the presence of chloride or other anions that are known to permeate through chloride channels, and they are competitively antagonized by picrotoxin. These phenomena have been correlated with the ability of barbiturates to compete for specific binding sites for dihydropicrotoxinin and with the relative potency of barbiturates to cause general depression of the CNS. Of particular interest is the fact that phenobarbital is an impotent competitor for dihydropicrotoxinin binding sites and a weak enhancer of the binding of benzodiazepines and GABA. Collectively, these observations suggest that a macromolecular complex composed of GABA-ergic receptors, chloride ionophores, and binding sites for benzodiazepines may be an important site of action for the depressant barbiturates (*see* Olsen, 1982). However, the relationship of these observations to the electrophysiological effects of the barbiturates is not at all clear, and they would appear to have little relevance to the anticonvulsant actions of phenobarbital.

While both barbiturates and benzodiazepines are capable of potentiating GABA-induced increases in chloride conductance, significant differences in their modes of action can be detected. In voltage-clamped spinal neurons grown in culture, pentobarbital appears to increase the lifetime of the open state of chloride channels that are regulated by GABA-ergic receptors; the magnitude of this effect more than offsets a barbiturate-induced decrease in the frequency of channel openings (Study and Barker, 1981). By contrast, high concentrations of diazepam (in excess of 1 μM) increase the frequency of channel openings with little effect on the lifetime of the open state. It has been suggested that barbiturates may prolong the activation of the channel by decreasing the rate of dissociation of GABA from its receptor.

The mechanisms of action of barbiturates have been reviewed by Nicoll (1979), Ho and Harris

(1981), Macdonald and McLean (1982), Olsen (1982), and Richter and Holman (1982).

Peripheral Nervous Structures. Barbiturates selectively depress transmission in *autonomic ganglia* and reduce nicotinic excitation by choline esters. This effect may account, at least in part, for the fall in blood pressure produced by intravenous oxybarbiturates and by severe barbiturate intoxication.

At *skeletal neuromuscular junctions,* the twitch response to a single electrical shock applied to the motor nerve may be augmented by subanesthetic concentrations of barbiturates. In toxic doses, barbiturates increase transmitter release but reduce the sensitivity of the postsynaptic membrane to the depolarizing effect of acetylcholine and decamethonium by an action within the ionophore. The neuromuscular blocking effects of both tubocurarine and decamethonium are enhanced during barbiturate anesthesia.

Respiration. Barbiturates depress both the respiratory drive and the mechanisms responsible for the rhythmic character of respiration; however, low doses of barbiturate occasionally enhance the response to CO_2 slightly. The neurogenic drive is diminished by hypnotic doses, but usually no more so than during natural sleep. *Neurogenic drive is essentially eliminated by a dose three times greater than that normally used to induce sleep.* Such doses also suppress the hypoxic and chemoreceptor drives; the hypoxic drive is affected by lower doses than is the chemoreceptor drive, but some function nevertheless persists after doses that obliterate the response to CO_2. Thus, with increasing depth of depression of the CNS, the dominant respiratory drive shifts to the carotid and aortic bodies. Eventually, if the dose is increased still further, the powerful hypoxic drive also fails. However, the margin between the lighter planes of surgical anesthesia and dangerous respiratory depression is sufficient to permit the ultrashort-acting barbiturates to be used, with suitable precautions, as anesthetic agents.

The barbiturates only slightly depress protective reflexes until the degree of intoxication is sufficient to produce severe respiratory depression. In animals, the cough reflex is depressed only by doses that seriously embarrass respiration, and, in this respect, the barbiturates differ from opioids and other antitussives that may exert a selective effect on cough reflexes. Coughing, sneezing, hiccoughing, and laryngospasm may occur when barbiturates are employed as intravenous anesthetic agents. Indeed, laryngospasm is one of the chief complications of barbiturate anesthesia.

Cardiovascular System. When given orally in sedative or hypnotic doses, the barbiturates do not produce significant overt cardiovascular effects, except for a slight decrease in blood pressure and heart rate such as occurs in normal sleep. During thiopental anesthesia, there is usually either no change or a fall in mean arterial pressure, the latter being more pronounced in hypertensive patients.

Hypotension is caused, in part, by partial inhibition of ganglionic transmission. When there is congestive heart failure or hypovolemic shock and reflexes are already operating maximally, barbiturates can cause an exaggerated fall in blood pressure. Because barbiturates impair reflex cardiovascular adjustments to inflation of the lung, positive-pressure respiration should be used cautiously and only when necessary to maintain adequate pulmonary ventilation in patients who are anesthetized or intoxicated with a barbiturate.

Apart from changes in blood pressure the following cardiovascular changes have often been noted when thiopental and other intravenous thiobarbiturates are administered after conventional preanesthetic medication: a decrease in cardiac output; considerable decrease in renal plasma flow; an increase in total calculated peripheral resistance; an increase or no change in heart rate; and a decrease in cerebral blood flow, with a marked fall in CSF pressure. Cardiac arrhythmias are observed only rarely in man (but frequently in animals) and do not result from sensitization of the myocardium to catecholamines. In general, the effects of thiopental anesthesia on the cardiovascular system are benign in comparison with those of other (volatile) anesthetic agents and do not constitute a hazard in normal clinical practice. Direct depression of cardiac contractility occurs only when doses several times those required to cause anesthesia are administered. This probably contributes to the cardiovascular depression that accompanies acute barbiturate poisoning, as does depression of vascular smooth muscle. Both cardiac glycosides and β-adrenergic agonists can overcome the myocardial depressant effect.

Gastrointestinal Tract. The oxybarbiturates tend to decrease the tonus of the gastrointestinal musculature and the amplitude of rhythmic contractions. The locus of action is partly peripheral and partly central, depending on the dose. A hypnotic dose does not significantly delay gastric emptying in man. The relief of various gastrointestinal symptoms by sedative doses is probably largely due to the central-depressant action.

Liver. The best-known effects of barbiturates on the liver are those on the microsomal drug-metabolizing system (*see* Chapter 1). The barbiturates combine with cytochrome P-450 and thus competitively interfere with the biotransformations of a number of substrates of this enzyme, which include other drugs as well as endogenous substrates, such as steroids. Thus, adverse drug interactions and potential endocrine imbalance can result from such inhibition. The other substrates may reciprocally inhibit barbiturate biotransformations. The nature of the inhibition is not simple, however, because barbiturates do not inhibit the biotransformations of all drugs that are substrates of the microsomal enzyme system. The barbiturates themselves do not necessarily have to be oxidized by the enzyme system in order to inhibit the biotransformations of other drugs.

The barbiturates cause a marked increase in the

enzyme, protein, and lipid content of the hepatic smooth endoplasmic reticulum. Their capacity to induce the synthesis of these components correlates with the plasma half-life of the drug but is unrelated to its metabolism by the enzyme system, since barbital is an effective inducer. Not only is the rate of metabolism of a number of drugs increased but also that of steroid hormones, cholesterol, bile salts, certain other endogenous substrates, and vitamin K and possibly vitamin D. Glucuronyl transferase activity is increased. Not all microsomal biotransformations of drugs and endogenous substrates are affected to the same degree, but a convenient rule of thumb is that, at maximal induction in man, the rates are approximately doubled. The inducing effect is not limited to the microsomal enzymes; for example, there is an increase in δ-aminolevulinic acid (ALA) synthetase, a mitochondrial enzyme, and aldehyde dehydrogenase, a cytoplasmic enzyme, and in the rate of conjugation of sulfobromophthalein with glutathione. The effect of barbiturates on ALA synthetase represents an action on feedback control of porphyrin synthesis, which provides heme for the induced cytochrome P-450. Excessive activation of the enzyme can cause dangerous exacerbations of porphyria in persons with intermittent porphyria. Barbiturates may also increase the rate of synthesis of certain proteins, such as the Y and Z proteins, which are believed to regulate the entry of anionic compounds into hepatic cells.

The effect of the barbiturates that are themselves metabolized by hepatic endoplasmic reticulum to increase the rate of their own metabolism accounts for part of the tolerance to the drugs. Many sedative-hypnotics, various anesthetics, and ethanol also are metabolized by and/or induce the microsomal enzymes, and cross-tolerance can occur on this basis. A number of other drugs, chlorinated hydrocarbon insecticides, lipid-rich foods, and certain food additives can also induce the microsomal enzymes, but only under exceptional circumstances have they been shown to increase the rate of elimination of barbiturates significantly in man.

Choleresis results from treatment with phenobarbital but not other barbiturates. Both bile salt–dependent flow and bile salt–independent flow are increased by barbiturates in persons with cholestasis. Biliary excretion of phospholipids, sulfobromophthalein, indocyanine green, rose bengal, and various drugs is also increased. The increase in bile salt secretion probably affects the absorption of various drugs and foodstuffs. Nevertheless, during chronic administration of phenobarbital, the biliary fluxes of phospholipids, bile acids, and cholesterol are not altered in normal subjects.

Genitourinary Tract. Anesthetic but not hypnotic doses of barbiturates decrease the force and frequency of uterine contractions. More important in the use of barbiturates during labor is their respiratory-depressant effect on the infant, since the placenta offers no significant barrier to their passage. Hypnotic doses do not affect the urinary bladder or ureter, but anesthetic doses may cause some depression of contraction.

Kidney. In the concentrations required to produce deep anesthesia, the barbiturates exert direct effects on renal tubular transport mechanisms. The maximal rate of secretion of p-aminohippurate may be depressed by as much as 15 to 25%. Pentobarbital also appears to depress the reabsorptive processes for sodium and glucose by a direct action on tubular cells. However, the direct effects may be overshadowed, at least in part, by the reflex vasoconstriction and decreased renal plasma flow consequent to systemic hypotension, and also by stimulation of the secretion of antidiuretic hormone (ADH). The net effect is a decrease in urine flow. The effect on electrolyte excretion varies, depending on the previous condition of the subject. Severe oliguria or anuria may occur in acute barbiturate poisoning, largely as a result of the marked hypotension.

Pharmacokinetics. *Absorption and Routes of Administration.* For hypnotic use, the barbiturates are usually administered orally. The intravenous route is usually employed for the management of convulsive emergencies or for general anesthesia; the rectal route is used occasionally in infants. Intramuscular injection is avoided, because the alkalinity of soluble preparations causes pain and necrosis at the site of injection.

By the oral route, the rate-limiting step in absorption from the empty stomach is that of dissolution and dispersal of the drug in the gastrointestinal contents. Absorption takes place mainly from the intestine, despite the favorable pH partition in the stomach. The sodium salts are more rapidly absorbed than are the free acids because of rapid dissolution. Food in the stomach decreases the rate of absorption but not the bioavailability.

Distribution. Barbiturates are bound to plasma albumin to various extents. Lipid solubility is the primary determinant of binding; thus, approximately 80% of thiopental but only 5% of barbital is bound. Weak acids, such as aspirin and warfarin, can displace barbiturates from albumin. The concentration of drug in CSF equals that of unbound barbiturate in plasma. Barbiturates partition into fat in proportion to their lipid solubility.

Highly lipid-soluble barbiturates, such as thiopental, methohexital, and thiamylal, undergo a rapid, flow-limited uptake into the most vascular areas of the brain, going first into the gray matter. Maximal uptake occurs within 30 seconds, and sleep may be induced within a few circulation times. Within 30 minutes there is then a redistribution into the less vascular areas of the brain and to other tissues; as little as 10% of the peak amount remains in the gray matter. The ultrashort duration of action is the result of this rapid distribution phase. For such drugs, there is no correlation between duration of action and elimination half-life. The highly vascular kidney, liver, and heart equilibrate almost as fast as does the brain, so that maximal tissue concentrations of thiopental, for example, occur within 1 minute to a few minutes after intravenous administration. Fifteen to 30 minutes is required for equilibration of resting muscle and skin, and more than an hour in the poorly vascular fat. The less lipid-soluble oxybarbiturates equilibrate much more slowly, since uptake is limited more by permeability and less by flow. As long as 20 minutes may be required for sleep to occur after intravenous administration of barbital or phenobarbital. Barbiturates also distribute to fetal blood, and concentrations approach those in maternal plasma.

Elimination. Those barbiturates with a high lipid:water partition coefficient not only are largely bound and consequently poorly filtered but are also readily reabsorbed from the lumen of the tubule. The burden of elimination is thus put on the drug-metabolizing systems. While a few barbiturates with low lipid:water partition coefficients (*e.g.,* aprobarbital and phenobarbital) are significantly excreted unchanged in the urine, this occurs slowly over a period of several days. About 25% of phenobarbital and nearly all of aprobarbital are so excreted. Renal excretion can be greatly increased by osmotic diuresis. Alkalinization of the urine also hastens excretion of those barbiturates with significant renal elimination because of the shift toward increased ionization of a weak organic acid.

When renal function is impaired, barbiturates that depend upon the kidney for elimination may cause severe CNS and cardiovascular depression and thereby may further diminish renal function.

The oxybarbiturates are metabolized only in the liver; thiobarbiturates are also biotransformed to a small extent in kidney, brain, and perhaps other tissues. The products are usually inactive, but demethylation of N-methyl congeners yields active products; thus, mephobarbital and metharbital give rise to phenobarbital and barbital, respectively. The metabolites are invariably more polar than the parent compounds and hence are excreted more rapidly.

Barbiturates are transformed by oxidation of radicals at C5 to alcohols, ketones, phenols, or carboxylic acids, which may appear in the urine as such or as glucuronic acid conjugates. Other biotransformations include N-hydroxylation, N-dealkylation of N-alkylbarbiturates to active metabolites, desulfuration of thiobarbiturates to oxybarbiturates, and opening of the barbituric acid ring. Side chain oxidation is the most important biotransformation responsible for the termination of biological activity. The biotransformations and pharmacokinetics of the barbiturates have been reviewed by Freudenthal and Carroll (1973) and by Breimer (1977).

The data on half-lives in Table 17–4 show that none of the barbiturates used for hypnosis in the United States appears to have an elimination half-life that is sufficiently short for virtually complete elimination to occur in 24 hours. *Thus, all of these barbiturates will accumulate during repetitive administration unless appropriate adjustments in dosage are made. Furthermore, the persistence of the drug in plasma during the day favors the development of tolerance and abuse.* There is, however, a defect in the application of all present pharmacokinetic data to the clinical situation, in that the half-lives are based on assays that determine both the

R(+) and S(−) enantiomers, yet the enantiomers have different half-lives as well as effects.

Half-lives are affected by various factors. With drugs that are metabolized, repetitive use shortens the half-life; for example, that of butabarbital is shortened by 20 to 25% during chronic administration of a single dose per day. Metabolic elimination is more rapid among young people than in the elderly and infants. Half-lives are increased during pregnancy, partly because of increased binding to plasma protein.

The effect of hepatic disease on the half-life is variable. Chronic liver disease increases the half-life of biotransformable barbiturates in some but not all patients. Cirrhosis increases both the half-life of certain barbiturates and the sensitivity of the patient to the CNS-depressant effects of the drugs. Because many alternative drugs are available, there seems to be little reason to use barbiturates in a patient with cirrhosis. If they must be employed, small doses should be tested. Barbiturates or other hypnotics should not be administered to patients showing premonitory signs of hepatic coma. The pharmacokinetics of barbiturates and the effects of hepatic and renal diseases have been reviewed by Breimer (1977).

Untoward Effects. *Aftereffects.* Drowsiness may last for only a few hours after a hypnotic dose of barbiturate, but residual depression of the CNS (hangover) is sometimes frankly evident the following day. Even in the absence of overt evidence of residual depression, subtle distortions of mood and impairment of judgment and fine motor skills may be demonstrable. For example, a 200-mg dose of secobarbital has been shown to impair performance of driving or flying skills for 10 to 22 hours. Therefore, users should be emphatically warned about piloting aircraft, driving automobiles, and operating dangerous machinery and also about potential deterioration of intellectual performance during the day following hypnotic use. Residual effects may also take the form of vertigo, nausea, vomiting, or diarrhea, especially in neurotic persons.

The aftereffects of barbiturates may sometimes be manifested as overt excitement. The user may awaken slightly intoxicated and feel euphoric and energetic; later, as the demands of his daytime activities challenge his possibly impaired faculties, he may display irritability and temper. It is not certain whether excitatory aftereffects are caused by persistence of the excitatory R(+) enantiomer or are withdrawal symptoms resulting from acute tolerance. Aftereffects such as nightmares and night terrors may be caused by deprivation of REM and/or stage-4 sleep, especially after several nights of use.

Paradoxical Excitement. In some persons, barbiturates repeatedly produce excitement rather than depression, and the patient may appear to be inebriated. This type of idiosyncrasy is relatively common among geriatric and debilitated patients and occurs most frequently with phenobarbital and N-methylbarbiturates.

Pain. Rarely, the use of barbiturates results in localized or diffuse myalgic, neuralgic, or arthritic pain, especially in psychoneurotic patients with insomnia. Like other nonanalgesic hypnotic drugs, barbiturates may cause restlessness, excitement, and even delirium when given in the presence of pain.

Hypersensitivity. Allergic reactions occur especially in persons who tend to have asthma, urticaria, angioedema, and similar conditions. Hypersensitivity reactions in this category include localized swellings, particularly of the eyelids, cheeks, or lips, and erythematous dermatitis. Rarely, exfoliative dermatitis may be caused by phenobarbital and can prove fatal; the skin eruption may be associated with fever, delirium, and marked degenerative changes in the liver and other parenchymatous organs.

Drug Interactions. Barbiturates combine with other CNS depressants to cause severe depression; ethanol is the most frequent offender, and interactions with antihistamines are also common. Isoniazid, methylphenidate, and monoamine oxidase inhibitors also increase the CNS-depressant effects.

The greatest number of drug interactions results from induction of hepatic microsomal enzymes. There is significant acceleration of the disappearance of corticosteroids, oral anticoagulants, digitoxin, β-adrenergic antagonists (metoprolol and propranolol), doxycycline, oral contraceptives, griseofulvin, quinidine, phenytoin, sulfadimethoxine, testosterone, tricyclic antidepressants, and zoxazolamine. In experimental animals, the metabolism of vitamins D and K is accelerated, and deficiencies in the coagulation factors II and VIII have also been shown. This finding may be pertinent to reported instances of coagulation defects in neonates whose mothers were taking phenobarbital. Elderly patients may have low concentrations of calcium in plasma as the probable result of accelerated elimination of vitamin D; barbiturates increase the incidence of fractures, probably in part because of an increased number of falls. Hepatic enzyme induction lowers endogenous steroid hormone concentrations, which may cause endocrine disturbances. Barbiturates also induce the hepatic generation of toxic metabolites of chlorocarbon anesthetics and carbon tetrachloride and consequently promote lipid peroxidation, which facilitates the periportal necrosis of the liver caused by these agents.

Barbiturates competitively inhibit the metabolism of certain other drugs. The most important interaction of this type is with tricyclic antidepressants.

Although barbiturates compete with other weak acids for binding to plasma albumin, the only clinically important displacement is that of thyroxine. The absorptions of dicumarol and griseofulvin are decreased by barbiturates, especially phenobarbital.

Other Untoward Effects. Because barbiturates enhance porphyrin synthesis, they are absolutely contraindicated in patients with acute intermittent porphyria or porphyria variegata. In hypnotic doses, the effects of barbiturates on the control of respiration are minor; however, in the presence of pulmonary insufficiency, serious respiratory depression may occur and the drugs are thus contra-

indicated. Rapid intravenous injection of a barbiturate may cause cardiovascular collapse before anesthesia ensues, so that the CNS signs of depth of anesthesia may fail to give an adequate warning of impending toxicity. Blood pressure can fall to shock levels; even slow intravenous injection of barbiturates often produces apnea and occasionally laryngospasm, coughing, and other respiratory difficulties.

BARBITURATE POISONING

In part because of the ready availability and promiscuous use of barbiturates, poisoning with these drugs is a major clinical problem; death occurs in 0.5 to 12% of cases. Most of the cases are the result of deliberate attempts at suicide, but some are from accidental poisonings in children or in drug abusers. A widely held concept is that poisoning often is the result of "drug automatism." This behavior relates to the patient who fails to fall asleep after the first or second dose of a hypnotic, becomes confused, and unwittingly ingests an overdose; on recovery, there is no memory of having taken the additional doses. The extent of poisoning from confusion during self-administration is controversial.

The *lethal dose* of barbiturate varies with many factors and cannot be stated with certainty. Severe poisoning is likely to occur when more than ten times the full hypnotic dose has been ingested at once. The barbiturates with short half-lives and high lipid solubility are more potent and more toxic than the more polar, long-acting compounds, such as phenobarbital and barbital. The potentially fatal dose of phenobarbital is 6 to 10 g, whereas that of amobarbital, secobarbital, or pentobarbital is 2 to 3 g. The lowest concentration of drug in plasma associated with lethal overdosage has been 6 mg/dl for phenobarbital and barbital but only 1 mg/dl for shorter-acting agents such as amobarbital and pentobarbital; if alcohol or other depressant drugs are also present, the concentrations that can cause death are lower. The finding of a high concentration in blood at necropsy does not in itself constitute *prima-facie* evidence of death from barbiturate poisoning. Patients with much higher blood concentrations than those mentioned above (*e.g.*, 120 mg/dl of barbital) have recovered satisfactorily, even without the use of hemodialysis. The highest blood concentration of phenobarbital from which a patient has recovered is 29 mg/dl.

The *signs and symptoms* of barbiturate poisoning are referable especially to the CNS and the cardiovascular system. Moderate intoxication resembles alcoholic inebriation. In severe intoxication, the patient is comatose, and the level of reflex activity conforms in a general way to the intensity of the central depression. The deep reflexes may persist for some time despite coexistent coma. The Babinski sign is often positive. The EEG may be of the burst-suppression type with brief periods of electrical silence. The pupils may be constricted and react to light, but late in the course of barbiturate poisoning hypoxic paralytic dilatation may appear. Respiration is affected early. Breathing may be either slow, or rapid and shallow; Cheyne-Stokes rhythm may be present. Superficial observation of respiration may be misleading with regard to actual minute volume and to the degree of respiratory acidosis and cerebral hypoxia; arterial P_{CO_2} and P_{O_2} must be determined. Eventually, blood pressure falls due to the direct effect of the drug and of hypoxia on medullary vasomotor centers with consequent arteriolar and venous dilatation; depression of cardiac contractility, sympathetic ganglia, and vascular smooth muscle also contribute. The patient thus develops shock, with a weak and rapid pulse, cold and sweaty skin, a rise in the hematocrit, and renal ischemia. Hypothermia, sometimes with temperatures as low as 32° C, often occurs. During recovery, hyperthermia may also occur. Pulmonary complications (atelectasis, edema, and bronchopneumonia) and renal failure are likely to be the fatal complications of severe barbiturate poisoning.

Not uncommonly, patients suffering from acute barbiturate intoxication develop necrosis of sweat glands and bullous cutaneous lesions, which are not due to hypersensitivity or hypothermia. These lesions heal slowly, sometimes requiring many weeks.

The optimal *treatment* of acute barbiturate intoxication is based upon general supportive measures and, often, the use of dialysis or hemoperfusion. A highly organized intensive care unit, prepared for around-the-clock effort with continuous monitoring of the patient, can reduce the mortality rate to less than 2%. Formerly, when CNS stimulants were used in attempts to antagonize barbiturates, mortality rates were as high as 40%. The present treatment is applicable in most respects for poisoning by any CNS depressant.

The depth of coma and adequacy of ventilation are first evaluated. If fewer than 24 hours have elapsed since ingestion, gastric lavage should be considered, even though little barbiturate is usually recovered from the stomach after 4 hours. Lavage or emesis should be attempted only after precautions have been taken to avoid aspiration. Apomorphine-induced emesis evacuates the stomach more rapidly and reliably than does ipecac. After lavage, a saline cathartic should be administered and repeated every 1 to 2 hours as long as bowel sounds are present. Activated charcoal placed in the stomach may adsorb some residual barbiturate.

Close and constant attention must be given to the maintenance of a patent airway and to the prevention of pneumonia; oxygen should be administered. Measures to prevent or treat atelectasis should be taken. Blood P_{CO_2} and pH should be monitored, and mechanical ventilation should be initiated when indicated. Fever or roentgenographic evidence of pneumonia calls for appropriate therapy.

Measures should be taken to prevent further loss of body heat, but it is not universally agreed that it is necessary to restore the body temperature to normal.

In severe acute barbiturate intoxication, circulatory collapse is a major threat. Often the patient is admitted to the hospital with severe hypotension or shock. The hypovolemic, vascular, and cardiodepressant factors are evaluated. Dehydration is often severe. Hypovolemia must be corrected, and, if necessary, the blood pressure can be supported with dopamine.

Renal failure consequent to shock and hypoxia accounts for perhaps one sixth of the deaths. Such failure also contributes to delayed elimination of long-acting barbiturates. Therefore, parameters of renal function and changes in the concentration of drug in plasma are assessed frequently. Anuria and uremia may ensue, even after the patient has recovered consciousness.

Should renal failure occur, the most effective method of disposing of the poison is hemodialysis or hemoperfusion. Elimination of the drug is achieved very much faster by these procedures than by endogenous mechanisms. Hemodialysis is more effective in removing long-acting than short-acting compounds because they are more water soluble and less protein bound. More effective extraction of the lipid-soluble, short-acting barbiturates can be achieved by the use of a lipid-containing dialysate or by hemoperfusion through activated charcoal, acrylic hydrogel-coated carbon, or ion-exchange resins. Perfusion through the lipid-adsorptive resin, AMBERLITE XAD-4, has been reported to clear the blood in 2.5 to 10 hours. Peritoneal dialysis is only 25% as rapid as hemodialysis in removing barbiturates from the body. If renal and cardiac function are satisfactory and the patient is hydrated, forced diuresis and alkalinization of the urine will significantly hasten the excretion of some but not all barbiturates. The likelihood of success is increased if the drug is only partly bound to plasma protein, has a relatively low pK_a, and is relatively slowly reabsorbed. These are characteristics of the long-acting barbiturates. It is desirable to achieve a diuresis of 8 to 14 liters per day. Because of elevated ADH levels, hypotonic solutions are usually less effective than osmotic or high-ceiling diuretics. When diuresis of this magnitude is achieved, it is absolutely necessary to maintain water and electrolyte balance. Even though forced diuresis and alkalinization can increase the renal clearance of pentobarbital by as much as 15 times, the total rate of detoxication is increased by only 15 to 25%, since little of this drug is usually excreted in the urine. In contrast, the rates of detoxication of barbital, phenobarbital, aprobarbital, and allobarbital—barbiturates for which renal excretion is a significant fraction of total elimination—are increased 30 to 180%; this can shorten the duration of coma substantially. Intoxication by barbiturates and its management have been reviewed by Gary and Tresnewsky (1983).

THERAPEUTIC USES

The use of barbiturates as sedative-hypnotic drugs is justifiably on the decline because they lack specificity of effect in the CNS, they have a lower therapeutic index than do the benzodiazepines, tolerance occurs more frequently than with benzodiazepines, the liability for abuse is greater, and there is a considerable number of drug interactions.

CNS Uses. The use of barbiturates as hypnotics is included in the general discussion on page 367.

Barbiturates may be used in large doses in the management of acute maniacal states, delirium, and certain psychoneurotic disorders, although they are being superseded by newer agents.

The era when barbiturates (particularly phenobarbital) were virtually the only drugs recommended for daytime sedation has long passed, and they have largely been replaced by benzodiazepines and other compounds. However, phenobarbital and butabarbital are still available as "sedatives" in a host of inefficacious combinations for the treatment of functional gastrointestinal disorders, urethral inflammation, hypertension, asthma, and coronary artery disease. They are also included in analgesic combinations, possibly counterproductively. Although they may effectively decrease hyperactivity in hyperthyroidism, benzodiazepines are preferred. The barbiturates still have valid uses as sedatives to decrease restlessness during illnesses in children such as colic, whooping cough, pylorospasm, and nausea and vomiting of functional origin, to suppress excitement of various abnormal origins, and to decrease apprehension preparatory to minor medical and dental procedures.

Barbiturates are sometimes used to antagonize unwanted CNS-stimulant effects of various drugs, such as ephedrine, dextroamphetamine, and theophylline; butabarbital and phenobarbital are most commonly used for such purposes. In these uses, they are probably superior to benzodiazepines.

Barbiturates are still employed for their rapid onset of action in the *emergency treatment* of *convulsions,* such as occur in tetanus, eclampsia, status epilepticus, cerebral hemorrhage, and poisoning by convulsant drugs; however, benzodiazepines are generally superior in these uses. Some representative dose ranges for intravenous administration are as follows: phenobarbital sodium, 100 to 300 mg; pentobarbital sodium, 100 to 500 mg; amobarbital sodium, 65 to 500 mg; thiopental sodium, 100 to 200 mg. The injection should be made slowly, with the usual precautions necessary for intravenous administration. Phenobarbital sodium is frequently used because of its anticonvulsant efficacy; however, even when administered intravenously, 15 minutes or more may be required for it to attain peak concentrations in the brain. Thus, the practice of continuing to administer phenobarbital until convulsions stop results in brain concentrations that continue to rise and may eventually exceed that required to control the seizures. The subsequent barbiturate-induced depression may summate with postictal depression. Administration of phenobarbital requires restraint and patience until the anticonvulsant effect develops before deciding whether a second dose is necessary. While the rapidity of onset of the ultrashort- and short-acting barbiturates would seem to have appeal, these drugs have a low ratio of anticonvulsant to hypnotic action. Diazepam offers many advantages for the emergency treatment of certain convulsive disorders, particularly for *status epilepticus.* The use of phenobarbital and mephobarbital in the symptomatic therapy of epilepsy is discussed in Chapter 20.

The barbiturates are being replaced by benzodiazepines for preanesthetic medication and basal anesthesia. The ultrashort-acting agents continue to be employed as intravenous anesthetics (Chapter 14). Short- and ultrashort-acting barbiturates are occasionally used as adjuncts to other agents in the production of obstetrical anesthesia. Although several studies have failed to affirm gross depression of respiration in the neonate at birth, evaluation of the effects on the fetus and neonate is difficult; it is prudent to avoid the use of barbiturates in obstetrics.

The barbiturates are employed as diagnostic and therapeutic aids in psychiatry, in *narcoanalysis* and *narcotherapy.* They are used to activate latent abnormalities in the EEG. In low concentrations, amobarbital has been administered directly into the carotid artery as a means of identifying the dominant cerebral hemisphere for speech prior to neurosurgery.

Anesthetic doses of barbiturates attenuate cerebral edema resulting from surgery, head injury, or cerebral ischemia, and they decrease infarct size and increase survival. The death rate from head injuries among juveniles and adults has been reported to be reduced by 80% and 50%, respectively. General anesthetics do not provide protection. The procedure is not without serious danger, however, and the ultimate benefit to the patient has been questioned (*see* Marshall and Bowers, 1982; Michenfelder, 1982; Steer, 1982).

Hepatic Metabolic Uses. Because hepatic glucuronyl transferase and the bilirubin-binding Y protein are increased by the barbiturates, phenobarbital has been successfully used to treat *hyperbilirubinemia* and *kernicterus* in the neonate; complete failure of this treatment can probably be attributed to premature discontinuation of the drug. The nondepressant barbiturate phetharbital (N-phenylbarbital) works equally well. Phenobarbital may improve the hepatic transport of bilirubin in patients with hemolytic jaundice. The effect of phenobarbital on bile salt metabolism and excretion has been employed in the treatment of selected cases of *cholestasis.*

Preparations and Dosage. Barbiturates are marketed in a vast array of preparations. In the United States, phenobarbital is an ingredient in more than 25 proprietary remedies, which are best ignored in favor of nonproprietary preparations. Extended-release forms are pointless and potentially dangerous in view of the long half-lives among available barbiturates, and they are disadvantageous in hypnotic use.

The hypnotic and sedative doses of the barbiturates are listed in Table 17–4.

CHLORAL DERIVATIVES

The pharmacology and uses of the chloral derivatives that are employed clinically are essentially the same, because they are all converted in the body to the same active intermediate. Two such compounds remain available in the United States. What is said below about *chloral hydrate* applies equally well to *triclofos sodium*, unless otherwise indicated.

Chemistry. *Chloral* is 2,2,2-trichloroacetaldehyde, an unstable, disagreeable oil that does not lend itself well to pharmaceutical formulations. Therefore, it was introduced into medicine in the form of its hydrate, formed by adding one molecule of water to the carbonyl group. The formula of chloral hydrate is $CCl_3CH(OH)_2$.

Chloral can form hemiacetals of the general formula $CCl_3CH(OH)(OR)$, of which *chloral alcoholate*, *chloral betaine*, *α-chloralose*, and *dichloralphenazone* are examples. They generate chloral hydrate *in vivo*. Their metabolite, *trichloroethanol* (CCl_3CH_2OH), is an excellent hypnotic, but it is not conveniently used as such, owing to its physical and irritant properties; instead, it is used as the monosodium salt of the phosphate ester, *triclofos sodium*, $CCl_3CH_2OPO_3H^- \cdot Na^+$.

Local Actions. Chloral hydrate is quite irritating to the skin and mucous membranes. Gastrointestinal side effects are particularly likely to occur if the drug is insufficiently diluted or if it is taken on an empty stomach. Triclofos generates some chloral in the stomach and hence causes some gastrointestinal irritation. It lacks the disagreeable taste of chloral hydrate.

Systemic Actions. Like the barbiturates, chloral hydrate has little analgesic activity, and excitement or delirium may be initiated by pain. It is effective against experimentally induced convulsions produced by strychnine, pentylenetetrazol, and electroshock and has been used in the treatment of eclampsia and tetanus; however, the ratio of anticonvulsant to sedative effects is low, and diazepam, clonazepam, or barbiturates are preferable in the treatment of acute convulsive disorders. The margin of safety is too narrow to permit the drug to be used as a general anesthetic agent.

During the first week of use of chloral hydrate, there is a decrease in the sleep latency and the number of awakenings, a variable change in total sleep time, and a slight decrease in SWS. In only one of seven studies in which the dose ranged between 0.5 and 1.5 g was REM sleep suppressed (*see* Kay *et al.*, 1976). Similarly, 1 g of triclofos has a negligible effect on sleep stages. There are claims that during repetitive nightly use, the effects on sleep disappear within 2 weeks; however, Hartmann (1976) has reported that total sleep time and REM latency remain elevated, even though the number of awakenings is increased. After discontinuation of the drug, a significant rebound in REM sleep does not occur.

In therapeutic doses, chloral hydrate has little effect on respiration and blood pressure. Toxic doses produce severe respiratory depression and hypotension. In large doses, chloral hydrate depresses cardiac contractility and shortens the refractory period, as do many hydrocarbon anesthetics. Untoward cardiac effects may occur when toxic doses are administered, especially to patients with heart disease; however, there is no evidence of deleterious effects on the heart from the continued use of the compound in therapeutic doses.

The pharmacological properties of *trichloroethanol* closely resemble those of chloral hydrate. Chloral hydrate is very rapidly reduced to trichloroethanol with a half-time of a few minutes, and significant amounts of chloral hydrate have not been detected in the blood after its oral administration; therefore, its central-depressant effects are probably caused by trichloroethanol.

Distribution and Fate. Chloral hydrate and trichloroethanol are sufficiently lipid soluble to permeate plasma membranes and enter cells throughout the body. Triclofos is rapidly hydrolyzed to trichloroethanol and is comparably distributed.

Chloral hydrate is reduced to trichloroethanol, largely by alcohol dehydrogenase in the liver. Ethanol accelerates the reduction, because its own oxidation provides NADH to drive the reduction of chloral hydrate. Chloral inhibits alcohol dehydrogenase. A small but variable amount of chloral hydrate and a larger fraction of trichloroethanol are oxidized to trichloroacetic acid, mainly in the smooth endoplasmic reticulum of the liver and kidney. Trichloroethanol is mainly conjugated with glucuronic acid, and the product (urochloralic acid) is excreted mostly into the urine and to a limited extent into the bile. The plasma half-life of trichloroethanol ranges from 4 to 12 hours. The pharmacokinetics of chloral hydrate and trichloroethanol have been reviewed by Breimer (1977).

Untoward Effects. The irritant actions of chloral hydrate give rise to an unpleasant taste, epigastric distress, nausea, occasional vomiting, and flatulence. Gastric necrosis has occurred after intoxicating doses. Undesirable CNS effects include light-headedness, malaise, ataxia, and nightmares. "Hangover" may also occur, although it is less common than with most barbiturates and some benzodiazepines. The tendency of hypnotics to cause persistent effects in the elderly is less pronounced with chloral hydrate than with agents that are metabolized by the hepatic microsomal enzyme system.

Rarely, patients exhibit *idiosyncratic reactions* to chloral hydrate. Occasionally, a patient becomes somnambulistic after receiving the drug, and may be disoriented and incoherent and show paranoid behavior. *Allergic reactions* include erythema, scarlatiniform exanthems, urticaria, and eczematoid dermatitis. Eosinophilia and leukopenia may also occur. Chloral hydrate is contraindicated in patients with marked hepatic or renal impairment, and it should perhaps be avoided in patients with severe cardiac disease. If gastritis is present, the drug should not be given orally but may be administered in olive oil as a retention enema.

Chloral hydrate causes displacement of oral anticoagulants from binding sites on albumin, thereby enhancing hypoprothrombinemia transiently. It also appears to both inhibit and enhance the metabolism of some drugs in man. The final effect on the action of other drugs may be complicated by the fact that trichloroacetic acid formed by the metabolism of chloral hydrate displaces acidic drugs from plasma-protein binding sites. The combination of chloral hydrate and furosemide in some persons may cause vasodilatation and flushing, tachycardia, hypotension or hypertension, and sweating. Chloral derivatives probably should be avoided in patients with intermittent porphyria.

There is a popular belief that chloral hydrate and ethanol in combination (the "Mickey Finn") are supra-additive; experimental studies in several species have confirmed the existence of an interaction between these drugs. Its basis is presumed to be inhibition of the metabolism of ethanol by chloral and enhancement of the generation of trichloroethanol by ethanol, in addition to the combined depressant effect of the two drugs.

Acute Intoxication. The toxic oral dose of chloral hydrate for adults is approximately 10 g, although death has been reported from as little as 4 g and individuals have survived after ingesting as much as 30 g. Poisoning by chloral hydrate resembles acute barbiturate intoxication, and the same supportive treatment is indicated. Gastric irritation may result in initial vomiting and even gastric necrosis. Pinpoint pupils may be seen, as in morphine poisoning. If the patient survives, icterus due to hepatic damage and albuminuria from renal irritation may appear. Treatment is the same as that for intoxication with other CNS depressants (*see* Barbiturate Poisoning, page 358); hemodialysis and hemoperfusion are effective.

Abuse and Chronic Intoxication. The habitual use of chloral hydrate may result in the development of tolerance, physical dependence, and addiction. Chloral addicts may take enormous doses of the drug. The chloral habit is similar to alcohol addiction, and sudden withdrawal may result in delirium and seizures with a high frequency of death, when untreated. The chloral habitué may suddenly exhibit what was formerly termed a "break in tolerance," and death may occur, either as a result of an overdose or a failure of the detoxication mechanism due to hepatic damage. In patients suffering from chronic intoxication, gastritis is common and skin eruptions may develop. Parenchymatous renal injury may also occur.

Dosage and Preparations. The dosage and preparations of *chloral hydrate* are listed in Table 17–4. Only brief comment is made here. The often-recommended dose of 0.5 to 1 g has only a slight effect on sleep, at best. Many individuals require as much as 2 g of chloral hydrate. To minimize irritation, solutions of the drug should be taken well diluted with water or milk. It is too irritating to be given parenterally. A dose of *triclofos sodium* of 1.5 g will yield a blood concentration of trichloroethanol approximately equal to that from 900 mg of chloral hydrate.

ETHCHLORVYNOL

Ethchlorvynol is a sedative-hypnotic drug with a rapid onset and short duration of action. It has the following structure:

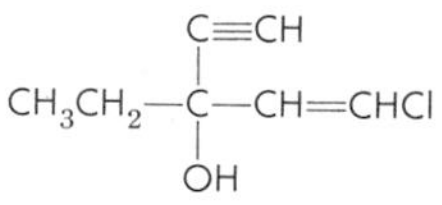

$$CH_3CH_2\!-\!\underset{\underset{OH}{|}}{\overset{\overset{C\equiv CH}{|}}{C}}\!-\!CH\!=\!CHCl$$

Ethchlorvynol

CNS Effects. Ethchlorvynol has anticonvulsant and muscle relaxant properties as well as sedative-hypnotic activity. Although the drug is said to produce less initial excitement than do the barbiturates, valid clinical confirmation is needed. The EEG pattern following ethchlorvynol resembles that seen after barbiturates. Ethchlorvynol administered to two subjects for 2 weeks decreased sleep latency, wake time, REM sleep, and stage-4 time and increased stage-2 and total sleep time (Kripke *et al.*, 1978); after withdrawal, rebound occurred in sleep latency and REM latency, wake time, and time spent in stage 2, but not in REM sleep or stage-4 sleep. If ethchlorvynol is taken along with ethanol, an exaggerated hypnotic effect may occur.

Absorption and Fate. Oral ethchlorvynol acts within 15 to 30 minutes. The maximal concentration in blood is attained in 1 to 1.5 hours. The apparent volume of distribution is about 4 liters per kilogram. The drug passes the placental barrier. Two-compartment kinetics is manifested, with a distribution half-life of about 1 to 3 hours and an elimination half-life of 10 to 25 hours. After intoxicating doses, dose-dependent rates of elimination may be seen. Approximately 90% of the drug is destroyed in the liver.

Side Effects, Intoxication, and Abuse. The most common side effects caused by ethchlorvynol are mintlike aftertaste, dizziness, nausea, vomiting, hypotension, and facial numbness. In persons in whom absorption is especially rapid, giddiness and ataxia frequently occur; these effects can be controlled by giving the drug with food. Mild "hangover" is also relatively common. An occasional patient responds with profound hypnosis, muscular weakness, and syncope unrelated to marked hypotension. Positional nystagmus or diplopia may occur, especially after overdoses. Idiosyncratic responses range from mild stimulation to marked excitement and hysteria. Ethchlorvynol should not be used with antidepressants, because delirium may result. Hypersensitivity reactions include urticaria, rare but sometimes fatal thrombocytopenia, and occasionally cholestatic jaundice. Because of a reported effect to suppress the anticipated response to dicumarol, the drug should be used cautiously in combination with drugs metabolized by the liver, and it is contraindicated in intermittent porphyria.

The therapeutic index of ethchlorvynol is probably about the same as that of barbiturates with an intermediate duration of action. Acute intoxication is characterized by prolonged deep coma, severe respiratory depression, hypotension, bradycardia, hypothermia, bullae, and sometimes pulmonary edema and the adult respiratory-distress syndrome. Death has occurred with a blood concentration of 14 mg/dl. The lethal dose usually ranges from 10 to 25 g, but death has followed a dose of 2.5 g (ethanol was also present), and one patient survived 50 g (with intensive care) after a coma lasting 7 days. Treatment is similar to that for acute barbiturate intoxication. Substantial amounts of ethchlorvynol have been recovered from the stomach by lavage as late as 5 hours after ingestion. Detoxication is best achieved by hemoperfusion with activated charcoal, cellulose acetate–coated activated charcoal, or resins. Dialysis against oil is also somewhat effective.

Chronic abuse of ethchlorvynol results in tolerance and physical dependence. Abusers may take up to 4 g of drug per day. Usually they show signs of intoxication, such as incoordination, tremors, ataxia, slurred speech, confusion, asthenia, hyperreflexia, nystagmus, diplopia, and sometimes toxic amblyopia, dichromatism, scotoma, and reversible peripheral or optic neuritis. Withdrawal symptoms may resemble delirium tremens and are sometimes suggestive of a schizophrenic reaction. They are especially severe in elderly patients.

Preparations and Dosage. These are listed in Table 17–4. A dose of 770 mg of ethchlorvynol is approximately equivalent to 100 mg of secobarbital.

GLUTETHIMIDE

Glutethimide is 3-ethyl-3-phenyl-2,6-piperidine-dione and is similar to methyprylon (*see* below). Their structures are as follows:

Glutethimide   Methyprylon

Glutethimide has little to recommend its continued use as a sedative-hypnotic drug. Its addiction liability and the severity of withdrawal symptoms are equal to those of the barbiturates, and certain features of acute intoxication make its treatment more difficult.

Pharmacological Actions. The pharmacology of glutethimide is like that of barbiturates in that it can induce hypnosis without selective analgesic, antitussive, or anticonvulsant actions. It is also similar in its effects on the EEG pattern and in its suppression of REM sleep. The drug exhibits pronounced anticholinergic activity, which is most prominent in the iris but which also is manifested by inhibition of salivary secretion and intestinal motility.

Absorption and Fate. Glutethimide is quite erratically absorbed from the gastrointestinal tract. The drug has a high lipid:water partition coefficient, so that following intravenous injection it quickly penetrates the brain and then redistributes. About 50% of the drug is bound to plasma proteins. More than 95% of glutethimide is metabolized in the liver; the half-life ranges from 5 to 22 hours. Active metabolites may accumulate after repetitive administration and during intoxication. Glutethimide induces hepatic microsomal enzymes.

Adverse Effects. With therapeutic doses, toxic side effects are rare and consist in "hangover," excitement, blurring of vision, gastric irritation, headache, and, infrequently, skin rashes, including exfoliative dermatitis. Thrombocytopenia, aplastic anemia, and leukopenia may also occur.

Acute Intoxication. The symptoms of acute intoxication are similar to those of barbiturate poisoning. Respiratory depression is usually less severe than with barbiturate intoxication, but circulatory failure is at least equally severe. The antimuscarinic actions cause xerostomia, ileus, atony of the urinary bladder, and long-lasting mydriasis and hyperpyrexia, which may persist for hours after the patient regains consciousness. In some cases of glutethimide poisoning, occasional bouts of tonic muscular spasms, twitching, and even convulsions occur. Patients also tend to show cyclic variations in the level of intoxication. A dose of 5 g is sufficient to produce severe intoxication. The lethal dose is between 10 and 20 g; plasma concentrations associated with lethality range from 2 to 80 μg/ml. In acute intoxication, the plasma half-life may exceed 100 hours but averages about 40 hours; hemodialysis shortens the half-life to about 14 hours. The fall in the plasma concentration of the drug may be followed by increased absorption from the intestinal tract, resulting in a rapid, secondary rise in the blood concentration following the initial dialysis. When hydrogel-coated charcoal or silicone oil is used, elimination is greatly accelerated.

Chronic Use and Abuse. Excessive use of glutethimide leads to tolerance and psychic and physical dependence. The abstinence syndrome includes tremulousness, nausea, tachycardia, fever, tonic muscle spasms, and generalized convulsions. The same symptoms occasionally occur in patients who have been taking glutethimide regularly in moderate doses (0.5 to 3 g daily) even when there is no evidence of abstention, and also in patients being treated for acute intoxication who have no previous history of drug abuse. In the latter case, tonic muscular spasms and, infrequently, generalized convulsions are seen. Catatonia and dyskinesias may be observed after abusers are withdrawn from a combination of glutethimide and an antihistamine. Chronic use may cause osteomalacia.

Preparations and Dosage. These are listed in Table 17–4. Considering the lack of any specific utility of glutethimide and the complications of treatment of its acute or chronic abuse, it is difficult to justify the continued use of this agent.

METHYPRYLON

Methyprylon is 3,3-diethyl-5-methyl-2,4-piperidinedione. Its structure is shown with that of glutethimide on page 363.

In a dose of 300 mg, the hypnotic effect of methyprylon is indistinguishable from that of 200 mg of secobarbital, but it is not as effective as the benzodiazepine triazolam. This dose also suppresses REM sleep as much as does 100 mg of pentobarbital.

Approximately 97% of methyprylon appears to be metabolized. The metabolites are partly conjugated to glucuronides. Only 60% of the free metabolites and glucuronides is recoverable from urine. The plasma half-life is 4 hours, but it is longer in acute intoxication. Methyprylon stimulates the hepatic microsomal enzyme system and δ-ALA synthetase; it should probably be avoided in patients with intermittent porphyria.

Untoward effects of methyprylon are not frequent, but include "hangover," nausea, vomiting, epigastric distress, diarrhea, esophagitis, headache, and rash. Neutropenia and thrombocytopenia of unproven origin have been reported in persons taking methyprylon. An idiosyncratic excitement occasionally occurs.

Acute intoxication resembles that caused by barbiturates, and the general principles of management are the same. Hypotension, shock, and pulmonary edema are more conspicuous features than is respiratory depression. Hemodialysis is an effective component of treatment. Peritoneal dialysis may also be effective; at pH 7.4, methyprylon is quite water soluble, which facilitates dialysis. The lethal dose is unknown; death has occurred after ingestion of 6 g, but recovery has occurred after 27 g. Coma may last for up to 5 days.

Habituation, tolerance, physical dependence, and addiction can occur. The abstinence syndrome is like that of the barbiturates and includes insomnia, confusion, hallucinations, and convulsions.

The dosage and preparations are shown in Table 17–4.

MEPROBAMATE

Meprobamate is a *bis*-carbamate ester with the following structural formula:

$$H_2N-\overset{\overset{\displaystyle O}{\|}}{C}-OCH_2-\overset{\overset{\displaystyle C_3H_7}{|}}{\underset{\underset{\displaystyle CH_3}{|}}{C}}-CH_2O-\overset{\overset{\displaystyle O}{\|}}{C}-NH_2$$

Meprobamate

Meprobamate was introduced as an antianxiety agent in 1955. However, it also became popular as a sedative-hypnotic drug. In the United States it is approved for use only in the treatment of anxiety. Meprobamate is discussed here mainly because of the continuing practice to use this drug for sedative-hypnotic purposes and because of precedence. The question of whether its sedative and antianxiety actions differ remains unanswered.

Pharmacological Actions. The properties of meprobamate might be characterized as being somewhere between those of the barbiturates and the benzodiazepines. Although meprobamate can cause widespread depression of the CNS, it does so unevenly; there is considerable selectivity in its influence on various CNS functions, and it does not cause anesthesia.

Meprobamate can depress polysynaptic reflexes in the spinal cord without affecting monosynaptic reflexes, and it is more selective than barbiturates in this respect. This effect is thought to contribute to its muscle relaxant properties, although supra-segmental loci of action cannot be discounted. With clinical doses in man, the muscle relaxant effects are negligible, although there may be some decrease in spasm as a result of a lessening of anxiety. Meprobamate does not appear to modify the effects of GABA-ergic inhibitory pathways and does not affect presynaptic inhibition in the spinal cord.

Although meprobamate may sometimes produce modest hyperalgesia, it appears to have a mild analgesic effect when there is musculoskeletal pain, and it enhances the analgesic effects of other drugs.

As an anticonvulsant, meprobamate antagonizes pentylenetetrazol and raises the electroshock seizure threshold in laboratory animals but does not prevent seizures from maximal electroshock. In man, meprobamate suppresses absence seizures, but it may aggravate tonic-clonic and myoclonic epilepsy. Generalized seizures frequently occur as the result of abrupt withdrawal from chronic use of large doses.

Aggressive animals become tame and docile when given doses of meprobamate that cause negligible impairment of locomotor and general activity. Behavior patterns that have been previously suppressed by punishment are restored ("released") by meprobamate. Naloxone blocks the effect of meprobamate on suppressed behavior. The drug inhibits a variety of responses to hypothalamic stimulation and shortens electrical afterdischarges in the limbic system; it also suppresses amygdalohippocampal-evoked potentials in doses that do not affect the arousal response evoked by stimulation of the reticular formation of the brain stem. Despite these selective experimental effects, which are usually thought to correlate with antianxiety effects in man, clinical proof of efficacy as a selective antianxiety agent is lacking. Usual clinical doses of meprobamate do not affect the EEG. Only two studies have been made on the effect of meprobamate on the stages of sleep (*see* Kay *et al.*, 1976). In one, the drug decreased stage-1 sleep and increased the time spent in stage-2 and REM sleep without affecting SWS.

Absorption, Fate, and Excretion. Meprobamate is well absorbed when administered orally; when tablets are taken, peak concentrations are reached in plasma in 1 to 3 hours. During chronic administration of sedative doses, concentrations in blood usually range between 5 and 20 μg/ml. There is little binding to plasma proteins. Eighty to 92% of the drug is metabolized in the liver, mainly to a side chain hydroxy derivative and a glucuronide; the remainder is excreted unchanged in the urine. The half-life of a single dose in plasma ranges from 6 to 17 hours, but it has been reported to be as long as 24 to 48 hours during chronic administration; the kinetics of elimination may be dependent on the dose. Meprobamate can induce some hepatic microsomal enzymes. It is not clear whether the drug induces the enzymes responsible for its own metabolism.

Adverse Effects and Intoxication. The major unwanted effects of sedative doses of meprobamate are drowsiness and ataxia. A single dose of 400 mg has little effect on the performance of psychometric tests; however, there is considerable impairment of learning and motor coordination and prolongation of reaction time when doses of 1600 mg are given.

Hypotension may occur in response to meprobamate. Allergic reactions have been reported in from 0.2 to 3.4% of different series of patients and appear most frequently in those with a history of dermatological or allergic conditions. Urticaria or an erythematous rash is the most common manifestation. Acute nonthrombocytopenic purpura has also been reported, and angioedema and bronchospasm have occurred occasionally.

Ethanol and meprobamate appear to be additive in their effects. Tricyclic antidepressants and monoamine oxidase (MAO) inhibitors increase the CNS-depressant effects of meprobamate. It is prudent to assume that the CNS-depressant effect of any drug will be exaggerated by therapeutic doses of meprobamate.

Within a year of the introduction of meprobamate into medicine, abuse was reported, and this soon became a major problem; it has continued despite a substantial decrease in the clinical use of the drug. After chronic medication with doses usually in excess of 2.4 g a day for several weeks, abrupt discontinuation evokes a withdrawal syndrome usually characterized by anxiety, insomnia, tremors, gastrointestinal disturbances, and, frequently, hallucinations; generalized seizures occur in about 10% of cases. Allgulander (1978) reported 40% of drug habitués with serious withdrawal syndromes had been using meprobamate, a considerably higher percentage than had been taking barbiturates. Mild symptoms sometimes occur after withdrawal from chronic doses of as low as 1.6 g a day.

Poison control centers continue to report a significant incidence of intoxication with meprobamate. Moderate overdosage, which results in blood concentrations in the range of 30 to 100 μg/ml, may cause vertigo, ataxia, slurred speech, impaired stance, stupor, or light coma. Ingestions that result in concentrations of 100 to 200 μg/ml cause coma, hypotension, respiratory depression, shock, pulmonary edema, and heart failure. Although a single dose of 12 g has been fatal, lethal doses usually exceed 40 g. The principles of the management of intoxication are essentially those described for barbiturate intoxication (*see* above). Hemodialysis or hemoperfusion is indicated only if brain stem functions are inadequate. Hemoperfusion with AMBERLITE XAD-4 resin or charcoal is superior to hemodialysis. Elimination can be considerably enhanced by diuresis promoted by the administration of saline and furosemide.

Conflicting reports have appeared on the effects of exposure of the fetus to meprobamate; it is recommended that meprobamate not be taken during pregnancy, especially during the first trimester.

Induction of hepatic microsomal enzymes by meprobamate may result in exacerbation of intermittent porphyria and may also be the cause of various drug interactions. The elimination of warfarin, estrogens, and oral contraceptives is increased by large doses of meprobamate, but interactions appear to be slight when usual doses are taken.

Therapeutic Uses. Even though meprobamate is currently approved for use only as an antianxiety agent, it is also employed as a hypnotic agent in the treatment of insomnia. It has especially been advocated for hypnotic use in geriatric patients, for whom it has been reported to be as effective as flurazepam and flunitrazepam (Keston and Brocklehurst, 1974; Brocklehurst *et al.*, 1978), more predictable than chloral hydrate, and subject to fewer dosage problems than barbiturates and probably flurazepam. The sedative and hypnotic doses are listed in Table 17–4.

METHAQUALONE

Methaqualone, a 2,3-disubstituted quinazoline, has been withdrawn from the market in the United States. Discussion is retained here because the drug is abused widely. Additional information can be found in *previous editions* of this textbook.

In addition to sedative-hypnotic properties, methaqualone possesses anticonvulsant, antispasmodic, local anesthetic, and weak antihistaminic properties. It also has antitussive activity comparable to that of codeine. Methaqualone may possess tranquilizing properties, but it is not clear that these are distinct from its sedative effects. Drug culturists contend that it causes a dissociative "high" achieved without the drowsiness caused by barbiturates; in fact, many abusers liken the effects of methaqualone to those of heroin. Abusers employ doses of 75 mg to 2 g a day, with an average of about 725 mg. Severe tonic-clonic convulsions may occur after abrupt withdrawal from such high doses.

Absorption and Fate. In man, 99% of methaqualone is absorbed in 2 hours. In the plasma, 70 to 90% is bound to albumin. More than 99% of the drug is metabolized by the hepatic microsomal system, and 4'-hydroxymethaqualone and the N'-oxide are the major primary metabolites. The pharmacokinetics is that of a two-compartment system, with a distribution half-life of less than 1 hour and an elimination half-life of 10 to 40 hours. Methaqualone causes a moderate degree of induction of hepatic cytochrome P-450 and UDP-glucuronyltransferase activity.

Side Effects, Intoxication, and Dependence. During sedation with methaqualone, fatigue and occasionally dizziness and torpor may occur. With hypnotic doses, there may be transient paresthesias preceding the onset of sleep. Persisting paresthesias and other signs of peripheral neuropathy that last for months to years may also occur. Occasionally, restlessness and anxiety are observed instead of sedation and sleep. Excessive dreaming and somnambulism also sometimes occur. "Hangover" is frequent. Other side effects include xerostomia, anorexia, nausea, vomiting, diarrhea, epigastric discomfort, sweating, bromidrosis, urticaria, and exanthems. Rarely, aplastic anemia has developed, but the relationship to methaqualone has not been proven. Severe CNS depression may occur when methaqualone is taken in combination with ethanol or other CNS depressants.

Mild overdosage usually causes excessive central depression much like that from barbiturates, but restlessness and excitement sometimes result instead. With severe overdosage, delirium, pyramidal signs (such as hypertonicity, hyperreflexia, and myoclonus), and frank convulsions may occur. Myoclonic episodes and amnesia have been reported, in one case with a dose as low as 400 mg. During coma, cardiovascular and respiratory depression are less severe than with barbiturates. Coma has been noted after 2.4 g and death after 8 g. In a review of 246 fatalities that were associated with methaqualone, Wetli (1983) reported that 72% of the deaths were the result of accidents caused by somnolence, poor judgment, and impulsive behavior, rather than from the direct toxic effects of overdosage. Treatment of intoxication is mainly supportive and may include the use of hemoperfusion through activated charcoal, oil, or cation-exchange resins. The biochemistry, experimental and clinical pharmacology, and toxicity of methaqualone have been reviewed by Brown and Goenechea (1973).

PARALDEHYDE

Paraldehyde is a polymer of acetaldehyde, but it is perhaps best regarded as a polyether of cyclic structure, as follows:

Paraldehyde

Because of some limited virtues and despite its disadvantages, paraldehyde has managed to survive a century of use; it deserves to be retired.

Pharmacological Actions. Paraldehyde is a rapidly acting hypnotic; after a therapeutic oral dose, sleep usually ensues in 10 to 15 minutes. The drug does not possess analgesic properties, and it may produce excitement or delirium in the presence of pain. In large doses, it is effective against all types of convulsions and against delirium.

Paraldehyde has little effect on respiration and blood pressure in ordinary therapeutic doses. In large doses, it produces respiratory depression and hypotension.

Pharmacokinetics. Oral paraldehyde is rapidly absorbed. With hypnotic doses, 70 to 80% is metabolized in the liver, most of the remainder is exhaled, and a small amount is excreted in urine. In hepatic insufficiency, the rate of elimination is slowed, and the proportion excreted in the expired air is increased. It is believed that paraldehyde is depolymerized to acetaldehyde in the liver and then oxidized by aldehyde dehydrogenase to acetic acid, which is ultimately metabolized to carbon dioxide and water.

The drug readily crosses the placental barrier. Some delay in onset of respiratory movements has been observed in the neonate following its administration to the mother during labor.

Untoward Effects and Poisoning. Paraldehyde has a strong aromatic odor and a disagreeable taste. Orally, it is irritating to the throat and stomach, and intramuscularly it may cause necrosis and also nerve injury. Intravenously it may cause cyanosis, cough, pulmonary edema, venous thrombosis, and hypotension.

Adverse effects and intoxication with paraldehyde are uncommon only because its use has been essentially restricted to hospitalized or institutionalized patients. The lethal dose is difficult to ascertain; death has occurred from 25 g, but one person has survived 150 g. According to one estimate, the minimal lethal blood concentration is about 50 mg/dl.

Patients poisoned by paraldehyde commonly exhibit very rapid, labored respiratory movements, possibly due to the injurious effect of paraldehyde or its decomposition products on the lungs and possibly, in some cases, due to acidosis. Acidosis, bleeding gastritis, muscular irritability, azotemia, oliguria, albuminuria, leukocytosis, fatty changes in the liver and kidney with toxic hepatitis and nephrosis, pulmonary hemorrhages and edema, and dilatation of the right ventricle have all been observed in cases of severe acute or chronic paraldehyde poisoning.

Chronic paraldehyde intoxication results in *tolerance* and *dependence*. The paraldehyde addict may become acquainted with the drug when it is used in the treatment of alcoholism and then, surprisingly in view of its disagreeable taste and odor, prefer it to alcohol. Paraldehyde addiction resembles alcoholism, and sudden withdrawal may result in delirium tremens and vivid hallucinations. Some paraldehyde habitués suffer from metabolic acidosis of unknown etiology, but it is in excess of that consequent to the oxidation of paraldehyde-derived acetaldehyde.

Therapeutic Uses. Paraldehyde has been used chiefly for the treatment of abstinence phenomena and other psychiatric states characterized by excitement; for the emergency treatment of convulsive episodes arising from tetanus, eclampsia, status epilepticus, and poisoning by convulsive drugs; and for basal and obstetrical anesthesia. Its most persisting use has been in the treatment of delirium tremens. Advocates point out that it may be administered more easily—as a retention enema—to restrained, difficult-to-manage patients (including children) than are intravenous or oral CNS depressants or anticonvulsants.

Dosage and Preparations. The hypnotic dose is shown in Table 17–4. When given rectally as a retention enema, the drug is usually added to 2 volumes of olive oil. In no case should paraldehyde be taken from partially empty containers, since an appreciable proportion of the drug may have been oxidized to acetic acid and other decomposition products. Because paraldehyde reacts rapidly with certain plastics, it should be measured with glass syringes.

MISCELLANEOUS SEDATIVE-HYPNOTIC DRUGS

Ethinamate. *Ethinamate* is a urethane with the following structure:

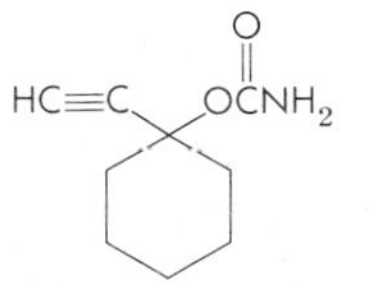

Ethinamate

It has a rapid onset and a short duration of action. Its effect on REM sleep is unknown. Ethinamate is inactivated at least partly by the liver, by hydroxylation of the cyclohexyl ring; the product is conjugated and excreted as the glucuronide. Side effects of ethinamate include nausea, occasional vomiting, and infrequently rash. Idiosyncratic excitement may be noted, especially in children. Fever and thrombocytopenia occur rarely. The lethal dose is unknown; death has resulted from the ingestion of 15 g, but there has been recovery after 28 g. Chronic use of larger-than-recommended doses may lead to psychic and physical dependence. The abstinence syndrome is similar to that for the barbiturates. It is often stated that 500 mg is equivalent to 100 mg of secobarbital, but some studies have found this dose to be little better than a placebo.

Others. *Etomidate* (AMIDATE) is used in the United States and other countries as an intrave-

nous anesthetic, often in combination with fentanyl. It is advantageous because of a lack of pulmonary- and vascular-depressant activity, although it has a negative inotropic effect on the heart. Its pharmacology and anesthetic uses are described in Chapter 14. It is also employed abroad as a sedative-hypnotic drug in intensive care units, during intermittent positive-pressure breathing, in epidural anesthesia, and in other situations. Because it is administered only intravenously, its use is limited to hospital settings. The myoclonus seen after anesthetic doses is not seen after sedative-hypnotic doses.

Clomethiazole has sedative, muscle relaxant, and anticonvulsant properties. It is used outside the United States for hypnosis in elderly and institutionalized patients, for preanesthetic sedation, and, especially, in the management of withdrawal from ethanol. Given alone, its effects on respiration are slight, and the therapeutic index is high. However, deaths from adverse interactions with ethanol are relatively frequent.

Nonprescription Hypnotic Drugs. An advisory review panel of the United States Food and Drug Administration has recommended that, except for certain antihistamines (doxylamine, phenyltoloxamine, and pyrilamine), all putative active ingredients be eliminated from nonprescription sleep aids that are currently marketed. It was also recommended that these antihistamines, as well as diphenhydramine, be subjected to additional clinical evaluation before further action is taken. Despite the prominent sedative side effects encountered during their use in the treatment of allergic diseases (*see* Chapter 26), these antihistamines have not been consistently effective in the treatment of sleep disorders. Contributory factors may include the rapid development of tolerance and the inadequacy of the doses that are currently approved. Nevertheless, these doses sometimes produce prominent residual daytime CNS depression. The elimination half-life of doxylamine is about 9 hours. The values for pyrilamine and phenyltoloxamine are not known, but clinical observations suggest that they may be longer than are optimal for useful hypnotic drugs. Diphenhydramine, with a half-life of about 4 hours, might have a theoretical advantage with regard to residual effects.

MANAGEMENT OF INSOMNIA

Few clinical disorders have been more casually and carelessly treated than insomnia. Insomnia has many causes, and an accurate differential diagnosis is required before treatment should be considered. Prescription of a hypnotic without regard to the underlying disturbance subjects the patient to the risk of abuse, may mask the signs and symptoms of a pernicious pathology, and may dangerously exacerbate an unrecognized sleep apnea. Furthermore, behavioral therapy, psychotherapy, or nonhypnotic drugs may be superior to hypnotic drugs when there is a specific cause of the insomnia. For example, dextroamphetamine or similar drugs may improve sleep in some hyperkinetic patients and those with Parkinson's disease; other examples include antidepressants for those with endogenous depression, phenothiazines or haloperidol for psychotics, phenytoin when there are paroxysmal nightmares, analgesics when sleep is impaired by (even subliminal) pain, and so forth.

Even when no specific pathological etiology can be identified, insomnia may nevertheless relate to identifiable causes, such as ingestion of food or coffee near bedtime, various drugs, or a host of other factors known to many. Only when specific causes cannot be eliminated or compensated for should a nonspecific, hypnotic drug be considered.

Nature does not compel man to sleep 8 hours a day, and many persons function well on much less sleep. Sometimes simple assurance of this fact is sufficient to improve sleep or at least to decrease the concern about nocturnal sleeplessness. A relaxing activity before bedtime is often efficacious.

When insomnia is expected to be *transient,* as in minor situational stress or jet lag, the use of hypnotic drugs may be justifiable, depending upon assessment of the situation and of personality factors. Unless there is a need for concurrent daytime sedation, a drug with a short half-life is indicated. In this setting, treatment should be limited to one to three nights.

In *short-term* insomnia, as when there is grief, short-term illness, a change in occupational status, or temporary family or occupational stress, a drug can be prescribed and the patient should be counseled. The antianxiety action of the benzodiazepines assists in such situations. Treatment should begin with a small dose, to be increased gradually if necessary. The drug should be discontinued for at least one or two nights after one or two nights of acceptable sleep have been obtained. Treatment should not exceed 3 weeks. Discontinuation should be accomplished gradually. Whether a hypnotic drug with a short half-life or an anti-anxiety drug with a longer half-life is prescribed depends upon the perceived contribution of anxiety to the insomnia and the acceptability of diminished daytime alertness. During the course of treatment, there should be surveillance to assess problems resulting from accumulation of drug, alterations in sleep pattern, and tolerance.

The use of sedative-hypnotic drugs in the treatment of *long-term insomnia* is controversial, not only because of the likelihood of tolerance and potential drug abuse but also because this condition is often secondary to disorders that are manageable by psychotherapy, physical therapy, chronotherapy, or nonhypnotic drugs. When there is no specific identifiable pathology, psychosocial-behavioral therapies are indicated; hypnotic drugs may be used in the early stages in conjunction with such treatment. A hypnotic drug should be administered no more frequently than every third night in order to avoid adverse alterations in sleep pattern, drug accumulation, and tolerance. The drug should be discontinued gradually after 3 to 6 months, or even earlier. Upon discontinuation, drugs that have relatively slow rates of elimination produce a lower incidence or intensity of symptoms of withdrawal, including rebound insomnia. However, such drugs may also produce more residual daytime effects than do those with shorter half-lives of elimination. The latter drugs may thus offer advantages if used on an intermittent schedule or in elderly patients, in whom residual cognitive impairment is especially frequent. However, the incidence and severity of residual daytime sequelae do not always correlate with the half-life of the hypnotic drug or its active metabolites. The responses in patients with severe, chronic insomnia are often quite erratic (*see* Nicholson, 1981; Linnoila *et al.,* 1982).

Much has been made of the importance of prescribing a short-acting hypnotic drug for patients who have prolonged sleep latency but who sleep well once sleep ensues, and a drug with a longer duration of action for those who awaken early and have difficulty in returning to sleep. For the former, triazolam has both a short onset and duration of action. For the latter, temazepam has acceptable properties, although flurazepam also suffices. However, for the elderly early waker, sleep counseling may often be sufficient. For those who awaken early with feelings of panic, psychotherapy and/ or antidepressant drugs are probably more appropriate. The actual prolongation of total sleep time by shortening latency or decreasing the number of "mini-awakenings" often does not amount to more than 20 to 40 minutes; this is not an appreciable amount of sleep. Consequently, the most important role of the physician may be to convince the patient that a short period of wakefulness is less serious than are the potential complications of dependence on hypnotics.

There has been an emphasis on the effects of drugs on the stages of sleep and especially on reductions in REM sleep. However, except for the number of "mini-awakenings," the sleep pattern often fails to relate to the sense of refreshing sleep. Thus, the emphasis has shifted to the patient's subjective evaluation of sleep and of the impact of the drug on daytime performance. Various tests have been devised to evaluate both the daytime effects of inadequate sleep and the residual depressant effects of a hypnotic drug (*see* Dement *et al.*, 1982).

There are situations in which alterations in sleep pattern during and after use of hypnotic drugs may have special relevance. Since night terrors and somnambulism most frequently occur during stage 4 of sleep, drugs that shorten or lighten this stage may be indicated. However, caution is in order, since, with some hypnotics, rebound effects on stage 4 may be quite severe or protracted. Furthermore, strong suppression of stage 4 may cause the emergence of day terrors or of suicidal ideation. Similarly, nightmares that normally occur during REM sleep may transfer to stage 2. Nocturnal enuresis may be prevented by drugs that suppress REM sleep. Suppression of REM sleep may also improve endogenous depression.

Except when specific drug therapy or nonpharmacological interventions are indicated, *benzodiazepines should be considered to be the hypnotic drugs of choice*, since they have better therapeutic indices, fewer drug interactions, less effect on respi-ration, and probably lower abuse liability than do the barbiturates and the other prescription hypnotic drugs available in the United States. The treatment of insomnia and related sleep disorders has been reviewed by Mendelson (1980), Borkovec (1982), Kales and coworkers (1982), Seidel and Dement (1982), Wincor (1982), and Kales and Kales (1983).

Alger, B. E., and Nicoll, R. A. Feed-forward dendritic inhibition in rat hippocampal pyramidal cells studied *in vitro. J. Physiol. (Lond.)*, **1982**, *328*, 105–123.

Al-Khudhairi, D.; Whitwam, J. G.; Chakrabarti, M. K.; Askitopoulou, H.; Grundy, E. M.; and Powrie, S. Haemodynamic effects of midazolam and thiopentone during induction of anaesthesia for coronary artery surgery. *Br. J. Anaesth.*, **1982**, *54*, 831–835.

Bliwise, D.; Seidel, W.; Karacan, I.; Mitler, M.; Roth, T.; Zorick, F.; and Dement, W. Daytime sleepiness as a criterion in hypnotic medication trials: comparison of triazolam and flurazepam. *Sleep*, **1983**, *6*, 156–163.

Borbély, A. A.; Mattmann, P.; Loepfe, M.; Fellman, I.; Gerne, M.; Strauch, I.; and Lehmann, D. A single dose of benzodiazepine hypnotics alters the sleep EEG in the subsequent drug-free night. *Eur. J. Pharmacol.*, **1983**, *89*, 157–161.

Brocklehurst, J. C.; Carty, M. H.; and Skorecki, J. The use of a kymograph in a comparative trial of flunitrazepam and meprobamate in elderly patients. *Curr. Med. Res. Opin.*, **1978**, *5*, 663–668.

Brown, S. S., and Goenechea, S. Methaqualone: metabolic, kinetic, and clinical pharmacological observations. *Clin. Pharmacol. Ther.*, **1973**, *14*, 314–324.

Carlen, P. L.; Gurevich, N.; and Polc, P. Low-dose benzodiazepine neuronal inhibition: enhanced Ca^{2+}-mediated K^+-conductance. *Brain Res.*, **1983**, *271*, 358–364.

Carskadon, M. A.; Seidel, W. F.; Greenblatt, D. J.; and Dement, W. C. Daytime carryover of triazolam and flurazepam in elderly insomniacs. *Sleep*, **1982**, *5*, 361–371.

Feinberg, I.; Hibi, S.; Cavness, C.; and March, J. Absence of REM rebound after barbiturate withdrawal. *Science*, **1974**, *185*, 534–535.

Greenblatt, D. J.; Allen, M. D.; Noel, B. J.; and Shader, R. I. Acute overdosage with benzodiazepine derivatives. *Clin. Pharmacol. Ther.*, **1977**, *4*, 497–514.

Gross, J. B.; Zebrowski, M. E.; Carel, W. D.; Gardner, S.; and Smith, T. C. Time course of ventilatory depression after thiopental and midazolam in normal subjects and in patients with chronic obstructive pulmonary disease. *Anesthesiology*, **1983**, *58*, 540–544.

Hall, R. C., and Zisook, S. Paradoxical reactions to benzodiazepines. *Br. J. Clin. Pharmacol.*, **1981**, *11*, Suppl. 1, 99S–104S.

Hartmann, E. Long-term administration of psychotropic drugs: effects on human sleep. In, *Pharmacology of Sleep.* (Williams, R. L., and Karacan, I., eds.) John Wiley & Sons, Inc., New York, **1976**, pp. 211–223.

Ikram, H.; Rubin, A. P.; and Jewkes, R. F. Effect of diazepam on myocardial blood flow of patients with and without coronary artery disease. *Br. Heart J.*, **1973**, *35*, 626–630.

Kales, A.; Soldatos, C. R.; Bixler, E. O.; and Kales, J. D. Early morning insomnia with rapidly eliminated benzodiazepines. *Science*, **1983a**, *220*, 95–97.

Keston, M., and Brocklehurst, J. C. Flurazepam and meprobamate: a clinical trial. *Age Ageing*, **1974**, *3*, 54–58.

Kripke, D. F.; Lavie, P.; and Hernandez, J. Polygraphic evaluation of ethchlorvynol (14 days). *Psychopharmacology*, **1978**, *56*, 221–223.

Lader, M., and Petursson, H. Long-term effects of benzodiazepines. *Neuropharmacology*, **1983**, *22*, 527–533.

Linnoila, M.; Ervin, C. W.; and Brendle, A. Efficacy and side-effects of flunitrazepam and pentobarbital in severely insomniac patients. *J. Clin. Pharmacol.*, **1982**, *22*, 14–19.

Michenfelder, J. D. Barbiturates for brain resuscitation: yes and no. *Anesthesiology*, **1982**, *57*, 74–75.

Nugent, M.; Artru, A. A.; and Michenfelder, J. D. Cerebral metabolic, vascular and protective effects of midazolam maleate. Comparison to diazepam. *Anesthesiology*, **1982**, *56*, 172–176.

O'Brien, C. P.; Cole, J. D.; Orzack, M. H.; Benes, F. M.; Beake, B. J.; Bird, M.; Tel, Y. B.; and Ionescu-Pioggia, M. Benzodiazepine abuse: what are the data? *Psychopharmacol. Bull.*, **1982**, *18*, 87–96.

Rao, S.; Sherbaniuk, R. W.; Prasad, K.; Lee, S. J. K.; and Sproule, B. J. Cardiopulmonary effects of diazepam. *Clin. Pharmacol. Ther.*, **1973**, *14*, 182–189.

Richter, S. A.; Harris, P.; and Hanford, P. Similar development of tolerance to barbital-induced inhibition of avoidance behavior and loss of righting reflex in rats. *Pharmacol. Biochem. Behav.*, **1982**, *16*, 467–471.

Rosenberg, L.; Mitchell, A. A.; Parsells, J. L.; Pashayan, H.; Louik, C.; and Shapiro, S. Lack of relation of oral clefts to diazepam use during pregnancy. *N. Engl. J. Med.*, **1983**, *309*, 1282–1285.

Roth, T.; Zorick, F.; Sickelsteel, J.; and Stepanski, E. Effects of benzodiazepines on sleep and wakefulness. *Br. J. Clin. Pharmacol.*, **1981**, *11*, Suppl. 1, 31S–35S.

Seitz, W.; Hempelman, G.; and Piepenbrock, S. Zur kardiovaskulären Wirkung von Flunitrazepam (ROHYPNOL, Ro-5-4200). *Anaesthesist*, **1977**, *26*, 249–256.

Smith, R. B.; Divoll, M.; Gillespie, W. R.; and Greenblatt, D. J. Effect of subject age and gender on the pharmacokinetics of oral triazolam and temazepam. *J. Clin. Psychopharmacol.*, **1983**, *3*, 172–176.

Study, R. E., and Barker, J. L. Diazepam and (-)-pentobarbital: fluctuation analysis reveals different mechanisms for potentiation of γ-aminobutyric acid responses in cultured central neurons. *Proc. Natl Acad. Sci. U.S.A.*, **1981**, *11*, 7180–7184.

Monographs and Reviews

Allgulander, C. Dependence on sedative and hypnotic drugs. *Acta Psychiatr. Scand.*, **1978**, Suppl. 270, 1–120.

Bellantuono, C.; Reggi, V.; Tognoni, G.; and Garattini, S. Benzodiazepines: clinical pharmacology and therapeutic use. *Drugs*, **1980**, *19*, 195–219.

Borkovec, T. D. Insomnia. *J. Consult. Clin. Psychol.*, **1982**, *50*, 880–895.

Breimer, D. D. Clinical pharmacokinetics of hypnotics. *Clin. Pharmacokinet.*, **1977**, *2*, 93–109.

———. Pharmacokinetics and metabolism of various benzodiazepines used as hypnotics. *Br. J. Clin. Pharmacol.*, **1979**, *8*, Suppl. 1, 7S–13S.

Dement, W.; Seidel, W.; and Carskadon, M. Daytime alertness, insomnia, and benzodiazepines. *Sleep*, **1982**, *5*, Suppl. 1, S28–S45.

Dubnick, B.; Lippa, A. S.; Klepner, C. A.; Coupet, J.; Greenblatt, E. N.; and Beer, B. The separation of 3H-benzodiazepine binding sites in brain and of benzodiazepine pharmacological properties. *Pharmacol. Biochem. Behav.*, **1983**, *18*, 311–318.

Freudenthal, R. I., and Carroll, F. I. Metabolism of certain commonly used barbiturates. *Drug Metab. Rev.*, **1973**, *2*, 265–278.

Gary, N. E., and Tresnewsky, O. Clinical aspects of drug intoxication: barbiturates and a potpourri of other sedatives, hypnotics, and tranquilizers. *Heart Lung*, **1983**, *12*, 122–127.

Greenblatt, D. J.; Divoll, M.; Abernethy, D. R.; Ochs, H. R.; and Shader, R. I. Benzodiazepine kinetics: implications for therapeutics and pharmacogeriatrics. *Drug Metab. Rev.*, **1983a**, *14*, 251–292.

———. Clinical pharmacokinetics of the newer benzodiazepines. *Clin. Pharmacokinet.*, **1983b**, *8*, 233–252.

Greenblatt, D. J.; Divoll, M.; Abernethy, D. R.; and Shader, R. I. Benzodiazepine hypnotics: kinetic and therapeutic options. *Sleep*, **1982**, *5*, 518–527.

Greenblatt, D. J., and Shader, R. I. *Benzodiazepines in Clinical Practice.* Raven Press, New York. **1974.**

Greenblatt, D. J.; Shader, R. I.; and Abernethy, D. R. Current status of benzodiazepines. *N. Engl. J. Med.*, **1983c**, *309*, 354–358, 410–416.

Greenblatt, D. J.; Shader, R. I.; Divoll, M.; and Harmatz, J. S. Benzodiazepines: a summary of pharmacokinetic properties. *Br. J. Clin. Pharmacol.*, **1981**, *11*, Suppl. 1, 11S–16S.

Haefely, W.; Pieri, L.; Polc, P.; and Schaffner, R. General pharmacology and neuropharmacology of benzodiazepine derivatives. In, *Psychotropic Agents.* (Hoffmeister, F., and Stille, G., eds.) *Handbook of Experimental Pharmacology*, Vol. 55, Pt. II. Springer-Verlag, Berlin, **1981**, pp. 13–262.

Ho, I. K., and Harris, R. A. Mechanism of action of barbiturates. *Annu. Rev. Pharmacol. Toxicol.*, **1981**, *21*, 83–111.

Kales, A., and Kales, J. Sleep laboratory studies of hypnotic drugs: efficacy and withdrawal effects. *J. Clin. Psychopharmacol.*, **1983**, *3*, 140–150.

Kales, A.; Kales, J.; and Soldatos, C. R. Insomnia and other sleep disorders. *Med. Clin. North Am.*, **1982**, *66*, 971–991.

Kales, A.; Soldatos, C. R.; Bixler, E. O.; and Kales, J. D. Rebound insomnia and rebound anxiety: a review. *Pharmacology*, **1983b**, *26*, 121–137.

Kay, D. C.; Blackburn, A. B.; Buckingham, J. A.; and Karacan, I. Human pharmacology of sleep. In, *Pharmacology of Sleep.* (Williams, R. L., and Karacan, I., eds.) John Wiley & Sons, Inc., New York, **1976**, pp. 83–210.

MacDonald, J. F., and Barker, J. L. Multiple actions of picomolar concentrations of flurazepam on the excitability of cultured mouse spinal neurons. *Brain Res.*, **1982**, *246*, 257–264.

Macdonald, R. L., and McLean, M. J. Cellular bases of barbiturate and phenytoin anticonvulsant drug action. *Epilepsia*, **1982**, *23*, Suppl. 1, S7–S18.

McElnay, J. C.; Jones, M. E.; and Alexander, B. Temazepam (RESTORIL, Sandoz Pharmaceuticals). *Drug Intell. Clin. Pharm.*, **1982**, *16*, 650–656.

MacKinnon, G. L., and Parker, W. A. Benzodiazepine withdrawal syndrome: a literature review and evaluation. *Am. J. Drug Alcohol Abuse*, **1982**, *9*, 19–33.

Marks, J. *The Benzodiazepines: Use, Overuse, Misuse, Abuse.* MTP Press, Ltd., Lancaster, **1978**, pp. 1–111.

Marshall, L. F., and Bowers, S. A. Medical management of head injury. *Clin. Neurosurg.*, **1982**, *29*, 312–325.

Mendelson, W. B. *The Use and Misuse of Sleeping Pills: A Clinical Guide.* Plenum Medical Book Co., New York, **1980.**

Mendelson, W. B.; Gillin, J. C.; and Wyatt, R. J. *Human Sleep and Its Disorders.* Plenum Press, New York, **1977.**

Mennini, T., and Garattini, S. Benzodiazepine receptors: correlation with pharmacological responses in living animals. *Life Sci.*, **1982**, *31*, 2025–2035.

Meyer, B. R. Benzodiazepines in the elderly. *Med. Clin. North Am.*, **1982**, *66*, 1017–1035.

Mitler, M. M. Evaluation of temazepam as a hypnotic. *Pharmacotherapy*, **1981**, *1*, 3–13.

Nicholson, A. N. Hypnotics: rebound insomnia and residual sequelae. *Br. J. Clin. Pharmacol.*, **1980**, *9*, 223–225.

————. The use of short- and long-acting hypnotics in clinical medicine. *Ibid.*, **1981**, *11*, 615–695.

Nicoll, R. A. Differential postsynaptic effects of barbiturates on chemical transmission. In, *Neurobiology of Chemical Transmission*. (Otsuka, M., and Hall, Z. W., eds.) John Wiley & Sons, Inc., New York, **1979**, pp. 267–278.

Olsen, R. W. Drug interactions at the GABA receptor-ionophore complex. *Annu. Rev. Pharmacol. Toxicol.*, **1982**, *22*, 245–247.

Owen, R. T., and Tyrer, P. Benzodiazepine dependence. *Drugs*, **1983**, *25*, 385–398.

Petursson, H., and Lader, M. H. Benzodiazepine dependence. *Br. J. Addict.*, **1981**, *76*, 133–145.

Richter, J. A., and Holman, J. R. Barbiturates: their *in vivo* effects and potential biochemical mechanisms. *Prog. Neurobiol.*, **1982**, *18*, 275–319.

Rickels, K. Clinical trials of hypnotics. *J. Clin. Psychopharmacol.*, **1983**, *3*, 133–139.

Roth, T.; Roehrs, T. A.; and Zorick, F. J. Pharmacology and hypnotic efficacy of triazolam. *Pharmacotherapy*, **1983**, *3*, 137–148.

Schöpf, J. Withdrawal phenomena after long-term administration of benzodiazepines. A review of recent investigations. *J. Pharmacopsychiatria*, **1983**, *16*, 1–8.

Schütz, H. *Benzodiazepines—A Handbook: Basic Data, Pharmacokinetics, and Comprehensive Literature.* Springer-Verlag, Berlin, **1982**.

Seidel, W. F., and Dement, W. C. Sleepiness in insomnia: evaluation and treatment. *Sleep*, **1982**, *5*, Suppl. 2, S182–S190.

Skolnick, P., and Paul, S. M. Benzodiazepine receptors in the central nervous system. *Int. Rev. Neurobiol.*, **1982**, *23*, 103–140.

Steer, C. R. Barbiturate therapy in the management of cerebral ischemia. *Dev. Med. Child Neurol.*, **1982**, *24*, 219–231.

Symposium. (Various authors.) *The Benzodiazepines.* (Garattini, S.; Mussini, E.; and Randall, L. O.; eds.) Raven Press, New York, **1973**.

Symposium. (Various authors.) *Psychopharmacology of Sleep.* (Wheatly, D., ed.) Raven Press, New York, **1981**.

Symposium. (Various authors.) *Pharmacology of Benzodiazepines.* (Usdin, E.; Skolnick, P.; Tallman, J. F.; Greenblatt, D.; and Paul, S. M.; eds.) Macmillan Press, Ltd., London, **1982**.

Symposium. (Various authors.) *The Benzodiazepines: From Molecular Biology to Clinical Practice.* (Costa, E., ed.) Raven Press, New York, **1983a**.

Symposium. (Various authors.) *Benzodiazepines Divided: A Multidisciplinary Review.* (Trimble, M. R., ed.) John Wiley & Sons, Ltd., Chichester, **1983b**.

Symposium. (Various authors.) *Anxiolytes: Neurochemical Behavioral and Clinical Perspectives.* (Malick, J. B.; Enna, S. J.; and Yamamura, H. I.; eds.) Raven Press, New York, **1983c**.

van der Kleijn, E.; Vree, T. B.; Baars, A. M.; Wijsman, R.; Edmunds, L. C.; and Knop, H. J. Factors influencing the activity and fate of benzodiazepines in the body. *Br. J. Clin. Pharmacol.*, **1981**, *11*, Suppl. 1, 85S–98S.

Wetli, C. V. Changing patterns of methaqualone abuse. A survey of 246 fatalities. *J.A.M.A.*, **1983**, *249*, 621–626.

Wikler, A. Review of research on sedative drug dependence at the addiction research center and University of Kentucky. In, *Predicting Dependence Liability of Stimulant and Depressant Drugs.* (Thompson, T., and Unna, K. R., eds.) University Park Press, Baltimore, **1976**, pp. 147–163.

Wincor, M. Z. Insomnia and the new benzodiazepines. *Clin. Pharm.*, **1982**, *1*, 425–432.

18 THE ALIPHATIC ALCOHOLS

J. Murdoch Ritchie

ETHYL ALCOHOL

Alcoholic beverages have been used since the dawn of history, and the opinions and traditions of the past often cloud the discussion of this subject. The oldest alcoholic drinks were fermented beverages of relatively low alcohol content, that is, the beers and wines. When the Arabs introduced the then recent technic of distilling into Europe in the Middle Ages, the alchemists believed that alcohol was the long-sought elixir of life. Alcohol was therefore held to be a remedy for practically all diseases, as indicated by the term *whisky* (Gaelic: *usquebaugh,* meaning "water of life"). It is now recognized that the therapeutic value of alcohol is much more limited than its social value.

PHARMACOLOGICAL PROPERTIES

Local Actions. Alcohol precipitates and dehydrates protoplasm and can therefore act as an astringent. It is also an irritant to denuded surfaces and to mucosae. The more concentrated the alcohol, the more pronounced are its effects.

Skin. Alcohol cools the skin by evaporation, and so alcohol sponges are commonly used in fever. Alcohol rubbed on the skin produces mild redness and burning, and it is therefore employed as a counterirritant and rubefacient. It is often used in bedridden patients to prevent bedsores and decubitus ulcers, for it hardens and cleans the skin and helps to prevent sweating.

Mucous Membranes. The irritant action of alcohol is particularly marked on mucosae. High concentrations may produce considerable inflammation of the gastric mucosa, for example.

Subcutaneous Tissues. Alcohol injected hypodermically causes considerable pain followed by anesthesia. If the injection is made close to nerves, neuritis and nerve degeneration may occur. Injections in or near nerves are deliberately used to cause anesthesia of protracted or even permanent character in the treatment of severe pain, for example, in *tic douloureux.*

Action on Bacteria. The bactericidal action of alcohol is discussed in Chapter 41.

Peripheral Nerves. Alcohol blocks conduction in peripheral nerve by decreasing the maximal values of both the sodium and the potassium conductances. The resting potential usually becomes slightly less negative. The concentrations required for blockade of peripheral nerve conduction (about 5 to 10%) are greatly in excess of those needed to produce the central effects (*see* Wallgren and Barry, 1970).

Central Nervous System. The central nervous system (CNS) is more obviously affected by alcohol than any other system of the body. Laymen in particular view alcoholic drinks as stimulating. However, alcohol, like other general anesthetics, is a primary and continuous depressant of the CNS. The apparent stimulation results from the unrestrained activity of various parts of the brain that have been freed from inhibition as a result of the depression of inhibitory control mechanisms. Alcohol depresses both excitatory and inhibitory postsynaptic potentials, is more effective in inhibiting synaptic (particularly polysynaptic) function than impulse propagation, potentiates presynaptic inhibition, and has a variety of effects on transmitter systems (*see* Klemm, 1979).

Electrophysiological studies suggest that alcohol, like other general anesthetics, exerts its first depressant action upon those parts of the brain involved in the most highly integrated functions. The polysynaptic structures of the reticular activating system and certain cortical sites are particularly susceptible (Himwich and Callison, 1972). The cortex is thus released from its integrating control. As a result, the various processes related to thought occur in a jumbled, disorganized fashion and the smooth operation of motor processes becomes disrupted. The first mental processes to be affected are those that depend on training and previous experience and that usually make for sobriety and self-restraint. The finer grades of discrimination, memory, concentration, and insight are dulled and then lost. Confidence abounds, the personality becomes expansive and vivacious, and speech may become eloquent and occasionally brilliant. Mood swings are uncontrolled and emotional outbursts frequent. These psychic changes are accompanied by sensory and motor disturbances. For example, spinal reflexes are at first enhanced because they have been freed from central inhibitions; as intoxication becomes more advanced, however, this first phase of enhanced reflex activity is succeeded by a general impairment of nervous function and a condition of general anesthesia ultimately prevails. However, there is little margin between the full surgical anesthetic dose and that which is dangerous to respiration.

In general, the effects of alcohol on the CNS are proportional to the concentration of alcohol in the blood. However, the effects are more marked when the concentration is rising than when it is falling. If the rate of absorption of alcohol from the gastrointestinal tract is rapid, a relatively high blood concentration may result from the ingestion of quite a small amount of alcohol. The same applies if the fraction of the cardiac output delivered to tissues such as muscle is low compared to brain; an effect on the CNS is then rapidly obtained. However, redistribution of the alcohol soon occurs and the effects, as a result, are relatively brief. The neurological and physiological effects of alcohol have been reviewed by Wallgren and Barry (1970), Kissin and Begleiter (1974), and Gross (1977); in a report by the U.S. Department of Health, Education, and Welfare (1978); and by Majchrowicz and Noble (1979).

Chronic excessive ingestion of ethanol is directly associated with serious neurological and mental disorders (*e.g.*, brain damage, memory loss, sleep disturbances, and psychoses). In addition, nutritional and vitamin deficiencies, incident to the poor food intake or the faulty gastrointestinal function of the alcoholic (*see* Hillman, 1974), seem to cause many neuropsychiatric syndromes that are common in alcoholics, such as Wernicke's encephalopathy, Korsakoff's psychosis, polyneuritis, and nicotinic acid deficiency encephalopathy (*see* Turner *et al.*, 1977; Chapter 66).

Respiration. Moderate amounts of alcohol in man may stimulate or depress respiration; the ventilatory response to carbon dioxide is, however, always depressed. Large amounts (sufficient to produce a blood concentration of 400 mg/dl or more) produce dangerous or lethal depression of respiration.

EEG. Alcohol produces a slowing of the alpha rhythm of the brain, and this effect becomes particularly prominent as intoxication develops. Chronic alcoholics, however, show no consistent, permanent pathological changes in rhythm (Turner *et al.*, 1977).

Sleep. Acute and chronic administration of alcohol produces a variety of effects on sleep (*see* Mendelson, 1979). Favorable effects of alcohol on sleep patterns have often been cited (*see* Turner *et al.*, 1981), but its effectiveness over the long term has not been demonstrated (Weitzman, 1981). Excessive use of alcohol seems to have a deleterious effect on nocturnal breathing (Issa and Sullivan, 1982).

Cardiovascular System. The *immediate* effects of alcohol on the circulation are relatively minor (Wallgren and Barry, 1970). The blood pressure, cardiac output, and force of myocardial contraction do not change greatly after a moderate amount of alcohol. The pulse rate may increase, but this is usually due to muscular activity or reflex stimulation. The cardiovascular depression that is observed in acute severe alcoholic intoxication is due mainly to central vasomotor factors and to the respiratory depression. However, *chronic* excessive use of alcohol has a clearly deleterious effect on the heart and may be the major cause of cardiomyopathy in the Western world (*see* Rubin, 1979; Altura, 1982). Electron-microscopic observations reveal characteristic intracellular lesions in the myocardium, associated with congestive heart failure; prognosis for return of muscle function is guarded. Conduction defects and rhythm disturbances are frequently seen in chronic alcoholics (Graboys and Lown, 1983), some of whom may have normal rhythm during abstinence but develop arrhythmias after acute consumption of alcohol (Greenspon and Schaal, 1983).

Alcohol in moderate doses causes vasodilatation, especially of the cutaneous vessels, and produces a warm and flushed skin. The vasodilatation results partly from central vasomotor depression and partly from a direct vasodilating action of alcohol on blood vessels (Altura and Altura, 1982). In laboratory animals moderate doses of alcohol dilate the coronary arteries and increase coronary blood flow. However, no beneficial increase in coronary blood flow occurs in man. Indeed, in individuals with classical stable angina and proven coronary artery disease, alcohol decreases the duration of exercise required to precipitate angina and to produce changes in the ECG that are characteristic of myocardial ischemia (Regan, 1982).

Alcohol administered to human subjects in doses sufficient to produce facial vasodilatation and mild inebriation causes no change in cerebral blood flow, cerebral metabolism, or cerebral vascular resistance. A plasma concentration associated with severe alcoholic intoxication (300 mg/dl) does indeed markedly increase mean cerebral blood flow and diminish cerebrovascular resistance. However, cerebral oxygen uptake is much reduced (*see* Wallgren, 1971). Experiments on laboratory animals have shown that alcohol constricts isolated cerebral and basilar arteries, as well as microvessels. This might lead to local areas of cerebral hypoxia, even in the absence of a general decrease in cerebral blood flow (Altura and Altura, 1982). There is no rational basis for the use of alcohol as a vasodilator in patients with cerebrovascular disease. Furthermore, several studies indicate that regular use of large amounts of alcohol is a risk factor for development of hypertension and stroke (*see* Klatsky *et al.*, 1981).

Plasma Lipoproteins. In contrast to the potential deleterious effects of alcohol on the cardiovascular system described above, several studies show a clear negative correlation between chronic ingestion of small amounts of ethanol and the incidence of coronary heart disease. This protective effect seems to occur because ethanol increases the concentration of high-density lipoproteins and decreases that of low-density lipoproteins in plasma (*see* Taskinen *et al.*, 1982; Hartung *et al.*, 1983). Apparently the lower the concentration of high-density lipoprotein in blood, the greater is the risk of coronary heart disease (*see* Chapter 34). It is not clear if the increase in high-density lipoprotein produced by alcohol and that which results from exercise are additive (*see* Willett *et al.*, 1980; Hartung *et al.*, 1983).

Skeletal Muscle. The total amount of work accomplished by an individual under the influence of small doses of alcohol may increase. This is chiefly the result of the central action of the alcohol and is caused by a lessened appreciation of fatigue. Large doses of alcohol cause CNS depression and thereby decrease the amount of muscular work accomplished. Such doses also directly damage the muscle (Rubin, 1979), causing an alcoholic skeletal myopathy similar in many respects to the alcoholic cardiomyopathy. There is a marked increase in the activity of creatine phosphokinase in plasma, indicative of muscle damage. Most patients with chronic alcoholism show electromyographical changes; about half show histological damage of varying severity (Rubin, 1979).

Body Temperature. After ingestion of alcohol, there is a feeling of warmth because alcohol enhances cutaneous and gastric blood flow. Increased sweating may also occur. Heat is therefore lost more rapidly, and the internal temperature consequently falls. With large amounts of alcohol, the central temperature-regulating mechanism itself becomes depressed and the fall in body temperature may become pronounced. The action of alcohol in lowering body temperature is naturally greater when the environmental temperature is low, or when the mechanisms for dissipating heat are disturbed, as during fever. Although moderate amounts of ethanol (0.2 to 1 g/kg) may have beneficial effects during exposure to cold, heavy intoxication is clearly dangerous.

Gastrointestinal Tract. The effects of alcoholic beverages on the gastrointestinal motor and secretory functions are influenced by a number of factors. Among these are the state of the digestive processes, the presence or absence of gastrointestinal disease, the amount and type of food present, the degree of tolerance for alcohol, accompanying psychological factors, and so forth.

Gastric secretions, like salivary secretions, are usually stimulated *psychically* by alcohol, especially if the individual likes it. The gastric juice produced in this way is rich in acid and normal in pepsin content. Alcohol may also *reflexly* stimulate the secretion of salivary and gastric juice by exciting sensory endings in the buccal and gastric mucosae. Finally, alcohol may evoke gastric secretion through a more *direct* action on the stomach, possibly involving the release of gastrin. The release of histamine has also been implicated. The various physiological mechanisms involved have been reviewed by Glass and colleagues (1979). Alcohol is a very effective stimulus for gastric acid secretion, and, clearly, the drinking of alcoholic beverages is inadvisable in patients with peptic ulcer.

The presence in the stomach of alcohol in concentrations of about 10% results in a gastric secretion rich in acid, but it is poor in pepsin unless psychic secretion is also elicited. Although the pepsin content is decreased, there is no interference with peptic digestion, and gastric motility is not reduced. As the concentration of alcohol in ingested beverages is raised above about 20%, gastric secretion tends to be inhibited and peptic activity is depressed. Strong alcoholic drinks, of 40% concentration and over, are quite irritating to the mucosa and cause congestive hyperemia and inflammation, with an accompanying loss of plasma protein into the gastrointestinal lumen. In such high concentrations alcohol produces an erosive gastritis (*see* Lorber *et al.*, 1974; Glass *et al.*, 1979). This may explain why one out of three heavy drinkers suffers from chronic gastritis. Aspirin can produce severe gastric damage and brisk gastric bleeding in dogs. This effect is much enhanced by alcohol. It is interesting that the prolongation of the bleeding time caused by aspirin is also enhanced by ethanol (Deykin *et al.*, 1982).

The habitual use of immoderate amounts of alcohol may lead to constipation, due probably to an inadequate food intake and an insufficient bulk residue. On the other hand, diarrhea may occur, as a result of the irritant action of certain flavoring oils; in the chronic inebriate, however, it may signify vitamin deficiency or a reduction in intestinal absorption of Na^+ and water (Mekhjian and May, 1977). Alcohol taken in moderate amounts does not significantly influence the motor activity of the colon, but taken to the point of intoxication it results in virtual cessation of gastrointestinal secretory and motor functions. Absorption is delayed, and pylorospasm and vomiting may occur independently of any reflex due to local irritation.

Alcohol contributes to the production of lesions of the esophagus and duodenum and is also an etiological factor in acute and chronic pancreatitis (Pirola and Lieber, 1974; Turner *et al.*, 1977). The pancreatitis appears to occur because ethanol produces not only increased secretion but also an obstruction of the pancreatic duct (*see* Wallgren and Barry, 1970), perhaps as a result of increased plasma concentrations of secretin that have been observed to follow the ingestion of alcohol by normal human subjects (Straus *et al.*, 1975).

Liver. Acute alcoholic intoxication in man is probably not associated with any great change in hepatic function. Alcohol increases the rate at which isolated liver slices synthesize fat. It also causes mobilization of fat from peripheral tissue. Fat thus accumulates in the liver of normal individuals after the ingestion of relatively small amounts of alcohol (*see* Feinman and Lieber, 1974). Alcohol inhibits the secretion of protein from hepatic cells, and its prolonged use results in the accumulation of protein (Baraona and Lieber, 1982). The accumulation of fat and protein may be benign at first, and the associated hepatic disorders are reversible on abstinence. However, these processes can become irreversible and proceed eventually to the characteristic cirrhosis seen in many alcoholics (Lieber, 1978). Malnutrition and vitamin deficiency may also contribute to the he-

patic and gastrointestinal disorders in man, particularly if alcoholic liver disease is present. For example, hepatic concentrations of vitamin A may be low even in the presence of normal levels in plasma (Leo and Lieber, 1982); the pattern of storage and release of folate by the liver may be disrupted (Hillman and Steinberg, 1982); and thiamine deficiency is so common that consideration should be given to its routine administration to alcoholics (Camillo *et al.*, 1981). Patients who abuse alcohol chronically may also develop hypoglycemia because of poor nutrition and depletion of hepatic glycogen.

Moderate or heavy daily drinking significantly increases concentrations of lead in the blood. This is caused not by an increased intake of lead but rather by impaired excretion that results from damage to the liver (Shaper *et al.*, 1982).

Teratogenic Effects. Although suspected for centuries, the *fetal alcohol syndrome* has only recently been fully described. The abnormality consists in CNS dysfunction (such as low IQ and microcephaly), slowness in growth, a characteristic cluster of facial abnormalities (such as short palpebral fissures, hypoplastic upper lip, and short nose), and a variable set of major and minor malformations. These features may be due, at least in part, to a direct action of ethanol to inhibit embryonic cellular proliferation early in gestation (Brown *et al.*, 1979). In addition to their characteristic morphological and neurological abnormalities, children with the fetal alcohol syndrome have a greatly increased susceptibility to both life-threatening and minor infectious diseases. Such children have extensive impairment of their immune system, which might well explain this susceptibility (Johnson *et al.*, 1981).

Ethanol seems to be the most frequent cause of teratogenically induced mental deficiency that is known in the Western world; even moderate drinking of alcohol is clearly contraindicated during pregnancy. Depending on the population studied, the incidence of the *full-blown* fetal alcohol syndrome ranges from 1 in 300 to 1 in 2000 live births; it is 1 in 3 in infants of alcoholic mothers (Council Report, 1983). The smallest quantity of alcohol ingestion reported to be associated with the fetal alcohol syndrome is about 75 ml (2.5 oz) daily (*see* Council Report, 1983). Although it is not clear if there is any safe lower limit, there is no evidence for any adverse effects associated with very modest consumption of alcohol (*e.g.*, a single daily glass of wine; 15 ml [0.5 oz] of alcohol). Reduction of the mother's drinking early in pregnancy seems to reduce the severity of the syndrome (Rossett *et al.,* 1981). Animal studies suggest that paternal alcohol ingestion may also have an adverse influence on the fetus, but the data are far from conclusive (Council Report, 1983).

Other effects on the fetus occur with excessive drinking (Council Report, 1983). For example, stillbirths and spontaneous abortions are two to three times as frequent in women who have three or more drinks daily as in those who have less than one drink a day. The pattern of wakefulness and sleep in the newborn may also be disturbed. There may be a decrease in birth weight, and various minor physical abnormalities are found (Tennes and Blackard, 1980).

Sexual Functions. It is a popular notion that alcohol is an aphrodisiac; indeed, aggressive sexual behavior is often seen after alcohol, usually as a result of a loss of inhibition and restraint. Shakespeare, however, realized that inebriation interferes with coitus. In *Macbeth*, for example, the following conversation occurs (Act 2, scene 3):

MACDUFF: What three things does drink especially provoke?
PORTER: Marry, sir, nose-painting, sleep, and urine. Lechery, sir, it provokes, and unprovokes; it provokes the desire, but it takes away the performance. . . .

The experiments of Gantt (1952) on the effects of alcohol on the sexual reflexes of normal dogs support the observations of Shakespeare; in neurotic dogs, alcohol has some therapeutic value. Objective measurements of penile tumescence and vaginal pressure show that ethanol significantly decreases sexual responsiveness in both men and women (Wilson, 1977).

In men, chronic ingestion of alcohol may lead to impotence, sterility, testicular atrophy, and gynecomastia. This feminization in alcoholic men has a dual origin. First, alcohol-induced hepatic injury leads to a hyperestrogenization and a reduced rate of production of testosterone; second, by increasing the activity of the enzymes of the hepatic endoplasmic reticulum, ethanol markedly increases the rate of metabolic inactivation of testosterone (Van

Thiel and Lester, 1976; Turner *et al.,* 1977). This alcohol-induced dysfunction is reversible in some abstinent alcoholics, but only if there is no gonadal atrophy (Van Thiel *et al.,* 1983).

Kidney. That alcohol exerts a *diuretic effect* has been established by a number of investigators and by most consumers. Although the large amounts of fluid ordinarily ingested with alcoholic beverages undoubtedly contribute to the increased urine flow, alcohol in itself can be demonstrated to produce a marked diuretic response in man by virtue of a decrease in renal tubular reabsorption of water. Considerable evidence indicates that alcohol causes this diuresis by acting on the supraopticoneurohypophyseal system to inhibit the secretion of antidiuretic hormone. The diuretic effect is roughly proportional to the blood alcohol concentration and occurs when the concentration is rising but not when it is stationary or falling (*see* Wallgren and Barry, 1970). Indeed, alcohol in repeated doses may have an antidiuretic effect. (*See* Beard and Sargent, 1979, for a review.)

Although the kidneys of habitual heavy drinkers may not be normal, this cannot necessarily be attributed to alcohol as such. With the possible exception of some individuals with arteriosclerotic renal disease, the ingestion of varying amounts of alcohol has no deleterious action on renal function either in normal subjects or in patients with acute or chronic nephritis.

Biogenic Amines. Concentrations of catecholamines in blood are elevated by alcohol. The increased concentration of norepinephrine in plasma is due, at least in part, to a decrease in its clearance from the blood, possibly because of inhibition of neuronal re-uptake (Eisenhofer *et al.,* 1983). The increased concentration of circulating catecholamines might be partly responsible for the transient hyperglycemia, the pupillary dilatation, and the slight rise in blood pressure that often occur during the early stages of intoxication. It has been suggested that the altered CNS distribution of biogenic amines, particularly 5-hydroxytryptamine, mediates both the sleep and the tolerance associated with alcohol ingestion (*see* Truitt, 1973). Furthermore, the biogenic amines have been implicated in ethanol addiction: opioid-like alkaloids are supposedly formed in the brain by a condensation between biogenic amines and acetaldehyde, a metabolite of ethanol (*see* Wajda, 1979). Indeed, it has been suggested that the actions of opioids and alcohol are mediated by similar mechanisms (Eidelberg, 1977). This might explain why naloxone both prevents and reverses some of the manifestations of alcohol intoxication (*see* Lyon and Anthony, 1982).

Endocrinological Effects. Alcohol exerts substantial effects on virtually every endocrine system in the body, and drug-induced alterations in their functions are significantly involved in the actions of alcohol (*see* Kakihana and Butte, 1979). Many of these effects (*e.g.*, those on the gonads, adrenals, and thyroid) are mediated by the direct actions of alcohol on the hypothalamus and pituitary (*see* Cicero, 1981, for review). Alcohol also interferes with the release of prolactin, growth hormone, and antidiuretic hormone.

Blood. Alcohol produces a number of hematological effects (*see* Lindenbaum, 1974). Some, such as sideroblastic and megaloblastic anemias, occur because alcohol interferes with several aspects of folate metabolism and transport, as well as with its normal pattern of storage and release from the liver (*see* Hillman and Steinberg, 1982). These effects are rapidly reversible with the onset of abstinence. Other effects, such as thrombocytopenia and vacuolization of the precursors of red and white cells, occur even when the diet is adequate and seem to result from a direct depressant action of alcohol on the bone marrow. There is also a depression of leukocyte migration into inflamed areas, which may partly account for the poor resistance of alcoholics to infection.

Geriatric Use of Alcohol. A number of studies have shown that alcohol, in moderate amounts, is a useful therapeutic agent for the elderly. Social interaction, alertness, and a variety of physical indices can improve (Turner *et al.*, 1981). However, the elderly may be particularly vulnerable to malnutrition, vitamin deficiencies, and the fluid and electrolyte imbalances that may accompany alcoholism. Furthermore, they may tolerate gastrointestinal bleeding and infection less well than do younger individuals. Finally, alcohol-induced peripheral neuropathy and cerebral degeneration will be superimposed on the normal loss of neurons that occurs with age. Thus, even casual use of alcohol may be a problem for the elderly, particularly if they are taking medications that interact with ethanol. There is little dependence of hepatic metabolism of alcohol on age (*see* Vestal, 1981).

Alcohol and Longevity. Compared to the general population, heavy drinkers show a markedly excessive mortality from a variety of diseases. Deaths from cancer of the mouth, pharynx, larynx, esophagus, liver, and lung are significantly more numerous among drinkers (*see* report by U.S. Department of Health, Education, and Welfare, 1978; Mezey, 1980; Klatsky *et al.*, 1981; Petersson *et al.*, 1982). Cirrhosis, accidents, and nonmalignant respiratory conditions also contribute significantly to the increased mortality of the heavy drinker. An epidemiological study suggests that the risk rises sharply at six or more drinks daily (Klatsky *et al.*, 1981). Total abstinence is associated with an increased mortality compared to light-to-moderate drinking. This might reflect the protection against coronary artery disease afforded by the increased plasma concentration of high-density lipoprotein.

Mechanism of Action. At least two major mechanisms may be involved in the diverse effects that occur in response to ethanol. First, many of the toxic effects of alcohol seem to be a consequence of the biochemical pathway by which it is degraded (*see* Christensen and Higgins, 1979; Higgins, 1979). As the alcohol is converted first to acetaldehyde and then to acetate, there is a large increase in the concentration of the reduced form of nicotinamide adenine dinucleotide (NADH) at the expense of nicotinamide adenine dinucleotide (NAD). The acetate is metabolized further to acetyl coenzyme A (CoA), a step that involves the conversion of adenosine triphosphate (ATP) to adenosine monophosphate (AMP). Many of the changes that follow the consumption of alcohol, such as the increased production of lactate and fatty acids and, possibly, the decreased hepatic citric acid cycle metabolism and fatty acid oxidation, appear to be a direct consequence of the increased NADH:NAD ratio produced by the oxidation of the alcohol (*see* Lieber *et al.*, 1975). Furthermore, ethanol-induced hyperuricemia seems to result from the accelerated turnover of AMP, some of which enters the pathway for degradation of purine nucleotides (Faller and Fox, 1982).

Secondly, ethanol has a membrane-disordering or membrane-fluidizing effect (*see* Chin and Goldstein, 1981; Lyon *et al.*, 1981; Goldstein *et al.*, 1982). This correlates well with the known pharmacology of ethanol. Thus, synaptosomal and erythrocyte plasma membranes from an alcohol-resistant strain of mice are less strongly disordered by ethanol *in vitro* than are the corresponding membranes from a related strain of ethanol-sensitive mice (Goldstein *et al.*, 1982). Furthermore, there is a clear relationship between the degree of intoxication and the disordering of membranes produced by a series of short-chain alcohols (Lyon *et al.*, 1981). The hypothesis that underlies many current studies is that the disordering of membranes is responsible for many of the abnormalities in function that are mediated by membrane-bound proteins. For example, changes in membrane-bound Na^+,K^+-ATPase activity are suggested to reflect ethanol-induced changes in membrane fluidity (Ricci *et al.*, 1981), and Rabin and Molinoff (1981) have shown that pharmacologically relevant concentrations of ethanol increase the activity of membrane-bound dopamine-activated adenylate cyclase. Furthermore, related effects may be at the basis of tolerance to alcohol (Johnson *et al.*, 1980). Thus, membranes and phospholipids of hepatic mitochondria from chronic alcoholic rats are more resistant to membrane disordering by alcohol; this is associated with a change in the composition of the membrane phospholipids (Waring *et al.*, 1981).

Interaction with Other Drugs. The impairment of muscular coordination and of judgment that is associated with ingestion of a moderate amount of alcohol (sufficient to produce a blood concentration of up to 50 mg/dl) may be very much enhanced in a person who has also taken sedatives, hypnotics, anticonvulsants, antidepressants, antianxiety drugs, or analgesic agents such as propoxyphene or opioids. *Psychopharmacological agents are now so widely used that it is important for the physician to* *warn patients given such medication of the enhanced effects of alcohol and of the consequent increased danger of driving an automobile after drinking alcohol.*

Unusual side effects may occur when alcohol is taken in association with other drugs. For example, patients treated with oral hypoglycemic agents may experience unpleasant symptoms similar to those experienced by patients who take disulfiram after the ingestion of alcohol (*see* below). Similar interactions can occur with metronidazole or cephalosporins. The combination of alcohol and an oral hypoglycemic agent may also cause unpredictable fluctuations of plasma glucose concentrations, apparently because of an additive hypoglycemic effect of alcohol and because chronic consumption of ethanol can decrease the half-life of tolbutamide. The hypoglycemic effect of insulin may also be markedly increased. Alcohol can interfere with the therapeutic actions of a wide variety of drugs by altering their metabolism. For example, acute ingestion of ethanol reduces the clearance of phenytoin because both drugs compete for the same hepatic microsomal oxidase system (*see* below; Sandor *et al.,* 1981). However, in the chronic drinker, enzyme induction by alcohol occurs, with the result that a period of abstinence leads to an enhanced rate of clearance of phenytoin. (For review, *see* Kissin, 1974; Hoyumpa and Schenker, 1982.)

Absorption, Fate, and Excretion. *Absorption.* Alcohol is rapidly absorbed from the stomach, small intestine, and colon. Vaporized alcohol can be absorbed through the lungs, and fatal intoxication has occurred as a result of its inhalation. It can also be absorbed from subcutaneous sites; however, if the concentration is excessive the astringent action of alcohol prevails, with the result that the local blood supply is effectively shut off and, in consequence, absorption is limited. Absorption of alcohol through the human skin is negligible.

Many factors modify the absorption of alcohol from the *stomach*. At first absorption is rapid, but then it decreases to a very slow rate although the gastric concentration is still high. If the emptying of the stomach is delayed, for example, by pylorospasm due to high concentrations of alcohol, the subsequent absorption of alcohol from the intestine will also be delayed. The volume, character, and dilution of the alcoholic beverage, the presence of food, the period of time taken to ingest the drink, and individual peculiarities are major influences on the rate at which the stomach empties. Depending on these factors, complete absorption may require from 2 to 6 hours or more. With increasing concentration of ingested alcohol, absorption is facilitated until concentrations are reached that impede absorption. Most foods in the stomach tend to retard absorption, milk being especially efficacious. Beer exerts a retarding action, like that of food.

Absorption from the *small intestine* is extremely rapid and complete, and it is largely independent of the presence of food in the stomach or intestine. Some carbohydrates have actually been noted to augment the rate of intestinal absorption of ethanol (Broitman *et al.,* 1976). The rapidity of absorption of alcohol from the small intestine is probably the reason why patients who have undergone gastrectomy may complain that they become intoxicated by amounts of alcohol that would have been innocuous prior to the operation. Indeed, the time of gastric emptying and, consequently, of the onset of the phase of extremely rapid intestinal absorption may well be the prime factor that determines the wide variety of rates of absorption of ingested alcohol that is seen in different individuals and under different conditions.

Distribution in the Body. After absorption, alcohol is fairly uniformly distributed throughout all tissues and all fluids of the body. The plasma concentration is somewhat higher than that in erythrocytes. The placenta is permeable to alcohol; thus, alcohol gains free access to the fetal circulation. Inasmuch as alcohol affects primarily the CNS, much attention has been focused on the concentration in the brain, where, as a result of a large blood supply, the concentration of alcohol quickly approaches that of the blood. The amount of alcohol in brains of persons dying of alcoholic intoxication varies from 300 to 600 mg/100 g. Alcohol is also present in cerebrospinal fluid, at a concentration lower than that in the blood when the blood concentration is rising and higher when the blood concentration is falling.

Metabolism. Ninety to 98% of the alcohol that enters the body is completely oxidized. The metabolism of alcohol differs from that of most substances in that the rate of oxidation is constant with time, and it is little increased by raising the concentration in the blood (zero-order kinetics). The amount of alcohol oxidized per unit of time is roughly proportional to body weight and probably to liver weight. In the adult, the *average* rate at which alcohol can be metabolized is about 30 ml (1 oz) in 3 hours. Direct determination in man indicates that the *maximal* daily metabolism of alcohol is about 450 ml (*see* Kalant, 1971; *see also* Appendix II). Various dietary, hormonal, and pharmacological factors can alter the metabolism of alcohol. For example, starvation lowers and insulin increases the rate of oxidation of alcohol. However, such effects are slight and probably have little significance in the treatment of acute alcoholic intoxication (*see* Stokes, 1971).

The initial oxidation of alcohol occurs chiefly in the liver, and the rate of metabolism is considerably reduced in hepatectomized animals. The primary step is the oxidation of alcohol to acetaldehyde by *alcohol dehydrogenase,* which is a zinc-containing enzyme of molecular weight about 85,000 that utilizes NAD as the hydrogen acceptor (*see* Sytkowski and Vallee, 1979). The acetaldehyde is converted to acetyl CoA, which is then oxidized through the citric acid cycle or utilized in the various anabolic reactions involved in the synthesis of cholesterol, fatty acids, and other tissue constituents.

Alcohol can also be metabolized to acetaldehyde by another system of enzymes, namely, the microsomal mixed-function oxidases that occur in the smooth endoplasmic reticulum of the liver. The extent to which this system metabolizes ethanol in man is probably very small, but it provides one basis for the known interactions between ethanol and the host of other drugs also metabolized by this system (*see* Teschke *et al.,* 1977; Pirola, 1978). For example, ethanol first decreases and then increases the activity of the enzymes of the hepatic endoplasmic reticulum.

Alcohol as a Food. Alcohol is a ready, albeit expensive, source of energy that is utilized more rapidly than most foods because it is quickly absorbed from the gastrointestinal tract and requires no preliminary digestion. The energy released per gram of ethyl alcohol is approximately 7 kcal. Some alcoholic beverages also contain protein and carbohydrate; for example, beer contains about 500 kcal per liter, only half of which is provided by its alcohol content. In contrast, distilled spirits contain no such foodstuffs, and their calories are derived purely from alcohol. Chronic alcoholics may supply one half or more of their daily caloric requirements by drinking alcohol and neglect to eat other foods that would balance their diet; consequently, vitamin and other dietary deficiencies may develop.

Excretion. Normally about 2% of ingested alcohol escapes oxidation; under special circumstances, such as when large doses of alcohol have been consumed, this value may be as high as 10%. Although small amounts of alcohol can be detected in various secretions, most of the alcohol that escapes oxidation is excreted through the kidneys and lungs. Simple arithmetic explains why attempts to hasten significantly the emergence from intoxication by the use of diuretics or agents inducing hyperpnea are doomed to failure. At most, the concentration in the urine is slightly greater than, and the concentration in the alveolar air only 0.05%, that of the blood.

Tolerance and Addiction to Alcohol. The repeated use of alcohol results in the development of tolerance, so that larger doses must be taken in order to produce characteristic effects. However, the degree of tolerance is not as marked as for morphine and nicotine. Tolerance and addiction to alcohol are discussed in Chapter 23.

Acute Alcoholic Intoxication. The characteristic signs and symptoms of alcoholic intoxication are well known. Nevertheless, the erroneous diagnosis of drunkenness is often made in patients who appear inebriated, but who have not ingested alcohol. Diabetic coma, for example, may be mistaken for severe alcoholic intoxication. Drug intoxications, cardiovascular accidents, and fractured skulls seem to be common causes for the diagnostic errors (*see* Morgan and Cagan, 1974). The odor of the breath, which is *not* due to any alcohol vapor but to impurities in the alcoholic beverages or to other causes, is a notoriously unreliable guide and may often be seriously misleading. For medicolegal purposes, the concentration of alcohol in the blood, exhaled air, or urine should be determined.

Treatment. The patient should be kept warm. The stomach may be lavaged, but care must be taken to prevent pulmonary aspiration of the return flow. Analeptics such as pentylenetetrazol or caffeine have no value. If significant respiratory depression is present, steps should be taken to protect the airway from aspiration and to provide ventilatory assistance if indicated. Increased intracranial pressure due to cerebral edema is treated by the usual medical measures, such as hypertonic mannitol solution intravenously. Since ethanol is so freely miscible in water, it lends itself ideally to removal by hemodialysis (*see* Morgan and Cagan, 1974). In general, the therapy of the type of acute alcoholic intoxication where the patient is somnolent or comatose does not differ significantly from that of acute central depression caused by conventional general anesthetics or hypnotics. Reference should be made to the treatment of acute barbiturate intoxication for further measures (*see* Chapter 17).

Acute alcoholic intoxication is not always associated with coma. Usually therapy is not required, and it is sufficient for the patient to wait while his tissues metabolize the ingested alcohol at the characteristic constant rate until sobriety ensues. However, in some individuals the release of central inhibitory control may lead to hyperactivity of an extremely violent nature. Sedatives and antipsychotic agents have been extensively employed to quiet such patients. Great care must be taken, however, when sedatives are used to treat a patient who has already treated himself to an excessive amount of a CNS depressant, namely, alcohol. The subject of acute alcoholic intoxication has been extensively reviewed by various authors (*e.g.*, Morgan and Cagan, 1974).

Concentration of Alcohol in Body Fluids in Relation to Alcoholic Intoxication. It is generally agreed that threshold effects (such as an increased reaction time, diminished fine motor control, and an impaired critical faculty) appear when the concentration of alcohol in the blood is 20 to 30 mg/dl; more than 50% of persons are grossly intoxicated when the concentration is 150 mg/dl. The average concentration in fatal cases is about 400 mg/dl (Committee on Medicolegal Problems, 1968).

The determination of alcohol in body fluids is often important for medicolegal purposes to establish how much alcohol was ingested. Methods of determining the concentration of alcohol are given by Harger (1974) and by Erickson (1979). The concentration of alcohol in the blood may be determined directly. Alternatively it can be estimated from the concentration either in expired air, which is about 0.05% that in the blood or, less frequently, in the urine, which is about 130% that in the blood.

Diagnosis of Intoxication. All but a few states have passed laws embodying the recommendations of the National Safety Council and the American Medical Association concerning the driving of motor vehicles by persons who are drunk. If the defendant's blood has a concentration of alcohol of 100 mg/dl or over, he should be considered as being under the influence of intoxicating beverages; if 50 mg/dl or under, not under the influence; if between 50 and 100 mg/dl, this fact must be considered only with other competent positive evidence with regard to the guilt or innocence of the defendant. The importance of such legislation is emphasized by the fact that the average person with a blood alcohol concentration of 100 or 150 mg/dl is 7 or 25 times, respectively, more likely to have a fatal accident than the driver with no alcohol in his blood (*see* reports by U.S. Department of Health, Education, and Welfare, 1974, 1978).

From the medicolegal point of view the major factor in judging the degree of intoxication is the concentration of alcohol in the blood. The individual, on the other hand, is often concerned more with the *quantity* of alcohol he can safely drink. Unfortunately for him this is not a simple question because many factors, such as his weight and the rate of absorption from the gastrointestinal tract, determine the concentration of alcohol in the blood produced by the ingestion of a given amount of alcohol (*see* Wallgren and Barry, 1970). On the aver-

age, ingestion of 44 g of alcohol taken as whisky (4 oz) or martini cocktail (5.5 oz) on an empty stomach results in a maximal blood concentration of 67 to 92 mg/dl; after a mixed meal, 30 to 53 mg/dl. Ingestion of the same amount of alcohol taken as conventional-strength beer (1.2 liters) on an empty stomach results in a maximal blood concentration of 41 to 49 mg/dl; after a mixed meal, 23 to 29 mg/dl. After gastrointestinal absorption is complete, the concentration in the blood at any time after ingestion can be estimated from the volume of distribution of the alcohol, which averages 0.54 liter/kg, and the rate of metabolism, which is about 120 mg/kg per hour (*see* Appendix II; Committee on Medicolegal Problems, 1968).

Contraindications. Contraindications to the use of alcohol largely follow from toxicological considerations. Patients with hepatic disease should not use alcohol, and gastrointestinal ulcers are also contraindications. Alcohol should be avoided by patients with alcoholic skeletal or cardiac myopathy. Clearly, it should be taken only in great moderation, or not at all, by pregnant women, and alcohol should usually be forbidden to patients who were once addicted to it (*see* Chapter 23). In general, the use of alcohol in the presence of any particular disease is a matter that the physician and patient must decide in each individual case.

Preparations. The official preparation of *alcohol* (*ethanol, ethyl alcohol*) contains not less than 94.9% and not more than 96.0% by volume of C_2H_5OH. *Dehydrated alcohol* contains not less than 99.5% by volume of C_2H_5OH. *Rubbing alcohol* contains about 70% (by volume) of ethanol, the remainder being perfume oils, water, and denaturants, with or without color additives.

Therapeutic Uses of Alcohol. Alcohol and alcoholic beverages are widely used by the laity for numerous ailments; their legitimate uses in medicine are few.

External. Alcohol is an excellent *solvent* for many drugs and is frequently employed for medicinal mixtures as a vehicle. Alcohol is a solvent for the *toxicodendrol* causing ivy poisoning; early and thorough washing of the affected parts with alcohol may abort or lessen the severity of the dermatitis. In *phenol skin burns* alcohol should be used immediately as a wash if castor oil is not available; it is not to be employed for gastric lavage, however, when phenol has been swallowed. Alcohol *cools* the skin when it is allowed to evaporate, and alcohol sponges are therefore used to treat fever. It is also *rubefacient* and is included in liniments. Alcohol (50 to 70% by volume) is employed as a rubbing agent on the skin of bedridden patients in order to prevent *decubitus ulcers.* It is also used to *decrease sweating,* and is an ingredient of many anhidrotic and astringent lotions. Ethyl alcohol still remains the most popular *skin disinfectant (see* Chapter 41).

Alimentary Tract. Alcoholic beverages, if enjoyed by the patient, may be given before meals as a *stomachic* to improve appetite and digestion, especially in convalescent and debilitated or elderly patients (Turner *et al.,* 1981).

Injection for Relief of Pain. Dehydrated alcohol may be injected in the close proximity of nerves or sympathetic ganglia for the relief of the long-lasting pain that occurs in *trigeminal neuralgia, inoperable carcinoma,* and other conditions. Epidural, subarachnoid, and lumbar paravertebral injections of alcohol have also been employed in appropriate circumstances. For example, lumbar paravertebral injections of alcohol may destroy sympathetic ganglia and thereby produce vasodilatation, relieve pain, and promote healing of lesions in patients with vascular disease of the lower extremities.

Systemic Uses. Alcohol acts as a *hypnotic* and *antipyretic,* and is widely employed for these purposes by lay persons. Alcoholic beverages are sometimes valuable during convalescence as rapidly assimilable sources of energy or as remedies for insomnia. Although sometimes used for this purpose, alcohol is ineffective in causing vasodilatation in persons with peripheral vascular disease or coronary artery disease; any benefits that may be noted from the ingestion of alcoholic beverages in such patients are probably due to a central-depressant action rather than to an increase in peripheral or coronary blood flow.

For generations alcoholic beverages have been used to check impending *"head colds."* Perhaps the greatest therapeutic advantage of such therapy is to make the patient drowsy and sleepy so that he stays in bed, whereas otherwise he would be ambulant to the detriment of at least his associates. Hamburger (1936) humorously advised the following therapy, culled from an old English book, to be instituted at the first inkling of a cold, namely, to hang one's hat on the bedpost, drink from a bottle of good whisky until two hats appear, and then get into bed and stay there.

The use of ethanol in the therapy of methyl alcohol poisoning is discussed below.

METHYL ALCOHOL

Methyl alcohol (CH$_3$OH), also called *methanol, wood alcohol,* and *Columbian spirit,* is the simplest of the alcohols. The pharmacology, biochemistry, toxicology, and clinical aspects of methyl alcohol have been extensively reviewed by Morgan and Cagan (1974) and by Tephly and colleagues (1979). It is widely employed industrially as a solvent. It is also used as an adulterant to "denature," and thereby make unfit to drink, the ethyl alcohol that is used for cleaning purposes, paint removal, and a variety of other uses. Such alcohol, being tax free, is considerably less expensive than more conventional alcoholic beverages and, unless denatured,

offers considerable temptation to the derelict. Methyl alcohol is purely of toxicological interest. Poisoning results from its ingestion as a substitute for, or as an adulterant of, ethyl alcohol. For example, 6% of all blindness in the United States Armed Forces during World War II was caused by methanol. Serious or fatal poisoning can also occur from industrial exposure.

Fate in the Body. After absorption, methyl alcohol is widely distributed in body tissues. While small amounts of the alcohol are then excreted in the urine and in the expired air, methyl alcohol is largely oxidized in the body to formaldehyde and formic acid. Animals differ in their ability to oxidize methanol to formic acid and to oxidize formic acid itself. In the rabbit only 1% is excreted as formic acid in the urine, compared with 20% in the dog; an intermediate value is obtained in man.

The oxidation of methanol, like that of ethanol, proceeds independently of the concentration in the blood. The rate, however, is only one seventh that of ethanol, so that complete oxidation and excretion of methyl alcohol usually require several days. Oxidation occurs mainly in the liver and kidney.

Relation of Methanol to Ethanol Oxidation. Although experiments with isolated rat tissue slices have emphasized the importance of catalase in the oxidation of methanol, it is still generally agreed that in man alcohol dehydrogenase is involved in the first step of oxidation. The fact that it is this same enzyme that is responsible for the oxidation of ethyl alcohol is presumably the explanation for the finding *in vitro* that ethanol very considerably depresses the rate of oxidation of methanol. The common biochemical pathway of oxidation of both alcohols also accounts for the clinical observations that simultaneous administration of ethanol may ameliorate the toxic sequelae of methanol poisoning *(see* Bergeron *et al.,* 1982). This is because the products of oxidation of methanol are toxic rather than methanol itself, and, therefore, the degree of poisoning is minimized if the rate of oxidation of methanol is reduced as much as possible.

Methyl Alcohol Poisoning. Poisoning due to methyl alcohol results from a combination of the following: (1) a minor factor of CNS depression, similar to that produced by ethyl alcohol; (2) a major factor of acidosis due to the production of formic acid (Clay *et al.,* 1975); and (3) a specific toxicity of the oxidation products of methanol for the retinal cells.

Symptoms. Methanol is less inebriating than ethanol; indeed, inebriation is not a prominent symptom of methanol intoxication unless a very large amount is consumed or ethanol is also ingested. An asymptomatic latent period of 8 to 36 hours may precede the onset of symptoms; if ethanol is simultaneously imbibed in sufficient amount, methanol poisoning may be considerably delayed, or, on occasion, even averted. In such cases ethanol intoxication is prominent, and methanol ingestion may not be suspected.

Symptoms and *signs* of methanol poisoning consist in headache, vertigo, vomiting, severe upper abdominal pain, back pain, dyspnea, motor restlessness, cold clammy extremities, blurring of vision, hyperemia of the optic disc, and, occasionally, diarrhea. Blood pressure is usually unaffected. The pulse is slow in severely ill patients, and bradycardia constitutes a grave prognostic sign. The visual disturbance can proceed to blindness, and the pupils then do not react to light. Restlessness and delirium may be marked. Despite the severe acidosis, Kussmaul respiration is not common. Coma can develop with amazing rapidity in relatively asymptomatic subjects. In moribund patients the respiration is slow, shallow, gasping, and "fish mouth" in type. Death may be sudden, or it may occur only after many hours of coma. Death occurs in inspiratory apnea, with terminal opisthotonos and convulsions.

Laboratory findings include evidence of severe acidosis, methanol and formic acid in blood and urine, moderate ketonemia, normal serum sodium and potassium concentrations, albuminuria, and slight or moderate acetonuria. The ketonemia and acetonuria are mild in comparison with the severity of the acidosis. Cerebral blood flow and cerebral oxygen consumption are both markedly reduced during methanol poisoning. Serum amylase is elevated as a result of pancreatitis; indeed, pancreatic injury probably accounts for the violent epigastric pain. Cerebrospinal fluid pressure is often elevated.

Death from methanol is nearly always preceded by blindness. As little as 4 ml of methanol has caused blindness, and ingestion of 80 to 150 ml is usually fatal. The formic acid produced is probably the cause of the selective injury to the retinal cells (see Tephly et al., 1979).

Treatment and Prognosis. The cardinal feature of methanol poisoning is the acidosis, and the correction of acidosis is the keystone of proper therapy if the patient is to survive. It is also believed that the prognosis with respect to salvage of vision is directly dependent on the rapidity and the completeness of the correction of the acidosis. However, acidosis itself is not the cause of the ocular disturbances, because these phenomena are not observed in other types of acidosis. Indeed, retinal changes may occur in methanol poisoning despite seemingly adequate therapy with alkali. Because of the slow oxidation of methanol the risk of recurrence of acidosis after a period of successful treatment is great, and hence close observation and proper therapy should be continued for several days to prevent sudden relapse and death. The metabolic acidosis is treated with alkali (see Chapter 35); hypokalemia from alkali therapy may require administration of potassium salts. In general, water and electrolyte balance and nutrition must be maintained. The use of hemodialysis or peritoneal dialysis will hasten the removal of methanol from the body. The patient should be kept warm and his eyes protected from strong light.

The administration of ethanol is recommended on the basis that it retards the oxidation of methanol, as explained above, and is a specific measure for the prevention of blindness that may otherwise follow. Ethanol administration may also be a life-saving procedure if alkali therapy must be postponed for any reason. Neurological damage, giving rise to a permanent motor dysfunction, may follow methanol poisoning; the rigidity and hypokinesis may be relieved by levodopa (Guggenheim *et al.*, 1971).

DISULFIRAM

History. *Tetraethylthiuram disulfide* (*disulfiram*) was used in the rubber industry as an antioxidant. Workers exposed to disulfiram developed a hypersensitivity to ethanol. Two Danish physicians, who had taken disulfiram in the course of an investigation of its potential anthelmintic usefulness and who became ill at a cocktail party, were quick to realize that the disulfiram had altered their response to alcohol. They then initiated a series of pharmacological and clinical studies that provided the basis for the use of disulfiram as an adjunct in the treatment of chronic alcoholism. Similar sensitization is produced by various congeners of disulfiram, cyanamide, eating the fungus *Coprinus atramentarius,* the hypoglycemic sulfonylureas, metronidazole, cephalosporins, and the ingestion of *animal charcoal* (*see* Kitson, 1977; Eneanya *et al.,* 1981).

Mechanism of Action. Disulfiram, given by itself, is a relatively nontoxic substance, and few untoward effects are observed when it is administered alone in reasonable doses in animals or man. However, disulfiram markedly alters the intermediary metabolism of alcohol. When ethanol is given to an animal or to an individual previously treated with disulfiram, the blood acetaldehyde concentration rises five to ten times higher than in an untreated animal or individual. This effect is accompanied by marked signs and symptoms, known as the *acetaldehyde syndrome.* Within about 5 to 10 minutes the face feels hot, and soon afterwards it is flushed and scarlet in appearance. As the vasodilatation spreads over the whole body, intense throbbing is felt in the head and neck, and a pulsating headache may develop. Respiratory difficulties, nausea, copious vomiting, sweating, thirst, chest pain, considerable hypotension, orthostatic syncope, marked uneasiness, weakness, vertigo, blurred vision, and confusion are observed. The facial flush is replaced by pallor, and the blood pressure may fall to shock level. As little as 7 ml of alcohol will cause mild symptoms in sensitive persons, and the effect, once elicited, lasts between 30 minutes (in mild cases) and several hours (in severe cases). After the symptoms wear off, the patient is exhausted and may sleep for several hours, after which he is well again.

Most of the signs and symptoms observed after the ingestion of disulfiram plus alcohol are attributable to the resulting increase in the concentration of acetaldehyde in the body. They can, in fact, be produced in normal humans by the intravenous injection of acetaldehyde. Acetaldehyde is produced as a result of the initial oxidation of ethanol by the alcohol dehydrogenase of the liver. It does not accumulate in the tissues because it is further oxidized almost as soon as it is formed, primarily by the enzyme aldehyde dehydrogenase. In the presence of disulfiram, however, the concentration of acetaldehyde rises because disulfiram appears to react with crucial sulfhydryl groups in both the cytosolic and the mitochondrial forms of this enzyme, thereby producing irreversible inactivation. Recovery of activity is not achieved by removal of the drug and must await synthesis of new molecules of enzyme (see Kitson, 1977). It is not clear whether diethyldithiocarbamate, the major metabolite of disulfiram, is involved in this action to any extent, even though it combines extensively with proteins in blood and tissues. Diethyldithiocarbamate is an avid chelator of copper and other metals and thereby inhibits the activity of several metalloenzymes, including dopamine β-hydroxylase and alcohol dehydrogenase. The latter action would account for the increased concentration of ethanol in blood sometimes reported during treatment with disulfiram. Inhibition of dopamine β-hydroxylase, with a consequent reduction of norepinephrine synthesis in sympathetic nerve terminals, may provide an explanation for the hypotension that is characteristic of the disulfiram-ethanol reaction. Injection of acetaldehyde into animals usually causes hypertension, which is mediated by the sympathetic nervous system, despite the fact that acetaldehyde has a direct vasodilating effect. Many aspects of the disulfiram-ethanol reaction remain to be explained, although inhibition of aldehyde dehydrogenase with resultant accumulation of acetaldehyde is probably the primary cause (see Kitson, 1977; Eneanya et al., 1981).

Disulfiram can inhibit most enzymes with crucial sulfhydryl groups, and it thus has a wide spectrum of biological effects. It inhibits hepatic microsomal drug-metabolizing enzymes and thereby interferes with the metabolism of phenytoin, chlordiazepoxide, barbiturates, and other drugs (Eneanya et al., 1981).

Absorption, Fate, and Excretion. About 80% of an oral dose of disulfiram is absorbed rapidly from the human gastrointestinal tract. However, only small amounts of disulfiram appear in blood because of its rapid reduction to diethyldithiocarbamate, principally by the glutathione reductase system in erythrocytes. This product is metabolized further in the liver, primarily by conjugation with glucuronic acid; small amounts of carbon disulfide and sulfate ion are also produced (see Eneanya et al., 1981). In the rat, no free disulfiram or diethyldithiocarbamate can be detected 4 hours after subcutaneous injection of disulfiram.

Toxic Reactions and Contraindications. Disulfiram by itself is largely, but not completely, innocuous. It may cause acneform eruptions, allergic dermatitis, urticaria, lassitude, fatigue, tremor, restlessness, reduced sexual potency, headache, dizziness, a garlic-like or metallic taste, and mild gastrointestinal disturbances. Hepatotoxicity, peripheral neuropathies, psychosis, and acetonemia have also been reported (see Eneanya et al., 1981).

Disulfiram may be teratogenic and should not be used during pregnancy. Alarming reactions may result from the ingestion of even small amounts of alcohol in persons being treated with disulfiram. Marked respiratory depression, cardiovascular collapse, cardiac arrhythmias, myocardial infarction, acute congestive heart failure, unconsciousness, convulsions, and sudden and unexplained fatalities have occurred. Obviously the use of disulfiram as a therapeutic agent is not without danger, and it should be attempted only under careful medical and nursing supervision. The patient must be warned that, as long as he is taking disulfiram, the ingestion of alcohol in any form will make him sick and may endanger his life. He must learn to avoid disguised forms of alcohol, such as sauces, fermented vinegar, cough syrups, and even aftershave lotions and backrubs.

Chemistry and Preparation. The chemical structure of disulfiram is as follows:

Disulfiram

Disulfiram (ANTABUSE) is available in the form of oral, scored tablets that contain 250 or 500 mg of the drug.

Administration and Dosage. Disulfiram should be administered only by a physician, and therapy is usually commenced in the hospital. The drug should never be administered until the patient has abstained from alcohol for at least 12 hours. In the initial phase of treatment, a maximal daily dose of 500 mg is given for 1 to 2 weeks. Maintenance dosage then ranges from 125 to 500 mg daily, depending on tolerance to side effects. Unless sedation is prominent, the daily dose should be taken in the morning, the time when the resolve not to drink may be strongest. Sensitization to alcohol may last for as long as 6 to 14 days after the last ingestion of disulfiram because of the slow rate of restoration of aldehyde dehydrogenase.

Therapeutic Use. The only therapeutic use of disulfiram is in the treatment of *chronic alcoholism*. Disulfiram is not a cure for alcoholism, but merely affords the volunteer a crutch by which the sincere desire to stop drinking can be fortified. The rationale for its use is that the patient knows that if he is to avoid the devastating experience of the "acetaldehyde syndrome" he cannot drink for at least 3 or 4 days after taking disulfiram. *Calcium carbimide* (*citrated calcium cyanamide;* TEMPOSIL) has similar but briefer effects. It is not available in the United States. This subject is further discussed in Chapter 23, which deals with the therapy of drug abuse.

Altura, B. M., and Altura, B. T. Microvascular and vascular smooth muscle actions of ethanol, acetaldehyde, and acetate. *Fed. Proc.*, **1982**, *41*, 2447–2451.

Bergeron, R.; Cardinal, J.; and Geadah, D. Prevention of methanol toxicity by ethanol therapy. *N. Engl. J. Med.*, **1982**, *307*, 1528.

Broitman, S. A.; Gottlieb, L. S.; and Vitale, J. J. Augmentation of ethanol absorption by mono- and disaccharides. *Gastroenterology*, **1976**, *70*, 1101–1107.

Brown, N. A.; Goulding, E. H.; and Fabro, S. Ethanol embryotoxicity: direct effects on mammalian embryos in vitro. *Science*, **1979**, *206*, 573–575.

Camillo, M. E.; Morgan, M. Y.; and Sherlock, S. Erythrocyte transketolase activity in alcoholic liver disease. *Scand. J. Gastroenterol.*, **1981**, *16*, 273–279.

Chin, J. H., and Goldstein, D. B. Membrane-disordering action of ethanol. *Mol. Pharmacol.*, **1981**, *19*, 425–431.

Clay, K. L.; Murphy, R. C.; and Watkins, W. D. Experimental methanol toxicity in the primate: analysis of metabolic acidosis. *Toxicol. Appl. Pharmacol.*, **1975**, *34*, 49–61.

Deykin, D.; Janson, P.; and McMahon, L. Ethanol potentiation of aspirin-induced prolongation of the bleeding time. *N. Engl. J. Med.*, **1982**, *306*, 852–854.

Eidelberg, E. On the possibility that opiate and ethanol actions are mediated by similar mechanisms. In, *Alcohol Intoxication and Withdrawal*, Vol. 3B. (Gross, M. M., ed.) Plenum Press, New York, **1977**, pp. 87–94.

Eisenhofer, G.; Lambie, D. G.; and Johnson, R. H. Effects of ethanol on plasma catecholamines and norepinephrine clearance. *Clin. Pharmacol. Ther.*, **1983**, *34*, 143–147.

Faller, J., and Fox, I. H. Ethanol-induced hyperuricemia. *N. Engl. J. Med.*, **1982**, *307*, 1598–1602.

Gantt, W. H. Effect of alcohol on the sexual reflexes of normal and neurotic male dogs. *Psychosom. Med.*, **1952**, *14*, 174–181.

Goldstein, D. B.; Chin, J. H.; and Lyon, R. C. Ethanol disordering of spin-labeled mouse brain membranes: correlation with genetically determined ethanol sensitivity of mice. *Proc. Natl Acad. Sci. U.S.A.*, **1982**, *79*, 4231–4233.

Graboys, T. B., and Lown, B. Coffee, arrhythmias, and common sense. *N. Engl. J. Med.*, **1983**, *308*, 835–837.

Greenspon, A. J., and Schaal, S. F. The "holiday heart": electrophysiologic studies of alcohol effects in alcoholics. *Ann. Intern. Med.*, **1983**, *98*, 135–139.

Guggenheim, M. A.; Couch, J. R.; and Weinberger, W. Motor dysfunction as a permanent complication of methanol ingestion. *Arch. Neurol.*, **1971**, *24*, 550–554.

Hamburger, L. P. Some minor ailments: their importance in the medical curriculum. *Yale J. Biol. Med.*, **1936**, *8*, 365–386.

Hartung, G. H.; Foreyt, J. P.; Mitchell, R. E.; Mitchell, J. E.; Reeves, R. S.; and Gotto, A. M. Effect of alcohol intake on high-density lipoprotein in runners and inactive men. *J.A.M.A.*, **1983**, *249*, 747–750.

Issa, F. G., and Sullivan, C. E. Alcohol, snoring and deep apnea. *J. Neurol. Neurosurg. Psychiatry*, **1982**, *45*, 353–359.

Johnson, D. A.; Lee, N. M.; Cooke, R.; and Loh, H. Adaptation to ethanol-induced fluidization of brain lipid bilayers: cross-tolerance and reversibility. *Mol. Pharmacol.*, **1980**, *17*, 52–55.

Johnson, S.; Knight, R.; Marmar, D. J.; and Steele, R. W. Immune deficiency in fetal alcohol syndrome. *Pediatr. Res.*, **1981**, *15*, 908–911.

Kakihana, R., and Butte, J. C. Ethanol and endocrine function. In, *Biochemistry and Pharmacology of Ethanol*, Vol. 2. (Majchrowicz, E., and Noble, E. P., eds.) Plenum Press, New York, **1979**, pp. 147–164.

Leo, M. A., and Lieber, C. S. Hepatic vitamin A depletion in alcoholic liver injury. *N. Engl. J. Med.*, **1982**, *307*, 597–601.

Lyon, L. J., and Anthony, J. Reversal of alcoholic coma by naloxone. *Ann. Intern. Med.*, **1982**, *96*, 464–465.

Lyon, R. C.; McComb, J. A.; Schreurs, J.; and Goldstein, D. B. A relationship between alcohol intoxication and the disordering of brain membrane by a series of short-chain alcohols. *J. Pharmacol. Exp. Ther.*, **1981**, *218*, 669–675.

Mekhjian, H. S., and May, E. S. Acute and chronic effects of ethanol on fluid transport in the human small intestine. *Gastroenterology*, **1977**, *72*, 1280–1286.

Mezey, Y. E. Alcohol consumption and mortality. *Gastroenterology*, **1980**, *79*, 1344–1345.

Petersson, B.; Trell, E.; and Kristenson, H. Alcohol abstention and premature mortality in middle-aged men. *Br. Med. J. [Clin. Res.]*, **1982**, *285*, 1457–1460.

Pohorecky, L. A. Influence of alcohol on peripheral neurotransmitter function. *Fed. Proc.*, **1982**, *41*, 2452–2455.

Rabin, R. A., and Molinoff, P. B. Activation of adenylate cyclase by ethanol in mouse striatal tissue. *J. Pharmacol. Exp. Ther.*, **1981**, *216*, 129–134.

Regan, T. J. Regional circulatory responses to alcohol and its congeners. *Fed. Proc.*, **1982**, *41*, 2438–2442.

Ricci, R. L.; Crawford, S. S.; and Miner, P. B. The effect of ethanol on hepatic sodium plus potassium activated ATPase activity in the rat. *Gastroenterology*, **1981**, *80*, 1445–1450.

Rossett, H. L.; Weiner, L.; and Edelin, K. C. Strategy for prevention of fetal alcohol effects. *Obstet. Gynecol.*, **1981**, *57*, 1–7.

Rubin, E. Alcoholic myopathy in heart and skeletal muscles. *N. Engl. J. Med.*, **1979**, *301*, 28–33.

Sandor, P.; Sellers, E. M.; Dumbrell, M.; and Khouw, V. Effect of short- and long-term alcohol abuse on phenytoin kinetics in chronic alcoholics. *Clin. Pharmacol. Ther.*, **1981**, *30*, 390–397.

Shaper, A. G.; Pocock, S. J.; Walker, M.; Wale, C. J.; Clayton, B.; Delves, H. D.; and Hinks, L. Effects of alcohol and smoking on blood lead in middle-aged British men. *Br. Med. J. [Clin. Res.]*, **1982**, *284*, 298–302.

Straus, E.; Urbach, H.-J.; and Yalow, R. S. Alcohol-stimulated secretion of immunoreactive secretin. *N. Engl. J. Med.*, **1975**, *293*, 1031–1032.

Taskinen, M.-R.; Valimaki, M.; Nikkila, E. A.; Kuusi, T.; Enholm, C.; and Ylikhri, R. High density protein subfractions and postheparin plasma lipases in alcoholic men before and after ethanol withdrawal. *Metabolism*, **1982**, *31*, 1168–1174.

Tennes, K., and Blackard, C. Maternal alcohol consumption, birthweight, and minor physical abnormalities. *Am. J. Obstet. Gynecol.*, **1980**, *138*, 774–780.

Teschke, R.; Matsuzaki, S.; Ohnishi, K.; Hasumura, Y.; and Lieber, C. S. Metabolism of alcohol at high concentrations: role and biochemical nature of the hepatic microsomal oxidizing system. *Adv. Exp. Med. Biol.*, **1977**, *85A*, 257–280.

Van Thiel, D. H.; Gavaler, J. S.; and Sanghvi, A. Recovery of sexual function in abstinent alcoholic men. *Gastroenterology*, **1983**, *84*, 677–682.

Van Thiel, D. H., and Lester, R. Sex and alcohol: a second peek. *N. Engl. J. Med.*, **1976**, *295*, 835–836.

Waring, A. J.; Rottenberg, H.; Ohnishi, T.; and Rubin, E. Membranes and phospholipids of liver mitochondria from chronic alcoholic rats are resistant to membrane disordering by alcohol. *Proc. Natl Acad. Sci. U.S.A.*, **1981**, *78*, 2582–2586.

Willett, W.; Hennekens, C. H.; Siegel, A. J.; Adner, M. M.; and Castelli, W. P. Alcohol consumption and high-density lipoprotein cholesterol in marathon runners. *N. Engl. J. Med.*, **1980**, *303*, 1159–1161.

Wilson, G. T. Alcohol and human sexual behavior. *Behav. Res. Ther.*, **1977**, *15*, 239–252.

Monographs and Reviews

Altura, B. T. Cardiovascular effects of alcohol and alcoholism. *Fed. Proc.*, **1982**, *41*, 2437–2477.

Baraona, E., and Lieber, C. S. Effects of alcohol in hepatic transport of proteins. *Annu. Rev. Med.,* **1982,** *33,* 281–292.

Beard, J. D., and Sargent, W. Q. Water and electrolyte metabolism following ethanol intake and during acute withdrawal from ethanol. In, *Biochemistry and Pharmacology of Ethanol,* Vol. 2. (Majchrowicz, E., and Noble, E. P., eds.) Plenum Press, New York, **1979,** pp. 3–16.

Christensen, E. L., and Higgins, J. J. Effect of acute and chronic administration of ethanol on the redox states of brain and liver. In, *Biochemistry and Pharmacology of Ethanol,* Vol. 1, (Majchrowicz, E., and Noble, E. P., eds.) Plenum Press, New York, **1979,** pp. 191–247.

Cicero, T. J. Neuroendocrinological effects of alcohol. *Annu. Rev. Med.,* **1981,** *31,* 123–142.

Committee on Medicolegal Problems. *Alcohol and the Impaired Driver: A Manual on the Medicolegal Aspects of Chemical Tests for Intoxication.* American Medical Association, Chicago, **1968.**

Council Report. Fetal effects of maternal alcohol use. *J.A.M.A.,* **1983,** *249,* 2517–2521.

Eneanya, D. L.; Bianchine, J. R.; Duran, D. O.; and Andresen, B. D. The actions and metabolic fate of disulfiram. *Annu. Rev. Pharmacol. Toxicol.,* **1981,** *21,* 575–596.

Erickson, C. K. Factors affecting the distribution and measurement of ethanol in the body. In, *Biochemistry and Pharmacology of Ethanol,* Vol. 1. (Majchrowicz, E., and Noble, E. P., eds.) Plenum Press, New York, **1979,** pp. 9–26.

Feinman, L., and Lieber, C. S. Liver disease in alcoholism. In, *The Biology of Alcoholism.* Vol. 3, *Clinical Pathology.* (Kissin, B., and Begleiter, H., eds.) Plenum Press, New York, **1974,** pp. 303–338.

Glass, G. B. J.; Slomiany, B. L.; and Slomiany, A. Biochemical and pathological derangements of the gastrointestinal tract following acute and chronic digestion of ethanol. In, *Biochemistry and Pharmacology of Ethanol,* Vol. 1. (Majchrowicz, E., and Noble, E. P., eds.) Plenum Press, New York, **1979,** pp. 551–586.

Gross, M. M. (ed.). *Alcohol Intoxication and Withdrawal.* Vols. A and B, *Advances in Experimental Medicine and Biology.* Plenum Press, New York, **1977.**

Harger, R. H. Recently published analytical methods for determining alcohol in body materials. Alcohol countermeasures literature review. *Report to Department of Transportation (DOT-HS-031-3-722).* National Technical Information Service, Springfield, Va., **1974.**

Higgins, J. J. Control of ethanol oxidation and its interaction with other metabolic systems. In, *Biochemistry and Pharmacology of Ethanol,* Vol. 1. (Majchrowicz, E., and Noble, E. P., eds.) Plenum Press, New York, **1979,** pp. 249–351.

Hillman, R. S., and Steinberg, S. E. The effects of alcohol on folate metabolism. *Annu. Rev. Med.,* **1982,** *33,* 345–354.

Hillman, R. W. Alcoholism and malnutrition. In, *The Biology of Alcoholism.* Vol. 3, *Clinical Pathology.* (Kissin, B., and Begleiter, H., eds.) Plenum Press, New York, **1974,** pp. 513–586.

Himwich, H. E., and Callison, D. A. The effects of alcohol on evoked potentials of various parts of the central nervous system of the cat. In, *The Biology of Alcoholism.* Vol. 2, *Physiology and Behavior.* (Kissin, B. and Begleiter, H., eds.) Plenum Press, New York, **1972,** pp. 67–84.

Hoyumpa, A. M., and Schenker, S. Major drug interactions: effect of liver disease, alcohol and malnutrition. *Annu. Rev. Med.,* **1982,** *33,* 113–149.

Kalant, H. Absorption, diffusion, distribution, and elimination of ethanol: effects on biological membranes. In, *The Biology of Alcoholism.* Vol. 1, *Biochemistry.* (Kissin, B., and Begleiter, H., eds.) Plenum Press, New York, **1971,** pp. 1–62.

Kissin, B. Interactions of ethyl alcohol and other drugs. In, *The Biology of Alcoholism.* Vol. 3, *Clinical Pathology.* (Kissin, B., and Begleiter, H., eds.) Plenum Press, New York, **1974,** pp. 109–161.

Kissin, B., and Begleiter, H. (eds.). *The Biology of Alcoholism.* Vol. 3, *Clinical Pathology.* Plenum Press, New York, **1974.**

Kitson, T. M. The disulfiram-ethanol reaction. *J. Stud. Alcohol,* **1977,** *38,* 96–113.

Klatsky, A. L.; Friedman, G. D.; and Siegelaub, A. B. Alcohol and mortality. A ten-year Kaiser-Permanente experience. *Ann. Intern. Med.,* **1981,** *95,* 139–145.

Klemm, W. R. Effects of ethanol on nerve impulse activity. In, *Biochemistry and Pharmacology of Ethanol,* Vol. 2. (Majchrowicz, E., and Noble, E. P., eds.) Plenum Press, New York, **1979,** pp. 243–267.

Lieber, C. S. Pathogenesis and early diagnosis of alcoholic liver injury. *N. Engl. J. Med.,* **1978,** *298,* 888–893.

Lieber, C. S.; Teschke, R.; Hasumura, Y.; and Decarli, L. M. Differences in hepatic and metabolic changes after acute and chronic alcohol consumption. *Fed. Proc.,* **1975,** *34,* 2060–2074.

Lindenbaum, J. Hematologic effects of alcohol. In, *The Biology of Alcoholism.* Vol. 3, *Clinical Pathology.* (Kissin, B., and Begleiter, H., eds.) Plenum Press, New York, **1974,** pp. 461–480.

Lorber, S. H.; Dinoso, V. P., Jr.; and Chey, W. Y. Diseases of the gastrointestinal tract. In, *The Biology of Alcoholism.* Vol. 3, *Clinical Pathology.* (Kissin, B., and Begleiter, H., eds.) Plenum Press, New York, **1974,** pp. 339–357.

Majchrowicz, E., and Noble, E. P. (eds.). *Biochemistry and Pharmacology of Ethanol,* Vols. 1–3. Plenum Press, New York, **1979.**

Medical Letter. Interactions of drugs with alcohol. **1981,** *23,* 33–34.

Mendelson, W. B. Pharmacologic and electrophysiologic effects of ethanol in relation to sleep. In, *Biochemistry and Pharmacology of Ethanol,* Vol. 2. (Majchrowicz, E., and Noble, E. P., eds.) Plenum Press, New York, **1979,** pp. 467–484.

Morgan, R., and Cagan, E. J. Acute alcohol intoxication, the disulfiram reaction, and methyl alcohol intoxication. In, *The Biology of Alcoholism.* Vol. 3, *Clinical Pathology.* (Kissin, B., and Begleiter, H., eds.) Plenum Press, New York, **1974,** pp. 163–189.

Pirola, R. C. *Drug Metabolism and Alcohol.* University Park Press, Baltimore, **1978.**

Pirola, R. C., and Lieber, C. S. Acute and chronic pancreatitis. In, *The Biology of Alcoholism.* Vol. 3, *Clinical Pathology.* (Kissin, B., and Begleiter, H., eds.) Plenum Press, New York, **1974,** pp. 359–402.

Stokes, P. E. Alcohol-endocrine relationships. In, *The Biology of Alcoholism.* Vol. 1, *Biochemistry.* (Kissin, B., and Begleiter, H., eds.) Plenum Press, New York, **1971,** pp. 397–436.

Sytkowski, A. J., and Vallee, B. L. Metalloenzymes and ethanol metabolism. In, *Biochemistry and Pharmacology of Ethanol,* Vol. 1. (Majchrowicz, E., and Noble, E. P., eds.) Plenum Press, New York, **1979,** pp. 43–63.

Tephly, T. R.; Makar, A. B.; McMartin, K. E.; Hayreh, S. S.; and Martin-Amat, G. Methanol: its metabolism and toxicity. In, *Biochemistry and Pharmacology of Ethanol,* Vol. 1. (Majchrowicz, E., and Noble, E. P., eds.) Plenum Press, New York, **1979,** pp. 145–164.

Truitt, E. B. A biogenic amine hypothesis for alcohol tolerance. *Ann. N.Y. Acad. Sci.,* **1973,** *215,* 177–182.

Turner, T. B.; Bennett, V. L.; and Hernandez, H. The beneficial side of moderate alcohol use. *Johns Hopkins Med. J.,* **1981,** *148,* 53–63.

Turner, T. B.; Mezey, E.; and Kimball, A. W. Measurement of alcohol-related effects in man: chronic effects in relation to levels of alcohol consumption. *Johns Hopkins Med. J.,* **1977,** *5,* 235–248, 273–286.

U.S. Department of Health, Education, and Welfare. *Alcohol and Health*. (Second and Third Special Reports to the Congress from the Secretary of Health, Education, and Welfare.) The Department, Washington, D. C., **1974, 1978.**

Vestal, R. E. Alcohol use as a health problem in aging: biological perspective. In, *Health and Behavior: A Research Agenda Interim Report*, No. 5. (Parron, D. L.; Solomon, F.; and Rodin, J.; eds.) National Academy Press, Washington, D.C., **1981**, pp. 41–45.

Wajda, I. J. Comparison of the effects of ethanol and those of opioid drugs on the metabolism of biogenic amines. In, *Biochemistry and Pharmacology of Ethanol*, Vol. 2. (Majchrowicz, E., and Noble, E. P., eds.) Plenum Press, New York, **1979**, pp. 187–295.

Wallgren, H. Effect of ethanol on intracellular respiration and cerebral function. In, *The Biology of Alcoholism*. Vol. 1, *Biochemistry*. (Kissin, B., and Begleiter, H., eds.) Plenum Press, New York, **1971**, pp. 103–125.

Wallgren, H., and Barry, H., III. *Actions of Alcohol*, Vols. I and II. American Elsevier Publishing Co., Inc., New York, **1970.**

Wartburg, J. P. von. The metabolism of alcohol in normals and alcoholics: enzymes. In, *The Biology of Alcoholism*. Vol. 1, *Biochemistry*. (Kissin, B., and Begleiter, H., eds.) Plenum Press, New York, **1971**, pp. 63–102.

Weitzman, E. D. Sleep and its disorders. *Annu. Rev. Neurosci.*, **1981**, *4*, 381–417.

CHAPTER
19 DRUGS AND THE TREATMENT OF PSYCHIATRIC DISORDERS

Ross J. Baldessarini

The use of drugs with well-demonstrated efficacy in psychiatric disorders has become widespread since the mid-1950s. Today, about 20% of prescriptions written in the United States are for medications intended to affect mental processes, namely, to sedate, stimulate, or otherwise change mood, thinking, or behavior. This practice reflects both the high frequency of primary emotional disorders and the nearly inevitable emotional, psychological, and social reactions of persons with medical illnesses. In addition, many drugs used for other purposes also modify emotions and cognition either as part of their usual actions or as toxic effects of overdosage. In this chapter, agents used primarily for the treatment of psychiatric disorders are discussed.

Other drugs may so alter the function of the central nervous system (CNS) as to warrant their designation as *psychotoxic*. These include useful substances with particular abuse liability (*e.g.*, opioids, sedatives, stimulants); agents without established therapeutic use, including many natural products that have arisen from popular or folk practices (*e.g.*, alcohol, coffee, tobacco, marihuana, hallucinogens); and agents with accepted medical indications that can produce psychiatric side effects (*e.g.*, antihypertensives, sedatives, stimulants, steroids, cardiac glycosides). Discussion of these agents is beyond the scope of this chapter, and the reader is referred to other sections dealing with CNS drugs and their potential behavioral toxicity. (*See* especially Chapter 23 and specialized reviews by Efron *et al.*, 1967; Shader, 1972; Usdin and Efron, 1972; Schultes, 1978.) Drugs used in the treatment of psychiatric disorders as well as psychotoxic agents are often collectively called *psychoactive* or *psychotropic*. Over 1500 compounds classified primarily as psychotropic agents have been described (Usdin and Efron, 1972; Usdin, 1978).

In the presentation of each drug group, a prototypical agent is sometimes used to exemplify the characteristics of the class. Important differences from the prototype are discussed when appropriate. An attempt is also made to define the characteristics of treatable conditions and to indicate how drugs are used in psychiatric patients. Although several alternative schemes exist, the psychotherapeutic agents described in this chapter are placed into three major categories. *Antipsychotic* or *neuroleptic* drugs are those used to treat the most severe psychiatric illnesses, the psychoses; they have beneficial effects on mood and thought but carry the risk of producing neurotoxic effects that mimic neurological diseases. *Mood-stabilizing* drugs (notably, lithium salts) and *antidepressants* (mood-elevating agents) are those used to treat affective disorders and related conditions. *Antianxiety-sedative* agents, particularly the benzodiazepines, are those used for the drug therapy of anxiety states.

The use of drugs in the treatment of psychiatric disorders is complicated by diagnostic uncertainties characteristic of clinical psychiatry. However, psychiatric diagnosis continues to gain objectivity, coherence, and reliability. The association between specific clinical syndromes and predictable responses to psychotropic drugs has supported the impressive recent progress in this area. Testable hypotheses about possible biological bases of severe psychiatric illnesses have been stimulated by knowledge of the mechanisms of action of psychotropic agents, assisted by the emergence of a medical discipline commonly known as *biological psychiatry*. Although there is sometimes disagreement among psychiatrists concerning diagnosis and the indications for various treatments, these uncertainties do not invalidate the many salutary effects of drugs on mental symptoms. The diagnostic terminology and criteria currently employed in the United States are well described in the *Diagnostic and Statistical Manual of Mental Disorders* of the American Psychiatric Association (1980).

History. Modification of behavior, mood, and emotion by drugs has always been a favorite indulgence of mankind. The use of psychoactive drugs evolved along two related paths. The first was in the use of drugs to modify normal behavior and to produce altered states of feeling for religious, ceremonial, or recreational purposes. The second was to alleviate mental ailments. A fascinating account of the early history and characteristics of many psychoactive compounds is presented by Lewin (1924). More modern reviews are those of Efron and associates (1967), Caldwell (1978), and Schultes (1978). In 1845, Moreau proposed that hashish intoxication provided a model psychosis useful in the study of insanity. Three decades later, Freud presented his study of cocaine and suggested its potential uses in pharmacotherapy. Soon thereafter, Kraepelin founded the first laboratory of clinical psychopharmacology in Dorpat. Later, in Munich he evaluated psychological effects of drugs in man. In 1931, Sen and Bose published the first report of the use of *Rauwolfia serpentina* in the treatment of insanity (*see* Shore and Giachetti, 1978). Insulin shock, pentylenetetrazol-induced convulsions, and electroconvulsive therapy followed in 1933, 1934, and 1937, respectively. Treatment of both major depression and schizophrenia thus became available. Amphetamine was the first synthetic drug to provide a model psychosis. In 1943, Hofmann purposefully ingested a minute amount of lysergic acid diethylamide (LSD) to experience its psychic effects. His report of the high potency of LSD made the concept that a toxic metabolic product might be the cause of mental illness more popular. Accounts of this and other early experiments in psychopharmacology have been presented by the original participants (*see* Ayd and Blackwell, 1970).

The first report on the treatment of psychotic excitement or mania with *lithium* was that of Cade (1949). This discovery was slow in gaining general acceptance by the medical community. In 1950, *chlorpromazine* was synthesized in France. The recognition of the unique effects of chlorpromazine by Laborit and colleagues (1952) and its use in psychiatric patients by Delay and Deniker (1952) marked the beginnings of modern psychopharmacology. The history of this revolutionary era in psychiatric therapy is recounted by Ayd and Blackwell (1970), Swazey (1974), and Caldwell (1978). The term *tranquilizer* was introduced in the early 1950s by Yonkman to characterize the psychic effect of reserpine. Despite its popularity, this ambiguous and misleading term is not used in this chapter.

A report on *meprobamate* by Berger (1954) marked the beginning of investigations of modern sedatives with useful antianxiety properties. An antitubercular drug, *iproniazid*, was introduced in the early 1950s and was soon recognized as a monoamine oxidase inhibitor and antidepressant (Kline, 1958; Crane, 1959); in 1958, Kuhn recog-

nized the antidepressant effect of *imipramine*. *Chlordiazepoxide*, the first of the antianxiety benzodiazepines, was developed by Sternbach in 1957. In the following year Janssen discovered the antipsychotic properties of *haloperidol*, a butyrophenone, and thus still another class of antipsychotic agents became available. During the 1960s there was a rapid expansion of psychopharmacological research, and many new theories of psychoactive drug effects were introduced. The clinical efficacy of many of these agents was firmly established during this decade.

In recent years, emphasis has centered on biogenic amines and their receptors in the CNS, their probable mediation of many effects of psychotropic drugs, and their possible causal involvement in mental illness. In addition, much attention is now being paid to the liabilities of treatment with psychotherapeutic drugs, especially their limited efficacy in severe or chronic mental illnesses, their risk of serious toxic effects, and the limitations of screening and testing methods used to develop new agents, most of which offer few advantages over drugs available for nearly 3 decades. A balanced view of their advantages and disadvantages is emerging. While not nearly the curative "wonder drugs" they promised to be initially, antipsychotic and antidepressant agents used to treat the most severe mental illnesses have had a remarkable impact on psychiatric practice and theory—an impact that can legitimately be called revolutionary.

Nosology.   The several classes of therapeutic psychotropic agents are fairly selective in their ability to modify the symptoms of mental illnesses. The optimal use of such drugs thus requires experience in the differential diagnosis of psychiatric conditions (American Psychiatric Association, 1980). A few salient aspects of psychiatric nosology are summarized briefly, and some further information is provided in the discussion of the specific classes of drugs.

A most important distinction is made between the *psychoses* and the less severe conditions commonly called the *neuroses* (or psychoneuroses). The psychoses are the most severe psychiatric disorders, in which there is not only a marked impairment of behavior but also a serious inability to think coherently, to comprehend reality, or to gain insight into the abnormality; these conditions often include *delusions* and *hallucinations*. The psychotic disorders include *organic* conditions (notably, *delirium* and *dementia*), which are typically associated with definable toxic, metabolic, or neuropathologic changes and are characterized by confusion, disorientation, and memory disturbances as well as behavioral disorganization, and *idiopathic* (or "functional") disorders, for which underlying causes remain obscure. The latter are characterized by the retention of orientation and memory in the presence of severely disordered emotion, thought, and behavior, except in unusually severe stuporous states sometimes encountered in these illnesses. Those primary disorders characterized by abnormal emotion or *mood* (disorders of *affect* with depression, dysphoria, elation, or mania) are called *major affective* or *manic-depressive* disorders (Winokur *et al.,* 1969; Pope and Lipinski, 1978; Baldessarini, 1983). These may ("bipolar" illnesses) or may not ("nonbipolar" illnesses) include periods of elation or excitement alternating with severe depression and autonomic changes, notably anergy, insomnia, anorexia, and altered daily rhythms of mood or activity. In addition, depression can occur as a milder disorder or as a symptom associated with other psychiatric or medical illnesses. The idiopathic psychoses characterized mainly by chronically disordered thinking and emotional withdrawal and often associated with paranoid delusions and auditory hallucinations are called *schizophrenia.* Acute idiopathic psychoses also occur that bear an uncertain relationship to schizophrenia or the major affective disorders. In addition, there are disorders marked by more or less isolated delusions; these may represent a separate category of illness called *delusional disorder* or *paranoia.*

Antipsychotic drugs exert beneficial effects in virtually all classes of psychotic illness, and, contrary to a common misconception, are *not* selective for schizophrenia. Moreover, antidepressant drugs that are especially beneficial in severe depression can also exert useful effects on less severe depressive syndromes and on conditions that are not obviously depressive in nature (*e.g.,* panic attacks, eating disorders, chronic pain, obsessive-compulsive disorders). Thus, in general, psychotropic drugs are not disease specific; they provide clinical benefit for specific syndromes or complexes of symptoms.

The less pervasive psychiatric disorders are the *neuroses.* While the ability to comprehend reality is retained, suffering and disability are sometimes very severe. Neuroses may be acute and transient or, more commonly, persistent or recurrent. They involve abnormal symptoms that may include mood changes (anxiety, panic, depression) or limited abnormalities of thought (obsessions, irrational fears) or of behavior (rituals or compulsions, pseudoneurological or "hysterical" conversion signs). In such disorders, drugs may have some beneficial effects for short periods, particularly by modifying associated anxiety and depression.

Other so-called characterological disorders may or may not respond to medical intervention; these conditions include characteristic personality styles (*e.g.,* paranoid, withdrawn, psychopathic, hypochondriacal) or behavior patterns (*e.g.,* abuse of alcohol or other substances, socially deviant or perverse behavior) that may run counter to societal expectations. Typically, drugs are not effective in such chronic conditions except when episodes of anxiety or depression occur or in cases of withdrawal from addicting substances (*see* Chapter 23).

Biological Hypotheses in Mental Illness. The introduction of relatively effective and selective drugs for the management of schizophrenic and manic-depressive patients in the 1950s encouraged formulation of biological concepts of the pathogenesis of these mental illnesses. This was followed by increased understanding of the actions of psychopharmacological agents. In addition, other agents were discovered that mimic some of the symptoms of severe mental illnesses. These include the induction of paranoid states by the abuse of amphetamines, the induction of hallucinations and altered emotional states by synthetic agents such as LSD or by natural products that can be formed in mammalian tissues (notably, N,N-dimethyltryptamine), and the occasional association of depression with antihypertensive agents (notably, reserpine and methyldopa) that alter the metabolism of biogenic amines in the CNS.

The leading hypothesis to arise from such considerations was based on data that indicated that antidepressants enhance the biological activity of monoamine neurotransmitters in the CNS and that antiadrenergic compounds may induce depression. It then seemed reasonable to speculate that a deficiency of amine neurotransmission in the CNS might be causative of depression or that an excess could result in mania. Further, since antipsychotic agents antagonize the actions of dopamine as a neurotransmitter in the forebrain, it was proposed that there may be a state of functional overactivity of dopamine in the limbic system or cortex in schizophrenia or mania. Alternatively, an endogenous psychotomimetic compound might be produced either uniquely or in excessive quantities in psychotic patients. This "pharmacocentric" approach to the construction of hypotheses is appealing in its seeming rationality, and it has gained abundant support from studies of the actions of antipsychotic and antidepressant drugs over the past 3 decades. In turn, the plausibility of such biological hypotheses has encouraged interest in genetic and family studies, as well as in clinical and biochemical studies. Despite extensive efforts, the attempts to document metabolic changes in human subjects predicted by these hypotheses have not, on balance, provided consistent or compelling corroboration (Matthysse and Sugarman, 1978; Murphy *et al.,* 1978; Praag, 1978; Baldessarini, 1983). Simultaneously, genetic studies have provided evidence that inheritance can account for only a *portion* of the causation of mental illnesses, leaving room for environmental and psychological hypotheses. Thus, the hopes of the 1950s and 1960s for the discovery of clearly defined, genetically determined inborn errors of metabolism to explain psychiatric disease have not been realized.

Moreover, there may be an oversimplification in the attempt to formulate hypotheses about the causes of mental illness from the tenets of psychopharmacology. Thus, it was commonly hoped that knowledge of the mechanisms of action of antipsychotic or antidepressant drugs would point the way to the discovery of underlying pathophysiological changes in schizophrenia or manic-depressive illness that are functionally opposite to the effects of the drugs. This has not proven to be the case.

The antipsychotic, antimanic, and antidepressant drugs have effects on cortical, limbic, hypothalamic, and brain stem mechanisms that are of fundamental importance for the regulation of arousal, consciousness, affect, and autonomic functions. It is entirely possible that physiological and pharmacological modification of these brain regions might have important behavioral consequences and useful clinical effects regardless of the fundamental nature or cause of the mental disorder in question. Moreover, the relatively poor temporal correlations between the known effects of most psychotropic drugs, which for the most part occur rapidly, and their clinical effects suggest that secondary or even more indirect changes brought about by the drugs may mediate their clinical actions.

Even if the most generous interpretations of the actions of psychotropic drugs could be taken to provide insights into the clinical pathophysiology or the etiology of mental illnesses, many other serious problems remain. They include biological heterogeneity, even within groups of the most carefully diagnosed patients. In addition, the already discussed lack of disease specificity of psychotropic drugs tends to minimize the chances of finding a discrete metabolic correlate for a specific disease. Finally, the technical problems associated with attempts to study changes in the metabolism or the post-mortem chemistry of the human CNS are awesome. Among these are artifacts introduced by drug treatment itself.

Nevertheless, the efforts of the past 3 decades have not been without reward. Thus, the introduction of pharmacologically oriented hypotheses concerning biological bases of the serious mental illnesses has encouraged critical research in psychiatry. These efforts have led to marked improvements in clinical investigative technics, fostered improved methods of differential diagnosis, and encouraged difficult and sophisticated genetic and family studies (such as natural "cross-fostering" experiments among adopted children as a method of separating genetic and environmental influences). In short, psychiatry has drawn closer to the mainstream of modern medicine. Much of the research in this complex field has been reviewed critically elsewhere, starting with a masterful critique by Kety in 1959. (More recent articles on research in schizophrenia and manic-depressive illness are listed under Monographs and Reviews at the end of this chapter.)

In *summary*, the available information does not permit a conclusion as to whether crucial, discrete biological lesions are the basis of the most severe mental illnesses (other than the deliria and dementias). Moreover, it is not necessary to presume that such a basis is operative in order to provide effective treatment for psychiatric patients with medications. Furthermore, it would be clinical folly to underestimate the importance of psychological and social factors in the manifestations of mental illnesses or to overlook psychological aspects of the conduct of biological therapies (Baldessarini, 1985).

Animal Experiments and Psychopharmacology. Because the essential characteristics of human mental disorders cannot be reproduced in animals, studies of etiology and treatment are greatly hampered. In man, psychiatric illness can manifest itself by disturbances in interpersonal relationships and communication. Internal conflict, anxiety, and depression are often revealed only through verbalization. Cognition, communication, and social structure in subhuman animals are difficult to compare with human achievements in this area. Although the study of animal behavior has not yet yielded much information concerning the mode of action of drugs in abnormal human behavior, such studies have led to screening procedures for the selection of drugs in the treatment of mental illness. The usefulness of many compounds in the treatment of psychiatric disorders was discovered fortuitously in patients receiving them for other purposes. However, many psychiatrically useful phenothiazines and drugs such as haloperidol, chlordiazepoxide, and others were discovered by means of animal screening technics. Once a therapeutically useful drug has been found, its properties in animal and other laboratory tests can be ascertained and new compounds with similar actions can be synthesized. The chance of discovering a unique therapeutic agent with this method is small, but variations in efficacy and toxicity may be found.

Clinical Evaluation of Psychotropic Drugs. Although there are problems in the evaluation of the efficacy of any drug, the difficulties in evaluating psychoactive drugs are particularly severe. Assessment of change and improvement in psychiatric illness has never been easy. The most striking example of this problem is found in literature concerning the efficacy of psychotherapy. Although psychotherapy seems to have salutary effects in individual patients, few studies have demonstrated this in a scientifically acceptable way. The problem should be simpler in the evaluation of pharmacotherapy, for here one presumes that the agent is uniform and administered to all patients in the same way. Unfortunately, results are still frequently equivocal. Evaluation of new psychotropic agents presents additional problems, which include the tendency to "rediscover" agents with actions and limitations similar to those of older agents and the ethical issues raised by conducting placebo-controlled trials in seriously ill subjects. The latter factor may account for an emphasis on studies that compare a new agent with a standard drug without a placebo control group. Reviews of the principles and problems in establishing the efficacy and safety of psychotropic drugs are available (Levine *et al.,* 1971;

Hardesty and Burdock, 1978; Baldessarini, 1983, 1985).

The discussions of psychotropic drugs in the following sections place major emphasis on the results of carefully controlled studies whenever these are available. Unfortunately, in many areas adequately controlled studies have never been done. Since the literature is so vast, reference is often made to review articles. As with all classes of drugs, the prudent physician will employ only a limited number of proven agents and become thoroughly familiar with their use.

I. Drugs Used in the Treatment of Psychoses

Several classes of drugs are effective in the symptomatic treatment of psychoses. They are most appropriately used in the therapy of schizophrenia, organic psychoses, the manic phase of manic-depressive illness, and other acute idiopathic psychotic illnesses. Their occasional use may be indicated in depression or in severe anxiety. These classes include compounds such as the phenothiazines, the structurally similar thioxanthenes, and the dibenzodiazepines and dibenzoxazepines; butyrophenones (phenylbutylpiperidines) and the newer diphenylbutylpiperidines; indolones and other heterocyclic compounds; and the rauwolfia alkaloids and related synthetic heterocyclic amine-depleting agents. Since these chemically dissimilar drugs share many properties, information about their pharmacology and clinical uses will be presented for the group as a whole. Particular attention will be paid to chlorpromazine, the oldest representative of the phenothiazine-thioxanthene class of drugs, and haloperidol, the original butyrophenone and representative of several related classes of aromatic butylpiperidine derivatives.

The use of these antipsychotic agents is extremely widespread, as is evident from the fact that hundreds of millions of patients have been treated with them since their introduction in the 1950s. While the antipsychotic drugs have had a revolutionary, beneficial impact on medical and psychiatric practice, their liabilities, especially their almost relentless association with ex-trapyramidal neurological effects, must also be emphasized (*see* Marsden *et al.*, 1975; Baldessarini *et al.*, 1980). The antipsychotic effects of these drugs appear to be unique; in the present chapter, they will be referred to as antipsychotic or neuroleptic agents.

PHENOTHIAZINES AND OTHER ANTIPSYCHOTIC AGENTS

The phenothiazines as a class, and especially chlorpromazine, the prototype, are among the most widely used drugs in medical practice. Chlorpromazine and the many other related agents that have been developed in the last 3 decades are primarily employed in the management of patients with serious psychiatric illnesses. In addition, many members of the group have other clinically useful properties, including antiemetic, antinausea, and antihistaminic effects and the ability to potentiate analgesics, sedatives, and general anesthetics; many of these actions are discussed elsewhere in this text (*see* Index). At the present time, there are more than 30 phenothiazine drugs that are used in psychiatric conditions and still others that are primarily intended for other uses.

History. The history of the antipsychotic agents is especially well summarized by Swazey (1974) and Caldwell (1978). Historical precedence should be given to the introduction of lithium salts for mania in 1949 (*see* page 427), and even earlier to the description of hypotensive and sedating properties of *Rauwolfia* plant extracts in the Indian medical literature (Sen and Bose, 1931; Shore and Giachetti, 1978). Plant products have been a part of Hindu medicine since ancient times, but there was little interest in their systematic use in Western psychiatry until the 1950s. In the early 1950s, some encouraging results were obtained with natural extracts of *Rauwolfia* and then with pure *reserpine,* which was isolated, characterized, and synthesized by Woodward. While reserpine and related compounds that share its ability to deplete monoamines from their vesicular storage sites in neurons exert antipsychotic effects, these are relatively weak and are typically associated with severe side effects, including profound hypotension, excessive salivation, diarrhea, and sedation. Thus, the clinical utility of reserpine is primarily as an antihypertensive agent (*see* Chapters 9 and 32).

Phenothiazine compounds were synthesized in Europe in the late nineteenth century as part of the development of aniline dyes such as methylene blue. In the late 1930s a derivative of phenothiazine, promethazine, was found to have antihistaminic properties and a strong sedative effect. Attempts to treat agitation in psychiatric patients with promethazine and other antihistamines followed in the period 1940–1950, but with little success.

Meanwhile, the ability of promethazine to prolong barbiturate sleeping time in rodents was discovered, and the drug was introduced into clinical anesthesia as a potentiating agent (Laborit *et al.*, 1952). This work prompted a search for other phenothiazine derivatives with anesthesia-potentiating actions as well as greater central activities, and in 1949–1950 Charpentier synthesized chlorpromazine. Soon thereafter, Laborit and colleagues described the ability of this compound to potentiate anesthetics and produce "artificial hibernation." They noted that chlorpromazine by itself did not cause a loss of consciousness but produced only a tendency to sleep and a lack of interest in what was going on. These central actions became known as *ataractic* or *neuroleptic* soon thereafter.

Courvoisier and associates (1953) described an amazingly large number of actions manifested by chlorpromazine. These included gangliolytic, adrenolytic, antifibrillatory, antiedematous, antipyretic, antishock, anticonvulsant, and antiemetic properties. In addition, chlorpromazine was found to enhance the activity of a number of analgesic and central depressant drugs.

The first attempts to treat mental illness with chlorpromazine alone were made in Paris in 1951 and early 1952 by Paraire and Sigwald. In 1952, Delay and Deniker began their important early work with chlorpromazine. They were convinced that chlorpromazine achieved more than symptomatic relief of agitation or anxiety and that it had an ameliorative effect upon psychotic processes with diverse symptomatology. In 1954, Lehmann and Hanrahan reported, for the first time in North America, the use of chlorpromazine in the treatment of psychomotor excitement and manic states. Subsequently, the drug was released for marketing in the United States. Clinical studies soon revealed that the most important use of chlorpromazine was in the treatment of psychotic states.

In the years that followed, a large number of structural analogs of chlorpromazine and other more novel compounds were prepared, tested on animal behavior, and reached clinical trial or application. Particularly important in this regard was the research of Janssen (1974), who worked in the late 1950s in Belgium with a series of derivatives of normeperidine in the hope of developing an improved analgesic agent. He found that propiophenones had analgesic effects, but that the addition of one methylene group to produce a butyrophenone led either to unexpected neuroleptic effects in animals or to a mixture of analgesic and neuroleptic effects. Modification of the butyrophenone structure led to virtually pure neuroleptic activity with potency seen previously only with some piperazine phenothiazines or thioxanthenes. The first of these new substances to be made available for clinical use in psychiatry was haloperidol (1958).

Chemistry and Structure-Activity Relationship. This topic has been reviewed by Zirkle and Kaiser (1970) and, more recently, by Biel and coworkers (1978). Phenothiazine has a three-ring structure in which two benzene rings are linked by a sulfur and a nitrogen atom (*see* Table 19–1, page 403). If the nitrogen at position 10 is replaced by a carbon atom with a double bond to the side chain, the compound becomes a thioxanthene. Other modifications of the middle ring have included substitution of a nitrogen atom for the sulfur in position 5 and a carbon atom for the nitrogen at position 10 to yield the still-experimental *acridanes,* such as clomacran.

Substitution of an electron-withdrawing group at position 2 (but not positions 3 or 4) increases the efficacy of phenothiazines and other tricyclic congeners. The nature of the substituent at position 10 also influences pharmacological activity. As can be seen in Table 19–1 (page 403), the phenothiazines and thioxanthenes can be divided into groups on the basis of substitution at this site. The group with an *aliphatic* side chain includes chlorpromazine and triflupromazine among the phenothiazines; these compounds are relatively low in potency (but *not* in clinical efficacy). A second group, with similar or somewhat greater potency, contains a *piperidine* moiety in the side chain; it includes thioridazine, mesoridazine, and piperacetazine. There appears to be a lower incidence of extrapyramidal side effects with this substitution, at least in the case of thioridazine, possibly due to increased antimuscarinic activity. The most potent phenothiazine and thioxanthene antipsychotic compounds are those of a third group, which have a *piperazine* (or piperazinyl) group; fluphenazine is an example. Use of these potent compounds entails a greater risk of inducing acute extrapyramidal effects but less tendency to produce sedation or autonomic side effects such as hypotension, unless unusually large doses are employed. Several piperazine phenothiazines and thioxanthenes have been esterified with long-chain fatty acids (enanthic [heptanoic] or decanoic) to produce slowly absorbed and hydrolyzed, long-acting, lipophilic prodrugs. Fluphenazine enanthate and decanoate are the only such derivatives currently available in the United States; the decanoate of haloperidol is in advanced clinical trials.

The thioxanthenes are similarly available with aliphatic and piperazine substituents; piperidines are not available. The analog of chlorpromazine among the thioxanthenes is chlorprothixene. The piperazine-substituted thioxanthenes include clopenthixol, flupentixol, and thiothixene; they are all highly potent and effective antipsychotic agents, although to date only thiothixene is available in the United States. Since thioxanthenes have an olefinic double bond between the central-ring carbon atom at position 10 and the side chain, geometric isomers exist; the *cis* (or α) isomers are the more active.

All of the phenothiazines and thioxanthenes used in psychiatry have three carbon atoms interposed between position 10 of the central ring and the first amino nitrogen atom of the side chain at this position; in addition, the amine is always tertiary. This structure of neuroleptic compounds contrasts with that of antihistaminic phenothiazines (*e.g.*, promethazine) or strongly anticholinergic phenothiazines (*e.g.*, ethopropazine, diethazine), which have only two carbon atoms separating the amino group from position 10 of the central ring; addition of a fourth carbon atom similarly results in a loss of neuroleptic activity. When one or two of the methyl or other substituents of the tertiary amino group of the side chain are removed (as can occur in the natural metabolism of chlorpromazine), there is an increasing loss of activity; in addition, increasing the size of amino N-alkyl substituents leads to a reduction of activity.

The structure-activity relationship has also been studied in detail for butyrophenones and their congeners. More than 20 of these compounds have been prepared and characterized; many have been used in clinical trials, for the most part in Europe. The largest group of butyrophenones includes substituted piperidine compounds that are analogs of haloperidol. Among these is spiperone, one of the most potent neuroleptics yet discovered. In addition, there are several investigational piperazine-substituted butyrophenones and a short-acting tetrahydropyridine derivative, droperidol, which is used almost exclusively in anesthesia.

More recently a second and closely related family of interesting drugs has been developed, the *diphenylbutylpiperidines*. These compounds include pimozide, fluspirilene, and penfluridol; pimozide was approved recently for general use in the United States. These agents are both extraordinarily potent and very long acting (several days to a week or more) even after *oral* administration, unlike any other type of neuroleptic agent. Further discussion of the structure-activity relationship of the butyrophenones and diphenylbutylpiperidines can be found in the review articles cited above.

Several other classes of heterocyclic compounds have neuroleptic or antipsychotic effects, but too few are available or sufficiently well characterized to permit conclusions regarding structure-activity relationship. These include a small number of *indole* compounds (notably, molindone and oxypertine) and several piperazine-substituted tricyclic compounds with various seven-membered central rings. These latter agents bear some resemblance to the imipramine-like antidepressant drugs and include *dibenzoxazepines* (notably, loxapine, a typical neuroleptic) and *dibenzodiazepines* (notably, clozapine, a most interesting antipsychotic agent that seems to have minimal central antidopaminergic activity; although the clinical utility of clozapine may be limited by sedative and antimuscarinic activity and a possible capacity to cause bone-marrow toxicity, other congeners, such as fluperlapine, are in clinical trials).

Other heterocyclic compounds include butaclamol, a pentacyclic compound with active (dextrorotatory) and inactive enantiomeric forms that have been useful in characterization of the stereochemistry of the sites of action of neuroleptic agents. Sulpiride is one of a series of substituted *benzamides* (which includes metoclopramide) with some neuroleptic activity. However, their hydrophilic properties may account for their limited penetration into the CNS and their low potency. The availability of drugs such as clozapine, sulpiride, and, to some

extent, thioridazine is encouraging, since they represent at least partial exceptions to the formerly almost-inevitable association of neurotoxic with antipsychotic effects.

PHARMACOLOGICAL PROPERTIES

The antipsychotic drugs share many pharmacological effects and therapeutic applications. Chlorpromazine is commonly taken as a prototype for the group. Many antipsychotic drugs, and especially chlorpromazine and other agents of low potency, have sedative effects. These are especially conspicuous early in treatment, although tolerance to this effect is typical; sedation may not be noticeable when very agitated psychotic patients are treated. Antipsychotic drugs also have antianxiety effects. However, this class of agents is not generally used for such a purpose, largely because of their neurological and autonomic side effects.

The term *neuroleptic,* which was introduced to characterize the effects of chlorpromazine and reserpine on psychiatric patients, was intended to contrast the effects of these agents with those of classical CNS depressants such as the general anesthetics, sedatives and hypnotics, and opioids. The neuroleptic syndrome consists in suppression of spontaneous movements and complex behavior, while spinal reflexes and unconditioned nociceptive-avoidance behaviors remain intact. In man, the neuroleptic drugs reduce initiative and interest in the environment, and they reduce displays of emotion or affect. Initially, there may be some slowness in response to external stimuli and drowsiness. However, subjects are easily aroused, capable of giving appropriate answers to direct questions, and seem to have intact intellectual functions; there is no ataxia, incoordination, or dysarthria at ordinary doses. Psychotic patients become less agitated and restless, and withdrawn or autistic patients sometimes become more responsive and communicative. Aggressive and impulsive behavior diminishes. Gradually (usually over a period of days), psychotic symptoms of hallucinations, delusions, and disorganized or incoherent thinking tend to disappear. In addition, early clinical reports of the effects of chlorpromazine described neurological effects, including bradykinesia, mild rigidity, some tremor, and occasional subjective restlessness (akathisia), that resemble those of Parkinson's disease (paralysis agitans). Formerly, some clinicians believed that the neurological and antipsychotic actions were inevitably, and perhaps causally, associated and even advocated their provocation as a test of the effectiveness of treatment.

While the original use of the term *neuroleptic* appears to have encompassed the whole unique syndrome just described, and to this day is commonly used as a synonym for *antipsychotic* in Europe, there is now a tendency to use the term *neuroleptic* to emphasize the more neurological aspects of the syndrome (*i.e.,* the extrapyramidal, parkinsonian effects) and to consider these as nonessential and undesirable. The description of drugs such as clozapine that are clearly antipsychotic and have little extrapyramidal action has reinforced this trend. At the present time, virtually all of the drugs with antipsychotic activity that are available in the United States also have effects on movement and posture and can thus be called neuroleptic. However, the more general and hopeful term *antipsychotic* is commonly used and may be preferable.

General Psychophysiological and Behavioral Effects.   In animals and in man, the most prominent observable effects of typical neuroleptic agents are strikingly similar. In low doses, operant behavior is reduced but spinal reflexes are unchanged. Exploratory behavior is diminished, and responses to a variety of stimuli are fewer, slower, and smaller, although the ability to discriminate stimuli is retained. Conditioned avoidance behaviors are selectively inhibited, while unconditioned escape or avoidance responses are not. The highly reinforcing self-stimulation of the animal brain (typically with electrodes placed in the monoamine-rich median forebrain bundle) is blocked, although the capacity to press the stimulation-inducing lever is not lost. Behavioral activation, stimulated environmentally or pharmacologically, is blocked. Feeding is inhibited. Most neuroleptics block the emesis and aggression induced by

apomorphine—a dopaminergic agonist. In high doses, most neuroleptic agents induce characteristic cataleptic immobility that allows the animal to be placed in abnormal postures that persist. Muscle tone is altered, and ptosis is typical. The animal appears to be indifferent to most stimuli, although it continues to withdraw from those that are noxious or painful. Many learned tasks can still be performed if sufficient stimulation and motivation are provided. Even very high doses of most neuroleptics do not induce coma, and the lethal dose is extraordinarily high. Many of these effects are well summarized by Fielding and Lal (1978).

Effects on Motor Activity.   Nearly all of the neuroleptic agents used in psychiatry can diminish spontaneous motor activity in every species of animal studied, including man. However, one of the more disturbing side effects of chlorpromazine, *akathisia,* is manifested by an increase in restless activity (page 405). The cataleptic immobility of animals treated with phenothiazines, described above, resembles the *catatonia* seen in some psychotic patients and in a variety of metabolic and neurological disorders affecting the CNS. In man, catatonic signs, along with other features of schizophrenia, are sometimes relieved by antipsychotic agents. However, rigidity and bradykinesia, which can mimic catatonia, can be induced in patients, especially by large doses of the more potent neuroleptic agents, and reversed by removal of the drug or the addition of an antiparkinsonian agent (*see* Fielding and Lal, 1978; Janssen and Van Bever, 1978).

Chlorpromazine causes skeletal muscular relaxation in some types of spastic conditions. Since it has little effect at spinal levels, actions on motor activity must be mediated at a higher level, perhaps in the basal ganglia. The drug does not produce blockade of the neuromuscular junction.

Phenothiazines and other antipsychotic drugs often produce parkinsonism and other extrapyramidal effects. Theories concerning the mechanisms underlying these extrapyramidal reactions, as well as descriptions of their clinical presentations and management, are given below.

Effects on Sleep. The effect of antipsychotic drugs on sleep patterns is not consistent, but they tend to normalize sleep disturbances characteristic of many psychoses. The ability to prolong and enhance the effect of opioid and hypnotic drugs appears to parallel the sedative rather than the neuroleptic potency of the particular agent. Thus, the more potent neuroleptic agents that do not cause drowsiness also do not enhance hypnosis produced by other drugs.

Effects on Conditioned Responses. Chlorpromazine impairs the ability of animals to make a conditioned avoidance response to a learned sensory cue that signals the onset of punishing shock avoidable by moving to a safe place in an experimental chamber. Under the influence of small doses of the drug, animals ignore the warning signal but still attempt to escape once the shock is applied. General CNS depressants, including barbiturates, and meprobamate affect both avoidance (the conditioned response) and escape (the unconditioned response) to approximately the same extent, and only in doses that produce ataxia or hypnosis. Many variations on this paradigm utilize operant conditioning technics in which the avoidance behavior requires bar pressing, which can be evaluated quantitatively and automatically. Passive avoidance behavior, requiring immobility, is also suppressed by neuroleptic drugs, in contrast to what might be expected in the case of drugs that suppress locomotion nonspecifically.

Since correlations between antipsychotic effectiveness and conditioned avoidance tests are quite good for many types of neuroleptic agents, they have become an important basis for screening procedures in pharmaceutical psychopharmacology laboratories. Despite their empirical utility and quantitative characteristics, effects on conditioned avoidance have not provided important insights into the basis of antipsychotic effects in man. For example, the effects of neuroleptic drugs on conditioned avoidance are subject to tolerance and are blocked by anticholinergic agents, while their clinical antipsychotic actions are not. Moreover, the extraordinarily close correlation between the potencies of drugs in

conditioned avoidance tests and their ability to block the behavioral effects of dopaminergic agonists such as amphetamine or apomorphine suggests that such avoidance tests may be specifically *selective* for drugs with extrapyramidal and other neurological effects. The inability of the atypical and more selective antipsychotic drugs, such as clozapine and sulpiride, to antagonize dopamine agonists or to block conditioned avoidance responses in animal behavioral tests also supports this interpretation. (*See* Barchas *et al.,* 1978; Fielding and Lal, 1978; Janssen and Van Bever, 1978.)

Effects on Complex Behavior. Antipsychotic drugs impair vigilance in human subjects performing a variety of tasks, such as continuous rotor-pursuit and tapping-speed tests. The drugs produce relatively little impairment of digit-symbol substitution, a test of intellectual functioning. On the other hand, secobarbital causes greater impairment in performance in digit-symbol substitution than in continuous performance and other vigilance tests. In normal subjects, neuroleptic agents of low potency may inhibit the performance of complex intellectual tasks such as story writing, but such experiments are difficult to design and interpret.

Effects on Specific Areas of the Nervous System. The effects of antipsychotic drugs are apparent at all levels in the nervous system. Although the actions underlying the antipsychotic and many of the neurological effects of antipsychotic drugs remain unknown, theories based on their ability to antagonize the actions of dopamine as a neurotransmitter in the basal ganglia and limbic portions of the forebrain have become most prominent and are supported by a large body of data.

Cortex. Since psychosis involves a disorder of higher functions and thought processes, cortical effects of antipsychotic drugs are of great interest. Much attention has been drawn to the effects of neuroleptics on dopaminergic projections to the mesiofrontal and deep-temporal (limbic) regions of the cerebral cortex and to the relative sparing of these areas from adaptive changes in dopamine metabolism that are suggestive of tolerance to actions of neuroleptics. However, there is little information available about specific effects on the cortex that sheds light on the mechanisms of action of antipsychotic drugs.

EEG. When neuroleptic drugs are given to animals, there is slowing and decreased variability of frequencies (*synchronization*) and a decrease in arousal-induced changes in the EEG; these effects are reversed by dopaminergic agonists, which also tend to induce arousal and desynchronization of the EEG (Longo, 1978). Similarly, when chlorpromazine is administered to man, there is a slowing of the EEG, with an increase in the occurrence of theta waves and, to a lesser degree, delta waves, a decrease in alpha waves and fast-beta activity, and some increase in burst activity and spiking (*see* Itil, 1978). The increased synchronization is accompanied by an increase in voltage. There is also a reduction of the arousing effects of sensory stimuli (*e.g.*, blocking of alpha rhythm). Studies on the effects of antipsychotic drugs on sensory-evoked EEG potentials have usually suggested either decreases in amplitudes and increases in latencies or a tendency toward "normalization" of aberrant responses, perhaps especially in patients who respond favorably to treatment (Shagass and Straumanis, 1978).

Seizure Threshold. Many neuroleptic drugs can lower the seizure threshold and induce discharge patterns in the EEG that are associated with epileptic seizure disorders. Aliphatic phenothiazines with low potency (particularly chlorpromazine) seem particularly able to do this, while the more potent neuroleptic piperazine phenothiazines and thioxanthenes (notably, fluphenazine and thiothixene) seem least likely to have this effect (Itil, 1978). The butyrophenones have variable and unpredictable effects on seizure activity; molindone may have the least activity of this type among neuroleptic agents. Overt seizures associated with the administration of antipsychotic drugs are more likely to be seen in patients who have either a history of epilepsy or a condition that predisposes to seizures. Neuroleptic agents, especially low-potency phenothiazines and thioxanthenes, should be used with *extreme caution*, if at all, in untreated epileptic patients and in patients undergoing withdrawal from central depressants such as alcohol or barbiturates. Antipsychotic drugs, especially the piperazines, can be used safely in epileptics if moderate doses are attained gradually and if concomitant anticonvulsant drug therapy is maintained (*see* Chapter 20).

Basal Ganglia. Because the extrapyramidal effects of nearly all of the clinically used antipsychotic drugs are prominent, a great deal of interest has centered on the actions of these drugs in the basal ganglia, notably the caudate nucleus, putamen, globus pallidus, and allied nuclei, which are believed to play a crucial role in the control of posture and the involuntary (extrapyramidal) aspects of movement. Current understanding of the role of a deficiency of dopamine in this region in the pathogenesis of Parkinson's disease, the modest success of levodopa or dopaminergic agonists (apomorphine, bromocriptine) in treating this disease, and the striking resemblance between the clinical manifestations of Parkinson's disease and the neurological effects of neuroleptic drugs have all focused attention on the possible role of a deficiency of dopamine activity in neuroleptic-induced extrapyramidal effects.

The hypothesis that interference with the transmitter function of dopamine in the mammalian forebrain might contribute to the neurological and possibly also the antipsychotic effects of the neuroleptic drugs arose from observations that neuroleptic drugs consistently increased the concentrations of the metabolites of dopamine, but had variable effects on the metabolism of other neurotransmitters. The importance of dopamine was also supported by histochemical studies, which indicated a preferential distribution of dopamine-containing fibers between midbrain and the basal ganglia (notably, the nigroneostriatal tract), and within the hypothalamus (*see* Chapters 12 and 21). Other dopamine-containing neurons project from midbrain tegmental nuclei to forebrain regions associated with the limbic system, as well as to temporal and mesio-prefrontal cerebral cortical areas closely interlinked with the limbic system. A somewhat simplistic, but attractive, concept arose: many extrapyramidal neurological effects of the antipsychotic drugs might be mediated by antidopaminergic effects in the basal ganglia. Their antipsychotic effects might be mediated by antagonism of dopaminergic neurotransmission in the limbic, mesocortical, and hypothalamic systems.

A compelling body of data has accumulated to support the theory that antagonism of dopamine-mediated synaptic neurotransmission is an important action of neuroleptic drugs (Carlsson, 1978; Creese *et al.,* 1978; Baldessarini and Tarsy, 1979). Thus, antipsychotic drugs with neuroleptic actions, but not their inactive congeners, increase the rate of production of dopamine metabolites (notably, 3-methoxytyramine and dihydroxyphenylacetic and homovanillic acids), the rate of conversion of the precursor amino acid tyrosine to dopamine and its metabolites (Sedvall, 1975), and the rate of firing of putative dopamine-containing cells in the midbrain (Bunney *et al.,* 1973). These effects have usually been interpreted to represent adaptive responses of neuronal systems that would reduce the impact of the presumed interruption of synaptic transmission at dopaminergic terminals in the caudate nucleus and other areas of the forebrain. Supporting evidence for such an interpretation includes observations that small doses of neuroleptic drugs block behavioral or neuroendocrine effects of dopaminergic agonists. Examples are stereotypical gnawing behavior in the rat induced by apomorphine; locomotor excitement induced by the injection of dopamine into limbic terminal fields, such as the nucleus accumbens septi; and the inhibition of prolactin secretion by apomorphine or levodopa, believed to be mediated by receptors for dopamine on mammotropic cells of the anterior pituitary. Notably, atypical antipsychotic drugs such as clozapine are characterized by their very weak actions or inactivity in such tests.

Neuroleptic drugs inhibit a dopamine-sensitive adenylate cyclase system in homogenates of caudate or limbic tissue (Clement-Cormier *et al.*, 1974) and interfere with electrophysiological responses to dopamine or apomorphine applied iontophoretically to receptive cells in the caudate nucleus. This latter effect can be overcome by the iontophoresis of analogs of adenosine 3',5'-monophosphate (cyclic AMP) (Siggins *et al.*, 1976), presumably by circumventing the blockade of receptor sites on the cell surface.

Radioligand-binding assays for dopaminergic receptors have also been employed. These assays use membrane fractions from mammalian caudate tissue as a source of receptors and tritiated neuroleptic drugs (particularly haloperidol or spiperone) or dopaminergic agonists as ligands (*see* Creese *et al.*, 1978; Snyder *et al.*, 1978). The correlation is generally excellent between the potency *in vitro* of antipsychotic drugs of *all types* to interfere with the binding of these ligands and estimates of their clinical potency or of their ability to block the effects of dopaminergic agonists in animals (Creese *et al.*, 1978). Analogs and isomers of the antipsychotic drugs that are inactive clinically lack the ability to compete for relevant ligand binding sites. This correlation is best with respect to a subset of dopaminergic receptor sites (D_2) (*see* Chapter 12).

Together, these findings strongly support the theory that antipsychotic drugs interfere with the actions of dopamine as a neurotransmitter. At the same time, they do not prove that antidopaminergic effects are either necessary or sufficient to account for the diverse extrapyramidal effects of the neuroleptic drugs, let alone their antipsychotic actions.

Limbic System. Dopaminergic projections from the midbrain terminate on septal nuclei, the olfactory tubercle, the amygdala, and other structures within the temporal and prefrontal lobes of the cerebrum. Because of the dopamine hypothesis just reviewed, much attention has also been given to the mesolimbic and mesocortical systems as possible sites of mediation of at least some of the antipsychotic effects of these agents. Speculations about the pathophysiology of the idiopathic psychoses such as schizophrenia have centered around the limbic area for many years. These have been given some indirect encouragement by repeated "natural experiments" that have associated psychotic mental phenomena with lesions of the temporal lobe and other portions of the limbic

system (*see* Meltzer and Stahl, 1976; Barchas *et al.*, 1978).

Many of the behavioral, neurophysiological, biochemical, and pharmacological findings about the dopaminergic system of the basal ganglia have been extended to mesolimbic and mesocortical tissue. Certain of the effects of antipsychotic drugs are very similar in extrapyramidal and limbic regions, including those on ligand-binding assays for dopaminergic receptors (Creese *et al.*, 1978). However, there are a number of differences in the extrapyramidal and antipsychotic actions of the neuroleptic drugs. For example, while several of the acute extrapyramidal effects of the neuroleptic drugs tend to diminish or to disappear with time or when anticholinergic drugs are administered concurrently, neither of these is characteristic of the antipsychotic effects. This difference may be accounted for by observations that suggest that not all dopaminergic systems are similar, either functionally or in their manner of physiological regulation of response to drugs (*see* Bunney and Aghajanian, 1978; Moore and Kelly, 1978; Sulser and Robinson, 1978). For example, while anticholinergic agents block the increase in turnover of dopamine in the basal ganglia induced by neuroleptic agents, they seem not to do so in limbic areas containing dopaminergic terminals. Further, the development of tolerance to the effect of antipsychotic drugs to enhance the turnover of dopamine is not as prominent in limbic as in extrapyramidal areas. For further discussions of this topic, *see* Carlsson (1978) and other references already cited.

Hypothalamus. In addition to neurological and antipsychotic effects that appear to be mediated in part by antidopaminergic actions of the neuroleptic drugs, there are endocrine changes that have been related to effects of these agents on the hypothalamus or pituitary that may also involve dopamine. Prominent among these is the ability of most neuroleptic drugs to increase the rate of secretion of prolactin in man.

The effect of neuroleptic agents on prolactin secretion is probably due to a blockade of the tuberoinfundibular dopaminergic system that projects from the arcuate nucleus of the hypothalamus to the median eminence by a direct antagonistic action at dopaminergic receptors localized on cells of the anterior pituitary. The existence of dopaminergic receptors in the pituitary itself, as well as morphological evidence of an intimate relationship between dopamine-containing neurosecretory terminals in the median eminence and the small blood vessels of the hypophyseal portal system, supports the hypothesis that dopamine is the prolactin release-inhibiting hormone known to exist in the hypothalamus (*see* Reichlin and Boyd, 1978; Chapter 59).

Correlations between the potencies of neuroleptic drugs to stimulate prolactin secretion and to cause behavioral effects are excellent in both animals and man. They prevail for many classes of drugs (Meltzer et al., 1978; Sachar, 1978). There are, however, a few discrepancies. The effects of neuroleptic drugs on prolactin secretion tend to occur at lower doses than do their antipsychotic effects; this may reflect their action outside the blood-brain barrier in the inferior hypothalamus or in the pituitary gland. There is little or no tolerance to the effect of antipsychotic drugs on prolactin, even after years of treatment. However, the effect is rapidly reversible when the drugs are discontinued (Overall, 1978). It seems likely that this effect of antipsychotic agents is responsible for the breast engorgement and galactorrhea that is sometimes associated with their use, even in male patients.

The effects of neuroleptics on other hypothalamic neuroendocrine functions are much less well characterized, although they do inhibit the release of growth hormone (Martin et al., 1978) and chlorpromazine may reduce the secretion of corticotropin-regulatory hormone in response to stress (Frohman, 1972). In addition to neuroendocrine effects, it is likely that the other autonomic effects of some antipsychotic drugs may be mediated by the hypothalamus. An important example is the *poikilothermic effect* of chlorpromazine, which is sometimes used to facilitate the induction of surgical hypothermia.

Brain Stem. Ordinarily clinical doses of the neuroleptics have little effect upon *respiration*. However, *vasomotor reflexes* mediated by either the hypothalamus or the brain stem are depressed by relatively low doses of chlorpromazine. This effect might occur at many points in the reflex pathway, and the net result is a centrally mediated fall in blood pressure. Even when there is acute overdosage with suicidal intent, the phenothiazines usually do not cause life-threatening coma or suppression of vital functions; this contributes importantly to their safety.

Chemoreceptor Trigger Zone (CTZ). Most neuroleptic agents have a marked protective action against the nausea- and emesis-inducing effects of apomorphine and certain ergot alkaloids, all of which can interact with central dopaminergic receptors in the CTZ of the medulla. The antiemetic effect of most neuroleptics occurs with very low doses. However, thioridazine, uniquely, has no clinical efficacy as an antiemetic in man. Drugs or other stimuli that cause emesis by an action on the nodose ganglion or locally on the gastrointestinal tract are not antagonized by antipsychotic drugs, but potent piperazines and butyrophenones are sometimes effective against nausea due to vestibular stimulation. Several antipsychotic agents have become especially popular for the treatment of nausea and vomiting (*see* below).

Spinal Cord. For the antipsychotic drugs as a group, the current consensus is that depressant actions on the spinal cord are minor, if present at all, and contribute little to the actions of these drugs.

Peripheral Nerves. Chlorpromazine is an effective local anesthetic, but the drug is not used for this purpose. Indeed, most of the antipsychotic drugs and even their clinically ineffective congeners exert local anesthetic or so-called membrane-stabilizing effects, especially at high concentrations (typically above 10 μM); these probably have little to do with the important actions of the drugs (Seeman, 1972; *see also* Creese et al., 1978).

Autonomic Nervous System. Since various antipsychotic agents have peripheral cholinergic blocking activity, α-adrenergic blocking actions, and adrenergic activity (secondary to the block of neuronal re-uptake of amines), their effects on the autonomic nervous system are complex and unpredictable. Antihistaminic and antitryptaminergic effects of these agents further complicate the picture.

Chlorpromazine does have significant α-adrenergic antagonistic activity and can either block or reverse the pressor effects of epinephrine. Based on the extent of antagonism of the effects of norepinephrine *in vivo* and competition for binding sites with radioligands selective for α-adrenergic receptors, the relative potencies of several antipsychotic drugs as α-adrenergic antagonists can be ranked as follows: relatively strong (piperacetazine > droperidol > triflupromazine > chlorpromazine); moderate (thioridazine > fluphenazine > haloperidol); relatively weak (trifluoperazine > clozapine ≫ pimozide). Since piperazines and haloperidol are used in low doses to produce antipsychotic effects, it follows that they should show little antiadrenergic activity in patients; indeed, this seems to be true (*see* Creese et al., 1978; Janssen and Van Bever, 1978; Snyder et al., 1978).

The cholinergic blocking effects of antipsychotic drugs are relatively weak, but the blurring of vision commonly experienced with chlorpromazine may be due to an anticholinergic action on the ciliary muscle. Chlorpromazine regularly produces miosis in man, which can be due to α-adrenergic blockade. Other phenothiazines can cause mydriasis, and this is especially likely to occur with thioridazine, which is the most potent muscarinic antagonist of the group. Chlorpromazine has intermediate antimuscarinic potency and can cause constipation and decreased gastric secretion and motility. Doses of 1 to 3 mg/kg can block the effects of physostigmine on intestinal tone and peristalsis, presumably as a result of cholinergic blockade. Decreased sweating and salivation are probably additional manifestations of the anticholinergic effects of the phenothiazines. Urinary retention is rare, but can occur in males with prostatism. Anticholinergic effects are least frequently caused by piperazines and other potent neuroleptics, including haloperidol (*see* Snyder et al., 1978). The anticholinergic status of clozapine remains controversial. It is very potent in several tests *in vitro* but does not seem to be active *in vivo* (*see* Carlsson, 1978).

The phenothiazines inhibit ejaculation without interfering with erection. Thioridazine produces this effect with some regularity, sometimes limiting its acceptance by male patients. Attribution of this effect to adrenergic blockade is logical but unsubstantiated inasmuch as thioridazine is less potent than chlorpromazine in its antiadrenergic effects.

For further discussion of the autonomic pharmacology of the phenothiazines, the exhaustive monographs by Gordon (1967, 1974) should be consulted. Reviews by Sigg (1968), Shader and DiMascio (1970), and Klein and colleagues (1980) also describe the autonomic side effects of numerous psychotropic drugs.

Endocrine System. The effects of neuroleptic drugs on hypothalamic regulatory hormones result in profound changes in the endocrine system, as mentioned above with respect to increased secretion of prolactin. Chlorpromazine can also reduce urinary concentrations of gonadotropins, as well as those of estrogens and progestins. As a result of these derangements, galactorrhea and gynecomastia can occur. Amenorrhea is also seen with chlorpromazine, but relatively infrequently. In animals, the drug can block ovulation, suppress the estrous cycle, cause infertility and pseudopregnancy, and maintain an endometrial decidual reaction. Inhibition of secretion of gonadotropin also can decrease testicular weight.

Since antipsychotic drugs are used chronically and thus cause prolonged elevations of concentrations of prolactin, there has been concern over a possible increased risk of carcinoma of the breast. To date, there is no evidence that the use of antipsychotic agents entails this risk (Overall, 1978; Schyve *et al.*, 1978). Nevertheless, neuroleptic and other agents that stimulate the secretion of prolactin should be avoided in patients with established carcinoma of the breast.

Nonreproductive endocrinological functions are also affected. Chlorpromazine may cause a decrease in the secretion of adrenocorticosteroids as a result of diminished release of corticotropin. It interferes with the secretion of pituitary growth hormone, an effect utilized for a while in the treatment of acromegaly. Neuroleptics are in fact poor therapy for acromegaly (Dimond *et al.*, 1973). There is no evidence that they retard growth or development of children. In addition, chlorpromazine can decrease the secretion of neurohypophyseal hormones. Weight gain and an increase in appetite occur with all phenothiazines but not with haloperidol. Chlorpromazine may also impair glucose tolerance and insulin release to a clinically appreciable degree in some "prediabetic" patients (Erle *et al.*, 1977); however, this effect is not known to occur with other neuroleptic agents. Peripheral edema occurs in 1 to 3% of patients and may be of endocrine origin.

Kidney. Chlorpromazine may have weak diuretic effects in animals and man, due either to a depressant action upon the secretion of antidiuretic hormone (ADH) or to inhibition of reabsorption of water and electrolytes by a direct action on the renal tubule, or both. The slight fall in blood pressure that occurs with chlorpromazine is not associated with a significant change in glomerular filtration rate; indeed, there is a tendency toward an increase in renal blood flow.

Cardiovascular System. The actions of chlorpromazine on the cardiovascular system are complex because the drug produces direct effects on the heart and blood vessels, and also indirect ones through actions on CNS and autonomic reflexes. In normal man, the intravenous administration of chlorpromazine causes *orthostatic hypotension,* due to a combination of central actions and peripheral α-adrenergic blockade, and reflex *tachycardia.* Oral therapy causes mild hypotension, systolic blood pressure being affected more than diastolic. Tolerance develops to the hypotensive effect, so that after several weeks of chronic administration the pressures return toward normal (Sakalis *et al.,* 1972). However, some degree of orthostatic hypotension may persist indefinitely. The orthostatic hypotension occurs more frequently with chlorpromazine and thioridazine, and less so with piperazine derivatives, haloperidol, loxapine, and molindone. Chlorpromazine also has a direct depressant action on the heart; cat papillary muscle shows a negative inotropic response to relatively low concentrations of chlorpromazine. The drug has a vasodilating action due to both its effects on the autonomic nervous system and a direct action on blood vessels; it may increase coronary blood flow.

Chlorpromazine has an antiarrhythmic effect upon the heart, which may be due either to a quinidine-like action or to a local anesthetic effect. ECG changes include prolongation of the Q-T and P-R intervals, blunting of T waves, and depression of the S-T segment. Thioridazine, in particular, causes a high incidence of T wave changes. Cardiotoxicity of a more severe nature has been reported in young patients (Alexander and Nino, 1969). These effects are uncommon when potent antipsychotic agents are administered.

Liver. Aside from the hypersensitivity reactions occasionally seen after administration of the antipsychotic drugs, such as an obstructive form of jaundice (*see* below), these agents have no characteristic hepatic effects. The drugs may be used in patients with hepatic disease, but caution is advisable. Since their metabolism may be delayed or modified, they may compromise an already diseased liver.

Miscellaneous Pharmacological Effects. There are reports of interactions of antipsychotic drugs with central neurohumors other than dopamine that may contribute to their antipsychotic effects or other actions (*see* Carlsson, 1978). For example, many neuroleptics enhance the turnover of acetylcholine, especially in the basal ganglia, perhaps secondary to the blockade of dopamine receptors on cholinergic neurons. In addition, as already discussed above, there is an inverse relationship between antimuscarinic potency of antipsychotic drugs in the brain and the likelihood of extrapyramidal effects (Snyder *et al.*, 1978). Although chlorpromazine and a few other low-potency phenothiazines have mild antagonistic actions at receptors for histamine and 5-hydroxytryptamine (5-HT), these effects are not shared by all antipsychotic drugs and are unlikely to contribute in an important way to their major actions.

Absorption, Fate, and Excretion. The study of the pharmacokinetics and metabolism of the antipsychotic drugs is an active aspect of their evaluation, although few conclusions with clinical relevance can be drawn. This situation is due in part to limitations of the laboratory technics involved, the complex metabolism of some antipsychotic agents, and, very importantly, inadequate attention to crucial clinical pharmacological aspects of the experimental design in many published reports on the topic (Cohen, 1984).

A few generalizations can be made. Most antipsychotic drugs tend to have erratic and unpredictable patterns of absorption, particularly with oral administration and even when liquid preparations are used. Parenteral (intramuscular) administration can increase the availability of active drug by four to ten times. The drugs are highly lipophilic, highly membrane or protein bound, and accumulate in the brain, lung, and other tissues with a high blood supply; they also enter the fetal circulation quite easily. It is virtually impossible (and usually not necessary) to remove these agents by dialysis.

The pharmacokinetics of antipsychotic drugs follows a multiphasic pattern. The usually stated elimination half-lives with respect to total concentrations in plasma are typically 20 to 40 hours. The biological effects of single doses usually persist for at least 24 hours; this encourages the common practice of giving the entire daily dose at one time, once the patient has accommodated to the initial side effects of the drug. Elimination from the plasma may be more rapid than from sites of high lipid content and binding, notably in the CNS. Direct pharmacokinetic studies on this issue are few and inconclusive. Nevertheless, metabolites of some agents have been detected in the urine for as long as several months after the drug has been discontinued. Slow removal of drug may contribute to the typically slow rate of exacerbation of psychosis after stopping drug treatment. Repository preparations of esters of neuroleptic drugs are absorbed and eliminated much more slowly than are oral preparations. For example, whereas half of an oral dose of fluphenazine hydrochloride is eliminated in about 20 hours, a depot of the enanthate or the decanoate ester requires 2 to 3 or 7 to 10 days, respectively. It is important to realize that the elimination of neuroleptics is much slower than that of antiparkinsonian compounds commonly administered concurrently to treat extrapyramidal effects. Thus, simultaneous interruption of the administration of both types of agents increases the risk of acute extrapyramidal reactions.

The main routes of metabolism of the antipsychotic drugs are by oxidative processes mediated largely by hepatic microsomal and other drug-metabolizing enzymes. Conjugation with glucuronic acid is a prominent route of metabolism. Hydrophilic metabolites of these drugs are excreted in the urine and, to some extent, in the bile. Most oxidized metabolites of antipsychotic drugs are also biologically *inactive*, but a few are not (notably, 7-hydroxychlorpromazine, mesoridazine, and several N-demethylated metabolites) and may contribute to the biological activity of the parent substance, as well as complicate the problem of correlating assays of drug in blood with clinical effects. A biological assay which detects active metabolites that can compete for binding of a radioligand may help to simplify this problem (*see* Creese *et al.*, 1978). The less potent antipsychotic drugs may induce their own hepatic metabolism or conjugation, since concentrations of chlorpromazine and other phenothiazines in blood are lower after several weeks of treatment with the same dosage; it is also possible that alterations of gastrointestinal motility are partially responsible. The fetus, the infant, and the elderly have diminished capacity to metabolize and eliminate antipsychotic agents;

children tend to metabolize these drugs more rapidly than do adults (Morselli, 1977; Popper, 1985).

The pharmacokinetics of antipsychotic drugs has been reviewed by Cooper and associates (1976), Morselli (1977), May and Van Putten (1978), Baldessarini (1984b), and Cohen (1984).

Detailed comments on the pharmacokinetics can be offered for only a few agents, such as chlorpromazine, that have been well studied. However, the complex metabolism of chlorpromazine limits its usefulness as a model agent (*see* May and Van Putten, 1978). The absorption of tablets of chlorpromazine is erratic, although the bioavailability seems to be increased somewhat by the use of liquid concentrates, as is true for many of the antipsychotic agents. However, these preparations tend to be expensive and inconvenient to use. Peak concentrations in plasma are attained in about 2 to 4 hours. Intramuscular administration of the drug avoids much of the first-pass metabolism in the liver (and possibly also the gut) and provides measurable concentrations in plasma within 15 to 30 minutes; bioavailability may be increased up to tenfold, but the clinical dose usually decreases by three- to fourfold. The gastrointestinal absorption of chlorpromazine is modified unpredictably by food and is probably decreased by antacids. There is controversy as to whether the concurrent administration of anticholinergic antiparkinsonian agents diminishes the intestinal absorption of some neuroleptic agents (Simpson *et al.*, 1980). Chlorpromazine and other antipsychotic agents bind significantly to membranes and to plasma proteins. Typically, over 85% of the drug in plasma is bound to albumin. Concentrations of some neuroleptics (*e.g.*, haloperidol) in brain can be up to ten times those in the blood, and their apparent volume of distribution may be as high as 20 liters per kilogram. Disappearance of chlorpromazine from plasma includes a rapid distribution phase ($t_{1/2}$ about 2 hours) and a slower elimination phase ($t_{1/2}$ about 30 hours), but markedly variable values have been reported; the half-life of elimination from human brain is unknown.

Attempts to correlate plasma concentrations of chlorpromazine or of its metabolites with clinical responses have not been especially successful until recently (*see* Cooper *et al.*, 1976; May and Van Putten, 1978; Cohen, 1984). They indicate that wide variations (at least tenfold) in plasma concentrations occur among individuals. These are not eliminated by controlling the dose, timing, and prior exposure to the drug, suggesting that individual genetic determinants may be responsible. Although it appears that plasma concentrations of chlorpromazine below 30 ng/ml are not likely to produce an adequate antipsychotic response and that levels above 750 ng/ml are likely to be associated with unacceptable toxicity (*see* Rivera-Calimlin and Hershey, 1984), it is not yet possible to state the concentrations in plasma that are likely to be associated with optimal clinical responses.

There may be as many as 10 or 12 metabolites of chlorpromazine that occur in man in *appreciable* quantities (Morselli, 1977). The most important metabolites, quantitatively, are nor$_2$-chlorpromazine (doubly demethylated), chlorophenothiazine (removal of entire side chain), methoxy and hydroxy products, and glucuronide conjugates of the hydroxylated compounds. In the urine, 7-hydroxylated and dealkylated (nor$_2$) metabolites and their conjugates predominate.

There is less information about other antipsychotic drugs. Thioridazine has been studied relatively well (Gottschalk *et al.*, 1975). Its pharmacokinetics and metabolism are similar to those of chlorpromazine, but the strong anticholinergic action of thioridazine on the gut may modify its own absorption. Major metabolites include sulfoxy products at ring-position 5 (inactive) or at the substituent at position 2 (including the *active* metabolite, mesoridazine). Demethylation of the piperidine ring is very rapid, but the activity of this metabolite is unknown. It is known that concentrations of thioridazine in plasma are relatively high (100s of nanograms per milliliter), possibly due to its relative hydrophilicity, and it is suspected that mesoridazine is an important contributor to neuroleptic activity.

The thioxanthenes are similar to chlorpromazine, except that metabolism to sulfoxides is common and ring-hydroxylated products are uncommon. Piperazine derivatives of the phenothiazines and thioxanthenes are also handled much like chlorpromazine, although metabolism of the piperidine ring itself occurs. Haloperidol and other butyrophenones are metabolized by an N-dealkylation reaction; the resultant fragments can be conjugated with glucuronic acid, and it is believed that all of the metabolites of haloperidol are inactive (Forsman and Öhman, 1974), with the possible exception of a reduced (but otherwise intact) metabolite (Korpi *et al.*, 1983). Typical plasma concentrations of haloperidol that are encountered clinically are about 10 to 15 ng/ml.

Tolerance and Physical Dependence. The antipsychotic drugs are not addicting, as the term is defined in Chapter 23. However, some degree of physical dependence may occur. There are reports of muscular discomfort and difficulty in sleeping that develop several days after abrupt discontinuation. EEG changes upon sudden withdrawal have not been detected. Monkeys given the human equivalent of nearly 600 mg of chlorpromazine daily for over a month showed no obvious withdrawal symptoms when the drug was discontinued.

Tolerance develops to the sedative effects of chlorpromazine and other phenothiazines over a period of days or weeks. Tolerance to antipsychotic drugs and cross-tolerance among the agents are also demonstrable in behavioral and biochemical experiments in animals, particularly those directed toward evaluation of the blockade of dopaminergic receptors in the basal ganglia (*see* Baldessarini and Tarsy, 1979). This form of tolerance may be less prominent in limbic and cortical areas of forebrain. One correlate of tolerance in forebrain dopaminergic systems is the development of *disuse supersensitivity* of those systems, possibly mediated by changes in the receptors for the neurotransmitter. This mechanism may underlie the clinical phenomenon of *withdrawal-emergent dyskinesias* (choreoathetosis on abrupt discontinuation of antipsychotic agents, especially following prolonged use of high doses of potent agents) (Baldessarini *et al.*, 1980). Although there may be cross-tolerance among neuroleptic drugs for some effects, clinical problems occur in making rapid changes from high doses of one type of agent to another; sedation, hypotension, and other autonomic effects or acute extrapyramidal reactions can result.

Preparations, Routes of Administration, and Dosage. Since there are a large number of agents with known neuroleptic or antipsychotic effects, Table 19–1 summarizes only those that are currently marketed in the United States. A few available agents are excluded that are now known to have inferior antipsychotic effects or that are no longer commonly used in psychiatric patients. These include promazine (SPARINE) and reserpine and other rauwolfia alkaloids. Prochlorperazine (COMPAZINE) has questionable utility as an antipsychotic agent and produces acute extrapyramidal reactions frequently; it is thus not commonly employed in psychiatry, although it is used as an antiemetic. An agent deserving of specific comment is thiethylperazine (TORECAN), which is currently marketed only as an antiemetic, although it is a potent dopaminergic antagonist with many neuroleptic-like properties; at high doses it is an efficacious antipsychotic agent (Rotrosen *et al.*, 1978). The United States has been slow to accept many psychotropic agents that are in common use in other countries; thus, there are many more thioxanthenes, butyrophenones, diphenylbutylpiperidines, and long-acting repository preparations of neuroleptic agents available in Europe.

Toxic Reactions and Side Effects. The antipsychotic drugs have a high therapeutic index and are remarkably safe agents. Fur-

thermore, most phenothiazines have a relatively flat dose-response curve and they can be used over a wide range of dosages. Although occasional deaths from overdosage have been reported, this is a rare event if the patient is given medical care and if an overdosage is not complicated by the concurrent ingestion of alcohol or other drugs. Based on animal data, the therapeutic index is lowest for thioridazine (20) and chlorpromazine (200) and is in excess of 1000 for the more potent agents (Janssen and Van Bever, 1978). Adult patients have survived doses of chlorpromazine up to 10 g, and deaths due to haloperidol appear to be unknown.

Side effects are often extensions of the many pharmacological actions of the drugs, which have already been discussed. The most important are those on the *CNS, cardiovascular system, autonomic nervous system,* and *endocrine functions.* The *extrapyramidal effects,* which are of great importance, are discussed in detail below (*see also* Shader and DiMascio, 1970). Other dangerous effects are agranulocytosis and pigmentary degeneration of the retina, both of which are extremely rare (*see* below).

Therapeutic doses of phenothiazines may cause faintness, palpitation, nasal stuffiness, dry mouth, blurred vision, some slight constipation, and, in males with prostatism, urinary retention. The patient may complain of being cold, drowsy, or weak. The most troublesome side effect is *orthostatic hypotension,* which may result in syncope. A fall in blood pressure is most likely to occur from administration of the phenothiazines with aliphatic side chains. Congeners of the piperazine type, as well as other potent neuroleptic agents, produce less hypotension and may be used when this side effect is to be avoided. A mild elevation of temperature may be seen during the first few days, particularly if the drug is given parenterally. On the other hand, hypothermia can occur and may be due both to the action on the heat-regulating center and to direct peripheral vasodilatation. Sensitivity and adaptation to changes of environmental temperature are impaired so that fatal hyperthermia and heat stroke are possible complications.

Table 19–1. SELECTED ANTIPSYCHOTIC DRUGS: CHEMICAL STRUCTURES, DOSES, DOSAGE FORMS, AND SIDE EFFECTS [1]

NONPROPRIETARY NAME / TRADE NAME	DOSE AND DOSAGE FORMS [2]			SIDE EFFECTS		
Phenothiazines 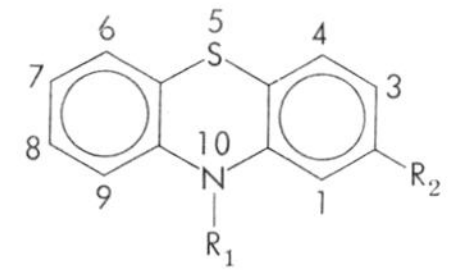	Antipsychotic Dose Range— Daily Dosage		Single Intramuscular Dose [3]	Sedative Effects	Extra-pyramidal Effects	Hypotensive Effects
	Usual (mg)	Extreme [4] (mg)	(mg)			
Chlorpromazine hydrochloride —(CH$_2$)$_3$—N(CH$_3$)$_2$ R_1; —Cl R_2 THORAZINE	300–800	25–2000 O,SR,L,I,S	25–50	+++	++	I.M. +++ Oral ++
Triflupromazine hydrochloride —(CH$_2$)$_3$—N(CH$_3$)$_2$ —CF$_3$ VESPRIN	100–150	25–300 L,I	20–60	++	+++	++
Mesoridazine besylate —(CH$_2$)$_2$ (piperidine N—CH$_3$) —SCH$_3$ ‖ O SERENTIL	75–300	25–400 O,L,I	25	+++	+	++
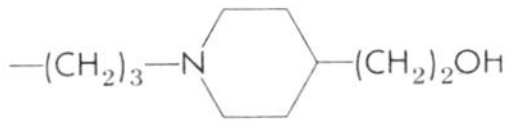 Piperacetazine —(CH$_2$)$_3$—N (piperidine)—(CH$_2$)$_2$OH —COCH$_3$	20–160	5–200 O		++	++	+
Thioridazine hydrochloride —(CH$_2$)$_2$ (piperidine N—CH$_3$) —SCH$_3$ MELLARIL	200–600	20–800 O,L		+++	+	++
Acetophenazine maleate —(CH$_2$)$_3$—N(piperazine)N—(CH$_2$)$_2$—OH —COCH$_3$ TINDAL	60–120	20–600 O		++	++	+
Fluphenazine hydrochloride Fluphenazine enanthate Fluphenazine decanoate 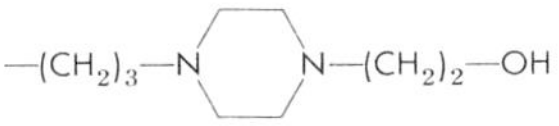 —(CH$_2$)$_3$—N(piperazine)N—(CH$_2$)$_2$—OH —CF$_3$ PERMITIL and PROLIXIN (HYDROCHLORIDES) (PROLIXIN ENANTHATE) and DECANOATE)	1–20	0.5–30 O,L,I	1.25–2.5 (decanoate or enanthate: 12.5–50 every 1–3 weeks)	+	+++	+

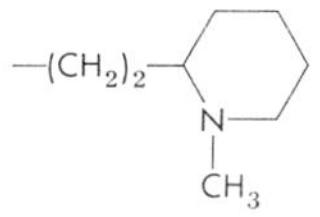

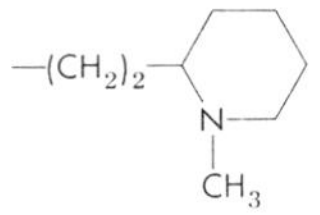

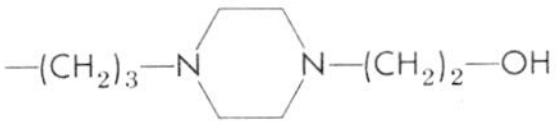

NONPROPRIETARY NAME	TRADE NAME	DOSE AND DOSAGE FORMS [2]			SIDE EFFECTS		

Phenothiazines

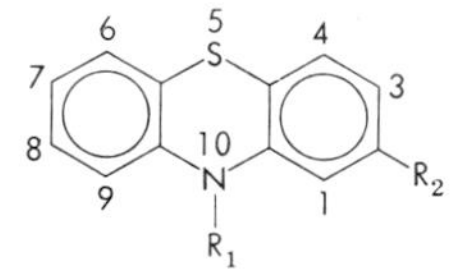

R₁ / R₂		Antipsychotic Dose Range— Daily Dosage		Single Intramuscular Dose [3]	Sedative Effects	Extra-pyramidal Effects	Hypotensive Effects
		Usual (mg)	Extreme [4] (mg)	(mg)			
Perphenazine 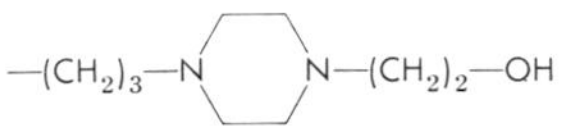 —(CH₂)₃—N⟩N—(CH₂)₂—OH TRILAFON	—Cl	8–32	4–64	5–10	++	++	+
		O,SR,L,I					
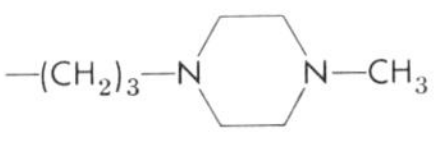 Trifluoperazine hydrochloride —(CH₂)₃—N⟩N—CH₃ STELAZINE	—CF₃	6–20	2–60	1–2	+	+++	+
		O,L,I					

Thioxanthenes [5]

R₁ / R₂		Antipsychotic Dose Range— Daily Dosage		Single Intramuscular Dose [3]	Sedative Effects	Extra-pyramidal Effects	Hypotensive Effects
		Usual (mg)	Extreme [4] (mg)	(mg)			
Chlorprothixene 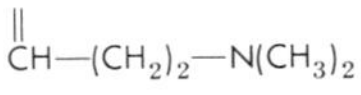 ‖ CH—(CH₂)₂—N(CH₃)₂ TARACTAN	—Cl	50–400	30–600	25–50	+++	++	++
		O,L,I					
Thiothixene hydrochloride ‖ CH(CH₂)₂—N⟩N—CH₃ NAVANE	—SO₂ | N(CH₃)₂	6–30	6–60	2–4	+ to ++	++	++
		O,L,I					

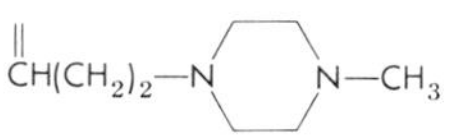

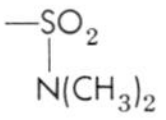

Other Heterocyclic Compounds

Haloperidol 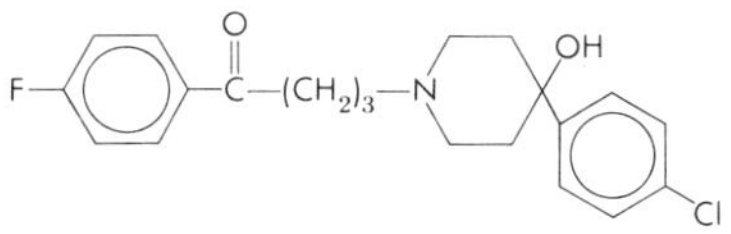 HALDOL		6–20	1–100	2–5	+	+++	+
		O,L,I					
Loxapine succinate 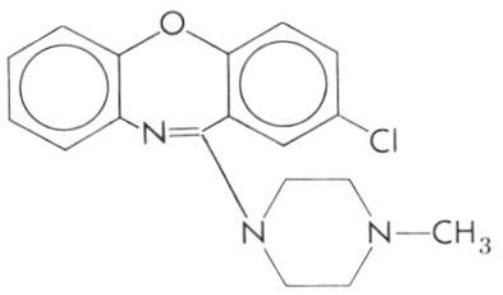 LOXITANE		60–100	20–250	12.5–50	+	++	+
		O,L,I					

Table 19–1.   SELECTED ANTIPSYCHOTIC DRUGS: CHEMICAL STRUCTURES, DOSES, DOSAGE FORMS, AND SIDE EFFECTS [1] **(Continued)**

NONPROPRIETARY NAME	TRADE NAME	DOSE AND DOSAGE FORMS [2]			SIDE EFFECTS		
Other Heterocyclic Compounds		*Antipsychotic Dose Range— Daily Dosage*	*Single Intramuscular Dose* [3]		*Sedative Effects*	*Extra- pyramidal Effects*	*Hypotensive Effects*
Molindone hydrochloride		Usual (mg)	Extreme [4] (mg)	(mg)			
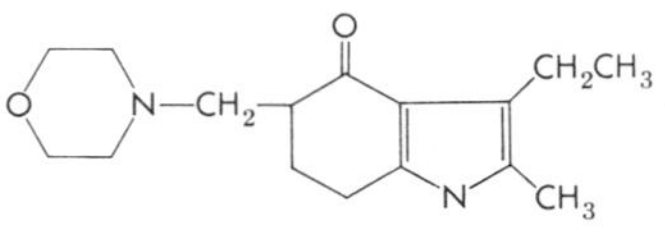		50–100	15–225		++	+	0
MOBAN			O,L				

[1] Antipsychotic agents for use in children under age 12 years include chlorpromazine, chlorprothixene (>6 years), thioridazine, and triflupromazine (among agents of low potency); and fluphenazine (not intramuscular), perphenazine, prochlorperazine, and trifluoperazine (>6 years) (among agents of high potency). Haloperidol has also been used extensively in children. *See* page 411.

[2] Dosage forms are indicated as follows: O = oral solid; L = oral liquid; SR = oral, sustained release; I = injection; S = suppository.

[3] Except for the enanthate and decanoate forms of fluphenazine, dosage can be given intramuscularly up to every 6 hours for agitated patients. Haloperidol decanoate is being used experimentally at intervals of 3 to 4 weeks, intramuscularly. Haloperidol lactate has been given intravenously in small doses; this is experimental.

[4] Extreme dosage ranges are occasionally exceeded cautiously and only when other appropriate measures have failed.

[5] Carbon replaces nitrogen in position 10 of the general formula for the phenothiazines.

Neurological Side Effects of Neuroleptic Drugs. A variety of neurological syndromes, involving particularly the extrapyramidal system, occur following the use of almost all antipsychotic drugs. These reactions are particularly prominent during treatment with the high-potency neuroleptic agents (tricyclic piperazines and butyrophenones). There is less likelihood of acute extrapyramidal side effects with thioridazine and with several other agents (notably, clozapine, fluperlapine, and sulpiride) that are not available in the United States. Neurological effects associated with antipsychotic drugs are described in detail by Marsden and associates (1975), Baldessarini and coworkers (1980), and Baldessarini (1984b).

There are probably six varieties of extrapyramidal syndromes associated with the use of antipsychotic drugs. Four of these usually appear concomitantly with the administration of the drug, and two are late-appearing syndromes that occur following prolonged treatment for many months or years. The clinical features of these syndromes and guidelines for their management are summarized in Table 19–2.

A *parkinsonian syndrome* that may be indistinguishable from idiopathic parkinsonism may develop during administration of antipsychotic drugs. Its incidence varies with different agents (Table 19–1), and in some patients it may not be seen at all. Clinically, there is a generalized slowing of volitional movement (akinesia) with mask facies and a reduction in arm movements. The most noticeable signs are *rigidity* and *tremor at rest*, especially involving the upper extremities. "Pill-rolling" movements may be seen, although this is not as prominent in neuroleptic-induced as in idiopathic parkinsonism. Parkinsonian side effects may be mistaken for depression since the flat facial expression and retarded movements resemble signs of depression. This reaction is usually managed by use of either antiparkinsonian agents with anticholinergic properties or amantadine; the use of levodopa incurs the risk of inducing agitation and worsening of the psychotic illness (*see* Chapter 21).

A rarer syndrome, *neuroleptic malignant syndrome,* resembles a very severe form of parkinsonism with catatonia, additional signs of autonomic instability (labile pulse and blood pressure, hyperthermia), stupor, and sometimes myoglobinemia. In its most severe form, this syndrome may persist for more than a week after stopping the offending agent. Since there is a high mortality (over 10%), immediate medical attention is required. This reaction has been associated with various types of neuroleptics, but its prevalence may be greater when relatively high doses of the more potent agents are used. Aside from immediate cessation of neuroleptic treatment and provision of supportive care, specific treatment is unsatisfactory; it has been suggested that administration of dantrolene or the dopaminergic agonist bromocriptine may be helpful (Caroff, 1980). While dantrolene is also used to manage a similar reaction to general anesthetics, there is no evidence that the neuroleptic-induced form of catatonia and hyperthermia is associated with a defect in calcium metabolism in skeletal muscle (Caroff *et al.*, 1983; *see also* Chapter 14).

Another extrapyramidal effect seen during antipsychotic drug therapy is *akathisia.* This term re-

Table 19–2. NEUROLOGICAL EFFECTS OF NEUROLEPTIC DRUGS

REACTION	FEATURES	TIME OF MAXIMAL RISK	PROPOSED MECHANISM	TREATMENT
Acute dystonia	Spasm of muscles of tongue, face, neck, back; may mimic seizures; *not* hysteria	1 to 5 days	Unknown	Many treatments can alter, but effects of antiparkinsonian agents are diagnostic and curative [1]
Parkinsonism	Bradykinesia, rigidity, variable tremor, mask facies, shuffling gait	5 to 30 days	Antagonism of dopamine	Antiparkinsonian agents helpful [2]
Malignant syndrome	Catatonia, stupor, fever, unstable blood pressure, myoglobinemia; can be fatal	Weeks; can persist for days after stopping neuroleptic	Antagonism of dopamine may contribute	Stop neuroleptic immediately; dantrolene or bromocriptine may help; [3] antiparkinsonian agents not effective
Akathisia	Motor restlessness; *not* anxiety or "agitation"	5 to 60 days	Unknown	Reduce dose or change drug; antiparkinsonian agents, [2] benzodiazepines, or propranolol [4] may help
Tardive dyskinesia	Oral-facial dyskinesia; widespread choreoathetosis	After months or years of treatment (worse on withdrawal)	Excess function of dopamine hypothesized	Prevention crucial; treatment unsatisfactory
Perioral tremor ("rabbit" syndrome)	Perioral tremor (may be a late variant of parkinsonism)	After months or years of treatment	Unknown	Antiparkinsonian agents often help [2]

[1] Many drugs have been claimed to be helpful for acute dystonia. Among the most commonly employed treatments are diphenhydramine hydrochloride, 25 or 50 mg intramuscularly, or benztropine mesylate, 1 or 2 mg intramuscularly or slowly intravenously, followed by oral medication with the same agent for a period of days to perhaps several weeks thereafter.

[2] For details regarding the use of oral antiparkinsonian agents, *see* the text and Chapter 21.

[3] Despite the response to dantrolene, there is no evidence of an abnormality of calcium transport in skeletal muscle; with lingering neuroleptic effects, bromocriptine may be tolerated in large doses (over 10 mg per day).

[4] Propranolol is often effective in relatively low doses (20 to 60 mg per day). Selective β_1-adrenergic antagonists are less effective.

fers to strong subjective feelings of distress or discomfort, often referred to the legs, as well as to a compelling need to be in constant movement rather than to any specific movement pattern. The patient feels that he must get up and walk or continuously move about, and he may be unable to keep this under control. Akathisia can be mistaken for agitation in psychotic patients; the distinction is critical, since agitation might be treated appropriately with an increase in dosage. Parenteral administration of benztropine sometimes allows a differential diagnosis between the two conditions, inasmuch as psychotic agitation usually does not respond to this drug; however, in most cases, the clinical response is equivocal. Due to the frequently unsatisfactory response of akathisia to antiparkinsonian or other drugs, treatment typically requires reduction of antipsychotic drug dosage. Antianxiety agents may help partially, and moderate doses of propranolol have been reported to be very beneficial in some

cases (Lipinski *et al.*, 1984). This syndrome is commonly not diagnosed and frequently interferes with the acceptance of neuroleptic treatment.

Acute dystonic reactions are occasionally seen with the initiation of antipsychotic drug therapy. Facial grimacing and torticollis can occur and may be associated with oculogyric crisis. These syndromes may be mistaken for hysterical reaction or seizures, but they respond dramatically to parenteral administration of anticholinergic antiparkinsonian drugs.

Tardive dyskinesia is a late-appearing neurological syndrome associated with antipsychotic drug use. It occurs more frequently in older patients, and an incidence that averages about 10 to 20% has been reported in chronically institutionalized patients. It may be more common in those with a history of prior brain damage. Its incidence with specific drug groups is not known, but it has been associated with every class of neuroleptic agents in common clinical use. The incidence appears to be very low with the experimental antipsychotic agent clozapine. Tardive dyskinesia is characterized by stereotypical involuntary movements consisting in sucking and smacking of the lips, lateral jaw movements, and fly-catching dartings of the tongue. There may be choreiform or purposeless, quick movements of the extremities. Slower, more dystonic, athetoid movements and postures of the extremities, trunk, and neck may also be seen, especially in younger males. All of these movements disappear during sleep, as they do in parkinsonism. Although the tardive dyskinesias may be masked by the administration of large doses of antipsychotic drugs, this form of treatment is considered dangerous and is employed only in very compelling circumstances, such as severely incapacitating dyskinesia, particularly with continuing psychosis. Symptoms may persist indefinitely after discontinuation of the medication, although sometimes tardive dyskinesias will disappear with time (weeks or as long as 1 to 3 years), especially in younger patients. Antiparkinsonian drugs typically exacerbate tardive dyskinesias and other forms of choreoathetosis, such as in Huntington's disease, and no adequate therapy has as yet been devised (Jeste and Wyatt, 1982); the best approach is preventive (*see* below).

A rare movement disorder that can appear late in treatment of chronically ill patients with antipsychotic agents is *perioral tremor,* sometimes referred to as the "rabbit" syndrome (Jus *et al.,* 1974) due to the peculiar movements that characterize this condition. While sometimes categorized with other tardive (late or slowly evolving) dyskinesias, the latter term is usually reserved for choreoathetotic reactions. The "rabbit" syndrome, in fact, shares many features with parkinsonism, since the tremor has a frequency of about 5 to 7 Hz and there is a favorable response to anticholinergic agents.

Histological examination of brains of patients who had signs of tardive dyskinesia or of brains of animals exposed to high doses of neuroleptic agents for prolonged periods has not revealed a clear or consistent lesion. Moreover, the pathophysiology of tardive dyskinesia remains obscure, although it is hypothesized that compensatory increases in the function of dopamine as a neurotransmitter in the basal ganglia may be involved. This idea is supported by comparison of therapeutic responses in patients with Parkinson's disease to those with tardive dyskinesia or other choreoathetotic dyskinesias such as Huntington's disease. Thus, antidopaminergic drugs tend to ameliorate tardive dyskinesia, while dopaminergic agonists worsen the condition; antimuscarinic agents tend to worsen tardive dyskinesia, and cholinergic agents sometimes help. In addition, there are now abundant data to support the concept of *disuse supersensitivity* of dopaminergic systems in the animal brain. Since supersensitivity to dopaminergic agonists tends not to persist for more than a few weeks after exposure to antagonists of the transmitter, this phenomenon is most likely to play a role in those variants of tardive dyskinesia that re-

solve rapidly; these are usually referred to as *withdrawal-emergent dyskinesias.* The theoretical and clinical aspects of this complex and troublesome problem have been reviewed in detail elsewhere (Baldessarini and Tarsy, 1979; Baldessarini *et al.,* 1980; Jeste and Wyatt, 1982).

It is important to prevent the neurological syndromes that complicate the use of antipsychotic drugs. Certain therapeutic guidelines should be followed. Thus, the routine use of antiparkinsonian agents in an attempt to *avoid* early extrapyramidal reactions is usually unnecessary and adds complexity, side effects, and expense to the treatment regimen. Antiparkinsonian agents should be reserved for cases of *overt* extrapyramidal reactions that respond favorably to such intervention, and the need for such agents ordinarily diminishes with time. The thoughtful and conservative use of antipsychotic drugs in patients with chronic or frequently recurrent psychotic disorders almost certainly can reduce the risk of tardive dyskinesia. Although reduction of the dose of an antipsychotic agent is the best way to minimize its neurological side effects, this may not be practical in a patient with uncontrollable psychotic illness. The best preventive practice is to use minimally effective doses of antipsychotic drugs for long-term therapy and to discontinue treatment as soon as it seems reasonable to do so or if a satisfactory response cannot be obtained.

Jaundice. Jaundice was observed in patients shortly after the introduction of chlorpromazine into medical practice and was the cause for some alarm. The incidence of this complication is very low and has decreased since the 1960s, presumably due to improved quality of the products or to the increased use of more potent agents, which tend to have less systemic toxicity than do the low-potency phenothiazines. Commonly occurring during the second to fourth week of therapy, the jaundice is generally mild, and patients rarely complain of pruritus. The jaundice following administration of phenothiazines is probably a manifestation of hypersensitivity. Eosinophilic infiltration of the liver as well as eosinophilia are frequently present. There is no correlation between the dose administered and the appearance of jaundice. Desensitization to chlorpromazine may occur with repeated administration in individuals exhibiting jaundice, and it may or may not recur if the same neuroleptic agent is given again. If jaundice is not observed within the first month of treatment with a phenothiazine, the chance of its later occurrence decreases with time. In cases of neuroleptic-induced jaundice when the psychiatric disorder calls for uninterrupted drug therapy, it is probably safest to use low doses of a potent, dissimilar agent.

Blood Dyscrasias. Mild leukocytosis, leukopenia, and eosinophilia occasionally occur with phenothiazine medication. It is difficult to determine whether a leukopenia occurring during the administration of a phenothiazine is a forewarning of impending *agranulocytosis.* This serious but rare complication occurs in not more than 1 in 10,000 patients receiving chlorpromazine or other low-potency agents, particularly in high doses; it usually appears within the first 8 to 12 weeks of treatment (DuComb and Baldessarini, 1977). Since the onset of blood dyscrasia may be sudden, the appearance of an apparent upper respiratory infection in a patient being treated with an antipsychotic drug should be followed immediately by a complete blood count.

Skin Reactions. Dermatological reactions to the phenothiazines are common. Urticaria or dermatitis occurs in about 5% of patients receiving chlorpromazine. Three types of skin disorders are associated with the use of phenothiazines. The first is a hypersensitivity reaction that may be urticarial, maculopapular, petechial, or edematous. It usually occurs between the first and eighth week of treatment. The skin clears following discontinuation of the drug and may remain so even if drug therapy is reinstituted. Secondly, contact dermatitis may occur in personnel who handle chlorpromazine, and there may be a certain degree of cross-sensitivity to the other phenothiazines. Thirdly, photosensitivity occurs, and the reaction resembles that seen with severe sunburn. This complication may be prevented simply by keeping the patient well covered. An effective sunscreen preparation should be prescribed for outpatients during the summer.

Abnormal gray-blue pigmentation induced by long-term administration of phenothiazines in high doses to chronic schizophrenics has been reported, but it is rare with current practices. Ultraviolet light with wavelengths above 320 nm seems to be primarily responsible for the effects.

Epithelial keratopathy is often observed in patients on long-term therapy with chlorpromazine, and opacities in the cornea and in the lens of the eye have also been noted. In extreme cases the deposits in the lens may result in impairment of vision. Active treatment of this condition (*e.g.,* with penicillamine) has not been especially helpful, and the deposits tend to disappear spontaneously, although slowly, following discontinuation of the low-potency drug usually implicated. Pigmentary retinopathy, which has been reported particularly following the use of high doses of thioridazine, may be a closely related toxic effect of the phenothiazines (Prien *et al.,* 1970); thus far it has been reported only with doses of thioridazine in excess of 1000 mg per day. A maximal daily dose of 800 mg is therefore currently recommended.

Metabolic Effects. Chlorpromazine may raise plasma cholesterol concentrations (Clark *et al.,* 1967). Other antipsychotic drugs are not known to have this effect.

Interactions with Other Drugs. The phenothiazines and thioxanthenes, especially those of low potency, affect the actions of a number of other drugs, sometimes with important clinical consequences (*see* Kaufman, 1976). Chlorpromazine was originally introduced to potentiate central depressants, and it and some of its congeners have

continued to be used for this purpose, especially in anesthesiology. In addition, such drugs can strongly potentiate sedatives and analgesics prescribed for medical purposes, as well as nonprescription sedatives and hypnotics, antihistamines, and cold remedies. Patients should also be warned to expect enhancement of the effects of alcohol. Chlorpromazine increases the miotic and sedative effects of morphine and is believed also to increase its analgesic actions. Furthermore, the drug markedly increases the respiratory depression produced by meperidine and can be expected to have similar effects when administered concurrently with other opioid analgesics. As should be clear from the discussion of the actions of neuroleptic drugs, they inhibit the actions of direct dopaminergic agonists and of levodopa.

Other interactive effects can be manifest on the cardiovascular system. Chlorpromazine and some other antipsychotic drugs, as well as their N-demethylated metabolites, may block the antihypertensive effects of guanethidine. The mechanism appears to involve blockade of uptake of guanethidine into sympathetic nerves. The more potent antipsychotic agents, especially molindone, seem to be much less likely to cause this effect. On the other hand, the phenothiazines can promote postural hypotension, possibly due to their α-adrenergic blocking properties. Thus, the interaction between phenothiazines and antihypertensives can be unpredictable.

Thioridazine may partially nullify the inotropic effect of digitalis by its quinidine-like action that can cause myocardial depression, decreased efficiency of repolarization, and increased risk of tachyarrhythmias. The antimuscarinic action of thioridazine can cause tachycardia and enhance the peripheral and central effects (confusion, delirium) of other anticholinergic agents, such as the tricyclic antidepressants and antiparkinsonian agents.

Drugs such as phenobarbital and other sedatives or anticonvulsants (*e.g.,* phenytoin, carbamazepine) that induce microsomal drug-metabolizing enzymes can enhance the metabolism of antipsychotic agents (Loga *et al.,* 1975); this effect may sometimes have significant clinical consequences.

DRUG TREATMENT OF PSYCHOSES

The antipsychotic drugs are not specific for the diagnostic type of psychosis to be treated. They are clearly effective in acute psychoses of unknown etiology, including mania, acute idiopathic psychoses, and acute exacerbations of schizophrenia, although most controlled clinical data exist for the acute and chronic phases of schizophrenia. In addition, antipsychotic drugs are used empirically in many other disorders, whether idiopathic or organic, in which psychotic symptoms and severe agitation are prominent. Unfortunately, for disorders other than schizophrenia and mania, there have been but few controlled comparisons with a placebo or sedatives, and well-designed, systematic studies of dose-response relationships are meager.

The fact that phenothiazines and other neuroleptic agents are indeed antipsychotic was slow to gain acceptance. However, many clinical trials have established that these agents are effective and that they are superior to agents such as the barbiturates or the benzodiazepines, or to alternatives such as electroconvulsive shock or other medical or psychological therapies (*see* Donaldson *et al.,* 1983). The "target" symptoms for which the neuroleptic agents seem to be especially effective include tension, hyperactivity, combativeness, hostility, negativism, hallucinations, acute delusions, insomnia, poor self-care, excessive fasting, anorexia, and sometimes withdrawal and seclusiveness; less likely is improvement in insight, judgment, memory, and orientation. The most favorable prognosis is for patients with relatively acute illnesses of brief duration who had relatively healthy personalities prior to the illness.

Despite the great success of the antipsychotic drugs, their use alone does not constitute optimal care of psychotic patients. The acute care, protection, and support of acutely psychotic patients, as well as mastery of technics employed in their long-term care and rehabilitation, continue to be important medical skills. Many detailed reviews of the clinical use of antipsychotic drugs are available (May, 1968; Davis and Garver, 1978; Klein *et al.,* 1980; Bassuk *et al.,* 1983; Baldessarini, 1984b, 1985).

In order to assess changes in the patient's condition, an accurate evaluation of his mental and physical status at the start of therapy is necessary. Treatment goals should then be defined. Although rating scales for symptom complexes are available (*see* Levine *et al.,* 1971), the physician can define treatable symptoms on the basis of clinical examination.

No one drug or combination of drugs has a selective effect on a particular symptom complex in groups of psychotic patients, although individual patients appear to do better with one agent than another; this can only be determined by trial and error. Since compliance with medication schedules can be poor on both inpatient and outpatient services, it is important to simplify the treatment regimen and to try to ensure that the patient is receiving the drug. In cases of severe and dangerous noncompliance, the patient can be treated with injections of fluphenazine decanoate or other long-acting preparations. Since delusional paranoid patients frequently believe that the medicine is "poison," this group is often given long-acting injectable preparations.

Since the choice of a drug cannot be made on the basis of anticipated therapeutic effect, the *selection* of a particular medication for treatment often depends on side effects. If a patient has responded well to a drug in the past, it should probably be used again. If the patient has a history of cardiovascular disease or stroke and the threat from hypotension is serious, a potent neuroleptic should be used in the smallest dose that is effective (*see* Table 19–1). If it seems important to minimize the risk of acute extrapyramidal symptoms, thioridazine should be considered. Small doses of potent antipsychotic drugs may be safest in the elderly. If the patient would be seriously discomforted by interference with ejaculation or if there are serious risks of cardiovascular or other autonomic toxicity, thioridazine should be avoided. If sedative effects are undesirable, a potent agent is preferable. If the patient has compromised hepatic function or if there is a potential threat of jaundice, high-potency agents may be used. The physician's experience with a particular drug may outweigh all other considerations. Skill in the use of antipsychotic drugs depends on selection of an adequate dosage, knowledge of what to expect, and judgment as to when to stop therapy or change drugs.

Some patients do not respond satisfactorily to antipsychotic drug treatment, and many chronically disorganized schizophrenic patients, while helped during periods of acute exacerbation of their disease, may show unsatisfactory responses between the more acute phases of illness. The individual nonresponder cannot be identified beforehand with certainty, and a small subgroup of patients do poorly or even become worse on medication, at least during some phases of their illness. If a patient does not improve after a course of adequate treatment and if he fails to respond to another drug given in adequate dosage, therapy should be discontinued and the diagnosis reevaluated.

The *time course of response* to antipsychotic drugs is such that 3 weeks or more is required to demonstrate positive effects in hospitalized schizophrenics. Full effect may require 6 weeks to 6 months. In contrast, improvement of some acutely psychotic patients can be seen within 48 hours. Aggressive parenteral administration of an antipsychotic drug at the start of an acute psychosis has not been found to increase the rate of appearance of therapeutic responses (Cole, 1982). Sedative or anxiolytic agents, such as the benzodiazepines, can be used for brief periods during the initiation of therapy with neuroleptic drugs; they are not effective in the chronic treatment of psychotic and, especially, schizophrenic patients.

After the initial response, drugs are frequently used in conjunction with other psychological and supportive treatments. Although there is no clear statistical evidence that formal psychotherapy greatly affects prognosis (Grinspoon *et al.,* 1968; May, 1968; Feinsilver and Gunderson, 1972; Hogarty and Ulrich, 1977), psychotherapy and other rehabilitative efforts are believed to assist the patient in adjusting to his environment.

There is no convincing evidence that combinations of antipsychotic drugs offer any advantage. A combination of an antipsychotic drug and an antidepressant may be useful in some cases, especially in depressed psychotic patients or in cases of agitated depression. However, the suggestion that a tricyclic antidepressant can reduce apathy and withdrawal in schizophrenia is not proven, and the hypothesis that diphenylbutylpiperidines are uniquely valuable against such "negative" symptoms of schizophrenia requires further study.

The *duration of treatment* has received a great deal of attention. In a review of 30 controlled prospective studies involving nearly 3500 schizophrenic patients, the mean overall relapse rate was 55% for those patients who were withdrawn from antipsychotic drugs and given a placebo, compared to only 17% of those who continued on drug therapy (Davis, 1975; Baldessarini *et al.,* 1980). It is sometimes found, at least for short periods (weeks or a few months), that dosage in chronic cases can be lowered to 50 to 200 mg of chlorpromazine (or its equivalent) per day without signs of relapse, although the average lowest effective dose for long-term maintenance treatment in schizophrenia is still not known (Davis and Garver, 1978; Baldessarini, 1984a; Baldessarini *et al.,* 1984). Intermittent therapy can be useful, particularly in reducing the incidence of side effects. Effective maintenance with monthly injections of a fluphenazine ester is well established and commonly practiced (Hirsch *et al.,* 1973; Kane *et al.,* 1983).

Optimal dosage of antipsychotic drugs is difficult to determine because of the variable dose-response curves and the difficulties in defining an end point of therapeutic response. In the treatment of acute psychoses, one should increase the dose of antipsychotic drug as rapidly as feasible, over a few days at most, to achieve control of symptoms. The dose is then adjusted during the next several weeks as the patient's condition warrants. Parenteral medication is often indicated for acutely agitated patients. Small doses (25 to 50 mg of chlorpromazine, 5 mg of haloperidol, or comparable doses of another agent) are given *intramuscularly* (and almost never by other routes); these can be repeated as frequently as hourly to obtain the desired response. Similar results can usually be obtained by additional doses at intervals of 4 to 8 hours for the first 24 to 72 hours. One must remain alert for hypotension or acute dystonic reactions, which are especially likely with such treatment. The desired effect

may be delayed for several hours. Some antipsychotic drugs, including fluphenazine, other piperazines, and haloperidol, have been given in doses of several hundred milligrams a day orally without disaster, although such high doses of potent agents do not yield significantly superior results (Quitkin *et al.,* 1974; Aubree and Lader, 1980; Cole, 1982). After an initial period of stabilization, regimens based on a single daily dose are effective and safe; they may also allow some degree of selection of the time at which unwanted effects occur so as to minimize the patient's discomfort.

Table 19–1 (page 403) gives usual and extreme ranges of dosage for antipsychotic drugs employed in the United States. These ranges are only guidelines, and they have been established, for the most part, in the treatment of schizophrenic patients. Higher doses have been used, but are considered experimental. While acutely disturbed inpatients may require higher doses of an antipsychotic drug than do more stable outpatients, the concept that a low-maintenance dose will suffice during follow-up care of a partially recovered or chronic psychotic patient is only starting to obtain support from appropriately controlled trials (Kane *et al.,* 1983). The typical dose to achieve clear antipsychotic effects is approximately 300 to 400 mg of chlorpromazine daily or the equivalent amount of another agent (Davis and Garver, 1978); as mentioned, daily doses as low as 50 to 200 mg are effective for some patients (Cole, 1982; Cohen, 1984). Careful observation of the patient's changing response is the best guide to dosage.

The treatment of *organic mental syndromes* (*i.e.,* delirium or dementia) is another accepted use of the antipsychotic drugs. They may be administered temporarily, while a specific and correctable structural, infectious, metabolic, or toxic cause is vigorously sought. They are sometimes used chronically when no correctable cause can be found. Once again, there are no drugs of choice or clearly established dosage guidelines (*see* Prien, 1973). In patients with acute "brain syndromes" without likelihood of seizures, frequent small doses (perhaps 2 to 6 mg) of a piperazine or haloperidol may be effective in controlling agitation. Agents with low potency should be avoided because of their greater tendency to produce sedation, hypotension, and seizures. The potent antipsychotic drugs are much less likely to cause excitement or additional confusion, as is common when barbiturates or other sedatives are given to such patients. This is also true for demented patients in whom use of small doses of potent antipsychotic drugs can be helpful.

The use of antipsychotic drugs in *mania* and *depression* has met with some success. Haloperidol and chlorpromazine are both effective in the treatment of mania and are often used concomitantly with the institution of lithium therapy (*see* below). In fact, it is often impractical to attempt to manage a manic patient with lithium alone during the first week of illness, when the antipsychotic drugs are usually required; sedative or anxiolytic agents may also be used. There is no controlled study of possible long-term preventive effects of antipsychotic drugs in manic-depressive illness. The treatment of depression with neuroleptics is more controversial. Controlled studies have demonstrated the efficacy of several antipsychotic drugs in some depressed patients, especially those with striking agitation or psychotic delusions (*see* Nelson and Bowers, 1978; Baldessarini *et al.*, 1980).

Anxiety is considered by some to be an indication for the use of antipsychotic drugs. In view of the wide range of disturbing and serious side effects, the routine use of these drugs for such a purpose is inappropriate. However, for patients who have crippling anxiety that does not respond to sedative-antianxiety drugs, a brief trial of an antipsychotic agent might be warranted. (An antidepressant drug could be appropriate if panic attacks are present.) The long-term utility of antipsychotic drugs for the treatment of anxiety is not established, nor is it known at what rate tolerance to their antianxiety effects may occur. Patients who require or demand medication for anxiety for prolonged periods require careful medical and psychiatric evaluation. The physician should recall that the risk of tardive dyskinesia is *not* clearly related to the dose of antipsychotic drugs (Baldessarini *et al.*, 1980). Thus, their use for prolonged periods, even in relatively small doses, can be expected to carry such a risk.

The status of the drug treatment of *childhood psychosis* and other behavioral disorders of children is confused by diagnostic inconsistencies and a paucity of controlled studies. Neuroleptics can benefit children with disorders that are characterized by some of the features that occur in adult psychoses. Low doses of the more potent agents seem to be preferred in an attempt to avoid interference with daytime activities or performance in school (Campbell, 1975). Due to the wide range of behavioral disorders of children that are sometimes called psychoses, one can expect a proportion of children so treated to respond unfavorably to these agents. In evaluating the behavioral disorders of children, it is important to consider the syndrome of "minimal brain dysfunction" or "hyperactivity," now designated *attention-deficit disorder;* this responds poorly to antipsychotic agents but uniquely well to certain stimulant drugs, especially dextroamphetamine and methylphenidate (*see* De La Cruz *et al.*, 1973). Information on dosages of antipsychotic drugs for children is very limited, as is the number of drugs currently approved in the United States for use in preadolescents. The recommended doses of antipsychotic agents for school-aged children with moderate degrees of agitation are lower than those for acutely psychotic children, who may require doses similar to those used in adults (total milligrams per day) (*see* Anders and Ciaranello, 1977; Werry, 1978; Popper, 1985; *see also* Table 19–1). Most relevant experience is with chlorpromazine, for which the recommended daily doses are approximately 2 mg/kg of body weight. A suggested limit is 200 mg per day (orally) for preadolescents, 40 mg per day (intramuscularly) for children under 5 years of age or 23 kg of body weight, and 75 mg per day (intramuscularly) under age 12 years or 45 kg. Usual daily doses for other agents of relatively low potency

are: triflupromazine, 2 mg/kg; thioridazine, 0.5 to 3 mg/kg; and chlorprothixene, 30 to 100 mg (over the age of 6). For neuroleptics of high potency, daily doses are: trifluoperazine, 1 to 15 mg (over 6 years of age) and 1 to 30 mg (over 12 years of age); fluphenazine, up to 10 mg; prochlorperazine, 10 mg; and perphenazine, 6 mg. Haloperidol, which is utilized to treat the rare syndrome of Gilles de la Tourette in children and adolescents (Shapiro *et al.*, 1973), is recommended at doses of 2 to 16 mg per day in children over 12 years of age; clonidine may also be of value (Cohen *et al.*, 1980).

For patients at the other end of the age spectrum, poor tolerance of the side effects of the antipsychotic drugs often limits the doses of drugs that can be given. One should proceed cautiously, using small, divided doses, with the expectation that the very elderly will require doses that are one half or less of those needed for young adults (*see* Prien and Cole, 1978; Raskin *et al.*, 1981).

MISCELLANEOUS MEDICAL USES FOR NEUROLEPTIC DRUGS

Neuroleptic drugs have a variety of uses in addition to the treatment of psychiatric patients. Predominant among these are the treatment of nausea and vomiting (Table 19–3), alcoholic hallucinosis, certain neuropsychiatric diseases marked by movement disorders (notably, Gilles de la Tourette's syndrome and Huntington's disease), and, occasionally, intractable hiccough and pruritus (for which trimeprazine is recommended).

Nausea and Vomiting. Chlorpromazine, in relatively low, nonsedative doses, can prevent vomiting of certain etiologies. The potent and selective antiemetic action of the drug has found useful clinical application in various disorders characterized by vomiting, such as uremia, gastroenteritis, carcinomatosis, radiation sickness, and emesis caused by drugs including estrogens, the tetracyclines, opioid analgesics, agents used in the chemotherapy of malignancy, and disulfiram. Chlorpromazine has also been used in nausea and vomiting of pregnancy, but pregnant patients should not be given the drug for this purpose (*see* Morselli, 1977; Goldberg and DiMascio, 1978). Chlorpromazine does not appear to control motion sickness. Although prochlorperazine is a potent antiemetic agent, it produces a high incidence of dystonias, especially when given intramuscularly, and hence should be used with caution. The same precautions should be observed in the use of phenothiazines for nausea and vomiting as with the use of potent analgesics in the treatment of pain, because they may mask diagnostic symptoms in acute surgical conditions or neurological syndromes. Not all the phenothiazines are equally effective as antiemetics, and thioridazine is a notable exception to the general rule that most neuroleptic agents have antiemetic effects. It should be remembered that this action of most antipsychotic agents may thwart attempts to induce emesis pharmacologically (*e.g.*, with apomorphine) in the management of cases of acute drug overdos-

Table 19–3. PHENOTHIAZINES USED IN THE TREATMENT OF NAUSEA AND VOMITING OR PRURITUS

NONPROPRIETARY NAME AND TRADE NAME	ROUTE, DOSAGE FORM, * AND ADULT DOSE		
	Oral	*Suppository*	*Intramuscular*
Chlorpromazine (THORAZINE)	O,SR,L 10–25 mg every 4–6 hr	25–100 mg every 6–8 hr	25–50 mg every 3–4 hr
Perphenazine (TRILAFON)	O,SR,L 8–16 mg/day	—	5 mg
Prochlorperazine (COMPAZINE)	O,SR,L 5–10 mg 3–4 times/day 10 mg twice a day (SR)	25 mg twice a day	5–10 mg every 3–4 hr (up to 40 mg/day)
Promethazine † (PHENERGAN)	O,L 12.5–25 mg every 4–6 hr	12.5–25 mg every 4–6 hr	12.5–25 mg every 4–6 hr
Thiethylperazine (TORECAN)	O 10–30 mg/day	10–30 mg/day	10 mg 1–3 times/day
Triflupromazine (VESPRIN)	L 20–30 mg/day	—	5–15 mg every 4–6 hr (up to 60 mg/day)
Trimeprazine † (TEMARIL)	O,SR,L 2.5 mg 4 times/day 5 mg twice a day (SR)	—	—

* Dosage forms: O = oral solid; SR = oral, sustained release; L = oral liquid.

† Promethazine and trimeprazine are not known to have antipsychotic effects; both have relatively strong anticholinergic and antihistaminic actions. Promethazine is sedative and antiemetic, while trimeprazine is antipruritic.

age. The preparations and dosages of phenothiazines that are effective in the treatment of nausea and vomiting (or pruritus) are listed in Table 19–3. Surprisingly, nausea is occasionally seen as a side effect of antipsychotic drugs.

Hiccough. An interesting use of chlorpromazine is in the control of *intractable hiccough.* The mechanism of action in this disorder is unknown.

Withdrawal Syndromes. Antipsychotic drugs are *not* useful in the management of withdrawal from opioids, and their use in the management of withdrawal from barbiturates and other nonbarbiturate sedatives is *contraindicated,* due to the high risk of seizures. This risk also precludes the use of neuroleptics during withdrawal from alcohol. However, they can be employed safely and effectively in certain psychoses associated with chronic alcoholism—especially the syndrome known as *alcoholic hallucinosis* (*see* Freedman *et al.,* 1980).

Other Neuropsychiatric Disorders. Antipsychotic drugs are useful in the management of several rare syndromes with psychiatric features that are also characterized by movement disorders. These include, in particular, Gilles de la Tourette's syndrome (marked by tics, other involuntary movements, grunts, and vocalizations that are fre-

quently obscene) (*see* Shapiro *et al.,* 1973; Van Woert *et al.,* 1976) and Huntington's disease (marked by severe and progressive choreoathetosis, psychiatric symptoms, and a clear genetic basis) (*see* Chase, 1976). Haloperidol is currently regarded as a drug of choice for these conditions, although it is probably not unique in its antidyskinetic actions.

II. Drugs Used in the Treatment of Disorders of Mood

Affective disorders—*major depression* and *mania* (or bipolar, *manic-depressive illness*)—are characterized by changes in mood as the primary clinical manifestation. Either extreme of mood may be associated with psychosis, characterized by disordered or delusional thinking and perceptions, often congruent with the predominant mood. Conversely, psychotic disorders may have associated or secondary changes in mood; the same is true of many medical illnesses. This overlap of disorders may lead to errors in diagnosis and clinical management. *Major depression* is the most common of the major mental illnesses, and it must be distinguished from normal grief, sadness and disappointment, and the dysphoria or demoralization often associated with medical illness. The condition is underdiagnosed and frequently undertreated (Keller *et al.*, 1982). Major depression is characterized by feelings of intense sadness and despair, mental slowing and loss of concentration, pessimistic worry, agitation, and self-deprecation. Physical changes also occur; these include insomnia, anorexia and weight loss, decreased energy and libido, and disruption of hormonal circadian rhythms. Perhaps 15% of individuals with this disorder display suicidal behavior during their lifetime. The condition responds well to tricyclic or other antidepressant drugs, monoamine oxidase inhibitors, or, in severe or treatment-resistant cases, electroconvulsive shock treatment (ECT). The decision to treat with an antidepressant drug is guided by the presenting clinical syndrome and its severity, and by the patient's personal and family history. Most of the antidepressant agents exert important actions on the metabolism of monoamine neurotransmitters and their receptors. This, together with strong evidence for genetic predisposition, has led to speculation that the biological basis of major mood disorders may include abnormal function of monoamine neurotransmission. However, there is little direct evidence for this view, and it is not clear whether actions on monoaminergic systems are crucial for the clinical effects of most antidepressant drugs (*see* Murphy *et al.*, 1978; Praag, 1978; Baldessarini, 1983).

Mania and the alternation of mania and depression (*bipolar affective disorder*) are less common than nonbipolar major depression. Mania and its milder form (*hypomania*) are treated with antipsychotic drugs or lithium salts in the short term and lithium for longer-term prevention of recurrences. Mania is characterized by excessive elation, typically tinged with dysphoria and irritability, marked insomnia, hyperactivity, uncontrollable speech and activity, and impaired judgment. The selection and management of appropriate treatment for depression and mania are discussed below.

TRICYCLIC ANTIDEPRESSANTS

Imipramine (a dibenzazepine derivative), *amitriptyline* (a dibenzocycloheptadiene derivative), and other closely related compounds are the drugs currently most widely used for the treatment of major depression. Because of their structure (*see* below), they are often referred to as the tricyclic antidepressants. Their efficacy in alleviating depression is well established, and support for their use in other psychiatric disorders is growing.

History. In the late nineteenth century, Thiele and Holzinger synthesized iminodibenzyl and described its chemical characteristics in detail. The pharmacological properties were not investigated until the late 1940s, when Häfliger and Schindler synthesized a series of more than 40 derivatives of iminodibenzyl for possible uses as antihistamines, sedatives, analgesics, and antiparkinsonian drugs. One of these was *imipramine,* a dibenzazepine compound, which differs from the phenothiazines only by replacement of the sulfur with an ethylene linkage to produce a seven-membered central ring. Following screening in animals, a few compounds, including imipramine, were selected on the basis of sedative or hypnotic properties for therapeutic trial.

During clinical investigation of these phenothiazine analogs, Kuhn (1958) found fortuitously that, unlike the phenothiazines, imipramine was relatively ineffective in quieting agitated psychotic patients. Instead, it apparently bestowed remarkable benefit upon certain depressed patients. Since then, indisputable evidence for the effectiveness of this compound has accumulated (*see* Klerman, 1972; Hollister, 1978; Klein *et al.*, 1980; Herrington and Lader, 1981).

Chemistry and Structure-Activity Relationship. The search for compounds related chemically to imipramine has yielded, to date, nine analogs that are in common clinical use in the United States. In addition to the dibenzazepines, *imipramine* and its secondary-amine congener (and major metabolite) *desipramine*, there are *amitriptyline* and its N-demethylated product *nortriptyline* (dibenzocycloheptadienes), as well as *doxepin* (a dibenzoxepine) and *protriptyline* (a dibenzocycloheptatriene). Three additional agents have recently been approved for general use in the United States: *trimipramine* (a dibenzazepine); *maprotiline* (containing an additional ethylene bridge across the central six-carbon ring); and *amoxapine* (*norloxapine;* a dibenzoxazepine with mixed antidepressant and neuroleptic properties) (Cohen *et al.*, 1982). Since these agents all have a three-ring molecular core and produce therapeutic responses in most patients with major depression, the trivial name *tricyclic antidepressants* is used for this group. To varying degrees, these agents also share the capability to inhibit the neuronal uptake of nor-epinephrine. Some of the newer antidepressant agents that are in clinical use in Europe have a variety of chemical structures and pharmacological properties that differ from the tricyclic antidepressants. These are sometimes referred to as "atypical antidepressants" to distinguish them from both the monoamine oxidase inhibitors and the tricyclic antidepressants. One of these, *trazodone,* is currently marketed in the United States. *Carbamazepine,* a derivative of iminostilbene with a carbamyl group at the 5 position, is an important antiepileptic agent (*see* Chapter 20). This drug is being evaluated for the treatment of bipolar affective disorders (*see* Post *et al.,* 1983).

The structures of the tricyclic antidepressant compounds and of trazodone are given in Table 19–4. Although dibenzazepines seem to be similar to the phenothiazines chemically, the ethylene group of imipramine's middle ring imparts dissimilar stereochemical properties and prevents conjugation among the rings, as occurs with the phenothiazines. The demethylated congener of imipramine, the secondary amine desipramine, has similar activity to that of imipramine as an antidepressant, although there are some pharmacological dissimilarities as discussed below. While it has been suggested that desipramine might be the agent responsible for therapeutic responses to imipramine, it is now certain that desipramine is no more

effective or rapidly acting than imipramine. The same generalizations can be made from the comparison between amitriptyline and nortriptyline. The latter pair are the structural homologs of the thioxanthenes among the antipsychotic drugs (*cf.* Tables 19–4 and 19–1); however, unlike the thioxanthenes, they do not occur as geometric isomers since there is no center of asymmetry. Geometric isomers of doxepin do exist; both are active and are included in available products. The 3-chloro analog of imipramine (the homolog of chlorpromazine), called clomipramine (ANAFRANIL), is quite sedative and is in common clinical use in Europe and Canada as an antidepressant. In further contrast to the phenothiazines, compounds with only two carbon atoms separating the amino nitrogen of the side chain from the central ring retain some activity. Except for these few facts, the structure-activity relationship of the tricyclic antidepressants remains poorly understood. The chemistry and structure-activity relationship of a variety of experimental antidepressant agents are discussed in more detail by Kaiser and Zirkle (1970) and Usdin (1978).

PHARMACOLOGICAL PROPERTIES

There are many gaps in our understanding of the pharmacological properties of

Table 19–4. **TRICYCLIC ANTIDEPRESSANTS AND TRAZODONE**

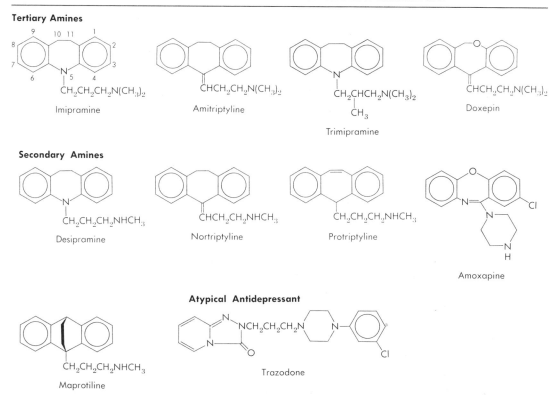

Tertiary Amines

Imipramine — $CH_2CH_2CH_2N(CH_3)_2$

Amitriptyline — $CHCH_2CH_2N(CH_3)_2$

Trimipramine — $CH_2CHCH_2N(CH_3)_2$; CH_3

Doxepin — $CHCH_2CH_2N(CH_3)_2$

Secondary Amines

Desipramine — $CH_2CH_2CH_2NHCH_3$

Nortriptyline — $CHCH_2CH_2NHCH_3$

Protriptyline — $CH_2CH_2CH_2NHCH_3$

Amoxapine

Atypical Antidepressant

Maprotiline — $CH_2CH_2CH_2NHCH_3$

Trazodone — $NCH_2CH_2CH_2N$

this class of agents, and systematic comparisons of large numbers of agents under identical conditions have been uncommon. Since it is the oldest and best studied, imipramine will be discussed as the prototype.

Central Nervous System. One might expect an effective antidepressant drug to have a stimulating or mood-elevating effect when given to a normal subject. Although this may occur with the monoamine oxidase (MAO) inhibitors, it is not true of the tricyclic antidepressants.

If a dose of 100 mg of imipramine is given to a normal subject, he feels sleepy and tends to be quieter, his blood pressure falls slightly, and he feels light-headed. Often unpleasant anticholinergic effects (dry mouth and blurred vision) appear. There is little, if any, change in pupillary size. Gait may become unsteady, and the subject feels tired and clumsy. These drug effects are usually perceived as unpleasant, and cause a feeling of "unhappiness" and an *increase* in anxiety. There may be a deterioration in tests of performance. These acute drug effects thus resemble those seen with certain phenothiazines.

Repeated administration for several days may lead to accentuation of these symptoms and, in addition, to difficulty in concentrating and thinking, comparable to that experienced during the course of similar treatment with chlorpromazine (Grunthal, 1958). Imipramine seems to produce greater impairment of cognitive and affective processes and lesser reduction in physical movement than does chlorpromazine.

In contrast, if the drug is given over a period of time to depressed patients, an elevation of mood occurs. *About 2 to 3 weeks must pass before the therapeutic effects of the drug are evident.* For this reason, the tricyclic antidepressants are not prescribed on an "as-needed" basis. The explanation of the slow onset of effects remains a matter of conjecture. Moreover, advertising claims notwithstanding, it has not been demonstrated that any agent of the tricyclic antidepressant group acts more rapidly on the core symptoms of major depression than does imipramine; although sedative or antianxiety effects may appear within a few days of treatment, all of these agents require several weeks to exert clinically important antidepressant actions.

The manner in which imipramine relieves the signs and symptoms of depression is not clear. Its effect has been described as a dulling of depressive ideation rather than as euphoric stimulation. However, reports of manic excitement as well as of euphoria and insomnia indicate that imipramine (and, indeed, virtually all effective antidepressant treatments) does have stimulant-like actions under certain circumstances (Bunney *et al.*, 1972).

Effects on Sleep. The tricyclic antidepressants occasionally have been used as hypnotics because of their sedative property. Although this effect may be useful in the initial therapy of a depressed patient who is not sleeping well, their general use to promote sleep in mild or primary insomnia is not recommended. In adequate doses they cause hangover and are not as effective as a conventional hypnotic. The drugs decrease the number of awakenings, increase stage-4 sleep, and markedly decrease time in rapid-eye-movement (REM) sleep, which is typically more prominent in the sleep of depressed patients. Indeed, the ability of a tricyclic antidepressant to suppress the onset of REM sleep early in treatment has been suggested to be predictive of whether a therapeutic effect will emerge later (Kupfer *et al.*, 1981). Amitriptyline and clomipramine appear to be especially sedative, while the secondary-amine antidepressants are less so.

EEG Effects. EEG studies in animals and man have revealed many complex effects, some of which change with the dose. Low doses of tricyclic antidepressants tend to have synchronizing effects that resemble those of sedatives or the phenothiazines; sometimes, particularly with amitriptyline, alpha rhythm is suppressed. High doses tend to produce stimulation and arousal and can induce seizure activity (*see* Itil, 1978; Longo, 1978).

Effects on Animal Behavior. Despite its clinical antidepressant effects, imipramine produces depression of spontaneous motor activity in laboratory animals. It impairs both acquisition and performance of conditioned avoidance responses. In all these tests, it is far less potent than chlorpromazine, although it bears some similarities to diazepam. Effects on hexobarbital- or alcohol-induced sedation are unpredictable; ataxia and mild hypothermia are usual.

Although imipramine decreases spontaneous motor activity in animals, it is also capable of stimulating a great variety of behavior patterns. Blockade of the reserpine-induced sedative or "depressive" patterns in animals is a characteristic of all the tricyclic antidepressants. The latter drugs must be given before the reserpine because an intact CNS store of amines must be present for this blocking effect to become evident. Since reserpine depletes the brain of both 5-HT and norepinephrine, it is not clear which amine, if not both, is important for this action. Although this interaction has been favored as a screening test for antidepressant agents and has helped to provide support for the "amine hypothesis" of affective disorders, the relationship between these animal tests and clinical depression is tenuous. Other effects in animals have been described that seem to represent stimulant-like activity. These include potentiation of adrenergic agonists, notably amphetamine, methylphenidate, and levodopa, and augmentation of some operant behaviors, food-reward reinforced behavior, and self-stimulation of the brain. Aggressive behavior induced by hypothalamic lesions can also be increased, as can shock-induced aggression in rodents after prolonged treatment with imipramine (*see* Lowe *et al.*, 1978). Many of these behavioral effects seem to be related to potentiation of amine-mediated (particularly noradrenergic) synaptic transmission in the CNS.

Actions on Brain Amines. All tricyclic antidepressants in current use in the United States potentiate the actions of biogenic amines in the CNS by blockade of their major means of physiological inactivation—re-uptake at nerve terminals. However, the potency and selectivity for inhibition of the neuronal transport (uptake) of norepinephrine, 5-HT, and dopamine vary greatly among the agents. For example, desipramine is one of the most potent of the group in blocking norepinephrine transport, but it is 100- to 1000-fold less potent as an inhibitor of 5-HT transport. In contrast, amitriptyline inhibits the uptake of 5-HT and norepinephrine equally well, even though it is about 20-fold less potent than desipramine in blocking norepinephrine transport. Clomipramine is a potent and rather selective blocker of 5-HT transport, while trazodone is less potent but more selective. None of these agents is very effective as an inhibitor of dopamine transport; this contrasts with the rather nonselective inhibitory actions of cocaine, amphetamine, and methylphenidate on the uptake of both norepinephrine and dopamine. The latter drugs are poor antidepressants, despite the fact that they have stimulant and even euphoriant effects in some people.

A few tentative generalizations may be made from these observations, together with the clinical and behavioral effects of antidepressant drugs. First, blockade of dopamine transport seems to be associated with stimulant rather than antidepressant activity. Second, inhibition of 5-HT uptake may have sedative as well as antidepressant consequences. Finally, inhibitory actions on the uptake of norepinephrine seem to correspond with antidepressant activity. However, there is increasing doubt that inhibition of the uptake of norepinephrine or 5-HT *per se* is either a necessary or sufficient explanation for the antidepressant action of these drugs. These doubts have been reinforced by the advent of so-called atypical antidepressant agents (*e.g.,* iprindole) that have little ability to interfere with the uptake of monoamines. Further, even though blockade of amine uptake is established promptly, the appearance of antidepressant effects requires administration of the drugs for several weeks. Thus, it is clear that potentiation of monoaminergic neurotransmission may be only an early event in a potentially complex cascade of events that eventually results in antidepressant activity (*see* Symposium, 1981; Baldessarini, 1983).

The administration of a tricyclic antidepressant produces an immediate reduction in the firing rate of neurons containing norepinephrine; with some agents, tryptaminergic neurons are also affected. There is a corresponding decrease in the turnover of the amines. These changes are thought to be a consequence of blockade of monoamine uptake, with a resultant increase in their action upon presynaptic autoreceptors that serve to regulate the excitability of and transmitter release from monoaminergic neurons. With continued treatment, neuronal firing and monoamine turnover return to or exceed pretreatment values, despite persistent blockade of uptake. These adaptive changes may involve in part a desensitization of presynaptic α_2-adrenergic receptors (Crews and Smith, 1978; Svensson and Usdin, 1978). By contrast, prolonged administration of tricyclic antidepressants (as well as of iprindole or MAO inhibitors) results in increased neuronal responsiveness to α_1-adrenergic agonists; this is associated with increased potency of such agonists in inhibiting the binding of prazosin, a specific α_1-adrenergic antagonist (Menkes *et al.*, 1983). Chronic administration of tricyclic antidepressants, iprindole, or MAO inhibitors also causes increased neuronal sensitivity to 5-HT (DeMontigny and Aghajanian, 1978), but a decreased capacity to bind radioactive spiperone in the cerebral cortex, suggesting a reduced number of 5-HT$_2$ receptors (Peroutka and Snyder, 1980). Finally, chronic administration of tricyclic antidepressants, atypical antidepressants, MAO inhibitors, or maximal electric shock reduces the number of β-adrenergic binding sites and the responsiveness of brain tissue to β-adrenergic agonists (*see* Sulser and Mobley, 1980). The relationship of these adaptive changes to the emergence of therapeutic responses is not known, but it seems clear that the various modalities useful in the treatment of major depression can produce similar alterations in the function of monoaminergic systems by a variety of pharmacological mechanisms.

Tricyclic antidepressants also act as antagonists at receptors for various neurohormones both *in vivo* and *in vitro;* these include muscarinic cholinergic (Snyder and Yamamura, 1977), α_1-adrenergic (U'Prichard *et al.*, 1978), and both H$_1$- and H$_2$-histaminergic receptors (Richelson, 1979). Both the pattern and potency of these effects differ widely among the various agents. For example, amitriptyline is one of the most potent of the group in blocking muscarinic cholinergic, H$_1$-histaminergic, and α_1-adrenergic receptors, while desipramine is 10- to 100-fold less potent than amitriptyline. Thus, these actions do not correlate with antidepressant potency, but they may be related to various untoward effects, such as sedation, confusion, and postural hypotension.

Autonomic Nervous System. The principal effects of the tricyclic antidepressants on the function of the autonomic nervous system are those that result from inhibition of norepinephrine transport into adrenergic nerve terminals and from antagonism of muscarinic cholinergic and α_1-adrenergic responses to the autonomic neurotransmitters. For example, the blurred vision, dry mouth, constipation, and urinary retention produced by therapeutic doses of tricyclic antidepressants are manifestations of anticholinergic actions. Amitriptyline causes the highest incidence of these effects, while desipramine is much less prone to do so (Blackwell *et al.*, 1978); trazodone and other atypical antidepressants have very weak anticholinergic properties (*see* Baldessarini, 1983). Since the autonomic changes that accompany depression may include some of these symptoms, the determination of what is a true autonomic side effect of a tricyclic antidepressant must rest on a careful physical examination and history obtained before the initiation of drug therapy.

Cardiovascular System. In therapeutic doses, the tricyclic antidepressants have significant effects on the cardiovascular system; with overdose these effects are life threatening (*see* Jefferson, 1975; Burrows *et al.*, 1976; Cassem, 1982). Imipramine lowers the blood pressure in anesthetized dogs and obtunds various cardiovascular reflexes, including the carotid occlusion reflex, the Bezold-Jarisch reflex, and postural responses. In man, the most common manifestation of such effects is *postural hypotension,* arising in part from peripheral α-adrenergic blockade. Mild sinus tachycardia is also frequently observed, probably as a consequence of both inhibition of norepinephrine uptake and blockade of muscarinic receptors. The most prominent ECG changes found during the use of imipramine and its congeners include inversion or flattening of the T waves and evidence of prolonged conduction times at all levels of the intracardiac conduction system. Direct depression of the myocardium can also be prominent. While these actions resemble those of quinidine and can produce antiarrhythmic effects when the ventricle is irritable, potentially dangerous interactions may occur when there are preexisting conduction defects (Glassman and Bigger, 1981). Dangerous ventricular arrhythmias can be precipitated, particularly when bundle-branch block is present. In addition, tricyclic antidepressants enhance the effects of other cardiac depressant drugs. Acute studies in animals suggest that the newer antidepressants (trazodone, in particular) have less intense depressant effects on cardiac conduction. Moreover, clinical studies indicate that trazodone has minimal effects on cardiac conduction and usually produces a slight sinus bradycardia instead of tachycardia (*see* Van De Merwe *et al.*, 1984). However, the relative safety of trazodone and similar agents during chronic administration to patients with cardiac disease requires further evaluation.

Since the tricyclic antidepressants can cause orthostatic hypotension, produce arrhythmias, and interact in deleterious ways with other drugs (*see* below), great caution must be observed in their use in patients with cardiac disease. Unfortunately, since many depressed patients fall in an age group where cardiac problems are common and coexistence of depressive illness and cardiovascular disease is frequent, the physician is faced with a dilemma. Milder cases may be self-limited, or treatment for anxiety and insomnia may suffice. In more severe cases, antidepressants can be utilized. Moderate, divided doses of the secondary amines (desipramine, nortriptyline) are currently preferred. For some severely depressed cardiac patients, ECT may be an option.

Respiration.   Imipramine in usual therapeutic doses produces little effect on respiration. Respiratory depression has been observed following poisoning with imipramine and with amitriptyline (*see* below).

Absorption, Distribution, Fate, and Excretion.   Imipramine and other tricyclic antidepressants are fairly well absorbed after oral administration. While they are usually initially used in divided doses, their relatively long half-lives and rather wide range of tolerated concentrations permit a gradual transition toward a single daily dose given at bedtime. This is most safely done for doses up to the equivalent of 150 mg of imipramine. High doses of these strongly anticholinergic agents can slow gastrointestinal activity and gastric emptying time, resulting in slower or erratic absorption of these and other drugs taken concomitantly; this can complicate the management of acute overdosage. Concentrations in plasma typically peak within 2 to 8 hours, but this can be delayed for over 12 hours. Intramuscular administration of some tricyclic antidepressants can be performed under unusual circumstances, particularly with severely depressed, anorexic patients who may refuse oral medication. The pharmacokinetic properties of these agents are discussed by Morselli (1977) and Amsterdam and associates (1980); *see also* Appendix II.

Once absorbed, these lipophilic drugs are widely distributed; their pharmacokinetic properties are similar to those of the phenothiazines. They are strongly bound to plasma protein and to constituents of tissues. The latter fact accounts for their large volumes of apparent distribution, which are typically 10 to 50 liters per kilogram. The

concentrations of these drugs in plasma that have been suggested to correlate best with satisfactory antidepressant responses range between 50 and 300 ng/ml or, more narrowly, between 100 and 200 ng/ml (50 to 140 ng/ml for nortriptyline). Toxic effects of these drugs can be expected when their concentrations in plasma rise above 1 μg/ml and can occur at even half this value (*see* Åsberg, 1976; Cooper *et al.*, 1976; Glassman and Perel, 1978; Amsterdam *et al.*, 1980; Baldessarini, 1983).

The tricyclic antidepressants are oxidized by hepatic microsomal enzymes, followed by conjugation with glucuronic acid. The major route of metabolism of imipramine is to the active drug desipramine; inactivation of either compound occurs largely by oxidation to 2-hydroxy metabolites (which retain some ability to block the uptake of amines) and conjugation with glucuronic acid. In contrast, amitriptyline (while mainly demethylated to nortriptyline) and nortriptyline undergo preferential oxidation at the 10 position, followed by glucuronidation; the 10-hydroxy metabolites may have some biological activity. While the demethylated metabolites of imipramine and amitriptyline possess antidepressant activity, it is not known to what extent they account for the activity of the parent drugs. These demethylated products can accumulate in concentrations approaching, or even exceeding, those of their precursors. Doxepin also appears to be converted to an active metabolite, nordoxepin, by N-demethylation (Ziegler *et al.*, 1978). There is relatively little published information on the metabolism of the newer antidepressants in man. Amoxapine is primarily converted to the active 8-hydroxy metabolite. In rats, trazodone is cleaved to form *m*-chlorophenylpiperazine, a substance with tryptaminergic agonist and antagonist properties similar to those of the parent compound. In man, neither the extent of formation nor the biological activity of this metabolite is known.

There is marked variation among subjects (up to 50-fold) in the ratio of methylated to demethylated molecules following administration of imipramine or amitriptyline in man (Nagy and Johansson, 1975). This variation, as well as that of the concentrations of the drug in blood, appears to be characteristic of the individual and is presumably under genetic control (Alexanderson and Sjöqvist, 1971). These characteristics can be assessed quite reliably by the administration of a small test dose and a single measurement of the concentration in plasma (Cooper *et al.*, 1976; Brunswick *et al.*, 1979).

The inactivation and elimination of tricyclic antidepressants occur over a period of several days, and half-lives range from about 16 hours for amitriptyline to an extreme of about 80 hours for protriptyline; the other agents have intermediate values (*see* Appendix II). It follows that most tricyclic antidepressants should be inactivated and excreted within a week after termination of treatment, with notable exceptions being ordinary doses of protriptyline and overdosage with the other agents (Spiker and Biggs, 1976). As with many other drugs, antidepressants are metabolized more rapidly by children and more slowly by patients over 60 years of age compared to young adults (*see* Nies *et al.*, 1977; Popper, 1985); dosages should be adjusted accordingly.

Tolerance and Physical Dependence. Tolerance to the anticholinergic effects, such as dry mouth, constipation, blurred vision, and tachycardia, tends to develop with continued use of imipramine. Occasional patients show physical or psychic dependence on the tricyclic antidepressants (Shatan, 1966). A withdrawal syndrome consisting in malaise, chills, coryza, and muscle aching has been reported to follow abrupt discontinuation of high doses of imipramine. Thus it is wise to discontinue a tricyclic antidepressant gradually over a week or longer. Despite these occasional problems, it is important to emphasize that tricyclic antidepressants have frequently been used for prolonged periods (years) by patients with severe recurring depression without evidence of tolerance to their desirable effects (*see* Davis, 1976).

Preparations, Routes of Administration, and Dosage. These are presented in Table 19–5. A further consideration of dosage and the use of antidepressant drugs appears below.

Toxic Reactions and Side Effects. Significant toxic effects of tricyclic antidepressant drugs are relatively common, and estimates of prevalence have run as high as 5% (Boston Collaborative Drug Surveillance Program, 1972). Most of these reactions involve antimuscarinic effects of the drugs and cerebral toxicity, but cardiac toxicity also represents a serious problem. Clinical consequences of the antimuscarinic effects include dry mouth and a sour or metallic taste, epigastric distress, constipation, dizziness, tachycardia, palpitations, blurred vision, and urinary retention. Special precautions should be taken in men with prostatic hypertrophy. Paradoxically, excessive sweating is a fairly common complaint; the mechanism of this response is not known. Weakness and fatigue are attributable to central effects of the drugs. There are marked individual differences in the type and the frequency of these side effects, and

Table 19–5. **ANTIDEPRESSANT DRUGS: DOSAGE FORMS AND DOSES**

NONPROPRIETARY NAME	TRADE NAMES	DOSAGE FORMS *	USUAL DAILY DOSE (*mg*)	EXTREME DAILY DOSE (*mg*) †
Tricyclics				
Amitriptyline HCl ‡	AMITRIL, ELAVIL	O,I	75–150	40–300
Amoxapine	ASENDIN	O	200–300	50–600
Desipramine HCl	NORPRAMIN, PERTOFRANE	O	75–200	25–300
Doxepin HCl	ADAPIN, SINEQUAN	O,L	75–150	25–300
Imipramine HCl	JANIMINE, TOFRANIL	O,I	50–200	30–300
Maprotiline HCl	LUDIOMIL	O	75–150	25–300
Nortriptyline HCl	AVENTYL, PAMELOR	O,L	75–100	20–150
Protriptyline HCl	VIVACTIL	O	15–40	15–60
Trimipramine maleate	SURMONTIL	O	50–150	50–300
Atypical				
Trazodone HCl	DESYREL	O	150–200	50–600
Monoamine Oxidase Inhibitors				
Isocarboxazid	MARPLAN	O	10–30	10–30
Phenelzine sulfate	NARDIL	O	15–30	15–90
Tranylcypromine sulfate	PARNATE	O	20–30	10–30

* Dosage forms: O = oral solid; L = oral liquid; I = injection.

† Extreme doses are for very young and very elderly patients at the low end and for hospital use in severe or treatment-resistant depression at the high end. In addition, due to the long biological half-life of MAO inhibition, small doses of MAO inhibitors are used after several days to weeks of treatment.

‡ Amitriptyline is also available in fixed-dose combinations with perphenazine (ETRAFON, TRIAVIL) and with chlordiazepoxide (LIMBITROL).

they may be related to concentrations of active drug in plasma. Older patients suffer more from dizziness, postural hypotension, constipation, delayed micturition, edema, and muscle tremors. Very rarely, amitriptyline may cause inappropriate secretion of ADH. Trazodone, but not the other antidepressant agents, can cause priapism and permanent impotence (Lansky and Selzer, 1984).

Another undesirable effect of antidepressant drugs (and apparently of all effective forms of medical treatment of depression) is a transition in certain patients from depression to hypomanic or *manic excitement*. This striking feature of so-called bipolar manic-depressive illness is sometimes referred to as the "switch process" (Bunney *et al.*, 1972; Goodwin, 1983). In addition to manic reactions to tricyclic antidepressants, confusion or delirium is common. These may be seen in approximately 10% of treated patients (and in over 30% of patients over age 50) (Davies *et al.*, 1971). These drug-related problems are frequently overlooked or misinterpreted as being part of the primary illness, particularly in the elderly. Small doses of physostigmine may aid in the diagnosis in some cases (*see* Granacher and Baldessarini, 1975). Among the CNS problems associated with tricyclic antidepressants, extrapyramidal reactions are rare, although *tremor* is not unusual. A fine tremor occurs in about 10% of those receiving a tricyclic agent; the prevalence of this effect is much higher in elderly patients, particularly when high doses of drug are administered. Tremor may respond to small doses of propranolol. In the therapy of CNS-based toxic or psychiatric reactions to tricyclic antidepressants, *antipsychotic drugs* are to be *avoided*, except for the management of manic reactions or severe agitation. They may exacerbate toxic confusional states, rather than help them. In any of these reactions, whether manic or toxic-organic, the best first step is to *stop the antidepressant*. Physostigmine may be effective in some cases, and, if sedation is urgently required, small doses of a benzodiazepine may be considered. Another toxic effect of tricyclic antidepressants is an increased risk of tonic-clonic seizures. This risk appears to

be especially great with maprotiline in doses above 250 mg per day (Rotblatt, 1982). There is some evidence that desipramine may have relatively less effect on seizure thresholds. In cases of overdosage, the incidence of seizures is markedly greater with amoxapine than with any other tricyclic antidepressant (Litovitz and Troutman, 1983).

Although *loss of accommodation* is a common ophthalmological side effect of any strongly anticholinergic agent, including tricyclic antidepressants, the precipitation of *glaucoma*, while frequently mentioned, is actually a rare event. The risk is probably highest in elderly patients with the narrow-angle type of glaucoma. They require emergency treatment with a miotic agent if an attack is precipitated. Tricyclic antidepressants can still be used in patients with glaucoma, provided that pilocarpine eyedrops or an equivalent medication is continued (Nouri and Cuendet, 1971). The most rational choice of an antidepressant in such a case would be desipramine or, especially, trazodone, due to the relatively low anticholinergic potency of these agents.

Various types of *cardiovascular difficulties* have already been discussed. In the absence of cardiac disease, the principal problem associated with imipramine-like agents is postural hypotension, which can be severe. There is risk of ischemic damage to the heart or brain in vulnerable individuals. Dihydroergotamine (10 mg per day) has been used safely to treat such hypotension (Bojanovsky and Tölle, 1974). However, it is often helpful to change medication to an agent (such as desipramine) with less α-adrenergic blocking activity, to reduce or divide doses, and to instruct patients in the need to rise slowly from a recumbent position. Tricyclic antidepressants, especially the tertiary amines and protriptyline, are to be avoided in the period following an acute myocardial infarction, in the presence of defects in bundle-branch conduction, or when other cardiac depressants are being administered. Mild congestive heart failure and the presence of many cardiac arrhythmias are not necessarily contraindications to the use of an antidepressant when depression and its associated medical risks are severe and appropriate medical care is provided (*see* Glassman and Bigger, 1981; Cassem, 1982; Veith *et al.,* 1982).

Children seem to be especially vulnerable to cardiotoxic and seizure-inducing effects of high doses of tricyclic compounds (Morselli, 1977). Deaths have occurred in children after accidental or deliberate overdosage with only a few hundred milligrams of drug.

Miscellaneous toxic effects of tricyclic antidepressants include jaundice, agranulocytosis, and rashes, but these are very infrequent. Weight gain has been described; while its mechanism is obscure, increased appetite and caloric intake are usually implicated. Delay of orgasm and *orgasmic impotence* have been described in men and women. The safety of antidepressants during pregnancy and lactation or in the treatment of young children is not well established. Epidemiological evidence concerning the possibility of *teratogenic effects* of the tricyclic agents is unconvincing (*see* Goldberg and DiMascio, 1978). Nevertheless, the possibility of toxic effects on the fetus remains (Morselli, 1977). For severe depression during pregnancy and lactation, ECT may be a relatively safe and effective alternative.

Acute poisoning with tricyclic antidepressants is not uncommon and, unlike acute overdosage with antipsychotic drugs, is life threatening. Unfortunately, most of the drugs used in the treatment of severe disorders of mood (tricyclic agents, MAO inhibitors, and lithium salts) are potentially lethal in doses that are available to patients with a high risk of suicide. While the margin of safety for the tricyclic antidepressants is not accurately known for man, deaths have been reported with doses of approximately 2000 mg of imipramine (or the equivalent of another drug), and severe intoxication can be expected at doses above 1000 mg. As a general rule, *it is unwise to dispense more than a week's supply of an antidepressant to an acutely depressed patient.*

The presentation of symptoms and the course of events in acute poisoning due to a tricyclic antidepressant is often complex (Nobel and Matthew, 1969; Nicotra *et al.,* 1981). A typical pattern is a brief phase of excitement and restlessness, sometimes with myoclonus, tonic-clonic seizures, or dystonia, followed by rapid development of coma, often with depressed respiration, hypoxia, depressed reflexes, hypothermia, and hypotension. There is striking evidence of anticholinergic effects, with mydriasis, flushed dry skin and dry mucosae, decreased bowel sounds, urinary retention, and tachycardia or other cardiac arrhythmias.

At this crucial stage the patient must be treated in an intensive care unit that provides constant cardiac monitoring and defibrillation and resuscitation when necessary. The most urgent needs are to support vital functions. Gastric lavage is sometimes used early in treatment, but this is best done only with a cuffed endotracheal tube safely in place. Although dialysis and diuresis are useless in such cases, administration of activated charcoal to adsorb the drug in the gut has some demonstrated utility (Crome *et al.,* 1977). The comatose phase disappears gradually, usually over 1 to 3 days, depending on the severity of the poisoning. A period of excitement and delirium is then very typical, again with prominent anticholinergic signs. Even when this phase of delirious intoxication has passed, the risk of life-threatening cardiac arrhythmias continues for at least several days, requiring close medical supervision and continued cardiac monitoring.

The efficacy and safety of various pharmacological interventions to counter tricyclic poisoning remain unsettled. Although physostigmine salicylate can sometimes produce dramatic effects to alleviate many of the antimuscarinic, cardiotoxic, and neurotoxic features of this syndrome, its safety and efficacy seem to be greater in cases of mild intoxication, characterized by confusion and delirium but with stable vital functions and the absence of coma, seizures, or life-threatening cardiac arrhythmias (Granacher and Baldessarini, 1975). In any event, physostigmine should not substitute for the aggressive use of other life-supporting measures (Krenzelok *et al.,* 1981).

Cardiac toxicity and hypotension in such poisonings can be especially difficult to manage. The heart is usually hyperactive, with supraventricular tachycardia and a high cardiac output. The QRS complex of the ECG is moderately responsive to tricyclic antidepressants, and in acute overdosage it is typically prolonged to over 100 milliseconds. Generally, cardiac glycosides and depressants such as quinidine or procainamide are contraindicated, but phenytoin has been given safely and may simultaneously be useful to suppress the convulsive seizures that are often present. In addition, propranolol has been recommended (*see* Vohra and Burrows, 1974). Diazepam has been used to control seizures and myoclonic and dystonic features of tricyclic antidepressant poisoning. Aside from the problems of management created by the specific effects of tricyclic antidepressants, serious hypoxia, hypertension or hypotension, and metabolic acidosis may have to be treated. In the presence of high concentrations of tricyclic antidepressants, the effects of α-adrenergic agonists, used as pressor agents, may be inhibited, and maintenance of intravascular volume may be difficult to achieve.

Interactions with Other Drugs. The tricyclic antidepressants are involved in several clinically important drug interactions (*see* Kaufman, 1976). The binding of tricyclic antidepressants to plasma albumin can be reduced by competition with phenytoin, phenylbutazone, aspirin, aminopyrine, scopolamine, and phenothiazines (*see* Gram *et al.*, 1973; Morselli, 1977). Other interactions that may also potentiate the effects of tricyclic drugs can result from interference with their metabolism in the liver. This effect has been associated with neuroleptic drugs (Linnoila *et al.*, 1982), methylphenidate, and certain steroids, including oral contraceptives (*see* Morselli, 1977). In the opposite direction, barbiturates and certain other sedatives, as well as cigarette smoking, can increase the hepatic metabolism of the antidepressants by inducing microsomal enzyme systems; benzodiazepines do not seem to have this effect.

Antidepressants potentiate the effects of alcohol, and probably other sedatives (Seppälä *et al.*, 1975). The anticholinergic activity of tricyclic antidepressants makes it important to monitor the results if the drugs must be used simultaneously with antiparkinsonian agents, antipsychotic drugs (especially thioridazine), or other compounds with antimuscarinic activity. The tricyclic antidepressants have prominent and potentially dangerous potentiative interactions with biogenic amines, such as norepinephrine, which normally are removed from their site of action by neuronal uptake. However, they block the effects of indirectly acting amines, such as tyramine, which must be taken up by sympathetic neurons to cause the release of norepinephrine (*see* Chapter 8). Presumably by a similar mechanism, the action of adrenergic neuron blocking agents such as guanethidine is prevented by the tricyclic antidepressants. This effect may be somewhat less noticeable with trimipramine and trazodone, which are less potent blockers of re-uptake of norepinephrine by sympathetic neurons. While its peripheral effects are blocked, the CNS stimulation produced by amphetamine may be potentiated by tricyclic antidepressants. This results from the inability of these drugs to interfere with amphetamine-induced release of dopamine from CNS neurons, combined with inhibition of the hepatic metabolism of amphetamine by tricyclic antidepressants (*see* Sulser, in Symposium, 1978).

Tricyclic agents and trazodone can block the centrally mediated antihypertensive action of clonidine. A particularly severe, but rare, interaction has been noted following the concurrent administration of an MAO inhibitor and a tricyclic antidepressant. The resultant syndrome can include severe CNS toxicity, marked by hyperpyrexia, convulsions, and coma. Although this reaction is rare and the two classes of antidepressant agents have been combined safely (*see* White and Simpson, 1981), this use should be regarded as unusual and controversial, since the interaction has a potentially catastrophic outcome. There is insufficient evidence that treatment with tricyclic agents plus MAO inhibitors is more efficacious than a tricyclic antidepressant alone. Tricyclic antidepressants can be used safely during ECT.

Therapeutic Uses. The use of tricyclic antidepressants in depressed patients is discussed below (*see* page 431).

Several other possible indications for these drugs have been suggested (Klein *et al.*, 1980; Baldessarini, 1983). *Enuresis* in children over 6 years of age has been accepted as a possible use for imipramine (in doses up to 2.5 mg/kg, or 50 mg total, daily), but such treatment produces only temporary effects (*see* Popper, 1985). Since there is increased recognition of the incidence of major depression in children, the use of imipramine and other antidepressants in this age group is becoming more accepted (Puig-Antich *et al.*, 1978). Because of the more efficient clearance of tricyclic antidepressants in children, effective doses may be up to twice the adult doses on a mg/kg basis (*see* Popper, 1985).

Other areas of suggested use that remain investigational include certain syndromes that may mimic depression, overlap diagnostically with depression, or be accompanied by or complicated by secondary depression. These include *alcoholism*, eating disorders (especially bulimia; *see* Hudson *et al.*, 1985), and the neuroses, especially *anxiety syndromes* that are characterized by *panic* reactions (Klein *et al.*, 1980) and some cases of *obsessive-compulsive disorder*. The latter is difficult to treat by any method, and it remains unclear if the occasional benefit seemingly provided by antidepressant drugs reflects an action on the primary disorder or on secondary depression that frequently accompanies it. *Chronic pain, neuralgias, migraine*, and *sleep apnea* are other syndromes that may belong in the same category and that sometimes respond favorably to tricyclic agents or to other treatments used for depression. There is also suggestive evidence that some antidepressants, notably amitriptyline and doxepin, may be of benefit in the treatment of patients with *peptic ulcer*. It is not certain whether the blockade of muscarinic and H_2-histaminergic receptors by these agents can account completely for these effects.

MONOAMINE OXIDASE (MAO) INHIBITORS

The MAO inhibitors comprise a chemically heterogeneous group of drugs that have in common the ability to block oxidative deamination of naturally occurring monoamines. However, the relationship between MAO inhibition and some of the ancillary therapeutic actions of these drugs is not firmly established. These drugs have numerous other effects, many of which are still poorly understood. For example, they lower blood pressure and were at one time used to treat hypertension. Their use in psychiatry has also become very limited as the tricyclic antidepressants have come to dominate the treatment of depression and allied conditions. Thus, MAO inhibitors are used most often when tricyclic antidepressants give an unsatisfactory result and when ECT is inappropriate or refused. In addition, it has been repeatedly suggested, with some scientific support, that whereas severe depression may not be the primary indication for these agents, certain neurotic illnesses with depressive features, and also with anxiety and phobias, may respond especially favorably. (*See* Robinson *et al.,* 1978; Klein *et al.,* 1980; Baldessarini, 1983.) The early record of success of MAO inhibitors in controlled trials in comparison with tricyclic antidepressants or ECT was not good (Klein *et al.,* 1980). Insufficient dosage may have caused this poor record, since recent studies and experience with larger doses have yielded benefits in major depression comparable to those obtained with imipramine and its congeners. These results have led to increased interest in these agents and to increases in the recommended dosages. Nevertheless, the complex, sometimes severe, and often unpredictable interactions between MAO inhibitors and many drugs and food-derived amines, as well as their tendency to damage the hepatic parenchyma, have made their medical use difficult and potentially hazardous.

History. In 1951, *isoniazid* and its isopropyl derivative, *iproniazid,* were developed for the treatment of tuberculosis. It was soon found that iproniazid had mood-elevating effects in tuberculous patients. In 1952, Zeller and coworkers found that iproniazid, in contrast to isoniazid, was capable of inhibiting the enzyme MAO. Following investigations by Kline and colleagues and by Crane it was applied in psychiatry for the treatment of depressed patients. MAO inhibitors had an important impact on the development of modern biological psychiatry. (For reviews of this topic, *see* Weil-Malherbe, 1967; Ayd and Blackwell, 1970; Baldessarini, 1983.) Because of toxicity, there has been a great deal of flux in the introduction and withdrawal of MAO inhibitors. At present, the MAO inhibitors available for use in depression are *isocarboxazid, phenelzine,* and *tranylcypromine.*

Chemistry and Structure-Activity Relationship. The first MAO inhibitors to be used in the treatment of depression were derivatives of hydrazine, a highly hepatotoxic substance. *Phenelzine* is the hydrazine analog of phenylethylamine, a substrate for MAO; *isocarboxazid* is a hydrazide derivative that probably must be converted to the corresponding hydrazine in order to produce long-lasting inhibition of MAO. Subsequently, compounds unrelated to hydrazine were found to be potent MAO inhibitors. Several of these agents were structurally related to amphetamine and were synthesized in an attempt to enhance central stimulant properties. Cyclization of the side chain of amphetamine resulted in the MAO inhibitor *tranylcypromine.* Details of the structure-activity relationship and the chemistry of these agents can be found elsewhere (*see* Kaiser and Zirkle, 1970; Biel *et al.,* 1978). Structures of the MAO inhibitors currently available in the United States for psychiatric patients are as follows:

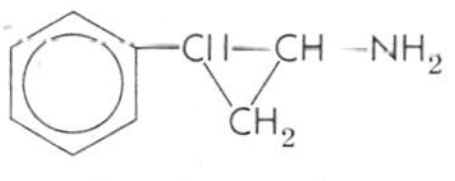

Tranylcypromine

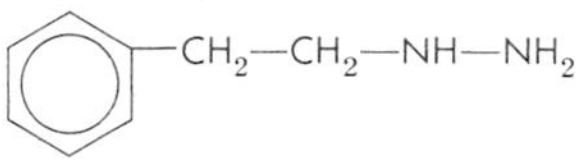

Phenelzine

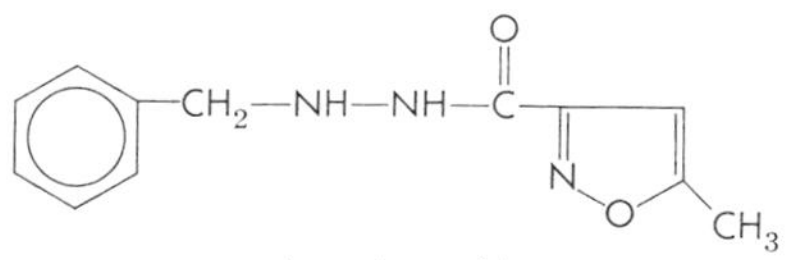

Isocarboxazid

PHARMACOLOGICAL PROPERTIES

MAO inhibitors exert their effects mainly on organ systems influenced by sympathomimetic amines and 5-HT. These agents inhibit not only MAO but other enzymes as well, and *they interfere with the hepatic metabolism of many drugs.* In addition, they are believed to exert effects not directly related to enzyme inhibition. MAO is a flavin-containing enzyme that is localized in mitochondrial membranes, whether in nerve terminals, the liver, or other organs. It is biochemically dissimilar to other nonspecific amine oxidases found, for example, in plasma. It is closely linked functionally with an aldehyde reductase in all tissues, but the products of these reactions can be carboxylic acids *or* alcohols, depending on the substrate and the tissue. MAO is important in regulating the metabolic degradation of catecholamines and 5-HT in neural or target tissues, and hepatic MAO has a crucial defensive role in inactivating circulating monoamines or those, such as tyramine, that originate in the gut and are absorbed into the portal circulation.

There are at least two types of MAO that display dissimilar preferences for substrates and differential sensitivities to selective inhibitors; these were originally defined by sensitivity to *clorgiline* and preference for 5-HT (MAO-A) and by sensitivity to *deprenyl* and preference for phenylethylamine (MAO-B). While direct biochemical evidence is incomplete, the two types appear to be distinct molecular entities that exist in various proportions in different tissues. For example, human placenta contains only MAO-A, and this type appears to be predominant in the peripheral noradrenergic nerve terminals of the rat. In contrast, human platelets contain only MAO-B, while about equal amounts of both types are found in the liver and brain of most species. The MAO inhibitors currently in therapeutic use are relatively nonselective, but selective inhibitors may offer advantages in certain clinical settings. Extensive discussions of these and other aspects of MAO and its inhibitors are provided in a symposium (*see* Symposium, 1979). (*See also* Chapters 4, 8, 9, and 21.)

The MAO inhibitors in clinical use are site-directed, irreversible ("suicide") inhibitors (*see* Singer, in Symposium, 1979). The hydrazines (phenelzine and the putative active metabolite of isocarboxazid) and the acetylenic agents (pargyline, clorgiline, and deprenyl) attack and inactivate the flavin prosthetic group following their oxidation to reactive intermediates by MAO. The chemistry of inhibition by cyclopropylamines (tranylcypromine) is less certain, but appears to involve the reaction of a sulfhydryl group in the active center of the enzyme following the formation of an *imine* by the action of MAO. In the clinical setting, maximal inhibition is usually achieved within a few days, although the antidepressant effect of these drugs may be delayed for 2 or 3 weeks. Up to 2 weeks may be required to restore amine metabolism to normal following withdrawal of the drugs, presumably because of the necessity for synthesis of new molecules of the enzyme; reversal following tranylcypromine is more rapid, possibly reflecting slow, spontaneous decomposition of the enzyme-inhibitor adduct. Behavioral effects of tranylcypromine are also produced more rapidly, perhaps due to amphetamine-like stimulant actions.

The enzyme-inhibitory effects of these drugs can be evaluated in human subjects by assay of urinary amines and their deaminated metabolites, sometimes after a test dose of an amine, or by direct assay of MAO activity in conveniently biopsied tissues, such as skin or jejunum, or, more commonly, in platelets. The platelet technic (which provides an index of the inhibition only of MAO-B) is currently favored as a means of monitoring the actions of MAO inhibitors and has led to the impression that favorable clinical responses are likely to occur when platelet MAO is inhibited by at least 85% (Robinson *et al.*, 1978). This relationship is best established for phenelzine, although it may also obtain with isocarboxazid; it sometimes has been a useful guide for therapy when large doses of tranylcypromine have proven to be clinically ineffective. However, clinical responses to clorgiline (which is selective for MAO-A) can be obtained with little or no reduction in MAO activity in platelets (*see* Murphy *et al.*, in Symposium, 1979).

The capacity of MAO inhibitors to act as antidepressants has most often been assumed to reflect the increased availability of one or more monoamine in the CNS or sympathetic nervous system, although this assumption has been difficult to prove. One problem is that the acute biochemical and pharmacological actions of MAO inhibitors precede the palliative effects in psychiatric illnesses by as long as 2 or more weeks. Reasons for this delay of therapeutic effects remain unexplained, but they are reminiscent of the comparable properties of the tricyclic antidepressants.

Effects on Sleep and the EEG. MAO inhibitors are among the most effective suppressors of REM sleep that are known. This effect has been used therapeutically in the treatment of narcolepsy. Moreover, when they are effective in the treatment of depression, MAO inhibitors correct the accompanying disorder of sleep, whether it is an increase or decrease of sleep time. In man, the effects of the MAO inhibitors upon the EEG are slight. Tranylcypromine does, however, have stimulant-like effects on the EEG.

Animal Behavior. The administration of single doses of an MAO inhibitor produces either minor changes in the behavior of animals or none at all, even when biochemical studies reveal marked alteration in the activity of the enzymes in the brain and significant elevations of concentrations of dopamine, norepinephrine, and 5-HT in the brain. However, when these drugs are combined with other agents, marked effects upon behavior and CNS function may be seen. Thus, in animals pretreated with MAO inhibitors, reserpine and tetrabenazine produce excitement rather than sedation (probably because of protection of monoamines released from intracellular storage); hexobarbital sleeping time is prolonged, and the actions of many other CNS depressants and stimulants may be augmented.

Cardiovascular System. The predominant cardiovascular effect associated with the use of MAO inhibitors in the treatment of depression is orthostatic hypotension, with little effect on basal diastolic pressure. In hypertensive patients, MAO inhibitors lower blood pressure and provide symptomatic relief in angina pectoris. Their use as antihypertensive agents, now obsolete, is described in *previous editions* of this textbook (*see also* Chapters 8 and 9).

Absorption, Fate, and Excretion. All the currently employed MAO inhibitors are readily absorbed when given by mouth. They are not given parenterally. These drugs produce maximal inhibition of MAO in biopsy samples from man within 5 to 10 days. There is little information on their pharmacokinetics. However, their biological activity is prolonged due to the characteristics of their interaction with the enzyme.

The hydrazide MAO inhibitors are thought to be cleaved, with resultant liberation of active products (*e.g.*, hydrazines). They are inactivated primarily by acetylation. About one half the population in the United States and Europe (and more in other populations, such as Eskimos and certain Orientals) are "slow acetylators" of hydrazine-type drugs, including phenelzine, and this may contribute to the exaggerated effects observed in some patients given conventional doses of phenelzine (Vesell, 1972).

Preparations and Dosage. These are presented in Table 19–5. A further consideration of dosage and the clinical use of these agents appears below.

Toxic Reactions and Side Effects. Toxic reactions from *overdosage* may occur in a matter of hours despite the long delay in onset of a therapeutic response. Reported effects of overdosage include agitation, hallucinations, hyperreflexia, hyperpyrexia, and convulsions. Both hypotension and hypertension have been reported. Treatment of such intoxication presents a problem. Sympathomimetic amines and barbiturates should be used with extreme caution. Conservative treatment aimed at maintaining normal temperature, respiration, blood pressure, and proper fluid and electrolyte balance has often been successful. Since the inhibition of the enzyme is irreversible, late toxic effects may appear. Patients with known overdosage of MAO inhibitors should be observed in the hospital for at least a week after the poisoning.

The potential toxic effects of the MAO inhibitors are more varied and potentially more serious than are those of any other group of therapeutic agents used in the treatment of psychiatric patients. The most dangerous are those involving the liver, the brain, and the cardiovascular system. Hepatotoxicity does not seem to be related to dosage or duration of therapy, and the incidence with currently used MAO inhibitors is low. Nevertheless, when it does occur, it can be serious because the hydrazine compounds cause cellular damage to the hepatic parenchyma. This problem led to discontinuation of use of several MAO inhibitors.

Excessive central stimulation consisting in tremors, insomnia, and hyperhidrosis may occur and might be considered extensions of the pharmacological effects. Agitation and hypomanic behavior may also occur, and on rare occasions hallucinations and confusion are observed. *Convulsions* have also been reported. Peripheral *neuropathy* following the use of hydrazines may possibly be related to a pyridoxine deficiency.

Orthostatic hypotension occurs with the use of all the MAO inhibitors currently employed. The immediate condition readily yields to recumbency, but the dose may have to be reduced or the medication withdrawn.

A variety of other less serious side effects have been reported, including dizziness and vertigo (perhaps related to orthostatic hypotension), headache, inhibition of ejaculation, difficulty in urination, weakness, fatigue, dry mouth, blurred vision, and skin rashes. Constipation is common, but the cause is not known. Phenelzine seems especially likely to exert such effects, even though significant antimuscarinic activity has not been detected *in vitro*.

Interactions with Other Drugs. The paucity of grossly observable signs following the administration of MAO inhibitors is deceptive, for major changes have occurred in the body's capacity to handle endogenous or exogenous biogenic amines and to respond normally to a wide spectrum of pharmacological agents. When MAO is inhibited, biogenic amines are not deaminated but remain active and produce behavioral and pharmacodynamic effects.

Because of their interference with various enzymes, the MAO inhibitors prolong and intensify the effects of other drugs and interfere with the metabolism of various naturally occurring substances. There is considerable evidence that administration of *precursors of biogenic amines* may cause marked effects when administered following MAO inhibitors. Thus, the administration of levodopa or 5-hydroxytryptophan (but not tryptophan) increases the concentrations of catecholamines or 5-HT, respectively, in brain and produces signs of central excitation in animals. The concurrent administration of levodopa and an MAO inhibitor to patients can be expected to produce agitation and hypertension.

The actions of *sympathomimetic amines* are potentiated following the use of MAO inhibitors. The effect is greater with indirectly acting amines (*e.g.*, amphetamine and tyramine) than with directly acting amines, which are potentiated in man to a greater degree by the tricyclic antidepressants. Since administered catecholamines are largely inactivated by catechol-O-methyltransferase and by neuronal re-uptake, the MAO inhibitors have less effect in prolonging and intensifying their action. On the other hand, inasmuch as certain sympathomimetic amines such as amphetamine and tyramine act peripherally, primarily by releasing the stores of catecholamines in nerve endings, and since the concentration of amines is raised by MAO inhibitors, profound potentiation of effects such as pressor responses may be expected (*see* below).

MAO inhibitors also interfere with detoxication mechanisms for certain other drugs. They prolong and intensify the effects of central-depressant agents, such as general anesthetics, sedatives, antihistamines, alcohol, and potent analgesics; of anticholinergic agents, particularly those used in the treatment of parkinsonism; and of antidepressant agents, especially imipramine and amitriptyline. A serious *hyperpyrexic* reaction occurs after the concomitant use of *meperidine*. This reaction may be mediated by the release of 5-HT, since it does not occur in experimental animals if they are pretreated with an inhibitor of 5-HT synthesis (*see* Kaufman, 1976).

Hypertensive crisis is a most serious toxic effect of MAO inhibitors related to drug interaction. Hypertensive crises were noted to be associated with the ingestion of cheese in patients receiving MAO inhibitors, particularly tranylcypromine and phenelzine but also other agents in this class. Acting on the suggestion of an alert pharmacist, Blackwell suggested that certain cheeses might contain a pressor amine or substance capable of liberating stored catecholamines (*see* Ayd and Blackwell, 1970). *Tyramine* was soon implicated as the culpable substance. The average meal of natural or aged cheeses contains enough tyramine to provoke a marked rise in blood pressure and other cardiovascular changes. As a result of inhibition of MAO, tyramine and other monoamines in food or produced by bacteria in the gut escape oxidative deamination in the liver and other organs and release catecholamines that are present in supranormal amounts in nerve endings and the adrenal medulla. Other foods implicated in this syndrome include beer, wine, pickled herring, snails, chicken liver, yeast, large quantities of coffee, citrus fruits, canned figs, broad beans (which contain dopa), and chocolate and cream or their products. Realistically, since more than 10 mg of tyramine seems to be required to produce significant hypertension, the most dangerous foods are aged cheeses and yeast products used as food supplements (*see* Folks, 1983). Patients being treated with an MAO inhibitor and their families should be given a list of foods to be avoided and a general warning about the use of *any* medication by the patient without permission. Care must even be exercised here, since certain depressed patients have used such a list as a compilation of potential suicidal agents.

In certain instances, intracranial bleeding has occurred, and death has sometimes followed. Headache is a common symptom, and fever frequently accompanies the hypertensive episode. Opioids should never be used for such headaches, and blood pressure should be evaluated immediately when a patient taking an MAO inhibitor reports a severe throbbing headache. There is a clinical similarity of the hypertensive syndrome to that seen in pheochromocytoma. Such episodes may also be encountered when MAO inhibitors are used with sympathomimetic amines, methyldopa, and dopamine. Acute increases in blood pressure can also follow the initial doses of reserpine and adrenergic neuron blocking agents such as guanethidine, when these are given concurrently with an MAO inhibitor. It should be noted that tranylcypromine can cause a reaction if administered when the effect of phenelzine is still present.

Switching a patient from one MAO inhibitor to another or to a tricyclic antidepressant requires that a rest period of 2 weeks intervenes.

Treatment of the hypertensive crisis is directed at lowering the blood pressure. For this purpose a short-acting α-adrenergic blocking agent (*e.g.*, phentolamine, 2 to 5 mg, intravenously) is recommended. In an emergency, chlorpromazine (50 to 100 mg, intramuscularly) can be used if phentolamine is not at hand. Fever may be reduced by external cooling.

The actual incidence of serious side effects is difficult to determine. It has been estimated that by 1970 3.5 million patients had used tranylcypromine and, of these, 50 persons sustained cerebrovascular accidents and 15 died. Coincidental presence of nondrug-induced pathology probably plays an important role. There is no evidence that the relative incidence of hypertensive crises is any greater with tranylcypromine than with the other agents in this class. However, tranylcypromine is not recommended for use in patients over 60 years of age, or in those with cardiac disease or hypertension or at risk of stroke; it is questionable whether *any* MAO inhibitor should be used by patients in these categories.

It is important to distinguish between the hypertensive interaction of MAO inhibitors and pressor amines and the potentially catastrophic interaction between MAO inhibitors and tricyclic antidepressants. The latter reaction is characterized by high fever and cerebral excitation, with variable degrees of hypertension; its mechanism is obscure. There is evidence that tricyclic antidepressants protect against the pressor effects of indirectly acting sympathomimetic amines such as tyramine, which must be transported into sympathetic nerve terminals to exert their action.

Therapeutic Uses. The MAO inhibitors have been used primarily in the treatment of *depression* and certain *phobic-anxiety* states. They also may be of value in the treatment of *bulimia, posttraumatic* reactions, and other *obsessive-compulsive*, ruminative disorders. Their possible use in *narcolepsy* is mentioned above. Since specific indications for their use are still evolving and their potential toxicity is relatively great, they have been reserved mainly for patients refractory to other treatments. They were at one time employed in the therapy of hypertension. The use of MAO inhibitors in psychiatry is discussed below, with other drug treatments for disorders of mood (page 431).

LITHIUM SALTS

Lithium salts were introduced into psychiatry in 1949 for the treatment of mania. However, they were not accepted in the United States for this use until 1970, in part due to reluctance of American physicians to accept the safety of this treatment. This was the result of reports of severe intoxication with lithium chloride from its use as a sodium substitute. Evidence for both the safety and the efficacy of lithium salts in the treatment of mania and the prevention of recurrent attacks of manic-depressive illness is now highly impressive. Many details of the pharmacology and uses of lithium salts in psychiatry and medicine are reviewed elsewhere (Baldessarini and Lipinski, 1975; Jefferson and Greist, 1977; Johnson, 1980; Herrington and Lader, 1981; Jefferson *et al.*, 1983).

History. Lithium urate is quite soluble, and, accordingly, lithium salts were used as a treatment of gout in the nineteenth century. The bromide of lithium was employed in that era as a sedative and anticonvulsant as well. Thereafter, lithium salts were little used until the late 1940s, when lithium chloride was employed as a salt substitute for cardiac and other chronically ill patients. This ill-advised usage led to several reports of severe intoxication and death and to considerable notoriety concerning lithium salts within the medical profession. Cade in Australia, while looking for toxic nitrogenous substances in the urine of mental patients for testing in guinea pigs, administered lithium salts to the animals in an attempt to increase the solubility of urates. Lithium carbonate made the animals lethargic, and, in an inductive leap, Cade gave lithium carbonate to several agitated or manic psychiatric patients. In 1949, he reported that this treatment seemed to have a specific effect in mania. For a more detailed account of the early development of lithium salts in psychiatric therapeutics, *see* Schou (1957, 1968) and Ayd and Blackwell (1970).

Chemistry. Lithium is the lightest of the alkali metals (group Ia); the salts of this monovalent cation share some characteristics with those of sodium and potassium, but not others. It is readily assayed in biological fluids by flame-photometric and atomic-absorption spectrophotometric methods. Traces of lithium ion occur in animal tissues, but it has no known physiological role. It is abundant in some alkaline mineral-spring waters. Both lithium carbonate and lithium citrate are currently in therapeutic use in the United States.

PHARMACOLOGICAL PROPERTIES

Therapeutic concentrations of lithium have almost no discernible psychotropic effects in normal man. It is not a sedative, depressant, or euphoriant, and this characteristic differentiates lithium from other psychotropic agents. The general biology and pharmacology of the lithium ion have been reviewed in detail by Schou (1957). The mechanism of action of lithium as a mood-stabilizing agent remains unknown, although effects on biological membranes are suspected.

An important characteristic of the lithium ion is that it has a relatively small gradient of distribution across biological membranes, unlike sodium and potassium; while it can replace sodium in supporting a single action potential in a nerve cell, it is not an adequate "substrate" for the sodium pump and it cannot, therefore, maintain membrane potentials. It is uncertain if important interactions occur between lithium (at therapeutic concentrations of about 1 mEq per liter) and the transport of other monovalent or divalent cations by nerve cells.

Central Nervous System. In addition to speculations about altered distribution of ions in the CNS, much attention has centered on the effects of low concentrations of lithium ion on the metabolism of the biogenic monoamines that have been implicated in the pathophysiology of mood disorders.

In animal brain tissue, lithium ion at concentrations of 1 to 10 mEq per liter inhibits the depolarization-provoked and calcium-dependent release of norepinephrine and dopamine, but *not* 5-HT, from nerve terminals. The release of 5-HT may even be enhanced by lithium, especially in the hippocampus (Treiser *et al.*, 1981). It may also slightly alter the re-uptake and presynaptic storage of catecholamines in directions consistent with increased inactivation of the amines. The ion has little effect on catecholamine-sensitive adenylate cyclase activity or on the binding of ligands to putative adrenergic receptors in brain tissue, although there is some evidence that lithium can inhibit the effects of receptor blocking agents to cause supersensitivity in such systems (Pert *et al.*, 1978; Bloom *et al.*, 1983). Lithium has been noted to modify hormonal responses mediated by adenylate cyclase in other tissues (*see* below). The effects of lithium on the distribution of sodium, calcium, and magnesium and on glucose metabolism have all been suggested to contribute to the antimanic or mood-stabilizing effects of the ion, but none of these hypotheses has been substantiated.

In recent years, evidence has accumulated for an important second-messenger role for inositol triphosphate and diacylglycerides (*see* Chapter 2). These compounds are released by hydrolysis of membrane phosphatidylinositides as a result of activation of receptors for numerous neurohormones. Lithium ion (at a concentration of 1 mM) severely inhibits the hydrolysis of *myo*-inositol-l-phosphate in brain and other tissues. As a result, lithium can decrease the content of phosphatidylinositides of cells that are stimulated intensely and that are insulated from exogenous sources of inositol (*e.g.*, neurons in the CNS). Depletion of phosphatidylinositides may reduce the responsiveness of neurons to muscarinic cholinergic, α-adrenergic, or other stimuli. Hypothetically, treatment with lithium ion could selectively modulate the function of hyperactive neurons that contribute to the manic state (*see* Berridge *et al.*, 1982; Berridge, 1984).

When given to manic patients who characteristically sleep very little, lithium corrects the sleep disorder as the mania abates. However, there are no well-established primary effects of lithium salts on sleep, except for some suppression of REM phases. Treatment with lithium also produces high-voltage slow waves in the human EEG, sometimes with superimposed fast-beta activity. Changes similar to those associated with ECT are occasionally observed and can include marked degrees of epileptiform discharge, even in subjects without a prior history of a seizure disorder (*see* Itil, 1978).

Absorption, Distribution, and Excretion. Lithium ions are readily and almost completely absorbed from the gastrointestinal tract. Complete absorption occurs in about 8 hours, with peak concentrations in plasma occurring 2 to 4 hours after an oral dose. Slow-release preparations of lithium carbonate provide a slower rate of absorption and thereby minimize fluctuations in plasma concentrations of the ion. However, absorption is variable and incomplete, and the incidence of lower intestinal tract symptoms may be increased. Lithium is initially distributed in the extracellular fluid and then gradually accumulated in various tissues to different degrees. The concentration gradients across cellular membranes are much smaller than those for sodium and potassium. The final volume of distribution (0.7 to 0.9 liter per kilogram) approaches that of total body water. Passage through the blood-brain barrier is slow, but when a steady state is achieved the concentration of lithium in the cerebrospinal fluid is about 40% of the concentration in plasma. There is no evidence of the ion binding to plasma proteins.

Approximately 95% of a single dose of lithium is eliminated in the urine. About one third to two thirds of an acute dose is excreted during a 6- to 12-hour initial phase of excretion, followed by a slow excretion over the next 10 to 14 days. The half-life averages 20 to 24 hours. With repeated administration, lithium excretion increases during the first 5 to 6 days until equilibrium is reached between ingestion and excretion. When therapy with lithium is stopped, there is a rapid phase of renal excretion followed by a slow 10- to 14-day phase. Since 80% of the filtered lithium is reabsorbed by the renal tubules, lithium clearance by the kidney is about 20% of that for creatinine, ranging between 15 and 30 ml per minute. This is somewhat lower in elderly patients (10 to 15 ml per minute) and higher in young persons. Sodium loading produces a small enhancement of lithium excretion, but *sodium depletion* promotes a clinically important degree of *retention of lithium*.

Because of the *low therapeutic index* for the lithium ion (as low as 2 or 3), concentrations in plasma or serum must be determined to facilitate the safe use of the drug. This is usually done daily in the treatment of acutely manic patients. Indeed, the risks of such early treatment are sufficiently great that one can postpone treatment with lithium until some degree of behavioral control and metabolic stability have been attained with antipsychotic drugs or sedatives. Although the concentration of lithium in blood is usually measured at a trough of the oscillations that result from repetitive administration, the peaks can be two or three times higher than the steady-state concentration. When the peaks are reached, intoxication may result. (This can occur even when concentrations in morning samples of plasma are in the acceptable range of 1 mEq per liter.) Because of the very low margin of safety of the lithium ion and because of its short half-life during initial distribution, *divided daily doses are used in man,* and even slow-release formulations are typically given twice daily.

While the pharmacokinetics of lithium varies considerably between subjects, it is relatively stable in the individual patient. However, well-established regimens can be complicated by occasional periods of sodium loss, as may occur with an intercurrent medical illness, or with losses or restrictions of fluids and electrolytes; heavy sweating may be an exception (*see* Jefferson *et al.*, 1982). Hence, all patients should have plasma concentrations checked at least occasionally. The relatively stable and characteristic pharmacokinetics of the lithium ion in single patients makes it possible to predict dosage requirements of an individual based on the results of administration of a single test dose of lithium carbonate, followed by a single plasma assay 24 hours later (Cooper and Simpson, 1978).

Most of the renal tubular reabsorption of the lithium ion seems to occur in the proximal tubule. Nevertheless, its retention can be increased by any diuretic that leads to sodium depletion (*e.g.*, furosemide, ethacrynic acid, and thiazides) (Himmelhoch *et al.*, 1977; DePaulo *et al.*, 1981). Renal excretion can be increased somewhat by the administration of osmotic diuretics, acetazolamide, or aminophylline, although this is of little help in the management of lithium-induced toxicity. Triamterene may increase excretion of lithium, suggesting that some reabsorption of the ion may occur in the distal nephron; however, spironolactone does not increase the excretion of lithium. Some nonsteroidal anti-inflammatory agents (*e.g.*, indomethacin and phenylbutazone) can facilitate renal proximal tubular resorption of lithium ion and thereby increase concentrations in plasma (*see* DePaulo *et al.*, 1981).

Less than 1% of ingested lithium leaves the human body in the feces, and 4 to 5% is excreted in the sweat (where it is secreted in relative excess compared to sodium) (*see* Jefferson *et al.*, 1982). Lithium is secreted in saliva in concentrations about twice those in plasma, while its concentration in tears is about equal to that in plasma. It is feasible to analyze these fluids instead of plasma in order to monitor lithium concentrations (Brenner *et al.*, 1982; Selinger *et al.*, 1982). Since the ion is also secreted in human milk, women receiving lithium should not breast-feed infants.

Preparations, Route of Administration, and Dosage. Preparations currently used in the United States are 300-mg tablets or capsules of Li_2CO_3. There are also slow-release preparations of lithium carbonate, as well as liquid preparations of lithium citrate. In Europe and elsewhere different quantities are sometimes prepared (*e.g.*, a 250-mg tablet), and salts other than the carbonate have been used. The carbonate salt is favored for tablets and capsules because it is relatively less hygroscopic and less irritating to the gut than other salts, especially the chloride. Parenteral administration is never employed.

Unlike most other drugs, the lithium ion is not prescribed merely by dose. Instead, due to the very low therapeutic index, determination of the concentration of the drug in blood is crucial, and lithium cannot be used with adequate safety in patients who cannot be tested regularly. The concentra-

tion that is currently considered to be optimal is between 0.8 and 1.25 mEq per liter; the range of 1.0 to between 1.25 and 1.5 mEq per liter is favored for treatment of manic or hypomanic patients. Somewhat lower values (0.75 to 1.0 mEq per liter) are considered adequate and safer for long-term use for prevention of recurrent manic-depressive illness; some patients may not relapse at concentrations as low as 0.5 to 0.75 mEq per liter. These concentrations refer to blood samples obtained at 10 ± 2 hours after the last oral dose of the day. The recommended concentration is often attained by doses of 900 to 1500 mg of lithium carbonate per day in outpatients and 1200 to 2400 mg per day in hospitalized manic patients; the optimal dose tends to be larger in younger and heavier individuals.

Toxic Reactions and Side Effects. Lithium therapy is associated initially with a transient increase in the excretion of 17-hydroxycorticosteroids, sodium, potassium, and water. This effect is usually not sustained beyond 24 hours. In the subsequent 4 to 5 days of lithium therapy, the excretion of potassium becomes normal, sodium is retained, and, in some cases, pretibial edema forms. Sodium retention has been associated with increased aldosterone secretion and responds to administration of spironolactone. Edema and sodium retention frequently disappear spontaneously after several days.

A small number of patients treated with lithium develop a benign, diffuse, nontender thyroid enlargement, suggestive of compromised thyroid function. In patients treated with lithium, thyroid ^{131}I uptake is increased, plasma protein-bound iodine and free thyroxine tend to be slightly low, and thyroid-stimulating hormone (TSH) secretion may be moderately elevated. These effects appear to result from interference with the iodination of tyrosine and, therefore, the synthesis of thyroxine. However, patients usually remain euthyroid and obvious hypothyroidism is rare. In patients who do develop goiter, discontinuation of lithium or treatment with thyroid hormone results in shrinkage of the gland. In rats, the ion inhibits thyrotropin activation of thyroid adenylate cyclase; inhibitory effects of lithium have been noted on the synthesis of cyclic AMP in several other situations (Forrest, 1975). Although it is unknown if there is a cause-and-effect relationship between this action of lithium and its subsequent effects, inhibition of adenylate cyclase could account for the antithyroid activity of the ion.

Polydipsia and polyuria occur in patients treated with lithium, occasionally to a disturbing degree. Cases of acquired nephrogenic diabetes insipidus have been reported in patients maintained at therapeutic plasma concentrations of the ion. Typically, mild polyuria appears early in treatment and then disappears. Late-developing polyuria is an indication to evaluate renal function, lower the dose of lithium, or consider addition of a thiazide diuretic to counteract the polyuria (*see* DePaulo *et al.*, 1981). The polyuria disappears with termination of lithium therapy. The mechanism of this effect may involve inhibition of the action of antidiuretic hormone (ADH) on renal adenylate cyclase, resulting in decreased ADH stimulation of renal reabsorption of water. However, there is also evidence that lithium may exert an action at steps beyond cyclic AMP synthesis to alter both thyroid and renal function. While there is uncertainty about the precise site of action of the cation, its effectiveness in blocking the renal response to ADH has aroused interest in its potential therapeutic usefulness in treatment of the syndrome of inappropriate secretion of ADH (White and Fetner, 1975). Evidence of chronic inflammatory changes in biopsied renal tissue has been found in a minority of patients given lithium for prolonged periods. Since there is little indication of progressive, clinically significant impairment of renal function, these are considered incidental findings by most experts; nevertheless, plasma creatinine and urine volume should be monitored during long-term use of lithium (*see* DePaulo *et al.*, 1981, and references therein).

The lithium ion also has a weak action on carbohydrate metabolism that resembles somewhat that of insulin. In intact rats, lithium causes an increase in skeletal muscle glycogen accompanied by severe depletion of glycogen from the liver. The mechanisms of action of insulin and lithium probably differ inasmuch as maximal amounts of the two agents produce additive effects on glucose metabolism in the isolated rat diaphragm (Haugaard *et al.*, 1974).

The prolonged use of lithium causes a benign and reversible depression of the T wave of the ECG, an effect not related to depletion of sodium or potassium (Demers and Heninger, 1971).

Lithium causes EEG changes characterized by diffuse slowing, widened frequency spectrum, and potentiation with disorganization of background rhythm. There are conflicting reports with regard to lithium and convulsive disorders. Seizures have been reported in nonepileptic patients with plasma lithium concentrations in the therapeutic range.

A benign, sustained increase in circulating polymorphonuclear leukocytes occurs during the chronic use of lithium and is reversed within a week after termination of treatment.

Allergic reactions such as dermatitis and vasculitis can occur with lithium administration.

The occurrence of toxicity is related to the plasma lithium concentration and its rate of rise following administration. Acute intoxication is characterized by vomiting, profuse diarrhea, coarse tremor, ataxia, coma, and convulsions. Symptoms of milder toxicity that are most likely to occur at the absorptive peak of lithium include nausea, vomiting, abdominal pain, diarrhea, sedation, and fine tremor. The more serious effects involve the nervous system and consist in mental confusion, hyperreflexia, gross tremor, dysarthria, seizures, and cranial-nerve and focal neurological signs, progressing to coma and death (Saron and Gaind, 1973). Other toxic effects are cardiac arrhythmias, hypotension, and albuminuria. In pregnancy, concomitant use of natriuretics and low-sodium diets can contribute to maternal and neonatal lithium intoxication (Goldfield and Weinstein, 1973), and during post-partum diuresis one can anticipate potentially toxic retention of lithium by the mother.

The use of lithium in pregnancy has been associated with neonatal goiter, CNS depression, hypotonia, and cardiac murmur. All these conditions reverse with time. More ominously, however, epidemiological data suggest that the use of lithium in early pregnancy may be associated with a severalfold increase in the incidence of cardiovascular anomalies of the newborn (especially Ebstein's malformation) (*see* Goldberg and DiMascio, 1978). For these reasons, the safety of lithium salts in pregnancy is at least uncertain, and such use is not recommended.

Treatment of Lithium Intoxication. Since there is no specific antidote for lithium intoxication, treatment is supportive. If renal function is adequate, excretion can be accelerated slightly with osmotic diuresis and intravenous sodium bicarbonate solution. Dialysis is probably the most effective means of removing the ion from the body and should be considered in severe poisonings. When the concentration of lithium in plasma is lowered by dialysis or other means, recovery is still slow. This suggests that the intracellular concentration of lithium may be the prime determinant of the appearance of clinical toxicity.

Interactions with Other Drugs. Interactions between lithium and diuretics have been discussed above. Lithium may decrease the pressor response to norepinephrine in man, as well as the subjective euphoria induced by cocaine or other stimulants. Thiazide diuretics may correct the nephrogenic diabetes insipidus caused by lithium (*see* Chapter 37). Lithium is often used in conjunction with antipsychotic, sedative, and antidepressant drugs. A few case reports have suggested a risk of increased CNS toxicity of lithium when it is combined with haloperidol; this is, however, at variance with more than a decade of experience with this combination (*see* Tupin and Schuller, 1978). The antipsychotic drugs may prevent nausea, which can be a sign of lithium toxicity. Urinary retention due to the anticholinergic effects of the tricyclic antidepressants can become particularly uncomfortable in the presence of a lithium-induced diuresis. There is, however, no absolute contraindication to the concurrent use of lithium and other psychotropic drugs. Nevertheless, extra caution is required in the simultaneous use of agents that have the potential to cause CNS toxicity. There are a few reports of confusional states following the use of ECT in patients who previously tolerated treatment with lithium (Mandel *et al.*, 1980).

Therapeutic Uses. The use of lithium in *manic-depressive illness* is discussed below. Lithium treatment is ideally conducted only in patients with normal sodium intake and with normal cardiac and renal function. Very occasionally, patients with severe systemic illnesses can be treated with lithium, provided there are sufficiently compelling indications. Its use in otherwise-healthy *adults or adolescents* for *acute mania* or the prevention of *recur-*

rences of bipolar manic-depressive illness are the only indications currently approved in the United States. In addition, based on compelling evidence of efficacy, it is also sometimes used as an alternative to tricyclic antidepressants in severe recurrent depression (nonbipolar manic-depressive illness) and as a supplement to antidepressant treatment in acute, major depression (*see* Davis, 1976; Ramsey and Mendels, 1981; Nelson and Byck, 1982). These beneficial effects may be associated with the presence of clinical features also found in bipolar affective disorder (*see* Baldessarini, 1983). There is also a growing clinical experience that suggests the utility of lithium in the management of disorders of childhood that are marked by episodic changes in mood and behavior and that bear an uncertain relationship to bipolar disorder in adults (*see* Popper, 1985).

Lithium salts have also been tried, with very mixed results, to treat a variety of disorders characterized by a recurrent or episodic course. These include premenstrual tension, drug-abuse syndromes including alcoholism, episodic aggression or anger, irregularity of food intake (notably in anorexia nervosa and the Klein-Levin syndrome with hypersomnia and hyperphagia), periodic catatonia (Gjessing's syndrome), and a variety of other neurotic, psychotic, or other behavioral disorders. In addition, lithium has undergone limited evaluation in several neurological disorders (especially Huntington's chorea and tardive dyskinesia), has been tried as an antithyroid agent, and has been used in the syndrome of inappropriate secretion of ADH. These trials have all had inconsistent or unconvincing results, and have not led to generally accepted treatments for any of the conditions listed (*see* Johnson and Johnson, 1978).

DRUG TREATMENT OF DISORDERS OF MOOD

Disorders of mood (*affective* disorders) are extremely common in general medical practice, as well as in psychiatry. The severity of these conditions covers an extraordinarily broad range, from normal grief reactions to death of a loved one, to severe, incapacitating, and frequently fatal psychosis. The lifetime risk of suicide in major affective disorders is about 15%, but this statistic does not begin to represent the morbidity of and cost from this group of severe and underdiagnosed illnesses. Clearly, not all of the grief, misery, and dis-appointments of the human condition are indications for medical treatment, and even severe affective disorders have a high rate of spontaneous remission, provided that sufficient time (perhaps only a matter of months) passes. The antidepressant agents or lithium salts are thus generally reserved for the more severe and incapacitating disorders of mood, and the most satisfactory results tend to occur in patients who have the more severe illnesses with the most "endogenous" or "melancholic" characteristics (*see* American Psychiatric Association, 1980; Baldessarini, 1983). The data from clinical research in support of the efficacy of antidepressant agents and of lithium are totally convincing (*see* Klerman, 1972; Klein *et al.*, 1980; Herrington and Lader, 1981; Baldessarini, 1983). Nevertheless, many shortcomings and problems continue to be associated with all drugs used to treat affective disorders. In addition to less-than-dramatic efficacy in some cases, virtually all of the drugs used to treat disorders of mood are potentially lethal when acute overdosage occurs and can cause an appreciable degree of less severe morbidity even with careful clinical use.

Despite their recognized limitations, the antidepressants and lithium salts have a well-established and important place in medical practice. Currently the tricyclic agents are the most widely used antidepressants. They are all apparently similar in efficacy for depression, provided that adequate doses are used for a sufficient period of time. Effective doses, calculated in terms of imipramine or its equivalent of a similar drug, are currently estimated to exceed 125 mg per day, and doses above 250 mg per day are best reserved for severely ill inpatients. Since the onset of action of all antidepressant drugs is delayed for up to 2 or 3 weeks, a trial of treatment with an adequate dose cannot be judged a failure for at least 1 month.

Secondary considerations govern the selection of a specific antidepressant. If some sedation seems desirable early in treatment, amitriptyline, doxepin, or trazodone is usually selected. If anticholinergic side effects are to be avoided, desipramine or trazodone may be a rational choice. Prior success with a specific agent is an additional consideration. The tertiary-amine tricyclic antidepressants are highly effective and commonly used; however, if they fail to produce satisfactory results, it is probably best to increase the dose, ideally with knowledge of the concentration of drug in plasma, before changing to other agents, such as the secondary-amine tricyclic antidepressants. This advice is based on research that indicates a complex biphasic relationship between the concentration of drug in blood and the clinical response for the *de-*methylated tricyclic agents (*see* Baldessarini, 1983).

Disappointing responses to antidepressant therapy usually result from the use of inadequate doses or too short a therapeutic trial. Unless a patient is very debilitated or unusually sensitive to the side effects of a tricyclic antidepressant, it is best to begin treatment with about 50 mg per day and to increase the dose rapidly to the equivalent of 150 mg per day or more of imipramine. For severely ill hospitalized patients, the dose can be raised to 300 mg per day, although little added benefit and much more toxicity are likely to result from these or higher doses. It is also wise to avoid single doses above 150 mg in outpatients. Due to the high rate of relapse within the first year following recovery from an acute, severe depressive illness, treatment is usually continued for at least several months. In this phase of treatment, doses below 100 mg per day of imipramine or its equivalent are less likely to be effective, and, as an approximate guideline, 100 to 150 mg per day for at least 3 to 6 months can be tried. Some physicians have attempted to discontinue treatment gradually over several months, in accordance with the clinical response observed. In addition to this approach to the management of the post-recovery phase of acute depression, there is increasing evidence that the prolonged use of a tricyclic agent can have important ameliorative or preventive effects on recurrent, nonbipolar depression. This treatment can be considered as an alternative to the use of lithium carbonate to prevent recurrent depression (*see* Davis, 1976; Klein *et al.*, 1980; Bialos *et al.*, 1982). While formal, controlled studies of long-term use of antidepressants have rarely exceeded 1 year, clinical experience indicates that many patients continue to obtain clinical benefit, safely, with imipramine-like agents for several years. There are a few case reports of possible "tolerance" to the antidepressant effects of MAO inhibitors after prolonged use.

While acute mania is a primary indication for the use of lithium carbonate, it is, in actual practice, an inferior agent for the management of severe manic attacks. These episodes represent a serious medical problem and require urgent hospitalization for the protection and careful medical management of the patient. While a few mildly hypomanic patients can be managed successfully as outpatients with lithium alone, it is more common to begin treatment of severely manic patients with antipsychotic doses of a neuroleptic drug (the type selected makes little difference). A benzodiazepine can also be used for sedation. As the intake of food and fluids becomes stable and the patient becomes more cooperative over 5 to 10 days, lithium can be introduced gradually and safely. While long-term benefits of antipsychotic drugs in bipolar disorders of mood have yet to be proven, the preventive effects of lithium carbonate have become its most compelling clinical indication. This is most clear with bipolar affective disorders, but lithium is probably also efficacious in the prevention of the emergence of recurrent depression. Tricyclic antide-

pressants, given alone, are usually contraindicated in bipolar illness, except to treat acute depressive phases, because of their tendency to provoke a "switch" to mania or hypomania. Even in acute depressive phases, bipolar patients are probably best managed with an antidepressant plus lithium. In view of the very low therapeutic index for lithium salts, it is important to be circumspect when advising a patient or family to embark on a prolonged regimen involving lithium. Factors that enter into this decision include the severity of the illness, the frequency of recurrence, and the probable reliability of the patient.

Other forms of treatment of depression have not been well established or are no longer regularly employed, with the important exception of ECT. This remains the most rapid and effective treatment for severe acute depression and is sometimes life-saving for acutely suicidal patients (*see* Avery and Winokur, 1977; Freeman *et al.*, 1978). The MAO inhibitors are generally considered drugs of second choice for the treatment of severe depression, even though the evidence for efficacy of adequate doses of tranylcypromine or phenelzine is convincing. The efficacy of isocarboxazid is uncertain, and the use of this agent is virtually extinct. Despite the favorable results obtained with tranylcypromine and with doses of phenelzine above 60 mg per day, the potential for unwanted reactions in their clinical use has limited their acceptance by many clinicians and patients. Nevertheless, MAO inhibitors are sometimes tried when a vigorous trial of a tricyclic antidepressant (*e.g.*, 200 to 300 mg daily of imipramine or its equivalent for 4 weeks) has been unsatisfactory and when ECT is refused. In addition, MAO inhibitors may have selective benefits for conditions other than depression, including neurotic illnesses marked by phobias and anxiety as well as dysphoria. Similar benefits may, however, be found with imipramine-like agents; thus, indications for the MAO inhibitors are limited and must be weighed against their potential toxicity and their complex interactions with many other drugs. Stimulants, with or without added sedatives, are an outmoded treatment for severe depression; not only are they ineffective compared to a placebo, but they worsen dysphoria and agitation in some patients. Some clinicians continue to find utility and safety in the short-term treatment of selected patients with a stimulant such as methylphenidate or amphetamine. These include patients with mild dysphoria or anergy associated with medical illnesses, as well as some geriatric patients; however, none of these possible indications has been investigated systematically.

III. Drugs Used in the Treatment of Anxiety

Sedatives with useful antianxiety effects are consistently among the most commonly prescribed drugs. The appropriate generic term for this group of agents remains uncertain, and terms such as *antianxiety agents, anxiolytics,* and *tranquilizers* represent to some extent wishful thinking and the impact of advertising. Drugs used to treat anxiety are sedatives or at least have many properties in common with traditional sedatives, such as the barbiturates. Even the benzodiazepines have sedative properties, particularly when relatively high doses are given. The wide diversity of compounds used to treat anxiety greatly complicates attempts to make generalizations about them. Many of these drugs are discussed in other chapters of this text (*see* Chapters 17, 18, 20, 21, 23, and 26). This section covers only a limited group of agents that are commonly used to treat anxiety and mild dysphoria, and only this use is emphasized. Since the benzodiazepines now dominate this field, they are given the most attention. Several reviews of the pharmacology of these drugs, particularly the benzodiazepines, are available (*see* Hollister *et al.,* 1980; Rosenbaum, 1982; Symposium, 1982; Greenblatt *et al.,* 1983b; Lader, 1984; Chapter 17).

History. Man has sought chemical agents to modify the effects of stress and the feelings of discomfort, tension, anxiety, and dysphoria throughout recorded history. Many of these efforts have led to the development of agents that are often classed as sedatives, and the single most widely used of these is one of the oldest—*ethanol.* In the last century, *bromide* salts and the *barbiturates* were introduced into medical practice as sedatives, along with compounds similar in effect to alcohol, including *paraldehyde* and *chloral hydrate.* By the 1930s it became apparent that bromides had cumulative toxic effects on the CNS, and their use in medical practice has largely disappeared. Throughout the early decades of this century, the barbiturates were the dominant antianxiety agents in medical practice; however, by the 1950s, there was concern with their propensity to induce tolerance, sometimes followed by physical dependence and potentially lethal reactions during withdrawal. These problems strongly colored professional and popular attitudes about sedatives and encouraged the search for safer agents. This experience probably contributed to the use of new terms that emphasize putative dissimilarities of newer agents from the barbiturates and related sedatives. Studies of derivatives of aliphatic polyalcohols led to the development of mephenesin, the *o*-methyl-phenyl derivative of propanetriol; this agent was found to have muscle relaxant and sedative properties, but was impractically short acting. Its chemical modifications led directly to the introduction of the *propanediol carbamates* (*meprobamate* and conge-

ners) in the early 1950s, along with a variety of other analogs of barbiturates or derivatives of higher alcohols.

Throughout the 1950s, despite the popularity of some of these compounds for daytime sedation or for hypnotic effects, an increasing awareness developed that they shared many of the undesirable properties of barbiturates. These included an unclear separation between their useful antianxiety effects and excessive sedation and an impressive propensity to cause physical dependence and severe acute intoxication on overdosage. This set the scene for the discovery of *chlordiazepoxide* in the late 1950s and the introduction of more than a dozen *benzodiazepine* congeners since that time. This class of sedatives has come to dominate the market and medical practice; in recent years, diazepam and its congeners have been among the frontrunners in terms of numbers of prescriptions written for all drugs used in medical practice.

BENZODIAZEPINES

Eight benzodiazepine derivatives are presently recommended for the treatment of anxiety. In their order of introduction, they are *chlordiazepoxide, diazepam, oxazepam, clorazepate, lorazepam, prazepam, alprazolam,* and *halazepam.* Although commonly used for treating anxiety, they share other therapeutic indications—notably sedation and induction of sleep. While other benzodiazepines are advertised with an emphasis on sedative or hypnotic effects, the differences between them and the eight recommended for anxiety are subtle and possibly insignificant in some cases (*see* Greenblatt *et al.,* 1983b). These other indications are discussed elsewhere (*see* Index).

History. Compounds of this type were initially synthesized in the 1930s. The first successful benzodiazepine, *chlordiazepoxide,* was developed by Sternbach's group at the Roche Laboratories in the late 1950s. Tests in animals indicated that chlordiazepoxide had interesting muscle relaxant, antistrychnine, and spinal reflex–blocking properties. It also produced "taming" of a number of species of animals in doses much lower than those producing ataxia or measurable hypnosis. This "taming" effect in monkeys led to the clinical trial of the drug in man for the determination of antianxiety effects. (For further details, *see* Symposium, 1982.)

Chemistry and Structure-Activity Relationship. Over 2000 benzodiazepines have been synthesized. The structure-activity relationship of this group has been reviewed by Sternbach (in Symposium, 1982). Chlordiazepoxide was the first compound introduced for clinical use, but several useful congeners have been developed. The structures of the eight benzodiazepines that are commonly recommended for treatment of anxiety are shown in Chapter 17 (Table 17–1, page 341).

Pharmacological Properties

Chlordiazepoxide and diazepam can be considered prototypical drugs for their class. They have achieved wide use as antianxiety agents.

Central Nervous System. *Behavioral and Neurophysiological Effects.* The effects of the benzodiazepines in the relief of anxiety can readily be demonstrated in experimental animals. In conflict punishment procedures, benzodiazepines greatly reduce the suppressive effects of punishment. Positive effects in this experimental model are not seen with antidepressants and antipsychotics. The behavioral effects of antianxiety agents are reviewed by Sepinwall and Cook (1978).

Difficulties in evaluating the therapeutic efficacy of psychotropic drugs in man are particularly great in the case of the antianxiety drugs, owing largely to the contribution of nonpharmacological factors to the treatment of anxiety; disparate results have thus been obtained. Many studies have shown that benzodiazepines are more effective than a placebo in the treatment of varied groups of anxious neurotic patients. However, negative results have also been reported (*see* Klein *et al.,* 1980). The clinical popularity of these drugs apparently is the result of a combination of their pharmacological actions, their relative safety, and an extraordinary demand for agents of this type by both doctors and patients.

In common with barbiturates, chlordiazepoxide blocks EEG arousal from stimulation of the brain stem reticular formation. Central-depressant actions of diazepam and other benzodiazepines on spinal reflexes occur and are in part mediated by the brain stem reticular system. Like meprobamate and the barbiturates, chlordiazepoxide depresses the duration of electrical afterdischarge in the limbic system, including the septal region, the amygdala, the hippocampus, and the hypothalamus. These and other limbic and autonomic effects are the focus of particular theoretical interest at the present time.

There is also much interest in the effects of benzodiazepines on neurotransmission in the CNS that is mediated by gamma-aminobutyrate (GABA). This has been stimulated by electrophysiological observations of their potentiation of the inhibitory effects of GABA, as well as by the discovery of specific binding sites for benzodiazepines in various brain regions. The binding of benzodiazepines can be modulated by both GABA and chloride ions even after solubilization and extensive purification of the binding sites. Compounds have been found that can competitively inhibit both the binding and the biological actions of the benzodiazepines, and endogenous substances are being sought that might be physiological ligands for such binding sites and that may either mimic or antagonize the actions of benzodiazepines. At concentrations in the therapeutic range, benzodiazepines can also reduce the excitability of some neurons by actions that involve neither GABA nor alterations in the permeability to chloride ions. Thus, the cellular mechanisms responsible for the behavioral effects of benzodiazepines remain to be clarified (*see* Tallman *et al.,* 1980; Yamamura, 1980; Mennini and Garattini, 1982; Skolnick and Paul, 1982; Study and Barker, 1982; Symposium, 1982; Chapters 17 and 20).

Effects on Sleep. Benzodiazepines can be used effectively as hypnotics in conjunction with their use as antianxiety drugs (Chapter 17). They seem to have only mild effects to suppress REM periods, but they do have a tendency to suppress the deeper phases of sleep, especially stage 4 (while *increasing* total sleep time). The significance of this is not known, but diazepam has been used in the treatment of "night terrors" that arise out of stage-4 sleep.

EEG Effects. The benzodiazepines cause an increase in fast-beta activity with an increase in amplitude of the EEG. This is a pattern similar to that of meprobamate and other sedatives. Virtually all benzodiazepines increase *seizure threshold* and are anticonvulsant. Diazepam and clorazepate are used clinically for this purpose (*see* Chapter 20).

Cardiovascular and Respiratory Systems. The cardiovascular effects of the benzodiazepines are mild, and this encourages their frequent use in cardiac patients. Diazepam, in an intravenous dose of 5 to 10 mg, causes a slight decrease in respiration, blood pressure, and left ventricular stroke work. Increase in heart rate and decrease in cardiac output can also occur. The effects are minimal, and it is unlikely that there is significant depression of cardiovascular function when the benzodiazepines are given in usual therapeutic doses by the oral route.

Skeletal Muscle. Diazepam and other benzodiazepines are widely used as muscle relaxants, although controlled studies have been inconsistent in showing an advantage of benzodiazepines over either placebo or aspirin. Some muscle relaxation occurs after administration of any of the CNS depressants, and the advantages of the benzodiazepines appear to be small when given by the oral route. (*See* Chapter 21.)

Absorption, Fate, and Excretion. Chlordiazepoxide, oxazepam, lorazepam, alprazolam, and halazepam are absorbed relatively slowly following oral administration, and peak concentrations in plasma may not be attained for hours. In contrast, diazepam is absorbed rapidly, reaching peak concentrations in about an hour in adults, and as quickly as 15 to 30 minutes in children. Clorazepate and prazepam do not appear as such in the blood. Clorazepate is quickly decarboxylated in the gastrointestinal tract, and the product, N-desmethyldiazepam (*nordazepam*), is rapidly absorbed; prazepam is absorbed slowly and is transformed primarily to nordazepam by the liver before reaching the systemic circulation (*see* Greenblatt *et al.*, 1981). With the exception of lorazepam, the benzodiazepines are unpredictably absorbed following intramuscular injection (*see* Greenblatt *et al.*, 1983b). Most of the benzodiazepines are bound to plasma protein to a great extent (85 to 95%)—a factor that limits the efficacy of dialysis in the treatment of acute poisonings. The apparent volumes of distribution for most benzodiazepines are high—about 1 to 3 liters per kilogram. Secondary peaks in the plasma concentration have been described for several benzodiazepines, for example, at 6 to 12 hours after an oral dose of diazepam. These are most likely due to enterohepatic recirculation (*see* Morselli, 1977).

The pharmacokinetic parameters that have been reported for these agents may be somewhat misleading for several reasons. Assay technics have not all been of high specificity, and active metabolites can markedly alter the actual biological half-life. For example, the formation of nordazepam from diazepam can extend biological half-life by twofold or threefold. Even more striking is the fact that halazepam (half-life in plasma of 2 to 4 hours) is metabolized principally to nordazepam, which has a half-life of up to 100 hours (*see* Greenblatt *et al.*, 1983a). Active compounds, including nordazepam, are also produced during the metabolism of chlordiazepoxide. Nordazepam is hydroxylated to oxazepam, which is inactivated by conjugation with glucuronic acid. Lorazepam, like oxazepam, is primarily converted to an inactive glucuronide. The metabolism of the benzodiazepines is described in more detail in Chapter 17 and is summarized in Table 17–3 (page 348).

The actual kinetics for some benzodiazepines is complex and is not easily analyzed by simple mathematical models. Thus, the usually stated half-life for the elimination phase of the drug does not adequately depict the kinetics of the early distributive phase, which can be important clinically. For example, the distributive (alpha) half-life of diazepam is about 1 hour, while the elimination (beta) half-time is about 1.5 days initially and even longer after prolonged treatment. Moreover, while correlations between plasma concentrations of benzodiazepines and clinical effects are imperfect (*see* Gottschalk, 1978), it is apparent that concentrations in plasma that border on twice the values usually considered to be effective are associated with undesirable degrees of sedation (*see* Morselli, 1977). For this reason, the benzodiazepines are *not* effectively or safely given once a day, despite their relatively long elimination half-lives; doses should be divided into two to four portions for the treatment of daytime anxiety.

The benzodiazepines as a class tend to have minimal pharmacokinetic interactions with other drugs, although their metabolism may be inhibited by cimetidine, disulfiram, isoniazid, and oral contraceptives, while it appears to be increased by rifampin. The *premature neonate* and the *elderly* may have half-lives for diazepam that are three or four times longer than those of young adults, children, or even full-term neonates. In addition, severe hepatic disease can increase the half-life of diazepam by a factor of two to five. Since formation of glucuronide is not restricted to hepatic microsomes, oxazepam, lorazepam, and possibly alprazolam may be safer agents for those with severely impaired hepatic function if they are given in small divided doses. Oxazepam may be safer for elderly patients because of its relatively short duration of action. Most of the benzodiazepines are excreted almost entirely in the urine and in the form of oxidized and glucuronide-conjugated metabolites.

Information on the pharmacokinetic properties and metabolism of the benzodiazepines is described by Morselli (1977), Gottschalk (1978), Hollister (1978), and Greenblatt and coworkers (1983b); *see also* Symposium (1982) and Appendix II.

Tolerance and Physical Dependence. High doses of benzodiazepines must be given for long periods of time and then abruptly withdrawn before marked withdrawal symptoms, occasionally including seizures, appear (*see* Allquander, 1978). Habituation can occur; however, because of the long half-lives and conversion to active metabolites, *withdrawal symptoms* after chronic use may not appear for a week after abrupt discontinuation of the drug. Propranolol has been used to counteract autonomic symptoms associated with withdrawal from a benzodiazepine (*see* Greenblatt *et al.*, 1983b). In most instances after usual doses, there is no withdrawal syndrome.

Toxic Reactions and Side Effects. The expected side effects of CNS depressants of drowsiness and ataxia are extensions of the pharmacological actions of these drugs.

With diazepam, antianxiety effects can be expected at blood concentrations of 300 to 400 ng/ml, while some sedative effects and psychomotor impairment begin at similar concentrations and gross CNS intoxication can be expected at concentrations over 900 to 1000 ng/ml (*see* Morselli, 1977). Therapeutic concentrations of chlordiazepoxide approximate 700 to 1000 ng/ml.

An *increase* in hostility and irritability, and vivid or disturbing dreams are sometimes associated with the benzodiazepines, with the possible exception of oxazepam. Equally paradoxical is an *increase* in anxiety. Such a response is especially likely to occur in patients who feel threatened by being dulled by the sedative effects of antianxiety agents. In addition, one of the most common causes of reversible *confusional states in the elderly* is surely the *overuse of sedatives* of all kinds, including what would ordinarily be referred to as "small" doses of benzodiazepines.

In general, the clinical toxicity of the benzodiazepines is low. Weight gain, which may be the result of renewed appetite, occurs in some patients. Many of the side effects reported for these drugs so overlap with symptoms of anxiety that unless a careful history is taken one is hard put to ascribe these effects to the drug. Among the other toxic reactions seen with chlordiazepoxide are skin rash, nausea, headache, impairment of sexual function, vertigo, and light-headedness. Agranulocytosis and hepatic reactions have been reported rarely. Menstrual irregularities have been noted, and women may fail to ovulate while taking benzodiazepines.

Overdosage with the benzodiazepines is frequent, but serious sequelae are rare unless other drugs or ethanol are also administered. A few deaths have been reported at doses greater than 700 mg of diazepam or chlordiazepoxide. The striking advantage of this group of drugs is the remarkable margin of safety. Treatment for overdosage is purely supportive of respiratory and cardiovascular function. The discovery that certain imidazobenzodiazepines have selective, antagonistic effects against the benzodiazepines might herald the development of clinically useful antidotes for states of intoxication (*see* Hunkeler *et al.*, 1981).

The question of teratogenic effects of benzodiazepines or other toxic effects on the fetus is controversial (*see* Safra and Oakley, 1975; Morselli, 1977; Goldberg and DiMascio, 1978). The most persistent, but unproven, suggestion has been that there may be a small increase in the risk of midline cleft deformities of the lip or palate, although these remain well below the overall risk of birth defects (about 2% in the general population) and are correctable by surgery. Benzodiazepines depress CNS function in the neonate, and especially in the premature newborn. Concentrations of these drugs in umbilical cord blood may exceed those in the maternal circulation; as mentioned, the fetus and newborn are much less able to metabolize benzodiazepines than are adults.

Interactions with Other Drugs. These are infrequent with the benzodiazepines, and, except for an additive effect with other CNS depressants, they are usually not significant. Minor pharmacokinetic interactions have been mentioned above. Heavy cigarette smoking may decrease the effectiveness of usual doses of these drugs. The ability of benzodiazepines to induce the hepatic metabolism of other agents is much smaller than that of many other sedatives, especially the barbiturates.

Preparations, Routes of Administration, and Dosage. These are presented in Table 19–6.

Therapeutic Uses. The benzodiazepines are used in the treatment of *anxiety* (*see* below). In addition, chlordiazepoxide has been widely employed in the treatment of *alcohol withdrawal syndromes* (*see* Chapter 23). The substitution of an antianxiety agent for alcohol in chronic alcoholism is sometimes attempted, but this does not appear to reduce alcohol intake significantly or in any way to be an effective treatment of alcoholism. Other uses

Table 19–6. BENZODIAZEPINES USED FOR ANXIETY: DOSAGE FORMS AND DOSES

NONPROPRIETARY NAME	TRADE NAME	DOSAGE FORMS *	USUAL DAILY DOSE (*mg*) †	EXTREME DAILY DOSE (*mg*)
Alprazolam	XANAX	O	0.75–1.5	0.5–4
Chlordiazepoxide	LIBRIUM	O,I	15–40	10–100
			25–100 (parenteral; may repeat in 2–4 hr)	25–300 (parenteral)
Clorazepate	TRANXENE	O ‡	30	7.5–90
Diazepam	VALIUM	O ‡,I	4–40	2–40
			2–20 (parenteral; may repeat in 3–4 hr)	
Halazepam	PAXIPAM	O	60–160	20–160
Lorazepam	ATIVAN	O,I	2–6	1–10
			2–4 (parenteral)	
Oxazepam	SERAX	O	30–60	30–120
Prazepam	CENTRAX	O	20–40	10–60

* Dosage forms: O = oral solid; I = injection.

† The daily doses are given as total milligrams per day, assuming doses are divided into two or four portions per day. Single parenteral doses are given for chlordiazepoxide and diazepam. All doses are for adults or adolescents. For children 6 to 12 years of age, chlordiazepoxide may be given in divided daily doses of 10 to 30 mg. Diazepam may be given in divided daily doses of 3 to 10 mg to children over 6 months of age. For younger children, consult the manufacturer's instructions.

‡ Clorazepate is also available as slow-release tablets (TRANXENE-SD) to be taken once daily. Diazepam is also available in slow-release capsules (VALRELEASE).

are as premedication in *anesthesia,* and in *obstetrics* during labor (*see* Chapters 13 and 14).

Diazepam has also been employed as a skeletal muscle relaxant. It has been used successfully in the treatment of *tetanus* in the intravenous dose of 2 to 20 mg at intervals of 2 to 8 hours. In conventional doses it has been claimed, but not proven, to relieve the muscular spasticity of *upper motoneuron* disorders. On the other hand, there is evidence from controlled studies that diazepam is effective in relieving spasticity and athetosis in patients with *cerebral palsy.* The use of diazepam in *cardioversion* is well documented. Diazepam is also employed in the management of *seizure disorders* and a number of other medical, neurological, and surgical conditions, about which there is further information in Chapters 17, 20, and 21 (*see also* Greenblatt *et al.,* 1983b).

OTHER SEDATIVES USED FOR ANXIETY

Many other classes of drugs that act on the CNS have been used in the past for daytime sedation and the treatment of anxiety. Many of these uses are now virtually obsolete. Such drugs include the propanediol carbamates (notably, *meprobamate*), the barbiturates (*see* Chapter 17), and many other pharmacologically similar nonbarbiturates (*e.g., chlormezanone*). The dosage forms and the usual sedative-hypnotic doses of many of these drugs are provided in Table 17–4 (page 352). The demise of these agents in modern psychiatric practice is due primarily to their tendency to cause unwanted degrees of sedation or frank intoxication at the dosage required to alleviate anxiety; meprobamate and the barbiturates present additional problems, particularly their liability to produce tolerance, physical dependence, and severe withdrawal reactions.

Other drugs that have been used in the treatment of anxiety include certain anticholinergic agents and antihistamines. Among these is *hydroxyzine,* an antihistamine that is widely prescribed for the treatment of anxiety. The popularity of hydroxyzine is surprising in view of studies that suggest that it is not an effective antianxiety agent unless given in doses (400 mg per day) that produce marked sedation (*see* Rickels, 1977; Goldberg, 1984). Hydroxyzine is also used intramuscularly as a preanesthetic medication for its sedative, anticholinergic, and antiemetic effects (*see* Chapter 13).

An entirely new class of drugs with potential utility in the treatment of anxiety are the azaspirodecanediones, currently represented by *buspirone* (BUSPAR). Originally developed as a potential antipsychotic agent, buspirone has a pattern of pharmacological properties that is distinct from that of the benzodiazepines, including an inability to influence the binding of either the benzodiazepines or GABA, a lack of anticonvulsant activity, and minimal interaction with CNS depressants (*see* Eison, 1984). At the present time, clinical studies indicate that buspirone is an effective antianxiety agent that produces distinctly less sedation than various benzodiazepines (*see* Goldberg, 1984).

DRUG TREATMENT OF ANXIETY

Anxiety is not only a cardinal symptom of many psychiatric disorders but also an almost-inevitable component of many medical and surgical conditions. Indeed, it is a universal human emotion, closely allied with appropriate fear, and often serving psychobiologically adaptive purposes. A most important clinical generalization is that anxiety is rather infrequently a "disease" in itself. The anxiety that is typically associated with the "psychoneurotic" disorders cannot be readily explained in biological or psychological terms (*see* Hoehn-Saric, 1982). In addition, symptoms of anxiety are commonly associated with depression and especially with dysthymic disorder ("neurotic" depression) and many personality disorders. Also, anxiety is a ubiquitous symptom associated with medical as well as psychiatric disorders, some of which can readily be diagnosed and effectively treated. Sometimes, despite a thoughtful evaluation of a patient, no treatable primary illness is found, or, if one is found and treated, it may be desirable to deal directly with the anxiety at the same time. In such situations, antianxiety medications are frequently and appropriately used (*see* Hollister *et al.*, 1980; Rosenbaum, 1982; Bassuk *et al.*, 1983; Greenblatt *et al.*, 1983b; Lader, 1984).

Currently, the most useful drugs seem to be the benzodiazepines. The specific drug chosen seems to make little difference. The older agents, because of their long tenure, have been more thoroughly investigated. In patients with impaired hepatic function or in the elderly, oxazepam is currently favored; since lorazepam and alprazolam have similar characteristics, they may be suitable alternatives if administered in small, divided doses. Chlordiazepoxide and diazepam have been used extensively in children.

Clinical experience strongly indicates that the most favorable responses to the benzodiazepines are obtained in situations that involve relatively acute anxiety reactions in medical or psychiatric patients who have either modifiable primary illnesses or primary anxiety disorders. However, this group of anxious patients also has a high response rate to placebo and is likely to undergo spontaneous improvement. Antianxiety drugs are also used in the management of more persistent or recurrent anxiety associated with the neuroses; guidelines for their appropriate use are less clear in these situations. Although there has been concern about the potential for habituation and abuse of sedatives, recent studies suggest that physicians tend to be conservative and may even *undertreat* patients with anxiety. They may either withhold drug unless symptoms or dysfunction are severe or interrupt treatment within a few weeks, causing a high pro-

portion of relapses. However, patients with very long-lasting or persistent patterns of dissatisfaction or insecurity or those who have diagnosable personality disorders (*see* American Psychiatric Association, 1980) may be particularly difficult to treat successfully with antianxiety agents. They may be at higher risk of a gradual escalation of dose, physical dependence, or impulsive overdosing. Nevertheless, the few data available suggest that such abuses are relatively infrequent or, when one considers the millions of patients using such drugs, even rare (*see* Greenblatt *et al.*, 1983b). Moreover, sustained benefits of benzodiazepine treatment can be demonstrated for at least several months (*see* Fabre *et al.*, 1981; Hollister *et al.*, 1981).

An important recent advance is the separation of various types of anxiety disorders, including those characterized by *panic* and *phobias* as well as other, more *generalized anxiety disorders*. Among features that help to make such distinctions are apparently preferential responses of panic disorder and some phobias to tricyclic antidepressants or to an MAO inhibitor (*see* Sheehan *et al.*, 1980; Pohl *et al.*, 1982; Shader *et al.*, 1982). There is also some evidence to suggest that alprazolam, perhaps uniquely, may have useful effects in panic disorder and major depression that are similar to those of imipramine and different from the antianxiety (or nonspecific) effects of benzodiazepines in mild anxious depression (*see* Sheehan, 1980; Chouinard *et al.*, 1982).

Other agents have been tried experimentally in anxiety. β-Adrenergic antagonists have been used in an attempt to block the peripheral autonomic manifestations of anxiety, but controlled trials are few and generally do not show better results than those obtained with the benzodiazepines (*see* Kathol *et al.*, 1980). Other methods of treatment, including psychotherapy and behavioral technics, are discussed by Lader (1984). There are important, nonpharmacological factors that bear on the use and effects of antianxiety drugs. Discussions of the nonspecific and placebo aspects of such treatment are provided by Rickels and associates (1978). The general topic of the evaluation and treatment of anxiety is well reviewed by Rickels and associates (1978), Rosenbaum (1982), Greenblatt and colleagues (1983b), and Lader (1984). Aspects of the abuse of sedatives are reviewed by Cole and colleagues (1981). The current status of some of the effective sedative-antianxiety agents as federally *controlled substances* is reviewed in Appendix I.

Alexander, C. S., and Nino, A. Cardiovascular complications in young patients taking psychotropic drugs. *Am. Heart J.*, **1969**, *78*, 757–769.

Alexanderson, B., and Sjöqvist, F. Individual differences in the pharmacokinetics of monomethylated tricyclic antidepressants: role of genetic and environmental factors and clinical importance. *Ann. N.Y. Acad. Sci.*, **1971**, *179*, 739–751.

American Medical Association Committee on Alcoholism and Drug Dependence. Barbiturates and barbiturate-like drugs. Considerations in their medical use. *J.A.M.A.*, **1974**, *230*, 1440–1441.

Amsterdam, J.; Brunswick, D.; and Mendels, J. The clinical application of tricyclic antidepressant pharmacokinetics and plasma levels. *Am. J. Psychiatry,* **1980,** *137,* 653–662.

Aubree, J. C., and Lader, M. H. High and very high dosage antipsychotics: a critical review. *J. Clin. Psychiatry,* **1980,** *41,* 341–350.

Avery, D., and Winokur, G. The efficacy of electroconvulsive therapy and antidepressants in depression. *Biol. Psychiatry,* **1977,** *12,* 507–523.

Baldessarini, R. J. Treatment of depression by altering monoamine metabolism: precursors and metabolic inhibitors. *Psychopharmacol. Bull.,* **1984a,** *20,* 224–239.

Baldessarini, R. J.; Katz, B.; and Cotton, P. Dissimilar dosing with high-potency and low-potency neuroleptics. *Am. J. Psychiatry,* **1984,** *141,* 748–752.

Bassuk, E. L.; Schoonover, S. C.; and Gelenberg, A. J. *The Practitioner's Guide to Psychoactive Drugs,* 2nd ed. Plenum Medical Book Publishing Co., New York, **1983.**

Berger, F. M. The pharmacological properties of 2-methyl-2-*n*-propyl-1,3 propanediol dicarbamate (MILTOWN), a new interneuronal blocking agent. *J. Pharmacol. Exp. Ther.,* **1954,** *112,* 413–423.

Berridge, M. J. Inositol trisphosphate and diacylglycerol as second messengers. *Biochem. J.,* **1984,** *220,* 345–360.

Berridge, M. J.: Downes, C. P.; and Hanley, M. R. Lithium amplifies agonist-dependent phosphatidylinositol responses in brain and salivary glands. *Biochem. J.,* **1982,** *206,* 587–595.

Bialos, D.; Giller, E.; and Jatlow, P. Recurrence of depression after the discontinuation of long-term amitriptyline treatment. *Am. J. Psychiatry,* **1982,** *139,* 325–329.

Blackwell, B.; Stefopoulos, A.; and Enders, P. Anticholinergic activity of two tricyclic antidepressants. *Am. J. Psychiatry,* **1978,** *135,* 722–724.

Bloom, F. E.; Baetge, G.; Deyo, S.; Ettenberg, A.; Koda, L.; Magisretti, P. J.; Shoemaker, W. J.; and Staunton, D. A. Chemical and physiological aspects of the actions of lithium and antidepressant drugs. *Neuropharmacology,* **1983,** *22,* 359–365.

Bojanovsky, J., and Tölle, R. Dihydroergotamin gegen die Kreislaufwirkungen der Thymoleptika. *Dtsch. Med. Wochenschr.,* **1974,** *99,* 1064–1065.

Boston Collaborative Drug Surveillance Program. Adverse reactions to tricyclic-antidepressant drugs. *Lancet,* **1972,** *1,* 529–530.

Braestrup, C., and Squires, R. Specific benzodiazepine receptors in the rat brain characterized by high-affinity ³H-diazepam binding. *Proc. Natl. Acad. Sci. U.S.A.,* **1977,** *74,* 3805–3809.

Brenner, R.; Cooper, T. B.; Yablonski, M. E.; Lieberman, J. A.; Lesser, M.; Siris, S. G.; and Rifkin, A. E. Measurement of lithium concentrations in human tears. *Am. J. Psychiatry,* **1982,** *139,* 678–679.

Brunswick, D. J.; Amsterdam, J. D.; Mendels, J.; and Stern, S. L. Prediction of steady-state imipramine and desmethylimipramine plasma concentrations from simple-dose data. *Clin. Pharmacol. Ther.,* **1979,** *25,* 605–610.

Bunney, B. S., and Aghajanian, G. K. Mesolimbic and mesocortical dopaminergic systems: physiology and pharmacology. In, *Psychopharmacology: A Generation of Progress.* (Lipton, M. A.; DiMascio, A.; and Killam, K. F.; eds.) Raven Press, New York, **1978,** pp. 159–169.

Bunney, B. S.; Walters, J. R.; Roth, R. H.; and Aghajanian, G. K. Dopaminergic neurons: effect of antipsychotic drugs and amphetamine on single cell activity. *J. Pharmacol. Exp. Ther.,* **1973,** *185,* 560–571.

Bunney, W. E., Jr.; Murphy, D. L.; and Goodwin, F. K. The "switch process" in manic-depressive illness. *Arch. Gen. Psychiatry,* **1972,** *27,* 295–302.

Burrows, G. D.; Vohra, J.; Hunt, D.; Sloman, J. G.; Soggins, B. A.; and Davies, B. Cardiac effects of different

tricyclic antidepressant drugs. *Br. J. Psychiatry,* **1976,** *129,* 335–341.

Cade, J. F. J. Lithium salts in the treatment of psychotic excitement. *Med. J. Aust.,* **1949,** *2,* 349–352.

Campbell, M. Psychopharmacology in childhood psychosis. *Int. J. Ment. Health,* **1975,** *4,* 238–254.

Carlsson, A. Mechanism of action of neuroleptic drugs. In, *Psychopharmacology: A Generation of Progress.* (Lipton, M. A.; DiMascio, A.; and Killam, K. F.; eds.) Raven Press, New York, **1978,** pp. 1057–1070.

Caroff, S. The neuroleptic malignant syndrome. *J. Clin. Psychiatry,* **1980,** *41,* 79–83.

Caroff, S.; Rosenberg, H.; and Gerber, J. C. Neuroleptic malignant syndrome and malignant hyperthermia. *J. Clin. Psychopharmacol.,* **1983,** *3,* 120–121.

Cassem, N. Cardiovascular effects of antidepressants. *J. Clin. Psychiatry,* **1982,** *43,* 22–28.

Chouinard, G.; Annable, L.; Fontaine, R.; and Solyom, L. Alprazolam in the treatment of generalized anxiety and panic disorders. *Psychopharmacology (Berlin),* **1982,** *77,* 229–233.

Chouinard, G., and Jones, B. D. Neuroleptic-induced supersensitivity psychosis: clinical and pharmacologic characteristics. *Am. J. Psychiatry,* **1980,** *137,* 16–21.

Clark, M. L.; Ray, T. S.; Paredes, A.; Ragland, R. E.; Costilee, J. P.; Smith, C. W.; and Wolf, S. Chlorpromazine in women with chronic schizophrenia: the effects on cholesterol levels and cholesterol behavioral relationships. *Psychosom. Med.,* **1967,** *29,* 634–642.

Clement-Cormier, Y. C.; Kebabian, J. W.; Petzold, G. L.; and Greengard, P. Dopamine-sensitive adenylate cyclase in mammalian brain: a possible site of action of antipsychotic drugs. *Proc. Natl. Acad. Sci. U.S.A.,* **1974,** *71,* 1113–1117.

Cohen, B. J.; Harris, P. Q.; Altesman, R. I.; and Cole, J. O. Amoxapine: a neuroleptic as well as an antidepressant? *Am. J. Psychiatry,* **1982,** *139,* 1165–1167.

Cohen, D. J.; Detlor, J.; and Young, J. G. Clonidine ameliorates Gilles de la Tourette syndrome. *Arch. Gen. Psychiatry,* **1980,** *37,* 1350–1357.

Cole, J. O. Antipsychotic drugs: is more better? *McLean Hosp. J.,* **1982,** *7,* 61–87.

Cole, J. O.; Haskell, D. S.; and Orzack, M. H. Problems with the benzodiazepines: an assessment of the available evidence. *McLean Hosp. J.,* **1981,** *6,* 46–74.

Cooper, T. B., and Simpson, G. M. Kinetics of lithium and clinical response. In, *Psychopharmacology: A Generation of Progress.* (Lipton, M. A.; DiMascio, A.; and Killam, K. F.; eds.) Raven Press, New York, **1978,** pp. 923–931.

Courvoisier, S.; Fournel, J.; Ducrot, R.; Kolsky, M.; and Koetschet, P. Propiérties pharmacodynamiques du chlorhydrate de chloro-3(dimethylamino-3′propyl)-10 phenothiazine (4560 RP). *Arch. Int. Pharmacodyn. Ther.,* **1953,** *92,* 305–361.

Crane, G. E. Iproniazid (MARSILID) phosphate, a therapeutic agent for mental disorders and debilitating disease. *Psychiatr. Res. Rep.,* **1959,** *8,* 142–152.

Creese, I.; Burt, D.; and Snyder, S. H. Biochemical actions of neuroleptic drugs: focus on dopamine receptor. In, *Handbook of Psychopharmacology,* Vol. 10. (Iversen, L. L.; Iversen, S. D.; and Snyder, S. H.; eds.) Plenum Press, New York, **1978,** pp. 37–89.

Crews, F. T., and Smith, C. B. Presynaptic alpha-receptor subsensitivity after long-term antidepressant treatment. *Science,* **1978,** *202,* 322–324.

Crome, P.; Dawling, S.; and Braithwaite, R. A. Effect of activated charcoal on absorption of nortriptyline. *Lancet,* **1977,** *1,* 1203–1205.

Davies, R. K.; Tucker, G. J.; Harrow, M.; and Detre, T. P. Confusional episodes and antidepressant medication. *Am. J. Psychiatry,* **1971,** *128,* 127.

Delay, J., and Deniker, P. Trente-huit cas de psychoses traitées par la cure prolongée et continue de 4560 RP.

Le Congrès des Al. et Neurol. de Langue Fr. In, *Compte rendu du Congrès*. Masson et Cie, Paris, **1952**.

Demers, R. G., and Heninger, G. R. Electrocardiographic T-wave changes during lithium carbonate treatment. *J.A.M.A.*, **1971**, *218*, 381–386.

DeMontigny, C., and Aghajanian, G. K. Tricyclic antidepressants: long-term treatment increases responsivity of rat forebrain neurons to serotonin. *Science*, **1978**, *202*, 1303–1305.

DePaulo, J. R., Jr.; Correa, E. I.; and Sapir, D. G. Renal toxicity of lithium and its implications. *Johns Hopkins Med. J.*, **1981**, *149*, 15–21.

Dimond, R. C.; Brammer, S. R.; Atkinson, R. L., Jr.; Howard, W. J.; and Earll, J. M. Chlorpromazine treatment and growth hormone secretory responses in acromegaly. *J. Clin. Endocrinol. Metab.*, **1973**, *36*, 1189–1195.

Donaldson, S. R.; Gelenberg, A. J.; and Baldessarini, R. J. The pharmacologic treatment of schizophrenia: a progress report. *Schizophr. Bull.*, **1983**, *9*, 504–527.

DuComb, L., and Baldessarini, R. J. Timing and risk of bone marrow depression by psychotropic drugs. *Am. J. Psychiatry*, **1977**, *134*, 1294–1295.

Erle, G.; Basso, M.; Federspil, G.; Sicolo, N.; and Scandellari, C. Effect of chlorpromazine on blood glucose and plasma insulin in man. *Eur. J. Clin. Pharmacol.*, **1977**, *11*, 15–18.

Fabre, L. F.; McLendon, D. M.; and Stephens, A. G. Comparison of the therapeutic effect, tolerance and safety of benzodiazepines administered for six months to out-patients with chronic anxiety neurosis. *J. Int. Med. Res.*, **1981**, *246*, 1568–1570.

Feinsilver, D., and Gunderson, J. Psychotherapy for schizophrenics—is it indicated? *Schizophr. Bull.*, **1972**, *6*, 11–23.

Folks, D. G. Monoamine oxidase inhibitors: reappraisal of dietary considerations. *J. Clin. Psychopharmacol.*, **1983**, *3*, 249–252.

Forrest, J. J., Jr. Lithium inhibition of cAMP-mediated hormones: a caution. *N. Engl. J. Med.*, **1975**, *292*, 423–424.

Forsman, A., and Öhman, R. On the pharmacokinetics of haloperidol. *Nord. Psykiatr. Tidskr.*, **1974**, *28*, 441–448.

Freeman, C. P.; Basson, J. V.; and Crighton, A. Double-blind controlled trial of electroconvulsive therapy (ECT) and simulated ECT in depressive illness. *Lancet*, **1978**, *1*, 738–740.

Frohman, L. A. Clinical neuropharmacology of hypothalamic releasing factors. *N. Engl. J. Med.*, **1972**, *286*, 1391–1398.

Glassman, A. H., and Bigger, J. T., Jr. Cardiovascular effects of therapeutic doses of tricyclic antidepressants. *Arch. Gen. Psychiatry*, **1981**, *38*, 815–820.

Goldberg, H. L., and DiMascio, A. Psychotropic drugs in pregnancy. In, *Psychopharmacology: A Generation of Progress*. (Lipton, M. A.; DiMascio, A.; and Killam, K. F.; eds.) Raven Press, New York, **1978**, pp. 1047–1055.

Goldfield, M. D., and Weinstein, M. R. Lithium carbonate in obstetrics: guidelines for clinical use. *Am. J. Obstet. Gynecol.*, **1973**, *116*, 15–22.

Goodwin, F. K. The impact of tricyclic antidepressants and lithium on the course of recurrent affective disorders. *McLean Hosp. J.*, **1983**, *8*, 1–16.

Gottschalk, L. A. Pharmacokinetics of the minor tranquilizers and clinical response. In, *Psychopharmacology: A Generation of Progress*. (Lipton, M. A.; DiMascio, A.; and Killam, K. F.; eds.) Raven Press, New York, **1978**, pp. 975–985.

Gottschalk, L. A.; Biener, R.; Noble, E.; Birch, H.; Wilbert, D.; and Heizer, J. Thioridazine plasma levels and clinical response. *Compr. Psychiatry*, **1975**, *16*, 323–337.

Gram, L. F.; Christiansen, J.; and Overo, K. F. Pharmacokinetic interaction between tricyclic antidepressants and other psychopharmaca. *Acta Psychiatr. Scand.* [*Suppl.*], **1973**, *243*, 52–53.

Granacher, R. P., and Baldessarini, R. J. Physostigmine in the acute anticholinergic syndrome associated with antidepressant and antiparkinson drugs. *Arch. Gen. Psychiatry*, **1975**, *32*, 375–380.

Greenblatt, D. J.; Divoll, M.; Abernethy, D. R.; Ochs, H. R.; and Shader, R. I. Clinical pharmacokinetics of the newer benzodiazepines. *Clin. Pharmacokinet.*, **1983a**, *8*, 233–252.

Greenblatt, D. J.; Shader, R. I.; and Abernethy, D. R. Current status of benzodiazepines. *N. Engl. J. Med.*, **1983b**, *309*, 354–358, 410–416.

Greenblatt, D. J.; Shader, R. I.; Divoll, M.; and Harmatz, J. S. Benzodiazepines: a summary of pharmacokinetic properties. *Br. J. Clin. Pharmacol.*, **1981**, *11*, 11S–16S.

Grinspoon, L.; Ewalt, J. R.; and Shader, R. Psychotherapy and pharmacotherapy in chronic schizophrenia. *Am. J. Psychiatry*, **1968**, *124*, 1645–1652.

Grunthal, E. Untersuchungen über die besondere psychologische Wirkung des Thymolepticums TOFRANIL. *Psychiatr.-Neurol. Wochenschr.*, **1958**, *136*, 402–408.

Hardesty, A. S., and Burdock, E. I. Quantitative clinical evaluation in psychopharmacology. In, *Psychopharmacology: A Generation of Progress*. (Lipton, M. A.; DiMascio, A.; and Killam, K. F.; eds.) Raven Press, New York, **1978**, pp. 871–878.

Haugaard, E. S.; Mickel, R.; and Haugaard, N. Actions of lithium ions and insulin on glucose utilization, glycogen synthesis and glycogen synthase in the isolated rat diaphragm. *Biochem. Pharmacol.*, **1974**, *23*, 1675–1685.

Himmelhoch, J. M.; Poust, R. I.; and Mallinger, A. G. Adjustment of lithium dose during lithium-chlorothiazide therapy. *Clin. Pharmacol. Ther.*, **1977**, *22*, 225–227.

Hirsch, S. R.; Gaind, R.; Rohde, P. D.; Stevens, B. C.; and Wing, J. K. Outpatient maintenance of chronic schizophrenic patients with long-acting fluphenazine: double blind placebo trial. *Br. Med. J.*, **1973**, *1*, 633–637.

Hoehn-Saric, R. Neurotransmitters in anxiety. *Arch. Gen. Psychiatry*, **1982**, *39*, 735–742.

Hogarty, G. E., and Ulrich, R. F. Temporal effects of drug and placebo in delaying relapse in schizophrenic outpatients. *Arch. Gen. Psychiatry*, **1977**, *34*, 297–301.

Hollister, L. E.; Conley, F. K.; Britt, R. H.; and Shuer, L. Long-term use of diazepam. *J.A.M.A.*, **1981**, *246*, 1568–1570.

Hollister, L. E.; Greenblatt, D. J.; Rickels, K.; Ayd, F. J.; and Greiner, G. E. Benzodiazepines: current update. *Psychosomatics*, **1980**, *21*, Suppl., 1–32.

Hudson, J. I.; Pope, H. G., Jr.; Jonas, J. M.; and Yurgelun-Todd, D. Treatment of anorexia nervosa with antidepressants. *J. Clin. Psychopharmacol.*, **1985**, *5*, 17–23.

Hunkeler, W.; Möhler, H.; Pieri, L.; Polc, P.; Bonetti, E. P.; Cumin, R.; Schaffner, R.; and Haefely, W. Selective antagonists of benzodiazepines. *Nature*, **1981**, *290*, 514–516.

Jefferson, J. W.; Greist, J. H.; Clagnaz, P. J.; Eischens, R. R.; Marten, W. C.; and Eversen, M. A. Effect of strenuous exercise on serum lithium level in man. *Am. J. Psychiatry*, **1982**, *139*, 1593–1595.

Jus, K.; Jus, A.; Gautier, J.; Villeneuve, A.; Pires, P.; Pineau, R.; and Villeneuve, R. Studies of the actions of certain pharmacological agents on tardive dyskinesia and on the rabbit syndrome. *Int. J. Clin. Pharmacol.*, **1974**, *9*, 138–145.

Kane, J. M.; Rifkin, A.; Woerner, M.; Reardon, G.; Sarantoakos, S.; Schiebel, D.; and Ramos-Lorenzi, J. Low-dose neuroleptic treatment of outpatient schizophrenics. *Arch. Gen. Psychiatry*, **1983**, *40*, 893–896.

Kathol, R. G.; Noyes, R., Jr.; Sylmen, D. J.; Crowe,

R. R.; Clancy, J.; and Kerber, R. E. Propranolol in chronic anxiety disorders. *Arch. Gen. Psychiatry*, **1980**, *37*, 1361–1365.

Keller, M. B.; Klerman, G. L.; Lavori, P. W.; Fawcett, J. A.; Coryell, W.; and Endicott, J. Treatment received by depressed patients. *J.A.M.A.*, **1982**, *248*, 1848–1855.

Klerman, G. L. Drug therapy of clinical depressions. *J. Psychiatr. Res.*, **1972**, *9*, 253–270.

Kline, N. S. Clinical experience with iproniazid (MARSILID). *J. Clin. Exp. Psychopathol.*, **1958**, *19*, Suppl., 72–78.

Korpi, E. R.; Phelps, B. H.; Granger, H.; Chang, W.-H.; Linnoila, M.; Meek, J. L.; and Wyatt, R. J. Simultaneous determination of haloperidol and its reduced metabolite in serum and plasma by isocratic liquid chromatography with electrochemical detection. *Clin. Chem.*, **1983**, *29*, 626–628.

Krenzelok, E. P.; North, D. S.; and Elkins, B. R. Physostigmine's use questioned for amoxapine overdose. *Am. J. Hosp. Pharm.*, **1981**, *38*, 1882–1889.

Kuhn, R. The treatment of depressive states with G22355 (imipramine hydrochloride). *Am. J. Psychiatry*, **1958**, *115*, 459–464.

Kupfer, D. J.; Spiker, D. G.; Coble, P. A.; Neil, J. F.; Ulrich, R.; and Shaw, D. H. Sleep and treatment prediction in endogenous depression. *Am. J. Psychiatry*, **1981**, *138*, 429–434.

Laborit, H.; Huguenard, P.; and Alluaume, R. Un nouveau stabilisateur vegetatif, le 4560 RP. *Presse Méd.*, **1952**, *60*, 206–208.

Lansky, M. R.; and Selzer, J. Priapism associated with trazodone therapy: case report. *J. Clin. Psychiatry*, **1984**, *45*, 232–233.

Lehmann, H. E.; and Hanrahan, G. E. Chlorpromazine, a new inhibiting agent for psychomotor excitement and manic states. *Arch. Neurol. Psychiatry*, **1954**, *71*, 227–257.

Linnoila, M.; George, L.; and Guthrie, S. Interaction between antidepressants and perphenazine in psychiatric patients. *Am. J. Psychiatry*, **1982**, *139*, 1329–1331.

Lipinski, J. F.; Zubenko, G.; Cohen, B. M.; and Barreira, P. Propranolol in the treatment of neuroleptic-induced akathisia. *Am. J. Psychiatry*, **1984**, *141*, 412–415.

Litovitz, T. L.; and Troutman, W. G. Amoxapine overdose: seizures and fatalities. *J.A.M.A.*, **1983**, *250*, 1069–1071.

Loga, S.; Curry, S.; and Lader, M. Interactions of orphenadrine and phenobarbitone with chlorpromazine: plasma concentrations and effects in man. *Br. J. Clin. Pharmacol.*, **1975**, *2*, 197–208.

Mandel, M. R.; Madsen, J.; Miller, A. L.; and Baldessarini, R. J. Intoxication associated with lithium and ECT. *Am. J. Psychiatry*, **1980**, *137*, 1107–1109.

Matthysse, S.; and Sugarman, J. Neurotransmitter theories of schizophrenia. In, *Handbook of Psychopharmacology*, Vol. 10. (Iversen, L. L.; Iversen, S. D.; and Snyder, S. H.; eds.) Plenum Press, New York, **1978**, pp. 211–242.

May, P. R. A. *Treatment of Schizophrenia: A Comparative Study of Five Treatment Methods*. Science House, New York, **1968**.

May, P. R. A.; and Van Putten, T. Plasma levels of chlorpromazine in schizophrenia: a critical review of the literature. *Arch. Gen. Psychiatry*, **1978**, *35*, 1081–1087.

Meltzer, H. Y.; Goode, D. J.; and Fang, V. S. The effect of psychotropic drugs on endocrine function. In, *Psychopharmacology: A Generation of Progress*. (Lipton, M. A.; DiMascio, A.; and Killam, K. F.; eds.) Raven Press, New York, **1978**, pp. 509–529.

Meltzer, H. Y.; and Stahl, S. M. The dopamine hypothesis of schizophrenia: a review. *Schizophr. Bull.*, **1976**, *2*, 19–76.

Menkes, D. B.; Aghajanian, G. K.; and Gallager, D. W. Chronic antidepressant treatment enhances agonist affinity of brain α_1-adrenoreceptors. *Eur. J. Pharmacol.*, **1983**, *87*, 35–41.

Mennini, T.; and Garattini, S. Benzodiazepine receptors: correlation with pharmacological responses in living animals. *Life Sci.*, **1982**, *31*, 2025–2035.

Moore, K. E.; and Kelly, P. H. Biochemical pharmacology of mesolimbic and mesocortical dopaminergic neurons. In, *Psychopharmacology: A Generation of Progress*. (Lipton, M. A.; DiMascio, A.; and Killam, K. F.; eds.) Raven Press, New York, **1978**, pp. 221–234.

Morselli, P. L. Psychotropic drugs. In, *Drug Disposition during Development*. (Morselli, P. L., ed.) Spectrum Publications, Inc., New York, **1977**, pp. 431–474.

Nagy, A.; and Johansson, R. Plasma levels of imipramine and desipramine in man after different routes of administration. *Naunyn Schmiedebergs Arch. Pharmacol.*, **1975**, *290*, 145–160.

Nelson, J. C.; and Bowers, M. B., Jr. Delusional unipolar depression: description and drug response. *Arch. Gen. Psychiatry*, **1978**, *35*, 1321–1328.

Nelson, J. C.; and Byck, R. Rapid response to lithium in phenelzine nonresponders. *Br. J. Psychiatry*, **1982**, *141*, 85–86.

Nicotra, M. B.; Rivera, M.; Pool, J. L.; and Noall, M. W. Tricyclic antidepressant overdose: clinical and pharmacological observations. *Clin. Toxicol.*, **1981**, *18*, 599–613.

Nies, A.; Robinson, D. S.; Friedman, M. J.; Green, R.; Cooper, T. B.; Ravaris, C. L.; and Ives, J. O. Relationship between age and tricyclic antidepressant plasma levels. *Am. J. Psychiatry*, **1977**, *134*, 790–793.

Noble, J.; and Matthew, H. Acute poisoning by tricyclic antidepressants: clinical features and management of 100 patients. *Clin. Toxicol.*, **1969**, *2*, 403–421.

Nouri, A.; and Cuendet, J. F. Atteintes oculaires au coures des traitements aux thymoleptiques. *Schweiz. Med. Wochenschr.*, **1971**, *101*, 1178.

Olphe, H. R.; and Schellenberg, A. Reduced sensitivity of neurons to noradrenaline after chronic treatment with antidepressant drugs. *Eur. J. Pharmacol.*, **1980**, *63*, 7–13.

Overall, J. E. Prior psychiatric treatment and the development of breast cancer. *Arch. Gen. Psychiatry*, **1978**, *35*, 898–899.

Peroutka, S. J.; and Snyder, S. H. Long-term antidepressant treatment decreases spiroperidol-labeled serotonin receptor binding. *Science*, **1980**, *210*, 88–90.

Pert, A.; Rosenblatt, J. E.; Sivit, C.; Pert, C. B.; and Bunney, W. E., Jr. Long-term treatment with lithium prevents the development of dopamine receptor supersensitivity. *Science*, **1978**, *201*, 171–173.

Pohl, R.; Berchou, R.; and Rainey, J. M. Tricyclic antidepressants and monoamine oxidase inhibitors in the treatment of agoraphobia. *J. Clin. Psychopharmacol.*, **1982**, *2*, 399–407.

Prien, R. F.; Delong, S. L.; Cole, J. O.; and Levine, J. Ocular changes occurring with prolonged high dose chlorpromazine therapy. *Arch. Gen. Psychiatry*, **1970**, *23*, 464–468.

Puig-Antich, J.; Blau, S.; Marx, N.; Greenhill, L. L.; and Chambers, W. Prepubertal major depressive disorder. *J. Am. Acad. Child Psychiatry*, **1978**, *17*, 695–707.

Quitkin, F.; Rifkin, A.; and Klein, D. F. Very high dosage vs. standard dosage fluphenazine in schizophrenia. *Arch. Gen. Psychiatry*, **1974**, *32*, 1276–1281.

Richelson, E. Tricyclic antidepressants and H_1 receptors. *Mayo Clin. Proc.*, **1979**, *54*, 669–674.

Robinson, D. S.; Nies, A.; Ravaris, C. L.; Ives, J. O.; and Bartlett, D. Clinical pharmacology of phenelzine. *Arch. Gen. Psychiatry*, **1978**, *35*, 629–635.

Rosenbaum, J. F. The drug treatment of anxiety. *N. Engl. J. Med.*, **1982**, *306*, 401–404.

Rotblatt, M. D. Antidepressants and seizures. *Drug Intell. Clin. Pharm.*, **1982**, *16*, 749–750.

Rotrosen, J.; Angrist, B. M.; Gershon, S.; Aronson, M.; Gruen, P.; Sachar, E.; Denning, R. K.; Matthysse, S.; Stanley, M.; and Wilk, S. Thiethylperazine. *Arch. Gen. Psychiatry*, **1978**, *35*, 1112–1118.

Sachar, E. J. Neuroendocrine responses to psychotropic drugs. In, *Psychopharmacology: A Generation of Progress*. (Lipton, M. A.; DiMascio, A.; and Killam, K. F.; eds.) Raven Press, New York, **1978**, pp. 499–507.

Safra, M. J., and Oakley, G. P., Jr. Association between cleft lip with or without cleft palate and prenatal exposure to diazepam. *Lancet*, **1975**, *2*, 478–480.

Sakalis, G.; Curry, S. H.; Mould, G. P.; and Lader, M. H. Physiologic and clinical effects of chlorpromazine and their relationship to plasma level. *Clin. Pharmacol. Ther.*, **1972**, *13*, 931–946.

Saron, B. M., and Gaind, R. Lithium. *Clin. Toxicol.*, **1973**, *6*, 257–269.

Schou, M. Lithium in psychiatric therapy and prophylaxis. *J. Psychiatr. Res.*, **1968**, *6*, 67–95.

Schyve, P. M.; Smithline, F.; and Meltzer, H. Y. Neuroleptic-induced prolactin level elevation and breast cancer: an emerging issue. *Arch. Gen. Psychiatry*, **1978**, *35*, 1291–1301.

Sedvall, G. Receptor feedback and dopamine turnover in CNS. In, *Handbook of Psychopharmacology*, Vol. 6. (Iversen, L. L.; Iversen, S. D.; and Snyder, S. H.; eds.) Plenum Press, New York, **1975**, pp. 127–177.

Selinger, D.; Simmons, S.; Hailer, A. W.; Nurnberger, J. I., Jr.; and Gershon, E. S. An effective method for measuring salivary lithium in patients on anticholinergic drugs. *Biol. Psychiatry*, **1982**, *17*, 1145–1155.

Sen, G., and Bose, K. C. *Rauwolfia serpentina*, a new Indian drug for insanity and high blood pressure. *Indian Med. World*, **1931**, *2*, 194–201.

Seppälä, T.; Linnoila, M.; Elonen, E.; Mattita, M. J.; and Mäki, M. Effect of tricyclic antidepressants and alcohol on psychomotor skills related to driving. *Clin. Pharmacol. Ther.*, **1975**, *17*, 515–522.

Shader, R. I.; Goodman, M.; and Gever, J. Panic disorders: current perspectives. *J. Clin. Psychopharmacol.*, **1982**, *2*, Suppl., 2–10.

Shagass, C., and Straumanis, J. J. Drugs and human sensory evoked potentials. In, *Psychopharmacology: A Generation of Progress*. (Lipton, M. A.; DiMascio, A.; and Killam, K. F.; eds.) Raven Press, New York, **1978**, pp. 699–709.

Shapiro, A. K.; Shapiro, E.; and Wayne, H. L. Treatment of Tourette's syndrome with haloperidol. Review of 34 cases. *Arch. Gen. Psychiatry*, **1973**, *28*, 92–97.

Shatan, C. Withdrawal symptoms after abrupt termination of imipramine. *Can. Psychiatr. Assoc. J.*, **1966**, *2*, 150–157.

Sheehan, D. V. Panic attacks and phobias. *N. Engl. J. Med.*, **1980**, *307*, 156–158.

Sheehan, D. V.; Ballenger, J.; and Jacobson, G. Treatment of endogenous anxiety with phobic, hysterical, and hypochondriacal symptoms. *Arch. Gen. Psychiatry*, **1980**, *37*, 51–59.

Simpson, G. M.; Cooper, T. B.; Bark, N.; Sud, I.; and Lee, H. J. Effect of antiparkinsonian medication on plasma levels of chlorpromazine. *Arch. Gen. Psychiatry*, **1980**, *37*, 205–208.

Skolnick, P., and Paul, S. M. Benzodiazepine receptors in the central nervous system. *Int. Rev. Neurobiol.*, **1982**, *23*, 103–140.

Snyder, S. H.; U'Prichard, D.; and Greenberg, D. A. Neurotransmitter receptor binding in the brain. In, *Psychopharmacology: A Generation of Progress*. (Lipton, M. A.; DiMascio, A.; and Killam, K. F.; eds.) Raven Press, New York, **1978**, pp. 361–370.

Snyder, S. H., and Yamamura, H. Antidepressants and the muscarinic acetylcholine receptor. *Arch. Gen. Psychiatry*, **1977**, *34*, 236–239.

Spiker, D. G., and Biggs, J. T. Tricyclic antidepressants: prolonged plasma levels after overdose. *J.A.M.A.*, **1976**, *236*, 1711–1712.

Study, R. E., and Barker, J. L. Cellular mechanisms of benzodiazepine action. *J.A.M.A.*, **1982**, *247*, 2147–2151.

Sulser, F., and Robinson, S. E. Clinical implications of pharmacological differences among antipsychotic drugs. In, *Psychopharmacology: A Generation of Progress*. (Lipton, M. A.; DiMascio, A.; and Killam, K. F.; eds.) Raven Press, New York, **1978**, pp. 943–954.

Svenssen, T. H., and Usdin, T. Feedback inhibition of brain noradrenaline neurons by tricyclic antidepressants: α-receptor mediation. *Science*, **1978**, *202*, 1089–1091.

Treiser, S. L.; Cascio, C. S.; O'Donohue, T. L.; Thoa, N. B.; Jacobowitz, D. M.; and Kellar, K. J. Lithium increases serotonin release and decreases serotonin receptors in the hippocampus. *Science*, **1981**, *213*, 1529–1531.

Tupin, J. P., and Schuller, A. B. Lithium and haloperidol incompatibility reviewed. *Psychiatr. J. Univ. Ottawa*, **1978**, *3*, 245–251.

U'Prichard, D. C.; Greenberg, D. A.; Sheehan, P. P.; and Snyder, S. H. Tricyclic antidepressants: therapeutic properties and affinity for alpha-noradrenergic receptor binding sites in the brain. *Science*, **1978**, *199*, 197–198.

Van De Merwe, T. J.; Silverstone, T.; Ankier, S. I.; Warrington, S. J.; and Turner, P. A double-blind non-crossover placebo-controlled study between group comparison of trazodone and amitriptyline on cardiovascular function in major depressive disorder. *Psychopathology*, **1984**, *17*, Suppl. 2, 64–76.

Veith, R. C.; Raskind, M. A.; and Caldwell, J. H. Cardiovascular effects of tricyclic antidepressants in depressed patients with chronic heart disease. *N. Engl. J. Med.*, **1982**, *306*, 954–959.

Vohra, J., and Burrows, G. D. Cardiovascular complications of tricyclic antidepressant overdosage. *Drugs*, **1974**, *8*, 432–437.

White, K., and Simpson, G. Combined MAOI–tricyclic antidepressant treatment: a reevaluation. *J. Clin. Psychopharmacol.*, **1981**, *1*, 264–282.

White, M. G., and Fetner, C. D. Treatment of the syndrome of inappropriate secretion of antidiuretic hormone with lithium carbonate. *N. Engl. J. Med.*, **1975**, *292*, 390–392.

Yamamura, H. I. (ed.). The mechanism of action of the benzodiazepines. *Fed. Proc.*, **1980**, *39*, 3016–3055.

Ziegler, V. E.; Biggs, J. T.; and Wylie, L. T. Doxepin kinetics. *Clin. Pharmacol. Ther.*, **1978**, *23*, 573–579.

Monographs and Reviews

Allquander, C. Dependence on sedative and hypnotic drugs. *Acta Psychiatr. Scand.* [*Suppl.*], **1978**, *270*, 1–120.

American Psychiatric Association. *Diagnostic and Statistical Manual of Mental Disorders*, 3rd ed. APA Press, Inc., Washington, D.C., **1980**.

Anders, T. F., and Ciaranello, R. Psychopharmacology of childhood disorders. In, *Psychopharmacology: From Theory to Practice*. (Barchas, J. D.; Berger, P. A.; Ciaranello, R.; and Elliott, G. R.; eds.) Oxford University Press, New York, **1977**, pp. 407–447.

Åsberg, M. Treatment of depression with tricyclic drugs: pharmacokinetic and pharmacodynamic aspects. *Pharmakopsychiatrie*, **1976**, *9*, 18–26.

Ayd, F. J., Jr., and Blackwell, B. (eds.). *Discoveries in Biological Psychiatry*. J. B. Lippincott Co., Philadelphia, **1970**.

Baldessarini, R. J. *Chemotherapy in Psychiatry*, 2nd ed. Harvard University Press, Cambridge, Mass., **1985**.

——. *Biomedical Aspects of Depression*. American Psychiatric Press, Inc., Washington, D.C., **1983**.

——. Antipsychotic agents. In, *Report of the Ameri-*

can *Psychiatric Association Commission on Psychiatric Therapeutics.* (Karasu, B., ed.) American Psychiatric Association, Washington, D.C., **1984b**, pp. 119–170.

Baldessarini, R. J.; Cole, J. O.; Davis, J. M.; Gardos, G.; Simpson, G.; and Tarsy, D. *Tardive Dyskinesia.* Task Force Report No. 18, American Psychiatric Association, Washington, D.C., **1980.**

Baldessarini, R. J., and Lipinski, J. F. Lithium salts: 1970–1975. *Ann. Intern. Med.,* **1975,** *83,* 527–533.

Baldessarini, R. J., and Tarsy, D. Relationship of the actions of neuroleptic drugs to the pathophysiology of tardive dyskinesia. *Int. Rev. Neurobiol.,* **1979,** *21,* 1–45.

Barchas, J. D.; Berger, P. A.; Matthysse, S.; and Wyatt, R. J. The biochemistry of affective disorders and schizophrenia. In, *Principles of Psychopharmacology,* 2nd ed. (Clark, W. G., and del Guidice, J., eds.) Academic Press, Inc., New York, **1978,** pp. 105–132.

Biel, J. H.; Bopp, B.; and Mitchell, B. D. Chemistry and structure-activity relationships of psychotropic drugs. In, *Principles of Psychopharmacology,* 2nd ed. (Clark, W. G., and del Guidice, J., eds.) Academic Press, Inc., New York, **1978,** pp. 140–168.

Caldwell, A. E. History of psychopharmacology. In, *Principles of Psychopharmacology,* 2nd ed. (Clark, W. G., and del Guidice, J., eds.) Academic Press, Inc., New York, **1978,** pp. 9–40.

Chase, T. N. Rational approaches to the pharmacotherapy of chorea. In, *The Basal Ganglia.* Association for Research in Nervous and Mental Disease Publications, Vol. 55. (Yahr, M. D., ed.) Raven Press, New York, **1976,** pp. 337–350.

Clark, W. G., and del Guidice, J. (eds.). *Principles of Psychopharmacology,* 2nd ed. Academic Press, Inc., New York, **1978.**

Cohen, B. M. The clinical utility of plasma neuroleptic levels. In, *Guidelines for the Use of Psychotropic Drugs.* (Stancer, H., ed.) Spectrum Publications, Inc., New York, **1984,** pp. 245–260.

Cooper, T. B.; Simpson, G. M.; and Lee, H. J. Thymoleptic and neuroleptic drug plasma levels in psychiatry: current status. *Int. Rev. Neurobiol.,* **1976,** *19,* 269–309.

Davis, J. M. Overview: maintenance therapy in psychiatry. I. Schizophrenia. *Am. J. Psychiatry,* **1975,** *132,* 1237–1245.

———. Overview: maintenance therapy in psychiatry. II. Affective disorders. *Ibid.,* **1976,** *133,* 1–13.

Davis, J. M., and Garver, D. L. Neuroleptics: clinical use in psychiatry. In, *Handbook of Psychopharmacology,* Vol. 10. (Iversen, L. L.; Iversen, S. D.; and Snyder, S. H.; eds.) Plenum Press, New York, **1978,** pp. 129–164.

De La Cruz, F. F.; Fox, B. H.; and Roberts, R. H. (eds.). Minimal brain dysfunction. *Ann. N.Y. Acad. Sci.,* **1973,** *205,* 1–396.

Efron, D. H.; Holmstedt, B.; and Kline, N. S. (eds.). *Ethnopharmacologic Search for Psychoactive Drugs.* Public Health Service Publication No. 67–1645, U.S. Government Printing Office, Washington, D.C., **1967.**

Eison, M. S. Use of animal models: toward anxioselective drugs. *Psychopathology,* **1984,** *17,* Suppl. 1, 37–44.

Fielding, S., and Lal, H. Behavioral actions of neuroleptics. In, *Handbook of Psychopharmacology,* Vol. 10. (Iversen, L. L.; Iversen, S. D.; and Snyder, S. H.; eds.) Plenum Press, New York, **1978,** pp. 91–128.

Freedman, A. M.; Kaplan, H. I.; and Sadock, B. J. (eds.). *Comprehensive Textbook of Psychiatry,* 3rd ed. The Williams & Wilkins Co., Baltimore, **1980.**

Glassman, A. H., and Perel, J. M. Tricyclic blood levels and clinical outcome: a review of the art. In, *Psychopharmacology: A Generation of Progress.* (Lipton, M. A.; DiMascio, A.; and Killam, K. F.; eds.) Raven Press, New York, **1978,** pp. 917–921.

Goldberg, H. L. Benzodiazepine and nonbenzodiazepine anxiolytics. *Psychopathology,* **1984,** *17,* Suppl. 1, 45–55.

Gordon, M. *Psychopharmacological Agents,* Vols. II and III. Academic Press, Inc., New York, **1967** and **1974.**

Herrington, R. N., and Lader, M. H. Chap. 1, Antidepressant drugs. Chap. 2, Lithium. In, *Handbook of Biological Psychiatry.* Pt. V, *Drug Treatment in Psychiatry—Psychotropic Drugs.* (Praag, H. M. van, ed.) Marcel Dekker, Inc., New York, **1981,** pp. 1–72.

Hollister, L. E. Tricyclic antidepressants. *N. Engl. J. Med.,* **1978,** *299,* 1106–1109, 1168–1172.

Irwin, S. Psychoactive drug evaluation. In, *Search for New Drugs.* (Rubin, A. A., ed.) Marcel Dekker, Inc., New York, **1972,** pp. 201–232.

Itil, T. M. Effects of psychotropic drugs on qualitatively and quantitatively analyzed human EEG. In, *Principles of Psychopharmacology,* 2nd ed. (Clark, W. G., and del Guidice, J., eds.) Academic Press, Inc., New York, **1978,** pp. 261–277.

Janssen, P. A. Butyrophenones and diphenylbutylpiperidines. In, *Psychopharmacological Agents,* Vol. 3. (Gordon, M., ed.) Academic Press, Inc., New York, **1974,** pp. 128–158.

Janssen, P. A., and Van Bever, W. F. Preclinical psychopharmacology of neuroleptics. In, *Principles of Psychopharmacology,* 2nd ed. (Clark, W. G., and del Guidice, J., eds.) Academic Press, Inc., New York, **1978,** pp. 279–295.

Jefferson, J. W. A review of the cardiovascular effects and toxicity of tricyclic antidepressants. *Psychosom. Med.,* **1975,** *37,* 160–179.

Jefferson, J. W., and Greist, J. H. *Primer of Lithium Therapy.* The Williams & Wilkins Co., Baltimore, **1977.**

Jefferson, J. W.; Greist, J. H.; and Ackerman, D. L. *Lithium Encyclopedia for Clinical Practice.* Lithium Information Center, Department of Psychiatry, University of Wisconsin, Madison, **1983.**

Jeste, D. V., and Wyatt, R. J. *Understanding and Treating Tardive Dyskinesia.* The Guilford Press, New York, **1982.**

Johnson, F. N. (ed.). *Handbook of Lithium Therapy.* University Park Press, Baltimore, **1980.**

Johnson, F. N., and Johnson, S. *Lithium in Medical Practice.* University Park Press, Baltimore, **1978.**

Kaiser, G., and Zirkle, C. L. Antidepressant drugs. In, *Medicinal Chemistry,* 2nd ed. (Burger, A., ed.) John Wiley & Sons, Inc., New York, **1970,** pp. 1470–1497.

Kaufman, J. S. Drug interactions involving psychotherapeutic agents. In, *Drug Treatment of Mental Disorders.* (Simpson, L. L., ed.) Raven Press, New York, **1976,** pp. 289–309.

Kety, S. S. Biochemical theories of schizophrenia. *Science,* **1959,** *29,* 1528–1532, 1590–1596.

Klein, D. F.; Gittelman, R.; Quitkin, F.; and Rifkin, A. *Diagnosis and Drug Treatment of Psychiatric Disorders: Adults and Children,* 2nd ed. The Williams & Wilkins Co., Baltimore, **1980.**

Lader, M. Antianxiety drugs in the psychiatric therapies. In, *Report of the American Psychiatric Association Commission on Psychiatric Therapeutics.* (Karasu, B., ed.) American Psychiatric Association, Washington, D.C., **1984,** pp. 53–84.

Levine, J.; Schiele, B. C.; and Bouthilet, L. (eds.). *Principles and Problems in Establishing the Efficacy of Psychotropic Agents.* Public Health Service Publication No. 2138, U.S. Government Printing Office, Washington, D.C., **1971.**

Lewin, L. *Phantastica, Narcotic and Stimulating Drugs; Their Use and Abuse.* Berlin, **1924;** English translation, London, **1931;** E. P. Dutton & Co., New York, **1931.**

Lipton, M. A.; DiMascio, A.; and Killam, K. F. (eds.). *Psychopharmacology: A Generation of Progress.* Raven Press, New York, **1978.**

Longo, V. G. Effects of psychotropic drugs on the EEG of animals. In, *Principles of Psychopharmacology*, 2nd ed. (Clark, W. G., and del Guidice, J., eds.) Academic Press, Inc., New York, **1978**, pp. 247–260.

Lowe, M. C.; Horita, A.; Gelenberg, A. J.; and Klerman, G. L. Preclinical pharmacology of antidepressants. In, *Principles of Psychopharmacology*, 2nd ed. (Clark, W. G., and del Guidice, J., eds.) Academic Press, Inc., New York, **1978**, pp. 311–323.

Marsden, C. D.; Tarsy, D.; and Baldessarini, R. J. Spontaneous and drug-induced movement disorders in psychiatric patients. In, *Psychiatric Aspects of Neurologic Disease*. (Benson, D. F., and Blumer, D., eds.) Grune & Stratton, Inc., New York, **1975**, pp. 219–265.

Martin, J. B.; Brazeau, P.; Tannenbaum, G. S.; Willoughby, J. O.; Epelbaum, J.; Terry, L. C.; and Durand, D. Neuroendocrine organization of growth hormone regulation. In, *The Hypothalamus*. Association for Research in Nervous and Mental Disease Publications, Vol. 56. (Reichlin, S.; Baldessarini, R. J.; and Martin, J. B.; eds.) Raven Press, New York, **1978**, pp. 329–357.

Murphy, D. L.; Campbell, I.; and Costa, J. L. Current status of the indoleamine hypothesis of the affective disorders. In, *Psychopharmacology: A Generation of Progress*. (Lipton, M. A.; DiMascio, A.; and Killam, K. F.; eds.) Raven Press, New York, **1978**, pp. 1235–1248.

Pope, H. G., and Lipinski, J. F. Diagnosis in schizophrenia and manic-depressive illness. *Arch. Gen. Psychiatry*, **1978**, *35*, 811–828.

Popper, C. W. Child and adolescent psychopharmacology. In, *Psychiatry*. (Cavenar, J. O., ed.) J. B. Lippincott Co., Philadelphia, **1985**.

Post, R. M.; Uhde, T. W.; Rubinow, D. R.; Ballenger, J. C.; and Gold, P. W. Biochemical effects of carbamazepine: relationship to its mechanisms of action in affective illness. *Prog. Neuropsychopharmacol. Biol. Psychiatry*, **1983**, *7*, 263–271.

Praag, H. M. van. Amine hypotheses of affective disorders. In, *Handbook of Psychopharmacology*, Vol. 13. (Iversen, L. L.; Iversen, S. D.; and Snyder, S. H.; eds.) Plenum Press, New York, **1978**, pp. 187–297.

Prien, R. F. Chemotherapy in chronic organic brain syndrome—a review of the literature. *Psychopharmacol. Bull.*, **1973**, *9*, 5–20.

Prien, R. F., and Cole, J. O. The use of psychopharmacological drugs in the aged. In, *Principles of Psychopharmacology*, 2nd ed. (Clark, W. G., and del Guidice, J., eds.) Academic Press, Inc., New York, **1978**, pp. 593–605.

Ramsey, T. A., and Mendels, J. Lithium as an antidepressant. In, *Antidepressants: Neurochemical, Behavioral and Clinical Perspectives*. (Enna, S. J.; Malick, J. B.; and Richelson, E; eds.) Raven Press, New York, **1981**, pp. 175–182.

Raskin, A.; Robinson, D. S.; and Levine, J. *Age and the Pharmacology of Psychoactive Drugs*. Elsevier-North Holland, Inc., New York, **1981**.

Reichlin, S., and Boyd, A. E., III. Neural control of prolactin secretion in man. *Psychoneuroendocrinology*, **1978**, *3*, 113–130.

Rickels, K. Drug treatment of anxiety. In, *Psychopharmacology in the Practice of Medicine*. (Jarvik, M. E., ed.) Appleton-Century-Crofts, New York, **1977**, pp. 309–324.

Rickels, K.; Downing, R. W.; and Winokur, A. Antianxiety drugs: clinical use in psychiatry. In, *Handbook of Psychopharmacology*, Vol. 13. (Iversen, L. L.; Iversen, S. D.; and Snyder, S. H.; eds.) Plenum Press, New York, **1978**, pp. 395–430.

Rivera-Calimlin, L., and Hershey, L. Neuroleptic concentrations and clinical response. *Annu. Rev. Pharmacol. Toxicol.*, **1984**, *24*, 361–386.

Schou, M. Biology and pharmacology of the lithium ion. *Pharmacol. Rev.*, **1957**, *9*, 17–58.

———. The biology and pharmacology of lithium: a bibliography. *Psychopharmacol. Bull.*, **1969**, *5*, 33–62.

Schultes, R. E. Ethnopharmacological significance of psychotropic drugs of vegetal origin. In, *Principles of Psychopharmacology*, 2nd ed. (Clark, W. G., and del Guidice, J., eds.) Academic Press, Inc., New York, **1978**, pp. 41–70.

Seeman, P. The membrane actions of anesthetics and tranquilizers. *Pharmacol. Rev.*, **1972**, *24*, 583–655.

Sepinwall, J., and Cook, L. Behavioral pharmacology of antianxiety drugs. In, *Handbook of Psychopharmacology*, Vol. 13. (Iversen, L. L.; Iversen, S. D.; and Snyder, S. H.; eds.) Plenum Press, New York, **1978**, pp. 345–393.

Shader, R. I., and DiMascio, A. *Psychotropic Drug Side Effects: Chemical and Theoretical Perspectives*. The Williams & Wilkins Co., Baltimore, **1970**.

Shader, R. J. (ed.). *Psychiatric Complications of Medical Drugs*. Raven Press, New York, **1972**.

Shore, P. A., and Giachetti, A. Reserpine: basic and clinical pharmacology. In, *Handbook of Psychopharmacology*, Vol. 10. (Iversen, L. L.; Iversen, S. D.; and Snyder, S. H.; eds.) Plenum Press, New York, **1978**, pp. 197–219.

Sigg, E. B. Autonomic side-effects induced by psychotherapeutic agents. In, *Psychopharmacology: A Review of Progress, 1957–1967*. (Efron, D. H.; Cole, J. O.; Levine, J.; and Wittenborn, J. R.; eds.) U.S. Government Printing Office, Washington, D.C., **1968**, pp. 581–588.

Siggins, G. R.; Hoffer, B. J.; Bloom, F. E.; and Ungerstedt, U. Cytochemical and electrophysiological studies of dopamine in the caudate nucleus. In, *The Basal Ganglia*. Association for Research in Nervous and Mental Disease Publications, Vol. 55. (Yahr, M., ed.) Raven Press, New York, **1976**, pp. 227–248.

Sulser, F., and Mobley, P. L. Biochemical effects of antidepressants in animals. In, *Psychotropic Agents: Antipsychotics and Antidepressants*. Vol. 55, Pt. I, *Handbook of Experimental Pharmacology*. (Hoffmeister, F., and Stille, G., eds.) Springer-Verlag, Berlin, **1980**, pp. 471–490.

Swazey, J. P. *Chlorpromazine in Psychiatry: A Study in Therapeutic Innovation*. M.I.T. Press, Cambridge, Mass., **1974**.

Symposium. (Various authors.) Affective disorders: drug actions in animals and man. In, *Handbook of Psychopharmacology*, Vol. 14. (Iversen, L. L.; Iversen, S. D.; and Snyder, S. H.; eds.) Plenum Press, New York, **1978**.

Symposium. (Various authors.) *Monoamine Oxidase: Structure, Function and Altered Functions*. (Singer, T. P.; Von Korff, D. W.; and Murphy, D. L.; eds.) Academic Press, Inc., New York, **1979**.

Symposium. (Various authors.) *Antidepressants: Neurochemical, Behavioral, and Clinical Perspectives*. (Enna, S. J.; Malick, J. B.; and Richelson, E.; eds.) Raven Press, New York, **1981**.

Symposium. (Various authors.) *Pharmacology of Benzodiazepines*. (Usdin, E.; Skolnick, P.; Tallman, J. F., Jr.; Greenblatt, D.; and Paul, S. M.; eds.) Macmillan Press Ltd., London, **1982**.

Tallman, J. F.; Paul, S. M.; Skolnick, P.; and Gallager, D. W. Receptors for the age of anxiety: pharmacology of the benzodiazepines. *Science*, **1980**, *207*, 274–281.

Usdin, E. Classification of psychotropic drugs. In, *Principles of Psychopharmacology*, 2nd ed. (Clark, W. G., and del Guidice, J., eds.) Academic Press, Inc., New York, **1978**, pp. 193–246.

Usdin, E., and Efron, D. H. *Psychotropic Drugs and Related Compounds*, 2nd ed. Public Health Service

Publication No. 72-9074, U.S. Government Printing Office, Washington, D. C., **1972.**

Van Woert, M. H.; Jutkowitz, R.; Rosenbaum, D.; and Bowers, M. B., Jr. Gilles de la Tourette's syndrome: biochemical approaches. In, *The Basal Ganglia*. Association for Research in Nervous and Mental Disease Publications, Vol. 55. (Yahr, M. D., ed.) Raven Press, New York, **1976,** pp. 459–465.

Vesell, E. S. Pharmacogenetics. *N. Engl. J. Med.*, **1972,** *287,* 904–909.

Weil-Malherbe, H. The biochemistry of the functional psychoses. *Adv. Enzymol.,* **1967,** *29,* 479–553.

Werry, J. S. (ed.). *Pediatric Psychopharmacology: The Use of Behavior Modifying Drugs in Children.* Brunner/ Mazel, Inc., New York, **1978.**

Winokur, G.; Clayton, P. J.; and Reich, T. *Manic-Depressive Illness.* C. V. Mosby Co., St. Louis, **1969.**

Zirkle, C. L., and Kaiser, C. Antipsychotic drugs. In, *Medicinal Chemistry,* 2nd ed. (Berger, A., ed.) John Wiley & Sons, Inc., New York, **1970,** pp. 1410–1469.

20 DRUGS EFFECTIVE IN THE THERAPY OF THE EPILEPSIES

Theodore W. Rall and Leonard S. Schleifer

GENERAL CONSIDERATIONS

Classification of Epileptic Seizures. The term *epilepsies* is a collective designation for a group of central nervous system (CNS) disorders having in common the occurrence of sudden and transitory episodes (seizures) of abnormal phenomena of motor (convulsion), sensory, autonomic, or psychic origin. The seizures are nearly always correlated with abnormal and excessive discharges in the electroencephalogram (EEG).

The prevalence of epilepsy is between 3 and 6 per 1000 population (Hauser, 1978). The term *primary* or *idiopathic epilepsy* denotes those cases where no cause for the seizures can be identified. *Secondary* or *symptomatic epilepsy* designates the disorder when it is associated with such factors as trauma, neoplasm, infection, developmental abnormalities, cerebrovascular disease, or various metabolic conditions. The detection of factors that contribute to secondary epilepsy has been facilitated by the advent of improved diagnostic procedures, such as computerized axial tomography and nuclear magnetic resonance scanning of the brain.

For purposes of drug treatment, it is more useful to classify patients according to the type of seizure they experience. A simplified form of the proposal from the Commission on Classification and Terminology of the International League Against Epilepsy (1981), based on the clinical manifestations of the attacks and the pattern of the EEG, is presented in Table 20–1. Accurate diagnosis is important, since pharmacotherapy is selective for a particular type of seizure (*see* below). A more complete description of the various types of seizures has been provided by Browne (Symposium,

1983a) and by Delgado-Escueta and coworkers (1983).

Nature and Mechanisms of Seizures. Almost a century ago John Hughlings Jackson, the father of modern concepts of epilepsy, proposed that seizures were caused by "occasional, sudden, excessive, rapid and local discharges of gray matter," and that a generalized convulsion resulted when normal brain tissue was invaded by the seizure activity initiated in the abnormal focus. In the intervening years little has been added to Jackson's concepts except for the electrical proof of their correctness. The EEG amply demonstrates that seizures are associated with abnormal and sometimes massive electrical discharges in the brain and serves as the basic method of differential diagnosis of the epilepsies.

Various experimental models have been used to investigate the mechanisms responsible for the genesis of epileptic seizures (*see* Symposium, 1972, 1981). For example, application of alumina cream to the motor cortex of the monkey produces chronically recurring, spontaneous convulsive seizures of focal onset. While a focus of groups of neurons that discharge synchronously at high frequency can be found near the original site of instillation, independent secondary epileptic foci can also develop in areas that are richly innervated by efferents from the primary lesion produced by alumina cream (*see* Wilder, in Symposium, 1972). These secondary foci persist after the surgical removal of the primary focus; they are not associated with any consistent changes in histological characteristics.

A potentially more informative model is that produced in a variety of animal species by a procedure termed *kindling* (*see* Symposium, 1981). This involves delivery of brief, localized trains of electrical stimuli to various areas of the brain at widely spaced intervals. With time, progressively longer and more intense periods of afterdischarge are produced at sites both near to and remote from the point of stimulation. Motor seizures of increasing degrees of severity can then be elicited regularly, even when several months have elapsed between

Table 20–1. CLASSIFICATION OF EPILEPTIC SEIZURES *

SEIZURE TYPE †		CHARACTERISTICS
I. *Partial Seizures* (Focal, Local Seizures)	A. Simple partial seizures	Various manifestations, without impairment of consciousness, including convulsions confined to a single limb or muscle group (*Jacksonian motor epilepsy*), specific and localized sensory disturbances (*Jacksonian sensory epilepsy*), and other limited signs and symptoms depending upon the particular cortical area producing the abnormal discharge
	B. Complex partial seizures	Attacks of confused behavior, with impairment of consciousness, with a wide variety of clinical manifestations, associated with bizarre generalized EEG activity during the seizure but with evidence of anterior temporal lobe focal abnormalities even in the interseizure period in many cases
	C. Partial seizures secondarily generalized	
II. *Generalized Seizures* (Convulsive or Nonconvulsive)	A.1. Absence seizures	Brief and abrupt loss of consciousness associated with high-voltage, bilaterally synchronous, 3-per-second spike-and-wave pattern in the EEG, usually with some symmetrical clonic motor activity varying from eyelid blinking to jerking of the entire body, sometimes with no motor activity
	A.2. Atypical absence seizures	Attacks with slower onset and cessation than is usual for absence seizures, associated with a more heterogeneous EEG
	B. Myoclonic seizures	Isolated clonic jerks associated with brief bursts of multiple spikes in the EEG
	C. Clonic seizures	Rhythmic clonic contractions of all muscles, loss of consciousness, and marked autonomic manifestations
	D. Tonic seizures	Opisthotonus, loss of consciousness, and marked autonomic manifestations
	E. Tonic-clonic seizures (*grand mal*)	Major convulsions, usually a sequence of maximal tonic spasm of all body musculature followed by synchronous clonic jerking and a prolonged depression of all central functions
	F. Atonic seizures	Loss of postural tone, with sagging of the head or falling

* Modified from the proposal from the Commission on Classification and Terminology of the International League Against Epilepsy (1981).

† Additional seizure types are presently unclassified due to incomplete data.

stimulations. In the advanced stages of kindling in the rat, the seizure consists of a running fit, sometimes including periods of tonus at the beginning and end of the seizure (*see* Pinel, in Symposium, 1981). After the evoked seizures display these characteristics, continued delivery of the kindling stimuli results in the emergence of spontaneous seizures that progressively become more severe. While this condition is associated with an increased frequency of interictal discharges that can be recorded from the original site of stimulation, the spontaneous seizures usually arise from remote sites. Thus, it appears that the process of epileptogenesis begins with a source of electrical discharges of sufficient intensity or frequency to produce adaptive changes in groups of neurons that are connected synaptically to the source, and it evolves by the progressive recruitment of neuronal circuits. These secondary foci can then discharge either spontaneously or in response to stimuli from other sources (*e.g.*, sensory stimuli) and can initiate generalized seizures.

Neither the nature of the adaptive changes involved in the development of secondary foci nor the mechanisms responsible for the sporadic precipitation of spontaneous generalized convulsions are clearly understood. The adaptive changes may be related to the phenomenon of *long-term potentiation* (LTP), which can be produced by high-frequency stimulation of inputs to the hippocampus, even in slices incubated *in vitro* (*see* Goddard, in Symposium, 1981). LTP appears to involve increases both in the size of excitatory synaptic potentials in response to a given stimulus and in the excitability of postsynaptic neurons in the presence of a given magnitude of synaptic potential. These changes persist for many hours after the application of a single train of electrical stimuli, thus distinguishing LTP from *posttetanic potentiation* (PTP), which involves a short-lived increase in the release of neurotransmitter following high-frequency stimulation of individual synapses.

It is also not clear what anatomical pathways are involved in the progression from focal to generalized seizures. For example, bilateral seizures can be elicited in kindled animals in whom the corpus callosum has been severed (*see* Burnham *et al.*, in Symposium, 1981). While there is evidence for the participation of the mesencephalic reticular formation in such circumstances, the relative contribution of ascending versus descending impulses to the lateral spread of seizure activity has not been determined.

Other experimental models utilize animals that are genetically susceptible to convulsive seizures precipitated by appropriate sensory stimuli (*see* Symposium, 1972). These include audiogenic seizures in certain strains of mice and seizures elicited by intermittent photic stimulation, prevalent in a specific group of baboons. More recently, two inbred strains of mice have been developed, one characterized by spontaneous tonic-clonic convulsions and the other by behavioral and electrocorticographic evidence of spontaneous absence seizures (Heller *et al.*, 1983; Maxson *et al.*, 1983). In addition to providing opportunities for the evaluation of antiepileptic drugs, these models call attention to inherited factors that are suspected to play a role in the genesis of human epilepsy.

Many observations made in patients with epilepsy are congruent with the picture of epileptogenesis provided by the kindling model in animals. For example, years may elapse after a penetrating head wound before the emergence of convulsive symptoms. Further, excision of relatively large amounts of brain tissue is required to ameliorate the symptoms of patients who undergo surgery for the relief of medically refractory focal epilepsy. In a study of the minority of patients who become free of seizures following removal of portions of the frontal lobe, a wide variety of patterns of attack were displayed prior to surgery; these ranged from absences to generalized tonic-clonic convulsions, both with and without focal onset (Rasmussen, 1983). While antiepileptic medication was eventually withdrawn from some of these patients without return of convulsive symptoms, the cortical EEG of the majority showed evidence of epileptiform discharges for many years after surgery. Finally, in a small proportion of these patients, neither macroscopic nor microscopic abnormalities were found in the excised tissue.

These and other observations suggest that the seizure disorder of most patients with epilepsy begins with and is sustained by the synchronous firing at high frequency of a relatively localized group of neurons. Individual attacks may arise from this primary focus or may emerge from diverse areas in which functional abnormalities have been induced. While there is as yet no definitive explanation for the paroxysmal discharges in primary foci, a reduction in inhibitory components of neuronal circuits is a leading candidate among the possible mechanisms. Several lines of evidence support this idea. For example, the small neurons with short axons that function in local inhibitory loops are known to be especially vulnerable to ischemia. In addition, groups of neurons display epileptiform discharges in the presence of a variety of drugs that interfere with the function of gamma-aminobutyric acid (GABA), the major inhibitory neurotransmitter in the brain; these include bicuculline, picrotoxin, pentylenetetrazol, and certain beta-lactam antibiotics. As recorded by intracellular electrodes, these neuronal bursts arise from a sudden, large depolarization, termed a *paroxysmal depolarizing shift* (PDS). The PDS displays the characteristics of a "giant" excitatory postsynaptic potential and appears to result from synchronous activity within a neural network (*see* Johnston and Brown, 1984). It can occur spontaneously or be triggered by external stimuli.

The pathological origins of primary seizure foci in man include congenital defects, head trauma and hypoxia at birth, inflammatory vascular changes subsequent to infectious illnesses of childhood, concussion or depressed skull fracture, abscess, neoplasm, and vascular occlusion of whatever etiology. Although these different lesions have somewhat different predilections for various brain areas, the type of chronic stable focus appears to be similar, and the type of seizure pattern shown by the patient seems more related to the anatomical connections of the focus than to the original etiology.

As revealed by the surface EEG, focal epileptiform discharges may occur only intermittently and may not be associated with any signs or symptoms. Presumably, the spread of convulsive activity to neighboring normal cells is restrained by inhibitory mechanisms. However, physiological changes that cannot in themselves cause seizures may trigger the focus or facilitate spread of abnormal electrical activity to normal tissue. Among such factors are changes in blood glucose concentration, blood gas tensions, plasma pH, and electrolyte composition of extracellular fluid; endocrine changes, fatigue, emotional stress, and nutritional deficiencies may also contribute. Many factors can interact to precipitate seizures in a brain predisposed by injury or inherited defect, and the physician should not be perplexed when some patients with seemingly identical seizure patterns respond quite differently to drug therapy.

Mechanisms of Action of Antiepileptic Agents. There are two general ways in which drugs might abolish or attenuate seizures: effects on pathologically altered neurons of seizure foci to prevent or reduce their excessive discharge, and effects that would reduce the spread of excitation from seizure foci and prevent detonation and disruption of function of normal aggregates of neurons. Most, if not all, antiepileptic agents that are presently available act at least in part by the second mechanism, since all modify the ability of the brain to respond to various seizure-evoking stimuli. While a variety of neurophysiological effects of such drugs have been noted, especially effects on inhibitory systems that involve GABA, investigators frequently fail to define those effects that might be prominent at therapeutic concentrations of free drug in plasma or those that are not characteristic of local anesthetics or sedatives. Thus, it must be admitted that mechanisms of action of antiepileptic agents are only poorly understood. Useful anticpileptic agents may be capable of causing some mixture of mutually reinforcing actions that permits therapeutic responses without undue disruption of normal function. With these general considerations in mind, the more plausible hypotheses of the action of antiepileptic agents will be discussed in the sections that deal with the individual drugs.

Chemical Structure and Antiepileptic Selectivity. The useful antiepileptic agents belong to several chemical classes. Most of the drugs introduced before 1965 are closely related in structure to phenobarbital, the oldest member of this therapeutic class. These include the hydantoins, the deoxybarbiturates, the oxazolidinediones, and the succinimides. The agents introduced after 1965 include benzodiazepines (*clonazepam* and *clorazepate*), an iminostilbene (*carbamazepine*), and a branched-chain carboxylic acid (*valproic acid*). The structure-activity relationships of these and other classes of compounds have been summarized (*see* Symposium, 1977). Several new compounds

structurally related to GABA (*e.g., progabide*) are currently being evaluated (*see* Lloyd and Morselli, in Symposium, 1982a).

The laboratory screening tests for potential antiepileptic drugs have relied heavily on the capacity to modify the effects of maximal electric shock (inhibition of tonic hindlimb extension) and to elevate the dose of pentylenetetrazol required to precipitate tonic-clonic convulsions (*see* Krall *et al.,* 1978). While the former test usually predicts activity against generalized tonic-clonic and cortical focal convulsions and the latter against absence seizures, there are a number of important exceptions to this generalization. There is a need for continued development of model systems for the detection and evaluation of potential therapeutic agents, and emphasis has recently been placed on the use of genetically based or kindling models.

Therapeutic Aspects. The ideal antiepileptic drug would obviously suppress all seizures without causing any unwanted effects. Unfortunately, the drugs used currently not only fail to control seizure activity in some patients, but they frequently cause side effects that range in severity from minimal impairment of the CNS to death from aplastic anemia or hepatic failure. The physician who treats patients with epilepsy is thus faced with the task of selecting the appropriate drug or combination of drugs that best controls seizures in an individual patient at an acceptable level of untoward effects. It is generally held that complete control of seizures can be achieved in up to 50% of patients and possibly another 25% can be improved significantly. The *degree of success* is largely dependent on the type of seizure and the extent of associated neurological abnormalities (*see* below).

For the purposes of drug therapy the classification of seizures given above may be further condensed. *Absence* seizures respond well to one group of drugs, and *generalized tonic-clonic* convulsions are usually adequately controlled by another. *Complex partial* seizures tend to be refractory to therapy but may respond to agents in the second group. *Infantile spasms* and *akinetic, atonic,* and *myoclonic* seizures are a group for which therapy is generally unsatisfactory. Multiple-drug therapy is often required, since two or more seizure types may occur in the same patient. However, *benign focal epilepsy of childhood* (Rolandic epilepsy), an inherited condition, often requires therapy with a single drug for only a limited period of time.

The general principles of the drug therapy of the epilepsies are summarized below, following discussion of the individual agents. Details of diagnosis and therapy can be found in the monographs and reviews listed at the end of the chapter.

Plasma Concentrations of Antiepileptic Drugs. Measurement of drug concentrations in plasma greatly facilitates antiepileptic medication, especially multiple-drug therapy (*see* Symposium, 1978, 1982a). However, clinical effects do not correlate well with concentrations in plasma for some drugs, and recommended concentrations are only guidelines for therapy. The ultimate therapeutic regimen must be determined by clinical assessment of effect and toxicity. Factors that contribute to this problem include the variability that has been noted in the chemical analysis of certain compounds and the fact that the values determined usually represent total concentrations in plasma. For many antiepileptic drugs, the concentration of free drug is only a small fraction of the total and may be variable. Plasma drug concentrations recommended for maintenance therapy, as well as other pharmacokinetic characteristics essential for interpretation of measured concentrations and for devising drug dosage schedules, are discussed with the individual agents and in Appendix II. The value of monitoring plasma concentrations of the antiepileptic agents is discussed further at the end of the chapter.

HYDANTOINS

PHENYTOIN

Phenytoin is a primary drug for all types of epilepsy except absence seizures. It has been more thoroughly studied in the laboratory and clinic than any other antiepileptic agent.

History. Phenytoin was first synthesized in 1908 by Biltz, but its anticonvulsant activity was not discovered until 1938 (Merritt and Putnam, 1938a). In contrast to the earlier accidental discovery of the anticonvulsant properties of bromide and phenobarbital, phenytoin was the product of a search among nonsedative structural relatives of pheno-

barbital for agents capable of suppressing electroshock convulsions in laboratory animals. It was introduced for the symptomatic treatment of epilepsy in the same year (Merritt and Putnam, 1938b). The discovery of phenytoin was a signal advance. Since this agent is not a sedative in ordinary doses, it established that antiepileptics need not impair consciousness and encouraged the search for drugs with selective anticonvulsant action.

Structure-Activity Relationship. Phenytoin has the following structural formula:

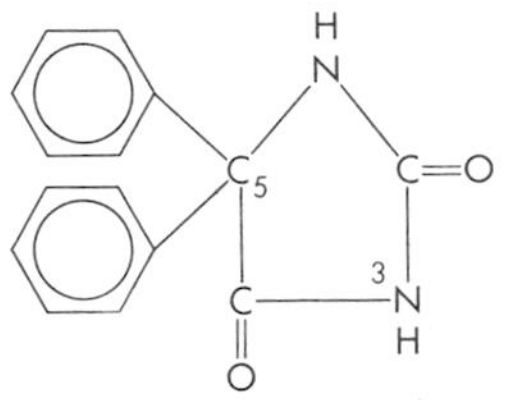

Phenytoin

A 5-phenyl or other aromatic substituent appears essential for activity against clinical generalized tonic-clonic seizures and for abolition of the maximal electroshock seizure pattern in laboratory animals. Alkyl substituents in position 5 contribute to sedation, a property absent in phenytoin. The 5 carbon permits asymmetry, as in mephenytoin, but there appears to be little difference in activity between isomers. (*See* Vida and Gerry, in Symposium, 1977.)

Pharmacological Effects. *Central Nervous System.* Phenytoin exerts antiepileptic activity without causing general depression of the CNS. In toxic doses it may produce excitatory signs and at lethal levels a type of decerebrate rigidity. The most easily demonstrated properties of phenytoin are its ability to limit the development of maximal seizure activity and to reduce the spread of the seizure process from an active focus. Both features are undoubtedly related to its clinical usefulness. Phenytoin can induce complete remission of generalized tonic-clonic and certain partial seizures but does not completely eliminate the sensory aura or other prodromal signs.

The anticonvulsant properties of phenytoin have been reviewed by Woodbury (Symposium, 1980). Unlike phenobarbital, phenytoin does not elevate the threshold for seizures induced by injection of such convulsant drugs as strychnine, picrotoxin, or pentylenetetrazol. It also has only limited ability to elevate threshold for electroshock seizures. Phenytoin does, however, restore abnormally increased excitability toward normal.

Probably the most significant effect of phenytoin

is its ability to modify the pattern of maximal electroshock seizures. The characteristic tonic phase can be abolished completely, but the residual clonic seizure may be exaggerated and prolonged. The drug produces similar alterations in the convulsions of psychiatric patients undergoing electroconvulsive therapy and in maximal seizures induced in animals by picrotoxin and pentylenetetrazol. This seizure-modifying action is observed also with other typical antiepileptics effective against generalized tonic-clonic seizures.

In various species, as revealed by a variety of stimulation-recording technics, the ability of phenytoin to reduce the duration of afterdischarge and to limit the spread of seizure activity is more prominent than its effect on threshold for stimulation. It is thus surprising that phenytoin does not consistently retard the process of kindling in various animal species; this is in contrast to results with phenobarbital, carbamazepine, valproate, and various benzodiazepines (*see* Wada, 1977). The prophylactic effect of phenytoin in human posttraumatic epilepsy has also been variable and difficult to evaluate (*see* Mutani, in Symposium, 1983b).

An *excitatory* effect on the cerebellum, to activate inhibitory pathways that extend to the cerebral cortex, has been suggested to contribute to the anticonvulsant effect of phenytoin (*see* Laxer *et al.,* in Symposium, 1980). Although phenytoin increases the discharge of cerebellar Purkinje cells and removal of the cerebellum decreases the effectiveness of the drug, this hypothesis remains controversial.

Mechanism of Action. A stabilizing effect of phenytoin is apparent on all neuronal membranes, including those of peripheral nerves, and probably on all excitable as well as nonexcitable membranes (*see* Woodbury, in Symposium, 1980; *see also* Chapter 31). In a variety of systems, phenytoin has been observed to decrease resting fluxes of sodium ions as well as sodium currents that flow during action potentials or chemically induced depolarizations (*see* Jones and Wimbish, 1985). In addition, influx of calcium ion during depolarization is decreased, either independently or as a consequence of reduced intracellular concentration of sodium. Phenytoin can also delay the activation of outward potassium current during an action potential, leading to an increased refractory period. Episodes of repetitive firing that result from the passage of current intracellularly are especially sensitive to suppression by phenytoin (*see* Macdonald and McLean, 1982). Although these ionic effects can usually be distinguished both quantitatively and qualitatively from those produced by local anesthetics, they seldom have been demonstrated at concentrations of phenytoin at or below 10 μM, the maximal plasma concentration of free drug that usually can be tolerated during therapy.

Absorption, Distribution, Biotransformation, and Excretion. The pharmacokinetic characteristics of phenytoin are markedly influenced by its limited aqueous solubility and its dose-dependent elimination. Its inactivation by the hepatic microsomal enzyme system is susceptible to alteration by other drugs.

Phenytoin is a weak acid with a pK_a of about 8.3; its aqueous solubility is limited, even in the intestine. Upon intramuscular injection, the drug precipitates at the injection site and is slowly absorbed, as if it had been administered in a repository preparation.

Absorption of phenytoin after oral ingestion is slow, sometimes variable, and occasionally incomplete. Significant differences in bioavailability of oral pharmaceutical preparations have been detected (Melikian *et al.,* 1977). Peak concentration after a single dose may occur in plasma as early as 3 hours or as late as 12 hours. Slow absorption during chronic medication blunts the fluctuations of drug concentration between doses. After absorption, phenytoin is rapidly distributed into all tissues and concentrations in plasma and brain are equal within minutes of intravenous injection (*see* Levy, in Symposium, 1980).

Phenytoin is extensively (about 90%) bound to plasma proteins, mainly albumin (*see* Goldberg, in Symposium, 1980). A greater fraction remains unbound in the neonate, in patients with hypoalbuminemia, and in uremic patients (*see* Appendix II). Fractional binding in tissues, including brain, is about the same as in plasma. Thus, the apparent volume of distribution of phenytoin is about 0.6 to 0.7 liter per kilogram but would be about ten times larger if calculated on the basis of unbound drug. The concentration in the cerebrospinal fluid (CSF) is equal to the unbound fraction in plasma.

Less than 5% of phenytoin is excreted unchanged in the urine. The remainder is metabolized primarily by the hepatic microsomal enzymes. The major metabolite, the parahydroxyphenyl derivative, is inactive. It accounts for 60 to 70% of a single dose of the drug and a somewhat smaller fraction during chronic medication. It is excreted initially in the bile and subsequently in the urine, in large part as the glucuronide. Other apparently inactive metabolites include the dihydroxy catechol and its 3-methoxy derivative, and the dihydrodiol. At plasma concentrations below 10 μg/ml, elimination is exponential (first order); plasma half-time ranges between 6 and 24 hours. At higher concentrations, dose-dependent elimination is apparent; plasma half-time increases with concentration (dose), perhaps because the hydroxylation reaction approaches saturation or is inhibited by the metabolites. A genetically determined limitation in ability to metabolize phenytoin has been detected. The pharmacokinetic properties of phenytoin have been reviewed by Richens (1979) and by Chang and Glazko (Symposium, 1982a).

Toxicity.   The toxic effects of phenytoin depend upon the route and duration of exposure as well as dosage. When it is administered intravenously at an excessive rate in the emergency treatment of cardiac arrhythmias or status epilepticus, the most notable toxic signs are *cardiac arrhythmias,* with or without *hypotension,* and/or *CNS depression.* Although *cardiac toxicity* occurs more frequently in older patients and those with known cardiac disease, it can also develop in young, healthy patients (Earnest *et al.,* 1983). These complications can be minimized by slow administration of dilute solutions of the drug. Acute overdosage by the oral route features primarily signs referable to the cerebellum and vestibular system. Toxic effects associated with chronic medication are also primarily dose-related *cerebellar-vestibular effects* but include *other CNS effects, behavioral changes, increased frequency of seizures, gastrointestinal symptoms, gingival hyperplasia, osteomalacia,* and *megaloblastic anemia. Hirsutism* is an annoying untoward effect in young females. Usually, these phenomena can be made bearable by proper adjustment of dosage. Serious adverse effects, including those on the skin, bone marrow, and liver, are probably manifestations of *drug allergy.* Although rare, they necessitate withdrawal of the drug. Moderate elevation of the concentrations of enzymes in plasma that are used to assess hepatic function are sometimes observed; since these changes are transient and may result in part from induced synthesis of the enzymes, they do not necessitate withdrawal of the drug (Aiges *et al.,* 1980). The

toxicity of phenytoin has been extensively reviewed in a symposium (1982a).

Central and peripheral nervous system toxicity is the most consistent effect of phenytoin overdosage. *Nystagmus, ataxia, diplopia,* and *vertigo* and other cerebellar-vestibular effects are common. *Blurred vision, mydriasis, ophthalmoplegia,* and *hyperactive tendon reflexes* also occur. *Behavioral* effects include *hyperactivity, silliness, confusion, dullness, drowsiness,* and *hallucinations.* While phenytoin has been implicated in the irreversible cerebellar damage noted in some epileptic patients, similar findings were described before the introduction of this agent. This condition may thus be a consequence of repeated seizures (*see* Dam, in Symposium, 1982a). While electrophysiological evidence of *peripheral neuropathy* can occur in up to 30% of patients receiving phenytoin, this phenomenon is rarely of clinical significance.

Gingival hyperplasia occurs in about 20% of all patients during chronic therapy and is probably the most common manifestation of phenytoin toxicity in children and young adolescents. The overgrowth of tissue appears to involve altered collagen metabolism (Hassell and Gilbert, 1983). Toothless portions of the gums are not affected. The condition does not necessarily require withdrawal of medication, and it can be minimized by good oral hygiene.

Gastrointestinal disturbances, including *nausea, vomiting, epigastric pain,* and *anorexia,* can be reduced by taking the drug with meals or in more frequent divided doses.

A variety of *endocrine* effects have been reported. Inhibition of release of *antidiuretic hormone* (ADH) has been observed in patients with inappropriate ADH secretion. *Hyperglycemia* and *glycosuria* appear to be due to inhibition of insulin secretion. *Osteomalacia,* with hypocalcemia and elevated alkaline phosphatase activity, has been attributed to both altered metabolism of vitamin D and inhibition of intestinal absorption of calcium. Phenytoin also increases the metabolism of vitamin K and reduces the concentration of vitamin K–dependent proteins that are important for normal calcium metabolism in bone (Keith *et al.,* 1983). This may explain why the osteomalacia is not always ameliorated by the administration of vitamin D.

Hypersensitivity reactions include *morbilliform rash* in 2 to 5% of patients and occasionally more serious skin reactions, including *Stevens-Johnson syndrome. Systemic lupus erythematosus* and potentially fatal *hepatic necrosis* have been reported rarely. *Hematological* reactions include *neutropenia* and *leukopenia.* A few instances of *red-cell aplasia, agranulocytosis,* and mild *thrombocytopenia* have also been reported. *Aplastic anemia* has been associated with hydantoins other than phenytoin (*see* Pisciotta, in Symposium, 1982a). *Megaloblastic anemia* has been attributed to altered folate absorption but probably also involves altered folate metabolism. It is rare and responds to administration of folic acid. Similar effects have been reported during medication with phenobarbital, primidone, and mephenytoin. *Lymphadenopathy,* resembling Hodgkin's disease and malignant lymphoma, is associated with reduced immunoglobulin A (IgA) production. *Hypoprothrombinemia* and *hemorrhage* have occurred in the newborn of mothers who received phenytoin during pregnancy; vitamin K is effective treatment or prophylaxis.

Preparations, Routes of Administration, and Dosage. *Phenytoin sodium (diphenylhydantoin sodium;* DILANTIN) is available as 30- and 100-mg capsules for oral use, and as a sterile solution of 50 mg/ml, with a special solvent, for parenteral use. Preparations of *phenytoin* include 50-mg tablets and oral suspensions. The latter must be thoroughly mixed before administration to avoid inaccuracies in dosage. There are significant differences in bioavailability among various preparations of phenytoin, and patients should thus be treated with the drug product of a single manufacturer (*see* Melikian *et al.,* 1977).

Choice and adjustment of the dosage of phenytoin and interpretation of measured concentrations of the drug in plasma must be dominated by recognition of the dose-dependent kinetics of elimination of the drug. As dosage is increased, plasma half-life and the time required to attain the plateau state increase. *Plasma drug concentration increases disproportionately as dosage is increased.* Nomograms based on Michaelis-Menten models of drug elimination have been of limited utility.

Initial daily dosage for adults is 3 to 5 mg/kg (300 mg daily). Dosage is subsequently adjusted, preferably with monitoring of plasma concentration, as needed for control of seizures or as limited by toxicity. Increments in dosage may be made at 1-week intervals at low dosage but at 2-week intervals when dosage exceeds 300 mg daily. Doses greater than 500 mg daily are rarely tolerated if taken regularly, although they may be necessary in occasional patients. Because of its relatively long half-life and slow absorption, a single daily dose is often satisfactory for adults, but gastric intolerance or the use of rapidly absorbed formulations may dictate divided dosage. Divided dosage is recommended for children (4 to 7 mg/kg per day). If loading dosage is deemed necessary, 600 to 1000 mg, in divided portions over 8 to 12 hours, will provide effective plasma concentrations within 24 hours in most patients.

Intravenous administration of phenytoin should not exceed 50 mg per minute. A slower rate is preferred, especially in elderly patients. Intramuscular administration is not recommended. Phenytoin tends to precipitate in a variety of solutions; if necessary, it can be diluted in normal saline solution and then used immediately.

Plasma Drug Concentrations. A good correlation is usually observed between the total concentration of phenytoin in plasma and the clinical effect. Thus, control of seizures is generally obtained with concentrations above 10 μg/ml, while toxic effects such as nystagmus develop around 20 μg/ml. Ataxia is apparent at 30 μg/ml and lethargy at about 40 μg/ml.

The degree of protein binding of phenytoin and, therefore, the concentration of drug that is free in plasma at any given total concentration vary from patient to patient. Such factors can confuse interpretation of measured concentrations of the drug. Since clinical signs of toxicity are correlated with the concentration of unbound drug, some patients will achieve adequate control of seizures without evidence of toxicity only when the total concentration of phenytoin is above the usual therapeutic range.

Drug Interactions. Well-documented *increase* in the concentration of phenytoin in plasma, by inhibition of its inactivation, has occurred during concurrent administration of *chloramphenicol, dicumarol, disulfiram, isoniazid, cimetidine,* or certain *sulfonamides.* Less well-documented or variable increase has been reported for a variety of other drugs. Inhibition of inactivation of phenytoin should be suspected for other agents that are also hydroxylated by the microsomal enzyme system. *Sulfisoxazole, phenylbutazone, salicylates,* and *valproate* can compete for binding sites on plasma proteins. Since this can increase the metabolic clearance and lower the total concentration of phenytoin, there may be little effect on the concentration of free drug in plasma at steady state (*see* Perucca and Richens, in Symposium, 1982a).

A well-documented *decrease* in phenytoin concentration is caused by *carbamazepine,* which may enhance the metabolism of phenytoin. Conversely, the concentration of carbamazepine may be reduced by phenytoin. Phenytoin increases the rate of clearance of *theophylline,* and plasma concentrations of phenytoin are also reduced when the two drugs are given concurrently. The latter effect may be due to enhanced metabolism and/or decreased absorption of phenytoin.

Interaction between phenytoin and *phenobarbital* is variable. Phenobarbital may increase the biotransformation of phenytoin by induction of the hepatic microsomal enzyme system, but may also decrease its inactivation, apparently by competitive inhibition. In addition, phenobarbital may reduce the oral absorption of phenytoin. Conversely, the phenobarbital concentration is sometimes increased by phenytoin. *Ethanol* has similar opposing effects on the inactivation of phenytoin.

Phenytoin has been demonstrated to enhance the metabolism of *corticosteroids* and may decrease the effectiveness of *oral contraceptives.* The suggested mechanism for this effect is an induction of metabolizing enzymes, although phenytoin is only a weak inducer of the hepatic microsomal enzyme system in man.

Therapeutic Uses. *Epilepsy.* Phenytoin is one of the more widely used antiepileptic agents, and it is effective in most forms of epilepsy except absence seizures. The use of phenytoin and other agents in the therapy of epilepsies is discussed further at the end of the chapter.

Other Uses. Some cases of *trigeminal and related neuralgias* respond well to phenytoin, but carbamazepine is the preferred agent. The use of phenytoin in the treatment of *cardiac arrhythmias* is discussed in Chapter 31.

OTHER HYDANTOINS

Mephenytoin. *Mephenytoin* (MESANTOIN), 3-methyl-5,5-phenylethylhydantoin, is N-demethylated to 5,5-phenylethylhydantoin. During chronic administration of mephenytoin, this active metabolite constitutes most of the total hydantoins in plasma and probably accounts, at least in part, for the therapeutic benefit and toxicity of chronic medication with mephenytoin (*see* Kupferberg, in Symposium, 1982a).

Pharmacological Effects and Metabolism. Mephenytoin is active in most anticonvulsant tests in animals. Unlike phenytoin, it antagonizes the effects of pentylenetetrazol, elevates seizure threshold, and is a sedative. Also unlike phenytoin, mephenytoin is rapidly absorbed after oral administration. Both mephenytoin and its N-demethylated metabolite are converted to inactive hydroxylated products in a stereospecific fashion by hepatic microsomal enzymes (Küpfer *et al.,* 1984). As a result of the hydroxylation, conjugation, and excretion of the S-enantiomer, the active R-enantiomer, 5,5-phenylethylhydantoin, accumulates in plasma. It is possible that the serious toxicity associated with mephenytoin results from the formation of arene oxide intermediates during the hydroxylation reaction.

Therapeutic Uses and Toxicity. Mephenytoin was introduced in 1945 for the treatment of epilepsy. Its antiepileptic spectrum is similar to that of phenytoin, and it may exacerbate absence seizures. The half-life of the active metabolite is about 95 hours in patients previously exposed to various other anticonvulsants (*see* Troupin *et al.,* 1979). Although mephenytoin causes less ataxia, gingival hyperplasia, gastric distress, and hirsutism than does phenytoin and less sedation than does phenobarbital, serious toxicity is common. These adverse effects include morbilliform rash (in 10% of patients), fever, lymphadenopathy, aplastic anemia, leukopenia, pancytopenia, agranulocytosis, hepatotoxicity, periarteritis nodosa, and lupus erythematosus. Consequently, mephenytoin is generally used only in patients who fail to respond to or do not tolerate safer agents.

Preparations and Dosage. Typical daily dosage is 200 to 600 mg in adults and 100 to 400 mg in children. The drug is available in 100-mg tablets.

Ethotoin. *Ethotoin* (PEGANONE) is 3-ethyl-5-phenylhydantoin. Introduced in 1957, it appeared to be of some value in the treatment of complex partial as well as generalized tonic-clonic seizures and to be relatively free of the typical adverse effects of phenytoin (*see* Kupferberg, in Symposium, 1982a). However, because of its low efficacy, it is employed only occasionally, mostly as an adjunct to other agents, in the therapy of generalized tonic-clonic seizures. The usual daily dose for adults is 2 to 3 g. Ethotoin is available in 250- and 500-mg tablets.

Skin rash, gastrointestinal distress, and drowsiness are the common adverse effects of ethotoin. Lymphadenopathy has also been reported. Metabolites, produced by the hepatic microsomal enzymes, include the N-dealkyl and parahydroxyphenyl derivatives and 5-hydroxy-5-phenylhydantoin (*see* Jones and Wimbish, 1985). The half-life in plasma is about 5 hours and does not appear to change with increasing dosage.

ANTICONVULSANT BARBITURATES

The pharmacology of the barbiturates as a class is considered in Chapter 17; discussion in this chapter is limited to the two barbiturates employed for therapy of the epilepsies. Although still marketed, a third barbiturate (*metharbital*) has virtually disappeared from the therapeutic scene.

PHENOBARBITAL

Phenobarbital was the first effective organic antiepileptic agent (Hauptmann, 1912). It has relatively low toxicity, is inexpensive, and is still one of the more effective and widely used drugs for this purpose.

Structure-Activity Relationship. The structural formula of phenobarbital (5-phenyl-5-ethylbarbituric acid) is shown in Table 17–5 (page 353). The structure-activity relationship of the barbiturates has been studied extensively and summarized by Vida and Gerry (in Symposium, 1977). Maximal anticonvulsant activity is obtained when one substituent at position 5 is a phenyl group. The 5,5-diphenyl derivative has less anticonvulsant potency than phenobarbital but is virtually devoid of hypnotic activity. By contrast, 5,5-dibenzyl barbituric acid causes convulsions.

Anticonvulsant Properties. Most barbiturates have anticonvulsant properties. However, the capacity of some of these agents, such as phenobarbital, to exert maximal anticonvulsant action at doses below those required for hypnosis determines their clinical utility as antiepileptics. Phenobarbital is active in most anticonvulsant tests in animals but is relatively nonselective. It limits the spread of seizure activity and also elevates seizure threshold.

The ability of some barbiturates to be selective anticonvulsants suggests that different mechanisms of action are involved in the anticonvulsant and hypnotic effects. Based on the electrophysiological effects of various barbiturates in dissociated cell cultures of mammalian spinal cord neurons, Mac-donald and McLean (1982) have proposed that the low potency of phenobarbital (relative to that of pentobarbital) both in producing GABA-like increases in the conductance of chloride ions and in reducing calcium-dependent release of neurotransmitters may account for the relatively selective effects of anticonvulsant barbiturates. Further, the ability of phenobarbital at therapeutic concentrations to reduce the excitatory effects of glutamate and to augment the inhibitory effects of GABA may be important to its anticonvulsant activity. Other distinctions between hypnotic and anticonvulsant barbiturates have been noted with respect to effects on the ability of preparations of brain cell membranes to bind certain drugs. Phenobarbital is much less potent than pentobarbital in displacing dihydropicrotoxinin and in enhancing the binding of GABA and various benzodiazepines (see Olsen, 1982; Thyagarajan et al., 1983). The relationship of these observations to the electrophysiological effects of barbiturates is not clearly understood.

Absorption, Distribution, Biotransformation, and Excretion. Oral absorption of phenobarbital is complete but somewhat slow; peak concentrations in plasma occur several hours after a single dose. It is 40 to 60% bound to plasma proteins and bound to a similar extent in tissues, including brain. The volume of distribution is approximately 0.5 liter per kilogram. The pK_a of phenobarbital is 7.3, and up to 25% of a dose is eliminated by pH-dependent renal excretion of the unchanged drug; the remainder is inactivated by hepatic microsomal enzymes. One major metabolite, the parahydroxyphenyl derivative, is inactive and is excreted in the urine partly as the glucuronide conjugate. Another major metabolite has been identified recently as the N-glucoside derivative (see Maynert, in Symposium, 1982a). The plasma half-life of phenobarbital is about 100 hours in adults; it is somewhat longer in neonates, while it is shorter and more variable in children.

Toxicity. The adverse effects of phenobarbital have been reviewed by Mattson and Cramer (Symposium, 1982a). Sedation, the most frequent undesired effect of phenobarbital, is apparent to some extent in all patients upon initiation of therapy, but tolerance develops during chronic medication. Nystagmus and ataxia occur at excessive dosage. Phenobarbital sometimes produces irritability and hyperactivity in children, and agitation and confusion in the elderly.

Scarlatiniform or morbilliform rash, possibly with other manifestations of drug allergy, occurs in 1 to 2% of patients. Exfoliative dermatitis is rare. Hypoprothrombinemia with hemorrhage has been observed in the newborn of mothers who have received phenobarbital during pregnancy; vitamin K is effective for treatment or prophylaxis. Megaloblastic anemia that responds to folate and osteomalacia that responds to high doses of vitamin D occur during chronic phenobarbital therapy of epilepsy, as they do during phenytoin medication. Other adverse effects of phenobarbital are discussed in Chapter 17.

Preparations, Routes of Administration, and Dosage. Phenobarbital and phenobarbital sodium are available in a variety of dosage forms for oral and parenteral use. The usual oral daily dose for adults is 1 to 5 mg/kg (60 to 250 mg). Since plasma half-life averages 100 hours, weeks are required to attain the plateau state. Double dosage for the initial 4 days provides an effective plasma drug concentration more promptly, but sedation will be prominent. The usual initial daily dose for children is 3 to 6 mg/kg, in two divided portions. Dosage is subsequently increased or adjusted, as required for control of seizures or as limited by toxicity.

Plasma Drug Concentrations. During chronic medication in adults, plasma concentration of phenobarbital averages 10 μg/ml per daily dose of 1 mg/kg; in children, the value is 5 to 7 μg/ml per 1 mg/kg. Although a precise relationship between therapeutic results and concentration of drug in plasma does not exist, plasma concentrations of 10 to 25 μg/ml are usually recommended for control of epilepsy; 15 μg/ml is the minimum for prophylaxis against febrile convulsions.

The relationship between plasma concentration of phenobarbital and adverse effects varies with the development of tolerance. Sedation, nystagmus, and ataxia are usually absent at concentrations below 30 μg/ml during chronic medication, but adverse effects may be apparent for several days at lower concentrations when therapy is initiated or whenever dosage is increased. Concentrations greater than 60 μg/ml may be associated with marked intoxication in the nontolerant individual.

Since significant behavioral toxicity may be present despite the absence of overt signs of toxicity, the tendency to maintain patients, particularly children, on excessively high doses of phenobarbital should be resisted. Plasma phenobarbital concentration should be increased above 30 to 40 μg/ml only if the increment is adequately tolerated and only if it contributes significantly to control of seizures. (See Booker, in Symposium, 1982a.)

Drug Interactions. Interactions between phenobarbital and other drugs usually involve induction of the hepatic microsomal enzyme system by phenobarbital (*see* Chapters 1 and 17). The variable interaction with phenytoin has been discussed previously (page 453). Concentrations of phenobarbital in plasma may be elevated by as much as 40% during concurrent administration of valproic acid (*see* below).

Therapeutic Uses.   Phenobarbital is an effective agent for *generalized tonic-clonic* and *partial seizures*. Its efficacy, low toxicity, and low cost make it a primary agent for these types of epilepsy, particularly in children. The use of phenobarbital in the therapy of the epilepsies is discussed further at the end of the chapter.

OTHER BARBITURATES

Mephobarbital.   *Mephobarbital* (MEBARAL) is N-methylphenobarbital. It is N-demethylated by the hepatic microsomal enzymes, and most of its activity during chronic medication can be attributed to the accumulation of phenobarbital. Consequently, the pharmacological properties, toxicity, and clinical uses of mephobarbital are the same as those for phenobarbital. However, oral absorption of mephobarbital is usually incomplete, and its dose is approximately twice that of phenobarbital. The plasma concentration of phenobarbital provides a guide to adjustment of mephobarbital dosage. (*See* Eadie, in Symposium, 1982a.)

DEOXYBARBITURATES

PRIMIDONE

Primidone is an effective agent for treatment of all types of epilepsy except absence seizures.

Chemistry.   Primidone may be viewed as a congener of phenobarbital in which the carbonyl oxygen of the urea moiety is replaced by two hydrogen atoms:

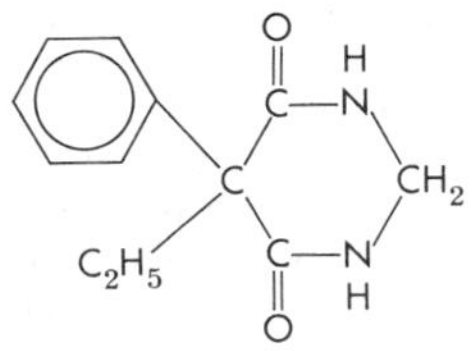

Primidone

Anticonvulsant Effects.   Primidone resembles phenobarbital in many laboratory anticonvulsant effects, but it is much less potent than phenobarbital in antagonizing seizures induced by pentylenetetrazol (*see*

Woodbury and Pippenger, in Symposium, 1982a). The anticonvulsant effects of primidone in animals are attributed to both the drug and its active metabolites, principally phenobarbital (*see* Frey, 1985).

Absorption, Distribution, Biotransformation, and Excretion.   Primidone is rapidly and almost completely absorbed after oral administration, although individual variability can be great. Peak concentrations in plasma are usually observed approximately 3 hours after ingestion. The plasma half-life of primidone is variable; mean values ranging from 7 to 14 hours have been reported (*see* Schottelius, in Symposium, 1982a).

Primidone is converted to two active metabolites, phenobarbital and phenylethylmalonamide (PEMA). Primidone and PEMA are bound to plasma proteins to only a small extent, whereas about half of phenobarbital is so bound. The half-life of PEMA in plasma is 16 hours; both it and phenobarbital accumulate during chronic medication. The appearance of phenobarbital in plasma may be delayed several days upon initiation of therapy with primidone. Approximately 40% of the drug is excreted unchanged in the urine; unconjugated PEMA and, to a lesser extent, phenobarbital and its metabolites constitute the remainder.

Toxicity.   The toxicity of primidone has been reviewed by Leppik and Cloyd (in Symposium, 1982a). The more common complaints are *sedation, vertigo, dizziness, nausea, vomiting, ataxia, diplopia,* and *nystagmus*. There may also be an *acute feeling of intoxication* immediately following administration of primidone. This occurs before there is any significant metabolism of the drug. The relationship of adverse effects to dosage is complex, since they result from both the parent drug and its two active metabolites and since tolerance develops during chronic medication. Side effects are occasionally quite severe when therapy is initiated.

Serious adverse effects are relatively uncommon, but *maculopapular* and *morbilliform rash, leukopenia, thrombocytopenia, systemic lupus erythematosus,* and *lymphadenopathy* have been reported.

Acute *psychotic reactions,* usually in patients with complex partial seizures, have also occurred. *Hemorrhagic disease* in the neonate, *megaloblastic anemia,* and *osteomalacia* similar to those discussed previously in connection with phenytoin and phenobarbital have also been described.

Preparations and Dosage. *Primidone* (MYSOLINE) is available as 50- and 250-mg tablets and as an oral suspension (250 mg/5 ml). The usual daily dose for adults is 750 to 1500 mg, given in divided doses; for children, 10 to 25 mg/kg. Therapy should be initiated at lower dosage (*e.g.,* 100 to 125 mg per day for adults) and increased gradually. Lower dosage may be possible or necessary when the drug is used concurrently with phenytoin.

Plasma Drug Concentrations. The relationship between the dose of primidone and the concentration of the drug and its active metabolites in plasma shows marked individual variability. During chronic medication, the plasma concentrations of primidone and phenobarbital average 1 μg/ml and 2 μg/ml, respectively, per daily dose of 1 mg/kg of primidone. The plasma concentration of PEMA is usually intermediate between those of primidone and phenobarbital. There is no clear relationship between the concentrations of primidone or its metabolites in plasma and therapeutic effect. As an initial guide, dosage of primidone may be adjusted primarily with reference to the concentration of phenobarbital, as outlined previously for administered phenobarbital, and secondarily with reference to the concentration of the parent drug. Concentrations of primidone greater than 10 μg/ml are usually associated with significant toxic side effects. A disproportionately high primidone:phenobarbital concentration ratio during chronic medication usually implies that medication has not been taken regularly. (*See* Fincham and Schottelius, in Symposium, 1982a.)

Drug Interactions. *Phenytoin* has been reported to *increase* the conversion of primidone to phenobarbital. *Isoniazid* has been demonstrated in one patient to *decrease* the conversion of primidone to phenobarbital and PEMA. Other drug interactions to be anticipated are those for phenobarbital.

Therapeutic Uses. Clinical antiepileptic efficacy of primidone was first reported in 1952 (*see* Fincham and Schottelius, in Symposium, 1982a). It is useful against *generalized tonic-clonic* and both *simple* and *complex partial seizures.* While it may be effective alone in patients who are refractory to other medications, primidone is generally used concurrently with phenytoin or carbamazepine. Its use in combination with phenobarbital is illogical. Primidone is ineffective against absence seizures but is sometimes useful against myoclonic seizures in young children. The therapeutic use of primidone and other antiepileptic agents is discussed further at the end of the chapter.

IMINOSTILBENES

CARBAMAZEPINE

Carbamazepine was approved in the United States for use as an antiepileptic agent in 1974. It has been employed since the 1960s for the treatment of trigeminal neuralgia (*see* Suria and Killam, in Symposium, 1980). It is now considered to be a primary drug for the treatment of all types of epilepsy except absence seizures.

Chemistry. Carbamazepine is related chemically to the tricyclic antidepressants. It is a derivative of iminostilbene with a carbamyl group at the 5 position; this moiety is essential for potent antiepileptic activity. The structural formula of carbamazepine is as follows:

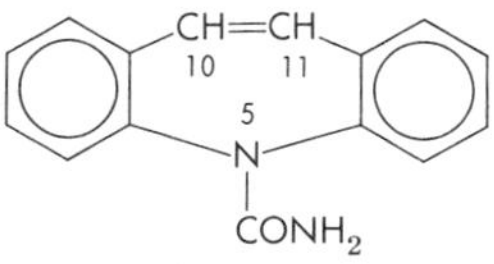

Carbamazepine

Pharmacological Effects. While the effects of carbamazepine in animals and man resemble those of phenytoin in many ways, there are a number of potentially important differences between the two drugs (*see* Julien, in Symposium, 1982a). For example, carbamazepine is more effective than phenytoin in reducing stimulus-induced discharges in the amygdala of kindled rats (Albright, 1983) and in blocking pentylenetetrazol-induced seizures (*see* Schmutz, 1985). Further, it has produced therapeutic responses in manic-depressive patients, including some in whom lithium carbonate was not effective (*see* Post *et al.,* 1983). Finally, carbamazepine has antidiuretic effects that are sometimes associated with *reduced* concentrations of ADH in plasma (*see* Masland, in Symposium, 1982a). The mechanisms responsible for these effects of carbamazepine are not clearly understood.

Both carbamazepine and phenytoin selectively facilitate the effects of activating certain inhibitory inputs to spinal trigeminal neurons in the cat. For example, under conditions in which high-frequency stimulation of the maxillary nerve and the periventricular gray matter produce equal reduction in the neuronal discharge that is evoked by single shocks delivered to the maxillary nerve, the administration of these drugs causes further reduction of only those responses evoked after prior stimulation of the maxillary nerve (Fromm *et al.*, 1982). While these observations resemble superficially the facilitation of the effects of activating GABA-ergic inhibitory circuits that are produced in many regions of the CNS by phenobarbital or the benzodiazepines, the identity of the inhibitory neurotransmitters that may function in this system is not known.

Therapeutic doses of carbamazepine increase the rate of firing of noradrenergic neurons in the locus ceruleus of the rat (Olpe and Jones, 1983). Since phenytoin does not have similar effects, the relationship of this observation to the therapeutic effects of carbamazepine is not clear. However, both clonidine (which inhibits discharge of noradrenergic neurons) and selective depletion of norepinephrine in the brain antagonize the anticonvulsant effects of carbamazepine. Thus, the capacity to increase discharge of noradrenergic neurons may contribute to the antiepileptic actions of the drug.

Because it can inhibit the binding of analogs of adenosine to brain cell membranes, carbamazepine has been postulated to be a partial agonist at adenosine receptors (Skerritt *et al.*, 1983). However, theophylline, an adenosine antagonist, inhibits anticonvulsant responses to carbamazepine only inconsistently (*see* Post *et al.*, 1983), and the relative potency of analogs of carbamazepine as inhibitors of binding to adenosine receptors does not correspond to their relative potency in inhibiting convulsions induced by electroshock (Marangos *et al.*, 1983). Although adenosine can exert powerful presynaptic and postsynaptic inhibitory effects on neurons (*see* Chapter 25), the role of any action on adenosine receptors in the pharmacological effects of carbamazepine cannot be deduced at this time.

Absorption, Distribution, Biotransformation, and Excretion. The pharmacokinetic characteristics of carbamazepine are complex. They are influenced by its limited aqueous solubility and by the ability of many antiepileptic drugs, including carbamazepine itself, to increase its conversion to an active metabolite by hepatic oxidative enzymes.

Carbamazepine is absorbed slowly and erratically after oral administration. Peak concentrations in plasma are usually observed 4 to 8 hours after oral ingestion but may be delayed by as much as 24 hours, especially following the administration of a large dose (*see* Morselli and Bossi, in Symposium, 1982a). The drug distributes rapidly into all tissues. Binding to plasma proteins occurs to the extent of about 75%, and concentrations in the CSF appear to correspond to the concentration of free drug in plasma.

The predominant pathway of metabolism in man involves conversion to the 10,11-epoxide (*see* Faigle and Feldman, in Symposium, 1982a). This metabolite is as active as the parent compound in various animals, and its concentrations in plasma and brain may reach about 50% of those of carbamazepine, especially during the concurrent administration of phenytoin or phenobarbital. The 10,11-epoxide is metabolized further to inactive compounds, which are excreted in the urine principally as glucuronides. Carbamazepine is also inactivated by conjugation and hydroxylation. Less than 3% of the drug is recovered in the urine as the parent compound or the epoxide. During long-term therapy, the half-life of carbamazepine in plasma averages between 10 and 20 hours. Because of induction of drug-metabolizing enzymes, the half-life is much longer in individuals who have received only a single dose. In patients who are receiving phenobarbital or phenytoin, the average half-life is reduced to 9 to 10 hours. The half-life of the 10,11-epoxide is somewhat shorter than that of the parent compound.

Toxicity. Acute intoxication with carbamazepine can result in *stupor* or *coma, hyperirritability, convulsions,* and *respiratory depression* (*see* Masland, in Symposium, 1982a). During chronic administration, the more frequent untoward effects of the drug include *drowsiness, vertigo, ataxia, diplopia,* and *blurred vision.* The frequency of *seizures* may increase especially with overdosage. Other adverse effects include *nausea, vomiting,* serious hematological toxicity (*aplastic anemia, agranulocytosis*), and hypersensitivity reactions (*dermatitis, eosinophilia, lymphadenopathy, splenomegaly*). A late complication of therapy with carbamazepine is *retention of water,* with decreased osmolality and concentration of sodium in plasma, especially in elderly patients with cardiac disease.

Some tolerance develops to the neurotoxic effects of carbamazepine, and they can be minimized by gradual increase in dosage or adjustment of maintenance dosage. A transient mild *leukopenia* occurs in about 10% of patients during initiation of therapy and usually resolves within the first 4 months of continued treatment; transient *thrombocytopenia* has also been noted. In about 2% of patients, a *persistent leukopenia* may develop that requires withdrawal of the drug. The initial concern that *aplastic anemia* might be a frequent complication of chronic therapy with carbamazepine has not materialized. The total number of cases reported is less than 25; however the outcome has been fatal in about 50%. In the majority of cases, the administration of multiple drugs or other underlying disease has made it difficult to establish a causal relationship. In any event, the prevalence of aplastic anemia appears to be about 1 in 50,000 patients who are treated with the drug. It is not clear whether monitoring of hematological function can avert the development of irreversible aplastic anemia (*see* Hart and Easton, 1982; Pisciotta, in Symposium, 1982a). While carbamazepine is carcinogenic in rats, it remains to be determined if it is carcinogenic or teratogenic in man.

Preparations and Dosage. *Carbamazepine* (TEGRETOL) is available in 100- and 200-mg tablets for oral administration. Therapy for *epilepsy* is usually started at a dosage of 200 mg, taken twice daily to minimize side effects. Dosage is then increased gradually to 600 to 1200 mg per day for adults and 20 to 30 mg/kg for children. Division of the daily intake into three doses is usually recommended in order to minimize fluctuations in plasma concentrations.

Therapy for *trigeminal neuralgia* is generally started at a dose of 200 mg per day; dosage may be increased gradually, as needed, to a level of 1200 mg per day if this is tolerated.

Plasma Drug Concentrations. There is no simple relationship between the dose of carbamazepine and concentrations of the drug in plasma (*see* Cereghino, in Symposium, 1982a). Therapeutic concentrations are reported to be 6 to 12 μg/ml, although there is considerable variation. Side effects referable to the CNS are frequent at concentrations above 9 μg/ml.

Drug Interactions. Phenobarbital and phenytoin may increase the metabolism of carbamazepine; the biotransformation of phenytoin as well as the conversion of primidone to phenobarbital may be enhanced by carbamazepine. Administration of carbamazepine may lower concentrations of valproate given concurrently. The metabolism of carbamazepine may be inhibited by propoxyphene and erythromycin (*see* Levy and Patlick, in Symposium, 1982a).

Therapeutic Uses. Carbamazepine is useful in patients with *generalized tonic-clonic* and both *simple* and *complex partial*

seizures. When it is employed, renal and hepatic function and hematological parameters should be monitored. The therapeutic use of carbamazepine is discussed further at the end of the chapter.

Neuralgia. Carbamazepine was introduced by Blom in the early 1960s and is now the primary agent for treatment of *trigeminal* and *glossopharyngeal neuralgias.* It is also effective for *lightning tabetic pain.* Most patients with neuralgia are benefited initially, but only 70% obtain continuing relief. Adverse effects have required discontinuation of medication in 5 to 20% of patients. The therapeutic range of plasma concentrations for antiepileptic therapy serves as a guideline for its use in neuralgia. Concurrent medication with phenytoin may be useful when carbamazepine alone is not satisfactory.

SUCCINIMIDES

ETHOSUXIMIDE

The succinimides evolved from a systematic search for effective agents less toxic than the oxazolidinediones for the treatment of absence seizures. Ethosuximide is a primary agent for this type of epilepsy.

Structure-Activity Relationship. Ethosuximide has the following structural formula:

Ethosuximide

The structure-activity relationship of the succinimides is in accord with that for other anticonvulsant classes. Methsuximide and phensuximide have phenyl substituents and are more active against maximal electroshock seizures. Ethosuximide, with alkyl substituents, is the most active against seizures induced by pentylenetetrazol and is the most selective for clinical absence seizures.

Anticonvulsant Properties. The anticonvulsant spectrum of ethosuximide in animals resembles that of trimethadione. The most prominent characteristic of both drugs is protection against the convulsant action of pentylenetetrazol. Ethosuximide also elevates threshold for electroshock seizures, but it abolishes the tonic extensor component of maximal electroshock seizures only in anesthetic doses (*see* Ferrendelli and Klunk, in Symposium, 1982a).

While it blocks focal neuronal discharges and the associated clonic seizure activity produced by the application of cobalt to the frontal cortex of the rat, ethosuximide appears to be inactive against seizures produced by application of aluminum hydroxide. The drug also has little effect on stimulus-induced afterdischarges in the kindled rat (Albright and Burnham, 1980). While phenytoin is totally inactive, ethosuximide suppresses spontaneous seizures in the *tottering* mutant mouse (Heller *et al.,* 1983).

Guberman and colleagues (1975) studied the effects of ethosuximide and phenytoin in acute penicillin-induced epilepsy in the cat. Epileptic bursts in the EEG, often resembling the spike-and-wave pattern of absence seizures, were reduced more effectively by ethosuximide than by phenytoin. Furthermore, there was a good correlation between the concentration of ethosuximide in plasma and effect, and concentrations were similar to those associated with therapeutic effects in patients with absence seizures. Because of these observations, together with the specific capacity of ethosuximide to antagonize seizures induced by gamma-hydroxybutyrate, it has been postulated that absence seizures involve paroxysmal activity in inhibitory neural systems and that ethosuximide has special antagonistic actions in such systems. This view lacks direct supporting evidence, although it might explain the emergence of generalized tonic-clonic seizures in some patients during treatment with ethosuximide.

Absorption, Distribution, Biotransformation, and Excretion. Absorption of ethosuximide appears to be complete, and peak concentrations occur in plasma within about 3 hours after a single oral dose. Ethosuximide is not significantly bound to plasma proteins; during chronic medication, the concentration in the CSF is similar to that in plasma. The apparent volume of distribution averages 0.7 liter per kilogram. In animals, it is relatively evenly distributed in all tissues and does not accumulate in fat (*see* Glazko and Chang, in Symposium, 1982a).

In man, 25% of the drug is excreted unchanged in the urine. The remainder is metabolized by hepatic microsomal enzymes. The major metabolite, the hydroxyethyl derivative, accounts for about 40% of administered drug, is inactive, and is excreted as such and as the glucuronide in the urine. Other metabolites include other hydroxylated products. The plasma half-life of ethosuximide averages between 40 and 50 hours in adults and is significantly shorter in children (approximately 30 hours).

Toxicity. The toxicity of ethosuximide has been reviewed by Dreifuss (Symposium, 1982a). The most common dose-related side effects are *gastrointestinal* complaints (*nausea, vomiting,* and *anorexia*) and *CNS* effects (*drowsiness, lethargy, euphoria, dizziness, headache,* and *hiccough*). Some tolerance to these effects develops. *Parkinson-like symptoms* and *photophobia* have also been reported. *Restlessness, agitation, anxiety, aggressiveness, inability to concentrate,* and other behavioral effects have occurred primarily in patients with a prior history of psychiatric disturbance.

Urticaria and other skin reactions, including *Stevens-Johnson syndrome,* as well as *systemic lupus erythematosus, eosinophilia, leukopenia, thrombocytopenia, pancytopenia,* and *aplastic anemia* have also been attributed to the drug. The leukopenia may be transient, despite continuation of the drug, but several deaths have resulted from bone-marrow depression. Renal or hepatic toxicity has not been reported.

Preparations and Dosage. *Ethosuximide* (ZARONTIN) is available for oral administration as 250-mg capsules and as a syrup (250 mg/5 ml). An initial daily dose of 250 mg in children (3 to 6 years old) and 500 mg in older children and adults is increased by 250-mg increments at weekly intervals until seizures are adequately controlled or toxicity intervenes. Divided dosage is occasionally required to prevent nausea or drowsiness associated with single daily dosage. Usual maintenance dosage is 20 to 40 mg/kg. Increased caution is required if daily dosage exceeds 1500 mg in adults or 750 to 1000 mg in children.

Plasma Drug Concentrations. During chronic medication, the plasma concentration of ethosuximide averages about 2 μg/ml per daily dose of 1 mg/kg. However, because of variation, concentrations in plasma cannot be predicted accurately. The plateau state is attained in 4 to 6 days in children; longer times are required in adults. A plasma concentration of 40 to 100 μg/ml is required for satisfactory control of absence seizures in most patients (*see* Sherwin, in Symposium, 1982a). However, some patients may be completely controlled at lower concentrations, and others are incompletely controlled at higher concentrations. A relationship between plasma concentration and adverse effects has not been established. Concentrations as high as 160 μg/ml have been tolerated without excessive toxicity.

Drug Interactions. Clinically significant interactions between ethosuximide and other drugs are rare. Increased toxicity should be anticipated with other drugs having similar dose-related adverse effects.

Therapeutic Uses. Ethosuximide is more effective than trimethadione against *absence seizures* and has a lower risk of serious adverse effects; it is an important therapeutic agent for this type of epilepsy. The use of ethosuximide and the other antiepileptic agents is discussed further at the end of the chapter.

OTHER SUCCINIMIDES

Methsuximide. Methsuximide, N,2-dimethyl-2-phenylsuccinimide, was introduced in 1956 for the therapy of absence seizures (*see* Porter and Kupferberg, in Symposium, 1982a). Ethosuximide subsequently proved more effective. Methsuximide, particularly when given concurrently with other drugs, may also be useful in the treatment of complex partial seizures. Adverse gastrointestinal and central effects are similar in pattern to those of ethosuximide. Severe depression, skin rash, fever, periorbital edema, leukopenia, aplastic anemia, nephropathy, and hepatotoxicity have also been reported.

Methsuximide (CELONTIN) is available as 150- and 300-mg capsules. Medication is initiated with 300 mg, given daily. The usual daily dose for adults is 600 to 1200 mg. Patients receiving higher doses, especially in multiple-drug therapy, should be carefully monitored.

Methsuximide is rapidly absorbed and metabolized by hepatic microsomal enzymes to the N-demethyl and various parahydroxyphenyl derivatives. The half-life of methsuximide in plasma is less than 2 hours, while that of the active N-demethyl metabolite is about 40 hours. During chronic administration of methsuximide, therapeutic responses are associated with plasma concentrations of 20 to 40 μg/ml of the metabolite or 0.04 to 0.08 μg/ml of the parent drug.

Phensuximide. The first succinimide introduced for the therapy of absence seizures was phensuximide (N-methyl-2-phenylsuccinimide). Low efficacy has relegated it to secondary status. Adverse gastrointestinal and central effects are similar to those for ethosuximide. A dreamlike state, skin rash, fever, granulocytopenia, leukopenia, and reversible nephropathy have also been reported.

Phensuximide (MILONTIN) is available as 500-mg capsules. The usual daily dose is 1 to 3 g, regardless of age. Phensuximide is rapidly absorbed and converted to the N-demethyl and various hydroxylated metabolites. The N-demethyl derivative, which is suspected of being an active species, has a half-life in plasma similar to that of the parent drug (about 8 hours) and is metabolized to 2-phenylsuccinamic acid. At steady state, the plasma concentration of the N-demethyl derivative is about 30% of that of phensuximide (*see* Porter and Kupferberg, in Symposium, 1982a).

VALPROIC ACID

Valproic acid was approved for use in the United States in 1978 after more than a decade of use in Europe. The antiepileptic properties of valproate were discovered serendipitously when it was employed as a vehicle for other compounds that were being screened for antiepileptic activity (*see* Symposium, 1982a).

Chemistry. Valproic acid (*n*-dipropylacetic acid) is a simple branched-chain carboxylic acid; its structural formula is as follows:

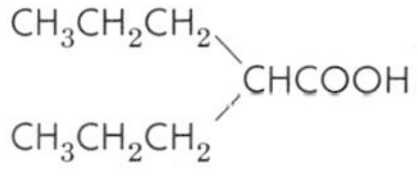

$$\begin{array}{c} CH_3CH_2CH_2 \\ \diagdown \\ CH_3CH_2CH_2 \end{array} CHCOOH$$

Valproic Acid

Certain other branched-chain carboxylic acids have potencies similar to that of valproic acid in antagonizing pentylenetetrazol-induced convulsions. However, increasing the number of carbon atoms to nine introduces marked sedative properties. Straight-chain acids have little or no activity. The primary amide of valproic acid has been reported to be about twice as potent as the parent compound (*see* Murray and Kier, in Symposium, 1977; Keane *et al.*, 1983).

Pharmacological Effects. Valproic acid has antiepileptic activity against a variety of types of seizures while causing only minimal sedation and other CNS side effects. It prevents pentylenetetrazol-induced seizures in mice with a potency greater than that of ethosuximide but less than that of phenobarbital. It also eliminates hindlimb extension in mice subjected to maximal electroshock but only at relatively high doses. These results suggest that valproate would be more useful in absence than in generalized tonic-clonic seizures.

While the drug is effective in a variety of other model systems considered useful for predicting efficacy in absence seizures, it also reduces the frequency and severity of spontaneous seizures in monkeys rendered epileptic by implantation of alumina cream. Furthermore, valproate can prevent induced convulsions in kindled rats and, at lower doses, can prevent the establishment of the kindling phenomenon in cats (*see* Wada, 1977).

The mechanism of action of valproate is unknown. Several investigators have proposed a possible interaction with the metabolism of GABA in the brain (*see* Chapman *et al.*, 1982). It has been suggested that selective increases in concentrations of GABA in synaptic regions may be promoted by inhibition of GABA transaminase or succinic semialdehyde dehydrogenase, inhibition of re-uptake by glial cells and nerve endings, or some combination of these actions. However, evidence is lacking for enhancement of the release of GABA under these circumstances. A postsynaptic site of action is suggested by a number of studies that demonstrate augmented responses to GABA after application of valproate by iontophoresis. However, exposure of neurons to known concentrations of valproate (up to 1 mM), both *in situ* and *in vitro*, is without effect on responses to GABA. Since an anticonvulsant effect that far outlasts the sojourn of the drug in plasma is observed following chronic administration and withdrawal of valproate, it is possible that either long-lived active metabolites or adaptive changes in neuronal function are important facets of its mechanism of action.

Absorption, Distribution, Biotransformation, and Excretion. Valproic acid is rapidly and almost completely absorbed after oral administration. Peak concentrations in plasma are observed in 1 to 4 hours, although this can be delayed for several hours if the drug is administered in enteric-coated tablets or is ingested with meals. The apparent volume of distribution for valproate is between 0.1 and 0.4 liter per kilogram. Its extent of binding to plasma proteins is usually about 90%, but the fraction bound is reduced as the total concentration of valproate is increased through the therapeutic range. Concentrations of valproate in CSF suggest equilibration with free drug in the blood.

Less than 3% of valproate is excreted unchanged in the urine and feces. When given in therapeutic doses, most of the drug is converted to the conjugate ester of glucuronic acid, while mitochondrial metabolism, principally by means of β-oxidation, accounts for the remainder. Some of these metabolites, notably 2-propyl-2-pentenoic acid and 2-propyl-3-oxopentanoic acid, have anticonvulsant activity and accumulate to a small extent in plasma during therapy. The half-life of valproate is approximately 15 hours but is reduced in patients taking other antiepileptic drugs (*see* Chapman *et al.*, 1982; Appendix II).

Toxicity. The toxicity of valproic acid has been reviewed by Dreifuss (Symposium, 1983c). The most common side effects are *gastrointestinal symptoms*, including anorexia, nausea, and vomiting in about 16% of patients. Effects on the CNS include *sedation, ataxia,* and *tremor;* these symptoms usually respond to a decrease in dosage. *Rash, alopecia,* and *stimulation of appetite* have been observed infrequently. Valproic acid has several effects on hepatic function. Elevation of hepatic enzymes in plasma is observed in 15 to 30% of patients and often occurs asymptomatically during the first several months of therapy. A rare complication is a *fulminant hepatitis* that is frequently fatal. Approximately 60 deaths from hepatic failure have been associated with valproic acid, and the incidence appears to be 1 in 20,000 to 40,000 patients using the drug. Approximately 85% of the cases have been in patients taking multiple drugs. Pathological examination reveals a microvesicular steatosis without evidence of inflammation or hypersensitivity reaction. Two deaths occurred in a single family, suggesting a predisposition for the formation of a toxic metabolite. The occurrence of fulminant hepatitis is not consistently preceded by abnormal tests of hepatic function, making advanced detection difficult. Acute pancreatitis and hyperammonemia have also been frequently associated with the use of valproic acid. (*See* Coulter and Allen, 1981; Zimmerman and Ishak, 1982; Mattson and Cramer, in Symposium, 1983a.)

Preparations and Dosage. *Valproic acid* (DEPA-KENE) is available in 250-mg capsules and in a syrup containing 250 mg/5 ml of the sodium salt. The usual daily doses are 1000 to 3000 mg in adults and 15 to 60 mg/kg in children (*see* Medical Letter, 1983); dosage is usually started at a lower level, and divided doses are given.

Divalproex sodium is a stable coordination compound containing equal proportions of valproic acid and sodium valproate. It reportedly causes a lower incidence of gastrointestinal side effects. Divalproex sodium (DEPAKOTE) is available in 250- and 500-mg tablets.

Plasma Drug Concentrations. The concentration of valproate in plasma that appears to be associated with therapeutic effects is approximately 50 to 100 μg/ml (Appendix II). However, the correlation between this concentration and efficacy is poor. There appears to be a threshold at about 50 μg/ml; this is the concentration at which binding sites on plasma albumin begin to become saturated (*see* Chapman *et al.*, 1982).

Drug Interactions. There is well-documented interaction between valproate and phenobarbital. Concentrations of phenobarbital in plasma rise by as much as 40% when valproate is given concurrently. The underlying mechanism appears to involve reduced hydroxylation of the phenobarbital. Total concentrations of phenytoin in plasma may fall when patients receive valproate and phenytoin concurrently. This may be due to enhanced metabolism as a consequence of displacement from plasma protein, and the concentration of free phenytoin is probably not changed (*see* Mattson, in Symposium, 1982a). The concurrent administration of valproate and clonazepam has been associated with the development of *absence status epilepticus;* however, this complication appears to be rare (Browne, 1980).

Therapeutic Uses. The therapeutic uses of valproic acid in epilepsy have been reviewed by Dreifuss (*see* Symposium, 1983c). The drug is particularly effective in *absence seizures,* and it has been shown to be helpful in a variety of other types of epilepsy, including *myoclonic* and *tonic-clonic* seizures. It is less effective in controlling partial seizures. The therapeutic uses of valproate in epilepsy are discussed further at the end of this chapter.

OXAZOLIDINEDIONES

TRIMETHADIONE

Although no longer the clinical agent of choice, trimethadione has been extensively studied in the laboratory and clinic, and, in this regard, it may still be considered the prototype for agents useful against absence seizures.

History. The demonstration by Perlstein and the confirmation by many others of the selectivity of trimethadione in the treatment of absence seizures was an important advance in the therapy of the epilepsies (*see* Withrow, in Symposium, 1980). It provided the first clear indication that drugs could be selective for the various types of epilepsy and spurred research on the basic physiological mechanism of the absence seizures, which previously had been refractory to therapy. Moreover, it provided a new pharmacological tool for such investigations.

Structure-Activity Relationship. Trimethadione has the structural formula as shown.

Trimethadione

The alkyl substituents on the carbon in position 5 appear important for the selectivity of the oxazolidinediones both as antagonists of pentylenetetrazol in animals and as clinically useful agents in the therapy of absence seizures. The same is true for the succinimides. The structure-activity relationship for these compounds has been reviewed by Toman and Goodman (1948) and by Close and Spielman (1961).

Pharmacological Effects. The outstanding anticonvulsant property of trimethadione in laboratory animals is its protective effect against pentylenetetrazol seizures, in which property it differs markedly from phenytoin (Toman and Goodman, 1948). Conversely, it is far inferior to phenytoin in its ability to modify the maximal electroshock seizure pattern. Dimethadione, the N-demethyl metabolite of trimethadione, is active and resembles the parent drug in most respects.

As is the case for ethosuximide, investigation of the mechanism of action of trimethadione has revealed little beyond demonstration of its selective effects in clinical and experimental seizures and of the differences between its electrophysiological effects and those of phenytoin. Ethosuximide has largely replaced trimethadione in the laboratory, as it has in the clinic. Further discussion of the actions of trimethadione can be found in *previous editions* of this textbook.

Absorption, Distribution, Biotransformation, and Excretion. Trimethadione is rapidly absorbed from the gastrointestinal tract; the peak plasma concentration after a single dose occurs in 0.5 to 2 hours. It is not bound significantly to plasma proteins and is uniformly distributed in tissues; its apparent volume of distribution is 60% of body weight. Trimethadione is largely demethylated by the hepatic microsomal enzymes to the active metabolite dimethadione. Dimethadione is not further metabolized but is excreted unchanged in the urine with a half-life of 6 to 13 days. During chronic medication, the metabolite accumulates and is largely responsible for the anticonvulsant effects. (*See* Symposium, 1982a.)

Toxicity. The most common undesired effects of trimethadione are *sedation* and *hemeralopia* (blurring of vision in bright light or glare effect). Hemeralopia does not usually require discontinuation of medication and can be overcome by the use of tinted glasses. Children are not as susceptible as adults. Drowsiness tends to diminish with continued medication.

Less common but more serious untoward effects include *exfoliative dermatitis* and other *skin rashes, blood dyscrasias, hepatitis,* and *nephrosis.* Fatalities have been reported. Moderate *neutropenia* is not uncommon (incidence as high as 20%); fulminating *pancytopenia* and *aplastic anemia* have occurred. *Lupus erythematosus* and *lymphadenopathy* have been observed. A *myasthenic syndrome* has also been reported. (*See* Booker, in Symposium, 1982a.)

Preparations and Dosage. *Trimethadione* (TRIDIONE) is available for oral use as 300-mg capsules, 150-mg sweetened tablets, and a flavored solution (40 mg/ml). The usual daily dose is 900 to 2400 mg for adults and 20 to 60 mg/kg (300 to 900 mg) for children. However, larger doses are sometimes necessary.

Plasma Drug Concentrations. During chronic medication, the plasma concentration of trimethadione averages 0.6 μg/ml per daily dose of 1 mg/kg. Plasma concentrations of the active metabolite dimethadione are 20 times higher (12 μg/ml per 1 mg/kg) and provide the guide for adjustment of dosage. Several weeks are required to attain the plateau state when therapy is initiated and when dosage is changed. A disproportionately high trimethadione:dimethadione concentration ratio usually implies that the patient has not been taking medication regularly. The plasma concentration of dimethadione must usually be maintained above 700 μg/ml for control of seizures. The relationship between plasma concentration and adverse effects has not been established. (*See* Booker, in Symposium, 1982a.)

Drug Interactions. Interactions between trimethadione and other drugs have not been reported.

Therapeutic Uses. Trimethadione is employed only in the treatment of *absence seizures,* and usually only in patients who are inadequately controlled by or do not tolerate other agents. Because of its potential for serious toxicity, treatment with trimethadione necessitates close medical supervision of the patient, especially during the initial year of therapy. The therapeutic use of trimethadione and other agents in the treatment of absence seizures is discussed further at the end of the chapter.

PARAMETHADIONE

Paramethadione differs from trimethadione only in the replacement of one of the methyl groups on the carbon in the 5 position by an ethyl substituent. Its pharmacological properties, therapeutic uses, dosage, and toxicity are similar to those of trimethadione.
Paramethadione (PARADIONE) is available in capsules and in a flavored solution.
Although the undesired effects of paramethadione and trimethadione are similar, the reported incidence of serious adverse effects may be less for paramethadione (*see* Symposium, 1982a). More importantly perhaps, individuals who do not tolerate one of the oxazolidinediones may tolerate the other.
Paramethadione is N-demethylated by the hepatic microsomal enzymes to an active metabolite that is slowly excreted in the urine. The metabolite accumulates during chronic medication and is probably responsible for most of the anticonvulsant activity of the parent drug.

BENZODIAZEPINES

The benzodiazepines are employed clinically primarily as sedative-antianxiety drugs; their pharmacology is presented in detail in Chapters 17 and 19. Discussion in this chapter is limited to consideration of their usefulness in the therapy of the epilepsies. A large number of benzodiazepines have broad antiepileptic properties, but only *clonazepam* and *clorazepate* have been approved in the United States for the chronic treatment of certain types of seizures. *Nitrazepam* is currently being evaluated for the therapy of *infantile spasms.* *Diazepam* has a well-defined role in the management of *status epilepticus,* while the utility of *lorazepam* is under investigation.

Chemistry. The structures of the benzodiazepines are presented in Table 17–1 (page 341). The structure-activity relationship for the anticonvulsant effect of the benzodiazepines has been summarized by Popp (Symposium, 1977).

Anticonvulsant Properties. In animals, prevention of pentylenetetrazol-induced seizures by the benzodiazepines is much more prominent than their modification of the maximal electroshock seizure pattern. Clonazepam is unusually potent in antagonizing the effects of pentylenetetrazol, but it is almost without action on seizures induced by maximal electroshock (Swinyard and Castellion, 1966). Nevertheless, in experimental models of epilepsy, benzodiazepines, including clonazepam, suppress the spread of seizure activity produced by epileptogenic foci in the cortex, thalamus, and limbic structures but do not abolish the abnormal discharge of the focus. Further, both diazepam and clonazepam suppress stimulus-induced generalized convulsions in kindled rats, but they produce little or no reduction in stimulus-induced afterdischarges (Albright and Burnham, 1980). In agreement with these observations in animals, clonazepam has anticonvulsant activity in patients with a wide variety of seizure disorders, with the notable exception of generalized tonic-clonic seizures (*see* Browne, in Symposium, 1983a).

A large body of electrophysiological and biochemical observations has linked the actions of benzodiazepines to the functions of receptor-chloride ionophore systems that are regulated by GABA (*see* Olsen, 1982; Symposium, 1982b). The evidence includes the ability of various benzodiazepines to potentiate the effects of exogenous GABA or to enhance GABA-mediated presynaptic and postsynaptic inhibitory pathways. Further, specific sites for benzodiazepines have been characterized in cell membranes from brain, and their properties can be modified by GABA and by chloride or related ions that are known to carry current through channels that are regulated by GABA. Both binding sites for GABA and the ability of GABA to enhance the binding of benzodiazepines are retained after extensive purification of binding sites for benzodiazepines from detergent-solubilized preparations of membranes. This suggests a close molecular association of sites of action for GABA and the benzodiazepines. There is also substantial agreement between the relative binding affinity and the relative potency to block pentylenetetrazol-induced convulsions for a large series of benzodiazepines.

While this body of evidence is impressive, it is largely circumstantial and does not provide clear explanations for the sedative, anxiolytic, or anticonvulsant effects of benzodiazepines. Nor does it explain how potentiation of responses to GABA by both barbiturates and benzodiazepines can lead to the differing pattern of antiepileptic effects that are displayed by these two groups of drugs. However, recent studies have revealed complexities both in the functions of receptors for GABA and in the electrophysiological effects of the benzodiazepines that may be important to the clarification of these issues. For example, Alger and Nicoll (1982) have detected two different types of receptors for GABA in hippocampal pyramidal cells; diazepam potentiates somatic responses to GABA that involve increases in chloride conductance, while barbiturates preferentially potentiate dendritic responses to GABA that include changes in the conductance to ions other than chloride. Furthermore, potentiation of responses to GABA requires concentrations of benzodiazepines 10- to 100-fold greater than those achieved in the CSF during therapy; at these lower concentrations, direct inhibitory effects on neuronal excitability are produced that appear to involve increases in a calcium-dependent conductance for potassium ions (MacDonald and Barker, 1982; Carlen *et al.*, 1983b). As the concentration of benzodiazepine approaches that required to observe potentiation of responses to GABA, the magnitude of these effects diminishes, and they ultimately disappear. These observations suggest that the anticonvulsant effects of the benzodiazepines may not depend entirely upon actions on GABAergic neurotransmission or on channels for chloride ions.

Recently, certain analogs of the imidazobenzodiazepines have been synthesized that both inhibit binding and reverse the effects of benzodiazepines, including those produced by low concentrations of benzodiazepines on hippocampal neurons (Carlen *et al.*, 1983a). The antagonist that has been most intensively investigated (Ro 15-1788) seldom produces obvious effects when administered by itself. However, it has definite anticonvulsant effects in kindled rats at doses that completely block the ataxia induced by diazepam (Robertson and Riives, 1983). Since the antagonist also reduces the magnitude of the anticonvulsant effects of diazepam to some degree, it is hypothesized to be a "partial agonist" with respect to sites that function in the anticonvulsant actions of the benzodiazepines. Together with other evidence that indicates the existence of multiple populations of binding sites for benzodiazepines, this suggests that it may be possible to develop anticonvulsant drugs with less sedative-ataxic effects than those currently available.

Absorption, Distribution, Biotransformation, and Excretion. Benzodiazepines are well absorbed after oral administration, and concentrations in plasma are usually maximal within 1 to 4 hours (*see* Symposium, 1982a; Browne, in Symposium, 1983a). After intravenous administration, they are redistributed in a manner typical of that for highly lipid-soluble agents (*see* Chapter 1). Central effects develop promptly but wane rapidly as the drugs move to other tissues. Diazepam is redistributed especially rapidly, with a half-time of about 1 hour. The extent of binding of benzodiazepines to plasma proteins correlates with lipid solubility, ranging from approximately 99% for diazepam to about 85% for clonazepam (*see* Appendix II).

The major metabolite of diazepam, N-desmethyldiazepam, is about as active as the parent drug. This metabolite is also produced by the rapid decarboxylation of clorazepate following its ingestion. Both diazepam and N-desmethyldiazepam are slowly hydroxylated to other active metabolites, such as oxazepam. The half-life of diazepam in plasma averages between 1 and 2 days, while that of N-desmethyldiazepam is about 60 hours. Both clonazepam and nitrazepam are metabolized principally by reduction of the nitro group to produce inactive 7-amino derivatives. Less than 1% of each drug is recovered unchanged in the urine. The half-life of clonazepam and nitrazepam in plasma averages about 1 day. Lorazepam is metabolized chiefly by conjugation with glucuronic acid; its half-life in plasma averages between 10 and 20 hours.

Toxicity. The acute toxicity of benzodiazepines is low relative to usual clinical dosage. For example, oral ingestion of as much as 60 mg (small child) or 100 mg (adult) of clonazepam has occurred without permanent sequelae (*see* Pinder *et al.,* 1976); therapy consisted in gastric lavage and supportive measures. *Cardiovascular* and *respiratory depression* may occur after the *intravenous* administration of diazepam, clonazepam, or lorazepam, particularly if other anticonvulsants or central depressants have been administered previously (*see* Symposium, 1983d).

The principal side effect of chronic oral medication with clonazepam is the syndrome of drowsiness, somnolence, fatigue, and lethargy. This occurs in about 50% of patients initially, but tends to subside with continued administration. *Muscular incoordination* and *ataxia* are common but less frequent. While these symptoms can usually be kept to tolerable levels by reduction in the dosage or the rate at which it is increased, they sometimes force discontinuation of the drug. Other side effects include *hypotonia, dysarthria,* and *dizziness. Behavioral disturbances,* especially in children, can be very troublesome; these include aggression, hyperactivity, irritability, and difficulty in concentration. Both anorexia and hyperphagia have been reported. *Increased salivary* and *bronchial secretions* may cause difficulties in children. *Seizures* are sometimes exacerbated (*see* Browne, in Symposium, 1983a), and *status epilepticus* may be precipitated if the drug is discontinued abruptly. Other aspects of the toxicity of the benzodiazepines are discussed in Chapters 17 and 19.

Preparations, Routes of Administration, and Dosage. *Clonazepam* (CLONOPIN) is available as 0.5-, 1-, and 2-mg tablets. The initial dose for adults should not exceed 1.5 mg per day, and for children it is 0.01 to 0.03 mg/kg per day. The dose-depen-dent side effects are reduced if two or three divided doses are given each day. Dosage may be increased every 3 to 7 days by 0.25 to 0.5 mg per day in children and 0.5 to 1 mg per day in adults. The maximal recommended dosage is 20 mg per day for adults and 0.2 mg/kg per day for children. In children, each 0.05 mg/kg per day produces an increase in the concentration of clonazepam in plasma of about 25 ng/ml.

Clorazepate dipotassium (TRANXENE) is available as 3.75-, 7.5-, and 15-mg tablets and capsules and in slow-release tablets. The maximal initial dose is 22.5 mg per day in three portions for adults and 15 mg per day in two doses for children. Daily doses should be increased by no more than 7.5 mg in any given week. The maximal recommended dose is 90 mg per day for adults and 60 mg per day for children. Clorazepate is not recommended for children under the age of 9.

Diazepam (VALIUM) is available as 2-, 5-, and 10-mg tablets, as 15-mg sustained-release capsules, and in solution for injection. For *status epilepticus,* diazepam is administered intravenously and at a rate of no more than 5 mg per minute. The usual dose for adults and older children is 5 to 10 mg, as required; this may be repeated at intervals of 10 to 15 minutes, up to a maximal dose of 30 mg. If necessary, this regimen can be repeated in 2 to 4 hours, but no more than 100 mg should be administered in a 24-hour period. An alternate regimen has recently been recommended (*see* Symposium, 1983d); initial therapy includes the infusion of 20 mg of diazepam over a period of 10 minutes or until seizures stop.

Plasma Drug Concentrations. Effective concentrations of clonazepam in plasma range from 5 to 70 ng/ml. The values for N-desmethyldiazepam formed by the decarboxylation of clorazepate range from 0.5 to 1.9 μg/ml. However, similar ranges of concentrations are observed in patients who have poor therapeutic responses or various side effects (*see* Browne, in Symposium, 1983a). Thus, neither clear-cut minimal therapeutic concentrations nor usually toxic concentrations can be stated.

Drug Interactions. Significant drug interactions with the benzodiazepines have not been reported. However, it must be remembered that benzodiazepines are known to potentiate the action of CNS-depressant drugs such as ethanol and barbiturates.

Therapeutic Uses. Clonazepam is useful in the therapy of *absence seizures* as well as *myoclonic seizures* in children. However, tolerance to its antiepileptic effects usually develops after 1 to 6 months of administration, and some patients will no longer respond to clonazepam at any dosage. While diazepam is currently the agent of choice for the treatment of *status epilepticus,* its relatively short duration of action is a disadvantage. Although diazepam is not useful as an oral agent for the treatment of seizure disorders, clorazepate is effective in combination with certain other drugs in the treatment of *partial seizures*. These applications are discussed further at the end of the chapter. Other uses of the benzodiazepines are described primarily in Chapters 17 and 19.

OTHER ANTIEPILEPTIC AGENTS

Phenacemide. Introduced in 1949, phenacemide (phenylacetylurea) is the straight-chain analog of 5-phenylhydantoin. Even if its efficacy remained unchallenged, its clinical value and use would be severely limited by its potential for serious toxicity. Adverse reactions include behavioral effects, gastrointestinal symptoms, rash, hepatitis, aplastic anemia, and nephritis. Phenacemide can be used as adjunctive therapy in the treatment of complex partial seizures refractory to other agents. Periodic assessment of hepatic, renal, and bone-marrow function is mandatory. The patient and his family must be alerted to the possible hazards of the drug.

Phenacemide (PHENURONE) is available as 500-mg tablets. Usual daily dosage in adults has varied from 1.5 to 5 g. Phenacemide is almost completely absorbed from the gastrointestinal tract. Biotransformation by hepatic microsomal enzymes includes inactivation by *p*-hydroxylation of the phenyl substituent; ring closure to form a hydantoin does not occur. Unchanged drug is not excreted in the urine. Plasma concentrations associated with efficacy and safety have not been established (*see* Browne, in Symposium, 1983a).

Acetazolamide. Acetazolamide, the prototype for the carbonic anhydrase inhibitors, is discussed with the saluretic agents in Chapter 36. Its anticonvulsant actions have been discussed in *previous editions* of this textbook and have been reviewed by Woodbury and Kemp (Symposium, 1982a). While it is sometimes effective against absence seizures, its usefulness is limited by the rapid development of tolerance. *Acetazolamide* (DIAMOX) is available as tablets and as a powder for solution for parenteral use.

Acetazolamide is rapidly absorbed from the gastrointestinal tract, is highly bound to plasma proteins, and is eliminated unchanged in the urine. Adverse effects are minimal when it is employed in moderate dosage for limited periods. Drowsiness and paresthesias may occur at high doses and during prolonged medication. Skin rash and other allergic reactions are not common.

Progabide. Progabide (4-[(4-chlorophenyl)(5-fluoro-2-hydroxyphenyl)-methylene] aminobutanamide) is an analog of the amide derivative of GABA. This compound behaves as an agonist at receptors for GABA, and it was developed as a result of hypotheses concerning the role of GABA in epileptogenesis and in the anticonvulsant actions of a number of antiepileptic drugs (Worms *et al.*, 1982). Progabide and its principal metabolite, the deamidated derivative, display anticonvulsant activity in a wide variety of animal models, including antagonism of pentylenetetrazol and modification of seizures induced by maximal electroshock. Progabide is currently undergoing clinical trials in both Europe and the United States. Although early reports of open trials were encouraging, the limited number of published studies that involve double-blind crossover protocols do not yet provide evidence of substantial efficacy (Dam *et al.*, 1983; Loiseau *et al.*, 1983). However, it should be noted that ethical considerations dictate that any new antiepileptic drug must first prove to be efficacious in patients in whom conventional therapy has failed.

GENERAL PRINCIPLES AND CHOICE OF DRUGS FOR THE THERAPY OF THE EPILEPSIES

Accurate evaluation of the type of seizure is essential for the rational pharmacotherapy of epilepsy. This requires a thorough examination of the patient, including the EEG. Epilepsy is a chronic condition, and long-term treatment is the rule; patients with conditions that might be mistaken for epilepsy (*e.g.*, withdrawal from chronic use of a sedative-hypnotic agent) or those who have experienced a single seizure precipitated by a reversible abnormality (*e.g.*, hypoglycemia) should not be treated continuously. Furthermore, an attempt should be made to ascertain the cause of the epilepsy with the hope of discovering a correctable lesion, either structural or metabolic. This is more likely in the very young patient or when the first seizure appears during adulthood. Once the decision has been made to use drugs to control the seizures, and this is often the case even if a specific etiology is found, the goal of therapy is to keep the patient free of seizures without interfering with normal function.

Even when it is anticipated that multiple-drug therapy will be required, *medication is initiated with a single drug. Initial dosage* is usually that expected to provide a plasma drug concentration during the plateau state at least in the lower portion of the range associated with clinical efficacy. However, to minimize dose-related adverse effects, therapy with some drugs is initiated at reduced dosage, and the clinically effective amount is attained gradually. Loading dosage is employed only if the urgency for control of seizures exceeds the risk of adverse effects during the initial therapy.

The results of the initial medication should be assessed with appropriate regard for the time required to attain the plateau state, the usual variability of incidence of seizures, and the anticipation that some tolerance usually develops to the sedative and other minor adverse effects of these drugs. Dosage is increased at appropriate intervals, as required for control of seizures or as limited by toxicity, and such adjustment is preferably assisted by monitoring of drug concentrations in plasma.

If a single drug fails to provide adequate control of seizures in maximal tolerated dosage, *another drug should be substituted or a second drug may be added.* The choice between these alternatives is usually determined by consideration of the adverse effects of the drug in the individual patient. Unless serious adverse effects of the drug dictate otherwise, *dosage should always be reduced gradually* when a drug is being discontinued, to minimize the risk of precipitating status epilepticus. No drug should be discarded as useless unless toxicity prevents increased dosage.

Essential to optimal management of epilepsy is the *filling-out of a seizure chart* by the patient or a relative; *frequent visits to the physician or seizure clinic,* particularly in the early period of treatment, since hematological and other possible somatic side effects require consideration of change in medication; and *long-term follow-up,* including repetition of EEG and neurological examination. Most crucial for successful management is *regularity of medication.*

Common *causes of failure* of antiepileptic medication are improper diagnosis of the type of seizure, incorrect choice of drug, inadequate or excessive dosage, too frequent changes in medication without regard for the time required for transition between plateau states, failure to utilize fully the advantages of multiple-drug medication, inattention to ancillary aspects of therapy, and poor compliance by the patient. Poor compliance may take the form of erratic medication, with only partial control of seizures; consistent failure to take medication, with failure ever to attain adequate drug concentration; or excessive medication, with needless toxicity. Poor compliance sometimes persists despite the best efforts of the physician, but it can usually be corrected. Similarly, failure of therapy because of inattention to recommendations about

diet, rest, avoidance of alcohol, and similar ancillary factors can usually be prevented.

Measurement of *plasma drug concentration* at appropriate intervals greatly facilitates the *initial adjustment* of dosage for individual differences in drug elimination and the *subsequent adjustment* of dosage to minimize dose-related adverse effects without sacrifice of seizure control. Periodic monitoring during *maintenance therapy* can detect failure of the patient to take the medication as prescribed; for the patient with infrequent seizures and apparent control, periodic monitoring can provide assurance that seizure control is, in fact, being maintained. Knowledge of plasma drug concentration can be especially helpful during *multiple-drug therapy.* If toxicity occurs, monitoring helps to identify the particular drug responsible, and, if pharmacokinetic drug interaction occurs, it can guide readjustment of dosage. In general, monitoring of drug concentrations in plasma during antiepileptic therapy is likely to be an aid whenever therapy is less than satisfactory or whenever it is associated with toxicity or an unexpected or atypical clinical response.

Duration of Therapy. In an attempt to provide guidelines for withdrawal of anticonvulsant drugs, Thurston and coworkers (1982) studied the effects of withdrawing treatment from 148 children who had been free of seizures for 4 years; 28% of the children had a recurrence of seizures during the next 15 to 23 years. Most of these were children who had focal seizures. The recurrence rates were lowest in children who had only tonic-clonic (14%) or absence (12%) seizures. Neurological dysfunction was associated with a high rate of recurrence (46%).

Other studies have suggested that the rate of recurrence for adults is around 40% (*see* Meinardi *et al.,* 1977). A history of a single recent seizure may interfere with employment or the right to have a driver's license; these are important considerations in adult patients.

If a decision to withdraw antiepileptic drugs is made, such withdrawal should be done gradually over a period of months. The risk of *status epilepticus* is great with abrupt cessation of therapy.

Generalized Tonic-Clonic and Simple Partial Seizures. Phenytoin and phenobarbital are the principal agents used to treat generalized tonic-clonic seizures. Phenobarbital is generally the agent of choice in children under the age of 5, while phenytoin is usually used first for older children and adults. Carbamazepine is as effective as phenytoin in the treatment of generalized tonic-clonic and simple partial seizures. Although it may involve a greater risk of serious toxicity, carbamazepine is sometimes recommended along with phenytoin as a drug of choice in these disorders (*see* Medical Letter, 1983).

Although valproic acid has not yet been approved for use in the United States in the treatment of generalized tonic-clonic seizures, clinical experience has shown that it is an effective agent for such patients. Some investigators have gone so far as to recommend valproate as the preferred drug for this disorder (Delgado-Escueta *et al.*, 1983). However, the availability of other effective drugs and the risk of serious hepatic toxicity argue against such a recommendation (Coulter, 1983).

Primidone alone may be effective in patients who are refractory to phenytoin and phenobarbital. However, it is more commonly employed concurrently with phenytoin. Since it is metabolized in part to phenobarbital, primidone is logically a substitute for, not a supplement to, phenobarbital. Mephenytoin is sometimes dramatically superior to phenytoin, but the advantage is offset by the greater risk of serious toxicity.

Absence Seizures. Trimethadione was the first agent of selective benefit against absence seizures in children. However, ethosuximide is more effective and has a lower risk of serious toxicity. Complete control of absence seizures can be attained in about 50% of patients, and significant reduction in seizure frequency is achieved in another 25%.

Numerous controlled studies have demonstrated the effectiveness of valproic acid in absence seizures. It may be possible to achieve a 75% reduction in the frequency of such seizures in approximately two thirds of patients by administration of this drug (*see* Mattson and Cramer, in Symposium, 1983a). Some investigators suggest that valproate might offer the advantage of preventing the emergence of tonic-clonic seizures without the need for additional therapy. Despite the efficacy of valproic acid, ethosuximide remains the drug of choice for treatment of absence seizures because of the propensity of valproate to cause serious hepatic toxicity.

Clonazepam is also effective in the treatment of absence seizures, particularly those with a myoclonic component. However, because tolerance may develop to the antiepileptic effects, other agents are generally preferred.

Phenytoin, phenobarbital, and primidone are ineffective against absence seizures and may increase their frequency, but medication with one of these agents is often required as additional therapy against the generalized tonic-clonic seizures that may appear in these patients.

Complex Partial Seizures. The treatment of complex partial seizures is generally less effective than is that of generalized or absence seizures. Essential to appropriate therapy is differentiation between absence seizures and complex partial seizures. The latter are characterized by an aura, a duration of 1 to 2 minutes, and postictal confusion. Absence seizures are characterized by an abrupt onset of loss of consciousness, a duration of 5 to 20 seconds, and a characteristic 3-per-second spike-and-wave activity in the EEG (*see* Solomon *et al.*, 1983). The agents used to treat absence seizures are generally ineffective for complex partial seizures.

Drugs that are effective for generalized tonic-clonic seizures are also employed for control of complex partial seizures. Phenytoin is often preferred, particularly if there are associated tonic-clonic seizures. Primidone is generally used in

preference to phenobarbital, although both are employed. Carbamazepine is also a very useful agent in the treatment of complex partial seizures and may be effective in cases that are refractory to other agents. Its use has been limited by fear of hematological side effects. Some investigators maintain that the risks of cautious treatment with carbamazepine are very low and consider it to be a drug of first choice in this disorder.

Febrile Convulsions. Two to four percent of children experience a convulsion associated with a febrile illness. About 33% of these children will have another febrile convulsion, and 2 to 3% become epileptic in later years. This is a sixfold increase in risk compared to the general population.

The treatment, if any, of febrile seizures is controversial (*see* Fishman, 1979). Several alternatives have been proposed, including no treatment, regular treatment with phenobarbital, or initiation of phenobarbital at the onset of a febrile illness. The latter course of action is doomed to failure because of the pharmacokinetic properties of phenobarbital. It takes several days to reach effective concentrations in blood, and the use of a sufficient loading dose results in toxic effects.

One approach to the problem of febrile seizures is to institute chronic therapy in those children who are at greatest risk for a recurrence of seizures. This includes children who have their first seizure before 18 months of age, those who have significant neurological abnormalities, and those in whom the seizures last more than 15 minutes or are complex in nature. The presence of two of these risk factors increases the likelihood of developing epilepsy to 13%. However, there is no evidence that prophylactic treatment reduces this risk. When a decision to treat is made, phenobarbital is the drug of choice. If the child has experienced no seizures for 30 months and is otherwise normal, therapy is usually discontinued (*see* Fishman, 1979; Freeman, 1980).

Seizures in Infants and Young Children. *Infantile myoclonic spasms* with *hypsarhythmia* are refractory to the usual antiepileptic agents; corticotropin or the adrenocorticosteroids are the agents of choice. Valproic acid has been used successfully in some patients. Clonazepam may be a useful adjunct, but tolerance often develops.

Valproate may be effective against *myoclonic, akinetic,* and *atonic* seizures in young children and is considered by some experts to be the agent of choice. Clonazepam is also useful in such cases. Phenytoin is relatively ineffective and may produce restlessness and hyperactivity when employed in young children.

Posttraumatic Epilepsy. Head injuries can predispose to the development of epilepsy; with penetrating wounds the risk may be as high as 30 to 40%. There is some clinical evidence to suggest that prophylactic therapy may be effective in preventing the development of a seizure disorder in such cases. This would be consistent with the kindling model of epilepsy, discussed above. The agents effective for treatment of focal seizures and generalized tonic-clonic convulsions are employed.

Status Epilepticus and Other Convulsive Emergencies. *Status epilepticus* is a neurological emergency; untreated it may be fatal. In addition to specific drug therapy, supportive care is essential. Attention must be paid to electrolyte abnormalities, cardiac arrhythmias, dehydration, hypoglycemia, and the possibility of hypotensive shock. Diazepam, administered intravenously, is the agent of choice for control of status epilepticus; the dosage is discussed above. It is effective in 80 to 90% of cases, largely independent of seizure type or etiology, but is least likely to work when the seizures are symptomatic of acute brain lesions. The use of either lorazepam or clonazepam as alternatives to diazepam is being evaluated. Lorazepam appears to offer the advantage of persistence of effective concentrations in plasma and brain for several hours, without appreciable delay in onset of action. Phenytoin, administered intravenously at a maximal rate of 50 mg per minute, may also be employed; however, a response usually occurs only after 15 to 20 minutes have elapsed. For this reason, some investigators advocate the *simultaneous* intravenous administration of both diazepam and phenytoin (*see* Symposium, 1983d). Therapy may also be initiated by the rapid intravenous infusion of phenobarbital (10 to 20 mg/kg) at the rate of 60 mg per minute. Whatever agent is employed, equipment for maintenance of an airway and for mechanical support of ventilation must be immediately available. If seizures continue despite treatment, general anesthesia may be required. After seizures are controlled, appropriate chronic antiepileptic therapy should be initiated.

Convulsive emergencies associated with *drug poisoning* and *drug-induced seizures* in previously nonepileptic patients during medication with agents such as the local anesthetics may also be controlled by diazepam and phenobarbital or another barbiturate. The control of *drug-withdrawal seizures* associated with abuse of alcohol, barbiturates, or related sedative-hypnotics is discussed in Chapter 23.

Antiepileptic Therapy and Pregnancy.
Children of epileptic mothers who received anticonvulsant medication during the early months of pregnancy have an increased incidence of a variety of birth defects. The risk is approximately 7%, compared to 2 to 3% for the general population. It is difficult to differentiate the effects of repeated seizures, teratogenic effects of anticonvulsants, and genetic factors. Evidence for a teratogenic effect is greatest for trimethadione (Zackai *et al.*, 1975). Although a "fetal hydantoin syndrome" has been described (Hanson and Smith, 1975), its existence as a direct consequence of exposure to phenytoin is controversial (*see* Janz, in Sympo-

sium, 1982c). Spina bifida has been associated with maternal use of valproate (Bjerkedal *et al.*, 1982). There is also evidence that the combined use of carbamazepine, valproate, and either phenytoin or phenobarbital is associated with an unusually high incidence of fetal abnormalities (Lindhout *et al.*, 1984). Abrupt discontinuation of antiepileptic medication incurs a definite risk of status epilepticus and its hazards for the fetus and mother. For these reasons, antiepileptic medication should *not* be discontinued in pregnant epileptic women for whom the medication is necessary for the prevention of major seizures. However, depending upon the frequency and severity of seizures in the *individual patient,* cautious reduction of dosage to a minimum may be feasible and advisable, particularly in the first trimester. Therapeutic abortion should be considered when trimethadione has been used during pregnancy. Folic acid deficiency, if present, should be corrected. Monitoring of anticonvulsant drug concentrations should be performed to detect alterations of drug metabolism during pregnancy (*see* Symposium, 1982c). The therapy of seizure disorders during pregnancy has been reviewed by Dalessio (1985).

The newborn of mothers who received phenobarbital, primidone, or phenytoin during pregnancy may also develop a deficiency of vitamin K–dependent clotting factors, and serious hemorrhage may occur during the first 24 hours of life. Bleeding can be prevented by administration of vitamin K.

Aiges, H. W.; Daum, F.; Olson, M.; Kahn, E.; and Teichberg, S.   The effects of phenobarbital and diphenylhydantoin on liver function and morphology. *J. Pediatr.,* **1980,** *97,* 22–26.

Albright, P. S.   Effects of carbamazepine, clonazepam, and phenytoin on seizure threshold in amygdala and cortex. *Exp. Neurol.,* **1983,** *79,* 11–17.

Albright, P. S., and Burnham, W. M.   Development of a new pharmacological seizure model: effects of anticonvulsants on cortical- and amygdala-kindled seizures in the rat. *Epilepsia,* **1980,** *21,* 681–689.

Alger, B. E., and Nicoll, R. A.   Feed-forward dendritic inhibition in rat hippocampal pyramidal cells studied *in vitro. J. Physiol.* (*Lond.*), **1982,** *328,* 105–123.

Bjerkedal, T.; Czeizel, A.; Goujard, J.; Kallen, B.; Mastroicova, P.; Nevin, N.; Oakley, G.; and Robert, E.   Valproic acid and spina bifida. *Lancet,* **1982,** *2,* 1096.

Browne, T. R.   Valproic acid. Medical intelligence. *N. Engl. J. Med.,* **1980,** *302,* 661–666.

Carlen, P. L.; Gurevich, N.; and Polc, P. The excitatory effects of the specific benzodiazepine antagonist Ro14-7437, measured intracellularly in hippocampal CA1 cells. *Brain Res.*, **1983a**, *271*, 115–119.

———. Low-dose benzodiazepine neuronal inhibition: enhanced Ca^{2+}-mediated K^+-conductance. *Ibid.*, **1983b**, *271*, 358–364.

Commission on Classification and Terminology of the International League Against Epilepsy. Proposal for revised clinical and electroencephalographic classification of epileptic seizures. *Epilepsia*, **1981**, *22*, 489–501.

Coulter, D. L. The treatable epilepsies. *N. Engl. J. Med.*, **1983**, *309*, 1456.

Coulter, D. L., and Allen, R. J. Hyperammonemia with valproic acid therapy. *J. Pediatr.*, **1981**, *99*, 317–319.

Dam, M.; Gram, L.; Philbert, A.; Hansen, B. S.; Lyon, B. B.; Christensen, J. M.; and Angelo, H. R. Progabide: a controlled trial in partial epilepsy. *Epilepsia*, **1983**, *24*, 127–134.

Earnest, M. P.; Marx, J. A.; and Drury, L. R. Complications of intravenous phenytoin for acute treatment of seizures. *J.A.M.A.*, **1983**, *249*, 762–765.

Fishman, M. A. Febrile seizures: the treatment controversy. *J. Pediatr.*, **1979**, *94*, 174–184.

Freeman, J. M. Febrile seizures: a consensus of their significance, evaluation, and treatment. *Pediatrics*, **1980**, *66*, 1009–1012.

Fromm, G. H.; Chattha, A. S.; Terrence, C. F.; and Glass, J. D. Do phenytoin and carbamazepine depress excitation and/or facilitate inhibition? *Eur. J. Pharmacol.*, **1982**, *78*, 403–409.

Guberman, A.; Gloor, P.; and Sherwin, A. L. Response of generalized penicillin epilepsy in the cat to ethosuximide and diphenylhydantoin. *Neurology (Minneap.)*, **1975**, *25*, 758–764.

Hanson, J. W., and Smith, D. W. The fetal hydantoin syndrome. *J. Pediatr.*, **1975**, *87*, 285–290.

Hart, R. G., and Easton, J. D. Carbamazepine and hematological monitoring. *Ann. Neurol.*, **1982**, *11*, 309–312.

Hassell, T. M., and Gilbert, G. H. Phenytoin sensitivity of fibroblasts as the basis for susceptibility to gingival enlargement. *Am. J. Pathol.*, **1983**, *112*, 218–223.

Hauptmann, A. LUMINAL bei Epilepsie. *Munch. Med. Wochenschr.*, **1912**, *59*, 1907–1909.

Hauser, W. A. Epidemiology of epilepsy. *Adv. Neurol.*, **1978**, *19*, 313–339.

Heller, A. H.; Dichter, M. A.; and Sidman, R. L. Anticonvulsant sensitivity of absence seizures in the *tottering* mutant mouse. *Epilepsia*, **1983**, *24*, 25–33.

Keane, P. E.; Simiand, J.; Mendes, E.; Santucci, V.; and Morre, M. The effects of analogues of valproic acid on seizures induced by pentylenetetrazol and GABA content in brain of mice. *Neuropharmacology*, **1983**, *22*, 875–879.

Keith, D. A.; Gundberg, C. M.; Japour, A.; Aronoff, J.; Alvarez, N.; and Gallop, P. M. Vitamin K–dependent proteins and anticonvulsant medication. *Clin. Pharmacol. Ther.*, **1983**, *34*, 529–532.

Krall, R. L.; Penry, J. K.; Kupferberg, H. J.; and Swinyard, E. A. Antiepileptic drug development. I. History and a program for progress. *Epilepsia*, **1978**, *19*, 393–408.

Küpfer, A.; Lawson, J.; and Branch, R. A. Stereoselectivity of the arene epoxide pathway of mephenytoin hydroxylation in man. *Epilepsia*, **1984**, *25*, 1–6.

Lindhout, D.; Höppener, R.; and Meinardi, H. Teratogenicity of antiepileptic drug combinations with special emphasis on epoxidation (of carbamazepine). *Epilepsia*, **1984**, *25*, 77–83.

Loiseau, P.; Bossi, L.; Guyot, M.; Orofiamma, B.; and Morselli, P. L. Double-blind crossover trial of progabide versus placebo in severe epilepsies. *Epilepsia*, **1983**, *24*, 703–714.

MacDonald, J. F., and Barker, J. L. Multiple actions of picomolar concentrations of flurazepam on the excitability of cultured mouse spinal neurons. *Brain Res.*, **1982**, *246*, 257–264.

Marangos, P. J.; Post, R. M.; Patel, J.; Zander, K.; Parma, A.; and Weiss, S. Specific and potent interactions of carbamazepine with brain adenosine receptors. *Eur. J. Pharmacol.*, **1983**, *93*, 175–182.

Maxson, S. C.; Fine, M. D.; Ginsburg, B. E.; and Koniecki, D. L. A mutant for spontaneous seizures in C57BL/10Bg mice. *Epilepsia*, **1983**, *24*, 15–24.

Medical Letter. Drugs for epilepsy. **1983**, *25*, 81–84.

Melikian, A. P.; Straughn, A. B.; Slywka, G. W. A.; Whyatt, P. L.; and Meyer, M. C. Bioavailability of 11 phenytoin products. *J. Pharmacokinet. Biopharm.*, **1977**, *5*, 133–146.

Merritt, H. H., and Putnam, T. J. A new series of anticonvulsant drugs tested by experiments on animals. *Arch. Neurol. Psychiatry*, **1938a**, *39*, 1003–1015.

———. Sodium diphenyl hydantoinate in treatment of convulsive disorders. *J.A.M.A.*, **1938b**, *111*, 1068–1073.

Olpe, H. R., and Jones, R. S. G. The action of anticonvulsant drugs on the firing of locus coeruleus neurons: selective, activating effect of carbamazepine. *Eur. J. Pharmacol.*, **1979**, *51*, 107–110.

Rasmussen, T. Characteristics of a pure culture of frontal lobe epilepsy. *Epilepsia*, **1983**, *24*, 482–493.

Richens, A. Clinical pharmacokinetics of phenytoin. *Clin. Pharmacokinet.*, **1979**, *4*, 153–169.

Robertson, H. A., and Riives, M. L. A benzodiazepine antagonist is an anticonvulsant in an animal model for limbic epilepsy. *Brain Res.*, **1983**, *270*, 380–382.

Skerritt, J. H.; Johnston, G. A. R.; and Chen Chow, S. Interactions of the anticonvulsant carbamazepine with adenosine receptors. 2. Pharmacological studies. *Epilepsia*, **1983**, *24*, 643–650.

Swinyard, E. A., and Castellion, A. W. Anticonvulsant properties of some benzodiazepines. *J. Pharmacol. Exp. Ther.*, **1966**, *151*, 369–375.

Thurston, J. H.; Thurston, L. D.; Hixon, B. B.; and Keller, A. J. Prognosis in childhood epilepsy. Additional follow-up of 148 children 15 to 23 years after withdrawal of anticonvulsant therapy. *N. Engl. J. Med.*, **1982**, *306*, 831–836.

Thyagarajan, R.; Ramanjaneyulu, R.; and Ticku, M. K. Enhancement of diazepam and γ-aminobutyric acid binding by (+)etomidate and pentobarbital. *J. Neurochem.*, **1983**, *41*, 578–585.

Worms, P.; Depoortere, H.; Durand, A.; Morselli, P. L.; Lloyd, K. G.; and Bartholini, G. γ-Aminobutyric acid (GABA) receptor stimulation. 1. Neuropharmacological profiles of progabide (SL 76002) and SL 75102, with emphasis on their anticonvulsant spectra. *J. Pharmacol. Exp. Ther.*, **1982**, *220*, 660–671.

Zackai, E. H.; Mellman, W. J.; Neiderer, B.; and Hanson, J. W. The fetal trimethadione syndrome. *J. Pediatr.*, **1975**, *87*, 280–284.

Zimmerman, H. J., and Ishak, K. G. Valproate-induced hepatic injury: analysis of 23 fatal cases. *Hepatology*, **1982**, *2*, 591–597.

Monographs and Reviews

Chapman, A.; Keane, P. E.; Meldrum, B. S.; Simiand, J.; and Vernieres, C. Mechanism of anticonvulsant action of valproate. *Prog. Neurobiol.*, **1982**, *19*, 315–359.

Close, W. J., and Spielman, M. A. Anticonvulsant drugs. In, *Medicinal Chemistry*, Vol. 5. (Hartung, W. H., ed.) John Wiley & Sons, Inc., New York, **1961**.

Dalessio, D. J. Current concepts: seizure disorders and pregnancy. *N. Engl. J Med.*, **1985**, *312*, 559–563.

Delgado-Escueta, A. V.; Treiman, D. M.; and Walsh, G. O. The treatable epilepsies. *N. Engl. J. Med.*, **1983**, *308*, 1508–1514, 1576–1584.

Frey, H.-H. Primidone. In, *Antiepileptic Drugs*. (Frey, H.-H., and Janz, D., eds.) *Handbook of Experimental Pharmacology*, Vol. 74. Springer-Verlag, Berlin, **1985**, pp. 283–289.

Frey, H.-H., and Janz, D. (eds.) *Antiepileptic Drugs. Handbook of Experimental Pharmacology*, Vol. 74. Springer-Verlag, Berlin, **1985**.

Johnston, D., and Brown, T. H. Mechanisms of neuronal burst generation. In, *Electrophysiology of Epilepsy*. (Schwartzkroin, R. A., and Wheal, H. V., eds.) Academic Press, Inc., New York, **1984**, pp. 277–301.

Jones, G. L., and Wimbish, G. H. Hydantoins. In, *Antiepileptic Drugs*. (Frey, H.-H., and Janz, D., eds.) *Handbook of Experimental Pharmacology*, Vol. 74. Springer-Verlag, Berlin, **1985**, pp. 351–419.

Macdonald, R. L., and McLean, M. J. Cellular bases of barbiturate and phenytoin anticonvulsant drug action. *Epilepsia*, **1982**, *23*, Suppl. 1, 7–18.

Meinardi, H.; van Heycop ten Ham, M. W.; Meijer, J. W. A.; and Bongers, E. Long-term control of seizures. In, *Epilepsy: The Eighth International Symposium*. (Penry, J. K., ed.) Raven Press, New York, **1977**, pp. 17–26.

Olsen, R. W. Drug interactions at the GABA receptor-ionophore complex. *Annu. Rev. Pharmacol. Toxicol.*, **1982**, *22*, 245–277.

Pinder, R. M.; Brogden, R. N.; Speight, T. M.; and Avery, G. S. Clonazepam: a review of its pharmacological properties and therapeutic efficacy in epilepsy. *Drugs*, **1976**, *12*, 321–361.

Post, R. M.; Uhde, T. W.; Rubinow, D. R.; Ballenger, J. C.; and Gold, P. W. Biochemical effects of carbamazepine: relationship to its mechanisms of action in affective illness. *Prog. Neuropsychopharmacol. Biol. Psychiatry*, **1983**, *7*, 263–271.

Schmutz, M. Carbamazepine. In, *Antiepileptic Drugs*. (Frey, H.-H., and Janz, D., eds.) *Handbook of Experimental Pharmacology*, Vol. 74. Springer-Verlag, Berlin, **1985**, pp. 479–506.

Solomon, G. E.; Kutt, H.; and Plum, F. *Clinical Management of Seizures: A Guide for the Physician*, 2nd ed. W. B. Saunders Co., Philadelphia, **1983**.

Symposium. (Various authors.) *Experimental Models of Epilepsy: A Manual for the Laboratory Worker*. (Purpura, D. P.; Penry, J. K.; Tower, D.; Woodbury, D. M.; and Walter, R.; eds.) Raven Press, New York, **1972**.

Symposium. (Various authors.) *Anticonvulsants*. (Vida, J. A., ed.) Academic Press, Inc., New York, **1977**.

Symposium. (Various authors.) *Antiepileptic Drugs: Quantitative Analysis and Interpretation*. (Pippenger, C. E.; Penry, J. K.; and Kutt, H.; eds.) Raven Press, New York, **1978**.

Symposium. (Various authors.) *Antiepileptic Drugs: Mechanisms of Action. Advances in Neurology*, Vol. 27. (Glaser, G. H.; Penry, J. K.; and Woodbury, D. M.; eds.) Raven Press, New York, **1980**.

Symposium. (Various authors.) *Kindling 2*. (Wada, J. A., ed.) Raven Press, New York, **1981**.

Symposium. (Various authors.) *Antiepileptic Drugs*, 2nd ed. (Woodbury, D. M.; Penry, J. K.; and Pippenger, C. E.; eds.) Raven Press, New York, **1982a**.

Symposium. (Various authors.) *Pharmacology of Benzodiazepines*. (Usdin, E.; Skolnick, P.; Tallman, J. F., Jr.; Greenblatt, D.; and Paul, S. M.; eds.) Macmillan Press, Ltd., London, **1982b**.

Symposium. (Various authors.) *Epilepsy, Pregnancy, and the Child*. (Janz, D.; Dam, M.; Richens, A.; Bossi, L.; Helgo, H.; and Schmidt, D.; eds.) Raven Press, New York, **1982c**.

Symposium. (Various authors.) *Epilepsy: Diagnosis and Management*. (Browne, T. R., and Feldman, R. G., eds.) Little, Brown & Co., Boston, **1983a**.

Symposium. (Various authors.) *Epilepsy: An Update on Research and Therapy. Progress in Clinical and Biological Research*, Vol. 124. (Nistico, G.; Perri, R. D.; and Meinardi, H.; eds.) Alan R. Liss, Inc., New York, **1983b**.

Symposium. (Various authors.) *Recent Advances in Epilepsy. I*. (Pedley, T. A., and Meldrum, B. S., eds.) Churchill Livingston, Inc., New York, **1983c**.

Symposium. (Various authors.) *Status Epilepticus: Mechanisms of Brain Damage and Treatment. Advances in Neurology*, Vol. 34. (Delgado-Escueta, A. V.; Wasterlain, C. G.; Treiman, D. M.; and Porter, R. J.; eds.) Raven Press, New York, **1983d**.

Toman, J. E. P., and Goodman, L. S. Anticonvulsants. *Physiol. Rev.*, **1948**, *28*, 409–432.

Troupin, A. S.; Friel, P.; Lovely, M. P.; and Wilensky, A. J. Clinical pharmacology of mephenytoin and ethotoin. *Ann. Neurol.*, **1979**, *6*, 410–414.

Wada, J. A. Pharmacological prophylaxis in the kindling model of epilepsy. *Arch. Neurol.*, **1977**, *34*, 389–395.

21 DRUGS FOR PARKINSON'S DISEASE, SPASTICITY, AND ACUTE MUSCLE SPASMS

Joseph R. Bianchine

Most of the drugs described in this chapter have in common the ability to improve skeletal muscle function by primary actions on the central nervous system (CNS). These drugs fall into two distinct categories on the basis of their pharmacological properties and their therapeutic uses. The first group acts primarily on the basal ganglia; its members exert either dopaminergic or anticholinergic effects, and they are useful for the treatment of Parkinson's disease and related disorders. *Levodopa* is the prototype of central-dopaminergic drugs, while *trihexyphenidyl* is the prototypical central-anticholinergic agent. Most members of the second group of drugs, those used to treat spasticity and acute muscle spasms, depress with varying degrees of selectivity certain neuronal systems that control muscle tone; dantrolene, however, acts directly on skeletal muscle.

Research on basic and clinical aspects of Parkinson's disease and the success of its treatment have advanced rapidly during the past 20 years. Consequently, the major emphasis of this chapter is placed on drugs that are effective in this condition. Similar dramatic advances have not been made in the development of effective agents for the treatment of chronic spasticity or acute muscle spasms.

I. Drugs for Parkinson's Disease

Parkinsonism: Clinical Overview. Parkinson's disease, first described by James Parkinson in 1817 as *paralysis agitans,* is a prevalent, serious neurological disease. It afflicts approximately one-half million persons in the United States alone, and more than 90% of the time the disease becomes manifest after the age of 55. The annual incidence of Parkinson's disease has re-

mained constant over the past 20 years. This suggests that the number of cases related to latent neurological manifestations of von Economo's encephalitis pandemic of the early 1920s may be less than previously hypothesized (Rajput *et al.*, 1984). Genetic factors do not appear to play an important role in most cases of Parkinson's disease, although familial cases have been documented (Ward *et al.*, 1983; Barbeau and Roy, in Symposium, 1984). The lack of evidence that Parkinson's disease is a genetically determined loss of neuronal function has prompted vigorous searches for environmental causes (*e.g.*, infections and toxins). Although no such agent has been documented for the vast majority of cases, a toxin has recently been shown to be responsible for the appearance of Parkinson's disease in exposed individuals.

MPTP (N-methyl-4-phenyl-1,2,3,6-tetrahydropyridine), a commercial compound used in organic synthesis, causes a syndrome that resembles Parkinson's disease when administered to primates (Burns *et al.*, 1983). Development of this animal model of the disease followed observation of the occurrence of irreversible parkinsonism in a number of drug addicts and a chemist; they were exposed to the compound because of its presence (as a side product) in a preparation of a meperidine analog that was used illegally in California (Langston *et al.*, 1983). MPTP-induced parkinsonism is similar to the idiopathic disease, pathologically and biochemically, and it responds favorably to the administration of levodopa. Substances like MPTP may be widespread in the environment, and there is concern that repeated exposure to small quantities of such chemicals, combined with the effects of aging, may be an etiological factor in the development of parkinsonism (Blume, 1983).

A parkinsonism-like syndrome may also arise as an untoward effect of certain drugs. Agents that produce such a syndrome have in common the capacity to prevent the action of dopamine in the basal ganglia of the brain (Calne *et al.*, 1979). For example, antipsychotic drugs such as the phenothiazines and butyrophenones block postsynaptic receptors for dopamine and cause extrapyramidal symptoms that resemble parkinsonism, especially in older patients (*see* Chapter 19). In contrast, reserpine produces a parkinsonism-like syndrome by depleting dopamine available for release by the presynaptic neuron. Progressive supranuclear palsy, olivopontocerebellar degeneration, Shy-Drager syndrome, carbon monoxide poisoning, manganese poisoning, and Wilson's disease commonly are associated with certain symptoms that are characteristic of Parkinson's disease. However, in these rare disorders, parkinsonism is only one aspect of a more widespread cerebral disorder. With the exception of manganese poisoning, dopaminergic drugs induce little improvement in these conditions.

Parkinson's disease, independent of specific etiology, usually appears insidiously in the latter decades of life and produces a slowly increasing disability in movement (Pearce, 1978). The disease is usually characterized by four major clinical features: tremor, bradykinesia, rigidity, and a disturbance of posture. In addition, as many as 30% of patients may have an accompanying dementia.

Tremor results from rhythmically alternating, "pill-rolling" contractions (three to five per second) of a muscle group and its antagonist. Distal muscles are more commonly involved than proximal muscles. Tremor can be present during rest, often disappears on purposeful movement (or during sleep), and usually increases remarkably with anxiety or stress. Tremor is commonly superimposed on the hypertonicity of mutually antagonistic groups of skeletal muscles. Initiation of movements becomes increasingly difficult, ponderous, and extremely inefficient and fatiguing.

Bradykinesia is characterized by three components—marked poverty of spontaneous movement, loss of normal associated movements, and slow initiation of all voluntary movements. It remains unclear if the major deficit is in planning the movement or in its execution. The "masked" facial expression in parkinsonism classically demonstrates all these features.

Rigidity is due to increased muscle tone; a "cog-

wheel" or "ratchet" resistance to passive movement of an extremity characterizes this feature.

A *postural defect* appears late in the progression of the disease. The patient is unable to maintain an upright position of the trunk while standing or walking. Consequently, a progressively stooped position is assumed and a festinating gait may occur.

In advanced stages of parkinsonism, loss of motor function causes a variety of other signs and symptoms, such as impairment of postural reflexes, reduced blinking, micrographia, microphonia, and impaired ocular convergence.

Parkinsonism: A Striatal Dopamine-Deficiency Syndrome. The basal ganglia contain a large number of putative neurotransmitters. To date, however, the bulk of interest has centered around two of these, dopamine and acetylcholine, that are present in high concentrations (*see* Lloyd, 1978). A simplistic, but useful, neurochemical model of the functions of the basal ganglia suggests that the striatal tracts, important for the smooth control of voluntary movements, normally contain balanced dopaminergic (inhibitory) and cholinergic (excitatory) components (*see* Calne, 1978; for more detailed models, *see* McGeer *et al.*, in Symposium, 1984). It is now clear that any imbalance in these individual systems produces specific disorders of movement. For example, the hyperkinetic locomotion and the behavior that are characteristic of Huntington's chorea may be the result of excessive dopaminergic activity in the basal ganglia (Klawans *et al.*, 1977). In contrast, there is a marked deficiency in the dopaminergic component of the basal ganglia in parkinsonism, attributed to loss of neurons in the substantia nigra. This deficiency of dopamine results in the signs and symptoms noted above. Consequently, the theoretical goal of the treatment of parkinsonism is to balance striatal activity by reducing cholinergic activity or enhancing dopaminergic function with centrally acting anticholinergic and dopaminergic drugs, respectively. Often, these two classes of drugs are combined effectively. The existence of other neurotransmitter systems in the basal ganglia provides a theoretical basis for novel therapeutic approaches to the treatment of Parkinson's disease (*see* Lang, in Symposium, 1984).

The understanding that parkinsonism is a syndrome of dopamine deficiency and the discovery of levodopa as an important drug for the treatment of the disease were the logical culmination of a series of related basic and clinical observations (*see* review by Hornykiewicz, 1973b). The first may have been the clinical finding that reserpine could induce a parkinsonism-like syndrome as a dose-dependent side effect. Reserpine was later shown to release and thereby deplete stores of 5-hydroxytryptamine (5-HT) and catecholamines in the brain. Subsequently, Carlsson and coworkers (1957) found that the akinesia and sedation produced by reserpine in mice could be reversed by the administration of dopa but not of 5-hydroxytryptophan, the precursor of 5-HT. The relevant clinical observation that the phenothiazines also may induce symptoms of parkinsonism provided another clue that helped focus on the basal ganglia as a site of action for this important class of drugs. The presence of dopamine in the brain, first reported by Montagu (1957), was confirmed by Carlsson and coworkers, who also showed depletion of the putative neurotransmitter by reserpine and its replenishment by dopa (Carlsson *et al.*, 1958).

Measurements of regional concentrations of dopamine in human brains provided the basic link between laboratory studies and clinical applications. Bertler and Rosengren (1959) and Carlsson (1959) found that about 80% of the dopamine in the human brain is concentrated in the basal ganglia, mostly in the caudate nucleus and putamen (corpus striatum). The pivotal discovery by Ehringer and Hornykiewicz (1960) that there is a marked deficiency of striatal dopamine (10% or less of normal) in the basal ganglia of patients with parkinsonism furnished the crucial evidence. The degree of deficiency correlated with the loss of melanin-containing neurons in the pars compacta of the substantia nigra, the most consistent pathological finding of parkinsonism. Mann and Yates (1983) found that the cells in the substantia nigra with the highest melanin content were the most reduced in number in brains of patients with Parkinson's disease. Recent studies have also demonstrated a moderate deficiency of dopamine in several regions of the cerebral cortex of such patients (Hornykiewicz and Kish, in Symposium, 1984). Parkinson's disease may be caused by an aggravation of the normal aging process, to which dopamine-containing neurons are especially sensitive (Rinne, 1982; Mann and Yates, 1983; Calne, 1984).

Since dopamine does not pass the blood-brain barrier when administered systemically, it has no therapeutic effect in parkinsonism. However, levodopa, the immediate metabolic precursor of dopamine, does permeate into striatal tissue, where it is decarboxylated to dopamine. Initial clinical trials with small intravenous doses of D,L-dopa provided encouraging results, but the drug caused prominent adverse reactions. Cotzias and associates (1967) first clearly demonstrated that small, gradual increments in oral dosage minimized unwanted effects of D,L-dopa. These clinical studies demonstrated the value of replenishment of depleted stores of dopamine in parkinsonism and fulfilled the predic-

tion made by the basic scientists in the previous decade. The clinical findings were quickly confirmed and extended in a number of trials with the active isomer, levodopa, which proved more effective than the racemic mixture. Several symposia and extensive reviews on the use of levodopa in parkinsonism have been published (*see* Bianchine, 1976; Yahr, 1978; Symposium, 1980; Rose and Capildeo, 1981; Fahn *et al.*, 1983; Symposium, 1984). The introduction of levodopa has been critically important not only for the care of the majority of patients with Parkinson's disease but also because it provided the first outstanding example of the successful therapeutic application of biochemically derived information to a chronic degenerative neurological disorder. The very reasonable expectation is that similar neurochemical approaches will lead to advances in therapy of other debilitating diseases of the nervous system (Klawans *et al.*, 1977; Calne *et al.*, 1979; Symposium, 1980).

LEVODOPA

The introduction of levodopa, L-3,4-dihydroxyphenylalanine, for the treatment of Parkinson's disease was followed by prompt and enthusiastic recognition of its remarkable therapeutic action in the majority of cases. The later introduction of "potentiators" of levodopa (dopa decarboxylase inhibitors) has further augmented the clinical value of this drug.

Chemistry. Levodopa is formed from L-tyrosine as an intermediary in the enzymatic synthesis of catecholamines. Dopamine is synthesized directly from levodopa by a cytoplasmic enzyme, aromatic L-amino acid decarboxylase. The structures of levodopa and dopamine are shown in Figure 21–1 (page 478).

There is a continuing search to find specific and useful analogs of dopamine for the treatment of Parkinson's disease (*see* Goldberg *et al.*, 1978). Two such classes of dopaminergic agonists, the aporphines and the ergolines, are described briefly below. Structural similarities between dopamine and prototypes of these classes of dopaminergic agonists are shown in Figure 21–2 (page 482). As expected, these agonists share many pharmacological properties with levodopa.

PHARMACOLOGICAL PROPERTIES

The main effects of levodopa are produced by the product of its decarboxylation, dopamine; levodopa, as such, is practically inert pharmacologically. Since about 95% of orally administered levodopa is rapidly decarboxylated in the periphery to dopamine, which does not penetrate the blood-brain barrier, large doses must be taken to allow sufficient accumulation of levodopa in the brain, where its decarboxylation raises the central dopamine concentration. Alternatively, the concurrent administration of peripherally acting inhibitors of dopa decarboxylase can reduce the required dose of levodopa (*see* below). Tolerance to therapeutic doses of levodopa is achieved only by gradual upward titration over a period of weeks until a maximal clinical response is obtained or until unacceptable side effects emerge.

Approximately 75% of patients with parkinsonism respond at least reasonably well to levodopa. Therapeutic response in some patients is seemingly "miraculous," especially at the outset. Essentially all signs and symptoms of parkinsonism except dementia can respond to the administration of this agent (Barbeau, 1981).

Central Nervous System. The pharmacological effects of levodopa on muscle tone and movement are not seen in normal individuals. Bradykinesia and rigidity usually respond more quickly and consistently than does tremor, but a significant reduction in tremor is often obtained with continued therapy. Amelioration of these primary neurological symptoms is accompanied by similar improvements in overall functional ability. Secondary motor manifestations such as disturbances in posture, gait, associated movements, facial expression, speech, handwriting, swallowing, and respiration are also proportionately improved.

Psychic Effects. In many patients, levodopa at least partially relieves the changes in mood that are characteristic of Parkinson's disease. Early in therapy, feelings of apathy are generally replaced by increased vigor and a sense of well-being. The result is described as a general alerting response characterized by apparent improvement in mental function and an increased interest in self, surroundings, and family. However, a significant number of patients develop serious behavioral side effects, which are dis-

cussed below. As mentioned, there is no evidence that levodopa improves the symptoms of dementia, present in up to one third of patients with Parkinson's disease.

Cardiovascular System. Peripheral decarboxylation of levodopa markedly increases the concentration of dopamine in blood. Dopamine is a pharmacologically active catecholamine with prominent effects on α- and β-adrenergic receptors, although its potency is much less than that of epinephrine, norepinephrine, or isoproterenol (Goldberg *et al.*, 1978). The reluctance of early investigators to test the effects of high doses of levodopa for parkinsonism rested largely on the expectation of potentially toxic cardiovascular effects, particularly hypertension and cardiac dysrhythmias. Contrary to such expectation, therapeutic doses of levodopa frequently cause only modest and asymptomatic *orthostatic hypotension;* tolerance to this effect develops within a few weeks of chronic treatment. The mechanism by which levodopa produces hypotension is not fully understood.

Therapeutic doses of levodopa produce *cardiac stimulation* by an action of dopamine on β-adrenergic receptors. Transient tachycardia and other cardiac arrhythmias may occur in some patients, and myocardial contractility may be increased for several hours after a large dose of levodopa, especially early in therapy. Tolerance to these effects also develops after several weeks of chronic treatment. The cardiac effects of levodopa mediated by dopamine are usually blocked by β-adrenergic antagonists such as propranolol.

Oral administration of levodopa to patients with severe congestive heart failure can cause a sustained improvement in cardiac function (Rajfer *et al.*, 1984). Peak hemodynamic responses occur 1 hour after ingestion of the drug; these include an increase in cardiac index and a decrease in systemic vascular resistance. The effects may be due to the activation of β_1-adrenergic and dopaminergic receptors.

Metabolic and Endocrine Effects. The tuberoinfundibular neurons of the hypothalamus comprise a major central dopaminergic system. These neurons play an important and as yet incompletely defined role in the modulation of hypothalamic-pituitary function (*see* Chapter 59). Dopamine inhibits the secretion of prolactin in man; it acts directly on the relevant cells of the adenohypophysis and may also stimulate the release of a prolactin inhibitory factor. Thus, levodopa and other dopaminergic agonists decrease the secretion of prolactin, while dopaminergic antagonists have an opposite effect. However, studies suggest that hypothalamic regulation of the adenohypophysis may be abnormal in Parkinson's disease (Langston and Forno, 1978). Consequently, the release of growth hormone that is noted in response to the administration of levodopa in normal subjects (*see* Chapter 59) is minimal or absent when levodopa is administered to patients with Parkinson's disease (Eddy *et al.*, 1971). A hypothalamic defect in the regulation of growth hormone might explain why earlier predictions of the production of acromegaly (or diabetes mellitus) in patients receiving levodopa have proven to be false (Sirtori *et al.,* 1972). Inhibition of prolactin secretion is useful in a variety of clinical situations.

Mechanism of Action. Since abundant evidence suggests that parkinsonism is a syndrome of deficiency of striatal dopamine, it follows that the immediate metabolic precursor of dopamine, levodopa, would act by replenishing these depleted stores. Evidence in favor of this mechanism includes a positive correlation between the symptoms of Parkinson's disease and loss of nigrostriatal neurons. Furthermore, the brains of patients with Parkinson's disease who had received high doses of levodopa until death contain concentrations of dopamine in the striatum that are five to eight times higher than those in untreated patients and that appear to be correlated with their clinical response to the drug. These findings indicate that dopamine storage capacity of the terminals of the nigrostriatal fibers is not completely lost in patients with parkinsonism. The striatal concentration of aromatic L-amino acid decarboxylase, the enzyme that converts levodopa to dopamine, is markedly reduced in parkinsonism, but sufficient enzymatic activity remains to account for the replenishment of dopamine following the administration of levodopa (*see* Hornykiewicz, 1973a, 1973b).

The actions of dopamine have been studied at the molecular level, and receptors for dopamine have been studied with ligand-binding technics. While the interpretation of much of the data is difficult, the general conclusion is that there are at least two types of receptors for dopamine, designated D_1 and D_2. D_1 receptors can be preferentially labeled with thioxanthenes or certain phenothiazines and appear to stimulate adenylate cyclase activity; D_2 receptors are preferentially labeled with butyrophenones and are thought to inhibit adenylate cyclase in some cases or to be unlinked to the enzyme in others. Despite the fact that dopamine clearly *stimulates* adenylate cyclase activity in homogenates of the basal ganglia, most investigators believe that the beneficial effects of levodopa (and bromocriptine; *see* below) in parkinsonism are mediated via D_2 receptors. Furthermore, the capacity of certain antipsychotic drugs to induce symptoms of the disease is also thought to be an effect exerted predominantly at D_2 receptors. In view of the facts that these brain regions probably contain both D_1 and D_2 receptors (and perhaps others) and that these receptors can have important

presynaptic and postsynaptic functions, it is possible to reconcile the body of information gathered to date. However, it is clear that such reconciliation does not provide the necessary information on the functions of dopamine in the basal ganglia (*see* Leff and Creese, 1983; Kebabian *et al.,* in Symposium, 1984; Snyder, 1984). Other crucial questions, such as how dopamine modulates striatal output and the cause of degeneration of the striatal nerve cells in Parkinson's disease, also remain largely unanswered.

Absorption, Distribution, Fate, and Excretion. Levodopa is rapidly absorbed from the small bowel by an active transport system for aromatic amino acids. Concentrations of the drug in plasma usually peak between 0.5 and 2 hours after an oral dose. The half-life in plasma is short—only 1 to 3 hours. The rate of absorption of levodopa is greatly dependent upon the rate of gastric emptying, the pH of gastric juice, and the length of time the drug is exposed to the degradative enzymes of the gastric mucosa and intestinal flora. For example, sluggish gastric emptying (caused either by intrinsic factors or by anticholinergic drugs), hyperacidity of gastric juice, and competition for absorption sites in the small bowel by amino acids each may interfere with the bioavailability of levodopa (Bianchine and Shaw, 1976). Thus, Nutt and associates (1984) found that administration of levodopa with meals delayed absorption of the drug and reduced peak concentrations in plasma by 30%.

More than 95% of levodopa is decarboxylated in the periphery by the widely distributed aromatic L-amino acid decarboxylase. The drug is extensively decarboxylated in its first passage through the liver, which is rich in decarboxylase, so that relatively little unchanged drug reaches the cerebral circulation and probably less than 1% penetrates into the CNS. Inhibition of peripheral decarboxylase markedly increases the fraction of administered levodopa that remains unmetabolized and available to cross the blood-brain barrier.

The principal metabolic pathways for levodopa are depicted in Figure 21–1. A small amount is methylated to 3-O-methyldopa, which accumulates in the CNS due to its long half-life. Most is converted to dopamine, small amounts of which in turn are metabolized to norepinephrine and epi-

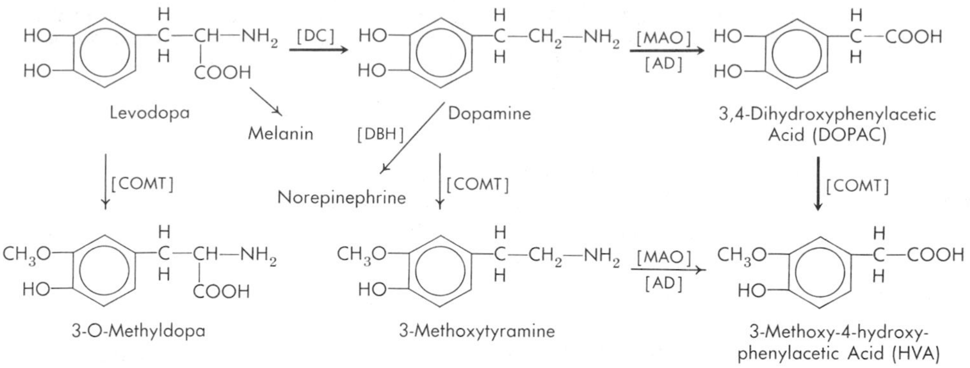

Levodopa   [DC]   Dopamine   [MAO] [AD]   3,4-Dihydroxyphenylacetic Acid (DOPAC)

Melanin   [DBH]   Norepinephrine

[COMT]   [COMT]   [COMT]

3-O-Methyldopa   3-Methoxytyramine   [MAO] [AD]   3-Methoxy-4-hydroxy-phenylacetic Acid (HVA)

Figure 21–1. *Important catabolic pathways of levodopa (L-dopa).*

Major pathways are shown by heavy arrows; minor pathways, by light arrows. *AD,* aldehyde dehydrogenase; *COMT,* catechol-O-methyltransferase; *DBH,* dopamine β-hydroxylase; *DC,* aromatic L-amino acid decarboxylase; *MAO,* monoamine oxidase. (For biosynthetic pathway, *see* Figure 4–3, p. 82.)

nephrine. Biotransformation of dopamine proceeds rapidly to yield the principal excretion products, 3,4-dihydroxyphenylacetic acid (DOPAC) and 3-methoxy-4-hydroxyphenylacetic acid (homovanillic acid, HVA). At least 30 metabolites of levodopa have been identified (Goodall and Alton, 1969). Several of these have powerful pharmacological effects that contribute to the spectrum of toxicity. Some evidence indicates that the metabolism of levodopa may be accelerated during prolonged therapy, possibly due to enzyme induction.

Metabolites of dopamine are rapidly excreted in the urine; about 80% of a radioactively labeled dose is recovered within 24 hours. The principal metabolites, DOPAC and HVA, account for up to 50% of the administered dose. These metabolites, as well as small amounts of levodopa and dopamine, also appear in the cerebrospinal fluid. Negligible amounts are found in the feces. After prolonged therapy with levodopa, the ratio of DOPAC to HVA excreted may increase, probably reflecting a depletion of methyl donors necessary for metabolism by catechol-O-methyl transferase; it is estimated that about three fourths of dietary methionine is utilized for the metabolism of large therapeutic doses of levodopa.

Side Effects and Toxicity. Careful and judicious administration of levodopa to an informed and cooperative patient is essential to optimize the ratio of benefit to toxicity (Marx, 1979; Fahn *et al.,* 1983). The majority of patients with Parkinson's disease who are treated with levodopa experience side effects. Their intensity and type vary greatly at different stages of therapy. Although many are relatively innocuous, others are troublesome and necessitate reduction in dosage or complete withdrawal of the drug. Side effects are generally dose dependent and reversible. Elderly patients are especially intolerant of large doses. The concurrent administration of levodopa and a peripheral inhibitor of dopa decarboxylase is the most effective means of decreasing the extracerebral side effects of levodopa (*see* below).

The most common side effects *early* in therapy with levodopa are nausea and vomiting. Cardiac arrhythmias occur in some patients, especially those with preexisting disturbances in cardiac conduction. The majority of patients on *long-term* therapy develop abnormal involuntary movements, which vary considerably in pattern and severity and often limit the tolerated dosage of levodopa. Psychiatric disturbances are produced by levodopa in a significant proportion of patients and frequently limit the dose that can be tolerated. All side effects are reversible and can generally be controlled by a reduction in dosage.

Because of these potential side effects, it is important to exercise very special care in the administration of levodopa to patients with coronary insufficiency, cardiac arrhythmias, occlusive cerebrovascular disease, affective disorders, or major psychoses.

Gastrointestinal. About 80% of patients experience anorexia, nausea, vomiting, or epigastric distress early in the course of treatment with levodopa. This is caused partially by stimulation of the medullary emetic center and is most likely to occur if dosage is increased too rapidly, if individual doses are too large, or if the drug is taken without food. Anorexia may result in transient weight loss in some patients. These symptoms are controlled by concurrent administration of food or by lowering of the dosage administered. Although certain phenothiazines are highly effective antiemetic drugs, they should not be used for the control of nausea in this situation, since they interfere with the action of dopamine at striatal receptor sites. Gastrointestinal side effects tend to disappear with continuing therapy as tolerance develops. Bleeding and perforation of peptic ulcers have been reported in a few patients.

Hypotension. About 30% of patients develop slight orthostatic hypotension early in therapy. It is usually asymptomatic, but some patients experience dizziness and, rarely, syncope. Careful regulation of dosage is necessary in such individuals, and the usual measures for controlling orthostatic hypotension should be employed. Despite continuation of therapy, blood pressure tends to return to values that obtained prior to treatment. The mechanism that underlies this effect remains unclear.

Cardiac Irregularities. Cardiac arrhythmias are not uncommon in the older-age group of patients with Parkinson's disease; consequently, a direct association between the development of an arrhythmia and therapy with levodopa is difficult to establish. However, the β-adrenergic action of dopamine on the heart, as well as direct β-adrenergic receptor stimulation by other catecholamine metabolites of the drug, presents a potentially serious side effect of levodopa. Fortunately, the incidence of arrhythmias is low. Sinus tachycardia, atrial and ventricular extrasystoles, atrial flutter and fibrillation, and ventricular tachycardia have been reported. These cardiac arrhythmias, which are more likely to occur in patients with coronary artery disease, can usually be controlled by the administration of a β-adrenergic antagonist.

Abnormal Involuntary Movements. These movements appear in approximately 50% of patients within 2 to 4 months after the initiation of treatment with levodopa. Unfortunately, they often coincide temporally with what would otherwise be optimal improvement. They appear with increasing frequency as drug administration continues and are directly related to the dose of the drug and to the degree of clinical improvement. About 80% of patients on full therapeutic doses for a year or longer will develop some abnormal movements (Fahn *et al.*, 1983).

The abnormal involuntary movements are variable in type and include faciolingual tics, grimacing, head bobbing, and various oscillatory and rocking movements of the arms, legs, or trunk. Rarely, exaggerated respiratory movements can produce an irregular gasping pattern or hyperventilation. Tolerance does not develop to this side effect; in fact, the symptoms tend to increase in severity if the dosage is not reduced (Fahn *et al.*, 1983). Although such movements are abolished by a decrease in the dose of levodopa or by the administration of pyridoxine, it is unfortunate that both these maneuvers reduce the therapeutic efficacy of levodopa as well. Therefore, the physician must carefully titrate the dose and time of administration of levodopa to maximize the therapeutic benefit while minimizing side effects. These abnormal involuntary movements are the most important side effect of levodopa that limits the dose that can be given. No satisfactory means, pharmacological or otherwise, has yet been found to antagonize this side effect selectively.

Behavioral Disturbances. Levodopa can cause hallucinations, paranoia, mania, insomnia, anxiety, nightmares, and emotional depression, particularly in elderly patients (Yahr, 1978). The actions of levodopa on the hypothalamus may cause renewed sexual interest, and this can cause additional behavioral changes.

Serious behavioral disturbances occur in about 15% of patients who receive levodopa and usually require reduction of dosage or, for some, complete withdrawal of the drug. One of the more common disturbances resembles an organic brain syndrome and is characterized by confusion, sometimes progressing to frank delirium. Although the mental depression of many patients is often improved by levodopa, some appear to develop a more severe depression, which in a few cases has led to suicidal gestures. Tricyclic antidepressant drugs have been helpful in some cases. Fully developed psychotic reactions with paranoid delusions or hallucinations are most likely to occur in patients with a history of mental disorder, organic brain syndrome including dementia, or postencephalitic parkinsonism (Sacks *et al.*, 1972). A few patients develop classical symptoms of hypomania, one manifestation of which may be inappropriate or excessive sexual behavior.

Abnormalities of Laboratory Tests. Urinary metabolites of levodopa cause false-positive tests for ketoacidosis by the dip-stick test; they also color the urine red, then black, on exposure to air or alkali.

Interactions with Other Drugs. Decarboxylation of levodopa to dopamine is catalyzed by the pyridoxine-dependent enzyme L-amino acid decarboxylase, and doses of *pyridoxine* that are only modestly in excess of the recommended dietary allowance enhance the extracerebral metabolism of levodopa. Consequently, when administered with levodopa, pyridoxine may completely reverse its therapeutic effect or promptly reduce its toxic side effects, depending on the clinical circumstances. Patients should be aware that pyridoxine is present in many *multivitamin preparations* in amounts in excess of 5 mg. A multivitamin preparation that does not contain pyridoxine is available. It is important to note that, when levodopa is coadministered with an inhibitor of L-amino acid decarboxylase, the interactive antagonistic effect of pyridoxine is lost (Yahr, 1975).

Antipsychotic drugs, such as *phenothiazines, butyrophenones,* and *reserpine,* can produce a parkinsonism-like syndrome. Reserpine acts by depleting stores of central dopamine, while the other agents block receptors for dopamine. Since these drugs nullify the therapeutic effects of levodopa, they are contraindicated. This possible etiological drug factor should be considered in every newly diagnosed case of parkinsonism. If the exposure to these antipsychotic drugs was short, it is likely that their prompt withdrawal alone will cause disappearance of symptoms of parkinsonism. As previously mentioned, the phenothiazines should not be used to combat the emetic effect of levodopa.

Nonspecific monoamine oxidase inhibitors, such as *phenelzine* and *isocarboxazid,* interfere with inactivation of dopamine, norepinephrine, and other catecholamines. Hence, they exaggerate, unpredictably, the central effects of levodopa and its catecholamine metabolites; hypertensive crisis and hyperpyrexia are very real and dangerous sequelae of their administration with levodopa. A monoamine oxidase inhibitor should be withdrawn at least 14 days prior to the administration of levodopa. It is interesting to note that a selective inhibitor of monoamine oxidase B has been under investigation as a drug for Parkinson's disease (*see* below).

Anticholinergic drugs, such as *trihexyphenidyl, benztropine, procyclidine,* and others, act synergistically with levodopa to improve certain symptoms of parkinsonism, especially tremor. However, large doses of anticholinergic drugs can slow gastric emptying sufficiently to cause a delay in the absorption of levodopa by the small bowel. This effect can be so pronounced as to detract from the therapeutic benefit of levodopa (Bianchine and Sunyapridakul, 1973).

Preparations and Dosage. *Levodopa* (DOPAR, LARODOPA) is available for oral use as tablets or capsules containing 100, 250, or 500 mg of the drug.

The optimal maintenance dosage of levodopa is determined by careful titration in each patient. When levodopa is given alone, the usual initial dose is 0.5 to 1 g daily, divided into two or more equal portions. The total daily dosage is then gradually increased by increments of 100 to 750 mg, every 3 to 7 days. The rate of increase in dosage is determined primarily by the patient's tolerance to nausea and vomiting. Significant objective improvement may appear during the second or third week as the daily dosage reaches 2 to 3 g. Further benefit accrues gradually with increasing dosage, even after the dose is stabilized at an apparently optimal level. Good therapeutic responses are not reached in some patients for as long as 1 to 6 months. Therefore, levodopa should not be considered ineffective until full doses have been administered for such periods. In general, younger patients with less severe symptoms derive greater benefit than do severely debilitated, elderly patients in whom maximal tolerated doses are often limited by side effects. The usual daily maintenance dose ranges from 3 to 8 g, taken in three or more divided doses. More frequent administration of smaller doses may reduce side effects and yield better results.

INHIBITORS OF AROMATIC L-AMINO ACID DECARBOXYLASE

Concurrent administration of levodopa with an inhibitor of aromatic L-amino acid (dopa) decarboxylase that is unable to penetrate into the CNS readily diminishes the decarboxylation of levodopa in peripheral tissues. Such reduction allows a greater proportion of levodopa to reach the desired receptor sites in the nigrostriatum. Concentrations of levodopa in plasma are higher and the half-life is longer after concurrent administration of a decarboxylase inhibitor and levodopa than when levodopa is given alone (Bianchine and Shaw, 1976). At present, *carbidopa* is the only such inhibitor that is clinically available in the United States, and it is supplied in combination with levodopa. *Benserazide* has similar properties and is marketed in Europe and Canada (Palfreyman *et al.,* 1978). Carbidopa has the following structure:

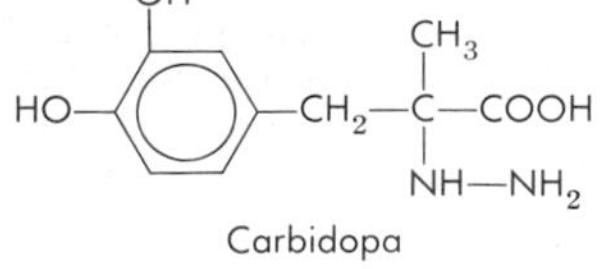

Carbidopa

Several clinical studies have clearly demonstrated distinct advantages of combined therapy with a decarboxylase inhibitor and levodopa. These may be summarized as follows: (1) The optimally effective dose of levodopa can be reduced by about 75%. (2) Nausea and vomiting from stimulation of receptors for dopamine in the medullary emetic center are largely eliminated. Likewise, the cardiac side effects are diminished or prevented. (3) Effective dosage of levodopa can be achieved much more quickly during initial therapy since the necessity to develop tolerance to the peripheral effects of dopamine is minimized. (4) Antagonism of the therapeutic efficacy of levodopa by pyridoxine is avoided. (5) The frequency and intensity of diurnal variations in control of symptoms by levodopa are reduced, presumably by avoidance of large fluctuations of the concentration of dopamine in the CNS. The number of divided doses per day may often be reduced without loss of control. (6) The percentage of patients who are improved and the degree of improvement appear to be somewhat greater than with levodopa alone (Yahr, 1978; Calne, 1984).

However, some of the problems of therapy with levodopa are not resolved by the concomitant use of peripheral decarboxylase inhibitors. Abnormal involuntary movements not only occur with the same frequency but also tend to develop earlier in therapy and may be more severe. Adverse mental effects also occur with about the same frequency but appear earlier in the course of therapy.

Untoward Effects. In recommended doses the peripheral decarboxylase inhibitors that are currently employed are essentially devoid of pharmacological activity when administered alone, and toxic effects have not been observed (Chase and Watanabe, 1972; Papavasiliou *et al.*, 1972). However, when administered in combination with levodopa, carbidopa generally will enhance, quantitatively, the pharmacological action of levodopa. In this sense, the side effects of carbidopa when administered with levodopa are those associated with enhancement of the effects of levodopa.

Preparations and Dosage. Carbidopa is available in scored tablets that contain 10 or 25 mg of the drug in combination with 100 mg of levodopa (SINEMET 10/100 or 25/100) or that contain 25 mg of carbidopa and 250 mg of levodopa (SINEMET 25/250). Physicians can obtain carbidopa as a single agent (LODOSYN) upon request of the manufacturer.

Generally, therapy is initiated with three or four tablets (100 mg of levodopa, 10 or 25 mg of carbidopa) daily in divided doses. This provides an amount of carbidopa sufficient to inhibit peripheral dopa decarboxylase activity maximally in most patients. If a greater therapeutic effect is needed, the dose can be increased progressively to a daily maximum of about 2000 mg of levodopa and 200 mg of carbidopa. For patients treated previously with levodopa alone, dosage with levodopa must be withheld overnight (8 hours) before starting the combination of levodopa and carbidopa. As a first approximation, the total daily dosage of levodopa must be reduced by approximately 75%.

AMANTADINE

Amantadine, introduced as an antiviral agent for the prophylaxis of A_2 influenza (*see* Chapter 54), was unexpectedly found to cause symptomatic improvement of patients with parkinsonism (Schwab *et al.*, 1972). This drug probably acts by releasing dopamine from intact dopaminergic terminals that remain in the nigrostriatum of patients with Parkinson's disease. Because of this facilitated release of dopamine, it appears that the therapeutic efficacy of amantadine is enhanced by the concurrent administration of levodopa. However, patients receiving near-maximal benefit from levodopa generally experience little additional improvement from amantadine.

Many studies confirm that amantadine is clearly less efficacious than levodopa but slightly more so than the anticholinergic drugs (Parkes *et al.*, 1970; Mawdsley *et al.*, 1972). Amantadine acts maximally within a few days but usually loses a portion of its efficacy within 6 to 8 weeks of continuous treatment. Consequently, many physicians use amantadine episodically for short (2- to 3-week) intervals whenever the patient requires additional therapeutic assistance.

Amantadine is readily absorbed from the gastrointestinal tract and has a relatively long duration of action. It is excreted unchanged in the urine and, therefore, can accumulate in the body when renal function is inadequate.

Mechanism of Action. Amantadine was observed to release dopamine from peripheral neuronal storage sites of animals who have received infusions of the transmitters; this peripheral effect suggested that amantadine might exert a similar action on the residual, intact dopaminergic terminals in the striatum of patients with parkinsonism. Amantadine causes release of dopamine from central neurons and facilitates its release by nerve impulses. Release of dopamine by amantadine may also occur from central sites other than nigrostriatal neurons. Amantadine has also been shown to delay the re-uptake of dopamine by neural cells, and it may have anticholinergic effects as well (*see* Lang, in Symposium, 1984).

Untoward Effects. Compared to levodopa or anticholinergic agents, amantadine is relatively free of side effects. They are generally mild, often transient, and always reversible. Their incidence and severity increase markedly when the daily dosage exceeds 200 mg. Hallucinations, confusion, and nightmares are more common when the drug is administered concurrently with anticholinergic agents or when the patient has an underlying psychiatric disorder. Insomnia, dizziness, lethargy, drowsiness, and slurred speech have also been reported. Nausea, vomiting, anorexia, and constipation occur infrequently (Forssman *et al.*, 1972).

Long-term use of amantadine may result in the appearance of *livedo reticularis* in the lower extremities. Although this complication is often cosmetically unacceptable, it merely reflects the local release of catecholamines with resultant vasoconstriction (Pearce *et al.*, 1974).

Preparations and Dosage. *Amantadine hydrochloride* (SYMMETREL) is available as 100-mg capsules and in a syrup containing 50 mg/5 ml. The usual dose is 100 mg, given twice daily.

APORPHINES

Apomorphine, commonly used as an emetic in the management of oral ingestion of certain poisons or oral drug overdosage, was the first dopaminergic agonist reported to have beneficial effects in Parkinson's disease. Because of renal damage associated with the chronic administration of large doses of apomorphine, Cotzias and associates (1976) shifted their investigations to N-propylnoraporphine, an analog of apomorphine. Compounds of this type remain under investigation.

ERGOLINES

Several ergot derivatives demonstrate dopaminergic activity in animal models of parkinsonism and mimic the neuroendocrinological effects of dopamine on the secretion of prolactin and growth hormone (*see* Chapter 39). These derivatives include bromocriptine, lisuride, pergolide, and mesulergine. Clinical trials of another derivative, lergotrile, were terminated because of hepatotoxicity. Bromocriptine has been studied most thoroughly and hence logically serves as a prototype for the ergolines. Its structure is shown in Figure 21–2. Bromocriptine is a derivative of lysergic acid (*see* Table 39–1). The addition of the bromine atom renders this alkaloid a potent dopaminergic agonist, with preference for D_2 receptors. Virtually all the pharmacological actions of bromocriptine result from stimulation of dopamine receptors in the CNS, cardiovascular system, pituitary-hypothalamic axis (Chapter 59), and gastrointestinal tract.

The following observations on the use of bromocriptine in parkinsonism have been established: (1)

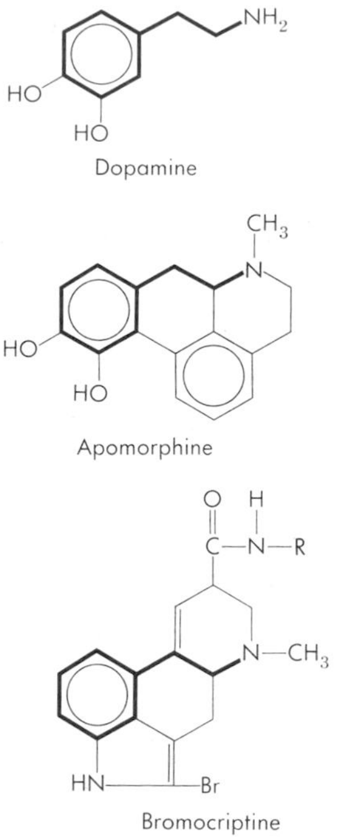

Figure 21–2. *Structural similarities (heavy lines) between dopamine, apomorphine, and bromocriptine.*

The complete structure of bromocriptine is shown in Table 39–1.

Patients with parkinsonism who experience excessive "on-off" phenomenon (*see* below) or who are not reasonably controlled with levodopa (or by the combination of levodopa and carbidopa) may be managed more smoothly when bromocriptine is added to the therapeutic regimen. This may be the main clinical value of bromocriptine. (2) In many patients with Parkinson's disease, high doses of bromocriptine (50 to 100 mg) elicit therapeutic responses that are equivalent to those obtained with levodopa. (3) Optimal clinical results may be achieved by a combination of submaximal doses of bromocriptine and levodopa (Lieberman *et al.*, 1979; Stern and Lees, 1983). (4) Visual and auditory hallucinations are more frequent with bromocriptine than with levodopa. (5) Symptomatic hypotension and cutaneous *livedo reticularis* are far more common with bromocriptine than with levodopa. (6) Bromocriptine induces less dyskinesia than does levodopa. (7) Similar to levodopa, bromocriptine induces a nonspecific arousal of the CNS that may be effective in treating patients who are comatose because of hepatic encephalopathy (Jellinger, 1982).

Bromocriptine is rapidly but only partially (about 30%) absorbed from the gastrointestinal tract. First-pass metabolism is extensive, such that systemic bioavailability is only a small fraction of the administered dose. Peak concentrations in plasma are found 1.5 to 3 hours after oral administration, and the half-life in plasma is about 3 hours. Many of the metabolites of bromocriptine have not been identified, but they do not appear to be active (Aellig and Neuesch, 1977); most are excreted in the bile.

Adverse effects of bromocriptine are generally related to its activity as a dopaminergic agonist. As with levodopa, these effects can be separated into two major groups—those effects noted with initiation of therapy, and those associated with long-term treatment. Initial side effects include nausea, vomiting, and postural hypotension. Unlike levodopa, there is a "first-dose phenomenon," manifested by sudden cardiovascular collapse (Linch et al., 1978). With long-term treatment constipation, erythromelalgia, psychiatric reactions, dyskinesia, alcohol intolerance, and digital vasospasm may be noted.

Bromocriptine mesylate (PARLODEL) is available in 2.5-mg tablets and 5-mg capsules. It is used as an adjunct to levodopa for the treatment of Parkinson's disease (with or without a peripheral decarboxylase inhibitor) (Keller and Daprada, 1979; Lieberman et al., 1979; Fahn et al., 1983). The initial dose of bromocriptine is 1.25 mg, given twice daily with meals. This is increased every 2 to 4 weeks by 2.5 mg per day. The maximal dose is 100 mg per day. Bromocriptine is also indicated for the therapy of hyperprolactinemia in a variety of clinical situations, including lactation, infertility, and amenorrhea-galactorrhea. In addition, it has been used as an adjunctive agent in the treatment of pituitary tumors associated with hyperprolactinemia or acromegaly (*see* Chapter 59). The initial dose of bromocriptine in the therapy of hyperprolactinemia is 2.5 mg, and most patients respond to a total daily dose of 5 to 7.5 mg. The use of bromocriptine has been reviewed by Vance and associates (1984).

SELEGILINE (DEPRENYL)

There are two isoenzymes that oxidize monoamines. While both isoenzymes (monoamine oxidase [MAO] A and B) are present in the periphery and inactivate monoamines of intestinal origin, the isoenzyme MAO-B predominates in certain regions of the CNS (*see* Chapter 19). Selegiline (deprenyl; phenylisopropyl-N-methylpropynylamine) is a highly selective inhibitor of MAO-B (Birkmayer et al., 1977; Yahr, 1978; Eisler et al., 1981; Riederer et al., 1983). In striking contrast to the known nonspecific MAO inhibitors (*e.g.*, phenelzine and isocarboxazid), selegiline does not cause profound and potentially lethal potentiation of the effects of catecholamines when administered concurrently with a centrally effective amine. For example, a patient receiving selegiline may eat cheeses (that contain tyramine) or take levodopa without danger. However, administration of selegiline inhibits the intracerebral metabolic degradation of dopamine. The resultant preservation of dopamine in the basal ganglia appears to enhance the therapeutic efficacy of levodopa. Consequently, when selegiline is added to the therapeutic

regimen, the dose of levodopa can be reduced without loss of therapeutic benefit. While clinical trials with this compound indicate beneficial effects, the improvement may be brief. The drug is unfortunately of very limited value in patients with advanced disease. Selegiline is not approved for general use in the United States.

ANTICHOLINERGIC DRUGS

Anticholinergic agents were the most effective drugs for treatment of Parkinson's disease for more than a century. However, the introduction of levodopa and, more recently, the availability of decarboxylase inhibitors such as carbidopa have relegated anticholinergics to a supportive role in the treatment of the disorder. Nonetheless, the anticholinergic drugs are still very useful for patients with minimal symptoms, for those unable to tolerate levodopa because of side effects or contraindications, and for those who are not benefited by levodopa. Furthermore, more than half the patients who derive therapeutic benefit from levodopa experience further amelioration of symptoms after supplemental treatment with an anticholinergic drug. These drugs are also useful to alleviate the parkinsonism-like syndrome induced by antipsychotic drugs.

The deficiency of dopamine in the striatum of patients with parkinsonism intensifies the excitatory effects of the cholinergic system within the striatum. Anticholinergics aid such patients by blunting this component of the nigrostriatal pathway (Calne, 1978).

PHARMACOLOGICAL PROPERTIES

Trihexyphenidyl, the prototype of this group of drugs, qualitatively resembles the belladonna alkaloids in its pharmacological actions and side effects (*see* Chapter 7). The drug favorably influences the tremor that is characteristic of parkinsonism. It is less effective in improving rigidity and bradykinesia. Among the secondary symptoms of parkinsonism, the anticholinergic agents improve excessive sialorrhea by inhibiting salivary secretion. Although the peripheral anticholinergic actions of the synthetic compounds selected for use in Parkinson's disease are less prominent than are those of the natural antimuscarinic alkaloids such as atropine, side effects of cycloplegia, constipation, and urinary retention may become troublesome, especially for the aged patient.

Side effects referable to the CNS, such as mental confusion, delirium, somnolence, and hallucinations, may also limit the utility of these drugs. Although there are essentially no pharmacological differences among the anticholinergic agents commonly used in parkinsonism, certain patients clearly appear to tolerate one preparation better than another.

The anticholinergic drugs used for the treatment of Parkinson's disease are listed in Table 21–1, as are certain antihistamines. The antihistamines listed in Table 21–1 are structurally related to diphenhydramine, possess some central anticholinergic properties, and are well tolerated, especially by elderly patients. While these antihistamines produce fewer side effects, they are not as efficacious as are the anticholinergic agents. Their sedative effect may be helpful in certain patients.

Preparations and Dosage. Patients should be started at the lower end of the range of daily dosage listed in Table 21–1, and this should be divided into two to four equal portions. Dosage should then be gradually increased until there is maximal improvement or, more likely, until the onset of intolerable side effects. It is especially important to tailor the medication to achieve the optimal balance between control of the disabling symptoms and the adverse reactions to the drugs. The optimal dose of a given drug for a particular individual cannot be stated. In general, elderly patients are less able to tolerate large doses of the drugs than are young patients. The drugs with prominent peripheral anticholinergic effects must be used with great caution in individuals suffering from narrow-angle glaucoma or urinary retention secondary to disorders of the prostate.

THERAPEUTIC USES OF DRUGS FOR PARKINSON'S DISEASE

Many aspects of the clinical use of levodopa, the combination of levodopa and carbidopa, and other dopaminergic drugs have been described in the preceding pages. The relative importance of these drugs is still not certain. Most neurologists agree that the combination of levodopa with the decarboxylase inhibitor is now the most effective preparation available for treatment of Parkinson's disease (Calne, 1984). A major controversy in the treatment of Parkinson's disease centers around the timing of initiation of treatment with levodopa. Some favor delaying such therapy, since there is evidence that relates drug-induced dyskinesias and fluctuations of response ("on-off" phenomenon) to the duration of therapy with levodopa (Fahn *et al.,* in Symposium, 1984). However, a number of investigators have concluded that drug-induced dyskinesias and fluctuations of response are a manifestation of the progression of the underlying disease, as opposed to the duration of levodopa therapy. This would support the view that treatment with levodopa should be initiated early in the course of the illness (Meunter, in Symposium, 1984).

Yahr (1978) distinguished two phases of treatment with levodopa. There is an initial induction phase that lasts several weeks and a subsequent, long-term maintenance phase. During the induction phase, the daily dosage of levodopa is increased slowly to minimize the likelihood of side effects such as insomnia, nausea, and anorexia. *One critical factor in successful therapy during this phase is the careful and slow titration of dosage for each patient.* This point can hardly be overemphasized. Too rapid an increase in dosage generally results in a therapeutic failure because of side effects and toxicity. The full benefits of treatment with levodopa become apparent in the maintenance phase; this level of improvement generally lasts for about 2 years. However, careful monitoring of the patient and judicious modification of all the therapeutic measures are required to maintain a desirable response. Attempts to eradicate every vestige of symptoms of parkinsonism with levodopa usually require doses that cause unacceptable side effects. Two major limiting factors of long-term therapy with levodopa are the development of abnormal involuntary movements and the "on-off" phenomenon. As mentioned above, it is not clear why both these undesirable effects are so delayed in appearance. Day-to-day and even within-the-day variations in the severity of symptoms have always been among the most characteristic features of parkinsonism. Treatment with levodopa has greatly increased their complexity and importance (Calne, 1984). The swings from "on" and "off" periods essentially represent a marked change from mobility to relative immobility. These fluctuations may occur many times a day and often with startling rapidity. "On" periods are usually associated with high or rising concentrations of levodopa in plasma, whereas "off" periods often correlate with low or falling values.

Nutt and associates (1984) carefully evaluated

Table 21–1. MISCELLANEOUS DRUGS FOR PARKINSONISM

DRUG CLASS, NONPROPRIETARY NAME, AND TRADE NAME	CHEMICAL STRUCTURE	DOSAGE FORMS *	RANGE OF AVERAGE DAILY DOSE
Anticholinergic Agents			
Benztropine mesylate (COGENTIN)		T,I	0.5–6 mg
Trihexyphenidyl hydrochloride (ARTANE, others)		T,C(S),E	1–15 mg
Procyclidine hydrochloride (KEMADRIN)		T	7.5–20 mg
Biperiden hydrochloride (AKINETON)		T,I †	2–8 mg
Ethopropazine hydrochloride ‡ (PARSIDOL)		T	50–600 mg
Antihistamines			
Diphenhydramine hydrochloride (BENADRYL, others)	*See* Chapter 26	C,T,E,S,I	75–400 mg
Orphenadrine hydrochloride (DISIPAL)		T	150–250 mg

* T = tablet; I = injection; C(S) = sustained-release capsule; E = elixir; C = capsule; S = syrup.
† As biperiden lactate.
‡ Ethopropazine is a phenothiazine with significant anticholinergic activity.

the clinical responses to oral and intravenous levodopa in patients with the "on-off" phenomenon. They found that meals reduced peak concentrations of levodopa in plasma by about 30% after oral administration of the drug. When intestinal absorption of levodopa was bypassed by constant intravenous infusion, the same patients exhibited a stable clinical state for at least 12 hours. Oral administration of certain hydrophobic amino acids reversed the therapeutic effect of intravenous levodopa, although concentrations of the drug in plasma remained unchanged. These data and others suggest that competition between levodopa and certain amino acids for intestinal absorption and for transport into the brain may contribute to "on-off" phenomena. However, this is unlikely to be the sole explanation.

It is not necessary to discontinue previous anticholinergic medication upon initiation of treatment with levodopa, although the dose of the former drug may need reduction. There is ample evidence that the judicious combination of levodopa and anticholinergic drugs may be beneficial.

Effects of Long-Term Treatment. The result of the initial therapy (1 or 2 years) is usually more impressive than the therapeutic benefit derived from long-term treatment (more than 3 years). Sweet and McDowell (1975) reviewed the outcome of 100 patients 5 years after starting levodopa. The adjusted death rate among patients receiving levodopa was less than that reported before the drug was available. However, the average "functional" status of the patients approaches pretreatment levels after 5 years despite remarkable improvement, particularly between 0.5 and 2 years of therapy. Yahr (1978) postulated that this slow loss of efficacy reflects advancement of the underlying disease (slow but progressive loss of neurons), rather than a specific loss of the effect of levodopa *per se*. Abnormal involuntary movements, rapid oscillations in motor performance ("on-off" phenomena), and postural instability are the major adverse effects of long-term treatment with levodopa or with the combination of levodopa and carbidopa (Barbeau and Pourcher, 1982). Thus, while levodopa does not cure Parkinson's disease, it does provide symptomatic relief for a long time and remains the most effective treatment available for this illness. It makes possible a more self-sufficient existence for a longer time than was possible before the drug became available (Joseph *et al.*, 1978).

Drug Holidays. Desensitization of receptors for dopamine has been hypothesized to account for some of the loss of therapeutic efficacy of dopaminergic agents in the treatment of patients with Parkinson's disease. This has prompted attempts at drug withdrawal (drug holidays), with the goal of allowing receptors to become "resensitized." This practice frequently requires hospitalization of patients to manage the complications associated with a severe exacerbation of symptoms. The benefits of drug holidays have yet to be clearly established (Kofman, in Symposium, 1984).

Drug-Induced Parkinsonism. Parkinsonism, acute dyskinesia, and dystonias that are induced by the phenothiazines and other antipsychotic agents usually respond readily to low doses of anticholinergic drugs. There is some controversy over whether anticholinergic agents should be administered routinely upon the initiation of chronic treatment with antipsychotic drugs in an attempt to prevent or delay the appearance of these symptoms of parkinsonism (*see* Chapter 19).

Miscellaneous Uses of Drugs for Parkinson's Disease. The efficacy of levodopa in Parkinson's disease has prompted clinical trials of the drug for a number of other neurological conditions characterized by disordered extrapyramidal function, such as torsion dystonia, cerebral palsy, and progressive supranuclear palsy. The results have been unimpressive. Administration of levodopa may provoke a nonspecific "awakening" of patients in hepatic coma (Morgan *et al.*, 1977) or coma associated with encephalitis or Reye's syndrome (Chandra, 1978). Levodopa has not been found to be useful for the treatment of any psychiatric disorder; in fact, the drug tends to exacerbate latent or active psychotic states, both organic and functional. In addition, dopaminergic agents are not useful in controlling or reversing the extrapyramidal side effects induced by antipsychotic drugs such as the phenothiazines and butyrophenones, since the latter agents presumably block the activation of dopaminergic receptors.

II. Drug Therapy of Spasticity and Acute Muscle Spasms

Spasticity. Spasticity is not a single disorder. The term is applied relatively globally to abnormalities of regulation of skeletal muscle that result from lesions at various levels in the CNS. A predominant component of such conditions is hyperexcitability of tonic stretch reflexes (heightened muscle tone). Tendon jerks are exaggerated, painful flexor spasms may occur, muscle weakness can be prominent, and there is a loss of dexterity.

The pathophysiology of these disorders is poorly understood but usually appears to include dysfunction of descending pathways (*e.g.*, corticospinal, vestibulospinal, reticulospinal) that exert control over the motoneurons. Disease is rarely limited to the primary corticospinal (pyramidal) tract. The peripheral reflex arcs, although hyperactive because of abnormal control from higher centers, do not appear to be primarily involved in the pathological process. Nevertheless, sites in these arcs, which include afferent fibers from the skin and muscle spindles, interneurons within the spinal cord, and efferent fibers to intrafusal and extrafusal muscle fibers, may be targets for pharmacological intervention to control spasticity. The most effective agents for control of spasticity include two that act predominantly within the CNS, *baclofen* and *diazepam*, and one, *dantrolene*, that acts directly on skeletal muscle. An excellent review of the drug therapy of spasticity is that written by Young and Delwaide (1981).

BACLOFEN

Baclofen is a derivative of the inhibitory neurotransmitter gamma-aminobutyric acid (GABA), and experimentation on its mechanism of action has been guided by this fact. Its structural formula is as follows:

$$Cl-\langle \text{benzene ring} \rangle-CHCH_2COOH$$
$$| $$
$$CH_2NH_2$$

Baclofen

Baclofen is particularly useful to reduce the frequency and severity of flexor or extensor spasms and to reduce increased flexor tone. Since it is effective in patients with complete spinal transections, its primary site of action appears to be in the spinal cord.

Baclofen is believed to exert its antispastic effects by depressing monosynaptic and polysynaptic transmission in the spinal cord. The drug reduces excitatory postsynaptic potentials in motoneurons in the ventral horn without affecting their membrane potential or input resistance (Fukuda et al., 1977). These effects superficially resemble those of GABA, which is released by interneurons in the spinal cord and depolarizes the axonal terminals of primary afferent fibers; this results in presynaptic inhibition of motoneurons. While bicuculline blocks these actions of GABA, the effects of baclofen are not so antagonized. Moreover, baclofen does not cause depolarization of primary afferent nerve terminals. While the underlying mechanisms are not clearly understood, observations of neurons in various regions of the CNS suggest that baclofen can hyperpolarize some cells by increasing potassium conductance (Newberry and Nicoll, 1984) and can inhibit the function of calcium channels in others (Dunlap, 1981). One or both of these actions could contribute to decreased release of excitatory transmitters from primary afferent terminals. There is no evidence that baclofen can increase chloride conductance, the most prominent action of GABA. Since both GABA and baclofen can produce similar bicuculline-insensitive effects under some circumstances, two classes of receptors for GABA (GABA-A and GABA-B) have been proposed. This hypothesis is supported by the demonstration of stereospecific binding sites for l-baclofen; such binding is inhibited by GABA but not by bicuculline or many GABA-mimetic compounds (Bowery et al., 1983). Thus, baclofen may act as an agonist at GABA-B (bicuculline-insensitive) receptors. However, the synaptic functions of such receptors are not yet appreciated.

Baclofen is absorbed rapidly after oral administration, and it has a half-life in plasma of about 3 to 4 hours. It is largely excreted unchanged by the kidney. The use of baclofen may be limited by its adverse effects, which include drowsiness, insomnia, dizziness, weakness, ataxia, and mental confusion. Sudden withdrawal of baclofen after chronic administration may cause auditory and visual hallucinations, anxiety, and tachycardia. Coma, respiratory depression, and seizures have been reported following significant overdosage. The threshold for initiation of seizures may be lowered in patients with epilepsy.

Preparations and Dosage. *Baclofen* (LIORESAL) is available in 10- and 20-mg tablets. Determination of optimal dosage in individual patients requires careful titration. Treatment is initiated with an oral dose of 5 mg, given two or three times daily, and after 3 days the individual dose is increased to 10 mg. The usual maximal dosage is 20 mg, four times daily. Occasionally, total doses of 100 to 150 mg per day may be beneficial. Abrupt withdrawal of the drug should be avoided. Baclofen should be administered cautiously and in decreased dosage to patients with impaired renal function.

Therapeutic Uses. Baclofen is most effective in the treatment of spasticity caused by multiple sclerosis or other diseases of the spinal cord, particularly traumatic lesions. Similar to other muscle relaxants, it may impair the ability of the patient to walk or stand. It is not recommended for the management of the spasticity in rheumatic disorders, stroke, or cerebral palsy, or the muscular rigidity of parkinsonism (Young and Delwaide, 1981).

DIAZEPAM

Diazepam and the other benzodiazepines are discussed in detail in Chapters 17 and 19. The presumed mechanism of action of the benzodiazepines is to enhance the efficiency of GABA-ergic transmission, as discussed in Chapter 17. At the level of the spinal cord, this may be manifest by enhancement of presynaptic inhibition of afferent neuronal terminals in the primary reflex arc. Diazepam is particularly useful for treatment of patients with spinal cord lesions, although it is probably not as effective as baclofen in relieving intermittent flexor spasms (Young and Delwaide, 1981). The drug may occasionally be useful in patients with cerebral palsy. Sedation can limit the efficacy of diazepam as a muscle relaxant, although its sedative and anxiolytic properties may be of value in certain patients (Lossius et al., 1980). The dose of diazepam should be titrated upward gradually to minimize unwanted effects, particularly sedation.

DANTROLENE

Dantrolene is unique in comparison with baclofen and diazepam, in that it exerts its effects by direct actions on skeletal muscle (Van Winkle, 1976; Davidoff, 1978). Dantrolene has the following chemical structure:

$$O_2N-\langle \text{ring} \rangle-\langle \text{furan} \rangle-CH=N-N\langle \text{ring} \rangle$$

Dantrolene

Pharmacological Properties. Dantrolene reduces contraction of skeletal muscle by a direct action on excitation-contraction coupling, apparently by decreasing the amount of calcium released from the sarcoplasmic reticulum (Van Winkle, 1976). Although the drug does depress the CNS, it does not appear to produce antispastic effects by actions on neurons. Dantrolene diminishes the force of electrically induced twitches in man without altering muscle action potentials, and it reduces reflex more than voluntary contraction (Herman *et al.,* 1972). The latter effect appears to be due to preferential actions on "fast" as compared to "slow" skeletal muscle fibers. Dantrolene does not affect neuromuscular transmission, nor does it change the electrical properties of skeletal muscle membranes (Davidoff, 1978).

In patients with upper motoneuron lesions, spasticity is generally diminished by treatment with dantrolene, and functional capacity is often improved. Unfortunately, the drug also tends to cause a generalized muscle weakness that negates functional improvement.

Dantrolene is also effective in alleviating the signs of malignant hyperthermia in susceptible animals and in patients. This rare, genetically determined syndrome is usually precipitated by the administration of neuromuscular blocking agents and inhalational anesthetics during surgery (*see* Chapter 11). Contraction of skeletal muscle apparently occurs as a result of excessive release of calcium from the sarcoplasmic reticulum.

Absorption of dantrolene from the gastrointestinal tract is slow and incomplete but sufficiently consistent to provide dose-related concentrations in plasma. The mean half-life of the drug in adults is about 9 hours after a 100-mg dose. It is slowly metabolized by the liver, and the 5-hydroxy and acetamido metabolites are excreted with unchanged drug in the urine.

Untoward Effects and Precautions. Dantrolene has a serious potential to cause hepatotoxicity. Fatal hepatitis has been reported in approximately 0.1 to 0.2% of patients treated with the drug for 60 days or longer. Symptomatic hepatitis may occur in 0.5% of patients treated with dantrolene for more than 60 days, while chemical abnormalities of hepatic function are noted in up to 1%. In view of this potential for hepatic injury, chronic administration of dantrolene should be halted if clear benefits are not evident within 45 days, and hepatic function should be monitored. The most common major side effect of dantrolene is weakness, an extension of its effect on skeletal muscle. Although weakness may be transient or mild, its persistence in some ambulatory patients may compromise therapeutic benefit. Euphoria, light-headedness, dizziness, drowsiness, and fatigue often occur early in treatment, but these side effects are generally transient; nevertheless, patients should be cautioned against driving or participating in hazardous occupations. Although the diarrhea that occurs in some patients can usually be controlled by a more gradual increase in dosage, it may necessitate withdrawal of the drug.

Preparations and Dosage. *Dantrolene sodium* (DANTRIUM) is available for oral use in capsules containing 25, 50, or 100 mg of the drug. The starting dose of 25 mg once a day is gradually increased by increments of 25 mg every 4 to 7 days to a maximal dose of 400 mg daily, given in four divided doses. For children, the recommended starting dose of 0.5 mg/kg twice a day is gradually increased to a maximum of 3 mg/kg four times a day, but not to exceed 400 mg daily. Dantrolene is also available for intravenous administration.

Therapeutic Uses. Dantrolene can relieve spasticity, but the weakness it produces may handicap the patient more than the spasticity it relieves. In view of its mechanism of action, it would appear to make little difference as to the cause of spasticity. Dantrolene provides significant and sustained reduction of spasticity and improves functional capacity for the majority of paraplegic and hemiplegic patients; clonus, mass-reflex movements, and abnormal resistance to passive stretch are reduced. About one half of patients with athetoid cerebral palsy and a smaller fraction of those with multiple sclerosis are also sufficiently improved to warrant continued treatment. Because of the muscle weakness caused by dantrolene, it is particularly useful for nonambulatory patients whose nursing care is made difficult by muscle contraction (Symposium, 1974; Pinder *et al.,* 1977; Davidoff, 1978; Young and Delwaide, 1981).

Dantrolene should be administered intravenously as soon as the syndrome of malignant hyperthermia is recognized; the initial dose is 1 mg/kg, and this may be repeated as necessary to a total of 10 mg/kg. Supportive measures are also important. These include discontinuation of anesthetics, administration of oxygen, management of acidosis and fever, and attention to urine output and water and electrolyte balance. Oral administration of dantrolene (1 to 2 mg/kg four times a day) may be necessary for 1 to 3 days to prevent recurrence of the condition.

THERAPEUTIC STATUS

There is no completely satisfactory form of therapy for alleviation of skeletal muscle spasticity (Davidoff, 1978; Young and Delwaide, 1981). While drugs such as baclofen, diazepam, and dantrolene are capable of providing variable relief of spasticity in given circumstances, troublesome muscle weakness, adverse effects on gait, and a variety of other side effects minimize their overall usefulness. These drugs may temporarily abate some of the symptoms of cerebral palsy, but they have a minor role in the overall management of this disorder. Muscle relaxants are of little value in Parkinson's disease or in other dysfunctions resulting from diseases of the brain.

DRUG THERAPY OF ACUTE MUSCLE SPASMS

A variety of conditions (*e.g.,* trauma, inflammation, anxiety, and pain) can be associated with acute muscle spasms. Several drugs have been employed in attempts to alleviate such spasms, including *mephenesin, carisoprodol* (SOMA), *chlorphenesin carbamate* (MAOLATE), *chlorzoxazone* (PARAFLEX), *metaxalone, methocarbamol* (ROBAXIN), *orphenadrine* (NORFLEX), and *cyclobenzaprine hydrochloride* (FLEXERIL). The efficacy of these compounds is difficult to assess because of the lack of well-controlled clinical studies. It is not clear that these agents offer any advantage over diazepam, sedatives, or analgesics. While some of these drugs have been vaguely characterized as interneuronal blocking agents, their limited efficacy may be due solely to general depression of the CNS. The pharmacological properties of these drugs are described in *earlier editions* of this textbook (*see also* Elenbaas, 1980). Such agents are not useful in the treatment of spasticity associated with chronic neurological disease.

Aellig, W. H., and Neuesch, E. Comparative pharmacokinetic investigations with tritium-labelled ergot alkaloids after oral and intravenous administration in man. *Int. J. Clin. Pharmacol.*, **1977**, *15*, 106–112.

Barbeau, A. The use of L-DOPA in Parkinson's disease: a 20 year follow-up. *Trends Pharmacol. Sci.*, **1981**, *2*, 297–299.

Barbeau, A., and Pourcher, E. New data on the genetics of Parkinson's disease. *Can. J. Neurol. Sci.*, **1982**, *9*, 53–60.

Bertler, A., and Rosengren, E. Occurrence and distribution of dopamine in brain and other tissues. *Experientia*, **1959**, *15*, 10–11.

Bianchine, J. R., and Shaw, G. M. Clinical pharmacokinetics of levodopa in Parkinson's disease. *Clin. Pharmacokinet.*, **1976**, *1*, 313–358.

Birkmayer, W.; Riederer, P.; Ambrozi, L.; and Youdim, M. B. H. Implications of combined treatment with "MODAPAR" and L-deprenyl in Parkinson's disease. *Lancet*, **1977**, *1*, 439–440.

Blume, E. Street drugs yield Parkinson's model. *J.A.M.A.*, **1983**, *250*, 13–14.

Bowery, N. G.; Hill, D. R.; and Hudson, A. L. Characteristics of GABA$_B$ receptor binding sites on rat whole brain synaptic membranes. *Br. J. Pharmacol.*, **1983**, *78*, 191–206.

Burns, R. S.; Chiueh, C. C.; Markey, S. P.; Ebert, M. H.; Jacobwitz, D. M.; and Kopin, I. J. A primate model of parkinsonism: selective destruction of dopaminergic neurons in the pars compacta of the substantia nigra by N-methyl-4-phenyl-1,2,3,6-tetrahydropyridine. *Proc. Natl. Acad. Sci. U.S.A.*, **1983**, *80*, 4546–4550.

Calne, D. B. Parkinsonism, clinical and neuropharmacologic aspects. *Postgrad. Med.*, **1978**, *64*, 82–88.

———. Progress in Parkinson's disease. *N. Engl. J. Med.*, **1984**, *310*, 523–524.

Calne, D. B., and Langston, J. W. The etiology of Parkinson's disease. *Lancet*, **1983**, *2*, 1457–1459.

Carlsson, A. The occurrence, distribution, and physiological role of catecholamines in the nervous system. *Pharmacol. Rev.*, **1959**, *11*, 490–493.

Carlsson, A.; Lindqvist, M.; and Magnusson, T. 3,4-Dihydroxyphenylalanine and 5-hydroxytryptophan as reserpine antagonists. *Nature*, **1957**, *180*, 1200.

Carlsson, A.; Lindqvist, M.; Magnusson, T.; and Waldeck, B. On the presence of 3-hydroxytyramine in brain. *Science*, **1958**, *127*, 471.

Chandra, B. Treatment of disturbances of consciousness caused by measles encephalitis with levodopa. *Eur. Neurol.*, **1978**, *17*, 265–270.

Chase, T. N., and Watanabe, A. M. Methyldopahydrazine as an adjunct to L-dopa therapy in parkinsonism. *Neurology (Minneap.)*, **1972**, *22*, 384–392.

Cotzias, G. C.; Papavasiliou, P. S.; Tolosa, E. S.; Mendez, J. S.; and Bell-Midura, M. Treatment of parkinsonism with aporphines: possible role of growth hormone. *N. Engl. J. Med.*, **1976**, *294*, 567–572.

Cotzias, G. C.; Van Woert, M. H.; and Schiffer, L. M. Aromatic amino acids and modification of parkinsonism. *N. Engl. J. Med.*, **1967**, *276*, 374–379.

Dunlap, K. Two types of γ-aminobutyric acid receptor on embryonic sensory neurones. *Br. J. Pharmacol.*, **1981**, *74*, 579–585.

Eddy, R. L.; Jones, A. L.; Chakmakjian, Z. H.; and Silverthorne, M. C. Effect of levodopa (L-dopa) on human hypophyseal trophic hormone release. *J. Clin. Endocrinol. Metab.*, **1971**, *33*, 709–712.

Ehringer, H., and Hornykiewicz, O. Verteilung von Noradrenalin und Dopamin (3-hydroxytyramin) im Gehirn des Menschen und ihr Verhalten bei Erkrankungen des extrapyramidalen Systems. *Klin. Wochenschr.*, **1960**, *38*, 1236–1239.

Eisler, T.; Teravainen, H.; Nelson, R.; Krebs, H.; Weise, V.; Lake, C. R.; Ebert, M. H.; Whetzel, N.; Murphy, D. L.; Kopin, I. J.; and Calne, D. B. Deprenyl in Parkinson's disease. *Neurology (N.Y.)*, **1981**, *31*, 19–23.

Forssman, B.; Kihlstrand, S.; and Larsson, L. E. Amantadine therapy in parkinsonism. *Acta Neurol. Scand.*, **1972**, *48*, 1–18.

Fukuda, T.; Kudo, Y.; and Ono, H. Effects of β-(p-chlorophenyl)-GABA (baclofen) on spinal synaptic activity. *Eur. J. Pharmacol.*, **1977**, *44*, 17–24.

Goldberg, L. I.; Volkman, P. H.; and Kohli, J. D. A comparison of the vascular dopamine receptor with other dopamine receptors. *Annu. Rev. Pharmacol. Toxicol.*, **1978**, *18*, 57–79.

Goodall, M. C., and Alton, H. Dopamine (3-hydroxytyramine) metabolism in parkinsonism. *J. Clin. Invest.*, **1969**, *48*, 2300–2308.

Herman, R.; Mayer, N.; and Mecomber, S. A. Clinical pharmaco-physiology of dantrolene sodium. *Am. J. Phys. Med.*, **1972**, *51*, 296–311.

Hornykiewicz, O. Dopamine in the basal ganglia. *Br. Med. Bull.*, **1973a**, *29*, 172–178.

Jellinger, R. Adjuvant treatment of Parkinson's disease with dopamine agonists: open trial with bromocriptine and CU 32-085. *J. Neurol.*, **1982**, *227*, 75–88.

Joseph, C.; Chassan, J. B.; and Koch, M. L. Levodopa in Parkinson's disease. *Ann. Neurol.*, **1978**, *3*, 116–118.

Keller, H. H., and Daprada, M. Central dopamine agonistic activity and microsomal biotransformation of lisuride, lergotrile and bromocriptine. *Life Sci.*, **1979**, *24*, 1211–1222.

Klawans, H. L.; Goetz, C.; Nausieda, P. A.; and Weiner, W. J. Recent advances in the biochemical pharmacology of extrapyramidal movement disorders. *Adv. Exp. Med. Biol.*, **1977**, *90*, 21–47.

Langston, J. W.; Ballard, P.; Tetrud, J. W.; and Irwin, I. Chronic parkinsonism in humans due to a product of meperidine-analog synthesis. *Science*, **1983**, *219*, 979–980.

Langston, J. W., and Forno, L. S. The hypothalamus in Parkinson's disease. *Ann. Neurol.*, **1978**, *3*, 129–133.

Lieberman, A. N.; Kupersmith, M.; Gopinathan, G.; Estey, E.; Goodgold, A.; and Goldstein, M. Bromocriptine in Parkinson's disease: further studies. *Neurology (Minneap.)*, **1979**, *29*, 363–369.

Linch, D. C.; Shaw, K. M.; Muhlemann, M. F.; and Ross, E. J. Bromocriptine-induced postural hypotension in acromegaly. *Lancet*, **1978**, *1*, 320.

Lloyd, K. G. Neurochemical compensation in Parkinson's disease. In, *Parkinson's Disease, Concepts and Prospects*. (Lakke, J. P. W. F.; Korf, J.; and Wesseling, H.; eds.) Excerpta Medica, Amsterdam, **1978**, pp. 61–72.

Lossius, R.; Dietrichson, P.; and Lunde, P. K. M. Effect of diazepam and desmethyl-diazepam in spasticity and rigidity: a quantitative study of reflexes and plasma concentrations. *Acta Neurol. Scand.*, **1980**, *61*, 378–383.

Mann, D. M. A., and Yates, P. O. Possible role of neuromelanin in the pathogenesis of Parkinson's disease. *Mech. Ageing Dev.*, **1983**, *21*, 193–203.

Marx, J. L. Parkinson's disease: search for better therapies. *Science*, **1979**, *203*, 737–738.

Mawdsley, C.; Williams, I. R.; Pullar, I. A.; Davidson, D. L.; and Kinloch, N. E. Treatment of parkinsonism by amantadine and levodopa. *Clin. Pharmacol. Ther.*, **1972**, *13*, 575–583.

Montagu, K. A. Catechol compounds in rat tissues and in brains of different animals. *Nature*, **1957**, *180*, 244–245.

Morgan, M. Y.; Jakobovits, A.; Elithorn, A.; James, I. M.; and Sherlock, S. Successful use of bromocriptine in the treatment of a patient with chronic portasystemic encephalopathy. *N. Engl. J. Med.*, **1977**, *296*, 793–794.

Newberry, N. R., and Nicoll, R. A. Direct hyperpolarizing action of baclofen on hippocampal pyramidal cells. *Nature*, **1984**, *308*, 450–452.

Nutt, J. G.; Woodward, W. R.; Hammerstad, J. P.; Carter, J. H.; and Anderson, J. L. The "on-off" phenomenon in Parkinson's disease. *N. Engl. J. Med.*, **1984**, *310*, 483–488.

Palfreyman, M. G.; Danzin, C.; Bey, P.; Jung, M. J.; Riberbeau-Gayon, G.; Aubry, M.; Vevert, J. P.; and Sjoerdsma, A. Difluoromethyl dopa, a new enzyme-activated irreversible inhibitor of aromatic L-amino acid decarboxylase. *J. Neurochem.*, **1978**, *31*, 927–932.

Papavasiliou, P. S.; Cotzias, G. C.; Duby, S. E.; Steck, A. J.; Fehling, C.; and Bell, M. A. Levodopa in parkinsonism; potentiation of central effects with a peripheral inhibitor. *N. Engl. J. Med.*, **1972**, *285*, 8–14.

Parkes, J. D.; Zilkha, K. J.; Calver, D. M.; and Knill-Jones, R. P. Controlled trial of amantadine hydrochloride in Parkinson's disease. *Lancet*, **1970**, *1*, 259–262.

Pearce, J. M. S. Aetiology and natural history of Parkinson's disease. *Br. Med. J.*, **1978**, *2*, 1664–1666.

Pearce, L. A.; Waterbury, L. D.; and Green, H. D. Amantadine hydrochloride: alteration in peripheral circulation. *Neurology (Minneap.)*, **1974**, *24*, 46–48.

Rajfer, S. I.; Anton, A. H.; Rossen, J. D.; and Goldberg, L. I. Beneficial hemodynamic effects on oral levodopa in heart failure. *N. Engl. J. Med.*, **1984**, *310*, 1357–1362.

Riederer, P.; Jellinger, K.; Danielczyk, W.; Seemann, D.; Ulm, G.; Reynolds, G. P.; Birkmayer, W.; and Koppel, H. Combination treatment with selective monoamine oxidase inhibitors and dopaminergic agonists in Parkinson's disease: biochemical and clinical observations. In, *Experimental Therapeutics of Movement Disorders.* (Fahn, S.; Calne, D. B.; and Shoulson, I.; eds.) Vol. 37, *Advances in Neurology.* Raven Press, New York, **1983**, pp. 159–176.

Sacks, O. W.; Kohl, M. S.; Messeloff, C. R.; and Schartz, W. F. Effects of levodopa in parkinsonian patients with dementia. *Neurology (Minneap.)*, **1972**, *22*, 516–519.

Schwab, R. S.; Poskanzer, D. C.; England, A. C.; and Young, R. R. Amantadine in Parkinson's disease. Review of more than two years' experience. *J.A.M.A.*, **1972**, *222*, 792–795.

Sirtori, C. R.; Bolme, P.; and Azarnoff, D. L. Metabolic responses to acute and chronic L-dopa administration in patients with parkinsonism. *N. Engl. J. Med.*, **1972**, *287*, 729–733.

Stern, G. M., and Lees, A. J. Sustained bromocriptine therapy in 50 previously untreated patients with Parkinson's disease. In, *Experimental Therapeutics of Movement Disorders.* (Fahn, S.; Calne, D. B.; and Shoulson, I.; eds.) Vol. 37, *Advances in Neurology.* Raven Press, New York, **1983**, pp. 17–21.

Van Winkle, W. B. Calcium release from skeletal muscle sarcoplasmic reticulum: site of action of dantrolene sodium? *Science*, **1976**, *193*, 1130–1131.

Ward, C. D.; Duvoisin, R. C.; Ince, S. E.; Nutt, J. G.; Eldridge, R.; and Calne, D. B. Parkinson's disease in 65 pairs of twins and in a set of quadruplets. *Neurology (N.Y.)*, **1983**, *33*, 815–824.

Yahr, M. D. Overview of present day treatment of Parkinson's disease. *J. Neural Transm.*, **1978**, *43*, 227–238.

Monographs and Reviews

Bernheimer, H.; Birkmayer, W.; Hornykiewicz, O.; Jellinger, K.; and Seitelberger, F. Brain dopamine and the syndromes of Parkinson and Huntington. *J. Neurol. Sci.*, **1973**, *20*, 415–455.

Bianchine, J. R. Drug therapy of parkinsonism. *N. Engl. J. Med.*, **1976**, *295*, 814–818.

Bianchine, J. R., and Sunyapridakul, L. Interactions between levodopa and other drugs: significance in the treatment of Parkinson's disease. *Drugs*, **1973**, *6*, 364–388.

Calne, D. B.; Kebabian, J.; Silbergeld, E.; and Evarts, E. Advances in the neuropharmacology of parkinsonism. *Ann. Intern. Med.*, **1979**, *90*, 219–229.

Davidoff, R. A. Pharmacology of spasticity, *Neurology (Minneap.)*, **1978**, *28*, 46–51.

Elenbaas, J. K. Centrally acting oral skeletal muscle relaxants. *Am. J. Hosp. Pharm.*, **1980**, *37*, 1313–1323.

Fahn, S.; Calne, D. B.; and Shoulson, I. (eds.). *Experimental Therapeutics of Movement Disorders.* Vol. 37, *Advances in Neurology.* Raven Press, New York, **1983**.

Greenblatt, D. J.; Shader, R. I.; and Abernathy, D. R. Drug therapy: current status of benzodiazepines. *N. Engl. J. Med.*, **1983**, *309*, 354–358, 410–416.

Hornykiewicz, O. Parkinson's disease: from brain homogenate to treatment. *Fed. Proc.*, **1973b**, *32*, 183–190.

Leff, S. E., and Creese, I. Dopamine receptors re-explained. *Trends Pharmacol. Sci.*, **1983**, *4*, 463–467.

Pinder, R. M.; Brogden, R. N.; Speight, T. M.; and Avery, G. S. Dantrolene sodium: a review of its pharmacological properties and therapeutic efficacy in spasticity. *Drugs*, **1977**, *3*, 3–23.

Quinn, N. P. Anti-parkinsonian drugs today. *Drugs*, **1984**, *28*, 236–262.

Rajput, A. H.; Offord, K. P.; Beard, C. M.; and Kurland, L. T. Epidemiology of parkinsonism: incidence, classification, and mortality. *Ann. Neurol.*, **1984**, *16*, 278–282.

Rinne, U. K. Parkinson's disease as a model for changes in dopamine receptor dynamics with aging. *Gerontology*, **1982**, *28*, Suppl. 1, 35–52.

Rose, F. C., and Capildeo, R. (eds.). *Research Progress in Parkinson's Disease.* Pitman Medical, Kent, England, **1981**.

Synder, S. H. Drugs and neurotransmitter receptors in the brain. *Science*, **1984**, *224*, 22–31.

Sweet, R. D., and McDowell, F. H. Five years' treatment of Parkinson's disease with levodopa: therapeutic results and survival of 100 patients. *Ann. Intern. Med.*, **1975**, *83*, 456–463.

Symposium. (Various authors.) Spasticity—its etiology, physiology and the pharmacology of a new agent. *Arch. Phys. Med. Rehabil.*, **1974**, *55*, 331–392.

Symposium. (Various authors.) *Parkinson's Disease: Concepts and Prospects.* (Lakke, J. P. W. F.; Korf, J.; and Wesseling, H.; eds.) Excerpta Medica, Amsterdam, **1977.**

Symposium. (Various authors.) *Parkinson's Disease: Current Progress, Problems, and Management.* Northern European Symposium on Parkinson's Disease. (Rinne, U. K.; Klinger, M.; and Stamm, G.; eds.) Elsevier, New York, **1980.**

Symposium. (Various authors.) Current concepts and controversies in Parkinson's disease. *Can. J. Neurol. Sci.*, **1984**, *11*, Suppl. 1, 89–240.

Vance, M. L.; Evans, W. S.; and Thorner, M. O. Bromocriptine. *Ann. Intern. Med.*, **1984**, *100*, 78–91.

Yahr, M. D. Levodopa. *Ann. Intern. Med.*, **1975**, *83*, 677–682.

Young, R. R., and Delwaide, P. J. Drug therapy: spasticity. *N. Engl. J. Med.*, **1981**, *304*, 28–33, 96–99.

22 OPIOID ANALGESICS AND ANTAGONISTS

Jerome H. Jaffe and William R. Martin

This chapter presents the pharmacological properties of the opioids (opioid agonists) and the opioid antagonists. The term *opioid* is used here to designate a group of drugs that are, to varying degrees, opium- or morphine-like in their properties. The opioids are employed primarily as analgesics, but they have many other pharmacological effects as well. Opioids interact with what appear to be several closely related receptors, and they share some of the properties of certain naturally occurring peptides, the *enkephalins*, the *endorphins*, and the *dynorphins*.

History. Although the psychological effects of opium may have been known to the ancient Sumerians, the first undisputed reference to poppy juice is found in the writings of Theophrastus in the third century B.C. The word *opium* itself is derived from the Greek name for juice, the drug being obtained from the juice of the poppy, *Papaver somniferum*. Arabian physicians were well versed in the uses of opium; Arabian traders introduced the drug to the Orient, where it was employed mainly for the control of dysenteries. Paracelsus (1493–1541) is credited with repopularizing the use of opium in Europe; it had fallen into disfavor because of its toxicity. By the middle of the sixteenth century, the uses of opium that are still valid were fairly well understood, and, in 1680, Sydenham wrote, ''Among the remedies which it has pleased Almighty God to give to man to relieve his sufferings, none is so universal and so efficacious as opium.''

In the eighteenth century opium smoking became popular in the Orient. At that time the use of opiates for their subjective effects was considerably more acceptable than it is at present. In Europe, the ready availability of opium led to some degree of overuse, but the problem of opium eating never became as prevalent or as socially destructive as the abuse of alcohol.

Opium contains more than 20 distinct alkaloids. In 1806, Sertürner reported the isolation of a pure substance in opium that he named morphine, after Morpheus, the Greek god of dreams. The discovery of other alkaloids in opium quickly followed that of morphine (codeine by Robiquet in 1832, papaverine by Merck in 1848). By the middle of the nineteenth century the use of pure alkaloids rather than crude opium preparations began to spread throughout the medical world.

The invention of the hypodermic needle and the parenteral use of morphine tended to produce a more severe variety of compulsive drug use. In the United States, the extent of the opioid-use problem was accentuated by the influx of opium-smoking Chinese laborers, the widespread use of morphine among wounded Civil War soldiers, and the unrestricted availability of opium that prevailed until the early years of this century. The history of opium and its alkaloids and the problems of addiction are described by Terry and Pellens (1928) and by Musto (1973).

The problem of addiction to opioids stimulated a search for potent analgesics that would be free of the potential to produce addiction. One compound, nalorphine, was shown to antagonize the effects of morphine. Eckenhoff and coworkers used it as an antidote for morphine poisoning in 1951. Two years later, Wikler and coworkers showed that it would precipitate acute abstinence in addicts; and in 1954, Lasagna and Beecher reported that nalorphine had analgesic actions in postoperative patients despite its antagonistic actions. Although nalorphine frequently produced anxiety and dysphoria and, hence, was not clinically useful as an analgesic, the discovery of its analgesic effects stimulated research that led to the development of new drugs, such as the relatively pure antagonist *naloxone* and compounds with mixed actions (*e.g., pentazocine, butorphanol,* and *buprenorphine*). Such agents not only have enlarged the range of available therapeutic entities but also, in conjunction with the subsequent discovery of receptors for opioids and endogenous peptides that bind to these receptors, have helped to change our views about the actions of the opioids.

By 1967, researchers had concluded that the complex interactions among morphine-like drugs, antagonists, and mixed agonist-antagonists could best be explained by postulating the existence of more than one type of receptor for the opioids and related drugs (Martin, 1967). In 1973, following a methodological approach developed by Goldstein and coworkers, three groups of investigators (Pert and Snyder; Simon, Hiller, and Edelman; and Terenius) independently described saturable, stereospecific binding sites for opioid drugs in the mammalian nervous system. In 1975, Hughes and Kosterlitz and their coworkers described the isolation from pig brain of two pentapeptides that exhibited morphine-like actions on the guinea pig ileum—actions that were specifically antagonized by naloxone. Within the same year, Goldstein and colleagues reported the presence of peptide-like substances in the pituitary gland with opioid activity. Over a remarkably brief period, subsequent research revealed that there are three distinct families of opioid peptides and multiple categories of opioid receptors. These developments have been reviewed by Simon and Hiller (1978), Terenius (1978), Bloom (1983), Akil and colleagues (1984), and Goldstein (1984).

Terminology. The term *opiate* was once used to designate drugs derived from opium—morphine, codeine, and the many semisynthetic congeners of morphine. Soon after the development of totally synthetic entities with morphine-like actions, the word *opioid* was introduced to refer in a generic sense to all drugs, natural and synthetic, with morphine-like actions. Some writers continued to use the term *opiate* in a generic sense, and in such contexts *opiate* and *opioid* are interchangeable. More recently, *opioid* has also been used to refer to antagonists of morphine-like drugs as well as to receptors or binding sites that combine with such agents.

The term *narcotic* was obsolete long before the discovery of endogenous opioid-like ligands and receptors for these substances. Derived from the Greek word for stupor and at one time applied to any drug that induced sleep, it was, for a number of years, used to refer to morphine-like strong analgesics. With the development of mixed agonist-antagonists, some of which do not suppress morphine-like physical dependence, and with the increasing use of the term in a legal context to refer to any substance that can cause dependence, the term *narcotic* is no longer useful in a pharmacological context. However, it is not likely to disappear soon.

Endogenous Opioid Peptides. Three distinct families of peptides have been identified thus far: the *enkephalins*, the *endorphins*, and the *dynorphins*. Each family is derived from a genetically distinct precursor polypeptide and has a characteristic anatomical distribution. These precursors are now commonly designated as proenkephalin (also proenkephalin A), pro-opiomelanocortin (POMC), and prodynorphin (also proenkephalin B). As shown in Figure 22–1, each of these precursors contains a number of biologically active peptides, both opioid and nonopioid, that have been detected in blood and various tissues. For example, POMC contains the amino acid sequence for melanocyte-stimulating hormone (γ-MSH), adrenocorticotropin (ACTH), and β-lipotropin (β-LPH); within

the 91 amino acid sequence of β-LPH are found β-endorphin and β-MSH (*see* Chapter 59). Although β-endorphin contains the sequence for met-enkephalin at its amino terminus, it is not converted to this peptide; instead, met-enkephalin is derived from the processing of proenkephalin. Leu-enkephalin and other opioid peptides are produced from both proenkephalin and prodynorphin. Prodynorphin yields five peptides that contain leu-enkephalin: dynorphin A(1–17), which can be cleaved further to dynorphin A(1–8); dynorphin B(1–13); and α- and β-neoendorphin, which differ from each other by only one amino acid.

The precursor molecules and the peptides derived therefrom are not confined to the central nervous system (CNS), and they are distributed in a specific fashion. The distribution of peptides from POMC is relatively limited. In the brain, they are found in the arcuate nucleus, which projects its fibers widely to limbic and brain stem areas; in the nucleus tractus solitarii; and in the nucleus commissuralis. Not surprisingly, an important location for peptides from POMC is the pituitary, where they occur in both the pars intermedia and the pars distalis. They are also contained in pancreatic islet cells.

The peptides from prodynorphin and proenkephalin are distributed widely throughout the CNS, where they are frequently found together in the same region; nevertheless, each family of peptides occurs in different groups of neurons. For example, in areas of the medulla that are involved in the modulation of pain, the prodynorphin peptides tend to be localized in neurons that are ventral to those containing peptides derived from proenkephalin. Of particular note, proenkephalin peptides are present in areas of the CNS that are presumed to be related to the perception of pain (*e.g.*, laminae I and II of the spinal cord, the spinal trigeminal nucleus, and the periaqueductal gray), to the modulation of affective behavior (*e.g.*, amygdala, hippocampus, locus ceruleus, and the cerebral cortex), and to the regulation of the autonomic nervous system (medulla oblongata) and neuroendocrinological functions (median eminence). While there are a few long enkephalinergic fiber tracts, these peptides are contained primarily in interneurons with short axons. The peptides from proenkephalin are also found in the adrenal medulla and in nerve plexuses and exocrine glands of the stomach and intestine. The anatomical distribution of opioid peptides has been reviewed by Bloom (1983) and by Akil and coworkers (1984).

Not all cells that make a given precursor polypeptide store and release the same mixture of active opioid peptides. For example, in the pituitary, more β-LPH than β-endorphin is stored in the anterior lobe, while the reverse is true in the intermedi-

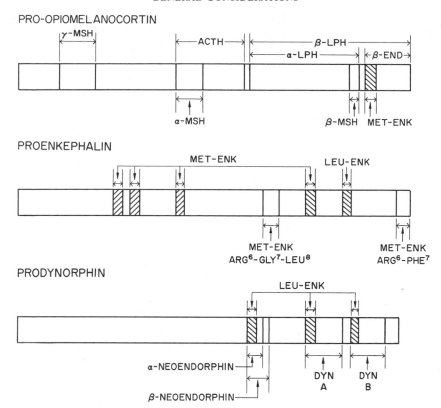

Figure 22–1. *Schematic representation of the structures of the protein precursors of the three families of opioid peptides.*

Abbreviations: ENK = enkephalin; DYN = dynorphin; END = endorphin. Other abbreviations are defined in the text. The sequence of met-enkephalin is Tyr-Gly-Gly-Phe-Met, while that of leu-enkephalin is Tyr-Gly-Gly-Phe-Leu. (Modified from Akil *et al.*, 1984.)

ate lobe; in addition, the ratio of dynorphin A(1–17) to dynorphin A(1–8) can vary from one region of the brain to the next (*see* Akil *et al.*, 1984). These differences are thought to arise from variations in the cellular complement of peptidases that produce and degrade the active opioid fragments.

While the endogenous opioid peptides appear to function as neurotransmitters, modulators of neurotransmission, or neurohormones, their role in physiological processes is not completely understood; where information exists, it will be discussed in the appropriate sections of this chapter. The elucidation of the physiological role of the opioid peptides has been made more difficult by their frequent coexistence with other putative neurotransmitters within a given neuron. For example, neurons that originate in the paraventricular nucleus contain at least three distinct peptides: dynorphin A(1–8), antidiuretic hormone, and corticotropin-releasing factor (CRF) (Roth *et al.*, 1983); in the rostral medulla, there are cells that contain 5-hydroxytryptamine (5-HT) and either enkephalins or dynorphins (*see* Basbaum and Fields, 1984).

Multiple Opioid Receptors. Studies of the binding of opioid drugs and peptides to specific sites in brain and other organs have suggested the existence of perhaps as many as eight types of opioid receptors. In the CNS, there is reasonably firm evidence for four major categories of receptors, designated μ (mu), κ (kappa), δ (delta), and σ (sigma). To add confusion, there may well be subtypes of each of these receptors. Although there is considerable variation in binding characteristics and anatomical distribution among different species, inferences have been drawn from data that attempt to relate pharmacological effects to interactions with a particular constellation of receptors (*see* Chang and Cuatrecasas, 1981; Martin, 1983; Snyder, 1984). For example, analgesia has been associated with both μ and κ receptors, while dysphoria or psychotomimetic effects have been ascribed to σ receptors; based primarily on their localization in limbic regions of the brain, δ receptors are thought to be involved in alterations of affective behavior. With the important exception of at least some types of σ receptors, the antagonist naloxone has been found to bind with high affinity to all opioid receptors; however, its affinity for μ receptors is generally more than tenfold higher than for κ- or δ-receptor sites.

Observations in man are congruent with many aspects of this classification of opioid receptors. However, since the binding characteristics of met- and leu-enkephalin have been crucial in the identification of δ receptors and since there is as yet no opioid drug with a spectrum of properties similar to that of these peptides, it has not been possible to define pharmacological effects on the CNS in human subjects that may be associated predominantly with δ receptors. Thus, the actions of opioid drugs that are currently available have usually been interpreted with respect to the participation of only three types of receptors—μ, κ, and σ; at each, a given agent may act as an agonist, a partial agonist, or an antagonist. These relationships are summarized in Table 22–1.

While there is, at present, no entirely satisfactory classification of the opioids, in this chapter these substances have been divided into three groups: *morphine-like opioid agonists* (substances acting as agonists primarily at μ, κ, and perhaps δ receptors); *opioid antagonists* (substances such as naloxone that are essentially devoid of agonist activity at any receptor); and opioids with mixed actions. The last-named category includes the *agonist-antagonists* (substances such as nalorphine or pentazocine that appear to be agonists at some receptors and antagonists at others) and the *partial agonists* (such as buprenorphine or propiram); also included in this category is butorphanol, an agent that appears to have neither agonist nor antagonist actions at μ receptors.

The current classification of opioid receptors evolved in particular from studies of the effects of various opioid drugs in dogs with spinal transec-

Table 22–1. SUMMARY OF THE ACTIONS OF PROTOTYPICAL AGONISTS, ANTAGONISTS, AND AGONIST-ANTAGONISTS AT OPIOID RECEPTORS

COMPOUND	RECEPTOR TYPES *		
	μ	κ	σ
Morphine	Ag †	Ag	—
Naloxone ‡	Ant	Ant	§
Pentazocine	Ant	Ag	Ag
Butorphanol	—	Ag	Ag
Nalbuphine	Ant	pAg	Ag§
Nalorphine	Ant	pAg	Ag§
Buprenorphine	pAg	—	—
Propiram	pAg	—	—
N-allyl-normetazocine	Ant		Ag

* The μ receptor is thought to mediate supraspinal analgesia, respiratory depression, euphoria, and physical dependence; the κ receptor, spinal analgesia, miosis, and sedation; the σ receptor, dysphoria, hallucinations, and respiratory and vasomotor stimulation. Actions at the δ receptor have not been studied sufficiently to include in the table. Categorizations are based on best inferences about actions in man. *See* text for further explanation.

† Ag = agonist; Ant = competitive antagonist; pAg = partial agonist; the absence of an entry means that the compound has not yet been fully studied; — = no significant action. Two drugs acting at the same receptors can still have different profiles of action because their relative affinities for the various receptors may differ.

‡ Naloxone is more potent in antagonizing the effects of μ agonists than κ or σ agonists and is thus thought to have the highest affinity for the μ receptor.

§ Some effects of σ agonists are antagonized by naloxone; others are not. The reason for this is not understood but may indicate that there are several subtypes of σ receptors. Curiously, nalorphine produces σ-like effects but does not have high affinity for the σ receptor. With nalbuphine, σ-like effects are minimal.

tions; some of these animals had been treated chronically with morphine and displayed tolerance and dependence (Martin *et al.*, 1976). The existence of three distinct opioid receptors was postulated: the μ receptor, which mediates the suppression of the opioid-withdrawal syndrome, analgesia, miosis, and respiratory depression produced by morphine-like drugs; the κ receptor, where drugs such as ketocyclazocine produce spinal analgesia but fail to suppress opioid withdrawal; and the σ receptor, responsible for the pupillary dilatation, tachypnea, and symptoms of mania produced by N-allylnormetazocine. Subsequently, the existence of δ receptors was proposed, based on the relative potencies of various opioid peptides and drugs to inhibit contractions of the isolated guinea pig ileum and mouse vas deferens (Lord *et al.*, 1977). This nomenclature has been used to categorize receptor sites in the CNS and gastrointestinal tract after evaluation of the binding characteristics of various opioids, including antagonists, analgesics, and either synthetic or naturally occurring peptides. Such studies have also provided evidence for the existence of other types or subtypes of opioid receptors. For example, binding sites for dextromethorphan have been identified in areas of the brain stem that are known to be involved in cough reflexes; these sites display a markedly different stereoselectivity for opioid drugs and have a low affinity for naloxone (*see* Snyder, 1984). Investigations employing an irreversible antagonist, naloxonazine, have suggested the existence of two types of μ receptors; the subtype with the lower affinity for morphine-like drugs (designated μ_2) is postulated to mediate respiratory depression (*see* Pasternak *et al.*, 1980). Finally, the drug phencyclidine (PCP) displaces N-allylnormetazocine from specific binding sites that are found predominantly in the hippocampus; these so-called σ opioid receptors may be an important site of action of PCP and related drugs (*see* Chapter 23). Since naloxone antagonizes very few of the actions of PCP and only some of the effects of opioids that are thought to act at σ receptors, there may be subtypes of these receptors as well (*see* Chang and Cuatrecasas, 1981; Martin, 1983; Snyder, 1984).

Studies on the binding of various opioids have shown that the affinity of agonists is markedly reduced by sodium ions and certain guanine nucleotides. In contrast, the affinity of "pure" antagonists is not altered, while that of agonist-antagonists is influenced to a lesser degree (*see* Snyder, 1984). This behavior is presumably related to the mechanism of action of the opioids (*see* below) and has been used extensively in industrial drug-screening procedures.

The endogenous opioid peptides display a variety of relative affinities for different types of receptors. For example, while met-enkephalin–arg^6–gly^7–leu^8 has equal affinity for μ and δ binding sites, other peptides derived from proenkephalin show a marked preference for δ sites. All the peptides from prodynorphin bind predominantly to κ sites; dynorphin B and dynorphin A(1–8) (a fragment from dynorphin A) also bind to μ and δ sites, respectively. In the CNS and peripheral tissues, β-endorphin binds to both μ and δ receptors, but it also appears to interact with more specialized sites (designated ϵ receptors) in the rat vas deferens (*see* Akil *et al.*, 1984).

The ability of one opioid drug to either intensify or ameliorate withdrawal signs and symptoms in human subjects who are physically dependent on another drug has been one important method for the categorization of the effects of these agents in man. Such data provide clues with regard to both the types of receptors and the mode of action at a given receptor (*e.g.*, agonist, antagonist, partial agonist) that are involved in the spectrum of pharmacological effects produced by an opioid drug. Details of such observations will be included in the discussions of the individual agents.

MORPHINE AND RELATED OPIOIDS

There are now many compounds that produce analgesia and other effects similar to those produced by morphine. Some of these may have some special properties, but none has proven to be clinically superior in relieving pain. Morphine remains the standard against which new analgesics are measured. Because the laboratory synthesis of morphine is difficult, the drug is still obtained from opium or extracted from poppy straw.

Source and Composition of Opium. Opium is obtained from the milky exudate of the incised unripe seed capsules of the poppy plant, *Papaver somniferum*. Once indigenous to Asia Minor, the plant is now grown legally and illegally in many parts of the world. The milky juice is dried in the air and forms a brownish, gummy mass. This is further dried and powdered to make the official powdered opium, containing a number of alkaloids. Only a few—morphine, codeine, and papaverine—have clinical usefulness. The alkaloids constitute about 25% by weight of opium and can be divided into two distinct chemical classes, *phenanthrenes* and *benzylisoquinolines*.

The principal phenanthrenes are morphine (10% of opium), codeine (0.5%), and thebaine (0.2%). The principal benzylisoquinolines are papaverine (1.0%), which is a smooth muscle relaxant (*see* Chapter 33), and noscapine (6.0%).

Chemistry of Morphine and Related Opioids. The structure of morphine, originally proposed by Gulland and Robinson in 1925, is as follows:

Morphine

Many semisynthetic derivatives are made by relatively simple modifications of the morphine or thebaine molecule. *Codeine* is methylmorphine, the methyl substitution being on the phenolic OH. *Thebaine* differs from morphine only in that both OH groups are methylated and that there are two double bonds in the ring ($\Delta^{6,7}$, $\Delta^{8,14}$). It has little analgesic action and produces seizures at a relatively low dosage. However, thebaine is a precursor of several important 14-OH compounds, such as *oxycodone* and *naloxone*. Certain derivatives of thebaine are more than 1000 times as potent as morphine (*e.g.*, *etorphine*). *Diacetylmorphine*, or *heroin*, is made from morphine by acetylation at the 3 and 6 positions. *Apomorphine*, which can also be prepared from morphine, is a potent emetic and dopaminergic agonist (*see* Chapter 21). *Hydromorphone*, *oxymorphone*, *hydrocodone*, and *oxycodone* are also made by modifying the morphine molecule. The structural relationship between morphine and some of its surrogates and antagonists is shown in Table 22–2.

Table 22–2. STRUCTURES OF OPIOIDS AND OPIOID ANTAGONISTS CHEMICALLY RELATED TO MORPHINE

NONPROPRIETARY NAME	CHEMICAL RADICALS AND POSITIONS			OTHER CHANGES †
	3 *	*6* *	*17* *	
Morphine	—OH	—OH	—CH$_3$	—
Heroin	—OCOCH$_3$	—OCOCH$_3$	—CH$_3$	—
Hydromorphone	—OH	=O	—CH$_3$	(1)
Oxymorphone	—OH	=O	—CH$_3$	(1),(2)
Levorphanol	—OH	—H	—CH$_3$	(1),(3)
Levallorphan	—OH	—H	—CH$_2$CH=CH$_2$	(1),(3)
Codeine	—OCH$_3$	—OH	—CH$_3$	—
Hydrocodone	—OCH$_3$	=O	—CH$_3$	(1)
Oxycodone	—OCH$_3$	=O	—CH$_3$	(1),(2)
Nalorphine	—OH	—OH	—CH$_2$CH=CH$_2$	—
Naloxone	—OH	=O	—CH$_2$CH=CH$_2$	(1),(2)
Naltrexone	—OH	=O	—CH$_2$–▷ 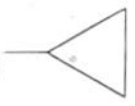 (cyclopropyl)	(1),(2)
Buprenorphine	—OH	—OCH$_3$	—CH$_2$–▷ 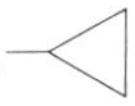 (cyclopropyl)	(1),(2),(4)
Butorphanol	—OH	—H	—CH$_2$–◇ 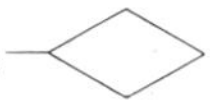 (cyclobutyl)	(2),(3)
Nalbuphine	—OH	—OH	—CH$_2$–◇ 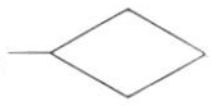 (cyclobutyl)	(1),(2)

* The numbers 3, 6, and 17 refer to positions in the morphine molecule, as shown above.

† Other changes in the morphine molecule are as follows:
  (1) Single instead of double bond between C7 and C8.
  (2) OH added to C14.
  (3) No oxygen between C4 and C5.
  (4) *Endo*etheno bridge between C6 and C14; 1-hydroxy-1,2,2-trimethylpropyl substitution on C7.

Structure-Activity Relationship of the Morphine-Like Opioids. In addition to morphine, codeine, and the semisynthetic derivatives of the natural opium alkaloids, there are a number of other structurally distinct chemical classes of drugs with pharmacological actions similar to those of morphine. These diverse groups share the capacity to produce analgesia, respiratory depression, gastrointestinal spasm, and morphine-like physical dependence. Clinically useful compounds include the morphinans, benzomorphans, methadones, phenylpiperidines, and propionanilides. In addition, *thiambutene* and *benzimidazole* derivatives possess morphine-like activity. Although the flat two-dimensional representations of these chemically diverse compounds appear to be quite different, molecular models show certain common characteristics; these are indicated by the heavy lines in the structure of morphine shown above. Among the important properties of the opioids that can be altered by structural modification are their affinity for various species of opioid receptors, agonist versus antagonistic activity, lipid solubility, resistance to metabolic breakdown, and binding to albumin in plasma (*see* Barnett *et al.*, 1978).

The discovery of endogenous peptides with preferential affinities for various types of opioid receptors has added new dimensions to the study of structure-activity relationships of opioid agonists and antagonists. In some instances, because of rapid hydrolysis or inability to penetrate into the CNS, the pharmacological properties of these peptides can only be demonstrated *in vitro* or by intracerebral injection, and their binding characteristics can only be determined with accuracy in the presence of protease inhibitors. However, due to their relatively simple structure, modern technics have led to the synthesis of scores of congeners, many of which are relatively resistant to enzymatic hydrolysis and share the binding characteristics and pharmacological actions of opioid alkaloids (including the capacity to induce tolerance and physical dependence). Structural modification of the peptides has yielded relatively selective agonists. For example, D-ala[2]-D-leu[5]-enkephalin (DADLE) and metkephamid are synthetic peptides that bind preferentially to δ receptors; morphiceptin (NH$_2$-tyr-pro-phe-pro-CONH$_2$) is a selective μ agonist. The development of selective antagonists has proven to be more difficult. Developments in this area have been reviewed recently (*see* Morley, 1980; Chang and Cuatrecasas, 1981; Martin, 1983; Akil *et al.*, 1984; Goldstein, 1984).

PHARMACOLOGICAL PROPERTIES

Morphine and related opioids produce their major effects on the CNS and the bowel. The effects are remarkably diverse and include analgesia, drowsiness, changes in mood, respiratory depression, decreased gastrointestinal motility, nausea, vomiting, and alterations of the endocrine and autonomic nervous systems. For reviews and references, *see* Martin and Sloan (1977), Duggan and North (1983), and Martin (1983). For older references, *see* Reynolds and Randall (1957) and *earlier editions* of this textbook.

Sites and Mechanism of Action. Morphine-like drugs behave as agonists, interacting with stereospecific and saturable receptors in the CNS and other tissues that are also the sites of action of a number of endogenous peptides (*see* above). These drugs appear to act preferentially at μ receptors, but they also have appreciable affinity for other types of opioid receptors.

Opioid drugs and peptides (especially μ and δ agonists) can produce naloxone-sensitive decreases in the spontaneous activity of neurons in the myenteric plexus of the gastrointestinal tract and in diverse areas of the CNS. These areas include those known to be involved in the regulation of functions that are affected by morphine-like drugs, such as respiration, pain perception, and affective behavior. Perhaps of greater interest are observations that opioids can selectively inhibit certain excitatory inputs to identified neurons. For example, the iontophoretic administration of morphine into the substantia gelatinosa suppresses the discharge of spinal neurons in lamina IV of the dorsal horn that is evoked by noxious stimuli (*e.g.*, heat) without changing responses to other inputs (*see* Duggan and North, 1983). While a postsynaptic action at discrete dendritic sites cannot be excluded, these findings suggest that opioids selectively inhibit the release of excitatory transmitters from terminals of nerves carrying nociceptive stimuli. In other situations, postsynaptic actions of opioids appear to be important. For example, application of opioids to neurons in the locus ceruleus reduces both spontaneous discharge and responses evoked by noxious stimuli. However, excitation of the neurons by antidromic stimulation is also suppressed, and the cells are hyperpolarized by the drugs (*see* Duggan and North, 1983).

At the cellular level, actions that result in increased potassium conductance and/or decreased calcium currents have been implicated in the electrophysiological effects of the opioids. However, the interrelationship between these actions and the underlying mechanisms is not clearly understood.

In some circumstances (*e.g.*, locus ceruleus neurons *in vitro*), the suppression of calcium currents is abolished by maneuvers that prevent hyperpolarizing responses to morphine; this suggests that the hyperpolarization that is produced by an increased potassium conductance causes a decrease in the voltage-dependent calcium conductance. In other circumstances (*e.g.*, myenteric plexus neurons), morphine prolongs the afterhyperpolarization that follows a train of action potentials; this effect occurs at concentrations that do not hyperpolarize the resting membrane. Since this afterhyperpolarization results from the activation of a potassium current that is caused by the entry of calcium during excitation, it appears that morphine may enhance the accumulation of free intracellular calcium, thereby causing an increased potassium conductance. Thus, it is possible that one primary action of opioids may be to increase the intracellular concentration of calcium; the ensuing hyperpolarization evidently decreases membrane excitability, either postsynaptically or presynaptically, to an extent sufficient to decrease the response to or the release of excitatory neurotransmitters, respectively. While this interpretation seems to be contradicted by the fact that elevation of the extracellular concentration of calcium frequently reduces the effects of opioids, such an increase in calcium does abolish morphine-induced hyperpolarization in myenteric neurons, for reasons that are not understood (*see* Duggan and North, 1983).

Opioids have been observed to inhibit prostaglandin-induced increases in the accumulation of adenosine $3',5'$-monophosphate (cyclic AMP) in homogenates of brain tissue and in cultured cell lines. This effect is specifically antagonized by naloxone and is dependent upon the presence of guanosine-triphosphate; the latter requirement is common to all known instances of receptor-mediated regulation of adenylate cyclase. Of potential relevance to mechanisms that underlie the phenomena of tolerance and withdrawal, the responses to prostaglandins recover in the continued presence of opioids and are then exaggerated upon the subsequent addition of naloxone (*see* Chapter 23). However, the relationship of such actions on the metabolism of cyclic AMP to the electrophysiological effects of opioids is not clear, and the administration of derivatives of cyclic AMP or inhibitors of cyclic nucleotide phosphodiesterase does not reduce responses to morphine (*see* Duggan and North, 1983). Nevertheless, there is one theoretical relationship that has not been explored. This stems from the demonstration that increased concentrations of cyclic AMP in hippocampal pyramidal neurons result in the reduction of calcium-dependent potassium conductances; this occurs without evidence of changes in stimulus-induced calcium currents (Madison and Nicoll, 1982). It follows that any morphine-induced decrease in cyclic AMP might tend to increase the impact of calcium upon potassium conductance.

Central Nervous System. In man, morphine-like drugs produce *analgesia, drowsiness, changes in mood,* and *mental clouding.* A significant feature of the analgesia is that it occurs without loss of consciousness. When therapeutic doses of morphine are given to patients with pain, they report that the pain is less intense, less discomforting, or entirely gone. Drowsiness occurs commonly both in volunteers and in patients with clinical pain. The extremities feel heavy and the body warm, the face (especially the nose) may itch, and the mouth becomes dry. In addition to relief of distress, some patients experience euphoria.

When morphine in the same dose is given to a presumably normal, pain-free individual, the experience is not always pleasant. Nausea is common, and vomiting may also occur. Feelings of drowsiness and inability to concentrate, difficulty in mentation, apathy, lessened physical activity, reduced visual acuity, and lethargy may ensue. In post-addict volunteers, mental clouding is less prominent than in normal subjects, and the euphoria is more pronounced. As the dose is increased, the subjective, analgesic, and toxic effects become more pronounced. In individuals who experience euphoria, the euphoric effect is accentuated; patients with severe pain that is not adequately relieved by smaller doses of morphine are usually relieved by larger doses (15 to 20 mg). The incidence of nausea and vomiting is also increased, and respiratory depression, the major toxic effect of morphine-like drugs, may become pronounced; but even large doses are not anticonvulsant and do not cause slurred speech or significant motor incoordination.

Analgesia. The relief of pain by morphine-like opioids is relatively selective, in that other sensory modalities (touch, vibration, vision, hearing, *etc.*) are not obtunded. Patients frequently report that the pain is still present but that they feel more comfortable (*see* below). Continuous dull pain is relieved more effectively than sharp intermittent pain, but with sufficient amounts of morphine it is possible to relieve even the severe pain associated with renal or biliary colic.

The selectivity of opioid-induced analgesia is greater than that of many other drugs that act on the CNS. Thus, the inhalation of nitrous oxide (20 to 40 volumes %), while producing analgesia that is approximately equivalent to 15 mg of morphine, also produces an overall impairment of consciousness, marked drowsiness, alterations in judgment, impairment of immediate and delayed memory, and nausea. Similarly, low concentrations of ether or gross intoxication with alcohol produce significant analgesia, but only in association with sedation and impairment of motor coordination, intellectual acuity, emotional control, and judgment. For a given degree of analgesia, the mental clouding produced by therapeutic doses of morphine is considerably less pronounced and of a qualitatively different character; morphine and related drugs rarely produce the garrulous, silly, and emotionally labile behavior frequently seen during intoxication with alcohol or a barbiturate. The subjective effects produced by opioids have been extensively studied in patients and nonaddict volunteers (*see* Bonica, 1980; Martin, 1983).

Any meaningful discussion of the action of analgesic agents must include some distinction between *pain as a specific sensation,* subserved by distinct neurophysiological structures, and *pain as suffering* (the original sensation plus the reactions evoked by the sensation). There is general agreement that all types of painful experiences, whether produced with experimental technics or occurring clinically as a result of pathology, include both the *original sensation* and the *reaction to that sensation* (*see* Sternbach, 1978).

In contrast to experimentally produced pain, pathological pain cannot be terminated at will, and the meaning of the sensation and the distress it engenders are markedly affected by the individual's previous experiences and current expectations. In experimentally produced pain, measurements of the effects of morphine on *pain threshold* have not always been consistent; some workers find that opioids reliably elevate the threshold, while many others do not obtain consistent changes. By contrast, moderate doses of morphine-like analgesics are quite effective in relieving clinical pain and increasing the capacity to *tolerate* experimentally induced pain. Opioids obtund the response to painful stimuli at several loci in the CNS. Not only is the sensation of pain altered by opioid analgesics, but the affective response is changed as well. This latter effect is best assessed by asking patients with clinical pain about the degree of relief produced by the drug administered. When pain does not evoke its usual responses (anxiety, fear, panic, and suffering), *a patient's ability to tolerate the pain may be markedly increased even when the capacity to perceive the sensation is relatively unaltered.* It is clear, however, that alteration of the emotional reaction to painful stimuli is not the sole mechanism of analgesia. Intrathecal administration of opioids can produce profound segmental analgesia without causing significant alteration of motor or sensory functions or subjective effects (*see* Yaksh, 1981).

Mechanisms and Sites of Opioid-Induced Analgesia. Opioid-induced analgesia is due to actions at several sites within the CNS and involves several systems of neurotransmitters. Although opioids do not alter the threshold or responsivity of afferent nerve endings to noxious stimulation or impair the conduction of the nerve impulse along peripheral nerves, they may decrease conduction of impulses of primary afferent fibers when they enter the spinal cord and decrease activity in other sensory endings. There are opioid binding sites (μ receptors) on the terminal axons of primary afferents within laminae I and II (substantia gelatinosa) of the spinal cord and in the spinal nucleus of the trigeminal nerve. Morphine-like drugs acting at this site are thought to decrease the release of neurotransmitters, such as substance P, that mediate transmission of pain impulses. Enkephalinergic nerve fibers in the dorsal horn of the spinal cord, which appear to come from interneurons, are usually inhibitory to dendrites and soma of nerves whose cell bodies may be in deeper laminae (IV and V). Morphine is inactive at sites at which met-enkephalin (primarily a δ agonist) inhibits neuronal firing. It can be inferred, therefore, that in the spinal cord, separate μ and δ receptors participate in inhibiting transmission of pain impulses. Agonists that interact with κ receptors also depress nociceptive spinal cord reflexes, but their spinal sites of action are less well understood. Stimulation of pain fibers activates enkephalinergic neurons in the spinal cord; these neurons may play a role in the gating of pain impulses and in mediating the effect of descending medullary analgesic pathways. Other neurotransmitters, such as 5-HT and norepinephrine, are also involved (*see* below).

There is a remarkable capacity to modulate the perception of pain in the CNS. Modulation of nociception involves neurons in the periventricular and periaqueductal gray matter that project to medullary nuclei (*e.g.*, raphe magnus and gigantocellularis); these nuclei send fibers in several distinct pathways to the spinal cord. There are also large inputs to the periaqueductal gray matter from the cortex, amygdala, and hypothalamus. Electrical stimulation of the periaqueductal gray matter produces analgesia by mechanisms that involve both opioid-like peptides and biogenic amines (*e.g.*,

5-HT and norepinephrine). There also appears to be an opioid system in the CNS that enhances susceptibility to painful stimuli (Wu *et al.*, 1983). Nociceptive modulatory systems can be activated by inputs from peripheral sensory nerves and possibly from higher centers. Part of the analgesic response to placebos may represent activation of such systems based on learning and experience with previous relief of pain.

As mentioned, there is evidence that nonopioid pathways also participate in the modulation of nociception. For example, the analgesic effects of stimulation at supraspinal sites are reduced by intrathecal administration of α-adrenergic and tryptaminergic antagonists; conversely, such administration of α-adrenergic (*e.g.*, clonidine) or tryptaminergic agonists produces an increase in nociceptive thresholds that is not reduced by naloxone or in subjects that have become tolerant to the effects of opioids. In addition, the effects of opioids and α-adrenergic agonists are additive, and subanalgesic doses of each class of drugs produce measurable analgesia (*see* Yaksh, 1981). A potential role of histamine in the modulation of nociception is suggested by the capacity of a wide variety of H_1 antagonists to enhance the antinociceptive effects of morphine in mice (Sun *et al.*, 1985).

Mechanism of Other CNS Effects. High doses of opioids can produce *muscular rigidity* in man, and both opioids and endogenous peptides cause catalepsy, circling, and stereotypical behavior in rats and other animals. These effects are probably related to actions at opioid receptors in the substantia nigra and striatum, and involve interactions with both dopaminergic and GABA-ergic neurons.

The mechanism by which opioids produce *euphoria, tranquility,* and other alterations of mood remains unsettled. Microinjections of opioids into the ventral tegmentum activate dopaminergic neurons that project to the nucleus accumbens. Animals will work to receive such injections, and activation (or disinhibition) of these neurons has been postulated to be a critical element in the reinforcing effects of opioids and, by inference, opioid-induced euphoria. However, the administration of dopaminergic antagonists does not consistently prevent these reinforcing effects. The neural systems that mediate opioid reinforcement in the ventral tegmentum appear to be distinct from those involved in the classical manifestations of physical dependence and analgesia (Bozarth and Wise, 1984).

The *locus ceruleus* contains both noradrenergic neurons and high concentrations of opioid receptors and is postulated to play a critical role in feelings of alarm, panic, fear, and anxiety. Activity in locus ceruleus is inhibited by α-adrenergic agonists and by both exogenous opioids and endogenous opioid-like peptides (*see* Redmond and Krystal, 1984). The role of the locus ceruleus in opioid withdrawal is discussed in Chapter 23.

Effects on the Hypothalamus and on Pituitary Hormones. Morphine decreases the response of the hypothalamus to afferent stimulation, but does not significantly alter its response to direct electrical stimulation. In many species, opioids alter the equilibrium point of the hypothalamic heat-regulatory mechanisms so that an animal will maintain a lower body temperature. In man, body temperature falls slightly after single therapeutic doses of morphine, although it appears to be increased by chronic high dosage. In the cat and other animals in which morphine causes excitement and mania, body temperature is increased. The effects on the regulation of temperature appear to involve actions at several types of opioid receptors in the spinal cord, medullary raphe, and hypothalamus; not all of these actions are sensitive to naloxone (*see* Martin, 1983).

Opioids act in the hypothalamus to inhibit the release of gonadotropin-releasing hormone (GnRH) and corticotropin-releasing factor (CRF), thus decreasing circulating concentrations of luteinizing hormone (LH), follicle-stimulating hormone (FSH), ACTH, and β-endorphin; the last two of these peptides are derived from the same precursor and are usually released simultaneously from corticotrophs in the pituitary. As a result of the decreased concentration of pituitary trophic hormones, the concentrations of testosterone and cortisol in plasma decline. In some species, the release of thyroid-stimulating hormone (TSH) is also inhibited, but this effect does not appear to be prominent or consistent in human subjects.

The administration of opioids increases the concentration of prolactin and growth hormone in plasma, possibly by reducing the dopaminergic inhibition of their secretion; the available data suggest that the effects on the two hormones are not mediated by the same types of opioid receptor (*see* Morley, 1980; Spiegel *et al.*, 1982). With chronic administration, tolerance develops to effects on hypothalamic releasing factors. For example, in male patients maintained on methadone, circulating concentrations of cortisol, LH, and testosterone are usually within the normal range.

The endogenous opioid peptides may play a role in the normal regulation of the secretion of several pituitary hormones, since the administration of naloxone increases concentrations of LH and FSH in plasma and depresses those of prolactin and growth hormone (Beaumont and Hughes, 1979).

The effects of morphine and other opioids on the secretion of antidiuretic hormone (ADH) are controversial. Some workers find increased release of ADH that is inhibited by naloxone. Other studies suggest that the diuresis that is sometimes observed after opioids is due to renal or hemodynamic effects, with either no change or a reduction in the concentration of ADH.

EEG. In man, single therapeutic doses of morphine-like opioids produce a shift toward increased voltage and lower frequencies in the EEG. In post-addicts, single doses of morphine suppress the rapid-eye-movement (REM) or "paradoxical sleep" phase of the EEG; slow-wave sleep is also reduced, while light sleep and waking time are increased. With repeated administration, some tolerance develops to these effects (*see* Martin, 1983).

Pupil. Morphine and most μ and κ opioid agonists cause constriction of the pupil in man. Miosis is due to an excitatory action on the autonomic segment of the nucleus of the oculomotor nerve in the dog, and the same mechanism may be presumed in man. Following toxic doses of opioids, *the miosis is marked and pinpoint pupils are pathognomonic;* however, marked mydriasis occurs when asphyxia intervenes. Some tolerance to the miotic effect develops, but addicts with high circulating concentrations of opioids continue to have constricted pupils.

The pupillary effects of morphine vary with the species. Cats (excited by morphine) and monkeys (sedated by morphine) show mydriasis. Therapeutic doses of morphine increase accommodative power and lower intraocular tension in both normal and glaucomatous eyes.

Excitatory Effects. High doses of morphine and related opioids produce convulsions. Several mechanisms appear to be involved, and different types of opioids produce seizures with different characteristics. Naloxone is more potent in antagonizing convulsions produced by some opioids (*e.g.,* morphine, methadone, and *d*-propoxyphene) than those produced by others (*e.g.,* meperidine, normeperidine, and thebaine). Anticonvulsant agents may or may not suppress seizures induced by opioids. Morphine-like drugs excite certain groups of neurons, especially hippocampal pyramidal cells; these excitatory effects are antagonized by naloxone and may result from disinhibition (*i.e.,* inhibition of inhibitory interneurons) (*see* Bloom, 1983; Duggan and North, 1983). Such effects may contribute to the seizures that are produced by some agents at doses only moderately higher than those required for analgesia. However, with most opioids, convulsions occur only at doses far in excess of those required to produce profound analgesia. In this circumstance, nonspecific (naloxone-insensitive) excitation, such as that produced by the application of morphine to Renshaw cells, may be involved.

In some species, relatively low doses of morphine produce gross excitation and hyperthermia. In the cat, for example, suitable doses produce not only analgesia but also a state in which the animal is continually restless, seems frightened, and cowers and scrambles to avoid being handled. Larger doses lead to seizures and death. These effects can be antagonized by naloxone and prevented by phenytoin. Following high doses of opioids, mice show increased locomotor activity. Animals stimulated rather than sedated by morphine include pigs, cows, sheep, goats, lions, tigers, bears, and horses. (For references, *see* Martin, 1983.)

Respiration. Morphine-like opioids depress respiration, at least in part by virtue of a direct effect on the brain stem respiratory centers. The respiratory depression is discernible even with doses too small to disturb consciousness, and increases progressively as the dose is increased. In man, death from morphine poisoning is nearly always due to respiratory arrest. Therapeutic doses of morphine in man depress all phases of respiratory activity (rate, minute volume, and tidal exchange). The diminished respiratory volume is due primarily to a slower rate of breathing, and with toxic amounts the rate may fall to 3 or 4 per minute. Morphine and related opioids may also produce irregular and periodic breathing; in man, this is often seen even after therapeutic doses.

Maximal respiratory depression occurs within approximately 7 minutes after intravenous administration of morphine, but may not be seen for as long as 30 minutes after intramuscular administration or as long as 90 minutes following subcutaneous administration. Following therapeutic doses, respiratory minute volume may be reduced for as long as 4 to 5 hours.

The primary mechanism of respiratory depression by morphine involves a reduction in the responsiveness of the brain stem respiratory centers to increases in carbon dioxide tension (P_{CO_2}). Opioids also depress the pontine and medullary centers involved in regulating respiratory rhythmicity and the responsiveness of medullary respiratory centers to electrical stimulation (*see* Mueller *et al.*, 1982; Martin, 1983).

The influence of various afferent stimuli on the respiratory center is not affected to the same degree. Hypoxic stimulation of the chemoreceptors may still be effective when the respiratory center shows decreased responsiveness to CO_2. When the main stimulus to respiration is hypoxia, the inhalation of high tensions of O_2 may produce apnea. In addition to a marked depression of the automatic regulation of respiration, voluntary control of respiration may also be altered. After large doses of morphine or synthetic analogs, patients will breathe if instructed to do so, but without such instruction they may remain relatively apneic.

Because of the accumulation of CO_2, respiratory rate and sometimes even minute volume can be unreliable indicators of the degree of respiratory depression that has been produced by morphine. Natural sleep also produces a decrease in the sensitivity of the medullary center to CO_2, and the effects of morphine and sleep are additive.

Numerous studies have compared morphine and morphine-like opioids with respect to their ratios of analgesic to respiratory-depressant activities. It is clear that all these opioids are capable of producing respiratory depression, and most studies have found that, when equianalgesic doses are used, the degree of respiratory depression observed is not significantly different from that seen with morphine (*see* Eckenhoff and Oech, 1960). However, the agonist-antagonist opioids are less likely to cause severe respiratory depression and are far less commonly associated with death due to overdosage (*see* below).

High concentrations of opioid receptors, as well as endogenous peptides, are found in the medullary areas believed to be important in ventilatory control. As mentioned previously, respiratory depression may be mediated by a subpopulation of μ receptors (μ_2), distinct from those that are involved in the production of analgesia (μ_1); there is also evidence that κ and δ receptors play some part in the respiratory-depressant effects of morphine. Thus, a "pure" μ_1-opioid agonist could theoretically produce analgesia with little respiratory depression. Such a possibility remains to be proven.

Cough. Morphine and related opioids also depress the *cough reflex*, at least in part by a direct effect on a cough center in the medulla. There is, however, no obligatory relationship between depression of respiration and depression of coughing, and effective antitussive agents are available that do not depress respiration (*see* below). As mentioned previously, suppression of cough appears to involve opioid receptors in the medulla that are less stereospecific and less sensitive to naloxone than are those responsible for analgesia.

Nauseant and Emetic Effects. Nausea and vomiting produced by morphine and its derivatives are unpleasant side effects caused by direct stimulation of the chemoreceptor trigger zone (CTZ) for emesis, in the area postrema of the medulla. Apomorphine, a dopaminergic agonist, also causes vomiting by stimulation of the CTZ. The emetic effect of morphine is counteracted by some phenothiazine derivatives, particularly those with a potent dopamine-blocking action (*see* Chapter 19). Certain individuals never vomit after morphine, whereas others do so each time the drug is administered.

Nausea and vomiting are relatively uncommon in recumbent patients given therapeutic doses of morphine, but nausea occurs in approximately 40% and vomiting in 15% of ambulatory patients given 15 mg of the drug subcutaneously. This suggests that a vestibular component is also operative. Indeed, it has been shown that the nauseant and emetic effects of morphine in man are markedly enhanced by vestibular stimulation, and that morphine and related synthetic analgesics produce an increase in vestibular sensitivity. Drugs that are useful in motion sickness are sometimes helpful in reducing opioid-induced nausea in ambulatory patients.

After a therapeutic dose of morphine, subsequent doses are unlikely to produce vomiting; other emetics are also ineffective after morphine. All clinically useful opioids produce some degree of nausea and vomiting. Careful, controlled clinical studies usually demonstrate that in equianalgesic dosage the incidence of such side effects is not significantly lower than that seen with morphine.

Cardiovascular System. In the supine patient, therapeutic doses of morphine-like opioids have no major effect on blood pressure or cardiac rate and rhythm. Such doses do produce peripheral vasodilatation, reduced peripheral resistance, and an inhibition of baroreceptor reflexes. Therefore, when supine patients assume the head-up position, orthostatic hypotension and fainting may occur. The *peripheral arteriolar and venous dilatation* produced by morphine involves several mechanisms. Morphine and most opioids provoke the release of *histamine,* which sometimes plays a large role in the hypotension. While vasodilatation is usually only partially blocked by histamine-receptor (H_1) blocking agents, it is effectively reversed by naloxone. Morphine also blunts the reflex vasoconstriction caused by increased P_{CO_2}.

Effects on the myocardium are not significant in normal man; the cardiac rate is either unaffected or slightly increased, and there is no consistent effect on cardiac output. The ECG is not altered. In patients with coronary artery disease but no acute medical problems, 8 to 15 mg of morphine intravenously produces a decrease in oxygen consumption, left ventricular end-diastolic pressure, and cardiac work; effects on cardiac index are usually slight (Alderman *et al.,* 1972; Popio *et al.,* 1978; Sethna *et al.,* 1982). In patients with acute myocardial infarction, the cardiovascular responses to morphine are generally similar (Lee *et al.,* 1976); they may, however, be more variable than in normal subjects, and the magnitude of changes (*e.g.,* the decrease in blood pressure) may be more pronounced.

Very large doses of morphine can be used to provide anesthesia, particularly during cardiac surgery (*see* Chapter 14). The depressant effects of most anesthetics on cardiac performance are thus avoided.

Morphine-like opioids should be used with caution in patients who have a decreased blood volume, since these agents can aggravate hypovolemic shock (*see* below). Morphine should be used with great care in patients with cor pulmonale, since deaths following ordinary therapeutic doses have been reported. The concurrent use of certain phenothiazines may increase the risk of morphine-induced hypotension.

Cerebral circulation is not directly affected by therapeutic doses of morphine. However, respiratory depression and CO_2 retention result in cerebral vasodilatation and an increase in cerebrospinal fluid pressure; the pressure increase does not occur when P_{CO_2} is maintained at normal levels by artificial ventilation.

In addition to obtunding cardiovascular reflexes, opioids can alter cardiovascular function by diverse means, such as by stimulating central and peripheral chemoreceptors; when applied to different parts of the brain, they either increase or decrease blood pressure and heart rate. Thus, the relatively minor cardiovascular effects associated with the therapeutic use of opioids probably reflect cancellation of opposing actions. In shock due to endotoxin, hypovolemia, or spinal injury, the administration of opioids worsens the cardiovascular status. The release of endogenous opioid peptides probably occurs under these circumstances, and the administration of opioid antagonists may be beneficial (*see* below).

Gastrointestinal Tract. The use of opium for relief of diarrhea and dysentery preceded by many centuries its employment for analgesia. The effects of morphine-like opioids on the bowel may vary widely, depending on the species, the dose, and the experimental technics. Therefore, the present discussion will concentrate on the effects observed in man.

Stomach. Morphine and related opioids cause some decrease in the secretion of hydrochloric acid; this can be overcome by chemical or psychic stimulation. A more pronounced effect is the decrease in motility associated with an increase in the tone of the antral portion of the stomach. There is also an increase in the tone of the first part of the duodenum, which often makes therapeutic intubation exceedingly difficult, delays the passage of the gastric contents through the duodenum for as much as 12 hours, and retards the absorption of drugs that are administered orally.

Small Intestine. Both biliary and pancreatic secretions are diminished by morphine, and digestion of food in the small intestine is delayed. There is an increase in resting tone, and periodic spasms are observed. The amplitude of the nonpropulsive type of rhythmic, segmental contractions is usually enhanced, but *propulsive contractions are markedly decreased.* The upper part of the small intestine, particularly the duodenum, is affected more than the ileum. A period of relative atony may follow the hypertonicity. Water is more completely absorbed from the chyme because of the delayed passage of the bowel contents, and the viscosity of the chyme is thereby increased. The tone of the ileocecal valve is enhanced. Large doses of atropine may counteract, in part, the gastrointestinal responses to morphine, but resection of the extrinsic nerves and ganglionic blocking agents do not do so. These issues have been reviewed by Burks (1976).

In the presence of intestinal hypersecretion that may be associated with diarrhea, morphine-like drugs inhibit the transfer of fluid and electrolytes into the lumen by naloxone-sensitive actions on the intestinal mucosa. Such actions may play an important role in the antidiarrheal effects of opioids in some circumstances (*see* Awouters *et al.,* 1983).

Large Intestine. Propulsive peristaltic waves in the colon are diminished or abolished after morphine, and tone is increased to the point of spasm. The resulting delay in the passage of the contents causes considerable desiccation of the feces, which, in turn, retards its advance through the colon. The amplitude of the nonpropulsive type of rhythmic contractions of the colon is usually enhanced. The tone of the anal sphincter is greatly augmented, and this, combined with inattention to the normal sensory stimuli for the defecation reflex due to the central actions of the drug, further contributes to morphine-induced constipation.

Atropine partially antagonizes the spasmogenic action on the human colon, but it has little effect on the decreased propulsive activity produced by morphine.

Whereas the intestinal responses to opium and morphine are unpleasant side effects when the drugs are given for analgesia, they can be desirable therapeutic objectives in themselves, especially in patients with exhausting diarrhea or dysentery. In patients with chronic ulcerative colitis, opioids may stimulate colonic motility, and the use of opioids during acute episodes of the disease sometimes leads to a toxic dilatation of the colon (Garrett *et al.,* 1967). While all morphine-like opioids produce qualitatively similar effects on the motility of the bowel, there are important quantitative differences. Not all opioids are useful in the treatment of diarrheas and some (such as diphenoxylate and loperamide) have relatively selective actions on the bowel that provide an important therapeutic advantage (*see* below).

Mechanism of Action on the Bowel. Neither the administration of ganglionic blocking agents nor the removal of the extrinsic innervation of the bowel prevents the characteristic actions of morphine and its surrogates in the unanesthetized animal. Morphine has many effects on the myenteric plexus of the intestine, including actions on cholinergic, tryptaminergic, and enkephalinergic receptors (*see* Burks, 1976). However, the constipating and antidiarrheal actions of opioids may not be due entirely to local actions on the intestine. Injection of minute quantities of morphine into the cerebral ventricles inhibits gastrointestinal propulsive activity, an effect abolished by intraventricular administration of opioid antagonists or by vagotomy. The local application of morphine or opioid peptides to the spinal cord also decreases peristalsis (Porreca and Burks, 1983). Although some tolerance develops to the effects of opioids on gastrointestinal motility, patients who take opioids chronically remain constipated.

Biliary Tract. Therapeutic doses of morphine, codeine, and other morphine surrogates can cause a marked increase in pressure in the biliary tract. After the subcutaneous injection of 10 mg of morphine sulfate the pressure in the common bile duct may rise more than tenfold within 15 minutes; this effect may persist for 2 hours or more. Symptoms often accompany the increased pressure and vary from epigastric distress to typical biliary colic.

Some patients with biliary colic may experience exacerbation and not relief of pain when given these drugs. Furthermore, an occasional individual complains of pain in the epigastrium or right hypochondrium after morphine, probably due to duodenal or biliary tract spasm. Spasm of the biliary tract produced by morphine is evident roentgenographically as well as manometrically, and a sharp constriction becomes apparent at the lower end of the common bile duct (sphincter of Oddi). This spasm prevents emptying and thus causes the intraductal pressure to rise, and is probably responsible for the elevations of plasma amylase and lipase that are sometimes found after patients have been given morphine. Such elevations may persist for 24 hours after therapeutic doses and may confuse the diagnosis of intra-abdominal pathology, especially when acute pancreatitis is one of the diseases under consideration. Although increases in pressure may occur with as little as 2.5 mg of morphine given intravenously, biliary spasm is not consistently produced by therapeutic doses, and some patients show no changes in bile duct size or pressure. Atropine only partially prevents morphine-induced biliary spasm, but opioid antagonists prevent or relieve it. Nitroglycerin (0.6 mg) administered sublingually also decreases the elevated intrabiliary pressure. Some opioids such as meperidine, fentanyl, and all of the available agonist-antagonists seem to produce less pronounced increases in biliary pressure.

Other Smooth Muscle. *Ureter and Urinary Bladder.* Therapeutic doses of morphine increase the tone and amplitude of contractions of the *ureter,* especially of the lower third. The response of the ureters in man to opioids is quite variable. When the antidiuretic effects of the drugs are prominent and urine flow decreases, the ureter may become quiescent.

The tone of the detrusor muscle of the *urinary bladder* is augmented by morphine; this sometimes causes urinary urgency. The tone of the vesical sphincter is also enhanced by morphine; this effect may make urination difficult, and catheterization is sometimes required following therapeutic doses of morphine. Naloxone antagonizes this action. In addition, the central effects of these drugs may make the patient inattentive to the stimuli arising in the bladder and may play a role in morphine-induced urinary retention.

Uterus. Studies of the effects of therapeutic doses of morphine in women suggest that labor may be somewhat prolonged (*see* Campbell *et al.,* 1961). The mechanism involved is not clear; however, it has been noted that, if the uterus is made hyperactive by oxytocics, morphine tends to restore tone, frequency, and amplitude of contractions to normal. In addition, the central effects of morphine may affect the degree to which the parturient is able to cooperate in the delivery. Neonatal mortality may thus be increased by the injudicious use of opioids during labor as a result of these factors and the high sensitivity of the neonate to the respiratory-depressant effect of these drugs.

Bronchial Musculature. Although large doses of morphine and meperidine produce constriction of the bronchi, this effect is rarely seen with therapeutic doses in man. The possible role of morphine-induced bronchoconstriction in the aggravation of asthma is discussed below.

Skin. In man, therapeutic doses of morphine cause cutaneous blood vessels to dilate. The skin of the face, neck, and upper thorax frequently becomes flushed and warm. These changes in cutaneous circulation may, in part, be due to the release of histamine and may be responsible for the *pruritus* and the *sweating* that commonly follow the administration of morphine. Histamine release

probably accounts for the urticaria commonly seen at the site of injection. Pruritus may also be due to effects of opioids on neural systems, since it is provoked by opioids that do not release histamine and is quickly abolished by small doses of naloxone (*see* Scott and Fischer, 1982).

Immune System. In mice, morphine reduces the number and phagocytic function of macrophages and polymorphonuclear leukocytes, as well as the survival time of animals with bacterial and fungal infections. While dose related, these effects are not antagonized by naloxone (Tubaro *et al.,* 1983). Morphine causes a dose-related suppression of the activity of natural killer cells from rats, while β-endorphin and met-enkephalin (but not morphine) *enhance* killer-cell activity in blood taken from human volunteers. Reduced lymphoproliferative responses to stimulation with phytohemagglutinin have also been seen in human heroin addicts. The implications of these effects, as well as the underlying mechanisms, are not at all clear at this time.

Tolerance, Physical Dependence, and Liability for Abuse. The development of tolerance and physical dependence with repeated use is a characteristic feature of all the opioid drugs, and the possibility of developing psychological dependence on the effects of these drugs is one of the major limitations of their clinical use. It is important to emphasize that the overall liability for abuse of an agent is not established by any one single factor; rather, it is a composite based on a number of factors. These include: (1) the capacity of the drug to produce the kind of physical dependence in which drug withdrawal causes sufficient distress to bring about drug-seeking behavior; (2) its ability to suppress withdrawal symptoms caused by withdrawal of other agents; (3) the degree to which it induces euphoria similar to that produced by morphine and related opioids; (4) the patterns of toxicity that occur when the dose is increased beyond the usual therapeutic range; and (5) physical characteristics of the drug, such as water solubility, that may determine whether it is likely to be abused by the parenteral route. There is evidence to suggest that the overall abuse liability of some of the agonist-antagonist opioids is lower than that of morphine-like agents. The implications of the differences in abuse potential for the choice of agents in therapy are discussed below, and the subject of compulsive drug use is elaborated in detail in Chapter 23.

Absorption, Distribution, Fate, and Excretion. *Absorption.* The opioids are readily absorbed from the gastrointestinal tract; they are also absorbed from the nasal mucosa and the lung (as when heroin is used as snuff or opium is smoked), and after subcutaneous or intramuscular injection. With most opioids, including morphine, the effect of a given dose is less after oral than after parenteral administration, due to significant but variable first-pass metabolism in the liver. For example, the bioavailability of oral preparations of morphine ranges from 15 to 49% in cancer patients (Säwe *et al.*, 1981). The shape of the time-effect curve also varies with the route of administration, so that the duration of action is often somewhat longer with the oral route. If adjustment is made for variability of first-pass metabolism and clearance, it is possible to achieve adequate relief of pain by the oral administration of morphine. Satisfactory analgesia in cancer patients has been associated with a very broad range of steady-state concentrations of morphine in plasma (16 to 364 ng/ml) (Neumann *et al.*, 1982).

When morphine and most opioids are given intravenously, they act promptly. However, the more lipid-soluble compounds have a somewhat more rapid onset of action after subcutaneous administration due to differences in the rates of absorption and entry into the CNS. When opioids are given acutely, their durations of analgesic action show relatively little variation (*see* Table 22–3). Other effects may persist longer than analgesia.

Table 22–3. A COMPARISON OF OPIOID ANALGESICS WITH RESPECT TO DOSAGE, DURATION OF ACTION, WITHDRAWAL SYMPTOMS, AND DISTINGUISHING FEATURES

NONPROPRIETARY NAME	TRADE NAME	DOSE * (*mg*)	DURATION OF ACTION * (*hours*)	WITHDRAWAL SYMPTOMS	DISTIN- GUISHING FEATURES ▲
Morphine		10	4–5	*see* text	*see* text
Heroin (diacetyl- morphine)		4 (2–8)	3–4	like morphine	2
Hydromorphone (dihydromorphinone)	DILAUDID	1.5	4–5	like morphine	
Oxymorphone (dihydro- hydroxymorphinone)	NUMORPHAN	1.0–1.5	4–5	like morphine	
Metopon (methyldihydro- morphinone		3.5	4–5	like morphine	3
Codeine		120 (10–20)	(4–6)	*see* text	*see* text
Hydrocodone (dihydro- codeinone)	HYCODAN †	(5–10)	(4–8)	between morphine and codeine	4,8
Drocode (dihydrocodeine)	SYNALGOS-DC †	60	4–5	between morphine and codeine	
Oxycodone (dihydro- hydroxycodeinone)		10–15 (3–5)	4–5 (4–5)	close to morphine	8
Pholcodine (β-morph- olinylethylmorphine)		(5–15)	(4–5)	much less than codeine	3,4,5
Levorphanol	LEVO-DROMORAN	2	4–5	like morphine	6,8
Methadone	DOLOPHINE	8–10	3–5	*see* text	6,8
Dextromoramide	PALFIUM	5–7.5	4–5	like methadone	3,6,8
Dipipanone		20–25	4–5	like methadone	3,6,8,9
Phenadoxone		10–20	1–3	less than mor- phine	3,9
Meperidine	DEMEROL, *etc.*	75–100	2–4	*see* text	1,7
Alphaprodine	NISENTIL	40	1–2	like meperidine	1,7

* *Dose* shown is the amount given *subcutaneously* that produces approximately the same analgesic effects as 10 mg of morphine administered subcutaneously. The figures in *parentheses* are the *doses* and the *duration of action* for *oral, antitussive* doses; they are not necessarily equieffective doses. *Duration of action* shown is for analgesic effects after *subcutaneous* administration; after *intravenous* administration, peak effects are somewhat more pronounced but overall effects are of shorter duration. The doses and durations shown in this table are based primarily on papers reviewed by Eddy and coworkers (1957), Reynolds and Randall (1957), and Lasagna (1964), and are augmented by more recent studies of newer drugs.

▲ 1 = causes little or no constipation; 2 = manufacture or importation into the United States illegal; 3 = not available in the United States; 4 = by tradition used mainly as an antitussive; 5 = little or no analgesic or euphorigenic activity; 6 = may exhibit cumulative effects on repeated dosage; 7 = retains 25 to 40% of efficacy when given orally; 8 = retains 50% or more of its analgesic efficacy when given orally; 9 = marked irritation at injection sites.

† These opioids are marketed in the United States only in combination with additional ingredients.

Distribution and Fate. When therapeutic concentrations of morphine are present in plasma, about one third of the drug is protein bound. Free morphine rapidly leaves the blood and accumulates in parenchymatous tissues, such as the kidney, lung, liver, and spleen. Skeletal muscle has a somewhat lower level of morphine, but because of its mass it accounts for the major fraction of the drug in the body. Morphine does not persist in tissues, and 24 hours after the last dose tissue concentrations are quite low.

Although the primary site of action of morphine is in the CNS, in the adult only small quantities pass the blood-brain barrier. Compared to other more lipid-soluble opioids such as codeine, heroin, and methadone, morphine crosses the blood-brain barrier at a considerably lower rate (*see* Oldendorf *et al., 1972*). Transport of opioids by the choroid plexus has been noted, but its significance remains uncertain.

Very small amounts of opioids introduced epidurally or directly into the spinal canal produce profound analgesia that lasts up to 24 hours. Distribution and metabolism after intrathecal or epidural administration of opioids are markedly dependent on the drug used. With highly lipophilic agents, such as heroin or hydromorphone, rapid absorption by neural tissues produces very localized effects and segmental analgesia. With morphine, the least lipophilic of the opioids used clinically, there is rostral spread of the drug, and prominent untoward effects, including nausea, vomiting, and respiratory depression, can be produced (*see* Bromage *et al.*, 1982; Moore *et al.*, 1984).

The major pathway for the detoxication of morphine is conjugation with glucuronic acid. While N-demethylation of many opioids occurs in several mammalian species including man, this pathway does not appear to be important in the metabolism of morphine in man. In young adults, the half-life of morphine in plasma is about 2.5 to 3 hours; this value may be slightly shorter in younger patients and longer in older individuals (Dahlström *et al.*, 1979; Owen *et al.*, 1983). In older patients, the volume of distribution is considerably smaller and initial concentrations of morphine in plasma are correspondingly higher (Owen *et al.*, 1983).

Excretion. Very little morphine is excreted unchanged; it is eliminated by glomerular filtration, primarily as morphine-3-glucuronide. Although traces of morphine are detectable in the urine for well over 48 hours, 90% of the total excretion takes place during the first day. About 7 to 10% of administered morphine eventually appears in the feces, and this comes almost exclusively from the bile as conjugated morphine. Enterohepatic circulation of morphine and morphine glucuronide occurs, which probably accounts for the presence of small amounts of morphine in the urine for several days after the last dose.

Codeine, in contrast to morphine, is approximately two thirds as effective orally as parenterally, both as an analgesic and as a respiratory depressant. Very few opioids have so high an oral-parenteral potency ratio; levorphanol and oxycodone are also in this group. Their greater oral efficacy is due to less first-pass metabolism in the liver. Once absorbed, codeine is metabolized by the liver and excreted chiefly in the urine, largely in inactive forms. A small fraction (approximately 10%) of administered codeine is demethylated to form morphine, and both free and conjugated morphine can be found in the urine after therapeutic doses of codeine. Codeine has an exceptionally low affinity for opioid receptors, and the analgesic effect of codeine may be due to its conversion to morphine. However, its antitussive actions probably involve distinct receptors that bind codeine itself with high affinity. The half-life of codeine in plasma is 2.5 to 3 hours.

Heroin (diacetylmorphine) is rapidly hydrolyzed to monoacetylmorphine (MAM), which, in turn, is hydrolyzed to morphine. Both heroin and MAM are more lipid soluble than morphine and enter the brain more readily. Current evidence suggests that morphine and MAM are responsible for the pharmacological actions of heroin. Heroin is mainly excreted in the urine, largely as free and conjugated morphine.

The absorption, fate, and distribution of morphine-like drugs have been reviewed by Way (1968) and Misra (1978).

Idiosyncrasy, Variations in Response, and Precautions. Morphine and related opioids produce a wide spectrum of unwanted effects, such as nausea, vomiting, dizziness, mental clouding, dysphoria, pruritus, constipation, and increased pressure in the biliary tract. These occur so commonly that they cannot be considered idiosyncratic, even though there are many patients who do not experience such effects. Rarely, a patient may develop a delirium. *Increased sensitivity* to pain after the analgesia has worn off may also occur.

Allergic phenomena occur with opioid analgesics, but they are not common. They are usually manifested as urticaria and other types of skin rashes; contact dermatitis in nurses and pharmaceutical workers has been reported. Wheals at the site of injection of morphine, codeine, and related drugs are probably caused by the release of histamine. Anaphylactoid reactions have been reported after intravenous codeine and morphine, but such reactions are quite rare; however, it has been suggested, but not proven, that they are responsible for some of the sudden deaths, episodes of pulmonary edema, and other complications that occur among addicts who use heroin intravenously (*see* Chapter 23).

A number of factors may alter the sensitivity to opioid analgesics, including the integrity of the blood-brain barrier. For example, when morphine is administered to the mother prior to delivery, the newborn infant may exhibit respiratory depression even though the drug produced no significant depression in the mother (*see* Way *et al.,* 1965). Since the blood-brain barrier does not play as prominent a role in limiting the access of all opioids to the CNS, some, such as meperidine, cause relatively less respiratory depression in the newborn in doses that produce analgesia in the mother. In adults, the duration of the analgesia produced by morphine increases progressively with age; however, there is little change in the degree of analgesia that is obtained with a given dose (*see* Kaiko, 1980). Changes in pharmacokinetic parameters can only partially explain these observations.

The patient with severe pain may tolerate larger doses of morphine (three to four therapeutic doses over a period of a few hours) but may exhibit subjective symptoms and respiratory depression should the pain suddenly subside. *Illnesses* of various types may increase or decrease the sensitivity to morphine and related drugs. Patients with *myxedema* and *multiple sclerosis* are more sensitive to the depressant effects, whereas *hyperthyroid* patients seem more tolerant; controlled studies, however, are lacking. All the opioid analgesics are metabolized by the liver, and the drugs should be used with caution in patients with hepatic disease, since increased bioavailability after oral administration or cumulative effects may occur (*see* Novick *et al.,* 1981; Säwe *et al.,* 1981).

Patients with *reduced blood volume* are considerably more susceptible to the hypotensive effects of morphine and related drugs, and these agents must be employed cautiously in patients with hypotension from any cause. The basis for this susceptibility and the uses of opioid antagonists in shock are discussed below. The respiratory-depressant effects of morphine and the related capacity to elevate intracranial pressure may be markedly exaggerated in the presence of head injury or of an already elevated cerebrospinal fluid pressure produced by trauma. Therefore, while *head injury per se* does not constitute an absolute contraindication to the use of opioids, the possibility of exaggerated depression of respiration must be considered. In addition, opioids may aggravate the effects of cerebral and spinal ischemia (*see* below). Finally, since opioids produce mental clouding and side effects such as miosis and vomiting, which are important signs in following the clinical course of patients with head injuries, the advisability of their use must be carefully weighed. In patients with *prostatic hypertrophy*, morphine may precipitate acute urinary retention, requiring repeated catheterization.

Morphine and related opioids must be used with great caution in any situation in which there is decreased respiratory reserve, such as *emphysema, kyphoscoliosis,* or even severe *obesity*. In patients with chronic *cor pulmonale,* death has occurred following therapeutic doses of morphine. Although many patients with such conditions seem to be functioning within normal limits, they are already utilizing compensatory mechanisms, such as increased respiratory rate. Many have chronically elevated levels of plasma CO_2, and may be less sensitive to the stimulating actions of CO_2. The further imposition of the depressant effects of opioids can be disastrous.

Opioids can precipitate attacks of *asthma* in anesthetized patients, but the risk does not seem to be high. There is general agreement, however, that during an asthmatic attack morphine and related drugs should be avoided. All opioid analgesics depress the respiratory center; most release histamine, depress the cough reflex, and tend to dry secretions. Giving such agents to asthmatic patients, in whom the airway resistance may be many times greater than normal, invites disaster by producing a decrease in respiratory drive without a corresponding decrease in airway resistance.

Interactions with Other Drugs. The depressant effects of some opioids may be exaggerated and prolonged by phenothiazines, monoamine oxidase inhibitors, and tricyclic antidepressants; the mechanisms of these supra-additive effects are not fully understood, but may involve alterations in the rate of metabolic transformation of the opioid or alterations in neurotransmitters involved in the actions of opioids. Some, but not all, phenothiazines reduce the amount of opioid required to produce a given level of analgesia. However, depending on the specific agent, the respiratory-depressant effects seem also to be enhanced, the degree of sedation is increased, and the hypotensive effects of phenothiazines become an additional complication. *Some phenothiazine derivatives enhance the sedative effects, but at the same time seem to be antianalgesic* and increase the amount of opioid required to produce satisfactory relief from pain (Moore and Dundee, 1961). Small doses of amphetamine increase the effects of morphine substantially (Forrest *et al.*, 1977), as does the antihistamine hydroxyzine, when given intramuscularly (Beaver and Feise, 1976).

Preparations, Routes of Administration, and Dosage of Opium and Its Alkaloids. The official morphine content of powdered opium is 10.0 to 10.5% by weight; it is available as a hydroalcoholic solution, *opium tincture (laudanum, deodorized opium tincture)*, containing approximately 10% opium (1% morphine). The average adult dose is 0.6 ml (equivalent to 6 mg of morphine), taken orally. A preparation of purified opium alkaloids is available for injection (PANTOPON). *Paregoric (camphorated opium tincture)* is a hydroalcoholic preparation in which there is also benzoic acid, camphor, and anise oil. The usual adult dose is 5 to 10 ml, which corresponds to 2 to 4 mg of morphine. Paregoric represents a needlessly complex therapeutic survival of a former day.

Morphine. Morphine is prescribed only in the form of its water-soluble salt, *morphine sulfate.* Solutions of morphine sulfate are available for oral use (from 2 to 20 mg/ml) and for injection (from 2 to 15 mg/ml); tablets and rectal suppositories are also available.

Subcutaneously or *intramuscularly,* 10 mg/70 kg of body weight is generally considered to be an optimal initial dose of morphine and provides satisfactory analgesia in approximately 70% of patients with moderate-to-severe pain (*e.g.*, postoperative pain) with only a moderate incidence of side effects. Subsequent doses may be higher or lower, depending on the analgesic response and the side effects produced. The usual *oral* adult dose of morphine is 10 to 30 mg. However, controlled studies have shown that, on average, oral administration is only about one sixth as effective as parenteral administration. There is wide variability in first-pass metabolism, and the dose should be titrated to the patient's needs.

Occasionally morphine sulfate is given *intravenously,* and it has been employed by this route for the control of severe postoperative pain and restlessness, for preoperative medication, for minor surgical procedures when general anesthesia is not indicated, for severe cardiac pain, for renal colic,

and for pulmonary edema. The usual dose is 2.5 to 5 mg. Maximal respiratory depression is manifest within 10 minutes. This dose may be repeated in 1 to 2 hours if necessary.

The dose of morphine for *infants and children* is 0.1 to 0.2 mg/kg (maximum 15 mg), injected subcutaneously or intramuscularly.

Codeine. Codeine is available in the form of its salts, *codeine sulfate* and *codeine phosphate*; both are supplied as tablets (15 to 60 mg). Codeine phosphate is much more soluble in water than is the sulfate, and is available for injection. It is contained in numerous analgesic combinations (liquids, tablets, and capsules) and in various antitussive combinations (liquids, capsules, and tablets).

Although a dose of 120 mg of codeine, administered subcutaneously, produces analgesia equivalent to that resulting from 10 mg of morphine, the former drug has few advantages over morphine when used parenterally. However, codeine has a high oral-parenteral potency ratio; in terms of total analgesia, codeine is about 60% as potent when given orally as when injected intramuscularly. In this respect it has definite advantages over morphine. Orally, a dose of 30 mg of codeine is approximately equianalgesic with 325 to 600 mg of aspirin. While the analgesic effects of opioids and aspirin-like drugs are usually additive, the analgesia produced by a combination of these two drugs at this dosage level sometimes exceeds that of 60 mg of codeine. However, the variability of the analgesic response at this dosage level is considerable (*see* Beaver, 1966; Cooper and Beaver, 1976). The effects of 15 mg of codeine orally can be demonstrated by objective technics to reduce the frequency of pathological cough, and progressively greater cough suppression is seen as the dose is increased up to 60 mg (Sevelius *et al.*, 1971). The abuse liability of codeine is lower than that of morphine, as discussed more fully in Chapter 23.

Apomorphine. Apomorphine, a dopaminergic agonist, is obtained by exposure of morphine to strong mineral acids. Its analgesic properties are diminished, but it retains the capacity to stimulate the medullary CTZ and to produce a combination of CNS excitation and depression. It has been used therapeutically for the production of emesis; the usual dose is 5 mg, given subcutaneously.

Etorphine hydrochloride is an analog of thebaine used exclusively for immobilizing large animals. In man, it is 400 times as potent as morphine in producing subjective effects and suppressing opioid withdrawal. Its duration of action is relatively short. Poisoning with etorphine should be treated in the same way as morphine poisoning.

Other Semisynthetic Morphine and Codeine Derivatives. There are many drugs that can substitute for morphine and codeine. Their names, doses, and special characteristics are shown in Table 22–3.

Hydromorphone hydrochloride (DILAUDID) is available in tablets (1 to 4 mg) and in rectal suppositories. Solutions for injection (from 1 to 10 mg/ml) are also available. *Oxycodone hydrochloride* is about as potent as morphine and is nearly ten times more potent than codeine. Like codeine, it is about one half as potent orally as parenterally. It is available in 5-mg tablets, as a solution, and in combination with other analgesics. *Oxymorphone hydrochloride* (NUMORPHAN) is available as a solution for injection and in rectal suppositories. *Hydrocodone bitartrate* is used in combination with other ingredients in proprietary antitussive and analgesic-antipyretic mixtures.

Diacetylmorphine (heroin) is not available for therapeutic use in the United States. Given intramuscularly to cancer patients with postoperative pain, it is about twice as potent as morphine. While peak analgesic effects occur a few minutes earlier than with morphine, its duration of action is not significantly different. Heroin does not appear to have any unique therapeutic advantages over the available opioids (*see* Kaiko *et al.*, 1981).

ACUTE OPIOID POISONING

Acute opioid poisoning may result from clinical overdosage, accidental overdosage in addicts, or attempts at suicide. Occasionally, a delayed type of poisoning may occur from the injection of an opioid into chilled skin areas or in patients with low blood pressure and shock. The drug is not fully absorbed, and, therefore, a subsequent dose may be given. When normal circulation is established, an excessive amount may suddenly be absorbed. It is difficult to state the exact amount of any opioid that is toxic or lethal to man. Recent experiences with methadone indicate that in nontolerant individuals serious toxicity may follow the oral ingestion of 40 to 60 mg. Older literature suggests that, in the case of morphine, a normal, pain-free adult is not likely to die after oral doses of less than 120 mg, or to have serious toxicity with less than 30 mg parenterally.

Symptoms and Diagnosis. By the time he is seen by the physician, the patient who has taken an overdose of an opioid is usually asleep or stuporous. If a large overdose has been taken, he cannot be aroused and may be in a *profound coma.* The *respiratory rate* is quite low (sometimes only 2 to 4 per minute), and *cyanosis* may be present. As the respiratory exchange becomes poorer, *blood pressure,* at first maintained near normal, falls progressively. If adequate oxygenation is restored early, the blood pressure will improve; if hypoxia persists untreated, however, there may be capillary damage, and measures to combat *shock* may then be required. The *pupils* are symmetrical and pinpoint in size; however, if hypoxia is severe, they may be dilated. *Urine formation* is depressed. *Body temperature* falls, and the skin becomes cold and clammy. The *skeletal muscles* are flaccid, the jaw is relaxed, and the tongue may fall back and block

the airway. Frank convulsions may occasionally be noted in infants and children. When death occurs, it is nearly always due to respiratory failure. Sometimes, even if respiration is restored, death may still occur as a result of complications, such as pneumonia or shock, that develop during the period of coma. *Pulmonary edema* is commonly seen with opioid poisoning. It is probably not due to contaminants or to anaphylactoid reactions, and has been observed following toxic doses of morphine, methadone, propoxyphene, and uncontaminated heroin.

The triad of *coma, pinpoint pupils,* and *depressed respiration* strongly suggests opioid poisoning. Since deliberate or accidental overdosage is common among addicts, the finding of needle marks suggestive of addiction further supports the diagnosis. Mixed poisonings, however, are not uncommon. In such cases, other agents such as a barbiturate or alcohol may also be contributing to the clinical picture. Examination of the urine and gastric contents for various drugs may aid in diagnosis, but the results usually become available too late to influence treatment.

Treatment. The first step is to establish a patent airway and ventilate the patient. Opioid antagonists such as naloxone can produce dramatic reversal of the severe respiratory depression (*see* below), and the use of naloxone is now the treatment of choice. The safest approach is the administration of small intravenous doses (*e.g.,* 0.4 mg of naloxone); this dose may be repeated after 2 to 3 minutes. For children, the initial dose is 0.01 mg/kg. If no effect is seen after a total dose of 10 mg, one can reasonably question the accuracy of the diagnosis. Pulmonary edema sometimes associated with opioid overdosage may be countered by positive-pressure respiration. Tonic-clonic seizures, occasionally seen as part of the toxic syndrome with meperidine and propoxyphene, are ameliorated by treatment with naloxone.

Opioid antagonists, such as nalorphine and levallorphan, that also have agonistic actions should be used with care since they may further embarrass respiration that has been depressed by alcohol, barbiturates, or related CNS depressants. Since naloxone has no direct respiratory-depressant action, it is the drug of choice. The presence of alcohol or a barbiturate does not prevent the salutary effect of an antagonist, and in cases of mixed intoxications the situation will be improved largely due to antagonism of the respiratory-depressant effects of the opioid. However, there is some evidence that naloxone and naltrexone may also antagonize some of the depressant actions of sedative-hypnotics (*see* below). One need not attempt to restore the patient to full consciousness. The duration of action of antagonists is usually shorter than that of many opioids; hence, the patient must be carefully watched, lest he slip back into coma. This is particularly important when the overdosage is due to methadone or *l*-acetylmethadol. The depressant effects of these drugs may persist for 24 to 72 hours, and fatalities have occurred as a result of premature discontinuation of naloxone. In such cases, longer-acting antagonists such as naltrexone may be useful.

The use of an opioid antagonist to treat acute poisoning in an addict should be undertaken with care, since the antagonist may precipitate a severe withdrawal syndrome that cannot be readily suppressed during the period of action of the antagonist.

These principles are appropriate in treating acute poisoning with any of the opioid agonists. Toxicity due to overdose of pentazocine and other opioids with mixed actions can be alleviated by high doses of naloxone, which is more effective than agonist-antagonists such as nalorphine and levallorphan. The pharmacological actions of opioid antagonists are discussed in more detail below.

Therapeutic Uses

Sir William Osler referred to morphine as "God's own medicine." While morphine-like drugs remain of great importance in the treatment of severe pain and the pain of terminal illness, physicians now have other options for many conditions that involve moderate pain.

General Principles. When opioid analgesics are administered for the relief of pain, cough, or diarrhea, only symptomatic treatment is being provided and the underlying pathology remains. The physician must constantly weigh the benefits of this relief against its costs and risks to the patient. Such costs and risks are frequently quite different, depending upon whether the symptom is a manifestation of an acute or a chronic disease.

In acute problems, opioids may obscure the progress of the disease or the location or intensity of pain. However, relief of pain can also facilitate history taking and examination, and thereby aid in diagnosis.

The problems that arise in the *treatment of chronic conditions* involve more com-plex considerations. Repeated daily administration will eventually produce some tolerance to the therapeutic effects of the drug, and some degree of physical dependence as well. The degree will depend on the particular drug, the frequency of administration, and the quantity administered. The risk of developing psychological dependency is always present. Thus, a decision to relieve any chronic symptom, especially pain, by the parenteral administration of an opioid may be shortsighted and can be a disservice to the patient. Measures other than opioid drugs should be employed to relieve chronic pain when they are effective and available. Such measures include the use of local nerve block, antidepressant drugs, electrical stimulation, acupuncture, hypnosis, or behavioral modification (*see* Reuler *et al.*, 1980).

In the usual doses, morphine-like drugs relieve suffering by altering the emotional component of the painful experience as well as by producing analgesia. The physician who views his patient as a whole person responding to a physically and emotionally stressful illness, who realizes the importance of his own relationship to the patient, and who utilizes this relationship to provide psychological support will need to prescribe considerably less opioid than a physician who cannot offer this kind of support. In addition to emotional support, the physician should also take into account the substantial variability in both the capacity to tolerate pain and the response to opioids. These factors may depend in part on the ability of the patient to mobilize endogenous opioids and other antinociceptive systems (*see* Tamsen *et al.*, 1982). As a result, some patients may require considerably more than the average dose of a drug to experience any relief from pain; others, perhaps because of more rapid metabolic disposition, may require a drug at shorter intervals. Some clinicians, out of an exaggerated concern for the possibility of inducing addiction, tend to prescribe initial doses of opioids that are too low or too infrequent to alleviate pain, and then respond to the patient's continued complaints with an even more exaggerated concern about dependence, despite the high probability that the request for more drug is only the expected consequence of the inadequate dosage prescribed (*see* Sriwatanakul *et al.,* 1983). Children are probably more apt to receive inadequate treatment for pain than are adults; if an illness or procedure causes pain for an adult, there is no reason to assume that it will produce less pain for a child (*see* Schechter, 1985). It is useful to remember that the typical initial dose of morphine (10 mg/70 kg) relieves postoperative pain satisfactorily in only two thirds of patients.

Pain. *Selection of a Drug.* In equianalgesic doses, morphine and most of its μ-agonist surrogates produce approximately the same incidence and degree of unwanted side effects (*see* Table 22–3). Nevertheless, there are some patients who may have side effects with one agent and not with another. Some drugs have shorter durations of action, others are particularly efficacious when given by mouth, and a few are considered to have a lower risk for producing opioid dependence. The availability of a wide range of agents provides for therapeutic flexibility.

For many types of pain, aspirin or any of a number of aspirin-like anti-inflammatory drugs provides relief equivalent to 60 mg of oral codeine; in some instances, their effects are equivalent to 8 mg or more of parenteral morphine. In most situations where oral medication is feasible, aspirin-like drugs should be the first to be used. If relief of pain is insufficient, these drugs can then be combined with orally effective morphine-like agents, such as codeine, or with agonist-antagonist opioids. Because they exert their effects by different mechanisms, combinations of these two classes of drugs can usually achieve an analgesic effect that would otherwise require a higher dose of opioid, but with fewer side effects. In treating chronic pain not associated with terminal illness, the amount of the agonist-antagonist opioid component in such combinations should be increased until adverse side effects appear before changing to a morphine-like opioid.

The combination of an opioid with a small dose of amphetamine may augment analgesia while reducing the sedative effects. When the pain is associated with biliary spasm, meperidine or one of the agonist-antagonist opioids may produce less increase in the spasm than will an equianalgesic dose of morphine or a similar agent. When the pain is likely to be of short duration (*e.g.,* diagnostic procedures, cystoscopy, orthopedic manipulation, *etc.*), a drug with a shorter duration of action, such as meperidine or alphaprodine, might be preferable to morphine or oxycodone.

Pain of Terminal Illness. Although they are not requisite or even desirable in all cases of terminal illness, the euphoria, tranquility, and analgesia afforded by the use of opioids can make the final days far less distressing for the patient and his family. Some degree of physical dependence and tolerance develops whenever an opioid is given in thera-

peutic dosage several times a day over a prolonged period. In patients with painful terminal illnesses such considerations should not in any way prevent the physician from fulfilling his primary obligation to ease the patient's discomfort. The physician should not wait until the pain becomes agonizing; *no patient should ever wish for death because of his physician's reluctance to use adequate amounts of effective opioids.* Such patients, while they may be physically dependent, are not considered "addicts" even though they may need large doses on a regular basis; in states that require the reporting of addicts, patients with terminal illnesses should not be reported.

Many clinicians who are experienced in the management of terminal illness now recommend that opioids be administered not on demand, but at sufficiently short, fixed intervals so that pain is continually under control and patients do not dread its return. Less drug is needed to prevent the recurrence of pain than to relieve it. Morphine remains the opioid of choice in most of these situations, and the route and dose should be adjusted to the needs of the individual patient. Many clinicians find that oral morphine is adequate in most situations, but the use of continuous intravenous infusions has gained renewed respect. Since the duration of analgesia produced by methadone and levorphanol is shorter than the half-lives of these drugs would suggest, appropriate vigilance is needed to avoid toxicity that may be caused by accumulation of drug. Constipation is an exceedingly common problem when opioids are used, and the use of stool softeners and laxatives should be initiated early (*see* Beaver, 1980; McGivney and Crooks, 1984). Amphetamines have demonstrable mood-elevating and analgesic effects and enhance opioid-induced analgesia; similar effects might be expected from cocaine if the proper dose were used. However, not all terminal patients require the euphoriant effects of cocaine or amphetamine and some experience side effects. Routine use of mixtures containing an opioid and either amphetamine or cocaine (*e.g.,* "Brompton's mixture") has declined. Controlled studies demonstrate no superiority of oral heroin (with or without the addition of cocaine) over oral morphine. While tolerance does develop to oral opioids, many patients obtain relief from the same dosages for weeks or months.

When opioids and other analgesics are no longer satisfactory, nerve block, chordotomy, or other types of neurosurgical intervention such as neurostimulation may be required if the nature of the lesion permits. Epidural or intrathecal administration of opioids, which produces concentrations of drug in the cerebrospinal fluid many times higher than those achieved after parenteral administration, may be useful when administration of opioids by usual routes no longer yields adequate relief of pain (*see* Chapter 15). While tolerance may develop, the technic can be used with ambulatory patients over periods of weeks or months (*see* Coombs *et al.,* 1983; Crawford *et al.,* 1983).

Postoperative Pain. Opioid analgesics are commonly employed to control pain and discomfort in the immediate postoperative period, but they should be considered two-edged swords. If used excessively, they may prevent the early recognition of complications, decrease the effectiveness of coughing, decrease respiratory ventilation, predispose to pneumonitis, reduce bowel motility, and cause urinary retention. Used properly, however, the reduction of pain associated with movements of the chest increases the patient's ability to breathe deeply and to cough voluntarily, and can also facilitate early ambulation. On balance, opioids tend to be underutilized in postoperative patients (*see* Sriwatanakul *et al.*, 1983). The use of fixed doses given "as needed" without consideration of individual differences often leads to unnecessary suffering. When pain is not too severe, oral codeine or oxycodone combined with aspirin-like drugs often provides adequate analgesia without the side effects associated with the use of usual doses of morphine.

Headache. Headache is often a recurrent problem, sometimes reflecting emotional disturbances, and opioid analgesics, with the possible exception of codeine, should not be employed unless all other measures have failed. Even then, considerable care should be employed to minimize psychological dependence and addiction.

Obstetrical Analgesia. The use of morphine and its synthetic surrogates in obstetrical analgesia is a highly specialized field requiring experience and sound judgment to ensure effective analgesia, safety for the fetus, and minimal interference with the progress of labor. All the available morphine-like opioids are powerful respiratory depressants, and the fetus seems more susceptible to their respiratory-depressant effects than does the mother. In equianalgesic doses, morphine and methadone appear somewhat more depressant to the fetus than are meperidine and closely related drugs. The pharmacological basis for this difference has been discussed above. The differences are sufficient to justify the selection of meperidine-like drugs in preference to morphine for obstetrical use (*see* below).

Sedation and Sleep. Morphine-like drugs tend to reduce all stages of sleep and induce a fluctuating drowsy-waking state that is not dysphoric (*see* Pickworth *et al.*, 1981). Opioids should not be used as sedatives unless sleeplessness is due to *pain* or *cough.* Although long years of use have demonstrated the value of opioids as preanesthetic medication, controlled clinical studies suggest that preanesthetic medication with a sedative or an antianxiety agent is just as effective in reducing preoperative apprehension and does not cause vomiting. The routine use of opioids for preanesthetic sedation in pain-free patients is difficult to justify on the basis of available evidence.

Cough. The antitussive effect of opioid drugs can be demonstrated experimentally against the coughing induced by electrical stimulation of the medulla or by chemical or mechanical irritation of the respiratory tract. With several opioids, the dose required to suppress cough induced by these technics is lower than that required for analgesia; this

finding is consistent with other evidence that suggests that distinct receptors mediate the antitussive actions of opioids. A 15-mg oral dose of codeine, although ineffective for analgesia, produces a demonstrable antitussive effect, and higher doses of codeine produce even more suppression of chronic cough. Interestingly, the degree of relief reported by patients does not necessarily correlate with actual reduction in the frequency of coughing (Sevelius *et al.*, 1971). There are now a number of effective nonopioid, nonaddictive antitussives available for clinical use (*see* below).

Dyspnea. Certain forms of dyspnea may be markedly relieved by morphine. This is especially true of the dyspnea of *acute left ventricular failure* and *pulmonary edema,* in which the response to intravenous morphine may be dramatic. The mechanism underlying this relief is still not clear. It may involve an alteration of the patient's reaction to impaired respiratory function and an indirect reduction of the work of the heart due to reduced fear and apprehension. Direct effects on oxygen consumption could play a role, since morphine reduces the oxygen consumption at rest in normal subjects (Santiago *et al.*, 1979). However, it is more probable that the major benefit is due to cardiovascular effects, such as decreased peripheral resistance and an increased capacity of the peripheral and splanchnic vascular compartments (*see* Vismara *et al.*, 1976). In patients with normal blood gases but severe breathlessness due to chronic obstruction of airflow ("pink puffers"), drocode (dihydrocodeine), 15 mg orally before exercise, reduces the feeling of breathlessness and increases exercise tolerance (Johnson *et al.*, 1983). Opioids are contraindicated in pulmonary edema due to respiratory irritants unless severe pain is also present; contraindications to their use in asthma have already been discussed.

Constipating Effects. The morphine-like opioids remain effective agents for causing constipation or treating diarrhea. Mild constipation and a drier stool are often desirable after ileostomy or colostomy, and the constipating action is especially valuable in treating exhausting diarrhea and dysenteries due to a number of causes. As in the case for cough, it requires considerably less morphine to affect the gut than to produce analgesia. Traditionally, opium preparations (opium tincture, 0.5 to 1.0 ml; paregoric, 5 to 10 ml) rather than the pure alkaloids are used; the morphine content of these doses cannot provide significant analgesia (especially by the oral route), but such dosage is, nevertheless, effective treatment for diarrhea. Synthetic opioids also produce a decrease in bowel motility as well as counteract the excessive secretion that accompanies some forms of diarrhea; several of these, such as *diphenoxylate, loperamide,* and *difenoxin,* are used exclusively for this purpose.

Special Anesthesia. High doses of morphine or other opioids have been used as the primary anesthetic agents in certain surgical procedures. Although respiration is so depressed that physical assistance is required, patients can retain consciousness (*see* Chapter 14). Opioids can also be injected intrathecally or epidurally to relieve postoperative and chronic pain (*see* Chapter 15).

LEVORPHANOL AND CONGENERS

Levorphanol is the only commercially available opioid agonist of the morphinan series. The *d* isomer (*dextrorphan*) is relatively devoid of analgesic action and makes little contribution to the activity of the racemate (*racemorphan*). The structure of levorphanol is indicated in Table 22–2.

The *pharmacological effects* of levorphanol in all species including man closely parallel those of morphine. However, clinical reports suggest that it produces less nausea and vomiting. The nonanalgesic isomer *dextrorphan* possesses considerable antitussive activity (*see* below). Levorphanol is promptly absorbed from subcutaneous sites. Although it is less effective when given orally, its oral-parenteral potency ratio is comparable to that of codeine and oxycodone. The average dose, 2 to 3 mg subcutaneously, is approximately equianalgesic with 10 mg of morphine. Maximal analgesia occurs 60 to 90 minutes after subcutaneous injec-

tion. The initial dose of levorphanol produces analgesia for a period of time comparable to that for morphine. However, levorphanol is metabolized less rapidly and has a half-life of about 11 hours; repeated administration at short intervals may thus lead to accumulation of the drug in plasma (*see* Dixon *et al.*, 1983). Clinical studies of levorphanol have been reviewed by Eddy and coworkers (1957) and by Lasagna (1964). The drug is available as *levorphanol tartrate* (LEVO-DROMORAN) in 2-mg tablets and as an injection.

MEPERIDINE AND CONGENERS

History. Meperidine is a synthetic, analgesic drug introduced by Eisleb and Schaumann in 1939. Originally studied as an atropine-like agent, it was soon discovered to have considerable analgesic activity. Although it exhibits some of the pharmacological effects of morphine in man, it is chemically quite dissimilar.

Chemistry. The structural formulas of meperidine, a phenylpiperidine, and some of its congeners are shown in Table 22–4.

Table 22–4.   CHEMICAL STRUCTURES OF PHENYLPIPERIDINE ANALGESICS

COMPOUND	R_1	R_3
Meperidine	—CH_3	—$COCH_2CH_3$ (C=O)
Alphaprodine	—CH_3	—$OCCH_2CH_3$ (C=O)
Diphenoxylate	—CH_2CH_2C—CN (with two phenyl groups)	—$COCH_2CH_3$ (C=O)
Fentanyl	—CH_2CH_2—(phenyl)	—N—C—CH_2CH_3 † (C=O, with phenyl)

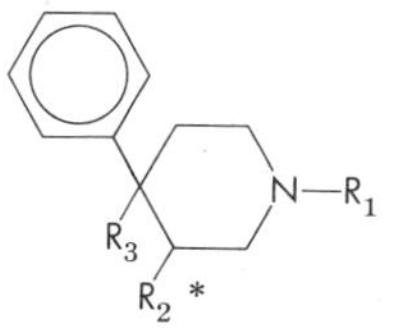

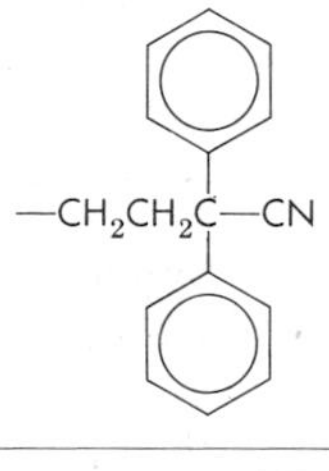

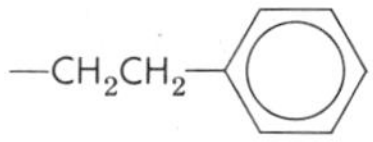

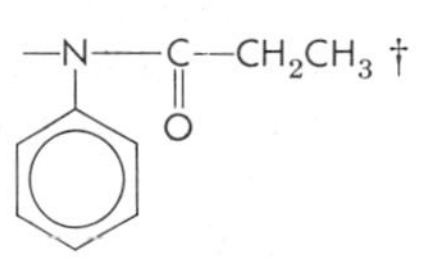

* R_2 = H, except in alphaprodine, where R_2 = CH_3.
† The sole *para* substitution on the piperidine ring is as shown.

PHARMACOLOGICAL PROPERTIES

Meperidine, like other opioids, binds to opioid receptors and exerts its chief pharmacological actions on the CNS and the neural elements in the bowel. Its profile of actions in man suggests that, compared to morphine, meperidine and/or its metabolites may interact more strongly with κ-opioid receptors.

Central Nervous System. Meperidine produces a pattern of effects similar but not identical to that described for morphine.

Analgesia. The analgesic effects of meperidine are detectable about 15 minutes after oral administration, reach a peak in about 2 hours, and subside gradually over several hours. The onset of analgesic effect is faster (within 10 minutes) after subcutaneous or intramuscular administration and reaches a peak in about 1 hour that corresponds closely to peak concentrations in plasma. In clinical use, the duration of effective analgesia is approximately 2 to 4 hours.

In general, 75 to 100 mg of meperidine given parenterally is approximately equivalent to 10 mg of morphine, and, in equianalgesic doses, meperidine produces as much sedation as does morphine and as much euphoria (10 to 20% of patients). Since neither morphine nor meperidine in these doses produces satisfactory analgesia in all patients in all situations, there are times when larger doses are appropriate. In terms of total analgesic effect, meperidine is less than one half as effective when given by mouth as when administered parenterally (*see* review by Lasagna, 1964). A few patients may experience dysphoria. Meperidine differs from morphine in that toxic doses sometimes cause CNS excitation, characterized by tremors, muscle twitches, and seizures; these effects are due largely to a metabolite, normeperidine (*see* below).

Respiration. In equianalgesic doses, meperidine depresses respiration to the same degree as does morphine. Peak respiratory depression is observed within 1 hour after intramuscular administration, and there is a return toward normal starting at about 2 hours, although minute volume is usually measurably depressed for as long as 4 hours (*see* Edwards *et al.*, 1982). The respiratory depression produced by meperidine can be antagonized by naloxone and other opioid antagonists.

Miscellaneous Effects on the Nervous System. After systemic administration, meperidine may obtund or abolish the corneal reflex. Like other opioids, meperidine causes pupillary constriction. Meperidine appears to increase the sensitivity of the labyrinthine apparatus in human subjects, a fact that may partially explain the higher incidence of dizziness, nausea, and vomiting encountered when the drug is given to ambulatory patients. Meperidine has effects on the secretion of pituitary hormones similar to those of morphine.

EEG. Upon continued administration of large doses at short intervals, slow waves appear in the EEG after a few days, and then become progressively slower and of greater amplitude. The slow waves persist even after tolerance has developed to the drug. The EEG record slowly returns to its original character about 48 hours after withdrawal of meperidine, a time course that probably parallels the elimination of normeperidine.

Cardiovascular System. In therapeutic doses, meperidine has no significant untoward effects on the cardiovascular system, particularly when patients are recumbent; myocardial contractility is not depressed, and the ECG is unaltered. Ambulatory patients given meperidine may experience syncope associated with a fall in blood pressure, but symptoms rapidly clear if the recumbent position is assumed. After the intravenous administration of meperidine, there is an increase in peripheral blood flow and a decrease in peripheral arterial and venous resistance, effects that are not blocked by prior oral administration of antihistamines. Intramuscular administration of meperidine does not significantly affect heart rate, but intravenous administration frequently produces an increased rate that is sometimes alarming. As with morphine, respiratory depression is responsible for an accumulation of CO_2, which, in turn, produces cerebrovascular dilatation, increase in cerebral blood flow, and elevation of cerebrospinal fluid pressure.

Smooth Muscle. Meperidine has a spasmogenic effect on certain smooth muscles; it is qualitatively similar to that observed with other opioids but less intense relative to its analgesic actions.

Gastrointestinal Tract. Clinical observations indicate that meperidine does not cause as much constipation when given over prolonged periods of time; this may be related to its shorter duration of action, which permits periods of normal function, or to a more favorable ratio of analgesic to gastrointestinal effects. After equianalgesic doses, the spasm in the biliary tract, as well as the rise in pressure in the common bile duct, induced by meperidine is less than that caused by morphine but greater than that by codeine. Clinical doses of meperidine slow gastric emptying sufficiently to delay absorption of other drugs significantly.

Uterus. The intact uterus of nonpregnant women is usually mildly stimulated by meperidine. Administered prior to an oxytocic, meperidine does not exert any antagonistic effect. Therapeutic doses given during active labor appear neither to delay the birth process nor to alter significantly the rhythmic uterine contractions, although the amplitude of contractions may sometimes be increased (Fishburne, 1982). The drug does not interfere with normal post-partum contraction or involution of the uterus, and it does not increase the incidence of post-partum hemorrhage.

Absorption, Fate, and Excretion. Meperidine is absorbed by all routes of administration, but absorption may be erratic after intramuscular injection. While peak concentrations in plasma are usually observed between the first and second hour after oral administration, only about 50% of the drug escapes first-pass metabolism to enter the circulation (Mather and Tucker, 1976).

Meperidine is metabolized chiefly in the liver. After intravenous administration, the rapid decline of the concentration in plasma due to distribution is followed by a slower phase with a half-time of about 3 hours. In patients with cirrhosis, the bioavailability of meperidine is increased to as much as 80% and the half-lives of both meperidine and normeperidine are prolonged. Approximately 60% of meperidine in plasma is protein bound. Heavy drinkers of alcohol have an increased apparent volume of distribution that leads to concentrations in plasma that are initially lower than would be found in nondrinkers. Older patients have higher concentrations in plasma and decreased binding to plasma proteins, both of which may account for their increased response to therapeutic doses.

In man, meperidine is hydrolyzed to meperidinic acid, which, in turn, is partially conjugated. Meperidine is also N-demethylated to normeperidine, which may then be hydrolyzed to normeperidinic acid and subsequently conjugated. The clinical significance of the formation of normeperidine is discussed further under toxicity. While very little meperidine is ordinarily excreted unchanged, up to 25% may be excreted unchanged when the urine is acidic. However, in such circumstances the overall clearance of meperidine from plasma is not substantially altered.

Preparations, Routes of Administration, and Dosage. Trade names for meperidine include DEMEROL and PETHADOL. The international nonproprietary name is *pethidine*. *Meperidine hydrochloride* is available for oral use in tablets (50 and 100 mg) and as a syrup, and in solutions for parenteral use. It is usually given intramuscularly. Although intravenous use may increase the incidence and severity of untoward effects, this route can be employed with safety (*see* below). Subcutaneous or intramuscular administration causes local irritation and tissue induration, and frequent repetition may lead to severe fibrosis of muscle tissue. The dose varies with the clinical situation. Most patients with moderate-to-severe pain are relieved by 100 mg parenterally. The effectiveness of the drug by the oral route is not reduced to the same degree as is that of morphine, but its oral-parenteral potency ratio is lower than that of codeine. Doses for infants and children average 1 to 1.8 mg/kg.

Alphaprodine hydrochloride (NISENTIL), a congener of meperidine, is available in solutions for injection. *Anileridine hydrochloride* is no longer available in the United States. Doses, durations of action, and distinguishing pharmacological features of alphaprodine are shown in Table 22–3.

Untoward Effects, Precautions, and Contraindications. The pattern and overall incidence of untoward effects that follow the use of meperidine are similar to those observed after equianalgesic doses of morphine, except that constipation and urinary retention are less common. Patients who experience nausea and vomiting with morphine may not do so with meperidine; the converse may also be true. As with other opioids, tolerance develops to some of these effects. The contraindications are the same as for other opioids. In patients or addicts who are tolerant to the depressant effects of meperidine, large doses repeated at short intervals produce tremors, muscle twitches, dilated pupils, hyperactive reflexes, and convulsions.

The excitatory symptoms that are observed with large doses of meperidine are due to the accumulation of normeperidine. Since normeperidine has a half-life of 15 to 20 hours, decreased renal or hepatic function increases the likelihood of such toxicity (Kaiko *et al.*, 1983). Opioid antagonists block the convulsant effect of normeperidine in the mouse.

Interaction with Other Drugs. There have been reports of severe reactions following the administration of meperidine to patients being treated with monoamine oxidase (MAO) inhibitors. These consisted in excitation, delirium, hyperpyrexia, and convulsions or severe respiratory depression. Chlorpromazine increases the respiratory-depressant effects of meperidine, as do tricyclic antidepressants; this is not true of diazepam. Concurrent administration of drugs such as promethazine or chlorpromazine may also greatly enhance meperidine-induced sedation without slowing clearance of the drug. Treatment with phenobarbital or phenytoin increases systemic clearance and decreases oral bioavailability of meperidine; this is associated with an elevation of the concentration of normeperidine in plasma (*see* Edwards *et al.*, 1982). As with morphine, concomitant administration of amphetamine has been reported to enhance the analgesic effects of meperidine and its congeners.

Tolerance, Physical Dependence, and Liability for Abuse. In situations where they are administered chronically, the duration of action of meperidine is shorter than that of morphine, and continuous depression of the CNS is usually attained only when the drug is used at less than 4-hour intervals. This may account for the slower development of tolerance to meperidine. Even when tolerance develops to the respiratory-depressant effects of meperidine, high doses given at frequent intervals may produce an excitatory syndrome, including hallucinations and seizures, probably as a result of the accumulation of normeperidine (*see* above; Chapter 23).

The pattern of withdrawal symptoms after abrupt discontinuation of meperidine differs from that after morphine in that there are fewer autonomic effects and the symptoms develop more rapidly and are of shorter duration. It should be emphasized that the degree of physical dependence that a drug induces is only one factor in determining its abuse liability (*see* above). Some congeners of meperidine can produce a marked degree of physical dependence, and withdrawal symptoms following abrupt discontinuation result in a severe morphine-like withdrawal syndrome. The abuse potential of the clinically available meperidine congeners is similar to that of meperidine.

THERAPEUTIC USES

The major use of meperidine is for analgesia. Unlike morphine and its congeners, meperidine is not useful for the treatment of cough or diarrhea.

Analgesia. Meperidine can be used in any situation where an opioid analgesic is required. However, there are a number of clinical conditions in which its lesser spasmogenic effects or its better oral efficacy make meperidine preferable to morphine. Because of concern about drug dependence, many clinicians prescribe doses of meperidine that are too low or too infrequent, thereby causing unnecessary suffering. This is discussed above, in the section on therapeutic uses of morphine.

The concentrations of meperidine in plasma required to produce satisfactory analgesia range from 100 to 800 ng/ml (average, 500 ng/ml); in any given patient, the analgesic concentration appears to remain relatively constant over time (Glynn and Mather, 1982). In some circumstances, a decrease in concentration of as little as 10% can result in a marked reduction in analgesia. As a result, some clinicians now recommend continuous intravenous infusion or parenteral administration "on demand" to reduce fluctuations in analgesic effects. The administration of about 25 mg of meperidine per hour will usually yield concentrations of 500 ng/ml in plasma (Edwards *et al.*, 1982).

Meperidine crosses the placental barrier and even in reasonable analgesic doses causes a significant increase in the percentage of babies who show delayed respiration, decreased respiratory minute volume, or decreased oxygen saturation, or who require resuscitation. Both fetal and maternal respiratory depression induced by meperidine can be treated with naloxone. Meperidine has been recovered from fetal blood within 2 minutes after administration to the mother. If delivery is prolonged, concentrations of meperidine in fetal blood at birth may be higher than those in maternal blood because fetal plasma has a slightly lower pH. In addition, the fraction of drug that is bound to protein is lower in the fetus; concentrations of free drug may thus be considerably higher than in the mother (Nation, 1981). Nevertheless, meperidine produces less respiratory depression in the newborn than does an equianalgesic dose of morphine or methadone and continues to be the preferred opioid for systemic analgesia during labor. Intravenous administration of small doses, repeated if necessary, is recommended (*see* Fishburne, 1982).

OTHER CONGENERS OF MEPERIDINE

Diphenoxylate. Diphenoxylate is a meperidine congener that has a definite constipating effect in man. While it has been proposed as a maintenance drug in the treatment of opioid dependence, its only recognized use is in the treatment of diarrhea. Although single doses in the therapeutic range (*see* below) produce little or no morphine-like subjective effects, at high doses (40 to 60 mg) the drug shows typical opioid activity, including euphoria, suppression of morphine abstinence, and a morphine-like physical dependence after chronic administration. Diphenoxylate is unusual in that even its salts are virtually insoluble in aqueous solution, thus obviating the possibility of abuse by the parenteral route. *Diphenoxylate hydrochloride* is available only in combination with atropine sulfate

(LOMOTIL, others), in tablets and as a liquid. Each tablet or 5 ml contains 2.5 mg of diphenoxylate and 25 μg of atropine sulfate. The recommended daily dosage for treatment of *diarrhea* in adults is 20 mg, in divided doses. It is a schedule-V preparation (*see* Appendix I). *Difenoxin* (diphenoxylic acid) is one of the metabolites of diphenoxylate; it has actions similar to those of the parent compound.

Loperamide. Loperamide, like diphenoxylate, is a piperidine derivative (4-[*p*-chlorophenyl]-4-hydroxy-N,N-dimethyl-α,α-diphenyl-1-piperidinebutyramide). It slows gastrointestinal motility by effects on the circular and longitudinal muscles of the intestine. It binds to opioid receptors in brain homogenates and intestinal strips; its constipating action is probably due, at least in part, to actions at these receptors. Some part of its antidiarrheal effect may be due to a reduction of gastrointestinal secretion produced by actions at opioid receptors in the intestinal mucosa. At higher, but still potentially relevant concentrations, loperamide binds to calmodulin and thereby reduces the activity of a number of calcium-dependent enzymes; this action is not antagonized by naloxone. It is not clear whether such an interaction with calmodulin contributes to the antisecretory or antidiarrheal effects of loperamide (*see* Awouters *et al.*, 1983).

In controlling chronic diarrhea, the drug is as effective as diphenoxylate. In clinical studies, the most common side effect is abdominal cramps. Little tolerance develops to its constipating effect.

In human volunteers taking large doses, concentrations of loperamide in plasma peak about 4 hours after ingestion; this long latency may be due to inhibition of gastrointestinal motility and to enterohepatic circulation of the drug. The apparent elimination half-time is 7 to 14 hours. Loperamide is not well absorbed after oral administration and, in addition, apparently does not penetrate well into the brain; these properties contribute to the selectivity of its action. A large proportion of the drug is excreted in the feces.

Even though high doses of loperamide suppress withdrawal symptoms in morphine-dependent monkeys, the drug is unlikely to be abused parenterally because of its low solubility; large doses of loperamide (18 to 54 mg) given to human volunteers do not elicit pleasurable effects typical of opioids. Its overall potential for abuse is probably lower than that of diphenoxylate (*see* Awouters *et al.*, 1983). The drug is available as *loperamide hydrochloride* (IMODIUM) in 2-mg capsules and as a liquid (1 mg/5 ml). The usual dosage is 4 to 8 mg per day; the daily dose should not exceed 16 mg.

FENTANYL

Fentanyl is a synthetic opioid related to the phenylpiperidines (Table 22–4). As an analgesic it is estimated to be 80 times as potent as morphine. It is primarily a μ agonist; a related agent, lofentanil, is 6000 times as potent as morphine in the dog. The respiratory-depressant effect of fentanyl is of shorter duration than that of meperidine; its

analgesic and euphoric effects are antagonized by opioid antagonists, but are not significantly prolonged or intensified by *droperidol,* a neuroleptic agent with which it is usually combined for use as an intravenous anesthetic (*see* Chapter 14). The subjective effects of the combination depend on the relative proportions of the two agents. High doses of fentanyl produce marked muscular rigidity, possibly as a result of the effects of opioids on dopaminergic transmission in the striatum; this effect can be antagonized by naloxone. Fentanyl is usually used only for anesthesia. *Fentanyl citrate* (SUBLIMAZE) is available as a solution for injection. It is also supplied as a fixed-dose combination with droperidol (INNOVAR). Newer congeners of fentanyl, such as *sufentanil citrate* (SUFENTA), are discussed in Chapter 14.

METHADONE AND CONGENERS

Methadone was synthesized by German chemists and came into clinical use at the end of World War II. It is primarily a μ agonist with pharmacological properties qualitatively similar to those of morphine.

Chemistry. Methadone has the following structural formula:

Methadone

In spite of the fact that the two-dimensional structure of methadone does not remotely resemble that of morphine, steric factors force the molecule to simulate the pseudopiperidine ring configuration that appears to be essential for opioid activity. The analgesic activity of the racemate is almost entirely the result of its content of *l*-methadone, which is 8 to 50 times more potent than the *d* isomer (depending upon the species and analgesic test employed). *d*-Methadone also lacks significant respiratory-depressant action and addiction liability, but it does possess antitussive activity.

Several structurally related congeners of methadone are in clinical use; as analgesics, these drugs have no demonstrable superiority over the parent compound. The dose, durations of action, and other effects of the congeners are compared to those of other opioid analgesics in Table 22–3.

Pharmacological Actions. The outstanding properties of methadone are its effective analgesic activity, its efficacy by the oral route, its extended duration of action in suppressing withdrawal symptoms in physically dependent individuals, and its tendency to show persistent effects with repeated administration.

Central Nervous System. After parenteral administration in man, a single dose of methadone is an effective analgesic, equal in potency and duration of action to morphine. However, miotic and respiratory-depressant effects can be detected for more than 24 hours (*see* Olsen *et al.,* 1981) and, upon repeated administration, marked sedation is seen in some patients (Martin *et al.,* 1973a). Effects on cough and on the secretion of pituitary hormones are qualitatively similar to those of morphine.

Smooth Muscle. Methadone, like morphine, increases intestinal tone, diminishes the amplitude of contractions, and produces a marked decrease in propulsive activity; it is constipating and causes biliary tract spasm.

Absorption, Fate, and Excretion. Appreciable concentrations of methadone can be found in the plasma within 10 minutes after its subcutaneous injection. It is also well absorbed from the gastrointestinal tract and can be detected in plasma within 30 minutes after oral ingestion; it reaches peak concentrations at about 4 hours. After therapeutic doses, about 90% of methadone is bound to plasma proteins. Peak concentrations occur in the brain within 1 or 2 hours after subcutaneous or intramuscular administration, and this correlates well with the intensity and duration of analgesia.

Methadone undergoes extensive biotransformation in the liver. The major metabolites, the results of N-demethylation and cyclization to form pyrrolidines and pyrroline, are excreted in the urine and the bile along with small amounts of unchanged drug. The amount of methadone excreted in the urine is increased when the urine is acidified. The half-life of methadone is about 1 to 1.5 days (*see* Appendix II).

Methadone appears to be firmly bound to protein in various tissues, including brain. After repeated administration there is gradual accumulation in tissues. When administration is discontinued, low concentrations are maintained in plasma by slow release from extravascular binding sites (*see* Kreek, 1979); this process probably accounts for the relatively mild but protracted withdrawal syndrome.

The use of methadone in the treatment of compulsive heroin users has revived interest in other methadone congeners, such as α-dl- and l-acetylmethadol (methadyl acetate). In subjects physically dependent on α-dl-acetylmethadol, opioid withdrawal symptoms are not perceived for 72 to 96 hours after the last oral dose, and most subjects are entirely comfortable when given a single dose of the drug as infrequently as every 72 hours (*see* Ling *et al.,* 1978). The relatively slow onset and protracted duration of action of this drug, which is probably inactive, are thought to be due in part to its conversion to active metabolites (noracetylmethadol, dinoracetylmethadol, and normethadol) that are slowly further metabolized or excreted (*see* Misra, 1978).

Preparations, Routes of Administration, and Dosage. *Methadone hydrochloride* (DOLOPHINE HCL) is available in tablets (5 and 10 mg) and in a solution for oral use, and as a solution for parenteral administration. The oral analgesic dose for adults is 5 to 15 mg, depending upon the severity of the pain and the response of the patient; the initial parenteral dose is usually 5 to 10 mg. After the oral administration of 15 mg, the average concentration in plasma is about 35 μg/ml; this has been suggested to be the minimal effective analgesic concentration (*see* Olsen *et al.,* 1981; Gourlay *et al.,* 1982).

In the United States, special controls on methadone have been enacted in an effort to prevent its unregulated large-scale use in the treatment of opioid addiction. Specialized dosage forms used in opioid addiction include tablets containing 40 mg of the drug.

Side Effects, Toxicity, Drug Interactions, and Precautions. Side effects, toxicity, and conditions that alter sensitivity to methadone are similar to those outlined for morphine, and the therapy of acute methadone intoxication is the same as for morphine. During chronic administration there may be excessive sweating, lymphocytosis, and increased concentrations of prolactin, albumin, and globulins in the plasma. Rifampin and phenytoin accelerate the metabolism of methadone and can precipitate withdrawal symptoms (*see* Kreek, 1979; Pond *et al.,* 1982).

Tolerance, Physical Dependence, and Liability for Abuse. Volunteer postaddicts who received subcutaneous or oral methadone daily developed partial *tolerance* to the nauseant, anorectic, miotic, sedative, respiratory-depressant, and cardiovascular effects of methadone. Tolerance develops more slowly to methadone than to morphine in some patients, especially with respect to the depressant effects. However, this may be related in part to cumulative effects of the drug or its metabolites. Sedation with concomitant slowing of the EEG occurs during experimental addiction (Martin *et al.,* 1973a). Tolerance to the constipating effect of methadone does not develop as fully as does tolerance to other effects. The behavior of the addicts who use methadone parenterally is strikingly similar to that of the morphine addict, but many former heroin users treated with oral methadone show virtually no overt behavioral effects (*see* Chapter 23).

Development of physical dependence during the chronic administration of methadone can be demonstrated by drug withdrawal or by administration of an opioid antagonist. Subcutaneous administration of 10 to 20 mg of methadone in former opioid addicts produces definite euphoria, equal in duration to that caused by morphine. On the basis of definitive studies, the overall abuse potential of methadone is rated comparable to that of morphine (Martin *et al.*, 1973a).

Therapeutic Uses. The primary uses of methadone are relief of pain, treatment of opioid abstinence syndromes, and treatment of heroin users. It is not widely used as an antiperistaltic agent. It should be employed with extreme caution, if at all, in labor.

Analgesia. The onset of analgesia occurs 10 to 20 minutes following parenteral administration and 30 to 60 minutes after oral medication. Despite its longer plasma half-life, the duration of the analgesic action of single doses is essentially the same as that of morphine. With repeated usage, some cumulative effects are seen, so that either lower dosage or longer intervals between doses become possible. In contrast to morphine, methadone and many of its congeners retain a considerable degree of their effectiveness when given orally. In terms of total analgesic effects, methadone given orally is about 50% as effective as the same dose administered intramuscularly; however, the oral-parenteral potency ratio is considerably lower when peak analgesic effect is considered (*see* Beaver, 1980). In equianalgesic doses, the pattern and incidence of untoward effects caused by methadone and morphine are similar.

PROPOXYPHENE

Of the four stereoisomers, only the alpha racemate, known as *propoxyphene,* has analgesic activity. Its analgesic effect resides in the dextrorotatory isomer, *d*-propoxyphene (dextropropoxyphene). However, levopropoxyphene seems to have some antitussive activity. As can be seen from the following formula, propoxyphene is related structurally to methadone.

Propoxyphene

Pharmacological Actions. Propoxyphene binds to opioid receptors and produces analgesia and other CNS effects that are similar to those seen with codeine and other opioids. It has no significant antipyretic or anti-inflammatory effects. It is likely that at equianalgesic doses the incidence of side effects such as nausea, anorexia, constipation, abdominal pain, and drowsiness would be similar to those of codeine.

As an analgesic, propoxyphene is about one half to two thirds as potent as codeine given orally. Because of the variability of response to analgesics, 30 to 60 mg of codeine given orally sometimes produces no more analgesia than placebo (*see* Cooper and Beaver, 1976). It is not surprising, therefore, that it has been difficult to show that 32 mg of the less potent propoxyphene hydrochloride is significantly superior to placebo. Beaver (1966) estimated that it requires 90 to 120 mg of propoxyphene hydrochloride administered orally to equal the analgesic effects of 60 mg of codeine, a dose that usually produces about as much analgesia as 600 mg of aspirin. Combinations of propoxyphene and aspirin (like combinations of codeine and aspirin) afford a higher level of analgesia than does either agent given alone.

Absorption, Fate, and Excretion. Propoxyphene is absorbed after oral or parenteral administration. After oral administration the water-soluble hydrochloride appears to be absorbed somewhat more rapidly than the relatively water-insoluble napsylate. However, differences in peak plasma concentrations between the two preparations are small. Following oral administration, concentrations in plasma reach their highest values at 1 to 2 hours. Estimates of the half-life of propoxyphene in plasma after single doses range from 3.5 to 15 hours, depending on the methodology used. There is great variability between subjects in terms of the rate of clearance and the plasma concentrations that are achieved. Bioavailability is limited by first-pass metabolism to between 30 and 70%. In man, the major route of metabolism is N-demethylation to yield norpropoxyphene. The half-life of norpropoxyphene is about 23 hours (*see* Gram *et al.*, 1979), and its concentration is severalfold higher in plasma than that of propoxyphene. The clearance of both the metabolite and the parent drug appears to slow with repeated administration and may be more rapid in smokers (Inturrisi *et al.*, 1982).

Toxicity. Given orally, propoxyphene is approximately one third as potent as orally administered codeine in depressing respiration. Moderately toxic doses usually produce CNS and respiratory depression, but with still-larger doses the clinical picture may be complicated by convulsions in addition to respiratory depression. Delusions, hallucinations, confusion, cardiotoxicity, and pulmonary edema have also been noted. Respiratory-depressant effects are significantly enhanced when alcohol or sedative-hypnotic agents are ingested concurrently, and deaths have occurred when excessive quantities of propoxyphene have been taken in conjunction with such agents. The excitatory and cardiotoxic effects may be due in part to norpropoxyphene. Naloxone antagonizes the respiratory-depressant, convulsant, and some of the cardiotoxic effects of propoxyphene.

Liability for Abuse. Very large doses (800 mg of the hydrochloride or 1200 mg of the napsylate per day) reduce the intensity of the morphine withdrawal syndrome somewhat less effectively than do 1500-mg doses of codeine. Maximal tolerated doses are equivalent to daily doses of 20 to 25 mg of morphine, given subcutaneously, or 10 mg of methadone. It does not appear to be longer acting than morphine in suppressing withdrawal. For most would-be abusers, use of higher doses of propoxyphene is prevented by untoward side effects and the occurrence of toxic psychoses. When very large doses are used in morphine-tolerant addicts, some respiratory depression is seen, suggesting that there is not a high degree of cross-tolerance between propoxyphene and morphine. Abrupt discontinuation of chronically administered propoxyphene hydrochloride (up to 800 mg per day, given for almost 2 months) results in mild abstinence phenomena, and large oral doses (300 to 600 mg) produce subjective effects that are considered pleasurable by postaddicts. Administered intravenously, it is recognized as an opioid; however, the drug is quite irritating when administered either intravenously or subcutaneously, so that abuse by these routes results in severe damage to veins and soft tissues, which limits the time the drug can be used parenterally.

Although propoxyphene has less potential for abuse than codeine, the incidence of abuse (corrected for the number of equianalgesic doses) has been approximately the same as with codeine. Further, some patients who have consumed very large overdoses of propoxyphene (about 1 g or more) have died. For these reasons, propoxyphene has been placed in schedule IV of the Federal Controlled Substances Act in the United States (*see* Appendix I).

Preparations, Route of Administration, Dosage, and Therapeutic Uses. Although it has been used experimentally for the suppression of withdrawal symptoms in cases of opioid addiction (*see* Jasinski *et al.*, 1977), the only recognized use of propoxyphene is for the treatment of mild-to-moderate pain that is not adequately relieved by aspirin. When appropriate doses are selected, combinations of aspirin and propoxyphene can be as effective as the combination of codeine and aspirin or aspirin-like anti-inflammatory agents. The wide popularity of propoxyphene in clinical situations in which codeine was once used seems to be largely a result of unrealistic overconcern about the addictive potential of codeine.

Propoxyphene hydrochloride (DARVON, DOLENE, others) is available in 32- and 65-mg capsules; *propoxyphene napsylate* (DARVON-N) is available in 100-mg tablets or as a suspension. Combinations of propoxyphene with aspirin or acetaminophen are also marketed in a variety of dosage forms.

OPIOIDS WITH MIXED ACTIONS: AGONIST-ANTAGONISTS AND PARTIAL AGONISTS

Most of the drugs to be discussed in this section presumably bind to the μ receptor and can therefore compete with other substances for these sites, but either they exert no actions (*i.e.*, they are *competitive antagonists* at the μ receptor) or they exert only limited actions (*i.e.*, they are *partial agonists* at the μ receptor). Drugs such as nalorphine, cyclazocine, and nalbuphine are competitive antagonists at the μ receptor (and block the effects of morphine-like drugs), yet they appear to exert partial agonistic actions at other receptors, including the κ and σ receptors. Pentazocine qualitatively resembles these three agents, but it appears to be a weaker antagonist at μ receptors and to have more powerful agonistic actions at κ receptors; buprenorphine and propriam behave as partial μ agonists (*see* Table 22–1). Studies in animals suggest that all opioids available clinically that display antagonistic properties at μ receptors also are relatively weak antagonists at δ receptors.

PENTAZOCINE

Pentazocine was synthesized as part of a deliberate effort to develop an effective analgesic with little or no abuse potential. It has both agonistic actions and weak opioid antagonistic activity. The pharmacology of pentazocine has been reviewed by Brogden and associates (1973).

Chemistry. Pentazocine is a benzomorphan derivative with the following structural formula:

Pentazocine

The compound has a large substituent on the nitrogen atom that is analogous to position 17 of morphine. This structural feature is common to a number of opioids with antagonist or agonist-antagonist activity. The analgesic and respiratory-depressant activity of the racemate is due mainly to the *l* isomer.

Pharmacological Actions. The pattern of CNS effects produced by pentazocine is generally similar to that of the morphine-like opioids, including analgesia, sedation, and respiratory depression. However, in experimental animals, pentazocine resembles drugs such as cyclazocine and nalorphine. It produces a type of analgesia that differs from that of morphine; it clearly interrupts nociceptive input in the spinal cord, while morphine also acts at supraspinal loci in producing analgesia. Thus, it is probable that the analgesic effects of pentazocine are due in part to agonistic actions at κ opioid receptors. A dose of approximately 20 mg, administered parenterally, produces the same degree of respiratory depression as does a 10-mg dose of morphine. Increasing the dose of pentazocine beyond 30 mg does not ordinarily produce proportionate increases in respiratory depression. However, at doses of 60 to 90 mg, nalorphine-like dysphoric and psychotomimetic effects may occur that can be readily antagonized by naloxone but not by nalorphine; these effects are probably due to actions at σ-opioid receptors.

The effects of low doses of pentazocine on the *gastrointestinal tract* are qualitatively similar to those of the opioids; relatively small intramuscular doses (15 mg) significantly decrease gastric emptying time. While higher doses (30 to 45 mg) increase the transit time through the intestinal tract, they produce less elevation of biliary pressure than do equianalgesic doses of morphine.

The *cardiovascular responses* to pentazocine differ from those seen with the morphine-like opioids, in that high doses cause an increase in blood pressure and heart rate. In normal subjects, pentazocine causes a decrease in effective renal plasma flow but no decrease in glomerular filtration rate. In patients with coronary artery disease, pentazocine (intravenously) elevates mean aortic pressure, left ventricular end-diastolic pressure, and mean pulmonary artery pressure, and causes an increase in cardiac work (Alderman *et al.*, 1972; Lee *et al.*, 1976). Pentazocine produces a rise in the concentrations of catecholamines in plasma; this may account for its effects on blood pressure.

The effects of pentazocine on *uterine contractility* do not appear to differ from those of meperidine.

Pentazocine behaves as a weak antagonist at μ-opioid receptors (approximately one fiftieth as potent as nalorphine). It does not antagonize the respiratory depression produced by morphine; however, when given to patients who have been receiving opioids on a regular basis, it may precipitate withdrawal symptoms. In patients tolerant to morphine-like opioids, pentazocine reduces the analgesia produced by their administration, even when clear-cut withdrawal symptoms are not precipitated.

Absorption, Fate, and Excretion. Pentazocine is well absorbed from the gastrointestinal tract and from subcutaneous and intramuscular sites. Concentrations in plasma coincide closely with the onset, duration, and intensity of analgesia; peak values occur 15 minutes to 1 hour after intramuscu-lar administration and 1 to 3 hours after oral administration. The half-life in plasma is 2 to 3 hours. First-pass metabolism in the liver is extensive, and somewhat less than 20% of pentazocine enters the systemic circulation (Ehrnebo *et al.*, 1977).

The action of the drug is terminated largely by biotransformation in the liver; the metabolites, products of the oxidation of the terminal methyl groups and glucuronide conjugates, are excreted by the kidney. There is considerable variability between individuals in terms of rate of pentazocine metabolism, and this may account for the variability of analgesic response. Pentazocine passes the placental barrier but to a lesser extent than does meperidine (*see* Brogden *et al.*, 1973).

Preparations, Routes of Administration, and Dosage. *Pentazocine lactate* (TALWIN) is available as solutions for injection, each milliliter of which contains the equivalent of 30 mg of the base. In an effort to reduce the use of tablets as a source of injectable pentazocine, tablets for oral use now contain *pentazocine hydrochloride* (equivalent to 50 mg of the base) and 0.5 mg of naloxone (TALWIN NX). After oral ingestion, naloxone is destroyed rapidly by the liver; however, if the material is dissolved and injected, the naloxone produces aversive effects in subjects dependent on opioids. Tablets containing mixtures of pentazocine with aspirin or acetaminophen are also available. Pentazocine is included under schedule IV of the Federal Controlled Substances Act (*see* Appendix I), but the drug is more strictly controlled in some states. In terms of analgesic effect, 30 to 60 mg of pentazocine given parenterally is approximately equivalent to 10 mg of morphine. An oral dose of about 50 mg of pentazocine results in analgesia equivalent to that produced by 60 mg of codeine orally. In terms of peak effect, pentazocine is approximately one fourth as potent orally as parenterally; in terms of total analgesic effect, one third as potent.

Side Effects, Toxicity, and Precautions. The most commonly reported untoward effects are sedation, followed by sweating, and dizziness or light-headedness; nausea also occurs, but vomiting is less common than with morphine. Nalorphine-like psychotomimetic effects such as uncontrollable or weird thoughts, anxiety, nightmares, and hallucinations have been reported. These are not common with doses in the therapeutic range but are seen with increasing frequency with parenteral doses above 60 mg. The clinical picture of overdosage has not been well defined, but epidemiological data suggest that overdose with pentazocine alone rarely causes death. High doses produce marked respiratory depression associated with increased blood pressure and tachycardia. The respiratory depression is antagonized by naloxone. Pentazocine is irritating when administered subcutaneously or intramuscularly. Repeated injections over long periods may cause extensive fibrosis of subcutaneous and muscular tissue. Patients who have been receiving opioids on a regular basis may experience abstinence signs and symptoms when given pentazocine. After an opioid-free interval of 1 to 2 days, it is usually possible to administer pentazocine without producing such withdrawal effects.

Tolerance, Physical Dependence, and Liability for Abuse. With frequent and repeated use, tolerance develops to the analgesic and subjective effects of pentazocine; however, it is not clear if the rate of development of this tolerance is comparable to that seen with morphine-like opioids or is the same for all effects of the drug. When given intravenously or subcutaneously to postaddicts, pentazocine (40 mg) produces essentially morphine-like effects; when the dose is increased to 60 mg, the effects begin to resemble the nervousness and loss of energy produced by nalorphine. In contrast to morphine and other μ agonists, pentazocine does not prevent or ameliorate the morphine withdrawal syndrome. Instead, when high doses of pentazocine are given to subjects dependent on morphine, it precipitates withdrawal symptoms because of its antagonistic actions at the μ receptor.

After chronic administration (60 to 90 mg every 4 hours), postaddicts develop physical dependence that can be demonstrated by abrupt withdrawal or by the administration of naloxone (but not of nalorphine). The withdrawal syndrome after chronic doses of more than 500 mg per day is similar in some respects to that seen after withdrawal of nalorphine, but it also has some of the characteristics of morphine withdrawal, including abdominal cramps, anxiety, chills, elevated temperature, vomiting, lacrimation, and sweating. Although milder in intensity, the syndrome is associated with drug-seeking behavior; that is, subjects request additional medicine to alleviate the withdrawal syndrome (Jasinski *et al.*, 1970).

On the basis of early testing, pentazocine was not believed to have a significant potential for abuse, and it was released for general use subject to no special controls. Subsequently, cases of compulsive self-administration primarily of *parenteral* pentazocine were reported. The availability of the oral preparation, greater appreciation of its potential for abuse, and more supervision by physicians and pharmacists have reduced the tendency to over-prescribe the parenteral form of pentazocine. Despite the absence of legal controls, pentazocine was not misused by heroin addicts to any significant extent until 1977, when the combination of pentazocine (usually extracted from the oral tablet) and the antihistamine tripelennamine, used intravenously, became popular in the addict subculture of several large urban areas. Pentazocine was then included under schedule IV of the Federal Controlled Substances Act. Administered intravenously to former addicts, tripelennamine produces euphoric effects that are additive to those of pentazocine. Pentazocine withdrawal symptoms can be managed by gradual reduction of pentazocine itself or by substitution of μ agonists, such as morphine or methadone. A syndrome of withdrawal from pentazocine has also been observed in neonates.

Therapeutic Uses. Pentazocine is used primarily as an analgesic. Because it is often employed in situations where there is chronic severe pain or in individuals who have drug-abuse problems, the risk of drug dependence definitely exists. However, the risk is lower than that associated with the use of morphine-like drugs in similar circumstances. Because abuse patterns appear to be less likely to develop with oral administration, this route should be used whenever possible. At present, it is not clear whether the dysphoric side effects of pentazocine are important to its relatively low potential for abuse.

NALBUPHINE

Nalbuphine is structurally related to both naloxone and oxymorphone (*see* Table 22–2). It is an agonist-antagonist opioid with a spectrum of effects that qualitatively resemble those of nalorphine and pentazocine; however, nalbuphine is a much more potent antagonist at μ receptors and is less likely to produce dysphoric side effects than is pentazocine.

Pharmacological Actions and Side Effects. Nalbuphine, like pentazocine, produces analgesia apparently by agonist actions at κ receptors; it has prominent antagonistic actions at μ receptors. An intramuscular dose of 10 mg causes analgesia equivalent to that which follows the administration of 10 mg of morphine; the onset and duration of both analgesic and subjective effects are similar to those of morphine. Nalbuphine depresses respiration as much as do equianalgesic doses of morphine; however, nalbuphine exhibits a ceiling effect, such that increases in dosage beyond 30 mg produce no further respiratory depression. In contrast to pentazocine and butorphanol, 10 mg of nalbuphine given to patients with stable coronary artery disease does not produce an increase in cardiac index, pulmonary arterial pressure, or cardiac work, and systemic blood pressure is not significantly altered (Romagnoli and Keats, 1978); these indices are also relatively stable when nalbuphine is given to patients with acute myocardial infarction (Lee *et al.*, 1981). Its gastrointestinal effects are probably similar to those of pentazocine. Nalbuphine produces few side effects at doses of 10 mg or less; sedation, sweating, and headache are the most common. At much higher doses (70 mg) side effects resemble those of nalorphine (dysphoria, racing thoughts, and distortions of body image). Nalbuphine is metabolized in the liver and has a half-life in plasma of about 5 hours. Given orally, nalbuphine is 20 to 25% as potent as when given intramuscularly (Beaver *et al.*, 1981).

Tolerance, Physical Dependence, and Liability for Abuse. Postaddicts "like" the effects of single (8-mg) doses of nalbuphine as much as they do those of low doses of morphine. When the dose of nalbuphine is increased to 72 mg, the degree of "liking" and euphoria is increased only slightly, and sedative as well as nalorphine-like side effects begin to occur. High doses of nalbuphine are more likely to be identified as a barbiturate than as an opioid.

In subjects dependent on low doses of morphine (60 mg per day), nalbuphine precipitates an abstinence syndrome. As an antagonist, it is one fourth as potent as nalorphine. During the first week of chronic administration, experimental subjects are relaxed and enjoy the drugged feeling; they usually identify nalbuphine as morphine-like, but occasionally as a barbiturate or an amphetamine. After 7 days (daily dose of 142 mg), subjects begin to complain of headache, difficulty in concentration, strange thoughts and dreams, irritability, and depression. Although complaints persist, some subjects continue to tolerate these effects; in these subjects, the administration of 4 mg of naloxone (but not 30 mg of nalorphine) produces an abstinence syndrome. Subjects describe this as morphine-like withdrawal and demand drugs for relief. The syndrome is similar in intensity to that seen with pentazocine, and symptoms are greatly diminished by the seventh day. The potential for abuse of parenteral nalbuphine in subjects not dependent on μ agonists is probably similar to that of parenteral pentazocine. However, in subjects who are dependent on such agonists, its abuse potential is probably lower than that of pentazocine because of the more potent antagonistic actions of nalbuphine at μ receptors. Since its release for use in 1979, there have been few reported cases of abuse of nalbuphine, and it has not been listed in any schedule of the Federal Controlled Substances Act.

Therapeutic Uses, Routes of Administration, Dosage, and Preparations. Nalbuphine can be used to produce analgesia in a variety of painful syndromes. However, because it is an agonist-antagonist, administration to patients who have been receiving morphine-like opioids may create difficulties unless a brief drug-free interval is interposed. *Nalbuphine hydrochloride* (NUBAIN) is supplied as an injectable solution (10 mg/ml) for intramuscular, subcutaneous, or intravenous use. The usual adult dose is 10 mg every 3 to 6 hours; this may be increased to 20 mg in nontolerant individuals, but no more than 160 mg per day should be administered.

BUTORPHANOL

Butorphanol is a morphinan congener with a profile of actions similar to those of pentazocine. The structural formula of butorphanol is shown in Table 22–2.

Pharmacological Actions and Side Effects. In postoperative patients, a parenteral dose of 2 to 3 mg of butorphanol produces analgesia and respiratory depression approximately equal to that produced by 10 mg of morphine or 80 mg of meperidine; the onset, peak, and duration of action are similar to those that follow the administration of morphine (*see* Gilbert *et al.*, 1976). The plasma half-life of butorphanol is about 3 hours. Like pentazocine and other drugs whose actions are hypothesized to be exerted primarily on κ and σ receptors, the increase in respiratory depression is much less pronounced as the dose is increased than it is with morphine and other μ-receptor agonists. Also like pentazocine, analgesic doses of butorphanol pro-

duce an increase in pulmonary arterial pressure and in the work of the heart; systemic arterial pressure is slightly decreased (Popio *et al.*, 1978).

The major side effects of butorphanol are drowsiness, weakness, sweating, feelings of floating, and nausea. While the incidence of psychotomimetic side effects is lower than that with equianalgesic doses of pentazocine, they are qualitatively similar (*see* above).

Tolerance, Physical Dependence, and Liability for Abuse. Single doses of butorphanol cause subjective effects that resemble those produced by cyclazocine, pentazocine, and nalorphine, rather than those by morphine. In subjects who are dependent on 60 mg of morphine per day, butorphanol neither suppresses nor precipitates a withdrawal syndrome. Such observations suggest that butorphanol has neither agonistic nor antagonistic actions at μ-opioid receptors (*see* Table 22–1). Postaddicts stabilized on 12 mg of butorphanol four times a day complain of drowsiness, constipation, difficulty in urinating, and inability to sleep. The drug is identified much more frequently as a barbiturate than as an opioid, and postaddicts express indifference or mild dislike for it. After chronic administration of butorphanol, the administration of 4 mg of naloxone or abrupt withdrawal of the drug produces a withdrawal syndrome characterized by discomfort and requests for medicine for relief. The peak intensity of withdrawal symptoms occurs 48 hours after discontinuation and is not as severe as that seen with equianalgesic doses of morphine; it resembles the syndrome that follows the use of cyclazocine and is largely over by the eighth day. Butorphanol is not included in any schedule of the Federal Controlled Substances Act, and there have been few reported cases of abuse since its introduction in 1978.

Therapeutic Uses, Routes of Administration, Dosage, and Preparations. Since butorphanol is available only in parenteral form, it is better suited for the relief of acute rather than chronic pain. Because of its side effects on the heart, it is less useful than morphine or meperidine in patients with congestive heart failure or myocardial infarction. The usual dose is between 1 and 4 mg of the tartrate given intramuscularly or 0.5 to 2 mg given intravenously; this may be repeated every 3 to 4 hours. *Butorphanol tartrate* (STADOL) is available in solutions containing 1 or 2 mg/ml for parenteral use.

BUPRENORPHINE

Buprenorphine is a semisynthetic, highly lipophilic opioid derived from thebaine (Table 22–2). It is 25 to 50 times more potent than morphine.

Pharmacological Actions and Side Effects. Buprenorphine produces analgesia and other CNS effects that are qualitatively similar to those of morphine. About 0.4 mg of buprenorphine is equianalgesic with 10 mg of morphine given intramuscularly. The duration of analgesia is reported in some studies to be more than 6 hours; in others it is said to be comparable to that of morphine (Ouellette, 1982). Some of the subjective and respiratory-depressant effects are unequivocally slower in onset and last longer than those of morphine. For example, peak miosis occurs about 6 hours after intramuscular injection, while maximal respiratory depression is observed at about 3 hours.

In receptor-binding studies, buprenorphine behaves like an antagonist (judged by the effect of Na^+ on affinity). In abstinent, morphine-dependent dogs, buprenorphine suppresses signs of withdrawal, while in stabilized opioid-dependent dogs, it precipitates withdrawal. Such behavior suggests that it is a partial μ agonist. Depending on dose, buprenorphine may cause symptoms of abstinence in patients who have been receiving morphine-like drugs (μ-receptor agonists) for several weeks (Houde, 1979). Although respiratory depression has not been a major problem in clinical trials, it is not clear whether there is a ceiling for this effect (as is seen with nalbuphine and pentazocine). While the respiratory depression and other effects of buprenorphine can be prevented by prior administration of naloxone, they are not readily reversed by high doses of naloxone once the effects have been produced. This suggests that buprenorphine dissociates very slowly from opioid receptors. Cardiovascular effects appear to be similar to those of morphine. Side effects are similar to those of other opioids and include sedation, nausea, vomiting, dizziness, sweating, and headache.

Buprenorphine is relatively well absorbed by most routes, including the sublingual; 0.4 to 0.8 mg of the drug administered sublingually produces satisfactory analgesia in postoperative patients. Concentrations in blood peak within 5 minutes after intramuscular injection and within 2 hours after oral or sublingual administration. While the half-life in plasma has been reported to be about 3 hours, this value bears little relationship to the rate of disappearance of effects. Both N-dealkylated and conjugated metabolites are detected in the urine, but most of the drug is excreted unchanged in the feces. About 96% of the circulating drug is bound to protein. The pharmacology of buprenorphine has been reviewed by Heel and coworkers (1980).

Tolerance, Physical Dependence, and Liability for Abuse. In postaddicts, subcutaneous doses of buprenorphine ranging from 0.2 to 2 mg produce typical morphine-like effects, including euphoria and pupillary constriction. Miosis is detectable for 72 hours. During chronic administration of 8 mg of buprenorphine per day, subjects identify the drug as morphine-like. However, naloxone, in doses sufficient to produce severe withdrawal in addicts who are dependent on morphine, pentazocine, or butorphanol, does not precipitate a withdrawal syndrome; at the same time, the subjective and physiological effects of subcutaneous morphine (in doses of up to 120 mg) are prevented or markedly attenuated. This attenuation or ''blockade'' persists for more than 30 hours after the last dose of buprenorphine.

When buprenorphine is discontinued, a withdrawal syndrome develops that is delayed in onset (some subjects do not report symptoms until after the fifteenth day); this consists in typical morphine-like withdrawal signs and symptoms, and it persists for about 1 to 2 weeks. Subjects describe the intensity as mild to moderate, and they demand drugs for relief (Jasinski et al., 1978). However, Mello and Mendelson (1980) reported that their subjects experienced no withdrawal symptoms upon abrupt withdrawal. Overall, the potential for abuse of buprenorphine is probably less than that of morphine.

Therapeutic Uses, Route of Administration, and Dosage. *Buprenorphine* may be used as an analgesic; its use as a maintenance drug for opioid-dependent subjects has also been proposed. The usual parenteral dose is 0.3 to 0.6 mg, given every 6 to 8 hours. Buprenorphine is not currently available in the United States.

OTHER AGONIST-ANTAGONISTS

Meptazinol is an agonist-antagonist opioid that is about one tenth as potent as morphine in producing analgesia. Its analgesic actions are antagonized by naloxone, and it can precipitate withdrawal in animals dependent on μ agonists. The potential for abuse of meptazinol has not been definitively assessed.

Dezocine, an aminotetralin, is another agonist-antagonist; its potency and duration of analgesic effect are similar to those of morphine. Increasing dosage above 30 mg/70 kg does not produce progressively more severe respiratory depression (*see* Romagnoli and Keats, 1984).

OPIOID ANTAGONISTS

Under ordinary circumstances, the drugs to be discussed in this section produce few effects unless opioids with agonistic actions have been administered previously. However, when the endogenous opioid systems are activated, as in shock or certain forms of stress, the administration of an opioid antagonist alone has visible consequences. These agents have obvious therapeutic utility in the treatment of overdosage with opioids. As the understanding of the role of endogenous opioid systems in pathophysiological states increases, additional therapeutic niches for these antagonists may develop.

Chemistry. Relatively minor changes in the structure of an opioid can convert a drug that is primarily an agonist into one with antagonistic actions at one or more types of opioid receptors. The most common such substitution is that of a larger moiety (*e.g.,* an allyl or methylcyclopropyl group) for the N-methyl group that is typical of the opioid agonists. Such substitutions transform morphine to *nalorphine,* levorphanol to *levallorphan,* and oxymorphone to *naloxone* or *naltrexone* (*see* Table 22–2). In some cases, congeners are produced that are competitive antagonists at μ receptors but that also have agonistic actions at κ and σ receptors. Nalorphine was the first such agent to be discovered, and its historical importance, both as an analgesic and as an opioid antidote, was mentioned previously; the more potent levallorphan has similar properties, but it is still in therapeutic use. Other congeners, especially naloxone and naltrexone, appear to be devoid of agonistic actions and probably interact with all types of opioid receptors, albeit with widely different affinities. (*See* Barnett and coworkers, 1978; Martin, 1983.)

PHARMACOLOGICAL PROPERTIES

The pharmacological actions of opioid antagonists depend upon whether an opioid agonist has been administered previously, the pharmacological profile of that opioid, and the degree to which physical dependence on that substance has developed.

Effects in the Absence of Opioid Drugs. *Naloxone* is a competitive antagonist at μ-, δ-, κ-, and σ-opioid receptors. In man, subcutaneous doses up to 12 mg produce no discernible subjective effects, and 24 mg causes only slight drowsiness. *Naltrexone* also appears to be a relatively pure antagonist, but with higher oral efficacy and a longer duration of action (Martin *et al.,* 1973b; Verebey *et al.,* 1976).

At high dosage, both naloxone and naltrexone may have some special agonistic effects. However, these are of little clinical significance. At doses in excess of 0.3 mg/kg of naloxone, normal subjects show increased systolic blood pressure and decreased performance on tests of memory (Cohen *et al.,* 1983). High doses of naltrexone appeared to cause mild dysphoria in one study but almost no subjective effects in several others (*see* Gritz *et al.,* 1976).

The subjective effects of *nalorphine* and *levallorphan* in man depend largely upon the dose, the subject, and the situation. For example, in patients with postoperative pain, a dose of 10 to 15 mg of nalorphine is about as effective as 10 mg of morphine in producing analgesia. This appears to be a result of agonistic actions at opioid receptors, similar to those of nalbuphine and pentazocine. At such dosage, a significant percentage of patients experience unpleasant reactions that range from anxiety and vivid, disturbing "unreal" daydreams to frank hallucinations. These dysphoric and psychotomimetic effects may reflect agonistic actions at σ-opioid receptors. While more potent in other respects, levallorphan may be less prone to produce dysphoria.

Nalorphine and levallorphan produce some degree of respiratory depression. However the relationship to dose is less clear than with morphine, and there appears to be a relatively low ceiling on the maximal respiratory depression that is observed. Nevertheless, these agents, especially levallorphan, can deepen the respiratory depression caused by low doses of morphine-like opioids, even though they reduce the effects on respiration of high doses of these opioids. This presumably reflects the independent participation of μ- and κ-opioid receptors in the production of respiratory depression. Both the dysphoric and respiratory-depressant effects of these agents can be antagonized by large doses of naloxone.

Although high doses of antagonists might be expected to alter the actions of *endogenous* opioid peptides, the detectable effects are both subtle and limited. There appear to be several explanations for this apparent paradox. For example, endogenous opioids both enhance and inhibit the perception of pain (Wu *et al.,* 1983). If antagonists interfere with both of these processes to the same degree, there may be little net change. However, when endogenous opioid systems are activated, the effects of opioid antagonists on endogenous peptides become measurable. Thus, although naloxone does not consistently alter tolerance of experimentally induced pain in human subjects, it does decrease tolerance in those who normally have high pain thresholds. Naloxone also antagonizes the analgesic effects of placebo medication and increases the pain that patients may be experiencing. The analgesia that is produced by low-frequency stimulation of acupuncture needles is antagonized by naloxone; such analgesia may involve activation of opioid peptidergic systems to some extent (Kiser *et al.,* 1983). In both man and animals, various forms of acute and chronic stress induce some degree of analgesia. The physiological systems that mediate this analgesia vary with the nature and duration of the stress; both opioid and nonopioid systems are involved. Some forms of stress-induced analgesia are antagonized by naloxone (*see* Takagi, 1982; Watkins and Mayer, 1982; Akil *et al.,* 1984).

Studies in animals have shown that the administration of naloxone will reverse or attenuate the hypotension associated with shock of diverse origin, including that caused by endotoxin, hypovolemia, and injury to the spinal cord. (For a review, *see* McNicholas and Martin, 1984.) Naloxone may act centrally by antagonizing the actions of endogenous opioids on neural systems that are involved in the regulation of blood pressure. These and other observations in animals have been followed by a few reports that suggest that naloxone may have beneficial effects in patients with prolonged hypotension or with cerebral ischemia of diverse origins. However, the therapeutic utility of naloxone in these conditions remains to be determined (*see* McNicholas and Martin, 1984).

Opioid antagonists prevent the overeating and obesity that is produced when rats are stressed; they also induce weight loss in genetically obese rats. Since these conditions are associated with an increase in the concentration of β-endorphin in the circulation and since opioid antagonists increase energy expenditure and interrupt hibernation in appropriate species, endogenous opioids have been hypothesized to have some role in the regulation of feeding or energy metabolism. This reasoning has led to the experimental use of opioid antagonists in the treatment of human obesity, especially that associated with stress-induced eating disorders. The observation that increases in the secretion of β-endorphin occur in runners as physical conditioning progresses has engendered speculation as to the relationship of endogenous opioids to such phenomena as the "runner's high" or the "exercise withdrawal syndrome." Additional evidence for the mobilization of endogenous opioids during physical conditioning stems from the observation that naloxone produces a prompt increase in the secretion of FSH and LH in amenorrheic female athletes and inhibits the exercise-induced release of prolactin and growth hormone (*see* Appenzeller, 1981; Carr *et al.*, 1981; Mandenoff *et al.*, 1982).

Antagonistic Actions. Small doses (0.4 to 0.8 mg) of *naloxone* given intramuscularly or intravenously in man prevent or promptly reverse the effects of μ-opioid agonists. In patients with respiratory depression, there is an increase in respiratory rate within 1 or 2 minutes. Sedative effects are reversed, and blood pressure, if depressed, returns to normal. One milligram of naloxone intravenously completely blocks the effects of 25 mg of heroin. Naloxone reverses the psychotomimetic and dysphoric effects of agonist-antagonists such as pentazocine, but higher doses (10 to 15 mg) are required. The duration of antagonistic effects depends on the dose but is usually 1 to 4 hours. Antagonism of opioid effects by naloxone is often accompanied by "overshoot" phenomena; for example, respiratory rate depressed by opioids transiently becomes higher than that prior to the period of depression. This "overshoot" is probably related to the "unmasking" of acute physical dependence (*see* below).

Effects in Physical Dependence. In subjects who are dependent on morphine-like opioids, small subcutaneous doses of naloxone (0.5 mg) precipitate a moderate-to-severe withdrawal syndrome that is very similar to that seen after abrupt withdrawal of opioids, except that the syndrome appears within minutes after administration and subsides in about 2 hours. The severity and duration of the syndrome are related to the dose of the antagonist and the degree and type of dependence. Higher doses of naloxone will precipitate a withdrawal syndrome in patients dependent on pentazocine, butorphanol, or nalbuphine.

Naloxone produces "overshoot" phenomena suggestive of early acute physical dependence 24 hours after a single large dose of morphine, and it precipitates withdrawal symptoms 5 days after a single 40-mg dose of methadone. Nalorphine and levallorphan do not precipitate withdrawal symptoms after chronic use of pentazocine, but do precipitate a morphine type of withdrawal syndrome following use of propiram.

Tolerance, Physical Dependence, and Liability for Abuse. Tolerance develops to the agonistic but not to the antagonistic effects of opioid agonist-antagonists and partial agonists. Tolerance to the subjective effects, including the dysphoric and the psychotomimetic responses to both nalorphine and cyclazocine, has been demonstrated in man; cross-tolerance between these agents has also been shown (*see* Martin, 1967). However, even in subjects highly tolerant to the dysphoric, sedative, and motor effects of cyclazocine, a small (4-mg) dose continues to prevent the euphoric, miotic, respiratory-depressant, and physical-dependence-producing properties of morphine and heroin.

Even after prolonged administration of high doses, discontinuation of naloxone is not followed by any recognizable withdrawal syndrome, and the withdrawal of naltrexone, another relatively pure antagonist, produces very few signs and symptoms. However, after chronic administration of high dosage, abrupt discontinuation of either nalorphine or cyclazocine causes a characteristic withdrawal syndrome that is similar for both drugs. Although the intensity of these withdrawal signs and symptoms in the nalorphine withdrawal syndrome is generally less than comparable manifestations of the morphine withdrawal syndrome, a more striking contrast is the absence of "craving" or drug-seeking behavior. Drug-seeking behavior is present in the syndromes that characterize withdrawal from agonist-antagonists such as pentazocine, butorphanol, or nalbuphine, which have characteristics of both the nalorphine- and the morphine-type withdrawal syndromes.

Since nalorphine, levallorphan, and naloxone (1) do not support physical dependence of the morphine type, (2) are viewed by postaddicts as either neutral or unpleasant drugs in terms of their subjective effects, and (3) do not produce a variety of physical dependence that leads to drug-seeking behavior, they are considered to have little or no potential for abuse (for references, *see* Martin, 1967; Jasinski *et al.*, 1971; Jasinski, 1973).

Absorption, Fate, and Excretion. The effects of *naloxone* are seen almost immediately after its intravenous administration. The drug is metabolized in the liver, primarily by conjugation with glucuronic acid; other metabolites are produced in small amounts. Following parenteral administration, the duration of action of naloxone is about 1 to 4 hours; its half-life in plasma is about 1 hour (*see* Misra, 1978). The drug is absorbed after oral administration, but it is metabolized so rapidly in its first passage through the liver that it is only one fiftieth as potent as when given parenterally. Oral doses of more than 1 g are almost completely metabolized in less than 24 hours.

After parenteral administration of nalorphine or levallorphan, the onset of action is prompt, but the half-life is short.

Unlike naloxone, *cyclazocine* and *naltrexone,* both of which have cyclopropylmethyl substitutions on the nitrogen, retain much of their efficacy by the oral route, and their durations of action are longer, approaching 24 hours after moderate oral doses (*see* Martin *et al.,* 1973b). In the treatment of patients addicted to opioids, naltrexone is used in large oral doses (over 100 mg) to prevent the euphorigenic effects of opioids. After such doses, peak concentrations in plasma are reached within 1 to 2 hours and then slowly decline with a half-life of 10 hours; this value does not change after chronic use. In man, naltrexone is metabolized to 6-naltrexol, which is a weak antagonist and has a longer half-life. Naltrexone is much more potent than naloxone, and 100-mg oral doses produce concentrations in tissues sufficient to block for 48 hours the effects of 25 mg of heroin (taken intravenously) (*see* Verebey *et al.,* 1976).

Preparations and Routes of Administration. *Naloxone hydrochloride* (NARCAN) is available in a solution for injection at a concentration of 0.4 mg/ml. It is the drug of choice in most situations where an opioid antagonistic effect is required. An injectable preparation for use in neonates (NARCAN NEONATAL) contains 0.02 mg/ml. *Levallorphan tartrate* (LORFAN) is available for injection in a solution containing 1 mg/ml. It is approximately ten times as potent as nalorphine, and its therapeutic indications are virtually identical. *Nalorphine hydrochloride* is no longer available in the United States. *Naltrexone hydrochloride* (TREXAN) is available in 50-mg tablets for the maintenance of the opioid-free state in former addicts. *Cyclazocine* is available only for investigational use.

THERAPEUTIC USES

Opioid antagonists have established uses in the treatment of opioid-induced toxicity, especially respiratory depression; in the diagnosis of physical dependence on opioids; and as therapeutic agents in the treatment of compulsive users of opioids, as discussed in Chapter 23. Their potential utility in the treatment of shock and other disorders that may involve mobilization of endogenous opioid peptides remains to be established.

Treatment of Opioid Overdosage. The dramatic effects of opioid antagonists in reversing opioid-induced respiratory depression in the adult have already been discussed. Opioid antagonists have also been effectively employed to decrease neonatal respiratory depression secondary to the administration of opioids to the mother. In the neonate, the initial dose is 10 μg/kg, given by way of the umbilical vein following delivery. There is overwhelming evidence that all known opioids, even in reasonable therapeutic doses (*e.g.,* 10 mg of morphine, 100 mg of meperidine), produce a significant increase in the incidence of depression of respiration in the neonate compared to deliveries in which no general anesthetic or opioid is used (Fishburne, 1982).

CENTRALLY ACTIVE ANTITUSSIVE AGENTS

Cough is a useful physiological mechanism serving to clear the respiratory passages of foreign material and excess secretions. It should not be suppressed indiscriminately. There are, however, many situations in which cough does not serve any useful purpose but may, instead, only annoy the patient or prevent rest and sleep. In such situations the physician should use a drug that will reduce the frequency or intensity of the coughing. The cough reflex is complex, involving the central and peripheral nervous systems as well as the smooth muscle of the bronchial tree. It has been suggested that irritation of the bronchial mucosa causes bronchoconstriction, which, in turn, stimulates cough receptors (which probably represent a specialized type of stretch receptor) located in tracheobronchial passages. Afferent conduction from these receptors is via fibers in the vagus nerve; central components of the reflex probably involve several mechanisms or centers that are distinct from the mechanisms involved in the regulation of respiration.

The drugs that can affect this complex mechanism directly or indirectly are quite diverse. For example, cough may be the first or only symptom in bronchial asthma or allergy, and in such cases bronchodilators (β-adrenergic agonists) have been shown to reduce cough without having any significant central effects; other drugs might act primarily on the central or the peripheral nervous system components of the cough reflex. The early literature on antitussives has been exhaustively reviewed by Eddy and associates (1969) and by Salem and Aviado (1970). This section describes a few of the many drugs that have been in clinical use and that are believed to act on the nervous system in modifying cough.

A number of drugs are known to reduce cough as a result of their central actions, although the exact mechanisms are still not entirely clear. Included among them are the opioid analgesics discussed above (codeine, hydrocodone, and hydromorphone are the opioids most commonly used to prevent cough) as well as a number of nonopioid agents. As mentioned previously, receptors distinct from the recognized μ and κ receptors probably mediate some of the antitussive actions of codeine, dextromethorphan, and related drugs.

In selecting a specific centrally active agent for a particular patient, the significant considerations are its antitussive efficacy against pathological cough and the incidence and type of side effects to be expected. While opioid addicts who cannot obtain their drug of choice, and occasionally adolescents seeking new experiences, may turn to cough preparations containing opioids or to paregoric, the number of persons who become dependent on them as a result of medical treatment is exceedingly small. In the overwhelming majority of situations requiring a cough suppressant, liability for abuse need not be the major consideration. Most of the nonopioid agents now offered as antitussives are effective against cough induced by a variety of experimental technics. However, the ability of these tests to predict clinical efficacy is limited.

Dextromethorphan. *Dextromethorphan* (*d*-3-methoxy-N-methylmorphinan) is the *d* isomer of the codeine analog of levorphanol; however, unlike the *l* isomer, it has no analgesic or addictive properties. The drug acts centrally to elevate the threshold for coughing. Its effectiveness in patients with pathological cough has been demonstrated in controlled studies; its potency is nearly equal to that of codeine. Compared to codeine, dextromethorphan produces fewer subjective and gastrointestinal side effects (Matthys *et al.*, 1983). In therapeutic dosage the drug does not inhibit ciliary activity, and its antitussive effects persist for 5 to 6 hours. Its toxicity is quite low, but extremely high doses may produce CNS depression.

The average adult dose of *dextromethorphan hydrobromide* is 15 to 30 mg, three to four times daily; however, as is the case with codeine, higher doses are often required. The drug is generally marketed for "over-the-counter" sale in syrups and lozenges, or in combinations with antihistamines and other agents.

Other Drugs. *Levopropoxyphene napsylate,* in doses of 50 to 100 mg orally, appears to suppress cough to about the same degree as does 30 mg of dextromethorphan. Unlike dextropropoxyphene, levopropoxyphene has little or no analgesic activity.

Noscapine is a naturally occurring opium alkaloid of the benzylisoquinoline group; except for its antitussive effect, it has no significant actions on the CNS in doses within the therapeutic range. In dogs, the drug is a potent releaser of histamine, and large doses cause bronchoconstriction and transient hypotension. Toxic doses produce convulsions in animals. The average adult dose is 15 to 30 mg, four to six times daily, but single doses of 60 mg have been used. It is available in tablets and is the primary ingredient in several proprietary mixtures.

Other drugs that have been used as centrally acting antitussives include *carbetapentane, caramiphen, chlophedianol, diphenhydramine,* and *glaucine.* Each is a member of a distinct pharmacological class unrelated to the opioids. The mechanism of action of diphenhydramine, an antihistamine, is unclear. Although sedative effects are common, paradoxical excitement may be seen in infants; dryness of mucous membranes due to anticholinergic effects and thickening of mucus may be a disadvantage. Glaucine, an alkaloid obtained from *Glaucium flavum* and used as an antitussive in Eastern Europe, appears to suppress cough in clinical studies. Its site of action is probably central (*see* Constant *et al.*, 1983). In general, the toxicity of these agents is low, but controlled clinical studies are still insufficient to determine whether they merit consideration as alternatives to more thoroughly studied agents.

Benzonatate (TESSALON) is a long-chain polyglycol derivative chemically related to procaine and believed to exert its antitussive action on stretch or cough receptors in the lung, as well as by a central mechanism. It has been administered by all routes; the oral dose is about 100 mg, but higher doses have been used.

Alderman, E. L.; Barry, W. H.; Graham, A. F.; and Harrison, D. C. Hemodynamic effects of morphine and pentazocine differ in cardiac patients. *N. Engl. J. Med.,* **1972,** *287,* 623–627.

Appenzeller, O. What makes us run? *N. Engl. J. Med.,* **1981,** *305,* 578–579.

Beaver, W. T., and Feise, G. Comparison of the analgesic effects of morphine, hydroxyzine, and their combination in patients with postoperative pain. In, *Advances in Pain Research and Therapy,* Vol. 1. (Bonica, J. J., and Albe-Fessard, D., eds.) Raven Press, New York, **1976,** pp. 553–557.

Beaver, W. T.; Feise, G. A.; and Robb, D. Analgesic effect of intramuscular and oral nalbuphine on postoperative pain. *Clin. Pharmacol. Ther.,* **1981,** *29,* 174–180.

Bozarth, M. A., and Wise, R. A. Anatomically distinct opiate receptor fields mediate reward and physical dependence. *Science,* **1984,** *224,* 516–517.

Bromage, P. R.; Camporesi, E. M.; Durant, P. A. C.; and Nielsen, C. H. Nonrespiratory side effects of epidural morphine. *Anesth. Analg.,* **1982,** *61,* 490–495.

Campbell, C.; Phillips, O. C.; and Frazier, T. M. Analgesia during labor: a comparison of pentobarbital, meperidine, and morphine. *Obstet. Gynecol.,* **1961,** *17,* 714–718.

Carr, D. B.; Bullen, B. A.; Skrinar, G. S.; Arnold, M. A.; Rosenblatt, M.; Beitins, I. Z.; Martin, J. B.; and McArthur, J. W. Physical conditioning facilitates the exercise-induced secretion of beta-endorphin and beta-lipotropin in women. *N. Engl. J. Med.,* **1981,** *305,* 560–562.

Chang, K.-J., and Cuatrecasas, P. Heterogeneity and properties of opiate receptors. *Fed. Proc.,* **1981,** *40,* 2729–2734.

Cohen, M. R.; Cohen, R. M.; Pickar, D.; Weingartner, H.; and Murphy, D. L. High-dose naloxone infusions in normals. *Arch. Gen. Psychiatry,* **1983,** *40,* 613–619.

Constant, O.; Slavin, B.; Lehane, J. R.; Jordan, C.; and Jones, J. G. Effect of the antitussive glaucine on bronchomotor tone in man. *Thorax,* **1983,** *38,* 537–542.

Coombs, D. W.; Saunders, R. L.; Gaylor, M. S.; Block, A. R.; Colton, T.; Harbaugh, R.; Pageau, M. G.; and Mroz, W. Relief of continuous chronic pain by intraspinal narcotics infusion via an implanted reservoir. *J.A.M.A.,* **1983,** *250,* 2336–2339.

Cooper, S. A., and Beaver, W. T. A model to evaluate mild analgesics in oral surgery outpatients. *Clin. Pharmacol. Ther.,* **1976,** *20,* 241–250.

Crawford, M. E., and others. Pain treatment on outpatient basis utilizing extradural opiates. A Danish multicentre study comprising 105 patients. *Pain,* **1983,** *16,* 41–47.

Dahlström, B.; Bolme, P.; Feychting, H.; Noack, G.; and Paalzow, L. Morphine kinetics in children. *Clin. Pharmacol. Ther.,* **1979,** *26,* 354–365.

Dixon, R.; Crews, T.; Inturrisi, C.; and Foley, K. Levorphanol: pharmacokinetics and steady-state plasma concentrations in patients with pain. *Res. Commun. Chem. Pathol. Pharmacol.,* **1983,** *41,* 3–17.

Edwards, D. J.; Svensson, C. K.; Visco, J. P.; and Lalka, D. Clinical pharmacokinetics of pethidine: 1982. *Clin. Pharmacokinet.,* **1982,** *7,* 421–433.

Ehrnebo, M.; Boréus, L.; and Lönroth, U. Bioavailability and first-pass metabolism of oral pentazocine in man. *Clin. Pharmacol. Ther.,* **1977,** *22,* 888–892.

Forrest, W. H., Jr.; Brown, B. W., Jr.; Brown, C. R.; Defalque, R.; Gold, M.; Gordon, H. E.; James, K. E.; Katz, J.; Mahler, D. L.; Schroff, P.; and Teutsch, G. Dextroamphetamine with morphine for the treatment of postoperative pain. *N. Engl. J. Med.,* **1977,** *296,* 712–715.

Garrett, J. M.; Sauer, W. G.; and Moertel, C. G. Colonic motility in ulcerative colitis after opiate administration. *Gastroenterology,* **1967,** *53,* 93–100.

Gilbert, M. S.; Hanover, R. M.; Moylan, B. S.; and Caruso, F. S. Intramuscular butorphanol and meperidine in postoperative pain. *Clin. Pharmacol. Ther.,* **1976,** *20,* 359–364.

Glynn, C. J., and Mather, L. E. Clinical pharmacokinetics applied to patients with intractable pain; studies with pethidine. *Pain,* **1982,** *13,* 237–246.

Gourlay, G. K.; Wilson, P. R.; and Glynn, C. J. Methadone produces prolonged postoperative analgesia. *Br. Med. J.,* **1982,** *284,* 630–631.

Gram, L. F.; Schou, J.; Way, W. L.; Heltberg, J.; and Bodin, N. O. *d*-Propoxyphene kinetics after single oral and intravenous doses in man. *Clin. Pharmacol. Ther.,* **1979,** *26,* 473–482.

Gritz, E. R.; Shiffman, S. M.; Jarvik, M. E.; Schlesinger, J.; and Charuvastra, V. C. Naltrexone: physiological and psychological effects of single doses. *Clin. Pharmacol. Ther.,* **1976,** *19,* 773–776.

Houde, R. W. Analgesic effectiveness of the narcotic agonist-antagonists. *Br. J. Clin. Pharmacol.,* **1979,** *1,* Suppl. 3, 297s–308s.

Inturrisi, C. E.; Colburn, W. A.; Verebey, K.; Dayton, H. E.; Woody, G. E.; and O'Brien, C. P. Propoxyphene and norpropoxyphene kinetics after single and repeated doses of propoxyphene. *Clin. Pharmacol. Ther.,* **1982,** *31,* 157–167.

Jasinski, D. R. Effects in man of partial morphine agonists. In, *Agonist and Antagonist Actions of Narcotic Analgesic Drugs.* (Kosterlitz, H. W.; Collier, H. O. J.; and Villarreal, J. E.; eds.) University Park Press, Baltimore, **1973,** pp. 94–103.

Jasinski, D. R.; Martin, W. R.; and Hoeldtke, R. D. Effects of short- and long-term administration of pentazocine in man. *Clin. Pharmacol. Ther.,* **1970,** *11,* 385–403.

———. Studies of the dependence-producing properties of GPA-1657, profadol, and propiram in man. *Ibid.,* **1971,** *12,* 613–649.

Jasinski, D. R.; Pevnick, J. S.; Clark, S. C.; and Griffith, J. D. Therapeutic usefulness of propoxyphene napsylate in narcotic addiction. *Arch. Gen. Psychiatry,* **1977,** *34,* 227–233.

Jasinski, D. R.; Pevnick, J. S.; and Griffith, J. D. Human pharmacology and abuse potential of the analgesic buprenorphine. *Arch. Gen. Psychiatry,* **1978,** *35,* 501–516.

Johnson, M. A.; Woodcock, A. A.; and Geddes, D. M. Dihydrocodeine for breathlessness in "pink puffers." *Br. Med. J.,* **1983,** *286,* 675–677.

Kaiko, R. F. Age and morphine analgesia in cancer patients with postoperative pain. *Clin. Pharmacol. Ther.,* **1980,** *28,* 823–826.

Kaiko, R. F.; Foley, K. M.; Grabinski, P. Y.; Heidrich, G.; Rogers, A. G.; Inturrisi, C. E.; and Reidenberg, M. M. Central nervous system excitatory effects of meperidine in cancer patients. *Ann. Neurol.,* **1983,** *13,* 180–185.

Kaiko, R. F.; Wallenstein, S. L.; Rogers, A. G.; Grabinski, P. Y.; and Houde, R. W. Analgesic and mood effects of heroin and morphine in cancer patients with postoperative pain. *N. Engl. J. Med.,* **1981,** *304,* 1501–1505.

Kiser, R. S.; Gatchel, R. J.; Bhatia, K.; Khatami, M.; Huang, X.-Y.; and Altshuler, K. Z. Acupuncture relief of chronic pain syndrome correlates with increased plasma met-enkephalin concentrations. *Lancet,* **1983,** *2,* 1394–1396.

Kreek, M. J. Methadone in treatment: physiological and pharmacological issues. In, *Handbook on Drug Abuse.* (Dupont, R. I.; Goldstein, A.; and O'Donnell, J.; eds.)

U.S. Government Printing Office, Washington, D. C., **1979,** pp. 57–86.

Lee, G.; DeMaria, A.; Amsterdam, E. A.; Realyvasquez, E.; Angel, J.; Morrison, S.; and Mason, D. T. Comparative effects of morphine, meperidine and pentazocine on cardiocirculatory dynamics in patients with acute myocardial infarction. *Am. J. Med.,* **1976,** *60,* 949–955.

Lee, G.; Low, R. I.; Amsterdam, E. A.; DeMaria, A. N.; Huber, P. W.; and Mason, D. T. Hemodynamic effects of morphine and nalbuphine in acute myocardial infarction. *Clin. Pharmacol. Ther.,* **1981,** *29,* 576–581.

Ling, W.; Klett, C. J.; and Gillis, R. D. A cooperative clinical study of methadyl acetate. *Arch. Gen. Psychiatry,* **1978,** *35,* 345–353.

Lord, J.; Waterfield, A. A.; Hughes, J.; and Kosterlitz, H. W. Endogenous opioid peptides: multiple agonists and receptors. *Nature,* **1977,** *267,* 495–499.

McGivney, W. T., and Crooks, G. M. Conference on the care of patients with severe chronic pain in terminal illness. *J.A.M.A.,* **1984,** *251,* 1182–1188.

Madison, D. V., and Nicoll, R. A. Noradrenaline blocks accommodation of pyramidal cell discharge in the hippocampus. *Nature,* **1982,** *299,* 636–638.

Mandenoff, A.; Fumeron, F.; Apfelbaum, M.; and Margules, D. L. Endogenous opiates and energy balance. *Science,* **1982,** *215,* 1536–1537.

Martin, W. R.; Eades, C. G.; Thompson, J. A.; Huppler, R. E.; and Gilbert, P. E. The effects of morphine- and nalorphine-like drugs in the non-dependent and morphine-dependent chronic spinal dog. *J. Pharmacol. Exp. Ther.,* **1976,** *197,* 517–532.

Martin, W. R.; Jasinski, D. R.; Haertzen, C. A.; Kay, D. C.; Jones, B. E.; Mansky, P. A.; and Carpenter, R. W. Methadone—a reevaluation. *Arch. Gen. Psychiatry,* **1973a,** *28,* 286–295.

Martin, W. R.; Jasinski, D. R.; and Mansky, P. A. Naltrexone, an antagonist for the treatment of heroin dependence. *Arch. Gen. Psychiatry,* **1973b,** *28,* 784–791.

Mather, L. E., and Tucker, G. T. Systemic availability of orally administered meperidine. *Clin. Pharmacol. Ther.,* **1976,** *20,* 535–540.

Matthys, H.; Bleicher, B.; and Bleicher, U. Dextromethorphan and codeine: objective assessment of antitussive activity in patients with chronic cough. *J. Int. Med. Res.,* **1983,** *11,* 92–100.

Mello, N. K., and Mendelson, J. H. Buprenorphine suppresses heroin use by heroin addicts. *Science,* **1980,** *207,* 657–659.

Moore, A.; Bullingham, R.; McQuay, H.; Allen, M.; Baldwin, D.; and Cole, A. Spinal fluid kinetics of morphine and heroin. *Clin. Pharmacol. Ther.,* **1984,** *35,* 40–45.

Moore, J., and Dundee, J. W. Alterations in response to somatic pain associated with anaesthesia. VII. The effect of nine phenothiazine derivatives. *Br. J. Anaesth.,* **1961,** *33,* 422–431.

Morley, J. E., and Levine, A. S. Stress-induced eating is mediated through endogenous opiates. *Science,* **1980,** *209,* 1259–1261.

Nation, R. L. Meperidine binding in maternal and fetal plasma. *Clin. Pharmacol. Ther.,* **1981,** *29,* 472–479.

Neumann, P. B.; Henriksen, H.; Grosman, N.; and Christensen, C. B. Plasma morphine concentrations during chronic oral administration in patients with cancer pain. *Pain,* **1982,** *13,* 247–252.

Novick, D. M.; Kreek, M. J.; Fanizza, A. M.; Yancovitz, S. R.; Gelb, A. M.; and Stenger, R. J. Methadone disposition in patients with chronic liver disease. *Clin. Pharmacol. Ther.,* **1981,** *30,* 353–363.

Oldendorf, W. H.; Hyman, S.; Braun, L.; and Oldendorf, S. Z. Blood-brain barrier penetration of morphine, codeine, heroin, and methadone after carotid injection. *Science,* **1972,** *178,* 984–986.

Olsen, G. D.; Wilson, J. E.; and Robertson, G. E. Respiratory and ventilatory effects of methadone in healthy women. *Clin. Pharmacol. Ther.,* **1981,** *29,* 373–380.

Ouellette, R. D. Buprenorphine and morphine efficacy in postoperative pain: a double-blind multiple-dose study. *J. Clin. Pharmacol.,* **1982,** *22,* 165–172.

Owen, J. A.; Sitar, D. S.; Berger, L.; Brownell, L.; Duke, P. C.; and Mitenko, P. A. Age-related morphine kinetics. *Clin. Pharmacol. Ther.,* **1983,** *34,* 364–368.

Pasternak, G. W.; Childers, S. R.; and Snyder, S. H. Opiate analgesia: evidence for mediation by a subpopulation of opiate receptors. *Science,* **1980,** *208,* 514–516.

Pickworth, W. B.; Neidert, G. L.; and Kay, D. C. Morphine-like arousal by methadone during sleep. *Clin. Pharmacol. Ther.,* **1981,** *30,* 796–804.

Pond, S. M.; Tong, T. G.; Benowitz, N. L.; Jacob, P., iii; and Rigod, J. Lack of effect of diazepam on methadone metabolism in methadone-maintained addicts. *Clin. Pharmacol. Ther.,* **1982,** *31,* 139–143.

Popio, K. A.; Jackson, D. H.; Ross, A. M.; Schreiner, B. F.; and Yu, P. N. Hemodynamic and respiratory depressant effects of morphine and butorphanol. *Clin. Pharmacol. Ther.,* **1978,** *23,* 281–287.

Porreca, F., and Burks, T. F. The spinal cord as a site of opioid effects on gastrointestinal transit in the mouse. *J. Pharmacol. Exp. Ther.,* **1983,** *227,* 22–27.

Reuler, J. B.; Girard, D. E.; and Nardone, D. A. The chronic pain syndrome: misconceptions and management. *Ann. Intern. Med.,* **1980,** *93,* 588–596.

Romagnoli, A., and Keats, A. S. Comparative hemodynamic effects of nalbuphine and morphine in patients with coronary artery disease. *Cardiovasc. Dis. Bull. Texas Heart Inst.,* **1978,** *5,* 19–24.

———. Ceiling respiratory depression by dezocine. *Clin. Pharmacol. Ther.,* **1984,** *35,* 367–373.

Roth, K. A.; Weber, E.; Barchas, J. D.; Chang, D.; and Chang, J.-K. Immunoreactive dynorphin-(1-8) and corticotropin-releasing factor in subpopulation of hypothalamic neurons. *Science,* **1983,** *219,* 189–191.

Santiago, T. V.; Johnson, J.; Riley, D. J.; and Edelman, N. H. Effects of morphine on ventilatory response to exercise. *J. Appl. Physiol.,* **1979,** *47,* 112–118.

Säwe, J.; Dahlström, B.; Paalzow, L.; and Rane, A. Morphine kinetics in cancer patients. *Clin. Pharmacol. Ther.,* **1981,** *30,* 629–635.

Scott, P. V., and Fischer, H. B. J. Intraspinal opiates and itching: a new relief? *Br. Med. J.,* **1982,** *284,* 1015–1016.

Sethna, D. H.; Moffitt, E. A.; Gray, R. J.; Bussell, J.; Raymond, M.; Conklin, C.; Shell, W. E.; and Matloff, J. M. Cardiovascular effects of morphine in patients with coronary arterial disease. *Anesth. Analg.,* **1982,** *61,* 109–114.

Sevelius, H.; McCoy, J. F.; and Colmore, J. P. Dose response to codeine in patients with chronic cough. *Clin. Pharmacol. Ther.,* **1971,** *12,* 449–455.

Spiegel, K.; Kourides, I. A.; and Pasternak, G. W. Prolactin and growth hormone release by morphine in the rat: different receptor mechanisms. *Science,* **1982,** *217,* 745–747.

Sriwatanakul, K.; Weis, O. F.; Alloza, J. L.; Kelvie, W.; Weintraub, M.; and Lasagna, L. Analysis of narcotic analgesic usage in the treatment of postoperative pain. *J.A.M.A.,* **1983,** *250,* 926–929.

Sun, C.-L. J.; Hui, F. W.; and Hanig, J. P. Effect of H_1 blockers alone and in combination with morphine to produce antinociception in mice. *Neuropharmacology,* **1985,** *24,* 1–4.

Takagi, H. Critical review of pain relieving procedures including acupuncture. In, *CNS Pharmacology, Neuropeptides,* Vol. 1. *Advances in Pharmacology and Therapeutics II.* (Yoshida, H.; Hagihara, Y.; and Ebashi, S.; eds.) Pergamon Press, Ltd., Oxford, **1982,** pp. 79–92.

Tamsen, A.; Sakurada, T.; Wahlström, A.; Terenius, L.; and Hartvig, P. Postoperative demand for analgesics in relation to individual levels of endorphins and substance P in cerebrospinal fluid. *Pain,* **1982,** *13,* 171–183.

Tubaro, E.; Borelli, G.; Croce, C.; Cavallo, G.; and Santiangeli, C. Effect of morphine on resistance to infection. *J. Infect. Dis.,* **1983,** *148,* 656–666.

Verebey, K.; Volavka, J.; Mule, S.; and Resnick, R. Naltrexone: disposition, metabolism, and effects after acute and chronic dosing. *Clin. Pharmacol. Ther.,* **1976,** *20,* 315–328.

Vismara, L. A.; Leamon, D. M.; and Zelis, R. The effects of morphine on venous tone in patients with acute pulmonary edema. *Circulation,* **1976,** *54,* 335–337.

Way, W. L.; Costley, E. C.; and Way, E. L. Respiratory sensitivity of the newborn infant to meperidine and morphine. *Clin. Pharmacol. Ther.,* **1965,** *6,* 454–461.

Wu, K. M.; Martin, W. R.; Kamerling, S. G.; and Wettstein, J. G. Possible medullary kappa hyperalgesic mechanism. I. A new potential role for endogenous opioid peptides in pain perception. *Life Sci.,* **1983,** *33,* 1831–1838.

Monographs and Reviews

Akil, H.; Watson, S. J.; Young, E.; Lewis, M. E.; Khachaturian, H.; and Walker, J. M. Endogenous opioids: biology and function. *Annu. Rev. Neurosci.,* **1984,** *7,* 223–255.

Awouters, F.; Niemegeers, C. J. E.; and Janssen, P. A. J. Pharmacology of antidiarrheal drugs. *Annu. Rev. Pharmacol. Toxicol.,* **1983,** *23,* 279–301.

Barnett, G.; Trsic, M.; and Willette, R. E. (eds.). *QuaSAR: Quantitative Structure Activity Relationships of Analgesics, Narcotic Antagonists, and Hallucinogens.* National Institute on Drug Abuse Research Monograph No. 22, U.S. Government Printing Office, Washington, D. C., **1978.**

Basbaum, A. I., and Fields, H. L. Endogenous pain control systems: brainstem spinal pathways and endorphin circuitry. *Annu. Rev. Neurosci.,* **1984,** *7,* 309–338.

Beaumont, A., and Hughes, J. Biology of opioid peptides. *Annu. Rev. Pharmacol. Toxicol.,* **1979,** *19,* 245–267.

Beaver, W. T. Mild analgesics, a review of their clinical pharmacology (Part II). *Am. J. Med. Sci.,* **1966,** *251,* 576–599.

———. Management of cancer pain with parenteral medication. *J.A.M.A.,* **1980,** *244,* 2653–2657.

Berger, P. A.; Akil, H.; Watson, S. J.; and Barchas, J. D. Behavioral pharmacology of the endorphins. *Annu. Rev. Med.,* **1982,** *33,* 397–415.

Bloom, F. E. The endorphins: a growing family of pharmacologically pertinent peptides. *Annu. Rev. Pharmacol. Toxicol.,* **1983,** *23,* 151–170.

Bonica, J. J. (ed.). *Pain.* Raven Press, New York, **1980.**

Brogden, R. N.; Speight, T. M.; and Avery, G. S. Pentazocine: a review of its pharmacological properties, therapeutic efficacy and dependence liability. *Drugs,* **1973,** *5,* 6–91.

Burks, T. F. Gastrointestinal pharmacology. *Annu. Rev. Pharmacol. Toxicol.,* **1976,** *16,* 15–31.

Chapman, D. B., and Way, E. L. Metal ion interactions with opiates. *Annu. Rev. Pharmacol. Toxicol.,* **1980,** *20,* 553–579.

Duggan, A. W., and North, R. A. Electrophysiology of opioids. *Pharmacol. Rev.,* **1983,** *35,* 219–282.

Eckenhoff, J. E., and Oech, S. R. The effects of narcotics and antagonists upon respiration and circulation in man. *Clin. Pharmacol. Ther.,* **1960,** *1,* 483–524.

Eddy, N. B.; Friebel, H.; Hohn, K.; and Halbach, H. Codeine and its alternates for pain and cough relief. *Bull. WHO,* **1969,** *40,* 639–719.

Eddy, N. B.; Halbach, H.; and Braenden, O. J. Synthetic substances with morphine-like effect. Clinical experience: potency, side-effects, addiction liability. *Bull. WHO,* **1957,** *17,* 569–863.

Fishburne, J. I. Systemic analgesia during labor. *Clin. Perinatol.,* **1982,** *9,* 29–53.

Goldstein, A. Opioid peptides: function and significance. In, *Opioids: Past, Present and Future.* (Collier, H. O. J.; Hughes, J.; Rance, M. J.; and Tyers, M. B.; eds.) Tayler & Frances Ltd., London, **1984,** pp. 127–143.

Heel, R. C.; Brogden, R. N.; Speight, T. M.; and Avery, G. S. Buprenorphine: a review of its pharmacological properties and therapeutic efficacy. *Drugs,* **1980,** *17,* 81–110.

Holaday, J. W. Cardiovascular effects of endogenous opiate systems. *Annu. Rev. Pharmacol. Toxicol.,* **1983,** *23,* 541–594.

Lasagna, L. The clinical evaluation of morphine and its substitutes as analgesics. *Pharmacol. Rev.,* **1964,** *16,* 47–83.

McNicholas, L. F., and Martin, W. R. New and experimental therapeutic roles for naloxone and related opioid antagonists. *Drugs,* **1984,** *27,* 81–93.

Martin, W. R. Opioid antagonists. *Pharmacol. Rev.,* **1967,** *19,* 463–521.

———. Pharmacology of opioids. *Ibid.,* **1983,** *35,* 283–323.

Martin, W. R., and Sloan, J. W. Neuropharmacology and neurochemistry of subjective effects, analgesia, tolerance, and dependence produced by narcotic analgesics. In, *Handbook of Experimental Pharmacology.* Vol. 45/I, *Drug Addiction I: Morphine, Sedative/Hypnotic and Alcohol Dependence.* (Martin, W. R., ed.) Springer-Verlag, Berlin, **1977,** pp. 43–158.

Misra, A. L. Metabolism of opiates. In, *Factors Affecting the Action of Narcotics.* (Adler, M. L.; Manara, L.; and Samanin, R.; eds.) Raven Press, New York, **1978,** pp. 297–343.

Morley, J. S. Structure-activity relationships of enkephalin-like peptides. *Annu. Rev. Pharmacol. Toxicol.,* **1980,** *20,* 81–110.

Mueller, R. A.; Lundberg, D. B. A.; Breese, G. R.; Hedner, J.; Hedner, T.; and Jonason, J. The neuropharmacology of respiratory control. *Pharmacol. Rev.,* **1982,** *34,* 255–285.

Musto, D. F. *The American Disease.* Yale University Press, New Haven, **1973.**

Redmond, D. E., Jr., and Krystal, J. H. Multiple mechanisms of withdrawal from opioid drugs. *Annu. Rev. Neurosci.,* **1984,** *7,* 443–478.

Reynolds, A. K., and Randall, L. O. *Morphine and Allied Drugs.* University of Toronto Press, Toronto, **1957.**

Salem, H., and Aviado, D. M. (eds.). *Antitussive Agents,* Vols. 1, 2, and 3. *International Encyclopedia of Pharmacology and Therapeutics,* Sect. 27. Pergamon Press, Ltd., Oxford, **1970.**

Schechter, N. L. Pain and pain control in children. *Curr. Probl. Pediatr.,* **1985,** *15.*

Simon, E. J., and Hiller, J. M. The opiate receptors. *Annu. Rev. Pharmacol. Toxicol.,* **1978,** *18,* 371–394.

Snyder, S. H. Drug and neurotransmitter receptors in the brain. *Science,* **1984,** *224,* 22–31.

Sternbach, R. A. (ed.). *The Psychology of Pain.* Raven Press, New York, **1978.**

Terenius, L. Endogenous peptides and analgesia. *Annu. Rev. Pharmacol. Toxicol.,* **1978,** *18,* 189–204.

Terry, C. E., and Pellens, M. *The Opium Problem.* Bureau of Social Hygiene, Inc., New York, **1928.**

Watkins, L. R., and Mayer, D. J. Organization of endogenous opiate and nonopiate pain control systems. *Science,* **1982,** *216,* 1185–1192.

Way, E. L. Distribution and metabolism of morphine and its surrogates. *Res. Publ. Assoc. Res. Nerv. Ment. Dis.,* **1968,** *46,* 13–31.

Yaksh, T. L. Spinal opiate analgesia: characteristics and principles of actions. *Pain,* **1981,** *11,* 347–354.

CHAPTER

23 DRUG ADDICTION AND DRUG ABUSE

Jerome H. Jaffe

As far back as recorded history, every society has used drugs that produce effects on mood, thought, and feeling. Moreover, there were always a few individuals who digressed from custom with respect to the time, the amount, and the situation in which these drugs were to be used. Thus, both the nonmedical use of drugs and the problem of drug abuse are as old as civilization itself.

Problems of Terminology. *Drug abuse* refers to the use, usually by self-administration, of any drug in a manner that deviates from the approved medical or social patterns within a given culture. The term conveys the notion of social disapproval, and it is not necessarily descriptive of any particular pattern of drug use or its potential adverse consequences.

Since this definition is largely a social one, it is not surprising that for any particular drug there is a great variation in what is considered abuse, not only from culture to culture but also from time to time and from one situation to another within the same culture. For example, in Western society, chronic intoxication with alcohol is considered drug abuse, yet on certain occasions gross intoxication with alcohol is not. The use of medically prescribed opioid analgesics for the relief of pain is quite proper; however, the self-administration of the same drugs, in the same dosages, for relief of depression or tension or to induce euphoria is considered flagrant abuse. Temporal variations are common. For example, several decades ago the use of psychedelic (hallucinogenic) compounds such as lysergic acid diethylamide (LSD) was a practice limited to a few college students and research workers in the United States; it was not illegal, and there was little social condemnation of the users. By the mid-1960s, experimentation with psychedelic drugs was widespread; the use of these drugs had become equivalent to abuse; and the possession, manufacture, or sale of such drugs had been made a criminal offense under federal law.

Nonmedical drug use is a less pejorative term but is so general that it encompasses behaviors ranging from the occasional use of alcohol to compulsive use of opioids, and includes behaviors that may or may not be associated with adverse effects. Nonmedical drug use may consist in *experimental use* of a drug on one or a few occasions, because of curiosity about its effects, or in order to conform to the expectations of peer groups. It may involve the *casual* or *"recreational" use* of modest amounts of a drug for its pleasurable effects, or *circumstantial use,* in which certain drug effects are sought because they are helpful in particular circumstances, as when students or truck drivers take amphetamines to alleviate fatigue. These various forms of nonmedical use may then lead to more intensive patterns of use in terms of frequency or amount and, in some cases, to patterns of *dependence* or *compulsive drug use*.

Compulsive Drug Use. One of the hazards in the use of drugs to alter mood and feeling is that some individuals eventually develop a dependence on the drug. They continue to take it in the absence of medical indications, often despite adverse social and medical consequences, and they behave as if the effects of the drugs are needed for continued well-being. The intensity of this "need" or dependence may vary from a mild desire to a "craving" or "compulsion" to use the drug, and, when the availability of the drug is uncertain, they may exhibit a preoccupation with its procurement. In extreme forms, the behavior exhibits the characteristics of a chronic relapsing disorder. Since intense reliance on the effects of self-administered drugs *per se* is generally a deviation from approved and expected patterns of use, the terms *compulsive drug use* and *compulsive abuse* are often interchangeable. However, there are often striking inconsistencies in the way the terms *drug dependence* and *drug abuse* are employed.

Dependence on a drug *per se* is not necessarily cause for concern. If the substance used has low toxicity and is relatively inexpensive (*e.g.*, caffeine), a drug-using behavior may meet the criteria for dependence but may not constitute a significant medical or social problem. More commonly, however, compulsive use of drugs is detrimental both to the user and to the society of which he is a part. However, in weighing detrimental effects, one must consider both the pattern of use by a given individual and the available alternatives. For example, if the most likely alternative to the use of opioids is the compulsive use of alcohol, there are many who would take the view that opioid dependence is far less destructive to the individual and society, and that some provision should be made to permit that particular individual to use opioid drugs.

Compulsive drug use is commonly, but not necessarily, associated with the development of tolerance and physical dependence. *Tolerance* has developed when, after repeated administration, a given dose of a drug produces a decreased effect or, conversely, when increasingly larger doses must be administered to obtain the effects observed with the original dose. *Physical dependence* refers to an altered physiological state (neuroadaptation) produced by the repeated administration of a drug, which necessitates the continued administration of the drug to prevent the appearance of a stereotypical syndrome, *the withdrawal or abstinence syndrome,* characteristic for the particular drug. The theoretical bases for the phenomena of tolerance and physical dependence are discussed below.

Addiction. It is possible to describe all known patterns of drug use without employing the terms *addict* or *addiction*. In many respects this would be advantageous, for the term *addiction*, like the term *abuse*, has been used in so many ways that it can no longer be employed without further qualification or elaboration. However, since it is not likely that the term will be dropped from the language, it is appropriate to make an effort to delimit its meaning. The definition used here is somewhat arbitrary, and it is not necessarily identical with other definitions of addiction or drug dependence (*see* World Health Organization, 1973; Edwards *et al.*, 1981). In this chapter, the term *addiction* will be used to mean *a behavioral pattern of drug use, characterized by overwhelming involvement with the use of a drug (compulsive use), the securing of its supply, and a high tendency to relapse after withdrawal*. Addiction is thus viewed as an extreme on a continuum of involvement with drug use and refers in a *quantitative* rather than a *qualitative* sense

to the degree to which drug use pervades the total life activity of the user and to the range of circumstances in which drug use controls his behavior. In most instances it will not be possible to state with precision at what point compulsive use should be considered addiction. Anyone who is addicted would be considered drug dependent within the WHO definitions, but *within the set of definitions used here the term* addiction *cannot be used interchangeably with* physical dependence. *It is possible to be physically dependent on drugs without being addicted and, in some special circumstances, to be addicted without being physically dependent* (*see* below).

The use of the terms *drug dependence,* to denote a behavioral syndrome, and *physical dependence,* to refer to biological changes that underlie withdrawal syndromes, causes confusion. To reduce some of this confusion, the term *neuroadaptation* has been proposed as a substitute for *physical dependence* (*see* Edwards *et al.*, 1981).

GENESIS OF DRUG USE AND DEPENDENCE

Whether the use of a drug is socially acceptable or subject to extreme disapproval, multiple factors determine who will experiment with the drug and experience its effects; other factors determine who will continue to use it casually or recreationally; and still other factors influence who will progress from casual to intensive or compulsive use.

Experimentation is largely a matter of availability, curiosity, the attitude and drug-using behavior of one's friends, the social acceptability of a given form of drug use, the risks believed to be associated with experimental use, and the tendency of the individual to respect social norms. Sometimes, drug experimentation may involve the use of substances that produce unpleasant effects. The host of materials ingested over the centuries for supposed aphrodisiac effects bears witness to this. However, from the thousands of substances that have been self-administered over the years, only a few have become staples in mankind's pharmacopoeia of drugs for nonmedical use; of these, still fewer give rise to serious problems of dependence. A full exploration of the interactions between man, environment, and drugs is beyond the scope of this chapter. (*See* National Commission, 1973; Edwards *et al.*, 1983.)

The emphasis here will be on the interactions of man and drug, and on those aspects of the interaction that are relevant to clinical situations and to the development of dependence.

Drugs as Reinforcers. Man's tendency to take drugs is shared with other mammals. Laboratory animals quickly learn to self-administer most of the drugs commonly used for nonmedical purposes, including opioids, barbiturates, alcohol, anesthetic gases, local anesthetics, volatile solvents, central nervous system (CNS) stimulants, phencyclidine, nicotine, and caffeine. Whether an animal will self-administer a drug depends on a number of factors, including the properties of the drug itself, the route of administration, the size of the individual dose, the amount of work required to obtain a dose and the time between the work and the drug administration (schedule of reinforcement), the presence of other drugs, and the kinds of drugs the animal has been given previously (*see* Kalant *et al.,* 1978; Johanson and Schuster, 1981). When given continuous access, animals show patterns of self-administration that are strikingly similar to those exhibited by human users of the same drug. Such observations suggest that preexisting psychopathology is not a requisite for initial or even continued drug taking, and that drugs themselves are powerful reinforcers, even in the absence of physical dependence.

Some drugs (*e.g.,* chlorpromazine) are never self-administered; they appear instead to have aversive properties, and animals learn to avoid behaviors that result in small injections of such drugs. On the other hand, animals will press a lever more than four thousand times to get a single injection of cocaine, and when given free access, they immediately begin self-administering high daily doses that may produce severe toxic effects and induce self-mutilating behavior. With stimulants such as amphetamine and cocaine, periods of self-imposed abstinence alternate with periods of drug administration; generally the animals die of toxic effects and inanition after a period of several weeks of continuous use. If saline solution is substituted for cocaine or amphetamine, there is a burst of rapid lever pressing for several hours, then abruptly all responding ceases and is not resumed. In contrast, animals self-administering morphine gradually raise the daily dose over a period of weeks, then self-administer the drug at a steady rate that avoids both gross toxicity and withdrawal symptoms. When saline solution is substituted for morphine, however, the animal continues to press the lever (except during the peak of withdrawal) and does so at a slow but steady rate over a period of weeks (*see* Woods, 1978; Johanson and Schuster, 1981).

Tolerance and Physical Dependence. In addition to the primary reinforcing effects, when drugs are used chronically other factors come into play that profoundly affect the pattern of use and the likelihood that the drug use will be continued. Among these are the capacities of some substances to produce *tolerance* and/or *physical dependence*. These phenomena, as previously defined, are often assumed to be inextricably linked to each other and to the problem of compulsive drug use. Neither of these assumptions is valid. Tolerance and physical dependence develop not only with opioids, alcohol, and hypnotics but also after chronic administration of a wide variety of drugs that are not self-administered by animals or used compulsively by man. Such drugs include anticholinergics, chlorpromazine, and imipramine. Nor does physical dependence invariably occur in every situation where tolerance develops. Tolerance is a very general phenomenon observed with a host of substances and involves many independent mechanisms.

In addition to *innate* tolerance to various classes of drugs, it is possible to distinguish two varieties of *acquired* pharmacological tolerance: dispositional and pharmacodynamic. Drug *dispositional tolerance* results from changes in the pharmacokinetic properties of the agent in the organism, such that reduced concentrations are present at the sites of drug action. The most common mechanism is an increased rate of metabolism. Dispositional tolerance has relatively little effect on the peak intensity of action and does not usually result in more than a threefold decrease in sensitivity. *Pharmacodynamic tolerance* results from adaptive changes within affected systems, such that the response is reduced in the presence of the same concentration of the drug. When a reduced effect of a drug on behavior is used as the measure of tolerance, it is a consistent finding that tolerance develops more rapidly and to a greater degree when the effect of the drug has a behavioral "cost" to the organism (*i.e.,* when it impairs its capacity to earn a reward or to avoid punishment) than when it does not. Thus, rats tested daily on a moving belt under the influence of alcohol develop more tolerance to the ataxic effects than rats receiving the same dose after the test, and both groups develop tolerance more rapidly than rats given an even larger dose of alcohol without daily testing. Similar relationships between behavioral conditions and the development of tolerance have been observed with opioids, marihuana, and amphetamines. (*See* Martin and Sloan, 1977a; Smith, 1977; Kalant, 1978; Tabakoff and Rothstein, 1983.)

Tolerance to Opioids. Tolerance does not develop uniformly to all the actions of opioid drugs. There may be complete tolerance to some actions, while responses to others are relatively unaltered. Tolerance to opioids is characterized by a shortened duration and decreased intensity of the analgesic, euphorigenic, sedative, and other CNS-depressant effects as well as by a marked elevation in the average lethal dose. While animals that are tolerant to opioids may metabolize them somewhat more rapidly, most of the tolerance seen with opioids is due to adaptation of cells in the nervous system to the drug's action.

Although tolerance itself does not necessarily affect the likelihood of continued use, it can affect patterns of use by increasing the amount of drug that must be taken to produce a given effect (*e.g.*, euphoria). The use of increased amounts may in turn enhance the risk of toxic effects or produce other problems if the drug is expensive or obtained illicitly.

Tolerance to opioid drugs can develop with remarkable rapidity. In the dog, considerable recovery from behavioral depression occurs during the course of a continuous 8-hour infusion of morphine (acute tolerance). Although such rapid changes do not occur in man, former morphine addicts can attain a dosage of 500 mg of morphine per day within 10 days. However, even with prolonged administration of opioids to experimental animals, there appears to be little tolerance to the facilitatory effect of such drugs on electrical self-stimulation of the brain or to their capacity to serve as discriminative stimuli (*see* Kornetsky *et al.*, 1979).

Associative processes akin to learning may be involved in the interactions between tolerance to opioids and the conditions under which they are given, as well as in certain forms of long-lasting residual tolerance (*see* Siegel *et al.*, 1982; Donegan *et al.*, 1983). Furthermore, animals and man previously dependent on opioids become physically dependent more rapidly on reexposure.

Tolerance to Alcohol, Barbiturates, and Related Hypnotics. Animals made tolerant to barbiturates or alcohol show significantly less sedation and ataxia than do nontolerant animals at the same blood

concentrations. However, as the blood concentrations are increased, there is progressively less difference between tolerant and nontolerant animals in the degree of CNS depression and, in contrast to the tolerance seen with opioids, animals tolerant to alcohol or barbiturates show only modest elevation of the lethal blood concentration. If the use of the CNS depressant has produced only ataxia and has been insufficient to depress respiration to some degree, there is little or no tolerance to the respiratory-depressant and lethal effects of the drug. It appears that only those systems that have been challenged or altered by the agent display tolerance to its effects (Okamoto *et al.*, 1978).

In the case of short-acting barbiturates (*e.g.*, pentobarbital), alcohol, and a number of nonbarbiturate hypnotics (glutethimide, meprobamate, *etc.*), a more rapid enzymatic degradation of the drug can also be demonstrated in tolerant animals. Thus, in the same animal, both *pharmacodynamic* tolerance and *dispositional* tolerance contribute to the decreased duration and intensity of the response to a given dose of drug.

With these groups of drugs, as with the opioids, tolerance does not directly increase the probability of continued or compulsive use. However, tolerance to toxic effects may not develop in parallel with tolerance to CNS depression and, in the case of alcohol particularly, the consumption of more drug in order to obtain CNS effects may increase the likelihood of direct drug-induced organ damage. Furthermore, the shortened duration of action may increase the frequency of drug taking, thereby increasing the number of times that drug-taking behavior will be reinforced.

Some aspects of tolerance to general CNS depressants develop with surprising rapidity. Thus, in man, when the blood concentration is falling after administration of a large dose of alcohol, the signs and symptoms of intoxication disappear at a concentration that was associated with gross intoxication when the blood level was rising. The degree of such *acute* CNS tolerance (as measured by the blood concentration of the drug when signs of ataxia disappear) seems directly related to the depth of the CNS depression that was produced by the drug. Acute tolerance also appears to develop with some benzodiazepines (Ellinwood *et al.*, 1983). It is not clear whether the mechanisms underlying acute tolerance are related to those involved in the tolerance that develops over longer periods. Tolerance to alcohol and related general CNS depressants has been reviewed by Kalant and associates (1971), Smith (1977), and Tabakoff and Rothstein (1983). Tolerance to CNS sympathomimetics, nicotine, cannabinoids, and psychedelics is also discussed under clinical characteristics of their abuse.

Physical Dependence. Physical dependence has been studied after chronic administration of opioids, CNS depressants (alcohol, barbiturates, related hypnotics, and benzodiazepines), amphetamines, cannabinoids, and nicotine. The withdrawal symptoms associated with many of these classes of agents are generally characterized by rebound effects in those same physiological systems that were modified initially by the drug (*rebound hyperexcitability*). For example, general depressants elevate the seizure threshold, but spontaneous seizures are seen during withdrawal. Amphetamines alleviate fatigue, suppress appetite, and elevate mood; amphetamine withdrawal is characterized by lack of energy, hyperphagia, and depression. However, it is not certain whether all the complex patterns of signs and symptoms seen during withdrawal from classical μ-agonist opioids or general depressants should be considered rebound effects, nor whether such a generalization is applicable to the syndromes observed after abrupt withdrawal of drugs such as nicotine, caffeine, clonidine, or opioids that do not act at μ receptors.

Time Required. The time required to produce physical dependence on any drug depends on a number of factors, but the most important seem to be the degree to which function in the CNS is altered by the drug and the continuity of this alteration. However, whether a withdrawal syndrome is clinically observable depends on (1) the criteria for withdrawal symptoms, (2) the sensitivity of technics used to detect withdrawal phenomena, and (3) the rate at which the drug is removed from its site of action.

Patients who have received therapeutic doses of morphine several times a day for 1 to 2 weeks will have only mild symptoms that may not be recognized as withdrawal symptomatology when the drug is stopped; symptoms are even less pronounced when the opioid is one that is slowly eliminated (such as methadone). However, if the drug is not simply discontinued but an opioid antagonist (naloxone) is used to induce withdrawal, it is possible to demonstrate withdrawal symptoms in man after therapeutic doses of morphine, methadone, or heroin given four times per day for as short a period as 2 to 3 days. In former heroin addicts naloxone precipitates mild withdrawal symptoms 1 week after a single 40-mg dose of methadone, indicating the presence of an otherwise-subclinical level of physical dependence. In short, the phenomenon of opioid physical dependence is initiated by the first dose, and this rapid development has important clinical implications (*see* below).

The time required to produce physical dependence with general CNS depressants or benzodiazepines is likewise short; when rapidly metabolized drugs are used, the earliest signs of rebound excitability can be detected after surprisingly brief periods of CNS depression. A single large dose of alcohol produces an elevation of the threshold for chemically induced seizures that is followed by a period of subnormal threshold. After 3 days of chronic exposure to ethanol, mice develop marked physical dependence, with spontaneous seizures upon abrupt withdrawal (*see* Tabakoff and Hoffman, 1983). In baboons, a withdrawal syndrome can be precipitated with a specific benzodiazepine antagonist after 3 to 7 days of administration of diazepam (Lukas and Griffiths, 1984). In man, it may require weeks of *mild intoxication* with short-acting barbiturates to produce clinically significant physical dependence, but some patients who are kept *deeply intoxicated* (semicomatose) for 16 to 20 hours per day, for 10 to 12 days, become so physically dependent that they develop seizures and delirium on abrupt withdrawal. If rebound changes in the EEG or insomnia are used as criteria, only 1 or 2 weeks of ordinary dosage at night is enough to induce low levels of physical dependence on CNS depressants and benzodiazepines (Kales *et al.*, 1983).

These observations indicate that the adaptational processes that eventually produce grossly observable withdrawal symptoms begin with the first dose. This has obvious implications not only for the problem of deciding just when physical dependence is present but also for the problem of determining the causes of compulsive drug use. It is quite conceivable that individuals who use short-acting drugs to induce euphoria or reduce tensions can perceive a relative dysphoria or an exacerbation of these same tensions (rebound effects) as the drug effects wane. Such increases in unpleasant feelings might then contribute to the motivation to repeat the use of the drug, and the alleviation of withdrawal phenomena might increase the effectiveness of the drug as a reinforcer of drug-using behavior. Similar subtle post-drug-use effects are also seen with amphetamines and cocaine and possibly with nicotine and short-acting benzodiazepines.

The relationship of tolerance and physical dependence to drug-seeking behavior and compulsive drug use is complex and differs with drug categories (*see* Cappell and LeBlanc, 1981). The notion that physical dependence increases drug-seeking behavior and the reinforcing effects of the drug is best established for the opioids, but even with this group of drugs other factors appear to be more potent determinants of behavior. For example, although some degree of physical dependence develops in medical patients who receive opioids regularly for more than a few days, the overwhelming majority of such patients do not exhibit drug-seeking behavior and do not become compulsive users. Even those who administer such drugs to themselves for brief periods discontinue the drug when the medical condition is relieved. A large proportion of the young men who served in the United States Army in Vietnam used heroin, and about half of this group became physically dependent. Nevertheless, a substantial percentage simply stopped their heroin use before their return to the United States, and many did so without benefit of any special treatment (*see* Robins, 1974). Thus, although some compulsive users attribute their drug problems entirely to "getting hooked" (either iatrogenically or in the course of using drugs illicitly), physical dependence is currently viewed not so much as a direct cause of compulsive use but as one of several factors that contribute to its development and to the tendency to relapse after withdrawal (*see* below).

Degree of Physical Dependence and Locus of Changes. Although it is possible to demonstrate changes in the biochemical and physiological properties of tissues (*e.g.*, brain, intestine) in dependent animals (*see* Tabakoff and Hoffman, 1983; Goldstein, 1984; Redmond and Krystal, 1984), the degree of physical dependence in the whole organism is still measured by the severity of the withdrawal syndrome produced either by abrupt withdrawal or by use of drug antagonists. In man, there appears to be an upper limit to the degree of physical dependence on opioids, such that increasing the daily dose in man beyond the equivalent of 500 mg of morphine does not significantly increase the severity of the withdrawal syndrome. Since the abrupt withdrawal of hypnotics or alcohol after high dosage produces seizures that can be fatal in man and animals, it is difficult to establish an upper limit of physical dependence on these agents.

In view of the distribution and widespread effects of endogenous opioid-like substances (*see* Chapters 12 and 22), it is not surprising that adaptive changes to the administration of exogenous opioids and withdrawal phenomena can be demonstrated throughout the autonomic and central nervous systems. Withdrawal hyperexcitability is observed in decerebrate animals, in the spinal cord of man, and in animals after cord transection. With local administration, the spinal cord or other structures can be made physically dependent on opioids with minimal involvement of the rest of the CNS (*see* Yaksh *et al.*, 1977). Neural structures that subserve the expression of the classical manifestations of physical dependence on opioids appear to be distinct from those that are critical for the reinforcing effects of these agents (*see* Wise, 1984). For example, opioids suppress activity in the locus ceruleus, an effect that is reversed by naloxone. Clonidine, an antihypertensive agent, also inhibits activity in these neurons, apparently by agonistic actions at α_2-adrenergic receptors. Clonidine also suppresses some of the signs and symptoms of withdrawal from opioids in rats and man and produces analgesia in rats. Tolerance develops to this analgesic effect, and there is cross-tolerance to morphine. Some of the affective and physiological aspects of the opioid withdrawal syndrome may thus be due to hyperactivity in the locus ceruleus or to increased sensitivity (supersensitivity) of structures that are innervated by noradrenergic neurons.

It is now quite clear that changes occur throughout the *entire* neuraxis during the development of physical dependence on CNS depressants, including, probably, alcohol (*see* Smith, 1977; Rosenberg and Okamoto, 1978). It is unclear whether there are distinct neural structures that subserve either the reinforcing effects of these agents or the phenomena that result from their withdrawal.

Cross-Dependence. The ability of one drug to suppress the manifestations of physical dependence produced by another and to maintain the physically dependent state is referred to as *cross-dependence.* Cross-dependence may be partial or complete, and the degree is more closely related to pharmacological effects than to chemical similarities.

In general, any potent morphine-like opioid will show cross-dependence with other opioids that act on the same receptors. Most sedative-hypnotics show a reasonable degree of cross-dependence with each other and with alcohol and barbiturates.

There is also some cross-dependence between barbiturates and volatile anesthetics.

If a long-acting drug such as methadone is substituted over several days for morphine, abrupt discontinuation produces a withdrawal syndrome characteristic of the long-acting drug rather than that of morphine. This aspect of cross-dependence has important clinical implications, since the withdrawal symptoms that occur with drugs with longer half-lives (methadone, phenobarbital, chlordiazepoxide) are generally less severe but more protracted. This phenomenon is the basis for the *substitution treatment* of physical dependence for both opioids and CNS depressants.

Mechanisms of Physical Dependence. Most theories postulate some form of CNS counteradaptation to the agonistic actions of the drugs and, in view of knowledge of negative-feedback control of the activities of regulatory molecules (such as receptors) and important metabolic pathways, it would be amazing if such did not occur. Counteradaptation results in the development of a "latent hyperexcitability" in neural systems affected by the drugs, which becomes manifest in the form of rebound or overshoot phenomena when the drugs are stopped or when an antagonist is administered. The theories differ largely in the level of explanation or in the mechanisms proposed to account for the counteradaptive changes; most involve models that account for the observation that physical dependence is generally accompanied by tolerance and that the two phenomena develop and decay at about the same rate. Complete explanations of the phenomena will be as complex as the interactions between neural systems in the CNS and the regulatory mechanisms that have evolved to control them.

For example, enzyme induction theories postulate that drugs that cause dependence could directly or indirectly inhibit an enzyme that synthesizes a product important for cell activity (*e.g.*, a neurotransmitter), and that the level of the enzyme itself is regulated by its product, the neurotransmitter. The initial drug effect is a result of the decrease in transmitter concentration, but this decrease also leads to increased synthesis of the enzyme and a new steady-state level that restores transmitter concentration, resulting in tolerance; when the drug is withdrawn there is excess enzyme, which then causes excess synthesis of transmitter, and this produces rebound effects until the enzyme activity falls to a new steady state (*see* Goldstein and Goldstein, 1968; Shuster, 1971).

At a somewhat higher level of neural organization, Martin (1968) has proposed a homeostatic and redundancy model in which tolerance is due to the opening of redundant pathways within the CNS when the primary pathway is blocked by the action of the drug. With drug withdrawal, activity in the primary pathway is restored, which in combination with continuing activity in the redundant pathway results in a rebound hyperexcitability of the pathways once depressed by the drug. While developed largely to account for opioid physical dependence, this theory is applicable to other drugs as well. Others have speculated that decreased neural activity in any functional system results in a "disuse supersensitivity" analogous to the denervation supersensitivity that develops in peripheral autonomic structures. The supersensitivity is thought to begin as soon as input is reduced and to account for decreased drug effect (tolerance); abrupt withdrawal of the drug or its displacement by an antagonist restores input to supersensitive elements, producing a "rebound" hyperactivity in the very systems that were depressed by the drug. Drugs that suppress similar final pathways should exhibit cross-dependence, even if they act on different receptors or by different mechanisms (*see* Jaffe and Sharpless, 1968).

Discussion of the many changes in the CNS that have been observed during the development of dependence, tolerance, or withdrawal is beyond the scope of this textbook. No single mechanism will account for all the complex phenomena that are seen. For additional discussion, *see* Martin and Sloan (1977a), Smith (1977), Chapman and Way (1980), Tabakoff and Hoffman (1983), Redmond and Krystal (1984), Terenius (1984), and Chapter 18.

Learning, Conditioning, and Relapse. Within the framework of learning theory, drug use, whether casual or compulsive, can be viewed as behavior that is maintained by its consequences; consequences that strengthen a behavior pattern are reinforcers. Drugs may reinforce the antecedent drug-taking behavior by inducing pleasurable effects (positive reinforcement) or by terminating some aversive or unpleasant situation (negative reinforcement), as when a drug alleviates pain or anxiety. Secondary or social reinforcement entirely independent of pharmacological effects may also play a role, as is the case when drug use results in special status, membership in a desired group, or the approval of friends. Sometimes social reinforcement maintains initial drug-using behavior until the individual comes to appreciate the primary drug effect or becomes tolerant to some initial aversive effects of the particular drug. This seems to be the case with many young people who do not like the initial effects of tobacco or who perceive nothing pleasurable about the initial effects of smoking marihuana. Although it is not as widely appreciated, many naive individuals find the effects of an initial dose of heroin, with its associated nausea and vomiting, somewhat unpleasant; however, social reinforcement may maintain the behavior until tolerance develops to these effects.

The development of physical dependence opens possibilities for another variety of reinforcement; each time drug use alleviates withdrawal distress the antecedent drug-using behavior is further reinforced. Even when tolerance attenuates the initial reinforcing effects, drugs that induce certain varieties of physical dependence produce a regularly recurring sense of distress that is immediately eliminated by another dose of the drug. During the withdrawal state, drug use can simultaneously alleviate distress and produce euphoria, a particularly powerful reinforcement (*see* Wikler, 1980; Donegan *et al.*, 1983).

There is not always a high correlation between the degree to which withdrawal from a given class of drugs causes dramatic symptoms or threatens physical well-being and the degree to which withdrawal generates aversive states and increases the reinforcing effects of the drug. Withdrawal from nicotine is undramatic and never threatens physical well-being, but it regularly motivates continued smoking. Some users of alcohol or hypnotics elect to stop such use abruptly, even though doing so may cause delirium and life-threatening seizures.

It is uncertain to what extent the primary reinforcing (euphorigenic) effects of drugs continue to contribute to their reinforcing effects once tolerance develops. After as little as 5 days of self-administration of alcohol or heroin in a laboratory setting, alcoholics or heroin addicts show more depression, dysphoria, and anxiety than a sense of well-being. In the case of opioids, however, there is a brief period immediately after each dose when mood is elevated (Meyer and Mirin, 1979). Patients tolerant to most of the effects of large doses of methadone still experience some positive effects on mood at about the time the concentration of methadone reaches peak values in plasma after each daily dose.

A *protracted opioid abstinence syndrome,* characterized by physiological and psychological abnormalities, commonly follows the acute syndrome due to withdrawal of opioids, and this condition can persist for weeks. Since the subjective sense of not being quite normal is immediately relieved by very small doses of opioid drugs, the protracted abstinence syndrome may predispose to relapse by creating a prolonged period of increased vulnerability, during which the effects of opioids are especially reinforcing (*see* Cushman and Dole, 1973; Martin *et al.*, 1973). Such a protracted state may also exist following withdrawal of other drugs that cause dependence. After withdrawal of alcohol, other CNS depressants, or benzodiazepines, sleep and mood may be disturbed for many weeks.

In both animals and man, drug effects, withdrawal phenomena, and relief of withdrawal symptoms by drugs can be conditioned to environmental stimuli. Such conditioning helps to explain how the rituals and circumstances surrounding drug use can act as secondary reinforcers, and how the mere taking of an inert pill or the use of a needle or syringe containing no drug can evoke the feelings (including relief of withdrawal symptoms) previously produced when the pill or syringe contained an active substance. The observation that withdrawal distress can become conditioned to the environment in which it occurs may underlie reports that former opioid addicts may experience sensations very similar to withdrawal symptoms, including an intensified craving for drugs, when they return to an environment where drugs are available. Alcoholics may have similar experiences, particularly when they are exposed to the sight and smell of alcohol. The conditions that elicit the most severe withdrawal and the most intense "craving" for opioids are those associated with the availability and use of the drug, rather than those associated with withdrawal (*e.g.*, being offered some heroin by a friend or watching someone else use the drug). Anecdotal reports suggest that these are also the circumstances that increase craving in recently abstinent alcoholics and cigarette smokers. (For references, *see* Wikler, 1980; Donegan *et al.*, 1983.)

Vulnerability. In man, drugs may produce effects experienced as pleasurable, novel, or tension reducing, but these effects are not such powerful reinforcers that repetitive drug use is inevitable. Much research has centered on why some individuals stop after experimentation, others continue drug use but do not become dependent, and still others become compulsive drug users.

Individuals who later become regular

users of socially disapproved drugs tend to be more impulsive, more rebellious with respect to social norms, and less tolerant of frustration. Certain psychiatric diagnostic categories are regularly overrepresented among those who seek treatment for alcoholism and drug dependency. These include depressive disorders, anxiety disorders, and antisocial personality (Rounsaville *et al.*, 1982; Hesselbrock *et al.*, 1985). Despite these findings, no single recognized addictive personality or constellation of traits has been identified that is equally applicable to all varieties of compulsive drug users. Indeed, given the different pharmacological effects of various drugs, it would be surprising if all compulsive drug users were similar.

There are many factors that could contribute to increased vulnerability to continued or compulsive drug use. Some individuals may experience a more intense response to the initial reinforcing properties of the drugs, such as a more intense euphoria or a more profound reduction of unpleasant feelings of anger, depression, or anxiety. Such intense reactions, in turn, could be due to differences in sensitivity to drug effects or to initially higher levels of distress. Thus, for some, drug use may be viewed as self-treatment for internal distress. Although the agent selected or the pattern of use may sometimes run counter to social norms, for some individuals the alternative may be a state of tension, anger, or depression that may be felt to be intolerable. On the other hand, the contributory factors may be entirely social, as in the case of young people who continue to smoke cigarettes more to conform to the pressures from friends than because of an especially intense need for the pharmacological effects of nicotine. Still other possibilities include differences in intensity of adverse effects of the drugs or in the intensity of withdrawal phenomena as experienced by different users (*see* above). For any given pattern of continued drug use the outcome is the result of an interaction between social, biological, and environmental factors. (*See* Platt and Labate, 1976; Dupont *et al.*, 1979; Deitrich and Spuhler, 1984.)

Sociological Factors. Social factors have a major influence on which individuals have access to various drugs, and social attitudes, as well as the laws of any given country, determine which drugs are acceptable for casual or "recreational" use, which may be used for relief of unpleasant feelings, and which are prohibited. In addition, the nature of a society often determines the kinds of unpleasant feelings induced in its members, as well as the kinds of behaviors that are viewed as socially acceptable. In general, when the use of a drug is widely accepted, the number of users tends to be large and their personal characteristics are quite diverse, including the characteristics of the small proportion who become compulsive users. When a particular form of drug use meets with severe disapproval, those who use it despite such sanctions tend to be very different from the average person in society in terms of attitudes and emotional adjustment even before use. Consequently, a high proportion may become intensive or compulsive users, sometimes leading to the conclusion that the particular drug is "more addicting" than those drugs used by larger and more diverse populations. Drugs may indeed differ in the degree to which they induce dependence, but the ratio of experimenters to addicts is not always a valid measure of the liability of a drug to cause dependence.

Users of any category of drug, whether legal or illegal, are more likely to employ other types of drugs than are nonusers. Thus, tobacco smokers are far more likely to use marihuana than are non-smokers. The use of more socially acceptable drugs precedes that of more disapproved agents in a predictable pattern. In the United States, the earlier the experimentation with marihuana, the greater the likelihood of later use of heroin and cocaine (Kandel and Maloff, 1983).

The acceptability of a drug may increase or decrease with time in a fadlike fashion, and there appear to be drug-specific social networks, each oriented toward particular drugs, rather than a general drug subculture. For some individuals, the use of a particular drug may symbolize acceptance of the values of a particular social network within a society. Conversely, belonging to such a network may require the use of its drug.

Chronic drug use may establish a complex equilibrium among family members, and abstinence on the part of the user, with its attendant changes in behavior and role, can also induce tension in other members of the family. Relapse to drugs or alcohol sometimes restores the previous pathological equilibrium. Cultural attitudes toward addicts and alcoholics and the legal or medical complications of drug use further increase the drug user's difficulties in obtaining realistic gratifications (alternative reinforcers) and simultaneously foster his return to an environment (the local bar or group of heroin addicts) where he is accepted, where the drug is available, and where its use is acceptable and has been repeatedly reinforced.

CLINICAL CHARACTERISTICS

Most of the pharmacological agents commonly used for subjective purposes (excluding caffeine) can be placed into eight major classes, as follows: (1) opioids, (2) CNS depressants, (3) CNS sympathomimetics (including cocaine), (4) nicotine and tobacco, (5) cannabinoids, (6) psychedelics (hallucinogens, psychotomimetics, psychotogens), (7) arylcyclohexylamines (*e.g.*, phencyclidine), and (8) inhalants (*e.g.*, nitrous oxide, ethyl ether, volatile solvents). Although the agents within each class have many actions in common, there are also differences, and the classification is offered merely for its didactic convenience.

OPIOIDS

Incidence and Patterns of Use. In the late 1960s the use of heroin increased considerably, in both the United States and Great Britain. Some of the reasons for the increase included changes in social attitudes toward drug use and toward established social norms in general, increased availability of drugs, and the substantial increase in the adolescent population (a result of the sharp increase in births following World War II), with its associated social changes. By the mid-1970s, heroin use in the United States had spread from urban areas to smaller communities. Members of racial and ethnic groups from lower socioeconomic strata continued to be overrepresented, but heroin was also used by more affluent members of society. In 1982, about 1.2% of young adults (age 18 to 25) reported having tried heroin at some time in their lives, although far fewer had used it on a daily basis.

In the United States there are three basic patterns of opioid use and dependence. One involves individuals whose drug use begins in the context of medical treatment and who obtain their initial supplies through medical channels. This group constitutes a very small percentage of the addicted population. Another pattern begins with experimental or "recreational" drug use, progresses to more intensive use, and involves primarily adolescents and young adults, with males far outnumbering females. Most of these users are introduced to the drug by other users. This is true both of the initial contact and of those subsequent contacts leading to relapse after periods of withdrawal. The way in which drug use spreads from one friend to another in epidemic fashion has been well documented (Hughes *et al.*, 1972). A third pattern involves users who begin in one or another of the preceding ways but later switch to oral opioids (methadone) obtained from organized treatment programs.

A user's first experience with opioids is often quite unpleasant, with nausea and vomiting as the outstanding features. Some may not try again for days or weeks; others, however, discover a new world of inner satisfaction with the first dose and make a conscious decision to continue to use the drug as frequently as their finances will permit. Some may struggle with the impulse to use it again and may do so only intermittently for many months or years before becoming regular users; some may never become compulsive users. The most common pattern may be to try the drug once or twice and then, with awareness of the dangers, to avoid it thereafter. Despite the medical and legal risks, where group values support opioid use and relatively pure drugs are easily available, a very high percentage of users may become physically dependent. In 1971, about 42% of United States Army enlisted men in Vietnam used opioids at least once, and about half of these users reported that at some time during their year in Vietnam they were physically dependent (*see* Robins, 1974).

The incidence of opioid addiction among physicians, nurses, and those in the related health professions is many times higher than in any group with comparable educational background. Most physician-addicts state that they first took the drug to overcome fatigue, depression, or to alleviate some bodily ailment, and few indicate that they were seeking thrills; the original motive, however, is not necessarily the major determinant of the consequences of the addiction that later develops. These are often related more to chance factors, such as whether they are prosecuted by enforcement agencies for their drug use. Considering the frequency with which opioid analgesics are used in clinical medicine, addiction as a complication of medical treatment is quite uncommon. When it does occur, the pattern it follows depends on both the emotional adjustment of the patient prior to involvement with opioids and the source of the drug. Those individuals who are not seriously disturbed emotionally and who continue to obtain it from physicians or treatment programs may avoid many of the problems associated with illicit drugs. Those who must obtain drugs from illicit traffic encounter the same problems that are faced by heroin users.

Rapid intravenous injection of an opioid produces a warm flushing of the skin and sensations in the lower abdomen described by addicts as similar in intensity and quality to sexual orgasm; this lasts for about 45 seconds and is known as a "rush," "kick," or "thrill." It is uncertain how much tolerance develops to this effect. Although heroin is the most commonly used illicit opioid, it has few special pharmacological properties that account for its popularity. Given subcutaneously, even experienced users cannot reliably distinguish heroin from morphine. This is understandable, since heroin is rapidly converted into morphine in the body. When these two drugs are given intravenously, addicts are better able to distinguish between them, probably because of the greater lipid solubility of heroin in comparison to morphine. This results in a higher rate of crossing the blood-brain barrier, and effects on the CNS are thus produced rapidly. In the brain, heroin is rapidly deacetylated to 6-monoacetyl morphine and then to morphine. In this sense, heroin carries morphine rapidly into the brain.

Symptoms and Effects of Compulsive Use. The behavior, social adjustment, and medical problems observed among opioid users and addicts are surprisingly varied. Experience with thousands of patients maintained on high daily doses of methadone for periods of up to 15 years has shown no direct injurious effects (Kreek, 1979, 1983). Good health and productive work are thus not incompatible with regular use of opioids. However, it is now clear that the behavior of the individual prior to opioid use and the purposes and patterns of use play a large role in determining the social and physiological consequences.

In England, where chronic opioid users may still obtain pure heroin from legitimate medical sources at no cost, the patterns of social adjustment are extremely varied. The majority of opioid users in Britain are young people who were introduced to drug use by friends, began out of curiosity, and continue because of the euphoric effects. The preferred route of administration is intravenous. The patterns of adjustment among the patients receiving treatment at London clinics are similar to those observed in the United States. Four major patterns have been noted: (1) "stables"—patients who are legitimately employed, do not engage in criminal activity, do not associate with other addicts, and do not buy extra heroin illicitly; (2) "junkies"—patients who are the opposite of the stable patients in these respects; (3) "loners"—patients who are on welfare rather than engaging in crime, do not associate with other addicts, but do use a wide variety of drugs not prescribed by the clinic; and (4) "two-worlders"—patients who are employed but associate with other addicts, buy extra drugs, and engage in criminal activities. The disorganized behavior and criminality of the "junkies" and the organized behavior of the "stables" antedate the addiction. Despite the legal source of drugs, those receiving heroin at London clinics had a high incidence of infections (due to neglect of hygienic procedures or to shared needles) and a surprisingly

high mortality rate, ranging from 2 to 6% per year. A follow-up study of young heroin addicts treated at London clinics revealed that 7 years later only 48% were still using opioids (43% obtained drugs from the clinics), 32% were abstinent and not abusing other drugs, and 12% were dead (*see* Stimson and Oppenheimer, 1982).

The health and social adjustment of patients maintained on oral methadone in the United States are equally varied. Many hold jobs, raise children, commit no crimes, and use no socially disapproved drugs. Yet other patients continue to commit crimes, do not obtain employment, and use other drugs or excessive amounts of alcohol. A substantial number experience significant depression (*see* Rounsaville *et al.,* 1982). The mortality rate among patients in maintenance programs is higher than that among others of comparable age and socioeconomic status, but the general consensus is that the high rate is not related to the effects of oral methadone *per se,* but directly or indirectly to problems that antedated methadone use or to the excessive use of alcohol and other drugs.

Similar variations in patterns of behavior, social adjustment, and impaired health have been noted among heroin addicts in the United States who utilize exclusively illegal sources for their drugs. Undoubtedly, the high cost and impurities of illicit drugs in the United States exact their toll. Many females earn their drug money through prostitution, and there is a high incidence of venereal disease among female heroin addicts. The average annual death rate among young-adult heroin addicts is several times higher than that for nonaddicts of similar age and ethnic backgrounds. In the younger group, much of this increase is due to fatal opioid overdosage that may be an accidental outcome of the dangerous fluctuations in the purity of illicit heroin or to combinations of opioids with alcohol or other CNS depressants. Considering the high prevalence of depression among opioid addicts, some apparent overdoses may be deliberate. Another frequent cause of sudden death has been termed an "anaphylactoid reaction," which probably results from the intravenous injection of a drug containing certain impurities. The suicide rate among addicts is considerably higher than that of the general population, and a surprisingly high percentage die violent deaths at the hands of others. The medical complications common among drug users include infections (*e.g.,* septicemia, endocarditis, hepatitis, acquired immune deficiency syndrome, tetanus, and pulmonary, cerebral, and subcutaneous abscesses) due to shared needles and unhygienic procedures, foreign-body emboli, granulomata due to injection of contaminants, and a variety of neurological, musculoskeletal, and other lesions that may be due to hypersensitivity reactions or to toxic impurities in drugs produced in illicit laboratories. (For references, *see* Richter, 1975.)

Opioids reduce pain, aggression, and sexual drives, and their use, therefore, is unlikely to induce crime. However, many individuals committed crimes prior to the use of opioids, and they do not necessarily stop when opioid use begins. In addition, many individuals who did not engage in crime previously may begin to do so in order to obtain money to buy opioids, since the cost is generally beyond the amount they can obtain legitimately. In general, the number of crimes goes up while addicts are using illicit opioids and goes down when they are abstinent or enter treatment (*see* McGlothlin, 1979; Anglin *et al.*, 1981).

Tolerance, Physical Dependence, and Withdrawal Symptoms. A remarkable degree of tolerance develops to the respiratory-depressant, analgesic, sedative, emetic, and euphorigenic effects of μ-agonist opioids; however, the rate at which this tolerance develops, in either the addict or the medical patient, depends in part on the pattern of use. With intermittent use, it is possible to obtain desired analgesic and sedative effects from doses in the therapeutic range for an indefinite period. It is only when there is a more or less continuous drug action that significant tolerance develops. Thus, if the drug is used frequently, the addict who is primarily seeking to get a "rush" or to maintain a state of dreamy indifference (a "high") must constantly increase the dose. In this way, some addicts can build up to phenomenally large doses (*e.g.*, 2 g of morphine intravenously over a period of 2.5 hours without significant change in blood pressure, pulse rate, or respiration). Although the lethal dose is greatly altered in tolerant individuals, a dose always exists that is capable of producing death from respiratory depression.

Tolerance does not develop equally or at the same rate to all the effects of opioids, and even users highly tolerant to respiratory-depressant effects continue to exhibit some degree of miosis and to complain of constipation. Addicts who self-administer heroin in an investigational laboratory setting develop tolerance to the euphorigenic effects within 1 to 2 weeks and thereafter seem dysphoric and depressed, except for a brief period following each intravenous dose (Meyer and Mirin, 1979). Subjects who are maintained on daily oral doses of 100 mg of methadone for more than 8

weeks still seem sedated and apathetic and have constricted pupils and decreased respiratory rates (Martin *et al.*, 1973). However, experience with thousands of patients maintained on methadone for periods of several years suggests that, while constipation is a continuing problem, substantial sedation and apathy are easily managed by reductions in dosage.

Even after several years of constant dosage of methadone, there is less than complete tolerance to several effects of the drug. In addition to constipation, insomnia and decreased sexual function persist in about 10 to 20% of patients, and about 50% complain of excessive sweating. Sensitivity of the CNS respiratory center to stimulation by CO_2 is diminished, as is the normal hyperventilation of late pregnancy. Increased plasma concentrations of albumin, total protein, and thyroid-binding globulin are also common findings. Altered hypothalamic-pituitary function may also persist, although most patients on high doses of methadone have normal concentrations of testosterone, follicle-stimulating hormone (FSH), and luteinizing hormone (LH). However, plasma concentrations of prolactin peak each day at about the same time as does the concentration of methadone, about 4 hours after an oral dose (*see* Kreek, 1983). Some patients may also perceive positive changes in mood and exhibit increases in skin temperature and decreases in pupillary size and heart rate a few hours after their daily dose (McCaul *et al.*, 1982).

Meperidine addicts may use large daily doses (3 to 4 g per day), but significant tolerance does not develop to the drug's excitant and atropine-like actions, which are due largely to a metabolite, normeperidine. When very high doses of meperidine are used, even the tolerant addict may show dilated pupils, increased muscular activity, twitching, tremors, mental confusion, and, occasionally, tonic–clonic seizures (*see* Chapter 22).

In general, there is a high degree of cross-tolerance and cross-dependence among opioids with actions at the same receptor type, but little or no cross-tolerance between opioids that act primarily at different receptors. Since most opioids are not completely selective and have some affinity for each of the various receptors, the extent of cross-tolerance between different opioids is variable.

Tolerance to opioids largely disappears when withdrawal has been completed, and many addicts have taken fatal overdoses by returning to their previous dosage immediately after undergoing withdrawal.

The character and the severity of the withdrawal symptoms that appear when an opioid is discontinued depend upon many factors, including the particular drug, the total daily dose used, the interval between doses, the duration of use, and the health and personality of the addict.

It is helpful to view the total clinical picture of the abstinence syndrome as made up of *purposive behavior,* which is goal oriented, highly dependent on the observer and the environment, and directed at getting more drug, and *nonpurposive behavior,* which is not goal oriented and which is relatively independent of the observer and the environment. The purposive phenomena, including complaints, pleas, demands, manipulations, and simulations, are as varied as the imagination of the drug-using population. In the hospital setting, they are considerably less pronounced when the patient is certain that his behavior does not affect the decision to give him a drug.

In the case of morphine, heroin, or μ agonists with similar durations of action, nonpurposive symptoms, such as lacrimation, rhinorrhea, yawning, and sweating, appear about 8 to 12 hours after the last dose. About 12 to 14 hours after the last dose, the addict may fall into a tossing, restless sleep known as the "yen," which may last several hours but from which he awakens more restless and more miserable than before. As the syndrome progresses, additional signs and symptoms appear, consisting in dilated pupils, anorexia, gooseflesh, restlessness, irritability, and tremor. With morphine and heroin, nonpurposive symptoms reach their peak at 48 to 72 hours. As the syndrome approaches peak intensity, the patient exhibits increasing irritability, insomnia, marked anorexia, violent yawning, severe sneezing, lacrimation, and coryza. Weakness and depression are pronounced. Nausea and vomiting are common, as are intestinal spasm and diarrhea. Heart rate and blood pressure are elevated. Marked chilliness, alternating with flushing and excessive sweating, is characteristic. Pilomotor activity resulting in waves of gooseflesh is prominent, and the skin resembles that of a plucked turkey. This feature is the basis of the expression "cold turkey" to signify abrupt withdrawal without treatment. Abdominal cramps and pains in the bones and muscles of the back and extremities are also characteristic, as are the muscle spasms and kicking movements that may be the basis for the expression "kicking the habit." Other signs of CNS hyperexcitability include ejaculation in men and orgasm in women. The respiratory response to CO_2, which is decreased during opioid administration, is exaggerated during withdrawal. Rebound phenomena are also observed in the endocrine system. Leukocytosis is common, and white-cell counts above 14,000/cu mm are often seen.

The failure to take food and fluids, combined with vomiting, sweating, and diarrhea, results in marked weight loss, dehydration, ketosis, and disturbance in acid-base balance. Occasionally there is cardiovascular collapse. At any point in the course of withdrawal, the administration of a suitable opioid will completely and dramatically suppress the symptoms of withdrawal. Obviously, administration of a drug cannot immediately restore body fluids or acid-base balance, and in this sense the syndrome is not completely reversible. Without treatment, the acute phase of the morphine withdrawal syndrome runs its course and most of the grossly observable symptoms disappear in 7 to 10 days, but it is not certain how long it takes to restore physiological equilibrium completely.

It is now clear that the recovery process is complex and protracted, and that the early opioid abstinence syndrome characterized by the signs and symptoms described above is followed by a *protracted abstinence syndrome,* during which a number of physiological variables attain subnormal values. For example, a period of hyposensitivity to the respiratory-stimulant effects of CO_2 persists for many weeks after the exaggerated sensitivity of the early abstinence period subsides. In addition, there seem to be subtle behavioral manifestations of protracted abstinence that include an incapacity to tolerate stress, a poor self-image, and overconcern about discomfort. It is not unreasonable to postulate that these altered states contribute to the tendency of compulsive opioid users to relapse after withdrawal (*see* Martin *et al.,* 1973).

The *abrupt withdrawal of methadone* produces a syndrome that is qualitatively similar to that of morphine, but it develops more slowly and is more prolonged, although usually less intense. The addict has few or no symptoms until 24 to 48 hours after the last dose, and then complains of weakness, anxiety, anorexia, insomnia, abdominal discomfort, headache, sweating, pain in muscles and bones, and hot and cold flashes. As with morphine withdrawal, there is nausea, vomiting, and an increase in body temperature, blood pressure, pulse, respiratory rate, and pupillary size. In general, after abrupt withdrawal, the primary or early abstinence syndrome reaches its maximal intensity by about the third day and may not begin to decrease until the third week, and apparent recovery may not occur until the sixth or seventh week. The early abstinence syndrome is followed by a secondary or protracted abstinence syndrome in which a number of previously elevated physiological parameters attain and remain at subnormal values through the twenty-fourth postwithdrawal week, and there are concomitant psychological disturbances such as tiredness, weakness, hypochondriasis, and feelings of lessened efficiency (Martin *et al.,* 1973). Even with very slow reduction in dosage, patients who have been maintained on high doses of methadone or acetylmethadol experience qualitatively similar withdrawal symptoms during and following the period of dosage reduction (Cushman and Dole, 1973; Senay *et al.*, 1977; Judson *et al.*, 1983).

The *meperidine abstinence syndrome* usually develops within 3 hours after the last dose, reaches its peak within 8 to 12 hours, and then declines, so that few symptoms are apparent after 4 to 5 days. Craving may be intense, but the nonpurposive autonomic signs, while present, are not as prominent; the pupils may not be widely dilated, and there is usually little nausea, vomiting, or diarrhea. However, at peak intensity the muscle twitching, restlessness, and nervousness may be worse than during morphine withdrawal.

Although *codeine* can partially suppress morphine withdrawal, withdrawal symptoms after codeine (1200 to 1800 mg per day), while qualitatively similar to those of morphine, are considerably less intense.

Withdrawal symptoms after semisynthetic and synthetic opioids are qualitatively similar to those after morphine, and they seem to follow the general rule that drugs with shorter durations of action tend to produce shorter, more intense abstinence syndromes while those drugs that are slowly eliminated produce withdrawal syndromes that are prolonged but mild. Some differences between the syndrome seen upon withdrawal of μ agonists and that seen with partial agonists and with agonist-antagonists are described in Chapter 22.

Withdrawal in the Newborn. Babies born to mothers who have been taking opioid agonists or agonist-antagonists regularly prior to delivery will be physically dependent. The signs of withdrawal include irritability and excessive and high-pitched crying, tremors, frantic sucking of fists, hyperactive reflexes, increased respiratory rate, increased stools, sneezing, yawning, vomiting, and fever. With heroin, signs most commonly appear within the first day of life; they may not appear for several days with methadone. The intensity of the syndrome does not always correlate with the duration of maternal opioid use or dose. There is no consensus on the best method of managing such withdrawal. Although clinicians have used paregoric, phenobarbital, diazepam, chlorpromazine, and clonidine, the use of paregoric (0.2 ml orally every 3 to 4 hours, increased as needed until symptoms are controlled) seems to be the most rational and effective approach when there is no question of simultaneous dependence on alcohol or other sedatives. While withdrawal symptoms when untreated are generally more severe in babies born to mothers who have been maintained on methadone, compared to those who have been using heroin, the greater opportunity to provide prenatal care to the mother maintained on methadone results in a significant decrease in overall fetal distress and mortality.

Babies fare better when the mother is maintained on low doses of methadone (*e.g.*, 20 to 30 mg), but any reduction of dosage must be gradual and the fetus must be monitored carefully; withdrawal of an opioid is potentially lethal for the fetus (*see* Finnegan, 1979; Stimmel *et al.*, 1983).

Opioid Antagonists. The abstinence syndromes described above are those seen when opioids are abruptly withdrawn. If, however, an antagonist such as naloxone is given, a withdrawal syndrome develops within a few minutes after parenteral administration and reaches its peak intensity within 30 minutes. Until the antagonist is eliminated, even large doses of previously used opioid cannot suppress the syndrome; partial suppression is possible, but only by using extremely large doses of opioid, which may then produce respiratory depression as the action of the antagonist wanes. Depending on the dose of the antagonist, precipitated withdrawal is usually more severe than that seen after abrupt withdrawal of the drug. Withdrawal from methadone produced by an antagonist is especially severe.

GENERAL CNS DEPRESSANTS: BARBITURATES AND RELATED SEDATIVE-HYPNOTIC DRUGS

In general, the subjective effects of barbiturates and related sedatives and antianxiety agents are similar but not identical to those of alcohol, and the effects vary considerably with the dose, the situation, and the personality of the user.

Prevalence, Agents Employed, and Patterns of Use. The incidence and prevalence of nonmedical and compulsive use of barbiturates, benzodiazepines, and related drugs cannot be stated with accuracy, but they are believed to exceed greatly that of the opioids. In 1982, 19% of young adults reported nonmedical use of sedatives, with 2.6% describing some use in the preceding month. About 15% indicated some experience with nonmedical use of tranquilizers. The incidence was relatively stable over the preceding 5 years (Miller *et al.*, 1983).

Opioid users frequently take barbiturates, benzodiazepines, or other sedatives to augment the effects of weak illicit heroin or to produce psychological effects when they have become tolerant to prescribed opioids. Many heroin users and patients maintained on methadone are physically dependent on both opioids and sedatives. Some alcoholics use these agents to relieve the alcohol withdrawal syndrome or to produce a state of intoxication devoid of the odor of alcohol. The short-acting barbiturates such as pentobarbital ("yellow jackets") or secobarbital ("red devils") are preferred to long-acting agents such as phenobarbital. Since the user is more interested in the pharmacological effects than in chemical classifications, it is not surprising that nonbarbiturates such as meprobamate, glutethimide, methyprylon, methaqualone, and some of the shorter-acting benzodiazepines are also abused. Paraldehyde and chloral hydrate, subject to considerable abuse in the past, have now been largely replaced by the other agents mentioned. Chlordiazepoxide and certain other benzodiazepines that have minimal euphoriant actions and relatively slow onset of effects are uncommon as drugs of abuse. While normal subjects do not find benzodiazepines to be particularly reinforcing, the more lipid-soluble agents, such as diazepam, have a more prompt onset of action and are used widely for nonmedical purposes; some sedative abusers prefer them over short-acting barbiturates (Griffiths et al., 1983).

The patterns of nonmedical use are exceedingly varied. They range from infrequent sprees of gross intoxication, lasting a few days, to the prolonged, compulsive, daily use of huge quantities and a preoccupation with securing and maintaining adequate supplies. Some users may never exhibit gross intoxication but may, nevertheless, take drugs several times a day. The original contact with the drug may have been through a physician's prescription or through illicit drug trade. In the medical patient, the development of the problem may be a gradual one, beginning with prolonged use for insomnia or anxiety and progressing through increased dosage at night to a few capsules for sedation in the morning. Eventually, the drug is a major part of the user's life. In such situations, what at one point could be considered a habituation at another is clearly an addiction. Neither the patient taking benzodiazepines over a period of months nor his physician may recognize the existence of dependence. Both may assume that the anxiety, tremulousness, and insomnia that

emerge when the drug is discontinued is a return of the original anxiety. There is no sharp line that can be drawn between appropriate use, abuse, habituation, and addiction. Most users take the drugs orally, but there are a few individuals who inject barbiturates intravenously or intramuscularly. Such users can be recognized by the large abscesses that cover the accessible areas of their bodies.

The combination of amphetamines and barbiturates produces more elevation of mood than either drug alone. The mechanisms of this supra-additive effect are not yet clear, but competition for the same microsomal enzyme system and hence production of higher blood concentrations of the drugs could be involved.

The amount of hypnotic that may be taken varies considerably, but an average daily dose of 1.5 g of short-acting barbiturate is not uncommon, and some individuals have consumed as much as 2.5 g daily over many months. Similar multiples of the usual daily therapeutic doses are taken by the compulsive users of meprobamate, glutethimide, methyprylon, and methaqualone. Abusers of benzodiazepines may ingest several hundred milligrams of diazepam or its equivalent every day. For references, see reviews by Smith (1977), Wesson and Smith (1977), and Mackinnon and Parker (1982).

Signs and Symptoms. Because tolerance develops to most of the actions of this group of drugs, there may be no apparent signs of chronic use. For the patient taking regular doses of sleeping pills the only manifestation may be a rebound insomnia when the drug is stopped. The patient taking benzodiazepines may experience insomnia and rebound increase in anxiety several days after stopping. Some users, however, attempt to maintain a state of intoxication. In these individuals, the acute and the chronic effects of mild intoxication with CNS depressants resemble those of intoxication with alcohol. The individual who is intoxicated with a barbiturate shows a general sluggishness, difficulty in thinking, slowness and slurring of speech, poor comprehension and memory, faulty judgment, narrowed range of attention, emotional lability, and exaggeration of basic personality traits. Irritability, quarrelsomeness, and moroseness are common. There may be laughing or crying without provocation, untidiness in personal habits, hostile and paranoid ideas, and suicidal tendencies (see Smith, 1977). Similar patterns of increasing irritability may be seen when sedative abusers are given high doses of diazepam chronically. Interestingly, such subjects seem less aware of their mood changes and behavioral impairments when taking diazepam than when ingesting high doses of barbiturates (Griffiths *et al.*, 1983). Chronic intoxication with all pharmacologically similar agents has not been studied in as controlled a manner, but the clinical descriptions of isolated cases of abuse of high doses of meprobamate, glutethimide, and methaqualone are quite similar to the picture of chronic barbiturate intoxication. Neurological effects described here are those for barbiturates. These effects include thick, slurred speech, nystagmus, diplopia, strabismus, difficulty in visual accommodation, vertigo, ataxic gait, positive Romberg's sign, hypotonia, dysmetria, and decreased superficial reflexes; deep reflexes, pupillary responses, and sensation are usually unaltered. Occasionally transient ankle clonus and Babinski's signs are elicitable. Nutrition is usually unimpaired. Skin rashes may develop; they may be erythematous, urticarial, purpuric, or scarlatiniform. The urine may contain albumin and casts.

Tolerance, Physical Dependence, and Withdrawal Symptoms. Chronic intoxication with short-acting barbiturates and related hypnotics results in both drug-disposition and pharmacodynamic tolerance. Pharmacodynamic tolerance also develops to most of the actions of benzodiazepines, but drug-disposition tolerance is less marked. Indeed, the slow accumulation of active metabolites of certain benzodiazepines tends to obscure the development of adaptive changes in the CNS. The overall tolerance that is attained has an upper limit that gives chronic intoxication with hypnotics a very characteristic picture. For example, an individual tolerant to 1.2 g of pentobarbital per day may show little evidence of intoxication on that dose; however, if the dose is raised by as little as 0.1 g per day, prolonged and perhaps cumulative intoxication may occur. It is also characteristic of adaptation to this class of agents that, while there may be considerable tolerance to the sedative and intoxicating effects, the lethal dose is not much greater in addicts than in normal individuals. Consequently, acute barbiturate or meprobamate poisoning may be accidentally or willfully superimposed on chronic intoxication at any time.

Benzodiazepines appear to be considerably safer than barbiturates and related sedatives, since acute overdosage is much less likely to produce fatal respiratory depression. Cross-tolerance between various agents in this group is common, but not all combinations have been studied.

There are marked similarities between the withdrawal syndromes seen with barbiturates and those seen with meprobamate, glutethimide, methaqualone, benzodiazepines, and related drugs. It seems justified, therefore, to use the term *general depressant withdrawal syndrome* to refer to the manifestations of withdrawal from any of these agents. In its mildest form, the general depressant withdrawal syndrome may consist in only paroxysmal EEG abnormalities, rebound increases in rapid-eye-movement (REM) sleep, insomnia, or anxiety. Somewhat greater degrees of physical dependence result in tremulousness and weakness, in addition to anxiety and insomnia. When the syndrome is severe, there may be, in addition, tonic-clonic seizures and delirium.

Former addicts can ingest 0.2 g of pentobarbital per day over many months without the development of any obvious manifestations of physical dependence on abrupt withdrawal. However, after a daily dose of 0.4 g for 3 months, abrupt withdrawal produces paroxysmal EEG changes without other significant symptoms in about 30% of subjects. After 0.6 g per day for 1 to 2 months, 50% of subjects show minor withdrawal symptoms such as insomnia, anorexia, tremor, and EEG changes, and 10% may have a single seizure. When subjects are continuously intoxicated (0.9 to 2.2 g per day) for several months, 75% may have seizures and 66% delirium, and all experience insomnia, tremor, and anorexia on abrupt withdrawal (Fraser *et al.*, 1958). Significant symptoms, similar to those described for barbiturates, are seen during withdrawal from meprobamate (3.2 to 6.4 g per day for 40 days).

If sleep patterns and electrical activity of the brain during sleep are used as measures of physical dependence, it becomes apparent that very little drug given over relatively short periods is sufficient to produce the effect. Subjects given hypnotic drugs in ordinary doses for several weeks show tolerance to the hypnotic effects. Rebound increases in percentage of REM sleep and insomnia are often seen when such drugs are discontinued. A similar rebound disturbance in sleep is seen upon withdrawal of shorter-acting benzodiazepines administered as a single dose at bedtime for as little as 1 to 2 weeks, although REM sleep does not rebound above baseline levels (*see* Kales *et al.*, 1983).

The typical course of withdrawal from large amounts of short-acting barbiturates is as follows: over the first 12 to 16 hours, as the concentration of the drug in blood declines and the intoxication clears, the patient seems to improve but then becomes increasingly restless, anxious, tremulous, and weak. There may be complaints of abdominal cramps, nausea, and vomiting. Orthostatic hypotension is characteristic and may produce fainting if the patient stands up quickly. Within the first 24 hours, he may become too weak to get out of bed; coarse tremors of the hands are prominent, deep reflexes may be hyperactive, and the blink reflex is increased. During this period, *purposive behavior* is prominent and the patient may plead for his drug. With the short-acting barbiturates and meprobamate, the symptoms usually reach their peak during the second and third days of abstinence; convulsions, when they occur, are usually seen within this period. The number of seizures varies from a single one to *status epilepticus*.

With the longer-acting barbiturates and the longer-acting benzodiazepines, symptoms may not begin until the second or third day and reach their peak more slowly. Seizures may not occur at all or may happen as late as the seventh to eighth day. When the rate of elimination of the barbiturate is slower than 20% per day, EEG changes and withdrawal symptoms may not be seen (Wulff, 1959). Thus, clinical studies are consistent with laboratory studies that show that the onset and intensity of withdrawal are related to the rate at which active drug leaves the CNS. However, this self-tapering effect does not assure that only trivial symptoms will follow the abrupt discontinuation of long-acting drugs. Some patients experience withdrawal phenomena even when the dose of benzodiazepines is tapered slowly, and there are reports of withdrawal syndromes when patients are switched from a long-acting benzodiazepine to a shorter-acting congener (Conell and Berlin, 1983). The benzodiazepine withdrawal syndrome commonly includes insomnia, restlessness, dizziness, nausea, abdominal pain, paresthesias, increased sensitivity to light and sound, headache, inability to concentrate, and muscle twitching. Seizures may occur but are uncommon. The syndrome may persist for 10 days to several weeks (*see* Hallstrom and Lader, 1981; Tyrer *et al.*, 1981).

Patients who have seizures as a result of withdrawal of a barbiturate may begin to show improvement after the third day, but more than half go on to develop delirium. Anxiety mounts with time, and frightening dreams may be succeeded by a refractory insomnia. Visual hallucinations, usually of a persecutory nature, may occur, generally at the same time that sensorial clouding begins. Disorientation for time and place completes the picture of a full-blown delirium. Once the delirium develops, even the administration of large doses of barbiturate may not suppress it immediately. This is also true of the delirium that develops during the withdrawal of alcohol. The reason for this relative irreversibility is not clear.

During the delirium, which usually occurs between the fourth and seventh day, agitation and hyperthermia can lead to exhaustion, cardiovascular collapse, and death. The withdrawal syndrome, even if untreated, usually clears by about the eighth day; this is generally preceded by a period of prolonged sleep. When hallucinations persist for several months, the situation would seem analogous to chronic alcoholic hallucinosis, which is felt by many investigators to be a manifestation of an underlying psychosis. Wulff (1959) has shown that photic stimulation will produce paroxysmal EEG changes in many patients who show no abnormalities in the resting EEG. Such changes were seen in over 90% of patients who exhibited abstinence phenomena. (For references, *see* Smith, 1977; Mackinnon and Parker, 1982.)

Babies born to mothers physically dependent on general CNS depressants or benzodiazepines will manifest withdrawal syndromes of varying severity. The signs are similar to those seen in the opioid withdrawal syndrome of the newborn; treatment involves the use of a general CNS depressant or a benzodiazepine, rather than an opioid or a phenothiazine (*see* Finnegan, 1979).

ALCOHOL

Prevalence and Patterns of Use. In Western society, alcohol has the unique distinction of being the only potent pharmacological agent with which obvious self-induced intoxication is socially acceptable. In the United States, two thirds of all adults use alcohol occasionally, and at least 12% of the users can be considered "heavy" drinkers. If cigarette smoking is excluded, alcoholism is by far the most serious drug problem in the United States and most other countries. Measured in terms of accidents, lost productivity, crime, death, or damaged health, the combined social costs of problem drinking in the United States were estimated for 1980 to exceed 89 billion dollars annually. The cost in broken homes, wasted lives, loss to society, and human misery is beyond calculation.

There are different patterns of alcoholism in which there are varying degrees of psychological and nutritional complications, physical dependence and withdrawal phenomena, "loss of control," and episodic use. In addition, problem drinkers may also abuse other drugs, such as sedatives, opioids, marihuana, and amphetamines. Sometimes these are used in combination with alcohol; at other times, such drugs are taken in preference to alcohol, and alcohol is used only when the drug of choice is not available.

The wide spectrum of alcohol use associated with adverse consequences makes it difficult to formulate any simple definition of problem drinking or alcoholism. Different people use alcohol for different reasons. For some it produces euphoria and releases emotions; for others it temporarily relieves depression or anxiety. However, other modes of reinforcement must come into play with chronic use since, after the first few days of drinking, alcoholics in laboratory settings often become more anxious and more depressed as drinking continues (*see* Mendelson and Mello, 1979).

Tolerance, Physical Dependence, and Special Complications. Chronic use of alcohol results in an increased capacity to metabolize alcohol, which declines after several weeks of abstinence, so that abstinent alcoholics and normal individuals metabolize alcohol at about the same rate. Chronic use of alcohol also produces pharmacodynamic tolerance, so that a higher blood concentration is necessary to produce intoxication in tolerant than in normal individuals. Some alcoholics can perform well on difficult tasks when their blood alcohol concentrations are above 200 mg/dl, twice the value that in most states is legally defined as significant intoxication. However, as is the case with barbiturates, there is no marked elevation of the lethal dose, and severe acute intoxication with respiratory depression may be superimposed on chronic alcoholic intoxication at any time (*see* Mendelson and Mello, 1979).

Cross-tolerance between alcohol and other drugs may be due to pharmacodynamic tolerance in the CNS or to more rapid metabolism, since the use of alcohol increases hepatic microsomal enzyme activity. Individuals tolerant to alcohol usually show cross-tolerance to general anesthetics; this cross-tolerance is probably a result of pharmacodynamic tolerance. There is also cross-tolerance to a variety of other sedative-hypnotics, including the benzodiazepines, which results from both pharmacodynamic (CNS) tolerance and from more rapid metabolism. However, cross-tolerance is seen only in the relatively sober alcoholic. When concentrations of alcohol in blood are high, the effects of other drugs are additive to those of alcohol. In addition, there is some mutual inhibition of metabolism as a result of competition for shared enzymatic systems (*see* Kalant *et al.*, 1971; Smith, 1977; Sellers and Busto, 1982). There is no obvious cross-tolerance between alcohol and opioid drugs.

Chronic maintenance of high concentrations of alcohol in blood produces a state of physical dependence. The signs and symptoms of the alcohol withdrawal syndrome are quite similar to those described for barbiturate withdrawal (*see* above). The intensity of the alcohol withdrawal syndrome correlates only partially with the amount of alcohol consumed and the duration of use. The low correlation is probably due to the way in which alcohol is metabolized. The body is able to metabolize the alcoholic content of about 30 ml (1 oz) of whisky in an hour (*see* Chapter 18). If the intake is sufficiently spread out over the day, each dose of alcohol may be metabolized without any substantial increase in blood concentration. On the other hand, the ingestion of only modestly larger amounts, but spaced so that the body's metabolic capacity is exceeded (*e.g.*, 120 ml [4 oz] of whisky every 3 hours), can produce much higher blood concentrations, which can induce clinically significant physical dependence in a matter of a few days (*see* above). Withdrawal phenomena most commonly appear within 12 to 72 hours after total cessation of drinking. However, even a relative decline in blood concentration (*e.g.*, from 300 to 100 mg/dl) may precipitate the syndrome, and such declines may occur with changes in the pattern of drinking, as well as with decreases in the total daily intake (*see* Mendelson and Mello, 1979).

With minimal levels of dependence, the entire syndrome may consist in disturbed sleep, nausea, weakness, anxiety, and mild tremors that last for less than a day. When dependence is severe, these symptoms are only prodromal.

The clinical picture of alcohol withdrawal in patients with severe physical dependence described by Victor and Adams (1953) is still the basis for the delineation of three somewhat distinct withdrawal states—the tremulous syndrome, alcohol-related seizure disorders, and delirium tremens. However, there is much *overlapping*, as the following description indicates.

Tremulousness, which appears within a few hours after the last drink, is often accompanied by nausea, weakness, anxiety, and sweating. Purposive behavior directed toward obtaining alcohol or a suitable substitute is prominent. There may be cramps and vomiting. Hyperreflexia is prominent. Tremors may be mild or so marked that the patient may be unable to lift a glass. The subject may begin to "see things," at first only when the eyes are closed but later even while the eyes are open. Insight is at first retained, and the subject remains oriented. The syndrome at this point is often referred to as *acute alcoholic hallucinosis*. However, some experts feel that hallucinosis is not necessarily an index of the severity of the withdrawal syndrome; it is sometimes seen while alcoholics are severely intoxicated (*see* Mendelson and Mello, 1979). Tonic-clonic seizures can occur, but they are less common in alcohol withdrawal than in barbiturate withdrawal. The spontaneous EEG shows mild but definite dysrhythmias, in contrast to the major alterations seen during withdrawal of short-acting barbiturates. As in the case of barbiturates, however, photic stimulation often reveals paroxysmal abnormalities, even when the spontaneous record appears normal. The REM phase of sleep that is depressed by alcohol shows a rebound increase during alcohol withdrawal.

The tremulous state reaches peak intensity within 24 to 48 hours, and seizures are most likely to occur within the first 24 hours after cessation of drinking. If the syndrome progresses further, insight is lost; the subject becomes weaker, more confused, disoriented, and agitated. He may be terrified by his persecutory hallucinations. They are often so vivid that the subject, even after recovery, sometimes doubts their unreality. At this stage, which appears around the third day of withdrawal, the picture is that of the *tremulous delirium,* which was described by Thomas Sutton in 1813. Hyperthermia is common, and exhaustion and cardiovascular collapse may occur.

The alcohol abstinence syndrome is self-limited. If the patient does not die, recovery usually occurs within 5 to 7 days, without treatment. Those patients in whom the sensorium is clear but hallucinations persist well beyond the usual period of recovery are frequently found to be paranoid schizophrenics.

Babies born to mothers who drink heavily during pregnancy not only experience alcohol withdrawal after delivery but also, in some cases, suffer from permanent mental retardation and other development abnormalities (*see* Finnegan, 1979; Chapter 18).

A number of special problems are seen in chronic alcoholism that are not apparent with other types of drug abuse. Many of these are thought to be related to multiple nutritional deficiencies, which are, in turn, the result of the capacity of alcohol to supply calories and depress appetite without supplying essential vitamins and amino acids. They include peripheral polyneuropathies, pellagra, nutritional amblyopia, Wernicke's encephalopathy, and some components of Korsakoff's psychosis. However, other disorders, such as fatty liver, cirrhosis of the liver, and damage to cardiac and skeletal muscle, once thought to be related to nutritional aberrations, are due, at least in part, to direct toxic effects of alcohol itself (*see* Mendelson and Mello, 1979; Chapter 18). Recently detoxified alcoholics frequently show some degree of cerebral atrophy and ventricular dilatation. Recently detoxified alcoholics also perform more poorly than age-matched controls on cognitive tests, especially those involving short-term memory. These cognitive deficits may indicate an early stage of Korsakoff's psychosis. There is reasonable consensus that these structural and functional changes are due, at least in part, to direct toxic effects of alcohol. Some recovery of both structure and function occurs with prolonged abstinence, but there is disagreement about its extent (*see* Brandt *et al.,* 1983; Grant *et al.,* 1984; Ron, 1984).

CNS Sympathomimetics: Amphetamine, Cocaine, and Related Drugs

The subjective effects of CNS sympathomimetics, like those of all centrally active drugs, are dependent on the user, the environment, the dose of the drug, and the route of administration. For example, moderate doses of amphetamine given orally to normal subjects commonly produce an elevation of mood, a sense of increased energy and alertness, and decreased appetite; task performance that has been impaired by fatigue or boredom is improved. Some individuals may become anxious, irritable, or loquacious. A few may experience transient drowsiness, but insomnia is more common. As the dose is increased toward toxic levels, the effects of individual experiences and of environment become less significant. The general pharmacology of these agents is described in Chapter 8. When equated for differences in potency, a number of other CNS sympathomimetics and related agents can produce subjective effects that resemble those of amphetamine. These drugs include dextroamphetamine, methamphetamine, phenmetrazine, methylphenidate, and diethylpropion.

Some congeners with substitutions in the aromatic ring (*e.g.,* fenfluramine) do not produce amphetamine-like subjective effects and have little or no potential for reinforcement (*see* Martin *et al.,* 1971; Griffiths *et al.,* 1978). Phenylpropanolamine suppresses appetite but is not self-administered by animals or recognized as amphetamine-like by human subjects, even at doses several times higher than those needed to produce anorexia. Mazindol also appears to be less reinforcing than amphetamine.

Cocaine addicts describe the euphoric effects of cocaine in terms that are almost indistinguishable from those used by amphetamine addicts. In the laboratory, subjects familiar with cocaine cannot distinguish between the subjective effects of 16 mg of cocaine and those of 10 mg of dextroamphetamine when both are given intravenously (Fischman and Schuster, 1982). Like amphetamine, cocaine reduces the sense of fatigue and the decrement in performance caused by sleep deprivation (*see*

Fischman, 1984). The toxic syndrome seen with cocaine seems clinically indistinguishable from that produced by amphetamines. In addition, animals exhibit similar patterns of self-administration of cocaine and amphetamine. While it is commonly assumed that the subjective effects of cocaine are more intense and its abuse potential more significant than those of the amphetamines, the similarities in terms of subjective behavioral, pharmacological, and toxic effects are more striking than the differences. Another distinct member of this group is (-)-cathinone, the active ingredient in freshly gathered leaves of the Khat shrub (*Catha edulis*); its actions are quite similar to those of amphetamine (*see* below). In this chapter, amphetamine is taken as the prototype of this group of drugs.

Consideration of these drugs as a class does not imply that they have identical mechanisms of action or that drug abusers cannot distinguish among them. For example, after intravenous administration of cocaine the effects are relatively brief, lasting only a matter of minutes, whereas those of methamphetamine may last for hours. With appropriately selected doses and tasks it is possible to demonstrate differences between the effects of amphetamine and cocaine on motor performance, aggression, and facilitation of self-stimulation with electrical current.

It is often assumed that cocaine is unique among the local anesthetics in possessing euphorigenic and reinforcing properties, but animals will also self-administer procaine and chloroprocaine (but not lidocaine). Human subjects who have had experience with cocaine are unable to distinguish lidocaine from cocaine when both are used intranasally (Van Dyke *et al.*, 1979). However, when given intravenously, cocaine (16 to 48 mg) produces a more clear-cut "high" than does procaine or lidocaine. Procaine does share some apparent stimulant properties with cocaine and has sometimes been mixed with or misrepresented as cocaine in illicit drug traffic. In terms of subjective effects, it appears to be one tenth as potent as cocaine; it is also metabolized more rapidly than cocaine, and this may account for its lack of popularity (*see* Fischman, 1984).

Elevation of mood is the typical, rather than the atypical, response to CNS sympathomimetics. Perhaps it is the capacity of so many normal individuals to experience the drug-induced mood elevation without becoming compulsive users that made it difficult fully to appreciate the potential for abuse

of the amphetamine-like drugs. This attitude changed as a result of both the waves of amphetamine abuse that have occurred throughout the United States and a number of Western European countries, and the belated appreciation of the significance of the epidemic of intravenous methamphetamine addiction that occurred in Japan immediately after World War II. Curiously, when the popularity of cocaine began to increase in the early 1970s, there was again a tendency to underestimate its toxicity and the seriousness of the dependence that it induces. More realistic and somber assessments now prevail. Amphetamines and several related drugs are now covered by the same federal regulations applicable to the opioids and cocaine, and illicit transactions are subject to the same penalties.

Incidence and Patterns of Use. Nonmedical use of CNS sympathomimetics fluctuates widely over time in response to cycles of availability and popularity. In the United States, the use of cocaine increased sharply during the late 1970s. By 1982, 28% of young adults (18 to 25 years old) reported having used cocaine at least once; 7% indicated use during the preceding month. Among this age group, 18% reported experience with stimulants, such as amphetamine (Miller *et al.*, 1983).

There are a number of different patterns of amphetamine abuse. One involves those who first obtain the drug from a physician in the course of treatment for obesity or depression and then pass through a phase of habituation as described for barbiturates. Truck drivers and students who use the drug to stay awake may also follow this pattern. Decreased prescribing of amphetamines has reduced the incidence of these patterns of dependence. More commonly, at present, the drug is obtained specifically for its euphoric effects. Those who inject the drugs intravenously may dissolve oral tablets or use crystalline methamphetamine ("crystal") manufactured in illegal laboratories. Used intravenously, amphetamine and methamphetamine are known as "speed."

During the early phases of intravenous use, three or four doses of 20 to 40 mg of amphetamine are usually considered sufficient. In addition to the marked euphoria, the user experiences a sense of markedly enhanced physical strength and mental capacity, and feels little need for either sleep or food. Difficult to substantiate by objective means is the claim made by many users that orgasm in both male and female is delayed, permitting extended periods of sexual activity finally culminating in orgasms reported to be more intense and pleasurable (*see* Kramer *et al.*, 1967). The sensation of "flash" or "rush" that immediately follows intravenous administration, while qualitatively distinct from the opioid "rush," is nevertheless described as being intensely pleasurable and somewhat akin to sexual orgasm. A similar "rush" also follows the intravenous use of cocaine, but it does not occur after oral or intranasal administration.

With time, tolerance develops to the euphorigenic effects of amphetamine; higher and more frequent doses are used, and toxic symptoms and signs then appear. These include bruxism, touching and picking of the face and extremities, suspiciousness, and a feeling of being watched. Perceptual changes and pseudohallucinations may also occur with cocaine. The most common of these are tactile ("cocaine bugs" in the skin) and visual ("snow lights"). In addition, the user seems fascinated or preoccupied with his own thinking processes and with philosophical concerns about "meanings" and "essences." Stereotypical, repetitious behavior is common. Many patients who later show a full-blown toxic psychosis exhibit a compulsion to take apart mechanical objects. They also have a compulsion to put them together, but are usually too disorganized to do so.

Both cocaine and amphetamine users commonly attempt to antagonize various toxic symptoms with other drugs. The mixture of an opioid (the preferred antagonist) and either cocaine or an amphetamine is known as a "speedball." Many amphetamine users simultaneously consume large amounts of barbiturates or alcohol. Interestingly, subjects taking high doses of amphetamine in experimental settings generally exhibit depression and irritability rather than euphoria (Griffith *et al.*, 1972). Nevertheless, the amphetamine user continues his drug in spite of the toxic effects. The drug may be injected every 2 to 3 hours around the clock for periods of several days, during which time he may eat little and remain awake continuously. Such an episode or "run" commonly ends when the user is out of drug or too disorganized or paranoid to continue. Stopping is followed within a few hours by a deep sleep, which usually lasts 12 to 18 hours but which may last longer if the "run" has been an unusually long one. Upon awakening, users are extremely hungry and lethargic. Some are depressed. Much of the paranoid ideation is gone. The lethargy may persist for many days; reinitiation of drug use eliminates the lethargy and also starts a new cycle. During a "run" some addicts are reported to use as much as 1 g of methamphetamine intravenously every few hours.

Patterns of *cocaine* use show similar variability. The leaves of the coca bush (*Erythroxylon coca*), from which cocaine is obtained, have been chewed by the natives living high in the Andes for untold generations. Used in this way, cocaine appears to produce a sense of decreased hunger and fatigue and increased well-being. Cases of acute overdosage, chronic toxicity, psychosis, or patterns of dependence in which users neglect responsibilities and focus on the use of coca are exceedingly rare. Andean natives appear to have little difficulty in discontinuing use of the drug when they move to lower altitudes. In contrast, the smoking of coca paste (60 to 80% cocaine sulfate) by younger people living in urban areas of Peru is associated with a variety of psychopathological states (euphoria, hypertalkativeness, irritability, stereotypical behaviors, insomnia, weight loss, and toxic psychosis), neglect of work, and a preoccupation with obtaining money to purchase coca paste. The paste is inexpensive, but it is reported that some users may smoke more than 40 g each day and engage in criminal activity to get money (*see* Jerí, 1980). The use of cocaine has increased in developed countries, where it is commonly taken intranasally ("snorted"), but is sometimes used intravenously. Cocaine (also called coke, snow, gold dust, and lady) is sold as a powder, often diluted with procaine, and varies greatly in purity. The powder is usually arranged on a glass in thin lines 3 to 5 cm long, each containing about 25 mg. The line is then inhaled into the nose through a straw or rolled paper. While the high price of the material limits daily use, users with sufficient funds or special access engage in "runs" or sprees of use like those described for amphetamine. More recently, the smoking of cocaine "free base" has become popular. Converted from the hydrochloride salt by alkalinization and extraction with organic solvents, cocaine base is volatilized at 90° C. When smoked, absorption of the free base from the lung is rapid and efficient, producing concentrations in plasma of more than 900 ng/ml; peak values of 150 to 200 ng/ml are reached 30 to 40 minutes after the inhalation of 96 mg of crystalline cocaine hydrochloride (*see* Fischman, 1984).

The euphoric effects of cocaine decay more rapidly after intravenous or intranasal administration than do concentrations of the drug in plasma, suggesting some form of acute tolerance (Fischman and Schuster, 1982; Van Dyke *et al.*, 1982). Cocaine users who try to maintain the euphoric state will take the drug repeatedly every 30 to 40 minutes if it is available.

Animals self-administering cocaine or amphetamines often show a cyclic pattern of use, with periods of spontaneous abstinence interposed between periods of use. A small priming dose during abstinence will reinitiate self-administration. With round-the-clock access to the drugs there is weight loss, self-mutilation, and death within about 2 weeks. Given a choice between cocaine and food over a period of 8 days, monkeys consistently select cocaine (Aigner and Balster, 1978).

Unlike the user of morphine, whose drives are usually decreased, the user of CNS sympathomimetics is hyperactive and during a toxic episode may act in response to persecutory delusions. Some individuals seem able to use the drug for months or years without developing a toxic paranoid syndrome, yet such symptoms can develop in the course of a single "run."

Many of those who use amphetamine and cocaine are best described as "recreational" or occasional users, but some become dependent. A small percentage of the latter (*e.g.*, those taking the drugs for control of obesity) seem able to restrict drug intake and function productively (stabilized addicts). Others show progressive social and occupational deterioration, punctuated by periods of hospitalization for toxic psychosis. In terms of the compulsion to continue use, the degree to which a drug pervades the life of the user, and the tendency to relapse following withdrawal, some compulsive users of amphetamine or cocaine are addicts. The risk of developing patterns of compulsive use is not limited to those who use drugs intravenously or smoke cocaine as the base. Severe dependence with psychological, physical, and vocational impairment is also seen among those who use cocaine intranasally. It is not clear whether the dependence syndromes caused by amphetamine or cocaine are as persistent as that produced by opioids. In the United States the waves of amphetamine use did not leave large numbers of chronic users in their wake. However, many intravenous users eventually became heroin users. Very little is known of the natural history of cocaine dependence (*see* Petersen and Stillman, 1977; Ellinwood, 1979; Jerí, 1980; Kleber and Gawin, 1984).

Mechanism of Reinforcing Effects. The reinforcing and euphorigenic effects of amphetamine, methylphenidate, and cocaine appear to involve the actions of catecholamines in the CNS, especially those of dopamine. They can be blocked, at least partially, by pimozide and other dopaminergic antagonists but are relatively unaffected by phenoxybenzamine. Furthermore, both amphetamine and apomorphine (a dopaminergic agonist) facilitate electrical self-stimulation of "reward" areas of the brain. Amphetamine and cocaine share with morphine the capacity to lower the amount of electrical current required to produce "rewarding" effects in these brain areas (Kornetsky and Esposito, 1981). The mechanisms of reinforcement are still uncertain. Amphetamine, methylphenidate, and cocaine all block the re-uptake of catecholamines, but so do the tricyclic antidepressants, which do not produce euphoria or stereotypy and are not abused. Amphetamine and phenmetrazine appear to release newly synthesized neurotransmitter selectively, and their effects can be blocked by inhibition of tyrosine hydroxylase, a procedure that does not block the central effects of methylphenidate or cocaine. Prior treatment with reserpine blocks the effects of the last-named drugs but not those of amphetamine (*see* Ellinwood, 1979). Microinjections of amphetamine into the nucleus accumbens, an area where ascending dopaminergic fibers terminate, are reinforcing. In contrast, microinjections of cocaine are reinforcing at medial prefrontal cortex, but not at nucleus accumbens. However, both drugs appear to depend on activation of dopaminergic neurons, since destruction of nucleus accumbens or microinjections of dopamine antagonists into cortex or nucleus accumbens reduce or eliminate their reinforcing effects (*see* Wise, 1984).

Cathinone is structurally similar to amphetamine and appears to act like the latter by releasing intra-

neuronal stores of dopamine. Its psychological, behavioral, cardiovascular, and toxic effects in animals and man are quite similar to those of amphetamine (*see* Kalix, 1984).

Tolerance, Toxicity, Physical Dependence, and Withdrawal Symptoms. Tolerance develops to some of the central effects of amphetamines (*e.g.*, its euphorigenic, anorectic, hyperthermic, and lethal actions), and the chronic user often increases the dose to continue to obtain the desired effect. Some users are able to take several hundred milligrams per day over prolonged periods. By suppressing appetite, high doses of amphetamine may foster ketosis; and, since amphetamine is excreted much more rapidly in acidic urine, some of the apparent tolerance may be due to more rapid elimination of the drug. At the same time there is increased sensitivity to other effects on the CNS (*see* below). Although tolerance to the convulsant and cardiorespiratory effects of cocaine has been reported, the preponderant view is that there is an increased sensitivity of the CNS to many of the effects of cocaine when the drug is administered repeatedly. The possibility of acute tolerance to some of the effects of cocaine was mentioned above. Cross-tolerance between the amphetamine-like sympathomimetic agents has been observed clinically, and cross-tolerance between the anorectic effect of cocaine and amphetamine has been demonstrated in rats (Woolverton *et al.*, 1978).

Tolerance does not develop to certain of the toxic effects of amphetamine on the CNS, and a toxic psychosis may occur after periods of weeks to months of continued use. Those who develop such a psychosis may have a lowered threshold during subsequent episodes if they resume use of amphetamine (*see* Ellinwood, 1979).

The fully developed toxic syndrome from amphetamine is characterized by vivid visual, auditory, and sometimes tactile hallucinations; picking and excoriation of the skin and delusions of parasitosis are not uncommon. There is also paranoid ideation, loosening of associations, and changes in affect occurring in association with a *clear sensorium*. In chronic users, there may be a striking paucity of sympathomimetic effects, and the blood pressure is not unduly elevated. It is often extremely difficult to differentiate this syndrome from a schizophrenic reaction. The syndrome may be seen as early as 36 to 48 hours after the ingestion of a single large dose of amphetamine; in apparently sensitive individuals, psychosis may be produced by 55 to 75 mg of dextroamphetamine. With high enough doses, psychosis can probably be induced in anyone. Unless the individual continues to use the drug, the psychosis usually clears within a week, the hallucinations being the first symptoms to disappear. Paranoid delusions and excitement are promptly suppressed by dopaminergic antagonists, such as haloperidol (Angrist *et al.*, 1974). Acidification of the urine, which facilitates excretion of amphetamine, also shortens the duration of the psychosis. The toxic syndrome observed with cocaine is almost identical to that caused by amphetamine and should also respond promptly to dopaminergic blocking agents.

Chronic use of high doses of amphetamines has been reported to produce microvascular damage, neuronal chromatolysis (primarily in brain areas rich in adrenergic neurons), and profound and longlasting (or permanent) depletion of dopamine in the caudate nucleus (*see* Ellinwood, 1979). Administration of large doses of methamphetamine to rats causes the appearance in the CNS of detectable concentrations of 6-hydroxydopamine, a substance that destroys adrenergic neurons (*see* Chapter 9; Seiden and Vosmer, 1984). In rats, continuous administration of amphetamine for 10 days can cause a significant decrease in the activity of tyrosine hydroxylase in the nigrostriatum that lasts for more than 3 months. After chronic use, animals (including man) begin to exhibit behaviors not seen after initial doses; these include exaggerated "startle" reactions, dyskinesias, and postural abnormalities. Chronic administration of cocaine also results in increased stereotypical behavior.

Four to 8 hours after a single intranasal dose of cocaine (96 mg), subjects report a decreased sense of energy and increased feelings of tiredness and sedation. After chronic administration of either cocaine or amphetamine, abrupt cessation is commonly followed by craving for the drug, prolonged sleep, general fatigue, lassitude, hyperphagia, and depression. Suppression of REM sleep and rebound after abrupt withdrawal have been reported. While these effects have not been consistently confirmed for amphetamine, they do appear to occur with cocaine. Such signs and symptoms appear to meet the criteria for a withdrawal syndrome. However, since abrupt discontinuation of the use of sympathomimetic amines or cocaine does not cause major, grossly observable, physiological disruption that necessitates the gradual withdrawal of the drug, there was, at one time, reluctance to accept the withdrawal syndrome as evidence of physical dependence on cocaine or amphetamine-like drugs. The role of withdrawal hyperphagia, lethargy, and depression in perpetuating the use of these drugs is unclear. Tricyclic antidepressants have been reported to produce prompt alleviation of dysphoria and hypersomnia, and they may reduce craving and the likelihood of relapse (*see* Gawin and Kleber, 1984).

Acute Toxicity. Because tolerance develops to the hyperthermic and cardiovascular effects of amphetamine, acute intoxication is more likely to occur in the neophyte. The syndrome includes dizziness, tremor, irritability, confusion, hallucinations, chest pain, palpitations, hypertension, sweating, and cardiac arrhythmias. There may be hyperpyrexia and convulsions. Death is usually preceded by hyperpyrexia, convulsions, and shock. Chlorpromazine will antagonize many of the effects of amphetamine and will also prevent shivering and reduce blood pressure. Diazepam is administered to control convulsions, and acidification of the urine is also indicated (*see* Chapter 8). Since cocaine is also a local anesthetic, acute intoxication is more frequently characterized by convulsions and cardiac arrhythmias. Death from acute intoxication with cocaine is no longer unusual and can occur after either intranasal or intravenous use. In nonhuman primates, dopaminergic antagonists substantially block the convulsive and lethal effects of cocaine. Clinically, chlorpromazine has been used to treat acute cocaine intoxication (*see* Kleber and Gawin, 1984); some clinicians prefer propranolol.

NICOTINE AND TOBACCO

The chemistry and the acute pharmacological effects of nicotine are considered in Chapter 10. In this section, the discussion centers on the use and effects of *tobacco products*.

History. Crewmen who accompanied Columbus to the New World were the first Europeans to observe the smoking of tobacco. In the following century the smoking of tobacco spread throughout the world, despite vigorous official opposition and, in some cases, draconian penalties. The tobacco plant was named *Nicotiana tabacum* in honor of Jean Nicot, who promoted its importation and cultivation in the belief that it had medicinal values. Nicotine was first isolated from the leaves by Posselt and Reiman in 1828. In the mid-nineteenth century, new varieties of tobacco, changes in the technology of curing the leaf, and machinery for mass production facilitated the spread of a new product—the cigarette—cheaper and neater than cigars and yielding a smoke so mild that it could be inhaled. In the United States, the consumption of cigarettes rose rapidly, and by the 1960s more than 600 billion cigarettes were consumed each year. *Per-capita* consumption of cigarettes is now level or declining slightly as older smokers die or give up smoking and fewer young people enter the ranks. In 1982, 33% of adults were still smokers, but only 20% of high school seniors were regular smokers, suggesting that the prevalence of smoking will continue to decline over the next decade.

Chemical Composition of Tobacco. About 4000 compounds are generated by the burning of tobacco; the smoke can be separated into gaseous and particulate phases. The composition of the actual smoke delivered to the smoker depends not only on the composition of the tobacco but also on how densely it is packed, the length of the column of tobacco, the characteristics of the filter and the paper, and the temperature at which the tobacco is burned. Rapid drawing of the smoke raises the temperature of the burning tip and changes the size of the particles and the composition of both the gaseous and particulate phases. These changes may in turn alter what is trapped in the filter. It is possible to specify the amounts of nicotine, "tar," and carbon monoxide delivered by a given cigarette when it is smoked by a machine under constant conditions, as is now done by governmental agencies in many countries. However, smokers do not usually conform to the smoking style of the machine.

Among the components of the gaseous phase that produce undesirable effects are carbon monoxide, carbon dioxide, nitrogen oxides, ammonia, volatile nitrosamines, hydrogen cyanide, volatile sulfur-containing compounds, nitriles and other nitrogen-containing compounds, volatile hydrocarbons, alcohols, and aldehydes and ketones (*e.g.*, acetaldehyde, formaldehyde, and acrolein). Some of the last-named substances are potent inhibitors of ciliary movement (Surgeon General, 1979, 1981). The particulate phase contains nicotine, water, and "tar"; "tar" is what remains after the moisture and nicotine are subtracted and consists primarily of polycyclic aromatic hydrocarbons, some of which are documented carcinogens. Among these are nonvolatile nitrosamines and aromatic amines, which are believed to play an etiological role in bladder cancer, and polycyclic hydrocarbons such as benzo[a]pyrene, an exceedingly potent carcinogen. The "tar" also contains numerous other compounds, including metallic ions and several radioactive compounds (*e.g.*, polonium 210). According to experts, the components most likely to contribute to the health hazards of smoking are carbon monoxide, nicotine, and "tar"; probable contributors to the health hazards of smoking are acrolein, hydrocyanic acid, nitric oxide, nitrogen dioxide, cresols, and amphenols; suspected hazards include a host of other chemicals (*see* Surgeon General, 1979).

When a cigarette is smoked on a standard machine, the delivery of "tar" varies from 0.5 to 35 mg and that of nicotine from 0.05 to 2.0 mg (1982 average, 1.0 mg). The actual content of nicotine in tobacco can vary from 0.2 to 5%, but is generally between 1 and 2% for smoking tobaccos. It is present in the protonated form in almost all cigarette tobaccos. Because of a more alkaline pH, it is present in the more readily absorbed, unprotonated form in cigars and in pipe tobaccos (*see* Surgeon General, 1979).

Effects on the CNS. Nicotine is self-administered by animals (*see* Goldberg *et al.*, 1981), but it is less powerful as a reinforcer than is amphetamine or cocaine. Nicotine appears to have very specific properties as a stimulus; its effects are not confused with those of other drugs. These properties appear to involve both stereospecific receptors for nicotine and dopaminergic pathways. They can be blocked with mecamylamine, but not with muscarinic cholinergic or adrenergic blocking agents (*see* Rosecrans, 1979; Schwartz and Kellar, 1983). Nicotine, as absorbed by the typical smoker, causes an increase in hand tremor and an alerting pattern in the EEG (low-voltage, fast activity); however, at the same time, there is decreased skeletal muscle tone, decreased amplitude in the electromyogram, and a decrease in deep-tendon reflexes. The latter effects may involve stimulation of the Renshaw cells in the spinal cord (*see* Domino, 1973). The smoking of one or two cigarettes after a few hours of abstinence produces a significant rise in the concentrations of several hormones and neurotransmitters in plasma. Nicotine causes nausea and vomiting, in part, by stimulating the chemoreceptor trigger zone of the medulla oblongata and by activating the vagal reflexes involved in the act of vomiting.

Animal studies indicate that nicotine stimulates the release of norepinephrine and dopamine from brain tissue and, depending on the dose, increases or inhibits the release of acetylcholine. Nicotine appears to facilitate memory and reduce aggression (*see* Jaffe and Jarvik, 1978).

Many of nicotine's effects could, in theory, be reinforcing. These include the alerting and muscle relaxant effects, the facilitation of memory or attention, and the decrease in appetite and irritability. However, in man, these effects may be incidental to some primary reinforcing action. When smokers are given nicotine intravenously in doses of about 1.5 mg, they report that the effects are pleasant and they show increased scores on scales devised to measure the euphorigenic effects of morphine and amphetamine (Henningfield *et al.*, 1983).

Absorption from Smoke. The nicotine in cigarette smoke, suspended on minute particles of "tar," is quickly absorbed from the lung, almost with the efficiency of intravenous administration. The compound reaches the brain within 8 seconds after inhalation. Nicotine in cigarette smoke, which is somewhat acidic, is not well absorbed from the mouth; pipe and cigar smoke, which is more alkaline (pH 8.5), is probably better absorbed, but the concentration of nicotine in the plasma of those who do not inhale cigars is still low compared to those who do inhale cigarettes (Armitage *et al.*, 1978). Peak concentrations of nicotine in plasma after a cigarette is smoked are typically 25 to 50 ng/ml (*see* Russell and Feyerabend, 1978).

The elimination of nicotine is multiexponential. Following a single cigarette, concentrations decline rapidly (over 5 to 10 minutes), primarily reflecting distribution. After chronic smoking, the elimination half-life of nicotine is approximately 2 hours (*see* Benowitz *et al.*, 1982). For the average smoker, concentrations of nicotine in plasma are somewhat higher at the end of the day. Nicotine is oxidized to its major metabolite, cotinine, which causes few or no cardiovascular or subjective effects. Since cotinine is cleared more slowly (half-life of about 19 hours), it is a better measure of overall intake than nicotine itself (Benowitz *et al.*, 1983).

Chronic Toxicity of Tobacco. Chronic use of tobacco is causally linked to a variety of serious diseases, ranging from coronary artery disease to lung cancer. The likelihood of developing any one of these disorders increases with the degree of exposure (measured in cigarettes per day, or "pack years"). For example, for all male smokers, the overall mortality ratio is about 1.7 compared to nonsmokers. The ratio is 2.0 for those who smoke two packs daily, and it is higher among inhalers than noninhalers. Cigar smoking increases mortality in proportion to the number smoked, but not as sharply as for cigarettes. Those who smoke pipes exclusively show a very slight increase in mortality. The differences between cigarette, pipe, and cigar smokers is probably related to the lesser inhalation among the latter two groups, which leads to lower exposure to all constituents of smoke. The smoking of tobacco continues to be described as the largest preventable cause of death in the United States.

Evidence indicates that the different diseases that are related to the use of tobacco may be caused, at least in part, by different constituents of tobacco or tobacco smoke. This raises the possibility that changes in the composition of cigarettes or selective filtration might lower the probability of one disorder, while having little effect on another. The catalog of tobacco-related diseases is extensive, and only the more important in terms of prevalence and seriousness can be mentioned here. Cardiovascular diseases related to tobacco include coronary artery disease, cerebrovascular disease, and peripheral vascular disease. Carbon monoxide (and related hypoxia) and the effects of nicotine on cardiac rhythm, free fatty acids in plasma, lipoproteins, and the coagulability of blood may play a role in the acceleration of atherosclerosis and in sudden cardiac death. Smoking shortens the survival time of arterial grafts and arteriovenous fistulas used to facilitate dialysis. Neoplastic diseases (cancer of the lung, larynx, oral cavity, esophagus, bladder, and pancreas) are probably due to one or more of the known carcinogens in the smoke, rather than to nicotine or carbon monoxide. Chronic obstructive lung disease is probably caused by effects on proteolytic enzymes, interference with immune mechanisms, and inhibition of clearance mechanisms. Impairment of respiratory function can be detected in young adults after only a few years of smoking (*see* Surgeon General, 1979, 1981). The ciliotoxic actions of tobacco smoke and its ability to inhibit pulmonary clearance mechanisms probably account for the remarkable synergism between tobacco smoke and such environmental carcinogens as asbestos in increasing mortality from lung cancer. The mechanisms by which smoking leads to an increased incidence of abortion, significantly reduces the birth weight of children born to women who smoke during pregnancy, and increases the likelihood of perinatal mortality and of sudden death of infants are unclear (*see* Surgeon General, 1981). Smokers have more sleep difficulties than do nonsmokers and tend to exhibit more depression, irritability, and anxiety. Recent studies suggest that nonsmokers who are passively exposed to tobacco smoke over prolonged periods may have an increased risk of pulmonary dysfunction and, perhaps, cancer (*see* Correa *et al.*, 1983). Passive inhalation of smoke may also aggravate angina.

The likelihood of development of a disorder related to smoking is reduced by cessation. Over a period of 5 to 10 years, the risk falls to a level only slightly above that of the nonsmoker. Destruction of lung tissue is not reversible, but, with cessation, the rate of decline in pulmonary function begins to resemble that of the nonsmoker.

Smokers metabolize a wide variety of drugs more rapidly than do nonsmokers, probably as a result of induction of enzymes in the intestinal mucosa or the liver by components of tobacco smoke. Among the drugs affected are theophylline, warfarin, phenacetin, propranolol, imipramine, caffeine, and antipyrine (*see* Vestal *et al.*,

1979). Smokers may require more opioids to obtain relief from pain, may be less sedated by benzodiazepines, and may obtain less antianginal effect from nifedipine, atenolol, or propranolol. Not all differences arise from altered rates of drug metabolism (*see* Deanfield *et al.*, 1984).

Tolerance, Physical Dependence, and Relapse. Tolerance develops to some of the effects of nicotine. Following one or two cigarettes, even the chronic smoker still exhibits an increase in blood pressure, pulse rate, and hand tremor; decreased skin temperature; and increases in the plasma concentrations of certain hormones. However, the dizziness, nausea, and vomiting experienced by nontolerant individuals do not occur unless the smoker's customary intake is exceeded substantially. Furthermore, while regular smokers report that injections of nicotine are pleasant, nonsmokers describe unpleasant reactions (*see* Jarvik, 1979; Henningfield *et al.*, 1983). Although smokers appear to metabolize nicotine more rapidly than do nonsmokers, it is likely that tolerance is due primarily to pharmacodynamic changes rather than to alterations in drug disposition. In rats, marked tolerance develops to the depressant effects of nicotine after a few closely spaced doses. There are conflicting reports on the duration of tolerance. In some studies of animals it appeared to disappear within 24 to 48 hours of abstinence; in others it persisted for months (*see* Jarvik, 1979; Surgeon General, 1979). In human smokers, some aspects of tolerance wax and wane rapidly. The first cigarette of the day produces a much greater cardiovascular and subjective response than do those that follow.

Cessation of the use of tobacco may be followed by a *withdrawal syndrome*, but it varies greatly from person to person in intensity and in specific signs and symptoms. There is uncertainty about what factors are responsible for its variability and virtually no information on what levels of exposure are required to induce physical dependence in man. The most consistent signs and symptoms (in addition to "craving" for tobacco, which subsides over a period of days to weeks) are irritability, anxiety, restlessness, and difficulty in concentrating (Hughes *et al.*, 1984). Drowsiness, headaches, increased appetite, sleep disturbances (insomnia), and gastrointestinal complaints are also common.

The syndrome is prompt in onset, usually within the first 24 hours, and some smokers complain that certain problems, such as increased appetite and inability to concentrate, persist for weeks or months. In some cases it is uncertain whether the specific problem represents an effect of withdrawal or a return to the *status quo* that existed before the individual started smoking. Among the objective findings that quickly follow cessation of smoking are changes in the EEG, with a decrease in high-frequency activity characteristic of arousal and an increase in low-frequency activity characteristic of drowsiness and hypoarousal. Decreases in performance on tests of vigilance and psychomotor performance and increases in hostility are detectable within hours. There is a decrease in heart rate and blood pressure, and peripheral blood flow increases. Weight gain is a common finding; it is postulated that this is due to increased activity of a lipoprotein lipase (Carney and Goldberg, 1984). Cough and other respiratory difficulties show improvement, and, over a period of weeks to months, smoking-induced acceleration in degradation of other drugs approaches the norm for nonsmokers. There is some evidence that a higher intake of nicotine is associated with more severe withdrawal and more difficulty in giving up cigarettes, but other factors are probably just as important. Women smokers report more symptoms than do men. Craving for cigarettes seems to exhibit a diurnal variation and is low on arising and rises to a peak in the evening. Unlike those who are dependent on opioids, individuals who try to cut down gradually may simply extend the period of discomfort as compared to those who stop abruptly. The syndrome of withdrawal from tobacco can be suppressed to some degree by nicotine, but related drugs such as lobeline appear to be ineffective (*see* Jaffe and Jarvik, 1978; Surgeon General, 1979). Use of buffered nicotine chewing gum reduces the irritability, anxiety, difficulty in concentrating, and somatic complaints that are associated with withdrawal, but it is less reliable or relatively ineffective in controlling insomnia, hunger, tremulousness, and craving for tobacco (Hughes *et al.*, 1984). To what degree the craving (either caused directly by withdrawal or elicited by environmental stimuli that have become conditioned to the use of tobacco) contributes to relapse among smokers is uncertain. Of those who seek some sort of formal help with their problem, about two thirds actually stop for at least a few days; but of these, only 20 to 40% are still abstinent 12 months later.

In the context of a formal cessation program, the use of nicotine gum, now available in several countries including the United States, significantly increased the number of smokers who remained abstinent for 1 year and was of greater help to those smokers who had the highest degree of dependence on nicotine (*see* Jarvik and Schneider, 1984). However, when nicotine gum was prescribed as an adjunct to a doctor's unsolicited advice to stop smoking, neither the nicotine gum nor a placebo added to the small impact of the admonition (Crofton *et al.*, 1983). A nasal spray containing nicotine has also been developed; its use results in plasma concentrations of nicotine that approach those achieved by smoking.

Gum containing nicotine (NICORETTE) is available in boxes of 96 pieces, each of which contains 2 mg of nicotine bound to an ion-exchange resin. The nicotine is released during chewing and is absorbed through the buccal mucosa. Chewed at a rate of one piece per hour, cardiovascular effects are minimal; however, the concentration of nicotine in blood does not reach the trough level obtained by smoking one cigarette per hour. At higher rates of chewing, the gum causes release of catecholamines and the expected cardiovascular effects. The drug is contraindicated or must be used with caution in patients with recent myocardial infarction, serious arrhythmias, or vasospastic disease. The most common side effects are hiccoughs, nausea, and vomiting. Not surprisingly, instances of dependence on nicotine gum have been reported.

Titration. Most heavy smokers behave as if they are attempting to adjust their concentration of nicotine within relatively narrow limits. When given cigarettes with a high content of nicotine, they reduce the number smoked and alter their puffing patterns, and thereby achieve concentrations of nicotine in plasma only slightly greater than those to which they are accustomed. When given cigarettes with exceedingly low nicotine content, they change patterns of puffing or increase the number of cigarettes smoked in order to avoid declines in plasma nicotine concentrations, but the regulation is less precise (*see* Benowitz *et al.*, 1984). Titration is of considerable clinical significance, since smokers who switch to "low tar and nicotine" cigarettes generally alter their puffing patterns in a manner that minimizes the potential benefit. Most "switchers" take in as much or more carbon monoxide than previously. Plasma concentrations of nicotine and cotinine may be somewhat lower, reflecting a slightly reduced intake of particulates, but there is little evidence of any benefit to health (*see* Ebert *et al.*, 1983; Benowitz and Jacob, 1984).

CANNABINOIDS (MARIHUANA)

History and Source. *Cannabis*, obtained from the flowering tops of *hemp* plants, is a very ancient drug. Other names for cannabis or its products include *hashish, charas, bhang, ganja, dagga,* and *marihuana*. The common hemp is an herbaceous annual, of which *Cannabis sativa* is the sole species and *Cannabis sativa* var. *indica* and var. *americana* are two varieties. While all parts of both the male and the female plant contain psychoactive substances (cannabinoids), the highest cannabinoid concentrations are found in the flowering tops. In the Middle East and North Africa the dried resinous exudate of the tops is called *hashish;* in the Far East it is called *charas*. The dried leaves and flowering shoots of the plant, containing smaller amounts of the active substance, are called *bhang,* and the resinous mass from the small leaves and brackets of inflorescence is called *ganja*. In the United States, the term *marihuana* is used to refer to any part of the plant or extract therefrom that induces somatic and psychic changes in man. Most commonly, the plant is cut, dried, chopped, and incorporated into cigarettes. Marihuana is sometimes contaminated with paraquat, an herbicide, and with *Salmonella* and *Aspergillus*.

Chemistry. The hemp plant synthesizes more than 60 cannabinoids, which include cannabinol, cannabidiol, cannabinolic acid, cannabigerol, cannabicyclol, and several isomers of tetrahydrocannabinol. The isomer believed responsible for most of the characteristic psychological effects of marihuana is l-Δ^9-tetrahydrocannabinol (Δ^9-THC), also referred to as l-Δ^1-THC. The effects of l-Δ^8-THC, which occurs in minute amounts in marihuana, are similar to those of l-Δ^9-THC.

Δ^9-THC has the following structure:

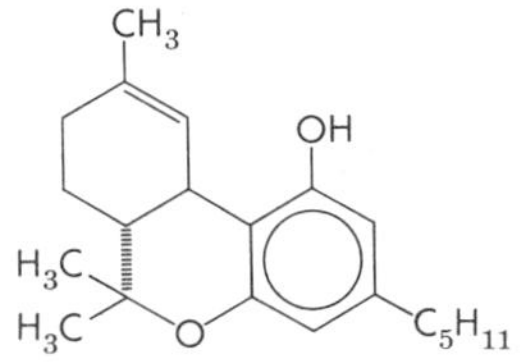

Tetrahydrocannabinol (Δ^9-THC)

Most other cannabinoids are not psychoactive, but they may interact with Δ^9-THC and alter its potency. Many derivatives of tetrahydrocannabinol have been synthesized and studied; some of these are more potent than the natural plant products and may have potential therapeutic uses. Hundreds of additional compounds are produced by pyrolysis when cannabis products are smoked. Several of these are also found in tobacco smoke, and they may be important in the long-term toxicity from use of cannabis (*see* Institute of Medicine, 1982; Fehr and Kalant, 1983).

Pharmacological Effects in Animals. In monkeys, both Δ^9-THC and Δ^8-THC produce sedation, decrease in aggressive behavior, loss of ability or motivation to perform complex tasks, and apparent hallucinations. Chronic high dosage produces a dose-related depression of ovarian function, decreases in concentrations of LH and FSH, and anovulatory cycles; tolerance may develop to these effects. Decreased spermatogenesis has also been reported. Δ^9-THC and several of its synthetic congeners have a number of actions not unlike those of the barbiturates. They prolong hexobarbital sleeping time, exhibit anticonvulsant activity, raise the threshold for EEG and behavioral arousal, and depress polysynaptic reflexes. Yet they may also prolong the stimulant action of amphetamine (*see* Harris *et al.*, 1977).

Pharmacological Effects in Man. Δ^9-THC exerts its most prominent effects on the CNS and cardiovascular system. Because of differences due to dose, route of administration, setting, and the experience and expectations of subjects, condensed descriptions of the behavioral responses to Δ^9-THC are sometimes misleading.

In the United States, the Δ^9-THC content of marihuana ranges broadly from 0.5 to 11%. Furthermore, as with tobacco, the amount of active material that reaches the blood stream is highly dependent on the smoking technic and the amount altered by pyrolysis.

An oral dose of 20 mg of Δ^9-THC or the smoking of a cigarette containing 2% Δ^9-THC produces effects on mood, memory, motor coordination, cognitive ability, sensorium, time sense, and self-perception. Most commonly there is an increased sense of well-being or euphoria, accompanied by feelings of relaxation and sleepiness when subjects are alone; where users can interact, sleepiness is less pronounced and there is often spontaneous laughter (for references, *see* Petersen, 1980; Institute of Medicine, 1982; Fehr and Kalant, 1983). The sleepiness contrasts with the effects of LSD and related hallucinogens, which induce a state of arousal. Short-term memory is impaired, and there is a deterioration in capacity to carry out tasks requiring multiple mental steps to reach a specific goal. This effect on memory-dependent, goal-directed behavior has been called "temporal disintegration," and is correlated with a tendency to confuse past, present, and future, and with depersonalization—a sense of strangeness and unreality about the self.

Balance and stability of stance are affected even at low doses, effects that are more apparent when the eyes are closed. Decreases in muscle strength and hand steadiness can be demonstrated. Performance of relatively simple motor tasks and simple reaction times are relatively unimpaired until higher doses are reached. More complex processes, including perception, attention, and information processing, which are involved in driving and flying, are impaired by doses equivalent to one or two cigarettes; the impairment persists for 4 to 8 hours, well beyond the time that the user perceives the subjective effects of the drug. The impairment produced by alcohol is additive to that induced by marihuana.

Marihuana smokers frequently report increased hunger, dry mouth and throat, more vivid visual imagery, and a keener sense of hearing. Subtle visual and auditory stimuli previously ignored may take on a novel quality, and the nondominant senses of touch, taste, and smell seem to be enhanced. Yet, in usual social doses, marihuana decreases empathy and the perception of emotions in others; clarity of sequential dialogue is impaired, and irrelevant ideas and words intrude into the stream of communication. Altered perception of time is a consistent effect of cannabinoids. Time seems to pass more slowly—minutes may seem like hours.

The effects of single doses of marihuana on the surface EEG are not prominent; an increased abundance of alpha waves is the effect reported most commonly. REM sleep is reduced. Some tolerance develops to these effects (*see* Petersen, 1980; Institute of Medicine, 1982; Fehr and Kalant, 1983). The surface EEGs of chronic users of marihuana or hashish are essentially normal. However, electrodes in deep brain structures of experimental animals reveal abnormalities that persist for months after cessation of exposure to Δ^9-THC.

Higher doses of Δ^9-THC can induce frank hallucinations, delusions, and paranoid feelings. Thinking becomes confused and disorganized; depersonalization and altered time sense are accentuated. Anxiety reaching panic proportions may replace euphoria, often as a result of the feeling that the drug-induced state will never end. With high enough doses, the clinical picture is that of a toxic psychosis with hallucinations, depersonalization, and loss of insight; this can occur acutely or only after months of use. Most users are able to regulate their intake in order to avoid the excessive dosage that produces these unpleasant effects. However, peak subjective effects of smoked cannabis occur 20 to 30 minutes after inhalation, and they lag somewhat behind concentrations of Δ^9-THC in plasma. Regulation of effect is thus imprecise (*see* Perez-Reyes *et al.*, 1982). Because of the high prevalence of marihuana use, dysphoric reactions and psychiatric emergencies as a result of smoking marihuana are no longer uncommon. Use of marihuana may also cause an acute exacerbation of symptomatology in stabilized schizophrenics, and it is one of the common precipitants of "flashbacks" in former users of LSD.

While there are similarities between the subjective effects of Δ^9-THC at high doses and those of LSD, there are also substantial differences. Cannabinoids should therefore be considered as a separate and distinct pharmacological class. The mechanism of action of Δ^9-THC is unknown, but effects on the CNS may involve some decrease in the activity of cholinergic neurons. The psychological effects are not prevented by pretreatment with α-methyltyrosine, which reduces brain concentrations of dopamine and norepinephrine, although such pretreatment does eliminate the euphoria produced by amphetamine and partially eliminates the euphoria produced by ethanol. Patients maintained on lithium or methadone continue to experience the effects of marihuana without apparent alteration.

The most consistent effects on the cardiovascular system are an increase in heart rate, an increase in systolic blood pressure while supine, decreased blood pressure while standing, and a marked reddening of the conjunctivae. Propranolol, a β-adrenergic blocking agent, prevents the tachycardia produced by Δ^9-THC, but it does not interfere with the subjective and behavioral effects. The increase in heart rate is dose related, and its onset and duration correlate well with concentrations of Δ^9-THC in blood. Increases of 20 to 50 beats per minute are usual, but a tachycardia of 140 beats per minute is not uncommon. Chronic use of cannabis causes an as-yet-unexplained increase in plasma volume.

Cannabis-induced inhibition of sweating leads to a rise of body temperature if the user is in a hot environment. There are no consistent changes in respiratory rate or deep-tendon reflexes. Pupillary size is not significantly altered, but intraocular pressure is decreased because of effects on the ocular vasculature. Δ^9-THC and selected synthetic congeners have antiemetic effects.

Cannabinoids suppress cellular and humoral immune responses in animals and *in vitro*. Cannabinoids can also impair synthesis of nucleic acids and proteins. The practical significance of these findings is unclear. There is little correlation between the potency of cannabinoids in producing psychic effects and their capability to suppress immune response or inhibit protein synthesis. While cannabis is teratogenic in high doses in some species, no such effects have been definitively linked to the use of cannabinoids by man.

Conflicting data have been reported on the effects of chronic high doses of marihuana on human sexual function. Anovulatory cycles, lowered concentrations of testosterone, and reversible inhibition of spermatogenesis have been reported. There is inhibition of the hypothalamic-pituitary axis in male and female monkeys. When the mother is exposed to cannabis during pregnancy, the offspring (in both man and animals) may exhibit persistent effects on behavior, which are most evident in terms of learning and responses to stimuli (*see* Petersen, 1980; Institute of Medicine, 1982; Fehr and Kalant, 1983; Jones, 1983).

Chronic smoking of marihuana and hashish has long been associated with bronchitis and asthma; such smoking adversely affects pulmonary function and the bronchial epithelium, even in young people. However, the acute response to Δ^9-THC (given orally, intravenously, or by aerosol) is a significant and relatively long-lasting bronchodilatation to which little tolerance develops (Gong *et al.*, 1984). This effect is seen in both normal subjects and asthmatics. The "tar" produced by pyrolysis of marihuana is more carcinogenic to animals than is that derived from tobacco (*see* Petersen, 1980; Institute of Medicine, 1982).

Chronic marihuana users may exhibit apathy; dullness; impairment of judgment, concentration, and memory; and loss of interest in personal appearance and pursuit of conventional goals. This has been called the "amotivational syndrome." It is clear that this may be due in part to factors other than the use of cannabis, and it is difficult to know the contribution of drug use in any given case. Cessation may lead to gradual improvement over a period of several weeks (*see* Petersen, 1980; Institute of Medicine, 1982; Fehr and Kalant, 1983; Jones, 1983). At present there is no evidence to suggest that any personality changes are due to irreversible organic brain damage. The possibility of an adverse effect of frequent or chronic low levels of intoxication on developing personality cannot be dismissed.

Absorption, Fate, and Excretion. It is estimated that no more than 60% of Δ^9-THC in a marihuana cigarette is actually absorbed. Thus, a 1-g cigarette containing 2% Δ^9-THC would deliver at most 10 mg of Δ^9-THC to the lungs. Pharmacological effects occur within minutes after smoking begins; plasma concentrations reach their peak at 7 to 10 minutes; physiological and subjective effects are not maximal for 20 to 30 minutes (Perez-Reyes *et al.*, 1982). The subjective effects of a cigarette seldom last longer than 2 or 3 hours. After oral administration, the onset of effects usually occurs at about 0.5 to 1 hour; peak effects may not occur until the second or third hour and correlate well with plasma concentrations. Effects may persist for 3 to 5 hours. Although gastrointestinal absorption is largely complete, Δ^9-THC is extensively metabolized as it passes through the liver. Bioavailability for Δ^9-THC administered orally ranges from 6 to 20% (*see* Institute of Medicine, 1982; Wall *et al.*, 1983).

Δ^9-THC is rapidly converted into an active metabolite, 11-hydroxy-Δ^9-THC, which produces effects identical to those of the parent compound. 11-Hydroxy-Δ^9-THC is, in turn, converted into more polar, inactive metabolites (of which 11-nor-Δ^9-THC-9-carboxylic acid is the most common), which are then excreted in the urine and feces. Metabolites excreted in the bile may be reabsorbed. Very little unmetabolized Δ^9-THC is found in the urine. After reaching their peaks, plasma concentrations of Δ^9-THC and 11-hydroxy-Δ^9-THC fall rapidly at first (half-time of minutes), reflecting the redistribution of these lipophilic compounds to lipid-rich tissues, including the CNS. This first phase of rapid decline is followed by a much slower phase (half-time of about 30 hours), reflecting the gradual metabolism and elimination of the drug from the body. Traces of Δ^9-THC and its metabolites persist in the plasma of man for several days or weeks. Consumption of repeated oral doses of Δ^9-THC by man for several days or its daily smoking for several weeks does not seem to produce clinically detectable evidence of accumulation, although accumulation of inactive metabolites is likely. Chronic marihuana smokers metabolize Δ^9-THC more rapidly than do nonsmokers. Marihuana also alters the metabolism of barbiturates, antipyrine, and ethanol (*see* Institute of Medicine, 1982).

Tolerance and Physical Dependence. In animals, tolerance develops to the lethal, hypothermic, and some of the behavioral effects of cannabinoids. While in certain species the degree of tolerance is remarkable, it may not develop to all the effects of the drug. Most of the tolerance is due to functional or pharmacodynamic adaptations of the CNS, rather than to a more rapid metabolic disposition (*see* Harris *et al.,* 1977; Fehr and Kalant, 1983).

Reports from many countries indicate that a number of regular users of hashish consume amounts of Δ^9-THC that would produce toxic effects in most Western users. When volunteers are given Δ^9-THC orally every 4 hours (maximal dose of 210 mg per day), tolerance develops to drug-induced changes of mood, tachycardia, decrease in skin temperature, increase in body temperature, decrease in intraocular pressure, changes in the EEG, and impairment of performance on psychomotor tests. Tolerance to the cardiac effects develops within a few days and decays relatively quickly (48 hours) (*see* Jones *et al.,* 1976). If, however, the total dosage used is low, subjects continue to experience a "high" after the first cigarette of the day. Experienced users may actually report more subjective effects from smoking marihuana than naive subjects. However, they generally show less impairment of perceptual and motor functions, as well as smaller increases in heart rate.

Some degree of cross-tolerance between alcohol and Δ^9-THC has been observed in rats. However, there is no cross-tolerance between cannabinoids and the psychedelics (hallucinogens).

Abrupt discontinuation of cannabinoids after chronic use of high dosage is followed by irritability, restlessness, nervousness, decreased appetite, weight loss, and insomnia. There is a rebound increase in REM sleep, which is suppressed by marihuana. Tremor, increased body temperature, and chills may also occur. This syndrome, observed under laboratory conditions when high doses of the drug have been used every few hours for several weeks, is relatively mild, begins within a few hours after cessation of drug administration, and lasts about 4 to 5 days. The relationship between this relatively mild syndrome and cannabis-seeking behavior, if any, is unclear (*see* Jones *et al.,* 1976; Fehr and Kalant, 1983; Jones, 1983).

Therapeutic Uses. Marihuana, Δ^9-THC, and certain synthetic analogs have several potential therapeutic applications. These include antiemetic effects, especially against nausea and vomiting caused by cancer chemotherapeutic agents. Some synthetic cannabinoids may find use as analgesics or anticonvulsants. The capacity of some natural and synthetic cannabinoids to lower intraocular pressure has had little clinical utility to date.

Δ^9-THC given orally or smoked has been shown to be equal or superior to prochlorperazine or metoclopramide in reducing nausea caused by cancer chemotherapy, and it may be especially useful for patients who are refractory to standard treatment. The most common serious side effects are depersonalization and dysphoria, which older patients may find especially disturbing. Other side effects are somnolence, conjunctivitis, and tachycardia. The tachycardia may be prevented by a β-adrenergic antagonist, and there is some suggestion that phenothiazines reduce the subjective effects of Δ^9-THC and, possibly, augment antiemetic effects. Δ^9-THC is available in the United States for oral use as an antiemetic in hundreds of teaching hospitals and cancer centers under special arrangement with the federal government. In addition, many states have authorized the use of marihuana and/or Δ^9-THC by any physician for treatment of nausea related to chemotherapy (*see* Poster *et al.,* 1981).

Work with synthetic compounds shows that the psychological effects (both euphorigenic and psychotogenic) can be separated to some degree from the potential therapeutic actions. *Nabilone* is a synthetic analog that is significantly better than prochlorperazine in reducing nausea and vomiting associated with cancer chemotherapy. Effects begin within 30 to 60 minutes of an oral dose of 2 mg and peak at about 2 hours; the duration of action is about 8 hours. Side effects include somnolence, dizziness, dry mouth, and some mild euphoria. At higher dosage nabilone produces euphoria, tachycardia, and, occasionally, dysphoria and depersonalization. Some tolerance develops to these effects. Nabilone also lowers intraocular pressure and appears to be effective when applied topically. Nabilone is now available in several countries for oral use as an antiemetic (*see* Weintraub and Standish, 1983). *Levonantradol* is another synthetic cannabinoid with antiemetic actions.

Patterns of Use. In the United States and in many other countries the smoking of marihuana (also known as grass, pot, tea, weed, and reefer) increased sharply between the early 1960s and the mid-1970s, but it has since begun to decline. In 1982, 64% of young adults in the United States reported some experience with marihuana. During the month prior to the survey 28% had used marihuana at least once, and 7% reported daily use; 11% of this age group had reported daily use 3 years earlier. While still common in large urban areas, marihuana is now used among all socioeconomic and ethnic groups and in rural as well as urban areas (Miller *et al.,* 1983). There is a growing recognition that the use of marihuana, particularly among adolescents, is associated with adverse effects on health and productivity that continue into young adulthood (*see* Kandel, 1984).

PSYCHEDELICS (HALLUCINOGENS, PSYCHOTOMIMETICS, PSYCHOTOGENS)

There is no sharp line that divides the psychedelics from other classes of centrally active drugs. Under certain conditions, or at toxic dosage, several classes of drugs (anticholinergics, bromides, antimalarials, opioid antagonists, cocaine, amphetamines, and corticosteroids) can induce illusions, hallucinations, delusions, paranoid ideations, and other alterations of mood and thinking that are observed in spontaneously occurring psychotic states. However, despite the legal terminology that defines lysergic acid diethylamide (LSD) and related drugs as hallucinogens, the production of hallucinations is not the most useful way to describe the very interesting pharmacological effects of this group of drugs.

The psychedelic drugs to be discussed here can, indeed, produce such pathological effects as the terms *hallucinogenic, psychotomimetic,* and *psychotogenic* imply, but the feature that distinguishes the psychedelic agents from other classes of drugs is their capacity reliably to induce states of altered perception, thought, and feeling that are not experienced otherwise except in dreams or at times of religious exaltation.

Most descriptions of the "psychedelic state" include several major effects. There is heightened awareness of sensory input, often accompanied by an enhanced sense of clarity, but a diminished control over what is experienced. Frequently there is a feeling that one part of the self seems to be a passive observer (a "spectator ego") rather than an active organizing and directing force, while another part of the self participates and receives the vivid and unusual sensory experiences. The environment may be perceived as novel, often beautiful, and harmonious. The attention of the user is turned inward, preempted by the seeming clarity and portentous quality of his own thinking processes. In this state the slightest sensation may take on profound meaning. Indeed, "meaningfulness" seems more important than what is meant, and the "sense of truth" more significant than what is true. Commonly, there is a diminished capacity to differentiate the boundaries of one object from another and of the self from the environment. Associated with the loss of boundaries there may be a sense of union with "mankind" or the "cosmos." The drug-induced sensation that the mind is capable of seeing more than it can tell and of experiencing more than it can explain has led some to apply the term *mind expanding* to these agents (Freedman, 1968).

As with any scheme of classification, the choice of agents to include or exclude is somewhat arbitrary. Most of the drugs that are generally included among the psychedelics are related either to the indolealkylamines, such as LSD, psilocybin,

psilocin, dimethyltryptamine (DMT), and diethyltryptamine (DET), or to the phenylethylamines (mescaline) or phenylisopropylamines, such as 2,5-dimethoxy-4-methylamphetamine (DOM, "STP"). However, even when a drug produces a profile of pharmacological effects that is quite similar to those of LSD at one dose level, it may produce other effects as the dose is raised. Thus, at low dosage, dimethoxyamphetamine (DMA) has primarily LSD-like effects, but it is more like amphetamine as the dose is raised. Martin and Sloan (1977b) have proposed three criteria for categorizing LSD-like drugs: (1) subjective effects and neurophysiological actions; (2) cross-tolerance between compounds; and (3) response to selective antagonists. By application of these criteria they have classified a variety of compounds that produce changes in perception and mood into five categories: (I) LSD-like: LSD, mescaline, psilocybin, psilocin; (II) probably LSD-like: DMA, DOM, tryptamine, DMT, numerous congeners of lysergic acid; (III) probably LSD-like but with other properties: 3,4-methylenedioxyamphetamine (MDA), 5-methoxy-3,4-methylenedioxyamphetamine (MMDA); (IV) probably not LSD-like: D-2-bromlysergic acid diethylamide (BOL), 5-hydroxytryptophan; and (V) not LSD-like: amphetamine, β-phenethylamine (PEA), 2,5-dimethoxy-4-ethylamphetamine (DOET), bufotenine, L-LSD, scopolamine, Δ^9-THC.

A number of compounds produce alterations of mood and perception that are so obviously distinct as to merit separate discussion. Included among these are phencyclidine, certain opioid agonist-antagonists (considered in Chapter 22), and inhalants such as nitrous oxide and certain volatile solvents.

LSD and Related Compounds. *History.* Drugs that induce psychedelic effects have been used for centuries. The peyote cactus (containing mescaline) and mushrooms (containing psilocin) were being used by the natives of Mexico and the Southwestern United States at the time of the Spanish conquest. There was a brief period of scientific interest in mescaline at the beginning of this century and again in the 1930s. However, Hoffman's discovery in 1943 of the psychedelic effects of LSD and its remarkable potency stimulated interest among scientists who felt its study might facilitate understanding of mental illness. In the 1950s hundreds of scientific papers were written on the effects of LSD on biological systems *in vitro*, animal behavior, patients with a wide range of physical and mental illnesses, and normal human volunteers. The effects of LSD then caught the attention of students, writers, and others more interested in its possibilities for self-exploration than for scientific investigation. Within a matter of a few years its use spread among young people, abetted by persuasive advocates who counseled young people to "turn on, tune in, and drop out." More conservative elements of society, made anxious as much by the unconventional life style associated with the use of LSD as by its known and suspected toxicities, passed laws and regulations designed to limit its availability. By 1970, LSD was included in the same regulatory category as heroin. Despite such laws the drug, which is relatively easy to manufacture, remains available and is still used. Chemists have also produced dozens of congeners of indoleamine and phenethylamine that cause subjective effects similar to those of LSD. The burdensome regulations and the recognition that LSD does not produce a "model psychosis" have markedly diminished its use in scientific investigations.

Chemistry. The structures of LSD, mescaline, psilocin, and several related compounds are shown in Table 23–1. The diversity of compounds included here precludes a consideration of structure-activity relationships (but *see* comments under Mechanism of Action).

Mechanism of Action. LSD and related psychedelic drugs have actions at multiple sites in the CNS, from the cortex to the spinal cord. Some of the best studied of these involve agonistic actions at presynaptic receptors for 5-hydroxytryptamine (5-HT) in the midbrain. An earlier view that the subjective effects were due to blockade of 5-HT now seems untenable. The firing rate of neurons in the dorsal raphe nuclei is sharply reduced after small doses of LSD are administered systemically. 5-HT itself is inhibitory when applied iontophoreti-

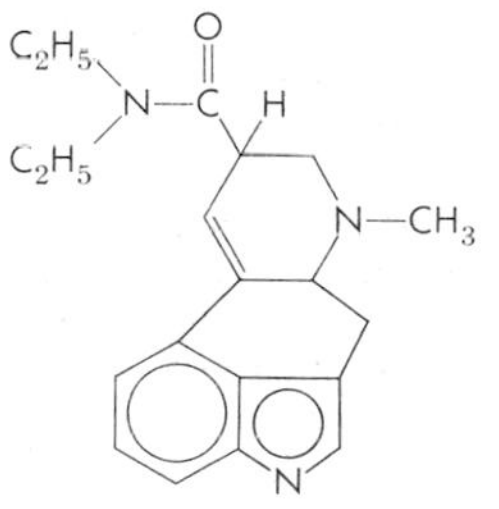

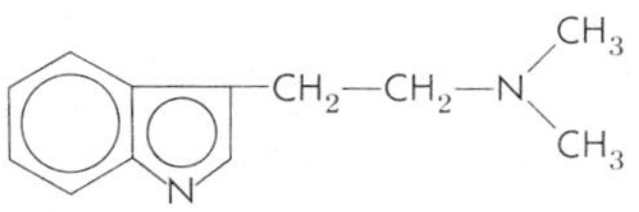

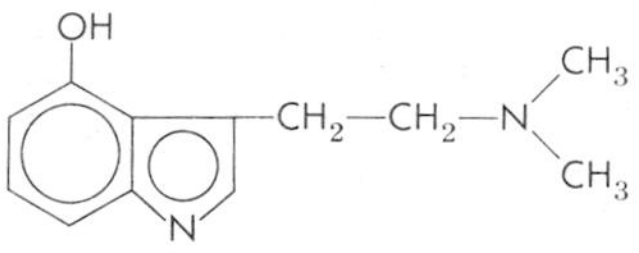

Table 23–1. STRUCTURAL FORMULAS AND CLASSIFICATION OF SELECTED PSYCHEDELIC DRUGS *

LSD-LIKE

Indoleamines

LSD

DMT

Psilocin

β-Phenethylamines

Mescaline

DOM

DMA

MIXED

MDA

MMDA

AMPHETAMINE-LIKE

Amphetamine

p-Methoxyamphetamine

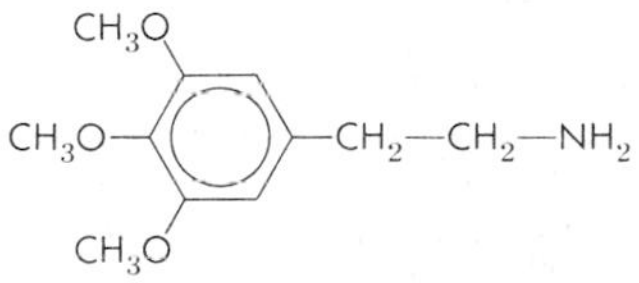

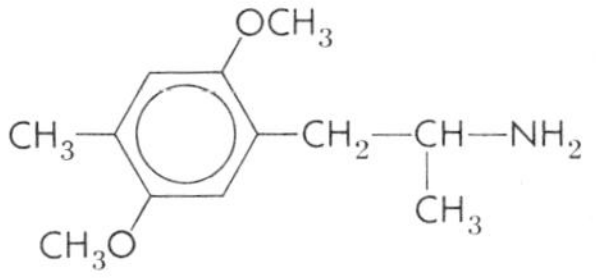

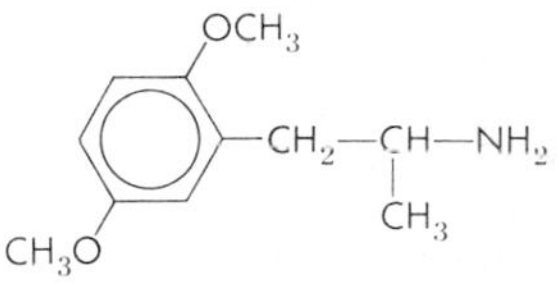

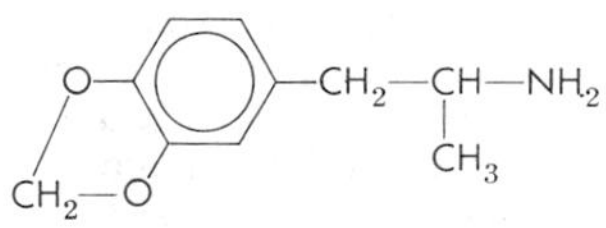

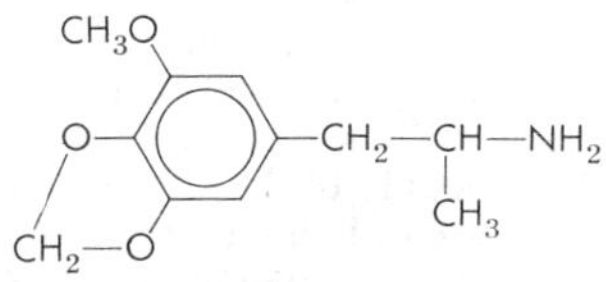

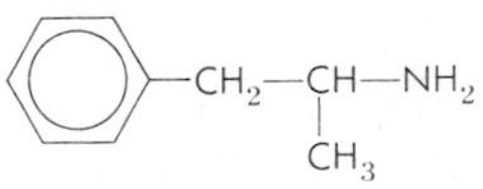

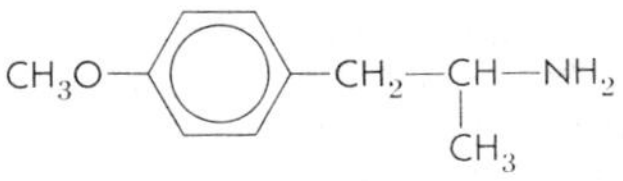

* Based on classification of Martin and associates, 1978.

cally to 5-HT-containing neurons in the dorsal raphe nuclei or to those neurons of the forebrain to which the dorsal raphe neurons project. While tryptamine produces inhibition about equally at both sites, LSD, psilocin, and DMT are considerably more potent in producing inhibition at the presumed presynaptic sites on the dorsal raphe neurons (Haigler and Aghajanian, 1977).

Based on ligand-binding studies, there are at least two distinct receptors for 5-HT in the CNS. However, neither of these appears to correspond to the presynaptic autoreceptor where LSD is hypothesized to exert important actions. LSD binds with approximately equal affinity to 5-HT$_1$ and 5-HT$_2$ receptors, as does the very potent but nonhallucinogenic ergot analog lisuride. Both drugs produce similar changes in the rate of firing of 5-HT-containing neurons. Haloperidol, which can block the hallucinogenic actions of LSD and mescaline, has a 400-fold greater affinity for the 5-HT$_2$ receptor than the 5-HT$_1$ receptor (Peroutka and Snyder, 1983). The precise mechanism by which LSD and related agents produce their subjective effects remains quite uncertain.

Pharmacological Effects. In man, oral doses of LSD as low as 20 to 25 μg produce CNS effects in susceptible individuals. At such doses there are few detectable effects on other organ systems.

Some of the features that distinguish the psychedelic state from other effects produced by drugs have already been described. In addition, LSD produces somatic effects largely sympathomimetic in nature, such as pupillary dilatation, increase in blood pressure, tachycardia, hyperreflexia, tremor, nausea, piloerection, muscular weakness, and increased body temperature.

Following oral doses of 0.5 to 2 μg/kg the somatic symptoms are usually perceived within a few minutes. These include dizziness, weakness, drowsiness, nausea, and paresthesias. They may be followed by a feeling of inner tension relieved by laughing or crying. Several feelings may seem to coexist at the same time, although euphoric effects tend to predominate. In the second or third hour, visual illusions, wavelike recurrences of perceptual changes (*e.g.*, micropsia, macropsia), and affective symptoms may occur. There may be difficulty in locating the source of a sound; the user may be hypervigilant or withdrawn, or may alternate between these states. With many subjects there is a fear of fragmentation or disintegration of the self. Afterimages are prolonged, and the overlapping of present and preceding perceptions occurs. Some subjects recognize these confluences, whereas others elaborate them into hallucinations. In contrast to naturally occurring psychoses, auditory hallucinations are rare. Synesthesias, the overflow from one sensory modality to another, may occur. Colors are heard and sounds may be seen. Subjective time is also seriously altered, so that clock time seems to pass extremely slowly. The loss of boundaries and the fear of fragmentation create a need for a structuring or supporting environment; and, in the sense that they create a need for experienced companions and an explanatory system, these drugs are "cultogenic." During the "trip,"

thoughts and memories can vividly emerge under self-guidance or unexpectedly, to the user's distress. Mood may be labile, shifting from depression to gaiety, from elation to fear. Tension and anxiety may mount and reach panic proportions. After about 4 to 5 hours, if a major panic episode does not occur, there may be a sense of detachment and the conviction that one is magically in control.

Between the dose ranges of 1 to 16 μg/kg, the intensity of the psychophysiological effects of LSD is proportional to the dose. The entire syndrome, including the pupillary dilatation, begins to clear after about 12 hours, although the half-life of the drug in man is approximately 3 hours (*see* Cohen, 1967; Freedman, 1969).

While the user may be greatly impressed with the drug experience and feel a greater sensitivity for art, music, human feelings, and the harmony of the universe, there is little evidence for long-term changes in personality, beliefs, values, or behavior.

Although the patterns of psychological and biochemical effects seen with other agents are quite similar to those with LSD, there are significant differences in potency, absorption, metabolism, duration of action, and the slope of the dose-response curves. DMT, for example, is inactive by mouth and must be injected, sniffed, or smoked to produce effects. LSD is longer acting and more than 100 times as potent as psilocybin and psilocin, the active alkaloids in the Mexican "magic mushroom"; it is 4000 times as potent as mescaline in producing altered states of consciousness. There may also be some differences in the frequency of somatic effects, such as more vomiting with mescaline. The effects of an oral dose of mescaline (about 5 mg/kg) persist for about 12 hours. DOM and DOET are particularly interesting in that at low doses they produce mild euphoria and enhanced self-awareness without perceptual distortion or hallucinogenic effects. At higher doses DOM has typical psychedelic activity, but with DOET there appears to be a rather wide dose range over which euphoria and self-awareness are produced without perceptual distortions. Infusions of tryptamine produce a profile of actions quite similar to those of LSD, including facilitation of spinal flexor reflexes, increases in respiratory rate, blood pressure, pulse, and pupillary diameter, wakefulness, desynchronization of the EEG, suppression of REM sleep, and perceptual distortions (*see* Martin and Sloan, 1977b). Most of the pharmacological actions of LSD, tryptamine, and, presumably, drugs with similar profiles are antagonized by chlorpromazine and cyproheptadine but not by α-adrenergic antagonists such as phenoxybenzamine.

Incidence and Patterns of Use. In the United States, the use of LSD ("acid") and related psychedelics reached a peak of popularity in the late 1960s and thereafter gradually declined. Psychedelic drugs are manufactured illegally and are still available through illicit channels. In 1982, approximately 21% of people in the United States aged 18 to 25 indicated use of hallucinogens at some time in their lives; only 1 or 2% had used such drugs during the preceding 30 days (Miller *et al.*, 1983).

In general, these drugs do not give rise to patterns of repetitive use over prolonged periods. The most common psychedelic-use pattern is the occasional "trip," separated by intervals of weeks or months during which marihuana is used with variable frequency. The "acid head," or chronic user, is quite uncommon, and even among this group "trips" are rarely more frequent than biweekly. Chronic users may complain of memory difficulties and seem to exhibit extreme passivity. For most users the "psychedelic scene" tends to become less interesting with time. Even though the smoking of marihuana may continue, the use of the potent psychedelics is generally discontinued.

Tolerance, Toxicity, and Physical Dependence. A high degree of tolerance to the behavioral effects of LSD develops after three or four daily doses; sensitivity returns after a comparable drug-free interval. Tolerance to the cardiovascular effects is less pronounced. There is considerable cross-tolerance between LSD, mescaline, and psilocybin, but none between LSD and the amphetamines or between LSD-like drugs and scopolamine or Δ^9-THC. Curiously, DMT induces little cross-tolerance to LSD, perhaps because of the short duration of action of DMT. Withdrawal phenomena are not seen after abrupt discontinuation of LSD-like drugs. In man, deaths attributable to *direct* effects of LSD are unknown, although fatal accidents and suicides during states of LSD intoxication have occurred. Death due to overdosage in animals results from respiratory failure, but in rabbits there is a marked hyperthermia as well. There appears to be a higher incidence of spontaneous abortion and fetal abnormalities among women who use illicit LSD, but the effects of pure LSD on pregnancy and the fetus remain uncertain (*see* Finnegan and Fehr, 1980). Among American Indian tribes that have used mescaline for several generations there appears to be no striking increase in genetic abnormalities or congenital malformations.

The evidence for significant psychological hazards in the use of psychedelic agents is unambiguous. The most common adverse effect is a temporary (24-hour) episode of panic—a "bad trip." This can be treated by reassurance in a supportive and familiar environment ("talking down"), antianxiety agents, or induction of sleep with barbiturates. Although phenothiazines antagonize the effects of LSD, they are usually not needed. Such "bad trips" cannot be reliably prevented and have been experienced even by users who had previous "good trips." Recurrences of drug effects without the drug, "flashbacks," are a puzzling phenomenon; they occur in more than 15% of users. Commonly precipitated by use of marihuana, anxiety, fatigue, or movement into a dark environment, "flashbacks" may persist intermittently for several years after the last exposure to LSD. They are exacerbated by the use of phenothiazines (*see* Abraham, 1983). In some individuals the use of psychedelics can precipitate serious depressions, paranoid behavior, or prolonged psychotic episodes. Whether such episodes would have occurred without the drug is not clear. Prolonged psychotic episodes following repeated use of LSD tend to resemble naturally occurring schizophreniform

psychotic states, and the prognosis appears to be similar (*see* Vardy and Kay, 1983). There is the possibility that repeated use of LSD can induce subtle deficits in the capacity for abstract thinking (Tucker *et al.*, 1972).

Therapeutic Uses. LSD has been proposed as an aid in psychotherapy, as an adjunct to the treatment of alcoholism and opioid addiction, and as a device to induce tranquility and reduce the need for opioid analgesics in cases of terminal cancer. In each situation, the use has been abandoned either because controlled studies have failed to demonstrate the value of LSD or because the elaborate precautions required to minimize adverse psychological reactions dampened enthusiasm and rendered its therapeutic use impractical.

ARYLCYCLOHEXYLAMINES

Phencyclidine and Related Compounds. *History and Source.* Phencyclidine, developed in the 1950s, was first used as an anesthetic for animals and, for a short time, as a general anesthetic in man. It fell into disuse quickly because patients experienced delirium when they emerged from anesthesia. Phencyclidine gained popularity in the early 1970s, when it became available as a drug to be smoked or "snorted." By the mid-1970s it was one of the most widely abused drugs in the United States; the prevalence of such use has declined sharply in the 1980s. The compound is relatively easy to synthesize, and it is known among drug abusers by a number of street names, among which are angel dust, crystal, horse tranquilizer, PCP, and peace pill. It is no longer used as a veterinary anesthetic, and the drug that is used illicitly is produced in clandestine laboratories and varies widely in purity. Phencyclidine is frequently misrepresented as LSD, mescaline, or Δ^9-THC. Many congeners with similar profiles of effects are now known, and some have been produced illicitly.

Chemistry. Phencyclidine is one of a group of arylcyclohexylamines. A related compound, ketamine, is still used as an anesthetic in man. The structural formula of phencyclidine is as follows:

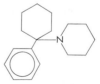

Phencyclidine

Pharmacological Actions. Phencyclidine and related arylcyclohexylamines have CNS-stimulant, CNS-depressant, hallucinogenic, and analgesic actions. The term *dissociative anesthetic* has been used to describe these drugs; they appear to represent a distinct category of agents in terms of their actions, as well as in terms of their properties in animal models.

In man, small doses produce a subjective sense of intoxication, with staggering gait, slurred speech, nystagmus, and numbness of the extremities. Users may exhibit sweating, catatonic muscular rigidity, and a blank stare; they may also experience changes in body image and disorganized thought, drowsiness, and apathy. There may be hostile and bizarre behavior. Amnesia for the episode may occur. With increasing dosage analgesia is more marked, and anesthesia, stupor, or coma may occur, although the eyes may remain open. Sensory impulses reach the cortex, but the individual experiences them in a distorted form. Heart rate and blood pressure are elevated; there is hypersalivation, sweating, fever, repetitive movements, and muscle rigidity on stimulation. At even higher doses prolonged coma, muscle rigidity, and convulsions may occur (for references, *see* Petersen and Stillman, 1978; Aniline and Pitts, 1982).

Monkeys with implanted catheters do not administer LSD to themselves, but they do self-administer phencyclidine. Few drugs seem to induce so wide a range of subjective effects. Among those effects that users seem to like are increased sensitivity to external stimuli, stimulation, mood elevation, and a sense of intoxication. Other effects, some of which appear to occur with every use, are described as unwanted; these include perceptual disturbances, restlessness, disorientation, and anxiety. The typical "high" from a single dose lasts 4 to 6 hours and is followed by an extended "coming-down" period.

At the cellular level, phencyclidine may interact with several neurotransmitter systems. It inhibits the re-uptake of dopamine, 5-HT, and norepinephrine by synaptosomes. However, its pharmacological effects are neither blocked nor mimicked by known transmitter agonists or antagonists. PCP and its psychoactive congeners exhibit saturable and stereospecific binding to distinct macromolecular sites in the CNS; the binding affinities of these compounds correlate well with psychoactive potencies, and the sites of interaction have a distinct distribution within the CNS. Recent evidence indicates that the PCP receptor may be related to the σ-opioid receptor, the binding site for N-allyl normetazocine. The latter drug has psychotomimetic actions and is also a μ-opioid antagonist. The μ-antagonist actions are due exclusively to the $(-)$ isomer of N-allyl normetazocine, while PCP-like actions and subjective effects are associated primarily with the $(+)$ isomer. The potency of PCP-like congeners to produce CNS effects appears to correlate with their ability to block K^+ conductance (*see* Lazdunski *et al.*, 1983; Quirion *et al.*, 1983; Zukin and Zukin, 1983).

Absorption, Fate, and Excretion. Phencyclidine is well absorbed following all routes of administration. The parent compound may be hydroxylated, and these metabolites are conjugated with glucuronic acid. While some of the metabolites are active, most of the pharmacological effects are due to phencyclidine itself. Only a small fraction of the drug is excreted unchanged. Phencyclidine is a weak base, and lowering urinary pH (to below 5.0) with ammonium chloride markedly accelerates its excretion. Decreases in plasma pH produce decreases in the concentration of the drug in the cerebrospinal fluid; signs of intoxication referable to

the CNS are thereby reduced. There is considerable gastroenteric recirculation, and continuous gastric suction can be of value in the treatment of overdosage. In cases of overdose, the half-life of phencyclidine appears to be about 3 days, but this value can be shortened to about 1 day by continuous gastric suction and acidification of the urine (Aronow and Done, 1978; Aniline and Pitts, 1982).

Patterns of Use, Tolerance, and Physical Dependence. Because phencyclidine and congeners are often misrepresented, the true extent of their use is uncertain and may be underestimated. About half of current users claim to take phencyclidine about once a week. "Runs" also occur and consist in use for 2 to 3 days, during which the users do not sleep and eat very little. There is then a prolonged sleep, from which the user often awakens depressed and disoriented. A few take the drug several times per day. Most commonly, several users participate; the drug is often sprinkled on tobacco, marihuana, or parsley and smoked after making the material into a cigarette. The drug may also be snorted or taken orally or intravenously. The amount of phencyclidine in a cigarette varies from 1 to 100 mg, and chronic users may ingest up to 1 g in 24 hours (*see* Aniline and Pitts, 1982).

In animals, tolerance develops to the behavioral and toxic effects of phencyclidine, but the extent varies with the species. Abrupt withdrawal after chronic use is followed by fearfulness, tremors, and facial twitches (*see* Balster and Wessinger, 1983). Clinical observations suggest that tolerance also develops in man; in addition, some chronic users make vague complaints about craving after stopping. Chronic users of large doses report persistent difficulties with recent memory, speech, and thinking that last from 6 months to 1 year after stopping. Personality changes ranging from social withdrawal and isolation to states of anxiety, nervousness, and severe depression have also been reported (*see* Petersen and Stillman, 1978).

Toxicity and Treatment of Overdose. The frequency of adverse effects is uncertain, but deaths due to direct toxicity, violent behavior, and accidents have been reported. Phencyclidine can cause acute behavioral toxicity (intoxication, aggression, brief confusional states), coma or convulsions (from severe overdosage), and psychotic states. The last-named condition may be long lasting. People with schizophrenia may be particularly vulnerable to the psychotogenic actions of phencyclidine.

Treatment of overdosage is symptomatic and is directed at protecting the patient and others from the effects of impaired behavior and judgment and at supporting vital functions. Hastening excretion by continuous gastric suction and acidification of the urine can substantially shorten the half-life of the drug but can also increase the risk of renal failure if there is significant rhabdomyolysis and myoglobinuria. Hypersalivation may require suction, respiratory depression may require artificial ventilation, and fever may require external cooling. Convulsions have been treated with diazepam and hypertension with hydralazine. "Talking down" is not helpful, and clinicians advise isolation of patients from external stimuli to the degree compatible with support of vital functions and control of violent or self-destructive behavior. Where possible, four or five burly aides are superior to mechanical restraints, since excessive muscle contractions may aggravate rhabdomyolysis. Coma may be preceded or followed by delirium, paranoia, and assaultive behavior, and clinical arrangements must take this into consideration. A psychotic phase may last for several weeks after a single dose of phencyclidine (see Aronow and Done, 1978; Petersen and Stillman, 1978; Aniline and Pitts, 1982).

MISCELLANEOUS SUBSTANCES USED FOR SUBJECTIVE EFFECTS

The catalog of agents that have been used to produce subjective changes is impressive, and each generation not only adds a few new substances but seems impelled to reevaluate the old.

Inhalants: Anesthetic Gases and Solvents. The intoxicating and euphorigenic effects of both nitrous oxide and ethyl ether were recognized before their potential as anesthetics was appreciated. In the nineteenth century, efforts to reduce alcoholism in Ireland by means of ether were markedly successful, but the use of ether became so widespread that it was necessary to take steps to reeducate the public to the use of alcohol. When access to alcohol or other intoxicants is restricted by finances, laws, or incarceration, substances with marked toxicity such as antifreeze, paint thinner, and other industrial solvents may be used. Since adolescents are usually prohibited from using alcoholic beverages, "glue sniffing" may fall into this category. However, prohibition of alcohol cannot fully explain such behavior. Physicians, dentists, and nurses with access to a wide variety of drugs have been known to inhale anesthetic gases, sometimes with catastrophic outcomes for themselves and their patients. The alkyl nitrites (butyl, isobutyl, and amyl), used medically as vasodilators, have become popular as aphrodisiacs. Inhalation of these agents is said to intensify and prolong orgasm. In 1980, about 17% of young adults (aged 18 to 25) indicated some experience with inhalants; a significantly higher percentage indicated experience with orgasms.

Animals will administer nitrous oxide, chloroform, and solvents (e.g., toluene) to themselves; however, only a few of the many compounds have been systematically studied. Mice made tolerant to nitrous oxide are not cross-tolerant to barbiturates, although cross-tolerance and cross-dependence between barbiturates and chloroform have been reported (see Sharp and Brehm, 1977). While high doses of these substances produce depression of the CNS, low doses of most of these "anesthetics" and solvents produce increased activity that is usually thought to be due to disinhibition.

Because toxicity varies greatly with the specific substance, it can be discussed only in general terms. The causes of fatalities are not clear; most appear to involve cardiac arrhythmias. Inhalation of volatile material from a plastic bag (a common practice) may result in hypoxia as well as an extremely high concentration of vapor. Aerosol propellants containing fluorinated hydrocarbons produce cardiac arrhythmias, and ischemia increases sensitivity to fluorocarbon-induced arrhythmias. Chlorinated solvents (e.g., trichloroethylene) depress myocardial contractility, and sympathetic activity is thereby increased reflexly. Ketones can produce pulmonary hypertension. Neurological impairment may occur with a variety of solvents. Peripheral neuropathies and progressive, fatal neurological deterioration have followed the "huffing" of lacquer thinner; however, because of the complexity of the mixture, the specific etiological agents are unknown. Studies of inhalers of aerosol paints have found indications of long-lasting brain damage (see Sharp and Brehm, 1977; Sharp and Carroll, 1978).

Other Agents. In large amounts, the common household spice nutmeg produces marked subjective changes. It is commonly used for this purpose by the inmates of prisons. The oral ingestion of the equivalent of two grated nutmegs produces, after a latency of several hours, leaden feelings in the extremities and a mental state that may include feelings of depersonalization and unreality. Agitation and apprehension are also common. Dry mouth, thirst, rapid heart rate, and red, flushed face are common and may mimic atropine poisoning (see Weil, 1967).

The medically inappropriate, excessive use of nonopioid analgesic mixtures (containing aspirin, phenacetin, caffeine, etc.) has been reported. Such use, however, is not characterized by extreme psychological dependence. Conceivably, excessive use of such drugs may be related to the mood-elevating effects of the caffeine, or to certain misconceptions about the capacity of such mixtures to relieve tension and increase the user's ability to concentrate on tedious tasks. Most investigators feel that tolerance and a limited degree of psychological dependence develop with caffeine and a withdrawal headache has been described repeatedly. Caffeine as a drug of abuse has been reviewed by Gilbert (1976) and Greden (1981).

For untold generations, peyote, ololiuqui (from the seeds of the morning glory, Rivea corymbosa), and "magic mushrooms" have been used to produce altered states of consciousness by the Indians of the North American continent. Throughout the world, many other substances are used for similar mind- and mood-changing effects. These include the use of kava in the South Pacific, indole-containing snuff among the Amazonian Indians in Brazil, and fly agaric among the Uralic-speaking tribes of Siberia. A discussion of the pharmacology and the use patterns of these substances is beyond the scope of this chapter. The interested reader should consult Efron and associates (1967).

TREATMENT

The indications for treatment vary with the drugs being used as well as with the social and cultural factors determining the particular pattern of drug use. Some patterns of drug use, such as the "recreational" (weekly or less frequent) use of marihuana, do not require treatment any more than does the occasional smoking of tobacco or the social use of alcohol. Such casual use is not without hazard, but this does not imply a treatable disorder. It is likely that changing views about drug use will continue to create gray areas where the indications for treatment are unclear. However, there is general agreement that treatment is appropriate for the adverse consequences of drug use and for the compulsive drug user who voluntarily seeks help.

WITHDRAWAL TECHNICS

Over the past decade, many views about withdrawal of drugs have been modified. No longer do all clinicians adhere to the view that drug withdrawal must be the first step in treatment of the drug-dependent individual or that treatment requires a carefully controlled, drug-free environment. Under appropriate circumstances successful withdrawal from opioids, alcohol, barbiturates, benzodiazepines, amphetamines, and cocaine has been accomplished on an ambulatory basis. However, successful ambulatory withdrawal requires the establishment of a positive therapeutic relationship and considerable clinical experience. Withdrawal from tobacco has been and remains an outpatient procedure. For the other drugs, withdrawal is usually more easily and more rapidly accomplished in an inpatient or residential setting where access to drugs can be controlled, the withdrawal syndrome observed, and appropriate treatment provided. When many addicted patients are being treated in the same treatment unit, drug smuggling can cause problems. However, when only an occasional patient is involved, it merely delays or prevents the completion of withdrawal; it should not unduly discourage attempts at treatment. Withdrawal in a controlled setting is obviously considerably more costly.

Certain general principles apply irrespective of the particular drug or drugs the patient has been using. (1) The *degree of physical dependence,* if any, that may have developed to each drug the patient has been using should be estimated. (2) A *medical history* should be taken and a physical examination carried out, to determine if there are any indications that the usual withdrawal technics should be modified. For example, a more gradual reduction of opioids would be appropriate in patients with angina pectoris, ulcerative colitis, pulmonary insufficiency, or other debilitating illness. Needless to say, patients who are experiencing severe pain from obvious causes are not appropriate candidates for withdrawal of opioid analgesics until some alternative method of managing the pain

is available. Clonidine, which has some analgesic properties, is sometimes particularly useful in this situation. (3) The patient should be given sufficient quantities of whichever *drugs* are necessary *to suppress severe withdrawal symptoms,* and the dose of these drugs is then gradually reduced.

Estimating the degree of physical dependence on opioids or on general CNS depressants from the history alone is difficult, since patients often distort their history of drug use. However, their motives vary widely, and so does the manner in which the history is distorted. For example, heroin users are usually unaware of the purity of the drugs they have been using. They tend to exaggerate their usage considerably and may also claim to be using large quantities of barbiturates or other sedatives in the hope that the doctor will then provide them with more generous amounts of opioids or hypnotics. Conversely, some individuals who use illicit drugs may completely deny the intake of barbiturates, even when they have been using a sufficient quantity to produce a dangerous degree of physical dependence. Others, who have used paregoric or cough medicines in an alcoholic vehicle, are often unaware of the large amounts of alcohol they consume. The possibility of physical dependence on general CNS depressants should always be considered when a patient who has had sufficient opioids to suppress withdrawal symptoms remains sleepless and jittery. In striking contrast are those addicts, such as physicians and nurses, who do not obtain their drugs through illicit traffic and who may attempt to minimize the extent of their use. The difficulty in getting an accurate history means that the physician must place great reliance on observation of the patient and on his familiarity with the symptoms of withdrawal from both opioids and general depressants.

While withdrawal syndromes are observed after abrupt cessation of other types of drugs (CNS stimulants, tobacco, arylcyclohexylamines, and cannabis), there is no consensus on how the syndromes are best managed. With the exception of the recent introduction of nicotine chewing gum, there is little evidence of benefit from treatment other than abrupt withdrawal.

Withdrawal of Opioids. Even with very gradual reduction in dosage, most patients will perceive some withdrawal symptoms. It may be possible, of course, to continue to give the patient the drug he was using (heroin, morphine, meperidine, *etc.*) and simply reduce the dose over a period of several days. However, for reasons already discussed, methadone is quite suitable for suppressing withdrawal symptoms and can be substituted for any of the natural or synthetic opioid analgesics currently in use. With *methadone substitution,* in an inpatient or residential setting, now considered the standard technic, the opioid withdrawal symptoms are rarely worse than those of a moderate "influenza-like" syndrome. There are, however, newer methods that use other drugs, settings, and time frames that may have advantages (*see* below).

The dose of methadone will vary with the degree of physical dependence and the medical condition of the patient. The patient is observed and, if significant withdrawal symptoms appear, an initial dose of methadone that rarely needs to exceed 15 to 20 mg is given orally. Additional methadone can be given if the symptoms are not suppressed or each time withdrawal symptoms reappear. It is rarely necessary to give more than 80 mg of methadone over the first 24 hours. After the patient has been observed for 24 to 36 hours and given methadone as described, it becomes a relatively simple matter to calculate a stabilization dose. Compared to its analgesic effects, methadone is more potent and acts longer to suppress withdrawal symptoms. Usually 1 mg of methadone can substitute for 4 mg of morphine, 2 mg of heroin, or 20 mg of meperidine. Reduction can be started as soon as the dose for stabilization has been determined. In hospitalized patients, reduction each day of 20% of the total daily dose is well tolerated and causes little discomfort. If the patient is not vomiting, methadone should be given by mouth and need not be given more frequently than twice a day. The majority of inpatients can be completely withdrawn from opioids in less than 10 days, although mild abstinence symptoms may persist for a number of days after the last dose of methadone. The protracted abstinence syndrome has been described above.

A number of clinicians have found that after a period of social stabilization (usually 6 to 18 months) many former heroin addicts maintained on methadone can be gradually withdrawn from methadone entirely on an ambulatory basis. Even though the dosage is reduced very slowly (*e.g.*, by less than 10% of the stabilization dose per week or by as little as 3 mg per week), many of these patients experience opioid withdrawal symptoms when the daily dosage of methadone is reduced to about 10 to 30 mg. Some patients are able to tolerate the discomfort and the psychological difficulties, complete the withdrawal process, and do not relapse to opioid use. Others complete the withdrawal process but later relapse to heroin use, and still others elect to discontinue withdrawal and remain on maintenance doses of methadone. Exceedingly gradual reduction of dosage is more likely to be successful for ambulatory patients (Senay *et al.*, 1977). Among the symptoms experienced over a period lasting up to several months after withdrawal are insomnia, irritability, restlessness, malaise, pain, fatigue, premature ejaculation, and gastrointestinal hyperactivity (Cushman and Dole, 1973).

Many nonopioids have been used for the opioid withdrawal syndrome; few have proven to have significant value. Certain drugs such as reserpine have a demonstrably aggravating effect on the course of withdrawal. The phenothiazines have not been demonstrated to be of significant help. Nighttime sedation with the barbiturates or related sedative-hypnotics is helpful, but complete suppression of opioid withdrawal symptoms with such agents alone cannot be achieved short of anesthetic doses. Clonidine, a centrally acting α_2-adrenergic agonist, can suppress some components of the opioid withdrawal syndrome in patients who are withdrawn from low-to-moderate doses of methadone. Methadone is abruptly discontinued, and clonidine is given for 7 to 10 days (10 to 25 $\mu g/kg$ per day) to suppress symptoms; clonidine is then withdrawn gradually over 3 to 4 days. The primary side effects are dry mouth, sedation, and orthostatic hypotension. Clonidine is more effective in suppressing autonomic signs and symptoms of withdrawal (*e.g.*, nausea, vomiting, diarrhea) than subjective discomfort or craving. Anxiety, restlessness, insomnia, and muscular aching are suppressed only minimally (*see* Charney *et al.*, 1982). Other α_2-adrenergic agonists, such as guanabenz, are also useful in ameliorating some aspects of the opioid withdrawal syndrome (Washton and Resnick, 1981). The theoretical basis for the use of clonidine has been discussed above.

Some patients have difficulty in tolerating the persistent low level of discomfort that is associated with slow withdrawal of methadone and express a preference to "get it over with faster." Once patients require only low doses of methadone (5 to 10 mg per day), this can be accomplished by administration of repeated doses (1.2 mg) of naloxone every 30 minutes for several hours. While the withdrawal can be quite uncomfortable, the severity of the syndrome subsides after the first 3 to 6 hours and it is then possible to give the patients a longer-acting antagonist such as naltrexone. Clonidine has also been used to ameliorate the symptoms of antagonist-precipitated withdrawal from opioids (*see* Charney *et al.*, 1982).

Withdrawal of General CNS Depressants (Barbiturates and Related Drugs). Abrupt withdrawal of general CNS depressants that have been used in high doses over prolonged periods can be fatal. Nevertheless, some European clinicians with considerable experience feel that abrupt withdrawal has its advantages; they administer sedatives only if a delirium develops or if the patient has more than one seizure. In the United States, where there is considerably more abuse of short-acting barbiturates, abrupt withdrawal is not considered a safe technic, and the administration of a suitable general CNS depressant is usually started before major withdrawal symptoms develop. Pentobarbital (orally) can be substituted for any barbiturate the patient has been using. Clinical observations suggest that it is also a suitable substitute for glutethimide, paraldehyde, chloral hydrate, and meprobamate and for the suppression of the alcohol withdrawal syndrome. Sufficient pentobarbital should be given to produce mild intoxication, that is, slight ataxia, nystagmus, and slurred speech. Most patients require from 0.2 to 0.4 g every 6 hours, but some may need up to 2.5 g over a 24-hour period. The daily dose can be estimated from the response to a 200-mg pentobarbital test dose. Once a level of mild intoxication has been achieved, the dosage of pentobarbital should be maintained for at least 24 to 36 hours. At this level, the patient should be free of tremulousness, irritability, and insomnia. The amount of barbiturate required for this initial period becomes the *stabilization level.*

Once the above-described stabilization level has been reliably established and the patient observed for 1 to 2 days, gradual withdrawal can be started. Clinical experience has shown that most patients can tolerate reductions of 0.1 g of pentobarbital per day without significant discomfort. With the use of the pentobarbital-substitution technic, withdrawal may take from 10 days to 3 weeks. It cannot safely be hurried. Patients who are taking large amounts of lesser-known sedatives or longer-acting benzodiazepines should probably be gradually withdrawn from the original drug of abuse without substitution therapy (*see* Wikler, 1968).

Some clinicians feel that the longer duration of action of phenobarbital has advantages for managing withdrawal of general CNS depressants, and use 30 mg of phenobarbital for each hypnotic dose of the drug of dependence (*e.g.,* for each 100 mg of pentobarbital), divided and given four times each day. Phenobarbital is then reduced by 30 mg per day (Wesson and Smith, 1977).

Other protocols have also been suggested (*see* Martin *et al.,* 1979).

Withdrawal of Alcohol. There are certain distinctions between the overall effects of chronic abuse of alcohol and those of other general CNS depressants, which necessitate differences in the therapeutic approach. Chronic ingestion of large amounts of alcohol is very frequently associated with various degrees of malnutrition and avitaminosis, especially vitamin B deficiencies. Some alcoholics may be severely dehydrated because of vomiting caused by alcoholic gastritis or withdrawal. Pneumonitis is also a frequent complication. Thus, injections of vitamins, attention to fluid balance, and administration of antibiotics are often a necessary part of treatment, but these are obviously not substitutes for measures that suppress the general-depressant withdrawal syndrome.

As is the case with mild degrees of physical dependence of any type, in the milder forms of alcohol withdrawal a wide variety of drugs (phenothiazines, sedatives, antianxiety agents) or simply nutritional supplements and good nursing care will provide some symptomatic relief. Indeed, although screening is a problem and the procedure involves risk for patients with medical problems or significant physical dependence, many alcoholics are now routinely withdrawn on an outpatient or day hospital basis without the use of any pharmacological agent (*see* Jaffe and Ciraulo, 1984).

When there is a significant degree of physical dependence, drugs that show cross-dependence with alcohol are demonstrably superior in reducing mortality and morbidity to those that do not show such cross-dependence. Unfortunately, the tremulousness, which in some patients may be the most severe manifestation of physical dependence, may in others be the prodrome of the more severe epileptiform and delirious states. It is not possible to know in advance which patients are only mildly physically dependent and which patients will develop delirium tremens. Since delirium tremens always carries with it a certain risk of a fatal outcome, it seems appropriate to treat all but the mildest cases of alcoholic withdrawal with agents that show cross-dependence with alcohol.

Theoretically, alcohol itself should be quite effective in the suppression of the alcohol withdrawal syndrome. However, its short duration of action and narrow range of safety make it a poor therapeutic agent. In practice, alcohol is usually abruptly stopped and longer-acting agents are substituted. If given in adequate quantities, pentobarbital, phenobarbital, chloral hydrate, paraldehyde, several benzodiazepines, and clomethiazole have all been shown to be effective in preventing the development of withdrawal symptoms or suppressing the syndrome once it develops. The general technic is similar to that used in the management of physical dependence on barbiturates, in that the patient is brought to a level of stabilization in which he exhibits either no withdrawal symptoms or only mild intoxication and the drug is then gradually withdrawn. Chlordiazepoxide, diazepam, and flurazepam are now the most widely used drugs for withdrawal in the United States, even though in some well-controlled studies they were not superior to a combination of paraldehyde and chloral hydrate; clomethiazole is commonly used in Europe and Australia. The long duration of action and slow elimination of most benzodiazepines make their use in the treatment of physical dependence on alcohol analogous to the use of methadone in the treatment of physical dependence on opioids. The rate at which the dosage of the benzodiazepine should subsequently be reduced has not been carefully studied; the clinician's adjustment of doses should be guided by the degree of intoxication and the appearance of tremulousness and insomnia. Some researchers have given diazepam at 2-hour intervals until all signs of withdrawal are suppressed. No further drug is given because desmethyl diazepam, the principal active metabolite, has a very long half-life (*see* Chapter 17; Sellers *et al.*, 1983). If seizures occur, diazepam should probably be given. Sodium valproate and clomethiazole are also effective. Some clinicians use phenytoin in alcohol withdrawal, but the value of this procedure in patients without a history of seizures unrelated to the use of alcohol is questionable. Dopaminergic antagonists, such as haloperidol, are still utilized to control hallucinations once the period of risk for seizures has passed (generally the first 48 hours of withdrawal) (*see* Gessner, 1979; Sellers and Kalant, 1982; Jaffe and Ciraulo, 1984).

Withdrawal of Benzodiazepines. The benzodiazepines can cause physical dependence of a type that resembles dependence on general CNS depressants. On theoretical grounds, the syndrome seen with the shorter-acting drugs, such as triazolam or temazepam, would be expected to be more rapid in onset, more intense, and of shorter duration than that seen with longer-acting agents, such as flurazepam or diazepam; the latter should be self-tapering.

In practice, however, it is often necessary to reduce dosage of even the longer-acting agents gradually over several weeks to prevent emergence of anxiety, tremulousness, or severe insomnia. Withdrawal of shorter-acting agents is best accomplished by switching to a longer-acting benzodiazepine, followed by tapering of that dosage over a period of days or weeks.

Withdrawal Technics in Mixed Patterns of Abuse. It is not uncommon to encounter individuals who are physically dependent on both opioids and general CNS depressants. The therapeutic regimen in such situations combines the procedures described above. General CNS depressants are given in sufficient quantity to produce mild intoxication, and a stabilization dose is determined. At the same time the patient is observed for the autonomic signs of opioid withdrawal, and sufficient methadone or another suitable opioid is given to suppress such symptoms. While the dose of the CNS depressant is held constant, the opioid is reduced as previously described. When withdrawal from opioids is complete, the dose of the CNS depressant is then reduced gradually. Simultaneous withdrawal of both classes of drugs at appropriate rates is not contraindicated, but this procedure requires considerable experience, since insomnia, weakness, and restlessness occur in both syndromes. Although the abrupt withdrawal of psychedelics, sympathomimetic drugs, and tobacco does not cause syndromes that require medical treatment, these syndromes do cause unpleasant physiological and psychological disturbances that may contribute to relapse. Administration of tricyclic antidepressants has been suggested for the treatment of the fatigue, irritability, depression, and hypersomnolence that may persist after withdrawal of amphetamines or cocaine (*see* Kleber and Gawin, 1984). However, such treatment may not reduce the desire to use the drug. Nicotine gum can reduce the severity of the tobacco withdrawal syndrome, and it also reduces the likelihood of relapse in highly dependent cigarette smokers (*see* above).

APPROACHES TO BEHAVIORAL MODIFICATION

A number of very different approaches are currently in use for modification of patterns of compulsive drug abuse. They differ not only in the way the problem is conceptualized but also in the goals given priority, the methods used, and the patterns of change induced. No longer do all approaches use total abstinence as the sole criterion of successful treatment. Instead, there is a growing emphasis on achieving productive and socially acceptable behavior and on improving physical health and interpersonal relationships. Sometimes marked changes occur in these areas even when the pattern of drug use has only been modified rather than eliminated.

Some treatments place emphasis on emotional problems that are believed to increase vulnerability to compulsive drug use; others aim at providing alternative gratifications or modifying life styles; still others use various forms of external pressure and threats of adverse consequences to change drug-use patterns; some employ pharmacological agents to modify the response to the drugs themselves. In practice, several of these methods may be combined in any one treatment program (see Glasscote et al., 1972; Lowinson and Ruiz, 1981). Although similar themes appear in programs designed to modify compulsive use of different drugs, the great differences in pharmacological effects and social attitudes make it convenient to discuss treatment approaches to each drug separately. The nonpharmacological methods can be only briefly summarized here.

In evaluating treatment it is essential to recognize that recovery, or at least periods of substantial improvement, commonly occurs for all forms of drug dependence even though there is little or no formal intervention (see Maddux and Desmond, 1982; Vaillant and Milofsky, 1982). For example, among United States Army personnel who began to use heroin in Vietnam, major changes in associates and environment led to rapid abandonment of illicit use of opioids (Robins, 1974). Cessation of opioid use does not necessarily mean total abstinence from all substances. Former users may be dependent on a variety of other drugs. It has been repeatedly observed that some alcoholics can drink alcohol after detoxication without immediately relapsing to pathological alcohol use. However, in general, such controlled use is observed only in those who have not been severely dependent. For the heavily dependent cigarette smoker, opioid addict, or alcoholic, any use regularly and quickly leads to compulsive use.

Hospitalization and Psychotherapy. Measured by the percentage of patients who remain abstinent, the results of prolonged hospital or institutional rehabilitation are disappointing, not only for opioid users but also for patients addicted to alcohol, barbiturates, or amphetamines. The use of prolonged hospitalization (more than 3 weeks) in traditional medical or psychiatric units is now on the decline, and questions have even been raised about the need for brief hospitalization for alcoholism or opioid use in the absence of medical complications.

There is little evidence to show that traditional individual *psychotherapy* alone is of any value in the treatment of the compulsive drug user, although such therapy has been reported to be bene-ficial for participants in methadone programs. Over the past 1 to 2 decades specialized forms of group psychotherapy have been developed, but there is no way of predicting the type of drug user who will be helped by one or another of the many technics now in use.

Voluntary Groups and Self-Regulatory Communities. Alcoholics Anonymous, Narcotics Anonymous, Phoenix House, Daytop Village, and similar groups have been helpful in the rehabilitation of certain types of compulsive drug users. Their efficacy may be due to a number of factors, including a reduction in the sense of isolation and a gratification of the need to belong. Equally important is the absence of a hard line between "patient" and "staff." The organizations are usually operated by former drug users, and the new member is immediately confronted by individuals who at once convey understanding and concern, and provide role models for responsible behavior. Also important is the participation itself, which keeps the individual away from the environment in which drug use occurred and in the company of people who share his concerns about drug use in a way that amounts to a ritualization of sobriety. Although a substantial proportion of treated alcoholics make contact with Alcoholics Anonymous at some point, it is not clear what proportion derive benefit. Only a small percentage of compulsive opioid users seem motivated to seek admission to self-regulating residential centers; fewer still actually enter after learning what is expected of members, and many leave within weeks after joining. Those who remain in residential programs do well while they are members, and many continue to do well after they leave, provided they have stayed for more than a few months. Indeed, the level of improvement seems directly related to the length of stay for up to 18 months.

Supervisory-Deterrent Approaches. Some approaches emphasize the maintenance of abstinence and involve a period in a hospital, prison, or special facility followed by careful supervision of the individual in the community. If the chemical analysis of urine specimens or other information indicates return to drug use, the supervisee, who has usually been paroled or civilly committed to the program, is reinstitutionalized. The critical element of the system is thought to be the deterrent effect of reinstitutionalization. In theory, this approach can be used with all types of compulsive drug abuse. While it is believed that this system was highly effective in Japan in controlling serious epidemics of amphetamine and heroin addiction and is still the major approach used in Singapore, the experience in the United States has been far less impressive. Very few individuals under such supervision who were dependent on opioids were able to remain totally abstinent, and by the end of the first year after discharge more than two thirds had been reinstitutionalized. The economic and social cost of such an approach has led to a major decline in its use for compulsive drug users. However, there is now increasing use of external pressure (e.g., threat of job loss) to motivate the working problem drinker to remain in treatment. The use of monitoring and external pressure with less draconian consequences for drug users who have been arrested or convicted of crimes appears to reduce the frequency of drug abuse. Enrollment of opioid-dependent parolees in methadone maintenance programs has also been associated with reductions in crime and illicit use of opioids (Anglin *et al.*, 1981).

Role of Pharmacological Agents. With every form of drug dependence, other drugs have been tried as therapeutic agents on a variety of theoretical grounds. Sometimes the therapeutic agents are directed at some postulated underlying psychological difficulty (*e.g.*, anxiety or depression) that is felt to contribute to the motivation to use the drug of dependence. Sometimes the therapeutic agent is intended to be a less toxic substitute, in whole or in part, for the effects of the drug being used, or at least to suppress any subclinical withdrawal phenomena (*e.g.*, oral nicotine for inhaled tobacco, oral methadone or acetylmethadol for injected heroin). Still other agents are intended to interfere in a variety of ways with the reinforcing or satisfying properties of the dependence-producing drug (*e.g.*, opioid antagonists), or to create situations where their use becomes unpleasant (*e.g.*, disulfiram).

Opioid Maintenance. Methadone maintenance was originally based on the hypothesis that, as a result of repeated use of opioids, the addict has sustained a metabolic alteration such that opioids produce a euphoria not experienced by nonaddicts, and that for months or years after withdrawal the addict experiences a feeling of abnormality (opioid hunger) relieved only by opioids. Since the original pilot studies of Dole and Nyswander, the use of this approach has been greatly expanded and the procedures and dosages have been substantially modified. Most commonly the procedure consists in the daily administration of 40 to 100 mg of methadone, orally in a flavored vehicle, combined with efforts at social rehabilitation. At the stabilization level (achieved by gradually increasing the dose over a period of several weeks), there is a high degree of cross-tolerance to all opioids so that the euphoric effects of even high doses of intravenous opioid are sharply diminished. While many patients report little or no craving for illicit opioids, in most treatment programs and under experimental conditions there are usually some patients who continue to seek out and use intravenous opioids despite the attenuated effects. This treatment explicitly emphasizes law-abiding and productive behavior rather than abstinence *per se*, and its relative effi-

cacy in reaching its goals is well documented (*see* Simpson *et al.*, 1982; Cooper *et al.*, 1983). The methadone-maintenance approach is subject to special regulations and is still criticized by some.

The use of methadone should not be confused with the British practice of prescribing heroin for self-administration. With methadone the route is exclusively oral, thus eliminating both the sharp ups and downs that characterize the effects of repeated doses of intravenous heroin and the complications that occur when addicts inject themselves without benefit of hygienic technic. Equally important, the duration of action of methadone is such that it need be given only once a day. Although the concentrations of methadone in plasma do change over the course of 24 hours (*see* Chapter 22), the decline is usually not great enough to produce perceptible withdrawal phenomena. Therefore, the ingestion of all medication can be supervised by scheduled visits to the clinic. Since nonmedical use of opioids seems to increase with greater availability of drugs, control of illicit redistribution from treatment programs is an important and controversial issue. In Great Britain, the prescribing of heroin for addicts is now restricted to clinics staffed by specialists, who are increasingly inclined to prescribe oral or parenteral methadone rather than injectable heroin. The existence of these clinics has not prevented the development of an illicit traffic in heroin that serves those who do not use the clinics and those who feel the clinics are not generous enough in their prescribing habits (*see* Stimson and Oppenheimer, 1982).

In one study of British addicts, new patients were randomly assigned to treatment with either intravenous heroin or oral methadone. After 1 year, those who had been given intravenous heroin were more likely to be in treatment at the clinic using prescribed intravenous drugs. Those originally assigned to oral methadone were more likely to have dropped out of treatment. Some of these dropouts stopped using opioids entirely, but a significant percentage was found to be using intravenous opioids obtained from the illicit drug traffic (Hartnoll *et al.*, 1980).

In practice, most methadone treatment programs in the United States permit patients to take some drug home, and there has been some illicit diversion. Concern about this has led to efforts to develop longer-acting opioids for clinical use. One such drug is methadyl acetate, which suppresses opioid withdrawal for up to 72 hours after a single dose and, theoretically, all doses can be ingested under direct supervision when patients come to the clinics three times per week. In clinical trials it appears to be similar to methadone in its overall effects. However, the dropout rate is somewhat greater than with methadone, and some patients experience stimulating side effects not associated with the use of methadone (*see* Judson *et al.*, 1983; Ling *et al.*, 1984). Methadyl acetate is still an investigational drug.

Opioid Antagonists. When the opioid receptors in the CNS are continuously occupied by antagonists, the effects of ordinary doses of opioids are attenuated or entirely blocked, and even the repeated administration of opioids for several weeks does not induce a significant degree of physical dependence.

Theoretically, the use of opioid antagonists might be helpful in several ways. If compulsive use of opioids is a result of the reinforcement of drug-seeking behavior due to drug effects, then the repeated use of opioids without effect (as would be the case if the patient were taking adequate amounts of an antagonist) would tend to produce extinction. Furthermore, if the development of physical dependence could be prevented, then conditioned abstinence phenomena should also be extinguished and the protracted abstinence syndrome should eventually subside. It is important to point out that, independent of the reinforcement model, prevention of the development of physical dependence in ambulatory patients may be of considerable value in that it may stop occasional illicit use from progressing quickly into regular and compulsive use. The patient who takes an antagonist behaves as if opioids are, for practical purposes, unavailable. This serves to decrease craving (Meyer and Mirin, 1979). A number of specific opioid antagonists (cyclazocine, naloxone, and naltrexone) have been subjected to clinical trial. Patients must first be withdrawn from opioids, since antagonists precipitate severe abstinence symptoms in individuals who are physically dependent.

Naloxone is virtually free of the psychotomimetic side effects associated with some agonist-antagonists (*see* Chapter 22), but its short duration of action and low oral efficacy make it impractical for treatment. *Naltrexone* is orally effective, seems relatively free of side effects, and, depending on the dose, can produce blockade for more than 24 hours. Given orally three times per week in doses of 100 to 150 mg, it provides almost continuous blockade of the subjective effects of exogenous opioids (*see* Chapter 22; Julius, 1979). Depot preparations of naltrexone have also been developed but have not yet been tested adequately. Clinical trials of oral naltrexone have shown that few patients continue to take naltrexone for more than 30 to 60 days. A few investigators have noted that the large doses commonly used produce subtle aversive side effects (*e.g.,* loss of energy), and hypothesize that such side effects could contribute to patients' reluctance to continue taking the drug (*see* Hollister *et al.,* 1981). Despite this difficulty, experienced clinicians believe that naltrexone is useful for selected patients during the immediate period after withdrawal.

Buprenorphine, a partial μ agonist (*see* Chapter 22), has also been suggested as a drug that may have advantages for maintenance purposes. Although clinical trials in ambulatory addicts have yet to be reported, laboratory studies have demonstrated that buprenorphine markedly attenuates the subjective effects of large doses of subcutaneous morphine and that addicts given buprenorphine sharply decrease self-administration of intravenous heroin (Mello and Mendelson, 1980). While buprenorphine produces morphine-like subjective

effects and respiratory depression at low doses, higher doses do not cause correspondingly more intense subjective or respiratory-depressant effects. Furthermore, it is a long-acting agent and withdrawal symptoms are minimal upon abrupt discontinuation (Jasinski *et al.,* 1978; Mello and Mendelson, 1980). Because of its partial agonist actions, it is possible to substitute buprenorphine for low doses of methadone or heroin without precipitating severe withdrawal symptoms (Lukas *et al.,* 1984).

Other Pharmacological Procedures. Maintenance approaches for compulsive users of general CNS depressants and amphetamine-like drugs have not been well studied. With the exception of patients dependent on very small doses of such drugs, most practitioners strive for total withdrawal. There have been occasional reports of behavioral improvement in compulsive cocaine users when given methylphenidate. Tricyclic antidepressants have been recommended for relief of lethargy following withdrawal of amphetamine or cocaine, but controlled clinical studies are lacking (*see* Kleber and Gawin, 1984). For the very heavy smoker, nicotine in the form of chewing gum appears to have some value in alleviating withdrawal and, in some cases, may serve as a less toxic substitute for nicotine inhaled in tobacco smoke.

Disulfiram and related agents have been used in the treatment of alcoholism for a number of years. When an individual who has been taking disulfiram ingests alcohol, a syndrome characterized by nausea, vomiting, flushing and hypotension, anxiety, and palpitations develops within minutes. The details of the administration and the potential hazards of disulfiram and related agents are discussed in Chapter 18. Disulfiram can be administered only with the patient's cooperation and, therefore, is useful only for selected patients. Other factors being equal, patients who take disulfiram relapse less rapidly than those who do not. Depot forms of disulfiram have also been employed. (For references, *see* Jaffe and Ciraulo, 1984.)

Conditioned aversion technics have been tried in alcoholism, smoking, and other forms of drug abuse. This usually involves the administration of an emetic agent (apomorphine or ipecac), followed shortly thereafter by a dose of the drug (*e.g.,* a small amount of whisky or other agent) so that nausea and vomiting occur soon after the drug is ingested. In this way, the taking of alcohol or the drug of abuse becomes a conditioned stimulus that produces a sensation of nausea. Enthusiasm for the aversion technics in the treatment of alcoholism has declined as their limitations have become clearer. However, there is a renewed interest in the use of apomorphine in subemetic doses as a dopaminergic agonist that reduces anxiety and craving for alcohol, and there have been several optimistic clinical reports (*see* Jaffe and Ciraulo, 1984). When smokers are encouraged to inhale more smoke than they are accustomed to, the smoke becomes aversive. This technic has been used in treatment with some reported success.

Drug Treatment of Postwithdrawal Mental Disturbances. As noted previously, the majority of alcoholics and opioid-dependent patients have diagnosable disorders in addition to drug dependence. The most common are various forms of depression, antisocial personality, anxiety disorders, alcoholism in opioid addicts, and drug dependence (usually involving sedatives or opioids) in alcoholics (Rounsaville *et al.,* 1982; Hesselbrock *et al.,* 1985). Depressive states, unstable mood, and insomnia are common during the months immediately following withdrawal of either alcohol or opioids. Because of the risk of dependence, most practitioners avoid the use of benzodiazepines or other sedatives in the management of alcoholism or other types of drug dependence. Although patients who abstain from the use of illicit drugs commonly experience some spontaneous improvement in mood, a significant percentage report persistent depression. Tricyclic antidepressants are frequently prescribed, but evidence for their efficacy is scant. Lithium has been reported to reduce the incidence of relapse in some alcoholics, but there is uncertainty about which alcoholics are most likely to benefit. (For references, *see* Jaffe and Ciraulo, 1984.)

ROLE OF THE MEDICAL PROFESSION IN PREVENTION

Since there is a relationship between availability of certain drugs and the prevalence of their self-administration, consideration must be given to regulation of the manufacture, prescription, and dispensing of those drugs considered to have a liability for abuse. Developing reasonable regulations requires efforts in several areas, including (1) methods for assessing the likelihood that a particular drug will be self-administered, (2) guidelines for classifying drugs in order to provide for different degrees of control at the levels of manufacturing, prescribing, and dispensing, and (3) general guidelines for medical practitioners who must prescribe these drugs for patients. The use of drugs with potential for abuse in the treatment of compulsive drug users creates special problems because of the belief that such individuals are particularly likely to sell or give some of their prescribed medication to others. While special concern about prescribing such drugs for this group is often based on moral and political issues, there is a core of legitimate concern linked to the effort to control availability of drugs used illicitly and to the belief that such drugs may aggravate and prolong the dependence syndrome.

Addicting and Nonaddicting Drugs: Assessing Liability for Abuse. Evaluation of the likelihood that a given drug will produce effects that might lead to its abuse is accomplished by determining whether animals will administer the new drug to themselves and how many properties it shares with prototypical drugs known to be abused. Both of these approaches have limitations. For example, animals do not self-administer psychedelics, but they will do so with caffeine, procaine, and apomorphine.

The technics used with opioid-like agents are well established. Thus, a drug is considered to be nonopioid with respect to liability for abuse (1) if it does not suppress the opioid withdrawal syndrome when tested in subjects physically dependent on morphine, (2) if it does not produce morphine-like physical dependence when given chronically, and (3) if postaddicts neither consistently identify it as "dope" (morphine-like) nor repeatedly request it when offered the opportunity to do so. On the other hand, if a compound is found to share all of these key characteristics with morphine, it is considered to have a high liability for abuse and is recommended for appropriate controls. However, some drugs share a few characteristics but not others. For example, cyclazocine produces a variety of physical dependence in which the withdrawal symptoms are not associated with drug-seeking behavior. Other drugs, such as nalbuphine, butorphanol, and loperamide, may be somewhat morphine-like with respect to one or two characteristics; however, because of differences in solubility or toxicity or because they appear to exhibit a ceiling effect in inducing euphoria, they are considered to present a lower order of risk. Such agents may be recommended for less stringent controls than those applied to the opioids. New drugs that have pharmacological actions similar to those of amphetamines or general CNS depressants are now required to be evaluated for potential for abuse prior to marketing for general use. The procedures for assessing potential for abuse have been summarized by Brady and Lukas (1984).

Treating the Compulsive Drug User. In the United States, the effort to control drug availability previously included severe restrictions on the use of opioids and certain other controlled drugs in the treatment of compulsive drug users. Musto (1973) has documented the history of the interactions between the medical profession and regulatory authorities. This situation has changed substantially since 1970, and opioids are now used both for easing withdrawal and for maintenance. However, it is likely that changes will continue to be made in laws and rules as practitioners and regulators strive for a balance between flexibility for treatment and control of illicit diversion. At present, continued administration of opioids to patients with chronic, incurable, and painful conditions is not considered "maintenance of an addiction" and, although the practice varies from state to state, such individuals are not generally reported to health authorities as opioid addicts.

The treatment of compulsive opioid users who

do not have an obvious medical problem is more complicated. Methadone and similar drugs for both the ambulatory withdrawal and maintenance treatment of heroin addiction are now used in the treatment of more than 80,000 individuals at several hundred separate centers throughout the United States. Federal and state governments have promulgated regulations that legitimize the use of methadone, but at the same time attempt to minimize the amount of take-home medication permitted in such programs and to reduce the likelihood that patients will obtain methadone from more than one source. It is still medically appropriate to administer an opioid to relieve acute withdrawal symptoms. However, it is expected that, where there are nearby specialized detoxication or maintenance programs, the patient will be referred to these specialized facilities. The use of opioid maintenance is restricted to specially licensed centers and to clinicians affiliated with them. Interested clinicians should contact the appropriate state and federal agencies for current regulations.

Thus far there are no specific regulations or constraints at the federal level that would prohibit the use of CNS stimulants or depressants in the treatment of compulsive users of nonopioid drugs. However, there is a prevalent view that with few exceptions chronic maintenance programs for these drugs are of little benefit to the patient, and a number of state medical boards have taken disciplinary actions against physicians who were too casual in prescribing CNS depressants and stimulants for purposes other than the traditional.

In practice, the physician must often administer opioids or sedatives even to persons who seem predisposed to develop dependence on such drugs. There are a few general rules applicable to opioids that, if followed in all cases, will reduce, but obviously not eliminate, the probability of such a complication. The patient should not be given an opioid when another drug of lower potential for abuse will suffice. The use of agonist-antagonists may be less risky where problems are anticipated. The patient who is not terminally ill should not be permitted to self-administer such drugs parenterally. Only a few days' supply should be dispensed at any given time, and a return to nonopioids should be undertaken as soon as the situation permits. If the drug has been administered repeatedly for more than a few weeks, a change to a long-acting drug a few days prior to discontinuation will minimize withdrawal symptomatology. On the other hand, the tendency to avoid the use of opioid analgesics should not be carried to unwarranted extremes; the patient who needs a potent analgesic should not be left in pain because of the physician's fear of causing addiction.

Most physicians exercise great care in prescribing potent opioids; many now exercise similar prudence in the prescription of sedatives, antianxiety agents, and CNS sympathomimetics. New regulations limiting the number of times a prescription order for controlled drugs can be renewed should result in more careful periodic reassessment of the need for such drugs.

Drugs given for the relief of fluctuating levels of pain, anxiety, or feelings of depression can be taken in several ways. They can be requested or taken by the patient each time the distress becomes too intense to tolerate, that is, for *relief* of distress; or they can be taken in anticipation of the recurrence of distress, that is, to *avoid* distress. With respect to inducing drug dependence, both ways carry risks. When used for *relief*, minimal amounts of drug will be used, since the time of drug action will correspond to the time when its action is required. However, each time relief is promptly obtained, the act of self-administration of the drug will be reinforced. Prescribing drugs with slower onset and longer duration of action may minimize this reinforcement process, but the likelihood of physical dependence is not reduced. Self-administration to *avoid* distress may be less reinforcing of each drug-taking act, but the patient never waits long enough to find out whether the drug is needed at all. Even the idea of discontinuing may cause anticipation of the return of distress. From a pharmacological viewpoint, the avoidance schedule leads to the regular and frequent use of unnecessary amounts of drug. Although there are no easy solutions to this therapeutic dilemma, the physician should be aware of the factors that may be operative and suggest to the patient the approach best suited to the individual situation. In the case of patients who are terminally ill, drugs should be given to prevent the recurrence of pain, rather than "as needed." Less drug is needed when it is given before pain becomes intense. Concerns about physical dependence in such cases should be secondary. It is also helpful if the physician takes advantage of his own relationship with the patient to reinforce efforts other than the use of drugs to cope with psychic and physical distress and advises the patient's family to do likewise.

A final caveat is in order. Undoubtedly, whether drugs are used for producing pleasure or for the avoidance or relief of depression or distress, it is the *self-administration* of drugs and the *self-induced* changes in mood that are the critical factors in the development of compulsive abuse. Physicians and other health professionals with easy access to potent drugs are at relatively high risk for developing drug dependence (Murray, 1978). Health-care professionals would do well to remember this, not only when treating patients but also whenever they consider treating themselves.

Abraham, H. D. Visual phenomenology of the LSD flash. *Arch. Gen. Psychiatry*, **1983**, *40*, 884–889.

Aigner, T. G., and Balster, R. L. Choice behavior in rhesus monkeys: cocaine versus food. *Science*, **1978**, *201*, 534–535.

Anglin, M. D.; McGlothlin, W. H.; and Speckart, G. The effect of parole on methadone patient behavior. *Am. J. Drug Alcohol Abuse*, **1981**, *8*, 153–170.

Angrist, B.; Sathananthan, G.; Wilk, S.; and Gershon, S. Amphetamine psychosis: behavioral and biochemical aspects. *J. Psychiatr. Res.*, **1974**, *11*, 13–23.

Armitage, A.; Dollery, C.; Houseman, T.; Kohner, E.; Lewis, P. J.; and Turner, D. Absorption of nicotine from small cigars. *Clin. Pharmacol. Ther.*, **1978**, *23*, 143–151.

Aronow, R., and Done, A. Phencyclidine overdose; an

emergency concept of management. *J.A.C.E.P.*, **1978**, *7*, 56–59.

Balster, R. L., and Wessinger, W. D. Central nervous system depressant effects of phencyclidine. In, *Phencyclidine and Related Arylcyclohexylamines: Present and Future Applications*. (Kamenka, J.-M.; Domino, E. F.; and Geneste, P.; eds.) NPP Books, Ann Arbor, **1983**, pp. 291–309.

Benowitz, N. L., and Jacob, P., III. Daily intake of nicotine during cigarette smoking. *Clin. Pharmacol. Ther.*, **1984**, *35*, 499–504.

Benowitz, N. L.; Jacob, P., III; Jones, R. T.; and Rosenberg, J. Interindividual variability in the metabolism and cardiovascular effects of nicotine in man. *J. Pharmacol. Exp. Ther.*, **1982**, *221*, 368–371.

Benowitz, N. L.; Kuyt, F.; and Jacob, P., III. Influence of nicotine on cardiovascular and hormonal effects of cigarette smoking. *Clin. Pharmacol. Ther.*, **1984**, *36*, 74–81.

Benowitz, N. L.; Kuyt, F.; Jacob, P., III; Jones, R. T.; and Osman, A.-L. Cotinine disposition and effects. *Clin. Pharmacol. Ther.*, **1983**, *34*, 604–611.

Brandt, J.; Butters, N.; Ryan, C.; and Bayog, R. Cognitive loss and recovery in long-term alcohol abusers. *Arch. Gen. Psychiatry*, **1983**, *40*, 435–442.

Carney, R. M., and Goldberg, A. P. Weight gain after cessation of cigarette smoking. *N. Engl. J. Med.*, **1984**, *310*, 614–616.

Chait, L. D., and Griffiths, R. R. Effects of caffeine on cigarette smoking and subjective response. *Clin. Pharmacol. Ther.*, **1983**, *34*, 612–622.

Charney, D. S.; Riordan, C. E.; Kleber, H. D.; Murburg, M.; Braverman, P.; Sternberg, D. E.; Heninger, G. R.; and Redmond, D. E. Clonidine and naltrexone. A safe, effective and rapid treatment of abrupt withdrawal from methadone therapy. *Arch. Gen. Psychiatry*, **1982**, *39*, 1327–1333.

Collier, H. O. J. Tolerance, physical dependence and receptors: a theory of the genesis of tolerance and physical dependence through drug-induced changes in the number of receptors. *Adv. Drug Res.*, **1966**, *3*, 171–188.

Conell, L. J., and Berlin, R. M. Withdrawal after substitution of a short-acting for a long-acting benzodiazepine. *J.A.M.A.*, **1983**, *250*, 2838–2840.

Correa, P.; Fontham, E.; Kickle, L. W.; Lin, Y.; and Haenszel, W. Passive smoking and lung cancer. *Lancet*, **1983**, *2*, 595–596.

Crofton, J.; Campbell, I. E.; Cole, P. V.; Friend, J. A. R.; Oldham, P. D.; Springett, V. H.; Berry, G.; and Raw, M. Comparison of four methods of smoking withdrawal in patients with smoking related diseases. Report by a Subcommittee of the Research Committee of the British Thoracic Society. *Br. Med. J. [Clin. Res.]*, **1983**, *286*, 595–597.

Cushman, P., and Dole, V. P. Detoxification of rehabilitated methadone-maintained patients. *J.A.M.A.*, **1973**, *226*, 747–752.

Deanfield, J.; Wright, C.; Krikler, S.; Ribeiro, P.; and Fox, K. Cigarette smoking and the treatment of angina with propranolol, atenolol, and nifedipine. *N. Engl. J. Med.*, **1984**, *310*, 951–954.

Dole, V. P.; Nyswander, M. E.; and Kreek, M. J. Narcotic blockade. *Arch. Intern. Med.*, **1966**, *118*, 304–309.

Ebert, R. V.; McNabb, McK. E.; McCusker, K. T.; and Snow, S. L. Amount of nicotine and carbon monoxide inhaled by smokers of low-tar, low-nicotine cigarettes. *J.A.M.A.*, **1983**, *250*, 2840–2842.

Ellinwood, E. H., Jr.; Linnoila, M.; Easler, M. E.; and Molter, D. W. Profile of acute tolerance to three sedative anxiolytics. *Psychopharmacology*, **1983**, *79*, 137–141.

Fischman, M. W., and Schuster, C. R. Cocaine self-administration in humans. *Fed. Proc.*, **1982**, *41*, 241–246.

Fraser, H. F.; Wikler, A.; Essig, C. F.; and Isbell, H.

Degree of physical dependence induced by secobarbital or phenobarbital. *J.A.M.A.*, **1958**, *166*, 126–129.

Freedman, D. X. The use and abuse of LSD. *Arch. Gen. Psychiatry*, **1968**, *18*, 300–347.

Gawin, F. H., and Kleber, H. D. Cocaine abuse treatment. Open pilot trial with desipramine and lithium carbonate. *Arch. Gen. Psychiatry*, **1984**, *41*, 903–909.

Goldberg, S. R.; Spealman, R. D.; and Goldberg, D. M. Persistent behavior at high rates maintained by intravenous self-administration of nicotine. *Science*, **1981**, *214*, 573–575.

Goldstein, A., and Goldstein, D. B. Enzyme expansion theory of drug tolerance and physical dependence. *Proc. Assoc. Res. Nerv. Ment. Dis.*, **1968**, *46*, 265–267.

Gong, H.; Tashkin, D. P.; Simmons, M. S.; Calvarese, B.; and Shapiro, B. J. Acute and subacute bronchial effects of oral cannabinoids. *Clin. Pharmacol. Ther.*, **1984**, *35*, 26–32.

Grant, I.; Adams, K. M.; and Reed, R. Aging, abstinence, and medical risk factors in the prediction of neuropsychologic deficit among long-term alcoholics. *Arch. Gen. Psychiatry*, **1984**, *41*, 710–718.

Griffith, J. D.; Cavanaugh, J.; Held, J.; and Oates, J. A. Dextroamphetamine. *Arch. Gen. Psychiatry*, **1972**, *26*, 97–100.

Griffiths, R. R.; Bigelow, G. E.; and Liebson, E. Differential effects of diazepam and pentobarbital on mood and behavior. *Arch. Gen. Psychiatry*, **1983**, *40*, 865–873.

Griffiths, R. R.; Brady, J. V.; and Snell, J. D. Progressive-ratio performance maintained by drug infusions: comparison of cocaine, diethylpropion, chlorphentermine, and fenfluramine. *Psychopharmacology*, **1978**, *56*, 5–13.

Haigler, H. J., and Aghajanian, G. K. Serotonin receptors in the brain. *Fed. Proc.*, **1977**, *36*, 2159–2164.

Hallstrom, C., and Lader, M. Benzodiazepine withdrawal phenomena. *Int. Pharmacopsychiatry*, **1981**, *16*, 235–244.

Hartnoll, R. L.; Mitcheson, M. C.; Battersby, A.; Brown, G.; Ellis, M.; Fleming, P.; and Hedley, N. Evaluation of heroin maintenance in controlled trial. *Arch. Gen. Psychiatry*, **1980**, *37*, 877–884.

Henningfield, J. E.; Miyasato, K.; and Jasinski, D. R. Cigarette smokers self-administer intravenous nicotine. *Pharmacol. Biochem. Behav.*, **1983**, *19*, 887–890.

Hesselbrock, M.; Meyer, R.; and Keener, J. Psychopathology in hospitalized alcoholics. *Arch. Gen. Psychiatry*, **1985**, in press.

Hollister, L. E.; Johnson, K.; Boukhabza, D.; and Gillespie, H. K. Aversive effects of naltrexone in subjects not dependent on opiates. *Drug Alcohol Depend.*, **1981**, *8*, 37–41.

Hughes, J. R.; Hatsukami, D. K.; Pickens, R. W.; Krahn, D.; Malin, S.; and Luknic, A. Effect of nicotine on the tobacco withdrawal syndrome. *Psychopharmacology*, **1984**, *83*, 82–87.

Hughes, P.; Barker, N.; Crawford, G.; and Jaffe, J. H. The natural history of a heroin epidemic. *Am. J. Public Health*, **1972**, *62*, 995–1001.

Jaffe, J. H., and Sharpless, S. K. Pharmacological denervation supersensitivity in the central nervous system: a theory of physical dependence. *Proc. Assoc. Res. Nerv. Ment. Dis.*, **1968**, *46*, 226–246.

Jarvik, M. E. Tolerance to the effects of tobacco. In, *Cigarette Smoking as a Dependence Process*. (Krasnegor, N. A., ed.) National Institute on Drug Abuse. Department of Health, Education, and Welfare Publication No. (ADM) 79-800, U.S. Government Printing Office, Washington, D. C., **1979**, pp. 150–157.

Jarvik, M. E., and Schneider, N. G. Degree of addiction and effectiveness of nicotine gum therapy for smoking. *Am. J. Psychiatry*, **1984**, *141*, 790–791.

Jasinski, D. R.; Pevnick, J. S.; and Griffith, J. D. Human

pharmacology and abuse potential of the analgesic buprenorphine. *Arch. Gen. Psychiatry,* **1978,** *35,* 501–516.

Jones, R. T.; Benowitz, N.; and Bachman, J. Clinical studies of cannabis tolerance and dependence. *Ann. N.Y. Acad. Sci.,* **1976,** *282,* 221–239.

Judson, B. A.; Goldstein, A.; and Inturrisi, C. E. Methadyl acetate (LAAM) in the treatment of heroin addicts. *Arch. Gen. Psychiatry,* **1983,** *40,* 834–840.

Julius, D. A. Research and development of naltrexone: a new narcotic antagonist. *Am. J. Psychiatry,* **1979,** *136,* 782–786.

Kalant, H.; Engel, J. A.; Goldberg, L.; Griffiths, R. R.; Jaffe, J. H.; Krasnegor, N. A.; Mello, N. K.; Mendelson, J. H.; Thompson, T.; and Van Ree, J. M. Behavioral aspects of addiction: group report. In, *The Bases of Addiction: Report of the Dahlem Workshop on the Bases of Addiction.* (Fishman, J., ed.) Abakon Verlagsgesellschaft, Berlin, **1978,** pp. 463–495.

Kandel, D. B. Marijuana users in young adulthood. *Arch. Gen. Psychiatry,* **1984,** *41,* 200–209.

Kornetsky, C., and Esposito, R. U. Reward and detection thresholds for brain stimulation: dissociative effects of cocaine. *Brain Res.,* **1981,** *209,* 496–500.

Kornetsky, C.; Esposito, R. U.; McLean, S.; and Jacobson, J. O. Intracranial self-stimulation thresholds. *Arch. Gen. Psychiatry,* **1979,** *36,* 289–292.

Kramer, J. C.; Fischman, V. S.; and Littlefield, D. C. Amphetamine abuse. *J.A.M.A.,* **1967,** *201,* 305–309.

Lazdunski, M.; Bidard, J.-N.; Romey, G.; Tourneur, Y.; Vignon, J.; and Vincent, J.-P. The different sites of action of phencyclidine and its analogues in nervous tissues. In, *Phencyclidine and Related Arylcyclohexylamines: Present and Future Applications.* (Kamenka, J.-M.; Domino, E. F.; and Geneste, P.; eds.) NPP Books, Ann Arbor, **1983,** pp. 83–106.

Ling, W.; Dorus, W.; Hargreaves, W. A.; Resnick, R.; Senay, E.; Tuason, V. B.; Blakis, M.; Holmes, E.; Klett, C. J.; Mejia, M.; and Weinberg, A. Alternative induction and crossover schedules for methadyl acetate. *Arch. Gen. Psychiatry,* **1984,** *41,* 193–199.

Lukas, S. E., and Griffiths, R. R. Precipitated diazepam withdrawal in baboons: effects of dose and duration of diazepam exposure. *Eur. J. Pharmacol.,* **1984,** *100,* 163–171.

Lukas, S. E.; Jasinski, D. R.; and Johnson, R. E. Electroencephalographic and behavioral correlates of buprenorphine administration. *Clin. Pharmacol. Ther.,* **1984,** *36,* 127–132.

McCaul, M. E.; Bigelow, G. E.; Stitzer, M. L.; and Liebson, I. Short-term effects of oral methadone in methadone maintenance subjects. *Clin. Pharmacol. Ther.,* **1982,** *31,* 753–761.

McGlothlin, W. H. Drugs and crime. In, *Handbook on Drug Abuse.* (Dupont, R. L.; Goldstein, A.; and O'Donnell, J.; eds.) National Institute on Drug Abuse, U.S. Government Printing Office, Washington, D. C., **1979,** pp. 357–364.

Maddux, J. F., and Desmond, D. P. Residence relocation inhibits opioid dependence. *Arch. Gen. Psychiatry,* **1982,** *39,* 1313–1317.

Martin, P. R.; Kapur, B. M.; Whiteside, E. A.; and Sellers, E. M. Intravenous phenobarbital therapy in barbiturate and other hypnosedative withdrawal reactions: a kinetic approach. *Clin. Pharmacol. Ther.,* **1979,** *26,* 256–264.

Martin, W. R. A homeostatic and redundancy theory of tolerance to and dependence on narcotic analgesics. *Proc. Assoc. Res. Nerv. Ment. Dis.,* **1968,** *46,* 206–225.

Martin, W. R.; Jasinski, D. R.; Haertzen, C. A.; Kay, D. C.; Jones, B. E.; Mansky, P. A.; and Carpenter, R. W. Methadone—a reevaluation. *Arch. Gen. Psychiatry,* **1973,** *28,* 286–295.

Martin, W. R.; Sloan, J. W.; Sapira, J. D.; and Jasinski, D. R. Physiologic, subjective, and behavioral effects

of amphetamine, methamphetamine, ephedrine, phenmetrazine, and methylphenidate in man. *Clin. Pharmacol. Ther.,* **1971,** *12,* 245–258.

Martin, W. R.; Vaupel, D. B.; Nozaki, M.; and Bright, L. D. The identification of LSD-like hallucinogens using the chronic spinal dog. *Drug Alcohol Depend.,* **1978,** *3,* 113–123.

Matsuzaki, M. Alteration in pattern of EEG activities and convulsant effect of cocaine following chronic administration in the rhesus monkey. *Electroencephalogr. Clin. Neurophysiol.,* **1978,** *45,* 1–15.

Mello, N. K., and Mendelson, J. H. Buprenorphine suppresses heroin use by heroin addicts. *Science,* **1980,** *207,* 657–659.

Mello, N. K.; Mendelson, J. H.; Sellers, M. L.; and Kuehnle, J. C. Effects of alcohol and marihuana on tobacco smoking. *Clin. Pharmacol. Ther.,* **1980,** *27,* 202–209.

Murray, R. M. The health of doctors: a review. *J. R. Coll. Physicians Lond.,* **1978,** *12,* 403–415.

Naranjo, C. A.; Sellers, E. M.; Chater, K.; Iversen, P.; Roach, C.; and Sykora, K. Non-pharmacological intervention in acute alcohol withdrawal. *Clin. Pharmacol. Ther.,* **1983,** *34,* 214–219.

Okamoto, M.; Boisse, N. R.; Rosenberg, H. C.; and Rosen, R. Characteristics of functional tolerance during barbiturate physical dependency production. *J. Pharmacol. Exp. Ther.,* **1978,** *207,* 906–915.

Perez-Reyes, M.; Di Guiseppi, S.; Davis, K. H.; Schindler, V. H.; and Cook, C. E. Comparison of effects of marihuana cigarettes of three different potencies. *Clin. Pharmacol. Ther.,* **1982,** *31,* 617–624.

Peroutka, S. J., and Snyder, S. H. Multiple serotonin receptors and their physiological significance. *Fed. Proc.,* **1983,** *42,* 213–217.

Pomerleau, O. F.; Fertig, J. B.; Seyler, L. E.; and Jaffe, J. Neuroendocrine reactivity to nicotine in smokers. *Psychopharmacology,* **1983,** *81,* 61–67.

Poster, D. S.; Penta, J. S.; Bruno, S.; and Macdonald, J. S. Δ^9-Tetrahydrocannabinol in clinical oncology. *J.A.M.A.,* **1981,** *245,* 2047–2051.

Quirion, R.; O'Donohue, T. L.; Everist, H.; Pert, A.; and Pert, C. B. Phencyclidine receptors and possible existence of an endogenous ligand. In, *Phencyclidine and Related Arylcyclohexylamines: Present and Future Applications.* (Kamenka, J.-M.; Domino, E. F.; and Geneste, P.; eds.) NPP Books, Ann Arbor, **1983,** pp. 667–684.

Ron, M. A. Assessment and significance of alcohol brain damage in the human subject. In, *Pharmacological Treatments for Alcoholism.* (Edwards, G., and Littleton, J., eds.) Croom Helm, London, **1984,** pp. 319–330.

Rosecrans, J. A. Nicotine as a discriminative stimulus to behavior: its characterization and relevance to smoking behavior. In, *Cigarette Smoking as a Dependence Process.* (Krasnegor, N. A., ed.) National Institute on Drug Abuse. Department of Health, Education, and Welfare Publication No. (ADM) 79-800, U.S. Government Printing Office, Washington, D. C., **1979,** pp. 58–69.

Rosenberg, H. C., and Okamoto, M. Loss of inhibition in the spinal cord during barbiturate withdrawal. *J. Pharmacol. Exp. Ther.,* **1978,** *205,* 563–568.

Rounsaville, B. J.; Weissman, M. M.; Kleber, H.; and Wilber, C. Heterogeneity of psychiatric diagnosis in treated opiate addicts. *Arch. Gen. Psychiatry,* **1982,** *39,* 161–166.

Schwartz, R. D., and Kellar, K. J. Nicotinic cholinergic receptor binding sites in the brain: regulation *in vivo. Science,* **1983,** *220,* 214–216.

Seiden, L. S., and Vosmer, G. Formation of 6-hydroxydopamine in caudate nucleus of the rat brain after a single large dose of methylamphetamine. *Pharmacol. Biochem. Behav.,* **1984,** *21,* 29–31.

Sellers, E. M., and Busto, U. Benzodiazepines and ethanol: assessment of the effects and consequences of psychotropic drug interactions. *J. Clin. Psychopharmacol.*, **1982**, *2*, 249–262.

Sellers, E. M.; Naranjo, C. A.; Harrison, M.; Devenyi, P.; Roach, C.; and Sykora, K. Diazepam loading: simplified treatment of alcohol withdrawal. *Clin. Pharmacol. Ther.*, **1983**, *34*, 822–826.

Senay, E. C.; Dorus, W.; Goldberg, F.; and Thornton, W. Withdrawal from methadone maintenance: rate of withdrawal and expectation. *Arch. Gen. Psychiatry*, **1977**, *34*, 361–367.

Siegel, S.; Hinson, R. E.; Krank, M. D.; and McCully, J. Heroin "overdose" death: contribution of drug-associated environmental cues. *Science*, **1982**, *216*, 436–437.

Simpson, D. D.; Joe, G. W.; and Bracy, S. A. Six-year follow-up of opioid addicts after admission to treatment. *Arch. Gen. Psychiatry*, **1982**, *39*, 1318–1326.

Snyder, S. H.; Weingartner, H.; and Faillace, L. A. DOET (2,5-dimethoxy-4-ethylamphetamine), a new psychotropic drug. Effects of varying doses in man. *Arch. Gen. Psychiatry*, **1971**, *24*, 50–55.

Stimmel, B.; Goldberg, J.; Reizman, A.; Murphy, R. J.; and Teets, K. Fetal outcome in narcotic-dependent women: the importance of the type of maternal narcotic used. *Am. J. Drug Alcohol Abuse*, **1983**, *9*, 383–395.

Tucker, G. J.; Quinlan, D.; and Harrow, M. Chronic hallucinogenic drug use and thought disturbance. *Arch. Gen. Psychiatry*, **1972**, *27*, 443–447.

Tyrer, P.; Rutherford, D.; and Huggett, T. Benzodiazepine withdrawal symptoms and propranolol. *Lancet*, **1981**, *2*, 520–522.

Vaillant, G. E., and Milofsky, E. S. Natural history of male alcoholism. IV. Paths to recovery. *Arch. Gen. Psychiatry*, **1982**, *39*, 127–133.

Van Dyke, C.; Jatlow, P.; Ungerer, J.; Barash, P.; and Byck, R. Cocaine and lidocaine have similar psychological effects after intranasal application. *Life Sci.*, **1979**, *24*, 271–274.

Van Dyke, C.; Ungerer, J.; Jatlow, P.; Barash, P.; and Byck, R. Intranasal cocaine: dose relationships of psychological effects and plasma levels. *Int. J. Psychiatry Med.*, **1982**, *12*, 1–13.

Vardy, M. M., and Kay, S. R. LSD psychosis or LSD-induced schizophrenia? *Arch. Gen. Psychiatry*, **1983**, *40*, 877–883.

Vestal, R. E.; Wood, A. J. J.; Branch, R. A.; Shand, D. G.; and Wilkinson, G. R. Effects of age and cigarette smoking on propranolol disposition. *Clin. Pharmacol. Ther.*, **1979**, *26*, 8–20.

Victor, M., and Adams, R. D. The effect of alcohol on the nervous system. *Res. Publ. Assoc. Res. Nerv. Ment. Dis.*, **1953**, *32*, 526–573.

Wall, M. E.; Sadler, B. M.; Brine, D.; Taylor, H.; and Perez-Reyes, M. Metabolism, disposition, and kinetics of delta-9-tetrahydrocannabinol in men and women. *Clin. Pharmacol. Ther.*, **1983**, *34*, 352–363.

Washton, A. M., and Resnick, R. G. Clonidine in opiate withdrawal: review and appraisal of clinical findings. *Pharmacotherapy*, **1981**, *1*, 140–146.

Weil, A. T. Nutmeg as a psychoactive drug. In, *Ethnopharmacologic Search for Psychoactive Drugs*. (Efron, D. H.; Holmstedt, B.; and Kline, N. S.; eds.) Public Health Service Publication No. 1645, U.S. Government Printing Office, Washington, D. C., **1967**, pp. 188–201.

Weintraub, M., and Standish, R. Nabilone: an antiemetic for patients undergoing cancer chemotherapy. *Hosp. Formulary*, **1983**, *18*, 1033–1035.

Wikler, A. Diagnosis and treatment of drug dependence of the barbiturate type. *Am. J. Psychiatry*, **1968**, *125*, 758–765.

Wise, R. W. Neural mechanisms of the reinforcing action of cocaine. In, *Cocaine: Pharmacology, Effects and Treatment of Abuse*. (Grabowski, J., ed.) National Institute on Drug Abuse Research Monograph Series,

Department of Health and Human Services Publication No. (ADM) 84-1326, U.S. Government Printing Office, Washington, D. C., **1984**, pp. 16–34.

Woolverton, W. L.; Kandel, D.; and Schuster, C. R. Tolerance and cross-tolerance to cocaine and *d*-amphetamine. *J. Pharmacol. Exp. Ther.*, **1978**, *205*, 525–535.

Yaksh, T. L.; Kohl, R. L.; and Rudy, T. A. Induction of tolerance and withdrawal in rats receiving morphine in the spinal subarachnoid space. *Eur. J. Pharmacol.*, **1977**, *41*, 275–284.

Zukin, R. S., and Zukin, S. R. A common receptor for phencyclidine and the *sigma* opiates. In, *Phencyclidine and Related Arylcyclohexylamines: Present and Future Applications*. (Kamenka, J.-M.; Domino, E. F.; and Geneste, P.; eds.) NPP Books, Ann Arbor, **1983**, pp. 107–124.

Monographs and Reviews

Aniline, O., and Pitts, F. N., Jr. Phencyclidine (PCP): a review and perspectives. *CRC Crit. Rev. Toxicol.*, **1982**, *10*, 145–177.

Brady, J. V., and Lukas, S. E. (eds.). *Testing Drugs for Physical Dependence Potential and Abuse Liability*. National Institute on Drug Abuse Research Monograph Series, Department of Health and Human Services Publication No. (ADM) 84-1332, U.S. Government Printing Office, Washington, D. C., **1984**.

Cappell, H., and LeBlanc, A. E. Tolerance and physical dependence: do they play a role in alcohol and drug self-administration? In, *Research Advances in Alcohol and Drug Problems*, Vol. 6. (Israel, Y.; Glaser, F. B.; Kalant, H.; Popham, R. E.; Schmidt, W.; and Smart, R. G.; eds.) Plenum Press, New York, **1981**, pp. 159–196.

Chapman, D. B., and Way, E. L. Metal ion interactions with opiates. *Annu. Rev. Pharmacol. Toxicol.*, **1980**, *20*, 533–579.

Cohen, S. Psychotomimetic agents. *Annu. Rev. Pharmacol.*, **1967**, *7*, 301–316.

Cooper, J. R.; Altman, F.; Brown, B. S.; and Czechowicz, D. (eds.). *Research on the Treatment of Narcotic Addiction: State of the Art*. National Institute on Drug Abuse Treatment Research Monograph Series, Department of Health and Human Services Publication No. (ADM) 83-1281, U.S. Government Printing Office, Washington, D. C., **1983**.

Deitrich, R. A., and Spuhler, K. Genetics of alcoholism and alcohol actions. In, *Research Advances in Alcohol and Drug Problems*, Vol. 8. (Smart, R. G.; Cappell, H. D.; Glaser, F. B.; Israel, Y.; Kalant, H.; Popham, R. E.; Schmidt, W.; and Sellers, E. M.; eds.) Plenum Press, New York, **1984**, pp. 47–98.

Domino, E. F. Neuropsychopharmacology of nicotine and tobacco smoking. In, *Smoking Behavior: Motives and Incentives*. (Dunn, W. L., Jr., ed.) V. H. Winston & Sons, Inc., Washington, D. C., **1973**, pp. 5–31.

Donegan, N. H.; Rodin, J.; O'Brien, C. P.; and Solomon, R. L. A learning-theory approach to commonalities. In, *Commonalities in Substance Abuse and Habitual Behavior*. (Levison, P. K.; Gerstein, D. R.; and Maloff, D. R.; eds.) Lexington Books, Lexington, Mass., **1983**, pp. 111–156.

Dupont, R. L.; Goldstein, A.; and O'Donnell, J. (eds.). *Handbook on Drug Abuse*. National Institute on Drug Abuse, U.S. Government Printing Office, Washington, D. C., **1979**.

Edwards, G.; Arif, A.; and Hodgson, R. Nomenclature and classification of drug- and alcohol-related problems: a WHO memorandum. *Bull. WHO*, **1981**, *59*, 225–242.

Edwards, G.; Arif, A.; and Jaffe, J. (eds.). *Drug Use and Misuse: Cultural Perspectives*. Croom Helm, London, **1983**.

Efron, D: H.; Holmstedt, B.; and Kline, N. S. (eds.). *Ethnopharmacologic Search for Psychoactive Drugs*.

Public Health Service Publication No. 1645, U.S. Government Printing Office, Washington, D. C., **1967.**

Ellinwood, E. H., Jr. Amphetamines/anorectics. In, *Handbook on Drug Abuse.* (Dupont, R. L.; Goldstein, A.; and O'Donnell, J.; eds.) National Institute on Drug Abuse, U.S. Government Printing Office, Washington, D. C., **1979,** pp. 221–231.

Fehr, K. O., and Kalant, H. (eds.). *Cannabis and Health Hazards.* The Addiction Research Foundation, Toronto, **1983.**

Finnegan, L. P. (ed.). *Drug Dependence in Pregnancy: Clinical Management of Mother and Child.* Department of Health, Education, and Welfare Publication No. (ADM) 79-678, U.S. Government Printing Office, Washington, D. C., **1979.**

Finnegan, L. P., and Fehr, K. O'B. The effects of opiates, sedative-hypnotics, amphetamines, cannabis, and other psychoactive drugs on the fetus and newborn. In, *Research Advances in Alcohol and Drug Problems,* Vol. 5. (Kalant, O. J., ed.) Plenum Press, New York, **1980,** pp. 653–723.

Fischman, M. W. The behavioral pharmacology of cocaine in humans. In, *Cocaine: Pharmacology, Effects and Treatment of Abuse.* (Grabowski, J., ed.) National Institute on Drug Abuse Research Monograph Series, Department of Health and Human Services Publication No. (ADM) 84-1326, U.S. Government Printing Office, Washington, D. C., **1984,** pp. 73–92.

Freedman, D. X. The psychopharmacology of hallucinogenic agents. *Annu. Rev. Med.,* **1969,** *20,* 409–418.

Gessner, P. K. Drug therapy of the alcohol withdrawal syndrome. In, *The Biochemistry and Pharmacology of Ethanol.* (Majchrowicz, E., and Noble, E., eds.) Plenum Press, New York, **1979,** pp. 375–435.

Gilbert, R. M. Caffeine as a drug of abuse. In, *Research Advances in Alcohol and Drug Problems,* Vol. III. (Gibbins, R. J.; Israel, Y.; Kalant, H.; Popham, R. E.; Schmidt, W.; and Smart, K. G.; eds.) John Wiley & Sons, Inc., New York, **1976,** pp. 49–176.

Glasscote, R.; Sussex, J. N.; Jaffe, J. H.; Ball, J.; and Brill, L. *The Treatment of Drug Abuse: Programs, Problems, Prospects.* Joint Information Service, Washington, D. C., **1972.**

Goldstein, D. B. The effects of drugs on membrane fluidity. *Annu. Rev. Pharmacol. Toxicol.,* **1984,** *24,* 43–64.

Greden, J. F. Caffeinism and caffeine withdrawal. In, *Substance Abuse: Clinical Problems and Perspectives.* (Lowinson, J. H., and Ruiz, P., eds.) The Williams & Wilkins Co., Baltimore, **1981,** pp. 274–286.

Greenblatt, D. J.; Shader, R. I.; and Abernethy, D. R. Current status of benzodiazepines. *N. Engl. J. Med.,* **1983,** *308,* 354–358, 410–416.

Harris, L. S.; Dewey, W. L.; and Razdan, R. K. Cannabis: its chemistry, pharmacology, and toxicology. In, *Drug Addiction II: Amphetamine, Psychotogen, and Marihuana Dependence.* (Martin, W. R., ed.) *Handbuch der Experimentellen Pharmakologie,* Vol. 45, Pt. 2. Springer-Verlag, Berlin, **1977,** pp. 371–429.

Institute of Medicine, National Academy of Sciences. (Various authors.) *Marijuana and Health: Report of Study.* National Academy Press, Washington, D. C., **1982.**

Jaffe, J. H., and Ciraulo, D. A. Drugs used in the treatment of alcoholism. In, *The Diagnosis and Treatment of Alcoholism.* (Mendelson, J. H., and Mello, N. K., eds.) McGraw-Hill Book Co., New York, **1984,** pp. 355–389.

Jaffe, J. H., and Jarvik, M. E. Tobacco use and tobacco use disorder. In, *Psychopharmacology: A Generation of Progress.* (Lipton, M. A.; DiMascio, A.; and Killam, K. F.; eds.) Raven Press, New York, **1978,** pp. 1665–1676.

Jasinski, D. R. Assessment of the abuse potentiality of morphine-like drugs (methods in man). In, *Drug Addiction I: Morphine, Sedative/Hypnotic and Alcohol Dependence.* (Martin, W. R., ed.) *Handbuch der Experimentellen Pharmakologie,* Vol. 45, Pt. 1. Springer-Verlag, Berlin, **1977,** pp. 179–258.

Jerí, F. R. (ed.). *Cocaine 1980.* Proceedings of the Interamerican Seminar on Medical and Sociological Aspects of Coca and Cocaine. Pacific Press, Lima, **1980.**

Johanson, C. E., and Schuster, C. R. Animal models of drug self-administration. In, *Advances in Substance Abuse; Behavioral and Biological Research,* Vol. II. (Mello, N. K., ed.) JAI Press, Inc., Greenwich, Conn., **1981,** pp. 219–297.

Jones, R. T. Cannabis and health. *Annu. Rev. Med.,* **1983,** *34,* 247–258.

Kalant, H. Behavioral criteria for tolerance and physical dependence. In, *The Bases of Addiction: Report of the Dahlem Workshop on the Bases of Addiction.* (Fishman, J., ed.) Abakon Verlagsgesellschaft, Berlin, **1978,** pp. 199–220.

Kalant, H.; LeBlanc, A. E.; and Gibbins, R. J. Tolerance to and dependence on some non-opiate psychotropic drugs. *Pharmacol. Rev.,* **1971,** *23,* 135–191.

Kalant, O. J. *The Amphetamines: Toxicity and Addiction.* Charles C Thomas, Publisher, Springfield, Ill., **1966.**

Kales, A.; Soldatos, C. R.; Bixler, E. O.; and Kales, J. D. Rebound insomnia and rebound anxiety: a review. *Pharmacology,* **1983,** *26,* 121–137.

Kalix, P. The pharmacology of Khat. *Gen. Pharmacol.,* **1984,** *15,* 179–187.

Kandel, D. B., and Maloff, D. R. Commonalities in drug use: a sociological perspective. In, *Commonalities in Substance Abuse and Habitual Behavior.* (Levison, P. K.; Gerstein, D. R.; and Maloff, D. R.; eds.) Lexington Books, Lexington, Mass., **1983,** pp. 3–27.

Kleber, H. D., and Gawin, F. H. Cocaine abuse: a review of current and experimental treatments. In, *Cocaine: Pharmacology, Effects and Treatment of Abuse.* (Grabowski, J., ed.) National Institute on Drug Abuse Research Monograph Series, Department of Health and Human Services Publication No. (ADM) 84-1326, U.S. Government Printing Office, Washington, D. C., **1984,** pp. 112–130.

Kreek, M. J. Methadone in treatment: physiological and pharmacological issues. In, *Handbook on Drug Abuse.* (Dupont, R. L.; Goldstein, A.; and O'Donnell, J.; eds.) National Institute on Drug Abuse, U.S. Government Printing Office, Washington, D. C., **1979,** pp. 57–86.

———. Health consequences associated with the use of methadone. In, *Research on the Treatment of Narcotic Addiction: State of the Art.* (Cooper, J. R.; Altman, F.; Brown, B. S.; and Czechowicz, D.; eds.) National Institute on Drug Abuse Treatment Research Monograph Series, Department of Health and Human Services Publication No. (ADM) 83-1281, U.S. Government Printing Office, Washington, D. C., **1983,** pp. 456–482.

Lewander, T. Effects of amphetamine in animals. In, *Drug Addiction II: Amphetamine, Psychotogen, and Marihuana Dependence.* (Martin, W. R., ed.) *Handbuch der Experimentellen Pharmakologie,* Vol. 45, Pt. 2. Springer-Verlag, Berlin, **1977,** pp. 33–246.

Lowinson, J. H., and Ruiz, P. (eds.). *Substance Abuse: Clinical Problems and Perspectives.* The Williams & Wilkins Co., Baltimore, **1981.**

Mackinnon, G. L., and Parker, W. A. Benzodiazepine withdrawal syndrome: a literature review and evaluation. *Am. J. Drug Alcohol Abuse,* **1982,** *9,* 19–33.

Martin, W. R., and Sloan, J. W. Neuropharmacology and neurochemistry of subjective effects, analgesia, tolerance, and dependence produced by narcotic analgesics. In, *Drug Addiction I: Morphine, Sedative/Hypnotic and Alcohol Dependence.* (Martin, W. R., ed.) *Handbuch der Experimentellen Pharmakologie,* Vol. 45, Pt. 1. Springer-Verlag, Berlin, **1977a,** pp. 43–158.

———. Pharmacology and classification of LSD-like hallucinogens. In, *Drug Addiction II: Amphetamine, Psychotogen, and Marihuana Dependence.* (Martin, W. R., ed.) *Handbuch der Experimentellen Pharmakologie,* Vol. 45, Pt. 2. Springer-Verlag, Berlin, **1977b,** pp. 305–368.

Mendelson, J. H., and Mello, N. K. Biologic concomitants of alcoholism. *N. Engl. J. Med., 1979, 301,* 912–921.

Meyer, R. E., and Mirin, S. M. *The Heroin Stimulus: Implication for a Theory of Addiction.* Plenum Press, New York, **1979.**

Miller, J. D.; Cisin, I. H.; Gardner-Keaton, H.; Harrell, A. V.; Wirtz, P. W.; Abelson, H. I.; and Fishburne, P. M. *National Survey on Drug Abuse: Main Findings 1982.* National Institute on Drug Abuse. Department of Health and Human Services Publication No. (ADM) 83-1263, U.S. Government Printing Office, Washington, D. C., **1983.**

Musto, D. F. *The American Disease.* Yale University Press, New Haven, **1973.**

National Commission on Marihuana and Drug Abuse. Second Report. *Drug Use in America: Problem in Perspective.* U.S. Government Printing Office, Washington, D. C., **1973.**

Petersen, R. C. (ed.). *Marijuana Research Findings: 1980.* National Institute on Drug Abuse Research Monograph Series, Department of Health and Human Services Publication No. (ADM) 80-1001, U.S. Government Printing Office, Washington, D. C., **1980.**

Petersen, R. C., and Stillman, R. C. (eds.). *Cocaine: 1977.* National Institute on Drug Abuse. Department of Health, Education, and Welfare Publication No. (ADM) 77-471, U.S. Government Printing Office, Washington, D. C., **1977.**

———. (eds.). Phencyclidine: an overview. In, *PCP (Phencyclidine) Abuse: An Appraisal.* National Institute on Drug Abuse. Department of Health, Education, and Welfare Publication No. (ADM) 78-728, U.S. Government Printing Office, Washington, D. C., **1978,** pp. 1–17.

Platt, J. J., and Labate, C. *Heroin Addiction. Theory, Research, and Treatment.* John Wiley & Sons, Inc., New York, **1976.**

Redmond, D. E., Jr., and Krystal, J. H. Multiple mechanisms of withdrawal from opioid drugs. *Annu. Rev. Neurosci., 1984, 7,* 443–478.

Richter, R. W. (ed.). *Medical Aspects of Drug Abuse.* Harper & Row, Hagerstown, Md., **1975.**

Robins, L. *The Vietnam Drug User Returns: Final Report, Sept. 1973.* Special Action Office Monograph, Ser. A, No. 2, U.S. Government Printing Office, Washington, D. C., **1974.**

Russell, M. A. H., and Feyerabend, C. Cigarette smoking: a dependence on high-nicotine boli. *Drug Metab. Rev.,* **1978,** *8,* 29–57.

Sellers, E. M., and Kalant, H. Alcohol withdrawal and delirium tremens. In, *Encyclopedic Handbook of Alcoholism.* (Pattison, E. M., and Kaufman, E., eds.) Gardner Press, Inc., New York, **1982,** pp. 147–166.

Sharp, C. W., and Brehm, M. L. (eds.). *Review of Inhalants: Euphoria to Dysfunction.* National Institute on Drug Abuse. Department of Health, Education, and Welfare Publication No. (ADM) 77-553, U.S. Government Printing Office, Washington, D. C., **1977.**

Sharp, C. W., and Carroll, L. T. (eds.). *Voluntary Inhalation of Industrial Solvents.* National Institute on Drug Abuse. Department of Health, Education, and Welfare Publication No. (ADM) 79-779, U.S. Government Printing Office, Washington, D. C., **1978.**

Shuster, L. Tolerance and physical dependence. In, *Narcotic Drugs: Biochemical Pharmacology.* (Clouet, D. H., ed.) Plenum Press, New York, **1971,** pp. 408–423.

Smith, C. M. The pharmacology of sedative/hypnotics, alcohol, and anesthetics: sites and mechanisms of action. In, *Drug Addiction I: Morphine, Sedative/Hypnotic and Alcohol Dependence.* (Martin, W. R., ed.) *Handbuch der Experimentellen Pharmakologie,* Vol. 45, Pt. 1. Springer-Verlag, Berlin, **1977,** pp. 413–587.

Stimson, G. V., and Oppenheimer, E. *Heroin Addiction: Treatment and Control in Britain.* Tavistock Publications, London, **1982.**

Surgeon General. *Smoking and Health.* (Office of Smoking and Health, eds.) Department of Health, Education, and Welfare Publication No. (PHS) 79-50066, U.S. Government Printing Office, Washington, D. C., **1979.**

———. *The Health Consequences of Smoking: The Changing Cigarette.* (Office of Smoking and Health, eds.) Department of Health and Human Services Publication No. (PHS) 81-50156, U.S. Government Printing Office, Washington, D. C., **1981.**

Tabakoff, B., and Hoffman, P. L. Neurochemical aspects of tolerance to and physical dependence on alcohol. In, *Biology of Alcoholism,* Vol. 7. (Kissin, B., and Begleiter, H., eds.) Plenum Press, New York, **1983,** pp. 199–252.

Tabakoff, B., and Rothstein, J. D. Biology of tolerance and dependence. In, *Medical and Social Aspects of Alcohol Abuse.* (Tabakoff, B.; Sutker, P. B.; and Randall, C. L.; eds.) Plenum Press, New York, **1983,** pp. 187–220.

Terenius, L. Opiate tolerance and dependence: roles of receptors and endorphins. In, *Research Advances in Alcohol and Drug Problems,* Vol. 8. (Smart, R. G.; Cappell, H. D.; Glaser, F. B.; Israel, Y.; Kalant, H.; Popham, R. E.; Schmidt, W.; and Sellers, E. M.; eds.) Plenum Press, New York, **1984,** pp. 1–21.

Thompson, T., and Unna, K. R. (eds.). *Predicting Dependence Liability of Stimulant and Depressant Drugs.* University Park Press, Baltimore, **1977.**

Wesson, D. R., and Smith, D. E. *Barbiturates: Their Use, Misuse, and Abuse.* Human Sciences Press, New York, **1977.**

Wikler, A. *Opioid Dependence: Mechanisms and Treatment.* Plenum Press, New York, **1980.**

Woods, J. H. Behavioral pharmacology of drug administration. In, *Psychopharmacology: A Generation of Progress.* (Lipton, M. A.; Di Mascio, A.; and Killam, K. F.; eds.) Raven Press, New York, **1978,** pp. 595–607.

World Health Organization. *Youth and Drugs.* Technical Report No. 516, WHO, Geneva, **1973.**

Wulff, M. H. The barbiturate withdrawal syndrome: a clinical and electroencephalographic study. *Electroencephalogr. Clin. Neurophysiol.,* **1959,** Suppl. 14, 1–173.

24 CENTRAL NERVOUS SYSTEM STIMULANTS

Strychnine, Picrotoxin, Pentylenetetrazol, and Miscellaneous Agents (Doxapram, Nikethamide, Methylphenidate)

Donald N. Franz

Stimulation of the central nervous system (CNS) can be produced in man and animals by a large number of natural and synthetic substances. Only a few have been used therapeutically. Some drugs exhibit prominent central stimulation at toxic levels, and others produce mild stimulation as a side effect. This chapter includes discussion of those drugs that produce central stimulation as their most prominent action and are generally classified as *analeptics* or *convulsants*.

Although some analeptics were formerly used in attempts to counteract severe intoxication by general depressants, *this practice has been overwhelmingly discredited* by the far greater success achieved with more conservative measures that stress intensive supportive care. All of the analeptics are capable of producing generalized convulsions in sufficient doses. Unfortunately, the margin of safety of doses for stimulation of central respiratory centers is generally very narrow and unpredictable. No safe, selective respiratory stimulant is currently available. Thus, only a few very specialized applications remain for these agents.

The excitability of the CNS reflects a balance between excitatory and inhibitory influences that is normally maintained within relatively narrow limits. Drugs can increase excitability either by blocking inhibition or by enhancing excitation. Strychnine and picrotoxin selectively block inhibition in the CNS; these drugs are important research tools employed to study inhibitory transmitters and receptor types (*see* Chapter 12). With the possible exception of pentylenetetrazol, the other analeptics described in this chapter do not affect inhibitory processes and, therefore, presumably act by enhancing excitation. The

pharmacology of analeptics has been reviewed by Hahn (1960), Esplin and Zablocka-Esplin (1969), and Wang and Ward (1977). The structure-activity relationship of convulsants that block inhibition has been reviewed by Smythies (1974).

STRYCHNINE

Strychnine has no demonstrated therapeutic value, despite a long history of unwarranted popularity. However, the mechanism of action of strychnine is thoroughly understood, and it is a valuable pharmacological tool for studies of inhibition in the CNS. Poisoning with strychnine results in a predictable sequence of dramatic symptoms that may be lethal unless interrupted by established therapeutic measures.

Source and Chemistry. Strychnine is the principal alkaloid present in *nux vomica*, the seeds of a tree native to India, *Strychnos nux-vomica*. The term *nux vomica* has been erroneously translated as "emetic nut." Actually, strychnine is not an emetic, and the word *vomica* means depression or cavity, a feature of the strychnos seed attributed by legend to the digital imprint of the Creator.

Nux vomica was introduced into Germany in the sixteenth century as a poison for rats and other animal pests. Its use as a pesticide persists to this day and is a source of accidental strychnine poisoning of children. Strychnine was first employed in medicine in 1540, but it did not gain wide usage until 200 years later.

In addition to strychnine, the closely related alkaloid *brucine* is found in nux vomica. Brucine is much less potent than strychnine. The structural formula of strychnine is as follows:

Strychnine

Pharmacological Actions. *Central Nervous System.* Strychnine produces excitation of all portions of the CNS. This effect, however, does not result from direct synaptic excitation. Strychnine increases the level of neuronal excitability by selectively blocking inhibition. Nerve impulses are normally confined to appropriate pathways by inhibitory influences. When inhibition is blocked by strychnine, ongoing neuronal activity is enhanced and sensory stimuli produce exaggerated reflex effects.

Strychnine is a powerful convulsant, and the convulsion has a characteristic motor pattern. Inasmuch as strychnine reduces inhibition, including the reciprocal inhibition existing between antagonistic muscles, the pattern of convulsion is determined by the most powerful muscles acting at a given joint. In most laboratory animals, this convulsion is characterized by tonic extension of the body and of all limbs. Tonic extension is preceded and followed during the phase of postictal depression by phasic *symmetrical* extensor thrusts that may be initiated by any modality of sensory stimulus. The sloth presents an interesting exception. In this animal, the powerful antigravity muscles are flexors, and the strychnine convulsion is characterized by tonic flexion of all limbs (Esplin and Woodbury, 1961). The pattern of the strychnine convulsion therefore contrasts sharply with that produced by drugs that directly excite central neurons.

Typical strychnine convulsions also occur in spinal animals. For this reason the effects of strychnine are often ascribed to a spinal locus of action, and the convulsion is frequently termed a *spinal convulsion*. In fact, other portions of the CNS are also excited by doses that produce the characteristic motor manifestations in a spinal animal. The tonic extensor convulsion reflects the action of strychnine to reduce inhibition, rather than the characteristic response of the spinal cord to a convulsant drug. Convulsions in spinal animals produced by drugs that directly excite neurons are asymmetrical and incoordinated, in contrast to the pattern observed with strychnine. The medulla, likewise, is affected by strychnine at dosages that produce hyperexcitability throughout the CNS. However, strychnine does not selectively stimulate the medulla, and the drug is not therapeutically useful as a respiratory analeptic.

Cardiovascular System. The complex changes in blood pressure that occur during strychnine convulsions are related to the effects of the drug on vasomotor centers, including those in the spinal cord.

Gastrointestinal Tract. Strychnine was at one time employed for atonic constipation and as a stomachic and bitter. It produces no selective gastrointestinal effects and has no place in the therapy of any gastrointestinal disorder.

Skeletal Muscle. Convulsive doses of strychnine have no detectable effect on skeletal muscle. Increased muscle tone is the result purely of the central actions of the drug. In supraconvulsive doses, a curariform action on the neuromuscular junction is observed.

Mechanism of Action. Strychnine has been the object of many experimental investigations. The convulsant action of the drug is due to interference with postsynaptic inhibition that is mediated by *glycine*. Glycine is an important inhibitory transmitter to motoneurons and interneurons in the spinal cord, and strychnine acts as a selective, competitive antagonist to block the inhibitory effects of glycine at all glycine receptors (Kuno and Weakly, 1972). Well-known examples of this type of postsynaptic inhibition are the inhibitory influences existing between the motoneurons of antagonistic muscle groups and recurrent spinal inhibition mediated by the Renshaw cell. Renshaw cells are excited by intraspinal collaterals of motoneuron axons that liberate acetylcholine. Strychnine blocks recurrent inhibition at the Renshaw cell–motoneuron synapse by antagonizing the action of glycine released by the Renshaw cell. The specificity of the binding of strychnine to glycine receptors has been used to demonstrate their dense localizations in the gray matter of the spinal cord, brain stem, and thalamus by autoradiographic technics (Zarbin *et al.*, 1981). Competitive receptor-binding studies indicate that both strychnine and glycine interact with the same receptor complex, although possibly at different sites (*see* Johnston, 1978). Tetanus toxin also blocks postsynaptic inhibition, but it acts by preventing release of glycine from inhibitory interneurons. Strychnine-sensitive postsynaptic inhibition in higher centers of the CNS is also mediated by glycine. The pharmacology of postsynaptic inhibition has been reviewed by Curtis (1969).

Absorption, Fate, and Excretion. Strychnine is rapidly absorbed from the gastrointestinal tract, mucous membranes, and parenteral sites of injection. It is readily metabolized, mainly by the enzymes of hepatic microsomes (Adamson and Fouts, 1959). Approximately 20% of the alkaloid escapes into the urine. The rate of destruction of strychnine is such that approximately two lethal doses can be given over a period of 24 hours without noticeable toxic symptoms or cumulative effects.

Toxicology. Despite the fact that strychnine preparations are less available than formerly, poisoning by strychnine still occurs from rodenticides and sugar-coated proprietary cathartic and tonic tablets. An increasing source of unwitting poisoning stems from the adulteration of "street drugs" with strychnine. There is no pharmacological rationale for this dangerous practice.

Many cases of accidental poisoning are in children, who may succumb to as little as 15 mg. The fatal adult oral dose is about 50 to 100 mg, but 30 mg has been lethal (Gosselin *et al.*, 1984).

Symptoms of Strychnine Poisoning. The effects of strychnine in man closely resemble those described above for laboratory animals. The first effect that is noticed is stiffness of the face and neck muscles. Heightened reflex excitability soon becomes evident. Any sensory stimulus may produce a violent motor response. In the early stages this is a coordinated extensor thrust, and in the later stages it may be a full tetanic convulsion. In this convulsion, the body is arched in hyperextension (opisthotonos) so that only the crown of the head and the heels of the patient may be touching the ground. All voluntary muscles, including those of the face, are in full contraction. Respiration ceases due to the contraction of the diaphragm and the thoracic and abdominal muscles. Convulsive episodes may recur repeatedly with intermittent periods of depression; the frequency and severity of the convulsions are increased by sensory stimulation. Death results from medullary paralysis, which is due primarily to the hypoxia resulting from the periods of impaired respiration. In the early stages the patient not only is conscious but also is acutely perceptive to all stimuli. The muscle contractions are quite painful, and the patient is extremely apprehensive and fearful of impending death as he awaits the next tetanic spasm. If untreated, death from strychnine often occurs after the second to fifth full convulsion, but the first may be fatal if sustained. The combination of impaired respiration and intense muscular contractions can produce severe respiratory and metabolic acidosis, the latter due to elevated concentrations of lactate in plasma (Boyd *et al.*, 1983).

Treatment of Strychnine Poisoning. The most urgent objectives in the treatment of strychnine poisoning are the prevention of convulsions and the support of respiration. *Diazepam* is the most useful agent for this purpose. It antagonizes the convulsions without potentiating postictal depression, as may be the case with barbiturates or other nonselective depressants of the CNS (Maron *et al.*, 1971; Gosselin *et al.*, 1984). In adults, convulsions may be terminated by 10 mg of diazepam, intravenously, which should be repeated as subsequent prodromal symptoms appear. Children may require smaller doses. Anesthesia or neuromuscular blockade may be necessary to control resistant convulsions in severely intoxicated patients. All forms of sensory stimulation should be minimized. If adequate respiratory ventilation is not restored by the termination of convulsions, intubation and mechanical assistance are essential. After convulsions are controlled, activated charcoal is an effective method of reducing absorption when used as a slurry in gastric lavage. Iodine tincture diluted with water (1:250), tannic acid solution (2.0%, or in the form of strong tea), or potassium permanganate (1:5000) may also be employed. Severe metabolic acidosis may require intravenous administration of sodium bicarbonate (Boyd *et al.*, 1983).

Therapeutic Uses. Strychnine had an undeserved reputation as a useful therapeutic agent. To the drug have been ascribed properties that it does not possess or that it exhibits only when administered in toxic doses. There is no current justification for its presence in any medication. Judicious treatment with strychnine may modify the neurological deterioration in some infants with *nonketotic hyperglycinemia,* a rare metabolic disorder characterized by abnormally high concentrations of glycine in the brain and cerebrospinal fluid. However, clinical improvement in severe forms of this condition is limited and transient (Sankaran *et al.*, 1982).

PICROTOXIN

Picrotoxin is obtained from *Anamirta cocculus,* a climbing shrub indigenous to Malabar and the East Indies. The drug is present in the seeds of the plant, commonly known as fishberries, a name derived from the practice of throwing the bruised berries upon the water as a means of catching fish. The fish, after devouring the berries, are incapacitated and rise to the surface.

Chemistry. Picrotoxin is a nonnitrogenous neutral compound that can be broken down into two dilactones, *picrotoxinin* and *picrotin;* the latter is inactive. Picrotoxinin, the active component, has the following structural formula:

Picrotoxinin

Pharmacological Actions. Picrotoxin is a powerful stimulant and affects all portions of the CNS. Larger doses of picrotoxin are required to produce convulsions in a spinal animal than in an intact animal; in this respect picrotoxin differs strikingly from strychnine.

No appreciable effect of picrotoxin is seen until convulsive doses are given. The resultant convulsion is clonic and incoordinated, and the pattern resembles that produced by pentylenetetrazol (*see* below). With large doses of picrotoxin a tonic-clonic seizure may occur in which tonic flexion precedes tonic extension. Accompanying the convulsive movements are salivation, elevation of blood pressure due to vasomotor stimulation, and frequently emesis. Respiratory stimulation with picrotoxin is quite evident, but only in doses approaching convulsant levels.

Mechanism of Action. In mammals it has been shown that picrotoxin blocks *presynaptic* inhibition and strychnine-resistant *postsynaptic* inhibition in the CNS. Picrotoxin selectively antagonizes the effects of the predominant inhibitory transmitter, *gamma-aminobutyric acid (GABA),* at all levels of the CNS. Current information indicates that GABA receptors are coupled to ionophores that permit the influx of chloride with resultant hyperpolarization of neuronal membranes. Picrotoxin antagonizes the effects of GABA, perhaps by interacting with sites closely associated with the ionophore (*see* Chapter 17). A similarly acting convulsant drug, *bicuculline,* interacts directly with the GABA receptor and is therefore a true antagonist (*see* Johnston, 1978; Olsen, 1981). Both drugs produce convulsions by blocking the inhibitory pathways mediated by GABA. The relative importance of blockade of presynaptic or postsynaptic inhibition for their convulsant activity is unknown (*see* Davidson, 1976).

Toxicology. Although picrotoxin is absorbed by all routes, the full effect on the CNS is not seen for several minutes, even when the drug is administered intravenously. Its duration of action is relatively brief. Picrotoxin is a highly toxic substance, and a dose of 20 mg may produce symptoms of severe poisoning. The fatal dose for man is unknown. *Diazepam* is an effective antidote for poisoning by picrotoxin and should be given as described above in the discussion of strychnine.

Therapeutic Uses. Formerly employed in the treatment of poisoning by CNS depressants, picrotoxin is not a selective respiratory stimulant (Hirsh and Wang, 1975) and is not regarded as a useful therapeutic agent.

PENTYLENETETRAZOL

Pentylenetetrazol (pentamethylenetetrazol) is a synthetic compound with the following structural formula:

Pentylenetetrazol

Pharmacological Actions. Pentylenetetrazol has been widely studied in man and experimental animals. The actions of the drug are exerted primarily on the CNS. All levels of the cerebrospinal axis are stimulated by the drug; however, the dose required to produce convulsive movements in an animal with the spinal cord transected is several times that needed in the intact animal.

Pentylenetetrazol is a useful laboratory tool for screening anticonvulsant drugs (*see* Chapter 20). In experimental animals, threshold convulsive doses of the drug produce motor activity characterized by forelimb and jaw clonus. This convulsion resembles that produced by electrical stimulation of the brain with current of just threshold intensity. With slightly larger doses of pentylenetetrazol, generalized, asynchronized clonic movements are observed. This phase is usually superseded by a tonic convulsion; such a convulsion resembles that produced by maximal brain stimulation in that the movements of the limbs consist in flexion followed by extension. Thus, the pentylenetetrazol convulsion contrasts markedly with that produced by strychnine (*see* above), which is characterized by extension only.

Mechanism of Action. The mechanism of action of pentylenetetrazol has been studied less extensively than that of other convulsants, such as picrotoxin or penicillin. However, its electrophysiological effects resemble those of the latter agents in a number of respects. These include the capacity to reduce the impact of GABA on chloride ion conductance at concentrations that do not alter resting neuronal membrane conductance in the absence of GABA (Scholfield, 1982). In addition, pentylenetetrazol appears to interact with binding sites for picrotoxinin and to block the enhanced binding of GABA and benzodiazepines that is produced by hypnotic barbiturates (*see* Olsen, 1982). While direct excitatory effects have not been excluded, it would appear that a major action of pentylenetetrazol may be to reduce GABA-ergic inhibition, thereby enhancing CNS excitability.

Absorption, Fate, and Excretion. Pentylenetetrazol is readily absorbed from all sites of administration and is rapidly and equally distributed throughout the tissues. It is rapidly metabolized by the liver to inactive products, 75% of which are excreted in the urine (Rowles *et al.*, 1971).

Therapeutic Uses. Pentylenetetrazol, administered intravenously, was formerly used to activate the EEG as a diagnostic aid in *epilepsy*. Subconvulsive doses of the drug, alone or together with stroboscopic light, will often activate latent epileptogenic foci.

Pentylenetetrazol has received extensive trial in the management of regressed geriatric patients. However, there is no convincing evidence that either pentylenetetrazol or any other CNS stimulant is of value in treating mental symptoms associated with senility.

Pentylenetetrazol has no selective action on respiratory centers (Hirsh and Wang, 1974) and is no longer used as a respiratory stimulant.

DOXAPRAM AND NIKETHAMIDE

A few pharmacological agents remain in use because of their supposedly selective ability to stimulate central respiratory centers that are sufficiently depressed to impair respiratory function. However, the potential value of this approach has not been fulfilled, and it is apparent that direct, supportive measures, such as mechanical ventilation and maintenance of cardiovascular functions, are more useful.

The chemical structures of doxapram and nikethamide are as follows:

Doxapram

Nikethamide

Pharmacological Actions. Doxapram and nikethamide stimulate all levels of the cerebrospinal axis. Tonic-clonic convulsions, similar to those that follow the administration of pentylenetetrazol, can be produced readily. These drugs appear to act by enhancing excitation rather than by blocking central inhibition.

Respiration can be stimulated by each of these agents in doses that produce little generalized excitation. Doxapram administered intravenously in low doses selectively stimulates respiration and increases tidal volume by activating carotid chemoreceptors and central respiratory neurons (Calverley *et al.*, 1983), but higher doses stimulate both respiratory and nonrespiratory neurons in the medulla oblongata of the cat about equally (Hirsh and Wang, 1974). Nikethamide appears to have little selectivity. These distinctions have also been observed in man (*see* Winnie, 1973). The duration of respiratory stimulation by these drugs is transient after a single intravenous dose and seldom lasts for more than 5 or 10 minutes. The brief duration of action may reflect a "bolus effect," in which a large fraction of the drug is initially delivered to the CNS followed by redistribution to other organs and tissues. This may in part account for the greater likelihood of seizures after repeated doses, since the convulsant dose is generally not much larger than that required to stimulate respiration. Limited clinical experience indicates that the margin of safety is greater and the incidence of side effects is less for doxapram than for nikethamide (Winnie, 1973). However, side effects indicative of subconvulsive CNS stimulation are common with both drugs: hypertension, tachycardia, arrhythmias, coughing, sneezing, vomiting, itching, tremors, muscle rigidity, sweating, flushing, and hyperpyrexia. Excessive CNS stimulation or convulsions may be controlled by intravenous administration of diazepam. Where needed most, in deeply comatose patients, analeptics are virtually ineffective in doses below those producing convulsions; postictal depression following convulsions further intensifies the coma (*see* Mark, 1967).

Preparations and Dosage. *Doxapram hydrochloride* (DOPRAM) is supplied for injection. Single or divided intravenous doses in the range of 0.5 to 1.5 mg/kg are employed to attempt to produce the desired effect. The drug may also be given by intravenous infusion at an initial rate of 5 mg per minute, later reduced 50% or more. The recommended maximal dosage is 4 mg/kg (or 3 g).

Nikethamide (CORAMINE) is available in aqueous solution for oral use and for parenteral administration. Intravenous or intramuscular doses range from 1 to 15 ml of the 25% parenteral solution.

Therapeutic Uses and Status. Successful treatment of *acute sedative-hypnotic intoxication* emphasizes an orderly regimen of supportive therapy *without* the use of respiratory stimulants (Clemmesen and Nilsson, 1961; *see* Chapter 17). Systematic improvements in physiological support have reduced mortality rates from 25% during the height of analeptic therapy to a present rate of less than 1%. Mechanical assistance to depressed respiration is established as being far safer, more reliable, and more effective than erratic stimulation by drugs. Present opinion is unanimous in the condemnation of analeptics for the management of poisoning from any sedative-hypnotic drug (Mark, 1967; Lawson and Proudfoot, 1971).

Doxapram and nikethamide have been used as temporary measures to correct acute respiratory insufficiency in patients with *chronic obstructive pulmonary disease*. Intermittent or continuous infusion is necessary for sustained respiratory stimulation and reduction in carbon dioxide tension; however, potential improvement in oxygen tension is offset by a disproportionate increase in oxygen consumption. Typical side effects are common. Consequently, the value of analeptics in the therapy of pulmonary disease is very limited (Bader and Bader, 1965; Bickerman and Chusid, 1970). They may be of some short-term value to alleviate respiratory depression induced by oxygen therapy in these patients (Moser *et al.*, 1973). Recommended oral doses of analeptics are ineffective.

METHYLPHENIDATE

Methylphenidate is a piperidine derivative that is structurally related to amphetamine and has the following formula:

Methylphenidate

Pharmacological Actions. In contrast to the other drugs discussed in this chapter, methylphenidate is a mild CNS stimulant with more prominent effects on mental than on motor activities. However, large doses produce signs of generalized CNS stimulation that may lead to convulsions in man and animals. Its pharmacological properties are essentially the same as those of the amphetamines. Methylphenidate also shares the abuse potential of the amphetamines.

Absorption, Fate, and Excretion. Methylphenidate is readily absorbed after oral administration and reaches peak concentrations in plasma in about 2 hours. Its half-life in plasma is 1 to 2 hours, but concentrations in the brain exceed those in plasma. The main urinary metabolite is a deesterified product, ritalinic acid, which accounts for 80% of the dose; microsomal oxidation in man is minimal (Faraj *et al.*, 1974).

Preparations and Dosage. *Methylphenidate hydrochloride* (RITALIN) is available as tablets that contain 5, 10, or 20 mg of drug. The usual adult dose is 10 mg, given two or three times daily. The initial dosage recommended for children with attention-deficit disorder is 0.25 mg/kg daily (Millichap, 1968). This dose is doubled each week, if untoward effects are not observed, until the optimal daily dosage of 2 mg/kg is reached. The drug is given in equal portions before breakfast and lunch. Sustained-release tablets that contain 20 mg of the drug have a duration of action of approximately 8 hours and may be useful to reduce the frequency of dosage for some patients.

Therapeutic Uses and Status. Methylphenidate has received extensive trial in various types of mental depression, in the treatment of overdosage from depressant drugs, and in relieving lassitude from various causes. Its effectiveness for these uses is doubtful.

Methylphenidate and dextroamphetamine are important adjuncts in the therapy of *hyperkinetic syndromes* in both children (Barkley, 1977; Weiss and Hechtman, 1979) and adults (Wender *et al.*, 1981) who are characterized as having *attention-deficit disorder* (ADD; formerly called "minimal brain dysfunction"). Double-blind studies with placebo control have clearly demonstrated that methylphenidate can improve behavior, concentration, and learning ability in 70 to 80% of children with ADD; dextroamphetamine is equally effective (Barkley, 1977; Weiss, 1981). However, indiscriminate use of these drugs for "problem" children and sole dependence on drug therapy for ADD should be discouraged (Sroufe and Stewart, 1973; Weiss, 1981). Both drugs have been shown to suppress growth during chronic therapy, but this effect appears to be less with methylphenidate (Mattes and Gittelman, 1983). Other side effects of methylphenidate (insomnia, anorexia, irritability, abdominal pain, headache, and increased heart rate) are often only temporary and may be controlled by reduction of dosage. Acute episodes of hallucinosis early in therapy with methylphenidate may represent rare idiosyncratic reactions. Although it has been generally assumed that the effects of methylphenidate and dextroamphetamine on the behavior and the mental concentration of patients with ADD are selective for this condition, these effects are also produced in normal subjects and may reflect an increase of attention in both groups (Rapoport *et al.*, 1978).

Methylphenidate may be effective in the treatment of *narcolepsy*, either alone or in combination with a tricyclic antidepressant (Zarcone, 1973).

Pemoline. *Pemoline* (CYLERT) is structurally dissimilar to methylphenidate but elicits similar changes in CNS function with minimal effects on the cardiovascular system. It is employed in treating ADD and can be given once daily because of its long half-life. However, clinical improvement is delayed by 3 to 4 weeks.

Adamson, R. H., and Fouts, J. R. Enzymatic metabolism of strychnine. *J. Pharmacol. Exp. Ther.*, 1959, *127*, 87–91.

Bader, M. E., and Bader, R. A. Respiratory stimulants in obstructive lung disease. *Am. J. Med.*, 1965, *38*, 165–171.

Bickerman, H. A., and Chusid, E. L. The case against the use of respiratory stimulants. *Chest*, 1970, *58*, 53–56.

Boyd, R. E.; Brennan, P. T.; Deng, J.-F.; Rochester, D. F.; and Spyker, D. A. Strychnine poisoning: recovery from profound lactic acidosis, hyperthermia, and rhabdomyolysis. *Am. J. Med.*, 1983, *74*, 507–512.

Calverley, P. M. A.; Robson, R. H.; Wraith, P. K.; Prescott, L. F.; and Flenley, D. C. The ventilatory effects of doxapram in normal man. *Clin. Sci.*, 1983, *65*, 65–69.

Clemmesen, C., and Nilsson, E. Therapeutic trends in the treatment of barbiturate poisoning—the Scandinavian method. *Clin. Pharmacol. Ther.*, 1961, *2*, 220–229.

Esplin, D. W., and Woodbury, D. M. Spinal reflexes and seizure patterns in the two-toed sloth. *Science*, 1961, *133*, 1426–1427.

Faraj, B. A.; Israili, Z. H.; Perel, J. M.; Jenkins, M. L.; Holtzman, S. G.; Cucinell, S. A.; and Dayton, P. G. Metabolism and disposition of methylphenidate-^{14}C: studies in man and animals. *J. Pharmacol. Exp. Ther.*, 1974, *191*, 535–547.

Gosselin, R. E.; Smith, R. P.; and Hodge, H. H. *Clinical Toxicology of Commercial Products*, 5th ed., Sect. III. The Williams & Wilkins Co., Baltimore, 1984, pp. III 375–III 379.

Hirsh, K., and Wang, S. C. Selective respiratory stimulating action of doxapram compared to pentylenetetrazol. *J. Pharmacol. Exp. Ther.*, 1974, *189*, 1–11.

———. Respiratory stimulant effects of ethamivan and picrotoxin. *Ibid.*, 1975, *193*, 657–663.

Kuno, M., and Weakly, J. N. Quantal components of the inhibitory synaptic potential in spinal motoneurones of the cat. *J. Physiol. (Lond.)*, 1972, *224*, 287–303.

Lawson, A. A. H., and Proudfoot, A. T. Medical management of acute barbiturate poisoning. In, *Acute Barbiturate Poisoning*. (Matthew, H., ed.) Excerpta Medica, Amsterdam, 1971, pp. 175–193.

Mark, L. C. Analeptics: changing concepts, declining status. *Am. J. Med. Sci.*, 1967, *254*, 296–302.

Maron, B. J.; Krupp, J. R.; and Tune, B. Strychnine poisoning successfully treated with diazepam. *J. Pediatr.*, 1971, *78*, 697–699.

Mattes, J. A., and Gittelman, R. Growth of hyperactive children on maintenance regimen of methylphenidate. *Arch. Gen. Psychiatry*, 1983, *40*, 317–321.

Millichap, J. G. Drugs in management of hyperkinetic and perceptually handicapped children. *J.A.M.A.*, 1968, *206*, 1527–1530.

Moser, K. M.; Luchsinger, P. C.; Adamson, J. S.; McMahon, S. L.; Schlueter, D. P.; Spivack, M.; and Weg, J. G. Respiratory stimulation with intravenous doxapram in respiratory failure. *N. Engl. J. Med.*, 1973, *288*, 427–431.

Rapoport, J. L.; Buchsbaum, M. S.; Zahn, T. P.; Weingartner, H.; Ludlow, C.; and Mikkelsen, E. J. Dextroamphetamine: cognitive and behavioral effects in normal prepubertal boys. *Science*, 1978, *199*, 560–563.

Rowles, S. G.; Born, G. S.; Russell, H. T.; Kessler, W. V.; and Christian, J. E. Biological disposition of pentylenetetrazol-10-^{14}C in rats and humans. *J. Pharm. Sci.*, 1971, *60*, 725–727.

Sankaran, K.; Casey, R. E.; Zaleski, W. A.; and Mendelson, I. M. Glycine encephalopathy in a neonate: treatment with intravenous strychnine and sodium benzoate. *Clin. Pediatr. (Phila.)*, 1982, *21*, 636–637.

Scholfield, C. N. Antagonism of γ-aminobutyric acid and muscimol by picrotoxin, bicuculline, strychnine, bemegride, leptazol, *d*-tubocurarine and theophylline in the isolated olfactory cortex. *Arch. Pharm. (Weinheim)*, 1982, *318*, 274–280.

Sroufe, L. A., and Stewart, M. A. Treating problem children with stimulant drugs. *N. Engl. J. Med.*, 1973, *289*, 407–413.

Wender, P. H.; Reimherr, F. W.; and Wood, D. R. Attention deficit disorder ('minimal brain dysfunction') in adults. *Arch. Gen. Psychiatry*, 1981, *38*, 449–456.

Winnie, A. P. Chemical respirogenesis: a comparative

study. *Acta Anaesthesiol. Scand.*, **1973**, Suppl. 51, 1–32.

Zarbin, M. A.; Wamsley, J. K.; and Kuhar, M. J. Glycine receptor: light microscopic autoradiographic localization with [³H] strychnine. *J. Neurosci.*, **1981**, *1*, 532–547.

Zarcone, V. Narcolepsy. *N. Engl. J. Med.*, **1973**, *288*, 1156–1166.

Monographs and Reviews

Barkley, R. A. A review of stimulant drug research with hyperactive children. *J. Child Psychol. Psychiatry*, **1977**, *18*, 137–165.

Curtis, D. R. The pharmacology of postsynaptic inhibition. *Prog. Brain Res.*, **1969**, *31*, 171–189.

Davidson, N. *Neurotransmitter Amino Acids*. Academic Press, Inc., New York, **1976**.

Esplin, D. W., and Zablocka-Esplin, B. Mechanisms of action of convulsants. In, *Basic Mechanisms of the Epilepsies*. (Jasper, H. H.; Ward, A. A., Jr.; and Pope, A.; eds.) Little, Brown & Co., Boston, **1969**, pp. 167–183.

Hahn, F. Analeptics. *Pharmacol. Rev.*, **1960**, *12*, 447–530.

Johnston, G. A. R. Neuropharmacology of amino acid inhibitory transmitters. *Annu. Rev. Pharmacol. Toxicol.*, **1978**, *18*, 269–289.

Olsen, R. W. The GABA postsynaptic membrane receptor-ionophore complex: site of action of convulsant and anticonvulsant drugs. *Mol. Cell. Biochem.*, **1981**, *39*, 261–279.

————. Drug interactions at the GABA receptor-ionophore complex. *Annu. Rev. Pharmacol. Toxicol.*, **1982**, *22*, 245–277.

Smythies, J. R. Relations between the chemical structure and biological activity of convulsants. *Annu. Rev. Pharmacol.*, **1974**, *14*, 9–21.

Wang, S. C., and Ward, J. W. Analeptics. *Pharmacol. Ther. [B]*, **1977**, *3*, 123–165.

Weiss, G. Controversial issues of the pharmacotherapy of the hyperactive child. *Can. J. Psychiatry*, **1981**, *26*, 385–392.

Weiss, G., and Hechtman, L. The hyperactive child syndrome. *Science*, **1979**, *205*, 1348–1354.

25 CENTRAL NERVOUS SYSTEM STIMULANTS
[*Continued*]

The Methylxanthines

Theodore W. Rall

THEOPHYLLINE, CAFFEINE, AND THEOBROMINE

Source and History. Theophylline, caffeine, and theobromine are three closely related alkaloids that occur in plants widely distributed geographically. It is believed that paleolithic man discovered the principal caffeine-containing plants throughout the world and made beverages from them. In South America, caffeine-containing beverages of great antiquity include *guaraná* (from the seeds of either *Paullinia cupana* or *Paullinia sorbilis*), *yoco* (from the bark of *Paullinia yoco*), and *maté* (from *Ilex paraguariensis*, a species of holly). At least half the population of the world consumes *tea* (containing caffeine and small amounts of theophylline and theobromine), prepared from the leaves of *Thea sinensis*, a bush native to southern China and now extensively cultivated in other countries. Cocoa and chocolate, from the seeds of *Theobroma cacao*, contain theobromine and some caffeine. *Coffee*, the most important source of caffeine in the American diet, is extracted from the fruit of *Coffea arabica* and related species. Cola-flavored drinks usually contain considerable amounts of caffeine, in part because of their content of extracts of the nuts of *Cola acuminata* (the guru nuts chewed by the natives of the Sudan) and in part because of the addition of caffeine as such in their production (*see* Graham, 1978).

The basis for the popularity of all the caffeine-containing beverages has been the ancient belief that these beverages had stimulant and antisoporific actions that elevated mood, decreased fatigue, and increased capacity for work. For example, legend credits the discovery of coffee to a prior of an Arabian convent. Shepherds reported that goats that had eaten the berries of the coffee plant gamboled and frisked about all through the night instead of sleeping. The prior, mindful of the long nights of prayer that he had to endure, instructed the shepherds to pick the berries so that he might make a beverage from them.

Classical pharmacological studies, principally of caffeine, during the first half of this century have confirmed these beliefs and have revealed that methylxanthines possess other important pharmacological properties as well. These properties were exploited for a number of years in a variety of therapeutic applications; many of these have now been replaced by more effective agents. However, in recent years there has been a resurgence of interest in the therapeutic use of the natural methylxanthines and synthetic derivatives thereof, principally as a result of increased knowledge of their cellular basis of action and their pharmacokinetic properties.

Chemistry. Caffeine, theophylline, and theobromine are methylated xanthines. They are often spoken of as *xanthine derivatives, methylxanthines*, or merely *xanthines*. Xanthine itself is dioxypurine and is structurally related to uric acid. Caffeine is 1,3,7-trimethylxanthine; theophylline, 1,3-dimethylxanthine; and theobromine, 3,7-dimethylxanthine. The structural formulas of xanthine and the three naturally occurring xanthine derivatives are as follows:

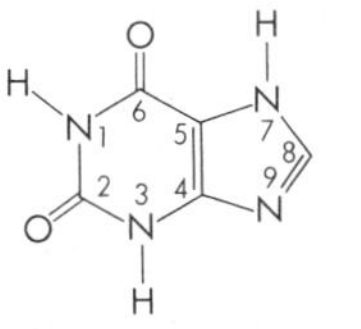

Xanthine

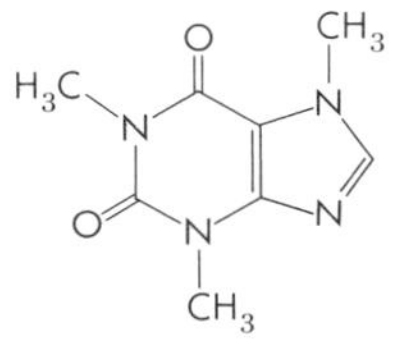

Caffeine

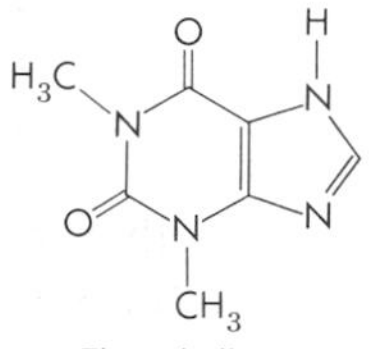

Theophylline

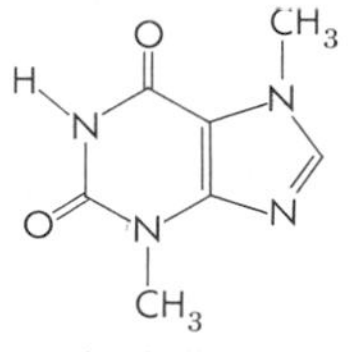

Theobromine

The solubility of the methylxanthines is low and is much enhanced by the formation of complexes (usually 1:1) with a wide variety of compounds. The most notable of such complexes is that between theophylline and ethylenediamine (to form *aminophylline*). The formation of complex double salts (*e.g.*, caffeine and sodium benzoate) or true salts (*e.g.*, *choline theophyllinate, oxtriphylline*) also enhances aqueous solubility. These salts or complexes dissociate to yield the parent methylxanthines when dissolved in biological fluids and should not be confused with covalently modified derivatives such as *dyphylline* (1,3-dimethyl-7-(2,3-dihydroxypropyl)-xanthine).

Studies of the actions of congeners of the methylxanthines in whole animals or other relatively complex biological systems have revealed a struc-

589

ture-activity relationship that is difficult to interpret. On the other hand, studies of the inhibition of cyclic nucleotide phosphodiesterases and the antagonism of receptor-mediated actions of adenosine (the best-characterized cellular actions of the methylxanthines) have revealed that the order of potency is theophylline > caffeine > theobromine. Congeners of theophylline that possess larger nonpolar substituents at positions 1 and 3 or additional alkyl groups at position 8 of the xanthine ring usually display enhancement of both activities; derivatives that lack a substituent at position 1 and those that have substitutions at positions 7 or 9 generally have reduced activity. Addition of an aromatic group at position 8 markedly increases potency as an antagonist at adenosine receptors but reduces inhibition of cyclic nucleotide phosphodiesterase. A number of nonxanthine compounds are much more potent than theophylline as inhibitors of cyclic nucleotide phosphodiesterase but lack the ability to antagonize actions of adenosine. These include papaverine, dipyridamole, and a variety of benzodiazepines. Other cellular actions of the methylxanthines require higher concentrations for detection than those enumerated above. These include mobilization of intracellular calcium ions and inhibition of binding of benzodiazepines to specific sites in brain tissue. The limited information available on these actions indicates that caffeine is somewhat more potent than theophylline.

PHARMACOLOGICAL PROPERTIES

Theophylline, caffeine, and theobromine share in common several pharmacological actions of therapeutic interest. They stimulate the central nervous system (CNS), act on the kidney to produce diuresis, stimulate cardiac muscle, and relax smooth muscle, notably bronchial muscle. Because the various xanthines differ markedly in the intensity of their actions on various structures, one particular xanthine has been used more than another for a particular therapeutic effect. Since theobromine displays a low potency in these pharmacological actions, it has all but disappeared from the therapeutic scene.

Central Nervous System. Theophylline and caffeine are potent stimulants of the CNS; theobromine is virtually inactive in this respect. Traditionally, caffeine has been considered the most potent of the methylxanthines; however, theophylline produces more profound and potentially more dangerous CNS stimulation than does caffeine.

Persons ingesting caffeine or caffeine-containing beverages usually experience less drowsiness, less fatigue, and a more rapid and clearer flow of thought. While caffeine produces an increased capacity for sustained intellectual effort and decreases reaction time, tasks involving delicate muscular coordination and accurate timing or arithmetic skills may be adversely affected (*see* Curatolo and Robertson, 1983). The above-mentioned effects may be produced by the administration of 85 to 250 mg of caffeine, the amount contained in 1 to 3 cups of coffee. Comparable effects of theophylline have not been carefully investigated, owing in part to the fact that CNS stimulatory actions of this agent have been observed principally as side effects in the therapy of bronchial asthma, in which the adult dose is above 250 mg. As the dose is increased, methylxanthines produce nervousness, restlessness, insomnia, tremors, hyperesthesia, and other signs of CNS stimulation. At still higher doses, focal and generalized convulsions are produced; theophylline is clearly more potent than caffeine in this regard. Such seizures, occasionally refractory to anticonvulsant agents, have sometimes occurred in patients when the blood concentration of theophylline was only about 50% above the top of the accepted therapeutic range.

Methylxanthines also stimulate the *medullary respiratory centers*. This action is particularly prominent in certain pathophysiological states, such as in Cheyne-Stokes respiration and in apnea of preterm infants, and when respiration is depressed by certain drugs, such as opioids. The methylxanthines appear to increase the sensitivity of medullary centers to the stimulatory actions of CO_2, and respiratory minute volume is increased at any given value of alveolar P_{CO_2}. Both methylxanthines may produce nausea and vomiting; this probably involves CNS actions, at least in part. Theophylline-induced emesis is common when concentrations in plasma exceed 15 μg/ml, which includes the upper part of the recommended range of therapeutic concentrations.

The relative potencies of caffeine and theophylline as CNS stimulants appear to vary depending on the species and experimental parameter studied. However, in preterm infants, the frequency and duration of episodes of apnea are reduced by both agents over similar ranges of concentration in plasma (*see* Symposium, 1981). Stimulatory effects are evident at low doses of the methylxanthines in individuals whose CNS function has been depressed by certain agents. For example, caffeine at 0.5 mg/kg is sufficient to produce respiratory stimulation in human subjects given 10 mg of morphine (Bellville *et al.*, 1962), while aminophylline (2 mg/kg) can rapidly reverse the narcosis induced by as much as 100 mg of morphine given intravenously to produce anesthesia (Stirt, 1983). Similar doses of aminophylline can also accelerate the recovery from a state of deep sedation produced intraoperatively by the intravenous administration of diazepam (0.4 mg/kg) (Arvidsson *et al.*, 1982). By contrast, there is little evidence to support the popular belief that caffeine can improve mental function during intoxication with ethanol (*see* Curatolo and Robertson, 1983).

A controversy has emerged as to whether the increase in respiratory minute volume produced by methylxanthines results largely from an increase in diaphragmatic contractility. On the one hand, the transdiaphragmatic pressure produced by stimulation of the phrenic nerve in anesthetized dogs is increased by theophylline at concentrations that include those achieved during therapy of asthma in man (Aubier *et al.*, 1983). Infusion of theophylline into the cerebral ventricles is without effect. On the other hand, administration of therapeutic doses of theophylline to cats increases phrenic nerve activity even after decerebration or sectioning of the spinal cord at various levels (Eldridge *et al.*, 1983). Furthermore, changes in diaphragmatic contractility would not explain the ability of dopaminergic antagonists to attenuate the respiratory stimulation induced by theophylline.

Cardiovascular System. Caffeine and theophylline, especially the latter, have prominent actions on the circulatory system. The capacity of theophylline to produce modest decreases in peripheral vascular resistance, sometimes powerful cardiac stimulation, increased perfusion of most organs, and diuresis has been exploited for the emergency treatment of congestive heart failure. However, the unpredictable absorption and disposition of theophylline in patients with compromised circulatory function led all too often to serious CNS and cardiac toxicity (Piafsky *et al.*, 1977). More effective vasodilators, specific inotropic agents, and diuretics are now preferred (*see* Cohn and Franciosa, 1977).

The actions of the methylxanthines on the circulatory system are complex and sometimes antagonistic, and the resultant effects largely depend upon the conditions prevailing at the time of their administration and the dose used. In addition to the traditional but poorly documented view that methylxanthines have appreciable capability to stimulate vagal and vasomotor centers in the brain stem, there is an array of more or less direct actions on vascular and cardiac tissues in combination with indirect peripheral actions that are mediated by catecholamines and possibly by the renin-angiotensin system. Therefore, the observation of a single function, for example, the blood pressure, is deceiving because the drugs may act on a variety of circulatory factors in such a way that the blood pressure may remain essentially unchanged.

Heart. At therapeutic plasma concentrations (10 to 20 μg/ml), theophylline produces a modest increase in heart rate in normal individuals (Ogilvie *et al.*, 1977; Vestal *et al.*, 1983). Low concentrations of caffeine may produce small decreases in heart rate (Starr *et al.*, 1937), presumably a consequence of stimulation of the medullary vagal nuclei. At higher concentrations, both methylxanthines produce definite tachycardia; sensitive individuals may experience other arrhythmias, such as premature ventricular contractions. Arrhythmias may also be encountered in persons who use caffeine-containing beverages to excess. Theophylline at 10 to 20 μg/ml in plasma also reduces the left ventricular ejection time index and isovolumetric contraction time, consistent with an increase in contractile force and a decrease in cardiac preload (Ogilvie *et al.*, 1977). The decrease in the venous filling pressure may be caused in part by the more complete emptying of the heart. In normal individuals, any rise in cardiac output may be brief and may be followed by a fall below the initial level. In patients with heart failure, however, the venous pressure is initially rather high; consequently the cardiac stimulation, together with the lowering of venous pressure produced by theophylline, leads to a marked increase in cardiac output that occurs almost immediately and persists for 30 minutes or more after intravenous administration.

The effects of theophylline at therapeutic plasma concentrations may be mediated in part by the augmented release of catecholamines from the sympathoadrenal system. For example, the infusion of graded doses of theophylline into normal human subjects increases the concentration of epinephrine in plasma by about 100% when theophylline concentrations reach 10 to 15 μg/ml (Vestal et al., 1983). Norepinephrine is affected to a lesser extent. The ingestion of 250 mg of caffeine, leading to concentrations in plasma of about 10 μg/ml, produces similar changes in circulating catecholamines (Robertson et al., 1978). The intravenous administration of as little as 200 mg of theophylline in human subjects can enhance the exocytosis of storage granules for catecholamines, as evidenced by an increase in dopamine β-hydroxylase activity in plasma (Aunis et al., 1975). Although both theophylline and caffeine at these concentrations produce increases in systolic blood pressure and plasma renin activity, only caffeine appears to raise the diastolic blood pressure significantly. The hemodynamic responses to the administration of caffeine are reduced following chronic ingestion (Robertson et al., 1981); parallel observations during the chronic administration of theophylline have not been made.

There are also studies in animals that indicate the importance of catecholamines in mediating the effects of methylxanthines on the heart. For example, the positive inotropic and chronotropic responses to the infusion of aminophylline (10 mg/kg) into dogs are markedly reduced following the administration of propranolol (Rutherford et al., 1981). However, prior treatment of dogs with propranolol does not prevent the ability of intravenous aminophylline (5 mg/kg) to reverse the impaired atrioventricular nodal conduction produced by decreasing the blood supply to this structure (Belardinelli et al., 1981). This action may be a consequence of the capacity of methylxanthines to antagonize the effects of adenosine released locally during ischemia (see below). Theophylline potentiates the inotropic response to norepinephrine in isolated atria (Rall and West, 1963). Since a concentration of at least 0.2 mM (36 μg/ml) is required, this interaction may be a consequence of the ability of methylxanthines to inhibit the degradation of adenosine 3',5'-monophosphate (cyclic AMP) (see below). At still higher concentrations of methylxanthines (1 to 10 mM), a variety of effects has been noted on myocardial tissue in vitro; alterations in the cellular metabolism of calcium may be involved (see below).

Blood Vessels.   After therapeutic doses of caffeine or theophylline in man, the peripheral vascular resistance declines, regardless of the change, if any, of arterial blood pressure (Starr et al., 1937; Ogilvie et al., 1977). Oncometric studies in animals show that there is a definite increase in organ volume following the administration of xanthines. Vasodilatation, coupled with an augmented cardiac output, results in an increased blood flow. However, in man the

increase in peripheral blood flow is short lived.

In contrast to their dilating effect upon the systemic blood vessels, the xanthines cause a marked increase in *cerebrovascular resistance* with an accompanying decrease in cerebral blood flow and in the oxygen tension of the brain (Wechsler et al., 1950; Moyer et al., 1952). It is this vasoconstriction, rather than the decrease in cerebrospinal fluid pressure that may also occur, that is believed to be responsible for the relief of hypertensive headache by the xanthines.

Experimentally, it can be demonstrated that the xanthines dilate coronary arteries and increase coronary blood flow. This led to their use in the treatment of coronary artery disease. However, opinion as to their value is divided and the evidence in this field is controversial. There seems to be general agreement in the studies on man that under certain conditions the xanthines increase coronary blood flow. There is also abundant evidence that the drugs increase the work of the heart. The outstanding question is whether the blood supply to the myocardium increases to a greater extent than does the oxygen demand. In spite of the controversial claims and disappointing clinical results, the xanthines unfortunately continue to be employed by some physicians in the treatment of coronary insufficiency.

In vitro, it has generally been found that methylxanthines (about 0.5 mM or above) cause relaxation of vascular smooth muscle in the presence of various stimulators of contraction (e.g., norepinephrine, angiotensin, K^+). While relaxation probably results from a reduction of the cytosolic concentration of Ca^{2+}, it is not clear to what extent the methylxanthines alter calcium binding and transport directly or influence these functions indirectly by means of changes in cyclic nucleotide metabolism. However, at concentrations close to those in the therapeutic range, the effects of methylxanthines are variable and depend upon the locale of the vascular bed and the experimental conditions employed. For example, theophylline (18 μg/ml) inhibits the vasoconstriction produced by nerve stimulation or by infusion of norepinephrine in the isolated, perfused rabbit kidney (Hedqvist et al., 1978). This occurs despite the fact that theophylline promotes release of norepinephrine during nerve stimulation. These effects appear to involve specific antagonism of the actions of adenosine. On the other hand, caffeine and theophylline (1 to 10 μg/ml) *augment* contractions of aortic strips in the presence of epinephrine (Kalsner, 1971). A similar potentiation of the effects of catecholamines is observed with bovine coronary artery (Kalsner *et al.*, 1975); however, in this case it is β-adrenergic receptor-mediated *relaxation* that is enhanced by methylxanthines. These effects appear to involve reduction in the extraneuronal uptake and metabolism of catecholamines. Lammerant and Becsei (1975) infused theophylline into the coronary artery of dogs and noted no changes in coronary blood flow until the heart rate was elevated to approximately 150 beats per minute by right atrial pacing. The *reduction* of coronary blood flow that was then caused by the methylxanthines may be due to antagonism of the coronary-dilating action of endogenously released adenosine (*see* Berne and Rubio, 1974). Infusion of aminophylline (7 mg/kg) into intact dogs potentiates the hypotensive effects of sodium nitroprusside (Pearl *et al.*, 1984); this is consistent with the possibility that theophylline can augment the accumulation of guanosine 3′,5′-monophosphate (cyclic GMP) (*see* Chapter 33).

Smooth Muscle.   The xanthines relax various smooth muscles other than those of blood vessels. The most important action in this respect is their ability to relax the smooth muscles of the *bronchi*, especially if the bronchi have been constricted either experimentally by histamine or clinically in asthma. Theophylline is the most effective and produces a definite increase in vital capacity. It is, therefore, of value in the treatment of bronchial asthma.

It is not clear to what extent therapeutic responses that occur when concentrations of theophylline in plasma are 5 to 20 μg/ml involve the release of or synergistic interactions with β-adrenergic agonists. In general, the concentrations of methylxanthines that produce bronchodilatation *in vivo* are considerably lower than those required to relax various preparations of airway muscle studied *in vitro*. Furthermore, prior adrenalectomy or administration of β-adrenergic antagonists causes a fivefold increase in the dose of theophylline required to reduce the bronchoconstriction induced by acetylcholine in guinea pigs (James, 1967). While augmented responses to β₂-adrenergic agonists have sometimes been noted in studies conducted *in vitro* in the presence of therapeutic concentrations of theophylline (Bertelli *et al.*, 1973), numerous investigations in man have failed to indicate that such combinations produce synergistic therapeutic responses (*see* Handslip *et al.*, 1981). It is also not clear to what extent theophylline-induced bronchodilatation might involve blockade of adenosine receptors. Administration of adenosine by inhalation to asthmatic (but not normal) subjects produces marked bronchoconstriction (Cushley *et al.*, 1983).

Theophylline (4 to 8 mg/kg) also inhibits the canine ureter *in situ*, relaxes the bladder, and, in relatively high concentrations, abolishes spontaneous contractions of the rat uterus and guinea pig taenia coli (Wein *et al.*, 1972; Pfaffman and McFarland, 1978). This last-named effect may account for the observation that intravenous injection of theophylline in man causes a transient suppression of motility in the large and small bowel.

Skeletal Muscle.   It has long been known that caffeine increases the capacity for muscular work in man. For example, the ingestion of caffeine (6 mg/kg) improves the racing performance of cross-country skiers, particularly at high altitudes (Berglund and Hemmingsson, 1982). However, it is not clear to what extent this effect involves direct actions of caffeine on neuromuscular transmission or whether therapeutic doses of theophylline produce similar effects. Administration of caffeine to human subjects increases the tension developed in the adductor pollicis muscle produced by stimulation of the ulnar nerve (Lopes *et al.*, 1983); similar concentrations of theophylline appear to have no significant effect (Wiles *et al.*, 1983). However, caffeine and theophylline increase about equally the transdiaphragmatic pressure generated by stimulation of the phrenic nerve in dogs (Aubier *et al.*, 1983). At higher concentrations (0.5 to 1 mM), caffeine and, to a lesser extent, theophylline clearly augment the contractility of striated muscle. The possible role of the translocation of Ca^{2+} in these effects is discussed below.

Diuretic Actions.   Methylxanthines, especially theophylline, increase the production of urine, and the patterns of enhanced excretion of water and electrolytes are very similar to those produced by the thiazides (Maren, 1961). In normal man, the infusion of aminophylline (3.5 mg/kg) appears to inhibit solute reabsorption in both the proximal nephron and the diluting segment without changing appreciably either rate of total renal blood flow or glomerular filtration; no additional effects are produced in the presence of furosemide (Brater *et al.*, 1983). However, the actions of theophylline are less clearly defined in patients with congestive heart failure during chronic treatment with high-ceiling diuretic agents. In this setting, the administration of aminophylline (400 mg) produces additional excretion of sodium, chloride, and potassium ions (Sigurd and Olesen, 1978). The diuretic actions of the xanthines are also mentioned in Chapter 36.

Secretion.   Methylxanthines augment release of the secretory products of a number of endocrine and exocrine tissues. One exception to this general statement is the ability of methylxanthines to inhibit secretion by mast cells and possibly other sources of mediators of inflammation. A number of the therapeutic and toxic properties of methylxanthines probably involve actions on secretory processes. However, the quantitative contribution of such actions has not often been delineated.

Gastric Secretion. The pattern of effects of methylxanthines on gastric secretion is dependent upon the species and conditions employed. Man is relatively sensitive, and moderate oral or parenteral doses of caffeine cause secretion of both acid and pepsin (*see* Debas *et al.*, 1971). Although never directly compared, theophylline would appear to be at least as potent as caffeine in this regard (Krasnow and Grossman, 1949). While atropine may partially inhibit caffeine-induced secretion of acid, the prior administration of cimetidine, an H_2-receptor antagonist, completely prevents the response to even relatively high doses of caffeine (Cano *et al.*, 1976).

It has been long known (and perhaps forgotten) that beverages made from roasted grain containing no caffeine stimulate acid secretion in man as much as does coffee (Öhnell and Berg, 1931); similarly, decaffeinated coffee is only slightly less potent than the natural product, and both are about twice as effective as is an equivalent amount of caffeine (Cohen and Booth, 1975). In view of the responsiveness of the human gastric mucosa to caffeine and other substances in various beverages, cognizance must be taken of the ubiquitous use of coffee and colas in the pathogenesis of peptic ulcer and in the management of the patient with an ulcer.

Secretion of Other Substances. As noted above, therapeutic concentrations of methylxanthines can increase the concentration of circulating catecholamines and can augment dopamine β-hydroxylase and renin activity in the plasma in man. Since propranolol does not prevent the increase in plasma renin activity, catecholamines are probably not involved in this response (Zehner *et al.*, 1975). Administration of theophylline results in increases in the plasma concentrations of gastrin (Feurle *et al.*, 1976) and parathyroid hormone (Bowser *et al.*, 1975). Epinephrine can also produce the latter effect, and thus it is not clear whether this represents a direct action of the methylxanthine. While high concentrations of theophylline cause significant increases in circulating insulin, therapeutic concentrations are usually without effect (Vestal *et al.*, 1983). Theophylline can also potentiate the insulinemic responses to infusions of secretin and cholecystokinin-pancreozymin (Serrano-Ríos *et al.*, 1974).

The release of histamine from rat peritoneal mast cells produced by a variety of stimuli can usually be inhibited only by relatively high concentrations of theophylline (0.2 to 2.5 mM). However, much lower concentrations (below 0.1 mM) are effective in antagonizing the augmentation of histamine release produced by adenosine acting in concert with antigen or a calcium ionophore (Marquardt *et al.*, 1978; Sydbom and Fredholm, 1982). These observations may relate to some of the therapeutic actions of theophylline in bronchial asthma, as well as to the observations that caffeine displays anti-inflammatory activity in various model systems (Vinegar *et al.*, 1976). Small doses of caffeine (5 to 10 mg/kg) also appear to reduce the ED50 for aspirin, indomethacin, and phenylbutazone by more than threefold.

Metabolism. The administration of caffeine (4 to 8 mg/kg) to normal or obese human subjects elevates the concentration of free fatty acids in plasma and increases the basal metabolic rate (Acheson *et al.*, 1980); therapeutic concentrations of theophylline produce similar effects on free fatty acids (Vestal *et al.*, 1983). It is not clear if the release and action of catecholamines are essential for the production of these metabolic responses.

Cellular Basis for the Action of Methylxanthines. Three basic cellular actions of the methylxanthines have received major attention in studies to explain their diverse effects. Listed in order of their increasing sensitivity to methylxanthines, they are: (1) those associated with translocations of intracellular calcium; (2) those mediated by increasing accumulation of cyclic nucleotides, particularly cyclic AMP; and (3) those mediated by blockade of receptors for adenosine. Of particular importance is the question of what types of actions contribute appreciably to the effects of methylxanthines in the therapeutic dose range. The concentration of free theophylline in plasma rarely exceeds 50 μM during therapy. At the present state of knowledge, this fact alone appears to limit severely the possible contribution of the first two categories of actions to the therapeutic effects of theophylline and leaves the anti-adenosine action as the leading candidate (*see* Rall, 1982). There are also several other types of actions that have received relatively little attention to date but that might prove to be very important in certain effects of the methylxanthines. These include their potentiation of inhibitors of prostaglandin synthesis (*see* Vinegar *et al.*, 1976), and the possibility that methylxanthines reduce the uptake and/or metabolism of catecholamines in nonneural tissues (*see* Kalsner, 1971; Kalsner *et al.*, 1975). Further investigation will be required to establish the contribution of these actions to both the immediate effect of the methylxanthines and those involving the release of catechol-amines.

Studies of the actions of methylxanthines on translocation of intracellular Ca^{2+} have involved principally those of caffeine on skeletal muscle. Caffeine (0.5 to 1 mM) augments the twitch response of the isolated frog sartorius muscle to stimulation of the motor nerve. The twitch is increased in height and is more rapid in onset and duration, probably because of sensitization of the mechanism for the release of Ca^{2+} from the terminal cisternae of the sarcoplasmic reticulum. Higher concentrations of caffeine produce contracture without nerve stimulation, owing probably to an increase in Ca^{2+} permeability of the sarcoplasmic reticulum, which normally participates in the termination of the contractile process by active uptake and sequestration of Ca^{2+} (see Bianchi, 1975). Under certain circumstances, effects of caffeine on Ca^{2+} release by preparations of skeletal muscle sarcoplasmic reticulum can be observed at concentrations as low as 0.25 mM (Katz et al., 1977). Similar mechanisms may be important in the actions of methylxanthines upon certain secretory processes, notably the release of catecholamines from the adrenal medulla. In this case, theophylline (1 mM) can induce some secretion in the absence of extracellular Ca^{2+} (Peach, 1972). Since the threshold for phenomena related to alterations in the permeability to or binding of Ca^{2+} in intracellular organelles appears to be considerably greater than maximal therapeutic concentrations for methylxanthines, it is doubtful that these mechanisms play an important role in their desirable pharmacological actions.

A large number of hormones, neurotransmitters, and autacoids have been found to accelerate the synthesis of cyclic AMP and cyclic GMP in their target tissues, and the methylxanthines, especially theophylline, have been used to evaluate the role of cyclic nucleotides in the actions of a particular hormone on its target tissue. Accordingly, one important indication that cyclic nucleotides function as intracellular mediators is evidence that methylxanthines potentiate both the effects of the hormone in question and the accumulation of cyclic AMP or cyclic GMP. As a corollary, it often has been proposed that a variety of actions of methylxanthines, particularly those in which theophylline is more potent than caffeine, are also mediated by cyclic nucleotides that accumulate as a consequence of inhibition of phosphodiesterase. However, theophylline at 50 μM and caffeine at 100 μM (the maximal therapeutic concentrations of free drug in plasma) produce minimal inhibition of phosphodiesterase activity and only rarely potentiate hormone-induced effects that are known to be mediated by cyclic AMP (see Rall, 1982). Thus, until more convincing data become available, it would seem prudent to be skeptical about the frequently expressed view that a given therapeutic action of a methylxanthine is achieved by inhibition of cyclic nucleotide phosphodiesterase. However, therapeutic doses of theophylline can enhance the effects of agents that stimulate cyclic GMP synthesis, and inhibition of phosphodiesterase may be important in such circumstances (Pearl et al., 1984).

In recent years, evidence has accumulated that adenosine functions as an autacoid. Its actions are mediated by specific receptors that are present in the plasma membrane of a wide variety of cells (see Symposium, 1983). Adenosine dilates blood vessels, particularly in the coronary and cerebral circulation, and slows the rate of discharge of cardiac pacemaker cells and of neurons in the CNS. In addition, it strongly inhibits hormone-induced lipolysis, reduces the release of norepinephrine from autonomic nerve endings, and inhibits the release of neurotransmitters in the CNS. Adenosine can also potentiate certain α-adrenergic actions of norepinephrine, leading to increased contraction of some smooth muscles or to augmented accumulation of cyclic AMP in brain tissue.

Receptors for adenosine should not be confused with the putative purinergic receptors of the gastrointestinal tract and other tissues that are characterized by much greater sensitivity to adenosine triphosphate (ATP) than to adenosine and by insensitivity to methylxanthines. At least two types of adenosine receptors have been characterized on the basis of both their relative sensitivity to various adenosine analogs and whether their activation produces stimulation or inhibition of cyclic AMP synthesis. The naturally occurring methylxanthines behave as competitive antagonists of adenosine, and they display nearly equal affinity for both types of receptors. Complete antagonism of adenosine-induced effects can usually be achieved with about a 20-fold molar excess of theophylline. Thus, depending upon the sensitivity of the particular system to adenosine and upon the amount of endogenous adenosine present in the experimental preparation, marked effects of theophylline are observed at concentrations ranging from 20 to 100 μM. Hence, the anti-adenosine effects of methylxanthines must be considered seriously even in those instances in which a regulatory function for adenosine has yet to be established.

The possibility that therapeutic responses to theophylline in asthmatic patients may involve antagonism at adenosine receptors is currently being challenged because of the properties of enprofylline (3-propylxanthine). This agent appears to be about fivefold more potent than theophylline as a bronchodilator in man and other species (see Persson, 1983), although it lacks the ability to produce diuresis or convulsions in rodents. Enprofylline is much less effective than theophylline in reducing responses to adenosine in all tissues examined, except for the rat hippocampus, where the reverse is true (Fredholm and Persson, 1982). Thus, it is not clear to what extent the two xanthines share common cellular actions or whether blockade of adenosine receptors has an important role in producing therapeutic responses to theophylline in asthmatic patients.

Toxicology.   Fatal poisoning in man by the ingestion of caffeine is rare (see Curatolo and Robertson, 1983). While emesis and convulsions are usually prominent consequences of caffeine overdosage, neither symptom was observed in at least one case of fatal poisoning. The concentration of caffeine in post-mortem blood has ranged from 80 μg/ml to over 1 mg/ml. While the acute lethal dose of caffeine in adults appears to be about 5 to 10 g, untoward reactions may be observed following the ingestion of 1 g (15 mg/kg; plasma concentrations above 30 μg/ml). These are mainly referable to the central nervous and circulatory systems. Insomnia, restlessness, and excitement are the early symptoms, which may progress to mild delirium. Sensory disturbances such as ringing in the ears and flashes of light are common. The muscles become tense and tremulous. Tachycardia and extrasystoles are frequent, and respiration is quickened.

Fatal intoxications with theophylline have been much more frequent than with caffeine. Rapid intravenous administration of therapeutic doses of *aminophylline* (500 mg) sometimes results in sudden death that is probably due to cardiac arrhythmias. Most toxicity is the result of repeated administration of the drug by both oral and parenteral routes. Aminophylline should be injected slowly over 20 to 40 minutes to avoid severe toxic symptoms, which include headache, palpitation, dizziness, nausea, hypotension, and precordial pain. Additional symptoms of toxicity are tachycardia, severe restlessness, agitation, and emesis; these effects are associated with plasma concentrations of more than 20 μg/ml. Focal and generalized seizures can also happen, sometimes without prior signs of toxicity. Seizures usually occur when concentrations in plasma exceed 40 μg/ml, although convulsions and death have resulted at plasma concentrations as low as 25 μg/ml (*see* Hendeles and Weinberger, 1982). Seizures caused by intoxication with methylxanthines can usually be treated with diazepam. However, in some cases of theophylline toxicity, the seizures have been refractory to intravenous diazepam, phenytoin, and phenobarbital. In a unique case a patient with a plasma concentration of theophylline of 190 μg/ml was reported to have survived, albeit with permanent neurological deficits; in this case, hemoperfusion through charcoal cartridges was probably lifesaving (Ehlers *et al.*, 1978). Premature infants may be relatively

resistant to poisoning by theophylline; concentrations in plasma of up to 80 μg/ml have resulted in sustained tachycardia as the only sign of toxicity (Cole and Davies, 1980).

Mutagenic and Carcinogenic Effects. Caffeine induces chromosomal abnormalities both in plant cells and in mammalian cells in culture and has potent mutagenic effects on microorganisms either alone or in combination with other mutagens (*see* Timson, 1977). These effects seem to be associated with inhibition of DNA-repair processes. They are observed only with concentrations of caffeine that are much in excess of those that follow the ingestion of beverages and medications. Furthermore, available evidence suggests that caffeine is neither mutagenic by itself nor in combination with known mutagens in mammals. At very high doses, caffeine appears to have some teratogenic activity in mammals. However, the information about human subjects is not clear-cut. While the United States Food and Drug Administration issued a warning in 1980 advising pregnant women to limit their exposure to caffeine, recent studies have found no association between maternal consumption of caffeine and the incidence of malformations in the offspring (*see* Curatolo and Robertson, 1983). Thus, while mutagenic effects would seem to pose little hazard in man, potential developmental toxicity for the human fetus and neonate warrants further investigation.

Epidemiological studies have suggested that consumption of coffee is associated with cancer of the pancreas, kidney, and lower urinary tract. However, these studies contain serious flaws, such as the selection of inappropriate groups of patients for controls and the failure to exclude smoking as a confounding variable (*see* Curatolo and Robertson, 1983). There is no clear evidence that the consumption of caffeine is causally related to the development of cancer in these organs. Similarly, the postulated association of benign fibrocystic disease of the breast with the consumption of methylxanthines has not been validated by recent investigations (*see* Curatolo and Robertson, 1983).

Relation to Myocardial Infarction. There has been controversy over a possible deleterious effect of caffeine in the etiology of acute myocardial infarction. Recent data indicate that coffee drinking is associated with little, if any, increased incidence of coronary heart disease (*see* Curatolo and Robertson, 1983).

Absorption, Fate, and Excretion. The methylxanthines are readily absorbed after oral, rectal, or parenteral administration. The oral absorption of theophylline is of particular importance because of its use in the treatment of chronic asthma. Theophylline administered in liquids or uncoated tablets is rapidly and completely absorbed. Absorption is also complete from some, but not all, sustained-release formulations (*see* Hendeles and Weinberger, 1982). Neither the presence of alcohol in solutions nor the use of more soluble salts (*e.g.*, theophylline sodium glycinate, choline theophyllinate) increases the rate or extent of absorption of theophylline. Parenteral or rectal administration does *not* obviate production of gastrointestinal distress, nausea, and vomiting. These symptoms are clearly a function of the concentration of theophylline in plasma. Any propensity of oral preparations to produce symptoms caused by local irritation of the gastrointestinal tract can probably be avoided by their administration with food, which slows but does not reduce absorption. In the absence of food, solutions or uncoated tablets of theophylline produce maximal concentrations in plasma within 2 hours; caffeine is more rapidly absorbed, and maximal plasma concentrations are achieved within 1 hour. Theophylline is completely and very rapidly absorbed when small volumes of *solutions* of aminophylline are administered as an enema (Bolme *et al.*, 1979). Use of rectal suppositories results in slow and erratic absorption. Intramuscular injection of soluble preparations of theophylline (*e.g.*, aminophylline) produces long-lasting local pain; this route of administration should not be used.

Methylxanthines are distributed into all body compartments; they cross the placenta and pass into breast milk. The apparent volume of distribution is similar for both caffeine and theophylline and usually is between 400 and 600 ml/kg. These values are considerably higher in premature infants. Theophylline is bound to plasma proteins to a greater extent than is caffeine, and the fraction bound declines as the concentration of methylxanthine increases. At therapeutic concentrations, the protein binding of theophylline averages about 60%, but it is decreased to about 40% in newborn infants and in adults with hepatic cirrhosis (*see* Hendeles and Weinberger, 1982).

Methylxanthines are eliminated primarily by metabolism in the liver. About 10% and 1% of administered theophylline and caffeine, respectively, are recovered in the urine unchanged. Caffeine has a half-life in plasma of 3 to 7 hours; this increases by about twofold in women during the later stages of pregnancy or the chronic use of oral contraceptive steroids (*see* Symposium, 1981). While there is considerable variability, the half-life of theophylline in young children averages about 3.5 hours, while values of 8 or 9 hours are more typical of adults (*see* Hendeles and Weinberger, 1982). In patients with hepatic cirrhosis or acute pulmonary edema, the rate of elimination is variable and much slower; values of more than 60 hours have been observed. In premature infants, the rate of elimination of both methylxanthines is markedly reduced. The average half-life for caffeine is more than 50 hours, while the mean values for theophylline obtained in various studies range between 20 and 36 hours. However, the latter values include the extensive conversion of theophylline to caffeine in these infants (*see* Symposium, 1981).

In addition to developmental and genetic factors, disposition of methylxanthines appears to be accelerated by smoking and by other agents that increase the capacity of drug-metabolizing systems in the liver. For example, the clearance of theophylline is increased nearly twofold during the administration of phenytoin (Marquis *et al.*, 1982). In contrast, disposition of theophylline is slowed in patients receiving certain macrolide antibiotics or cimetidine or after a single injection of influenza vaccine (*see* Hendeles and Weinberger, 1982). Furthermore, the elimination kinetics for theophylline displays dose dependency. Thus, increases in dosage sometimes produce concentrations in plasma that are higher than those predicted from the rate of elimination determined previously for a given patient. Adjustments in dosage should therefore be made in small increments. In cases of theophylline overdosage or poisoning, the decline in plasma concentration to nontoxic levels may require a protracted period of time (*see* Ehlers *et al.*, 1978).

The principal metabolites of caffeine in the urine are 1-methyluric acid and 1-methylxanthine. Much smaller amounts of 1,3-dimethyluric acid, 7-methylxanthine, and 1,7-dimethylxanthine are detected (Cornish and Christman, 1957). While the chief urinary metabolite of theophylline is 1,3-dimethyluric acid, considerable amounts of 1-methyluric acid and 3-methylxanthine are also excreted. The latter compound accumulates in plasma to concentrations that approximate 25% of that of theophylline (Thompson *et al.*, 1974). Since 3-methylxanthine is about 50% as potent as theophylline in relaxing airway smooth muscle *in vitro* (Williams *et al.*, 1978), it may contribute to some extent to the therapeutic effects of theophylline.

The hepatic metabolism of theophylline in preterm infants not only is reduced in rate but also results in a different pattern of products. Most notable is the conversion of theophylline to caffeine, which accumulates in plasma to a concentration of 20 to 35% of that of theophylline. About 50% of theophylline appears in the urine unchanged in such infants, while caffeine and 1-methyluric acid account for around 10% each; nearly all of the remainder is excreted as 1,3-dimethyluric acid (*see* Symposium, 1981). These developmental differences suggest that multiple cytochrome P-450 systems are involved in the metabolism of theophylline.

The administration of allopurinol to adult human subjects receiving theophylline decreases the excretion of 1-methyluric acid (and increases the excretion of 1-methylxanthine) without altering the appearance of 1,3-dimethyluric acid; this suggests that xanthine oxidase also participates in the metabolism of theophylline (*see* Symposium, 1981). Clearance of theophylline may be slowed modestly when allopurinol is given concurrently. There is no evidence that the methylxanthines are converted to uric acid or that their ingestion exacerbates gout.

Preparations and Routes of Administration. The xanthines are weakly basic alkaloids. For oral administration either the free base or one of the salts may be used; for parenteral administration, however, it is necessary to employ one of the salts. *Caffeine* is available in tablets (100, 150, and 200 mg) and in capsules containing pellets for timed release (200 and 250 mg). *Citrated caffeine* is a mixture of equal parts of caffeine and citric acid and is available in 65-mg tablets. *Caffeine and sodium benzoate injection* is a mixture of approximately equal parts of caffeine and sodium benzoate. It is available for intramuscular injection. *Theophylline* is available in a wide range of dosages (50 to 500 mg) in tablets, tablets designed for timed release, capsules, and capsules containing coated pellets for timed release. The bioavailability of some timed-release preparations has not been documented. Elixirs, liquids, syrups, and suspensions are also available.

Aminophylline (theophylline ethylenediamine) is the most widely used of the soluble theophylline salts. It contains 85% anhydrous theophylline. It is available as solutions for intravenous or intramuscular injection, tablets, sustained-release tablets, elixirs, solutions for both oral and rectal administration, and rectal suppositories.

Oxtriphylline, also called *choline theophyllinate*, contains 64% anhydrous theophylline. Tablets (partially enteric coated) and an elixir are available, as are sustained-release tablets and a syrup.

Theophylline sodium glycinate contains 50% anhydrous theophylline and is freely soluble in water. It is available as an elixir for oral administration.

Dyphylline is 7-(2,3-dihydroxypropyl) theophylline. This substance is a chemical entity distinct from theophylline, and *no* evidence exists for its transformation to theophylline to *any* degree after administration. Unfortunately, this substance is often considered as "a theophylline" and is sometimes mistakenly assigned a theophylline "equiva-

lence" of 70% (*see* Webb-Johnson and Andrews, 1977). Since its introduction in 1946, dyphylline has been extensively used in the treatment of asthma; however, investigation of its efficacy and pharmacokinetic properties has begun only recently (*see* Hendeles and Weinberger, 1982). Oral formulations are incompletely absorbed, and the half-time of elimination is about 2 hours. Since dyphylline appears to be only about one fifth as potent as theophylline as a bronchodilator in patients, both the doses recommended and the claims made for this compound seem unjustified. Nevertheless, dyphylline is marketed extensively.

Pentoxifylline (1-[5-oxohexyl]-3,7-dimethylxanthine) has recently been approved in the United States for use in the treatment of patients with intermittent claudication due to chronic occlusive arterial disease. Clinical studies indicate that pentoxifylline can lengthen the distance walked before the onset of claudication; there is also more direct evidence for increased blood flow in the ischemic limbs of such patients (*see* Dettelbach and Aviado, 1985). The clinical response is thought to result primarily from an improvement in the subnormal flexibility of the erythrocytes of these patients; a decreased concentration of fibrinogen in plasma may also contribute to the observed reduction in blood viscosity. Clinical responses to chronic oral administration of pentoxifylline have not been associated with changes in peripheral vascular resistance, heart rate, or cardiac output, and the drug is not thought to act as a vasodilator to any significant degree. Nevertheless, the mechanism of action of pentoxifylline is poorly defined, and studies of the structure-activity relationship have not yet appeared. While enhanced flexibility and a variety of other changes in the properties of erythrocytes can be produced *in vitro*, the concentration of pentoxifylline that is required for such effects is more than 40-fold that observed in the plasma of patients. Furthermore, 2 weeks or more usually elapse after onset of oral therapy before any beneficial effects (and the associated changes in blood viscosity) are evident. Pentoxifylline (TRENTAL) is available in 400-mg controlled-release tablets. The usual dose is 400 mg, taken three times a day with meals.

THERAPEUTIC USES

The diverse pharmacological actions of the methylxanthines have found many therapeutic applications. Caffeine has been incorporated into a number of "over-the-counter" preparations that are widely used for analgesia. Its use as a stimulant of the CNS in the treatment of overdosage with barbiturates or opioids has markedly diminished. Theophylline preparations are primarily employed to relax bronchial smooth muscle in the treatment of asthma and chronic obstructive pulmonary disease, and they are of particular importance in the treatment of *status asthmaticus* refractory to the inhalation of adrenergic agonists. In recent years, both caffeine and theophylline have been used in the treatment of the prolonged apnea sometimes observed in preterm infants. The use of theophylline to stimulate the myocardium in the treatment of acute episodes of congestive heart failure has become virtually extinct. The use of the diuretic actions of the methylxanthines is principally confined to the inclusion of caffeine in subtherapeutic amounts in "over-the-counter" preparations.

Bronchial Asthma. Theophylline compounds, particularly aminophylline, play an important role in the management of the asthmatic patient. They are useful as prophylactic drugs and are valuable adjuncts in the treatment of prolonged attacks and in the management of status asthmaticus. Although adrenocorticosteroids may be necessary for the treatment of prolonged attacks of asthma, bronchodilator drugs occupy a dominant place in therapy. The successful treatment of status asthmaticus calls for a variety of measures, including the use of oxygen, sympathomimetic drugs, expectorants, sedatives, and bronchial aspiration (*see* Webb-Johnson and Andrews, 1977). One of the most effective bronchodilating agents is theophylline.

Studies on asthmatic subjects reveal that therapeutic effects of theophylline require a plasma concentration of at least 5 to 8 μg/ml. Toxic effects become apparent at about 15 μg/ml and are frequent above 20 μg/ml. Accordingly, most therapeutic strategies are aimed at achieving and maintaining average concentrations in plasma of about 10 μg/ml. In view of the wide range of rates of elimination of theophylline, this is a difficult task without careful titration of dosage against therapeutic and toxic effects and the aid of periodic determination of concentrations of drug in plasma. For treatment of episodes of severe bronchospasm and status asthmaticus, aminophylline is administered intravenously. A loading dose of 6 mg/kg (equivalent to about 5 mg/kg of theophylline) is infused over 20 to 40 minutes. In the absence of the desired therapeutic response and signs or symptoms of toxicity, an additional 3 mg/kg of aminophylline can be slowly infused. Continued therapy for acute symptoms can be maintained initially by the infusion of 0.5 mg/kg per hour of aminophylline to otherwise-healthy adults who are nonsmokers (*see* Hendeles and Weinberger, 1982). Children below the age of 12 and adults who are smokers will require higher infusion rates of 0.8 to 0.9 mg/kg per hour to maintain therapeutic concentrations. Patients with reduced hepatic function or perfusion should receive lower maintenance doses. In any event, infusions should not be continued beyond 6 hours without knowledge of the concentration of the drug in plasma. Hendeles and Weinberger (1982) provide detailed guidelines for the initiation and maintenance of oral therapy with theophylline. These include using small initial doses (*e.g.*, 400 mg per day for adults) with increments of about 25% at intervals of 3 days, until maximal doses are achieved that range from 13 mg/kg per day (healthy adults) to 24 mg/kg per day (children between 1 and 9 years of age). Adjustments in the dosage regimen are guided by the appearance of signs of toxicity (*e.g.*, nausea, vomiting, headache), by clinical response, and by determination of the concentration of theophylline in plasma. The interval between doses also presents a problem in individuals who have high rates of elimination of theophylline. For example, when an 8-hour interval is used for compatibility with a reasonably normal sleep schedule in young children, doses determined to produce mean concentrations in plasma that are within the therapeutic range could also produce cyclical overdosage and underdosage in a significant fraction of patients. Sustained-release formulations that are completely absorbed would provide considerable therapeutic advantage for such patients (*see* Hendeles and Weinberger, 1982). However, the rate of absorption varies considerably among different formulations, and changing products after establishing a successful regimen may result in excessive fluctuations in the concentration of theophylline in plasma. While rectal instillation of solutions of aminophylline represents an alternative to oral or intravenous administration, the limited data available indicate that the extent of absorption is too variable to permit continuous use by this route; rectal suppositories also provide erratic results.

The administration of the β_2-adrenergic agonists metaproterenol or terbutaline concurrently with doses of theophylline that result in *peak* concentrations in plasma of no greater than 10 μg/ml can provide therapeutic responses that are at least as great as those achieved with higher doses of theophylline. Such regimens apparently do not increase the incidence of adverse effects above that observed with theophylline alone (Wolfe *et al.*, 1978; Billing *et al.*, 1982). Although evidence for *greater-than-additive* therapeutic responses to combinations of β_2-adrenergic agonists and theophylline is not convincing (Wolfe *et al.*, 1978; Handslip *et al.*, 1981), individualized regimens of combinations of these two classes of agents may well achieve effective bronchodilatation with reduced risk of toxicity. Although there is some controversy, the combined use of ephedrine and theophylline appears to offer no therapeutic advantage over theophylline alone (*see* Hendeles and Weinberger, 1982). The use of preparations with fixed-dose combinations of components is irrational unless they happen by chance to correspond to an optimized regimen previously established with the individual agents. The addition of barbiturates in order to counteract the CNS effects of theophylline entails the risk of increasing the rate of elimination of theophylline, as well as possible interference with the determination of concentrations of the xanthine in plasma by certain analytical procedures. Common sense interdicts the use of caffeine-containing beverages and proprietary medications during therapy with theophylline. The following interactions would thereby be avoided: the additive CNS, cardiovascular, and gastrointestinal effects of caffeine; the effects of caffeine on the elimination of theophylline by competition for common metabolic enzymes; and the interference by caffeine with the determination of theophylline by certain analytical procedures.

Chronic Obstructive Pulmonary Disease. Theophylline is also used in the treatment of this disorder. The therapeutic approach is similar to that for asthma. However, the treatment of cardiovascular sequelae of chronic obstructive pulmonary disease (pulmonary hypertension, cor pulmonale, and right-heart failure) is more complex, and theophylline does not appear to play a prominent role in current approaches (*see* Fishman, 1976). It is probable that theophylline does not have appreciable direct dilating effects on pulmonary arteries, but perhaps can assist in reducing the hypoxemia that apparently is the primary cause of pulmonary hypertension.

Apnea of Preterm Infants. Episodes of prolonged apnea, lasting more than 15 seconds and accompanied by bradycardia, are not infrequent occurrences in premature infants. They pose the threat of recurrent hypoxemia and neurological damage. While they are often associated with serious systemic illness, no specific cause is found in many instances. Beginning with the work of Kuzemko and Paala (1973), methylxanthines have undergone clinical trials for the treatment of apnea of undetermined origin. A number of studies have shown that oral or intravenous administration of aminophylline eliminates episodes of apnea that last more than 20 seconds and markedly reduces those of shorter duration (*see* Symposium, 1981). Satisfactory responses occur with concentrations of theophylline in plasma of 3 to 5 μg/ml; higher concentrations may produce a more regular pattern of respiration without further reduction in the frequency of episodes of apnea and bradycardia. Therapeutic concentrations are achieved with loading doses of 2.5 to 5 mg/kg of theophylline and can be maintained with as little as 2 mg/kg per day. While used less than theophylline, the available data indicate that caffeine is equally effective over the same range of concentrations in plasma; the slower rate of elimination usually requires maintenance doses that are about one half of those for theophylline. Since the administration of theophylline leads to the accumulation of caffeine in these infants (*see* above), there may be no advantage to the use of theophylline. Although effects on growth or development of infants following treatment with methylxanthines have not been detected, the evidence is far from definitive. Therapy is thus continued for as brief a period as possible, usually only a few weeks.

The relationship of apnea of preterm infants to "sleep apnea" or sudden infant death that occurs in apparently healthy term infants during the first year of life is not known. In any event, theophylline also decreases the incidence of apnea and periodic breathing in full-term infants who display these respiratory abnormalities (Kelly and Shannon, 1981). Effective doses range from 6 to 12 mg/kg of theophylline per day, leading to concentrations in plasma of 6 to 19 μg/ml.

Miscellaneous Uses. Caffeine is rarely used in treating cases of poisoning by central depressants. The drug is given by intramuscular injection, usually as caffeine and sodium benzoate (0.5 g). Other approaches are preferred (*see* Chapters 17 and 68).

Caffeine in combination with an analgesic, such as aspirin, is widely employed in the treatment of ordinary types of headache. There are few data to substantiate this use. Caffeine is also used in combination with an ergot alkaloid in the treatment of migraine. The ability of methylxanthines to produce constriction of cerebral blood vessels may improve the therapeutic response.

After the claim that coffee could substitute for amphetamine or methylphenidate in the treatment of children with attention-deficit disorder (Schnackenberg, 1973), there have been a number of reports both confirming and denying the original observations. However, most have failed to detect a significant effect of caffeine in the treatment of such children (*see* Curatolo and Robertson, 1983).

XANTHINE BEVERAGES

Various means of estimation lead to the conclusion that the *per-capita* intake of caffeine in the United States averages above 200 mg daily (*see* Graham, 1978). About 90% of this amount results from drinking coffee. Depending upon the alkaloid content of the coffee bean and the method of brewing, 1 cup of coffee contains about 85 mg of caffeine, while 1 cup of tea contains about 50 mg of caffeine and 1 mg of theophylline; cocoa contains about 250 mg of theobromine and 5 mg of caffeine per cup. A 12-oz (360-ml) bottle of a cola drink contains about 50 mg of caffeine, half of which is added by the manufacturer as the alkaloid.

The xanthine beverages present a medical problem in that a large fraction of the population consumes enough caffeine to produce substantial effects on a number of organ systems. Accordingly, the physician should be aware of the caffeine intake of patients and should secure a dietary history. Due consideration should be given to the possible contribution of caffeine to the presenting signs and symptoms, as well as to its potential interaction with any contemplated therapeutic regimen. Patients with active peptic ulcer should restrict their intake of both caffeine-containing and roasted-grain beverages. It is puzzling that a substance that can produce seizures in sufficient dosage is sometimes urged upon patients to counteract the sedative effects of some anticonvulsant agents (*see* Stephenson, 1977).

There is little doubt that the popularity of the xanthine beverages depends on their stimulant action, although most people are unaware of any stimulation. The degree to which an individual is stimulated by a given amount of caffeine varies. For example, some persons boast of their ability to drink several cups of coffee in the evening and yet "sleep like a log." On the other hand, there are rare persons who are so sensitive to caffeine that even a single cup of coffee will cause a response bordering on the toxic.

Overindulgence in xanthine beverages may lead to a condition that might be considered one of chronic poisoning. Central nervous stimulation results in restlessness and disturbed sleep; myocardial stimulation is reflected in premature systoles and tachycardia. The essential oils of coffee may cause some gastrointestinal irritation, and diarrhea is a common symptom. The high tannin content of tea, on the other hand, is apt to cause constipation.

There is no doubt that a certain degree of tolerance (Colton *et al.*, 1968; Robertson *et al.*, 1981) and of psychic dependence (*i.e.*, habituation) develops to the xanthine beverages. This is probably true even in those individuals who do not partake to excess. However, the morning cup of coffee is so much a part of American and European dietary habit that one seldom looks upon its consumption as a drug habit. The feeling of well-being and the increased performance it affords, although possibly obtained at the expense of decreased efficiency later in the day, are experiences that few individuals would care to give up.

Acheson, J. J.; Zahorska-Markiewiez, B.; Pittet, P.; Anantharaman, K.; and Jéquier, E. Caffeine and coffee: their influence on metabolic rate and substrate utilization in normal weight and obese individuals. *Am. J. Clin. Nutr.*, **1980**, *33*, 989–997.

Arvidsson, S. B.; Ekstrom-Jodal, B.; Martinell, S. A. G.; and Niemand, D. Aminophylline antagonises diazepam sedation. *Lancet*, **1982**, *2*, 1467.

Aubier, M.; Murciano, D.; Viires, N.; Lecocguic, Y.; and Pariente, R. Diaphragmatic contractility enhanced by aminophylline: role of extracellular calcium. *J. Appl. Physiol.*, **1983**, *54*, 460–464.

Aunis, D.; Mandel, P.; Miras-Portugal, M. T.; Coquillat, G.; Rohmer, F.; and Warter, J. M. Changes of human plasma dopamine-beta-hydroxylase activity after intravenous administration of theophylline. *Br. J. Pharmacol.*, **1975**, *53*, 425–427.

Belardinelli, L.; Mattos, E. C.; and Berne, R. M. Evidence for adenosine mediation of atrioventricular block in the ischemic canine myocardium. *J. Clin. Invest.*, **1981**, *68*, 195–205.

Bellville, J. W.; Escarraga, L. A.; Wallenstein, S. L.; Wang, K. C.; Howland, W. S.; and Houde, R. W. Antagonism by caffeine of the respiratory effects of codeine and morphine. *J. Pharmacol. Exp. Ther.*, **1962**, *136*, 38–42.

Berglund, B., and Hemmingsson, P. Effects of caffeine ingestion on exercise performance at low and high altitudes in cross-country skiers. *Int. J. Sports Med.*, **1982**, *3*, 234–236.

Berne, R. M., and Rubio, R. Regulation of coronary blood flow. *Adv. Cardiol.*, **1974**, *12*, 303–317.

Bertelli, A.; Bianchi, C.; and Beani, L. Interaction between β-adrenergic stimulant and phosphodiesterase inhibiting drugs on the bronchial muscle. *Experientia*, **1973**, *29*, 300–302.

Billing, B.; Dahlqvist, R.; Garle, M.; Hornblad, Y.; and Ripe, E. Separate and combined use of terbutaline and theophylline in asthmatics. Effects related to plasma levels. *Eur. J. Respir. Dis.*, **1982**, *63*, 399–409.

Bolme, P.; Edlund, P.-O.; Eriksson, M.; Paalzow, L.; and Winbladh, B. Pharmacokinetics of theophylline in young children with asthma: a comparison of rectal enema and suppositories. *Eur. J. Clin. Pharmacol.*, **1979**, *16*, 133–139.

Bowser, E. W.; Hargis, G. K.; Henderson, W. J.; and Williams, G. A. Parathyroid hormone secretion in the rat: effect of aminophylline. *Proc. Soc. Exp. Biol. Med.*, **1975**, *148*, 344–346.

Brater, D. C.; Kaojaren, S.; and Chennavasin, P. Pharmacodynamics of the diuretic effects of aminophylline and acetazolamide alone and combined with furosemide in normal subjects. *J. Pharmacol. Exp. Ther.*, **1983**, *227*, 92–97.

Cano, R.; Isenberg, J. I.; and Grossman, M. I. Cimetidine inhibits caffeine-stimulated gastric acid secretion in man. *Gastroenterology*, **1976**, *70*, 1055–1057.

Cohen, S., and Booth, G. H. Gastric acid secretion and lower-esophageal-sphincter pressure in response to coffee and caffeine. *N. Engl. J. Med.*, **1975**, *293*, 897–899.

Cole, G. F., and Davies, D. P. Theophylline poisoning. *Br. Med. J.*, **1980**, *280*, 52.

Colton, T.; Gosselin, R. E.; and Smith, R. P. The tolerance of coffee drinkers to caffeine. *Clin. Pharmacol. Ther.*, **1968**, *9*, 31–39.

Cornish, H. H., and Christman, A. A. A study of the metabolism of theobromine, theophylline, and caffeine in man. *J. Biol. Chem.*, **1957**, *228*, 315–323.

Cushley, M. J.; Tattersfield, A. E.; and Holgate, S. T. Adenosine antagonism as an alternative mechanism of action of methylxanthines in asthma. *Agents Actions* [*Suppl.*], **1983**, *13*, 109–113.

Debas, H. T.; Cohen, M. M.; Holubitsky, I. B.; and Harrison, R. C. Caffeine-stimulated gastric acid and pepsin secretion: dose-response studies. *Scand. J. Gastroenterol.*, **1971**, *6*, 453–457.

Ehlers, S. M.; Zaske, D. E.; and Sawchuk, R. J. Massive theophylline overdose; rapid elimination by charcoal hemoperfusion. *J.A.M.A.*, **1978**, *240*, 474–475.

Eldridge, F. L.; Millhorn, D. E.; Waldrop, T. G.; and Kiley, J. P. Mechanism of respiratory effects of methylxanthines. *Respir. Physiol.*, **1983**, *53*, 239–261.

Feurle, G.; Arnold, R.; Helmstädter, V.; and Creutzfeldt, W. The effect of intravenous theophylline ethylenediamine on serum gastrin concentration in control subjects and patients with duodenal ulcers and Zollinger-Ellison syndrome. *Digestion*, **1976**, *14*, 227–231.

Fredholm, B. B., and Persson, C. G. A. Xanthine derivatives as adenosine receptor antagonists. *Eur. J. Pharmacol.*, **1982**, *81*, 673–676.

Handslip, P. D. J.; Dart, A. M.; and Davies, B. H. Intravenous salbutamol and aminophylline in asthma: a search for synergy. *Thorax*, **1981**, *36*, 741–744.

Hedqvist, P.; Fredholm, B. B.; and Ölundh, S. Antagonistic effects of theophylline and adenosine on adrenergic neuroeffector transmission in the rabbit kidney. *Circ. Res.*, **1978**, *43*, 592–598.

James, G. W. L. The role of the adrenal glands and of α- and β-adrenergic receptors in bronchodilatation of guinea-pig lungs *in vivo*. *J. Pharm. Pharmacol.*, **1967**, *19*, 797–802.

Kalsner, S. Mechanism of potentiation of contractor responses to catecholamines by methylxanthines in aortic strips. *Br. J. Pharmacol.*, **1971**, *43*, 379–388.

Kalsner, S.; Frew, R. D.; and Smith, G. M. Mechanism of methylxanthine sensitization of norepinephrine responses in a coronary artery. *Am. J. Physiol.*, **1975**, *228*, 1702–1707.

Katz, A. M.; Repke, D. I.; and Hasselbach, W. Dependence of ionophore- and caffeine-induced calcium release from sarcoplasmic reticulum vesicles on external and internal calcium ion concentrations. *J. Biol. Chem.*, **1977**, *252*, 1938–1949.

Kelly, D. H., and Shannon, D. C. Treatment of apnea and excessive periodic breathing in the full-term infant. *Pediatrics*, **1981**, *68*, 183–186.

Krasnow, S., and Grossman, M. I. Stimulation of gastric secretion in man by theophylline ethylenediamine. *Proc. Soc. Exp. Biol. Med.*, **1949**, *71*, 335–336.

Kuzemko, J. A., and Paala, J. Apnoeic attacks in the newborn treated with aminophylline. *Arch. Dis. Child.*, **1973**, *48*, 404–406.

Lammerant, J., and Becsei, I. Inhibition of pacing-induced coronary dilation by aminophylline. *Cardiovasc. Res.*, **1975**, *9*, 532–537.

Lopes, J. M.; Aubier, M.; Jardini, J.; Aranda, J. V.; and Macklem, P. T. Effect of caffeine on skeletal muscle function before and after fatigue. *J. Appl. Physiol.*, **1983**, *54*, 1303–1305.

Maren, T. H. The additive renal effect of oral aminophylline and trichlormethiazide in man. *Clin. Res.*, **1961**, *9*, 57.

Marquardt, D. L.; Parker, C. W.; and Sullivan, T. J. Potentiation of mast cell mediator release by adenosine. *J. Immunol.*, **1978**, *120*, 871–878.

Marquis, J.-F.; Carruthers, S. G.; Spence, J. D.; Brownestone, Y. S.; and Toogood, J. H. Phenytoin-theophylline interaction. *N. Engl. J. Med.*, **1982**, *307*, 1189–1190.

Moyer, J. H.; Tashnek, A. B.; Miller, S. I.; Snyder, H.; and Bowman, R. O. The effect of theophylline with ethylenediamine (aminophylline) and caffeine on cerebral hemodynamics and cerebrospinal fluid pressure in patients with hypertension headaches. *Am. J. Med. Sci.*, **1952**, *224*, 377–385.

Ogilvie, R. I.; Fernandez, P. G.; and Winsberg, F. Cardiovascular response to increasing theophylline concentrations. *Eur. J. Clin. Pharmacol.*, **1977**, *12*, 409–414.

Öhnell, H., and Berg, H. Zur Frage über die Ventrikelfunktion nach verabreichung verschiedener Arten von Kaffee. *Acta Med. Scand.*, **1931**, *76*, 491–520.

Peach, M. J. Stimulation of release of adrenal catecholamine by adenosine 3′5′-cyclic monophosphate and theophylline in the absence of extracellular Ca^{2+}. *Proc. Natl. Acad. Sci. U.S.A.*, **1972**, *69*, 834–836.

Pearl, R. G.; Rosenthal, M. H.; Murad, F.; and Ashton, J. P. A. Aminophylline potentiates sodium nitroprusside–induced hypotension in the dog. *Anesthesiology*, **1984**, *61*, 712–715.

Pfaffman, M. A., and McFarland, S. A. Relationship between theophylline-induced relaxation and excitation-contraction coupling in intestinal smooth muscle. *Arch. Int. Pharmacodyn. Ther.*, **1978**, *232*, 180–191.

Piafsky, K. M.; Sitar, D. S.; Rango, R. E.; and Ogilvie, R. I. Theophylline kinetics in acute pulmonary edema. *Clin. Pharmacol. Ther.*, **1977**, *21*, 310–316.

Rall, T. W., and West, T. C. The potentiation of cardiac inotropic responses to norepinephrine by theophylline. *J. Pharmacol. Exp. Ther.*, **1963**, *139*, 269–274.

Robertson, D.; Jürgen, C.; Frölich, M. D.; Carr, R. K.; Watson, J. T.; Hollifield, J. W.; Shand, D. G.; and Oates, J. A. Effects of caffeine on plasma renin activity, catecholamines and blood pressure. *N. Engl. J. Med.*, **1978**, *298*, 181–186.

Robertson, D.; Wade, E.; Workman, R.; Woosley, R. L.; and Oates, J. A. Tolerance to the humoral and hemodynamic effects of caffeine in man. *J. Clin. Invest.*, **1981**, *67*, 1111–1117.

Rutherford, J. D.; Vatner, S. F.; and Braunwald, E. Effects and mechanism of action of aminophylline on cardiac function and regional blood flow distribution in conscious dogs. *Circulation*, **1981**, *63*, 378–387.

Schnackenberg, R. Caffeine as a substitute for schedule II stimulants in hyperkinetic children. *Am. J. Psychiatry*, **1973**, *130*, 796–798.

Serrano-Ríos, M.; Hawkins, F. G.; Esobar-Jiménez, F.; and Rodriguez-Miñón, J. L. The effect of aminophylline on insulin release induced by secretin and cholecystokinin-pancreozymin in normal humans. *J. Clin. Endocrinol. Metab.*, **1974**, *38*, 194–199.

Sigurd, B., and Olesen, K. H. Comparative naturetic and diuretic efficacy of theophylline ethylenediamine and of bendroflumethiazide during long-term treatment with the potent diuretic bumetanide. *Acta Med. Scand.*, **1978**, *203*, 113–119.

Starr, I.; Gamble, C. F.; Margolies, A.; Donal, J. S.; Joseph, N.; and Eagle, E. A clinical study of the action of 10 commonly used drugs on cardiac output, work and size; on respiration, on metabolic rate and on the electrocardiogram. *J. Clin. Invest.*, **1937**, *16*, 799–823.

Stephenson, P. E. Physiologic and psychotropic effects of caffeine on man. *J. Am. Diet. Assoc.*, **1977**, *71*, 240–247.

Stirt, J. A. Aminophylline may act as a morphine antagonist. *Anaesthesia*, **1983**, *38*, 275–278.

Sydbom, A., and Fredholm, B. B. On the mechanism by which theophylline inhibits histamine release from rat mast cells. *Acta Physiol. Scand.*, **1982**, *114*, 243–251.

Thompson, R. D.; Nagasawa, H. T.; and Jenne, J. W. Determination of theophylline and its metabolites in human urine and serum by high-pressure liquid chromatography. *J. Lab. Clin. Med.*, **1974**, *84*, 584–593.

Vestal, R. E.; Eriksson, C. E.; Musser, B.; Ozaki, L. K.; and Halter, J. B. Effect of intravenous aminophylline on plasma levels of catecholamines and related cardiovascular and metabolic responses in man. *Circulation*, **1983**, *67*, 162–171.

Vinegar, R.; Truax, J. F.; Selph, J. L.; Welch, R. M.; and White, H. L. Potentiation of the anti-inflammatory and analgesic activity of aspirin by caffeine in the rat. *Proc. Soc. Exp. Biol. Med.*, **1976**, *151*, 556–560.

Wechsler, R. L.; Kleiss, L. M.; and Kety, S. S. The effects of intravenously administered aminophylline on cerebral circulation and metabolism in man. *J. Clin. Invest.*, **1950**, *29*, 28–30.

Wein, A. J.; Gregory, J. G.; Sansone, T. C.; and Schoenberg, H. W. The effects of aminophylline on ureteral and bladder contractility. *Invest. Urol.*, **1972**, *9*, 290–293.

Wiles, C. M.; Moxham, J.; Newham, D.; and Edwards, R. H. Aminophylline and fatigue of adductor pollicis in man. *Clin. Sci.*, **1983**, *64*, 547–550.

Williams, J. F.; Lowitt, S.; Polson, J. B.; and Szentivanyi, A. Pharmacological and biochemical activities of some monomethylxanthines and methyluric acid derivatives of theophylline and caffeine. *Biochem. Pharmacol.*, **1978**, *27*, 1545–1550.

Wolfe, J. D.; Tashkin, D. P.; Calvarese, B.; and Simmons, M. Bronchodilator effects of terbutaline and aminophylline alone and in combination in asthmatic patients. *N. Engl. J. Med.*, **1978**, *298*, 363–367.

Zehner, J.; Klaus, D.; Klumpp, F.; and Lemke, R. The influence of propranolol, practolol, and theophylline on the plasma renin activity. *Res. Exp. Med. (Berl.)*, **1975**, *166*, 275–282.

Monographs and Reviews

Bianchi, C. P. Cellular pharmacology of contraction of skeletal muscle. In, *Cellular Pharmacology of Excitable Tissues.* (Narahashi, T., ed.) Charles C Thomas, Publisher, Springfield, Ill., **1975**, pp. 485–519.

Cohn, J. N., and Franciosa, J. A. Vasodilator therapy of cardiac failure. (Second of two parts.) *N. Engl. J. Med.*, **1977**, *297*, 254–258.

Curatolo, P. W., and Robertson, D. The health consequences of caffeine. *Ann. Intern. Med.*, **1983**, *98*, 641–653.

Dettelbach, H. R., and Aviado, D. M. Clinical pharmacology of pentoxifylline with special reference to its hemorrheologic effect for the treatment of intermittent claudication. *J. Clin. Pharmacol.*, **1985**, *25*, 8–26.

Fishman, A. P. State of the art—chronic cor pulmonale. *Am. Rev. Respir. Dis.*, **1976**, *114*, 775–794.

Graham, D. M.   Caffeine—its identity, dietary sources, intake and biological effects. *Nutr. Rev.*, **1978**, *36*, 97–102.

Hendeles, L., and Weinberger, M.   Improved efficacy and safety of theophylline in the control of airway hyperreactivity. *Pharmacol. Ther.*, **1982**, *18*, 91–105.

Persson, C. G. A.   The profile of action of enprofylline, or why adenosine antagonism seems less desirable with xanthine antiasthmatics. *Agents Actions [Suppl.]*, **1983**, *13*, 115–129.

Rall, T. W.   Evolution of the mechanism of action of methylxanthines: from calcium mobilizers to antago-

nists of adenosine receptors. *Pharmacologist*, **1982**, *24*, 277–287.

Symposium. (Various authors.)   Developmental pharmacology of the methylxanthines. (Soyka, L. F., ed.) *Semin. Perinatol.*, **1981**, *5*, 303–408.

Symposium. (Various authors.)   *Regulatory Function of Adenosine*. (Berne, R. M.; Rall, T. W.; and Rubio, R.; eds.) Martinus Nijhoff, Boston, **1983.**

Timson, J.   Caffeine. *Mutat. Res.*, **1977**, *47*, 1–52.

Webb-Johnson, D. C., and Andrews, J. L., Jr.   Bronchodilator therapy. *N. Engl. J. Med.*, **1977**, *297*, 476–482, 758–764.

SECTION
IV
Autacoids

INTRODUCTION

William W. Douglas

Assembled for consideration in this section are a number of substances with widely differing structures and pharmacological activities; although disparate in these respects, they are grouped together here because they have in common a natural occurrence in the body. At the same time, the opportunity is taken to discuss drugs antagonizing their actions, wherever such drugs are available. The oldest and most familiar substances in the group, *histamine* and the histamine antagonists, are dealt with in Chapter 26. The same chapter is concerned with another endogenous amine, *5-hydroxytryptamine (5-HT, serotonin, enteramine)*, and its antagonists. Chapter 27 is devoted to the polypeptides—*angiotensin, bradykinin, kallidin,* and others. Chapter 28 is concerned with *prostaglandins* and other derivatives of arachidonic acid. The section thus includes a motley of substances of intense pharmacological activity that are normally present in the body or may be formed there, and that cannot conveniently be classed with other members of this broad group, such as the neurohumors and hormones. These different substances have been variously described as *local hormones, autopharmacological agents,* and the like; but a generic term that is at once shorter, more accurate, and euphonious is *autacoid,* a word derived from the Greek *autos* (''self'') and *akos* (''medicinal agent'' or ''remedy''). This term was devised by Sir Edward Schäfer (1916), later Sharpey-Schafer, as a substitute for Starling's word *hormone,* which, being derived from the Greek *hormaein* (meaning ''to stir up''), is a misnomer for the inhibitory substances that also came to be embraced by this designation. However, Starling's term *hormone,* albeit unsatisfactory from the etymological standpoint, has won the day, and Schäfer's has passed into limbo. Such a good word deserves a better fate, and hence it was revived here, now 2 decades ago. Most of the substances described in this section can probably lay claim to the title without distortion of its sense.

What of the significance of this group of autacoids? What is their role in the body? What is their value as drugs and what is their place in therapeutics? In certain cases, only rather imprecise answers can be given to these questions. The very fact that the substances have been classified under the noncommittal title of *autacoids* is, in a sense, a confession that the evidence does not at present permit a more precise functional classification such as, for example, hormone or neurohumor. This is not to say that such functions are foreign to the autacoids. On the contrary, as the evidence concerning their possible roles in the body is unfolded, it will be apparent to the reader that both such functions may be displayed by the substances under consideration. But the core of the matter is that, while the autacoids possess an astonishingly wide range of pharmacological activities and in vanishingly small amounts, there are comparatively few instances where a physiological role can be stated with assurance. After the example of Pirandello, who named one of his plays *Six Characters in Search of an Author,* portions of the present section might well have been entitled ''Various Autacoids in Search of a Function.'' The problem, as will become clear from what follows, is not so much with a dearth of hypotheses as with a surfeit of them. But while scientists dispute the rival claims of the different hypotheses, there is general agreement that each of the autacoids to be discussed is of importance in the body's economy. All are agents that the body employs in the execution of various functions in health and disease; they are clearly part and parcel of the physiological and pathological phenomena that provide the rationale for drug therapy; and their existence provides numerous possibilities for therapeutic intervention by the use of drugs that mimic or antagonize their action or interfere in one way or another with their metabolism. Together these facts thrust the autacoids squarely to the center of interest for those who are concerned with the pharmacological basis of therapeutics.

CHAPTER

26 HISTAMINE AND 5-HYDROXYTRYPTAMINE (SEROTONIN) AND THEIR ANTAGONISTS

William W. Douglas

HISTAMINE

History. The history of β-aminoethylimidazole, or histamine, shows several close parallels with that of acetylcholine (ACh). Both compounds were synthesized as chemical curiosities before their biological significance was recognized; both were first detected as uterine stimulants in extracts of ergot, from which they were subsequently isolated; and both proved to be casual contaminants of ergot, resulting from bacterial action.

When Dale and Laidlaw (1910, 1911) subjected histamine to intensive pharmacological study, they discovered, *inter alia,* that it stimulated a host of smooth muscles and had an intense vasodepressor action. With rare acumen they drew attention to the observation that the pharmacological activity of histamine resembled that of many tissue extracts and, further, that the immediate symptoms with which an animal responds to an injection of a normally inert protein, to which it has been sensitized, are to a large extent those of poisoning by β-aminoethylimidazole (histamine). Their prescient comments anticipated by many years the events that were to thrust histamine to the center of physiological interest, namely, the discovery of its occurrence in the body and its release during immediate hypersensitivity (allergic) reactions and upon cellular injury. Although histamine had been identified chemically in tissue extracts previously, it was suspected that it might have arisen from putrefaction. It was not until 1927 that Best, Dale, Dudley, and Thorpe isolated histamine from impeccably fresh samples of liver and lung, thereby establishing beyond doubt that this amine is a natural constituent of the body. Demonstrations of its presence in a variety of other tissues soon followed—

hence the name *histamine* after the Greek word for tissue, *histos*.

Meanwhile, Lewis and his colleagues, in a series of brilliant experiments, had amassed evidence that a substance with the properties of histamine ("H-substance") was liberated from the cells of the skin by injurious stimuli, including the reaction of antigen with antibody (Lewis, 1927). Given the chemical evidence of histamine's presence in the body, there remained little impediment to supposing that Lewis' "H-substance" was histamine itself. This conception was advanced with telling force by Dale in his Croonian lectures of 1929 and stimulated the growth of interest in histamine to a rare luxuriance. Now, more than half a century later, it is evident that endogenous histamine is involved in diverse physiological processes quite apart from allergic reactions and injury. Thus, histamine clearly participates in the physiological regulation of gastric secretion, and there are strong indications that it serves as a chemical transmitter or modulator within the brain. Early suspicions that histamine acts through more than one receptor have now been borne out, and it is clear that two distinct subclasses of histamine receptor exist, H_1 (Ash and Schild, 1966) and H_2 (Black *et al.*, 1972). The former type of receptor is blocked selectively by the classical "antihistamines" (such as pyrilamine) developed around 1940 and the latter by the H_2-blocking drugs introduced in the early 1970s. The discovery of H_2 antagonists has contributed enormously to the current resurgent interest in histamine in biology and clinical medicine.

Chemistry. Histamine is 2-(4-imidazolyl)ethylamine (or β-aminoethylimidazole). It is a hydrophilic molecule comprised of an imidazole ring and an amino group connected by two methylene groups. The pharmacologically active form at both H_1 and H_2 receptors is the monocationic $N\gamma$—H tautomer, that is, the charged form of the species depicted in Table 26–1, although different chemical properties of this monocation may be involved at these two different receptor sites (Ganellin, in Ganellin and Parsons, 1982).

There are many drugs with histamine-like properties, and most contain the following fragment:

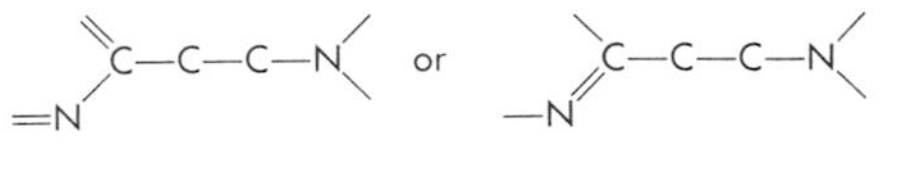

However, there are a number of exceptions, and one can say only that compounds with appreciable histamine-like activity generally consist of small, nitrogen-containing heterocyclic rings to which are attached 2-aminoethyl side chains. Among such agonists there is a striking lack of correlation between their action on gastric secretion and their other histamine-like actions. This reflects the existence of two subclasses of receptor for the amine, termed H_1 and H_2, that show different structural requirements for both binding and activation. Some H_1 and H_2 agonists are shown in Table 26–1. Structure-activity relationships are discussed by Ganellin, in Ganellin and Parsons (1982).

Table 26–1.   STRUCTURE OF HISTAMINE AND SOME H₁ AND H₂ AGONISTS

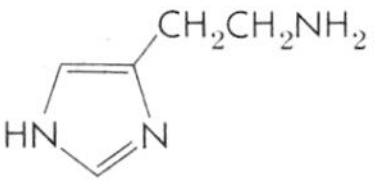

Histamine

H₁-Receptor Agonists   *H₂-Receptor Agonists*

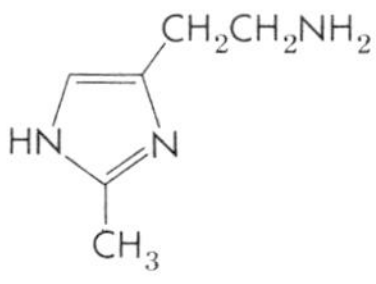

2-Methylhistamine   (8:1) *   4(5)-Methylhistamine   (170:1)

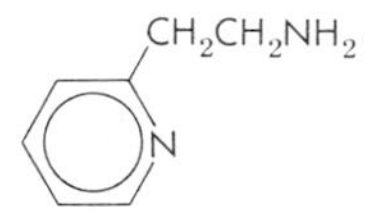

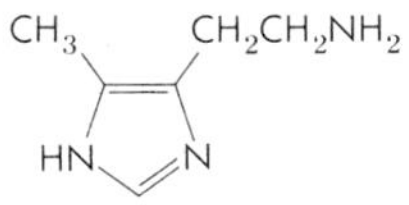

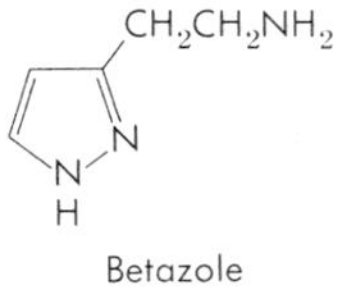

2-Pyridylethylamine   (30:1)   Betazole   (10:1)

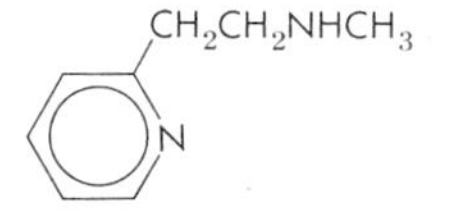

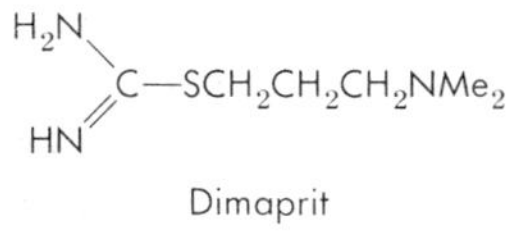

Betahistine   (40:1)   Dimaprit   (2000:1)

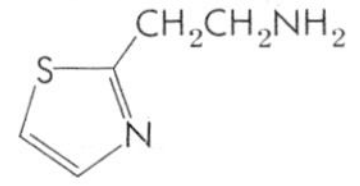

2-Thiazolylethylamine   (90:1) 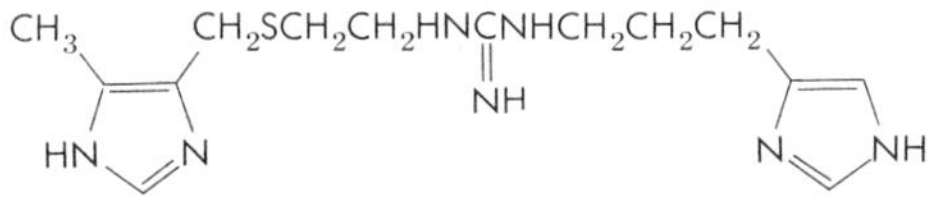   Impromidine   (10,000:1)

* The ratios in parentheses indicate approximate relative activities of the various compounds at the two receptor types ($H_1:H_2$ for the H_1 agonists; $H_2:H_1$ for the H_2 agonists). Only impromidine is more potent than histamine on a molar basis (about 40-fold). The other agonists are less potent. For further details, *see* Ganellin, in Ganellin and Parsons (1982).

PHARMACOLOGICAL EFFECTS:
H$_1$ AND H$_2$ RECEPTORS

Histamine contracts many smooth muscles, such as those of the bronchi and gut, but powerfully relaxes others, including those of fine blood vessels. It is also a very potent stimulus to gastric acid production. Effects attributable to these actions dominate the overall response to the drug; however, there are several others, of which edema formation and stimulation of sensory nerve endings are perhaps the most familiar. Some of these effects, such as bronchoconstriction and contraction of the gut, are mediated by one type of histamine receptor, the H$_1$ receptors (Ash and Schild, 1966), which are readily blocked by pyrilamine and other such classical antihistamines, now more properly described as histamine H$_1$-receptor blocking drugs or simply H$_1$ blockers. Other effects, most notably gastric secretion, are completely refractory to such antagonists, involve activation of H$_2$ receptors, and are susceptible to inhibition by the more recently developed histamine H$_2$-receptor blocking drugs (Black *et al.*, 1972). Still others, such as the hypotension resulting from vascular dilatation, are evidently mediated by receptors of both H$_1$ and H$_2$ types, since they are annulled only by a combination of H$_1$ and H$_2$ blockers.

The two classes of histamine receptors also reveal themselves by differential responses to various histamine-like agonists. Thus, 2-methylhistamine preferentially elicits responses mediated by H$_1$ receptors, whereas 4-methylhistamine has a correspondingly preferential effect mediated through H$_2$ receptors (Black *et al.*, 1972). These compounds are representatives of two classes of histamine-like drugs, the H$_1$- and H$_2$-receptor agonists. The structures of some are indicated in Table 26–1. The availability of these H$_1$ and H$_2$ agonists and of the corresponding antagonists has greatly enriched understanding of the pharmacology and physiology of histamine and has allowed new therapeutic approaches (*see* Rocha e Silva, 1966, 1978; Beaven, 1978; Hirschowitz, 1979; Ganellin and Parsons, 1982).

Cardiovascular System. Histamine in man and most other animals characteristically exerts a predominantly dilator effect on the vasculature that involves the finer blood vessels; this results in flushing, lowered total peripheral resistance, and a fall in systemic blood pressure. In addition, histamine tends to increase capillary permeability. Its effects on the heart are generally less important. Extensive reviews on the complex cardiovascular effects of histamine are available (*see* Rocha e Silva, 1966, 1978; Levi *et al.*, in Ganellin and Parsons, 1982).

Vasodilatation. Loosely referred to as "capillary dilatation," this is the characteristic action of histamine on the vascular tree, and it is by far the most important in man. It involves both H$_1$ and H$_2$ receptors distributed throughout the resistance vessels in most vascular beds. Activation of either type of receptor can elicit maximal vasodilatation, but the responses differ somewhat. H$_1$ receptors have the higher affinity for histamine, are activated at lower concentrations of the drug, and mediate a dilator response that is relatively rapid in onset and short lived. By contrast, activation of H$_2$ receptors causes dilatation that develops more slowly and is more sustained. As a result, H$_1$ blocking agents given alone effectively counter small dilator responses to low doses of histamine but only blunt the initial phase of larger dilator responses to higher doses. The effects of such large doses of histamine obviously then are completely blocked only by a combination of H$_1$ and H$_2$ antagonists. Following injection of histamine in man, vasodilatation is most apparent in the skin of the face and upper part of the body, the so-called blushing area, which becomes hot and flushed.

Increased "Capillary" Permeability. This is the second of the classical effects of histamine on the fine vessels and results in outward passage of plasma protein and fluid into the extracellular spaces, an increase in the flow of lymph and its protein content, and formation of edema. H$_1$ receptors are clearly important for this response; participation of H$_2$ receptors is uncertain.

While it is traditional to ascribe each of the two classical vascular effects of histamine to an action on "capillaries," it should be understood that, when so used, the word is a generic term for the vessels of the microcirculation. *Dilator responses* are mainly attributable to inhibitory effects of histamine on the smooth muscle of metarterioles, arterioles, and precapillary sphincters upstream, and muscular venules downstream. Such dilatation as occurs in the true capillaries and smallest postcapillary venules, both of which are devoid of smooth muscle, is passive, due both to the fall in resistance upstream (and increased blood flow) and to a rise in pressure in larger veins, which histamine tends to constrict. Within the microcirculation, vessels larger than about 80 μm, both arterioles and venules, tend to constrict in response to histamine, and these effects are mainly mediated by H_1 receptors.

Increased permeability results mainly from actions of histamine on postcapillary venules, where histamine causes the endothelial cells to contract and separate at their boundaries and thus to expose the basement membrane, which is freely permeable to plasma protein and fluid. The gaps between endothelial cells may also permit passage of particles such as platelets or injected colloidal drugs and dyes that become trapped between the cells and the basement membrane. The active separation of the endothelial cells is favored by the dilatation of the small venules. An additional factor favoring increased transcapillary movement of fluid and macromolecules may be increased transcapillary vesicular transport (*see* Altura and Halevy, 1978).

Triple Response. When histamine is injected intradermally, it elicits a characteristic triad of phenomena known as the "triple response" (Lewis, 1927). This is comprised of the following: (1) a localized red spot, extending for a few millimeters around the site of injection, appearing within a few seconds, reaching a maximum in about a minute, and soon acquiring a bluish tint; this results from the direct, vasodilatory effect of histamine on the minute blood vessels; (2) a brighter red flush or "flare," of irregular outline, extending about 1 cm or so beyond the original red spot and developing more slowly; this is due to histamine-induced axon reflexes that cause vasodilatation indirectly; and (3) a wheal that is discernible in 1 to 2 minutes and occupies the same area as the original small red spot at the injection site; this reflects histamine's effect to increase "capillary" permeability, thereby causing edema.

Endothelium-Dependent Vasodilatation. Various autacoids can elicit vasodilatation in an indirect manner by an action on vascular endothelial cells; this results in the release of a substance that, in turn, relaxes the vascular smooth muscle cells. The chemical identity of this endothelially derived relaxing factor (EDRF) is unknown, but it may act on the smooth muscle cells by increasing guanosine 3',5'-monophosphate (cyclic GMP) concentrations

and, ultimately, by decreasing the state of phosphorylation of the light chains of myosin (*see* Rapoport and Murad, 1983; Chapter 33). The extent to which vasodilator effects of histamine can be explained by this indirect action is presently uncertain; however, at least some such effects of histamine appear to involve endothelium-dependent vasodilatation (*see* Furchgott, 1984).

Constriction of Larger Vessels. Histamine tends to constrict larger blood vessels, in some species more than in others. In rabbits and other rodents the effect extends to the level of the arterioles and may, with higher doses of histamine, overshadow dilatation of the finer blood vessels. A net increase in total peripheral resistance and an elevation of blood pressure can then be observed.

Heart. Histamine has direct actions on the heart that affect both contractility and electrical events. It increases the force of contraction of both atrial and ventricular muscle by promoting calcium flux, and it speeds heart rate by hastening diastolic depolarization in the S-A node. It also acts directly to slow A-V conduction, to increase automaticity, and, in high doses especially, to elicit diverse arrhythmias. With the exception of slowed A-V conduction, which involves mainly H_1 receptors, all of these effects are largely attributable to H_2 receptors. However, this varies with species, as does the sensitivity of the heart to histamine.

With conventional doses of histamine given intravenously, direct cardiac effects of histamine are not prominent and tend to be overshadowed by baroreceptor reflexes elicited by the reduced blood pressure, which stimulate heart rate and force of contraction through enhanced sympathetic outflow. Such effects, coupled with some constriction of the large veins and augmented venous return, may cause a prompt but transient rise in cardiac output; thereafter, cardiac output is generally little altered or may even fall as blood pools in the periphery.

Systemic Blood Pressure. In man and most other species, histamine lowers blood pressure by reducing total peripheral resistance. Because this involves both H_1 and H_2 receptors in the complex manner already described, the fall in blood pressure has two components: the first is attributable to H_1 receptors (rapid in onset but not well sustained), while the second is mediated by H_2 receptors (higher threshold, slower to develop but well sustained). The effects of H_1 and H_2 blockers are entirely predictable.

Histamine Shock. Histamine in large doses causes a profound and progressive fall in blood pressure. As the minute blood vessels dilate, they trap large amounts of blood and, as their permeability increases, plasma escapes from the circulation. These effects diminish effective blood volume, reduce venous return, and greatly lower cardiac output. The condition resembles surgical or traumatic shock (*see* Symposium, 1982).

Regional Vascular Responses. In addition to interspecies differences, responses to histamine vary in different vascular beds within a single species. For the most part, the differences are quantitative and reflect varying degrees of dilatation in the skeletal, mesenteric, coronary, cerebral, and renal beds. But sometimes, even where the overall response is clearly vasodilatation (*e.g.*, in cats), vasoconstriction is evident in liver, spleen, and skin. Within the pulmonary circulation, both constrictor and dilator effects (involving H_1 and H_2 receptors, respectively) have been demonstrated. Gastric blood vessels are strongly dilated by events that are initiated at both H_1 and H_2 receptors; the H_2 component is, in part, indirect and due to increased metabolic activity that results from stimulation of gastric acid secretion (*see* Eyre and Chand and also Levi *et al.*, in Ganellin and Parsons, 1982).

Vascular Tissue in Vitro. Isolated blood vessels from various species and regions (cranial, mesenteric, aortic, and umbilical arteries as well as umbilical vein and other large veins, including vena cava) commonly show constrictor responses to histamine *in vitro*. Under such conditions the vessels usually have little of the tone that is evident *in vivo*, a tone that facilitates demonstration of dilator effects. Furthermore, minimal injury to the intima during preparation of vessels can prevent the endothelium-dependent vasodilatation described above. These constrictor responses, which are mediated by H_1 receptors, are thus of doubtful relevance to conditions *in vivo* (*see* Levi *et al.*, in Ganellin and Parsons, 1982; Furchgott, 1984).

Extravascular Smooth Muscle. Histamine stimulates, or more rarely relaxes, various smooth muscles. Contraction is due to activation of H_1 receptors and relaxation (for the most part) to activation of H_2 receptors. Responses of different tissues, species, and even individuals vary widely (*see* Parsons, in Ganellin and Parsons, 1982). *Bronchial muscle* of guinea pigs is exquisitely sensitive, and bronchoconstriction leads to death. Minute doses of histamine will also evoke intense bronchocon-

striction in patients with bronchial asthma and certain other pulmonary diseases. In normal man and many animals, the effect is much less pronounced and exceptionally, as in the sheep bronchus or cat trachea, histamine causes relaxation. Although the spasmogenic influence of H_1 receptors is dominant in human bronchial muscle, H_2 receptors with dilator function are also present. Thus, histamine-induced bronchospasm *in vitro* is potentiated slightly by H_2 blockade. In asthmatic subjects in particular, histamine-induced bronchospasm may involve an additional, reflex component that arises from irritation of afferent vagal nerve endings (*see* Eyre and Chand, in Ganellin and Parsons, 1982; Nadel and Barnes, 1984).

The *uterus* of some species contracts to histamine while that of the rat relaxes; in the human uterus, gravid or not, the response is negligible. Responses of *intestinal muscle* also vary with species and region, but the classical effect is contraction. *Bladder, ureter, gallbladder, iris,* and many other smooth muscle preparations are affected little or inconsistently by histamine.

Exocrine Glands. *Gastric Glands.* Histamine is a remarkably powerful gastric secretagogue and evokes a copious secretion of gastric juice of high acidity in doses below those that influence the blood pressure. Its effect on the composition of gastric juice varies somewhat with species and dose, but in man the output of pepsin and intrinsic factor of Castle is increased along with that of acid. The principal effect, to increase the production of acidic gastric juice, is well sustained during a prolonged infusion of histamine. It results from a direct stimulant effect on the parietal cells where, acting upon H_2 receptors that are linked to adenylate cyclase, histamine drives a membrane pump (H^+,K^+-ATPase) that extrudes protons. The potent secretagogue activity of histamine reflects the dominant function of this autacoid in the physiological stimulation of gastric acid production (*see* below). Physiological stimulation also involves ACh, released by vagal activity, and the hormonal secretagogue, gastrin. There are important, mutually supportive interactions between the three secretagogues, and some of these appear to operate at the level of the parietal cell. For example, reduction in vagal influence, by vagotomy or administration of atropine, depresses the effect of histamine. In addition, blockade of H_2 receptors not only inhibits acid production in response to histamine but also reduces the effect of gastrin or vagal stimulation (*see* Soll and Grossman, 1981; Code, in Ganellin and Parsons, 1982; Berglindh, 1984; and below).

Other Exocrine Glands. The effects of histamine on glands outside the stomach are relatively unimportant. The drug has some stimulant actions on salivary, pancreatic, intestinal, bronchial, and lacrimal secretions, but these are generally inconstant, fleeting, and feeble. In salivary glands, where the action of histamine has been most closely studied, it is possible to show some stimulation after chronic denervation, which is thus direct; however, in normally innervated glands, much of the effect seems to be mediated through the nerves. Histamine stimulates secretion of bile even after removal of the stomach.

Nerve Endings: Pain, Itch, and Indirect Effects. Histamine can stimulate various nerve endings. Thus when introduced into the epidermis, it causes itch; when delivered more deeply into the dermis, it evokes pain, sometimes accompanied by itching. Stimulant actions on one or another type of nerve ending, including autonomic afferents and efferents, have been mentioned above as factors that contribute to the ''flare'' component of the triple response and to indirect effects of histamine on the heart, bronchi, and other organs. The neuronal receptors for histamine are generally of the H_1 type (*see* Rocha e Silva, 1966, 1978; Ganellin and Parsons, 1982).

Adrenal Medulla and Ganglia. Histamine stimulates ganglion cells and chromaffin cells when it is administered in large amounts or by close arterial injection, but not when conventional doses are given intravenously. Nevertheless, a secondary rise in blood pressure attributable to adrenal medullary stimulation is seen in experimental animals given large doses of histamine intravenously and in patients with pheochromocytoma given modest doses.

Central Nervous System. Histamine does not penetrate the blood-brain barrier to any significant degree, and effects on the central nervous system (CNS) are not usually evident in response to parenteral injections of the autacoid. However, when injected directly into the cerebral ventricles or given by iontophoretic application into certain regions of the brain, histamine may elicit behavioral responses, elevate blood pressure, increase heart rate, lower body temperature, increase secretion of antidiuretic hormone, cause arousal or emesis, increase or decrease firing of neurons, and stimulate or inhibit the secretion of several adenohypophyseal hormones. These central effects seem to involve both H_1 and H_2 receptors, and some, at least, may reflect the existence of central histaminergic nerves and neuroendocrine mechanisms (*see* Chapter 12; Schwartz *et al.*, in Ganellin and Parsons, 1982).

Cells Mediating Inflammatory and Immune Responses. Histamine has an inhibitory effect on the secretory activities of mast cells and basophils, which are themselves the principal sources of the histamine and the other inflammatory substances that are released during immediate hypersensitivity reactions (*see* below). Histamine similarly depresses secretion of lysosomal enzymes from neutrophils and secretion of antibodies and lymphokines from lymphocytes. It also reduces cytolytic activity. For the most part, these diverse ''anti-inflammatory'' effects, which are mediated by H_2 receptors on the various cells, are of modest intensity and are perhaps of limited clinical significance (*see* Plaut and Lichtenstein, in Ganellin and Parsons, 1982).

Mechanism of Action. Receptors for histamine, which are almost certainly components of the cell surface, have not yet been isolated or identified by physical or chemical means. Knowledge of their structural properties is restricted to such inferences as can be drawn from pharmacological studies of structure-activity relationships of histaminergic agonists and antagonists (*see* Ganellin, in Ganellin and Parsons, 1982). How interaction of histamine with its receptors elicits the appropriate cellular responses is also uncertain.

Broadly speaking, there are two principal lines of evidence that bear on the problem of stimulus-response coupling for histamine, as well as for most other autacoids and many drugs. Inorganic ions are the focus of the first of these mechanisms. Alterations in membrane permeability allow sodium or calcium ions, for example, to flow down their electrochemical gradients into the cell, thereby altering its electrical properties and ionic composition. Breakdown of phosphatidylinositides and generation of polyphosphorylated derivatives of inositol (such as inositol triphosphate) may participate in the regulation of calcium channels. Calcium ions are also mobilized from intracellular sites. The importance of the intracellular concentration of free calcium for the regulation of contraction, secretion, and various other cellular responses is well established (*see* Chapter 2). Changes in membrane permeability to ions in response to histamine are reflected in the smooth muscle depolarizing responses that accompany contraction, in the depolarization of chromaffin cells, in the generation of nerve impulses, and in an increased calcium component of the cardiac action potential during the positive inotropic effect. It should be noted, however, that both contraction and relaxation can be induced with histamine (as with other substances) in smooth muscles that are fully depolarized by potassium. Here, changes in tension reflect an effect of histamine that is clearly not dependent on voltage but that presumably involves the opening of calcium channels in the membrane to allow influx of calcium ions or the mobilization of calcium from cellular sources. Contractile responses to histamine in the absence of extracellular calcium must be explained by such utilization of intracellular calcium.

The second line of evidence concerning stimulus-response coupling relates to effects of extracellular regulators on adenylate cyclase and, perhaps, on guanylate cyclase. Several effects of histamine, including gastric acid secretion, stimulation of cardiac contraction, and inhibition of secretion from basophils, have all been associated with elevated concentrations of adenosine 3',5'-monophosphate (cyclic AMP). These responses are all mediated through H_2 receptors. Histamine also stimulates accumulation of cyclic AMP in brain and other neural tissue through H_2 receptors. Relaxation of some smooth muscles, which again involves H_2 receptors, has also been associated with a rise in cyclic AMP concentrations. Contraction, on the other hand, which involves H_1 receptors, may be accompanied by accumulation of cyclic GMP. However, this may be secondary to effects on calcium. Moreover, accumulation of cyclic GMP has, in general, been linked with relaxation of smooth muscle. Additional complications have been noted above; thus, relaxation of vascular smooth muscle in response to histamine may require the intermediacy of endothelial cells. It should be evident that much uncertainty surrounds the nature of histamine receptors, their mode of operation, and the details of stimulus-response coupling (*see* Rasmussen, 1981; Ganellin and Parsons, 1982; Johnson, in Ganellin and Parsons, 1982).

ENDOGENOUS HISTAMINE: DISTRIBUTION AND BIOSYNTHESIS

Distribution. Histamine is widely, if unevenly, distributed throughout the animal kingdom and is present in many venoms, noxious secretions, bacteria, and plants (Reite, 1972). Almost all mammalian tissues contain preformed histamine, in amounts ranging from less than 1 to more than 100 μg/g. Concentrations in plasma and other body fluids are generally very low, but human cerebrospinal fluid contains significant amounts (Khandelwal *et al.*, 1982). The concentration is particularly high in the skin, intestinal mucosa, and lungs. Of no less importance than concentration, and often unrelated to it, is histamine-synthesizing capacity. Some tissues synthesize and turn over histamine at a remarkably high rate.

Origin, Synthesis, and Storage. Histamine that is ingested or formed by bacteria in the gastrointestinal tract does not contribute significantly to the endogenous pool. Most histamine that is absorbed is catabolized in the gut wall or liver and eliminated in the urine (*see* below). Every mammalian tissue that contains histamine is capable of synthesizing it from histidine by virtue of its content of L-histidine decarboxylase, an enzyme specific for histidine, to be distinguished from the less specific aromatic amino acid decarboxylase. In most tissues the chief site of histamine *storage* is the mast cell or, in the blood, its circulating counterpart, the basophil. These cells synthesize histamine and store it in secretory granules. The turnover rate of histamine here is slow, and, when tissues rich in mast cells are depleted of their stores of histamine, it may take weeks before concentrations of the autacoid return to normal. Nonmast-cell sites of histamine formation or storage include cells of the human epidermis, cells in the gastric mucosa, neurons within the CNS, and cells in regenerating or rapidly growing tissues. At these sites turnover is rapid, since the histamine is continuously released rather than stored. This contributes significantly to the daily excretion of histamine and its metabolites in the urine. Since L-histidine decarboxylase is an inducible enzyme, the histamine-forming capacity at such nonmast-cell sites is subject to regulation by various physiological and other factors. Conjecture on the functions of nonmast-cell histamine is therefore abundant (*see* Beaven, in Ganellin and Parsons, 1982).

ENDOGENOUS HISTAMINE: FUNCTIONS

Histamine Release in Anaphylaxis and Allergy. Although Dale and Laidlaw had drawn attention to the close correspondence between the effects of poisoning with histamine and anaphylactic shock as early as 1910, many years elapsed before the meaning of this correspondence became apparent. Three major clues were provided by (1) the work of Dale (1913), which showed convincingly that the hypersensitivity phenomenon involved a reaction of antigen with cell-fixed antibody; (2) the work of Lewis (1927), demonstrating that a histamine-like agent ("H-substance") was liberated in the skin during the local anaphylactic reaction; and (3) the work of Best and associates (1927), establishing beyond doubt that histamine is a natural constituent of the tissues of the body. The first two clues prompted Lewis (1927) to enunciate the hypothesis that the antigen-antibody reaction caused the cells to liberate a substance with the properties of histamine that was responsible for the characteristic physiological accompaniments of the phenomenon, that is, vasodilatation, itching, and edema formation. The third clue allowed Dale (1929) to argue forcibly that this "H-substance" was histamine itself. Within a few years, the release of histamine during the antigen-antibody reaction had been demonstrated, and the histamine hypothesis of the mediation of hypersensitivity phenomena won wide acceptance. When, following World War II, the newly discovered histamine antagonists were found to reduce the intensity of various hypersensitivity reactions, the involvement of histamine was established beyond all reasonable doubt. During this same period, however, it became increasingly evident from the failure of these antagonists to suppress the reactions completely that histamine was not the only factor involved.

Mechanism. The principal target cells of the hypersensitivity reactions of the immediate type are the mast cells and basophils. Within the secretory granules of these cells, the histamine is stored along with a heparin-protein complex to which it is loosely bound by ionic forces; several hydrolytic enzymes and various other pharmacologically active substances are also present (*see* below). The secretion (or "release") of histamine from sensitized mast cells or basophils in response to specific antigen is believed to be initiated when the antigen combines with and bridges adjacent molecules of reaginic antibodies (IgE) that have become attached to the cell surface. The ensuing perturbation seemingly sets in motion a series of reactions that show a critical requirement for calcium and metabolic energy and terminate in the extrusion of the contents of secretory granules by the process of exocytosis. In these several respects the secretory behavior of mast cells and basophils is identical with that of various gland cells, endocrine and exocrine, and conforms to a rather general pattern of stimulus-secretion coupling in which a secretagogue-induced rise in the intracellular concentration of calcium ions apparently serves to initiate exocytosis (Douglas, 1968, 1978). Allergic "release" of histamine is thus an active secretory process to be clearly distinguished from cytolysis. The two unusual features of the allergic secretory response are, firstly, that the secretagogue is a specific antigen and, secondly, that the membrane receptor through which it acts requires the prior at-

tachment of reaginic immunoglobulin (IgE) molecules to become functional. Despite intense experimentation, the details of stimulus-secretion coupling in mast cells, basophils, and other secretory cells are still obscure. Among the events that have been implicated in the response are: activation of proteases, methylation of phospholipids, opening of membrane calcium channels and mobilization of calcium ions, activation of phospholipase A_2 and arachidonate metabolism, altered cyclic AMP synthesis, and enhanced protein phosphorylation.

Significant *inhibition* of the secretory response of mast cells during the acute hypersensitivity reaction can be achieved with epinephrine and related drugs that act through β-adrenergic receptors on these cells. In this instance the effect seems to be the result of cyclic AMP accumulation. The beneficial effects of β-adrenergic agonists in allergic states such as asthma are, however, mainly due to their relaxant effect on bronchial smooth muscle. Cromolyn, on the other hand, owes its clinical usefulness largely to an inhibitory effect on mast-cell secretion (*see* below). Histamine itself, acting through H_2 receptors on mast cells and basophils, can also reduce the secretory response somewhat; however, the functional significance of this negative feedback is uncertain (*see* Foreman, 1981; Metcalfe *et al.*, 1981; Symposium, 1981; Plaut and Lichtenstein, in Ganellin and Parsons, 1982; Symposium, 1982; Lagunoff *et al.*, 1983; Larsen and Henson, 1983; Ishizaka, 1984).

Limitations of the Histamine Hypothesis of Hypersensitivity Reactions: Involvement of Other Autacoids. The classical histamine hypothesis provides only a partial explanation for the spectrum of effects that results from immediate hypersensitivity reactions. Beside histamine, a broad array of biologically active substances of a proinflammatory nature is synthesized and/or released.

Histamine is expelled along with all of the other constituents of the secretory granules, including heparin, proteins, and peptides. These include an eosinophil chemotactic factor (ECF-A); a neutrophil chemotactic factor (NCF-A); and enzymes, such as β-glucuronidase and other exoglycosidases, neutral proteases, superoxide dismutase, and peroxidase. In rodents, but not in man, 5-hydroxytryptamine is also secreted. Moreover, in addition to these preformed substances, there appear various newly synthesized compounds. These arise in part from the mast cells or basophils themselves, as a consequence of the metabolic events that accompany stimulation. They are also formed secondarily from neighboring tissue by the enzymes and other substances discharged from the mast cells and basophils. The list includes a host of metabolites of arachidonic acid (*see* Chapters 28 and 29), a platelet-activating factor (PAF; an ether lipid of uncertain metabolic origin) (*see* Benveniste and Arnoux, 1983), and kinins. Many of these substances have potent biological activities and contribute importantly to the allergic response; indeed, their effects may in some situations, such as allergic asthma, dominate the clinical picture (*see*

Mathews, 1982; Dahlén *et al.*, 1983; Editorial, 1983a).

Histamine Release by Drugs, Peptides, Venoms, and Other Agents.

Numerous drugs and other substances in clinical use have antigenic activity and may, on a second or subsequent exposure, trigger the release of histamine and other autacoids from mast cells and basophils by the immediate hypersensitivity reaction. In addition, many compounds, including a large number of therapeutic agents, can stimulate histamine release directly without prior sensitization. Responses of this sort are most likely to occur in response to intravenous injections and to certain categories of substances, particularly those that are organic bases. Among these bases are amides, amidines, quaternary ammonium compounds, pyridinium compounds, piperidines, alkaloids, and antibiotic bases. *Radiocontrast media* and certain *plasma expanders* may also elicit the response. The phenomenon is one of clinical concern, for it accounts for many unexpected reactions of anaphylactoid nature (*see* Lorenz *et al.*, 1981; Symposium, 1982; Weck and Bundgaard, 1983).

Although such release of histamine is generally encountered as a side effect of drugs administered for some therapeutic purpose, there are certain compounds of experimental interest for which the ability to release histamine is the dominant pharmacological characteristic. Such drugs are commonly referred to as *histamine liberators*. The archetype is the polybasic substance known as compound 48/80. This is a mixture of low-molecular-weight polymers of *p*-methoxy-N-methylphenethylamine (*see* Paton, 1957), of which the hexamer is most active (*see* Lagunoff *et al.*, 1983). The decision to classify a drug as a histamine liberator is, however, arbitrary. Some antibiotic bases and many peptides with other activities are among the most active histamine-releasing substances known.

Basic polypeptides are commonly effective histamine releasers, and their potency generally increases with the number of basic groups over a limited range. Polymyxin B is very active and is the best studied; others include bradykinin, substance P, neurotensin, protamine, and somatostatin. Since basic polypeptides are released upon tissue injury or are present in stings and venoms (*e.g.*, mast-cell degranulating protein in bees), they seemingly constitute pathophysiological stimuli to secretion for mast cells and basophils. Also to be viewed in the same way are the *anaphylotoxins* (*C3a* and *C5a*), which are low-molecular-weight peptides that are cleaved from the complement system. Some *enzymes,* notably *phospholipase A$_2$* and *chymotrypsin,* also have pronounced histamine-releasing activity of possible pathophysiological relevance. Of experimental interest are the histamine-releasing activities of lectins such as concanavalin A and calcium ionophores such as A23187.

Within seconds of the intravenous injection of a histamine liberator, human subjects experience a burning, itching sensation, as if a bundle of nettles had been placed on the skin. This effect, most marked in the palms of the hand and in the face, scalp, and ears, is soon followed by a feeling of intense warmth. The skin reddens, and the color rapidly spreads over the trunk. Blood pressure falls, and the heart rate accelerates, and the subject complains of headache, often intense. After a few minutes, blood pressure recovers, and edema and crops of giant hives appear in the skin, particularly over the thorax and abdomen. There is colic, nausea, hypersecretion of acid with acid vomitus, and moderate bronchospasm (Lecomte, 1957). The effect becomes less intense with successive injections as the mast-cell stores of histamine are depleted. Histamine liberators do not deplete tissues of nonmast-cell histamine.

Mechanism. Each of the above-mentioned classes of histamine-releasing substances can set in motion the classical, energy-dependent secretory response of the mast cells or basophils, and they may produce this effect in each instance by causing a rise in the intracellular concentration of calcium ions. Some are ionophores and transport calcium into the cell; others, such as the anaphylotoxins, seemingly act like specific antigens to increase membrane permeability to calcium; basic histamine releasers, such as compound 48/80 and polymyxin B, act principally by mobilizing calcium from cellular sources. Numerous reviews of this complex field are available (*see* Goth, 1978; Pepys and Edwards, 1979; Metcalfe *et al.*, 1981; Lagunoff *et al.*, 1983).

Histamine Release by Other Means.

Some clinical conditions in which release of histamine occurs in response to other forms of stimulation include *cold urticaria, cholinergic urticaria,* and *solar urticaria.* Some of these involve specific secretory responses of the mast cells and, indeed, cell-fixed IgE (*see* Salvaggio, 1982). However, histamine release also occurs whenever there is nonspecific cell damage from any cause. The redness and urticaria that follow scratching of the skin is a familiar example.

Injury, Stress, "Induced Histamine," and Microcirculation.

Schayer (1963) suggested that "induced histamine," which is not stored but immediately freed, has a role in regulating the microcirculation to satisfy locally increased requirements for blood resulting from injurious stimuli. Such histamine was also proposed to account for the delayed phase of vasodilatation occurring in inflammation. However, many other proinflammatory autacoids have since been identified, and these may contribute to this phase of inflammation. Whether histamine has any physiological role in the regulation of the microcirculation is uncertain (Altura, 1982).

Tissue Growth and Repair. A conspicuously high histamine-forming capacity is present in many tissues undergoing rapid growth or repair, such as embryonic tissue, regenerating liver, bone marrow, wound and granulation tissue, and malignant growths. Newly formed ''nascent histamine'' may have some function in anabolic processes (*see* Kahlson and Rosengren, 1971).

Gastric Secretion. In 1920, Keeton and associates and also Popielski reported that histamine stimulates gastric secretion, and the former investigators proposed that endogenous histamine might mediate some of the stimulatory effects of the vagus. MacIntosh, in 1938, showed that histamine was released from the stomach during vagal stimulation and thus provided essential experimental support for the idea. Nearly 50 years were to pass, however, before sufficient evidence accumulated to allow Code (1965), Kahlson and Rosengren (1971), and others to mount persuasive arguments that histamine has an important physiological function in evoking gastric secretion. Because no drug then existed that would block the effect of histamine on gastric secretion and thereby allow a critical test of the possibility, the idea was vigorously challenged. With the development of the H_2 antagonists, the importance of histamine could no longer be doubted, since these drugs were found to inhibit not only gastric secretion elicited by injected histamine but also basal secretion and that elicited by various physiological stimuli (whether mediated by the vagus or by gastrin). The major problems that remain are to identify the cells that synthesize, store, and release histamine in the stomach; to learn how these cells are activated; and to characterize the action of histamine and the nature of its interactions with ACh and with gastrin. Cells that contain histamine, ''histaminocytes,'' have been found in the gastric mucosa in more-or-less close proximity to the gastric glands; they resemble enterochromaffin cells in some rodents, while they are similar to mast cells in dogs and other species. However, little is known of the regulation of histamine release. Histamine itself acts directly on the parietal cells through H_2 receptors, apparently linked to adenylate cyclase, to activate a proton pump in the parietal cell membrane (*see* below). ACh and gastrin can also stimulate the parietal cells directly through different receptors. They activate the same pump, but their efficacies as secretagogues show a considerable dependence on the level of concomitant stimulation by histamine, which seems to sensitize the cells or amplify the intracellular signals. This apparently explains the inhibitory effects of H_2 antagonists on acid secretion evoked by gastrin or ACh (*see* below). The efficacy of histamine is similarly influenced, but to a much lesser extent, by the presence or absence of the other secretagogues. Whether there is merit in the old conjecture that secretagogues such as gastrin act, at least in part, by releasing histamine is still uncertain. The primacy of histamine in the physiological control of gastric acid secretion is, however, now accepted (*see* reviews by Beaven and by Code, in Ganellin and Parsons, 1982).

Nerves and Brain. *Afferent Nerves.* Histamine, released by one means or another, is frequently involved in initiation of sensory impulses evoking *pain and itch.*
Efferent Nerves. The possibility that *''active reflex vasodilatation''* may be mediated by histamine liberated by efferent nervous function continues to be debated. There is, as yet, no convincing evidence of peripheral histaminergic nerves.
Brain. Evidence supports the idea that histamine serves as a chemical transmitter of certain histaminergic nerves in the brain, some of which may be involved in the control of the anterior pituitary gland (*see* Schwartz *et al.,* in Ganellin and Parsons, 1982; *see also* Chapter 12).

Headache. Endogenous histamine has been implicated in the genesis of headaches, particularly the syndrome named *histaminic cephalalgia.* There is little evidence to support this idea (*see* Lecomte, 1957; Burland and Mills, in Ganellin and Parsons, 1982).

Growths of Mast Cells and Basophils. In *urticaria pigmentosa* (mastocytosis), mast cells aggregate in the upper corium and give rise to pigmented cutaneous lesions that urticate when stroked. In *systemic mastocytosis,* similar aggregates are also found in other organs. Patients with these syndromes suffer a constellation of signs and symptoms attributable to excessive histamine release, including, in addition to urticaria and dermographism, pruritus, headache, weakness, hypotension, flushing of the face, and a variety of gastrointestinal effects such as peptic ulceration. The signs and symptoms are precipitated or exacerbated by a variety of stimuli—the friction of toweling the skin or exposure to drugs that release histamine directly or to which patients are allergic. Excessive numbers of basophils are present in the blood in *myelogenous leukemia* and raise its histamine content to high levels. *Gastric carcinoid* tumors secrete histamine, and this apparently contributes to the patchy ''geographical'' flush.

ADDITIONAL CONSIDERATIONS

Absorption, Fate, and Excretion. Histamine is readily absorbed after parenteral injection and acts rapidly when given by the subcutaneous or intramuscular route. Its action is evanescent, since it diffuses into tissues and is rapidly metabolized. Very large amounts of histamine can be given orally, however, without causing effects, since much is converted by intestinal bacteria to inactive N-acetylhistamine, and the free histamine absorbed is mostly inactivated as it traverses the intestinal wall or circulates through the liver.

In man, there are two major paths of histamine metabolism. The more important one involves ring methylation and is catalyzed by the enzyme histamine-N-methyltransferase, which is specific for histamine and is widely distributed. Most of the product, N-methylhistamine, is converted by monoamine oxidase (MAO) to N-methyl imidazole acetic acid. In the other path, histamine undergoes oxidative deamination catalyzed mainly by the nonspecific enzyme diamine oxidase (DAO). The products are imidazole acetic acid and, eventually, its riboside. The various metabolites, which have little or no pharmacological activity, are excreted in the urine. The relative roles of these enzymes in the metabolism of endogenous histamine have not yet been established. Some inhibitors of histamine synthesis and degradation are known, but these are of little clinical interest (*see* Schayer, 1978; Wetterquist, 1978; Beaven, in Ganellin and Parsons, 1982; Khandelwal *et al.*, 1982).

Toxicity. Overdosage with histamine is rare, and symptoms are generally not dangerous. However, massive doses cause intense headache, flushing, profound fall of blood pressure, bronchospasm, dyspnea, a metallic taste, vomiting, and diarrhea. The prompt injection of histamine antagonists will suppress these reactions.

Preparations. *Histamine phosphate* is available for injection in preparations containing 0.275 or 0.55 mg/ml (equivalent to 0.1 or 0.2 mg of histamine base per milliliter).

CLINICAL USES

The practical applications of histamine are limited to its use as a diagnostic agent. Histamine has been much used to assess the ability of the stomach to secrete acid and to determine parietal cell mass. Thus, anacidity or hyposecretion in response to histamine may reflect *pernicious anemia, atrophic gastritis,* or *gastric carcinoma,* whereas a hypersecretory response may be found in patients with *duodenal ulcer* or with the *Zollinger-Ellison syndrome.* Administered by itself, histamine causes distressing side effects; but these can be greatly reduced by giving beforehand an H_1 antagonist. However, there are other, more suitable stimulants of gastric secretion (*see* below).

The fact that intradermal histamine causes a "flare" that is mediated by axon reflexes allows a test for the *integrity of sensory nerves,* of value in certain neurological conditions.

The stimulant effect of histamine on chromaffin cells has been applied in a provocative test for *pheochromocytoma.* Histamine (administered by inhalation) has also been used to assess *bronchial reactivity.*

H_1 and H_2 Agonists. Drugs with histamine-like activity that act preferentially or selectively on H_1 or H_2 receptors not only are valuable experimental tools but also offer some advantage over histamine in the clinic (*see* Ganellin, in Ganellin and Parsons, 1982).

H_1 Agonists. Clinical uses of histamine that depend on activation of H_1 receptors are limited, and it is not known whether H_1 agonists (Table 26–1) are more suitable for diagnostic tests of bronchial reactivity, integrity of nerves, or the presence of pheochromocytoma. A moderately selective drug, *betahistine,* has had some very limited clinical use as a vasodilator and is available for investigational use.

H_2 Agonists. These agents have a clear place in tests of gastric secretory function, since they allow a more selective stimulation with reduced adverse effects. *Betazole* (3-pyrazolylethylamine; Table 26–1) was found to stimulate gastric acid secretion preferentially in the early 1950s (Rosière and Grossman, 1951). Although it has only 2% of the potency of histamine at H_2 receptors, its potency at H_1 receptors is still less (about 0.2%). This degree of selectivity, although modest, has led to the common use of betazole as a gastric acid secretagogue in man (*see* Figure 26–1, page 625). However, the residual H_1 activity still results in some adverse effects, such as flushing, weakness, syncope, and headache. The use of the drug in atopic individuals is not advised. Other, newer H_2 agonists (Table 26–1) are much more selective and may prove more suitable. Most noteworthy is *impromidine,* which has activity at H_2 receptors more than 10,000 times that at H_1 receptors. In man, impromidine elicits maximal gastric acid secretion with only minor circulatory effects (Hunt *et al.*, 1980).

Preparations. *Betazole hydrochloride* (HISTALOG) is available in ampuls containing 50 mg in 1 ml. The usual adult dose is 50 mg, given intramuscularly or subcutaneously. *Impromidine* is only available for investigational use.

PENTAGASTRIN

The potent physiological gastric secretagogue, *gastrin,* which is released from the pyloric antrum by vagal and local gastric responses to feeding, is a heptadecapeptide. The full spectrum of gastrin-like activity is also present in smaller fragments of the peptide, the smallest effective compound being the C-terminal tetrapeptide amide: Trp-Met-Asp-Phe-NH_2. This has about 10% of the potency of gastrin. A synthetic pentapeptide derivative, *pentagastrin,* is still more active and has been adopted for gastric function tests as an alternative to histamine or betazole; pentagastrin causes fewer and less severe reactions.

Chemistry. Pentagastrin is N-*t*-butyloxycarbonyl - β - alanyl - L - tryptophanyl - L - methionyl - L-aspartyl-L-phenylalanine amide. It has the structural formula:

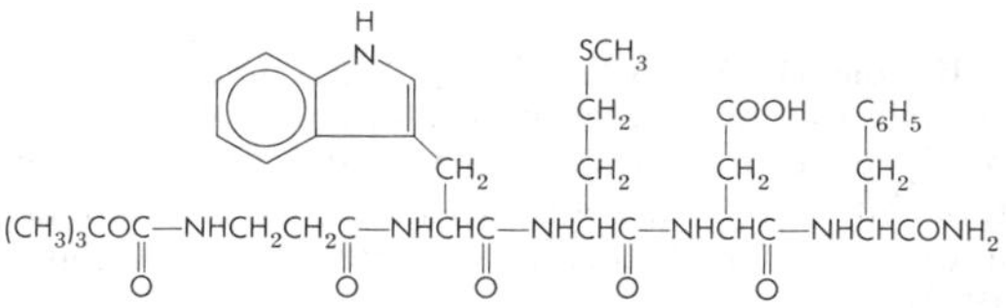

Pentagastrin

Pharmacological Effects. The most prominent action of pentagastrin is to stimulate the secretion of gastric acid, pepsin, and intrinsic factor; additionally, it stimulates pancreatic secretion, inhibits absorption of water and electrolytes from the ileum, contracts the smooth muscle of the lower esophageal sphincter and stomach (but delays gastric emptying time), relaxes the sphincter of Oddi, increases blood flow in the gastric mucosa, and, *in high doses,* stimulates a variety of smooth muscles in different species. It also mimics or blocks the effects of the polypeptides pancreozymin-cholecystokinin, secretin, and caerulein, a naturally occurring decapeptide that, together with pancreozymin-cholecystokinin, shares a common C-terminal heptapeptide sequence with gastrin. The half-life of pentagastrin in the circulation appears to be about 10 minutes.

Clinical Use. Pentagastrin elicits reproducible gastric secretory responses comparable to those induced by histamine or betazole and offers several advantages. The pentagastrin test requires only a single subcutaneous injection; it is relatively short in duration of action, and side effects are usually minor and transient. These may include various gastrointestinal phenomena, such as nausea, borborygmi, and the urge to defecate, and circulatory effects, including flushing, tachycardia, faintness, and dizziness. Allergic reactions are rare. Gastric secretion begins within 10 minutes, reaches a maximum within 30 minutes, and lasts for about an hour (*see* Baron, 1972).

Preparation. *Pentagastrin* (PEPTAVLON) is marketed in ampuls containing 0.25 mg/ml. The diagnostic dose is 6 μg/kg, administered by subcutaneous injection.

INHIBITION OF ALLERGIC RELEASE OF HISTAMINE AND OTHER AUTACOIDS

Therapy aimed at controlling the symptoms of immediate hypersensitivity reactions with antagonists of histamine is useful but only partially effective. This is because histamine is but one of a battery of autacoids released or formed during the reaction, which together elicit the symptoms (*see* above). To suppress the effects of all these agents would require a corresponding battery of blocking agents; even if these were all available, such an approach would be cumbersome. It is for this reason that treatment of allergic reactions often necessitates the use of nonspecific "physiological antagonists" such as epinephrine, which essentially counter responses to the antigen-induced flood of autacoids by eliciting responses of an opposite nature. But this approach, like the use of blocking drugs, does not address the underlying cause. An attractive and advantageous procedure, uniquely applicable to *prophylaxis,* is to prevent production or release of the autacoids by inhibiting responses of sensitized mast cells and basophils to specific antigens. Adrenergic drugs and theophylline, beside their many other actions, tend to inhibit such allergic responses; this may contribute to their clinical utility. A much more specific inhibition is possible, however, with the type of antiallergic drug exemplified by *cromolyn.* This agent inhibits antigen-induced secretion of histamine from human pulmonary mast cells and from mast cells at certain other sites. Although the usefulness of cromolyn is circumscribed (human basophils, curiously, are not protected), the drug is a valuable adjunct in the prophylactic management of certain cases of asthma and certain other atopic states.

CROMOLYN SODIUM

History. Cromolyn was synthesized after a long search, the initial purpose of which was to enhance the smooth muscle relaxant, particularly bronchodilator, properties of the drug khellin, a chromone (benzopyrone) of plant origin. Successive modifications in structure yielded *bis*-chromones, the most important being cromolyn. This lacked bronchodilator activity but, unexpectedly, prevented allergic bronchospasm. Analysis revealed a novel mechanism of action, namely, inhibition of release of histamine and other autacoids (Altounyan, 1967; Cox *et al.*, 1970).

Chemistry. Cromolyn sodium, the disodium salt of 1,3-*bis*(2-carboxychromone-5-yloxy)-2-hydroxypropane, has the following structure:

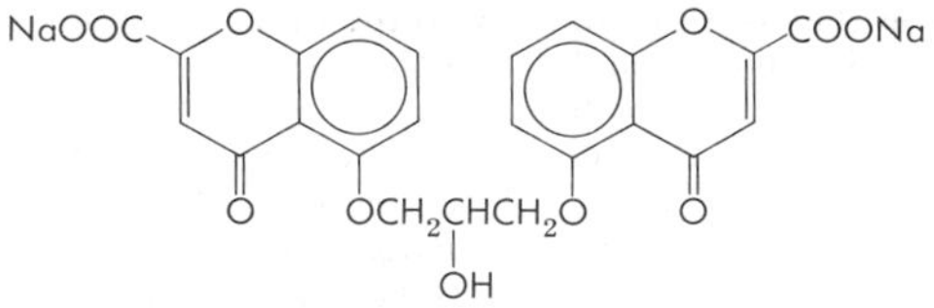

Cromolyn Sodium

Pharmacological Effects. Cromolyn does not relax bronchial or other smooth muscle. Nor does it inhibit significantly responses of these muscles to any of a variety of pharmacological spasmogens. It does, however, inhibit the release of histamine and other autacoids (including leukotrienes) from human lung during allergic responses mediated by IgE and thereby reduces the stimulus for bronchospasm. Inhibition of the liberation of leukotrienes is particularly important in allergic bronchial asthma, where these products appear to be the principal cause of bronchoconstriction (Dahlén *et al.,* 1983; *see* Chapter 28). Cromolyn is believed to act on the pulmonary mast cells, the primary target cells for the immediate hypersensitivity reaction. Inhibition of antigen-induced release of histamine and production of leukotrienes can readily be demonstrated in mast cells isolated from the rat peritoneal cavity. Cromolyn does not inhibit the binding of IgE to mast cells nor the interaction between cell-bound IgE and specific antigen; rather, it suppresses the secretory response to this reaction. How it does so is uncertain. The effect is not restricted to the antigen-antibody reaction, although this may be preferentially affected. It can also be observed when secretion of histamine is elicited by drugs such as 48/80, whose action is independent of cell-fixed IgE (*see* above).

Attempts to explain the action of cromolyn in terms of changes in concentrations of cyclic nucleotides have been unrewarding and have prompted statements that cromolyn has a "membrane-stabilizing" action or reduces calcium fluxes. Cromolyn has been shown to promote the phosphorylation of a single mast-cell protein, and this action has been advanced as a further possible explanation for its effect (Theoharides *et al.,* 1980). There are remarkable species and tissue differences in responsiveness to cromolyn.

Absorption, Fate, and Excretion. Cromolyn is very poorly absorbed after oral administration and is therefore given, for asthma, by inhalation. A special turbo inhaler is used to disperse the finely powdered drug (mixed with lactose). By this route, some 10% penetrates deep into the lungs and is absorbed into the blood, where its half-life is about 80 minutes. The drug is not metabolized and is excreted unchanged, about half in the urine and half in the bile. Aqueous solutions are available for nasal and ophthalmic uses.

Toxicity. Cromolyn is generally well tolerated by patients; adverse reactions are infrequent and minor, even during continuous use over several years. The most common reactions, probably related to the direct irritant effect of the powder, include bronchospasm, wheezing, cough, nasal congestion, and pharyngeal irritation. Sometimes dizziness, dysuria, joint swelling and pain, nausea, headache, and rash are encountered. More serious and rare effects, probably attributable to hypersensitivity to the drug, include laryngeal edema, angioedema, urticaria, and anaphylaxis.

Preparations and Dosage. *Cromolyn sodium for inhalation* (INTAL) is available in capsules that contain 20 mg of the finely powdered drug mixed with lactose. The contents of the capsule are inhaled by means of a special turbo inhaler, usually four times daily. Alternatively, a solution of the drug can be used with a power-operated nebulizer. A 4% liquid nasal spray (NASALCROM) is available in a pump that delivers a metered spray containing 5.2 mg with each compression. The recommended dose is one spray in each nostril three to six times a day. A 4% ophthalmic solution (OPTICROM) is also available; 1 to 2 drops are used four to six times daily.

Clinical Use. The main use of cromolyn is in the *prophylactic treatment* of bronchial asthma. This is based on the experimental observation that, when given before an antigenic challenge, it will inhibit bronchoconstriction and prevent the objective signs and the symptoms of the acute asthmatic attack. This protective effect can last for hours. By contrast, if cromolyn is administered even as soon as 1 minute after the antigenic challenge, it has little effect on the course of the response. For this reason, *cromolyn has no place in the treatment of the acute asthmatic attack, nor in status asthmaticus.*

When given prophylactically, cromolyn benefits many asthmatic patients, especially children, by improving pulmonary function and reducing the frequency and intensity of asthmatic episodes; the need for administration of corticosteroids or bronchodilators is thus diminished. The beneficial effect may take several weeks to become evident. Tolerance does not develop. Patients of different ages and with various types of asthma may be benefited. The effectiveness of the drug is not restricted to patients with extrinsic, atopic, IgE-mediated asthma; intrinsic asthma and dust- and exercise-induced asthmas may also be benefited. However, the drug is ineffective in many patients.

Other clinical conditions in which beneficial effects of cromolyn may occur include *allergic rhinitis,* various *atopic diseases of the eye,* and *giant papillary conjunctivitis,* which may result from the use of contact lenses (*see* Berman, 1983; Medical Letter, 1983).

HISTAMINE ANTAGONISTS: H₁- AND H₂-BLOCKING AGENTS

History. It was long obvious that drugs able to antagonize the actions of histamine would be of great interest both as investigative tools and as therapeutic agents. Histamine-blocking activity was first detected in 1937 by Bovet and Staub in one of a series of amines with a phenolic ether function synthesized by Fourneau. This substance, 2 - isopropyl - 5 - methylphenoxyethyldiethylamine, protected guinea pigs against several lethal doses of histamine, antagonized histamine-induced spasms of various smooth muscles, and, most significantly, lessened the symptoms of anaphylactic shock. This drug was too toxic for clinical use, but by the early 1940s some derivatives were proven to be acceptable. One of these, *pyrilamine maleate,* described by Bovet and his colleagues in 1944, is still one of the most specific and effective histamine blockers of this category. While these developments were taking place in wartime France, the leads offered by the original Fourneau compounds were also being followed in the United States and resulted in the discovery of the highly effective histamine antagonists *diphenhydramine* and *tripelennamine* (*see* Bovet, 1950; Ganellin, in Ganellin and Parsons, 1982).

By the early 1950s many compounds with histamine-blocking activity had been described and were available to the physician. However, none of these drugs blocked all of the many effects of histamine. While they effectively inhibited many important responses to histamine, which were later ascribed to a population of histamine receptors termed H₁ receptors by Ash and Schild in 1966, they uniformly failed to inhibit others, most conspicuously gastric acid secretion. It was thus of very considerable interest when, in 1972, Black and colleagues described a new and chemically distinct class of drugs that selectively blocked the stimulant effect of histamine on gastric acid secretion; these agents also suppressed the other responses to hista-

mine that were refractory to the older antagonists. This discovery established the existence of a second population of histamine receptors, H₂ receptors; it provided powerful new pharmacological tools with which to explore the functions of endogenous histamine; and it ushered in a major new class of therapeutic agents (*see* Black *et al.* and also Ganellin, in Ganellin and Parsons, 1982).

Terminology and Mechanism of Action. Depending on the receptors with which they interact, antagonists of histamine are currently classified as H₁ or H₂ antagonists (or blockers). There are already some indications that subpopulations of histamine receptors exist, and a further elaboration of this scheme seems not unlikely (*see* Black *et al.,* in Ganellin and Parsons, 1982). All of the available antagonists are reversible, competitive inhibitors of the actions of histamine.

H₁-BLOCKING AGENTS

Structure-Activity Relationship. Like histamine, most H₁ antagonists contain a substituted ethylamine moiety, $-\overset{|}{\underset{|}{C}}-\overset{|}{\underset{|}{C}}-N\diagup$; unlike histamine, which has a primary amino group and a single aromatic ring, most H₁ blockers have a tertiary amino group linked by a two- or three-atom chain to two aromatic substituents and conform to the general formula:

$$\begin{array}{c} Ar_1 \\ \diagdown \\ X-\overset{|}{\underset{|}{C}}-\overset{|}{\underset{|}{C}}-N\diagup \\ Ar_2 \diagup \end{array}$$

where Ar is aryl and X is a nitrogen or carbon atom or a $-C-O-$ ether linkage to the β-aminoethyl side chain. Sometimes the two aromatic rings are bridged, as in the tricyclic derivatives, or the ethylamine may be part of a ring structure. Other variations are also possible (*see* Table 26–2 and the structure of cyproheptadine, below). Extensive reviews of this complex field are available (*see* Ganellin, in Ganellin and Parsons, 1982).

Pharmacological Properties. Most H₁ blockers have similar pharmacological actions and therapeutic applications and can be conveniently discussed together. Their characteristic pharmacological activity is largely predictable from the foregoing presentation of the responses to histamine that involve interaction with H₁ receptors.

Smooth Muscle. H₁-blocking drugs inhibit most responses of smooth muscle to histamine. Within the *gastrointestinal*

Table 26–2.   REPRESENTATIVE H₁-RECEPTOR BLOCKING DRUGS

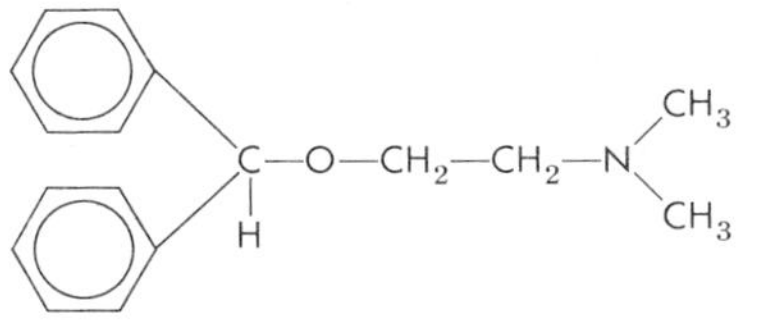

Diphenhydramine * (an ethanolamine)

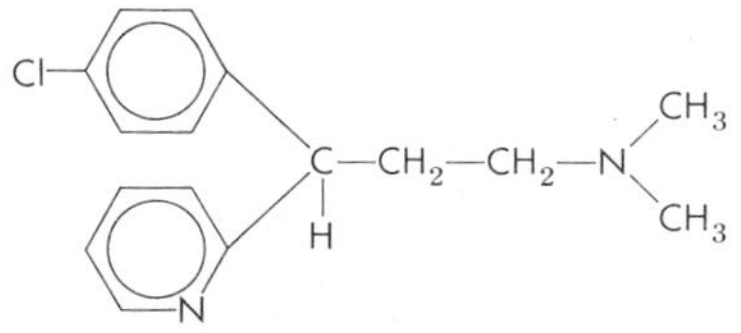

Chlorpheniramine ‡ (an alkylamine)

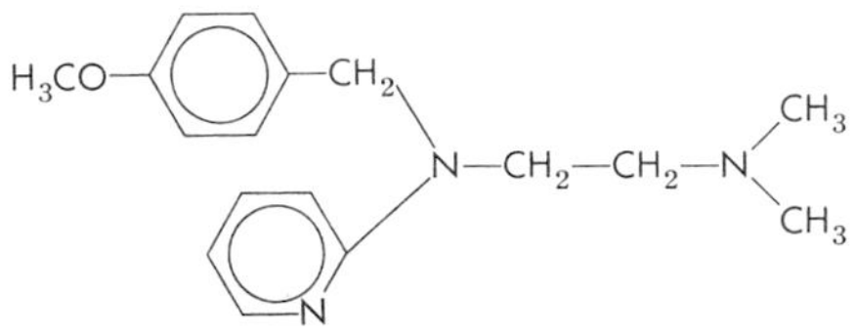

Pyrilamine † (an ethylenediamine)

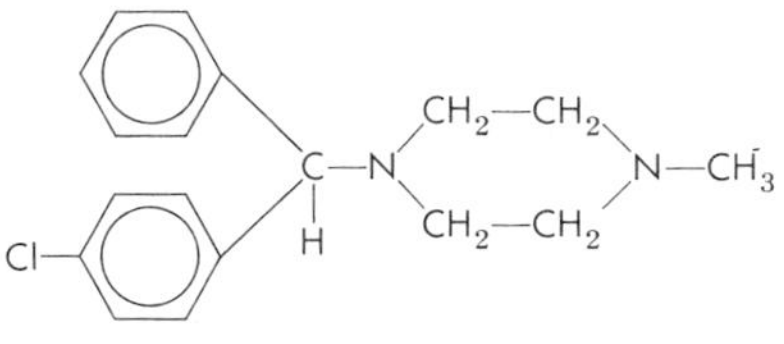

Chlorcyclizine § (a piperazine)

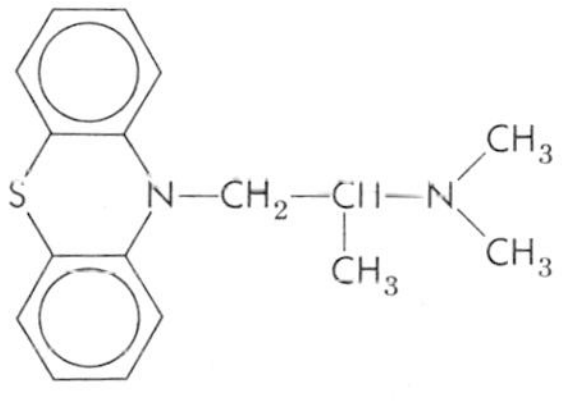

Promethazine (a phenothiazine)

* Dimenhydrinate is a combination of diphenhydramine and 8-chlorotheophylline in equal molecular proportions.
† Tripelennamine is the same less H₃CO.   ‡ Pheniramine is the same less Cl.   § Cyclizine is the same less Cl.

tract, the guinea pig ileum has been extensively studied *in vitro*. This preparation illustrates the competitive and surmountable nature of the block as well as its specificity. Similar antagonism is also readily demonstrable *in vivo* and in other regions of the gastrointestinal tract.

Antagonism of the constrictor action of histamine on *respiratory smooth muscle* is easily shown *in vivo*, in isolated lungs, or in strips of tracheal, bronchial, or bronchiolar muscle of various species including man. In guinea pigs, death by asphyxia follows quite small doses of histamine, yet the animal may survive a hundred lethal doses of histamine if given an H₁-blocking drug. In the same species, striking protection is also afforded against anaphylactic bronchospasm, but this is not so in man, in whom allergic bronchoconstriction is mediated mainly by leukotrienes.

Within the *vascular tree*, the H₁-blocking drugs inhibit both the vasoconstrictor effects of histamine and, to a degree, the more important vasodilator effects. Residual vasodilatation reflects the involvement of H₂ receptors and can only be suppressed by the concurrent administration of an H₂ blocker. Effects of the histamine antagonists on histamine-induced changes in systemic blood pressure parallel these vascular effects.

Capillary Permeability. H₁-blocking drugs strongly antagonize the action of histamine that results in increased capillary permeability and formation of edema and wheal.

"Flare" and Itch. The "flare" component of the triple response and the itching caused by intradermal injection of histamine are two different manifestations of a stimulant action of histamine on nerve endings. H₁-blocking drugs suppress both. Although most H₁ blockers have local anesthetic properties, they act, at relatively low concentrations, by blocking histamine receptors, presumably on the nerve endings.

Adrenal Medulla and Autonomic Ganglia. H₁-blocking drugs selectively suppress the stimulant effects of histamine on adrenal chromaffin cells and autonomic ganglia.

Failure to Inhibit Gastric Secretion. Gastric secretion is *not* inhibited at all by H₁-blocking agents; indeed, H_1 blockers are used in conjunction with histamine in diagnostic tests of gastric secretory function to lessen circulatory and other side effects (*see* above).

Other Exocrine Glands. H_1-blocking drugs inconstantly suppress histamine-evoked salivary, lacrimal, and other exocrine secretions. The atropine-like properties of many of these agents may, however, contribute to lessened secretion in cholinergically innervated glands and reduce ongoing secretion in, for example, the respiratory tree.

Immediate Hypersensitivity Reactions: Anaphylaxis and Allergy. During such hypersensitivity reactions, histamine is but one of many potent autacoids that are released (*see* above), and its relative importance for the ensuing symptoms varies widely with species and tissue. It follows that the protection afforded by histamine antagonists, which do not prevent responses to these other autacoids, is also variable with species and tissue. In man, some phenomena, including edema formation and itch, are fairly well controlled; others, such as hypotension, are less so; and bronchoconstriction is reduced little, if at all, since leukotrienes are the principal cause of allergic bronchoconstriction (*see* Dahlén *et al.*, 1983). In guinea pigs, by contrast, allergic bronchoconstriction is mediated mainly by histamine, and H_1 antagonists offer considerable protection.

Central Nervous System. The H_1 blockers can both stimulate and depress the CNS. Stimulation is occasionally encountered in patients given conventional doses, who become restless, nervous, and unable to sleep. Moreover, quite small doses may evoke EEG activation and epileptiform seizures in patients with focal lesions of the CNS. Central excitation is also a striking feature of poisoning, which not uncommonly results in convulsions, particularly in infants. Central depression, on the other hand, is the usual accompaniment of therapeutic doses of the H_1 antagonists. Diminished alertness, slowed reaction times, and somnolence are common manifestations. Some of the H_1 blockers are more likely to depress the CNS than others, and patients vary in their susceptibility and responses to individual drugs. The ethanolamines (Table 26–3, p. 622) are particularly prone to depress. Diphenhydramine, for example,

causes somnolence in about half of those taking the drug (*see* Carruthers *et al.*, 1978; Faingold, 1978). An antitussive effect reflects another and, perhaps, unrelated central action.

An interesting and useful property of *certain* H_1 blockers is the ability to counter *motion sickness*. This effect was first observed with dimenhydrinate and subsequently with diphenhydramine (the active moiety of dimenhydrinate), promethazine, and various piperazine derivatives.

Mechanism of Central Action. How the various H_1-blocking drugs produce their depressant and stimulant effects is uncertain. The effects may reflect antagonism of endogenous histamine released by central histaminergic neurons. The drugs bind with high affinity to H_1 receptors in brain (*see* Schwartz *et al.*, in Ganellin and Parsons, 1982). Whether the anti–motion sickness activity of some of the H_1 blockers is related to their ability to block muscarinic receptors (*see* below) is also unclear. Scopolamine is the most potent drug in prevention of motion sickness (*see* Chapter 7), and promethazine, which is perhaps the H_1-blocking drug with the strongest ACh-blocking action, is one of the most effective in combating motion sickness (*see* below).

Anticholinergic Effects. Many of the H_1 antagonists tend to inhibit responses to ACh that are mediated by muscarinic receptors. These antimuscarinic or atropine-like actions are sufficiently prominent in some of the drugs to be manifest during clinical usage (*see* below). Among the H_1 blockers, pyrilamine is one of the *least* liable to produce this effect. Its relatively high degree of specificity has rendered it a favorite pharmacological tool (*see* Rocha e Silva and Antonio, 1978).

Local Anesthetic Effect. The H_1-blocking drugs possess local anesthetic activity. Some are more potent than procaine. Promethazine and pyrilamine are especially active. However, the concentrations required for this effect are several orders higher than those that antagonize histamine.

Absorption, Fate, and Excretion. The H_1 blockers are well absorbed from the gastrointestinal tract. Following oral administration, the effects develop within 30 minutes, are maximal within 1 to 2 hours, and last about 3 to 6 hours, although some of the drugs are much longer acting (Table 26–3, page 622).

Extensive studies of the metabolic fate of H_1-blocking drugs have been limited to a few compounds. *Diphenhydramine,* given orally, reaches a maximal concentration in the blood in about 2 hours, remains at about this level for another 2 hours, and then falls exponentially with a plasma elimination half-time of about 4 hours. The drug is widely distributed throughout the body, including the CNS. Little, if any, is excreted unchanged in the urine; most appears there as degradation products that are almost completely excreted within 24 hours. The main site of metabolic transformation is the liver. *Tripelennamine* and the other H$_1$ blockers appear to be eliminated in much the same way (*see* review by Witiak and Lewis, 1978).

Information on the concentrations of these drugs achieved in the skin and mucous membranes is lacking. However, significant inhibition of "wheal-and-flare" responses to the intradermal injection of histamine or allergen may persist for 36 hours or more after treatment with some longer-acting H$_1$ blockers, even when concentrations of the drugs in plasma are very low. Hydroxyzine is a case in point (*see* Simons *et al.*, 1984a). Such results emphasize the need for flexibility in the interpretation of the recommended dosage schedules (Table 26–3). Less frequent dosage may suffice. Like many other drugs that are metabolized extensively, H$_1$ blockers such as chlorpheniramine and hydroxyzine are eliminated more rapidly by children than by adults (*see* Simons *et al.*, 1984b). H$_1$ blockers are among the many drugs that induce hepatic microsomal enzymes, and they may facilitate their own metabolism.

Side Effects. In therapeutic doses, all H$_1$ blockers elicit side effects. Although these are rarely serious and often disappear with continued therapy, they are sometimes so troublesome that the drug must be withdrawn. Some difference in the incidence and severity of the side effects with different preparations is discernible, but there is marked variation in the responses of individual subjects.

The side effect with the highest incidence, and the one common to all drugs in this group, is *sedation* (*e.g., see* Carruthers *et al.*, 1978). Although this may be a desirable adjunct in the treatment of some patients, it interferes with the patient's daytime activities. Concurrent ingestion of alcohol or other CNS depressants heightens the danger of accident. Other untoward

reactions referable to *central actions* include dizziness, tinnitus, lassitude, incoordination, fatigue, blurred vision, diplopia, euphoria, nervousness, insomnia, and tremors.

The next most frequent side effects involve the *digestive tract* and include loss of appetite, nausea, vomiting, epigastric distress, and constipation or diarrhea. Their incidence may be reduced by giving the drug with meals. Other side effects include dryness of the mouth, throat, and respiratory passages, sometimes inducing cough; urinary retention or frequency and dysuria; palpitation; hypotension; headache; tightness of the chest; and tingling, heaviness, and weakness of the hands. The atropine-like actions of many of the H$_1$ blockers clearly account for some of these side effects.

Drug allergy may develop when H$_1$ blockers are given orally, but more commonly it results from topical application. Allergic dermatitis is not uncommon; other hypersensitivity reactions include drug fever and photosensitization. Grave hematological complications such as *leukopenia, agranulocytosis,* and *hemolytic anemia* are very rare. *Teratogenic effects* have been noted in response to piperazine compounds, but extensive clinical studies have not demonstrated any association between the use of such H$_1$ blockers and fetal anomalies in man. Nevertheless, it would seem prudent to avoid such drugs during pregnancy, especially in the first trimester. Since H$_1$ blockers interfere with skin tests for allergy, they must be withdrawn well beforehand.

Acute Poisoning. Although the H$_1$-blocking drugs have a relatively high margin of safety, acute poisoning with them is common. These drugs are frequently found in medicine cabinets, and all too often they are the cause of accidental poisoning in young children.

The central effects of the H$_1$ blockers constitute their greatest danger. In the small child, the dominant effect is excitation, and the syndrome of poisoning includes *hallucinations, excitement, ataxia, incoordination, athetosis,* and *convulsions.* The convulsions, sometimes heralded by muscular tremors and athetoid movements, are of the intermittent tonic-clonic type and difficult to control. *Fixed, dilated pupils* with a *flushed face*, together with *sinus tachycardia, urinary retention, dry mouth*, and *fever*, lend the syndrome a remarkable similarity to that of atropine poisoning. Terminally, there is deepening coma with cardiorespiratory collapse and death, usually within 2 to 18 hours. In the adult, fever and flushing are not usually in evidence, and the phase of excitement leading to convulsions and postictal depression is not uncommonly preceded by drowsiness and coma. There is no specific therapy for poisoning with H$_1$ blockers, and treatment is along general symptomatic and supportive lines.

Preparations. There is a needlessly large number of H$_1$ blockers. Since there are many advan-

tages to using the older and well-tried drugs, it would seem wise for the physician to become familiar with a few representative compounds from the different classes, and to base his therapy upon these. Few, if any, of the "newer" drugs have any conspicuous therapeutic advantage, and most are more costly. Each is invariably introduced with claims of greater efficacy or reduced toxicity; experience often forces reevaluation. The most recent entry, *terfenadine*, is said to lack significant sedative effect (*see* Editorial, 1983b). The physician should, however, bear in mind that patients respond differentially to the different H$_1$ blockers and that failure with one does not preclude success with another. The brief discussion that follows is intended to provide only an indication of the different classes of H$_1$-blocking drugs and their properties. Preparations are listed in Table 26–3.

Table 26–3.   PREPARATIONS AND DOSAGE OF REPRESENTATIVE H$_1$-BLOCKING AGENTS *

CLASS AND NONPROPRIETARY NAME	TRADE NAME	DURATION OF ACTION (HOURS)	PREPARATIONS †	SINGLE DOSE (ADULT)
Ethanolamines				
Diphenhydramine hydrochloride	BENADRYL and others	4–6	O,L,I,T	25–50 mg
Dimenhydrinate	DRAMAMINE and others	4–6	O,L,I	50 mg
Carbinoxamine maleate	CLISTIN	3–4	O	4–8 mg
Ethylenediamines				
Tripelennamine hydrochloride	PBZ	4–6	O,T	25–50 mg; 100 mg (sustained release)
Tripelennamine citrate	PBZ		L	37.5–75 mg
Pyrilamine maleate		4–6	O	25–50 mg
Alkylamines				
Chlorpheniramine maleate	CHLOR-TRIMETON and others	4–6	O,L,I	4 mg 8–12 mg (sustained release) 5–20 mg (injection)
Brompheniramine maleate	DIMETANE and others	4–6	O,L,I	4 mg 8–12 mg (sustained release) 5–20 mg (injection)
Piperazines				
Hydroxyzine hydrochloride	ATARAX and others	6–24	O,L,I	25 mg
Hydroxyzine pamoate	VISTARIL	6–24	O,L	25 mg
Cyclizine hydrochloride	MAREZINE	4–6	O	50 mg
Cyclizine lactate	MAREZINE	4–6	I	50 mg
Meclizine hydrochloride	ANTIVERT and others	12–24	O	25–50 mg
Phenothiazines				
Promethazine hydrochloride	PHENERGAN and others	4–6	O,L,I,S	25 mg

* For a discussion of phenothiazines, *see* Chapter 19.

† Preparations are designated as follows: O = oral solids; L = oral liquids; I = injection; S = suppository; T = topical. Many H$_1$-blocking agents are also available in preparations that contain multiple drugs.

Ethanolamines (Prototype: Diphenhydramine). The drugs in this group are potent and effective H₁ blockers that possess significant antimuscarinic activity and have a pronounced tendency to induce sedation. With conventional doses, about half of those who are treated with these drugs experience somnolence, although with carbinoxamine the proportion is less. The incidence of gastrointestinal side effects, however, is low in this group.

Ethylenediamines (Prototype: Pyrilamine). These include some of the most specific H₁ antagonists. Although their central effects are relatively feeble, somnolence occurs in a fair proportion of patients. Gastrointestinal side effects are quite common. This group contains some of the oldest and best-known H₁-blocking drugs.

Alkylamines (Prototype: Chlorpheniramine). These are among the most potent H₁-blocking agents and are generally effective in relatively low doses. The drugs are not so prone to produce drowsiness and are among the more suitable agents for daytime use; but again, a significant proportion of patients do experience this effect. Side effects involving CNS stimulation are more common in this than in other groups.

Piperazines (Prototype: Chlorcyclizine). The oldest member of this group, chlorcyclizine, is an H₁ blocker with prolonged action and a comparatively low incidence of drowsiness. Hydroxyzine is a long-acting compound that is widely used for skin allergies; its considerable central-depressant activity may contribute to its prominent antipruritic action. Cyclizine and meclizine have been used primarily to counter motion sickness, although other H₁ blockers, promethazine and diphenhydramine (dimenhydrinate), are more effective (as is scopolamine; *see* below).

Phenothiazines (Prototype: Promethazine). Most drugs of this class are H₁ blockers and also possess considerable anticholinergic activity. The prototype, promethazine, was introduced in 1946 for the management of allergic conditions. The prominent sedative effects of this compound and its value in motion sickness were early recognized. Promethazine and its many congeners are now used primarily for their antiemetic effects (*see* Chapter 19).

Therapeutic Uses.

H₁-blocking drugs have an established and valued place in the symptomatic treatment of various immediate hypersensitivity reactions, in which their usefulness is attributable to their antagonism of endogenously released histamine, one of several autacoids that together elicit the allergic response. In addition, the central properties of *some* of the series are of considerable therapeutic value, particularly in suppressing motion sickness.

Diseases of Allergy. H₁ antagonists are most useful in acute exudative types of allergy such as *pollinosis* and *urticaria.* Their effect, however, is purely palliative and confined to the suppression in varying degree of symptoms attributable to the pharmacological activity of histamine released by the antigen-antibody reaction. The drugs do not diminish the intensity of this reaction, which is the root cause of the various hypersensitivity diseases. This can be achieved only by other means, such as the removal or avoidance of allergen, specific desensitization, suppression of the reaction by corticosteroids, or, in restricted instances, use of cromolyn. This limitation must be clearly recognized. In *bronchial asthma,* histamine blockers are singularly ineffectual. They have no role in the therapy of the severe attack, in which chief reliance must be placed on "physiological antagonists" such as epinephrine, isoproterenol, and theophylline. Equally, in the treatment of *systemic anaphylaxis,* in which autacoids other than histamine are again important, the mainstay of therapy is once more epinephrine, with histamine antagonists having only a subordinate and adjuvant role. The same is true for severe *angioedema,* in which laryngeal swelling constitutes a threat to life.

Other allergies of the respiratory tract are more amenable to therapy with H₁ blockers. The best results are obtained in *seasonal rhinitis* and *conjunctivitis* (hay fever, pollinosis), in which these drugs relieve the sneezing, rhinorrhea, and itching of eyes, nose, and throat. A gratifying response is obtained in most patients, especially at the beginning of the season when pollen counts are low; however, the drugs are less effective when the allergens are in abundance, when exposure to them is prolonged, and when nasal congestion has become prominent. In *perennial vasomotor rhinitis,* H₁ blockers are of limited value. Although H₁-blocking drugs have long been used in elixirs and syrups for controlling *cough,* especially in asthmatic children, any benefit from their specific antiallergic action or sedation may be offset by the anticholinergic properties of these drugs, which, by excessive drying of the respiratory tree, can render bronchial secretion viscid and make expectoration difficult.

Certain of the *allergic dermatoses* respond favorably to H₁ blockers. Benefit is most striking in *acute urticaria,* although the itching in this condition is perhaps better controlled than are the edema and the erythema. *Chronic urticaria* is less responsive, but some measure of benefit may be had in a fair proportion of patients. *Angioedema* is also responsive to treatment with H₁ blockers, but the paramount importance of epinephrine in the severe attack must be reemphasized, especially in the life-threatening involvement of the larynx. Here, however, it may be appropriate to administer *additionally* an H₁ antagonist by the intravenous route. H₁ blockers also have a place in the treatment of *itching pruritides.* Some relief may be obtained in many patients suffering from *atopic dermatitis* and *contact dermatitis,* although topical corticosteroids seem to be more valuable, and in such diverse conditions as *insect bites* and *ivy poisoning.* Various other pruritides without allergic basis sometimes respond to antihistamine therapy, usually when the drugs are applied topically but sometimes when they are given orally. However, the considerable danger of producing allergic dermatitis with local application of H_1 blockers must be recognized. Since these drugs inhibit allergic dermatoses, *they should be withdrawn well before skin testing for allergies.*

The urticarial and edematous lesions of *serum sickness* respond to H_1 blockers, but fever and arthralgia often do not. *Gastrointestinal allergies* are seldom benefited significantly by these drugs.

Many *drug reactions* attributable to allergic phenomena respond to therapy with H_1 blockers, particularly those characterized by itch, urticaria, and angioedema; reactions of the serum-sickness type also respond to intensive treatment. However, explosive release of histamine generally calls for treatment with epinephrine, with H_1-blocking drugs being accorded a subsidiary role. Nevertheless, prophylactic treatment with an H_1 blocker may suffice to reduce symptoms to a tolerable level when a drug known to be a powerful histamine liberator is to be given. Extensive discussion of the effects of H_1 antagonists in allergic and related conditions may be found in the articles by Beaven (1978), Hahn (1978), Burland and Mills (in Ganellin and Parsons, 1982), Salvaggio (1982), and Symposium (1982).

Common Cold. Despite early claims and persistent popular belief, H_1-blocking drugs are without value in combating the common cold. Their weak anticholinergic effects may tend to lessen rhinorrhea, but this drying effect may do more harm than good, as may also their tendency to induce somnolence (*see* West *et al.*, 1975).

Motion Sickness, Vertigo, and Sedation. Although scopolamine, given orally, parenterally, or transdermally, is the most effective of all drugs for the prophylaxis and treatment of *motion sickness,* some H_1 blockers are useful in a broad range of milder conditions and offer the advantage of fewer adverse effects. These include dimenhydrinate and the piperazines (cyclizine, meclizine, and others). Promethazine is more potent and more effective and its additional antiemetic properties may be of value in reducing vomiting, but its pronounced sedative action is usually disadvantageous (*see* Graybiel *et al.*, 1975; Wood, 1979). Whenever possible, the various drugs should be administered an hour or so before the anticipated motion.

Some H_1 blockers, notably dimenhydrinate and meclizine, are often of benefit in vestibular disturbances, such as *Ménière's disease*, and in other types of *true vertigo* (*see* Cohen and deJong, 1972). The same drugs and promethazine have some lesser usefulness in treating the nausea and vomiting subsequent to chemotherapy or radiation therapy for malignancies; however, more effective antiemetic drugs are available (*see* Chapter 19).

The tendency of certain of the H_1 blockers to produce somnolence has led to their use as *hypnotics.* They are nonaddicting, but tolerance tends to limit their period of usefulness. They are by no means as powerful or effective as the benzodiazepines, for example, but they may have some value in selected patients. H_1 blockers, particularly diphenhydramine and pyrilamine, are often present in various proprietary remedies for insomnia that are sold "over the counter." While these remedies are generally ineffective in the recommended doses, some singularly sensitive individuals may derive benefit (*see* Faingold, 1978; Chapter 17). The sedative and mild antianxiety activities of hydroxyzine and diphenhydramine have contributed to their use as weak anxiolytics.

H_2-BLOCKING AGENTS

The search for drugs to oppose the several actions of histamine that are resistant to block by H_1 antagonists was lent special impetus by the many indications of involvement of endogenous histamine in gastric secretion and the clinical evidence that hypersecretion of gastric acid and peptic ulceration account for much illness (as many as 4,000,000 hospital days per year in the United States alone). The discovery and introduction of such drugs, the histamine H_2-receptor blocking drugs, soon provided incontrovertible evidence of the importance of endogenous histamine in the physiological control of gastric secretion. They have also provided a new and effective therapeutic approach to the treatment of gastric hypersecretory states.

Chemistry. The synthesis of H_2 antagonists was achieved by stepwise modifications of the histamine molecule, which resulted, some 200 compounds later, in the first highly effective drug with potent H_2-blocking activity, *burimamide* (Black *et al.*, 1972). This, like later compounds, retained the imidazole ring of histamine but possessed a much bulkier side chain. Subsequent modifications of this structure produced compounds that were well absorbed orally and that had acceptable levels of toxicity. *Cimetidine*, the first H_2 blocker to be introduced for general clinical use, won rapid acceptance for the treatment of duodenal ulcers and other gastric hypersecretory conditions and soon became one of the most widely prescribed of all drugs. This success led to the synthesis of numerous congeners and to the discovery of many other effective H_2 blockers. One such agent is *ranitidine.* The structures of cimetidine and ranitidine are as follows:

Cimetidine

Ranitidine

Unlike the H_1 blockers, H_2 blockers such as cimetidine and ranitidine are polar, hydrophilic molecules. Like histamine, cimetidine and some other H_2 blockers are imidazole derivatives; however, this ring structure is not essential. Ranitidine possesses a substituted furan ring, and still other ring structures appear in other highly effective agents (*see* Ganellin, in Ganellin and Parsons, 1982).

Pharmacological Properties. The H_2 blockers are reversible, competitive antagonists of the actions of histamine on H_2 receptors. They are highly selective in their action and are virtually without effect on H_1 receptors or, indeed, on receptors for other autacoids or drugs. The most prominent of the effects of histamine that are mediated by H_2 receptors is stimulation of gastric acid secretion, and it is the ability of the H_2 blockers to inhibit this effect that explains much of their importance. Despite the widespread distribution of H_2 receptors in the body, H_2 blockers interfere remarkably little with physiological functions other than gastric secretion, implying that the extragastric H_2 receptors are of minor physiological importance. However, like the H_1 blockers, the H_2 blockers do inhibit those effects on the cardiovascular and other systems that are elicited through the corresponding receptors by exogenous or endogenous histamine (*see* Brogden *et al.*, 1982; Burland and Mills, in Ganellin and Parsons, 1982; Ganellin and Parsons, 1982).

Gastric Secretion. H_2 blockers inhibit gastric acid secretion elicited by histamine or other H_2 agonists in a dose-dependent, competitive manner; the degree of inhibition parallels the plasma concentration of the drug over a wide range (Figure 26–1). In addition, the H_2 blockers inhibit gastric secretion elicited by muscarinic agonists or by gastrin, although this effect is not always complete. This breadth of inhibitory effect is not due to nonspecific actions at the receptors for these other secretagogues. Rather, this effect, which is noncompetitive and indirect, appears to indicate either that these two classes of secretagogues utilize histamine as the final common mediator or, more probably, that ongoing histaminergic stimulation of the parietal cell is important for amplification of the stimuli provided by ACh or gastrin when they act on their own discrete receptors. Receptors for all three

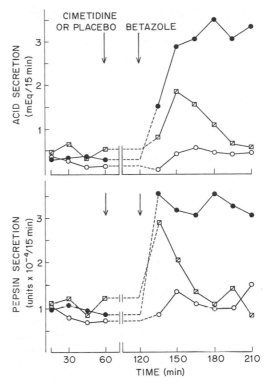

Figure 26–1. *Effect of cimetidine on betazole stimulation of secretion of acid (upper panel) and of pepsin (lower panel) in man.*

A placebo (•) or cimetidine (200 mg, ▨; 300 mg, ○) was given orally 1 hour before the subcutaneous administration of betazole (1.5 mg/kg). (Modified from Binder and Donaldson, 1978.)

secretagogues are present on the parietal cell (*see* Soll and Grossman, 1981; Code, in Ganellin and Parsons, 1982; Berglindh, 1984). Whatever the explanation, the ability of H_2 blockers to suppress responses to all three physiological secretagogues makes them potent inhibitors of all phases of gastric acid secretion. Thus, these drugs will inhibit basal (fasting) secretion and nocturnal secretion and also that stimulated by food, sham feeding, fundic distention, insulin, or caffeine. The H_2 blockers reduce both the volume of gastric juice secreted and its hydrogen ion concentration. Output of pepsin, which is secreted by the chief cells of the gastric glands (mainly under cholinergic control), generally falls in parallel with the reduction in volume of the gastric juice (Figure 26–1). Secretion of intrinsic factor is also reduced, but it is normally secreted in great excess, and absorption of vitamin B_{12} is usually adequate even during long-term therapy with H_2 blockers. Concentrations of gastrin in plasma are not significantly altered under fasting conditions; however, the normal prandial elevation of gastrin concentration may be augmented, apparently as a consequence of a reduction in the negative feedback that is normally provided by acid. The reduction of gastric acid secretion caused by H_2 blockers protects experimental animals from gastric ulceration induced by stress, pyloric ligation, aspirin and related compounds, or histaminergic and cholinergic drugs. The H_2 blockers also counter peptic ulceration in man, as will be described below. They have no consistent effect on the rate of gastric emptying, lower-esophageal sphincter pressure, or pancreatic secretion.

Absorption, Fate, and Excretion. Both cimetidine and ranitidine are rapidly and virtually completely absorbed by the oral route. Absorption is little impaired by food or by antacids. Peak concentrations in plasma are attained in about 1 to 2 hours. Hepatic first-pass metabolism results in bioavailabilities of about 60% for cimetidine and 50% for ranitidine. The elimination half-life is about 2 to 3 hours for each drug. However, since ranitidine is some four to ten times more potent than cimetidine and is usually administered at one half the dose, ranitidine is effective for a relatively long time (8 to 12 hours). Both drugs are eliminated primarily by the kidneys, and 60% or more may appear in the urine unchanged; much of the rest is oxidation products. Small amounts are recovered in the stool.

Adverse Reactions and Side Effects. Some tens of millions of patients have been treated with cimetidine, and the number who have received ranitidine is already very large. This explains the fact that the list of adverse reactions that have been reported is long. However, it is evident that *the incidence of adverse reactions is low and that the reactions encountered are generally minor.* In part this may be attributed to the relative absence of physiologically important mechanisms that utilize H_2 re-

ceptors in organs other than the stomach; in part it reflects the poor penetration of the drugs across the normal blood-brain barrier. Some side effects are clearly not due to specific blockade of H_2 receptors. Thus, certain disturbing responses to cimetidine have not been observed with ranitidine.

Among the side effects associated with both drugs are headache, dizziness, malaise, myalgia, nausea, diarrhea or constipation, skin rashes, pruritus, loss of libido, and impotence. Cimetidine binds to androgen receptors, and this contributes to the sexual dysfunctions mentioned and also to gynecomastia. Ranitidine lacks antiandrogenic activity and, when substituted for cimetidine, gynecomastia and impotence may disappear (Jansen *et al.,* 1983). Cimetidine, given intravenously, stimulates the secretion of prolactin, and elevated concentrations of the hormone have been reported during chronic oral treatment. The mechanism is not clear, and ranitidine has relatively little effect in this regard. Cimetidine binds to cytochrome P-450 and thereby diminishes the activity of the hepatic microsomal mixed-function oxidases. As a result, various other therapeutic agents may accumulate during treatment with cimetidine. Among the many drugs whose metabolism is affected are warfarin, phenytoin, theophylline, phenobarbital, diazepam, propranolol, and imipramine (*see* Sedman, 1984). Ranitidine binds less avidly to the P-450 system and interferes little with its function. Both cimetidine and ranitidine tend to reduce hepatic blood flow, which can slow the clearance of drugs such as lidocaine. Cimetidine can cause various CNS disturbances, particularly in elderly patients and in individuals with hepatic or renal disease; these include slurred speech, somnolence, lethargy, restlessness, confusion, disorientation, agitation, hallucinations, and seizures. Such reactions are less frequent with ranitidine, possibly because of its even poorer ability to pass the blood-brain barrier. In rare instances, cimetidine use has been associated with thrombocytopenia, granulocytopenia, hepatotoxicity, or renal toxicity. Small increments in plasma creatinine concentrations are not uncommon, and this may simply reflect competition between cimetidine and creatinine for renal excretion. Cimetidine, but not ranitidine, has been noted to enhance some cell-mediated immune responses, particularly in immunologically depressed individuals. Given by rapid intravenous injection, both cimetidine and ranitidine have occasionally produced profound bradycardia and other cardiotoxic effects. Such injection may also cause histamine release in susceptible individuals. The profoundly hypochlorhydric stomach favors both the formation of bezoars and the survival of bacteria. The former has followed treatment with cimetidine, and the latter may explain rare cases of candidal peritonitis. (For reviews of the adverse effects of H_2 blockers, *see* McGuigan, 1981; Freston, 1982b; Zeldis *et al.*, 1983.)

Preparations, Routes of Administration, and Dosage. *Cimetidine* (TAGAMET) is available for *oral* use as tablets containing 200, 300, or 400 mg. Recommended dosage for adults with duodenal ulcer is 300 mg four times a day with meals and at bedtime; alternatively, 200 mg can be given with meals and 400 mg at bedtime. A liquid formulation containing 300 mg/5 ml is available. Where oral administration is impractical, cimetidine may be given parenterally (intramuscularly or intravenously), and an injection (300 mg/2 ml) is available.

Ranitidine (ZANTAC) is available for oral use as tablets containing 150 mg. The usual dosage schedule is 150 mg twice daily. An injection containing 25 mg/ml is also available; 50 mg can be given intramuscularly or intravenously every 6 to 8 hours.

Therapeutic Uses. The clinical use of H_2 blockers centers on their capacity to inhibit the secretion of gastric acid in hypersecretory states, particularly those involving peptic ulceration. As a rough guide, a 50% inhibition of acid secretion is achieved with plasma concentrations of 800 ng/ml for cimetidine or 100 ng/ml for ranitidine. More important are the effects of these drugs on the secretion of acid over a 24-hour period. Cimetidine (1000 mg per day) causes about a 50% reduction, while ranitidine (300 mg per day) effects about a 70% reduction. The corresponding inhibitions of nocturnal secretion are about 70% and 90%.

Duodenal Ulcer. Cimetidine and ranitidine have proven value in the treatment of duodenal ulcer disease in which most, but not all, patients show hypersecretion of gastric acid. They profoundly lower basal and nocturnal secretion and that stimulated by meals and other factors, reduce both daytime and nighttime pain and the consumption of antacids, and hasten healing. The incidence of healing in 4- to 6-week periods is, in some trials, more than twice that of patients taking a placebo. Most (85 to 90%) duodenal ulcers are healed after 8 weeks of therapy. Healing rates of this order can be achieved by the use of highly efficacious antacids given at short intervals (*see* Chapter 42), but H_2 blockers have the advantage of convenience in administration and lack of effect on the motility of the bowel. Both H_2 blockers reduce the rate of recurrence of ulcer if given in maintenance doses after the acute episode. Whereas ulcers recur within a year in somewhat more than half of patients given a placebo, they recur in only some 20% of patients who receive bedtime doses of cimetidine or ranitidine.

Gastric Ulcer. Cimetidine and ranitidine both accelerate the healing of benign gastric ulcers: healing rates of 50% and 75% at 8 weeks have been observed. Moreover, given prophylactically, the drugs markedly reduce rates of relapse.

Zollinger-Ellison Syndrome. In this disease, in which gastrin produced by the tumor may increase secretion of gastric acid to life-threatening levels, the H_2 blockers have provided a valuable treatment. Nevertheless, very high doses of these agents may be needed, with a consequent high incidence of side effects, especially with cimetidine (Jansen *et al.*, 1983). Furthermore, high doses may fail to control acid secretion adequately. For these reasons, the more recently discovered and efficacious "acid pump" blockers (*see* below) may be of particular value in this condition.

Other Conditions. Clearly, H_2 blockers may be useful whenever it is appropriate to reduce the output of gastric acid. Among the applications are *reflex esophagitis, stress ulcers* in the severely ill or burned patient, *upper gastrointestinal bleeding* (although this use is controversial), *preanesthetic use* in emergency operations (to lower the incidence of acid aspiration syndrome), *short-bowel (anastomosis) syndrome,* and hypersecretory states associated with *systemic mastocytosis* or *basophilic leukemia with hyperhistaminemia* (Baron, 1981; Brogden *et al.*, 1982; Freston, 1982a; Misiewicz and Wormsley, 1982; Riley and Salmon, 1982; Zeldis *et al.*, 1983).

OTHER APPROACHES TO CONTROL GASTRIC SECRETION

H_2 blockers are not, of course, the only drugs that are useful in gastric hypersecretory states. Antacids and other agents are discussed in Chapter 42, and anticholinergic agents are described in Chapter 7. These agents, particularly antacids, are commonly used in conjunction with H_2 blockers. Adequate control of acid secretion is not always achieved with H_2 blockers. Where stimulation by gastrin is very intense, as in many patients with Zollinger-Ellison syndrome, the H_2 blockers may not provide adequate control. Intense pathophysiological stimulation due to histamine or other agents may likewise be refractory to treatment with these drugs. Moreover, a small percentage of patients with peptic ulcer (up to about 10%) with seemingly conventional levels of gastric hypersecretion are poorly controlled or derive little benefit from H_2 blockers. Finally, with conventional dosage regimens of the drugs, acid secretion is by no means completely suppressed. Indeed, even if one could block completely the receptors for all secretagogues, some secretion of acid would persist as a result of the autonomous basal activity of the parietal cells. For these various reasons much interest is centered on the recent discovery of a new class of drugs that powerfully suppresses gastric acid secretion, whether basal or evoked by any of the three physiological secretagogues, by blocking the ultimate step in acid secretion in the parietal cell, namely, extrusion of protons.

Gastric Acid (Proton) Pump Inhibitors. The parietal cells secrete acid by means of a membrane pump, identified as an H^+,K^+-ATPase, that exchanges hydrogen ions for potassium ions. By analogy with the familiar Na^+,K^+-ATPase, whose function can be inhibited by digitalis and related drugs, this proton pump can likewise be inhibited by a newly discovered family of drugs, a group of substituted benzimidazoles. The unique feature of these agents is that their site of action involves the final, common process in acid production. Thus, they inhibit secretion of acid, be it basal or stimulated. These agents are singularly effective in suppressing gastric acid secretion, and virtual anacidity can be achieved *in vivo*. They are effective orally as well as intravenously, they have a prolonged duration of action, and they appear to be well tolerated.

Omeprazole, the prototypical "acid pump" inhibitor, is not available for general clinical use in the United States. It has the following structure:

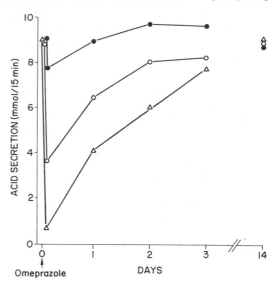

Omeprazole

Omeprazole blocks gastric acid secretion by inhibiting the H^+,K^+-ATPase in the parietal-cell membrane (Fellenius *et al.*, 1981; Lamers *et al.*, 1984; Sachs, 1984). Although the drug is largely cleared from the plasma in a few hours, it inhibits acid secretion *in vivo* for much longer. This is apparently because omeprazole is concentrated in the parietal cells; inhibition of the ATPase is reversible. The powerful, sustained inhibitory effect of single oral doses of omeprazole on gastric acid secretion is illustrated in Figure 26–2.

Study of the effects of "acid pump" inhibitors in patients is still limited but encouraging. In those with duodenal ulcers, a single oral dose of omeprazole causes a more profound reduction of daily secretion of gastric acid than is obtained with cimetidine or ranitidine given four times or twice a day, respectively (Walt *et al.*, 1983); ulcers have

Figure 26–2. *Inhibitory effect of omeprazole on secretion of gastric acid in man.*

Maximal secretory responses were elicited in six healthy human subjects by infusing pentagastrin (91 μg) over a 1-hour period before and at various intervals after a *single oral dose* of omeprazole (○, 20 mg; △, 40 mg) or placebo (●). Note the profound and prolonged inhibition. (Modified from Lind *et al.*, 1983.)

healed promptly (Gustavsson *et al.*, 1983). Moreover, in patients with severe gastric acid hypersecretion due to Zollinger-Ellison syndrome who were resistant to H_2 blockers, a single daily dose of omeprazole (30 to 80 mg orally) profoundly inhibited gastric acid secretion and led to prompt disappearance of symptoms and to rapid healing of peptic ulcers. The beneficial effects were sustained throughout the treatment, which lasted for an average of 14 months. The drug was well tolerated, and no laboratory abnormalities were noted (Lamers *et al.*, 1984). It is evident that inhibitors of H^+,K^+-ATPase offer a promising and singularly effective therapeutic approach to the suppression of excess secretion of gastric acid (*see* Sachs, 1984).

5-HYDROXYTRYPTAMINE (SEROTONIN)

History. Mammalian physiologists have known for about a century that a vasoconstrictor material appears in serum when blood is allowed to clot. This unidentified vasoconstrictor material, which went by a variety of names, such as *vasotonin,* was a frequent nuisance in perfusion experiments in which defibrinated blood was used. In the late 1940s, the substance appeared in another context during a search for humoral pressor agents such as angiotensin that might explain arterial hypertension. In this work the serum vasoconstrictor was a "pest," to be eliminated before the other enquiry could proceed. In 1948, investigators at the Cleveland Clinic isolated this vasoconstrictor substance as a crystalline complex and named it *serotonin* (Rapport *et al.,* 1948); shortly thereafter, Rapport (1949) deduced that the active moiety was 5-hydroxytryptamine (5-HT). This compound, when prepared synthetically in 1951, proved to have all the properties of natural serotonin.

Quite independently, work was begun in the 1930s by Erspamer and colleagues, whose original purpose was to extract and characterize the substance that imparts peculiar histochemical properties to enterochromaffin cells of the gastrointestinal mucosa. Their experiments led them to discover, first in the mucosa and later in other tissues, a gut-stimulating factor of basic nature, which they termed *enteramine.* By the late 1940s, Erspamer had shown that it was present in many tissues of vertebrates and invertebrates and had suggested that it was an indole alkylamine. In 1952, Erspamer and Asero identified enteramine as 5-hydroxytryptamine (*see* Erspamer, 1954, 1966a, 1966b).

Thus, by the time 5-HT had been recognized as such, there already existed a mass of evidence indicating that it was widely distributed in nature and possessed a variety of pharmacological actions. It is therefore not surprising that the introduction of synthetic 5-HT in 1951 touched off an explosion of research. This was further fueled when 5-HT was discovered in the brain (Twarog and Page, 1953; Amin *et al.,* 1954), when lysergic acid diethylamide (LSD) and other potent hallucinogens were recognized to be structurally similar to 5-HT and were found to block smooth muscle responses to 5-HT (Gaddum, 1953; Woolley and Shaw, 1954), and when the potent tranquilizing drug reserpine was observed to lower concentrations of 5-HT in brain (*see* Brodie and Shore, 1957). All this suggested that 5-HT serves as a neurotransmitter, a function now established, and focused attention on a possible role of 5-HT in mental illnesses (*see* Woolley, 1962). These events, as much as any other, contributed greatly to the development of the subdiscipline of psychopharmacology (*see* Chapter 19).

Source and Chemistry. 5-HT (serotonin) is 3-(β-aminoethyl)-5-hydroxyindole. Like histamine, it is widely distributed in the animal and plant kingdoms. It occurs, for example, in vertebrates; in tunicates, mollusks, arthropods, and coelenterates; in fruits such as pineapples, bananas, and plums; and in various nuts. It is also present in numerous stings and venoms, including those of the common stinging nettle, cowhage (the prankster's "itching powder"), wasps, and scorpions. It is formed enzymatically from the amino acid tryptophan by hydroxylation, followed by decarboxylation (*see* below).

Numerous synthetic or naturally occurring congeners of 5-HT have varying degrees of peripheral and central pharmacological activity. Particularly noteworthy are the "tryptamines" of plant origin with potent effects on brain function. For example, N,N-dimethyltryptamine (DMT) and its 5-hydroxy derivative (bufotenine) are active principles of the cahobe bean found along the shores of the Carib-

bean and used in aboriginal rites to induce mental changes. Both of these compounds can be formed in the mammal by N-methylation of tryptamine and 5-HT, respectively. Also, the active ingredients of various Mexican hallucinogenic mushrooms (*e.g., Psilocybe mexicana*) used for related purposes are 4-substituted tryptamine derivatives (*psilocin* is 4-hydroxy-N,N-dimethyltryptamine, and *psilocybin* is 4-phosphoryloxy-N,N-dimethyltryptamine). Furthermore, a 4-substituted tryptamine moiety can be recognized in the most potent known psychotomimetic drug, LSD. (*See* Woolley, 1962; Mantegazzini, 1966; Symposium, 1968a, 1973, 1974a, 1974b; Weil-Malherbe, 1978; Ho *et al.,* 1982; *see also* Chapters 12, 19, and 23.)

PHARMACOLOGICAL ACTIONS

5-HT stimulates or inhibits a variety of smooth muscles and nerves. These and other actions result in a wide spectrum of responses involving, in particular, the cardiovascular, respiratory, and gastrointestinal systems. Characteristically, responses to 5-HT are variable. This is attributable in large part to two factors: (1) many of the effects of 5-HT are reflexly mediated and hence subject to influences such as pattern of innervation, route and speed of injection, anesthetic state, and spontaneous tone; and (2) tachyphylaxis is common when tests are made at frequent intervals. What follows is a description of some of the more prominent effects of 5-HT. For detailed accounts, *see* Erspamer (1966b), Essman (1977, 1978a, 1978b, 1978c), De Clerck and Vanhoutte (1982), and Ho and colleagues (1982).

Respiratory System. *Stimulation of Afferent Nerves.* Intravenous injection of 5-HT commonly causes a short-lived increase in respiratory minute volume and rate. With lower doses, the effect is due to stimulation of carotid and aortic chemoreceptors. With higher doses, other ill-defined effects contribute. Sometimes respiratory movements are inhibited through stimulation of vagal afferent fibers.

Bronchoconstriction. 5-HT causes bronchoconstriction in many animals, but rarely in man, except in asthmatic patients. The effect is partly reflex but mainly due to direct stimulation of bronchial smooth muscle.

Cardiovascular System. The effects of 5-HT on this system are uniquely complex. By acting directly on vascular smooth muscle, the drug may evoke vasoconstriction or vasodilatation, depending on the vascular bed, its resting tone, and the dose given. By its actions on a variety of sensory nerve endings, it activates pressor and depressor reflexes; by direct and reflex mechanisms, it either stimulates or depresses cardiac output; and in high doses it influences ganglionic transmission, adrenal medullary secretion, and transmitter release from nerve endings.

Blood Vessels. Direct *vasoconstriction* is the classical effect of 5-HT that is responsible for the synonyms *vasotonin* and *serotonin*. In animals, such vasoconstriction is revealed in its purest form after pithing the spinal cord or performing other maneuvers to obviate indirect effects. The effect of 5-HT is then to cause a prompt, uncomplicated rise in blood pressure lasting several minutes. The splanchnic and renal beds are particularly affected. Cerebral blood vessels are constricted powerfully in several species. Pulmonary vasoconstriction is prominent in dogs and cats but less so in man. Placental, uterine, and umbilical vessels also constrict.

Vasodilatation occurs in skeletal muscle, especially with lower doses of 5-HT. The drug acts directly on the smooth muscle, but it can also reduce the output of norepinephrine from sympathetic nerve terminals (*see* below). In the forearm, where muscle is preponderant, vasodilatation tends to increase blood flow. Superficial vessels of the human skin also dilate following intradermal or intra-arterial injection of 5-HT. The resulting flush, at first bright red, assumes a dusky hue indicating stagnation, probably as a result of venoconstriction. However, the overall response to 5-HT given intra-arterially is a rise in cutaneous vascular resistance. In the hand, where skin is preponderant, this effect reduces blood flow. *Capillary permeability* is not much affected by 5-HT, except in rats, where it increases.

Heart. 5-HT has positive inotropic and chronotropic effects of varying intensity, which result from direct actions on cardiac tissue and indirect actions mediated by the release of norepinephrine from sympathetic nerve terminals. *In vivo,* such effects are commonly blunted or overshadowed by autonomic reflexes arising from changes in blood pressure or direct actions of 5-HT on baroreceptors, chemoreceptors, and vagal endings in the coronary bed. The last-mentioned action is particularly noteworthy. It initiates the coronary chemoreflex (Bezold-Jarisch reflex), characterized by inhibition of sympathetic outflow and increased activity of the cardiac (efferent) vagus, leading to profound bradycardia and hypotension. No significant changes in the electrical properties of the heart have been attributed to 5-HT.

Blood Pressure. In contrast to the pithed animal (*see* above), the intact animal responds to an intravenous injection of 5-HT with changes in blood pressure that are notoriously variable, since they represent the outcome of several opposed and capricious influences, direct and reflex. In most species, including man, it is nevertheless possible to discern three successive phases: a brief depressor phase; a succeeding pressor phase; and finally, within 1 or 2 minutes of the injection, a prolonged depressor phase. The *early depressor phase* results from the coronary chemoreflex. The *pressor phase* is due mainly to the direct effects of 5-HT to increase total peripheral resistance and cardiac output. The *late depressor phase* is attributable mainly to the direct vasodilator effects of 5-HT, principally in skeletal muscle.

Veins are strongly constricted by 5-HT, and intense venospasm commonly accompanies intravenous infusions.

Platelets. 5-HT weakly promotes platelet aggregation without inducing the "release reaction."

Smooth Muscle. *Alimentary Tract.* Intravenous injections of 5-HT stimulate motility of the small intestine. Man is particularly sensitive and often responds to doses insufficient to affect the cardiovascular or respiratory system. Motility of the stomach and large intestine may also be increased, but the usual response is inhibition. Segments of gastrointestinal tract *in vitro* generally exhibit responses qualitatively similar to those obtained *in vivo,* namely, contraction, inhibition, or mixtures of these. The complexity of the pattern is in large measure due to the variety of elements, neural and muscular, responding to 5-HT. In the isolated guinea pig ileum, 5-HT contracts the longitudinal muscle partly by acting directly upon it and partly by exciting intramural ganglion cells. In addition, 5-HT can increase peristaltic activity by stimulating or sensitizing intramural nerve endings.

The inhibitory actions of 5-HT in guinea pig stomach are due mainly to excitation of ganglion cells that have an inhibitory function. Inhibition in isolated human colon is more complex; ganglion cells in both muscle layers participate, and, in addition, both muscle layers, circular and longitudinal, are directly relaxed.

Other Smooth Muscle. In addition to the actions on bronchi, blood vessels, and gut, 5-HT stimulates numerous other smooth muscles. The isolated uterus of the estrous rat is exquisitely sensitive, but isolated strips of human uterus in various functional states are not, and large doses of 5-HT given intravenously have minor and equivocal actions on the contractile activity of the human pregnant uterus.

Exocrine Glands. Intravenous infusion of 5-HT in the dog reduces the volume, acidity, and pepsin content of *gastric juice* secreted spontaneously or in response to vagal activation, cholinergic drugs, or histamine, but it increases the production of mucus. Somewhat similar effects have been described in man and apparently involve reflex as well as direct actions. Variable effects on salivary, pancreatic, and other exocrine secretions have been reported.

Nerve Endings. The stimulatory effects of 5-HT on sensory nerve endings, mentioned above in connection with respiratory and circulatory reflexes, are but illustrations of a general property of 5-HT, shown also by its tendency, upon intravenous administration, to produce pain at the site of injection, gasping, hyperventilation, substernal "pressure," coughing, and "tingling and pricking all over." Stimulant effects of 5-HT on *autonomic efferent nerves,* with release of norepinephrine or ACh, seem to participate in the responses of some tissues, for example, the heart and gut. However, inhibition of transmitter output of nerve endings has also been noted.

Autonomic Ganglia. In high dose, 5-HT elicits firing of ganglion cells; lower doses facilitate or inhibit ganglionic transmission, depending on experimental conditions.

Adrenal Medulla and Other Endocrine Glands. High doses of 5-HT cause secretion of catecholamines from the adrenal gland by depolarizing chromaffin cells. The drug has capricious stimulatory or inhibitory effects on many other endocrine systems, including the adrenal cortex, pancreatic β cells, and adenohypophyseal cells (*see* below).

Central Nervous System. Although 5-HT serves as a neurotransmitter within the brain, and sites responsive to 5-HT are abundant and easily demonstrated by microiontophoretic application of the drug, central effects are not usually encountered when 5-HT is given parenterally, for it poorly penetrates the blood-brain barrier. When injected into the cerebral ventricles, 5-HT elicits a variety of behavioral responses; it also disrupts motor function and temperature regulation (*see* Feldberg, 1968). Applied by microiontophoresis to randomly encountered neurons throughout the CNS from neocortex to spinal cord, 5-HT inhibits some cells and stimulates others. However, when similarly applied to neurons known to receive tryptaminergic input, 5-HT has so far been observed only to inhibit. Moreover, it is inhibitory to the same neurons that release it by acting through autoreceptors (*see* Aghajanian, in Ho *et al.*, 1982). The hallucinogenic effects of some 5-HT-like drugs, such as LSD, have been briefly alluded to above. For discussion of these and other diverse responses of the CNS that have been attributed to agents with tryptaminergic activity, *see* Ho and colleagues (1982), Marwaha and Anderson (1984), and Chapters 12, 19, and 23.

Mode of Action. Receptors for 5-HT, located on the cell surface, are less well characterized than are those for histamine. That distinct types of receptors for 5-HT exist is evident from their wide range of susceptibilities to different blocking drugs (*see* below). As with histamine, transduction of receptor occupancy into a functional response seems to involve changes in membrane permeability to inorganic ions, which thereby influence ion fluxes; membrane potential, excitability, and spiking activity; or changes in the intracellular concentrations of second messengers such as calcium ions or cyclic nucleotides (*see* Berridge, 1975; Rasmussen, 1981; Kennedy, 1983).

ENDOGENOUS 5-HYDROXYTRYPTAMINE:
DISTRIBUTION AND BIOSYNTHESIS

Distribution. About 90% of the 5-HT present in the body, which in an adult human probably amounts to 10 mg, is lodged in the gastrointestinal tract, mainly in enterochromaffin cells. A few similar 5-HT–containing cells are also present in other tissues. Of the remaining 5-HT, most is present in platelets and the CNS. Mast cells of rodents and cattle contain 5-HT, but mast cells of other species, including man, do not (*see* Erspamer, 1966a, 1966b; Essman, 1978d).

Origin, Synthesis, Uptake, Storage, and Metabolism. Although considerable amounts of 5-HT are present in the diet (*see* above), much is metabolized as it crosses the intestinal wall and the rest is destroyed by the liver and lungs. The 5-HT found in enterochromaffin cells, neurons, and most other 5-HT–containing cells is synthesized *in situ* from tryptophan. Platelets, an important exception, acquire 5-HT from their environment (*see* below). In cells that synthesize 5-HT, tryptophan is first hydroxylated to 5-hydroxytryptophan (5-HTP) by the enzyme tryptophan-5-hydroxylase (the activity of which is rate limiting), and is then decarboxylated to 5-HT by the nonspecific aromatic L-amino acid decarboxylase. In the cytoplasm, 5-HT, whether synthesized or acquired, is taken up into secretory granules and stored therein as a nondiffusible complex with adenosine triphosphate (ATP) and other substances. The molecular events involved in pumping the amine into its granular storage sites and sequestering it there are very similar to those involved in the storage of the catecholamines. Drugs that disrupt the storage of catecholamines, such as reserpine, impair that of 5-HT similarly. Platelets take up 5-HT during their passage through the intestinal blood vessels, where they encounter relatively high concentrations of 5-HT that result from its secretion by enterochromaffin cells and possibly other sources. The important mechanism is a high-affinity uptake that allows accumulation of 5-HT against an enormous concentration gradient. A high-affinity uptake mechanism like that of platelets is also present in tryptaminergic nerve endings, thereby permitting them to recapture released transmitter. These uptake mechanisms are also similar to those for re-uptake of catecholamines by adrenergic and dopaminergic neurons; for example, both are influenced by many of the tricyclic antidepressant drugs.

An amount of 5-HT roughly equal to that present in the body is synthesized each day. Turnover times of 5-HT in brain and gastrointestinal tract have been estimated at about 1 and 17 hours, respectively. However, 5-HT in rodent mast cells turns over very slowly and that bound in platelets appears to be released only on their destruction or during the "release reaction" induced by thrombin or other agents. (For reviews on the metabolism of 5-HT and drugs affecting it, *see* Erspamer, 1966b; Bosin, 1978; Garattini and Samanin, 1978; Ahlman and Dahlström, Polak *et al.*, and Schächter and Grahame-Smith, in De Clerck and Vanhoutte, 1982; and Fernstrom, Fuller, Ho and Estevez, Lovenberg and Kuhn, Maitre *et al.*, and Sanders-Bush, in Ho *et al.*, 1982.)

ENDOGENOUS 5-HYDROXYTRYPTAMINE:
FUNCTIONS

A major function of 5-HT is to serve as the chemical transmitter of neurons within the brain that are referred to as "tryptaminergic" (or "serotonergic"). In addition, 5-HT serves as a precursor for the pineal hormone, *melatonin*. Less evident is its function in platelets, enterochromaffin cells, and other cells with established or suspected endocrine function.

Nervous System. Within the CNS the cell bodies of the 5-HT–containing neurons are located almost exclusively in the raphe nuclei of the brain stem, from which axons project extensively to other portions of the brain stem, to the spinal cord, and to the forebrain (*see* Aghajanian, in Ho *et al.*, 1982). Among the many functions in which endogenous 5-HT has been implicated are pain perception, sleep, and various kinds of behaviors, both normal and abnormal; the latter in particular include affective disorders. It may also participate in the regulation of temperature and blood pressure, as well as in neuroendocrine regulation (*see* Chapters 12 and 19; *see also* Ho *et al.*, 1982; Robinson, 1984). Some tryptaminergic fibers also seem to be present in the peripheral nervous system, particularly in the gut (*see* Gershon, 1981; Ahlman and Dahlström, in De Clerck and Vanhoutte, 1982).

Hypothalamic–Anterior Pituitary Function. The hypothalamic neuroendocrine cells that release hypophysiotropic hormones seem to be controlled, in part, by tryptaminergic neurons. Thus, 5-HT has been implicated as a possible physiological factor in the release of ACTH, growth hormone, prolactin, luteinizing hormone, follicle-stimulating hormone, and thyroid-stimulating hormone (*see* Krieger, 1978; Gudelsky *et al.*, in Marwaha and Anderson, 1984). At the level of the adenohypophysis itself, the only prominent effects are on the pars intermedia, where 5-HT can diminish or increase the secretion of melanocyte-stimulating hormone, depending on species, and can inhibit or stimulate action potentials (Taraskevich and Douglas, 1984; Douglas and Taraskevich, 1985).
Storage with Peptides in Endocrine Cells and Neurons. In various species, 5-HT (or another arylethylamine such as dopamine or histamine) may occur in a host of cells known or believed to secrete polypeptide hormones, for example, the parafollicular cells (C cells) of the thyroid, α and β cells of the endocrine pancreas, and other cells of the neuroendocrine series (*see* Pearse, 1977; Polak *et al.*, in De Clerck and Vanhoutte, 1982). Whereas the amine is stored and released along with the polypeptide hormone in the secretory granules, its function is unknown. Coincidental storage of amines (including 5-HT) and peptides in neurons is also a common finding (*see* Symposium, 1983c).

Enterochromaffin System. The physiological function of enterochromaffin cells is still uncertain. Beside 5-HT, they may contain the peptides substance P and motilin, which are potent autacoids in their own right (*see* Polak *et al.*, in De Clerck and Vanhoutte, 1982). Many 5-HT–containing neurons in the CNS also contain substance P. Intestinal enterochromaffin cells show a basal release of 5-HT that is augmented by mechanical stimulation; by hypertonicity and acidity; by norepinephrine; and also by vagal influences, apparently mediated by adrenergic fibers (*see* Ahlman and Dahlström, in De Clerck and Vanhoutte, 1982).

Tumors of 5-HT–Forming Cells: Malignant Carcinoid. Tumors of enterochromaffin or related cells (*carcinoid tumors*) may synthesize and release large amounts of 5-HT along with other autacoids. The 5-HT contributes to diarrhea and abdominal cramps. With massive tumors, so much tryptophan may be diverted to 5-HT synthesis that niacin synthesis suffers and *pellagra* results.

Platelet 5-HT. The function of 5-HT in platelets is obscure. Platelets depleted of 5-HT by reserpine function normally, or nearly so; bleeding time, clotting time, and capillary resistance are little affected (*see* De Clerck and Herman, 1983). The old conjecture that efflux of 5-HT from platelets may be involved in regulation of vascular tone has attracted fresh interest in the light of the antihypertensive effect of certain 5-HT antagonists (*see* below; Van Nueten, 1983); however, support for the idea is slender.

ADDITIONAL CONSIDERATIONS

Absorption, Fate, and Excretion. For experimental purposes, 5-HT is usually given intravenously, but it is also well absorbed after intramuscular injection. Given orally, it is also fairly well absorbed but it is metabolized rapidly and is ineffective. In man, most 5-HT, endogenous or ingested, undergoes oxidative deamination by MAO to form 5-hydroxyindoleacetaldehyde. This is promptly degraded, mainly by further oxidation to 5-hydroxyindoleacetic acid (5-HIAA) by aldehyde dehydrogenase, but also in small part by reduction, by alcohol dehydrogenase, to 5-hydroxytryptophol (5-HTOL). The three enzymes are present in liver and in various tissues that contain 5-HT, including the brain. Following intravenous injection of 5-HT, its uptake and degradation by the lung are important; depending on the rate of infusion, 30 to 90% of 5-HT is taken up by pulmonary endothelial cells.

The principal metabolite, 5-HIAA, is excreted in the urine, along with much smaller amounts of 5-HTOL, mainly as the glucuronide or sulfate, and traces of other metabolites. About 2 to 10 mg of 5-HIAA is excreted daily by the normal adult as a result of metabolism of endogenous 5-HT. Larger amounts are excreted by patients with malignant carcinoid, a fact of diagnostic value. However, ingestion of 5-HT–containing foods also increases excretion of 5-HT metabolites (*see* Erspamer, 1966a; Brown, 1977; Bosin, 1978).

Ingestion of ethyl alcohol diverts 5-hydroxyindoleacetaldehyde from the normally predominant oxidative route to the reductive pathway because of the elevated concentration of NADH. This greatly increases excretion of 5-HTOL and correspondingly reduces that of 5-HIAA (*see* Bosin, 1978; Youdim and Ashkenazi, in Ho *et al.*, 1982).

Drugs Affecting Endogenous 5-HT. Many of these are described in other chapters. The following is but an outline. (1) The *precursor of 5-HT*, tryptophan, can increase endogenous concentrations of the amine and cause behavioral changes (*see* Fernstrom and also Lovenberg and Kuhn, in Ho *et al.*, 1982). It may be of value in phenylketonuria. (2) *Inhibitors of synthesis* include p-chlorophenylalanine (PCPA), which blocks the rate-limiting enzyme tryptophan hydroxylase. The compound is a valuable experimental tool but is too toxic for clinical use. (3) *Inhibitors of membrane uptake* include the tricyclic antidepressant drugs, which also inhibit catecholamine uptake. A more potent and selective inhibition of 5-HT uptake is obtained with fluoxetine, zimeldine, and some other antidepressant drugs (*see* Fuller, Ho, and Estevez and also Maitre *et al.*, in Ho *et al.*, 1982). (4) *Inhibitors of granule uptake and storage* include reserpine, tetrabenazine, and other benzoquinolizines, all of which deplete stores of 5-HT (as well as other amines). A long-lasting depletion of 5-HT can also be achieved with the anorectic drug fenfluramine and with p-chloroamphetamine and its analogs. (5) *Inhibitors of degradation* include principally the MAO inhibitors. (6) *Neurotoxins* that preferentially destroy 5-HT–containing neurons include 5,6-dihydroxytryptamine (5,6-DHT) and 5,7-DHT. (7) *Antagonists of 5-HT* at the level of the receptor are discussed below. (*See* Symposium, 1978; Fuller, 1980; Ho *et al.*, 1982; Fuller, in Marwaha and Anderson, 1984.)

5-HT ANTAGONISTS

Ergot alkaloids and related compounds were early recognized as antagonists at receptors for 5-HT, particularly on smooth muscle (*see* Chapter 39); in this group the *lysergic acid derivatives* such as the diethylamide (LSD), 2-bromo-LSD, and 1-methyl-d-lysergic acid butanolamide (methysergide, *see* below) are especially potent. Also, many *indole compounds* are 5-HT antagonists. Beside the ergot derivatives, many other drugs of diverse structure possess significant antagonistic activity at certain receptors for 5-HT. Among them are H_1 blockers of the ethylenediamine type and also, most notably, *cyproheptadine* (*see* below), *phenothiazines* (particularly chlorpromazine), and β-*haloalkylamines* such as phenoxybenzamine (*see* Gyermek, 1966; Garattini and Samanin, 1978; Ho *et al.*, 1982; Fuller, in Marwaha and Anderson, 1984). However, it has been difficult to discover highly selective 5-HT antagonists. The two drugs that are usually classified as 5-HT antagonists, *methysergide* and *cyproheptadine*, have other prominent pharmacological activities that dominate their clinical usefulness; the latter, for example, is very commonly used for its potent H_1 blocking activity. Perhaps the point can be best illustrated by the fact that a major class of 5-HT receptors ($5-HT_2$) has been defined by examination of the binding of the neuroleptic drug *spiperone (spiroperidol)*, which is also used to label dopamine receptors (*see* Peroutka and Snyder, 1983). While

all this calls for caution in interpreting effects of so-called 5-HT antagonists, it would be wrong to infer that such "cross-talk" is inevitable. Some experimental 5-HT antagonists are very selective (*see* Cohen *et al.*, 1983). Among the more familiar 5-HT antagonists that are commonly encountered in an experimental context are *metergoline, metitepine, mianserin, pizotyline (pizotifen)*, and *cinanserin*. Although these agents are among the most specific of their class, they all have significant activity at receptors for other autacoids (*see* Fuller, 1980; Ho *et al.*, 1982; Janssen, 1983; Fuller, in Marwaha and Anderson, 1984).

It has long been evident that 5-HT receptors are heterogeneous, and the picture has become increasingly complex; evidence suggests the existence of several subpopulations of receptors. Radioligand-binding studies, principally in brain tissue, have identified two broad 5-HT–binding sites: the first, preferentially labeled with $[^3H]5-HT$, are termed $5-HT_1$ receptors; the second, preferentially labeled with $[^3H]$spiperone, are termed $5-HT_2$ receptors (*see* Peroutka and Snyder, 1983). Paradoxically, it is receptors of the $5-HT_2$ variety, whose affinity for 5-HT is only about one thousandth that of the $5-HT_1$ receptors, that have been most frequently associated with functional responses. But it is clear that there are more than two types of 5-HT–binding sites, and much additional work remains. That a substance effective as an antagonist at one type of 5-HT–receptor site may fail to block at another is obvious from what has been said. What adds to confusion is that it may act in the opposite way, as an agonist. The best example is LSD—a potent antagonist of 5-HT on some smooth muscles, yet a potent agonist mimicking 5-HT at central synapses. In addition, most of the 5-HT antagonists listed at the end of the preceding paragraph have partial agonistic activity.

Ketanserin. This agent is the prototype of a novel series of 5-HT antagonists (*see* Van Nueten *et al.*, 1981; Janssen, 1983). It has the following structure:

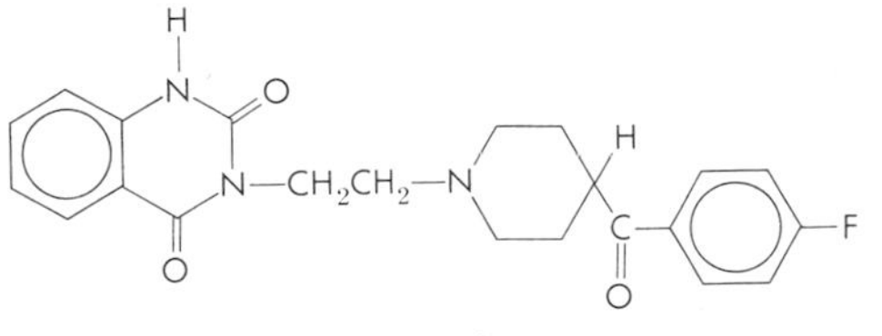

Ketanserin

Ketanserin blocks 5-HT receptors that apparently belong to the $5-HT_2$ category without having any significant effect on $5-HT_1$ receptors; because of this discrimination, it has been described as the first selective $5-HT_2$ blocker. To avoid misinterpretation, however, it is important to note that ketanserin is nonspecific in the sense that it has substantial affinity for α_1-adrenergic receptors, histamine H_1 receptors, and, to a lesser extent, dopamine receptors (*see* Janssen, 1983). However, in its action at 5-HT receptors, ketanserin has the merit of acting as a pure antagonist. It antagonizes vasoconstrictor effects of 5-HT on various vascular preparations and, interestingly, it converts the vasoconstrictor effect of 5-HT in the guinea pig stomach to a vasodilator response. It also blocks the contractile response of tracheal muscle to 5-HT and the aggregating effect of 5-HT on platelets. It does not block the classical, direct contractile responses of the guinea pig ileum or the rat stomach. The pharmacological profile is thus interesting and offers a further challenge for classification of 5-HT receptors.

It is, however, the ability of ketanserin to lower blood pressure in hypertensive animals and man that accounts for the considerable clinical interest in the compound. It has been viewed as a novel antihypertensive agent that may act through 5-HT$_2$ receptors and may have other therapeutic uses. (*See* De Clerck and Vanhoutte, 1982; Janssen, 1983; Symposium, 1983a, 1983b.) The mechanism of the antihypertensive action is, however, controversial. The drug has some α_1-blocking activity on human vasculature that is demonstrable at therapeutic concentrations (*see* Reimann and Frölich, 1983). Moreover, although ketanserin lowers blood pressure in certain hypertensive animals, a more selective 5-HT$_2$ antagonist (LY53857) does not; this latter drug has a very much lower affinity for α_1-adrenergic receptors (Cohen *et al.*, 1983). Blockade of α_1 receptors is, of course, a familiar antihypertensive mechanism. In addition, ketanserin appears to inhibit sympathetic outflow from the CNS (McCall and Schuette, 1984).

Methysergide. This drug (1-methyl-*d*-lysergic acid butanolamide) is a congener of methylergonovine and of LSD. Its structure is depicted in Table 39–1. It inhibits the vasoconstrictor and pressor effects of 5-HT as well as the action of the amine on a variety of extravascular smooth muscles and other cells. Unlike LSD, however, it has comparatively little action on the nervous system in usual doses. Although methysergide is an ergot derivative, it has only feeble vasoconstrictor and oxytocic activity.

Methysergide is useful for the *prophylactic treatment* of *migraine* and other *vascular headaches*, including Horton's syndrome. The protective effect of methysergide takes 1 to 2 days to develop and as long to pass off when treatment is terminated. Rebound headaches not uncommonly occur when the drug is withdrawn. Methysergide is without benefit when given during the acute attack. It is not clear why methysergide or any of the other effective agents should be of value in migraine or other vascular headaches. The mechanism of such headaches is unknown. For comparative evaluation of the prophylactic effects of methysergide and other agents, particularly β-adrenergic antagonists, *see* Diamond and Medina (1980), Paskin (1981), and Fozard (1982); *see also* Chapter 39.

Methysergide is useful in combating diarrhea and malabsorption in patients with *carcinoid* and may be beneficial in the *postgastrectomy dumping syn-*

drome. Both these conditions have a 5-HT–mediated component.

Untoward Effects. These are usually mild and transient, but may be severe enough to require withdrawal of the drug. The most common are gastrointestinal and include heartburn, diarrhea, cramps, nausea, and vomiting. Effects attributable to central actions include unsteadiness, drowsiness, weakness, light-headedness, nervousness, insomnia, confusion, excitement, euphoria, hallucinations, and even frank psychotic episodes. There may be either loss of appetite or weight gain. Reactions suggestive of vascular insufficiency have been observed in a few patients, and exacerbation of angina pectoris has been noted. One infrequent, but potentially serious, complication of prolonged treatment is *inflammatory fibrosis*. This gives rise to various syndromes, depending on the site, including retroperitoneal fibrosis, pleuropulmonary fibrosis, and coronary and endocardial fibrosis. Usually the fibrosis retrogresses after withdrawal of the drug, but this is not always so and persistent cardiac valvular damage has been reported. Because of this danger, treatment should be interrupted for 3 weeks or more every 6 months.

Preparation and Dosage. Methysergide maleate (SANSERT) is available in 2-mg tablets. The adult dose is about 4 to 8 mg daily, in divided doses taken with food.

Cyproheptadine. This compound has the following structural formula:

Cyproheptadine

Its structure resembles that of the phenothiazine H$_1$ antagonists, and, indeed, it is an effective H$_1$ blocker. It is discussed here because it also has prominent 5-HT–blocking activity on various smooth muscles. In addition, it has weak anticholinergic activity and possesses mild central-depressant properties.

Uses and Side Effects. Cyproheptadine shares the properties and uses of other H$_1$ blockers (*see* above). It appears to be about as effective as hydroxyzine in controlling *skin allergies*, particularly the accompanying *pruritus*. It also appears to be useful in *cold urticaria* (*see* Salvaggio, 1982). In allergic conditions its actions as a 5-HT antagonist are irrelevant, since 5-HT is not involved in human allergic responses. The 5-HT–antagonizing properties of cyproheptadine are, however, of benefit in the *postgastrectomy dumping syndrome, intestinal hypermotility of carcinoid,* and some other conditions that do involve the release of 5-HT.

Side effects of cyproheptadine include drowsiness, dry mouth, and many other effects common to H_1 blockers (*see* above). Weight gain and increased growth in children have been observed. The mechanism may involve interference with regulation of the secretion of growth hormone (*see* Fernstrom, in Ho *et al.*, 1982).

Preparations. *Cyproheptadine hydrochloride* (PERIACTIN) is available as tablets (4 mg) and as a syrup (2 mg/5 ml). The usual dose for adults is 4 mg, three or four times per day. The total dose should not exceed 0.5 mg/kg.

Altounyan, R. E. C. Inhibition of experimental asthma by a new compound, disodium cromoglycate, "INTAL." *Acta Allergol. (Kbh.)*, **1967**, *22*, 487–489.

Altura, B. M. Reticulo-endothelium cell function and histamine release in shock and trauma; relationship in microcirculation. *Klin. Wochenschr.*, **1982**, *60*, 882–890.

Amin, A. H.; Crawford, T. B. B.; and Gaddum, J. H. The distribution of substance P and 5-hydroxytryptamine in the central nervous system of the dog. *J. Physiol. (Lond.)*, **1954**, *126*, 596–618.

Ash, A. S. F., and Schild, H. O. Receptors mediating some actions of histamine. *Br. J. Pharmacol.*, **1966**, *27*, 427–439.

Baron, J. H. Gastric functions tests. In, *Chronic Duodenal Ulcer.* (Wastell, C., ed.) Appleton-Century-Crofts, New York, **1972**, pp. 82–114.

Best, C. H.; Dale, H. H.; Dudley, H. W.; and Thorpe, W. V. The nature of the vasodilator constituents of certain tissue extracts. *J. Physiol. (Lond.)*, **1927**, *62*, 397–417.

Binder, H. J., and Donaldson, R. M., Jr. Effect of cimetidine on intrinsic factor and pepsin secretion in man. *Gastroenterology*, **1978**, *74*, 371–375.

Black, J. W.; Duncan, W. A. M.; Durant, C. J.; Ganellin, C. R.; and Parsons, E. M. Definition and antagonism of histamine H_2-receptors. *Nature*, **1972**, *236*, 385–390.

Bovet, D.; Horclois, R.; and Walthert, F. Propriétés antihistaminiques de la N-*p*-méthoxybenzyl-N-diméthylaminoéthyl α amino-pyridine. *C. R. Soc. Biol. (Paris)*, **1944**, *138*, 99–100.

Bovet, D., and Staub, A. Action protectrice des éthers phénoliques au cours de l'intoxication histaminique. *C. R. Soc. Biol. (Paris)*, **1937**, *124*, 547–549.

Brodie, B. B., and Shore, P. A. A concept for a role of serotonin and norepinephrine as chemical mediators in the brain. *Ann. N.Y. Acad. Sci.*, **1957**, *66*, 631–642.

Carruthers, S. G.; Shoeman, D. W.; Hignite, C. E.; and Azarnoff, D. L. Correlation between plasma diphenhydramine level and sedative and antihistamine effects. *Clin. Pharmacol. Ther.*, **1978**, *23*, 375–382.

Cerletti, A.; Taeschler, M.; and Weidmann, H. Pharmacologic studies on the structure-activity relationship of hydroxyindole alkylamines. *Adv. Pharmacol.*, **1968**, *6B*, 233–246.

Cohen, B., and deJong, J. M. B. V. Meclizine and placebo in treating vertigo of vestibular origin. Relative efficacy in a double-blind study. *Arch. Neurol.*, **1972**, *27*, 129–135.

Cohen, M. L.; Fuller, R. W.; and Kurz, K. D. LY53857, a selective and potent serotonergic (5-HT_2) receptor antagonist, does not lower blood pressure in the spontaneously hypertensive rat. *J. Pharmacol. Exp. Ther.*, **1983**, *227*, 327–332.

Dahlén, S. E.; Hansson, G.; Hedquist, P.; Bjorck, T.; Granstrom, E.; and Dahlen, B. Allergen challenge of lung tissue from asthmatics elicits bronchial contraction that correlates with the release of leukotrienes C_4, D_4 and E_4. *Proc. Natl Acad. Sci. U.S.A.*, **1983**, *80*, 1712–1716.

Dale, H. H. The anaphylactic reaction of plain muscle in the guinea-pig. *J. Pharmacol. Exp. Ther.*, **1913**, *4*, 167–223.

——. Some chemical factors in the control of the circulation. *Lancet*, **1929**, *1*, 1179–1183, 1233–1237, 1285–1290.

Dale, H. H., and Laidlaw, P. P. The physiological action of β-imidazolylethylamine. *J. Physiol. (Lond.)*, **1910**, *41*, 318–344.

——. Further observations on the action of β-imidazolylethylamine. *Ibid.*, **1911**, *43*, 182–195.

——. Histamine shock. *Ibid.*, **1919**, *52*, 355–390.

De Clerck, F. F., and Herman, A. G. 5-Hydroxytryptamine and platelet aggregation. *Fed. Proc.*, **1983**, *42*, 228–232.

Douglas, W. W. Stimulus-secretion coupling: the concept and clues from chromaffin and other cells. The First Gaddum Memorial Lecture. *Br. J. Pharmacol.*, **1968**, *34*, 451–474.

——. Stimulus-secretion coupling: variations on the theme of calcium activated exocytosis involving cellular and extracellular sources of calcium. In, *Respiratory Tract Mucus.* Ciba Foundation Symposium, Vol. 54. Elsevier/Excerpta Medica/North Holland, Amsterdam, **1978**, pp. 61–90.

Editorial. Inflammatory mediators of asthma. *Lancet*, **1983a**, *2*, 829–831.

Editorial. No sneezing —or dozing—seen with new H_1 blocker. *J.A.M.A.*, **1983b**, *249*, 3151–3152.

Erspamer, V. Occurrence of indolealkylamines in nature. In, *5-Hydroxytryptamine and Related Indolealkylamines.* (Erspamer, V., ed.) *Handbuch der Experimentellen Pharmakologie*, Vol. 19. Springer-Verlag, Berlin, **1966a**, pp. 132–181.

Feldberg, W. The monoamines of the hypothalamus as mediators of temperature responses. In, *Recent Advances in Pharmacology*, 4th ed. (Robson, J. M., and Stacey, R. S., eds.) J. & A. Churchill, Ltd., London, **1968**, pp. 349–397.

Fellenius, E.; Berglindh, T.; Sachs, G.; Olbe, L.; Elander, B.; Sjostrand, S. E.; and Wallmark, B. Substituted benzimidazoles inhibit gastric acid secretion by blocking $(H^+ + K^+)ATPase$. *Nature*, **1981**, *290*, 159–161.

Gaddum, J. H. Antagonism between LSD and 5-hydroxytryptamine. *J. Physiol. (Lond.)*, **1953**, *121*, 15P.

Graybiel, A.; Wood, C. D.; Knepton, J.; Hoche, J. P.; and Perkins, G. F. Human assay of antimotion sickness drugs. *Aviat. Space Environ. Med.*, **1975**, *46*, 1107–1118.

Gustavsson, S.; Adami, H. D.; Loof, L.; Nybers, A.; and Nyren, D. Rapid healing of duodenal ulcers with omeprazole. *Lancet*, **1983**, *2*, 124–125.

Hunt, R. H.; Mills, J. G.; Beresford, J.; Billings, J. A.; Burland, W. L.; and Milton-Thompson, G. J. Gastric secretory studies in humans with impromidine (SK&F 92676)—a specific histamine H_2 receptor agonist. *Gastroenterology*, **1980**, *78*, 505–511.

Jansen, R. T.; Collen, M. J.; Pandol, S. J.; Allende, H. D.; Raufman, J.-P.; Bissonette, B. M.; Duncan, W. C.; Durgan, P. L.; Gillin, J. C.; and Gardner, J. D. Cimetidine-induced impotence and breast changes in patients with gastric hypersecretory states. *N. Engl. J. Med.*, **1983**, *308*, 883–888.

Janssen, P. A. J. 5-HT_2 receptor blockade to study serotonin-induced pathology. *Trends Pharmacol. Sci.*, **1983**, *5*, 198–206.

Khandelwal, J. K.; Hough, L. B.; and Green, J. P. Histamine and some of its metabolites in human body fluids. *Klin. Wochenschr.*, **1982**, *60*, 914–918.

Klein, G. L., and Galant, S. P. A comparison of the antipruritic efficacy of hydroxyzine and cyproheptadine in children with atopic dermatitis. *Ann. Allergy*, **1980**, *44*, 142–145.

Lamers, B. H. W.; Lind, T.; Moberg, S.; Jansen, J. B. M. J.; and Olbe, L. Omeprazole in Zollinger-Ellison syndrome. *N. Engl. J. Med.*, **1984**, *310*, 758–761.

Lecomte, J. Liberation of endogenous histamine in man. *J. Allergy*, **1957**, *28*, 102–112.

Lind, T.; Cederberg, C.; Ekenved, G.; Hagland, U.; and Olbe, L. Effect of omeprazole—a gastric proton pump inhibitor—on pentagastrin stimulated acid secretion in man. *Gut*, **1983**, *24*, 270–276.

McCall, R. B., and Schuette, M. R. Evidence for an alpha-1 receptor-mediated central sympathoinhibitory action of ketanserin. *J. Pharmacol. Exp. Ther.*, **1984**, *228*, 704–710.

Medical Letter. Cromolyn sodium nasal spray for hay fever. **1983**, *25*, 89–90.

Pearse, A. G. E. The diffuse neuro-endocrine system and the APUD concept; related "endocrine" peptides in brain, intestine, pituitary, placenta and anuran cutaneous glands. *Med. Biol.*, **1977**, *55*, 115–125.

Peroutka, S. J., and Snyder, S. H. Multiple serotonin receptors and their physiological significance. *Fed. Proc.*, **1983**, *42*, 213–217.

Popielski, L. β-Imidazolyläthylamin und die Organextrakte. Erster Teil: β-Imidazolyläthylamin als mächtiger Erreger der Magendrüsen. *Pflügers Arch. Ges. Physiol.*, **1920**, *178*, 214–236.

Rapport, M. M. Serum vasoconstrictor (serotonin). V. The presence of creatinine in the complex: a proposed study of the vasoconstrictor principle. *J. Biol. Chem.*, **1949**, *180*, 961–969.

Rapport, M. M.; Green, A. A.; and Page, I. H. Serum vasoconstrictor (serotonin). IV. Isolation and characterization. *J. Biol. Chem.*, **1948**, *176*, 1243–1251.

Reimann, I. W., and Frölich, J. C. Ketanserin. (Letter.) *Lancet*, **1983**, *1*, 703–704.

Robinson, S. E. Serotonergic-cholinergic interactions in blood pressure control in the rat. *Fed. Proc.*, **1984**, *43*, 21–24.

Rosière, C. E., and Grossman, M. I. An analog of histamine that stimulates gastric acid secretion without other actions of histamine. *Science*, **1951**, *113*, 651.

Sachs, G. Pump blockers and ulcer disease. *N. Engl. J. Med.*, **1984**, *310*, 785–786.

Schayer, R. W., and Cooper, J. A. D. Metabolism of C^{14} histamine in man. *J. Appl. Physiol.*, **1956**, *9*, 481–483.

Simons, F. E. R.; Simons, K. J.; Becker, M. D.; and Haydey, R. P. Pharmacokinetics and antipruritic effects of hydroxyzine in children with atopic dermatitis. *J. Pediatr.*, **1984a**, *104*, 123–127.

Simons, F. E. R.; Simons, K. J.; and Frith, E. M. The pharmacokinetics and antihistaminic effects of the H_1 receptor antagonist hydroxyzine. *J. Allergy Clin. Immunol.*, **1984b**, *73*, 69–75.

Soll, A. H., and Grossman, M. I. The interaction of stimulants on the function of isolated canine parietal cells. *Philos. Trans. R. Soc. Lond. [Biol.]*, **1981**, *296*, 5–15.

Theoharides, T. C.; Sieghart, W.; Greengard, P.; and Douglas, W. W. Antiallergic drug cromolyn may inhibit histamine secretion by regulating phosphorylation of a mast cell protein. *Science*, **1980**, *207*, 80–82.

Twarog, B. M., and Page, I. H. Serotonin content of some mammalian tissues and urine and a method for its determination. *Am. J. Physiol.*, **1953**, *175*, 157–161.

Vanhoutte, P. M.; Van Nueten, J. M.; Symoens, J.; and Janssen, P. A. J. Antihypertensive properties of ketanserin (R 41 468). *Fed. Proc.*, **1983**, *42*, 182–185.

Van Nueten, J. M. 5-Hydroxytryptamine and precapillary vessels. *Fed. Proc.*, **1983**, *42*, 223–227.

Van Nueten, J. M.; Janssen, P. A. J.; Van Beek, J.; Xhonneux, R.; Verbeuren, T. J.; and Vanhoutte, P. M. Vascular effects of ketanserin (R 41 468), a novel antagonist of $5-HT_2$ serotonergic receptors. *J. Pharmacol. Exp. Ther.*, **1981**, *218*, 217–230.

Walt, R. P.; Gomes, M. D.; Wood, E. C.; Losan, L. H.; and Pounder, R. E. Effect of daily oral omeprazole on 24 hour intragastric acidity. *Br. Med. J. [Clin. Res.]*, **1983**, *287*, 12–14.

Wenting, G. J.; Man in't Veld, A. J.; Woittiez, A. J.; Boomsma, F.; and Schalekamp, M. A. D. H. Treatment of hypertension with ketanserin, a new selective $5-HT_2$ receptor antagonist. *Br. Med. J. [Clin. Res.]*, **1982**, *284*, 537–539.

West, S.; Brandon, B.; Stolley, P.; and Rumrill, R. A review of antihistamines and the common cold. *Pediatrics*, **1975**, *56*, 100–107.

Woolley, D. W., and Shaw, E. A biochemical and pharmacological suggestion about certain mental disorders. *Science*, **1954**, *119*, 587–588.

Monographs and Reviews

Altura, B. M., and Halevy, S. Cardiovascular actions of histamine. In, *Histamine II and Anti-Histaminics: Chemistry, Metabolism and Physiological and Pharmacological Actions*. (Rocha e Silva, M., ed.) *Handbuch der Experimentellen Pharmakologie*, Vol. 18, Pt. 2. Springer-Verlag, Berlin, **1978**, pp. 1–39.

Baron, J. H. (ed.) *Cimetidine in the 80s*. Churchill Livingstone, Edinburgh, **1981**.

Beaven, M. A. *Histamine: Its Role in Physiological and Pathological Processes*. S. Karger, Basel, **1978**.

Becker, E. L.; Simon, A. S.; and Austen, K. F. (eds.). *Biochemistry of the Acute Allergic Reactions*. Fourth International Symposium. Alan R. Liss, Inc., New York, **1981**.

Benveniste, J., and Arnoux, B. A. (eds.). *Platelet-Activating Factor and Structurally Related Ether-Lipids*. Inserm Symposium Series, Vol. 23. Elsevier, New York, **1983**.

Berglindh, T. The mammalian gastric parietal cell *in vitro*. *Annu. Rev. Physiol.*, **1984**, *46*, 377–392.

Berman, B. A. Cromolyn: past, present and future. *Pediatr. Clin. North Am.*, **1983**, *30*, 915–930.

Berridge, M. J. The interaction of cyclic nucleotides and calcium in the control of cellular activity. *Adv. Cyclic Nucleotide Res.*, **1975**, *6*, 1–98.

Bosin, T. R. Serotonin metabolism. In, *Availability, Localization and Disposition*. Vol. 1, *Serotonin in Health and Disease*. (Essman, W. B., ed.) Spectrum Publications, Inc., New York, **1978**, pp. 181–300.

Bovet, D. Introduction to antihistamine agents and antergan derivatives. *Ann. N.Y. Acad. Sci.*, **1950**, *50*, 1089–1126.

Brogden, R. N.; Carmine, A. A.; Heel, R. C.; Speight, T. M.; and Avery, G. S. Ranitidine: a review of its pharmacology and therapeutic use in peptic ulcer disease and other allied diseases. *Drugs*, **1982**, *24*, 267–303.

Brown, H. Serotonin-producing tumors. In, *Clinical Correlates*. Vol. 4, *Serotonin in Health and Disease*. (Essman, W. B., ed.) Spectrum Publications, Inc., New York, **1977**, pp. 393–423.

Code, C. F. Histamine and gastric secretion: a later look, 1955–1965. *Fed. Proc.*, **1965**, *24*, 1311–1325.

Cox, J. S. C.; Beach, J. E.; Blair, A. M.; Clarke, A. J.; King, J.; Lee, T. B.; Loveday, D. E. E.; Moss, G. F.; Orr, T. S. C.; Ritchie, I. R.; and Sheard, P. Disodium cromoglycate (INTAL). *Adv. Drug Res.*, **1970**, *5*, 115–196.

De Clerck, F. F., and Vanhoutte, M. (eds.). *5-Hydroxytryptamine in Peripheral Reactions*. Raven Press, New York, **1982**.

Douglas, W. W., and Taraskevich, P. S. The electrophysiology of adenohypophyseal cells. In, *Electrophysiology of the Secretory Cell*. (Poisner, A. M., and Trifario, J. M., eds.) Elsevier, Amsterdam, **1985**, pp. 63–92.

Diamond, S., and Medina, J. L. Newer drug therapies for headache. *Postgrad. Med.*, **1980**, *68*, 125–140.

Erspamer, V. Pharmacology of indolealkylamines. *Pharmacol. Rev.*, **1954**, *6*, 425–487.

—— (ed.). *5-Hydroxytryptamine and Related Indolealkylamines. Handbuch der Experimentellen Pharmakologie*, Vol. 19. Springer-Verlag, Berlin, **1966b.**

Essman, W. B. (ed.). *Serotonin in Health and Disease*, Vol. 4. *Clinical Correlates*. Spectrum Publications, Inc., New York, **1977.**

——. *Serotonin in Health and Disease*, Vol. 1. *Availability, Localization and Disposition*. Spectrum Publications, Inc., New York, **1978a.**

——. *Serotonin in Health and Disease*, Vol. 2. *Physiological Regulation and Pharmacological Action*. Spectrum Publications, Inc., New York, **1978b.**

——. *Serotonin in Health and Disease*, Vol. 3. *The Central Nervous System*. Spectrum Publications, Inc., New York, **1978c.**

——. Serotonin distribution in tissues and fluids. In, *Availability, Localization and Disposition*. Vol. 1, *Serotonin in Health and Disease*. (Essman, W. B., ed.) Spectrum Publications, Inc., New York, **1978d,** pp. 15–179.

Faingold, C. L. Antihistamines as central nervous system depressants. In, *Histamine II and Anti-Histaminics: Chemistry, Metabolism and Physiological and Pharmacological Actions*. (Rocha e Silva, M., ed.) *Handbuch der Experimentellen Pharmakologie*, Vol. 18, Pt. 2. Springer-Verlag, Berlin, **1978,** pp. 561–573.

Foreman, J. C. The pharmacological control of immediate hypersensitivity. *Annu. Rev. Pharmacol. Toxicol.,* **1981,** *21,* 63–81.

Fozard, J. R. Basic mechanisms of antimigraine drugs. *Adv. Neurol.,* **1982,** *33,* 295–307.

Freston, J. W. Cimetidine. I. Developments, pharmacology and efficacy. *Ann. Intern. Med.,* **1982a,** *97,* 573–580.

——. Cimetidine. II. Adverse reactions and patterns of use. *Ibid.,* **1982b,** *97,* 728–734.

Fuller, R. W. Pharmacology of central serotonin neurons. *Annu. Rev. Pharmacol. Toxicol.,* **1980,** *20,* 111–127.

Furchgott, R. F. The role of endothelium in the responses of vascular smooth muscle to drugs. *Annu. Rev. Pharmacol. Toxicol.,* **1984,** *24,* 175–197.

Ganellin, C. R., and Parsons, M. E. (eds.). *Pharmacology of Histamine Receptors*. Wright/PSG, Bristol, **1982.**

Garattini, S., and Samanin, R. Drugs affecting serotonin: a survey. In, *Physiological Regulation and Pharmacological Action*. Vol. 2, *Serotonin in Health and Disease*. (Essman, W. B., ed.) Spectrum Publications, Inc., New York, **1978,** pp. 247–293.

Gershon, M. D. Enteric serotoninergic neurons. *Annu. Rev. Neurosci.,* **1981,** *4,* 227–272.

Goth, A. On the general problems of the release of histamine. In, *Histamine II and Anti-Histaminics: Chemistry, Metabolism and Physiological and Pharmacological Actions*. (Rocha e Silva, M., ed.) *Handbuch der Experimentellen Pharmakologie*, Vol. 18, Pt. 2. Springer-Verlag, Berlin, **1978,** pp. 57–74.

Gyermek, L. Drugs which antagonize 5-hydroxytryptamine and related indolealkylamines. In, *5-Hydroxytryptamine and Related Indolealkylamines*. (Erspamer, V., ed.) *Handbuch der Experimentellen Pharmakologie*, Vol. 19. Springer-Verlag, Berlin, **1966,** pp. 471–528.

Hahn, F. Antianaphylactic and antiallergic effects. In, *Histamine II and Anti-Histaminics: Chemistry, Metabolism and Physiological and Pharmacological Actions*. (Rocha e Silva, M., ed.) *Handbuch der Experimentellen Pharmakologie*, Vol. 18, Pt. 2. Springer-Verlag, Berlin, **1978,** pp. 439–504.

Hirschowitz, B. I. H-2 histamine receptors. *Annu. Rev. Pharmacol. Toxicol.,* **1979,** *19,* 203–244.

Ho, B. T.; Schoolar, J. C.; and Usdin, E. (eds.). *Serotonin in Biological Psychiatry. Adv. Biochem. Psychopharmacol.,* **1982,** *34.*

Ishizaka, K. (ed.). Mast cell activation and mediator release. *Prog. Allergy,* **1984,** *34,* 1–338.

Kahlson, G., and Rosengren, E. *Biogenesis and Physiology of Histamine*. Edward Arnold, Ltd., London, **1971.**

Keeton, R. W.; Luckhardt, A. B.; and Koch, F. C. Gastrin studies. IV. The response of the stomach mucosa to food and gastrin bodies as influenced by atropine. *Am. J. Physiol.,* **1920,** *51,* 469–481.

Kennedy, M. B. Experimental approaches to understanding the role of protein phosphorylation in the regulation of neuronal function. *Annu. Rev. Neurosci.,* **1983,** *6,* 493–525.

Kingsley, P. J., and Cox, J. S. G. Cromolyn sodium (sodium cromoglycate) and drugs with similar activities. In, *Allergy: Principles and Practice*, Vol. 1. (Middleton, E.; Reed, C.; and Ellis, E. F.; eds.) C. V. Mosby Co., St. Louis, **1978,** pp. 481–498.

Krieger, D. T. Endocrine processes and serotonin. In, *The Central Nervous System*. Vol. 3, *Serotonin in Health and Disease*. (Essman, W. B., ed.) Spectrum Publications, Inc., New York, **1978,** pp. 51–67.

Lagunoff, D.; Martin, T. W.; and Read, G. Agents that release histamine from mast cells. *Annu. Rev. Pharmacol. Toxicol.,* **1983,** *23,* 331–351.

Larsen, G. L., and Henson, P. M. Mediators of inflammation. *Annu. Rev. Immunol.,* **1983,** *1,* 335–359.

Lewis, T. *The Blood Vessels of the Human Skin and Their Responses*. Shaw & Sons, Ltd., London, **1927.**

Lorenz, W.; Doenicke, A.; Schoning, B.; and Neugebauer, E. The role of histamine in adverse reactions to intravenous agents. In, *Adverse Reactions to Anaesthetic Drugs*. (Thornton, J. A., ed.) Elsevier/North Holland, Amsterdam, **1981,** pp. 169–238.

McGuigan, J. E. A consideration of the adverse effects of cimetidine. *Gastroenterology,* **1981,** *80,* 181–192.

MacIntosh, F. C. Histamine as a normal stimulant of gastric secretion. *Q. J. Exp. Physiol.,* **1938,** *28,* 87–98.

Mantegazzini, P. Pharmacological actions of indolealkylamines and precursor amino acids on the central nervous system. In, *5-Hydroxytryptamine and Related Indolealkylamines*. (Erspamer, V., ed.) *Handbuch der Experimentellen Pharmakologie*, Vol. 19. Springer-Verlag, Berlin, **1966,** pp. 424–470.

Marwaha, J., and Anderson, W. J. (eds.). *Neuroreceptors in Health and Disease. Monogr. Neural Sci.,* **1984,** *10,* 1–256.

Mathews, K. P. Respiratory atopic disease. *J.A.M.A.,* **1982,** *248,* 2587–2610.

Metcalfe, D. D.; Kaliner, M.; and Donlon, M. A. The mast cell. *CRC Crit. Rev. Immunol.,* **1981,** *3,* 23–74.

Misiewicz, J. J., and Wormsley, K. G. (eds.). *The Clinical Use of Ranitidine*. Medical Publishing Foundation, Oxford, **1982.**

Nadel, J. A., and Barnes, P. J. Autonomic regulation of the airways. *Annu. Rev. Med.,* **1984,** *35,* 451–467.

Paskin, N. H. Pharmacology of migraine. *Annu. Rev. Pharmacol. Toxicol.,* **1981,** *21,* 463–478.

Paton, W. D. M. Histamine release by compounds of simple chemical structure. *Pharmacol. Rev.,* **1957,** *9,* 269–328.

Pepys, J., and Edwards, A. M. (eds.). *The Mast Cell: Its Role in Health and Disease*. Pitman Medical, Tunbridge Wells, **1979.**

Rapoport, R. M., and Murad, F. Endothelium-dependent and nitrovasodilator-induced relaxation of vascular smooth muscle: role for cyclic GMP. *J. Cyclic Nucleotide Protein Phosphorylation Res.,* **1983,** *9,* 281–296.

Rasmussen, H. *Calcium and cAMP as Synarchic Messengers*. John Wiley & Sons, Inc., New York, **1981.**

Reite, O. B. Comparative physiology of histamine. *Physiol. Rev.,* **1972,** *52,* 778–819.

Riley, A. J., and Salmon, P. R. (eds.). *Ranitidine*. Excerpta Medica, Amsterdam, **1982.**

Roberts, F., and Calcutt, C. R. Histamine and the hypothalamus. *Neuroscience,* **1983,** *9,* 721–739.

Rocha e Silva, M. (ed.). *Histamine: Its Chemistry, Metabolism and Physiological and Pharmacological Ac-*

tions. *Handbuch der Experimentellen Pharmakologie*, Vol. 18, Pt. 1. Springer-Verlag, Berlin, **1966**.

——— (ed.). *Histamine II and Anti-Histaminics: Chemistry, Metabolism and Physiological and Pharmacological Actions. Handbuch der Experimentellen Pharmakologie*, Vol. 18, Pt. 2. Springer-Verlag, Berlin, **1978.**

Rocha e Silva, M., and Antonio, A. Bioassay of antihistaminic action. In, *Histamine II and Anti-Histaminics: Chemistry, Metabolism and Physiological and Pharmacological Actions*. (Rocha e Silva, M., ed.) *Handbuch der Experimentellen Pharmakologie*, Vol. 18, Pt. 2. Springer-Verlag, Berlin, **1978**, pp. 381–438.

Salvaggio, J. E. (ed.). Primer on allergic and immunologic diseases. *J.A.M.A.*, **1982**, *248*, 2579–2772.

Schäfer, E. A. *The Endocrine Organs: An Introduction to the Study of Internal Secretion*. Longmans, Green & Co., New York, **1916.**

Schayer, R. W. Induced synthesis of histamine, microcirculatory regulation and the mechanism of action of the glucocorticoid hormones. *Prog. Allergy*, **1963**, *7*, 187–212.

———. Histamine and microcirculation. *Life Sci.*, **1974**, *15*, 391–401.

———. Biogenesis of histamine. In, *Histamine II and Anti-Histaminics: Chemistry, Metabolism and Physiological and Pharmacological Actions*. (Rocha e Silva, M., ed.) *Handbuch der Experimentellen Pharmakologie*, Vol. 18, Pt. 2. Springer-Verlag, Berlin, **1978**, pp. 109–129.

Sedman, A. J. Cimetidine—drug interactions. *Am. J. Med.*, **1984**, *76*, 109–114.

Symposium. (Various authors.) Biological role of indolealkylamine derivatives. (Garattini, S., and Shore, P., eds.) *Adv. Pharmacol.*, **1968a**, *6A*, 1–440; *6B*, 1–323.

Symposium. (Various authors.) 5-Hydroxytryptamine. (Paasonen, M. K., and Klinge, E., eds.) *Ann. Med. Exp. Biol. Fenn.*, **1968b**, *46*, 361–519.

Symposium. (Various authors.) *Serotonin and Behavior*. (Barchas, J. D., and Usdin, E., eds.) Academic Press, Inc., New York, **1973**, pp. 1–642.

Symposium. (Various authors.) Serotonin—new vistas: histochemistry and pharmacology. (Costa, E.; Gessa, G. L.; and Sandler, M.; eds.) *Adv. Biochem. Psychopharmacol.*, **1974a**, *10*, 1–329.

Symposium. (Various authors.) Serotonin—new vistas: biochemistry and behavioural and clinical studies. (Costa, E.; Gessa, G. L.; and Sandler, M.; eds.) *Adv. Biochem. Psychopharmacol.*, **1974b**, *11*, 1–428.

Symposium. (Various authors.) Serotonin neurotoxins. (Jacoby, J. H., and Lytle, L. D., eds.) *Ann. N.Y. Acad. Sci.*, **1978**, *305*, 1–702.

Symposium. (Various authors.) *Biochemistry of the Acute Allergic Reaction*. Fourth International Symposium. (Becker, E. L.; Simon, A. S.; and Austen, K. F.; eds.) Alan R. Liss, Inc., New York, **1981.**

Symposium. (Various authors.) *Histamine and Antihistamines in Anaesthesia and Surgery*. (Ahnefeld. F. W.; Doenicke, A.; and Lorenz, W.; eds.) *Klin. Wochenschr.*, **1982**, *60*, 871–1062.

Symposium. (Various authors.) New antihypertensive drugs. *Fed. Proc.*, **1983a**, *42*, 153–210.

Symposium. (Various authors.) 5-Hydroxytryptamine and the vascular system. *Fed. Proc.*, **1983b**, *42*, 211–237.

Symposium. (Various authors.) Coexistence of neuromodulators: biochemical and pharmacological consequences. *Fed. Proc.*, **1983c**, *42*, 2910–2952.

Taraskevich, P. S., and Douglas, W. W. Electrical activity in adenohypophyseal cells and effects of hypophysiotropic substances. *Fed. Proc.*, **1984**, *43*, 2373–2378.

Wallis, D. Neuronal 5-hydroxytryptamine receptors outside the central nervous system. *Life Sci.*, **1981**, *29*, 2345–2355.

Weck, A. L. D., and Bundgaard, H. (eds.). *Allergic Reactions to Drugs. Handbook of Experimental Pharmacology*, Vol. 63. Springer-Verlag, Berlin, **1983.**

Weil-Malherbe, H. Serotonin and schizophrenia. In, *The Central Nervous System*. Vol. 3, *Serotonin in Health and Disease*. (Essman, W. B., ed.) Spectrum Publications, Inc., New York, **1978**, pp. 231–291.

Wetterquist, H. Histamine metabolism and excretion. In, *Histamine II and Anti-Histaminics: Chemistry, Metabolism and Physiological and Pharmacological Actions*. (Rocha e Silva, M., ed.) *Handbuch der Experimentellen Pharmakologie*, Vol. 18, Pt. 2. Springer-Verlag, Berlin, **1978**, pp. 131–150.

Witiak, D. T., and Lewis, N. J. Absorption, distribution, metabolism, and elimination of antihistamines. In, *Histamine II and Anti-Histaminics: Chemistry, Metabolism and Physiological and Pharmacological Actions*. (Rocha e Silva, M., ed.) *Handbuch der Experimentellen Pharmakologie*, Vol. 18, Pt. 2. Springer-Verlag, Berlin, **1978**, 513–560.

Wood, C. D. Antimotion sickness and antiemetic drugs. *Drugs*, **1979**, *17*, 471–479.

Woolley, D. W. *The Biochemical Basis of Psychoses; or, the Serotonin Hypothesis about Mental Illness*. John Wiley & Sons, Inc., New York, **1962.**

Zeldis, J. B.; Friedman, L. S.; and Isselbacher, K. J. Drug therapy: ranitidine—a new H_2-receptor antagonist. *N. Engl. J. Med.*, **1983**, *309*, 1368–1373.

CHAPTER

27 POLYPEPTIDES—ANGIOTENSIN, PLASMA KININS, AND OTHERS

William W. Douglas

ANGIOTENSIN

History. In 1898, Tiegerstedt and Bergman found that crude saline extracts of the kidney contained a pressor principle, which they named *renin*. Their discovery had an obvious bearing on the problem of arterial hypertension and its relation to kidney disease that had been posed by Richard Bright's work some 60 years earlier; however, relatively little interest was generated until 1934, when Goldblatt and his colleagues showed convincingly that it was possible to produce persistent hypertension in dogs by constricting the renal arteries. Within a few years, several investigators had detected pressor activity in renal venous blood following renal artery constriction and had attributed the effect to renin. Renin thus came to occupy a central position in the field of experimental hypertension. In 1940, Braun-Menéndez and his colleagues in Argentina and Page and Helmer at the Cleveland Clinic reported independently that renin was an enzyme that acted on a plasma protein substrate to catalyze the formation of the actual pressor material, a peptide, which was named *hypertensin* by the former group and *angiotonin* by the latter. These two terms persisted for nearly 20 years, until it was agreed to rename the pressor substance *angiotensin* and to call the plasma substrate *angiotensinogen*. Meanwhile in the mid-1950s, Skeggs, Peart, and their respective colleagues determined the amino acid composition and sequence of the active material. Two forms of angiotensin were recognized, the first a decapeptide (angiotensin I) and the second an octapeptide (angiotensin II) formed from angiotensin I by enzymatic cleavage by another enzyme, termed *angiotensin converting enzyme*. The octapeptide was shown to be the more active form, and its synthesis in 1957 by Schwyzer and by Bumpus made the material available for intensive study (*see* Page and Bumpus, 1974; Skeggs, 1984).

A further impetus to research came in 1958, when Gross suggested that the renin-angiotensin system was involved in electrolyte balance and the regulation of aldosterone secretion by the adrenal cortex. It was soon shown that the kidneys are important for the increase in aldosterone secretion in response to hemorrhage; that saline extracts of kidney stimulate aldosterone release; and that synthetic angiotensin, in minute amounts, stimulates the output of aldosterone in man. Moreover, elevated rates of renin secretion were noted upon experimental reduction of sodium concentration in plasma (*see* Gross, 1968). Thus, the renin-angioten-

sin system came to be recognized as a mechanism to stimulate aldosterone secretion and thereby to conserve sodium and maintain blood volume. Such an action, clearly complementary to the long-familiar vasoconstrictor actions, led to a broadening of the concept of the renin-angiotensin system as an important physiological mechanism in the interrelated homeostatic functions concerned with the volume, pressure, and electrolyte composition of body fluids.

The development, in the 1970s, of pharmacological agents capable of acting effectively *in vivo* to inhibit the formation of angiotensins or to block their receptors provided the analytical tools with which to assess these postulated physiological and pathophysiological functions and to discover others. These inhibitors have illuminated the homeostatic functions of the renin-angiotensin system and have revealed, in a vivid manner, an involvement of the system in the maintenance of elevated blood pressure in diverse hypertensive states that is much more extensive than had been supposed. This has led to the development of a new and broadly efficacious class of antihypertensive drugs.

A further dimension of interest has been lent by demonstrations of renin and angiotensin in a wide variety of tissues, including the brain. It is thus no longer fitting to view these substances solely within the classical framework of the kidney and circulation. But what scope this broad distribution may offer for pharmacological intervention remains to be seen.

Chemistry. The synthesis and degradation of the angiotensins *in vivo* are complex processes that are outlined in Figure 27–1 and treated in greater detail below (*see* page 643). Briefly, the process is initiated when the enzyme renin acts on angiotensinogen (renin substrate), an α-globulin, to release the decapeptide angiotensin I (angiotensin-[1-10] decapeptide). This decapeptide has limited intrinsic pharmacological activity, but it is cleaved by angiotensin converting enzyme (ACE) to yield the highly active octapeptide angiotensin II (angiotensin-[1-8]octapeptide). This, in turn, undergoes hydrolysis by aminopeptidase to yield the heptapeptide angiotensin III (angiotensin-[2-8]heptapeptide), known alternatively as [des-Asp[1]] angiotensin II, which is also pharmacologically active. Further cleavage yields peptides with little activity. In an alternative (minor) path, converting enzyme and aminopeptidase act in the opposite sequence such that the decapeptide, angiotensin I, is hydrolyzed first to [des-Asp[1]]

639

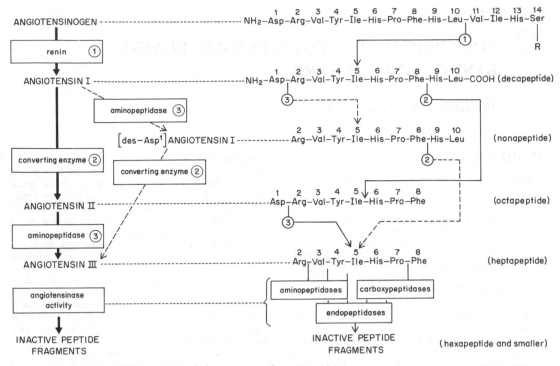

Figure 27-1. *Formation and destruction of angiotensins.*

The left-hand scheme is complemented by the diagram on the right of structures and sites of enzymatic cleavage (the numbers within circles correspond to those assigned to the enzymes within the boxes). The solid arrows show the classical paths, while the dashed arrows indicate an alternative (minor) path. The structures of the angiotensins shown are those found in man, horse, rat, and pig; the bovine form has valine in the 5 position. The sequence of human angiotensinogen is depicted (Tewksbury *et al.*, 1981).

angiotensin I, which, like the parent compound, has limited pharmacological activity. It is then cleaved by converting enzyme to form the active angiotensin III (*see* Skeggs, 1984).

Many analogs of angiotensin II have been synthesized, and considerable information on the structure-activity relationship is available. As is evident from the activity of angiotensin III, most of the essential information resides in the C-terminal heptapeptide. Phenylalanine in position 8 is critical. Its removal from any of the angiotensins abolishes *agonist* (but not necessarily antagonist) activity, which, however, can be restored to some extent by substituting other aromatic amino acids. The other aromatic residues in positions 4 and 6, the guanido group in position 2, and the C-terminal carboxyl are involved mainly in binding to the receptor site. Position 1 is not critical (thus the efficacy of angiotensin III), but replacement of aspartic acid in position 1 with sarcosine (N-methylglycine) enhances binding and slows hydrolysis by rendering the peptide refractory to an important subgroup of aminopeptidases that are specific for aspartic or glutamic acid ("Asp-aminopeptidase"; "angiotensinase A"). Such a substitution, combined with that of alanine in place

of phenylalanine in position 8, yields a potent angiotensin II blocking agent, *saralasin* (*see* below). Further information on the chemistry of the angiotensins is available in the reviews by Page and Bumpus (1974), Regoli and coworkers (1974), and Bumpus (1977).

PHARMACOLOGICAL PROPERTIES

The most familiar and best-studied effects of angiotensin II are vasoconstriction and stimulation of the synthesis and secretion of aldosterone by the adrenal cortex. However, the peptide has numerous other effects. Some involve stimulation of the heart and the sympathetic nervous system; these complement the direct vasomotor effects and contribute to the increase in blood pressure caused by angiotensin. Others, such as stimulation of drinking and increased secretion of antidiuretic hormone, complement the effects of aldosterone and contribute to retention of sodium and water. In the following discussion the description refers to the octapeptide angiotensin II. As will become apparent from a brief description of the effects of the other angiotensins, only the heptapeptide angiotensin III shares most of the effects of angiotensin II; with the possible exception of the effects on the adrenal cortex, angiotensin III is generally weaker (*see* Bell *et al.*, 1984). The decapeptide angiotensin I and its nonapeptide derivative, [des-Asp[1]]-angiotensin, are much more restricted in their actions (*see* reviews by Page and Bumpus, 1974; Regoli *et al.*, 1974; Peach, 1977; Fitzsimons, 1980; Ferrario, 1983).

Cardiovascular System. The strong pressor activity that led to the discovery of the renin-angiotensin system involves a constellation of effects, among which are direct stimulation of vascular and cardiac muscle, facilitation of sympathetic transmission in the periphery, and stimulation of central sympathetic outflow. Moreover, reflex responses, especially those involving baroreceptors, may obtund or mask the primary effects of angiotensin, such that the overall responses of the intact individual may be quite complex.

Blood Vessels. Vasoconstriction in response to angiotensin involves precapillary arterioles and, to a lesser but significant extent, postcapillary venules. The peptide has a direct action on the vascular smooth muscle and indirectly stimulates contraction by means of the sympathetic nervous system. The relative importance of the effects depends on species, vascular bed, route of injection, and dose of the compound. With intravenous infusions in man, the direct action seems to account for most of the increase in total peripheral resistance; however, in certain vascular beds, such as those of the hand and the foot, vasoconstriction has a large sympathetic component, since it is much reduced by α-adrenergic antagonists.

The vasoconstrictor effect of angiotensin given intravenously is strongest in the vessels of the skin, splanchnic region, and kidney; blood flow in these regions falls sharply. The effect is less in the vessels of the brain and still weaker in skeletal muscle. In both these regions blood flow may

actually increase, especially following low doses, since the relatively weak vasoconstrictor response is opposed by the elevated systemic blood pressure. Nevertheless, with high doses cerebral blood flow tends to fall. Vasoconstriction prejudicial to flow may also occur in coronary vessels.

Heart. Angiotensin acts directly on the membrane of atrial and ventricular muscle to prolong the plateau phase of the action potential and hence to increase inward calcium current and force of contraction. This effect is opposed by calcium channel blockers. Angiotensin has no direct effect on the heart rate but tends to increase heart rate and force of contraction by its central and peripheral stimulant and facilitatory actions on sympathetic outflow (*see* below). However, by increasing systemic blood pressure and baroreceptor discharge, angiotensin may initiate reflex vagal activity sufficient to slow the heart and raise end-diastolic pressure. The rise in central venous pressure is generally modest, since angiotensin has a comparatively feeble constrictor effect on the larger veins and hence reduces venous capacity much less than does, for example, norepinephrine. As a result of these various factors cardiac output generally falls. Despite this, the work of the heart often increases as a result of the elevated systemic blood pressure and increased mechanical load, and there may be coronary insufficiency.

Blood Pressure. Angiotensin is the most potent pressor agent known; on a molar basis, it is about 40 times more so than norepinephrine. When a single moderate dose is injected intravenously, systemic blood pressure begins to rise within about 10 seconds, rapidly reaches maximum, and returns to normal in a few minutes. When the drug is infused continuously, blood pressure is maintained at an elevated level for hours or days. Indeed, with such infusion the effectiveness of angiotensin may even increase with time. Angiotensin commonly causes a moderate rise in pulmonary arterial pressure that is due less, perhaps, to its feeble pulmonary vasoconstrictor action than to an increase of pressure in the pulmonary vein as end-diastolic pressure rises.

Blood Volume, Capillary Permeability, and Lymph Flow. Angiotensin appears to constrict postcapillary venules and thus increases filtration pressure in the capillaries. In addition, it increases vascular permeability by causing separation of the endothelial cells by some contractile response. There is a significant diminution in blood volume and increases in extravascular fluid and the flow of lymph.

Extravascular Smooth Muscle. Effects of angiotensin on smooth muscle other than that in blood vessels are generally weak, but contractions are readily elicited in preparations such as guinea pig ileum and rat uterus *in vitro*. Beside direct stimulation of the smooth muscle cells, angiotensin can elicit indirect effects, contraction or relaxation, by exciting cholinergic or adrenergic ganglion cells or nerve endings. An unusual, seemingly direct, relaxant effect of angiotensin has been noted on tracheal muscle contracted by 5-hydroxytryptamine in dogs and cats.

Central Nervous System. Because the blood-brain barrier is impermeable to peptides, the possibility that angiotensin might have central actions was overlooked for many years. However, angiotensin gains access to those specialized regions of the brain that lack a barrier (several periventricular regions) and thereby elicits a variety of responses (*see* Fitzsimons, 1980; Ferrario, 1983; Ganong, 1984).

Central Sympathetic Stimulation. Small amounts of angiotensin infused into the vertebral arteries, including those of man, cause a sustained rise in systemic blood pressure. This is mediated by sympathetic vasoconstriction and cardiac stimulation, and is due to effects of the drug on the medulla in the area postrema.

Drinking and Hydration. Angiotensin has a centrally mediated dipsogenic effect that can be observed following intravenous injection as well as after injection of the peptide into the third ventricle or surrounding areas. The preoptic region and subfornical organ seem particularly sensitive. Hunger for food is suppressed in favor of drinking (*see also* Fitzsimons, 1980; Elfont and Fitzsimons, 1983).

Release of Antidiuretic Hormone. Angiotensin increases activity in supraoptic neurons when injected into the brain or third ventricle and can thus stimulate secretion of antidiuretic hormone (ADH). It also enhances release of ADH from the neuro-

hypophysis *in vitro*. Increased secretion of ADH has been noted less consistently after intravenous injections. Responses of anterior pituitary cells are minor and capricious (*see* Ganong, 1984).

Peripheral Autonomic Nervous System. In addition to central enhancement of sympathetic outflow, angiotensin can facilitate peripheral sympathetic transmission, mainly by augmenting the output of norepinephrine from the nerve terminals but also apparently by amplifying the responses of the effector cells and by facilitating ganglionic transmission (*see* Langer, 1981). High concentrations of the peptide can stimulate ganglion cells directly.

Adrenal Medulla. Angiotensin stimulates the release of catecholamines from the adrenal medulla by directly depolarizing the chromaffin cells. Moderate doses of angiotensin given intravenously to normal subjects produce only a small effect that does not contribute substantially to the overall cardiovascular response. But intense and dangerous responses have been noted in individuals with pheochromocytoma (*see* below).

The Adrenal Cortex and Secretion of Aldosterone. Angiotensin directly stimulates the synthesis and secretion of aldosterone; its effects on the output of other corticosteroids are variable, usually minor, and dependent on species. Increased output of aldosterone is elicited by very low concentrations of angiotensin that have little or no effect on blood pressure. The effect begins within a few minutes of injection and may be maintained indefinitely by infusion; indeed, the response tends to increase somewhat with time, at least in part as the zona glomerulosa hypertrophies. Increased secretion of aldosterone, in turn, acts on the kidney to cause retention of sodium and excretion of potassium and hydrogen ions. The stimulant effect of angiotensin on the synthesis and release of aldosterone is enhanced when the concentration of sodium in plasma is low or when that of potassium is high. The peptide's effects are reduced when concentrations of these cations in plasma are altered in the opposite direction. Such changes in sensitivity are believed to be due to alterations of the number of receptors for angiotensin on the zona glomerulosa cells as well as to adrenocortical hyperplasia in the sodium-depleted state (*see* Davis and Freeman, 1976; Bell *et al.*, 1984).

The Kidney and Formation of Urine. Beside its indirect effects on renal tubular function, mediated by aldosterone, angiotensin influences urine formation through hemodynamic and intrarenal actions that interact in a complex way. Both the rise in systemic blood pressure, which increases renal perfusion pressure, and the vasoconstrictor effect on *efferent* glomerular arterioles tend to enhance glomerular filtration; vasoconstriction of the *afferent* arterioles has the opposite effect, as does the action of angiotensin on the glomerular capillaries, where a contractile response of mesangial cells (and possibly endothelial cells) shrinks the structure and reduces the surface area available for filtration. The outcome of all this depends on the concentration of angiotensin, as well as species and circulatory-renal status. In healthy man the typical response is a brisk antidiuresis and antinatriuresis, accompanied by reduced rates of effective renal plasma flow and glomerular filtration. However, certain hypertensive individuals and patients with hepatic cirrhosis and ascites or other cardiovascular-renal deficiencies respond in a contrary fashion with diuresis and natriuresis (*see* Gross and Mohring, 1973; Symposium, 1983a, 1984a; Ménard *et al.*, 1984).

Actions of the Other Angiotensins. The pharmacological properties so far described are those of angiotensin II. Angiotensin I has less than 1% of the intrinsic activity of angiotensin II on smooth muscle, heart, or adrenal cortex, for example, although its activity on the adrenal medulla and the sympathetic and central nervous systems may not be quite as weak. Little is known of the direct actions of [des-Asp¹]angiotensin I, save that its potency on vascular smooth muscle is very low. On the other hand, angiotensin III retains most of the activity of angiotensin II. In most instances it is somewhat weaker; its pressor activity, for example, is about 25 to 50% of that of angiotensin II, and its stimulant action on the adrenal medulla is perhaps only about 10% of that of angiotensin II; however, it is about as potent as angiotensin II in stimulating the secretion of aldosterone (Davis and Freeman, 1977; Peach, 1977; Bell *et al.*, 1984).

Mechanism of Action. The effects of angiotensin are exerted through specific receptors on cell surfaces, and these can be blocked selectively by certain analogs of the peptide (*see* below). How the action at the receptor level is translated into the appropriate cellular responses remains somewhat obscure. The peptide depolarizes the membranes of chromaffin, ganglion, and smooth muscle cells. However, smooth muscle continues to respond to angiotensin (as it does to several other agonists) when it has been depolarized by excess potassium, presumably due to both facilitation of the entry of calcium into cells and mobilization of stores of intracellular calcium. Prolongation of the action potential and increased influx of calcium ions may account for the augmented release of sympathetic transmitter and the positive inotropic effect. The stimulant action on the output of aldosterone is due to increased synthesis of the steroid. Again, angiotensin acts through a calcium-dependent mechanism that facilitates the initial reaction in the biosynthetic path, conversion of cholesterol to pregnenolone. Influx of calcium, with resultant activation of a phospholipase, may also account for increased production of eicosanoids by some cells. The role of prostaglandins and related compounds is uncertain, but sometimes (*e.g.*, with renal vasoconstriction) it is possible to reduce responses to angiotensin with indomethacin and other drugs that block their synthesis. Cyclic nucleotides have also been implicated in the mediations of responses to angiotensin. However, even for the best-studied effects, namely, increased secretion of aldosterone and cardiac stimulation, it is still quite uncertain that cyclic nucleotides are involved (*see* Capponi *et al.*, 1981).

ENDOGENOUS RENIN-ANGIOTENSIN SYSTEM

The renin-angiotensin system exists in each of the vertebrate classes studied (*see* Wilson, 1984). The main source of renin is the kidney, from which it is secreted by the granular juxtaglomerular (JG) cells that lie in the walls of the afferent arterioles as they enter the glomeruli. These are endocrine cells in the sense that they discharge their secretory product, renin, directly into the renal arterial blood stream. Their "peculiarity" lies in the fact that renin is not itself a hormone but is an enzyme that catalyzes the formation of the active hormones, the angiotensins. Renin and the other components of the renin-angiotensin system are also found at various extrarenal sites, including the brain (*see* below).

Synthesis and Catabolism of Elements of the Renin-Angiotensin System in Vivo. *Renin.* This enzyme, a protease with high substrate specificity, is both the initiating and the rate-limiting element in the production of the active peptides. It releases the decapeptide angiotensin I by cleaving the peptide bond between residues 10 and 11 of its substrate, angiotensinogen (Figure 27–1). Renin is a glycoprotein with a half-life in the circulation of about 15 minutes. Inactive forms of renin are present in the kidney and also in the plasma, where their concentration is about ten times greater than that of the active form. They are, at least in part, precursors (prorenins), but their physiological status is uncertain. Of practical concern in the estimation of plasma renin activity (PRA) is the fact that they may be activated by chilling or acidification. Both factors may act indirectly through activation of the protease, kallikrein (see Hsueh, 1982; Cordes, 1984; Haber, 1984; Skeggs, 1984). Renins in tissues other than the kidney (tissue renins or isorenins) are closely related to the renal renin. The mouse submaxillary gland is extraordinarily rich in renin and prorenin, and study of this tissue has provided critical biochemical information about their structures and processing (see Corvol et al., 1983).

Other Angiotensin-Generating Activities. A few other enzymes can also catalyze the synthesis of angiotensins from angiotensinogen. *Cathepsin D*, like renin and tissue isorenins, forms angiotensin I, whereas *cathepsin G* and *tonin* synthesize angiotensin II directly (see Genest, 1984).

Angiotensinogen(s). These are glycoproteins, present in abundance in the plasma globulin fraction and synthesized by the liver. The relevant portion of the proteins is the amino terminus, from which angiotensin I is cleaved (Figure 27–1). Human angiotensinogen serves as a substrate only for the renin of man or primates, whereas the angiotensinogens of other animals are substrates for the renins of all species examined, including man. The sequence at the cleavage site of human angiotensinogen is Leu-Val, but it is Leu-Leu in other species (Tewksbury et al., 1981).

Angiotensin Converting Enzyme (ACE; Kininase II; Dipeptidyl Carboxypeptidase). This enzyme was discovered serendipitously, in plasma, as the factor responsible for conversion of the decapeptide prohormone angiotensin I into the classical pressor agent, angiotensin II (see Skeggs, 1984). It is a rather nonspecific metalloenzyme (containing Zn) that cleaves dipeptide units from peptide substrates with diverse amino acid sequences. Preferred substrates have one free carboxyl group (but not two) in the C-terminal amino acid, and proline must not be the penultimate amino acid. Because of this latter restriction, the enzyme does not degrade angiotensin II. Furthermore, other peptides and related substances with penultimate prolines (or "proline surrogates") act as inhibitors of converting enzyme (see below). Among the many natural substrates is bradykinin; converting enzyme is identical with the activity designated as kininase II, which *inactivates* bradykinin and other potent *vasodilator* peptides (see below and Figure 27–3). Although slow conversion of angiotensin I to angiotensin II occurs in plasma, the very rapid metabolism that occurs *in vivo* is due largely to the activity of tissue-bound enzyme present on the luminal aspect of vascular endothelial cells. For example, in man the lung converts some 20 to 40%

of angiotensin I to angiotensin II in a single circulation. Extrapulmonary conversion is also brisk; thus, intra-arterial injection of angiotensin I into the forearm causes immediate distal vasoconstriction, attributable to local formation of angiotensin II (see Erdös, 1979; Ryan, 1982; Doyle and Bearn, 1984; Skeggs, 1984).

Angiotensins I, II, and III and Metabolites. When given intravenously, angiotensin I is so rapidly converted to angiotensin II that the pharmacological responses are indistinguishable—provided, of course, that converting enzyme has not been inhibited. Angiotensin II has a short half-life (a minute or so), and it is degraded by several peptidases (Figure 27–1). Of its metabolites, only the heptapeptide angiotensin III retains significant activity.

Angiotensinases. This term is applied to various peptidases that are involved in the degradation and inactivation of angiotensin II; none is specific. Among them are aminopeptidases, the activity of which may also contribute to the formation of active angiotensins. One aminopeptidase, "Asp-aminopeptidase" or "angiotensinase A," is specific for aspartic (or glutamic) acid, and its action terminates with the formation of the [des-Asp[1]] compounds. In some tissues a considerable portion of angiotensin I is converted to [des-Asp[1]]angiotensin I; in the adrenal gland the fraction is as large as one half. These and other reactions are shown in Figure 27–1.

Functions of the Renin-Angiotensin System. The renin-angiotensin system is an important component of the interrelated homeostatic mechanisms that regulate hemodynamics and water and electrolyte balance. Factors that lower blood volume, renal perfusion pressure, or the sodium concentration in plasma tend to stimulate the secretion of renin, while factors that increase these parameters tend to inhibit its secretion (see Figure 27–2).

Control of Renin Secretion. The secretion of renin from the juxtaglomerular (JG) cells is controlled by three influences—two acting locally within the kidney and the third acting through the central nervous system (CNS) and mediated by sympathetic secretomotor nerves.

The first intrarenal influence is mechanical; factors that tend to lower renal perfusion pressure elicit the secretion of renin. These include a fall in systemic blood pressure from any cause, such as diminished cardiac output, lowered total peripheral resistance, or reduction in blood volume through sodium deficiency or hemorrhage; local vascular effects, such as renal arterial or aortic stenosis, can also augment secretion. The immediate stimulus to secretion is believed to be reduction in the *tension* within the wall of the glomerular afferent arterial vessel.

The second intrarenal influence is ionic; reduction in sodium load to the kidney stimulates the secretion of renin. This effect is *not* exerted directly on the JG cells but is apparently mediated by events in the renal tubule of the same glomerulus, particularly the macula densa region located at the end of the loop of Henle and at the beginning of the

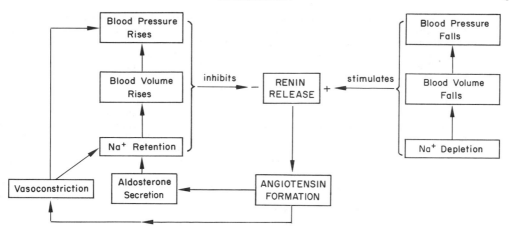

Figure 27–2. *A schematic portrayal of the possible homeostatic role of the renin-angiotensin system.*

distal tubule. It is generally believed that the macula densa somehow monitors the ionic environment in the tubular fluid and relays to the JG cells the stimulus for secretion. The macula densa cells abut the JG cells and constitute with the latter (and some other specialized cells) the "juxtaglomerular apparatus."

The third influence—the sympathetic nervous control of renin output—is secretomotor, as witness the increased output of renin when renal nerves are stimulated. The nerves innervate the JG cells directly and act through β-adrenergic receptors. The sympathetic secretomotor innervation mediates various central nervous influences on renin secretion that are determined by reflex and other factors. A fall in systemic blood pressure will, for example, activate sympathetic secretomotor activity through baroreceptors and volume receptors. The sympathetic outflow also stimulates release of renin in response to painful stimuli (including the cold pressor test) or certain stressful emotional states.

Other factors that can influence the release of renin include various autacoids. Among them are prostaglandins, which may participate in transduction or modulation of the physiological stimuli within the kidney, and angiotensin II itself, which has an inhibitory effect apparently indicative of a negative-feedback mechanism (*see* Davis and Freeman, 1982; Torretti, 1982; Freeman *et al.,* 1984; Gibbons *et al.,* 1984).

Role in Secretion of Aldosterone. The renin-angiotensin-aldosterone axis is an important element in the regulation of sodium balance. Not only does angiotensin stimulate the adrenal cortex directly to increase secretion of aldosterone, but also it exerts trophic and permissive influences on that tissue which reinforce and augment the other stimuli (*e.g.,* hormonal or ionic). The system is highly sensitive and is activated by small negative sodium balances that appear to be too subtle to be sensed by the kidney or the adrenal cortex. This high sensitivity seems to be mediated by the sympathetic

secretomotor system, for it is blunted by β-adrenergic blocking agents (*see* Peart, 1978; Davis and Freeman, 1982; Laragh, 1984).

Intrarenal Functions. Direct intrarenal regulation of glomerular filtration is a phylogenetically ancient function of the renin-angiotensin system that antecedes its involvement in regulation of adrenal secretion and blood pressure (*see* Nishimura and Bailey, 1982). In mammals, despite the persistent intimate association of the renin secretory system with the glomerulus, intrarenal functions are poorly delineated. However, angiotensin can clearly be formed locally. It may thereby modify glomerular filtration rate by hydraulic effects (differential constriction of the glomerular afferent and efferent arterioles) or by reduction of the glomerular capillary filtration area; in addition, there are indications that angiotensin may affect tubular reabsorption directly (*see* Wright and Briggs, 1979; Symposium, 1983b).

Although there are many unsettled questions about details of the role of the renin-angiotensin system in physiological control of renal function, it must be emphasized that in patients with poor renal perfusion (*e.g.,* because of stenosis of a renal artery), adequate renal function may be dependent on secretion of renin and angiotensin-induced constriction of the efferent glomerular arterioles. Renal failure can be precipitated by the removal of this prop, as may occur during treatment with inhibitors of converting enzyme (*see* below; *see also* Doyle and Bearn, 1984; Ménard *et al.,* 1984; Symposium, 1984a).

Involvement in Circulatory Responses and Homeostasis. As indicated in Figure 27–2, factors that *lower* blood pressure or volume tend to *stimulate* renin secretion, while factors that *raise* blood pressure or volume have the opposite effect. The renin-angiotensin system is thus one of the many layers of physiological controls of systemic blood pressure (*see* Guyton *et al.,* 1972). Its activation by mild postural changes has been mentioned in regard to aldosterone secretion. Its additional contribution to maintenance of systemic blood pressure is apparent from the small, but quite evident, reduction in blood pressure that is seen in normal individuals when the system is inhibited (*see* Hodsman and Robertson, 1983). Physiological stimuli act through the baroreceptor sympathetic reflex mechanism to stimulate renin release; facilitation of peripheral sympathetic outflow to blood vessels and heart may account in part for the response. Stronger, pathophysiological stimuli, such as hemorrhage, recruit in addition the local renal mechanisms for stimulation of renin secretion.

Involvement in Hypertensive States. The renin-angiotensin system contributes to hypertension in many individuals. There is, however, no simple relationship between renin secretion, as reflected by plasma renin activity (PRA), and blood pressure. Although elevated PRA is found in most individuals with *malignant hypertension* and is commonly found in patients with *hypertension resulting from stenosis of the renal artery,* most patients with hypertension do *not* have high PRA. Thus, in the great majority of hypertensive patients, those with *essential hypertension,* PRA and plasma concentrations of angiotensin II are generally distributed throughout the rather broad range of values found in normotensive individuals; indeed, a fair number of patients (about 25%) are at the low end of this range or below it. Nevertheless, as the homeostatic functions of the renin-angiotensin system have become increasingly apparent, suspicion has been aroused that many seemingly "normal" values of PRA encountered in most individuals with essential hypertension are indeed inappropriately high, given the fact that they occur in the presence of conditions (high blood pressure and perhaps sodium retention and expansion of blood volume) that should suppress the secretion of renin. Support for this view has come from several sources. For example, if PRA is examined as a function of sodium balance, then some 25% of patients with so-called essential hypertension have values above normal (*see* Laragh, 1984).

Such evidence, by itself, might suggest that the role of the renin-angiotensin system in essential hypertension, although greater than formerly postulated, is still rather limited. Nevertheless, there is other evidence that indicates much wider involvement. It has long been recognized that a more effective index than PRA might be provided by drugs that block the renin-angiotensin system. Now that such agents have been developed and tested (*see* below), they have been found to lower blood pressure in a broad range of hypertensive conditions, often where there is no evidence of elevated PRA. It is evident that the newly introduced therapeutic agents that inhibit one or another aspect of the renin-angiotensin system have dispelled the notion that this system is relevant only to a restricted group of hypertensive patients with grosser forms of the malady stigmatized by evident renal pathology; this notion was engendered by historical accident and the chronological capriciousness of discovery from Richard Bright to Goldblatt and beyond.

Possible Functions in the Central Nervous System. The brain contains all of the components of a renin-angiotensin system wholly independent of the classical renal system: renin-like activity (isorenin), angiotensinogen and angiotensin I, angiotensin I converting enzyme, angiotensin II, angiotensin II receptors, and angiotensinases. Moreover, histochemical methods have revealed angiotensin-like immunoreactivity at many sites within the CNS, including nerve terminals, thus raising the possibility that angiotensin II serves as a neurotransmitter or modulator. Conjecture concerning possible functions of angiotensin within the CNS has naturally stemmed from the various pharmacological effects of the peptide (all seemingly exerted by actions on periventricular structures or regions where there is no blood-brain barrier). These include *increased thirst, appetite for sodium, release of ADH (and possibly ACTH),* and *stimulation of central sympathetic outflow* resulting in pressor responses. Angiotensin is dipsogenic when given in minute amounts directly into the third ventricle and surrounding areas or when administered intravenously in concentrations that fall well within the physiological range observed during mild sodium depletion (Fitzsimons, 1980). Moreover, drinking responses have been attenuated by administration of antagonists of angiotensin II. Compulsive thirst in some patients with renal disease, even when they are edematous, may reflect high concentrations of angiotensin II in the blood (*see* Ganong, 1984).

Extrarenal Sources of Renin. Other tissues, beside the brain, that show renin-like (isorenin) activity include blood vessels, uterus, placenta, amniotic fluid, salivary glands, and adrenal cortex. The physiological meaning is as yet obscure (*see* Page and Bumpus, 1974; Genest, 1984).

Physiological Significance of the Other Angiotensins. The functions of angiotensins other than angiotensin II have yet to be defined. In the rat, concentrations of angiotensin III in plasma may approach those of angiotensin II; they are much lower in man and dog.

CLINICAL CONSIDERATIONS

Angiotensin itself is of limited therapeutic usefulness, and most clinical interest focuses on antagonists of angiotensin and inhibitors of other components of the renin-angiotensin system. Nevertheless, the peptide has occasionally been used as an alternative to sympathomimetic amines, where its unique properties offer some advantage—for example, in hypotensive crises encountered during the administration of halogenated anesthetics, where cardiac arrhythmias are a potential hazard. With the advent of potent drugs that inhibit endogenous formation of angiotensin II and precipitate grave hypotension in some patients, the use of angiotensin as an antidote may increase (*see* Hodsman and Robertson, 1983).

Angiotensin is a very potent pressor agent. Its effects are well sustained and are very unlikely to be accompanied by disturbing cardiac arrhythmias or to be followed by hypotension. Moreover, the peptide does not cause spasm of the vein into which it is infused. On the other hand, neither does it significantly constrict the capacitance vessels, increase venous return, or stimulate cardiac output. Too rapid infusion of angiotensin may raise systemic blood pressure to dangerous heights. Profound reflex bradycardia and, occasionally, ventricular arrhythmias may occur.

Preparation. *Angiotensin amide* (HYPERTENSIN), the amide of angiotensin II (1-L-asparaginyl-5-L-valyl angiotensin octapeptide), is the preparation that has been used clinically. It is not available commercially in the United States. The drug is given slowly by intravenous infusion at a rate of about 0.01 to 0.2 μg/kg per minute. Blood pressure must be monitored closely.

INHIBITORS OF THE RENIN-ANGIOTENSIN SYSTEM

Drugs that specifically inhibit actions of biologically active endogenous substances or prevent their formation have traditionally provided some of the most powerful probes with which to determine the function of these autacoids in physiological and pathological processes. Such drugs, moreover, are frequently found to have valuable therapeutic applications. For many years, therefore, inhibitors of the renin-angiotensin system have been sought, with a particular impetus provided by the possibility of discovering effective antihypertensive drugs.

In the 1970s, two distinct classes of effective inhibitors of the renin-angiotensin system were identified: *angiotensin II antagonists,* which block receptors for the peptide, and *converting-enzyme inhibitors,* which slow the rate of formation of angiotensin II from its inactive precursor. Their discovery and experimental application led to rapid advances in the field and to the introduction of a new category of clinically useful antihypertensive drugs, the orally effective converting-enzyme inhibitors. Drugs of the latter type, exemplified by *captopril,* have proven to be effective in a surprisingly broad range of patients with essential hypertension, as well as for those with the more classically recognized renin-dependent hypertensive conditions. This, in turn, has heightened interest in alternative approaches to inhibition of the renin-

angiotensin system. Some recent experimental results with *inhibitors of renin* appear promising (*see* below). Moreover, inhibition of sympathetic secretomotor control of renin secretion from the JG cells seems to contribute to the salutary effects of β-adrenergic antagonists and some other antihypertensive agents on blood pressure (*see* Chapters 9 and 32).

ANTAGONISTS OF ANGIOTENSIN II

The useful antagonists of angiotensin II are slightly modified congeners in which agonist activity is profoundly attenuated by replacement of phenylalanine in position 8 with some other amino acid; in addition, stability is enhanced by substitutions that slow degradation and thus prolong the life of a given compound in the circulation. The best studied of these antagonists of angiotensin II combines alanine in position 8 with sarcosine (N-methylglycine) in position 1; the "blocked" amino acid sarcosine not only slows degradation of the peptide but also increases its affinity for the receptor. This substance, $[Sar^1, Val^5, Ala^8]$angiotensin-(1-8)octapeptide or *saralasin,* was introduced by Pals and associates in 1971, who showed that it effectively antagonized the pressor effects of angiotensin II in rats and that it lowered blood pressure in renin-dependent hypertensive animals. They suggested that the drug could be used to assess the function of endogenous angiotensin II in the regulation of blood pressure. The possible utility of saralasin in man soon became apparent when it was shown not only to block pressor responses to injected angiotensin but also to lower blood pressure in certain renin-dependent hypertensive patients and even in normal subjects who were depleted of sodium (*see* Atlas *et al.,* 1983; Laragh, 1984).

Pharmacological Properties. Saralasin and related drugs compete with angiotensin II for its receptors. Because their residual agonist activity is only about 1% of that of angiotensin II, they behave as competitive inhibitors in the presence of the latter. However, qualitatively, they behave like angiotensin II itself in the absence of the peptide (*see* Bumpus, 1977; Peach, 1977); they are thus classified as partial agonists. When given by intravenous infusion to healthy individuals or to patients with hypertension, saralasin commonly causes a transient rise in blood pressure that lasts for 1 to 2 minutes and its action then evolves in different ways, depending largely on the concentration of endogenous angiotensin II. In the normal, sodium-replete individual, the pressor response tends to be relatively well sustained. In the sodium-depleted individual, the response is not sustained and there may be a depressor phase. In individuals with hypertension, there is a broad correspondence between the dependency of the condition on renin and the response. Thus, saralasin commonly causes a fall in systemic blood pressure in patients with renovascular hypertension, whereas sharp, sustained pressor responses may be encountered in patients with so-called low-renin essential hypertension. Saralasin has thus found clinical application as an aid in the differential diagnosis of hypertension and in the assessment of the involvement of renin. However, the blood pressure responses are complicated by the residual agonist activity of the compound and are so subject to sodium balance and other variables that false-positive and false-negative results are numerous. A better index of the participation of renin in hypertensive states is thus provided by inhibitors of converting enzyme (*see* Laragh, 1984).

Preparation and Dosage. *Saralasin acetate* (SARENIN) is available for intravenous infusion in 30-ml ampuls that contain 18 mg as the acetate. The possible hazards of exaggerated changes in blood pressure should be borne in mind.

Prior to evaluation of the response to saralasin, the patient is mildly depleted of sodium by the administration of furosemide (*e.g.*, 80 mg orally the evening before) or by adherence to a low-sodium diet for 3 to 5 days. Blood pressure is monitored frequently, and, when stable, saralasin can be given by intravenous infusion (18 mg over 20 to 30 minutes). Alternatively, for patients in whom a marked change in blood pressure would constitute a particular risk, the infusion can be initiated at a very low rate (0.05 μg/kg per minute); this is increased to 5, 10, and 20 μg/kg per minute at 10-minute intervals until a pressor or depressor response occurs. With either schedule, the test is terminated if there is a sustained change in blood pressure. Some patients who display a marked depressor response may exhibit rebound hypertension 1 to 3 hours later.

INHIBITORS OF ANGIOTENSIN CONVERTING ENZYME

The discovery of potent inhibitors of converting enzyme provides one of many illustrations of the utility of seemingly esoteric pharmacological enquiry on the properties of poisons of plant or animal origin. It arose from observations by Ferreira and colleagues in the 1960s that the venoms of pit vipers are not only capable of forming bradykinin (*see* below) but also contain factors that intensify responses to bradykinin. These bradykinin potentiating factors (BPFs) proved to be a family of peptides of 5 to 13 amino acid residues, which were identified and subsequently synthesized. They were shown to inhibit an enzyme that catalyzes the degradation and inactivation of bradykinin (now known as kininase II). In 1968, Bakhle observed that these same peptides also inhibit the converting enzyme responsible for forming angiotensin II. Soon thereafter Erdös and associates established that angiotensin converting enzyme and kininase II are one and the same enzyme, a peptidyl dipeptidase (or dipeptidyl carboxypeptidase). Thus, a single enzyme catalyzes both the *synthesis* of angiotensin II, the most potent pressor substance

known, and the *destruction* of bradykinin, the most potent vasodilator. This curious fact complicates interpretation of the mode of hypotensive action of drugs that inhibit the enzyme. Nevertheless, the principal pharmacological and clinical effects of these drugs seem to arise from suppression of synthesis of angiotensin II. This is understandable, since such synthesis is a specific and critical function of converting enzyme, whereas destruction of bradykinin is readily and rapidly achieved by other enzymes. In this light, there is some justification for reference to inhibitors of the enzyme as (angiotensin) converting-enzyme inhibitors (ACE inhibitors). However, this loose terminology should not be allowed to obscure the fact that the inhibitors, albeit specific at the level of the enzyme, act on an enzyme with many substrates, among which are potent autacoids, enkephalins, and others.

Following the discovery of the BPFs, the nonapeptide BPF$_{9a}$ became available in synthetic form (*teprotide*) and was tested in man. It was found, on intravenous administration, to lower blood pressure more consistently than did the angiotensin II antagonists and in a much broader spectrum of individuals, including many patients with essential hypertension. This was a signal event that implicated angiotensin still more widely in the pathogenesis of hypertension, showed the feasibility of treatment with this approach, and encouraged the search for compounds that, in contrast to peptides, would be effective orally. This search culminated in the introduction of the orally effective converting-enzyme inhibitor *captopril* and has provided a fresh and powerful type of drug therapy for hypertension and, as events have shown, for cardiac failure.

Chemistry. The most thoroughly studied of the peptide inhibitors of converting enzyme is the nonapeptide (BPF$_{9a}$) known as *teprotide;* it has the following structure: pyroGlu-Trp-Pro-Arg-Pro-Gln-Ile-Pro-Pro (*see* Cushman *et al.*, 1977). Teprotide (like other BPFs) acts as a competitive inhibitor of converting enzyme, with an affinity for the enzyme much higher than that of angiotensin I. It is not itself a substrate for the enzyme. Although converting enzyme will cleave many different C-terminal dipeptide residues, it will not cleave peptides with proline in the penultimate position, as with teprotide and other BPFs. As noted, the penultimate proline in angiotensin II is, indeed, responsible for its refractoriness to further cleavage by converting enzyme. Moreover, the presence of pyroGlu at the N terminus renders teprotide refractory to aminopeptidases; this confers further stability and effectiveness *in vivo*. Nevertheless, teprotide has a relatively short duration of action and must be given parenterally to be effective.

The orally effective converting-enzyme inhibitor *captopril* (Cushman *et al.*, 1977) was developed by a rational approach that involved analysis of the inhibitory action of teprotide; inferences about the action of converting enzyme on its substrates; and analogy with carboxypeptidase A, which was known to be inhibited by D-benzylsuccinic acid. Ondetti, Cushman, and their colleagues argued that inhibition of converting enzyme might be produced by succinyl amino acids that corresponded in length to the dipeptide cleaved by converting enzyme. This proved to be true and led ultimately to the synthesis of a series of carboxy alkanoyl or mercapto alkanoyl derivatives that acted as potent competitive inhibitors of the enzyme (*see* Petrillo and Ondetti, 1982). Most active (with a K_i of 1.7 nM) was D-3-mercapto-methylpropanoyl-L-proline or captopril, which has the following structure:

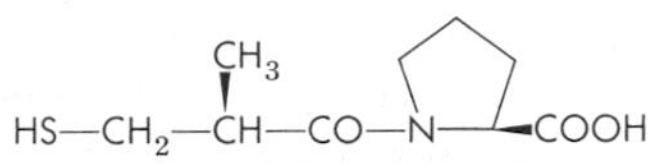

Captopril

Various other inhibitors of converting enzyme have since been synthesized. One such is *enalaprilic acid* (with a K_i of about 0.2 nM). It resembles captopril in containing a "proline surrogate," but it differs in that it is an analog of a tripeptide rather than a dipeptide. Enalaprilic acid itself is poorly absorbed orally; it is administered orally as the monoethyl ester, *enalapril*, which serves as a prodrug. The structure of enalapril is as follows:

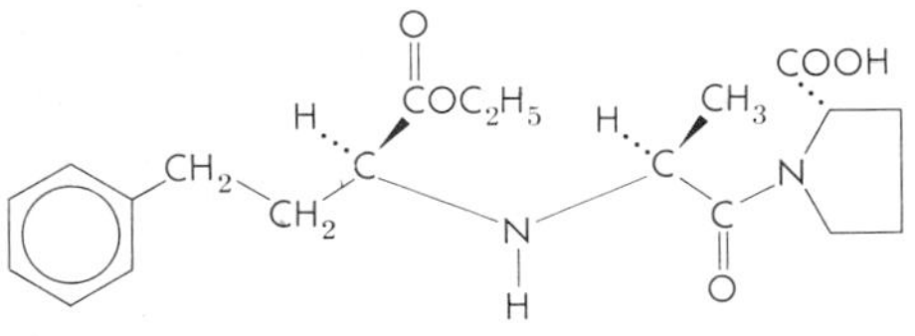

Enalapril

Pharmacological Effects. The essential effect of these agents on the renin-angiotensin system is to inhibit conversion of the relatively inactive angiotensin I to the active angiotensin II (or the conversion of [des-Asp[1]]angiotensin I to angiotensin III). In this way they attenuate or abolish responses to angiotensin I. The converting-enzyme inhibitors are highly specific drugs. They do not interact, directly, with other components of the renin-angiotensin system, including receptors for the peptide. For example, when tested on isolated smooth muscle preparations (*e.g.*, the guinea pig ileum) that possess membrane-bound converting-enzyme activity *in vitro*, they selectively reduce responsiveness to angiotensin I without influencing that to angiotensin II or, indeed, to any of many other pharmacological agents, with the notable exception of bradykinin, which, of course, is potentiated. Accounts of the biological activities of drugs of this class are presented in several reviews and symposia

(*see,* for example, Heel *et al.*, 1980; Antonaccio, 1982; Petrillo and Ondetti, 1982; Romankiewicz *et al.*, 1983; Doyle and Bearn, 1984; Symposium, 1984a).

Cardiovascular System. In vivo, the characteristic result of inhibition of converting enzyme is attenuation or loss of the pressor response to intravenous injection of angiotensin I; that to angiotensin II is unaffected (Collier *et al.*, 1973). A single, small oral dose (20 mg) of captopril in the human subject abolishes the pressor effect of angiotensin I for more than 2 hours, and about 4 hours are needed for 50% recovery (Ferguson *et al.*, 1977). The capacity of angiotensin I to stimulate secretion of aldosterone is likewise suppressed. These two phenomena are central to the *in-vivo* effects of the converting-enzyme inhibitors and explain much of the therapeutic utility of the compounds. However, the total response *in vivo* is more complex, and for a variety of reasons.

Because the renin-angiotensin system participates in homeostasis, it follows that suppression of the biosynthesis of angiotensin II might set compensatory adjustments in motion. Indeed, there is usually a striking increase in renin secretion, leading to very high concentrations of circulating renin and angiotensin I. Although in such circumstances formation of angiotensin II may still be low, these changes may not be devoid of other functional significance; knowledge is currently inadequate. A second complication is that, despite their apparent high selectivity of action, the enzyme they inhibit is less fastidious and hydrolyzes bradykinin among other biologically active peptides. While such effects may contribute to the broad spectrum of responses observed *in vivo*, present evidence indicates that the effects of clinical interest are due mainly to reduced concentrations of angiotensin II. Thirdly, one should bear in mind that most knowledge of the actions and functions of the renin-angiotensin system has come from acute experiments, whereas many of the unexpected and therapeutically useful responses to converting-enzyme inhibitors occur during long-term treatment. These unanticipated responses may point to unrecognized functions of the renin-angiotensin system that are exerted over a longer time frame—for example, there may be trophic or permissive influences on sympathetic outflow. Finally, it should be remembered that the components of the renin-angiotensin system are present in many tissues. Relevant in this context, for example, is the isorenin system present in the blood vessels themselves. It is against this complex background that one must view the effects of converting-enzyme inhibitors, which are much more extensive than had been expected.

In healthy, sodium-replete animals and man, a single oral dose of captopril (100 mg in man) lowers systemic blood pressure, supine or erect, but the effect is slight (Atlas *et al.,* 1983). With repeated doses over a period of several days, however, there is a more prominent reduction in blood pressure and a subtle blunting of compensatory postural reflexes. By contrast, even a single dose of captopril regularly lowers blood pressure substantially in normal subjects when they have been depleted of sodium. This effect is accompanied by a clear fall in total peripheral resistance; a small effect on vascular resistance may also be seen in sodium-replete subjects, even when no fall in blood pressure is evident.

Effects in Hypertension. Captopril lowers systemic arteriolar resistance and mean, diastolic, and systolic blood pressures in various hypertensive states. The effects are readily observed in animal models of renal hypertension, such as the classical Goldblatt hypertensive rat, and they are also seen in the spontaneously hypertensive rat, which is considered to be a more reasonable model of essential hypertension in man (and in which plasma renin activity is about the same as in normotensive rats). In human subjects with hypertension of most types, with the exception of that due to primary aldosteronism, captopril commonly lowers blood pressure. The initial reduction tends to be positively correlated with PRA and angiotensin II concentrations prior to treatment. However, as treatment with captopril is continued, a greater number of patients show a sizable reduction in blood pressure, and the antihypertensive effect then correlates poorly or not at all with pretreatment values of PRA. This result, which is as yet little understood, presents a challenge to current understanding of the mechanisms of hypertension. At the same time it confers on captopril and other drugs of this class a welcome breadth of clinical utility as antihypertensive agents.

The fall in systemic blood pressure observed in hypertensive individuals results from a reduction of total peripheral resistance in which there seems to be a somewhat variable participation by different vascular beds. The kidney is a notable exception to this variability, in that there is a prominent vasodilator effect and increased blood flow is a relatively constant finding (*see* Symposium, 1984a). This is perhaps not surprising, since the renal vessels are exceptionally sensitive to the vasoconstrictor actions of angiotensin II. Blood flow in cerebral and coronary beds, where autoregulatory phenomena are prominent, is generally well maintained.

Beside causing systemic arteriolar dilatation, captopril increases the compliance of large arteries, and this contributes to reduction of systolic pressure. Cardiac function in patients with uncomplicated hypertension is generally little changed, although there may be a slight increase in stroke volume and cardiac output with sustained treatment. Baroreceptor function and cardiovascular reflexes are not compromised, and responses to postural changes and exercise are litte impaired. Yet surprisingly, even when a substantial lowering of blood pressure is achieved, heart rate generally increases little. This perhaps reflects an alteration of baroreceptor function with increased arterial compliance.

Secretion of aldosterone in the general population of hypertensive individuals is reduced, but not seriously impaired, by inhibition of converting enzyme. The stimulation that results from postural changes, in which angiotensin plays a prominent role, is much attenuated. However, aldosterone output is maintained at adequate levels by other secretagogues, such as ACTH and potassium. The activity of these secretagogues on the zona glomerulosa of the adrenal cortex requires, at most, only very small trophic or permissive amounts of angiotensin II, which are always present since inhibition of converting enzyme is never complete. Excessive retention of potassium is encountered only occasionally.

Effects in Chronic Congestive Heart Failure. This condition presents a complex pathophysiological profile (*see* Chapter 30). Inhibition of converting enzyme by captopril commonly results in beneficial modification of many of the distorted parameters that contribute to the vicious cycle that is operative. Systemic arteriolar dilatation reduces afterload, and both cardiac output and cardiac index increase, as do indices of stroke work and stroke volume. Heart rate is generally reduced. Systemic blood pressure falls, sometimes steeply at the outset, but tends to return toward initial levels. Renovascular resistance falls sharply, and renal blood flow increases. There is a natriuresis as a result of the improved renal hemodynamics and the reduced stimulus to secretion of aldosterone by angiotensin II. The excess volume of body fluids contracts, which reduces venous return to the right heart. A further reduction results from venodilatation and an increased capacity of the venous bed. Venodilatation is another somewhat-unexpected effect of inhibition of converting enzyme, for angiotensin II has little acute venoconstrictor activity. Nevertheless, chronic infusion of angiotensin II has been reported to increase venous tone *in vivo,* perhaps by some central or peripheral interaction with the sympathetic nervous system (*see* Schwartz and Chatterjee, 1983). The response to the converting-enzyme inhibitor also involves reductions of pulmonary arterial pressure, pulmonary capillary wedge pressure, and left atrial and left ventricular filling pressure (preload). The better hemodynamic performance results in increased tolerance of exercise. Cerebral and coronary blood flows are usually well maintained, even when systemic blood pressure is very substantially reduced (*see* Symposium, 1982a, 1983c, 1984a; Romankiewicz *et al.,* 1983; Schwartz and Chatterjee, 1983).

Absorption, Fate, and Excretion. Captopril is rapidly absorbed when given orally. Bioavailability averages about 65% and is reduced significantly by food; the drug is thus generally given 1 hour before meals. Peak concentrations in plasma occur within an hour, and the drug is cleared rapidly (half-life of approximately 2 hours). About 95% of the drug is eliminated in the urine, about 50% as captopril itself and the rest as metabolites (disulfide dimer and cysteine disulfide). Excretion is slowed in patients with impaired renal function.

Precautions and Adverse Reactions. Untoward reactions occasionally appear to be a specific result of inhibition of converting enzyme. A steep fall in blood pressure may occur, for example, following the first dose of captopril in patients with severe hypertension who have been treated with multidrug regimens that include diuretics. A similar reaction may occur in patients with congestive heart failure, especially when they have been vigorously treated with diuretics. Care should be exercised in patients who are likely to be depleted of salt and water. Treatment should be initiated with very small doses of the inhibitor and preferably at an interval after withdrawal of the diuretic. The latter can be given again, subsequently, if necessary. Inhibition of converting enzyme can also induce renal insufficiency in patients with bilateral renal stenosis or with stenosis of the artery to a single remaining kidney. This is apparently caused by reduction of the concentration of angiotensin II, which is needed in such conditions to constrict the efferent glomerular arterioles and maintain adequate glomerular filtration. Despite some reduction in the concentration of aldosterone, significant retention of potassium is rarely encountered.

Captopril is generally well tolerated. In one large series of patients who received about 350 mg of captopril daily, the estimated 4-year cumulative frequency of discontinuation of the drug because of side effects was less then 12%. This compares favorably with the value for other standard antihypertensive agents (*e.g.,* the corresponding value is 15% for propranolol) (*see* Groel *et al.,* 1983). Subsequent studies with smaller doses of captopril (<150 mg per day) indicate a lower incidence of side effects. Among these are *erythematous and other rashes, disturbance or loss of the sense of taste, vertigo, headache, hypotension,* and various minor *gastrointestinal disturbances*. All of these may disappear with continued treatment. *Neutropenia* is a serious but relatively rare toxicity; the incidence is substantially increased in patients with renal insufficiency or autoimmune disease, such as lupus erythematosus or collagen vascular diseases. *Proteinuria* (>1.0 g per day) may occur, particularly in patients with a history of renal disease. Early suggestions of an association between captopril and membranous glomerulopathy have not been supported by more recent studies (*see* Groel *et al.*, 1983).

Preparation and Dosage. *Captopril* (CAPOTEN) is available in tablets containing 25, 50, or 100 mg. The drug should be taken 1 hour or so before meals. The recommended initial dose for adults is 25 mg three times a day. This is increased, as necessary, at intervals of 1 to 2 weeks to 50 mg and then to 100 mg. The maximal daily dose should not exceed 450 mg. Recent experience indicates that twice-daily dosage commonly suffices and that more than 150 mg daily is rarely needed. Very much smaller doses, 6.25 mg or less three times daily, are appropriate for initiation of therapy in patients with heart failure or in others who have received intensive therapy with diuretics. Reduced dosage is also indicated for patients with impaired renal function.

Therapeutic Uses. Converting-enzyme inhibitors were developed specifically to modify an identified pathogenic factor in arterial hypertension. Although captopril, the archetypal compound, has been in clinical use for only a few years, its ability to lower blood pressure in a majority of patients with *hypertension* of various types is well established. A whole new therapeutic approach to this major clinical problem has thus opened. In addition, these drugs have proven to be useful in the treatment of *congestive heart failure*.

Hypertension. In initial clinical studies, captopril was administered predominantly to severely ill patients with advanced hypertension who were refractory to standard multidrug antihypertensive regimens. The inhibitor was commonly given alone and, to obtain a rapid response, in high doses. While reduction of systemic blood pressure was generally achieved, several significant adverse reactions, including renal toxicity and neutropenia, were encountered. In the light of the perceived risk-to-benefit ratio, extension of the use of captopril to patients with less severe and uncomplicated forms of hypertension was judged to be inappropriate.

Subsequent clinical experience indicates that converting-enzyme inhibitors have a broader range of usefulness. It is now known that a maximal lowering of blood pressure may take some weeks to develop and that significant reduction in blood pressure may be achieved in many hypertensive patients with relatively low doses of captopril that cause relatively few adverse reactions; this is especially true when captopril is used concurrently with a diuretic. There is thus increasing interest in the use of captopril and other converting-enzyme inhibitors in mild-to-moderate essential hypertension. When used as the sole antihypertensive agent, captopril is roughly comparable in its activity to a thiazide diuretic or a β-adrenergic antagonist, and it lowers blood pressure significantly in

about half of patients in this group. When used with a thiazide diuretic, this fraction rises to more than 80%. The concurrent administration of a β-adrenergic blocking agent also enhances the response, but to a lesser extent. This is perhaps because the β-adrenergic blockers owe their efficacy, in part, to inhibition of renin release.

The precise place of captopril, or other inhibitors of converting enzyme such as enalapril, in the treatment of mild-to-moderate essential hypertension remains to be established. However, it is apparent that drugs of this class offer several advantages. Since they have no sympatholytic activity, cardiovascular reflexes are retained, responses to exercise and posture are not disrupted, and postural hypotension is rare. Unlike β-adrenergic antagonists, they are not contraindicated in patients with bronchial asthma or diabetes (*see* Chapter 9). In contrast to the thiazide diuretics, they do not cause hypokalemia, hyperuricemia, or hyperglycemia. Indeed, they oppose the secondary hyperaldosteronism produced by the diuretics and ameliorate or prevent the hypokalemia. Furthermore, they are well tolerated and have relatively little tendency to cause side effects such as lethargy, weakness, and sexual dysfunction that not uncommonly diminish the "quality of life" and undermine compliance of patients on standard multidrug antihypertensive therapy. Indeed, patients formerly treated with such standard regimens have reported an improved sense of well-being during treatment with a converting-enzyme inhibitor. (*See* Beyer and Peuler, 1982; Symposium, 1982a, 1983c, 1984a; Hodsman and Robertson, 1983; Johnston *et al.*, 1984.) These facts argue that converting-enzyme inhibitors will find increasing use in the treatment of mild-to-moderate hypertension.

Some less common hypertensive conditions in which converting-enzyme inhibitors appear to be particularly useful include *malignant hypertension, renovascular hypertension, hypertensive crisis of scleroderma*, and *dialysis-resistant hypertension* in end-stage renal failure (*see* reviews just cited; *see also* Chapter 32).

Chronic Congestive Heart Failure. Vasodilators have a valued place in the management of acute heart failure, but their utility in chronic congestive failure has been more limited (*see* Smith and Braunwald, 1984; *see also* Chapter 33). Converting-enzyme inhibitors not only induce systemic arteriolar dilatation, and thereby reduce afterload, but they also cause venodilatation, lessen fluid retention, and thus reduce preload. These and other beneficial effects described above lead to increased cardiac output, amelioration of signs and symptoms of congestion, increased exercise tolerance, and improved clinical status. Although initially indicated for patients inadequately controlled by digitalis and diuretics, converting-enzyme inhibitors are now being used at earlier stages of cardiac decompensation. (*See* Symposium, 1982a, 1983c, 1984a; Romankiewicz *et al.*, 1983; Schwartz and Chatterjee, 1983.)

Enalapril. This newer inhibitor of converting enzyme has a mechanism of action and spectrum of pharmacological effects and therapeutic applications that are characteristic of those described for captopril. Clinical experience has indicated that enalapril is efficacious in the same broad range of hypertensive conditions, although the main focus has been on essential hypertension (usually mild to moderate) and on chronic congestive heart failure. However, enalapril has several distinctive features. While of minor significance, it is considerably more potent than captopril. Of greater interest is the prolonged duration of action of enalapril; the drug binds more tightly to converting enzyme and persists longer in the plasma. This often allows effective treatment with a single daily dose, although twice-daily dosage may sometimes be more appropriate. Furthermore, in contrast to captopril, enalapril is not a sulfhydryl compound. Present evidence suggests that some of the side effects of captopril are due to the sulfhydryl group; these may thus be encountered less frequently. The incidences of rash and disturbance of taste appear to be lower; however, both neutropenia and proteinuria, although rare, have been encountered. The relative merits of captopril and enalapril (and other converting-enzyme inhibitors under development) will become clear only with the accumulation of a great deal more data.

Enalapril is rapidly absorbed when given orally, and bioavailability is little affected by food. Unlike captopril, enalapril is a prodrug that is not itself highly active, and it must be hydrolyzed to the active parent dicarboxylic acid, enalaprilate. Plasma concentrations of the latter reach a maximum only after 3 to 4 hours. The onset of action after oral administration is thus slower than with captopril, and peak reduction in blood pressure occurs some 4 to 6 hours after ingestion. By contrast, responses to enalaprilate given intravenously are apparent in 15 minutes (*see* Sweet, 1983; Symposium, 1983c; Doyle and Bearn, 1984; Joint National Committee, 1984).

Preparations and Dosage. Enalapril maleate (VASOTEC) is available for oral use as tablets containing 5, 10, or 20 mg. Daily dosage ranges from a total of 10 mg to 40 mg (occasionally 80 mg), given once or in divided doses. Enalaprilate (*enalaprilat injection*) is provided in solutions for injection that contain 1 or 5 mg/ml. Both drugs are for investigational use in the United States at the present time.

RENIN INHIBITORS

Inhibitors of renin are attracting increasing interest both as analytical tools and as possible therapeutic agents. Various highly active inhibitors have recently been described, and some have potent hypotensive activity in man when given intravenously. Inhibitors containing as few as three residues have been found, and it seems possible that compounds of clinical value may become available (*see* Fehrentz *et al.*, 1984; Haber, 1984).

PLASMA KININS (KALLIDIN, BRADYKININ)

History. The discovery of the plasma kinins had its origins in the old observation that urine, injected intravenously, lowers blood pressure. In the 1920s

and 1930s, Frey and his associates Kraut and Werle characterized the hypotensive substance and showed that similar material could be obtained from saliva, plasma, and a variety of tissues. Since the pancreas was a rich source, they named this material *kallikrein* after an old Greek synonym for that organ, *kallikréas*. By 1937, Werle, Götze, and Keppler had established that kallikreins have an indirect effect and, behaving as enzymes, split off a pharmacologically active substance from some inactive precursor present in plasma. Their discovery preceded by 2 years the analogous finding that renin acts similarly. In 1948, Werle and Berek named the active substance *kallidin* and showed it to be a polypeptide cleaved from a plasma globulin that they termed *kallidinogen* (*see* Werle, 1970).

Interest in the field intensified when Rocha e Silva and associates (1949) reported that the venoms of certain snakes, as well as the enzyme trypsin, acted on plasma globulin to produce a substance, probably a polypeptide, that also lowered blood pressure and caused a slowly developing contraction of the gut. Because of the slow response of the gut, they named this substance *bradykinin*, a term derived from the Greek words *bradys*, meaning "slow," and *kinein*, meaning "to move." Since bradykinin and kallidin were formed under similar conditions and had similar pharmacological actions, it was early suspected that they were closely related. Identification of the pure materials some 10 years later confirmed this suspicion. In 1960, bradykinin, formed by reacting trypsin with globulin, was isolated by Elliott and coworkers and synthesized by Boissonnas and associates. It proved to be a nonapeptide of the structure shown below. Shortly thereafter, this same nonapeptide was found to be a constituent of kallidin, which, however, also contained a pharmacologically similar decapeptide with the same sequence of amino acids but with an additional N-terminal lysine residue. These substances are now recognized to be but two of a large number of polypeptides that have related chemical structures and pharmacological properties and that are widely distributed in nature. For the whole group the generic term *kinins* has been adopted, and kallidin and bradykinin are referred to as *plasma kinins* (*see* Bertaccini, 1976; Erdös, 1979; Schachter and Barton, 1979; Fritz *et al.*, 1983).

Synthesis and Catabolism of Kinins and Other Chemical Considerations. Because two separate experimental paths led to the identification of the plasma kinins, nomenclature has been confused. The term *kallidin* (which formerly embraced both the nonapeptide and decapeptide) is now restricted to the decapeptide, while the term *bradykinin* has been retained for the nonapeptide. Bradykinin has the following amino acid sequence: Arg-Pro-Pro-Gly-Phe-Ser-Pro-Phe-Arg. Kallidin has an additional lysine residue in the N-terminal position and is sometimes referred to as lysyl-bradykinin. The two peptides are cleaved from precursors, referred to as *kininogens*, in the plasma α_2-globulin fraction (Figure 27–3). This cleavage may be effected by enzymes (serine proteases) collectively referred to as *kininogenases*. Among these the greatest inter-

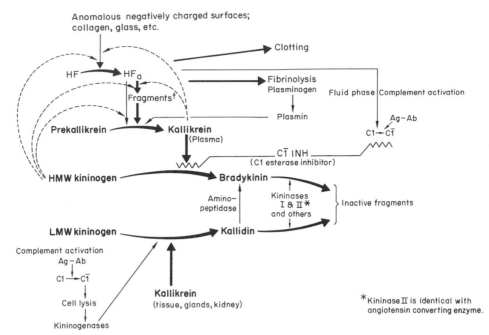

Figure 27–3. *Formation and destruction of the kinins.*

Bradykinin and kallidin are formed, respectively, by plasma and tissue kallikreins. Note the relationship of the plasma kinin–forming system to other Hageman factor (HF)–dependent processes, notably blood clotting and fibrinolysis. Observe that two components of the kinin cascade, prekallikrein and high-molecular-weight (HMW) kininogen, are essential for HF activation and function and hence are also clotting factors (*see* Chapter 58). Their points of interaction are indicated by the dashed arrows; note especially the strong positive feedback provided by kallikrein, which is a major HF activator in the fluid phase and mainly responsible for the formation of the HF fragments (†) that are potent "kallikrein activators." The kallikrein-inhibiting effect of complement C1 esterase inhibitor (C1 INH) is indicated; this is the primary inhibitor of plasma kallikrein. Other plasma protease inhibitors, α_2-macroglobulin and α_1-antitrypsin, act at the same site. The latter seems to be of more importance, however, with regard to inhibition of tissue kallikrein. The activation of complement by antigen-antibody complexes (Ag-Ab), leading to cell lysis liberating kininogenases, is indicated, along with fluid-phase activation of complement by HF$_a$. Negative-feedback, "restraining" mechanisms and many other complexities are omitted. Note that kininase II is the same enzyme (dipeptidyl carboxypeptidase) as angiotensin converting enzyme (*see* text and Figure 27–1.)

est attaches to the *kallikreins,* a group of enzymes of high substrate specificity that are present in plasma and in many other body fluids, cells, and tissues (*e.g.,* the kidney, various exocrine glands and their secretions, lymph, exudates, joint fluids, and urine). Some kallikrein is in the active form; some as the zymogen. Other kininogenases include trypsin, plasmin, and various proteolytic enzymes in certain snake and insect venoms and bacteria. Plasma kallikrein (like trypsin and snake venoms) releases the nonapeptide kinin *bradykinin* directly from a kininogen of high (~100,000) molecular weight (HMW kininogen). Glandular and other tissue kallikreins release the decapeptide kinin *kallidin* from a kininogen of lower (~50,000) molecular weight (LMW kininogen).

The kinins have an evanescent existence—their half-life in plasma is only about 15 seconds. Moreover, in a single passage through the pulmonary vascular bed some 80 to 90% of the kinins may be destroyed and as many as five peptide bonds may be cleaved (*see* Ryan, 1982). The principal catabolizing enzyme in the lung and in other vascular beds is the dipeptidyl carboxypeptidase known in this context as kininase II and in another (*see* above) as angiotensin converting enzyme. Removal of the carboxy-terminal dipeptide abolishes kinin-like activity. A slower-acting enzyme, arginine carboxypeptidase (carboxypeptidase-N; kininase I), removes the carboxy-terminal arginine. This too usually abolishes kinin-like activity; however, the des-Arg kinins that are formed may be active in some damaged tissues, where the characteristics of the receptor are apparently altered (*see* Marceau *et al.,* 1983).

Normal blood contains all essential ingredients for the formation of massive amounts of bradykinin. Usually, very little bradykinin is formed, mainly because plasma kallikrein is present in an inactive form, prekallikrein. Conversion of prekallikrein to kallikrein, with resultant formation of bradykinin, is, however, readily brought about by various factors. These include substantial changes in pH or temperature and contact with negatively charged surfaces, such as occur on glass and kaolin or on biological material such as collagen, which is readily exposed by tissue damage. A common triggering element is activation of Hageman factor (HF), which also sets in motion the coagulation cascade and fibrinolysis. (It is unclear why formation of kinins is integrated with these other phenomena.) Protease inhibitors present in plasma exert a restraining influence on the cascade. Prominent among them is the inhibitor of the activated first component of complement (C$\bar{1}$ INH), but α_2-macroglobulin is also potent. Another inhibitor, α_1-antitrypsin, acts slowly and may serve mainly to inactivate, preferentially, small amounts of circulating tissue (glandular) kallikreins; the latter kallikreins are resistant to inhibition by α_2-macroglobulin. The synthesis and destruction of kinins are schematized in Figure 27–3. Extensive discussion of this complex field can be found in various reviews (Erdös, 1970, 1979; Fujii et al., 1979; Schachter and Barton, 1979; Fritz et al., 1983).

The decapeptide kallidin is about as active as the nonapeptide bradykinin and need not be converted to the latter to exert its characteristic effects. Some conversion of kallidin to bradykinin occurs as the N-terminal lysine residue is removed by the activity of plasma aminopeptidase, as indicated in Figure 27–3. However, this reaction is slow relative to inactivation by hydrolysis at the carboxy terminus. The minimal effective structure required to elicit the classical responses is that of the nonapeptide. It is, however, interesting that in certain conditions that mainly involve damage to tissues, the normally inactive products of hydrolysis by kininase I, namely des-Arg^9-bradykinin and des-Arg^{10}-kallidin, possess considerable activity (see Marceau et al., 1983). Despite much effort, no effective antagonists that act at kinin receptors have been discovered (see Erdös, 1979; Regoli and Barabé, 1980; Marceau et al., 1983).

PHARMACOLOGICAL PROPERTIES

The plasma kinins possess an extraordinarily high degree of pharmacological activity. They are the most potent vasodilator autacoids of mammals, and in very low concentration they increase capillary permeability, produce edema, evoke pain and reflexes by acting on nerve endings, contract or relax various smooth muscles (directly or through short or longer nervous paths), and elicit sundry other responses. In all these respects bradykinin and kallidin behave very similarly (see Erdös, 1970, 1979; Schachter and Barton, 1979; Regoli and Barabé, 1980; Marceau et al., 1983).

Cardiovascular System. *Blood Vessels.* On a molar basis, kinins are about ten times more potent than histamine in causing vasodilatation. Intrave-

nously in man they cause flushing in the blush area and conjunctival injection. Blood vessels in muscle, kidney, viscera, and various glands are also dilated, as are coronary and cerebral vessels; throbbing headache may occur. Certain of these direct effects may be complemented by the ability of kinins to stimulate the release of histamine from mast cells. Effects on pulmonary vessels vary with dose, species, and state of development. Dilatation of systemic arterioles causes a sharp fall in systolic and diastolic blood pressures. In contrast, large arteries and most veins, large and small, tend to be contracted by the kinins; however, dilator responses may also be encountered, and kinins are among the agents that induce endothelium-dependent vasodilatation. Kinins promote dilatation of the fetal pulmonary artery, closure of the ductus arteriosus, and constriction of the umbilical vessels, all of which occur in the adjustment from fetal to neonatal circulation.

Heart. Cardiac muscle is not directly affected by bradykinin, but the fall in total peripheral resistance and systemic blood pressure due to vasodilatation, combined with contraction of the large veins and increased venous return, causes a reflex increase in heart rate and increased cardiac output.

Vascular Permeability and Edema Formation. The plasma kinins increase permeability in the microcirculation. The effect, like that of histamine and 5-hydroxytryptamine, is exerted on the small venules and involves separation of the junctions between endothelial cells. This, together with an increased hydrostatic pressure gradient, causes edema to form. Such edema, coupled with stimulation of nerve endings (see below), results in a "wheal-and-flare" response to intradermal injections in man.

Extravascular Smooth Muscle. Various smooth muscle preparations contract in response to the kinins. The rat uterus is especially sensitive. It was the characteristic, slowly developing contraction of the isolated guinea pig ileum that prompted the name *bradykinin*. Certain smooth muscles, such as the rabbit aorta, are little affected; still others, such as the rat duodenum, are relaxed. Tracheobronchial constriction is prominent in guinea pigs, but dilatation as well as constriction may occur in other species. In man, respiratory distress is encountered in asthmatics, especially when the kinins are inhaled.

Stimulation of Nerve Endings and Production of Pain. The plasma kinins are powerful algesic agents. They cause an intense, burning pain when applied to the exposed base of a blister, and a throbbing, burning pain in the hand when injected into the brachial artery. Nociceptive responses or pain occurs when the kinins are injected into animals or man either intraperitoneally or into arteries supplying skin, muscle, or various viscera. Such a nociceptive response can be elicited from the coronary vasculature and is accompanied by sympathetically mediated tachycardia and pressor effects.

Stimulation of Autonomic Ganglia and Chromaffin Cells.   The kinins, in relatively high concentration, stimulate ganglion cells and elicit discharge of catecholamines from the adrenal medulla, where they depolarize chromaffin cells. Such actions occasionally contribute significantly to the excitatory and inhibitory responses of the intestine and other organs.

Central Nervous System.   The injection of bradykinin into the cerebral ventricles causes a wide spectrum of behavioral, autonomic, and EEG effects.

Mechanism of Action.   Little is known of the receptors for bradykinin or other kinins, save that they may be distinguished pharmacologically from receptors for various other peptides. Some responses appear to be mediated by generation of eicosanoids, seemingly as a result of stimulation of phospholipase A_2. Release of prostaglandins in response to bradykinin in guinea pig lung contributes to bronchoconstriction. A similar mechanism may underlie the later phases of vasodilatation, the slowly developing nociceptive responses, and other effects of kinins that are reduced by inhibitors of prostaglandin synthesis, including the prominent renal vasodilator effects. Enhanced calcium fluxes, protein phosphorylation, adenosine 3',5'-monophosphate (cyclic AMP), and guanosine 3',5'-monophosphate (cyclic GMP) have all been implicated in the mediation of some kinin-induced responses (*see* reviews cited; *see also* Fritz *et al.*, 1983; Margolius, 1984).

FUNCTIONS OF ENDOGENOUS KALLIKREINS AND KININS

Despite decades of experimentation on these potent autacoids, the functions of endogenous kallikreins and kinins still elude definition. It is presently conventional to talk of two separate systems: the plasma system and the tissue, or glandular, system. Although these are distinguishable by locus, mode of activation, and chemical features (Figure 27–3), this may be misleading. On the one hand, there is clearly much overlap and some pathophysiological conditions result in activation of both systems. On the other hand, this classification may be an oversimplification that obscures a multiplicity of functions, particularly with regard to the tissue systems. Thus, it would seem unwise to assume that kallikreins in cells and tissues as diverse as kidney, basophils, salivary glands, and accessory sex glands subserve the same purpose. Furthermore, there are clear grounds for rejecting the view that kallikreins and kininogens exist only to generate kinins, although this is a most obvious role. Both plasma kallikrein and HMW kininogen are active in their own right, for example, as factors in the intrinsic clotting cascade. And kallikreins, in particular, are suspected of exerting various other physiological influences directly; these range from regulation of tissue growth and repair to reproductive functions (*see*, for example, Schachter, 1979; Fritz *et al.*, 1983).

With regard to the plasma system, it may be noted that familial deficiency of HMW kininogen (Fletcher trait) or prekallikrein (Fitzgerald, Flaujeac, or Williams traits), which results in defects in intrinsic clotting and fibrinolysis, leads to reduced formation of kinins. By contrast, deficiency of the plasma inhibitor of the activated first component of complement (C$\overline{1}$ INH, Figure 27–3), as in *hereditary angioneurotic edema,* leads to excess formation of kinins, which contributes to the episodic edema. A deficiency in kininase activity possibly underlies a syndrome characterized by bouts of *hyperbradykininemia* and flushing. Other pathological conditions that have been associated with excess kinin formation include *carcinoid* and *postgastrectomy dumping syndrome, septic* and *anaphylactic shock, allergic responses,* and *inflammatory reactions.* It has long been evident that kinins can elicit all of the cardinal signs of inflammation. In addition, they cause accumulation of leukocytes *in vivo* and interact with receptors on lymphocytes and phagocytes. On these various grounds the kallikrein-kinin systems have long been associated with *defense* and *repair responses.*

The physiological functions of glandular kallikreins are far from understood. Small amounts seem to find their way into the lymph, and the resulting formation of kinins and vasodilatation were early considered to contribute to functional hyperemia and to facilitate exocrine secretion. A minute fraction of the total kallikrein activity of blood and of urine seems to reflect this "leakage." But most of the glandular kallikreins pass into the various secretions of the sweat, salivary, pancreatic, intestinal, and accessory sex glands. One possibility, consistent with their cellular locus and their effects in various experimental situations, is that kallikreins participate in regulation of membrane movement of water and electrolytes. This idea seems attractive in the light of evidence from the kidney, where kinins can influence the electrolyte composition and volume of urine markedly. There also seems to be some interaction between aldosterone and endogenous renal kallikrein. The latter is lodged in and released from the distal tubules, which are the site of action of aldosterone; furthermore, secretion of kallikrein and urinary output of kallikrein and kinins are modulated by aldosterone. Since the kidney itself can stimulate synthesis of aldosterone by secreting renin, this has suggested that the kallikrein-kinin and the renin-angiotensin-aldosterone systems may interdigitate. There are also many observations that point to an inverse relationship between urinary concentrations of kallikrein and blood pressure (Fujii *et al.*, 1979; Schachter and Barton, 1979; Fritz *et al.*, 1983; Mayfield and Margolius, 1983; Margolius, 1984).

Therapeutic Considerations.   As with most other autacoids, therapeutic interest in the kinins focuses particularly on attempts to modulate their metabolism *in vivo.* The kinins themselves have an extremely short life, and no therapeutic use has been found for them. More interest is centered on the possibility of slowing the degradation of kinins formed endogenously. This is partially achieved with inhibitors of kininase II, such as captopril (*see* above). However, degradation of kinins usually proceeds sufficiently rapidly in the presence of such inhibitors, in part due to the activities of other enzymes, such as kininase I; physiological consequences are thus generally minor.

The opposite approach, that of blocking the endogenous kinin system, has potential applications because of the involvement of excess kinins in numerous clinical conditions. The lack of specific antagonists is a current frustration. Nevertheless, in certain conditions where kinins have been implicated, such as inflammatory states, some of the beneficial effects of aspirin and other nonsteroidal anti-inflammatory agents may reflect suppression of prostaglandin synthesis initiated by the kinins (*see* Chapter 28). Blockade of kinin formation with inhibitors of kallikrein is another option. This possibility was suggested by the work of Werle and colleagues, who discovered that various tissues contained a polypeptide inhibitor of kallikrein. Their discovery in 1930 was made before that of the classical trypsin inhibitor. But by 1965 it was evident that kallikrein inhibitor and trypsin inhibitor were one and the same. This polyvalent protease inhibitor has long been available commercially as *aprotinin* (TRASYLOL). It has been used with some success to treat acute pancreatitis, carcinoid syndrome, and certain other conditions involving excess kinin formation (*see* Haberland, 1978; Fritz *et al.*, 1983). Aprotinin has also been used as an experimental tool. For example, the demonstration that aprotinin does not suppress the antihypertensive activity of converting-enzyme inhibitors such as captopril provides evidence that this activity is unlikely to be explained by accumulation of endogenous kinins.

OTHER KININS AND VASODILATOR PEPTIDES

Many peptides of mammalian or nonmammalian provenance resemble bradykinin and kallidin in their structure, formation, and pharmacological activities. In addition, there are others that share the common feature of potent vasodilator activity or deserve consideration here for other reasons. Among such mammalian peptides, most have been discovered by pharmacological analysis of extracts of the gut or the brain, which has revealed the presence, in both tissues, of a variety of highly active peptides. These gut peptides and neuropeptides are believed to subserve a variety of local autacoid, endocrine, neuroendocrine, neurotransmitter, neuromodulator, and other roles and are the focus of intense interest in neurobiology (*see* Iversen, 1984; *see also* Chapter 12). Among them, two with potent vasodilator function are singled out for brief discussion here. *Substance P* was discovered more than half a century ago and is the prototype of the large group of peptides that is common to the brain and gut; *vasoactive intestinal peptide* (VIP) was discovered in the early 1970s. Vasodilator peptides that are produced by cells in the mammalian atrium are described in Chapter 36.

Substance P. This is an undecapeptide with the following structure: Arg-Pro-Lys-Pro-Gln-Gln-Phe-Phe-Gly-Leu-Met-NH$_2$. The peptide was originally detected by Euler and Gaddum in 1931 in extracts of gut and brain; these were prepared as powders, hence the appellation "P." The active principle was purified, characterized, and synthesized 40 years later. The pharmacological effects of substance P include vasodilatation; stimulation of intestinal, bronchial, and other smooth muscles; stimulation of salivary secretion; diuresis and natriuresis; and a variety of effects on the peripheral and central nervous systems apparently attributable to depolarization of neurons. Substance P has been localized within nerves in the peripheral and central nervous systems and is suspected of being a neurotransmitter, neuromodulator, or trophic factor. It is abundant in primary sensory afferent neurons of the small nonmyelinated type and has been associated with the transmission of pain sensation and with antidromic vasodilatation and related phenomena. *Capsaicin,* the irritant principle of capsicum (cayenne, tabasco pepper, *etc.*), releases substance P from these fibers and, administered chronically, causes them to degenerate. Substance P–containing fibers in the vagus have been implicated in neuronally mediated bronchoconstriction. Like other neuropeptides, substance P is sometimes present in neurons that also contain other transmitters, such as 5-hydroxytryptamine (5-HT) (*see* Chapters 12 and 26). It is also present, along with 5-HT and other autacoids, in enterochromaffin cells of the gastrointestinal and biliary tracts. It is therefore one of the autacoids secreted by tumors of these cells and contributes to the signs and symptoms of the carcinoid syndrome (*see* Symposium, 1982b; Pernow, 1983; Iversen, 1984).

Vasoactive Intestinal Polypeptide (VIP). This peptide, which contains 28 amino acid residues, was isolated from the small intestine by Said and Mutt in 1972. It was subsequently shown to be widely distributed in the CNS and in peripheral nerves. It is sometimes found in neurons, together with transmitters such as acetylcholine (*e.g.,* in cholinergic neurons to some exocrine glands). The range of effects produced by VIP is very broad. Beside being a very potent vasodilator, it directly stimulates cardiac contractility. It is a potent stimulator of glycogenolysis. It relaxes many smooth muscles and causes bronchodilatation. It stimulates secretion of several adenohypophyseal hormones (and is suspected of hypophysiotropic function). It also stimulates pancreatic, salivary, intestinal, and other exocrine secretions. Its overproduction by cells of the endocrine pancreas or ganglioneuromata, may explain the *chronic watery diarrhea syndrome (pancreatic cholera)*. Its release from "VIP-ergic" neurons is believed to be responsible for various nonadrenergic, noncholinergic responses to stimulation of the autonomic nervous system, and its concurrent release with acetylcholine from cholinergic nerves to salivary glands may explain the long-enigmatic, atropine-resistant component of salivary secretion in response to stimulation of these nerves. Extensive accounts of these and other effects of VIP and related peptides can be found in a recent symposium (Symposium, 1984b).

Nonmammalian Peptides. Kinins that resemble bradykinin and other mammalian kinins are found in wasp stings (along with kallikreins) and in other nonmammalian sources (*see* Bertaccini, 1976; Schachter and Barton, 1979; Fritz, *et al.*, 1983). In addition, comparative studies have led to the discovery of many biologically active peptides in diverse lower vertebrates and invertebrates. This work has revealed a variety of peptides with potent pharmacological activity and with immediate clinical utility, such as the pancreatic secretagogue *caerulein* (*ceruletide;* TYMTRAN). Moreover, it has provided valuable clues to novel actions and structure-activity relationships and has illustrated the power of the comparative approach in discerning evolutionary patterns in functional and biosynthetic processes. Several of the peptides have a close structural resemblance to substance P and are grouped with it as *tachykinins* (Erspamer, 1981).

Bell, J. B. G.; Chu, F. W.; Tait, J. F.; Tait, S. A. S.; and Khosla, M. The use of the superfusion approach with rat adrenal capsular cells to compare the steroidogenic potencies of angiotensin analogues, without the effects of peptide degradation. *Proc. R. Soc. Lond. [Biol.]*, **1984**, *221*, 21–30.

Collier, J. G.; Robinson, B. F.; and Vane, J. R. Reduction of pressor effects of angiotensin I in man by synthetic nonapeptide (B.P.P.9$_a$ or SQ 20,881) which inhibits converting enzyme. *Lancet,* **1973**, *1*, 72–74.

Cordes, E. H. Structure and function of carboxyl proteases. In, *Hypertension and the Angiotensin System: Therapeutic Approaches.* (Doyle, A. E., and Bearn, A. G., eds.) Raven Press, New York, **1984**, pp. 77–91.

Corvol, P.; Panthier, J. J.; Foote, S.; and Rougeon, F. Structure of the mouse submaxillary gland renin precursor and a model for renin processing. *Hypertension,* **1983**, *5*, Suppl. 1, 3–9.

Cushman, D. W.; Cheung, H. S.; Sabo, E. F.; and Ondetti, M. A. Design of potent competitive inhibitors of angiotensin-converting enzyme. Carboxyalkanoyl and mercaptoalkanoyl amino acids. *Biochemistry,* **1977**, *16*, 5484–5491.

Davis, J. O., and Freeman, R. H. Historical perspectives on the renin-angiotensin-aldosterone system and angiotensin blockade. *Am. J. Cardiol.*, **1982**, *49*, 1385–1389.

Elfont, R. M., and Fitzsimons, J. T. Renin dependence of captopril-induced drinking after ureteric ligation in the rat. *J. Physiol. (Lond.)*, **1983**, *343*, 17–30.

Fehrentz, J.-A.; Heitz, A.; Castro, B.; Cazaubon, C.; and Nisato, D. Aldehyde peptides inhibiting renin. *FEBS Lett.*, **1984**, *167*, 273–276.

Ferguson, R. K.; Brunner, H. R.; Turini, G. A.; Gavras, H.; and McKinstry, D. N. A specific orally active inhibitor of angiotensin-converting enzyme in man. *Lancet*, **1977**, *1*, 775–778.

Genest, J. Angiotensin-forming enzymes from extrarenal source. In, *Hypertension and the Angiotensin System: Therapeutic Approaches.* (Doyle, A. E., and Bearn, A. G., eds.) Raven Press, New York, **1984**, pp. 93–107.

Groel, J. T.; Tadros, S. S.; Dreslinski, G. R.; and Jenkins, A. C. Long-term antihypertensive therapy with captopril. *Hypertension*, **1983**, *5*, Suppl. III, III145–III151.

Haber, E. Control of renin action: inhibitors and antibodies. In, *Hypertension and the Angiotensin System: Therapeutic Approaches.* (Doyle, A. E. and Bearn,

A. G., eds.) Raven Press, New York, **1984**, pp. 138–148.

Laragh, J. H. Conceptual diagnostic and therapeutic dimensions of renin-system profiling of hypertensive disorders and of congestive heart failure: four new research frontiers. In, *Hypertension and the Angiotensin System: Therapeutic Approaches.* (Doyle, A. E., and Bearn, A. G., eds.) Raven Press, New York, **1984**, pp. 47–72.

Ménard, J.; Alhenc-Gelas, F.; Gardes, J.; Misumi, J.; and Corvol, P. Intrarenal formation of and role of angiotensins: practical implications. In, *Hypertension and the Angiotensin System: Therapeutic Approaches.* (Doyle, A. E., and Bearn, A. G., eds.) Raven Press, New York, **1984**, pp. 109–121.

Nishimura, H., and Bailey, J. R. Intrarenal renin-angiotensin system in primitive vertebrates. *Kidney Int.*, **1982**, *22*, Suppl., 185–192.

Patchett, A. A. The design of enalapril. In, *Hypertension and the Angiotensin System: Therapeutic Approaches.* (Doyle, A. E., and Bearn, A. G., eds.) Raven Press, New York, **1984**, pp. 155–165.

Rocha e Silva, M.; Beraldo, W. T.; and Rosenfeld, G. Bradykinin, a hypotensive and smooth muscle stimulating factor released from plasma globulin by snake venoms and by trypsin. *Am. J. Physiol.*, **1949**, *156*, 261–273.

Skeggs, L. T., Jr. Historical overview of the renin-angiotensin system. In, *Hypertension and the Angiotensin System: Therapeutic Approaches.* (Doyle, A. E., and Bearn, A. G., eds.) Raven Press, New York, **1984**, pp. 31–45.

Tewksbury, D. A.; Dart, R. A.; and Travis, J. The amino terminal amino acid sequence of human angiotensinogen. *Biochem. Biophys. Res. Commun.*, **1981**, *99*, 1311–1315.

Monographs and Reviews

Antonaccio, M. J. Angiotensin converting enzyme (ACE) inhibitors. *Annu. Rev. Pharmacol. Toxicol.*, **1982**, *22*, 57–87.

Atlas, S. A.; Niarchos, A. P.; and Case, D. B. Inhibitors of the renin-angiotensin system. Effects on blood pressure, aldosterone secretion and renal function. *Am. J. Nephrol.*, **1983**, *3*, 118–127.

Bertaccini, G. Active polypeptides of nonmammalian origin. *Pharmacol. Rev.*, **1976**, *28*, 127–177.

Beyer, K. H., and Peuler, J. D. Hypertension: perspectives. *Pharmacol., Rev.*, **1982**, *34*, 287–313.

Bumpus, F. M. Mechanisms and sites of action of newer angiotensin agonists and antagonists in terms of activity and receptor. *Fed. Proc.*, **1977**, *36*, 2128–2132.

Capponi, A.; Aguilera, G.; Fakunding, J. L.; and Catt, K. J. Angiotensin II. Receptors and mechanism of action. In, *Biochemical Regulation of Blood Pressure.* (Saffer, R. L., ed.) John Wiley & Sons, Inc., New York, **1981**, pp. 205–262.

Davis, J. O., and Freeman, R. H. Mechanisms regulating renin release. *Physiol. Rev.*, **1976**, *56*, 1–56.

———. The other angiotensins. *Biochem. Pharmacol.*, **1977**, *26*, 93–97.

Doyle, A. E., and Bearn, A. G. (eds.). *Hypertension and the Angiotensin System: Therapeutic Approaches.* Raven Press, New York, **1984**.

Erdös, E. G. (ed.). *Bradykinin, Kallidin and Kallikrein. Handbuch der Experimentellen Pharmakologie*, Vol. 25. Springer-Verlag, Berlin, **1970**.

——— (ed.). *Bradykinin, Kallidin and Kallikrein. Handbuch der Experimentellen Pharmakologie*, Vol. 25, Suppl. Springer-Verlag, Berlin, **1979**.

Erspamer, V. The tachykinin peptide family. *Trends Neurosci.*, **1981**, *4*, 267–269.

Ferrario, C. M. Neurogenic actions of angiotensin II. *Hypertension*, **1983**, *5*, Suppl. V, V73–V79.

Fitzsimons, J. T. Angiotensin stimulation of the central nervous system. *Rev. Physiol. Biochem. Pharmacol.*, **1980**, *87*, 117–167.

Freeman, R. H.; Davis, J. O.; and Villareal, D. Role of renal prostaglandins in the control of renin release. *Circ. Res.*, **1984**, *54*, 1–9.

Fritz, H.; Back, N.; Dietze, G.; and Haberland, G. L. (eds.). Kinins-III. *Adv. Exp. Med. Biol.*, **1983**, *156A*, 1–701; *156B*, 705–1222.

Fujii, S.; Moriya, H.; and Suzuki, T. (eds.). Kinins-II. *Adv. Exp. Med. Biol.*, **1979**, *120A*, 1–610; *120B*, 1–719.

Galen, C. On the anatomy of veins and arteries (*c.* 168). In, *Opera Medicorum Graecorum*, Vol. 2. (Kuhn, D. C. G., ed.) Offisina Libraria Cnoblochii, Lipsiae, **1821**, p. 781.

Ganong, W. F. The brain renin-angiotensin system. *Annu. Rev. Physiol.*, **1984**, *46*, 17–31.

Gibbons, G. H.; Dzau, V. J.; Farhi, E. R.; and Barger, A. C. Interaction of signals influencing renin release. *Annu. Rev. Physiol.*, **1984**, *46*, 291–308.

Gross, F. The regulation of aldosterone secretion by the renin-angiotensin system under various conditions. *Acta Endocrinol.* (*Kbh.*), **1968**, Suppl. 124, 41–64.

Gross, F., and Mohring, J. Renal pharmacology, with special emphasis on aldosterone and angiotensin. *Annu. Rev. Pharmacol.*, **1973**, *13*, 57–90.

Guyton, A. C.; Coleman, T. G.; and Granger, H. J. Circulation: overall regulation. *Annu. Rev. Physiol.*, **1972**, *34*, 13–46.

Haberland, G. L. The role of kininogenases, kinin formation and kininogenase inhibition in post traumatic shock and related conditions. *Klin. Wochenschr.*, **1978**, *56*, 325–331.

Heel, R. C.; Brogden, R. N.; Speight, T. M.; and Avery, G. S. Captopril: a preliminary review of pharmacological properties and therapeutic efficacy. *Drugs*, **1980**, *20*, 409–452.

Hodsman, G. P., and Robertson, J. I. S. Captopril: five years on. *Br. Med. J.* [*Clin. Res.*], **1983**, *287*, 851–852.

Hsueh, W. A. Inactive renin in human plasma. *Miner. Electrolyte Metab.*, **1982**, *7*, 169–178.

Iversen, L. L. Amino acids and peptides: fast and slow chemical signals in the nervous system? (The Ferrier Lecture, 1983.) *Proc. R. Soc. Lond.* [*Biol.*], **1984**, *221*, 245–260.

Johnston, C. I.; Arnolda, L.; and Hiwatari, M. Angiotensin-converting enzyme inhibitors in the treatment of hypertension. *Drugs*, **1984**, *27*, 271–277.

Joint National Committee. The 1984 Report of the Joint National Committee on Detection, Evaluation, and Treatment of High Blood Pressure. *Arch. Intern. Med.*, **1984**, *144*, 1045–1057.

Langer, S. Z. Presynaptic regulation of the release of catecholamines. *Pharmacol. Rev.*, **1981**, *32*, 337–362.

Laragh, J. H.; Case, D. B.; Wallace, J. M.; and Keim, H. Blockade of renin or angiotensin for understanding human hypertension: a comparison of propranolol, saralasin and converting enzyme blockade. *Fed. Proc.*, **1977**, *36*, 1781–1787.

Marceau, F.; Lussier, A.; Regoli, D.; and Giroud, J. P. Pharmacology of kinins: their relevance to tissue injury and inflammation. *Gen. Pharmacol.*, **1983**, *14*, 209–229.

Margolius, H. S. The kallikrein-kinin system and the kidney. *Annu. Rev. Physiol.*, **1984**, *46*, 309–326.

Mayfield, R. K., and Margolius, H. S. Renal kallikrein-kinin system. Relation to renal function and blood pressure. *Am. J. Nephrol.*, **1983**, *3*, 145–155.

Page, I. H., and Bumpus, F. M. (eds.). *Angiotensin. Handbuch der Experimentellen Pharmakologie*, Vol. 37. Springer-Verlag, Berlin, **1974**.

Peach, M. J. Renin-angiotensin system: biochemistry and mechanisms of action. *Physiol. Rev.*, **1977**, *57*, 313–370.

Peart, W. S. Renin release. *Gen. Pharmacol.*, **1978**, *9*, 65–72.

Pernow, B. Substance P. *Pharmacol. Rev.*, **1983**, *35*, 85–141.

Petrillo, E. W., and Ondetti, M. A. Angiotensin-converting enzyme inhibitors: medicinal chemistry and biological actions. *Med. Res. Rev.*, **1982**, *2*, 1–41.

Regoli, D., and Barabé, J. Pharmacology of bradykinin and related kinins. *Pharmacol. Rev.*, **1980**, *32*, 1–47.

Regoli, D.; Park, W. K.; and Rioux, F. Pharmacology of angiotensin. *Pharmacol. Rev.*, **1974**, *26*, 69–123.

Romankiewicz, J. A.; Brogden, R. N.; Heel, R. C.; Speight, T. M.; and Avery, G. S. Captopril: an update review of its pharmacological properties and therapeutic efficacy in congestive heart failure. *Drugs*, **1983**, *25*, 6–40.

Ryan, J. W. Processing of the endogenous polypeptides by the lungs. *Annu. Rev. Physiol.*, **1982**, *44*, 241–255.

Schachter, M. Kallikreins (kininogenases)—a group of serine proteases with bioregulatory actions. *Pharmacol. Rev.*, **1979**, *31*, 1–17.

Schachter, M., and Barton, S. Kallikreins (kininogenases) and kinins. In, *Endocrinology: Metabolic Basis of Clinical Practice*. (Cahill, G., Jr., and de Groot, L. J., eds.) Grune & Stratton, Inc., New York, **1979**.

Schwartz, A. B., and Chatterjee, K. Vasodilator therapy in chronic congestive heart failure. *Drugs*, **1983**, *26*, 148–173.

Smith, T. W., and Braunwald, E. The management of heart failure. In, *Heart Disease*, 2nd ed., Vol. I. (Braunwald, E., ed.) W. B. Saunders Co., Philadelphia, **1984**, pp. 503–559.

Sweet, C. S. Pharmacological properties of the converting enzyme inhibitor, enalapril maleate (MK-421). *Fed. Proc.*, **1983**, *42*, 167–170.

Symposium. (Various authors.) Captopril: worldwide clinical experience. *Br. J. Clin. Pharmacol.*, **1982a**, *14*, Suppl. 2, 65S–252S.

Symposium. (Various authors.) Substance P in the nervous system. *Ciba Found. Symp.*, **1982b**, *91*, 1–349.

Symposium. (Various authors.) The kidney in hypertension. *Am. J. Nephrol.*, **1983a**, *3*, 57–192.

Symposium. (Various authors.) Control of glomerular function by intrinsic contractile elements. *Fed. Proc.*, **1983b**, *42*, 3045–3085.

Symposium. (Various authors.) Symposium on the renin-angiotensin-aldosterone system: treatment of hypertension and heart failure. (Murphy, B., ed.) *J. Hyperten.*, **1983c**, *1*, Suppl. 1, 1–157.

Symposium. (Various authors.) Regional hemodynamics following captopril therapy. *Am. J. Med.*, **1984a**, *76*, 1–119.

Symposium. (Various authors.) First international symposium on VIP and related peptides. *Peptides*, **1984b**, *5*, 143–458.

Torretti, J. Sympathetic control of renin release. *Annu. Rev. Pharmacol. Toxicol.*, **1982**, *22*, 167–192.

Werle, E. Discovery of the most important kallikreins and kallikrein inhibitors. In, *Bradykinin, Kallidin and Kallikrein*. (Erdös, E. G., ed.) *Handbuch der Experimentellen Pharmakologie*, Vol. 25. Springer-Verlag, Berlin, **1970**, pp. 1–6.

Wilson, J. X. The renin-angiotensin system in non-mammalian vertebrates. *Endocr. Rev.*, **1984**, *5*, 45–61.

Wright, F. S., and Briggs, J. P. Feedback control of glomerular blood flow, pressure and filtration rate. *Physiol. Rev.*, **1979**, *59*, 958–1006.

28 PROSTAGLANDINS, PROSTACYCLIN, THROMBOXANE A₂, AND LEUKOTRIENES

Salvador Moncada, Roderick J. Flower, and John R. Vane

History. There are few substances that currently command more widespread interest in biological circles than do the prostaglandins and the related products of arachidonic acid metabolism. Although their history extends back to the early 1930s, it was the isolation, characterization, and synthesis of the representative compounds in the early 1960s that generated such intense interest. The reasons are not hard to find. The prostaglandins are among the most prevalent of autacoids and have been detected in almost every tissue and body fluid; their production increases in response to astonishingly diverse stimuli; they produce, in minute amounts, a remarkably broad spectrum of effects that embraces practically every biological function; and inhibition of their biosynthesis is now recognized as a mechanism of some of the most widely used therapeutic agents, the nonsteroidal anti-inflammatory drugs such as aspirin (*see* Chapter 29).

A harbinger of this remarkable development was the observation made in 1930 by two American gynecologists, Kurzrok and Lieb, that strips of human uterus relax or contract when exposed to human semen. A few years later, Goldblatt in England and Euler in Sweden independently reported smooth-muscle-contracting and vasodepressor activity in seminal fluid and accessory reproductive glands, and Euler identified the active material as a lipid-soluble acid, which he named "prostaglandin" (*see* Euler, 1973). More than 20 years were to pass before technical advances allowed the demonstration that prostaglandin was in fact a family of compounds of unique structure, permitted the isolation in crystalline form of two prostaglandins, prostaglandin E_1 (PGE_1) and $PGF_{1\alpha}$, and led to the elucidation of their structures in 1962 (*see* Bergström and Samuelsson, 1968). Soon, more prostaglandins were characterized and, like the others, proved to be 20-carbon unsaturated carboxylic acids with a cyclopentane ring.

When the general structure of the prostaglandins became apparent, their kinship with essential fatty acids was recognized, and in 1964 Bergström and coworkers and van Dorp and associates independently achieved the biosynthesis of PGE_2 from arachidonic acid using homogenates of sheep seminal vesicle (*see* Samuelsson, 1972).

Until recently it was believed that PGE_2 and $PGF_{2\alpha}$ were the most important prostaglandins. Indeed, thousands of analogs of these compounds were made in the largely frustrated hope that compounds of therapeutic value with a greater selectivity of action would emerge. However, since 1973, several discoveries have caused a radical shift in emphasis away from PGEs and PGFs. The first was the isolation and identification of two unstable cyclic endoperoxides, prostaglandin G_2 (PGG_2 or 15-OOH PGH_2) and prostaglandin H_2 (PGH_2) (*see* Flower, 1978). Later came the elucidation of the structure of thromboxane A₂ (TXA_2) and that of its degradation product, thromboxane B₂ (TXB_2) (Hamberg *et al.*, 1975), and then the discovery of prostacyclin (PGI_2) (Moncada *et al.*, 1976). These findings, coupled with the elucidation of a different enzymatic pathway (a lipoxygenase), which converts arachidonic acid to compounds such as 12-hydroperoxyeicosatetraenoic acid (HPETE) and 12-hydroxyeicosatetraenoic acid (HETE), have led to the realization that the "classically known" prostaglandins constitute only a fraction of the physiologically active products of arachidonic acid metabolism. Recently, the products of a pathway initiated by the action of a 5-lipoxygenase enzyme have been characterized; they have been named leukotrienes (LTs) because of their initial discovery in leukocytes and their conjugated triene structure (*see* Samuelsson, 1983). These include a 5,12-dihydroxy compound (LTB_4), which has potent chemotactic properties, and a 5-hydroxy derivative that is conjugated with glutathione (LTC_4). The latter is one of the components of the "slow-reacting substance of anaphylaxis" (SRS-A). The leukotrienes are believed to have important functions as mediators of inflammation.

Chemistry and Biosynthesis. The families of prostaglandins, leukotrienes, and related compounds are called eicosanoids because they are derived from 20-carbon essential fatty acids that contain three, four, or five double bonds: 8,11,14-eicosatrienoic acid (dihomo-γ-linolenic acid), 5,8,11,14-eicosatetraenoic acid (arachidonic acid) (*see* Figure 28–2), and 5,8,11,14,17-eicosapentaenoic acid. In man, arachidonic acid is the most abundant precursor, and it is either derived from dietary linoleic acid (octadecadienoic acid) or is ingested as a constituent of meat. Arachidonate is then esterified as a component of the phospholipids of cell membranes or is found in ester linkage in other complex lipids. The concentration of free arachidonic acid is low, and the biosynthesis of the eicosanoids depends primarily upon its release from cellular stores by various acyl hydrolases.

The enhanced biosynthesis of the eicosanoids that occurs in response to widely divergent physical, chemical, and hormonal stimuli is generally believed to involve activation of these enzymes caused by increases in the intracellular concentration of calcium. The prevailing view is that calmodulin, acting in concert with calcium, is important in the activation of these acyl hydrolases and that membrane-bound forms of both phospholipase A_2 and C are probably involved in the formation of precursor arachidonic acid (Craven and DeRubertis, 1983; Cooper and Malik, 1984). Once released, arachidonic acid and its congeners are rapidly metabolized to oxygenated products by several distinct enzyme systems; products that contain ring structures (prostaglandins, thromboxanes, and prostacyclin) result from the initial action of *cyclooxygenase*, while the hydroxylated derivatives of straight-chain fatty acids (*e.g.*, leukotrienes) result from the action of various lipoxygenases.

Prostaglandins, Thromboxanes, and Prostacyclin. The prostaglandins can be considered as analogs of an unnatural compound with the trivial name *prostanoic acid,* the structure of which is as follows:

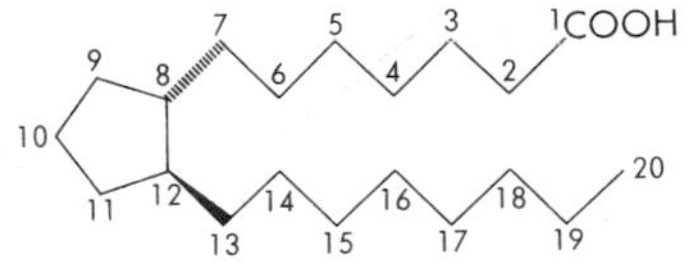

They fall into several main classes, designated by letters and distinguished by substitutions on the cyclopentane ring. These structures are shown in Figure 28–1. The main classes are further subdivided in accord with the number of double bonds in the side chains. This is indicated by subscript 1, 2, or 3, and reflects the fatty acid precursor. Thus, prostaglandins derived from 8,11,14-eicosatrienoic acid carry the subscript 1; those derived from arachidonic acid carry the subscript 2; and those derived from 5,8,11,14,17-eicosapentaenoic acid carry the subscript 3. In man, there is little evidence that prostaglandins of the 1 or 3 series are important. However, prostaglandins of the 3 series may have greater significance in fish and marine animals, where 5,8,11,14,17-eicosapentaenoic acid is the predominant precursor.

Prostaglandins of the E and F_α series are sometimes referred to as the "primary prostaglandins," even though they are products of the metabolism of prostaglandins of the G and H series. The As, Bs, and Cs are all derivatives of the corresponding Es. Thromboxanes contain a six-membered oxane ring instead of the cyclopentane ring of the prostaglandins and result from the metabolism of the Gs and Hs.

Synthesis of the primary prostaglandins is accomplished in stepwise manner by a ubiquitous complex of microsomal enzymes, the first of which is referred to as *fatty acid cyclooxygenase.* The unesterified precursor acids are oxygenated and cyclized to form the cyclic endoperoxide deriva-

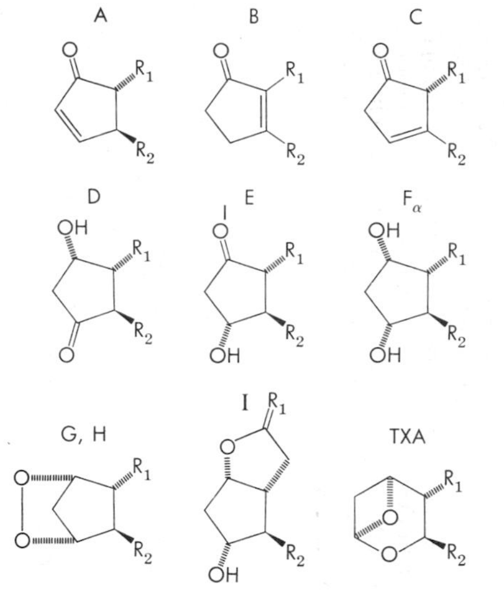

Figure 28–1. *Ring structures of the six "primary" prostaglandins* (A–F), *the cyclic endoperoxides* (G, H), *prostacyclin* (I), *and thromboxane A* (TXA).

In the stereochemical convention followed, the groups indicated by IIIIII lie behind the plane of the cyclopentane ring, while those indicated by ➞ lie in front of it.

tives, prostaglandin G (PGG) and prostaglandin H (PGH). There is an absolute requirement for heme as a cofactor for the formation of PGG, whereas the enzyme that converts PGG to PGH requires the addition of an antioxidant to prevent the progressive inactivation that occurs *in vitro.* These endoperoxides, which are chemically unstable (*e.g.*, PGG_2 and PGH_2 have half-lives of 5 minutes at 37° C and pH 7.5), are then isomerized enzymatically or nonenzymatically into different products, PGE, PGF, or PGD (*see* Figure 28–2; Flower, 1978). PGA, PGB, and PGC, which arise from the corresponding PGE by dehydration and isomerization, are formed chemically during extraction; probably none of them occurs biologically.

The endoperoxide PGH_2 is also metabolized into two unstable and highly biologically active compounds with structures that differ from those of the primary prostaglandins. One of these is thromboxane A_2 (TXA_2), formed by an enzyme, *thromboxane synthetase,* first isolated from human and equine platelets. TXA_2 has a very short chemical half-life ($t_{1/2} = 30$ seconds at 37° C and pH 7.5); it breaks down nonenzymatically into the stable thromboxane B_2 (TXB_2) (Figure 28–2).

The other route of metabolism of PGH_2 is to prostacyclin (PGI_2), yet another unstable compound ($t_{1/2} = 3$ minutes at 37° C and pH 7.5) formed by an enzyme, *prostacyclin synthetase,* first discovered in vascular tissue. PGI_2 has a double-ring structure, closed by an oxygen bridge between carbons 6 and 9. It is hydrolyzed nonenzymatically to a stable compound, 6-keto-$PGF_{1\alpha}$ (Figure 28–2).

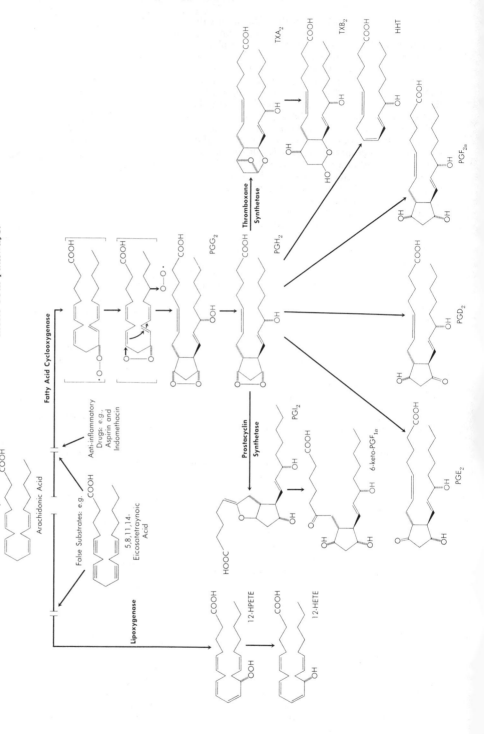

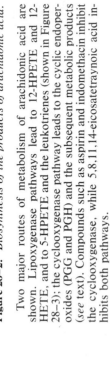

Figure 28–2. *Biosynthesis of the products of arachidonic acid.*

Two major routes of metabolism of arachidonic acid are shown. Lipoxygenase pathways lead to 12-HPETE and 12-HETE, and to 5-HPETE and the leukotrienes (shown in Figure 28–3); the cyclooxygenase pathway leads to the cyclic endoperoxides (PGG and PGH) and the subsequent metabolic products (*see* text). Compounds such as aspirin and indomethacin inhibit the cyclooxygenase, while 5,8,11,14-eicosatetraynoic acid inhibits both pathways.

The endoperoxides are also transformed into a 17-carbon hydroxy acid (HHT) with the concomitant formation of malondialdehyde, and, although HHT can be formed nonenzymatically, it is also generated by a purified preparation of thromboxane synthetase.

While tissues seem to be able to synthesize the intermediate prostaglandin endoperoxides from free arachidonic acid, the fate of these endoperoxides in each tissue depends on several factors that have not been clearly defined. Certainly, the presence of the different isomerases varies from tissue to tissue. For example, lung and spleen are able to synthesize the whole range of products, but other tissues cannot; platelets synthesize mainly TXA_2, whereas the blood vessel wall primarily produces PGI_2.

Even though PGE_2, PGD_2, and $PGF_{2\alpha}$ can be formed nonenzymatically, isomerases for the synthesis of PGE_2 and PGD_2 have been identified. In some tissues, there may be a reductase that catalyzes the interconversion of PGE_2 and $PGF_{2\alpha}$. Moreover, the biochemical conditions under which the enzymes are studied influence the range of products obtained. For example, the production of $PGF_{2\alpha}$ is enhanced in the presence of reducing agents, while certain proteins increase the rate of isomerization of the endoperoxide to PGD_2. Interestingly, glutathione favors the generation of PGE_2.

Products of Lipoxygenases. Despite extensive knowledge of lipid peroxidation and the identification of lipoxygenases in plants, the discovery of mammalian enzymes that catalyze the oxidation of polyunsaturated fatty acids to the corresponding hydroperoxides is relatively recent (*see* Nugteren, 1977). The first such enzyme was originally found in lung and platelets; it is responsible for the formation of lipid peroxides such as 12-HPETE and its degradation product, 12-HETE. Subsequently, a number of enzymes have been discovered that peroxidize arachidonic acid in different positions. The most important of these is a 5-lipoxygenase. The action of this enzyme results in the formation of a complex group of compounds known collectively as leukotrienes. The structures of these compounds and the 5-lipoxygenase pathway are shown in Figure 28–3.

The first step of the 5-lipoxygenase pathway is the formation of 5-hydroperoxyeicosatetraenoic acid (5-HPETE); this is converted either to the related monohydroxyeicosatetraenoic acid (5-HETE) or to a 5,6 epoxide, known as leukotriene A_4 (LTA_4). Leukotriene A_4 may itself be transformed either to 5,12-dihydroxyeicosatetraenoic acid, known as leukotriene B_4 (LTB_4), or to leukotriene C_4 (LTC_4); the latter is a glutathionyl derivative, formed by the action of a glutathione-S-transferase. Leukotriene D_4 (LTD_4) is synthesized by the removal of glutamic acid from LTC_4, and LTE_4 results from the subsequent cleavage of glycine. The final step of these transformations produces LTF_4 by the reincorporation of γ-glutamic acid into the molecule to form a γ-glutamyl, cysteinyl derivative (*see* Piper, 1983; Samuelsson, 1983). It is now generally accepted that a mixture of LTC_4 and LTD_4

makes up the material originally known as the "slow-reacting substance of anaphylaxis" (SRS-A), first described by Feldberg and Kellaway (1938).

Inhibitors of Prostaglandin Biosynthesis. The association between aspirin-like drugs and prostaglandins became clear in 1971 (Vane, 1971). In retrospect, several observations can be recognized as providing critical clues. It was discovered in 1969 that aspirin prevented the escape of an unknown autacoid from guinea pig lungs during anaphylaxis; this autacoid, which was called rabbit aorta contracting substance, was later identified as thromboxane A_2. During the following 2 years it was found that aspirin and related anti-inflammatory drugs interfered with the liberation of prostaglandins from spleen and platelets and prevented the synthesis of prostaglandins from arachidonic acid in tissue homogenates. It is now known that these drugs prevent production of the prostaglandin endoperoxides by the cyclooxygenase enzyme and, as a result, inhibit the synthesis of all of the products beyond this step in the metabolic pathway (*see* Flower, 1974). A clear-cut inhibition of prostaglandin synthesis, as measured by the prostaglandin content of synovial fluid, urine, or semen, is evident in man treated with conventional doses of these anti-inflammatory agents, and their therapeutic efficacy largely parallels their ability to inhibit fatty acid cyclooxygenase. Thus, inhibition of cyclooxygenase provides an important basis for understanding many of the therapeutic and other effects of aspirin-like drugs (*see* Chapter 29).

Since different metabolites of the prostaglandin endoperoxides sometimes produce opposite biological effects (*see* below), there would be a number of potential advantages in the development of compounds with preferential inhibitory actions on one or another of the enzymes that isomerize the endoperoxides (*see* Moncada and Vane, 1979; Moncada, 1982; Vane, 1982). For example, there is current interest in analogs of imidazole, such as *dazoxiben*, that appear to inhibit thromboxane synthetase preferentially (Patrignani *et al.*, 1984). Such compounds might have antithrombotic effects *in vivo* by selectively reducing the formation of TXA_2 (which promotes platelet aggregation and vasoconstriction) without interfering with the production of PGI_2 (which inhibits aggregation and produces vasodilatation).

One of the limitations of the aspirin-like drugs is their inability to inhibit the metabolism of arachidonic acid by lipoxygenases. In fact, inhibition of the cyclooxygenase can lead to *increased* formation of leukotrienes, perhaps by increasing the amount of arachidonic acid that is available to the lipoxygenases (*see* Piper, 1983). This effect may play a role in the production of symptoms of hypersensitivity in certain individuals (especially asthmatic patients) following the administration of aspirin and similar drugs (*see* Chapter 29). Analogs of the natural fatty acid precursors can serve as competitive inhibitors of the formation of both prostaglandins and the products of lipoxygenases. One such inhibitor is the acetylenic analog of arachidonic acid, 5,8,11,14-eicosatetraynoic acid (Figure

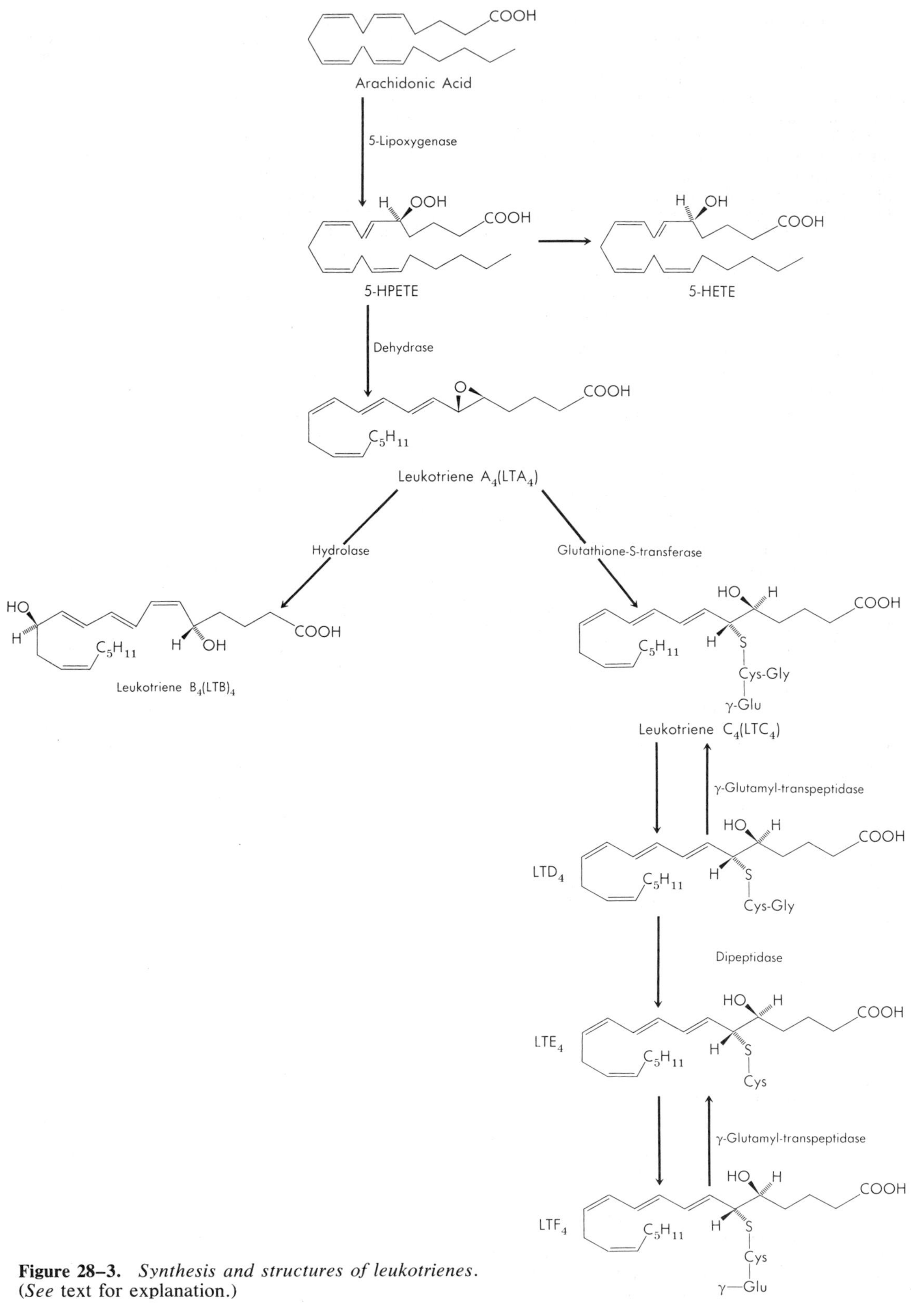

Figure 28–3. *Synthesis and structures of leukotrienes.*
(*See* text for explanation.)

28–2). Moreover, in many tissues calcium channel blockers (*e.g., nifedipine; see* Chapter 33) or inhibitors of calmodulin (*e.g., fluperazine*) can reduce the release of arachidonic acid, prostaglandins, and leukotrienes that is evoked by various stimuli. The therapeutic potential of such agents remains to be assessed, and investigation in this area is intense.

Catabolism. Efficient mechanisms exist for the catabolism and inactivation of most prostaglandins. For example, about 95% of infused PGE_2 is inactivated during one passage through the pulmonary circulation. Because of the unique position of the lungs between the venous and arterial circulation, the pulmonary vascular bed constitutes an important filter for many substances (including some prostaglandins) that might be released from tissues into the venous circulation. The clearance of these potent, vasoactive substances protects the cardiovascular system and other organs from their prolonged effects due to recirculation.

Broadly speaking, the enzymatic catabolic reactions are of two types: an initial (relatively rapid) step, catalyzed by prostaglandin-specific enzymes, wherein prostaglandins lose most of their biological activity, and a second (relatively slow) step in which these metabolites are oxidized by enzymes probably identical to those responsible for the β and ω oxidation of most fatty acids. This sequence of reactions, which leads to the appearance of the metabolites in the urine, has been investigated in man (Hamberg and Samuelsson, 1971); the degradation of PGE_2 is summarized in Figure 28–4.

The initial step is the oxidation of the 15-OH group to the corresponding ketone by prostaglandin 15-OH dehydrogenase (PGDH). The 15-keto compound is then reduced to the 13,14-dihydro derivative, a reaction catalyzed by prostaglandin Δ^{13}-reductase (Anggard *et al.*, 1971). While

these first two reactions occur very rapidly, subsequent steps are slower. These consist of β and ω oxidation of the side chains of the prostaglandins, giving rise to a polar dicarboxylic acid, which is excreted in the urine as the major metabolite of both PGE_1 and PGE_2.

Enzymes that catalyze the degradation of prostaglandins are widely distributed in the body and are present in the spleen, kidney, adipose tissue, intestine, liver, and testicle, as well as in the lung. The enzymes responsible for β or ω oxidation are found in the liver, lung, kidney, and intestine. The liver is probably the major site for side chain oxidation (*see* Samuelsson *et al.*, 1975; Flower, 1978).

The metabolism of TXA_2 in man has been inferred from investigation of the fate of TXB_2 (Roberts *et al.*, 1981). While up to 20 metabolites have been identified in urine, by far the most abundant is 2,3-dinor-TXB_2 (Figure 28–4).

The degradation of PGI_2 apparently begins with its spontaneous hydrolysis in blood to 6-keto-$PGF_{1\alpha}$. While the metabolism of this compound in man involves the same steps as those for PGE_2 and $PGF_{2\alpha}$, it has been suggested that β oxidation occurs prior to the actions of PGDH and prostaglandin Δ^{13}-reductase (Rosenkranz *et al.*, 1980).

PHARMACOLOGICAL PROPERTIES

No other autacoids show more numerous and diverse effects than do prostaglandins and other metabolites of arachidonic acid. Not only is the spectrum of actions broad, but also different compounds show different activities, both qualitatively and quantitatively. It would be confusing to present the myriad of pharmacological effects that have been ascribed to these substances and even more so to delve into the activities of their synthetic analogs. This discussion is limited to those activities that are thought to be the most important.

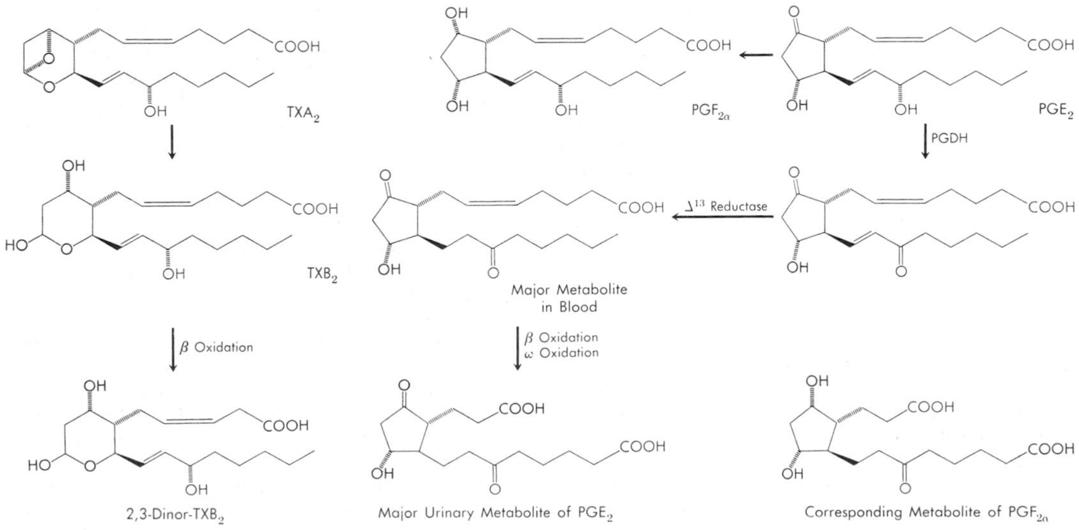

Figure 28–4. *Metabolism of PGE_2, $PGF_{2\alpha}$, and thromboxane A_2 (TXA_2).* (*See* text for explanation.)

Cardiovascular System. In most species and in most vascular beds PGEs and PGAs are potent vasodilators; when injected into the femoral arterial bed in dogs, their potency exceeds that of acetylcholine or histamine, although it is less than that of bradykinin. Responses to PGF$_{2\alpha}$ show species variation, but vasodilatation has been observed following injection into the human brachial artery of PGF$_{2\alpha}$ and PGs A$_1$, A$_2$, B$_1$, E$_1$, and E$_2$ (Robinson et al., 1973). Dilatation in response to prostaglandins seemingly involves arterioles, precapillaries, sphincters, and postcapillary venules. PGEs are not universally vasodilatory; constrictor effects have been noted at selected sites. Superficial veins of the hand are contracted by PGF$_{2\alpha}$, but not by PGEs. The behavior of other large-capacitance veins in various animals is similar (see Nakano, 1973).

Cardiac output is generally increased by PGs E, F, and A. Weak, direct inotropic effects have been noted in various isolated preparations. In the intact animal, however, increased force of contraction as well as increased heart rate is in large measure a reflex consequence of fall in total peripheral resistance. Systemic blood pressure generally falls in response to PGs E and A, and blood flow to most organs, including the heart and kidney, is increased. These effects are particularly striking in some patients with hypertensive disease (see Lee, 1974).

Prostaglandin endoperoxides (both being roughly equipotent) have variable effects in vascular beds ranging from vasodilatation to vasoconstriction, and sometimes they induce constriction followed by dilatation (see Dusting et al., 1979). Since the endoperoxides are substrates for conversion to other potent prostaglandins, their effects are a result of intrinsic vasoconstrictor activity coupled with some vasodilatation due to rapid conversion to a prostaglandin that is a vasodilator (most probably prostacyclin [PGI$_2$]). They are rapidly converted into PGI$_2$ during passage through the lungs; PGH$_2$ is thus less active as a hypotensive agent when injected intra-arterially than when given intravenously (Armstrong et al., 1976).

While very few studies have been performed with thromboxane A$_2$ (TXA$_2$) because of its intrinsic instability, it contracts all vascular smooth muscle strips tested. It appears to be a powerful vasoconstrictor in the whole animal and in isolated vascular beds (Dusting et al., 1978; Samuelsson et al., 1978; Whittle et al., 1981). TXB$_2$ is inactive when effects on the cardiovascular system are tested.

The intravenous administration of PGI$_2$ causes prominent hypotension in animals, including man. It is about five times more potent than PGE$_2$ in producing this effect. The compound causes dilatation in various vascular beds, including the coronary, renal, mesenteric, and skeletal muscle, and, of note, the pulmonary circulation. It relaxes essentially all isolated preparations of vascular smooth muscle that have been tested. Its degradation product, 6-keto-PGF$_{1\alpha}$, is at least 1000 times less active than PGI$_2$. Because it is not inactivated by the pulmonary circulation, PGI$_2$ is equipotent as a vasodilator when given either intra-arterially or intravenously (Moncada, 1982; Vane, 1982).

While there is marked species variation, the intra-arterial or intravenous administration of the leukotrienes (LTC$_4$ or LTD$_4$) produces an initial increase in the blood pressure; in most species, this is followed by prolonged hypotension (see Piper, 1983). These effects are usually attenuated by inhibitors of cyclooxygenase, but the hypotensive phase is prolonged by one such compound (indomethacin) in the guinea pig. Since relaxant effects have not been observed in vascular smooth muscle in vitro (Berkowitz et al., 1984), this hypotensive phase may result in large part from decreased cardiac contractility that is secondary to a marked, leukotriene-induced reduction in coronary blood flow. While LTC$_4$ and LTD$_4$ have little effect on most large arteries or veins in vitro, some arterial vessels, especially including distal segments of the pulmonary artery, are contracted by nanomolar concentrations of these agents; LTE$_4$ is much less potent (Berkowitz et al., 1984).

The leukotrienes have prominent effects on the microvasculature, where they appear to act on the endothelial lining of postcapillary venules to cause exudation of plasma; they are more than 1000-fold more potent than histamine in this regard (see Piper, 1983). While LTB$_4$ also causes exudation of plasma, this effect is indirect and requires the participation of leukocytes.

Blood. The prostaglandins and related products exert powerful actions on platelets. Some of them, like PGE$_1$ and PGD$_2$, are inhibitors of the aggregation of human platelets in vitro at concentrations around 0.1 μM. PGI$_2$ is some 30 to 50 times more potent, inhibiting aggregation at concentrations between 1 and 10 nM. This fact and the observation that PGI$_2$ is generated by the vascular wall (particularly by the vascular endothelium) have led to the suggestion that the substance controls the aggregation of platelets in vivo. PGE$_2$ exerts variable effects on platelets; it is a potentiator of some forms of aggregation at low concentrations (below 1 μM) and an inhibitor at higher concentrations.

One of the products of arachidonic acid metabolism in platelets, TXA$_2$, is a very powerful inducer of platelet aggregation and the platelet release reaction. The endoperoxides, although active, are much less so than TXA$_2$. Pathways of platelet aggregation that are dependent on the generation of TXA$_2$ are sensitive to the inhibitory action of aspirin (see Chapter 29; Moncada and Vane, 1979).

PGA$_2$, PGE$_1$, and PGE$_2$ induce erythropoiesis by stimulating the release of erythropoietin from the renal cortex (see Fisher and Gross, 1977). Moreover, PGE$_1$ and PGE$_2$ produce variable effects on the fragility of red cells; at very low concentrations (10 to 100 pM) they decrease fragility, while at higher concentrations (1 nM) they increase it (see Rasmussen and Lake, 1977).

The leukotriene LTB$_4$ is a potent chemotactic agent for polymorphonuclear leukocytes; other leukotrienes do not share this action (see Piper, 1983). Its potency is comparable to that of various chemotactic peptides and platelet-activating factor.

Chemoattraction of leukocytes appears to be the main effect of LTB_4 in the microvasculature.

The cyclooxygenase product PGD_2 and the lipoxygenase products 5-HPETE and 5-HETE can enhance the release of histamine from human basophils under a number of circumstances; in contrast, PGE_2 and PGI_2 inhibit histamine secretion (Peters *et al.*, 1984). These effects are modulatory, and the actions of PGD_2 and 5-HPETE appear to involve inhibition of adenylate cyclase that has been stimulated by such agents as PGE_2 or histamine (H_2-receptor effect).

Smooth Muscle. Eicosanoids contract or relax many smooth muscles beside those of the vasculature. The leukotrienes (*e.g.*, LTD_4) contract most smooth muscles. Again, responses may vary with species, type of prostaglandin, endocrine status of the tissue, and experimental conditions. However, few smooth muscles are uninfluenced, and many display intense and consistent responses.

Bronchial and Tracheal Muscle. In general, PGFs contract and PGEs relax bronchial and tracheal muscle from various species, including man. Asthmatic individuals are particularly sensitive, and $PGF_{2\alpha}$ has caused intense bronchospasm. In contrast, both PGE_1 and PGE_2 are potent bronchodilators when given to such patients by aerosol (*see* Cuthbert, 1973). Prostaglandin endoperoxides and TXA_2 are constrictors of guinea pig tracheal strips *in vitro*. TXA_2 is the more potent and induces bronchoconstriction in guinea pigs when given by aerosol (Hamberg *et al.*, 1976). PGI_2, on the other hand, is without effect or induces slight bronchodilatation; it antagonizes bronchoconstriction produced by other agents in man (Bianco *et al.*, 1978).

While there is considerable species variation, LTC_4 and LTD_4 are powerful bronchoconstrictors in many species, including man (*see* Piper, 1983). These agents appear to act directly on smooth muscle, especially that in peripheral airways, and are far more potent than histamine both *in vitro* and *in vivo*. When administered intravenously to guinea pigs, the bronchoconstrictor effects of the leukotrienes are mediated in part by TXA_2; the effects of LTB_4 appear to be due solely to the synthesis of TXA_2.

Uterus. Strips of nonpregnant human uterus are contracted by PGFs but relaxed by PGs E, A, and B. The contractile response is most prominent before menstruation, whereas relaxation is greatest at mid-cycle. Uterine strips from pregnant women are uniformly contracted by PGFs and by low concentrations of PGE_2; PGI_2 and high concentrations of PGE_2 produce relaxation. The intravenous infusion of PGE_2 or $PGF_{2\alpha}$ to pregnant human females produces a dose-dependent increase in the frequency and intensity of uterine contraction. Uterine responsiveness to prostaglandins increases somewhat as pregnancy progresses, but far less than does that to oxytocin (*see* Chapter 39). In some species (*e.g.*, guinea pig), products of the lipoxygenase pathway have uterine-stimulating effects.

Gastrointestinal Muscle. *In-vitro* responses vary widely with species, segment, type of muscle, and the particular eicosanoid. In the main, longitu-dinal muscle from stomach to colon is contracted by both PGEs and PGFs, while circular muscle generally relaxes to PGEs and contracts to PGFs. Prostaglandins of the A and D series generally have little activity. The *in-vivo* effects are also variable in man. Shortened transit times have been observed in the small intestine and colon. Diarrhea, cramps, and reflux of bile have been noted in response to oral PGE; these are common side effects (along with nausea and vomiting) in patients given prostaglandins for abortion (Bennett, 1977). Prostaglandin endoperoxides, TXA_2, and PGI_2 are less active than the PGEs or PGFs on gastrointestinal smooth muscle. The leukotrienes have potent contractile effects, and the guinea pig ileum has been used extensively in the bioassay of SRS-A.

Gastric and Intestinal Secretions. PGEs, PGAs, and PGI_2 inhibit gastric acid secretion stimulated by feeding, histamine, or gastrin. Volume of secretion, acidity, and content of pepsin are all reduced, probably by an action exerted directly on the secretory cells. In addition, these prostaglandins are vasodilators in the gastric mucosa, and PGI_2 may be involved in the local regulation of blood flow. Mucus secretion in the stomach and small intestine is increased by prostaglandins, and there is substantial movement of water and electrolytes into the intestinal lumen. Such effects may underlie the watery diarrhea noted in animals and man following the oral or parenteral administration of prostaglandins. In contrast to PGE_2 and $PGF_{2\alpha}$, PGI_2 does not induce diarrhea in animals or man; indeed, it prevents that provoked by other prostaglandins and inhibits the toxin-induced accumulation of intestinal fluid in experimental models.

Kidney and Urine Formation. PGE_2 and PGI_2 infused directly into the renal arteries of dogs increase renal blood flow and provoke diuresis, natriuresis, and kaliuresis; there is little change in the rate of glomerular filtration unless renal vasoconstriction is present (Dunn and Hood, 1977). TXA_2 decreases renal blood flow and the rate of glomerular filtration. PGEs inhibit water reabsorption induced by antidiuretic hormone (ADH) in the toad bladder and in rabbit collecting tubules (*see* Nakano and Koss, 1973). PGE_2 also inhibits chloride reabsorption in the thick ascending limb of the loop of Henle in the rabbit (Stokes, 1979). In addition, PGI_2, PGE_2, and PGD_2 can cause the release of renin from the renal cortex (Gerber *et al.*, 1979; Seymour *et al.*, 1979).

Central Nervous System. A large number of observations have been made on the effects of prostaglandins in the central nervous system (CNS). However, a convincing body of evidence for a particular physiological role has yet to emerge. Many stimulant and depressant effects of prostaglandins on the CNS have been reported (*see* Wolfe, 1982). Among them is sedation; stupor, catatonia, and other behavioral changes follow injection of PGEs (but not PGFs) into the cerebral ventricles in cats. PGEs also antagonize convulsions induced by pentylenetetrazol, penicillin, and picrotoxin. Many of these effects require rather high concentrations of prostaglandins. The firing rates of individual brain cells may be increased or decreased after application of PGE or PGF by microiontophoresis. The application of PGE$_2$ or PGD$_2$ inhibits the release of catecholamines from various areas of the brain and from sympathetic nerve endings. A great deal of attention has been focused on the fever that is caused in various species in response to intracerebroventricular injection of PGEs. Release of PGE$_2$ into the CNS has been proposed to explain the genesis of pyrogen-induced fever. However, there is considerable evidence that contradicts this hypothesis (*see* Wolfe, 1982).

Afferent Nerves and Pain.   In man, PGEs cause pain when injected intradermally, and they irritate the mucous membranes of the eyes and respiratory passages. These effects are generally not as immediate or intense as those caused by bradykinin or histamine, but they outlast those caused by the other autacoids and are accompanied by tenderness and hyperalgesia. PGEs and PGI$_2$ sensitize the afferent nerve endings to the effects of chemical or mechanical stimuli; the release of these prostaglandins during the inflammatory process thus serves as an amplification system for the pain mechanism (*see* Moncada *et al.*, 1978). The role of PGE$_2$ and PGI$_2$ in inflammation is discussed in Chapter 29.

Endocrine System.   A variety of endocrine tissues respond to prostaglandins. In a number of species, the systemic administration of PGE$_2$ increases circulating concentrations of ACTH, growth hormone, prolactin, and the gonadotropins; the last-named effect appears to involve a hypothalamic site of action (*see* Behrman, 1979). Other effects include stimulation of steroid production by the adrenals, stimulation of insulin release, thyrotropin-like effects on the thyroid, and LH-like effects on isolated ovarian tissue, causing increased progesterone secretion from the corpus luteum. This last effect, observed *in vitro,* contrasts with what is perhaps the most remarkable of all the effects of prostaglandins in the endocrine system, namely, luteolysis. This property is possessed especially but not uniquely by PGF$_{2\alpha}$.

Luteolysis.   Prompt subsidence of progesterone output and regression of the corpus luteum follows parenteral injection of PGF$_{2\alpha}$ in a wide variety of mammals. This effect interrupts early pregnancy, which is dependent on luteal rather than placental progesterone. The mechanism of luteolysis is uncertain, but it may involve block of the normal ovarian response to circulating gonadotropin. The abortifacient action of prostaglandins in early human pregnancy does not seem to be accompanied by any demonstrable fall in plasma progesterone concentrations, and luteolysis is not a significant factor (*see* Goldberg and Ramwell, 1975; Horton and Poyser, 1976).

Metabolic Effects.   PGEs, notably PGE$_1$, inhibit the basal rate of lipolysis from adipose tissue *in vitro* and also lipolysis stimulated by exposure to catecholamines or other lipolytic hormones. Such effects have also been noted *in vivo* in various species, including man, but are more capricious. Indeed, low doses of PGE$_1$ in man tend to stimulate lipolysis, seemingly by an indirect effect mediated by sympathetic stimulation. PGEs also have some insulin-like effects on carbohydrate metabolism (Nakano, 1973) and exert parathyroid hormone-like effects that result in mobilization of calcium from bone in tissue culture (Klein and Raisz, 1970).

Mechanism of Action.   The acidic lipid nature of prostaglandins, HETEs, and some of the leukotrienes places them in a unique chemical class of autacoids and raises the question whether their diverse actions can be accommodated within the familiar concept of specific membrane-bound receptors of the sort invoked to explain the actions of autacoids of the classical amine or peptide type. Nevertheless, in many tissues prostaglandins regulate the synthesis of adenosine 3',5'-monophosphate (cyclic AMP) by activating or inhibiting adenylate cyclase in a fashion that appears to be identical to that for hormones and other autacoids. Moreover, there is a growing body of evidence for the existence of specific membrane-bound receptors for prostaglandins, thromboxanes, and leukotrienes in many tissues.

The metabolites of arachidonic acid appear to exert their actions by utilizing a variety of receptor-mediated mechanisms. For example, PGE$_2$ stimulates steroid formation in the adrenal cortex by activating adenylate cyclase; it suppresses epinephrine-induced lipolysis by inhibiting adenylate cyclase; and it stimulates uterine contraction by increasing the intracellular concentration of free calcium. In the last-named case, there is no evidence for inhibition of adenylate cyclase. Other mechanisms are less well defined. These include the relationship between the release and metabolism of arachidonic acid, which involves calcium ions and peroxidative conditions, and the stimulation of guanylate cyclase (Mittal and Murad, 1982). It is also not clear whether guanosine 3',5'-monophosphate (cyclic GMP) might serve to mediate or to oppose the effects of one or more of the metabolites of arachidonic acid that are generated under these circumstances.

The mechanism of action of prostaglandins and related substances has been studied intensively in platelets (*see* Mittal and Murad, 1982). The prostaglandin endoperoxides and TXA$_2$ can cause platelet clumping and facilitate aggregation that has been induced by other agents. These effects are associated with the release of intracellular calcium (Owen and Le Breton, 1981). The increased calcium promotes aggregation and production of additional TXA$_2$. Platelet aggregation is inhibited by PGI$_2$ by increasing the concentration of cyclic AMP. A progressive increase in the sequestration of calcium is associated with the accumulation of the cyclic nucleotide (Owen and Le Breton, 1981). There is evidence for more than one population of receptors for PGI$_2$ in platelets. PGE$_1$ appears to interact with receptors that have a high affinity for PGI$_2$, while PGD$_2$ acts at sites with a lower affinity. Relatively high concentrations of PGE$_2$ inhibit aggregation and stimulate adenylate cyclase, apparently by acting upon one or both of these receptors for PGI_2.

Receptor Antagonists. There are presently no universally effective, potent antagonists of responses to the prostaglandins or the leukotrienes. However, some compounds are effective in selected *in-vitro* tests, and a few of these may be of practical value *in vivo*. The most important prostaglandin antagonists are of three types: the 7-oxa analogs of the prostaglandin molecule (*e.g.*, 7-oxa-13-prostanoic acid); the dibenzoxazepine hydrazide derivatives, of which SC-19220 is the most representative; and polyphloretin phosphate, a polyanionic polyester of phloretin and phosphoric acid, and related compounds. While these compounds block the effects of prostaglandins on certain cells, they fail to do so uniformly. This presumably reflects heterogeneity of receptors for this complex class of autacoids (*see* Sanner and Eakins, 1976).

Several compounds have been described that selectively antagonize responses to TXA_2 in platelets and smooth muscle from various tissues. The effects of endoperoxides (*e.g.*, PGH_2) are also inhibited, presumably because they interact with the same population of receptors. One group of compounds are prostanoids with a bicycloheptane ring (Sprague *et al.*, 1983); another antagonist is 13-azaprostanoic acid (Le Breton *et al.*, 1979). The biological effects of these compounds are currently under investigation, especially with regard to their potential to modify thrombotic phenomena *in vivo*. Recently, two additional antagonists of responses to TXA_2 have been developed. Both compounds also inhibit the bronchoconstriction that is produced by $PGF_{2\alpha}$ and PGD_2 (Carrier *et al.*, 1984; Chan *et al.*, 1984; Weichman *et al.*, 1984). The potential clinical utility of agents with this pharmacological spectrum remains to be determined.

A potent and specific antagonist of SRS-A has been available since 1973 (before its peptidoleukotriene components were identified) (Augstein *et al.*, 1973). This substance, a chromone carboxylic acid (FPL 55712), has been a valuable investigational tool, but it has a biological half-life (about 30 seconds) that is too short for clinical application. A structural analog of LTD_4 also antagonizes specific responses to the peptidoleukotrienes; its duration of action is also brief (Weichman *et al.*, 1983).

ENDOGENOUS PROSTAGLANDINS AND
LEUKOTRIENES: POSSIBLE FUNCTIONS IN
PHYSIOLOGICAL AND PATHOLOGICAL
PROCESSES

With some autacoids, the scope of permissible conjecture on their possible involvement in normal and abnormal functions is limited by their restricted distribution. This is not so with the metabolites of arachidonic acid. Because these substances can probably be formed by virtually every tissue and cell type, it is not unreasonable to suspect that each pharmacological effect observed may reflect a physiological or pathophysiological function. And such suspicions have been nurtured and presented in countless hypotheses bearing on just about every bodily function (*see* appended list of monographs and reviews).

Platelets. An area in which there has been considerable interest is the elucidation of the role played by prostaglandin endoperoxides and TXA_2 in platelet aggregation and by PGI_2 in the prevention of such aggregation. It is generally accepted that stimulation of platelets to aggregate leads to activation of membrane phospholipases with the consequent release of arachidonic acid and its transformation into prostaglandin endoperoxides and TXA_2. These substances induce platelet aggregation. However, this pathway is not the only mechanism for the induction of platelet aggregation, since, for example, thrombin aggregates platelets without the release of arachidonic acid. The importance of the thromboxane pathway is, however, implied by the fact that aspirin inhibits the second phase of platelet aggregation and induces a mild hemostatic defect in man (Jobim, 1978).

PGI_2 generated in the vessel wall may be the physiological antagonist of this system in platelets. According to this concept, PGI_2 and TXA_2 represent biologically opposite poles of a mechanism for regulating platelet–vessel wall interaction and the formation of hemostatic plugs and intra-arterial thrombi (*see* Moncada and Vane, 1979).

Reproduction and Parturition. Much interest is attached to the possible involvement of prostaglandins in reproductive physiology. Their very high concentrations in human semen, coupled with the substantial absorption of prostaglandins by the vagina, have encouraged speculation that prostaglandins deposited during coitus may facilitate conception by actions on the cervix, uterine body, Fallopian tubes, and transport of semen. While there does seem to be a correlation between lowered concentrations of prostaglandins in semen and some cases of male infertility, the role of the eicosanoids in semen remains obscure.

During pregnancy in the human female, the capacity of the fetal membranes to elaborate prostaglandins rises progressively. Concentrations of prostaglandins in blood and amniotic fluid are elevated during labor, but it is not certain whether this is a major determinant of the onset of labor or only serves to sustain uterine contractions that have been initiated by oxytocin. In any event, inhibitors of cyclooxygenase can increase the length of gestation, prolong the duration of spontaneous labor, and interrupt premature labor. The last-named effect has prompted clinical investigation of these agents for the prevention of premature delivery. While effective, their potential impact on fetal development (*e.g.*, premature closure of the ductus arteriosus), together with the availability of other tocolytic agents, has limited the use of cyclooxygenase inhibitors for this purpose (*see* Chapter 39).

$PGF_{2\alpha}$ produced in the uterus is the long-sought luteolytic hormone in some subprimate species.

This knowledge has led to the development of prostaglandin analogs for veterinary use in synchronizing estrus in farm animals such as sheep, cattle, pigs, and horses. This method has simplified breeding procedures and is used to provide safe, early abortions before the animals are sent to market. However, a luteolytic prostaglandin analog for human use has not been developed. The possible roles of prostaglandins in reproductive processes have been reviewed by Goldberg and Ramwell (1975) and by Horton and Poyser (1976).

Vascular and Pulmonary Smooth Muscle. Local generation of PGE$_2$ and PGI$_2$ has been implicated in the maintenance of patency of the ductus arteriosus. This hypothesis has been strengthened by the fact that aspirin-like drugs induce closure of a patent ductus in animals and neonates (*see* Chapter 29). Prostaglandins might also play a role in the maintenance of placental blood flow (*see* Rankin, 1978).

A complex mixture of autacoids is released when sensitized lung tissue is challenged by the appropriate antigen. Various prostaglandins and leukotrienes are prominent components of this mixture. While both bronchodilator (PGE$_2$) and bronchoconstrictor (*e.g.*, PGF$_{2\alpha}$, TXA$_2$, LTC$_4$) substances are released, responses to the peptidoleukotrienes probably dominate during allergic constriction of the airway (*see* Piper, 1983). Included in the evidence for this conclusion is the ineffectiveness of inhibitors of cyclooxygenase and of histaminergic antagonists in the treatment of human asthma. Moreover, the relatively slow metabolism of the leukotrienes in lung tissue contributes to the long-lasting bronchoconstriction that follows challenge with antigen and may be a factor in the high bronchial tone that is observed in asthmatics in periods between acute attacks.

Kidney. Prostaglandins probably modulate renal blood flow and may serve to regulate urine formation by both renovascular and tubular effects. Additional roles in the regulation of the secretion of renin are also likely. The elaboration of PGE$_2$ and PGI$_2$ is increased by factors that reduce renal blood flow (*e.g.*, stimulation of sympathetic nerves and angiotensin), and inhibitors of cyclooxygenase augment the renovasoconstriction that is produced by such stimuli (*see* Aiken and Vane, 1973). The effects of ADH on the reabsorption of water may be restrained by the concomitant production and action of PGE$_2$, and the negative-feedback effects of angiotensin on renin secretion are opposed by the stimulant actions of PGI$_2$, PGE$_2$, and PGD$_2$.

Increased biosynthesis of prostaglandins has been associated with Bartter's syndrome. This is a rare disease characterized by low-to-normal blood pressure, decreased sensitivity to angiotensin, high activity of renin in plasma, hyperaldosteronism, and excessive loss of potassium. There is also an increased granulation of renal medullary interstitial cells and an increased excretion of prostaglandins in the urine. After chronic administration of inhibitors of cyclooxygenase, sensitivity to angiotensin, plasma renin values, and the concentration of aldosterone in plasma return to normal. Although plasma potassium rises, it remains low, and urinary potassium wasting persists. Whether an increase in prostaglandin biosynthesis is the cause of Bartter's syndrome or a reflection of a more basic physiological defect is not known (*see* Ferris, 1978).

Inflammatory and Immune Responses. Prostaglandins and leukotrienes are released by a host of mechanical, thermal, chemical, bacterial, and other insults, and they contribute importantly to the genesis of the signs and symptoms of inflammation (*see* Moncada *et al.*, 1978; Larsen and Henson, 1983). The peptidoleukotrienes have powerful effects on vascular permeability, while LTB$_4$ is a potent chemoattractant for polymorphonuclear leukocytes and can promote exudation of plasma by mobilizing this source of additional inflammatory mediators. Although prostaglandins do not appear to have direct effects on vascular permeability, both PGE$_2$ and PGI$_2$ markedly enhance edema formation and leukocyte infiltration by promoting blood flow in the inflamed region. Moreover, they potentiate the pain-producing activity of bradykinin and other autacoids (*see* Chapter 27). The lipoxygenase products, such as 5-HPETE and 5-HETE, may be required for the release of histamine from basophils, and they promote the secretion of histamine and other substances from mast cells. However, PGEs suppress the secretion of mediators of inflammation by mast cells in anaphylactic reactions and inhibit the participation of lymphocytes in delayed hypersensitivity reactions. Moreover, they inhibit the release of hydrolases and lysosomal enzymes from human neutrophils as well as from mouse peritoneal macrophages.

Prostaglandins have also been implicated in the control of the immunological response. PGE$_1$ has been claimed to influence the functions of B lymphocytes selectively and to act synergistically with procarbazine to depress immune responsiveness. In addition, the humoral antibody response is decreased by PGE$_1$. Prostaglandins also affect T lymphocytes. The T ("killer") lymphocyte, active in slowing tumor growth and killing malignant cells, is inhibited by PGEs in its ability to reject allogenic thymus cells *in vitro*. Exogenously administered prostaglandins have been reported to prolong skin allograft survival. Concentrations of PGE in plasma increase in proportion to the hypersensitized state and return to normal with acceptance of the graft. It has thus been suggested that prostaglandins, by inhibiting T- and B-cell functions, might facilitate graft acceptance. Finally, PGE is also active in inhibiting production and release of lymphokines by sensitized T lymphocytes (*see* Bourne, 1974; Goldyne, 1977; Pelus and Strausser, 1977).

Some experimental tumors in animals and certain spontaneous human tumors (medullary carcinoma of the thyroid, renal-cell adenocarcinoma, carcinoma of the breast) are accompanied by increased concentrations of local or circulating prostaglandins, bone metastasis, and hypercalcemia. The immunosuppressive activity of certain of these tumors may be related to their ability to produce prostaglandins. Furthermore, since prostaglandins of the E series have potent osteolytic activity, it has been suggested that they are implicated in some cases of hypercalcemia. Recent studies have implicated platelet aggregation and the effects of prostaglandins thereon in the hematogenous metastasis of tumors. While pretreatment of animals with inhibitors of thromboxane synthetase reduces the formation of tumor colonies, the administration of such agents after the injection of tumor cells is without effect. However, the infusion of PGI$_2$ either before or after the injection of cells markedly inhibits the establishment of tumor colonies. These effects have been attributed to inhibition of platelet aggregation, rather than to vasodilatation (*see* Honn *et al.*, 1983).

THERAPEUTIC USES

As described above, there has been intense interest in the effects of the prostaglandins on the female reproductive system. Their action as *abortifacients* is already clearly established. Given early in pregnancy they are abortifacient, but initial hopes that they might provide a simple, convenient means of postimplantation "contraception," perhaps given as a vaginal suppository, have not yet been fulfilled. Moreover, the abortifacient action of prostaglandins in the early weeks of pregnancy is inconstant and often incomplete, and may be accompanied by distressing side effects. Nevertheless, prostaglandins appear to be of value in missed abortion and molar gestation, and they have been widely used for the induction of midtrimester abortion. While PGE$_2$ or PGF$_{2\alpha}$ can induce labor at term, they may have more value when used to facilitate labor by promoting ripening and dilatation of the cervix. These actions of prostaglandins are considered more fully in Chapter 39.

The capacity of several prostaglandins to suppress gastric ulceration in experimental animals is a property of potential therapeutic importance. Some markedly inhibit gastric secretion when given orally to man and have antiulcer activity. However, all the PGE analogs have caused undesirable side effects, especially diarrhea. Analogs of PGI$_2$, which appear to cause fewer side effects, are being developed for this use.

PGE$_1$ has been administered by intra-arterial or intravenous infusion to patients with severe peripheral vascular disease. In the absence of complete arterial occlusion, dramatic and long-lasting improvement has been observed after short-term infusion (Olsson and Carlsson, 1976; Clifford *et al.*, 1980; Pardy *et al.*, 1980). Similar results have been obtained with the use of PGI$_2$ (Belch *et al.*, 1983a, 1983b).

Although the use of drugs that inhibit platelet aggregation in the treatment of acute myocardial infarction is controversial, there is evidence that PGI$_2$ can reduce the ischemic damage that follows ligation of a branch of the coronary artery in cats by mechanisms other than those related to coronary vasodilatation or inhibition of platelet aggregation (Schrör *et al.*, 1982).

Both PGE$_1$ and PGI$_2$ have been valuable for improving the harvest and storage of blood platelets for therapeutic transfusion. Recent clinical experience in cardiopulmonary bypass, charcoal hemoperfusion, and renal dialysis has indicated that PGI$_2$ is also useful in the prevention of platelet aggregation in extracorporeal circulation systems. In addition, PGI$_2$ has been used in place of heparin during dialysis of patients with renal disease, and it may have advantages for those in whom the use of heparin is contraindicated (Zusman *et al.*, 1981).

The pulmonary blood vessels, and particularly the ductus arteriosus in neonates, are especially sensitive to the vasodilatory effect of PGE$_1$ and PGI$_2$. These prostaglandins have been used to increase pulmonary blood flow and oxygenation of blood in infants with congenital heart defects that restrict pulmonary or systemic blood flow. Under such circumstances, dilatation of the ductus arteriosus improves blood flow and tissue oxygenation. At present, only PGE$_1$ (*alprostadil*) is available for this purpose in the United States; PGI$_2$ (*epoprostenol*) is available in Europe. Alprostadil (PROSTIN VR PEDIATRIC) is marketed in 1-ml ampuls containing 0.5 mg. The drug is usually infused intravenously at an initial rate of 0.1 μg/kg per minute, with subsequent reductions to the lowest dosage that maintains the response. Apnea is observed in about 10% of neonates so treated, particularly in those who weigh less than 2 kg at birth. The treatment is considered palliative until corrective surgery can be performed.

Continuous, chronic intravenous infusion of PGI$_2$ in a patient with primary pulmonary hypertension decreased pulmonary vascular resistance and improved oxygenation and exercise tolerance in one investigational study (Higenbottam *et al.*, 1984).

Aiken, J. W., and Vane, J. R. Intrarenal prostaglandin release attenuates the renal vasoconstrictor activity of angiotensin. *J. Pharmacol. Exp. Ther.*, **1973**, *184*, 678–687.

Anggard, E.; Larsson, C.; and Samuelsson, B. The distribution of 15-hydroxyprostaglandin dehydrogenase and prostaglandin-Δ^{13}-reductase in tissues of the swine. *Acta Physiol. Scand.*, **1971**, *81*, 396–404.

Armstrong, J. M.; Boura, A. L. A.; Hamberg, M.; and Samuelsson, B. A comparison of the vasodepressor effects of the cyclic endoperoxides PGG$_2$ and PGH$_2$ with those of PGD$_2$ and PGE$_2$ in hypertensive and normotensive rats. *Eur. J. Pharmacol.*, **1976**, *39*, 251–258.

Augstein, J.; Farmer, J. B.; Lee, T. B.; Sheard, P.; and Tattersall, M. L. Selective inhibitor of slow reacting substance of anaphylaxis. *Nature* [*New Biol.*], **1973**, *245*, 215–217.

Belch, J. J. F.; Drury, J. K.; Capell, H.; Forbes, C. D.; Newman, P.; McKenzie, F.; Leiberman, P.; and Prentice, C. R. M. Intermittent epoprostenol (prostacyclin) infusion in patients with Raynaud's syndrome. *Lancet*, **1983a**, *1*, 313–315.

Belch, J. J. F.; McArdle, B.; Pollock, J. G.; Forbes, C. D.; McKay, A.; Leiberman, P.; Lowe, G. D. O.; and Prentice, C. R. M. Epoprostenol (prostacyclin) and severe arterial disease. A double-blind trial. *Lancet*, **1983b**, *1*, 315–317.

Berkowitz, B. A.; Zabko-Potapovich, B.; Valocik, R.; and Gleason, J. G. Effects of the leukotrienes on the vasculature and blood pressure of different species. *J. Pharmacol. Exp. Ther.*, **1984**, *229*, 105–112.

Bianco, S.; Robuschi, M.; Ceserani, R.; and Gandolfi, C. Prevention of aspecifically induced bronchoconstriction by prostacyclin (PGI$_2$) in asthmatic subjects. *Int. Res. Commun. Syst. Med. Sci.*, **1978**, *6*, 256.

Carrier, R.; Cragoe, E. J.; Ethier, D.; Ford-Hutchinson, A. W.; Girard, Y.; Hall, R. A.; Hamel, P.; Rokach, J.; Share, N. N.; Stone, C. A.; and Yusko, P. Studies on L-640,035: a novel antagonist of contractile prostanoids in the lung. *Br. J. Pharmacol.*, **1984**, *82*, 389–395.

Chan, C. C.; Nathaniel, D. J.; Yusko, P. J.; Hall, R. A.; and Ford-Hutchinson, A. W. Inhibition of prostanoid-mediated platelet aggregation *in vivo* and *in vitro* by 3-hydroxymethyldibenzo(b,f)thiepin 5,5-dioxide (L-640,035). *J. Pharmacol. Exp. Ther.*, **1984**, *229*, 276–282.

Clifford, P. C.; Martin, M. F. R.; Sheddon, E. J.; Kirby, J. D.; Baird, R. N.; and Dieppe, P. A. Treatment of vasospastic disease with prostaglandin E$_1$. *Br. Med. J.* [*Clin. Res.*], **1980**, *281*, 1031–1039.

Cooper, C. L., and Malik, K. U. Mechanism of action of vasopressin on prostaglandin synthesis and vascular function in the isolated rat kidney: effect of calcium antagonists and calmodulin inhibitors. *J. Pharmacol. Exp. Ther.*, **1984**, *229*, 139–147.

Craven, P. A., and DeRubertis, F. R. Ca^{2+} calmodulin-dependent release of arachidonic acid for renal medullary prostaglandin synthesis. *J. Biol. Chem.*, **1983**, *258*, 4814–4823.

Dusting, G. J.; Moncada, S.; and Vane, J. R. Vascular actions of arachidonic acid and its metabolites in the perfused mesenteric and femoral beds of the dog. *Eur. J. Pharmacol.*, **1978**, *49*, 65–72.

Feldberg, W., and Kellaway, C. H. Liberation of histamine and formation of lysocithin-like substances by cobra venom. *J. Physiol. (Lond.)*, **1938**, *94*, 187–226.

Gerber, J. G.; Keller, R. T.; and Nies, A. S. Prostaglandins and renin release. The effect of PGI$_2$, PGE$_2$, and 13,14-dihydro PGE$_2$ on the baroreceptor mechanism of renin release in the dog. *Circ. Res.*, **1979**, *44*, 796–799.

Hamberg, M., and Samuelsson, B. On the metabolism of prostaglandins E$_1$ and E$_2$ in man. *J. Biol. Chem.*, **1971**, *246*, 6713–6721.

Hamberg, M.; Svensson, J.; and Samuelsson, B. Thromboxane: a new group of biologically active compounds derived from prostaglandin endoperoxides. *Proc. Natl Acad. Sci. U.S.A.*, **1975**, *72*, 2994–2998.

Higenbottam, T.; Wheeldon, D.; Wells, F.; and Wallwork, J. Long-term treatment of primary pulmonary hypertension with continuous intravenous epoprostenol (prostacyclin). *Lancet*, **1984**, *1*, 1046–1047.

Klein, D. C., and Raisz, L. G. Prostaglandins: stimulation of bone resorption in tissue culture. *Endocrinology*, **1970**, *86*, 1436–1440.

Le Breton, G. C.; Venton, D. L.; Enke, S. E.; and Halushka, P. V. 13-Azaprostanoic acid: a specific antagonist of the human blood platelet thromboxane/endoperoxide receptor. *Proc. Natl Acad. Sci. U.S.A.*, **1979**, *76*, 4097–4101.

Moncada, S.; Gryglewski, R.; Bunting, S.; and Vane, J. R. An enzyme isolated from arteries transforms prostaglandin endoperoxides to an unstable substance that inhibits platelet aggregation. *Nature*, **1976**, *263*, 663–665.

Olsson, A. G., and Carlsson, A. L. Clinical, hemodynamic and metabolic effects of intraarterial infusions of prostaglandin E$_1$ in patients with peripheral vascular disease. *Adv. Prostaglandin Thromboxane Res.*, **1976**, *1*, 429–432.

Owen, N. E., and Le Breton, G. C. Ca^{2+} mobilization in blood platelets as visualized by chlortetracycline fluorescence. *Am. J. Physiol.*, **1981**, *241*, 613–619.

Pardy, B. J.; Lewis, J. D.; and Eastcott, H. H. G. Preliminary experience with prostaglandins E$_1$ and I$_2$ in peripheral vascular disease. *Surgery*, **1980**, *88*, 826–832.

Patrignani, P.; Filabozzi, P.; Catella, F.; Pugliese, F.; and Patrono, C. Differential effects of dazoxiben, a selective thromboxane-synthase inhibitor, on platelet and renal prostaglandin-endoperoxide metabolism. *J. Pharmacol. Exp. Ther.*, **1984**, *228*, 472–477.

Peters, S. P.; Kagey-Sobotka, A.; MacGlashan, D. W., Jr.; and Lichtenstein, L. M. Effect of prostaglandin D$_2$ in modulating histamine release from human basophils. *J. Pharmacol. Exp. Ther.*, **1984**, *228*, 400–404.

Roberts, L. J.; Sweetman, B. J.; and Oates, J. A. Metabolism of thromboxane B$_2$ in man. Identification of twenty urinary metabolites. *J. Biol. Chem.*, **1981**, *256*, 8384–8393.

Robinson, B. F.; Collier, J. G.; Karim, S. M. M.; and Somers, K. Effect of prostaglandins A$_1$, A$_2$, B$_1$, E$_2$ and F$_2$ on forearm arterial bed and superficial hand veins in man. *Clin. Sci.*, **1973**, *44*, 367–376.

Rosenkranz, B.; Fischer, C.; Weimer, K. E.; and Frolich, J. C. Metabolism of prostacyclin and 6-keto-prostaglandin F$_{1\alpha}$ in man. *J. Biol. Chem.*, **1980**, *255*, 10194–10198.

Schrör, K.; Darius, H.; Ohlendorf, R.; Matzky, R.; and Klaus, W. Dissociation of antiplatelet effects from myocardial cytoprotective activity during acute myocardial ischemia in cats by a new carbacyclin derivative (ZK 36 375). *J. Cardiovasc. Pharmacol.*, **1982**, *4*, 554–561.

Seymour, A. A.; Davis, J. O.; Freeman, R. H.; DeForrest, J. M.; Rowe, B. P.; and Williams, G. M. Renin release from filtering and nonfiltering kidneys stimulated by PGI$_2$ and PGD$_2$. *Am. J. Physiol.*, **1979**, *237*, 285–290.

Sprague, P. W.; Heikes, J. E.; Harris, D. N.; and Greenberg, R. 7-Oxabicyclo [2.2.1] heptane analogs as modulators of the thromboxane A$_2$ and prostacyclin receptors. *Adv. Prostaglandin Thromboxane Leukotriene Res.*, **1983**, *11*, 337–344.

Stokes, J. B. Effect of prostaglandin E$_2$ on chloride transport across the rabbit thick ascending limb of Henle: selective inhibition of the medullary portion. *J. Clin. Invest.*, **1979**, *64*, 495–502.

Vane, J. R. Inhibition of prostaglandin synthesis as a mechanism of action for aspirin-like drugs. *Nature* [*New Biol.*], **1971**, *231*, 232–235.

Weichman, B. M.; Wasserman, M. A.; Holden, D. A.; Osborn, R. R.; Woodward, D. F.; Ku, T. W.; and Gleason, J. G. Antagonism of the pulmonary effects of the peptidoleukotrienes by a leukotriene D$_4$ analog. *J. Pharmacol. Exp. Ther.*, **1983**, *227*, 700–705.

Weichman, B. M.; Wasserman, M. A.; and Gleason, J. G. SK&F 88046: a unique pharmacologic antagonist of bronchoconstriction induced by leukotriene D$_4$, thromboxane and prostaglandins F$_{2\alpha}$ and D$_2$ *in vitro*. *J. Pharmacol. Exp. Ther.*, **1984**, *228*, 128–132.

Whittle, B. J. R.; Kauffman, G. L.; and Moncada, S. Vasoconstriction with thromboxane A$_2$ induces ulceration of the gastric mucosa. *Nature*, **1981**, *292*, 472–474.

Zusman, R. M.; Rubin, R. H.; Cato, A. E.; Cocchetto, D. M.; Crow, J. W.; and Tolkoff-Rubin, N. Hemodialysis using prostacyclin instead of heparin as the sole antithrombotic agent. *N. Engl. J. Med.*, **1981**, *304*, 934–939.

Monographs and Reviews

Behrman, H. R. Prostaglandins in hypothalamo-pituitary and ovarian function. *Annu. Rev. Physiol.*, **1979**, *41*, 685–700.

Bennett, A. The role of prostaglandins in gastrointestinal tone and motility. In, *Prostaglandins and Thromboxanes*. (Berti, F.; Samuelsson, B.; and Velo, G. P.; eds.) Plenum Press, New York, **1977**, pp. 275–285.

Bergström, S., and Samuelsson, B. The prostaglandins. *Endeavour*, **1968**, *27*, 109–113.

Bourne, H. R. Immunology. In, *The Prostaglandins*.

(Ramwell, P. W., ed.) Plenum Press, New York, **1974**, pp. 277–292.

Cuthbert, M. F. Prostaglandins and respiratory smooth muscle. In, *The Prostaglandins: Pharmacological and Therapeutic Advances.* (Cuthbert, M. F., ed.) J. B. Lippincott Co., Philadelphia, **1973**, pp. 253–286.

Dunn, M. J., and Hood, V. L. Prostaglandins in the kidney. *Am. J. Physiol.*, **1977**, *233*, F169–F184.

Dusting, G. J.; Moncada, S.; and Vane, J. R. Prostaglandins, their intermediates and precursors, their cardiovascular actions and regulatory roles in normal and abnormal circulatory systems. *Prog. Cardiovasc. Dis.*, **1979**, *21*, 405–430.

Euler, U. S. von. Some aspects of the actions of prostaglandins. The First Heymans Memorial Lecture. *Arch. Int. Pharmacodyn. Ther.*, **1973**, *202*, Suppl., 295–307.

Ferris, T. F. Prostaglandins, potassium and Bartter's syndrome. *J. Lab. Clin. Med.*, **1978**, *92*, 663–668.

Fisher, J. W., and Gross, D. M. Effects of prostaglandins on erythropoiesis. In, *Prostaglandins in Hematology.* (Silver, M.; Smith, B. J.; and Kocsis, J. J.; eds.) Spectrum Publications, Inc., New York, **1977**, pp. 159–185.

Flower, R. J. Drugs which inhibit prostaglandin biosynthesis. *Pharmacol. Rev.*, **1974**, *26*, 33–67.

———. Prostaglandins and related compounds. In, *Handbook of Experimental Pharmacology*, Vol. 50. (Vane, J. R., and Ferreira, S. H., eds.) Springer-Verlag, Berlin, **1978**, pp. 374–422.

Goldberg, V. J., and Ramwell, P. W. Role of prostaglandins in reproduction. *Physiol. Rev.*, **1975**, *55*, 325–351.

Goldyne, M. E. Prostaglandins and the modulation of immunological responses. *Int. J. Dermatol.*, **1977**, *16*, 701–712.

Hamberg, M.; Svensson, J.; Hedqvist, P.; Strandberg, K.; and Samuelsson, B. Involvement of endoperoxides and thromboxanes in anaphylactic reactions. *Adv. Prostaglandin Thromboxane Res.*, **1976**, *1*, 495–501.

Harris, R. H.; Ramwell, P. W.; and Gilmer, P. J. Cellular mechanisms of prostaglandin action. *Annu. Rev. Physiol.*, **1979**, *41*, 653–668.

Honn, K. V.; Busse, W. D.; and Sloane, B. F. Prostacyclin and thromboxanes: implications for their role in tumor cell metastasis. *Biochem. Pharmacol.*, **1983**, *32*, 1–11.

Horton, E. W., and Poyser, N. L. Uterine luteolytic hormone. A physiological role for prostaglandin F$_{2\alpha}$. *Physiol. Rev.*, **1976**, *56*, 595–651.

Jobim, F. Acetylsalicylic acid, hemostasis and human thromboembolism. *Semin. Thromb. Hemostas.*, **1978**, *4*, 199–240.

Larsen, G. L., and Henson, P. M. Mediators of inflammation. *Annu. Rev. Immunol.*, **1983**, *1*, 335–359.

Lee, J. B. Cardiovascular renal effects of prostaglandins. *Arch. Intern. Med.*, **1974**, *133*, 56–76.

Mittal, C. K., and Murad, F. Guanylate cyclase: regulation of cyclic GMP metabolism. In, *Cyclic Nucleotides.*

Handbook of Experimental Pharmacology, Vol. 58. (Nathanson, J. A., and Kebabian, J. W., eds.) Springer-Verlag, Berlin, **1982**, pp. 225–260.

Moncada, S. Biological importance of prostacyclin. VIII Gaddum Memorial Lecture. *Br. J. Pharmacol.*, **1982**, *76*, 3–31.

Moncada, S.; Ferreira, S. H.; and Vane, J. R. Pain and inflammatory mediators. In, *Inflammation. Handbook of Experimental Pharmacology*, Vol. 50. (Ferreira,

Moncada, S., and Vane, J. R. Pharmacology and endogenous roles of prostaglandin endoperoxides, thromboxane A$_2$ and prostacyclin. *Pharmacol. Rev.*, **1979**, *30*, 293–331.

Nakano, J. General pharmacology of prostaglandins. In, *The Prostaglandins: Pharmacological and Therapeutic Advances.* (Cuthbert, M. F., ed.) J. B. Lippincott Co., Philadelphia, **1973**, pp. 23–124.

Nakano, J., and Koss, M. C. Pathophysiologic roles of prostaglandins and the action of aspirin-like drugs. *South. Med. J.*, **1973**, *66*, 709–721.

Nugteren, D. H. Arachidonate lipoxygenase. In, *Prostaglandins in Hematology.* (Silver, M.; Smith, B. J.; and Kocsis, J. J.; eds.) Spectrum Publications, Inc., New York, **1977**, pp. 11–25.

Pelus, L. M., and Strausser, H. R. Prostaglandins and the immune response. *Life Sci.*, **1977**, *20*, 903–914.

Piper, P. J. Pharmacology of leukotrienes. *Br. Med. Bull.*, **1983**, *39*, 255–259.

Rankin, J. H. G. Role of prostaglandins in the maintenance of the placental circulation. *Adv. Prostaglandin Thromboxane Res.*, **1978**, *4*, 261–269.

Rasmussen, H., and Lake, W. Prostaglandins and the mammalian erythrocyte. In, *Prostaglandins in Hematology.* (Silver, M.; Smith, B. J.; and Kocsis, J. J.; eds.) Spectrum Publications, Inc., New York, **1977**, pp. 187–202.

Samuelsson, B. Biosynthesis of prostaglandins. *Fed. Proc.*, **1972**, *31*, 1442–1460.

———. Leukotrienes: mediators of immediate hypersensitivity reactions and inflammation. *Science*, **1983**, *220*, 568–575.

Samuelsson, B.; Goldyne, M.; Granstrom, E.; Hamberg, M.; Hammarstrom, S.; and Malmsten, C. Prostaglandins and thromboxanes. *Annu. Rev. Biochem.*, **1978**, *47*, 997–1029.

Samuelsson, B.; Granstrom, E.; Green, K.; Hamberg, M.; and Hammarstrom, S. Prostaglandins. *Annu. Rev. Biochem.*, **1975**, *44*, 669–694.

Sanner, J. H., and Eakins, K. E. Prostaglandin antagonists. In, *Prostaglandins: Chemical and Biochemical Aspects.* (Karim, S. M. M., ed.) M. T. P. Press, Lancaster, England, **1976**, pp. 139–189.

Vane, J. R. Prostacyclin: a hormone with a therapeutic potential. *J. Endocrinol.*, **1982**, *95*, 3P–43P.

Wolfe, L. S. Eicosanoids: prostaglandins, thromboxanes, leukotrienes, and other derivatives of carbon-20 unsaturated fatty acids. *J. Neurochem.*, **1982**, *38*, 1–14.

SECTION

V

Drug Therapy of Inflammation

In this section drugs that are anti-inflammatory, analgesic, and antipyretic will be considered; their mechanisms of action differ from those of the anti-inflammatory steroids and the opioid analgesics. Also included are miscellaneous anti-inflammatory agents and drugs used in the treatment of gout, such as colchicine and allopurinol. Several other agents are employed to suppress the manifestations of inflammation but are considered more conveniently in other sections of the textbook. These especially include the adrenocorticosteroids; also in this category are immunosuppressive agents, chloroquine, and penicillamine.

CHAPTER

29 ANALGESIC-ANTIPYRETICS AND ANTI-INFLAMMATORY AGENTS; DRUGS EMPLOYED IN THE TREATMENT OF GOUT

Roderick J. Flower, Salvador Moncada, and John R. Vane

The anti-inflammatory, analgesic, and antipyretic drugs are a heterogeneous group of compounds, often chemically unrelated (although most of them are organic acids), which nevertheless share certain therapeutic actions and side effects. The prototype is aspirin; hence these compounds are often referred to as *aspirin-like drugs*.

There has been substantial progress in elucidating the mechanism of action of aspirin-like drugs, and it is now possible to understand why such heterogeneous agents have the same basic therapeutic activities and often the same side effects. Indeed, their therapeutic activity appears to depend to a large extent upon the inhibition of a defined biochemical pathway responsible for the biosynthesis of the prostaglandins and related autacoids. The mechanism of action of aspirin-like drugs and some of their shared properties will first be consid-

ered; then the more important drugs will be discussed in some detail.

History. The medicinal effect of the bark of willow and certain other plants has been known to several cultures for centuries. In England in the mid-eighteenth century, Reverend Edmund Stone described in a letter to the president of the Royal Society "an account of the success of the bark of the willow in the cure of agues" (fever). Edmund Stone had accidentally tasted the bark of the common white willow (*Salix alba vulgaris*), and the bitterness was, to him, strongly reminiscent of *Cinchona* bark (the source of quinine). He rationalized his finding on the grounds that since the willow grew in damp or wet areas "where agues chiefly abound," it would probably possess curative properties appropriate to that condition.

The active ingredient in the willow bark was a bitter glycoside called *salicin*, first isolated in a pure form in 1829 by Leroux, who also demonstrated its antipyretic effect. On hydrolysis, salicin yields *glucose* and *salicylic alcohol*. The latter can be converted into *salicylic acid*, either *in vivo* or by chemical manipulation. Salicylic acid was also prepared from *oil of gaultheria* (oil of wintergreen) and

674

from extracts of other plants, including *Spiraea ulmaria* (a relative of the rose). The synthetic manufacture of this acid from phenol was accomplished in 1860 by Kolbe and Lautemann. *Sodium salicylate* was first used for the treatment of rheumatic fever and as an antipyretic in 1875, and the discovery of its uricosuric effects and of its utility in the treatment of gout soon followed. The enormous success of this drug prompted Hoffman, a chemist employed by Bayer, to prepare acetylsalicylic acid based on the earlier, but forgotten, work of Gerhardt in 1853. After demonstration of its anti-inflammatory effects, this compound was introduced into medicine in 1899 by Dreser under the name of *aspirin*. The name is said to have been derived from *Spiraea*, the plant species from which salicylic acid was once prepared.

The synthetic salicylates soon displaced the more expensive compounds obtained from natural sources. By the early years of this century the chief therapeutic (antipyretic, anti-inflammatory, and analgesic) actions of aspirin were known. Toward the end of the nineteenth century, other drugs were discovered that shared some or all of these actions; among these, only derivatives of para-aminophenol (*e.g.*, *acetaminophen*) are used today, principally for antipyresis and analgesia. Beginning with *indomethacin*, a host of new agents has been introduced into medicine in various countries during the past 20 years. While deserving to be called aspirin-like, these drugs have been used primarily for their anti-inflammatory effects.

MECHANISM OF ACTION OF ASPIRIN-LIKE DRUGS

Although this class of drugs had been known to inhibit a wide variety of reactions *in vitro*, no convincing relationship could be established with their known anti-inflammatory, antipyretic, and analgesic effects. In 1971, Vane and associates and Smith and Willis demonstrated that low concentrations of aspirin and indomethacin inhibited the enzymatic production of prostaglandins (*see* Chapter 28). There was, at that time, some evidence that prostaglandins participated in the pathogenesis of inflammation and fever, and this reinforced the hypothesis that inhibition of the biosynthesis of these autacoids could explain a considerable number of the clinical actions of the drugs (*see* Higgs *et al.*, in Symposium, 1983a). In the subsequent years the following major points have been established: (1) All mammalian cell types studied (with the exception of the erythrocyte) have microsomal enzymes for the synthesis of prostaglandins. (2) Prostaglandins are always released when cells are damaged and have been detected in increased concentrations in inflammatory exudates. All available evidence indicates that cells do not store prostaglandins, and their release thus depends on biosynthesis *de novo*. (3) All aspirin-like drugs inhibit the biosynthesis and release of prostaglandins in all cells tested. (4) With the exception of the anti-inflammatory glucocorticoids, other classes of drugs generally do not affect the biosynthesis of prostaglandins.

Inflammation. While it is difficult to give an adequate description of the inflammatory phenomenon in terms of underlying cellular events in the injured tissue, there are certain features of the process that are generally agreed to be characteristic. These include fenestration of the microvasculature, leakage of the elements of blood into the interstitial spaces, and migration of leukocytes into the inflamed tissue. On a macroscopic level, this is usually accompanied by the familiar clinical signs of erythema, edema, tenderness (hyperalgesia), and pain. During this complex response, chemical mediators such as histamine, 5-hydroxytryptamine (5-HT), various chemotactic factors, bradykinin, leukotrienes, and prostaglandins are liberated locally. Phagocytic cells migrate into the area, and cellular lysosomal membranes may be ruptured, releasing lytic enzymes. All these events may contribute to the inflammatory response. However, aspirin-like drugs have little or no effect upon the release or activity of histamine, 5-HT, or lysosomal enzymes. Similarly, potent antagonists of 5-HT or histamine have little or no therapeutic effect in inflammation; consequently, the importance of these mediators in the initiation or maintenance of the inflammatory response is questionable.

Inflammation in patients with rheumatoid arthritis probably involves the combination of an antigen (gamma globulin) with an antibody (rheumatoid factor) and complement, causing the local release of chemotactic factors that attract leukocytes. The leukocytes phagocytose the complexes of antigen, antibody, and complement and also release the many enzymes contained in their lysosomes. These lysosomal enzymes then cause injury to cartilage and other tissues, and this furthers the degree of inflammation. Cell-mediated immune reactions may also be involved. Prostaglandins are also released during this process.

The effects produced by intradermal, intravenous, or intra-arterial injections of prostaglandins are strongly reminiscent of inflammation. In nanogram amounts, prostaglandin E_2 (PGE_2) and prostacyclin (PGI_2), which are likely to be generated in inflammation, cause erythema and increase local blood flow. Two important vascular effects of prostaglandins of the E series are not generally shared by other mediators of inflammation—a long-lasting vasodilator action and the capacity to counteract the vasoconstrictor effects of substances such as norepinephrine and angiotensin. The erythema induced by intradermal injection of prostaglandins clearly illustrates their long-lasting action (up to 10 hours). In contrast to their long-lasting effects upon cutaneous vessels and superficial veins, vasodilatation produced by prostaglandins in other vascular beds vanishes within a few minutes.

A number of putative mediators of inflammation increase vascular permeability (leakage) in the postcapillary and collecting venules. It is not clear whether prostaglandins can produce such effects without the participation of other inflammatory mediators. In fact, prostaglandins produce vasodilatation more effectively than they do edema. However, PGE_1, PGE_2, and PGA_2 (but not $PGF_{2\alpha}$) cause edema when injected into the hind paw of the rat. In addition, there is a clear synergism between PGE_1 and bradykinin when these two mediators are given together. Interestingly, some of the vascular effects of bradykinin appear to be due to stimulation of the synthesis of prostaglandins.

Migration of leukocytes into an inflamed area is an important aspect of the inflammatory process. The prostaglandins are unlikely to be directly involved in the chemotactic response; however, another product of the metabolism of arachidonic acid, leukotriene B_4, is a very potent chemotactic substance (*see* Chapter 28; Larsen and Henson, 1983). The lipoxygenase enzyme that generates the leukotrienes is insensitive to the aspirin-like drugs; thus, concentrations of these drugs that suppress the formation of prostaglandins do not generally decrease cell migration (Higgs *et al.*, 1980). At higher concentrations, a suppression of cell migration is usually observed, but inhibition of lipoxygenase does not appear to be involved. However, drugs that inhibit both lipoxygenase and cyclooxygenase do have superior anti-inflammatory actions (Higgs and Flower, 1981).

Pain. The aspirin-like drugs are usually classified as mild analgesics, but this is not altogether true. A consideration of the type of pain as well as its intensity is important in the assessment of analgesic efficacy. In postoperative pain, for example, the aspirin-like drugs can be superior to the opioid analgesics.

Prostaglandins are associated particularly with the development of pain that accompanies injury or inflammation. Large doses of PGE_2 or $PGF_{2\alpha}$, given to women by intramuscular or subcutaneous injection to induce abortion, cause intense local pain. Prostaglandins can also cause headache and vascular pain when infused intravenously in man. While the doses of prostaglandins required to elicit pain are high in comparison with the concentrations expected *in vivo*, induction of hyperalgesia (*i.e.*, a state in which pain can be elicited by normally painless mechanical or chemical stimulation) seems to be a typical response to low concentrations of prostaglandins. A long-lasting hyperalgesia occurs when minute amounts of PGE_1 are given intradermally to man. Furthermore, in experiments in man where separate subdermal infusions of PGE_1, bradykinin, or histamine (or a mixture of bradykinin and histamine) caused no overt pain, marked pain was experienced when PGE_1 was

added to bradykinin or histamine. When PGE_1 was infused with histamine, itching was also noted.

These and other observations indicate that prostaglandins have the ability to sensitize pain receptors to mechanical and chemical stimulation; this has been confirmed by electrophysiological measurement of sensory nerve discharge in the presence of prostaglandins. According to Perl (1976), prostaglandin-induced hyperalgesia results from a lowering of the threshold of the polymodal nociceptors of C fibers. The aspirin-like drugs do not affect the hyperalgesia or the pain caused by direct action of prostaglandins, consistent with the notion that it is their synthesis that is inhibited. A possible exception to this is the fenamates, which may have some antagonistic action against prostaglandins, as well as potent capability to inhibit their synthesis.

Fever. Regulation of body temperature requires a delicate balance between the production and loss of heat, and the hypothalamus regulates the set point at which body temperature is maintained. In fever, this set point is obviously elevated, and aspirin-like drugs promote its return to normal. These drugs do not influence body temperature when it is elevated by such factors as exercise or increases in the ambient temperature.

Fever may be a result of infection or one of the sequelae of tissue damage, inflammation, graft rejection, malignancy, or other disease states. A multitude of microorganisms can cause fever. There is evidence that bacterial endotoxins (lipopolysaccharides from the cell wall) act by stimulating the biosynthesis and release by neutrophils and other cells of an *endogenous pyrogen*, a protein with a molecular weight in the range of 10,000 to 20,000. The current view is that the endogenous pyrogen passes from the general circulation into the central nervous system (CNS), where it acts upon discrete sites within the brain, especially the preoptic hypothalamic area. There is evidence that the resultant elevation of body temperature is mediated by the release of prostaglandins and that aspirin-like drugs suppress the effects of endogenous pyrogen by inhibiting the synthesis of these substances. The evidence includes the ability of prostaglandins, especially PGE_2, to produce fever when infused into the cerebral ventricles or when injected into the hypothalamus. Fever is a frequent side effect of prostaglandins when they are administered to women as abortifacients. Moreover, some studies have demonstrated an increase in prostaglandin-like substances in the cerebrospinal fluid when endogenous pyrogen is injected intravenously. The fever produced by the administration of pyrogen, but not that by prostaglandins, is reduced by aspirin-like drugs (*see* Milton, 1982).

Inhibition of Prostaglandin Biosynthesis by Aspirin-like Drugs. There are now numerous systems *in vitro* and *in vivo* in which inhibition of prostaglandin biosynthesis by aspirin, indomethacin, or similar compounds has been demonstrated; this effect is not restricted to any one species or tissue. It is dependent only on the drug reaching the cyclooxygenase enzyme. The distribution and pharmacokinetic properties of each agent thus have an important bearing on the drug's activity.

Aspirin-like drugs inhibit or interfere with a variety of other enzymes and cellular systems. However, few other enzymes known to be susceptible to aspirin-like drugs are affected at concentrations that inhibit the cyclooxygenase, although inhibition of other enzymes may contribute to the toxic effects of these drugs, particularly with overdosage.

Any hypothesis that purports to explain the action of a drug in terms of inhibition of an enzyme must satisfy at least two basic criteria. First, the free concentrations achieved in plasma during therapy must be sufficient to inhibit the enzyme in question. Second, there must be a reasonable correlation between antienzyme activity and therapeutic potency.

Certainly, there is good evidence that therapeutic doses of aspirin-like compounds reduce prostaglandin biosynthesis in man. Such doses of aspirin or indomethacin inhibit the production of prostaglandins by human platelets and reduce the prostaglandin content of human semen. There is also a reduction of prostaglandin metabolites in urine (Hamberg, 1972) and of concentrations of prostaglandins in synovial fluid of arthritic knee joints (Higgs et al., 1974).

There is a reasonably good rank-order correlation between the antienzyme activity of these drugs and their anti-inflammatory activity (estimated by a popular laboratory model of inflammation, the carrageenin edema test in rat hind paw). The only outstanding exception is indomethacin, which is apparently more potent against paw edema than in the enzyme inhibition assay. Ham and associates (1972) found a similar correlation for individual members of structurally related groups of aspirin-like drugs (except for the fenamates). More interesting is that the high degree of stereospecificity for anti-inflammatory activity among several pairs of enantiomers of α-methyl arylacetic acids is also evident in their inhibitory effect on prostaglandin synthetase. In each instance the d isomer was more potent. Another example of this type of selectivity is provided by the drug sulindac. It is a prodrug that is only weakly active; it is metabolized in vivo to a highly active anti-inflammatory metabolite. Likewise, the drug itself has little ability to inhibit prostaglandin biosynthesis, but the sulfide metabolite is a potent inhibitor.

The degree to which microsomal preparations of cyclooxygenase from different tissues are inhibited by aspirin-like drugs also varies considerably, and it is possible that there are multiple forms of the enzyme. Investigation of this possibility may permit design of drugs with greater specificity.

Mode of Inhibitory Action. Aspirin-like drugs inhibit the conversion of arachidonic acid to the unstable endoperoxide intermediate, PGG_2, which is catalyzed by the cyclooxygenase (*see* Chapter 28). Individual agents have differing modes of inhibitory activity on the cyclooxygenase. Aspirin itself acetylates a serine at the active site of the enzyme (Roth and Siok, 1978). Platelets are especially susceptible to this action because (unlike most other cells) they are incapable of regenerating the enzyme, presumably because they have little or no capacity for protein biosynthesis. In practical terms this means that a single dose of aspirin will inhibit the platelet cyclooxygenase for the life of the platelet (8 to 11 days); in man, a dose as small as 40 mg per day is sufficient to produce this effect. In contrast to aspirin, salicylic acid has no acetylating capacity and is almost inactive against cyclooxygenase in vitro. Nevertheless, it is as active as aspirin in reducing the synthesis of prostaglandins in vivo (Hamberg, 1972). The basis of this action and, thus, of the anti-inflammatory effects of salicylic acid is not clearly understood. Since aspirin is rapidly hydrolyzed to salicylic acid in vivo (half-life in human plasma, approximately 15 minutes), the acetylated and the nonacetylated species probably act as pharmacologically distinct entities.

Most of the other common aspirin-like drugs are "irreversible" inhibitors of the cyclooxygenase, although there are some exceptions (*see* Flower, 1974). For indomethacin, the mode of inhibition is particularly complex and probably involves a site on the enzyme different from that which is acetylated by aspirin.

SHARED THERAPEUTIC ACTIVITIES AND SIDE EFFECTS OF ASPIRIN-LIKE DRUGS

All aspirin-like drugs are antipyretic, analgesic, and anti-inflammatory, but there are important differences in their activities. For example, acetaminophen is antipyretic and analgesic but is only weakly anti-inflammatory. The reasons for such differences are not clear; variations in the sensitivity of enzymes in the target tissues may be important.

When employed as *analgesics,* these drugs are usually effective only against pain of low-to-moderate intensity, particularly that associated with inflammation. They have much lower maximal effects than do the opioids. However, they do not cause dependence and are mainly free of the unwanted effects of the opioids on the CNS. Aspirin-like drugs do not change the perception of sensory modalities other than pain. As mentioned, the type of pain is important; chronic postoperative pain or pain arising from inflammation is particularly well controlled by aspirin-like drugs, whereas pain arising from the hollow viscera is usually not relieved.

As *antipyretics,* aspirin-like drugs reduce the body temperature in febrile states. Although all such drugs are antipyretics and analgesics, some are not suitable for either routine or prolonged use because of toxicity; phenylbutazone is an example.

This class of drugs finds its chief clinical application as *anti-inflammatory agents* in the treatment of musculoskeletal disorders, such as rheumatoid arthritis, osteoarthritis, and ankylosing spondylitis. In general, aspirin-like drugs provide only symptomatic relief from the pain and inflammation associated with the disease and do not arrest the progression of pathological injury to tissue.

In addition to sharing many therapeutic activities, aspirin-like drugs share several unwanted effects. The most common is a propensity to induce *gastric* or *intestinal ulceration* that can sometimes be accompanied by a secondary anemia from the resultant blood loss. Aspirin-like drugs vary considerably in their tendency to cause such erosions (*see* individual sections). Gastric damage by these agents can be brought about by at least two distinct mechanisms. While local irritation by the drugs in the stomach allows back diffusion of acid into the mucosa and induces tissue damage, the parenteral administration of these anti-inflammatory agents can also cause gastric damage and bleeding. This appears to be correlated with inhibition of the biosynthesis of gastric prostaglandins (*see* Whittle and Vane, 1983). The predominant prostaglandins synthesized by the gastric mucosa are PGI_2 and PGE_2; these eicosanoids inhibit acid secretion by the stomach and promote the secretion of cytoprotective mucus in the intestine. Such prostaglandins and their analogs can prevent mucosal damage, including that induced by anti-inflammatory drugs, in both experimental animals and man (*see* Robert, 1981). Thus, inhibition of the synthesis of endogenous prostaglandins may render the stomach more susceptible to damage.

There are other side effects of these drugs that probably depend upon their capacity to block endogenous prostaglandin biosynthesis; these include disturbances in platelet function and the prolongation of gestation or spontaneous labor. *Platelet function* appears to be disturbed because aspirin-like drugs prevent the formation by the platelets of thromboxane A_2 (TXA_2), a potent aggregating agent. This accounts for the tendency of these drugs to increase the

bleeding time. *Prolongation of gestation* by aspirin-like drugs has been demonstrated in both experimental animals and the human female. Furthermore, prostaglandins of the E and F series are potent uterotropic agents, and their biosynthesis by the uterus increases dramatically in the hours before parturition. It is thus hypothesized that prostaglandins play a major role in the initiation and progression of labor and delivery (*see* Chapter 39).

Aspirin-like drugs have little effect on renal function in normal human subjects; however, they decrease renal blood flow and the rate of glomerular filtration in patients with congestive heart failure or hepatic cirrhosis with ascites or in those who are hypovolemic for any reason (*see* Lifschitz, 1983; Clive and Stoff, 1984; Dunn, 1984). Similar effects occur in patients with chronic renal disease. Under these circumstances, acute renal failure may be precipitated. These effects appear to reflect the function of renal prostaglandins to mitigate the vasoconstrictive influences of norepinephrine and angiotensin II that result from the activation of pressor mechanisms.

In addition to their hemodynamic effects in the kidney, aspirin-like drugs promote the retention of salt and water by reducing the prostaglandin-induced inhibition of both the reabsorption of chloride and the action of antidiuretic hormone. This may cause edema in some patients with arthritis who are treated with an aspirin-like drug (*see* Clive and Stoff, 1984). These drugs also promote hyperkalemia, apparently by suppressing the prostaglandin-induced secretion of renin. This effect may account in part for the utility of aspirin-like drugs in the treatment of *Bartter's syndrome,* characterized by hypokalemia, hyperreninemia, hyperaldosteronism, juxtaglomerular hyperplasia, normotension, and resistance to the pressor effect of angiotensin II. Excessive production of renal prostaglandins may play an important role in the pathogenesis of this syndrome.

While nephropathy is uncommonly associated with the chronic use of individual aspirin-like drugs, the abuse of analgesic mixtures has been linked to the development of renal injury, including *papillary necrosis* and *chronic interstitial nephritis.* The injury is often insidious in onset, is usually manifest initially as reduced tubular function and concentrating ability, and may progress to irreversible renal insufficiency if misuse of analgesics continues. Females are involved more frequently than are males, and there is often a history of recurring urinary tract infection. Emotional disturbances are common, and other drugs may be abused concurrently. Despite numerous clinical observations and experimental studies in animals and man, crucial details of the problem remain uncertain. Phenacetin was suggested to be the nephrotoxic component of analgesic mixtures and, therefore, was removed from these products. While the incidence of analgesic nephropathy in some countries has subsequently declined, this has not been a universal result, especially in Australia. Indeed, there is evidence that the substitution of acetaminophen or salicylamide for phenacetin in such mixtures does not reduce the incidence of renal damage. It is possible that chronic abuse of any aspirin-like drug or analgesic mixture may cause renal injury in the susceptible individual (*see* Nanra, in Symposium, 1983b; Maher, 1984).

Several other features of aspirin-like drugs that depend upon their capacity to block prostaglandin biosynthesis also deserve mention. Prostaglandins have been implicated in the maintenance of patency of the *ductus arteriosus*, and indomethacin and related agents have been used with some success in neonates to close the ductus when it has remained patent. The release of prostaglandins by the endometrium during menstruation may be a cause of severe cramps and other symptoms of *primary dysmenorrhea*; treatment of this condition with aspirin-like drugs has met with considerable success (*see* Chan, 1983; Owen, 1984).

Certain individuals display intolerance to aspirin and most aspirin-like drugs; this is manifest by symptoms that range from vasomotor rhinitis with profuse watery secretions, angioneurotic edema, generalized urticaria, and bronchial asthma to laryngeal edema and bronchoconstriction, hypotension, shock, loss of consciousness, and complete vasomotor collapse. While rare in children, this syndrome may occur in 20 to 25% of middle-aged patients with asthma, nasal polyps, or chronic urticaria (*see* Settipane, in Symposium, 1983c). Despite the resemblance to anaphylaxis, the underlying mechanism does not appear to be immunological in nature. Moreover, an individual who is intolerant to one aspirin-like drug may react when exposed to any of a variety of such agents, despite their chemical diversity. The underlying mechanism is unknown, but a common factor among the drugs that provoke the reaction appears to be their ability to inhibit the cyclooxygenase. This has prompted the hypothesis that the reaction reflects the diversion of arachidonic acid metabolism toward the formation of increased amounts of leukotrienes and other products of the lipoxygenase pathway (*see* Szczeklik and Gryglewski, 1983). However, this view does not explain why only a minority of patients with asthma or other predisposing conditions display the reaction.

Choice of Drug to Be Prescribed. The choice of an agent as a simple antipyretic or analgesic is seldom a problem. It is in the field of *rheumatology* that the decision becomes complex. The choice between aspirin-like agents for the treatment of arthritides is largely empirical. A drug may be chosen and given for a week or more; if the therapeutic effect is adequate, treatment should be continued unless toxicity supervenes. There is a large variation in the response of individuals to different aspirin-like drugs, even when they are closely allied members of the same chemical family. Thus, a patient may do well on one propionic acid derivative (such as ibuprofen) but not on another. This may indicate that these drugs share (unequally) different types of therapeutic actions. Discussion of principles of the use of aspirin-like drugs is provided by Miller and associates (1978) and in several symposia (Symposium, 1983a, 1983b, 1984).

All the drugs in this chapter, with the exception of the *p*-aminophenol derivatives, have a tendency to cause gastrointestinal side effects, which may range from mild dyspepsia and heartburn to ulceration of the stomach or duodenum (or reactivation of latent ulcers), sometimes with fatal results. Generally speaking, the newer drugs such as the propionic acid derivatives are probably the best tolerated. *Hypersensitivity to aspirin* is a contraindication to therapy with any of the drugs discussed in this chapter; administration of any one of these could provoke a life-threatening hypersensitivity reaction reminiscent of anaphylactic shock (*see* above).

When dealing with a child or a pregnant woman, the choice of drugs is considerably restricted. Only drugs that have been extensively tested in children should be used; this commonly means that only aspirin, naproxen, or ibuprofen should be prescribed. However, neither naproxen nor ibuprofen is recommended for such use in the United States. If aspirin-like drugs must be given to a pregnant woman, low doses of aspirin are probably the safest. Although toxic doses of salicylates cause teratogenic effects in animals, there is no evidence to suggest that salicylates in moderate doses have teratogenic effects in humans. In any case, aspirin should be discontinued prior to the anticipated time of parturition in order to avoid prolonging labor, increasing post-partum hemorrhage, intrauterine closure of the ductus arteriosus, and other complications (*see* Collins, 1981).

Many aspirin-like drugs bind firmly to

plasma proteins and thus may displace other drugs from the binding sites. This can cause serious problems if the patient is receiving, for example, warfarin, a sulfonylurea hypoglycemic agent, or methotrexate; the dosage of such agents may require adjustment, or concurrent administration should be avoided. The problem with warfarin is accentuated because almost all of the aspirin-like drugs disturb normal platelet function (*see* Pullar and Capell, 1983).

Having determined that the likelihood of side effects is acceptably low, one can choose a drug regimen. Initially, fairly low doses of the agent chosen should be prescribed to determine the patient's reaction. Some investigators suggest that the patient should be allowed use of mild analgesics (*e.g.*, acetaminophen) to control sporadic pain. When the patient has problems with sleeping because of pain or morning stiffness, a larger single dose of the drug may be given at night; as an alternative, single doses of another drug (*e.g.*, 50 to 100 mg of indomethacin) may be given to supplement existing medication without much danger of serious side effects. A week is generally long enough to determine the effect of a given drug. If the drug is effective, treatment should be continued, reducing the dose if possible and stopping it altogether if it is no longer necessary. Side effects usually appear in the first weeks of therapy. If the patient does not respond, another compound should be tried, since there is a marked variation in the response of individuals to different but closely related drugs.

For mild arthropathies, the scheme outlined above, together with rest and physiotherapy, will probably be effective. However, patients with a more debilitating disease may not respond adequately. In such cases, more aggressive therapy should be initiated with aspirin or indomethacin. Continuous combination therapy with more than one aspirin-like drug is best avoided; there is little evidence of extra benefit to the patient, and the incidence of side effects is generally increased.

For the seriously debilitated patient who cannot tolerate these drugs or in whom they are not adequately effective, other forms of therapy should be considered (*see* O'Duffy and Luthra, 1984). Gold is discussed in a separate section of this chapter. Other relevant agents include chloroquine and hydroxychloroquine (Chapter 45), immunosuppressive agents (Chapter 55), glucocorticoids (Chapter 63), and penicillamine (Chapter 69).

A final important consideration is the cost of therapy, particularly since these agents are frequently used chronically. Generally speaking, aspirin is very inexpensive; phenylbutazone and indomethacin are more expensive; the cost of the newer drugs is very high.

THE SALICYLATES

Despite the introduction of many new drugs, aspirin (acetylsalicylic acid) is still the most widely prescribed analgesic-antipyretic and anti-inflammatory agent, and it is the standard for comparison and evaluation of the others.

As a therapeutic agent, aspirin presents something of a paradox. Prodigious amounts of the drug are consumed in the United States; some estimates place the quantity as high as 10 to 20 thousand tons annually. The layman relies upon it as the common household analgesic; yet, because the drug is so generally available, he often underrates its usefulness. Likewise, the pharmacologist and clinician praise the efficacy and safety of aspirin as an analgesic and antirheumatic agent; yet they find it necessary to warn constantly of its role as a common cause of lethal drug poisoning in young children and its potential for serious toxicity if it is used improperly.

The older literature on salicylates has been summarized by Hanzlik (1927). *See* Cohen (1976), Miller and coworkers (1978), and Symposium (1983a) for more recent reviews of some of the clinical pharmacology.

Chemistry. Salicylic acid (orthohydroxybenzoic acid) is so irritating that it can only be used externally, and, therefore, various derivatives of this acid have been synthesized for systemic use. These comprise two large classes, namely, *esters of salicylic acid* obtained by substitution in the carboxyl group, and *salicylate esters of organic acids* in which the carboxyl group of salicylic acid is retained and substitution is made in the OH group. For example, aspirin is an ester of acetic acid. In addition, there are salts of salicylic acid. The chemical relationships can be seen from the structural formulas shown in Table 29–1.

Table 29–1. **STRUCTURAL FORMULAS OF THE SALICYLATES**

Salicylic Acid

Aspirin

Diflunisal

Methyl Salicylate

Structure-Activity Relationship. Salicylates generally act by virtue of their salicylic acid content, although some of the effects of aspirin are due to its capacity to acetylate proteins (*see* below). Substitutions on the carboxyl or hydroxyl groups change the potency or toxicity of the compound. The *ortho* position of the OH group is an important feature for the action of salicylate. Benzoic acid, C_6H_5COOH, shares many of the actions of salicylic acid but is much weaker. The effects of simple substitutions on the benzene ring have been extensively studied, and new salicylate derivatives are still being synthesized. A difluorophenyl derivative, *diflunisal*, has recently been introduced for clinical use.

PHARMACOLOGICAL PROPERTIES

Analgesia. The types of pain usually amenable to relief by salicylates are those of low intensity, whether circumscribed or widespread in origin; particularly amenable are headache, myalgia, arthralgia, and other pains arising from integumental structures rather than from viscera. The salicylates are more widely used for pain relief than is any other class of drugs. Chronic use does not lead to tolerance or addiction, and toxicity is lower than that of more potent analgesics. The salicylates alleviate pain by virtue of a peripheral action (*see* above); direct effects on the CNS may also be involved.

Antipyresis. As discussed above, salicylates usually lower an elevated body temperature rapidly and effectively. However, moderate doses that produce this effect also increase oxygen consumption and metabolic rate. In toxic doses, these compounds have a pyretic effect that results in sweating; this enhances the dehydration that occurs in salicylate intoxication (*see* below).

Miscellaneous Neurological Effects. In high doses, salicylates have toxic effects on the CNS, consisting in stimulation (including convulsions) followed by depression. Confusion, dizziness, tinnitus, high-tone deafness, delirium, psychosis, stupor, and coma may occur. The *tinnitus* and *hearing loss* caused by salicylate poisoning are similar to those seen in Ménière's disease and are due to increased labyrinthine pressure or an effect on the hair cells of the cochlea. There is a close relation between the hearing loss in decibels and the concentration of salicylate in plasma. The loss is completely reversible within 2 or 3 days after withdrawal of the drug.

Nausea and *vomiting* are induced by salicylates and result from stimulation of sites that are accessible from the cerebrospinal fluid (CSF), probably in the medullary chemoreceptor trigger zone (CTZ). In man, centrally induced nausea and vomiting generally appear at plasma salicylate concentrations of about 270 μg/ml, but these same effects may occur at much lower plasma values as a result of local gastric irritation.

Respiration. The effects of salicylate on respiration are of paramount importance because they contribute to the serious acid-base balance disturbances that characterize poisoning by this class of compounds. Salicylates stimulate respiration directly and indirectly. Full therapeutic doses of salicylates increase oxygen consumption and CO_2 production in experimental animals and man. This effect of salicylate occurs primarily in skeletal muscle and is a result of salicylate-induced uncoupling of oxidative phosphorylation (*see* below). The increased production of CO_2 stimulates respiration. The increased alveolar ventilation balances the increased CO_2 production, and thus plasma CO_2 tension (P_{CO_2}) does not change. The *initial* increase in alveolar ventilation is characterized mainly by an increase in depth of respiration and only a slight increase in rate, a pattern similar to that produced by inhalation of CO_2 and by exercise. If the respiratory response to CO_2 has been depressed by the administration of a barbiturate or an opioid, salicylates will cause a marked increase in plasma P_{CO_2} and respiratory acidosis.

As salicylate gains access to the medulla, it directly stimulates the respiratory center. This results in marked hyperventilation, characterized by an increase in depth and a pronounced increase in rate. Patients with salicylate poisoning may have prominent increases in respiratory minute volume, and *respiratory alkalosis* ensues. Plasma salicylate concentrations of 350 μg/ml are nearly always associated with hyperventilation in man, and marked hyperpnea occurs when the level approaches 500 μg/ml.

A *depressant* effect of salicylate on the medulla appears after high doses or after prolonged exposure. Toxic doses of salicylates cause central respiratory paralysis as well as circulatory collapse secondary to vasomotor depression. Since enhanced CO_2 production continues, respiratory acidosis ensues (*see* below).

Acid-Base Balance and Electrolyte Pattern. Therapeutic doses of salicylate produce definite changes in the acid-base balance and electrolyte pattern. The initial event, as discussed above, is an extracellular and intracellular *respiratory alkalosis*. *Compensation* for the respiratory alkalosis promptly ensues. Renal excretion of bicarbonate accompanied by sodium and potassium is increased, plasma bicarbonate is thus lowered, and blood pH returns toward normal. This is the stage of *compensated respiratory alkalosis*. This stage is most often seen in adults given intensive salicylate therapy and seldom proceeds further.

Subsequent changes in acid-base status generally occur only when toxic doses of salicylates are ingested by infants and children and occasionally after large doses in adults. In infants and children, the phase of respiratory alkalosis may not be observed by the physician, since the child with salicylate intoxication is rarely seen early enough. The stage generally present is characterized by a decrease in blood pH, a low plasma bicarbonate concentration, and a normal or nearly normal plasma P_{CO_2}, changes consistent, except for P_{CO_2}, with the picture of metabolic acidosis. However, in reality there is a *combination of respiratory acidosis and metabolic acidosis* produced as follows. The respiratory depression from toxic doses of salicylate permits the enhanced production of CO_2 to outstrip its alveolar excretion; consequently, plasma P_{CO_2} increases and blood pH decreases. Since the concentration of bicarbonate in plasma is already low due to increased renal bicarbonate excretion, the acid-base status at this stage is essentially an uncompensated respiratory acidosis. Superimposed, however, is a true metabolic acidosis caused by accumulation of acids as a result of three processes. First, salicylic acid derivatives dissociate at plasma pH, and in toxic doses displace about 2 to 3 mEq per liter of plasma bicarbonate. Second, vasomotor depression caused by toxic doses of salicylate impairs renal function with consequent accumulation of strong acids of metabolic origin, namely, sulfuric and phosphoric acids. Third, organic acids accumulate secondary to salicylate-induced derangement of carbohydrate metabolism, especially pyruvic, lactic, and acetoacetic acids. Hence, metabolic acidosis is further enhanced.

The series of events that produce acid-base disturbances in salicylate intoxication also cause alterations of *water and electrolyte balance*. The low plasma P_{CO_2} leads to decreased renal tubular reabsorption of bicarbonate and increased renal excretion of sodium, potassium, and water (*see* introduction to Section VIII). In addition, water is lost by salicylate-induced sweating and by insensible water loss through the lungs during hyperventilation, and dehydration rapidly occurs. Since more water than electrolyte is lost by way of the sweat and lungs, the dehydration is associated with hypernatremia.

Prolonged exposure to high doses of salicylate also causes *potassium depletion* due to both renal and extrarenal factors.

Cardiovascular Effects. Ordinary therapeutic doses of salicylates have no important direct cardiovascular actions. The peripheral vessels tend to dilate after large doses, due to a direct effect on their smooth muscle. Toxic amounts depress the circulation directly and by central vasomotor paralysis.

In patients given large doses of sodium salicylate or aspirin, such as are used in acute rheumatic fever, the circulating plasma volume increases (about 20%), the hematocrit falls, and cardiac output and work are increased. Consequently, in patients with clear evidence of carditis, such alterations can cause congestive failure and pulmonary edema, and high doses are best avoided in such individuals.

Gastrointestinal Effects. The ingestion of salicylate may result in epigastric distress, nausea, and vomiting. The mechanism of the emetic effect is discussed above. Salicylate may also cause gastric ulceration and even hemorrhage in experimental animals and in man. Exacerbation of peptic ulcer symptoms (heartburn, dyspepsia), gastrointestinal hemorrhage, and erosive gastritis have all been reported in patients on high-dose therapy, but may rarely occur with low doses as a hypersensitivity response. The salicylate-induced gastric bleeding is painless and frequently leads to blood loss in the stool and occasionally to an iron-deficiency anemia. In most cases, however, blood loss is not significant.

The occurrence of these effects in *man* has been demonstrated by many investigators. For example, ingestion of 4 or 5 g of aspirin per day for 26 days, a dose that produces plasma salicylate concentrations in the usual range for anti-inflammatory therapy (120 to 350 μg/ml), results in an average fecal blood loss of about 3 to 8 ml per day as compared with approximately 0.6 ml per day in untreated subjects (Leonards and Levy, 1973). Gastroscopic or direct examination in salicylate-treated subjects reveals discrete ulcerative and hemorrhagic lesions of the gastric mucosa; in many cases, multiple hemorrhagic lesions with sharply demarcated areas of focal necrosis are observed. The incidence of bleeding is highest with salicylates that dissolve slowly and deposit as particles in the gastric mucosal folds. Occult blood loss might be reduced or prevented by administering aspirin in a solution that is made just before it is ingested or in a dosage form that provides reliable disintegration and dissolution.

As discussed above, the mechanisms by which salicylates injure gastric mucosal cells are complex. Deleterious effects result from local actions, which cause injury to the submucosal capillaries with subsequent necrosis and bleeding, and from effects on the secretion of acid and mucus, which appear to be due to systemic inhibition of the formation of prostaglandins. There may also be an increased bleeding tendency, secondary to impaired platelet aggregation.

Hepatic and Renal Effects. There is an increasing awareness that salicylates can produce hepatic injury. In general, the hepatotoxicity is dose dependent and is not associated with evidence of hypersensitivity; the concentration of salicylate in plasma has usually been maintained above 150 μg/ml. While the vast majority of cases occurs in patients with connective tissue disorders (*e.g.*, juvenile rheumatoid arthritis), hepatotoxicity has been observed in patients receiving salicylates for headaches or for various orthopedic problems (*see* Benson, in Symposium, 1983b). Symptoms are usually absent, and elevated enzyme activities in plasma (SGOT, SGPT) are the principal indications of hepatic damage. About 5% of the patients also have hepatomegaly, anorexia, and nausea, and jaundice may be present; in these instances, salicylates should be discontinued because of the potential hazard of fatal hepatic necrosis. For these and other reasons, restriction of salicylates has been advised in patients with chronic liver disease.

There is also concern that salicylates may be an important factor in the severe hepatic injury and encephalopathy observed in *Reye's syndrome* (*see* Committee on Infectious Diseases, 1982). This syndrome is a rare but often fatal consequence of infection with varicella and various strains of influenza virus. While there is a strong epidemiological association, a causal relationship with salicylates has not been established. Nevertheless, various agencies and the Surgeon General of the United States have advised against the use of salicylates in children with chickenpox or influenza.

As discussed above, salicylates and aspirin-like drugs can cause retention of salt and water as well as acute reduction of renal function in patients with congestive heart failure or hypovolemia. While chronic use of salicylates alone is rarely associated with nephrotoxicity, the prolonged and excessive

ingestion of analgesic mixtures containing salicylates in combination with acetaminophen or salicylamide can produce papillary necrosis and interstitial nephritis in certain individuals (Clive and Stoff, 1984).

Uricosuric Effects. Appropriate doses of salicylate increase the urinary excretion of urates, and the drug was once used in acute and chronic gout. The uricosuric action is markedly dependent on the dose. Low doses (1 or 2 g per day) may actually decrease urate excretion and elevate plasma urate concentrations; intermediate doses (2 or 3 g per day) usually do not alter urate excretion; large doses (over 5 g per day) induce uricosuria and lower plasma urate levels. Such large doses are poorly tolerated. Even small doses of salicylate should not be given concomitantly with probenecid and other uricosuric agents that decrease tubular reabsorption of uric acid, because it annuls their effect (*see* Chapter 38).

Effects on the Blood. Ingestion of aspirin by normal individuals causes a definite prolongation of the bleeding time; this is not due to hypoprothrombinemia and can occur with a dose as small as 0.3 g. For example, a single dose of 0.65 g of aspirin approximately doubles the mean bleeding time of normal persons for a period of 4 to 7 days. This effect is probably due to acetylation of platelet cyclooxygenase and the consequent reduced formation of TXA_2.

Aspirin should be avoided in patients with severe hepatic damage, hypoprothrombinemia, vitamin K deficiency, or hemophilia, because the inhibition of platelet hemostasis can result in hemorrhage. Also, aspirin therapy should be stopped at least 1 week prior to surgery, if conditions permit. Additionally, care should be exercised in the use of aspirin during long-term treatment with oral anticoagulant agents, because of the possible danger of blood loss from the gastric mucosa. However, the intentional use of aspirin and other drugs that inhibit platelet aggregation, in conjunction with oral anticoagulants, is being actively explored for the prophylaxis of coronary and cerebral arterial thrombosis (*see* Marcus, 1983; *see also* Chapter 58).

Salicylate medication does not ordinarily alter the *leukocyte* or *erythrocyte* count, the hematocrit, or the hemoglobin content, nor does it produce methemoglobinemia. The mechanism of the salicylate reduction in leukocytosis and in the elevated *erythrocyte sedimentation rate* in acute rheumatic fever is not understood. The *plasma iron concen-*

tration is markedly decreased and *erythrocyte survival time* shortened by doses of 3 to 4 g per day. Aspirin is included among the drugs that can cause a mild degree of hemolysis in individuals with a glucose-6-phosphate dehydrogenase deficiency.

Effects on Rheumatic, Inflammatory, and Immunological Processes, and on Connective Tissue Metabolism.

For almost 100 years the salicylates have retained their preeminent position in the treatment of the rheumatic diseases. Although they suppress the clinical signs and even improve the histological picture in acute rheumatic fever, subsequent tissue damage such as cardiac lesions and other visceral involvement is unaffected. In addition to their action on prostaglandin biosynthesis, the mechanism of action of the salicylates in rheumatic disease may also involve effects on other cellular and immunological processes in mesenchymal and connective tissues.

Because of the known relationship between rheumatic fever and immunological processes, attention has been directed to the effects of salicylates on *antigen-antibody* reactions. These agents suppress a variety of such reactions. Several different mechanisms are involved, including suppression of antibody production, interference with antigen-antibody aggregation, inhibition *in vitro* of antigen-induced release of histamine, and nonspecific stabilization of changes in capillary permeability in the presence of immunological insults. The concentrations of salicylates needed to produce these effects are high, and the relationship of the suppressive effects of salicylates on immunological processes to their antirheumatic efficacy in man is yet to be determined.

Drugs useful as antirheumatic and anti-inflammatory agents influence the metabolism of *connective tissue,* and these effects may be involved in their anti-inflammatory action. For example, salicylates can affect the composition, biosynthesis, or metabolism of connective tissue mucopolysaccharides concerned with the ground substance that provides barriers to spread of infection and inflammation.

Metabolic Effects. The salicylates have a multiplicity of effects on metabolic processes, some of which have already been discussed. Only a few pertinent aspects will be presented here.

Oxidative Phosphorylation. The uncoupling of oxidative phosphorylation by salicylate is similar to that induced by 2,4-dinitrophenol. The effect occurs in man with doses of salicylate used in the treatment of rheumatoid arthritis.

As a result of the uncoupling action of salicylates, a number of adenosine triphosphate (ATP)–dependent reactions are inhibited. Other consequences of this uncoupling action include the salicylate-induced increase in oxygen uptake and

carbon dioxide production described above, the depletion of hepatic glycogen, and the pyretic effect of toxic doses of salicylate. Salicylate in toxic doses may decrease aerobic metabolism as a result of inhibition of various dehydrogenases, by competing with the pyridine nucleotide coenzymes, and inhibition of some oxidases that require nucleotides as coenzymes, such as xanthine oxidase.

Carbohydrate Metabolism. The effects of salicylate on carbohydrate metabolism are complex. Multiple factors appear to be involved, some tending to lower and others to raise the blood glucose concentration. In both animals and man, large doses of salicylates may cause hyperglycemia and glycosuria and deplete liver and muscle glycogen; these effects are partly explained by the release of epinephrine, through activation of central sympathetic centers. Such large doses also reduce aerobic metabolism of glucose, increase glucose-6-phosphatase activity, and promote the secretion of glucocorticoids.

Nitrogen Metabolism. Salicylate in toxic doses causes a significant negative nitrogen balance, characterized by an aminoaciduria. Adrenocortical activation may contribute to the negative nitrogen balance by enhancing protein catabolism. The mechanism of the aminoaciduria produced by salicylates is not known.

Fat Metabolism. Salicylates reduce lipogenesis by partially blocking incorporation of acetate into fatty acids; they also inhibit epinephrine-stimulated lipolysis in fat cells and displace long-chain fatty acids from binding sites on human plasma proteins. The combination of these effects leads to increased entry and enhanced oxidation of fatty acids in muscle, liver, and other tissues, and to the lowering of concentrations of plasma free fatty acids, phospholipid, and cholesterol; the oxidation of ketone bodies is also increased.

Endocrine Effects. Salicylate directly or indirectly influences the function of a number of endocrine systems; such effects are in part responsible for some of the metabolic and pharmacological responses to the drug.

Adrenal Cortex. Very large doses of salicylate stimulate steroid secretion by the adrenal cortex through an effect on the hypothalamus and increase transiently the plasma concentrations of free adrenocorticosteroids by displacement from plasma proteins. However, there is abundant evidence that the anti-inflammatory effects of salicylate are independent of these effects on adrenocorticosteroids.

Thyroid Gland. Chronic administration of salicylate decreases the plasma protein–bound iodine and thyroidal uptake and clearance of iodine, but increases oxygen consumption and rate of disappearance of thyroxine and triiodothyronine from the circulation. These effects are probably due to the competitive displacement by salicylate of thyroxine and triiodothyronine from prealbumin and the thyroxine-binding globulin in plasma.

Salicylates and Pregnancy. There is no evidence that moderate therapeutic doses of salicylates cause fetal damage in human beings, although babies born to women who ingest salicylates chronically may have significantly reduced weights at birth. In addition, there is a definite increase in perinatal mortality, anemia, ante-partum and post-partum hemorrhage, prolonged gestation, and complicated deliveries (*see* above).

Local Irritant Effects. Salicylic acid is quite irritating to skin and mucosa and destroys epithelial cells. The keratolytic action of the free acid is employed for the local treatment of warts, corns, fungal infections, and certain types of eczematous dermatitis. The tissue cells swell, soften, and desquamate. The salts of salicylic acid are innocuous to the unbroken skin; however, if the free acid is released in the stomach, the gastric mucosa may be irritated. Methyl salicylate (oil of wintergreen) is irritating to both skin and gastric mucosa and is only used externally, in liniments as a counterirritant.

Pharmacokinetics and Metabolism. These important aspects of the salicylates have been reviewed by Davison (1971).

Absorption. Orally ingested salicylates are absorbed rapidly, partly from the stomach but mostly from the upper small intestine. Appreciable concentrations are found in plasma in less than 30 minutes; after a single dose, a peak value is reached in about 2 hours and then gradually declines. Rate of absorption is determined by many factors, particularly the disintegration and dissolution rates if tablets are given, the pH at the mucosal surfaces, and gastric emptying time.

Salicylate absorption occurs by passive diffusion primarily of the nondissociated lipid-soluble molecules (salicylic acid and acetylsalicylic acid) across gastrointestinal membranes and hence is influenced by gastric pH. If the pH is increased, salicylate is more ionized and this tends to decrease rate of absorption; however, a rise in pH also increases solubility of salicylate, enhancing its absorption. Actually, there is little meaningful difference between the rates of absorption of sodium salicylate, aspirin, and the numerous buffered preparations of salicylates. What differences do exist probably have no therapeutic significance, since the rate-limiting factor in the onset of effects is accumulation of these drugs at their sites of action. The presence of food delays absorption of salicylates.

Rectal absorption of salicylate is usually slower, incomplete, and unreliable; rectal administration is therefore not advisable when high plasma concentrations of the drug are required. Salicylic acid is rapidly absorbed from the intact *skin,* especially when applied in oily liniments or ointments, and systemic poisoning has occurred from its application to large areas of skin. Methyl salicylate is likewise speedily absorbed when applied cutaneously; its gastrointestinal absorption may be delayed many hours, and, therefore, gastric lavage should be performed even in cases of poisoning that are seen late.

When the nonionized salicylate molecules in the gastric lumen enter the mucosal cells, they dissociate predominantly to the ionized form at the intracellular pH of 7.0 and accumulate there in large amounts; for example, the concentration of salicylate anion in mucosal cells may be 15 to 20 times that in the gastric lumen. As a result, gastric mucosal damage may occur.

Distribution. After absorption, salicylate is distributed throughout most body tissues and most transcellular fluids, primarily by pH-dependent passive processes. For example, it can be detected in synovial, spinal, and peritoneal fluid, and in saliva and milk. Salicylate is actively transported by a low-capacity, saturable system out of the CSF across the choroid plexus. Salicylate crosses the blood-brain barrier only slowly because of the large fraction of drug in the ionized form. The drug readily crosses the placental barrier.

The volumes of distribution of aspirin and sodium salicylate in normal subjects average about 160 ml/kg of body weight. Ingested aspirin is mainly absorbed as such, but some enters the systemic circulation as salicylic acid, consequent to hydrolysis by esterases in the gastrointestinal mucosa and the liver. Aspirin can be detected in the plasma only for a short time; for example, 30 minutes after a dose of 0.65 g, only 27% of the total plasma salicylate is in the acetylated form. The absorbed ester is rapidly hydrolyzed to salicylic acid in plasma, liver, and erythrocytes, and more slowly in synovial fluid. As a result of the rapid hydrolysis, plasma concentrations of aspirin are always low and rarely exceed 20 μg/ml at ordinary therapeutic doses. Methyl salicylate is also rapidly hydrolyzed to salicylic acid, mainly in the liver.

At concentrations encountered clinically, from 80 to 90% of the salicylate is bound to plasma proteins, especially albumin. Hypoalbuminemia, as may occur in rheumatoid arthritis, is associated with a proportionately higher level of free salicylate in the plasma. Salicylate competes with thyroxine, triiodothyronine, penicillin, thiopental, phenytoin, sulfinpyrazone, bilirubin, tryptophan, certain peptides, possibly steroids, uric acid, and naproxen for plasma protein binding sites. Aspirin as such is bound to a more limited extent; however, it acetylates human plasma albumin *in vivo* by reaction with the ϵ-amino group of lysine. Hormones, DNA, platelets, and hemoglobin and other proteins are also acetylated. The binding of phenylbutazone and flufenamic acid to albumin is modified as a result of acetylation of this protein by aspirin. The acetylation of human plasma albumin by aspirin is inhibited by salicylate anion.

Biotransformation and Excretion. The biotransformation of salicylate takes place in many tissues, but particularly in hepatic endoplasmic reticulum and mitochondria. The three chief metabolic products are salicyluric acid (the glycine conjugate), the ether or phenolic glucuronide, and the ester or acyl glucuronide. In addition, a small fraction is oxidized to gentisic acid (2,5-dihydroxybenzoic acid) and to 2,3-dihydroxybenzoic and 2,3,5-trihydroxybenzoic acids. Wilson and associates (1978) found an additional metabolite of salicylic acid in man—gentisuric acid, the glycine conjugate of gentisic acid.

Salicylates are *excreted* mainly by the kidney. Studies in man indicate that salicylate is excreted in the urine as free salicylic acid (10%), salicyluric acid (75%), salicylic phenolic (10%) and acyl (5%) glucuronides, and gentisic acid (<1%). However, excretion of free salicylate is extremely variable and depends upon both the dose and the urinary pH. In alkaline urine, more than 30% of the ingested drug may be eliminated as free salicylate, whereas in acidic urine this may be as low as 2%.

The plasma half-life for aspirin is approximately 15 minutes; that for salicylate is 2 to 3 hours in low doses and about 12 hours at usual anti-inflammatory doses. The half-life of salicylate may be as long as 15 to 30 hours at high therapeutic doses or when there is intoxication. This dose-dependent elimination is the result of the limited ability of the liver to form salicyluric acid and the phenolic glucuronide.

The plasma concentration of salicylate is increased by conditions that decrease glomerular filtration rate or reduce the secretory Tm of the proximal tubules, such as renal disease or the presence of inhibitors that compete for the transport system (*e.g.*, probenecid). Changes in urinary pH also have significant effects on salicylate excretion. At a urinary pH of 6.0, a large fraction of salicylate is nonionized and readily back-diffuses. Thus, the clearance of salicylate is about four times as great at pH 8.0 as at pH 6.0, and it is well above the glomerular filtration rate at pH 8.0. High rates of urine flow decrease tubular back diffusion, whereas the opposite is true in oliguria. The conjugates of salicylic acid with glycine and glucuronic acid are water-soluble organic acids that do not readily back-diffuse across the renal tubular cells. Their excretion, therefore, is both by glomerular filtration and proximal tubular secretion and is not pH dependent.

Preparations, Routes of Administration, and Dosage. The two most commonly used preparations of salicylate for systemic effects are *sodium salicylate* and *aspirin (acetylsalicylic acid)*.

Sodium salicylate is available in tablets that contain 325 or 650 mg of drug and in an injectable solution for parenteral use. *Aspirin* is available in tablets ranging from 65 to 975 mg, capsules, and suppositories; timed-release tablets are also marketed.

Other salicylates that are available for systemic use include *salsalate* (salicylsalicylic acid), sodium thiosalicylate, choline salicylate, and magnesium salicylate. *Salicylamide*, which is not metabolized to salicylate *in vivo*, has antipyretic, analgesic, and anti-inflammatory effects similar to those of salicylate. It also has sedative and hypotensive effects. However, the drug is very rapidly inactivated during absorption and the initial circulation through the liver. *Diflunisal* is discussed below.

Methyl salicylate (sweet birch oil, wintergreen oil, gaultheria oil, betula oil) is employed only for cutaneous counterirritation in the form of salves, liniments, and other preparations. *Salicylic acid* is used for local application as a keratolytic agent, in plasters, liquids, creams, ointments, and other topical preparations.

The *dose* of salicylate depends on the condition being treated. The usual single dose of sodium salicylate or aspirin in adults is 300 mg to 1.0 g. This may be repeated every 4 hours. In acute rheumatic fever and rheumatoid arthritis more intensive medication is employed (*see* below).

The *route of administration* is practically always oral. There is rarely any necessity for parenteral administration. The *rectal* administration of aspirin suppositories may be necessary in infants or when oral medication is not retained. Salicylates are conveniently taken in tablets or capsules with a full glass of water to minimize gastric irritation. Aspirin is poorly soluble, has many chemical incompatibilities, and should be dispensed only in solid dry form.

Timed-release preparations are of limited value, since the half-time for elimination of salicylate is so long. Absorption from *enteric-coated* tablets is sometimes incomplete.

Preparations of aspirin containing alkali or buffer are sometimes better tolerated, but alkalinization of the urine, which may occur, can shorten the plasma half-life of salicylates considerably (*see* above).

TOXIC EFFECTS

Salicylates are widely used in medicine and are indiscriminately employed by the laity for every conceivable ailment. Over 10,000 cases of serious salicylate intoxication are seen in the United States every year. Some of them are fatal, and many occur in children. Considering their abuse and their availability, the high incidence of toxic reactions to salicylate is not surprising, and the drug should not be viewed as a harmless household remedy.

Hypersensitivity is also a cause of untoward responses to salicylate. Furthermore, renal or hepatic insufficiency or hypoprothrombinemia or other bleeding disorders enhance the possibility of salicylate toxicity. Children with fever and dehydration are particularly prone to intoxication from relatively small doses of salicylate. Many of the unwanted effects that are common to the aspirin-like drugs are discussed above.

Salicylate Intoxication. The *fatal dose* varies with the preparation of salicylate. From 10 to 30 g of sodium salicylate or aspirin has caused death in adults, but much larger amounts (130 g of aspirin, in one case) have been ingested without fatal outcome. The lethal dose of methyl salicylate is considerably less than that of sodium salicylate. As little as 4 ml (4.7 g) of methyl salicylate may be fatal in children.

Symptoms and Signs. Mild chronic salicylate intoxication is termed *salicylism*. When fully developed, the syndrome consists chiefly in headache, dizziness, ringing in the ears, difficulty in hearing, dimness of vision, mental confusion, lassitude, drowsiness, sweating, thirst, hyperventilation, nausea, vomiting, and occasionally diarrhea. A more severe degree of salicylate intoxication is characterized by CNS disturbances (including EEG abnormalities), skin eruptions, and marked alterations in acid-base balance. The above-mentioned CNS effects are more pronounced and generalized convulsions and coma may occur. Fever is usually prominent, especially in children. Dehydration often occurs as a result of hyperpyrexia, sweating, vomiting, and the loss of water vapor during hyperventilation. Gastrointestinal symptoms are often conspicuous, and approximately 50% of all individuals with plasma salicylate concentrations of more than 300 μg/ml experience nausea.

A most prominent feature of salicylate intoxication is the *disturbance in acid-base balance and electrolyte composition of the plasma*, the characteristics of which have already been presented. The most severe metabolic disturbances occur in infants and very young children who become intoxicated as the result of therapeutic overdosage; most of the acidotic patients seen with salicylate intoxication are in this group. Higher doses of the drug and a longer duration of intoxication intensify the metabolic effects and the acidosis.

Hemorrhagic phenomena are occasionally seen during salicylate poisoning, the mechanism and significance of which have been discussed. Petechial

hemorrhages are a prominent post-mortem feature. Thrombocytopenic purpura is a rare complication. While hyperglycemia may occur during salicylate intoxication, *hypoglycemia* may be a serious consequence of toxicity in young children. It should be seriously considered in any young child with coma, convulsions, or cardiovascular collapse.

Severe toxic *encephalopathy* may be a prominent feature of salicylate poisoning and may be difficult to differentiate from chorea or rheumatic encephalopathy. As poisoning progresses, central stimulation is replaced by increasing depression, stupor, and coma. Cardiovascular collapse and respiratory insufficiency ensue, and terminal asphyxial convulsions and pulmonary edema sometimes appear. Death usually results from respiratory failure after a period of unconsciousness.

Symptoms of poisoning by *methyl salicylate* differ little from those just described. Central excitation, intense hyperpnea, and hyperpyrexia are prominent features. The odor of the drug can easily be detected on the breath and in the urine and vomitus. Poisoning by *salicylic acid* differs only in the increased prominence of gastrointestinal symptoms due to the marked local irritation.

Treatment. Salicylate poisoning represents an acute medical emergency. The treatment is largely symptomatic. Death may result despite all recommended procedures. Salicylate medication is withdrawn as soon as intoxication is suspected. The patient should be hospitalized. Hospitalization is particularly advisable in the case of methyl salicylate poisoning because children have been known to succumb within a few hours after the parents had been informed that recovery seemed assured or that the intoxication was inconsequential. Blood should be obtained for plasma salicylate determinations and acid-base and electrolyte studies. The salicylate concentration is reasonably well correlated with clinical severity, when corrected for the duration of the intoxication, and is of value in assessing the type of therapy to be instituted. Absorption of salicylate from the gastrointestinal tract can be reduced by emesis, gastric lavage, administration of activated charcoal, or a combination of these.

Hyperthermia and dehydration are the immediate threats to life, and the initial therapy must be directed to their correction and to the maintenance of adequate renal function. External sponging with tepid water or alcohol should be provided quickly to any child with very high fever. Adequate amounts of intravenous fluids must be given promptly. The type and amount of solutions to be employed depend upon the interpretation of the laboratory data on acid-base balance. If the patient presents with an acidosis, correction of the low blood pH is essential, especially since acidosis results in a shift of salicylate from plasma into brain and other tissues. Bicarbonate solution should be infused intravenously, if possible, in sufficient quantity to maintain alkaline diuresis. Correction of ketosis and hypoglycemia by administration of glucose is also essential for complete control of the metabolic acidosis; however, the ketosis clears only slowly. If potassium deficiency occurs during salicylate intoxication, it should be treated by adding the cation to the intravenous fluids once it has been determined that urine formation is adequate. Plasma transfusion may be beneficial, especially if the shock syndrome intervenes. Any attempt to obtund the salicylate-induced hyperventilation by giving a barbiturate or an opioid is dangerous and may rapidly lead to respiratory acidosis and coma. Hemorrhagic phenomena may necessitate whole-blood transfusion and vitamin K (phytonadione).

Measures to rid the body rapidly of salicylate should be immediately undertaken. Forced diuresis with alkalinizing solution appears to be better than alkali alone. In severe intoxication, extrarenal measures such as exchange transfusion, peritoneal dialysis, hemodialysis, and hemoperfusion are the most effective measures available for the removal of salicylate. These measures should be considered seriously in all salicylate-intoxicated patients whose clinical condition is deteriorating despite otherwise-appropriate therapy and in those who have associated serious disease. (*See* Hill, 1973; Brenner and Simon, 1982; Proudfoot, in Symposium, 1983b.)

Aspirin Hypersensitivity. Aspirin hypersensitivity or intolerance is discussed above. While rather uncommon, it is important to recognize this syndrome, since the administration of aspirin and many other aspirin-like drugs may result in severe and possibly fatal reactions. Treatment of such responses to salicylates does not differ from that ordinarily employed in acute anaphylactic reactions. Epinephrine is the drug of choice and usually controls angioedema and urticaria without difficulty; asthma induced by aspirin may at times prove refractory to therapy.

THERAPEUTIC USES

There are many *systemic* and a few *local* uses of the salicylates. Several are based on tradition and empirical results rather than on a clear understanding of the mechanism of therapeutic benefit.

Systemic Uses. *Antipyresis.* Antipyretic therapy is reserved for patients in whom fever in itself may be deleterious, and for those who experience considerable relief when a fever is lowered. Little is known concerning the relationship between fever and the acceleration of immune processes; it may at times be a protective physiological mechanism. The course of the patient's illness may be obscured by the relief of symptoms and the reduction of fever from the use of antipyretic drugs; otherwise the effect of salicylate is nonspecific and does not influence the course of the underlying disease. The antipyretic dose of salicylate for adults is 325 to 650 mg orally every 4 hours; for children, 65 mg/kg per day in four to six divided doses, not to exceed a total daily dose of 3.6 g.

Analgesia. Salicylate is valuable for the nonspecific relief of certain types of pain, for example,

headache, arthritis, dysmenorrhea, neuralgia, and myalgia. For this purpose, it is prescribed in the same doses and manner as for antipyresis.

Acute Rheumatic Fever. In this disease, the salicylates suppress the acute exudative inflammatory process of the disease but do not affect the progression of the disease or the later phases of granulomatous inflammation or scar formation. Within 24 to 48 hours after adequate doses of salicylate, there is usually considerable or complete relief of pain, swelling, immobility, local heat, and redness of the involved joints; fever and pulse rate are lowered and the patient feels much improved. However, cardiac complications, chorea, encephalopathy, subcutaneous nodules, and other features are not prevented or benefited, and the duration of the disease is not shortened. Nevertheless, if a patient has severe carditis and heart failure, the nonspecific anti-inflammatory effect of salicylates and particularly of adrenocorticosteroids may be invaluable in reducing the burden upon the heart.

For maximal suppression of rheumatic inflammation, doses that provide a plasma salicylate concentration of 250 to 350 μg/ml should be maintained, but polyarthritis and fever usually respond to smaller amounts. For adults, a total daily dosage of 5 to 8 g, given at intervals in 1-g amounts, usually suffices. Children are given 100 to 125 mg/kg per day, in divided portions every 4 to 6 hours, for up to 1 week; the dose is then reduced in stepwise fashion at weekly intervals to 60 mg/kg per day (10 mg/kg every 4 hours, or 15 mg/kg every 6 hours) and maintained as long as necessary. Anorexia, tinnitus, nausea, and vomiting are common during the first 3 or 4 days of therapy, but tend to subside despite continuation of medication. Ordinarily, full doses are continued until at least 2 weeks after the patient is asymptomatic and all evidence of active inflammation has disappeared. The drug is then gradually discontinued over a period of 7 to 10 days. If symptoms and signs of the disease reappear, salicylate therapy is reinstituted. Aspirin is recommended and sodium salicylate should be avoided, because restricted sodium intake may be advisable if there is evidence of active cardiac involvement. Therapy with glucocorticoids does not yield overall results superior to those obtained with the salicylates; salicylate and glucocorticoids are additive in their effects. If carditis is not evident, salicylates and not steroids should be used. However, if acute severe carditis is present, most investigators believe adrenocorticosteroids should be given instead of salicylates, at least initially.

Rheumatoid Arthritis. Despite the development of the newer anti-inflammatory agents, salicylates are still regarded as the standard with which other drugs should be compared for the treatment of rheumatoid arthritis. In addition to the analgesia that allows more effective therapeutic exercises, there is improvement in appetite and a feeling of well-being. Salicylates also reduce the inflammation in joint tissues and surrounding structures. Damage to joints is the most difficult aspect of rheumatoid arthritis to manage, and any agent that reduces the inflammation is important in lessening or delaying the development of crippling. Salicylates can be shown to produce objectively measurable anti-inflammatory changes when given in large doses for long periods to patients with active rheumatoid disease. Fairly large doses of salicylate are advised (4 to 6 g daily), but some patients respond well to less.

The majority of patients with rheumatoid arthritis can be controlled with salicylates alone or with other aspirin-like anti-inflammatory agents. Some require more aggressive therapy with more toxic drugs, such as gold salts, hydroxychloroquine, penicillamine, adrenocorticosteroids, or immunosuppressive agents.

Other Uses. Because of the potent and long-lasting effect of low doses of aspirin on platelet function, it has been suggested that this drug could be of use in the treatment or prophylaxis of diseases associated with platelet hyperaggregability, such as coronary artery disease, myocardial infarction, and postoperative deep-vein thrombosis (*see* Chapter 58). The effects of aspirin (300 mg to 1.5 g daily) after myocardial infarction have been assessed in various clinical trials; little effect on morbidity or mortality has been noted (*see* Mustard *et al.* and Elwood, in Symposium, 1983c). However, a Veterans Administration Cooperative Study indicates that aspirin (324 mg per day) reduces the incidence of acute myocardial infarction and death in men with unstable angina (Lewis *et al.*, 1983). Similarly, studies of patients with atherosclerosis who experience transient ischemic attacks indicate that the administration of aspirin reduces the frequency of such attacks and the incidence of stroke and death (*see* Fields, in Symposium, 1983c); these studies employed a daily dose of 1.3 g, and the beneficial effects were confined to males. Clinical trials are in progress to assess the effects of lower doses of aspirin.

Relationship of Plasma Salicylate Concentration to Therapeutic Effect and Toxicity. For optimal anti-inflammatory effect for patients with rheumatic diseases, plasma salicylate concentrations of 150 to 300 μg/ml are required. In this range, the clearance of the drug is nearly constant (despite the fact that saturation of metabolic capacity is approached) because the fraction of drug that is free and thus available for metabolism or excretion increases as binding sites on plasma proteins are saturated. The total concentration of salicylate in plasma is thus a relatively linear function of dose (Furst *et al.*, 1979). Optimal intensive salicylate therapy can be achieved only by individualizing the total dose of aspirin. This is especially important since the range of plasma salicylate concentrations needed for optimal anti-inflammatory effects may overlap that at which tinnitus is noted. Tinnitus may be a reliable index of therapeutic plasma concentration in those patients with normal hearing, but not in those with a preexisting hearing loss. In the latter patients, plasma salicylate concentrations may be a more useful guideline. Hyperventilation generally occurs at concentrations greater than 350 μg/ml and other signs of intoxication, such as acidosis, at concentrations greater than 460 μg/ml.

Single analgesic-antipyretic doses of salicylate usually yield plasma concentrations below 60 μg/ml.

The plasma concentration of salicylate is generally little affected by other drugs, but concurrent administration of aspirin lowers the concentrations of indomethacin, naproxen, and fenoprofen, at least in part by displacement from plasma proteins. Important adverse interactions of aspirin with warfarin and methotrexate are mentioned above (page 680). Other interactions of aspirin include the antagonism of spironolactone-induced natriuresis and the blockade of the active transport of aminosalicylic acid and penicillin from CSF to blood.

Local Uses. *Salicylic acid* is applied topically as a *keratolytic agent*. In combination with benzoic acid, it is often prescribed for *epidermophytosis*. Salicylic acid is also employed as a *wart* and *corn* remover (10 to 20% in collodion). It is sometimes prescribed in talc (2 to 4%) for *hyperhidrosis*.

Methyl salicylate is reserved for external use as a *counterirritant*. It is employed for painful muscles or joints, in an ointment, liniment, or other preparation. Absorption of methyl salicylate can occur through the skin, and death has resulted from systemic poisoning from the local misapplication of the drug. It is a common *pediatric poison*, and its use should be strongly discouraged. It is also used as a *flavoring agent*.

DIFLUNISAL

Diflunisal is a difluorophenyl derivative of salicylic acid (*see* Table 29–1); it is not converted to salicylic acid *in vivo*. While diflunisal is more potent than aspirin in anti-inflammatory tests in animals, its relative efficacy as an anti-inflammatory agent in man has not been fully documented. It is largely devoid of antipyretic effects. The drug has been used primarily as an analgesic in the treatment of osteoarthritis and musculoskeletal strains or sprains; in these circumstances it is about three to four times more potent than aspirin. Diflunisal does not produce auditory side effects and appears to cause fewer and less intense gastrointestinal effects than does aspirin. Diflunisal increases the clearance of uric acid at therapeutic doses.

Diflunisal is almost completely absorbed after oral administration, and peak concentrations occur in plasma within 2 to 3 hours. It is extensively bound to plasma albumin (99%). Diflunisal appears in the milk of lactating women; its penetration into the CNS is uncertain. About 90% of the drug is excreted as glucuronides, and its rate of elimination is dependent upon dosage. At the usual analgesic dose (500 to 750 mg per day) the plasma half-life ranges between 8 and 12 hours. (For reviews, *see* Brogden *et al.*, 1980; Davies, 1983; van Winzum *et al.*, in Symposium, 1983a.)

Diflunisal (DOLOBID) is marketed in 250- and 500-mg tablets. For mild-to-moderate pain, the usual initial dose is 500 to 1000 mg, followed by 250 to 500 mg every 8 to 12 hours. For osteoarthritis, 250 to 500 mg is administered twice daily; maintenance dosage should not exceed 1.5 g per day.

PYRAZOLON DERIVATIVES

This group of drugs includes phenylbuta-zone, oxyphenbutazone, antipyrine, aminopyrine, dipyrone, and a more recent addition, apazone (azapropazone). With the exception of apazone, these drugs have been in clinical use for many years; phenylbutazone is the most important from the therapeutic viewpoint, while antipyrine, dipyrone, and aminopyrine are seldom used today. Apazone is not yet available in the United States.

PHENYLBUTAZONE

Phenylbutazone, employed originally as a solubilizing agent for aminopyrine, was introduced in 1949 for the treatment of rheumatoid arthritis and allied disorders. It is an effective anti-inflammatory agent, but serious toxicity limits its use in long-term therapy. Its structural formula is as follows:

Phenylbutazone

Pharmacological Properties. The anti-inflammatory effects of phenylbutazone are similar to those of the salicylates, but its toxicity differs significantly. Like aminopyrine, phenylbutazone can cause agranulocytosis. The pharmacology and toxicology of phenylbutazone and its metabolites and congeners have been reviewed in a symposium (Symposium, 1977) and by Fowler (in Symposium, 1983a).

Anti-inflammatory Effects. Phenylbutazone has prominent anti-inflammatory effects and is used frequently in, for example, race horses to enhance their performance; somewhat comparable effects are demonstrable in patients with rheumatoid arthritis and related disorders.

Antipyretic and Analgesic Effects. The antipyretic effect of phenylbutazone has been little studied in man. For pain of nonrheumatic origin, its analgesic efficacy is inferior to that of salicylates. *Because of its toxicity, phenylbutazone should not be used routinely as an analgesic or antipyretic.*

Uricosuric Effect. In doses of about 600 mg per day, phenylbutazone has a mild uricosuric effect in man, probably attributable to one of its metabolites. This results from diminished tubular reabsorption of uric acid. Low concentrations of the drug inhibit tubular secretion of uric acid and cause retention of urate. A congener, *sulfinpyrazone,* is much more effective than phenylbutazone as a uricosuric agent and is useful for the treatment of chronic gout (*see* below and Chapter 38).

Effects on Water and Electrolytes. Phenylbutazone causes significant retention of sodium and chloride, accompanied by a reduction in urine volume; edema may result. The excretion of potassium is not changed. Plasma volume frequently increases as much as 50%, and, as a result, cardiac decompensation and acute pulmonary edema have occurred in patients given the drug. The expansion of plasma volume accounts, in part, for the anemia observed during medication.

Other Effects. Phenylbutazone reduces the uptake of iodine by the thyroid gland, apparently secondary to inhibition of biosynthesis of organic iodine compounds. Goiter and myxedema may occasionally result from this effect.

Pharmacokinetics and Metabolism. Phenylbutazone is rapidly and completely absorbed from the gastrointestinal tract or the rectum, and the peak concentration in plasma is reached in 2 hours. After therapeutic doses, phenylbutazone is 96% bound to plasma proteins. The half-time of phenylbutazone in plasma is very long—50 to 65 hours. The drug penetrates into the synovial spaces and reaches a concentration about one half of that in the plasma; significant concentrations may persist in the joints for up to 3 weeks after treatment is discontinued.

Phenylbutazone undergoes extensive metabolic transformation in man. Contrary to early reports, the most significant primary reactions involve glucuronidation and hydroxylation of the phenyl rings or the butyl side chain. The conjugates are excreted in the urine and represent the bulk of the excreted drug. *Oxyphenbutazone,* a metabolite of phenylbutazone, has antirheumatic and sodium-retaining activities similar to those of the parent drug. Oxyphenbutazone is also extensively bound to plasma proteins and has a half-life in plasma of several days. It accumulates significantly during chronic administration of phenylbutazone and contributes to the pharmacological and toxic effects of the parent drug. Only a trace of unchanged phenylbutazone is excreted in the urine. Oxyphenbutazone is excreted mainly as the O-glucuronide.

Drug Interactions. Other *anti-inflammatory* agents, *oral anticoagulant* agents, *oral hypoglycemics, sulfonamides,* and other drugs may be displaced from binding to plasma proteins by phenylbutazone. The net result may be increased pharmacological or toxic effects of the displaced drug, depending upon the drug and its disposition after being displaced. The well-documented increased risk of bleeding associated with concurrent phenylbutazone-warfarin medication involves such displacement, but phenylbutazone also modifies the action of the oral anticoagulant agent and influences platelet function. The gastrointestinal effects of phenylbutazone also contribute to the hazard. Displacement of plasma protein–bound thyroid hormone complicates the interpretation of *thyroid function tests.*

Phenylbutazone may cause induction of hepatic microsomal enzymes, and it may also inhibit inactivation of other drugs that are hydroxylated by the microsomal system. It has been said to increase the effect of *insulin.*

Toxic Effects. Phenylbutazone is poorly tolerated by many patients. Some type of side effect is noted in 10 to 45% of patients, and medication may have to be discontinued in 10 to 15%. Nausea, vomiting, epigastric discomfort, and skin rashes are the most frequently reported untoward effects. Diarrhea, vertigo, insomnia, euphoria, nervousness, hematuria (enhanced by concomitant administration of an anticoagulant), and blurred vision have also been observed. In addition, water and electrolyte retention and edema formation occur.

More serious forms of adverse effects include peptic ulcer (or its reactivation) with hemorrhage or perforation, hypersensitivity reactions of the serum-sickness type, ulcerative stomatitis, hepatitis, nephritis, aplastic anemia, leukopenia, agranulocytosis, and thrombocytopenia. *A number of deaths have occurred, especially from aplastic anemia and agranulocytosis.*

When phenylbutazone is given, the patient should be closely supervised and his blood should be examined frequently; weight should also be checked to warn of undue retention of sodium. The drug should only be given for short periods (not more than 1 week). Even then, the incidence of disturbing side effects is about 10%. The patient must be told to discontinue the drug and promptly report to the physician if he develops fever, sore throat or other oral lesions, skin rash, pruritus, jaundice, weight increase, or tarry stools. The drug is contraindicated in patients with hypertension; cardiac, renal, or hepatic dysfunction; or a history of peptic ulcer or hypersensitivity to the drug. The toxic effects of the drug are more severe in elderly persons, and its use in this group is inadvisable.

Preparations, Route of Administration, and Dosage. *Phenylbutazone* (AZOLID, BUTAZOLIDIN) is available in 100-mg coated tablets and capsules for oral administration. Daily doses of 300 to 600 mg for brief periods provide maximal therapeutic effects (higher doses only increase toxicity), but the disease may subsequently be adequately controlled by doses of 100 to 400 mg per day. The drug should be taken with meals to lessen gastric irritation.

Therapeutic Uses. Phenylbutazone is used for the therapy of *acute gout* and for the treatment of *rheumatoid arthritis and allied disorders.* Acute exacerbations of these conditions respond particularly well to the drug, and its use should be reserved for such episodes. Phenylbutazone should be employed only after other drugs have failed and then only after careful consideration of the risks involved as compared with the advantage to the patient. Indiscriminate use of phenylbutazone in the therapy of trivial acute or chronic *musculoskeletal disorders* can only be condemned.

Phenylbutazone is an effective alternative to colchicine in *acute gout.* Excellent relief can be attained with a brief course of medication, and about 85 to 95% of acute attacks are controlled within 24 to 36 hours. Phenylbutazone causes fewer gastrointestinal side effects than does colchicine and is more reliable when initiation of medication has been delayed. Dosage recommendations have varied: 800 mg daily for 2 days; 800 mg the first day, followed by 300 mg daily for 3 days; or an initial dose of 400 mg, followed by 100 mg every 4 hours until articular inflammation subsides. The relative merits and dangers of phenylbutazone, compared with colchicine, have been discussed by Yü (1974). The drug should not be used prophylactically nor as a uricosuric agent.

Phenylbutazone has a *limited* role in the therapy of *rheumatoid arthritis,* primarily for relief of acute exacerbations of the disorder that are not relieved by other measures. Synovitis is often reduced by a brief regimen (600 mg on the first day, followed by 400 mg daily for 3 days). Because of the high incidence of adverse effects, long-term therapy is not recommended. Brief courses of the drug, *if justified,* may be of similar benefit for acute exacerbations of *ankylosing spondylitis* and *osteoarthritis.*

OXYPHENBUTAZONE

Oxyphenbutazone is a *p*-hydroxy analog of phenylbutazone (on the N-1 phenyl group) and one of the active metabolites of the parent drug. Various aspects of its pharmacology and metabolism are discussed above, in comparison with phenylbutazone. Oxyphenbutazone has the same spectrum of activity, therapeutic uses, interactions, and toxicity as the parent compound, and it shares the same indications, dangers, and contraindications for clinical use. Oxyphenbutazone is said to cause somewhat less gastric irritation.

Oxyphenbutazone (OXALID, TANDEARIL) is marketed in 100-mg tablets. It should be taken in three or four divided portions after meals to lessen gastric irritation. Dosage of oxyphenbutazone is the same as that of phenylbutazone.

ANTIPYRINE AND AMINOPYRINE

Antipyrine (phenazone) and *aminopyrine (amidopyrine)* were introduced into medicine in the late nineteenth century as antipyretics and subsequently were also widely used as analgesics and anti-inflammatory agents. However, clinical use of aminopyrine was sharply curtailed after its potentially fatal bone-marrow toxicity, *agranulocytosis,* was recognized, and antipyrine has also lost favor. Both drugs have disappeared from the therapeutic scene in the United States, but antipyrine is still employed in some countries, usually in analgesic mixtures. A variety of related pyrazolon derivatives has also enjoyed sporadic popularity, for example, *dipyrone.* It, too, can cause agranulocytosis. A full description of the pharmacological properties of these drugs may be found in *earlier editions* of this textbook.

APAZONE (AZAPROPAZONE)

Apazone is a relatively new pyrazolon, aspirin-like agent with a spectrum of activity very similar to that of phenylbutazone, although it is much less toxic. Thus, it is anti-inflammatory, analgesic, and antipyretic. In addition, apazone is a potent uricosuric agent and is particularly useful for the treatment of acute gout. The drug is not currently available in the United States. The structural formula of apazone is as follows:

Apazone

Apazone is rapidly and probably almost completely absorbed from the gastrointestinal tract following oral administration to man; peak concentrations in plasma are achieved 4 hours later. The compound is extensively bound to plasma proteins (>95%), and the biological half-life is about 20 to 24 hours. The drug penetrates slowly into the synovial fluid. Most of the drug (about 65%) is excreted in the urine unchanged; approximately 20% is present as the 6-hydroxy derivative. There may be significant enterohepatic cycling.

Clinical experience to date suggests that apazone is generally well tolerated. Gastrointestinal side effects occur in about 3% of patients, with nausea, epigastric pain, dyspepsia, and heartburn being the most frequent complaints. These are seldom sufficiently serious to compel withdrawal of the drug. Skin rashes are also observed in 3% of patients, while CNS effects (headache, vertigo) are reported less frequently. The overall incidence of untoward reactions is probably 6 to 10%.

Because apazone is an inhibitor of prostaglandin synthetase, all precautions discussed above for the group are applicable; it can be assumed that the drug is ulcerogenic. It should not be given to patients who have experienced aspirin-induced bronchospasm. Since the drug binds extensively to albumin, its adverse interactions with other agents may resemble those of phenylbutazone. There is no evidence that apazone causes agranulocytosis.

Apazone has been advocated for the treatment of rheumatoid arthritis, osteoarthritis, and gout. It is available outside the United States as *azapropazone* (RHEUMOX) in 300-mg capsules and 600-mg tablets. The usual dose is 1200 mg per day (in divided doses), but this may be reduced to 900 mg for maintenance therapy or increased to 1800 mg if required. For the treatment of acute gout, an initial dose of 2400 mg (in four portions) is given on the first day, followed by daily doses of 1800 mg until the acute attack has subsided; daily maintenance doses of 1200 mg are then administered until symptoms disappear. (For a review, *see* Templeton, in Symposium, 1983a.)

PARA-AMINOPHENOL DERIVATIVES

The so-called coal tar analgesics, *phenacetin* and its active metabolite, *acetaminophen,* are effective alternatives to aspirin as analgesic-antipyretics; however, unlike aspirin, their anti-inflammatory activity is weak and seldom clinically useful. Acetaminophen has less overall toxicity and is thus preferred to phenacetin.

Because acetaminophen is well tolerated, lacks many of the side effects of aspirin, and is available without prescription, it has earned a prominent place as a "common household analgesic." However, acute overdosage causes fatal hepatic damage, and the number of self-poisonings and suicides with acetaminophen has grown alarmingly in recent years. In addition, many individuals, physicians included, seem unaware of the poor anti-inflammatory activity of acetaminophen.

History. *Acetanilid* is the parent member of this group of drugs. It was introduced into medicine in 1886 under the name of *antifebrin* by Cahn and Hepp, who had accidentally discovered its antipyretic action. However, acetanilid proved to be excessively toxic, and the early reports of poisoning from acetanilid prompted the search for less toxic compounds. *Para-aminophenol* was tried in the belief that the body oxidized acetanilid to this compound. Toxicity was not lessened, however, and a number of chemical derivatives of para-aminophenol were then tested. One of the more satisfactory of these was *phenacetin (acetophenetidin)*. It was introduced into therapy in 1887 and was extensively employed in analgesic mixtures until it was implicated in analgesic-abuse nephropathy (*see* above).

Acetaminophen (paracetamol; N-acetyl-*p*-aminophenol) was first used in medicine by von Mering in 1893. However, it has gained popularity only since 1949, after it was recognized as the major active metabolite of both acetanilid and phenacetin. It has been available in the United States without a prescription since 1955.

Chemistry. The relationship between the drugs of this group and their metabolites is shown in Table 29–2. The antipyretic activity of the compounds resides in the aminobenzene structure. Introduction of other radicals into the hydroxyl group of para-aminophenol and into the free amino group of aniline reduces toxicity without loss of antipyretic action. Best results are obtained with phenolic alkyl ethers (ethyl in phenacetin) and with the amides (acetyl in phenacetin and acetaminophen).

Pharmacological Effects.
Acetaminophen and phenacetin have analgesic and antipyretic effects that do not differ significantly from those of aspirin. However, as mentioned, they have only weak anti-inflammatory effects. The pharmacological effects of phenacetin are a combination of its inherent activity and those of acetaminophen, its major metabolite. Minor metabolites contribute significantly to the toxic effects of both drugs. The pharmacological properties of acetaminophen have been reviewed by Ameer and Greenblatt (1977).

Exactly why acetaminophen is an effective analgesic-antipyretic but only a weak anti-inflammatory agent has not been satisfactorily explained. An anti-inflammatory effect can be demonstrated in animal models, but only at doses considerably in excess of those required for analgesia. Acetaminophen is only a weak inhibitor of prostaglandin biosynthesis, although there is some evidence to suggest that it may be more effective against enzymes in the CNS than those in the periphery. This fact may partly account for its well-documented ability to reduce fever and to induce analgesia, effects that involve actions on neural tissue.

Subjective Effects and Liability for Abuse. Phenacetin has been said to cause relaxation, drowsiness, euphoria, stimulation, and increased efficiency; such effects have been thought to contribute to its liability for abuse. In patients, minor subjective effects may well occur secondary to relief of pain or fever. Restlessness and excitement may occur for 3 or 4 days after discontinuation of chronic administration of phenacetin.

Other Effects. Single or repeated therapeutic doses of phenacetin or acetaminophen have no effect on the cardiovascular and respiratory systems. Acid-base changes do not occur. Neither drug produces the gastric irritation, erosion, or bleeding that may occur after salicylates. They have only a weak effect upon platelets and no effect on bleeding time or the excretion of uric acid.

Pharmacokinetics and Metabolism.
Acetaminophen and phenacetin are metabolized primarily by the hepatic microsomal enzymes. The metabolic pathways for the two drugs are rather different, except, of course, that a considerable proportion of phenacetin is dealkylated to acetaminophen.

Acetaminophen is rapidly and almost completely absorbed from the gastrointestinal tract. The concentration in plasma reaches a peak in 30 to 60 minutes, and the half-life in plasma is about 2 hours after therapeutic doses. Acetaminophen is relatively uniformly distributed throughout most body fluids. Binding of the drug to plasma proteins is variable; 20 to 50% may be bound at the concentrations encountered during acute intoxication. Following therapeutic doses, 90 to 100% of the drug may be recovered in the urine within the first day. However, practically no acetaminophen is excreted unchanged, and the bulk is excreted after hepatic conjugation with glucuronic acid (about 60%), sulfuric acid (about 35%), or cysteine (about 3%); small amounts of hydroxylated and deacetylated metabolites have also been detected. Children have less capacity for glucuronidation of the drug than do adults. When high doses are ingested, acetaminophen undergoes N-hydroxylation to form N-acetyl-benzoquinoneimine, a highly reactive intermediate (*see* Figure 1–4, page 18). This metabolite reacts with sulfhydryl groups in proteins and glutathione. When hepatic glutathione is depleted (*e.g.,* after the ingestion of large amounts of acetaminophen), reaction with hepatic proteins is increased and hepatic necrosis is the result.

In the normal individual, 75 to 80% of *phenacetin* is rapidly metabolized to acetaminophen (Table 29–2). The peak concentration of phenacetin in

Table 29–2. STRUCTURAL FORMULAS OF MAJOR PARA-AMINOPHENOL DERIVATIVES, AND THEIR INTERRELATIONS

Acetanilid → Acetaminophen ← Phenacetin

Aniline   Conjugated Acetaminophen   Para-Phenetidin
R = glucuronate (major)
sulfate (minor)

Methemoglobin-Forming and Other Toxic Metabolites

plasma usually occurs in about 1 hour and that of acetaminophen derived therefrom in 1 to 2 hours. Phenacetin is converted to at least a dozen other metabolites, by N-deacetylation to para-phenetidin and by hydroxylation and further metabolism of phenacetin and para-phenetidin. An unknown metabolite, but an oxidizing agent, is responsible for formation of methemoglobin and hemolysis of red blood cells. Individuals with a genetically determined limitation in their ability to metabolize phenacetin to acetaminophen convert a greater fraction of phenacetin to toxic metabolites, possibly with propensity for serious methemoglobin formation and hemolysis. Less than 1% of phenacetin is excreted unchanged in the urine.

Toxic Effects. In recommended therapeutic dosage, acetaminophen and phenacetin are usually well tolerated. *Skin rash* and other allergic reactions occur occasionally. The rash is usually erythematous or urticarial, but sometimes it is more serious and may be accompanied by *drug fever* and *mucosal lesions*. Patients who are sensitive to the salicylates may also exhibit sensitivity to these drugs. In a few isolated cases, the use of acetaminophen has been associated with *neutropenia, pancytopenia*, and *leukopenia*.

Despite the fact that acetaminophen is a metabolite of phenacetin, the signs and symptoms of acute intoxication with the two compounds are markedly different. The most serious adverse effect of acute overdosage of acetaminophen is a dose-dependent, potentially fatal *hepatic necrosis*. *Renal tubular necrosis* (also seen with phenacetin) and *hypoglycemic coma* may also occur. Phenacetin may cause *methemoglobinemia* and *hemolytic anemia* as a form of acute toxicity, but more commonly as a consequence of chronic overdosage. Lethal doses of phenacetin are not associated with hepatic damage, but with *cyanosis, respiratory depression*, and *cardiac arrest*. Acetaminophen is much less likely to cause the formation of methemoglobin and has not been incriminated in the hemolytic reactions, but it may cause thrombocytopenia. The nephrotoxicity associated with chronic abuse of acetaminophen, phenacetin, and other analgesics has been discussed above.

Hepatotoxicity. In adults, hepatotoxicity may occur after ingestion of a single dose of 10 to 15 g (200 to 250 mg/kg) of acetaminophen; a dose of 25 g

or more is potentially fatal. The mechanism of this effect is discussed above (*see also* Chapter 1). Symptoms during the first 2 days of acute poisoning by acetaminophen do not reflect the potential seriousness of the intoxication. Nausea, vomiting, anorexia, and abdominal pain occur during the initial 24 hours and may persist for a week or more. Clinical indications of hepatic damage become manifest within 2 to 4 days of ingestion of toxic doses. Initially, plasma transaminases are elevated, and the concentration of bilirubin in plasma may be increased; in addition, the prothrombin time is prolonged. Perhaps 10% of poisoned patients who do not receive specific therapy develop severe liver damage; of these, 10 to 20% eventually die in hepatic failure. Acute renal failure also occurs in some patients. Biopsy of the liver reveals centralobular necrosis with sparing of the periportal area. In nonfatal cases, the hepatic lesions are reversible over a period of weeks or months.

Severe liver damage (with levels of aspartate aminotransferase activity in excess of 1000 I.U. per liter of plasma) occurs in 90% of patients with plasma concentrations of acetaminophen greater than 300 μg/ml at 4 hours or 45 μg/ml at 15 hours after the ingestion of the drug. Minimal hepatic damage can be anticipated when the drug concentration is less than 120 μg/ml at 4 hours or 30 μg/ml at 12 hours after ingestion.

Treatment. Early diagnosis is vital in the treatment of overdosage with acetaminophen, and methods are available for the rapid determination of concentrations of the drug in plasma. Vigorous supportive therapy is essential when intoxication is severe. Procedures to limit continuing absorption of the drug must be initiated promptly; induction of vomiting or gastric lavage should be performed in all cases and should be followed by oral administration of activated charcoal. These measures are most likely to be of value when they are instituted within 4 hours of the ingestion.

A promising method of treatment is the administration of sulfhydryl compounds, which probably act, in part, by replenishing hepatic stores of glutathione. N-acetylcysteine is particularly effective and well tolerated when given orally. The drug is recommended if less than 24 hours has elapsed since ingestion of acetaminophen. A loading dose of 140 mg/kg is given, followed by the administration of 70 mg/kg every 4 hours for 17 doses. Dosage is terminated if assays of acetaminophen in plasma indicate that the risk of hepatotoxicity is low. *Acetylcysteine* (MUCOMYST) is available as a sterile 10 or 20% solution in vials containing 4, 10, and 30 ml. The solution is diluted with cola, fruit juice, or water to achieve a 5% solution and should be consumed within 1 hour of preparation. This use of N-acetylcysteine is considered experimental in the United States. Consultation may be obtained from the Rocky Mountain Poison Center, Denver, Colorado (Tel.: 800–525–6115). (For comprehensive discussions, *see* Prescott and Critchley, 1983; Rumack, in Symposium, 1983b.)

Other Toxic Effects. Phenacetin-induced *hemolytic anemia* and the *methemoglobinemia* that follows poisoning with acetanilid or phenacetin are discussed in *earlier editions* of this textbook.

Preparations, Routes of Administration, and Dosage. *Acetaminophen (paracetamol;* N-acetyl-*p*-aminophenol) is marketed under many trade names (*e.g.,* TEMPRA, TYLENOL). Preparations include tablets (160, 325, 500, 650 mg), capsules (325 and 500 mg), suppositories, chewable tablets, wafers, elixirs, and solutions. The conventional oral or rectal dose of acetaminophen is 500 to 1000 mg; the total daily dose should not exceed 4000 mg. For children, the single dose is 40 to 480 mg, depending upon age and weight; no more than five doses should be administered in 24 hours. A dose of 10 to 15 mg/kg may also be used. Acetaminophen should not be administered for more than 10 days or to young children except upon advice of a physician.

Phenacetin has been employed only in analgesic mixtures. In recent years it has been removed from almost all such mixtures. In some instances acetaminophen has been included to replace it.

Therapeutic Uses. Acetaminophen is a suitable substitute for aspirin for its analgesic or antipyretic uses in patients in whom aspirin is contraindicated (*e.g.,* those with peptic ulcer) or when the prolongation of bleeding time caused by aspirin would be a disadvantage.

INDOMETHACIN AND SULINDAC

Indomethacin was the product of a laboratory search for drugs with anti-inflammatory properties. It was introduced in 1963 for the treatment of rheumatoid arthritis and related disorders. Although indomethacin is widely used and is effective, toxicity often limits its use. Sulindac was developed in an attempt to find a less toxic but effective congener of indomethacin. The development, chemistry, and pharmacology of both drugs have been reviewed by Shen and Winter (1977) and by Rhymer and Gengos (Symposium, 1983a).

INDOMETHACIN

Chemistry. The structural formula of indomethacin, a methylated indole derivative, is as follows:

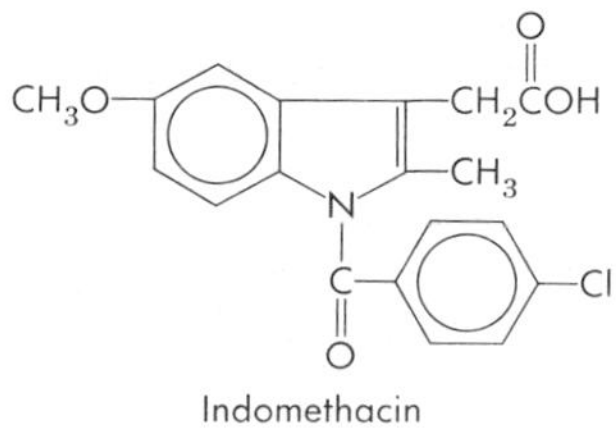

Indomethacin

Pharmacological Properties. Indomethacin has prominent anti-inflammatory and analgesic-antipyretic properties in experimental animals similar to those of the salicylates, and comparable effects have been demonstrated in man.

The anti-inflammatory effects of indomethacin are evident in patients with rheumatoid and other types of arthritis, including acute gout. Although indomethacin is more potent than aspirin, doses that are tolerated by patients with rheumatoid arthritis usually do not produce effects that are superior to those of salicylate. Contrary to early belief, indomethacin has *analgesic* properties distinct from its anti-inflammatory effects, and there is evidence for both a central and a peripheral effect. The *antipyretic* effect of indomethacin is also demonstrable in patients with fever.

Indomethacin is one of the most potent inhibitors of the prostaglandin-forming cyclooxygenase. Like colchicine, it inhibits motility of polymorphonuclear leukocytes. Like many other of the aspirin-like drugs, indomethacin uncouples oxidative phosphorylation in supratherapeutic concentrations and depresses the biosynthesis of mucopolysaccharides.

Pharmacokinetics and Metabolism. Indomethacin is rapidly and almost completely absorbed from the gastrointestinal tract following oral ingestion. The peak concentration in plasma is attained within 2 hours in the fasting subject but may be somewhat delayed when the drug is taken after meals. The concentrations in plasma required for an anti-inflammatory effect have not been accurately determined but are probably less than 1 μg/ml. Steady-state concentrations in plasma after chronic administration are approximately 0.5 μg/ml. Indomethacin is 90% bound to plasma proteins and also extensively bound to tissues. The concentration of the drug in the CSF is low, but its concentration in synovial fluid is equal to that in plasma within 5 hours of administration.

Indomethacin is largely converted to inactive metabolites. About half of a single oral dose is O-demethylated and about 10% is conjugated with glucuronic acid by the hepatic microsomal enzymes. A portion is also N-deacylated by a nonmicrosomal system. Some of these metabolites are detectable in plasma, and free and conjugated metabolites are eliminated in the urine, bile, and feces. There is enterohepatic cycling of the conjugates and probably of indomethacin itself. Ten to 20% of the drug is excreted unchanged in the urine, in part by tubular secretion. The half-life in plasma is extremely variable, perhaps because of enterohepatic cycling, and ranges between 2 and 11 hours.

Drug Interactions. The total plasma concentration of indomethacin plus its inactive metabolites is increased by concurrent administration of *probenecid*, possibly because of reduced tubular secretion of the former. However, it has not been determined whether the concentration of free indomethacin in plasma is altered or whether the dosage of indomethacin must be adjusted when the two drugs are employed together. Indomethacin does not interfere with the uricosuric effect of probenecid. Indomethacin is said not to modify the effect of the *oral anticoagulant agents*. However, concurrent administration could be hazardous because of the increased risk of gastrointestinal bleeding. Indomethacin antagonizes the natriuretic and antihypertensive effects of *furosemide;* the antihypertensive effects of thiazide diuretics or of β-adrenergic blocking agents may also be reduced. Acute renal failure associated with the concomitant administration of indomethacin and *triamterene* has been reported (*see* Clive and Stoff, 1984).

Toxic Effects. A very high percentage (35 to 50%) of patients receiving usual therapeutic doses of indomethacin experience untoward symptoms, and about 20% must discontinue its use. Most adverse effects are dose related.

Gastrointestinal complaints and complications consist in anorexia, nausea, and abdominal pain. Single ulcers or multiple ulceration of the entire upper gastrointestinal tract, sometimes with perforations and hemorrhage, has been reported. Occult blood loss may lead to anemia in the absence of ulceration. Acute pancreatitis has also been reported. Diarrhea may occur and is sometimes associated with ulcerative lesions of the bowel. Hepatic involvement has been rare, although some fatal cases of hepatitis and jaundice have been reported. The most frequent CNS effect (indeed, the most common side effect) is severe frontal headache, occurring in 25 to 50% of patients who take the drug chronically. Dizziness, vertigo, light-headedness, and mental confusion are also frequent. Severe depression, psychosis, hallucinations, and suicide have occurred. Early reports of corneal opacities and pallor of the optic disc seem to have been largely erroneous, but the signs should be sought in anyone taking the drug.

Hematopoietic reactions include neutropenia, thrombocytopenia, and, rarely, aplastic anemia. Deaths in children have occurred from what was probably overwhelming sepsis due to activation of latent infections. *Hypersensitivity* reactions are manifested as rashes, itching, urticaria, and, more seriously, acute attacks of asthma. Patients sensitive to *aspirin* may exhibit cross-reactivity to indomethacin. Indomethacin should not be used in pregnant women, nursing mothers, persons operating machinery, or patients with psychiatric disorders, epilepsy, or parkinsonism. It is also contraindicated in individuals with renal disease or ulcerative lesions of the stomach or intestines.

Preparations, Routes of Administration, and Dosage. *Indomethacin* (INDOCIN) is available for oral use in capsules containing 25 or 50 mg of the drug, and in sustained-release capsules (75 mg); it is also supplied in 50-mg suppositories.

The initial dose is 25 mg, two or three times daily, and this can be increased by 25-mg increments at weekly intervals until the total daily dose is 100 to 200 mg. Few patients tolerate more than 100 mg per day without severe side effects. Most patients respond within 4 to 6 days, but some require substantially longer treatment. The drug should be taken in divided portions with food or immediately after meals, to lessen gastric distress. A dose of indomethacin taken with milk at bedtime is said to reduce the incidence of morning headache.

Indomethacin is also available for intravenous injection as the sodium trihydrate (INDOCIN I.V.) to induce closure of a patent ductus arteriosus in neonates.

Therapeutic Uses. Because of the high incidence and severity of side effects associated with chronic administration, indomethacin must not be routinely used as an analgesic or antipyretic. However, it has proven useful as an antipyretic in Hodgkin's disease when the fever has been refractory to other agents. Indomethacin has become an accepted part of the rheumatologist's armamentarium and a standard (together with aspirin) against which to measure the activity of other, newer drugs.

Clinical trials of indomethacin as an anti-inflammatory agent have been reviewed by Shen and Winter (1977) and by Rhymer and Gengos (in Symposium, 1983a). The majority of these trials have demonstrated that indomethacin relieves pain, reduces swelling and tenderness of the joints, increases grip strength, and decreases the duration of morning stiffness. In these actions the drug is superior to placebo and equivalent to phenylbutazone; estimates of its potency relative to salicylates vary between 10 and 40 times. Overall, about two thirds of patients benefit from treatment with indomethacin; however, if 75 to 100 mg of the drug fails to provide benefit within 2 to 4 weeks, alternative therapy must be considered. The incidence and severity of side effects with indomethacin are particularly annoying, but a useful way of employing the undoubted potency of the drug, perhaps in combination with other and better-tolerated daytime therapy, is to give a large single dose (up to 100 mg) at bedtime. This enables the patient to obtain a better-quality sleep, reduces the severity and length of morning stiffness, and provides good analgesia until mid-morning. The side effects of indomethacin are apparently better tolerated when it is given at night.

Indomethacin is as effective as phenylbutazone and more effective than aspirin in the treatment of *ankylosing spondylitis* and *osteoarthrosis*. It is also very effective in the treatment of *acute gout,* although it is not uricosuric.

Patients with *Bartter's syndrome* have been successfully treated with indomethacin, as well as with other inhibitors of prostaglandin synthetase (*see* Clive and Stoff, 1984). The results are frequently dramatic; however, the condition of the patients may deteriorate rapidly when therapy is discontinued, and the long-term therapy necessary to control the disease requires administration of a drug that is better tolerated.

Cardiac failure in neonates caused by a *patent ductus arteriosus* may be controlled by the administration of indomethacin. A typical regimen involves administration of 0.2 mg/kg every 12 hours for three doses. While not an approved indication for indomethacin, successful closure can be expected in more than 70% of neonates who are treated with the drug, and such therapy is usually attempted before resorting to surgical ligation (*see* Evens, in Symposium, 1984). The primary limitation of this approach is potential renal toxicity, and restriction of fluids and diuretic therapy are often required. Renal failure, enterocolitis, thrombocytopenia, or hyperbilirubinemia contraindicates the use of indomethacin.

SULINDAC

Chemistry.   Sulindac is closely related to indomethacin; its structural formula is as follows:

Sulindac

It is unlikely, however, that sulindac itself has much therapeutic efficacy; most of its pharmacological activity resides in its sulfide metabolite.

Pharmacological Properties.   In laboratory studies, sulindac exhibits the classical activities of aspirin-like drugs. In all tests, sulindac is less than half as potent as indomethacin.

Because sulindac is a prodrug, it appears to be either inactive or relatively weak in many tests, whereas its sulfide metabolite may be very active. This especially applies to tests where little or no metabolism can occur. The sulfide metabolite is more than 500 times more potent than sulindac as

an inhibitor of cyclooxygenase (*see* Rhymer, in Symposium, 1983a). These observations may help to explain the somewhat lower incidence of gastrointestinal toxicity of sulindac, since the gastric or intestinal mucosa is not exposed to high concentrations of an active drug during oral administration. Sulindac is also unusual in that it does not alter the urinary excretion of prostaglandins or plasma renin activity in either normal human subjects or patients with Bartter's syndrome (*see* Rhymer, in Symposium, 1983a). This relative lack of effect on the kidney may involve limitations of the access of the sulfide metabolite to the renal cyclooxygenase and/or low potency to inhibit the renal enzyme.

Pharmacokinetics and Metabolism.   The metabolism and pharmacokinetics of sulindac are complex and vary enormously among species. After oral administration to man, about 90% of the drug is absorbed. Peak concentrations of sulindac in plasma are attained within 1 hour, while those of the sulfide metabolite occur about 2 hours after the oral administration of sulindac.

Sulindac undergoes two major biotransformations in addition to conjugation reactions. It is oxidized to the sulfone and then reversibly reduced to the sulfide. It is this latter metabolite that is the active moiety, although all three compounds are found in comparable concentrations in human plasma. The half-life of sulindac itself is about 7 hours, but the active sulfide has a half-life as long as 18 hours. Study of the pharmacokinetic properties of sulindac and its metabolites is complicated by extensive enterohepatic circulation (*see* Porter, in Symposium, 1984). There seems to be little or no placental transfer of the drug, but it is present in breast milk. Sulindac and the sulfone and sulfide metabolites are all more than 93% bound to plasma protein; the sulfone is the most highly bound, and sulindac is the least.

Little of the sulfide or its conjugates is found in urine. The principal components that are so excreted are the sulfone and its conjugate, which account for nearly 30% of an administered dose; sulindac and its conjugates account for about 20%. Up to 25% of an oral dose may appear as metabolites in the feces (*see* Rhymer, in Symposium, 1983a).

Preparations, Route of Administration, and Dosage.   *Sulindac* (CLINORIL) is available as 150- and 200-mg tablets. The most common dosage for adults is 150 to 200 mg twice a day, although dosage should be optimized for each individual. The maximal daily dose is 400 mg. The drug may be given with food if gastric discomfort is experienced, although this could delay absorption and reduce the concentration in plasma.

Toxic Effects.   While the incidence of toxicity is lower than with indomethacin, untoward reactions to sulindac are common. Some estimate the incidence to be 25% (*see* Rhymer, in Symposium, 1983a).

Gastrointestinal side effects are seen in nearly 20% of patients, although these are generally mild. Abdominal pain and nausea are the most frequent complaints, followed by constipation. Gastric bleeding appears to be relatively uncommon. CNS side effects are seen in up to 10% of patients, with drowsiness, dizziness, headache, and nervousness being those most frequently reported. Skin rash and pruritus occur in 5% of patients. Transient elevations of hepatic enzymes in plasma are less common. As with other aspirin-like drugs, there is a danger that sulindac could precipitate a severe reaction in patients who are sensitive to aspirin; platelet function may also be impaired and bleeding time prolonged.

Therapeutic Uses. Sulindac has been utilized mainly for the treatment of rheumatoid arthritis, osteoarthrosis, and ankylosing spondylitis. The drug has also been used with success in the treatment of periarticular disease and acute gout. The analgesic and anti-inflammatory effects exerted by sulindac (400 mg per day) are comparable to those achieved with aspirin (4 g per day), ibuprofen (1200 mg per day), indomethacin (125 mg per day), and phenylbutazone (400 to 600 mg per day) (*see* Rhymer, in Symposium, 1983a).

THE FENAMATES

The fenamates are a family of aspirin-like drugs that are derivatives of N-phenylanthranilic acid. The group includes mefenamic, meclofenamic, flufenamic, tolfenamic, and etofenamic acids.

Although the biological activity of this group of drugs was discovered in the 1950s, the fenamates have not gained widespread clinical acceptance. They cause side effects frequently; diarrhea, in particular, may be very severe. Therapeutically, they also have no clear advantages over several other aspirin-like drugs.

Mefenamic acid and *meclofenamate* are the only members of the series available in the United States. The use of mefenamic acid is indicated only for analgesia and for relief of the symptoms of primary dysmenorrhea. While meclofenamate is employed in the treatment of rheumatoid arthritis and osteoarthritis, it is not recommended as initial therapy. Flufenamic acid is used in many other countries, as is mefenamic acid, for its anti-inflammatory effects. Other members of the series will not be discussed further.

Chemistry. Mefenamic acid and meclofenamate are both N-substituted phenylanthranilic acids. Their structures are as follows:

Mefenamic Acid

Meclofenamate Sodium

Pharmacological Properties. In the tests of anti-inflammatory activity, mefenamic acid is about half as potent and flufenamic acid about 1.5 times as potent as phenylbutazone. Both drugs also have antipyretic and analgesic properties. In tests of analgesia, mefenamic acid was the only fenamate to display a central as well as a peripheral action.

The fenamates appear to owe these properties to their capacity to inhibit cyclooxygenase. Unlike the other aspirin-like drugs, certain of the fenamates (especially meclofenamic acid) appear to antagonize certain effects of prostaglandins, such as $PGF_{2\alpha}$-induced contraction of isolated bronchial smooth muscle (Collier and Sweatman, 1968).

Much of the basic pharmacology, pharmacokinetics, and early clinical experience with the fenamates has been summarized in a symposium (1966).

Pharmacokinetic Properties. Meclofenamate is more rapidly absorbed following a single oral dose than is mefenamic acid; peak concentrations in plasma are reached in 0.5 to 2 hours for the former and in 2 to 4 hours for the latter drug. The two agents have similar half-lives in plasma (2 to 4 hours). In man, approximately 50% of a dose of mefenamic acid is excreted in the urine. Of this, approximately half is the conjugated 3-hydroxymethyl metabolite, a little less than half is the 3-carboxyl metabolite and its conjugates, and the remaining few percent is mostly conjugated mefenamic acid. Twenty percent of the drug is recovered in the feces, mainly as the unconjugated 3-carboxyl metabolite.

Preparations, Route of Administration, and Dosage. *Mefenamic acid* (PONSTEL) is available in 250-mg capsules for oral administration. For acute pain, the initial dose for adults and children over 14 years of age is 500 mg; thereafter, 250 mg may be given every 6 hours with food. The drug is not recommended for use in children or pregnant women, nor should it be given for longer than 7 days. *Meclofenamate sodium* (MECLOMEN) is available in capsules containing the equivalent of 50 or 100 mg of meclofenamic acid. The usual daily dose is 200 to 400 mg in three or four portions. Dosage requires adjustment for the individual but should not exceed 400 mg per day. The drug is not recommended for children. *Flufenamic acid* is not available in the United States.

Toxic Effects and Precautions. The most common side effects (occurring in approximately 25% of all patients) involve the gastrointestinal system. Usually these take the form of dyspepsia or upper gastrointestinal discomfort, although diarrhea, which may be severe and associated with inflammation of the bowel, or constipation is also relatively common. There have also been reports of bleeding ulcers following treatment with mefenamic acid. Steatorrhea may also be associated with diarrhea.

Other reactions that have been noted less frequently include transient abnormalities of hepatic and renal function, CNS effects, and skin rashes. A potentially serious side effect seen in isolated cases is a hemolytic anemia, which may be of an autoimmune type.

The fenamates are contraindicated in patients with a history of gastrointestinal disease. If diarrhea or skin rash appears, the drug should be stopped at once. The physician and patient should watch for signs of hemolytic anemia. The fenamates can cause bronchoconstriction in patients who are sensitive to aspirin. Like all inhibitors of prostaglandin synthetase, these drugs affect platelet function.

Drug Interactions. The fenamates bind strongly to plasma proteins, and there is thus the possibility of displacement of other drugs from nonspecific binding sites on plasma albumin. This possibility has been confirmed for oral anticoagulants when mefenamic acid is administered.

Therapeutic Uses. As an *analgesic agent,* mefenamic acid has been used to relieve pain arising from rheumatic conditions, soft-tissue injuries, other painful musculoskeletal conditions and dysmenorrhea. While mefenamic acid clearly possesses analgesic activity, toxicity limits its utility. It appears to offer no advantage over other analgesic agents. As *anti-inflammatory agents,* mefenamic acid and meclofenamate have been mainly tested in short-term trials in the treatment of osteoarthritis and rheumatoid arthritis. While advantages of these agents are not apparent, meclofenamate may be of value in some patients who have not responded satisfactorily to other aspirin-like drugs.

TOLMETIN

Tolmetin is an anti-inflammatory, analgesic, and antipyretic agent that was introduced into clinical practice in the United States in 1976. Tolmetin, in recommended doses, appears to be approximately equivalent in efficacy to moderate doses of aspirin; it is usually better tolerated. The structural formula of tolmetin is as follows:

Tolmetin

Pharmacological Properties. Tolmetin is an effective anti-inflammatory agent; it is more potent than aspirin and less potent than indomethacin or phenylbutazone. Tolmetin also exerts antipyretic and analgesic effects in experimental animals and man. Like most of the other drugs considered in this chapter, tolmetin causes gastric erosions and prolongs bleeding time. The pharmacology of tolmetin has been reviewed by Brogden and associates (1978) and by Ehrlich (in Symposium, 1983a).

Pharmacokinetics and Metabolism. Tolmetin is rapidly and completely absorbed following its oral administration to man, and the concentrations achieved in plasma are not reduced by the concomitant administration of gastric antacids. Peak concentrations are achieved 20 to 60 minutes after oral administration, and the half-life in plasma is about 1 to 2 hours.

After absorption, tolmetin is extensively (99%) bound to plasma proteins. Virtually all of the drug can be recovered in the urine after 24 hours; some is unchanged but most is conjugated or otherwise metabolized. The major metabolic transformation involves oxidation of the para-methyl group to a carboxylic acid.

Preparations, Route of Administration, and Dosage. *Tolmetin sodium* (TOLECTIN) is supplied as 200-mg tablets and 400-mg capsules for oral use. The recommended initial dose is 400 mg three times daily, and it is suggested that one of these doses be taken on retiring and another on awakening. The response to the drug is usually seen within a week, and the dose can then be adjusted; the usual range is 600 to 1800 mg per day in divided doses. The maximal recommended dose is 2 g per day. The drug may be given with meals, milk, or antacids to lessen abdominal discomfort. The recommended initial daily dose for children (2 years and older) is 20 mg/kg per day in three or four divided doses. Maintenance dosage ranges from 15 to 30 mg/kg per day.

Toxic Effects. Some 25 to 40% of patients who take tolmetin experience side effects, and 5 to 10% discontinue use of the drug. Gastrointestinal side effects are the most common, with epigastric pain (15% incidence), dyspepsia, nausea, and vomiting being the chief manifestations. Gastric and duodenal ulceration has also been observed. CNS side effects, including nervousness, anxiety, insomnia, drowsiness, and visual disturbance, are less common and are said to be neither as frequent nor severe as those caused by indomethacin.

Similarly, the incidence of tinnitus, deafness, and vertigo is less than with aspirin. There is an occasional skin rash or urticaria. It should be assumed that tolmetin will probably precipitate bronchoconstriction in those patients who are hypersensitive to aspirin. In addition, there have been several reports of severe anaphylactoid reactions to tolmetin (and to its close relative *zomepirac*) in patients who are not sensitive to aspirin and other aspirin-like drugs (*see,* for example, Rake and Jacobs, 1983).

Drug Interactions. Despite its extensive binding to albumin, tolmetin does not interfere with concurrent treatment with warfarin or oral hypoglycemic agents. Tolmetin differs in this regard from many other drugs of this type.

Therapeutic Uses. Tolmetin is approved in the United States for the treatment of *osteoarthritis, rheumatoid arthritis,* and the *juvenile form of the disease;* it has also been used in the treatment of *ankylosing spondylitis.* In rheumatoid arthritis, many investigators have compared tolmetin (0.8 to 1.6 g per day) with aspirin (4 to 4.5 g per day) or indomethacin (100 to 150 mg per day). In general, there has been little difference in therapeutic efficacy. Tolmetin may be tolerated somewhat better than aspirin in equieffective doses. Similar results have been obtained with related arthritides and with soft-tissue injuries (*see* Ehrlich, in Symposium, 1983a).

ZOMEPIRAC

Zomepirac is closely related to tolmetin. Its analgesic activity in man is more prominent than its anti-inflammatory effect (*see* Morley *et al.,* 1982; Huskisson, in Symposium, 1983a). This drug was marketed briefly in the United States for the treatment of mild-to-moderate pain, but it was abruptly withdrawn by the manufacturer following reports of severe anaphylactoid reactions.

PROPIONIC ACID DERIVATIVES

These drugs represent a relatively new group of effective, useful aspirin-like agents. They may offer significant advantages over aspirin, indomethacin, and the pyrazolon derivatives for many patients, since they are usually better tolerated. Nevertheless, propionic acid derivatives share all of the detrimental features of the entire class of drugs. Furthermore, their rapid proliferation in number and heavy promotion have made difficult the physician's task of making a rational choice between members of the group and between propionic acid derivatives and the more established agents. The similarities between drugs in this class (and certain of the others discussed above) are far more striking than are the differences.

Ibuprofen, naproxen, and *fenoprofen* are described individually below. These drugs are currently available in the United States, but several additional agents in this class are in use in other countries. These include *fenbufen, flurbiprofen, indoprofen, ketoprofen,* and *suprofen.* Ibuprofen was the first member of this class to come into general use, and experience with this drug is correspondingly greater. It has recently been approved for sale without a prescription in the United States. The most distinctive feature among the others may probably be claimed by naproxen; its longer half-life makes twice-daily administration feasible. The structural formulas of these drugs are shown in Table 29–3.

Pharmacological Properties. The pharmacodynamic properties of propionic acid

Table 29–3.   STRUCTURAL FORMULAS OF ANTI-INFLAMMATORY PROPIONIC ACID DERIVATIVES

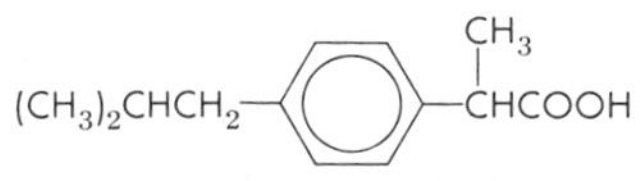

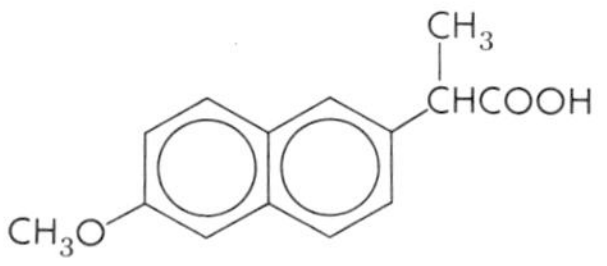

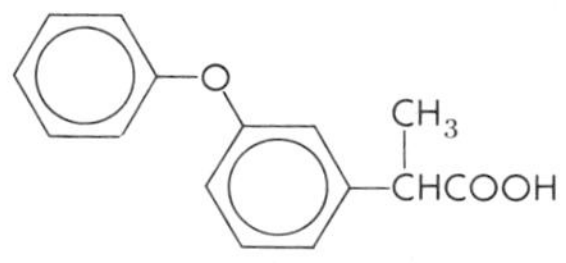

derivatives do not differ significantly. While they do vary in potency, this is not of obvious clinical significance. All are effective anti-inflammatory agents in various experimental models of inflammation in animals; all have useful anti-inflammatory, analgesic, and antipyretic activity in man.

All of these compounds can cause gastrointestinal erosions (gastric, duodenal, and intestinal) in experimental animals. All produce gastrointestinal side effects in man, although these are usually less severe than with aspirin.

The propionic acid derivatives are all effective inhibitors of the cyclooxygenase responsible for the biosynthesis of prostaglandins, although there is considerable variation in their potency. For example, naproxen is approximately 20 times more potent than aspirin, while ibuprofen, fenoprofen, and aspirin are roughly equipotent in this action. It is thus not surprising that all of these agents alter platelet function and prolong bleeding time, as described above. It should also be assumed that any patient who is intolerant of aspirin may also suffer a severe reaction following administration of one of these drugs.

Some of the propionic acid derivatives have prominent inhibitory effects on leukocyte migration. Naproxen is particularly potent in this regard. It is more active than colchicine *in vitro* and produces substantial effects at concentrations comparable to those achieved therapeutically (*see* Segre, in Symposium, 1983a).

Drug Interactions. The potential adverse drug interactions of particular concern with this group derive from their high degree of binding to albumin in plasma. However, none of the propionic acid derivatives has been found to alter the effects of the oral hypoglycemic drugs or warfarin (*see* Day *et al.*, in Symposium, 1983a). Nevertheless, the physician should be prepared to adjust the dosage of warfarin because these drugs impair platelet function and may cause gastrointestinal lesions.

As discussed above, the propionic acid derivatives can be expected to reduce the diuretic and natriuretic effects of furosemide as well as the antihypertensive effects of such agents as the thiazide diuretics,

β-adrenergic antagonists, prazosin, and captopril (*see* Day *et al.*, in Symposium, 1983a; Clive and Stoff, 1984). These effects probably result from the inhibition of the synthesis of renal prostaglandins (*see* above).

Simultaneous administration of aspirin and naproxen results in displacement of the latter from albumin and an increased rate of its clearance. However, this effect is of little clinical relevance.

IBUPROFEN

Ibuprofen has been discussed in detail by Kantor (1979) and by Adams and Buckler (in Symposium, 1983a).

Pharmacokinetics and Metabolism. Ibuprofen is rapidly absorbed following oral administration to man, and peak concentrations in plasma are observed after 1 to 2 hours. The half-life in plasma is about 2 hours. Absorption is also efficient, although slower, from suppositories.

Ibuprofen is extensively (99%) and firmly bound to plasma proteins, but the drug occupies only a fraction of the total drug-binding sites at usual concentrations. Ibuprofen passes slowly into the synovial spaces and may remain there in higher concentration as the concentrations in plasma decline. In experimental animals, ibuprofen and its metabolites pass easily across the placenta.

The excretion of ibuprofen is rapid and complete. Greater than 90% of an ingested dose is excreted in the urine as metabolites or their conjugates, and no ibuprofen *per se* is found in the urine. The major metabolites are a hydroxylated and a carboxylated compound.

Preparations, Route of Administration, and Dosage. *Ibuprofen* (MOTRIN, RUFEN) is supplied as 200-, 300-, 400-, and 600-mg tablets; only the 200-mg tablets (ADVIL, NUPRIN) are available without a prescription. A syrup containing 20 mg/ml is available outside the United States.

For rheumatoid arthritis and osteoarthritis, daily doses of up to 2400 mg in divided portions may be given, although the usual total dose is 1200 to 1600 mg. It may also be possible to reduce the dose for maintenance purposes. For mild-to-moderate pain, especially that of primary dysmenorrhea, the usual dose is 400 mg every 4 to 6 hours as needed. The drug may be given with food to minimize gastrointestinal side effects. The safety and efficacy of ibuprofen in children have not been established.

Toxic Effects. Ibuprofen has been used in patients with known peptic ulceration or a history of gastric intolerance to other aspirin-like agents. Nevertheless, therapy must usually be discontinued in 10 to 15% of patients because of intolerance to the drug.

Gastrointestinal side effects are experienced by 5 to 15% of patients taking ibuprofen; epigastric pain, nausea, heartburn, abdominal discomfort, and sensations of "fullness" in the gastrointestinal tract are the usual difficulties. However, the incidence of these side effects is less with ibuprofen than with aspirin or indomethacin. Occult blood loss is uncommon.

Other side effects of ibuprofen have been reported less frequently. They include thrombocytopenia, skin rashes, headache, dizziness and blurred vision, and, in a few cases, toxic amblyopia, fluid retention, and edema. Patients who develop ocular disturbances should discontinue the use of ibuprofen.

Ibuprofen is not recommended for use by pregnant women, nor by those who are breast-feeding their infants.

NAPROXEN

The pharmacological properties and therapeutic uses of naproxen have been reviewed by Brogden and associates (1979) and by Segre (in Symposium, 1983a).

Pharmacokinetics and Metabolism. Naproxen is fully absorbed when administered orally. The rapidity, but not the extent, of absorption is influenced by the presence of food in the stomach. Peak concentrations in plasma occur within 2 to 4 hours and may be achieved more rapidly after the administration of naproxen sodium. Absorption may be accelerated by the concurrent administration of sodium bicarbonate or reduced by magnesium oxide or aluminum hydroxide. Naproxen is also absorbed rectally, but peak concentrations in plasma are achieved more slowly. The half-life of naproxen in plasma is about 14 hours.

Naproxen and its metabolites are almost entirely excreted in the urine. About 30% of the drug undergoes 6-demethylation, and most of this metabolite, as well as naproxen itself, is excreted as the glucuronide or other conjugates.

Naproxen is almost completely (99%) bound to plasma protein following normal therapeutic doses. Naproxen crosses the placenta and appears in the milk of lactating women at approximately 1% of the maternal plasma concentration.

Preparations, Route of Administration, and Dosage. *Naproxen* (NAPROSYN) is available in 250-, 375-, and 500-mg tablets for oral administra-

tion. *Naproxen sodium* (ANAPROX) is marketed in tablets containing 275 mg of the salt (equivalent to 250 mg of naproxen). For rheumatoid arthritis, osteoarthritis, and ankylosing spondylitis, the usual dose of naproxen is 250 to 375 mg, given twice daily. The dose is adjusted depending on the clinical response, but long-term therapy with daily doses above 1000 mg has not been investigated. Favorable responses in patients with rheumatoid arthritis have been associated with dosage regimens that maintain a minimal concentration in plasma of greater than 50 μg/ml (*see* Porter, in Symposium, 1984). For acute gout, the usual initial dose of naproxen is 750 mg, followed by 250 mg every 8 hours until the attack has subsided. For mild-to-moderate pain, especially that associated with primary dysmenorrhea, bursitis, and acute tendonitis, the initial dose is 500 mg, followed by 250 mg every 6 to 8 hours. The drug may be given with meals if gastric discomfort is experienced.

Toxic Effects. The incidence of gastrointestinal and CNS side effects is about equal, although naproxen is better tolerated than indomethacin in both regards. Gastrointestinal complications have ranged from relatively mild dyspepsia, gastric discomfort, and heartburn to nausea, vomiting, and gastric bleeding. CNS side effects range from drowsiness, headache, dizziness, and sweating to fatigue, depression, and ototoxicity. Less common reactions include pruritus and a variety of dermatological problems. A few instances of jaundice, impairment of renal function, angioneurotic edema, thrombocytopenia, and agranulocytosis have been reported.

FENOPROFEN

The pharmacological properties and therapeutic uses of fenoprofen have been reviewed by Brogden and associates (1977) and by Burt and coworkers (Symposium, 1983a).

Pharmacokinetics and Metabolism. Oral doses of fenoprofen are readily, if incompletely (85%), absorbed. The presence of food in the stomach retards absorption and lowers peak concentrations in plasma, which are usually achieved within 2 hours. The concomitant administration of antacids does not seem to alter concentrations that are achieved.

After absorption, fenoprofen is almost completely (99%) bound to plasma albumin. The drug is extensively (>90%) metabolized and excreted almost entirely in the urine. Fenoprofen undergoes metabolic transformation to the 4-hydroxy analog. The glucuronic acid conjugate of fenoprofen itself and 4-hydroxy fenoprofen are formed in almost equal amounts and together account for 90% of the excreted drug. The half-life of fenoprofen in plasma is about 3 hours.

Preparations, Route of Administration, and Dosage. *Fenoprofen calcium* (NALFON) is available in capsules and tablets containing 200 to 600 mg of the active drug for oral administration. The recommended dosage to treat rheumatoid arthritis or osteoarthritis is 300 to 600 mg, given three to four times a day, but this may be increased to a maximum of 3.2 g per day. For mild-to-moderate pain, the usual dose is 200 mg every 4 to 6 hours. Fenoprofen may be administered with meals. The drug is not recommended for children.

Toxic Effects. Gastrointestinal side effects have been the most frequently reported; abdominal discomfort and dyspepsia occur in about 15% of patients. Constipation and nausea have also been reported. These side effects are almost always less intense than with equipotent doses of aspirin and force discontinuation of therapy in a few percent of patients. Nevertheless, care should be exercised when giving the drug to patients having a history of gastrointestinal ulceration or other pathology. Other side effects include skin rash and, less frequently, CNS effects, such as tinnitus, dizziness, lassitude, confusion, and anorexia.

THERAPEUTIC USES

The approved indications for the use of one or another of the propionic acid derivatives include the symptomatic treatment of *rheumatoid arthritis, osteoarthritis, ankylosing spondylitis,* and *acute gouty arthritis;* they are also utilized as *analgesics.*

Clinical studies indicate that the propionic acid derivatives are comparable to aspirin for the control of the signs and symptoms of rheumatoid arthritis and osteoarthritis. In patients with rheumatoid arthritis there is a reduction in joint swelling, pain, and duration of morning stiffness. By objective measurements, strength, mobility, and stamina are improved. In general, the intensity of untoward effects is less than that associated with the ingestion of indomethacin or high doses of aspirin. However, aspirin is considerably less expensive for those who can tolerate it.

While ibuprofen, naproxen, and fenoprofen may be of benefit in the treatment of ankylosing spondylitis, only naproxen has received approval for this use in the United States. As mentioned previously, naproxen appears to exert a prominent inhibitory effect on the migration of leukocytes; this may contribute to its efficacy in the treatment of acute attacks of gout. Clinical studies have indicated that these three agents may be as effective as aspirin in the treatment of juvenile rheumatoid arthritis. However, the data are as yet insufficient to establish their safety for chronic use in children.

These agents are also effective for symptomatic relief from pain associated with injuries to soft tissues, and they have been used to relieve pain post partum and following oral, ophthalmic, and other types of surgery. Both ibuprofen and naproxen are more effective than aspirin for relief of pain from dysmenorrhea. Indeed, the effectiveness of ibuprofen in this condition was one important reason for its release in 1984 for "over-the-counter" use.

It is difficult to find data on which to base a rational choice between the members of this group of drugs, if in fact one can be made. However, in studies that compared the activity of several members of this group, patients preferred naproxen (with fenoprofen next) in terms of analgesia and relief of morning stiffness (*see* Huskisson, in Symposium, 1983a; Hart and Huskisson, 1984). With regard to side effects, naproxen was the best tolerated, followed by ibuprofen and fenoprofen. There was considerable interpatient variation in the preference for a single drug and also between the designation of the best drug and the worst agent. Unfortunately, it is probably impossible to predict *a priori* which drug will be most suitable for any given individual. Nevertheless, more than 50% of patients with rheumatoid arthritis will probably achieve adequate symptomatic relief by the use of one or another of the propionic acid derivatives.

PIROXICAM

Piroxicam is the newest anti-inflammatory, analgesic, and antipyretic agent to be introduced into clinical practice in the United States. In recommended doses, piroxicam appears to be the equivalent of aspirin, indomethacin, or naproxen for the long-term treatment of rheumatoid arthritis or osteoarthritis. It is tolerated better than aspirin or indomethacin and thus far seems to be equivalent to the propionic acid derivatives in this regard. The principal advantage of piroxicam is its long half-life, which permits the administration of a single daily dose. The pharmacological properties and therapeutic uses of piroxicam have been reviewed in a symposium (Symposium, 1982) and by Wiseman (in Symposium, 1983a). The structural formula of piroxicam is as follows:

Piroxicam

Pharmacological Properties. Piroxicam is an effective anti-inflammatory agent; it is about equal in potency to indomethacin as an inhibitor of prostaglandin biosynthesis *in vitro*. Piroxicam also exerts antipyretic and analgesic effects in experimental animals and man. As with other aspirin-like drugs, piroxicam can cause gastric erosions and it prolongs the bleeding time.

Pharmacokinetics and Metabolism. Piroxicam is completely absorbed after oral administration; peak concentrations in plasma occur within 2 to 4 hours. Neither food nor antacids alter the rate or extent of absorption. There is enterohepatic cycling of piroxicam, and estimates of the half-life in plasma have been variable; a mean value appears to be about 45 hours (*see* Porter, in Symposium, 1984).

After absorption, piroxicam is extensively (99%) bound to plasma proteins. At steady state (*e.g.*, after 7 to 10 days), concentrations of piroxicam in plasma and synovial fluid are approximately equal. Less than 10% of the drug is excreted in the urine unchanged. The major metabolic transformation in man is hydroxylation of the pyridyl ring, and this compound and its glucuronide conjugate account for about 60% of the drug excreted in the urine and feces.

Preparations, Route of Administration, and Dosage. *Piroxicam* (FELDENE) is available in 10- and 20-mg capsules for oral administration. The usual daily dose for the relief of signs and symptoms of rheumatoid arthritis or osteoarthritis is 20 mg; if desired, this may be given in two portions. Since steady-state concentrations in plasma are not reached for 7 to 10 days, maximal therapeutic responses should not be expected for 2 weeks, even though they may be evident earlier. It has been suggested that satisfactory responses are associated with concentrations in plasma greater than 5 to 6 μg/ml.

Toxic Effects. The reported incidence of adverse effects in patients who take piroxicam has ranged from 11 to 46%; between 4 and 12% of patients stop using the drug because of side effects. Gastrointestinal reactions are the most common, but less than 5% of patients discontinue treatment because of these. The incidence of peptic ulcer is less than 1%. As with other aspirin-like drugs, piroxicam alters the function of platelets, and it should be assumed that piroxicam will precipitate bronchoconstriction in those patients who are hypersensitive to aspirin.

Therapeutic Uses. Piroxicam is approved in the United States for the treatment of rheumatoid arthritis and osteoarthritis. It has also been used in the treatment of ankylosing spondylitis, acute musculoskeletal disorders, and acute gout.

GOLD

Gold, in elemental form, has been employed for centuries as an antipruritic to relieve the itching palm. In more modern times, the observation by Robert Koch in 1890 that gold inhibited *Mycobacterium tuberculosis in vitro* led to trials in arthritis and lupus erythematosus, thought by some to be tuberculous manifestations. The favorable observations of Forestier (1929) were largely responsible for stimulating interest in gold therapy (chrysotherapy). At present, gold is employed in the treatment of rheumatoid arthritis; its use is usually reserved for those patients with rapidly progressive disease who do not obtain satisfactory relief from therapy with aspirin-like drugs. However, gold compounds are among a small number of agents that are capable of arresting the progress of the disease and inducing apparent remissions in some patients. Since degenerative lesions do not regress once formed, there is an increasing tendency to attempt to induce remission early in the course of the disease. Such therapy is most often initiated with gold.

Chemistry. The significant preparations of gold are all compounds in which the gold is attached to sulfur. The more water-soluble compounds employed in therapy contain hydrophilic groups in addition to the aurothio group. The structural formulas of *aurothioglucose, gold sodium thiomalate,* and *auranofin* are as follows:

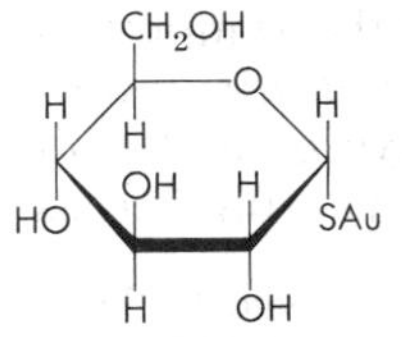

Aurothioglucose

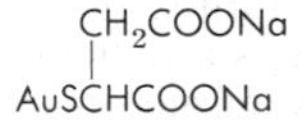

$$CH_2COONa$$
$$AuSCHCOONa$$

Gold Sodium Thiomalate

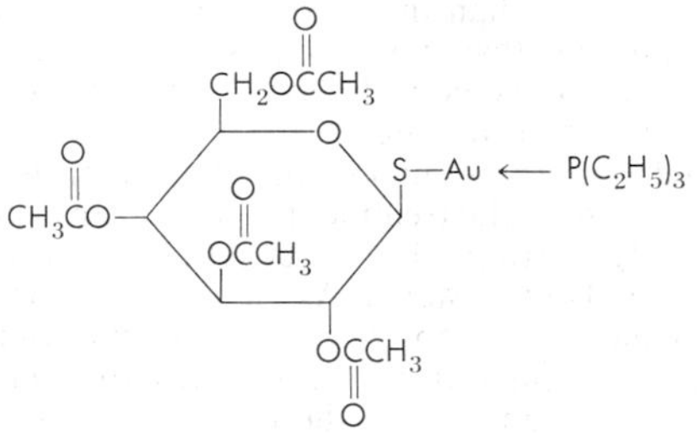

Auranofin

Monovalent gold has a relatively strong affinity for sulfur, weak affinities for carbon and nitrogen, and almost no affinity for oxygen, except in chelates. The strong affinity for sulfur and the inhibitory effect of gold salts on various enzymes have suggested that the therapeutic effects of gold salts might derive from inhibition of sulfhydryl systems. However, other sulfhydryl inhibitors do not appear to have therapeutic actions in common with gold.

Pharmacological Actions. Gold compounds can suppress or prevent, but not cure, experimental arthritis and synovitis due to a number of infectious and chemical agents. As with other agents that are thought to induce remission of rheumatoid arthritis, gold compounds have minimal anti-inflammatory effects in other circumstances and cause only a gradual reduction of the signs and symptoms of inflammation associated with rheumatoid arthritis. While many effects of gold compounds have been observed, which, if any, is related to the therapeutic effects of gold in rheumatoid arthritis is unknown. Perhaps the best hypotheses relate to the capacity of gold compounds to inhibit the function of mononuclear phagocytes, thereby suppressing immune responsiveness (*see* Lipsky, in Symposium, 1983d). Decreased concentrations of rheumatoid factor and immunoglobulins are often observed in patients who are treated with gold.

In experimental animals, gold is sequestered in organs that are rich in mononuclear phagocytes, and it selectively accumulates in the lysosomes of type-A synovial cells and other macrophages within the inflamed synovium of patients who are treated with gold compounds. Moreover, the administration of gold thiomalate to animals depresses the migration and phagocytic activity of macrophages in inflammatory exudates, and chrysotherapy reduces the augmented phagocytic capacity of blood monocytes from patients with rheumatoid arthritis. Other mechanisms of action of gold compounds have been suggested, but none is generally accepted. These include inhibition of prostaglandin synthesis, interference with complement activation, and inhibition of the activity of lysosomal and other enzymes.

Aurothioglucose, but not other compounds of gold, in toxic doses induces obesity in dogs and certain strains of mice. Gold-induced necrosis of the oligodendroglia in the ventromedial hypothalamus occurs in both rats and mice. Gold is deposited in the scar. The gold of gold thiomalate, which does not induce obesity, is not found in hypothalamic loci. These effects of gold are not observed in human subjects.

Absorption, Distribution, and Excretion. *Aurothioglucose and Gold Sodium Thiomalate.* These more water-soluble gold compounds are rapidly absorbed after intramuscular injection, and peak concentrations in blood are reached in 2 to 6 hours, unless the drug is suspended in oil. These agents are erratically absorbed by the oral route. Less is known about the distribution of gold in man than in animals. Tissue distribution depends not only on the type of compound administered but also on the time after administration and probably on the duration of treatment. Early in the course of therapy, several percent of the total body content of gold is in the blood, where it is first bound (about 95%) to albumin. During the course of the first week, a substantial fraction may be transferred to the erythrocytes in some patients. During treatment, the concentration in the synovial fluid is about half that in plasma.

With continued therapy, the concentration of gold in the synovium of affected joints is about ten times that of skeletal muscle, bone, or fat. Gold deposits are also found in macrophages of many tissues, as well as in renotubular epithelium, seminiferous tubules, hepatocytes, and adrenocortical cells.

The pharmacokinetic properties of gold in these compounds are complex and vary with the dose and the duration of treatment. The plasma half-life is about 7 days for a 50-mg dose. With successive doses the half-life lengthens, and values of weeks or months may be observed after prolonged therapy. After a cumulative dose of 1 g of gold, about 60% of the amount administered is retained in the body. After termination of treatment, urinary excretion of gold can be detected for as long as a year, even though concentrations in blood fall to the normal trace amounts in about 40 to 80 days. Substantial quantities of gold have been found in the liver and skin of patients many years after the cessation of therapy. Sulfhydryl agents, such as dimercaprol, penicillamine, and N-acetylcysteine, increase the excretion of gold.

The excretion of gold is 60 to 90% renal and 10 to 40% fecal, the latter probably mostly by biliary secretion. In the first day after injection the gold concentration in urine ranges from about equal to twice that in plasma; after 7 days it may be slightly above to slightly below the plasma concentration. Fecal excretion is erratic but tends to be low in the first day after injection and to increase during the next several days. The pharmacokinetics of gold has been reviewed by Gottlieb (1982).

Auranofin. Auranofin is a more hydrophobic gold-containing compound that is not yet available for general use in the United States. It is more readily absorbed after oral administration (to the extent of about 25%). While therapeutic doses of auranofin (6 mg per day) lead to concentrations of gold in plasma that are similar to that achieved with conventional parenteral therapy, the accumulation of gold during a 6-month course of treatment with auranofin is only about 20% of that found with injectable gold compounds (*see* Gottlieb, 1982). After cessation of treatment, the half-life of gold in the body is about 80 days (*see* Chaffman *et al.,* 1984). Auranofin is predominantly excreted in the feces.

Preparations, Route of Administration, and Dosage. *Aurothioglucose* (SOLGANAL) contains approximately 50% gold. Although it is water soluble, it is employed as a sterile suspension in a suitable fixed oil. Commercial preparations contain 50 mg/ml. *Gold sodium thiomalate* (MYOCHRYSINE) also contains approximately 50% gold and is very soluble in water. It is available as a sterile aqueous solution for injection.

The optimal intramuscular dosage schedule for the treatment of rheumatoid arthritis is still debated. Moreover, some rheumatologists use the same dosage regimen for either compound while others do not. The usual dose is 10 mg of either gold compound in the first week as a test dose, followed by 25 mg in the second and third weeks. Thereafter, either 25 to 50 mg (gold sodium thiomalate) or 50 mg (aurothioglucose) is administered at weekly intervals until the cumulative dose reaches 1 g. A favorable response is usually not evident for a few months. If a remission occurs, treatment is continued but the dose is reduced or the dosage interval is increased. For example, 25 to 50 mg may be administered every 2 weeks for up to 20 weeks, followed by a dose every 3 weeks for an additional 18 weeks; thereafter monthly intervals may be utilized for an indefinite period (*see* Sigler, in Symposium, 1983e). If neither significant toxicity nor clinical response is apparent after the administration of 1 g of gold sodium thiomalate, gradual increase in dosage may be considered; the weekly dose of this compound should not exceed 100 mg.

Clinical Toxicity. The most common toxic effects that are associated with the therapeutic use of gold are those that involve the skin and the mucous membranes, usually of the mouth. These occur in about 15% of all patients. While clearly dose related, these effects do not correlate well with the concentration of gold in plasma (*see* Rothermich, in Symposium, 1983a). Cutaneous reactions may vary in severity from simple *erythema* to severe *exfoliative dermatitis*. Lesions of the mucous membranes include *stomatitis, pharyngitis, tracheitis, gastritis, colitis,* and *vaginitis; glossitis* is fairly common. As with silver, a gray-to-blue pigmentation *(chrysiasis)* may occur in the skin and mucous membranes, especially in areas exposed to light.

The kidneys may be affected to some degree in 5 to 8% of patients receiving gold, and transient and mild proteinuria is frequent during therapy. Heavy albuminuria and microscopic hematuria occur in 1 to 3% of cases. The site of damage is usually the proximal tubules. Although there are only a few reports in the literature of gold-induced *nephrosis,* the number reported in some series suggests an incidence of several percent. The nephrosis is usually reversible, and the predominant lesion is membranous glomerulonephritis.

Severe *blood dyscrasias* may also occur. *Thrombocytopenia* is observed in about 1% of patients. Most often this appears to be an immunological disturbance that results in

an accelerated degradation of platelets. Occasionally the thrombocytopenia is a consequence of effects upon the bone marrow. In either case, withdrawal of the drug usually leads to recovery, but fatalities have occurred. *Leukopenia, agranulocytosis,* and *aplastic anemia* may also occur; aplastic anemia is rare but often fatal. When panmyelopathy results from aurotherapy, the concentrations of coproporphyrin and δ-aminolevulinic acid (δ-ALA) in urine may increase, as in lead poisoning. Eosinophilia is common, and many rheumatologists temporarily discontinue gold therapy when it occurs.

Gold may cause a variety of other severe toxic reactions, including *encephalitis, peripheral neuritis, hepatitis, pulmonary infiltrates,* and *nitritoid crisis* (*see* Gordon et al., 1975; Gottlieb, 1976–1977). Fortunately, the incidence of serious reactions is low, and they generally are the result of failure to discontinue therapy when earlier, less serious symptoms occur.

Auranofin appears to be better tolerated than are the injectable gold compounds, and the incidence and severity of mucocutaneous and hematological side effects are less. However, auranofin frequently produces gastrointestinal disturbances, which are sometimes troublesome, and the incidence of nephrotoxicity may be similar for auranofin and the parenteral preparations.

Avoidance and Treatment. Regular examination of the skin, buccal mucosa, urine, and blood, including cell and platelet counts, should be made. It is the practice in many arthritis clinics to initiate therapy with small doses of gold and to increase the dose gradually. Although untoward effects are not eliminated by this procedure, the severity of those reactions that occur early is somewhat reduced. If an untoward response occurs, therapy should be withheld until it subsides completely. If the reaction is a rash or stomatitis, antihistamines and glucocorticoids may be administered, the latter systemically and/or topically. Glucocorticoids are also indicated in gold-induced nephrosis. If gold therapy is initiated in a patient receiving a glucocorticoid, the latter should be withdrawn gradually when the accumulated dose of gold is 400 to 600 mg.

If the reaction to gold therapy is not of a serious type, injections may be cautiously resumed 2 or 3 weeks after the toxic reaction has subsided and the steroid has been withdrawn. Maintenance dosage should be two thirds to three fourths that previously planned. However, many experts decline to use the drug again, once toxicity has occurred.

If a severe reaction to gold occurs or if the above-mentioned steps fail to control the toxic effects, treatment with dimercaprol or penicillamine should be instituted. The administration of dimercaprol may shorten a therapeutic remission induced by gold.

Therapeutic Uses. Gold compounds find their chief therapeutic application in *rheumatoid arthritis*. Although the currently marketed compounds require intramuscular injection and can cause serious toxicity, they are among the most effective agents available for the treatment of rapidly progressive forms of the disease. Since other effective drugs (*e.g.,* penicillamine, cyclophosphamide) can produce significantly more toxicity during long-term therapy, gold compounds are usually chosen to initiate therapy of rheumatoid arthritis when the goal is to attempt to halt progression of the disease (*see* Kaye, 1982; Rothermich, in Symposium, 1983a; Lipsky, in Symposium, 1983d; Sigler, in Symposium, 1983e; O'Duffy and Luthra, 1984). While the place of auranofin in the therapy of rheumatoid arthritis is yet to be defined, its efficacy appears to approach that of gold sodium thiomalate. Auranofin appears to be a useful addition to the limited group of drugs with the potential to modify the course of rheumatoid arthritis (*see* Symposium, 1983e; Chaffman *et al.,* 1984).

At present, gold is used in early, active arthritis that progresses despite an adequate regimen of aspirin-like drugs, rest, and physical therapy. Both subjective and objective manifestations of rheumatoid arthritis are improved. Gold compounds often arrest the progression of the disease in involved joints, at least temporarily; prevent involvement of unaffected joints; improve grip strength and morning stiffness; and decrease the erythrocyte sedimentation rate and abnormal plasma glycoprotein and fibrinogen levels. Gold should not be used if the disease is mild and is usually of little benefit when the disease is advanced. It has been estimated that chrysotherapy will induce a protracted remission in about 15% of patients, improve symptoms in 60 to 70% of patients, and must be discontinued in 15 to 20% of patients because of toxicity (*see* Lorber *et al.,* 1975; Cats, 1976); about 10 to 15% of patients do not respond. The duration of the remission after discontinuation of treatment with gold is extremely variable (from 1 to 18 months). Although the recurrence is usually not as severe as the original disease and the majority of patients respond favorably to a second course of gold therapy, many rheumatologists now prefer to continue treatment indefinitely without waiting for a relapse to occur. After 3 to 6 years of either continuous or discontinuous therapy, more than 50% of patients who had responded initially have terminated their treatment because of relapse or delayed toxicity (*see* Pinals, in Symposium, 1983d). In addition, there is a high rate of dropout because of the long period of treatment, requirement for office visits, intramuscular administration, and laboratory tests.

Therapy with gold is sometimes beneficial in juvenile rheumatoid arthritis, palindromic rheumatism, psoriatic arthritis, Sjögren's syndrome, non-disseminated lupus erythematosus, and pemphigus (*see* Pennys *et al.,* 1973; Gordon *et al.,* 1975; Gottlieb, 1976–1977). Gold should not be used to treat patients with disseminated lupus.

Contraindications. Gold therapy is contraindicated in patients with *renal disease, hepatic dysfunction* or a *history of infectious hepatitis,* or *hematological disorders.* Gold should not be readministered to patients who have developed severe hematological or renal toxicity during a course of chrysotherapy. It is contraindicated during pregnancy or breast feeding. Patients who have recently had *radiation* should not receive gold because of its depressant action on hematopoietic tissue. Concomitant use of *antimalarials, immunosuppressants, phenylbutazone,* or *oxyphenbutazone* is contraindicated because of the potential of these drugs to cause blood dyscrasias. *Urticaria, eczema,* and *colitis* are also considered to be contraindications to the use of the metal. Finally, gold is poorly tolerated by aged individuals.

Other Therapy for Rheumatoid Arthritis.

In addition to aspirin-like drugs and gold, which have been discussed in this chapter, other agents are also used in the therapy of rheumatoid arthritis. These include glucocorticoids (Chapter 63), immunosuppressive agents (azathioprine and cyclophosphamide; Chapter 55), penicillamine (Chapter 69), and antimalarials (chloroquine and hydroxychloroquine; Chapter 45). Paradoxically, levamisole, an anthelmintic agent with immunostimulant properties, is also effective in rheumatoid arthritis and is being evaluated for this purpose (*see* Chapter 44). These drugs are generally reserved for patients who are refractory to therapeutic regimens that include rest, physiotherapy, and aspirin-like drugs.

Despite the dramatic symptomatic improvement in rheumatoid arthritis caused by glucocorticoids, they too do *not* arrest the progress of the disease and are at least as toxic as gold. Consequently, gold is usually used in preference to glucocorticoids. Penicillamine offers the advantage of oral therapy and may be as effective as gold; however, there is little or no radiological evidence of reduced progression of erosive lesions (*see* O'Duffy and Luthra, 1984). While immunosuppressants (*e.g.,* cyclophosphamide) may be somewhat more effective than gold, the use of such agents is frequently associated with serious toxicity, and such treatment should be reserved only for patients with rheumatoid arthritis and other collagen diseases who are refractory to other forms of therapy.

DRUGS EMPLOYED IN THE TREATMENT OF GOUT

An acute attack of gout occurs as a result of an inflammatory reaction to crystals of sodium urate (the end product of purine metabolism in man) that are deposited in the joint tissue. The inflammatory response involves local infiltration of granulocytes, which phagocytize the urate crystals. Lactate production is high in synovial tissues and in the leukocytes associated with the inflammatory process, and this favors a local decrease in pH that fosters further deposition of uric acid.

Several therapeutic strategies can be used to counter attacks of gout. *Uricosuric drugs* increase the excretion of uric acid, thus reducing concentrations in plasma. *Colchicine* has a specific efficacious action in gout, probably secondary to an effect on the mobility of granulocytes. *Allopurinol* is a selective inhibitor of the terminal steps of the biosynthesis of uric acid. Although prostaglandins may be implicated in the pain and inflammation, there is no evidence that they contribute to the pathogenesis of gout; nevertheless, *aspirin-like drugs* may afford symptomatic relief, and some of them are uricosuric as well.

The pharmacology of aspirin-like drugs is described in the previous section. Discussion in this section is limited to colchicine, allopurinol, and the clinical use of the uricosuric agents. The basic pharmacology of uricosuric drugs is presented in Chapter 38. A useful volume on uric acid that contains major sections on the pathogenesis and therapy of gout is that edited by Kelley and Weiner (1978).

COLCHICINE

Colchicine is a unique anti-inflammatory agent in that it is largely effective only against gouty arthritis. It provides dramatic relief of acute attacks of gout and is an effective prophylactic agent against such attacks.

History. Colchicine is an alkaloid of *Colchicum autumnale* (autumn crocus, meadow saffron), a plant so named because it grew in Colchis in Asia Minor. Although the poisonous action of colchicum was known to Dioscorides, preparations of the plant were not recommended for pain of articular origin until the sixth century A.D. Colchicum was introduced for the therapy of acute gout by von Störck in 1763, and its specificity for this syndrome soon resulted in its incorporation in a number of "gout mixtures" popularized by charlatans. Benjamin Franklin, himself a sufferer from gout, is reputed to have introduced colchicum therapy in the United States. The alkaloid *colchicine* was isolated from colchicum in 1820 by Pelletier and Caventou.

Chemistry. The structural formula of colchicine is as follows:

Colchicine

The structure-activity relationship of colchicine and related agents has been discussed by Wallace (1961).

Pharmacological Properties. The anti-inflammatory effect of colchicine in acute gouty arthritis is selective for this disorder. Colchicine is only occasionally effective in other types of arthritis; it is not an analgesic and does not provide relief of other types of pain.

Colchicine is also an antimitotic agent and is widely employed as an experimental tool in the study of normal and abnormal cell division and cell function.

Effect in Gout. Colchicine does not influence the renal excretion of uric acid, its concentration in blood, or the miscible pool of uric acid. By virtue of its ability to bind to microtubular protein, colchicine interferes with the function of the mitotic spindles and causes depolymerization and disappearance of the fibrillar microtubules in granulocytes and other motile cells. This action is apparently the basis of the long-accepted view of the beneficial effect of colchicine (*see* Malawista, 1975), namely, the inhibition of the migration of granulocytes into the inflamed area. This reduces the release of lactic acid and proinflammatory enzymes that occurs during phagocytosis and breaks the cycle that leads to the inflammatory response. However, there are a number of apparently contradictory observations that cannot be accommodated by this simple hypothesis (*see* Wallace and Ertel, 1978).

Neutrophils exposed to urate crystals ingest them and produce a glycoprotein, which may be the causative agent of acute gouty arthritis. Injected into joints, this substance produces a profound arthritis that is histologically indistinguishable from that caused by direct injection of urate crystals. Spilberg and associates (1979) found that colchicine does not prevent phagocytosis of urate crystals but appears to prevent either the production by or release from leukocytes of the glycoprotein that causes the joint pain and inflammation.

Effect on Cell Division. Colchicine can arrest plant and animal cell division *in vitro* and *in vivo.* Mitosis is arrested in the metaphase, due to failure of spindle formation. Bizarre and abnormal nuclear configurations ensue, and the cells often die. Cells with the highest rates of division are affected earliest. High concentrations may completely prevent cells from entering mitosis. The effect is not specific for colchicine and is exhibited by the vinca alkaloids (vincristine and vinblastine), podophyllotoxin, griseofulvin, and other agents.

Other Effects. Colchicine inhibits the release of histamine-containing granules from mast cells, the secretion of insulin from beta cells of pancreatic islets, and the movement of melanin granules in melanophores; all of these processes may involve the translocation of granules by the microtubular system.

Colchicine also exhibits a variety of other pharmacological effects. It lowers body temperature, increases the sensitivity to central depressants, depresses the respiratory center, enhances the response to sympathomimetic agents, constricts blood vessels, and induces hypertension by central vasomotor stimulation. It enhances gastrointestinal activity by neurogenic stimulation but depresses it by a direct effect, and alters neuromuscular function.

Absorption, Distribution, Biotransformation, and Excretion. Colchicine is rapidly absorbed after oral administration, and peak concentrations occur in plasma by 0.5 to 2 hours. Large amounts of the drug and metabolites enter the intestinal tract in the bile and intestinal secretions, and this fact, plus the rapid turnover of intestinal epithelium, probably explains the prominence of intestinal manifestations in colchicine poisoning. The kidney, liver, and spleen also contain high concentrations of colchicine, but it is apparently largely excluded from heart, skeletal muscle, and brain. The drug can be detected in leukocytes and in the urine for at least 9 days after a single intravenous dose.

Colchicine is metabolized to a mixture of compounds *in vitro.* Most of the drug is excreted in the feces; however, in normal individuals, 10 to 20% of the drug is excreted in the urine. In patients with liver disease, hepatic uptake and elimination are reduced and a greater fraction of the drug is excreted in the urine (*see* Wallace *et al.*, 1970).

Toxicity. Colchicine is tolerated well in moderate dosage. The most common side effects reflect the action of the drug on the rapidly proliferating epithelial cells in the gastrointestinal tract, especially in the jejunum. *Nausea, vomiting, diarrhea,* and *abdominal pain* are the most common and earliest untoward effects of colchicine overdosage. To avoid more serious toxicity, administration of the drug is discontinued as soon as these symptoms occur. A latent period of several hours or more occurs between the administration of the drug and the onset of symptoms. This interval is not altered by dosage or route of administration. For this reason, and because of individual variation, adverse effects may be unavoidable during an initial course of colchicine medication. However, the patient often remains relatively consistent in his response to the drug, and therefore toxicity can be minimized or avoided during subsequent courses of therapy. The drug is as effective when given intravenously as orally; the onset of the therapeutic effect may be faster, and the gastrointestinal side effects may be almost completely avoided when the drug is given intravenously.

In acute poisoning with colchicine, there is hemorrhagic gastroenteritis, extensive vascular damage, nephrotoxicity, muscular depression, and an ascending paralysis of the CNS.

Colchicine produces a temporary leukopenia that is soon replaced by a leukocytosis, sometimes due to a striking increase in the number of basophilic granulocytes. The site of action is apparently directly on the bone marrow. *Chronic administration* of colchicine entails some risk of *agranulocytosis, aplastic anemia, myopathy,* and *alopecia.* Azospermia has also been described.

Preparations. *Colchicine* is available as 0.5- and 0.6-mg tablets; they should be stored in tight, light-resistant containers. A sterile solution (0.5 mg/ml) is also available for injection.

Therapeutic Uses. Colchicine provides dramatic relief of *acute attacks* of gout. The effect is sufficiently selective that the drug has been used for diagnostic purposes, but the test is not infallible. Colchicine also has an established role to *prevent* and to *abort* acute attacks of gout. (*See* Gutman, 1973; Yü, 1974; Rodnan, 1982; Talbott, in Symposium, 1983a.)

Acute Attacks. When colchicine is given promptly within the first few hours of an attack, less than 5% of patients fail to obtain relief. A patient who is in helpless agony with a tumefied, red, hot joint is sufficiently relieved so that he can walk about in a few hours. Pain, swelling, and redness abate within 12 hours and are completely gone in 48 to 72 hours. While still advocated by some physicians (*see,* for example, Rodnan, 1982), the former practice of administering colchicine at hourly intervals is not uniformly recommended. An initial dose of 1 mg (or 1.2 mg) is usually followed by doses of 0.5 to 1.2 mg every 1 to 2 hours; drug administration is stopped as soon as the pain disappears or gastrointestinal symptoms develop. The total dose usually required to alleviate an attack is 4 to 10 mg, and the latter amount should not be exceeded. Opioids or other drugs may be required for the diarrhea. In subsequent attacks, the patient may be able to stop medication short of the amount causing toxic reactions. To avoid cumulative toxicity, the course of colchicine should not be repeated within 3 days. Colchicine may be administered intravenously, and there may be distinct advantages to this route of administration for some patients. A single dose of 2 mg, diluted in 10 to 20 ml of water or 0.9% sodium chloride solution, is usually adequate. The solution is very irritating if extravasation occurs.

Great care should be exercised in prescribing colchicine for aged or feeble patients, and for those with cardiac, renal, or gastrointestinal disease. In these patients and in those who do not tolerate or respond to colchicine, indomethacin is preferred (50 mg three times daily until the pain is alleviated). In fact, many physicians routinely use indomethacin instead of colchicine for acute gouty arthritis.

Prophylactic Uses. For patients with chronic gout, colchicine has established value as a prophylactic agent during the asymptomatic intercritical period. It has a preeminent place in the prevention of acute gout when there is frequent recurrence of attacks. The regular ingestion of colchicine effectively minimizes the frequency and the intensity of acute episodes; by reducing stiffness and aching, it often permits relatively normal activity in a person who otherwise would be incapacitated. Prophylactic medication is also indicated upon initiation of chronic medication with allopurinol or the uricosuric agents, since acute attacks often increase in frequency during the early months of such therapy.

The *prophylactic dose* of colchicine depends upon the frequency and severity of prior attacks. As little as 0.5 mg two to three times a week may suffice; as much as 1.8 mg per day may be required by some patients.

Colchicine should be taken in larger abortive doses immediately upon the first twinge of articular pain or the appearance of any prodrome of an acute attack. Thus, the patient should always have the drug with him. The judicious ingestion of colchicine during the premonitory, incipient, and inflorescent stages of acute gouty arthritis will abort paroxysms and prevent chronic gouty arthritis.

Prior to and following surgery in patients with gout, colchicine should be given for a few days (0.5 mg, three times a day); this greatly reduces the very high incidence of acute attacks of gouty arthritis precipitated by operative procedures.

Daily administration of colchicine is useful for the prevention of attacks of *familial Mediterranean fever* (familial paroxysmal polyserositis). Colchicine has also been employed to treat a variety of skin disorders, including psoriasis and Behçet's syndrome (*see* Aram, 1983).

ALLOPURINOL

Allopurinol is an effective drug for the therapy of both the primary hyperuricemia of gout and that secondary to hematological disorders or antineoplastic therapy. In contrast with the uricosuric agents that increase the renal excretion of urate, allopurinol inhibits the terminal steps in uric acid biosynthesis. Since overproduction of uric acid is a contributing factor in most patients with gout and a characteristic of most types of secondary hyperuricemia, allopurinol represents a rational approach to therapy.

History. The introduction of allopurinol by Hitchings, Elion, and associates provides an elegant example of the development of a drug on a rational biochemical basis. Originally synthesized as a candidate antineoplastic agent, allopurinol was found to lack antimetabolite activity but, by *in-vitro* test, it proved to be a substrate for and an inhibitor of xanthine oxidase. Inhibition of xanthine oxidase *in vivo* was initially established in leukemic patients receiving therapy with the antimetabolite 6-mercaptopurine. Allopurinol delayed inactivation of 6-mercaptopurine by xanthine oxidase and also reduced the plasma concentration and renal excretion of uric acid. Subsequent clinical trial for treatment of gout by Rundles and coworkers was successful and quickly confirmed (*see* Elion, 1978).

Chemistry and Pharmacological Effects. Allopurinol, an analog of hypoxanthine, has the following structural formula:

Allopurinol

Both allopurinol and its primary metabolite, alloxanthine (oxypurinol), are inhibitors of xanthine oxidase. Inhibition of this enzyme accounts for the major pharmacological effects of allopurinol (*see* Elion, 1978).

In man, uric acid is formed primarily by the xanthine oxidase–catalyzed oxidation of hypoxanthine and xanthine. At low concentrations, allopurinol is a substrate for and competitive inhibitor of the enzyme; at high concentrations, it is a noncompetitive inhibitor. Alloxanthine, the metabolite of allopurinol formed by the action of xanthine oxidase, is a noncompetitive inhibitor of the enzyme; the formation of this compound, together with its long persistence in tissues, is undoubtedly responsible for much of the pharmacological activity of allopurinol. Inhibition of the penultimate and ultimate steps in uric acid biosynthesis reduces the plasma concentration and urinary excretion of uric acid and increases the plasma concentrations and renal excretion of the more soluble oxypurine precursors.

Before allopurinol treatment of hyperuricemia, the urinary content of purines is almost solely uric acid. During such treatment, the urinary purines are divided among hypoxanthine, xanthine, and uric acid. Since each has its independent solubility, the concentration of uric acid in plasma is reduced without exposing the urinary tract to an excessive load of uric acid and the likelihood of calculus formation.

The alterations in purine metabolism produced by allopurinol explain its salutary effects in gout. By lowering the uric acid concentration in plasma below its limit of solubility, the dissolution of tophi is facilitated and the development or progression of chronic gouty arthritis is prevented. The formation of uric acid stones virtually disappears with therapy, and this prevents the development of nephropathy. The incidence of acute attacks of arthritis may increase during the early months of therapy but is subsequently reduced.

Tissue deposition of xanthine and hypoxanthine usually does not occur during allopurinol therapy because the renal clearance of the oxypurines is rapid; their plasma concentrations are only slightly increased and do not exceed their solubility. Although xanthine constitutes about 50% of total oxypurine excreted in the urine and is relatively insoluble, xanthine stone formation during allopurinol therapy has occurred only in an occasional patient with very high uric acid production prior to treatment. The risk can be minimized by alkalinization of the urine and by increasing the daily fluid intake during the administration of allopurinol. In some patients, the allopurinol-induced increase in excretion of oxypurines is less than the reduction in uric acid excretion; this disparity is primarily a result of reutilization of oxypurines and feedback inhibition of de-novo purine biosynthesis. Increased oxypurine excretion matches the reduction in uric acid excretion in patients with phosphoribosyltransferase deficiency; such individuals are unable to reutilize oxypurines.

Absorption, Distribution, Biotransformation, and Excretion. Allopurinol is relatively rapidly absorbed after oral ingestion, and peak plasma concentration is reached within 30 to 60 minutes. About 20% is excreted in the feces in 48 to 72 hours, presumably as unabsorbed drug. Allopurinol is rapidly cleared from plasma with a half-time of 2 to 3 hours, primarily by conversion to alloxanthine. Less than 10% of a single dose or about 30% of the drug ingested during chronic medication is excreted unchanged in the urine. Self-inhibition of the metabolism of allopurinol to alloxanthine explains this dose-dependent elimination. Alloxanthine is slowly excreted in the urine by the net balance of glomerular filtration and probenecid-sensitive tubular reabsorption. The plasma half-time of alloxanthine is 18 to 30 hours in patients with normal renal function and increases in proportion to the reduction of glomerular filtration in patients with renal impairment.

Allopurinol and its metabolite alloxanthine are distributed in total tissue water, with the exception of brain, in which their concentration is about one third that in other tissues. Neither compound is bound to plasma proteins.

Drug Interactions. Interactions between allopurinol and *probenecid* and other *uricosuric* agents and those between allopurinol and 6-*mercaptopurine* (and its derivative *azathioprine*) have been alluded to above. Allopurinol may also interfere with the hepatic inactivation of other drugs, including the *oral anticoagulant* agents. Although the effect is variable and of clinical significance only in some patients, increased monitoring of prothrombin activity is recommended in patients receiving both medications.

Whether the increased incidence of skin rash in patients receiving concurrent allopurinol-ampicillin medication, compared with that of these agents administered individually, should be ascribed to allopurinol or to hyperuricemia remains to be established. Hypersensitivity reactions have been reported in patients with compromised renal function who are receiving a combination of allopurinol and a thiazide diuretic. The concomitant administration of allopurinol and theophylline leads to increased accumulation of an active metabolite of theophylline, 1-methylxanthine; the concentration of theophylline in plasma may also be increased.

The reported interference by allopurinol with mobilization of hepatic iron has not been confirmed, and the proposed role of xanthine oxidase in iron metabolism remains unestablished. Nevertheless, concurrent administration of iron during allopurinol medication is not recommended.

Toxicity. Allopurinol is well tolerated by most patients. The most common adverse effects are hypersensitivity reactions. They may occur even after months or years of chronic medication. These usually subside within a few days after medication is discontinued. Serious reactions preclude further use of the drug.

Attacks of acute gout may occur more frequently during the initial months of allopurinol medication and may require concurrent prophylactic therapy with colchicine (*see* above).

The cutaneous reaction is predominantly a pruritic, erythematous, or maculopapular eruption, but occasionally the lesion is exfoliative, urticarial, or purpuric. Fever, malaise, and muscle aching may also occur. Such effects are noted in about 3% of patients with normal renal function but more frequently in those with renal impairment.

Transient leukopenia or leukocytosis and eosinophilia are rare reactions but may require cessation of therapy. A few cases of hepatomegaly and elevated levels of serum glutamic oxalacetic acid transaminase have been recorded, and there have been isolated reports of peripheral neuritis, bone-marrow depression, and cataract. Eosinophilia with epidermal necrolysis has resulted in renal failure.

Undesirable side effects such as headache, drowsiness, nausea, vomiting, vertigo, diarrhea, and gastric irritation occur occasionally but usually do not require that therapy be stopped.

Preparations, Route of Administration, and Dosage. *Allopurinol* (LOPURIN, ZYLOPRIM) is available as 100- and 300-mg tablets for oral use.

For control of hyperuricemia in gout, the aim of therapy is to reduce plasma uric acid concentration below 6 mg/dl. Medication must not be initiated during an acute attack of gouty arthritis, and it is started at low doses to minimize the risk of precipitating such attacks. Concurrent prophylactic colchicine therapy is also recommended during and sometimes beyond the initial months of therapy. Fluid intake should be sufficient to maintain daily urinary volume above 2 liters; slightly alkaline urine is preferred. An initial daily dose of 100 mg is increased by 100-mg increments at weekly intervals. The usual daily maintenance dose for adults is 200 to 300 mg for those with mild gout and 400 to 600 mg for patients with moderately severe tophaceous gout. Daily doses in excess of 300 mg should be given in divided portions. Dosage must be reduced in patients with renal impairment in proportion to the reduction in glomerular filtration (Hande et al., 1984); 100 mg daily or 300 mg twice weekly is often satisfactory.

In the treatment of secondary hyperuricemias, as for the prevention of uric acid nephropathy during vigorous therapy of certain neoplastic diseases, a dose of 200 to 800 mg daily for 2 to 3 days or longer is advisable, together with a high fluid intake. In children with secondary hyperuricemias associated with malignancies, the usual daily dose is 150 to 300 mg, depending upon age.

Therapeutic Uses. Allopurinol provides effective therapy for both the primary *hyperuricemia* of gout and that secondary to polycythemia vera, myeloid metaplasia, or other blood dyscrasias. (*See* Gutman, 1973; Yü, 1974; Kelley, 1975.)

Allopurinol is contraindicated in patients who have exhibited serious adverse effects from the medication, nursing mothers, and children, except those with malignancy.

In *gout,* allopurinol is generally used in the severe chronic forms characterized by one or more of the following conditions: gouty nephropathy, tophaceous deposits, renal urate stones, impaired renal function, or hyperuricemia not readily controlled by the uricosuric drugs. In the absence of these indications, the uricosuric agents should be favored.

When given in effective doses and over prolonged periods, allopurinol fosters resorption of tophi and improvement of joint function in patients with tophaceous gout; this occurs *pari passu* with the reduction in plasma uric acid concentration. By decreasing the amount of uric acid excreted and thereby preventing the development of nephrolithiasis, allopurinol eliminates the major cause of renal injury in patients with gout. It also appears likely that gouty nephropathy can be reversed by the drug if therapy is begun at a reasonably early stage, before renal function is severely compromised; however, there is little evidence of improvement in advanced renal disease.

Since attacks of acute gout occur in patients taking allopurinol, particularly during the initial stage of treatment, colchicine is used prophylactically when therapy is begun and continued if necessary to prevent such attacks. Concurrent allopurinol and uricosuric therapy is also employed occasionally, especially in patients with large tophaceous deposits in whom it is desirable both to reduce production and to increase elimination of uric acid. Such combined medication is valid, but interaction between these drugs is sometimes complex. The uricosuric agents increase the renal excretion of alloxanthine and thus cause a reduction in allopurinol effect. Conversely, allopurinol may delay elimination of probenecid and increase its concentration in plasma.

Allopurinol is also administered prophylactically to reduce the hyperuricemia and to prevent urate deposition or renal calculi in patients with leukemias, lymphomas, or other malignancies, particularly when *antineoplastic* or *radiation* therapy is initiated. Allopurinol inhibits the enzymatic inactivation of 6-mercaptopurine by xanthine oxidase. Thus, when allopurinol is used concomitantly with oral 6-mercaptopurine or azathioprine, dosage of the antineoplastic agent must be reduced to one fourth to one third of the usual dose. The risk of bone-marrow suppression is also increased when allopurinol is administered with cytotoxic agents that are not metabolized by xanthine oxidase, particularly cyclophosphamide.

The *iatrogenic hyperuricemia* sometimes induced by the thiazides and other drugs can be prevented or reversed by concurrent allopurinol medication, although this is rarely necessary. Allopurinol is also useful in lowering the high plasma concentrations of uric acid in patients with the *Lesch-Nyhan syndrome* and thereby prevents the complications resulting from hyperuricemia; there is no evidence that it alters the progressive neurological and behavioral abnormalities characteristic of the disease.

CLINICAL USE OF URICOSURIC AGENTS

As described in Chapter 38, the uricosuric agents act directly on the renal tubule to increase the rate of excretion of uric acid. While many agents share this property, only a few—probenecid, sulfinpyrazone, and benzbromarone—are used clinically as uricosuric agents. The last-named compound is not available for general use in the United States. In the clinical use of the available uricosuric drugs, it must be kept in mind that they can alter the plasma binding, distribution, and renal excretion of other organic acids, whether these be naturally occurring substances or drugs and drug metabolites.

Gout. The use of probenecid and sulfinpyrazone for the mobilization of uric acid in *chronic gout* is well established. In about two thirds of patients, these agents cause uric acid to be excreted at a rate sufficient to exceed that of formation and thereby promptly lower the plasma uric acid concentration. Although the intravenous administration of large doses of these drugs can cause a fivefold to sevenfold increase in the renal clearance of urate, continuous oral administration to patients with tophaceous gout approximately doubles the daily excretion of urates. In such patients, continued administration prevents the formation of new tophi and causes gradual shrinkage, or even disappearance, of old tophi. In gouty arthritis, there is a reduction in the swelling of chronically enlarged joints and a dramatic degree of rehabilitation may be achieved in patients who suffer severe pain and limitation of joint movement. In those patients who do not respond well to uricosuric agents because of impaired renal function, allopurinol is especially useful, as described above. In patients with gouty nephropathy, allopurinol offers the additional advantage over the uricosuric agents in that the daily excretion of uric acid is reduced rather than increased. Its administration is compatible with the simultaneous use of the uricosuric agents if necessary.

Neither the uricosuric agents nor allopurinol alters the course of acute attacks of gout or supplants the use of colchicine and anti-inflammatory agents in their management. Indeed, the acute attacks may increase in frequency or severity during the early months of therapy when urate is being mobilized from affected joints. Therefore, therapy with uricosuric agents should *not be initiated* during an acute attack but may be continued if already begun. Colchicine in small doses (0.5 to 2 mg per day) may be administered at this period (or at any time) to reduce the frequency of attacks. When an acute attack occurs, it is treated with full doses of colchicine or whatever agent has proven most satisfactory in the management of previous attacks (*e.g.,* indomethacin, naproxen). The use of salicylates is contraindicated because they antagonize the action of probenecid and sulfinpyrazone. Later in the course of therapy, acute attacks become less frequent or may cease altogether.

In the treatment of gout, the uricosuric drugs are given continually in the lowest dose that will maintain satisfactory plasma uric acid concentrations. Since the pK_a of uric acid is 5.6 and the solubility of the undissociated form is very low, maintaining the output of a large volume of alkaline urine minimizes its intrarenal deposition. This precaution is essential during the early weeks of therapy when uric acid excretion is large, especially in patients with a history of renal disease associated with the passage of urate stones or gravel. It is believed that renal disease of any etiology is a predisposing factor in the development of gouty nephropathy. Eventual improvement in renal function in patients with gouty nephropathy has been reported, but it is uncommon. The use of allopurinol permits a more favorable prognosis in such patients. (For detailed evaluations of uricosuric agents, *see* Yü, 1974; Boss and Seegmiller, 1979; Rodnan, 1982.)

Other Hyperuricemic States. Uricosuric agents are useful for the control of the hyperuricemia re-

sulting from the use of the cytotoxic antineoplastic agents or from diseases that involve accelerated formation and destruction of blood cells. The use of other drugs, such as diuretics, levodopa, and ethambutol, as well as certain disease states, including toxemia of pregnancy, diabetic ketosis, and uremia, may be accompanied by moderate-to-marked elevation of plasma uric acid. The hyperuricemia may remain asymptomatic, but attacks of gout or renal precipitation of urate may occur. The management of such hyperuricemic states has been outlined by Yü (1974).

Selection of Agents for the Treatment of Gout and Hyperuricemia. Acute attacks of gout are effectively treated with colchicine or indomethacin, as discussed above. After the acute arthritis has responded to therapy, the patient should be evaluated in order to select a rational regimen for long-term management. Elevated concentrations of uric acid in plasma and the observation of crystals of urate in the aspirated fluid from an affected joint establish the diagnosis of hyperuricemia and symptomatic gout. When evaluated on a diet that is low in purines, patients with hyperuricemia can be categorized with regard to quantities of uric acid excreted in the urine. About 80 to 90% of such individuals excrete less than 600 mg of uric acid daily; the remainder excrete more than this amount due to excessive synthesis of urate. The former group can be managed effectively with uricosuric agents; the latter, however, is logically treated with allopurinol. If deposits of urate are evident as tophi, renal stones, or renal insufficiency, allopurinol is generally the preferred drug. During the first several months of treatment with allopurinol, colchicine may be given simultaneously to prevent acute attacks of gout. Patients with mild-to-moderate hyperuricemia (7 to 9 mg/dl) who do not have arthritis should be advised to take liberal amounts of fluids and a diet low in purines. Drug-induced hyperuricemia is most commonly caused by diuretics (*see* Chapter 36); acute attacks of gout are only rarely caused by such agents. However, hyperuricemia that accompanies chemotherapy or radiotherapy for various neoplasms may be considerably more severe and is usually treated prophylactically with allopurinol and hydration.

Cats, A. A multicentre controlled trial of the effects of different dosages of gold therapy followed by a maintenance dosage. *Agents Actions,* **1976,** *6,* 355–363.

Collier, H. O. J., and Sweatman, W. J. F. Antagonism by fenamates of prostaglandin F$_{2\alpha}$ and of slow reacting substance on human bronchial muscle. *Nature,* **1968,** *219,* 864–865.

Collins, E. Maternal and fetal effects of acetaminophen and salicylates in pregnancy. *Obstet. Gynecol.,* **1981,** *58,* 57S–62S.

Committee on Infectious Diseases. Aspirin and Reye's syndrome. *Pediatrics,* **1982,** *69,* 810–812.

Forestier, J. L'aurothérapie dans les rhumatismes chronique. *Bull. Mém. Soc. Méd. Hôp. Paris,* **1929,** *53,* 323–327.

Furst, D. E.; Tozer, T. N.; and Melmon, K. L. Salicylate clearance, the resultant of protein binding and metabolism. *Clin. Pharmacol. Ther.,* **1979,** *26,* 380–389.

Gordon, M. H.; Tiger, L. H.; and Ehrlich, G. E. Gold

reactions are not more common in Sjögren's syndrome. *Ann. Intern. Med.*, **1975**, *82*, 47–49.

Gutman, A. B. The past four decades of progress in the knowledge of gout, with an assessment of the present status. *Arthritis Rheum.*, **1973**, *16*, 431–445.

Ham, E. A.; Cirrillo, V. J.; Zanetti, M.; Shen, T. Y.; and Kuehl, F. A., Jr. Studies on the mode of action of nonsteroidal anti-inflammatory agents. In, *Prostaglandins in Cellular Biology.* (Ramwell, P. W., and Pharris, B. B., eds.) Plenum Press, New York, **1972**, pp. 345–352.

Hamberg, M. Inhibition of prostaglandin synthesis in man. *Biochem. Biophys. Res. Commun.*, **1972**, *49*, 720–726.

Hande, K. R.; Noone, R. M.; and Stone, W. J. Severe allopurinol toxicity. Description and guidelines for prevention in patients with renal insufficiency. *Am. J. Med.*, **1984**, *76*, 47–56.

Higgs, G. A.; Eakins, K. E.; Mugridge, K. G.; Moncada, S.; and Vane, J. R. The effects of non-steroid anti-inflammatory drugs on leukocyte migration in carrageenin-induced inflammation. *Eur. J. Pharmacol.*, **1980**, *66*, 81–86.

Higgs, G. A., and Flower, R. J. Anti-inflammatory drugs and the inhibition of arachidonate lipoxygenase. In, *SRS-A and Leukotrienes.* (Piper, P. J., ed.) John Wiley & Sons, Ltd., London, **1981**, pp. 197–207.

Higgs, G. A.; Vane, J. R.; Hart, F. D.; and Wojtulewski, J. A. Effects of anti-inflammatory drugs on prostaglandins in rheumatoid arthritis. In, *Prostaglandin Synthetase Inhibitors.* (Robinson, H. J., and Vane, J. R., eds.) Raven Press, New York, **1974**, pp. 165–173.

Hill, J. B. Salicylate intoxication. *N. Engl. J. Med.*, **1973**, *288*, 1110–1113.

Kantor, T. G. Ibuprofen. *Ann. Intern. Med.*, **1979**, *91*, 877–882.

Leonards, J. R., and Levy, G. Gastrointestinal blood loss during prolonged aspirin administration. *N. Engl. J. Med.*, **1973**, *289*, 1020–1022.

Lewis, H. D., Jr., and others. Protective effects of aspirin against acute myocardial infarction and death in men with unstable angina. *N. Engl. J. Med.*, **1983**, *309*, 396–403.

Lifschitz, M. D. Renal effects of nonsteroidal anti-inflammatory agents. *J. Lab. Clin. Med.*, **1983**, *102*, 313–323.

Lorber, A.; Simon, T. M.; Leeb, J.; and Carroll, P. E., Jr. Chrysotherapy: pharmacological and clinical correlates. *J. Rheumatol.*, **1975**, *2*, 401–410.

Maher, J. F. Analgesic nephropathy. *Am. J. Med.*, **1984**, *76*, 345–348.

Malawista, S. E. The action of colchicine in acute gouty arthritis. *Arthritis Rheum.*, **1975**, *18*, Suppl. 6, 835–846.

Marcus, A. J. Aspirin as an anti-thrombotic medication. *N. Engl. J. Med.*, **1983**, *309*, 1515–1516.

Pennys, N. S.; Eaglestein, W. H.; Indgin, S.; and Frost, P. Gold sodium thiomalate treatment of pemphigus. *Arch. Dermatol.*, **1973**, *108*, 56–60.

Perl, E. R. Sensitization of nociceptors and its relation to sensation. *Advances in Pain Research and Therapy*, Vol. I. (Bonica, J. J., and Albe-Fersard, D., eds.) Raven Press, New York, **1976**, pp. 17–34.

Rake, G. W., Jr., and Jacobs, R. L. Anaphylactoid reactions to tolmetin and zomepirac. *Ann. Allergy*, **1983**, *50*, 323–325.

Roth, G. R., and Siok, C. J. Acetylation of the NH_2-terminal serine of prostaglandin synthetase by aspirin. *J. Biol. Chem.*, **1978**, *253*, 3782–3784.

Spilberg, I.; Mandell, B.; Mehta, J.; Simchowitz, L.; and Rosenberg, D. Mechanism of colchicine action in acute urate crystal-induced arthritis. *J. Clin. Invest.*, **1979**, *64*, 775–780.

Wallace, S. L. Colchicine: clinical pharmacology in acute gouty arthritis. *Am. J. Med.*, **1961**, *30*, 439–448.

Wallace, S. L.; Omokoku, B.; and Ertel, N. H. Colchi-

cine plasma levels: implications as to pharmacology and mechanism of action. *Am. J. Med.*, **1970**, *48*, 443–448.

Wilson, J. T.; Howell, R. L.; Holladay, M. W.; Brilis, G. M.; Chrastil, J.; Watson, J. T.; and Taber, D. V. Gentisuric acid; metabolic formation in animals and identification as a metabolite of aspirin in man. *Clin. Pharmacol. Ther.*, **1978**, *23*, 635–643.

Monographs and Reviews

Ameer, B., and Greenblatt, D. J. Acetaminophen. *Ann. Intern. Med.*, **1977**, *87*, 202–209.

Aram, H. Colchicine in dermatologic therapy. *Int. J. Dermatol.*, **1983**, *22*, 566–569.

Boss, G. R., and Seegmiller, J. E. Hyperuricemia and gout; classification, complications, and management. *N. Engl. J. Med.*, **1979**, *300*, 1459–1468.

Brenner, B. E., and Simon, R. R. Management of salicylate intoxication. *Drugs*, **1982**, *24*, 335–340.

Brogden, R. N.; Heel, R. C.; Pakes, G. E.; Speight, T. M.; and Avery, G. S. Diflunisal: a review of its pharmacological properties and therapeutic use in pain and musculoskeletal strains and sprains and pain in osteoarthritis. *Drugs*, **1980**, *19*, 84–106.

Brogden, R. N.; Heel, R. C.; Speight, T. M.; and Avery, G. S. Tolmetin: a review of its pharmacological properties and therapeutic efficacy in rheumatic diseases. *Ibid.*, **1978**, *15*, 429–450.

———. Naproxen up to date. *Ibid.*, **1979**, *18*, 241–277.

Brogden, R. N.; Pinder, R. M.; Speight, T. M.; and Avery, G. S. Fenoprofen: a review of its pharmacological properties and therapeutic efficacy in rheumatic diseases. *Drugs*, **1977**, *13*, 241–265.

Chaffman, M.; Brogden, R. N.; Heel, R. C.; Speight, T. M.; and Avery, G. S. Auranofin: a preliminary review of its pharmacological properties and therapeutic use in rheumatoid arthritis. *Drugs*, **1984**, *27*, 378–424.

Chan, W. Y. Prostaglandins and nonsteroidal anti-inflammatory drugs in dysmenorrhea. *Annu. Rev. Pharmacol. Toxicol.*, **1983**, *23*, 131–149.

Clive, D. M., and Stoff, J. S. Renal syndromes associated with nonsteroidal antiinflammatory drugs. *N. Engl. J. Med.*, **1984**, *310*, 563–572.

Cohen, L. S. Clinical pharmacology of acetylsalicylic acid. *Semin. Thromb. Hemostas.*, **1976**, *2*, 146–175.

Davies, R. O. Review of the animal and clinical pharmacology of diflunisal. *Pharmacotherapy*, **1983**, *3*, 9S–22S.

Davison, C. Salicylate metabolism in man. *Ann. N.Y. Acad. Sci.*, **1971**, *179*, 249–268.

Dunn, M. J. Nonsteroidal antiinflammatory drugs and renal function. *Annu. Rev. Med.*, **1984**, *35*, 411–428.

Elion, G. B. Allopurinol and other inhibitors of urate synthesis. In, *Uric Acid. Handbuch der Experimentellen Pharmakologie*, Vol. 51. (Kelley, W. N., and Weiner, I. M., eds.) Springer-Verlag, Berlin, **1978**, pp. 485–514.

Flower, R. J. Drugs which inhibit prostaglandin biosynthesis. *Pharmacol. Rev.*, **1974**, *26*, 33–67.

Gottlieb, N. L. Chrysotherapy. *Bull. Rheum. Dis.*, **1976–1977**, *27*, 912–917.

———. Comparative pharmacokinetics of parenteral and oral gold compounds. *J. Rheumatol.*, **1982**, *9*, Suppl. 8, 99–109.

Hanzlik, P. J. *Actions and Uses of the Salicylates and Cinchophen in Medicine.* The Williams & Wilkins Co., Baltimore, **1927**.

Hart, F. D., and Huskisson, E. C. Non-steroidal anti-inflammatory drugs. Current status and rational therapeutic use. *Drugs*, **1984**, *27*, 232–255.

Kaye, R. L. The current clinical status of gold therapy in rheumatic diseases. *J. Rheumatol.*, **1982**, *9*, Suppl. 8, 124–131.

Kelley, W. N. Effects of drugs on uric acid in man. *Annu. Rev. Pharmacol. Toxicol.*, **1975**, *15*, 327–350.

Kelley, W. N., and Weiner, I. M. (eds.). *Uric Acid. Handbuch der Experimentellen Pharmakologie*, Vol. 51. Springer-Verlag, Berlin, **1978.**

Larsen, G. L., and Henson, P. M. Mediators of inflammation. *Annu. Rev. Immunol.*, **1983**, *1*, 335–359.

Miller, R. L.; Insel, P. A.; and Melmon, K. L. Inflammatory disorders. In, *Clinical Pharmacology: Basic Principles in Therapeutics*, 2nd ed. (Melmon, K. L., and Morrelli, H. F., eds.) Macmillan Publishing Co., New York, **1978**, pp. 657–708.

Milton, A. S. Prostaglandins in fever and the mode of action of antipyretic drugs. In, *Pyretics and Antipyretics. Handbook of Experimental Pharmacology*, Vol. 60. (Milton, A. S., ed.) Springer-Verlag, Berlin, **1982**, pp. 257–303.

Morley, P. A.; Brogden, R. N.; Carmine, A. A.; Heel, R. C.; Speight, T. M.; and Avery, G. S. Zomepirac: a review of its pharmacological properties and analgesic efficacy. *Drugs*, **1982**, *23*, 250–275.

O'Duffy, J. D., and Luthra, H. S. Current status of disease-modifying drugs in progressive rheumatoid arthritis. *Drugs*, **1984**, *27*, 373–377.

Owen, P. R. Prostaglandin synthetase inhibitors in the treatment of primary dysmenorrhea. *Am. J. Obstet. Gynecol.*, **1984**, *148*, 96–103.

Prescott, L. F., and Critchley, J. A. J. H. The treatment of acetaminophen poisoning. *Annu. Rev. Pharmacol. Toxicol.*, **1983**, *23*, 87–101.

Pullar, T., and Capell, H. A. Interaction between oral anticoagulant drugs and non-steroidal anti-inflammatory agents: a review. *Scott. Med. J.*, **1983**, *28*, 42–47.

Robert, A. Current history of cytoprotection. International workshop on protective actions of prostaglandins on the gastro-intestinal mucosa. *Prostaglandins*, **1981**, *21*, Suppl., 89–96.

Rodnan, G. P. Treatment of the gout and other forms of crystal-induced arthritis. *Bull. Rheum. Dis.*, **1982**, *32*, 43–53.

Shen, T. Y., and Winter, C. A. Chemical and biological studies on indomethacin, sulindac and their analogues. *Adv. Drug Res.*, **1977**, *12*, 90–245.

Symposium. (Various authors.) *Fenamates in Medicine.* (Kendall, P. H., ed.) Baillière, Tindall & Cassell, London, **1966.**

Symposium. (Various authors.) Rheumatology workshop. A modern review of Geigy pyrazoles. *J. Int. Med. Res.*, **1977**, *5*, Suppl. 2, 2–120.

Symposium. (Various authors.) Pharmacology, efficacy, and safety of a new class of anti-inflammatory agents: a review of piroxicam. *Am. J. Med.*, **1982**, *72*, No. 2A, 1–90.

Symposium. (Various authors.) *Anti-Rheumatic Drugs.* (Huskisson, E. C., ed.) Praeger Publishers, New York, **1983a.**

Symposium. (Various authors.) Antipyretic analgesic therapy. Current world wide status. *Am. J. Med.*, **1983b**, *75*, No. 5A, 1–140.

Symposium. (Various authors.) New perspectives on aspirin therapy. *Am. J. Med.*, **1983c**, *74*, No. 6A, 1–109.

Symposium. (Various authors.) Management of rheumatoid arthritis and osteoarthritis. *Am. J. Med.*, **1983d**, *75*, No. 4B, 1–91.

Symposium. (Various authors.) Oral gold therapy in rheumatoid arthritis: auranofin. *Am. J. Med.*, **1983e**, *75*, No. 6A, 1–164.

Symposium. (Various authors.) Symposium for rational pharmacotherapy: the nonsteroidal antiinflammatory drugs (NSAIDs). *Drug Intell. Clin. Pharm.*, **1984**, *18*, 34–58.

Szczeklik, A., and Gryglewski, R. J. Asthma and anti-inflammatory drugs. Mechanisms and clinical patterns. *Drugs*, **1983**, *25*, 533–543.

Wallace, S. L., and Ertel, N. H. Pharmacology of drugs used in the treatment of acute gout. In, *Uric Acid. Handbuch der Experimentellen Pharmakologie*, Vol. 51. (Kelley, W. N., and Weiner, I. M., eds.) Springer-Verlag, Berlin, **1978**, pp. 525–555.

Whittle, B. J. R., and Vane, J. R. Prostacyclin, thromboxanes, and prostaglandins—actions and roles in the gastrointestinal tract. In, *Progress in Gastroenterology*. (Jerzy Glass, G. B., and Sherlock, P., eds.) Grune & Stratton, Inc., New York, **1983**, pp. 3–30.

Yü, T.-F. Milestones in the treatment of gout. *Am. J. Med.*, **1974**, *56*, 676–683.

SECTION VI

Cardiovascular Drugs

A major pharmacological action of a number of drugs is their ability to alter cardiovascular function; these agents will be considered in this section. Many additional drugs, however, also markedly influence the heart and blood vessels; they are described elsewhere in connection with their other important pharmacodynamic properties.

CHAPTER 30

DIGITALIS AND ALLIED CARDIAC GLYCOSIDES

Brian F. Hoffman and J. Thomas Bigger, Jr.

Digitalis and certain other cardiac glycosides have in common a powerful action on the myocardium that is unrivaled in value for the treatment of heart failure. These drugs are found in a number of plants, and a few also are present in the venom of certain toads. The preparations commonly employed are obtained from digitalis and strophanthus; older preparations also came from squill. In the following discussion, the term *digitalis* is used to designate the entire group of *cardiac glycosides* rather than only those obtained from digitalis. The general descriptions of the pharmacology and the uses of digitalis apply to all related cardiac glycosides unless otherwise stated.

History. A large number of plant extracts containing cardiac glycosides have been used by natives in various parts of the world as arrow and ordeal poisons. *Squill* was known as a medicine to the ancient Egyptians. The Romans employed it as a diuretic, heart tonic, emetic, and rat poison. *Strophanthus* was introduced into medicine in 1890 by Sir Thomas Fraser, who discovered its digitalis-like action while studying African arrow poisons. The dried skin of the common toad has been used for centuries as a drug by the Chinese. Digitalis, or foxglove, was mentioned in 1250 in the writings of Welsh physicians. It was described botanically 300 years later by Fuchsius, who gave it the name *Digitalis purpurea*.

In 1785, William Withering published his famous book, entitled *An Account of the Foxglove and Some of Its Medical Uses: with Practical Remarks on Dropsy and Other Diseases*. Withering was aware that digitalis was effective only in certain forms of dropsy (edema) but apparently did not associate this with the cardiac actions of the drug. He recognized that the heart was affected, however, for he wrote, "It has a power over the motion of the heart to a degree yet unobserved in any other medicine, and this power may be converted to salutary ends." Apparently, John Ferriar in 1799 was the first to ascribe to digitalis a primary action on the heart and to relegate the diuretic effect to a position of secondary importance. Whereas Withering recorded the benefits to be derived from the proper use of foxglove, his advice was not always heeded. Even during the nineteenth century, digitalis was used indiscriminately for many disorders, often in toxic doses. During the early twentieth century, as a result of the work of Cushny, Mackenzie, Lewis, and others, the drug gradually came to be looked upon as a specific in the treatment of atrial fibrillation. Only subsequently was it established that the main value of digitalis is in the therapy of congestive heart failure.

Sources and Composition of the Digitalis Principles. Official digitalis is the dried leaf of the foxglove plant, *Digitalis purpurea*. Seeds and leaves of a number of other digitalis species also contain active cardiac principles. *Digitalis lanata* leaves are used in Europe and are the source of certain purified preparations employed in the United States. The formerly official strophanthus is obtained from the seeds of the *Strophanthus Kombé* or *hispidus*. Official ouabain is derived from *Strophanthus gratus*. *Squill*, the dried, fleshy bulb of the "sea onion," comes from *Urginea (Scilla) maritima*. Other sources of cardiac glycosides are described in *earlier editions* of this textbook.

Chemical Nature and Properties of the Cardiac Glycosides. Each glycoside represents the combination of an *aglycone*, or *genin*, with from one to four molecules of sugar. Pharmacological activity resides in the aglycone, but the particular sugars attached to the aglycone modify water and lipid solubility and potency of the resulting glycoside. The major contributions to this field have been reviewed by Chen and Henderson (1954), Fieser and Fieser (1959), Tamm (1963), and Marshall (1970).

The aglycones can be released from the cardiac glycosides by hydrolysis. They are chemically related to bile acids, sterols, and sex and adrenocortical hormones. The basic structure is a cyclopentanoperhydrophenanthrene nucleus to which is attached an unsaturated lactone ring at C 17. In addition, methyl, hydroxyl, and aldehyde groups are attached in specific positions that vary with the particular aglycone. All the naturally occurring aglycones carry OH groups at position 14, and many have additional OH groups, particularly at position 3, where the sugar moieties usually are attached. The hydroxyl group at C 3 is highly reactive, and semisynthetic derivatives have been made by reaction of aglycones with organic acids, sugars, xanthine, and other agents. *Acetylstrophanthidin*, one such semisynthetic derivative, is usually not employed clinically but is widely used for experimental purposes because of its rapid onset and relatively short duration of action. The number and the position of other OH groups are important for determining aqueous versus lipid solubility, protein binding, metabolic disposition, and duration of action. In general, the aglycones have more transient and less potent myocardial actions than the glycosides but cause similar toxic effects.

The unsaturated lactone ring attached to C 17 possesses the $\Delta^{\alpha,\beta}$ structure, and may be five or six membered. Saturation of the lactone ring reduces activity by tenfold or more, and increases the speed of development of the cardiac actions (Vick *et al.*, 1957); opening of the ring completely abolishes activity.

The structural formulas of *digoxigenin* and *digitoxigenin* are as follows:

Digoxigenin

Digitoxigenin

Digoxin and digitoxin are the only cardiac glycosides used frequently and consist of the corresponding aglycone with three molecules of digitoxose, a 2,6-dideoxyhexose, joined in glycosidic linkage and attached at position 3. The chemical constituents of various other glycosides are described in *earlier editions* of this textbook.

PHARMACODYNAMICS

Digitalis is used most frequently to increase the adequacy of the circulation in patients with congestive heart failure and to slow the ventricular rate in the presence of atrial fibrillation and flutter. *The main pharmacodynamic property of digitalis is its ability to increase the force of myocardial contraction.* The beneficial effects of the drug in patients with heart failure—increased cardiac output; decreased heart size, venous pressure, and blood volume; diuresis and relief of edema—are all explained on the basis of increased contractile force, *a positive inotropic action.* The second important action of digitalis is to slow the ventricular rate in atrial fibrillation or flutter.

Because digitalis often dramatically slows the ventricular rate in atrial fibrillation, it was believed for many years that the main effect of the drug was to slow the heart rate. Starting perhaps with Wenckebach (1910) and as a result of numerous subsequent clinical studies, the conviction grew and finally became firmly established that digitalis is effective in congestive heart failure regardless of the cardiac rhythm, and that the beneficial effect is brought about *not* so much by virtue of cardiac slowing but by its direct action to increase the force of myocardial contraction. The mechanisms responsible for these beneficial effects of digitalis are complex. Digitalis exerts direct effects on the heart that modify both its mechanical and electrical activity. It also acts directly on the smooth muscle of the vascular system. In addition, digitalis exerts a number of effects on neural tissue and thus indirectly influences the mechanical and electrical activity of the heart and modifies vascular resistance and capacitance. Finally, changes in the circulation brought about by digitalis often result in reflex alterations in autonomic activity and hormonal balance that indirectly influence cardiovascular function. In describing the effects of digitalis on the heart and circulation, it is convenient to discuss the *direct and indirect actions* on the heart before considering the integrated effects of digitalis on the entire cardiovascular system.

DIRECT EFFECTS

Myocardial Contractility. Digitalis increases the contractility of cardiac muscle in a dose-dependent manner—a *positive inotropic effect*. The effects are similar for both atrial and ventricular muscle and are *qualitatively* the same for muscle obtained from either normal or failing hearts. The effects of digitalis on mechanical activity can be demonstrated for both isometric and isotonic contractions. If an isolated preparation of cardiac muscle is studied under *isometric conditions* and the resting length is set at the peak of the length-tension relationship, an appropriate concentration of digitalis increases the peak force developed. In addition, it increases the rate of development of force and decreases the time to peak tension. These changes occur without any alteration in resting tension. The effects are similar qualitatively at all points on the length-tension relationship; for any given end-diastolic fiber length, digitalis increases the tension that can be generated.

The extent to which digitalis increases isometric tension depends strongly on the initial condition of the muscle. If the capacity to develop force is severely depressed, the effect is much larger than would occur in normal muscle (*see* Figure 30–1).

If the preparation of cardiac muscle is studied under *isotonic conditions,* digitalis shifts the force-velocity curve upward. The maximal load and rate of shortening both increase. Digitalis thus increases the rate at which work can be done and also the maximal work that the muscle can perform.

Concentrations of digitalis considerably higher than those needed to demonstrate the positive inotropic effect cause an increase in resting tension

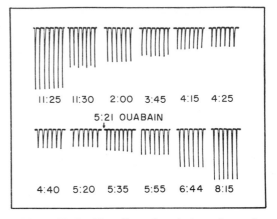

Figure 30–1. *The effect of ouabain on force of contraction of an isolated papillary muscle from the right ventricle of a cat heart.*

The muscle was prepared for isometric recording of contractions induced by rhythmic electrical stimulation. Systolic tension of the muscle, recorded as a downward deflection, decreased spontaneously during 6 hours of perfusion. The addition of ouabain in a concentration of 13 μg per liter (22 nM) restored the force of contraction. (After Gold and Cattell, 1940. Courtesy of the *Archives of Internal Medicine.*)

and partial *contracture.* Usually this is associated with a decrease in shortening velocity and peak isometric tension. It is almost certain that this effect is a toxic one and is unrelated to therapeutic actions.

The direct positive inotropic effect of digitalis also can be demonstrated in studies on the isolated supported mammalian heart or on the mammalian heart-lung preparation. These preparations present an advantage in that the effects of digitalis on the systemic vasculature and autonomic nervous system do not complicate the interpretation of its direct cardiac actions. With the isolated heart it is possible to keep heart rate and end-diastolic intraventricular pressures constant so that inotropic effects caused by changes in rate or end-diastolic fiber length need not be considered. Under these conditions, appropriate concentrations of digitalis increase the maximal rate of development of intraventricular pressure, decrease the duration of isovolumic contraction, increase ejection velocity, increase peak systolic pressure, and decrease the duration of contraction. Usually, stroke volume and aortic flow increase and, because the ventricle empties more completely during systole, end-systolic volume is reduced. In the canine heart-lung preparation, it is possible to demonstrate the major effects of digitalis on a failed heart. In this preparation failure can be induced by a variety of means; and among these, perhaps the simplest to study is failure induced by increasing resistance to aortic flow. A sufficient increase in aortic resistance reduces stroke volume; as a consequence, end-systolic volume is increased. With reasonably constant ventricular filling during diastole, end-diastolic pressure and volume increase. Because of the length-tension relationship, the increase in end-diastolic fiber length initially compensates for the elevated resistance to ejection. However, with time the contraction of the ventricle weakens; there is a progressive decrease in stroke volume and progressive increases in both end-diastolic pressure and volume. Because heart rate is constant and stroke volume decreased, aortic flow necessarily decreases. Under these conditions, administration of digitalis brings about most dramatic changes. Because digitalis increases the capacity of the fibers to develop tension and to shorten, the ventricle is able to develop sufficient pressure during systole to eject an increased stroke volume in spite of the increased aortic resistance. The increased stroke volume results in a decrease in end-*systolic* volume and a progressive decrease in end-*diastolic* volume and end-diastolic pressure. These changes in pressure and ventricular volume are demonstrated in Figure 30–2 in terms of intraventricular pressure-volume loops.

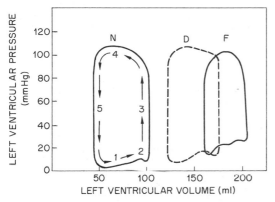

Figure 30–2. *Schematic representation of pressure-volume loops for the normal and failing left ventricle and the effects of digitalis.*

For the control loop (*N*), the arrows show the changes in ventricular pressure and volume with time during the single cardiac cycle. The numbers on the control loop indicate the phases of the cardiac cycle: *1* = diastasis, *2* = atrial systole, *3* = isovolumic contraction, *4* = ejection, *5* = isovolumic relaxation. End-diastolic pressure is relatively low, for the control curve pressure develops rapidly, and ejection is well maintained during systole. The loop labeled *F* shows the types of change that result from failure. End-systolic and end-diastolic volumes are greatly increased, as is end-diastolic pressure. During isovolumic contraction, pressure develops less rapidly and stroke volume is reduced. When digitalis has exerted its positive inotropic effect (*D*), the loop shifts to lower diastolic pressures and volumes and stroke volume increases.

Mechanism of Action. It appears that there are two components to the positive inotropic effect of digitalis: direct inhibition of the membrane-bound Na^+,K^+-activated adenosine triphosphatase (Na^+,K^+-ATPase), which leads to an increase in intracellular calcium concentration ($[Ca^{2+}]_i$), and an associated increase in a slow inward current (i_{si}) during the action potential (AP). This current is the result of movement of Ca^{2+} into the cell, and it contributes to the plateau of the AP. It seems clear that digitalis, in therapeutic concentrations, exerts no *direct* effect on the contractile proteins or on the interactions between them. Also, it seems most unlikely that the positive inotropic effect of digitalis is due to any action on the cellular mechanisms that provide the chemical energy for contraction. The hydrolysis of adenosine triphosphate (ATP) by the Na^+,K^+-ATPase provides the energy for the so-called sodium pump—the system in the sarcolemma of cardiac fibers that actively extrudes sodium and transports potassium into the fibers. Digitalis glycosides bind specifically to the Na^+,K^+-ATPase, inhibit its enzymatic activity, and impair the active transport of these two monovalent cations. As a result, there is a gradual increase in intracellular sodium ($[Na^+]_i$) and a gradual small decrease in $[K^+]_i$. These changes are small at therapeutic concentrations of the drug. It is the increase in $[Na^+]_i$ that at present is judged to be crucially related to the positive inotropic effect of digitalis. This is so because in cardiac fibers intracellular Ca^{2+} is exchanged for extracellular Na^+ by a transport system that is driven by the concentration gradients for these ions and the transmembrane potential (*see* Figure 30–3) (Reuter and Seitz, 1968; Mullins, 1979). When $[Na^+]_i$ is increased because of inhibition of the pump by digitalis, the exchange of extracellular Na^+ for intracellular Ca^{2+} is diminished, and $[Ca^{2+}]_i$ increases. The probable consequence of this is an increased store of Ca^{2+} in the sarcoplasmic reticulum (SR) and, with each AP, a greater release of Ca^{2+} to activate the contractile apparatus.

This exchange of ions presumably results from the operation of a carrier in the membrane. Through such a mechanism either an

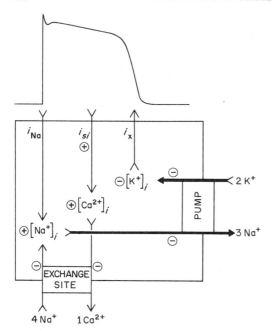

Figure 30–3. *Schematic representation of fluxes of Na^+, K^+, and Ca^{2+} across the cardiac cell membrane and the effects of digitalis thereon.*

During the transmembrane action potential, shown at the top, there is a net entry of Na^+ and Ca^{2+} and a net loss of K^+. The intracellular concentrations of Na^+ ($[Na^+]_i$) and K^+ ($[K^+]_i$) are maintained by the activity of the Na^+,K^+ pump, shown at the right. The intracellular concentration of calcium ($[Ca^{2+}]_i$) is in part regulated by exchange for sodium (exchange site). The effects of digitalis are shown as $\oplus$ or $\ominus$ next to the relevant process or parameter. Active extrusion of Na^+ is decreased; this leads to an increase in $[Na^+]_i$, which, in turn, causes an increase in $[Ca^{2+}]_i$. This, in turn, increases i_{si}.

increase in extracellular $[Ca^{2+}]$ ($[Ca^{2+}]_o$), a decrease in $[Na^+]_o$, or an increase in $[Na^+]_i$ would elevate $[Ca^{2+}]_i$ and cause a positive inotropic effect. This mechanism explains the well-known observation that force of cardiac contraction is roughly proportional to the extracellular ratio of $[Ca^{2+}]/[Na^+]^2$. The positive inotropic effect of a reduction in $[K^+]_o$ can also be explained, since a sufficient decrease in extracellular K^+ inhibits outward transport of Na^+ by the pump (Eisner *et al.*, 1983).

In addition, by mechanisms that are not clearly defined, the increase in $[Ca^{2+}]_i$ en-

hances ion movement through channels responsible for a slow inward current, i_{si}, that is carried by Ca^{2+}. Thus, more Ca^{2+} is delivered during the plateau of each AP to activate each contraction (*see* Figure 30–3).

Contraction of most mammalian hearts is initiated by and is proportional to the influx of Ca^{2+} that occurs during the transmembrane AP (Beeler and Reuter, 1970). This, in turn, causes the release of additional Ca^{2+} from the sarcoplasmic reticulum, as shown by Fabiato and Fabiato (1977) in chemically "skinned" cardiac fibers.

Evidence obtained in part through the use of voltage clamp technics and ion-selective intracellular electrodes has shown the following: digitalis decreases exchange of Na^+ for K^+ by the Na^+,K^+-ATPase; this inhibition of the pump is associated with a decrease in outward current (Gadsby and Cranefield, 1979); digitalis in reasonable concentration increases $[Na^+]_i$ (Deitmer and Ellis, 1978); other interventions that cause inhibition of the pump, such as a decrease in $[K^+]_o$, also result in an elevated $[Na^+]_i$ and stronger contraction (Eisner *et al.*, 1983); the elevation of $[Na^+]_i$ that results from inhibition of the pump is associated with an increase in $[Ca^{2+}]_i$ (Lee and Dagostino, 1982); and the positive inotropy caused by digitalis is associated with a greater increase in free myoplasmic calcium prior to and during contraction (Allen and Blinks, 1978; Blinks *et al.*, 1982). In other experiments (Weingart *et al.*, 1978; Lederer and Eisner, 1982; Marban and Tsien, 1982), voltage clamp has been employed to show that nontoxic concentrations of digitalis increase the magnitude of slow inward current and that this change parallels the positive inotropic action. The change in slow inward current is a consequence of the increase in $[Ca^{2+}]_i$ and not of the increase in $[Na^+]_i$. The mechanism of this effect is unclear. In sum, the data strongly support the sequence shown in Figure 30–3. Inhibition of the pump results in elevated $[Na^+]_i$; this reduces exchange of Na^+ for Ca^{2+} and elevates $[Ca^{2+}]_i$. This, in turn, augments i_{si} and the influx of Ca^{2+} during each AP. The relative importance to the positive inotropic effect of the increase in $[Ca^{2+}]_i$ that results from reduction in Na^+-for-Ca^{2+} exchange on the one hand, and the augmentation of i_{si} that results from elevated $[Ca^{2+}]_i$ on the other, remains to be established. Both effects would contribute to the increased $[Ca^{2+}]_i$, whereas the latter might also directly influence excitation-contraction coupling.

The mechanism described thus assumes that the Na^+,K^+-ATPase is the pharmacological receptor for digitalis and that when digitalis binds to this enzyme it induces a conformational change that decreases the active transport of sodium. Schatzman first described this enzymatic system in red-cell membranes and its specific inhibition by digitalis. In 1957, Skou prepared a Na^+,K^+-ATPase from crab nerve membrane. The enzyme was specifically inhibited by ouabain and appeared to be an integral part of the Na^+, K^+ pump. Wilbrandt proposed that the digitalis-induced positive inotropic effect on the myocardium was due to an increase in $[Ca^{2+}]_i$ and that this resulted from inhibition of Na^+ and K^+ transport. Many studies have provided evidence that digitalis binds to the ATPase in a specific and saturable manner, that the binding results in a conformational change of the enzyme, that the rate of binding is increased by $[Na^+]$ and decreased by $[K^+]$, and that the binding site for digitalis is probably on the external surface of the membrane (*see* Schwartz, 1976; Hess and Müller, 1982). Furthermore, the magnitude of the inotropic effect of digitalis is proportional to the degree of inhibition of the enzyme (Akera *et al.*, 1970; Hougen and Smith, 1978). Digitalis has little direct effect on the uptake or release of Ca^{2+} by SR or mitochondria (Besch *et al.*, 1970).

In spite of the evidence that the positive inotropy results from inhibition of the pump and a resultant elevation of $[Ca^{2+}]_i$, some data suggest other possible mechanisms of action of digitalis. First, a number of studies have shown that very low concentrations of glycosides cause *stimulation* of the pump and a concomitant positive inotropic effect (*see* Noble, 1980). Other studies attribute the effect of digitalis to an alteration in Ca^{2+} binding by sarcolemmal phospholipids (Gervais *et al.*, 1977). The question of alternative modes of action has been discussed (*see* Weingart, 1981; Marban and Tsien, 1982). It does seem clear that a positive inotropic effect is not prominent until there has been some inhibition of the active transport of Na^+ and K^+ (Hougen and Smith, 1978).

Electrical Activity. Because some of the therapeutic and most of the serious toxic effects of digitalis can be related to actions upon the electrophysiological properties of the heart, these actions of the drug have been studied extensively. Understanding of the cellular mechanisms involved has been greatly enhanced in recent years through the application of microelectrode technics to the study of isolated, superfused preparations of cardiac tissue. The results obtained have been supplemented by intracardiac records of the electrical activity of the heart *in situ,* both in experimental animals and in man, and by study of the response of the heart to electrical stimulation.

Purkinje Fibers. The direct effects of digitalis on the electrical activity of cardiac fibers will be described first in terms of the changes caused by digitalis in the transmembrane potentials of mammalian cardiac Purkinje fibers. These cells have been studied most intensively. In addition, most attempts to explain the toxic effects of digitalis on the electrical activity of the heart have been based on data for Purkinje fibers.

The effects of digitalis on the transmembrane AP and resting potential (RP) of the canine cardiac Purkinje fiber are dependent on both the time of exposure to digitalis and its concentration. The following sequence of changes can be observed (Vassalle *et al.*, 1962; Kassebaum, 1963; Müller, 1965; Rosen *et al.*, 1973a). Initially, if the preparation is stimulated at a low rate, there is a small increase in action potential duration (APD). This is not seen if the rate of stimulation is high. Subsequently, there is a decrease in APD that results largely from a shortening of the duration of the plateau (phase 2). Usually, this is associated with an increase in the slope of phase-4 depolarization. Later, there is a decrease in RP or maximal diastolic potential (MDP) and a further decrease in APD (*see* Figure 30–4). Largely because of the less negative RP, or because phase-4 depolarization causes the upstroke of the AP (phase 0) to start at a less negative potential, the maximal rate of rise of phase 0 ($\dot{V}_{max}$) decreases as does the amplitude of the AP (*see* Chapter 31). Finally, when toxic effects are fully developed, the RP is markedly reduced, there is a directly induced decrease in $\dot{V}_{max}$ (Kassebaum, 1963), conduction velocity is reduced, and ultimately the fibers become inexcitable.

The effects of digitalis on phase 4 vary as a function of $[K^+]_o$ and probably other factors. At low values of $[K^+]_o$, the most consistent effect is an increase in the slope of phase 4. This results in *increased automaticity* that can be demonstrated if the driving stimulus is terminated. At somewhat higher levels of $[K^+]_o$ (≥ 4 mM), a different change in the time course of membrane potential can be observed during phase 4. This is the appearance of *delayed afterdepolarizations* (Davis, 1973; Ferrier *et al.*, 1973; Rosen *et al.*, 1973b). This change in membrane potential also is called a transient depolarization (Ferrier *et al.*, 1973; Lederer and Tsien, 1976). The delayed afterdepolarization initially appears as a subthreshold depolarization early during phase 4 or as a damped train of afterdepolarizations (*see* Chapter 31). As toxicity progresses, the afterdepolarization increases in

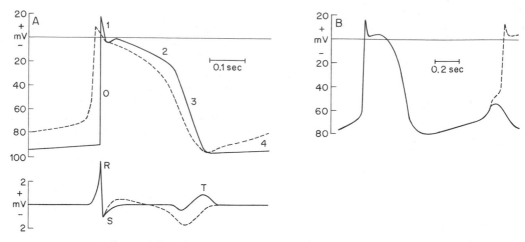

Figure 30–4. *Effects of digitalis on transmembrane potentials and electrograms.*

A. Schematic representation of a transmembrane action potential recorded from a cardiac Purkinje fiber (top trace) and a unipolar electrogram recorded from the same preparation (bottom trace) under control conditions (solid lines) and in the presence of digitalis (dashed lines). Phases 0, 1, 2, 3, and 4 have their usual meaning. After the effects of digitalis have developed, there is a decrease in maximal diastolic potential, an increase in the slope of phase-4 depolarization, and a decrease in action potential duration. Because of the increase in phase-4 depolarization, the fiber becomes automatic. Voltage at which activation occurs shifts to a more positive value, and the amplitude of the action potential decreases. Because of the change in the slope and duration of phases 2 and 3, there is a change in the S-T segment and T wave of the electrogram and a decrease in the R-T interval.

B. Schematic representation of the appearance of delayed afterdepolarizations caused by digitalis in the record of transmembrane potential from a Purkinje fiber. The delayed afterdepolarizations are shown as being subthreshold (solid line) and suprathreshold (dashed line); the latter initiates an extra action potential. *See* text for further explanation.

amplitude until it attains the threshold for initiation of an AP. When this occurs, the delayed afterdepolarization caused by the *extra* response is also quite likely to reach the threshold because, within limits, the amplitude of the delayed afterdepolarization increases as the interval between APs decreases. Clearly, then, digitalis can initiate ectopic impulses by two quite different means: enhancement of normal phase-4 depolarization or the development of delayed afterdepolarizations. At present, the clinical differentiation between these two mechanisms often is not possible.

As is the case for the mechanism by which digitalis increases cardiac contractility, there still is some uncertainty about the exact mechanisms by which direct effects of digitalis alter the transmembrane potentials of cardiac fibers (Rosen *et al.*, 1975b; Weingart, 1981; Hoffman, 1983). It may be helpful to consider changes in electrical activity in relation to the concentration of glycoside or the intensity of its effect. At low concentrations, digitalis does not significantly influence the fast inward channel for Na^+. The increase in APD seen at very low concentrations of drug might be due to changes in the passive properties of the membrane (Kassebaum, 1963), but it more likely reflects inhibition of the Na^+,K^+-ATPase and a resulting decrease in outward current that is independent of time (Isenberg and Trautwein, 1974; *see* Chapter 31). This occurs because the Na^+-for-K^+ exchange pump is electrogenic (Gadsby and Cranefield, 1979). Inhibition of the pump, through a decrease in outward current, would also result in a modest decrease in RP and an increase in the slope of diastolic depolarization. Failure to see the increase in APD at rapid rates might result from an associated increase in $[K^+]_o$. During each AP, $[K^+]_o$ in interfiber spaces undergoes a transient increase due to K^+ efflux from the fibers (Kline and Kupersmith, 1982); this increase would be augmented when the pump is inhibited. The elevated $[K^+]_o$ would directly speed the onset of repolarization by increasing permeability to K^+. Because of the small decrease in RP, conduction velocity may increase slightly (Peon *et al.*, 1978). At higher concentrations of digitalis the basis for the typical changes in transmembrane potentials may be as follows. The greater reduction in pump current further decreases RP; in addition, as $[K^+]_o$ rises (Miura and Rosen, 1978), both E_K (the potassium equilibrium potential) and RP decrease. The increase in $[Na^+]_i$ will decrease E_{Na} and tend to decrease AP amplitude. The augmentation of i_{si} (*see* above) will shift the plateau to more positive potentials. This change might also be expected to increase APD. Since the AP actually shortens, we must assume that toward the end of the plateau net outward current is increased enough to offset the change in i_{si}. Three factors probably contribute here. The elevation of $[Ca^{2+}]_i$ both speeds inactivation of i_{si} (Marban and Tsien, 1982) and augments outward K^+ current. Additionally, with more marked inhibition of the pump, $[K^+]_o$ will rise to a greater extent during each AP and speed the onset of repolarization. Finally, at very high concentrations of glycoside, effects associated with toxicity appear. Phase 0 of the AP will be depressed due to the greater loss of RP and resultant voltage-dependent inactivation of sodium channels (*see* Chapter 31), the greater increase in $[Na^+]_i$, and also a direct effect of digitalis that modifies the voltage dependence of sodium channel inactivation (Kassebaum, 1963). Conduction velocity will slow as the result of two factors: a decrease in the excitatory current that is provided by the smaller AP, and a decrease in the extracellular spread of current that results from a calcium-induced decrease in the conductance at gap junctions between fibers (DeMello, 1975; Weingart, 1977). These factors combine to reduce the amount of myocardial tissue that can be simultaneously excited by an AP at any given point (*see* below).

The cellular electrophysiological changes responsible for digitalis-induced arrhythmias are complex. A number of studies on the effects of cardiac glycosides on pacemaker activity were based on the assumption that automaticity in Purkinje fibers resulted from a voltage- and time-dependent decrease in a specific potassium current, i_{K_2} (*see* Weingart, 1981). It now is proposed that the pacemaker current is an inward current, i_f, carried mainly by Na^+ (DiFrancesco, 1981). The direct effects of digitalis on this current are uncertain. In contrast, the mechanism by which digitalis induces delayed afterdepolarizations (*see* Chapter 31; Figure 30–4) has been studied intensively (Lederer and Tsien, 1976; Kass *et al.*, 1978a, 1978b). Evidence indicates that with calcium overload there is an oscillatory release and re-uptake of Ca^{2+} by intracellular stores, most likely the SR. This oscillatory change in $[Ca^{2+}]_i$ results in aftercontractions and a coincident transient inward current (TI). The TI, in turn, causes the afterdepolarizations. The TI may result from a special sarcolemmal conductance or may reflect alterations in electrogenic exchange of Na^+ for Ca^{2+}. Any factor that increases $[Ca^{2+}]_i$ sufficiently will cause delayed afterdepolarizations and aftercontractions, and anything that reduces the influx of Ca^{2+}, such as blockade of slow inward channels or a reduction in $[Ca^{2+}]_o$, will tend to attenuate or abolish them.

The results of studies of effects of digitalis on isolated preparations of cardiac muscle (particularly Purkinje fibers) must be interpreted with care because some effects may be dependent on the nature of the preparation and can be modified by the experimental conditions. Nevertheless, Purkinje fibers are more sensitive to the toxic actions of digitalis than are ventricular muscle fibers (Vassalle *et al.*, 1962). For both, toxicity develops more rapidly if the fibers are stimulated at a more rapid rate. The development of toxicity is inhibited by an increase in $[K^+]_o$ and facilitated by an increase in $[Ca^{2+}]_o$. When toxicity has developed, it can to a certain extent be reversed by elevating $[K^+]_o$. The effect of rate is not surprising, since the active transport required of the Na^+,K^+-ATPase is a function of the number of APs per unit of time. The influence of increasing $[K^+]_o$ may result from the stimulatory effect of extracellular potassium on the pump, as well as from decreased binding of digitalis to the ATPase. The interaction between $[Ca^{2+}]_o$ and digitalis reflects the effect of a higher concentration of this ion on the sodium-calcium exchange process and on i_{si}, mentioned above.

Other Specialized Fibers. Digitalis exerts direct effects on the fibers of the sinoatrial (S-A) node and the atrioventricular (A-V) node, and on the specialized atrial fiber system. At concentrations that may obtain during clinical use, digitalis has little direct effect on the transmembrane potentials of the rabbit S-A node (Toda and West, 1966; Ten Eick and Hoffman, 1969a). Most of the clinically important effects of digitalis on the rate of formation of impulses by the S-A node are due to indirect effects that the drug exerts through the parasympathetic and sympathetic nervous systems (*see* below). Nevertheless, concentrations of digitalis that cause toxicity can partially depolarize S-A nodal fibers and stop the generation of impulses. High concentrations of digitalis directly depress conduction of impulses through the A-V node. However, as for the S-A node, the clinically important actions of cardiac glycosides on the A-V node are mediated by the autonomic nervous system. The direct actions decrease conduction velocity, increase the effective refractory period (ERP), and ultimately cause complete A-V block. These changes in conduction are associated with a decrease in MDP and in the rate of rise and amplitude of the A-V nodal AP. The *specialized atrial fibers* respond to digitalis in much the same manner as do Purkinje fibers. Most importantly, digitalis causes not only an increase in automaticity due to enhanced phase-4 depolarization but also generation of ectopic impulses due to production of delayed afterdepolarizations (Hashimoto and Moe, 1973).

Atrial and Ventricular Muscle Fibers. The direct effects of digitalis on the transmembrane potentials of ventricular muscle have been studied fairly extensively. The changes in the duration of the AP resemble those described for Purkinje fibers. The decrease in this value is not marked but probably accounts for the decrease in the Q-T interval of the ECG (*see* Figure 30–4 and below). The ventricular transmembrane APs also show an increase in slope of the plateau and a decrease in the slope of phase 3. These alterations in the transmembrane potential cause changes in the S-T segment and the T wave in the ECG (*see* Figure 30–4 and below). In sufficiently high concentration, digitalis decreases both the RP and the amplitude of the AP of atrial and ventricular fibers and decreases the maximal rate of depolarization during phase 0. High concentrations thus can decrease conduction velocity and ultimately cause inexcitability. These drastic effects are not seen in clinical settings. Digitalis does not cause phase-4 depolarization in atrial or ventricular muscle fibers, but delayed afterdepolarizations may occur (Ferrier, 1976).

INDIRECT EFFECTS

Electrical Activity. There is no doubt that many of the effects of digitalis on the electrical and mechanical activity of the mammalian heart result from glycoside-induced modification of both autonomic neural activity and the sensitivity of the heart to the vagal and sympathetic neurotransmitters. The decrease in sinus rate in the presence of heart failure is caused in large part by a glycoside-induced increase in efferent vagal impulses and a reflexly induced decrease in sympathetic tone; these changes are associated with improvement of the circulation. Other alterations of autonomic activity are more complex and less well understood (*see* Rosen *et al.,* 1975b; Mudge *et al., 1978*; Gillis and Quest, 1980).

Most experimental and clinical evidence supports the concept that efferent vagal activity is enhanced by digitalis; in both experimental animals and man, sinus slowing caused by therapeutic concentrations of a cardiac glycoside can be diminished by atropine. The increase in vagal activity appears to result from effects at several sites in the nervous system. The arterial baroceptors are sensitized, possibly because of an effect of digitalis on active transport of cations in the afferent nerve terminals (Saum *et al.,* 1976). Pace and Gillis (1976) have shown an increase in afferent impulse traffic in carotid sinus nerves in cats given digoxin. Digitalis also affects the central vagal nuclei and the nodose ganglion (Chai *et al.,* 1967) and may modify the excitability of efferent vagal fibers (Ten Eick and Hoffman, 1969b). Effects that modify transmission in autonomic ganglia also have been described. Studies on isolated preparations suggest that the sensitivity of the sinus node to the negative chronotropic effect of acetylcholine is increased by digitalis (Toda and West, 1966). Most data indicate that administration of digitalis will intensify the effects of the vagus on the heart through several or all of the mechanisms mentioned above as well as by effects on the heart and circulation that modify input to the autonomic nervous system (*see* below).

Changes in sympathetic activity caused by digitalis also have been described and are complex. Studies on both the S-A node and the A-V node indicate that sufficiently high concentrations of glycoside can decrease the sensitivity of these tissues to catecholamines and efferent sympathetic impulses. Other studies have shown enhancement of efferent sympathetic activity induced by toxic concentrations of digitalis (*see* Gillis and Quest, 1980). The enhanced efferent sympathetic activity may result from effects of digitalis that gains access to structures in the area postrema of the medulla oblongata via the choroid plexus (Mudge *et al.,* 1978). Digitalis also may inhibit re-uptake of norepinephrine by sympathetic terminals. The role of increased effects of norepinephrine in causing digitalis-induced arrhythmias has been reviewed by Gillis and Quest (1980) and by Rosen (1981). The importance of norepinephrine in promoting arrhythmias caused by digitalis is suggested by studies on isolated cardiac Purkinje fibers (Tse and Han, 1978) and also by the capacity of β-adrenergic blocking drugs to attenuate or prevent some digitalis-induced disturbances of ventricular rhythm.

The combined effects of these indirect actions of digitalis on the *normal* heart and circulation are reasonably clear. However, when the circulation is abnormal, as when a patient has congestive heart failure, the net effects may be quite different. When the heart is normal, the augmented vagal activity typically decreases the rate of generation of impulses in the S-A node; other effects of digitalis on this node probably are not significant with usual therapeutic concentrations of the drug. In normal man at rest, a decrease in sinus rate may not occur when digitalis is given. However, the vagal effect of digitalis is still present, since the maximal heart rate achieved during exercise is significantly diminished (Horwitz *et al.*, 1977). If the sinus rate is increased, as in heart failure, the negative chronotropic effect of digitalis is usually quite prominent. Here withdrawal of compensatory sympathetic activity contributes to the net effect.

Atrial fibers, both specialized and nonspecialized, are quite sensitive to the actions of acetylcholine. The indirect action of digitalis thus causes prominent changes in the electrical activity of the atrium in experimental animals. At what may be assumed to be therapeutic concentrations, the indirect effects predominate over the direct effects. The liberated acetylcholine causes an increase in RP, a decrease in latent automaticity of specialized atrial fibers, and a marked decrease in the duration of the atrial AP and ERP. The indirect effect of digitalis on conduction in normal atrial fibers cannot be predicted with certainty because conduction velocity is dependent on so many variables. Nevertheless, if hyperpolarization is significant, conduction is slowed. What should be remembered is that the indirect effects tend to oppose the direct effects of digitalis (decrease in RP, increase in APD) on the atrium. Also, the most significant effects at therapeutic concentrations of digitalis are the decrease in atrial APD and ERP. These changes permit the atria to respond to stimulation at much higher rates. Thus, if digitalis is given during atrial flutter or atrial

fibrillation, the net rate of atrial impulses may increase (*see* below).

If the RP of human atrial muscle is significantly decreased due to disease, digitalis can cause hyperpolarization and improvement in APs and conduction (Hordof *et al.*, 1978). This is due to liberation of acetylcholine, and the effect is abolished by atropine. If there is phase-4 depolarization, automaticity is decreased. Such findings demonstrate the importance of the initial condition of the tissue in relation to the net effect of digitalis. Toxic concentrations of ouabain cause delayed afterdepolarization in human atrial muscle fibers.

The *A-V node* is strongly influenced by the indirect actions of digitalis. The enhanced vagal activity and the decrease in sensitivity to catecholamines have pronounced effects on both the generation of the A-V nodal AP and the transmission of impulses through the node. Acetylcholine causes some hyperpolarization of certain fibers in the A-V node (Cranefield *et al.*, 1959) but, more importantly, decreases the rate of rise and amplitude of APs at these sites. Also, the recovery of excitability is delayed. Because of these changes, conduction is slowed and the ERP is greatly prolonged. The impairment of conduction may progress to complete heart block. A decreased sensitivity to norepinephrine would intensify these effects. In the A-V node, therefore, the direct and indirect effects of digitalis bring about similar changes. The most important result is to diminish the rate at which atrial impulses can be transmitted to the ventricles. Thus, in atrial tachycardias, atrial flutter, and atrial fibrillation, administration of digitalis will decrease the ventricular rate because of block of an increased fraction of atrial impulses in the A-V junction.

The effectiveness of the A-V block due to the direct and indirect effects on the A-V node is enhanced in atrial flutter and fibrillation because digitalis, through its indirect effect on the atria, usually *increases* the rate at which impulses enter the atrial margin of the node. Those impulses that enter the node but fail to propagate through it spread slowly and leave the tissue refractory in their wake (concealed conduction); this *repetitive concealed conduction* increases the fraction of time during which the node is effectively refractory (*see* below).

The *His-Purkinje system* is strongly influenced by the sympathetic nervous system but ordinarily is not particularly sensitive to changes in vagal activity. Thus, in contrast to the S-A node, atria, and A-V node, it is the indirect effects of digitalis mediated through the sympathetic nervous system that influence electrical activity of the specialized ventricular conducting system.

Acetylcholine clearly can have effects on the electrical activity of the His bundle (Bailey *et al.*, 1972) and cardiac Purkinje fibers; it causes an increase in RP, a decrease in automatic rate, and some effect on the duration of the AP (Danilo *et al.*, 1978; Gadsby *et al.*, 1978; Tse and Han, 1978). Also, when impulses arise from partially depolarized Purkinje fibers, acetylcholine may either slow the rate of impulse generation or increase the transmembrane potential toward the normal value. Finally, acetylcholine antagonizes the effects of isoproterenol on Purkinje fibers. However, it does not modify the effects of digitalis on the transmembrane AP (Bailey *et al.*, 1979). The enhanced vagal activity will, however, decrease the release of transmitter from sympathetic nerve terminals.

Enhanced efferent sympathetic activity may be important in relation to the drug-initiated arrhythmias that occur when the concentration of digitalis is high. If the heart is deprived of sympathetic innervation, toxic doses of digitalis usually cause cardiac arrest rather than ventricular arrhythmias and fibrillation (Erlij and Mendez, 1964; Ten Eick and Hoffman, 1969b). It seems reasonable to conclude, therefore, that the indirect and direct effects may at times act synergistically to cause disturbances of rhythm.

The indirect effects of digitalis probably result in only minor changes in the electrical activity of *ventricular fibers;* only extremely high concentrations of acetylcholine affect canine ventricular transmembrane RPs and APs. Similarly, catecholamines cause only small changes in the duration of the ventricular AP.

In *summary,* the indirect effects of digitalis, mediated primarily through the vagus, result in prominent changes in the activity of the sinus node, the atria, and the A-V node. At therapeutic concentrations, neurally mediated indirect effects on the functions of the specialized ventricular conducting system and the ventricles are much less important.

Mechanical Activity. The *direct* action of digitalis is primarily responsible for its positive inotropic effect on the heart. Nevertheless, certain of the drug's indirect effects do contribute to alterations of mechanical activity. For example, the decrease in heart rate due to sinus slowing influences contractility because of a change in end-diastolic fiber length; there is also a direct inotropic effect due to the change in rate. A decrease in ventricular rate caused by partial A-V block has similar effects. Enhanced vagal activity decreases the force of atrial contraction, but this negative inotropic effect, which might slightly reduce atrial transfer of blood, probably does not significantly attenuate the direct positive inotropic effect of digitalis on ventricular function.

Similarly, although vagal stimulation can decrease the force of ventricular contraction in experimental animals, particularly when contractility has been enhanced by sympathetic activation (Levy, 1971), it is not likely that acetylcholine liberated by enhanced vagal activity significantly attenuates the direct positive inotropic effect of cardiac glycosides. Interactions between digitalis and the sympathetic nervous system also are not crucially important in relation to the positive inotropic effect of digitalis. The glycoside can exert a strong positive inotropic effect after complete blockade of cardiac β-adrenergic receptors.

EFFECTS ON ELECTRICAL ACTIVITY OF THE HEART IN SITU

The effects of digitalis on the electrical activity of the heart *in situ* have been studied extensively. There is a reasonable correspondence between the toxic effects of digitalis on the canine and the human heart, and observations made on experimental animals have thus contributed importantly to our understanding of the therapeutic and toxic effects of digitalis in man.

The Canine Heart in Situ. Digitalis has a biphasic effect on the *electrical excitability* of both the atria and the ventricles. Low doses cause a slight increase in excitability, whereas higher doses decrease it (Mendez and Mendez, 1957). The enhanced excitability likely results from inhibition of Na^+,K^+-ATPase and a resultant small decrease in RP. The decreased excitability caused by very high concentrations of digitalis presumably results from the direct effect of digitalis on voltage-dependent inactivation of the fast inward channel (Kassebaum, 1963) and possibly also from a further reduction in RP sufficient to cause partial inactivation of the fast inward channel. Sufficiently high concentrations of digitalis can cause inexcitability of all cardiac tissues. The atria are more sensitive than ventricular muscle, and Purkinje fibers are much more sensitive than ventricular muscle to these toxic actions of digitalis (*see* Trautwein, 1963; Hoffman and Singer, 1964).

The effects of digitalis on *conduction velocity* in the different cardiac tissues is variable. First, one can consider how the direct effects of digitalis might modify conduction. Conduction velocity depends, among other factors, not only on the level of the RP but also on the degree of inactivation of the fast inward channel, the membrane resistance, and the resistance between cardiac cells at gap junctions. Since high concentrations of digitalis can decrease RP, shift the curve describing inactivation of the fast inward channel in a depolarizing direction, decrease membrane resistance, and increase the resistance of the gap junctions, toxic concentrations of the drug can decrease conduction velocity in atrial and ventricular muscle fibers and cardiac Purkinje fibers. In addition, the presence of delayed afterdepolarizations can slow and impair impulse propagation.

In the atrium, the direct effects of therapeutic concentrations of a cardiac glycoside usually are antagonized by the enhanced vagal effect (*see* above), although conduction slows with high toxic concentrations. In Purkinje fibers and ventricular muscle, low concentrations of glycoside slightly speed conduction, whereas very high concentrations cause slowing. Conduction in the Purkinje system is impaired at a lower concentration of drug than is required to affect ventricular muscle (Moe and Mendez, 1951; Swain and Weidner, 1957). Since digitalis typically does *not* prolong the QRS complex in the human ECG, the meaning of slowing of impulse propagation in the specialized conducting system of the canine heart is difficult to evaluate. The depression of conduction through the A-V node has been described in the previous section. Records of His bundle electrograms show that the prolongation of the P-R interval and the production of heart block are due

primarily to actions on the A-V node and not to direct effects on the His bundle or bundle branches.

The effects of digitalis on the *refractoriness* of atrial muscle depend upon the relative predominance of the indirect (vagal) effects and the direct effects. Ordinarily, because of the enhanced vagal effects, the atrial refractory period is shortened. This is paralleled by a decrease in the duration of the atrial transmembrane action potential. However, if the heart has been denervated or if atropine has been given, digitalis increases the duration of atrial refractory periods. The effects of digitalis on the *ERP of the A-V node* have been described in detail. The vagal effect, the antiadrenergic effect, and the direct effect all increase the effective and functional refractory periods of the A-V junction. In the *ventricle,* digitalis shortens the duration of refractoriness, in parallel with the decrease in duration of the transmembrane AP. The change is modest in magnitude and proportional to the change in the Q-T interval in the ECG. Digitalis also alters the response of ventricular muscle to a single stimulus applied after the end of the T wave, such that a single stimulus can elicit repetitive ventricular responses (Lown *et al.,* 1967).

The effects of digitalis on impulse generation and conduction in the canine heart *in situ* provide a reasonably good picture of the usual changes brought about by therapeutic and toxic concentrations of cardiac glycosides in man. If sequential doses of digitalis are given gradually to an anesthetized dog to increase the body store and concentration in cardiac tissues, first to therapeutic and then to toxic levels, the sequence of changes in electrical activity is reasonably reproducible. Small doses of drug decrease the sinus rate, minimally increase the P-R interval, and prolong the ERP of the A-V node. Also, if the vagus is stimulated to cause A-V block, it can be seen that digitalis increases the automaticity of the specialized ventricular conducting system. This is evidenced by a decrease in the interval between the block and the first ventricular escape beat and by an increase in the rate of the escape rhythm as the dose of digitalis increases. The escape rhythms that occur after administration of digitalis are particularly interesting in that they do not show the phenomenon of overdrive suppression. Rather, the rate of the ectopic pacemaker is usually increased after overdrive (Wittenberg *et al.*, 1972).

The Human Heart in Situ. Perhaps surprisingly, most studies of the human atrium have shown only minimal effects of digitalis on the duration of refractoriness. This is true of normal atria (Dhingra *et al.*, 1975; Wu *et al.*, 1975) and those that have been denervated by cardiac transplantation (Goodman *et al.*, 1975). Refractoriness of the A-V node is increased, and A-V nodal conduction is slowed. The mechanism for this is similar to that described for the dog. Refractoriness of the His-Purkinje system in man can be studied only by retrograde activation, because A-V nodal refractoriness usually prevents premature supraventricular impulses from propagating to the His bundle. When this method is used, intravenous ouabain in nontoxic doses does not cause any significant change in refractoriness or conduction in the His-Purkinje system (Gomes *et al.*, 1978). In contrast, the functional and effective refractory periods of ventricular muscle are decreased slightly but significantly. This may increase the interval during which ventricular premature depolarizations can induce reentrant excitation through the specialized conducting system.

Mechanism of Cardiac Slowing in Atrial Fibrillation. In typical atrial fibrillation the impulse spreads through the atrial syncytium in a manner that may best be described as random reentry. Most atrial fibers are reexcited as soon as they recover sufficiently from refractoriness. The impulses arriving at the A-V node as a result of this activity are rapid (as many as 500 per minute) and random in time. Most of these impulses either fail to enter the A-V node because it is refractory or propagate only partway through it and give rise to the phenomenon of concealed conduction. The concealed conduction of these impulses increases the time during which nodal tissues are partially or totally refractory. The minimal interval between ventricular responses is determined by the ERP of the A-V node. Longer ventricular cycles occur when one or more successive atrial impulses enter the node but fail to propagate to the His bundle. The average frequency of the ventricular contractions during atrial fibrillation thus is determined by the refractoriness of the A-V junction. When atrial

fibrillation is accompanied by congestive heart failure, the resulting reduction in vagal tone and increase in sympathetic tone increase the ventricular rate. In rapid atrial fibrillation, the ventricular rate is grossly irregular and frequently, after short R-R intervals, stroke volume may be very small. The major effect of digitalis on ventricular rate during atrial fibrillation results from its actions on the A-V node. The ERP of the A-V node is prolonged by the increase in vagal effects, the direct effect of the glycoside, and perhaps by the antiadrenergic effect of digitalis described above. The net result of these actions is to decrease ventricular rate and, very often, to improve ventricular function.

In addition to its effects on A-V transmission, digitalis reduces ventricular rate during atrial fibrillation by another mechanism that operates simultaneously. Through its indirect action on the atria, mediated by acetylcholine, digitalis decreases the duration of the atrial transmembrane AP and decreases the ERP of atrial fibers. The result is that there is an increase in the mean frequency at which atrial fibers are excited. Because of the increase in the rate at which impulses enter the atrial margin of the A-V node, a greater proportion of them are extinguished as a result of concealed conduction and a smaller proportion propagate to excite the ventricles.

Action in Atrial Flutter. A circus-movement flutter about an obstacle of crushed atrial tissue in the dog heart will sustain itself at a stable frequency for hours, provided the path length (perimeter of the obstacle) is long enough to permit expiration of the refractory period between circuits. When such a flutter is established in an animal in which the vagi have been blocked with atropine, the administration of digitalis slows the flutter frequency and eventually restores normal sinus rhythm. In similar preparations in which the vagus nerves are intact, digitalis often converts the atrial flutter to atrial fibrillation. Administration of atropine may now restore normal rhythm. The explanation of these results may be found in the direct and indirect effects of digitalis upon the atrial refractory period. When the vagi are blocked, digitalis prolongs the refractory period; however, when the nerves are not blocked, the ERP is abbreviated (Farah and Loomis, 1950). The vagal effects are not uniformly distributed; the atrial refractory period is greatly reduced at some points and not at all at others. As a result, the flutter wave front becomes fractionated and fibrillation occurs.

Effect in Patients with the Wolff-Parkinson-White Syndrome. Effects of digitalis on conduction in and refractoriness of anomalous A-V bypass tracts are variable. Wellens and Durrer (1973) found that ouabain *decreased* refractoriness of the accessory pathways but did not change refractoriness of atrial muscle. In contrast, Sellers and coworkers (1977) found variable effects among different subjects. The important point to remember is that digitalis can decrease the ERP of the bypass tract sufficiently so that rapid atrial impulses can cause *ventricular fibrillation*. This decrease in refractoriness is seen in about 30% of patients with Wolff-Parkinson-White syndrome given the drug.

This effect constitutes a clear *contraindication* to the use of digitalis.

Electrocardiographic Effects. Digitalis has characteristic effects on the ECG that may assist in determining whether a patient is taking digitalis. However, these changes cannot be used to estimate digitalis dosage or the degree of digitalization. Furthermore, the effects of digitalis are often superimposed on changes resulting from the basic cardiac disease. The ECG must be evaluated with these facts in mind. As mentioned previously, even toxic doses of digitalis typically do not cause an increase in the duration of the QRS complex.

Within 2 to 4 hours after a large oral dose of digitalis, definite alterations may appear in the ECG. Changes are first noted in the S-T segment or in the T wave itself. The normally upright T wave becomes diminished in amplitude, isoelectric, or inverted in one or more leads. The S-T segment may also show depression when the main QRS complex is upward; occasionally the S-T segment is elevated by digitalis when the main QRS deflection is downward. The changes in the S-T segment and the T wave may occur alone or may coincide. In precordial leads, these changes can simulate those resulting from coronary artery disease or recent coronary occlusion. After exercise in digitalized patients the J point may show depression similar to that caused by myocardial ischemia.

The P-R interval may be prolonged by digitalis. This effect occurs somewhat later than changes described above. The interval rarely becomes greater than 0.25 second, unless there is disease of the conduction system. Atropine can abolish lower degrees of A-V block produced by digitalis, but the direct (or antiadrenergic) actions of the drug are not overcome by atropine.

The Q-T interval is shortened by digitalis because ventricular repolarization is accelerated. Large doses occasionally cause changes in the size and the shape of the P wave. Digitalis can widen the abnormal QRS complex in the Wolff-Parkinson-White syndrome, probably by slowing A-V nodal propagation without affecting conduction time in the anomalous A-V pathway. This effect may be reversed by atropine. Almost every type of ECG tracing associated with cardiac disorders can be simulated by the effects of digitalis on the heart. However, if QRS widening occurs during normal sinus rhythm, it almost certainly is the result of concurrent disease, since digitalis does not cause this change.

EFFECTS ON THE
CARDIOVASCULAR SYSTEM

The overall effects of digitalis on the cardiovascular system not only are a composite of changes in the force of ventricular contraction and heart rate but also result from effects on the autonomic nervous system and on vascular smooth muscle; furthermore, reflex adjustments to the initial hemodynamic changes caused by the drug are also important. The effects of digitalis on cardiovascular function differ depending on whether the heart and circulation are normal or whether there is congestive heart failure.

The extent to which digitalis changes systemic arterial pressure, cardiac output, heart size, and end-diastolic and venous pressures depends on whether the measurements are made while the subject is at rest or during exercise, as well as on other variables such as the use of anesthetics, the presence or absence of stress, and the work required of the heart at the time of measurement. For these reasons, there has been disagreement and argument for many years about many of the effects of digitalis on both the normal circulation and the circulation during congestive heart failure. It probably is helpful to consider first the changes brought about by the administration of digitalis to a conscious experimental animal or to a normal human subject and then deal with the effects of the drug in the presence of heart failure.

The Normal Heart and Circulation. When a rapidly acting drug like ouabain is injected intravenously into a *normal* conscious dog, the effects are reasonably clear and consistent (McRitchie and Vatner, 1976; Horwitz *et al.*, 1977). Usually there are increases in both systolic and mean arterial pressures that reach their maxima in 5 minutes and decline slowly over 30 minutes. All indices of ventricular contractility increase, but not markedly; these include the maximal rate of development of left intraventricular systolic pressure and the maximal rate of fiber shortening during systole. The increase in contractility can be demonstrated after doses of propranolol that block cardiac β-adrenergic receptors. It occurs in the absence of an increase in end-diastolic ventricular pressure or diameter and thus does not result from increased fiber length. The increase in contractility thus clearly results from the direct positive inotropic effect of digitalis. Heart rate usually decreases moderately, stroke volume increases, end-systolic ventricular volume decreases somewhat, and cardiac output is diminished slightly. If ouabain is injected after denervation of the arterial baroreceptors, usually there is little decrease in sinus rate even though the vagus nerves are intact; this indicates that a major cause of the sinus slowing is a reflex response to both the rate of change and the extent of increase in arterial pressure. If heart rate is maintained at the pretreatment value by atrial pacing, ouabain does not cause a decrease in cardiac output; however, there often is a decrease in heart size from the control value. The demonstration that the left ventricle can maintain or increase stroke volume and maintain cardiac output without an increase in end-diastolic fiber length and in spite of an increase in aortic pressure provides additional evidence that ouabain exerts a direct positive inotropic effect.

Since mean systemic arterial pressure is elevated without an increase in cardiac output, there must be an *increase in systemic vascular resistance*. This results from a direct effect of digitalis to cause contraction of the smooth muscle in the arterial resistance vessels. Digitalis also augments sympathetic outflow from the CNS, but this probably causes only minimal change in arterial resistance. After baroreceptor denervation, the glycoside-induced increase in systemic arterial pressure is enhanced; reflexes are thus important in modulating but not in causing the vasopressor effect of digitalis.

Digitalis also acts directly on *smooth muscle in veins* to cause constriction; in the dog, this effect is quite prominent in the hepatic veins and may result in venous pooling in the portal vessels. This action has been thought to be responsible for the decrease in cardiac output that often is observed after intravenous injection of digitalis into normal subjects.

If the effects of ouabain are evaluated in dogs during exercise, it can be shown that digitalis decreases maximal running speed, maximal cardiac index, and heart rate but causes no significant modification of the changes in left ventricular contractility, stroke volume, or end-diastolic diameter that result from the exercise. If the decrease in maximal heart rate is prevented with atropine, ouabain causes no significant change in any of these variables during exercise. If the effects of norepinephrine on the heart are blocked by propranolol, ouabain increases the maximal rate of development of pressure during exercise and improves exercise capacity. These findings indicate that the bradycardia caused by digitalis limits the capacity of the normal heart to do work. Furthermore, in the presence of very high levels of sympathetic activity, the positive inotropic effect of digitalis is negligible (Horwitz *et al.*, 1977).

Studies of the effects of digitalis on the heart and circulation of *normal human subjects* show that, in general, the changes are similar to those described above for the dog (Mason *et al.*, 1969; Smith and Haber, 1973). Digitalis exerts a direct positive inotropic effect on the normal human heart (Braunwald *et al.*, 1961). It causes a modest increase in systemic arterial pressure, an increase in systemic vascular resistance, and some venous constriction (Mason and Braunwald, 1964). Usually there is either no increase in cardiac output or a modest decrease; cardiac slowing is not prominent (Dresdale *et al.*, 1959; Selzer *et al.*, 1959). Overall, the increase in ventricular contractility is countered by the combined effect of increased systemic vascular resistance and decreased heart rate. Thus, cardiac output remains constant. The effects of the drug on patients with heart failure are quite different.

Heart Failure. To understand the effects of digitalis in patients with congestive heart failure, it is important to consider the factors that regulate cardiac contractility and their alteration in this disease. Furthermore, it is essential to appreciate other changes that are secondary to heart failure, such as retention of salt and water and reflex adjustments to impaired cardiac function.

The force developed by the ventricles during systole is regulated both by extrinsic factors, such as the level of sympathetic tone, and intrinsic factors, which include the frequency of contraction and the length of the fibers just before the onset of systole. In addition, the external work done by the ventricles is determined by their volume and the interaction between the afterload (the impedance met by the ventricle during ejection) and the contracting ventricle.

To describe the effects of digitalis on the failed ventricle it is essential first to consider the *pressure-volume relationship* described by Patterson and Starling in 1914 and extended by others in the form of the cardiac function curve (*see* Figure 30–5). For any given state of the ventricles, when end-diastolic fiber length and end-diastolic volume increase because of an increase in filling pressure, the force of ventricular contraction increases, up to a limit. Usually this results in an increase in the force developed during systole and in the stroke volume and stroke work. The absolute value of stroke volume or work for a given end-diastolic volume depends on the inotropic state of the ventricles. In the failing heart, the capacity to develop force during systole is reduced and thus a greater end-diastolic volume is needed to perform any given level of external work. In cardiac failure, therefore, one can imagine the following sequence of events. Reduced systolic ejection, caused by a mismatch of work capacity and load, results in decreased systolic ejection and an increased end-systolic volume. With constant filling, end-diastolic pressure and volume increase. If this sequence progresses, the ventricular volume will increase progressively. At the same time, because of the Laplace relationship, the effectiveness of increased wall tension in developing intraventricular pressure and the extent to which fiber shortening results in systolic ejection will both diminish. Further dilatation thus may be needed to maintain aortic flow. (At an excessive end-diastolic fiber length the force of contraction decreases; whether this occurs in the failed human heart *in situ* is doubtful.)

If, by means of the pressure-volume relation, the heart is unable to compensate for the load imposed, other mechanisms must be recruited; these usually include increased sympathetic and decreased vagal activity. These changes increase heart rate, myocardial contractility, systemic vascular resistance, and venous tone. Retention of salt and water may increase circulating blood volume. The retention of salt and water is due to decreased renal blood flow, in part because of increased activity in efferent sympathetic nerves. The increase in venous pres-

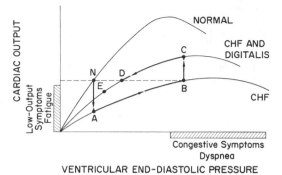

Figure 30–5. *Diagrammatic representation of the use of the Frank-Starling mechanism as a compensation for congestive heart failure.*

The three curves depict ventricular function in normal subjects and in those with congestive heart failure (*CHF*) and heart failure after treatment with digitalis. The points *N* through *D* represent in sequence: initial reduction of contractility due to congestive heart failure (*N* to *A*); use of Frank-Starling compensation to maintain cardiac output (*A* to *B*); increase in contractility when digitalis is administered (*B* to *C*); and reduction in the use of Frank-Starling compensation, which digitalis allows (*C* to *D*). Any factor that reduces ventricular filling pressure (decreased venous return) will lower cardiac output in spite of an inotropic effect (*D* to *E*). Of note is the fact that points *N*, *B*, and *D* all lie on the same line in the vertical axis and thus all represent the same cardiac output, but each is on a different end-diastolic pressure on the horizontal axis. The levels at which symptoms of congestion, such as dyspnea, and symptoms of low cardiac output, such as fatigue, occur are represented by the cross-hatched areas. (After Mason, 1973. Courtesy of *The American Journal of Cardiology*.)

sure is due in part to the venoconstriction, in part to the increased intravascular volume, and in part to the increase in end-diastolic right ventricular pressure.

If severe congestive heart failure involves both right and left ventricles, the following changes from normal usually will be found. Heart rate is elevated, end-diastolic ventricular pressures and volumes are increased, stroke volume is diminished, and end-systolic volume is increased. Cardiac output is decreased at rest and increases minimally with exertion. Systemic arterial resistance is elevated, primarily because of increased efferent sympathetic activity; tone in venous beds may be elevated. Because of the elevated diastolic left ventricular pressure, pulmonary capillary pressure is increased; if this capillary pressure exceeds a critical value, pulmonary edema develops. Because of edema and venous congestion, the lungs become stiffened and the work of breathing is increased;

this results in dyspnea, orthopnea, and tachypnea. Because of the elevated right ventricular diastolic pressure, systemic venous pressure is increased and there is peripheral congestion, hepatomegaly, and edema. The increased sympathetic effect on renal vessels decreases renal perfusion, and this directly and indirectly results in retention of salt and water, increases blood volume, and contributes to the formation of edema. Systemic arterial pressure usually is not changed markedly as a result of failure and may be normal or elevated. Because of the decrease in cardiac output, perfusion of tissue is inadequate; hepatic blood flow may be decreased enough to slow elimination of some drugs, and cerebral perfusion may be impaired and result in confusion and other abnormalities of function of the CNS.

When digitalis is administered to patients with heart failure, its beneficial effects are primarily due to its direct positive inotropic action. A second important effect is the indirect action to decrease sinus rate. Because of the direct positive inotropic effect, the ventricles shift from one ventricular function curve to another (*see* Figure 30–5). They are thus able to develop more tension, empty more adequately, and eject more blood against the existing afterload. The increased stroke volume causes a decrease in end-systolic volume; since the ventricles contain less blood at the onset of diastole, end-diastolic pressure and volume both decrease if filling is constant. In spite of the decrease in fiber length, the ventricles can still do enough work to increase stroke volume because of the improved inotropic state. The decrease in heart size and the increase in output occur in spite of the decrease in heart rate. The direct positive inotropic effect thus increases cardiac output, decreases cardiac filling pressures, and decreases heart size and venous and capillary pressures. The decrease in ventricular volume increases the efficiency of contraction. Because of the improvement in the circulation, sympathetic activity is reduced; this, in turn, results in a decrease in systemic arterial resistance and venous tone. The former change decreases the afterload on the left ventricle and permits a further improvement in cardiac function.

Many factors are likely involved in the retention of salt and water in heart failure, but their consideration is not essential to the present discussion. However, the

mechanism by which digitalization relieves edema is of interest. In addition to the fact that cardiac output is increased, the improved hemodynamic state that follows the administration of digitalis causes a reduction in efferent sympathetic nerve impulse traffic and thus improves renal perfusion. However, in large part, the decrease in sympathetic impulses to the kidney may result primarily from a direct effect of digitalis on afferent nerve fiber endings in the heart. Acetylstrophanthidin applied to the ventricular epicardium or injected into the coronary circulation of dogs causes an almost immediate decrease in sympathetic nerve activity in the kidneys (Thames, 1979). This action appears to be mediated through neural receptors in the heart with vagal afferent connections. This mechanism might account for a number of other responses to digitalis that are manifest before the positive inotropic action is fully developed.

Effects on the Veins. In spite of repeated demonstrations of the action of digitalis on the contractile force of the heart muscle in many varied experimental preparations, it took many years to overcome arguments that the salutary action of the drug in congestive heart failure in man is due to some other action of the drug. After all, Withering himself believed its primary effect was on the kidneys. Mention has already been made of the emphasis long placed upon cardiac slowing as the primary therapeutic action. Many studies, reviewed in *earlier editions* of this textbook, attempted to ascribe the beneficial effect of digitalis in heart failure primarily to an action to reduce venous tone, rather than to a direct positive inotropic effect. This clearly is not correct. Nevertheless, the effects of digitalis on venous tone and capacitance are important because they modify the pressure available to fill the ventricles. An understanding of this relationship is essential because treatment of congestive heart failure often includes, in addition to digitalis, the use of diuretics (which decrease blood volume and ventricular filling pressure) and vasodilators (which reduce afterload, preload, or both). This problem is considered in a subsequent section. However, it is clear from Figure 30–5 that a reduction in filling pressure (sufficient to shift ventricular function from *D* to *E*) would reduce cardiac output in spite of an improvement in contractility due to a direct positive inotropic effect.

Effects on the Coronary Circulation. The effects of digitalis on the coronary circulation depend on a number of actions, which can be described as direct and indirect. Digitalis glycosides constrict coronary arteries, presumably by a direct action on their smooth muscle. This effect may not be prominent when concentrations of drug in the plasma and tissues are kept at levels required to exert an optimal positive inotropic effect in heart failure.

Studies in man show no significant change in coronary blood flow or cardiac oxygen consumption in normal subjects or those with heart failure given strophanthus glycosides intravenously. Studies in conscious dogs demonstrate that ouabain can increase the perfusion of segments of the ventricle rendered ischemic by coronary occlusion and, in addition, can increase contractility of the ischemic parts of the myocardium.

Once again one faces the problem of discriminating between what digitalis can do and what it does do. This is quite important, because it may often be desirable to give digitalis to patients who have heart failure and reasonably severe coronary atherosclerosis. If the heart is dilated because of failure, it is likely that digitalis will improve the relationship between coronary flow and the needs of the myocardium for perfusion. The larger the heart during diastole, the greater the wall tension required to produce a given intraventricular pressure during systole. If digitalis decreases heart size during diastole, it is likely that this effect will more than compensate for any increase in oxygen consumption and requirement for perfusion that may result from the direct inotropic effect. If digitalis causes a decrease in heart rate and a decrease in the duration of systole, both of these changes will augment coronary perfusion. In *summary,* if the heart is dilated in failure, it seems most likely that the therapeutic effect of digitalis will improve the relationship between coronary flow and myocardial demand for perfusion.

In the case of regional ischemia, it probably is reasonable to assume that digitalis may exert its usual effect on the coronary vessels that provide blood to the nonischemic parts of the heart and cause constriction. At the same time the vessels that deliver blood to the ischemic regions may be less responsive to digitalis.

PHARMACOKINETICS

A detailed consideration of pharmacokinetics will be restricted to digoxin and digitoxin; these are the two most widely used preparations and have been studied most thoroughly in relation to clinical use. Some information on other preparations will be found below under Choice of Preparations. The significant data for digoxin and digitoxin are summarized in Table 30–1 (*see also* Appendix II).

Absorption. Absorption of *digoxin* after oral administration is somewhat variable; the fraction of the administered dose that is absorbed depends strongly on the type of preparation used and varies from 40 to 90%.

Absorption is best with the preparation in a hydroalcoholic vehicle. Variation in bioavailability with tablets has been recognized as a significant clinical problem. Absorption of some preparations may be as low as 40%; with others the fraction reaches 75%. This variability is most prominent with tablets from different manufacturers; this does not result from differences in the content of active glycoside but from differences in the rate and extent of dissolution (Lindenbaum et al., 1971). The problems of bioavailability of digoxin have been reviewed thoroughly (New York Heart Association Task Force on Digitalis Preparations, 1974). It is advisable for physicians to use a preparation with which they are familiar and to indicate the commercial source if the drug is prescribed by a nonproprietary name. Absorption of digoxin also can be retarded by the presence of food in the gastrointestinal tract, by delayed gastric emptying, and by malabsorption syndromes. In approximately 10% of patients, a substantial fraction of ingested digoxin is converted to inactive products, such as 2-hydroxydigoxin, by intestinal microorganisms (Lindenbaum et al., 1981). Antibiotics such as neomycin decrease absorption, as can steroid-binding resins (*see* below).

After oral administration, the concentration of digoxin in plasma typically reaches a peak in 2 to 3 hours; the maximal effect is apparent in 4 to 6 hours (Table 30–1). If a loading dose of digoxin is not given, up to 1 week can elapse before steady-state plasma concentrations are attained, since the half-life of the drug in the body is 1 to 2 days.

Absorption of *digitoxin* is much more complete (90 to 100%) than is that of digoxin because digitoxin is more lipid soluble. No significant problems with bioavailability have been noted for digitoxin, but its rate of absorption is also influenced by the factors mentioned above for digoxin. Because of its long half-life, steady-state concentrations in plasma are attained slowly and recovery from toxicity is protracted.

Distribution. The glycosides are distributed slowly in the body, in part due to their relatively large volume of distribution. As for other drugs, the presence of congestive heart failure can slow the rate at which steady-state distribution is attained. About 25% of digoxin in the plasma is bound to proteins; in contrast, most (95% or more) digitoxin is so bound. These differences in binding account in part for the differences in apparent volume of distribution of the glycosides and in the concentrations in plasma that are associated with therapeutic effects. Digitalis glycosides are distributed to most body tissues, including red blood cells, skeletal muscle, and heart. At equilibrium, the concentrations in cardiac tissue are 15 to 30 times those in the plasma; the concentration in skeletal muscle is about half that in the heart. Binding to tissue is decreased by an increase in extracellular concentration of potassium, and the volume of distribution may be altered in some disease states. The time required to attain peak concentrations of digitalis glycosides in the heart and plasma is usually *less* than the time required for maximal effect; peak effect may not occur until 1 hour or more after levels in the heart reach their maximal value.

Elimination. *Digoxin* is eliminated primarily by the kidney. The drug is both filtered at the glomerulus and secreted by the tubules. There is some reabsorption from the tubular lumen, and this may become significant when the rate of flow of tubular fluid is markedly reduced. A very few patients form an inactive metabolite of digoxin, dihydrodigoxin; it is almost impossible to obtain a therapeutic effect with digoxin in such individuals. Also, a rare patient seems to form antibodies to the glycoside, and this prevents its therapeutic effect. *Digitoxin* is actively metabolized by hepatic microsomal enzymes; one of the products is digoxin. Metabolism of digitoxin may be accelerated by drugs that induce microsomal enzymes, including phenylbutazone, phenobarbital, phenytoin, and rifampin; the magnitude of this effect is variable among patients.

The half-time for elimination of *digoxin,* which averages 1.6 days, is strongly dependent on renal function; in most instances, there is a close correlation between the decrease in creatinine clearance and the concentration of digoxin in plasma

that is attained with any given maintenance dose. Interventions that change renal perfusion, such as the administration of vasodilators, may cause significant change in the rate of elimination of digoxin. The half-time for elimination of *digitoxin* is nearly 7 days and is *not* appreciably changed by hepatic disease; this probably reflects the huge reserve capacity of the liver for metabolic degradation of this drug. There is an enterohepatic circulation of digitoxin, but only a minor fraction of unchanged drug is eliminated through the intestine.

Dosage and Administration. Digitalis is used almost exclusively for two purposes—either to restore an adequate circulation in patients with congestive heart failure or to slow ventricular rate in patients with atrial fibrillation or flutter. Other uses are much less frequent. Since both conditions require chronic therapy, it is necessary to establish and to maintain an adequate concentration of digitalis in the heart. If there is no urgent need for an immediate effect, a maintenance dose can be given daily by mouth and its effect evaluated after appropriate intervals. A maximal effect will be achieved in approximately four elimination half-lives. On the other hand, if it is desired to achieve a full therapeutic effect fairly rapidly, it is necessary to give a large initial dose because of the relatively long half-time for elimination (*see* Table 30–1).

By tradition, the initial loading dose is called the *digitalizing dose.* The size of this dose may be difficult to estimate. In theory, it is the steady-state total body store sufficient to cause the desired therapeutic effect. However, the estimate of the loading dose must be adjusted for the condition of the individual patient. Depending on the state of the heart and the cause of the cardiac abnormality, the "digitalizing" dose may be much less than the dose that is likely to cause toxicity or it may be almost equal to it.

In practice, the digitalizing dose is selected from prior estimates (Table 30–1), with consideration of factors that increase or decrease the requirement for the individual patient (*see* below). If the need for a partial effect of digitalis is urgent, the initial dose is often given intravenously. If it is certain that the patient has *not* been taking digitalis, 1.0 mg

Table 30–1. DOSAGES, TIME OF EFFECT, AND FATE OF DIGOXIN AND DIGITOXIN IN MAN *

	DIGOXIN	DIGITOXIN
Average digitalizing dose		
Oral	0.75–1.5 mg	0.8–1.2 mg
IV	0.5–1.0 mg	0.8–1.2 mg
Average daily maintenance dose		
Oral	0.125–0.5 mg	0.05–0.2 mg
IV	0.25 mg	0.10 mg
Onset of action		
Oral	1.5–6 hr †	3–6 hr
IV	5–30 min	30–120 min
Maximal effect		
Oral	4–6 hr	6–12 hr
IV	1.5–3 hr	4–8 hr
Intestinal absorption	< 40–90% ‡ (75%)	90–100%
Plasma protein binding	25%	95%
Disposition half-time	1.6 days	7 days
Route of elimination	Renal excretion of unchanged drug; limited hepatic metabolism	Hepatic degradation of molecule; renal excretion of metabolites
Enterohepatic circulation	Small	Large
"Therapeutic" plasma concentration	0.5–2.0 ng/ml	10–35 ng/ml

* *See also* Appendix II.

† Dependent on relationship of dose to meals, gastric emptying time, and type of preparation.

‡ About 90% of digoxin in an alcoholic elixir is absorbed from a normal enteric tract; about 75% of a tablet with high bioavailability is absorbed by a normal enteric tract. Absorption may be poor with certain tablets or when there is gastrointestinal malabsorption.

of digoxin can be given intravenously over a period of 10 to 20 minutes. Very often the loading dose is divided into two doses of 0.5 mg, given 3 to 4 hours apart. After the initial dose, a maintenance dose is administered daily and, after an appropriate interval, this may be increased or decreased as indicated by the therapeutic response and the concentration of drug in plasma. Because digitalis causes serious toxic effects so frequently and because digitalis toxicity is often lethal, it always is essential to observe the patient carefully, and it is frequently necessary to adjust the maintenance dose to achieve an optimal effect.

The maintenance dose must be equal to the daily loss. For *digoxin,* this is approximately 35% of the total body store; for *digitoxin,* approximately 10%. Regardless of the size of the initial dose, after a sufficient time (four to five times the $t_{1/2}$) the concentration in plasma and the total body store will be determined solely by the maintenance dose. Whether or not the desired effect has been obtained can be evaluated by careful and frequent observation of the patient. In patients with atrial fibrillation, the dose can be adjusted to produce the desired decrease in ventricular rate at rest and during exertion. Evaluation of effects in patients with heart failure is more difficult and should include quantification of changes in the signs and symptoms of failure, measurement of changes in body weight, venous pressure, and systolic time intervals, and evaluation of changes in exercise tolerance. The ECG and measurement of the concentration of cardiac glycoside in plasma may be helpful in adjusting the dosage.

Choice of Preparations and Routes of Administration. These decisions are made with consideration of the desired speed of onset of the therapeutic effect, the suitability of various routes of administration for the individual patient, the need for a stable concentration in plasma, and the likelihood of toxicity. *Digoxin* can be given intravenously or orally; after intravenous administration there will be an appreciable effect in 5 to 30 minutes and a maximal effect in 1.5 to 2 hours. Digoxin should not be given intramuscularly because it causes severe pain and muscle necrosis. After oral administration, an effect usually will be evident in 1 to 2 hours and the peak effect will occur in 4 to 6 hours. Because of its relatively short $t_{1/2}$, the steady-state concentration of digoxin in plasma can be changed reasonably rapidly. The disadvantage of the use of this drug is that the therapeutic effect may be greatly diminished or lost if the patient fails to take several doses. Its advantage is that toxic effects disappear relatively rapidly after the drug is discontinued. *Digitoxin* is not associated with problems of bioavailability. Absorption is virtually complete after oral administration, and, compared with digoxin, concentrations in plasma are better maintained, particularly if a patient's compliance is sporadic. Elimination of the parent drug is ordinarily independent of renal function, and at times this may be an important consideration. On the other hand, because of the long $t_{1/2}$ of digitoxin, it may take days after discontinuation of therapy for a sufficient fraction of the total body store to be eliminated if there is toxicity. The major active glycoside in *digitalis leaf* is digitoxin. The preparation is standardized by bioassay. Variability in the potency of the preparation is likely, and, in most cases, there is no compelling reason to use it.

Assay and Unitage of Digitalis Preparations. The USP requires spectrophotometric assay of digitoxin and digoxin against appropriate reference standards. *Powdered digitalis* requires bioassay, by determination of the lethal dose in pigeons in comparison with that of a reference standard. Tablets or capsules of digitalis powder are prescribed by weight or in units. The official USP unit represents the potency of 100 mg of the USP *Digitalis Reference Standard Powder* and is roughly equivalent to 0.1 mg of digitoxin.

Preparations Available for Clinical Use. *Digitoxin* (CRYSTODIGIN, PURODIGIN). As officially described, the drug is either pure digitoxin or a mixture of cardioactive glycosides obtained from *Digitalis purpurea, D. lanata,* or other species and consisting chiefly of digitoxin. *Digitoxin tablets* are available for oral use, each tablet containing 0.05, 0.1, 0.15, or 0.2 mg of drug. *Digitoxin injection* is available for *intravenous* administration and consists of a sterile solution of digitoxin in approximately 50% alcohol; glycerin may also be present. Each milliliter contains 0.2 mg of the drug. There is evidence that market preparations of crystalline digitoxin may differ somewhat in potency.

Digoxin (LANOXIN). This drug is a glycoside obtained from the leaves of *Digitalis lanata*. It is available for both oral and intravenous administration. *Digoxin tablets* contain 0.125, 0.25, or 0.5 mg each. *Digoxin solution in capsules* (LANOXICAPS) contains either 0.05, 0.1, or 0.2 mg of digoxin in stable solution in each capsule. Bioavailability is estimated to be 25% greater than for tablets, and the capsules provided are intended to be equivalent to 0.0625, 0.125, and 0.25 mg in tablet form. *Digoxin elixir* contains 0.05 mg/ml. *Digoxin injection* contains 0.1 mg/ml or 0.25 mg/ml. The appropriate dose can be diluted with 10 ml of sterile 0.9% sodium chloride solution before injection. The solution should be administered slowly (5 to 10 min-

utes), and care taken to avoid extravenous injection.

Deslanoside (desacetyl-lanatoside C; CEDILANID-D). This precursor glycoside is derived from lanatoside C by alkaline hydrolysis, and is more soluble than the parent substance. It is marketed as *deslanoside injection* for intramuscular or intravenous use, in a sterile solution containing 0.2 mg/ml of drug.

Powdered Digitalis. This powder is available in tablets or capsules containing 100 mg.

THERAPEUTIC USES

Heart Failure. By far the most important use of digitalis is to treat heart failure. Digitalis is useful regardless of whether the failure is predominantly of the left or right ventricle or involves both. With very few exceptions, the type of rhythm exhibited by the decompensated heart neither indicates nor contraindicates the use of digitalis. Nevertheless, arrhythmias may modify the response to the drug.

Although the treatment of heart failure frequently includes the administration of digitalis, a cardiac glycoside is not the only modality that is utilized (Williams and Fisch, 1983). Traditionally, treatment of chronic mild failure has included limitation of physical activity, restriction of salt intake, and the use of a natriuretic diuretic. If these measures were not sufficient, digitalis was typically added. More recently, systemic vasodilators (*see* Chapter 33) have been used, in conjunction with a diuretic, to treat *acute* cardiac failure of the type associated with shock secondary to myocardial infarction; subsequently, vasodilators or inhibitors of peptidyl dipeptidase (angiotensin converting enzyme) (*see* Chapter 27) were evaluated for *chronic* treatment of congestive failure in conjunction with a diuretic, digitalis, or both. A reduction in cardiac work, brought about by a reduction in afterload, coupled with elimination of excess salt and water and a reduction in ventricular filling pressures (caused by diuretics and venodilators), often is sufficient to relieve symptoms of heart failure. Digitalis is thus not *essential* for treatment of all cases of failure. Moreover, since chronic administration of digitalis is associated with significant toxicity (*see* below), the drug should not be used unless it is clearly indicated. The role of digitalis in treating heart failure is currently undergoing reevaluation.

In some studies, withdrawal of digitalis from patients who were also receiving diuretics or vasodilators or both did not result in significant worsening of cardiac function (Gheorghiade and Beller, 1983). In other studies, digitalis was found to be beneficial in treating failure in patients with normal sinus rhythm if failure was not relieved by diuretics (Lee *et al.,* 1982).

Until satisfactory data become available, it probably is best to adhere to tested practice and use digitalis for both the initial and chronic treatment of heart failure when restriction of activity, reduced salt intake, and diuresis are not sufficient. In many instances, if failure persists during this treatment, results can be improved by the addition of a drug that reduces afterload or both preload and afterload. The use of vasodilators and diuretics without digitalis may not be effective for chronic treatment because of development of tolerance to the effects of the vasodilator drugs on blood vessels. At the same time, if diuretics and vasodilators result in a satisfactory hemodynamic and clinical response without digitalis, and if there is reason to think that the patient is more likely than usual to suffer digitalis intoxication, chronic treatment without digitalis would be reasonable. If failure is associated with atrial fibrillation (*see* below), digitalis is still the drug of choice, although other means to control ventricular rate are available (*see* Chapter 31).

Effectiveness. The effectiveness of digitalis in treating heart failure depends in part on the cause of the failure and in part on the severity of the cardiac damage. Failure can result from an increase in the requirement for blood flow, as in patients with anemia or left-to-right shunts; from an increase in the impedance to flow, as in patients with hypertension or valvular stenosis; or from a decrease in the capacity of the heart to do work, as in patients with coronary artery disease. In the first two cases, digitalis might exert a strong positive inotropic effect but still not restore the circulation to normal. In the third case, even with a maximal inotropic effect, the performance of the heart may be limited. Since it seems that toxic effects of digitalis on the heart are more likely if the heart is severely damaged, it is important to estimate the degree of improvement in the circulation that can be expected from an optimal concentration of drug in plasma

and to recognize the need to correct abnormalities that increase the work required of the heart. Also, during maintenance therapy there may be changes in the condition of the patient that increase the concentration of digitalis in plasma or increase the sensitivity of the heart to its therapeutic or toxic effects (*see* below); usually it is desirable to use the lowest maintenance dose that provides the desired results.

Digitalis is particularly useful in patients with heart failure that results from an absolute or relative chronic overload (such as that caused by hypertension, valvular lesions, or atherosclerotic heart disease). Digitalis may not be of value in thyrotoxicosis, hypoxia, and severe thiamine deficiency. Experimental failure caused by poisons that reduce high-energy phosphate stores (cyanide, azide, dinitrophenol, *etc.*) is not relieved by digitalis.

Once digitalis has restored compensation, its continued use has traditionally been thought to prevent the recurrence of heart failure. Usually digitalis is given chronically to patients with diminished cardiac reserve who previously have experienced an episode of failure, even though they are subsequently free of symptoms (unless the cause of failure has been eliminated). In forms of reversible heart disease, such as that associated with infections, anemia, thyrotoxicosis, thiamine deficiency, and arteriovenous fistula, correction of the underlying disease is of greater import than the administration of digitalis. Poor response to digitalis is to be expected in cases of active rheumatic and other forms of infectious or toxic myocarditis, and in advanced cardiomyopathy. When shock and congestive failure exist together, as they may after myocardial infarction, digitalis may be indicated for therapy of the failure, in conjunction with drugs that decrease afterload. In the final analysis, improvement of cardiac function by digitalis depends on the cardiac reserve. In badly damaged hearts digitalis cannot provide much benefit.

There are two major clinical problems associated with the use of diuretics to treat congestive heart failure. Many decrease total body stores of potassium, and this increases the likelihood of digitalis toxicity (*see* below). Furthermore, potent diuretics can cause such a large decrease in circulating blood volume that end-diastolic ventricular pressure may decrease markedly. If the heart requires an elevated filling pressure to perform its external work, this may increase the severity of failure (*see* Figure 30–5). A similar problem may result from the use of vasodilators that decrease preload excessively.

Use of Digitalis to Prevent Heart Failure. Numerous studies have shown improved cardiac function in subjects with heart disease without overt clinical evidence of failure (Selzer and Malmborg, 1962). Also, it is possible that digitalization can decrease the rate of progression of cardiac damage in patients in whom the requirement for cardiac work, in relation to the work capacity of the heart, is such that a progressive increase in end-diastolic pressure and volume will occur. This may be particularly important in patients with inadequate coronary flow in whom the increase in ventricular volume and wall tension will decrease perfusion but increase the need for such perfusion. In all patients, if an increase in heart rate is needed to compensate for a diminished stroke volume, the energy requirement of the heart will be increased. Finally, it seems likely that marked overdistention of the ventricles causes structural changes that subsequently are not fully reversed by digitalization.

Atrial Fibrillation. Even in the absence of congestive heart failure, digitalis is indicated in many cases of atrial fibrillation (*see* below). The inappropriately rapid ventricular rate in this disorder results in palpitation that may cause great discomfort, and a reduction in cardiac work capacity that may lead to heart failure. The aim of digitalis therapy in patients with atrial fibrillation is to reduce the ventricular rate. The mechanism of ventricular slowing by digitalis in this disorder has been discussed. The fibrillation is rarely halted by digitalis, and the drug should not be employed with this objective. The dosage should be adjusted to maintain the ventricular rate in the range of 60 to 80 per minute at rest, and not to exceed 100 with moderate exercise. If digitalis fails to cause a sufficient decrease in ventricular rate, verapamil or a β-adrenergic blocking drug such as propranolol may also be used (*see* Chapter 31). Digitalis occasionally may be indicated as a prophylactic agent in patients in whom atrial fibrillation is likely.

Atrial Flutter. Digitalis can be used to manage atrial flutter. The primary effect of the drug is to increase the ERP of the A-V node. This almost always decreases the ventricular rate by increasing the degree of A-V block. Furthermore, digitalis prevents sudden increases in ventricular rate when exercise, excitement, or other factors decrease vagal and enhance sympathetic effects on A-V transmission. Digitalis can terminate atrial flutter. However, quite large doses are usually required, and cardioversion is preferable. Digitalis also may convert atrial flutter to fibrillation, and this, too, facilitates control of ventricular rate. Finally, if such conversion to fibrillation occurs, withdrawal of digitalis may result in the return of sinus rhythm. The change from flutter to fibrillation and the conversion to normal sinus rhythm probably result from digitalis-induced changes in vagal effects. If digitalis is used prior to attempts to convert atrial flutter to sinus rhythm with quinidine, there is an increased risk of digitalis toxicity (*see* below and Chapter 31).

Paroxysmal Tachycardia. Atrial and A-V nodal paroxysmal tachycardia are the most common tachyarrhythmias next to atrial fibrillation. Attacks are often abruptly terminated by measures that enhance vagal activity. Digitalis is often successful, probably by virtue of reflex vagal stimulation; intravenous administration of a rapidly acting preparation may be required. It should be remembered that *paroxysmal supraventricular tachycardia with partial A-V block may be a result of serious intoxication with digitalis.* It is extremely important to be

certain of the diagnosis and etiology of the tachyarrhythmia before digitalis is used.

Effects in Patients with the Sick Sinus Syndrome (Sinoatrial Dysfunction). In dogs, digoxin slows conduction into and out of the sinus node, increases the sinus escape interval after overdrive, and increases the likelihood of sinus node reentry. In man, however, digoxin decreases corrected sinus node recovery times and does not decrease sinus rate (Reiffel *et al.,* 1979). These findings suggest that digoxin does not have an adverse effect on the function of the sinus node in patients with the sick sinus syndrome. On the other hand, there has been one report (Margolis *et al.,* 1975) of severe toxicity in this condition. It would seem appropriate, if digitalization of such patients is required, to evaluate the effects of digitalis either by electrophysiological testing or by careful clinical monitoring.

Anomalous Atrioventricular Pathway. In patients with an anomalous A-V pathway, digitalis should *not* be used to treat atrial fibrillation unless it has been proven that digitalis will not increase the ventricular rate during fibrillation by shortening the ERP of the accessory pathway.

DIGITALIS INTOXICATION

Withering recognized many of the signs of digitalis toxicity: "The foxglove when given in very large and quickly repeated doses, occasions sickness, vomiting, purging, giddiness, confused vision, objects appearing green or yellow; increased secretion of urine, with frequent motions to part with it; slow pulse, even as low as 35 in a minute, cold sweats, convulsions, syncope, death."

Toxic effects of digitalis are frequent and can be severe or lethal. The overall incidence of digitalis toxicity is not certain, but estimates have been made for some populations (Beller *et al.,* 1971; Smith, 1975); approximately 25% of hospitalized patients taking digitalis show some signs of toxicity. The single most frequent cause of intoxication with digitalis is the concurrent administration of diuretics that cause potassium depletion. As might be expected from the mode of action of digitalis, the manifestations of toxicity are varied and can involve most organ systems in the body. The most important toxic effects, in terms of risk to the patient, are those that involve the heart. If unrecognized or improperly treated, such reactions frequently are fatal.

Digitalis is one of the most commonly prescribed drugs, and the number of patients for whom it is prescribed will increase as the proportion of older individuals in the population increases. Furthermore, all digitalis preparations have comparably low margins of safety and all can cause similarly severe toxic reactions. This is to be expected in view of their mechanism of action. The only difference among preparations is the duration of toxicity; for preparations that are more rapidly eliminated, the duration of toxicity will be comparatively short. *Because digitalis intoxication can be fatal and because it occurs frequently, physicians must exercise every precaution in prescribing digitalis; patients should be monitored carefully. Physicians must be familiar with the early signs of toxicity, the conditions or drugs likely to bring it about, and the means to treat intoxication. Patients should be educated about these matters as much as is deemed possible.*

Toxic Effects on the Heart. There is little evidence that excessive amounts of digitalis in patients have direct, deleterious effects on the mechanical activity of the heart. Concentrations in blood that are associated with toxicity typically cause abnormalities of cardiac rhythm and disturbances of A-V conduction, including complete A-V block. Ordinarily, abnormalities of conduction in the ventricular specialized conducting system and in the ventricles are not seen and, thus, digitalis does not directly prolong the QRS complex. Very high concentrations of the drug may impair conduction in the atria and prolong the P wave.

It is important to realize that all disturbances of rhythm associated with high concentrations of digitalis in plasma or tissues are *not* necessarily manifestations of digitalis toxicity and that low concentrations of the drug in plasma do not preclude the possibility of drug-induced arrhythmias or other toxicity. The concentrations measured in plasma serve only as crude, although useful, guides to the likelihood of efficacy and toxicity. Digitalis is used to treat patients with diseased hearts, and such hearts are likely to develop arrhythmias and conduction abnormalities. For example, an increase in the severity of heart failure often itself is a cause of atrial or ventricular arrhythmias. The demonstration that digitalis is the cause of such an arrhythmia or conduction abnormality depends on noting the response when administration of the drug is stopped, evaluation of the ECG, and measurement of the concentration of digitalis in plasma (Smith, 1975). In some instances, measurement of salivary Ca^{2+} and K^+ concentration may be of help (Wotman *et al.,* 1971).

Although digitalis toxicity can mimic almost any arrhythmia or disturbance of conduction, certain abnormalities are of special importance (Bigger, 1972; Bigger and Strauss, 1972). Digitalis can cause marked *sinus bradycardia* and can also bring about *complete S-A block.* Both abnormalities probably result from a combination of enhanced vagal effects, a decreased sympathetic influence, and the direct effects of the drug. The likelihood is greater in patients with disease involving the sinus node. Toxicity can also be manifested as *disturbances of atrial rhythm,* including premature depolarizations and paroxysmal and nonparoxysmal supraventricular tachycardias. These arrhythmias are most likely caused by delayed afterdepolarizations or by reentrant excitation due to depressed conduction in the A-V and S-A nodes, but enhancement of automaticity by digitalis is also a possible mechanism. Sufficiently precise tests are not yet available to identify each mechanism in patients.

The effects of digitalis on the *A-V junction* are important in relation to both its therapeutic and toxic effects. Toxicity is manifested by *high levels of A-V block* and by the appearance of *accelerated A-V junctional rhythms;* the most typical disturbances appear as either escape beats or as a nonparoxysmal *A-V junctional tachycardia.* This arrhythmia is almost always due to digitalis but occasionally can be caused by acute inferior myocardial infarction or acute myocarditis. The development of A-V block is due in part to the vagal effects of digitalis and sometimes can be overcome by atropine; at other times the depression of A-V conduction almost certainly results from the direct effect of digitalis on the A-V node, perhaps intensified by its antiadrenergic action.

The accelerated rhythms originating in the A-V junction usually have been assumed to result from enhanced phase-4 depolarization, but more recent studies support delayed afterdepolarizations as a cause of some types of escape beats (Rosen *et al.*, 1980). An A-V junctional tachycardia caused by toxic levels of digitalis may be quite difficult to recognize in patients with atrial fibrillation.

The *disturbances of ventricular rhythm* most frequently caused by digitalis are *premature depolarizations* that appear as coupled beats (bigeminy, trigeminy); these arrhythmias are not specific for digitalis. Digitalis toxicity also can cause *ventricular tachycardia* and *ventricular fibrillation*. The premature depolarizations usually are not caused by increased automaticity; some very likely are due to reentry and some to delayed afterdepolarizations. Persistent ventricular tachycardia probably results from increased automaticity of Purkinje fibers.

As mentioned above, digitalis decreases the ERP of human ventricular muscle but not that of the His-Purkinje system; it thus increases the interval during which reentrant excitation can be elicited (Gomes *et al.*, 1978). In addition, it has been shown in experiments on dogs that certain disturbances of rhythm caused by digitalis respond to alterations in the dominant heart rate and rhythm in a manner that suggests they are due to delayed afterdepolarizations (Wittenberg *et al.*, 1972). This makes it difficult to identify the mechanisms responsible for ventricular arrhythmias caused by digitalis. Sometimes, when digitalis causes a ventricular tachycardia, the polarity of the major QRS deflection in the ECG reverses for alternate complexes. This so-called *bidirectional tachycardia* once was thought to be a certain indication of excessive digitalis; however, the same ECG abnormality can be caused by other factors. The alternation in QRS polarity probably results from alternate excitation of the ventricles over one and then the other bundle branch.

Two further points about cardiac toxicity are of particular importance. First, the *likelihood* and probably also the *severity* of the arrhythmia are directly related to the severity of the underlying heart disease. If subjects with normal hearts ingest large but not lethal quantities of digitalis, either in an attempt at suicide or by accident, premature impulses and rapid arrhythmias are infrequent. The only typical findings are sinus

bradycardia and A-V block. These disturbances probably result in large part from the marked increase in the concentration of potassium in plasma that is caused by severe, acute intoxication with digitalis. Second, infants and children seem to tolerate higher concentrations of digitalis in their plasma and myocardium than do adults. Studies on preparations isolated from canine hearts indicate that this results, at least in part, from real differences in sensitivity of the young specialized fibers to toxic effects of digitalis (Rosen *et al.*, 1975a). Also, the volume of distribution and the half-time for elimination of digitalis may be age dependent (Glantz *et al.*, 1976; Berman *et al.*, 1977).

Other Untoward Effects. *Gastrointestinal Effects.* *Anorexia, nausea,* and *vomiting* are among the earliest evidences of digitalis overdosage if digitalis leaf is used. Anorexia is most common with digoxin, and this symptom is easily missed in the elderly or depressed patient. Vomiting may occasionally develop without preliminary anorexia or nausea. Nausea and vomiting may be transitory or entirely absent in some patients. *Diarrhea* may also be noted, and in rare cases it is the only gastrointestinal manifestation of digitalis toxicity. *Abdominal discomfort* or *pain* often accompanies the gastrointestinal symptoms. Once the drug is stopped, gastrointestinal symptoms disappear in a few days. The nausea and vomiting are due primarily to a direct action of digitalis to excite the chemoreceptor trigger zone (CTZ) in the area postrema of the medulla (*see* Borison and Wang, 1953) rather than to a direct irritant effect on the gastrointestinal tract, although the latter may be important when digitalis leaf is employed.

Neurological Effects. *Headache, fatigue, malaise,* and *drowsiness* are common symptoms and can occur early in the course of digitalis intoxication; generalized muscle weakness and easy fatigability may be particularly prominent. *Neuralgic pain,* usually involving the lower third of the face and simulating trigeminal neuralgia, may be the earliest, most severe, and even the sole manifestation of digitalis intoxication; the extremities and lumbar area may also be involved, and paresthesias often accompany the pain. *Mental symptoms* include disorientation, confusion, aphasia, and even delirium and hallucinations ("digitalis delirium"); rarely, *convulsions* have occurred. Neuropsychiatric effects are especially likely to develop in elderly patients with atherosclerotic disease. The exact role played by digitalis is uncertain.

Vision. Vision is often blurred. White borders or halos may appear on dark objects ("white vision"), and objects may appear frosted. Color vision can be disturbed; chromatopsia is most common for yellow and green, but less frequently red, brown, and blue vision can occur. Transitory amblyopia, diplopia, and scotomata may also ensue. It has also been reported that digitalis can affect the papillomacular fibers of the optic nerve and cause retrobulbar neuritis. In an epidemic of accidental digitoxin intoxication, 95% of 179 patients complained of visual disturbances; 95% complained of extreme fatigue and weakness. ECG signs considered characteristic of digitalis poisoning were observed in 70% of the subjects (Lely and Enter, 1970).

Other Effects. *Gynecomastia* may be induced in men by digitalis therapy; it has been suggested that the drug, on the basis of its chemical similarity to the sex hormones, may exert estrogenic activity in certain cases.

Factors Influencing the Likelihood of Toxicity. The most *obvious* cause of digitalis toxicity is the ingestion of too large a maintenance dose. The most *frequent* cause is concurrent administration of a diuretic that decreases body stores of potassium. Overdosage may result from the physician's decision, from the fact that the patient has independently increased the dose, or from improved absorption of the drug. The last-named cause might result from a change to a formulation with greater bioavailability. A decreased rate of elimination also could increase the concentration of drug in plasma to the toxic range. For digoxin, this can result from a decrease in renal function. Even quite marked abnormalities of hepatic function do not significantly decrease the metabolism of digitoxin. However, since one metabolite of digitoxin is digoxin, changes in renal elimination of the latter might contribute to toxicity when a patient is taking digitoxin.

Many factors are important in modifying the sensitivity of the heart to digitalis. A decrease in the plasma concentration of potassium is perhaps the most important cause of toxicity because many patients with congestive heart failure receive diuretics. Dialysis also can result in depletion of potassium. An abnormally high concentration of calcium in plasma can also contribute to toxicity. This could result from prolonged bed rest, myeloma, or parathyroid disease. A low concentration of magnesium in plasma has effects similar to those of high calcium. This change might result from diuretic therapy or dialysis. Hypothyroidism increases the likelihood of toxicity because elimination of digitalis is depressed and because in this condition the heart is more sensitive to cardiac glycosides. Conversely, hyperthyroid patients may require larger doses of digitalis to achieve a therapeutic effect. If hyperkalemia occurs in a patient taking maintenance doses of digitalis, complete A-V block may result.

Increased activity of the sympathetic nervous system (Gillis and Quest, 1980) and a number of pharmacological agents can increase the likelihood of arrhythmias due to digitalis intoxication; the latter are discussed in a subsequent section. In some patients, intestinal microorganisms convert much of ingested digoxin to an inactive metabolite, 2-hydroxydigoxin. If these patients take an antibiotic that suppresses the intestinal flora, the amount of parent drug absorbed will increase and may cause toxicity (Lindenbaum *et al.*, 1981).

It is important to remember that almost any worsening of the condition of the heart or circulation may increase the sensitivity of the heart to toxic actions of digitalis. Cardiac ischemia has this effect, as does an increase in the severity of congestive heart failure. With ischemia, there will very likely be a decrease in availability of chemical energy, and this can further depress the Na^+,K^+ pump. With severe impairment of ventilation or circulation there will be hypoxia and acidosis. The latter certainly contributes to toxicity, since a decrease in pH, like an increase in $[Ca^{2+}]_o$, depresses the Na^+,K^+ pump in cardiac tissues. With severe circulatory impairment, renal perfusion may be depressed. In addition, there likely will be an increase in heart rate in spite of the action of digitalis. The increase in rate can intensify the effects of digitalis by increasing the requirement for the pump to transport cations. Finally, with severe heart failure there may be either an increase in sympathetic activity or additional depletion of cardiac stores of norepinephrine. Both changes might contribute to toxicity.

Advanced age almost always decreases the required maintenance dose of digitalis, and, as suggested above, infants and children often require larger doses than would be estimated from body size. In contrast, premature infants may be unusually sensitive to digitalis. During the first 24 to 48 hours after the onset of myocardial infarction there may be an increased likelihood of toxic effects on rhythm and conduction.

Diagnosis of Digitalis Intoxication. Digitalis is often used in situations in which the toxic effects of the drug are difficult to distinguish from the effects of cardiac disease. The diagnostic problem arises most frequently with the hospital admission of a patient with serious arrhythmia and congestive failure from whom a history of recent digitalis therapy cannot be elicited. Administration of a loading dose of a cardiac glycoside to such a patient obviously could be lethal if the arrhythmia were caused by digitalis. Means to diagnose latent or overt toxicity have been suggested but not widely adopted. Introduction of a single electrical stimulus to the ventricles after the end of the T wave causes repetitive ventricular responses in patients who are marginally toxic (Lown *et al.*, 1967). The intravenous administration of edrophonium will cause A-V block and the appearance of ventricular premature depolarizations in patients on the verge of overt toxicity. However, these tests are not without risk.

The concentration of digitalis glycosides in plasma can be measured with specific radioimmunoassays, and this will show if digitalis has been taken and, if it has, whether the concentration is in a therapeutic or toxic range. However, these ranges overlap. *Careful and judicious clinical appraisal is still the most important diagnostic tool* (Smith, 1975).

Treatment of Digitalis Intoxication. The treatment of digitalis toxicity is almost always successful if appropriate means are used (Bigger and Strauss, 1972; Smith and Haber, 1973; Smith, 1975; Williams and Fisch, 1983). Thus, it is vitally important to make the correct diagnosis. The patient should be admitted to an intensive care unit and the ECG monitored. No additional digitalis should be given. Diuretics that cause potassium depletion should be withheld. If severe arrhythmias are present, additional treatment is needed. Phenytoin, lidocaine, and potassium salts are the most effective agents. Administration of K^+, either orally or intravenously, decreases the binding of

digitalis to the heart and directly antagonizes certain cardiotoxic effects of the glycoside. If intravenous infusions are utilized, the ECG must be monitored frequently. It is essential, in addition, to measure the concentration of K^+ in plasma before and during the administration of potassium. If this value is low or normal, an increase will usually suppress many ectopic beats and abnormal rhythms caused by digitalis and improve depressed A-V conduction. In contrast, if the initial concentration of potassium in plasma is high, a further increase will *intensify* A-V block and depress the automaticity of ventricular pacemakers. *The result may be complete A-V block and cardiac arrest.* Potassium is contraindicated if A-V block is severe.

Among the antiarrhythmic drugs, *phenytoin* and *lidocaine* are quite effective in suppressing *ventricular arrhythmias* caused by digitalis (*see* Chapter 31). Phenytoin is also effective for the treatment of *atrial arrhythmias* caused by digitalis. The other antiarrhythmic drugs (quinidine, procainamide, propranolol) are effective at times but are associated with a higher probability of producing new arrhythmias. In addition, quinidine can increase the concentration of digitalis in plasma (*see* below). *Atropine* will sometimes diminish sinus bradycardia, S-A arrest, and second- or third-degree A-V block. The use of electrical countershock to treat arrhythmias in digitalized patients is hazardous, because it may cause severe conduction abnormalities and ventricular arrhythmias. If it must be used, the energy of the shock should be as low as possible.

When toxicity is extreme, as when a very large amount has been taken in an attempt at suicide, it is possible to treat the toxicity with antibodies to the glycoside (Smith *et al.*, 1982). Very high doses of digitalis cause a progressive increase in the plasma concentration of potassium that is uniformly lethal. This can be reversed by administration of Fab fragments of digitalis-specific antibody for digoxin or digitoxin. These fragments are not too likely to cause allergic reactions, and they bind digitalis effectively. Thus, they decrease the concentration of free drug available to interact with the heart cell membrane. The Fab fragments have a very high affinity for the glycoside. After they are given, the total concentration of glycoside in plasma rises markedly because of binding to the antibody, but the fraction of drug in the plasma that is free is reduced to extremely low levels. The Fab-digitalis complex is eliminated readily in the urine. This is particularly important in settings where toxicity is caused by digitoxin.

Drug Interactions. Recent investigations have revealed a potentially important interaction between digoxin and *quinidine* (*see* Bigger, 1982). The administration of quinidine results in an increase in the plasma concentration of the glycoside in over 90% of digitalized patients. The degree of change is proportional to the dose of quinidine; however, there is marked individual variation in the magnitude. While the rise in the concentration of digoxin in plasma may be as great as fourfold, the average change is twofold. The concentration of digoxin in plasma apparently starts to rise within 24 hours after initiation of the administration of quinidine and reaches a new steady state in about 4 days. Thereafter it remains elevated for as long as quinidine is administered, unless the dose of digoxin is reduced appropriately. The effect of quinidine may be due, in part, to the displacement of digoxin from binding sites in tissues. A decrease in the volume of distribution of digoxin has also been reported. In addition, renal clearance is reduced by 40 to 50% in most patients. It seems likely that, when digoxin and quinidine are administered concurrently, the effects of the cardiac glycoside on the heart and CNS are intensified and toxicity will result. The digitalized patient who receives quinidine should be followed closely with respect to changes in the ECG and, if possible, the concentration of digoxin in plasma in order to make an appropriate adjustment of dosage; it may be advisable to reduce the dose of digoxin in anticipation of such changes. A similar interaction may occur with digitoxin, although this has not been well documented. The use of antiarrhythmic drugs in conjunction with digitalis is further discussed in Chapter 31. In addition to quinidine, concentrations of digoxin in plasma are also increased by quinine, verapamil, and amiodarone.

Interactions between cardiac glycosides and *diuretics* have been discussed above. *Amphotericin B*, which can also cause hypokalemia, may similarly provoke manifestations of digitalis intoxication. Administration of *β-adrenergic agonists* or *succinylcholine* may increase the likelihood of arrhythmias in digitalized patients. Several other drugs, including nifedipine, spironolactone, amiloride, and triamterene, have been reported to decrease renal clearance of digoxin. Phenylbutazone, phenobarbital, phenytoin, rifampin, and other drugs that increase hepatic microsomal enzyme activity may speed the metabolism of digitoxin. Agents that impair the absorption or alter the elimination of digitalis glycosides are mentioned elsewhere (*see* Appendix III).

AMRINONE AND MILRINONE

These two bipyridine derivatives have shown some promise as positive inotropic agents (Farah and Alousi, 1978; Alousi *et al.*, 1981). They have the following structural formulas:

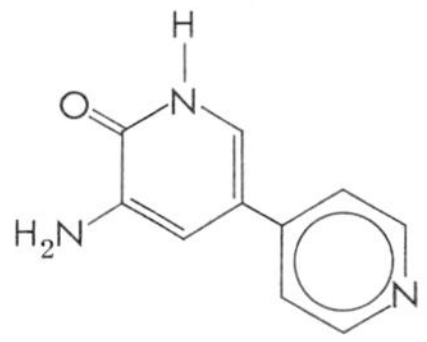

Amrinone

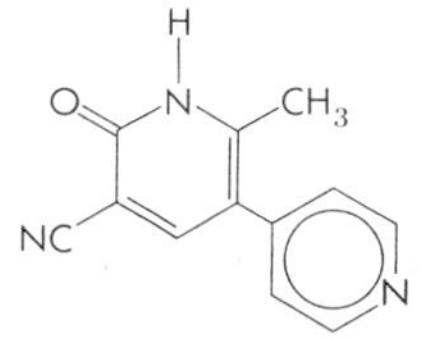

Milrinone

Both agents increase force of contraction and rate of shortening of cardiac muscle *in vitro;* milrinone is considerably more potent. Amrinone has no effects on transmembrane potentials of canine Purkinje fibers, but it augments slow responses. It is unlikely to cause afterdepolarizations but increases those caused by digitalis. Its inotropic effect appears to be age-dependent (Binah and Rosen, 1981) and may be associated with inhibition of a cyclic nucleotide phosphodiesterase (Endoh *et al.*, 1982). The positive inotropy is not prevented by α- or β-adrenergic blockade or by depletion of catecholamines, and it is not associated with inhibition of sarcolemmal Na^+,K^+-ATPase. Inotropic effects are additive to those of digitalis. Amrinone also relaxes vascular and tracheal smooth muscle. Both agents increase contractility of the normal canine heart *in situ* and cause a dose-dependent increase in heart rate and decrease in systemic vascular resistance. In experimental models of heart failure, both increase stroke volume, ejection fraction, and sinus rate, and both decrease systemic arterial pressure.

Amrinone has been evaluated in a number of patients with severe heart failure. It acts promptly after intravenous administration. When given orally, the peak effect is seen in 1 to 3 hours and the duration of action is 4 to 6 hours. When given to digitalized subjects in heart failure, amrinone increases cardiac index and stroke work index; decreases left ventricular end-diastolic pressure, wedge pressure, and systemic vascular resistance; and causes only minor changes in sinus rate and systemic arterial pressure. Exercise performance is increased, and benefits persist for weeks to months. Toxicity includes gastrointestinal intolerance, hepatotoxicity, fever, and reversible thrombocytopenia in 20% of patients. Amrinone has not been shown to be arrhythmogenic.

Amrinone has recently been approved for use in the United States for the short-term management of congestive heart failure. It is supplied as *amrinone lactate injection* (INOCOR) for intravenous administration. Therapy is initiated with a dose of 0.75 mg/kg given over 2 to 3 minutes, followed by a maintenance infusion of 5 to 10 μg/kg per minute. The recommended maximal daily dose is 10 mg/kg. Fluid balance, electrolyte concentrations, and renal function should be monitored carefully during treatment, and measurements of central venous pressure may also be useful. Milrinone is not yet available for general use in the United States.

During short trials in a limited number of patients, milrinone has also been shown to be effective in the treatment of severe heart failure by increasing cardiac contractility and decreasing systemic vascular resistance (Maskin *et al.*, 1983). Its actions are like those of amrinone, but it is better tolerated and seems not to cause thrombocytopenia.

Akera, T.; Larsen, F. S.; and Brody, T. M. Correlation of cardiac sodium- and potassium-activated adenosine triphosphatase activity with ouabain-induced inotropic stimulation. *J. Pharmacol. Exp. Ther.*, **1970**, *173*, 145–151.

Allen, D. G., and Blinks, J. R. Calcium transients in aequorin-injected frog cardiac muscle. *Nature*, **1978**, *273*, 509–513.

Alousi, A. A.; Helstosky, A.; Monenaro, M. J.; and Cicero, F. Intravenous and oral cardiotonic activity of WIN 47203, a potent amrinone analogue in dogs. *Fed. Proc.*, **1981**, *40*, 663.

Bailey, J. C.; Greenspan, K.; Elizari, M. V.; Anderson, G. J.; and Fisch, C. Effects of acetylcholine on automaticity and conduction in the proximal portion of the His-Purkinje specialized conduction system of the dog. *Circ. Res.*, **1972**, *30*, 210–216.

Bailey, J. C.; Watanabe, A. M.; Besch, H. R.; and Lathrop, D. A. Acetylcholine antagonism of the electrophysiological effects of isoproterenol on canine cardiac Purkinje fibers. *Circ. Res.*, **1979**, *44*, 378–383.

Beeler, G. W., and Reuter, H. The relationship between membrane potential, membrane currents and activation of contraction in ventricular myocardial fibers. *J. Physiol. (Lond.)*, **1970**, *207*, 211–229.

Beller, G. A.; Smith, T. W.; Abelman, W. H.; Haber, E.; and Hood, W. B., Jr. Digitalis intoxication. A prospective clinical study with serum level correlations. *N. Engl. J. Med.*, **1971**, *284*, 989–997.

Berman, W., Jr.; Ravenscroft, P. J.; Sheiner, L. B.; Hayman, M. A.; Melmon, K. L.; and Rudolph, A. M. Differential effects of digoxin at comparable concentrations in tissues of fetal and adult sheep. *Circ. Res.*, **1977**, *41*, 635–642.

Besch, H. R., Jr.; Allen, J. C.; Glick, G.; and Schwartz, A. Correlation between the inotropic action of ouabain and its effects on subcellular enzyme systems from canine myocardium. *J. Pharmacol. Exp. Ther.*, **1970**, *171*, 1–12.

Bigger, J. T., Jr., and Strauss, H. C. Digitalis toxicity: drug interactions promoting toxicity and the management of toxicity. *Semin. Drug Treat.*, **1972**, *2*, 147–177.

Binah, O., and Rosen, M. R. Developmental changes in the inotropic effects of amrinone. *Circulation*, **1981**, *64*, IV–22.

Braunwald, E.; Bloodwell, R. D.; Goldberg, L. I.; and Morrow, A. G. Studies on digitalis. IV. Observations in man on the effects of digitalis preparations on the contractility of the nonfailing heart and on total vascular resistance. *J. Clin. Invest.*, **1961**, *40*, 52–59.

Chai, C. Y.; Wang, H. H.; Hoffman, B. F.; and Wang, S. C. Mechanisms of bradycardia induced by digitalis substances. *Am. J. Physiol.*, **1967**, *212*, 26–34.

Cranefield, P. F.; Hoffman, B. F.; and Paes de Carvalho, A. Effects of acetylcholine on single fibers of the atrioventricular node. *Circ. Res.*, **1959**, *7*, 19–23.

Danilo, P.; Rosen, M. R.; and Hordof, A. J. Effects of acetylcholine on the ventricular specialized conducting system of neonatal and adult dogs. *Circ. Res.*, **1978**, *43*, 777–784.

Davis, L. D. Effect of changes in cycle length on diastolic depolarization produced by ouabain in canine Purkinje fibers. *Circ. Res.*, **1973**, *32*, 206–214.

Deitmer, J. W., and Ellis, D. The intracellular sodium activity of cardiac Purkinje fibers during inhibition and reactivation of the Na-K pump. *J. Physiol. (Lond.)*, **1978**, *284*, 241–259.

DeMello, W. C. Effect of intracellular injection of calcium and strontium on cell communication in heart. *J. Physiol. (Lond.)*, **1975**, *250*, 231–245.

Dhingra, R. C.; Amat-y-Leon, F.; Wyndham, C.; Wu, D.; Denes, P.; and Rosen, K. The electrophysiological effects of ouabain on sinus node and atrium in man. *J. Clin. Invest.*, **1975**, *56*, 555–562.

DiFrancesco, D. A new interpretation of the pace-maker current in calf Purkinje fibres. *J. Physiol. (Lond.)*, **1981**, *314*, 359–376.

Dresdale, P. T.; Yuceoglu, Y. Z.; Michton, R. J.; Schultz, M.; and Lunger, M. Effects of lanatoside C on cardiovascular hemodynamics—acute digitalizing doses in subjects with normal hearts and with heart disease without failure. *Am. J. Cardiol.*, **1959**, *4*, 88–99.

Eisner, D. A.; Lederer, W. J.; and Vaughan-Jones, R. D. The control of tonic tension by membrane potential and intracellular sodium activity in the sheep cardiac Purkinje fibre. *J. Physiol. (Lond.)*, **1983**, *335*, 723–743.

Endoh, M.; Yamashita, S.; and Taira, N. Positive inotropic effect of amrinone in relation to cyclic nucleotide metabolism in the canine ventricular muscle. *J. Pharmacol. Exp. Ther.*, **1982**, *221*, 775–783.

Erlij, D., and Mendez, R. The modification of digitalis intoxication by excluding adrenergic influences on the heart. *J. Pharmacol. Exp. Ther.*, **1964**, *144*, 97–103.

Fabiato, A., and Fabiato, F. Calcium release from the sarcoplasmic reticulum. *Circ. Res.*, **1977**, *40*, 119–129.

Farah, A. E., and Alousi, A. A. New cardiotonic agents: a search for a digitalis substitute. *Life Sci.*, **1978**, *22*, 1139–1148.

Farah, A. E., and Loomis, T. A. The action of cardiac glycosides on experimental auricular flutter. *Circulation*, **1950**, *2*, 742–748.

Ferrier, G. R. Effects of tension on acetylstrophanthidin-induced transient depolarizations and after-contractions in canine myocardial and Purkinje tissues. *Circ. Res.*, **1976**, *38*, 156–161.

Ferrier, G. R.; Saunders, J. H.; and Mendez, C.   A cellular mechanism for the generation of ventricular arrhythmias by acetylstrophanthidin. *Circ. Res.*, **1973**, *32*, 600–609.

Gadsby, D. C., and Cranefield, P. F.   Direct measurement of changes in sodium pump current in canine cardiac Purkinje fibers. *Proc. Natl. Acad. Sci. U.S.A.*, **1979**, *76*, 1783–1787.

Gadsby, D. C.; Wit, A. L.; and Cranefield, P. F.   The effects of acetylcholine on the electrical activity of canine cardiac Purkinje fibers. *Circ. Res.*, **1978**, *43*, 29–35.

Gervais, A.; Lane, L. K.; Annes, B. N.; Lindenmayer, G. E.; and Schwartz, A.   A possible molecular mechanism of action of digitalis: ouabain action on calcium binding to sites associated with a purified sodium-potassium-activated adenosine triphosphatase from kidney. *Circ. Res.*, **1977**, *40*, 8–14.

Gheorghiade, M., and Beller, G. A.   Effects of discontinuing maintenance digoxin therapy in patients with ischemic heart disease and congestive heart failure in sinus rhythm. *Am. J. Cardiol.*, **1983**, *51*, 1243–1250.

Glantz, J. A.; Kernoff, R.; and Goldman, R. H.   Age-related changes in ouabain pharmacology: ouabain exhibits a different volume of distribution in adult and young dogs. *Circ. Res.*, **1976**, *39*, 407–414.

Gold, H., and Cattell, M.   Mechanism of digitalis action in abolishing heart failure. *Arch. Intern. Med.*, **1940**, *65*, 263–278.

Gomes, J. A. C.; Dhatt, M. S.; Akhtar, M.; Carambas, C. R.; Rubenson, D. S.; and Damato, A.   Effects of digitalis on ventricular myocardial and His-Purkinje refractoriness and reentry in man. *Am. J. Cardiol.*, **1978**, *42*, 931–939.

Goodman, D. J.; Rossen, R. M.; Cannom, D. S.; Rider, A. K.; and Harrison, D. C.   Effects of digoxin on atrioventricular conduction. Studies in patients with and without cardiac autonomic innervation. *Circulation*, **1975**, *51*, 251–256.

Hashimoto, K., and Moe, G. K.   Transient depolarizations induced by acetylstrophanthidin in specialized tissues of dog atrium and ventricle. *Circ. Res.*, **1973**, *32*, 618–624.

Hess, P., and Müller, P.   Extracellular versus intracellular digoxin action on bovine myocardium, using a digoxin antibody and intracellular glycoside application. *J. Physiol. (Lond.)*, **1982**, *322,*, 197–210.

Hordof, A. J.; Spotnitz, A.; Mary-Rabine, L.; Edie, R. N.; and Rosen, M. R.   The cellular electrophysiologic effects of digitalis on human atrial fibers. *Circulation*, **1978**, *57*, 223–229.

Horwitz, L. D.; Atkins, J. M.; and Saito, M.   Effects of digitalis on left ventricular function in exercising dogs. *Circ. Res.*, **1977**, *41*, 744–749.

Hougen, T. J., and Smith, T. W.   Inhibition of myocardial cation active transport by subtoxic doses of ouabain in the dog. *Circ. Res.*, **1978**, *42*, 856–863.

Isenberg, G., and Trautwein, W.   The effect of dihydroouabain and lithium ions on the outward current in cardiac Purkinje fibers. Evidence for electrogenicity of active transport. *Pfluegers Arch.*, **1974**, *350*, 41–54.

Kass, R. S.; Lederer, W. J.; Tsien, R. W.; and Weingart, R.   Role of calcium ions in transient inward currents and aftercontractions induced by strophanthidin in cardiac Purkinje fibers. *J. Physiol. (Lond.)*, **1978a**, *281*, 187–208.

Kass, R. S.; Tsien, R. W.; and Weingart, R.   Ionic basis of transient inward current induced by strophanthidin in cardiac Purkinje fibers. *J. Physiol. (Lond.)*, **1978b**, *281*, 209–226.

Kassebaum, D. G.   Electrophysiological effects of strophanthin in the heart. *J. Pharmacol. Exp. Ther.*, **1963**, *140*, 329–338.

Kline, R. P., and Kupersmith, J.   Effects of extracellular potassium accumulation and sodium pump activation on automatic canine Purkinje fibers. *J. Physiol. (Lond.)*, **1982**, *324*, 517–533.

Lederer, W. J., and Eisner, D. A.   The effects of sodium pump activity on the slow inward current in sheep cardiac Purkinje fibres. *Proc. R. Soc. Lond. [Biol.]*, **1982**, *214*, 249–262.

Lederer, W. J., and Tsien, R. W.   Transient inward current underlying arrhythmogenic effects of cardiotonic steroids in Purkinje fibers. *J. Physiol. (Lond.)*, **1976**, *263*, 73–100.

Lee, C. O., and Dagostino, M.   Effect of strophanthidin on intracellular Na ion activity and twitch tension of constantly driven canine cardiac Purkinje fibers. *Biophys. J.*, **1982**, *40*, 185–198.

Lee, D. C. S.; Johnson, R. A.; Bingham, J. B.; Leahy, M.; Dinsmore, R. E.; Goroll, A. H.; Newell, J. B.; Strauss, H. W.; and Haber, E.   Heart failure in outpatients: a randomized trial of digoxin versus placebo. *N. Engl. J. Med.*, **1982**, *306*, 699–705.

Lely, A. H., and Enter, C. H. J. van.   Large scale digitoxin intoxication. *Br. Med. J.*, **1970**, *3*, 737–740.

Levy, M. N.   Sympathetic-parasympathetic interactions in the heart. *Circ. Res.*, **1971**, *29*, 437–445.

Lindenbaum, J.; Mellow, M. H.; Blackstone, M. O.; and Butler, V. P., Jr.   Variability in biological availability of digoxin from four preparations. *N. Engl. J. Med.*, **1971**, *285*, 1344–1347.

Lindenbaum, J.; Rund, D. G.; Butler, V. P.; Tse-Eng, D.; and Saha, J. R.   Inactivation of digoxin by the gut flora: reversal by antibiotic therapy. *N. Engl. J. Med.*, **1981**, *305*, 789–794.

Lown, B.; Cannon, R. L.; and Rossi, M. A.   Electrical stimulation and digitalis drugs: repetitive response in diastole. *Proc. Soc. Exp. Biol. Med.*, **1967**, *126*, 698–701.

McRitchie, R. J., and Vatner, S. F.   The role of the arterial baroceptors in mediating cardiovascular responses to cardiac glycosides in conscious dogs. *Circ. Res.*, **1976**, *38*, 321–326.

Marban, E., and Tsien, R. W.   Enhancement of calcium current during digitalis inotropy in mammalian heart: positive feed-back regulation by intracellular calcium? *J. Physiol. (Lond.)*, **1982**, *329*, 589–614.

Margolis, J. R.; Strauss, H. C.; Miller, H. C.; Gilbert, M.; and Wallace, A. G.   Digitalis and the sick sinus syndrome: clinical and electrophysiologic documentation of a severe toxic effect on sinus node function. *Circulation*, **1975**, *52*, 162–169.

Maskin, C. S.; Sinoway, L.; Chadwick, B.; Sonnenblick, E. H.; and LeJemtel, T. H.   Sustained hemodynamic and clinical effects of a new cardiotonic agent, WIN 47203, in patients with severe congestive heart failure. *Circulation*, **1983**, *67*, 1065–1070.

Mason, D. T.   Regulation of cardiac performance in clinical heart disease: interactions between contractile state mechanical abnormalities and ventricular compensatory mechanisms. *Am. J. Cardiol.*, **1973**, *32*, 437–448.

Mason, D. T., and Braunwald, E.   Studies on digitalis. X. Effects of ouabain on forearm vascular resistance and venous tone in normal subjects and in patients with heart failure. *J. Clin. Invest.*, **1964**, *43*, 532–543.

Mason, D. T.; Spann, J. F., Jr.; and Zelis, R.   New developments in the understanding of the actions of the digitalis glycosides. *Prog. Cardiovasc. Dis.*, **1969**, *11*, 443–478.

Mendez, C., and Mendez, R.   The action of cardiac glycosides on the excitability and conduction velocity of the mammalian atrium. *J. Pharmacol. Exp. Ther.*, **1957**, *121*, 402–413.

Miura, D. S., and Rosen, M. R.   The effects of ouabain on the transmembrane potentials and intracellular potassium activity of canine cardiac Purkinje fibers. *Circ. Res.*, **1978**, *42*, 333–338.

Moe, G. K., and Mendez, R. The action of several cardiac glycosides on conduction velocity and ventricular excitability in the dog heart. *Circulation*, **1951**, *4*, 729–734.

Mudge, G. H.; Lloyd, B. L.; Greenblatt, D. J.; and Smith, T. W. Inotropic and toxic effects of a polar cardiac glycoside derivative in the dog. *Circ. Res.*, **1978**, *43*, 847–854.

Müller, P. Ouabain effects on cardiac contraction, action potential and cellular potassium. *Circ. Res.*, **1965**, *17*, 46–56.

Mullins, L. J. The generation of electric currents in cardiac fibers by Na/Ca exchange. *Am. J. Physiol.*, **1979**, *236*, C103–C110.

New York Heart Association Task Force on Digitalis Preparations. What should the practicing physician know about digoxin bioavailability and how will FDA action affect him? *Circulation*, **1974**, *49*, 399–400.

Pace, D. B., and Gillis, R. A. Neuroexcitatory effects of digoxin in the cat. *J. Pharmacol. Exp. Ther.*, **1976**, *199*, 583–600.

Peon, J.; Ferrier, G. R.; and Moe, G. K. The relationship of excitability to conduction velocity in canine Purkinje tissue. *Circ. Res.*, **1978**, *43*, 125–135.

Reiffel, J. A.; Bigger, J. T., Jr.; and Cramer, M. The effects of digoxin on sinus nodal function before and after vagal blockade in patients with sinus nodal dysfunction: a clue to the mechanisms of the action of digitalis on the sinus node. *Am. J. Cardiol.*, **1979**, *43*, 983–989.

Reuter, H., and Seitz, N. The dependence of calcium efflux from cardiac muscle on temperature and external ion composition. *J. Physiol. (Lond.)*, **1968**, *195*, 451–470.

Rosen, M. R.; Fisch, C.; Hoffman, B. F.; Danilo, P.; Lovelace, D. E.; and Knoebel, S. B. Can accelerated atrioventricular junctional escape rhythms be explained by delayed afterdepolarizations? *Am. J. Cardiol.*, **1980**, *45*, 1272–1284.

Rosen, M. R.; Gelband, H.; and Hoffman, B. F. Correlation between effects of ouabain on the canine electrocardiogram and transmembrane potentials of isolated Purkinje fibers. *Circ. Res.*, **1973a**, *47*, 65–72.

Rosen, M. R.; Gelband, H.; Merker, C.; and Hoffman, B. F. Mechanisms of digitalis toxicity: effects of ouabain on phase 4 of canine Purkinje fiber transmembrane potentials. *Circ. Res.*, **1973b**, *47*, 681–689.

Rosen, M. R.; Hordof, A. J.; Hodess, A. B.; Verosky, M.; and Vulliemoz, Y. Ouabain-induced changes in electrophysiologic properties of neonatal, young and adult canine cardiac Purkinje fibers. *J. Pharmacol. Exp. Ther.*, **1975a**, *194*, 255–263.

Rosen, M. R.; Wit, A. L.; and Hoffman, B. F. Electrophysiology and pharmacology of cardiac arrhythmias. IV. Cardiac antiarrhythmic and toxic effects of digitalis. *Am. Heart J.*, **1975b**, *89*, 391–399.

Saum, R. W.; Brown, A. M.; and Tuley, F. H. An electrogenic sodium pump and baroceptor function in normotensive and spontaneously hypertensive rats. *Circ. Res.*, **1976**, *39*, 497–505.

Schwartz, A. Is the cell membrane Na^+,K^+-ATPase enzyme system the pharmacological receptor for digitalis? *Circ. Res.*, **1976**, *39*, 2–7.

Sellers, T. D., Jr.; Bashore, T. M.; and Gallagher, J. J. Digitalis in the preexcitation syndrome: analysis during atrial fibrillation. *Circulation*, **1977**, *56*, 260–270.

Selzer, A.; Hultgren, H. N.; Ebnother, C. L.; Bradley, H. W.; and Stone, A. O. Effects of digoxin on the circulation in normal man. *Br. Heart J.*, **1959**, *21*, 335–342.

Selzer, A., and Malmborg, R. O. Hemodynamic effects of digoxin in latent cardiac failure. *Circulation*, **1962**, *25*, 695–702.

Smith, T. W. Digitalis toxicity: epidemiology and clinical use of serum concentration measurements. *Am. J. Med.*, **1975**, *58*, 470–476.

Smith, T. W.; Butler, V. P., Jr.; Haber, E.; Fozzard, H.; Marcus, F. I.; Bremner, F.; Schulman, I. C.; and Phillips, A. Treatment of life-threatening digitalis intoxication with digoxin-specific Fab antibody fragments. *N. Engl. J. Med.*, **1982**, *307*, 1357–1362.

Smith, T. W., and Haber, E. Medical progress: digitalis. *N. Engl. J. Med.*, **1973**, *289*, 945–952, 1010–1015, 1063–1072, 1125–1129.

Swain, H. H., and Weidner, C. L. A study of substances which alter intraventricular conduction in isolated dog heart. *J. Pharmacol. Exp. Ther.*, **1957**, *120*, 137–146.

Ten Eick, R. E., and Hoffman, B. F. Chronotropic effect of cardiac glycosides in cats, dogs and rabbits. *Circ. Res.*, **1969a**, *25*, 365–378.

———. The effect of digitalis on the excitability of autonomic nerves. *J. Pharmacol. Exp. Ther.*, **1969b**, *169*, 95–108.

Thames, M. D. Acetylstrophanthidin-induced reflex inhibition of canine renal sympathetic nerve activity mediated by cardiac receptors with vagal afferents. *Circ. Res.*, **1979**, *44*, 8–15.

Toda, N., and West, T. C. Influence of ouabain on cholinergic responses in the sinoatrial node. *J. Pharmacol. Exp. Ther.*, **1966**, *153*, 104–113.

Tse, W., and Han, J. Interaction of epinephrine and ouabain on automaticity of canine Purkinje fibers. *Circ. Res.*, **1978**, *34*, 777–782.

Vassalle, M.; Karis, J.; and Hoffman, B. F. Toxic effects of ouabain on Purkinje fibers and ventricular muscle fibers. *Am. J. Physiol.*, **1962**, *203*, 433–439.

Vick, R. L.; Kahn, J. B., Jr.; and Acheson, G. H. Effects of dihydrodigoxin and dihydrodigitoxin on the heart-lung preparation of the dog. *J. Pharmacol. Exp. Ther.*, **1957**, *121*, 330–339.

Weingart, R. The actions of ouabain on intercellular coupling and conduction velocity in mammalian ventricular muscle. *J. Physiol. (Lond.)*, **1977**, *264*, 341–365.

Weingart, R.; Kass, R. S.; and Tsien, R. W. Is digitalis inotropy associated with enhanced slow inward calcium current? *Nature*, **1978**, *273*, 389–392.

Wellens, H. J., and Durrer, D. Effect of digitalis on atrioventricular conduction and circus movement tachycardias in patients with Wolff-Parkinson-White syndrome. *Circulation*, **1973**, *47*, 1229–1233.

Wenckebach, K. F. Discussion on the effects of digitalis on the human heart. *Br. Med. J.*, **1910**, *2*, 1600–1605.

Wittenberg, S. M.; Gandel, P.; Hogan, P. M.; Kreuger, W.; and Klocke, F. J. Relationship of heart rate to ventricular automaticity in dogs during ouabain administration. *Circ. Res.*, **1972**, *30*, 167–176.

Wotman, S.; Bigger, J. T.; Mandel, I. D.; and Bartelstone, H. J. Salivary electrolytes in the detection of digitalis toxicity. *N. Engl. J. Med.*, **1971**, *285*, 871–876.

Wu, D.; Wyndham, C.; Amat-y-Leon, F.; Denes, P.; Dhingra, R.; and Rosen, K. The effects of ouabain on induction of atrioventricular nodal re-entrant paroxysmal supraventricular tachycardia. *Circulation*, **1975**, *52*, 201–207.

Monographs and Reviews

Bigger, J. T., Jr. Mechanisms of digitalis toxic arrhythmias and the clinical recognition of toxicity. In, *Controversies in Clinical Pharmacology and Drug Development.* (Palmer, W., ed.) Futura Publishing Co., Inc., Mount Kisco, N.Y., **1972**.

———. The quinidine-digoxin interaction. *Mod. Concepts Cardiovasc. Dis.*, **1982**, *51*, 73–78.

Blinks, J. R.; Wier, W. G.; Morgan, J. P.; and Hess, P. Regulation of intracellular $[Ca^{2+}]$ by cardiotonic drugs. In, *Advances in Pharmacology and Therapeutics II. Vol. 3, Cardio-Renal and Cell Pharmacology.*

(Xoshida, H.; Hagiwara, Y.; and Ebashi, S.; eds.) Pergamon Press, Ltd., Oxford, **1982**, pp. 205–216.

Borison, H. L., and Wang, S. C. Physiology and pharmacology of vomiting. *Pharmacol. Rev.*, **1953**, *5*, 193–230.

Chen, K. K., and Henderson, F. G. Pharmacology of sixty-four cardiac glycosides and aglycones. *J. Pharmacol. Exp. Ther.*, **1954**, *111*, 365–383.

Fieser, L. F., and Fieser, M. *Steroids*. Reinhold Publishing Corp., New York, **1959**.

Gillis, R. A., and Quest, J. A. The role of the central nervous system in the cardiovascular effects of digitalis. *Pharmacol. Rev.*, **1980**, *31*, 19–97.

Hoffman, B. F. The pharmacology of cardiac glycosides. In, *Cardiac Therapy.* (Rosen, M. R., and Hoffman, B. F., eds.) Martinus Nijhoff, Boston, **1983**, pp. 387–412.

Hoffman, B. F., and Singer, D. H. Effects of digitalis on electrical activity of cardiac fibers. *Prog. Cardiovasc. Dis.*, **1964**, *7*, 226–260.

Marshall, P. G. Steroids: cardiotonic glycosides and aglycones: toad poisons. In, *Rodd's Chemistry of Carbon Compounds*, 2nd ed., Vol. 2 D. (Coffey, S., ed.) Elsevier Publishing Co., Amsterdam, **1970**, pp. 360–421.

Noble, D. Mechanism of action of therapeutic levels of cardiac glycosides. *Cardiovasc. Res.*, **1980**, *14*, 495–514.

Rosen, M. R. Interactions of digitalis with the autonomic nervous system and their relationship to cardiac arrhythmias. In, *Disturbances in Neurogenic Control of the Circulation.* (Abboud, F.; Fozzard, H.; Gilmore, J.; and Reis, D.; eds.) American Physiological Society, Bethesda, **1981**, pp. 251–263.

Tamm, C. The stereochemistry of the glycosides in relation to biological activity. In, *Proceedings of the First International Pharmacological Meeting.* Vol. 3, *New Aspects of Cardiac Glycosides.* (Wilbrandt, W., and Lindgren, P., eds.) Pergamon Press, Ltd., Oxford, **1963**, pp. 11–26.

Trautwein, W. Generation and conduction of impulses in the heart as affected by drugs. *Pharmacol. Rev.*, **1963**, *15*, 277–332.

Weingart, R. Influence of cardiac glycosides on electrophysiologic processes. In, *Cardiac Glycosides,* Pt. 1. *Handbook of Experimental Pharmacology*, Vol. 56/1. Springer-Verlag, Berlin, **1981**, 221–254.

Williams, E. S., and Fisch, C. Treatment of cardiac failure. In, *Cardiac Therapy.* (Rosen, M. R., and Hoffman, B. F., eds.) Martinus Nijhoff, Boston, **1983**, pp. 453–480.

31 ANTIARRHYTHMIC DRUGS

J. Thomas Bigger, Jr., and Brian F. Hoffman

Drug therapy of cardiac arrhythmias is based on a complex group of considerations. First, knowledge of the mechanism, consequences, and natural history of the arrhythmia to be treated is enormously helpful. The response of an arrhythmia to drugs is as much a function of pathophysiological condition as it is of drug action. Second, a clear understanding of the pharmacology of the drugs to be used is needed. This includes detailed knowledge of drug action on the electrophysiological properties of normal and abnormal cardiac tissues, of their effects on the mechanical properties of the heart and vasculature, and of their interactions with the autonomic nervous system and their effects on other organ systems. Optimal therapy of disturbances of cardiac rhythm requires considerable knowledge of the pharmacokinetics of antiarrhythmic drugs and how these parameters are affected by disease. Finally, a broad knowledge of adverse effects of the agents and their potential interactions with other drugs is necessary to monitor the course of therapy.

CARDIAC ELECTROPHYSIOLOGY

Resting Potential. There is a voltage difference across the surface membrane of all cardiac cells, the *resting transmembrane voltage* or potential (*Vm*). For most cardiac cells, the resting transmembrane voltage is about −80 to −90 mV relative to the extracellular fluid. The resting transmembrane concentration gradients for ions such as Na$^+$ and K$^+$ are established by active transport. Typical values for concentrations of ions in myocardial cells (*i*) and in extracellular fluid (*o*) (in millimoles per liter of water) are: [K]$_o$ = 4.0, [K]$_i$ = 150, [Na]$_o$ = 140, and [Na]$_i$ = 30. If there were no voltage gradient across the membrane and the membrane were semipermeable to an ion, such as K$^+$, K$^+$ would have diffused out of the cell until the concentrations inside and outside were equal. However, the Na$^+$-K$^+$ exchange pump counteracts diffusional forces. In addition, fixed negative charges in the cell attract K$^+$ and counteract the concentration gradient that promotes diffusion (Noble, 1975). When these forces are equal, no net flux of ions will occur. The Nernst equation can be solved for the voltage that will maintain the existing transmembrane concentration gradient at a constant value—the equilibrium voltage, E_X, for an ion, X:

$$E_X = \frac{RT}{F} \ln \frac{[X]_o}{[X]_i}$$

where [X]$_o$ is the concentration of the ion in extracellular fluid, [X]$_i$ is the intracellular concentration, R is the gas constant, T is the absolute temperature, and F is the Faraday constant. Given the ion concentrations listed above, E_K = −97 mV and E_{Na} = +40 mV. Since the resting membrane is permeable primarily to K$^+$, the resting transmembrane voltage is close to E_K. However, other ions, such as Na$^+$, do make a small contribution to resting transmembrane voltage.

Action Potentials. When cardiac cells are excited, a complex sequence of voltage changes occurs as a function of time and voltage, due to changes in ionic conductances across the membrane. A typical transmembrane *action potential* of a Purkinje fiber is diagrammed in Figure 31–1, *A*. The action potential is divided into *phases* for purposes of description and discussion. Phase 0 = rapid depolarization and reversal of transmembrane voltage; phase 1 = rapid repolarization to the plateau level of voltage; phase 2 = long-sustained depolarized level or the plateau of the action potential; phase 3 = rapid repolarization to resting (diastolic) levels of transmembrane voltage; and phase 4 = the diastolic voltage time course. Many cells in the normal heart have action potentials that differ substantially from those of the Purkinje fiber. For example, action potentials of sinus and A-V nodal cells have a very slowly rising phase 0, and phases 1, 2, and 3 are not clearly distinguished from one another. Also, many cells have a steady transmembrane voltage during phase 4, whereas others show spontaneous depolarization during this period. Automatic fibers in the sinus node and His-Purkinje system reach a maximal negative value of *Vm* at the end of phase-3 repolarization. Then, these fibers may begin progressive spontaneous depolarization. If *Vm* achieves the critical *threshold voltage*, excitation occurs. The firing rate of a normally automatic cell is determined by: (1) the value of maximal diastolic voltage, (2) the slope of phase-4 depolarization, and (3) the value of the threshold voltage. When a cell or group of cells undergoes self-excitation by this process and initiates an impulse that propagates to the rest of the heart, it is known as a *pacemaker*. Although many fibers may

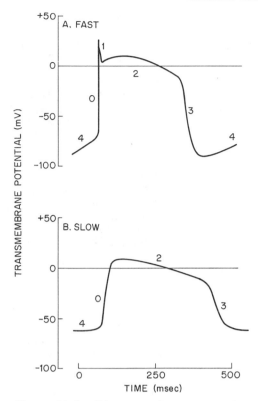

Figure 31–1. *Diagrammatic representation of fast and slow responses from mammalian cardiac Purkinje fibers.*

A. Fast Response. The phases of the normal fast response are shown: depolarization (*0*), repolarization (*1, 2, 3*), and the diastolic phase (*4*). Note the spontaneous phase-4 depolarization in this example. The rate of rise of phase 0 is rapid, and propagation will be rapid.

B. Slow Response. The slow response is initiated from a reduced (less negative) level of diastolic transmembrane voltage, shows slow depolarization, and has a long duration. Such an action potential propagates exceedingly slowly and leaves a long refractory wake.

undergo phase-4 depolarization, propagation of the cardiac impulse that originates in the sinus node will interrupt this process in most cells before they attain threshold; such cells are called *latent pacemakers*.

The ionic basis for the cardiac action potential is still a subject of debate and active study. Although the voltage clamp technic has revealed clearly the ionic basis of the action potential of nerve, there are serious technical problems in the application of this technic to cardiac muscle. It has been most successfully used in cardiac Purkinje fibers. Current concepts on the genesis of the cardiac action potential have been reviewed by Trautwein (1973), McAllister and associates (1975), and Noble (1975).

A summary of the important ionic currents is given in Table 31–1.

Phase 0. In most cardiac cells, phase 0 is generated by the movement of Na^+ through channels that selectively allow permeation of this ion; they are activated in a voltage-dependent manner when the propagating cardiac impulse or spontaneous phase-4 depolarization causes the so-called *m* gate in the channel to open. The inward Na^+ current, i_{Na}, is very intense but very brief; it is terminated by a process called *inactivation*—rapid closure of a hypothetical gate (the *h* gate) in the Na^+ channel. After inactivation, the Na^+ channel cannot be opened again until it is *reactivated* during and after phase-3 repolarization. Thus, the Na^+ channel can exist in one of three states: resting, active, or inactivated. A small fraction of the Na^+ channels may inactivate slowly or remain open during the plateau of the action potential, permitting a small residual Na^+ current to flow.

Phase 1. Quick repolarization to the plateau of the action potential is brought about by several factors: the passive electrical properties of Purkinje fibers; inactivation of i_{Na}; and activation of i_{qr}, a transient outward (K^+) current.

Phase 2. The plateau of the action potential is one of the most unusual characteristic features of the *cardiac* action potential. Membrane conductance is reduced during the plateau to values lower than those that obtain during diastole (phase 4). The Ca^{2+} or slow channel is activated during the plateau, which allows secondary inward current, i_{si}, to flow; i_{si} is inactivated in a manner analogous to the inactivation of i_{Na}, but the time constant for inactivation of i_{si} is much greater (50 milliseconds compared to 0.5 millisecond). Therefore, i_{si} declines slowly during the plateau.

Phase 3. A time-dependent outward current, i_{X_1}, plays an important role in terminating the plateau and causing the fiber to repolarize to normal diastolic values of *Vm*. This current is carried primarily by K^+, but also by another unspecified ion or ions. The i_{X_1} activates (*i.e.*, the X_1 channel opens) at about -40 mV, with a time constant of about 0.5 second. By the end of the plateau, i_{X_1} has waxed to a considerable value, while i_{si} has waned. Phase 3 is primarily the result of activated i_{X_1} in the presence of inactivating i_{si}. In the steady state, i_{X_1} is completely deactivated (*i.e.*, the X_1 channel is closed) at values of *Vm* more negative than -50 mV. This means that i_{X_1} deactivates quickly at the end of repolarization.

Phase 4. In many cells (*e.g.*, ordinary atrial or ventricular muscle), *Vm* is constant during diastole; these cells will rest indefinitely until activated by a propagating impulse or an external stimulus. However, as mentioned above, other cells exhibit spontaneous phase-4 depolarization and self-excitation (*see* Figure 31–1, *A*). This type of behavior is characteristic of the His-Purkinje system. Several ionic currents modulate normal automaticity: two time-independent currents—outward background current (i_{K_1}) and inward background current (i_{bi})—and a time-dependent current, the *pacemaker current* (which may be either i_{K_2} or i_f). Until recently, the time-dependent current was regarded as

Table 31–1. IONIC CURRENTS AND THE PURKINJE FIBER ACTION POTENTIAL

CURRENT	MAJOR ION RESPONSIBLE FOR THE CURRENT	PHASE OF ACTION POTENTIAL	REVERSAL VOLTAGE	DIRECTION OF CURRENT FLOW	PHYSIOLOGICAL ROLE
i_{Na}	Na^+	0	+40	Inward	Depolarizes fiber during phase 0
i_{qr}	K^+	1	? *	Outward	Rapid repolarization in phase 1; not present in ventricular muscle
i_{si}	Ca^{2+}	1, 2	+100	Inward	Contributes to plateau of action potential; triggers the release of internal Ca^{2+}
i_{X_1}	K^+, ?	3	−70	Outward	Repolarizes fiber during phase 3
i_{K_2}	K^+	4	−100	Outward	Deactivates, permitting spontaneous depolarization †
i_f	Na^+	4	?	Inward	Activates, promoting spontaneous depolarization †
i_{bi}	Na^+, Ca^{2+}	0, 1, 2, 3, 4	+40	Inward	Tends to depolarize fiber
i_{K_1}	K^+	0, 1, 2, 3, 4	−100	Outward	Tends to repolarize fiber

* While the reversal voltage is unknown, it is presumably more negative than −25 mV.

† There is controversy about whether the pacemaker current during phase 4 of the Purkinje fiber action potential is due to deactivation of a K^+ current (i_{K_2}) or to activation of an inward current (i_f).

an outward current, i_{K_2}, that is fully activated during the plateau of the action potential and is still almost fully activated at the beginning of phase 4. At diastolic values of Vm, i_{K_2} was thought to deactivate slowly (time constant of about 1 second). The progressive decrease in the outward current, i_{K_2}, during diastole was regarded as the cause of Purkinje fiber diastolic depolarization. However, there is recent evidence that the time-dependent current is an *inward* current, i_f, similar to the current responsible for pacemaker activity in the sinus node (DiFrancesco, 1981a). The i_f begins to activate when Vm falls below −50 mV and progressively activates during diastole to depolarize the fiber. The i_f is not a pure ionic current; Na^+ and K^+ both play a role in its genesis (DiFrancesco, 1981b). Electrogenic extrusion of Na^+ can be an important part of background outward current. Pacemaker activity in the sinus node may have an ionic mechanism that is similar to the i_f concept in Purkinje fibers (Brown and Noble, 1974; Noma and Irisawa, 1976; Brown and DiFrancesco, 1980). Background currents, i_{si}, and electrogenic Na^+ pumping also play a role in the automaticity of the sinus node. Spontaneous activity of sinus nodal cells is faster than that of Purkinje fibers because i_f activates at a faster rate.

Fast and Slow Responses. Cranefield and colleagues (1972) classified cardiac action potentials as *fast* and *slow* responses. Depolarization in the *fast response* (see Figure 31–1, *A*) is generated by an intense inward i_{Na}, has a large, fast-rising phase 0, propagates very rapidly, and has a large safety factor for conduction. Normal atrial, ventricular, and Purkinje fiber action potentials are examples of the fast response. The *slow response* has a slowly rising phase 0, propagates very slowly, and has a low safety factor for conduction (Figure 31–1, *B*). Action potentials of cells in the sinus node, pecti-

nate muscles, A-V node, and A-V rings are examples of slow responses seen under normal conditions. For a discussion of abnormal conditions that may generate slow responses, *see* the section on reentrant arrhythmias below.

Excitability and Refractoriness. *Excitability* is traditionally measured in terms of the strength of an electrical pulse required to excite the heart. The functional significance of changes in excitability is usually difficult to determine. Therefore, little emphasis is placed here on the effects of antiarrhythmic drugs on excitability. *Refractoriness* has been defined in many different ways; in this discussion, refractoriness is usually used to refer to the duration of the *effective refractory period* (ERP), which is the minimal interval between two propagating responses. In most cardiac cells the ERP is closely linked to action potential duration (APD), because recovery from inactivation of the Na^+ channel closely parallels repolarization. However, sinus and A-V nodal cells (slow responses) have strikingly different characteristics. In slow responses, refractoriness can outlast full repolarization, so that the ERP is much longer than the APD. Antiarrhythmic drugs prolong the ERP relative to APD in many types of cardiac cells.

A period often can be found during the latter part of repolarization when the threshold for electrical stimulation is less than the value found in diastole after full recovery; this period of *supernormal excitability* has been regarded as a paradoxical response. An explanation for supernormal excitability has been found for cardiac Purkinje fibers and may hold for some other types of cells as well. In Purkinje fibers, toward the end of repolarization, Vm is closer to the threshold voltage than it is after full repolarization. Therefore, a smaller electrical pulse can carry the membrane to threshold during phase-3 repolarization than would be required in diastole.

Responsiveness and Conduction. The term *membrane responsiveness* is used to describe the response of a cardiac fiber to a stimulus (*e.g.*, a propagating action potential or applied electrical pulse). Cardiac fibers do not regain their full ability to develop a normal response until repolarization is complete. Changes in the maximal rate of depolarization during phase 0 ($\dot{V}_{max}$) provide an index of changes in availability of the Na^+ conductance system or the degree of recovery from inactivation of the Na^+ channel. Phase-0 $\dot{V}_{max}$ is an important determinant of conduction velocity and block of premature impulses. In cardiac Purkinje fibers, the $\dot{V}_{max}$ of a response is very strongly dependent on Vm at the instant of excitation (*see* Figure 31–2). In normal fibers, the time constant for recovery from inactivation of the Na^+ channel is quite short, such that recovery of $\dot{V}_{max}$ is primarily a function of transmembrane voltage as repolarization occurs. Consequently, $\dot{V}_{max}$ is similar when a cardiac fiber is stimulated at a given level of Vm, regardless of whether the fiber is stimulated during phase-3 repolarization or during phase-4 depolarization. The time constant for recovery of Na^+ channels is significantly longer: (1) at low (more positive) values of Vm; (2) during treatment with antiarrhythmic

drugs; and (3) in membranes altered by disease. The S-shaped relationship between $\dot{V}_{max}$ and Vm (Figure 31–2) is typical not only of cardiac Purkinje fibers but also of atrial and ventricular muscle. Cells of the sinus node and the A-V node do not have this S-shaped relationship; like excitability, responsiveness does not return in nodal cells (slow responses) until well after repolarization is complete. There is a considerable safety factor in cardiac muscle (except in the S-A and A-V nodes), since $\dot{V}_{max}$ must be reduced to half or less of normal before conduction velocity decreases.

MECHANISMS RESPONSIBLE FOR CARDIAC ARRHYTHMIAS

An arrhythmia is an abnormality of rate, regularity, or site of origin of the cardiac impulse or a disturbance in conduction that causes an alteration in the normal sequence of activation of the atria and ventricles. Arrhythmias may arise because of alterations in impulse generation, impulse conduction, or both.

ARRHYTHMIAS DUE TO ABNORMALITIES OF IMPULSE GENERATION

There are many examples of arrhythmias that arise because of either enhancement or failure of normal automaticity. Mechanisms of abnormal automaticity are also subjects of ongoing experimental interest.

Altered Normal Automaticity. When considering arrhythmias due to abnormalities of automaticity, it is important to recall that only a few types of cardiac cells frequently develop normal automaticity: sinus node, distal A-V node, and the His-Purkinje system. Other cell types can develop automaticity as well, for example, specialized atrial fibers in the internodal tracts and fibers near the ostium of the coronary sinus (Wit and Cranefield, 1977).

Sinus Node. In the sinus node, rate can be altered by autonomic activity or intrinsic disease. Increased vagal activity can slow or stop sinus nodal pacemakers by increasing potassium conductance (g_K); this increases outward K^+ currents, hyperpolarizes the pacemaker cells, and slows or stops their depolarization. Increased sympathetic traffic to the sinus node increases the rate of phase-4 depolarization, probably by a combination of effects (*e.g.*, increased rate of activation of the pacemaker current, i_f; increased magnitude of i_{si}). Intrinsic disease of sinus nodal pacemaker cells seems to be responsible for faulty pacemaker activity in the sick sinus syndrome in man. The precise mechanism and pathogenesis are still unknown.

Purkinje Fibers. Augmented automaticity in the His-Purkinje system is a common cause of arrhythmias in human subjects. Increased sympathetic nerve activity can cause a substantial increase in the rate of spontaneous firing. This increase is brought about by an ionic mechanism that is similar to the changes causing sinus tachycardia. In cardiac Purkinje fibers, catecholamines enhance auto-

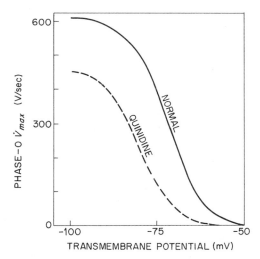

Figure 31–2. *Membrane responsiveness.*

Membrane responsiveness in a cardiac Purkinje fiber is depicted. The maximal rate of rise of depolarization during phase 0 is plotted as a function of transmembrane voltage at the time of activation. The solid line shows the relationship under normal conditions, and the dashed line depicts the effect of a moderate-to-high concentration of quinidine. Quinidine shifts the relationship on its voltage axis so that a reduced response is obtained at any given level of transmembrane voltage. Also, the maximal rate of depolarization is reduced.

maticity by increasing the rate of activation of i_f and shifting the voltage dependence for activation of i_f toward more positive (depolarized) values; current thus begins to flow earlier in the course of repolarization (phase 3) (Tsien, 1974; DiFrancesco, 1981a). The inward background current (i_{bi}), which flows in the diastolic voltage range, does not appear to be altered by catecholamines. It is possible for A-V junctional pacemakers to usurp control of the ventricles in the presence of a normal sinus node and normal A-V conduction. This could occur because of selectivity of traffic in sympathetic nerves (Randall, 1977) or increased release of catecholamines locally. Also, higher neural activity, including that associated with cardiovascular reflexes, alters cardiac rate and produces disturbances of rhythm primarily by changing the pattern of firing of various subunits of the cardiac autonomic nerves (Levitt *et al.*, 1976). The effect of the vagus on the His-Purkinje system in man is not well understood. The response of Purkinje fibers to acetylcholine varies with species; acetylcholine slows normal pacemaker activity in the dog but accelerates it in sheep. In addition, many questions about functional vagal innervation of the His-Purkinje system are unsettled; it appears that vagal innervation of the proximal system may be significant, whereas that of the peripheral system is more sparse (Levy, 1977). However, recent evidence suggests a significant physiological role for vagal activity in the ventricle.

In disease, automaticity in the His-Purkinje system may become reduced. In the sick sinus syndrome it is typical for the ventricular pacemakers to be depressed as well as the sinus node (*see* Bigger and Reiffel, 1979). Thus, very long pauses in cardiac rhythm may occur when the sinus node fails as a pacemaker. In A-V block due to widespread bundle-branch disease, the rate of ventricular pacemakers may also be abnormally slow. In neither of these examples has a mechanism been identified.

Abnormal Generation of Impulses. In addition to the arrhythmias caused by alterations of normal automaticity, numerous abnormal mechanisms for the generation of impulses have been observed in experimental preparations (Hoffman and Cranefield, 1960; Bigger, 1973; Cranefield, 1977). Many of these mechanisms appear to fit into one of two categories—abnormal automaticity or triggered activity. *Abnormal automaticity* is a term used to refer to spontaneous diastolic depolarization that occurs at a very low (relatively positive) value of Vm in a cell that normally has a much higher value of Vm in diastole. *Triggered activity* is the generation of impulses by afterdepolarizations that reach threshold (*see* below). Both of these mechanisms differ strikingly from those responsible for normal automaticity. Moreover, both of these mechanisms can cause the formation of impulses in fibers that ordinarily are incapable of automatic function (*e.g.*, ordinary atrial or ventricular muscle cells).
Abnormal Automaticity. Purkinje fibers, atrial cells, and ventricular cells can all show spontaneous diastolic depolarization and repetitive auto-

matic firing when their resting Vm is reduced substantially (*e.g.*, to -60 mV or less negative values). The ionic mechanisms for such abnormal automaticity are not known, but i_{X_1} and i_{si} may contribute to this behavior.
Early Afterdepolarizations. Early afterdepolarizations are secondary depolarizations that occur before repolarization is complete. Characteristically, the secondary depolarization commences at membrane potentials that are relatively close to those that obtain during the plateau of the action potential (*see* Figure 31–3, *A*). Often, a burst of depolarizations occurs followed by a few damped oscillations, until, finally, Vm either rests at the range of the plateau voltage (about -20 to -40 mV) or returns to a relatively high resting value. Experimentally, early afterdepolarizations have been produced in cardiac Purkinje fibers by a number of maneuvers, including stretching, hypoxia, and chemical alterations. Early afterdepolarizations are promoted by (and may result from) (1) decreased background outward current (i_{K_1}), (2) increased background inward current (i_{bi}), (3) increased residual i_{Na} during the plateau, (4) increased magnitude and/or duration of i_{si}, and (5) reduced magnitude of i_{X_1}. Cardiac Purkinje fibers

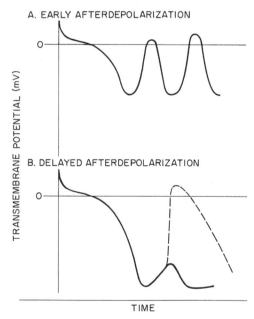

A. EARLY AFTERDEPOLARIZATION

B. DELAYED AFTERDEPOLARIZATION

TRANSMEMBRANE POTENTIAL (mV)

TIME

Figure 31–3. *Two forms of triggered activity in a cardiac Purkinje fiber.*

A. Early Afterdepolarization. Repolarization is interrupted by secondary depolarizations. Such responses may excite neighboring fibers and be propagated.
B. Delayed Afterdepolarization. After full repolarization is achieved, Vm again transiently depolarizes. If the delayed afterdepolarization reaches threshold, a propagating response can occur (dashed line).

tend to have two stable resting potentials, one at about -70 to -90 mV and another at -30 to -50 mV (Noble, 1975; Cranefield, 1977). Also, when the Vm of cardiac muscle fibers is in the range of the plateau voltage, the membrane conductance is low and tiny inward currents cause substantial depolarization.

Delayed Afterdepolarizations. A delayed afterdepolarization is a secondary depolarization occurring early in diastole, that is, after full repolarization has been achieved (*see* Figure 31–3, *B*). The delayed afterdepolarization is not self-initiated but is dependent on a prior action potential. Delayed afterdepolarizations may be seen when certain cell types are exposed to catecholamines (Wit and Cranefield, 1977), digitalis (Ferrier, 1977), low $[K]_o$ (Eisner and Lederer, 1979), or perfusates containing low $[Na]_o$ and high $[Ca]_o$ (Cranefield, 1977). Delayed afterdepolarizations can reach threshold and give rise to a single premature depolarization. If the premature depolarization is followed by a delayed afterdepolarization, a second impulse may result. In this way, delayed afterdepolarizations can cause either coupled extrasystoles or runs of tachyarrhythmias. A number of factors have been identified that tend to increase the amplitude of delayed afterdepolarizations, thus increasing the likelihood that they will reach threshold. They include increases in the basic driven or spontaneous rate, premature systoles, increased $[Ca]_o$, catecholamines, and other drugs, particularly digitalis. The mechanism for delayed afterdepolarizations that arise in digitalis toxicity is discussed at greater length in Chapter 30. Delayed afterdepolarizations can readily be induced by digitalis in the His-Purkinje system and, with more difficulty, in specialized atrial or ordinary ventricular cells (Ferrier, 1977). The delayed afterdepolarizations induced by digitalis in Purkinje fibers are associated with an abnormal transient inward current that is carried mainly by Na^+ (Lederer and Tsien, 1976). It is reasonable to speculate that some clinical arrhythmias caused by digitalis, for example, coupled ventricular premature depolarizations and atrial or ventricular tachycardias, result from delayed afterdepolarizations. Also, some supraventricular tachycardias that arise in the absence of drug therapy may be triggered activity that arises from delayed afterdepolarizations.

Triggered Arrhythmias. As mentioned, when a delayed afterdepolarization reaches threshold, a single extrasystole may result or sustained repetitive firing of the cell may be triggered. Activation by this mechanism must be initiated by an action potential; thus, it cannot arise *de novo,* as can a normal automatic rhythm. Although triggered activity cannot be self-initiated, it can be self-sustained. Triggered activity in cells that have delayed afterdepolarizations shares many characteristics that are often associated with reentrant tachyarrhythmias (*see* below). Both triggered activity and reentrant arrhythmias can be initiated by a single premature stimulus and may also be terminated by a single premature stimulus. These common characteristics make it difficult to assign a mechanism for a given clinical tachyarrhythmia. The attempt to

define mechanisms for arrhythmias in man becomes even more difficult when one considers that an action potential caused by normal automaticity may initiate triggered activity, or a single extrasystole caused by an afterdepolarization may initiate a reentrant rhythm.

ARRHYTHMIAS CAUSED BY ABNORMALITIES OF IMPULSE CONDUCTION

Arrhythmias may arise by *recirculating activation* that is incited by an initiating depolarization. Such arrhythmias (often referred to as *reentrant arrhythmias*), like triggered rhythms, are self-sustained but are not self-initiated. For reentry to be initiated, one-way block of conduction must occur, and there must be an anatomical or functional "barrier" to conduction that forms a circuit (Cranefield *et al.*, 1972; Bigger, 1973). Furthermore, the pathlength of the circuit must be greater than the wavelength of the cardiac impulse, where wavelength is the product of conduction velocity and the refractory period (*see* Figure 31–4). The principal difficulty in attributing cardiac arrhythmias to reentry is that, usually, the cardiac refractory period is very long, cardiac conduction is rapid, and the pathways available are reasonably

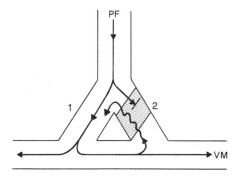

Figure 31–4. *Reentry.*

The diagram shows one of the forms of reentrant reexcitation in the ventricle (Schmitt and Erlanger, 1928–29). A branched Purkinje fiber *(PF)* terminates on a strip of ventricular muscle *(VM)*. The shaded area in branch 2 represents a depolarized area that is the site of a *one-way block;* thus, orthograde sinus impulses are blocked in this area, but retrograde responses are propagated successfully. Retrograde conduction in branch 2 is slow enough for cells in branch 1 to recover and respond to the reentering impulse. A single reactivation of branch 1 will produce a single ventricular premature depolarization; continuous conduction around the circuit will cause ventricular tachycardia.

Antiarrhythmic drugs can abolish such reentrant activity by producing *two-way block* in branch 2 or by improving conduction in branch 2, that is, by removing the one-way block.

short. For reentry to occur, normal conduction must be greatly slowed, refractoriness markedly shortened, or both. Nevertheless, reentry can serve as an explanation for cardiac arrhythmias. The sinus and A-V nodes are regions in which conduction is normally very slow; further slowing by premature activation or by disease easily creates conditions that permit reentry. Disease processes may also create conditions that permit reentry even in those types of fibers that usually conduct the cardiac impulse at very rapid rates, such as cardiac Purkinje fibers. Usually, marked slowing of conduction is the abnormality that permits reentry. However, marked abbreviation of action potentials and of refractoriness can play a role as well (Sasyniuk and Méndez, 1971). Conduction may be slowed due either to alterations in the *fast response* or development of *slow responses*.

Altered Fast Response. As mentioned in the discussion of responsiveness, the conduction velocity of impulses is critically dependent on the Vm at the time of activation (*see* Figure 31–2). When resting Vm is less than -75 mV (as with stretch or high $[K]_o$), V_{max} and conduction velocity decrease substantially because of voltage-dependent inactivation of the fast Na^+ channel. When resting Vm is between -50 and -65 mV, conduction velocity is greatly reduced and abnormal "fast responses" can propagate slowly enough to permit reentry. If Vm is more positive than -50 mV or so, the Na^+ channel will be almost totally inactivated and fast responses cannot be elicited. At such low values of Vm, fast responses may conduct decrementally; that is, the adequacy of the propagating response as a stimulus to resting tissue in its path lessens progressively as it propagates in depolarized tissues. Under such conditions, a delicate balance exists that determines whether conduction succeeds or fails.

Slow Responses and Very Slow Conduction. Slow action potentials were discovered in cardiac Purkinje fibers exposed to increased $[K]_o$ and catecholamines by Carmeliet and Vereeke (1969). In the voltage range at which slow potentials emerge, i_{Na} is inactivated and the pacemaker current, i_f, is fully deactivated; thus, these currents are unlikely to play a role in the genesis of the slow response. The inward current that causes the slow potential is i_{si}. Since i_{si} is relatively small in magnitude, slow responses are more likely to develop when background outward currents are decreased. Typically, slow responses are 40 to 80 mV in amplitude, depolarize at 1 to 2 V per second (*i.e.*, about 0.002 the rate of the fast response), and last for 0.4 to 1 second (*see* Figure 31–1, *B*). The small-amplitude and very low phase-0 V_{max} of slow responses lead to very slow conduction, which increases the likelihood of reentry. Slow responses can arise and propagate successfully in tissues too depolarized to generate a fast response. The slow response can easily overcome the chief difficulty for the production of reentry in heart muscle; it propagates so slowly that reentry can occur in very short pathways (Cranefield *et al.*, 1972; Wit *et al.*, 1972a, 1972b). Reentry in relatively small Purkinje fiber

circuits has been demonstrated directly (Wit *et al.*, 1972a, 1972b). As noted above, the duration of the action potential and refractoriness may shorten dramatically at the site of block due to local-circuit current flow (Sasyniuk and Méndez, 1971). Thus, premature stimulation can produce sufficient heterogeneity in the duration of the action potential and in refractoriness to permit reentry of subsequent impulses.

Significance of Reentry. Reentry may occur in many sites in the heart. The slow conduction in reentrant circuits may be due either to depressed fast responses or to slow responses. Reentry is relatively easy to elicit in the vicinity of the sinus or A-V nodes by the use of premature stimulation to slow conduction and to produce a functional one-way block, even in normal hearts (Weisfogel *et al.*, 1975). Clinically, reentry is the usual cause of paroxysmal supraventricular tachycardia. Reentry in the His-Purkinje system is thought to be one cause of coupled ventricular premature depolarizations and ventricular tachycardia in man. This idea is supported by extensive experimentation (Wit *et al.*, 1972a, 1972b; Wellens *et al.*, 1976). Durrer and coworkers (1971) and El-Sherif and associates (1977) have shown, in experimental acute myocardial infarction in the dog, that the cardiac impulse can meander through the infarcted region and emerge much later to produce ventricular premature depolarizations, ventricular tachycardia, or ventricular fibrillation. However, it should be mentioned again that reentrant arrhythmias are very difficult to distinguish from triggered arrhythmias in the clinical setting.

CLASSIFICATION OF ANTIARRHYTHMIC DRUGS

Antiarrhythmic drugs have been grouped together according to the pattern of electrophysiological effects that they produce and/or their presumed mechanisms of action. Classifications such as the one presented in Table 31–2 are commonly used in discussing antiarrhythmic drugs, and physicians should thus be conversant with them. However, it should also be recognized that drugs within a class do differ significantly, such that one member may be effective and safe in a particular patient while another may not.

Much of the information that is used to classify antiarrhythmic drugs comes from experimental studies in animals. For example, the classification in Table 31–2 relies heavily on observations made with preparations of canine or bovine cardiac Purkinje fibers. The agents in class I directly alter membrane conductances of cations, particularly those of Na^+ and K^+, to varying degrees during different phases of the cardiac action potential. It is

**Table 31–2. CLASSIFICATION OF ANTIARRHYTHMIC DRUGS
ACCORDING TO THEIR MECHANISM OF ACTION**

CLASS		ACTION	DRUGS
I.		*Sodium Channel Blockade*	
	A.	Moderate phase-0 depression and slow conduction (2+) *; prolong repolarization	Quinidine, procainamide, disopyramide
	B.	Minimal phase-0 depression and slow conduction (0 to 1+); shorten repolarization	Lidocaine, phenytoin, tocainide, mexiletine
	C.	Marked phase-0 depression and slow conduction (4+); little effect on repolarization	Encainide, lorcainide, flecainide
II.		*β-Adrenergic Blockade*	Propranolol, others
III.		*Prolong Repolarization*	Amiodarone, bretylium
IV.		*Calcium Channel Blockade*	Diltiazem, verapamil

* Relative magnitude of effect on conduction velocity indicated on a scale of 1+ to 4+.

useful to subcategorize these drugs in terms of their relative ability to depress $\dot{V}_{max}$ (by blockade of fast sodium channels) and to slow membrane repolarization. Class II includes agents that have primarily indirect effects on electrophysiological parameters by virtue of their ability to block β-adrenergic receptors. The agents in class III are mechanistically the least well defined. They appear to share the capacity to prolong the period of membrane repolarization (and thus of refractoriness) without appreciable effect on $\dot{V}_{max}$. Finally, class-IV agents have relatively selective depressant actions on calcium channels.

Such schemes can lead to ambiguities. Some drugs have multiple actions and are entitled to membership in more than one class. It may not be clear in a particular case which of the drug's actions is responsible for its efficacy. Moreover, when drugs are given to patients with heart disease and arrhythmias, their effects on the central and autonomic nervous systems, on hemodynamics, or on myocardial ischemia or metabolism may importantly influence their antiarrhythmic action.

USE-DEPENDENT BLOCKADE OF ION CHANNELS

An understanding of the effects of many antiarrhythmic drugs on the heart depends in part on knowledge of how those drugs interact with the gated channels that permit ionic currents across the sarcolemma (Hille, 1978; Courtney, 1980; Gintant and Hoffman, 1985). This question has been evaluated by studies on single channels with the patch clamp technic (Ogden *et al.*, 1981) and on populations of channels by voltage clamping (Hondeghem and Katzung, 1980; Bean *et al.*, 1983; Gintant and Hoffman, 1983). The simplest approach to understanding effects of local anesthetic antiarrhythmic agents on i_{Na} is to assume that the drug interacts with the channel and blocks it, such that the conductance falls to and remains at zero for as long as the drug interacts with the components of the channel. In terms of this scheme and the description of the fast channel given above, the interaction of drug and channel can be represented as shown in

Figure 31–5. *R, O,* and *I* represent the resting, open, and inactivated states of the channel, respectively; *D* is drug; and *R*, O*,* and *I** are the nonconducting forms of the channel to which drug is bound. *A* indicates the voltage- and time-dependent reactivation of the channel, and *A** any modification of this process caused by drug. The diagram is greatly simplified and, in particular, ignores the fact that there are probably a number of transition states for the channel, as between *R* and *O*.

In terms of this diagram, a drug such as lidocaine might interact with any or all of the three states of the channel. However, the drug may preferentially combine with channels in the *R, O,* or *I* state. In addition, the drug-channel complex need not undergo voltage-dependent transitions in the usual way. A more negative transmembrane potential might be needed for the *I* → R** transition than for *I → R* or, alternatively, the drug might have to dissociate from channels in the *I** state for the *I → R* transition to occur.

For most local anesthetic antiarrhythmic drugs, it appears as if channel blockade is most likely when the channel is in the *O* or *I* state and that reactivation is slowed or incomplete at usual transmembrane voltages. The consequences of this are important for the actions of antiarrhythmic drugs. A concentration of drug that exerted a minimal effect on a quiescent fiber at normal resting potential could block a significant fraction of channels during one action potential. Also, to the extent that the

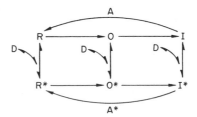

Figure 31–5. *Modulated-receptor hypothesis for the action of antiarrhythmic drugs. (See text for explanation.)*

$I^* \rightarrow R^*$ (or $I^* \rightarrow R$) transition is slowed, channels would accumulate in the I^* state during repeated action potentials and i_{Na} for each action potential would decrease until a steady state had been attained. This is the phenomenon of *use-dependent block,* and it has been described for all local-anesthetic antiarrhythmic drugs and for some slow-channel blocking drugs (*see* below; *see also* Chapter 33). In addition, some antiarrhythmic drugs appear to cause "tonic" (*i.e.,* not use-dependent) block of i_{Na} through interaction with channels in the R state.

If the association of drug with channel and dissociation of drug from channel are both relatively rapid, use-dependent block will reach a steady state during the course of a few action potentials and, if the interval between action potentials is reasonably long, little blockade will persist at the time of the upstroke of the action potential. If dissociation is quite slow, use-dependent block may not develop fully until there have been many action potentials, and a significant degree of block will be present at the time that each action potential is initiated. Finally, since a decrease in transmembrane voltage causes inactivation of fast channels, the effects of drugs on i_{Na} may be greatly enhanced in partially depolarized cells.

INDIVIDUAL ANTIARRHYTHMIC AGENTS

Discussion of the individual drugs that are most useful for the treatment or prophylaxis of cardiac arrhythmias follows. The effects of these agents on the electrophysiological properties of specialized cardiac fibers are summarized in Table 31–3, while drug-induced alterations in the ECG are listed in Table 31–4. The clinical utility of each agent is described in the text, and an overall estimate of their value in the management of specific arrhythmias is presented in Table 31–5. Pharmacokinetic parameters for the major agents are summarized in Appendix II.

QUINIDINE

Quinidine is the dextrostereoisomer of quinine; it shares all of the pharmacological actions of quinine, including its antimalarial, antipyretic, and oxytocic effects. However, the actions of quinidine on cardiac muscle are more intense than are those of quinine.

History. Quinidine, an optical isomer of quinine, was first described in 1848 by van Heyningen, and was prepared and given its present name by Pasteur in 1853. In the use of quinine and quinidine for malaria, it was noted many years ago that patients with malaria who also had atrial fibrillation would occasionally be cured of arrhythmia by these drugs.

Perhaps the earliest recorded reference to the use of cinchona in atrial fibrillation is that of the French physician Jean-Baptiste de Sénac of Paris, in 1749 (*see* Willius and Keys, 1942). Years later

Table 31–3. EFFECTS OF THERAPEUTIC CONCENTRATIONS OF ANTIARRHYTHMIC DRUGS ON ELECTROPHYSIOLOGICAL PROPERTIES OF SPECIALIZED CARDIAC FIBERS *

	QUINIDINE, PROCAINAMIDE, DISOPYRAMIDE	LIDOCAINE, PHENYTOIN	PROPRAN- OLOL	BRETY- LIUM	VERA- PAMIL
Sinus Node					
Automaticity	0	0	↓	↑ †, ↓	↓
A-V Node					
Effective Refractory Period (ERP) ‡	↓, 0, ↑	0, ↓	**↑**	↓, 0, ↑	**↑**
Purkinje Fibers					
Action Potential Amplitude	↓	0, ↓, ↑	0	0	0
Phase-0 $\dot{V}_{max}$	↓	0, ↓, ↑	0, ↓	0	0
Action Potential Duration (APD)	↑	↓	↓	↑	0, ↓
Effective Refractory Period (ERP)	↑	↓	↓	↑	0
ERP/APD	↑	↑	↑	0	0
Membrane Responsiveness	**↓**	↓	↓	0	0
Automaticity	↓	↓	↓	↑ †, ↓	0, ↓

* Changes are indicated as follows: ↓, decreased; 0, no change; ↑, increased; where multiple arrows are shown, there is variability in the direction of change. Boldface arrows indicate effects of greater magnitude.

† Due to release of catecholamines on initial exposure to the drug.

‡ Due to a complex balance of direct and indirect autonomic effects.

Table 31–4. EFFECTS OF THERAPEUTIC CONCENTRATIONS OF ANTIARRHYTHMIC DRUGS ON SINUS RATE AND ON ELECTROPHYSIOLOGICAL AND ELECTROCARDIOGRAPHIC INTERVALS *

DRUG	SINUS RATE	P-R	A-H	H-V	QRS	Q-T$_c$ †	VENTRICULAR RATE IN ATRIAL FIBRILLATION
Quinidine	0, ↑	0, ↑	↓, 0, ↑	0, ↑	↑	↑	0, ↑
Procainamide	0	0, ↑	↓, 0, ↑	0, ↑	↑	↑	0, ↑
Disopyramide	0	0	0, ↓	0, ↑	0, ↑	↑	↑, 0
Lidocaine	0	0	0, ↓	0	0	0	↑, 0, ↓
Phenytoin	0	0	0, ↓	0	0	0, ↓	↑, 0, ↓
Propranolol	↓	0, ↑	0, ↑	0	0	0, ↓	↓
Bretylium	0, ↓	0, ↑	0	0	0	0, ↑	↑, ↓
Verapamil	0, ↓	↑	↑	0	0	0	↓

* Changes are indicated as follows: ↓, decreased; 0, no change; ↑, increased; where multiple arrows are shown, there is variability in the direction of change.

† The Q-T$_c$ interval is the Q-T interval corrected for heart rate.

Wenckebach (1914) reported on the effect of quinine alkaloids in certain cardiac arrhythmias. Frey (1918), impressed by the report of Wenckebach, studied quinine, cinchonine, and quinidine in patients with atrial fibrillation and found quinidine to be the most effective. His observations were quickly confirmed by others, and the use of quinidine was extended to additional disorders of cardiac rhythm.

Chemistry. The chemistry of the cinchona alkaloids is presented in the discussion of quinine (Chapter 45). Quinidine differs from quinine only in the steric configuration of the secondary alcohol group.

PHARMACOLOGICAL PROPERTIES

Cardiac Electrophysiological Effects. Quinidine has powerful direct effects on most types of cells in the heart. In addition, drug-induced alterations of autonomic regulation of the heart also influence the electrical properties of cardiac cells.

Automaticity. Therapeutic concentrations of quinidine have little effect on the action potential or the firing rate of the isolated rabbit *sinus node;* in the human denervated heart, quinidine slows sinus rate very slightly. Indirect effects of quinidine can increase sinus rate by cholinergic blockade or by reflexly increasing sympathetic activity (*see* Mason *et al.*, 1977). Quinidine can also cause severe depression of the sinus node in patients with the *sick sinus syndrome* (*see* Bigger and Reiffel, 1979). Therapeutic concentrations of quinidine sub-

Table 31–5. RELATIVE UTILITY OF ANTIARRHYTHMIC DRUGS IN THE TREATMENT OF SPECIFIC CARDIAC ARRHYTHMIAS *

ARRHYTHMIA	QUINIDINE	PROCAINAMIDE	DISOPYRAMIDE	LIDOCAINE	PHENYTOIN	PROPRANOLOL	BRETYLIUM	VERAPAMIL
Supraventricular								
Atrial fibrillation, conversion	2	2	1	0	0	1	0	1
Atrial fibrillation, prophylaxis	3	3	3	0	0	2	0	2
Atrial fibrillation, rate control	0	0	0	0	0	2	0	3
Paroxysmal supraventricular tachycardia	2	2	2	0	1	3	0	4
Atrial premature depolarizations	3	3	3	0	1	3	0	2
Ventricular								
Ventricular premature depolarizations	3	3	3	4	2	1	1	2
Ventricular tachycardia	3	3	2	3	2	1	2	1
Digitalis-Induced Arrhythmias								
Atrial tachycardia with block	1	1	1	3	3	2	0	0
Nonparoxysmal A-V junctional tachycardia	1	1	1	3	3	2	0	0
Ventricular arrhythmias	1	1	1	3	3	2	0	0

* The relative utility score is based on an overall estimate of efficacy, convenience, and toxicity. The scale of relative utility is as follows: 0, none; 1, poor; 2, fair; 3, good; 4, excellent.

stantially decrease the firing rate of *cardiac Purkinje fibers* by a direct action; quinidine decreases the slope of phase-4 depolarization and shifts the threshold voltage toward zero. The shift in threshold is due to a shift in the i_{Na} reactivation curve and use-dependent blockade of some fast channels. The decrease in the slope of phase 4 is not yet explained. Quinidine can suppress arrhythmias caused by enhanced normal automaticity in the His-Purkinje system. The potent effect of quinidine on the normal automaticity in the His-Purkinje system also presents a hazard in the treatment of arrhythmias in the presence of A-V block. Therapeutic concentrations of quinidine have little effect on *abnormal automaticity* in markedly depolarized Purkinje fibers or on delayed afterdepolarizations. However, quinidine may prevent triggered activity by preventing the premature stimulus that initiates the process.

Excitability and Threshold. Quinidine increases the diastolic electrical current threshold in atrial and ventricular muscle and in Purkinje fibers; it also increases the fibrillation threshold in atria and ventricles (Wallace *et al.*, 1966a). As mentioned above, the threshold voltage is shifted by quinidine.

Responsiveness and Conduction. Quinidine decreases the amplitude, overshoot, and $\dot{V}_{max}$ of phase 0 in atrial, ventricular, and Purkinje cells. These effects become progressively more intense as the concentration of the drug is increased, and they are not accompanied by significant change in the resting Vm. The upstroke of premature responses is particularly depressed by quinidine because the drug causes changes in the voltage and time dependence of reactivation; for any steady-state value of Vm, $\dot{V}_{max}$ is reduced and, during dynamic changes in Vm, $\dot{V}_{max}$ takes longer to reach its steady-state value (*see* Figure 31–2). The time-dependent changes are most marked at low (less negative) values of Vm.

Duration of the Action Potential and Refractoriness. Quinidine causes small but significant increases in the duration of the action potential of ordinary atrial, ventricular, or Purkinje cells. The effective refractory period (ERP) of all of these cell types increases much more than would be

expected from the changes in the duration of the action potential. This finding is explained by the changes in responsiveness discussed above.

Effect on Reentrant Arrhythmias. Quinidine can abolish reentrant arrhythmias because of its effect on ERP, responsiveness, and conduction. For example, when ventricular premature depolarizations are caused by reentry in loops of Purkinje fibers, quinidine can convert one-way block to two-way block, thus making reentry impossible (*see* Figure 31–4).

The mechanism of its antiarrhythmic action in atrial flutter or fibrillation is more complex.

Atrial Flutter. Prolongation of the ERP of the atrium is commonly cited as the one desirable attribute of an "antiflutter" drug. The situation is by no means simple, for the effects of antiarrhythmic drugs upon ERP and upon conduction velocity are inextricably linked. When quinidine is administered to a dog in which a circus-movement flutter has been established, or to a patient with atrial flutter, the frequency invariably declines before reversion to sinus rhythm abruptly ensues. Quinidine slows conduction velocity in atrial muscle, which could account for the reduction of rate; but it also increases the atrial refractory period, which could reduce the rate by forcing the circulating impulse to travel in relatively refractory tissue. The two actions are opposed. If the predominant effect of quinidine were a primary reduction of conduction velocity, reversion to sinus rhythm would not be expected to occur until the flutter frequency diminished to less than the prevailing rate of the sinus node. But if the action is primarily upon the ERP, then the conduction velocity will be secondarily depressed until some minimal value is reached below which successful impulse propagation is no longer possible. This may well be the mechanism of action of quinidine in the experimental situation, but the details of the process are still not clearly defined. Méndez and associates (1969) have emphasized the importance of the "wavelength" (*i.e.*, the product of ERP and conduction velocity) in termination of circus-movement flutter. Agents that prolong the ERP without specifically depressing conduction velocity are more effective than those with both actions.

Atrial Fibrillation. If atrial fibrillation were due to a single circus movement about an obstacle so limited in size that activation of the surrounding tissue is irregular and fractionated, then the circuit pathway itself would be unstable. This mechanism seems unlikely, for fibrillation can be, and often is, a very stable arrhythmia. If, however, fibrillation is due to the random reentry of numerous fractionated wavelets, changing in breadth, direction, and number from moment to moment, then the persistence of the arrhythmia is critically related to the degree of inhomogeneity of the tissue and to the mean ERP. Vagal stimulation or cholinomimetic drugs should tend to perpetuate the arrhythmia by reducing the mean ERP and by increasing the range of variation of the ERPs. The action of quinidine here is twofold. By virtue of its direct and antivagal actions, quinidine may increase the mean ERP and also reduce the inhomogeneity. The action of quinidine, in terms of these concepts, is based not on its ability to snuff out a dominant circus movement but on its ability to reduce the number of wavelets possible in a given mass of tissue.

Electrocardiographic Effects. At therapeutic concentrations in man, quinidine causes a small increase in heart rate and in the P-R, QRS, and Q-T intervals. Clinical electrophysiological studies reveal that quinidine prolongs the ERP of the atrium, shortens the A-H interval (A-V nodal conduction), and usually prolongs the H-V interval slightly (His-Purkinje system conduction). QRS widening begins at low concentrations of quinidine in plasma and increases progressively as concentration increases. This effect is useful for monitoring the progress of therapy.

Autonomic Nervous System. In experimental animals, quinidine has a very significant atropine-like action, blocking the effects of vagal stimulation or acetylcholine. Quinidine also has α-adrenergic blocking properties. This action can cause vasodilatation and, via baroreceptors, activate sympathetic efferent activity. Together, the cholinergic blockade and increased β-adrenergic activity caused by quinidine can increase sinus rate and enhance A-V nodal conduction in some human subjects (Mason *et al.*, 1977).

Absorption, Distribution, and Elimination. When administered orally, quinidine sulfate is absorbed rapidly and peak concentrations in plasma are attained in 60 to 90 minutes. The absorption of quinidine gluconate is somewhat slower and less complete; peak concentrations in plasma are not reached until 3 or 4 hours after an oral dose. Although quinidine can be given intramuscularly, it causes pain at the injection site and a substantial increase in creatine kinase activity in plasma.

About 90% of quinidine in plasma is bound to proteins (alpha-1 acid glycopro-

tein and albumin). The drug enters erythrocytes and apparently binds to hemoglobin; at steady state, concentrations of quinidine in plasma and erythrocytes are approximately equal. Quinidine distributes rapidly to most tissues except brain, and the apparent volume of distribution is 2 to 3 liters per kilogram.

Quinidine is largely metabolized by the liver and excreted in the urine; the elimination half-time is about 6 hours. Renal excretion of the parent drug is also significant, and about 20% is eliminated by this route.

Although quinidine is extensively metabolized in man, knowledge about its metabolic fate is still incomplete. Most urinary metabolites are hydroxylated at only one site, either on the quinoline ring or on the quinuclidine ring; small amounts of dihydroxy compounds are also found (Drayer *et al.*, 1977). The fraction of a dose of quinidine that is metabolized and the metabolic pathway appear to vary considerably from patient to patient. There is some controversy about whether the concentration of quinidine in plasma rises in patients with renal failure or congestive heart failure (*see* Kessler *et al.*, 1974; Conrad *et al.*, 1977; Drayer *et al.*, 1977). The situation is complicated by the fact that some of quinidine's major metabolites are probably cardioactive (Drayer *et al.*, 1977).

Quinidine is both filtered at the glomerulus and secreted by the proximal renal tubule; passive back diffusion of the unchanged molecule occurs in the distal nephron. Since quinidine is a weak base, its excretion is enhanced if the urine is acidic. When the urinary pH is increased from the 6–7 range to the 7–8 range, renal clearance of quinidine decreases by as much as 50% and concentration in the plasma increases. This situation rarely occurs clinically unless the patient takes sodium bicarbonate or acetazolamide concurrently or has renal tubular acidosis.

Routes of Administration, Dosage, and Preparations. For practical purposes, quinidine is only given orally, although it can be administered either intramuscularly or intravenously under special circumstances. The usual oral dose of quinidine sulfate is 200 to 300 mg three or four times a day. In most patients, quinidine will reach a steady state on such a schedule in about 24 hours and its concentration in plasma will fluctuate less than 50% between doses. Because of the large interindividual variation, drug interactions, and other causes of variability, it is wise to examine the ECG carefully after the initial dose of quinidine and to measure the plasma concentration of the drug at steady state (*see* Appendix II). Adjustment of dosage is often necessary. If an effective concentration must be achieved rapidly, a loading dose of 600 to 1000 mg can be given.

Quinidine sulfate (CIN-QUIN, QUINORA, others) is available in tablets (100 to 300 mg), capsules (200 and 300 mg), and sustained-release tablets (300 mg), and as an injection (200 mg/ml). Preparations of the gluconate and polygalacturonate salts are also available.

THERAPEUTIC USES

Quinidine is a broad-spectrum drug; it is effective for acute and chronic treatment of supraventricular and ventricular arrhythmias. Quinidine is primarily used chronically to prevent recurrences of supraventricular tachyarrhythmias or to suppress ventricular arrhythmias. Individualization of dosage is usually required at the outset of therapy because plasma concentrations will vary substantially in different individuals, and the response of any given arrhythmia will vary in different patients. Because of this, several 24-hour Holter ECG recordings are often required to ensure adequate control of arrhythmias. Vigilance must be maintained to detect toxic reactions.

Supraventricular Arrhythmias. Quinidine is useful as chronic oral therapy for supraventricular arrhythmias. The objective of therapy usually is to prevent or to reduce the frequency of arrhythmic episodes.

Paroxysmal Supraventricular Tachycardia (PSVT). Quinidine can be effective against recurrent, aggravating PSVT, either the usual A-V nodal reciprocating tachycardia or the PSVT seen in the Wolff-Parkinson-White syndrome. In the A-V nodal form of PSVT, digitalis and other methods usually are tried before quinidine because of the very significant toxicity of the latter drug. The mode of action of quinidine in PSVT is not certain. It may suppress the atrial premature depolarizations that trigger the PSVT, or alter conduction and refractoriness of the atrium and A-V node so that PSVT no longer occurs. In the Wolff-Parkinson-White syndrome, quinidine often slows conduction and increases refractoriness in the accessory A-V connection and, therefore, prevents attacks of PSVT.

Atrial Flutter or Fibrillation. Quinidine was used for many years as the drug of choice for conversion of atrial flutter or atrial fibrillation to sinus rhythm. Since the advent of DC cardioversion, quinidine has been relegated to a supporting role in the management of these two arrhythmias. Patients scheduled for cardioversion are given oral maintenance doses of quinidine (*e.g.,* 400 mg every 6 hours) 1 or 2 days before the anticipated cardioversion. About one third of patients with atrial fibrillation and a similar proportion of patients with atrial flutter will convert to sinus rhythm on this dose of quinidine; others require DC shock. Maintenance of quinidine therapy helps to prevent recurrence of atrial fibrillation. If atrial premature depolarizations occur soon after cardioversion, the dose of quinidine should be increased until they are abolished or quinidine toxicity is encountered. If uninterrupted sinus rhythm resumes after cardioversion, the concentration of quinidine in plasma should be adjusted to steady-state values between 2 and 5 μg/ml.

Ventricular Arrhythmias. Quinidine is one of the most useful drugs for chronic treatment of ventricular arrhythmias (ventricular premature depolarization, ventricular tachycardia) or for the prevention of ventricular fibrillation.

Ventricular Premature Depolarizations and Nonsustained Ventricular Tachycardia. The ventricular premature depolarization (VPD) is a very common rhythm disturbance. VPDs are treated when they cause discomfort (palpitations), impair hemodynamic performance, or increase the likelihood of death. When treating VPDs or brief recurrent bursts of ventricular tachycardia, the dose of quinidine is adjusted while 24-hour Holter ECG recordings are analyzed to establish the intensity of drug effect. Usually, the dose of quinidine is increased until complex forms (pairs or runs of VPDs) are abolished and the frequency of VPDs is reduced by 70 to 80%; this dose is then maintained. When the arrhythmia is caused by an acute process, such as open-heart surgery, acute myocardial infarction, or acute myocarditis, quinidine can be discontinued when the acute process appears to be resolved. If the arrhythmia treated was life threatening, quinidine should be discontinued while the patient is in the hospital and can be monitored carefully for recurrence.

Sustained Ventricular Tachycardia. The treatment of sustained ventricular tachycardia is quite different. Prior to the advent of DC cardioversion, heroic and skilled dosage with quinidine was used to convert ventricular tachycardia to sinus rhythm. There were many problems associated with this approach, and the incidence of toxicity was high. This approach has been abandoned. Although sustained ventricular tachycardia can be relatively resistant to treatment with drugs, it usually responds readily to DC conversion. After conversion, drug therapy is guided by electrophysiological observations (Horowitz *et al.,* 1980; Swerdlow *et al.,* 1983).

Digitalis-Induced Arrhythmias. The complex rhythm disturbances that can attend digitalis toxicity are discussed in detail in Chapter 30. Although quinidine can be effective for the treatment of a variety of digitalis-induced arrhythmias, it is not the preferred drug, since adverse effects on cardiac rhythm are more likely to occur with quinidine than with other effective treatments (*e.g.*, phenytoin or lidocaine).

UNTOWARD EFFECTS

About one third of the patients who receive quinidine will have immediate adverse effects that necessitate discontinuation of therapy. If this initial hurdle is passed, few extracardiac adverse effects are encountered during chronic therapy. However, excessive concentration of the drug in plasma will cause adverse effects in any patient. Because quinidine has a low therapeutic ratio, constant vigilance is required in every patient taking this drug.

Cardiotoxicity. As the concentration of quinidine in plasma rises above 2 μg/ml, the QRS complex and the Q-T$_c$ interval will widen progressively (Heissenbuttel and Bigger, 1970). These changes are useful in monitoring quinidine therapy. If the duration of the QRS complex increases by 50% or more, a reduction in dosage should be considered. At high plasma concentrations of the drug, cardiac toxicity may become severe; S-A block or arrest, high-grade A-V block, ventricular tachyarrhythmias, or asystole may occur. Conduction is slowed tremendously in all parts of the heart. In addition, Purkinje fibers can become depolarized and develop abnormal automaticity. These changes are responsible for the bizarre arrhythmias seen in severe poisoning with quinidine. Polymorphic ventricular tachycardia caused by quinidine toxicity is a life-threatening event and must be treated with the utmost caution. Appropriate criteria that can separate arrhythmias due to drug toxicity from spontaneous worsening of the initial arrhythmia must be used. The ECG is one such aid and must be closely monitored in an intensive care unit. Sodium lactate, catecholamines, glucagon, and magnesium sulfate may be useful in counteracting ventricular tachyarrhythmias caused by quinidine (Bellet *et al.*, 1959; Wasserman *et al.*, 1959). Quinidine and its hydroxy metabolites can be removed by dialysis (Conrad *et al.*, 1977).

Quinidine Syncope. Occasionally patients taking quinidine experience syncope or sudden death. In some instances, this reaction may be the result of high concentrations of quinidine in plasma or the result of coexisting digitalis toxicity. However, ventricular tachyarrhythmias may occur in susceptible individuals while the concentrations of quinidine in plasma are low. Individuals with the long Q-T syndrome or those who respond to quinidine with marked lengthening of the Q-T interval appear to be particularly at risk and should not be treated with this drug (Koster and Wellens, 1976).

"Paradoxical" Ventricular Response to Atrial Fibrillation. A frequently mentioned complication of quinidine when the drug is used to treat atrial fibrillation is the so-called paradoxical increase in ventricular rate. Quinidine often causes a substantial decrease in the atrial rate in atrial fibrillation. If the atrial rate decreases sufficiently, the ventricular rate may increase abruptly because of the decrease in concealed conduction of atrial impulses in the A-V node. In some patients, quinidine may be anticholinergic as well. Paradoxical increase in ventricular rate is not common in patients treated only with quinidine. However, the effect is so dramatic in some patients that it is traditional to digitalize patients prior to administration of quinidine in order to avoid this event.

Blood Pressure. Quinidine can cause significant hypotension, particularly when given intravenously. This response is probably due to the α-adrenergic blocking effect of the drug. Hemodynamic studies indicate that hypotension due to quinidine is caused by vasodilatation without significant decrease in cardiac output; therapeutic concentrations of quinidine have no significant adverse effects on myocardial performance. Very high concentrations may adversely affect myocardial contractility.

Arterial Embolism. The risk of embolism following conversion of atrial fibrillation to sinus rhythm is a source of concern. The fibrillating atria do not contract, and thrombi often develop in the left atrium, particularly in the atrial appendage. After sinus rhythm resumes, atrial contraction may dislodge thrombi; stroke is the most dreaded sequela of the resultant arterial embolization. However, the long-term risk of systemic embolization is greater if atrial fibrillation persists than if conversion to sinus rhythm occurs. If cardioversion is performed as an elective procedure, patients are usually given anticoagulants for 1 to 2 weeks prior to conversion. The risk of embolization is reasonably small even without anticoagulation.

Cinchonism. Like other cinchona alkaloids and the salicylates, quinidine can cause cinchonism. Symptoms of mild cinchonism include tinnitus, loss of hearing, slight blurring of vision, and gastrointestinal upset. If toxicity is severe, headache, diplopia, photophobia, and altered color perception may occur, as can confusion, delirium, and psychosis. The skin may be hot and flushed; nausea, vomiting, diarrhea, and abdominal pain are likely.

Gastrointestinal Symptoms. The most common adverse reactions to quinidine are referable to the gastrointestinal tract—nausea, vomiting, and diarrhea. Gastrointestinal symptoms often occur, even when drug concentrations in plasma are low. This type of adverse reaction is apparent almost immediately after quinidine is first administered and forces early discontinuation of the drug in almost one third of patients so treated.

Hypersensitivity Reactions. Hypersensitivity to quinidine can cause *fever;* this reaction is rare and disappears when the drug is discontinued. Rarely, quinidine causes *anaphylactic reactions,* which require the usual emergency measures. *Thrombocytopenia* is an uncommon but potentially lethal outcome of treatment with quinidine. Thrombocytopenia usually occurs after several weeks or months of therapy and is due to formation of drug-platelet complexes that evoke a circulating antibody. When quinidine, platelets, and antibody are all present in the circulation, platelets agglutinate and lyse. Thrombocytopenia can be profound, and severe bleeding may ensue. If quinidine is stopped, the platelet count will return to near normal within days. Until the bleeding time is normal, patients should be kept in the hospital and, if neces-

sary, treated with adrenocorticosteroids and transfusions of platelets. Asthma-like *respiratory difficulty* or *vascular collapse* can occur as a result of hypersensitivity. Artificial ventilation and supportive measures are usually effective.

DRUG INTERACTIONS

Drugs such as phenobarbital or phenytoin that induce drug-metabolizing enzymes in the liver may significantly shorten the duration of action of quinidine by increasing its rate of elimination (Data *et al.,* 1976). Since patients vary tremendously in their susceptibility to enzyme induction, it is difficult to predict which individuals will be affected. When quinidine is given to patients who have stable concentrations of digoxin in plasma, the digoxin concentration usually doubles due to a decrease in its clearance (Bigger, 1982). Occasionally, patients who are receiving warfarin or other oral anticoagulants will have an increase in prothrombin time after quinidine is begun (Koch-Weser, 1968); the mechanism of this reaction is not clear. Since quinidine is an α-adrenergic blocking agent, it can interact additively with drugs that cause vasodilatation or decreased blood volume. For example, nitroglycerin can cause severe postural hypotension in patients who are taking quinidine. The effect of any given concentration of quinidine on the heart is greater when the concentration of K^+ in plasma is increased.

PROCAINAMIDE

Procainamide is useful for the treatment of a variety of arrhythmias, and it can be administered by several routes. Unfortunately its potency and versatility are marred by its short duration of action and a high incidence of adverse reactions when it is used chronically.

History. In 1936, Mautz demonstrated that direct application of procaine to the heart elevated the threshold of ventricular muscle to electrical stimulation. Extension of this observation by numerous workers established that the cardiac actions of procaine resemble those of quinidine. However, the therapeutic value of procaine as an antifibrillatory and antiarrhythmic agent is limited by rapid enzymatic hydrolysis and prominent adverse effects on the central nervous system. A systematic study of congeners and metabolites of procaine was undertaken to find a compound with clinically useful quinidine-like actions; procainamide was discovered as a result (Mark *et al.*, 1951).

Chemistry. Procainamide has the following structural formula:

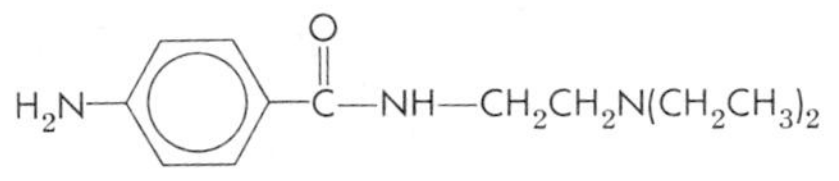

$$H_2N-\text{(ring)}-\overset{\overset{\displaystyle O}{\|}}{C}-NH-CH_2CH_2N(CH_2CH_3)_2$$

Procainamide

It differs from procaine merely by replacement of the ester linkage by the amide.

PHARMACOLOGICAL PROPERTIES

Cardiac Electrophysiological Effects. The direct effects of procainamide on the electrical activity of the heart are very similar to those produced by quinidine. However, its indirect effects, that is, those resulting from interaction with the autonomic nervous system, are significantly different. The effects of procainamide on automaticity, excitability, responsiveness, and conduction are virtually the same as those of quinidine (Table 31–3). As a result, the effects of procainamide on the ECG are also quite similar.

A metabolite of procainamide, N-acetylprocainamide (NAPA; *see* below), accumulates in plasma in significant concentrations during treatment. While NAPA is antiarrhythmic, it is less potent than procainamide, and some of its cardiac actions are qualitatively different. In canine Purkinje fibers, it has little effect on automaticity, phase-0 V_{max}, or action-potential amplitude, but it does prolong the duration of the action potential in a fashion similar to procainamide. NAPA has been assigned the nonproprietary name of *acecainide* and is being evaluated for the treatment of ventricular arrhythmias. The drug appears to be effective only in selected patients (*see* Keefe *et al.*, 1981).

Autonomic Nervous System. The anticholinergic action of procainamide is much weaker than that of quinidine. Procainamide does not produce α-adrenergic blockade, but, in the dog, it can block autonomic ganglia weakly and cause a measurable impairment of cardiovascular reflexes.

Absorption, Distribution, and Elimination. Procainamide is quickly and nearly completely absorbed following oral administration in normal subjects (Appendix II). The peak concentration in plasma is reached 45 to 75 minutes after ingestion of capsules, but somewhat later after administration of tablets. In the first week after acute myocardial infarction, oral absorption may be poor, the peak plasma concentration may be quite delayed, and concentrations of the drug may be inadequate to control arrhythmias (Koch-Weser *et al.*, 1969). Sustained-release formulations of procainamide have lower bioavailability than do standard capsules. Absorption of these formulations is delayed so much that the duration of action exceeds 8 hours.

About 20% of the procainamide in plasma is bound to proteins. Procainamide is rapidly distributed into most body tissues except the brain, and the apparent volume of distribution is about 2 liters per kilogram. However, this value can decrease to about 1.5 liters per kilogram in patients with cardiac failure or shock. Compensation for this change should be made in calculating dosage.

Procainamide is eliminated by renal excretion and hepatic metabolism. The biotransformation of procainamide has been intensively studied since the discovery that its major metabolic pathway is N-acetylation (Dreyfuss *et al.*, 1972). It is thought that there is bimodal genetic variation in the activity of the N-acetyltransferase for procainamide, similar to the situation for isoniazid, dapsone, and other drugs (Gibson *et al.*, 1975; Reidenberg *et al.*, 1975). However, there is another acetylase system that does not show such variation and that also may contribute to the metabolism of procainamide (Giardina *et al.*, 1977). In fast acetylators or in renal insufficiency, 40% or more of a dose of procainamide may be excreted as N-acetylprocainamide (NAPA), and concentrations of NAPA in plasma may equal or exceed those of the parent drug. Two other metabolites of procainamide, the structures of which are not yet known, account for 8 to 15% of a dose of procainamide (Giardina *et al.*, 1976). For optimal patient management, information should be available about the concentrations of both procainamide and NAPA in plasma.

A large fraction (up to two thirds) of a

dose of procainamide is eliminated unchanged in the urine. Procainamide is a weak base that is filtered, secreted by the proximal tubule, and reabsorbed by the distal tubule. Moderate changes in the pH of the urine cause little change in the renal excretion of procainamide. When intrinsic renal function or renal perfusion decreases, the concentration of procainamide in plasma rises significantly (Koch-Weser and Klein, 1971). However, as the blood urea nitrogen rises, the fraction of a dose of procainamide that is excreted unchanged decreases. The elimination of NAPA is almost entirely by renal excretion, and NAPA can accumulate to dangerous levels when renal failure or congestive heart failure is present.

Preparations, Dosage, and Routes of Administration. *Procainamide hydrochloride* (PRO-NESTYL, others) is available for oral administration as capsules and tablets (250 to 500 mg). Sustained-release tablets are also marketed (250 to 750 mg). *Procainamide hydrochloride injection* contains 100 or 500 mg/ml and is suitable for intramuscular and intravenous injection.

Procainamide is one of the most versatile of all antiarrhythmic drugs with respect to the variety of routes of administration that can be used and the flexibility of dosing schedules. Procainamide can be administered intravenously, intramuscularly, or orally. The concentration in plasma needed for antiarrhythmic effects is usually 3 to 10 μg/ml, occasionally much higher. The probability of toxicity becomes greater as the plasma concentration rises above 8 μg/ml. As with quinidine, the cardiac effects of procainamide are enhanced if the concentration of K^+ in plasma is elevated.

Intravenous Administration. In acute or unstable situations, intravenous administration is desirable for speed (injection or rapid infusion), precision (constant infusion), and reliability of effect. The total loading dose is *never* given as a single intravenous injection because it can cause hypotension. One rapid and safe method to establish effective concentrations in plasma is *intermittent intravenous administration:* 100 mg is injected over 2 to 4 minutes, and this dose is repeated every 5 minutes until the arrhythmia is controlled, adverse effects are seen, or the total size of the dose (about 1000 mg) suggests that the arrhythmia under treatment is resistant (Bigger and Heissenbuttel, 1969; Giardina *et al.,* 1973). The 5-minute dosing interval permits examination of the blood pressure and ECG after each dose. Serious hypotension or excessive widening of the QRS interval can thus be avoided. Alternatively, the same dose can be given over a similar period by *rapid intravenous infusion.* For example, 600 mg can be infused at a rate of 20 mg per minute (Bigger, 1975). The same precautions should be taken. When the arrhythmia is controlled, a *constant-rate intravenous infusion* is often used to maintain effective concentrations in plasma. The infusion rate can be estimated as the product of the desired concentration (3 to 10 μg/ml) and the estimated total clearance of procainamide (*see* Appendix II).

Oral Administration. For chronic therapy, oral administration is the only practical route. Total daily doses of 3 to 6 g or more usually are required for therapeutic efficacy. Because its elimination half-life is short (about 3 hours in normal subjects), the drug must be given fairly frequently. Fortunately, most patients can take procainamide orally at intervals of 6 or more hours because the elimination half-time is usually longer (5 to 8 hours) in patients with cardiac disease. Measurement of procainamide and NAPA concentrations in plasma can help to guide therapy.

When oral therapy is begun, a loading dose (12 mg/kg) is occasionally desirable. However, steady state is reached within 1 day without loading doses because of the short half-life of the drug.

One special circumstance is worthy of comment—the change from intravenous infusion to oral dosage. This transition often is required in the management of patients with acute myocardial infarction (Bigger, 1975). The infusion should be stopped and about one elimination half-time permitted to elapse before administration of the first oral dose; the oral dose can be chosen very precisely based on the previous intravenous dose.

Intramuscular Administration. Procainamide is rapidly and almost completely absorbed after intramuscular injection.

THERAPEUTIC USES

Procainamide is employed to treat a wide variety of cardiac arrhythmias. In general, the effectiveness of the drug parallels that of quinidine. However, procainamide is effective in some patients who have failed to respond to maximally tolerated doses of quinidine and *vice versa.*

Ventricular Arrhythmias. Procainamide is effective for most ventricular arrhythmias. Ventricular premature depolarizations and paroxysmal ventricular tachycardia are abolished in a large percentage of cases within a few minutes after intravenous injection or within an hour after oral or intramuscular administration. The best way to evaluate the efficacy of chronic oral regimens is quantitative analysis of 24-hour Holter ECG recordings. High doses of procainamide are often required to control sustained ventricular tachycardia (Greenspan *et al.,* 1980).

Arrhythmias in Digitalis Toxicity. Although ventricular premature depolarizations and ventricular tachycardia caused by digitalis intoxication can be suppressed by procainamide, its effects are unpredictable and fatalities have occurred. If ventricular tachycardia induced by digitalis is accompanied by marked disturbances of A-V conduction, procainamide can precipitate ventricular asystole or fibrillation. The complexities and dangers of the combined effects of digitalis and procainamide have been discussed by Zapata-Díaz and coworkers (1952).

Supraventricular Arrhythmias. The efficacy of procainamide against atrial arrhythmias is comparable to that of quinidine. Often, however, high doses (4 to 8 g per day) are required to control atrial arrhythmias. Like quinidine, procainamide is only moderately effective in converting atrial flutter or chronic atrial fibrillation to sinus rhythm. Procainamide can be used to prevent recurrences of atrial flutter or atrial fibrillation after cardioversion.

UNTOWARD EFFECTS

Cardiotoxicity. The incidence of adverse effects is high when procainamide is used clinically. Excessive concentrations in plasma produce ECG changes very similar to those seen during quinidine therapy. The same rules and precautions for using and discontinuing quinidine (*see* above) pertain to procainamide. High concentrations of procainamide in plasma can produce ventricular premature depolarizations, ventricular tachycardia, or ventricular fibrillation. Interestingly, the syndrome of marked Q-T prolongation and severe ventricular arrhythmias described for quinidine appears to be much less common with procainamide. Procainamide, like quinidine, will slow the atria in atrial fibrillation and can thereby cause a "paradoxical" increase in the ventricular response.

Blood Pressure. If procainamide is administered intravenously, it can cause hypotension. Intermittent or rapid intravenous infusion can be adjusted so that significant hypotension is unusual, provided that doses do not exceed 600 mg. Toxic concentrations of procainamide can diminish myocardial performance and promote hypotension.

Extracardiac Adverse Effects. During oral administration of procainamide, gastrointestinal symptoms (anorexia, nausea, vomiting, and, rarely, diarrhea) may occur; these symptoms are much less common than with quinidine. Although procainamide has fewer adverse effects on the cen-

tral nervous system than procaine or lidocaine, a variety of symptoms, including giddiness, psychosis, hallucinations, and mental depression, can result from the drug.

Hypersensitivity Reactions. This type of adverse effect is the most common and troublesome. Occasionally, *fever* occurs during the first few days of therapy and forces discontinuance of procainamide. *Agranulocytosis* may occur in the early weeks of therapy; fatal infections may follow. Leukocyte and differential blood counts should be done regularly during therapy, and complaints of sore throat should receive prompt evaluation. Myalgias, angioedema, skin rashes, digital vasculitis, and Raynaud's phenomenon have all been attributed to procainamide (*see* Bigger and Heissenbuttel, 1969).

Systemic Lupus Erythematosus–like Syndrome. Ladd (1962) described a syndrome caused by procainamide that superficially resembles authentic systemic lupus erythematosus (SLE). Arthralgia is the most common symptom; pericarditis, pleuropneumonic involvement, fever, and hepatomegaly are common signs. The most serious complication is hemorrhagic pericardial effusion with tamponade. Drug-induced SLE is different from the naturally occurring disease. In the drug-induced syndrome, there is no predilection for females; the brain and kidney are spared; leukopenia, anemia, thrombocytopenia, and hyperglobulinemia are rare; and false-positive serologic tests for syphilis do not occur. The drug-induced syndrome is reversible when procainamide is discontinued. About 60 to 70% of patients who receive procainamide will develop antinuclear antibodies after 1 to 12 months of therapy. Only 20 to 30% of those with antinuclear antibodies will develop the clinical symptoms and signs of the SLE syndrome if treatment is continued. When symptoms occur, LE-cell preparations are often positive. The development of antinuclear antibodies alone is insufficient reason to discontinue therapy with procainamide. However, procainamide usually should be stopped when patients become symptomatic. An exception should be made if the patient has a life-threatening arrhythmia for which alternative therapy is not available. In this circumstance, symptoms of SLE may be controlled with aspirin or adrenocorticosteroids. It is not yet clear if individuals who acetylate procainamide slowly have an increased risk of developing the SLE-like syndrome (Giardina *et al.*, 1977; Woosley *et al.*, 1978); it is known that slow acetylators are more susceptible to hydralazine-induced lupus. Furthermore, the use of acecainide (NAPA) has only rarely been associated with the development of antinuclear antibodies.

DISOPYRAMIDE

Disopyramide has been available in the United States since 1978 for oral treatment of some ventricular arrhythmias in adults.

Chemistry. Disopyramide has the following structural formula:

Disopyramide

PHARMACOLOGICAL PROPERTIES

Cardiac Electrophysiological Effects. Disopyramide has not yet been studied extensively. The drug slows the sinus rate by a direct effect (Sekiya and Vaughan Williams, 1963). In patients with the sick sinus syndrome, disopyramide can depress the automaticity of the sinus node (Seipel and Breithardt, 1976; LaBarre *et al.*, 1979). Therapeutic concentrations decrease the slope of phase-4 depolarization in Purkinje fibers and decrease their spontaneous rate of firing (Kus and Sasyniuk, 1975); the mechanism of the change in pacemaker activity is unknown. The effects of disopyramide on the duration of the action potential, refractoriness, and membrane responsiveness are very similar to the effects of quinidine or procainamide. Disopyramide reduces the differences in the duration of the action potential between normal and infarcted tissues by lengthening the action potential of normal cells (Sasyniuk and Kus, 1976). Disopyramide seems somewhat more potent than quinidine in increasing atrial or ventricular refractoriness and less potent in the His-Purkinje system.

Electrocardiographic Effects. Disopyramide usually causes little change in the sinus rate or the P-R interval. The QRS rarely increases by more than 20% at concentrations of the drug that are in the therapeutic range; the Q-T_c consistently lengthens by a small amount. Electrophysiological studies in man show that disopyramide shortens the recovery time of the sinus node. It consistently increases atrial refractoriness, but conduction and refractoriness in the A-V node do not change. Similarly, conduction in the His-Purkinje system is usually minimally changed. The effective refractory period (ERP) of the ventricle is increased (Marrott *et al.*, 1976). Birkhead and Vaughan Williams (1977) showed that after cholinergic blockade, disopyramide (2 mg/kg) substantially decreases sinus rate and increases the recovery time of the sinus node; the drug also increases the ERP of the atrium and the functional refractory period of the A-V node. Apparently, the atropine-like action of disopyramide nullifies some of its direct effects. Patients with bundle-branch disease are more likely to develop an increase in the H-V interval after disopyramide than are patients with normal intraventricular conduction (Desai *et al.*, 1979).

Autonomic Nervous System. Disopyramide has cholinergic blocking properties about 10% as potent as atropine (Mirro *et al.*, 1980). The drug is neither an α- nor a β-adrenergic antagonist.

Absorption, Distribution, and Elimination. About 90% of an oral dose of disopyramide is absorbed, of which a small fraction is subject to first-pass metabolism by the liver. Concentrations in plasma peak at 1 to 2 hours after a dose.

At normal therapeutic concentrations (3 μg/ml) about 30% of disopyramide is bound to plasma proteins; the bound fraction varies with the total concentration of drug in plasma. The apparent volume of distribution of disopyramide is about 0.6 liter per kilogram.

About 50% of a dose of disopyramide is excreted by the kidney unchanged, 20% as the mono-N-dealkylated metabolite, and another 10% as unidentified metabolites. The monodealkylated metabolite has less antiarrhythmic and atropine-like activity than does the parent compound. The half-time for elimination is 5 to 7 hours, and this value is markedly prolonged in patients with renal insufficiency (up to 20 hours or more).

Preparations, Dosage, and Route of Administration. In the United States, disopyramide is approved only for oral administration. It is available as *disopyramide phosphate* in capsules containing 100 or 150 mg of the base (NORPACE). The usual total daily dose is 400 to 800 mg; this amount is divided into four doses (most often 150 mg four times daily). Loading doses of 200 to 300 mg will rapidly produce effective concentrations. Maintenance doses must be carefully adjusted for patients with renal failure according to the creatinine clearance; efficacy, toxic manifestations, and plasma concentration should be carefully monitored in such patients.

In the United States, disopyramide is approved only for the treatment of ventricular arrhythmias in adults. Its efficacy against atrial and ventricular arrhythmias caused by digitalis has not been established by controlled trials. Experience in Europe indicates that disopyramide is about as efficacious as quinidine or procainamide in converting atrial arrhythmias to sinus rhythm and that it is useful for the maintenance of sinus rhythm after cardioversion (Hartel *et al.*, 1974; Luoma *et al.*, 1978). Intravenous and oral disopyramide is effective for reducing the frequency of VPD in acute myocardial infarction, but efficacy for sustained ventricular tachycardia or primary ventricular fibrillation has not yet been demonstrated.

UNTOWARD EFFECTS

The anticholinergic action of disopyramide produces a significant incidence of dry mouth, constipation, blurred vision, urinary hesitancy, and, occasionally, urinary retention. Disopyramide can cause nausea, abdominal pain, vomiting, or diarrhea, but gastrointestinal symptoms are significantly less common than when quinidine is used. Disopyramide reduces cardiac output and left ventricular performance by a direct depressant effect and peripheral arteriolar constriction. The adverse effects on ventricular function can be striking in patients who have preexisting ventricular failure (Jensen *et al.*, 1975; Podrid *et al.*, 1980). Great caution should be exercised in treating such patients with disopyramide. The *adverse hemodynamic effects* are more marked than those of quinidine, procainamide, lidocaine, or phenytoin. The *blood pressure* usually increases transiently after intravenous administration of disopyramide, even though the cardiac output falls; total peripheral vascular resistance thus increases markedly.

LIDOCAINE

Lidocaine is widely used as a local anesthetic (*see* Chapter 15). It has also achieved prominence as an antiarrhythmic agent and is now in common use, particularly as emergency treatment, for ventricular arrhythmias that are encountered after cardiac surgery or acute myocardial infarction. Its mechanism of action differs in some respects from that of quinidine and procainamide, and it possesses certain advantages over the older drugs. Chief among these, especially for use in the coronary care unit, is that its antiarrhythmic action can be established very rapidly and safely by intravenous administration, and its effects decline quickly when the infusion is terminated. This permits moment-to-mo-ment titration of ventricular ectopic activity.

PHARMACOLOGICAL PROPERTIES

Cardiac Electrophysiological Effects. Unlike quinidine and procainamide, lidocaine exerts most of its electrophysiological effects on the heart by a direct action; no important interactions between lidocaine and the autonomic nervous system have been described.

Automaticity. Therapeutic concentrations of lidocaine have no effect on action potentials or firing rate of the isolated sinus node of the rabbit (Mandel and Bigger, 1971). Depression of the human sinus node by lidocaine is distinctly unusual but can occur in subjects with preexisting disease of the sinus node (Bigger and Reiffel, 1979). Therapeutic concentrations of lidocaine decrease the slope of normal phase-4 depolarization in Purkinje fibers (Davis and Temte, 1969; Bigger and Mandel, 1970). This action is caused by a decrease in the pacemaker current (i_{K_2} or i_f) and an increase in time-independent outward current (i_{K_1}) (Weld and Bigger, 1976; Carmeliet and Saikawa, 1982). Lidocaine also can counteract automaticity in depolarized, stretched Purkinje fibers and delayed after-depolarizations caused by digitalis. This could result from an increase in i_{K_1} that overcomes small inward currents that cause depolarization or from a decrease in inward Na^+ current (Carmeliet and Saikawa, 1982; Colatsky, 1982).

Excitability and Threshold. Lidocaine causes an increase in the diastolic electrical current threshold in cardiac Purkinje fibers by increasing K^+ conductance (g_{K_1}) without changing resting Vm or the voltage threshold (Arnsdorf and Bigger, 1975). Lidocaine also increases the threshold for ventricular fibrillation (Gerstenblith *et al.*, 1972).

Responsiveness and Conduction. Lidocaine has complex effects on membrane responsiveness, and studies of this relationship have yielded conflicting results. The steady-state relationship between $\dot{V}_{max}$ and Vm is little altered in normal Purkinje fibers by therapeutic concentrations of lidocaine.

However, therapeutic concentrations of lidocaine prevent fast responses at low (less negative) values of Vm (Davis and Temte, 1969; Bigger and Mandel, 1970). This effect can be explained by an increase in i_{K_1} caused by lidocaine, which counteracts small inward-going excitatory currents, or by a decrease in inward Na^+ current. Also, the effect of lidocaine on responsiveness depends on $[K]_o$; at $[K]_o$ up to 4.5 mM, therapeutic concentrations have little effect on responsiveness (Obayashi *et al.*, 1975). At $[K]_o$ of 5.6 or 6.0, therapeutic concentrations of lidocaine reduce $\dot{V}_{max}$ at any level of Vm (Singh and Vaughan Williams, 1971; Obayashi *et al.*, 1975). Toxic concentrations clearly shift responsiveness in much the same way as quinidine (Bigger and Mandel, 1970). Abnormal ventricular muscle fibers that survive experimental infarction show reduced responsiveness when exposed to therapeutic concentrations of lidocaine (Kupersmith *et al.*, 1975). Even therapeutic concentrations of lidocaine will delay reactivation of i_{Na}. Responsiveness decreases because the effect of lidocaine is use dependent and is increased at fast heart rates (*see* above) (Hondeghem and Katzung, 1980; Bean *et al.*, 1983).

Because of the large safety factor for conduction, lidocaine usually has no effect on conduction velocity in normal tissues of the His-Purkinje system or ventricular muscle. Under abnormal circumstances, lidocaine may either decrease or increase conduction velocity in the His-Purkinje system or in ventricular muscle; in ischemic tissues, conduction velocity usually decreases substantially (Kupersmith *et al.*, 1975); in tissues depolarized by stretch or low $[K]_o$, lidocaine causes hyperpolarization and significant increases in conduction velocity (Arnsdorf and Bigger, 1972).

Duration of the Action Potential and Refractoriness. Lidocaine causes almost no change in the duration of the action potential of ordinary or specialized atrial fibers. It very substantially decreases the duration of the action potential in Purkinje fibers and ventricular muscle; this effect is attributed to blockade of small Na^+ currents that flow during the plateau of the action potential (Colatsky, 1982). The greatest change is seen in portions of the

His-Purkinje system, where the duration of the action potential is normally longest (Wittig *et al.*, 1973). Thus, lidocaine tends to reduce the temporal and spatial dispersion of refractoriness. The effective refractory period (ERP) shortens after exposure to lidocaine, but this effect is less pronounced than that on the duration of the action potential. This difference may be due to decreased responsiveness (because of delayed reactivation of i_{Na}) and/or the tendency for increased outward current to quell small responses.

Effect on Reentrant Arrhythmias. Lidocaine can abolish ventricular reentry, either by causing two-way block or by improving conduction. If one-way block occurs in ischemic, depolarized elements of a reentry circuit, lidocaine would be likely to abolish reentry by producing two-way block. Conduction can be improved by lidocaine if depolarization and slow conduction are due to decreased g_{K_1} (*e.g.*, stretch or low $[K]_o$) or if slow conduction depends on the long and unequal action potential durations in portions of the reentrant circuit. Lidocaine can increase resting Vm in the former case or selectively shorten the duration of the action potential in the latter case.

Lidocaine is much less effective than quinidine or procainamide in slowing the atrial rate in atrial flutter or atrial fibrillation or in converting these arrhythmias to sinus rhythm. This lack of effect is expected, since lidocaine has so little effect on either refractoriness or responsiveness in the atria.

Electrocardiographic Effects. In striking contrast to quinidine and procainamide, lidocaine causes negligible change in the ECG; the Q-T interval may shorten, but the QRS does not widen. Lidocaine has quite variable effects on the refractory period of the A-V node; there is usually no change, but some individuals show substantial shortening. The latter action is probably responsible for the marked increase in ventricular response that can occur in patients with atrial flutter and A-V block who are treated with lidocaine. Usually the effective refractory period in the His-Purkinje system shortens substantially during treatment with lidocaine. However, lidocaine can cause complete A-V block within the His-Purkinje system in patients with preexisting bundle-branch disease.

Autonomic Nervous System. In contrast to quinidine, procainamide, disopyramide, propranolol, and bretylium, lidocaine has no significant interaction with the autonomic nervous system.

Absorption, Distribution, and Elimination. Although lidocaine is well absorbed after oral administration, it is subject to extensive first-pass hepatic metabolism, and only about one third of the drug reaches the general circulation. Thus, the concentrations of drug in plasma are low and unpredictable. In addition, many patients experience nausea, vomiting, and abdominal discomfort after oral administration of lidocaine, and this route is thus not used. The drug is almost completely absorbed after intramuscular administration.

About 70% of lidocaine in plasma is bound to proteins, mostly alpha-1 acid glycoprotein. Distribution is rapid, and the apparent volume of distribution for lidocaine is normally about 1 liter per kilogram; this volume is substantially reduced in patients with heart failure (Thomson *et al.*, 1973).

Essentially no lidocaine is excreted unchanged in the urine. Deethylation in the liver results in the appearance of monoethylglycylxylidine and then glycine xylidide. The former metabolite has antiarrhythmic activity, while the latter has almost none (Burney *et al.*, 1974). Severe hepatic disease or reduced perfusion of the liver in heart failure decreases the rate of metabolism (Thomson *et al.*, 1973). The clearance of lidocaine approaches the rate of hepatic blood flow and is thus very sensitive to changes in this parameter (Nies *et al.*, 1976). The clearance of lidocaine also may decrease as a result of prolonged infusion (LeLorier *et al.*, 1977). The half-time for elimination is normally about 100 minutes.

Preparations, Dosage, and Routes of Administration. *Lidocaine hydrochloride injection* (XYLOCAINE) is available for intravenous administration in solutions containing 10 or 20 mg/ml; the injection contains no preservative, sympathomimetic, or other vasoconstrictor, and *it is thus the preparation of lidocaine that should be given intravenously.* Catastrophic arrhythmias can occur if preparations that contain sympathomimetic amines are used accidentally.

Lidocaine is only administered intravenously or intramuscularly. To achieve effective concentrations rapidly in plasma, intravenous administration of about 1 to 1.5 mg/kg of body weight is used. A second injection may be required in 5 minutes; this should be half the size of the first. Smaller doses should be used for patients who are in heart failure. Rapid infusion also may be employed to administer the loading dose. A constant rate of intravenous infusion is used to maintain an effective concentration. Infusions in the range of 1 to 4 mg per minute produce therapeutic concentrations in plasma of 1 to 5 μg/ml in 7 to 10 hours; in patients with heart failure or shock, the same rate of infusion will produce plasma concentrations two or more times higher (Appendix II). As the circulatory status changes, hepatic blood flow can change dramatically and shifts in the concentration of lidocaine in plasma will reflect these alterations (Nies *et al.*, 1976). Lidocaine can be given intramuscularly in emergencies to obtain effective concentrations in plasma quickly. A dose of 4 to 5 mg/kg will produce an effective concentration within 15 minutes, and this therapeutic level is maintained for about 90 minutes (Lie *et al.*, 1978).

THERAPEUTIC USES

Lidocaine has a narrow antiarrhythmic spectrum. It is used almost exclusively to treat ventricular arrhythmias, primarily in intensive care units. Lidocaine is effective against ventricular arrhythmias caused by acute myocardial infarction, open-heart surgery, and digitalis. After many negative studies (*see* Bigger *et al.*, 1977), Lie and coworkers (1974) demonstrated that infusions at a rate of 3 mg per minute provided effective prophylaxis for primary ventricular fibrillation in the acute phase of myocardial infarction. The utility of the intramuscular administration of lidocaine to prevent primary ventricular fibrillation while patients with acute myocardial infarction are being transported to a hospital is in dispute (Valentine *et al.*, 1974; Lie *et al.*, 1978).

UNTOWARD EFFECTS

Lidocaine has few undesirable cardiovascular effects, although it can adversely affect hemodynamics in patients who have severely compromised cardiac function. The main adverse effects are on the central nervous system. At concentrations in plasma near 5 μg/ml, symptoms are often subtle, such as feelings of dissociation, paresthesias (often perioral), mild drowsiness, or agitation. Higher concentrations may cause decreased hearing, disorientation, muscle twitching, convulsions, or respiratory arrest. The minor central nervous system effects are not dangerous but do severely disturb some patients. Such symptoms should prompt a decrease of the infusion rate. The more severe toxic manifestations are life threatening.

Few drug interactions have been reported with lidocaine. β-Adrenergic antagonists can decrease hepatic blood flow in patients with heart disease. This will cause a decrease in the rate of hepatic metabolism of lidocaine and an increase in its plasma concentration (Nies et al., 1976). Other basic drugs can displace lidocaine from its binding sites on alpha-1 acid glycoprotein (Routledge et al., 1980). Plasma concentrations of lidocaine are higher in patients who are receiving cimetidine concurrently. The mechanism of this interaction is complex, but the dose of lidocaine may require adjustment (Knapp et al., 1983). Lidocaine appears to potentiate the effects of succinylcholine.

PHENYTOIN

Phenytoin has been used since 1938 in the treatment of epileptic seizures (see Chapter 20). In 1950, Harris and Kokernot reported that phenytoin was an effective therapeutic agent for ventricular tachycardia in experimental acute myocardial infarction in the dog. Clinical studies have demonstrated its utility for ventricular arrhythmias in man; it is particularly noted for its efficacy against arrhythmias in patients with digitalis toxicity (see Damato, 1969; Atkinson and Davison, 1974). The history, chemistry, and preparations of phenytoin are discussed in Chapter 20.

PHARMACOLOGICAL PROPERTIES

Cardiac Electrophysiological Effects. The electrophysiological effects of phenytoin are very similar, but not identical, to those of lidocaine.

Automaticity. Therapeutic concentrations of phenytoin have no effect on the normal sinus node of the rabbit *in vitro;* toxic concentrations cause a modest slowing. Phenytoin can reverse sinoatrial

block produced by digitalis in the isolated rabbit atrium. Rarely, phenytoin causes depression of the sinus node in patients with sinus node disease (see Bigger and Reiffel, 1979). Phenytoin has the same effect on normal automaticity in cardiac Purkinje fibers as does lidocaine, probably by the same mechanism, that is, a marked increase in i_{K_1}. Phenytoin is effective in abolishing triggered activity due to digitalis-induced delayed afterdepolarizations in cardiac Purkinje fibers (Rosen et al., 1976; Peon et al., 1978). This action may underlie phenytoin's efficacy against certain arrhythmias caused by cardiac glycosides.

Excitability, Responsiveness, and Conduction. Phenytoin has effects on excitability that are virtually identical to those of lidocaine (Bigger et al., 1970). Its effects on responsiveness are also very similar to those of lidocaine. By increasing diastolic potassium conductance, phenytoin makes it difficult to obtain responses at very low levels of Vm. In addition, it can repolarize cells that are depolarized because of decreased membrane conductance. The effects of phenytoin on responsiveness have the same interaction with $[K]_o$ as described for lidocaine (Singh and Vaughan Williams, 1971; Rosen et al., 1976). The discussion of the effects of lidocaine on the duration of the action potential and on *reentrant ventricular arrhythmias* applies to phenytoin as well (see Wit et al., 1975).

Electrocardiographic Effects. Like lidocaine, phenytoin has little effect on the ECG; the Q-T interval often shortens slightly. Clinical electrophysiological studies show that phenytoin has quite variable effects on the A-H interval and the A-V nodal refractory period of patients with normal A-V conduction (Caracta et al., 1973). The A-V nodal refractory period usually shortens significantly when phenytoin is given to digitalized patients. The effective refractory period (ERP) of the His-Purkinje system shortens very significantly in man, presumably due to shortening of the duration of the action potential in Purkinje fibers (Damato, 1969; Bissett et al., 1974).

Autonomic Nervous System. Phenytoin has complex interactions with the autonomic nervous system; most of its effects are central. It has been shown that phenytoin decreases the efferent traffic in cardiac sympathetic nerves caused by ouabain toxicity (Gillis et al., 1971). Phenytoin also may modulate vagal efferent activity via a central action. Phenytoin has no peripheral cholinergic or β-adrenergic blocking activity.

Absorption, Distribution, and Elimination. Only a few points that are crucial to the use of phenytoin as an antiarrhythmic drug will be discussed here. A more detailed discussion is presented in Chapter 20.

Absorption of phenytoin from the gastrointestinal tract is slow and somewhat erratic. Absorption after intramuscular injection is also slow and may be incomplete. About 90% of phenytoin in plasma is bound to albumin; the fraction is less in patients with uremia. After intravenous administration, phenytoin is distributed to tissues reasonably rapidly. The drug is eliminated by hepatic hydroxylation. Since the major metabolites of phenytoin lack anticonvulsant properties, it is presumed that they have no antiarrhythmic activity. Metabolism is relatively slow and not substantially altered by changes in hepatic blood flow. In some patients, the enzyme system that metabolizes phenytoin becomes saturated by concentrations of the drug in the therapeutic range; hence, dose-dependent kinetics of elimination can result and can cause unexpected toxicity (see Chapter 20; Appendix II).

Dosage and Routes of Administration. Phenytoin should be given by intermittent intravenous injection or orally. The vehicle used for the injectable preparation has a pH of about 12, and causes severe phlebitis if infused. Critical arrhythmias should not be treated by the intramuscular route because absorption is too unreliable. The schedule for *intermittent intravenous injection* of phenytoin is almost identical to that described above for procainamide: 100 mg of phenytoin is given every 5 minutes until the arrhythmia is controlled or until adverse effects are encountered (Bigger *et al.*, 1968). The rate of injection should not exceed 50 mg per minute. Usually about 700 mg is required; doses above 1000 mg are rarely needed. *Oral treatment* of arrhythmias usually is initiated with loading doses because of phenytoin's long elimination half-time. A dose of 15 mg/kg is given the first day, 7.5 mg/kg on the second and third days, and 4 to 6 mg/kg per day for chronic maintenance (most often 400 mg per day). The oral maintenance dose can be given once a day or divided into two portions.

THERAPEUTIC USES

Phenytoin is used to treat ventricular arrhythmias, paroxysmal atrial flutter or fibrillation, and supraventricular arrhythmias caused by digitalis. Phenytoin is usually effective against ventricular arrhythmias seen after open-heart surgery and acute myocardial infarction, but lidocaine is equally effective and is easier to use. Phenytoin is relatively ineffective against recurrent, drug-resistant ventricular tachycardia in patients with chronic ischemic heart disease. Phenytoin reduces ventricular arrhythmias in the year following myocardial infarction if the concentration of the drug in plasma is kept above 10 μg/ml (Vajda *et al.*, 1973; *see also* Bigger *et al.*, 1977); such concentrations are readily attained with doses of 400 to 500 mg per day. Phenytoin is highly effective against multiform and complex ventricular premature depolarizations, ventricular tachycardia, and atrial tachycardia with A-V block induced by digitalis; often, small doses will yield striking effects. It is somewhat less effective against nonparoxysmal A-V junctional tachycardia; higher doses are needed, and a larger fraction of cases fails to respond. Phenytoin has been used effectively with electrophysiological guidance against sustained ventricular tachycardia in chronic coronary heart disease (Fisher *et al.*, 1977; Horowitz *et al.*, 1978) and

against ventricular tachyarrhythmias in the long Q-T syndrome, often in conjunction with a β-adrenergic blocking agent (Schwartz *et al.*, 1975). The effects of phenytoin on sinus arrest or sinoatrial block caused by digitalis in human subjects are unknown. Phenytoin is relatively ineffective against the common atrial arrhythmias, such as atrial flutter, atrial fibrillation, and supraventricular tachycardia (see Bigger *et al.*, 1968; Damato, 1969; Atkinson and Davison, 1974; Wit *et al.*, 1975).

UNTOWARD EFFECTS

The most prominent adverse effects of phenytoin during acute treatment of arrhythmias are referable to the central nervous system and include drowsiness, nystagmus, vertigo, ataxia, and nausea. The progression of such symptoms shows an orderly relationship to increasing concentrations in plasma. In acute treatment of arrhythmias, neurological signs usually indicate that plasma concentrations are in excess of 20 μg/ml. This information is useful; if an arrhythmia has not responded to phenytoin at concentrations of 20 μg/ml or more, it is unlikely to respond at higher concentrations. A myriad of adverse reactions and interactions with other drugs has been described during chronic therapy with phenytoin; these are discussed in Chapter 20.

TOCAINIDE AND MEXILETINE

Both tocainide and mexiletine are antiarrhythmic drugs that closely resemble lidocaine in their chemical structures, pharmacological properties, and therapeutic indications. In contrast to lidocaine, both drugs are effective after oral administration. Tocainide has recently been approved for general use in the United States, while mexiletine is available for investigational purposes.

The effects of tocainide on the electrophysiological properties of specialized cardiac fibers and on electrocardiographic intervals are virtually identical to those of lidocaine (see Tables 31–3 and 31–4); however, it has not been directly determined if tocainide shares the effects of lidocaine on ischemic or damaged myocardial fibers (*e.g.*, increased duration of the ERP) (see Holmes *et al.*, 1983). In general, the electrophysiological effects of mexiletine also resemble those of lidocaine. However, the capacity of mexiletine to reduce the automaticity of cardiac Purkinje fibers is more reminiscent of quinidine, in that a shift of the threshold voltage for firing toward more positive values of Vm plays an important role. In patients with impaired A-V nodal and ventricular conduction, mexiletine may be more apt to reduce conduction velocities in the affected regions than is lidocaine (see Keefe *et al.*, 1981).

Tocainide is completely absorbed after oral administration; peak concentrations in plasma occur within 1 to 2 hours. Up to 50% of a dose of tocainide is excreted as such in the urine. The half-life in plasma is 12 to 15 hours, and this value may increase twofold in patients with renal or hepatic disease (see Holmes *et al.*, 1983). Mexiletine is readily absorbed after oral administration, and its systemic bioavailability is about 90%. The drug is eliminated after hepatic metabolism; about 10% of a dose is found unchanged in the urine. The elimination half-life is approximately 10 hours.

Tocainide and mexiletine have been used for the intravenous and oral treatment of ventricular arrhythmias, especially those that arise acutely after myocardial infarction; responsiveness to lidocaine is quite predictive of a response to tocainide. Chronic oral therapy of ventricular ectopic beats with either drug has met with variable success. In some studies, the effectiveness of tocainide has appeared to approach that of procainamide or quinidine (*see* Holmes *et al.*, 1983). Mexiletine has been reported to suppress ventricular tachycardia in some patients who had not responded to other drugs. In contrast to lidocaine, tocainide prolongs the refractory period of the accessory pathway in patients with Wolff-Parkinson-White syndrome; however, its therapeutic value in this condition has not been established. While tocainide can suppress digitalis-induced arrhythmias in dogs, similar observations in man have not been reported.

Tocainide hydrochloride (TONOCARD) is available in 400- and 600-mg tablets. The usual oral dose is 400 to 600 mg, three times daily.

OTHER LOCAL ANESTHETIC ANTIARRHYTHMIC DRUGS

Three investigational agents—*encainide, flecainide,* and *lorcainide*—possess a pattern of electrophysiological effects that differs appreciably from those of drugs such as lidocaine and procainamide (*see* Table 31–2). This group of drugs may prove to have particular utility in suppressing premature ventricular contractions and potentially life-threatening ventricular tachycardias (*see* Keefe *et al.*, 1981; Eiriksson and Brogden, 1984; Kunze *et al.*, 1984; Meinertz *et al.*, 1984).

Encainide, flecainide, and lorcainide have rather selective depressant effects on fast sodium channels. Thus, they decrease the $\dot{V}_{max}$ and overshoot of action potentials in atrial, ventricular, and Purkinje fibers and slow conduction in these structures, most prominently in the His-Purkinje system. There are relatively small effects on repolarization, duration of action potentials, and the ERP in Purkinje fibers; the pattern of such effects appears to vary with the individual agent. A-V nodal conduction velocity and refractory period are usually unchanged by encainide and lorcainide; however, refractory periods in accessory pathways are often prolonged by these two drugs. The QRS complex is widened by all three agents in a dose-dependent fashion, and a marked effect on this parameter is one indication for reduced dosage.

While all three drugs are readily absorbed after oral administration, only flecainide is not subject to marked first-pass hepatic extraction. Encainide and lorcainide exhibit dose-dependent bioavailability, which can be greater than 80% during chronic administration of therapeutic doses. The half-life of encainide in plasma is about 4 hours. Two hepatic

metabolites accumulate in plasma during chronic administration, the O-demethylated compound and its 3-methoxy derivative. The former has appreciable antiarrhythmic activity, and it may have depressant effects on A-V nodal conduction that are not displayed by the parent drug. Estimates of the plasma half-life of lorcainide range from 8 to 13 hours. While aromatic hydroxylations are the principal routes of biotransformation, the active N-dealkylated derivative (*norlorcainide*) accumulates during chronic therapy to concentrations in plasma that exceed those of the parent drug. Estimates of the plasma half-life of flecainide range from 7 to 24 hours; published information on its pharmacokinetic properties is scarce.

Clinical investigations of these three drugs indicate that they may be particularly useful in the long-term management of premature ventricular beats, especially in those patients who have not responded to other agents. Successful suppression of ventricular tachycardia has been more variable. Encainide and lorcainide may also be beneficial in the treatment of some patients with the Wolff-Parkinson-White syndrome.

PROPRANOLOL

The pharmacology of the β-adrenergic blocking agents is discussed in Chapter 9. Only those properties of propranolol related to its use in the treatment of cardiac arrhythmias are considered here.

PHARMACOLOGICAL PROPERTIES

Cardiac Electrophysiological Effects. Most of the antiarrhythmic effects of propranolol can be explained by its selective β-adrenergic blocking action. Propranolol has two other direct actions that must be considered in connection with its antiarrhythmic activity: it increases background outward current (i_{K_1}) and, in high concentrations, it significantly depresses i_{Na}.

Automaticity. β-Adrenergic stimulation causes a marked increase in the slope of phase-4 depolarization and in the spontaneous firing rate in the *sinus node*. This effect is competitively blocked by propranolol. Propranolol has little effect on sinus rate when catecholamines are absent. The resting heart rate is only slightly affected by propranolol, but the acceleration of sinus rate during exercise or as a result of emotion is blunted (Seides *et al.*, 1974). Propranolol can cause severe slowing of sinus rate in patients with preexisting sinus node disease (Strauss *et al.*, 1976). Also, propranolol has significant effects on automaticity in cardiac Purkinje fibers. The ventricular rate slows somewhat when dogs with complete A-V block are given propranolol, due to blockade of background sympathetic activity (Wallace *et al.*, 1967). When the firing rate of Purkinje fibers is increased by high concentrations of catecholamines, propranolol will reverse this action and slow spontaneous firing. Under some conditions, cardiac Purkinje fibers require the action of catecholamines to sustain their spontaneous activity. In this case, propranolol can totally abolish normal automaticity in the His-Purkinje system. At low concentrations, propranolol increases outward background current, i_{K_1}, in Purkinje fibers, as do lidocaine and phenytoin; this action decreases automaticity as well (Stagg and Wallace, 1974).

Excitability and Threshold. The electrical threshold of the atria and ventricles of normal dogs is not much affected by propranolol, and the electrical threshold for ventricular fibrillation is not consistently increased (Wallace *et al.*, 1966b). However, propranolol increases the threshold for fibrillation after experimental infarction (Gang *et al.*, 1984). In Purkinje fibers, concentrations of propranolol that cause shortening of the action potential will increase slightly the electrical current threshold. Very high concentrations increase threshold in Purkinje fibers by an effect on i_{Na}.

Responsiveness and Conduction. Only very high concentrations of propranolol (*e.g.*, 1000 to 3000 ng/ml) affect responsiveness in Purkinje fibers (Davis and Temte, 1968). These concentrations are much greater than those needed for substantial β-adrenergic blockade (100 to 300 ng/ml). However, concentrations over 1000 ng/ml are often required for control of ventricular arrhythmias (Woosley *et al.*, 1977). Low-amplitude premature responses are abolished by propranolol (Davis and Temte, 1968). These effects are similar to those seen with lidocaine or phenytoin and are probably due to an increase in g_{K_1}. Different effects may occur in abnormal fibers. In the dog heart *in situ*, propranolol causes slowing of intramyocardial conduction in muscle that is made acutely ischemic. It has no such effect on normal portions of the ventricle (Kupersmith *et al.*, 1976). Slow

responses can be dependent on catecholamines, as can afterdepolarizations (Carmeliet and Vereeke, 1969; Wit and Cranefield, 1977); propranolol or other β-adrenergic blockers should ameliorate arrhythmias caused by these mechanisms.

Duration of the Action Potential and Refractoriness. Propranolol has little effect on the duration of action potentials in the sinus node, atrium, or A-V node. In ventricular muscle, action potentials shorten slightly; in Purkinje fibers, action potentials often shorten substantially (Davis and Temte, 1968). Propranolol has little effect on refractoriness of normal atrial or ventricular muscle. It causes a substantial increase in the *effective refractory period* (ERP) of the A-V node due to its β-adrenergic blocking action; *this action is the basis of the major uses of propranolol as an antiarrhythmic drug.* The ERP of Purkinje fibers is shortened substantially (Davis and Temte, 1968).

Effect on Reentrant Arrhythmias. Propranolol could interrupt reentrant activity in many ways. In paroxysmal supraventricular tachycardia due to A-V nodal reentry, the substantial increase in A-V nodal refractoriness may abolish reentry. In the ventricles, propranolol may abolish slow responses that are dependent on catecholamines, repolarize tissues depolarized by virtue of decreased g_{K_1} (*e.g.*, stretch or low $[K]_o$), or abolish depressed fast responses in ischemic ventricular muscle. In higher concentration, propranolol has "quinidine-like" effects on phase-0 depolarization and responsiveness of Purkinje fibers. In addition, propranolol may favorably influence arrhythmias by its effect on the relationship between oxygen supply and demand by decreasing myocardial oxygen utilization and thus the extent of ischemia.

Electrocardiographic Effects. Propranolol often causes an increase in the P-R interval and slight shortening of the Q-T_c without any effect on the duration of the QRS complex. Clinical electrophysiological studies reveal little effect of propranolol, except for the dramatic increase in the ERP of the A-V node; there is no increase in the H-V interval after conventional doses of the drug (Seides *et al.*, 1974).

Autonomic Nervous System. Propranolol causes β-adrenergic blockade and leaves vagal and α-adrenergic mechanisms intact. A detailed discussion of β-adrenergic antagonists is presented in Chapter 9.

Absorption, Distribution, and Elimination. Intestinal absorption of propranolol is excellent, but extensive first-pass metabolism reduces bioavailability considerably (*see* Chapter 9; Appendix II). As with lidocaine, the hepatic extraction of propranolol is very high and elimination is significantly reduced when hepatic blood flow decreases. Propranolol may decrease its own elimination rate by decreasing cardiac output and hepatic blood flow, particularly in patients with heart disease.

Dosage and Routes of Administration. Propranolol is given orally for long-term treatment of cardiac arrhythmias. Concentrations in plasma that are associated with therapeutic effects vary widely (20 to 1000 ng/ml) and depend on the arrhythmia being treated. The dose ranges from 40 to 80 mg per day for treatment of arrhythmias that are sensitive to effects of the drug. More than 1000 mg a day may be needed to treat resistant arrhythmias. Propranolol is usually effective when given four times a day. The duration of action can be prolonged by the administration of large doses, since propranolol has a greater margin of safety than do the other antiarrhythmic drugs. For emergency use, propranolol can be given intravenously; 1 to 3 mg is administered with very careful monitoring of the ECG, arterial blood pressure, and pulmonary arterial pressure (by means of a Swan-Ganz catheter); this dose may be repeated after a few minutes if necessary. Much lower doses are needed to achieve a given plasma concentration when given intravenously than after oral administration because first-pass hepatic extraction is avoided.

THERAPEUTIC USES

Supraventricular Arrhythmias. Propranolol is used primarily to treat supraventricular tachyarrhythmias such as atrial fibrillation, atrial flutter, or paroxysmal supraventricular tachycardia. For these arrhythmias, the objective of therapy usually is to slow the ventricular rate rather than to abolish the arrhythmia. Propranolol accomplishes this objective by blocking β-adrenergic influences on the A-V node, thereby increasing refractoriness of the A-V node. Only rarely does propranolol convert these supraventricular arrhythmias to sinus rhythm. Not infrequently, propran-

olol and digitalis will successfully control the ventricular rate in patients with atrial fibrillation or flutter when maximal doses of digitalis alone do not; this additive effect may result from the fact that digitalis increases vagal tone, while propranolol blocks β-adrenergic influences on the A-V node.

Combination therapy with quinidine and propranolol probably improves the likelihood of converting atrial fibrillation to sinus rhythm. Propranolol has been helpful in preventing paroxysmal supraventricular tachycardia due to A-V nodal reciprocation and the paroxysmal supraventricular tachycardia of the Wolff-Parkinson-White syndrome alone or in combination with quinidine (Gettes and Yoshonis, 1970; Wu *et al.*, 1974). In the latter condition, quinidine increases the refractoriness of the accessory A-V connection and propranolol can be relied upon to increase A-V nodal refractoriness.

Ventricular Arrhythmias. Conventional doses of propranolol (240 to 320 mg per day) are not likely to be effective against ventricular arrhythmias except in special circumstances. Propranolol is an excellent choice for treatment of symptomatic ventricular premature depolarizations in patients without structural heart disease; the drug often markedly reduces symptoms, even when the arrhythmia is not greatly affected. When ventricular arrhythmias are triggered by exercise or emotion, even small doses of propranolol (*e.g.*, 80 to 160 mg per day) are very likely to prevent them. In patients with ischemic heart disease, propranolol may ameliorate ventricular arrhythmias by preventing or reducing ischemia. However, most ventricular arrhythmias respond incompletely or not at all to conventional doses of propranolol. Large doses of propranolol (500 to 1000 mg a day) may be required to control ventricular arrhythmias (Woosley *et al.*, 1979). Propranolol is the drug of choice for severe ventricular arrhythmias in the prolonged Q-T syndrome; when propranolol fails, removal of the left stellate ganglion may be effective (Vincent *et al.*, 1974; Schwartz and Moss, 1981).

Two large, randomized, placebo-controlled trials, one with timolol (10 mg twice a day) and one with propranolol (60 or 80 mg three times a day), showed that treatment with these β-adrenergic antagonists was effective for reducing death and nonfatal myocardial infarction in the year after acute myocardial infarction (Beta-Blocker Heart Attack Study Group, 1981; Norwegian Multicenter Study Group, 1981). Treatment with metoprolol for 2 years after myocardial infarction has also been shown to reduce mortality (*see* Symposium, 1984a).

Digitalis-Induced Arrhythmias. Propranolol abolishes ventricular arrhythmias induced by digitalis by effects both directly on the heart and, probably, on the central nervous system (Gillis, 1969).

However, the incidence of adverse effects during treatment of digitalis-induced arrhythmias with propranolol is higher than with phenytoin or lidocaine.

UNTOWARD EFFECTS

Propranolol usually is well tolerated; most of its undesirable effects are related to β-adrenergic blockade. In patients with ventricular failure, the level of sympathetic activity is high and provides significant support to the ventricle. Therefore, when propranolol is used as an antiarrhythmic drug, particularly when it is given intravenously, significant hypotension or left ventricular failure can occur. Occasionally, propranolol will precipitate left ventricular failure in a patient who has not previously had heart failure. Many patients who have ventricular failure can tolerate chronic oral therapy with propranolol if digitalis, vasodilators, or diuretics are used concomitantly. The potent effect of propranolol on conduction in the A-V node can also lead to serious adverse effects, such as A-V block or asystole. Sudden withdrawal of propranolol in patients with angina pectoris can precipitate worsening of angina, cardiac arrhythmias, and acute myocardial infarction. Other untoward effects of propranolol are described in Chapter 9.

BRETYLIUM

Bretylium was introduced into medicine as an antihypertensive agent in the 1950s; however, for a number of reasons, it was supplanted by guanethidine (see Chapter 9). Bretylium also has antiarrhythmic properties and, in 1978, was approved in the United States for intramuscular or intravenous administration in emergency situations when other antiarrhythmic drugs prove to be ineffective.

Chemistry. Bretylium has the following structural formula:

Bretylium

PHARMACOLOGICAL PROPERTIES

Cardiac Electrophysiological Effects. Bretylium directly affects the electrical properties of heart muscle. In addition, it has important interactions with the autonomic nervous system (see Chapter 9).

Automaticity. The effects of bretylium on cardiac automaticity are complex and not fully understood. Bretylium has little direct effect on automaticity of the isolated perfused *sinus node*. It decreases the sinus rate slightly in dogs with surgically denervated hearts (Waxman and Wallace, 1972). Bretylium lacks potent effects on normal automaticity in the *His-Purkinje system*. Immediately after injection, the firing rate of Purkinje fibers *in vitro* increases and quiescent fibers may become automatic (Bigger and Jaffe, 1971; Allen *et al.*, 1972). These effects are probably caused by release of catecholamines from adrenergic nerve terminals and are abolished by pretreatment with either reserpine or propranolol.

Excitability and Threshold. Bretylium has little effect on the diastolic electrical current threshold. However, the drug does increase the ventricular fibrillation threshold significantly (Allen *et al.*, 1972; Kniffen *et al.*, 1975). This action probably does not depend on its adrenergic neuron blocking action. Other blockers of adrenergic neurons (such as guanethidine) do not elevate the ventricular fibrillation threshold.

Responsiveness and Conduction. Therapeutic concentrations of bretylium have no significant effect on membrane responsiveness or conduction in either Purkinje fibers or ventricular muscle. Toxic concentrations cause mild decreases of these parameters.

Duration of the Action Potential and Refractoriness. Bretylium causes no change in either the duration of action potentials or the effective refractory period (ERP) of isolated rabbit atria. However, atrial ERP increases after the administration of bretylium to both intact and sympathectomized dogs. Bretylium causes marked prolongation of action potentials in canine Purkinje and ventricular muscle fibers (Bigger and Jaffe, 1971; Waxman and Wallace, 1972). The distribution of this change within the conducting system is such that the normal disparity in the duration of the action potentials is reduced. Also, bretylium minimizes the disparity in the duration of the action potential and ERP between normal and infarcted regions in experimental models of acute myocardial infarction in dogs (Cardinal and Sasyniuk, 1978).

Effect on Reentrant Arrhythmias. Bretylium could terminate reentrant arrhythmias either by its capacity to prolong refractoriness markedly without affecting propagation of the cardiac impulse or by releasing catecholamines. The latter effect may cause repolarization and increased conductivity in abnormal depolarized tissues.

Electrocardiographic Effects. In human subjects, bretylium decreases the sinus rate and increases the P-R and Q-T intervals; the duration of the QRS complex does not increase. Initially, after intravenous doses, heart rate may increase. In dogs, bretylium causes the sinus rate and conduction in the A-V node to slow, due to a direct effect; conduction in the His-Purkinje system is not altered (Waxman and Wallace, 1972). In man, acute administration decreases the refractory periods in the A-V node and the ventricles (Anderson *et al.,* 1982).

Autonomic Nervous System. Bretylium has no effect on vagal reflexes and does not alter the responsiveness of cardiac cholinergic receptors. However, the drug profoundly affects the sympathetic nervous system. It is taken up and concentrated in adrenergic nerve terminals. Initially, as it is taken up, bretylium releases norepinephrine from nerve terminals; later, it prevents release of the transmitter (*see* Chapter 9). It does *not* depress preganglionic or postganglionic sympathetic nerve conduction, impair transmission across sympathetic ganglia, deplete the adrenergic neuron of norepinephrine, or decrease the responsiveness of adrenergic receptors. During chronic treatment with bretylium, the adrenergic receptors show increased responsiveness to circulating catecholamines.

Hemodynamic Effects. Even very high concentrations of bretylium do not decrease the contractility of the mammalian myocardium; contractility can increase as a result of release of catecholamines (Heissenbuttel and Bigger, 1979). Bretylium can cause hypotension due to its neuronal blocking action (Chatterjee *et al.,* 1973). Hypotension is accentuated by standing and is maximal during upright exercise, because bretylium blocks vital reflexes and prevents both vasoconstriction during standing and tachycardia during exercise.

Absorption, Distribution, and Elimination. There is a paucity of critically needed information on the pharmacokinetics of bretylium. Oral absorption of bretylium is notoriously poor (less than 40%), as would be expected of a quaternary amine. Bretylium is eliminated almost entirely by renal excretion without significant metabolism; 70 to 80% of an intramuscular dose is excreted unchanged in the urine. The average half-time for elimination is about 9 hours; longer half-times of 15 to 30 hours occur in patients with renal insufficiency (*see* Heissenbuttel and Bigger, 1979).

Preparation, Dosage, and Routes of Administration. In the United States, bretylium is approved only for short-term intravenous or intramuscular use. It is available as *bretylium tosylate* (BRETYLOL) in a solution containing 50 mg/ml. The contents of the 10-ml ampul should be diluted to a volume of 50 ml or more, and a dose of 5 to 10 mg/kg should be infused over 10 to 30 minutes every 6 hours. In extreme emergencies, such as during cardiac resuscitation, a dose of 5 mg/kg of the undiluted solution can be injected intravenously; this dose can be repeated at intervals of 15 to 30 minutes, not to exceed a total of about 30 mg/kg. For intramuscular administration, undiluted bretylium tosylate should be used, and doses are usually repeated every 6 to 8 hours. The patient should be kept supine during treatment or, if allowed up, carefully observed for postural hypotension.

THERAPEUTIC USES

Currently, bretylium tosylate is recommended only for treatment of life-threatening ventricular arrhythmias that fail to respond to adequate doses of a first-line antiarrhythmic drug, such as lidocaine or procainamide. Use of bretylium should be limited to intensive care facilities. Although experience with bretylium is limited and many published studies do not contain adequate controls, the response of severe, refractory ventricular arrhythmias has been impressive. Even ventricular fibrillation that has failed to respond to other drugs and repeated DC countershock may respond promptly to bretylium tosylate (*see* Heissenbuttel and Bigger, 1979; Symposium, 1984b). Ventricular tachycardia or ventricular premature depolarizations usually respond much later (*e.g.,* 6 hours or more after a dose).

UNTOWARD EFFECTS

Hypotension is the principal undesirable effect of bretylium tosylate when it is used intravenously to treat acute arrhythmias. Orthostatic hypotension of significant magnitude usually occurs, and supine hypotension is not rare. Hypotension is occasionally so severe that bretylium must be discontinued. Rapid intravenous administration may cause *nausea* and *vomiting*. During prolonged oral therapy, many patients develop tachyphylaxis to the hypotensive but not to the antiarrhythmic effects of bretylium. *Parotid pain* is a relatively common untoward effect during chronic oral therapy. Tricyclic antidepressant drugs can prevent uptake of bretylium by adrenergic nerve terminals and thus reduce its proclivity to cause orthostatic hypotension.

AMIODARONE

Amiodarone is an orally effective, investigational drug that shares some of the properties of bretylium. In particular, it slows repolarization in various types of myocardial fibers and increases the ventricular fibrillation threshold.

The electrophysiological effects of amiodarone have not yet been characterized in detail. In addition, the electrocardiographic alterations observed shortly after intravenous administration of the drug are often different from those seen after several days of oral treatment. Active metabolites of amiodarone may be involved, especially in view of its slow metabolism and elimination. Acutely, there is little increase of the refractory period in the His-Purkinje system and the ventricular myocardium; nevertheless, amiodarone suppresses ventricular tachycardia in most patients (Hariman *et al.,* 1984; Saksena *et al.,* 1984). It has been suggested that these effects result from a selective action on diseased cardiac tissue to lengthen the refractory period and slow conduction in a fashion similar to that of lidocaine. After chronic oral administration, amiodarone lengthens the ventricular ERP and increases the A-H and H-V intervals (Heger *et al.,* 1981). These effects may be associated with the capacity of the drug to slow A-V nodal conduction and increase the duration of ventricular action potentials (*see* Keefe *et al.*, 1981). The drug has been reported to antagonize α- and β-adrenergic effects noncompetitively; however, the potential role of such actions in the effects of amiodarone has not been defined. Amiodarone increases the ventricular fibrillation threshold in animal models.

The pharmacokinetic properties of amiodarone are complex and poorly characterized. Maximal therapeutic responses may be delayed for many weeks after starting oral administration of the drug at constant dosage; similarly, therapeutic and toxic effects may persist for weeks following discontinuation of amiodarone (*see* Keefe *et al.*, 1981; Wilkinson *et al.*, 1984). Its terminal elimination may be multiphasic, and estimates of plasma half-life have ranged from less than 10 to more than 50 days. Amiodarone is metabolized extensively in the liver. The desethyl derivative accumulates in plasma during chronic therapy; its biological activity has not been determined.

Clinical investigations suggest that amiodarone may be useful in the long-term treatment of patients with recurrent ventricular tachycardia and/or fibrillation (Heger *et al.*, 1981; Hariman *et al.*, 1984; Saksena *et al.*, 1984). It may also be of value in the management of some patients with atrial fibrillation associated with the Wolff-Parkinson-White syndrome (Kappenberger *et al.*, 1984). Even though optimal dosage regimens have not been established, the incidence of cardiovascular toxicity has been low. However, asymptomatic corneal microdeposits develop in nearly all patients treated with the drug, and peripheral neuropathy or disturbed thyroid function has been noted in some.

VERAPAMIL

Verapamil, a derivative of papaverine, was first used as a coronary vasodilator. Further studies showed that the drug has a novel mechanism of action: it blocks calcium channels in the membranes of smooth and cardiac muscle cells. In 1981, verapamil was approved in the United States for treatment of angina pectoris and supraventricular arrhythmias. The general discussion of calcium channel blockers appears in Chapter 33. Discussion here is confined to the use of verapamil to treat arrhythmias.

PHARMACOLOGICAL PROPERTIES

Cardiac Electrophysiological Effects. Verapamil has direct effects on the electrical and mechanical properties of heart muscle and vascular smooth muscle cells.

Impulse Formation. Verapamil slows substantially the spontaneous firing of pacemaker cells in the sinus node *in vitro* (Wit and Cranefield, 1974; Zipes and Fischer, 1974). However, in intact animals and in man heart rate slows only minimally because the direct effect of verapamil is partially nullified by increased sympathetic activity due to the arterial vasodilatation. In man, the usual net effect of verapamil is a 10 to 15% decrease in heart rate. Verapamil has no significant effect on intra-atrial conduction.

Verapamil decreases the rate of phase-4 spontaneous depolarization in cardiac Purkinje fibers (Danilo *et al.*, 1980) and can block the delayed afterdepolarizations and triggered activity seen in experimental digitalis toxicity (Rosen and Danilo, 1980).

Effect on Reentrant Rhythms. The most marked effect of verapamil is on the A-V node (Wit and Cranefield, 1974). In man, as well as other species, verapamil decreases the conduction velocity through the A-V node and significantly increases its functional refractory period. The effect on A-V nodal conduction is presumably a direct result of calcium channel blockade (Husaini *et al.*, 1973; Roy *et al.*, 1974). However, this effect is not prominent at concentrations of certain other calcium channel blockers (*e.g.*, nifedipine) that are achieved clinically. Treatment with atropine and β-adrenergic blocking agents does not prevent the effects of verapamil on the A-V node. The potent actions of verapamil on the A-V node are responsible for its effect on the ventricular response to atrial flutter or fibrillation and its ability to terminate paroxysmal supraventricular tachycardia.

Verapamil can abolish ventricular reentrant rhythms that are caused by slow responses in the ventricles. In addition, verapamil has the ability to protect ischemic cells and can reduce damage during brief periods of ischemia (Watts *et al.*, 1980). The depressed fast responses seen after ischemia can thus be prevented, and reentrant ventricular arrhythmias can be avoided.

Electrocardiographic Effects. Verapamil slows heart rate and increases the P-R interval in sinus rhythm. In patients with atrial fibrillation, verapamil slows ventricular rate substantially.

Autonomic Nervous System. Verapamil has no cholinergic or β-adrenergic blocking properties. However, it does have α-adrenergic blocking activity, which may explain its effect on the arrhythmias seen after release of experimental coronary occlusion.

Absorption, Distribution, and Elimination. The pharmacokinetic properties of verapamil are discussed in Chapter 33 (*see also* Appendix II). Using the ventricular response to atrial fibrillation as an indicator, the effects of verapamil persist after the concentration of the drug falls to unmeasurable levels in plasma, suggesting that an active metabolite might be present. One metabolite, norverapamil, can reach a steady-state concentration in plasma that is approximately equal to that of the parent drug; norverapamil has about 20% of the activity of the parent compound as a vasodilator.

Dosage and Routes of Administration. To convert PSVT to sinus rhythm, a dose of 5 to 10 mg of verapamil is given intravenously over at least 2 minutes. To obtain rapid control of the ventricular rate in atrial fibrillation or atrial flutter, 10 mg of verapamil can be given intravenously over 2 to 5 minutes, and this dose can be repeated in 30 minutes if necessary. To prevent recurrences of PSVT or to control the ventricular response to atrial fibrillation, an 80- to 120-mg dose is given orally four times a day.

THERAPEUTIC USES

Supraventricular Arrhythmias. Verapamil has become the drug of first choice for abolishing acute episodes of paroxysmal supraventricular tachycardia due to A-V nodal reentry or due to anomalous A-V connections (either the Wolff-Parkinson-White type or concealed bypass tracts). Verapamil is also very useful for immediate reduction of the ventricular response to atrial fibrillation or atrial flutter. In man, intravenous verapamil (75 μg/kg) slows the ventricular response to atrial fibrillation by about 30% (Aronow *et al.*, 1979). Atrial tachycardia with A-V block caused by digitalis toxicity may be a manifestation of delayed afterdepolarizations and triggered activity. Verapamil could be effective in abolishing this arrhythmia, but its use is too

risky because it can cause additional A-V block and suppress automaticity in the His-Purkinje system.

Ventricular Arrhythmias. Although verapamil has significant effects on ventricular arrhythmias, it does not play a major role in their treatment because of better alternatives. Verapamil is used to treat ventricular tachycardia and ventricular fibrillation caused by coronary artery spasm; it prevents the episodes of spasm and improves the tolerance of ventricular tissues to ischemia, rather than having a significant direct antiarrhythmic effect. Also, α-adrenergic blocking effects of verapamil may either prevent or reduce the intensity of arrhythmias that result when perfusion of myocardial tissue is restored.

UNTOWARD EFFECTS

The principal adverse effects of verapamil are cardiac and gastrointestinal. Because of its effects on sinus node automaticity, verapamil should be given with great caution to patients who have dysfunction of the S-A node. Because of its potent effect on A-V conduction, verapamil is contraindicated in patients who have preexisting block in the A-V node. Verapamil is also contraindicated in patients with severe left ventricular dysfunction, unless the failure is precipitated by high heart rate. Unexpected sinus bradycardia, A-V block, left ventricular failure, or hypotension can occur in elderly patients after intravenous administration of verapamil. Lower doses and a slower rate of injection should thus be used in patients over the age of 60. Verapamil can increase the ventricular rate when given intravenously to patients with the Wolff-Parkinson-White syndrome and atrial fibrillation; this is due to reflex increases in sympathetic nervous activity (Gulamhusein *et al.*, 1982). The major gastrointestinal effect of verapamil is constipation, but gastric upset and other upper gastrointestinal symptoms can occur as well.

Drug Interactions. Concurrent use of verapamil and β-adrenergic blocking agents or digitalis can lead to significant bradycardia or A-V block. The main reason for this is the additive effects of these drugs on the sinus or A-V nodes. In addition, verapamil interacts with digoxin in a manner similar to the quinidine-digoxin interaction. During treatment with verapamil, a substantial fraction of patients will show a significant increase in the concentration of digoxin in plasma due to a reduction in clearance of the cardiac glycoside. Concomitant use of verapamil with antihypertensive drugs that depress the sinus node, such as reserpine or methyldopa, can intensify sinus bradycardia.

Allen, J. D.; Zaidi, S. A.; Shanks, R. G.; and Pantridge, J. F. The effects of bretylium on experimental cardiac dysrhythmias. *Am. J. Cardiol.*, **1972**, *29*, 641–649.

Anderson, J. L.; Brodine, W. N.; Patterson, E.; Marshall, H. W.; Allison, S. D.; and Lucchesi, B. R. Serial electrophysiologic effects of bretylium in man and their correlation with plasma concentrations. *J. Cardiovasc. Pharmacol.*, **1982**, *4*, 871–872.

Arnsdorf, M. F., and Bigger, J. T., Jr. Effect of lidocaine hydrochloride on membrane conductance in mammalian cardiac Purkinje fibers. *J. Clin. Invest.*, **1972**, *51*, 2252–2263.

———. The effect of lidocaine on components of excitability in long mammalian cardiac Purkinje fibers. *J. Pharmacol. Exp. Ther.*, **1975**, *195*, 206–215.

Aronow, W. S.; Landa, D.; Plasencia, G.; Wong, R.; Karlsberg, R. P.; and Ferlinz, J. Verapamil in atrial fibrillation and atrial flutter. *Clin. Pharmacol. Ther.*, **1979**, *26*, 578–582.

Atkinson, A. J., and Davison, R. Diphenylhydantoin as an antiarrhythmic drug. *Annu. Rev. Med.*, **1974**, *25*, 99–113.

Bean, B. P.; Cohen, C. J.; and Tsien, R. W. Lidocaine block of cardiac sodium channels. *J. Gen. Physiol.*, **1983**, *81*, 613–642.

Bellet, S.; Hamdan, G.; Somlyo, A.; and Lara, R. The reversal of cardiotoxic effects of quinidine by molar sodium lactate: an experimental study. *Am. J. Med. Sci.*, **1959**, *237*, 165–176.

Beta-Blocker Heart Attack Study Group. The beta-blocker heart attack trial. *J.A.M.A.*, **1981**, *246*, 2073–2074

Bigger, J. T., Jr. Pharmacologic and clinical control of antiarrhythmic drugs. *Am. J. Med.*, **1975**, *58*, 479–488.

Bigger, J. T., Jr., and Heissenbuttel, R. H. The use of procaine amide and lidocaine in the treatment of cardiac arrhythmias. *Prog. Cardiovasc. Dis.*, **1969**, *11*, 515–534.

Bigger, J. T., Jr., and Jaffe, C. C. The effect of bretylium tosylate on the electrophysiologic properties of ventricular muscle and Purkinje fibers. *Am. J. Cardiol.*, **1971**, *27*, 82–92.

Bigger, J. T., Jr., and Mandel, W. J. Effects of lidocaine on the electrophysiological properties of ventricular muscle and Purkinje fibers. *J. Clin. Invest.*, **1970**, *49*, 63–77.

Bigger, J. T., Jr.; Schmidt, D. H.; and Kutt, H. Relationship between the plasma level of diphenylhydantoin sodium and its cardiac antiarrhythmic effects. *Circulation*, **1968**, *38*, 363–374.

Bigger, J. T., Jr.; Weinberg, D. I.; Kovalik, A. T. W.; Harris, P. D.; Cranefield, P. F.; and Hoffman, B. F. Effects of diphenylhydantoin on excitability and automaticity in the canine heart. *Circ. Res.*, **1970**, *26*, 1–15.

Birkhead, J. S., and Vaughan Williams, E. M. Dual effect of disopyramide on atrial and atrioventricular conduction and refractory periods. *Br. Heart J.*, **1977**, *39*, 657–660.

Bissett, J. K.; de Soyza, N. D. B.; Kane, J. J.; and Murphy, M. L. Improved intraventricular conduction of premature beats after diphenylhydantoin. *Am. J. Cardiol.*, **1974**, *33*, 493–497.

Brown, H. F., and DiFrancesco, D. Voltage clamp investigations of membrane currents underlying pace-maker activity in rabbit sino-atrial node. *J. Physiol. (Lond.)*, **1980**, *308*, 331–351.

Brown, H. F., and Noble, S. J. Effects of adrenaline on membrane currents underlying pacemaker activity in frog atrial muscle. *J. Physiol. (Lond.)*, **1974**, *238*, 51–53.

Burney, R. G.; DiFazio, C. A.; Peach, M. J.; Petrie, K. A.; and Silvester, M. J. Antiarrhythmic effects of lidocaine metabolites. *Am. Heart J.*, **1974**, *88*, 765–769.

Caracta, A. R.; Damato, A. N.; Josephson, M. E.; Ricciutti, M. A.; Gallagher, J. J.; and Lau, S. H. Electrophysiologic properties of diphenylhydantoin. *Circulation*, **1973**, *47*, 1234–1241.

Cardinal, R., and Sasyniuk, B. I. Electrophysiologic effects of bretylium tosylate on subendocardial Purkinje fibers from infarcted canine hearts. *J. Pharmacol. Exp. Ther.*, **1978**, *204*, 159–174.

Carmeliet, E., and Saikawa, T. Shortening of the action potential and reduction of pacemaker activity by lidocaine, quinidine, and procainamide in sheep cardiac Purkinje fibers. An effect on Na or K currents? *Circ. Res.*, **1982**, *50*, 257–272.

Carmeliet, E. E., and Vereeke, J. Adrenaline and the plateau phase of the cardiac action potential. *Pfluegers Arch.*, **1969**, *313*, 300–315.

Chatterjee, K.; Mandel, W. J.; Vyden, J. K.; Parmley, W. W.; and Forrester, J. S. Cardiovascular effects of bretylium tosylate in acute myocardial infarction. *J.A.M.A.*, **1973**, *223*, 757–760.

Colatsky, T. J. Mechanisms of action of lidocaine and quinidine on action potential duration in rabbit cardiac Purkinje fibers. An effect on steady state sodium currents? *Circ. Res.*, **1982**, *50*, 17–27.

Conrad, K. A.; Molk, B. L.; and Chidsey, C. A. Pharmacokinetic studies of quinidine in patients with arrhythmias. *Circulation*, **1977**, *55*, 1–7.

Courtney, K. R. Interval-dependent effects of small antiarrhythmic drugs on excitability of guinea-pig myocardium. *J. Mol. Cell. Cardiol.*, **1980**, *12*, 1273–1286.

Cranefield, P. F. Action potentials, afterpotentials, and arrhythmias. *Circ. Res.*, **1977**, *41*, 415–423.

Cranefield, P. F.; Wit, A. L.; and Hoffman, B. F. Conduction of the cardiac impulse. III. Characteristics of very slow conduction. *J. Gen. Physiol.*, **1972**, *59*, 227–246.

Damato, A. N. Diphenylhydantoin: pharmacological and clinical use. *Prog. Cardiovasc. Dis.*, **1969**, *12*, 1–15.

Danilo, P., Jr.; Hordof, A. J.; Reder, R. F.; and Rosen, M. R. Effects of verapamil on electrophysiologic properties of blood superfused cardiac Purkinje fibers. *J. Pharmacol. Exp. Ther.*, **1980**, *213*, 222–227.

Data, J. L.; Wilkinson, G. R.; and Nies, A. S. Interaction of quinidine with anticonvulsant drugs. *N. Engl. J. Med.*, **1976**, *294*, 699–702.

Davis, L. D., and Temte, J. V. Effects of propranolol on the transmembrane potentials of ventricular muscle and Purkinje fibers of the dog. *Circ. Res.*, **1968**, *22*, 661–667.

———. Electrophysiological actions of lidocaine on canine ventricular muscle and Purkinje fibers. *Ibid.*, **1969**, *24*, 639–655.

Desai, J. M.; Scheinman, M.; Peters, R. W.; and O'Young, J. Electrophysiological effects of disopyramide in patients with bundle branch block. *Circulation*, **1979**, *59*, 215–225.

DiFrancesco, D. A new interpretation of the pace-maker current in calf Purkinje fibers. *J. Physiol. (Lond.)*, **1981a**, *314*, 359–376.

———. A study of the ionic nature of the pace-maker current in calf Purkinje fibers. *Ibid.*, **1981b**, *314*, 377–393.

Drayer, D. E.; Restivo, K.; and Reidenberg, M. M. Specific determination of quinidine and (3S)-3-hydroxy-quinidine in human serum by high pressure liquid chromatography. *J. Lab. Clin. Med.*, **1977**, *90*, 816–822.

Dreyfuss, J.; Bigger, J. T., Jr.; Cohen, A. I.; and Schreiber, E. C. Metabolism of procainamide in rhesus monkey and man. *Clin. Pharmacol. Ther.*, **1972**, *13*, 366–371.

Durrer, D.; Van Dam, R. T.; Freud, G. E.; and Janse, M. J. Reentry and ventricular arrhythmias in local ischemia and infarction in the intact dog heart. *Proc. K. Ned. Akad. Wet. [Biol. Med.]*, **1971**, *74*, 321–334.

Eisner, D. A., and Lederer, W. J. Inotropic and arrhythmogenic effects of potassium-depleted solutions on mammalian cardiac muscle. *J. Physiol. (Lond.)*, **1979**, *294*, 255–277.

El-Sherif, N.; Scherlag, B. J.; Lazzara, R.; and Hope, R. R. Reentrant ventricular arrhythmias in the late myocardial infarction period. 1. Conduction characteristics in the infarction zone. *Circulation*, **1977**, *55*, 686–702.

Fisher, J. D.; Cohen, H. L.; Mehra, R.; Altschuler, H.; Escher, D. J. W.; and Furman, S. Cardiac pacing and pacemakers II. Serial electrophysiologic-pharmacologic testing for control of recurrent tachyarrhythmias. *Am. Heart J.*, **1977**, *93*, 658–668.

Frey, W. Weitere Erfährungen mit Chinidin bei absoluter Herzunregelmässigkeit. *Wien Klin. Wochenschr.*, **1918**, *55*, 849–853.

Gang, E. S.; Bigger, J. T., Jr.; and Uhl, E. W. Effects of timolol and propranolol on inducible sustained ventricular tachyarrhythmias in dogs with subacute myocardial infarction. *Am. J. Cardiol.*, **1984**, *53*, 275–281.

Gerstenblith, G.; Spear, J. F.; and Moore, E. N. Quantitative study of the effect of lidocaine on the threshold for ventricular fibrillation in the dog. *Am. J. Cardiol.*, **1972**, *30*, 242–247.

Gettes, L. S., and Yoshonis, K. F. Rapidly recurring supraventricular tachycardia; a manifestation of reciprocity tachycardia and an indication for propranolol therapy. *Circulation*, **1970**, *41*, 689–700.

Giardina, E. G. V.; Dreyfuss, J.; Bigger, J. T., Jr.; Shaw, J. M.; and Schreiber, E. C. Metabolism of procainamide in normal and cardiac subjects. *Clin. Pharmacol. Ther.*, **1976**, *19*, 339–351.

Giardina, E. G. V.; Heissenbuttel, R. H.; and Bigger, J. T., Jr. Intermittent intravenous procainamide to treat ventricular arrhythmias; correlation of plasma concentration with effect on arrhythmia, electrocardiogram, and blood pressure. *Ann. Intern. Med.*, **1973**, *78*, 183–193.

Giardina, E. G. V.; Stein, R. M.; and Bigger, J. T., Jr. The relationship between the metabolism of procainamide and sulfamethazine. *Circulation*, **1977**, *55*, 388–394.

Gibson, T. P.; Matusik, J.; Matusik, E.; Nelson, H. A.; Wilkinson, J.; and Briggs, W. A. Acetylation of procainamide in man and its relationship to isonicotinic acid hydrazide acetylation phenotype. *Clin. Pharmacol. Ther.*, **1975**, *17*, 395–399.

Gillis, R. A. Cardiac sympathetic nerve activity; changes induced by ouabain and propranolol. *Science*, **1969**, *166*, 508–510.

Gillis, R. A.; McClellan, J. R.; Sauer, T. S.; and Standaert, F. G. Depression of cardiac sympathetic nerve activity by diphenylhydantoin. *J. Pharmacol. Exp. Ther.*, **1971**, *179*, 599–610.

Gintant, G. A., and Hoffman, B. F. The influence of molecular form of local anesthetic-type antiarrhythmic agents on the maximum upstroke velocity of canine cardiac Purkinje fibers. *Circ. Res.*, **1983**, *52*, 735–746.

Greenspan, A. M.; Horowitz, L. N.; Spielman, S. R.; and Josephson, M. E. Large dose procainamide therapy for ventricular tachycardia. *Am. J. Cardiol.*, **1980**, *46*, 453–462.

Gulamhusein, S.; Ko, P.; Carruthers, S. G.; and Klein,

G. J. Acceleration of the ventricular response during atrial fibrillation in the Wolff-Parkinson-White syndrome after verapamil. *Circulation*, **1982**, *65*, 348–354.

Hariman, R. J.; Gomes, J. A. C.; Kang, P. S.; and El-Sherif, N. Effects of intravenous amiodarone in patients with inducible repetitive ventricular responses and ventricular tachycardia. *Am. Heart J.*, **1984**, *107*, 1109–1116.

Hartel, G.; Louhija, A.; and Konttinen, A. Disopyramide in the prevention of recurrence of atrial fibrillation after electroconversion. *Clin. Pharmacol. Ther.*, **1974**, *15*, 551–555.

Heger, J. J.; Prystowsky, E. N.; Jackman, W. M.; Naccarelli, G. V.; Warfel, K. A.; Rinkenberger, R. L.; and Zipes, D. P. Amiodarone: clinical efficacy and electrophysiology during long-term therapy for recurrent ventricular tachycardia or ventricular fibrillation. *N. Engl. J. Med.*, **1981**, *305*, 539–545.

Heissenbuttel, R. H., and Bigger, J. T., Jr. The effect of oral quinidine on intraventricular conduction in man. Correlation of plasma quinidine with changes in intraventricular conduction time. *Am. Heart J.*, **1970**, *80*, 453–462.

————. Bretylium tosylate: a newly available antiarrhythmic drug for ventricular arrhythmias. *Ann. Intern. Med.*, **1979**, *90*, 229–238.

Hondeghem, L. M., and Katzung, B. G. Test of a model of antiarrhythmic drug action. Effect of quinidine and lidocaine on myocardial conduction. *Circulation*, **1980**, *61*, 1217–1224.

Horowitz, L. N.; Josephson, M. E.; Farshidi, A.; Spielman, S. R.; Michelson, E. L.; and Greenspan, A. M. Recurrent sustained ventricular tachycardia. 3. Role of the electrophysiologic study in selection of antiarrhythmic regimens. *Circulation*, **1978**, *58*, 986–997.

Horowitz, L. N.; Josephson, M. E.; and Kastor, J. A. Intracardiac electrophysiologic studies as a method for the optimization of drug therapy in chronic ventricular arrhythmia. *Prog. Cardiovasc. Dis.*, **1980**, *23*, 81–98.

Husaini, M. H.; Kvasnicka, J.; Ryden, L.; and Holmberg, S. Action of verapamil on sinus node, atrioventricular, and intraventricular conduction. *Br. Heart J.*, **1973**, *35*, 734–737.

Jensen, G.; Sigurd, B.; and Uhrenholt, A. Hemodynamic effects of intravenous disopyramide in heart failure. *Eur. J. Clin. Pharmacol.*, **1975**, *8*, 167–173.

Kappenberger, L. J.; Fromer, M. A.; Steinbrunn, W.; and Shenasa, M. Efficacy of amiodarone in the Wolff-Parkinson-White syndrome with rapid ventricular response via accessory pathway during atrial fibrillation. *Am. J. Cardiol.*, **1984**, *54*, 330–335.

Kessler, K. M.; Lowenthal, D. T.; Warner, H.; Gibson, T.; Briggs, W.; and Reidenberg, M. M. Quinidine elimination in patients with congestive heart failure or poor renal function. *N. Engl. J. Med.*, **1974**, *290*, 706–709.

Knapp, A. B.; Maguire, W.; Keren, G.; Karmen, A.; Levitt, B.; Miura, D. S.; and Somberg, J. C. The cimetidine-lidocaine interaction. *Ann. Intern. Med.*, **1983**, *98*, 174–177.

Kniffen, F. J.; Lomas, T. E.; Counsell, R. E.; and Lucchesi, B. R. The antiarrhythmic and antifibrillatory actions of bretylium and its *o*-iodobenzyl trimethylammonium analog, UM-360. *J. Pharmacol. Exp. Ther.*, **1975**, *192*, 120–128.

Koch-Weser, J. Quinidine-induced hypoprothrombinemic hemorrhage in patients on chronic warfarin therapy. *Ann. Intern. Med.*, **1968**, *68*, 511–517.

Koch-Weser, J., and Klein, S. W. Procainamide dosage schedules, plasma concentrations, and clinical effects. *J.A.M.A.*, **1971**, *215*, 1454–1460.

Koch-Weser, J.; Klein, S. W.; Foo-Canto, L. L.; Kastor, J. A.; and DeSanctis, R. W. Antiarrhythmic prophylaxis with procainamide in acute myocardial infarction. *N. Engl. J. Med.*, **1969**, *281*, 1253–1260.

Koster, R. W., and Wellens, H. J. J. Quinidine-induced ventricular flutter and fibrillation without digitalis therapy. *Am. J. Cardiol.*, **1976**, *38*, 519–523.

Kunze, K.-P.; Kuck, K.-H.; Schlüter, M.; Kuch, B.; and Bleifeld, W. Electrophysiologic and clinical effects of intravenous and oral encainide in accessory atrioventricular pathway. *Am. J. Cardiol.*, **1984**, *54*, 323–329.

Kupersmith, J.; Antman, E. M.; and Hoffman, B. F. *In vivo* electrophysiological effects of lidocaine in canine acute myocardial infarction. *Circ. Res.*, **1975**, *36*, 84–91.

Kupersmith, J.; Shiang, H.; Litwak, R. S.; and Herman, M. V. Electrophysiological and antiarrhythmic effects of propranolol in canine acute myocardial ischemia. *Circ. Res.*, **1976**, *38*, 302–307.

Kus, T., and Sasyniuk, B. I. Electrophysiological actions of disopyramide phosphate on canine ventricular muscle and Purkinje fiber. *Circ. Res.*, **1975**, *37*, 844–854.

LaBarre, A.; Strauss, H. C.; Scheinman, M. M.; Evans, G. T.; Bashore, T.; Tiedeman, J. S.; and Wallace, A. G. Electrophysiologic effects of disopyramide phosphate on sinus node function in patients with sinus node dysfunction. *Circulation*, **1979**, *59*, 226–235.

Ladd, A. T. Procainamide-induced lupus erythematosus. *N. Engl. J. Med.*, **1962**, *267*, 1357–1358.

Lederer, W. J., and Tsien, R. W. Transient inward current underlying arrhythmogenic effects of cardiotonic steroids in Purkinje fibers. *J. Physiol. (Lond.)*, **1976**, *263*, 73–100.

LeLorier, J.; Moisan, R.; Gagne, J.; and Caille, G. Effect of the duration of infusion on the disposition of lidocaine in dogs. *J. Pharmacol. Exp. Ther.*, **1977**, *203*, 507–511.

Levitt, B.; Cagin, N.; Kleid, J.; Somberg, J.; and Gillis, R. A. Role of the nervous system in the genesis of cardiac rhythm disorders. *Am. J. Cardiol.*, **1976**, *37*, 1111–1113.

Levy, M. N. Parasympathomimetic control of the heart. In, *Neural Regulation of the Heart.* (Randall, W. C., ed.) Oxford University Press, New York, **1977**, pp. 95–130.

Lie, K. I.; Liem, K. L.; Louridtz, W. J.; Janse, M. J.; Willebrands, A. F.; and Durrer, D. Efficacy of lidocaine in preventing primary ventricular fibrillation within one hour after a 300 mg intramuscular injection. *Am. J. Cardiol.*, **1978**, *42*, 486–488.

Lie, K. I.; Wellens, H. J. J.; van Capelle, F. J.; and Durrer, D. Lidocaine in the prevention of primary ventricular fibrillation. A double-blind, randomized study of 212 consecutive patients. *N. Engl. J. Med.*, **1974**, *291*, 1324–1326.

Luoma, P. V.; Kujala, P. A.; Juustila, H. J.; and Takkunen, J. T. Efficacy of intravenous disopyramide in the termination of supraventricular arrhythmias. *J. Clin. Pharmacol.*, **1978**, *18*, 293–301.

McAllister, R. E.; Noble, D.; and Tsien, R. W. Reconstruction of the electrical activity of cardiac Purkinje fibers. *J. Physiol. (Lond.)*, **1975**, *251*, 1–59.

Mandel, W. J., and Bigger, J. T., Jr. Electrophysiologic effects of lidocaine on isolated canine and rabbit atrial tissue. *J. Pharmacol. Exp. Ther.*, **1971**, *178*, 81–93.

Mark, L. C.; Kayden, H. J.; Steele, J. M.; Cooper, J. R.; Berlin, I.; Rovenstine, E. A.; and Brodie, B. B. The physiological disposition and cardiac effects of procaine amide. *J. Pharmacol. Exp. Ther.*, **1951**, *102*, 5–15.

Marrott, P. K.; Ruttley, M. S. T.; Winterbottam, J. T.; and Muir, J. R. A study of the acute electrophysiological and cardiovascular action of disopyramide in man. *Eur. J. Cardiol.*, **1976**, *4*, 303–312.

Mason, J. W.; Winkle, R. A.; Rider, A. K.; Stinson, E. B.; and Harrison, D. C. The electrophysiologic effects of quinidine in the transplanted human heart. *J. Clin. Invest.*, **1977**, *59*, 481–489.

Meinertz, T.; Zehender, M. K.; Geibel, A.; Treese, N.;

Hofmann, T.; Kasper, W.; and Pop, T. Long-term antiarrhythmic therapy with flecainide. *Am. J. Cardiol.*, **1984**, *54*, 91–96.

Méndez, C.; Mueller, W. J.; Merideth, J.; and Moe, G. K. Interaction of transmembrane potentials in canine Purkinje fibers and at Purkinje fiber-muscle junctions. *Circ. Res.*, **1969**, *24*, 361–372.

Mirro, M. J.; Watanabe, A. M.; and Bailey, J. C. Electrophysiological effects of disopyramide and quinidine on guinea-pig atria and canine cardiac Purkinje fibers. Dependence on underlying cholinergic tone. *Circ. Res.*, **1980**, *46*, 660–668.

Nies, A. S.; Shand, D. G.; and Wilkinson, G. R. Altered hepatic blood flow and drug disposition. *Clin. Pharmacokinet.*, **1976**, *1*, 135–155.

Noma, A., and Irisawa, H. Membrane currents in the rabbit sinoatrial node cell as studied by the double microelectrode method. *Pfluegers Arch.*, **1976**, *364*, 45–52.

Norwegian Multicenter Study Group. Timolol-induced reduction in mortality and reinfarction in patients surviving acute myocardial infarction. *N. Engl. J. Med.*, **1981**, *304*, 801–807.

Obayashi, K.; Hayakawa, H.; and Mandel, W. J. Interrelationships between external potassium concentration and lidocaine: effects on canine Purkinje fiber. *Am. Heart J.*, **1975**, *89*, 221–226.

Ogden, D. C.; Siegelbaum, S.; and Colquhoun, D. Block of acetylcholine activated ion channels by an uncharged local anesthetic. *Nature*, **1981**, *289*, 596–598.

Peon, J.; Ferrier, G. R.; and Moe, G. K. The relationship of excitability to conduction velocity in canine Purkinje tissue. *Circ. Res.*, **1978**, *43*, 125–135.

Podrid, P. J.; Schoenberger, A.; and Lown, B. Congestive heart failure caused by oral disopyramide. *N. Engl. J. Med.*, **1980**, *302*, 614–617.

Randall, W. C. Sympathetic control of the heart. In, *Neural Regulation of the Heart.* (Randall, W. C., ed.) Oxford University Press, New York, **1977**, pp. 43–94.

Reidenberg, M. M.; Drayer, D. E.; Levy, M.; and Warner, H. Polymorphic acetylation of procainamide in man. *Clin. Pharmacol. Ther.*, **1975**, *17*, 722–730.

Rosen, M. R., and Danilo, P., Jr. Effects of tetrodotoxin, lidocaine, verapamil and AHR-2666 on ouabain-induced delayed afterdepolarizations in canine Purkinje fibers. *Circ. Res.*, **1980**, *46*, 117–124.

Rosen, M. R.; Danilo, P., Jr.; Alonso, M. B.; and Pippenger, C. E. Effects of therapeutic concentrations of diphenylhydantoin on transmembrane potentials of normal and depressed Purkinje fibers. *J. Pharmacol. Exp. Ther.*, **1976**, *197*, 594–604.

Routledge, P. A.; Barchowsky, A.; Bjornsson, T. D.; Kitchell, B. B.; and Shand, D. G. Lidocaine plasma protein binding. *Clin. Pharmacol. Ther.*, **1980**, *27*, 347–351.

Roy, P. R.; Spurrell, R. A. J.; and Sowton, E. The effect of verapamil on the cardiac conduction system in man. *Postgrad. Med. J.*, **1974**, *50*, 270–275.

Saksena, S.; Rothbart, S. T.; Shah, Y.; and Cappello, G. Clinical efficacy and electropharmacology of continuous intravenous amiodarone infusion and chronic oral amiodarone in refractory ventricular tachycardia. *Am. J. Cardiol.*, **1984**, *54*, 347–352.

Sasyniuk, B. I., and Kus, T. Cellular electrophysiologic changes induced by disopyramide phosphate in normal and infarcted hearts. *J. Int. Med. Res.*, **1976**, *4*, 20–25.

Sasyniuk, B. I., and Méndez, C. A mechanism for reentry in canine ventricular tissue. *Circ. Res.*, **1971**, *28*, 3–15.

Schmitt, F. O., and Erlanger, J. Directional differences in the conduction of the impulse through heart muscle and their possible relation to extrasystolic and fibrillary contractions. *Am. J. Physiol.*, **1928–29**, *87*, 326–347.

Schwartz, P. J., and Moss, A. J. Delayed repolarization

(QT or QTU prolongation) and malignant ventricular arrhythmias. *Mod. Concepts Cardiovasc. Dis.,* **1981,** *51,* 85–90.

Schwartz, P. J.; Periti, M.; and Malliani, A. The long Q-T syndrome. *Am. Heart J.,* **1975,** *89,* 378–390.

Seides, S. F.; Josephson, M. E.; Batsford, W. P.; Weisfogel, G. M.; Lau, S. H.; and Damato, A. N. The electrophysiology of propranolol in man. *Am. Heart J.,* **1974,** *88,* 733–741.

Seipel, L., and Breithardt, G. Sinus recovery time after disopyramide phosphate. *Am. J. Cardiol.,* **1976,** *37,* 1118.

Sekiya, A., and Vaughan Williams, E. M. A comparison of the antifibrillatory actions and effects on intracellular cardiac potentials of pronethalol, disopyramide and quinidine. *Br. J. Pharmacol.,* **1963,** *21,* 473–481.

Singh, B. N., and Vaughan Williams, E. M. Effect of altering potassium concentration on the action of lidocaine and diphenylhydantoin on rabbit atrial and ventricular muscle. *Circ. Res.,* **1971,** *29,* 286–295.

Stagg, A. L., and Wallace, A. G. The effect of propranolol on membrane conductance in canine cardiac Purkinje fibers. *Circulation,* **1974,** *50,* Suppl. III, 145.

Strauss, H. C.; Gilbert, M.; Svenson, R. H.; Miller, H. C.; and Wallace, A. G. Electrophysiological effects of propranolol on sinus node function in patients with sinus node dysfunction. *Circulation,* **1976,** *54,* 452–459.

Swerdlow, C. D.; Winkle, R. A.; and Mason, J. W. Determinants of survival in patients with ventricular tachyarrhythmias. *N. Engl. J. Med.,* **1983,** *308,* 1436–1442.

Thomson, P. D.; Melmon, K. L.; Richardson, J. A.; Cohn, K.; Steinbrunn, W.; Cudihee, R.; and Rowland, M. Lidocaine pharmacokinetics in advanced heart failure, liver disease, and renal failure in humans. *Ann. Intern. Med.,* **1973,** *78,* 499–508.

Tsien, R. W. Effects of epinephrine on the pacemaker potassium current of cardiac Purkinje fibers. *J. Gen. Physiol.,* **1974,** *64,* 293–319.

Vajda, F. J. E.; Prineas, R. J.; Lovell, R. R. H.; and Sloman, J. G. The possible effect of long-term high plasma levels of phenytoin on mortality after acute myocardial infarction. *Eur. J. Clin. Pharmacol.,* **1973,** *5,* 138–144.

Valentine, P. A.; Frew, J. L.; Mashford, M. L.; and Sloman, J. G. Lidocaine in the prevention of sudden death in the pre-hospital phase of acute infarction. A double-blind study. *N. Engl. J. Med.,* **1974,** *291,* 1327–1331.

Vincent, G. M.; Abildskov, J. A.; and Burgess, M. J. Q-T interval syndromes. *Prog. Cardiovasc. Dis.,* **1974,** *16,* 523–530.

Wallace, A. G.; Cline, R. E.; Sealy, W. C.; Young, W. G., Jr.; and Troyer, W. G., Jr. Electrophysiologic effects of quinidine. Studies using chronically implanted electrodes in awake dogs with and without cardiac denervation. *Circ. Res.,* **1966a,** *19,* 960–969.

Wallace, A. G.; Schaal, S. F.; Sugimoto, T.; Rozear, M.; and Alexander, J. A. The electrophysiologic effects of beta-adrenergic blockade and cardiac denervation. *Bull. N.Y. Acad. Med.,* **1967,** *43,* 1119–1137.

Wallace, A. G.; Troyer, W. G.; Lesage, M. A.; and Zotti, E. F. Electrophysiologic effects of isoproterenol and beta blocking agents in awake dogs. *Circ. Res.,* **1966b,** *18,* 140–148.

Wasserman, F.; Brodsky, L.; Kathe, J. H.; Rodensky, P. L.; Dick, M. M.; and Denton, P. S. The effect of molar sodium lactate in quinidine intoxication. *Am. J. Cardiol.,* **1959,** *3,* 294–299.

Watts, J. A.; Koch, C. D.; and LaNoue, K. F. Effects of Ca^{2+} antagonism on energy metabolism: Ca^{2+} and heart function after ischemia. *Am. J. Physiol.,* **1980,** *238,* H909–H916.

Waxman, M. B., and Wallace, A. G. Electrophysiologic effects of bretylium tosylate on the heart. *J. Pharmacol. Exp. Ther.,* **1972,** *183,* 264–274.

Weisfogel, G. M.; Batsford, W. P.; Paulay, K. L.; Josephson, M. E.; Ogunkelu, J. B.; Akhtar, M.; Seides, S. F.; and Damato, A. N. Sinus node re-entrant tachycardia in man. *Am. Heart J.,* **1975,** *90,* 295–304.

Weld, F. M., and Bigger, J. T., Jr. The effect of lidocaine on diastolic transmembrane currents determining pacemaker depolarization in cardiac Purkinje fibers. *Circ. Res.,* **1976,** *38,* 203–208.

Wellens, H. J. J.; Duren, D. R.; and Lie, K. I. Observations on mechanisms of ventricular tachycardia in man. *Circulation,* **1976,** *54,* 237–244.

Wenckebach, K. F. *Die unregelmässige Herztätigkeit und ihre klinische Bedeutung.* W. Engelmann, Leipzig, **1914.**

Wilkinson, P. R.; Rees, J. R.; Storey, G. C. A.; and Holt, D. W. Amiodarone: prolonged cessation of chronic therapy. *Am. Heart J.,* **1984,** *107,* 787–788.

Willius, F. A., and Keys, T. E. Cardiac clinics. XCIV. A remarkably early reference to the use of cinchona in cardiac arrhythmia. *Proc. Staff Meet. Mayo Clin.,* **1942,** *17,* 294–296.

Wit, A. L., and Cranefield, P. F. Effect of verapamil on the sinoatrial and atrioventricular nodes of the rabbit and the mechanism by which it arrests re-entrant atrioventricular tachycardia. *Circ. Res.,* **1974,** *35,* 413–425.

———. Triggered activity in cardiac muscle fibers of the simian mitral valve. *Ibid.,* **1976,** *38,* 85–98.

———. Triggered and automatic activity in the canine coronary sinus. *Ibid.,* **1977,** *41,* 435–445.

Wit, A. L.; Cranefield, P. F.; and Hoffman, B. F. Slow conduction and reentry in the ventricular conducting system. II. Single and sustained circus movement in networks of canine and bovine Purkinje fibers. *Circ. Res.,* **1972a,** *30,* 11–22.

Wit, A. L.; Hoffman, B. F.; and Cranefield, P. F. Slow conduction and reentry in the ventricular conducting system. I. Return extrasystole in canine Purkinje fibers. *Circ. Res.,* **1972b,** *30,* 1–10.

Wit, A. L.; Rosen, M. R.; and Hoffman, B. F. Electrophysiology and pharmacology of cardiac arrhythmias. VIII. Cardiac effects of diphenylhydantoin. *Am. Heart J.,* **1975,** *90,* 265–272, 397–404.

Wittig, J.; Harrison, L. A.; and Wallace, A. G. Electrophysiological effects of lidocaine on distal Purkinje fibers of canine heart. *Am. Heart J.,* **1973,** *86,* 69–78.

Woosley, R. L.; Drayer, D. E.; Reidenberg, M. M.; Nies, A. S.; Carr, K.; and Oates, J. A. Effect of acetylator phenotype on the rate at which procainamide induces antinuclear antibodies and the lupus syndrome. *N. Engl. J. Med.,* **1978,** *298,* 1157–1159.

Woosley, R. L.; Kornhauser, D.; Smith, R.; Reele, S.; Higgins, S. B.; Nies, A. S.; Shand, D. G.; and Oates, J. A. Suppression of chronic ventricular arrhythmias with propranolol. *Circulation,* **1979,** *60,* 819–827.

Woosley, R. L.; Shand, D.; Kornhauser, D.; Nies, A. S.; and Oates, J. A. Relation of plasma concentration and dose of propranolol to its effect on resistant ventricular arrhythmias. *Clin. Res.,* **1977,** *25,* 262A.

Wu, D.; Denes, P.; Dhingra, R.; Kahn, A.; and Rosen, K. M. The effects of propranolol on induction of A-V nodal reentrant paroxysmal tachycardia. *Circulation,* **1974,** *50,* 665–677.

Zapata-Díaz, J.; Cabrera, C. E.; and Méndez, R. An experimental and clinical study on the effects of procaine amide (PRONESTYL) on the heart. *Am. Heart J.,* **1952,** *43,* 854–870.

Zipes, D. P., and Fischer, J. C. Effects of agents which inhibit the slow channel on sinus node automaticity and atrioventricular conduction in the dog. *Circ. Res.,* **1974,** *34,* 184–192.

Monographs and Reviews

Bigger, J. T., Jr. Electrical properties of cardiac muscle and possible causes of cardiac arrhythmias. In, *Cardiovascular Arrhythmias.* (Dreifus, L. S., and Likoff, W., eds.) Grune & Stratton, Inc., New York, **1973**, pp. 13–34.

———. The quinidine-digoxin interaction. *Mod. Concepts Cardiovasc. Dis.*, **1982**, *51*, 73–78.

Bigger, J. T., Jr.; Dresdale, R. J.; Heissenbuttel, R. H.; Weld, F. M.; and Wit, A. L.   Ventricular arrhythmias in ischemic heart disease: mechanism, prevalence, significance and management. *Prog. Cardiovasc. Dis.*, **1977**, *19*, 255–300.

Bigger, J. T., Jr., and Reiffel, J. A.   Sick sinus syndrome. *Annu. Rev. Med.*, **1979**, *30*, 91–118.

Boura, A. L. A., and Green, A. F.   Adrenergic neurone blocking agents. *Annu. Rev. Pharmacol.*, **1965**, *5*, 183–212.

DiPalma, J. R., and Schults, J. E.   Antifibrillatory drugs. *Medicine (Baltimore)*, **1950**, *29*, 123–168.

Eiriksson, C. E., and Brogden, R. N.   Lorcainide: a preliminary review of its pharmacodynamic properties and therapeutic efficacy. *Drugs*, **1984**, *27*, 279–300.

Ferrier, G. R.   Digitalis arrhythmias: role of oscillatory afterpotentials. *Prog. Cardiovasc. Dis.*, **1977**, *19*, 459–474.

Gintant, G. A., and Hoffman, B. F.   The role of local anesthetic effects in the actions of antiarrhythmic drugs. In, *Local Anesthetics*. (Strichartz, G. R., ed.) *Handbook of Experimental Pharmacology*. Springer-Verlag, Berlin, **1985** (in press).

Hille, B.   Local anesthetic action on inactivation of the Na channel in nerve and skeletal muscle: possible mechanisms for antiarrhythmic agents. In, *Biophysical Aspects of Cardiac Muscle*. (Morad, M., ed.) Academic Press, Inc., New York, **1978**, pp. 55–74.

Hoffman, B. F., and Cranefield, P. F.   *Electrophysiology of the Heart*. McGraw-Hill Book Co., New York, **1960**.

Holmes, B.; Brogden, R. N.; Heel, R. C.; Speight, T. M.; and Avery, G. S.   Tocainide: a review of its pharmacological properties and therapeutic efficacy. *Drugs*, **1983**, *26*, 93–123.

Keefe, D. L. D.; Kates, R. E.; and Harrison, D. C.   New antiarrhythmic drugs: their place in therapy. *Drugs*, **1981**, *22*, 363–400.

Lucchesi, B. R.   Antiarrhythmic drugs. Key references. *Circulation*, **1979**, *59*, 1076–1078.

Noble, D.   *The Initiation of the Heartbeat*. Clarendon Press, Oxford, **1975**.

Symposium. (Various authors.)   The Göteborg metoprolol trial in acute myocardial infarction. (Roberts, W. C., ed.) *Am. J. Cardiol.*, **1984a**, *53*, 1D–50D.

Symposium. (Various authors.)   Symposium on the management of ventricular dysrhythmias. (Roberts, W. C., ed.) *Am. J. Cardiol.*, **1984b**, *54*, 1A–36A.

Trautwein, W.   Membrane currents in cardiac muscle fibers. *Physiol. Rev.*, **1973**, *53*, 793–835.

32 ANTIHYPERTENSIVE AGENTS AND THE DRUG THERAPY OF HYPERTENSION

Peter Rudd and Terrence F. Blaschke

During the past 3 decades, effective pharmacological treatment of high blood pressure has replaced radical therapy of malignant hypertension and therapeutic indifference toward "benign essential hypertension." Morbidity and mortality have fallen with the development of effective agents to reduce blood pressure. Guidelines for management of hypertension have been derived logically, and effective therapy has been implemented widely. Although antihypertensive agents interfere with normal homeostatic mechanisms, the elucidation of their mechanisms of action has thus far failed to answer many important questions about the pathogenesis of essential hypertension. Yet, a thorough understanding of their properties is crucial to optimal use of these drugs, particularly in rational combinations that enhance effectiveness and minimize toxicity.

Hypertension is one of the few common diseases for which successful treatment has improved long-term morbidity and mortality (Veterans Administration Cooperative Study Group, 1967, 1970; Hypertension Detection and Follow-up Cooperative Group, 1979). Accumulated experience with antihypertensive medications has also led to better recognition of the potential risks and benefits of treatment with specific agents in particular subpopulations of patients.

Hypertension is generally defined as an elevation of systolic and/or diastolic arterial blood pressure, and a value of 140/90 mm Hg is generally accepted as the upper limit of normotension. Certain risk factors (*e.g.,* hypercholesterolemia, diabetes, smoking, and a family history of vascular disease) in conjunction with hypertension predispose to arteriosclerosis and consequent cardiovascular morbidity and mortality. Patient populations with sustained diastolic blood pressures in the range of 105 to 129 mm Hg are unequivocally benefited by ef-

fective reduction of blood pressure (Veterans Administration Cooperative Study Group, 1967, 1970). Even suboptimal reduction of blood pressure may benefit the moderately to severely hypertensive patient (Taguchi and Freis, 1974). Treatment of patients with diastolic blood pressures in the range of 90 to 104 mm Hg should be individualized, especially at the lower end of this range when other cardiovascular risk factors are absent. The benefits of antihypertensive treatment are the avoidance of accelerated or malignant hypertension, a lower incidence of hypertensive renal failure, and a decrease in the incidence of hemorrhagic stroke and cardiac failure. Only recently has it been demonstrated that aggressive care of patients with mild diastolic hypertension (90 to 104 mm Hg) can apparently reduce the incidence of myocardial infarction (Hypertension Detection and Follow-up Cooperative Group, 1979; Stamler and Stamler, 1984).

I. Pharmacology of Specific Antihypertensive Agents

Several antihypertensive agents that act predominantly on the peripheral sympathetic nervous system, at adrenergic receptors, on autonomic ganglia, and on the renin-angiotensin system are described in more detail in Chapters 4, 9, 10, and 27. The present chapter focuses on additional important agents not discussed in those chapters and on the therapeutic utility of the entire group of drugs. One classification of antihypertensive drugs, based on their primary site or mechanism of action, is shown in Table 32–1. Any such scheme necessarily oversimplifies the mechanisms of action, and the predominant hypotensive mechanism may differ with the duration of treatment.

The acute and chronic hemodynamic consequences of treatment with antihypertensive agents are presented in Table 32–2; this provides a framework for potential

Table 32–1. CLASSIFICATION OF ANTI-HYPERTENSIVE DRUGS BY THEIR PRIMARY SITE OR MECHANISM OF ACTION

A. *Diuretics* (Chapter 36)
   1. Thiazides and related agents (hydrochlorothiazide, chlorthalidone, *etc.*)
   2. Loop diuretics (furosemide, bumetanide, ethacrynic acid)
   3. Potassium-sparing diuretics (triamterene, spironolactone, amiloride)

B. *Sympatholytic Drugs* (Chapters 9, 10)
   1. Centrally acting agents (methyldopa, clonidine, guanabenz, guanfacine)
   2. β-Adrenergic antagonists (propranolol, metoprolol, *etc.*)
   3. α-Adrenergic antagonists (prazosin, phenoxybenzamine, phentolamine)
   4. Mixed antagonists (labetalol)
   5. Adrenergic neuron blocking agents (guanethidine, guanadrel, reserpine)
   6. Ganglionic blocking agents (trimethaphan)

C. *Vasodilators*
   1. Arterial (hydralazine, minoxidil, diazoxide, calcium channel blockers)
   2. Arterial and venous (nitroprusside)

D. *Angiotensin Converting Enzyme Inhibitors* (Chapter 27) (captopril, enalapril)

complementary effects of concurrent therapy with two or more antihypertensive agents. The similarity of hemodynamic consequences that result from use of drugs in a single class has important implications. There is little benefit from concurrent use of two or more agents in a single class, since compensatory mechanisms and/or side effects are likely to be augmented without improving the antihypertensive effect.

DIURETICS

The thiazides and the closely related phthalimidine derivatives (*e.g.*, chlorthalidone) have become a mainstay of antihypertensive therapy. Details of their pharmacology are presented in Chapter 36. Although the term *diuretic* is used, their major hypotensive effect during chronic administration appears to be due to vasodilatation, rather than to saluresis or loss of free water *per se*. However, their effect on peripheral vascular resistance may be secondary to diuretic-induced changes in sodium balance.

BENZOTHIADIAZINES AND RELATED COMPOUNDS

Thiazides and related compounds comprise the most frequently used antihypertensive agents in the United States (Cypress, 1982). Despite the large number of related compounds, the drugs in the benzothiadiazine group have a similar pattern of pharmacological effects and are generally interchangeable (with appropriate adjustment of dosage). When given acutely and in reasonably large doses (*e.g.*, 50 to 100 mg of hydrochlorothiazide), they decrease plasma volume, cardiac output, glomerular filtration rate, renal blood flow, and mean arterial pressure. Chronically, however, the hypotensive effect of thiazides is observed at doses far less than those needed for saluresis, kaluresis, or loss of free water. The urinary filtration fraction, renal vascular resistance, and plasma renin activity all rise modestly. With chronic administration, some of the plasma volume initially lost is recovered, but it remains about 5% below pretreatment values. The cardiac output and glomerular filtration rate return to near normal, while mean arterial pressure remains reduced and systemic vascular resistance falls (De Carvalho *et al.*, 1977; Van Brummelen *et al.*, 1979). Since the thiazides potentiate the antihypertensive effect of other agents that have different mechanisms of action, their use with other antihypertensive drugs is rational and common. There is no way to predict the hypotensive response to thiazides from the duration or severity of hypertension in a given patient, although they are unlikely to be effective when used alone in severe hypertension.

The hemodynamic effects of thiazides raise questions about the nature of their mechanism of action as antihypertensive agents. Their effects are probably multiple and include reduction in interstitial fluid volume with consequent decrease in vascular wall stiffness and increase in vascular compliance. Since plasma renin activity and concentrations of norepinephrine and aldosterone in plasma all rise as compensatory reactions to the use of thiazides, reduced availability of these substances is not responsible for the hypotensive effects.

Table 32–2. HEMODYNAMIC EFFECTS OF COMMONLY USED ANTIHYPERTENSIVE AGENTS *

| | DIURETICS | | SYMPATHOLYTIC AGENTS | | | VASODILATORS | ANGIOTENSIN CONVERTING ENZYME INHIBITORS |
	Acute	Chronic	Methyldopa, Reserpine, Clonidine, Guanethidine	Prazosin	β Blockers		
Heart rate	↑	↔	↓	↑	↓	↑	↔
Cardiac output	↓	↔	↓	↑	↓	↑	↔
Total peripheral resistance	↑	↓	↓	↓	↔	↓	↓
Plasma volume	↓↓	↓	↑	↑	↑	↑	↑
Plasma renin activity	↑	↑	↓	↓	↓	↑	↑
Renal blood flow	↓	↓	↓	↔	↓	↑	↑

* Changes are indicated as follows: ↑, increased; ↓, decreased; ↑, increased or no change; ↓, decreased or no change; ↔, unchanged.

Anephric patients do not show a reduction of blood pressure when given thiazides (Bennett *et al.*, 1977). Ultimately, the drug-induced saluresis appears to be critical, since a saline infusion but not a dextran infusion returns blood pressure to pretreatment levels (Tobian, 1967).

Most patients will respond to thiazides within 2 to 4 weeks, although a minority may require up to 12 weeks to achieve the maximal hypotensive response to a given dosage (Soghikian and Bartenbach, 1977). Therefore, increasing the dosage of a thiazide at intervals of less than 4 weeks may lead to unnecessary toxicity, including otherwise-avoidable potassium depletion. The antihypertensive effect of thiazides lasts longer and occurs at lower doses than does the diuretic effect (Lutterodt *et al.*, 1980). Moreover, the dose-response curve for lowering blood pressure reaches a maximum at relatively low doses in most patients. Thus, there is little additional hypotensive effect from daily doses of hydrochlorothiazide above 50 mg or chlorthalidone above 25 mg (Materson *et al.*, 1978). Higher doses do, however, increase the incidence and severity of undesirable metabolic side effects, especially hyperlipoproteinemia, hypokalemia, hyperuricemia, and hyperglycemia (Tweeddale *et al.*, 1977). Since many hypertensive patients will require at least one other drug in addition to a thiazide to control their blood pressure, the use of a high dose of a thiazide for the sake of single-drug therapy is unjustified.

The thiazides and chlorthalidone can elevate plasma lipid concentrations to comparable degrees (Grimm *et al.*, 1981), although intersubject variability is considerable. Chlorthalidone may increase total cholesterol by 5%, total triglyceride by 10%, and low-density-lipoprotein cholesterol by 10%, compared to placebo-treated subjects (Goldman *et al.*, 1980). The mechanisms of these effects are unknown (Perez-Stable and Caralis, 1983). Although the clinical importance of such changes remains uncertain, they do raise concern about the most appropriate initial therapy for hypertension and emphasize the importance of using the lowest effective dose (Dollery, 1981; Kaplan, 1983).

The thiazides cause a number of other side effects, including headache, fatigue, vertigo, palpitations, and rash; impotence may also occur. Less common side effects include acute cholecystitis, interstitial nephritis, necrotizing vasculitis, hemolytic anemia, allergic pneumonitis or noncardiogenic pulmonary edema, anaphylaxis, and potentiation of myelosuppression caused by cancer chemotherapeutic agents.

OTHER DIURETIC
ANTIHYPERTENSIVE AGENTS

The thiazides and related compounds are more effective antihypertensive agents than are the loop diuretics, such as *furosemide* and *bumetanide*, in patients without edema (Ram *et al.*, 1981). As with thiazides, the change in plasma concentrations of

potassium caused by loop diuretics correlates with the diuretic effect but not with the hypotensive effect over a dose range of 40 to 80 mg of furosemide twice daily. The loop diuretics produce hypercalciuria, rather than the hypocalciuria associated with thiazides.

While *spironolactone* in doses up to 100 mg per day is equivalent to hydrochlorothiazide in its hypotensive effect, doses above 100 mg per day produce an unacceptable incidence of side effects (Schrijver and Weinberger, 1979). Spironolactone may be particularly useful for individuals with clinically significant hyperuricemia, hypokalemia, or glucose intolerance, and it is the agent of choice for primary hyperaldosteronism. In contrast to thiazide diuretics, spironolactone does not affect plasma concentrations of calcium, total cholesterol, low-density-lipoprotein cholesterol, or glucose, but it may reduce high-density-lipoprotein cholesterol up to 33% after 12 months of treatment (Falch and Schreiner, 1983). Other potassium-sparing agents, such as *triamterene* or *amiloride*, are not effective antihypertensive agents, but they are quite useful in reducing kaluresis and potentiating hypotensive effects in combination with a thiazide (De Carvalho *et al.*, 1980; Multicenter Diuretic Cooperative Study Group, 1981). These agents should be used cautiously with measurements of potassium concentrations in plasma in patients predisposed to hyperkalemia. Renal insufficiency is a relative contraindication to the use of potassium-sparing diuretics.

When glomerular filtration rates are reduced by 50% or more, thiazides lose most of their effectiveness as both diuretics and antihypertensive agents. Selection of a loop diuretic may then be particularly useful. Concurrent use of a thiazide and a loop diuretic may control refractory edema in azotemic, hypertensive patients (Wollam *et al.*, 1982).

Diuretic-Associated Drug Interactions. Among the many drug interactions associated with the treatment of hypertension with diuretics, those related to nonsteroidal anti-inflammatory drugs and to potassium homeostasis predominate.

Prostaglandins have an important role in the regulation of renal blood flow, glomerular filtration, renin secretion, tubular ion transport, and water metabolism (*see* Chapter 28). Not surprisingly, when nonsteroidal anti-inflammatory agents inhibit the biosynthesis of prostaglandins and related compounds, their renal actions are compromised, especially when there is renal dysfunction or hemodynamic alterations such as may occur during aggressive treatment with diuretics (*see* Chapter 29; *see also* Clive and Stoff, 1984). Sodium retention is almost a universal side effect of treatment with aspirin-like drugs (Brater, 1979). These agents thus attenuate the efficacy of diuretics, and fluid retention may occur, although rarely in massive amounts (Schooley *et al.*, 1977). Loss of control of blood pressure occurs in many hypertensive patients treated concurrently with nonsteroidal anti-inflammatory agents and diuretics. The above-described impairment of renal function caused by aspirin-like drugs may also cause hyperkalemia.

Potassium homeostasis is impaired by diuretics, and the interactions can become exceedingly complex when sympatholytic agents are utilized concurrently. Catecholamines and insulin have important effects on cellular uptake and release of potassium, particularly in muscle and liver. In addition, catecholamines control the secretion of insulin and *vice versa* (directly or indirectly). Many sequences of events can be envisioned, depending on the drugs being utilized, but severe hypokalemia is the most feared consequence (*see* Holland *et al.*, 1981; Brown *et al.*, 1983).

The need for routine potassium supplementation for hypertensives receiving diuretic therapy remains controversial (Harrington *et al.*, 1982). Patients at high risk for complications of hypokalemia include those with ischemic heart disease, arrhythmias, severe hepatic disease, major gastrointestinal fluid losses, and diabetes mellitus; also at risk are elderly patients and those who are receiving cardiac glycosides or corticosteroids concurrently (Lawson, 1981). In the majority of otherwise-healthy hypertensives, the hypokalemia that results from diuretics is of little clinical consequence.

Dietary sources of potassium are notoriously high in calories (averaging about 9 kcal/mEq of potassium). Pharmacological supplementation, most commonly with potassium chloride, is often recommended when plasma potassium concentrations fall below 3.0 to 3.3 mEq per liter. In standard doses, potassium-sparing diuretics are somewhat more effective than potassium supplements when hypokalemia already exists (Kohvakka *et al.*, 1979; Morgan and Davidson, 1980).

SYMPATHOLYTIC AGENTS

Since the first demonstration in 1940 that bilateral excision of the thoracic sympathetic chain could lower blood pressure, the search for effective, chemical sympatholytic agents has been intensive. Many compounds that have been tested are tolerated poorly because they produce substantial orthostatic hypotension, tachycardia, and diarrhea. In addition, their utility is sometimes limited because of the development of tolerance to their antihypertensive action and increased secretion of renin. However, newer agents and the development of rational schemes for concurrent drug therapy have overcome many of these difficulties. The subgroups of sympatholytic agents are shown in Table 32–1.

METHYLDOPA

Methyldopa is one of the oldest and most widely used antihypertensive agents. This derivative of phenylalanine was first synthesized as an inhibitor of L-aromatic amino acid (dopa) decarboxylase and was found to have hypotensive activity. Its structural formula is as follows:

Methyldopa

Mechanism of Action. Earlier theories on the mechanism of action of methyldopa focused on the possibility that the drug interfered with neurotransmission in peripheral sympathetic nerves by causing depletion of norepinephrine. These views were based on the capacity of the drug to inhibit the decarboxylation of dopa *in vitro*. Subsequent emphasis was placed on the conversion of methyldopa to α-methylnorepinephrine in adrenergic neurons, where it could be stored and released as a "false neurotransmitter" in place of norepinephrine. However, numerous observations were inconsistent with these theories, especially the fact that responses to sympathetic nerve stimulation are only slightly inhibited at the time of the maximal hypotensive response to methyldopa.

Currently, methyldopa is thought to exert its hypotensive effect within the central nervous system (CNS) by virtue of its conversion to α-methylnorepinephrine, a potent α_2-adrenergic agonist. By analogy with the actions of clonidine, this would lead to a decrease in sympathetic outflow from the CNS (*see* Langer *et al.*, 1980; *see also* Chapter 9). This hypothesis is supported by the following observations. Inhibition of the decarboxylation of methyldopa centrally, but not in the periphery, blocks the hypotensive effect of the drug. Pretreatment with phentolamine (an α-receptor antagonist) also blocks methyldopa's hypotensive effect. Furthermore, the effects of methyldopa on blood pressure do not correlate with reductions in the concentration of norepinephrine in the CNS. While additional central or peripheral mechanisms cannot be ruled out, they probably play only a minor role.

Hemodynamic Effects. Methyldopa reduces total peripheral resistance without causing much change in cardiac output or heart rate. The fall in blood pressure is maximal 4 to 6 hours after an oral dose. Arterial pressure generally falls more when the patient is standing than when supine. Although orthostatic hypotension can occur, it is usually less severe than that seen with drugs that act on the peripheral autonomic nervous system. Secretion of renin decreases, but this is neither the dominant effect of the drug nor is it necessary. If methyldopa is used alone, fluid retention, weight gain, and loss of its antihypertensive effect are common.

In older patients, methyldopa may decrease cardiac output and heart rate. All patients show decreased concentrations of norepinephrine in plasma; this reduction correlates directly with the mean change in arterial pressure but not with changes in renal blood flow or plasma or total blood volumes. Of interest, treatment with methyldopa may significantly reduce left ventricular hypertrophy within 12 weeks without any apparent relationship to the degree of change in blood pressure (Fouad *et al.,* 1982).

Absorption, Metabolism, and Excretion. Absorption of oral methyldopa is variable and incomplete. Bioavailability after oral administration averages 25%. Peak concentrations in plasma occur at 2 to 3 hours, and elimination of the drug is biphasic regardless of the route of administration. Renal excretion accounts for about two thirds of drug clearance from plasma. Slow elimination of unidentified active metabolites occurs in patients with renal failure, and dosage should be reduced in patients with hepatic or renal dysfunction; the hypotensive response should also be titrated carefully (Myhre *et al.,* 1982).

Preparations, Routes of Administration, and Dosage. *Methyldopa* (ALDOMET) is available in oral tablets containing 125, 250, or 500 mg and in an oral suspension (250 mg/5 ml). The usual initial dose is 250 mg twice daily, and there appears to be little additional effect with daily doses in excess of 2 g. Once-daily administration of methyldopa at night minimizes the effects of sedation and postural hypotension (Wright *et al.,* 1977). A parenteral preparation, *methyldopate hydrochloride* (ALDOMET ESTER HYDROCHLORIDE), is also available (50 mg/ml). It is usually given by intermittent intravenous infusion of 250 to 1000 mg every 6 hours, adjusted to the needs of the individual patient. Methyldopate is the ethyl ester of methyldopa, and the rate of deesterification can be variable among patients. If this rate is slow, a paradoxical hypertensive effect can occur.

Toxicity and Precautions. The most commonly reported side effects with methyldopa are sedation, postural hypotension, dizziness, dry mouth, and headache. Sedation may wane after the first week of therapy, but it can recur with any major increase in dosage. Decreased mental acuity is a common, although subtle, problem. Other undesirable effects include sleep disturbances, depression, impotence, anxiety, blurred vision, and parkinsonian signs. Dry mouth and nasal stuffiness may also occur.

More worrisome but rarer toxic reactions include hemolytic anemia, thrombocytopenia, leukopenia, hepatitis, and lupus-like syndromes. With prolonged therapy, 10 to 20% of patients develop a positive direct Coombs test; hemolytic anemia occurs in less than 5% of these patients. While the development of a positive direct Coombs test need not alter therapy, frank hemolysis requires immediate cessation of methyldopa. The Coombs test may remain positive for months after treatment is stopped. Severe hemolysis may be limited by treatment with corticosteroids. Drug fever may occur and may be confused with sepsis. Transient abnormalities of liver function develop in up to 3% of patients and may progress to hepatic necrosis, although the hepatitis is usually reversible. Hepatitis may occur as late as 3 years after initiation of therapy, but it usually appears within the first 2 months of treatment.

A variety of less common toxic reactions include lichenoid and granulomatous skin eruptions, myocarditis, retroperitoneal fibrosis, and carotid sinus hypersensitivity with bradycardia, hypotension, and syncope. Even more rarely methyldopa has been associated with pancreatitis, biliary carcinoma, colitis, and hyperprolactinemia.

Important drug interactions include enhancement of the hypotensive effects of methyldopa by concomitant use of diuretics or general anesthetics and reduction of the antihypertensive effect by tricyclic antidepressants, barbiturates, and sympathomimetic amines. The toxicity of lithium and haloperidol may be increased by concurrent administration of methyldopa.

Sudden withdrawal of methyldopa may rarely cause an abrupt rise in blood pressure. Treatment of this rebound phenomenon consists in reinstitution of therapy or, if severe, parenteral administration of a potent vasodilator such as sodium nitroprusside.

Therapeutic Uses. Methyldopa is an effective antihypertensive agent when given in conjunction with a thiazide, but frequent side effects have limited its usefulness. The therapy of hypertension is discussed in more detail below.

CLONIDINE

First used as a nasal decongestant, clonidine was found serendipitously to have hypotensive effects. The central antihypertensive effects of this agent have focused attention on the role of α-adrenergic receptors in the CNS and the functional interactions between central and peripheral adrenergic activities (Sambhi and Villarreal, 1983). The structural formula of clonidine is as follows:

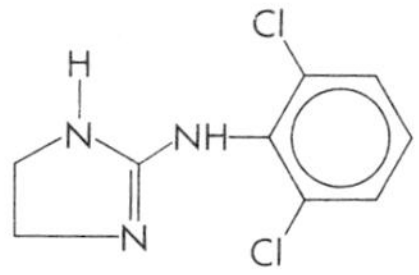

Clonidine

Locus and Mechanism of Action. The actions of clonidine are complex. Its major actions are those of a centrally acting α_2-adrenergic agonist, and it thereby resembles methyldopa. In addition, clonidine is clearly only a partial agonist, and its effects at a given site are thus dependent on the endogenous concentration of norepinephrine. Thus, if the concentration (*i.e.*, rate of release) of norepinephrine is high, clonidine may appear to act as an antagonist. Since agonist or partial agonist effects may be exerted at presynaptic or postsynaptic receptors at multiple sites in the CNS, interpretation is obviously difficult. There is evidence for effects of the drug in both the hypothalamus and the medulla oblon-

gata. The net result of these actions is clearly a diminished sympathetic outflow from the CNS (*see* Isaac, 1980; *see also* Chapter 9).

After intravenous administration, clonidine causes a transient rise in blood pressure followed by a more prolonged fall. The initial hypertension results from stimulation of postsynaptic vascular α receptors. The later generalized depression of the cardiovascular system, which leads to hypotension, bradycardia, and decreased cardiac output, results from clonidine-induced reductions in spontaneous discharges from the splanchnic and cardiac nerves. Evidence for clonidine's central site of action includes the following: intracisternal administration produces typical hypotensive and cardiodepressant effects; obliterative neurosurgical procedures in animals eliminate these effects; and the drug decreases spontaneous presynaptic sympathetic nerve activity without affecting circulatory reflexes. α_2-Adrenergic blocking agents antagonize the effects of clonidine when they are administered centrally.

Peripherally, clonidine impairs adrenergic neurotransmission by activating inhibitory presynaptic α_2 receptors (Langer *et al.*, 1980). Impairment of peripheral noradrenergic transmission by clonidine is most pronounced at low frequencies of nerve stimulation.

Pharmacological Effects. Acute oral administration of clonidine results in a reduction in heart rate and stroke volume in supine patients; total peripheral resistance is also reduced if the patient is standing. Sympathetic tone in different parts of the cardiovascular system thus determines the net effects on the heart and resistance vessels. Inconsistent results have been observed in long-term hemodynamic studies: the cardiac index and heart rate usually decrease more than does total peripheral resistance. Hypotensive effects generally parallel reductions in the concentration of circulating norepinephrine. There is poor correlation with plasma renin activity or concentrations of aldosterone. Clonidine does not block sympathetic reflexes that are activated by standing. The drug lowers coronary vascular resistance, independently of effects on heart rate or myocardial contractility. Bradycardia is rarely severe, and significant arrhythmias are infrequent.

Clonidine reduces renovascular resistance without changing renal blood flow or glomerular filtration rate. The capacity of clonidine to decrease the release of renin is lost if the kidneys are denervated. However, after the administration of clonidine in normal subjects, salt depletion or postural changes may still stimulate renin secretion. Clonidine is an effective antihypertensive agent in patients with renal failure, including those who are undergoing chronic hemodialysis.

Absorption, Metabolism, and Excretion. Clonidine is rapidly and almost completely absorbed after oral administration, and bioavailability is high. Peak concentrations in plasma occur in 1 to 3 hours; the terminal plasma half-life averages 9 hours (Reid, 1981). Plasma concentrations correlate with decreases in blood pressure up to values of 1.5 to 2.0 ng/ml. Higher concentrations produce no additional or even reduced antihypertensive effects. Since maximally effective concentrations in plasma may occur after a dose of as little as 0.3 mg, there appears to be little justification for oral doses greater than 0.3 mg twice daily for the majority of patients (Pettinger, 1980). Clonidine is very soluble in lipid and easily penetrates into the CNS. Nearly one half of an oral dose of clonidine is degraded in the liver, but none of the metabolites has significant pharmacological activity. The remainder of the drug is excreted unchanged in the urine (Arndts *et al.*, 1983). In patients with renal dysfunction, the half-life increases to 18 to 41 hours, and reduction of dosage is necessary (Lowenthal, 1980).

Preparations, Route of Administration, and Dosage. *Clonidine hydrochloride* (CATAPRES) is marketed in 0.1-, 0.2-, and 0.3-mg tablets. The usual total daily dosage is 0.2 to 0.8 mg, administered in two or more doses. The administration of two unequal doses, with the larger dose given at bedtime, can limit unwanted drowsiness caused by clonidine and still permit control of blood pressure (Jain *et al.*, 1977). Parenteral administration of clonidine has been effective in hypertensive crises, but suitable preparations are not generally available (Russ *et al.*, 1983).

Toxicity and Precautions. Xerostomia and sedation are the most frequently encountered side effects of clonidine. They occur in up to 50% of patients but may diminish in 2 to 4 weeks despite continued use of the drug. Up to 10% of patients must discontinue clonidine because of persistence of sedation, dizziness, dry mouth, nausea, indigestion, or impotence. The xerostomia is often accompanied by dry eyes, dry nasal mucosa, parotid gland swelling, and anorexia. When clonidine is used as the sole drug for treatment of hypertension, fluid retention, weight gain, and loss of the hypotensive effect may occur; all are correctable by administration of diuretics. CNS side effects include vivid dreams or nightmares, insomnia, restlessness, anxiety, and depression. Rash, angioneurotic edema, urticaria, alopecia, and pruritus are dermatological toxicities. Other rare reactions include hyperglycemia, elevated creatine phosphokinase, gynecomastia, urinary retention, and increased sensitivity to alcohol. Concurrent use of tricyclic antidepressants and clonidine has been associated with reduction in the antihypertensive effect.

Sudden withdrawal of clonidine may produce a hypertensive crisis, which may be life threatening. Nervousness, headache, abdominal pain, tachycardia, and sweating, consistent with sympathetic overactivity, accompany the crisis. The same constellation has been reported after sudden cessation of a variety of other antihypertensive agents, including methyldopa, guanabenz, guanadrel, and β-adrenergic antagonists. The symptoms of sympathetic overactivity may sometimes occur without return of blood pressure to pretreatment or higher values. The syndrome has been reported in patients who were receiving as little as 0.6 mg of clonidine per day. It usually begins 18 to 20 hours after the last dose. Hypertension above pretreatment levels may persist for up to 7 to 10 days, and this is generally associated with elevated concentrations of catecholamines in plasma and urine. The exact incidence of the syndrome is uncertain; however, given the large number of patients who have received clonidine and the high probability of poor compliance with dosage regimens, the syndrome is probably rare. However, it has occurred even when the dosage of clonidine was reduced gradually.

Individuals who exhibit severe withdrawal hypertension should be treated parenterally with vasodilators such as sodium nitroprusside or with a combination of α- and β-adrenergic antagonists (*e.g.*, phentolamine and propranolol). Treatment with a β blocker alone may exaggerate the hypertensive effect from high concentrations of circulating catecholamines. Alternatively, the withdrawal syndrome may be treated by readministration of clonidine. All patients who receive clonidine as well as α- and β-blocking agents should be warned of the possibility of severe withdrawal reactions, and rapid discontinuation of clonidine for any reason should be discouraged.

Prominent signs of overdosage with clonidine include depression of sensorium, blood pressure, heart rate, and respiration. The combination of respiratory depression and miosis may simulate overdosage with opioids. Treatment consists in ventilatory support for apnea; chronotropic support with atropine, epinephrine, or dopamine; and intravenous fluids, dopamine, or α-adrenergic antagonists (*e.g.*, tolazoline) for refractory hypotension.

Therapeutic Uses. Clonidine has generally been used in conjunction with diuretics for the treatment of hypertension. It may also be substituted for other sympatholytic agents in standard three-drug therapy with a diuretic and a vasodilator. The treatment of hypertension is considered in greater detail below.

GUANABENZ AND GUANFACINE

Guanabenz and guanfacine are centrally acting α2-adrenergic agonists with pharmacological properties (including side effects) that are similar to those of clonidine.

The antihypertensive effect of guanabenz is maximal approximately 2 to 4 hours after oral dosage and dissipates over the next 10 hours. Bioavailability is good, the half-life in plasma is approximately 6 hours, and most of the drug is metabolized. *Guanabenz acetate* (WYTENSIN) is available in 4- and 8-mg tablets. The initial dose is 4 mg, taken twice daily. The maximal dose, which is only rarely required, is 32 mg twice a day.

Guanfacine, which is not yet available for general use in the United States, has a relatively long half-life (14 to 18 hours) and is largely eliminated by renal excretion (of the unchanged drug and a hydroxylated metabolite). Once-daily administration of guanfacine (1 to 3 mg) appears to provide effective control of blood pressure (*see* Beevers *et al.*, 1981; Jerie and Lasance, 1981; Hedner *et al.*, 1984).

PRAZOSIN

Prazosin is the first member of a class of peripheral α1-adrenergic antagonists derived from quinazoline. A related compound, trimazosin, is under clinical investigation (*see* Chapter 9). Prazosin has the following structural formula:

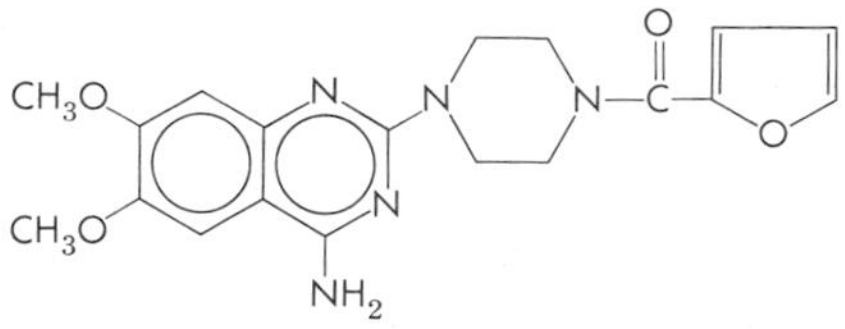

Prazosin

Locus and Mechanism of Action. The major, if not the sole, mechanism of action of prazosin is competitive blockade of the vascular postsynaptic α1-adrenergic receptor (Stanaszek *et al.*, 1983). Both α1 and α2 receptors may be found postsynaptically in vascular smooth muscle, and the ratio of these receptor subtypes appears to determine the net effect of the drug at a given site. The relative affinity of prazosin for α1 compared to α2 receptors is very high (Davey, 1980); this selectivity is not shared by classical α-adrenergic antagonists such as phentolamine. The selectivity allows prazosin to block the contractile response of vascular smooth muscle to norepinephrine without interfering with its activity at α2 sites. Activation of prejunctional α2 receptors by norepinephrine is inhibitory to further release of the transmitter (*see* Chapters 4 and 9).

Pharmacological Effects. At rest, prazosin reduces mean arterial pressure and peripheral resistance but produces little or no tachycardia, in contrast to direct peripheral vasodilators, which cause a reflex increase in sympathetic tone. At clinically effective doses of prazosin, cardiovascular responses to exercise, exposure to cold, and changes in pressure imposed on the carotid sinus are largely unchanged, even though blood pressure and peripheral resistance remain reduced (Mancia *et al.*, 1980). Nevertheless, the hypotensive effect of prazosin is greater when the patient is standing, and a mild reflex tachycardia can result.

This effect may be more dramatic after the first dose of the drug than after subsequent administrations, despite similar concentrations in plasma. This suggests the development of a relative tolerance to the hypotensive effect, perhaps due to reflex sympathetic compensation to the reduced blood pressure. However, marked tachyphylaxis does not generally occur during long-term treatment (Walker *et al.*, 1981).

Patients appear to fall into two groups based on their response to prazosin. One group experiences a marked reduction of blood pressure after the first dose of the drug, exhibits no tachycardia, and usually requires only a small dose to maintain adequate reduction of blood pressure. The other group exhibits only a minimal reduction of blood pressure after the first dose, usually has a significant tachycardia, and requires a higher dose of prazosin to maintain control of blood pressure. Measurement of pharmacokinetic parameters in these two groups has revealed no differences. The long-term response to prazosin and the maintenance dose can be predicted from analysis of the response to the first dose (Larochelle *et al.*, 1982).

Absorption, Fate, and Elimination. Prazosin undergoes first-pass metabolism by the liver, but there is a linear correlation between dose and the steady-state concentration achieved in plasma. Peak concentrations occur 1 to 3 hours after oral administration, and these values vary widely among subjects. Over 90% of the drug is bound to α_1-acid glycoprotein, and only a small fraction is bound to albumin. The plasma half-life is 2 to 3 hours. Only a small amount of prazosin is found unaltered in the urine, and dealkylated metabolites are predominantly eliminated in the bile. In patients with chronic renal failure or congestive heart failure, the unbound fraction of prazosin in plasma is increased and the half-life of prazosin is prolonged (Baughman *et al.*, 1980; Rubin and Blaschke, 1980). The antihypertensive effect of prazosin persists for longer than expected (up to 10 to 12 hours), presumably because of active metabolites (Stanaszek *et al.*, 1983).

Preparations and Dosage. *Prazosin hydrochloride* (MINIPRESS) is available in 1-, 2-, or 5-mg capsules. The usual initial dose of prazosin is 1 mg two or three times daily; this is then increased as necessary. While total daily doses as high as 20 to 40 mg have been given, benefit is marginal beyond doses of 6 to 10 mg per day.

Toxicity and Precautions. Prazosin may cause a so-called first-dose phenomenon, characterized by hypotension with sudden loss of consciousness, typically 30 to 90 minutes after the initial dose. This is particularly likely to occur in individuals who are depleted of sodium or who are taking other antihypertensive medications. Frank syncope may occur in up to 1% of patients who receive 2 mg or more of prazosin initially; this is avoidable if the first dose is limited to 1 mg and is given just prior to bedtime. Faintness and dizziness have been reported in up to one half of patients receiving prazosin (Stanaszek *et al.*, 1983). The symptoms are generally accompanied by pronounced falls in standing blood pressure and may recur with re-treatment after a hiatus of a few days. Less common side effects include palpitations, tachycardia, headache, lassitude, dry mouth, diarrhea, weight gain, peripheral edema, nausea, urinary urgency, nasal stuffiness, constipation, polyarthritis, eosinophilia, hypersensitivity, and priapism. Plasma concentrations of glucose, free fatty acids, and uric acid may also be elevated.

Therapeutic Uses. The efficacy of prazosin for the treatment of mild-to-moderate hypertension is well documented. Prazosin is more effective when combined with a diuretic and/or a β blocker than when used alone. Although prazosin has been used in patients with severe congestive heart failure, pheochromocytoma, or hypertensive crisis, there are better alternatives.

β-Adrenergic Antagonists

Since they were introduced in the 1960s, β-adrenergic blocking agents have become the most commonly used drugs for cardiovascular diseases. Most of their features are discussed in Chapter 9, but characteristics particularly relevant to their use in hypertension will be mentioned here.

Pharmacodynamic Properties. Despite differences in pharmacological properties (which include membrane-stabilizing activity, partial-agonist activity, and ability to penetrate the CNS), all of the β-adrenergic antagonists have comparable capacities to lower blood pressure in doses that are equipotent for the production of β blockade (Frishman, 1981a). However, the exact mechanism by which such blockade lowers blood pressure during chronic administration has been controversial. While many mechanisms have been proposed, the more plausible appear to be a combination of reduction of cardiac output and inhibition of renin secretion. Both of these effects result from blockade of β_1-adrenergic receptors (see Chapters 4 and 9).

A major difference among β-blocking agents is their selectivity for β_1 as compared to β_2 receptors. While such selectivity is clearly advantageous in at least certain patients (e.g., those with obstructive pulmonary disease), it is only relative with the drugs that are currently available. Since standard doses of β blockers produce widely varied concentrations in plasma, it is not always possible to realize the inherent selectivity of a given agent in a particular patient.

Of particular concern is the effect of these antagonists on renal function. Stimulation of renin secretion is mediated by β_1 receptors, while β_2 receptors appear to mediate catecholamine-induced renal vasodilatation. In most acute studies, β blockers reduce renal plasma flow and the rate of glomerular filtration without regard to their selectivity for β_1 receptors. After chronic administration, nonselective β blockers appear to reduce glomerular filtration rate and effective renal plasma flow more than do cardioselective agents. However, most studies have shown these differences to be insignificant clinically.

One feature that may deserve additional study and consideration is that of the intrinsic sympathomimetic (or partial agonist) activity of these agents (see Chapter 9). While certain advantages of such activity have been suggested (e.g., less bradycardia, pulmonary obstruction, or hypersensitivity to catecholamines upon withdrawal of the antagonist), significant clinical advantages of the use of partial agonists remain to be demonstrated.

Pharmacokinetic Properties. Most of the differences in the pharmacokinetic proper-

ties of these drugs can be explained on the basis of their relative lipophilicity. The more lipid-soluble agents (particularly propranolol; also metoprolol) are quite rapidly and completely absorbed from the gastrointestinal tract, extensively metabolized in the liver, substantially distributed to the CNS, and rapidly eliminated (Cruickshank, 1980). In view of their extensive first-pass metabolism, their bioavailability is sensitive to changes in hepatic blood flow (see Williams, 1983) and to drug interactions with agents that alter such flow (e.g., hydralazine; Schneck and Vary, 1984) or that inhibit hepatic drug metabolism (e.g., cimetidine).

β Blockers with low lipophilicity (atenolol and nadolol) are not metabolized appreciably; they have longer half-lives, and their dosage must be reduced in patients with renal failure. The last-named fact is also true of propranolol because it has active metabolites that are excreted by the kidney (see Wilkinson, 1982). Atenolol and nadolol cross the blood-brain barrier to a limited extent and may be particularly useful if CNS side effects are troublesome (see Frishman et al., 1979a).

Untoward Effects. Sudden withdrawal of β blockers may cause a syndrome characterized by ventricular arrhythmias, severe angina, myocardial infarction, and even death. The incidence appears to be as high as 5%, especially with relatively short-acting agents like propranolol (Shand and Wood, 1978). The incidence and intensity of such reactions are lower with longer-acting agents like atenolol. Gradual discontinuation of a β-adrenergic antagonist over a period of 7 to 14 days has been recommended (Rangno, 1981).

The safety of β blockers in pregnancy remains controversial (Rubin, 1981). However, atenolol was shown to be safe and effective in hypertension associated with pregnancy (Rubin et al., 1983). Neonatal bradycardia has been noted as a rare complication. Elderly patients with hypertension appear to tolerate β blockers well, despite fears of precipitating heart failure (Wikstrand and Berglund, 1982). These agents should be avoided or used with caution in patients with asthma, chronic obstructive pulmonary disease, peripheral vascular disease, congestive heart failure, or insulin-dependent diabetes.

RESERPINE AND RAUWOLFIA ALKALOIDS

The pharmacological properties of reserpine are presented in Chapter 9. Reserpine is an effective antihypertensive agent, particularly when used concurrently with other agents, such as thiazides. Its low cost, once-daily administration, and minimal change in effect when compliance is erratic make it useful as an agent for long-term treatment of patients with uncomplicated, mild hypertension. However, reserpine causes mental depression in as many as 25% of patients, and the drug should be discontinued at the first sign of despondency. Drug-induced depression may persist for months after cessation of therapy, and it may be severe enough to provoke suicide. *Reserpine is contraindicated in patients with a history of depression.*

GUANETHIDINE

The pharmacological properties of guanethidine and its congener guanadrel are described in Chapter 9. Guanethidine is usually employed only in patients with severe hypertension, and it is used less frequently now that alternative vasodilators and sympatholytic agents are available. Guanethidine is particularly likely to cause severe orthostatic hypotension. The drug does not enter the CNS in significant amounts, and it is thus an alternative for patients who are intolerant of the central effects of other sympatholytics.

TRIMETHAPHAN

Trimethaphan, a ganglionic blocking agent, is discussed in Chapter 10. It has been largely supplanted by other agents because of a high incidence of adverse reactions. However, it is still occasionally useful in the treatment of hypertension associated with dissecting aneurysms.

VASODILATORS

HYDRALAZINE

Although hydralazine was introduced into clinical practice over 30 years ago, it fell into disfavor because of excessive side effects when it was given alone or in conjunction with a ganglionic blocking agent. However, hydralazine now enjoys new popularity, since many of its unwanted effects are minimized when it is used concurrently with a diuretic and a β-adrenergic antagonist. Hydralazine has the following structural formula:

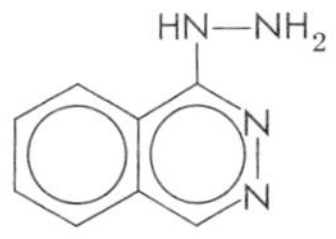

Hydralazine

Locus and Mechanism of Action. Hydralazine causes direct relaxation of arteriolar vascular smooth muscle. The mechanism of this effect may be similar to that of organic nitrates, in that it appears to involve activation of guanylate cyclase and accumulation of guanosine 3′,5′-monophosphate (cyclic GMP) (*see* Chapter 33). However, other actions may also contribute to the vasodilatation. Prominent compensatory reactions to such vasodilatation include increased heart rate and contractility, increased plasma renin activity, and fluid retention, all of which counteract the antihypertensive effect of the drug.

Pharmacological Effects. Most of the effects of hydralazine are confined to the cardiovascular system. The drug decreases diastolic more than systolic blood pressure by lowering peripheral vascular resistance, and it increases heart rate, stroke volume, and cardiac output. Because of preferential dilatation of arterioles rather than veins, postural hypotension is uncommon. Peripheral vasodilatation is widespread but not uniform; blood flow usually increases in the splanchnic, coronary, cerebral, and renal vascular beds unless the fall in blood pressure is very marked.

Absorption, Fate, and Excretion. Hydralazine is quickly and almost totally absorbed from the gastrointestinal tract. However, it is subject to significant first-pass metabolism in the liver, the extent of which is determined by the patient's acetylator phenotype. Genetically determined "slow acetylators" achieve higher concentrations in plasma than do "fast acetylators" who receive the same dose. The incidence of excessive hypotension and other toxicities is higher in patients with the slow-acetylator phenotype, and these individuals should generally not receive more than 200 mg of hydralazine daily. Acetylation phenotype has little effect on plasma concentrations after parenteral administration.

Peak concentrations of hydralazine occur in plasma within 30 to 120 minutes after ingestion, and these correlate with peak hypotensive effects; the duration of effect is 6 to 8 hours. After parenteral administration, hypotensive effects are seen in 10 to 20 minutes and last for 2 to 4 hours. About 85% of circulating hydralazine is bound to albumin. In addition to acetylation, hydralazine is also subjected to ring hydroxylation and conjugation with glucuronic acid.

Preparations and Dosage. *Hydralazine hydrochloride* (APRESOLINE HCL) is available in 10-, 25-, 50-, and 100-mg tablets and in 1-ml ampuls containing 20 mg of the drug. The usual oral dosage is 25 to 100 mg twice daily, although the elderly and those with impaired renal function may require smaller doses administered up to four times daily. Twice-daily administration of hydralazine has been found to be as effective as administration four times a day for control of blood pressure, regardless of acetylator phenotype.

Toxicity. The overall incidence of adverse reactions to hydralazine may be as high as 20%. The most common reactions include headache, nausea, vomiting, tachycardia, palpitations, dizziness, weakness, fatigue, and postural hypotension. Less commonly, patients may exhibit diarrhea, constipation, anxiety, sleep disturbances, angina, and nasal congestion. Fewer than 10% of patients receiving hydralazine develop a lupus-like syndrome, consisting in myalgia, arthralgia, fever, antinuclear antibodies, and, more rarely, rash, lymphadenopathy, chest pain, asthenia, and hepatosplenomegaly. The syndrome usually occurs after more than 2 months of administration, in those who acetylate the drug slowly, in the summer season, and when dosage exceeds 200 mg per day. The syndrome generally disappears within 6 months of discontinuation of the drug. However, rheumatoid symptoms have been reported to persist for up to 8 years. Patients who develop only antinuclear antibodies without other clinical features of the syndrome need not discontinue the medica-

tion. The exact mechanism of the lupus-like syndrome is unknown. Most of the autoantibodies are of the IgG type, although IgM antibodies may also be found. Periodic determination of antinuclear antibody is probably not justified if there are no symptoms (Mansilla-Tinoco *et al.*, 1982).

Therapeutic Uses. Hydralazine is especially useful when combined with a diuretic *and* a β blocker or other sympatholytic agent. Reflex tachycardia in response to vasodilatation and other side effects usually limit the usefulness of the drug when it is used alone. It must be administered carefully to older patients or to those with underlying heart disease, since it may precipitate angina or myocardial ischemia. Hydralazine has been widely used in severe hypertension during pregnancy. In patients with hypertensive crises, it reduces blood pressure rapidly, but it must be employed with caution to avoid excessive hypotension. The drug should be given intravenously in such situations to avoid unpredictable absorption; small, incremental doses are given to minimize precipitous hypotension.

Minoxidil

Minoxidil is a potent vasodilator. It acts directly on vascular smooth muscle cells, and its mechanism of action is probably similar to that of hydralazine. The chemical structure of minoxidil is as follows:

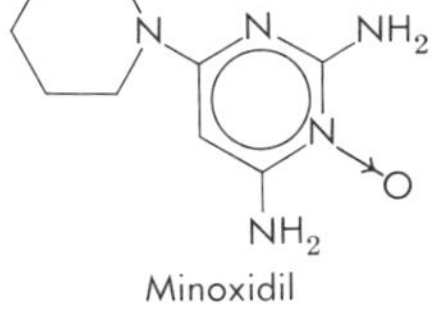

Minoxidil

Pharmacological Effects. Minoxidil produces arteriolar dilatation, decreased peripheral vascular resistance, and lowered systolic and diastolic blood pressures. The magnitude of its antihypertensive response is proportional to the initial level of the blood pressure, and it has minimal hypotensive activity in normal subjects (Lowenthal and Affrime, 1980). The hypotensive effect of minoxidil is accompanied by reflex increases in heart rate and cardiac index.

Plasma concentrations of norepinephrine, renin, and aldosterone also rise, especially during acute administration. There may be some decline in renal function in patients with renal parenchymal disease. In contrast, there is often improvement in renal function in patients with previously uncontrolled malignant hypertension.

Absorption, Metabolism, and Excretion. Minoxidil is rapidly and completely absorbed from the gastrointestinal tract. Peak concentrations in plasma are observed in 1 hour, and its maximal pharmacological effect occurs in 2 to 3 hours. While the average half-life in plasma is 3 hours, the antihypertensive effect may persist for 1 to 3 days. Sequestration in tissues may explain its prolonged effect (Campese, 1981).

Minoxidil is metabolized predominantly by the liver, especially by conjugation with glucuronic acid. The metabolites have reduced pharmacological activity. While both minoxidil and its metabolites are primarily excreted by the kidneys (Lowenthal and Affrime, 1980), only 12% of the drug is excreted unchanged in the urine. In patients with end-stage renal disease, renal excretion is reduced and excretion in the feces may increase to 20%.

Preparations and Dosage. *Minoxidil* (LONITEN) is supplied in 2.5- and 10-mg tablets. The initial daily dosage is usually 5 mg; this can be gradually increased to 40 mg in one or two daily doses. Although doses of up to 100 mg a day have been used, most patients require no more than 10 to 40 mg per day in one or two divided doses. In situations that require a prompt reduction of blood pressure, a loading dose of minoxidil (5 to 20 mg) may be administered, and additional doses of 2.5 to 10 mg can be given at 4-hour intervals, depending on the initial response (Alpert and Bauer, 1982).

Toxicity. While the hypotensive efficacy of minoxidil is impressive, adverse reactions prompt withdrawal of the drug in up to 70% of patients. The most common side effects are *fluid retention* and *hypertrichosis*. The degree of sodium and water retention is correlated with the dose and the duration of administration and, if present, the degree of renal impairment. The drug increases sodium reabsorption in the proximal tubule, and potent diuretics such as furosemide may be required to avoid weight gain, loss of the antihypertensive effect, and cardiac decompensation. Hypertrichosis occurs in nearly all patients treated with minoxidil for more than 4 weeks. The hair growth commonly involves the temples, forehead, face, ear pinnae, eyebrows, forearms, and all hairy body surfaces. Many patients thus refuse to use the drug. The hypertrichosis does not have an endocrine basis, and the effect is presumed to be due to enhanced cutaneous blood flow. Extemporaneously prepared topical preparations of minoxidil have been used to treat severe alopecia (Weiss *et al.,* 1981).

Cardiovascular effects include tachycardia and palpitations from reflex sympathetic stimulation. The tachycardia is often associated with a decrease in the S-T segment, T wave flattening, or T wave inversion; these changes may revert after months of continued treatment (Campese, 1981). Pericardial effusion may occur, especially in patients with renal insufficiency, although it is usually insignificant hemodynamically. All of these effects can usually be minimized with diuretics and/or β-blocking agents. There have been rare reports of myocardial fibrosis and hydropic vacuolization in a few elderly patients who received minoxidil for severe hypertension. Even more rarely, skin rashes, Stevens-Johnson syndrome, glucose intolerance, serosanguinous bullae, antinuclear antibody formation, and thrombocytopenia may occur.

Rebound hypertension may rarely follow the withdrawal of minoxidil, especially in patients who have been taking large doses. Gradual reduction of the dose or pretreatment with an α-blocking agent such as prazosin seems to prevent this problem.

Therapeutic Uses. Because it is effective in nearly all patients, minoxidil is useful in treating *severe* hypertension that is refractory to the conventional three-drug regimens that consist of a diuretic, a sympatholytic, and another vasodilator.

CALCIUM CHANNEL BLOCKERS

The calcium channel blockers have emerged as a new class of drugs with great potential for manipulation of the function of smooth muscle. Of the many agents in various stages of development, three are available in the United States at the present time: *nifedipine, verapamil,* and *diltiazem* (*see* Henry, 1980; Spivack *et al.*, 1983). The approved indications for use of these drugs include the treatment of angina (*see* Chapter 33) and specific arrhythmias (Chapter 31). The general pharmacology of the calcium channel blockers is discussed in Chapter 33. Although these drugs are not currently approved in the United States for the treatment of hypertension, they are being used experimentally for this purpose; features that are particularly relevant to such use will be mentioned briefly here.

As a group, the calcium channel blockers are potent arterial vasodilators. In contrast to agents like hydralazine, calcium channel blockers cause dilatation of coronary arteries, accelerate relaxation of the ventricles, and improve subendocardial perfusion (Braunwald, 1982). However, these agents also suppress the automaticity of the S-A node and depress conduction through the A-V node. Nifedipine is the most potent arteriolar dilator of the three drugs, and it appears to do so at concentrations that have little direct effect on the heart. Thus, nifedipine in therapeutic doses produces more reflex activation of the sympathetic nervous system than do verapamil and diltiazem. The direct negative inotropic and chronotropic effects of verapamil and diltiazem limit reflex sympathetic activation of myocardial function that occurs as peripheral vascular resistance falls; these two agents are also more likely to disturb A-V conduction, particularly in patients with conduction disorders.

Nifedipine causes a modest reduction in plasma concentrations of potassium (Murphy *et al.*, 1983). Concomitant use of a diuretic is frequently necessary to avoid fluid retention, and this could well increase the hypokalemia.

Additional information is needed before the role of calcium channel blockers in the treatment of hypertension can be defined.

SODIUM NITROPRUSSIDE

Sodium nitroprusside was approved for medical use in the United States in 1974, 45 years after it was first shown to lower blood pressure. It directly relaxes both arteriolar and venous smooth muscle, decreasing preload and afterload. Its mechanism of action appears to be the same as that of the organic nitrates (*see* Chapter 33). The structural formula of sodium nitroprusside is as follows:

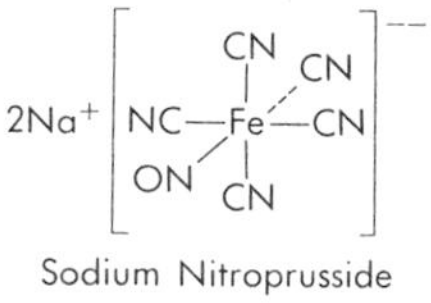

$$2Na^+ \left[\begin{array}{c} CN \\ | \quad CN \\ NC-Fe-CN \\ | \quad CN \\ ON \quad CN \end{array} \right]^{--}$$

Sodium Nitroprusside

Pharmacological Properties. The hypotensive effect of nitroprusside occurs whether the patient is supine or standing, but venous pooling is more extensive when the patient is upright. Renal blood flow and glomerular filtration rate are maintained, and plasma renin activity increases. By reducing preload, myocardial workload is decreased, and ischemic changes, including angina, are less likely than with more selective arteriolar vasodilators, such as diazoxide, hydralazine, and minoxidil.

Nitroprusside must be given parenterally. Its onset of action is maximal in 1 to 2 minutes, and the effect dissipates quickly when an intravenous infusion is stopped. Arterial pressure can easily be titrated to almost any level by altering the rate of infusion, and tolerance or resistance to the drug is rare. The ferrous ion in the nitroprusside molecule reacts promptly with sulfhydryl-containing compounds in the red blood cells; cyanide ion is produced, but it is reduced to thiocyanate in the liver. Thiocyanate is excreted in the urine with a half-life of 3 to 4 days.

The acute toxicity of nitroprusside is entirely secondary to excessive vasodilatation and hypotension. Close monitoring of blood pressure is necessary to avoid nausea, vomiting, sweating, restlessness, headache, palpitations, and substernal distress. After prolonged administration, thiocyanate may accumulate and cause an acute toxic psychosis, especially if the patient has renal impairment or hyponatremia. The plasma concentration of thiocyanate should be monitored and should not be allowed to exceed 10 mg/dl. Excessive concentrations of thiocyanate can also interfere with thyroid function. In patients with renal failure, thiocyanate is readily removed by hemodialysis.

Sodium nitroprusside (NIPRIDE, NITROPRESS) is utilized to treat hypertensive emergencies and, experimentally, to manage severe, refractory congestive heart failure. The drug is available in 5-ml vials that contain 50 mg. The contents of the vial should be dissolved in 2 to 3 ml of 5% dextrose in water. Addition of this solution to 500 ml of 5% dextrose in water produces a concentration of 100 μg/ml. Because the compound decomposes in light, only fresh solutions should be used and the bottle should be covered with an opaque wrapping. The freshly prepared solution has a very faint, brownish tint; any highly colored solution should be discarded. The usual rate of infusion is 0.5 to 10 μg/kg per minute, and average doses of 3 μg/kg per minute reduce diastolic blood pressure by 30 to

40%. If infusion rates of 10 μg/kg per minute do not produce adequate reduction of blood pressure within 10 minutes, administration of nitroprusside should be stopped to minimize potential toxicity.

DIAZOXIDE

Diazoxide is closely related chemically to the thiazide diuretics. Its structural formula is as follows:

Diazoxide

The pharmacological effects of diazoxide include both an antidiuretic action and the capacity to relax arteriolar smooth muscle directly. Striking increases in heart rate and cardiac output may accompany the hypotensive effect. In contrast to nitroprusside, diazoxide has no substantial effect on venous capacitance, and it can cause marked retention of sodium and water. This compensatory reaction may blunt the hypotensive effects of diazoxide, but it can be countered by the use of potent diuretics.

Absorption, Metabolism, and Excretion. The half-life of diazoxide in plasma is 20 to 60 hours. The hypotensive effect is proportional to the concentration of unbound drug in plasma, which is 10% of the total. Patients with renal dysfunction exhibit decreased binding of diazoxide to albumin (O'Malley *et al.*, 1975), and such patients are thus likely to have a greater-than-ordinary hypotensive effect following its administration. Urinary excretion of the unchanged drug accounts for about one third of its elimination. Diazoxide also is metabolized by the liver to inactive derivatives.

Preparation, Route of Administration, Therapeutic Use, and Dosage. *Diazoxide* (HYPERSTAT I.V.) is available for intravenous use in 20-ml ampuls that contain 300 mg of the drug. The drug is employed primarily in hypertensive emergencies. It works rapidly, and invasive monitoring of arterial pressure is not required. Rapid, intravenous administration of large doses of diazoxide, which was recommended previously, may cause severe hypotension. More predictable, controlled hypotensive effects may be obtained from administration of the drug by slow infusion over 15 to 30 minutes. Bolus injections of 0.5 to 1.0 mg/kg over 5 to 10 seconds may produce maximal reductions in mean arterial pressure after 2 minutes, and this dose may be repeated every 5 to 10 minutes (Ogilvie *et al.*, 1982). If a β blocker and a diuretic are administered prior to diazoxide, it can be given by slow infusion of 5 to 10 mg/kg over 15 to 30 minutes; blood pressure is usually lowered with few side effects (Garrett and Kaplan, 1982). Diazoxide should not be used to treat hypertension associated with aortic coarctation, arteriovenous shunts, or aortic dissection. Similarly, risks outweigh benefits in its use for intracerebral hemorrhage or acute pulmonary edema.

Toxicity and Precautions. Diazoxide produces both fluid retention and hyperglycemia. If diazoxide is used for more than 12 to 24 hours, administration of a potent diuretic or restriction of sodium may be necessary. Mild, transient hyperglycemia usually requires no special treatment, except in diabetic patients (*see* Chapter 64). Other side effects include tachycardia, myocardial and cerebral ischemia caused by hypotension, azotemia, and hypersensitivity reactions. Diazoxide may interrupt labor by causing uterine relaxation and, therefore, is not the agent of choice in most obstetrical settings. Rare side effects include gastrointestinal disturbances, flushing, local pain and inflammation after extravasation, altered taste and smell, excessive salivation, and dyspnea.

INHIBITORS OF THE RENIN-ANGIOTENSIN SYSTEM

A search for clinically useful inhibitors of the renin-angiotensin system began when its pathogenic role in hypertension was first noted. While peptide antagonists of angiotensin II have been synthesized and studied extensively, only one such agent, *saralasin*, is available clinically, and its utility is very limited. Of much greater interest are the pharmacological effects and the therapeutic utility of inhibitors of angiotensin converting enzyme. The prototypical compound, *captopril*, has now been used widely, and its sphere of usefulness for the treatment of hypertension appears to be expanding. A second such agent, *enalapril*, is expected to be available for general clinical use in the United States in the near future. These agents are discussed in detail in Chapter 27.

II. Therapy of Hypertension

NONPHARMACOLOGICAL THERAPY OF HYPERTENSION

Of the nonpharmacological treatments of hypertension, weight reduction and salt restriction are the most successful (Frumkin *et al.*, 1978; Andrews *et al.*, 1982; Stamler and Stamler, 1984). Blood pressure reductions from loss of weight can average 2 to 3 mm Hg per kilogram of weight loss, up to a total of 10 kg. Weight loss has been associated with a significant fall in total circulating and cardiopulmonary blood volumes, venous return, cardiac output, and plasma concentrations of norepinephrine (Reisin *et al.*, 1983). These results are achievable even without salt restriction (Maxwell *et al.*, 1984).

Moderate salt restriction (consumption of 70 to 100 mEq per day; half of the usual American dietary intake) can reduce diastolic blood pressure by 7 mm Hg and may be comparable to treatment with thiazides or β blockers (Morgan *et al.*, 1978). However, salt restriction does not decrease blood pressure in all hypertensive patients and commonly is effective in only about half of such individuals. Gradual reduction of salt consumption may enhance compliance; traditional dietary instructions have low rates of success (Nugent *et al.*, 1984). There have been few direct comparisons of the effects of weight reduction and sodium restriction on blood pressure. The effect of modest weight reduction (5 kg) versus restriction of salt intake to about 80 mEq per day is probably similar (Gillum *et al.*, 1983).

Weight reduction should be attempted routinely in the treatment of obese, borderline hypertensives, and it obviously becomes definitive therapy if blood pressure is thereby maintained at normal levels. Weight loss should be gradual, with emphasis on long-term maintenance of ideal weight and blood pressure. Similarly, sodium restriction should be encouraged and used as definitive therapy if effective. Moreover, ingestion of large quantities of sodium should certainly be avoided during pharmacological therapy since such ingestion can negate or reduce the effect of diuretics on blood pressure and may increase the loss of potassium. Other factors that should be addressed include moderation in alcohol consumption (2 oz [60 ml] or less of ethanol daily), modification of dietary fats, avoidance of tobacco, and exercise.

DRUG THERAPY OF HYPERTENSION

Drug therapy for hypertension is reserved for those whose blood pressure cannot be maintained in an acceptable range by nonpharmacological means. The initial goal of antihypertensive therapy is to achieve and maintain diastolic blood pressure below 90 mm Hg without compromising renal, cerebral, or myocardial function or producing intolerable symptoms (Joint National Committee, 1984).

In recent years, most national advisory groups have advocated the use of a *stepped-care approach* when treatment is necessary. One such approach is outlined in Table 32–3 (*see* Joint National Committee, 1984). Therapy is initiated with small doses of a single agent, either a thiazide-type diuretic or a β-adrenergic antagonist. Subsequently, the dose of that drug is increased gradually until the desired blood pressure is achieved, the side effects become intolerable, or the maximal recommended dose is reached. At that point, an additional antihypertensive agent is added in stepwise fashion. Such an approach leaves room for flexibility and individualization, and it permits the use of complementary interactions of various agents to minimize the required dosages of each drug and to reduce anticipated toxicities.

Although the use of such step-care regimens may lead to overly standardized treatment, there is a sound pharmacological basis for most of the recommended sequences and combinations. Before proceeding to the next step in such a regimen,

Table 32–3.   STEPPED-CARE APPROACH TO DRUG THERAPY OF HYPERTENSION *

Step 1   Therapy with a single drug (either a thiazide-type diuretic or a β-adrenergic antagonist). Dosage is increased until desired blood pressure is reached or unwanted side effects are evident, up to maximal recommended dose.

Step 2   Therapy with two drugs by addition of either a thiazide-type diuretic or certain sympatholytic agents (usually a β antagonist, but clonidine, guanabenz, methyldopa, prazosin, guanadrel, or reserpine may be used). Captopril or enalapril may be substituted if other agents are ineffective or if side effects limit their use.

Step 3   Therapy with three drugs by addition of a vasodilator (usually hydralazine; minoxidil for resistant cases). Captopril or enalapril may be substituted as in step 2. While not yet approved for therapy of hypertension, calcium channel blocking agents may prove useful in step 2 or step 3.

Step 4   Therapy with four drugs by addition of guanethidine (or of captopril or enalapril).

* Modified from Joint National Committee (1984).

the clinician should evaluate possible reasons for inadequate response. These include considerations of compliance, dosage, salt intake, drug interactions, and the presence of secondary hypertension. Causes of secondary hypertension that should be considered include pheochromocytoma, primary aldosteronism, Cushing's syndrome, renal parenchymal disease, and renal arterial stenosis to name a few. Whenever possible, the regimen should be simplified such that drugs are not taken more than once or twice daily. In patients whose blood pressure has been controlled for 6 to 12 months, gradual reduction of drug dosages and/or cautious stepwise withdrawal of antihypertensive medication may be attempted. In this way, maximal advantage may be taken of changes in hypotensive drug interactions or in nonpharmacological factors, and drug dosages can be reduced to the minimal amount necessary to achieve the desired effect (Joint National Committee, 1984).

MILD HYPERTENSION

As previously discussed, the data that support treatment with antihypertensive agents are firm for patients who have diastolic blood pressures that consistently exceed 105 mm Hg (Cressman and Gifford, 1983). However, the value of reduction of diastolic blood pressure from the range of 90 to 104 mm Hg is a subject of controversy; pharmacological treatment is obviously not justified unless it favorably alters prognosis despite the cost, inconvenience, and potential toxicities of antihypertensive agents. Because epidemiological evidence that relates mild hypertension to premature mortality is strong, many authorities recommend drug therapy if a trial of dietary modification for several months fails to produce reduction of diastolic blood pressure to below 90 mm Hg (Cressman and Gifford, 1983; World Health Organization, 1983). In contrast, others have advocated that drug therapy be delayed (especially in patients below the age of 50 years) if blood pressures are not consistently above 94 mm Hg and if there is no evidence of target organ disease or of major risk factors for cardiovascular disease (Alderman, 1980; Freis, 1982; World Health Organization, 1982).

There is also controversy about optimal initial therapy; this involves not only the choice between thiazide diuretics and β blockers but also the possible use of certain other sympatholytic agents as alternative step-1 treatment. Current data suggest that β-adrenergic antagonists are about as effective as thiazides in lowering blood pressure; extensive comparisons of the two drugs used separately are in progress (Wilhelmsen et al., 1981). In the meantime, in the absence of specific contraindications (e.g., asthma or other chronic pulmonary disease), some authorities favor the use of β blockers as initial therapy in patients who are less than 50 years of age, especially those who are white and who have a rapid resting pulse rate but no evidence of peripheral vascular disease; the presence of ischemic heart disease is another indication for the use of a β-adrenergic antagonist. There is a very low but disturbing incidence of sudden death associated with the use of thiazides alone (Morgan et al., 1980). Therapy with low doses of hydrochlorothiazide (25 mg daily) minimizes the risk of hypokalemia and is inexpensive (Licht et al., 1983). While abnormalities of plasma lipoproteins accompany the use of thiazides, these may be minimized by diets that lower concentrations of cholesterol in plasma (Grimm et al., 1981) or they may be prevented by the concomitant use of β blockers (Meier et al., 1982; Weidmann et al., 1983). Centrally acting α agonists (e.g., clonidine, guanabenz) or peripheral α antagonists (e.g., prazosin) may be considered for initial therapy in selected cases; however, it is currently difficult to decide which of these agents should be chosen in a given circumstance (Kaplan, 1983).

MODERATE AND SEVERE HYPERTENSION

The severity of hypertension is determined not only by its magnitude but also by the evidence of resultant damage to various organs. In general, when diastolic pressure exceeds 105 mm Hg, it cannot be brought to the desired level (e.g., ≤90 mm Hg) by the administration of a single antihypertensive agent without unacceptable adverse effects. Since most antihypertensive medications elicit compensatory reactions, combinations of drugs are needed to minimize resistance (see Table 32–2). The use of sympatholytic or vasodilator agents by themselves is commonly associated with fluid retention and loss of hypotensive effect; this prompts the administration of a diuretic. Vasodilators that affect the arteriolar circulation in preference to the capacitance vessels predictably cause reflex tachycardia and elevation of plasma renin activity (Zsoter, 1983). Both of these compensatory changes can be blocked with sympatholytic drugs. Concurrent therapy with a diuretic, a sympatholytic agent, and a vasodilator may thus be necessary to control moderate-to-severe hypertension. Except in true emergencies (see below), it is generally preferable to reduce blood pressure over a period of several weeks with oral therapy. Renal function may decline transiently when therapy is initiated, but it usually improves thereafter.

HYPERTENSIVE EMERGENCIES

Hypertensive emergencies are clinical syndromes that result from or are complicated by sustained elevations of blood pressure, usually exceeding 200 mm Hg systolic and/or 120 mm Hg diastolic. The seriousness of the clinical situation (and thus the aggressiveness of treatment) is determined by evidence of new or progressive damage to end organs caused by the elevation of blood pressure. Examples of emergencies in which blood pressure must be lowered immediately include hypertensive encephalopathy, intracranial hemorrhage, acute congestive heart failure, dissecting aortic aneurysm, and severe hypertension associated with toxemia of pregnancy, unstable angina pectoris, acute myocardial infarction, head trauma, or extensive burns (Joint National Committee, 1984). However, the blood pressure must not be reduced precipitously, since the perfusion of critical organs can be compromised. Cerebrovascular insufficiency may be especially exacerbated. During severe hypertension, the autoregulatory behavior of cerebral blood vessels usually maintains cerebral perfusion at a reasonably constant level by intense vasoconstriction. However, appropriate vasodilatation may not occur promptly when blood pressure is reduced; establishment of normal autoregulation may require hours to days. Accordingly, blood pressure should not be lowered to normal levels within a few hours. A more reasonable goal is to reduce mean arterial pressure by 15% in the first hour, followed by a gradual decline in blood pressure toward normal over 24 to 48 hours. Controlled reductions of blood pressure are most easily achieved with titratable infusions, such as with nitroprusside or trimethaphan, or with small boluses or prolonged infusions of diazoxide. Oral antihypertensive medication (*e.g.*, with minoxidil, clonidine, β blockers) should be started as soon as possible. Unless there is clear evidence of intravascular fluid overload, such as in acute left ventricular failure, diuretics should not be used. They may exacerbate hypovolemia if present and cause severe vasoconstriction. However, the use of diuretics may become necessary during the course of treatment with agents that promote sodium retention, such as diazoxide or minoxidil.

Hypertensive crises in pediatric patients are generally treated with the same drugs as used in adults, with appropriate modification of dose (Pruitt, 1981). The treatment of hypertension during lactation is discussed by White (1984) and its management during pregnancy is described by Wilson and Matzke (1981). Preoperative control of hypertension, including the choice of anesthesia, has been reviewed by Goldman and Caldera (1979).

TREATMENT OF ISOLATED SYSTOLIC HYPERTENSION

One of the most difficult questions in the management of hypertension is whether isolated systolic hypertension should be treated. When defined as a systolic pressure of >160 mm Hg and a diastolic pressure of <95 mm Hg, isolated systolic hypertension may occur in more than 20% of the population over age 70. Although the associations of isolated systolic hypertension with increased morbidity and mortality from coronary heart disease, cerebrovascular insufficiency, and congestive heart failure are well known, clinical and physiological manifestations of the condition may be different in older versus younger patients (Adamopoulos *et al.*, 1975). Previous attempts to treat isolated systolic hypertension with standard antihypertensive medications have often produced unacceptable side effects, especially in older patients prone to dizziness, fainting, and excessive lability of arterial pressure (Tarazi, 1978).

The question remains as to whether treatment confers a net benefit despite the risks and inconvenience. There has been no conclusive demonstration of an acceptable risk-to-benefit ratio in treating isolated systolic hypertension. Because the elderly are more likely to have increased total peripheral resistance rather than increased cardiac output, thiazides are generally recommended as initial treatment, despite the high incidence of postural hypotension (Kirkendall and Hammond, 1980; Niarchos and Laragh, 1984). Alternative agents include β blockers (O'Malley and O'Brien, 1980) and prazosin (Caris, 1982). Dosages and frequency of administration of these agents are often decreased in the elderly to minimize side effects (Wood and Feely, 1981).

Adamopoulos, P. N.; Chrysanthakopoulis, S. G.; and Frohlich, E. D. Systolic hypertension: nonhomogeneous diseases. *Am. J. Cardiol.*, **1975**, *36*, 697–701.

Alpert, M. A., and Bauer, J. H. Rapid control of severe hypertension with minoxidil. *Arch. Intern. Med.*, **1982**, *142*, 2099–2104.

Andrews, G.; MacMahon, S. W.; Austin, A.; and Byrne, D. G. Hypertension: comparison of drug and non-drug treatments. *Br. Med. J.* [*Clin. Res.*], **1982**, *284*, 1523–1526.

Arndts, D.; Doevendans, J.; Kirsten, R.; and Heintz, B. New aspects of the pharmacokinetics and pharmacodynamics of clonidine in man. *Eur. J. Clin. Pharmacol.*, **1983**, *24*, 21–30.

Baughman, R. A.; Arnold, S.; and Benet, L. Z. Altered prazosin pharmacokinetics in congestive heart failure. *Eur. J. Clin. Pharmacol.*, **1980**, *17*, 425–428.

Beevers, D. G.; Bloxham, C. A.; and Walker, J. M. Guanfacine: a new centrally-acting anti-hypertensive agent. *Pharmacotherapy*, **1981**, *2*, 513–516.

Bennett, W. M.; McDonald, W. J.; Kuehnel, E.; Hartnett, M. N.; and Porter, G. A. Do diuretics have antihypertensive properties independent of natriuresis? *Clin. Pharmacol. Ther.*, **1977**, *22*, 499–504.

Brater, D. C. Effect of indomethacin on salt and water homeostasis. *Clin. Pharmacol. Ther.*, **1979**, *25*, 322–330.

Brown, M. J.; Brown, D. C.; and Murphy, M. B. Hypokalemia from beta$_2$-receptor stimulation by circulating epinephrine. *N. Engl. J. Med.*, **1983**, *309*, 1414–1419.

Cypress, B. K. Medication therapy in office visits for hypertension: National Ambulatory Medical Care Survey, 1980. *Advance Data from Vital and Health Statistics*, No. 80. DHHS Publication No. (PHS) 82–1250, Public Health Service, Hyattsville, Md., **1982**, pp. 1–11.

Davey, M. J. Aspects of the pharmacology of prazosin. *Med. J. Aust.*, **1980**, *2*, Suppl., 4–8.

De Carvalho, J. G. R.; Dunn, F. G.; Lohmoller, G.; and Frohlich, E. D. Hemodynamic correlates of prolonged thiazide therapy: comparison of responders and nonresponders. *Clin. Pharmacol. Ther.*, **1977**, *22*, 875–880.

De Carvalho, J. G. R.; Emery, A. C.; and Frohlich, E. D. Spironolactone and triamterene in volume-dependent essential hypertension. *Clin. Pharmacol. Ther.*, **1980**, *27*, 53–56.

Falch, D. K., and Schreiner, A. The effect of spironolactone on lipid, glucose and uric acid levels in blood during long-term administration to hypertensives. *Acta Med. Scand.*, **1983**, *213*, 27–30.

Fouad, F. M.; Nakashima, Y.; Tarazi, R. C.; and Salcedo, E. E. Reversal of left ventricular hypertrophy in hypertensive patients treated with methyldopa; lack of association with blood pressure control. *Am. J. Cardiol.*, **1982**, *49*, 795–801.

Frumkin, K.; Nathan, R. J.; Prout, M. F.; and Cohen, M. C. Nonpharmacologic control of essential hypertension in man: a critical review of the experimental literature. *Psychosom. Med.*, **1978**, *40*, 294–320.

Garrett, B. N., and Kaplan, N. M. Efficacy of slow infusion of diazoxide in the treatment of severe hypertension without organ hypoperfusion. *Am. Heart J.*, **1982**, *103*, 390–394.

Gillum, R. F.; Prineas, R. H.; Jeffery, R. W.; Jacobs, D. R.; Elmer, P. J.; Gomez, O.; and Blackburn, H. Nonpharmacologic therapy of hypertension: the independent effects of weight reduction and sodium restriction in overweight borderline hypertensive patients. *Am. Heart J.*, **1983**, *105*, 128–133.

Goldman, A. I.; Steele, B. W.; Schnaper, H. W.; Fitz, A. E.; Frohlich, E. D.; and Perry, H. M. Serum lipoprotein levels during chlorthalidone therapy. A Veterans Administration–National Heart, Lung, and Blood Institute Cooperative Study on antihypertensive therapy: mild hypertension. *J.A.M.A.*, **1980**, *244*, 1691–1695.

Grimm, R. H.; Leon, A. S.; Hunninghake, D. B.; Lenz, K.; Hannan, P.; and Blackburn, H. Effects of thiazide diuretics on plasma lipids and lipoproteins in mildly hypertensive patients. *Ann. Intern. Med.*, **1981**, *94*, 7–11.

Hedner, T.; Nyberg, G.; and Mellstrand, T. Guanfacine in essential hypertension: effects during rest and isometric exercise. *Clin. Pharmacol. Ther.*, **1984**, *35*, 604–609.

Holland, O. G.; Nixon, J. V.; and Kuhnert, L. Diuretic-induced ventricular ectopic activity. *Am. J. Med.*, **1981**, *70*, 762–768.

Hypertension Detection and Follow-up Program Cooperative Group. Five-year findings of the Hypertension Detection and Follow-up Program. I. Reduction in mortality of persons with high blood pressure, including mild hypertension. *J.A.M.A.*, **1979**, *242*, 2562–2571.

Jain, A. K.; Ryan, J. R.; Vargas, R.; and McMahon, F. G. Efficacy and acceptability of different dosage schedules of clonidine. *Clin. Pharmacol. Ther.*, **1977**, *21*, 382–387.

Jerie, P., and Lasance, A. Guanfacine in the treatment of hypertension: two years' experience with low dose monotherapy. *Int. J. Clin. Pharmacol. Ther. Toxicol.*, **1981**, *19*, 279–287.

Kohvakka, A.; Eisalo, A.; and Manninen, V. Maintenance of potassium balance during diuretic therapy. *Acta Med. Scand.*, **1979**, *205*, 319–324.

Larochelle, P.; Du Souich, P.; Hamet, P.; Larocque, P.; and Armstrong, J. Prazosin plasma concentration and blood pressure reduction. *Hypertension*, **1982**, *4*, 93–101.

Licht, J. H.; Haley, R. J.; Pugh, B.; and Lewis, S. B. Diuretic regimens in essential hypertension; a comparison of hypokalemic effects, BP control, and cost. *Arch. Intern. Med.*, **1983**, *143*, 1694–1699.

Lowenthal, D. T., and Affrime, M. B. Pharmacology and pharmacokinetics of minoxidil. *J. Cardiovasc. Pharmacol.*, **1980**, *2*, Suppl. 2, S93–S106.

Lutterodt, A.; Nattel, S.; and McLeod, P. J. Duration of antihypertensive effect of a single daily dose of hydrochlorothiazide. *Clin. Pharmacol. Ther.*, **1980**, *27*, 324–327.

Mancia, G.; Ferrari, A.; Gregorini, L.; Ferrari, M. C.; Bianchini, C.; Terzoli, L.; Leonetti, G.; and Zanchetti, A. Effects of prazosin on autonomic control of circulation in essential hypertension. *Hypertension*, **1980**, *2*, 700–707.

Mansilla-Tinoco, R.; Harland, S. J.; Ryan, P. J.; Bernstein, R. M.; Dollery, C. T.; Hughes, G. R. V.; Bulpitt, C. J.; Morgan, A.; and Jones, J. M. Hydralazine, antinuclear antibodies, and the lupus syndrome. *Br. Med. J. [Clin. Res.]*, **1982**, *284*, 936–939.

Materson, B. J.; Oster, J. R.; Michael, U. F.; Bolton, S. M.; Burton, Z. C.; Stambaugh, J. E.; and Morledge, J. Dose response to chlorthalidone in patients with mild hypertension; efficacy of a lower dose. *Clin. Pharmacol. Ther.*, **1978**, *24*, 192–198.

Maxwell, M. H.; Kushiro, T.; Dornfeld, L. P.; Tuck, M. L.; and Waks, A. U. BP changes in obese hypertensive subjects during rapid weight loss; comparison of restricted v. unchanged salt intake. *Arch. Intern. Med.*, **1984**, *144*, 1581–1584.

Meier, A.; Weidmann, P.; Mordasini, R.; Riesen, W.; and Bachmann, C. Reversal or prevention of diuretic-induced alterations in serum lipoproteins with betablockers. *Atherosclerosis*, **1982**, *41*, 415–419.

Morgan, T.; Adam, W.; Gillies, A.; Wilson, M.; Morgan, G.; and Carney, S. Hypertension treated by salt restriction. *Lancet*, **1978**, *1*, 227–230.

Morgan, T. O.; Adams, W. R.; Hodgson, M.; and Gibberd, R. W. Failure of therapy to improve prognosis in elderly males with hypertension. *Med. J. Aust.*, **1980**, *2*, 27–31.

Multicenter Diuretic Cooperative Study Group. Multiclinic comparison of amiloride, hydrochlorothiazide, and hydrochlorothiazide plus amiloride in essential hypertension. *Arch. Intern. Med.*, **1981**, *141*, 482–486.

Murphy, M. B.; Scriven, A. J. I.; and Dollery, C. T. Role of nifedipine in treatment of hypertension. *Br. Med. J. [Clin. Res.]*, **1983**, *287*, 257–259.

Myhre, E.; Rugstad, H. E.; and Hansen, T. Clinical pharmacokinetics of methyldopa. *Clin. Pharmacokinet.*, **1982**, *7*, 221–233.

Niarchos, A. P., and Laragh, J. H. Effects of diuretic therapy in low-, normal- and high-renin isolated systolic systemic hypertension. *Am. J. Cardiol.*, **1984**, *53*, 797–801.

Nugent, C. A.; Carnahan, J. E.; Sheehan, E. T.; and Myers, C. Salt restriction in hypertensive patients; comparison of advice, education, and group management. *Arch. Intern. Med.*, **1984**, *144*, 1415–1417.

Ogilvie, R. I.; Nadeau, J. H.; and Sitar, D. S. Diazoxide concentration-response relation in hypertension. *Hypertension*, **1982**, *4*, 167–173.

O'Malley, K.; Velasco, M.; Pruitt, A.; and McNay, J. L. Decreased plasma protein binding of diazoxide in uremia. *Clin. Pharmacol. Ther.*, **1975**, *18*, 53–58.

Pettinger, W. A. Pharmacology of clonidine. *J. Cardiovasc. Pharmacol.*, **1980**, *2*, Suppl. 2, S21–S28.

Ram, C. V. S.; Garrett, B. N.; and Kaplan, N. M. Moderate sodium restriction and various diuretics in the treatment of hypertension; effects of potassium wastage and blood pressure control. *Arch. Intern. Med.*, **1981**, *141*, 1015–1019.

Rangno, R. E. Propranolol withdrawal; practical considerations. *Arch. Intern. Med.*, **1981**, *141*, 161–162.

Reid, J. L. The clinical pharmacology of clonidine and related central antihypertensive agents. *Br. J. Clin. Pharmacol.*, **1981**, *12*, 295–302.

Reisin, E.; Frohlich, E. D.; Messerli, F. H.; Dreslinksi, G. R.; Dunn, F. G.; Jones, M. M.; and Batson, H. M. Cardiovascular changes after weight reduction in obesity hypertension. *Ann. Intern. Med.*, **1983**, *98*, 315–319.

Rubin, P., and Blaschke, T. Prazosin protein binding in health and disease. *Br. J. Clin. Pharmacol.*, **1980**, *9*, 177–182.

Rubin, P. C.; Butters, L.; Clark, D. M.; Reynolds, B.; Sumner, D. J.; Steedman, D.; Low, R. A.; and Reid,

J. L. Placebo-controlled trial of atenolol in treatment of pregnancy-associated hypertension. *Lancet,* **1983,** *1,* 431–434.

Russ, G. R.; Whitworth, J. A.; and Kincaid-Smith, P. Comparison of intramuscularly and intravenously administered clonidine in the treatment of severe hypertension. *Med. J. Aust.,* **1983,** *2,* 229–231.

Schneck, E. W., and Vary, J. E. Mechanism by which hydralazine increases propranolol bioavailability. *Clin. Pharmacol. Ther.,* **1984,** *35,* 447–453.

Schooley, R. T.; Wagley, P. F.; and Lietman, P. S. Edema associated with ibuprofen therapy. *J.A.M.A.,* **1977,** *237,* 1716–1717.

Schrijver, G., and Weinberger, M. H. Hydrochlorothiazide and spironolactone in hypertension. *Clin. Pharmacol. Ther.,* **1979,** *25,* 33–42.

Soghikian, K., and Bartenbach, D. E. Influence of dosage and duration of therapy on the rate of response to methyclothiazide in essential hypertension. *South. Med. J.,* **1977,** *70,* 1397–1404.

Taguchi, J., and Freis, E. D. Partial reduction of blood pressure and prevention of complications in hypertension. *N. Engl. J. Med.,* **1974,** *291,* 329–331.

Tweeddale, M. G.; Ogilvie, R. I.; and Ruedy, J. Antihypertensive and biochemical effects of chlorthalidone. *Clin. Pharmacol. Ther.,* **1977,** *22,* 519–527.

Van Brummelen, P.; Woerlee, M.; and Schalekamp, M. A. D. H. Long-term versus short-term effects of hydrochlorothiazide on renal haemodynamics in essential hypertension. *Clin. Sci.,* **1979,** *56,* 463–469.

Veterans Administration Cooperative Study Group on Hypertensive Agents. Effects of treatment on morbidity in hypertension: results in patients with diastolic blood pressure averaging 115 through 129 mm Hg. *J.A.M.A.,* **1967,** *202,* 1028–1034.

———. Effects of treatment on morbidity in hypertension. II. Results in patients with diastolic blood pressure averaging 90 through 114 mm Hg. *Ibid.,* **1970,** *213,* 1143–1152.

Walker, R. G.; Whitworth, J. A.; Saines, D.; and Kincaid-Smith, P. Prazosin: long-term treatment of moderate and severe hypertension and lack of "tolerance." *Med. J. Aust.,* **1981,** *2,* 146–147.

Weidmann, P.; Gerber, A.; and Mordasini, R. Effects of antihypertensive therapy on serum lipoproteins. *Hypertension,* **1983,** *5,* Suppl. III, 120–131.

Weiss, V. C.; West, D. P.; and Mueller, C. E. Topical minoxidil in alopecia areata. *J. Am. Acad. Dermatol.,* **1981,** *5,* 224–226.

White, W. B. Management of hypertension during lactation. *Hypertension,* **1984,** *6,* 297–300.

Wikstrand, J., and Berglund, G. Antihypertensive treatment with beta-blockers in patients aged over 65. *Br. Med. J. [Clin. Res.],* **1982,** *285,* 850.

Wilhelmsen, L.; Berglund, G.; Elmfeldt, D.; and Wedel, H. Beta-blocker versus saluretics in hypertension. Comparison of total mortality, myocardial infarction, and sudden death: study design and early results on blood pressure reduction. *Prev. Med.,* **1981,** *10,* 38–49.

Wollam, G. L.; Tarazi, R. C.; Bravo, E. L.; and Dustan, H. P. Diuretic potency of combined hydrochlorothiazide and furosemide therapy in patients with azotemia. *Am. J. Med.,* **1982,** *72,* 929–938.

World Health Organization/International Society of Hypertension. Mild Hypertension Liaison Committee. Trials of the treatment of mild hypertension; an interim analysis. *Lancet,* **1982,** *1,* 149–156.

———. Guidelines for the treatment of mild hypertension; memorandum from a WHO/ISH meeting. *Hypertension,* **1983,** *5,* 394–397.

Wright, J. M.; McLeod, P. J.; and McCullough, W. Antihypertensive efficacy of a single bedtime dose of methyldopa. *Clin. Pharmacol. Ther.,* **1977,** *20,* 733–737.

Monographs and Reviews

Alderman, M. H. Mild hypertension: new light on an old controversy. *Am. J. Med.,* **1980,** *69,* 653–655.

Brass, E. P. Effects of antihypertensive drugs on endocrine function. *Drugs,* **1984,** *27,* 447–458.

Braunwald, E. Mechanism of action of calcium-channel-blocking agents. *N. Engl. J. Med.,* **1982,** *307,* 1618–1627.

Campese, V. M. Minoxidil: a review of its pharmacological properties and therapeutic use. *Drugs,* **1981,** *22,* 257–278.

Caris, T. N. Hypertension in older patients: what drugs to use and when. *Geriatrics,* **1982,** *37,* 38–43.

Clive, D. M., and Stoff, J. S. Renal syndromes associated with nonsteroidal anti-inflammatory drugs. *N. Engl. J. Med.,* **1984,** *310,* 563–572.

Cressman, M. D., and Gifford, R. W. Controversies in hypertension: mild hypertension, isolated systolic hypertension, and the choice of a step one drug. *Clin. Cardiol.,* **1983,** *6,* 1–10.

Cruickshank, J. M. The clinical importance of cardioselectivity and lipophilicity in beta blockers. *Am. Heart J.,* **1980,** *100,* 160–178.

Dollery, C. T. Does it matter how blood pressure is reduced? *Clin. Sci.,* **1981,** *61,* 413S–420S.

———. Hypertension and new antihypertensive drugs: clinical perspectives. *Fed. Proc.,* **1983,** *42,* 207–210.

Epstein, F. H., and Rosa, R. M. Adrenergic control of serum potassium. *N. Engl. J. Med.,* **1983,** *309,* 1450–1451.

Freis, E. D. Should mild hypertension be treated? *N. Engl. J. Med.,* **1982,** *307,* 306–309.

Frishman, W. Clinical pharmacology of the new beta-adrenergic blocking drugs. Part 1. Pharmacodynamic and pharmacokinetic properties. *Am. Heart J.,* **1979,** *97,* 663–670.

Frishman, W. H. β-Adrenoceptor antagonists: new drugs and new indications. *N. Engl. J. Med.,* **1981a,** *305,* 500–506.

———. Nadolol: a new β-adrenoceptor antagonist. *Ibid.,* **1981b,** *305,* 678–682.

———. Drug therapy: atenolol and timolol, two new systemic beta-adrenoceptor antagonists. *Ibid.,* **1982,** *306,* 1456–1462.

Frishman, W.; Jacob, H.; Eisenberg, E.; and Ribner, H. Clinical pharmacology of the new beta-adrenergic blocking drugs. Part 8. Self-poisoning with beta-adrenoceptor blocking agents: recognition and management. *Am. Heart J.,* **1979a,** *98,* 798–811.

Frishman, W., and Silverman, R. Clinical pharmacology of the new beta-adrenergic blocking drugs. Part 2. Physiologic and metabolic effects. *Am. Heart J.,* **1979,** *97,* 797–807.

Frishman, W.; Silverman, R.; Strom, J.; Elkayam, U.; and Sonnenblick, E. Clinical pharmacology of the new beta-adrenergic blocking drugs. Part 4. Adverse effects. Choosing a β-adrenoceptor blocker. *Am. Heart J.,* **1979b,** *98,* 256–262.

Frohlich, E. D. Methyldopa; mechanisms and treatment 25 years later. *Arch. Intern. Med.,* **1980,** *140,* 954–959.

Frohlich, E. D.; Cooper, R. A.; and Lewis, E. J. Review of the overall experience of captopril in hypertension. *Arch. Intern. Med.,* **1984,** *144,* 1441–1444.

Gifford, R. W. Isolated systolic hypertension in the elderly; some controversial issues. *J.A.M.A.,* **1982,** *247,* 781–792.

Gifford, R. W., and Tarazi, R. C. Resistant hypertension: diagnosis and management. *Ann. Intern. Med.,* **1978,** *88,* 661–665.

Goldman, L., and Caldera, D. L. Risks of general anesthesia and elective operation in the hypertensive patient. *Anesthesiology,* **1979,** *50,* 285–292.

Harrington, J. T.; Isner, J. M.; and Kassirer, J. P. Our

national obsession with potassium. *Am. J. Med.,* **1982,** *73,* 155–159.

Henry, P. D.   Comparative pharmacology of calcium antagonists: nifedipine, verapamil and diltiazem. *Am. J. Cardiol.,* **1980,** *46,* 1047–1058.

Isaac, L.   Clonidine in the central nervous system: site of mechanism of hypotensive action. *J. Cardiovasc. Pharmacol.,* **1980,** *2,* Suppl. 1, S5–S19.

Jaillon, P.   Clinical pharmacokinetics of prazosin. *Clin. Pharmacokinet.,* **1980,** *5,* 365–376.

Johnston, C. I.; Arnolda, L.; and Hiwatari, M.   Angiotensin-converting enzyme inhibitors in the treatment of hypertension. *Drugs,* **1984,** *27,* 271–277.

Joint National Committee on Detection, Evaluation, and Treatment of High Blood Pressure.   The 1984 Report. U.S. Department of Health and Human Services, Public Health Service, National Institutes of Health Publication No. 84–1088, Bethesda, Md., **1984.** (The reader is also referred to *Arch. Intern. Med.,* **1984,** *144,* 1045–1057.)

Kaplan, N. M.   New choices for the initial drug therapy of hypertension. *Am. J. Cardiol.,* **1983,** *51,* 1786–1788.

Kirkendall, W. M., and Hammond, J. J.   Hypertension in the elderly. *Arch. Intern. Med.,* **1980,** *140,* 1155–1161.

Langer, S. Z.; Cavero, I.; and Massingham, R.   Recent developments in noradrenergic neurotransmission and its relevance to the mechanism of action of certain antihypertensive agents. *Hypertension,* **1980,** *2,* 372–382.

Lawson, A. A. H.   Potassium replacement: when is it necessary? *Drugs,* **1981,** *21,* 354–361.

Lowenthal, D. T.   Pharmacokinetics of clonidine. *J. Cardiovasc. Pharmacol.,* **1980,** *2,* Suppl. 1, S29–S37.

McDevitt, D. G.   β-Adrenoceptor blocking drugs and partial agonist activity; is it clinically relevant? *Drugs,* **1983,** *25,* 331–338.

Morgan, D. B., and Davidson, C.   Hypokalemia and diuretics: an analysis of publications. *Br. Med. J. [Clin. Res.],* **1980,** *280,* 905–908.

O'Malley, K., and O'Brien, E.   Management of hypertension in the elderly. *N. Engl. J. Med.,* **1980,** *302,* 1397–1401.

Perez-Stable, E., and Caralis, P. V.   Thiazide-induced disturbances in carbohydrate, lipid, and potassium metabolism. *Am. Heart J.,* **1983,** *106,* 245–251.

Pruitt, A. W.   Pharmacologic approach to the management of childhood hypertension. *Pediatr. Clin. North Am.,* **1981,** *28,* 135–144.

Robertson, J. I. S.; Kaplan, N. M.; Caldwell, A. D. S.; and Speight, T. M. (eds.).   β-Blockade in the 1980s: focus on atenolol. *Drugs,* **1983,** *25,* Suppl. 2, 1–340.

Rubin, P. C.   Beta-blockers in pregnancy. *N. Engl. J. Med.,* **1981,** *305,* 1323–1326.

Sambhi, M. P., and Villarreal, H.   Central alpha-adrenoceptors: basic mechanisms and clinical applications in cardiovascular disease. *Chest,* **1983,** *83,* Suppl., 293–440.

Shand, D. G., and Wood, A. J. J.   Propranolol withdrawal syndrome—why? *Circulation,* **1978,** *58,* 202–203.

Spivack, C.; Ocken, S.; and Frishman, W. H.   Calcium antagonists; clinical use in the treatment of systemic hypertension. *Drugs,* **1983,** *25,* 154–177.

Stamler, J., and Stamler, R.   Intervention for the prevention and control of hypertension and atherosclerotic diseases: United States and international experience. *Am. J. Med.,* **1984,** *77,* Suppl. 2, 13–36.

Stanaszek, W. F.; Kellerman, D.; Brogden, R. N.; and Romankiewicz, J. A.   Prazosin update; a review of its pharmacological properties and therapeutic use in hypertension. *Drugs,* **1983,** *25,* 339–384.

Tarazi, R. C.   Clinical importance of systolic hypertension. *Ann. Intern. Med.,* **1978,** *88,* 426–427.

Tobian, L.   Why do thiazide diuretics lower blood pressure in essential hypertension? *Annu. Rev. Pharmacol.,* **1967,** *7,* 399–408.

Weinshilboum, R. M.   Series on pharmacology in practice. 8. Antihypertensive drugs that alter adrenergic function. *Mayo Clin. Proc.,* **1980,** *55,* 390–402.

Wilkinson, R.   β-Blockers and renal function. *Drugs,* **1982,** *23,* 195–206.

Williams, R. L.   Drug administration in hepatic disease. *N. Engl. J. Med.,* **1983,** *309,* 1616–1622.

Wilson, A. L., and Matzke, G. R.   The treatment of hypertension in pregnancy. *Drug Intell. Clin. Pharm.,* **1981,** *15,* 21–26.

Wood, A. J., and Feely, J.   Management of hypertension in the elderly. *South. Med. J.,* **1981,** *74,* 1503–1508.

Zsoter, T. T.   Vasodilators. *Can. Med. Assoc. J.,* **1983,** *129,* 424–428.

33 DRUGS USED FOR THE TREATMENT OF ANGINA: ORGANIC NITRATES, CALCIUM CHANNEL BLOCKERS, AND β-ADRENERGIC ANTAGONISTS

Philip Needleman, Peter B. Corr, and Eugene M. Johnson, Jr.

Angina pectoris is the principal symptom of ischemic heart disease. Both the typical and variant forms of angina may be manifested by sudden, severe, pressing substernal pain that often radiates to the left shoulder and along the flexor surface of the left arm. The pain of typical angina is commonly induced by exercise, emotion, or eating and is often associated with depression of the S-T segment of the ECG. The underlying pathology is usually advanced atherosclerosis of the coronary vasculature. In contrast, variant (Prinzmetal's) angina is apparently caused by vasospasm of the coronary vessels and may or may not be associated with severe atherosclerosis. Patients with variant angina develop chest pain while at rest and exhibit elevation of the S-T segment of the ECG.

Anginal attacks may recur for years. They result from temporary and relative ischemia of the myocardium, such that blood flow is insufficient to maintain oxygenation, nutrition, and removal of metabolites. This can be due to a decrease in myocardial blood flow, an increase in the requirement of the myocardium for oxygen, or both.

This chapter deals with the pharmacological agents that are used for the treatment of angina pectoris. The primary drugs include organic nitrates, calcium channel blockers, and β-adrenergic antagonists. The strategy for pharmacological relief of angina is based on improvement of the balance between myocardial oxygen supply and demand. For typical exertional angina, this necessitates increasing the blood flow to the heart or decreasing its work load. Treat-ment of variant (Prinzmetal's) angina is directed at reduction of vasospasm of the coronary vessels.

Until recently, many of the drugs used to prevent anginal attacks were no more effective than a placebo. In fact, the use of placebos has been reported to relieve symptoms in as many as 50% of patients with angina pectoris. For over a century, however, nitroglycerin has been known to be useful to prevent or relieve acute anginal attacks. More recently, the efficacy of β-adrenergic antagonists and calcium channel blockers has been established for the long-term prophylaxis of typical angina. In addition, the calcium channel blockers appear to be effective for the treatment of vasospastic angina. While antianginal agents provide only symptomatic treatment, administration of β-adrenergic antagonists (and other agents) does appear to decrease the incidence of sudden death associated with myocardial ischemia and infarction (*see* Chapters 9 and 31).

ORGANIC NITRATES

History. Nitroglycerin was first synthesized by Sobrero in 1846, and he observed that a small quantity of the oily substance placed on the tongue elicited a severe headache. Constantin Hering, in 1847, developed the sublingual dosage form for nitroglycerin, which he advocated for a number of diseases. The eminent English physician, T. Lauder Brunton, was unable to relieve severe recurrent anginal pain except when he bled his patient, and he believed that phlebotomy provided relief by lowering arterial blood pressure. In 1857, Brunton administered amyl nitrite, a known vasodepressor, by inhalation, and he noted that anginal pain was relieved within 30 to 60 seconds. The action of amyl nitrite was transitory, however, and the dosage was difficult to adjust. In 1879, William Murrell decided that the action of nitroglycerin mimicked that of amyl nitrite, and he established the use of sublingual nitroglycerin for relief of the acute anginal attack and as a prophylactic agent to be taken prior to exertion. The empirical observation that organic nitrates could be used safely for the rapid and dramatic alleviation of the symptoms of angina pectoris led to their widespread acceptance by the medical profession (*see* Krantz, 1975).

Chemistry. Organic nitrates are polyol esters of nitric acid, whereas organic nitrites are esters of nitrous acid (Table 33–1, page 813). Nitrate esters (—C—O—NO$_2$) and nitrite esters (—C—O—NO) are characterized by a sequence of carbon-oxygen-nitrogen, whereas nitro compounds (which are not vasodilators) possess carbon-nitrogen bonds (C—NO$_2$). Thus, glyceryl trinitrate is not a nitro compound, and it is erroneously called nitroglycerin; however, this nomenclature is both widespread and official. Amyl nitrite is a highly volatile liquid that is administered by inhalation. Organic nitrates of low molecular weight (such as nitroglycerin) are moderately volatile, oily liquids, whereas the high-molecular-weight nitrate esters (*e.g.*, erythrityl tetranitrate, pentaerythritol tetranitrate, isosorbide dinitrate) are solids. The fully nitrated polyols are lipid soluble, whereas incompletely nitrated compounds (which are metabolites) are more soluble in water. In the pure form (without an inert carrier such as lactose), nitroglycerin is explosive.

PHARMACOLOGICAL PROPERTIES

Cardiovascular Effects. *Hemodynamic Effects in Normal Individuals.* The organic nitrates and nitrites are dilators of arterial and venous smooth muscle. The mechanism by which they produce relaxation of smooth muscle is discussed below. Low concentrations of nitroglycerin produce dilatation of the veins that predominates over that of arterioles. The venodilatation results in decreased left and right ventricular end-diastolic pressures, which are greater on a percentage basis than is the decrease in systemic arterial pressure. Net systemic vascular resistance is usually relatively unaffected; heart rate is unchanged or slightly increased; and pulmonary vascular resistance is consistently reduced (Ferrer *et al.*, 1966). In normal individuals or those with coronary artery disease (in the absence of heart failure), sublingual administration of nitroglycerin decreases cardiac output. Doses of nitroglycerin that do not alter systemic arterial pressure often produce arteriolar dilatation

in the face and neck, resulting in a flush. The same doses may also cause headache, presumably due to dilatation of meningeal arterial vessels.

Rapid administration of high doses of organic nitrates decreases systolic and diastolic blood pressure and cardiac output, resulting in pallor, weakness, dizziness, and activation of compensatory sympathetic reflexes. The resultant tachycardia and peripheral arteriolar vasoconstriction tend to maintain peripheral resistance; this is superimposed on sustained venous pooling. Coronary blood flow increases transiently due to coronary vasodilatation but subsequently falls as arterial blood pressure decreases and cardiac output falls. A marked hypotensive effect may occasionally follow sublingual administration of nitroglycerin. This is especially likely when the individual is in the upright position, which augments venous pooling and further decreases cardiac output.

Mechanism of Relief of Symptoms of Angina Pectoris. Typical attacks of angina are usually precipitated by exercise, stress, cold, or meals, which increases cardiac work and myocardial demand for oxygen. Effective drugs could correct the inadequacy of myocardial oxygenation by (1) increasing the supply of oxygen to ischemic myocardium by direct dilatation of the coronary vasculature, or (2) decreasing the oxygen demand secondary to a reduction of cardiac work. Brunton ascribed the relief of anginal pain afforded by nitrates to a decrease in cardiac work secondary to the fall in systemic blood pressure. After demonstration of direct coronary vasodilatation in experimental animals, it became generally accepted that nitrates relieved anginal pain by dilating coronary arteries and thereby increasing coronary blood flow. This hypothesis was questioned by Gorlin and associates (1959), who were unable to demonstrate increases in coronary blood flow in patients with coronary insufficiency following the administration of nitroglycerin. Although the mode of action of organic nitrates to relieve typical angina is not fully understood, the preponderance of evidence favors a reduction in the myocardial requirement for oxygen as the major action. In contrast, the ability of nitrates to dilate large coronary vessels selectively may be the primary mechanism by which they benefit patients with angina caused by coronary spasm (*see* below).

Effects on Total and Regional Coronary Blood Flow. Increases in the myocardial requirement for oxygen are normally met by increasing blood flow, rather than by more complete extraction of oxygen from the blood. Ischemia is a powerful stimulus to coronary vasodilatation, and regional blood flow is adjusted by autoregulatory mechanisms that alter the tone of small resistance vessels. When there is atherosclerotic coronary occlusion, ischemia distal to the lesion is a stimulus for marked vasodilatation, and, if the degree of occlusion is severe, much of the *capacity* to dilate is utilized to maintain resting blood flow to the compromised area. When situations arise that increase demand, further dilatation may not be possible.

As mentioned, organic nitrates do not increase *total* coronary blood flow in patients with typical angina due to atherosclerosis. However, these drugs do appear to cause redistribution of blood flow in the heart when there is partial occlusion of the coronary circulation. Under these circumstances, there is a disproportionate reduction in blood flow in subendocardial regions of the heart, which are subjected to the greatest extravascular compression during systole, and organic nitrates tend to restore blood flow in these regions toward normal. For example, nitroglycerin increases the rate of washout of radioactive xenon injected directly into diseased regions of the ventricular wall of angina patients (Horwitz *et al.,* 1971), indicating that blood flow to regions of poorly perfused myocardium has been improved. Nitrates also increase endocardial blood flow (Becker *et al.,* 1971) and the oxygenation of tissue (Winbury *et al.,* 1971) relative to epicardial regions in ischemic canine ventricle.

The hemodynamic mechanisms responsible for these effects are not entirely clear. Most hypotheses have focused on the ability of organic nitrates to cause dilatation of large epicardial vessels without impairing autoregulation in the small vessels, which are responsible for about 90% of the overall coronary vascular resistance. Experimental

evidence in animals (Cohen and Kirk, 1973) and in patients during coronary bypass surgery indicates that nitrates do have a selective effect on large coronary vessels. Moreover, analyses of coronary angiograms in human subjects have shown that sublingual nitroglycerin can dilate epicardial stenoses and reduce the resistance to flow through such areas (Brown *et al.,* 1981; Feldman *et al.,* 1981). The resultant increment in blood flow would be distributed preferentially to ischemic myocardial regions as a consequence of vasodilatation induced by autoregulation. To the extent that organic nitrates decrease myocardial requirements for oxygen (*see* below), the increased blood flow in ischemic regions could be balanced by decreased flow in nonischemic areas, and an overall increase in coronary blood flow need not occur. Redistribution of blood flow to subendocardial tissue is *not* typical of all vasodilators. Dipyridamole, for example, dilates resistance vessels nonselectively by distorting autoregulation; it is ineffective in patients with typical angina.

Effects on Myocardial Oxygen Requirements. The organic nitrates reduce the requirement of the myocardium for oxygen by their effects on the systemic circulation. The major determinants of myocardial oxygen consumption include the stress on the ventricular wall during systole, the heart rate, and the state of contractility of the myocardium. The stress on the ventricular wall is affected by a number of factors that are generally considered under the categories of "preload" and "afterload." *Preload* is determined by the diastolic pressure that distends the relaxed ventricular wall (left ventricular end-diastolic pressure). Increasing end-diastolic pressure and volume augment the ventricular tension required to eject blood (by the law of Laplace, tension = pressure × radius). Decreasing venous resistance (which increases venous capacitance) decreases venous return to the heart, ventricular end-diastolic pressure and volume, and thereby oxygen consumption. An additional benefit of reducing left ventricular filling pressure is to increase the pressure gradient for perfusion across the ventricular wall; this favors endocardial perfusion (Parratt, 1979).

Afterload, or ventricular systolic wall tension, is the force distributed in the ventricular wall during ejection of blood. It is related to the radius of the ventricle and to the aortic pressure (and therefore to peripheral resistance). Decreasing peripheral arteriolar resistance reduces afterload and thus myocardial consumption of oxygen.

Organic nitrates do not directly alter the inotropic or chronotropic state of the heart. The drugs do decrease both preload and afterload as a result of respective dilatation of venous capacitance and arteriolar resistance vessels. Since the primary determinants of oxygen demand are reduced by the nitrates, their net effect usually is to decrease myocardial consumption of oxygen.

Paradoxically, however, high doses of organic nitrates may reduce diastolic blood pressure to such an extent that reflex tachycardia and adrenergic enhancement of contractility may override the salutary action of the drugs. The resultant negative effect on oxygen balance can aggravate ischemia and, potentially, initiate an anginal attack.

Relative Importance of the Actions of Organic Nitrates. Of the two general mechanisms by which nitrates can reduce myocardial ischemia, their ability to reduce the demand for oxygen (by reducing preload and afterload) appears to be the most important for patients with typical angina. When nitroglycerin is injected or infused directly into the coronary circulation of patients with coronary artery disease, anginal attacks (induced by electrical pacing) are not aborted, even when coronary blood flow is increased. Sublingual administration of nitroglycerin does relieve anginal pain in the same patients (Ganz and Marcus, 1972). Furthermore, venous phlebotomy that is sufficient to reduce left ventricular end-diastolic pressure can mimic the beneficial effect of nitroglycerin (Parker *et al.*, 1970; Strauer and Scherpe, 1978).

Patients are able to exercise for considerably longer periods after the administration of nitroglycerin. Nevertheless, angina occurs, with or without nitroglycerin, at the same value of the "triple product" (aortic pressure × heart rate × ejection time). The triple product can be determined experimentally and is proportional to the myocardial consumption of oxygen. The observation that angina occurs at the same level of myocardial oxygen consumption suggests that the beneficial effects of nitroglycerin are the result of a reduced cardiac oxygen demand, rather than the result of an increase in the delivery of oxygen to ischemic regions of myocardium. However, these results do not preclude the possibility that a favorable redistribution of blood flow to ischemic subendocardial myocardium contributes to the relief of pain in a typical anginal attack, nor do they preclude the possibility that direct coronary vasodilatation may *not* be the major effect of nitroglycerin in situations where vasospasm compromises myocardial blood flow.

Other Effects. The organic nitrates and nitrites act on almost all smooth muscle structures. *Bronchial* smooth muscle is relaxed irrespective of the cause of the preexisting tone. The muscles of the *biliary tract,* including those of the gallbladder, biliary ducts, and sphincter of Oddi, are effectively relaxed. In patients with T-tube drainage, a nitrate can rapidly reduce biliary pressure, whether elevated spontaneously or in response to morphine, and can induce rapid emptying of biliary contents into the duodenum. Pain and other symptoms incident to increased pressure are transiently relieved. Smooth muscle of the *gastrointestinal tract,* including that of the esophagus, can be relaxed and its spontaneous motility decreased by nitrate both *in vivo* and *in vitro.* The effect may be transient and incomplete *in vivo,* but abnormal "spasm" is frequently reduced. Similarly, nitrate can relax *ureteral* and *uterine* smooth muscle, but these effects are somewhat unpredictable. Organic nitrates are singularly devoid of actions on tissues other than smooth muscle.

Mechanism of Action. Nitrites, organic nitrates, nitroso compounds, and a variety of other nitrogen oxide–containing substances (including nitroprusside; *see* Chapter 32) can activate guanylate cyclase and increase the synthesis of guanosine $3',5'$-monophosphate (cyclic GMP) in smooth muscle and other tissues (*see* Mittal and Murad, 1982; Rapaport and Murad, 1983). These agents all lead to the formation of the reactive free radical nitric oxide (NO), which interacts with and activates guanylate cyclase. A cyclic GMP–dependent protein kinase is thus stimulated, with resultant alteration of the phosphorylation of various proteins in smooth muscle. This eventually leads to the *de*phosphorylation of the light chain of myosin (Rapaport *et al.*, 1983). This protein is thought to play an important role in the contractile process in its phosphorylated form. Analogs of cyclic GMP can also relax vascular and bronchial smooth muscle. The nitrogen oxide–containing vasodilators and related agents that give rise to nitric oxide and utilize this mechanistic pathway have come to be called *nitrovasodilators.*

Absorption, Fate, and Excretion. The biotransformation of organic nitrates is the result of reductive hydrolysis catalyzed by the hepatic enzyme glutathione–organic nitrate reductase. The enzyme converts the lipid-soluble organic nitrate esters into more water-soluble denitrated metabolites and inorganic nitrite. The partially and fully denitrated metabolites are considerably less potent vasodilators than are the parent compounds. However, under certain conditions their activity may become important. Since the liver has an enormous capacity to catalyze this reaction, the biotransformation of organic nitrates is a major factor in determining their duration of action *in vivo* and the relative efficacy of the drugs when given by various routes of administration. The pharmacokinetic properties of nitroglycerin and isosorbide dinitrate have been studied in the greatest detail.

Nitroglycerin. Investigation of biotransformation of organic nitrates began with the observation that inorganic nitrite was formed when organic nitrate esters were incubated with homogenates of rabbit liver. Studies in a variety of systems indicate that the reductive hydrolysis requires glutathione and is rapidly catalyzed by glutathione–organic nitrate reductase (Needleman, 1975). One molecule of nitroglycerin reacts with two of reduced glutathione to release one inorganic nitrite ion from either the 2 or 3 position; the products are 1,3- or 1,2-glyceryl dinitrate and oxidized glutathione. A comparison of the maximal velocities of metabolism of the clinically used nitrates by this reductase indicates that erythrityl tetranitrate is degraded three times faster than is nitroglycerin, while isosorbide dinitrate and pentaerythritol nitrate are denitrated at one sixth and one tenth of the rate of nitroglycerin.

In man, peak concentrations of nitroglycerin are found in plasma within 4 minutes of sublingual administration; the compound has a half-life of 1 to 3 minutes. Dinitrate metabolites, which are about ten times less potent as vasodilators, appear to have a half-life of approximately 40 minutes (*see* Appendix II).

Isosorbide Dinitrate. The major route of metabolism of isosorbide dinitrate in man is by enzymatic denitration followed by formation of glucuronides. Sublingual administration produces maximal concentrations of the drug in plasma by 6 minutes, and the fall in concentration is rapid (half-life approximately 45 minutes). The primary initial metabolites, isosorbide-2-mononitrate and isosorbide-5-mononitrate, have longer half-lives (2 to 5 hours) and are presumed to be responsible, at least in part, for the therapeutic efficacy of isosorbide dinitrate. There is considerable interest in the therapeutic potential of isosorbide-5-mononitrate, since its bio-availability is excellent after oral administration and it has a significantly longer half-life than does isosorbide dinitrate.

Correlation of Plasma Concentrations of Drug and Biological Activity. Intravenous administration of nitroglycerin or the long-acting nitrates (isosorbide dinitrate, pentaerythritol tetranitrate, and erythrityl tetranitrate) in anesthetized animals produces the same transient decrease (1 to 4 minutes) in blood pressure (Needleman *et al.*, 1972). Relative to nitroglycerin, the potency of erythrityl tetranitrate as a vasodepressor in dogs is about 12%, and isosorbide dinitrate 3.5% (Parker *et al.*, 1975). Since denitration markedly reduces the activity of the organic nitrates, their rapid clearance from blood indicates that the transient duration of action under these conditions correlates with the concentrations of the parent compounds (Needleman *et al.*, 1972; Yap and Fung, 1978). The kinetics of hepatic denitration is characteristic of each nitrate. In addition, it appears to be influenced by hepatic blood flow or the presence of hepatic disease. In experimental animals, injection of moderate amounts of organic nitrates into the portal vein results in little or no vasodepressor activity (Needleman *et al.*, 1972; Commarato *et al.*, 1973). A substantial amount of drug can be metabolized during its first circulation through the liver.

Routes of Administration. When relief of acute anginal pain is the objective, rapid onset of action is essential and duration of effect is less important. In contrast, for prevention of ischemia, duration of action and predictability of effect are the main issues. The rapidity of onset and the duration of action of any nitrate are directly related to the method of administration. In addition, new formulations are available that permit sustained release of organic nitrate.

Sublingual Administration. The sublingual route of administration of organic nitrates is rational and effective for the treatment of acute attacks of angina pectoris. Most of the drug bypasses the hepatic circulation initially, since only about 15% of the cardiac output is delivered to the liver. A transient but effective concentration of drug appears in the circulation. The onset of action is in 1 to 2 minutes, but the effects fall off rapidly and are undetectable within 1 hour.

One expects and finds little difference in the *duration* of action of the various nitrates when relatively small doses are taken sublingually, since the metabolic capacity is high. Under this condition, their half-lives depend only on the rate at which they are delivered to the liver. Indeed, when equieffective doses of nitroglycerin and isosorbide dinitrate are given sublingually, there is no significant difference in their duration of action; effects on exercise tolerance wane with a half-time of about 20 minutes (Goldstein *et al.*, 1971). Erythrityl tetranitrate is also able to prolong exercise tolerance and prevent depression of the S-T segment in the ECG when administered sublingually to patients with typical angina. However, the duration of action of this agent is also short when it is given in this way (10 to 45 minutes). *Thus, the sublingual administration of organic nitrates is most appropriate to alleviate acute attacks of angina and for the immediate prophylaxis of such attacks.*

Oral Administration. Organic nitrates have been administered orally in an attempt to provide convenient and prolonged prophylaxis against attacks of angina. Under these circumstances, the drugs must be given in sufficient dosage to saturate the liver's capacity to degrade them; otherwise, insufficient nitrate will reach the systemic circulation. These formulations generally have a slow onset of action. Peak effects occur at 60 to 90 minutes, and the duration of action is 3 to 6 hours.

The efficacy of *low doses* of organic nitrates (*e.g.*, 5 mg of isosorbide dinitrate) given orally for prophylaxis of angina is questionable. A review of 59 studies wherein low doses of oral nitrates were administered demonstrated that the majority of the investigations failed to include adequate controls, crossover protocols, double-blind design, and valid statistical analysis (Stipe and Fink, 1973). When only properly designed investigations were evaluated, oral nitrates were usually no more effective than placebos.

High doses of nitrates given orally can cause a small decrease in arterial blood pressure, a substantial decrease in left ventricular filling pressure, and an increase in the exercise tolerance of patients with angina (Franciosa *et al.*, 1974). High doses of isosorbide dinitrate (30 mg orally, given four times daily) produce sustained hemodynamic and antianginal effects (Danahy *et al.*, 1977). Under these circumstances the activities of less potent metabolites may also contribute to the therapeutic effect. Chronic oral administration of isosorbide dinitrate (120 to 720 mg daily) has resulted in persistence of the parent compound and higher concentrations of metabolites in plasma (Shane *et al.*, 1978). However, such high doses are more likely to cause troublesome side effects and tolerance.

Significant, prolonged (up to 4 hours) improvement of exercise tolerance can also be demonstrated in patients with angina pectoris who are given a sustained-release oral form of nitroglycerin (Winsor and Berger, 1975). Again, high doses (6.5 mg) of nitroglycerin are required to elicit prolonged hemodynamic responses.

Intravenous Nitroglycerin. The intravenous administration of nitroglycerin permits rapid attainment of high concentrations of drug in the systemic circulation and prompt initiation of therapy. Because of its rapid degradation, the concentration can be titrated quickly and safely. The antianginal effects of intravenous nitroglycerin are useful in the treatment of coronary vasospasm and unstable angina pectoris, and this route of administration may become the preferred approach for the urgent treatment of congestive heart failure and acute ischemic syndromes (*see* Jaffe and Roberts, 1982). Intravenous nitroglycerin has been shown to be effective in the control of hypertension during and after coronary artery bypass surgery, and it may be efficacious in controlling pulmonary hypertension associated with acute respiratory failure.

Nitroglycerin Ointment. The topical administration of nitroglycerin in an ointment has been used to provide gradual absorption of the drug for prolonged prophylactic purposes. Effects are apparent within 60 minutes, and they persist for 4 to 8 hours. Doses of nitroglycerin ointment are large (often up to 30 mg), and absorption is quite variable. Patients with angina who used 2% nitroglycerin ointment (average dose of 5 mg) experienced improved and prolonged exercise capacity and showed decreased ischemic S-T segment changes in the ECG (Reichek *et al.,* 1974). Slow-release preparations of nitroglycerin for cutaneous use, for example, nitroglycerin discs (transdermal systems), represent an innovative attempt to produce sustained concentrations of the drug in plasma. The preparations utilize a nitroglycerin reservoir (impregnated into a polymer bonded to an adhesive bandage), which permits gradual absorption over 24 hours. The onset of action is slow, and peak effects occur after 1 to 2 hours. Such therapy, when adequately evaluated, may provide a simple and effective once-daily method for long-term prophylaxis of myocardial ischemia.

Transmucosal or Buccal Nitroglycerin. The patient inserts this formulation under the upper lip, adherent to the gingiva. Dissolution of the tablet proceeds in a gradual, uniform manner. This formulation appears to act as promptly as does sublingual nitroglycerin (hemodynamic alterations occur in 2 to 5 minutes), and it is therefore useful for short-term prophylaxis of angina. The tablet continues to release nitroglycerin into the circulation for a prolonged period, and exercise tolerance may be enhanced for up to 5 hours (Abrams, 1983).

Tolerance. Sublingual organic nitrates are usually taken by the patient at the time of an anginal attack or in anticipation of exercise or stress. Such intermittent treatment results in reproducible cardiovascular effects. However, frequently repeated exposure of experimental animals to high doses of organic nitrates leads to a decrease in the magnitude of most of the pharmacological effects of these agents (*see* Needleman and Johnson, 1975). The therapeutic significance of this phenomenon is likely to increase as the oral administration of higher doses of organic nitrates (and use of the sustained-release preparations) becomes more prevalent. For example, the chronic oral use of isosorbide dinitrate (120 mg per day) led to the development of partial tolerance to the hemodynamic effects of the drug and to cross-tolerance to the venodilatation produced by sublingual nitroglycerin (Zelis and Mason, 1975). However, clinical experience with high-dose nitrate therapy is limited, and other studies have demonstrated undiminished therapeutic activity in response to the administration of long-acting nitrates for 10 months (Abrams, 1980).

A special aspect of tolerance has been observed among individuals exposed to nitroglycerin in the manufacture of explosives. If protection is inadequate, workers may experience severe headaches, dizziness, and postural weakness during the first several days of employment. Tolerance then develops, but headache and other symptoms may reappear after a few days away from the job, the "Monday disease." The most serious effect of chronic exposure is a form of *organic nitrate dependence.* Individuals without demonstrable organic vascular disease have died suddenly or developed myocardial infarctions after a few days' break in chronic exposure, and there are now well-documented cases with typical subjective and objective findings of severe myocardial ischemia, relieved by nitroglycerin, during withdrawal from chronic exposure to an organic nitrate. Coronary and digital arteriospasm during withdrawal and its relaxation by nitroglycerin have also been demonstrated radiographically. Because of the potential problem of nitrate dependence, it seems prudent not to withdraw nitrates abruptly from a patient who has received such therapy chronically.

The mechanism of initiation and maintenance of tolerance to these drugs is due neither to an alteration of the biotransformation of organic nitrates nor to changes in sympathetic function. When blood vessels are removed from animals that have been made tolerant to organic nitrates, they too are hyposensitive to the effects of the agents, suggesting alteration in the activation of the guanylate cyclase–cyclic GMP system discussed above.

Toxicity and Untoward Responses. Untoward responses to the therapeutic use of organic nitrates are almost all secondary to actions on the cardiovascular system. *Headache* is common and can be severe. It usually decreases over a few days if treatment is continued, and often can be controlled by decreasing the dose. Transient episodes of *dizziness, weakness,* and other manifestations of the cerebral ischemia associated with *postural hypotension* may develop occasionally in many patients, particularly if standing immobile, and may occasionally progress to loss of consciousness. This reaction appears to be accentuated by alcohol. Even in the most severe nitrate syncope, positioning and other procedures to facilitate venous return are the only therapeutic measures required. It was widely believed that nitrates can increase intraocular pressure and precipitate glaucoma, but this fear appears to be completely unfounded. Drug *rash* is occasionally produced by all the organic nitrates, but it appears to occur most commonly with pentaerythritol tetranitrate.

Preparations and Dosage. Data for the nitrites and organic nitrates available for clinical use are given in Table 33–1. Sodium nitrite is obsolete except as an intravenous solution for use in the treatment of cyanide poisoning (*see* Chapter 70). Amyl nitrite acts very rapidly after inhalation and is occasionally used for very brief effects. Nitroglycerin is sufficiently unstable and volatile for the tablets to lose activity rapidly unless kept in a tightly sealed, dark-tinted glass container (without a cotton plug); plastic is unsatisfactory. Active tablets should produce a distinct burning sensation when placed under the tongue. Only nitroglycerin, erythrityl tetranitrate, and isosorbide dinitrate are available in sublingual tablets.

THERAPEUTIC USES

Angina. Diseases that predispose to angina should be treated as part of a comprehensive therapeutic program. Such conditions as hypertension, anemia, thyrotoxicosis, obesity, heart failure, and chronic and acute anxiety can precipitate anginal

Table 33–1.   ORGANIC NITRATES AVAILABLE FOR CLINICAL USE

NONPROPRIETARY NAME AND TRADE NAMES	CHEMICAL STRUCTURE	PREPARATIONS, DOSES, AND ROUTES OF ADMINISTRATION *
Amyl nitrite (isoamyl nitrite)	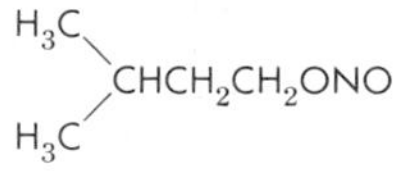 H_3C $CHCH_2CH_2ONO$ H_3C	Inh: 0.18 or 0.3 ml, inhalation
Nitroglycerin (glyceryl trinitrate; NITRO-BID, NITROSTAT, others)	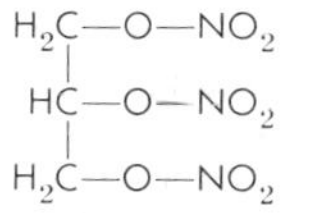 $H_2C-O-NO_2$ $HC-O-NO_2$ $H_2C-O-NO_2$	T: 0.15 to 0.6 mg C: 2.5 to 9 mg every 8 to 12 hr B: 1 to 2 mg every 3 to 8 hr O: 1.25 to 5 cm (1/2 to 2 in.), topical to skin, every 4 to 8 hr D: 1 disc (2.5 to 15 mg/24 hr) every 24 hr IV: 5 μg/min; increments of 5 μg/min
Isosorbide dinitrate (ISORDIL, SORBITRATE, others)	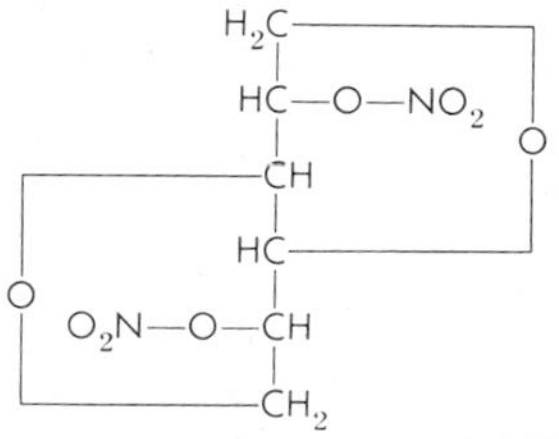 H_2C $HC-O-NO_2$ CH O HC $O_2N-O-CH$ CH_2 O	T: 2.5 to 10 mg every 4 to 6 hr T(C): 5 to 10 mg every 2 to 3 hr T(O): 5 to 30 mg every 6 hr C: 40 mg every 6 to 12 hr
Erythrityl tetranitrate (CARDILATE)	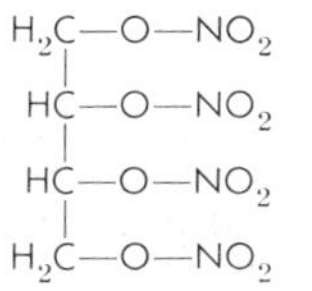 $H_2C-O-NO_2$ $HC-O-NO_2$ $HC-O-NO_2$ $H_2C-O-NO_2$	T: 5 to 10 mg three times daily T(C): 10 mg three times daily
Pentaerythritol tetranitrate (PENTRITOL, PERITRATE, others)	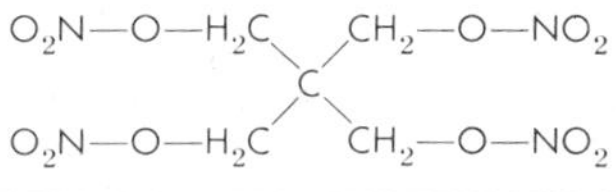 O_2N-O-H_2C CH_2-O-NO_2 C O_2N-O-H_2C CH_2-O-NO_2	T(O): 10 to 40 mg four times daily C: 30 to 80 mg every 12 hr

* B = buccal (transmucosal) tablets; C = sustained-release capsule or tablet; D = transdermal disc; Inh = inhalant; IV = intravenous injection; O = ointment; T = tablet for sublingual use; T(C) = chewable tablet; T(O) = oral tablet.

symptoms in many patients. The patient should be asked to stop smoking, overeating, and exercising shortly after meals, and he should avoid exposure to certain sympathomimetic agents (*e.g.*, those used in nasal decongestants) that increase myocardial oxygen demand. The use of drugs that modify the perception of pain is a poor approach to the treatment of angina, since the underlying myocardial ischemia is not relieved.

Sublingual Administration. Because of its rapid action, long-established efficacy, and low cost, nitroglycerin is the most useful drug among the organic nitrates that can be given sublingually. An initial dose of 0.3 mg of nitroglycerin will often relieve pain within 3 minutes. Pain may be prevented when the drug is used prophylactically immediately prior to exercise or stress. The smallest effective dose should be prescribed. Patients should be taught to contact their physicians when more than three tablets taken over a 15-minute period do not relieve a sustained attack, since this situation may be indicative of myocardial infarction. The patient should be advised that there is no virtue in trying to avoid taking the sublingual nitroglycerin tablets for anginal pain. Other nitrates that can be taken sublingually do not appear to be longer acting or more effective than nitroglycerin. They are often more expensive (Goldstein *et al.*, 1971).

Oral Administration. Oral nitrates employed at usual dose (*e.g.*, 5 to 10 mg of isosorbide dinitrate) are no more effective than placebo in decreasing the frequency of angina or increasing the patient's exercise tolerance. Clinical studies that have used higher doses either of isosorbide dinitrate (*e.g.*, 20 mg or more orally every 4 hours) or sustained-release preparations of nitroglycerin (Winsor and Berger, 1975) indicate that such regimens decrease the frequency of attacks of angina, improve exercise tolerance, and favorably alter the determinants of myocardial oxygen demand. However, these high doses increase the risk of hypotension, tachycardia, and tolerance.

Topical Administration. Application of nitroglycerin ointment can relieve angina for 4 hours or more. Usually 2% nitroglycerin ointment is applied to the skin (2.5 to 5 cm [1 to 2 in.] as it is squeezed from the tube; it is then spread in a uniform layer); the dosage must be adjusted for each patient. The ointment is particularly useful for controlling nocturnal angina, which commonly develops within 3 hours after the patient goes to sleep. A transdermal nitroglycerin disc applied once every 24 hours produces a continuous concentration of nitrate in blood and provides a simple and effective method for long-term prophylaxis of angina pectoris.

Congestive Heart Failure. The goal of treatment of congestive heart failure is to increase cardiac output and reduce pulmonary and peripheral edema. Conventional therapy of heart failure involves the use of positive inotropic agents and diuretics (*see* Chapters 30 and 36). Vasodilators can improve cardiovascular function in congestive heart failure, even in some patients who are unresponsive to conventional therapy (*see* Symposium, 1978; 1983; 1984).

Acute Heart Failure. The utility of vasodilators to relieve pulmonary congestion and to increase cardiac output in acute congestive heart failure is well established. The acceptance of these drugs for such treatment has been aided by the development of bedside technics that allow frequent measurement of ventricular filling pressure and cardiac output. Thus, the effects of the drug can be objectively evaluated, and their doses and intervals of administration can be optimized for the ability to improve left ventricular performance. Initial use of vasodilators was aimed at reduction of preload by producing venodilatation, which reduced end-diastolic pressure and relieved pulmonary congestion. The utility of reduction of afterload (by dilatation of arterioles and reduction of peripheral resistance) to increase cardiac output has been described more recently (Franciosa *et al.*, 1972).

The response of the cardiovascular system to vasodilators is different in patients with congestive failure than in normal individuals. In a normal subject the administration of a vasodilator produces venodilatation, which decreases preload and results in decreased cardiac output. The drugs also reduce afterload, which causes only a small increase in stroke volume. The net effect of vasodilators in a normal individual is a marked decrease in blood pressure and tachycardia.

Patients with congestive heart failure have elevated peripheral vascular resistance due to compensatory increases in adrenergic tone. Some patients also have enhanced activity of the renin-angiotensin system. These factors act to maintain blood pressure and redistribute blood flow to vital organs, despite low cardiac output. Arteriolar resistance may be elevated to a degree that is greater than optimal to maintain maximal cardiac output (Ross, 1976). Drugs that reduce peripheral resistance in patients with congestive heart failure significantly increase the ejection fraction, stroke volume, cardiac output, and tissue perfusion. The increases in cardiac output may counterbalance the fall in peripheral resistance, and little or no change in the patient's blood pressure and heart rate may occur. If the reduction of preload is excessive (to below-normal levels), the cardiac output will fall. The hemodynamic effects of the drugs must, therefore, be monitored carefully. When this is done, the treatment can be individualized so that preload and afterload are appropriately reduced and cardiac output is increased in the face of a net reduction of myocardial oxygen demand. The use of conventional positive inotropic agents may allow a similar increase in cardiac output, but at the cost of increased consumption of oxygen.

Many of the vasodilators used in other clinical conditions (*e.g.*, angina and hypertension) have also been utilized to improve left ventricular function and provide relief of symptoms in acute heart failure. Classification of these drugs is usually based on their major site of action. Thus, agents such as nitroglycerin and isosorbide dinitrate are described as primarily relaxing venous smooth muscle. They would be expected to decrease venous return, lower ventricular filling pressures, and relieve pulmonary congestion. Small decreases in preload would result in little effect on cardiac output, but excessive decreases in preload will reduce cardiac output. A second group of agents (*e.g.*, hydralazine, minoxidil) is designated as primarily arterial vasodilators; they decrease afterload and increase cardiac output with little change in filling pressure or preload. There are also drugs that act on both arterial and venous beds to similar degrees. These include nitroprusside, α-adrenergic antagonists, and angiotensin converting enzyme inhibitors. Termed "balanced" vasodilators, they tend to decrease both filling pressure and pulmonary congestion and increase cardiac output as a result of a decrease in arterial resistance. Although this description of the effects of these agents is useful clinically, it is clearly an oversimplification from the point of view of the pharmacological actions of the drugs and the physiological responses to arterial and venous dilatation in the complex and heterogeneous conditions that are manifest as congestive heart failure.

Directly acting agents (nitrates, minoxidil, hydralazine, nitroprusside) cause arteriolar dilatation and/or venodilatation of all regional vascular beds rather uniformly. They require widely varying doses in different individuals, and these doses are usually higher than those necessary to treat angina or hypertension. In contrast, α-adrenergic blocking agents and angiotensin converting enzyme inhibitors would be expected to reverse the inappropriately high vasoconstrictive effects of norepinephrine and angiotensin on specific vascular beds. Doses of these agents that produce vasodilatation in heart failure are comparable to those used in the treatment of hypertension (Packer, 1982).

Most of the adverse effects of vasodilator therapy in acute heart failure relate to excessive vasodilatation, which results in excessively reduced filling pressures and hypotension, decreased ventricular performance, and decreased perfusion of tissues. These problems can be avoided by careful attention to changes in ventricular filling pressures and cardiac output, especially with the directly acting vasodilators.

Chronic Heart Failure. In contrast to their well-established efficacy in acute failure, the results of treatment of chronic heart failure with vasodilators are less satisfactory. The objectives of long-term vasodilator therapy are to reduce morbidity and mortality and to produce sustained improvement of left ventricular function at rest and during exercise.

Unfortunately, the initial improvement in left ventricular function produced by vasodilators does not persist in many patients. In most cases, even sustained increases in cardiac output and improved ventricular function have not been associated with demonstrable increases in exercise capacity or relief of symptoms (Packer, 1982). Moreover, the abrupt withdrawal of an infusion of nitroprusside from patients with severe chronic heart failure may be associated with a rebound in hemodynamic effects that produce a transient deterioration in cardiac performance. Presumably, this is due to the activation of baroreceptor reflexes, and its magnitude is related to the degree of preservation of compensatory vasoconstrictive mechanisms in individual patients (Packer *et al.*, 1979). At present, neither the mechanisms that underlie the tolerance to vasodilator therapy nor the reasons why increases in ventricular function fail to increase exercise capacity are clearly understood. Considerably more study will be required to optimize long-term therapy with vasodilators and to assess the effects of such treatment on morbidity and mortality in this complex and heterogeneous disorder.

Myocardial Infarction. Some therapeutic maneuvers are directed at reducing the size of a myocardial infarction and preserving or retrieving viable tissue by reducing the oxygen demand of the myocardium. A drug that favorably alters the oxygen balance could decrease the area of myocardial damage if it were given soon after infarction.

In the past, nitroglycerin was considered to be contraindicated for use in patients with acute myocardial infarction. Its ability to induce hypotension and trigger a reflex tachycardia was feared. However, when the effects of nitroglycerin were carefully monitored, they were found to decrease left ventricular filling pressure, thus relieving pulmonary congestion in patients with heart failure following acute myocardial infarction. Since the effects of sublingual nitroglycerin are transient, investigators have tested the usefulness of intravenous infusions of the drug. When the dose is adjusted such that tachycardia does not occur, intravenous nitroglycerin can reduce the elevation of the S-T segment that follows acute coronary occlusion in both normal dogs and in those with preexisting multivessel coronary occlusive disease (Epstein *et al.*, 1975). Other vasodilators, such as nitroprusside or phentolamine, have been tested for their capacity to diminish ischemic injury but appear to have no advantage over nitroglycerin. The frequency of elevation of the S-T segment during acute coronary occlusion in dogs was reduced by nitroglycerin but increased by nitroprusside, and regional coronary blood flow was increased by nitroglycerin but reduced by nitroprusside (Chiariello *et al.*, 1976). Furthermore, nitroglycerin is more effective than nitroprusside in reducing coronary collateral resistance, whereas phentolamine may have a deleterious effect (Capurro *et al.*, 1977).

Intravenous infusion of nitroglycerin in patients with acute myocardial infarction at doses that maintain or improve stroke work can relieve pulmonary congestion by decreasing left ventricular filling pressure; there is also a reduction of myocardial oxygen demand. Additional clinical evidence demonstrates that nitroglycerin can decrease the electrophysiological signs of ischemic injury in patients with acute myocardial infarction. In a randomized, prospective study of 85 patients with acute myocardial infarction, intravenous nitroglycerin caused a decrease in the size of the affected zone in patients with inferior infarcts, but the drug had no effect in patients with anterior infarcts (Roberts, 1983). However, there have been contradictory reports, and additional experience with larger experimental groups and with careful monitoring of hemodynamic parameters is required to define the utility of organic nitrates in myocardial infarction.

Variant (Prinzmetal's) Angina. Numerous studies of experimental animals have demonstrated that coronary blood flow can be modulated by neurogenic stimulation of the large coronary arteries. These vessels normally contribute little to coronary resistance. However, stimulation of the large vessels may cause marked coronary constriction, resulting in reduced blood flow and ischemic pain. Variant angina is now believed to be the result of coronary vasospasm, possibly resulting from such stimulation. Transmitters that have been hypothesized to be involved in the initiation of vasospasm include catecholamines, 5-hydroxytryptamine, and histamine. It has also been postulated that endothelial-cell injury may promote contraction because of the deficiency of vasodilators that originate from these cells. Ergonovine maleate, a vasoconstrictor (*see* Chapter 39), has been utilized intravenously during coronary arteriography as a provocative diagnostic test to induce coronary artery vasospasm and identify patients with variant angina. Ergonovine-induced coronary artery spasm is reversed by nitroglycerin.

CALCIUM CHANNEL BLOCKERS

Hass and Hartfelder reported in 1962 that verapamil, a coronary vasodilator, possessed negative inotropic and chronotropic effects that were not seen with other, apparently similar vasodilatory agents, such as nitroglycerin. The mechanism of action of verapamil was initially thought to be due to coronary vasodilatation and blockade of myocardial β-adrenergic receptors. However, Fleckenstein suggested that the mechanism of action of these agents was not related to β-adrenergic blockade, but to inhibition of the movement of calcium ions into cells with resultant inhibition of excitation-contraction coupling (Fleckenstein *et al.*, 1967). Fleckenstein termed such agents *calcium antagonists*.

Rougier, Coraboeuf, and colleagues subsequently presented definitive evidence that depolarization in atrial tissue was mediated by two inwardly directed ionic currents (Rougier *et al.*, 1969). When a cardiac cell potential reaches threshold, the membrane permeability for sodium increases rapidly and markedly. The so-called *fast channel* is responsible for this influx of sodium, and it is blocked by tetrodotoxin (*see* Chapter 15). The time required for the second inward current to reach maximal values is much longer. This current is caused in large part by the movement of calcium ions into the cell through a membrane pore that is thus termed the *slow channel*. The movement of calcium through this slow channel is inhibited by Mn^{2+}, but not by tetrodotoxin, and it contributes to the maintenance of the plateau phase of the cardiac action potential (Rougier *et al.*, 1969). A derivative of verapamil, D-600, was subsequently shown to block the movement of calcium through the slow channel and thereby alter the plateau phase of the cardiac action potential (Kohlhardt *et al.*, 1972).

Although these agents were termed *calcium antagonists*, they do not directly antagonize the effects of calcium. Rather, they inhibit the entry of calcium into cells or its mobilization from intracellular stores and, as such, have been termed *calcium channel blockers*.

Chemistry. The three calcium channel blockers presently approved for clinical use in the United States have markedly different chemical structures. *Verapamil* is a benzeneacetonitrile; its methoxy derivative, designated D-600, was one of the first of these agents to be evaluated pharmacologically. *Nifedipine* is a dihydropyridine, while *diltiazem* is a benzothiazepine. Their structural formulas are as follows:

Verapamil

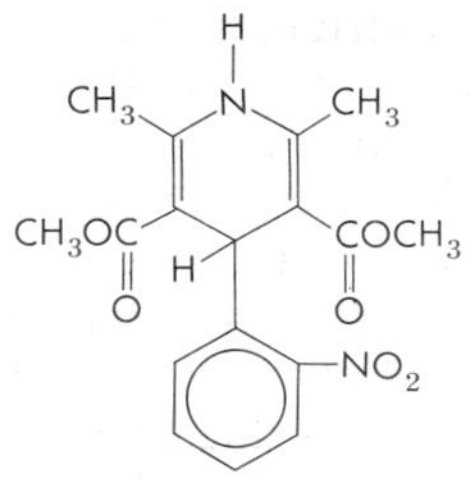

Nifedipine

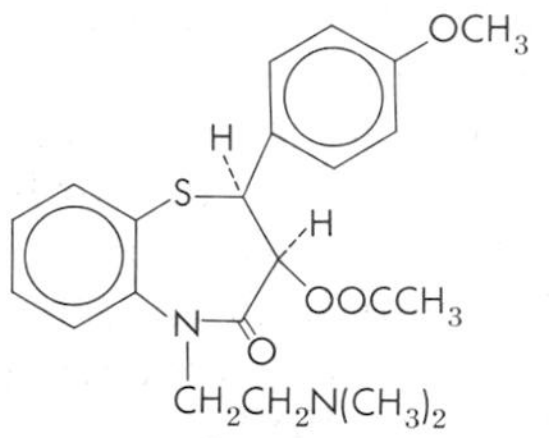

Diltiazem

All three agents are optically active, and the *l* isomers are five to ten times more potent than the *d* isomers as blockers of calcium channels. Both verapamil and diltiazem are water soluble, whereas nifedipine is soluble only in organic solvents such as alcohol or polyethylene glycol.

PHARMACOLOGICAL PROPERTIES

Actions in Vascular Tissue. Depolarization in vascular smooth muscle is dependent on the inward movement of Ca^{2+}, rather than Na^+, and is insensitive to tetrodotoxin (Bolton, 1979). Furthermore, contraction of vascular smooth muscle is regulated by the cytoplasmic concentration of Ca^{2+}. At least two different mechanisms appear to be responsible for contraction in vascular smooth muscle cells (Bolton, 1979). The first mechanism, termed *electromechanical coupling,* is mediated by voltage-sensitive calcium channels, which open in response to depolarization of the membrane. Extracellular calcium moves down its electrochemical gradient into the cell to initiate the contractile process. After closure of the calcium channels, a finite period of time is required before the channel can open again in response to a stimulus. The second mechanism, termed *pharmacomechanical coupling,* involves an agonist-induced contraction that occurs without depolarization of the membrane. It results from the release of intracellular calcium

from sarcoplasmic reticulum (Somlyo and Somlyo, 1968). Subsequently, this receptor-mediated effect also results in an increase in the influx of extracellular calcium. An increase in the cytosolic concentration of calcium by either mechanism results in enhanced binding of calcium to calmodulin. The Ca^{2+}-calmodulin complex activates myosin light-chain kinase, with resultant phosphorylation of the light chain of myosin. Such phosphorylation appears to promote interaction between actin and myosin and the contraction of smooth muscle. Although the calcium channel blockers can interfere with mobilization of calcium and reduce the elevation of intracellular calcium that occurs by either mechanism, these agents block the voltage-dependent calcium channels in vascular smooth muscle at significantly lower concentrations than are required to interfere with the receptor-mediated mechanism. The calcium channel blockers relax arterial smooth muscle, but they have little effect on most venous beds and hence do not affect cardiac preload.

Actions in Cardiac Cells. The mechanisms involved in excitation-contraction coupling in the heart differ from those in vascular smooth muscle. Membrane depolarization in atrial and ventricular conducting tissue and in myocytes of the atria and ventricles occurs as a result of two inward currents, one carried by sodium through the fast channel and the second by calcium through the slow channel (Coraboeuf, 1978). In the sinoatrial and atrioventricular nodes, depolarization is very largely dependent on the movement of calcium through the slow channel. Within the cardiac myocyte, calcium binds to troponin, the inhibitory effect of troponin on the contractile apparatus is relieved, and actin and myosin interact to cause contraction. Thus, blockade of the slow channel by calcium channel blockers can result in a negative inotropic effect.

The effect of a calcium channel blocker on atrioventricular conduction and on the rate of the sinus node pacemaker appears to be dependent in part on whether the agent delays the recovery of the slow channel

(Henry, 1983). Recovery is the process whereby a channel regains its capacity to carry calcium in response to activation. Although nifedipine reduces the slow inward current in a dose-dependent manner, it does not affect the rate of recovery of the slow calcium channel (Kohlhardt and Fleckenstein, 1977). The channel blockade caused by nifedipine and related dihydropyridines also shows little dependence on the frequency of stimulation. At doses used clinically, nifedipine does not affect conduction through the node. In contrast, verapamil not only reduces the magnitude of the calcium current through the slow channel but also decreases the rate of recovery of the channel (Ehara and Kaufmann, 1978). In addition, channel blockade caused by verapamil (and to a lesser extent by diltiazem) is enhanced as the frequency of stimulation increases. Verapamil slows A-V conduction and depresses the rate of the sinus node pacemaker. The slowing of atrioventricular conduction with verapamil or diltiazem is the basis for their use in the treatment of supraventricular tachyarrhythmias (*see* Chapter 31).

Hemodynamic Effects. All three of the calcium channel blockers discussed herein decrease coronary vascular resistance and increase coronary blood flow. Nifedipine is a more potent vasodilator *in vivo* and *in vitro* than is verapamil, which is usually more potent than diltiazem. Since the hemodynamic effects of each of these three agents vary depending on the route of administration and the extent of left ventricular dysfunction, each will be presented separately.

Nifedipine given intravenously increases forearm blood flow with little effect on venous pooling; this indicates a selective dilatation of arterial resistance vessels (Robinson *et al.*, 1980). The decrease in arterial blood pressure elicits sympathetic reflexes, with resultant tachycardia and positive inotropy. Nifedipine also has direct negative inotropic effects *in vitro*. However, nifedipine relaxes vascular smooth muscle at significantly lower concentrations than those required for prominent direct effects on the heart (Ono and Hashimoto, 1983). Thus, blood pressure is lowered, contractility and

segmental ventricular function are improved (Serruys *et al.*, 1981), and heart rate and cardiac output are increased modestly. After oral administration of nifedipine, peripheral blood flow increases due to arterial dilatation; there is no change in venous tone (Robinson *et al.*, 1980). The increase in cardiac output is due to a decrease in arteriolar resistance coupled with the positive inotropic effect that results from the expected sympathetic reflexes (Theroux *et al.*, 1980). Recent evidence suggests that sublingual nifedipine produces a more marked improvement in cardiac performance in patients with poor ventricular function (but without failure) than it does in patients with normal ventricular function (Ludbrook *et al.*, 1982).

Verapamil is a less potent vasodilator *in vivo* than nifedipine; however, as with nifedipine, verapamil causes little effect on venous resistance vessels at concentrations that produce arteriolar dilatation (Robinson *et al.*, 1980). However, the cardiac actions of verapamil are more prominent than are those of nifedipine. With doses of verapamil sufficient to produce peripheral arterial vasodilatation, there are more direct negative chronotropic, dromotropic, and inotropic effects than with nifedipine. Intravenous verapamil causes a decrease in arterial blood pressure due to a decrease in vascular resistance, but the reflex tachycardia can be blunted by the direct negative chronotropic effect of the drug (Singh and Roche, 1977). The intrinsic negative inotropic effect of verapamil is partially offset by both a decrease in afterload and the reflex increase in adrenergic tone. Thus, in patients without congestive heart failure, ventricular performance is not impaired and may actually improve (Hecht *et al.*, 1981). In contrast, in patients with congestive heart failure, intravenous verapamil can lead to a marked decrease in contractility and left ventricular function (Chew *et al.*, 1981). Oral administration of verapamil results in reduction of peripheral vascular resistance and blood pressure with no change in heart rate (Theroux *et al.*, 1980).

Intravenous administration of diltiazem can result initially in a marked decrease in peripheral vascular resistance and arterial blood pressure, which elicits a reflex increase in heart rate and cardiac output. Heart rate then falls below initial levels because of the direct negative chronotropic effect of the agent. Oral administration of diltiazem results in a sustained fall in both heart rate and mean arterial blood pressure (Theroux *et al.,* 1980).

ABSORPTION, FATE, AND EXCRETION

Pharmacokinetic parameters for the calcium channel blockers are presented in Appendix II.

Nifedipine. Nifedipine is rapidly and almost completely absorbed after sublingual administration. Bioavailability is about 50% after oral administration, and peak concentrations in plasma are attained in 1 to 3 hours. The drug is extensively (98%) bound to plasma proteins, and it is metabolized to inactive products with a half-time of 3 to 4 hours. The metabolites are predominantly excreted by the kidney; nifedipine itself does not appear in the urine.

Verapamil. Verapamil is efficiently absorbed after oral administration, but bioavailability is low (about 20%) due to extensive first-pass metabolism in the liver. The extent of metabolism decreases with prolonged oral treatment, and bioavailability improves (Kates *et al.,* 1981). Effects of verapamil are evident 1 to 2 hours after oral administration and peak by 5 hours. The half-life in plasma averages 5 hours, but it is increased after prolonged administration and in children and older individuals. In patients with hepatic cirrhosis, the half-life of verapamil may be increased fourfold, and bioavailability is also increased. Oral doses of verapamil should thus be reduced by 80% and intravenous doses by 50% for such patients (Somogyi *et al.,* 1981). Norverapamil, a metabolite produced by N-demethylation, is biologically active but is a less potent vasodilator. It accumulates to concentrations that are equal to those of verapamil after prolonged oral administration (Kates *et al.,* 1981). The half-life of norverapamil is 8 to 10 hours and can increase to 13 hours after continued dosage. After intravenous administration of verapa-

mil, peak effects are evident in 10 to 15 minutes.

Diltiazem. The bioavailability of diltiazem is about 50% after oral administration; effects of the drug are noticeable within 15 minutes and peak within 30 minutes. Diltiazem is metabolized with a half-time of 3 to 4 hours. It is initially deacetylated and then O- or N-demethylated; phenolic metabolites have also been detected. Desacetyl diltiazem appears to possess 40 to 50% of the pharmacological activity of the parent compound, although concentrations in plasma remain low (15 to 30% of the parent drug).

Preparations, Routes of Administration, and Dosages. *Nifedipine.* Nifedipine (PROCARDIA) is supplied in 10-mg capsules. The initial oral dose is 10 mg, given three times daily, and this should then be titrated over a period of 7 to 14 days to control symptoms of angina. The usual effective dose is 10 to 20 mg three times daily, but 20 to 30 mg taken three or four times daily may be necessary. The total daily dose should not exceed 180 mg.
Verapamil. Verapamil hydrochloride (CALAN, ISOPTIN) is supplied as 80- or 120-mg tablets and as an injection (5 mg/2 ml). The drug is given intravenously to interrupt supraventricular arrhythmias, and arterial pressure and the ECG must be monitored. An initial intravenous dose of 5 to 10 mg (or 75 to 150 μg/kg) is given over 2 minutes. This can be repeated 30 minutes later if necessary. The initial oral dose of verapamil for the treatment of angina is 80 mg three or four times daily. Dosage is then titrated at daily or weekly intervals. The optimal daily dose for most patients is between 320 and 480 mg.
Diltiazem. Diltiazem hydrochloride (CARDIZEM) is supplied in 30- or 60-mg tablets. Oral administration of diltiazem is initiated at doses of 30 mg four times daily, and the dose can be increased as necessary to 60 mg taken three or four times each day.

TOXICITY AND UNTOWARD RESPONSES

In general, the major toxicities associated with the use of calcium channel blockers involve excessive vasodilatation, negative inotropy, depression of the sinus nodal rate, and A-V nodal conduction disturbances.

Nifedipine. The predominant difficulty with this agent is excessive vasodilatation, which results most commonly in peripheral edema and dizziness and less commonly in headaches, hypotension, digital dysesthesia, flushing, nausea, vomiting, and sedation. These side effects, which occur in 20% of patients, are usually benign and may abate with time or with adjustment of the dose. Aggravation of myocardial ischemia has been reported, potentially due to excessive hypotension and decreased coronary perfusion, selective coronary vasodilatation in nonischemic regions of the myocardium (*i.e.*, coronary steal, since vessels perfusing ischemic regions may already be maximally dilated), or an increase in oxygen demand due to excessive tachycardia. At therapeutic doses, verapamil and diltiazem are less likely to aggravate myocardial ischemia because of their lower capacity to induce excessive peripheral arteriolar dilatation.

Verapamil. Although bradycardia, transient asystole, hypotension, and exacerbation of heart failure have been reported, these responses have usually occurred after intravenous administration, or in patients with disease of the S-A node or atrioventricular conduction disturbances, or in the presence of β-adrenergic blockade. The use of intravenous verapamil with a β-adrenergic antagonist is contraindicated because of the increased propensity for atrioventricular block and/or severe depression of ventricular function. Verapamil is well tolerated orally. A small percentage of patients experience headache, dizziness, constipation, a flushing rash, peripheral edema, or first- or second-degree A-V nodal block and hypotension. Patients with ventricular dysfunction, sinoatrial or atrioventricular nodal conduction disturbances, and systolic blood pressures below 90 mm Hg should not be treated with verapamil, particularly intravenously. Verapamil can cause an increase in the concentration of digoxin in plasma, although toxicity from the cardiac glycoside rarely develops (Schwartz *et al.*, 1982). The use of verapamil to treat digitalis toxicity is thus contraindicated; A-V nodal conduction disturbances may be exacerbated, particularly if paroxysmal atrial tachycardia with atrioventricular block is present.

Diltiazem. There are few reports about the adverse effects of this agent, but caution should be used in the presence of β-adrenergic antagonists. Side effects are minor, but diltiazem has effects on the S-A and A-V nodes that are very similar to those of verapamil, particularly when the daily dose approaches 360 mg.

THERAPEUTIC USES

Variant Angina. This form of angina is a direct result of a reduction in flow, not of an increase in oxygen demand. A number of controlled clinical trials have demonstrated the efficacy of the three calcium channel blocking agents discussed above for the treatment of variant angina. These drugs can attenuate ergonovine-induced vasospasm in patients with variant angina, which suggests that protection in variant angina is due to coronary dilatation rather than to alterations in peripheral hemodynamics (Waters *et al.*, 1981). In a large multicenter study, nifedipine eliminated attacks of variant angina in 63% of patients. The incidence of attacks was greatly reduced in most patients; in only 7% of those studied was the agent ineffective (Antman *et al.*, 1980a). Although some reports indicate that verapamil is equally effective (Severi *et al.*, 1980), others have reported that verapamil is less effective than nifedipine (Kimura and Kishida, 1981). Diltiazem also appears to be highly effective, although only a few studies have been reported to date (Yasue *et al.*, 1979). Unfortunately, the relatively short duration of action of nifedipine limits its effectiveness throughout the night, and attacks of variant angina often occur during sleep (Yasue *et al.*, 1979).

Exertional Angina. Calcium channel blockers are also effective in the treatment of exertional or exercise-induced angina. The utility of the calcium channel blockers could result from an increase in blood flow due to coronary arterial dilatation or from a decrease in myocardial oxygen demand, secondary to a decrease in arterial blood pressure, heart rate, or contractility. Numerous studies with double-blind, placebo-controlled protocols have shown that nifedipine in a single sublingual dose of 10 to 20 mg will decrease the number of anginal attacks and attenuate exercise-induced depression of the S-T segment (Moskowitz *et al.*, 1979). Beneficial effects are also apparent after long-term oral administration of any of the three agents (Neumann and Luisada, 1966; Wagniart *et al.*, 1982).

The double product, which is calculated as heart rate × systolic blood pressure, is an indirect measure of myocardial oxygen demand. Since the level of the double product (or oxygen demand) at a given external work load is reduced by these agents, and the value of the double product at peak exercise is not altered, the beneficial effect of calcium channel blockers is likely due to a decrease in oxygen demand rather than to an increase in nutritional coronary flow (Moskowitz *et al.*, 1979; Wagniart *et al.*, 1982; Rouleau *et al.*, 1983). The fixed obstruction present in the patient with exertional angina appears to be unresponsive to dilatation by any of the calcium channel blockers.

In approximately 10% of patients, nifedipine may aggravate anginal symptoms. This may be caused by increased sympathetic tone secondary to peripheral vasodilatation, a marked decrease in coronary perfusion pressure, or coronary steal. This adverse effect is not prominent with verapamil or diltiazem because of their limited ability to induce marked peripheral vasodilatation and reflex tachycardia. Concurrent therapy with nifedipine and propranolol has proven more effective than either agent given alone in exertional angina, presumably because the β-adrenergic antagonist suppresses reflex tachycardia (Bassan et al., 1982). This concurrent drug therapy is particularly attractive, since nifedipine, unlike verapamil and diltiazem, does not delay atrioventricular conduction and will not enhance the negative dromotropic effects associated with β-adrenergic blockade. Although concurrent administration of verapamil or diltiazem with a β-adrenergic antagonist is also more effective, the potential for atrioventricular block, severe bradycardia, and decreased left ventricular function negates any advantage. This is particularly important if left ventricular function is compromised prior to therapy.

Unstable Angina. Although described by a number of terms, including preinfarction angina or crescendo angina, unstable angina can best be defined as angina of recent onset associated with minimal exertion. It is prolonged and frequent; both elevation and depression of the S-T segment are observed, as is inversion of the T wave. There is severe restriction of coronary flow, and it is likely that vasospasm also occurs in some patients (Hugenholtz et al., 1981). Medical therapy for unstable angina involves administration of nitrates and β-adrenergic blocking agents, which are effective in controlling pain. However, mortality after 1 year is nearly 7%, and 20% of patients have a myocardial infarction (Multicenter Study, 1978). Calcium entry blockers offer a unique approach to the treatment of unstable angina. Experience is currently limited, but nearly all studies to date demonstrate benefit (Nakamura and Koiwaya, 1979; Hugenholtz et al., 1981). These agents may be particularly effective if the underlying mechanism is vasospasm with S-T segment elevation (Nakamura and Koiwaya, 1979). However, there is insufficient evidence to assess whether such treatment actually improves morbidity or mortality. By contrast, therapy directed toward reduction of platelet function and thrombotic episodes does appear to decrease morbidity and mortality in patients with unstable angina (see Chapters 29 and 58).

Other Uses. The use of calcium channel blockers as antiarrhythmic agents is discussed in Chapter 31, and their use for the treatment of hypertension is discussed in Chapter 32.

β-ADRENERGIC ANTAGONISTS

The β-adrenergic antagonists are effective in reducing the severity and frequency of attacks of exertional angina. In contrast, these agents are not useful for vasospastic angina and may, on occasion, worsen the condition. This deleterious effect is likely due to an increase in coronary resistance caused by the unopposed effects of catecholamines acting at α-adrenergic receptors. Although propranolol has been the agent evaluated most extensively in the treatment of angina, all β-adrenergic antagonists appear to be equally effective in the treatment of exertional angina (Thadani et al., 1980). The effectiveness of β-adrenergic antagonists in the treatment of exertional angina is attributable to a fall in myocardial oxygen consumption at rest and during exertion (Hamer and Sowton, 1966; Elliott and Stone, 1969). The decrease in myocardial oxygen consumption is due to a negative chronotropic effect (particularly during exercise) and to a negative inotropic effect. While β-adrenergic antagonists increase total peripheral resistance by blocking vascular receptors in skeletal muscles that mediate vasodilatation, arterial pressure falls due to the decrease in heart rate and myocardial contractility. Not all of the actions of propranolol are beneficial. The decrease in heart rate and contractility causes an increase in the systolic ejection period and an increase in left ventricular end-diastolic volume; this tends to increase oxygen consumption (Parker et al., 1968). However, the net effect of β-adrenergic blockade is usually to decrease myocardial oxygen consumption, particularly during exercise. Nevertheless, in patients with limited cardiac reserve who are critically dependent on adrenergic stimulation, β-adrenergic blockade can result in profound decreases in left ventricular function.

Currently there are six β-adrenergic blocking agents approved for clinical use in the United States. For a detailed consideration of these agents, see Chapter 9.

COMBINATION THERAPY

Since nitrates, calcium channel blockers, and β-adrenergic antagonists are each useful in the treatment of exertional angina and reduce oxygen consumption by different means, concurrent therapy has been advocated.

Nitrates and β-Adrenergic Antagonists. The concurrent use of organic nitrates and β-adrenergic antagonists can be very effective in the treatment of typical exertional angina. The additive efficacy is primarily a result of one drug blocking the adverse effects of the other agent on net myocardial oxygen consumption. β-Adrenergic antagonists can block the reflex tachycardia and positive inotropic effects that are sometimes associated with nitrates. Nitrates can attenuate the increase in left ventricular end-diastolic volume associated with β-adrenergic blockade by increasing venous capacitance. β-Adrenergic antagonists may also increase coronary vascular resistance, and this too may be alleviated in part by concurrent administration of nitrates.

Calcium Channel Blockers and β-Adrenergic Antagonists. In patients with exertional angina that is not controlled adequately with nitrates and β-adrenergic antagonists, the administration of a calcium channel blocker can provide improvement. Most studies to date have evaluated the combined use of nifedipine and a β-adrenergic blocker since the latter agent will attenuate the reflex increase in heart rate caused by nifedipine. During exercise, the combined use of propranolol and nifedipine results in a lower heart rate and blood pressure than are observed with either agent alone. As mentioned above, nifedipine does not depress the S-A node, A-V nodal conduction, or ventricular inotropy *in vivo* and, therefore, does not enhance the adverse effects of propranolol. However, close monitoring is required during adjustment of dosage, since severe hypotension may ensue. Verapamil and diltiazem should be used cautiously, if at all, if a β-adrenergic blocking agent is being taken concurrently. Verapamil or diltiazem must not be administered intravenously under such circumstances.

Calcium Channel Blockers and Nitrates. In severe vasospastic or exertional angina, the combination of a nitrate and a calcium channel blocker may provide additional relief over that obtained with either type of agent alone. Since nitrates reduce preload whereas calcium channel blockers reduce afterload, the net effect on reduction of oxygen demand should be additive. However, excessive vasodilatation can occur. The concurrent administration of a nitrate and nifedipine has been advocated in particular for patients with exertional angina with heart failure, the sick sinus syndrome, or atrioventricular conduction disturbances. The combined use of a calcium channel blocker and β-adrenergic antagonist would not be appropriate in such situations.

Calcium Channel Blockers, β-Adrenergic Antagonists, and Nitrates. In patients with exertional angina that is not controlled by the administration of two types of antianginal agents, the use of all three may provide improvement. Nifedipine decreases afterload, nitrates decrease preload, and β-adrenergic antagonists decrease heart rate and myocardial contractility. Only nifedipine (and *not* verapamil or diltiazem) should be used in conjunction with a β-adrenergic antagonist under these circumstances.

DIPYRIDAMOLE

Dipyridamole (2,6-*bis*-[diethanolamino]-4,8-dipiperidinopyrimido-[5,4-*d*]-pyrimidine) is similar to papaverine in many of its pharmacological properties (*see* below). In therapeutic doses, dipyridamole usually produces only slight alteration of systemic blood pressure or peripheral blood flow. The drug does decrease coronary vascular resistance and increases coronary blood flow and oxygen tension in coronary sinus blood. However, dipyridamole appears to act predominantly on small resistance vessels of the coronary bed, and it alters transcapillary exchange in the same way as does severe hypoxemia. Thus, it appears to have little effect on vascular resistance in ischemic areas where small vessels are already maximally dilated.

The actions of dipyridamole seem to be linked, at least in part, to the metabolism and transport of adenosine and adenine nucleotides; in particular, dipyridamole inhibits the uptake of adenosine by erythrocytes and other cells. Adenosine, which is released from the hypoxic myocardium, is a coronary vasodilator and appears to be an important signal for the autoregulation of coronary blood flow.

In the doses usually employed clinically, dipyridamole is quite nontoxic. Gastrointestinal intolerance with nausea, vomiting, and diarrhea occurs occasionally, as do headache and vertigo. Excessive doses can cause peripheral vasodilatation and hypotension.

Dipyridamole has been used predominantly for the prophylaxis of *angina pectoris*. Although many conflicting observations have been reported, there is no convincing evidence that either acute or chronic administration decreases the frequency or severity of anginal attacks. There is no improvement of performance during standardized exercise tolerance tests. The effects of dipyridamole on platelets are described in Chapter 58.

Dipyridamole (PERSANTINE) is available in tablets. The usual dosage is 50 mg three times daily, taken at least 1 hour before meals.

VASODILATORS IN THE TREATMENT OF VASCULAR INSUFFICIENCY

Vasodilator drugs have been used in an attempt to increase peripheral blood flow to areas where perfusion is compromised by acute or chronic arterial obstruction or vasospasm. The drugs that have been used can be divided into agents that interfere with adrenergically mediated vasoconstriction (Chapter 9) and drugs that directly dilate vascular smooth muscle, such as *papaverine, isoxsuprine, nylidrin, cyclandelate,* and *niacin derivatives.* The pharmacological properties of this latter group are described briefly below and in more detail in *earlier editions* of this textbook.

Despite the fact that these drugs continue to be promoted and widely prescribed for the treatment of chronic occlusive vascular diseases of skeletal muscle (arteriosclerosis obliterans, thromboangiitis obliterans), there is no acceptable evidence that they are efficacious (Medical Letter, 1978; Coffman, 1979). Likewise, the utility of vasodilators in reversing or delaying the deleterious effects of acute or chronic cerebrovascular insufficiency is controversial, and the case for clinical efficacy is unimpressive. Direct-acting vasodilators can increase blood flow in normal resting skeletal muscle and in brain. However, it is unlikely that any vasodilator drug can significantly increase blood flow distal to a physical occlusion. Autoregulatory mechanisms in skeletal muscle and cerebral vascular beds produce dilatation in response to ischemia; hence vasodilators will increase blood flow primarily to nonischemic areas.

Vasospastic conditions affecting cutaneous circulation (*e.g.*, Raynaud's syndrome) may be responsive to α-adrenergic antagonists, but drug therapy is usually reserved for the most severe cases.

Papaverine. Papaverine (6,7-dimethoxy-1-veratrylisoquinoline) is an alkaloid present to the extent of about 1% in crude opium. It is, however, unrelated chemically or pharmacologically to the opioid alkaloids. Papaverine is a nonspecific smooth muscle relaxant. It has been suggested that vasodilatation is related to its ability to inhibit cyclic nucleotide phosphodiesterase, an action for which it has been widely used as an experimental tool. Papaverine is capable of producing arteriolar dilatation in the systemic, coronary, and cerebral circulations. Large doses can depress A-V nodal and intraventricular conduction and produce arrhythmias. These direct effects on the myocardium are seen only after parenteral administration of high doses. Papaverine has not been demonstrated to be of therapeutic value in any condition. Furthermore, at least some of the widely promoted sustained-release preparations produce very low and erratic concentrations in blood when compared to conventional preparations. Side effects associated with the use of papaverine include facial flushing, tachycardia, drowsiness, and gastrointestinal symptoms. Papaverine also frequently causes elevation of the activities of alkaline phosphatase and transaminases in plasma, indicative of hepatic toxicity.

Papaverine hydrochloride is marketed in a large number of preparations. Despite lack of proof of efficacy, the compound is sold by more than 20 pharmaceutical companies. *Dioxyline phosphate* is a synthetic derivative of papaverine; *ethaverine* is also closely related to papaverine and has similar actions.

Cyclandelate. *Cyclandelate* (3,3,5-trimethylcyclohexyl mandelate) is a musculotropic vasodilator; although quite different chemically, it appears to exert actions similar to those of papaverine. However, its pharmacological properties are scantily characterized. Cyclandelate appears to be a more potent vasodilator *in vitro* than is papaverine. As with the other vasodilators, reports in the literature are contradictory, and the therapeutic value of cyclandelate has never been convincingly demonstrated for any condition.

Cyclandelate is available in tablets and capsules. Side effects include flushing, tachycardia, headache, a feeling of weakness, and gastrointestinal symptoms.

Isoxsuprine. Isoxsuprine is similar chemically to the sympathomimetic amines and has often been described as a β-adrenergic agonist. However, the drug appears to act as a musculotropic vasodilator, and its effects are not blocked by propranolol (Manley and Lawson, 1968). Objective studies do not support the use of this drug in obstructive arterial disease or in any other condition.

Isoxsuprine hydrochloride is available in tablets and as an injection. Side effects include hypotension, tachycardia, nausea, vomiting, dizziness, abdominal distress, and severe rash.

Nylidrin. The vasodilator activity of this compound appears to be a combination of direct musculotropic and β-adrenergic agonistic activity. It has been and is used in a variety of vascular disorders without proof of efficacy. Side effects include dizziness, weakness, palpitations, trembling, nervousness, and vomiting. *Nylidrin hydrochloride* is available in tablets.

Nicotinic Acid and Nicotinyl Alcohol. These drugs (*see* Chapters 34 and 66) produce more dilatation of the vessels of the blush areas than of the extremities. There is no consistent increase in skin or muscle blood flow in patients with obstructive vascular disease. There is no basis for the use of these agents in such conditions, despite their promotion for this purpose.

Abrams, J. Nitrate tolerance and dependence. *Am. Heart J.*, **1980**, *99*, 113–123.

——. Nitroglycerin and long-acting nitrates in clinical practice. *Am. J. Med.*, **1983**, *74*, Suppl., 85–94.

Antman, E., and others. Nifedipine therapy for coronary-artery spasm: experience in 127 patients. *N. Engl. J. Med.*, **1980a**, *302*, 1269–1273.

Bassan, M.; Weiler-Raveil, D.; and Shalev, O. The additive anti-anginal action of oral nifedipine in patients receiving propranolol. *Circulation*, **1982**, *66*, 710–716.

Becker, L. C.; Fortuin, N. J.; and Pitt, B. Effect of ischemia and antianginal drugs on the distribution of radioactive microspheres in the canine left ventricle. *Circ. Res.*, **1971**, *28*, 263–269.

Bolton, T. B. Mechanisms of action of transmitters and other substances on smooth muscle. *Physiol. Rev.*, **1979**, *59*, 606–718.

Brown, B. G.; Bolson, E.; Petersen, R. B.; Pierce, C. D.; and Dodge, H. T. The mechanism of nitroglycerin action: stenosis vasodilation as a major component of the drug response. *Circulation*, **1981**, *64*, 1089–1097.

Capurro, N. L.; Kent, K. M.; and Epstein, S. E. Comparison of nitroglycerin-, nitroprusside-, and phentolamine-induced changes in coronary collateral function in dogs. *J. Clin. Invest.*, **1977**, *60*, 295–301.

Chew, C. Y. C.; Hecht, H. S.; Collett, J. T.; McAllister, R. G.; and Singh, B. N. Influence of severity of ventricular dysfunction on hemodynamic responses to intravenously administered verapamil in ischemic heart disease. *Am J. Cardiol.*, **1981**, *47*, 917–922.

Chiariello, M.; Gold, H. K.; Leinbach, R. C.; Davis, M. A.; and Maroko, P. R. Comparison between the effects of nitroprusside and nitroglycerin on ischemic injury during acute myocardial ischemia. *Circulation*, **1976**, *54*, 766–773.

Cohen, M. V., and Kirk, E. S. Differential response of large and small coronary arteries to nitroglycerin and angiotensin: autoregulation and tachyphylaxis. *Circ. Res.*, 1973, *33*, 445–453.

Commarato, M. A.; Winbury, M. M.; and Kaplan, H. R. Glyceryl trinitrate and pentrinitrol (pentaerythritol trinitrate); comparative cardiovascular effects in dog, cat and rat by different routes of administration. *J. Pharmacol. Exp. Ther.*, 1973, *187*, 300–307.

Coraboeuf, E. Ionic basis of electrical activity in cardiac tissues. *Am. J. Physiol.*, 1978, *234*, H101–H116.

Danahy, D. T.; Burwell, D. T.; Aronow, W. S.; and Prakash, R. Sustained hemodynamic and antianginal effect of high dose oral isosorbide dinitrate. *Circulation,* 1977, *55*, 382–387.

Ehara, T., and Kaufmann, R. The voltage- and time-dependent effects of (-)-verapamil on the slow inward current in isolated cat ventricular myocardium. *J. Pharmacol. Exp. Ther.*, 1978, *207*, 49–55.

Elliott, W. C., and Stone, J. M. Beta-adrenergic blocking agents for the treatment of angina pectoris. *Prog. Cardiovasc. Dis.*, 1969, *12*, 83–92.

Epstein, S. E.; Kent, K. M.; Goldstein, R. E.; Borer, J. S.; and Redwood, D. R. Reduction of ischemic injury by nitroglycerin during acute myocardial infarction. *N. Engl. J. Med.*, 1975, *292*, 29–35.

Feldman, R. L.; Pepine, C. J.; and Conti, C. R. Magnitude of dilation of large and small coronary arteries by nitroglycerin. *Circulation,* 1981, *64*, 324–333.

Ferrer, M. I.; Bradley, S. E.; Wheeler, H. O.; Enson, Y.; Preiseg, R.; Brickner, P. W.; Conroy, R. J.; and Harvey, R. M. Some effects of nitroglycerin upon the splanchnic, pulmonary, and systemic circulations. *Circulation,* 1966, *33*, 357–373.

Fleckenstein, J. A.; Kammermeier, H.; Doring, H.; and Freund, H. J. Zum Wirkungs—Mechanismus neuartiger Koronardilalatoren mit gleichzeitig Sauerstoff—einsparenden, myokard—Effekten. Prenylamin und Iproveratril. *Z. Kreislaufforsch,* 1967, *56*, 716–744, 839–853.

Franciosa, J. A.; Limas, C. J.; Guiha, N. H.; Rodriguera, E.; and Cohn, J. N. Improved left ventricular function during nitroprusside infusion in acute myocardial infarction. *Lancet,* 1972, *1*, 650–654.

Franciosa, J. A.; Mikulic, E.; Cohn, J. N.; Jose, E.; and Fabie, A. Hemodynamic effects of orally administered isosorbide dinitrate in patients with congestive heart failure. *Circulation,* 1974, *50*, 1020–1024.

Ganz, W., and Marcus, H. S. Failure of intracoronary nitroglycerin to alleviate pacing-induced angina. *Circulation,* 1972, *46*, 880–889.

Goldstein, R. E.; Douglas, M. D.; Rosing, M. D.; Redwood, D. R.; Beiser, G. D.; and Epstein, S. E. Clinical and circulatory effects of isosorbide dinitrate. Comparison with nitroglycerin. *Circulation,* 1971, *43*, 629–640.

Gorlin, R.; Brachfield, N.; MacLeod, C.; and Bopp, P. Effect of nitroglycerin on the coronary circulation in patients with coronary artery disease or increased left ventricular work. *Circulation,* 1959, *19*, 705–718.

Hamer, J., and Sowton, E. Effects of propranolol on exercise tolerance in angina pectoris. *Am. J. Cardiol.,* 1966, *18*, 354–363.

Hecht, H. S.; Chew, C. Y. C.; Burnam, M. H.; Hopkins, J.; Schnugg, S.; and Singh, B. N. Verapamil in chronic stable angina: amelioration of pacing-induced abnormalities of left ventricular ejection fraction, regional wall motion, lactate metabolism and hemodynamics. *Am. J. Cardiol.,* 1981, *50*, 536–544.

Horwitz, L. D.; Gorlin, R.; Taylor, W. J.; and Kemp, H. G. Effects of nitroglycerin on regional myocardial blood flow in coronary artery disease. *J. Clin. Invest.,* 1971, *50*, 1578–1584.

Hugenholtz, P. G.; Michels, H. R.; Serruys, P. W.; and Brower, R. W. Nifedipine in the treatment of unstable angina, coronary spasm and myocardial ischemia. *Am. J. Cardiol.,* 1981, *47*, 163–173.

Jaffe, A. S., and Roberts, R. The use of intravenous nitroglycerin in cardiovascular disease. *Pharmacotherapy,* 1982, *2*, 273–280.

Johnson, E. M., Jr.; Harkey, A. B.; Blehm, D. J.; and Needleman, P. Clearance and metabolism of organic nitrates. *J. Pharmacol. Exp. Ther.*, 1972, *182*, 56–62.

Kates, R. E.; Keefe, D. L. D.; Schwartz, J.; Harapat, S.; Kirsten, E. B.; and Harrison, D. C. Verapamil disposition kinetics in chronic atrial fibrillation. *Clin. Pharmacol. Ther.*, 1981, *30*, 44–51.

Kimura, E., and Kishida, H. Treatment of variant angina with drugs: a survey of 11 cardiology institutes in Japan. *Circulation,* 1981, *63*, 844–848.

Kohlhardt, M.; Bauer, B.; Krause, H.; and Fleckenstein, A. Differentiation of the transmembrane Na and Ca channels in mammalian cardiac fibres by the use of specific inhibitors. *Pflugers Arch.,* 1972, *335*, 309–322.

Kohlhardt, M., and Fleckenstein, A. Inhibition of the slow inward current by nifedipine in mammalian ventricular myocardium. *Naunyn Schmiedebergs Arch. Pharmacol.,* 1977, *298*, 267–272.

Ludbrook, P. A.; Tiefenbrunn, A. J.; Reed, F. A.; and Sobel, B. E. Acute hemodynamic responses to sublingual nifedipine: dependence on left ventricular function. *Circulation,* 1982, *65*, 489–498.

Manley, E. S., and Lawson, J. W. Effect of beta adrenergic receptor blockade on skeletal muscle vasodilation produced by isoxsuprine and nylidrin. *Arch. Int. Pharmacodyn. Ther.,* 1968, *175*, 239–250.

Medical Letter. Drugs for ischemic peripheral arterial disease. 1978, *20*, 11.

Moskowitz, R. M.; Piccini, P. A.; Nacarelli, G.; and Zelis, R. Nifedipine therapy for stable angina pectoris: preliminary results of effects on angina frequency and treadmill exercise response. *Am. J. Cardiol.,* 1979, *44*, 811–816.

Multicenter Study. Unstable angina pectoris: national cooperative study group to compare surgical and medical therapy. II. In-hospital experience and initial follow-up results in patients with one, two, and three vessel disease. *Am. J. Cardiol.,* 1978, *42*, 839–848.

Nakamura, M., and Koiwaya, Y. Beneficial effect of diltiazem, a new antianginal drug, on angina pectoris at rest. *Jpn. Heart J.,* 1979, *20*, 613–621.

Needleman, P.; Lang, S.; and Johnson, E. M., Jr. Organic nitrates: relationship between biotransformation and rational angina pectoris therapy. *J. Pharmacol. Exp. Ther.,* 1972, *181*, 489–497.

Neumann, M., and Luisada, A. A. Double blind evaluation of orally administered iproveratril in patients with angina pectoris. *Am J. Med. Sci.,* 1966, *251*, 552–556.

Ono, H., and Hashimoto, K. *In vitro* tissue effects of calcium flux inhibition. In, *Calcium Channel Blocking Agents in the Treatment of Cardiovascular Disorders.* (Stone, P. H., and Antman, E. M., eds.) Futura Publishing Co., Mount Kisco, N.Y., 1983, pp. 155–175.

Packer, M.; Meller, J.; Medina, N.; Gorlin, R.; and Herman, M. V. Rebound hemodynamic events after the abrupt withdrawal of nitroprusside in patients with severe chronic heart failure. *N. Engl. J. Med.,* 1979, *301*, 1193–1197.

Parker, J. C.; Di Carlo, F. J.; and Davidson, I. W. F. Comparative vasodilator effects of nitroglycerin, pentaerythritol trinitrate and biometabolites, and other organic nitrates. *Eur. J. Pharmacol.,* 1975, *31*, 29–37.

Parker, J. O.; Case, R. B.; Khaja, F.; Ledwich, J. R.; and Armstrong, P. W. The influence of changes in blood volume on angina pectoris: a study of the effect of phlebotomy. *Circulation,* 1970, *16*, 593–604.

Parker, J. O.; West, R. O.; and Digiorgi, S. Hemodynamic effects of propranolol in coronary heart disease. *Am. J. Cardiol.,* 1968, *21*, 11–19.

Rapaport, R. M.; Draznin, M. B.; and Murad, F. Endothelium-dependent vasodilator- and nitrovasodilator-induced relaxation may be mediated through cyclic GMP formation and cyclic GMP–dependent protein phosphorylation. *Trans. Assoc. Am. Physicians*, **1983**, *96*, 19–30.

Reichek, N.; Goldstein, R. E.; and Redwood, D. R. Sustained effects of nitroglycerin ointment in patients with angina pectoris. *Circulation*, **1974**, *50*, 348–352.

Roberts, R. Intravenous nitroglycerin in acute myocardial infarction. *Am. J. Med.*, **1983**, *74*, Suppl., 45–52.

Robinson, B. F.; Dobbs, R. J.; and Kelsey, C. R. Effects of nifedipine on resistance vessels, arteries and veins in man. *Br. J. Clin. Pharmacol.*, **1980**, *10*, 433–438.

Rougier, O.; Vossort, G.; Garnier, D.; Gargouil, Y. M.; and Coraboeuf, E. Existence and role of a slow inward current during the frog atrial action potential. *Pflugers Arch.*, **1969**, *308*, 91–110.

Rouleau, J.-L.; Chatterjee, K.; Ports, T. A.; Doyle, M. B.; Hiramatsu, B.; and Parmley, W. W. Mechanism of relief of pacing-induced angina with oral verapamil: reduced oxygen demand. *Circulation*, **1983**, *67*, 94–100.

Schwartz, J. B.; Keefe, D.; Kates, R. E.; Kirsten, E. B.; and Harrison, D. C. Acute and chronic pharmacodynamic interaction of verapamil and digoxin in atrial fibrillation. *Circulation*, **1982**, *65*, 1163–1170.

Serruys, P. W.; Brower, R. W.; Ten Katen, H. J.; Bom, A. H.; and Hugenholtz, P. G. Regional wall motion from radiopaque markers after intravenous and intracoronary injections of nifedipine. *Circulation*, **1981**, *63*, 584–591.

Severi, S.; Davies, G.; Maseri, A.; Marzullo, P.; and L'Abbate, A. Long-term prognosis of "variant" angina with medical treatment. *Am. J. Cardiol.*, **1980**, *46*, 223–232.

Shane, S. J.; Iazzetta, J. J.; Chisholm, A. W.; Berka, J. F.; and Leung, D. Plasma concentrations of isosorbide dinitrate and its metabolites after chronic oral dosage in man. *Br. J. Clin. Pharmacol.*, **1978**, *6*, 37–41.

Singh, B. N., and Roche, A. H. G. Effects of intravenous verapamil on hemodynamics in patients with heart disease. *Am. Heart J.*, **1977**, *94*, 593–599.

Somlyo, A. V., and Somlyo, A. P. Electromechanical and pharmacomechanical coupling in vascular smooth muscle. *J. Pharmacol. Exp. Ther.*, **1968**, *159*, 129–145.

Somogyi, A.; Albrecht, M.; Kliems, G.; Shafer, K.; and Eichelbaum, M. Pharmacokinetics, bioavailability and ECG response of verapamil in patients with liver cirrhosis. *Br. J. Clin. Pharmacol.*, **1981**, *12*, 51–60.

Stine, A. A., and Fink, G. B. Prophylactic therapy of angina pectoris with organic nitrates: relationship of drug efficacy and clinical experimental design. *J. Clin. Pharmacol.*, **1973**, *13*, 244–250.

Strauer, B. E., and Scherpe, A. Ventricular function and coronary hemodynamics after intravenous nitroglycerin in coronary artery disease. *Am. Heart J.*, **1978**, *95*, 210–219.

Thadani, U.; Davidson, C.; Singleton, W.; and Taylor, S. H. Comparison of five beta-adrenoreceptor antagonists with different ancillary properties during sustained twice daily therapy in angina pectoris. *Am. J. Med.*, **1980**, *68*, 243–250.

Theroux, P.; Waters, D. D.; DeBaisieux, J. C.; Szlachcic, J.; Mizgala, H. F.; and Bourassa, M. G. Hemodynamic effects of calcium ion antagonists after acute myocardial infarction. *Clin. Invest. Med.*, **1980**, *3*, 81–85.

Wagniart, P.; Ferguson, R. J.; Chaitmann, B. R.; Achard, F.; Benacerraf, A.; Delanguenhagen, B.; Morin, B.; Pasternac, A.; and Bourassa, M. G. Increased exercise tolerance and reduced electrocardiographic ischemia with diltiazem in patients with stable angina pectoris. *Circulation*, **1982**, *66*, 23–28.

Waters, D. D.; Theroux, P.; Szlachcic, J.; and Dauwe, F. Provocative testing with ergonovine to assess the efficacy of treatment with nifedipine, diltiazem and verapamil in variant angina. *Am. J. Cardiol.*, **1981**, *48*, 123–130.

Wendt, R. L. Systemic and coronary vascular effects of the 2- and the 5-mononitrate esters of isosorbide. *J. Pharmacol. Exp. Ther.*, **1972**, *180*, 732–742.

Winbury, M. M.; Howe, B. B.; and Weiss, H. R. Effect of nitroglycerin and dipyridamole on epicardial and endocardial oxygen tension—further evidence for redistribution of myocardial blood flow. *J. Pharmacol. Exp. Ther.*, **1971**, *176*, 184–199.

Winsor, T., and Berger, H. J. Oral nitroglycerin as a prophylactic antianginal drug: clinical, physiologic, and statistical evidence of efficacy based on a three-phase experimental design. *Am. Heart J.*, **1975**, *90*, 611–626.

Yap, P. S. K., and Fung, H. L. Pharmacokinetics of nitroglycerin in rats. *J. Pharm. Sci.*, **1978**, *67*, 584–586.

Yasue, H.; Omote, S.; Takizowa, A.; Nagao, M.; Miwa, K.; and Tanaka, S. Circadian variation of exercise capacity in patients with Prinzmetal's variant angina: role of exercise-induced coronary arterial spasm. *Circulation*, **1979**, *59*, 938–948.

Zelis, R., and Mason, D. T. Isosorbide dinitrate. Effect on the vasodilator response to nitroglycerin. *J.A.M.A.*, **1975**, *234*, 166–170.

Monographs and Reviews

Antman, E. M.; Stone, P. H.; Muller, J. E.; and Braunwald, E. Calcium channel blocking agents in the treatment of cardiovascular disorders. Part I: Basic and clinical electrophysiologic effects. *Ann. Intern. Med.*, **1980b**, *93*, 875–885.

Chatterjee, K., and Parmley, W. W. The role of vasodilator therapy in heart failure. *Prog. Cardiovasc. Dis.*, **1977**, *19*, 301–325.

Coffman, J. D. Vasodilator drugs in peripheral vascular disease. *N. Engl. J. Med.*, **1979**, *300*, 713–717.

Di Carlo, F. J. Nitroglycerin revisited: chemistry, biochemistry, interactions. *Drug Metab. Rev.*, **1975**, *4*, 1–38.

Henry, P. D. Mechanisms of action of calcium antagonists in cardiac and smooth muscle. In, *Calcium Channel Blocking Agents in the Treatment of Cardiovascular Disorders.* (Stone, P. H., and Antman, E. M., eds.) Futura Publishing Co., Mount Kisco, N.Y., **1983**, pp. 107–154.

Johnson, E. M., Jr. Chemistry of organic nitrates. In, *Organic Nitrates.* (Needleman, P., ed.) *Handbuch der Experimentellen Pharmakologie*, Vol. 40. Springer-Verlag, Berlin, **1975**, pp. 16–23.

Krantz, J. C., Jr. Historical background. In, *Organic Nitrates.* (Needleman, P., ed.) *Handbuch der Experimentellen Pharmakologie*, Vol. 40. Springer-Verlag, Berlin, **1975**, pp. 1–12.

Mittal, C. K., and Murad, F. Guanylate cyclase: regulation of cyclic GMP metabolism. In, *Cyclic Nucleotides.* (Nathanson, J. A., and Kebabian, J. W., eds.) *Handbook of Experimental Pharmacology*, Vol. 58. Springer-Verlag, Berlin, **1982**, pp. 225–260.

Murad, F.; Arnold, W. P.; Mittal, C. K.; and Braughler, J. M. Properties and regulation of guanylate cyclase and some proposed functions for cyclic GMP. *Adv. Cyclic Nucleotide Res.*, **1979**, *11*, 175–204.

Needleman, P. Biotransformation of organic nitrates. In, *Organic Nitrates.* (Needleman, P., ed.) *Handbuch der Experimentellen Pharmakologie*, Vol. 40. Springer-Verlag, Berlin, **1975**, pp. 57–96.

Needleman, P., and Johnson, E. M., Jr. The pharmacological and biochemical interaction of organic nitrates with sulfhydryls. In, *Organic Nitrates.* (Needleman, P., ed.) *Handbuch der Experimentellen Pharmakologie,* Vol. 40. Springer-Verlag, Berlin, **1975,** pp. 97–114.

Opie, L. H. (ed.). *Calcium Antagonists and Cardiovascular Disease.* Vol. 6, *Perspectives in Cardiovascular Research.* Raven Press, New York, **1984.**

Packer, M. Selection of vasodilator drugs for patients with severe chronic heart failure: an approach based on a new classification system. *Drugs,* **1982,** *24,* 64–74.

Parratt, J. R. Nitroglycerin—the first one hundred years: new facts about an old drug. *J. Pharm. Pharmacol.,* **1979,** *31,* 801–809.

Rapaport, R. M., and Murad, F. Endothelium-dependent and nitrovasodilator-induced relaxation of vascular smooth muscle: role for cyclic GMP. *J. Cyclic Nucleotide Protein Phosphorylation Res.,* **1983,** *9,* 281–296.

Ross, J. Afterload mismatch and preload reserve: a conceptual framework for the analysis of ventricular function. *Prog. Cardiovasc. Dis.,* **1976,** *18,* 255–264.

Stone, P. H., and Antman, E. M. (eds.). *Calcium Channel Blocking Agents in the Treatment of Cardiovascular Disorders.* Futura Publishing Co., Mount Kisco, N. Y., **1983.**

Stone, P. H.; Antman, E. M.; Muller, J. E.; and Braunwald, E. Calcium channel blocking agents in the treatment of cardiovascular disorders. Part II: Hemodynamic effects and clinical applications. *Ann. Intern. Med.,* **1980,** *93,* 886–904.

Symposium. (Various authors.) Vasodilator and inotropic therapy of heart failure. (Mason, D. T., ed.) *Am. J. Med.,* **1978,** *62,* 101–216.

Symposium. (Various authors.) First North American conference on nitroglycerin therapy: perspectives and mechanisms. (Abrams, J., and Roberts, R., eds.) *Am. J. Med.,* **1983,** *74,* 1–93.

Symposium. (Various authors.) Second North American conference on nitroglycerin: perspectives and mechanisms. (Roberts, R., ed.) *Am. J. Med.,* **1984,** *76,* 1–83.

Warren, S. E., and Francis, G. S. Nitroglycerin and nitrate esters. *Am. J. Med.,* **1978,** *65,* 53–62.

34 DRUGS USED IN THE TREATMENT OF HYPERLIPOPROTEINEMIAS

Michael S. Brown and Joseph L. Goldstein

The *hyperlipoproteinemias* are conditions in which the concentration of cholesterol- or triglyceride-carrying lipoproteins in plasma exceeds an arbitrary normal limit, typically defined as the ninety-fifth percentile of a random population. Clinical concern arises because an elevated concentration of lipoproteins can accelerate the development of atherosclerosis, with its dual sequelae of thrombosis and infarction. About half of the deaths in the United States are a result of such events. Recent clinical evidence strongly suggests that reduction of the concentration of lipoproteins in plasma can diminish the increased risk of atherosclerosis that accompanies hyperlipoproteinemia. Therapy is thus recommended, particularly for individuals with a family history of premature atherosclerosis. Certain types of hypertriglyceridemia can also cause life-threatening pancreatitis, and in this case a reduction of lipoprotein concentrations has clearly been shown to be beneficial.

NORMAL PATHWAYS OF LIPOPROTEIN TRANSPORT

Plasma cholesterol and triglyccrides are transported in lipoproteins, which are large, globular particles that contain an oily core of nonpolar lipid (cholesteryl esters or triglycerides) surrounded by a polar coat of phospholipids, free (*i.e.*, unesterified) cholesterol, and apoproteins. There are six classes of lipoproteins that differ from one another in size and density, in the relative proportions of triglycerides and cholesteryl esters in the core, and in the nature of the apoproteins on the surface (Table 34–1). Each class of lipoproteins has a specific tissue (or tissues) of origin and catabolism, and each plays a defined role in the transport of lipids. The pathway for transport of lipoproteins, shown schematically in Figure 34–1, can be divided into two components: one for transport of exogenous lipids (*i.e.*, lipids that enter the circulation from the intestine) and another for the transport of endogenous lipids (*i.e.*, lipids that enter the circulation from the liver and tissues other than the intestine) (Havel *et al.*, 1980; Brown *et al.*, 1981; Goldstein *et al.*, 1983).

Exogenous Pathway. Exogenous lipid transport begins with intestinal incorporation of dietary triglycerides and cholesterol into large lipoprotein particles called *chylomicrons* (diameter, 80 to 500 nm), which are secreted into the lymph and subsequently enter the blood stream. When chylomicrons reach the capillaries of adipose tissue and muscle, they are digested by an enzyme, lipoprotein lipase, that is bound to the surface of the endothelial cells. Lipoprotein lipase hydrolyzes the triglycerides in the core of the chylomicrons, and the liberated fatty acids cross the endothelium and enter the underlying adipocytes or muscle cells; they are then either esterified again to form triglycerides for storage or oxidized to provide energy.

After most of the triglycerides have been removed in this fashion, the chylomicron dissociates from the capillary endothelium and enters the circulation again. Its size has been reduced and its content of triglycerides diminished, but its cholesteryl esters remain intact. The particle is now designated as a *chylomicron remnant* (diameter, 30 to 50 nm). When the remnant reaches the liver, it is cleared from the circulation by a receptor that recognizes two protein components of the chylomicron remnant, apoproteins E and B-48. The receptor-bound remnant is taken into the hepatic cell by a process termed *receptor-mediated endocytosis*. Within the cell the remnant is digested in lysosomes, and the cholesteryl esters are cleaved to generate free cholesterol. The free cholesterol has several fates: it can be used for membrane synthesis, it can be stored by the liver cell as cholesteryl esters, it can be excreted into the bile either as cholesterol or after conversion to bile acids, or it can be used to form endogenous lipoproteins that are secreted into plasma.

Endogenous Pathway. Endogenous lipid transport begins when the liver secretes triglycerides and cholesterol into the plasma in *very-low-density lipoproteins* (VLDL; diameter, 30 to 80 nm). The

Table 34–1.   **CHARACTERISTICS OF THE MAJOR CLASSES OF LIPOPROTEINS
IN HUMAN PLASMA**

LIPOPROTEIN CLASS *	MAJOR CORE LIPIDS	MAJOR APOPROTEINS	ORIGIN OF APOPROTEINS	TRANSPORT FUNCTION	MECHANISM OF LIPID DELIVERY
Chylomicrons	Dietary trigly-cerides	A-1, A-2, A-4, B-48	Small intestine	Dietary triglyceride	Hydrolysis by lipoprotein lipase
Chylomicron remnants	Dietary cholesteryl esters	B-48, E	Chylomicrons	Dietary cholesterol	Receptor-mediated endocytosis in liver
VLDL	Endogenous triglycerides	B-100, C, E	Liver and small intestine	Endogenous triglyceride	Hydrolysis by lipoprotein lipase
IDL	Endogenous cholesteryl esters and triglycerides	B-100, E	VLDL	Endogenous cholesterol	Receptor-mediated endocytosis in liver (50%) or conversion to LDL (50%)
LDL	Endogenous cholesteryl esters	B-100	IDL	Endogenous cholesterol	Receptor-mediated endocytosis in liver or extrahepatic tissues
HDL	Endogenous cholesteryl esters	A-1, A-2	Liver and small intestine	Facilitates removal of cholesterol from extrahepatic tissues	Cholesteryl ester transfer to IDL and LDL

* VLDL denotes very-low-density lipoprotein; IDL, intermediate-density lipoprotein; LDL, low-density lipoprotein; HDL, high-density lipoprotein.

major stimulus for such secretion is a high-calorie intake (especially a high-carbohydrate intake), which induces the liver to assemble triglycerides for export and storage in adipose tissue. The triglycerides of VLDL are cleaved in capillaries by the same lipoprotein lipase that digests chylomicrons. Digestion produces a VLDL remnant (analogous to the chylomicron remnant) that is designated as *intermediate-density lipoprotein* (IDL; diameter, 25 to 35 nm). After release from the endothelium, the IDL particles have two metabolic fates. Some of the particles are cleared rapidly by the liver, again by receptor-mediated endocytosis. The receptor that acts on the IDL particle is called the *low-density lipoprotein* (LDL) receptor. It binds lipoproteins that contain apoprotein E or B-100, and it therefore interacts with both IDL and LDL particles (*see* below).

About half of the IDL particles are not cleared rapidly by the liver. Rather, they remain in the circulation, where most of the remaining triglycerides are removed, and the density of the particle increases further, until it becomes LDL (diameter, 18 to 28 nm). LDL circulates for a relatively long time in man (half-life of about 1.5 days). The particles are eventually degraded by binding to LDL receptors in liver and certain extrahepatic tissues. Circulating LDL constitutes the major reservoir of cholesterol in human plasma, accounting for 60 to 70% of the total. When liver or extrahepatic tissues require cholesterol for the synthesis of new membranes, steroid hormones, or bile acids, they synthesize LDL receptors and obtain cholesterol by

the receptor-mediated endocytosis of LDL. Conversely, when tissues no longer require cholesterol for cell growth or metabolic purposes, they decrease the synthesis of LDL receptors. This phenomenon of feedback regulation can be exploited in the design of drugs that reduce plasma concentrations of LDL by stimulating production of LDL receptors (*see* below).

As cells of the body die and as cell membranes undergo turnover, free cholesterol is continually released into the plasma. This cholesterol is immediately adsorbed onto *high-density lipoproteins* (HDL; diameter, 5 to 12 nm), and in this location it is esterified with a long-chain fatty acid by an enzyme in plasma, lecithin:cholesterol acyltransferase (LCAT). The newly formed cholesteryl esters are rapidly transferred from HDL to VLDL or LDL particles by a cholesteryl ester transfer protein in plasma. This completes the cycle by which LDL delivers cholesterol to tissues, and the cholesterol is returned to new LDL particles by means of the combined actions of HDL, LCAT, and the transfer protein (Figure 34–1).

In addition to degradation by specific receptors, lipoproteins are also disposed of by less specific pathways, some of which operate in macrophages and other scavenger cells. When the concentration of a lipoprotein in plasma rises, the rate of its degradation by such pathways increases. This contributes to the deposition of cholesterol in such abnormal locations as arterial walls (producing atheromas) and macrophages of tendons and skin (producing xanthomas) (Brown and Goldstein, 1983).

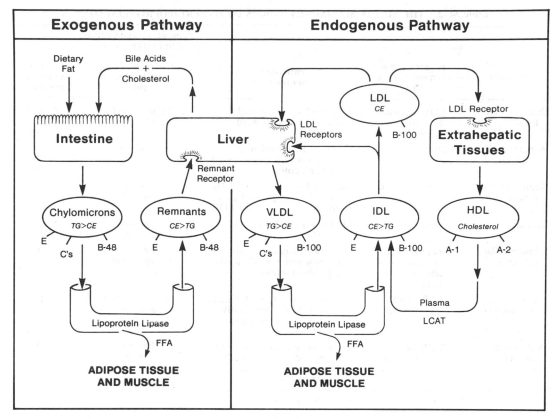

Figure 34–1. *Model for the metabolism of plasma lipoproteins, showing the separate pathways for transport of endogenous and exogenous lipids.*

CE denotes cholesteryl esters; *FFA*, free fatty acids; *TG*, triglycerides; *HDL*, high-density lipoprotein; *IDL*, intermediate-density lipoprotein; *LCAT*, lecithin:cholesterol acyltransferase; *LDL*, low-density lipoprotein; and *VLDL*, very-low-density lipoprotein. *A-1, A-2, B-48, B-100, C's,* and E represent the apoproteins associated with the indicated lipoprotein particle. For further explanation, *see* the text. (Modified from Goldstein, Kita, and Brown, 1983.)

DISEASES THAT CAUSE HYPERLIPOPROTEINEMIA

The hyperlipoproteinemias can be designated as either primary or secondary. Secondary hyperlipoproteinemias are complications of a more generalized metabolic disturbance, such as diabetes mellitus, hypothyroidism, or excessive intake of ethanol (Table 34–2). The primary hyperlipoproteinemias can be divided into two major groups: those that are caused by an inherited single-gene defect (so-called monogenic hyperlipoproteinemias) and those that appear to be caused by a combination of multiple subtle genetic factors that act together with environmental insults (so-called multifactorial or polygenic hyperlipoproteinemias) (Table 34–3). The monogenic disorders are inherited in a predictable Mendelian fashion; each family member can be classified as either affected or unaffected. In multifactorial hyperlipoproteinemia, the plasma lipid concentrations of an entire family are shifted slightly toward the upper range of normal, and those relatives with values at the high end of the family spectrum are above the ninety-fifth percentile for the population as a whole. Of all individuals in the population with hyperlipoproteinemia, the majority have the multifactorial type. Individuals with the monogenic forms of hyperlipoproteinemia generally have much higher concentrations of lipid than do those with the polygenic type.

Table 34–2. THE MAJOR SECONDARY FORMS OF HYPERLIPOPROTEINEMIA

DISORDER	PLASMA LIPO-PROTEIN ELEVA-TION	PROPOSED MECHANISM	TYPICAL PLASMA LIPID CONCENTRATIONS T = Triglyceride C = Cholesterol (mg/dl)	TYPICAL CLINICAL FINDINGS *
Diabetes mellitus	VLDL (occasionally chylomicrons)	Increased secretion and delayed catabolism of VLDL	T: 300–10,000 C: 200–300	X, P, A
Hypothyroidism	LDL	Decreased catabolism of LDL, owing to suppressed LDL receptors	T: 100–400 C: 300–400	A
Nephrotic syndrome	VLDL and LDL	Increased secretion of VLDL and LDL; decreased catabolism of VLDL and LDL	T: 100–500 C: 300–500	A
Uremia	VLDL	Decreased catabolism of VLDL	T: 300–800 C: 200–300	A
Primary biliary cirrhosis	Lipoprotein X (↑ cholesterol and phospholipid)	Diversion of biliary cholesterol and phospholipids into blood stream	T: 100 C: 300–2000	X, A
Alcoholic hyperlipidemia	VLDL (usually chylomicrons)	Increased secretion of VLDL in individuals genetically predisposed to hypertriglyceridemia	T: 300–10,000 C: 200–300	X, P
Oral contraceptives	VLDL (occasionally chylomicrons)	Increased secretion of VLDL in individuals genetically predisposed to hypertriglyceridemia	T: 300–10,000 C: 200–300	X, P

* X = xanthomas; P = pancreatitis; A = premature atherosclerosis.

Tables 34–2 and 34–3 summarize the characteristics of the diseases that cause hyperlipoproteinemia. The monogenic disorders range from extremely common autosomal dominant diseases, such as the heterozygous forms of familial hypercholesterolemia (prevalence of 1 in 500 in the population) and multiple lipoprotein–type hyperlipoproteinemia (prevalence of 1 in 250 in the population), to rare diseases, such as familial lipoprotein lipase deficiency (1 in 1,000,000 in the population). The mutant gene product has been identified in three of the monogenic disorders. In familial lipoprotein lipase deficiency, affected homozygotes fail to produce lipoprotein lipase, and they are thus unable to catabolize dietary triglyceride contained within chylomicrons. In familial hypercholesterolemia, the gene for the LDL receptor is defective, and LDL cannot be removed from the circulation at a normal rate (Goldstein and Brown, 1983). In familial dysbetalipoproteinemia (also called type-3 hyperlipoproteinemia), patients inherit two mutant genes at the locus for apo E, the apoprotein that is necessary for binding of chylomicron remnants and IDL to hepatic receptors (Mahley and Angelin, 1983). The defective molecules of apoprotein E fail to bind to either chylomicron remnant receptors or LDL receptors. Surprisingly, homozygosity for the abnormal apo-E gene is necessary, but not sufficient, to produce hyperlipoproteinemia. In addition to such homozygosity (which occurs in 1 in 100 in-

dividuals in the population), the development of hyperlipoproteinemia (which occurs in only 1 in 100 homozygotes) requires another aggravating factor, such as hypothyroidism or the simultaneous inheritance of a second genetic defect in lipoprotein metabolism.

The causes of the multifactorial hyperlipoproteinemias are not established. The postulated subtle genetic abnormalities that predispose to these forms of disease are often aggravated by obesity and by diets that are high in saturated fats and cholesterol. For this reason, patients with the multifactorial diseases often respond better to dietary manipulation than do patients with the monogenic defects (see below).

EVALUATION OF HYPERLIPOPROTEINEMIA

By arbitrary definition, individuals with hyperlipoproteinemia have a concentration of cholesterol and/or triglyceride in plasma that is above the ninety-fifth percentile for the population; this limit varies with age and sex (see Rifkind and Segal, 1983).

Knowledge of the plasma concentrations of cholesterol and triglyceride usually reveals the class of lipoprotein that is elevated, and this in turn is useful in making a genetic diagnosis. An elevated concentration of cholesterol in the presence of a nor-

Table 34–3. THE MAJOR PRIMARY FORMS OF HYPERLIPOPROTEINEMIA

DISORDER AND PATTERN OF INHERITANCE *	BIOCHEMICAL DEFECT	PLASMA LIPOPROTEIN ELEVATION	PROPOSED MECHANISM	TYPICAL PLASMA LIPID CONCENTRATIONS T = Triglyceride C = Cholesterol (mg/dl)	TYPICAL CLINICAL FINDINGS †	DRUG THERAPY First Choice	DRUG THERAPY Other
Monogenic							
Familial lipoprotein lipase deficiency; R	Deficiency of lipoprotein lipase	Chylomicrons	Decreased hydrolysis of triglycerides in chylomicrons	T: 10,000 C: 500	X, P	None	None
Familial type-III hyperlipoproteinemia (dysbetalipoproteinemia); R ‡	Abnormal form of apo E	Chylomicron remnants and IDL	Decreased catabolism of chylomicron remnants and IDL	T: 350 C: 350	X, A	Clofibrate	Nicotinic acid
Familial hypercholesterolemia (heterozygous form); D	Deficiency of LDL receptor	LDL	Decreased catabolism of LDL; decreased catabolism of IDL with increased conversion to LDL	T: 100 C: 350	X, A	Bile acid resin plus nicotinic acid	Probucol; D-thyroxine; β-sitosterol; neomycin
Familial hypertriglyceridemia; D	Unknown	VLDL (rarely chylomicrons)	Decreased catabolism or increased production of VLDL	T: 500 C: 200	X, A, P	Nicotinic acid; gemfibrozil	Clofibrate
Multiple lipoprotein–type hyperlipidemia (familial combined hyperlipidemia); D	Unknown	VLDL and LDL (rarely chylomicrons)	Increased production of VLDL	T: 100–500 C: 250–400	X, A, P	Nicotinic acid; gemfibrozil	Clofibrate; bile acid resin
Multifactorial							
Polygenic hypercholesterolemia; complex	Unknown	LDL	Unknown	T: 100 C: 280	A	Bile acid resin plus nicotinic acid	Probucol; D-thyroxine; β-sitosterol; neomycin
Hypertriglyceridemia; complex	Unknown	VLDL	Unknown	T: 500 C: 200	—	Nicotinic acid; gemfibrozil	Clofibrate

* All of the monogenic disorders are autosomal. R = recessive; D = dominant.

† X = xanthomas; P = pancreatitis; A = premature atherosclerosis.

‡ Requires homozygosity for apo-E abnormality plus additional factor(s) for clinical expression.

mal value for triglyceride is almost always due to an excessive concentration of LDL. If one defines an elevated LDL concentration as that which exceeds the ninety-fifth percentile, then most individuals with an elevation of LDL will have polygenic hypercholesterolemia. About 1 in 25 of such individuals will have the heterozygous form of familial hypercholesterolemia. This disease can usually be diagnosed by a constellation of clinical findings: an extremely high concentration of plasma cholesterol (typically 350 to 450 mg/dl), the presence of tendon xanthomas (present in 75% of affected adults), and a strong family history of hypercholesterolemia and premature heart disease. Heterozygotes express about one half the normal number of LDL receptors and manifest hypercholesterolemia from the time of birth. This is in contrast to the polygenic form of hypercholesterolemia, which does not usually become manifest until adulthood. About 1 in 1,000,000 individuals in the population inherits two abnormal genes for the LDL receptor. Such homozygotes have a distinct syndrome that is characterized by severe hypercholesterolemia of 600 to 1000 mg/dl (LDL concentrations eight to ten times normal), a unique form of cutaneous planar xanthomas, and clinical signs of coronary atherosclerosis beginning as early as 5 years of age and typically ending in death from myocardial infarction by 20 to 30 years of age (Goldstein and Brown, 1983).

A triglyceride concentration in the range of 200 to 800 mg/dl with a normal or near-normal cholesterol concentration almost always indicates a simple elevation of VLDL. Triglyceride concentrations greater than 1000 mg/dl usually indicate the presence of chylomicrons, either alone or in addition to elevated VLDL. This distinction can be made by allowing such severely hyperlipemic plasma (which is usually either turbid or milky) to stand in the refrigerator at 4° C overnight. If chylomicrons are present, a creamy layer will form on top. If the plasma below the creamy layer is turbid, then VLDL is also elevated. If the plasma below the creamy layer is clear, then the VLDL is not elevated. The distinction between a primary and a secondary form of hypertriglyceridemia is often a difficult one, especially since many hypertriglyceridemic individuals with a genetically determined predisposition (*see* Table 34–3) can have their disease aggravated by the simultaneous presence of one of several common conditions, such as diabetes mellitus, excessive intake of alcohol, or use of oral contraceptives (*see* Table 34–2).

A moderate elevation of both cholesterol and triglyceride usually indicates that an individual has an elevation of both LDL and VLDL; this occurs frequently in familial multiple lipoprotein-type hyperlipoproteinemia and less commonly in familial hypercholesterolemia. Such a combined elevation might also be a sign of familial dysbetalipoproteinemia. The latter disease can be suspected if tuberous or palmar xanthomas are found. If doubt exists, the presence of dysbetalipoproteinemia can be confirmed by ultracentrifugation and electrophoretic technics in specialized laboratories (Mahley and Angelin, 1983).

INDICATIONS FOR TREATMENT OF HYPERLIPOPROTEINEMIA

Abundant circumstantial evidence indicates that treatment of hyperlipoproteinemia will diminish or prevent atherosclerotic complications. For example, numerous population studies have shown that an elevated concentration of total cholesterol or LDL-cholesterol in plasma constitutes a major risk factor for the occurrence of atherosclerotic events (Goldstein et al., 1973; Keys, 1975). Moreover, in the monogenic disorders, family studies have documented a markedly increased risk of vascular disease among affected members (Stone et al., 1974; Brunzell et al., 1976). Nevertheless, treatment of hyperlipoproteinemia was, until recently, a controversial issue, mainly because the lowering of plasma lipids had not been shown prospectively to prolong life or diminish the clinical complications of atherosclerosis. In 1984, the results of the Lipid Research Clinics Coronary Primary Prevention Trial, a multicenter, randomized, double-blind study, provided strong evidence that a reduction in plasma concentrations of LDL-cholesterol can reduce the risk of coronary heart disease (Lipid Research Clinics Program, 1984a, 1984b).

The design of this major study was as follows. A large number (3806) of asymptomatic middle-aged men with primary forms of hypercholesterolemia were divided into control and treatment groups. The treatment group received cholestyramine, a bile acid–binding resin, and the control group received a placebo for an average of 7.4 years. Both groups followed a moderate cholesterol-lowering diet. In the cholestyramine group, plasma LDL-cholesterol concentrations were reduced by 20%, which was 13% greater than that obtained in the control group (p < 0.001). The cholestyramine group experienced a 24% reduction in death by myocardial infarction and a 19% reduction in nonfatal myocardial infarction (p < 0.05). In addition, the incidence rates for newly positive exercise tests (indicative of myocardial ischemia), angina pectoris, and coronary bypass surgery were reduced by 25%, 20%, and 21%, respectively, in the cholestyramine group. No serious adverse effects of cholestyramine were noted. One or more gastrointestinal symptoms (e.g., gas, heartburn, bloating, and constipation) were noted in 29% of the cholestyramine group and 26% of the placebo group.

These results provide the long-sought evidence

that reduction of LDL-cholesterol concentrations can diminish the incidence of morbidity and mortality of coronary heart disease. The implications of these results for the treatment of hyperlipoproteinemia and for prevention of atherosclerosis are compelling. Analysis of the relationship between reduction of cholesterol and coronary heart disease suggests that the incidence of coronary heart disease in patients with hyperlipoproteinemia would be reduced by nearly 50% for individuals who achieved a 25% reduction in plasma total cholesterol or a 35% fall in plasma LDL-cholesterol (Lipid Research Clinics Program, 1984b).

In deciding how to treat an individual with hypercholesterolemia, the physician must bear in mind that the normal values for plasma lipid and lipoprotein concentrations (*i.e.*, within the ninety-fifth percentile) are arbitrary. The population studies suggest that an increased risk of coronary artery disease begins at a total plasma cholesterol concentration of about 200 mg/dl in a 40-year-old man, which is close to the *median* value for the United States population. Thus, in some individuals, a total plasma cholesterol concentration of 250 mg/dl, although statistically within the ninety-fifth percentile, may still be high enough to predispose to atherosclerosis. In this context, knowledge of the family history is helpful. If there is a high incidence of atherosclerosis in first-degree relatives, then common sense would dictate a more aggressive approach to therapy.

The role of hypertriglyceridemia (in the range of 300 to 1000 mg/dl) as an independent risk factor for coronary atherosclerosis has not been established unequivocally, although several epidemiological studies have revealed a correlation (Carlson and Bottiger, 1981). The decision about drug treatment in this group of patients should be influenced by the presence of other risk factors for coronary heart disease (*see* below) and the family history of premature atherosclerosis. Patients with triglyceride concentrations approaching 1000 mg/dl are subject to sudden and precipitous increases in plasma VLDL and chylomicrons, which can lead to acute pancreatitis. Drug treatment for this group is clearly indicated.

Epidemiological studies have revealed a negative correlation between the plasma concentration of HDL, which normally accounts for 20 to 30% of the total plasma cholesterol, and the risk of coronary heart disease (Miller, 1980). The basis of this association is not yet clear. It is not known whether high concentrations of HDL are themselves protective or whether they are an indication of some other beneficial aspect of lipid metabolism. For example, hypertriglyceridemic individuals frequently have a low concentration of HDL-cholesterol. When these patients are treated with drugs that lower VLDL concentrations, the HDL will often return to the normal range. Since there is no evidence that increasing the plasma concentration of HDL-cholesterol in itself decreases the risk of coronary heart disease, the use of drugs for the specific purpose of increasing concentrations of HDL is currently not recommended.

THERAPEUTIC STRATEGIES

Diet. The first principle for treatment of all hyperlipoproteinemias is the provision of a diet that maintains a normal body weight and that minimizes concentrations of lipids in plasma. Individuals who are overweight should initially consume a weight-reducing diet. Thereafter, they should be placed on a diet that is low in cholesterol and saturated animal fats and relatively (but not absolutely) high in polyunsaturated vegetable oils, which reduce concentrations of plasma LDL-cholesterol. Many experienced clinicians and nutritionists now agree that virtually all patients with hyperlipoproteinemia, either primary or secondary, can be treated with a single diet. For specific details of such diets, *see* Connor and Connor (1982). Rare individuals with extreme sensitivity to dietary triglycerides (*i.e.*, those with familial lipoprotein lipase deficiency) must be placed on a diet that is severely reduced in total fat.

Elimination of Aggravating Factors. If an individual has a hyperlipoproteinemia that is exacerbated by some other illness (such as diabetes mellitus, alcoholism, or hypothyroidism), the exacerbating disease must be treated. In addition, individuals with hyperlipoproteinemia should be encouraged to reduce all other risk factors that might potentiate the development of atherosclerosis. These include cessation of smoking, treatment of hypertension, maintenance of a good exercise and physical fitness program, and careful control of blood glucose in diabetics.

Drugs. The final aspect of therapy for hyperlipoproteinemia involves the administration of drugs that lower plasma concentrations of lipoproteins, either by diminishing the production of lipoproteins or by enhancing the efficiency of their removal from plasma. The drugs that exist for this purpose are reviewed below. The concept has now arisen that a combination of drugs may have synergistic effects in lowering plasma lipid concentrations, especially that of LDL. The first successful combination was one of *nicotinic acid* and a *bile acid–*

binding resin, which effectively lowers LDL concentrations in patients with heterozygous familial hypercholesterolemia (Kane *et al.,* 1981). *Probucol* and, more recently, *mevinolin* (or *compactin*) have also been given concurrently with bile acid–binding resins for their effect on LDL.

DRUGS THAT LOWER CONCENTRATIONS OF PLASMA LIPOPROTEINS

NICOTINIC ACID

Nicotinic acid was discovered as a hypolipidemic drug in 1955 (Altschul *et al.,* 1955). The lipid-lowering property of nicotinic acid is not shared by nicotinamide and has nothing to do with the role of these substances as vitamins. Pharmacological doses of nicotinic acid are useful in the treatment of most forms of hyperlipoproteinemia, but this usefulness is limited by the frequent occurrence of side effects. The chemistry of nicotinic acid and its function as a vitamin are discussed in Chapter 66.

Effects on Plasma Lipids and Lipoproteins. Large doses of nicotinic acid rapidly reduce the concentrations of triglycerides in plasma by lowering concentrations of VLDL; effects are noted in 1 to 4 days. Plasma concentrations of triglycerides may be reduced by 20% to over 80%; the degree of reduction is directly related to the initial concentration of VLDL (Carlson and Olsson, 1979). Concentrations of LDL-cholesterol fall more slowly, but a drop is clearly apparent within 5 to 7 days of the initiation of therapy. The magnitude of the fall in LDL is related to the dose, and the maximal effect is usually achieved 3 to 5 weeks after an appropriate dosage regimen has been established. When nicotinic acid is used alone, a 10 to 15% reduction in plasma LDL-cholesterol is typically seen; when it is used in combination with a bile acid–binding resin, a 40 to 60% reduction may occur (Kane *et al.,* 1981). Administration of nicotinic acid usually results in a mild-to-moderate increase in the concentration of HDL-cholesterol. Eruptive, tuboeruptive, tuberous, and tendon xanthomas regress after prolonged therapy.

Mechanism of Action. Nicotinic acid decreases the production of VLDL, which in turn results in a decreased production of its daughter particles, IDL and LDL (Grundy *et al.,* 1981). The mechanism by which nicotinic acid lowers VLDL production remains uncertain, but it is likely related to several of the drug's diverse actions, including inhibition of lipolysis in adipose tissue, decreased esterification of triglycerides in the liver, and increased activity of lipoprotein lipase (Gey and Carlson, 1971). Nicotinic acid does not produce any detectable changes in total body synthesis of cholesterol nor does it significantly alter excretion of bile acids in man (Grundy *et al.,* 1981).

Adverse Effects. Nicotinic acid produces an intense cutaneous flush and pruritus, involving the face and the upper part of the body. While these reactions decrease in intensity in most individuals after they have been on therapy for several weeks, they are unpleasant and may result in poor patient compliance. One aspirin (0.3 g) taken 30 minutes beforehand can markedly reduce the flushing, which appears to be mediated by a prostaglandin (Andersson *et al.,* 1977; Olsson *et al.,* 1983). Slow upward adjustment of dosage also appears to ameliorate this problem. Gastrointestinal disturbances such as vomiting, diarrhea, and dyspepsia are also common, and peptic ulceration has been reported. Hyperpigmentation, acanthosis nigricans, and dry skin may occur after prolonged therapy in rare instances.

Abnormalities of hepatic function occur in patients taking large doses of nicotinic acid. These include jaundice, a decrease in the excretion of bromosulfophthalein, and increases of plasma transaminase activities. Hyperglycemia and abnormal glucose tolerance occur in many nondiabetic patients taking nicotinic acid. Plasma concentrations of uric acid may also be elevated, and the incidence of acute gouty arthritis is increased. The drug should therefore be used with extreme caution, if at all, in patients who have hepatic disease, diabetes mellitus, or gout. The abnormalities of plasma glucose and uric acid and hepatic function are reversible when the drug is discontinued. Nicotinic acid may increase the vasodilatation and postural hypotension caused by antihypertensive agents. Toxic amblyopia (one case) and reversible cystoid edema of the macula (three cases) have also been reported.

Nicotinic acid should not be used in pregnancy unless it is absolutely essential to prevent life-threatening pancreatitis due to hypertriglyceridemia. Children receiving combination therapy for heterozygous familial hypercholesterolemia (bile acid–binding resin plus nicotinic acid) should not be given nicotinic acid until after puberty.

Preparations, Dosage, and Therapeutic Uses. Preparations of *nicotinic acid* (*niacin*) are described in Chapter 66. The usual dosage of nicotinic acid is 2 to 8 g daily. The daily dose is divided into three or four portions, taken orally with or just after meals. There are other preparations of nicotinic acid that produce sustained concentrations of the drug in blood, but they appear to cause gastrointestinal irritation and hepatotoxicity. To reduce gastric irritation and to enhance absorption of nicotinic acid, the drug is best given at mealtimes, initially in small doses (three 100-mg tablets per day). Over a 1- to 3-week period, additional tablets are added to the regimen until the maintenance dose is reached. This is usually considerably lower in children (55 to 87 mg/kg per day) than in adults.

Nicotinic acid fell into relative disrepute because of the variety of troublesome untoward effects associated with its use, but it has regained popularity as a result of its ability to reduce elevated concentrations of both VLDL and LDL. Because of these effects, nicotinic acid is useful in the management of all types of hyperlipoproteinemia except familial lipoprotein lipase deficiency. In particular, nicotinic acid is the drug of choice for patients with severe hypertriglyceridemia associated with elevated chylomicrons (type-V hyperlipoproteinemia).

The combination of nicotinic acid and a bile acid–binding resin may allow effective reduction of the concentration of LDL with more conservative doses of each drug than would be required if either was given alone. In severe cases of familial hypertriglyceridemia associated with elevated chylomicrons (in subjects without gout or diabetes), a maintenance dosage of 3 g of nicotinic acid per day can prevent the recurrent bouts of pancreatitis and eruptive xanthomas that occur in this disorder.

In two different trials of secondary prevention, the long-term use of nicotinic acid significantly decreased the incidence of recurrent myocardial infarction. In both trials, however, there was no definitive effect on cardiovascular or overall mortality (Coronary Drug Project, 1975; Carlson *et al.*, 1977). Moreover, in the Coronary Drug Project, an increased incidence of atrial fibrillation and other cardiac arrhythmias was observed, in addition to the aforementioned gastrointestinal and dermatological effects. Nicotinic acid should thus be used with caution and primarily in high-risk patients with hyperlipoproteinemia who have not responded dramatically to dietary measures.

Clofibrate

As a result of screening tests in rats, Thorp and Waring (1962) found that a series of aryloxyisobutyric acids was effective in reducing plasma concentrations of total lipid and cholesterol. The compound that combined maximal effectiveness with minimal toxicity was clofibrate. Since then, it has been widely used in man. However, its use has become increasingly circumscribed because its effectiveness for the primary or secondary prevention of atherosclerosis and its clinical sequelae have come into question (Coronary Drug Project, 1975; Oliver *et al.*, 1978); furthermore, awareness of latent adverse effects of clofibrate has grown (Oliver *et al.*, 1978; Palmer, 1978). At present, clofibrate is used almost exclusively for the treatment of familial dysbetalipoproteinemia (type-III hyperlipoproteinemia). It is occasionally useful in patients with severe hypertriglyceridemia who do not respond to nicotinic acid or gemfibrozil.

Chemistry. Clofibrate, the ethyl ester of *p*-chlorophenoxyisobutyric acid, has the following structural formula:

Clofibrate

Several derivatives of clofibrate have been synthesized and used effectively in Europe for the treatment of hypertriglyceridemia. In general, these drugs, which include bezafibrate, ciprofibrate, and fenofibrate, appear to be more potent than clofibrate and can be used in much lower doses (Carlson and Olsson, 1979; Rossner and Oro, 1981).

Effects on Plasma Lipids and Lipoproteins. Clofibrate characteristically reduces the plasma triglyceride concentration by lowering the levels of VLDL within 2 to 5 days after initiation of therapy. In most patients, plasma cholesterol and LDL concentrations also fall. However, a large fall in VLDL may be accompanied by a *rise* in LDL, such that the net effect on cholesterol may be slight. The mean value of plasma cholesterol was reduced only 6% in men treated chronically with clofibrate (1.8 g per day) during the Coronary Drug Project (1975); the reduction in plasma triglyceride was 22%.

In a similar trial of primary prevention involving asymptomatic men with hypercholesterolemia, clofibrate lowered the plasma cholesterol concentration by only 6 to 11% (Oliver *et al.*, 1978). This very modest effect in unselected patients can be contrasted with that in familial dysbetalipoproteinemia, where concentrations of cholesterol and triglycerides may be lowered by approximately 50% and by as much as 80%, respectively (Levy *et al.*, 1972). In such patients, administration of clofibrate results in the mobilization of deposits of cholesterol in tissues, accompanied by regression and disappearance of xanthomas. Clofibrate has no effect on hyperchylomicronemia, nor does it affect concentrations of HDL (except in some hypertriglyceridemic subjects in whom marked reduction of VLDL may be accompanied by modest increments in HDL). Thus, clofibrate appears to have specific efficacy only in patients with familial dysbetalipoproteinemia.

The clinical evidence for the efficacy of clofibrate in preventing deaths from coronary artery disease is not encouraging. A number of clinical trials have now been completed, and none has shown a clear-cut beneficial effect. A double-blind study conducted by the World Health Organization compared clofibrate with placebo in 10,000 men in the upper third of the distribution of plasma cholesterol concentrations (Oliver *et al.*, 1978). There was a decrease in nonfatal myocardial infarction in those treated with clofibrate but no decrease in fatal myocardial infarctions. Moreover, clofibrate-treated patients had a higher noncardiac mortality rate than did control subjects, due mainly to an increased incidence of malignant neoplasms and complications of cholecystectomy.

Mechanism of Action. The sites of action of clofibrate are only partially established,

and the details of its mechanism of action are largely lacking (*see* Havel and Kane, 1973). Its primary effect is to increase the activity of lipoprotein lipase, which in turn enhances the rate of intravascular catabolism of VLDL and IDL to LDL (Boberg *et al.*, 1977). In some cases, it may also hasten the rate of removal of these lipoproteins from plasma. Hepatic synthesis and release of VLDL are not altered consistently.

Absorption, Fate, and Excretion. In man, clofibrate is completely absorbed from the intestine, but it appears in the plasma as the deesterified *p*-chlorophenoxyisobutyric acid (CPIB); peak concentrations of the acid occur in the plasma within 4 hours after the oral administration of clofibrate. The major fraction of CPIB is bound to plasma albumin. The elimination of CPIB proceeds in two kinetic phases, with the slower exponential phase having a mean half-time of nearly 15 hours. Essentially all the acid is excreted in the urine, about 60% as the glucuronide.

Adverse Effects and Drug Interactions. Clofibrate is usually well tolerated, but occasionally patients experience nausea, diarrhea, or weight gain (apparently related to increased appetite). Skin rash, alopecia, weakness, impotence, breast tenderness, and decreased libido also have been reported to occur occasionally. A more disturbing effect is a now well-characterized flulike syndrome, associated with severe muscle cramps and tenderness, stiffness, and weakness. The syndrome recurs whenever the drug is taken and is associated with elevated activities of creatine phosphokinase and glutamic-oxaloacetic transaminase in the plasma. These same enzymatic activities are sometimes elevated even in asymptomatic patients who are receiving clofibrate. Administration of clofibrate also increases the lithogenicity of bile and has thus been associated with an increased incidence of cholelithiasis and cholecystitis (Palmer, 1978).

Patients with existing or suspected coronary artery disease may be at risk from drug-induced cardiac arrhythmias, cardiomegaly, increased angina, claudication, and thromboembolic phenomena (Coronary

Drug Project, 1975). The drug enhances the effect (and toxicity) of other acidic drugs such as phenytoin and tolbutamide, presumably by displacing them from their binding sites on albumin. This same effect may in part explain the enhancement of the effects of coumarin anticoagulants by clofibrate. A reduction in the dosage of oral anticoagulants and frequent determinations of prothrombin time are usually required to control patients who are receiving both medications. Concentrations of the active metabolite of clofibrate are increased in patients taking probenecid concurrently, while they are decreased during administration of rifampin. Administration of high doses of clofibrate to mice and rats resulted in a higher frequency of benign and malignant hepatic tumors than in control animals. Long-term use of clofibrate in man may be associated with a slightly increased incidence of various tumors (Oliver *et al.*, 1978). The drug is contraindicated in patients with impaired renal or hepatic function and in pregnant or nursing women.

Preparation, Dosage, and Therapeutic Uses. *Clofibrate* (ATROMID-S) is available as capsules containing 500 mg. The drug is administered orally in a dose of 2 g daily, in two or four portions. Increase in dosage above 2 g per day does not appear to increase its effects on lipids but does greatly increase the incidence of side effects. In all cases, its effects on lipids are enhanced by proper diet. Clofibrate is indicated only in subjects with increased concentrations of VLDL and IDL who have failed to respond adequately to dietary therapy alone. It is the drug of choice in familial dysbetalipoproteinemia and may also be useful in certain patients with other forms of hypertriglyceridemia or multiple lipoprotein-type hyperlipoproteinemia. Because clofibrate has only a modest effect on LDL and since there exist other more effective agents for lowering the concentration of LDL, the drug is of limited utility for patients with either familial hypercholesterolemia or polygenic hypercholesterolemia. Furthermore, since clofibrate may *increase* the concentration of LDL in some patients with elevations of VLDL, the effects of the drug should be monitored by sequential measurements of plasma lipoproteins. A shift from an excess of VLDL to one of LDL suggests the necessity to discontinue the drug.

GEMFIBROZIL

Gemfibrozil is the newest drug to be marketed in the United States for the treatment of hyperlipoproteinemia. It was synthesized in 1968 as a structural congener of clofibrate. When tested as one of 8700 other compounds for lipid-lowering properties in animals, gemfibrozil proved to be the most effective and the least toxic; it was first used in clinical trials in 1971 (Marks, 1982). Gemfibrozil is effective in reducing the plasma concentration of VLDL in hypertriglyceridemic patients who do not respond to diet. The drug has the interesting (and perhaps beneficial) property of raising the plasma concentration of HDL. Clinical experience with gemfibrozil is relatively limited, and its long-term safety has not been established.

Chemistry. Gemfibrozil has the following structural formula:

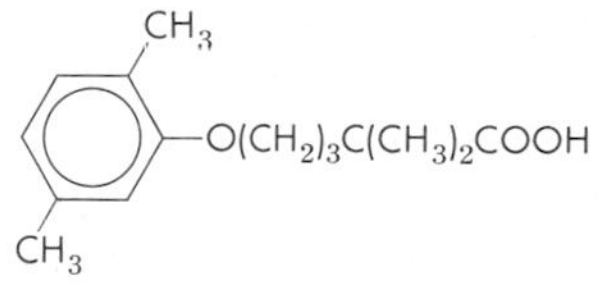

$$\text{CH}_3\text{-ring-O(CH}_2)_3\text{C(CH}_3)_2\text{COOH}$$

Gemfibrozil

Effects on Plasma Lipids and Lipoproteins. In hypertriglyceridemic patients, gemfibrozil characteristically decreases the plasma concentration of triglycerides by 40 to 55% by lowering the level of VLDL. A maximal effect is usually achieved within 3 to 4 weeks. The drug also lowers VLDL-cholesterol concentrations to a comparable degree. This is accompanied by an increase in the plasma concentrations of HDL-cholesterol, such that the total cholesterol may be lowered only slightly. The drug is much less effective in lowering LDL, and it reduces plasma LDL-cholesterol by less than 10% in hypercholesterolemic patients. Gemfibrozil raises plasma concentrations of HDL-cholesterol by about 20 to 25% in patients with either hypertriglyceridemia or hypercholesterolemia (Samuel, 1983).

The effects of gemfibrozil and clofibrate were compared in the treatment of hyperlipoproteinemia in patients with maturity-onset diabetes mellitus; plasma triglycerides were reduced by 40% by gemfibrozil, compared to only 5% by clofibrate (Marks, 1982). Gemfibrozil also effectively lowers VLDL-triglyceride concentrations in patients with nephrotic syndrome and uremia (Marks, 1982).

Mechanism of Action. Knowledge of the mechanism by which gemfibrozil lowers plasma VLDL is limited. It is not known whether the drug influences the production or the removal of VLDL or both. The effect of gemfibrozil on plasma lipoprotein lipase activity is much smaller than that of clofibrate, suggesting that the drug acts primarily to inhibit hepatic secretion of VLDL (*see* Symposium, 1976). Gemfibrozil has been shown to inhibit lipolysis of stored triglyceride in adipose tissue and to decrease the uptake of fatty acid by the liver (Symposium, 1976). Theoretically, both of these actions should lead to a decreased delivery of fatty acids to the liver, with a consequent reduction in the synthesis and secretion of VLDL-triglyceride. The mechanism by which gemfibrozil raises HDL concentrations is not known.

Absorption, Fate, and Excretion. Gemfibrozil is rapidly and completely absorbed from the gastrointestinal tract. Peak concentrations in blood occur 1 to 2 hours after oral administration. The drug then undergoes an enterohepatic circulation. After administration of a single dose of 600 mg, the plasma concentration is about 15 μg/ml in 2 hours and 5 μg/ml after 9 hours. Final excretion occurs primarily through the kidneys, mainly as the glucuronide.

Adverse Effects and Drug Interactions. Gemfibrozil is generally well tolerated, but it has not been subjected to the same scrutiny as has clofibrate. Mild gastrointestinal distress (abdominal pain, diarrhea, nausea) is the most frequent side effect and occurs in about 5% of patients. Eosinophilia, skin rash, musculoskeletal pain, blurred vision, mild anemia, and leukopenia have been reported occasionally. Gemfibrozil potentiates the effect of oral anticoagulants, presumably by displacing them from their binding sites on albumin. The drug may also have a mild hyperglycemic effect. Diabetic patients may require a slight increase in their dosage of insulin or an oral hypoglycemic agent if they are taking one of these drugs concurrently with gemfibrozil.

Like clofibrate, gemfibrozil may enhance the formation of gallstones. Several studies in which patients were treated for 1 year have shown a 1 to 1.5% incidence of new or enlarged gallstones, a frequency that is only slightly higher than that in untreated controls. Until further data become available, the drug should not be given to individuals with disease of the gallbladder. A significant increase in benign liver nodules, hepatic carcinomas, and Leydig-cell tumors has been observed in male rats treated chronically with high doses of gemfibrozil.

The safety of gemfibrozil for children or pregnant women has not been established. Although gemfibrozil is effective in the treatment of hypertriglyceridemia secondary to nephrotic syndrome and uremia, its long-term safety in patients with renal dysfunction is unknown. One preliminary study found no toxicity or deterioration of renal function in 12 patients with nephrotic syndrome and 12 patients with uremia who were treated for 6 months with a standard dose of gemfibrozil (Marks, 1982).

Preparation, Dosage, and Therapeutic Uses. *Gemfibrozil* (LOPID) is available as 300-mg capsules. The recommended dosage (for adults only) is 600 mg twice daily, taken 30 minutes before the morning and evening meals. Gemfibrozil should be reserved for the treatment of patients with severe hypertriglyceridemia whose plasma concentrations of VLDL cannot be lowered by diet and more conventional drugs. The drug is not effective in the treatment of hyperchylomicronemia due to familial lipoprotein lipase deficiency, nor is it usually effective in patients with elevated plasma LDL concentrations.

PROBUCOL

Probucol was initially described 15 years ago as a cholesterol-lowering agent in animals (Barnhart *et al.*, 1970), and it was recently marketed for use in man as an agent that causes a moderate reduction in plasma concentrations of LDL-cholesterol. Probucol has several properties that set it apart from other lipid-lowering drugs. Two of these properties may limit its clinical utility: it is a highly hydrophobic compound, and it thus persists in adipose tissue for months after patients stop taking it; and it causes a substantial lowering of plasma HDL-cholesterol concentrations in addition to its effects on LDL. Experience with the drug is limited, and the long-term effects are not known.

Chemistry. Probucol has no apparent structural similarity to other agents that lower cholesterol concentrations. It is a sulfur-containing *bis*-phenol with the following structural formula:

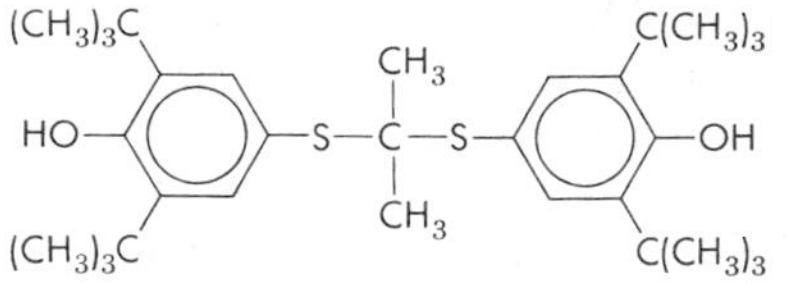

$(CH_3)_3C$ CH_3 $C(CH_3)_3$

HO—⬡—S—C—S—⬡—OH

$(CH_3)_3C$ CH_3 $C(CH_3)_3$

Probucol

Effects on Plasma Lipids and Lipoproteins. Probucol lowers concentrations of LDL-cholesterol in plasma by 10 to 15% when used in conjunction with an appropriate diet. The drug also consistently lowers plasma HDL-cholesterol concentrations, often to an extent that is proportionately greater than its effect on LDL. In most studies, the maximal effect on plasma cholesterol (LDL plus HDL) occurred after 1 to 3 months of treatment. The effects on plasma concentrations of VLDL and triglycerides are minimal.

Mechanism of Action. Studies on the mechanism of action of probucol are limited, and the results have been inconsistent. It is thus not known whether probucol acts to decrease synthesis of LDL or to stimulate its catabolism. No studies of the effect of probucol on LDL receptor activity *in vivo* or *in vitro* have been reported. The effect of the drug to lower plasma concentrations of HDL appears to be associated with a suppression of the synthesis of apo A-1, the major protein component of HDL (Nestel and Billington, 1981; Atmeh *et al.*, 1983).

Absorption, Fate, and Excretion. Despite its lipid solubility, less than 10% of an oral dose of probucol is absorbed. The majority of the drug is excreted in the feces. Peak concentrations in blood are higher and less variable when the drug is taken with food. Probucol accumulates slowly in adipose tissue, and it may persist in fat and blood for 6 months or longer after the last dose is taken. The major pathway of elimination is via the bile and feces; renal clearance is negligible.

Adverse Effects. Probucol is well tolerated, and there is little short-term toxicity. Diarrhea, flatulence, abdominal pain, and nausea are the most troublesome side effects, occurring in about 10% of patients. Other adverse effects reported occasionally include eosinophilia, paresthesias, and angioneurotic edema. The safety of probucol has not been established for children or during pregnancy. Because of its persistence in the body, it is recommended that patients discontinue probucol and practice contraception for at least 6 months before attempting to become pregnant.

Probucol has caused fatal cardiac arrhythmias in experimental animals, especially those that had received a diet high in cholesterol and saturated fat. Although prolongation of the Q-T interval can occasionally occur in patients treated with the drug, there have been no reports of other arrhythmias or unexplained syncope. Nevertheless, patients should be advised to adhere to a low-cholesterol, low-fat diet throughout treatment, and an ECG should be obtained prior to therapy, 6 months later, and every year thereafter. Probucol should not be given to patients with evidence of recent myocardial damage or with ECG findings suggestive of ventricular irritability.

Preparation, Dosage, and Therapeutic Uses. *Probucol* (LORELCO) is available as 250-mg tablets. The recommended dosage (for adults only) is 500 mg twice daily, taken with morning and evening meals. Probucol should be reserved for the treatment of hypercholesterolemia in patients with excessive plasma LDL concentrations who cannot be controlled with dietary management and more conventional drugs. Because of its potentially undesirable effect to lower HDL concentrations, probucol is not widely recommended. Specifically, its use should be restricted to patients with heterozygous familial hypercholesterolemia in whom elevated LDL concentrations do not respond to combined therapy with a bile acid–binding resin and nicotinic acid. The drug is not generally effective in lowering LDL in patients with familial multiple lipoprotein–type hyperlipoproteinemia, nor is it of known benefit in patients with hypertriglyceridemia. There is as yet no evaluation of the efficacy of probucol for prevention or control of atherosclerosis or its clinical sequelae.

BILE ACID–BINDING RESINS:
CHOLESTYRAMINE AND COLESTIPOL

The first of these agents, *cholestyramine,* was originally used to control pruritus in patients with elevated concentrations of plasma bile acid due to cholestasis. While this remains a valid use of the drug, greater interest now centers on the ability of this and similar agents to lower concentrations of plasma LDL-cholesterol (Hashim and

Van Itallie, 1965). Inasmuch as the bile acid–binding resins are not absorbed from the gastrointestinal tract, they are perhaps the safest drugs currently available for the treatment of hyperlipoproteinemia.

Chemistry. Cholestyramine is the chloride salt of a basic anion-exchange resin. The ion-exchange sites are provided by trimethylbenzylammonium groups in a large copolymer of styrene and divinylbenzene. The average polymeric molecular weight is greater than 10^6. Cholestyramine has the following structural formula:

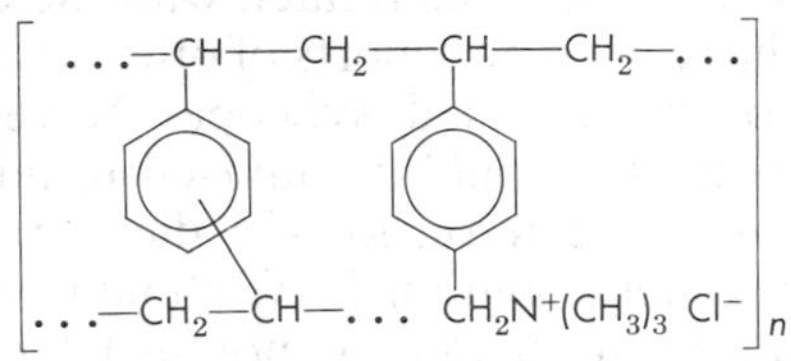

Cholestyramine

A second resin, colestipol hydrochloride, is a copolymer of diethyl pentamine and epichlorohydrin. The structural formula of colestipol is as follows:

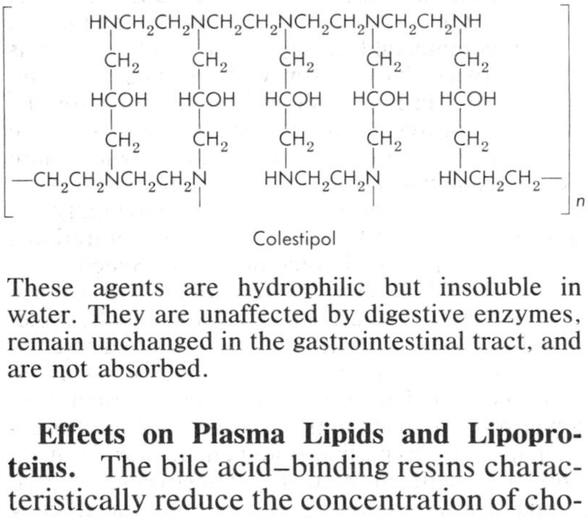

Colestipol

These agents are hydrophilic but insoluble in water. They are unaffected by digestive enzymes, remain unchanged in the gastrointestinal tract, and are not absorbed.

Effects on Plasma Lipids and Lipoproteins. The bile acid–binding resins characteristically reduce the concentration of cholesterol in plasma by lowering the level of LDL. The fall in the concentration of LDL is usually apparent in 4 to 7 days and approaches 90% of the maximal effect within 2 weeks. The magnitude of the effect on LDL is related to the dose and is usually in the range of 20%. In most patients, concentrations of triglyceride in plasma (VLDL) increase by 5 to 20% during the first weeks of therapy with a bile acid–binding resin; this increase usually then disappears gradually, and, within 4 weeks, concentrations of VLDL and triglyceride return to pretreatment values. In patients with elevated concentrations of VLDL and IDL, the increase

of triglycerides that follows the initiation of therapy with these agents may be greater and the increase in VLDL and IDL may be more sustained. For these reasons, bile acid–binding resins are most effective when only LDL is in excess, as in familial hypercholesterolemia or polygenic hypercholesterolemia. Bile acid–binding resins have no predictable effect on the concentration of HDL. When therapy with the resin is discontinued, plasma concentrations of lipids rise rapidly and then slowly approach the pretreatment values over a period of 3 to 4 weeks.

Mechanism of Action. These resins, administered orally, are not absorbed. They bind bile acids in the intestine, and there is thus a large increase in the fecal excretion of the acids. Since bile acids suppress the microsomal hydroxylase that catalyzes the rate-limiting step in the conversion of cholesterol to bile acids, their removal increases production of bile acids from cholesterol (Grundy et al., 1971). Furthermore, since bile acids are required for the intestinal absorption (and enterohepatic reabsorption) of cholesterol, there is some additional fecal loss of neutral sterol. The net loss of bile acids and neutral sterol from the liver leads to two compensatory changes in hepatic metabolism: an increase in the number of cell-surface LDL receptors and an increase in the activity of 3-hydroxy-3-methylglutaryl CoA (HMG CoA) reductase, the rate-controlling enzyme in cholesterol synthesis (Brown and Goldstein, 1981). Both of these compensatory changes restore homeostasis to the liver by the provision of increased amounts of cholesterol for conversion to bile acid. The increased number of hepatic LDL receptors leads to an increased uptake of LDL from plasma, resulting in a lower plasma LDL-cholesterol concentration (Shepherd et al., 1980; Kovanen et al., 1981). The effectiveness of the resin depends on the ability of hepatic cells to increase the number of active LDL receptors. Thus, individuals with the homozygous form of familial hypercholesterolemia, who lack LDL functional receptors, do not respond to such therapy (Goldstein and Brown, 1983). However, heterozygotes, who have one normal gene for the receptor, do respond. Body pools of cholesterol are decreased after long-term therapy with bile acid–binding resins, and there is also regression of tendon xanthomas.

Adverse Effects and Drug Interactions. These preparations often have an unpleasant sandy or gritty quality, and patients may complain of this. Nausea, abdominal discomfort, indigestion, and constipation are frequent difficulties. Impaction may occur, and hemorrhoids are frequently aggravated. The addition of bran cereal to the diet is usually sufficient to minimize the constipation. Beside increasing concentrations of triglycerides in plasma, the bile acid–binding resins often transiently increase activities of alkaline phosphatase and transaminases as well. Since cholestyramine is a chloride form of an anion-exchange resin, hyperchloremic acidosis can occur, especially in younger and smaller patients in whom the relative dosage is higher.

With high doses of resins steatorrhea may occur, and preexisting steatorrhea is aggravated by conventional doses. In such cases, the absorption of fat-soluble vitamins is also impaired and vitamin supplementation is recommended. Hypoprothrombinemia has been observed.

The resins obviously may also bind other compounds in the intestine, including drugs administered concurrently. This has been noted particularly with chlorothiazide, phenylbutazone, phenobarbital, anticoagulants, thyroxine, and various digitalis preparations. As a general rule, it is recommended that other drugs taken orally should be ingested at least 1 hour before or 4 hours after the resin.

Bile acid–binding resins should probably not be administered during pregnancy. Children with heterozygous familial hypercholesterolemia should not begin therapy with resins until 6 years of age (Kane and Malloy, 1982).

Preparations, Dosage, and Therapeutic Uses. *Cholestyramine resin* (QUESTRAN) is available in packets that contain 9 g of powder (equivalent to 4 g of resin) or in cans that contain 378 g. *Colestipol hydrochloride* (COLESTID) is available in packets containing 5 g of resin and in bottles containing 500 g of drug. Both resins must be mixed with water or other fluids or pulpy fruits before ingestion. They should never be swallowed in the dry form. They are usually administered in daily dosages of 12 to 16 g (cholestyramine) or 15 to 30 g (colestipol), divided into two to four portions to be taken either before or during meals and at bedtime.

Cholestyramine or colestipol is the drug of choice in patients with elevated concentrations of LDL (heterozygous familial hypercholesterolemia and polygenic hypercholesterolemia). When administered with a diet low in both cholesterol and saturated fats, the resins lower plasma LDL by 15 to 20%. When cholestyramine or colestipol is administered in conjunction with either nicotinic acid or an inhibitor of HMG CoA reductase (compactin or mevinolin), a reduction of LDL concentrations

in the range of 50% can be achieved (Kane *et al.*, 1981; Bilheimer *et al.*, 1983; Illingworth, 1983; Mabuchi *et al.*, 1983). The bile acid–binding resins are of no known benefit to patients with excessive concentrations of chylomicrons, VLDL, or IDL, and they may indeed exacerbate the excess of triglycerides. Thus, they should not be used to treat disorders characterized primarily by hypertriglyceridemia.

A recent long-term prospective study, the Lipid Research Clinics Coronary Primary Prevention Trial, has provided conclusive evidence for the efficacy and safety of cholestyramine in lowering LDL-cholesterol concentrations and in reducing the morbidity and mortality of coronary heart disease (Lipid Research Clinics Program, 1984a, 1984b). A summary of the results of this study is reviewed above.

HMG CoA REDUCTASE INHIBITORS: COMPACTIN AND MEVINOLIN

The most encouraging recent development in the treatment of hypercholesterolemia has been the introduction of a new class of fungal metabolites that are potent competitive inhibitors of HMG CoA reductase, the rate-controlling enzyme in the cholesterol biosynthetic pathway. These drugs are extremely effective in lowering plasma concentrations of LDL-cholesterol. They appear to act by inhibiting cholesterol synthesis in the liver, which in turn triggers a compensatory increase in the synthesis of hepatic LDL receptors and thereby causes a reduction in the concentration of plasma LDL (Brown and Goldstein, 1981). Compactin (or ML-236B), the first HMG CoA reductase inhibitor to be discovered, was isolated in Japan by Endo in 1976. The compound was obtained from cultures of *Penicillium* species (Endo *et al.*, 1976). Several years later, a structurally related compound, mevinolin (or monacolin K), was independently isolated from cultures of *Aspergillus* and *Monascus* species by workers at the Merck Sharp and Dohme Research Laboratories and by Endo, respectively. Although compactin and mevinolin appear to be the most effective drugs for the treatment of hypercholesterolemia in man, they have not yet been subjected to full clinical or toxicological testing. Mevinolin is currently under study in the United States as an investigational drug. It is well tolerated and without adverse effects in short-term studies. The long-term safety of mevinolin and compactin has not been assessed.

Chemistry. Compactin and mevinolin differ from each other by one methyl group, and they both resemble HMG CoA, the natural substrate of HMG CoA reductase. HMG CoA, compactin, and mevinolin have the following structural formulas:

HMG CoA

Compactin   R = H
Mevinolin   R = CH₃

The total organic syntheses of compactin and mevinolin have been accomplished, and dozens of congeners have been synthesized. Several of these synthetic agents have more potent inhibitory effects *in vitro* on HMG CoA reductase than do the parent compounds.

Effects on Plasma Lipids and Lipoproteins. In healthy subjects with normal plasma concentrations of cholesterol and triglyceride, mevinolin decreases the plasma LDL-cholesterol by 35 to 45% without affecting the concentration of VLDL or HDL (Tobert *et al.*, 1982). In patients with heterozygous familial hypercholesterolemia or other forms of hypercholesterolemia (*i.e.*, polygenic hypercholesterolemia or familial multiple lipoprotein–type hyperlipoproteinemia), compactin and mevinolin lower plasma LDL-cholesterol concentrations by about 30%. A maximal effect is usually achieved within 2 weeks. When patients with heterozygous familial hypercholesterolemia are treated with either compactin or mevinolin in combination with a bile acid–binding resin, plasma LDL-cholesterol concentrations are lowered by 50% without any reduction in plasma HDL-cholesterol or VLDL-triglyceride (Bilheimer *et al.*, 1983; Illingworth, 1983; Mabuchi *et al.*, 1983).

Mechanism of Action. In keeping with the structural resemblance between these compounds and HMG CoA, inhibition of HMG CoA reductase by compactin or mevinolin is competitive, reversible, and highly specific. The drugs have an affinity for the enzyme (K_i = 1 nM) that is 10,000-fold greater than that of the natural substrate, HMG CoA (K_m = 10 μM). In cell-free systems compactin and mevinolin inhibit sterol synthesis from [^{14}C]acetate by 50% at nanomolar concentrations. The mechanism by which an inhibition of cholesterol synthesis lowers plasma concentrations of LDL has been examined in animals and man. In patients with heterozygous familial hypercholesterolemia and in normal dogs, mevinolin lowers plasma LDL by enhancing the receptor-mediated degradation of the lipoprotein (Kovanen *et al.*, 1981; Bilheimer *et al.*, 1983).

A theoretical basis for the ability of mevinolin or compactin to stimulate receptor-mediated catabolism of LDL comes from studies of human and animal cells in tissue culture. Like most cells in the body, these cells have a dual source of the cholesterol that is required for synthesis of new mem-

branes. They can synthesize cholesterol *de novo* by a pathway that requires the action of HMG CoA reductase or they can obtain cholesterol from plasma LDL through endocytosis mediated by the LDL receptor (Goldstein and Brown, 1977). When human fibroblasts or cultured hepatocytes are incubated with compactin or mevinolin, HMG CoA reductase is inhibited competitively and the *de novo* synthesis of cholesterol is blocked. This block triggers a regulatory response that seems designed to provide more cholesterol for the cell: there is a simultaneous increase in the synthesis of both HMG CoA reductase and LDL receptors (Brown *et al.*, 1978; Brown and Goldstein, 1981; Pangburn *et al.*, 1981).

Mevinolin seems to have the same effect *in vivo* as it does in cultured cells. An increase in hepatic LDL receptors has been demonstrated directly in dogs treated with the drug (Kovanen *et al.*, 1981). An increase in LDL receptors in man has been inferred from the observation that the rate of removal of radiolabeled LDL from the blood stream increases after therapy (Bilheimer *et al.*, 1983). Studies of cholesterol balance performed on patients treated with mevinolin have shown that the drug enhances LDL receptor activity without lowering total body synthesis of cholesterol below the normal range (Grundy and Bilheimer, 1984).

In dogs and in man, the combination of a bile acid–binding resin and an inhibitor of HMG CoA reductase produces a much greater decrease of plasma LDL concentrations than can be obtained with either drug alone. This is due to a synergistic effect of the two types of drugs to stimulate receptor-mediated removal of LDL from plasma (Kovanen *et al.*, 1981; Bilheimer *et al.*, 1983). The bile acid–binding resins increase the liver's demand for cholesterol for conversion to bile acids. The HMG CoA reductase inhibitor prevents the liver from synthesizing additional cholesterol to meet this need; the liver is forced to rely on LDL receptors, and compensatory mechanisms drive the synthesis of receptors upward. In dogs, the combined treatment can lead to a threefold increase in both the number of hepatic LDL receptors and the rate of removal of LDL from plasma, with a concomitant 75% reduction of plasma concentrations of LDL (Kovanen *et al.*, 1981).

Absorption, Fate, and Excretion. Information on the pharmacokinetics of the HMG CoA reductase inhibitors is limited. In animals, 5 to 30% of an oral dose of compactin or mevinolin is rapidly absorbed from the gastrointestinal tract and taken up by the liver, which is the major site of cholesterol synthesis in the body. Compactin and mevinolin undergo extensive metabolism within the liver, but the products have not yet been characterized. The major route of excretion is through the biliary tract, with virtually none of the drug or its metabolites appearing in the urine.

Adverse Effects. Compactin and mevinolin are well tolerated acutely, but the long-term toxicity of these drugs has not been evaluated. No significant adverse effects were observed when patients were treated for 1 to 3 months. The safety of these drugs for children has not been established. During embryogenesis, HMG CoA reductase plays a crucial role in providing cholesterol and other nonsterol compounds to the developing fetus. Hence, compactin and mevinolin should not be administered to pregnant women, and the drugs should be withheld for several months before pregnancy is planned.

Preparation and Therapeutic Uses. *Mevinolin* is under study in the United States as an investigational drug. Until the long-term safety of mevinolin and compactin is established, these drugs should be reserved for the experimental treatment of patients with the heterozygous form of familial hypercholesterolemia. When combined with a bile acid–binding resin, mevinolin or compactin can lower plasma concentrations of LDL by 50% in such patients. Patients with homozygous familial hypercholesterolemia who lack functional LDL receptors are unresponsive. However, some homozygotes do have a capacity to produce a small number of receptors, and they may respond. Compactin and mevinolin are not useful for the treatment of hypertriglyceridemia.

OTHER DRUGS

Dextrothyroxine sodium (CHOLOXIN), the optical isomer of the naturally occurring hormone L-thyroxine, lowers plasma concentrations of LDL by about 20% in hypercholesterolemic patients. The drug is believed to exert its action by stimulating hepatic synthesis of LDL receptors, which in turn leads to an enhanced removal of LDL from plasma (Thompson *et al.,* 1981). Plasma concentrations of VLDL and HDL are not changed significantly. The drug is available as scored tablets. The initial oral dose for adults is 1 to 2 mg daily for 1 month. This dose is increased by 1 to 2 mg at intervals of 1 month until a satisfactory effect is achieved or until a maximal daily dose of 8 mg is reached. For children, the initial daily dose is 0.05 mg/kg and the maximal dose is 4 mg. The most serious adverse effect of this drug is an increase in frequency or severity of anginal attacks in patients with coronary heart disease. The incidence increases with the dose, so that at doses of 10 mg per day the occurrence of angina is frequent whereas at 4 mg per day it is uncommon. Other adverse effects are cardiac arrhythmias and the hypermetabolic effects associated with administration of thyroid hormones, such as nervousness, sweating, tremor, and insomnia. The drug potentiates the effect of concurrently administered oral anticoagulants. The use of dextrothyroxine should be restricted to young patients with familial hypercholesterolemia or polygenic hypercholesterolemia who are known to be free of coronary artery disease and who do not respond to diet and more conventional drugs.

The antibiotic *neomycin* (*see* Chapter 51) has a hypolipidemic effect only when administered orally. The effect is not dependent on its antimicrobial activity but appears to be secondary to the formation of insoluble complexes with bile acids in the intestine. Its mechanism of action might thus be similar to that of the sequestrants of bile acids. Small doses of neomycin reduce the plasma concentration of LDL; effects on VLDL are variable. Neomycin is administered in divided doses of 0.5 to 2 g per day. While the drug is absorbed only to a minor extent, ototoxicity and nephrotoxicity may occur in patients with impaired renal function. Diarrhea and malabsorption are other complications. Neomycin should be considered only for patients with familial hypercholesterolemia or polygenic hypercholesterolemia who are unable or unwilling to follow other regimens.

β-Sitosterol is a plant sterol with a structure similar to that of cholesterol, except for the substitution of an ethyl group at C 24 of its side chain. Like most plant sterols, it is not absorbed by man. β-Sitosterol lowers plasma concentrations of LDL but has no effect on VLDL. Its mechanism of action is not known but may relate to an inhibition of the absorption of dietary cholesterol. It is indicated only for treatment of excess LDL in patients with polygenic hypercholesterolemia who appear to be extremely sensitive to small amounts of dietary cholesterol (Kane and Malloy, 1982). The long-term effects of β-sitosterol are unknown. Adverse reactions include a mild laxative effect and occasional nausea and vomiting. The recommended dose is 6 g (usually mixed with coffee, tea, fruit juice, or milk to increase palatability), taken 30 minutes before meals and at bedtime.

Altschul, R.; Hoffer, A.; and Stephen, J. D. Influence of nicotinic acid on serum cholesterol in man. *Arch. Biochem. Biophys.,* **1955,** *54,* 558–559.

Andersson, R. G. G.; Gunnar, A.; Brattsand, R.; Ericsson, E.; and Lundholm, L. Studies on the mechanism of flush induced by nicotinic acid. *Acta Pharmacol. Toxicol.* (*Copenh.*), **1977,** *41,* 1–10.

Atmeh, R. F.; Stewart, J. M.; Boag, D. E.; Packard, C. J.; Lorimer, A. R.; and Shepherd, J. The hypolipidemic action of probucol: a study of its effects on high and low density lipoproteins. *J. Lipid Res.,* **1983,** *24,* 588–595.

Barnhart, J. W.; Sefranka, J. A.; and McIntosh, D. D. Hypocholesterolemic effect of 4,4'-(isopropylidene-dithio)-*bis*(2,6-di-*t*-butylphenol) (probucol). *Am. J. Clin. Nutr.,* **1970,** *23,* 1229–1233.

Bilheimer, D. W.; Grundy, S. M.; Brown, M. S.; and Goldstein, J. L. Mevinolin and colestipol stimulate receptor-mediated clearance of low density lipoprotein from plasma in familial hypercholesterolemia heterozygotes. *Proc. Natl Acad. Sci. U.S.A.,* **1983,** *80,* 4124–4128.

Boberg, J.; Boberg, M.; Gross, R.; Grundy, S.; Augustin, J.; and Brown, V. The effect of treatment with clofibrate on hepatic triglyceride and lipoprotein lipase activities of post heparin plasma in male patients with hyperlipoproteinemia. *Atherosclerosis,* **1977,** *27,* 499–503.

Brown, M. S.; Faust, J. R.; Goldstein, J. L.; Kaneko, I.; and Endo, A. Induction of 3-hydroxy-3-methylglutaryl coenzyme A reductase activity in human fibroblasts incubated with compactin (ML-236B), a competitive inhibitor of the reductase. *J. Biol. Chem.,* **1978,** *253,* 1121–1128.

Brunzell, J. D.; Schrott, H. G.; Motulsky, A. G.; and Bierman, E. L. Myocardial infarction in the familial forms of hypertriglyceridemia. *Metabolism,* **1976,** *25,* 313–320.

Carlson, L. A., and Bottiger, L. E.   Serum triglycerides, to be or not to be a risk factor for ischaemic heart disease? *Atherosclerosis*, **1981**, *39*, 287–291.

Carlson, L. A.; Danielson, M.; Ekberg, I.; Klintemar, B.; and Rosenhamer, G.   Reduction of myocardial reinfarction by the combined treatment with clofibrate and nicotinic acid. *Atherosclerosis*, **1977**, *28*, 81–86.

Coronary Drug Project.   Clofibrate and niacin in coronary heart disease. *J.A.M.A.*, **1975**, *231*, 360–381.

Endo, A.; Kuroda, M.; and Tanzawa, K.   Competitive inhibition of 3-hydroxy-3-methylglutaryl coenzyme A reductase by ML-236A and ML-236B, fungal metabolites having hypocholesterolemic activity. *F.E.B.S. Lett.*, **1976**, *72*, 323–326.

Goldstein, J. L.; Schrott, H. G.; Hazzard, W. R.; Bierman, E. L.; and Motulsky, A. G.   Hyperlipidemia in coronary heart disease. II. Genetic analysis of lipid levels in 176 families and delineation of a new inherited disorder, combined hyperlipidemia. *J. Clin. Invest.*, **1973**, *52*, 1544–1568.

Grundy, S. M.; Ahrens, E. H., Jr.; and Salen, G.   Interruption of the enterohepatic circulation of bile acids in man: comparative effects of cholestyramine and ileal exclusion on cholesterol metabolism. *J. Lab. Clin. Med.*, **1971**, *78*, 94–121.

Grundy, S. M., and Bilheimer, D. W.   Inhibition of 3-hydroxy-3-methylglutaryl-CoA reductase by mevinolin in familial hypercholesterolemia heterozygotes: effects on cholesterol balance. *Proc. Natl Acad. Sci. U.S.A.*, **1984**, *81*, 2538–2542.

Grundy, S. M.; Mok, H. Y. I.; Zech, L.; and Berman, M.   Influence of nicotinic acid on metabolism of cholesterol and triglycerides in man. *J. Lipid Res.*, **1981**, *22*, 24–36.

Hashim, S. A., and Van Itallie, T. B.   Cholestyramine resin therapy for hypercholesterolemia: clinical and metabolic studies. *J.A.M.A.*, **1965**, *192*, 289–293.

Illingworth, D. R.   Mevinolin in the therapy of heterozygous familial hypercholesterolemia. *Arteriosclerosis*, **1983**, *3*, 479a.

Kane, J. P., and Malloy, M. J.   Treatment of hypercholesterolemia. *Med. Clin. North Am.*, **1982**, *66*, 537–550.

Kane, J. P.; Malloy, M. J.; Tun, P.; Phillips, N. R.; Freedman, D. D.; Williams, M. L.; Rowe, J. S.; and Havel, R. J.   Normalization of low-density-lipoprotein levels in heterozygous familial hypercholesterolemia with a combined drug regimen. *N. Engl. J. Med.*, **1981**, *304*, 251–258.

Kovanen, P. T.; Bilheimer, D. W.; Goldstein, J. L.; Jaramillo, J. J.; and Brown, M. S.   Regulatory role for hepatic low density lipoprotein receptors *in vivo* in the dog. *Proc. Natl Acad. Sci. U.S.A.*, **1981**, *78*, 1194–1198.

Levy, R. I.; Fredrickson, D. S.; Shulman, R.; Bilheimer, D. W.; Breslow, J. L.; Stone, N. J.; Lux, S. E.; Sloan, H. R.; Kraus, R. M.; and Herbert, P. N.   Dietary and drug treatment of primary hyperlipoproteinemia. *Ann. Intern. Med.*, **1972**, *77*, 267–294.

Lipid Research Clinics Program.   The lipid research clinics coronary primary prevention trial results. I. Reduction in incidence of coronary heart disease. *J.A.M.A.*, **1984a**, *251*, 351–364.

———.   The lipid research clinics coronary primary prevention trial results. II. The relationship of reduction in incidence of coronary heart disease to cholesterol lowering. *Ibid.*, **1984b**, *251*, 365–374.

Mabuchi, H.; Sakai, T.; Sakai, Y.; Yoshimura, A.; Watanabe, A.; Wakasugi, T.; Koizumi, J.; and Takeda, R.   Reduction of serum cholesterol in heterozygous patients with familial hypercholesterolemia: additive effects of compactin and cholestyramine. *N. Engl. J. Med.*, **1983**, *308*, 609–613.

Nestel, P. J., and Billington, T.   Effects of probucol on low density lipoprotein removal and high density lipoprotein synthesis. *Atherosclerosis*, **1981**, *38*, 203–209.

Oliver, M. F.; Heady, J. A.; Morris, J. N.; and Cooper, M. J.   A co-operative trial in the primary prevention of ischaemic heart disease using clofibrate. *Br. Heart J.*, **1978**, *40*, 1069–1118.

Olsson, A. G.; Carlson, L. A.; Anggard, E.; and Ciabattoni, G.   Prostacyclin production augmented in the short term by nicotinic acid. *Lancet*, **1983**, *2*, 565–566.

Palmer, R. H.   Prevalence of gallstones in hyperlipidemia and incidence during treatment with clofibrate and/or cholestyramine. *Trans. Assoc. Am. Physicians*, **1978**, *91*, 424–432.

Pangburn, S. H.; Newton, R. S.; Chang, C.-M.; Weinstein, D. B.; and Steinberg, D.   Receptor-mediated catabolism of homologous low density lipoproteins in cultured pig hepatocytes. *J. Biol. Chem.*, **1981**, *256*, 3340–3347.

Rifkind, B. M., and Segal, P.   Lipid research clinics program reference values for hyperlipidemia and hypolipidemia. *J.A.M.A.*, **1983**, *250*, 1869–1872.

Rossner, S., and Oro, L.   Fenofibrate therapy of hyperlipoproteinaemia. *Atherosclerosis*, **1981**, *38*, 273–282.

Samuel, P.   Effects of gemfibrozil on serum lipids. *Am. J. Med.*, **1983**, *74*, 23–27.

Shepherd, J.; Packard, C. J.; Bicker, S.; Lawrie, T. D. V.; and Morgan, H. G.   Cholestyramine promotes receptor-mediated low-density-lipoprotein catabolism. *N. Engl. J. Med.*, **1980**, *302*, 1219–1222.

Stone, N. J.; Levy, R. I.; Fredrickson, D. S.; and Verter, J.   Coronary artery disease in 116 kindred with familial type II hyperlipoproteinemia. *Circulation*, **1974**, *49*, 476–488.

Thompson, G. R.; Soutar, A. K.; Spengel, F. A.; Jadhav, A.; Gavigan, S. J. P.; and Myant, N. B.   Defects of receptor-mediated low density lipoprotein catabolism in homozygous familial hypercholesterolemia and hypothyroidism *in vivo*. *Proc. Natl Acad. Sci. U.S.A.*, **1981**, *78*, 2591–2595.

Thorp, J. M., and Waring, W. S.   Modification and distribution of lipids by ethyl chlorophenoxyisobutyrate. *Nature*, **1962**, *194*, 948–949.

Tobert, J. A.; Bell, G. D.; Birtwell, J.; James, I.; Kukovetz, W. R.; Pryor, J. S.; Buntinx, A.; Holmes, I. B.; Chao, Y.-S.; and Bolognese, J. A.   Cholesterol-lowering effect of mevinolin, an inhibitor of 3-hydroxy-3-methylglutaryl–coenzyme A reductase, in healthy volunteers. *J. Clin. Invest.*, **1982**, *69*, 913–919.

Monographs and Reviews

Assmann, G.   *Lipid Metabolism and Atherosclerosis.* F. K. Schattauer Verlag GmbH., Stuttgart, **1982.**

Brown, M. S., and Goldstein, J. L.   Lowering plasma cholesterol by raising LDL receptors. (Editorial.) *N. Engl. J. Med.*, **1981**, *305*, 515–517.

———.   Lipoprotein metabolism in the macrophage: implications for cholesterol deposition in atherosclerosis. *Annu. Rev. Biochem.*, **1983**, *52*, 223–261.

Brown, M. S.; Kovanen, P. T.; and Goldstein, J. L.   Regulation of plasma cholesterol by lipoprotein receptors. *Science*, **1981**, *212*, 628–635.

Carlson, L. A., and Olsson, A. G.   Effect of drugs on lipoprotein metabolism. *Prog. Biochem. Pharmacol.*, **1979**, *15*, 238–257.

Connor, W. E., and Connor, S. L.   The dietary treatment of hyperlipidemia. Rationale, technique and efficacy. *Med. Clin. North Am.*, **1982**, *66*, 485–518.

Gey, K. F., and Carlson, L. A. (eds.).   *Metabolic Effects of Nicotinic Acid and Its Derivatives.* Hans Huber Publishers, Bern, **1971.**

Goldstein, J. L., and Brown, M. S.   The low-density lipoprotein pathway and its relation to atherosclerosis. *Annu. Rev. Biochem.*, **1977**, *46*, 897–930.

———.   Familial hypercholesterolemia. In, *The Metabolic Basis of Inherited Disease*, 5th ed. (Stanbury,

J. B.; Wyngaarden, J. B.; Fredrickson, D. S.; Goldstein, J. L.; and Brown, M. S.; eds.) McGraw-Hill Book Co., New York, **1983,** pp. 672–712.

Goldstein, J. L.; Kita, T.; and Brown, M. S. Defective lipoprotein receptors and atherosclerosis: lessons from an animal counterpart of familial hypercholesterolemia. *N. Engl. J. Med.,* **1983,** *309,* 288–295.

Havel, R. J.; Goldstein, J. L.; and Brown, M. S. Lipoproteins and lipid transport. In, *Metabolic Control and Disease,* 8th ed. (Bondy, P. K., and Rosenberg, L. E., eds.) W. B. Saunders Co., Philadelphia, **1980,** pp. 393–494.

Havel, R. J., and Kane, J. P. Drugs and lipid metabolism. *Annu. Rev. Pharmacol.,* **1973,** *13,* 287–308.

Keys, A. Coronary heart disease. The global picture. *Atherosclerosis,* **1975,** *22,* 149–192.

Mahley, R. W., and Angelin, B. Type III hypercholesterolemia: recent insights into the genetic defect of familial dysbetalipoproteinemia. *Adv. Intern. Med.,* **1983,** *29,* 385–441.

Marks, J. (ed.). *Dyslipoproteinaemia—Aspects of Gemfibrozil Therapy,* Vol. 4. *Research and Clinical Forums,* Kent, England, **1982.**

Miller, G. J. High density lipoproteins and atherosclerosis. *Annu. Rev. Med.,* **1980,** *31,* 97–108.

Symposium. (Various authors.) Gemfibrozil: a new lipid lowering agent. *Proc. R. Soc. Med.,* **1976,** *69,* Suppl. 2, 1–120.

SECTION VII

Water, Salts, and Ions

Normal inorganic constituents of the body may be considered as pharmacological agents when they are administered to repair either acute or chronic states of depletion or deficiency. These compounds fall into several groups. Those that contribute to the osmolality, the pH, or the volume of the body fluids are considered in this section (Chapter 35), while those that have a more unique relationship to the function of specific organs are discussed in the appropriate organ-related sections of the text. Thus, calcium and phosphate are considered together with the agents that are primarily responsible for their regulation—vitamin D, parathyroid hormone, and calcitonin (Chapter 65); iodide is presented with other agents that are relevant to the function of the thyroid gland (Chapter 60), and the salts of iron are discussed in the context of hematopoiesis (Chapter 56). Drugs that are inorganic ions, such as lithium (Chapter 19), are described in chapters most appropriate to their therapeutic utility, while metallic ions that are primarily of toxicological importance are grouped in Chapter 69. It is not within the scope of this textbook to consider the role of trace elements in nutrition.

CHAPTER

35 AGENTS AFFECTING VOLUME AND COMPOSITION OF BODY FLUIDS

Gilbert H. Mudge

The volume and composition of the body fluids vary tremendously from one compartment to another and from one cell type to another, and are maintained remarkably constant despite the vicissitudes of daily life and the stresses imposed by disease. This remarkable system has developed over millions of years and permits the efficient regulation of homeostasis. The responsible mechanisms reside in a variety of organs and tissues, which include the central nervous system (CNS), the heart, the lungs, the gastrointestinal tract, and the kidneys. The failure of the kidney to repair a disordered state is more commonly related to the unavailability of adequate raw material rather than to some primary renal disturbance *per se*. To the extent that this is true, it follows that the wisdom with which the raw materials are supplied may be crucial.

Disturbances in fluid and electrolyte metabolism involve four major properties of the body fluids—volume, osmolality, hydrogen ion concentration (pH), and the concentrations of specific ions. In some diseases an abnormality in one property may dominate the picture. However, severely ill patients often have multiple disturbances that coexist and interact.

Throughout this chapter, guidelines for therapy are suggested. The reader should be aware that these represent an approach that is an approximation for an average patient. The physician must examine the details of management as carefully as in any other therapeutic regimen in clinical medicine.

DISTURBANCES OF VOLUME AND OSMOLALITY

THE DISTRIBUTION AND THE COMPOSITION OF BODY FLUIDS

Distribution of Body Fluids. Total body water in man varies from 50% of body weight in the obese to 70% in the lean. This total volume is divided into two major compartments, the intracellular and the extracellular, and a smaller compartment, the transcellular. This last-named includes fluids within the tracheobronchial tree, the gastrointestinal tract, the excretory system of the kidneys and glands, the cerebrospinal fluid, and the aqueous humor of the eye.

The volumes of these compartments may be estimated with the use of agents that distribute themselves uniformly throughout a particular compartment. One can estimate the total volume of body water, the extracellular volume, and the plasma volume. The volume of the intracellular compartment can be calculated as the difference between total body water and the volume of the extracellular compartment (*see* Table 35–1).

Composition of Body Fluids. There are vast differences in the composition of the two major compartments. An average composition for *plasma* is as follows:

CATIONS		ANIONS	
	(*mEq/liter*)		
Sodium	135–145	Chloride	98–106
Potassium	3.5–5.0	Bicarbonate	24–28
Calcium	4.5–5.3	Phosphate and	
		sulfate	2–5
Magnesium	1.5–2.0	Organic anions	3–6
		Protein	15–20

The concentration of the filterable ions in the *interstitial fluid* can be calculated from the values in serum with a correction for serum water (SW) and the Donnan ratio. Both of these corrections are necessary because of the contribution of protein. The Donnan ratio is 0.95 for cations and 1.05 for anions, and the calculation is made according to the following equations:

$$Na_{IF} = \frac{Na_S}{SW} \times 0.95$$

$$Cl_{IF} = \frac{Cl_S}{SW} \times 1.05$$

where the subscripts IF and s refer to interstitial fluid and serum, respectively. A clinical laboratory usually reports the concentration in whole serum. The water content of serum is normally about 92%. Since the composition of the interstitial fluid is very similar to that of serum, these two fluids are often considered as the same and are grouped together as *extracellular fluid*.

The composition of *intracellular fluid* is quite different. The major cations are potassium and magnesium with little sodium; the major anions are phosphate and protein with some bicarbonate and, in most cells, very little chloride. Because muscle tissue represents the largest segment of intracellular fluid, its composition has often been considered as representative of this compartment. However, the intracellular fluids of various tissues differ from each other; furthermore, intracellular fluid is not homogeneous within a given tissue, but varies in the several cellular organelles. The data for *muscle-cell fluid* are as follows:

CATIONS		ANIONS	
	(*mEq/liter*)		
Sodium	10	Bicarbonate	10
Potassium	150	Phosphate and	
Magnesium	40	sulfate	150
		Protein	40

Table 35–1. THE MEASUREMENT AND DISTRIBUTION OF BODY WATER

COMPARTMENT	% TOTAL BODY WATER	AGENT USED FOR ESTIMATE *
Total Body Water (TBW)	100	DHO, THO, antipyrine
Intracellular Water (ICW)	55	By difference between TBW and ECW
Extracellular Water (ECW)	35	Inulin, SO_4^{2-}, Cl^-, Br^-
Plasma Volume (PV)	7.5	T1824, ^{131}I-albumin
Interstitial Fluid (IF)	27.5	By difference between ECW and PV
Inaccessible Bone Water	7.5	Special technics
Transcellular Water	2.5	Special technics

* DHO = deuterated water; THO = tritiated water; T1824 = plasma protein–bound dye.

The composition of the body can also be studied by the use of radioactive isotopes and by calculation of the *total exchangeable quantity* of a given ion. The method involves the administration of a known quantity of radioactive material, the equilibration of the isotope with all the stable element with which it will readily equilibrate (usually 24 hours), the determination of the specific activity in serum, and the calculation of the total quantity of the ion that is exchangeable. Normal values for adults are:

	MALE	FEMALE
	(mEq/kg of Body Weight)	
Sodium	40	38
Potassium	48	39
Chloride	29	29

It is known from other analyses that about 75% of total body sodium and 85% of total body potassium are exchangeable.

Cellular Mechanisms of Electrolyte Control. The manner by which the major compositional differences of the intracellular and extracellular fluids are maintained has been studied extensively. These ions are not at equilibrium but exist in a steady state away from equilibrium; this demands an energy-requiring series of operations, referred to in general as "active transport." In the steady-state condition, the concentration of sodium and potassium within the cell is dependent on the rate of pumping of sodium out and potassium in (by the Na^+, K^+-activated adenosine triphosphatase system) and the rates at which these ions move by passive diffusion along the established electrochemical gradients. These ionic transport mechanisms are partially responsible for the regulation of cell volume. In addition, they serve to establish and maintain the electrical potential gradients across the cell membrane that are essential for the generation and propagation of action potentials in excitable cells.

Osmotic Pressure. The chief determinant of the passage of fluid from one compartment to another is osmotic pressure (activity of water molecules). Those solutes that *cannot* freely permeate membranes by diffusion contribute an *effective osmotic pressure* and one that promotes a redistribution of water. Those solutes that *can* freely permeate a cell membrane influence the *total osmotic pressure* but do not generate effective osmotic gradients and hence do not lead to the net movement of water between compartments.

INTERNAL EXCHANGES OF WATER AND SOLUTE

Intracellular and Extracellular Fluid Volumes. Almost all cell membranes are freely permeable to water. Exceptions include the sweat glands and the distal nephron. However, as a consequence of free diffusion of water in the major tissues of the body, it follows that the extracellular and intracellular fluids are of equal osmolality, and that any transient alteration in the effective osmolality of one fluid must cause a redistribution of water until the two fluids are once again of equal osmolality. Primary changes in osmolality occur most often in the extracellular fluid; under some circumstances intracellular osmolality may be directly altered by marked changes in cell metabolism.

The principal determinant of the effective osmolality of the extracellular fluid is the concentration of sodium salts. These ions represent more than 90% of all extracellular solutes that contribute an *effective osmolality*.

Addition of Water. If a subject drinks water faster than he can excrete it, he develops a positive water balance. This water gains access initially to the extracellular space, where it expands the volume and dilutes the solutes (*hyponatremia*). The decrease in effective osmolality (increase in the activity of water) is accompanied by a net movement of water molecules from the extracellular space to the intracellular fluid. Obviously, this will cease when the two fluids are once again of equal osmolality, albeit lower than initially. The result is the distribution of the increment of water through the volume of total body water.

Addition of Salt. If a subject is administered a sodium salt in a concentration in excess of that in extracellular fluid, the concentration of sodium in the extracellular space will increase (*hypernatremia*). Although more sodium tends to enter cells, the rate of extrusion will match the enhanced entry. Thus, the increment of salt is effectively confined to the extracellular compartment. The addition of solute diminishes the activity of the molecules of extracellular water, and fewer water molecules enter intracellular fluid than leave it. Water thus redistributes from cells to extracellular space until the two fluids are once again of equal osmolality, albeit higher than initially.

The above effects on intracellular volume are observed if *hypo*natremia results from a loss of salt in excess of water, or if *hyper*natremia results as a consequence of the loss of water in excess of salt. However, in these two circumstances, in addition to a redistribution of water between the two major compartments, total body fluid will have been diminished.

The corollary is, of course, that a gain (or loss) of a saline fluid that is isosmotic with body fluids will cause no shift of water between the cells and the extracellular compartments, but it will expand (or contract) extracellular volume.

Interstitial and Plasma Volumes. The same basic principles apply to the steady-state distribution of volume between these two components of the extracellular space. The vascular endothelium is permeable to water and to *most* of the solutes. However, it is relatively *im*permeable to the larger molecular species such as proteins. The segregation of these molecules within the vascular component tends to diminish the activity of the water molecules, and if there were no counteracting force all the extracellular fluid would move into the plasma. In the regulation of fluid distribution between the vascular and interstitial fluids, the counteracting force is the hydrostatic pressure within the vascular system. This increases the activity of the molecules of water to such an extent as virtually to nullify the opposite effect exerted by the plasma proteins. In addition, there is a small colloidal osmotic force operating in the interstitial fluid and a minor pressure force referred to as "tissue tension." The *balance* of these forces—the Starling forces—is the determinant of the steady-state distribution of volume between the two compartments.

There is an additional influence that operates owing to the fact that the plasma proteins are charged molecules. Since they are unable to penetrate the endothelial membrane, an equilibrium is set up (the Gibbs-Donnan equilibrium) such that there is a slightly greater concentration of diffusible ions in the fluid associated with the charged impermeant anion. The total influence of the protein on the activity of plasma water is referred to as the "colloidal *oncotic* pressure."

All the above-described Starling forces are usually so adjusted that about one fourth of the extracellular fluid is within the confines of the vascular system and the remainder is in the interstitial space. Furthermore, these forces operate in such a fashion that there is a tendency for water and diffusible solutes to leave the vascular bed at the arteriolar end of the capillaries and return at the same rate at the venous end. In this fashion, there is a large turnover of water and diffusible solutes between the two compartments without a net change in volume. The importance of this turnover is obvious, because this is how the circulation can efficiently bring oxygen and nutrients to the cell and remove carbon dioxide and other end products of metabolism without relying solely on diffusion.

Net shifts do occur, however, when there is a dislocation of these Starling forces. An increase in the hydrostatic pressure transmitted to the capillaries may permit a greater rate of transudation than reabsorption. The same effect may be noted when there is hypoproteinemia and the colloidal oncotic pressure is thereby diminished. In both circumstances, there is a net movement of volume to the interstitial fluid compartment. The overall effect may be mitigated partially by another system of vessels, namely, the lymphatic system.

One of the important therapeutic implications is that the plasma volume cannot specifically be increased unless the administered fluid contains a colloidal agent. The administration of saline solution to a subject who has lost blood will reexpand the extracellular fluid volume, but most of the expansion will occur in the interstitial compartment.

EXTERNAL EXCHANGES OF WATER AND SOLUTE

The Balance Principle. In the early decades of this century a great deal of research involved measuring the intake and output of various nutrients and their metabolites.

While this method has properly become archaic for the study of intermediary metabolism, it nevertheless provides the conceptual basis for our understanding of the pathogenesis and proper therapy of many disturbances of fluid and electrolyte metabolism. With the exceptions that are noted below, one may consider that water and the major solutes do not undergo metabolic alteration. Hence, concentrations within the body fluids represent the balance between intake and output, both for water and the solute in question. By general usage, if a patient gains or loses something, he is in *positive* or *negative* balance, respectively; if there are no significant changes, the balance is *neutral*. The latter is often referred to as "being in balance," and this is the condition of the normal subject who is neither gaining nor losing weight (Table 35–2).

In general, the greater the change in external balance and the more acutely it occurs, the more accurate is the estimate of the change itself. With large changes, insensible, unmeasured, or unestimated losses assume relatively less importance. Also, with large external changes, analytical errors become less important. This applies both to direct chemical analysis and to clinical estimates based on history and physical examination. It is possible to get independent estimates that serve as checks—for example, the change in weight that accompanies a large change in fluid balance. The proper management of many patients includes an accurate record of *intake and output* and daily weights. This is particularly true of severely ill patients with complex disturbances. Intake includes oral intake, infusions, transfusions, and so forth. Output includes urine, vomitus, and fecal and other intestinal losses. Except for research purposes, insensible losses through the lungs and skin are not measured, but they should be estimated. Solid food is rarely included in the estimate of intake even though it provides some water of oxidation. In acute renal failure, this assumes importance.

The *initial state* may have two connotations. It may refer to the value presumed to have been present in the state of health (*e.g.,* body water estimated from a patient's normal weight), or it may refer to any state during an illness prior to the initiation of a specific treatment.

From an accurate knowledge of the external balance, or even from a thoughtful guess as to its probable value, it is possible to deduce many pathophysiological mechanisms. Changes in the balance of water and solute may occur simultaneously, but their independent contributions should be evaluated separately.

It should be emphasized that the effect of a change in external balance on the composition of the body fluids is independent of the discrete physiological mechanisms that may be involved. For example, the loss of 10 liters of water has essentially the same effect on the residual body fluids, whether due to excessive losses through the skin or to the passage of very dilute urine in uncontrolled diabetes insipidus. Because of this, the "black box" mechanisms of fluid and electrolyte balance warrant reemphasis.

Table 35–2. REPRESENTATIVE "NORMAL" VALUES OF FLUID AND ELECTROLYTE INTAKE AND OUTPUT *

	INTAKE		OUTPUT		
	Oral	*Metabolism*	*Urine*	*Feces*	*Insensible*
Water as fluid, ml	1200	0	1500	100	900
Water in food, ml	1000	300			
Nitrogen, g	13	0	12	1.0	0
Sodium, mEq	75	0	74	0.5	0.5
Potassium, mEq	50	0	45	5.0	0
Chloride, mEq	75	0	74	0.5	0.5
Nonvolatile acid, mEq	0	70	70	0	0
Volatile acid, mEq	0	14,000	0	0	14,000

* A single value is selected for each entry to facilitate comparison of intake and output, and all are adjusted to depict a zero net external balance. Nonvolatile acids are largely phosphoric and sulfuric acid residues of metabolism. Volatile acid is exclusively carbon dioxide. All values refer to the amount per 24 hours.

Fixed and Labile Ions and Solutes. Provided the definitions are not extended too far or applied too rigidly, it is useful to bear in mind the distinction between fixed and labile solutes. This is based on physiological considerations. In the case of charged particles, a *fixed ion* is one that exists in the ionic form under all physiological circumstances. This holds true for strong electrolytes such as sodium, potassium, and chloride. Through metabolic alterations, *labile ions* may either be generated from nonionic precursors or converted to nonionic end products. Thus, labile ions may be added to or removed from the body fluids in a form other than that of the charged ion. For example, the ammonium cation (NH_4^+) can be converted to urea in the liver, and also synthesized from amino acids in the kidney. Bicarbonate ion (HCO_3^-) is labile since at the proper pH it can be converted to H_2CO_3, and thence to its volatile form, CO_2. Another example would be the formation of lactate from glucose. In addition, the ion of a weak acid or base may be buffered so as to change its ionic equivalence (*e.g.*, monobasic and dibasic phosphate). Of course, this is not metabolic alteration in the usual sense, but it does denote a degree of lability.

The same considerations apply to nonelectrolytes. Mannitol does not undergo metabolic change and may be considered fixed. However, glucose, which has the same osmotic characteristics as mannitol, is highly labile.

It is a truism that in electrolyte metabolism the most important attribute of any solute relates to its actual concentration in solution in the body fluids. For many solutes, this is directly related to their external balance. However, this does not apply to those that may be either formed or catabolized within the body. It should be apparent that metabolism may change either ionic or osmotic characteristics.

Consideration of Basal Requirements. A summary of average values for the intake and output of water and the major electrolytes is given in Table 35–2. These values presuppose average diet and physical activity, a normal state of metabolism, and no abnormal losses. There is considerable variation from one individual to another and moderate variation from day to day. The composition of important fluids that may be lost from the body is given in Table 35–3.

Insensible Perspiration. Water is continuously lost from the surface of the skin and from the air that is exhaled by the lungs. This is pure water with no solute.

Sweat. This is a hypotonic solution. The rate of sweating is responsive to internal heat, and, therefore, it is difficult to assign a "daily average." Furthermore, it is exceedingly difficult to estimate, and in some circumstances represents a large and unidentifiable loss.

Table 35–3. PRODUCTION RATES AND COMPOSITION OF VARIOUS BODY FLUIDS *

	VOLUME	COMPOSITION			
		Na^+	K^+	Cl^-	HCO_3^-
	ml/24 hr	mEq/liter			
Cutaneous sweat	100–200	50–80	5	40–85	—
Gastrointestinal					
Saliva	1500	10	30	10	10–20
Gastric fluid	2500	10–115	1–35	90–150	0–15
Bile	500	130–160	3–12	90–120	40–50
Pancreatic fluid	700	115–150	3–8	55–95	60–120
Intestinal fluids	3000				
Jejunum	—	85–150	2–10	45–125	—
Ileum	—	85–120	3–10	60–130	—
Ileostomy (old)	—	40–50	3–5	20–30	—
Cecostomy	—	45–135	5–45	20–90	—
Feces					
Normal	100	5	50	5	—
Diarrhea (cholera)	—	130	20	100	50

* Data are summarized from the literature for both average values and their ranges, and refer to an adult in a temperate climate engaging in mild physical activity.

Gastrointestinal. Although there is a large turn-over of ions and water between the gut lumen and the body fluid, the *net* loss from the gastrointestinal tract in the feces is usually trivial.

Urine. A liter of urine per day is adequate to contain the solutes destined for excretion.

Endogenous Water. A certain amount of water is produced by the body each day from the metabolism of nutrients.

Sodium Chloride. The average diet contains 4 to 10 g of NaCl a day. This value varies widely due to personal tastes. If salt is removed from the diet, the normal kidney excretes urine that is virtually free of sodium chloride within 3 to 5 days.

Potassium. In the face of reduced intake this cation is not quite so well conserved by the kidney as is sodium, and with chronic reduction of dietary intake it is important to guard against a deficit.

Magnesium. Renal and gastrointestinal conservation of magnesium is excellent.

Summary. These approximate daily basal requirements may be summarized as follows:

Water	1500–2000 ml
Potassium chloride	30–60 millimoles
Sodium chloride	75 millimoles
Magnesium salts	8 millimoles

These amounts relate specifically to the adult. Since the requirements for water and electrolytes are related more closely to the rate of metabolism than to age or body size, the following values may be helpful:

	PER 100 KCAL
Water	100 ml
Sodium	2–3 mEq
Potassium	2–3 mEq
Chloride	4–6 mEq

The probable average caloric expenditure per 24 hours may be estimated from the following:

KG	KCAL
0–10 kg	100/kg
11–20 kg	1000 + 50/kg, for each kg in excess of 10
> 20 kg	1500 + 20/kg, for each kg in excess of 20

CLINICAL DISTURBANCES OF VOLUME AND OSMOLALITY

For purposes of classification, several points warrant emphasis. The terms *dehydration* and *overhydration* are often inadequate. For an appropriate description, as well as for correct therapy, each condition should be described with two independent terms—*volume* and *osmolality* (Table 35–4). (1) The reference point for the classification system is the extracellular fluid. This is justified for two reasons. First, it is the plasma that is available for chemical analysis. Second, it is the extracellular compartment, or its close relative the transcellular compartment, from which abnormal fluid losses occur. (2) The classification is valid for acute changes occurring over hours or days. With more chronic disturbances, compensatory physiological adjustments make the classification less accurate. (3) These conditions may or may not be associated with disturbances in acid-base bal-

Table 35–4. TYPES OF ACUTE CHANGES IN VOLUME AND OSMOLALITY *

ACUTE EXTRACELLULAR CHANGE	CLINICAL EXAMPLE	Δ VOLUME		Δ CONC. PLASMA SODIUM	Δ HEMATOCRIT	Δ CONC. PLASMA PROTEIN
		Δ ECW	Δ ICW			
Isotonic contraction	Cholera	↓	0	0	↑	↑
Hypertonic contraction	Excess sweating	↓	↓	↑	0	↑
Hypotonic contraction	Adrenal insufficiency	↓	↑	↓	↑	↑
Isotonic expansion	Isotonic saline	↑	0	0	↓	↓
Hypertonic expansion	Hypertonic saline	↑	↓	↑	↓	↓
Hypotonic expansion	Water intoxication	↑	↑	↓	0	↓

* For discussion of hematocrit, *see* text. Direction of change is shown by arrows. 0 = no change; ECW = extracellular water; ICW = intracellular water. Under clinical examples, isotonic and hypertonic saline refer to infusions.

ance. (4) The primary classification refers to changes in *extracellular* volume. If, in response to changes in osmolality, there are secondary changes in *intracellular* volume, these may be in the same or opposite direction to those in the extracellular compartment. (5) The classification is based on external changes in water or solute balance, but without any change in red-blood-cell mass or total circulating protein.

It is rare in clinical situations to find pure examples of the categories listed in Table 35–4. This is not surprising since each depends on two factors, which may be influenced by partially independent mechanisms.

Sodium Concentration as an Index of Plasma Osmolality. Since sodium is the major extracellular solute, its concentration may be used as an index of osmolality, directly for the extracellular fluid and indirectly for the intracellular. As a first approximation, osmolality is twice the sodium concentration. This estimate is not valid in two instances.

Pseudohyponatremia. This is a condition in which the concentration of sodium in the plasma is abnormally low when analyzed by conventional methods (which depend on aliquots measured volumetrically), but in which the concentration would be normal if referred to plasma water. The discrepancy occurs when there is an abnormally high concentration of large molecules and hence an abnormally low percentage of plasma water, most commonly with hyperlipemia or marked hyperproteinemia. A clue to the former is afforded by the lactescence of the serum; the latter occurs particularly in multiple myeloma but also with severe volume depletion.

Sodium as a False Index. This occurs, even with corrections for plasma water, when there is an abnormally high concentration of another solute that is an effective extracellular osmotic particle. It may be seen with severe *hyperglycemia* in diabetes mellitus or following the infusion of large amounts of glucose. It is also seen after the administration of a nonmetabolizable extracellular solute such as *mannitol*. Glucose slowly gains access to the intracellular space by carrier-mediated transport. Thus, if the concentration in plasma rises abruptly, glucose acts at least transiently as if it were confined to the extracellular space. This may lead to hyperosmolality without hypernatremia and, indeed, due to shifts of water from the intracellular to the extracellular space, may be associated with hyponatremia. The simplest method of evaluation is to determine the concentrations of sodium and glucose separately, convert these to osmolar terms, and add them together. If hyperglycemia is rapidly corrected under the influence of insulin, a significant amount of extracellular solute may in effect disappear. This is accompanied by a redistribution of water between the extracellular and intracellular compartments. (*See* Katz, 1973.)

Isotonic Contraction. This occurs when *sodium and water are lost in isotonic proportions*. The most common example is the loss of fluid from the gastrointestinal tract, and cholera is the classical disease. This type of disturbance may be complicated by acid-base changes. Loss of strongly acidic fluid from the stomach leads to metabolic alkalosis; loss of alkaline bile and pancreatic fluid, or the less alkaline fluid of severe diarrhea, leads to metabolic acidosis. The characteristic of this type of dehydration is a normal value for the concentration of sodium in serum. Therefore, regardless of the volume deficit of the extracellular phase, so long as the *concentration* of plasma sodium is normal, there will be no redistribution of water to the cellular compartment. The repair of the dehydration requires an expansion of the extracellular fluid volume with a solution that approximates the composition of that fluid. Although in many instances simple restoration of the volume of the extracellular space will serve to replace the plasma volume proportionately, there are occasions when more prompt and specific attention must be directed to plasma volume by providing a colloidal solution that will specifically ensure its expansion.

Hypertonic Contraction. This type of dehydration is observed in any circumstance in which there is a *loss of water in excess of sodium*. The classical example involves survival on a life raft under the unremitting impact of the tropical sun (Gamble, 1947). In more common clinical conditions it occurs when the patient is unable to drink water owing to a clouded sensorium and too little water has been provided parenterally. Other circumstances include diabetes insipidus, excessive sweating (of a hypotonic fluid), and osmotic diuresis. When this occurs in uncontrolled diabetes mellitus, the effect of high concentrations of glucose (a labile solute) is additive to the negative external balance of water in causing extracellular hypertonicity. Less commonly the disturbance may be produced by a high dietary intake of protein if unaccompanied by sufficient water intake. The external loss of sodium and water decreases extracellular fluid volume, but there is partial compensation for this reduction because of simultaneous extracellular hypertonicity, which results in redistribution of water from the intracellular to the extracellular compartment. On theoretical grounds there should be no change in hematocrit if there were a pure loss of water, since this would occur proportionately from the plasma and the erythrocytes. In most clinical examples, there is also a negative balance of sodium and the hematocrit would therefore rise.

Hypotonic Contraction. This occurs when there is a *loss of sodium in excess of water*. Chief among these conditions are chronic renal insufficiency and adrenocortical insufficiency. It also occurs commonly when isotonic fluid losses are treated with water (isotonic glucose solution) and too little or no salt. Essentially the same mechanism is involved when physical exercise in a hot, dry climate is associated with the drinking of water but without the ingestion of salt tablets to replace the loss of salt that occurred through perspiration. In this type of dehydration the concentration of sodium in the plasma is reduced. This reduction in effective extracellular osmolarity results in the movement of water from extracellular fluid into the cells. Thus, the extracellular fluid is reduced by loss to both the external environment and the cells. In most instances the intensity of the dehydration is of significant magnitude and warrants prompt and aggressive attention.

Isotonic Expansion. This is the *proportional retention of sodium and water* and is the basis of generalized edema. The extracellular compartment may also be expanded by the injudicious use of isotonic saline solution in the overtreatment of dehydration. Even major fluctuations of dietary salt intake rarely give rise to isotonic expansion, at least in the adult. Normal renal function quite rapidly compensates for dietary changes. The changes described in Table 35–4 are most applicable to the rapid and excessive infusion of isotonic saline solution, since with spontaneous disease the slower development of edema is accompanied by changes in red-blood-cell mass and plasma protein. Indeed, the hypoproteinemia of hepatic and renal disease may be an important cause of edema. By definition, in all these examples the concentration of sodium in the plasma is normal, although a slight degree of hyponatremia is not uncommon.

Hypertonic Expansion. This occurs when *sodium is retained in excess of water*. In its simplest form, it results from the rapid and excessive infusion of hypertonic saline solution. The most common clinical example probably occurs in infants improperly treated for diarrhea and involves the balance between input and output. When treatment consists in oral administration of salt and water, the concentration of salt may be erroneously excessive, or the total quantity administered may be too great to be excreted by the kidneys. Accidental salt poisoning has been reported in infants following the addition of sodium chloride instead of sugar to the formula. In these instances, hypertonicity is extreme, but volume expansion is more variable and dependent upon fluid intake and excretion (Finberg *et al.*, 1963). Fatality from severe hypernatremia is due primarily to damage to the CNS. Osmotically induced water shifts decrease intracellular volume. This contributes to the fall in hematocrit; expansion of plasma volume is obviously also involved.

Hypotonic Expansion. This occurs with *retention of water in excess of sodium*. The simplest example is water intoxication due to the excessive ingestion of water. The concentrations of sodium and protein in the plasma fall by dilution. Since water distributes itself throughout the body fluids in proportion to the compartment size, there is an increase in both the extracellular and the intracellular volumes. It is for this reason that on theoretical grounds the hematocrit does not change since the erythrocytes gain water and enlarge. In a sense, the hematocrit measures the nonproportional distribution of water between the two compartments. Careful studies provide data that are in close agreement with the theory (Wynn, 1955). Excessive ingestion of water is sometimes encountered in emotionally disturbed patients. The dominant symptoms are weakness and confusion or other signs of CNS dysfunction. This may progress from confusion and apathy to stupor, coma, and generalized seizures.

Another more complicated example of hypotonic expansion is seen in some patients with edema. In rare instances, during its spontaneous development, edema is associated with a significantly greater retention of water than of salt, often referred to as dilutional hyponatremia. Far more frequently this results from the excessive use of diuretics, which may produce an imbalance between the losses of salt and water. The syndrome of the inappropriate secretion of antidiuretic hormone (ADH) also produces hypotonic expansion.

TREATMENT OF FLUID AND ELECTROLYTE DEFICITS

The basic objective of therapy is to restore the volume and composition of the body fluids to normal. However, this requires extensive qualification insofar as priorities are concerned. The present discussion is limited to water and salt balance. The more complex derangements involving blood loss and protein depletion will be considered separately.

Volume Contraction. This is life threatening because it impairs the circulation. Blood volume decreases, cardiac output falls, and the integrity of the microcirculation is compromised. This occurs whether volume contraction is isotonic, hypertonic, or hypotonic, even though, as outlined above, there are important differences between them. Given volume depletion of sufficient magnitude to threaten life, the prompt infusion of *isotonic sodium chloride solution is indicated;* indeed, it is difficult to contrive a contraindication.

The volume of fluid that needs to be replaced varies enormously. As an extreme example, intravenous therapy at the rate of 100 ml per minute for the first 1000 ml is considered necessary for the successful treatment of cholera (Carpenter, 1966). Most conditions require far less dramatic treatment. Attention should also be directed to the speed with which the volume depletion developed. For example, a 4-kg weight loss due to the loss of gastrointestinal fluids is far more debilitating if it occurs over 2 to 3 hours than over a period of days or weeks. *A general rule is to replace one half of the estimated volume loss in the first 12 to 24 hours of treatment.*

Disorders of Osmolality. Even with moderately severe hyponatremia or hypernatremia, frequently the disorder may be satisfactorily corrected with isotonic saline solution, provided there is normal renal function. Given an adequate supply of raw materials the kidney is a remarkably effective regulator of the osmolality of the body. This is accomplished by the excretion of urine at a concentration appropriate to correct the underlying disturbance.

However, if the disturbance in osmolality is severe, it is proper to treat this directly. Clinical judgment should be based on the actual physiological consequences of the disorder, and not on blood chemistry values considered in isolation. As is the case with disturbances of volume, a change in osmolality varies in importance depending on the speed of its development. Extreme hyponatremia may be asymptomatic if it develops slowly over months but not if it occurs in a few hours. If the plasma sodium concentration is lowered rapidly in infants with hypernatremia, seizures due to water intoxication may develop even when the plasma is still hypernatremic.

In addition to the diffusion of water, intracellular osmolality within the CNS is regulated by mechanisms specific for brain tissue. These involve both the gain and loss of ions and the formation and degradation of "idiogenic osmoles" (Melton and Nattie, 1983). Since both of these processes are slow relative to the diffusion of water, it is not advisable to correct osmolality immediately (as measured by plasma concentrations) in either hypoosmotic or hyperosmotic states. *A reasonable goal is to restore the extracellular osmolality one third to one half of the way toward normal within 1 day.* Except in extreme circumstances, this leads to major symptomatic and physiological improvement. In some cases of dilutional hyponatremia, it is often debatable whether specific therapy is justified, either because of the absence of any detectable harm or because of the ineffectiveness of such measures (*see* Chapter 36).

Requirements to Correct Disturbances in Osmolality. As an example, given a plasma sodium concentration of 120 mEq per liter, how much salt would be required to elevate this to 130 mEq per liter? For a 70-kg subject without gross volume deficits or excesses, one may assume a total body water of 50 liters. Although the administered sodium will be distributed in the volume of the extracellular fluid, it will exert an osmotic effect to move fluid into that compartment from the intracellular space. This will diminish the increment in extracellular osmolality and will increase intracellular osmolality. The concentration of sodium in the plasma will not rise by the desired increment of 10 mEq per liter until the osmolality of both the intracellular and extracellular compartments has been raised to a similar extent. Thus, 50 liters × 10 mEq per liter equals 500 mEq of sodium. In this example the volume that is added with the hypertonic saline solution is ignored. A calculation based exclusively on the extracellular volume would be in error. Using TBW for total body water, [Na] for sodium concentration in plasma, and subscripts 1 and 2 for the initial and final states, if TBW is kept constant and one solves for electrolyte balance, then:

$$(TBW_1 \times [Na]_1) + Na \text{ Balance} = TBW_2 \times [Na]_2$$
$$50 \times 120 \quad + 500 \quad = 50 \quad \times 130$$

The same principle applies to the calculation of water requirements for the treatment of hypernatremia. Thus, for the same subject, if the initial concentration of sodium in the plasma was 175 mEq per liter and one desired to dilute this to 160 mEq per liter, this would require a positive water balance of 4.7 liters; with the same equation, now keeping electrolyte content constant, and solving for the change in fluid balance, then:

$$TBW_1 \times [Na]_1 = TBW_2 \times [Na]_2$$
$$50 \times 175 \quad = 54.7 \quad \times 160$$

Simple modifications of these equations may be used to estimate requirements involving changes in both volume and osmolality.

Technics of Administration of Fluid. While fluids can be administered by mouth, gavage, hypodermoclysis, or vein, acute emergencies dictate that fluid replacement be initiated *intravenously*. With intravenous administration, due consideration must be given to the status of the cardiovascular system in relation to the volume infused. If cardiac function is impaired and large volumes of fluid are thought to be indicated, either the central venous or pulmonary venous pressure should be monitored. If the venous pressure rises substantially, the rate of infusion should be decreased or it should be terminated.

Oral intake and administration by *gavage* should obviously be avoided when there is nausea or vomiting or when the patient is unconscious and likely to aspirate. Until recently the oral route was ineffective when large volumes of fluid had to be given. However, modern technics of *oral rehydration therapy* have had a dramatic impact, especially in areas where diarrhea from cholera and other causes is a major public health problem. The new technics are based on the fact that the addition of glucose to electrolyte solutions greatly increases the intestinal absorption of electrolyte and water. In cases of cholera, once initial dehydration has been corrected intravenously, it has been possible to provide further replacement orally. This has major implications with regard to cost and other practical matters related to the preparation of sterile intravenous solutions under less-than-optimal conditions. Enhancement of sodium absorption by glucose probably involves both the provision of an energy source for active transport as well as the cotransport of sugar and electrolyte in a manner analogous to that of the renal tubule (*see* Introduction to Section VIII). Carbohydrates other than glucose may also be effective but have been used less widely (*see* McQuestion, 1983). The solution recommended by the World Health Organization contains 2% dextrose, 0.35% NaCl, 0.25% $NaHCO_3$, and 0.15% KCl.

Fluids Available for the Repair of Dehydration. A plethora of commercially prepared solutions is now available for replacement of fluid deficits. Some that are in frequent use include (1) 0.225%, 0.45%, 0.9%, and 5% NaCl in water; (2) 2.5%, 5%, and 10% dextrose in water; (3) mixtures of dextrose and NaCl in varying concentrations; (4) 5% $NaHCO_3$ in water; (5) mixtures of KCl (0.075 to 0.3%) with NaCl and/or with dextrose; and (6) Ringer's injection with or without lactate or lactate plus dextrose. Several points warrant emphasis: (1) These solutions consist of simple compounds that are chemically compatible in virtually all proportions, with the exception of calcium salts, which have limited solubility. (2) The pH range may extend from 3.5 to 8. However, the solutions are not buffered and, therefore, the pH in this range has no effect on systemic acid-base balance, except when bicarbonate or its precursors are included. The pH of the solution may affect the stability and possible compatibility of other drugs that are added to it. (3) Of prime pharmacological importance is the actual composition of the infused fluid, expressed either as millimoles (mmol), milliequivalents (mEq), or milliosmoles (mOsmol) per liter. However, for pharmaceutical formulation, gravimetric terminology is essential. (4) Unfortunately, by common usage a trivial and inconsistent nomenclature has become widespread. The original term *normal physiological saline* has evolved to *normal saline*, which is 154 mEq per liter. (5) Actual measurements of osmolality are usually made in terms of milliosmoles per kilogram of water; calculations of osmolarity, which are derived from molar concentrations, are expressed in milliosmoles per liter, without correction for activity coefficients or other factors. For most pharmacological purposes, the differences between these two terminologies are sufficiently small that they may be ignored. (6) Repair solutions consist of both fixed and labile solutes. The latter are of two types. For example, in the metabolism of precursors of bicarbonate (*e.g.,* lactate), one anion is replaced by another and there is no change in osmolality. However, in the metabolism of glucose to CO_2 and water, the osmolality attributable to glucose disappears. In these situations the CO_2 and water, which are end products of metabolism, are inconsequential with regard to effective osmolality.

Due to the flexibility and effectiveness of physiological homeostatic mechanisms, the repair solution utilized need not be identical to the calculated deficit if the disturbance is minor or short lived. However, for major disturbances, especially those in which large volumes of intake and output may be anticipated, the composition of the repair solution should resemble that of the calculated imbalance quite closely. The incorporation of glucose into intravenous solutions has become increasingly popular. This is a useful source of calories. Nevertheless, when there is a high turnover of fluid, the total amount of glucose infused must be monitored. As an approximation for adults, if the amount infused exceeds 500 g per day, persistent hyperglycemia, glycosuria, and polyuria may result. An advantage of fructose is its rapid removal from the extracellular space; urinary excretion is thereby minimized.

Solutions of less than 110 mOsmol per liter should not be infused into peripheral veins, since they may cause hemolysis. (Solutions of 0.9% NaCl or 5% dextrose in water are isosmotic with plasma.) Very hypertonic infusions are best given into large central veins, where they become diluted rapidly.

CORRECTION OF PLASMA AND BLOOD VOLUME

When the plasma volume is contracted as the result of simple loss of fluid and electrolyte, as in cholera, the defect may be corrected in many patients by the simple replacement of saline. When the initial losses are of a more complex nature, as in hemorrhagic shock, these same solutions also have the capacity to improve cardiovascular function transiently. In such a setting, the volume of saline (or equivalent) that is required is far greater than the initial loss of whole blood (Cervera and Moss, 1975). Nevertheless, *saline should be employed as an initial emergency measure.* The best substitute for the loss of whole blood is obviously suitable and adequately crossmatched whole blood. However, when plasma volume is critically jeopardized, the use of colloid-containing solutions is an-

other interim measure that is more efficacious than saline.

Natural Products. There are several types of solutions that contain natural colloids. Products of human origin carry the risk of transmitting hepatitis (hepatitis virus B) or the viral agent responsible for acquired immune deficiency syndrome (AIDS). For units of plasma derived from a single donor, this risk is no greater than for a single transfusion of whole blood. Preparations of pooled plasma are heated during manufacture to minimize this risk. Some commercial preparations of plasma proteins contain low concentrations of prekallikrein activators (Hageman-factor fragments). These have a hypotensive action, which may worsen the condition for which plasma proteins are prescribed (Colman, 1978).

Synthetic Products. The search for synthetic substitutes for plasma or blood has been stimulated by the limited availability of natural products. Substances that are specifically designed to restore plasma volume must have an oncotic pressure comparable to plasma. Replacements for whole blood must in addition have adequate capacity to carry oxygen. These products also have various applications in the preparation of organs for transplantation and in the operation of various bypass machines required in cardiovascular surgery.

In addition to the properties just mentioned, desirable characteristics of a plasma expander include: (1) adequate time in the circulation; (2) absence of other pharmacological actions; (3) absence of antigenic, allergenic, or pyrogenic effects; (4) absence of interference with typing or cross-matching blood; (5) stability during long periods of storage and under wide variations of environmental temperature; (6) ease of sterilization; and (7) viscosity characteristics suitable for infusion. A number of substances have been studied in the past. Those of current interest are briefly described below.

Dextran. This compound was first isolated from solutions of beet sugar, where it is formed by the action of a contaminating bacterium, *Leuconostoc mesenteroides.* It has suitable oncotic properties but no oxygen-carrying capacity.

Chemistry. In its original form, dextran is a branched polysaccharide of about 200,000 glucose units, with a molecular weight of approximately 40 million. The glucose units in the main chain are bound together through 1:6 glucosidic linkages; those in the shorter branches, through 1:4 linkages. By partial hydrolysis and fractionation, dextran can be converted to polysaccharides of any desired molecular weight.

There are two forms of dextran currently available. One has an average molecular weight of either 70,000 or 75,000 (depending on the pharmaceutical preparation), and the other has an average molecular weight of 40,000. Both agents expand plasma volume. The lower-molecular-weight dextran may well have advantages; its administration not only corrects hypovolemia but also appears to improve the microcirculation independently of simple volume expansion. It minimizes the sludging of blood that may accompany shock.

Hemodynamic Action. When dextran is given to normal individuals, there is a temporary increase in venous pressure, right atrial pressure, stroke volume, and cardiac output. As a result of the hypervolemia, urine flow is increased. In an individual who has sustained a loss of whole blood or plasma, a single infusion of dextran increases the circulating blood volume and improves the hemodynamic status for 24 hours or longer.

Effects on Blood. Dextran may interfere with typing, cross-matching, or Rh determinations, but this is unpredictable. It may produce a hemostatic defect described as an acquired form of von Willebrand's disease. The uses of dextran for its antiplatelet and antithrombotic effects are mentioned in Chapter 58.

Antigenic Action. Dextran is a potent antigen. This is true of the native polysaccharide and the hydrolysis products. Furthermore, dextran occurs in commercial sugar, and dextran-producing organisms can be found in the human gastrointestinal tract. Therefore, a small percentage of individuals who have never received dextran have precipitins to the polysaccharide in the circulation.

The antigenic activity of dextran would seem to preclude its repeated use. However, when given in the massive doses that are employed for infusion, antibody production does not occur, due presumably to the phenomenon of "immunological paralysis." Indeed, the incidence of anaphylactoid reactions to colloidal volume expanders such as plasma protein solutions, dextran, and hetastarch is remarkably low and is significantly less than that for transfusions or for many drugs (Ring and Messmer, 1977).

Distribution, Metabolic Fate, and Excretion. Following the infusion of dextran, the molecules of smaller molecular weight are excreted by the kidney. However, the remainder traverses the capillary wall very slowly and is slowly oxidized over a period of a few weeks. The persistence of dextran and its ultimate metabolic disposal are desirable features.

Untoward Reactions. Dextran appears to have no significant deleterious effects on renal, hepatic, or other vital functions. However, when glomerular filtration rate is reduced, the excessive tubular reabsorption of water may increase the concentration of dextran in the tubular fluid, such that viscosity impedes the flow of fluid through the tubule.

The incidence of sensitivity reactions is extremely variable, depending upon the preparation employed. As the technic of manufacture has improved, the number of untoward responses has diminished. These consist in itching, urticaria, joint pains, and other side effects, and are relatively mild in character. Their incidence in normal individuals is less than 10%.

Clinical Status. Dextran possesses most of the attributes of an ideal plasma expander, its chief defect being antigenicity. It has been successfully employed in the treatment of the circulatory inadequacies associated with the hypovolemia attending the loss of both whole blood and plasma. It must be realized that the use of a plasma expander is a temporary measure in the treatment of blood loss.

Hetastarch. This synthetic polymer, also known as hydroxyethyl starch, is prepared from amylopectin by the introduction of hydroxyethyl ether groups into its glucose residues. The purpose of the modification is to retard the rate of degradation of the polymer. This preparation bears many similarities to dextran. Hetastarch has an average molecular weight of 450,000, with a range from 10,000 to 1,000,000. Molecules with the lower molecular weights are readily excreted in the urine, and, with the usual preparation, about 40% of the dose is excreted within 24 hours. The molecules of higher molecular weight are metabolized slowly; only about 1% of a dose persists after 2 weeks.

Like dextran, hetastarch is used for its oncotic properties; it has no oxygen-carrying capacity. In the management of shock and in postoperative cardiac patients, hetastarch has the same efficacy as albumin as far as major hemodynamic effects are concerned (Puri *et al.*, 1983). The significance of any effect on blood coagulation is uncertain, and such effects are uncommon (Diehl *et al.*, 1982). Although hetastarch is said to have fewer antigenic properties than dextran, this assertion is not supported by clinical experience (Ring and Messmer, 1977).

Hemoglobin Solutions. Stroma-free solutions of hemoglobin are well tolerated, and they can expand plasma volume and increase oxygen-carrying capacity in experimental animals. A major problem is the short period of intravascular retention of hemoglobin due to renal excretion. Another problem involves the excessively high affinity for oxygen when hemoglobin is free in solution. These undesired effects are being approached by chemical modification and polymerization of the protein (Symposium, 1982; Cerny *et al.*, 1983).

Perfluorochemicals. These compounds dissolve oxygen rather than binding it as a chelate. Emulsions of two perfluorochemicals together with hetastarch (FLUOSOL-DA) act as oncotic agents with oxygen-carrying capacity. In a clinical trial of severely anemic patients, untoward reactions were minimal and as much as 24% of the oxygen consumed was furnished by the preparation. These agents are still in an experimental stage (Tremper *et al.*, 1982).

Preparations. *Plasma protein fraction* (PLAS-MANATE, PLASMA-PLEX) is a sterile aqueous solution containing 5% human plasma proteins in sodium chloride solution, of which not less than 83% is albumin and the remainder is α- and β-globulins; it is osmotically equivalent to plasma. The risk of transmitting hepatitis B virus is minimized by manufacturers by heating at 60° C for 10 hours. The initial dose may be 250 or 500 ml for treatment of shock.

Albumin human (ALBUMINAR, ALBUTEIN) is a sterile preparation of 5 or 25% serum albumin obtained by fractionating blood from human donors. The 5% solution is osmotically equivalent to plasma. Risk of hepatitis B virus is minimized by heating in the same manner as described above. These preparations have 130 to 160 mEq of sodium chloride per liter.

Dextran. Two forms of dextran, which differ in molecular size, are available for use as plasma expanders. *Dextran 70 injection* (MACRODEX) contains 6% *dextran* (average molecular weight 70,000) in 0.9% sodium chloride solution or 5% dextrose in water. *Dextran 75 injection* (DEXTRAN 75, GENTRAN 75) is virtually identical but with an average molecular weight of 75,000. *Dextran 40 injection* (GENTRAN 40, 10% LMD, RHEOMACRODEX) contains 10% *dextran 40* (average molecular weight 40,000) in 0.9% sodium chloride solution or 5% dextrose in water. The molecular weight of the former preparation approximates that of human plasma albumin; the smaller molecular size of the latter preparation is said to have the advantage of retarding rouleau formation and sludging of red blood cells. Both preparations are available in units of 500 ml.

Hetastarch injection (HESPAN) is prepared as a 6% solution in 0.9% sodium chloride in units of 500 ml.

PROBLEMS OF CARBOHYDRATES, FATS, AND PROTEINS

In the absence of the normal dietary intake of foodstuffs, intravenous glucose protects against the development of ketosis and minimizes the wasting of protein. On a short-term basis, one should administer approximately 100 g of glucose per day to an adult. For more prolonged treatment, there are available a number of preparations designed specifically for administration by mouth or gavage. These contain carbohydrates, fats, either protein hydrolysates or pure amino acids, and trace nutrients.

Intravenous Hyperalimentation. This technic is important in the management of patients with severe intestinal dysfunction, trauma, or various surgical complications, in both children and adults. Its success justifies its use, but complications are serious and can be avoided only by meticulous attention to detail by the pharmacist, nurse, and physician. A positive nitrogen balance can be achieved and maintained for as long as several months.

The basic nutrient solution consists of hypertonic dextrose (20 to 25% or more) and amino acids in addition to electrolytes, vitamins, and trace elements. The need for hypertonic solutions is dictated by the limits of water intake. Long-term tactical planning is required for a number of details; these include intravenous technics, blood chemical determinations, and day-to-day estimates of requirements for water, electrolytes, and nutritional components.

The infusion is given through a percutaneous catheter inserted into a large branch of the superior vena cava. Delivery into a large vein permits prompt adjustment of osmolality by dilution. Rigid sterile surgical technic is essential. A peristaltic pump should be used to drive the infusion through the tubing, which contains a microfilter. Both tubing and filter should be changed frequently. Ancillary medications should be given by another route. Pharmaceutical incompatibilities must be avoided. These include incompatibilities with electrolytes such as bicarbonate, calcium, phosphate, and sulfate (for other details, *see* Fischer, 1977; Grant, 1980; Committee on Nutrition, 1983).

Mechanical complications related to the insertion of the catheter are infrequent. Infection is the most serious complication; the incidence is greatly reduced by in-line filters. The regimen should be initiated gradually, then kept constant from day to day and carefully monitored. Mild *glycosuria* is common but may subside after stimulation of endogenous insulin production as a result of the hyperglycemia. However, severe glycosuria may lead to excessive water loss and hypertonic contraction of body fluids. With adequate amounts of sodium, potassium, magnesium, chloride, and bicarbonate, electrolyte imbalance may be avoided. Prolonged *hypophosphatemia* may lead to serious neurological and hematological complications, and phosphate is a requirement. *Hyperammonemia* may occur, particularly in infants, and can be prevented by reducing the nitrogenous components of the infusion. The rationale for the parenteral administration of fat does not involve total caloric requirements as much as it does the fact that certain lipids are essential nutrients, particularly for the synthesis of various components of cellular membranes. Most formulations provide more-than-adequate quantities of trace elements and vitamins. However, unexpected instances of deficiencies have been reported in patients who have been maintained by intravenous hyperalimentation for very long periods of time.

Preparations. In addition to the solutions of electrolytes and simple sugars, which have been previously mentioned, the following solutions are used in parenteral alimentation.

Amino Acids. Amino acid injection (AMINOSYN, TRAVASOL) consists of approximately 15 amino acids (both essential and nonessential), with total amino acid content from 3 to 11.4%. Formulations vary as to total osmolality and are available with or without electrolytes. The proportion of amino acids also varies slightly between preparations. A solution of 3.5% amino acids is only slightly hypertonic and may be administered by peripheral vein; more concentrated solutions are intended for infusion by central vein and are usually mixed with hypertonic glucose solution to provide additional caloric intake. Other preparations of amino acids (*e.g.*, NEPHRAMINE, which contains primarily essential amino acids) are designed for patients with renal failure. Additional formulations are available for use in hepatic failure (HEPATAMINE) or high metabolic stress (FREAMINE HBC).

Fat Emulsion. Emulsions of 10 and 20% fat (INTRALIPID, others) are prepared from refined soybean or safflower oil, egg-yolk phospholipids, and glycerin. The major fatty acids are linoleic, oleic, palmitic, stearic, and linolenic. The preparation is isotonic and may be administered into a peripheral vein. It should not be mixed with other solutions employed in parenteral alimentation.

ACID-BASE DISTURBANCES

Abnormalities of the pH of body fluids are frequently encountered and are of major clinical importance.

An *acid* may be defined as a substance that can provide a hydrogen ion (proton donor) and a *base* is a substance that can accept a hydrogen ion, as follows:

$$\text{Acid} \rightleftharpoons \text{Base} + \text{H}^+$$

The negative logarithm of the equilibrium constant for this reversible reaction is termed the pK_a. This is a measure of the intrinsic tendency of the proton donor to dissociate and to form the acceptor. Proton donors with low values of pK_a have the greatest tendency to dissociate and are commonly referred to as strong acids. The Henderson-Hasselbalch equation expresses the pH of a solution as a function of the concentrations of the acid-base pair and the value of pK_a:

$$pH = pK_a + \log \frac{[\text{Base}]}{[\text{Acid}]}$$

This equation makes clear the fact that the pH is determined by the pK_a and the *ratio* of the concentrations of the acid-base pair. Since many different substances may coexist in solution, and since a solution can have only a single hydrogen ion concentration or pH, it follows that the ratios of each buffer pair must vary in order to satisfy the general equation:

$$pH = pK_{a_\text{I}} + \log \frac{[\text{Base}]_\text{I}}{[\text{Acid}]_\text{I}} = pK_{a_\text{II}} + \log \frac{[\text{Base}]_\text{II}}{[\text{Acid}]_\text{II}}$$

in which I and II refer to different chemical entities.

Classification. The following conventions are now generally accepted. *Acidemia* and *alkalemia* refer, respectively, to an abnormal increase or decrease in the hydrogen ion concentration of the blood, regardless of cause. *Acidosis* and *alkalosis* refer, respectively, to clinical states that can lead to either acidemia or alkalemia. However, in each condition the extent to which there is an actual change in the hydrogen ion concentration depends on both the magnitude of the initiating disturbance and the degree of compensation. For example, acidosis results in acidemia if there is only partial compensation; if fully compensated, there is no acidemia and hydrogen ion concentration is normal. In most clinical disturbances there is a variable extent of partial compensation.

For reasons that will be amplified, it is most convenient to evaluate clinical disturbances of pH by reference to the HCO_3^-:H_2CO_3 system rather than to other proton acceptors or donors. It is also conventional to refer to the partial pressure of carbon dioxide (P_{CO_2}) rather than to the concentration of H_2CO_3.

There are four primary types of alteration of the ratio of HCO_3^- to P_{CO_2}. These are summarized in Table 35–5. They involve respiratory disorders in which the initial disturbance is either a decrease in P_{CO_2} (*respiratory alkalosis*) or an increase in P_{CO_2} (*respiratory acidosis*) and metabolic disorders in which the initial disturbance is either a decrease in HCO_3^- (*metabolic acidosis*) or an increase in HCO_3^- (*metabolic alkalosis*).

Mechanisms of Compensation. The responses that tend to minimize any deviation in pH are both chemical and physiological in nature.

Table 35–5. PLASMA VALUES IN ACID-BASE DISORDERS: SUMMARY OF PROMPT AND DELAYED CHANGES

CONDITION	INITIAL ABNORMALITY	DIRECTION OF CHANGE IN PLASMA COMPOSITION					
		Prompt				Delayed *	
		P_{CO_2}	HCO_3^-	pH	Cl^-	HCO_3^-	Cl^-
Respiratory alkalosis	↓ P_{CO_2}	↓	↓ †	↑	0	↓	↑
Acute respiratory acidosis	↑ P_{CO_2}	↑	↑ †	↓	0	—	—
Chronic respiratory acidosis	↑ P_{CO_2}	↑	↑ †	↓	↓	↑	↓
Metabolic acidosis	↓ HCO_3^-	↓ ‡	↓	↓	0, ↑	↑	± or ↑
Metabolic alkalosis	↑ HCO_3^-	↑ ‡	↑	↑	↓	↓	↑

* The delayed changes are the result of renal compensatory mechanisms that alter the rate of excretion of bicarbonate, titratable acid, ammonium, or chloride. Renal compensation is usually maximally effective after several days but varies with the nature of the abnormality. In metabolic alkalosis, the delayed change also includes the development of organic acidemia. In metabolic acidosis, the plasma chloride concentration varies depending on the cause of the acidosis, *i.e.*, a gain of HCl or of other acids.

† Chemical effect of P_{CO_2} on nonbicarbonate buffers (*see* text).

‡ Physiological effect of change in ventilation.

Buffers. For significant buffering to occur in biological fluids, the pK_a of the compound in question must be within the pH range of those fluids. Buffering is maximally efficient when the ratio of proton acceptor to donor is unity, and this occurs when $pH = pK_a$. Total buffering capacity also depends on the concentration of the buffer itself. The role of true buffer reactions is often inadequately appreciated, particularly in the extent to which the intracellular buffers (principally proteins) are involved in the regulation of bicarbonate concentration in the presence of changing concentrations of carbon dioxide. In the following example, the diffusion reactions between the extracellular and intracellular spaces have been omitted.

$$H^+ + HCO_3^- + K^+Buf^- \rightleftharpoons HBuf + K^+ + HCO_3^-$$
$$\Updownarrow$$
$$H_2CO_3$$

K^+Buf^- is principally the potassium salt of intracellular proteins. Note that the concentration of bicarbonate is altered without any change in its external balance, such as intake or renal excretion. This buffer reaction contributes to the changes in bicarbonate concentration that occur promptly in primary respiratory disorders (Table 35–5).

The Bicarbonate–Carbonic Acid System. This system has unique importance when compared to other buffers, particularly because the bicarbonate–carbonic acid system is the major buffer system in the body that is subject to physiological regulation. Carbonic acid is the principal acidic end product of metabolism (Table 35–2). Unlike other proton donors, H_2CO_3 is converted to a volatile form (CO_2) that is exhaled through the lungs; unlike the macromolecular buffers, HCO_3^- and H_2CO_3 can be excreted by the kidney and their ratio in the urine can be regulated physiologically. This system accounts for a major portion of the direct chemical buffering of extracellular fluid. In addition, the buffer pair can be administered separately as "drugs": the proton acceptor, HCO_3^-, as a simple salt, usually sodium, and the proton donor as CO_2 gas by inhalation. With a change in the ratio between proton donor and acceptor in this system, other buffers in the same fluid must also change. The nonbicarbonate buffers include principally hemoglobin, other proteins, and phosphate. The ratio of the bicarbonate–carbonic acid system at a pH of 7.4 is 20:1. Although a buffer pair is more efficient when the ratio is close to 1, the unique qualities of this particular system make it highly effective even at a ratio of 20:1.

Ion Exchange. Cations such as sodium and potassium, and perhaps magnesium and calcium, from muscle, bone, and other tissues can exchange for hydrogen ions in the extracellular fluid, and this plays a significant role in the moderation of alterations in acid-base equilibrium. The exchange of anions probably plays a much less important role, except for the shift of chloride and bicarbonate that occurs across the red-cell membrane.

Respiratory Regulation. In terms of quantity alone, the lungs play the major role in the daily excretion of acid. Approximately 10 mmol of CO_2 are generated and expired each minute. The CNS is responsive to P_{CO_2} and pH and regulates the rate and depth of respiratory activity. A depression in pH or an elevation of P_{CO_2} increases alveolar ventilation, which, in turn, serves to eliminate more acid as CO_2. The change in ventilation in response to acid-base disturbances is normally very prompt.

Renal Regulation. The renal mechanisms contribute to acid-base regulation by varying the net rate of excretion of hydrogen ions and by selectively reabsorbing and rejecting cations and anions. In terms of combating an acidosis, one can view the major role of the kidney as reabsorbing all the filtered bicarbonate and, in addition, generating new bicarbonate that is formed by the excretion of hydrogen ion as either ammonium or titratable acid. Since the normal diet gives rise to nonvolatile acids that must be eliminated by the kidney, this mechanism is normally in operation. In the renal compensation for alkalosis, particularly metabolic alkalosis produced by the excessive intake of sodium bicarbonate, the amount of filtered bicarbonate is increased and is only partially reabsorbed. Thus, bicarbonate is excreted in the urine, mainly as the sodium salt. Details are presented in the Introduction to Section VIII.

Laboratory Diagnosis of Acid-Base Disturbances. The most common laboratory measurements are the pH and P_{CO_2} of the blood, and the total CO_2 content of the serum. Determination of the pH of freshly voided urine specimens is useful and simple. The calculation of the *anion gap* is also exceedingly helpful and may provide important insight into etiology. In normal plasma (with all values in milliequivalents per liter) the difference between the concentration of sodium (140) and the sum of the concentrations of bicarbonate (25) and chloride (105) is 10. A normal range is 8 to 12. Since the anion gap represents the difference between two relatively large num-

bers, it is subject to accumulative analytical error. If the concentration of a normal anion, other than chloride or bicarbonate, is abnormally high, or if an abnormal anion has accumulated, this may be detected by the anion gap. Major anions that are involved include β-hydroxybutyrate, acetoacetate, lactate, phosphate, and sulfate. Much less commonly, and unrelated to acid-base disturbances, the anion gap may be decreased (Oh and Carroll, 1977).

The *potassium* ion plays a complex role in many acid-base disturbances. This will be discussed in a separate section below.

MAJOR ACID-BASE DISORDERS

Respiratory Alkalosis. This is caused by primary hyperventilation, which increases the elimination of CO_2 by the lungs and thus lowers the P_{CO_2} and raises the pH of the blood. Mild respiratory alkalosis is encountered in a number of different situations. These include mechanical hyperventilation, hypoxia, sepsis, hepatic failure, pulmonary disease, and drug administration (particularly salicylates). More severe alkalosis with tetany, paresthesias, or confusion may be seen with hysterical overbreathing and lesions of the CNS.

Mild asymptomatic alkalosis requires no specific treatment. With hysterical hyperventilation, symptoms may be alleviated by rebreathing into a paper bag. Sedation may also be employed in combination with breathing a gas mixture containing CO_2 (usually 5%). The special case of respiratory alkalosis that occurs during recovery from metabolic acidosis is considered below.

Respiratory Acidosis. The primary disorder is the retention of carbon dioxide because of impaired ventilation. The increase in P_{CO_2} lowers the ratio of $HCO_3^-:P_{CO_2}$ and hence decreases pH. The accumulation of CO_2 is partially buffered by the tissues. The kidney responds slowly by increasing the reabsorption of bicarbonate at the expense of chloride. Thus, after several days, acute and chronic respiratory acidosis may be distinguished from each other by the concentration of HCO_3^- in plasma.

Retention of carbon dioxide results from two main causes: depression of the respiratory center in the medulla and pathological changes in the alveoli or airways. In both instances respiratory minute volume may decline progressively due to diminishing responsiveness of the medulla to changes in P_{CO_2} and pH. Respiratory drive may become inadequate and totally dependent on impulses arising from the hypoxic carotid body. The administration of oxygen may result in apnea (*see* Chapter 16). This does not mean that patients with respiratory acidosis should not receive oxygen, but that artificial respiration is essential in the presence of inadequate respiratory drive. If ventilatory assistance is not available and oxygen is required, it should be administered very cautiously.

Obviously, the most important aspects of therapy relate to an improvement in the basic cause underlying the hypoventilation. However, in severe respiratory acidosis, particularly in asthmatic patients, it may be essential to correct the derangement of pH directly. This can be accomplished by the infusion of sodium bicarbonate solution. At a more normal pH the bronchodilator drugs become more effective and the basic pulmonary disorder may be alleviated (Menitove and Goldring, 1983).

Metabolic Acidosis. This disturbance commonly results from a loss of proton acceptors (such as bicarbonate during severe diarrhea) or from the accession of proton donors (such as keto acids, lactic acid) that either appear during metabolic or circulatory disorders or arise from the administration of an acidifying salt (such as ammonium chloride). Insight into the etiology may be gained from the anion gap; this is increased by the keto acids and lactic acid. In renal insufficiency the abnormally large anion gap is attributable to phosphate and sulfate. If acidosis is the result of the administration of ammonium chloride, the anion gap is normal since the increased chloride anion is accounted for in the measurement. Respiratory compensation involves hyperventilation, which occurs promptly. Renal compensation involves the increased excretion of hydrogen ions in the form of titratable acidity and ammonium. The latter is generated *in vivo* from amino acid precursors.

No effort is made herein to detail the specific therapy for the many types of acidosis. However, the role of adequate renal function should be emphasized. Since metabolic acidosis is often accompanied by volume depletion, renal blood flow may be compromised and the kidneys may be unable to excrete appropriate amounts of titratable acid and ammonium. This may be corrected by the administration of isotonic sodium chloride solution. When it is considered advisable to employ an alkalinizing salt, the use of a solution of sodium bicarbonate instead of sodium lactate is recommended. When sodium lactate is employed, it is converted to bicarbonate by cellular oxidative activity. If this is deficient, the therapeutic goal will not have been achieved.

When metabolic acidosis is acute and severe, cautious treatment with sodium bicarbonate is warranted. The goal of therapy is to restore the plasma concentration of HCO_3^- approximately halfway to normal. Because of the persistently high rate of lactic acid production in lactic acidosis, undertreatment is more likely to occur in this condition than in other forms of metabolic acidosis. Overtreatment is to be avoided, since the rapid conversion from acidosis to alkalosis may be harmful. Even a partial correction of the plasma HCO_3^- may produce a disequilibrium between the pH of the plasma and that of the cerebrospinal fluid. This results from the slow rate at which HCO_3^- crosses the blood-brain barrier. As a consequence, the fluids that influence the respiratory center directly remain more acidic than normal and hyperventilation is maintained. The resultant hypocapnia, combined with the partially corrected HCO_3^- concentration in the peripheral blood, may lead to alkalosis.

The dose of HCO_3^- is usually calculated on the empirical assumption that the ion is distributed in a volume equivalent to 50% of body weight. This is an approximation that includes diverse buffer reactions in both extracellular and intracellular fluids. In more chronic diseases, such as chronic renal insufficiency, the metabolic acidosis can be ameliorated with the use of sodium bicarbonate or preparations of sodium citrate. The dose must be found empirically, and small doses should be used initially so as not to overtreat.

Metabolic Alkalosis. This is characterized by an increase in the concentration of bicarbonate in the extracellular fluid, unassociated with a proportionate increase in the P_{CO_2}. Metabolic alkalosis can be induced by the loss of hydrogen ions, as in vomiting acidic gastric secretions, or by the administration of alkalinizing salts, such as sodium bicarbonate. Respiratory compensation consists in hypoventilation. Despite considerable variation between patients, the degree of hypoventilation is approximately proportional to the initial increment in plasma HCO_3^-. The respiratory response significantly blunts the increase in pH but may also produce mild hypoxia. However, the latter is usually not sufficient to counteract the hypoventilation. Renal compensation involves the urinary excretion of sodium bicarbonate, a response that is well documented when alkalosis is produced by the administration of sodium bicarbonate and is associated with expansion of extracellular fluid volume. However, when metabolic alkalosis is accompanied by volume depletion, little or no sodium bicarbonate may be excreted by the kidney and the pH of the urine may be acidic. The renal excretion of the bicarbonate anion requires the obligatory excretion of an accompanying fixed cation, principally sodium. When volume is reduced or sodium is depleted, mechanisms to promote the retention of sodium are implemented. Bicarbonate is retained simultaneously despite persistent alkalosis. It should be emphasized that sodium depletion during metabolic alkalosis is the most frequent cause of paradoxical aciduria. This situation should be monitored by the frequent determination of urinary pH. There is a third compensatory mechanism in metabolic alkalosis, which involves the accumulation of organic acids in the plasma. These may be estimated by the anion gap. Such acids lower the concentration of bicarbonate in plasma to a significant extent (*see* Madias *et al.*, 1979).

In most cases acute metabolic alkalosis

may be corrected by the administration of adequate amounts of sodium chloride solution. The ability of a neutral salt to correct an acid-base disturbance is based on physiological rather than chemical mechanisms. In the case of alkalosis due to vomiting, the body is depleted of water, hydrogen ion, chloride, and, to a lesser extent, sodium. Once an adequate extracellular volume is reestablished, normal renal mechanisms become effective and sodium, along with bicarbonate, is excreted in the urine. The complex relationship of *potassium* to alkalosis is considered in a separate section below.

Severe metabolic alkalosis may be life threatening. In rare instances, the severity of symptoms requires direct correction of the abnormal pH itself. This can be accomplished with an acidifying salt such as ammonium chloride since, in the presence of normal hepatic function, the alkalosis can be corrected without waiting for renal mechanisms to come into play. Hepatic failure is a contraindication to the administration of ammonium chloride. The administration of 0.1 N hydrochloric acid by catheter into a large central vein may be employed in instances in which it is desired to lower the systemic pH promptly and directly without reliance on either renal or hepatic mechanisms. The infused acid is immediately buffered by the circulating blood, although mild hemolysis may occur; if administered into a peripheral vein, severe thrombophlebitis can result. This procedure should be considered as a heroic measure that is to be used only when more conventional therapy has failed (Abouna *et al.*, 1974).

Alkalinization or Acidification of the Urine. There are situations in which the primary purpose of therapy is to change the pH of the urine. This is readily accomplished, when renal function is normal, by the administration of either alkalinizing or acidifying salts. Such a maneuver produces only a modest distortion in systemic acid-base balance. However, in edema-forming states, when the renal reabsorption of sodium is inappropriately high, alkalinizing salts are poorly excreted. Furthermore, in the presence of renal insufficiency, there is a diminished capacity of the kidney to compensate for acidosis, and acidifying salts may have harmful systemic effects.

One goal of alkalinization of the urine (to a pH greater than 7.4) is to increase the solubility of certain weak acids that are more soluble as salts than as undissociated acids. This is indicated when there is an excessively high concentration of the acid in the urine. Examples include cystine, in cystinuria; uric acid, in spontaneous hyperuricemia or following the administration of oncolytic or uricosuric agents; methotrexate, in high-dosage therapy; and the administration of certain sulfonamides. A second goal is to increase the excretory rate of lipid-soluble organic acids whose reabsorption is accomplished by diffusion of the nonionized species. Examples include the treatment of overdosage of salicylate or phenobarbital.

An alternate approach to the administration of an alkalinizing salt is to utilize an inhibitor of carbonic anhydrase such as acetazolamide (*see* Chapter 36). When sodium bicarbonate is administered, large doses (10 to 15 g per day) are required to keep the urine persistently alkaline throughout the 24-hour period. When acetazolamide increases bicarbonate excretion, it depletes the body stores of the anion, which tends to reduce the efficacy of the drug. It thus may be logical to prescribe both acetazolamide and sodium bicarbonate. Their actions on the pH of the urine are complementary. However, it should be kept in mind that acetazolamide may competitively inhibit the tubular secretion of other organic acids.

The urine is purposely rendered more *acidic* than normal either to increase the renal excretion of lipid-soluble organic bases or to provide conditions appropriate for a specific pharmacological effect. There are no examples in which acidification is required to increase the solubility of a basic drug. A low urinary pH is required for the activation of methenamine, a urinary tract antiseptic; some other antimicrobials (*e.g.*, nitrofurantoin) are more potent in an acidic urine (Milne, 1978).

Preparations for the Treatment of Acid-Base Disturbances. *Sodium bicarbonate* has been discussed above. Precursors of bicarbonate include *lactate* and *acetate*.

Citrate and citric acid oral solutions are a palatable form in which to prescribe an alkalinizing agent. A typical formulation (BICITRA) contains 500 mg of sodium citrate and 334 mg of citric acid per 5 ml (1 mEq/ml of sodium).

Tromethamine (THAM) is a synthetic buffer (*tris*-[hydroxymethyl]aminomethane); it is available as a 0.3 M solution adjusted to pH 8.6 with acetic acid. It is also supplied as a powder (THAM-E) to be dissolved in 1 liter of sterile water. Each liter contains 300 mmol (36 g) of tromethamine, 30 mmol of sodium chloride, and 5 mmol of potassium chloride. The use of tromethamine is contraindicated in pregnant women or patients with uremia or chronic respiratory acidosis. It should not be given for longer than 1 day.

AMMONIUM AND ACID-FORMING SALTS

The ammonium ion is toxic in high concentrations, but it serves a major role in the maintenance of acid-base balance. It is a proton donor that dissociates to H^+ and NH_3, and the dissociation constant (pK_a 9.3) is such that, in the pH range of blood, NH_4^+ constitutes about 99% of the total ammonia ($NH_3 + NH_4^+$).

Endogenous Metabolism. Ammonia in the body represents that which is liberated from the deamination of amino acids and the deamidation of amides. Portal venous blood contains a high concentration of ammonia. Normally about 20% of the urea produced in the body diffuses into the gut, where it is converted by bacteria to ammonia and carbon dioxide. Intestinal bacteria also produce ammonia from dietary proteins. The ammonia is absorbed and converted back to urea in the liver by way of the ornithine (urea) cycle. Another significant role of ammonia is in the synthesis of glutamine.

Renal Excretion. Normal renal venous blood contains a high concentration of ammonia synthesized from glutamine and other amino acids in the kidney. The ammonia that is formed by the kidney is excreted when the urine is acidic, but is largely returned to the systemic circulation if the urine is alkaline. In an acidic urine, NH_3 accepts a proton and exists almost entirely as NH_4^+. Under normal states of metabolism, about 70 mEq of nonvolatile acid is generated per day (Table 35–2); about one half of this is excreted in the urine in conjunction with NH_4^+, and the remainder is excreted as titratable acid. Renal production of ammonia is stimulated by acidosis; ammonia buffers urinary acid and allows further secretion of protons into the tubular fluid. Potassium depletion also results in a primary increase in the renal synthesis of ammonia, sometimes accompanied by slight alkalinization of the urine (Tannen, 1977). This may increase the amount of ammonia that is returned to the circulation via the renal vein and have a deleterious effect when potassium depletion coexists with hepatic failure.

Normal physiological mechanisms are designed to keep the concentration of ammonia in blood as low as possible. Thus, ammonia added to the venous circulation by the kidney or gastrointestinal tract is converted to urea by the liver.

Toxicity. Patients with severe hepatic disease and portal hypertension often develop derangements of the CNS (hepatic encephalopathy) which are manifested by disturbance of consciousness, asterixis, and EEG abnormalities. Since the syndrome is most often associated with elevated concentrations of ammonia in blood, and since it can be provoked by feeding of protein as well as by ingestion of ammonium salts, it is thought to represent, in part, ammonia toxicity to the brain. The occurrence of hyperammonemia in children and infants has been associated with defects of enzymes of the urea cycle. Hyperammonemia due to defects of ornithine transcarbamylase or carbamylphosphate synthetase may be related to cyclic vomiting and to at least one form of migraine. The mechanisms by which ammonia induces changes in the CNS are currently unknown.

Pharmacological Actions. *Diuresis from Ammonium Salts.* Following the absorption of ammonium chloride, the conversion of the ammonium ion to urea frees hydrogen ion and bicarbonate is dissipated. This may result in severe acidosis.

Acid-forming salts were formerly employed as primary diuretics, but they have become obsolete.

Correction of Metabolic Alkalosis. Ammonium chloride is useful for this purpose, particularly when sodium chloride is contraindicated in the edematous patient. The acidifying action depends on the conversion of the ammonium ion to urea by the liver, and ammonium salts are thus contraindicated in hepatic insufficiency. Ammonium chloride, which has a *fixed* anion, is an acidifying salt; ammonium carbonate and ammonium bicarbonate, which have a *labile* anion, are not acidifying.

Expectorant Action. The ammonium ion supposedly exerts an expectorant action, and its salts are sometimes used for this purpose.

Local Actions. Solutions of ammonium hydroxide are local irritants. When applied to the skin in low concentration, they have a rubefacient action, and in high concentrations they are vesicant. Ammonia gas is very irritating, but when inhaled in dilute form it can stimulate reflexly the medullary respiratory and vasomotor centers through irritation of the sensory endings of the trigeminal nerve. High concentrations of ammonia vapor are injurious to the lungs, and death may result from pulmonary edema. Long exposure to low concentrations of ammonia may lead to chronic pulmonary irritation. The maximal concentration of ammonia vapor that can be tolerated without harmful effect is probably less than 250 ppm. High concentrations of neutral ammonium salts are irritating to the gastric mucosa and may produce nausea and vomiting.

Preparations. *Ammonium chloride* is available as an injection or tablets. *Aromatic ammonia spirit* is a solution of ammonia, ammonium carbonate, and various essential oils in 70% alcohol, and is employed as a reflex stimulant. It is given by mouth in a dose of 2 ml, well diluted in water, or it is used as an inhalant.

Reversal of Intoxication with Ammonia. Several measures have been advocated for the management of encephalopathy associated with hepatic failure. Dietary intake of protein should be curtailed. *Neomycin* may be used to reduce the number of ammonia-producing microorganisms in the intestine. *Lactulose* is a disaccharide that is metabolized by intestinal bacteria to organic acids in the lower intestinal tract. The acidification of the intestinal contents retards the nonionic diffusion of ammonia from the colon to the blood. Although lactulose is theoretically incompatible with neomycin because of the latter's action on the intestinal flora, clinical results suggest that the two agents may be administered concomitantly (Fischer and Baldessarini, 1976). Therapy with *arginine* has been advocated because it acts as a precursor of ornithine in the urea cycle in the liver; *glutamate* has been advocated because it reacts with ammonia in the enzymatic synthesis of glutamine. While these two amino acids have been used singly and in combination to attempt to lower plasma concentrations of ammonia, there is no proof of efficacy.

POTASSIUM

Potassium is the predominant intracellular cation. Disorders of potassium homeostasis are particularly evident because of the vital role that the ion assumes in the maintenance of electrical excitability of nerve and muscle. Potassium also plays an important role in the genesis and correction of imbalances of acid-base metabolism. Potassium salts are thus important therapeutic agents, but they are extremely dangerous if used improperly.

Physiological Regulation

Absorption and Distribution. Active ion transport systems maintain a high gradient of potassium across the plasma membrane; while the plasma concentration is 4 to 5 mEq per liter, the intracellular concentration is approximately 150 mEq per liter, with modest variation from one cell type to another. Almost all the dietary potassium is absorbed from the gastrointestinal tract, and in the steady state the amount of potassium excreted in the urine is thus essentially equal to that in the diet. In the fluids within the intestinal tract the potassium concentration is two to three times greater than that in the plasma (Table 35–3). In the adult, the daily intake varies with dietary habits and is usually in the range of 50 to 100 mEq.

Potassium is accumulated by cells by an energy-dependent mechanism that extrudes sodium. There is a high concentration gradient for potassium from cell to extracellular fluid, and a high gradient for sodium in the opposite direction. Rapid and selective changes in the permeability to these ions is of particular importance in excitable tissues.

Excretion. Renal mechanisms are of paramount importance in maintaining both the total body potassium and its concentration in the plasma within narrow limits. Potassium is freely filtered at the glomerulus and is almost completely reabsorbed in the proximal tubule. The amount excreted in the urine, which is normally equivalent to 10% of the amount filtered, gains access to the tubular fluid by tubular secretion. This occurs in the distal convoluted tubule and, under some circumstances, in the collecting duct. The secretory process has two steps: active uptake of potassium from plasma to tubular cell and passive diffusion down an electrochemical gradient from cell to tubular fluid. There is variable reabsorption of potassium in the same segments of the nephron (Stanton and Giebisch, 1982).

Tubular reabsorption of sodium has a dual impact on the secretion of potassium. First, sodium reabsorption is active and thereby the tubular fluid becomes negative relative to the cell. This increases the electrical gradient for potassium secretion. Second, increased amounts of fluid may be delivered to the secretory segment as the result of inhibition of sodium reabsorption in the more proximal segment, regardless of cause. The increased volume of distal fluid tends to lower the concentration of potassium within it, thus increasing the gradient for diffusion. This increases the total amount of potassium that is secreted. These two factors, both related to sodium, play an important role in the regulation of potassium homeostasis. For example, any condition in which there is an acute increase in sodium excretion is associated with an increase in potassium excretion as well. In contrast, when little sodium is available to the distal tubule for reabsorption, potassium secretion is minimal.

Aldosterone stimulates distal sodium reabsorption and potassium secretion. Clinical conditions that enhance the secretion of aldosterone are characterized by potassium loss.

The normal renal response to changes in intake is different for sodium and potassium. For illustration, assume that the intake of each ion is 100 mEq per day and that the kidneys and adrenals are normal. What then is the kinetics of renal adjustment when intake is increased or decreased by 100 mEq, that is, either doubled or reduced to zero? In this example, the intake of the other cation is assumed to remain constant. The increased amount of dietary sodium will be excreted rather slowly over several days. When sodium intake is reduced to zero, the urine will become sodium free within 3 to 4 days. In the case of potassium, the increased intake will be excreted more rapidly—in a matter of hours. When potassium intake is reduced, the amount of potassium excreted in the urine will fall, but this is a gradual process and even after weeks of reduced intake the urine will not become potassium free.

Adaptation to Potassium Loads. When the intake of potassium is increased, the resultant degree of hyperkalemia depends on the prior intake of potassium. If this has been low, the degree of hyperkalemia is far greater than if it has been high. Since ingested potassium is virtually *completely* absorbed in the upper intestinal tract, it is apparent that adaptation involves mechanisms of excretion and redistribution.

The increased rate of urinary excretion is achieved by increased tubular secretion of potassium. Hyperkalemia directly enhances the Na^+,K^+-ATPase activity in the kidney, and this enzyme is critically involved in the adaptive response (Hayslett and Binder, 1982). When other physiological variables are kept constant, potassium loading normally produces an enormous increase in potassium excretion at the expense of only slight hyperkalemia (Young, 1982).

The major extrarenal adaptation involves the uptake of potassium by tissues, principally muscle and liver. The amount of potassium that is involved is relatively small compared to endogenous intracellular stores and hence cannot readily be detected by analyses of tissue. However, the operation of these processes is readily discerned by their effect on extracellular concentrations of potassium. A number of endocrine systems are involved. Hyperkalemia stimulates the release of insulin, which in turn facilitates the cellular uptake of potassium in muscle independently of any action of the hormone on carbohydrate metabolism. Stimulation of Na^+,K^+-ATPase and a consequent effect on sodium efflux may be involved. Insulin also enhances sequestration of potassium in liver and muscle by mechanisms that are related to the concurrent uptake and/or metabolism of glucose. Hyperkalemia also stimulates the secretion of glucagon. Although this hormone increases plasma potassium by an action on the liver, it also has a hypokalemic effect that results from its stimulation of the renal excretion of potassium. Thus, both the adrenals and the pancreas have an endocrine function in the adaptation to potassium loads. When the function of both glands is compromised, subjects may be predisposed to hyperkalemia. This may occur when potassium loads are given to patients with diabetes mellitus who, at the same time, are subject to either spontaneous hypoaldosteronism or its iatrogenic equivalent in the form of potassium-sparing diuretics (Goldfarb *et al.,* 1975). Conversely, when a high-potassium intake is suddenly terminated, adrenocortical hyperfunction may persist, leading to hypokalemia that can cause paralysis (Duggin and Price, 1974).

The sympathetic nervous system is also involved in the regulation of cellular and plasma concentrations of potassium. With the increasing use of specific sympathetic blocking agents, these relationships are assuming greater clinical importance. Epinephrine causes an initial rise in plasma potassium due to the release of the ion from liver, followed by a decrease due to uptake of potassium by both liver and skeletal muscle. The rise in plasma potassium is mediated by α receptors, the fall by β receptors. These adrenergic effects do not depend on insulin (Bia and DeFronzo, 1981; Vick, 1981). When the plasma potassium is slightly elevated by other factors, it is possible that the effects of β-adrenergic receptor blockade may be additive and lead to hyperkalemia of a dangerous degree.

During excessive intake of potassium the amount of the ion secreted into the colon increases; this is excreted in the feces. As in the distal tubule of the kidney, Na^+,K^+-ATPase is involved. As a mechanism of physiological compensation, the intestinal excretion of potassium is far less important in the normal subject than in the patient with chronic renal insufficiency, in whom a major fraction of dietary potassium may be eliminated by this route.

Potassium Metabolism and Acid-Base Balance. This subject is complicated by the fact that it involves both ion-exchange mechanisms across the membranes of many types of cells and the excretory function of the kidney. In addition, the physiological disposition of the hydrogen and potassium ions may be influenced, at least in part independently of each other, by the balance of other cations and anions.

Cellular Equilibria. The intracellular concentrations of both potassium *and hydrogen* ions are higher than those of the extracellular fluid. When the extracellular hydrogen ion concentration is increased, as in acidosis, there is a shift of potassium from cells to extracellular fluid. When the extracellular concentration of hydrogen ion is decreased, potassium moves into cells. Thus, extracellular acidosis produces hyperkalemia, and extracellular alkalosis produces hypokalemia. A change of 0.1 unit in plasma pH can be accompanied by a change of opposite sign of 0.6 mEq per liter in the plasma concentration of potassium.

When a change in the concentration of potassium is the initiating event, the distribution of hydrogen ion may also be affected. In severe potassium depletion, when K^+ leaves the cell it exchanges with extracellular Na^+ and H^+ to preserve electroneutrality. This redistribution of hydrogen ion results in extracellular alkalosis and intracellular acidosis. The opposite tends to occur in hyperkalemia (Adler and Fraley, 1977).

Renal Mechanisms. Deprivation of dietary potassium initially increases urinary pH slightly and also stimulates the renal synthesis of ammonia (Tannen, 1977). Since urinary pH controls the excretion of both titratable acid and ammonia, the immediate overall effect is to diminish net acid excretion. If the concomitant loss of potassium is mild, the decreased elimination of acid results in metabolic acidosis. However, if potassium depletion becomes more extensive, systemic metabolic alkalosis and intracellular acidosis develop. These results appear contradictory. The phenomenon has been observed in several species, including man (Cooke *et al.*, 1952; Mudge and Hardin, 1956). Because of its strong kaliuretic action, aldosterone, combined with a low-potassium diet, has been used to produce this condition experimentally; the production of aldosterone is increased in its clinical counterparts. However, there is no absolute requirement for increased secretion of aldosterone.

Considered together, the data suggest that near the normal range of potassium balance, the potassium ion has a regulatory role in the determination of urinary pH and ammonia synthesis, but that with severe potassium depletion, additional mechanisms supervene.

The exact nature of these mechanisms continues to remain obscure for several reasons. First, accurate counterparts of many clinical syndromes have not been reproduced experimentally. Second, an extraordinary number of factors appear to play a role. These include the balance of chloride, the relative balance of sodium and potassium, the concentrations of renin and aldosterone in plasma, the role of other adrenocortical hormones, and the rates of production of prostaglandins. Third, the complex functions of the distal tubule involve the reabsorption of chloride and sodium along with the secretion of potassium and hydrogen ions.

In early studies it was suggested that a key mechanism might involve competition between potassium and hydrogen ions for secretion by the distal tubule and that the rate of secretion for each ion might be primarily determined by its own concentration within the cells of the tubule. Thus, in potassium depletion the intracellular concentration of potassium would be low while that of hydrogen ion would be high, due to the concomitant intracellular acidosis. If these concentrations determined rates of secretion, this would lead to an acidic urine, complete reabsorption of bicarbonate, and persistence of extracellular alkalosis. The correction of the potassium deficit would increase intracellular potassium concentration and decrease that of intracellular hydrogen ion. This would lead to decreased hydrogen ion secretion, decreased bicarbonate reabsorption, increased urine pH, increased bicarbonate excretion, and correction of the extracellular alkalosis.

While a number of observations are consistent with the above mechanism, direct micropuncture studies of distal tubule function have revealed a complex relationship between hydrogen ion and potassium. The salient features are as follows: (1) Alkalemia stimulates and acidemia inhibits the tubular secretion of potassium. (2) Inhibition of fluid reabsorption in the proximal tubule during acidosis enhances delivery of fluid to the distal segment and thus increases potassium secretion. This counteracts the direct inhibitory effect of low plasma pH. (3) Potassium secretion appears not to be influenced by the pH of the tubular fluid itself. (4) The augmentation of potassium secretion in alkalosis may involve two additional factors: the increased delivery of sodium and water to the distal segment and the inhibition of distal potassium *reabsorption* as the result of a low tubular fluid concentration of chloride (Stanton and Giebisch, 1982).

PATHOLOGICAL CONDITIONS

The metabolism of the potassium ion may be considered pathological when its concentration in either the extracellular or intracellular fluid is above or below normal. The concentration in both compartments must be appraised for a complete understanding of potassium imbalance.

Measurement of Extracellular Potassium. The concentration of potassium in the plasma is readily measured directly. *Pseudohypokalemia* may be encountered in the same conditions that produce pseudohyponatremia, that is, when the plasma water content is abnormally low. *Pseudohyperkalemia* occurs with marked thrombocytosis or leukocytosis. Potassium leaks from the cells during the clotting process; true values are obtained with plasma from blood that is harvested with anticoagulants. Falsely high values are also obtained in the absence of hemolysis with samples of venous blood from patients with sickle-cell anemia. Hemolysis in shed blood also produces falsely high estimates of the plasma concentration. However, an elevated potassium concentration in serum or plasma from patients with intravascular hemolysis may be a true representation of the concentration *in vivo*.

Since both hypokalemia and hyperkalemia directly influence the electrical activity of the heart, the ECG may be employed as a guide. This is particularly useful when there is a diagnostic emergency and when the concentration must be monitored sequentially during therapy to replace potassium.

As a first approximation, the concentration of potassium in the fluids of the gastrointestinal tract is about three times that of plasma (Table 35–3). Direct measurement of fecal potassium is useful only in the exceptional case. Measurement of the urinary concentration of potassium is often uninterpretable unless many factors are taken into account, such as the concentration in plasma, previous or simultaneous drug treatment, dietary intake, and the rate of urine flow. Under normal circumstances the amount of potassium excreted in the urine shows less diurnal variation than does sodium.

Measurement of Intracellular Potassium. Measurement of the intracellular concentration of potassium is virtually synonymous with measurement of total body potassium. Skeletal muscle obviously accounts for the bulk of the total intracellular store, but it is not necessarily representative of all types of cells. For example, in potassium depletion skeletal muscle shows a major loss of the ion while myocardial potassium remains virtually normal.

Attempts to obtain accurate measurements of intracellular stores have been frustrating. The concentration of potassium in the plasma is an index of only limited value. In those conditions in which extracellular and intracellular concentrations change in the same direction, that is, in otherwise-uncomplicated potassium depletion, there may be only a slight fall in the plasma concentration while the intracellular concentration may vary from almost normal to clearly low values. There are other conditions in which the extracellular and intracellular concentrations diverge because of the movement of potassium from one compartment to the other. Examples include acute alkalosis or acidosis, untreated diabetic ketoacidosis, and hypokalemic periodic paralysis. Since the erythrocyte and leukocyte may be readily sampled, their potassium content may be measured directly. However, these data correlate poorly with total body stores. The total amount of potassium in the body may also be directly measured with the naturally occurring isotope, ^{40}K. However, this is a research procedure and the errors are sufficiently great that small but physiologically important changes may not be detected. Although usually considered to be investigational procedures, careful determination of metabolic balance and biopsy of skeletal muscle may provide the most accurate means to assess intracellular stores (Patrick, 1977).

In the usual clinical situation, an evaluation of total body potassium must depend on other sources of information. A careful analysis of the patient's history is probably the single most important step. Particular attention must be given to the quantitative aspects of dietary intake and abnormal fluid losses, especially from the gastrointestinal tract, with the realization that significant changes in external balance rarely occur acutely but require days or weeks.

Hyperkalemia. *Causes.* Hyperkalemia results from a variety of causes: a sudden increase in potassium intake, either by mouth or by vein; severe tissue trauma; acute rhabdomyolysis; acute acidosis, but sometimes also chronic acidosis; untreated Addison's disease; the rare metabolic disorder hyperkalemic periodic paralysis; an acute increase in osmolality, as after the infusion of hypertonic mannitol or, in a more special case, with the induction of hyperglycemia in diabetic patients who are also deficient in aldosterone; the action of glucagon; the acute stimulation of α-adrenergic receptors; β-adrenergic receptor blockade; and the improper use of potassium-sparing diuretics (Goldfarb et al., 1975; Knochel, 1977). Hyperkalemia is *not* observed during chronic renal failure, except as an almost terminal event (due to the effectiveness of both the renal and intestinal adaptive mechanisms). However, in each of the above-listed conditions the degree of hyperkalemia will be accentuated by renal insufficiency.

Consequences. Deleterious effects on the electrical activity of the heart are by far the most important consequences of hyperkalemia. At modest levels of elevation (plasma potassium 5 to 7 mEq per liter), the T waves become increased in height or "tented"; the P-R interval lengthens; and the P wave ultimately disappears. At higher concentrations of potassium (8 to 9 mEq per liter) there is a profound depression in impulse generation and conduction in all cardiac tissues, widening of the QRS complex, and eventual asystole, sometimes preceded by ventricular tachycardia or fibrillation (*see* Ettinger et al., 1974). There is a moderate variation in the absolute concentration of potassium in plasma at which these changes occur.

Increase in Total Body Potassium. As indicated above in the discussion of adaptation to high-potassium intake, it is not possible to increase total body potassium significantly above normal.

Hypokalemia. *Causes.* The most common cause of hypokalemia is depletion of total body potassium. However, the plasma concentration may also fall without any change in external balance, and hence without depletion, as a result of acute alkalosis, treatment with insulin, hypokalemic periodic paralysis, and stimulation of β-adrenergic receptors.

Consequences. Since hypokalemia and depletion of potassium often coexist, it is difficult to attribute the sequelae specifically to one condition or the other. It is probable that the abnormalities associated with neuromuscular dysfunction are primarily correlated with the degree of hypokalemia. These include impaired neuromuscular function, which may vary from minimal weakness to frank paralysis; intestinal dilatation and ileus; and abnormalities of myocardial function with disturbed ECG patterns such as prolongation of the Q-T interval, a broad and flat T wave, depression of the S-T segment, and defects in conduction (Perez-Stable and Caralis, 1983).

Decrease in Total Body Potassium. *Types of Potassium Depletion.* Three subgroups have important implications for guidelines to therapy. First, *simple depletion* occurs when extracellular and intracellular concentrations are reduced to approximately the same extent. Transmembrane potentials are unchanged, and conduction abnormalities are not observed. Second, the intracellular stores may be excessively lowered relative to extracellular concentrations when there is a *disturbance in membrane function.* And third, a diminished capacity for potassium, or *pseudodepletion,* may occur when the total cellular mass is reduced with little or no change in the composition of the residual cells (Patrick, 1977).

This classification is admittedly an oversimplification, but it provides a useful framework. For example, mild starvation may lead to pseudodepletion, but severe starvation causes all three types. The inability of cell membranes to maintain normal gradients is seen in uremia, thyrotoxicosis, severe and prolonged hypoxia, and simultaneous deficiencies in pancreatic and adrenocortical function. Cardiac glycosides also produce this type of defect. As a more complex example, depletion of potassium may produce rhabdomyolysis. If the depletion is sufficiently severe (approximately 25 to 30% of normal body stores), the integrity of the membrane of the muscle cell becomes secondarily impaired. This leads to a further loss of intracellular potassium (Knochel, 1978).

Causes of Potassium Depletion. The most common causes of potassium depletion are associated with an increased rate of excretion by either the kidneys or the gastrointestinal tract. Increased renal excretion occurs in the following conditions: therapy with diuretics; the administration of large doses of anionic drugs that achieve high concentrations in the urine (*e.g.,* aminosalicylic acid and penicillin G and related antibiotics); primary disorders of renal function, such as renal tubular acidosis; secondary disorders of tubular function induced by amphotericin B or by deficiency of magnesium; primary hyperaldosteronism; and excessive ingestion of licorice or other compounds with mineralocorticoid activity. Secondary hyperaldosteronism markedly enhances the potassium loss, particularly with the use of diuretics. The administration of sodium bicarbonate acutely increases potassium excretion, but the effect may be short lived since both hypokalemia and expansion of extracellular volume suppress production of aldosterone (Sanderson, 1954).

Increased elimination of potassium via the gastrointestinal tract occurs with the loss of any gastrointestinal fluid (vomitus, diarrhea, or surgical drainage), chronic abuse of laxatives, the malabsorption syndromes, and mucus-secreting villous adenomas of the small intestine. Aldosterone accentuates some of these losses, but this is less well documented than those from the kidney. Malabsorption syndromes frequently cause hypocalcemia, which tends to counterbalance the effect of hypokalemia on neuromuscular function.

Although the concentration of potassium in perspiration is only about 10 mEq per liter, cutaneous losses from excessive exercise in a hot environment can result in significant depletion (Knochel, 1978).

Relationship to Metabolic Alkalosis. The popular term *hypokalemic hypochloremic metabolic alkalosis* is an unfortunate collection of redundancies that no longer denotes what was originally intended. First, except in the most contrived experimental situation, all instances of metabolic alkalosis are hypochloremic. And second, due to shifts of potassium from the extracellular to intracellular space, all instances of alkalosis are hypokalemic.

The phrase was originally used to describe cases of metabolic alkalosis in which the acid-base imbalance could be corrected only after repair of the simultaneous depletion of both potassium and chloride. As an example, consider the metabolic alkalosis that results from the loss of chloride and hydrogen ions in the vomitus. There may also be a substantial loss of potassium in the urine and gastric juice with the production of hypokalemia. Even with potassium deficits as high as 500 mEq (in adults), the underlying acid-base deficit may be corrected by administration of sodium chloride without repair of the potassium deficit (Kassirer and Schwartz, 1966). This can be accomplished even though moderate hypokalemia may persist. However, when potassium depletion is more severe, potassium salts are required to correct the alkalosis; administration of sodium chloride will only repair depletion of extracellular fluid volume without correcting the alkalosis (Cooke *et al.,* 1952).

The renal tubular interaction between potassium and hydrogen ions has been discussed above. Metabolic alkalosis can be divided into two categories: chloride responsive and chloride resistant. The preferred terminology is *sodium chloride responsive* and *sodium chloride resistant.* Two separate but related factors are involved: the renal conservation of chloride during alkalosis and the requirement for sodium chloride compared to potassium chloride for repair. Sodium chloride–responsive alkaloses include those caused by loss of gastric juice, diuretic therapy, the posthypercapnic state, and excessive fecal losses of chloride (congenital chloridorrhea or villous adenoma). In these instances the kidney effectively conserves chloride by reducing the urinary concentration to 10 mEq per liter. Acid-base balance can be corrected with sodium chloride. To minimize concomitant hypokalemia, the administration of small amounts of potassium chloride may or may not be considered desirable. The sodium chloride–resistant alkaloses include several disorders of adrenocortical function (primary aldosteronism, Cushing's syndrome, ACTH-secreting tumors, licorice poisoning), Bartter's syndrome, and potassium depletion from other causes, if severe. The kidney fails to conserve chloride effectively and, despite the often severe hypochloremia, the concentration of chloride in the urine is greater than 10 mEq per liter. When sodium chloride is administered, extracellular fluid volume may be repaired temporarily, but the sodium and chloride are promptly jettisoned in the urine. *Chloride-wasting nephropathy* is an appropriate descriptive term (Garella *et al.,* 1970). The acid-base disorder is ameliorated or corrected by the administration of potassium chloride. The time required for correction depends on the nature of the underlying disorder. Prior to treatment, both types of alkalosis are characterized by hypochloremia, hypokalemia, and paradoxical aciduria. The single test that distinguishes between the two categories is determination of the concentration of chloride in urine (in the absence of diuretic drugs). It is also important to make a clinical estimate of the magnitude of potassium loss and of its duration.

Paradoxical aciduria is the excretion of an acidic urine in the presence of metabolic alkalosis. Its relationship to contraction of extracellular volume and sodium depletion has been discussed previously. Paradoxical aciduria also occurs in posthypercapnic alkalosis with inadequate replenishment of sodium chloride. With alkalosis induced by the high-ceiling diuretics, the urine is acidic during the diuretic phase, when sodium and chloride are excreted, as well as in the postdiuretic phase, when sodium is conserved. Thus, severe potassium depletion is only one of the conditions that produce paradoxical aciduria.

Effect of Diuretics. As described in Chapter 36, several classes of diuretics increase the excretion of potassium. This is regularly observed acutely, but the consequences of chronic therapy with diuretics are more controversial. In patients with uncomplicated hypertension, the daily administration of diuretics produces a slight reduction in plasma potassium concentration and either little or no change in total body potassium. In edematous patients the results are more variable. One might anticipate that to the extent that these patients have secondary hyperaldosteronism, they would also be more prone to diuretic-induced losses of potassium. The validity of this concept is amply supported by the high incidence of severe potassium deficiency in a series of patients treated simultaneously with diuretics and carbenoxolone, an agent with mineralocorticoid activity (Knochel, 1978). In this group, chlorthalidone appeared particularly prone to produce potassium depletion.

The problem is further complicated by the effects of diuretics on acid-base balance. When edema fluid is rapidly mobilized by high-ceiling diuretics, the resulting alkalosis is largely of the subtraction type. When the same diuretics are used chronically to maintain the patient free of edema, persistence of the alkalosis must involve the negative chloride balance itself, as well as the associated response of the renal acidification mechanisms. With chronic diuretic therapy, despite the association of alkalosis and hypokalemia, there is no evidence in the vast majority of patients that potassium depletion itself is a cause of the alkalosis. However, exceptions have been noted (Knochel, 1978).

Consequences of Potassium Depletion. The effects of hypokalemia, listed above, are also seen when there is depletion of intracellular potassium. The changes in acid-base balance are also discussed above. In addition, there is reduced tolerance to carbohydrate and a deficiency in glycogen deposition. Polyuria that is resistant to antidiuretic hormone is a prominent symptom. A deficit of potassium appears to increase the renal synthesis of prostaglandins, which in turn decrease the permeability of the distal nephron to water. The disorder is responsive to indomethacin, an inhibitor of prostaglandin synthesis (Galvez *et al.*, 1977).

Morphological Changes. In skeletal muscle, so-called waxy degeneration is observed, which may progress to severe rhabdomyolysis. In the heart, patchy necrosis occurs, especially in the subendocardial region. In the kidney, there is vacuolization of the epithelium of the proximal convolution, along with hyperplasia of cells in the medulla.

PHARMACOLOGICAL CONSIDERATIONS

Transient Volume of Distribution. When potassium is administered as a drug, the factors that govern its distribution are of major importance. It is not possible to increase the total body content of potassium significantly above normal. However, it is very easy to raise the extracellular concentration excessively. For example, if mild hypokalemia is treated injudiciously, one may suddenly find that the plasma concentration of potassium has risen alarmingly (*e.g.*, from 3 to 9 mEq per liter). This does not represent a significant increment in total body potassium, of which only about 2% is located extracellularly. However, *it is the concentration in the extracellular fluid that determines life-threatening toxicity.* Therefore, even though the administered potassium is eventually destined either to be excreted or taken up by cells, knowledge of the transient concentration achieved in the plasma must govern the use of potassium as a therapeutic agent.

Indications and Rationale for Treatment with Potassium. As a practical matter one should distinguish between prophylaxis and replacement and, in states of potassium depletion, between acute and chronic conditions. In addition, it is essential to consider as a separate group those patients who are receiving cardiac glycosides.

Indications. The unequivocal indication for the therapeutic administration of potassium is profound muscular weakness associated with hypokalemia, with or without corresponding abnormalities in cardiac conduction. One should include hypokalemia of all origins, including the specific disease entity of hypokalemic periodic paralysis. Also to be considered are those conditions, particularly diabetic ketoacidosis, in which standard treatment may be *anticipated* to produce acute and severe hypokalemia. In these conditions, the rationale for treatment is to correct a life-threatening disturbance of neuromuscular function.

Replacement of potassium is also indicated in those cases of metabolic alkalosis with potassium depletion that are classified as resistant to sodium chloride.

In either acute or chronic disorders of acid-base or fluid balance, potassium may be indicated either to correct or prevent the disturbances attributable to hypokalemia. The goal of therapy is to elevate the plasma concentration of the ion to the low normal range. Potassium supplementation should be considered if: (1) the concentration of potassium in plasma is less than 2.5 mEq per liter on repeated occasions, even if the patient is asymptomatic; (2) the concentration of potassium is between 2.5 and 3.0 mEq per liter with symptoms or ECG findings suggestive of hypokalemia; or (3) the plasma potassium concentration is consistently between 3.0 and 3.5 mEq per liter and there are clear-cut symptoms or ECG signs of hypokalemia.

Since digitalis and potassium have competitive affinities for myocardial Na^+,K^+-ATPase, the actions of digitalis are accentuated by hypokalemia. Therefore, the criteria for supplementation with potassium are altered for patients who are receiving a digitalis glycoside. In such individuals it is advisable to maintain the plasma potassium concentration at 3.2 mEq per liter or higher. Although digitalis-related arrhythmias are accentuated by hypokalemia, there is no evidence that they are influenced by the absolute concentration of potassium within the normal range for plasma (*i.e.,* from 3.5 to 5.0 mEq per liter). The role of potassium in the treatment of digitalis intoxication is considered in Chapter 30.

The prophylactic administration of potassium cannot be justified when the plasma concentration is normal, except for patients with hypokalemic periodic paralysis. In this disorder the concentration of potassium is often normal during asymptomatic periods, but the frequency of attacks may be diminished by high-potassium intake.

Contraindications. Supplementation with potassium is contraindicated when potassium-sparing diuretics are prescribed, with the possible exception of patients with Bartter's syndrome. Chronic renal insufficiency is a contraindication, probably for two reasons. First, the urinary excretion of potassium normally provides a fortunate safety mechanism in the event of transient hyperkalemia. Second, cellular uptake of potassium may be defective during chronic renal insufficiency. In acute renal failure, potassium intake should be reduced to the lowest possible level. Tubular secretion of potassium may be defective in patients with sickle-cell anemia, and supplementation can induce dangerous hyperkalemia (DeFronzo *et al.,* 1979).

Potassium salts have a somewhat unpleasant taste, and they can be irritating to the gastrointestinal tract; many patients do not take the prescribed dose. This assumes particular importance when an ambulatory noncompliant patient requires hospitalization and the same dose that was prescribed is continued under supervision that assures compliance. In addition, salt substitutes that contain potassium may be prescribed at the same time. Instances of severe hyperkalemia have resulted from such a sequence.

Misleading Indications. In the common situation in which diuretics are chronically prescribed, patients may also receive digitalis for underlying heart failure. As indicated above, alkalosis and hypokalemia may result. Potassium supplementation is warranted to control the plasma concentration of potassium; small doses of ammonium chloride should be considered as a means to replenish chloride without sodium. In the vast majority of patients, potassium is not indicated for the correction of alkalosis. If this distinction were more clearly kept in mind, the incidence of iatrogenic hyperkalemia might be reduced. However, there have been rare instances of an exceptional degree of alkalosis, hyponatremia, and potassium depletion acutely induced by thiazides (Fichman *et al.,* 1971).

Oral Administration of Potassium. Potassium chloride is the preferred salt for most situations because of the frequency with which deficits of potassium and chloride coexist. This salt has a moderately unpleasant taste. For the prophylaxis of hypokalemia during chronic diuretic therapy, a total oral dose of potassium of 20 to 50 mEq per day in divided portions is effective for most patients. This is given in addition to dietary intake, which may be quite variable.

Intravenous Administration of Potassium. In acute illness when the oral administration of potassium is not possible, it may be administered intravenously. A number of factors must be considered. All doses are for adults.

Since the normal potassium intake is 50 to 100 mEq per day, it is rare that a larger amount is warranted. In patients with potassium depletion this amount slowly but adequately corrects the deficit. With extreme depletion or with high rates of ongoing loss, larger doses may be required. The recommended maximal rate of administration varies from 10 to 30 mEq per hour. If an infusion rate of greater than 30 mEq per hour is considered to be essential, the ECG should be monitored continuously so that the earliest indication of hyperkalemia may be detected. When infused into a peripheral vein, concentrations of potassium chloride up to 40 mEq per liter are usually tolerated and do not produce localized pain. If higher concentrations are required because of the concomitant need to minimize fluid intake, a central vein should be employed. When high concentrations are used, even brief errors in the rate of administration can cause cardiotoxicity. It is therefore recommended that, when the potassium concentration in the infusion is 80 mEq per liter or higher, the *total amount* of ion in the infusion system should not exceed 10 mEq. In this case a fluid volume up to 100 ml can be conveniently administered by SOLUSET or similar device with a very low rate of infusion of fluid. The available dose of potassium may be renewed as indicated by the clinical situation.

Toxicity of Potassium Salts. The cardiac toxicity of hyperkalemia, which has been discussed above, is one of the leading causes of iatrogenic morbidity and mortality. Enteric-coated tablets of potassium chloride and other slow-release formulations can be irritating to the gastrointestinal tract and cause ulceration. The rather bad-tasting solutions of KCl may limit the patient's compliance.

Treatment of Hyperkalemia. The acute management of this problem includes, first and foremost, the termination of the administration of potassium, if this is the cause. Additional treatment includes the intravenous administration of a calcium salt, glucose, insulin, and sodium bicarbonate. Ion-exchange resins such as sodium polystyrene sulfonate, administered by mouth or by rectum, are also useful (*see* below). If the above measures fail, either peritoneal or extracorporeal dialysis may be lifesaving.

Preparations to Repair Potassium Depletion and to Control Hyperkalemia. Preparations of potassium chloride for oral administration are supplied in a vast array of formulations (liquids, powders, and effervescent tablets) and flavors, a reflection of their lack of palatability. Liquids generally contain from 10 to 40 mEq per 15 ml. Enteric-coated tablets, tablets that contain a wax matrix, and controlled-release capsules are also available. *Potassium chloride injection* is a sterile solution of potassium chloride in water. It is usually marketed as a 15% (2 mEq/ml) solution. This solution should never be administered as such but must be suitably diluted. Various other potassium salts are also available.

Cation-Exchange Resins. Exchange resins are useful to lower concentrations of potassium in plasma and other body fluids. One of the most efficient is *sodium polystyrene sulfonate* (KAYEXALATE), which exchanges sodium for potassium. It may be given by mouth, instilled as an enema, or inserted in the rectum in a dialysis bag to facilitate recovery. The resin should be retained in the rectum for 30 to 60 minutes. When administered orally, a laxative should be given concurrently to avoid fecal impaction. The use of resins by mouth is often avoided because there is nausea and vomiting. The usual oral dose is 15 g of the resin one to four times daily. It should be suspended in a palatable vehicle.

When used as an enema, 30 to 50 g of the resin in 100 ml of a suitable vehicle is inserted through a large Foley catheter with the 30-ml Foley bag inflated. The rectal tube is clamped and the material left in the rectum for the period indicated above. The clamp is then released and the material expelled by the patient. Such enemas are given at 6-hour intervals until the potassium concentration is within a safe range.

Calcium Gluconate. Calcium gluconate may be a very useful agent in combating the deleterious effects of hyperkalemia on the heart. It may be administered directly intravenously as a 10% solution while the ECG is monitored. The usual dose is 10 to 20 ml, but as much as 50 ml of a 10% solution can be administered safely if given slowly. Following this, another 50 ml of the calcium gluconate (10%) can be placed in a larger volume of fluid (dextrose injection, *etc.*) and administered more slowly. Available preparations are described in Chapter 65.

MAGNESIUM

Magnesium is the second most plentiful cation of the intracellular fluids. It is essential for the activity of many enzymes and plays an important role in neurochemical transmission and muscular excitability. Deficits are accompanied by a variety of structural and functional disturbances (*see* Mordes and Wacker, 1978; Rude and Singer, 1981).

The average 70-kg adult has about 2000 mEq of magnesium in his body. About 50% of this is in bone, 45% exists as an intracellular cation, and 5% is in the extracellular fluid. Intracellular concentrations of magnesium range from 5 to 30 mEq/kg. The concentration in plasma is 1.5 to 2.2 mEq of magnesium per liter, with about two thirds as free cation and one third bound to plasma proteins. Intracellular and extracellular concentrations of magnesium can vary independently, and a deficit in one compartment may not be accompanied by a significant change in the other. About 30% of the magnesium in the skeleton represents an exchangeable pool. Mobilization of the cation from this pool in bone is fairly rapid in children but not in adults.

Absorption and Excretion. The average adult in the United States ingests about 20 to 40 mEq of magnesium a day, and of this approximately one third is absorbed from the gastrointestinal tract. Absorption occurs in the upper small bowel by means of an active process closely related to the transport system for calcium. Ingestion of low amounts of magnesium results in increased absorption of calcium and *vice versa*.

Magnesium is excreted principally by the kidney, and, under normal conditions, 3 to 5% of the filtered ion is excreted in the urine. Most of the reabsorption of magnesium occurs in the proximal tubule (Massry, 1977). Renal excretion of magnesium is increased by many diuretic agents, and hypomagnesemia can occur as a complication of diuretic therapy (Sheehan and White, 1982). Small amounts of magnesium are excreted in milk and saliva.

PHYSIOLOGICAL AND PHARMACOLOGICAL ACTIONS

Enzyme Systems. Magnesium is a cofactor of all enzymes involved in phosphate transfer reactions that utilize adenosine triphosphate (ATP) and other nucleotide triphosphates as substrates. Many other enzymes are also influenced by this ion.

Magnesium plays a vital role in the reversible association of intracellular particles and in the binding of macromolecules to subcellular organelles. For example, the binding of mRNA to ribosomes is magnesium dependent, as is the functional integrity of ribosomal subunits.

Central Nervous System. Certain of the effects of magnesium on the nervous system are similar to those of calcium. Hypomagnesemia causes increased CNS irritability, disorientation, convulsions, and psychotic behavior (Shils, 1969).

The flaccid, anesthesia-like state that is produced by the intravenous administration of high doses of magnesium sulfate is probably due to peripheral neuromuscular blockade. In a carefully monitored study of two subjects in whom the plasma concentration of magnesium was raised to 15 mEq per liter, the ensuing profound muscular paralysis was unaccompanied by any significant loss of sensation or consciousness (Somjen *et al.*, 1966).

Neuromuscular System. Magnesium has a direct depressant effect on skeletal muscle. In addition, excess magnesium decreases acetylcholine release by motor-nerve impulses, reduces the sensitivity of the motor end-plate to applied acetylcholine, and decreases the amplitude of the motor end-plate potential. The most critical of these effects is inhibition of acetylcholine release (Hubbard, 1973). The actions of increased magnesium on neuromuscular function are antagonized by calcium. The administration of magnesium sulfate in preeclampsia and eclampsia potentiates neuromuscular blockade produced by *d*-tubocurarine, decamethonium, and succinylcholine (Ghoneim and Long, 1970). Abnormally low concentrations of magnesium in the extracellular fluid result in increased acetylcholine release and increased muscle excitability that can produce tetany.

Cardiovascular System. Certain of the cardiac effects of excess magnesium are similar to those of the potassium ion. High concentrations of magnesium (10 to 15 mEq per liter) cause increased conduction time with lengthened P-R and QRS intervals of the ECG. Magnesium slows the rate of S-A nodal impulse formation. Higher concentrations of magnesium (greater than 15 mEq per liter) produce cardiac arrest in diastole. Magnesium may abolish digitalis-induced premature ventricular contractions (Sodeman, 1965), but it is rarely used for this purpose unless hypomagnesemia is also present. States of magnesium deficiency may or may not be associated with decreased potassium in cardiac cells and enhanced toxicity to cardiac glycosides (Seller *et al.*, 1970). The ECG changes seen with magnesium depletion are similar to those seen with hypercalcemia (Seelig, 1969).

Excess magnesium causes vasodilatation by both a direct action on blood vessels and ganglionic blockade.

ABNORMALITIES OF MAGNESIUM METABOLISM

Hypomagnesemia. The *pathology* of magnesium depletion includes changes in skeletal and cardiac muscle and striking nephrocalcinosis. The latter is unique in that it consists in the formation of tiny microliths within the lumen of the nephron, almost entirely confined to the thick ascending limb of Henle's loop. Damage to tubular cells occurs when the microliths grow sufficiently large to cause obstruction. In the course of several months on a magnesium-deficient regimen, volunteer subjects have developed hypomagnesemia, with inconsistent occurrence of hypokalemia and hypocalcemia. They may exhibit neuromuscular disorders akin to those seen in hypocalcemia.

Magnesium deficiency can occur in diarrhea and steatorrhea; in chronic alcoholism; with prolonged intravenous feeding with magnesium-free solutions; during hemodialysis; and in diabetes mellitus, pancreatitis, postdiuretic electrolyte imbalance, renal tubular damage, and primary aldosteronism. Magnesium deficiency is therefore often associated with hypokalemia and hypocalcemia.

Hypomagnesemia, as well as a decrease in total body stores of magnesium, frequently occurs in chronic alcoholic patients. The factors responsible probably include increased renal excretion of magnesium, decreased dietary intake of magnesium, vomiting and diarrhea, and hyperaldosteronism in the presence of hepatic cirrhosis. This observation and the similarity between the signs and symptoms of experimental magnesium deficiency in experimental animals and those of delirium tremens have led to the hypothesis that hypomagnesemia is a causative factor in the latter condition. However, convincing evidence of this is lacking. As part of the total treatment program for chronic alcoholism, the plasma concentrations of magnesium and of calcium, which is also frequently decreased, should be determined and corrected if found to be low (*see* Rude and Singer, 1981).

When deficits of magnesium and potassium coexist, repletion of the magnesium deficit may be necessary in order to correct that of potassium. This interaction of the two ions is thought to be mediated by the effect of adrenal steroids on renal excretion (Güllner *et al.*, 1981).

During rapid growth periods in newborns and children, hypomagnesemia has been associated with poor intake or excessive losses. A low concentration of magnesium in plasma in newborns who are fed cow's milk or artificial formulas is apparently related to a high phosphate:magnesium ratio in these diets. In infancy the symptoms reliably associated with hypomagnesemia are seizures, hyperirritability, exaggerated tendon reflexes, and increased muscle tone. There is frequently a concomitant hypocalcemia that is resistant to therapy with calcium and vitamin D. Symptoms may be corrected by the replacement of magnesium (Cockburn *et al.*, 1973). Magnesium therapy also appears to be important in correcting hypocalcemia in infants. Oral administration of calcium for treatment of hypocalcemia without regard to decreased magnesium may only exacerbate a magnesium deficiency by reducing intestinal absorption of the cation. This is consistent with the proposed common transport mechanism for magnesium and calcium in the gastrointestinal tract.

Hypomagnesemia in protein-calorie malnutrition is well documented. Conflicting reports exist on the significance of magnesium therapy in reducing the mortality rate in such patients (Rosen *et al.*, 1970).

Magnesium deficiency, particularly if severe, can lead to a form of hypocalcemia that persists despite increased calcium intake until the deficit of magnesium is repaired. Several factors may be involved, including parathyroid dysfunction and an altered equilibrium between calcium in bone and extracellular fluid (Massry, 1977). If tetany is present, it is reversed by the administration of magnesium but not of calcium. Other interrelationships between magnesium, calcium, and the parathyroid glands are discussed in Chapter 65.

A high proportion of patients who form oxalate and phosphate renal stones have low excretion rates of magnesium. When compared to normal subjects, patients with primary hyperparathyroidism and renal stones have a low urinary magnesium concentration relative to calcium excretion. Hyperparathyroid patients with osteitis fibrosa excrete relatively high concentrations of magnesium, and it has been suggested that magnesium excretion may be a factor in the rarity of urinary calculi in these patients.

Conflicting reports exist regarding changes in magnesium metabolism in women taking oral contraceptive hormones (Simpson and Dale, 1972).

Hypomagnesemia is treated with parenteral fluids containing magnesium sulfate or chloride.

Hypermagnesemia. An elevated magnesium concentration in plasma is usually due to renal insufficiency. The use of magnesium sulfate as a cathartic in patients with impaired renal function can lead to severe toxicity, as can chronic ingestion of magnesium-containing antacids by such individuals. Magnesium cathartics may undergo excessively rapid absorption in patients with large gastrojejunal stomas. Hypermagnesemia is manifested by muscle weakness, hypotension, ECG changes, sedation, and confusion. As plasma concentrations of magnesium begin to exceed 4 mEq per liter, the deep-tendon reflexes are decreased and may be absent at levels approaching 10 mEq per liter. At 12 to 15 mEq per liter respiratory paralysis is a potential hazard; the respiratory effects can be antagonized to some extent by the intravenous administration of calcium salts. The concentration of magnesium in the plasma at which complete heart block occurs may be quite variable (*see* Mordes and Wacker, 1978).

Plasma concentrations of magnesium increase in the fetus and approach the maternal blood values after magnesium sulfate administration in eclampsia and preeclampsia. The neonate may be drowsy and exhibit respiratory difficulties and diminished muscle tone. However, Stone and Pritchard (1970) found no relationship between the plasma magnesium concentration of blood collected from the umbilical cord and the Apgar score. In infants who suffer hypoxia during delivery, hypermagnesemia can result, and the plasma magnesium concentration is inversely correlated with the Apgar score (Engel and Elin, 1970).

Preparations. Magnesium citrate, sulfate, and hydroxide are the preparations usually employed for their action on the gastrointestinal tract. There are many magnesium preparations used as antacids. For parenteral medication, magnesium sulfate is usually employed. The dosage is expressed in terms of the hydrated salt, $MgSO_4 \cdot 7H_2O$. One gram of this salt is equivalent to 4.06 mmol (8.12 mEq) of magnesium. *Magnesium sulfate injection* is available in concentrations ranging from 10 to 50%.

Therapeutic Uses. *Gastrointestinal Uses.* The uses of magnesium salts as cathartics (Chapter 43) and as antacids (Chapter 42) are discussed elsewhere.

Local Use. Skin burns from hydrofluoric acid are a serious industrial hazard. Infiltration of the contaminated area with magnesium salts has been recommended on the basis of animal experiments (Harris and Rumack, 1981).

Central Depression. Magnesium sulfate is used in the treatment of seizures associated with acute nephritis and with eclampsia of pregnancy. The dose for children is 0.1 to 0.2 ml/kg of body weight (0.16 to 0.32 mEq/kg) of a 20% solution administered intramuscularly. In the treatment of patients with toxemia of pregnancy, Rogers and associates (1969) have developed a system of initial and sustaining dosage, based on body weight. It is possible to attain unduly high plasma concentrations, and the patient must be carefully monitored both clinically and chemically. If magnesium therapy of this sort is to be used, a preparation of a calcium salt should be readily available for intravenous injection to counteract the potential serious hazard of magnesium intoxication. A clinical sign of significance is the presence of deep-tendon reflexes. As long as these are active, it is probable that the patient will not develop respiratory paralysis.

Hypomagnesemia. Intravenous administration of magnesium sulfate is the treatment for severe magnesium deficiency; it should be injected extremely slowly with observance of the same precautions as described above. Two to 4 g may be given daily in divided doses (16 to 32 mEq).

Abouna, G. M.; Veazey, P. R.; and Terry, D. B., Jr. Intravenous infusion of hydrochloric acid for treatment of severe metabolic alkalosis. *Surgery*, **1974**, *75*, 194–202.

Adler, S., and Fraley, D. S. Potassium and intracellular pH. *Kidney Int.*, **1977**, *11*, 433–442.

Bia, M. J., and DeFronzo, R. A. Extrarenal potassium homeostasis. *Am J. Physiol.*, **1981**, *240*, F257–F268.

Carpenter, C. C. J. Clinical studies in Asiatic cholera. VI. Overall clinical observations. *Bull. Johns Hopkins Hosp.*, **1966**, *118*, 243–245.

Cerny, L. C.; Cerny, E. L.; Cerny, M. E.; Baldwin, J. E.; and Gill, B. Mixtures of whole blood and hydroxyethyl starch-hemoglobin polymers. *Crit. Care Med.*, **1983**, *11*, 739–743.

Cervera, A. L., and Moss, G. Progressive hypovolemia leading to shock after continuous hemorrhage and 3:1 crystalloid replacement. *Am. J. Surg.*, **1975**, *129*, 670–674.

Cockburn, F.; Brown, J. K.; Belton, N. R.; and Forfar, J. O. Neonatal convulsions associated with primary disturbances of calcium, potassium, and magnesium metabolism. *Arch. Dis. Child.*, **1973**, *48*, 99–108.

Colman, R. W. Paradoxical hypotension after volume expansion with plasma protein fraction. *N. Engl. J. Med.*, **1978**, *299*, 97–98.

Cooke, R. E.; Segar, W. E.; Cheek, D. B.; Coville, F. E.; and Darrow, D. C. Extrarenal correction of alkalosis associated with potassium deficiency. *J. Clin. Invest.*, **1952**, *31*, 798–805.

DeFronzo, R. A.; Taufield, P. A.; Black, H.; McPhedran, P.; and Cooke, C. R. Impaired renal tubular potassium secretion in sickle cell disease. *Ann. Intern. Med.*, **1979**, *90*, 310–316.

Dell, R. B.; Lee, C. E.; and Winters, R. W. Influence of body composition on the *in vivo* response to acute hypercapnia. *Pediatr. Res.*, **1971**, *5*, 523–538.

Diehl, J. T.; Lester, J. L., III; and Cosgrove, D. M. Clinical comparison of hetastarch and albumin in postoperative cardiac patients. *Ann. Thorac. Surg.*, **1982**, *34*, 674–679.

Duggin, G. G., and Price, M. A. Hypokalemic muscular paresis in migratory Papua/New Guineans. *Lancet*, **1974**, *1*, 649–651.

Engel, R. R., and Elin, R. J. Hypermagnesemia from birth asphyxia. *J. Pediatr.*, **1970**, *77*, 631–637.

Ettinger, P. O.; Regan, T. J.; and Oldewurtel, H. A. Hyperkalemia, cardiac conduction, and the electrocardiogram: a review. *Am. Heart J.*, **1974**, *88*, 360–371.

Fichman, M. P.; Vorherr, H.; Kleeman, C. R.; and Telfer, N. Diuretic-induced hyponatremia, *Ann. Intern. Med.*, **1971**, *75*, 853–863.

Finberg, L.; Kiley, J.; and Luttrell, C. N. Mass accidental salt poisoning in infancy. A study of a hospital disaster. *J.A.M.A.*, **1963**, *184*, 187–190.

Fischer, J. E., and Baldessarini, R. J. Pathogenesis and therapy of hepatic coma. *Prog. Liver Dis.*, **1976**, *5*, 363–397.

Galvez, O. G.; Bay, W. H.; Roberts, B. W.; and Ferris, T. F. The hemodynamic effects of potassium deficiency in the dog. *Circ. Res.*, **1977**, *40*, Suppl. I, 11–16.

Gamble, J. L. Physiological information gained from studies on the life raft ration. *Harvey Lect.*, **1947**, *62*, 247–273.

Garella, S.; Chazan, J. A.; and Cohen, J. J. Saline-resistant metabolic alkalosis or "chloride-wasting nephropathy." *Ann. Intern. Med.*, **1970**, *73*, 31–38.

Ghoneim, M. M., and Long, J. P. The interaction between magnesium and other neuromuscular blocking agents. *Anesthesiology*, **1970**, *32*, 23–27.

Goldfarb, S.; Strunk, B.; Singer, I.; and Goldberg, M. Paradoxical glucose-induced hyperkalemia. Combined aldosterone-insulin deficiency. *Am. J. Med.*, **1975**, *59*, 744–750.

Güllner, H.-G.; Gill, J. R., Jr.; and Bartter, F. C. Correction of hypokalemia by magnesium repletion in familial hypokalemic alkalosis with tubulopathy. *Am. J. Med.*, **1981**, *71*, 578–582.

Harris, J. C., and Rumack, B. H. Comparative efficacy of injectable calcium and magnesium salts in the therapy of hydrofluoric acid burns. *Clin. Toxicol.*, **1981**, *18*, 1027–1032.

Kassirer, J. P., and Schwartz, W. B. Correction of metabolic alkalosis in man without repair of potassium deficiency. *Am. J. Med.*, **1966**, *40*, 19–26.

Katz, M. A. Hyperglycemia-induced hyponatremia—calculation of sodium depression. *N. Engl. J. Med.*, **1973**, *289*, 843–844.

Knochel, J. P. Role of glucoregulatory hormones in potassium homeostasis. *Kidney Int.*, **1977**, *11*, 443–452.

———. Rhabdomyolysis and effects of potassium deficiency on muscle structure and function. *Cardiovasc. Med.*, **1978**, *3*, 247–261.

Madias, N. E.; Ayus, J. C.; and Adrogué, H. J. Increased anion gap in metabolic alkalosis. The role of plasma-protein equivalency. *N. Engl. J. Med.*, **1979**, *300*, 1421–1423.

Melton, J. E., and Nattie, E. E. Brain and CSF water and ions during dilutional and isosmotic hyponatremia in the rat. *Am. J. Physiol.*, **1983**, *244*, R724–R732.

Menitove, S. M., and Goldring, R. M. Combined ventricular and bicarbonate strategy in the management of status asthmaticus. *Am. J. Med.*, **1983**, *74*, 898–901.

Milne, M. D. Influence of acid base balance on efficacy and toxicity of drugs. In, *Nephrotoxicity.* (Fillastre, J.-P., ed.) Masson Publishing USA, Inc., New York, **1978**, pp. 53–61.

Mudge, G. H., and Hardin, B. Response to mercurial diuretics during alkalosis: a comparison of acute metabolic and chronic hypokalemic alkalosis in the dog. *J. Clin. Invest.*, **1956**, *35*, 155–163.

Oh, M. S., and Carroll, H. J. The anion gap. *N. Engl. J. Med.*, **1977**, *297*, 814–817.

Patrick, J. Assessment of body potassium stores. *Kidney Int.*, **1977**, *11*, 476–490.

Perez-Stable, E., and Caralis, P. V. Thiazide-induced disturbances in carbohydrate, lipid, and potassium metabolism. *Am. Heart J.*, **1983**, *106*, 245–251.

Puri, V. K.; Howard, M.; Paidipaty, B. B.; and Singh, S. Resuscitation in hypovolemia and shock: a prospective study of hydroxyethyl starch and albumin. *Crit. Care Med.*, **1983**, *11*, 518–523.

Ring, J., and Messmer, K. Incidence and severity of anaphylactoid reactions to colloid volume substitutes. *Lancet*, **1977**, *1*, 466–469.

Rogers, S. F.; Flowers, C. E., Jr.; and Alexander, J. A. Aggressive toxemia management. *Obstet. Gynecol.*, **1969**, *33*, 724–728.

Rosen, E. U.; Campbell, P. G.; and Moosa, G. M. Hypomagnesemia and magnesium therapy in protein-calorie malnutrition. *J. Pediatr.*, **1970**, *77*, 709–714.

Sanderson, P. H. Renal response to massive alkali loading in the human subject. In, *Ciba Foundation Symposium on the Kidney.* (Lewis, A. A. G., and Wolstenholme, G. E. W., eds.) Little, Brown & Co., Boston, **1954**, pp. 165–174.

Seelig, M. S. Electrographic patterns of magnesium depletion appearing in alcoholic heart disease. *Ann. N.Y. Acad. Sci.*, **1969**, *162*, 906–917.

Seller, R. H.; Cangiano, J.; Kim, K. E.; Mendelssohn, S.; Brest, A. N.; and Swartz, C. Digitalis toxicity and hypomagnesemia. *Am. Heart J.*, **1970**, *79*, 57–68.

Sheehan, J., and White, A. Diuretic-associated hypomagnesaemia. *Br. Med. J.*, **1982**, *285*, 1157–1159.

Shils, M. E. Experimental human magnesium depletion. *Medicine (Baltimore)*, **1969**, *48*, 61–85.

Simpson, G. R., and Dale, E. Serum levels of phosphorus, magnesium, and calcium in women utilizing combination oral or long-acting injectable progestational contraceptives. *Fertil. Steril.*, **1972**, *23*, 326–330.

Sodeman, W. A.   Diagnosis and treatment of digitalis toxicity. *N. Engl. J. Med.,* **1965,** *273,* 35–37, 93–95.

Somjen, G.; Hilmy, M.; and Stephen, C. R.   Failure to anesthetize human subjects by intravenous administration of magnesium sulfate. *J. Pharmacol. Exp. Ther.,* **1966,** *154,* 652–659.

Stone, S. R., and Pritchard, J. A.   Effects of maternally administered magnesium sulfate on the neonate. *Obstet. Gynecol.,* **1970,** *35,* 574–577.

Tannen, R. L.   Relationship of renal ammonia production and potassium homeostasis. *Kidney Int.,* **1977,** *11,* 453–465.

Tremper, K. K.; Freidman, A. E.; Levine, E. M.; Lapin, R.; and Camarillo, D.   The preoperative treatment of severely anemic patients with a perfluorochemical oxygen-transport fluid, fluosol-DA. *N. Engl. J. Med.,* **1982,** *307,* 277–283.

Vick, R. L.   Extra-renal control of body potassium. *Cardiovasc. Res. Cent. Bull.,* **1981,** *19,* 105–112.

Wynn, V.   A metabolic study of acute water intoxication in man and dogs. *Clin. Sci.,* **1955,** *14,* 669–680.

Young, D. B.   Relationship between plasma potassium concentration and renal potassium excretion. *Am. J. Physiol.,* **1982,** *242,* F599–F603.

Monographs and Reviews

Cohen, J. J., and Kassirer, J. P.   *Acid-Base.* Little, Brown & Co., Boston, **1982.**

Committee on Nutrition, American Academy of Pediatrics.   Commentary on parenteral nutrition. *Pediatrics,* **1983,** *71,* 547–552.

Fischer, J. E.   Hyperalimentation. *Adv. Surg.,* **1977,** *11,* 1–69.

Grant, J. P.   *Handbook of Total Parenteral Nutrition.* W. B. Saunders Co., Philadelphia, **1980.**

Hayslett, J. P., and Binder, H. J.   Mechanism of potassium adaptation. *Am. J. Physiol.,* **1982,** *243,* F103–F112.

Hubbard, J. I.   Microphysiology of vertebrate neuromuscular transmission. *Physiol. Rev.,* **1973,** *53,* 674–723.

McQuestion, M. J. (ed.).   *Oral Rehydration Therapy: An Annotated Bibliography.* Pan American Health Organization, Washington, D. C., **1983.**

Massry, S. G.   Pharmacology of magnesium. *Annu. Rev. Pharmacol. Toxicol.,* **1977,** *17,* 67–82.

Mordes, J. P., and Wacker, W. E. C.   Excess magnesium. *Pharmacol. Rev.,* **1978,** *29,* 273–300.

Narins, R. G., and Emmett, M.   Simple and mixed acid-base disorders: a practical approach. *Medicine (Baltimore),* **1980,** *59,* 161–187.

Rude, R. K., and Singer, F. R.   Magnesium deficiency and excess. *Annu. Rev. Med.,* **1981,** *32,* 245–259.

Stanton, B. A., and Giebisch, G. H.   Regulation of potassium homeostasis. In, *Functional Regulation at the Cellular and Molecular Levels.* (Corradino, R. A., ed.) Elsevier North Holland, Inc., New York, **1982,** pp. 259–283.

Symposium. (Various authors.)   Acellular oxygen-delivery resuscitation fluids. (DeVenuto, F., ed.) *Crit. Care Med.,* **1982,** *10,* 237–293.

VIII

Drugs Affecting Renal Function and Electrolyte Metabolism

INTRODUCTION

Gilbert H. Mudge and Irwin M. Weiner

The important homeostatic role of the kidney in maintaining the volume and the composition of the body fluids has already been stressed in the preceding chapter. It is not surprising, therefore, to find that drugs that alter renal function comprise a major and indispensable group of therapeutic agents. The most widely used drugs in this group are the diuretics, which may be classified according to their chemical constitution or, preferably, according to the physiological functions that they affect. Some of the diuretics have therapeutic applications in addition to those that result from alterations of excretory function. It should also be noted that the kidney is the major excretory organ for many therapeutic agents and their metabolites. A knowledge of renal mechanisms is important, therefore, in evaluating the pattern of drug excretion, particularly since alteration of renal function may markedly affect the rate of excretion and hence the duration of drug action or the extent of drug toxicity.

PHYSIOLOGICAL CONSIDERATIONS

The majority of excretory products appear in the glomerular filtrate and are incompletely reabsorbed by the renal tubules. Other substances can also be secreted by the renal tubular cells into the tubular urine and in this manner be eliminated from the body. Certain substances, moreover, undergo both reabsorption and secretion. It should be emphasized that the terms *reabsorption* and *secretion* refer to the direction of net transport without any implication as to underlying cellular mechanisms. Therefore, the factors that are important in the determination of volume and composition of urine are: (1) glomerular filtration, (2) tubular reabsorption, and (3) tubular secretion.

Glomerular Filtration. The glomerulus of the kidney is similar to other capillary beds, and filtration is subject to the same physical laws that govern the transport of fluid and permeable solutes across any capillary membrane. The filtering force is the hydrostatic pressure of the blood derived from the work of the heart. The plasma proteins do not penetrate the normal glomerular membrane to an appreciable extent. All the plasma constituents gain access to the glomerular capsule with the exception of the proteins, lipids, and substances bound to proteins.

Although the rate of glomerular filtration is a very important aspect of renal function, drugs that affect the rate of filtration will not be discussed in this section. A common cause of reduction in the filtration rate is organic change in the renal vascular bed. There is no drug available to correct this abnormality. Another common cause of reduction in filtration rate is the reduced renal blood flow secondary to heart failure. For its correction, attention is directed to the heart rather than to the kidney. Many drugs used in the treatment of hypertension reduce renal blood flow and filtration rate, but these represent undesirable side effects. Drugs with marked hemodynamic action, such as epinephrine, alter filtration rate and urine flow by affecting arterial pressure and afferent and efferent renal arteriolar resistance, but no therapeutic application is made of these actions. Finally, there are a few agents, such as dopamine, that significantly increase renal blood flow and filtration rate. Experience has demonstrated that one can alter the rate of excretion of many substances much more effectively by drugs that alter tubular function than by those that change filtration rate.

Tubular Transport of Inorganic Compounds. The importance of the reabsorptive function of the renal tubules to the body economy cannot be overemphasized and can best be illustrated by a few numerical considerations. The rate of glomerular filtration in the average adult is approximately 125 ml per minute. In such an individual, the total extracellular fluid volume is approximately 12.5 liters. Thus, a volume equivalent to that of the extracellular fluid is filtered across the glomerular capillary bed within a period of 100 minutes. During this time approximately 100 ml of urine reaches the bladder. Therefore, the tubules normally reabsorb over 99% of the glomerular filtrate. Obviously the composition of the tubular reabsorbate must closely approximate that of the extracellular fluid; otherwise, extreme distortions in the composition of the extracellular fluid would soon result. Reabsorption is largely achieved by active transport of electrolyte and other solutes from tubular fluid to tubular cell and thence to the extracellular fluid. This involves the expenditure of energy derived from metabolic activity. Physical forces involving the oncotic pressure of the peritubular plasma may also contribute to the reabsorption of water. The magnitude of this component is relatively small and uncertain.

Tubular Reabsorption of Sodium. It is convenient to consider the overall relationship between the reabsorption of solute and of water in terms of a single solute, the sodium ion (*see* Figure VIII–1). Sodium salts constitute by far the largest fraction of the filtered solutes and are reabsorbed in almost all segments of the nephron. The movement of sodium across the tubular epithelium occurs in large part through the epithelial cells, the transcellular route. In addition, a portion of sodium reabsorption occurs in the spaces between cells, the paracellular pathway. Transcellular transport may be divided into two processes: (1) the movement of sodium from the tubular fluid into the tubular cells and (2) the extrusion of sodium from the cells into the peritubular or extracellular fluid. The latter process involves the active transport of sodium against an electrochemical gradient. This gradient is the result of the negative intracellular potential of the tubular cell and the relatively low concentration of sodium in the intracellular fluid. This transport mechanism is essentially similar in all segments of the nephron (Figure VIII–1, *F*). The energy for active extrusion is derived from the hydrolysis of adenosine triphosphate (ATP), and the pump is a Na^+,K^+-ATPase. This enzyme is located in the basolateral membrane of the epithelial cell and is often referred to as the "sodium pump." The cardiac glycosides are potent inhibitors of Na^+,K^+-ATPase and, under experimental conditions, can block active reabsorption of sodium in all segments of the nephron.

In contrast to the single mechanism for extrusion of sodium, a number of separate mechanisms are involved in the movement of sodium across the luminal membrane from the tubular fluid into the tubular cells. These mechanisms differ by several criteria: localization to more discrete segments of the nephron, relationship to transport of other solutes, sensitivity to drugs, and biophysical and biochemical aspects of the transport process. Thus far, four major mechanisms for sodium entry have been identified: *A*, The direct entry of sodium ions *per se* along a favorable electrochemical gradient; *B*, the entry of sodium, coupled to the entry of an organic solute or phosphate; *C*, the entry of sodium in exchange for a cation (*e.g.*, H^+) moving in the opposite direction; and *D*, the entry of sodium coupled to the entry of chloride (*see* Figure VIII–1). In *B*, the entry of sodium may be coupled to that of a nonelectrolyte (*e.g.*, glucose) or to an ion, such as phosphate or an amino acid, lactate,

MECHANISMS OF SODIUM TRANSPORT
ACROSS TUBULAR EPITHELIUM

FUNCTIONAL ORGANIZATION OF THE
NEPHRON

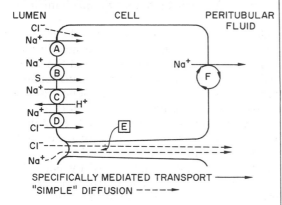

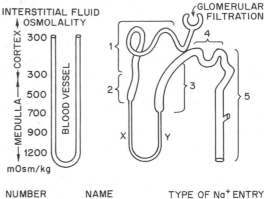

SPECIFICALLY MEDIATED TRANSPORT ⟶
"SIMPLE" DIFFUSION ----→

A Na^+ entry *per se*

B Na^+ cotransport with glucose or organic acids

C $Na^+ - H^+$ exchange

D $Na^+ - Cl^-$ cotransport

E Cl^- diffusion, Na^+ following

F   Active Na^+ extrusion (Na^+, K^+-ATPase)

NUMBER	NAME	TYPE OF Na^+ ENTRY
1	Proximal convoluted tubule	A, B, C
2	Late proximal tubule	A, E
3	Thick ascending limb of Henle's loop	D
4	Distal convolution	?
5	Late distal tubule and collecting system	A, C

Figure VIII–1. *Schematic summary of the major mechanisms for the renal tubular reabsorption of sodium and the relationship of these to the functional organization of the kidney.*

In the left panel the mechanisms of Na^+ uptake and extrusion are shown in simplified fashion as if all the mechanisms existed in a single hypothetical cell. In the right panel the regions of the nephron are shown (denoted numerically), as are the sites at which the various transport processes are localized. The right panel also shows the *countercurrent system*. The vertical axis depicts the isosmotic cortex and the hyperosmotic medulla. Region 3 is the site of cotransport of sodium and chloride, but it is impermeable to water. This generates interstitial hyperosmolarity. The osmolarity of this space is also influenced by passive processes in the thin descending limb (*X*) and thin ascending limb (*Y*) of the loop of Henle, as well as by active and passive processes in the collecting duct (lower part of region 5).

The active ATP-dependent extrusion of Na^+ is localized to the basolateral membrane. To avoid confusion, this diagram excludes the buffer reactions consequent to $Na^+ - H^+$ exchange, the movements of K^+, and the movements of anions at the basolateral membrane. Quantitatively, reabsorption of Na^+ in each region is approximately in the rank order $1 > 2 = 3 > 4 > 5$. It is unknown exactly to what extent this order fluctuates in disease states.

The principal natriuretic actions of the major classes of diuretics can be summarized according to the segmental site (numerical) and to the susceptible cellular mechanism (alphabetical): osmotic diuretics, 1-A, 2-A, 2-E, and 3-D; inhibitors of carbonic anhydrase, 1-C; high-ceiling diuretics, 3-D. Thiazides act on region 4, but the cellular mechanism is unknown.

or other organic anion. Sodium entry by *D* is not yet fully characterized with respect to the ratio of sodium and chloride ions, the possible involvement of potassium in the coupled mechanism, and the possibility of active transport of chloride (for general reviews, *see* Burg, 1981; Burg and Good, 1983).

These mechanisms for entry of sodium differ in the extent to which they are electrogenic (*i.e.*, capable of generating a current). For example, the movement of sodium ions *per se* (*A*) is electrogenic, as is also the cotransport of sodium with glucose (*B*). However, the cotransport of a sodium ion with a monovalent anion and the exchange of sodium ions for protons (*C*) are not electrogenic. With respect to the inward movement of sodium *per se*, it should be recalled that only a very small degree of charge separation can occur in physiological solutions. Thus, the electrogenic movement of sodium (*A*) results in secondary or compensatory flow of other ions, which maintains electroneutrality. This is primarily accomplished by the separate entry of the chloride anion into the cell. In this instance, sodium and chloride move in the same direction but by different mechanisms. This is to be distinguished from the cotransport of sodium and chloride (D), for which a single mechanism is involved.

A striking characteristic of the proximal tubule is the isosmotic nature of reabsorption. As much as 80% of the filtered solute is reabsorbed in this segment, and the permeability to water is so high that osmotically proportional amounts of water are reabsorbed at the same time. However, it has been possible to show that the tubular fluid does in fact become slightly hypoosmotic (Schafer, 1984). This important observation provides evidence for the sequence of events that has long been postulated—namely, active reabsorption of solute (principally sodium), decrease in total solute concentration in the tubular fluid, establishment of an osmotic gradient for the diffusion of water, passive reabsorption of water, and continued maintenance of tubular fluid osmolality at essentially isosmotic values.

As will be amplified later, most of the filtered bicarbonate is reabsorbed by Na^+-H^+ exchange very early in the proximal tubule (Figure VIII–1, 1–C). The cotransport of sodium with anions other than chloride also occurs in approximately the same segment (1–B). As a result of these two processes and because of the nature of isosmotic proximal tubular reabsorption, there is a marked increase in the concentration of chloride in the tubular fluid, while the concentration of sodium does not change. This results in an electrochemical gradient that is favorable for the passive reabsorption of chloride. Sodium is available to move secondarily in order to preserve electroneutrality. These ion movements, the paracellular pathway (E), occur in the late proximal tubule through the intercellular spaces (Burg and Good, 1983). In this instance sodium transport does not require active extrusion by the Na^+,K^+-ATPase. While the immediate steps in reabsorption by this mechanism are passive in nature, it should be appreciated that the favorable gradient for diffusion of chloride is generated by active transport mechanisms at upstream sites in the early proximal segment. The quantitative importance of this so-called passive reabsorption of sodium and chloride remains uncertain, particularly in relation to clinical conditions in which the overall rate of sodium chloride excretion may be abnormal. Osmotic diuretics such as mannitol dilute the concentrations of sodium and chloride in the tubular fluid, and some of their natriuretic action may be attributed to interference with such "passive" reabsorption.

In the thick ascending limb (region 3) the tubule is relatively impermeable to water, despite the active reabsorption of solute. This has two consequences. First, there is a fall in the concentration of sodium and chloride in the tubular fluid, reaching a minimal value usually in the first portion of the distal convolution; second, the concentrations of sodium and chloride become elevated in the interstitial fluid. A concentration gradient across the tubular epithelium is thus established by active transport at the site of low water permeability. This gradient then becomes multiplied in a longitudinal direction by the countercurrent mechanism, so that within the interstitial fluid a large osmotic gradient becomes established between the isosmotic renal cortex and the hyperosmotic medulla and papilla. The osmotic gradients are partly maintained by the relatively meager blood flow to the medullary region. The contribution of sodium reabsorption in the segments indicated as region 5 in Figure VIII–1 is probably less significant than the others in terms of the total amount of sodium reabsorbed, but is of unique importance in being associated with the area of the nephron susceptible to the antidiuretic hormone (ADH). In the presence of ADH, there is a high permeability to water in this segment. As a result, the tubular fluid, particularly within the collecting ducts, equilibrates with the hyperosmotic interstitium and is then discharged at the end of the collecting duct as a hypertonic or concentrated solution. In the absence of ADH, this portion of the nephron is relatively impermeable to water. Thus, the reabsorption of sodium chloride in regions 3, 4, and 5 progressively lowers the osmolality of the tubular fluid. Under this condition, the tubular fluid does not reach osmotic equilibration with the adjacent interstitium. As a result, in the absence of ADH, the voided urine is characteristically hypoosmotic, or dilute.

There are two other features that characterize distal sodium reabsorption. First, the absolute amount reabsorbed in this area is determined not only by the amount filtered but also by the proportion of the filtrate that has already undergone reabsorption at more proximal sites. This fraction may vary over a wide range, particularly in pathological conditions associated with edema formation or oliguria. Second, the distal mechanisms may have discrete sensitivities to the action of some drugs, including the adrenocortical hormones.

Free-Water Production. By definition, this term refers to the amount of solute-free water that would have to be added to, or subtracted from, the urine voided over a period of time (usually calculated on a minute basis) in order to render that urine specimen isosmotic with a simultaneous sample of plasma. In arithmetical terms, free-water production equals urine volume (V) minus the osmolal clearance (C_{OSM}). The latter term has the usual dimensions of clearance (UV/P) and refers to the sum of the concentrations of all osmotically active solutes in plasma and urine. When the urine is more dilute than plasma, free-water production is positive; when the urine is more concentrated, free-water production is negative. In the first instance, solute-free water is actually excreted as part of the voided urine; in the latter instance, solute-free water can be considered as being returned to the body from the kidney. When the urine has the same osmolality as plasma, free-water production is zero regardless of the rate of urine flow.

Free-water production is an operational concept. At no time, and in no place, does solute-free water exist as such within the kidney. The concept is important in that it takes into account more than just the concentration of osmotically active solute in the urine. By introducing the dimensions of volume per unit time, the net rate at which either the concentrating or diluting mechanism is operating may be accurately described. It should be emphasized that free-water production is *not* synonymous with diuresis. Some of the most efficacious diuretics may produce a massive diuresis of almost isosmotic urine, and hence with a minimal rate of free-water production.

The concept of free-water production has played an interesting role in localizing the site of diuretic action within the nephron. In order to infer intrarenal sites of action on the basis of the excretion of solute and water, observations must be made under one or the other of two physiological extremes—either in the absence of ADH or under its maximal influence. The former condition is obtained during unequivocal water diuresis or in patients with diabetes insipidus of posterior pituitary origin; the latter condition may be achieved by restriction of water, infusion of hypertonic solute, or administration of exogenous ADH.

Figure VIII–2 shows the pattern obtained with three different diuretics in the presence and absence of ADH; these can be evaluated in terms of Figure VIII–1. The interpretations that have been advanced are essentially as follows. If sodium reabsorption is inhibited in the proximal tubule (*i.e.,* regions 1 and 2), an increased amount of solute will be delivered to the more distal segments, including the ascending limb (region 3). With the greater load to this latter site, an increased amount of sodium will be reabsorbed along with chloride, leading to an increase in either the positive or negative free-water production in the absence or presence of ADH, respectively. This is the result obtained with *mannitol.* In addition, in the case of positive free-water production, some of the increase might also be attributed to augmented delivery and reabsorption of sodium in the most distal nephron (regions 4 and 5). A second pattern is illustrated by *ethacrynic acid,* a high-ceiling diuretic. If chloride and sodium reabsorption were to be inhibited predominantly in the ascending limb (region 3), the urine would tend to remain isosmotic. Despite the resultant diuresis, the production of both positive and negative free water would be impaired. A third possibility is illustrated with *chlorothiazide.* The findings have been interpreted in terms of the inhibition of sodium reabsorption at a distal site (region 4). Since the rate of negative free-water production (in the presence of ADH) is normal, it is inferred that there is no inhibition of transport in the ascending limb (region 3). However, since positive free-water production (in the absence of ADH) is partially inhibited, it has been proposed that the drug acts at some distal site of sodium reabsorption.

Although there is uncertainty about some of these interpretations, there can be no doubt

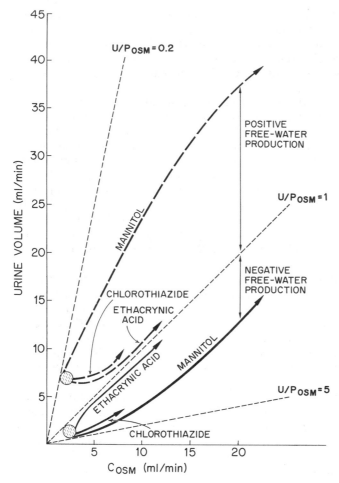

Figure VIII–2. *Relation of urine volume to osmolar clearance (C_{OSM}).*

The diuretic agents were given during a maximal water diuresis, that is, in the absence of ADH (dash lines), or to dehydrated subjects under maximal influence of ADH (solid lines). The magnitude of free-water production is given graphically as the vertical distance between any observed point and the isosmotic line ($U/P_{OSM} = 1$). The shaded circles indicate normal rates of solute excretion (*i.e.*, without diuretics) at extremes of ADH activity. Note that the maximal and minimal urinary osmolalities (as indicated by U/P_{OSM}) are achieved only at normal rates of solute excretion. These data from the literature were obtained in normal man.

that different diuretics act by distinct and separate mechanisms as judged by free-water production. Of course, the demonstration of an action at one site does not invariably exclude an action elsewhere. By these criteria, osmotic diuretics and acetazolamide act proximally (regions 1 and 2), high-ceiling diuretics act on the ascending limb (region 3), and chlorothiazide acts on the distal segment (region 4). These localizations of action are in general agreement with those obtained with a variety of micropuncture technics.

Hydrogen Ion Secretion. It has long been known that the kidney plays an important role in maintaining acid-base balance. This applies to normal conditions but increases in importance as a homeostatic compensation to metabolic acidosis. The renal response to this condition can be described in four separate parameters, as follows: (1) the complete reabsorption of filtered sodium bicarbonate, (2) the acidification of the urinary buffers (*i.e.*, the production of titratable acid), (3) the excretion of fixed anions in combination with NH_4^+ rather than Na^+, and (4) the adjustment of urinary pH or H^+ ion concentration. Each process can be considered in terms of the same underlying mechanism, H^+ secretion. The source of the secreted protons is carbonic acid derived from the intracellular hydration of carbon dioxide.

In normal circumstances most of bicarbonate reabsorption occurs early in the proximal tubule. In this process H^+ is secreted into the tubular fluid while Na^+ is simultaneously reabsorbed, largely if not entirely by the Na^+-H^+ exchange mechanism (*see* Aronson,

1983). The Na^+ combines with the HCO_3^- in the tubular cell and is returned to the extracellular fluid as $Na^+HCO_3^-$. The H^+ in the tubular urine combines with HCO_3^- to form H_2CO_3, which is rapidly broken down to CO_2 and H_2O. This CO_2 then readily back-diffuses across the tubular epithelium to become admixed with the carbonic acid–bicarbonate pool of the body. The overall reaction is the reabsorption of Na^+ and HCO_3^-.

When all the bicarbonate in the tubular urine has been removed, H^+ will be added to the buffer systems in the urine, primarily phosphate, with the conversion of HPO_4^{2-} to $H_2PO_4^-$. The reabsorbed Na^+ will be returned to the extracellular fluid as $Na^+HCO_3^-$ and thus contribute to the available fixed cation of the extracellular fluid. If secretion of H^+ proceeds at a rate insufficient to reabsorb the filtered bicarbonate, an alkaline urine containing large amounts of bicarbonate will be excreted. On the other hand, at maximal rates of H^+ transport, not only will all the bicarbonate disappear from the urine but also the titratable acidity of the urine will rise as a result of protonation of the buffer systems and more $Na^+HCO_3^-$ will be returned to extracellular fluid than was filtered at the glomerulus.

If bicarbonate and phosphate buffers were not present in the tubular urine, secretion of H^+ would increase the hydrogen ion concentration of the urine to such an extent that further transport of H^+ would be blocked because of the concentration gradient of H^+ thereby established between tubular cell and tubular urine. (The minimal pH that can be achieved in the urine of man is 4.4 to 4.5.) However, in response to the need for conservation of fixed cation, the kidney synthesizes ammonia. When ammonia is formed in the renal tubular cells, it diffuses readily into the tubular urine. If the urine is acidic, the ammonia that diffuses immediately reacts with H^+ to form NH_4^+. The renal tubule is impermeable to the charged particle (NH_4^+), and hence it does not diffuse back out of the tubular fluid. There are two important consequences of this reaction: first, H^+ is removed, and this permits further secretion of H^+ to occur; second, NH_3 is removed, and this permits more NH_3 to diffuse from tubular cell to tubular urine. In short, the two processes occur concurrently and can continue only by aiding and abetting each other. By this sequence of events, large amounts of Na^+ can be retrieved from neutral salts and returned to the extracellular fluid as sodium bicarbonate.

The above discussion is of pharmacological significance because the rate of H^+ secretion in the renal tubule can be greatly decreased by drugs that inhibit carbonic anhydrase. This enzyme catalyzes both the hydration of CO_2 and dehydration of H_2CO_3 and thus determines the relative concentrations of these molecular species. This, in turn, is an important determinant of both the availability of hydrogen ion for secretion and the disposition of the hydrogen ion within the tubular fluid (*see* Warnock and Rector, 1981).

Potassium Reabsorption and Secretion. Potassium is an unusual fixed cation in that it undergoes both tubular reabsorption and secretion. Reabsorption occurs largely in the proximal tubule, secretion in the distal tubule. Since the major fraction of the filtered potassium is reabsorbed, and since this process is relatively inflexible, it follows, therefore, that variations in the amount of potassium actually excreted may be attributed to the distal secretory mechanism (region 5 of Figure VIII–1). As judged by the action of many diuretic agents, the volume of unreabsorbed glomerular filtrate that flows through the distal tubule is one of the determinants of the rate of secretion of potassium. Thus, some drugs have the dual effect of increasing the urinary excretion of both sodium and potassium, the former by inhibition of reabsorption and the latter by augmentation of secretion (*see* Giebisch *et al.*, 1981).

Reabsorption of Calcium. In general, the reabsorption of calcium resembles that of sodium in the various segments of the nephron. Indeed, in short-term experiments in which sodium excretion is manipulated, calcium excretion follows in a closely parallel manner. However, reabsorption of calcium and sodium can be dissociated to meet the separate needs to regulate the concentration of each ion. For example, parathyroid hormone enhances calcium reabsorption relative to that of sodium. This enhancement occurs in the distal tubule and the immediately succeeding segment. The thiazide diuretics decrease sodium reabsorption in the distal tubule (region 4) while they simultaneously increase calcium reabsorption (Edwards *et al.*, 1973). This action appears to be independent of parathyroid hormone.

Tubular Transport of Organic Compounds.   In the preceding discussion the number of different chemical compounds (*i.e.*, inorganic electrolytes) that were considered is small compared to the total number of organic compounds that are present in the plasma and therefore are candidates for renal tubular transport.

In general, endogenous substances such as glucose, amino acids, and other essentials are filtered and then reabsorbed. They do not appear in the voided urine unless presented to the tubules in unusually large amounts so that transport capacity is exceeded. While reabsorption of such compounds occurs by highly specific mechanisms that can be affected experimentally by a variety of agents, these compounds have no application in therapeutics. Indeed, drug-induced glucosuria or aminoaciduria is a manifestation of nephrotoxicity.

Two major mechanisms for secretion of organic compounds have been identified—one for organic acids, the other for organic bases; both are localized in the proximal tubule. In general, substances that affect one system do not affect the other. Whereas the processes of filtration and secretion increase the amount of a substance presented to the tubular fluid, the amount ultimately excreted depends on the degree of reabsorption. This may occur both in the proximal tubule and in more distal segments.

In order to encompass all the foreign organic compounds that have been studied, it is essential to consider two separate mechanisms for their reabsorption. The first, diffusion, proceeds at a rate that is primarily dependent on the lipid solubility of the compound in question. If the molecule is an acid or a base, the pK_a of the compound and the pH of the tubular fluid are also important, since the nonionized form may be far better able to permeate the tubular epithelium. The rate of formation of urine (time available for reabsorption) is another important variable. These factors are fully discussed in Chapter 1. A carrier-mediated mechanism of *reabsorption* has been clearly shown for a few foreign compounds; this is usually difficult to demonstrate because of the quantitatively more important role of diffusion. In fact, little distinction need be made between endogenous and exogenous organic solutes with respect to carrier-mediated reabsorption and secretion. For example, uric acid, an endogenous product of metabolism, is both secreted and reabsorbed by the same carrier-mediated mechanisms as are many organic acids. The complications that arise from the effects of a drug on one or both components of a bidirectional transport system are discussed in Chapter 38.

Aronson, P. S. Mechanisms of active H^+ secretion in the proximal tubule. *Am. J. Physiol.*, **1983**, *14*, F647–F659.

Burg, M. B. Renal handling of sodium, chloride, water, amino acids, and glucose. In, *The Kidney*, 2nd ed., Vol. 1. (Brenner, B. M., and Rector, F. C., Jr., eds.) W. B. Saunders Co., Philadelphia, **1981**, pp. 328–370.

Burg, M., and Good, D. Sodium chloride coupled transport in mammalian nephrons. *Annu. Rev. Physiol.*, **1983**, *45*, 533–547.

Edwards, B. R.; Baer, P. G.; Sutton, R. A. L.; and Dirks, J. H. Micropuncture study of diuretic effects on sodium and calcium reabsorption in the dog nephron. *J. Clin. Invest.*, **1973**, *52*, 2418–2427.

Giebisch, G.; Malnic, G.; and Berliner, R. W. Renal transport and control of potassium excretion. In, *The Kidney*, 2nd ed., Vol. 1. (Brenner, B. M., and Rector, F. C., Jr., eds.) W. B. Saunders Co., Philadelphia, **1981**, pp. 408–439.

Schafer, J. A. Mechanisms coupling the absorption of solutes and water in the proximal nephron. *Kidney Int.*, **1984**, *25*, 708–716.

Warnock, D. G., and Rector, F. C., Jr. Renal acidification mechanisms. In, *The Kidney*, 2nd ed., Vol. 1. (Brenner, B. M., and Rector, F. C., Jr., eds.) W. B. Saunders Co., Philadelphia, **1981**, pp. 440–494.

36 DIURETICS AND OTHER AGENTS EMPLOYED IN THE MOBILIZATION OF EDEMA FLUID

Irwin M. Weiner and Gilbert H. Mudge

Diuretics are agents that increase the rate of urine formation. By common usage the term *diuresis* has two separate connotations: one refers to the increase in urine volume *per se*, the other to the net loss of solute and water. Under some conditions, the maintenance of an adequate urine volume in itself justifies the use of diuretic agents. However, by far the most important indication is the mobilization of edema fluid, that is, the production of a negative fluid balance such that extracellular volume is returned toward normal. The use of some of these agents in the therapy of hypertension is discussed in Chapter 32.

Localization of Site of Drug Action. Most diuretics act directly on the kidney and, with few exceptions, on tubular rather than glomerular function. There are a number of factors that complicate the analysis of tubular localization of drug action. First, a drug may act on separate transport mechanisms at different sites. Second, there may be important species differences, most marked in the case of uricosuric agents but also observed with some diuretics. Third, although popularly simplified in terms of a single schematic nephron, the operation of the kidney is actually accomplished by millions of individual units that may respond differently both to physiological stress and to the action of diuretics. Fourth, modern concepts of renal function emphasize the architectural integrity of the nephron as an entire unit. This applies to many discrete functions, including solute reabsorption, the operation of the countercurrent system, and the determinants of bidirectional transport, that is, secretion in one segment and reabsorption in another. In the case of the countercurrent mechanism, for example, the magnitude of water reabsorption from the collecting duct is determined primarily by solute reabsorption in the ascending limb. And, fifth, particularly in the case of the quantitative interpretation of sodium and water reabsorption, a drug action at one site may be accompanied by secondary and compensatory changes in transport at another segment. These secondary effects may be mediated by normal mechanisms, rather than by drug action at both sites. The compensatory changes may obscure the primary action. It has long been recognized that changes in solute reab-

sorption in one segment may influence tubular function at more distal sites that are "downstream." However, there is increasing evidence that the reverse may also be true. Distal events may influence more proximal transport. The mechanisms are both intrarenal and extrarenal in nature. Since sodium, the major solute of the tubular fluid, is reabsorbed throughout most portions of the nephron, it is quite possible that many drugs that inhibit its reabsorption act at more than a single site. The apparent localization of drug action to a particular locus may in large part be determined by experimental conditions, as well as by quantitative differences between the actions of the diuretic agent at different sites (*see* Reineck and Stein, 1981). Despite the above complexities, it is now possible to identify the sites in the nephron at which the major classes of diuretics have their principal actions (*see* Introduction to Section VIII).

Extrarenal Sites of Drug Action. Many of the newer diuretics have proven to be useful in the investigation of electrolyte transport in organs other than the kidney, particularly under *in-vitro* conditions. Not surprisingly, these studies have revealed fundamental mechanisms common to many tissues. However, these are not reviewed systematically in this chapter unless the action at the extrarenal site occurs with reasonable dosages and is of sufficient magnitude to be clinically important.

OSMOTIC DIURETICS

The term *osmotic diuretic* is used for certain solutes that have the following attributes in common: (1) they are freely filterable at the glomerulus; (2) they undergo limited reabsorption by the renal tubule; (3) they are pharmacologically inert by conventional criteria; and (4) they are usually resistant to metabolic alteration. These characteristics permit the administration of such agents in sufficiently large quantities to contribute significantly to the osmolality of the plasma, the glomerular filtrate, and the tubular fluid.

Mechanism of Diuretic Action. Sodium salts are the major solutes in proximal tubular fluid. During their reabsorption water diffuses passively, such that the concentration of sodium in tubular fluid remains essentially constant (*see* Introduction to Section VIII). However, in the presence of non-reabsorbable solute, the diffusion of water is reduced relative to that of sodium. As a consequence, the concentration of sodium (and chloride) decreases to less than that of the extracellular fluid. The net reabsorption of sodium diminishes because of two factors: the concentration of sodium in the tubular fluid becomes abnormally low, and the rate of entry of this ion into the tubular cell diminishes; in addition, there is an increased flux of sodium from the peritubular fluid back into the lumen as a result of the abnormal concentration gradient that becomes established in that direction (Gennari and Kassirer, 1974). These factors reduce the net reabsorption of sodium salts, probably throughout the nephron. The segments that are quantitatively the most important are the proximal tubule and the thick ascending limb. The overall consequence is an enhanced rate of urine flow associated with a relatively smaller increment in the excretion of sodium salts. It is the increase in urine flow that is the primary basis of therapeutic efficacy.

The same general considerations apply to all osmotic diuretics, even though they may be handled slightly differently by the renal tubule. Mannitol undergoes very little reabsorption. About 50% of the urea filtered at the glomerulus is not reabsorbed. This fraction tends to increase with elevated loads of urea. In severe hyperglycemia the mechanism for reabsorption of glucose becomes saturated and the unreabsorbed portion acts as an osmotic diuretic. Urographic and angiographic radiocontrast agents have all the attributes of osmotic diuretics described above. The renal tubule is impermeable to the iodinated organic moiety that provides radioopacity. With most radiological procedures, the induced diuresis is abrupt and short lived and has relatively little impact on fluid and electrolyte balance.

When the rate of glomerular filtration is acutely reduced (*e.g.*, in hypotension, hypovolemic shock, dehydration, or trauma) the solutes of the glomerular filtrate undergo more complete reabsorption so that there is a disproportionately large fall in the rate of urine flow and solute excretion. The administration of a normal solute, such as sodium chloride, may restore renal excretory function, but only if there is improvement in renal hemodynamics. If the rate of glomerular filtration remains severely reduced, administration of sodium chloride fails to augment urine flow because of its virtually complete tubular reabsorption. Under these conditions, diuretics that normally act by directly inhibiting tubular transport may also be ineffective because they do not reduce tubular reabsorptive capacity sufficiently to compensate for the diminished filtered load.

However, under the same conditions, the osmotic diuretics usually retain their efficacy. To take mannitol as an example— even though the filtration rate is reduced, mannitol is still filtered at the glomerulus. The tubular impermeability to mannitol is not altered by acute renal ischemia of short duration. Hence, the mannitol that is filtered is also excreted in the voided urine. Unreabsorbed solute limits the back diffusion of water. As a consequence, urine volume can be maintained even in the presence of decreased glomerular function. As a first approximation, urine volume is proportional to the rate of solute excretion, which under these circumstances may be composed largely of the administered osmotic diuretic. Nephrotoxic agents and prolonged, severe renal ischemia may damage the tubular epithelium and produce acute tubular necrosis with oliguria. The tubule is then no longer selectively impermeable, and osmotic diuretics become ineffective.

The intestinal and renal tubular epithelia have many permeability characteristics in common. Most osmotic diuretics, which, by definition, are poorly reabsorbed by the renal tubules, are also not absorbed from the gastrointestinal tract. Thus, these agents must be administered parenterally in order to achieve effective concentrations in plasma. While urea is absorbed from the intestine, it is not given by this route. Glycerin and isosorbide are effective when administered orally. However, the onset of their action is slower and the extent of diuresis is less. These agents are particularly used to elevate the osmolality of plasma and thereby to decrease intraocular pressure, since they penetrate the eye poorly.

Therapeutic Uses. *Mannitol* is the agent most extensively employed. Perhaps one of the clearest and most important indications is the *prophylaxis of acute renal failure* in conditions as diverse as cardiovascular operations, severe traumatic injury, operations in the presence of severe jaundice, and management of hemolytic transfusion reactions. In each of these conditions, a precipitous fall in the flow of urine may be anticipated either as the result of an acutely reduced filtration rate or from acute changes in tubular permeability. The latter may be the consequence of the presence of a noxious agent within the tubular fluid in excessively high concentrations. In these situations, mannitol exerts an osmotic effect within the tubular fluid, inhibits water reabsorption, and maintains the rate of urine flow. As a consequence, the concentration of the toxic agent within the tubular fluid does not reach the excessively high levels that otherwise would have been achieved by the more complete reabsorption of water. The early use of osmotic diuretics protects the kidney against damage. The maintenance of an adequate flow of relatively dilute urine is probably the single most important factor. In the presence of hypotension mannitol is more effective than saline solution in maintaining glomerular filtration. If given in sufficiently large amounts, mannitol increases extracellular osmolality, which results in a shift of water from the intracellular to the extracellular compartment.

Mannitol is also used for the *reduction of the pressure and volume of the cerebrospinal fluid.* By elevating the osmolality of the plasma, one is able to enhance the diffusion of water from this fluid back into the plasma. However, the degree of success is quite variable (*see* Prockop, 1976). Mannitol, glycerin, and isosorbide are also used for the short-term reduction of intraocular pressure, particularly preoperatively and postoperatively in patients who require ocular surgery. They are also useful in certain other ophthalmological procedures.

Toxicity. Mannitol is distributed in the extracellular fluid, and consequently, the acute administration of hypertonic solutions in amounts sufficient to make a significant contribution to extracellular osmolarity will inevitably be accompanied by an acute expansion of extracellular fluid volume. In the patient with cardiac decompensation, this represents an undesirable hazard. A variety of signs and symptoms suggestive of hypersensitivity reactions has occurred in occasional patients. Urea is more irritating to tissues and may cause thrombosis or pain if extravasation occurs. Glycerin is metabolized and can cause hy-

perglycemia and glycosuria. Headache, nausea, and vomiting are relatively common sequelae of the administration of any osmotic diuretic.

Preparations and Dosage. *Mannitol* (OSMITROL) is available for intravenous administration in concentrations of 5 to 25% in volumes ranging from 50 to 1000 ml of water. The adult dose for promotion of diuresis ranges from 50 to 200 g over a 24-hour period of infusion; the rate is generally adjusted to maintain a urinary output of at least 30 to 50 ml per hour. It should be preceded by a test dose in patients with marked oliguria or questionable adequacy of renal function. Plasma volume should also be assessed by determination of central venous or pulmonary arterial pressure, since correction of plasma volume should precede or accompany the use of these agents for oliguria. The recommended test dose is 200 mg/kg, infused over 3 to 5 minutes; if the first or a second test dose fails to promote a urinary flow greater than 30 ml per hour for 2 to 3 hours, the patient's status should be reevaluated prior to continuation of therapy. When used for the prevention of acute renal failure during various types of surgery or for the treatment of oliguria, the total dose is 50 to 100 g of mannitol for an adult patient. The dose for the reduction of intracranial pressure and brain mass prior to or after neurosurgery, or for the reduction of intraocular tension during an acute attack of congestive glaucoma or for ophthalmic surgery, is 1.5 to 2 g/kg, given as a 15 or 20% solution over a period of 30 to 60 minutes. Contraindications to the administration of mannitol include renal disease of sufficient severity to produce anuria, marked pulmonary congestion or edema, marked dehydration, and intracranial hemorrhage unless craniotomy is to be performed. The infusion of mannitol should be terminated if the patient develops signs of progressive renal dysfunction, heart failure, or pulmonary congestion.

Urea is a white crystalline powder, with a slightly bitter taste, freely soluble in water. A sterile preparation (UREAPHIL) is available that may be reconstituted for intravenous use. When administered in this manner, the solution may contain up to 30% urea and an isosmotic concentration of dextrose or invert sugar (equal parts of dextrose and levulose), the latter substances being necessary to prevent the hemolysis produced by pure solutions of urea. Intravenous doses of 1 to 1.5 g of urea per kilogram of body weight are optimal in preparation for neurosurgical procedures.

Glycerin (GLYROL, OSMOGLYN) is given orally, particularly for use prior to ophthalmological procedures. Since the agent is rapidly metabolized, it produces relatively little diuresis. The dose for adults is 1 to 1.5 g/kg, and it is given as a 50 or 75% solution. The total daily dose should not exceed 120 g. Maximal reduction of intraocular pressure occurs 1 hour after its administration, and the effect disappears after 5 hours.

Isosorbide (ISMOTIC) is also used orally for ophthalmological purposes. The effects observed are generally similar to those of glycerin, although diuresis is greater and hyperglycemia does not occur. Dosage may range from 1 to 3 g/kg and may be given two to four times daily.

INHIBITORS OF CARBONIC ANHYDRASE

Acetazolamide is the prototype of a class of agents that have had limited usefulness as diuretics but have played a major role in the development of fundamental renal physiology and pharmacology.

History. In the early 1930s, Roughton discovered the enzyme carbonic anhydrase in erythrocytes. The activity has subsequently been found in many sites—including the renal cortex, gastric mucosa, pancreas, eye, and central nervous system (CNS). When sulfanilamide was introduced as a chemotherapeutic agent, metabolic acidosis was recognized as a side effect. The drug was found to inhibit carbonic anhydrase *in vitro* and to inhibit the normal acidification of the urine *in vivo*. Subsequent studies with more potent inhibitors established the role of carbonic anhydrase in renal transport (Maren, 1967).

Chemistry and Structure-Activity Relationship. Among the enormous number of sulfonamides that have been synthesized and tested, acetazolamide has been studied the most extensively as an inhibitor of carbonic anhydrase. The other drugs of this class that are available in the United States are dichlorphenamide and methazolamide. Their structural formulas are as follows:

Acetazolamide

Dichlorphenamide

Methazolamide

The most striking structure-activity relationship is that carbonic anhydrase inhibitory activity is abolished by N-sulfamyl substitutions (Maren, 1976).

Mechanism of Action. Acetazolamide is a potent, reversible inhibitor of carbonic anhydrase. The concentration of the drug required for 50% inhibition of the enzyme from the renal cortex is about 10 nM. The enzyme catalyzes the hydration of carbon dioxide and the dehydration of carbonic acid (reactions 1 and 2, respectively):

$$H_2O + CO_2 \underset{2}{\overset{1}{\rightleftharpoons}} H_2CO_3 \rightleftharpoons HCO_3^- + H^+$$

These reactions can occur, of course, in the absence of the enzyme, but the rates are too slow to allow normal physiological function. In general, the enzyme is normally present in tissues in huge excess. More than 99% of enzyme activity in the kidney must be inhibited before physiological effects become apparent. The enzyme itself is the dominant tissue component to which the inhibitors become bound.

Action on the Kidney. Following the administration of acetazolamide, the urine volume promptly increases. The normally acidic pH becomes alkaline. The urinary concentration of the bicarbonate anion increases and is matched by sodium and substantial amounts of potassium. (*See* Table 36–1.) The urinary concentration of chloride falls. The increased alkalinity of the urine is necessarily accompanied by a decrease in the excretion of titratable acid and of ammonia.

The above sequence of events may be attributed to the inhibition of H^+ secretion by the renal tubule. This inhibition is indirect and, in the proximal tubule, is the consequence of inhibition of cytoplasmic carbonic anhydrase, which decreases the availability of protons for Na^+-H^+ exchange. In addition, carbonic anhydrase bound to the brush-border membrane is also inhibited. This slows the dehydration of carbonic acid in the lumen and, thereby, the diffusion of CO_2 into the tubular cell. The overall effect is that bicarbonate reabsorption in the proximal tubule is reduced by some 80% (Lucci *et al.*, 1983). More than half of this rejected bicarbonate is reabsorbed in later segments

Table 36–1. URINARY ELECTROLYTE COMPOSITION DURING DIURESIS *

	VOLUME (ml/min)	pH	Na^+	K^+	Cl^-	HCO_3^-
				(mEq/l)		
Control	1	6	50	15	60	1
Mannitol	10	6.5	90	15	110	4
Mercurial	7	6	150	8	160	1
Acetazolamide	3	8.2	70	60	15	120
Benzothiadiazides (thiazides)	3	7.4	150	25	150	25
High-ceiling diuretics	8	6	140	10	155	1
Potassium-sparing diuretics	2	7.2	130	5	110	15
Aminophylline	3	6	150	15	160	1

* Data are representative of results that would be observed in man or dog during normal hydration and acid-base balance. Such findings are readily reproducible during the peak of diuresis and following a single maximally effective dose. However, a significant range of urinary values may be anticipated; *a single value is given here solely to facilitate comparison of one drug with another*. Excretion rates are obtainable as the product of urinary volume and composition.

of the nephron by mechanisms that do not involve carbonic anhydrase and that are not yet fully characterized. Acetazolamide also inhibits H^+ secretion by some segments of the distal nephron. These distal mechanisms, which have a lower capacity than do those in the proximal tubule, apparently depend on the cytoplasmic form of carbonic anhydrase but not on the membrane-bound form of the enzyme (Warnock and Rector, 1981).

Effect on Plasma Composition. Acetazolamide increases the urinary excretion of bicarbonate and fixed cation, mostly sodium. As a result, the concentration of bicarbonate in the extracellular fluid decreases and metabolic acidosis results. In metabolic acidosis, the renal response to acetazolamide is greatly reduced; conversely, it is enhanced with metabolic alkalosis. Factors other than the amount of filtered bicarbonate must be determinants of drug action since the extracellular alkalosis of potassium depletion (with presumed intracellular acidosis) decreases the diuretic response.

Acetazolamide produces a marked increase in potassium excretion, attributable to enhanced secretion in the distal nephron. The effects on potassium are most prominent in acute experiments.

Eye. The presence of carbonic anhydrase in a number of intraocular structures, including the ciliary processes, and the high concentration of bicarbonate in the aqueous humor have focused attention on the role that the enzyme might play in the secretion of aqueous humor. Acetazolamide reduces the rate of aqueous humor formation; intraocular pressure in patients with glaucoma is correspondingly reduced. This action of the drug appears to be independent of systemic acid-base balance (*see* review by Maren, 1967).

Gastrointestinal Tract. Under appropriate experimental conditions, it is possible to implicate carbonic anhydrase in the formation of gastric and pancreatic juice and to block secretion by enzyme inhibition. These processes are relatively insensitive to ordinary doses of carbonic anhydrase inhibitors, and their pharmacological effect has no therapeutic applications.

Central Nervous System. An action of acetazolamide on the CNS was first suggested by the frequency of paresthesias and somnolence as side effects. Subsequently, the drug was found to inhibit epileptic seizures and to decrease the rate of formation of spinal fluid. Metabolic acidosis from ketogenic diets diminishes epileptic seizures, and acetazolamide, by virtue of its action on the kidney, leads to the production of a systemic acidosis. However, there is undoubtedly a more direct action on CNS function. An increase in local CO_2 tension may result from inhibition of the enzyme in the brain, the choroid plexus, or the erythrocytes of the cerebral blood. The exact role of carbonic anhydrase in brain function remains unknown. The concentration of the enzyme varies from one site to another within the brain. Acetazolamide may reduce the rate of cerebrospinal fluid formation by the choroid plexus, but it may also transiently elevate cerebrospinal fluid pressure as a result of an increase in intracranial blood flow (Maren, 1967; Laux and Raichle, 1978).

Respiration. The dynamic state of CO_2 in the blood and its transport between the blood and both the alveoli and the peripheral tissues are related to the carbonic anhydrase activity of the circulating erythrocytes. Acetazolamide may create a disequilibrium in the CO_2 transport system, giving rise to increased CO_2 tensions in the tissues and a decreased tension in the expired gas. A decrease in the rate of elimination of CO_2 may therefore result from acetazolamide administration, but this appears to be transient due to compensatory mechanisms.

Absorption, Fate, and Excretion. Acetazolamide is readily absorbed from the gastrointestinal tract. Peak concentrations in plasma occur within 2 hours. The drug is excreted by the kidney, and both active tubular secretion and passive reabsorption are involved. Excretion is complete within 24 hours. Acetazolamide is tightly bound to carbonic anhydrase and, consequently, is present in greater amounts in those tissues in which the enzyme is present in high concentration, particularly the erythrocytes and the renal cortex. Some carbonic anhydrase inhibitors do not penetrate the erythrocyte. Thus, renal and systemic drug actions may be dissociated on the basis of drug distribution (*see* Maren, 1967). Acetazolamide is not metabolized.

Preparations and Dosage. *Acetazolamide* (DIAMOX) is available as 125- or 250-mg tablets and as sustained-release capsules containing 500 mg. An effective single oral dose is 250 to 500 mg. Vials of *acetazolamide sodium* are available for parenteral administration. When used as a diuretic, it should be given once daily or every other day. To achieve a sustained metabolic acidosis, the drug should be given at intervals of 8 hours. Doses of 250 to 1000 mg per day (divided for amounts over 250 mg) are utilized for treatment of chronic simple glaucoma. *Dichlorphenamide* (DARANIDE) is available as 50-mg tablets. Optimal effects have been achieved with doses of 200 mg per day. *Methazolamide* (NEPTAZANE) is available as 50-mg tablets; the usual dose is 100 to 300 mg per day.

Clinical Toxicity. Serious toxic reactions are infrequent. With large doses, many patients exhibit drowsiness and paresthesias. In hepatic cirrhosis, episodes of disorientation may be induced; it has been postulated that urinary alkalinization diverts ammonia of renal origin from the urine into the systemic circulation. Hypersensitivity reactions are relatively rare. They consist in fever, skin reactions, bone-marrow depression, and sulfonamide-like renal lesions. Calculus formation and ureteral colic have been attributed to the marked reduction in urinary citrate produced by acetazolamide associated with either no change or even a rise in urinary calcium. Acetazolamide depresses the uptake of iodine by the thyroid gland. However, drugs of this class are not therapeutically useful as antithyroid agents. Teratogenic effects have been demonstrated in animals, and it is recommended that these drugs not be administered during pregnancy. Since carbonic anhydrase inhibitors alkalinize the urine, they interfere with the action of methenamine as a urinary tract antiseptic. Drug-induced osteomalacia has been reported in conjunction with the use of phenytoin.

Therapeutic Uses. Inhibitors of carbonic anhydrase are not used frequently as therapeutic agents. Their most common application is to reduce intraocular pressure (in the treatment of glaucoma); their value in the management of absence seizures is limited by the rapid development of tolerance. Acetazolamide is rarely administered as a diuretic but may be useful for alkalinization of the urine. The clinical situations in which such alkalinization is appropriate are discussed in Chapter 35. Acetazolamide appears to have a beneficial effect in the management of *periodic paralysis* even when associated with hypokalemia (Griggs *et al.*, 1970). It has been postulated that the induced acidosis raises the extracellular potassium concentration locally in the microcirculation of muscle. Acetazolamide is also effective in ameliorating the symptoms of *acute mountain sickness* (Larson *et al.*, 1982).

BENZOTHIADIAZIDES AND RELATED AGENTS

History. This class of diuretics has an interesting history and provides an instructive example of the manner in which newly synthesized agents may be endowed with unanticipated efficacious properties. They were synthesized as an outgrowth of studies on inhibitors of carbonic anhydrase. In the examination of certain benzenedisulfonamides, ring closure was found to occur between an acylamino group and the sulfamyl group *ortho* to it. This changed fundamental characteristics of the diuresis. The voided urine contained increased amounts of chloride, a response significantly different from that evoked by the parent compounds (*see* Beyer, 1958). Subsequent studies indicated that the benzothiadiazides have a direct effect on the renal tubular transport of sodium and chloride that is independent of any effect on carbonic anhydrase.

Chlorothiazide provided the first serious challenge to the *mercurial diuretics*, a class of organometallic compounds that dominated therapy in this area for over 30 years. The pharmacology of the mercurials, which are now obsolete, is presented in *earlier editions* of this textbook.

Chemistry and Structure-Activity Relationship. Most compounds of this group are analogs of 1,2,4-benzothiadiazine-1,1-dioxide (*see* Table 36–2 for the parent structural formula and the substituents of the analogs that have received the most intensive study). As a group they can be designated as the "benzothiadiazide," or "thiazide," diuretics. The relationship between structure and activity is complex and is influenced by physiological and pharmacokinetic factors. The problem has been re-

viewed by Beyer and Baer (1961). Some compounds have hyperglycemic activity, for which the structural requirements differ from those for diuresis (Wales *et al.*, 1968).

It should be emphasized that all thiazides thus far carefully examined have parallel dose-response curves and comparable maximal chloruretic effects. This implies that they have a similar mechanism of action. The various analogs differ primarily in the dose required to produce a given effect and not necessarily in their optimal therapeutic response.

There are some other sulfonamide diuretics that differ chemically from the thiazides by the nature of the heterocyclic ring. However, their pharmacological action is indistinguishable from that of the thiazides. They have the following structures:

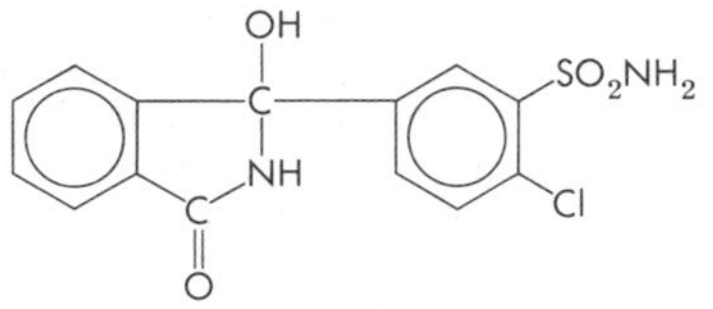

Chlorthalidone

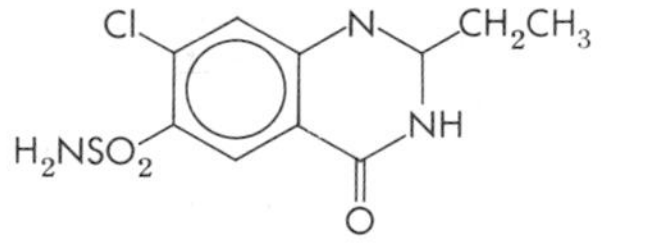

Quinethazone

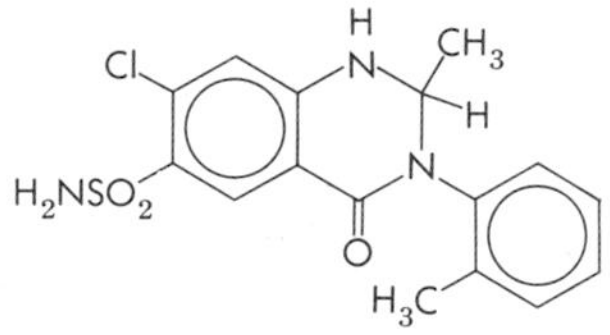

Metolazone

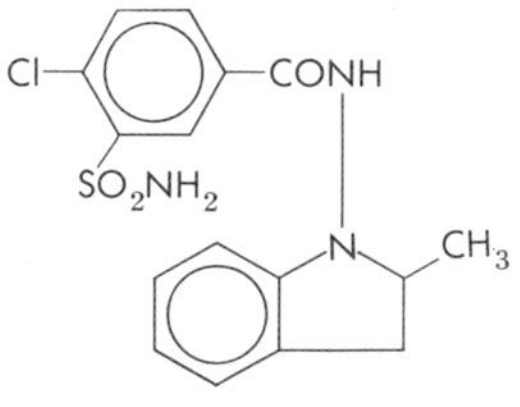

Indapamide

Mechanism of Renal Action. Thiazides act directly on the kidney to increase the excretion of sodium chloride and an accompanying volume of water; they also increase excretion of potassium. The thiazides vary widely in their potency as carbonic anhydrase inhibitors. Those that are active in this respect may, at sufficient dosage, have the same effect on bicarbon-

Table 36–2. SUMMARY OF CHEMICAL STRUCTURES AND DIURETIC PROPERTIES OF THE BENZOTHIADIAZIDES AND RELATED AGENTS *

Agent †	R_2	R_3	R_6	RANGE OF OPTIMALLY EFFECTIVE ORAL DIURETIC DOSE IN MAN (mg/day)	RELATIVE ORAL NATRIURETIC MAXIMAL RESPONSE IN MAN	EQUIEFFECTIVE CHLORURETIC I.V. DOSE IN THE DOG (mg/kg)	CARBONIC ANHYDRASE 50% INHIBITION IN VITRO (M)	DURATION OF ACTION (Hours)
Chlorothiazide ‡	H	H	Cl	500–2000	1	1.25	2×10^{-6}	6–12
Hydrochlorothiazide	H	H	Cl	25–100	1.8	0.05	2×10^{-5}	6–12
Hydroflumethiazide	H	H	CF_3	25–200	1.6	0.25	2×10^{-4}	6–12
Bendroflumethiazide	H	CH_2—(phenyl)	CF_3	2.5–15	2.3	0.01	3×10^{-4}	6–12
Benzthiazide ‡	H	CH_2—S—CH_2—(phenyl)	Cl	50–200	1.6	0.01–0.05	$ca.\ 10^{-7}$	6–12
Trichlormethiazide	H	$CHCl_2$	Cl	1–4	2.1	0.01	6×10^{-5}	24
Methyclothiazide	CH_3	CH_2Cl	Cl	2.5–10	2.3			24
Polythiazide	CH_3	$CH_2SCH_2CF_3$	Cl	1–4	2.5	0.01–0.03	5×10^{-7}	24–48
Cyclothiazide	H	(norbornenyl-CH_2)	Cl	1–2	—			18–24
Chlorthalidone	—	—	—	25–200	2.3	0.25	3×10^{-7}	24–72
Quinethazone	—	—	—	50–200	1			18–24
Metolazone	—	—	—	2.5–20	1	0.1	5×10^{-5}	12–24
Acetazolamide	—	—	—	250–375	0.3		7×10^{-8}	
Indapamide	—	—	—	2.5–5	1	0.3		24–36

* Note the general agreement between the optimal oral dosage for man relative to the equieffective dosage by intravenous administration in the dog. The relative oral natriuretic response in man is based on the method of Ford (1961), who used careful metabolic regimens and doses in the general range indicated. The numerical values refer to potency ratios, with the natriuretic response to a standard dose of chlorothiazide being given the value of 1. Despite the extremely wide range of effective oral dosage, the usual natriuretic response by this assay varies less than threefold.

† The above-listed agents are available under the following nonproprietary and selected trade names: Chlorothiazide: DIURIL. Hydrochlorothiazide: ESIDRIX, HYDRODIURIL, ORETIC. Hydroflumethiazide: SALURON. Bendroflumethiazide: NATURETIN. Benzthiazide: EXNA. Trichlormethiazide: METAHYDRIN. Methyclothiazide: ENDURON. Polythiazide: RENESE. Cyclothiazide: ANHYDRON. Chlorthalidone: HYGROTON. Quinethazone: HYDROMOX. Metolazone: DIULO. Acetazolamide: DIAMOX. Indapamide: LOZOL.

‡ Unsaturated between C 3 and N 4.

ate excretion as does acetazolamide. However, this phenomenon is seldom encountered clinically. The use of thiazides as antihypertensive agents is considered in Chapter 32. In patients with diabetes insipidus, the thiazides actually *decrease* urinary volume (*see* Chapter 37).

Like many other organic acids, the thiazides are actively secreted in the proximal tubule. This secretion may be curtailed by competitors such as probenecid (*see* Chapter 38). In some circumstances, probenecid can inhibit the diuretic response to a thiazide, suggesting that the diuretic must be in the tubular fluid in order to exert its effect (Beyer and Baer, 1961). The major, if not exclusive, site of action of thiazides is the distal tubule. In distal tubular microperfusion studies, sodium reabsorption was inhibited when chlorothiazide was added only to the fluid perfusing the lumen, a result consistent with the effects of probenecid (Costanzo and Windhager, 1978). The mechanism of sodium reabsorption in the early distal tubule is obscure, and, thus, so is the detailed mechanism of action of the thiazides. The maximal rate of sodium excretion induced by thiazides is modest relative to that achievable with some other types of diuretics. This is attributable to the fact that about 90% of filtered sodium is reabsorbed before the tubular fluid reaches the site of action of the thiazides.

Thiazide-induced increases in *potassium* excretion are most readily seen in acute studies; they may be negligible during chronic administration (*see* Table 36–1). The nephron segments responsible for secretion of potassium are distal to the site of action of thiazides, and the drug-induced enhancement of flow through these distal segments is a stimulant to potassium secretion (Giebisch *et al.*, 1981). Another factor that determines potassium secretion, the transepithelial electrical potential, is not influenced by thiazides (Costanzo and Windhager, 1978). Although minor differences in the kaliuresis caused by different thiazides have been observed in special circumstances, these have no practical consequences.

The *glomerular filtration* rate may be reduced by the thiazides, particularly with intravenous administration. This is presumably the result of a direct action on the renal vasculature. It has little significance in the interpretation of primary drug action but may be of clinical importance, particularly in patients with diminished renal reserve.

Thiazides may increase the concentration of *urate* in plasma. Two factors are involved. The first is an enhanced reabsorption of urate in the proximal tubule; this is secondary to enhanced reabsorption of fluid caused by a diuretic-induced contraction of extracellular fluid volume. Second, thiazides may inhibit the tubular excretion of urate (*see* Chapter 38). The increase in uric acid concentration may have little significance, since the incidence of acute attacks of gout is primarily related to the concentration of uric acid in plasma before treatment with a thiazide.

Unlike some other natriuretic agents, the thiazides decrease the renal excretion of *calcium*. This is a result of a direct action on the distal tubule (Costanzo and Windhager, 1978). The excretion of *magnesium* is enhanced by the thiazides, leading to hypomagnesemia.

Iodide and *bromide* are excreted by renal mechanisms qualitatively similar to those for chloride. Diuretic agents that produce chloruresis fail to modify the discriminatory function of the tubule for the different halides. Thus, all chloruretic agents may be useful in the management of bromide intoxication. In addition, increased excretion of iodide, particularly with prolonged diuretic therapy, may produce slight iodine depletion.

Effect on Composition of Extracellular Fluid. The thiazides tend to produce less distortion of the composition of the extracellular fluid than do other diuretic agents. This may be the result of the relatively modest intensity of diuresis produced by these drugs.

Absorption, Fate, and Distribution. Chlorothiazide is poorly absorbed from the gastrointestinal tract, to the extent of about 10%. The other drugs in this class that have been studied have much greater bioavailability (*see* Appendix II; Beermann and Groschinsky-Grind, 1980). Bile acid–binding resins (colestipol and cholestyramine) may impair absorption of the thiazides. Most of these agents cause a demonstrable diuretic effect within an hour after oral administration. However, the persistence of the drugs in the body varies greatly; for example, the half-life of chlorothiazide in plasma is 1.5 hours, while that for chlorthalidone is 44 hours. The durations of action of the thiazides and related agents are summarized in Table 36–2. Differences are due to variation in rates of renal tubular secretion and clearance, metabolism, and enterohepatic circulation. The range of volumes of distribution is also great. Several of the drugs in this class are known to be highly concentrated in erythrocytes, probably as a result of binding to carbonic anhydrase (Beermann and Groschinsky-Grind, 1980). Binding to plasma proteins varies considerably among these agents; there is no correlation of this factor with half-life.

Clinical Toxicity.   In animals the demonstrable toxic dose of all the thiazides is manyfold that required for their pharmacological action. For example, large acute doses can depress CNS function. Clinical toxicity is relatively rare and usually results from unexpected hypersensitivity. Cases of purpura, dermatitis with photosensitivity, depression of the formed elements of the blood, and necrotizing vasculitis have been reported.

Thiazide-induced *hypokalemia* is discussed in Chapter 35 along with the indications for potassium supplementation. Alternatively, the thiazides have been prescribed in combination with a potassium-sparing diuretic (*see* below) in order to obtain an additive diuretic effect with maintenance of potassium balance. The plasma *uric acid* is frequently elevated. For reasons that are unexplained, prolonged therapy with thiazides on rare occasions gives rise to hypercalcemia and hypophosphatemia that simulate hyperparathyroidism (Reineck and Stein, 1981).

Borderline *renal* and/or *hepatic insufficiency* may be unpredictably aggravated by the thiazides. In patients, particularly those with hypertensive disease and decreased renal reserve, the manifestations of renal insufficiency may be aggravated after inten-

sive or prolonged courses of thiazides that lead to excessive depletion of fluid and electrolyte. In patients with cirrhosis of the liver, deterioration of mental function, including the onset of coma, has been attributed to thiazide therapy. Many observers have noted a correlation with hypokalemia and alkalosis. Increased concentrations of ammonia in the blood have been reported. Cholestatic hepatitis has also been observed.

The thiazides may induce *hyperglycemia* and aggravate preexisting diabetes mellitus; the pharmacological effect of the oral hypoglycemic agents may also be reduced. Three apparently relevant factors have been identified in the rat: diminished insulin secretion in response to elevation of plasma glucose, enhanced glycogenolysis, and diminished glycogenesis (Hoskins and Jackson, 1978). Clinical studies suggest that potassium depletion plays a role in glucose intolerance, perhaps by inhibiting the conversion of proinsulin to insulin (for review *see* Perez-Stable and Caralis, 1983). The disturbance in carbohydrate metabolism is relatively common and is probably unrelated to the much rarer toxic reaction of acute pancreatitis. Thiazides cause increases in the concentrations of cholesterol and triglycerides in plasma by unknown mechanisms. It is not known if this effect enhances the risk of atherosclerosis (Perez-Stable and Caralis, 1983).

Preparations and Dosage.   The thiazides are available as tablets for oral administration. The wide range of dosage is indicated in Table 36–2. In a few instances, preparations of a sodium salt are available for intravenous administration when that route is required.

The shorter-acting thiazides are often given in divided daily doses. The longer-acting compounds have a duration of action of 24 hours or more and need be given only once daily (*see* Table 36–2). A single daily dose is often preferable to improve patient compliance to a regimen of antihypertensive therapy. Fixed-dose preparations of a thiazide with an aldosterone antagonist or other potassium-sparing diuretic are available and can be employed to advantage when the maintenance of potassium balance presents a problem (*see* below).

Therapeutic Uses.   The thiazides are the diuretics of choice in the management of *edema* due to mild-to-moderate congestive heart failure. Edema due to chronic hepatic or renal disease may also respond favorably. The use of the thiazides to treat *hypertensive disease* is discussed in Chapter 32. Less common usage includes the treatment of *diabetes insipidus* (*see* Chapter 37) and the management of *hypercalciuria* in patients who have recurrent urinary calculi composed of calcium salts (Yendt and Cohanim, 1978).

HIGH-CEILING DIURETICS

The term *high-ceiling* has been used to denote a group of diuretics that have a distinctive action on renal tubular function. The peak diuresis is far greater than that observed with other agents. The main site of action is the thick ascending limb of the loop of Henle. The agents are thus sometimes referred to as *loop diuretics*. Three drugs of this class are in clinical use in the United States: ethacrynic acid, furosemide, and bumetanide. There are a number of other such compounds, some of which are in clinical use in other countries—for example, muzolimine and etozolin.

Chemistry and Structure-Activity Relationship. The agents available in the United States have the following structures:

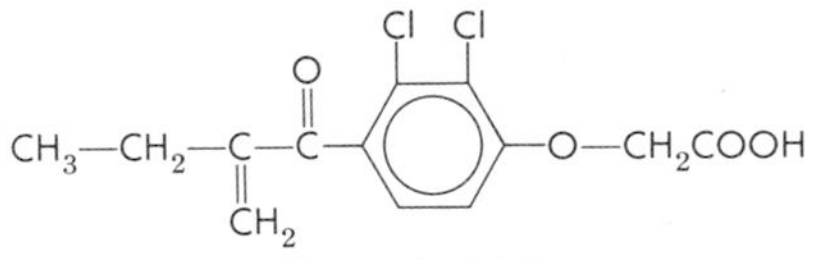

Ethacrynic Acid

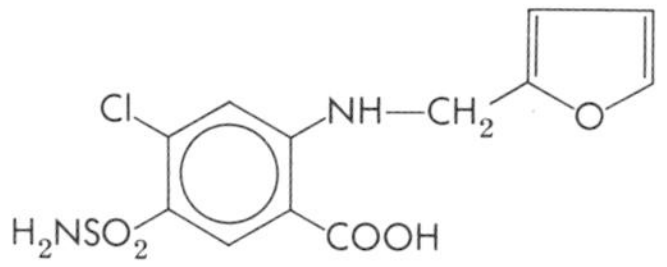

Furosemide

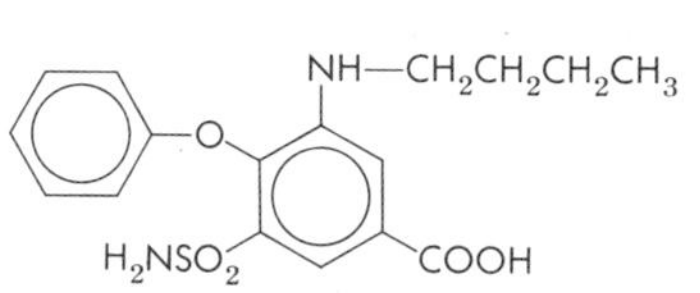

Bumetanide

These drugs share few structural features, and they constitute a pharmacological rather than a chemical class. Of the five agents mentioned above, three are carboxylic acids and a fourth, etozolin, is an ester that is hydrolyzed to an active carboxylic acid *in vivo*. Only two of the drugs are sulfonamides.

Ethacrynic acid contains an α,β-unsaturated ketone moiety, which confers on it a high degree of reactivity toward sulfhydryl groups. It was synthesized in an attempt to mimic the sulfhydryl reactivity of the mercurial diuretics (Schultz *et al.*, 1962). It is clear from the other structures shown above that this is not a prerequisite for diuretic activity. However, it remains unsettled whether such reactivity is crucial for the action of ethacrynic acid (Koechel, 1981). *Furosemide* is one of a series of anthranilic acid derivatives. Congeners differ in milligram potency but exhibit the same pharmacological spectrum. *Bumetanide* is a 3-aminobenzoic acid derivative. Several analogs, which have various substituents, are about equally active in test animals (Feit, 1971). Bumetanide has a higher milligram potency than furosemide, but in other respects the compounds are similar (Flamenbaum and Friedman, 1982).

Mechanism of Diuretic Action. In general, the time of onset and the duration of diuresis achieved with the agents in this class are shorter than those with the thiazides. The brevity of action is determined in large part by pharmacokinetic factors; the intensity of diuresis also calls compensatory mechanisms into play.

The high-ceiling diuretics act primarily to inhibit electrolyte reabsorption in the thick ascending limb of the loop of Henle. There are three major lines of evidence for this contention. First, these agents virtually eliminate both positive and negative free-water production, in which the ascending limb plays a central role (*see* Figure VIII–2). Second, micropuncture experiments demonstrate a greatly enhanced delivery of sodium and chloride to the beginning of the distal tubule. Third, in microperfusion experiments *in vitro* there is complete inhibition of sodium chloride transport in the thick ascending limb at luminal concentrations of drug in the range expected to occur *in vivo* (for reviews *see* Reineck and Stein, 1981; Flamenbaum and Friedman, 1982). The drugs act at the luminal face of the epithelial cells to inhibit the cotransport mechanism for the entry of sodium and chloride (*see* Figure VIII–1; Imai, 1977; Stoner and Trimble, 1982).

These agents tend to increase renal blood flow without increasing filtration rate, especially after intravenous injection. Such a change in renal hemodynamics reduces fluid and electrolyte reabsorption in the proximal tubule and may augment the initial diuretic response (*see* below). The increase in renal blood flow is relatively short lived. With the reduction of extracellular fluid volume that is induced by diuresis, there is a tendency for renal blood flow to decrease; this sets the stage for increased reabsorption from the proximal tubule. The latter phenomenon may be thought of as a compensatory mechanism that limits delivery of solute to the thick ascending limb, thereby diminishing the diuresis. The question of a minor direct action of high-ceiling diuretics on the proximal tubule remains controversial (Reineck and Stein, 1981). Both furosemide and bumetanide are inhibitors of carbonic anhydrase (both are sulfonamides), but these activities are too weak to contribute to a proximal diuresis except when massive doses are employed (Østergaard et al., 1972). Ethacrynic acid is not a carbonic anhydrase inhibitor. Actions of high-ceiling diuretics in segments distal to the thick ascending limb have not been firmly established. However, the magnitude of the diuresis engendered by these drugs suggests that there may be multiple secondary sites of action (see Table 36-1).

The increase in *potassium* excretion and the elevation in the concentration of *uric acid* in plasma are reminiscent of similar phenomena encountered with the thiazide diuretics; they probably result from the same mechanisms as those discussed for the thiazides.

Diuretics of this class enhance the excretion of both *calcium* and *magnesium* to an extent approximately proportional to the increase in sodium excretion. Unlike the thiazides, high-ceiling diuretics do not increase calcium reabsorption in the distal tubule (Edwards et al., 1973). The calciuric action of these agents is the basis for their use in symptomatic hypercalcemia (Suki et al., 1970).

High-ceiling diuretics increase the excretion of *titratable acid* and *ammonia*. This phenomenon, which is thought to be due to effects on the distal nephron, is one of the factors in the genesis and maintenance of diuretic-induced metabolic alkalosis (Bosch et al., 1977).

Hemodynamic Actions. The ability of high-ceiling diuretics to enhance renal blood flow has already been mentioned. However, this effect is not always obtained. Depending on the experimental conditions, including the dose and rate of administration of the diuretic, either an increase or decrease in renal blood flow may occur. These changes are of interest, since they indicate that the renal actions are more complicated than simply to increase the excretion of solute. When furosemide increases renal blood flow, there is a redistribution of flow from medulla to cortex and within the cortex. Acute diuresis increases intraluminal pressure and transiently reduces the filtration rate (Mudge et al., 1975). This raises the possibility that diuretic-induced redistribution of blood flow might be directly mediated by changes in pressure. However, many studies have indicated a more complicated mechanism that involves both prostaglandins and renin. The renal secretion of these substances is increased by the high-ceiling diuretics. Stimulation of renin release results from both the effect of vascular dilatation on the juxtaglomerular apparatus and that of elevated sodium concentration in the region of the macula densa. Indomethacin, in doses adequate to inhibit the synthesis of prostaglandins, blocks the increase in renal blood flow and the increased secretion of prostaglandins and renin produced by furosemide. Although the effect is relatively small, it is clear that treatment with indomethacin blunts the natriuretic response to furosemide and that this is not mediated by a pharmacokinetic interaction (Brater, 1983).

In patients with pulmonary edema high-ceiling diuretics increase venous capacitance, thereby decreasing left ventricular filling pressure. This is an acute action, and it can be of benefit before the onset of diuresis (Dikshit et al., 1973). It is thought that this is mediated by a metabolite of arachidonic acid, perhaps prostacyclin.

Extrarenal Sites of Action. In isolated systems and with high doses, these agents act upon electrolyte transport in a variety of tissues. For example, there may be a slight decrease in bile flow (Erlinger et al., 1970) or changes in the ionic fluxes of isolated erythrocytes (Dunn, 1973). These actions have no known clinical implications. An exception is the action on the inner ear, consisting in a depression of the cochlear microphonic and neural potentials, and a transient increase in the sodium and potassium concentrations in the endolymph. This may result from a direct toxic action on the hair cells (Rybak, 1982).

Effect on Composition of Extracellular Fluid. Metabolic alkalosis may result from the use of the high-ceiling diuretics. When the mobilization of edema fluid is rapid, the alkalosis largely results from a contraction of extracellular fluid volume. With chronic therapy, the dietary intake of salt and the urinary excretion of hydrogen ions and potassium become important factors. This is discussed in Chapter 35. Alkalosis is frequently accompanied by hyponatremia, but each is produced by separate mechanisms.

Absorption, Distribution, and Excretion. The high-ceiling diuretics are readily absorbed from the gastrointestinal tract, although to variable degrees. For example, the bioavailability of furosemide is about 65%, while that of bumetanide is nearly 100% (Beermann and Groschinsky-Grind, 1980). Ethacrynic acid, furosemide, and bumetanide are extensively bound to plasma proteins, but they are rapidly secreted by the organic acid transport system of the proximal tubule. In this manner they gain access to the tubular fluid and eventually to their site of action more distally. Furosemide has been particularly well studied in this context. Probenecid inhibits the secretion of furosemide into the tubular urine, and the dose-response curve for furosemide is shifted to the right when expressed in terms of the concentration of the diuretic in plasma (Figure 36–1). When the response is plotted as a function of the rate of excretion of furosemide, it is unchanged. Thus, the interaction between these two compounds occurs at the level of tubular secretion and not at the site of action of the diuretic. There is a complex interplay of several factors, including duration of action, that determines the extent to which inhibition of secretion influences the overall diuretic response (Brater, 1983).

About two thirds of an intravenous dose of ethacrynic acid is excreted by the kidneys, the remainder by the liver. The major urinary products are the unchanged drug and conjugates with sulfhydryl compounds, mainly cysteine and N-acetylcysteine (Koechel, 1981). A large fraction of furosemide is excreted as such and a lesser fraction as a glucuronide (Beermann and Groschinsky-Grind, 1980). About half of bumetanide is excreted unchanged in the urine; metabolites are also observed (Flamenbaum and Friedman, 1982).

Clinical Toxicity. Two generalizations may be made from extensive experience with ethacrynic acid and furosemide: abnormalities of fluid and electrolyte imbalance are the most common forms of clinical toxicity (*see* discussion at end of this chapter), and side effects unrelated to the primary action of these drugs are quite rare.

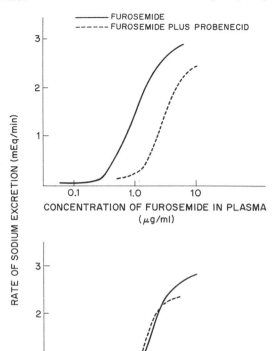

Figure 36–1. *The effect of probenecid on diuretic response curves for furosemide in human subjects.*

The upper panel depicts response as a function of the concentration of furosemide in plasma, while the lower panel is expressed as a function of the rate of excretion of furosemide. Probenecid inhibits the secretion of furosemide, such that at any concentration of furosemide in plasma the quantity of furosemide delivered to its site of action is diminished. This phenomenon accounts for the shift in the concentration-response curve (upper panel). On the other hand, probenecid does not directly interfere with the action of furosemide. Consequently, the curves in the lower panel are virtually superimposable. (Modified from Brater, 1983.)

Hyperuricemia is relatively common, but in most patients it represents little more than a chemical abnormality. Other reactions include gastrointestinal disturbances (with or without bleeding), depression of formed elements in the blood, skin rashes, paresthesias, and hepatic dysfunction. Cross-sensitivity may occur between furosemide and other sulfonamides. Gastrointestinal side effects are much more frequent with ethacrynic acid than furosemide. Furosemide and the thiazides have been implicated as causes of allergic interstitial nephritis, leading to reversible renal failure (Lyons *et al.*, 1973). A decrease in tolerance to carbohydrate may occur, but to a lesser extent than with the thiazides. Acute hypoglycemia of unexplained origin has been reported as a manifestation of overdosage. Because of their effect on offspring in experimental animals, the high-ceiling diuretics should not be prescribed during pregnancy unless absolutely necessary.

The development of deafness, either transient or permanent, is a serious and rare complication of treatment with ethacrynic acid. Transient deafness has also been reported with furosemide; it may be less frequent with bumetanide (Flamenbaum and Friedman, 1982). Drug-induced changes in the electrolyte composition of the endolymph represent a possible mechanism (Rybak, 1982). Due to the rarity of this complication it is difficult to evaluate the contention that it is more common in the presence of renal insufficiency and that it occurs with one drug more often than with another. From available data, it appears that ototoxicity from diuretics is unique to this class of drugs. If another potentially ototoxic drug, such as an aminoglycoside antibiotic, is being administered and concurrent diuretic therapy is indicated, it is advisable to use a diuretic agent from another class, for example, a thiazide.

The high-ceiling diuretics may interact adversely with other drugs. Ethacrynic acid and furosemide are significantly bound to plasma albumin and may compete for sites on the protein with drugs such as warfarin and clofibrate (Sellers and Koch-Weser, 1970; Prandota and Pruitt, 1975). The renal clearance of lithium is decreased during chronic therapy with diuretics (when there is depletion of sodium), and their concurrent use should be avoided unless concentrations of lithium in plasma can be monitored very carefully. The nephrotoxicity produced by cephaloridine is increased by

furosemide, and one should be judicious in the use of any cephalosporin in conjunction with furosemide or ethacrynic acid (Dodds and Foord, 1970).

Preparations. *Ethacrynic acid* (EDECRIN) is available for oral use as 25- and 50-mg tablets. The usual dose for adults is from 50 to 200 mg per day. The optimal dose should be determined for each patient, starting with minimal amounts. The sodium salt of ethacrynic acid is available for intravenous use; the usual dose is 50 mg.

Furosemide (LASIX) is available as 20-, 40-, and 80-mg tablets and in an oral solution. In adults, the usual initial dosage ranges from 20 to 80 mg daily. Dosage may be repeated after 6 to 8 hours and titrated carefully to a maximum of 600 mg per day. The usual pediatric dose is 2 mg/kg, which may be titrated up to 6 mg/kg. A preparation is also available for parenteral administration, either intravenously or intramuscularly. The recommended adult dose by this route is 20 or 40 mg, repeated if necessary after not less than 2 hours. Once the desired effect is obtained, the dose should be given once or twice daily to control edema. The usual pediatric dose is 1 mg/kg, which may be titrated to a maximum of 6 mg/kg.

Bumetanide (BUMEX) is available for oral use as 0.5- and 1.0-mg tablets. The usual dose for adults ranges from 0.5 to 2.0 mg, generally given once daily. A second or third dose may be given at 4- to 5-hour intervals up to a maximum of 10 mg daily. Alternate-day therapy or intermittent dosing for 3 to 4 days followed by 1- to 2-day rest periods may be the safest and most effective method for continued control of edema. In patients with hepatic failure, the dosage should be kept to a minimum and adjusted very carefully. Bumetanide is also available for parenteral administration. The usual dose is 0.5 to 1.0 mg, intravenously or intramuscularly. A second or third dose may be given at 2- to 3-hour intervals, up to a maximum of 10 mg daily.

Therapeutic Uses. Due to the lower incidence of gastrointestinal reactions and a less precipitous dose-response curve, furosemide is prescribed much more frequently than is ethacrynic acid. The extent to which bumetanide will be used is not yet known. The high-ceiling diuretics are effective for the treatment of *edema* of cardiac, hepatic, or renal origin. The oral route should be used unless impractical or the clinical situation demands a very prompt diuresis, in which case intravenous or intramuscular administration may be employed. This applies particularly to the management of *acute pulmonary edema*. In this condition the favorable hemodynamic changes and the rapid reduction of the volume of extracellular fluid are of sufficient magnitude to reduce venous return and right ventricular output. In the management of refractory edema, the high-ceiling agents may be used in conjunction with other types of diuretics, particularly the potassium-sparing drugs, but there is no rationale for administering two high-ceiling agents concomitantly.

In the presence of *nephrosis* or *chronic renal failure*, doses of furosemide far higher than usual may be required (Muth, 1973). The reason for this is not well established. It has been suggested that the high protein content in the tubular fluid inhibits diuresis by binding the diuretic (Green and Mirkin, 1981). In addition, patients with uremia have a decreased rate of tubular secretion (Rose *et al.*, 1976). Furosemide is metabolized to a reactive intermediate that produces hepatic necrosis in experimental animals. At the usual clinical dose hepatic toxicity is not observed, but the possible occurrence of this undesirable effect should be kept in mind when the massive doses sometimes employed in renal failure must be given (Mitchell *et al.*, 1974). By conventional measurements, renal function is not compromised by high doses. However, the incidence of undesirable side effects may be increased (Allison and Kennedy, 1971). The high-ceiling diuretics have also been used in patients with early *acute renal failure*, but results are inconclusive. The drugs are contraindicated once anuric renal failure is unequivocally established. In symptomatic *hypercalcemia*, the high-ceiling diuretics may lower the concentration of calcium in plasma by increasing its urinary excretion. When employed for this purpose, the replacement of urinary losses of sodium and chloride is required (Suki *et al.*, 1970).

ALDOSTERONE ANTAGONISTS

The role of adrenocorticosteroids in the regulation of electrolyte and water balance is discussed in Chapter 63. With insight into the chemistry of the steroids and with more complete knowledge of their physiological function, it has been possible to synthesize competitive antagonists that are useful as diuretics.

SPIRONOLACTONE

Chemistry. A number of 17-spirolactone steroids have been employed, of which *spironolactone* appears to have the greatest selectivity and efficacy. Its structural formula is as follows:

Spironolactone

Mechanism of Diuretic Action. Compounds of this type are competitive antago-

nists of the actions of mineralocorticoids, of which aldosterone is the most potent naturally occurring compound. The aldosterone receptor is a soluble, cytoplasmic protein that appears to exist in two allosteric forms. Spironolactone binds to the receptor and prevents it from assuming the active conformation. As a consequence, the entire chain of biochemical events that leads to the synthesis of physiologically active transport proteins is aborted (*see* Corvol *et al.*, 1981).

Aldosterone receptors are present in several tissues, including the salivary glands, colon, and several segments of the nephron. In the present context, the most important target cells are those of the late distal tubule and collecting system. The overall action of aldosterone is to enhance sodium reabsorption and potassium secretion. Implicit in the foregoing description of mechanism are two phenomena that are amply supported by experimental evidence: first, spironolactone is effective only in the presence of either endogenous or exogenous aldosterone; second, the action of the antagonist may be overcome by increasing the concentration of aldosterone (Kagawa *et al.*, 1959; Liddle, 1961).

Under controlled conditions the urinary $Na^+:K^+$ ratio serves as an indirect index of aldosterone activity. The ratio can be greatly increased in response to the administration of spironolactone. Spironolactone also increases calcium excretion through a direct effect on tubular transport (Wills *et al.*, 1969).

At relatively high concentrations, spironolactone can inhibit the biosynthesis of aldosterone. Theoretically, such an action could result in diuretic activity. However, it is unlikely that this action occurs at therapeutic concentrations (Corvol *et al.*, 1981).

Absorption, Distribution, and Excretion. About 70% of an oral dose of spironolactone is absorbed. The compound is metabolized to a significant extent during its first passage through the liver, and there is considerable enterohepatic circulation. Binding to plasma proteins is extensive. Virtually no unmetabolized drug appears in the urine (Beermann and Groschinsky-Grind, 1980).

Canrenone is a major metabolite of spironolactone, and it can be interconverted enzymatically with its hydrolytic product, *canrenoate*. Their structures are as follows:

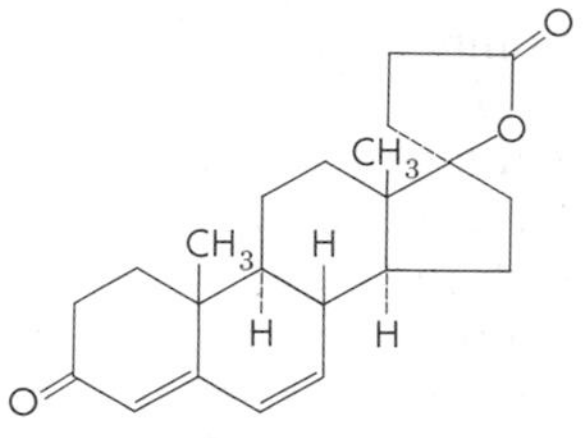

Canrenone

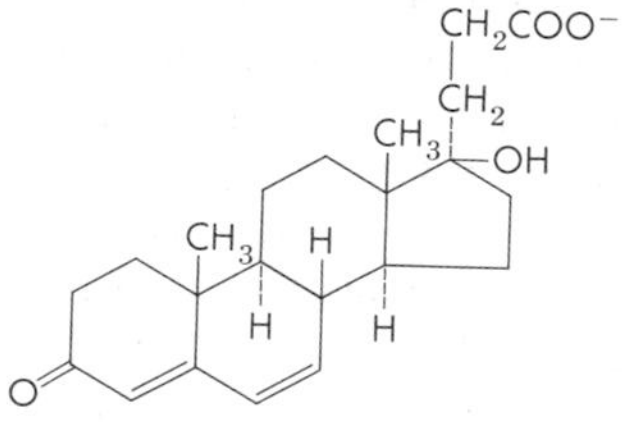

CH_2COO^-

Canrenoate

Canrenone is an active aldosterone antagonist, and its formation contributes to, but does not account fully for, the biological activity of spironolactone. Canrenoate has no intrinsic activity, but it can exert biological effects by virtue of its interconversion with canrenone. Salicylates may interfere with the tubular secretion of canrenone and thereby decrease the effectiveness of spironolactone. The potassium salt of canrenoate is a water-soluble substance that can be administered parenterally. Both canrenone and potassium canrenoate are utilized clinically in some countries, but they are not available in the United States (Beermann and Groschinsky-Grind, 1980; Corvol et al., 1981).

Clinical Toxicity. The most serious toxic effects of spironolactone result from hyperkalemia. Although hyperkalemia is almost certain to occur when the drug is injudiciously administered in conjunction with a high intake of potassium, it may also happen even when ordinary doses are given simultaneously with a thiazide to patients with severe renal insufficiency. A number of minor reactions have also been reported that are usually reversible when the drug is discontinued. Of these, the most common are gynecomastia, androgen-like side effects, and minor gastrointestinal symptoms. Spironolactone has been shown to be tumorigenic when administered to rats chronically and in high doses.

Preparations and Dosage. *Spironolactone* (ALDACTONE) is available in 25-, 50-, and 100-mg oral tablets. It is effective in an average daily dose of 100 mg, given in single or divided doses. The dose may range from 25 to 200 mg daily in adults. Dosage in children should be initiated at 3.3 mg/kg. Spironolactone may also be given in doses of 400 mg per day as a diagnostic test for primary aldosteronism and in doses of 100 to 400 mg daily in preparation for surgery after such a diagnosis. A fixed-dose combination of either 25 or 50 mg of both hydrochlorothiazide and spironolactone is also available (ALDACTAZIDE). Dosage should be determined by titration of the individual agents.

Therapeutic Uses. The aldosterone antagonists are widely used in the treatment of *hypertension* and in the management of *refractory edema*. Frequently, they have been employed in conjunction with other diuretic agents rather than as the sole drug. On theoretical grounds, the potassium loss that occurs secondary to the use of other diuretics may be decreased by the coadministration of aldosterone antagonists. In general, this has been substantiated by clinical experience in the treatment of congestive heart failure, cirrhosis of the liver, and the nephrotic syndrome. However, the quantitative effects are not exactly predictable, due to the complex interactions of the primary disease, the degree of secondary hyperaldosteronism, and the actions of the diuretics given concomitantly.

Competitive aldosterone antagonists, as well as other potassium-retaining agents, are also useful in both the diagnosis and the management of those rare metabolic and renal diseases associated with hypokalemia and potassium depletion (*see* Liddle, 1966).

OTHER POTASSIUM-SPARING DIURETICS

During the last several decades, the introduction of new natriuretic agents has been paralleled by studies on the secretion of potassium. These have established (1) that potassium excretion is achieved by distal tubular secretion, (2) that excessive potassium losses may constitute an unfavorable consequence of diuretic action, (3) that the excretion of potassium can be influenced by steroids with mineralocorticoid activity, and (4) that the loss of potassium may also be influenced by drugs that act directly on the distal nephron independently of adrenal steroids. While it is true that triamterene and amiloride possess moderate natriuretic activity, their major importance lies in their effect on potassium excretion (Baer and Beyer, 1972).

Chemistry. Both triamterene and amiloride are organic bases. They have the following structures:

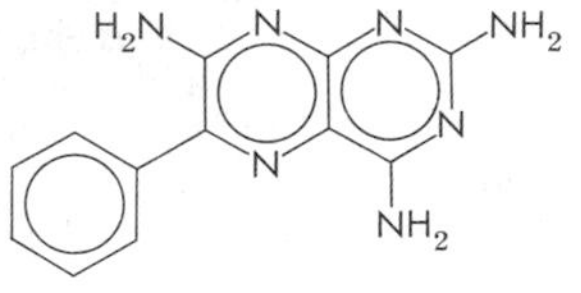

Triamterene

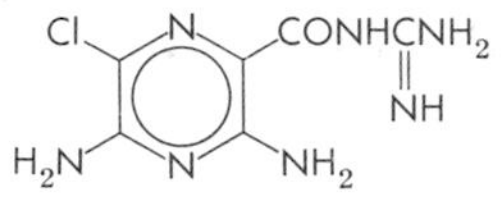

Amiloride

Triamterene is a pteridine with structural resemblance to folic acid and some of the inhibitors of dihydrofolate reductase. It is a weak inhibitor of the enzyme *in vivo*. Amiloride is a pyrazinoylguanidine. It is one of a large series of pyrazine derivatives examined for the ability to prevent loss of potassium (Cragoe, 1983).

Mechanism of Diuretic Action. Although triamterene is the older of the two drugs in this therapeutic class, amiloride has been studied more thoroughly in terms of mechanisms. This is in large part attributable to the fact that amiloride is much more soluble in aqueous solution. To the extent that comparable studies are available, both drugs seem to have identical actions.

These agents interfere with transport in the late segments of the nephron. They induce a modest increase in the excretion of sodium, mostly accompanied by chloride as the anion (*see* Table 36–1). Under ordinary circumstances there is little change in the excretion of potassium, although sometimes there is a slight increase. However, when excretion of potassium is high because of increased intake, administration of another diuretic, or an excess of mineralocorticoid, these drugs cause a sharp decrease in its excretion (*see,* for example, Wiebelhaus *et al.*, 1967). In many respects these effects resemble those of spironolactone, but it is quite clear that these drugs are not aldosterone antagonists. Their primary action is to inhibit the electrogenic entry of sodium (*see* Figure VIII–1, 5–A).

This mechanism for permeation of sodium is quite widespread, and amiloride has been particularly useful in studies of sodium transport in a wide variety of systems (Benos, 1982). In some of these, amiloride acts as a competitive inhibitor of sodium transport; in others, the inhibition does not conform to competitive kinetics. This issue is not settled for the mammalian nephron.

Because of the interruption of electrogenic sodium transport by these agents, the electrical potential across the tubular epithelium falls. The reduction or elimination of this potential, which is one of the driving forces for secretion of potassium, is probably the basis of the potassium-sparing effect (Giebisch *et al.*, 1981). The potassium-sparing diuretics may also cause slight alkalinization of the urine, which is attributable to inhibition of hydrogen secretion in the distal nephron. The mechanism of this inhibition is not known. These compounds are not inhibitors of carbonic anhydrase. Amiloride is an inhibitor of the Na^+-H^+ exchange mechanism of the proximal tubule and of the Na^+,K^+-ATPase. These latter actions require much higher concentrations of the drug than can be achieved *in vivo*. Amiloride decreases calcium excretion, an action which is additive to that of chlorothiazide (Costanzo and Weiner, 1976).

Absorption, Distribution, and Excretion. Amiloride and triamterene are available only for oral use. About 50% of an oral dose of each agent is absorbed. Triamterene is bound to plasma proteins to the extent of about 60%; amiloride is not bound. Both drugs have apparent volumes of distribution that are greater than body water (*see* Appendix II). Amiloride is not metabolized. The metabolism of triamterene is very extensive, and some of the metabolites have diuretic activity. Both drugs are secreted in the proximal tubule, presumably by the organic cation secretory mechanism.

Clinical Toxicity. The most serious toxic effect is hyperkalemia, which is a direct consequence of the major action of the drugs. Triamterene produces relatively few other side effects. The most common are nausea, vomiting, leg cramps, and dizziness. Slight-to-moderate azotemia is relatively common. This does not appear to be directly related to electrolyte and water imbalance and is reversible. Megaloblastic anemia has been reported in patients with alcoholic cirrhosis, presumably due to inhibition of dihydrofolate reductase in patients with reduced stores and intake of folic acid.

The most common side effects of amiloride, aside from hyperkalemia, are nausea, vomiting, diarrhea, and headache.

Preparations. *Triamterene* (DYRENIUM) is administered only by the oral route. It is marketed in capsules containing 50 or 100 mg. The usual initial dose is 100 mg, given twice daily. The maximal daily dose is 300 mg. The maintenance dose should be determined for the individual patient and may be as low as 100 mg every other day. The fixed-dose combination of triamterene (50 mg) and hydrochlorothiazide (25 mg) (DYAZIDE) is available in capsules, one or two of which are usually given twice daily.

Amiloride hydrochloride (MIDAMOR) is available for oral use as 5-mg tablets. The usual dose is 5 to 10 mg per day. The maintenance dose should be determined for each patient individually. The fixed-dose combination of amiloride hydrochloride (5 mg) and hydrochlorothiazide (50 mg) (MODURETIC) is available in tablets. The usual dose is one or two tablets per day.

Therapeutic Uses. Some patients with *edema* have a satisfactory diuretic response to a potassium-sparing diuretic alone. However, the available clinical data suggest that the greatest usefulness of these drugs may be in conjunction with other diuretic agents. In general, the administration of a potassium-sparing diuretic with another natriuretic compound augments natriuresis and reduces potassium loss. With concurrent drug therapy, it is this latter effect that is more consistently observed. Therefore, the rationale of concomitant drug therapy is primarily in relation to potassium metabolism. Hansen and Bender (1967) summarized the experience obtained from several hundred patients maintained on long-term regimens with triamterene alone, hydrochlorothiazide alone, and both drugs together, and showed that both drugs together provided the highest incidence of normal values of potassium in plasma. Because of the real possibility of inducing serious hyperkalemia, patients treated with a potassium-sparing diuretic should *not* receive supplements of potassium. These drugs and spironolactone should *not* be prescribed together; an unexpectedly high degree of hyperkalemia has occurred when this was done.

XANTHINES

The xanthines have long been known for their diuretic action. Their additional pharmacological properties are discussed in Chapter 25. Of the xanthines, theophylline has the greatest action on the kidney.

Mechanism of Diuretic Action. The stimulatory effect of the xanthines on cardiac function has raised the possibility that diuresis may result, in part, from the increased renal blood flow and glomerular filtration rate. However, all drugs of this class appear to have a direct action on the renal tubule. The urinary response involves an increase in the rate of excretion of sodium and chloride, with no significant effect on urinary acidification. Diuretic action is only slightly affected by changes in acid-base balance but is potentiated by the coadministration of carbonic anhydrase inhibitors. It has been postulated that intracellular pH directly affects the intrarenal action of these agents. Augmentation of potassium excretion is not remarkable. Theophylline has been a useful agent in the study of water and electrolyte metabolism and the role of adenosine 3′,5′-monophosphate (cyclic AMP) to regulate these processes (Strewler and Orloff, 1977).

Clinical Application. The xanthines are rarely employed as primary diuretics. However, when used for other purposes, particularly as bronchodilators, the coexistence of their diuretic action should be kept in mind.

URICOSURIC DIURETICS

Interest in the development of diuretics that are simultaneously uricosuric stems from several considerations. Many of the currently available diuretics commonly lead to urate retention, hyperuricemia, and, in the rare subject, attacks of gout. Furthermore, hyperuricemia may itself be a risk factor for the development of cardiovascular disease, carbohydrate intolerance, and urate-induced nephropathy. One such diuretic, *ticrynafen*, was used only briefly in the United States. Its pharmacology is reviewed in the *sixth edition* of this textbook. Another, *indacrinone*, is not yet available for therapeutic use.

INDACRINONE

Indacrinone has the following structural formula:

Indacrinone

The carbon bearing the methyl and phenyl groups is asymmetrical, and there are two enantiomers. Both are potent uricosuric agents, but the (-)-enantiomer is the much more potent diuretic. Hence, it is possible to optimize the ratio of uricosuric and diuretic activities by manipulating the ratio of the two enantiomers (Blaine *et al.*, 1982). A mixture of the isomers of indacrinone (90% [+] and 10% [−])

is now in clinical trial. Of considerable theoretical interest is the discovery of another uricosuric diuretic, one of whose optical isomers is diuretic but not uricosuric, while the other is uricosuric but not diuretic (Fanelli *et al.*, 1980).

Indacrinone is effective orally in small doses. The agent undergoes tubular secretion, which is inhibited by probenecid, and is reabsorbed by nonionic diffusion. The diuretic action of indacrinone is prompt and more prolonged than that of furosemide or ethacrynic acid. Micropuncture studies indicate that indacrinone inhibits urate reabsorption in the proximal tubule and sodium chloride reabsorption in the ascending limb of the loop of Henle. Uricosuria is blunted but not abolished by pyrazinoate; this has no effect on diuresis (*see* Weinman *et al.*, 1976; Fanelli *et al.*, 1977a, 1977b; Stoner and Trimble, 1982).

THE CLINICAL USE OF DIURETICS

Pathological Physiology of Edema Formation. In a healthy subject, changes in dietary intake or variations in the extrarenal loss of fluid and electrolytes are accompanied by fine adjustments in the rate of renal excretion. Edema can obviously result either from an abnormally high intake of water and electrolyte or from abnormally low rates of their excretion. When fluids are administered parenterally with excessive vigor, edema can certainly be produced. However, when cardiac and renal function are normal, the condition is short lived. In the usual edematous states encountered in clinical medicine, the underlying abnormality involves a decreased rate of renal excretion, and the regulation of sodium excretion is the mechanism that is primarily disturbed. The retention of this cation is accompanied by retention of extracellular anion and a proportional amount of water and, as a result, the increased volume of extracellular fluid is usually of normal composition and osmolality. However, in patients with severe cardiac or hepatic decompensation, retention of water may be relatively greater than that of electrolyte, and hypoosmolality results.

The exact mechanisms by which the kidney retains excessive amounts of sodium have been intensively examined. In many edematous states, increased rates of aldosterone secretion have been correlated with increased tubular reabsorption of sodium. In addition, particularly in cardiac decompensation, the glomerular filtration rate may be reduced. However, quantitative studies, both in disease and under experimental conditions, have failed to provide a predictable relationship between the rate of sodium excretion and either the amount of sodium filtered or the activity of aldosterone. For this reason, additional factors have been postulated that might regulate sodium reabsorption and excretion.

These hypotheses have recently been strengthened greatly by the characterization of two different types of endogenous agents that promote natri-

uresis and diuresis. Atria are known to contain secretory granules, and their number changes during water deprivation. Furthermore, intravenous injection of extracts from atria into rats causes natriuresis and diuresis (de Bold, 1982). Peptides have now been purified from mammalian atria that promote the excretion of sodium and water and that relax vascular and intestinal smooth muscle. The sequences of two of these peptides (*atriopeptins* or *atrial natriuretic factors*) have been determined, and it is thought that they may be derived from a common precursor (*atriopeptigen*) (Currie *et al.*, 1984). Hypothetically, elevation of extracellular fluid volume and/or sodium concentration will stimulate the synthesis and secretion of these interesting putative hormones. Another factor, termed *endoxin*, has been characterized partially. It is not a peptide, it binds to antidigoxin antibodies, and it appears to promote natriuresis by inhibition of Na^+,K^+-ATPase. The source of endoxin is not known (*see* Grantham and Edwards, 1984).

The normal relationship between the volumes of interstitial fluid and the circulating plasma depends on dynamic equilibria across the capillary membrane (*see* Chapter 35). In diseases of hepatic origin, particularly cirrhosis, the pressure relationships are disturbed primarily within the portal circulation, and the formation of edema becomes manifest as ascites. In congestive heart failure, pressure-flow relationships may be disturbed relatively more in either the systemic or the pulmonary circulation, and edema may be localized accordingly. In the nephrotic syndrome or other hypoproteinemic states, the equilibrium across all capillary membranes tends to be altered and edema fluid accumulates in a variety of tissues. However, in each instance the formation of significantly increased amounts of extracellular fluid is either preceded or accompanied by decreased rates of renal excretion.

Indications for the Use of Diuretics. When edema accumulates, three therapeutic approaches are available to mobilize the fluid and thereafter maintain the constancy of the extracellular fluid volume. The first is to correct the primary disease. This is, of course, the most desirable goal. The second is to suppress renal tubular reabsorptive capacity by the use of drugs. The third is to reduce the amount of sodium salts absorbed from the gastrointestinal tract. This is achieved primarily by a low-salt diet.

In most patients with *cardiac decompensation*, digitalis should be administered in full, adequate dosage and should be considered the primary therapeutic agent. Diuretic drugs acting directly on the kidney, irrespective of their potency or effectiveness, must be considered to have a secondary, albeit important, role.

The diuretics are extensively employed in the management of ascites, especially when associated with *cirrhosis* of the liver. Periodic administration either eliminates the necessity for or reduces the interval between paracenteses. Not only does a diuretic regimen contribute to the comfort of the patient, but also his meager protein reserves are spared inasmuch as significant amounts of protein are lost when ascitic fluid is mechanically withdrawn. With mild, asymptomatic, or residual ascites, no useful purpose is served in attempting to make the patient completely free of edema if this involves the persistent administration of diuretics and the production of hypovolemia or electrolyte imbalances.

As a general rule, *chronic renal disease* that causes edema may be treated in the same manner as other edematous states, with the recognition that these patients are more subject to electrolyte imbalance. In the presence of primary renal disease there is often a lesser effect of the diuretic on tubular function. In the case of the high-ceiling diuretics, particularly furosemide, an increased dose is required (Muth, 1973). The thiazides are relatively less effective and in high doses may decrease the glomerular filtration rate.

In the *nephrotic syndrome,* the response to diuretic agents is often disappointing. Although hypoproteinemia is a major etiological factor, the administration of albumin produces a minimal and unpredictable diuretic response. The important role of the corticosteroids in the management of the nephrotic syndrome is discussed in Chapter 63.

In incipient *acute renal failure,* diuretics have been used in the hope of diminishing further renal damage. Protection has been obtained in experimental models, and several intrarenal mechanisms may be involved. Unfortunately such administration of diuretics has been of limited clinical utility (Tiller and Mudge, 1980).

Complications of Diuretic Therapy. With the availability of powerful diuretics, there has been an increased incidence of complications in the management of the edematous state that may be directly attributed to the diuresis itself. It should be remembered that the goal of diuretic therapy is the mobilization of edema fluid in such a manner that the extracellular fluid is restored toward normal, in terms of both volume and composition. The *excessively rapid mobilization* of edema may lead to malaise and asthenia. Rapid changes in the pressure-flow relationships in the cardiovascular system may, even in the presence of an expanded extracellular fluid volume, give rise to symptoms usually associated with hypovolemia. In *intensive long-term therapy,* the diuretic-induced renal loss of sodium chloride may lead to *extracellular fluid depletion,* with or without hyponatremia. The condition usually responds to discontinuation of the diuretic agent and the liberalization of sodium chloride intake in the diet. Both these conditions are relatively rare.

A far more common condition, particularly in congestive heart failure and hepatic cirrhosis, is *chronic dilutional hyponatremia.* This is associated with persistent edema and expanded extracellular volume. It may occur solely as a result of the underlying disease, but is most often seen as a consequence of diuretic therapy. The physiological defect results from the inability of the patient to excrete an adequately dilute urine. The distal generation of positive free water is defective. This is attributed to an inadequate sodium load to this segment of the nephron. Water restriction is the most direct therapeutic approach, but may be complicated by uncontrollable thirst.

The problems of diuretic-induced *alkalosis* and *potassium depletion* are discussed above and in Chapter 35. In addition, *hyperkalemia* may result if potassium-sparing diuretics are used injudiciously or if potassium supplements are administered simultaneously.

Both extracellular and intracellular *magnesium depletion* may result from the use of diuretics. Since magnesium and potassium deficits may interact, the problem is complex and warrants extensive evaluation (*see* Chapter 35). Depending on the type of diuretic employed, concentrations of calcium in plasma may increase or decrease, as discussed above.

Refractory Edema. The increasing attention being given to so-called refractory edema is, in fact, partly attributable to the high degree of success in the management of the less severely ill patient. This has enabled many patients with cardiac decompensation to survive longer in an edema-free state. With the progression of the underlying disease, these patients consequently tend to become edematous at a time when their cardiac reserve is significantly more impaired than in the earlier years of their illness.

With many drugs, diuretic efficacy is decreased by hyponatremia. An additional factor in drug refractoriness is the reduction in glomerular filtration rate. It should also be emphasized that diuresis is limited in an overall sense by the extracellular fluid volume. As edema subsides, the response to an individual dose of most drugs diminishes until, as the edema-free state is approached, the magnitude of diuresis is necessarily smaller than at the height of the edema.

When a patient becomes refractory to a diuretic, the entire regimen should be reevaluated. In some instances, minor adjustments of dosage may suffice. Bed rest itself may restore drug responsiveness, due to improvement in the renal circulation. Abnormalities of extracellular fluid composition should be sought for and corrected. The administration of additional diuretics may be appropriate. As a general rule, patients who are refractory to a diuretic of moderate efficacy, such as the thiazides, will show a more satisfactory response to high-ceiling diuretics.

Use of Multiple Diuretics and Adjuvant Agents. The availability of many different types of diuretics and many different compounds of the same type has provided the temptation to alter the diuretic regimen at frequent intervals. In the *initial management* of the edematous subject, when *mobilization* of edema fluid is the primary goal of therapy, the changing status of the patient warrants appropriate adjustments in dosage schedules and also in the agents selected for use. However, in the *chronic management* of edema, the best therapeutic results are often correlated with a purposefully constant therapeutic regimen.

Despite the widespread use of high-ceiling diuretics for the treatment of chronic edema, especially of cardiac origin, one may properly raise the question of their overuse in situations in which other diuretics, although less effective by conventional standards, might equally well achieve the desired therapeutic goal with less risk of overtreatment.

In the severely edematous patient, it is becoming apparent that, if a single diuretic agent proves ineffective, it is proper to use more than one type of diuretic agent. Of course, nothing is to be gained by the administration of two drugs of the same type, such as two different thiazides. Specific examples of rational concurrent therapy with diuretics have been cited in the discussion of individual drugs.

Allison, M. E. M., and Kennedy, A. C. Diuretics in chronic renal disease: a study of high dosage furosemide. *Clin. Sci.*, **1971**, *41*, 171–187.

Beyer, K. H. The mechanism of action of chlorothiazide. *Ann. N.Y. Acad. Sci.*, **1958**, *71*, 363–379.

Blaine, E. H.; Fanelli, G. M., Jr.; Irvin, J. D.; Tobert, J. A.; and Davies, R. O. Enantiomers of indacrinone: a new approach to producing an isouricemic diuretic. *Clin. Exp. Hypertens.* [A], **1982**, *4*, 161–176.

Bosch, J. P.; Goldstein, M. H.; Levitt, M. F.; and Kahn, T. Effect of chronic furosemide administration on hydrogen and sodium excretion in the dog. *Am. J. Physiol.*, **1977**, *232*, F397–F404.

Costanzo, L. S., and Weiner, I. M. Relationships between clearances of Ca and Na: effect of distal diuretics and PTH. *Am. J. Physiol.*, **1976**, *230*, 67–73.

Costanzo, L. S., and Windhager, E. E. Calcium and sodium transport by the distal convoluted tubule of the rat. *Am. J. Physiol.*, **1978**, *235*, F492–F506.

Currie, M. G.; Geller, D. M.; Cole, B. R.; Siegel, N. R.; Fok, K. F.; Adams, S. P.; Eubanks, S. R.; Galluppi, G. R.; and Needleman, P. Purification and sequence analysis of bioactive atrial peptides (atriopeptins). *Science*, **1984**, *223*, 67–69.

de Bold, A. J. Atrial natriuretic factor of the rat heart.

Studies on isolation and properties. *Proc. Soc. Exp. Biol. Med.*, **1982**, *170*, 133–138.

Dikshit, K.; Vyden, J. K.; Forrester, J. S.; Chatterjee, K.; Prakash, R.; and Swan, H. J. C. Renal and extrarenal hemodynamic effects of furosemide in congestive heart failure after acute myocardial infarction. *N. Engl. J. Med.*, **1973**, *288*, 1087–1090.

Dodds, M. G., and Foord, R. D. Enhancement by potent diuretics of renal tubular necrosis induced by cephaloridine. *Br. J. Pharmacol.*, **1970**, *40*, 227–236.

Dunn, M. J. Diuretics and red blood cell transport of cations. In, *Modern Diuretic Therapy in the Treatment of Cardiovascular and Renal Disease.* (Lant, A. F., and Wilson, G. M., eds.) Excerpta Medica, Amsterdam, **1973**, pp. 196–208.

Edwards, B. R.; Baer, P. G.; Sutton, R. A. L.; and Dirks, J. H. Micropuncture study of diuretic effects on sodium and calcium reabsorption in the dog nephron. *J. Clin. Invest.*, **1973**, *52*, 2418–2427.

Erlinger, S.; Dhumeaux, D.; Berthelot, P.; and Dumont, M. Effect of inhibitors of sodium transport on bile formation in the rabbit. *Am. J. Physiol.*, **1970**, *219*, 416–422.

Fanelli, G. M., Jr.; Bohn, D. L.; Scriabine, A.; and Beyer, K. H., Jr. Saluretic and uricosuric effects of (6,7 - dichloro - 2 - methyl - 1 - oxo - 2 - phenyl - 5 - indanyloxy) acetic acid (MK-196) in the chimpanzee. *J. Pharmacol. Exp. Ther.*, **1977a**, *200*, 402–412.

Fanelli, G. M., Jr.; Bohn, D. L.; and Zacchei, A. G. Renal excretion of a saluretic-uricosuric agent (MK-196) and interaction with a urate-retaining drug, pyrazinoate, in the chimpanzee. *J. Pharmacol. Exp. Ther.*, **1977b**, *200*, 413–419.

Fanelli, G. M., Jr.; Watson, L. S.; Bohn, D. L.; and Russo, H. F. Diuretic and uricosuric activity of 6,7 - dichloro - 2,3 - dihydro - 5 - (2 - thienylcarbonyl)benzofuran-2-carboxylic acid and stereoisomers in chimpanzee, dog and rat. *J. Pharmacol. Exp. Ther.*, **1980**, *212*, 190–197.

Feit, P. W. Aminobenzoic acid diuretics. 2. 4-Substituted-3-amino-5-sulfamylbenzoic acid derivatives. *J. Med. Chem.*, **1971**, *14*, 432–439.

Ford, R. V. The new diuretics. *Med. Clin. North Am.*, **1961**, *45*, 961–972.

Gennari, F. J., and Kassirer, J. P. Osmotic diuresis. *N. Engl. J. Med.*, **1974**, *291*, 714–720.

Green, T. P., and Mirkin, B. L. Furosemide disposition in normal and proteinuric rats: urinary drug-protein binding as a determinant of drug excretion. *J. Pharmacol. Exp. Ther.*, **1981**, *218*, 122–127.

Griggs, R. C.; Engel, W. K.; and Resnick, J. S. Acetazolamide treatment of hypokalemic periodic paralysis. Prevention of attacks and improvement of persistent weakness. *Ann. Intern. Med.*, **1970**, *73*, 39–48.

Hansen, K. B., and Bender, A. D. Changes in serum potassium levels occurring in patients treated with triamterene and triamterene-hydrochlorothiazide combination. *Clin. Pharmacol. Ther.*, **1967**, *8*, 392–399.

Hoskins, B., and Jackson, C. M., III. The mechanism of chlorothiazide-induced carbohydrate intolerance. *J. Pharmacol. Exp. Ther.*, **1978**, *206*, 423–430.

Imai, M. Effect of bumetanide and furosemide on the thick ascending limbs of Henle's loop of rabbits and rats perfused *in vitro. Eur. J. Pharmacol.*, **1977**, *41*, 409–416.

Kagawa, C. M.; Sturtevant, F. M.; and Van Arman, C. G. Pharmacology of a new steroid that blocks salt activity of aldosterone and desoxycorticosterone. *J. Pharmacol. Exp. Ther.*, **1959**, *126*, 123–130.

Kloner, R. A.; Reimer, K. A.; Willerson, J. T.; and Jennings, R. B. Reduction of experimental myocardial infarct size with hyperosmolar mannitol. *Proc. Soc. Exp. Biol. Med.*, **1976**, *151*, 677–683.

Larson, E. B.; Roach, R. C.; Schoene, R. B.; and

Hornbein, T. F. Acute mountain sickness and acetazolamide. *J.A.M.A.*, **1982**, *248*, 328–332.

Laux, B. E., and Raichle, M. E. The effect of acetazolamide on cerebral blood flow and oxygen utilization in the rhesus monkey. *J. Clin. Invest.*, **1978**, *62*, 585–592.

Liddle, G. W. Specific and non-specific inhibition of mineralocorticoid activity. *Metabolism*, **1961**, *10*, 1021–1030.

Lucci, M. S.; Tinker, J. P.; Weiner, I. M.; and DuBose, T. D., Jr. Function of proximal tubule carbonic anhydrase defined by selective inhibition. *Am. J. Physiol.*, **1983**, *245*, F443–F449.

Lyons, H.; Pinn, V. W.; Cartell, S.; Cohen, J. J.; and Harrington, J. T. Allergic interstitial nephritis causing reversible renal failure in four patients with idiopathic nephrotic syndrome. *N. Engl. J. Med.*, **1973**, *288*, 124–128.

Maren, T. H. Relations between structure and biological activity of sulfonamides. *Annu. Rev. Pharmacol. Toxicol.*, **1976**, *16*, 309–327.

Mitchell, J. R.; Potter, W. Z.; Hinson, J. A.; and Jollow, D. J. Hepatic necrosis caused by furosemide. *Nature*, **1974**, *251*, 508–511.

Mudge, G. H.; Cooke, W. J.; and Berndt, W. P. Electrolyte excretion and free-water production during onset of acute diuresis. *Am. J. Physiol.*, **1975**, *228*, 1304–1312.

Muth, R. G. Diuretics in chronic renal insufficiency. In, *Modern Diuretic Therapy in the Treatment of Cardiovascular and Renal Disease.* (Lant, A. F., and Wilson, G. M., eds.) Excerpta Medica, Amsterdam, **1973**, pp. 294–305.

Østergaard, E. H.; Magnussen, M. P.; Nielsen, C. K.; Eilertsen, E.; and Frey, H.-H. Pharmacological properties of 3-*n*-butylamino-4-phenoxy-5-sulfamylbenzoic acid (bumetanide), a new potent diuretic. *Arzneim. Forsch.*, **1972**, *22*, 66–72.

Prandota, J., and Pruitt, A. W. Furosemide binding to human albumin and plasma of nephrotic children. *Clin. Pharmacol. Ther.*, **1975**, *17*, 159–166.

Prockop, L. D. The pharmacology of increased intracranial pressure. In, *Clinical Neuropharmacology.* (Klawans, H. L., ed.) Raven Press, New York, **1976**, pp. 147–171.

Rose, H. J.; Pruitt, A. W.; Dayton, P. G.; and McNay, J. L. Relationship of urinary furosemide excretion rate to natriuretic effect in experimental azotemia. *J. Pharmacol. Exp. Ther.*, **1976**, *199*, 490–497.

Schultz, E. M.; Cragoe, E. J., Jr.; Bicking, J. B.; Bolhofer, W. A.; and Sprague, J. A. Alpha, beta-unsaturated ketone derivatives of aryloxyacetic acids, a new class of diuretics. *J. Med. Pharm. Chem.*, **1962**, *5*, 660–662.

Sellers, E. M., and Koch-Weser, J. Displacement of warfarin from human albumin by diazoxide and ethacrynic, mefenamic, and nalidixic acids. *Clin. Pharmacol. Ther.*, **1970**, *11*, 524–529.

Stoner, L. C., and Trimble, M. E. Effects of MK-196 and furosemide on rat medullary thick ascending limbs of Henle *in vitro*. *J. Pharmacol. Exp. Ther.*, **1982**, *221*, 715–720.

Suki, W. N.; Yium, J. J.; Von Minden, M.; Saller-Hebert, C.; Eknoyan, G.; and Martinez-Maldonado, M. Acute treatment of hypercalcemia with furosemide. *N. Engl. J. Med.*, **1970**, *283*, 836–840.

Wales, J. K.; Krees, S. V.; Grant, A. M.; Viktora, J. K.; and Wolff, F. W. Structure-activity relationships of benzothiadiazine compounds as hyperglycemic agents. *J. Pharmacol. Exp. Ther.*, **1968**, *164*, 421–432.

Weinman, E. J.; Knight, T. F.; McKenzie, R.; and Eknoyan, G. Dissociation of urate from sodium transport in the rat proximal tubule. *Kidney Int.*, **1976**, *10*, 295–300.

Wiebelhaus, V. D.; Brennan, F. T.; Sosnowski, G.; Maass, A. R.; Weinstock, J.; and Bender, A. D. The natriuretic and diuretic characteristics of triamterene in the dog. *Arch. Int. Pharmacodyn. Ther.*, **1967**, *169*, 429–451.

Wills, M. R.; Gill, J. R., Jr.; and Bartter, F. C. The interrelationships of calcium and sodium excretions. *Clin. Sci.*, **1969**, *37*, 621–630.

Yendt, E. R., and Cohanim, M. Prevention of calcium stones with thiazides. *Kidney Int.*, **1978**, *13*, 397–409.

Monographs and Reviews

Baer, J. E., and Beyer, K. H. Subcellular pharmacology of natriuretic and potassium-sparing drugs. *Prog. Biochem. Pharmacol.*, **1972**, *7*, 59–93.

Beermann, B., and Groschinsky-Grind, M. Clinical pharmacokinetics of diuretics. *Clin. Pharmacokinet.*, **1980**, *5*, 221–245.

Benos, D. J. Amiloride: a molecular probe of sodium transport in tissues and cells. *Am. J. Physiol.*, **1982**, *242*, C131–C145.

Beyer, K. H., and Baer, J. E. Physiological basis for the action of newer diuretic agents. *Pharmacol. Rev.*, **1961**, *13*, 517–562.

Brater, D. C. Pharmacodynamic considerations in the use of diuretics. *Annu. Rev. Pharmacol. Toxicol.*, **1983**, *23*, 45–62.

Corvol, P.; Claire, M.; Oblin, M. E.; Geering, K.; and Rossier, B. Mechanism of the antimineralocorticoid effects of spirolactones. *Kidney Int.*, **1981**, *20*, 1–6.

Cragoe, E. J., Jr. (ed.). *Diuretics: Chemistry, Pharmacology, and Medicine.* John Wiley & Sons, Inc., New York, **1983**.

Flamenbaum, W., and Friedman, R. Pharmacology, therapeutic efficacy, and adverse effects of bumetanide, a new "loop" diuretic. *Pharmacotherapy*, **1982**, *2*, 213–222.

Giebisch, G.; Malnic, G.; and Berliner, R. W. Renal transport and control of potassium excretion. In, *The Kidney*, 2nd ed., Vol. 1. (Brenner, B. M., and Rector, F. C., Jr., eds.) W. B. Saunders Co., Philadelphia, **1981**, pp. 408–439.

Grantham, J. J., and Edwards, R. M. Natriuretic hormones: at last, bottled in bond? *J. Lab. Clin. Med.*, **1984**, *103*, 333–336.

Koechel, D. A. Ethacrynic acid and related diuretics: relationship of structure to beneficial and detrimental actions. *Annu. Rev. Pharmacol. Toxicol.*, **1981**, *21*, 265–293.

Liddle, G. W. Aldosterone antagonists and triamterene. *Ann. N.Y. Acad. Sci.*, **1966**, *139*, 466–470.

Maren, T. H. Carbonic anhydrase: chemistry, physiology, and inhibition. *Physiol. Rev.*, **1967**, *47*, 595–781.

Perez-Stable, E., and Caralis, P. V. Thiazide-induced disturbances in carbohydrate, lipid, and potassium metabolism. *Am. Heart J.*, **1983**, *106*, 245–251.

Reineck, H. J., and Stein, J. H. Mechanisms of action and clinical uses of diuretics. In, *The Kidney*, 2nd ed., Vol. 1. (Brenner, B. M., and Rector, F. C., Jr., eds.) W. B. Saunders Co., Philadelphia, **1981**, pp. 1097–1131.

Rybak, L. P. Pathophysiology of furosemide ototoxicity. *J. Otolaryngol.*, **1982**, *11*, 127–133.

Strewler, G. J., and Orloff, J. The role of cyclic nucleotides in the transport of water and electrolytes. *Adv. Cyclic Nucleotide Res.*, **1977**, *8*, 311–361.

Tiller, D. J., and Mudge, G. H. Pharmacologic agents used in the management of acute renal failure. *Kidney Int.*, **1980**, *18*, 700–711.

Warnock, D. G., and Rector, F. C., Jr. Renal acidification mechanisms. In, *The Kidney*, 2nd ed., Vol. 1. (Brenner, B. M., and Rector, F. C., Jr., eds.) W. B. Saunders Co., Philadelphia, **1981**, pp. 440–494.

37 AGENTS AFFECTING THE RENAL CONSERVATION OF WATER

Richard M. Hays

ANTIDIURETIC HORMONE

Evolutionary Considerations. The earliest forms of life in the Cambrian sea had little concern with water balance. They were probably close to equilibrium with their environment with respect to both its osmolality and its ionic composition. With time, however, the environment changed; the salinity of the oceans increased manyfold, and, at the same time, fresh-water lakes and rivers formed. Primitive marine forms, such as the hagfish, simply maintained equilibrium with sea water. More imaginative species, notably the fish, employed their gills as well as their kidneys to retain their extracellular fluid near its original Cambrian composition. Salt-water species developed efficient pumps for sodium chloride in the gill, as well as renal pumps for magnesium and sulfate to excrete these ions. Fresh-water forms, threatened by salt loss, made the opposite adaptation and developed the capacity to reabsorb sodium chloride across their gills. Those species that alternate between fresh and salt water as part of their life cycle acquired the ability to switch their gill transport systems from salt reabsorption to salt secretion.

Although gill-mediated salt transport was the primary mechanism for the regulation of volume, *vasotocin,* the evolutionary precursor of the antidiuretic peptides, was already present in the central nervous system (CNS) of the early aquatic species. Its role in fish is not completely understood, but includes such actions as modification of blood flow through the gill and control of glomerular filtration rate.

With the emergence of life on land, antidiuretic hormone (ADH) became the mediator of a remarkable regulatory system for the conservation of water. ADH is released by the posterior pituitary under conditions of water deprivation (when plasma osmolality is elevated) or when extracellular volume is depleted (irrespective of the level of plasma osmolality). In amphibia, the target organs for ADH are skin and the urinary bladder; in other vertebrates, including man, the site of action is the renal collecting duct. In each of these target tissues, ADH acts by increasing the permeability of the cell membrane to water, thus permitting water to move passively down an osmotic gradient across skin, bladder, or collecting duct into the extracellular compartment.

In view of the long evolutionary history of the hormone, it is not surprising that ADH acts at sites in the nephron other than the collecting duct and on tissues other than the kidney. It is a potent vasopressor; indeed, the name *vasopressin* was originally chosen on the basis of its vasoconstrictor action. It is a neurotransmitter, and, among its actions in the CNS, it appears to play a role in the secretion of adrenocorticotropic hormone (ACTH) and in the regulation of circulation, temperature, and other visceral functions. ADH is also believed to promote the release of coagulation factors by the vascular endothelium. These renal and nonrenal actions of ADH will be discussed in this chapter.

Chemistry. duVigneaud and coworkers (1953, 1954) determined the structures of ADH and oxytocin and accomplished the complete synthesis of each. This was an unprecedented achievement at a time when the synthesis of even small peptides required years of effort, and duVigneaud was awarded the Nobel Prize in 1955. Studies in his laboratory established principles of the structure-activity relationship that underlie much of the current effort to design peptides for therapeutic purposes. The structures of 8-arginine vasopressin (the neurohypophyseal peptide found in all mammals except swine), 8-lysine vasopressin (*lypressin,* the swine peptide), and oxytocin (the oxytocic and milk-ejecting peptide, *see* Chapter 39) are shown in Table 37–1. All are nonapeptides with two cysteine residues forming a bridge between positions 1 and 6. Integrity of the disulfide bond is essential for biological activity, and amino acid substitutions dictate specific physiological actions. Thus, a basic amino acid residue in position 8 confers antidiuretic activity, while isoleucine in position 3 promotes oxytocic activity.

The natural hormones are subjected to rapid enzymatic degradation *in vivo.* Four sites of cleavage have been identified, the most important of which appear to be at positions 7–8 and 8–9 in the linear portion of the peptide; the disulfide bond and position 1–2 are also sites of modification by a variety of enzymes in kidney, brain, liver, and uterus (*see* Walter and Simmons, 1977). The kidney and liver are the major sites of metabolic clearance.

The development of technics for solid-phase peptide synthesis made it possible to synthesize and screen great numbers of analogs of ADH, and, in 1967, Zaoral and coworkers announced the synthesis of 1-deamino-8-D-arginine vasopressin (dDAVP, *desmopressin;* Table 37–1), now the preferred drug for the treatment of ADH-sensitive diabetes insipidus (Zaoral *et al.,* 1967). Deamination at position 1 renders the molecule less subject to the action of

Table 37–1. CHEMICAL STRUCTURES AND ACTIVITIES OF NATIVE AND SYNTHETIC ANTIDIURETIC PEPTIDES

	ACTIVITY * (Relative to Arginine Vasopressin)	
	Antidiuretic	*Pressor*

Native Peptides

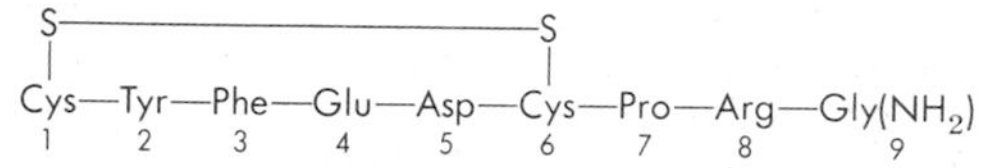

```
S————————————S
|            |
Cys—Tyr—Phe—Glu—Asp—Cys—Pro—Arg—Gly(NH₂)
 1   2   3   4   5   6   7   8    9
```
8-Arginine Vasopressin
(ADH, AVP; mammals)

100	100

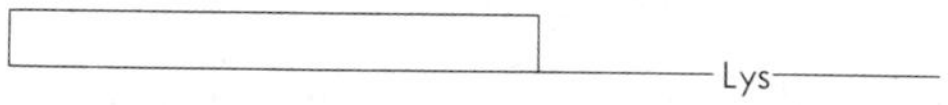

```
┌──────────────┐
│              │————Lys————
```
8-Lysine Vasopressin
(lypressin, LVP; swine)

80	60

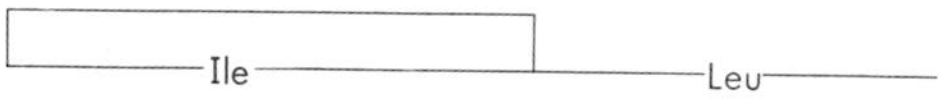

```
┌──────────────┐
│      Ile     │————Leu————
```
Oxytocin

1	1

Synthetic Antidiuretic Peptide

```
    S————————————┐
    |            │
H—C—H           │
    |            │
H—C—H           │
    |            │
O=C—————————————D-Arg————
```
1-Deamino-8-D-Arginine Vasopressin
(desmopressin, dDAVP)

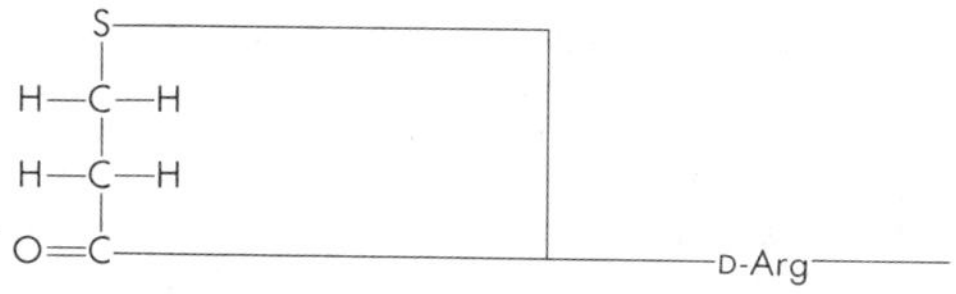

1200	0.39

Synthetic ADH Antagonists

Analogs

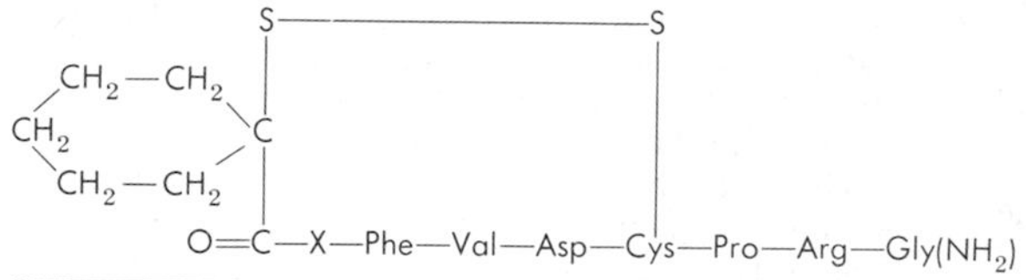

```
        S————————————S
        |            |
CH₂—CH₂ |            |
|      C|            |
CH₂     |            |
|      /|            |
CH₂—CH₂ |            |
        |            |
    O=C—X—Phe—Val—Asp—Cys—Pro—Arg—Gly(NH₂)
```

1. X † = D-Tyr
2. X   = O-Ethyl-tyr
3. X   = D-Phe
4. X   = D-Ile

* Assayed in the rat.

† X refers to substituent shown in position 2 of structure to the left.

peptidases; it is this resistance to degradation that is the most important factor in the superior antidiuretic activity of desmopressin. The substitution of D- for L-arginine in position 8 sharply decreases pressor activity and thus greatly increases the ratio of antidiuretic to pressor effects. Synthetic peptides that have selective pressor activity have also been designed; one example, 2-phenylalanine-8-lysine vasopressin (*felypressin*), is in use in Europe as a vasoconstrictor.

Recently, a series of potent and specific antagonists of the antidiuretic action of ADH has been synthesized (Sawyer and Manning, 1982). Initially, substitution of a β-mercapto-β,β-cyclopentamethylene propionic acid residue at position 1 and O-alkyltyrosine residues at position 2 of 4-valine, 8-arginine vasopressin yielded antagonists that were effective in inhibiting the action of exogenous or endogenous ADH in rats (Sawyer and Manning, 1982; Ishikawa and Schrier, 1983). Two examples (analogs 1 and 2) are shown in Table 37–1. The antagonists were shown to inhibit binding of ADH to its receptor and activation of adenylate cyclase by ADH in membrane preparations from a number of species (Stassen *et al.*, 1982). However, analogs in this initial series retained some antidiuretic agonistic activity and antagonized vasopressor and oxytocic responses. A new series, in which D-amino acids were substituted for tyrosine in position 2 (Table 37–1, analogs 3 and 4), has, in several instances, shown no agonistic activities and greatly reduced antivasopressor and antioxytocic activities (Sawyer and Manning, 1984). The antagonists have the potential of clinical utility in a number of pathological states in which water has accumulated due to the action of ADH.

Antidiuresis in the mammal involves a hypothalamiconeurohypophyseal system for the synthesis, storage, and release of ADH and a renal system for hormonally regulated concentration of the urine. At almost every point, pharmacological agents, as well as disease, can modify the normal chain of events.

Anatomy. The hypothalamiconeurohypophyseal tract is an extended neurosecretory system; the perikarya are located in specific hypothalamic nuclei, and their long axons traverse the supraopticohypophyseal tract to terminate in the median eminence and pars nervosa of the posterior pituitary. Interruption of the tract at any level produces retrograde degeneration of the cell bodies and axons. However, interruption below the level of the median eminence does not result in clinical diabetes insipidus, since axons terminating in the median eminence are spared and secrete adequate amounts of ADH. Lesions above this level generally result in diabetes insipidus.

Synthesis. In man, ADH and oxytocin are synthesized primarily at two hypothalamic sites: the supraoptic and paraventricular nuclei. However, studies with antisera to ADH have identified sites of synthesis outside these two major nuclei (Rhodes *et al.*, 1981). There is good evidence that ADH and oxytocin are synthesized predominantly in separate neurons.

Synthesis itself occurs in the perikaryon of the neuron and appears to follow the pattern established for many hormones. Thus, a relatively large and biologically inactive precursor (prohormone) containing ADH, a neurophysin (proteins that bind ADH and oxytocin), and a glycopeptide is synthesized on ribosomes; incorporated into large (0.1 to 0.3 μm), membrane-enclosed granules; and then split into several moieties (ADH-neurophysin, intact and truncated glycopeptides) during the movement of the granules from the perikaryon down the axon to their storage position in the terminal bulbs of the axons (*see* Brownstein, 1983; North *et al.*, 1983).

Transport and Storage. The process of axonal transport of the granules is relatively rapid; newly synthesized neurohypophyseal hormones arrive at the posterior lobe within 30 minutes of a stimulus such as hemorrhage. The axons involved in transport of granules may be of two types, carrying vasopressin and neurophysins not only to the classical terminations in the neurohypophysis but also to the external zone of the median eminence, where they may enter the adenohypophyseal portal circulation and play a role as corticotropin-releasing factors (*see* Zimmerman *et al.*, 1977; *see also* below). Once the granules have arrived at the bulbous axonal terminations, they are stored until the need for secretion.

Secretion. Much of our current understanding of the secretion of ADH comes from the morphological studies of Douglas and associates (Douglas, 1973) and from technics for the study of the hypothalamiconeurohypophyseal system in organ culture (*see* Sladek and Knigge, 1977). Briefly, the neurosecretory system functions as a conventional neuron. Incoming impulses from osmoreceptors, higher cerebral centers, vascular baroreceptors, and other sites converge on the nerve bodies in the supraventricular or paraventricular nuclei. Stimulation leads to depolarization of the nerve membrane, which is propagated to the terminal bulb. The resultant influx of Ca^{2+} promotes fusion of granules with the membrane of the bulb and exocytosis of the granular contents. Neurophysins, as well as ADH or oxytocin, are released.

Physiological Stimuli for the Secretion of ADH. The two principal physiological stimuli for the secretion of ADH are an increase in plasma osmolality and a decrease in extracellular volume. Other stimuli include pain, nausea, and hypoxia.

Hyperosmolality. The classical experiments of Verney (1947) showed that an increase of less than 2% in the osmolality of blood perfusing the hypothalamus produced a sharp antidiuresis in dogs. Antidiuresis was stimulated by hypertonic saline or sucrose solution, but not by hypertonic urea, suggesting that actual osmotic shrinkage of some receptor cell was necessary. This concept of an "osmoreceptor" that communicates with the nerve bodies is still retained by physiologists; current candidates for the osmoreceptor include the organum vasculosum of the lamina terminalis and the subfornical organ; both of these structures lack a blood-brain barrier (Andersson, 1978).

The pattern of secretion of ADH in response to hyperosmolality is shown in Figure 37–1, *A*. The threshold for secretion is approximately 280 mOsm/kg; below this level, ADH is barely detectable in plasma. Above threshold, the concentration of ADH in plasma rises rapidly as osmolality increases. Patients with fully developed ADH-sensitive diabetes insipidus are unable to increase the rate of secretion of ADH, while patients with partial disease show a range of concentrations in plasma. Subjects with nephrogenic diabetes insipidus (failure of the kidney to respond to ADH) or psychogenic polydipsia secrete ADH normally in response to hyperosmolality.

There is also evidence for a direct functional interplay between the neural centers that regulate thirst and those that control the secretion of ADH. Drinking appears to suppress ADH secretion before there is any decrease in plasma osmolality.

Volume Depletion. The second major stimulus for the secretion of ADH is depletion of extracellular fluid volume. Hemorrhage, sodium depletion, or other acute causes of reduction of extracellular volume, irrespective of plasma osmolality, produce a discharge of ADH into the circulation. Secretion occurs from what appears to be a readily releasable

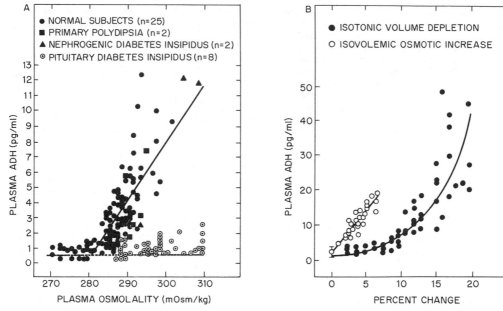

Figure 37–1. *Patterns of secretion of ADH.*

A. Effect of osmolality on the concentration of ADH in plasma. (After Robertson, Mahr, Athar, and Sinha, 1973. Courtesy of *Journal of Clinical Investigation.*)

B. Comparison of the effects of an increase in osmolality and a decrease in extracellular volume (both expressed as percent change) on the concentration of ADH in plasma. (After Dunn, Brennan, Nelson, and Robertson, 1973. Courtesy of *Journal of Clinical Investigation.*)

"pool" of hormone, representing about 10 to 20% of the total ADH in the gland. Subsequent release takes place at a considerably slower rate. In addition to these acute stimuli, more chronic conditions in which effective circulating volume is reduced (*e.g.,* cardiac failure, hepatic cirrhosis with ascites, adrenal insufficiency, hypothyroidism, and excessive use of diuretics) may also be associated with abnormally high concentrations of ADH in plasma.

The receptors that mediate this type of release differ completely from those involved in the response to hyperosmolarity. They include the baroreceptors of the left atrium and pulmonary veins, as well as those in the carotid sinus and aorta. Impulses from these receptors are relayed to the hypothalamus via afferent pathways in the vagus and the glossopharyngeal nerves. Secretion of ADH is believed to be under tonic inhibitory control by the baroreceptors, so that hormone is released when blood pressure falls and release is inhibited when blood pressure rises. Secretion in response to hypoxia, nausea, and pain may also be mediated by baroreceptors in the aortic arch and carotid sinus (Sklar and Schrier, 1983).

The pattern of release of ADH during volume depletion in the rat is shown in Figure 37–1, *B.* Isotonic contraction of volume causes little change in plasma ADH until the loss approaches 10%, after which concentrations of ADH increase exponentially. This response eventually exceeds that of hypertonicity. The resultant concentrations of

ADH are high enough to exert a direct pressor effect on arterioles and may help to maintain blood pressure under such conditions.

Other Mediators of ADH Secretion. There is now a large and often contradictory literature on mediators of ADH secretion in the CNS. The problem of evaluating the action of a given agent in the CNS is made difficult by simultaneous peripheral actions of many agents, which may trigger baroceptor responses, and by the increasing recognition that neurotransmission may involve multiple, rather than single agents at synaptic sites (Swanson, 1983). Agents for which there is good evidence for a stimulatory action include dopamine, angiotensin II, prostaglandins, and endogenous opioids; inhibitors include gamma-aminobutyric acid. (*See* Sklar and Schrier, 1983, for a detailed review.) Of the agents listed, a few deserve comment.

Angiotensin II is a potent dipsogen, and there is evidence that it plays a role in thirst related to volume depletion. Angiotensin II can be synthesized in the brain, as well as peripherally, and is thought to be a neurotransmitter. There has been a long-standing controversy over the role of angiotensin II in secretion of ADH. Circulating angiotensin II has not been shown consistently to stimulate ADH secretion in hydrated animals; however, it does appear to do so under conditions of dehydration (Claybaugh, 1976). There is evidence, again controversial, that angiotensin II mediates release of

ADH in response to volume depletion in uremic patients (Benmansour *et al.*, 1980). Nevertheless, angiotensin II can produce calcium-dependent secretion of ADH in cultures of hypothalamico-neurohypophyseal tissue from the rat (Ishikawa and Schrier, 1983). In addition, angiotensin II can be detected immunocytochemically in magnocellular neurons of the supraoptic and paraventricular nuclei; in most instances it is localized in the same cell bodies that contain ADH (Kilcoyne *et al.*, 1980). Thus, angiotensin II may be a mediator of ADH secretion under certain conditions, either at a central site, via the circulation, or both.

There is an elaborate system of *endogenous opioids* within the mammalian brain (*see* Chapters 12 and 22). Evidence exists for both inhibitory and stimulatory effects of leu-enkephalin on the secretion of ADH (Sklar and Schrier, 1983). *Prostaglandins* may play a role in both the osmotic (Ishikawa *et al.*, 1981) and the nonosmotic (Sklar and Schrier, 1983) secretion of ADH.

Pharmacological Agents and the Secretion of ADH. A number of pharmacological agents alter the osmolality of urine, and, in many cases, it has been hypothesized that their action involves stimulation or inhibition of the secretion of ADH. Direct renal effects may be present as well; this complicates interpretation of mechanism of action (*see* Hays and Levine, 1981).

Stimulators. These include *vincristine, vinblastine, cyclophosphamide, clofibrate, tricyclic antidepressants, carbamazepine, nicotine,* and *colchicine.* Diuretics, notably the *loop diuretics* and the *thiazides,* may produce hyponatremia if administered chronically. Secretion of ADH, mediated by baroreceptors in response to volume depletion, and intrinsic renal mechanisms contribute to retention of water. Diuretics are probably the most common causes of hyponatremia.

Inhibitors. Ethanol and *phenytoin* inhibit the secretion of ADH. Both *mineralocorticoids* and *glucocorticoids* exert an inhibitory role, but for different reasons. Mineralocorticoids are essential for the maintenance of normal extracellular volume; their absence results in volume depletion and baroreceptor-mediated secretion of ADH. Glucocorticoids may inhibit secretion of ADH by a central action, but they may also reduce cardiac stroke volume, triggering secretion of ADH mediated by baroreceptors (*see* Schrier and Bichet, 1981).

Pathophysiology. *ADH-Sensitive Diabetes Insipidus.* ADH-sensitive diabetes insipidus, also referred to as central or neurogenic diabetes insipidus, results from the failure to secrete adequate quantities of ADH. The result is polyuria and the excretion of a dilute urine (specific gravity, 1.001 to 1.005). Any lesion that interrupts the supraopticoneurohypophyseal system and reduces the secretion of ADH to levels that are less than approximately 7% of normal will produce clinically apparent diabetes insipidus. Trauma or surgery in the region of the pituitary and hypothalamus, malignancy, and infiltrative lesions are well-recognized causes of this condition; there are also famil-

ial and idiopathic varieties of the disease. Acute, postoperative diabetes insipidus may be transient in nature.

The appropriate diagnosis of ADH-sensitive diabetes insipidus requires differentiation from other causes of polyuria (*e.g.,* diabetes mellitus, various natriuretic syndromes, primary polydipsia, *etc.*). The diagnosis of diabetes insipidus is confirmed by showing that the patient is unable to reduce urine volume and increase urine osmolality after a period of carefully observed fluid deprivation. Finally, it is necessary to distinguish the ADH-sensitive condition from nephrogenic diabetes insipidus (failure of the kidney to respond to ADH) by administration of the hormone. Patients with ADH-sensitive diabetes insipidus show a prompt increase in urine osmolality (to levels significantly above that of plasma) if given vasopressin intravenously (1 ml per minute of a solution containing 5 units per liter of aqueous vasopressin). Patients with nephrogenic diabetes insipidus show little or no response. For a more complete discussion of diagnostic procedures, *see* Hays and Levine (1981).

While the traditional diagnostic approach will differentiate the cause of polyuria in the great majority of patients, it has become clear from direct determination of concentrations of ADH in plasma by radioimmunoassay that incorrect diagnoses can be made (*see* Zerbe and Robertson, 1981).

Nephrogenic Diabetes Insipidus. Nephrogenic diabetes insipidus, a failure of the renal tubule to respond to ADH, has many etiologies. As discussed above, drugs can interfere with the ability to produce a concentrated urine. Renal disease may cause hyposthenuria and polyuria especially when the structure or function of the distal tubule and collecting duct are disproportionately affected. Congenital forms of the disease are also well known, although rare (*see* Hays and Levine, 1981). *Diuretics* are the mainstay of treatment, since exogenous ADH is ineffective (*see* below).

Inappropriate Secretion of ADH. Excessive production of ADH, with resultant retention of water and dilutional hyponatremia, may occur in patients with a variety of tumors or head injuries, meningitis or encephalitis, pulmonary infections, and other diseases. ADH is produced ectopically in the case of tumors and pulmonary disease, or by abnormal stimulation of the hypothalamico-neurohypophyseal system (head injury, meningitis, *etc.*). Concentrations of the hormone may be exceedingly high, as determined by radioimmunoassay, and unresponsive to normal control mechanisms. Drugs that stimulate the secretion of ADH (*e.g.,* vincristine, cyclophosphamide) or that sensitize the kidney to ADH (*e.g.,* chlorpropamide) may also produce abnormal water retention and dilutional hyponatremia.

Action of ADH on the Kidney. Upon release from the pituitary, ADH circulates in the vascular space with a half-time of disappearance of 17 to 35 minutes in the human adult. Several factors are responsible for removal of the hormone from the circulation. Enzymatic cleavage by peptidases has been mentioned above; in addition, there is some binding to receptors on smooth muscle. These receptors, as well as those found on hepatocytes, have been termed V_1 receptors (Michell *et al.*, 1979). Their affinity for ADH is far less than is that of the receptors of the renal distal tubule (V_2 receptors). It is believed that V_1 receptors utilize polyphosphoinositides and Ca^{2+} as second messengers. V_2 receptors interact with adenylate cyclase and stimulate the synthesis of adenosine 3',5'-monophosphate (cyclic AMP) (*see* below). ADH is bound by receptors on the basolateral (nutrient) surface of the cortical and medullary portions of the collecting duct. The critical role of the collecting duct in the conservation of water is described in the Introduction to Section VIII (*see* page 882). By the time tubular fluid arrives at the cortical segment of the collecting duct, it has been rendered hypotonic by the action of the chloride pump of the loop of Henle. In the well-hydrated subject, where concentrations of ADH are low, the entire collecting duct remains relatively impermeable to water; the urine thus remains dilute. A minimal osmolality of 50 mOsm/kg can be achieved, and as much as 15% of the filtered water can escape into the urine, virtually free of electrolytes. Under conditions of dehydration or volume depletion, on the other hand, concentrations of ADH are significantly elevated, and the cortical and medullary segments of the collecting duct become permeable to water. There is an osmotic gradient between the dilute tubular urine and the peritubular interstitial fluid, which becomes more pronounced in the medullary and papillary segments. Water moves passively down this concentration gradient and is reabsorbed from the tubule; the final osmolality of the urine may be as high as 1200 mOsm/kg in man and 4000 mOsm/kg in certain rodents. A significant saving of water is thus possible.

Cellular Action of ADH. The binding of ADH to cellular receptors initiates a sequence of steps that eventually increases the permeability of the opposite (luminal) cell surface to water. The sequence of steps is one of many examples in which cyclic AMP appears to serve as the intracellular mediator of the actions of a hormone on its target cell. ADH activates adenylate cyclase at the basolateral membrane, with resultant accumulation of cyclic AMP intracellularly. Cyclic AMP, in turn, initiates a series of events that ultimately increases the permeability of the luminal membrane. The exact nature of these events and their relationship to one another are not completely understood. However, the following is hypothesized: (1) a cyclic AMP–dependent protein kinase is activated; (2) a phosphoprotein phosphatase may also be activated; (3) microtubules and microfilaments appear to be important in the initiation and maintenance of the action of ADH (Taylor, 1977); and (4) aggregates of membrane-associated proteins appear on the luminal membrane surface. These aggregates were first described in freeze-fracture electron micrographic studies by Chevalier and associates (1974), and a series of observations has established their role in the movement of water across the membrane. Water may move through narrow protein-associated channels that are close to the size of the water molecule and can exclude solutes even as small as urea (Rosenberg and Finkelstein, 1978; Carvounis *et al.*, 1979). The aggregates are components of cytoplasmic vesicles that become inserted into the luminal membrane in response to ADH by a process that resembles exocytosis (Wade, 1980). The changes in the cell membrane induced by ADH have been reviewed (Hays, 1983).

Endogenous Modulators of the Renal Response. Prostaglandins appear to be important inhibitors of the renal response to ADH. The extent to which ADH increases prostaglandin synthesis, thereby limiting its hydroosmotic action, is not yet established (*see* Zusman *et al.*, 1977a; Bisordi *et al.*, 1980). Another system that appears to modulate the renal response is the kallikrein-kinin system, which inhibits ADH-stimulated water flow in the amphibian bladder (Carvounis *et al.*, 1981).

Other Renal Sites of ADH Action. ADH has recently been shown to exert important effects on the glomerulus and on the thick ascending limb of the loop of Henle. ADH decreases the glomerular ultrafiltration coefficient (Brenner, 1983), possibly by inducing contraction of glomerular mesangial cells (Ausiello *et al.*, 1980). ADH also stimulates active reabsorption of NaCl by the medullary thick ascending limb (Hall and Varney, 1980). The latter action augments the effect of ADH on the permeability of the collecting duct to water by increasing the tonicity of the medullary interstitial fluid; this provides a more favorable osmotic gradient for reabsorption of water.

Pharmacological Agents That Modify the Renal Response to ADH. *Chlorpropamide, acetaminophen,* and *indomethacin* enhance the action of ADH. This may be explained in part by inhibition of renal prostaglandin synthesis (*see*, for example, Zusman *et al.*, 1977b). Thus, these agents "sensitize" the kidney to concentrations of ADH that ordinarily would be too low to stimulate reabsorption of water. Kusano and associates (1983) have shown that chlorpropamide stimulates reabsorption of NaCl by the thick ascending limb, an action that would also promote water reabsorption (*see* above).

A number of pharmacological agents inhibit the antidiuretic action of the hormone to the point of producing ADH-resistant polyuria (nephrogenic diabetes insipidus). *Lithium carbonate,* used in the treatment of manic-depressive disorders, can cause a reversible polyuria (*see* Chapter 19). *Methoxyflurane,* an anesthetic now in limited use, causes severe renal failure and associated polyuria, both of which may be irreversible. The antibiotic *demeclocycline* causes defects in the ability of the kidney to produce a concentrated urine in a high percentage of patients and can produce symptomatic polyuria and polydipsia. The ability of demeclocycline to antagonize the action of ADH has been used successfully to promote diuresis in patients with water intoxication due to inappropriate secretion of ADH (Forrest *et al.,* 1978). These and other inhibitory effects have been reviewed by Forrest and Singer (1977).

Nonrenal Actions of ADH. As mentioned, ADH and related peptides are old hormones in evolutionary terms, and they are found in species that have no mechanisms for the concentration of urine. It is thus not surprising that there are actions of ADH in mammals in addition to those on the kidney.

Cardiovascular System. Reference has already been made to the pressor effect of ADH and to evidence that the concentrations of hormone that can be generated in response to volume depletion are high enough to exert a vasoconstrictor effect in man. This occurs only at concentrations that are significantly higher than those required for maximal antidiuresis. The pressor effect of ADH is a general one, and smooth muscle of all parts of the vasculature can be affected. Circulation in the skin and the gastrointestinal tract is markedly reduced. The coronary vessels are not exempt from the vasoconstrictor effects of vasopressin, and pulmonary arterial pres-

sure also rises. Given the vasoconstrictor effects of ADH, it is not surprising that there have been numerous studies of its role in the maintenance of vascular tone and in human hypertension. ADH may indeed be important in the maintenance of vascular tone. Dogs with diabetes insipidus, for example, have an impaired ability to maintain blood pressure following blood loss (Frieden and Keller, 1954); more recent studies have also supported this view (Schwartz and Reid, 1981). However, the evidence for a role of ADH in human hypertension is very tenuous. Elevation of ADH secretion has been observed in some patients with essential hypertension, but neither the level of secretion nor the vascular sensitivity to ADH has appeared to be sufficient to explain the condition (*see* Share and Crofton, 1984).

The effects of vasopressin on the *heart* are indirect and are the result of decreased coronary blood flow and of reflexly induced alterations in vagal and sympathetic tone.

The effects of ADH on the coronary blood flow can readily be demonstrated in man, especially if large doses are employed. In patients with coronary insufficiency, ECG changes similar to those seen after exercise can be observed. The cardiac actions of the hormone are of more than academic interest. Some patients with coronary insufficiency experience anginal pain even in response to the relatively small amounts of ADH required to control diabetes insipidus. ADH-induced myocardial ischemia has led to severe reactions and even death. This is an important consideration in relation to the use of ADH in the control of gastrointestinal hemorrhage (*see* below).

Other Smooth Muscle. The stimulatory effects of ADH on smooth muscle also occur in the *enteric tract.* The response is elicited only by large doses. The smooth muscle of the *uterus* is stimulated by large doses of ADH at all stages of the menstrual cycle and during gestation.

Blood Coagulation. An unexpected action of ADH and its analogs was described by Mannucci and colleagues (1977), who noted that ADH or desmopressin was effective in the management of moderately severe hemophilia and von Willebrand's disease. Both peptides increase the level of factor VIII, possibly by stimulating its release from the vascular endothelium. ADH or desmopressin can thus be administered prophylactically during surgical procedures on such patients to prevent bleeding. Recently, desmopressin was shown to be effective in reducing bleeding time in uremic patients (Mannucci *et al.*, 1983).

Central Nervous System. There is growing recognition of the possible role of ADH as a neurotransmitter. Immunohistochemical studies have shown the existence of vasopressinergic pathways originating in the paraventricular nucleus and going to the forebrain, hindbrain, spinal cord, and (via the median eminence) the hypophyseal portal system and the anterior pituitary (*see* Zimmerman *et al.*, 1984). *Autonomic effects* that may result from the actions of ADH in the CNS include bradycardia, increase in respiratory rate, suppression of fever, and modulation of sleep patterns. Pathways to the brain stem and spinal cord may be involved in the central autonomic regulation of the circulation (Schmid *et al.*, 1984). *Learned behavior* may be influenced by ADH (deWied, 1976), although recent studies have suggested that visceral autonomic effects of ADH, rather than direct modulation of memory processes, may be involved (Gash and Thomas, 1983). *Secretion of ACTH* is enhanced by ADH that arrives at the anterior pituitary via a pathway that secretes the peptide into the hypophyseal portal blood (Zimmerman *et al.*, 1977). However, ADH is not the principal corticotropin-releasing factor (*see* Chapter 59).

Water Circulation in the Brain. ADH introduced into the lateral ventricle of the monkey has been reported to increase the permeability of the brain to water (Raichle and Grubb, 1978). Noto and coworkers (1979) found that ADH and cyclic AMP accelerated diffusion of water across the arachnoid villi in the cat. This observation could be important in our understanding of the regulation of cerebrospinal fluid circulation.

For a discussion of the CNS actions of ADH, *see* Meisenberg and Simmons (1983).

Absorption, Fate, and Excretion. When ADH, lypressin, and their congeners are given orally, they are quickly inactivated by trypsin, which cleaves the 8–9 peptide link. ADH in aqueous solution may be given by the intravenous, intramuscular, or subcutaneous route and by the nasal insufflation of powders or sprays. Due to rapid inactivation by a number of enzymes that cleave the peptide at several sites (*see* above), the effects are brief after intravenous administration unless the hormone is given by continuous infusion. An exception is desmopressin, which is found in the circulation for a prolonged period when absorbed from the nasal mucous membranes. After intramuscular or subcutaneous injection, the effects last only a few hours. Repository forms, such as *vasopressin tannate in oil*, are effective for 24 to 96 hours after intramuscular injection.

The half-life of ADH in the circulation is 17 to 35 minutes, due particularly to inactivation by peptidases in various tissues. The kidney and the liver are of major importance in the removal of ADH from the circulation, accounting for one third to one half of the clearance. In the rat, approximately 50% of the clearance of ADH is apparently by glomerular filtration, and the remainder is removed at peritubular sites beyond the glomerulus (Rabkin *et al.*, 1979). Thus, both the luminal and contraluminal surfaces are exposed to the hormone. Less than 20% of the total ADH removed from the circulation is excreted in the urine, indicating that most of the hormone is degraded within the kidney.

Preparations, Bioassay, and Unitage. ADH is available in two types of preparations. One is an extract in which no separation of the antidiuretic and oxytocic principles has been made. It is assayed for its oxytocic activity, which parallels antidiuretic activity. Activity is compared to that of a USP bovine pituitary standard and is expressed in terms of USP *posterior pituitary units. Posterior pituitary* consists of desiccated posterior pituitary powder that contains approximately 1 USP posterior pituitary unit in each milligram; it is marketed as capsules for inhalation containing 45 units of antidiuretic activity. *Posterior pituitary injection* (PITUITRIN-S) is a sterile aqueous extract of the gland that contains the equivalent of 20 USP posterior pituitary units per milliliter.

Vasopressin injection (PITRESSIN) is prepared from the posterior pituitary glands of domestic animals by separation of ADH from the oxytocic hormone, or by synthesis. It is assayed for pressor activity rather than antidiuretic activity, but these are identical, unit for unit. The test method is the blood pressure of the rat. Activity is designated as *pressor units* and is determined by comparison with a USP standard. Theoretically, there should be no difference in antidiuretic activity between a USP posterior pituitary unit and a USP pressor unit. Vasopressin injection contains 20 pressor units and not more than 1 oxytocic unit per milliliter.

Desmopressin acetate (DDAVP) is marketed as a clear liquid solution containing 0.1 mg/ml of the synthetic peptide. The preparation is available in a screw-top vial containing 2.5 ml; it includes an applicator tube for intranasal administration. A solution for injection is also marketed.

Lypressin (DIAPID) is available as a nasal spray containing 0.185 mg/ml, equivalent to 50 USP posterior pituitary units (pressor) per milliliter. One spray into a nostril provides approximately 2 pressor units.

Vasopressin tannate (PITRESSIN TANNATE IN OIL) is a water-insoluble tannate of the antidiuretic principle. It is marketed suspended in peanut oil. Each milliliter contains 5 pressor units.

THERAPEUTIC USES

The actions of ADH on the kidney and the circulation provide the basis for therapeutic applications of the hormone. ADH is also used in the control of certain bleeding disorders.

Antidiuretic Action. Once the diagnosis of ADH-sensitive diabetes insipidus has been made, the administration of vasopressin provides effective and immediate therapy, with reduction of urine volume to normal. With the exception of patients who experience transient diabetes insipidus as a result of head injury or surgery in the area of the pituitary, therapy is lifelong. Until relatively recently, the principal mode of therapy was intramuscular administration of *vasopressin tannate*. Desmopressin, administered intranasally, has now become the drug of choice.

Numerous clinical trials (*see* Cobb *et al.*, 1978) have confirmed the initial reports that *desmopressin* is an effective agent in both adults and children and has few side effects. The duration of effect from a single intranasal dose is from 6 to 20 hours, and twice-daily administration has proven to be effective in the majority of patients. There is considerable variability in the dose of desmopressin required to maintain normal urine volume (2.5 to 20 μg twice daily), and the dosage must be tailored to the needs of the individual patient. In view of the high cost of the drug and the importance of avoiding water intoxication, it has been suggested that the schedule of administration be adjusted to determine the minimal amount required (Cobb *et al.*, 1978). An initial dose of 2.5 μg can be used, and therapy should first be directed toward the control of nocturia. An equivalent or higher morning dose controls daytime polyuria in most patients, although a third dose may occasionally be needed in the afternoon. Resistance to desmopressin may develop (Cobb *et al.*, 1978). Administration of more than 40 to 50 μg may cause headache.

Vasopressin tannate in oil suspension was the standard therapy for vasopressin-sensitive diabetes insipidus, and this preparation is still useful for the treatment of patients who are refractory to desmopressin or who experience significant side effects. Given as an intramuscular injection (2 to 5 units every 2 or 3 days), it produces a satisfactory antidiuresis in virtually all patients. Care must be used in preparing the ampul for use; it should be warmed in the hand and mixed until the hormone is distributed in the solution. In view of the inconvenience of intramuscular injection and its side effects (*see* below), vasopressin tannate is less desirable than desmopressin, especially in children.

Vasopressin injection, the aqueous form of ADH, has no place in the chronic therapy of diabetes insipidus. Given intramuscularly, its rate of absorption and its duration of action are unpredictable. Given intravenously, it has two uses: in the initial diagnostic evaluation of patients with suspected diabetes insipidus and to control polyuria in the patient with diabetes insipidus who has experienced recent surgery (*e.g.*, hypophysectomy) or head trauma. Under these circumstances polyuria may be transient, and long-acting agents may produce water intoxication.

Lypressin, synthetic lysine vasopressin administered as a nasal spray, produces antidiuresis if administered approximately every 4 hours. Its short duration of action limits its effectiveness, especially in cases of severe diabetes insipidus.

Pressor Action. Despite its name, *vasopressin should not be employed as a pressor agent*. If it is desired to produce systemic peripheral vasoconstriction, preference should be given to appropriate sympathomimetic amines that can increase peripheral resistance without reducing coronary blood flow. However, justifiable exception may be made for the use of vasopressin as an adjunct in the control of bleeding *esophageal varices* and during abdominal surgery in patients with portal hypertension. When large doses (20 units in 5 minutes) are infused in normal subjects or in patients with cirrhosis and portal hypertension, there is a marked decrease in portal blood flow and pressure lasting approximately 30 minutes (Edmunds and West, 1962). Only a moderate rise in arterial pressure occurs. This effect on portal circulation is attributable to marked splanchnic vasoconstriction. As an alternative to systemic administration, infusion of vasopressin directly into the superior mesenteric artery has been advocated (Nusbaum *et al.*, 1968). Unfortunately and despite many years of experience, there is no uniform agreement about the effectiveness of such treatment, especially in the case of intravenous administration (Fogel *et al.*, 1982). Simultaneous administration of nitroglycerin has been reported to reverse the cardiotoxic effects, while enhancing the beneficial splanchnic effects of vasopressin (Groszmann *et al.*, 1982).

Bleeding Disorders. Reference has been made above to the unexpected action of ADH and desmopressin in von Willebrand's disease and moderately severe hemophilia (Mannucci *et al.*, 1977). The beneficial effect of the peptides appears to be related to an increase in factor-VIII activity.

Untoward Reactions and Contraindications. Following the injection of large doses of vasopressin, marked facial pallor as a result of cutaneous vasoconstriction is commonly observed. Increased intestinal activity is likely to cause nausea, belching, cramps, and an urge to defecate. Women are apt to experience uterine cramps of a menstrual character. Most serious, however, is the effect on the coronary circulation. Individuals suffering from vascular disease, especially disease of the coronary arteries, should never receive vasopressin, except in the small doses needed for the treatment of diabetes insipidus. Sometimes even these small doses may cause myocardial ischemia. Other cardiac complications include arrhythmias and decreased cardiac output. Peripheral vasoconstriction and gangrene have been encountered in patients receiving large doses of vasopressin.

When posterior pituitary powder is applied to the nasal mucosa, local irritation is common and hypersensitivity reactions may occur. Allergic reactions, ranging from urticaria to anaphylaxis, may also occur in patients receiving vasopressin.

Complications of the administration of vasopressin tannate include sterile abscesses and abdominal pain. Many of the untoward effects described above are not encountered with desmopressin, although headache and elevations of blood pressure may occur in patients taking large (40-μg) doses of the drug (Cobb et al., 1978). As mentioned, there is a possibility of water intoxication with the use of any of these antidiuretic agents.

BENZOTHIADIAZIDES

Chlorothiazide and other benzothiadiazide (thiazide) diuretics paradoxically cause a reduction in the polyuria of patients with diabetes insipidus (Crawford and Kennedy, 1959). Their clinical use for this purpose is now well established. Other potent natriuretic agents, such as ethacrynic acid, have also been successfully employed.

Since effective agents are available for the treatment of ADH-sensitive diabetes insipidus, the principal use of the thiazide diuretics is in the treatment of the ADH-resistant (nephrogenic) disease. Here, the change from a copious polyuria to the excretion of a smaller volume of urine can reduce or eliminate the handicap of the patient in the pursuit of daily activities. In infants with diabetes insipidus resistant to ADH, the antidiuretic effect may be of more crucial importance since the uncontrolled polyuria may exceed the child's capacity to imbibe and absorb fluids.

The mechanism of the antidiuretic effect is not yet completely understood. Most investigators agree that the natriuretic action of the thiazides

plays an important role and that depletion of salt is essential for antidiuresis. Under these conditions, there is excessive reabsorption of sodium chloride in the proximal tubule, with resultant reduction of volume delivered to the distal tubule. Consequently, less free water can be formed, and the polyuria is diminished (see DeFronzo and Thier, 1981).

Therapeutic Use. Chlorothiazide and its congeners are less effective than vasopressin in the treatment of pituitary diabetes insipidus but are useful for patients who experience undesirable side effects or allergic reactions after vasopressin and invaluable for those who have nephrogenic diabetes insipidus. Since their antidiuretic effects appear to parallel their ability to cause natriuresis, they are given in doses similar to those used for the mobilization of edema fluid. Chlorothiazide, 1.0 to 1.5 g, or hydrochlorothiazide, 50 to 150 mg, in daily divided doses, have been most frequently employed. Reduction of urine volume to 50% or less of pretreatment volumes is considered to be a good response. Moderate restriction of sodium chloride intake has been shown to enhance the antidiuretic effect.

Among the most common of the side effects encountered is potassium depletion. Other untoward effects of the thiazides are described in Chapter 36, as are the chemistry, pharmacology, and preparations of these agents.

OTHER DRUGS

Chlorpropamide, an oral hypoglycemic agent, is effective in reducing polyuria in patients with ADH-sensitive diabetes insipidus (Arduino et al., 1966). It appears to sensitize the kidney to the low concentrations of ADH still in circulation in many patients with diabetes insipidus (Ingelfinger and Hays, 1969). It is ineffective in patients with a total absence of ADH and, of course, is ineffective in nephrogenic diabetes insipidus. Recent studies (Kusano et al., 1983) have shown that chlorpropamide also stimulates reabsorption of NaCl by the thick ascending limb of the loop of Henle, promoting reabsorption of water as discussed above.

Chlorpropamide impairs free-water excretion, and a number of cases of hyponatremia and water intoxication have resulted from its use. Webster and Bain (1970) reported an average reduction in urine volume of 70% in patients with diabetes insipidus, with urine becoming hypertonic during periods of low fluid intake. The major problem with chlorpropamide therapy is the incidence of hypoglycemic reactions, especially among children; its use is thus not advised (see Webster and Bain, 1970; Cobb et al., 1978). Other agents (e.g., clofibrate) may directly stimulate the secretion of ADH by the pituitary. The untoward effects that accompany the chronic administration of clofibrate should also be considered in those situations in which an oral agent must be employed (see Chapter 34). However, given the availability of desmopressin and the incidence of untoward side effects of agents such as chlorpropamide and clofibrate, the importance of these oral agents has declined (*see* Hays and Levine, 1981).

ADH ANTAGONISTS

Attempts to design a synthetic peptide antagonist to ADH have been discussed above. These agents, when available, may provide relief to patients with water intoxication; they will also provide an important investigative tool for study of the entire spectrum of action of ADH. *Demeclocycline* is effective in producing a water diuresis in patients with water intoxication due to inappropriate secretion of ADH. At a dosage of 600 to 1200 mg per day, demeclocycline restores the concentration of Na^+ in plasma to normal within 5 to 14 days and affords symptomatic relief, according to the report of Forrest and coworkers (1978). Patients with cirrhosis may show a deterioration of renal function when demeclocycline is administered (Oster *et al.*, 1976). Demeclocycline appears to be superior to lithium carbonate in the treatment of inappropriate secretion of ADH.

Arduino, F.; Ferraz, F. P. J.; and Rodrigues, J. Antidiuretic action of chlorpropamide in idiopathic diabetes insipidus. *J. Clin. Endocrinol. Metab.*, **1966**, *26*, 1325–1328.

Ausiello, D. A.; Kreisberg, J. I.; Roy, C.; and Karnovsky, M. J. Contraction of cultured rat glomerular cells of apparent mesangial origin after stimulation with angiotensin II and arginine vasopressin. *J. Clin. Invest.*, **1980**, *65*, 754–760.

Benmansour, M.; Caillens, H.; and Ardaillou, R. The effect of inhibition of angiotensin II synthesis on the response of plasma antidiuretic hormone (ADH) to the osmotic and volume-dependent stimuli in uremic patients. *Nephrologie*, **1980**, *1*, 109–112.

Bisordi, J. E.; Schlondorff, D.; and Hays, R. M. Interaction of vasopressin and prostaglandins in the toad urinary bladder. *J. Clin. Invest.*, **1980**, *66*, 1200–1210.

Brenner, B. M. Control of glomerular function by intrinsic contractile elements: introductory remarks. *Fed. Proc.*, **1983**, *42*, 3045.

Carvounis, C. P.; Carvounis, G.; and Arbeit, L. A. Role of the endogenous kallikrein-kinin system in modulating vasopressin-stimulated water flow and urea permeability in the toad urinary bladder. *J. Clin. Invest.*, **1981**, *67*, 1792–1796.

Carvounis, C. P.; Levine, S. D.; Franki, N.; and Hays, R. M. Membrane pathways for water and solutes in the toad bladder. II. Reflection coefficients of the water and solute channels. *J. Membr. Biol.*, **1979**, *49*, 269–281.

Chevalier, J.; Bourguet, J.; and Hugon, J. S. Membrane associated particles: distribution in frog urinary bladder epithelium at rest and after oxytocin treatment. *Cell Tissue Res.*, **1974**, *152*, 129–140.

Claybaugh, J. R. Effect of dehydration on stimulation of ADH release by heterologous renin infusions in conscious dogs. *Am. J. Physiol.*, **1976**, *231*, 655–660.

Cobb, W. E.; Spare, S.; and Reichlin, S. Neurogenic diabetes insipidus: management with dDAVP (1-desamino-8-D-arginine vasopressin). *Ann. Intern. Med.*, **1978**, *88*, 183–188.

Crawford, J. D., and Kennedy, G. C. Chlorothiazide in diabetes insipidus. *Nature*, **1959**, *183*, 891–892.

DeFronzo, R. A., and Thier, S. O. Inherited disorders of renal tubule function. In, *The Kidney*, 2nd ed. (Brenner, B. M., and Rector, F. C., Jr., eds.) W. B. Saunders Co., Philadelphia, **1981**, pp. 1816–1871.

Dunn, F. L.; Brennan, T. J.; Nelson, A. E.; and Robertson, G. L. The role of blood osmolality and volume in regulating vasopressin secretion in the rat. *J. Clin. Invest.*, **1973**, *52*, 3212–3219.

duVigneaud, V.; Gish, D. T.; and Katsoyannis, P. G. A synthetic preparation possessing biological properties associated with arginine vasopressin. *J. Am. Chem. Soc.*, **1954**, *76*, 4751–4752.

duVigneaud, V.; Ressler, C.; Swan, J. M.; Roberts, C. W.; Katsoyannis, P. G.; and Gordon, S. The synthesis of an octapeptide amide with the hormonal activity of oxytocin. *J. Am. Chem. Soc.*, **1953**, *75*, 4879–4880.

Edmunds, R., and West, S. P. A study of the effect of vasopressin on portal and systemic blood pressure. *Surg. Gynecol. Obstet.*, **1962**, *114*, 458–462.

Fogel, M. R.; Kinauer, C. M.; Andres, L. L.; Mahal, A. S.; Stein, O. E.; Kiemeny, M. J.; Rinki, M. M.; Walter, J. E.; Siegmund, D.; and Gregory, P. B. Continuous intravenous vasopressin in active upper gastrointestinal bleeding. *Ann. Intern. Med.*, **1982**, *96*, 565–569.

Forrest, J. N., Jr.; Cox, M.; Hong, C.; Morrison, G.; Bia, M.; and Singer, I. Superiority of demeclocycline over lithium in the treatment of chronic syndrome of inappropriate antidiuretic hormone. *N. Engl. J. Med.*, **1978**, *298*, 173–177.

Frieden, J., and Keller, D. Decreased resistance to hemorrhage in neurohypophysectomized dogs. *Circ. Res.*, **1954**, *2*, 214–220.

Gash, D. M., and Thomas, G. J. What is the importance of vasopressin in memory processes? *Trends Neurosci.*, **1983**, *6*, 197–198.

Groszmann, R. J.; Kravetz, D.; Bosdch, J.; Glickman, M.; Brunix, J.; Bredfeldt, J.; Conn, H. O.; Rodes, J.; and Storer, E. H. Nitroglycerin improves the hemodynamic response to vasopressin in portal hypertension. *Hepatology*, **1982**, *2*, 757–762.

Hall, D. A., and Varney, D. M. Effect of vasopressin on electrical potential difference and chloride transport in mouse thick ascending limb of Henle's loop. *J. Clin. Invest.*, **1980**, *66*, 792–802.

Ingelfinger, J. R., and Hays, R. M. Evidence that chlorpropamide and vasopressin share a common site of action. *J. Clin. Endocrinol. Metab.*, **1969**, *29*, 738–740.

Ishikawa, S.; Saito, T.; and Yoshida, S. The effect of prostaglandins on the release of arginine vasopressin from the guinea pig hypothalamoneurohypophyseal complex in organ culture. *Endocrinology*, **1981**, *108*, 193–198.

Ishikawa, S., and Schrier, R. W. Role of calcium in osmotic and nonosmotic release of vasopressin from rat organ culture. *Am. J. Physiol.*, **1983**, *244*, R703–R708.

Kilcoyne, M. M.; Hoffman, D. L.; and Zimmerman, E. A. Immunocytochemical localization of angiotensin II and vasopressin in rat hypothalamus; evidence for production in the same neuron. *Clin. Sci.*, **1980**, *59*, 57S–60S.

Kusano, E.; Braun-Werness, D. J.; Keller, M. J.; and Dousa, T. P. Chlorpropamide action on renal concentrating mechanism in rats with hypothalamic diabetes insipidus. *J. Clin. Invest.*, **1983**, *72*, 1298–1313.

Mannucci, P. M.; Pareti, F. I.; Ruggeri, Z. M.; and Capitano, A. 1-Deamino-8-D-arginine vasopressin: a new pharmacological approach to the management of haemophilia and von Willebrand's disease. *Lancet*, **1977**, *1*, 869–872.

Mannucci, P. M.; Remuzzi, G.; Pusineri, F.; Lombardi, R.; Valsecchi, C.; Mecca, G.; and Zimmerman, T. S. Deamino-8-D-arginine vasopressin shortens the bleeding time in uremia. *N. Engl. J. Med.*, **1983**, *308*, 8–12.

Meisenberg, G., and Simmons, W. H. Centrally mediated effects of neurohypophyseal hormones. *Neurosci. Biobehav. Rev.*, **1983**, *7*, 263–280.

Michell, R. H.; Kirk, C. J.; and Billah, M. M. Hormonal stimulation of phosphatidylinositol breakdown with particular reference to the hepatic effects of vasopressin. *Biochem. Soc. Trans.*, **1979**, *7*, 861–865.

North, W. G.; Mitchell, T. I.; and North, G. M. Characteristics of a precursor to vasopressin-associated bovine neurophysin. *FEBS Lett.*, **1983**, *152*, 29–34.

Noto, T.; Nakajima, T.; Jaji, Y.; and Nagawa, Y. Effect of vasopressin and cyclic AMP on water transport at arachnoid villi of cats. *Endocrinol. Jpn.*, **1979**, *26*, 239–244.

Nusbaum, M.; Baum, S.; Kuroda, K.; and Blakemore, W. S. Control of portal hypertension by selective mesenteric arterial drug infusion. *Arch. Surg.*, **1968**, *97*, 1005–1013.

Oster, J. R.; Epstein, M.; and Ulano, H. B. Deterioration of renal function with demeclocycline administration. *Curr. Ther. Res.*, **1976**, *20*, 794–801.

Rabkin, R.; Share, L.; Payne, P. A.; Young, J.; and Crofton, J. The handling of immunoreactive vasopressin by the isolated perfused rat kidney. *J. Clin. Invest.*, **1979**, *63*, 6–13.

Raichle, M. E., and Grubb, R. L. Regulation of brain water permeability by centrally-released vasopressin. *Brain Res.*, **1978**, *143*, 191–194.

Rhodes, C. H.; Morrell, J. I.; and Pfaff, D. W. Immunohistochemical analysis of magnocellular elements in rat hypothalamus: distribution and numbers of cells containing neurophysin, oxytocin, and vasopressin. *J. Comp. Neurol.*, **1981**, *198*, 45–64.

Robertson, G. L.; Mahr, E. A.; Athar, S.; and Sinha, T. Development and clinical application of a new method for the radioimmunoassay of arginine vasopressin in human plasma. *J. Clin. Invest.*, **1973**, *52*, 2340–2352.

Rosenberg, P. A., and Finkelstein, A. Water permeability of gramicidin A–treated lipid bilayer membranes. *J. Gen. Physiol.*, **1978**, *72*, 341–350.

Sawyer, W. H., and Manning, M. The development of vasopressin antagonists. *Fed. Proc.*, **1984**, *43*, 87–90.

Schmid, P. G.; Sharabi, F. M.; Guo, G. B.; Ahbound, F. M.; and Thames, M. D. Vasopressin and oxytocin in the neural control of the circulation. *Fed. Proc.*, **1984**, *43*, 97–102.

Schwartz, J., and Reid, I. A. Effect of vasopressin blockade on blood pressure regulation during hemorrhage in conscious dogs. *Endocrinology*, **1981**, *109*, 1778–1780.

Share, L., and Crofton, J. T. The role of vasopressin in hypertension. *Fed. Proc.*, **1984**, *43*, 103–106.

Sladek, L., and Knigge, M. Osmotic control of vasopressin release by rat hypothalamus—neurohypophysial explants in organ culture. *Endocrinology*, **1977**, *101*, 1834–1838.

Stassen, F. L.; Erickson, R. W.; Huffman, W. F.; Stefankiewicz, J.; Sulat, L.; and Wiebelhaus, V. D. Molecular mechanisms of novel antidiuretic antagonists: analysis of the effects on vasopressin binding and adenylate cyclase activation in animal and human kidney. *J. Pharmacol. Exp. Ther.*, **1982**, *223*, 50–54.

Swanson, L. W. Neuropeptides—new vistas on synaptic transmission. *Trends Neurosci.*, **1983**, *6*, 294–295.

Webster, B., and Bain, J. Antidiuretic effect and complications of chlorpropamide therapy in diabetes insipidus. *J. Clin. Endocrinol. Metab.*, **1970**, *30*, 215–227.

Zaoral, M.; Kole, J.; and Sorm, F. Amino acids and peptides. LXXI. Synthesis of 1-deamino-8-D-aminobutyrine-vasopressin, 1-deamino-8-D-lysine vasopressin, and 1-deamino-8-D-arginine vasopressin. *Coll. Czech. Chem. Commun.*, **1967**, *32*, 1250–1257.

Zerbe, R. L., and Robertson, G. L. A comparison of plasma vasopressin measurements with a standard indirect test in the differential diagnosis of polyuria. *N. Engl. J. Med.*, **1981**, *305*, 1539–1546.

Zimmerman, E. A.; Nilaver, G.; Hou-Yu, A.; and Silverman, A. J. Vasopressinergic and oxytocinergic pathways in the central nervous system. *Fed. Proc.*, **1984**, *43*, 91–96.

Zimmerman, E. A.; Stillman, M. A.; Recht, L. D.; Antures, J. L.; and Carmill, P. W. Vasopressin and corticotropin releasing factor. An axonal pathway to portal capillaries in the zona externa of the median eminence containing vasopressin and its interaction with adrenal corticoids. *Ann. N.Y. Acad. Sci.*, **1977**, *297*, 405–419.

Zusman, R. M.; Keiser, H. R.; and Handler, J. S. Vasopressin-stimulated prostaglandin E biosynthesis in the toad urinary bladder. *J. Clin. Invest.*, **1977a**, *60*, 1339–1347.

———. Inhibition of vasopressin-stimulated prostaglandin E biosynthesis by chlorpropamide in the toad bladder. *Ibid.*, **1977b**, *60*, 1348–1353.

Monographs and Reviews

Andersson, B. Regulation of water intake. *Physiol. Rev.*, **1978**, *58*, 582–603.

Brownstein, M. J. Biosynthesis of vasopressin and oxytocin. *Annu. Rev. Physiol.*, **1983**, *45*, 129–135.

deWied, D. Hormonal influences on motivation, learning and memory processes. *Hosp. Pract.*, **1976**, *11*, 123–131.

Douglas, W. W. How do neurons secrete peptides? Exocytosis and its consequences, including "synaptic vesicle" formation in the hypothalamoneurohypophyseal system. *Prog. Brain Res.*, **1973**, *39*, 21–39.

Forrest, J. N., Jr., and Singer, I. Drug-induced interference with action of antidiuretic hormone. In, *Disturbances in Body Fluid Osmolality*. (Andreoli, T. E.; Grantham, J. J.; and Rector, F. C., Jr.; eds.) American Physiological Society, Bethesda, **1977**, pp. 309–340.

Hays, R. M. Alteration of luminal membrane structure by antidiuretic hormone. *Am. J. Physiol.*, **1983**, *245*, C289–C296.

Hays, R. M., and Levine, S. D. Pathophysiology of water metabolism. In, *The Kidney*, 2nd ed. (Brenner, B. M., and Rector, F. C., Jr., eds.) W. B. Saunders Co., Philadelphia, **1981**, pp. 777–840.

Sawyer, W. H., and Manning, M. Effective antagonists of the antidiuretic action of vasopressin in rats. *Ann. N.Y. Acad. Sci.*, **1982**, *394*, 464–472.

Schrier, R. W., and Bichet, D. G. Osmotic and nonosmotic control of vasopressin release and the pathogenesis of impaired water excretion in adrenal, thyroid, and edematous disorders. *J. Lab. Clin. Med.*, **1981**, *98*, 1–15.

Sklar, A. H., and Schrier, R. W. Central nervous system mediators of vasopressin release. *Physiol. Rev.*, **1983**, *63*, 1243–1280.

Symposium. (Various authors.) *Neurohypophysis: International Conference on the Neurohypophysis*. (Moses, A. M., and Share, L., eds.) S. Karger, Basel, **1977**.

Taylor, A. Role of microtubules and microfilaments in the action of vasopressin. In, *Disturbances in Body Fluid Osmolality*. (Andreoli, T. E.; Grantham, J. J.; and Rector, F. C., Jr.; eds.) American Physiological Society, Bethesda, **1977**, pp. 97–124.

Verney, E. B. Croonian lecture: The antidiuretic hormone and the factors which determine its release. *Proc. R. Soc. Lond. [Biol.]*, **1947**, *135*, 25–106.

Wade, J. B. Hormonal modulation of epithelial structure. In, *Current Topics in Membranes and Transport*, Vol. 13. (Bronner, F., and Kleinzeller, A., eds.) Academic Press, Inc., New York, **1980**, pp. 123–147.

Walter, R., and Simmons, W. H. Metabolism of neurohypophyseal hormones: considerations from a molecular viewpoint. In, *Neurohypophysis: International Conference on the Neurohypophysis*. (Moses, A. M., and Share, L., eds.) S. Karger, Basel, **1977**, pp. 167–188.

Zimmerman, E. A. Localization of hypothalamic hormones by immunocytochemical techniques. In, *Frontiers in Neuroendocrinology*, Vol. 4. Raven Press, New York, **1976**, pp. 25–62.

38 INHIBITORS OF TUBULAR TRANSPORT OF ORGANIC COMPOUNDS

Irwin M. Weiner and Gilbert H. Mudge

The physiological factors that influence the renal excretion of organic compounds have been considered in Chapter 1 and in the Introduction to Section VIII. Pharmacological agents can change the rate of excretion by affecting (1) the glomerular filtration rate, (2) the extent of binding to plasma proteins, (3) the rate of urine flow, (4) the pH of urine, or (5) the activity of tubular transport mechanisms. This chapter describes a class of agents that act on the tubular transport of certain drugs and of urate, all of which are organic anions. Thus far there are no therapeutic agents specifically designed to inhibit the renal transport of organic cations (Rennick, 1981).

The transport mechanisms for organic anions are located only in the proximal tubule. The most thoroughly studied is that for the secretion of para-aminohippurate (PAH) and a great variety of other organic anions (Møller and Sheikh, 1982). The overall process of secretion requires, first, the uptake of PAH from interstitial fluid across the basolateral membrane into the cell and, second, the subsequent movement of PAH from the cell across the brush-border membrane into the tubular fluid. As a result of the first step the concentration of PAH in intracellular fluid is driven to levels much higher than that in the interstitial fluid. This process is mediated by an integral constituent of the basolateral membrane that can be saturated and inhibited competitively, a so-called *transporter*. The driving force for this transport is derived, at least in part, from two separate mechanisms. Since the sodium concentration in the interstitial fluid is much higher than within the cell, the gradient for diffusion of sodium is in a secretory direction. This can influence the movement of an anion such as PAH. In addition, there may be an exchange of PAH for another anion from within the cell (Tune *et al.,* 1969; Sheikh and Møller, 1982; Kasher

et al., 1983). In the second step of PAH secretion, PAH moves from a high intracellular concentration to a lower concentration in the tubular fluid. In some species this is specifically mediated by a transporter in the brush-border membrane that is saturable and subject to competitive inhibition (Guggino *et al.,* 1983).

Many anionic drugs and metabolites of drugs are secreted by this two-step mechanism, and such compounds, when present simultaneously, may interfere with the secretion of one another. The competition for secretion observed *in vivo* is a reflection of events at the basolateral membrane. The transporter in this membrane has a smaller capacity and a higher affinity for its substrates than does that in the brush-border membrane (Ross and Holohan, 1983). Although competition for secretion occurs frequently, it is not always apparent *in vivo.* To illustrate this point, consider the action of probenecid, the prototypical inhibitor of secretion, on the renal excretion of two organic anions—penicillin and salicylate. Probenecid itself is a highly lipid-soluble carboxylic acid. It is completely reabsorbed in an acidic urine, while net tubular secretion is apparent in an alkaline urine. Penicillin is also secreted by the tubule, but it is a much more polar compound and, therefore, is not reabsorbed. The effect of probenecid is to decrease the excretion of penicillin by inhibition of its secretion, regardless of whether the urine is acidic or alkaline. In contrast, the action of probenecid on the excretion of salicylate is apparent only when the urine is alkaline. When the urine is acidic, the passive reabsorption of both salicylate and probenecid is virtually complete and thus any interaction between the two at the secretory level is not reflected in the voided urine. It is possible to take advantage of competition for secretion in order to prolong the action of a therapeutic agent (*see* below). In other instances the retention of one drug that is induced by another is potentially dangerous (Nierenberg, 1983).

Action of Uricosuric Agents. A uricosuric agent is a drug that increases the rate of excretion of uric acid. There is perhaps no other class of therapeutic agents for which the observations in their entirety appear so inconsistent and at times contradictory. This results from the complexity of the transport mechanisms, as well as the marked species variation of individual mechanisms and their sensitivity to drug action. Birds, reptiles, and some mammals demonstrate net secretion of urate; in some mammalian species both net secretion and net reabsorption can be observed; and in others, including man, net reabsorption is found almost invariably. In those animals that demonstrate net secretion, the mechanism is analogous, and in some instances identical, to the mechanism for the secretion of PAH. In man and other species that demonstrate net reabsorption, the reabsorptive process is mediated by a specific transporter and it is inhibitable. Finally, in all species that have been studied thoroughly, the major transport mechanism, either secretion or reabsorption, is opposed by a smaller flux operating in the opposite direction; that is, there is bidirectional transport. In most instances the smaller flux is specifically mediated (Mudge *et al.*, 1973; Roch-Ramel and Weiner, 1980). As a consequence of all of these factors, a drug that is uricosuric in one species may produce urate retention in another; within one species a drug may cause either urate retention or uricosuria, depending on the dose; and one uricosuric drug may either add to or inhibit the action of another.

In man, uric acid is largely reabsorbed; the amount excreted is usually about 10% of that filtered. Studies with brush-border membranes from other animals that also demonstrate net reabsorption of urate indicate that the first step in reabsorption is the uptake of urate from tubular fluid by the same transporter that allows PAH to move from cell to lumen. This transporter can act as an anion exchanger. Thus, urate in the tubular fluid can be exchanged for either an organic or an inorganic anion moving in the opposite direction. It has been suggested that the anionic compositions of luminal and intracellular fluids are such that reabsorption of urate is favored. In the case of PAH, the high intracellular concentration produced by the transporter in the basolateral membrane is sufficient to overcome the reabsorptive tendency of the brush-border transporter (Guggino *et al.*, 1983). The exit step for urate at the basolateral membrane has not yet been characterized. Probenecid and other uricosuric drugs, when present in the lumen, compete with urate for the brush-border transporter, thereby inhibiting its reabsorption. Thus, the same drug, probenecid, inhibits the secretion of one anion (*e.g.*, PAH) by an action at the basolateral membrane and inhibits the reabsorption of another anion (*e.g.*, urate) by an action at the luminal membrane.

The *paradoxical effect of uricosuric agents* refers to the fact that, depending on dosage, a drug may either decrease or increase the excretion of uric acid. Decreased excretion usually occurs at a low dose, while increased excretion is observed at a higher dose. Not all agents show this phenomenon. With some drugs, such as salicylate, the biphasic effect may be seen within the normal dose range; with pyrazinamide, reduction of the excretion of uric acid is the dominant action except at extremely high (experimental) doses (Fanelli and Weiner, 1973). Two mechanisms for a drug-induced *decrease* in excretion of urate have been advanced; they are not mutually exclusive. The first presumes that the small secretory movement of urate is mediated by a mechanism separate from that for the secretion of PAH. This secretory mechanism is thought to be extremely sensitive to low concentrations of compounds such as salicylate and pyrazinamide (Fanelli and Weiner, 1973). Higher concentrations of these substances may inhibit urate reabsorption in the usual manner. The second proposal suggests that the urate-retaining anionic drug gains access to the intracellular fluid by an independent mechanism and promotes reabsorption of urate across the brush border by anion exchange (Guggino *et al.*, 1983).

There are two mechanisms by which one drug may nullify the uricosuric action of another. First, the drug may inhibit the secretion of the uricosuric agent, thereby denying it access to its site of action, the luminal aspect of the brush border. Second, the inhibition of urate secretion by one drug may counterbalance the inhibition of urate reabsorption by the other (Fanelli and Weiner, 1979). There are situations in which two uricosuric agents administered together almost completely nullify each other's actions (see, for example, Yü et al., 1963). In such an instance one of the drugs (A) must have a strong paradoxical action. Drug B inhibits the secretion of A, thereby preventing its uricosuric action but not its urate-retaining action. The latter effect balances the uricosuric action of drug B.

There are a great many compounds that have uricosuric activity, but only a few are prescribed for this purpose. Some have other primary pharmacological actions, and their ability to increase urate excretion is either incidental or unexpected. In all instances the active compound is probably either an anionic drug or an anionic metabolite. On the other hand, there are a number of drugs and toxins that cause retention of urate. Both classes of compounds have been reviewed by Emmerson (1978). Uricosuric diuretics are described in Chapter 36.

PROBENECID

History. Probenecid was developed as a result of a planned approach to achieve a specific objective. When penicillin was first introduced, it was in critically short supply and the rapid renal excretion of the antibiotic was thus of practical significance. For this reason, Beyer and associates began a study to find an organic acid that would depress the tubular secretion of penicillin in the manner described above. The first compound to be evaluated clinically was CARINAMIDE. It proved to be effective, but the drug was secreted by the renal tubules fairly rapidly and it was necessary to give frequent doses. This problem was overcome with the discovery of probenecid (Beyer et al., 1951).

Chemistry. Probenecid is a highly lipid-soluble benzoic acid derivative (pK_a 3.4) with the following structural formula:

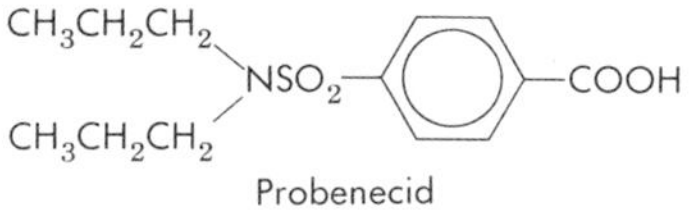

$$CH_3CH_2CH_2 \atop CH_3CH_2CH_2 > NSO_2 - \bigcirc - COOH$$

Probenecid

Various congeners of probenecid have been studied. Increasing the size of the N-alkyl substitution results in more efficient compounds. Optimal activity appears in probenecid, the N-dipropyl derivative. Gutman (1966) has reviewed the structure-activity relationship of probenecid congeners and that of other uricosuric drugs.

Pharmacological Actions. The actions of probenecid are largely confined to inhibition of the transport of organic acids across epithelial barriers. This is most important for the renal tubule, in which tubular secretion of many drugs and drug metabolites is inhibited (Weiner et al., 1964; Diamond, 1978). The renal action of probenecid reduces the concentrations of certain compounds in the urine and raises them in the plasma. This is a desirable therapeutic effect in the case of penicillin and related antibiotics that have a beneficial systemic action, but it may be undesirable with an agent such as nitrofurantoin when it is employed as a urinary antiseptic. When tubular secretion of a substance is inhibited, its final concentration in the urine is determined by the degree of filtration, which in turn is a function of binding to plasma protein, and by the degree of reabsorption. The significance of each of these factors varies widely with different compounds.

Uric Acid. Uric acid is the only important endogenous compound whose excretion is known to be increased by probenecid. This results from inhibition of its reabsorption (see above). The uricosuric action of probenecid is blunted by the administration of salicylates.

Miscellaneous Substances. Probenecid inhibits the tubular secretion of a number of drugs, such as indomethacin, methotrexate, dyphylline, and the active metabolite of clofibrate, but there is no clinical indication for the coadministration of probenecid. In the case of a number of endogenous or exogenous organic acids whose rate of excretion is determined for diagnostic purposes, misleading values may be obtained if the patient is receiving probenecid. Substances of interest include para-aminohippurate (PAH), phenolsulfonphthalein (PSP), and 5-hydroxyindoleacetic acid (5-HIAA). In contrast to the older agent iodopyracet, the excretion of modern urographic contrast agents, such as diatrizoate, is not inhibited by probenecid since tubular secretion is not involved.

Cerebrospinal Fluid. Probenecid inhibits the transport of 5-HIAA and other acidic metabolites of cerebral monoamines from the subarachnoid space to the plasma. This has been the subject of interest in psychopharmacology (see Van der Poel et al., 1977). The transport of drugs such as penicillin G may also be affected (Spector and Lorenzo, 1974; see Chapter 50).

Biliary Excretion. Since probenecid and some of its metabolites may be secreted into the bile, it is not surprising that probenecid depresses the biliary secretion of other compounds, including the diagnostic agents indocyanine green and sulfobromophthalein (BSP). The inhibition of biliary secretion also has implications in the use of rifampin for the treatment of tuberculosis. Higher concentrations of the antibiotic are achieved in plasma if probenecid is administered concurrently (Guarino and Schanker, 1968; Kenwright and Levi, 1973).

Absorption, Fate, and Excretion. Probenecid is completely absorbed after oral administration. Peak concentrations in plasma are reached in 2 to 4 hours. The half-life of the drug in plasma is dose dependent and varies from less than 5 hours to more than 8 hours over the therapeutic range (*see* Appendix II). Between 85 and 95% of the drug is bound to plasma albumin. The small unbound portion gains access to the glomerular filtrate; a much larger portion is actively secreted by the proximal tubule. The high lipid solubility of the undissociated form results in virtually complete absorption by back diffusion unless the urine is markedly alkaline. A small amount of probenecid glucuronide appears in the urine. It is also hydroxylated to metabolites that retain their carboxyl function and have uricosuric activity (Israeli *et al.*, 1972).

Preparation and Dosage. Probenecid (BENEMID) is a white crystalline, odorless powder. The free acid is insoluble in water, but the sodium salt is freely soluble. The compound is marketed as oral tablets (500 mg). The dosage schedule depends upon the objectives of therapy. To block effectively the renal excretion of penicillin, a total daily dose of 2 g is employed in adults. This is administered in four divided doses. For children, an initial dose of 25 mg/kg is followed by maintenance doses of 10 mg/kg given four times daily. In the treatment of chronic gout, 250 mg is given twice daily for 1 week, following which 500 mg is administered twice daily. In some patients it may be necessary to increase the daily dose gradually to a maximum of 2 g, given in four divided portions.

Adjunct in Penicillin Therapy. The oral administration of probenecid in conjunction with penicillin G results in higher and more prolonged concentrations of the antibiotic in plasma than when penicillin is given alone. The elevation in the plasma level is at least twofold and sometimes much greater. Although the reduction of a daily dose of penicillin G from 1 million to 500,000 units has very little significance, a reduction by 50% or more may be of importance for convenience in the treatment of resistant infections that may require the administra-

tion of penicillin G in very large doses. This combined regimen may also be useful to minimize the amount of potassium that is administered to some patients who receive very large doses of penicillin.

Probenecid is also included in regimens that can be completed during one visit to the physician for the treatment and prophylaxis of gonococcal infections (*see* Chapter 50).

Untoward Reactions and Precautions. Probenecid is well tolerated by most patients. Some degree of gastrointestinal irritation is experienced by at least 2% of patients; the incidence is considerably higher after large doses. Cautious administration is advised in patients with a history of peptic ulcer. Most reports place the incidence of hypersensitivity reactions, usually mild skin rashes, between 2 and 4%. More serious hypersensitivity reactions occur, but they are rare. The nephrotic syndrome has been reported as a toxic reaction. The appearance of a rash during the concurrent administration of probenecid and penicillin G or a congener presents the physician with an awkward diagnostic dilemma. The compound also increases to some degree the concentration of sulfonamide in the blood. Huge overdosage of probenecid results in stimulation of the central nervous system, convulsions, and death from respiratory failure.

SULFINPYRAZONE

History. Despite its therapeutic efficacy as an anti-inflammatory and uricosuric agent, phenylbutazone (*see* Chapter 29) has undesirable side effects severe enough to preclude its continuous use. For this reason, a number of congeners were evaluated for uricosuric and anti-inflammatory activity. One of these, in which a phenyl-thioethyl configuration replaces the butyl side chain of the parent compound, displayed promising activity. When the metabolites of the new compound were studied, it was found that side chain oxidation *in vivo* led to the formation of the sulfoxide, *sulfinpyrazone,* which was a potent uricosuric agent (Gutman *et al.*, 1960).

Chemistry. The chemical structure of sulfinpyrazone is as follows:

Sulfinpyrazone

It is a strong organic acid (pK_a 2.8) that readily forms soluble salts. Burns and coworkers (1958) studied a number of congeners; they found that a low pK_a and polar side chain substitutions favor uricosuric activity (*see also* Gutman, 1966).

Pharmacological Actions. Sulfinpyrazone in sufficient dosage is a potent inhibitor of the renal tubular reabsorption of uric acid. As with other uricosuric agents, small doses may reduce the excretion of uric acid. Like probenecid, sulfinpyrazone reduces the renal tubular secretion of many other organic anions. The drug may induce hypoglycemia by inhibiting the metabolism of the sulfonylurea oral hypoglycemic agents; hepatic metabolism of warfarin is also impaired. The uricosuric action of sulfinpyrazone is additive to that of probenecid and phenylbutazone but is mutually antagonistic to that of the salicylates (Yü et al., 1963).

Sulfinpyrazone lacks the anti-inflammatory and analgesic properties of its congener, phenylbutazone.

Platelet Aggregation. The effect of sulfinpyrazone on platelet function is discussed in Chapter 58.

Absorption, Fate, and Excretion. Sulfinpyrazone is well absorbed after oral administration. It is strongly bound to plasma albumin to the extent of 98 to 99% and displaces other anionic drugs that have their highest affinity for the same binding site (site I) (Sudlow et al., 1975). The half-life of the drug in plasma after its intravenous injection is about 3 hours. After oral administration, however, its uricosuric effect may persist for as long as 10 hours. Although little sulfinpyrazone is available for filtration at the glomerulus, it is secreted by the proximal tubule and undergoes little passive back diffusion. Approximately half of the orally administered dose appears in the urine within 24 hours. Most of the drug (90%) in the urine is unchanged; the remainder is eliminated as the N^1-*p*-hydroxyphenyl metabolite, which also is a potent uricosuric substance (*see* Gutman et al., 1960; Dayton et al., 1961).

Preparations and Dosage. *Sulfinpyrazone* (ANTURANE) is available as 100-mg tablets and 200-mg capsules. For the treatment of *chronic gout*, the initial dosage is 100 to 200 mg given twice daily. After the first week, the dose may be gradually increased until a satisfactory lowering of plasma uric acid is achieved and maintained. This may require from 200 to 800 mg per day, divided in two to four doses and preferably given with meals. Larger doses are poorly tolerated and unlikely to produce a further uricosuric effect in the resistant patient.

Untoward Reactions and Precautions. *Gastrointestinal irritation* occurs in 10 to 15% of all patients receiving sulfinpyrazone, and an occasional patient may require discontinuance of its use. Gastric distress is lessened when the drug is taken in divided doses with meals. Sulfinpyrazone should be given to patients with a history of peptic ulcer only with the greatest caution. *Hypersensitivity* reactions, usually a rash with fever, do occur, but less frequently than with probenecid. The severe blood dyscrasias and salt and water retention, hazards of phenylbutazone therapy (*see* Chapter 29), have not been observed during sulfinpyrazone therapy. However, depression of hematopoiesis has been demonstrated experimentally, and periodic blood-cell counts are therefore advised during prolonged therapy.

BENZBROMARONE

This is a potent uricosuric agent that is used in Europe. It has the following structural formula:

Benzbromarone

The drug is readily absorbed after oral ingestion, and peak concentrations in blood are achieved in about 4 hours. It is metabolized to the monobromine and dehalogenated derivatives, both of which have uricosuric activity, and is principally excreted in the bile. The uricosuric action is blunted by aspirin or sulfinpyrazone and is abolished by pyrazinamide. No paradoxical retention of urate has been observed. At clinically effective doses there is no effect on the synthesis of urate. Therefore, benzbromarone probably reduces the concentration of urate in plasma solely by inhibiting its tubular reabsorption. Its action on the tubular transport of other organic acids has not been systematically examined.

Benzbromarone is of interest as a member of a newer chemical class of uricosuric agents. As the micronized powder it is effective in a single daily dose of 40 to 80 mg, which makes it significantly more potent than other uricosuric drugs. It may be useful clinically in patients who are either allergic or refractory to other drugs used for the treatment of gout (Diamond, 1978).

THE CLINICAL USE OF URICOSURIC AGENTS

This subject is described in Chapter 29 in conjunction with the discussion of other types of drugs that are also used for the treatment of gout and other syndromes characterized by hyperuricemia.

Beyer, K. H.; Russo, H. F.; Tillson, E. K.; Miller, A. K.; Verwey, W. F.; and Gass, S. R. BENEMID, *p*-(di-*n*-propylsulfamyl)-benzoic acid: its renal affinity and its elimination. *Am. J. Physiol.*, **1951**, *166*, 625–640.

Burns, J. J.; Yü, T.-F.; Dayton, P. G.; Berger, L.; Gutman, A. B.; and Brodie, B. B. Relationship between pK_a and uricosuric activity in phenylbutazone analogues. *Nature*, **1958**, *182*, 1162–1163.

Dayton, P. G.; Sicam, L. E.; Landrau, M.; and Burns, J. J. Metabolism of sulfinpyrazone and other thio analogues of phenylbutazone in man. *J. Pharmacol. Exp. Ther.*, **1961**, *132*, 287–390.

Fanelli, G. M., Jr., and Weiner, I. M. Pyrazinoate excretion in the chimpanzee: relation to urate disposition and the actions of uricosuric drugs. *J. Clin. Invest.*, **1973**, *52*, 1946–1957.

————. Urate excretion: drug interactions. *J. Pharmacol. Exp. Ther.*, **1979**, *210*, 186–195.

Guarino, A. M., and Schanker, L. S. Biliary excretion of probenecid and its glucuronide. *J. Pharmacol. Exp. Ther.*, **1968**, *164*, 387–395.

Guggino, S. E.; Martin, G. J.; and Aronson, P. S. Specificity and modes of the anion exchanger in dog renal microvillus membranes. *Am. J. Physiol.*, **1983**, *244*, F612–F621.

Gutman, A. B.; Dayton, P. G.; Yü, T.-F.; Berger, L.; Chen, W.; Sicam, L. E.; and Burns, J. J. A study of the inverse relationship between pK_a and rate of renal excretion of phenylbutazone analogues in man and dogs. *Am. J. Med.*, **1960**, *29*, 1017–1033.

Israeli, Z. H.; Perel, J. M.; Cunningham, R. F.; Dayton, P. G.; Yü, T.-F.; Gutman, A. B.; Long, K. R.; Long, R. C., Jr.; and Goldstein, J. H. Metabolites of probenecid. Chemical, physical, and pharmacological studies. *J. Med. Chem.*, **1972**, *15*, 709–716.

Kasher, J. S.; Holohan, P. D.; and Ross, C. R. Na$^+$ gradient–dependent *p*-aminohippurate (PAH) transport in rat basolateral membrane vesicles. *J. Pharmacol. Exp. Ther.*, **1983**, *227*, 122–129.

Kenwright, S., and Levi, A. J. Impairment of hepatic uptake of rifamycin antibiotics by probenecid and its therapeutic implications. *Lancet*, **1973**, *2*, 1401–1405.

Nierenberg, D. W. Competitive inhibition of methotrexate accumulation in rabbit kidney slices by nonsteroidal anti-inflammatory drugs. *J. Pharmacol. Exp. Ther.*, **1983**, *226*, 1–6.

Sheikh, M. I., and Møller, J. V. Na$^+$ gradient–dependent stimulation of renal transport of *p*-aminohippurate. *Biochem. J.*, **1982**, *208*, 243–246.

Spector, R., and Lorenzo, A. V. The effects of salicylate and probenecid on the cerebrospinal fluid transport of penicillin, aminosalicylic acid and iodide. *J. Pharmacol. Exp. Ther.*, **1974**, *188*, 55–65.

Sudlow, G.; Birkett, D. J.; and Wade, D. N. The characterization of two specific drug binding sites on human serum albumin. *Mol. Pharmacol.*, **1975**, *11*, 824–832.

Tune, B. M.; Burg, M. B.; and Patlak, C. S. Characteristics of *p*-aminohippurate transport in proximal renal tubules. *Am. J. Physiol.*, **1969**, *217*, 1057–1063.

Monographs and Reviews

Diamond, H. S. Uricosuric drugs. In, *Uric Acid*. (Kelley, W. N., and Weiner, I. M., eds.) Springer-Verlag, Berlin, **1978**, pp. 459–484.

Emmerson, B. T. Abnormal urate excretion associated with renal and systemic disorders, drugs, and toxins. In, *Uric Acid*. (Kelley, W. N., and Weiner, I. M., eds.) Springer-Verlag, Berlin, **1978**, pp. 287–324.

Gutman, A. B. Uricosuric drugs, with special reference to probenecid and sulfinpyrazone. *Adv. Pharmacol.*, **1966**, *4*, 91–142.

Kelley, W. N., and Weiner, I. M. (eds.). *Uric Acid*. Springer-Verlag, Berlin, **1978**.

Møller, J. V., and Sheikh, M. I. The renal organic anion transport system: pharmacological, physiological, and biochemical aspects. *Pharmacol. Rev.*, **1982**, *34*, 315–358.

Mudge, G. H.; Berndt, W. O.; and Valtin, H. Tubular transport of urea, glucose, phosphate, uric acid, sulfate, and thiosulfate. In, Sect. 8, *Renal Physiology. Handbook of Physiology*. (Orloff, J., and Berliner, R. W., eds.) American Physiological Society, Washington, D. C., **1973**, pp. 587–652.

Rennick, B. R. Renal tubule transport of organic cations. *Am. J. Physiol.*, **1981**, *240*, F83–F89.

Roch-Ramel, F., and Weiner, I. M. Renal excretion of urate: factors determining the actions of drugs. *Kidney Int.*, **1980**, *18*, 665–676.

Ross, C. R., and Holohan, P. D. Transport of organic anions and cations in isolated renal plasma membranes. *Annu. Rev. Pharmacol. Toxicol.*, **1983**, *23*, 65–85.

Van der Poel, F. W.; Van Praag, H. M.; and Korf, J. Evidence for a probenecid-sensitive transport system of acid monoamine metabolites from the spinal subarachnoid space. *Psychopharmacology*, **1977**, *52*, 35–40.

Weiner, I. M. Transport of weak acids and bases. In, Sect. 8, *Renal Physiology. Handbook of Physiology*. (Orloff, J., and Berliner, R. W., eds.) American Physiological Society, Washington, D. C., **1973**, pp. 521–554.

Weiner, I. M.; Blanchard, K. C.; and Mudge, G. H. Factors influencing renal excretion of foreign organic acids. *Am. J. Physiol.*, **1964**, *207*, 953–963.

Yü, T.-F.; Dayton, P. G.; and Gutman, A. B. Mutual suppression of the uricosuric effects of sulfinpyrazone and salicylate: a study in interactions between drugs. *J. Clin. Invest.*, **1963**, *42*, 1330–1339.

Drugs Affecting Uterine Motility

In this section, only the uterine-stimulating (or oxytocic) and uterine-relaxing (or tocolytic) agents are discussed. The effects of estrogens, androgens, and anterior pituitary hormones on the reproductive system are presented in Section XV.

CHAPTER

39 OXYTOCIN, PROSTAGLANDINS, ERGOT ALKALOIDS, AND OTHER DRUGS; TOCOLYTIC AGENTS

Theodore W. Rall and Leonard S. Schleifer

Drugs that modify the progress of labor and delivery have obvious utility in modern obstetrics. Historically, the ergot alkaloids (now represented by *ergonovine* and *methylergonovine*) were the first agents to be employed to initiate or accelerate parturition. In modern practice, *oxytocin* has displaced these drugs for this purpose, and their use is now confined to the post-partum period. The utility of oxytocin and the ergot alkaloids in obstetrics, as well as their general pharmacological properties, will be described below. The prostaglandins are the latest group of uterine-stimulating agents to be studied. Discussion in this chapter will be limited to the effects of prostaglandins of the E and F types on the uterus and their potential for use as abortifacients and to facilitate delivery at term. The general discussion of the prostaglandins appears in Chapter 28.

Several classes of drugs, notably β_2-adrenergic agonists and alcohol, have been used to inhibit uterine contractility and to delay parturition. The general discussion of the pharmacology of these compounds appears in Chapters 8 and 18, respectively. Only their therapeutic use in obstetrics is discussed below.

Physiological and Anatomical Considerations. Uterine smooth muscle is characterized by a high degree of spontaneous electrical and contractile activity. Waves of decreased membrane potential with superimposed spike activity are associated with contraction. Cell-to-cell spread of excitation occurs, but electrical conduction is slow and decremental in nature. Low-resistance contacts between cells (gap junctions) greatly facilitate the spread of excitation. The number of such junctions is regulated by steroid hormones and increases in the later stages of pregnancy. Increased frequency and duration of spike activity in "pacemaker" areas and more extensive spread of excitation are associated with increases in force of contraction. In most species (including the human female), the influx of sodium ions appears to play the primary role in depolarization. However, the duration of spike potentials is relatively long, and depolarization is not affected by tetrodotoxin. This indicates the lack of participation of so-called fast sodium channels in this process.

Even in those species in which most of the depolarizing current appears to be carried by calcium ions, the amount of calcium that crosses the plasma membrane during excitation is insufficient to cause contraction directly. Nevertheless, the availability of extracellular calcium ion (and thus the presence of blockers of calcium channels) strongly influences the response of uterine smooth muscle to various physiological and pharmacological stimuli. Evidently, extracellular calcium plays an important role in triggering the release of much larger amounts of calcium from intracellular stores. As in cardiac and skeletal muscle, the interaction of actin and myosin that results in muscle contraction is instigated by calcium. However, the anatomical arrangement and biochemical properties of contractile proteins are much different in smooth muscle, including that of the uterus. Of particular importance in smooth muscle is the fact that contraction appears to be initiated by the relatively slow process of phosphorylation of the light chains of myosin, a reaction that is catalyzed by a calcium- and calmodulin-dependent enzyme. (*See* Kao, 1977; Huszar, in Symposium, 1981; Huszar and Roberts, 1982.)

The uterus has parasympathetic and sympathetic innervation, the former by way of the pelvic nerve and the latter by way of postganglionic fibers from the inferior mesenteric and hypogastric ganglia. Both can elicit increased activity in the mature human uterus, but denervation causes little change in uterine motor activity. Both α_1-(excitatory)- and β_2-(inhibitory, hyperpolarizing)-adrenergic receptors are clearly demonstrable in the myometrium of mammals. The inhibitory effects of β_2-adrenergic agonists on uterine contractility are mediated by adenosine $3',5'$-monophosphate (cyclic AMP); the cyclic nucleotide functions intracellularly to lower the concentration of cytosolic calcium. Excitatory receptors for oxytocin have also been demonstrated. Prostaglandins E_2 and $F_{2\alpha}$ and, in some species, 5-hydroxytryptamine (5-HT) increase uterine contractile activity.

Uterine smooth muscle is unusually susceptible to endocrine influence, especially that of the estrogens. Thus, spontaneous activity, as well as responsiveness to neurogenic, hormonal, and pharmacological stimulation, increases greatly at puberty and varies thereafter with the ovulatory cycle. In some species, progesterone markedly inhibits uterine activity. Whether progesterone has an important physiological role in regulating the motor activity of the human uterus has yet to be clearly demonstrated.

In addition to such factors as endocrinological status, contractile responses of uterine smooth muscle are strongly influenced by variables such as the period of gestation, the degree of stretch, and the region of the uterus under consideration. Thus, it is not surprising that there are many conflicting reports of the effects of drugs on this organ. Unless otherwise stated, the effects of the drugs to be discussed are those that have been confirmed in the human female.

Human Parturition. The physiological processes that are involved in the onset and progression of labor in human beings are complex and have been defined only to a limited degree; it has been particularly difficult to establish the sequence of events that leads to the initiation of labor. The views of most investigators have centered on the complementary and sometimes synergistic actions of oxytocin and the prostaglandins, and the changes in their capacity to exert effects that can result from developmental events in the fetus, placenta, and fetal membranes.

Oxytocin has stimulatory effects on the smooth muscle of the uterus that are so potent and selective as to suggest that the polypeptide serves a true hormonal function at this site. Oxytocin elicits contractions of the fundus that are indistinguishable in amplitude, duration, and frequency from those seen in late pregnancy and during spontaneous labor. However, a direct link between endogenous oxytocin and the onset of labor has been difficult to establish. Parturition still occurs in the complete absence of oxytocin; however, labor is prolonged. While the concentration of oxytocin in plasma is elevated at the onset of spontaneous labor, the increase is only about twofold (Fuchs *et al.*, 1983). In addition, the induction of labor by artificial rupture of the membranes is not associated with a sustained increase in the concentration of oxytocin in the circulation (Husslein *et al.*, 1983). However, the sensitivity of the uterus to oxytocin increases as pregnancy progresses (*see* below), and the number of receptors for oxytocin in the myometrium and decidua is markedly elevated in the later stages of pregnancy (Fuchs *et al.*, 1982). While it is not certain that oxytocin triggers the onset of labor, it can be considered, at least, to play an important facilitatory role in parturition.

Prostaglandins also appear to have important functions in human parturition. Inhibitors of prostaglandin synthesis can delay the onset of or prolong spontaneous labor (*see* Chapter 29). Although uterine sensitivity to the prostaglandins changes relatively little during pregnancy, the specific activity of phospholipases that catalyze the rate-limiting step in the formation of prostaglandins increases in human amnion late in gestation (Okazaki *et al.*, 1981). This fetal membrane also possesses large amounts of both cyclooxygenase and phospholipids that contain arachidonic acid (*see* Okita *et al.*, 1983). The formation of prostaglandins by the amnion may increase progressively during the later stages of pregnancy as a result of the accumulation of substances derived from the fetus, such as surfactant or catecholamines; eventually, the amount of prostaglandins that reaches the myometrium may be sufficient to initiate labor (Sbarra *et al.*, 1983; Di Renzo *et al.*, 1984). Although increased concentrations of prostaglandins or their metabolites are not observed in plasma until there has been substantial cervical dilatation (Fuchs *et al.*, 1983), it is possible that such measurements do not reflect events that are taking place within the uterine cavity.

The views just presented are not mutually exclusive, and it is likely that both oxytocin and prostaglandins play direct roles in the initiation and maintenance of uterine contractions during labor. In addition, the entire process of human parturition is under the influence of steroidal hormones. Most attention has been focused on the increasing concentrations of estrogens in the plasma and amniotic fluid during the later stages of pregnancy, especially the marked changes in the final 2 to 3 weeks. Progesterone concentrations may decrease at the same time; furthermore, a progesterone-binding protein accumulates in the fetal membranes and may serve to decrease the effective concentration of the hormone in these structures. In any event, the progressive domination by estrogen has been held responsible for the increases in myometrial excitability (due to increases in slow sodium channels and gap junctions), the myometrial sensitivity to oxytocin, and the capacity to elaborate prostaglandins in the fetal membranes. The changing hormonal milieu may also be responsible for the so-called ripening of the uterine cervix during pregnancy; among other changes, there is a marked, progressive decrease in the content of collagen (Uldbjerg *et al.*, 1983). These alterations are thought to be crucial in preparation for the softening, dilatation, and effacement that occurs in normal labor and delivery. (*See* Huszar and *see also* Challis and Mitchell, in Symposium, 1981; Liggins, in Symposium, 1983.)

OXYTOCIN

The structure, formation, storage, and release of the neurohypophyseal hormones, oxytocin and antidiuretic hormone (ADH), and a comparison of their biological activities have been presented in Chapter 37. The following discussion will deal in more detail with the physiological and pharmacological properties of oxytocin. This hormone has slight, but not insignificant, antidiuretic and vascular activity that may become manifest when large doses are used (*see* below).

Biosynthesis and Physiological Role of Oxytocin. Oxytocin is synthesized in the supraoptic and paraventricular nuclei of the hypothalamus within neurons that are distinct from those that contain ADH. It is formed by the processing of a larger precursor molecule that also contains a specific binding protein for the hormone, termed oxytocin-neurophysin. Oxytocin-neurophysin contains a sequence of more than 90 amino acid residues that is identical with a region in ADH-neurophysin (Land *et al.*, 1983). The two neurophysins can bind either hormone (Rholam *et al.*, 1982). The dimeric complex of oxytocin and its neurophysin is stored in and released from secretory granules in nerve endings, especially in the neurohypophysis.

Sensory stimuli arising from the cervix and vagina initiate secretion of oxytocin from the posterior pituitary. Stimulation of the breast also results in secretion of oxytocin; the hormone causes contraction of the myoepithelium that surrounds aveolar channels in the mammary gland. This milk-ejection reflex fails to occur in the complete absence of oxytocin. The secretion of both ADH and oxytocin is provoked by increases in the osmolality of plasma and is suppressed by ethanol; the latter effect forms the basis for the use of ethanol as a tocolytic agent (*see* below). While the peripheral actions of oxytocin appear to play no significant role in responses to dehydration or hypovolemia, neurons that contain oxytocin project to regions in the hypothalamus, brain stem, and spinal cord that are known to be involved in the regulation of the autonomic nervous system (*see* Buijs, 1983). Thus, such release from the neurohypophysis might reflect activation of oxytocinergic neurons that may participate in the central regulation of blood pressure.

Oxytocin has also been implicated in the modulation of memory, primarily on the basis of the amnestic effects that follow its injection into the cerebral ventricles. Studies of such phenomena have revealed the capacity of synaptic membranes to convert oxytocin to a specific peptide fragment that has greatly enhanced amnestic potency but is devoid of uterine-stimulating properties (Burbach *et al.*, 1983).

Substantial amounts of oxytocin and its neurophysin have been detected in the gonads of a variety of mammals, including man (*see* Pickering *et al.*, 1983). The physiological correlates of this finding are yet to be determined.

Pharmacological Properties

Uterus. Oxytocin stimulates both frequency and force of contractile activity in uterine smooth muscle. With higher concentrations, sustained decreases in resting membrane potential occur. At threshold concentrations, where there is no change in membrane potential, oxytocin initiates spike discharges, increases the frequency and number of spikes in a burst discharge, and increases the amplitude of spike discharges (*see* Kao, 1977). These effects are highly dependent on the presence of estrogen, and the immature uterus is quite resistant. Although progesterone antagonizes the stimulant effect of oxytocin *in vitro*, the corresponding effect in the pregnant human uterus has been difficult to demonstrate.

A very low level of motor activity prevails in the human uterus during the first and second trimesters of pregnancy. During the third trimester, spontaneous motor activity increases progressively until the sharp rise that constitutes the initiation of labor and delivery. The responsiveness of the uterus to oxytocin roughly parallels the increase in spontaneous activity. Oxytocin can initiate or enhance rhythmic contractions at any time, but in early pregnancy only very high doses elicit a response. Approximately an eightfold increase in responsiveness occurs between the twentieth and thirty-ninth week. Most of this increase takes place during the last 9 weeks. Thus, slow intravenous infusion of a few units of oxytocin usually is effective in initiating labor at term. However, there is considerable variability among individuals and labor has been initiated by the infusion of as little as 25 milliunits (0.05 μg) of oxytocin (*see* below).

Mechanism of Action. The demonstration of specific receptors for oxytocin in human myometrium and the progressive increase in their number that occurs during pregnancy have been discussed above. While such sites appear to mediate the actions of oxytocin, the mechanism for translation of receptor binding into increased frequency and force of contraction is unknown. While oxytocin causes the release of prostaglandins in several species, it is unclear if this effect is primary or if it is a result of uterine contraction. There are conflicting reports as to whether inhibitors of prostaglandin synthesis can alter the contractile effect of oxytocin on the human myometrium *in vitro* (Garrioch, 1978; Wikland *et al.*, 1982). The effects of prostaglandins on uterine muscle are discussed below.

Mammary Gland. The alveolar ramifications of the mammary gland are surrounded by a network of modified smooth muscle, the myoepithelium. Contraction of these cells forces milk from the alveolar channels into the large sinuses, where it is easily available to the suckling infant. This function is known as milk ejection (milk letdown, in domestic animals). The myoepithelium is highly responsive to oxytocin. Although the catecholamines inhibit milk ejection, the contraction of the myoepithelium is not believed to be dependent on autonomic innervation, but is considered to be under the control of oxytocin and the reflex pathways that initiate the release of the hormone. Oxytocin is occasionally employed to promote milk ejection when this component of lactation appears to be inefficient in nursing mothers.

Cardiovascular System. Oxytocin has a marked but transient, direct relaxing effect on vascular smooth muscle when large amounts are administered to man. A decrease in systolic and especially diastolic blood pressure, flushing, reflex tachycardia, and an increase in limb blood flow are observed. The amounts of oxytocin administered for most obstetrical purposes are insufficient to pro-duce marked alterations of blood pressure. However, large doses may produce a marked fall in arterial pressure, particularly in deeply anesthetized patients (*see* Nakano, 1973).

When studied *in vitro,* oxytocin has a weak constricting effect on renal, splanchnic, and skeletal muscle arteries of various species, including man; however, relaxation will often occur if the vessel is first constricted by another agent. By contrast, oxytocin is a powerful constrictor of umbilical arteries and veins; its potency on human vessels is sufficient to suggest a role for oxytocin in effecting their closure at birth (*see* Altura and Altura, 1984).

Other Actions. Oxytocin usually produces an increase in sodium excretion in experimental animals, although this effect may depend on the presence of ADH in the circulation. Such effects are minor in man. However, when large doses of oxytocin are administered for therapeutic purposes, an antidiuretic effect can occur, and signs of water intoxication have been observed when excessive volumes of intravenous fluids have been administered concurrently (Saunders and Munsick, 1966). Oxytocin can suppress the secretion of ACTH (Legros *et al.*, 1984).

Absorption, Fate, and Excretion. Oxytocin is effective after administration by any parenteral route. A less efficient but convenient route is the intranasal application of a spray. The ready absorption of oxytocin from buccal lozenges also permits the use of the oral mucosa as a route of administration. The nasal route of administration is reserved for uses post partum.

The distribution and fate of oxytocin in the body are much like those of ADH (*see* Chapter 37). While there is evidence for passage of oxytocin through the primate placenta, the extent to which the hormone crosses the human placenta is not certain (*see* Roy and Karim, 1983). Oxytocin is found in increasing concentrations in the fetal circulation and the amniotic fluid during the later stages of pregnancy and labor, but the relative fetal and maternal contribution has not been determined. The half-life of oxytocin ranges from 12 to 17 minutes; similar values are obtained in females during labor and in males (Amico *et al.*, 1984). Its removal from plasma is accomplished largely by the kidney and the liver. During pregnancy, the concentration of an aminopeptidase (oxytocinase or cystyl-aminopeptidase) in plasma increases about tenfold (Majkić-Singh *et al.*, 1982). This enzyme is capable of degrading both oxytocin and ADH and is apparently derived from the placenta. While it may serve to regulate the local concentration of oxytocin in the uterus, this enzyme evidently has little to do with the disappearance of oxytocin from plasma (Amico *et al.*, 1984).

Bioassay and Unitage. The uterine-stimulating potency of posterior pituitary extracts is determined by bioassay of their avian vasodepressor activity, which parallels uterine-stimulating activity. Activity is expressed in terms of *USP units*. The strength of the preparations of synthetic oxytocin now in use is still expressed in these units, each unit being the equivalent of approximately 2 μg of the pure hormone.

Preparations and Routes of Administration. *Oxytocin injection* (PITOCIN, SYNTOCINON) contains 10 USP units per milliliter and may be administered intravenously or intramuscularly. All commercial preparations of oxytocin are now synthetic. Oxytocin is also available in the form of a nasal spray, containing 40 USP units per milliliter.

THERAPEUTIC USES

The uses of oxytocin in *obstetrics* are discussed below.

Use during Lactation. Theoretically oxytocin should be of value for the relief of engorgement of the breasts during lactation and in cases of inadequacy of breast feeding in which insufficient milk ejection is felt to be a contributing factor. The hormone is administered most conveniently by the intranasal route. In cases of inadequacy of breast feeding, it is given by a single burst of the nasal spray in each nostril 2 to 3 minutes before a feeding is to begin. The procedure is often not successful. However, it is simple and without risk to the patient, and when effective it resolves a frustrating and sometimes painful problem for the patient. Oxytocin is not useful when inadequate production of milk is the underlying problem.

PROSTAGLANDINS

The sources, chemistry, and physiological actions of this ubiquitous group of autacoids are presented in Chapter 28. In the female reproductive system, prostaglandins are found in the ovary, myometrium, and menstrual fluid in concentrations that vary with the ovulatory cycle. Following coitus, accessible portions of the female reproductive tract are also exposed to prostaglandins, which occur in high concentrations in seminal fluid. The fetal membranes are an important source of these and other products of the metabolism of arachi-donic acid in the pregnant uterus. At term and during labor, prostaglandin concentrations rise in amniotic fluid, umbilical cord blood, and maternal blood. The physiological role of the prostaglandins in human parturition has been discussed above.

In spite of the clearly demonstrable effectiveness of the prostaglandins in stimulating (or, in a few instances, relaxing) smooth muscle in reproductive organs, their physiological role in menstruation and conception remains debatable. The semen of a number of mammalian species is devoid of prostaglandins. Although the widely used drugs aspirin and indomethacin profoundly depress prostaglandin synthesis, their use has not yet been clearly shown to influence menstruation or reproduction in patients receiving therapeutic doses. However, aspirin-like drugs are effective in the treatment of uterine hypercontractility and cramping pain in women with primary dysmenorrhea (*see* Owen, 1984; Chapters 29 and 61). These agents can also delay the onset of or prolong spontaneous labor (*see* below).

PHARMACOLOGICAL PROPERTIES

The prostaglandins can be considered to be local hormones since, with few exceptions, they exert their effects and are inactivated principally in the tissues or organs in which they are synthesized. Those found most abundantly in the uterus, and in the menstrual and amniotic fluid, are of the E and F types. Prostacyclin (PGI_2) is confined largely to the uterine, umbilical, and fetal vasculature, where it may serve to ensure an adequate flow of blood and a patent ductus arteriosus. Clinical investigation for obstetrical use has been limited almost entirely to PGE_2, $PGF_{2\alpha}$, and the synthetic derivative, 15-methyl $PGF_{2\alpha}$.

Myometrium. During the last two trimesters of pregnancy, the administration of either PGE_2 or $PGF_{2\alpha}$ causes strong uterine contractions and can induce delivery of the fetus (*see* Andersson *et al.*, in Symposium, 1983). As with oxytocin, the sensitivity of the uterus to prostaglandins increases as gestation progresses. However, the changes are less pronounced, and prostaglandins are much more effective than is oxytocin in the earlier months. The higher doses that are required to produce abortion in the first few weeks after conception result in serious systemic effects. There is no information on alterations in the number or function of myometrial receptors for the prostaglandins during pregnancy, and the increasing sensitivity may primarily reflect changes in the excitability of uterine smooth muscle that are induced by steroids (*see* above).

When studied *in vitro*, $PGF_{2\alpha}$ consistently stimulates contractions of myometrial tissue from both pregnant and nonpregnant women, while PGE_2 often causes relaxation. As a result, the formation of disproportionately large amounts of $PGF_{2\alpha}$ has generally been held responsible for the uterine hypercontractility that occurs in primary dysmenorrhea. However, PGE_2 is as effective as $PGF_{2\alpha}$ for the induction of labor at term. This apparent discrepancy between observations *in vivo* and *in vitro* may be explained by the biphasic effects of PGE_2 on strips of uterine muscle from women late in pregnancy; low concentrations of PGE_2 regularly increase contractions, while higher concentrations produce a brief or weak excitatory response followed by a long period of quiescence (Wikland *et al.*, 1982). Since PGI_2 consistently inhibits myometrial contractions *in vitro*, the effects of high doses of PGE_2 may reflect interaction with receptors for PGI_2, a circumstance that has been observed elsewhere (*e.g.*, in platelets; *see* Chapter 28).

Cervix. The local instillation of prostaglandins can induce cervical ripening at doses that do not affect uterine motility (*see* Symposium, 1983). These agents can also produce softening of the cervix late in the first trimester of pregnancy, by which time a major change in the structure of cervical collagen has occurred. The mechanisms underlying these effects are not known, and the role of endogenous prostaglandins in cervical ripening during normal, spontaneous labor is yet to be established. However, it is likely that they are important in the ripening that is produced by the insertion of various devices (*e.g.*, bougies) into the cervix to induce such changes.

Clinical Toxicity. The principal side effects that attend the use of the prostaglandins are caused by their stimulatory action on the smooth muscle of the alimentary tract. In addition, transient pyrexia is experienced by many patients who have received PGE_2 or 15-methyl $PGF_{2\alpha}$. This is probably due to actions on thermoregulatory centers in the hypothalamus. Large doses of $PGF_{2\alpha}$ or 15-methyl $PGF_{2\alpha}$ may cause hypertension by constriction of vas-

cular smooth muscle, while large doses of PGE_2 may produce vasodilatation.

Preparations and Routes of Administration. *Dinoprost tromethamine* (PROSTIN F2 ALPHA) is a solution containing the equivalent of 5 mg of $PGF_{2\alpha}$ per milliliter; it is available for intra-amniotic administration to induce abortion. *Dinoprostone* (PROSTIN E2) is available in vaginal suppositories containing 20 mg of PGE_2. It is used to induce abortion, to evacuate the uterus in the management of missed abortion, and for treatment of benign hydatidiform mole. *Carboprost tromethamine* (PROSTIN/15M) is a solution containing 0.25 mg of carboprost (15-methyl $PGF_{2\alpha}$) per milliliter for intramuscular administration. It is used to induce abortion or to aid in the expulsion of the fetus during the course of abortion by another method. Dosage of these preparations is discussed below.

THERAPEUTIC USES

The major use of PGE_2, $PGF_{2\alpha}$, and 15-methyl $PGF_{2\alpha}$ that is currently approved in the United States is for the performance of midtrimester abortions. This is discussed below. In addition, there have been numerous investigations of their potential use as cervical ripening agents to facilitate normal or induced labor (*see* Symposium, 1983; Lange *et al.*, 1984); also under investigation is the use of these agents to soften the cervix prior to performance of first-trimester abortions by the method of dilatation and evacuation (Kent *et al.*, 1983; Arias, 1984).

ERGOT AND THE ERGOT ALKALOIDS

The dramatic effect of ergot ingested during pregnancy has been recognized for over 2000 years, and it was first used by physicians as a uterine-stimulating agent almost 400 years ago. In the early years of this century, the isolation and chemical identification of the active principles of ergot were accomplished and detailed study of their biological activity was begun. The elucidation of the constituents of ergot and their complex actions comprises a most important chapter in the evolution of modern pharmacology. The ergot alkaloids are therefore discussed in some detail in this and other chapters, even though the very complexity of their actions limits their therapeutic uses.

Source. *Ergot* is the product of a fungus (*Claviceps purpurea*) that grows upon rye and other grains. Rye is the most susceptible. The parasite can be found in the grainfields of North America and Europe. Rye destined for commercial sale is subject to government inspection and is rejected if it contains more than 0.3% infected grain. In dry years the rejection rate is usually less than 1%, but in other years it has been as high as 36%. Infection of other edible grain by *Claviceps purpurea* or other fungi that produce pharmacologically active alkaloids occurs, but it is less common.

The spores are carried by insects or the wind to the ovaries of young rye, where they germinate into hyphal filaments. As the hyphal filaments penetrate deep into the ovary of the rye, a dense tissue forms. This tissue gradually consumes the entire substance of the grain and hardens into a purple, curved body called the *sclerotium*. This sclerotium is still a major commercial source of ergot alkaloids.

Ergot has been termed a "veritable treasure house of pharmacological constituents." The substances isolated from ergot were divided by Barger (1931) into two main groups. In the first group are those products peculiar to ergot and not obtainable from any other source. Among these are the ergot alkaloids. The second group consists of a heterogeneous collection of compounds, including several amines of pharmacological importance (*e.g.*, histamine, tyramine, *etc.*).

History. The contamination of an edible grain by a poisonous, parasitic fungus spread death and destruction for centuries. As early as 600 B.C., an Assyrian tablet alluded to a "noxious pustule in the ear of grain"; and in one of the sacred books of the Parsees (400 to 300 B.C.) the following pertinent passage occurs, "Among the evil things created by Angro Maynes are noxious grasses that cause pregnant women to drop the womb and die in childbed." It was fortunate for the ancient Greeks that they objected to the "black malodorous product of Thrace and Macedonia," and therefore did not eat rye. Rye was also comparatively unknown to the early Romans, for it was not introduced into Southwest Europe until after the beginning of the Christian era. Consequently, there is no undisputed reference to ergot poisoning in the early Greek and Roman literature. It was not until the Middle Ages that written descriptions of ergot poisoning first appeared, although it is probable that the disease was prevalent long before this time. Strange epidemics were described in which the characteristic symptom was gangrene of the feet, legs, hands, and arms. In severe cases, the tissue became dry and black and the mummified limbs separated off without loss of blood. Limbs were said to be consumed by the Holy Fire and blackened like charcoal. Mention was also made of agonizing burning sensations in the extremities. The disease was called Holy Fire or St. Anthony's fire, the latter name being in honor of the saint at whose shrine relief was said to be obtained. The relief that followed migration to the shrine of St. Anthony was probably real, for the sufferers received a diet free of contaminated grain

during their sojourn at the shrine. The symptoms of ergot poisoning were not restricted to the limbs. Indeed, a frequent complication of ergot poisoning was abortion. A convulsive type of ergotism was also known. The effects of ergot poisoning were described most effectively in paintings and woodcuts during the late Middle Ages (*e.g.*, Grünewald's altar paintings, now located in the museum at Colmar, France).

Ergot was known as an obstetrical herb before it was identified as the cause of St. Anthony's fire. It was mentioned as early as 1582 by Lonicer as a proven means of producing pains in the womb. It was used by midwives long before it was recognized by the medical profession. The first physician to employ ergot was Desgranges, but he did not publish his observations until 1818. Ten years before, a letter published by John Stearns in the *Medical Repository* of New York, entitled "Account of the Pulvis Parturiens, a Remedy for Quickening Childbirth," marked the official introduction of ergot into medicine (Thoms, 1931). This communication is of sufficient historical interest to quote certain pertinent portions of it:

It [pulvis parturiens] expedites lingering parturition and saves to the accoucheur a considerable portion of time, without producing any bad effects on the patient. . . . Previous to its exhibition it is of the utmost consequence to ascertain the presentation . . . as the violent and almost incessant action which it induces in the uterus precludes the possibility of turning. . . . If the dose is large it will produce nausea and vomiting. In most cases you will be surprised with the suddenness of its operation; it is, therefore, necessary to be completely ready before you give the medicine. . . . Since I have adopted the use of this powder I have seldom found a case that detained me more than three hours. . . .

The use of ergot spread rapidly in the United States, but its adoption in Europe was delayed, perhaps, as Barger (1931) has suggested, because the Old World had suffered too much from the poisonous properties of ergot. The dangers attending the use of the drug, however, were soon recognized. In 1824, Hosack wrote that the number of stillborn children had increased so greatly since the introduction of ergot that the Medical Society of New York instituted an inquiry. Said Hosack, "The ergot has been called . . . *pulvis ad partum;* as it regards the child, it may, with almost equal truth be denominated the *pulvis ad mortem.*" This astute observer recommended that the drug be used only to control post-partum hemorrhage. Thus, more than a century and a half ago, the indications and contraindications of ergot were accurately defined.

Chemistry. The ergot alkaloids can all be considered to be derivatives of the tetracyclic compound 6-methylergoline. The naturally occurring alkaloids contain a substituent in the β configuration at position 8 and a double bond in ring D (Table 39–1). The natural alkaloids of therapeutic interest are amide derivatives of *d-lysergic acid;* these compounds contain a double bond between C 9 and C 10 and thus belong to the family of 9-ergolene compounds. Many alkaloids, containing either a

Table 39–1. NATURAL AND SEMISYNTHETIC ERGOT ALKALOIDS

A. AMINE ALKALOIDS AND CONGENERS

ALKALOID	X	Y
d-Lysergic acid	$-COOH$	$-H$
d-Isolysergic acid		$-COOH$
d-Lysergic acid diethylamide (LSD)	$-C(=O)-N(CH_2CH_3)_2$	$-H$
Ergonovine (ergometrine)	$-C(=O)-NH-CH(CH_3)-CH_2OH$	$-H$
Methylergonovine	$-C(=O)-NH-CH(CH_2CH_3)-CH_2OH$	$-H$
Methysergide [1]	$-C(=O)-NH-CH(CH_2CH_3)-CH_2OH$	$-H$
Lisuride	$-H$	$-NH-C(=O)-N(CH_2CH_3)_2$
Lysergol	$-CH_2OH$	$-H$
Lergotrile [2,3]	$-CH_2CN$	$-H$
Metergoline [1,2]	$-CH_2-NH-C(=O)-O-CH_2-phenyl$	$-H$

B. AMINO ACID ALKALOIDS

ALKALOID [4]	R(2')	R'(5')
Ergotamine	$-CH_3$	$-CH_2-phenyl$
Ergosine	$-CH_3$	$-CH_2CH(CH_3)_2$
Ergostine	$-CH_2CH_3$	$-CH_2-phenyl$
Ergotoxine group:		
Ergocornine	$-CH(CH_3)_2$	$-CH(CH_3)_2$
Ergocristine	$-CH(CH_3)_2$	$-CH_2-phenyl$
α-Ergocryptine	$-CH(CH_3)_2$	$-CH_2CH(CH_3)_2$
β-Ergocryptine	$-CH(CH_3)_2$	$-CHCH_2CH_3$
Bromocriptine [5]	$-CH(CH_3)_2$	$-CH_2CH(CH_3)_2$

[1] Contains methyl substitution at N 1.
[2] Contains hydrogen atoms at C 9 and C 10.
[3] Contains chlorine atom at C 2.
[4] Dihydro derivatives contain hydrogen atoms at C 9 and C 10.
[5] Contains bromine atom at C 2.

methyl or a hydroxymethyl group at position 8, are present in ergot in small quantities. These have been called *clavine alkaloids* and consist principally of both 9-ergolenes (*e.g., lysergol*) and 8-ergolenes (*e.g., elymoclavine,* the 8-ergolene isomer of lysergol). A crystalline, pharmacologically active preparation was first isolated from ergot in 1906 by Barger, Carr, and Dale as well as by Kraft. This material was called *ergotoxine.* It is now known to be a mixture of four alkaloids, *ergocornine, ergocristine, α-ergocryptine,* and *β-ergocryptine.* The first pure ergot alkaloid, *ergotamine,* was obtained by Stoll in 1920. Moir reported the discovery of the "water soluble uterotonic principle of ergot" in 1932. This was subsequently determined to be *ergonovine* (also designated *ergometrine*).

The chemical structures of the alkaloids of ergot have been elucidated primarily by Stoll and associates and by Jacobs and Craig and their coworkers (*see* Rutschmann and Stadler, 1978). Optical isomerism is due to the presence of two asymmetrical carbon atoms (positions 5 and 8) in the lysergic acid portion of the molecule. Derivatives of *l*-lysergic acid (the epimer at position 5) and of *d*-isolysergic acid (the epimer at position 8) display relatively little biological activity. Upon hydrolysis, ergonovine and its derivatives yield lysergic acid and an amine; consequently they are designated as *amine alkaloids.* The alkaloids of higher molecular weight yield lysergic acid, ammonia, pyruvic acid (or a derivative thereof), proline, and one other amino acid (either phenylalanine, leucine, isoleucine, or valine) and are thus known as *amino acid alkaloids* or *ergopeptines.*

Numerous semisynthetic derivatives of the ergot alkaloids have been prepared, and several are of therapeutic interest (*see* Rutschmann and Stadler, 1978). The earliest derivatives were prepared by the catalytic hydrogenation of the natural alkaloids, yielding a series of compounds that are saturated in ring D of lysergic acid. These have been designated *dihydroergotamine, dihydroergocristine,* and so forth, and possess somewhat different pharmacological properties than do the parent alkaloids. Another ergopeptine derivative is *bromocriptine* (2-bromo-α-ergocryptine). In addition, it is possible to prepare different amides of lysergic acid. Two products of this series, lysergic acid diethylamide (LSD; Chapter 23) and lysergic acid hydroxybutylamide (*methylergonovine*), are of pharmacological interest. Methylation of the indole nitrogen of the latter compound yields 1-methylmethylergonovine (*methysergide;* Chapter 26). A large number of related compounds that are not derivatives of lysergic acid have also been prepared. These include *lisuride* (N-[6-methyl-8α-(9-ergolenyl)]-N′,-N′-diethylurea), *lergotrile* (2-chloro-6-methyl-8β-cyanomethyl-ergoline), and *metergoline* (1,6-dimethyl-8β-carbobenzoxyaminomethyl-ergoline) (*see* Chapter 21).

PHARMACOLOGICAL PROPERTIES

The pharmacological actions of the ergot alkaloids are varied and complex; some actions are completely unrelated, and some are even mutually antagonistic. The marked effects of ergotamine on the cardiovascular system, for example, are due to simultaneous peripheral vasoconstriction, depression of vasomotor centers, and peripheral adrenergic blockade. The following presentation will be concerned primarily with the responses of the smooth muscle of the uterus and blood vessels. The actions on adrenergic receptors and vasomotor reflexes are discussed in Chapter 9; CNS effects are discussed in Chapters 21 and 23. The use of bromocriptine to control the secretion of prolactin is described in Chapter 59. A summary of the actions of representative ergot alkaloids is presented in Table 39–2.

The stimulation of vascular and uterine smooth muscle by ergot alkaloids was once thought to reflect an action that was exerted independently of receptors for other substances that cause such contractile responses. However, there is now convincing evidence that mediation by α-adrenergic receptors, tryptaminergic receptors, or both is involved (*see* Berde and Stürmer, 1978; Müller-Schweinitzer and Weidmann, 1978). In general, the effects of all the ergot alkaloids appear to result from their actions as partial agonists or antagonists at adrenergic, dopaminergic, and tryptaminergic receptors (Table 39–2). The spectrum of effects depends on the agent, dosage, species, tissue, and experimental or physiological conditions. However, there are some aspects of the actions of ergot alkaloids that are not entirely compatible with this view: (1) while agonistic effects are generally apparent only at concentrations that are lower than those required to observe antagonism, this is not always the case (*e.g.,* the action of methysergide on cerebral blood vessels); (2) the effects of full agonists (*e.g.,* norepinephrine) are usually augmented by low concentrations of ergot alkaloids, even those with weak efficacy as partial agonists (*e.g.,* the action of ergonovine on arterioles); and (3) the contractile responses to other agents, such as acetylcholine or angiotensin, are sometimes also augmented by low concentrations of ergot alkaloids, and such synergistic effects are not always prevented by adrenergic or tryptaminergic blocking agents. These and other observations emphasize the importance of the physiological or pathophysiological state in determining the spectrum and intensity of effects produced in animals or patients. An emerging body of biochemical data suggests that ergot alkaloids and chemically related compounds interact to varying degrees with subtypes of receptors for the biogenic amines (Gundlach *et al.,* 1983; McPherson and Beart, 1983; Markstein *et al.,* 1983). This type of information may eventually provide more complete explanations for the complex patterns of effects produced by these agents.

Table 39-2. PHARMACOLOGICAL ACTIONS OF SELECTED ERGOT ALKALOIDS

COMPOUND	Interactions with Tryptaminergic Receptors	Interactions with Dopaminergic Receptors	Interactions with α-Adrenergic Receptors	Uterine Stimulation
		PHARMACOLOGICAL ACTIONS		
Ergotamine	Partial agonist in certain blood vessels; nonselective antagonist in various smooth muscles; poor agonist/antagonist in CNS	No notable actions on central or peripheral structures, but high emetic potency after intravenous administration	Partial agonist and antagonist in blood vessels and various smooth muscles; mainly antagonist in peripheral and central nervous systems	Highly active
Dihydroergotamine	Partial agonist and antagonist in a few smooth muscles; may be agonist in lateral geniculate nucleus	Nonselective antagonist in sympathetic ganglia; low emetic potency	Partial agonist in veins; antagonist in blood vessels, various smooth muscles, and peripheral and central nervous systems	Active on pregnant human uterus
Bromocriptine	Only a few weak antagonistic actions reported	Partial agonist and antagonist in various areas of CNS; presumed agonist in inhibiting secretion of prolactin; less emetic potency than ergotamine	No agonistic effects; somewhat less potent antagonist than dihydroergotamine in various tissues	Inactive
Ergonovine and methylergonovine	Partial agonists in human umbilical and placental blood vessels; selective and fairly potent antagonists in various smooth muscles; partial agonists and antagonists in some areas of CNS	Weak antagonists in certain blood vessels; partial agonists and antagonists in various areas of CNS; less potent than bromocriptine in producing emesis or inhibiting secretion of prolactin	Partial agonists in blood vessels (less than ergotamine); little antagonistic action	Very highly active
Methysergide	Partial agonist in certain blood vessels and areas of CNS; selective and very potent antagonist in many tissues and areas of CNS	Little evidence for agonistic or antagonistic activity; no emetic activity	Little or no agonistic or antagonistic action	Very little activity

935

Aside from the stereochemical considerations mentioned above, few rules governing structure-activity relationships have emerged. In general, small amide derivatives of lysergic acid are potent and relatively selective antagonists of 5-HT, while the amino acid alkaloids are usually less selective and show similar affinities as blocking agents at α-adrenergic and tryptaminergic receptors. Dihydrogenated derivatives usually have fewer and less intense agonistic actions than do the parent alkaloids. Finally, insertion of a methyl group at position 1 usually results in compounds with less affinity for receptors for catecholamines and with more selective ability to block tryptaminergic receptors.

Uterus.   All the natural alkaloids of ergot markedly increase the motor activity of the uterus. After small doses, contractions are increased in force or frequency, or both, but are followed by a normal degree of relaxation. As the dose is increased, contractions become more forceful and prolonged, resting tonus is markedly increased, and sustained contracture can result. Although this characteristic precludes their use for induction or facilitation of labor, it is quite compatible with their use post partum or post abortion to control bleeding and maintain uterine contraction. The sensitivity of the uterus to ergot alkaloids varies, especially with the degree of maturity and the stage of gestation, but even an immature uterus is stimulated. The gravid uterus is very sensitive, and small doses of ergot alkaloids can be given immediately post partum to obtain a marked uterine response, usually without significant side effects.

Although all natural ergot alkaloids have qualitatively the same effect on the uterus, they exhibit marked differences in potency. Ergonovine is the most active and is less toxic than is ergotamine, the most potent of the amino acid alkaloids; unlike ergotamine, it is also effective after oral administration. For these reasons, ergonovine and its semisynthetic derivative, methylergonovine, have replaced other ergot preparations as uterine-stimulating agents in obstetrics.

Methylergonovine differs little from ergonovine in its uterine actions. The dihydrogenated alkaloids do not have the uterine-stimulating properties of the parent alkaloids when tested in experimental animals. However, they are capable of exerting a marked uterine-stimulating action on the pregnant human uterus at term.

The uterine-stimulating effect of ergot alkaloids apparently involves interactions with receptors for biogenic amines, in that cyproheptadine blocks the effects of both 5-HT and ergonovine in the rat uterus (Hashimoto *et al.*, 1977), while phentolamine blocks the effects of both norepinephrine and ergotamine, but not of oxytocin, in the rabbit uterus (*see* Berde and Stürmer, 1978).

Cardiovascular System.   Ergotamine, the other natural amino acid alkaloids, and the dihydrogenated derivatives exert complex actions on the cardiovascular system. These are discussed further in Chapter 9.

The natural amino acid alkaloids, particularly ergotamine, produce constriction of both arteries and veins. While dihydroergotamine retains appreciable vasoconstrictor activity, it is far more effective on capacitance than on resistance vessels. This property is the basis for investigation of its usefulness in the treatment of postural hypotension. The dihydrogenated derivatives of the ergotoxine group are considerably less active and usually produce hypotension because of effects in the CNS. In doses used in the treatment of migraine, ergotamine usually produces only small increments in blood pressure but does increase peripheral vascular resistance and decrease blood flow in various organs (Tfelt-Hansen *et al.*, 1983). These effects result in part from reduced flow through nonnutritive arteriovenous anastomoses (*see* Saxena, 1978). While less potent than ergotamine, the amine alkaloids can also raise blood pressure slightly and decrease blood flow in the extremities when administered in therapeutic doses. The intensity of pressor effects is greater when the blood pressure is elevated.

Ergot alkaloids that produce peripheral vasoconstriction can also damage the capillary endothelium. The mechanism of this toxic action is not clearly understood. Vascular stasis, thrombosis, and gangrene result and are prominent features of ergot poisoning. The propensity of these alkaloids to cause gangrene appears to parallel their vasoconstrictor activity.

Vascular Responses Related to the Therapy of Migraine.   Ergotamine is effective in relieving migraine headaches, even though it is neither sedative nor analgesic. The etiology of migraine is complex and poorly understood, and there are multiple forms of the syndrome that may involve different pathophysiological processes. Those attacks that are associated with a subjective "aura" or objective prodromal neurological signs and symptoms have been classified as "classical" migraine. Such attacks begin with a period of unexplained diminished blood flow in some region of the cerebrum (Sakai and Meyer, 1978); this was believed to produce localized ischemia and result in the prodromal symptoms. The dominant view has been that the reduced flow was caused by vasospasm, perhaps as a consequence of the release of 5-HT from platelets. Attacks without prodromal symptoms (classified as "common" migraine) were thought to begin in a similar, but less intense fashion. However, recent studies that have employed sophisticated technics for the measurement of regional cerebral blood flow have not detected areas of reduced flow at the onset of attacks of common migraine (Olesen *et al.*, 1982). Moreover, attacks of classical migraine appear to begin with a spreading wave of reduced blood flow that is usually preceded by focal hyperemia at some site (Lauritzen *et al.*, 1983). The pattern and progression of oligemia do not seem to be consistent with a vasospastic episode in a major cerebral vessel, and the degree of hypoperfusion is not thought to be sufficient to produce signs and symptoms of ischemia. Thus, it appears that oligemia may be caused by events in adjacent brain tissue, perhaps analogous to the phenomenon of "spreading depression" that ensues after local injury or the local application of potassium chloride to cerebral tissue.

Following the oligemic phase in classical migraine, and at some undefined point in common migraine, there is a prolonged period during which the flow of blood is increased in both intracerebral and extracranial vessels (Sakai and Meyer, 1978). The resultant increased amplitude of pulsations of the cranial arteries, chiefly the meningeal branches of the external carotid, is believed to be the chief source of the pain. Factors that decrease the amplitude of pulsation, for example, digital pressure on the carotid artery, reduce the intensity of the headache, and there is a parallel decline in arterial pulsation when ergotamine provides relief from pain (*see* Wolff, 1972; Saper, 1978a). In addition to reducing extracranial blood flow, ergotamine can decrease hyperperfusion of regions served by the basilar artery without decreasing cerebral hemispheric flow (Sakai and Meyer, 1978). There is also some evidence that opening of arteriovenous anastomoses during an attack contributes to the marked decrease in resistance to flow in areas served by the carotid artery (*see* Saxena, 1978). Therapeutic doses of ergotamine, acting perhaps as a tryptaminergic agonist, cause decreased shunting of blood from the carotid artery to the jugular vein in experimental animals.

Absorption, Fate, and Excretion. The amino acid alkaloids, such as ergotamine, are slowly and incompletely absorbed from the gastrointestinal tract. Peak concentrations in plasma are achieved in 2 hours. For unexplained reasons, the concurrent administration of caffeine (100 mg per 1 mg of ergotamine) increases both the rate of absorption and the peak plasma concentration about twofold; oral and rectal preparations used in the treatment of migraine often contain such a combination. The effective intramuscular dose of ergotamine is about 10% of the oral dose, but absorption from the site of injection is slow, as judged by a latent period of about 20 minutes before the onset of the uterine response. The effective intravenous dose is about 50% of the intramuscular dose, and a uterine-stimulating effect is observed within 5 minutes.

The rate of clearance from plasma is approximately equal to that of hepatic blood flow; this may explain the very low bioavailability of ergotamine when administered orally (Ibraheem *et al.*, 1983).

Ergotamine is metabolized in the liver by largely undefined pathways, and 90% of the metabolites are excreted in the bile (*see* Eckert *et al.*, 1978). Only traces of unmetabolized drug can be found in urine and feces. There is evidence that ergotamine is sequestered in various tissues. This probably accounts for its long-lasting therapeutic and toxic actions, despite a half-time of about 2 hours for disappearance from plasma.

Bromocriptine is absorbed more completely after oral administration and is eliminated more slowly than is ergotamine. Dihydroergotamine and dihydroergotoxine are much less completely absorbed and are eliminated more rapidly than is ergotamine. The low bioavailability of dihydroergotamine is also apparently due primarily to rapid hepatic clearance (Little *et al.*, 1982). The amine alkaloids are rapidly and virtually completely absorbed after oral administration and reach peak concentrations in plasma within 60 to 90 minutes that are more than tenfold those achieved with an equivalent dose of ergotamine. A uterotonic effect can be observed within 10 minutes after oral administration of 0.2 mg of ergonovine to women post partum. Judging from the relative duration of action, ergonovine is metabolized and/or eliminated more rapidly than is ergotamine. The half-life of methylergonovine in plasma ranges between 0.5 and 2 hours (Mantyla and Kanto, 1981). Studies on animals indicate that the principal metabolites of the amine alkaloids are hydroxylated in the A ring, while the metabolism of the amino acid alkaloids primarily involves alterations in the tricyclopeptide moiety. Nearly all of the metabolites recovered after the administration of methysergide to human subjects are devoid of the methyl group at position 1.

Ergot Poisoning. The ergot alkaloids are highly toxic and may cause acute or chronic poisoning. The former is rare and usually results from large amounts of ergot ingested in attempts at abortion. The symptoms consist in vomiting, diarrhea, unquenchable thirst, tingling, itching, and coldness of the skin, a rapid and weak pulse, confusion, and unconsciousness. The natural amino acid alkaloids are many times more toxic than their dihydrogenated derivatives. Fatal poisoning has occurred after the oral administration of 26 mg of ergotamine over a period of several days, and also following single injections of only 0.5 to 1.5 mg.

At present the epidemic form of chronic ergot poisoning arising from the ingestion of contaminated grain is seldom seen. However, poisoning from the injudicious therapeutic administration of ergot alkaloids is not rare. Although poisoning is usually due to overdosage, increased sensitivity to ergot alkaloids may accompany febrile and septic states and disease of the liver. Several fatalities from gangrene have occurred in patients with hepatic damage who received ergotamine for relief of the accompanying pruritus. Patients with occlusive peripheral vascular disease are extremely susceptible to the vascular complications of ergotamine therapy.

In chronic ergotism, whether due to overdosage or to unusual susceptibility, striking circulatory changes develop. The feet and legs, and somewhat less frequently the hands, become cold, pale, and numb. Muscle pain occurs while walking and later at rest. Arterial pulses in the affected limbs become faint or even disappear. Eventually gangrene develops, beginning usually in the toes but sometimes in the fingers. Two factors are involved in the impairment of the circulation, vasoconstriction and intimal lesions; the latter may result in thrombi that completely occlude the smaller arteries. Additional circulatory disturbances may include anginal pain, tachycardia or bradycardia, and elevation or lowering of the blood pressure.

The most common other symptoms are *headache, nausea, vomiting, diarrhea,* and *dizziness.* Also, there may be noticeable weakness, formication, itching, and coldness of the skin. Symptoms particularly referable to the CNS are confusion, depression, drowsiness, and rarely, convulsions, hemiplegia, tabetic manifestations, and a fixed miosis.

Methysergide has been implicated in the initiation and exacerbation of fibrotic disease of several types (*see* Chapter 26).

Complications of Ergotamine Therapy. When ergotamine is prescribed in correct dosage in the absence of contraindications, it is a safe and useful drug; few serious complications have been reported from its use in the migraine syndrome.

Nausea and vomiting occur in approximately 10% of patients after oral administration and in about twice that number after parenteral administration; there is a direct effect of the drug on CNS emetic centers. However, severe nausea is common during attacks of migraine regardless of treatment. Weakness in the legs is common, and muscle pains, which occasionally are quite severe, may occur in the extremities. Numbness and tingling of the fingers and toes are other reminders of the ergotism that this alkaloid may cause. Precordial distress and pain suggestive of angina pectoris, as well as transient tachycardia or bradycardia, have also been noted. Localized edema and itching may occur in an occasional hypersensitive patient. Most of these effects are not alarming and ordinarily do not necessitate interruption of ergotamine therapy.

Treatment. The treatment of ergotism consists in complete withdrawal of the offending drug and symptomatic measures. The latter include attempts to maintain an adequate circulation to the affected parts. Pharmacological agents that have been employed include anticoagulants, low-molecular-weight dextran, and potent vasodilator drugs. Carliner and associates (1974) have reported the successful treatment of a severe case of ergotism by the intravenous infusion of sodium nitroprusside. Nausea and vomiting may be relieved by atropine or by antiemetic compounds of the phenothiazine type.

Preparations and Routes of Administration. Only a few of the purified ergot alkaloids are available for therapeutic application. *Ergotamine tartrate* (ERGOMAR, others) is available in tablets that contain 2 mg (sublingual) of the salt. The drug is also available as a suspension for inhalation; each dose delivers 0.36 mg of the salt. Preparations containing mixtures of *ergotamine tartrate and caffeine* (CAFERGOT, others) are also available; tablets and capsules contain 1 mg of ergotamine tartrate and 100 mg of caffeine, and the corresponding suppositories contain 2 mg and 100 mg, respectively. *Dihydroergotamine mesylate* (D.H.E. 45) is supplied as a solution (1 mg/ml) for injection. *Methysergide maleate* (SANSERT) is available as oral tablets containing 2 mg.

Ergonovine maleate (ERGOTRATE MALEATE) is available in solution for injection (0.2 mg/ml) and in oral 0.2-mg tablets. *Methylergonovine maleate* (METHERGINE) is marketed for injection (0.2 mg/ml) and in 0.2-mg oral tablets.

Ergoloid mesylates (dihydrogenated ergot alkaloids; HYDERGINE, others) are available in 0.5- or 1.0-mg tablets. Each 0.5-mg tablet contains 0.167 mg each of dihydroergocornine, dihydroergocristine, and dihydroergocryptine (dihydro-α-ergocryptine and dihydro-β-ergocryptine in the proportion of 2:1) as the mesylates. A liquid containing 1 mg/ml and liquid-filled capsules are also available.

Bromocriptine mesylate (PARLODEL) is supplied in 2.5-mg tablets and in 5-mg capsules.

THERAPEUTIC USES

The major therapeutic uses of the ergot alkaloids fall into two categories: (1) applications in obstetrics (discussed later in this chapter), and (2) treatment of migraine. The use of bromocriptine in the treatment of Parkinson's disease is discussed in Chapter 21, while the uses related to the suppression of the secretion of prolactin are presented in Chapter 59.

Migraine. Ergotamine remains an important agent for symptomatic relief of the pain of migraine, particularly in those patients for whom aspirin-like drugs provide incomplete relief. However, before reliance is placed on ergotamine or other medications, it is important that the physician attempt to assess and correct any underlying emotional or physical stresses, dietary or hormonal factors, or ingestion of drugs that may influence the incidence and severity of attacks (*see* Saper, 1978b).

Dosage and Route of Administration. Ergotamine is usually administered *orally* or *sublingually;* the dose is 2 mg, given as soon as the headache starts. Doses of 2 mg may be given at intervals of 30 minutes thereafter, if necessary, until a total of 6 mg has been taken. No more than 10 mg should be ingested per week.

Ergotamine may also be administered by inhalation. A single inhalation (about 0.36 mg) is used at the onset of an attack, and this may be repeated at intervals of 5 minutes to a total of six doses in 24 hours. The maximal dosage in 1 week is 5.4 mg (about 15 inhalations).

If a patient cannot tolerate ergotamine orally, rectal administration of a mixture of caffeine and ergotamine tartrate may be attempted. At the onset of an attack, one-half to one suppository (1 to 2 mg) may be used, and another suppository may be used in 1 hour, if necessary. No more than two suppositories per attack or five suppositories per week should be administered.

Dihydroergotamine mesylate can be administered by intramuscular injection (1 mg, repeated at 1-hour intervals to a total of 3 mg) or, in some circumstances, intravenously (2 mg, maximum). No more than 6 mg should be given intravenously in 1 week.

Since overdosage is the chief cause of untoward effects from ergotamine, the smallest amount effective for relief of the headache should be employed. The speed and thoroughness of the relief from pain are directly proportional to the promptness with which medication is started after the onset of an attack. If the drug is given early, the dose may be decreased considerably. If the headache has reached its peak, larger amounts of ergotamine are needed. Not only is a longer time then required for effective action but also unpleasant side effects from medication are more pronounced. Some investigators recommend that ergotamine be used with caution during the period in which patients with classical migraine are experiencing neurological disturbances.

Efficacy. Ergotamine is effective in the vast majority of cases. The specificity of the drug for migraine is indicated by the fact that only occasionally are other types of headaches influenced. Relief is often dramatic. After parenteral injection of ergotamine, the headache may disappear in 15 minutes, but sometimes only after 2 hours or more. Oral medication is much slower in bringing relief, an average of 5 hours being required, and it may fail in severe attacks. The drug is not useful in preventing attacks. Observance of the specified maximal weekly doses is important, not only to minimize the untoward effects of the drug but also to avoid possible dependence. Patients who take ergotamine daily for prolonged periods may require increased dosage to achieve relief and may experience rebound attacks of migraine.

Dihydroergotamine has also been used for the treatment of migraine, but fewer patients respond to it than to ergotamine.

Caffeine enhances the action of the ergot alkaloids in the treatment of migraine, a discovery that must be credited to the sufferers from the disease who observed that strong coffee gave symptomatic relief, especially when combined with the ergot alkaloids. As mentioned, caffeine increases the oral and rectal absorption of ergotamine, and it is widely believed that this accounts for the enhancement of therapeutic effects. Caffeine may also contribute to vasoconstriction in both extracranial and intracranial vessels by its capacity to increase the release of catecholamines and to antagonize adenosine-induced vasodilatation, respectively (*see* Chapter 25). Whatever the contributing factors, some physicians prefer to obtain the augmented therapeutic response by administration of caffeine and ergotamine separately, rather than by use of fixed-dose combinations.

Contraindications. Because gangrene due to ergotamine has occurred in a number of patients with infection, sepsis is a definite contraindication. It should not be used in patients with vascular disease, such as syphilitic arteritis, marked atherosclerosis, coronary artery disease, thrombophlebitis, and Raynaud's or Buerger's syndrome. Diseases of the liver or kidney are also contraindications. Serious toxicity has been reported from the use of ergotamine in patients with pruritus, especially when the symptom is secondary to hepatic disease. Although very large amounts of ergotamine are required to produce abortion, pregnancy constitutes an objection to use.

Other Uses. The mixture of ergoloid mesylates has been widely employed in the treatment of senile dementias. In a few apparently well-controlled studies, patients treated with dihydroergotoxine have displayed slight improvement in some behavioral or other psychological measure (*see* Loew and Weil, 1982). The mechanisms that could possibly underlie any beneficial responses are not understood, and the subject remains controversial.

Ergonovine has been used as a provocative agent during coronary arteriography to aid in the diagnosis of angina pectoris secondary to coronary artery spasm (*Prinzmetal's variant angina*) (*see* Chapter 33).

Prophylaxis of Migraine. Because of the putative role of 5-HT in the genesis of attacks of migraine, attention was focused initially on tryptaminergic antagonists for use in prophylactic treatment. However, only a few such antagonists (notably methysergide) have been found to be effective. In recent years, there has been a proliferation of agents that either are, or appear to be, effective in reducing the number and/or severity of attacks. One of the most important problems in making such a judgment is the occurrence of a prominent placebo response. In addition, the studies usually do not make a distinction between effects in classical migraine and those in common migraine. In no instance has a drug been found to eliminate attacks of migraine in any patient or to produce at least some beneficial effects in all patients.

Propranolol. Propranolol is currently the preferred drug for the prophylaxis of migraine. Its beneficial effects were first noted incidental to its use in the treatment of angina (*see* Chapter 9). In a long-term study, about 70% of patients with either classical or common migraine experienced fewer or less intense attacks during the administration of 80 to 160 mg of propranolol per day (Diamond *et al.,* 1982); the level of benefit remained constant for up to 12 months and was maintained in about 45% of the patients for 1 to 2 months after discontinuation of the medication. The mechanisms that underlie this effect are not known, and the relevance of β-adrenergic blockade has been questioned. While some other β-adrenergic antagonists (*e.g.,* atenolol and nadolol) also appear to be effective (Forssman et al., 1983; Ryan et al., 1983), a number of similar agents are not (see Peatfield, 1983).

Methysergide. While methysergide is not useful for the treatment of acute attacks of migraine, it was the first agent found to be effective prophylactically. The proportion of patients who respond to methysergide (4 to 8 mg per day) is somewhat less than that for propranolol (see Saper, 1978b). The major disadvantage to therapy with this drug is the danger of retroperitoneal fibrosis; drug-free periods of 3 to 4 weeks are recommended every 6 months. The relevance of tryptaminergic blockade to the beneficial effects of methysergide has been questioned because, with the exception of pizotyline (see Capildeo and Rose, 1982), no other such antagonist has been found to be effective.

Amitriptyline. Amitriptyline in doses up to 100 mg per day appears to be about as effective as methysergide for the prophylaxis of migraine (Couch and Hassanein, 1979). This effect seems relatively independent of antidepressant responses to the drug since nondepressed patients with severe migraine have experienced improvement most frequently. The mechanisms that underlie this effect are not known.

Calcium Channel Antagonists. Among this group of drugs are several agents that have shown promise for the prophylactic treatment of migraine and a related syndrome known as cluster headaches (see Peroutka, 1983). While older representatives (e.g., verapamil and nifedipine) appear to be effective, newer agents, such as flunarizine and nimodipine, may prove to be more useful (Amery, 1983; Diamond and Schenbaum, 1983; Gelmers, 1983; Meyer and Hardenberg, 1983). It has been proposed that calcium channel antagonists may be relatively selective in reducing vasospastic episodes in cerebral blood vessels because contractile responses of these vessels display a greater dependence on *extracellular* calcium than do those in blood vessels from other regions of the body (Peroutka et al., 1984). There also appear to be differences in the degree of tissue selectivity among various drugs in this group. A general discussion of the pharmacology of calcium channel antagonists appears in Chapter 33.

THE CLINICAL USE OF DRUGS THAT STIMULATE UTERINE MOTILITY

There are many indications for, and contraindications to, the clinical use of agents that stimulate uterine contractions. In brief, the clearest indications are: (1) to induce or augment labor in *selected* individuals, (2) to control post-partum uterine atony and hemorrhage, (3) to cause uterine contraction after cesarean section or during other uterine surgery, and (4) to induce therapeutic abortion.

Induction of Labor. The use of uterine-stimulating agents for the induction of labor is reserved for those cases where continuation of the pregnancy is considered to be a greater risk to the mother or fetus than the concomitant risks of pharmacological induction.

When it is determined that a medical indication exists for the termination of pregnancy (e.g., maternal diabetes, isoimmunization, hypertensive states, anemia, prolonged pregnancy with placental insufficiency), a careful assessment of the clinical variables must be made. Objective determination of fetal maturity must also be made, and the possibility of fetopelvic disproportion should be considered. Other potential contraindications to induction of labor include abnormal fetal position, evidence of fetal distress, placental abnormalities, and previous uterine surgery.

The drug of choice for the induction of labor is oxytocin. For all ante-partum indications except abortion, oxytocin should be given by intravenous infusion of a dilute solution, preferably by means of a variable-speed infusion pump. A suitable concentration for use in induction of labor at term is 10 milliunits per milliliter (10 units added to 1 liter of 5% dextrose). The infusion is started at the rate of 0.1 to 0.2 ml (1 to 2 milliunits) per minute. If no response is obtained within 15 minutes, the rate of administration can be increased at 15- to 30-minute intervals in increments of 0.1 to 0.2 ml per minute to a maximum of 2.0 ml (20 milliunits) per minute. The total dose required to initiate labor ranges from 600 to 12,000 milliunits, with an average of 4000. Seitchik and Castillo (1982, 1983) have recommended a specific regimen for the administration of oxytocin. This includes an initial dose of 1 milliunit per minute, escalation of the dose at a rate no greater than 1 milliunit per minute every 30 minutes, and maintenance of a dose of 4 milliunits per minute (if attained) for at least 1 hour before increasing the dose further. In their hands, no patient has required a dose greater than 9 milliunits per minute.

During the entire procedure trained personnel must be present and uterine activity should be carefully monitored. If contractions become too forceful or frequent or resting tone is elevated, the infusion should be immediately discontinued. Changes in fetal heart rate are useful indicators of fetal distress. Occasionally, even the cautious use of oxytocin will stimulate the uterus to a sustained tetanic contraction, which may so interfere with the placental circulation that it may be necessary to administer a general anesthetic to effect uterine relaxation. As labor progresses, it may be necessary to decrease the dosage of oxytocin or to terminate the infusion. The infusion should be maintained at the lowest possible rate that will allow adequate progression of labor (Baxi et al., 1980).

When employed at term, oxytocin induces labor in the majority of cases. If amniotomy is also used, as it is by many obstetricians, successful induction occurs in 80 to 90% of cases.

The prostaglandins ($PGF_{2\alpha}$ and PGE_2) are potential alternatives to oxytocin for the induction of labor. Although investigation of their use as a sole inducing agent continues (*see*, for example, Ueland and Conrad, in Symposium, 1983), the prostaglandins and their synthetic derivatives may prove to be more valuable as adjunctive therapy in the management of spontaneous or induced labor for their effects on cervical ripening (*see* Symposium, 1983; Lange *et al.*, 1984). Such use of prostaglandins is currently investigational in the United States.

The prostaglandins have the potential advantage of stimulating uterine contractions at any stage of pregnancy; thus, they are useful for the treatment of most cases of missed abortion, late intrauterine death, molar gestation, and premature rupture of the membranes (*see* Thiery and Amy, 1977).

Augmentation of Labor. In most circumstances, oxytocin should not be used for the augmentation of labor if labor is progressing, albeit slowly. The type of contraction produced often is too forceful and sustained to be compatible with the safety of mother and fetus. When the uterus, under the stimulus of a drug, contracts too forcibly against an incompletely dilated and rigid cervix, the following accidents may occur: (1) the force of the contraction may drive the presenting part through the incompletely dilated cervical tissues and cause severe laceration of the mother and trauma to the infant; (2) if the soft tissues are unyielding, the uterus may rupture; and (3) the forceful tetanic contraction of the uterus may compromise placental exchange and fetal oxygenation.

There are occasions, however, when oxytocin can be used advantageously by the experienced obstetrician to manage *dysfunctional labor*. Cases must be selected carefully and dosage regulated continuously. Oxytocin is usually effective in those patients where there is a very prolonged latent phase of cervical dilatation as well as in those cases where there is a significant arrest of dilatation or descent. When there is protracted dilatation or descent without actual arrest, a response to uterine-stimulating agents will generally not be obtained (*see* Friedman, 1978). In patients who are receiving epidural anesthesia, the reflexly stimulated release of oxytocin during the second stage of labor may be impaired (Goodfellow *et al.*, 1983). The cautious use of oxytocin may reduce the need to employ forceps for delivery under these circumstances.

Third Stage of Labor and Puerperium. After delivery of the fetus, it is desirable to have the uterus firm and active. This reduces greatly the incidence and extent of post-partum hemorrhage. The use of uterine-stimulating agents for this purpose has declined in recent years, in part because of the decreased utilization of general anesthetics during delivery. When used, the usual procedure is to await delivery of the placenta before the administration of a uterine-stimulating agent. In any case, it is necessary to exclude the possibility of a multiple pregnancy before the drug is given. Ergonovine (or methylergonovine) is preferred for this use because of its sustained duration of action. The intramuscular injection of 0.2 to 0.3 mg produces a rapid and lasting response. Either alkaloid may also be given intravenously in a dose of 0.2 mg if immediate action is desirable.

In the normal individual, the period of uterine involution is 8 to 10 weeks, but the process is most rapid during the first 10 days. If involution is delayed, stimulation of the uterus is definitely helpful because delayed involution is usually associated with uterine atony. Under such conditions, either ergonovine (0.2 to 0.4 mg, two to four times daily) or methylergonovine (0.2 mg, three to four times daily) may be given orally for as long a period as is necessary to accomplish the desired results (usually 2 to 7 days). If infection develops in the postpartum uterus, there is evidence that the use of ergonovine may limit its spread. Caution must be observed in the use of ergonovine for an extended period of time. The possibility of interference with lactation must be considered with the use of either alkaloid.

Therapeutic Abortion. Abortion during the *first trimester* is most commonly accomplished by means of suction curettage. No satisfactory form of drug-induced abortion during this period is yet available, although the use of synthetic prostaglandins applied intravaginally has met with some success in the termination of pregnancies at 6 to 7 weeks gestation (Brenner *et al.*, 1983). Beyond the first few weeks of the *second trimester* several alternative procedures for abortion are available. Intra-amniotic injection of a hypertonic (20%) solution of sodium chloride has been employed, but numerous failures occur and the procedure entails serious potential hazards for the patient. Oxytocin is not generally effective, even with infusion of relatively large doses (20 to 30 units). The *prostaglandins* have been used effectively for second-trimester abortion. While vaginal suppositories of dinoprostone (PGE_2) inserted at intervals of 3 to 5 hours have been used effectively, there has been more experience with the cautious intra-amniotic instillation of 40 mg of dinoprost tromethamine ($PGF_{2\alpha}$). If the fetal membranes are still intact 24 hours later, an additional 10 to 40 mg may be administered. In other circumstances, especially when the uterine contents have not been eliminated but the membranes are ruptured, the intramuscular administration of 0.25 mg of carboprost tromethamine (15-methyl $PGF_{2\alpha}$) has been effective; subsequent doses may be administered at approximately 2-hour intervals. Nausea, vomiting, and diarrhea are frequent side effects of the use of these prostaglandins. The intra-amniotic instillation of low doses of $PGF_{2\alpha}$ (5 to 10 mg) in combination with a hyperosmolar solution of urea has recently been investigated and compared with the widely used method of dilatation and evacuation (Kafrissen *et al.*, 1984). The principal conclusion was that dilatation and evacuation remains the safest and most effective procedure available for abortion at 13 to 20 weeks gestation.

After spontaneous or therapeutic abortion or premature delivery, the post-partum indications for ergonovine and oxytocin to control bleeding and maintain uterine tone are similar to those after delivery at term.

Oxytocin-Challenge Test. Oxytocin has been used for an ante-partum test of uteroplacental insufficiency in high-risk pregnancies. Oxytocin is infused initially at the rate of 0.5 milliunit per minute; this rate is increased slowly until uterine contractions occur every 3 to 4 minutes. Concurrent monitoring of the pattern of the fetal heart rate indicates whether the contractions result in signs of fetal distress. The outcome of the oxytocin-challenge test is helpful in determining whether there exists adequate placental reserve for continuation of a high-risk pregnancy (Freeman, 1975).

THE CLINICAL USE OF DRUGS THAT INHIBIT UTERINE MOTILITY

There are several indications for, and contraindications to, the clinical use of agents that inhibit uterine contractions. The clearest indications are: (1) to delay or prevent premature parturition in *selected* individuals and (2) to slow or arrest delivery for brief periods in order to undertake other therapeutic measures. Tocolytic agents that are currently in use include β_2-adrenergic agonists, magnesium sulfate, and ethanol. The use of tocolytic agents has been reviewed in recent symposia (Symposium, 1981, 1982) and by Caritis (1983).

Premature Labor. Premature births account for a large fraction of perinatal morbidity and mortality. Despite major advances in neonatal care, retention of the fetus *in utero* is preferred in most instances. It is often difficult to determine if premature birth is imminent, and 50% or more of patients who present with regular uterine contractions will respond to bed rest and hydration. If this fails, a tocolytic agent may be administered. However, the desire to prolong intrauterine development must be balanced against the risks of continued pregnancy to both the mother and fetus, as well as the risks of pharmacological intervention. In general, the use of tocolytic agents is reserved for those pregnancies where the gestational age is greater than 20 weeks and less than 34 to 36 weeks; at the more advanced gestational ages, definite evidence for immaturity of the fetus is usually sought. When the decision to use a tocolytic agent is made, therapeutic success is most likely if cervical dilatation is less than 4 cm and cervical effacement is less than 80%; tocolysis is usually not attempted if the membranes have ruptured, since there is risk of infection. Other contraindications include eclampsia or severe preeclampsia, chorioamnionitis, premature detachment of the placenta, and fetal distress.

β_2-Adrenergic Agonists. These agents are preferred for the treatment of premature labor. Currently, only *ritodrine* is approved for this use in the United States. *Ritodrine hydrochloride* (YUTOPAR) is available in a solution (10 mg/ml) for intravenous administration and in 10-mg oral tablets. Treatment is initiated by the intravenous infusion of a solution of ritodrine (0.3 mg/ml) at the rate of 0.1 mg per minute. If tolerated, the dose is gradually increased (0.05 mg per minute every 10 minutes) to a maximum of 0.35 mg per minute or until labor is controlled. Once contractions cease, the infusion is usually continued for 12 hours at the rate attained. Oral therapy is begun 30 minutes before termination of the infusion by the administration of 10 mg every 2 hours for the first 24 hours, followed by 10 to 20 mg every 4 to 6 hours; the total daily dose should not exceed 120 mg.

As might be expected, the administration of ritodrine or other β_2-adrenergic agonists produces a number of cardiovascular and metabolic side effects in the mother (*see* Chapter 8). Although mean arterial pressure changes very little, there is a dose-related tachycardia and increase in cardiac output that probably results from a reflex response to the lowered diastolic blood pressure combined with direct actions on β_1-adrenergic receptors in the heart. The secretion of renin is enhanced, and this presumably contributes to the decreased renal excretion of sodium, potassium, and water that occurs. If hydration during therapy is overly vigorous, pulmonary edema may result, either with or without evidence of myocardial failure. Total fluid intake should be restricted to less than 2 liters in 24 hours, and ECG monitoring before and during therapy has been advocated (Benedetti, 1983). Evidence of cardiac disease is a contraindication to the use of these agents.

Ritodrine and similar drugs can cause marked hyperglycemia. While this usually does not require treatment, persistent hyperglycemia (>200 mg/dl) may result in reactive hypoglycemia in the infant should parturition proceed. The use of β_2-adrenergic agonists in patients with insulin-dependent diabetes is hazardous and is usually considered to be contraindicated. In most cases, the concomitant infusion of insulin is required to prevent the development of diabetic ketoacidosis. Hypokalemia is another consequence of the administration of ritodrine. Since this reflects the movement of potassium to the intracellular compartment, total body stores are not reduced and treatment is not indicated.

A number of other selective β_2-adrenergic agonists have also been employed for the management of preterm labor; these include *terbutaline* and *fenoterol*. The indications, contraindications, and side effects associated with the use of any of these agents are similar to those for ritodrine.

Magnesium Sulfate. The major indication for the administration of magnesium sulfate to pregnant women is for the prevention or control of seizures associated with eclampsia or severe preeclampsia. At doses somewhat higher than those useful in these conditions, uterine contractions can be effectively inhibited. In the presence of normal renal function, magnesium sulfate may be a useful alternative when the use of a β_2-adrenergic agonist is contraindicated. A variety of protocols has been used. The regimen recommended by Petrie (Symposium, 1981) involves the intravenous administration of a loading dose of 6 g of magnesium sulfate over a period of 20 minutes, followed by an infusion at the rate of 2 g per hour until the frequency of uterine contractions is reduced to less than 1 every 10 minutes. Thereafter, the rate of infusion is reduced to 1 g per hour, and therapy is continued for 24 to 72 hours. If cervical dilatation progresses beyond 5 cm, the drug is discontinued. Effective inhibition of uterine contractions has been associated with concentrations of magnesium in plasma between 4 and 8 mg/dl (3.3 to 6.6 mEq/liter). Higher concentrations produce progressive inhibition of cardiac conduction and neuromuscular transmission and can lead to respiratory depression and cardiac arrest (*see* Chapter 35). Neonatal depression can also occur; this may be alleviated by the administration of calcium. Attempts to use combinations of magnesium sulfate and ritodrine have resulted in a marked increase in the incidence of cardiovascular side effects, especially myocardial ischemia, even though lower doses of ritodrine were effective (Ferguson *et al.*, 1984). However, the oral administration of a β_2-adrenergic agonist following the arrest of labor by magnesium sulfate has been beneficial in the management of a few diabetic patients (Hill *et al.*, 1984).

Ethanol. Ethanol has been used for nearly 2 decades for the prevention of premature labor. While ethanol may be nearly as effective as ritodrine in prolonging gestation, it does not produce a corresponding reduction in the incidence of fetal respiratory distress (*see* Fuchs and Fuchs, in Symposium, 1981). As a result, it has been largely supplanted by β_2-adrenergic agonists. Nevertheless, there remain circumstances in which other agents are contraindicated (*e.g.*, cardiac disease) and in which ethanol may be useful. Inhibition of uterine contractions is associated with concentrations of ethanol in plasma of 0.12 to 0.18%. These are achieved by the intravenous infusion of a 10% solution at a rate of 7.5 ml/kg per hour for 2 hours and maintained by infusion at a rate of 1.5 ml/kg per hour for up to 10 hours.

Other Agents. Calcium channel antagonists are known to relax the myometrium *in vitro* and to inhibit markedly the amplitude (but not the frequency) of oxytocin-induced contractions. One such agent, *nifedipine,* appears to be effective in delaying parturition for 4 to 27 days. However, the available data are limited, and the potential usefulness of nifedipine or related agents cannot be estimated at this time (*see* Forman *et al.*, in Symposium, 1981). While inhibitors of prostaglandin synthesis, such as *indomethacin,* can prolong gestation in both term and preterm pregnancies, their use in the management of premature labor has been curtailed because of concern for their potential to cause adverse effects in the fetus. Of particular importance is the possibility of premature closure of the ductus arteriosus and the production of pulmonary hypertension. However, this class of drugs may be much less hazardous if employed for brief periods at earlier gestational ages, when there is less possibility of premature closure of the ductus (*see* Niebyl, in Symposium, 1981).

Other Uses. There are a number of circumstances in which inhibition of uterine contractions for brief periods would provide the opportunity to initiate other therapeutic measures under more favorable conditions. Among the more obvious of these is the alleviation of fetal distress during transport of the mother to hospital or during preparation for operative delivery that might be necessitated by such complications as a breech presentation, prolapsed cord, or partial premature detachment of the placenta (*see* Lipshitz, in Symposium, 1981). Both β_2-adrenergic agonists and magnesium sulfate have been employed successfully for the management of these and other complications of both spontaneous and induced labor.

Amery, W. K. Flunarizine, a calcium channel blocker: a new prophylactic drug in migraine. *Headache,* **1983,** *23,* 70–74.

Amico, J. A.; Seitchik, J.; and Robinson, A. G. Studies of oxytocin in plasma of women during hypocontractile labor. *J. Clin. Endocrinol. Metab.,* **1984,** *58,* 274–279.

Arias, F. Efficacy and safety of low-dose 15-methyl prostaglandin $F_{2\alpha}$ for cervical ripening in the first trimester of pregnancy. *Am. J. Obstet. Gynecol.,* **1984,** *149,* 100–101.

Barger, G.; Carr, F. H.; and Dale, H. H. An active alkaloid from ergot. *Br. Med. J.,* **1906,** *2,* 1792.

Baxi, L. V.; Petrie, R. H.; and Caritis, S. N. Induction of labor with low-dose prostaglandin $F_{2\alpha}$ and oxytocin. *Am. J. Obstet. Gynecol.,* **1980,** *136,* 28–31.

Benedetti, T. J. Maternal complications of parenteral β-sympathomimetic therapy for premature labor. *Am. J. Obstet. Gynecol.,* **1983,** *145,* 1–6.

Brenner, P. F.; Marrs, R. P.; Roy, S.; and Mishell, D. R., Jr. Methods to determine success of attempts to terminate early gestation pregnancies with prostaglandin vaginal suppositories. *Contraception,* **1983,** *28,* 111–124.

Burbach, J. P. H.; Bohus, B.; Kovacs, G. L.; Van Nispen, J. W.; Greven, H. M.; and De Wied, D. Oxytocin is a precursor of potent behaviourally active neuropeptides. *Eur. J. Pharmacol.,* **1983,** *94,* 125–131.

Capildeo, R., and Rose, F. C. Single-dose pizotifen, 1.5 mg nocte: a new approach in the prophylaxis of migraine. *Headache,* **1982,** *22,* 272–275.

Carliner, N. H.; Denune, D. P.; Finch, C. S., Jr.; and Goldberg, L. I. Sodium nitroprusside treatment of ergotamine-induced peripheral ischemia. *J.A.M.A.,* **1974,** *227,* 308–309.

Couch, J. R., and Hassanein, R. S. Amitriptyline in migraine prophylaxis. *Arch. Neurol.,* **1979,** *36,* 695–699.

Diamond, S.; Kudrow, L.; Stevens, J.; and Shapiro, D. B. Long-term study of propranolol in the treatment of migraine. *Headache,* **1982,** *22,* 268–271.

Diamond, S., and Schenbaum, H. Flunarizine, a calcium channel blocker, in the prophylactic treatment of migraine. *Headache,* **1983,** *23,* 39–42.

Di Renzo, G. C.; Venincasa, M. D.; and Bleasdale, J. E. The identification and characterization of β-adrenergic receptors in human amnion tissue. *Am. J. Obstet. Gynecol.,* **1984,** *148,* 398–405.

Ferguson, J. E., II; Hensleigh, P. A.; and Kredenster, D. Adjunctive use of magnesium sulfate with ritodrine for preterm labor tocolysis. *Am. J. Obstet. Gynecol.,* **1984,** *148,* 166–171.

Forssman, B.; Lindblad, C. J.; and Zbornikova, V. Atenolol for migraine prophylaxis. *Headache,* **1983,** *23,* 188–190.

Freeman, R. K. The use of the oxytocin challenge test for antepartum clinical evaluation of uteroplacental respiratory function. *Am. J. Obstet. Gynecol.*, **1975**, *121*, 481–489.

Fuchs, A.-R.; Fuchs, F.; Husslein, P.; Soloff, M. S.; and Fernström, M. J. Oxytocin receptors and human parturition: a dual role for oxytocin in the initiation of labor. *Science*, **1982**, *215*, 1396–1398.

Fuchs, A.-R.; Goeschen, K.; Husslein, P.; Rasmussen, A. B.; and Fuchs, F. Oxytocin and the initiation of human parturition. III. Plasma concentrations of oxytocin and 13,14-dihydro-15-keto-prostaglandin $F_{2\alpha}$ in spontaneous and oxytocin-induced labor at term. *Am. J. Obstet. Gynecol.*, **1983**, *147*, 497–502.

Garrioch, D. B. The effect of indomethacin on spontaneous activity in the isolated human myometrium and on the response to oxytocin and prostaglandin. *Br. J. Obstet. Gynaecol.*, **1978**, *85*, 47–52.

Gelmers, H. J. Nimodipine, a new calcium antagonist, in the prophylactic treatment of migraine. *Headache*, **1983**, *23*, 106–109.

Goodfellow, C. F.; Hull, M. G. R.; Swaab, D. F.; Dogterom, J.; and Buijs, R. M. Oxytocin deficiency at delivery with epidural analgesia. *Br. J. Obstet. Gynaecol.*, **1983**, *90*, 214–219.

Gundlach, A. L.; Krstich, M.; and Beart, P. M. Guanine nucleotides reveal differential actions of ergot derivatives at D-2 receptors labelled by [^{3}H]spiperone in striatal homogenates. *Brain Res.*, **1983**, *278*, 155–163.

Hashimoto, H.; Hayashi, M.; Nakahara, Y.; Niwaguchi, T.; and Ishii, H. Actions of D-lysergic acid diethylamide (LSD) and its derivatives on 5-hydroxytryptamine receptors in the isolated uterine smooth muscle of the rat. *Eur. J. Pharmacol.*, **1977**, *45*, 341–348.

Hill, W. C.; Katz, M.; Kitzmiller, J. L.; and Burr, R. E. Tocolysis for the insulin-dependent diabetic woman. *Am. J. Obstet. Gynecol.*, **1984**, *148*, 1148–1150.

Husslein, P.; Kofler, E.; Rasmussen, A. B.; Sumulong, L.; Fuchs, A.-R.; and Fuchs, F. Oxytocin and the initiation of human parturition. IV. Plasma concentrations of oxytocin and 13,14-dihydro-15-keto-prostaglandin $F_{2\alpha}$ during induction of labor by artificial rupture of the membranes. *Am. J. Obstet. Gynecol.*, **1983**, *147*, 503–507.

Ibraheem, J. J.; Paalzow, L.; and Tfelt-Hansen, P. Low bioavailability of ergotamine tartrate after oral and rectal administration in migraine sufferers. *Br. J. Clin. Pharmacol.*, **1983**, *16*, 695–699.

Kafrissen, M. E.; Schulz, K. F.; Grimes, D. A.; and Cates, W., Jr. Midtrimester abortion. Intra-amniotic instillation of hyperosmolar urea and prostaglandin $F_{2\alpha}$ v dilatation and evacuation. *J.A.M.A.*, **1984**, *251*, 916–919.

Kent, D. R.; Goldstein, A. I.; and Milokovich, D. Preoperative cervical dilatation with a single long-acting prostaglandin analog suppository. *J. Reprod. Med.*, **1983**, *28*, 778–780.

Kraft, F. Über das Mutterkorn. *Arch. Pharm.*, **1906**, *244*, 336–359.

Land, H.; Grez, M.; Ruppert, S.; Schmale, H.; Rehbain, M.; Richter, D.; and Schütz, G. Deduced amino acid sequence from the bovine oxytocin—neurophysin I precursor cDNA. *Nature*, **1983**, *302*, 342–344.

Lange, I. R.; Collister, C.; Johnson, J.; Cote, D.; Torchia, M.; Freund, G.; and Manning, F. A. The effect of vaginal prostaglandin E_2 pessaries on induction of labor. *Am. J. Obstet. Gynecol.*, **1984**, *148*, 621–629.

Lauritzen, M.; Olsen, T. S.; Lassen, N. A.; and Paulson, O. B. Regulation of regional cerebral blood flow during and between migraine attacks. *Ann. Neurol.*, **1983**, *14*, 569–572.

Legros, J. J.; Chiodera, P.; Geenen, V.; Smitz, S.; and von Frenckell, R. Dose-response relationship between plasma oxytocin and cortisol and adrenocorticotropin concentrations during oxytocin infusion in normal men. *J. Clin. Endocrinol. Metab.*, **1984**, *58*, 105–109.

Little, P. J.; Jennings, G. L.; Skews, H.; and Bobik, A. Bioavailability of dihydroergotamine in man. *Br. J. Clin. Pharmacol.*, **1982**, *13*, 785–790.

McPherson, G. A., and Beart, P. M. The selectivity of some ergot derivatives for α_1 and α_2-adrenoceptors of rat cerebral cortex. *Eur. J. Pharmacol.*, **1983**, *91*, 363–369.

Majkić-Singh, N.; Vuković, A.; Spasić, S.; Ruzic, A.; Stojanov, M.; and Berkés, I. Oxytocinase (CAP) activity in serum during normal pregnancy. *Clin. Biochem.*, **1982**, *15*, 152–153.

Mantyla, R., and Kanto, J. Clinical pharmacokinetics of methylergometrine (methylergonovine). *Int. J. Clin. Pharmacol. Ther. Toxicol.*, **1981**, *19*, 386–391.

Markstein, R.; Closse, A.; and Frick, W. Interaction of ergot alkaloids and their combination (co-dergocrine) with α-adrenoceptors in the CNS. *Eur. J. Pharmacol.*, **1983**, *93*, 159–168.

Meyer, J. S., and Hardenberg, J. Clinical effectiveness of calcium entry blockers in prophylactic treatment of migraine and cluster headaches. *Headache*, **1983**, *23*, 266–277.

Moir, C. The action of ergot preparations on the puerperal uterus. *Br. Med. J.*, **1932**, *1*, 1119–1122.

Okazaki, T.; Sagawa, N.; Bleasdale, J. E.; Okita, J. R.; MacDonald, P. C.; and Johnston, J. M. Initiation of human parturition. XIII. Phospholipase C, phospholipase A_2 and diacylglycerol lipase activities in fetal membranes and decidua vera tissues from early and late gestation. *Biol. Reprod.*, **1981**, *25*, 103–109.

Okita, J. R.; Johnston, J. M.; and MacDonald, P. C. Source of prostaglandin precursor in human fetal membranes: arachidonic acid content of amnion and chorion laeve in diamnionic-dichorionic twin placentas. *Am. J. Obstet. Gynecol.*, **1983**, *147*, 477–482.

Olesen, J.; Lauritzen, M.; Tfelt-Hansen, P.; Henriksen, L.; and Larsen, B. Spreading cerebral oligemia in classical- and normal cerebral blood flow in common migraine. *Headache*, **1982**, *22*, 242–248.

Peroutka, S. J.; Banghart, S. B.; and Allen, G. S. Relative potency and selectivity of calcium antagonists used in the treatment of migraine. *Headache*, **1984**, *24*, 55–58.

Rholam, M.; Nicolas, P.; and Cohen, P. Binding of neurohypophyseal peptides to neurophysin dimer promotes formation of compact and spherical complexes. *Biochemistry*, **1982**, *21*, 4968–4973.

Ryan, R. E., Sr.; Ryan, R. E., Jr.; and Sudilovsky, A. Nadolol: its use in the prophylactic treatment of migraine. *Headache*, **1983**, *23*, 26–31.

Sakai, F., and Meyer, J. S. Regional cerebral hemodynamics during migraine and cluster headaches measured by the ^{133}Xe inhalation method. *Headache*, **1978**, *18*, 122–132.

Saunders, W. G., and Munsick, R. A. Antidiuretic potency of oxytocin in women post partum. *Am. J. Obstet. Gynecol.*, **1966**, *95*, 5–11.

Sbarra, A. J.; Selvaraj, R. J.; Cetrulo, C. L.; Thomas, G.; Louis, F.; and Kennison, R. Phagocytosis and onset of human labor. *Am. J. Obstet. Gynecol.*, **1983**, *146*, 622–629.

Seitchik, J., and Castillo, M. Oxytocin augmentation of dysfunctional labor. I. Clinical data. *Am. J. Obstet. Gynecol.*, **1982**, *144*, 899–905.

———. Oxytocin augmentation of dysfunctional labor. III. Multiparous patients. *Ibid.*, **1983**, *145*, 777–780.

Stoll, A. Zur Kenntnis der Mutterkornalkaloide. *Verh. Naturf. Ges. (Basel)*, **1920**, *101*, 190–191.

Tfelt-Hansen, P.; Kanstrup, I.-L.; Christensen, N. J.; and Winkler, K. General and regional haemodynamic effects of intravenous ergotamine in man. *Clin. Sci.*, **1983**, *65*, 599–604.

Thoms, H. John Stearns and pulvis parturiens. *Am. J. Obstet. Gynecol.*, **1931**, *22*, 418–423.

Uldbjerg, N.; Ekman, G.; Malmström, A.; Olsson, K.; and Ulmsten, U. Ripening of the human uterine cervix related to changes in collagen, glycosaminoglycans, and collagenolytic activity. *Am. J. Obstet. Gynecol.*, **1983**, *147*, 662–666.

Wikland, M.; Lindblom, B.; Wilhelmsson, L.; and Wiqvist, N. Oxytocin, prostaglandins, and contractility of the human uterus at term pregnancy. *Acta Obstet. Gynecol. Scand.*, **1982**, *61*, 467–472.

Monographs and Reviews

Altura, B. M., and Altura, B. T. Actions of vasopressin, oxytocin, and synthetic analogs on vascular smooth muscle. *Fed. Proc.*, **1984**, *43*, 80–86.

Barger, G. *Ergot and Ergotism.* Gurney & Jackson, Edinburgh, **1931**.

Berde, B., and Stürmer, E. Introduction to the pharmacology of ergot alkaloids and related compounds as a basis of their therapeutic application. In, *Ergot Alkaloids and Related Compounds.* (Berde, B., and Schild, H. O., eds.) *Handbuch der Experimentellen Pharmakologie,* Vol. 49. Springer-Verlag, Berlin, **1978**, pp. 1–28.

Buijs, R. M. Vasopressin and oxytocin—their role in neurotransmission. *Pharmacol. Ther.*, **1983**, *22*, 127–141.

Caritis, S. N. Treatment of preterm labour: a review of the therapeutic options. *Drugs*, **1983**, *26*, 243–261.

Eckert, H.; Kiechcl, J. R.; Rosenthaler, J.; Schmidt, R.; and Schreier, E. Biopharmaceutical aspects: analytical methods, pharmacokinetics, metabolism and bioavailability. In, *Ergot Alkaloids and Related Compounds.* (Berde, B., and Schild, H. O., eds.) *Handbuch der Experimentellen Pharmakologie,* Vol. 49. Springer-Verlag, Berlin, **1978**, pp. 719–803.

Friedman, E. A. *Labor: Clinical Evaluation and Management,* 2nd ed. Appleton-Century-Crofts, New York, **1978**.

Huszar, G., and Roberts, J. M. Biochemistry and pharmacology of the myometrium and labor: regulation at the cellular and molecular levels. *Am. J. Obstet. Gynecol.*, **1982**, *142*, 225–237.

Kao, C. Y. Electrophysiological properties of the uterine smooth muscle. In, *Biology of the Uterus.* (Wynn, R. M., ed.) Plenum Press, New York, **1977**, pp. 423–496.

Loew, D. M., and Weil, C. Hydergine in senile mental impairment. *Gerontology*, **1982**, *28*, 54–74.

Müller-Schweinitzer, E., and Weidmann, H. Basic pharmacological properties. In, *Ergot Alkaloids and Related Compounds.* (Berde, B., and Schild, H. O., eds.) *Handbuch der Experimentellen Pharmakologie,* Vol. 49. Springer-Verlag, Berlin, **1978**, pp. 87–232.

Nakano, J. Cardiovascular actions of oxytocin. *Obstet. Gynecol. Surv.*, **1973**, *28*, 75–92.

Owen, P. R. Prostaglandin synthetase inhibitors in the treatment of primary dysmenorrhea. *Am. J. Obstet. Gynecol.*, **1984**, *148*, 96–103.

Peatfield, R. Migraine: current concepts of pathogenesis and treatment. *Drugs*, **1983**, *26*, 364–371.

Peroutka, S. J. The pharmacology of calcium channel antagonists: a novel class of anti-migraine agents? *Headache*, **1983**, *23*, 278–283.

Pickering, B. T.; Swann, R. W.; and González, C. B. Biosynthesis and processing of neurohypophysial hormones. *Pharmacol. Ther.*, **1983**, *22*, 143–161.

Roy, A. C., and Karim, S. M. M. Significance of the inhibition by prostaglandins and cyclic GMP of oxytocinase activity in human pregnancy and labour. *Prostaglandins*, **1983**, *25*, 55–70.

Rutschmann, J., and Stadler, P. A. Chemical background. In, *Ergot Alkaloids and Related Compounds.* (Berde, B., and Schild, H. O., eds.) *Handbuch der Experimentellen Pharmakologie,* Vol. 49. Springer-Verlag, Berlin, **1978**, pp. 29–85.

Saper, J. R. Migraine. I. Classification and pathogenesis. *J.A.M.A.*, **1978a**, *239*, 2380–2383.

———. Migraine. II. Treatment. *Ibid.*, **1978b**, *239*, 2480–2484.

Saxena, P. R. Arteriovenous shunting and migraine. *Res. Clin. Stud. Headache*, **1978**, *6*, 89–102.

Symposium. (Various authors.) Preterm parturition. (Creasy, R. K., ed.) *Semin. Perinatol.*, **1981**, *5*, 191–302.

Symposium. (Various authors.) Beta-receptor agonists in obstetrics. (Ingemarsson, I., ed.) *Acta Obstet. Gynecol. Scand.*, **1982**, *108*, Suppl. 1, 13–72.

Symposium. (Various authors.) The forces of labor: uterine contractions and the resistance of the cervix. (Ulmsten, U., and Ueland, K., eds.) *Clin. Obstet. Gynecol.*, **1983**, *26*, 1–106.

Thiery, M., and Amy, J. Spontaneous and induced labor: two roles for the prostaglandins. *Obstet. Gynecol. Annu.*, **1977**, *6*, 127–171.

Wolff, H. G. *Wolff's Headache and Other Pain,* 3rd ed. (Dalessio, D. J., rev.) Oxford University Press, New York, **1972**.

Locally Acting Drugs

CHAPTER

40 SURFACE-ACTING DRUGS

Ewart A. Swinyard and Madhu A. Pathak

A large number of drugs act locally in a purely mechanical or physical manner. Although they possess both therapeutic and pharmaceutical usefulness, their pharmacological properties warrant only brief discussion. Their effects are confined to the site of application when the compounds are employed in reasonable dosage. These effects are described adequately by the names that are applied to the groups into which the drugs can be classified, namely, *demulcents, emollients, protectives, adsorbents,* and *absorbable hemostatics.* Other drugs act primarily at the site of application but have a chemical rather than a physical basis of action; they are *astringents, irritants, sclerosing agents, caustics, keratolytics, antiperspirants* and *deodorants, antiseborrheics, melanizing* and *demelanizing agents, sunscreening agents, mucolytics,* and certain *enzymes.*

DEMULCENTS

The demulcents comprise a group of compounds of high molecular weight that form aqueous solutions having the ability to alleviate irritation, particularly of mucous membranes or abraded surfaces. When applied locally to irritated or abraded tissues, the demulcents tend to coat the surface and, by mechanical means, protect the underlying cells from stimuli that result from contact with air or irritants in the environment. The demulcents are applied to the skin in the form of lotions, ointments, or wet dressings; to the eyes in the form of artificial tears and in wetting agents for contact lenses; to the gastrointestinal tract in the form of demulcent drinks or enemas; and to the throat in the form of lozenges or gargles. The demulcents also have valuable pharmaceutical properties. They mask the obnoxious taste of certain drugs, and solutions of demulcents are often used as vehicles for this purpose. They are also employed to provide stable emulsions or suspensions of drugs immiscible with or insoluble in aqueous vehicles. Chemically, the more important demulcents are either gums, synthetic cellulose derivatives, or polyhydroxy compounds; their principal uses will be briefly described.

The two most commonly employed demulcent gums are *acacia* and *tragacanth. Acacia* (gum arabic), either in the form of the powder or as *acacia syrup* (a vanilla-flavored syrup that contains 10% acacia), is employed chiefly to suspend or emulsify drugs. It is also incorporated in lozenges. *Tragacanth* (gum tragacanth), a gum that in the presence of sufficient water swells to 50 times its original volume, is used as a demulcent base for cutaneous medication, a suspending agent for insoluble powders, and an emulsifying agent for oils administered orally. Other natural plant hydrocolloids used to a lesser extent than acacia and tragacanth include *agar, glycyrrhiza,* and *sodium alginate.*

The synthetic cellulose derivatives—*methylcellulose, carboxymethylcellulose sodium,* and others—are widely used in contact-lens solutions, artificial tears, other ophthalmic preparations, and toothpastes, and as suspending agents for nosedrops and other drugs that act locally. In addition, they are also used as hydrophilic colloid laxatives (*see* Chapter 43).

The demulcent polyhydroxy compounds include *glycerin (glycerol), propylene glycol,* and the *polyethylene glycols.* Glycerin is a trihydric alcohol. It is miscible with water and alcohol, and is extensively employed as a vehicle for many drugs applied to the skin. Diluted with rose water it is an effective lotion for chapped and roughened hands. In combination with starch it forms a jelly base known as *starch glycerite,* a preparation sometimes employed as an emollient and a vehicle. Glycerin is frequently used in moisturizing creams (*e.g.,* ACID MANTLE, AQUACARE, LUBRIDERM); it is a hygroscopic agent that, when absorbed into the skin, can moisten the stratum corneum.

Glycerin absorbs water, and, therefore, in high concentration it is somewhat dehydrating and irritating to exposed tissue. The irritant action of glycerin accounts for its efficacy in promoting evacuation of the bowel when used rectally in the form of a suppository. It is also available as *glycerin oral solution* (50 and 75%). When given orally, glycerin may be used for the management of cerebral edema, to lower ocular tension in glaucoma, and to decrease cerebrospinal fluid pressure (*see* Chapter 36). It may be employed as a sweetening agent or vehicle in place of syrups.

Various congeners of glycerin are much more toxic than the parent compound. They exert a nephrotoxic effect and also may damage the liver. Indeed, deaths have resulted from the ingestion of drugs dissolved in *diethylene glycol* for oral administration (Bowie and McKenzie, 1972), and poisonings from *ethylene glycol* continue to occur (Parry and Wallach, 1974); *propylene glycol* is said to be less toxic (however, *see* Genel, 1978).

Propylene glycol is a clear, colorless, viscous liquid with a slightly acrid taste. It is completely miscible with water and dissolves many essential oils. It is used as a solvent for oral and injectable drugs, and is also employed in cosmetics, lotions, and ointments, as in the water-washable *hydrophilic ointment*. The topical application of a 40 to 60% aqueous solution of propylene glycol with occlusion has been reported to clear the skin in X-linked ichthyosis and ichthyosis vulgaris (Goldsmith and Baden, 1972).

Polyethylene glycols are high-molecular-weight polymers produced by reacting ethylene oxide with ethylene glycol or water. They have the general formula $H(OCH_2CH_2)_nOH$. The n may range from 1 to a large number; hence, the molecular weights of these substances range from 150 to about 20,000. Substances with molecular weights up to 600 are liquids at room temperature and resemble highly refined petroleum oils in appearance and consistency. Those with molecular weights of 1000 to 9000 are solids at room temperature and resemble petroleum waxes such as paraffin. The polyethylene glycols are of growing importance to the drug industry because of their blandness, water solubility, wide compatibility, and low order of toxicity. They are employed as water-soluble ointment bases, as ingredients of lotions and suppositories, and as tablet coatings. As emulsifying and dispersing agents, they provide stability and homogeneity to formulations containing oily components and water. In addition, related compounds, such as polyoxyl 40 stearate, polysorbate 80, and sodium lauryl sulfate, are also used as emulsifying and dispersing agents.

Several proprietary water-miscible (oil-in-water) ointment bases, such as CETAPHIL and UNIBASE, are also available. These bases can be readily removed from the skin by washing and are valuable when large quantities of liquid are to be incorporated into an ointment.

Urea, in concentrations of 2 to 20%, is used to promote hydration and removal of excess keratin in dry skin and hyperkeratotic conditions. In concentrations of 40%, it may be employed to remove dystrophic and potentially disabling nails without local anesthesia and surgery.

EMOLLIENTS

Emollients are fats or oils used for their local action on the skin and, occasionally, the mucous membranes. These oleaginous substances, also known as occlusive agents and humectants, are employed as protectives and as agents for softening the skin and rendering it more pliable, but chiefly as vehicles for more active drugs. Emollients soften the skin by forming an occlusive oil film on the stratum corneum, thus preventing drying from evaporation of the water that diffuses to the surface from the underlying layers of skin. Only the commonly employed emollients are described below.

Vegetable Oils. Vegetable oils include *olive oil, cottonseed oil, corn oil, almond oil, peanut oil, persia oil,* and *cocoa butter*. With the exception of the last-named preparation, all are fluids. When taken internally, they act as mild cathartics and as protectives for the gastrointestinal tract in cases of corrosive poisoning. When applied externally, they are emollient to the skin and mucous membranes. They also provide the vehicles for many drugs that are injected in oily solution or suspension. Cocoa butter is a solid that melts at body temperatures. It is widely used as a suppository and an ointment base.

Animal Fats. The animal fat of particular pharmacological interest is *anhydrous lanolin (wool fat)*. This is a yellow, unctuous mass obtained from the wool of sheep. Wool fat is usually employed mixed with 25 to 30% water, in which form it is known as *lanolin (hydrous wool fat)*. These two semisolids are used principally as bases for ointments. Because certain individuals are allergic to wool fat, it has been deleted from many formulations.

Hydrocarbons. The important emollient hydrocarbons are *paraffin, petrolatum, white petrolatum, mineral oil,* and *light mineral oil*. Hydrophilic *petrolatum* is an ointment (water-in-oil) base characterized by the capacity to take up large amounts of water; it contains cholesterol, stearyl alcohol, white wax, and white petrolatum. Many ointments have a base composed of either white wax (5%) and white petrolatum (95%) or yellow wax (5%) and petrolatum (95%). The former combination is termed *white ointment;* the latter, *yellow ointment*. *Paraffin* is used mainly in ointments to raise their melting points. *White petrolatum* is a common ointment base and also is employed as an emollient and a lubricant. *Light mineral oil* has been used as a vehicle for drugs to be applied to the nasal mucous membranes; however, aqueous vehicles are preferred for this purpose. The more viscous *mineral oil* is an ingredient in various pharmaceutical preparations and is used also as a laxative.

Waxes. *White wax (bleached beeswax)* and *yellow wax (beeswax)* are employed to harden ointment bases. A base composed of lard hardened with wax is known as a *cerate*. *Spermaceti*, a waxy substance obtained from the head of the sperm whale, was used to raise the melting point of ointments; *cetyl esters wax* is a synthetic substitute. A mixture of oil and wax is sometimes used as a vehicle for drugs when slow absorption and sustained effect are desired.

A widely employed, pleasant-smelling, soft emollient preparation is *rose water ointment*. It consists essentially of cetyl esters wax, white wax, almond oil, rose water, and rose oil. Most of the commercial *cold creams* are modifications of this basic preparation. Cold creams are pleasant-smelling, water-in-oil, soft, emulsion-base creams. Because of the lubricating, emollient, and cooling effects, a cold cream serves as a vehicle or a base in many cosmetic products, such as cleansing, night, moisturizing, and eye creams.

Other proprietary water-miscible (water-in-oil) bases, such as AQUAPHOR and HYDROPHILIC PETROLATUM, are also available. Although large amounts of liquids can be incorporated in these bases, they cannot be readily removed from the skin by washing.

PROTECTIVES AND ADSORBENTS

Protectives are designed to cover the skin or mucous membranes in order to prevent contact with possible irritants. Although demulcents and emollients are also protective, common usage restricts the term to certain insoluble and chemically inert substances in a very fine state of subdivision, for example, *dusting powders*, and to the several materials that form an adherent, continuous, flexible or semirigid coat when applied to the skin. Some chemically inert powders also adsorb dissolved or suspended substances, such as gases, toxins, and bacteria; these are known as *adsorbents*. Substances used internally for this purpose are described below, under *gastrointestinal protectives and adsorbents*. Unfortunately, there are no all-purpose effective protective agents; it is essential, therefore, to choose a particular substance for protection against a specific hazard.

Dusting Powders. Powders increase evaporation, reduce friction, and provide antipruritic and cooling effects. These relatively innocuous (inert and insoluble) substances are used to cover and to protect epithelial surfaces, ulcers, and wounds. Those with a smooth surface act mainly by preventing friction; those with a porous structure, by absorbing moisture. The absorption of skin moisture also decreases friction and discourages growth of certain bacteria. The more important dusting powders include *talc, zinc oxide, zinc stearate, magnesium stearate, starch, boric acid,* and *insoluble salts of bismuth*. Water-absorbent powders should not be used on raw surfaces with profuse exudate, as they tend to cake and form adherent crusts. Starch may be metabolized by microorganisms on the skin; consequently, its use may result in the overgrowth of *Candida*. It also becomes doughy when it absorbs moisture and requires the addition of an antiseptic to prevent fermentation. Zinc stearate and magnesium stearate are not wetted by moisture, and thus they permit seepage and evaporation and do not crust.

Medicated or perfumed *talc* (mainly magnesium silicate) is widely used as a dusting powder under the name *talcum powder*. Although *talc* is a benign substance when applied to the intact skin, it can induce severe granulomatous reactions when introduced into wounds or an operative field. For this reason, *talc* should never be used as a dusting powder for surgical gloves. *Absorbable dusting powder* (BIO-SORB) is an absorbable powder prepared from cornstarch. The resulting product is mixed with 2% magnesium oxide and contains residual amounts of sodium sulfate and sodium chloride. It is used as a dusting powder for surgical gloves. It appears to produce no appreciable reaction in tissues and is absorbed completely in a short time. This product is used only in surgery and does not replace the other uses of talc.

Dextranomer (DEBRISAN) is used for the debridement of secreting wounds, such as *venous stasis ulcers, decubitus ulcers, infected traumatic* and *surgical wounds,* and *infected burns*. It consists of spherical hydrophilic beads of dextranomer, 0.1 to 0.3 mm in diameter; the paste is a mixture of beads and polyethylene glycol. The beads, composed of a three-dimensional network of macromolecular chains of cross-linked dextran, allow substances with a molecular weight of less than 1000 to enter freely; those with a molecular weight of 1000 to 5000 enter less freely, and higher-molecular-weight substances are excluded from the beads. Each gram of dextranomer absorbs approximately 4 ml of water; this action is continuous as long as unsaturated beads or paste are in proximity to the wound. The rapid and continuous removal of exudate from the surface of the wound results in a marked reduction in *inflammation, edema,* and *pain* and appears to enhance the formation of granulation tissue and reduce the time for wound healing. The application and/or removal of the beads may cause transitory pain, bleeding, blistering, and erythema in some patients.

Mechanical Protectives. Agents in this category are used to provide occlusive protection from the external environment, to give mechanical support, and as vehicles for various medicaments. *Collodion* (5% pyroxylin in an ether-alcohol vehicle) and *flexible collodion*, composed of collodion with camphor (2%) and castor oil (3%), are occasionally used to seal small wounds and as vehicles for medicated collodions. *Absorbable gelatin film* (GEL-FILM) is used as a mechanical protective and as a temporary supportive and replacement matrix in surgical repair. It is also a component of STOMAHESIVE, which is placed around an ostomy. *Zinc gelatin*, a smooth jelly composed of zinc oxide (10%) and gelatin (15%) in a glycerin-water vehicle, is spread between layers of bandage and used as a protective dressing and support for varicosities and similar lesions. The dressing may be removed by soaking with warm water.

Dimethicone, a relatively inert silicone, is used in ointments, sprays, lotions, and creams. It is an excellent water-protective agent. Because of its low surface tension, dimethicone ointment penetrates crevices in the skin to form a plastic barrier. It is nontoxic, stable, inert, and water repellent; as such, it is useful as a "barrier cream" in industry when skin may be frequently exposed to irritant aqueous compounds. Dimethicone sprays are not helpful against organic solvents.

Gastrointestinal Protectives and Adsorbents. The principal gastrointestinal protectives and adsorbents include *magnesium trisilicate, aluminum hydroxide, activated charcoal, kaolin,* and *pectin.*

Magnesium trisilicate, a relatively weak antacid, is an effective gastrointestinal adsorbent. The gelatinous silicon dioxide, formed by the reaction of magnesium trisilicate with the gastric contents, is said to protect ulcerated mucosal surfaces and favor healing. The salt also interferes with the absorption of tetracyclines, anticholinergics, and other drugs. It is usually given orally suspended in water, in a dose of 1 g four times a day. Chronic use may rarely result in silica kidney stones.

A number of aluminum compounds, such as *aluminum hydroxide gel, dried aluminum hydroxide gel,* and *aluminum phosphate gel,* are used as adsorbents. These substances also decrease the absorption of tetracyclines, anticholinergics, and other drugs. Since they neutralize hydrochloric acid so efficiently, they are discussed under the gastric antacids (Chapter 42).

Activated charcoal, an odorless, tasteless, fine black powder, is the residue from the destructive distillation of various organic materials, treated to increase its adsorptive power. The adsorptive capacity of various brands of activated charcoal differs enormously; a finely powdered activated charcoal with a high adsorptive capacity is satisfactory. Activated charcoal, because of its broad spectrum of adsorptive activity and its rapidity of action, is considered to be the most valuable single agent for the emergency treatment of oral drug poisoning (*see* Chapter 68).

Kaolin is a native, hydrated aluminum silicate, powdered and freed from gritty particles by elutriation. It is used internally and externally for its adsorbent properties.

Pectin is a purified carbohydrate product obtained from the acid extraction of the rind of citrus fruits or from apple pomace. Chemically, it consists chiefly of polygalacturonic acid, some of the hydroxyl groups of which are methylated. It dissolves in 20 parts of water; the resulting colloidal solution is viscous, opalescent, and acidic. Pectin may be administered simply and conveniently in the form of ground raw apple. Kaolin with pectin (KAOPECTATE) usually contains 5.85 g of kaolin and 130 mg of pectin per 30 ml. It is claimed to act as an adsorbent and demulcent in the treatment of diarrhea. However, adequately controlled clinical studies that demonstrate the efficacy of these popular but minimally effective antidiarrheal mixtures are lacking.

Simethicone (GAS-X, MYLICON), a light-gray, translucent liquid of greasy consistency, is a mixture of liquid dimethylpolysiloxanes with antifoaming and water-repellent properties. It is promoted as an adjunct in the treatment of conditions in which gas is a problem, such as flatulence, functional gastric bloating, and postoperative gaseous distention. It has also been used to reduce gas shadows in radiography of the bowel and to improve visualization in gastroscopy. Clinical studies in support of these recommendations are not convincing. Simethicone is available as an oral suspension and in tablets. The usual adult oral dose is 40 to 80 mg after each meal and at bedtime. Simethicone is also used in combination with antacids, antispasmodics, sedatives, and digestants.

ANTIPERSPIRANTS AND DEODORANTS

Antiperspirants and *deodorants,* applied as aerosol sprays, pads, sticks, and roll-on creams, liquids, or semisolids, are vigorously promoted to the public for the control of excessive perspiration and body odor. Under normal conditions perspiration is odorless. The unpleasant odor sometimes associated with skin secretions results from chemical and bacterial degradation of the components of perspiration. Consequently, proper skin hygiene is essential to the control of body odors. Many individuals find skin hygiene inadequate and utilize preparations that decrease the flow and/or inhibit the degradation of perspiration.

Antiperspirants. Four topical antiperspirants (*aluminum chlorohydrates, aluminum chloride, buffered aluminum sulfate,* and *aluminum zirconium chlorohydrates*) have been classified by a United States Food and Drug Administration advisory review panel as safe and effective when used in the appropriate concentration. *Aluminum chlorohydrates* are available in forms that differ in the ratio of aluminum to chlorine, and they are also available as complexes with polyethylene glycol or propylene glycol. They are less acidic than aluminum chloride. These salts are used in a concentration of 25% (anhydrous) or less. *Aluminum chloride* hydrolyzes in water to aluminum hydroxide and hydrochloric acid; it is thus acidic and irritating to the skin. Aluminum chloride is considered to be safe and effective if used in concentrations of 15% or less. *Buffered aluminum sulfate* (an 8% solution buffered with 8% sodium aluminum lactate) is also effective and is virtually nonirritating to the skin. Because of the propensity of zirconium to elicit allergic reactions and sarcoidlike granulomas when inhaled, *aluminum zirconium chlorohydrates* are not used in aerosol-type antiperspirants. They are applied topically to the axillae in a concentration not to exceed 20% (as the anhydride) in nonprescription products. *Glutaraldehyde* (as a 2% buffered solution) is used to treat hyperhydrosis of the palms of the hands and soles of the feet. It should not be applied to the axillae.

Antiperspirants differ in their ability to prevent wetness. During normal use, only 20 to 40% reduction can be expected. There is individual variation in the response to antiperspirants; some people actually perspire more after the application of certain products.

Deodorants. *Deodorants* reduce the number of resident bacteria on the skin and thus inhibit bacterial decomposition of perspiration. The agents most commonly employed include *benzalkonium chloride, methylbenzethonium chloride,* and *neomycin sulfate.* These agents are not devoid of untoward side effects. Quaternary ammonium compounds such as benzalkonium are inactivated by soaps and irritate the skin if used in concentrations exceeding 1%, and the use of antibiotics may sensitize the individual and/or result in the production of resistant strains of bacteria.

Available proprietary preparations are either antiperspirant or deodorant or both, depending on the ingredients in the formulation. Consequently, allergic reactions may be induced by any of the abovementioned agents as well as by the perfume used to scent the preparations. Diagnosis of allergic manifestations is usually not difficult, inasmuch as the allergic response is usually confined to the axilla.

ABSORBABLE HEMOSTATICS

The absorbable hemostatics arrest bleeding either by the formation of an artificial clot or by providing a mechanical matrix that facilitates clotting when applied directly to denuded or bleeding surfaces. Since they are absorbed from the site of application after varying periods of time, they are referred to as absorbable hemostatics. The agents to be described are used to *control oozing from minute vessels* and will not effectively combat bleeding from arteries or veins when there is appreciable intravascular pressure. The absorbable hemostatics include *absorbable gelatin sponge, oxidized cellulose,* and *thrombin.*

Absorbable gelatin sponge is a sterile, absorbable, water-insoluble, gelatin-base sponge. It is used for the control of capillary oozing and frank hemorrhage, particularly from highly vascular areas that are difficult to suture. For this purpose it is frequently moistened with sterile isotonic sodium chloride solution or with thrombin solution before use. When implanted in tissues it is absorbed completely in 4 to 6 weeks without inducing excessive formation of scar tissue. When applied to bleeding areas of skin or to nasal, rectal, or vaginal mucosa it completely liquefies within 2 to 5 days. It is available as absorbable gelatin sponge (GELFOAM) (cones, packs, and sponges), absorbable gelatin film (GELFILM), and absorbable gelatin powder (GELFOAM).

Oxidized cellulose (OXYCEL) is a specially treated form of surgical gauze or cotton that promotes clotting by a physical effect, rather than by any alteration of the normal clotting mechanism. It is used in surgical procedures to control capillary, venous, and small arterial hemorrhage when ligation or other conventional methods of control are impractical or ineffective. It is also employed in oral surgery and exodontia. Oxidized cellulose should not be used in combination with thrombin because the low pH interferes with the activity of the thrombin. Moreover, it should not be employed for permanent packing or implantation in fractures because it interferes with bone regeneration and may result in cyst formation. The preparation may inhibit epithelialization and hence should not be used as a surface dressing except for the immediate control of hemorrhage. It is marketed as sterile cotton pledgets, gauze pads, and gauze strips.

Thrombin (THROMBINAR, THROMBOSTAT) is applied topically to control capillary oozing in operative procedures and to shorten the duration of bleeding from punctured sites in heparinized patients (*e.g.*, after hemodialysis). Thrombin should never be injected, particularly intravenously, because of the possibility of thrombosis and death. Thrombin is dusted on as a powder, applied as a solution, or combined with a suitable sponge matrix (*e.g.*, absorbable gelatin sponge).

ASTRINGENTS

Astringents are locally acting drugs that precipitate proteins but have so little penetrability that only the surface of cells is affected. Many germicidal protein precipitants exert an astringent effect in high dilutions. Certain metallic ions, such as those of zinc and aluminum, are primarily astringent. Zinc sulfate (0.25%) is the only astringent recommended for use in nonprescription ophthalmic products. *Tannic acid* is also astringent. However, there are few if any legitimate medical uses for this substance. Sufficient tannic acid may be absorbed from the gastrointestinal tract, denuded surfaces, and mucous membranes to cause severe centralobular necrosis of the liver (*see* Eshchar and Friedman, 1974).

IRRITANTS

The irritants are chemicals that act locally on cutaneous or mucosal tissue to produce "inflammation." The first response to local irritation is an increased circulation to the injured part. The localized vasodilatation, mediated by way of an axon reflex, is attended by the feeling of comfort, warmth, and sometimes itching. Localized hyperesthesia also occurs. Drugs that evoke only reactive hyperemia are known as *rubefacients.* If the irritant action progresses, the capillaries dilate widely and become more permeable. Plasma escapes into the extracellular spaces, fluid collects under the epidermis, and blisters are formed. Drugs capable of causing this degree of irritation are known as *vesicants.* Drugs are the *least* useful means available for producing hyperemia and irritation. Heat is often the rubefacient of choice.

Camphor is employed exclusively for its local actions. The compound is a rubefacient when rubbed on the skin. When not vigorously applied, however, it may produce a feeling of coolness. Camphor also has a mild local anesthetic action, and its application to the skin may be followed by numbness. Camphor has a hot, bitter taste and, when taken in small amounts, produces a feeling of warmth and comfort in the stomach. In large doses it is irritating and causes nausea and vomiting; convulsions may also occur.

Camphor, an aromatic crystalline substance, is an ingredient in *paregoric* and a number of proprietary preparations for external application. Preparations of camphor for local application include *camphor spirit* (10% in alcohol) and *camphorated parachlorophenol* (35% parachlorophenol and 65% camphor). Camphor spirit is used as a local irritant. Camphor, applied topically as a 0.1 to 3% lotion or ointment, is used as an antipruritic and a surface anesthetic. Camphorated parachlorophenol has local *antibacterial* properties and is used in dentistry for the treatment of infected root canals.

Cantharidin, the active irritant in cantharides (*Spanish flies, Russian flies*), is used locally only for its irritant and vesicant action on the skin; it causes intradermal vesiculation. It is available as *cantharidin collodion* (CANTHARONE), cantharidin (0.7%) in a film-forming vehicle containing flexible collodion. It is used for the removal of benign epithelial growths: warts (ordinary, periungal, subungal, plantar, and palpebral) and molluscum contagiosum. Thick hyperkeratotic lesions should be pared down, painted with cantharidin collodion, allowed to dry, and covered with a nonporous occlusive tape. The blisters induced by this agent heal rapidly, without leaving a scar. Despite the lore, it is not an aphrodisiac.

SCLEROSING AGENTS

Sclerosing agents are irritating substances that are used to obliterate varicose veins in the lower extremities and fibrose uncomplicated hemorrhoids. Numerous irritants have been used as sclerosing agents. Only two, however, warrant even the brief description given below. These agents are contraindicated in acute thrombophlebitis or when there is significant valvular or deep-venous incompetence.

Morrhuate sodium injection is a sterile solution of the sodium salts of the fatty acids of cod liver oil. It is marketed as a 5% aqueous solution; the intravenous dose is 1 to 5 ml injected into a localized segment of vein. Hypersensitivity reactions occasionally occur, and appropriate measures should be taken to avoid such effects. Pulmonary embolism has also occurred. *Sodium tetradecyl sulfate* (SOTRADECOL) is an anionic surface-active agent used to sclerose varicose veins. The preparation for this purpose is a 1 or 3% aqueous solution. Not more than 0.5 to 2.0 ml should be injected at any one site; total volume for a single treatment should not exceed 10 ml of a 3% solution (*see* Perchuk, 1974). The drug may cause pain at the site of the injection and sloughing of the tissue if the solution is allowed to extravasate. Allergic reactions, including anaphylaxis, have been reported. Sodium tetradecyl sulfate should not be employed in pregnant women unless clearly needed. The use of these agents to sclerose esophageal varices in patients with hepatic disease and portal hypertension is considered investigational, and the efficacy of this procedure remains to be established.

CAUSTICS, ESCHAROTICS, KERATOLYTICS, AND ANTISEBORRHEICS

Caustics and Escharotics. A *caustic* (or *corrosive*) is a topical agent that causes destruction of tissues at the site of application. If the agent also precipitates cell proteins and the inflammatory exudate forms a scab (or eschar) that is later organized into a scar, it is also known as an *escharotic* (or *cauterizant*). Most, but not all, caustics are also escharotics. Certain caustics, especially the alkalis, redissolve precipitated proteins, partly by hydrolysis, so that no scab or only a soft scab forms; such agents penetrate deeply and are generally unsuitable for therapeutic use. Caustics are used to destroy *warts, condylomata, keratoses, certain moles,* and *hyperplastic tissue.* They have also been used in the management of *fungal infections* and *eczematoid dermatitis.* Agents commonly classified in this category include the following: *glacial acetic acid, exsiccated alum, podophyllum, podophyllum resin, phenol, silver nitrate,* and *trichloroacetic acid.* Trichloroacetic acid (10 to 35%) is the most useful caustic generally employed.

Keratolytics (Desquamating Agents). *Benzoic acid, salicylic acid, resorcinol,* various thiols, and certain other substances are frequently used as keratolytic agents. Salicylic acid produces desquamation by solubilizing the intercellular cement that binds scales in the stratum corneum. An effective keratolytic therapy involves the use of 60% propylene glycol under plastic occlusion. The addition of 6% salicylic acid to the former results in a very effective keratolytic preparation (KERALYT) that is effective in a variety of skin diseases associated with hyperkeratosis (*e.g., ichthyosis, seborrheic dermatitis, psoriasis, chronic eczematous dermatitis, hyperkeratosis* of the palms and soles, *keratosis pilaris, warts, actinic keratosis, etc.*).

Antiseborrheics. Seborrheic dermatitis is an inflammatory, erythematous, and scaling eruption that occurs primarily in those areas with a large number and high activity of sebaceous glands, such as the scalp, face, and trunk. It is often associated with itching. The antiseborrheic and antidandruff medicated shampoos contain a variety of agents, including quaternary ammonium surfactants, chlorinated phenols, salicylic acid, sulfur, zinc pyrithione, selenium sulfide, and tar. Only single entities prepared in pharmaceutical forms especially designed for the treatment of seborrheic dermatitis are considered here.

Selenium sulfide is a bright-orange, insoluble powder that is used externally for control of seborrheic dermatitis, dandruff, and nonspecific dermatoses. Its antidandruff effectiveness is thought to result from its antimitotic activity and substantivity (residual adherence after shampoo and rinse) to the skin (Kligman *et al.*, 1976). The toxicity of insoluble selenium sulfide contrasts sharply with the highly toxic soluble selenites, selenates, and organic selenium compounds. In rats, the oral LD50 for the insoluble selenium sulfide is quite comparable to that for other substances commonly employed in shampoos. Comparatively little absorption occurs after local application of selenium sulfide to normal skin, but the drug is absorbed more readily from inflamed or damaged epithelium. Prolonged contact with skin surfaces may result in burns and dermatitis venenata. Selenium sulfide is employed as *selenium sulfide lotion* (EXSEL, SELSUN), a therapeutic shampoo containing 2.5% of the active ingredient in a detergent vehicle. It is also available as a nonprescription drug in a 1% suspension (SELSUN BLUE) in a scented, detergent vehicle. The preparation should not be used more frequently than required to maintain control. Adverse effects include chemical conjunctivitis if the preparation enters the eyes, increased oiliness or dryness of the hair, and orange tinting of gray hair. The latter effect may be minimized by thoroughly rinsing the hair immediately after each treatment.

Zinc pyrithione is widely used in nonprescription formulations (DANEX, HEAD AND SHOULDERS, others) that are temporarily effective for the management of dandruff. Like selenium sulfide, zinc pyrithione is thought to act by reducing the turnover of epidermal cells (Kligman *et al.*, 1976); the two agents are equally effective and more effective than a nonmedicated shampoo. Zinc pyrithione has little or no toxicity when applied as directed to normal skin and hair.

MELANIZING AGENTS

Many characteristics of normal and abnormal skin pigmentation and achromasia are of importance in pharmacology. Skin alterations resulting from untoward effects of drugs are discussed in connection with the agents responsible for such changes. The drugs discussed in this and the following section have clinically useful melanizing (hyperpigmenting) or demelanizing (hypopigmenting and depigmenting) properties. Many details relating to the etiology and management of vitiliginous and lentiginous skin disorders are presented in the reviews by Mosher and associates (1979, 1983), as well as in the monograph edited by Kawamura and associates (1971).

TRIOXSALEN

Trioxsalen (4,5′,8-trimethylpsoralen), a congener of methoxsalen, is used to facilitate repigmentation in vitiligo, increase tolerance to solar exposure, and enhance pigmentation. Recently, it has also been used as a photochemotherapeutic agent in the treatment of psoriasis, but it is less effective than

methoxsalen. The structural formula of this furocoumarin is shown below.

Trioxsalen

Pharmacological Actions. The mode of action of trioxsalen in inducing repigmentation of the vitiliginous skin is not yet known. It is believed, however, that its action depends upon the presence of functional melanocytes and their proliferation (mitotic activation) by the photoactivated trioxsalen. Well-controlled exposure of the skin either to sunlight or to ultraviolet radiation from artificial sources (320 to 400 nm) is essential for the stimulation of melanin pigmentation. Repigmentation may begin after a few weeks; however, significant results may take as long as 6 to 9 months to occur. The drug activates the few functional melanocytes present in the vitiliginous skin area that retain the capacity to form dihydroxyphenylalanine (DOPA) (Mosher *et al.*, 1983) and evokes a mitotic response in these cells; the latter is indicated by the autoradiographic studies of Africk and Fulton (1971) and the light- and electron-microscopic studies of Pathak and associates (1974, 1976b). The increase in perifollicular and epidermal pigment is thought to occur by one or more of the following mechanisms: (1) an increase in the number of functional melanocytes and also, possibly, by activation of dormant or resting melanocytes; (2) the augmentation of melanosome (melanin granule) synthesis; (3) an increase in the activity of tyrosinase, the enzyme that catalyzes the conversion of tyrosine to DOPA, a precursor of melanin; and (4) the hypertrophy of melanocytes and increased arborization of their dendrites. The metabolism of trioxsalen has been studied by Mandula and Pathak (1979).

Side Effects and Contraindications. Side effects are minimal; an occasional patient may experience gastric irritation and nausea. The drug is contraindicated in patients with photosensitizing diseases, such as erythropoietic protoporphyria or acute lupus erythematosus. No other photosensitizing drug should be administered with trioxsalen. The safety of this drug in children under 12 years of age has not been established.

Preparation. *Trioxsalen* (TRISORALEN) is available in 5-mg tablets. The usual oral dose is 10 mg daily, taken 2 hours before exposure to sunlight or ultraviolet light. Higher doses (0.6 mg/kg and above) have, however, been used in the treatment of vitiligo (Mosher *et al.*, 1983). If a patient is treated on alternate days and follicular repigmentation is not apparent after 3 to 4 months, the drug should be discontinued as a failure. Exposure times should be limited to the manufacturer's recommended schedule, except at low latitudes (0 to 20°), where exposure times should be reduced. When used to increase tolerance to sunlight, treatment should be limited to 14 days.

Therapeutic Uses. Trioxsalen is used in *idiopathic vitiligo,* to *increase tolerance to sunlight,* and to enhance *skin pigmentation* (tanning). The drug is a potent skin photosensitizing agent and should be used only under medical supervision. Its effectiveness in the photochemotherapy of psoriasis after oral administration remains to be established (Mosher *et al.,* 1983).

METHOXSALEN

Methoxsalen (8-methoxypsoralen) is used in combination with exposure to ultraviolet radiation (320 to 400 nm) to increase skin tolerance to sunlight, to facilitate repigmentation in vitiligo, and to treat skin diseases such as psoriasis, eczema, and mycosis fungoides. The chemistry of the psoralens has been reviewed by Fowlks (1959) and by Pathak and associates (1974, 1976a). Methoxsalen has the following structural formula:

OCH$_3$
Methoxsalen

The combination-treatment regimen of psoralen (P) and ultraviolet radiation (320 to 400 nm, commonly referred to as UV-A) is known by the acronym PUVA (Fitzpatrick *et al.,* 1976). Skin reactivity to ultraviolet radiation is markedly enhanced by the ingestion of methoxsalen.

Pharmacological Actions. Methoxsalen is a potent photosensitizer of the skin, particularly to long-wavelength (320 to 400 nm) ultraviolet light (Pathak *et al.,* 1967). Patients with psoriasis are treated with methoxsalen orally (0.3 to 0.6 mg/kg) and approximately 2 hours later are exposed to a measured dose of UV-A radiation (320 to 400 nm; 0.5 to 3.0 joules/cm^2). Exposure is carried out with a specially designed ultraviolet lamp system. After oral ingestion, increased sensitivity of the skin to such radiation appears in 1 hour, reaches a maximum in 2 hours, and disappears in about 8 hours. Treatments are not given more often than once every other day. Methoxsalen is metabolized rapidly. Approximately 90 to 95% of the drug (as metabolites) is excreted in the urine within 24 hours. The therapeutic effect in psoriasis is believed to result from the photochemically induced covalent binding of methoxsalen to pyrimidine bases. This photoconjunction appears to involve first the formation of monofunctional C-4 cycloadducts of methoxsalen at the 5,6 double bond of pyrimidine bases in DNA. Subsequently, bifunctional adducts involving interstrand cross-links between two pyrimidine bases on opposite strands of DNA are formed (Cole, 1970; Dall'Aqua *et al.,* 1972; Pathak *et al.,* 1974). The light-dependent conjugation of

epidermal DNA with psoralens is believed to inhibit DNA synthesis and cell division, thereby leading to clinical improvement in diseases such as psoriasis.

Exposure of methoxsalen-treated patients to ultraviolet light thickens the stratum corneum, induces an inflammatory reaction in the skin, and increases the amount of melanin in the exposed area. Repigmentation persists for 8 to 14 years without further treatment. Topical therapy is recommended for the repigmentation of small macules of vitiligo. The topical application of methoxsalen (0.1 to 1%) renders the skin very sensitive to ultraviolet radiation; blistering occurs frequently, and photosensitivity may persist for several days. The mechanism of repigmentation or hyperpigmentation in patients with vitiligo appears to be similar to that of trioxsalen, as discussed above.

Side Effects and Contraindications. The most common side effects after oral therapy include excessive erythema (burns), nausea, pruritus, edema, vesiculation, and formation of bullae. Although abnormal hepatic function was originally reported in a few patients taking methoxsalen, this apparently is not a danger (*e.g., see* Melski *et al.,* 1977). It would seem prudent, however, to perform tests of hepatic function prior to the initiation of therapy and at intervals thereafter. Exposure to large doses of UV-A can cause cataracts in albino mice, and this effect may be enhanced by the administration of methoxsalen. While ocular effects have not been reported in man, annual ophthalmic examinations are recommended in patients who are receiving long-term therapy with methoxsalen. Patients should be told emphatically to wear UV-A absorbing, wraparound sunglasses. The potential long-term side effects of methoxsalen plus UV-A treatment are the same as those known to occur from ultraviolet exposure; they include actinic alterations of the skin (aging), skin cancer, and cataracts.

Stern and associates (1979) have evaluated the risk of cutaneous carcinoma in a 2-year prospective study of nearly 1400 patients receiving photochemotherapy with 8-methoxypsoralens for psoriasis. Their data suggested that patients having skin types I and II (who sunburn easily and tan poorly) and a previous history of receiving ionizing radiation were at a high risk for the development of cutaneous carcinoma. A higher-than-expected proportion of squamous-cell carcinomas that arose in areas not habitually exposed to the sun was seen (Epstein, 1979).

Preparations. *Methoxsalen* (OXSORALEN) is available in 10-mg capsules and as a 1% lotion. For vitiligo the capsules are given orally to adults in a dose of 20 mg once a day, followed in 2 hours with a 5-minute exposure to sunlight or UV-A radiation (1 to 2 joules/cm^2); exposure may be gradually increased to 30 minutes (15 to 20 joules/cm^2). If the 1% lotion is used, it is applied by a physician at weekly intervals to well-defined vitiliginous lesions, followed by one half the minimal dose of ultraviolet light predicted to produce erythema. Subsequent exposures should be increased with caution. *The topical preparation should never be dispensed to the patient for home use.* The beneficial effects of orally administered methoxsalen photochemotherapy can be achieved in patients with either vitiligo or psoriasis by well-controlled exposure to ultraviolet light that is less than that which produces grossly observable phototoxic reactions in skin.

Therapeutic Uses. Methoxsalen should be used only under strict medical supervision. It may be effective for the treatment of *idiopathic vitiligo* when employed in conjunction with exposure of affected areas of the skin to ultraviolet light. If the vitiligo is extensive and is associated with total destruction of melanocytes, the drug is ineffective. It may be effective when used to enhance skin tolerance to sunlight. Well-controlled clinical studies suggest that oral methoxsalen, followed by exposure to high-intensity, long-wavelength ultraviolet light, is effective in the management of *psoriasis* (Parrish *et al.*, 1974; Melski *et al.*, 1977). Its use should be reserved for those with severe, recalcitrant psoriasis that is not adequately responsive to other forms of therapy.

DEMELANIZING AGENTS

Some of the well-known demelanizing (depigmenting) agents include various derivatives of hydroquinone and catechol. The cutaneous depigmentation caused by the topical application of these chemicals appears to result from the selective cytotoxic action of the reactive free radicals that are generated during the oxidation of these substances by the enzyme tyrosinase. Chemical depigmentation of the skin thus involves a decrease in the number of functional melanocytes and the inhibition of the process of pigmentation.

MONOBENZONE

Monobenzone, the monobenzyl ether of hydroquinone, is an amelanotic agent used topically for the induction of complete, often irreversible depigmentation of severely affected patients with pigmentary problems. The use of monobenzone should be restricted to situations in which it is desired to achieve *complete* amelanosis. Monobenzone (*p*-benzyloxyphenol) has the following structural formula:

Monobenzone

Pharmacological Actions. The mechanism of action of monobenzone is not fully understood. The histology of the skin after depigmentation is the same as that seen in vitiligo; the epidermis is normal except for the absence of identifiable melanocytes. Electron microscopy reveals the absence of melanocytes and melanosomes. The selective destruction of melanocytes is accompanied by

increased degradation of melanosomes, destruction of membranous organelles, and inhibition of the enzyme tyrosinase, which catalyzes the oxidation of tyrosine to dihydroxyphenylalanine, a precursor of melanin. Response to therapy is usually not apparent for 1 to 4 months, and complete depigmentation may require 9 to 12 months of treatment. Untoward effects, including mild erythema, dermatitis, and eczematous reactions, have been reported. Unless carefully applied, unsightly depigmented patches may result from its use. Systemic toxicity has not been observed after its local application.

Preparation. *Monobenzone* (BENOQUIN) is marketed as a 20% ointment. It is applied to hyperpigmented areas two or three times daily. Depigmentation is usually observed after 1 to 4 months of therapy. Treated areas should not be exposed to sunlight; the depigmenting site should be protected with a topical sunscreen. If a satisfactory response is not observed within 4 months, treatment should be discontinued.

Therapeutic Uses. Monobenzone is a potent depigmenting chemical, more effective than hydroquinone, and is a useful agent for permanent depigmentation in patients with generalized vitiligo who are unresponsive to methoxsalen or trioxsalen photochemotherapy and who wish to be one color (Mosher *et al.*, 1977, 1983). Monobenzone should *not* be used as a hypopigmenting agent in melasma or in hyperpigmentation caused by the excessive formation of melanin, such as occurs in generalized lentigo, severe freckling, or melasma of pregnancy, or in hyperpigmentation that follows inflammation of the skin. Monobenzone is of no value in the treatment of *café au lait* spots, pigmented nevi, malignant melanoma, or pigmentation resulting from substances other than melanin.

HYDROQUINONE

Hydroquinone (*p*-dihydroxybenzene) is a safe but weak depigmenting agent used topically in the treatment of hypermelanosis (*e.g.*, circumscribed brown hypermelanotic macules of melasma, in women taking progestational agents, in Berlock dermatitis caused by certain perfumes, in postinflammatory hyperpigmentation, severe freckling, and melasma of pregnancy). Although percutaneous application does not, in most instances, completely remove the hyperpigmentation, results are good enough to help the majority of patients become less self-conscious about their abnormality.

Pharmacological Actions. Histochemical and electron-microscopic studies reveal that hydroquinone affects the nonfollicular and follicular melanocyte system. It decreases the formation and increases the degradation of melanosomes, causes structural changes in the membranous organelles of the melanocytes, and inhibits tyrosinase (Jimbow *et al.*, 1974). Depigmentation is not immediate, since hydroquinone interferes only with the formation of new melanin. Cutaneous depigmentation is reversible, since the production of melanin is resumed when the drug is discontinued. It should be emphasized that hydroquinone does not produce the confettilike depigmentation often seen after the application of monobenzone.

Side Effects and Contraindications. Side effects are usually mild; burning, stinging, rash, and irritation have been reported. Possible allergic reactions have been noted. Therefore, patients should be patch-tested for sensitivity before initiating therapy. The drug should not be used near the eyes, on open cuts, or on children under 12 years of age.

Preparations. *Hydroquinone* is marketed in the form of creams (2%, 4%) with or without sunscreens; it is also available in lotions (2%) and solutions (3%). These preparations are applied to the area to be lightened twice daily and rubbed in well, for up to 2 to 3 months. Hydroquinone lotion (2%) in propylene glycol, in combination with retinoic acid (0.05%), appears to be more effective in the treatment of melasma than is hydroquinone cream.

Therapeutic Uses. Hydroquinone is used to bleach and lighten localized areas of darkened skin (melasma, postinflammatory hyperpigmentation, and severe freckling).

SUNSCREENING AGENTS

Sunscreens are formulated to protect the user against the sunburn reaction normally evoked by ultraviolet radiation (290 to 320 nm) and are also used to prevent skin cancer, premature aging of the skin (*actinic elastosis*), and various forms of photosensitivity diseases (*e.g.,* polymorphic light eruptions, drug-induced phototoxic and photoallergic reactions). Sunscreens protect the viable cells of the skin by absorbing and reflecting the solar radiation that impinges upon them. Topical sunscreens that absorb and filter the solar radiation exhibit a wide range of effectiveness, depending upon the ultraviolet absorption spectrum and the extinction coefficient of the agent itself, its concentration, the vehicle in which it is formulated, and its substantivity to remain on the skin after sweating or swimming. The sunscreens may be grouped into three broad categories. (1) Para-aminobenzoic acid and its derivatives are common constituents of many preparations. Lotions containing 5% para-aminobenzoic acid (PABA) offer a particularly high degree of protection. Those containing 2.5 to 7% concentrations of derivatives of PABA, such as pentyl *p*-dimethylaminobenzoate (padimate A) and ethylhexyl *p*-dimethylaminobenzoate (padimate O), are also effective. (2) Sunscreens that rely on the absorptive capacity of other compounds include those that contain benzophenones and cinnamates. These agents are also highly effective against UV-A radiation (320 to 400 nm) when present in adequate concentrations. (3) Physical sunscreens include heavy creams or pastes containing such compounds as titanium dioxide, zinc oxide, and red petrolatum. While they reflect and scatter radiation and are opaque to light of all wavelengths, they lack cosmetic appeal.

Sunscreen products available in the United States are rated according to the degree of protection they can provide. The rating numbers are referred to as SPF (sun protection factor) and range from 2 to 15. The SPF is defined as the ratio of the ultraviolet exposure required to produce a minimally perceptible sunburn on protected skin to the exposure that will produce the same erythema on the adjacent, unprotected skin (Pathak, 1982).

In prescribing sunscreen agents, the most important consideration should be the individual's reactivity to sunlight. People with fair skin and blue eyes, who burn easily and tan poorly or minimally (skin types I and II), should use sunscreens that are highly protective. Most formulations are not water resistant and should be reapplied after swimming or during prolonged sunbathing. Drug-induced photosensitization reactions can be prevented by prescribing topical sunscreens containing benzophenones. To avoid cross-sensitization reactions, individuals who have experienced phototoxic or allergic reactions to drugs such as sulfonamides, thiazide diuretics, or local anesthetics that are derivatives of para-aminobenzoic acid should not utilize sunscreens that contain PABA or its derivatives. Patients who are sensitive to ultraviolet radiation (290 to 400 nm) and also to visible radiation (400 to 760 nm) should use opaque sunscreens that contain zinc oxide and other light-scattering agents. Artificial tanning preparations containing dihydroxyacetone provide no protection against sunburn unless a sunscreen is also incorporated in the formulation.

MUCOLYTICS

Although iodides, ammonium chloride, and other drugs have been used orally for many years to loosen viscid sputum and to improve expectoration, the use of nebulized mucolytic agents for this purpose is a comparatively recent development. A number of substances have been reported to be effective mucolytic agents, but more definitive studies have shown them to be either ineffective or undesirable for a variety of clinical reasons. Only acetylcysteine will be mentioned here.

Acetylcysteine (MUCOMYST) liquefies mucus and DNA (the component of pus responsible for its viscosity) but has no effect on fibrin, blood clots, or living tissue. It exerts its mucolytic activity through its free sulfhydryl group, which acts directly on the mucoproteins to open the disulfide bonds and lower the viscosity of the mucus. The mucolytic activity is greatest at pH 7 to 9. Liquefaction after inhalation is apparent within 1 minute; maximal effect occurs in 5 to 10 minutes; after direct application, the effect is immediate. It is used by inhalation and direct application as adjunct therapy in patients with abnormal, viscid, or inspissated mucous secretions. The agent is marketed as a 10 or 20% sterile solution. A nebulized solution, 1 to 10 ml of a 20% solution or 2 to 20 ml of a 10% solution, is inhaled every 2 to 6 hours. By direct instillation, 1 or 2 ml of a 10 or 20% solution is used every 1 to 4 hours. Untoward effects are not common but include bronchospasm, stomatitis, severe rhinorrhea and bronchorrhea, nausea, and vomiting. Consequently, asthmatic patients under treatment with acetylcysteine should be watched closely. Acetylcysteine is also used in the treatment of poisoning with acetaminophen (*see* Chapter 29).

ENZYMES

This discussion is limited to enzymes that act at local sites after either topical application or hypodermic injection. The uses of streptokinase and urokinase for thrombosis and embolism are discussed in Chapter 58. The uses of oral preparations of enzymes in cystic fibrosis and pancreatic insufficiency are discussed in Chapter 42.

Chymopapain

Pharmacological Action. Chymopapain is a proteolytic enzyme derived from the crude latex of *Carica papaya.* It is used for chemonucleolysis—the removal of the *nucleus pulposus* of prolapsed intervertebral discs. The enzyme attacks the proteoglycan portion of the *nucleus pulposus* but does not affect collagenous components. Injection into the central portion of human lumbar intervertebral discs results in an increase in the urinary concentration of glycosaminoglycans of the type known to occur in human intervertebral discs; in addition, chymopapain or its immunologically reactive fragments are detectable in plasma within 30 minutes and decline after 24 hours.

Therapeutic Use. Chymopapain is used for the treatment of documented herniated lumbar intervertebral discs that have not responded to an adequate period of conservative therapy. The enzyme has not been studied in the treatment of herniated discs in areas other than the lumbar spine. Chymopapain is contraindicated in patients sensitive to the enzyme, in cases of severe spondylolisthesis or progressive paralysis, and in those previously injected with chymopapain (*see* Gunby, 1983). The recommended dosage is 2000 to 5000 units per disc in a volume of 1 to 2 ml. The maximal dose in a single patient with multiple disc herniation is 10,000 units. *Chymopapain* (CHYMODIACTIN, DISCASE) is marketed as a powder to be dissolved for injection.

Hyaluronidase

Hyaluronidase is a soluble enzyme product prepared from mammalian testes.

Pharmacological Actions. Hyaluronidase hydrolyzes hyaluronic acid by splitting the glucosaminidic bond between C 1 of the glucosamine moiety and C 4 of glucuronic acid. This temporarily decreases the viscosity of the cellular cement, promotes diffusion of injected fluids or of localized transudates or exudates, and in this way facilitates their absorption. Sensitivity to hyaluronidase occurs, although infrequently; a test for sensitivity should be conducted prior to administration.

Therapeutic Uses. *Hyaluronidase* (WYDASE) is effective for enhancing the dispersion and absorption of other injected drugs, for hypodermoclysis, as an adjunct in subcutaneous urography, for improving resorption of radiopaque agents, and to enhance absorption of drugs in tissue spaces and in transudates of fluids. It is available as a powder to be dissolved for injection or in a stabilized solution for injection.

Proteolytic Enzymes

Chymotrypsin for ophthalmic solution (ALPHA CHYMAR, CATARASE) is a proteolytic enzyme used to dissolve the zonules of the lens (zonulysis) during surgery for intracapsular cataracts. It diffuses behind the iris into the posterior chamber, where the equatorial pericapsular membrane of the lens is dissolved within 5 minutes, zonular fibers are lysed within 10 to 15 minutes, and complete lysis of the entire zonular membrane occurs within 30 minutes. Enzymatic zonulysis is indicated primarily in young adults (over 25 years of age) and in patients with traumatic cataracts or a history of repair of retinal detachment. The zonules of elderly patients are fragile, and the enzyme may not be required. Chymotrypsin is contraindicated in patients under 20 years of age because of probable adhesion of the lens to the vitreous; this is not responsive to lysis with chymotrypsin. Adverse reactions include transient increases in intraocular pressure, moderate uveitis, corneal edema, striation, and possible delayed healing of the incisions. Since blood inactivates the enzyme, the anterior chamber of the eye should be free of blood before the chymotrypsin is administered. From 0.25 to 2 ml of a freshly prepared solution of chymotrypsin (75 to 150 units per milliliter) is injected slowly behind the iris into the posterior chamber. A second application of the enzyme may be required if the zonules are resistant. Following extraction, the pupils may be contracted with a miotic agent.

Collagenase is an enzymatic debriding agent derived from the fermentation of *Clostridium histolyticum.* It has the capacity to digest native collagen as well as the denatured protein. Since collagen accounts for approximately 75% of the dry weight of skin, the enzyme is utilized for debridement for severely burned areas and dermal lesions. The usefulness of this agent in other necrotic skin lesions remains to be determined. The enzyme's optimal pH range is 6 to 8. Detergents, hexachlorophene, and ions of heavy metals (mercury and silver) inhibit enzymatic activity; cleansing materials such as hydrogen peroxide, Dakin's solution, and buffered (pH 7.0 to 7.5) normal saline solution do not. Collagenase, as an ointment containing 250 units per gram (BIOZYME-C, SANTYL), is applied to the lesion every day (or more frequently if the dressing becomes soiled) and is covered with a sterile dressing. Should infection intervene, appropriate antimicrobial therapy should be used. The collagenase is discontinued when sufficient debridement of necrotic tissue has taken place.

Fibrinolysin-deoxyribonuclease (ELASE) is a topical debriding agent composed of two hydrolytic enzymes: fibrinolysin, derived from bovine plasma, and deoxyribonuclease, isolated from bovine pancreas. The former acts principally on fibrin of blood clots and fibrinous exudates, whereas the latter hydrolyzes deoxyribonucleic acid (DNA). This combination of enzymes is indicated for topical use as a debriding agent in general surgical wounds, ulcerative lesions, and second- and third-degree burns, and following circumcision and episiotomy; it is also used intravaginally in cervicitis (benign, post-partum, and postconization) and vaginitis and as an irrigating agent in infected wounds, otorhinolaryngological wounds, and superficial hematomas. Adverse reactions are usually minimal and include local irritation with hyperemia after higher concentrations. The agent should not be used in patients with a history of hypersensitivity reactions to either of the components. Fibrinolysindeoxyribonuclease is available as a lyophilized powder (25 units of fibrinolysin and 15,000 units of deoxyribonuclease per 30-ml vial) and as an ointment containing fibrinolysin (1 unit per gram) and deoxyribonuclease (667 units per gram).

Sutilains is a proteolytic enzyme elaborated by *Bacillus subtilis*. At body temperature it has optimal activity at a pH range of 6.0 to 6.8. It is available as *sutilains ointment* (TRAVASE), 1 g of which contains approximately 82,000 casein units of proteolytic activity. The ointment is used for wound debridement as adjunct therapy to established methods of wound care. It is indicated in second- and third-degree burns; decubitus ulcers; incisional, traumatic, and pyogenic wounds; and ulcers secondary to peripheral vascular disease. Patients should be warned to keep the enzyme away from the eyes. Untoward local effects include mild and transient pain, paresthesia, bleeding, and dermatitis; if bleeding or dermatitis occurs, therapy should be discontinued. Systemic toxicity has not been observed from the topical application of the ointment.

Papain is used for the enzymatic debridement and the promotion of healing of surface lesions, particularly where healing is retarded by local infection, necrotic tissue, fibrinous or purulent debris, or eschar. It is marketed for topical use as an ointment containing 10% papain and 10% urea (PANAFIL WHITE). It is applied directly to the lesion at least twice daily and covered with gauze. It should not be used in the eyes.

Trypsin is employed in the form of an aerosol that contains trypsin, balsam Peru, and castor oil (GRANULEX). It is used for the management of decubitus ulcers and varicose ulcers and for debridement of eschar and sunburn. The aerosol is applied a minimum of twice daily.

Africk, J., and Fulton, J.   Treatment of vitiligo with topical trimethylpsoralen and sunlight. *Br. J. Dermatol.,* **1971,** *84,* 151–156.

Bowie, M. D., and McKenzie, D.   Diethylene glycol poisoning in children. *S. Afr. Med. J.,* **1972,** *46,* 931–934.

Cole, R. S.   Light-induced cross-linking of DNA in the presence of a furocoumarin (psoralen). *Biochim. Biophys. Acta,* **1970,** *217,* 30–39.

Dall'Aqua, F.; Marciani, S.; Vedaldi, D.; and Rodighiero, G.   Formation of interstrand cross-linkings on DNA of guinea pig skin after application of psoralen and irradiation at 365 nm. *FEBS Lett.,* **1972,** *27,* 192–194.

Epstein, J. H.   Risks and benefits of the treatment of psoriasis. *N. Engl. J. Med.,* **1979,** *300,* 852–853.

Eschar, J., and Friedman, G.   Acute hepatotoxicity of tannic acid added to barium enemas. *Am. J. Dig. Dis.,* **1974,** *19,* 825–829.

Fitzpatrick, T. B.; Parrish, J. A.; Pathak, M. A.; and Tanenbaum, L.   The risks and benefits of oral PUVA photochemotherapy and psoriasis. In, *Psoriasis: Proceedings of the Second International Symposium.* (Farber, E. M., and Cox, A. J., eds.) Yorke Medical Books, New York, **1976,** pp. 320–327.

Fowlks, W. L.   The chemistry of the psoralens. *J. Invest. Dermatol.,* **1959,** *32,* 249–254.

Genel, M.   Central nervous system toxicity associated with ingestion of propylene glycol. *J. Pediatr.,* **1978,** *93,* 515–516.

Goldsmith, L. A., and Baden, H. P.   Propylene glycol with occlusion for treatment of ichthyosis. *J.A.M.A.,* **1972,** *220,* 579–580.

Gunby, P.   Chymopapain: tropical tree to surgical suite. *J.A.M.A.,* **1983,** *249,* 1115–1120.

Jimbow, K.; Pathak, M. A.; Obata, H.; and Fitzpatrick, T. B.   Mechanism of depigmentation by hydroquinone. *J. Invest. Dermatol.,* **1974,** *62,* 436–449.

Kawamura, T.; Fitzpatrick, T. B.; and Seiji, M. (eds.). *Biology of Normal and Abnormal Melanocytes.* University of Tokyo Press, Tokyo, **1971.**

Kligman, A. M.; McGinley, K. J.; and Leyden, J. J.   The nature of dandruff. *J. Soc. Cosmet. Chem.,* **1976,** *27,* 111–139.

Mandula, B. B., and Pathak, M. A.   Metabolic reactions *in vitro* of psoralens with liver and epidermis. *Biochem. Pharmacol.,* **1979,** *28,* 127–132.

Medical Letter.   Sunscreens. **1979,** *21,* 46–48.

Melski, J. W.; Tanenbaum, L.; Parrish, J. A.; Fitzpatrick, T. B.; Bleich, H. L.; and 28 Participating Investigators.   Oral methoxsalen photochemotherapy for the treatment of psoriasis: a cooperative clinical trial. *J. Invest. Dermatol.,* **1977,** *68,* 328–335.

Mosher, D. B.; Fitzpatrick, T. B.; and Ortonne, J.-P.   Abnormalities of pigmentation. In, *Dermatology in General Medicine.* (Fitzpatrick, T. B.; Eisen, A. Z.; Wolff, K.; Freedberg, I. M.; and Austen, K. F.; eds.) McGraw-Hill Book Co., New York, **1979,** pp. 568–629.

Mosher, D. B.; Parrish, J. A.; and Fitzpatrick, T. B.   Monobenzyl ether of hydroquinone: a retrospective study of treatment of 18 vitiligo patients and a review of the literature. *Br. J. Dermatol.,* **1977,** *97,* 669–679.

Mosher, D. B.; Pathak, M. A.; and Fitzpatrick, T. B.   Vitiligo: etiology, pathogenesis, diagnosis, and treatment. In, *Update: Dermatology in General Medicine.* (Fitzpatrick, T. B.; Eisen, A. Z.; Wolff, K.; Freedberg, I. M.; and Austen, K. F.; eds.) McGraw-Hill Book Co., New York, **1983,** pp. 205–225.

Parrish, J. A.; Fitzpatrick, T. B.; Tanenbaum, L.; and Pathak, M. A.   Photochemotherapy of psoriasis with oral methoxsalen and long-wave ultraviolet light. *N. Engl. J. Med.,* **1974,** *291,* 1207–1211.

Parry, M. F., and Wallach, R.   Ethylene glycol poisoning. *Am. J. Med.,* **1974,** *57,* 143–150.

Pathak, M. A.   Topical and systemic approaches to protection of human skin against harmful effects of solar radiation. *J. Am. Acad. Dermatol.,* **1982,** *7,* 285–312.

Pathak, M. A.; Fitzpatrick, T. B.; and Parrish, J. A.   Pharmacologic and molecular aspects of psoralen photochemotherapy. In, *Psoriasis: Proceedings of the Second International Symposium.* (Farber, E. M., and

Cox, A. J., eds.) Yorke Medical Books, New York, **1976a**, pp. 262–271.

Pathak, M. A.; Jimbow, K.; Parrish, J. A.; Kaidbey, K. H.; Kligman, A. L.; and Fitzpatrick, T. B. In, *Pigment Cell—Unique Properties of Melanocytes: Proceedings of the Ninth International Pigment Cell Conference*. Pt. II, Vol. 3. (Riley, V., ed.) S. Karger, Basel, **1976b**, pp. 291–298.

Pathak, M. A.; Kramer, D. M.; and Fitzpatrick, T. B. Photobiology and photochemistry of furocoumarins (psoralens). In, *Sunlight and Man*. (Pathak, M. A.; Harber, L. C.; Seiji, M.; and Kukita, A.; eds.) University of Tokyo Press, Tokyo, **1974**, pp. 335–368.

Pathak, M. A.; Worden, L. R.; and Kaufman, K. D. Effect of structural alterations on the photosensitizing potency of furocoumarins (psoralens) and related compounds. *J. Invest. Dermatol.*, **1967**, *48*, 103–118.

Perchuk, E. Injection therapy of varicose veins. A method of obliterating huge varicosities with small doses of sclerosing agent. *Angiology*, **1974**, *25*, 393–405.

Stern, R. S.; Thibodeau, L. A.; Kleinerman, R. A.; Parrish, J. A.; Fitzpatrick, T. B.; and 22 Participating Investigators. Risk of cutaneous carcinoma in patients treated with oral methoxsalen photochemotherapy for psoriasis. *N. Engl. J. Med.*, **1979**, *300*, 809–813.

CHAPTER

41 ANTISEPTICS AND DISINFECTANTS; FUNGICIDES; ECTOPARASITICIDES

Stewart C. Harvey

I. Antiseptics and Disinfectants

Topical anti-infective agents have a number of indispensable uses for which they are widely employed. Every invasive procedure, whether it is a simple hypodermic injection or major surgery, is preceded by the application of an *antiseptic*. These agents are also applied prophylactically to the hands of surgeons, nurses, dentists, and others in their routine practice. Neonates are partially or completely bathed with antiseptic solutions. Hospital gowns, linens, catheters, and instruments are treated with sterilants, and the hospital premises are washed with disinfectant solutions. Antiseptic agents are in home medicine cabinets and in deodorant soaps. *Disinfectants* play a major role in water treatment and in public health sanitation. They are used as preservatives in pharmaceutical preparations, cosmetics, and even foodstuffs. Beyond these various prophylactic uses, antiseptics are sometimes still of value in treating local infections, even though systemic antimicrobial drugs have superseded topical anti-infective agents in the treatment of many superficial infections. Topical antifungal drugs are especially useful.

From the above, it is clearly important that health professionals be knowledgeable about topical anti-infective agents. Nevertheless, many individuals are inadequately informed about these agents and use them in a sometimes casual, sometimes ritual manner that is largely irrational, often ineffective, and occasionally harmful. For example, in a survey of ophthalmological surgical practice, Apt and Isenberg (1982) found an improper preoperative antiseptic in use by about two thirds of responders. Although the subject lacks great inherent interest, it is incumbent upon the health professional to choose wisely from the many available agents and to be aware of their advantages and limitations.

History. Centuries before the existence of microorganisms was appreciated, chemicals were used to control the suppuration of wounds and the spread of contagious disease. The earliest written records of man contain references to the use of germicidal agents. Egyptian embalmers found excellent preservatives among the spices, vegetable oils, and gums, as attested by the fine state of preservation of Egyptian mummies. Persian laws instructed the populace to store drinking water in bright copper vessels. The practice of salting, smoking, and spicing foods is older than recorded history. The use of wine and vinegar in the dressing of wounds dates back at least to Hippocrates.

During the nineteenth century, the agents used empirically for their germicidal action included several compounds still employed. For example, iodine was used in treating wounds several decades before the bacterial etiology of suppuration was suspected. Because it was then believed that there was an association between putrefaction and the spread of disease, chlorine occupied a prominent place due to the fact that it was a deodorant. Semmelweiss decreased the incidence of puerperal fever in the obstetrical ward of the Allgemeines Krankenhaus of Vienna from about 10 to 1% by ordering the medical students (who were prone to come directly from the autopsy room to the obstetrical ward) to wash their hands in chlorinated lime before examining patients. Following the introduction of the technic of aseptic surgery by Lister in 1867, the importance of disinfection of the skin of the patient, the hands of the surgeon, the instruments, and the hospital environment was readily appreciated. Some of the early drugs employed for these purposes are still valuable today. During the early part of this century, the use of germicides in purification of water supplies and in the sanitization of utensils and containers in multiple use by the public became widespread. An interesting review of the ancient and modern uses of germicidal substances is given by Block (1983).

Terminology. The terminology used to describe the actions of drugs on microorganisms is unfortunately confusing due to the discrepancy between the strict definitions of the terms employed and their usage in loose medical parlance.

Antiseptics are substances that kill or prevent the growth of microorganisms. This term is used especially for preparations *applied to living tissue.* The definition derives from the original meaning of the term *antiseptic* as a substance that opposes sepsis, putrefaction, or decay. A *disinfectant* is an agent that prevents infection by the destruction of pathogenic microorganisms. It is commonly used in reference to substances *applied to inanimate objects.* A *sanitizer* represents a particular kind of disinfectant; it is an agent that reduces the number of bacterial contaminants to levels judged safe by public health requirements. *Sterilization,* in contrast to *sanitization,* refers to the complete destruction of all forms of life, especially microorganisms, by some chemical or physical process. Under appropriate conditions, a disinfectant may produce complete sterilization. A *germicide,* in the broad and most useful sense, is an agent that destroys microorganisms. Germicides may be further defined by the appropriate use of self-evident terms such as *bactericide, fungicide, virucide,* and *amebicide.*

Properties Desirable in Topical Anti-infective Agents. *Germicidal* rather than germistatic activity is important to antiseptics, disinfectants, and sterilants. If pathogenic microorganisms are not killed, they may resume growth and potentially cause infections once the drug has been diluted or inactivated in body fluids or exudates. A high degree of *germicidal* potency is also desirable in order that anatomical barriers to diffusion, interaction with tissue constituents, and dilution in biological fluids not prevent effective concentrations from being reached. In contrast to the systemic antimicrobial drugs, a *broad spectrum* of germicidal activity rarely favors superinfections (at most sites) and hence is highly desirable. Disinfectants and sterilants, especially, should have bactericidal, sporicidal, fungicidal, protozoacidal, and virucidal activities. The importance of virucidal activities in disinfectants for excreta is obvious; virucidal activity is also important in antiseptic handwashes for health care personnel. *Rapid onset* and *sustained activity* are also important, especially for antiseptics. The degree and incidence of resistance should be low.

A topical anti-infective agent should possess certain physical and chemical properties. *Lipid solubility* favors germicidal activity. For agents applied to the intact skin, lipid solubility favors penetration through the outer epidermal barrier, but a lipid/water distribution coefficient of 1 to 3 favors penetration of both barriers. *Dispersibility* is important for disinfectants and sterilants and for antiseptics applied to wounds and abraded surfaces. Penetrance through eschars is more or less a function of dispersibility. Dispersibility largely depends upon a low surface tension. Strong adsorption to biological materials or to various inanimate objects can interfere with activity. A universal disinfectant should be *nondestructive* to other materials. Offensive odor, color, and staining properties should be absent or minimal.

The therapeutic index is of course a prime consideration in determining the usefulness of an antiseptic. Germicidal concentrations should not produce local cellular damage, nor should they interfere with the body defenses or impair healing. There should be no systemic toxicity from topical application.

Importance of Germicidal Kinetics. The rate of germicidal action approximates first-order kinetics and is dependent upon the concentration, temperature, pH, and vehicle in which the drug is applied. On the skin of the hands and arms, the time necessary for a 50% reduction in bacterial count is about 0.6 minute for 70% ethanol and 7 minutes for 1:1000 benzalkonium chloride. Obviously, where time is a critical factor, the kinetics are of the utmost importance. The medical and promotional literature frequently neglects this important aspect of the pharmacology of antiseptics.

The conditions in which antiseptics are used are usually much more complex than implied above, because of diffusion, penetration, binding, redistribution, and other factors. The rate of action is often not directly proportional to the concentration, and for many antiseptics there is an optimal concentration. Furthermore, many antiseptics fall far short of complete antisepsis; neither of the two agents used in the example above can reduce the bacterial count of the skin by much more than 90%. The pharmacokinetics of antifungal drugs in relation to efficacy has been reviewed by Drouhet (1978).

Requirements for Germicidal Efficacy. The surface bacterial population on glabrous skin ranges from 100 to 5000/cm^2; it is 200,000/cm^2 on the face and scalp. In the axilla it is about 3,000,000/cm^2. By inoculation, it takes over 5,000,000 *Staphylococcus aureus* cells to cause an infection in a healthy adult. Thus, for needle punctures and small incisions in healthy subjects, antiseptic prophylaxis is more ritualistic than necessary, and a very high percentage of killing is unnecessary. However, in shock, trauma, general anesthesia, hypothermia, or immunosuppression, a threshold inoculum may be several magnitudes smaller. Furthermore, with some pathogens, such as *Salmonella typhi* and hepatitis B virus, fewer than 10 microorganisms may cause infection. In such instances, essentially 100% killing is required. Successful treatment of infections also requires a high percentage of killing.

Status of Antiseptics in Relation to Systemic Chemotherapeutic Agents. Most germicides have been employed at one time or another in the local treatment of *wounds* and *infections.* Because of tissue toxicity, inadequate penetration into foci of infection, and reduced activity in the presence of body fluids, dramatic benefit from this use of germicides is the exception rather than the rule. The importance of antiseptics in treating infections is now secondary to that of systemic antimicrobial agents. In experienced hands, selected germicides may be useful in cleansing wounds and in reducing bacterial contamination. However, the common belief that substantial benefit is obtained from the application of antiseptics to wounds, cuts, and abrasions is not supported by the considerable evidence in this field. The various applications of surgical antiseptics have been considered in detail by Price (1968) and Altemeier (1983).

In *dermatological infections,* systemic treatment will usually provide more dramatic results than topical therapy. Nevertheless, there are also barriers to the outward movement of systemic drugs, especially into the stratum corneum, so that both systemic and topical treatment may be of value. Also, where resistance or intolerance to systemic antimicrobial drugs exists, topical antiseptics may be indicated. Burns and superficial fungal infections are examples in which topical treatment may be superior to systemic treatment. Nevertheless, even superficial dermatomycoses are sometimes better treated with systemic, rather than topical, drugs (*see* Symposium, 1980; Chapter 54). Topical therapy is not the only recourse; debridement and various cleansing, dressing, and surgical procedures are vital to good management.

Value of Prophylactic Antisepsis. Since the time of Semmelweiss, an enormous body of evidence has accumulated that hospital disinfection, the sterilization of instruments, and the antiseptic surgical handwash usually greatly diminish the incidence and severity of postoperative infections. A greater emphasis is placed upon the suppression of environmental sources of pathogens than upon preoperative antisepsis of patients (*see* Haley, 1983; Simmons, 1983a). It appears that preoperative disinfection of the patient does not always decrease the incidence of infection, even though the surface population of potential pathogens may be markedly suppressed. For example, Wells and coworkers (1983) found that infections after cardiothoracic surgery were mainly caused by Enterobacteriaceae not originally present at the site of incision. Body bathing with hexachlorophene was reported not to affect the postoperative infection rate among 5760 patients, despite a substantial reduction in the cutaneous bacterial population (Ayliffe *et al.,* 1983; Leigh *et al.,* 1983). Antiseptic showers that markedly decreased the number of staphylococci on the scrotum were not found to alter the incidence of infections after vasectomy (Randall *et al.,* 1983). Disinfection of the urethral meatus and the inclusion of antiseptics in catheter bags do not seem to prevent urinary tract infections from catheterization (*see* Wong, 1983); however, a concerted regimen of total urethral antisepsis with an antiseptic lubricant gel, perineal antisepsis, and antiseptics in catheter bags does (Southampton Infection Control Team, 1982). A number of other failures of topical prophylaxis are cited in the section on iodophors.

ACIDS

Hydrogen ion is bacteriostatic at pH approximately 3 to 6 and bactericidal at pH below 3. Small, lipid-soluble weak acids both penetrate into the bacterial cell and disrupt the cell membrane; hence, they exert a greater effect than do mineral acids. Acids have been used in the preservation of food since antiquity. At present, several are used as antiseptics, fungicides, spermatocides, or cauterizing agents.

ACETIC ACID

This acid in 5% concentration is bactericidal to many types of microorganisms, and it is bacteriostatic at lower concentrations. It is applied prophylactically as a 1% solution in surgical dressings and as a 0.25% solution during bladder catheterization and for bladder irrigation. Otitis externa caused by *Pseudomonas, Candida,* or *Aspergillus* is treated with 2 to 5% solutions. Concentrations of 5% are applied to extensive burns to suppress the growth of *Pseud. aeruginosa,* which is quite susceptible. Vaginal douches with 0.25 and 1% solutions are used to treat infections caused by *Candida* and *Trichomonas* and also as spermatocides. These solutions can be irritating to the vagina, and higher concentrations are irritating to the skin.

BENZOIC ACID

This compound has been widely used as a *food preservative.* In a concentration of 0.1% it prevents bacterial and fungal growth if the medium is slightly acidic. Benzoic acid is relatively nontoxic and almost tasteless. A daily intake of 4 to 6 g does not cause toxic symptoms aside from slight gastric irritation. Larger doses have systemic effects not unlike those of the salicylates. After ingestion, the benzoic acid is conjugated with glycine and excreted in the urine as hippuric acid.

Benzoic acid is a component of *benzoic and salicylic acids ointment,* which is discussed with the antifungal drugs (*see* below). Benzoic acid can be safely applied to the skin in high concentrations.

BORIC ACID

Boric acid has an unwarranted reputation as a germicide. It is primarily bacteriostatic, even in saturated aqueous solution, and its action is very slow. There is little to warrant its continued use in an era of potent antiseptics.

LACTIC ACID

Lactic acid is less volatile than acetic acid; solutions applied topically thus persist longer on the skin or in the vagina. In the United States, lactic acid has been used in spermatocides in concentrations of 1 to 2%, but it is employed more widely elsewhere as a mild antiseptic. It can be used for the same purposes as acetic acid. A 10.5% solution is sometimes used to suppress pathogenic bacteria on the skin of neonates and thus to decrease the rate of infection. The acid can be corrosive to tissues after prolonged contact; in a 16.7% concentration in flexible collodion it is combined with salicylic acid for the removal of warts and benign epithelial tumors.

MISCELLANEOUS ACIDS

Propionic, salicylic, and undecylenic acids are discussed under Antifungal Drugs.

ALCOHOLS

The aliphatic alcohols are germicidal in varying degree, roughly in logarithmic proportion to their lipid solubility. Thus, potency increases with chain length up to amyl, after which micelle formation limits the availability of free alcohol. Branching and additional hydroxyl groups diminish potency.

ETHANOL

Ethanol is an antimicrobial drug of low potency but moderate efficacy in appropriate concentrations. It is bactericidal to all of the common pathogenic bacteria, but some rare species survive and can grow in otherwise-optimal concentrations of the chemical. It is erratic as a fungicide and virucide; it is virtually inactive against dried spores. The mechanisms of action appear to be precipitation of bacterial proteins and dissolution of membrane lipids.

Against staphylococci, concentrations between 40 and 60% are the most effective, but they act more slowly than 70% ethanol (*rubbing alcohol*). On the skin, 70% ethanol kills nearly 90% of the cutaneous bacteria within 2 minutes, provided the area is kept moist during that time. The user deludes himself if he expects more than a 75% reduction in cutaneous bacterial count when 70% ethanol is applied by a single wipe of ethanol-wetted cotton and left to evaporate. An ethanol foam not only prevents premature evaporation but also does not seem to cause the residual dry sensation that a soap wash does. Concentrations above 80% have a low efficacy.

The germicidal activities of chlorhexidine, iodine, iodophors, quaternary ammonium antiseptics, and hexachlorophene are increased by ethanol. Alcohol is also combined with acetone to make an effective antiseptic and cleansing mixture.

Briefly applied to the skin, 70% ethanol does no damage, but it is irritating if left on for long periods of time. As the result of removal of cutaneous lipids, frequent use causes dry skin and scaliness. Irritation is sometimes caused by denaturants in ethanol. Applied to wounds or raw surfaces, ethanol not only increases the injury but also forms a coagulum under which bacteria may subsequently thrive. It is thus not used to disinfect open lesions.

Ethanol is mainly used prophylactically before needle insertions and minor surgical procedures; the commonly used strength is 70%. It is also still widely used for disinfection and "sterilization" in private practice, but its limited efficacy against viruses and spores indicates that such uses should be abandoned. Aerosols of 70% ethanol appear to be satisfactory disinfectants of respiratory equipment. Other uses of ethanol are described in Chapter 18.

ISOPROPANOL

In concentrations above 70%, isopropanol is slightly more germicidal than ethanol, and it is effective in undiluted form. It causes vasodilatation beneath the surface of application, so that needle punctures and incisions at the site bleed more than with ethanol. It defats and dries the skin and is more irritating than ethanol. The odor is more offensive than that of ethanol. Isopropanol is used in any strength from 70% by volume (*isopropyl rubbing alcohol*) to 100%. Isopropanol is used as a vehicle for other germicidal compounds, and it increases their efficacies.

MISCELLANEOUS ALCOHOLS

Benzyl alcohol was once used as an antiseptic, but presently it is employed mainly as a preservative. It is used at a concentration of 0.9% in heparinized bacteriostatic sodium chloride solution for flushing intravenous catheters. In neonates, this has led to central nervous system (CNS) depression, apnea, convulsions and/or coma, intracranial hemorrhages, hyperbilirubinemia, leukopenia, thrombocytopenia, hepatic dysfunction, dermatologic abnormalities, metabolic acidosis, and death (Gershanik *et al.*, 1982). Adverse effects also probably occur in adults.

Octoxynol and *nonoxynol 9* have antiseptic properties but are used only as spermatocides, for which nonoxynol 9 appears to be the agent of choice.

ALDEHYDES

Several aldehydes possess microbicidal, sporicidal, and virucidal activity. The aldehyde group condenses with amino groups to form azomethines, and other types of linkages are also formed. In low concentrations, a toxic action is exerted on cells, including microorganisms; in higher concentrations, proteins are precipitated.

FORMALDEHYDE

Formaldehyde is effective against bacteria, fungi, and viruses, but the action is slow. In a concentration of 0.5%, 6 to 12 hours is required to kill bacteria and 2 to 4 days to kill spores; even in 8% concentration, 18 hours is required to kill spores. Organic matter interferes with the effectiveness of formaldehyde; the aldehyde is inactivated by proteins, especially, and a large excess of formaldehyde must be applied to compensate for depletion. In sufficient concentrations, proteins are precipitated.

As a germicide, formaldehyde is mainly used in 2 to 8% concentration to disinfect inanimate objects, such as surgical instruments and gloves. To sterilize tuberculous sputum, it is employed as an 8% solution in 65 to 70% isopropanol. Formaldehyde cannot be applied safely to the mucous membranes or most of the skin in concentrations high enough to kill microbes rapidly; hence it is seldom used as an antiseptic. Several compounds that slowly release formaldehyde are under investigation. The urinary antiseptic methenamine (Chapter 49) is effective because of the formaldehyde released. Some areas of the skin can tolerate fungicidal concentrations. The noncorrosive properties of formaldehyde make it a popular disinfectant for hemodialyzers and endoscopes.

The astringent properties of 20 to 30% formaldehyde are employed in the treatment of hyperhidrosis; the soles of the feet and palms of the hands can usually tolerate these concentrations. The protein-precipitant action is used in the fixation of histological specimens and in the alteration of bacterial toxins to toxoids for vaccines.

Alteration of tissue proteins by formaldehyde causes local toxicity and promotes allergic reactions. Repeated contact with solutions of formaldehyde may cause an eczematoid dermatitis. Dermatitis from clothing treated with formaldehyde for crease resistance has occurred.

GLUTARALDEHYDE

Glutaraldehyde is superior to formaldehyde as a sterilizing agent. It is effective against all microorganisms, including viruses and spores. It is less volatile than formaldehyde and hence causes less odor and irritant fumes, although it can cause contact dermatitis. It has been marketed as a 2% alkaline solution in 70% isopropanol, which is promoted as rapidly acting. However, a period of 3 to 10 hours is necessary to sterilize dried spores. In neutral or alkaline solution, glutaraldehyde polymerizes and thus has a useful shelf-life of less than 14 days. An acid-stabilized solution not only polymerizes more slowly but also kills dried spores in 20 minutes. Neutral emulsifying agents, such as polyethylene glycol and poloxamers, stabilize and increase the activity of both acidic and alkaline solutions of glutaraldehyde. One such preparation, which contains 0.74% glutaraldehyde has been reported to be considerably superior to 1.1% formaldehyde for the disinfection of hemodialysis systems (Petersen et al., 1982). Neither alkaline nor acidic solutions are damaging to most surgical instruments and endoscopes. As a sterilizing agent for endoscopes, it is superior to iodophors and hexachlorophene. In the gas-aerosol phase, glutaraldehyde is effective against airborne and surface resident microorganisms. A glutaraldehyde-phenate preparation (0.13% glutaraldehyde) has been shown to be highly effective for disinfection of respiratory tubing (Bageant et al., 1981). *Succinic dialdehyde* is also effective as a disinfectant.

CHLORHEXIDINE

Chlorhexidine is one of a number of biguanides with potent antiseptic activity. Its structure is as follows:

Chlorhexidine

Chlorhexidine is one of the three most important surgical antiseptics, and it is the most important dental antiseptic in current use.

Chlorhexidine is rapidly bactericidal to both gram-positive and gram-negative bacteria, although some gram-negative bacilli are relatively resistant. It is not virucidal. It has good substantivity, and 26% remains on the skin after 29 hours; this residue is active. Chlorhexidine is effective in the presence of soaps, blood, and pus, although activity may be somewhat reduced. It has a very high therapeutic index.

Minimal inhibitory concentrations of chlorhexidine *in vitro* range from about 1 to 1000 μg/ml, according to the bacterium and type of culture medium. A 0.1% aqueous solution will kill 99.99% of *Staph. aureus*, *Escherichia coli*, and *Pseud. aeruginosa* within 15 seconds. However, 84% of hospital strains of *Pseud. aeruginosa* have been reported to be resistant to 50 μg/ml, as are certain other species (Nakahara and Kozukue, 1982). In general, chlorhexidine appears to be somewhat more effective than povidone-iodine when used on the skin. Alcohols enhance the efficacy of chlorhexidine.

Chlorhexidine has a low toxicity. Accidental intravenous injection has occurred, which resulted in some hemolysis in one instance and no effect in another. In ordinary preoperative use, chlorhexidine rarely causes adverse skin reactions, but prolonged, repetitive use may cause contact dermatitis and photosensitivity in as many as 8% of users. Constant use in a mouthwash can favor gingival bleeding after brushing the teeth (Ainamo et al., 1982); it also stains the teeth. Nosocomial infections and pseudoinfections by *Pseudomonas* species have occurred from the use of contaminated aqueous chlorhexidine solutions in which the bacteria persisted (*see* Anyiwo et al., 1982; Sobel et al., 1982).

Chlorhexidine gluconate in a 4% emulsion ("skin cleanser") is used as a surgical scrub, as a handwash for health-care personnel, for preoperative preparation of patients, and as a general antiseptic for prophylaxis (such as bathing of the neonate); it is also applied to wounds. A 0.5% solution in 70% isopropanol with emollients is used as a handrinse. In Europe, the hydrochloride is used for burns, as a nasal cream for staphylococcal carriers, and for general antiseptic purposes. Both the gluconate and acetate are used for irrigation of the bladder and body cavities, suppression of dental plaque, and treatment of aphthous ulcers and periodontal infections.

HALOGENS AND HALOGEN-CONTAINING COMPOUNDS

CHLORINE AND CHLOROPHORS

Chlorine became widely used in the sterilization of water supplies during the first decade of the twentieth century, and in World War I chlorine-containing compounds became extensively employed in medicine and surgery. Today, they are used mainly as sanitizing agents.

CHLORINE

Elemental chlorine is a potent germicidal agent. It exerts its antibacterial action in both the elemental form and as undissociated hypochlorous acid (HOCl), which is formed by the hydrolysis of chlorine. The concentration of undissociated HOCl and hence the bactericidal activity of chlorine are pH dependent. Thus, the bactericidal action of chlorine is ten times greater at pH 6.0 than at pH 9.0. At pH 7.0, the concentration of chlorine necessary to kill most microorganisms in 15 to 30 seconds varies between 0.10 and 0.25 ppm. However, mycobacteria are uniquely resistant to chlorine; 500 times the concentrations cited are necessary to destroy *Mycobacterium tuberculosis*. Chlorine is also fungicidal, protozoacidal, and virucidal.

Chlorine is a highly reactive element and thus can be bound by organic material, which decreases bactericidal efficacy. In the presence of excessive organic matter, chlorine is not the disinfectant of choice. In the disinfection of water, the uptake of chlorine by the organic matter present is known as the *chlorine demand*. It is generally considered that a residual chlorine content of 0.2 to 0.4 ppm of water affords a generous margin of safety. In order to attain this concentration of chlorine in relatively pure water, it is sufficient to add only 0.5 ppm; in grossly polluted waters, 20 ppm is scarcely sufficient.

Elemental chlorine has no medical uses. Its principal relevance to public health is its use in the treatment of community water supplies, although chlorinated lime or chlorine bromide is often used instead.

CHLOROPHORS

Chlorine itself has limited usefulness as an antiseptic because of difficulties in handling the element in its gaseous state and because chlorine water is very unstable. Many compounds, however, slowly yield hypochlorous acid, and these can be employed for the disinfection of inanimate objects and in surgery. Such compounds may be regarded as chlorophors, even though the ultimate product is hypochlorous acid. The germicidal efficiency of such compounds is related to the ease and extent of the liberation of HOCl.

Chloramines. The chloramines are amines, amides, or imides containing an N-chloro substituent. They are unstable in water and slowly release chlorine. Some chloramines also have a direct germicidal action. Since the early 1960s the use of chloramines has mostly been limited to the emergency sterilization of water. In the United States, *halazone* is used for this purpose. Chloramines may be more effective in preventing the growth of cutaneous bacteria than is chlorhexidine (Selk *et al.*, 1982). Concentrations 1000 times the minimal bactericidal concentration were required to irritate the skin. A renewal of the use of chloramines for skin and wound antisepsis and for disinfection is likely.

Chlorinated Lime. Chlorinated lime consists of a mixture of calcium chloride and calcium hypochlorite and should contain a minimum of 30% available chlorine. It is too irritating to be used on tissues, but it is widely employed for the disinfection of inanimate objects and drinking water. Chlorinated lime is relatively unstable, even in solid form, and loses much of its activity over a period of a year.

Chlorine Dioxide. In water, ClO_2 yields Cl_2 and HOCl. A concentration of 0.0001% at pH 7 will kill *E. coli* in 6 seconds and poliovirus in 1 minute. Because it has two and one-half times the oxidizing capacity of Cl_2, ClO_2 is especially used to treat effluent wastes; it is also used to treat municipal water in many cities in the United States. There is an increasing use of ClO_2 for disinfection of nonoxidizable objects in hospitals.

Hypochlorite Solutions. *Sodium hypochlorite* is regaining its former status as a useful antiseptic, disinfectant, and sterilant. *Sodium hypochlorite solution* contains 4 to 6% NaClO, a concentration too high to be applied to tissues except in root canal therapy. For surgical purposes, *diluted sodium hypochlorite solution* is used; it contains 0.45 to 0.5% NaClO and it may be further diluted 1:3. The preparation is bactericidal, sporicidal, fungicidal, protozoacidal, and virucidal. Hypochlorite is inactivated by organic matter. It is used to loosen and help dissolve and deodorize necrotic tissue. However, at the same time, it dissolves clots and delays clotting. It is irritating to the skin unless rinsed off promptly. Because hypochlorite solutions are unstable, they should be freshly prepared.

Diluted sodium hypochlorite solutions may be used to irrigate ragged or dirty wounds, as an antiseptic in certain peritoneal dialysis systems (*see* Maiorca *et al.*, 1983), and to disinfect or sterilize certain instruments or other objects. The Centers for Disease Control recommends 0.1% NaClO for high-level sterilization (*see* Simmons, 1983a).

Oxychlorosene sodium (CLORPACTIN) is a mixture of hypochlorous acid and the sodium salt of dodecylbenzenesulfonic acid; the latter component promotes penetration and the germicidal actions of the hypochlorite.

IODINE

Tincture of iodine was first used as an antiseptic by a French surgeon in 1839, and it was employed in treating battle wounds in the U.S. Civil War. Despite the present wide choice of antiseptics, iodine is still among the most valuable agents. The drug has survived on the basis of efficacy, economy, and low toxicity to tissues.

Chemistry. The solubility of iodine in water at pH 7.5 is about 0.15%. It is several times more soluble in 70% ethanol. In order to increase the iodine content of solutions and tinctures, NaI is included;

I^- combines with I_2 to yield I_3^-. Nevertheless, whatever the total iodine concentration, the concentration of the free form, which is the active form, cannot exceed 0.15%. The I_3^- ion is thus only a reservoir (iodophor) from which I_2 can be released. There are seven species of iodine in solution, of which HOI is the predominant one. Iodine forms reversible complexes with amino and heterocyclic nitrogen, oxidizes sulfhydryl groups, and irreversibly saturates double bonds and iodinates tyrosine residues.

Germicidal Actions. Iodine is bactericidal, sporicidal, fungicidal, protozoacidal, cysticidal, and virucidal; gram-positive and gram-negative bacteria are about equally affected. In the absence of organic matter, the vast majority of most bacteria are killed within 10 minutes by a 0.0002% solution and in 10 seconds by a 1% solution; amebic cysts, enteric viruses, and wet spores are susceptible to concentrations of 0.15% or less, but several hours may be needed for dry spores, even at much higher concentrations. Ethanol enhances germicidal activity and also increases dispersibility and penetrance. The action of iodine will persist on the surgeon's gloved hands for several hours, although it gradually diminishes after 15 minutes.

Preparations. *Iodine tincture* contains approximately 2% iodine and 2.4% sodium iodide diluted in 50% ethanol. Aqueous solutions of iodine are *strong iodine solution (compound iodine solution, Lugol's solution)* and *iodine topical solution.* The former contains approximately 5% iodine and 10% potassium iodide; the latter, 2% iodine and 2.4% sodium iodide.

Toxicity. The toxicity of iodine to intact skin is quite low compared to its germicidal potency. Most of the iodine burns that gave iodine a bad reputation were caused by a 7% tincture. Iodine tinctures sting strongly when applied to raw surfaces, but iodine solution stings only slightly. However, the reputation that aqueous iodine has for low toxicity in wounds may be undeserved. Rodeheaver and coworkers (1982) reported that in guinea pigs the incidence of infection in wounds seeded with 1000 or more *E. coli* was increased by irrigation with 1% iodine solution.

In rare instances, an individual may exhibit hypersensitivity to iodine and react markedly to moderate amounts of the element applied to the skin. Symptoms usually take the form of fever and generalized skin eruptions of various types.

Oral ingestion usually causes fatalities only when large amounts (30 to 150 ml) of iodine tincture have been taken. Little free iodine is absorbed from the gastrointestinal tract; the systematic effects are largely the result of shock due to massive loss of fluid from the gastrointestinal tract, tissue hypoxia, and sometimes ethanol intoxication. Iodine can be inactivated in the stomach by gastric lavage with solutions of starch or 5% sodium thiosulfate.

Therapeutic Uses. The chief use of solutions of elemental iodine is in the *disinfection of the skin.* In this regard iodine is probably superior to any other agent. It is best employed in the form of the tincture. Iodine may also be employed in the treatment of *wounds* and *abrasions.* Applied to abraded tissue, aqueous solutions are less irritating than the tincture. Aqueous solutions of 0.5 to 2% iodine with iodide are suitable for wounds and abrasions and a 0.1% solution may be used for irrigations. These concentrations can readily be made by proper dilution of the official solutions with water. For application to *mucous membranes,* a 2% solution of iodine in glycerin is the preparation of choice. In the treatment of *cutaneous infections* due to bacteria and fungi, the tincture or solution of iodine may be employed. Strong iodine solution has keratolytic properties, probably because of the iodide content, and it is sometimes used in the treatment of keratoscleritis.

Iodine may be used to render contaminated water safe for drinking. The addition of 5 drops of iodine tincture to each quart of water will kill not only amebae but also bacteria within 15 minutes without making the water unpalatable. Twelve drops and 1 hour may be needed for *Giardia.*

Iodine has been reviewed by Gershenfeld (1977) and Gottardi (1983).

IODOPHORS

An iodophor is a loose complex of elemental iodine with a carrier molecule, which serves as a sustained-release reservoir of iodine. The definition embraces the solutions and tinctures with their carrier, NaI (*see* above), but in common use it is restricted to preparations in which the carrier is a neutral, amphipathic organic compound. The organic carrier augments dispersibility and penetrance.

Chemistry. In povidone-iodine, I_2 is complexed mainly with the pyrrolidone nitrogen of polyvinylpyrrolidone. In 10% povidone-iodine (which contains 1% "available" iodine) the *free* iodine concentration is only 8 μM (0.001% free iodine). As povidone-iodine is diluted to 0.1%, the free iodine concentration rises (because of dissociation of the complex) to a peak of 80 μM; however, this is only 7% of that achieved when NaI is the carrier (*see* Gottardi, 1983). Bactericidal activity is thus higher at 0.1% than at 10% concentration. Thus, povidone-iodine should be diluted for use, and at no concentration of povidone-iodine can the germicidal activity equal that of NaI-based preparations of iodine. *Pseud. cepacia* and even *Staph. aureus* can grow in 10% povidone-iodine (*see,* for example, Craven *et al.,* 1981).

Germicidal Actions. Povidone-iodine is bacteriostatic at 640 μg/ml and bactericidal at 960 μg/ml against *Staph. aureus in vitro.* However, *Mycobacterium tuberculosis* is generally resistant. There have been few investigations of the antiseptic efficacy of diluted iodophors. A standard surgical scrub with 10% povidone-iodine will decrease the cutaneous bacterial population by about 85%, which leaves a residual population very much higher than does 1% iodine tincture or chlorhexidine solution. The population returns to normal in 6 to 8 hours, but effective control is lost in about 1 hour, which is no longer than can be achieved with iodine tincture and much less than with chlorhexidine or hexachlorophene. However, when the hands are contaminated by gram-negative bacteria, povidone-iodine is a more effective scrubbing disinfectant than is aqueous chlorhexidine (Dineen, 1978). It is not as effective as 1% tincture of iodine. Blood on the hands moderately decreases its efficacy.

Toxicity. Repetitive application of iodophors to the skin may cause contact dermatitis (Marks, 1982). The incidence of allergic reactions when solutions are employed is perhaps 12 to 20% (Kunze *et al.*, 1983); they may occur in the absence of sensitivity to iodine solutions, although cross-sensitivity is common. There have been a number of reports of povidone-iodine-induced thyroid suppression from the bathing of neonates, continual disinfection for peritoneal dialysis, and the topical treatment of burns. Descriptions of toxic effects in various model systems *in vitro* and *in vivo* are difficult to evaluate.

Therapeutic Uses. The principal use of iodophors is in the prophylaxis of postoperative infection. Iodophors are one of three antiseptics recommended by the Centers for Disease Control (*see* Simmons, 1983b). However, more properly controlled prospective studies are needed to establish the true prophylactic value of these agents compared to others. Even accepting the consensus that preoperative scrubbing-rinsing of the hands of health personnel with iodophors decreases the incidence of nosocomial infections, the effects of povidone-iodine on skin flora are not as marked as with 1% iodine tincture or 0.5% chlorhexidine (*see* Berry *et al.*, 1982), and the duration of action is much less than with chlorhexidine. The common belief that disinfection of the skin, mouth, or wounds with povidone-iodine protects against postoperative infections does not seem to be supported by a number of recent studies (*see*, for example, de Jong *et al.*, 1982; Galland *et al.*, 1983; Rogers *et al.*, 1983). Topical povidone-iodine is considered to be effective in the management of burns, provided that treatment starts early before the poorly penetrable eschar forms (Pegg, 1982). Povidone-iodine may be of benefit in the presence of some active infections or known bacterial contamination (*see*, for example, Dattani *et al.*, 1982; Bapat *et al.*, 1983; Knight *et al.*, 1983).

Povidone-iodine is widely used in office and emergency chemosterilization, for which it is generally inferior to various other sterilants. If used, it should be diluted. Since the agent has poor efficacy against *M. tuberculosis*, it should not be used to sterilize bronchoscopes.

Povidone-iodine is available in a wide variety of preparations for applications to the skin and mucous membranes and for use as a disinfectant.

HEAVY METALS

MERCURY COMPOUNDS

Mercuric chloride was the first mercurial to be used as an antiseptic and disinfectant. Because of its toxicity it was supplanted by other agents, among which were a number of organic mercurials. Unlike mercuric chloride, these antiseptics are only bacteriostatic and fungistatic. After a long period of medical use, the inadequacies of the organic mercurials became recognized, and they are now generally considered obsolete. However, *merbromin* and *thimerosal* remain available. Several mercury compounds are used as preservatives in drugs and cosmetics and are a common cause of sensitization to such products. Thimerosal in soft-contact-lens solutions is the principal cause of delayed hypersensitivity to such solutions. *Ammoniated mercury ointment* is still used occasionally as an antiseptic in *impetigo contagiosa* and *superficial pyodermas*, for scaling in *psoriasis*, for *pruritus ani*, and in *pinworm* and *crab louse* infestations. Not only can ammoniated mercury cause dermatitides but also rare systemic mercury intoxication. For further details about mercurial antiseptics, see the *sixth edition* of this textbook and the treatise by Block (1983).

SILVER COMPOUNDS

Inorganic silver salts are highly germicidal in solution. For example, silver nitrate destroys most microorganisms in a concentration of 0.1%. Lower concentrations are bacteriostatic. Silver nitrate is toxic to tissue cells in bactericidal concentrations. Silver ions combine with sulfhydryl, amino, phosphate, and carboxyl groups. Interactions with such groups on proteins cause denaturation, which is the basis of the astringent and caustic effects. Such actions cause disruption of the microbial cell membrane and death of the organism. However, other mechanisms also appear to be involved, since insoluble silver compounds and even metallic silver exert germicidal actions. Silver-protein complexes formed when high concentrations of silver ion are applied to tissue provide a reservoir for the sustained release of silver ion.

Silver Nitrate. Silver nitrate is used as a caustic, antiseptic, and astringent agent. The degree of action depends upon the concentration employed and the period of time during which the compound is allowed to act. The silver ion is precipitated by chloride; consequently, solutions of ionizable salts of silver do not readily penetrate into tissue. Silver salts stain tissue black due to the deposition of reduced silver. Most of the stain slowly disappears spontaneously, but some may persist indefinitely at some sites.

Gonococci and *Pseudomonas* are quite sensitive to silver ions. Consequently, *silver nitrate ophthalmic solution* (1%) is routinely employed for the *pro-*

phylaxis of ophthalmia neonatorum and a 0.5% solution is applied topically in *extensive burns,* especially when silver sulfadiazine is contraindicated. It causes neither pain nor hypersensitivity. Because it penetrates the eschar poorly, it is only effective before the eschar becomes dry. An appreciable proportion of hospital isolates of various gram-negative bacteria presently show plasmid-mediated resistance to silver. In the burn exudate, silver ion reacts with chloride to form insoluble silver chloride, which may cause hypochloremia and, indirectly, hyponatremia. Absorbed nitrate can cause methemoglobinemia. For the treatment of *aphthous ulcers,* a 10% solution is applied. The solid form, *toughened silver nitrate (lunar caustic)* is used for the cauterization of wounds and for removing granulation tissue and warts. It is conveniently dispensed in pencils that should be moistened before use.

Silver Sulfadiazine. This compound (SILVA-DENE) was introduced to replace silver nitrate in the topical treatment of *extensive burns.* Like silver nitrate, it penetrates the eschar poorly, and treatment should be initiated before the eschar becomes firm and dry. The solubility is low enough that insufficient silver ion is released to precipitate significant amounts of chloride ion or proteins. Hypochloremia, hyponatremia, and eschars that adhere to dressings are thus avoided. Despite its low solubility, silver sulfadiazine exerts a prominent antibacterial action against *Pseudomonas.* The compound is painless upon application. Furthermore, unlike silver nitrate, it does not cause argyrial staining of wounds or bed linens. Insufficient sulfadiazine is absorbed to cause crystalluria. Bacterial resistance to sulfonamides can result from the use of silver sulfadiazine. Allergies to sulfadiazine occur in about 1.3% and leukopenia in 3 to 5% of cases.

Mild Silver Protein. The concentration of free silver ion is quite low in mild silver protein (ARGYROL), despite the fact that the complex is 19 to 23% silver. The silver does not interact with other proteins and hence is nonirritating and nonastringent. However, it is only bacteriostatic. It is surprising that some ophthalmologists still use this obsolete antiseptic for preoperative preparation of the patient.

ZINC COMPOUNDS

Zinc compounds are employed as astringents, antiperspirants, styptics, corrosives, and mild antiseptics. They probably owe their action to the ability of the zinc ion to precipitate protein, but other mechanisms may be involved in the effect on bacteria. The highly ionizable, soluble salts, such as zinc chloride, are quite irritating and can be used as escharotics.

Zinc sulfate is used as *zinc sulfate ophthalmic solution* (EYE-SED, 0.217%; OP-THAL-ZIN, 0.25%) in angular (diplobacillary) *conjunctivitis.* For application to the skin, zinc sulfate is used in a concentration of 4%. It is often incorporated with sulfurated

potash in equal concentration in a lotion known as *white lotion.* Zinc sulfate has been used in such skin diseases and infections as *acne, ivy poisoning, lupus erythematosus,* and *impetigo.* The compound also forms the basis for some deodorant anhidrotics. Zinc sulfate is used in vaginal deodorants in concentrations of 0.25 to 4%. The compound accelerates the rate of healing of leg ulcers, other lesions, and acrodermatitis enteropathica, especially in patients with low plasma concentrations of zinc; the salt has been applied topically or given orally in a dose of 220 mg three times a day.

Zinc chloride is occasionally used as an astringent in solutions of 0.2 to 2%. *Zinc acetate* is used as an astringent and styptic.

Zinc oxide is incorporated in powders, ointments, and pastes. It has a mild astringent and antiseptic action. It is used in skin diseases and infections such as *eczema, impetigo, ringworm, varicose ulcers, pruritus,* and *psoriasis.* Zinc oxide can alter skin pigmentation. Preparations containing zinc oxide include *zinc oxide ointment* (20 or 25% zinc oxide), *zinc oxide paste* (25% zinc oxide), and *zinc oxide and salicylic acid paste* (2% salicylic acid in zinc oxide paste). *Calamine* consists of a pink powder containing zinc oxide (not less than 98%) and a small amount of ferric oxide. It is incorporated into *calamine lotion* (8% calamine and 8% zinc oxide) and *phenolated calamine lotion (compound calamine lotion)* (1% phenol in calamine lotion). *Zinc stearate* and *zinc oleate* have actions similar to those of zinc oxide.

Zinc pyrithione, in concentrations of 1 to 2%, is employed in the treatment of *seborrhea* and *dandruff.*

NITROFURAZONE

Nitrofurazone is one of several nitrofurans with antimicrobial activity. Its structure is:

Nitrofurazone

Nitrofurazone affects a variety of gram-positive and gram-negative bacteria and some protozoa. A bacteriostatic action is exerted upon most bacteria in the concentration range of 1:100,000 to 1:200,000. Bactericidal concentrations are approximately twice as great. Certain strains of bacteria, however, are insensitive to concentrations of the agents far in excess of those mentioned. Bacteria slowly develop only a limited degree of resistance to nitrofurazone. Interaction with blood constituents and pus is limited, and penetration into fissures is thus relatively good. Nitrofurazone is not significantly absorbed from the intact or burned skin or from mucous membranes. Topically, the drug causes no pain and is not cytotoxic, but pustular contact dermatitis occurs in 0.5 to 2% of cases.

In the United States, *nitrofurazone* (FURACIN) is used in the form of a 0.2% cream, topical solution, or soluble dressing, but elsewhere it is also employed in ointments and powders. It is highly efficacious in the treatment of *burns*. It is stated to provide effective *prophylaxis against nosocomial infections* (*see* review by Hooper and Covarrubias, 1983). It may be used to promote the rapid closure of small granulating wounds and the healing of donor skin-graft sites, for the prevention of peritoneal adhesion, and as an antiseptic lubricant for transurethral resection. In Africa, it is used in the treatment of trypanosomiasis.

OXIDIZING AGENTS

Oxidants are especially deleterious to anaerobic and microaerophilic microorganisms, but they have general germicidal activity. The halogens discussed previously act in part through oxidation. The only other germicidal oxidants of clinical significance are the peroxides. However, the use of ozone for treatment of municipal water supplies is increasing.

HYDROGEN PEROXIDE

Hydrogen peroxide once had an undeserved reputation as a surgical and domestic antiseptic, but it almost slipped into oblivion, mainly because of decomposition on storage. However, there is a resurgence in the use of *stabilized hydrogen peroxide*. The lethal action is mediated by the hydroxyl free radical and not by peroxide or superoxide. Although the antimicrobial spectrum is broad, there is a wide range in the rate of killing of various microorganisms. Furthermore, tissue catalase causes rapid decomposition of hydrogen peroxide, which protects the cells but prematurely terminates germicidal action. Consequently, it is futile to attempt antisepsis with this substance. Hydrogen peroxide at a concentration of 1.5% is used as a mouthrinse, but the contact time is too short for the preparation to be effective. At a concentration of 3 to 6%, the substance is an excellent disinfectant and sterilant; it is noncorrosive to many materials and leaves no residue. Hydrogen peroxide (1.5%) in isotonic saline solution is used to dissolve cerumen. Hydrogen peroxide has been reviewed by Turner (1983).

BENZOYL PEROXIDE

Hydrous benzoyl peroxide slowly releases oxygen and hence is bactericidal, especially to anaerobic and microaerophilic bacteria. It is also keratolytic, antiseborrheic, and irritant. Benzoyl peroxide is used in the treatment of *acne vulgaris* and *acne rosacea*. The bactericidal action on *Propionibacterium acnes* decreases the production of irritating fatty acids in sebum, and the keratolytic action helps peel the caps from the comedones. After application, there may be transient stinging or burning sensations, which disappear after continued use. Vasodilatation and perivascular lymphocytic infiltration occur. It is especially irritating to skin on the neck and circumoral areas. It must be kept away from the eyes. Excess dryness of the skin and desquamation may occur after 1 to 2 weeks of use. Benzoyl peroxide can cause contact dermatitis. It also bleaches clothing. Benzoyl per-

oxide is available as a cleansing bar, in cleansing liquids, creams, gels, lotions, sticks, and pads.

PHENOLS

Phenol was not the first antiseptic to be used as such, but the dramatic demonstration of its efficacy by Lister in 1867 made it not only the antiseptic and disinfectant of choice for several decades but also the standard to which other antiseptics were compared. Even today, the phenol coefficient (the ratio of the minimal inhibitory concentration of an antiseptic against a standard bacterial strain to that of phenol) is often used as an index of activity, although other measures are also now in use. Subsequent to 1867, numerous other phenols were introduced, some with phenol coefficients of several thousand. The principal chemical categories are the alkyl and aryl phenols, *p*-hydroxybenzoates (parabens), halophenols, and *bis*-phenols.

HEXACHLOROPHENE

Hexachlorophene is a polychlorinated *bis*-phenol with the following structure:

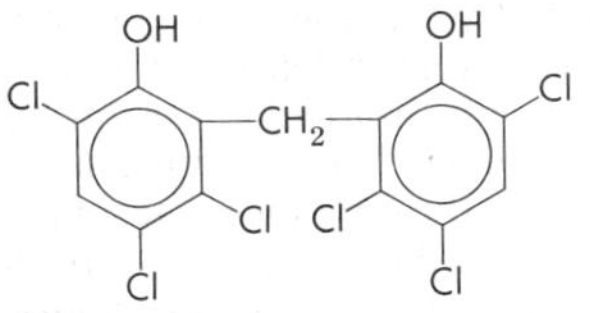

Hexachlorophene

Germicidal Actions. The actions of low concentrations of hexachlorophene appear to include interruption of the bacterial electron-transport chain and inhibition of other membrane-bound enzymes. Higher concentrations actually rupture bacterial membranes. Hexachlorophene is more effective against gram-positive than gram-negative bacteria. The drug exhibits high bacteriostatic activity, but considerable time is required to kill microorganisms and there is little effect on spores. A 3% solution may kill *Staph. aureus* within 15 to 30 seconds, but as long as 24 hours or more may be required for some gram-negative bacteria. Indeed, *E. coli*, *Klebsiella*, and *Pseud. aeruginosa* have occasionally been found as contaminants in hexachlorophene-containing products and have been the cause of epidemics in hospitals. Furthermore, repeated use of the agent favors overgrowth and superinfections by gram-negative bacteria. Consequently, 4-chloro-3,5-xylenol (parachlorometaxylenol) or 4-chloro-3-cresol (parachlorometacresol) is included in some preparations. Nevertheless, such combinations may still require as long as 3 hours to kill gram-negative bacteria. The additives enhance the efficacy against gram-positive bacteria.

Development of resistance of microorganisms to hexachlorophene has not been reported. The presence of organic matter such as pus or serum reduces the efficiency of hexachlorophene, but activity is retained in the presence of soaps, oils, and vehicles for topical application.

Hexachlorophene accumulates in the skin. Immediately after a hand scrub with 3% hexachlorophene, the cutaneous bacterial population may be decreased by only 30 to 50%; however, 60 minutes later the population surviving hexachlorophene will have fallen further to about 4%. Under surgical gloves, hexachlorophene decreases the cutaneous bacterial population less effectively than does chlorhexidine, iodine, or povidone-iodine. Repeated daily applications over a period of 2 to 4 days create a steady-state reservoir of drug in the skin that maintains the bacterial population at about 1 to 5% of normal during the 24-hour interval between applications, but this residual population is considerably greater than that which survives repetitive application of chlorhexidine. Removal of the hexachlorophene residue and regrowth of the normal flora begin promptly after a wash with non-medicated soap or alcohol rinse.

Toxicity. Although hexachlorophene and the other *bis*-phenols are less toxic to tissue than is phenol, hexachlorophene causes moderate histological damage in experimental models; solutions containing detergents are the most toxic. Hexachlorophene is toxic by the oral route. Systemic toxicity can also occur from topical use when the drug is applied daily to the skin of underweight, premature infants or infants with excoriated skin, or several times a day to the skin or vagina of adults. Confusion, diplopia, lethargy, twitching, convulsions, respiratory arrest, and death have occurred. Diffuse status spongiosus of the brain has been demonstrated, especially in the brain stem reticular formation. Endoneurial pressure is increased. In experimental animals this condition appears to be slowly reversible, but damage in some children appears to be permanent. The routine use of hexachlorophene by pregnant nurses has been reported to be teratogenic (*see* Janerich, 1979). Details of the toxicity of hexachlorophene may be found in references cited in the *sixth edition* of this textbook.

Therapeutic Uses. Since most of the potentially pathogenic bacterial residents of the skin are gram positive, hexachlorophene is commonly used by health-care personnel and others who are in a position to spread contaminants from their own hands. The drug is also used to degerm the skin of patients scheduled for certain surgical procedures. However, several days of preoperative treatment are necessary to decrease the cutaneous flora to the maximal extent. Since chlorhexidine acts within a few minutes, decreases the bacterial population to a greater extent than does hexachlorophene, and has equal substantivity and approximately the same antibacterial spectrum, it would seem appropriate to use chlorhexidine in lieu of hexachlorophene.

Routine use of hexachlorophene preparations is effective in reducing the incidence and severity of pyogenic skin infections. However, when hexachlorophene is the only antibacterial drug in the preparation, an excess of gram-negative microorganisms appears in about a week, and the incidence of infections with such bacteria increases. Candidal infections also occur with greater frequency during chronic use of hexachlorophene.

The use of hexachlorophene in the nursery has diminished sharply since the discovery that the daily bathing of neonates with 3% hexachlorophene emulsion could result in serious neurotoxicity. In hospitals in which the drug is still used, the practice is to employ a low concentration (0.25%), which is less effective than 3%, or delay the hexachlorophene bath until the third day. Sometimes only the umbilical stump, the most common site for initial colonization by staphylococci, is bathed. The practice of subsequently rinsing off the hexachlorophene residue with an alcohol or bathing the neonate with nonmedicated soap, in order to prevent absorption of hexachlorophene through the skin, defeats the original purpose of the use of the antiseptic. Since chlorhexidine suppresses the bacterial population on the skin more effectively and is not absorbed, it is a more rational choice of antiseptic for the purpose.

Hexachlorophene is available as an emulsion, foam-tincture, solution, or sponge.

PARABENS

The term *paraben* is derived from *para*-hydroxybenzoate, and the parabens are all esters of *p*-hydroxybenzoic acid. They include *butylparaben, ethylparaben, methylparaben,* and *propylparaben.* These agents are used as preservatives in a great variety of pharmaceutical preparations. Their actions are both those of phenols and an antimetabolite effect of parahydroxybenzoic acid. They have antifungal properties. All are effective in low concentrations (usually 0.1 to 0.3%) that are devoid of systemic toxic effects. However, as constituents of antibacterial ointments, dermatological preparations, and proprietary lotions and skin creams, they are recognized causes of severe and intractable contact dermatitis.

Parabens have been identified as the cause of chronic dermatitis in numerous instances. Patients sensitive to one paraben show cross-sensitivity to the others. The first step in treatment is to eliminate contact with parabens, a difficult task since they are so widely used in proprietary preparations, and their presence is often not indicated on the label.

PHENOL

Phenol is an obsolete antiseptic that has nevertheless managed to persist, in part because of other properties. Its use as a disinfectant is valid, depending upon the bacterium and duration of exposure. It is bacteriostatic in concentrations of about 0.02 to 1%, bactericidal to some microorganisms in concentrations as low as 0.04% and to all above 1.6%, and fungicidal above 1.3%. It is not sporicidal. Its activity is decreased or abolished in lipids and soaps. The protein-phenol complex is a loose one, such that phenol penetrates into tissues and can denature tissue proteins. Application of moderate concentrations to the skin causes epidermal separation, and a severe exposure causes deep necrosis. Concentrations above 0.5% cause a depolarizing local anesthesia. Oral ingestion can result in mucocutaneous and gastrointestinal corrosion, with severe pain and vomiting. Both oral ingestion and extensive application to skin can cause systemic toxicity, manifest by transient CNS stimulation followed by CNS and cardiovascular depression; death may result. There is concern that phenol may be carcinogenic. Fatal neonatal hyperbilirubinemia from inhalation of phenolic vapors has occurred in poorly ventilated nurseries in which phenol was used to disinfect mattresses and bassinets.

Phenol is not available as a single-entity antiseptic product. It is a component (0.1 to 4.5%) of various liquids, gels, ointments, and lotions (including *phenolated calamine lotion;* compound calamine lotion), throat sprays, gargles, and lozenges. In most of these, phenol is included as a local anesthetic for pruritus, stings, bites, burns, or sore throat, but some preparations are labeled for antiseptic use. Phenol is still used for disinfection in some hospitals. Because of its penetrance, it is an effective fecal disinfectant. Aerosols are used to "sterilize" bags and other containers for drugs, instruments, foodstuffs, and so forth. The caustic actions are used for facial skin peels.

RESORCINOL

Resorcinol, *m*-dihydroxybenzene, is both bactericidal and fungicidal but is only about one third as active as phenol. Locally, resorcinol is a protein precipitant. It also has keratolytic properties. The compound resembles phenol in its systemic actions. Central stimulation is more prominent than with phenol. Resorcinol is employed in the treatment of *acne, ringworm, eczema, psoriasis, seborrheic dermatitis,* and other cutaneous lesions. Its mild irritant and keratolytic properties may be important to whatever erratic efficacy resorcinol has in these disorders. It is usually applied as an ointment, cream, or lotion in concentrations of 1 to 10%. It is also used as *compound resorcinol ointment,* which contains 6% resorcinol. *Resorcinol monoacetate* gradually liberates resorcinol and, therefore, exerts a milder but more lasting action. It is used for the same purposes as resorcinol. Resorcinol monoacetate is compounded with sulfur in preparations for seborrhea.

TARS

The medicinal tars are sometimes considered to be antiseptic because of various phenolic components. However, whatever efficacy they have in their uses mainly results from a mild irritant effect. The tars are used in the treatment of diseases of the skin, such as *psoriasis* and *eczema-dermatitis*. *Coal tar, coal tar solution,* and *juniper tar* are available in a wide variety of topical preparations for these purposes.

MISCELLANEOUS PHENOLS

Clorophene (*o*-benzyl-*p*-chlorophenol) is bactericidal to gram-positive and gram-negative bacteria and is virucidal to lipid-containing viruses. Its phenol coefficients range from 71 to 225. It is used as a hospital and a household disinfectant. It is an ingredient of VESTAL LPH and one form of LYSOL.

Cresol is a mixture of the three isomers of methylphenol. It is three to ten times as potent as phenol. Although it has a higher therapeutic index than phenol, it is used in a very high concentration, and intoxications have occurred. It is very irritating. It is formulated as *saponated cresol solution* (50% cresol) in order to be miscible with water. It is only used for disinfection. Cresol is an excellent agent for the disinfection of excrement.

Hexylresorcinol is a useful antiseptic that is relatively odorless and does not stain. It is employed in a 1:1000 solution of glycerite in mouthwashes or pharyngeal antiseptic preparations. It is quite irritating to tissue, and an occasional individual exhibits marked sensitivity to its local application. Nevertheless, hexylresorcinol is used as a cleanser for skin wounds.

Orthophenylphenol is a broad-spectrum germicide with phenol coefficients that range from 71 to 500. It is used as a hospital and household disinfectant. It is an ingredient of VESTAL LPH and one form of LYSOL.

Chloroxylenol (parachlorometaxylenol) is a broad-spectrum germicide with an objectionable odor. It is active at alkaline pH. It is partially inactivated by some tissue constituents. It is incorporated at concentrations of 0.1 to 2% into preparations for the treatment of superficial burns, acne vulgaris, eczema, seborrheic dermatitis, tinea pedis, and diaper rash. It is also used in combination with hexachlorophene to enhance its antimicrobial spectrum and to prevent contamination by gram-negative bacteria. The drug is irritant and is utilized in some counterirritant products. It is also allergenic.

Parachlorophenol is similar to phenol in its properties and uses. It is a more potent antiseptic than phenol, but the toxicity and caustic actions are also greater. *Camphorated parachlorophenol,* a mixture of approximately 1 part parachlorophenol to 2 parts camphor, is used in root canal therapy; however, it is inferior to sodium hypochlorite and locally instilled antibiotics for this purpose. Blood and necrotic tissue markedly decrease its efficacy.

Para-tertiary-amylphenol is germicidal to gram-positive and gram-negative bacteria and *Candida*. The phenol coefficient usually lies between 30 and 100, but it is much lower for *Pseud. aeruginosa*. This agent is used only in combination with others. In VESTAL LPH it is used at a concentration of 3% in combination with 0.64% clorophene and 0.5% orthophenylphenol. This product has been implicated in epidemics of neonatal hyperbilirubinemia (*see* Wysowski *et al.,* 1978).

Thymol is both antiseptic and antifungal, with phenol coefficients from 27 to 44. It is used in lotions for acne vulgaris, ointments for hemorrhoids, ointments and lotions for topical analgesia, cough drops, and vaginal douches. In mouthwashes and gargles (*e.g.,* LISTERINE) it is used in a concentration too low to be effective within any practical contact time.

Triclosan (2[2,4-dichlorophenoxy]-5-chlorophenol) has broad-spectrum bactericidal activity, except that it has a low efficacy against *Pseud. aeruginosa*. Its substantivity is like that of hexachlorophene. A 0.5% tincture has been reported to be superior to 4% chlorhexidine emulsion or 60% iso-propanol for disinfection of the hands (Bartzokas *et al.*, 1983). It occasionally causes contact dermatitis. It is incorporated into antiseptic bar soaps at concentrations up to 1% and in various products for the treatment of minor burns, abrasions, insect bites, and so forth, at a concentration of 0.1 to 0.2%. In countries other than the United States it is employed as a surgical scrub and preoperative antiseptic and as a disinfectant, but its limited efficacy against *Pseudomonas* is a drawback. It has been reported to be effective in the treatment of acne vulgaris.

QUATERNARY AMMONIUM COMPOUNDS

Most detergents have germicidal activity, but it is weak and erratic. There is a misconception that soaps and other anionic detergents are somewhat germicidal as skin cleansers. Washing can remove germ-laden soil from the skin and bacteria attached to the shedding layer of the stratum corneum, but vigorous scrubbing actually increases the number of bacteria at the surface; therefore, strong germicides must be added to surgical scrubs and hospital skin cleansers. The washing of wounds with soaps and detergents increases the incidence of infections. An exception is poloxamer 188, which can be used safely as a wound cleanser at a 20% concentration (Rodeheaver *et al.*, 1980). Certain quaternary ammonium detergents themselves have strong bactericidal activity *in vitro* and sometimes are effective germicides on the skin and mucous membranes. Structures of the three most important quaternary ammonium antiseptics are shown below.

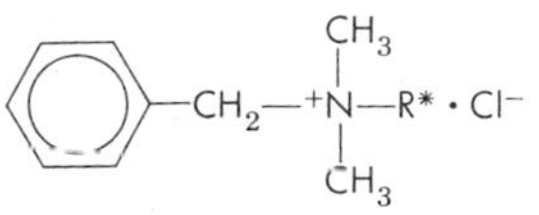

Benzalkonium Chloride

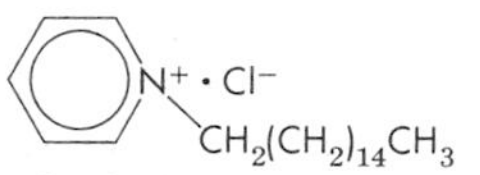

Cetylpyridinium Chloride

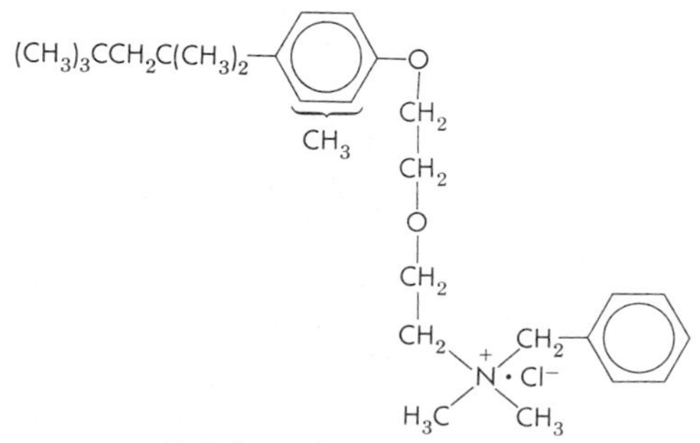

Methylbenzethonium Chloride †

---

* *R* represents any alkyl from C_8H_{17} to $C_{18}H_{37}$; the preparation is thus a mixture of molecules in which the alkyls differ.

† Benzethonium differs from methylbenzethonium in lacking the CH_3 in the position indicated by the brace.

Germicidal Properties. Quaternary ammonium agents in low concentrations are bactericidal *in vitro* to a wide variety of gram-positive and gram-negative bacteria; the gram-positive microorganisms are the more sensitive. Some gram-negative bacteria, especially *Pseud. cepacia,* are resistant, and epidemics have been caused by using instruments supposedly sterilized by quaternary ammonium agents or by contaminated commercial preparations. *Mycobacterium tuberculosis* is also relatively resistant. Many fungi, lipid-containing viruses, and spermatozoa are susceptible. Ethanol enhances the germicidal activity, so that tinctures are more effective than aqueous solutions. The major site of action of these compounds appears to be the cell membrane, where the agents cause changes in permeability.

Anionic surface-active agents antagonize the effect of cationic agents. Thus, within certain time limits, bacteriostatic actions of cationic compounds can be reversed by soaps and other anionic agents. Germicidal activity of the cationic compounds is reduced by organic matter and by other reactive substances; Lawrence (1968) lists the more important chemicals that are incompatible with cationic agents. Of special importance is the fact that these agents are adsorbed to a significant degree by cotton, rubber, and other porous materials. This adsorption reduces the effective concentration of the agent and thereby decreases its germicidal efficiency (*see* below).

Preparations. Compounds in use include *benzalkonium chloride* (ZEPHIRAN, others), *benzethonium chloride, cetyldimethylbenzylammonium chloride, cetylpyridinium chloride* (CEPACOL, others), and *methylbenzethonium chloride.* They are available in a large number of preparations for application to the skin and mucous membranes and for use as disinfectants.

Actions and Uses. Quaternary ammonium agents are detergents as well as sanitizers, and they were once widely used in sanitation before it was realized how many substances can inactivate them. In medicine they have been overly employed as all-purpose antiseptics for application to skin, tissue, and mucous membranes and as disinfectants for medical and surgical materials.

Antiseptic Uses. Quaternary ammonium antiseptics are relatively nonirritating to tissue in effective concentrations. They have a rapid onset of action. They wet and penetrate tissue surfaces and possess detergent, keratolytic, and emulsifying actions. They have a relatively low systemic toxicity, but poisoning from oral ingestion has occurred. Nevertheless, certain serious shortcomings must be kept in mind. Their activity is antagonized by soaps, tissue constituents, and pus. Also, when applied to the skin, they tend to form a film under which bacteria may remain viable; the inner surface of the film has low bactericidal power whereas the outer surface is strongly bactericidal. They do not kill spores. Their action is rather slow when compared to that of iodine. A 0.1% solution of benzalkonium chloride applied to the human skin requires about 7 minutes to decrease the bacterial population by a mere 50%; a 0.1% tincture has a slower action than 70% ethanol. Even in the absence of antagonistic tissue constituents, a 0.002% solution requires 9 hours to kill 98% of *E. coli;* this poorly effective concentration is close to that advocated for irrigation and lavage of the urinary tract. The cationic surfactants interact with keratin and cause epidermal damage, although this is minor except during continued use. Lastly, these drugs can cause occasional allergic responses with chronic use, as with certain deodorant preparations and diaper washes; cutaneous necrosis has been reported. In aggregate, the disadvantages would appear greatly to outweigh the advantages. Since superior agents are available, there seems little reason to use the cationic surfactants as antiseptics. Despite this fact, their use as antiseptics persists. Benzalkonium and benzethonium chlorides are effective spermatocides.

Disinfectant Uses. Surface-active agents have been widely used for the sterilization of instruments and other materials such as cotton pledgets and rubber gloves. However, skin, rubber gloves, surgical sponges of various materials, endoscopes, and objects made of polyethylene or polypropylene adsorb quaternary ammonium antiseptics to such a degree that the concentration of the solution may be materially reduced. Thus, repeated use of the same solution for disinfection of porous materials can reduce the concentration of the agent below the bactericidal limit. Hospital infections have been traced to materials stored in ineffective solutions of benzalkonium chloride. The chemistry, actions, uses, and abuses of quaternary ammonium antiseptics have been reviewed by Dixon and coworkers (1976) and Petrocci (1983).

MISCELLANEOUS GERMICIDES

Anthralin. *Anthralin* (1,8,9-anthratriol) is a mild irritant with weak antimicrobial activity. The compound is employed in the treatment of *psoriasis* and *chronic dermatoses.* Anthralin is available as *anthralin cream,* in concentrations of 0.1 to 1%, and as *anthralin ointment,* in concentrations of 0.1 to 1%. The weakest preparation is first employed, and the strength is then increased according to the tolerance of the patient. Anthralin is sometimes quite effective in cases of psoriasis that do not respond to other treatment. It should be kept away from the eyes and other sensitive surfaces. Anthralin stains the skin reddish-brown.

Ethylene and Propylene Oxides. *Ethylene oxide* is a gaseous alkylating germicide with a broad spectrum of activity. It is sporicidal and virucidal. It is used to disinfect and sterilize heat-labile equipment and surgical instruments. It alkylates tissue constituents and is thus toxic. Inhalation causes nausea, vomiting, neurological disorders, and even death. Traces of the gas in gloves or clothing may cause burns. Desorption for 8 hours at 50° C is much more effective than for 24 hours at room temperature. Residues in vascular catheters can cause thrombophlebitis; in endotracheal tubes, tracheitis.

The gas is explosive in concentrations above 3% and must be mixed with CO_2 or fluorocarbons. The optimal humidity is 30 to 40%. An exposure of 3 hours is used to guarantee killing of desiccated spores. For further information, *see* Block (1983).

Propylene oxide, a liquid, is also an effective sterilizing agent (*see* Block, 1983).

Ichthammol. *Ichthammol (ammonium ichthosulfonate)* is the product obtained from sulfonating and neutralizing with ammonia, the distillate of certain bituminous schists. The compound contains approximately 10% sulfur in the form of organic sulfonates. It is a brown, viscous fluid with a strong characteristic odor and is soluble in both aqueous and organic solvents. Ichthammol is mildly irritant and somewhat antiseptic. It is used alone, or in combination with other antiseptics, for the treatment of cutaneous disorders and to promote healing in chronic inflammations. The drug is employed in the form of *ichthammol ointment* (10% in a petrolatum base). At one time the drug was used widely, but it has deservedly lost much popularity.

Propiolactone. *Propiolactone* is the lactone of beta-hydroxypropionic acid. Like most four-membered rings, it is labile. Consequently, it acylates many important nucleophils. The ability to react with adenine in DNA is probably the basis of its virucidal, mutagenic, and carcinogenic actions. Its most important use is in the treatment of blood products and certain vaccines to kill hepatitis and other viruses. Propiolactone is used in liquid or vapor form for sterilization in the pharmaceutical and food industries and to some extent in hospitals. It is as much as 4000 times more active than ethylene oxide and 25 times more active than formaldehyde. However, it is not as penetrating. Like ethylene oxide and formaldehyde, the vapors or unreacted liquid residues are irritant, and a thorough decontamination of sterilized objects is required before use.

Sulfur. Sulfur must be converted to pentathionic acid ($H_2S_5O_6$) in order to exert germicidal action. Presumably the oxidation of sulfur to pentathionic acid is accomplished by certain microorganisms or by epidermal cells when the element is applied to the skin. Sulfur possesses a keratolytic property, which may be the basis for the therapeutic action of the element in certain cutaneous disorders unassociated with infection.

Sublimed sulfur (flowers of sulfur) is a fine, yellow crystalline, water-insoluble powder. *Precipitated sulfur* is a much finer powder and, therefore, has a greater reactive surface than sublimed sulfur. It is the form of sulfur most often used in topical preparations. It is available in bar soaps, shampoos, gels, lotions, and creams. *Colloidal sulfur* is the most active form of sulfur and is available in various products for acne and seborrhea. Sublimed sulfur is used in the preparation of *sulfurated lime topical solution. White lotion* contains sulfurated potash, which is a complex polysulfide and thiosulfate.

Sulfur is used as a fungicide and parasiticide (*see*

below). Sulfur alone, or in combination with other keratolytic agents (often 2% salicylic acid, resorcinol, or coal tar), is widely used in the treatment of cutaneous disorders such as *psoriasis, seborrhea, acne,* and *eczema-dermatitis*. The percentage of sulfur employed may be that of the full-strength ointment, or less if the patient's skin exhibits intolerance. Prolonged local use of sulfur may result in a characteristic dermatitis venenata.

Triclocarban. *Triclocarban* has broad-spectrum antibacterial and antifungal activity. It is one of several anilides that have been incorporated into antiseptic soaps and disinfectants. When hexachlorophene was withdrawn from nonprescription products, it was replaced in bar soaps by one or more of the halogenated salicylanilides (dibromsalan and tribromsalan) or triclocarban. The salicylanilides were subsequently withdrawn because they caused occasional photosensitization. *Triclosan* has superseded them.

II. Antifungal Drugs

In temperate climates, fungal infections comprise a minor fraction of human diseases caused by microorganisms. Nevertheless, the incidence, particularly of superficial infections such as tinea pedis, is appreciable. The list of chemicals reputed to have some degree of antifungal activity is long, and a number of preparations of low efficacy are successfully foisted upon both the lay public and the medical profession, despite the existence at the present time of drugs that are demonstrably beneficial in dermatophytosis.

Many antibacterial agents possess fungistatic or fungicidal properties. Therefore, many of the drugs discussed under antiseptics and disinfectants have been employed in the local treatment of fungal infections, and their uses in such mycoses have already been noted in some instances. The present discussion will be restricted to *nonsystemic antifungal drugs;* systemic antifungal drugs are discussed in Chapter 54. Various aspects of the discovery, actions, and uses of antifungal drugs have been reviewed by Drube (1972), Kobayashi and Medoff (1977), Drouhet (1978), Borgers (1980), and Ryley and associates (1981).

Mechanisms of Antifungal Action. Drugs exert fungistatic and fungicidal actions by a variety of mechanisms (*see* references cited above). In addition, many agents used in the treatment of superficial mycoses are virtually devoid of either fungi-

static or fungicidal actions in the concentrations employed, and their beneficial effects probably depend upon factors not related to any direct effect on fungi. The keratolytic agents exert their effect mainly by promoting desquamation of the stratum corneum, especially in hyperkeratotic locations. The fungus resides in the stratum corneum, where keratin is its substrate, not in the toxin-induced lesion. Thus, keratolysis removes the offending fungus as well as aids in the penetration of drugs. Drugs that prevent hyperhidrosis indirectly retard proliferation of the fungus by altering the conditions of growth. Astringent drugs exert a palliative effect by allaying the symptoms of acute inflammation and irritation and by anhidrotic actions.

BENZOIC ACID AND SALICYLIC ACID

Benzoic and salicylic acids ointment is known as *Whitfield's ointment*. It combines the fungistatic action of benzoate with the keratolytic action of salicylate. It contains benzoic acid and salicylic acid in a ratio of 2:1 (usually 6%:3%). It is used mainly in the treatment of *tinea pedis*. Since benzoic acid is only fungistatic, eradication of the infection occurs only after the infected stratum corneum is shed, and continuous medication is required for several weeks to months. The salicylic acid accelerates the desquamation. The ointment is also sometimes used to treat *tinea capitis*. Mild irritation may occur at the site of application.

CICLOPIROX OLAMINE

Ciclopirox olamine (LOPROX) has broad-spectrum antifungal activity. The chemical structure is:

Ciclopirox Olamine

It is fungicidal to *Candida albicans, Epidermophyton floccosum, Microsporum canis, Trichophyton mentagrophytes,* and *T. rubrum*. It also inhibits the growth of *Pityrosporum obiculare (Malassezia furfur)*. After application to the skin, it penetrates through the epidermis into the dermis, but even under occlusion less than 1.5% is absorbed into the systemic circulation. Since the half-life is 1.7 hours, no systemic accumulation occurs. The drug penetrates into hair follicles and sebaceous glands. It can sometimes cause hypersensitivity. It is available as a 1% cream for the treatment of cutaneous candidiasis and tinea corporis, cruris, pedis, and versicolor. Cure rates in the dermatomycoses and candidal infections have been variously reported to be 81 to 94%. No topical toxicity has been noted.

PROPIONIC AND CAPRYLIC ACIDS

Sodium and calcium propionates have long been incorporated into bread dough as nontoxic inhibitors of mold growth. *Propionic acid* and *sodium propionate* are promoted for the treatment of the dermatomycoses. They are relatively weak and possess only fungistatic activity; both *in vitro* and in human infections, viable fungi can be recovered after exposure to them. Both their low efficacy and exaggerated price make them irrational choices for treatment. They may be compounded together or with salicylic acid, sodium caprylate, or other agents. Sodium propionate is used in proprietary preparations in concentrations of 1 to 5%.

UNDECYLENIC ACID

Undecylenic acid is 10-undecenoic acid, an 11-carbon, unsaturated compound. It is a yellow liquid with a characteristic rancid odor. It is primarily fungistatic, although fungicidal activity may be observed with long exposure to high concentrations of the agent. The drug is active against a variety of fungi, including the common pathogens in superficial mycoses. *Undecylenic acid* (DESENEX, others) is available in a foam, ointment, powder, soap, and solution. *Zinc undecylenate* is marketed as a cream or powder. The zinc provides an astringent action that aids in the suppression of inflammation. *Compound undecylenic acid ointment* (DESENEX, UNDOGUENT) contains both undecylenic acid (about 5%) and zinc undecylenate (about 20%). *Calcium undecylenate* (CALDESENE) is available as a powder. *Copper undecylenate* is compounded with undecylenic acid, salicylic acid, propionic acid, sodium propionate, and sodium caprylate.

Undecylenic acid preparations are employed in the treatment of various *dermatomycoses*, especially *tinea pedis*. Concentrations of the acid as high as 10%, as well as in the compound ointment, may be applied to the skin. The preparations as formulated are usually not irritating to tissue, and sensitization to them is uncommon. It is of undoubted benefit in retarding fungal growth in *tinea pedis*, but the infection frequently persists despite intensive treatment with preparations of the acid and the zinc salt. At best, the clinical "cure" rate is about 50% (Smith *et al.*, 1977) and is thus much lower than that obtained with the imidazoles, haloprogin, or tolnaftate. The efficacy in the treatment of *tinea capitis* is marginal, and the drug is no longer used for that purpose. Undecylenic acid preparations are also approved for use in the treatment of diaper rash, tinea cruris, and other minor dermatological conditions.

HALOPROGIN

Haloprogin is a halogenated phenolic ether with the following structure:

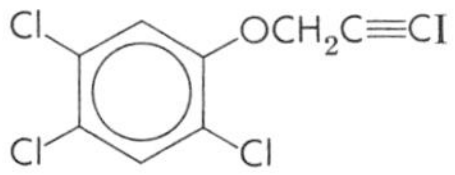

Haloprogin

It is fungicidal to various species of *Epidermophyton, Pityrosporum, Microsporum, Trichophyton,* and *Candida*. During treatment with this drug, irritation, pruritus, burning sensations, vesiculation, increased maceration, and "sensitization" (or exacerbation of the lesion) occasionally occur, especially on the foot if occlusive footgear is worn. It is possible that the sensitization indicates a rapid therapeutic response in which the release of toxins makes the lesion temporarily worse. Haloprogin is poorly absorbed through the skin; it is converted to trichlorophenol in the body. The systemic toxicity from topical application appears to be low.

Haloprogin (HALOTEX) is available as a 1% cream or solution. It is applied twice a day for 2 to 4 weeks. Its principal use is against *tinea pedis*, for which the cure rate is about 80%; it is thus approximately equal in efficacy to tolnaftate. It is also used against *tinea cruris, tinea corporis, tinea manuum,* and *tinea versicolor*.

IMIDAZOLES

There are a number of related imidazoles that have broad-spectrum antifungal activity *in vitro* and which are effective topically against nearly all of the fungi of clinical interest. In addition, they are active against certain bacteria and protozoa. Four of the imidazoles are currently available in the United States and a fifth, tioconazole, is in an advanced phase of development. Three—clotrimazole, econazole, and miconazole—are used topically in the treatment of the superficial mycoses; two—ketoconazole and miconazole—are used to treat systemic mycoses (*see* Chapter 54). There are several others under intensive investigation.

Antifungal Activity. All the members of the group have essentially the same spectrum of activity, although there are differences in relative activities against specific microorganisms. They are fungicidal if the concentration is sufficiently high. The drugs inhibit a broad spectrum of fungi, including epidermophytes, yeasts, *Aspergillus, Cladiosporum, Coccidioides immitis, Histoplasma capsulatum, Madurella mycetomi, Mucor, Paracoccidioides brasiliensis,* and *Phialophora*. Actinomycetes, gram-positive bacteria, certain anaerobes (such as *Bacteroides fragilis*), and *Trichomonas vaginalis* are also inhibited. Acquired resistance to imidazoles occurs rarely and has been seen only with *Candida albicans*.

Ergosterol is important to the integrity and function of the fungal cell membrane. The imidazoles inhibit the incorporation of acetate into ergosterol, and they also inhibit lanosterol demethylase. There is disorganization and thickening of the plasmalemma. The uptake of essential nutrients is impaired. Such a mechanism would explain the selectivity for fungi and low toxicity for mammalian cells, but it does not explain the actions on gram-positive bacteria, anaerobes, and trichomonads.

Strains of yeast that do not synthesize their own ergosterol are nevertheless inhibited by clotrimazole and miconazole (Taylor *et al.,* 1983). The mechanisms of action of the imidazoles have been reviewed by Borgers (1980).

Clotrimazole. Clotrimazole has the following structure:

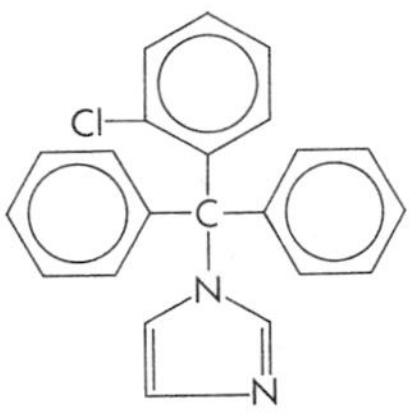

Clotrimazole

Most strains of dermatophytes and *Candida* species are inhibited by concentrations of less than 2 μg/ml. Most strains of fungi isolated in otomycosis are sensitive to 0.1 μg/ml. Sensitive strains of *Candida* are killed by concentrations above 5 μg/ml. Clotrimazole also has activity against *Trichomonas* and the ameba *Naegleria fowleri.*

Absorption of clotrimazole is less than 0.5% after application to the intact skin; from the vagina, it is 3 to 10%. Fungicidal concentrations remain in the vagina for as long as 3 days after application of the drug (Ritter *et al.,* 1982). The small amount absorbed is metabolized in the liver and excreted in bile. In adults, an oral dose of 200 mg per day will give rise to plasma concentrations of 0.2 to 0.35 μg/ml.

On the skin, in a small fraction of recipients, clotrimazole may cause stinging, erythema, edema, vesication, desquamation, pruritus, and urticaria. Applied to the vagina, about 1.6% of recipients complain of a mild burning sensation and, rarely, of lower abdominal cramps, slight increase in urinary frequency, or skin rash. Occasionally, the sexual partner may experience penile or urethral irritation. By the oral route, clotrimazole causes gastrointestinal irritation. In patients using troches, the incidence is about 5%.

Clotrimazole is available as a 1% cream, lotion, or solution (LOTRIMIN, MYCELEX), 1% vaginal cream or 100-mg vaginal tablets (GYNE-LOTRIMIN, MYCELEX-G), and 10-mg troches (MYCELEX). On the skin, applications are made twice a day. For the vagina, the standard regimens are one tablet once a day at bedtime for 7 days or 5 g of cream once a day for 7 to 14 days; however, alternative regimens are gaining prominence (*see* below). Troches are to be dissolved slowly in the mouth five times a day for 14 days.

Clotrimazole has been reported to cure dermatophyte infections in 60 to 100% of cases. Tinea corporis and tinea cruris require about 3 or 4 weeks of treatment, but tinea pedis may require as long as 8 weeks. Tinea capitis and tinea favosa are difficult to cure, the average cure rate from several studies being only about 12%. In erythasma, a bacterial infection, the cure rate is 83 to 100%. From a number of studies, the cure rates in cutaneous candidiasis are 80 to 100%. In vulvovaginal candidiasis, the cure rate is usually above 90% when the 7-day regimen is used. A 3-day regimen of 200 mg once a day appears to be similarly effective, as does single-dose treatment (500 mg) (*see* Goormans *et al.,* 1982; Krause, 1982; Milsom and Forssman, 1982). Recurrences usually do not reflect failure of any regimen but rather reinfection from the anus, and concomitant enteric therapy has been proposed. The cure rate with oral troches for oral and pharyngeal candidiasis may be as high as 100%.

The details of the pharmacology and clinical uses of clotrimazole may be found in a symposium (Symposium, 1974) and in the review by Sawyer and associates (1975b).

Econazole. Econazole nitrate (SPECTAZOLE), the deschloro derivative of miconazole, has the following structure:

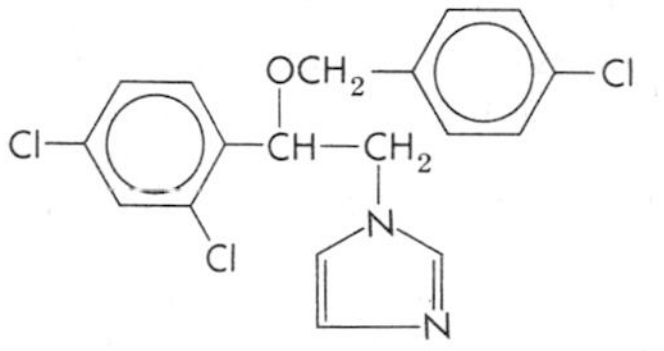

Econazole

Econazole has been variously reported on the one hand to be less active than miconazole against the yeasts and on the other to be the most active of the topical imidazoles (Bergen and Vangdal, 1983). Minimal inhibitory concentrations range from 0.12 to 25 μg/ml. It is two to eight times more active than miconazole against filamentous fungi; minimal inhibitory concentrations lie between 0.025 and 12.5 μg/ml. Econazole is especially active against the mycelial forms.

Econazole readily penetrates the stratum corneum and is found in effective concentrations down to the mid-dermis. However, less than 1% of an applied dose appears to be absorbed into the blood.

Approximately 3% of recipients have local erythema, burning, stinging, or itching. Oral toxicity in animals is very low.

Econazole is available as a water-miscible cream (1%) to be applied twice a day. It is approved for the treatment of tinea pedis, tinea cruris, tinea corporis, tinea versicolor, and cutaneous candidiasis. Relief may begin within 1 to 2 days after the start of treatment, and a significant mycological improvement may be evident within a few days. Tinea versicolor responds more slowly and may require 2 weeks for substantial improvement. At least a month of therapy is recommended for tinea pedis and tinea versicolor in order to prevent recurrences, but 2 weeks is sufficient with other tineas. Mixed infections of the scalp may require treatment for over 5 weeks. Econazole has been used successfully in the treatment of various mycoses (mostly candidiasis) of the ear, nose, and throat. It is also effective in oculomycosis (Oji and Clayton, 1982). The status of econazole among the topical imidazoles remains to be determined. However, in the treatment of vaginal candidiasis it appears to be slightly less effective than or equieffective with clotrimazole (*see* Stettendorf *et al.*, 1982; Gabriel and Thin, 1983).

Miconazole Nitrate. Miconazole is a very close chemical congener of econazole, with the following structure:

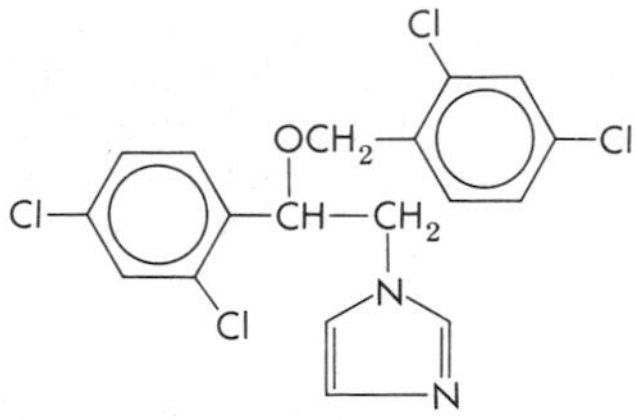

Miconazole

The minimal inhibitory concentration varies from as low as 0.001 μg/ml for *Paracoccidioides* to 32 μg/ml for some strains of *Cladiosporum* and *Phialophora*. Dermatophytes, *Candida albicans*, and most common fungal pathogens are inhibited by 0.2 to 10 μg/ml.

Miconazole readily penetrates the stratum corneum of the skin and persists there for more than 4 days after application. Less than 1% is absorbed into the blood. Absorption is no more than 1.3% from the vagina.

Adverse effects from topical application to the vagina include burning, itching, or irritation in about 7% of recipients and infrequently pelvic cramps (0.2%), headache, hives, or skin rash. Irritation, burning, and maceration are rare after cutaneous application. Miconazole is considered safe for use during pregnancy, although vaginal use should be avoided during the first trimester.

Miconazole nitrate is available as a 2% dermatological cream, spray, powder, or lotion (MICATIN, MONISTAT-DERM), to be applied twice daily for 14 days in the treatment of superficial dermatomycoses. To avoid maceration, only the lotion should be applied to intertriginous areas. It is available as a 2% vaginal cream, 100-mg suppositories (MONISTAT 7), to be applied high in the vagina at bedtime for 7 days, and 200-mg vaginal suppositories (MONISTAT 3) for 3-day therapy. It is also available for intravenous use (*see* Chapter 54).

In the treatment of *tinea pedis,* topical miconazole relieves itching within a few days; vesicles and fissures heal rapidly, but desquamation may continue for several weeks. The mycological cure rate may be over 90%. In the treatment of *tinea cruris,* the drug is comparably effective. *Tinea versicolor, ringworm, onychomycosis,* and *cutaneous candidiasis* also respond to topical miconazole. In the treatment of *vulvovaginal candidiasis,* the mycological cure rate at the end of 1 month is about 80 to 95%. In one double-blind study, the cure rates with miconazole and clotrimazole were almost identical (Lebherz *et al.,* 1983). Pruritus sometimes is relieved after a single application. Some vaginal infections caused by *T. glabratus* also respond. The

free base is used to treat ophthalmic mycoses (*see* Jones, 1978). The actions and uses of miconazole have been reviewed by Sawyer and associates (1975a), Kobayashi and Medoff (1977), and Heel and associates (1980).

TOLNAFTATE

Tolnaftate is a thiocarbamate with the following structure:

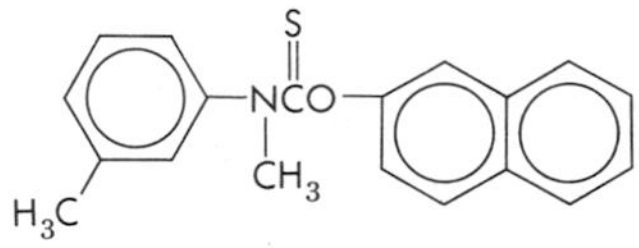

Tolnaftate

Tolnaftate is effective in the treatment of the majority of cutaneous mycoses caused by *T. rubrum, T. mentagrophytes, T. tonsurans, E. floccosum, M. canis, M. audouini, M. gypseum,* and *Pityrosporum obiculare,* but it is ineffective against *Candida.* The drug is less effective in the presence of hyperkeratotic lesions, and these should be treated with 10% salicylic acid ointment alternating with tolnaftate. In tinea pedis the cure rate is around 80%, compared to about 95% for miconazole. Lesions on the scalp due to *T. tonsurans* and *M. audouini* do not respond. The drug does not alter the course of onychomycosis. Relapse may occur after cessation of therapy and approximates the rate observed when griseofulvin is employed; it is not due to development of drug resistance in the microorganisms. Re-treatment is usually successful. Toxic or allergic reactions to tolnaftate have not been reported.

Tolnaftate (AFTATE, TINACTIN) is available in 1% concentration as a cream, gel, powder, aerosol powder, and topical solution, or as a topical aerosol solution. The preparations are applied locally twice a day. When pruritus is present, it is usually relieved in 24 to 72 hours. Involution of interdigital lesions due to susceptible fungi is very often complete in 7 to 21 days.

MISCELLANEOUS ANTIFUNGAL AGENTS

Acrisorcin (AKRINOL; 9-aminoacridinium 4-hexylresorcinolate) is effective against *Pityrosporum obiculare* and is used in the treatment of *tinea versicolor* (*pityriasis versicolor*). The drug is available as *acrisorcin cream* (0.2%). It is applied twice daily to the affected areas; application is continued for 6 weeks after clearing of the lesions. Relapses sometimes occur. Occasionally it causes hives, blisters, and erythematous vesicles. The drug may cause burning sensations when applied to eczematous lesions. Its use may result in photo-induced pruritus. It should be kept away from the eyes.

Natamycin (NATACYN) is a pentaenic macrolide. It has a broader antifungal spectrum than does amphotericin B, especially against ocular pathogens. It is also much less irritating to the eye and hence is used to treat fungal keratitis, especially when caused by myceliating fungi. It is the drug of choice in infections caused by *Fusarium solani.* However, it penetrates poorly and may not reach deep corneal mycoses. It is used as a 5% suspension.

Carbol-fuchsin topical solution contains 0.3% basic fuchsin, 4.5% phenol, 10% resorcinol, 5% acetone, and 10% ethanol. It is still marketed for the treatment of *tinea pedis* and *tinea cruris.*

Sulfur still offers a useful alternative to other drugs, and its value in the treatment of the superficial cutaneous mycoses is probably underrated. Sulfur is used in combination with salicylic acid or resorcinol.

The uses of *selenium sulfide* are described in Chapter 40. It is effective in the treatment of *tinea versicolor* and *tinea capitis.*

Aminacrine hydrochloride exerts germicidal actions against bacteria, fungi, and trichomonads. It is incorporated into suppositories and creams for the treatment of vaginal infections.

Many of the agents discussed in the section on antiseptics and disinfectants are antifungal, and the antimycotic uses of some are mentioned in that section. *Acetic acid* requires no further discussion. *Gentian violet* (1.35%) is still used for the topical treatment of *vaginal candidiasis.* The excellent fungicidal properties of *iodine* are usually overlooked. The tincture can be used to treat various dry forms of cutaneous superficial mycoses, and the solution may be applied to wet forms.

Iodoquinol (diiodohydroxyquin) and *clioquinol (iodochlorhydroxyquin)* are incorporated into vaginal preparations to suppress candidal and monilial infections and into dermatological preparations for the treatment of various dermatomycoses and other skin diseases; as amebicides, they are discussed in Chapter 46.

III. Ectoparasiticides

The ectoparasiticides are both ectozoic and ectophytic. In common usage, however, the term *ectoparasiticides* connotes only those drugs that are used against the animal parasites. In the human, these are primarily pediculocides and miticides.

LINDANE (GAMMA BENZENE HEXACHLORIDE)

Lindane is the gamma isomer of hexachlorocyclohexane. It is lipid soluble, is absorbed through chitin, and is insecticidal by producing seizures. It can also cause convulsions in humans, even by the topical route (*see* Chapter 70); in children, especially, the seizures are of the grand mal type. Diazepam is an appropriate antagonist. Nervousness, irritability, insomnia, vertigo, amblyopia, stupor, and coma have also been observed following excessive cutaneous application. The drug can sensitize the heart to arrhythmias. It is irritant to the skin, eyes, and mucosae, and care must be taken to keep the drug away from the face and eyes. Fatal cases of aplastic anemia have resulted from prolonged exposure to vaporized lindane. The compound is readily absorbed through the skin, even of adults, and about 10% ultimately appears in the urine.

Lindane (gamma benzene hexachloride; KWELL, SCABENE) is an excellent miticide in the treatment of *scabies.* It is employed in 1% concentration in a vanishing cream, lotion, or shampoo. The mixture is applied in a thin layer over the entire cutaneous surface (15 to 25 g of cream for an adult) and is not removed for 8 to 12 hours. Pruritus is usually relieved within 24 hours, and the great majority of patients do not require a second treatment. If necessary, however, second and third applications can be made at weekly intervals.

The drug is also a very active pediculocide and is effective in the treatment of *pediculosis pubis, capitis,* and *corporis.* A single application of the 1% cream, lotion, or shampoo usually suffices to eradicate the ectoparasite. Lindane is also used to treat infestation by *Phthirus pubis* (crab lice).

MALATHION

Malathion is an anticholinesterase; its structure is shown in Table 6–2 (page 115). The general pharmacology of the anticholinesterases is discussed in Chapter 6.

Malathion is rapidly pediculocidal and niticidal; lice and their eggs (nits) are killed within 3 seconds by 0.003% and 0.06% malathion in acetone, respectively. The pharmaceutical preparation contains 78% isopropanol.

Malathion is very rapidly metabolized by man but only slowly by insects; thus, there is very high selectivity for lice and no toxicity to the patient with the amounts and schedule employed.

Malathion (PRIODERM) is available as a 0.5% lotion for the treatment of head lice and nits. It is gently rubbed onto the scalp and left for 8 to 12 hours, after which the hair is shampooed and combed. A second application may be made after 7 to 9 days, if necessary.

MISCELLANEOUS ECTOPARASITICIDES

Benzyl benzoate is a relatively harmless substance that in high concentration is toxic to *Acarus scabiei.* The compound has been widely employed in the treatment of *scabies* and is also useful in the treatment of *pediculosis. Benzyl benzoate* is used as a 26 to 30% lotion. In the treatment of *scabies,* the lotion is applied to the entire body, except the face, after thorough cleansing. When the first application is dry, a second coat is applied. After 24 hours, the residue is then washed off.

Pyrethrins, which are discussed in Chapter 70, are moderately effective as pediculocides. Commercial preparations contain piperonyl butoxide, which enhances the effectiveness by inhibiting enzymatic destruction in the insect. Commercial preparations contain 0.165 to 0.333% pyrethrins, 2 to 4% piperonyl butoxide, and up to 5.5% petroleum distillate. They are available as a gel, shampoo, and various liquids. Preparations should be kept away from the eyes and mucous membranes.

Crotamiton (N-ethyl-*o*-crotonotoluidide; EURAX) is an effective scabicide. It is available as a cream or lotion containing 10% crotamiton. It occasionally causes irritation, especially on inflamed skin or when applied over a prolonged period of time. It can cause sensitization. Paradoxically, the preparations also have antipruritic properties.

An emulsion of 31% *tetrahydronaphthalene* and 0.03% *copper oleate* (CUPREX) is promoted as a pediculocide and niticide, but its true efficacy remains to be determined.

Sulfur ointment and other preparations containing sulfur are employed in the treatment of *scabies* and, less frequently, of *pediculosis*. *Sulfurated lime topical solution* (16.5% lime, 25% sublimed sulfur) is also used in both types of infestations.

Thiabendazole (MINTEZOL) can be applied to the skin as a 10% suspension in the treatment of cutaneous *larva migrans*. It has scabicidal activity, for which it is used outside of the United States. It is also reputed to be mildly antifungal.

Ainamo, J.; Askainen, S.; and Paloheimo, L. Gingival bleeding after chlorhexidine mouthrinses. *J. Clin. Periodontol.*, **1982,** *9,* 337–345.

Anyiwo, C. E.; Coker, A. O.; and Daniel, S. O. *Pseudomonas aeruginosa* in postoperative wounds from chlorhexidine solutions. *J. Hosp. Infect.*, **1982,** *3,* 189–191.

Apt, L., and Isenberg, S. Chemical preparation of skin and eye in ophthalmic surgery: an international survey. *Ophthalmic Surg.*, **1982,** *13,* 1026–1029.

Ayliffe, G. A.; Noy, M. F.; Babb, J. R.; Davies, J. G.; and Jackson, J. A comparison of pre-operative bathing with chlorhexidine-detergent and non-medicated soap in the prevention of wound infection. *J. Hosp. Infect.*, **1983,** *3,* 237–244.

Bageant, R. A.; Marsik, F. J.; Kellogg, V. A.; Hyler, D. L.; and Groschel, D. H. M. In-use testing of our glutaraldehyde disinfectants in the cidemic washer. *Respir. Care*, **1981,** *26,* 1255–1261.

Bapat, R. D.; Supe, A. N.; and Sathe, M. J. Management of small bowel perforation with intra- and post-operative lavages with povidone iodine. (A prospective study.) *J. Postgrad. Med.*, **1983,** *29,* 29–33.

Bartzokas, C. A.; Gibson, M. F.; Graham, R.; and Pinder, D. C. A comparison of triclosan and chlorhexidine preparations with 60 per cent isopropyl alcohol for hygienic hand disinfection. *J. Hosp. Infect.*, **1983,** *4,* 245–255.

Bergen, T., and Vangdal, M. In vitro activity of antifungal agents against yeast species. *Chemotherapy*, **1983,** *29,* 104–110.

Berry, A. R.; Watt, B.; Goldacre, M. J.; Thomson, J. W.; and McNair, T. J. A comparison of the use of povidone-iodine and chlorhexidine in the prophylaxis of postoperative wound infection. *J. Hosp. Infect.*, **1982,** *3,* 55–63.

Craven, D. E.; Moody, B.; Connolly, M. G.; Kollish, N. R.; Strottmeier, K. D.; and McCabe, W. R. Pseudobacteremia caused by povidone-iodine solution contaminated with *Pseudomonas cepacia*. *N. Engl. J. Med.*, **1981,** *305,* 621–623.

Dattani, I. M.; Gerken, A.; and Evans, B. A. Aetiology and management of non-specific vaginitis. *Br. J. Vener. Dis.*, **1982,** *58,* 32–35.

de Jong, T. E.; Vierhout, R. J.; and van Vroonhoven, T. J. Povidone-iodine irrigation of the subcutaneous tissue to prevent surgical wound infections. *Surg. Gynecol. Obstet.*, **1982,** *155,* 221–224.

Dineen, P. Hand-washing degerming: a comparison of

povidone-iodine and chlorhexidine. *Clin. Pharmacol. Ther.*, **1978,** *23,* 63–67.

Gabriel, G., and Thin, R. N. Clotrimazole and econazole in the treatment of vaginal candidosis. A single-blind comparison. *Br. J. Vener. Dis.*, **1983,** *59,* 56–58.

Galland, R. B.; Karlowski, T.; Midwood, C. J.; Madden, M. V.; and Carmalt, H. Topical antiseptics in addition to preoperative antibiotics in preventing post-appendicectomy wound infections. *Ann. R. Coll. Surg. Engl.*, **1983,** *65,* 397–399.

Gershanik, J.; Boecler, B.; Ensley, H.; McClosky, S.; and George, W. The gasping syndrome and benzyl alcohol poisoning. *N. Engl. J. Med.*, **1982,** *307,* 1384–1388.

Goormans, E.; Bergstein, N. A.; Loendersloot, E. W.; and Branolte, J. H. One-dose therapy of *Candida* vaginitis. I. Results of an open multicentre trial. *Chemotherapy*, **1982,** *28,* Suppl. 1, 106–109.

Jones, D. B. Therapy of postsurgical fungal endophthalmitis. *Ophthalmology (Rochester)*, **1978,** *85,* 357–373.

Knight, C. D., Jr.; Farnell, M. B.; and Hollier, L. H. Treatment of aortic graft infection with povidone-iodine irrigation. *Mayo Clin. Proc.*, **1983,** *58,* 472–475.

Krause, U. Results of a single-dose treatment of vaginal mycoses with 500 mg CANESTEN vaginal tablets. *Chemotherapy*, **1982,** *28,* Suppl. 1, 99–105.

Kunze, J.; Kaiser, H. J.; and Petres, J. Relevanz einer Jodallergie bei handelsüblichen Polyvidon-Jod-Zubereitungen. *Z. Hautkr.*, **1983,** *58,* 255–261.

Lebherz, T. B.; Goldman, L.; Wiesmeier, E.; Mason, D.; and Ford, L. C. A comparison of the efficacy of two vaginal creams for vulvovaginal candidiasis, and correlations with the presence of *Candida* species in the perianal area and oral contraceptive use. *Clin. Ther.*, **1983,** *5,* 409–416.

Leigh, D. A.; Stronge, J. L.; Marriner, J.; and Sedgwick, J. Total body bathing with HIBISCRUB (chlorhexidine) in surgical patients: a controlled trial. *J. Hosp. Infect.*, **1983,** *4,* 229–235.

Maiorca, R.; Cantaluppi, A.; Cancarini, G. C.; Scalamongna, A.; Broccoli, R.; Graziani, G.; Brasa, S.; and Ponticelli, C. Prospective controlled trial of a Y-connector and disinfectant to prevent peritonitis in continuous ambulatory peritoneal dialysis. *Lancet*, **1983,** *2,* 642–644.

Marks, J. G., Jr. Allergic contact dermatitis to povidone-iodine. *J. Am. Acad. Dermatol.*, **1982,** *6,* 473–475.

Milsom, I., and Forssman, L. Treatment of vaginal candidosis with a single 500-mg clotrimazole pessary. *Br. J. Vener. Dis.*, **1982,** *58,* 124–126.

Nakahara, H., and Kozukue, H. Isolation of chlorhexidine-resistant *Pseudomonas aeruginosa* from clinical lesions. *J. Clin. Microbiol.*, **1982,** *15,* 166–168.

Oji, E. O., and Clayton, Y. M. The role of econazole in the management of oculomycosis. *Int. Ophthalmol.*, **1982,** *4,* 137–142.

Petersen, N. J.; Carson, L. A.; Doto, I. L.; Aguero, S. M.; and Favero, M. S. Microbiologic evaluation of a new glutaraldehyde-based disinfectant for hemodialysis systems. *Trans. Am. Soc. Artif. Intern. Organs*, **1982,** *28,* 287–290.

Randall, P. E.; Ganguli, L.; and Marcuson, R. W. Wound infection following vasectomy. *Br. J. Urol.*, **1983,** *55,* 564–567.

Ritter, W.; Patzschke, K.; Krause, U.; and Stettendorf, S. Pharmacokinetic fundamentals of vaginal treatment with clotrimazole. *Chemotherapy*, **1982,** *28,* Suppl. 1, 37–42.

Rodeheaver, G.; Bellamy, W.; Kody, M.; Spatafora, G.; Fitton, L.; Leyden, K.; and Edlich, R. Bactericidal activity and toxicity of iodine-containing solutions in wounds. *Arch. Surg.*, **1982,** *117,* 181–186.

Rodeheaver, G. T.; Kurtz, L.; Kircher, B. J.; and Edlich,

R. F. Pluronic F-68: a promising new skin wound cleanser. *Ann. Emerg. Med.*, **1980**, *9*, 572–576.

Rogers, D. M.; Blouin, G. S.; and O'Leary, J. P. Povidone-iodine wound irrigation and wound sepsis. *Surg. Gynecol. Obstet.*, **1983**, *157*, 426–430.

Selk, S. H.; Pogány, S. A.; and Higuchi, T. Comparative antimicrobial activity, *in vitro* and *in vivo*, of soft N-chloramine systems and chlorhexidine. *Appl. Environ. Microbiol.*, **1982**, *43*, 899–904.

Smith, E. B.; Powell, R. F.; Graham, J. L.; and Ulrich, J. A. Topical undecylenic acid in tinea pedis: a new look. *Int. J. Dermatol.*, **1977**, *16*, 52–56.

Sobel, J. D.; Hashman, N.; Reinherz, G.; and Merzbach, D. Nosocomial *Pseudomonas cepacia* infection associated with chlorhexidine contamination. *Am. J. Med.*, **1982**, *73*, 183–186.

Southampton Infection Control Team. Evaluation of aseptic techniques and chlorhexidine on the rate of catheter-associated urinary-tract infection. *Lancet*, **1982**, *1*, 89–91.

Stettendorf, S.; Benijts, G.; Vignali, M.; and Kreysing, W. Three-day therapy of vaginal candidiasis with clotrimazole vaginal tablets and econazole ovules: a multicenter comparative study. *Chemotherapy*, **1982**, *28*, Suppl. 1, 87–91.

Taylor, F. R.; Rodriguez, R. J.; and Parks, L. W. Relationship between antifungal activity and inhibition of sterol biosynthesis in miconazole, clotrimazole, and 15-azasterol. *Antimicrob. Agents Chemother.*, **1983**, *23*, 515–521.

Wells, F. C.; Newsom, S. W.; and Rowlands, C. Wound infection in cardiothoracic surgery. *Lancet*, **1983**, *1*, 1209–1210.

Wysowski, D. K.; Flynt, J. W., Jr.; Goldfield, M.; Altman, R.; and Davis, A. T. Epidemic neonatal hyperbilirubinemia and use of a phenolic disinfectant detergent. *Pediatrics*, **1978**, *61*, 165–170.

Monographs and Reviews

Altemeier, W. A. Surgical antiseptics. In, *Disinfection, Sterilization, and Preservation*, 3rd ed. (Block, S. S., ed.) Lea & Febiger, Philadelphia, **1983**, pp. 493–504.

Block, S. S. (ed.). *Disinfection, Sterilization, and Preservation*, 3rd ed. Lea & Febiger, Philadelphia, **1983**.

Borgers, M. Mechanism of action of antifungal drugs, with special reference to the imidazole derivatives. *Rev. Infect. Dis.*, **1980**, *2*, 520–534.

Dixon, R. E.; Kaslow, R. A.; Mackel, D. C.; Fulkerson, C. C.; and Mallison, G. F. Aqueous quaternary ammonium antiseptics and disinfectants. Use and misuse. *J.A.M.A.*, **1976**, *236*, 2415–2417.

Drouhet, E. Antifungal agents. *Antibiot. Chemother.*, **1978**, *25*, 253–288.

Drube, C. G. Antifungal agents. In, *Annual Reports in Medicinal Chemistry*, Vol. 8. (Heinzelman, R. V., ed.) Academic Press, Inc., New York, **1972**, pp. 116–127.

Gershenfeld, L. Iodine. In, *Disinfection, Sterilization, and Preservation*, 2nd ed. (Block, S. S., ed.) Lea & Febiger, Philadelphia, **1977**, pp. 196–218.

Gottardi, W. Iodine and iodine compounds. In, *Disinfection, Sterilization, and Preservation*, 3rd ed. (Block, S. S., ed.) Lea & Febiger, Philadelphia, **1983**, pp. 183–196.

Haley, R. W. The epidemiology and prevention of nosocomial infections. In, *Disinfection, Sterilization, and Preservation*, 3rd ed. (Block, S. S., ed.) Lea & Febiger, Philadelphia, **1983**, pp. 556–564.

Heel, R. C.; Brogden, R. N.; Carmine, A.; Morley, P. A.; Speight, T. M.; and Avery, G. S. Ketoconazole: a review of its efficacy in superficial and fungal infections. *Drugs*, **1982**, *23*, 1–36.

Heel, R. C.; Brogden, R. N.; Pakes, G. E.; Speight, T. M.; and Avery, G. S. Miconazole: a preliminary review of its therapeutic efficacy in systemic fungal infections. *Drugs*, **1980**, *19*, 7–30.

Hooper, G., and Covarrubias, J. Clinical use and efficacy of FURACIN: an historical perspective. *J. Int. Med. Res.*, **1983**, *11*, 289–293.

Janerich, D. T. Environmental causes of birth defects: the hexachlorophene issue. (Editorial.) *J.A.M.A.*, **1979**, *241*, 830–831.

Kobayashi, G. S., and Medoff, G. Antifungal agents: recent developments. *Annu. Rev. Microbiol.*, **1977**, *31*, 291–308.

Lawrence, C. A. Quaternary ammonium surface-active disinfectants. In, *Disinfection, Sterilization, and Preservation*. (Lawrence, C. A., and Block, S. S., eds.) Lea & Febiger, Philadelphia, **1968**, pp. 430–452.

Pegg, S. P. The role of drugs in management of burns. *Drugs*, **1982**, *24*, 256–260.

Petrocci, A. N. Surface-active agents: quaternary ammonium compounds. In, *Disinfection, Sterilization, and Preservation*, 3rd ed. (Block, S. S., ed.) Lea & Febiger, Philadelphia, **1983**, pp. 309–329.

Price, P. B. Surgical antiseptics. In, *Disinfection, Sterilization, and Preservation*. (Lawrence, C. A., and Block, S. S., eds.) Lea & Febiger, Philadelphia, **1968**, pp. 532–542.

Ryley, J. F.; Wilson, R. G.; Gravestock, M. B.; and Poyser, J. P. Experimental approaches to antifungal chemotherapy. *Adv. Pharmacol. Chemother.*, **1981**, *18*, 49–176.

Sawyer, P. R.; Brogden, R. N.; Pinder, R. M.; Speight, T. M.; and Avery, G. S. Miconazole: a review of its antifungal activity and therapeutic efficacy. *Drugs*, **1975a**, *9*, 406–423.

———. Clotrimazole: a review of its antifungal activity and therapeutic efficacy. *Ibid.*, **1975b**, *9*, 424–447.

Simmons, B. P. CDC guidelines for the prevention and control of nosocomial infections. Guideline for hospital environmental control. *Am. J. Infect. Control*, **1983a**, *11*, 97–120.

———. CDC guidelines for prevention and control of nosocomial infections. Guideline for prevention of surgical wound infections. *Ibid.*, **1983b**, *11*, 133–143.

Symposium. (Various authors.) Clotrimazole. *Postgrad. Med. J.*, **1974**, *50*, Suppl. 1, 1–108.

Symposium. (Various authors.) First international symposium on ketoconazole. Session III. *Rev. Infect. Dis.*, **1980**, *2*, 578–598.

Turner, F. J. Hydrogen peroxide and other oxidant disinfectants. In, *Disinfection, Sterilization, and Preservation*, 3rd ed. (Block, S. S., ed.) Lea & Febiger, Philadelphia, **1983**, pp. 240–250.

Wong, E. S. Guideline for prevention of catheter-associated urinary tract infections. *Am. J. Infect. Control*, **1983**, *11*, 28–33.

CHAPTER

42 GASTRIC ANTACIDS, MISCELLANEOUS DRUGS FOR THE TREATMENT OF PEPTIC ULCERS, DIGESTANTS, AND BILE ACIDS

Stewart C. Harvey

GASTRIC ANTACIDS

Antacids are basic compounds that neutralize acid in the gastric contents. They are employed by physicians chiefly in the treatment of reflux esophagitis and peptic ulcer, and by the laity in self-medication for a wide variety of symptoms.

The gastric antacids are an abused group of drugs. As a result of excessive advertising, the public has come to believe that man is constantly fighting a battle against acidity. The substantial incidence of placebo responsiveness of individuals with minor gastrointestinal upsets, and even with peptic ulcer, further deludes the laity and often the physician into inappropriate use of antacids. Yet when indicated, they may be used too casually to be of optimal value.

Chemistry. Antacids are compared quantitatively in terms of their *acid-neutralizing capacity* (ANC), defined as the number of milliequivalents of 1 N HCl that can be brought to pH 3.5 in 15 minutes. The time limit reflects the fact that some formulations may react with acid so slowly that a negligible amount is neutralized during the sojourn of the preparation in the stomach.

Among the bases that are responsible for neutralization of acid, hydroxide is most commonly employed. Other basic anions used in antacids include carbonate, bicarbonate, citrate, and trisilicate. However, the antacid properties and therapeutic suitability of a product are also greatly influenced by the metallic cation. Aluminum and magnesium hydroxides are the usual preparations. The hydroxides of the alkali metals are completely ionized in water and are thus too strongly basic for clinical use. The solubility of magnesium hydroxide is very low. Consequently, the free concentration of OH^- is too low for $Mg(OH)_2$ to be corrosive. Nevertheless, $Mg(OH)_2$ is quite reactive with H_3O^+, and it thus quickly neutralizes acid to the end point of pH 3.5. It is the most rapidly acting of the insoluble antacids. Magnesium carbonate is much more soluble, yet it reacts much less rapidly with H_3O^+ because of its crystalline structure. Magnesium trisilicate is too insoluble and unreactive to be useful as an antacid.

Calcium carbonate neutralizes acid at about the same rate as $MgCO_3$. The rate of neutralization depends on the particle size and the crystal structure of the preparation.

Aluminum hydroxide is also very insoluble, and the solubility-product constant has an indefinite value because $Al(OH)_3$ polymerizes to a number of products of different composition and chemical reactivity (*see* Carlson and Malagelada, 1982). The rate of neutralization of acid by $Al(OH)_3$ is considerably slower than that achieved with $Mg(OH)_2$, $MgCO_3$, or $CaCO_3$, and it varies with the method of preparation. Because of complexities of the chemistry of the hydrated aluminum ion, even the most reactive $Al(OH)_3$ cannot elevate the pH much above 4.5.

PHARMACOLOGICAL PROPERTIES

Gastrointestinal Effects. *Intragastric pH.* The acid-neutralizing properties of antacids in the stomach more or less parallel those observed *in vitro*. However, mucoproteins and other substances tend to slow the rate of neutralization and decrease the ANC, especially of $Al(OH)_3$. In addition, for the treatment of duodenal ulcers, the rate of neutralization of gastric acid by $Al(OH)_3$ is usually too slow relative to gastric emptying time to neutralize gastric acid when the stomach is empty. The concurrent use of $Mg(OH)_2$ and $Al(OH)_3$ provides both a fast-acting component, which can achieve neutralization within a few minutes, and a more sustained effect. Food in the stomach delays emptying and allows more time for $Al(OH)_3$ to react.

Antipeptic Effects. Partial neutralization of human gastric juice can *increase* its peptic activity. At pH 2, peptic activity is nearly four times that at pH 1.3. Activity remains elevated until the pH exceeds 4 (*see* Berstad, 1982a), and, when the pH exceeds 6 to 7, pepsin becomes irreversibly inactivated.

There has been confusion about the possible direct antipeptic activity of aluminum-containing antacids. Early reports indicated that $Al(OH)_3$ had antipeptic activity, whereas later ones did not. The discrepancy resulted from a procedural artifact (*see* Berstad, 1982a). At a pH above 3, particles of $Al(OH)_3$ adsorb pepsin and remove it from solution; active pepsin is released when the pH falls below 3. An important function of $Mg(OH)_2$ in mixtures of $Mg(OH)_2$ and $Al(OH)_3$ may be to keep the pH sufficiently high such that pepsin remains adsorbed to the $Al(OH)_3$.

Effects on Acid Secretion. Elevation of the pH in the gastric antrum causes hypersecretion of acid and pepsin. In patients with duodenal ulcer, the effect of $NaHCO_3$ is quite pronounced. If the pH is maintained above 4 in such patients, daily acid secretion is increased 6 to 20 times; a continuous pH over 5.5 will double the acid secretion caused by a meal. The effect is usually attributed to the release of gastrin. However, Peters and associates (1983) reported that the increase in the plasma concentration of gastrin caused by continuous alkalinization with $NaHCO_3$ is small compared to that caused by a steak meal. In normal individuals, the effect of gastric alkalinization on acid secretion after a meal appears to be small; for example, the increase in acid secretion caused by $Al(OH)_3$ and $Mg(OH)_2$ is only 16% (Carlson and Malagelada, 1982). In man, chronic concurrent administration of $Al(OH)_3$ and $Mg(OH)_2$ does not affect gastrin concentrations in plasma (Herzog *et al.*, 1982).

Acid Rebound. Once the intragastric pH has been increased by $Al(OH)_3$, $CaCO_3$, $Mg(OH)_2$, or $NaHCO_3$, there is a persistence of gastric acid secretion even after the pH has returned to a value that should terminate the antral secretion of gastrin. The continuation of secretion ("rebound") is brief and of a low degree after $Al(OH)_3$, $Mg(OH)_2$, or $NaHCO_3$, but it is prolonged and relatively intense after large doses (*e.g.*, more than 1 g) of $CaCO_3$. While alkalinization of the proximal jejunum causes an increase in acid secretion, the cations also have effects. For example, $AlCl_3$, $CaCl_2$, or $MgCl_2$ evokes the secretion of gastrin when instilled into the gastric antrum. The greater acid rebound after $CaCO_3$ may result from two actions: a prominent action in the small intestine to stimulate secretion of gastrin and a response of the parietal cells to the transient hypercalcemia that results from administration of $CaCO_3$. The subject of acid rebound has been reviewed by Holtermüller (1982) and by Holtermüller and Dehdaschti (1982).

Gastrointestinal Motor Activity. Alkalinization of the gastric contents increases gastric motility through the action of gastrin. However, Al^{3+} can relax the smooth muscle of the stomach and delay gastric emptying. The relaxant effect is less in the presence of Mg^{2+}, and $Al(OH)_3$ and $Mg(OH)_2$ taken concurrently have little effect on gastric emptying (Lux *et al.*, 1982). Alkalinization of the gastric contents also increases lower esophageal pressure and esophageal clearance by a mechanism that is independent of gastrin.

Antacids affect bowel motility and secretions. Magnesium hydroxide causes laxation and is sometimes used for that effect (*see* Chapter 43). Laxation is sometimes attributed to an osmotic effect, but Mg^{2+} also stimulates the secretion of cholecystokinin, which may contribute to the increased motor activity. Aluminum compounds cause constipation. Calcium carbonate is usually believed to cause constipation, but Clemens and Feinstein (1977) have indicated that it may sometimes be laxative. Ca^{2+} in the duodenum also causes the release of cholecystokinin. The effects of antacids on the release of intestinal hormones and the effects on intestinal and pancreatic secretions have been reviewed by Holtermüller and Dehdaschti (1982); the effects of antacids on bowel habits have been discussed by Ström (1982).

Miscellaneous Gastrointestinal Effects. Mucus secretion is said to be stimulated by Al^{3+}, an effect that would enhance the mucosal barrier to acid (*see* Caspary, 1982). It was once thought that $Al(OH)_3$ itself affords mechanical protection by adhering to the ulcer crater. The substance is somewhat adhesive and demulcent, but careful endoscopic studies indicate that coating of ulcer craters is not a consistent finding.

In the gut, antacids form insoluble compounds with numerous substances. Interactions are especially prominent with aluminum-containing antacids. Aluminum forms insoluble $AlPO_4$, which decreases the bioavailability of phosphate. Although aluminum fluoride is somewhat soluble, aluminum-containing antacids interfere with the absorption of fluoride, probably through the formation of more complex compounds, such as fluoroapatite. Aluminum-containing antacids adsorb bile acids, lysolecithin, and various proteins. The action to adsorb pepsin was noted above. Furthermore, Al^{3+} is strongly astringent and precipitates many proteins. It also reacts with fatty acids to form hydrophobic soaps. Calcium carbonate and $Mg(OH)_2$ have weaker adsorptive activity than $Al(OH)_3$, and Ca^{2+} and Mg^{2+} are also less astringent than Al^{3+}. However, CaF_2 is insoluble, and $CaCO_3$ probably interferes with the absorption of fluoride. Insoluble calcium phosphates are also retained in the gut. Ingestion of large doses of $CaCO_3$ can cause depletion of phosphate, even though small doses of calcium promote positive phosphate balance.

There has been concern that chronic alkalinization may permit the growth of microorganisms in the stomach, from which the microorganisms may colonize the upper airway and lungs. Treatment with antacids does increase the number of microorganisms in the gastric aspirate (*see* DuMoulin *et al.*, 1982).

Absorption, Distribution, and Excretion. *Effect of Absorption on Acid-Base Balance.* Antacids vary in the extent to which they are absorbed. Unneutralized $NaHCO_3$ and sodium citrate are completely absorbed and cause transient metabolic alkalosis. Even bicarbonate and citrate that are neutralized in the stomach disturb systemic acid-base balance as though the antacid had been absorbed intact. In order to understand this seeming paradox, one need only reflect on the fact that, in the absence of exogenous antacid, gastric HCl is neutralized by enteric $NaHCO_3$, such that there is no effect on the overall acid-base balance. Exogenous antacid upsets this cycle by intercepting HCl. The spared enteric $NaHCO_3$ is absorbed, and excess $NaHCO_3$ is thus delivered into the plasma. Sodium citrate has an identical effect, since citrate is rapidly metabolized to HCO_3^- in the liver.

Aluminum, calcium, and magnesium ions are not completely absorbed, and antacids containing these metals thus do not alter acid-base balance to the extent that $NaHCO_3$ and sodium citrate do. Unreacted insoluble antacids pass through the intestines largely as such and are eliminated in the feces. The reacted portion of these antacids enters the intestines in the form of the cation. In the intestine, some of the cation is absorbed; that which is absorbed has the same effect on the systemic bicarbonate pool as an equivalent amount of $NaHCO_3$,

since the spared enteric HCO_3^- returns to the systemic bicarbonate pool. Unabsorbed cation does not spare enteric $NaHCO_3$, because an equivalent amount of HCO_3^- or CO_3^{2-} is consumed in the formation of insoluble hydroxides or carbonates. For example, Ca^{2+} reacts with CO_3^{2-} in the small intestine to form $CaCO_3$. The equivalent of $2HCO_3^-$ is thus retained in the gut, and there is no net change in overall acid-base balance. Similarly, Al^{3+} may be thought of as reacting with CO_3^{2-} to form an unstable $Al_2(CO_3)_3$ intermediate, which is then transformed into basic aluminum carbonates, aluminum hydroxide, and oxyaluminum hydroxide. Some of Mg^{2+} is eliminated in the feces as $Mg(OH)_2$; the remainder of unabsorbed Mg^{2+} is eliminated mostly as soluble salts, such as the chloride and bicarbonate. There is an increase in the systemic HCO_3^- pool in proportion to the amount of Cl^- lost in the feces. Small amounts of the cations from the insoluble antacids are also eliminated as sundry other insoluble compounds, such as soaps, phosphates, and so forth.

Aluminum-Containing Antacids. The fraction of aluminum absorbed from aluminum-containing antacids is small. Dietary aluminum intake is normally about 3 to 25 mg daily, of which about 15 μg or about 0.1% is absorbed. However, about 0.1 to 0.5 mg of the cation may be absorbed from a standard daily dose of an aluminum-containing antacid. In persons with normal renal function, this leads to about a doubling of the average concentration of aluminum in plasma, which is normally 5 to 20 μg per liter; however, in some persons it may be increased tenfold (*see*, for example, Herzog *et al.*, 1982; Lembcke *et al.*, 1982). Aluminum is eliminated in the urine, and the renal clearance has been estimated to be 5.6 ml per minute in persons with normal renal function. Plasma concentrations rise in renal failure, and values in excess of 300 μg per liter have been reported (Griswold *et al.*, 1983). The accumulation of aluminum may not be simply the result of a decreased glomerular filtration; uremic patients often have hyperparathyroidism, and parathyroid hormone has been shown to increase aluminum absorption in rats (Mayer and Burnatowska-Hledin, 1983). The absorption, distribution, and excretion of aluminum have been reviewed by Alfrey (1983).

Calcium-Containing Antacids. The amount of calcium absorbed from $CaCO_3$ is usually stated to be 10%, but it probably depends upon the amount of gastric acid; in one study, 0 to 2% of a single 2-g dose was found to be absorbed in achlorhydric persons, 9 to 16% in normal subjects, and 11 to 37% in patients with peptic ulcer. Similar fractions are absorbed when $CaCO_3$ is given chronically in daily doses of 20 g. A dose-absorption relationship has not been established for $CaCO_3$; however, by analogy with other forms of calcium, the amount absorbed probably reaches a plateau at a dose of about 20 g. Dietary fat decreases absorption.

After a single 4-g dose in normal subjects, the concentration of calcium in plasma rises and may be maintained for nearly 3 hours; after an 8-g dose, the hypercalcemia is more persistent. A normal individual can ingest 20 g per day without developing chronic hypercalcemia, but clinically dangerous hypercalcemia may follow the administration of as little as 3.4 g per day to patients with uremia. Bicarbonate ion that accompanies the absorption of calcium from $CaCO_3$ causes a slight-to-moderate metabolic alkalosis after each dose, but a clinically significant persistent alkalosis develops only slowly during a maintenance regimen.

The main route of elimination of absorbed calcium is by urinary excretion, and excretion of calcium varies with the creatinine clearance. Persons with normal renal function excrete an average of 7% of a daily dose of 50 mg/kg of calcium (approximately equivalent to 8 g of $CaCO_3$ per day). The amount excreted thus falls far short of the amount absorbed even after weeks of treatment, and it takes months to achieve a new steady state. (*See* Ivanovich *et al.*, 1967; Makoff *et al.*, 1969.)

Magnesium-Containing Antacids. As with calcium, the bioavailability of magnesium from antacids appears to be dose dependent. When large antacid doses are employed, about 5% is absorbed from $Mg(OH)_2$ (*see* Herzog *et al.*, 1982). The chronic ingestion of antacid doses of $Mg(OH)_2$ causes only slight increases in plasma concentrations of magnesium in persons with normal renal function. Since renal excretion is the principal route of elimination, toxic concentrations may occur in persons with renal failure.

Adverse Effects. Adverse effects of antacids may be classified into those that are dependent on the magnitude of change in pH or acid-base balance and those that are dependent upon a particular chemical entity.

pH-Dependent Effects. Although metabolic alkalosis has long been considered to be an adverse effect of antacids, the potential for adverse effects from alkalosis *per se* has probably been exaggerated. Distortions of acid-base balance that accompany the absorption of cations from antacids (*see* above) are usually transient and clinically insignificant in persons with normal renal function.

At the time when large doses of $NaHCO_3$ and/or $CaCO_3$ were commonly administered with milk and cream for the management of peptic ulcer, a condition known as the *milk-alkali syndrome* occurred relatively frequently. The condition is characterized by hypercalcemia, alkalosis, nephrocalcinosis and other calcinoses, and azotemia. Although the disorder occurred most often when $CaCO_3$ and $NaHCO_3$ were used in combination, it has happened with either agent alone or with $Mg(OH)_2$. The ingestion of large amounts of milk, renal dysfunction, gastrointestinal hemorrhage, and loss of gastric juice by suction or vomiting seem to predispose to the disorder. Factors in addition to metabolic acidosis thus appear to be responsible.

Alkaluria from chronic use of antacids predisposes to nephrolithiasis. As the pH increases, so does the ionization of phosphate, and the formation of calcium phosphate stones is favored. Hypercalciuria from the ingestion of $CaCO_3$ increases the probability of calcific nephroliths. Alkaluria is not thought to increase the incidence of calcium oxalate stones. Concerns about increased bacterial colonization of the stomach and upper airway as a result of chronic neutralization of the gastric contents are mentioned above.

Composition-Dependent Effects. Antacids affect bowel habits. Aluminum hydroxide causes constipation in rough proportion to the dose. The effect is greater in elderly patients. Aluminum compounds have caused ileus and colonic perforation, possibly as extensions of the constipating effect. Obstruction from bezoars formed from masses of $Al(OH)_3$ and blood or other intestinal contents have also been reported. In contrast, the most frequent side effect of $Mg(OH)_2$ is loose stools or frank diarrhea. With preparations that contain both $Al(OH)_3$ and $Mg(OH)_2$ the net effect is somewhat dependent on the ratio of $Al(OH)_3$ to $Mg(OH)_2$. However, if the dose of $Mg(OH)_2$ is large enough, diarrhea will prevail regardless of the ratio of aluminum to magnesium; approximately two thirds of users of products with various ratios experience diarrhea when the dose of $Mg(OH)_2$ exceeds 8.5 g per day. Magnesium trisilicate and $MgCO_3$ also cause laxation. Constipation from $CaCO_3$ is more frequent than is diarrhea.

The release of CO_2 from carbonate-containing antacids causes belching, abdominal distention, flatulence, and occasional nausea. Bicarbonate is usually neutralized in the stomach or absorbed, such that only belching results. Gastroesophageal reflux may be exacerbated during episodes of belching.

Aluminum-containing antacids are usually thought not to cause adverse effects in persons with normal renal function, although severe hypophosphatemia can sometimes occur. In persons with renal impairment, chronic administration of aluminum compounds can exacerbate or even initiate osteodystrophy, proximal myopathy, and encephalopathy. The severity of these complications correlates with plasma concentrations of aluminum. The sequence of events is not clear. Hyperaluminumemia is at least in part the result of the diminished renal clearance of aluminum; as mentioned above, it may be exacerbated by increased absorption of aluminum as a result of hyperparathyroidism associated with uremia (*see* Cannata *et al., 1983*). However, some investigators attribute the hyperparathyroidism to hyperaluminumemia, since high concentrations of aluminum are found in parathyroid tissue from patients treated with aluminum hydroxide (*see* Cann *et al., 1979*). The osteodystrophy is thought to be the result of aluminum deposition in bone (*see* Cannata *et al., 1983*), but hyperparathyroidism may be a factor. The encephalopathy is almost certainly the result of high concentrations of aluminum in the brain. The use of aluminum compounds to decrease absorption of phosphate in uremic patients would seem to be hazardous and inappropriate. Suitable doses of calcium carbonate similarly suppress plasma phosphate concentrations and parathyroid hormone concentrations without causing hypercalcemia (*see* Bournerias *et al., 1983*; Gokal *et al., 1983*). Other phosphate-binding substitutes for aluminum compounds are $Mg(OH)_2$ and certain resins. The relationship of renal function to aluminum metabolism has been reviewed by Mayer and Burnatowska-Hledin (1983). For reviews of aluminum toxicity, *see* Liss (1980) and Alfrey (1983).

The sodium content of various antacids can be important, particularly for patients with heart failure or hypertension; sodium content is on the label.

Drug Interactions. Antacids may alter the rate of absorption, bioavailability, and/or renal elimination of a number of drugs. Aluminum compounds delay gastric emptying, which can slow the rate of absorption of many drugs; the inclusion of $Mg(OH)_2$ in combination products partially offsets this effect. The absorption of several drugs is probably accelerated by magnesium compounds. In general, there is little clinical significance to interference with the rate of absorption, as long as bioavailability is not also affected. Alkalinization of the gastric contents does decrease the bioavailability of iron and tetracyclines. When the antacid contains aluminum, the bioavailability of

iron may be decreased even if the iron is administered well in advance of the antacid. Aluminum compounds also decrease the bioavailability of antimuscarinic drugs, phenothiazines, diflunisal, digoxin, fluoride, indomethacin (but not aspirin or tolmetin), isoniazid, phosphate, prednisone, prednisolone, ranitidine, sulfadiazine, tetracyclines, and fat-soluble vitamins. Some have indicated that the bioavailability of cimetidine is decreased (Steinberg *et al., 1982*), while others found no change (Allgayer *et al., 1983*). The bioavailability of propranolol is said to be diminished. Calcium carbonate decreases the bioavailability of antimuscarinic agents, fluoride, iron, phenothiazines, phosphate, quinidine, and tetracyclines; magnesium-containing antacids have similar effects on the bioavailability of dicumarol, digoxin, prednisone (but not prednisolone), and tetracyclines. While the clinical significance of certain of these interactions is uncertain, it is prudent to avoid the concurrent use of antacids and drugs intended for systemic absorption.

Alkalinization of the urine can obviously affect renal clearance. The rates of elimination of salicylates and phenobarbital are enhanced, whereas those of amphetamine, ephedrine, mecamylamine, pseudoephedrine, and quinidine are decreased. A curious effect of antacids on elimination kinetics is to decrease the hepatic metabolism of ranitidine.

Thiazide diuretics cause calcium retention, and this may exacerbate hypercalcemia from $CaCO_3$.

PREPARATIONS AND DOSAGE

Antacid products vary widely in their chemical composition, acid-neutralizing capacity (ANC), and sodium content. Table 42–1 is provided for quick comparison of the common oral suspensions. Comparable data on solid dosage forms can be found below. In general, the composition and ANC of a tablet are close to those of 5 ml of the corresponding oral suspension.

The contents of simethicone in the oral suspensions are indicated in Table 42–1; there is usually a simethicone-containing tablet that corresponds to the suspension of the same name. Simethicone, a surface-active agent, is included to disperse foam and to diminish gastroesophageal reflux and thus some dyspeptic symptoms.

Aluminum Compounds. *Aluminum Hydroxide Gel.* So-called aluminum hydroxide is actually a

Table 42–1. COMPOSITION AND NEUTRALIZING CAPACITY OF REPRESENTATIVE PROPRIETARY ANTACID SUSPENSIONS *

PRODUCT	CONTENT (mg/5 ml)					ACID-NEUTRALIZING CAPACITY [2] (per 5 ml)
	$Al(OH)_3$	$Mg(OH)_2$	$CaCO_3$	Si [1]	Na	
DELCID	600	665	0	0	<15	42
MAALOX TC [3]	600	300	0	0	0.8	28
MYLANTA-II	400	400	0	30	1.1	25
KUDROX	565	180	0	0	<15	25
GELUSIL-II	400	400	0	30	1.3	24
BASALJEL XS [3]	$Al(OH)CO_3$ equivalent to 1000 $Al(OH)_3$ [4]			0	23	22
SIMECO	365	300	0	30	7–14	22
TITRALAC	0	0	1000	0	11	19
CAMALOX	225	200	250	0	2.5	18
DI-GEL	282	87	0	20	8.5	18
MARBLEN	400 $MgCO_3$ + 520 $CaCO_3$ [4]			0	3	18
ALTERNAGEL	600	0	0	0	<2	16
SILAIN-GEL	282	285	0	25	4.8	15
RIOPAN	540 magaldrate [4]			0 [5]	<0.1	15
GELUSIL-M [3]	300	200	0	25	1.2	15
ALUDROX	307	103	0	0	1.1	14
BASALJEL	$Al(OH)CO_3$ equivalent to 400 $Al(OH)_3$ [4]			0	2.3	14
milk of magnesia	0	388	0	0	0.12	14
MAALOX	225	200	0	0 [5]	1.3	13
MYLANTA	200	200	0	20	0.7	13
GELUSIL	200	200	0	25	0.7	12
WINGEL	180	160	0	0	2.5	12
KOLANTYL GEL	150	150	0	0	<4.6	10
AMPHOJEL	320	0	0	0	<7	7
GAVISCON	31.7 $Al(OH)_3$ + 137 $MgCO_3$ + Na alginate [4]			0	13	1

* Solid dosage forms (mostly tablets) are also available for most preparations. Their compositions, contents, and acid-neutralizing capacities per unit are similar to those of the suspensions.
[1] Si = simethicone.
[2] In milliequivalents. In some cases, a 60-minute rather than a 15-minute test was performed.
[3] TC = therapeutic concentrate; XS = extra strength; M = medium strength.
[4] Indicated composition is in lieu of $Al(OH)_3$, $Mg(OH)_2$, and/or $CaCO_3$.
[5] MAALOX PLUS contains 25 mg and RIOPAN PLUS 20 mg of simethicone.

mixture of aluminum hydroxide and aluminum oxide hydrates; it usually contains some carbonate. Aluminum hydroxide is marketed mostly in combination with $Mg(OH)_2$ (see Table 42–1). Loss of ANC during storage is greater with $Al(OH)_3$ than with any other antacid. Loss from the solid dosage forms exceeds that from the suspensions.

Basic Aluminum Carbonate Gel. The chemical composition of this substance is indefinite. In Table 42–1 it is represented by $Al(OH)CO_3$. It is marketed in the form of a suspension that contains the equivalent of 400 or 1000 mg of $Al(OH)_3$ per 5 ml or in the form of tablets or capsules, each of which contains 500 mg of equivalent.

Dihydroxyaluminum Aminoacetate. This is a complex basic salt of aluminum and glycine. It has an ANC of 7 mEq/500 mg.

Dihydroxyaluminum Sodium Carbonate. This product is in essence a combination of $Al(OH)_3$ and $NaHCO_3$. The carbonate reacts rapidly with acid, and the dihydroxyaluminum moiety provides a slower, more sustained effect. Each tablet (ROLAIDS) contains 334 mg of the compound, including 53 mg of Na^+, and has an ANC of 8 mEq.

Aluminum Phosphate Gel. This compound, marketed as PHOSPHALJEL, has an insignificant capacity to act as an antacid.

Magnesium Compounds. *Magnesium Hydroxide.* The only single-entity preparation of $Mg(OH)_2$ is *milk of magnesia* (see Table 42–1). Magnesium hydroxide is frequently incorporated with $Al(OH)_3$ in a variety of products.

Magaldrate. Magaldrate is a complex hydroxymagnesium aluminate with the approximate formula $[Mg(OH)^+]_4 [Al_2(OH)_{10}^{4-}] \cdot 2H_2O$. It reacts with acid in stages. The hydroxymagnesium is relatively rapidly converted to magnesium ion and the aluminate to hydrated aluminum hydroxide; the aluminum hydroxide then reacts more slowly to give a sustained antacid effect. Magaldrate does not simply simulate physical mixtures of magnesium and aluminum hydroxides, since the aluminum hydroxide freshly generated in the gastric acid does not have time to convert to less reactive forms. Magaldrate (RIOPAN) is available as a suspension (see Table 42–1) and as tablets either to chew or to swallow; each tablet contains 480 mg of magaldrate and not more than 0.1 mg of Na^+, and has an ANC of 13.5 mEq.

Sodium Compounds. *Sodium Bicarbonate.* Sodium bicarbonate is available in tablets that contain 325 to 650 mg of $NaHCO_3$. One gram neutralizes 12 mEq of acid. For continuous nasogastric irrigation during surgery or in intensive care, a 0.05 N solution may be used.

Sodium Citrate. As an antacid, sodium citrate is used in the form of a 0.3 M solution, which can be made extemporaneously in hospital pharmacies. Shohl's solution (BICITRA), which has citric acid in addition to sodium citrate, has about the same ANC and is sometimes used.

Calcium Compounds. *Calcium carbonate* is available as a single-entity preparation under a variety of proprietary names (*e.g.,* TUMS). Tablets contain from 350 to 750 mg. The ANC is approximately 10 mEq for a 500-mg tablet.

Antacid Mixtures. Antacids are used in combination for three primary purposes: to combine fast- and slow-reacting compounds to give a preparation a relatively even, sustained action; to lower the dose of each component; and to use one component to antagonize one or more side effects of another (*e.g.,* laxation versus constipation).

The most common combination is that of $Al(OH)_3$ and $Mg(OH)_2$. Several oral suspensions containing this combination are listed in Table 42–1. Most of the preparations are also available as tablets with composition and ANC similar to those of 5 ml of the corresponding suspension. In the various mixtures, the ratio of $Al(OH)_3$ to $Mg(OH)_2$ varies from about 1:1 to 3:1. Other combinations include $CaCO_3$ and $Mg_2Si_3O_8$.

Dosage. Dosage regimens for the treatment of peptic ulcer have ranged from the ridiculously casual to the compulsively intense. It was once calculated that a dose of 50 mEq per hour (1200 mEq per day) would be required to neutralize continuously the gastric acid of 90% of patients with duodenal ulcer. The estimate took into account the effect of antacids to increase gastric secretion and the rate of emptying of the stomach. However, preparations containing $Al(OH)_3$ and $Mg(OH)_2$ do not greatly increase gastric secretion and antacids are not rapidly emptied from the stomach when administered *post cibum*. When a high dose of antacid (*e.g.,* 144 mEq) is taken 1 and 3 hours after a standard steak meal, the gastric contents remain buffered for about 4 hours after that meal. A dose taken at bedtime will buffer for a much shorter time unless gastric emptying is retarded with an antimuscarinic drug. These observations have led to the seven-times-a-day regimen, in which antacids are given at 1 and 3 hours *post cibum* and at bedtime. The regimen does not provide around-the-clock buffering and has not been adequately studied, but it apparently protects the mucosa enough of the time to promote healing. In contrast, the casual, take-as-needed schedule is clearly inadequate.

Unfortunately, there is no standard dose in terms of number of tablets or milliliters of suspension; this is because of product-to-product differences in ANC and other properties. In the early clinical studies in which the seven-times-a-day regimen was used, each dose was approximately 144 mEq (about 1000 mEq per day). There is presently much revision in the dosage, and doses as low as 280 mEq per day have been reported to be effective in the treatment of duodenal ulcer. Certainly, concomitant administration of antisecretory drugs lowers the requirement. However, in Zollinger-Ellison syndrome, more than 1000 mEq per day will probably continue to be required, even in conjunction with antisecretory drugs.

THERAPEUTIC USES

The clinical status of antacids is in a state of evolution. There were predictions that the availability of cimetidine would eliminate antacids from among the antiulcer drugs, yet that has not happened. H_2-blocking agents are not universally effective, and there are conditions, such as Zollinger-Ellison syndrome, giant duodenal ulcers, and others, in which an H_2 blocker alone is not optimally effective. The continued use of antacids also results from the conservative practice to employ them in combination with an H_2 blocker, even when there is no evidence that such a combination is superior to either drug alone. The effect of newer antiulcer drugs on the use of antacids remains to be seen. Antacids will undoubtedly continue to be used as nonprescription drugs.

Peptic Ulcer. Reports from several trials indicate that high doses (860 to 1000 mEq per day) of $Al(OH)_3$ and $Mg(OH)_2$ suspension have an efficacy comparable to that of cimetidine in the treatment of both *duodenal* and *gastric ulcers*. After 4 weeks of treatment, the percentage of healed *duodenal ulcers* ranged from 52 to 78% (*see,* for example, Ippoliti *et al.,* 1983). The percentage is usually slightly higher with cimetidine than with antacids, but statistically significant differences have not been demonstrated. Paradoxically, with antacids there is a poor correlation between healing and the disappearance of pain (*see* Isenberg, 1982). High doses of $Al(OH)_3$ alone have been reported to result in the healing of 71% of duodenal ulcers, 12% less than with ranitidine. The time to relapse after healing is the same with antacids as with cimetidine. However, Gotthard and associates (1982) reported that when *l*-hyoscyamine was combined with antacids, the time to relapse after healing was more than double that after cimetidine. Nevertheless, continuous use of antacids for prophylaxis is not recommended. High doses of antacids in conjunction with cimetidine are usually required for the effective treatment of giant duodenal ulcers (*see* Jaszewski *et al.*, 1983) and the Zollinger-Ellison syndrome.

There have been several trials of "low-dose" antacids for the treatment of duodenal ulcer. In one study (*see* Berstad, 1982b), a rate of healing of 81% was achieved after 4 weeks with a daily dose of Al(OH)$_3$ and Mg(OH)$_2$ as low as 280 mEq (consumed as chewable tablets in a seven-times-a-day schedule). When a comparably low daily dose was divided into only four portions, the rate of cure was distinctly lower than that with cimetidine (Isenberg *et al.*, 1983).

In the treatment of *gastric ulcer*, daily doses of antacids of about 330 mEq per day have resulted in a rate and incidence of healing comparable to that achieved with cimetidine. In contrast to the situation in duodenal ulcer, antacids are apparently equal to cimetidine in relief of nocturnal pain from gastric ulcers. There has been little exploration of different dose regimens and combinations.

Further information on the use of antacids for the treatment of peptic ulcer may be found in the reviews by Morris and Rhodes (1979), Holtermüller and Herzog (1982), Ippoliti (1982), and Petersen and Richardson (1983). (*See also* Halter, 1982; Symposium, 1982d.) Earlier references may be found in *previous editions* of this textbook.

Reflux Esophagitis. Antacids were used for the treatment of "heartburn" and related disorders long before reflux esophagitis was recognized as a clinical entity. The effects of antacids to neutralize gastric acid and hence to reduce the erosive activity of the refluence, to enhance the competence of the lower-esophageal sphincter, and to increase esophageal clearance of acid provide a rationale for their use. However, there is a general clinical impression that antacids suppress symptoms and promote healing in mild-to-moderate reflux esophagitis only about as well as do placebos (*see* Saco *et al.*, 1982; Graham and Patterson, 1983). Nevertheless, the seven-times-a-day regimen is usually employed for mild-to-moderate reflux esophagitis. In more severe cases, hourly doses or even continuous intraesophageal drip has been used.

The alginate-containing product, GAVISCON, has been reported to decrease the amount of refluence and increase esophageal acid clearance, even though it has no demonstrable effect on lower-esophageal sphincter pressure. The product is widely used in the treatment of mild-to-moderate reflux esophagitis. Its efficacy may tentatively be said to be that of antacids or a placebo. However, findings from various clinical trials vary widely (from no effect on either symptoms or healing to symptomatic improvement and endoscopically verified healing in 75% and 50% of patients, respectively). Reports of trials with antacid-free alginate are also contradictory. For additional information, *see* Richter and Castell (1982), Teilum (1982), Wesdorp (1982), Bachman (1983), Frazier and Fendler (1983), Jamieson and associates (1983), and Wu and Castell (1983).

Miscellaneous Uses. During anesthesia, coma, cesarean section, or endoscopy, aspiration of gastric contents may occur and cause pneumonitis or pneumonia. Prior neutralization of gastric acid provides some protection. The aim should be to keep the pH above 3.5 (possibly as high as 5, to suppress peptic activity). Various antacids may be given just prior to and during the procedure. However, if aspirated, the particulate antacids themselves can cause pulmonary damage, which makes the use of sodium citrate (15 ml of a 0.3 M solution) attractive (*see* Wrobel *et al.*, 1982). There seems to be little advantage of sodium citrate over NaHCO$_3$, and the latter is sometimes used prior to endoscopy. Because conventional antimuscarinic drugs decrease the competency of the lower-esophageal sphincter, their use is not advised. The prophylaxis of aspiration pneumonia has been reviewed by Coombs (1983). The effects of drugs often used during anesthesia on the lower-esophageal sphincter have been reviewed by Cotton and Smith (1984).

Antacids and cimetidine are both effective in the prophylaxis of stress ulceration and consequent acute upper-gastrointestinal hemorrhage. They appear to be more effective in the prevention of complications than of the initial erosions. Antacids are administered hourly or by continuous nasogastric instillation. It is also common practice to administer antacids in the treatment of upper-gastrointestinal bleeding, except that which originates in the esophagus. Results have been inconsistent. Antacids appear to be superior to cimetidine but inferior to somatostatin, secretin, or tranexamic acid. The use of antacids and other drugs in the prophylaxis and treatment of upper-gastrointestinal bleeding has been reviewed by Berstad (1982c) and Priebe (1982).

Aluminum hydroxide is sometimes used as an antidiarrheal agent, especially when diarrhea is thought to be caused by bile acids. Basic aluminum carbonate or Al(OH)$_3$ is used to decrease absorption of phosphate in calcinosis universalis, recurrent phosphatic nephrolithiasis, hyperphosphatemia, or renal failure with hyperparathyroidism. The adverse effects of aluminum compounds in renal failure have been discussed above. Magnesium hydroxide is used as a laxative (*see* Chapter 43) and to decrease the formation of calcium oxalate kidney stones (by decreasing calcium absorption). Antacids are often administered in acute pancreatitis to decrease the delivery of acid into the duodenum. However, Maisto and Bremner (1983) found them to have no effect on the course of the disease.

H$_2$-BLOCKING AGENTS AND PROTON PUMP INHIBITORS

Cimetidine has had an extraordinary impact on the treatment of peptic ulcer and reflux esophagitis. The pharmacological properties of cimetidine and related H$_2$ antagonists are discussed in Chapter 26. Proton pump inhibitors such as omeprazole appear to have the potential to be the most effective drugs for the treatment of peptic ulcer and related conditions. These novel agents are also described in Chapter 26.

MUSCARINIC ANTAGONISTS

These agents are discussed in Chapter 7. While conventional atropinelike compounds have only a modest ability to reduce the secretion of gastric acid in doses that do not cause annoying or severe side effects, newer agents that selectively antagonize M_1-muscarinic receptors are more promising. Pirenzepine is such a drug. The effects of muscarinic antagonists may interfere with the secretion of gastrin in addition to that of acid, and they can influence the gastric mucosal secretion of HCO_3^- and mucus. These drugs may thus influence several systems that modulate both acid secretion and the mucosal barrier. The efficiency of pirenzepine for the treatment of duodenal ulcer appears to be approximately that of cimetidine, particularly when the dose of pirenzepine is 100 mg per day or more. In one large trial of pirenzepine, less than 1% of the subjects discontinued treatment because of side effects (Giorgi-Conciato *et al.,* 1982). Pirenzepine is not yet available in the United States. For additional information on pirenzepine, *see* Chierichetti and associates (1979), Symposium (1980a, 1982c), Halter (1982), Pfeiffer (1982), and Petersen and Richardson (1983). Perspectives on the role of antimuscarinic drugs in the treatment of peptic ulcer may be found in the reviews by Walan (1982), Peppercorn (1983), and Piper (1983).

SUCRALFATE

Sucralfate is a complex substance formed from a sulfated disaccharide (sucrose) and polyaluminum hydroxide. Its primary unit may be represented by $C_{12}H_6O_{11}[SO_3^-Al_2(OH)_5^+]_8 \cdot nH_2O$. When the pH is below 4, there is extensive polymerization and cross-linking of sucralfate. The condensed polymer is a very sticky, viscid yellow-white gel. Continued reaction with acid gradually consumes $Al_2(OH)_5^+$ until some sucrose octasulfate moieties are entirely freed of aluminum. The reaction is very slow and is incomplete during the sojourn of the substance in the stomach. Sucralfate has no practical ANC. Even though the pH in the duodenum is well above 4, the gel retains its viscid, demulcent properties. The gel adheres strongly to epithelial cells and to the base of ulcer craters. The affinity for the crater base is much higher than that for the epithelial surface, and it is difficult to wash the gel from the crater. In man, the gel remains adherent to ulcerated epithelium for longer than 6 hours. It is of interest that the gel is more adherent to duodenal than to gastric ulcers. Antacids and food do not appear to affect the integrity of the adherent gel, but proteins in foodstuffs adsorb to its luminal surface, thus adding an additional layer. The gel interacts very little with mucin. Investigations *in vitro* show that the gel coating on the mucosa is considerably less permeable to H_3O^+ than are mucin and aluminum hydroxide. The gel prevents the exudation of proteins from an ulcer crater. It also adsorbs pepsin, trypsin, and bile acids.

The incidence and severity of side effects from sucralfate are very low. Only the reported incidences of constipation in 2.3% and a sense of dry mouth in 0.7% of recipients appear to be significant. Sherman and coworkers (1983) found that sucralfate lowers concentrations of phosphate in plasma toward normal in uremic patients. The use of sucralfate also results in elevated plasma concentrations of aluminum in uremic patients (*see* Leung *et al.,* 1983).

Sucralfate (CARAFATE) is available as 1-g tablets. The dose is one tablet 1 hour before each meal and at bedtime. Treatment should be continued for 4 to 8 weeks unless healing has been proven. Since the preparation is activated by acid, antacids should not be taken for 30 minutes before or after sucralfate.

There have been a number of prospective trials of sucralfate in the treatment of peptic ulcer. In all studies sucralfate has been effective against both duodenal and gastric ulcers. Administration before meals was found to be distinctly more effective than after meals. In several trials in which sucralfate and cimetidine were compared, the percentage of healed ulcers after sucralfate treatment was about the same as that after cimetidine. After remission, continued treatment with sucralfate markedly postpones relapse, and the drug is considerably more effective in this regard than is cimetidine. However, after discontinuation of treatment, relapses occur sooner than with cimetidine. The rate of healing of gastric ulcer is less than for duodenal ulcer. For details of the chemistry, actions, and clinical uses of sucralfate, *see* Symposium (1981, 1983), Garnett (1982), and Spiro (1982).

BISMUTH COMPOUNDS

Bismuth subgallate, subnitrate, and subsalicylate once were called antacids, although they have no measurable ANC. They have some antipeptic activity and demulcent properties. *Bismuth subcitrate,* formerly called tripotassium dicitrato bismuthate, is the most recent of the bismuth subsalts to be tested clinically. The composition may be represented approximately by $[Bi_3(OH)_3(C_6H_5O_7)_2]_n$. The substance is a stable colloidal suspension when the pH is above 3.5 to 4.0; it forms a white precipitate in gastric acid. Bismuth subcitrate has a strong affinity for mucosal glycoproteins, especially in the necrotic tissue in ulcer craters. Ulcer craters become preferentially and visibly coated with a white layer of polymer-glycoprotein complex. One or 2 hours after administration, the layer is about 300 μm thick. The complex is only slowly permeated by H_3O^+, such that the layer constitutes a diffusion barrier to gastric acid. During treatment, plasma concentrations of bismuth usually rise to 10 to 20 μg per liter. A concentration of 100 μg per liter is stated to be the minimal toxic value. Absorbed bismuth is mostly excreted in the urine. No significant adverse effects of bismuth subcitrate have thus far been reported. However, the chronic use of other bismuth salts has caused encephalopathy and osteodystrophy.

Bismuth subcitrate is not yet available in the United States. It is marketed in other countries as tablets and an oral suspension. The bismuth content is 120 mg per tablet or 5 ml of suspension. The dose is one tablet or 5 ml of suspension four times a day, to be taken before meals and at bedtime. Bismuth subcitrate is used to treat both duodenal and gastric ulcers, and in these uses it appears to be as effective as cimetidine. In addition, the relapse rate has been reported to be less with bismuth subcitrate than with cimetidine. The two agents are approximately equieffective in the relief of pain. For detailed information on clinical trials, *see* Symposium (1982b), Glover and associates (1983), Kellow and associates (1983), and Shreeve and associates (1983).

CARBENOXOLONE SODIUM

Carbenoxolone has been in general use as an antiulcer drug in Europe since 1962. It is an oleandane derivative obtained from glycyrrhiza. The drug has a steroidlike structure, and it possesses significant mineralocorticoid activity. While other mineralocorticoids do not have antiulcer properties, the concurrent administration of spironolactone interferes with the therapeutic effect of carbenoxolone.

Carbenoxolone alters the composition of mucus and enhances the mucosal barrier to diffusion of acid. There is an augmentation of glycoprotein synthesis in experimental animals, but this has not yet been demonstrated in man. Additional effects of carbenoxolone are perhaps mediated by prostaglandins, and the drug may inhibit enzymes that inactivate these autacoids. Carbenoxolone also suppresses the activation of pepsinogen. While this agent may be as effective as cimetidine in the treatment of peptic ulcers, adverse effects result fairly frequently from its mineralocorticoid actions. These include hypokalemia, fluid retention, and hypertension. Impaired glucose tolerance has also been observed. These effects would appear to constitute major deterrents to the use of carbenoxolone. For additional information, *see* Symposium (1980b, 1981) and Barrowman and Pfeiffer (1982).

PROSTAGLANDINS

Prostaglandins E_2 and I_2, the predominant prostaglandins synthesized by the gastric mucosa, inhibit the secretion of acid and stimulate the secretion of mucus (*see* Chapters 28 and 29). Prostaglandins can protect against ulceration caused by aspirin, indomethacin, bile, ethanol, thermal insult, and NaOH; this has been attributed to strengthening of the mucosal barrier. Attempts are thus being made to take advantage of these properties for the treatment of peptic ulcer, and several clinical trials have been undertaken with PGE_2 and derivatives thereof. While such drugs are effective in promoting healing, the agents that are currently available cause a considerable incidence of diarrhea. In the United States, no prostaglandin has yet been approved for use in the treatment of peptic ulcers, and no appropriate dosage forms are available.

The gastrointestinal actions and clinical uses of prostaglandins have been reviewed by Cohen (1982), Sixma (1982), Konturek (1983), and Somerville and Langman (1983).

MISCELLANEOUS DRUGS FOR PEPTIC ULCER

There are a number of other drugs in use or under investigation as antiulcer agents. Only one, *deglycyrrhizinized liquorice* (CAVED-S), is marketed (in Canada and Europe) for this purpose. Its actions on the gastroduodenal mucosae are like those of carbenoxolone, but the drug lacks mineralocorticoid activity. *Metoclopramide* has been used in the treatment of peptic ulcer with the intention of augmenting normal peristalsis and abolishing the enterogastric reflux of bile, which is thought to be a factor in the pathogenesis of many gastric and some duodenal ulcers. It is of some value in the treatment of gastric ulcer, but its efficacy has been poor in duodenal ulcer. It tends to prevent gastroesophageal reflux, and it is employed in the management of reflux esophagitis. The pharmacology and uses of metoclopramide have been discussed by Albibi and McCallum (1983). *Tricyclic antidepressants* can suppress the secretion of gastric acid (*see* Berardi and Caplan, 1983), and there have been clinical trials of both *trimipramine* and *doxepin* for the treatment of peptic ulcer. Mangla and Pereira (1982) reported success with doxepin for the treatment of ulcers that had been refractory to cimetidine and antacids. *Somatostatin* may become the drug of choice to arrest hemorrhage from peptic ulcers (*see* Berstad, 1982c). It is strikingly more effective than cimetidine.

DIGESTANTS

Digestants are drugs that supposedly promote the process of digestion in the gastrointestinal tract in conditions characterized by a lack of one or more of the specific substances that function in the digestion of food. While a number of products are marketed, including many bizarre mixtures of components, the only preparations that merit consideration here are those of pancreatic enzymes.

PANCREATIC ENZYMES

The enzymes of the pancreas are obtainable in preparations known as *pancreatin* and *pancrelipase*. They contain principally amylase, trypsin (protease), and lipase. Pancrelipase is of porcine origin and has relatively more lipase activity than does pancreatin. Pancreatin is prepared from porcine or bovine pancreas. These preparations are employed for the treatment of conditions in which the secretion of pancreatic juice is deficient, for example, pancreatitis and mucoviscidosis. Their administration can significantly reduce the nitrogen and fat content of the stool, and these parameters can be monitored as a guide to dosage, which should be individualized. Since acid and peptic activity in the stomach can destroy the pancreatic enzymes, enteric-coated tablets are sometimes used. However, the coating may prevent delivery of the enzymes in the duodenum. Supplementation of the regimen with an H_2-blocking agent may help to overcome gastric inactivation. Adverse effects of pancreatic enzymes are few. High doses may cause nausea and diarrhea; the administration of these preparations may also cause hyperuricemia.

BILE ACIDS

The bile acids and their conjugates are important constituents of bile. The important bile acids in human bile are cholic acid (3,7,12-trihydroxy-cholanic acid) and chenodeoxycholic acid ($3\alpha,7\alpha$-dihydroxycholanic acid); these are mainly present as the glycine and taurine conjugates (glycocholic, taurocholic, glycochenodeoxycholic, and tauro-chenodeoxycholic acids), the salts of which are often referred to as the *bile salts*. The structure of cholanic acid is as follows:

Cholanic Acid

Bile salts are strongly amphiphilic and, with the aid of biliary phospholipids, they readily form micelles with and emulsify lipids. They are important not only for the emulsification of cholesterol and other lipids in bile but also for the emulsification of dietary lipids preparatory to digestion and absorption.

Pharmacological and Toxic Effects. Bile acids increase the output of bile and hence are called *choleretic* drugs; the bile salts have little choleretic activity. Dehydrocholic acid, a semisynthetic cholate, is especially active and evokes the secretion of a bile of low specific gravity; it is therefore called a *hydrocholeretic drug*. The increase in bile flow is not the result of true cholepoiesis, since the augmented flow is only that necessary to secrete the increased load of bile acid imposed by that administered. The secretion of preformed bile pigment is not increased, and any increase in bile pigments in the intestine is the result of its flushing from dead spaces and/or the hemolytic actions of the drugs themselves. Dehydrocholate actually decreases the excretion of bilirubin. Therefore, bile acids are ineffective in attenuating jaundice.

Chenodiol (chenodeoxycholic acid) and ursodeoxycholic acid, but not cholic acid, decrease the cholesterol content of bile. If the bile is super-saturated with cholesterol, it will become unsaturated when the content of chenodiol reaches approximately 70% of the total bile acids. The mechanism is twofold: (1) absorption of cholesterol by the small intestine is impaired, possibly as the result of a decrease in the output of bile salts, and (2) synthesis of cholesterol is diminished through inhibition of hydroxymethylglutaryl-CoA reductase. The agent also inhibits cholesterol 7α-hydroxylase and thus decreases the synthesis of the other bile acids and, *pari passu,* their conjugates. The decrease in cholesterol concentration in bile may not only halt the formation of cholesterolic gallstones but also promote their dissolution during sustained treatment. These agents have no effect on calcified stones or on radiolucent bile pigment stones. In addition, therapy is successful only in those with functional gallbladders.

Prolonged treatment with chenodiol causes patchy loss of microvilli in the biliary epithelium and an increase in sinusoidal lipocytes (Bateson *et al.,* 1977). Dehydrocholic and taurocholic acids cause similar effects. Some patients have increases in plasma SGOT and aspartate aminotransferase activities. Hepatotoxicity has been attributed to the conversion of chenodiol to lithocholic acid by intestinal microorganisms; lithocholic acid is a hepatotoxin. Diarrhea may also occur. Bile salts can impair the resistance to acid of the mucosal barrier of the stomach and esophagus and probably also the upper duodenum. This fact is thought to have pathophysiological implications in gastritis, peptic ulcer, and reflux esophagitis.

Preparations and Dosage. *Dehydrocholic acid* (DECHOLIN) is available in tablets containing 244 or 250 mg. The usual dose is 244 to 500 mg, three times daily after meals. *Ox bile extract* resembles that from human bile and is available in tablets. The bile acid content is equivalent to about 45% cholic acid. The usual dose is 150 to 600 mg. *Chenodiol* (CHENIX) is available in 250-mg tablets. It is given initially in divided doses that total 8 to 10 mg/kg per day; this is then adjusted upward to 13 to 17 mg/kg.

Therapeutic Uses. Because of their physiological role in the absorption of dietary lipids, the bile salts were once used widely for so-called replacement therapy in pathological conditions in which the concentration of bile acids in the upper intestine is low (such as biliary fistula, disease or resection of the ileum, hepatic or extrahepatic cholestasis). However, the usual preparations are generally ineffective and sometimes harmful. They are little used today. Hydrocholeretic drugs are sometimes used after gallbladder surgery to facilitate T-tube drainage.

The National Cooperative Gallstone Study established the safety and efficacy of chenodiol for the dissolution of gallstones (*see* Schoenfield *et al.,* 1981). However, the overall response rate was not high and appropriate selection of patients for such treatment is thus important. At a daily dose of 750 mg of chenodiol (the highest dose tested), there was confirmed complete dissolution of radiolucent gallstones in only 13% of patients during 2 years of treatment. Partial or complete dissolution occurred in 41% of this group. Therapy was most successful in women, in thin patients, and in those with small or floating gallstones or with cholesterol concentrations in plasma above 227 mg/dl. The incidence of significant hepatotoxicity was 3% among patients who received 750 mg of chenodiol daily; biochemical abnormalities disappeared spontaneously in all of these patients after cessation of treatment. Diarrhea occurred in 40% of patients, but it was mild and never caused termination of treatment. The mean plasma cholesterol concentration was elevated slightly. Ursodeoxycholic acid may be more effective than chenodiol, and it appears to have much less tendency to cause hepatotoxicity or diarrhea (Tint *et al.*, 1982). Studies indicate that gallstones will recur in a relatively high percentage of patients after cessation of treatment with bile acids.

Allgayer, H.: Rollinghoff, W.; and Baumgartner, G. Absence of *in vivo* and *in vitro* interactions of magnesium hydroxide containing antacid with cimetidine in peptic ulcer. *Z. Gastroenterol.*, **1983**, *21*, 351–354.

Bateson, M. C.; Hopwood, D.; and Bouchier, I. A. D. Effect of gallstone-dissolution therapy on human liver structure. *Am. J. Dig. Dis.*, **1977**, *22*, 293–299.

Berstad, A. Antacids and pepsin. *Scand. J. Gastroenterol.*, **1982a**, *17*, Suppl. 75, 13–15.

————. Antacid therapy of duodenal ulcer. Effects of smaller doses. *Ibid.*, **1982b**, *17*, Suppl. 75, 97–99.

Bournerias, F.; Monnier, N.; and Reveillaud, R. J. Risk of orally administered aluminum hydroxide and results of withdrawal. *Proc. Eur. Dial. Transplant Assoc.*, **1983**, *20*, 207–212.

Cann, C. E.; Prussin, S. G.; and Gordan, G. S. Aluminum uptake by the parathyroid glands. *J. Clin. Endocrinol. Metab.*, **1979**, *49*, 543–545.

Cannata, J. B.; Briggs, J. D.; Junor, B. J.; Beastall, G.; and Fell, G. S. The influence of aluminum on parathyroid hormone levels in haemodialysis patients. *Proc. Eur. Dial. Transplant Assoc.*, **1983**, *19*, 244–247.

Caspary, W. F. Measurement of intragastric potential difference. In, *Antacids in the Eighties.* (Halter, F., ed.) Urban & Schwarzenberg, Munich, **1982**, pp. 64–69.

DuMoulin, G. C.; Hedley-Whyte, J.; Paterson, D. G.; and Lisbon, A. Aspiration of gastric bacteria in antacid-treated patients: a frequent cause of postoperative colonization of the airway. *Lancet*, **1982**, *1*, 242–245.

Giorgi-Conciato, M.; Daniotti, S.; Ferrari, P. A.; Gaetani, M.; Petrini, G.; Sala, P.; and Valentino, P. Efficacy and safety of pirenzepine in peptic ulcer and in non ulcerous gastroduodenal diseases. A multicentre controlled clinical trial. *Scand. J. Gastroenterol.*, **1982**, *17*, Suppl. 81, 1–41.

Glover, S. C.; Cantlay, J. S.; Weir, J.; and Mowat, N. A. Oral tripotassium-dicitratobismuthate in gastric and duodenal ulceration. A double-blind controlled trial. *Dig. Dis. Sci.*, **1983**, *28*, 13–17.

Gokal, R.; Ramos, J. M.; Ellis, H. A.; Parkinson, I.; Sweetman, V.; Dewar, J.; Ward, M. K.; and Kerr, D. N. Histological renal osteodystrophy and 25-hydroxycholecalciferol and aluminum levels in patients on continuous ambulatory peritoneal dialysis. *Kidney Int.*, **1983**, *23*, 15–21.

Gotthard, R.; Ström, M.; Bodemar, G.; and Walan, A. Treatment of active prepyloric and duodenal ulcers with antacid/anticholinergic, cimetidine and placebo. *Scand. J. Gastroenterol.*, **1982**, *17*, Suppl. 75, 86–96.

Graham, D. Y., and Patterson, D. J. Double-blind comparison of liquid antacid and placebo in the treatment of symptomatic reflux esophagitis. *Dig. Dis. Sci.*, **1983**, *28*, 559–563.

Griswold, W. R.; Reznik, V.; Mendoza, S. A.; Trauner, D.; and Alfrey, A. C. Accumulation of aluminum in a nondialyzed uremic child receiving aluminum hydroxide. *Pediatrics*, **1983**, *71*, 56–58.

Herzog, P.; Schmitt, K. F.; Grendahl, T.; and van der Linden, J., Jr. Evaluation of serum and urine electrolyte changes during therapy with a magnesium-aluminum containing antacid: results of a prospective study. In, *Antacids in the Eighties.* (Halter, F., ed.) Urban & Schwarzenberg, Munich, **1982**, pp. 123–135.

Ippoliti, A.; Elashoff, J.; Valenzuela, J.; Cano, R.; Frankl, H.; Samloff, M.; and Koretz, R. Recurrent ulcer after successful treatment with cimetidine or antacid. *Gastroenterology*, **1983**, *85*, 875–880.

Isenberg, J. I.; Peterson, W. L.; Elashoff, J. D.; Sanderfeld, M. A.; Reedy, T. J.; Ippoliti, A. F.; Van Deventer, G. M.; Frankl, H.; Longstreth, G. F.; and Anderson, D. S. Healing of benign gastric ulcer with low-dose antacid or cimetidine. A double-blind, randomized, placebo-controlled trial. *N. Engl. J. Med.*, **1983**, *308*, 1319–1324.

Ivanovich, P.; Fellows, H.; and Rich, C. The absorption of calcium carbonate. *Ann. Intern. Med.*, **1967**, *66*, 917–923.

Jaszewski, R.; Crane, S. A.; and Cid, A. A. Giant duodenal ulcers. Successful healing with medical therapy. *Dig. Dis. Sci.*, **1983**, *28*, 486–489.

Kellow, J. E.; Barr, G. D.; Middleton, W. R.; and Piper, D. W. Comparison of colloidal bismuth subcitrate tablets and liquid in duodenal ulcer healing. *J. Clin. Gastroenterol.*, **1983**, *5*, 417–420.

Lembcke, B.; Fuchs, C.; Hesch, R. D.; and Caspary, W. F. Effects of long-term antacid administration on mineral metabolism. In, *Antacids in the Eighties.* (Halter, F., ed.) Urban & Schwarzenberg, Munich, **1982**, pp. 112–122.

Leung, A. C.; Henderson, I. S.; Halls, D. J.; and Dobbie, J. W. Aluminum hydroxide versus sucralfate as a phosphate binder in uraemia. *Br. Med. J.*, **1983**, *30*, 1379–1381.

Lux, G.; Hartog, C.; Ruppin, H.; and Rösch, W. Combined acid secretion and gastric emptying under antacid and pirenzepine. In, *Antacids in the Eighties.* (Halter, F., ed.) Urban & Schwarzenberg, Munich, **1982**, pp. 57–63.

Maisto, O. E., and Bremner, C. G. Antacids in the treatment of acute alcohol-induced pancreatitis. *S. Afr. Med. J.*, **1983**, *63*, 351–352.

Makoff, D. L.; Gordon, A.; Franklin, A. S.; and Gerstein, A. R. Chronic calcium carbonate therapy in uremia. *Arch. Intern. Med.*, **1969**, *123*, 15–21.

Mangla, J. C., and Pereira, M. Tricyclic antidepressants in the treatment of peptic ulcer disease. *Arch. Intern. Med.*, **1982**, *142*, 273–275.

Peters, M. N.; Feldman, M.; Walsh, J. H.; and Richardson, C. T. Effect of gastric alkalinization on serum gastrin concentrations in humans. *Gastroenterology*, **1983**, *85*, 35–39.

Saco, L. S.; Orlando, R. C.; Levinson, S. L.; Bozymski, E. M.; Jones, J. D.; and Frakes, J. T. Double-blind controlled trial of bethanechol and antacid versus placebo and antacid in the treatment of erosive esophagitis. *Gastroenterology*, **1982**, *82*, 1369–1373.

Schoenfield, L. J., and others. Chenodiol (chenodeoxycholic acid) for dissolution of gallstones: The National Cooperative Gallstone Study. *Ann. Intern. Med.*, **1981**, *95*, 257–282.

Sherman, R. A.; Hwang, E. R.; Walker, J. A.; and Eisinger, R. P. Reduction in serum phosphorus due to sucralfate. *Am. J. Gastroenterol.*, **1983**, *78*, 210–211.

Shreeve, D. R.; Klass, H. J.; and Jones, P. E. Comparison of cimetidine and tripotassium dicitrato bismuthate in healing and relapse of duodenal ulcers. *Digestion*, **1983**, *28*, 96–101.

Steinberg, W. M.; Lewis, J. H.; and Katz, D. M. Antacids inhibit absorption of cimetidine. *N. Engl. J. Med.*, **1982**, *307*, 400–404.

Tint, G. S.; Salen, G.; Colalillo, A.; Graber, D.; Verga, D.; Speck, J.; and Shefer, S. Ursodeoxycholic acid: a safe and effective agent for dissolving cholesterol gallstones. *Ann. Intern. Med.*, **1982**, *97*, 351–356.

Walan, A. Treatment of peptic ulcer with small doses of an antacid and an anticholinergic compared with cimetidine and placebo. In, *Antacids in the Eighties.* (Halter, F., ed.) Urban & Schwarzenberg, Munich, **1982**, pp. 83–86.

Wrobel, J.; Koh, T. C.; and Saunders, J. M. Sodium citrate: an alternative antacid for prophylaxis against aspiration pneumonitis. *Anaesth. Intensive Care*, **1982**, *10*, 116–119.

Monographs and Reviews

Albibi, R., and McCallum, R. W. Metoclopramide: pharmacology and clinical application. *Ann. Intern. Med.*, **1983**, *98*, 86–95.

Alfrey, A. C. Aluminum. *Adv. Clin. Chem.*, **1983**, *23*, 69–91.

Bachman, B. A. Gastroesophageal reflux. Simple measures often suffice. *Postgrad. Med.*, **1983**, *74*, 133–141.

Barrowman, J. A., and Pfeiffer, C. J. Carbenoxolone: a critical analysis of its clinical value in peptic ulcer. In, *Drugs and Peptic Ulcer*, Vol. 1. (Pfeiffer, C. J., ed.) CRC Press, Boca Raton, **1982**, pp. 123–132.

Berardi, R. R., and Caplan, N. B. Agents with tricyclic structures for treatment of peptic ulcer disease. *Clin. Pharm.*, **1983**, *2*, 425–431.

Berstad, A. Management of acute upper gastrointestinal bleeding. *Scand. J. Gastroenterol.*, **1982c**, *17*, Suppl. 75, 103–108.

Carlson, G. L., and Malagelada, J. R. Chemistry of the antacids: its relevance to antacid therapy. In, *Antacids in the Eighties.* (Halter, F., ed.) Urban & Schwarzenberg, Munich, **1982**, pp. 7–16.

Chierichetti, S. M.; Gaetani, M.; and Petrini, G. (eds.). Pharmacokinetic and clinical studies on pirenzepine, new antiulcer drug. *Scand. J. Gastroenterol.*, **1979**, *14*, Suppl. 47, 1–67.

Clemens, J. D., and Feinstein, A. R. Calcium carbonate and constipation: an historical review of medical mythopoeia. *Gastroenterology*, **1977**, *72*, 957–961.

Cohen, M. M. Gastric mucosal protection with prostaglandins. In, *Drugs and Peptic Ulcer*, Vol. 1. (Pfeiffer, C. J., ed.) CRC Press, Boca Raton, **1982**, pp. 133–146.

Coombs, D. W. Aspiration pneumonia prophylaxis. (Editorial.) *Anesth. Analg.*, **1983**, *62*, 1055–1058.

Cotton, B. R., and Smith, G. The lower oesophageal sphincter and anaesthesia. *Br. J. Anaesth.*, **1984**, *56*, 37–46.

Frazier, J. L., and Fendler, K. J. Current concepts in the pathogenesis and treatment of reflux esophagitis. *Clin. Pharm.*, **1983**, *2*, 546–557.

Garnett, W. R. Sucralfate—alternative therapy for peptic-ulcer disease. *Clin. Pharm.*, **1982**, *1*, 307–314.

Halter, F. (ed.). *Antacids in the Eighties.* Symposium on antacids. Urban & Schwarzenberg, Munich, **1982**, pp. 1–53.

Holtermüller, K. H. Acid rebound: fact or fiction. *Hepatogastroenterology*, **1982**, *29*, 135–137.

Holtermüller, K. H., and Dehdaschti, M. Antacids and hormones. *Scand. J. Gastroenterol.*, **1982**, *17*, Suppl. 75, 24–31.

Holtermüller, K. H., and Herzog, P. Antacids: pharmacology and clinical efficacy—a critical evaluation. In,

Drugs and Peptic Ulcer, Vol. 1. (Pfeiffer, C. J., ed.) CRC Press, Boca Raton, **1982**, pp. 105–122.

Ippoliti, A. F. Antacid therapy for duodenal and gastric ulcer: the experience in the United States. *Scand. J. Gastroenterol.*, **1982**, *17*, Suppl. 75, 82–85.

Isenberg, J. I. Effects of antacids on dyspeptic symptoms. In, *Antacids in the Eighties.* (Halter, F., ed.) Urban & Schwarzenberg, Munich, **1982**, pp. 75–79.

Jamieson, G. G.; Beauchamp, G.; and Duranceau, A. C. The physiologic basis for the medical management of gastroesophageal reflux. *Surg. Clin. North Am.*, **1983**, *63*, 841–850.

Kauffman, G. L., Jr. Drug therapy for peptic ulcer: drugs that act on the gastric mucosa. *J. Clin. Gastroenterol.*, **1981**, *3*, Suppl. 2, 95–101.

Konturek, S. J. Pharmacologic control of gastric acid secretion in peptic ulcer. *Mt. Sinai J. Med.*, **1983**, *50*, 457–467.

Lewis, J. H. Treatment of gastric ulcer. What is old and what is new. *Arch. Intern. Med.*, **1983**, *143*, 264–274.

Liss, L. (ed.). *Aluminum Neurotoxicity.* Chem-Orbital, Park Forest South, Ill., **1980**.

Marks, I. N. Current therapy in peptic ulcer. *Drugs*, **1980**, *20*, 283–299.

Mayer, G. H., and Burnatowska-Hledin, M. A. Impaired renal function and aluminum metabolism. *Fed. Proc.*, **1983**, *42*, 2979–2983.

Morgan, M. Control of intragastric pH and volume. *Br. J. Anaesth.*, **1984**, *56*, 47–57.

Morris, T., and Rhodes, J. Antacids and peptic ulcer—a reappraisal. *Gut*, **1979**, *20*, 538–545.

Nutrition Reviews. Silicon overdosage in man. **1982**, *40*, 208–209.

Peppercorn, M. A. Drug therapy of peptic ulcer disease. *Compr. Ther.*, **1983**, *9*, 47–52.

Petersen, W. L., and Richardson, C. T. Pharmacology and side effects of drugs used to treat peptic ulcer. In, *Gastrointestinal Disease: Pathophysiology, Diagnosis, and Management*, 3rd ed. (Sleisinger, M. H., and Fordtran, J. S., eds.) W. B. Saunders Company, Philadelphia, **1983**, pp. 708–725.

Pfeiffer, C. J. (ed.). *Drugs and Peptic Ulcer.* Vol. 1, *Therapeutic Agents for Peptic Ulcer Disease.* CRC Press, Inc., Boca Raton, **1982**.

Piper, D. W. Drugs for the prevention of peptic ulcer recurrence. *Drugs*, **1983**, *26*, 439–453.

Priebe, H.-J. Prophylactic use of antacids or cimetidine in the prevention of acute gastric hemorrhage. In, *Antacids in the Eighties.* (Halter, F., ed.) Urban & Schwarzenberg, Munich, **1982**, pp. 93–98.

Pries, J. M. Coping with reflux esophagitis in the aged. *Geriatrics*, **1982**, *37*, 57–59, 64, 67.

Richter, J. E., and Castell, D. O. Gastroesophageal reflux. Pathogenesis, diagnosis, and therapy. *Ann. Intern. Med.*, **1982**, *97*, 93–103.

Sixma, J. J. Prostaglandins and prostaglandin inhibitors in clinical practice. *Neth. J. Med.*, **1982**, *25*, 2–5.

Soll, A. H. Pharmacology of inhibitors of parietal cell function. *J. Clin. Gastroenterol.*, **1981**, *3*, Suppl. 2, 85–90.

Somerville, K. W., and Langman, M. J. Newer antisecretory agents for peptic ulcer. *Drugs*, **1983**, *25*, 315–330.

Spiro, H. M. Pharmacology, clinical efficacy, and adverse effects of sucralfate, a nonsystemic agent for peptic ulcer. *Pharmacotherapy*, **1982**, *2*, 67–71.

Ström, M. Antacid side-effects on bowel habits. *Scand. J. Gastroenterol.*, **1982**, *17*, Suppl. 75, 54–56.

Symposium. (Various authors.) Advances in the basic and clinical pharmacology of pirenzepine. Proceedings of the Second International Symposium on Pirenzepine. (Baron, J. H., and Londong, W., eds.) *Scand. J. Gastroenterol.*, **1980a**, *15*, Suppl. 66, 1–114.

Symposium. (Various authors.) Carbenoxolone symposium. XI International Congress of Gastroenterology. (Jones, F. A.; Hunt, T. C.; and Reed, P. I.; eds.) *Scand. J. Gastroenterol.*, **1980b**, *15,* Suppl. 65, 1–121.

Symposium. (Various authors.) Gastritis, duodenitis, and peptic ulcer disease. Fourth International Symposium. (Samloff, I. M., ed.) *J. Clin. Gastroenterol.*, **1981**, *3,* Suppl. 2, 1–184.

Symposium. (Various authors.) *Antacids in the Eighties.* (Halter, F., ed.) Urban & Schwarzenberg, Munich, **1982a.**

Symposium. (Various authors.) DE-NOL in the treatment of peptic ulcer. Proceedings of the DE-NOL symposium at the 7th World Congress of Gastroenterology. (Tytgat, G. N. J., and Paul, Z. M., eds.) *Scand. J. Gastroenterol.*, **1982b**, *17,* Suppl. 80, 1–60.

Symposium. (Various authors.) On the selectivity of antimuscarinic compounds. Proceedings of the Third International Symposium on Pirenzepine. (Dotevall, G.; Jaup, B. H.; and Stockbrügger, R. W.; eds.) *Scand. J. Gastroenterol.*, **1982c**, *17,* Suppl. 72, 1–273.

Symposium. (Various authors.) Symposium on antacids. Proceedings from an International Symposium. (Forssell, H., and Walan, A., eds.) *Scand. J. Gastroenterol.*, **1982d**, *17,* Suppl. 75, 1–120.

Symposium. (Various authors.) Proceedings of the World Congress of Gastroenterology. (Marks, I. N.; Samloff, I. M.; Äärimaa, M.; and Siurale, M.; eds.) *Scand. J. Gastroenterol.*, **1983**, *18,* Suppl. 83, 1–82.

Teilum, D. Reflux esophagitis. *Scand. J. Gastroenterol.*, **1982**, *17,* Suppl. 75, 161–165.

Wesdorp, I. C. Treatment of reflux oesophagitis. *Scand. J. Gastroenterol.*, **1982**, *17,* Suppl. 79, 106–119.

Wu, W. C., and Castell, D. O. Gastroesophageal reflux. *Compr. Ther.*, **1983**, *9,* 57–63.

CHAPTER
43 LAXATIVES

Laurence L. Brunton

Laxatives are drugs that promote defecation. Their zealous overuse by a self-prescribing public, fostered by advertisements for these agents, reflects a misconception of what frequency of bowel movement is normal, desirable, or necessary, and demonstrates the acceptance of Meredith's dictum that one "is not altogether fit for the battle of life who is in a perpetual contention with his dinner" (Meredith, 1859). In fact, there are few valid indications for the use of laxatives since constipation can generally be resolved by increasing the fiber content of the diet, exercise, and bowel training. In some instances, constipation may result from important underlying causes, such as adverse reactions to drugs or toxins (Table 43–1), metabolic disorders, and disorders of the large intestine (*see* Devroede, 1983); in these cases the cause rather than the symptom should be treated.

GENERAL CONSIDERATIONS

Colonic Function. Like the small intestine, the colon is normally an organ of absorption. Daily, the colon receives approximately 1500 ml of fluid and absorbs all but 150 ml. The absorptive capacity of the colon is even greater, approaching 5 to 6 liters per day. This uptake of fluid is secondary to active transport of Na^+; the luminal equilibrium concentration for net uptake of Na^+ is 25 to 30 mM. The mechanism responsible for colonic absorption of Na^+ is primarily electrogenic Na^+ transport, which relies on a Na^+,K^+-ATPase activity in the basolateral membrane of the colonic epithelium; neutral absorption of NaCl may also be involved. The colon absorbs Cl^- by an electrically neutral mechanism that involves exchange of Cl^- for HCO_3^- and by neutral uptake of NaCl. Agents that elevate intracellular concentrations of adenosine 3',5'-monophosphate (cyclic AMP) in colonic enterocytes apparently stimulate electrogenic secretion of Cl^- and may inhibit neutral NaCl uptake. This causes net fluid secretion. The colon also secretes K^+, probably by means of an active mechanism that is stimulated by cyclic AMP.

The colon absorbs relatively few nutrients; it does, however, absorb short-chain fatty acids (two to four carbon atoms in length) by diffusion. The absorption of these fatty acids increases that of fluid and electrolytes. This is in contrast to the effects of longer-chain fatty acids (≥ 12 carbons) and dihydroxy bile acids (*see* below; *see also* Binder, 1983; Symposium, 1983).

Colonic function is subject to complex sets of regulatory influences. In contrast to the small intestine, electrolyte transport in the colon is susceptible to regulation by mineralocorticoids. The response of the colon to aldosterone is similar to that of the kidney: uptake of Na^+ and H_2O is enhanced, while K^+ is secreted. Other hormones and neurotransmitters that influence colonic fluxes of water and electrolyte include somatostatin, opioids, antidiuretic hormone, and dopaminergic and adrenergic agonists, all of which enhance absorption or inhibit secretion; vasoactive intestinal peptide (VIP) and prostaglandins, which are secretagogues; and cholinergic agonists, which cause net secretion of NaCl and H_2O (*see* Racusen and Binder, 1979; Binder, 1983; Bridges *et al.*, 1983; Donowitz *et al.*, 1983). In some systems, these agents act to inhibit adenylate cyclase (somatostatin and opiate peptides) or to stimulate the enzyme (prostaglandins E and I_2 and VIP). Some of their effects may thus be due to cyclic AMP–dependent regulation of Cl^- secretion. Cholera toxin, "the ultimate laxative," clearly stimulates intestinal secretion in the small intestine and the colon by its ability to activate adenylate cyclase in the mucosa. The effects of adrenergic and cholinergic agents do not fit well with

Table 43–1. SOME COSTIVE (CONSTIPATING) AGENTS

Analgesics (inhibitors of prostaglandin synthesis)
Antacids (containing calcium carbonate or aluminum hydroxide)
Anticholinergic agents
Antidiarrheal agents
Antihistamines (H_1 blockers; anticholinergic effect)
Antiparkinsonian drugs (anticholinergic effect)
Barium sulfate
Clonidine
Diuretics that cause hypokalemia
Ganglionic blocking agents
Heavy metals (especially lead)
Iron
Laxatives (used chronically)
Monoamine oxidase inhibitors
Muscle relaxants
Opioids
Phenothiazines (anticholinergic effect)
Polystyrene resins
Tricyclic antidepressants (anticholinergic effect)
Verapamil

such a theory, however; both α_2- and β-adrenergic agonists cause net uptake of fluid, whereas muscarinic cholinergic stimulation causes net fluid secretion. Coordinate adrenergic and cholinergic control of colonic function likely involves the integration of cyclic AMP– and Ca^{2+}–dependent pathways, and several cellular loci are probably involved, including enterocytes, components of the enteric nervous system, smooth muscle, and mucus-secreting goblet cells. Superposed on local hormonal regulation of fluid and electrolyte fluxes are the effects of neurohumors and sensory and reflex pathways that involve the lumbar spinal cord, pelvic nerves, and higher inhibitory centers, through which poorly quantifiable factors such as stress and other psychological variables affect colonic function.

Defecation and Constipation. Normal size, frequency, and consistency of fecal output are difficult to quantify and are subject to personal variation and to sociological patterning, of which the makers of laxatives take full advantage. There is no distinct advantage in frequent bowel movements. While once daily may be average, between three times weekly and three times daily may be considered normal (*see* Devroede, 1983). Patients' fears of "autointoxication" due to retention of colonic contents are unfounded if hepatic function is normal.

Reduced frequency and bulk and increased hardness of feces surely do occur, mainly due to dehydration of material that stays too long in the colon before expulsion. The bulk, softness, and hydration of feces are very dependent on the fiber content of the diet; thus, sufficient dietary fiber and water are mainstays in any regimen for the treatment of constipation.

Mechanisms of Laxative Action. Precise mechanisms of action of many laxatives remain uncertain because of the complex factors that affect colonic function, prominent variations of water and electrolyte transport among experimental species and preparations, and a certain costiveness of research in this area. Such lack of movement notwithstanding, three general mechanisms of laxative action can be described. (1) By their hydrophilic or osmotic properties, laxatives may cause retention of fluid in colonic contents, thereby increasing bulk and softness and facilitating transit. (2) Laxatives may act, both directly and indirectly, on the colonic mucosa to decrease net absorption of water and NaCl, possibly by some of the mechanisms mentioned above. (3) Laxatives may increase intestinal motility, causing decreased absorption of salt and water secondary to decreased transit time. The role of abnormal colonic motility as a causative factor in constipation is not certain (Meunier *et al.*, 1979); however, the interactions of motility with absorptive and secretory functions are topics of current research. More detailed information on putative mechanisms of action of individual agents appears below.

Classification and Choice of Laxatives. In this chapter, laxatives are classified by their general mechanisms of action. However, commonly used agents may also be arranged according to the pattern of laxative effects produced by the usual clinical dosage (Table 43–2). Note that the latency and effect of all laxatives vary with dosage.

Table 43–2. CLASSIFICATION AND COMPARISON OF REPRESENTATIVE LAXATIVES

LAXATIVE EFFECT AND LATENCY IN USUAL CLINICAL DOSAGE

Softening of Feces, 1 to 3 Days	*Soft or Semifluid Stool, 6 to 8 Hours*	*Watery Evacuation, 1 to 3 Hours*
Bulk-forming laxatives Bran Psyllium preparations Methylcellulose	Diphenylmethane derivatives Phenolphthalein Bisacodyl	Saline cathartics * Sodium phosphates Magnesium sulfate Milk of magnesia
Docusates Lactulose	Anthraquinone derivatives Senna Cascara sagrada Danthron	Castor oil

* Also employed in lower dosage for laxative effect.

In high enough dosage, many laxatives promote catharsis, which implies purgation and a more fluid evacuation. While the major group of agents (*e.g.*, bulk-forming agents, docusates) frequently have distinguishing characteristics that limit or indicate their usefulness in a particular patient, agents within each group usually share utility and limitations.

DIETARY FIBER AND BULK-FORMING LAXATIVES

The most satisfactory prophylactic and treatment for functional constipation is a diet rich in fiber. Dietary fiber will also benefit patients who need to avoid straining at the stool and patients with irritable bowel disease and diverticular disease of the colon. There are various bulk-forming agents that can be utilized as supplements to dietary fiber; these include both natural and semisynthetic polysaccharides and celluloses derived from grains, seed husks, or kelp, including *bran, psyllium, methylcellulose,* and *carboxymethylcellulose,* as well as the synthetic resin *polycarbophil*.

Dietary fiber is plant cell wall that escapes digestion by the secretions of the human gastrointestinal tract. Usual sources of dietary fiber are whole grains, bran, vegetables, and fruit. Plant cell walls consist of varying quantities of fibrillar polysaccharides (mainly cellulose), matrix polysaccharides (pectins, hemicelluloses), lignins, cutin, waxes, and some glycoproteins (*see* Selvendran, 1984). Dietary fiber acts as a laxative by virtue of binding water and ions in the colonic lumen, thereby softening the feces and increasing their bulk. Some components of dietary fiber (*e.g.*, pectins) are digested by colonic bacteria to metabolites that contribute to laxative action by adding to the osmotic activity of the luminal fluid. They also support the growth of colonic bacteria, thereby increasing fecal mass (*see* Stephen and Cummings, 1980). It is also possible that bacterial fermentation of dietary fiber produces metabolites that influence colonic mechanisms of fluid and electrolyte transport directly. Dietary fibers and bulk-forming agents from different sources vary in their composition, and thus in their water-holding capacity, and in the

relative contribution of these different modes of action. The fiber contents of common foods are now listed in numerous textbooks and diet plans. On the basis of satisfactory laxation as judged from patients' comments, 20 to 60 g of dietary fiber daily is sufficient (*see* Mendeloff, 1977; Bingham *et al.*, 1979).

Effects on the Intestinal Tract; Systemic Effects. Dietary fiber and bulk-forming agents increase the mass of stool, its water content, and the rate of colonic transit. These effects are usually apparent within 24 hours and, with repeated administration, reach a maximum after several days. Dietary fiber alone, in the form of a diet rich in fruit, vegetables, and whole grains, can increase the daily fecal mass markedly (*see* Symposium, 1983). The lignin and pectin in dietary fibers will bind bile acids, thereby protecting them from bacterial degradation and increasing their excretion in the feces. The consequent enhancement of hepatic synthesis of bile acids from cholesterol may reduce plasma concentrations of cholesterol in low-density lipoproteins. The effects of dietary fiber on plasma cholesterol and lipoproteins are variable and depend on the type of fiber studied (*see* Anderson and Chen, 1979; Symposium, 1983). Refined gums and pectin, for instance, are hypocholesterolemic in man, primarily by reducing the plasma low-density lipoprotein fraction, whereas cellulose is not (Behall *et al.*, 1984). The mechanisms of such effects are not known.

When used over several months, bran and other bulk-forming agents reduce intraluminal rectosigmoid pressure and relieve symptoms in patients with irritable bowel disease and diverticular disease of the colon (*see* Brodribb, 1977). Whether a lack of dietary fiber contributes to disorders of the large bowel and other diseases remains to be established (*see* Painter and Burkitt, 1975; Mendeloff, 1977).

Their ability to absorb water and to provide an emollient intestinal mass makes the bulk-forming laxatives useful for the symptomatic relief of *acute diarrhea* and to regulate the effluent in patients with an *ileostomy* or *colostomy*. However, loss of sodium, potassium, and water may be increased in such patients. The alleged effectiveness of the bulk-forming agents as appetite suppressants in the management of *obesity* has *not* been substantiated.

Adverse Effects. Bulk-forming laxatives have few side effects and minimal systemic effects. Allergic reactions may occur, especially with use of plant gums. Flatulence and borborygmi occur occasionally. Possible alterations in Ca^{2+} metabolism are incompletely defined, as are effects on glucose tolerance. The latter may be related to the dextrose content of some preparations and is a consideration in the treatment of diabetic patients. Cellulose can bind many drugs and reduce their intestinal absorption; these include cardiac glycosides, salicylates, and nitrofurantoin. Psyllium may bind coumarin derivatives. While specific information is sparse, the potential for this interaction is great and warrants monitoring and discussion with the patient. Carboxymethylcellulose sodium and psyllium colloid may contain significant quantities of sodium and should not be used when retention of Na^+ and H_2O could present a problem.

Intestinal obstruction and impaction may occur after the administration of bulk-forming agents, especially when there is preexisting gastrointestinal pathology. One should avoid the use of these agents in individuals with stenosis, ulceration, or adhesions. Esophageal and intestinal obstruction can occur when these substances are taken dry. Patients may avoid these problems by drinking a glass of water concurrently.

Bran, Whole Grains, and Other Dietary Fiber. Bran contains more than 40% dietary fiber and is a convenient source of intestinal bulk. Bran-rich cereals contain 25% dietary fiber. Crude bran may be added to cereals, salads, and baked goods. Approximately 6 g of crude miller's bran daily produces a noticeable enhancement in the bulk and softness of stools. Fresh fruits, vegetables, and legumes contribute generously to dietary fiber. Burkitt and Meisner (1978) have provided a helpful guide to the fiber content of foods. *Malt soup extract* (MALTSUPEX), 12 g daily in four divided doses (as tablets), provides an adult with a fiber and maltose supplement derived from barley.

Psyllium (Plantago). *Plantago seed* has been replaced by refined preparations from psyllium seeds that are enriched in mucilloid, a hydrophilic substance that forms a gelatinous mass when mixed with water. Typical brand-name preparations are EFFERSYLLIUM, KONSYL, METAMUCIL, and MODANE BULK. Some of these preparations contain dextrose as a dispersing agent. The usual dose is 3 to 3.6 g, once to thrice daily, in 250 ml of fruit juice or water. Chronic administration of the psyllium preparations may produce modest reduction of plasma cholesterol concentration, apparently by interference with reabsorption of bile acids. Sensitization, with asthmatic symptoms upon inhalation of psyllium powder, has been reported in atopic individuals chronically exposed to the powder during its manufacture.

Semisynthetic Celluloses and Gums. *Methylcellulose* (COLOGEL) and *carboxymethylcellulose sodium* are hydrophilic derivatives of cellulose. These indigestible and unabsorbable compounds form a bulky colloid when mixed with water, leading to a softening of the stool within 1 to 3 days. Such celluloses have also been employed to increase the bulk and consistency of stools in patients who suffer from chronic watery diarrhea. The sodium content of carboxymethylcellulose preparations may lead to fluid retention. Capsules (which also contain other ingredients) and oral solutions of these agents are available; all should be administered with ample water, and the usual dose is 4 to 6 g daily in two or three portions (1.0 to 1.5 g for children).

Other Bulk-Forming Agents. *Polycarbophil* and *calcium polycarbophil* (MITROLAN) are nonabsorbed hydrophilic polyacrylic resins with more water-binding capacity than the aforementioned agents. They absorb 60 to 100 times their weight in water and thereby add soft bulk to feces. These preparations have the advantage of a low sodium content. Calcium polycarbophil releases Ca^{2+} in the gastrointestinal tract and should thus be avoided by patients who must restrict their intake of calcium or who are taking tetracyclines. Calcium polycarbophil is available as chewable tablets that contain the equivalent of 500 mg of polycarbophil. The recommended adult dose is 1 g, four to six times daily; each dose should be taken with 250 ml of water. *Karaya gum (sterculia gum)* is a powder that contains relatively stable, poorly absorbed hydrophilic polysaccharides. In a daily dosage of 5 to 10 g with water, it acts similarly to the other bulk-forming agents. Allergic reactions, characterized by urticaria, rhinitis, dermatitis, and asthma, have occasionally been reported.

SALINE AND OSMOTIC LAXATIVES

These agents include various magnesium salts; the sulfate, phosphate, and tartrate salts of sodium or potassium; the disaccharide lactulose; glycerin; and sorbitol. They are poorly and slowly absorbed and act by their osmotic properties in the luminal fluid. Magnesium salts can, in addition, cause duodenal secretion of cholecystokinin (Harvey and Read, 1975), a hormone whose pharmacological actions include stimulation of fluid secretion and motility; it is possible that this mechanism contributes to their laxative activity. The primary osmotic effect of lactulose, which is not absorbed in the upper intestine, may be augmented in the distal ileum and colon by bacterial metabolism of the disaccharide to lactate and other organic acids that are only partially absorbed. There is speculation that the concomitant reduction in luminal pH enhances motility and secretion.

Effects on the Intestinal Tract. Full cathartic doses of saline laxatives (15 g of $MgSO_4$ or the equivalent with 250 ml of water) produce a thorough, semifluid or water evacuation in 3 hours or less. Lower doses produce a laxative effect with a latency of 6 to 8 hours. The cathartic effect is most prominent if the laxative is taken when the stomach is empty. These agents are useful for emptying the bowel prior to surgical, radiological, and colonoscopic procedures and can help eliminate parasites following appropriate therapy (*see* Chapter 44) and toxic material in some cases of poisoning (*see* Chapter 68).

The increased osmotic activity in the lumen that follows administration of lactulose results in modest accumulation of fluid and passage of soft, formed feces in 1 to 3 days. Another important aspect of the action of lactulose is reduction of intestinal absorption of ammonia, presumably because of reduced production and increased utilization of ammonia by intestinal bacteria and enhanced excretion of ammonia in the feces. These effects account for the efficacy of lactulose in lowering concentrations of ammonia in blood in 75% of patients with portal hypertension and hepatic encephalopathy associated with chronic liver disease. With a latency of 1 to 7 days, lactulose reduces blood ammonia in these patients by 25 to 50% (Avery *et al.,* 1972; Conn, 1978).

Adverse Effects. Some absorption of the component ions of the saline laxatives does occur, and in certain instances they may produce systemic toxicity. In an individual with impaired renal function, the accumulation of magnesium ions in the body fluids may be sufficient to cause intoxication (*see* Chapter 35). Magnesium laxatives should thus be administered only if renal function is adequate. Similarly, sodium salts may be contraindicated in patients with congestive heart failure or renal disease, and phosphate salts may reduce the concentration of ionized calcium in plasma. Hypertonic solutions of the saline laxatives can produce significant dehydration. For this reason, these salts should be administered with sufficient water by mouth to ensure that no net loss of body water occurs.

Lactulose may cause flatulence, cramps, and abdominal discomfort, especially when therapy is initiated; these symptoms occur in about 20% of patients receiving full doses of the drug. Nausea and vomiting have also been reported, particularly with higher dosage. Excessive dosage can cause diarrhea, loss of fluid and potassium, and exacerbation of hepatic encephalopathy. Since lactulose is a disaccharide of galactose and fructose, its use is contraindicated in patients who require a galactose-free diet, and it must be used cautiously in diabetics. The preparation also contains some lactose.

Magnesium Salts. The usual dose of *magnesium sulfate (Epsom salt)* is 15 g, but 5 g (about 40 mEq of magnesium ion) produces a significant laxative effect when administered in dilute solution to a fasting individual or to a child. The intensely bitter taste may induce nausea and should be masked by taking the salt in citrus juices. *Milk of magnesia* is a 7.0 to 8.5% aqueous suspension of magnesium hydroxide. The usual adult dose is 30 to 60 ml (about 80 to 160 mEq of magnesium ion); the dose for children is 0.5 ml/kg. *Magnesium hydroxide* is also available as tablets. The usual dose is 1.8 to 3.6 g (62 to 124 mEq). Other magnesium salts commonly employed as gastric antacids have similar laxative properties (*see also* Chapter 42). *Magnesium citrate oral solution* provides the equivalent of 4 g of magnesium hydroxide in the usual 240-ml dose.

Sodium Phosphates. Phosphate salts are relatively pleasant tasting. The most frequently employed preparation is *sodium phosphates oral solution* (PHOSPHO-SODA), which contains 1.8 g of dibasic sodium phosphate and 4.8 g of monobasic sodium phosphate in 10 ml. The usual dose is 10 to 40 ml, taken with ample water. *Sodium phosphates enema,* in a dose of 118 ml, is employed for rectal administration.

Other Saline Laxatives. The other saline laxatives, such as *sodium sulfate (Glauber's salt)* and *potassium sodium tartrate (Rochelle salt),* are now little used and have no advantage over the preparations listed above.

Lactulose. This agent is a semisynthetic disaccharide with the following structure:

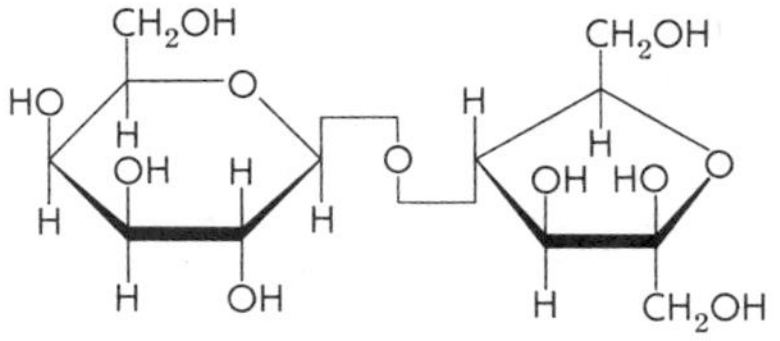

Lactulose

Lactulose (CEPHULAC, CHRONULAC) is available as a syrup; each 15 ml contains 10 g of lactulose and not more than 2.2 g of galactose, 1.2 g of lactose, and 1.2 g of other sugars. The sweet taste can be masked by mixing the syrup with fruit juice. The drug should be taken with ample water.

The daily maintenance dose for management of constipation varies widely but may be as low as 7 to 10 g, as a single dose or divided. Larger doses (up to 40 g) are sometimes required initially, and the full effect of lactulose may not be attained for a few days.

For management of *chronic portal hypertension* and *hepatic encephalopathy,* the usual maintenance dose is 20 to 30 g (30 to 45 ml), three or four times daily; this is adjusted such that there are two or three soft stools daily and a fecal pH of 5 to 5.5. Therapy can be initiated with hourly doses of 20 to 30 g if indicated. Lactulose can also be given rectally if necessary. Maintenance of the proper fecal pH is essential for appropriate effects on intestinal elimination of ammonia. Excessive diarrhea must be avoided. Other laxatives should not be employed concurrently in order to avoid inadequate acidification of the stool. For additional aspects of the management of this disease, *see* Avery and colleagues (1972).

Glycerin. *Glycerin* acts mainly by its osmotic effect to soften and lubricate the passage of inspissated feces. It may also stimulate rectal contraction. Rectal suppositories promote colonic evacuation in 30 minutes. The usual rectal dosages are 3 g for adults and 1 to 1.5 g for children under 6 years.

Sorbitol. *Sorbitol* (D-glucitol), a polyalcohol of sorbose, acts as an osmotic agent when administered rectally as an enema (120 ml of a 25 to 30% solution for adults; 30 to 60 ml for children). It can also be given orally (*e.g.*, 30 ml of a 70% solution). When sodium polystyrene sulfonate is utilized in the therapy of hyperkalemia, sorbitol is frequently included to combat the constipating effect of the cation-exchange resin.

STIMULANT LAXATIVES

These agents stimulate accumulation of water and electrolytes in the colonic lumen, and they also enhance intestinal motility. This group includes *diphenylmethane* derivatives, *anthraquinones*, and *castor oil*, as well as the surfactants, *docusates*, *poloxamers*, and *bile acids*. Docusates and poloxamers are also known as stool softeners. Despite some similarities in their mechanisms of action, the clinical uses and limitations of these agents vary sufficiently to require separate description. The medical importance of the stimulant laxatives stems more from their popularity and abuse than from their valid therapeutic applications.

The effects of the stimulant laxatives on intestinal fluxes of electrolytes and water are readily demonstrated *in vitro* or *in situ* under conditions in which effects on motility are excluded. Concentrations of these agents that reduce net absorption of electrolytes and water also increase the permeability of the mucosa, possibly by making tight junctions leaky. The stimulant laxatives may inhibit intestinal Na^+,K^+-ATPase; this action could account for at least a portion of their laxative effect (*see* above). Many of the stimulant laxatives also increase the synthesis of prostaglandins and cyclic AMP, and this may contribute to increased secretion of water and electrolytes. Inhibition of prostaglandin synthesis with indomethacin does reduce the effects of many of these agents on net water flux (*see* Symposium, 1983). Fairbairn and Moss (1970) have summarized structure-activity relationships among the stimulant laxatives.

DIPHENYLMETHANE DERIVATIVES

The primary diphenylmethane laxatives are *phenolphthalein* and *bisacodyl*. These agents have similar pharmacological characteristics and clinical uses.

Laxative Effects. Individual effective doses of the diphenylmethane derivatives vary as much as fourfold to eightfold. Consequently, recommended doses that promote laxation in the majority of patients may be relatively ineffective in some patients but may produce griping and excessively fluid evacuation in others. Since the diphenylmethane derivatives act primarily on the colon, laxative effects are not usually produced in less than 6 hours. They are frequently taken at bedtime to produce their effect the next morning. Use of these agents should be limited to 10 consecutive days (*see* below).

Absorption and Excretion. As much as 15% of a therapeutic dose of phenolphthalein is absorbed and eliminated by the kidney, most of it in conjugated form. The urine becomes pink or red if it is sufficiently alkaline. Some absorbed drug is also excreted in the bile, and the resulting enterohepatic cycle may contribute to prolongation of the laxative effect.

Bisacodyl is rapidly converted by intestinal and bacterial enzymes to its active desacetyl metabolite. As much as 5% of an orally administered dose is absorbed and excreted in the urine as the glucuronide. This inactive metabolite is also excreted in the bile and may be hydrolyzed to active drug in the colon.

Adverse Effects. The major dangers of overdosage of the diphenylmethane derivatives are fluid and electrolyte deficits resulting from excessive laxative effect. Moreover, allergic reactions, including fixed-drug eruption, Stevens-Johnson syndrome, a syndrome that resembles lupus erythematosus, osteomalacia, and protein-losing gastroenteropathy, have been reported to follow the use of *phenolphthalein*. Laxatives containing phenolphthalein are additionally undesirable because of their potential for abuse (*see* below).

Phenolphthalein. The laxative effect of phenolphthalein was discovered in 1902 by Vamossy, during a study undertaken for the Hungarian government to determine its safety as an additive for identification of artificial wines. It has since been widely employed as a laxative, but not as an additive to wines. The structural formula of phenolphthalein is as follows:

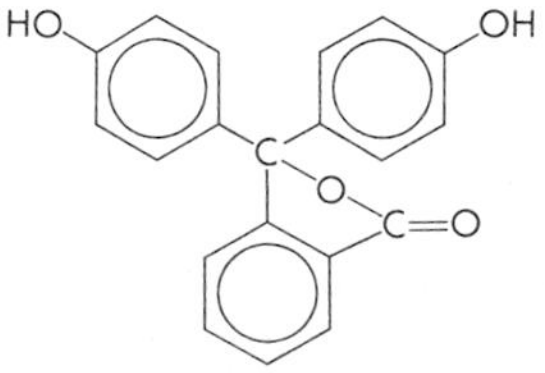

Phenolphthalein

Phenolphthalein is available as tablets and a liquid and in numerous proprietary preparations. The usual dose is 30 to 195 mg for adults and 15 to 60 mg for children. Phenolphthalein usually acts in

6 to 8 hours. The patient should be warned of possible pink coloring of the urine and feces.

Bisacodyl. Bisacodyl, 4,4'-(2-pyridylmethylene) diphenol diacetate, was introduced as a laxative in 1953 on the basis of structure-activity studies of compounds related to phenolphthalein. Bisacodyl has the following structural formula:

CH₃OCO   OCOCH₃

Bisacodyl

Bisacodyl (DULCOLAX, others) is available as 5-mg enteric-coated tablets for oral administration and as 10-mg suppositories and in suspension (10 mg/30 ml) for rectal administration. It is also supplied in kits, with other agents, for evacuation of the bowel prior to diagnostic procedures or surgery.

The usual *oral dosage* is 10 to 15 mg for adults and 5 to 10 mg for children (0.3 mg/kg). To avoid gastric irritation, patients should swallow tablets without chewing or crushing and should not take bisacodyl within 1 hour of milk or antacid medication. One or two soft, formed stools are usually produced within 6 to 12 hours. Recommended *rectal dosage* is 10 mg for adults and for children over 2 years, and 5 mg for children under 2 years. After rectal administration, the drug usually acts in 15 to 60 minutes. Bisacodyl suppositories may produce a burning sensation in the rectum; mild proctitis and sloughing of epithelium have been reported after use of the suppositories for several weeks. Hence, prolonged use should be discouraged.

Isatin Derivatives. *Oxyphenisatin acetate* is a laxative with pharmacological properties similar to those of bisacodyl. However, oxyphenisatin acetate, particularly when administered with the docusates, has been incriminated as a cause of hepatic injury (*see* Goldstein *et al.,* 1973) and has been withdrawn from the market in many countries; it should no longer be used.

ANTHRAQUINONE LAXATIVES

The anthraquinone laxatives include 1,8-dihydroxyanthraquinone (*danthron*) and its glycosides, which are contained in *senna* and *cascara.* Their clinical uses and limitations are similar to those of the diphenylmethane derivatives.

Absorption, Metabolism, and Excretion. Following an oral dose, the naturally occurring anthraquinone glycosides are poorly absorbed from the small intestine. After removal of the sugar (D-glucose or L-rhamnose) and reduction to the anthrol by colonic bacteria, the agents are absorbed to a moder-

ate degree. Absorbed material may be excreted in the bile, with possible effects on the small bowel, and in saliva, milk, and urine. As an aglycone, danthron may be absorbed in the small intestine without the need for bacterial metabolism.

Laxative Effects. The major active constituents of this class of laxatives are derivatives related to 1,8-dihydroxyanthraquinone. The effects of the individual preparations vary, depending upon their anthraquinone content and the ease of liberation of the active constituents from their inactive precursor glycosides by the intestinal microflora. These agents do increase colonic motility, an effect attributed to stimulation of Auerbach's plexus by anthraquinone. The galenical preparations often employed may contain other active ingredients. Since the laxative effect of the anthraquinone is limited mainly to the large intestine, these agents are generally effective 6 hours or more after oral administration.

Adverse Effects. The undesirable properties of anthraquinone laxatives are mainly an excessive laxative effect. Following a normal laxative dose, the quantity appearing in milk during lactation may be sufficient to affect a nursing infant; nursing mothers should be warned of the possibility and encouraged to avoid these agents. Renal excretion of the compounds may cause abnormal color of the urine (yellowish brown turning red with increasing pH). Large doses may produce nephritis. A melanotic pigmentation of the colonic mucosa (*melanosis coli*) has been observed in individuals who have taken anthraquinone laxatives over extended periods of time. The pigmentation is benign and is usually reversible within 4 to 12 months after medication is discontinued. Its presence may help confirm a suspicion of laxative abuse.

Senna. Senna is obtained from the dried leaflets or pods of *Cassia acutifolia* or *Cassia angustifolia.* Preparations of senna leaf—*senna, senna fluidextract,* and *senna syrup*—usually produce a single, thorough bowel evacuation within 6 hours, but with considerable griping. This reflects the effect of the drug on colonic motility.

Concentrates of senna pods, standardized by chemical or biological assay, are usually preferred. They are more stable and more reliable than the preparations of senna leaf and are alleged to cause less cramping and griping than does crude senna. Preparations of senna pods are available as granules, syrup, suppositories, and tablets. The dosage is as labeled.

Cascara Sagrada. *Cascara sagrada* (*sacred bark*) is obtained from the bark of the buckthorn tree, *Rhamnus purshiana.* The most commonly employed preparation is *aromatic cascara fluidextract.* A 5-ml dose usually causes a single soft or semifluid evacuation of the bowel in approximately 8 hours. Proprietary preparations that contain the anthranol glycosides from cascara sagrada (*casanthranol*) are also available. The adult dose is 30 mg.

Danthron. *Danthron* (DORBANE, MODANE) is 1,8-dihydroxyanthraquinone. Its structural formula is as follows:

Danthron

Although danthron is a free anthraquinone, its pharmacological properties, uses, and limitations are similar to those of the anthraquinone glycosides. Danthron is available as 37.5- and 75-mg tablets and in solution (37.5 mg/5 ml). The usual adult dose of 37.5 to 150 mg produces a soft or semifluid stool in 6 to 8 hours.

Other Anthraquinone Preparations. Proprietary preparations contain anthraquinone derivatives from a number of other plant sources. None is superior to the preparations described; most should be abandoned.

CASTOR OIL

The bean of the castor plant, *Ricinus communis,* contains two well-known noxious ingredients: an extremely toxic protein, *ricin,* and an oil composed chiefly of the triglyceride of *ricinoleic acid* (12-hydroxyoleic acid). The objectionable taste and purgative qualities of the oil, ascribable to the ricinoleic acid, have been dreaded by children since the time of the early Egyptians. The cathartic effect is too strong to warrant use of this agent for common constipation.

Metabolism, Catharsis, and Adverse Effects. Used externally, castor oil is a bland emollient. Within the small intestine, however, pancreatic lipases hydrolyze the oil to glycerol and ricinoleic acid. Ricinoleate, like other anionic surfactants, reduces net absorption of fluid and electrolytes and stimulates intestinal peristalsis. Ricinoleic acid is also absorbed and metabolized like other fatty acids.

Because ricinoleate acts in the small intestine, accumulation of fluid and evacuation are prompt and thorough, such as desired before radiological examination. Colonic emptying is so complete that several days may pass before feces do.

The altered intestinal permeability caused by castor oil may reflect grosser morphological damage to the intestinal mucosa. The strong purgative action can cause colic as well as dehydration with electrolyte imbalance. For these reasons and because of possible reduction of the absorption of nutrients, chronic use of castor oil must be avoided. The stimulant effects of this agent are reportedly sufficient to cause uterine contraction in pregnant women, who should, therefore, avoid using castor oil.

Preparations and Dosage. Castor oil is usually administered when the stomach is empty. As little as 4 ml may produce a laxative effect in the fasting adult. However, the usual dose for a cathartic effect is 15 to 60 ml for adults, 5 to 15 ml for children over 2 years of age, and 1 to 5 ml for younger children. Full doses of castor oil cause the evacuation of one or two copious, semifluid stools within 1 to 6 hours; thus, this laxative should not be taken late in the day with the expectation of sleeping.

Preparations include *castor oil* and *aromatic castor oil.* Although the objectionable taste of the oil is partially masked in the latter preparation, flavored *castor oil emulsions* are somewhat more palatable.

DOCUSATES

Docusate sodium, the prototype for this group of anionic surfactants, is widely employed in the pharmaceutical industry as an emulsifying, wetting, and dispersing agent. It has the following structural formula:

Docusate Sodium

In recommended dosage, the docusates have minimal laxative effects; their clinical usefulness is limited to keeping the feces soft such that straining at the stool can be avoided. Many details of their pharmacology remain uncertain.

Laxative Effects. In recommended oral dosage, the docusates produce minimal softening of the feces with a latency of 1 to 3 days. These surfactants apparently hydrate and soften the stool by emulsifying feces, water, and fat. *In vitro* and *in situ,* docusate sodium also alters net intestinal absorption of electrolytes and water and has effects on the *intestinal mucosa* similar to those of other stimulant laxatives (Donowitz, 1979).

Adverse Effects. The docusates are well tolerated. Cramping pains have been reported occasionally, and the liquid preparations sometimes cause nausea. Docusates increase the intestinal absorption of other drugs administered concurrently and may increase their toxicity. Of particular concern are the observations that docusate sodium is absorbed, appears in the bile in significant concentration, has cytotoxic effects on liver cells in tissue culture, and may contribute to the hepatotoxicity of danthron.

Preparations and Dosage. *Docusate sodium (dioctyl sodium sulfosuccinate;* COLACE, DOXINATE), *docusate calcium (dioctyl calcium sulfosuccinate;* SURFAK), and *docusate potassium (dioctyl* *potassium sulfosuccinate;* KASOF) are available as capsules. Docusate sodium is also available in tablets, solution, and as a syrup. The usual *oral* dose for adults is 50 to 300 mg daily, as a single or divided dose; for children, 1.25 mg/kg, up to four times daily. The solutions should be administered in milk or fruit juice to mask the bitter taste. The usual *rectal* dose of the liquid is 50 to 100 mg, as a 0.1% solution.

POLOXAMERS

Poloxamers are polyoxyethylene-polyoxypropylene polymers that are nonionic surfactants and, when ingested, have many of the properties of the docusates. *Poloxamer 188* is a water-soluble powder with an average molecular weight of 8350. A dosage of 240 to 480 mg of poloxamer 188 (ALAXIN), once daily, softens the stool in 3 to 5 days.

DEHYDROCHOLIC ACID

Bile acids have effects on the intestine that are similar to those of other anionic surfactants and stimulant laxatives; they reduce net absorption of water and electrolytes and cause diarrhea if they escape ileal absorption. *Dehydrocholic acid* is considered safe and effective as an oral laxative when administered to adults in a dosage of 750 mg to 1.5 g daily in three doses. Dehydrocholate is also an effective hydrocholeretic in this dosage range (*see* Chapter 42).

OTHER LAXATIVES

MINERAL OIL

Mineral oil is a mixture of aliphatic hydrocarbons obtained from petroleum. The oil is indigestible and absorbed only to a limited extent. When taken for 2 or 3 days, it penetrates and softens the stool and may also interfere with absorption of water. The adverse effects that may result from the use of mineral oil as a laxative argue against its use. These include interference with the absorption of essential fat-soluble substances, elicitation of foreign-body reactions in the intestinal mucosa and in other tissues, and leakage of the oil past the anal sphincter. Lipid pneumonitis can also follow oral ingestion of mineral oil.

MIXTURES AND COMBINATIONS

There is no evidence that mixtures of several laxatives have advantages over single agents used judiciously. Indeed, the use of a mixture of laxatives can have serious drawbacks, such as the enhanced absorption of other agents by docusates. It would be prudent to avoid these mixtures.

USES AND ABUSES OF LAXATIVES

Laxatives are of secondary importance to a fiber-rich diet and other nonpharmacological means for the prevention and treatment of constipation. Laxatives have no role in the management of constipation that results from intestinal pathology. Valid uses of these agents are few and include maintenance of soft feces, prevention of straining at the stool, and evacuation of the bowel prior to diagnostic or surgical procedures. *All laxatives are contraindicated in a patient with cramps, colic, nausea, vomiting, or other symptoms of appendicitis or any undiagnosed abdominal pain.*

Constipation. Many of the causes of functional constipation are simple to correct without the use of drugs. A fiber-rich diet, bowel training, the reminder that "haste does not make waste," adequate fluid intake, appropriate physical activity, reassurance to overcome emotional factors, and similar measures are often successful. Correction of underlying disease must not be neglected. In cases of drug-induced constipation, correction by readjustment of drug dosage or by use of alternative drugs should be attempted before resorting to concurrent laxative medication.

If nonpharmacological measures alone are inadequate, they may be supplemented by the bulk-forming agents. Stimulant laxatives should be used only in refractory cases. When laxatives are employed in the treatment of constipation, they should be administered in the lowest effective dosage as infrequently as possible, and they should be discontinued promptly and completely upon termination of the need.

Other Valid Uses. The use of laxatives is justified to prevent straining at the stool by patients with *hernia* or *cardiovascular disease*. In addition, they are frequently indicated, both before and after surgery, to maintain soft feces in patients with *hemorrhoids and other anorectal disorders*. For these purposes, dietary fiber or the bulk-forming agents are generally satisfactory and should be preferred. A fiber-rich diet and related drugs also have an established role in the management of *diverticular disease* of the colon and *irritable bowel disease*.

Stimulant or saline laxatives at cathartic doses are frequently employed prior to *radiological examination* of the gastrointestinal tract, kidneys, or other abdominal or retroperitoneal structures and prior to *elective bowel surgery*. Stimulant laxatives, taken either orally or rectally, may replace enemas for emptying the large bowel prior to *proctological examination*.

In the treatment of drug overdosage and poisoning, cathartic doses of saline laxatives (*e.g.,* sodium phosphate, 16 g; magnesium sulfate, 30 g) may be administered to remove agents from the intestine (*see* Chapter 68). Stimulant laxatives must be avoided, as must castor oil, which may enhance absorption of chlorinated hydrocarbons. Laxatives should not be used in patients who show signs of electrolyte imbalance or impaired renal function (Dreisbach, 1983). Laxatives may also be employed with certain *anthelmintics* (*see* Chapter 44).

Cathartic Colon. The prolonged and habitual use of laxatives is deplorable and unhealthy. Many individuals have unusual notions regarding the frequency, quantity, and consistency of stools necessary for health, and they readily resort to self-prescribed laxatives to achieve these goals. Even the casual use of these drugs can develop into the cathartic habit. After a thorough evacuation of the colon by a laxative, several days may elapse before a normal bowel movement can again occur. In the interim, the patient becomes convinced of constipation and again turns to the favorite remedy. After a time, bowel habits become so abnormal that there is total reliance on a daily dose of a laxative for a bowel movement.

The patient suffering from cathartic colon presents a difficult therapeutic problem. Initially, all laxatives should be discontinued, and the patient should be informed not to expect a bowel movement for several days. The underlying cause for constipation, if one exists, must be found and eliminated, and the patient's misconceptions pertaining to bowel function must be corrected. Proper diet, exercise, and bowel training must be undertaken. If necessary, a mild stimulant laxative in minimally effective dosage may be employed during the period in which reestablishment of normal colonic function and defecatory reflexes is being attempted (*see* Devroede, 1983).

Dangers of Laxative Abuse. In addition to perpetuating dependence upon drugs, the laxative habit may provide the basis for serious *gastrointestinal disturbances.* Spastic colitis and other functional ills have been traced to the habitual use of stimulant laxatives; after prolonged abuse, the appearance of the digestive tract by x-ray examination may resemble that of enterocolitis. Surreptitious ingestion of laxatives can cause signs and symptoms that are mistaken for gastrointestinal disease and lead to unnecessary surgery.

Repeated misuse of stimulant laxatives may also result in excessive *loss of water and electrolytes;* secondary aldosteronism may occur if volume depletion is prominent. Steatorrhea and protein-losing gastroenteropathy with hypoalbuminemia have been observed, as have excessive excretion of calcium in the stools and osteomalacia of the vertebral column.

Much more dangerous than the laxative habit is the practice of taking a laxative for the relief of abdominal pain. An inflamed appendix can be ruptured by the resulting intestinal motor activity, and the mortality rate of the condition is vastly increased.

Anderson, J. W., and Chen, W.-J. L. Plant fiber: carbohydrate and lipid metabolism. *Am. J. Clin. Nutr.,* **1979,** *32,* 346–363.

Behall, K. M.; Lee, K. H.; and Moser, P. B. Blood lipids and lipoproteins in adult men fed four refined fibers. *Am. J. Clin. Nutr.,* **1984,** *39,* 209–214.

Bingham, S.; Cummings, J. H.; and McNeil, N. I. Intakes and sources of dietary fiber in the British population. *Am. J. Clin. Nutr.,* **1979,** *32,* 1313–1319.

Bridges, R. J.; Nell, G.; and Rummel, W. Influence of vasopressin and calcium on electrolyte transport across isolated colonic mucosa of the rat. *J. Physiol. (Lond.),* **1983,** *338,* 463–475.

Brodribb, A. J. M. Treatment of symptomatic diverticular disease with a high-fibre diet. *Lancet,* **1977,** *1,* 664–666.

Burkitt, D. P., and Meisner, P. How to manage constipation with high-fiber diet. *Geriatrics,* **1979,** *34,* No. 2, 33–40.

Conn, H. O. Lactulose: a drug in search of a modus operandi. *Gastroenterology,* **1978,** *74,* 624–626.

Donowitz, M. Current concepts of laxative action: mechanisms by which laxatives increase stool water. *J. Clin. Gastroenterol.,* **1979,** *1,* 77–84.

Donowitz, M.; Elta, G.; Battisti, L; Fogel, R.; and Label-Schwartz, E. Effect of dopamine and bromocriptine on rat ileal and colonic transport. *Gastroenterology,* **1983,** *84,* 516–523.

Fairbairn, J. W., and Moss, M. J. R. The relative purgative activities of 1,8-dihydroxyanthracene derivatives. *J. Pharm. Pharmacol.,* **1970,** *22,* 584–593.

Goldstein, G. B.; Lam, K. C.; and Mistilis, S. P. Drug-induced active chronic hepatitis. *Am. J. Dig. Dis.,* **1973,** *18,* 177–184.

Harvey, R. F., and Read, A. E. Mode of action of the saline purgatives. *Am. Heart J.,* **1975,** *89,* 810–812.

Mendeloff, A. I. Dietary fiber and human health. *N. Engl. J. Med.,* **1977,** *297,* 811–814.

Meunier, P.; Rochas, A.; and Lambert, R. Motor activity of the sigmoid colon in chronic constipation: comparative study with normal subjects. *Gut,* **1979,** *20,* 1095–1101.

Painter, N. S., and Burkitt, D. P. Diverticular disease of the colon, a 20th century problem. *Clin. Gastroenterol.,* **1975,** *4,* 3–21.

Selvendran, R. R. The plant cell wall as a source of dietary fiber: chemistry and structure. *Am. J. Clin. Nutr.,* **1984,** *39,* 320–337.

Stephen, A. M., and Cummings, J. H. Mechanism of action of dietary fibre in the human colon. *Nature,* **1980,** *284,* 283–284.

Monographs and Reviews

Avery, G. S ; Davies, E. F.; and Brogden, R. N. Lactulose: a review of its therapeutic and pharmacological properties with particular reference to ammonia metabolism and its mode of action in portal systemic encephalopathy. *Drugs,* **1972,** *4,* 7–48.

Binder, H. J. Absorption and secretion of water and electrolytes by small and large intestine. In, *Gastrointestinal Disease,* 2nd ed. (Sleisenger, M. H., and Fordtran, J. S., eds.) W. B. Saunders Co., Philadelphia, **1983,** pp. 811–829.

Devroede, G. Constipation: mechanisms and management. In, *Gastrointestinal Disease,* 2nd ed. (Sleisenger, M. H., and Fordtran, J. S., eds.) W. B. Saunders Co., Philadelphia, **1983,** pp. 288–308.

Dreisbach, R. H. *Handbook of Poisoning,* 11th ed. Lange Medical Publications, Los Altos, Calif., **1983,** pp. 1–632.

Meredith, G. A. *The Ordeal of Richard Feverel.* (**1859;** revised in **1878.**) New American Library of World Literature, New York, **1961,** p. 13.

Racusen, L. C., and Binder, H. J. Adrenergic interaction with ion transport across colonic mucosa: role of both α- and β-adrenergic agonists. In, *Mechanisms of Intestinal Secretion.* (Binder, H. J., ed.) *Kroc Foundation Series,* Vol. 12. Alan R. Liss, Inc., New York, **1979,** pp. 201–216.

Symposium. (Various authors.) Symposia of the Giovanni Lorenzini Foundation. In, *New Trends in Pathophysiology and Therapy of the Large Bowel,* Vol. 17. (Barbara, L.; Miglioli, M.; and Phillips, S. F.; eds.) Elsevier Science Publishers, Amsterdam, **1983.**

Chemotherapy of Parasitic Diseases

INTRODUCTION

Leslie T. Webster, Jr.

Parasitic infections are a major worldwide health problem; this is particularly true in less developed countries, where these diseases also cause a substantial economic burden. The global prevalence of human parasitic infection already exceeds 50% and is increasing. Diverse factors are responsible, including population crowding; poor sanitation and health education; inadequate control of parasite vectors and reservoirs of infection; introduction of water control projects and water supply systems for agriculture; increased world travel, population migration, and military operations; and development of resistance to agents used for chemotherapy or control of vectors. Certain infections, for example, malaria, cannot be ignored because of high morbidity and mortality, but others, such as the most prevalent helminthic infections, remain neglected because their effects on human health are more subtle.

Effective and practical antiparasitic vaccines have yet to be devised, and chemotherapy is thus the most efficient and inexpensive single method to control most parasitic infections. To achieve optimal results, this approach must be combined with other measures that are appropriate for the particular infection, environment, and host populations. Effective and safe drugs are still needed to prevent or treat some major parasitic infections, for example, leishmaniasis and trypanosomiasis; other pharmaceuticals, for example, the antimalarials, are losing their utility because of the development of drug resistance. Continuous research and clinical surveillance are thus required to provide a steady supply of improved antiparasitic agents and to detect possible drug interactions, long-term drug toxicity, rare but serious drug-associated reactions, and resistance to drugs.

To be used for chemotherapy in human populations, an ideal antiparasitic agent would have a high therapeutic ratio; be easily given, preferably by the oral route in a single dose or divided doses on the same day; be chemically stable for long periods under climatic conditions encountered in regions of use; be free of problems such as the development of resistance; and be inexpensive. Few antiparasitic drugs meet all of these criteria.

Most antiparasitic agents have been discovered and developed by the synthesis and screening of many compounds for efficacy against pathogenic parasites in appropriate animal models. Attempts have also been made to identify and exploit important biological differences between parasite and host. The latter approach demands increased understanding of the basic biochemistry, physiology, and cell and molecular biology of parasites and of their interactions with their hosts. Improvement of methods to maintain parasites *in vitro* and to screen compounds *in vitro* and *in vivo* for antiparasitic activity has accelerated this process. However, the crucial test remains the demonstration of efficacy and safety of a given drug in man. Careful clinical pharmacological and pharmacokinetic studies of rela-

Table XI–1. DRUGS FOR CHEMOTHERAPY OF PARASITIC INFECTIONS

The recommendations presented here represent the best judgment not only of the author but also of several authorities in the United States and abroad. However, this field is a dynamic one; in time, certain of these recommendations will require modification not only in the order of choice but also in the specific drugs that are recommended.

INFECTION AND PARASITE	DRUG ORDER OF CHOICE		COMMENTS
	1st	*2nd*	
I. PROTOZOAN INFEC-TIONS			
Amebiasis			
Entamoeba histolytica Asymptomatic ame-biasis	Diloxanide furoate [1]	—	Although effective, iodo-quinol is *not* recom-mended because of potential toxicity (*see* Chapter 46)
Intestinal and sys-temic amebiasis, including amebic abscesses	Metronidazole plus diloxanide furoate [1] subsequently	—	
Balantidiasis			
Balantidium coli	Tetracycline	—	—
Giardiasis			
Giardia lamblia	Quinacrine or metronida-zole [3]	—	Tinidazole [2], in a single dose of 2 g for adults, is also effective
Leishmaniasis			
Leishmania brazili-ensis and *L. mexicana* American mucocuta-neous and cutane-ous leishmaniasis	Stibogluconate sodium [1]	Amphotericin B	Amphotericin B is used when antimonials are ineffective or contrain-dicated
L. donovani Visceral leishmania-sis (kala azar)	Stibogluconate sodium [1]	Pentamidine isethionate	Pentamidine is used when antimonials are ineffec-tive or contraindicated
L. tropica Cutaneous leishman-iasis (oriental sore)	Stibogluconate sodium [1]	—	—
Malaria			
Infections with chlo-roquine-sensitive *Plasmodium fal-ciparum; P. ma-lariae; P. ovale; P. vivax*	Chloroquine phosphate	—	Used for both prophy-laxis and treatment of uncomplicated attacks; chloroquine HCl can be used parenterally in adults who cannot take oral medication
Infections with *P. vivax* and *P. ovale*	Primaquine phosphate after chloroquine phos-phate	—	Used to prevent attacks after departure from an endemic area or to ef-fect a "radical" cure
Infections with chlo-roquine-resistant or multidrug-resis-tant *P. falciparum*			
a. Prophylaxis	Pyrimethamine-sul-fadoxine and chloro-quine phosphate	Mefloquine [2,3,4] and pyri-methamine-sulfadoxine	Some strains are resistant to pyrimethamine-sul-fadoxine; use of chlo-roquine is controversial (*see* Chapter 45)

Table XI–1. DRUGS FOR CHEMOTHERAPY OF PARASITIC INFECTIONS (Continued)

INFECTION AND PARASITE	DRUG ORDER OF CHOICE		COMMENTS
	1st	*2nd*	
b. Treatment	Quinine sulfate orally or quinine dihydrochloride [1] intravenously, plus pyrimethamine-sulfadiazine	Quinine plus tetracycline [3] or mefloquine [2,3,4] plus pyrimethamine-sulfadiazine	In an emergency, quinidine [3,4] may be substituted for quinine dihydrochloride; mefloquine [2,3,4] can only be given orally (*see* Chapter 45)
Pneumocystosis			
Pneumocystis carinii	Trimethoprim-sulfamethoxazole	Pentamidine isethionate	Trimethoprim-sulfamethoxazole appears safer and more effective than pentamidine
Trichomoniasis			
Trichomonas vaginalis	Metronidazole	—	Both sexual partners should be treated
Trypanosomiasis			
Trypanosoma cruzi South American trypanosomiasis (Chagas' disease)	Nifurtimox [1]	—	More effective in acute than in chronic infection
T. rhodesiense; T. gambiense African trypanosomiasis (sleeping sickness)			
a. No CNS involvement (early stage)	Suramin [1]	Pentamidine isethionate	Pentamidine is used only for *T. gambiense*
b. CNS involvement (late stage)	Suramin [1] followed by melarsoprol [1]	—	
II. METAZOAN (HELMINTH) INFECTIONS			
A. NEMATODE (ROUNDWORM) INFECTIONS			
Ascariasis			
Ascaris lumbricoides	Mebendazole or pyrantel pamoate or levamisole [2]	Piperazine citrate	Mebendazole is preferred for polyinfections with *Ascaris*, hookworms, and *Trichuris*
Capillariasis			
Capillaria philippinensis	Mebendazole [3,4]	—	—
Dracunculiasis			
Dracunculus medinensis (guinea worm infection)	Niridazole [1]	Metronidazole [3,4]	Niridazole is contraindicated in patients with CNS disturbances or severe hepatic disease
Enterobiasis			
Enterobius (Oxyuris) vermicularis (pinworm infection)	Mebendazole or pyrantel pamoate	—	Mebendazole is preferred for polyinfections with *Ascaris*, hookworms, and *Trichuris*

Table XI–1. DRUGS FOR CHEMOTHERAPY OF PARASITIC INFECTIONS (Continued)

INFECTION AND PARASITE	DRUG ORDER OF CHOICE		COMMENTS
	1st	*2nd*	
Filariasis			
Wuchereria bancrofti, Brugia (W.) malayi, Dipetalonema perstans, Loa loa	Diethylcarbamazine	—	—
Onchocerca volvulus	Diethylcarbamazine followed by suramin	Mebendazole [4]	Benzimidazole carbamates may be combined with diethylcarbamazine [4]
Hookworm Infections			
Necator americanus Ancylostoma duodenale	Mebendazole or pyrantel pamoate [3]	—	Mebendazole is preferred for polyparasitic infections; levamisole appears to be effective against *A. duodenale* [4]
Cutaneous larva migrans	Thiabendazole	—	—
Strongyloidiasis			
Strongyloides stercoralis	Thiabendazole	Mebendazole [4]	Immunosuppressed patients are especially at risk
Toxocariasis			
Toxocara species Visceral larva migrans	Thiabendazole or diethylcarbamazine	—	Efficacy is questionable
Trichinosis			
Trichinella spiralis	Thiabendazole	Mebendazole [3,4]	In man, efficacy is questionable, particularly against larvae in tissue
Trichuriasis			
Trichuris trichiura (whipworm infection)	Mebendazole	Oxantel [2] or pyrantel [2] pamoate; thiabendazole	Mebendazole is preferred for polyparasitic infections
B. Cestode (Tapeworm) Infections			
Taeniasis			
Taenia saginata (beef tapeworm)	Niclosamide or praziquantel [3]	—	—
Taenia solium (pork tapeworm)	Praziquantel [3]	Niclosamide	Praziquantel is preferred for *T. solium* because of the danger of cysticercosis
Diphyllobothriasis			
Diphyllobothrium latum (fish tapeworm)	Niclosamide or praziquantel [3]	—	—
Hymenolepiasis			
Hymenolepis nana (dwarf tapeworm)	Niclosamide or praziquantel [3]	—	—

Table XI–1. DRUGS FOR CHEMOTHERAPY OF PARASITIC INFECTIONS (Continued)

INFECTION AND PARASITE	DRUG ORDER OF CHOICE		COMMENTS
	1st	*2nd*	
Echinococcosis			
Echinococcus granulosus Cystic hydatid disease or hydatidosis	Mebendazole [4]	—	Surgical resection is recommended first
Echinococcus multilocularis Alveolar hydatid disease	Mebendazole [4]	—	Surgical resection is recommended first; mebendazole is *not* larvicidal, and efficacy is questionable
C. TREMATODE (FLUKE) INFECTIONS			
Blood Fluke Infections (Schistosomiasis)			
Schistosoma haematobium	Praziquantel	Metrifonate [1]	Niridazole is contraindicated in patients with CNS disturbances or severe hepatic disease
S. japonicum	Praziquantel	Niridazole [1]	
S. mansoni	Praziquantel	Oxamniquine	
S. mekongi	Praziquantel	—	
S. intercalatum	Praziquantel	—	
Intestinal Fluke Infections			
Fasciolopsis buski, Heterophyes heterophyes, Metagonimus yokogawai	Praziquantel [3,4]	—	—
Liver Fluke Infections			
Clonorchis sinensis, Opisthorchis felineus, Opisthorchis viverrini	Praziquantel [3]	—	—
Fasciola hepatica	Praziquantel [3,4]	—	—
Lung Fluke Infections (Paragonimiasis)			
Paragonimus species, *P. westermani, P. kellicotti*	Praziquantel [3,4]	—	—

[1] Available from the Parasitic Disease Drug Service, Center for Infectious Disease, Centers for Disease Control, Atlanta, Georgia 30333. *Telephone:* 404-329-3670; 404-329-2888 (evenings, weekends, holidays).
[2] Not available in the United States.
[3] Considered investigational for this use in the United States.
[4] Limited data.

tively few patients in major endemic areas of infection should be conducted to determine the feasibility and optimal dosage regimens for chemotherapy. Population-based chemotherapy would ideally be instituted only after appropriate parasitological and epidemiological studies have been conducted to determine patterns of transmission and both the age-specific prevalence and intensity of infection as these variables relate to disease. Analysis of such patterns after periodic follow-up observations should improve the chemotherapy of parasitic infections.

The major parasitic infections of man and the agents currently favored for their prophylaxis or treatment are listed in Table XI–1; the pharmacology of anthelmintic and antiprotozoal drugs is presented in Chapters 44 to 47. Treatment of infections with ectoparasites is not considered, nor is comprehensive or exhaustive coverage of the chemotherapy of human parasitic infections intended. In addition to the current medical and scientific literature, authoritative information about this subject can be obtained from the Centers for Disease Control, Atlanta, Georgia 30333, and the World Health Organization.

Albert, A. *Selective Toxicity: The Physico-Chemical Basis of Therapy*, 6th ed. Chapman & Hall, Ltd., London, **1979.**

Anderson, R. M., and May, R. M. Population dynamics of human helminth infections: control by chemotherapy. *Nature*, **1982,** *297,* 557–563.

Martindale: The Extra Pharmacopoeia, 28th ed. The Pharmaceutical Press, London, **1982.**

Warren, K. S., and Mahmoud, A. A. F. *Tropical and Geographic Medicine*. McGraw-Hill Book Co., New York, **1984.**

World Health Organization. *Intestinal Protozoan and Helminthic Infections*. Technical Report No. 666, WHO, Geneva, **1981.**

CHAPTER

44 DRUGS USED IN THE CHEMOTHERAPY OF HELMINTHIASIS

Leslie T. Webster, Jr.

Anthelmintics are drugs used to rid the body of parasitic worms known as helminths. These drugs are of great importance because helminthiasis is the most common disease in the world. More than 2 billion people are hosts to various types of worms, and this number is increasing. For example, with increased agricultural use of land and artificial irrigation, multiplication of aquatic snails has occurred in endemic areas. This has led to a marked increase in the number of people infected with schistosomes. Infection with more than one type of helminth is common in many tropical regions. Furthermore, as a result of human migration and travel, worms may appear in geographical locations where previously they had been unknown.

The term *anthelmintic* is not restricted to drugs that act locally to expel worms from the *gastrointestinal tract*. Several types of worms penetrate *tissues*, and drugs used to combat such systemic infections are also termed *anthelmintics*.

Worms parasitic for man are Metazoa that belong to widely different zoological species. These organisms vary with respect to bodily structure, physiology, habitat in the human host, and susceptibility to chemotherapy. Because of substantial progress in the discovery and development of drugs, particularly in veterinary medicine, the physician now has effective agents that will cure or control most human infections caused by intestinal helminths. Improved drugs are still badly needed to treat several types of systemic helminthiasis, for example, *echinococcosis, filariasis*, and *trichinosis*. The availability of more selective and safer anthelmintics places greater responsibility on the physician to make an accurate diagnosis and prescribe proper therapy. Physicians and technicians who lack experience in the analysis of biological specimens for pathogenic parasites should have their findings corroborated by an expert.

In the following presentation, individual anthelmintics are presented in *alphabetical order,* without regard to their relative importance or therapeutic application. Treatment of specific common helminthic infections is then discussed briefly.

ANTIMONY COMPOUNDS

Trivalent antimonial compounds, such as *antimony potassium tartrate,* are no longer recommended for the treatment of helminth infections because of their unacceptable toxicity and difficulty of administration in comparison with newer chemotherapeutic agents. The pharmacology of these drugs is presented in *earlier editions* of this textbook. *Sodium stibogluconate,* a pentavalent antimonial used to treat *leishmaniasis,* is discussed in Chapter 47.

BEPHENIUM HYDROXYNAPHTHOATE

Bephenium, originally developed for the treatment of hookworm infections, has largely been replaced by other chemotherapeutic agents for this purpose (*see* Table XI–1). The drug has reported clinical efficacy against infections with *Ascaris lumbricoides* and *Trichostrongylus orientalis.* The pharmacology of bephenium is presented in *earlier editions* of this textbook.

DIETHYLCARBAMAZINE

During World War II, over 15,000 cases of filariasis occurred in American military personnel quartered on the islands of the Western Pacific. This stimulated the search for effective filaricides. The most promising group of antifilarial compounds to emerge were piperazine derivatives, of which *diethylcarbamazine* is the most important (Hewitt *et al.,* 1948; Hawking, 1979; Van den Bossche, 1981).

Chemistry. *Diethylcarbamazine* has the following structural formula:

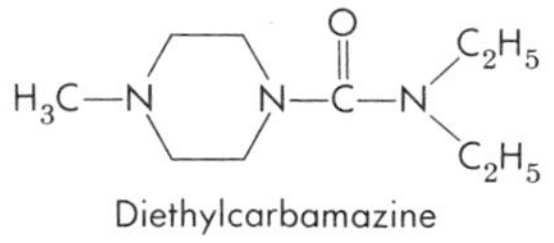

Diethylcarbamazine

The drug is marketed as the dicitrate salt, a colorless, crystalline solid, highly soluble in water.

Anthelmintic Action. Diethylcarbamazine causes rapid disappearance of microfilariae of *Wuchereria bancrofti, W. (Brugia) malayi,* and *Loa loa* from the blood of man. The drug causes microfilariae of *Onchocerca volvulus* to disappear from the skin but does not kill microfilariae in nodules that contain the adult (female) worms. It does not affect the microfilariae of *W. bancrofti* in a hydrocele, despite penetration into the fluid. The drug has two types of action on susceptible microfilariae. The first is to decrease the muscular activity and eventually immobilize the organisms; this may result from a hyperpolarizing effect of the piperazine moiety, and it causes dislocation of the parasites from their normal habitat in the host (Langham and Kramer, 1980). The second action is to produce alterations in the microfilarial surface membranes, thereby rendering them more susceptible to destruction by host defense mechanisms (*see* Hawking, 1979; Van den Bossche, 1981). There is definite evidence that diethylcarbamazine kills adult worms of *Loa loa* and presumptive evidence that it kills adult *W. bancrofti* and *W. malayi.* However, it has little action against adult *O. volvulus.* The mechanism of the filaricidal action of diethylcarbamazine is unknown (*see* Hawking, 1979).

Absorption, Fate, and Excretion. Diethylcarbamazine is readily absorbed from the gastrointestinal tract. After a single oral dose of 200 to 400 mg, the concentration in plasma peaks in 1 to 2 hours; the plasma half-life is about 8 hours after a 200-mg dose and 12 hours after an 800-mg dose (Ree *et al.,* 1978). Metabolism of diethylcarbamazine is both rapid and extensive (Faulkner and Smith, 1972). Excretion is nearly all urinary, and more than 70% of the drug appears as metabolites. The compound is distributed almost equally throughout all body compartments with the exception of fat. Little accumulation occurs when repeated doses are given.

Preparation, Route of Administration, and Dosage. *Diethylcarbamazine citrate* (HETRAZAN) is available as tablets, each containing 50 mg. The product is stable even under conditions of high temperature and humidity. The dosage of diethylcarbamazine used to treat filarial disease has varied considerably, and suggested dosage regimens may be modified effectively according to local experience.
Wuchereria bancrofti, W. malayi. For mass treatment with the objective of reducing microfilaremia to subinfective levels for mosquitoes, the dose is 2 mg/kg, three times daily after meals, for 7 days; for treatment directed toward possible cure, this dosage regimen is carried out for 10 to 30 days. Much experience has shown that, if people can be

persuaded to take an adequate amount of diethyl-carbamazine, the microfilariae and probably some of the adult worms will be destroyed. For practical purposes, an adequate amount seems to be a total dose of about 72 mg/kg of the citrate salt. The period over which this amount is administered has varied from area to area; spaced, low weekly doses of 6 mg/kg for prolonged periods produce as good an effect as high daily or monthly doses, and are less likely to cause adverse reactions (World Health Organization, 1967; Partono *et al.*, 1981).

Loa loa. A dose of 2 mg/kg should be given three times daily after meals for 2 to 3 weeks. If repeated courses are required to produce cure, they should be separated by periods of 3 to 4 weeks.

Onchocerca volvulus. Treatment is effective in removing microfilariae from the skin; however, they usually return after some weeks because the adult worms are not killed. It may be possible to hold both forms in check by periodic short courses of treatment. When lesions of the eye are present, the initial dose of diethylcarbamazine should not exceed 0.5 mg/kg. This is given once on the first day and twice on the second. The dose is then increased to 1 mg/kg, three times daily for the third day, and therapy is continued up to a total of 14 days with a dose of 2 to 3 mg/kg in two divided doses each day.

In patients infected with *O. volvulus* or *W. malayi,* and to a lesser extent in those infected with *W. bancrofti* and *Loa loa,* the initial systemic reactions provoked by the massive destruction of microfilariae, macrofilariae, or both during treatment may be severe. In such cases the dosage should be lowered or the drug stopped temporarily. Relief of these symptoms in heavily infected individuals may be afforded by pretreatment with corticosteroids, for example, dexamethasone (2 to 4 mg twice daily) (Greene, 1984). Once the initial reactions have subsided, continued treatment should not provoke a further series of reactions.

Toxicity and Side Effects. Untoward direct reactions to diethylcarbamazine, although fairly frequent, are not severe and usually disappear within a few days despite continuation of therapy. These include headache, general malaise, weakness, joint pains, anorexia, nausea, and vomiting. Other adverse effects result directly or indirectly from destruction of the parasites. These are especially severe in patients heavily infected with *O. volvulus.* In *W. malayi* or *Loa loa* infections, reactions are usually milder, although the drug may induce severe encephalitis in *Loa loa.* In patients with onchocerciasis, there is usually a typical reaction within 16 hours after the first oral dose. This consists in intense itching and skin rashes, enlargement and

tenderness of the inguinal lymph nodes, sometimes a fine papular rash, hyperpyrexia, tachycardia, and headache. These symptoms persist for 3 to 7 days and then subside, after which quite high doses can be tolerated. Ocular complications include limbitis, punctate keratitis, uveitis, and atrophy of the retinal pigment epithelium (Rivas-Alcala *et al.*, 1981; Dominguez-Vazquez *et al.*, 1983). Nodular swellings may occur along the course of the lymphatics, and there is often an accompanying lymphadenitis. This reaction also subsides within a few days. Almost all patients receiving therapy exhibit a leukocytosis, first evident on the second day, reaching its peak on the fourth or fifth day, and gradually subsiding over a period of a few weeks. Reversible proteinuria may occur, and the eosinophilia frequently observed in patients with filariasis can be intensified by drug therapy.

Precautions and Contraindications. There are no contraindications to the use of diethylcarbamazine, other than the fact that low doses should be used for initial therapy, especially in onchocerciasis and infection due to *Loa loa* (to minimize adverse reactions to destruction of the parasites). As mentioned, pretreatment with corticosteroids may be undertaken to minimize such reactions (Greene, 1984). These may be especially severe in patients with mixed infections due to *O. volvulus* and *Loa loa.*

Therapeutic Uses. Diethylcarbamazine can be used effectively to treat infections caused by *W. bancrofti, W. malayi, Loa loa,* and *O. volvulus.* In the first three, radical cure can be achieved by either single or multiple courses of treatment. In onchocerciasis, radical cure is unlikely because the drug fails to kill the adult worms. Control can be achieved by short periodic courses of treatment. The drug has also been used effectively to treat filariasis due to *Tetrapetalonema perstans* or *Tetrapetalonema streptocerca* (Ottesen, 1984). In patients with *eosinophilic lung (tropical eosinophilia),* treatment with diethylcarbamazine causes a rapid disappearance of symptoms. This, and the finding of microfilariae in lung biopsies, suggest an association between filariasis and certain pulmonary syndromes. Diethylcarbamazine is also effective in clearing *Ascaris* infections, but it has been replaced by other agents for this purpose.

HYCANTHONE

Hycanthone, a thioxanthone analog developed from *lucanthone,* is effective in treating human schistosomiasis caused by the trematodes *Schistosoma haematobium* and *S. mansoni*. However, clinical use of this compound has been sharply reduced because of reports that it is mutagenic and carcinogenic (*see* Batzinger and Bueding, 1977). Hycanthone is not discussed further because it has been replaced by other effective antischistosomal agents (*see* Table XI–1). Information about hycanthone is available in *previous editions* of this textbook.

LEVAMISOLE

Tetramisole evolved from an extensive search of over 2700 heterocyclic compounds for a novel broad-spectrum anthelmintic for veterinary use. Modification of the chemical structure of the active metabolite of a compound that produced positive results in anthelmintic screens led to the identification of tetramisole. *Levamisole,* the S(-) isomer of tetramisole, accounts for most of the anthelmintic activity of the racemate (*see* Janssen, 1976). It has the following structural formula:

Levamisole

Anthelmintic and Immunomodulatory Actions. Levamisole is toxic to a broad range of gastrointestinal and systemic nematodes that infect man and animals (*see* Janssen, 1976). Of particular clinical interest in man is the drug's action against *Ascaris*; the compound also has activity against hookworm species, *Strongyloides* larvae, and microfilariae. It shows little effect on infections with *Trichuris* and *Enterobius*. Levamisole produces contraction of nematodes, succeeded by tonic paralysis. Reversible stimulation of ganglionic structures is followed by a depolarizing type of neuromuscular blockade (Van Neuten, 1972; Coles *et al.,* 1974). Levamisole also increases the resting potential of isolated muscle from *Ascaris* (Van den Bossche, 1980). Levamisole inhibits fumarate reductase from *Ascaris* muscle; the racemate, tetramisole, is less potent in this respect. Such inhibition is compatible with the greater anthelmintic potency of levamisole and may contribute to its antiparasitic effect. Levamisole (1 μM) also causes a stereospecific inhibition of human alkaline phosphatases, except for those in the intestine and placenta (Van Belle, 1976).

Levamisole has been shown to be an immunostimulant in both experimental animals and man (*see* Renoux, 1980), and it has been used as an adjunct for therapy of certain chronic and recurrent infections, rheumatoid arthritis, and immunosuppressed states, including those associated with malignancies (*see* reviews by Brugmans, 1978; Chirigos, 1978). It appears to act by restoring cell-mediated immune mechanisms of peripheral leukocytes; precursor T lymphocytes are also stimulated to differentiate into mature T cells (Symoens and Rosenthal, 1977; Renoux, 1980).

Absorption, Fate, and Excretion. After a 150-mg oral dose in an adult, levamisole is rapidly and completely absorbed, reaching peak concentrations in plasma of about 0.7 μg/ml after 1 to 2 hours. The drug is extensively metabolized by the liver and completely eliminated in the urine and feces within 48 hours. The half-life of levamisole in plasma is about 4 hours, while that of its metabolites averages 16 hours (Symoens and Rosenthal, 1977). Urinary excretion of unchanged levamisole is low and is inversely proportional to pH, as expected for a weak base. A major metabolite that results from opening of the thiazole ring may account for some of the immunopharmacological effects of levamisole (*see* Symoens *et al.,* 1979; Renoux, 1980).

Toxicity and Side Effects. At the low doses used for *Ascaris* infections, levamisole produces few side effects in otherwise-normal individuals. Minor drug-associated disturbances referable to the gastrointestinal tract and central nervous system (CNS) include nausea, vomiting, abdominal distress, fatigue, headache, dizziness, insomnia, and confusion. More significant adverse reactions include reversible agranulocytosis, skin rashes, and febrile illnesses. These are more likely to occur at the higher doses that are used for immunoprophylaxis or immunotherapy (*see* Symoens *et al.,* 1978).

Therapeutic Uses and Dosage. The antiparasitic uses of levamisole have been reviewed by Miller (1980). It is a good drug for the treatment and control of *Ascaris* infections, where a single dose of 50 to 150 mg may eliminate all parasites in 90 to 100% of infected patients. Although clinical efficacy has been demonstrated against hookworms, particularly with multiple-dose regimens, an optimal dosage schedule has yet to be established. The use of this drug in strongyloidiasis, filariasis, and leishmaniasis is still investigational. Levamisole is available as the hydrochloride in certain countries; the drug is not approved for clinical use in the United States.

MEBENDAZOLE

Mebendazole was introduced for the treatment of roundworm infections as a result of research carried out by Brugmans and collaborators (1971). It is the prototype of a number of benzimidazole derivatives, including *albendazole* and *flubendazole,* which were developed as broad-spectrum anthelmintics for animal and human use (*see* review by Van den Bossche *et al.,* 1982).

Chemistry. *Mebendazole* has the following structural formula:

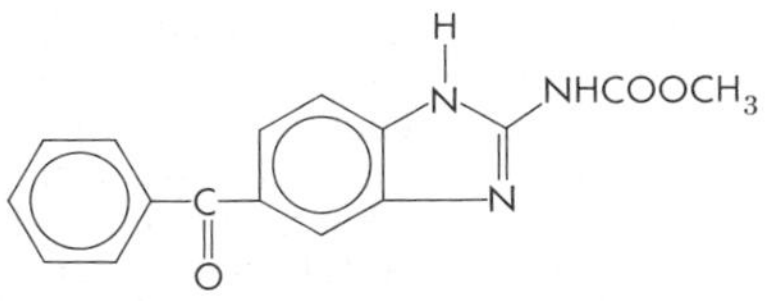

Mebendazole

It is a yellowish amorphous powder, very slightly soluble in water and most organic solvents, and not unpleasant to taste.

Anthelmintic Action.   Mebendazole is an extremely versatile anthelmintic agent. It is highly effective against *ascariasis, intestinal capillariasis, enterobiasis, trichuriasis,* and *hookworm infection* as single or mixed infections. Variable results have been obtained against *Strongyloides stercoralis.* It has shown promise in the treatment of *hydatid disease, trichinosis,* and *onchocerciasis;* in infections with the filarial worm *Tetrapetalonema perstans;* and with both beef and pork tapeworms (Keystone and Murdoch, 1979; Wahlagren and Frolov, 1983). The drug causes selective disappearance of cytoplasmic microtubules in the tegumental and intestinal cells of affected worms. Secretory substances accumulate in Golgi areas, secretion of acetylcholinesterase and uptake of glucose are impaired, and glycogen is depleted. These effects of the drug are not noted in host cells. Although mebendazole has a high affinity for parasite tubulin *in vitro,* the drug also binds to host tubulin; the biochemical basis for its selective action is thus unclear (*see* Van den Bossche, 1981; Watts *et al.,* 1982).

Immobilization and death of the parasites occur slowly, and clearance from the gastrointestinal tract may not be complete until 3 days after treatment with mebendazole. The drug inhibits the development of larval hookworms *in vitro* at a concentration of 50 μg/ml, but much higher concentrations have no effect on fully formed larvae. Shortly after treatment is started, eggs of *Trichuris* and hookworms fail to develop to the larval stage (Wagner and Chavarria, 1974). (*See also* Miller *et al.,* 1974; Wolfe and Wershing, 1974.)

Absorption, Fate, and Excretion.   Only a small fraction of an oral dose of mebendazole is absorbed, concentrations in plasma are low, and up to 10% may be recovered in the urine within 48 hours. Most of the material excreted in the urine is the decarboxylated metabolite.

Preparation, Route of Administration, and Dosage. *Mebendazole* (VERMOX) is available as chewable tablets, each containing 100 mg of the drug. Mebendazole is given orally, and the same dosage schedule applies to adults and children. For control of enterobiasis, a single 100-mg tablet is given; a second should be given after 2 weeks. For control of ascariasis, trichuriasis, and hookworm infection, 100 mg is administered morning and evening on 3 consecutive days. If the patient is not cured 3 weeks after treatment, a second course should be given. Fasting or purging is not required.

Infections with *Capillaria philippinensis* are more resistant to treatment; 400 mg of the drug should be given per day in divided doses for at least 20 days. The drug has caused complete regression of intrahepatic hydatid cysts when given in a course of 400 to 600 mg three times a day for 21 to 30 days.

Toxicity and Side Effects.   Probably as a result of its poor absorption, mebendazole has not caused systemic toxicity in routine clinical use, even in the presence of anemia and malnutrition. Transient symptoms of abdominal pain and diarrhea have occurred in cases of massive infestation and expulsion of worms. Side effects in a few patients treated with high doses include allergic reactions, alopecia, and reversible neutropenia (*see* Schantz *et al.,* 1982). Embryotoxic and teratogenic effects may occur in pregnant rats at single oral doses as low as 10 mg/kg. *Flubendazole,* a related effective anthelmintic, has no teratogenic effects in rats or in rabbits (Thienpont *et al.,* 1978).

Precautions and Contraindications.   Mebendazole should not be given to pregnant women, nor should it be used in patients who have experienced allergic reactions to the agent.

Therapeutic Uses. Mebendazole is the drug of choice in the treatment of *Trichuris trichiura.* It produces a large proportion of cures and, in those not cured with a first course of treatment, a marked reduction in egg production. It is also the drug of choice for infection with *Ancylostoma duodenale.* It is particularly valuable in the treatment of double or triple infections since it also has high activity, and is a highly recommended alternative to pyrantel pamoate, against *ascariasis, enterobiasis,* and *Necator americanus* infection (Chavarria *et al.,* 1973; Sargent *et al.,* 1974). In the Philippines, mebendazole has been used in high dosage successfully in the treatment of intestinal capillariasis (Singson *et al.*, 1975). In even higher dosage successful cure of hydatid disease has been achieved, but surgery is often required and additional clinical evaluation is necessary (Schantz *et al.*, 1982). Drugs of the benzimidazole class are currently being tested clinically for treatment of *onchocerciasis*.

METRIFONATE

Metrifonate (BILARCIL) is an organophosphorus inhibitor of cholinesterases, used first as an insecticide (DIPTEREX, DYLOX) and later as an anthelmintic. The original trials in man arose from the hope that the anticholinesterase activity of organophosphorus compounds in arthropods would extend to other invertebrates, including the helminths. Metrifonate was selected for trial on the basis of *in-vitro* tests carried out with *Ascaris lumbricoides*. In 1962 it was shown to have high anthelmintic activity in several different human infections. The substance has the following structural formula:

Metrifonate

Metrifonate undergoes extensive metabolism *in vivo*, and it also rearranges spontaneously at physiological pH to form *dichlorvos* (2,2-dichlorovinyl dimethyl phosphate, DDVP); this metabolite is probably responsible for inhibition of acetylcholinesterase (Reiner *et al.*, 1975; Symposium, 1981b). This effect alone is unlikely to explain the antischistosomal properties of metrifonate (Bloom, 1981). *In vitro*, the drug is about equipotent as an inhibitor of acetylcholinesterase in *S. mansoni* and *S. haematobium*, yet clinically it is effective only against infeçtion with *S. haematobium*. Location of *S. haematobium* in the vesical plexus rather than in the mesenteric venous plexus in man may be an important determinant of the clinical efficacy of metrifonate (Omer and Teesdale, 1978; Feldmeier *et al.*, 1982).

Peak concentrations in plasma of metrifonate (30 μM) and of dichlorvos (0.3 μM) are reached within an hour after a single oral dose of metrifonate (10 mg/kg). The half-life of both compounds in plasma is about 1.5 hours (Nordgren *et al.*, 1981); this value is similar to that found for the spontaneous disappearance of metrifonate at physiological pH (Reiner, 1981). Once formed, dichlorvos is rapidly metabolized in the plasma as well as by schistosomal arylesterases (Reiner *et al.*, 1980).

Given in therapeutic doses, metrifonate produces rapid and almost complete inhibition of plasma cholinesterase activity of the host; this recovers to almost normal levels within a few weeks of stopping treatment. Erythrocyte acetylcholinesterase is inhibited to a lesser degree but recovers more slowly (Nordgren *et al.*, 1981). Despite these

changes, the drug is well tolerated. Side effects such as mild vertigo, lassitude, nausea, and colic are dose related and occur infrequently. Treated individuals should, of course, be free from recent exposure to insecticides that might add to the anticholinesterase effect and not receive depolarizing neuromuscular blocking agents for at least 48 hours after treatment.

Metrifonate is recommended only for the treatment of *S. haematobium* infection. Its low cost, effectiveness, and ready acceptance have given it an important role in the treatment of urinary schistosomiasis in North and East Africa. The dose employed is 5 to 15 mg/kg, given orally three times at intervals of 2 weeks. Successful prophylaxis has been carried out in a highly endemic area with a dosage of 7.5 mg/kg, given once every 4 weeks (Jewsbury *et al.*, 1977). In the United States, metrifonate is available only from the Parasitic Disease Drug Service of the Centers for Disease Control.

NICLOSAMIDE

Niclosamide is a halogenated salicylanilide derivative that was introduced as a taeniacide after laboratory trials in rats with *Hymenolepis diminuta* (Gönnert and Schraufstätter, 1960). Impressive evidence of its high activity and safety has accumulated, and it is generally regarded as a very effective agent for treating most infections with cestodes in animals and man (Keeling 1968).

Chemistry. Niclosamide has the following structural formula:

Niclosamide

It is tasteless, odorless, and insoluble in water.

Anthelmintic Action. Niclosamide has prominent activity against most of the cestodes that infect man; *Enterobius (Oxyuris) vermicularis* is also susceptible. Little drug enters *H. diminuta in vitro*, unless a homogenate of intestine is added. At low concentrations, niclosamide stimulates oxygen uptake by *H. diminuta*, but at higher concentrations respiration is inhibited and glucose uptake is blocked. The principal action of the drug may be to inhibit anaerobic phosphorylation of adenosine diphosphate (ADP) by the mitochondria of the parasite, an energy-producing process that is dependent on CO_2 fixation (Scheibel and Saz, 1966; Scheibel *et al.*, 1968). Worms affected by the drug either in the gut or *in vitro* deteriorate, such that the scolex and segments may be partially digested and unrecognizable.

Preparation, Route of Administration, and Dosage. *Niclosamide* (NICLOCIDE) is supplied in 500-mg chewable tablets. The drug is given orally in a single dose, usually after fasting; those with chronic constipation should be given a laxative before administering the drug. The recommended dose for an adult is 2 g, the tablets to be chewed thoroughly and washed down with a small amount of water. The dosage for children who weigh between 11 and 34 kg is 1 g and for children under 2 years, 0.5 g. For small children it is advisable to grind the tablets as finely as possible and to mix the powder with a little water. A purge may be given 2 hours after the dose in the hope of obtaining less damaged lengths of the worm and an identifiable scolex.

In infections with *H. nana*, which are usually multiple, the recommended dose of 2 g should be taken once daily for 7 days after breakfast. Discharge of intestinal mucus can be promoted by the administration of sour fruit juices. Worms lodging under accumulations of mucus thus become more readily accessible to the drug.

Toxicity and Side Effects. Niclosamide is quite free of undesirable effects other than very occasional gastrointestinal upset. Very little is absorbed from the gastrointestinal tract, and the drug has no direct irritant effect. No side effects were observed when niclosamide was given to debilitated or pregnant patients (Gönnert and Schraufstätter, 1960). Follow-up studies showed no alteration in hepatic or renal function or in blood counts of treated patients (Abdallah and Saif, 1961).

Precautions and Contraindications. There are no contraindications to the use of niclosamide as a taeniacide. However, it is important to note that the lethal action of the drug against the adult worm does not extend to the ova. Thus, use of niclosamide in *Taenia solium* infections may expose the patient to the risk of *cysticercosis*, since, following digestion of the dead segments, viable ova will be liberated into the lumen of the gut. It is mandatory to give an adequate purge within 1 to 2 hours after the drug has been given, to clear the bowel of all dead segments before they can be digested. In *T. saginata* infections in which there is no risk of cysticercosis, purging is unnecessary unless immediate proof of cure by finding the scolex is desired.

Therapeutic Uses. Niclosamide can be considered an agent of choice in the treatment of *Diphyllobothrium latum, H. nana, T. saginata,* and most other human intestinal cestode infections (Brown, 1968; Jones, 1979). It is also very effective in the treatment of *T. solium* infection, but the danger of cysticercosis following its administration makes praziquantel the preferred drug for this condition. The ready acceptance of niclosamide by patients, together with the fact that fasting is not necessary, makes it valuable, particularly in the treatment of children.

NIRIDAZOLE

Chemistry. *Niridazole* was developed from the synthesis of a large number of nitrothiazole derivatives. The nitrothiazole nucleus was chosen because heterocyclic compounds bearing a nitro group as a characteristic substituent occupy an important position in chemotherapy. Niridazole has the following structural formula:

Niridazole

The substance is a yellow crystalline powder that is odorless and tasteless. It is sparingly soluble in water and most organic solvents.

Antiparasitic Action. Niridazole is schistosomicidal and amebicidal and also acts against a variety of anaerobic and facultatively anaerobic bacteria. Female schistosomes are more susceptible to the drug than are males; pathological effects are first noted in the gonads of both sexes. Enzymatic reduction of the nitro group of niridazole by the organism is required for antiparasitic activity. Chemically reactive forms of niridazole bind covalently to macromolecules of *S. mansoni,* and the nonprotein thiol content of the parasite becomes decreased (Tracy *et al.,* 1983).

Other Actions. Treatment with niridazole reduces the inflammatory responses to infection with the guinea worm (*D. medinensis*) and to *S. mansoni* eggs deposited in the tissues. This action is probably due to the formation of 1-thiocarbamoyl-2-imidazolidinone, a metabolite of niridazole that suppresses cell-mediated immune reactions (Mahmoud *et al.,* 1975; Tracy *et al.,* 1980; Gautam *et al.,* 1982; Tracy *et al.,* 1982).

Niridazole is also a bacterial mutagen (Connor et al., 1974). This and its bactericidal effect are dependent on enzymatic reduction of the nitro group of the compound, a process carried out physiologically by facultative anaerobes or anaerobes in the host intestine (Blumer et al., 1980; Tracy and Webster, 1981). Given in sufficiently high doses for prolonged periods, niridazole is carcinogenic in mice and hamsters (Bulay et al., 1977). However, this effect may be due to oxidative rather than to reductive metabolism of the drug (Webster et al., 1984).

Absorption, Fate, and Excretion. After oral administration niridazole is absorbed almost entirely over a period of several hours. The drug is largely metabolized during its first passage through the liver. Owing to slow absorption and rapid metabolism, only low concentrations of the drug are achieved in the plasma. A number of metabolites attain higher concentrations in plasma, and some persist for long periods due to binding to albumin (Symposium, 1969a; Valencia et al., 1984). The drug is eliminated largely as metabolites, which appear about equally in the urine and feces. The urine becomes dark in color and has an unpleasant odor. Because the schistosomicidal activity of niridazole is attributable to the parent compound, part of its effectiveness may be due to the high concentration achieved in the portal blood. Except for S. haematobium, species of Schistosoma live mainly or exclusively in the mesenteric venous system.

Preparations, Route of Administration, and Dosage. Niridazole (AMBILHAR) is supplied in scored tablets of 100 and 500 mg. In the United States it is available from the Parasitic Diseases Division, Centers for Disease Control. Niridazole is taken orally. The usual daily dose for schistosomiasis and dracunculiasis is 25 mg/kg (maximum of 1.5 g) for 7 days.

Toxicity and Side Effects. Niridazole may produce changes in the EEG and cause agitation, confusional states, visual and auditory hallucinations, and localized or generalized convulsions. CNS toxicity is more common and pronounced in patients with impaired hepatic function, for example, in hepatosplenic schistosomiasis. The drug causes T wave abnormalities in the ECG that disappear 1 to 2 weeks after cessation of therapy. Transitory reduction in sperm production without impairment of fertility has also been described. Treatment with niridazole can provoke hemolysis in individuals with red cells deficient in glucose-6-phosphate dehydrogenase (Doyen et al., 1967).

Niridazole also causes the following less specific effects: abdominal spasm and discomfort, nausea, vomiting, diarrhea, loss of appetite, and headache. Less frequently encountered are insomnia, skin rash, and paresthesias. The incidence and the severity of these side effects are considerably less in children. Effects of niridazole are described in more detail in a symposium (Symposium, 1969a).

Precautions and Contraindications. Impairment of hepatic function demands close attention to patients who receive niridazole; reduction of drug dosage may be necessary. Some consider the drug to be contraindicated when there is hepatocellular disease. Niridazole may also be contraindicated in patients with epilepsy, psychotic or severe neurotic behavior, or marked debilitation. Hemolytic anemia is a possible complication in patients with genetically determined glucose-6-phosphate dehydrogenase deficiency. Because of its possible carcinogenicity, niridazole should not be used indiscriminately.

Therapeutic Uses. Although it has no direct effect on the worms, niridazole is now used primarily to treat dracunculiasis or guinea worm infection (D. medinensis) (Kothari et al., 1968). It is also employed as an alternative to praziquantel for chemotherapy of schistosomiasis due to S. japonicum.

OXAMNIQUINE

Oxamniquine is a metabolite of the most active of a novel series of 2-aminomethyltetrahydroquinoline compounds that showed promising schistosomicidal activity and low toxicity in laboratory animals (see Foster, 1973). It is prepared by microbial (Aspergillus sclerotiorum) hydroxylation of its synthetic precursor.

Chemistry. Oxamniquine has the following structural formula:

Oxamniquine

It is a light-orange crystalline solid.

Anthelmintic Action. Schistosoma mansoni is highly susceptible to oxamniquine; therapeutically useful activity has not been demonstrated against either S. haematobium or japonicum. Effective treatment with the drug causes a shift of worms from the mesentery to the liver within a few days. Later, surviving unpaired females return to the mesentery but do not lay eggs. Egg loads in primate hosts have been found to be due to only one or two surviving pairs of worms. Male worms are retained in the liver by tissue reactions, and the vast majority are dead. The primary mechanism of action of oxamniquine is unknown, even though the drug exhibits anticholinergic properties. The latter are evidenced by stimulation of motor activity in S. mansoni and inhibition of carbachol-induced paralysis; acetylcholinesterase activity is not affected (Kaye, 1984).

Absorption, Fate, and Excretion. Oxamniquine is readily absorbed following oral ingestion, and a peak concentration in plasma occurs within about 3 hours. The presence of food significantly delays absorption and limits the concentration achieved in plasma during the first several hours after administration. Most of an administered dose is excreted in the urine. Only a small proportion is excreted unchanged; up to 70% appears as a single metabolite, a 6-carboxyl derivative, and there are traces of a second compound, a 2-carboxylic acid. The major metabolite is formed by the intestine during absorption and is present in the plasma at concentrations more than tenfold greater than those of oxamniquine. The metabolite is predominantly excreted in the first 12 hours and is devoid of schistosomicidal activity (Kaye and Woolhouse, 1976; Kaye and Roberts, 1980; Kaye, 1984).

Preparation, Route of Administration, and Dosage. *Oxamniquine* (VANSIL) is available as capsules, each of which contains 250 mg of the drug. Because of severe local pain following intramuscular injection, oxamniquine is taken orally; the dosage depends on the geographical location. For the treatment of all forms of *S. mansoni* infections in Brazil, the recommended dose is 12 to 15 mg/kg, given as a single dose. For children weighing less than 30 kg, the dose is 20 mg/kg (in two doses of 10 mg/kg with an interval of 2 to 8 hours between them). The drug is tolerated better after food. In Africa, the recommended total dose ranges from 15 to 60 mg/kg, given over 1 to 3 days. The most appropriate regimen within this range is determined by the geographical location and the particular strain of *S. mansoni*. Intrinsic differences in the susceptibility of parasites to the drug seem to account for most of the variation in dosage, although pharmacokinetic factors may play a role (Kaye, 1984).

Toxicity and Side Effects. Dizziness and drowsiness have been reported after the administration of oxamniquine. Convulsions have occurred in a small number of patients, particularly in individuals with a history of epilepsy. Minor and transient elevation of transaminase activities may be of little clinical significance, since oxamniquine has been used safely in patients with severe hepatosplenic disease. The mild eosinophilia that occurs after treatment is likely due to the host's reaction to dead and dying worms. Orange-to-red discoloration of the urine may follow therapy.

Therapeutic Uses. Oxamniquine is currently used in the treatment of infections with *Schistosoma mansoni*. Its value as an orally administered, readily accepted, and inexpensive schistosomicide has been proven, both for the treatment of individual patients and in mass-treatment and control programs (*see* Clarke *et al.,* 1976; Katz *et al.,* 1977; Pedro *et al.,* 1977; Bassily *et al.,* 1978; Omer, 1978). It is effective in all stages of infection and in patients with hepatosplenic involvement. Recommended dosages differ in various geographical areas (*see* above). Oxamniquine has been used successfully in combination with *metrifonate* for the treatment of mixed *mansoni* and *haematobium* infections.

PIPERAZINE

The discovery of the anthelmintic properties of *piperazine* is usually credited to Fayard (1949), but these were first observed by Boismare, a Rouen pharmacist, whose recipe is quoted in Fayard's thesis. Clinically, the drug is highly effective against both *Ascaris lumbricoides* and *Enterobius (Oxyuris) vermicularis*. A large number of substituted piperazine derivatives exhibit anthelmintic activity, but apart from diethylcarbamazine none has found a place in human therapeutics (*see* Standen, 1963).

Chemistry. Piperazine has the following structural formula:

Piperazine

It is available as the hexahydrate, which contains about 44% of base, and as various salts. These occur as stable, nonhygroscopic, white crystals, freely soluble in water.

Anthelmintic Action. The predominant effect of piperazine on *Ascaris* is to cause a flaccid paralysis that results in expulsion of the worm by peristalsis. Affected worms recover if incubated in drug-free medium. Piperazine blocks the response of *Ascaris* muscle to acetylcholine, apparently by altering the permeability of the cell membrane to ions that are responsible for the maintenance of the resting potential. The drug causes hyperpolarization and suppression of spontaneous spike potentials with accompanying paralysis (*see* Saz and Bueding, 1966). The basis for its selectivity of action is not entirely clear.

Absorption, Fate, and Excretion. Piperazine is readily absorbed from the gastrointestinal tract. A portion of the absorbed drug is degraded, and the remainder is excreted in the urine. Rogers (1958) observed no significant difference between the rates of urinary excretion of the citrate, phosphate, and adipate. However, there was a wide variation in the rates at which piperazine was excreted by different individuals.

Preparations, Route of Administration, and Dosage. Piperazine salts are available as tablets, each containing 250 or 500 mg, and as syrups containing 100 mg/ml, calculated as the hexahydrate. Of the various preparations, one is probably as good as another. The liquid formulations are more acceptable for children. *Piperazine citrate* is the salt available in the United States (ANTEPAR, VERMIZINE).

Piperazine preparations are always given orally. Prior fasting or supplementary treatment with cathartics or enemas is unnecessary. Many different dosage schedules have been investigated, and all have resulted in a considerable measure of success. In *ascariasis*, accepted therapy is to give 75 mg/kg (maximum of 3.5 g) as a single daily dose for 2 consecutive days. Children should be treated in the same way. This dosage schedule will cure nearly all patients. A single dose of 4 g has been shown to cure about 50% of patients and to reduce markedly the worm burden in the remainder (Goodwin and Standen, 1958). In *oxyuriasis*, single daily doses of 65 mg/kg, with a maximum of 2.5 g, given for 7 days, will result in 95 to 100% cure. One study in hospital patients showed that a single dose of 4 g of piperazine cured more than 90% of patients (White and Scopes, 1960). Because of the possibility of autoinfection, a second dose should be given to ambulatory patients 2 weeks after the first.

Toxicity and Side Effects. There is a wide range between effective therapeutic and overtly toxic doses of piperazine. Laboratory studies on patients receiving treatment for several days have showed no abnormality. Very occasionally gastrointestinal upset, transient neurological effects, and urticarial reactions have attended its use. Piperazine has been used without ill effect during pregnancy. Lethal doses cause convulsions and respiratory depression.

Precautions and Contraindications. Piperazine is contraindicated in patients with a history of epilepsy. Neurotoxic effects have occurred in individuals with renal dysfunction because urinary excretion is the main route of elimination of the drug.

Therapeutic Uses. Piperazine is particularly useful in treating combined *ascariasis* and *oxyuriasis*. In the treatment of *ascariasis*, piperazine has the advantage of greatly reducing the motility of the worms, thereby reducing the hazard of migration. Since the worms are usually alive when passed, there is little chance of absorption of disintegration products. Where partial intestinal obstruction is a complication of infection, conservative management together with the administration of piperazine syrup through a drainage tube may obviate the need for surgical intervention.

Treatment of *oxyuriasis* is complicated by the readiness with which reinfection may occur. Many authorities advocate the simultaneous treatment of the entire household with piperazine in lieu of investigation of each member by anal swabs. The palatability of the various preparations, ease of administration to children, and low toxicity make piperazine a good agent for pinworm infections. Its main disadvantage is the requirement for multiple doses over a prolonged period.

PRAZIQUANTEL

Praziquantel is a pyrazinoisoquinoline derivative that was developed after this class of compounds was discovered to have anthelmintic activity in 1972. It is clinically effective against a wide spectrum of cestode and trematode infections in animals and humans (*see* Symposium, 1981a, and comprehensive review by Andrews *et al.*, 1983).

Chemistry. Praziquantel has the following structural formula:

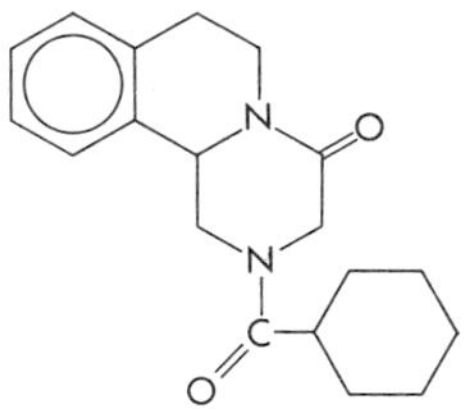

Praziquantel

It is a colorless crystalline powder with a bitter taste.

Anthelmintic Action. Praziquantel is rapidly and reversibly taken up but not metabolized by helminths *in vitro*. The drug has two primary and immediate actions in susceptible organisms. At the lowest effective concentrations it causes increased muscular activity, followed by contraction and spastic paralysis. It is this potentially reversible effect that probably causes the worms to lose their attachment to host tissues, resulting, for example, in the rapid shift of *Schistosoma mansoni* and *S. japonicum* from the mesenteric veins to the liver or in the expulsion of intestinal cestodes into the environment. At higher but still therapeutic concentrations, praziquantel causes vacuolization and vesiculation of the tegument of susceptible parasites. If sufficiently pronounced, this effect results in release of the contents of the parasite, activation of host defense mechanisms, and destruction of the worms. Comparisons of the stage-specific resistance of *S. mansoni* to praziquantel *in vitro* and *in vivo* indicate that the clinical efficacy of this drug correlates well with its tegumental action (Xiao *et al.*, 1985).

The molecular basis of the actions of praziquantel is not yet understood. The drug causes increased membrane permeability to certain monovalent and divalent cations, particularly calcium (Pax *et al.*, 1978). Drug-induced muscular contraction and tegumental damage of *S. mansoni* are both dependent on calcium, but praziquantel acts differently than do potassium ions or calcium ionophores in mammalian systems. Mammalian membranes are relatively resistant to this agent. Other biochemical effects have been observed, but their relationship to the mode of action of praziquantel is not clear (*see* Andrews *et al.*, 1983).

Absorption, Fate, and Excretion. In man, praziquantel is readily absorbed after oral administration. Maximal concentrations in plasma occur in 1 to 2 hours. Rapid metabolism to a number of hydroxylated and conjugated products limits the half-life of praziquantel in plasma to 1.5 hours, and only traces of unchanged drug are recovered in the urine. Plasma concentrations of metabolites are at least 100-fold that of praziquantel. About 80% of a dose of praziquantel is recovered as metabolites in the urine after 4 days; 90% of this amount is excreted within 24 hours.

Preparation, Route of Administration, and Dosage. To date, *praziquantel* (BILTRICIDE) is approved in the United States only for the treatment of all species of human schistosomiasis. The same preparation is used elsewhere to treat other infections with trematodes (*see* Table XI–1). A single oral dose of 40 mg/kg is sufficient for *S. haematobium* and *S. mansoni* infections, whereas two oral doses of 30 mg/kg several hours apart are recommended for *S. japonicum* infections. The single dosage regimen is also appropriate for mixed infections with *S. haematobium* and *S. mansoni*. Praziquantel, given in three oral doses of 25 mg/kg each on the same day, has also allowed high rates of cure of infections with the liver flukes, *Clonorchis sinensis* and *Opisthorchis viverrini*. Preliminary studies have indicated that *Fasciola hepatica* may

respond to more prolonged treatment, even though the trematode is quite refractory to praziquantel in animal hosts and *in vitro*. Infections with the lung fluke, *Paragonimus westermani*, may require high doses of praziquantel (three doses of 25 mg/kg per day for 2 days). Lower single doses are recommended for treatment of infections with adult cestodes, for example, 25 mg/kg for *Diphyllobothrium latum* or *Hymenolepis nana* and 10 mg/kg for *Taenia saginata* or *T. solium*. Although low doses of praziquantel are effective in eliminating juvenile and adult stages of *Echinococcus granulosus* and *E. multilocularis* from dogs and cats, these infections and hydatid disease in man appear quite resistant to the drug. The use of prolonged high-dose therapy with praziquantel for human cysticercosis is promising but still investigational (Sotelo *et al.*, 1984). The clinical uses of praziquantel have been reviewed recently (Andrews *et al.*, 1983; Pearson and Guerrant, 1983).

Toxicity and Side Effects. Abdominal discomfort, particularly pain, and headache and dizziness may occur shortly after administration of the drug; these effects are transient and appear to be dose related. The skin rashes noted occasionally may have an allergic basis. Extensive tests for mutagenesis, carcinogenesis, and teratogenicity have been negative (*see* review by Frohberg and Schencking, 1981).

Therapeutic Uses. Praziquantel is well tolerated, safe, and effective when given in one or two doses during the same day for single or mixed infections with all species of schistosomes that infect man. It thus appears to have ideal properties for individual or population-based chemotherapy. The drug also appears to be extremely useful against other trematode infections and cestodes that affect man; this even includes *cysticercosis* caused by the larval stage of *Taenia solium*.

PYRANTEL PAMOATE

Pyrantel pamoate was introduced first into veterinary practice as a broad-spectrum anthelmintic effective against pinworm, roundworm, and hookworm (Austin *et al.*, 1966). Its effectiveness and lack of toxicity led to its trial against related intestinal helminths in man (Bumbalo *et al.*, 1969). Successful clinical trials have resulted in its acceptance for the treatment of infections with various nematodes. *Oxantel pamoate*, an *m*-oxyphenol analog of pyrantel, has been used successfully for single-dose treatment of trichuriasis.

Chemistry. Pyrantel is employed as the pamoate salt. It has the following structural formula:

Pyrantel

The pamoate is a white crystalline salt practically insoluble in either alcohol or water. It is tasteless and stable.

Anthelmintic Action. Pyrantel and its analogs are depolarizing neuromuscular blocking agents. They induce marked, persistent nicotinic activation, which results in spastic paralysis of the worm. Pyrantel also inhibits cholinesterases. It causes a slowly developing contracture of preparations of *Ascaris* at $\frac{1}{100}$ the concentration of acetylcholine required to produce the same effect. In single muscle cells of the helminth, pyrantel causes depolarization and increased spike-discharge frequency, accompanied by increase in tension. In contrast, piperazine causes hyperpolarization with reduction in spike-discharge frequency and relaxation in identical preparations. In the *Ascaris* preparations, pyrantel and piperazine are mutually antagonistic (Aubry *et al.*, 1970; Eyre, 1970). Pyrantel is effective against hookworm, pinworm, and roundworm; however, unlike its analog oxantel, it is ineffective against *Trichuris trichiura*.

Absorption, Fate, and Excretion. Pyrantel pamoate is poorly absorbed from the gastrointestinal tract, a property that contributes to its selective action on gastrointestinal nematodes. Less than 15% is excreted in the urine as parent drug and metabolites. The major proportion of an administered dose is recovered in the feces.

Preparation, Route of Administration, and Dosage. *Pyrantel pamoate* (ANTIMINTH) is supplied as an oral suspension (50 mg of the base per milliliter). The drug is given orally at any time without regard to ingestion of food or beverages. A single dose of 11 mg/kg, to a maximum of 1 g, should be used to treat infections with *Ascaris lumbricoides, Enterobius (Oxyuris) vermicularis, Ancylostoma duodenale, Necator americanus,* or *Trich-*

ostrongylus. In the case of pinworm, it is wise to repeat the treatment after an interval of 2 weeks.

Toxicity and Side Effects. When given parenterally to rabbits, pyrantel can produce complete neuromuscular blockade; if given orally, toxic effects are produced only by very large doses. Transient and mild gastrointestinal symptoms are occasionally observed in man, as are headache, dizziness, and fever.

Precautions and Contraindications. Pyrantel pamoate has not been studied in pregnant women. Thus, its use in pregnant patients and children less than 2 years of age is not recommended. Because pyrantel pamoate and piperazine appear to be mutually antagonistic, it would be unwise to use them together.

Therapeutic Uses. Pyrantel pamoate may be regarded as an agent of choice in the treatment of *ascariasis* and *enterobiasis*. High cure rates have been achieved after single-dose treatment. Similarly, high rates of cure have been achieved against *Ancylostoma, Necator americanus,* and *Trichostrongylus*. The drug should be used in combination with oxantel for mixed infections with *Trichuris trichiura*.

PYRVINIUM PAMOATE

The use of pyrvinium pamoate has declined markedly for the treatment of pinworm infections, since more effective agents are now available (*i.e.*, mebendazole and pyrantel pamoate). Pyrvinium pamoate is discussed in *earlier editions* of this textbook.

THIABENDAZOLE

Thiabendazole was the product of investigation of several hundred substituted benzimidazole compounds. Some of these are among the most potent chemotherapeutic agents known, complete larvicidal activity being manifested *in vitro* at 10 pg/ml. This potency, coupled with the absence of activity toward other microorganisms and relatively low mammalian toxicity, suggests an interference with metabolic pathways essential to a variety of helminths (Brown *et al.*, 1961). The drug has been reviewed extensively (*see* Symposium, 1969b).

Chemistry. Thiabendazole has the following structural formula:

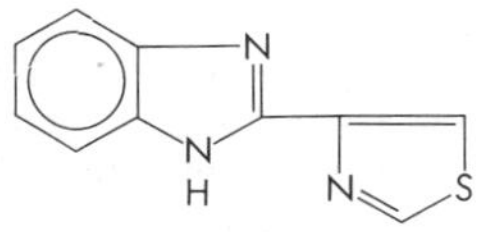

Thiabendazole

The drug occurs as a stable, white crystalline compound. It is almost insoluble in water but readily soluble in dilute acid or alkali.

Anthelmintic Action.

Thiabendazole has a high degree of activity against a wide range of nematodes that infect the gastrointestinal tract of domestic animals; it is also larvicidal *in vitro* at very high dilution (Brown *et al.*, 1961; Standen, 1963). A concentration of 1 ppm prevents the embryonic development of *Ascaris* eggs *in vitro* (Egerton, 1961). Its primary mechanism of action is unknown, although the compound inhibits the helminth-specific mitochondrial fumarate reductase system, possibly by interacting with an endogenous quinone (Kohler and Bachmann, 1978). In *Strongyloides,* thiabendazole may suppress assembly of microtubules, leading to inhibition of secretion of parasite acetylcholinesterase and dislodgment of the worm (Watts *et al.,* 1982). Of particular interest are reports that thiabendazole kills larvae in the muscle of pigs experimentally infected with *Trichinella spiralis.* Several early cases of human trichinosis treated with thiabendazole have shown marked clinical improvement. Generally the drug seems to allay symptoms and reduce eosinophilia, but its effect on larvae that have migrated to muscle is questionable. Anti-inflammatory, antipyretic, and analgesic effects, demonstrated in laboratory animals, may have contributed to the clinical responses. Thiabendazole has no effect on *filariasis.* It is active *in vitro* against a variety of *saprophytic and pathogenic fungi,* particularly against strains of *Trichophyton* and *Microsporum.* Clinically, however, response to treatment of superficial fungal infections has been equivocal.

Absorption, Fate, and Excretion.

After oral administration of thiabendazole in man, absorption is rapid. Peak concentrations in plasma occur about 1 hour after treatment. Most of the drug is excreted in the urine within 24 hours as 5-hydroxy-thiabendazole, conjugated either as the glucuronide or as the sulfate.

Preparations, Route of Administration, and Dosage. *Thiabendazole* (MINTEZOL) is available as an oral suspension containing 500 mg/5 ml and in 500-mg chewable tablets. The drug is preferably given after meals. The maximal daily recommended dose is 3 g. The standard dose for treating all roundworm infections is 25 mg/kg. This is taken twice daily for 1 day for pinworms, and for 2 successive days for all other infections. Single-day courses have been utilized quite successfully for all but the treatment of cutaneous larva migrans and trichinosis. A 2-day course is required in treating the former and may be repeated in 2 days if active lesions are still present; the condition has been treated successfully by topical application of thiabendazole. In early trichinosis infection, treatment may be continued for 2 or 3 additional days, according to the response of the patient. Treatment with thiabendazole for disseminated strongyloidiasis should be continued for at least 5 days. Thiabendazole may be tried in the treatment of visceral larva migrans at the usual dosage until either the symptoms subside or toxic effects intervene. Since this is usually a self-limiting disease, however, treatment should be restricted to severe cases.

Toxicity and Side Effects.

Side effects frequently encountered are anorexia, nausea, vomiting, and dizziness. Less frequently, diarrhea, epigastric distress, pruritus, weariness, drowsiness, giddiness, and headache occur. Rarer side effects include tinnitus, collapse, abnormal sensation in the eyes, numbness, hyperglycemia, xanthopsia, enuresis, decrease in pulse rate and systolic blood pressure, and transitory changes in liver function tests. Fever, facial flush, chills, conjunctival injection, angioneurotic edema, lymphadenopathy, perianal rash, and skin rash occur infrequently, but it is not certain whether these represent hypersensitivity to the drug, hypersensitivity to the parasite, or manifestations of the disease. Some patients may excrete a metabolite that imparts an odor to urine, much like that occurring after ingestion of asparagus. Crystalluria without hematuria has been reported on occasion; it promptly subsides with discontinuation of therapy. Transient leukopenia has been noted in a few patients on thiabendazole therapy.

Up to one third of patients treated with the recommended dosage have been incapacitated for several hours by one or more symptoms; half were incapacitated for as long as 24 hours by doses of about 50 mg/kg.

Precautions and Contraindications. There are no absolute contraindications to the use of thiabendazole. Because CNS side effects occur quite frequently, activities requiring mental alertness should be prohibited during therapy. Since thiabendazole has hepatotoxic potential, it should be used with caution in patients with hepatic disease or decreased hepatic function.

Therapeutic Uses. Administration of thiabendazole is a major advance in the therapy of *S. stercoralis* infections and of *cutaneous larva migrans*. A 2- to 5-day course of treatment produces a better-than-90% cure rate in strongyloidiasis. Pseudohookworm infection (*trichostrongyliasis*) also responds well, but its use for this purpose is considered investigational in the United States. The majority of patients experience marked relief of symptoms of creeping eruption. Progression of the disease should cease after 2 successive days of treatment. If active lesions persist after a 2-day interval, a second course of treatment is recommended. There is circumstantial evidence that the drug is also beneficial in the treatment of *visceral larva migrans*. Although thiabendazole is effective against *trichinosis* in animals, its value in the human disease remains unproven. It seems to allay symptoms and to reduce eosinophilia early in the infection, but its effect on larvae that have migrated to muscle is open to doubt. Thiabendazole produces a cure rate of more than 90% in *enterobiasis* and a lesser, and more variable, rate in *ascariasis* and *hookworm disease*. The efficacy of the drug against *whipworm* varies greatly, depending on the size of the dose and the duration of treatment. A single 2-day course of treatment produces up to 35% cures. An advantage of thiabendazole is its effectiveness against *Ascaris, Enterobius, Strongyloides,* and *Trichuris* and, consequently, its usefulness in patients with multiple infections.

TREATMENT OF HELMINTH INFECTIONS

NEMATODES (ROUNDWORMS)

Ascaris lumbricoides. *Ascaris lumbricoides,* known as the "roundworm," is cosmopolitan and affects about 25% of the world's population. Although cases of ascariasis are not infrequent in temperate climates, the parasite flourishes best in warm localities. In tropical countries, from 70 to 90% of the population may be infected. In the rural southern United States, the incidence of ascariasis is high in the children of poorer families.

Treatment. The older, less efficient, and more toxic ascaricides have largely been replaced by more active, less toxic compounds. Both *mebendazole* and *pyrantel pamoate* are preferred agents. *Piperazine* is effective but used less often because of occasional neurotoxicity and hypersensitivity reactions. Cure with any of these drugs can be achieved in nearly 100% of cases. *Levamisole,* although not approved for use in the United States, has been successfully employed abroad for *Ascaris* control programs. If ascariasis is a complication of hookworm infection, great care should be taken in treating the latter to avoid promoting unusual activity of the ascarids. Under such circumstances, the roundworms may block the lumen of the appendix and produce symptoms of appendicitis. They often occlude the common bile duct and occasionally invade the hepatic parenchyma. Perforation of the intestinal wall with subsequent peritonitis may rarely occur. If the worms are unusually active, they may form a tangled mass and cause intestinal obstruction. In the treatment of such mixed infections the advantage lies with mebendazole and pyrantel pamoate, because these agents are effective against *Ascaris* and both species of hookworms. Mebendazole offers a further advantage in that it is also effective against *Trichuris*. Preference should probably be given to pyrantel pamoate, however, because single-dose treatment is effective and it does not possess the teratogenic potential of mebendazole. Pyrantel pamoate is also effective against *Ancylostoma duodenale,* but this use is considered investigational in the United States. In addition to its ascaricidal effect, levamisole reduces excretion of *A. duodenale* eggs and *Strongyloides* larvae. However, this drug has little efficacy against *Trichuris*.

Hookworm: Necator americanus, Ancylostoma duodenale. *N. americanus* predominates in the United States, whereas *A. duodenale* occurs nearly exclusively in other parts of the world. These related species affect over 20% of the human population and flourish chiefly between latitudes 30° south and 40° north. Distribution much further north, into areas where a similar environment prevails, has been brought about by carriers. Such conditions occur in mines and large mountain tunnels, hence the terms *miner's disease* and *tunnel disease*.

Treatment. Treatment of hookworm disease involves two related objectives. The first is to restore the blood values to normal, and the second is to expel the intestinal parasites. Proper diet and treatment with iron are usually sufficient for the first objective, but blood transfusion may occasionally be required. *Mebendazole* and *pyrantel pamoate* are now agents of first choice against both *A. duodenale* and *N. americanus*, and have the advantage of effectiveness against other roundworms when there is multiple infection. *Thiabendazole*, while not a drug of first choice for hookworm because of its toxicity, has the advantage of being effective in the treatment of ascariasis, trichuriasis, oxyuriasis, and strongyloidiasis, and hence is of special value in patients with multiple infections. It is the drug of choice for treating *larva migrans* or "creeping eruption," due most commonly to penetration of the skin of man by larvae of the dog hookworm, *Ancylostoma braziliense*.

Trichuris trichiura. *Trichuris* (whipworm) infection is encountered throughout the world, especially in warm, humid climates. It is frequently found along with *Ascaris* and *hookworms*. The worm does not usually cause appreciable trouble except in heavily infected young children, who may exhibit mild toxicity and some degree of anemia. Rarely, worms may lodge in the appendix or may penetrate the bowel wall and give rise to peritonitis.

Treatment. *Mebendazole* in a dosage of 100 mg twice daily for 3 days is considered the safest and most effective treatment against whipworm, either alone or in combination with *Ascaris* and hookworm. *Thiabendazole* is also effective in an appreciable proportion of cases.

Strongyloides stercoralis. *Strongyloides stercoralis*, sometimes called the threadworm or dwarf threadworm, is frequently found in tropical and subtropical regions, often together with other intestinal helminths. Infection with this worm is common in parts of the southern United States. Similar environmental conditions often exist underground in mines, even in temperate zones, where the worm is occasionally found. Multiplication of the parasite and autoinfection account for persistence of the infection.

Treatment. *Thiabendazole* is highly effective and is considered to be the drug of choice. A 2-day course of therapy is normally prescribed; in *disseminated strongyloidiasis*, thiabendazole should be taken for at least 5 days.

Enterobius (Oxyuris) vermicularis. *Oxyuris*, the pinworm, is cosmopolitan and the most common helminthic infection in the United States, especially in school children. This parasite rarely causes serious clinical problems; pruritus in the perianal and perineal regions, however, can be severe and irritating, and scratching may cause infection. In female patients, worms may wander into the genital tract and penetrate into the peritoneal cavity. Salpingitis or even peritonitis may occur. Because the infection may easily be distributed throughout members of a family, a school, or an institution, the physician must decide whether to treat all persons in close contact with an infected person, and more than one course of therapy may be required.

Treatment. Both *mebendazole* and *pyrantel pamoate* are highly effective. When their use is allied with rigid standards of personal hygiene, a very high proportion of cures can be obtained. Treatment is simple and almost devoid of side effects. Mebendazole should not be used during pregnancy because of its teratogenic potential. Daily doses of *piperazine* for 1 week are also effective. Pyrantel pamoate, mebendazole, and piperazine have the added advantage of successfully clearing concurrent *Ascaris* infection.

Trichinella spiralis. The trichina worm is ubiquitous, regardless of climate, and does live outside a host. It is found frequently in Canada, Eastern Europe, and the United States. The only mode of infection is by eating raw, or insufficiently cooked, flesh of trichinous animals. All pork, not forgetting pork sausages, should be thoroughly cooked before being eaten. The encysted larvae are killed by exposure to 60° C for 5 minutes.

Treatment. *Thiabendazole*, in well-tolerated doses, has been shown to kill *Trichinella* larvae in the muscle of experimental animals. In human cases, results have been variable. It appears to allay symptoms and to reduce eosinophilia in early cases, but its effect on larvae that have migrated to muscle is questionable. *Corticosteroids* may be of considerable value in controlling the acute and dangerous manifestations of established infection. *Mebendazole* has been shown to kill encysted larvae in experimental animals, but clinical experience with this drug and other benzimidazoles is very limited.

Filariae: Wuchereria bancrofti. Infection with this species is especially a risk in Central Africa, South America, India, and southern China, although it is also widely distributed throughout the tropics. *Wuchereria (Brugia) malayi* is restricted to

Indonesia, the Malay peninsula, Vietnam, southern China, central India, and Sri Lanka. The migrating filaria, *Loa loa,* is a purely African species. It is found chiefly in the large river regions of western Central Africa, from Sierra Leone to Angola.

Treatment. Although drugs of the benzimidazole class may have therapeutic potential, *diethylcarbamazine* is now the only agent used for both suppression and cure. It is advisable to start with a small initial dose to diminish allergic reactions that result from destruction of microfilariae, particularly those of *Loa loa. Corticosteroids* may be required to control acute reactions. In rare instances, serious cerebral allergic reactions have been observed in the treatment of loiasis, probably due to destruction of microfilariae in the brain. If headache is severe and there is other evidence of an adult *Loa loa* near the orbit, extra care is advisable in initial dosing. The most satisfactory results are achieved in *W. bancrofti* and *W. malayi* infections if treatment is started early, before obstructive lesions of the lymphatics have occurred. Even in late cases, however, improvement may result. In longstanding *elephantiasis,* surgical measures are required to improve lymph drainage and remove redundant tissue.

Onchocerca volvulus. This filarial worm is very common all over West and Central Africa. It was presumably imported from there into Mexico, northeastern Venezuela, and Guatemala.

Treatment. Migrating microfilariae in the skin in onchocerciasis can readily be eliminated by treatment with *diethylcarbamazine.* Allergic reactions, however, are likely to be even more severe than those occurring in the treatment of *Loa loa.* Great care should be exercised in initial dosing, particularly in cases where lesions of the eye are present (*see* above). The adult worms have little susceptibility to this drug. Elimination of adult worms can be achieved by the administration of *suramin* (*see* Chapter 47). A test dose of 100 to 200 mg of suramin is first given intravenously. This is followed by 1 g given intravenously every week for 5 weeks. The reaction to suramin is similar to that provoked by diethylcarbamazine, but it appears much later and is more prolonged and less severe. Suramin is therefore used after a course of diethylcarbamazine to destroy the adult worms and eradicate the infection. However, benzimidazoles (*e.g.,* mebendazole) or other compounds may eventually replace the relatively toxic suramin for therapy of onchocerciasis.

Dracunculus medinensis. Known as the *guinea, dragon,* or *Medina* worm, this parasite occurs in East and West Africa, India, Pakistan, Bangladesh, Arabia, and Iraq.

Treatment. Traditional treatment is to draw the adult worm out alive. Natives do this by rolling it onto a small piece of wood, drawing out a little of it day by day. If the worm is ruptured, severe secondary infections may occur. It is therefore recommended that the site at which the worm has broken through should be continuously washed with water to cause the worm to discharge all the larvae. After this it may be more easily extracted. Alternatively the worm may be removed by incisions along its course, under local anesthetic. Satisfactory healing with either extrusion of the worm or, if no worm was extruded, complete symptomatic and functional relief has been obtained by the administration of *niridazole.* No local reactions occur if the worm is ruptured on extrusion (*see* Kothari *et al.,* 1968). Similar results have been obtained with *metronidazole.* However, more credit is given to the anti-inflammatory properties of these drugs than to a direct effect on the adult female worm.

CESTODES (FLATWORMS)

Taenia saginata. Man is the definitive host for *Taenia saginata,* known as the beef tapeworm. This most common form of tapeworm is usually detected after passage of proglottids from the intestine. It is cosmopolitan and rarely produces serious clinical disease. However, the infection must be distinguished from that produced by *Taenia solium.*

Treatment. Niclosamide and praziquantel are the drugs of choice for treatment of infection by *Taenia saginata.* They are very effective, simple to administer, and comparatively free from side effects. Assessment of cure can be difficult because the worm, segments as well as scolex, is usually passed in a partially digested state. Cure can be assumed only if no further segments have been passed by the end of 4 months. If parasitological diagnosis is uncertain, praziquantel is the preferred drug because of the danger of cysticercosis (*see* below).

Taenia solium. *Taenia solium,* or pork tapeworm, is also cosmopolitan. A danger unique to *T. solium* infection is *cysticercosis,* the harboring of the cysticerci (larvae) in the tissues of the human host. This autoinfection by parasite eggs usually results either from ingestion of fecally contaminated infected material or from eggs, liberated from a gravid segment, passing upward into the duodenum, where the outer layers are digested. In either case, the free larvae gain access to the circulation and the tissues exactly as in their cycle in the intermediate host, the pig. The seriousness of the disease that results depends upon the particular tissue invaded. The usual sites are the brain, orbit, muscles, liver, and lungs.

Treatment. The treatment of infection with *T. solium* is the same as that with *T. saginata,* except that praziquantel is preferred to avoid the danger of cysticercosis. Repeated therapy may be required if parasitological cure is not obtained.

Diphyllobothrium latum. *Diphyllobothrium latum,* the fish tapeworm, is a common parasite in many European countries, the Near East, Siberia, northern Manchuria, Japan, and the lake regions of Canada and the United States. In North America the pike is the most common second intermediate host. The eating of inadequately cooked infested fish introduces the larvae into the human intestine. The tasting of foods containing fish during their preparation is another common cause of infection. In countries where infection with fish tapeworm is common, there is a high incidence of megaloblastic anemia, which resembles addisonian pernicious anemia in all respects. This syndrome, which has been termed "bothriocephalus anemia," is especially prevalent in Finland, where in the past, 90% of the population of certain provinces harbored worms. Expulsion of the worm results in a hematological remission.

Treatment. Treatment is again the same as that for *T. saginata,* that is, niclosamide or praziquantel. The presence of eggs in the stool 18 or more days after treatment is indicative of drug failure or reinfection.

Hymenolepis nana. *Hymenolepis nana,* the dwarf tapeworm, is the smallest of the tapeworms found in the small intestine of man. Children are infected more often than adults. It is cosmopolitan, but infection is more common in warm climates. It is the most frequently occurring tapeworm disease in the southern United States. *Hymenolepis nana* can develop from ovum to mature adult in man without an intermediate host. The cysticerci develop in the villi of the intestine for 3 to 4 days and then regain access to the intestinal lumen. Treatment must therefore be adapted to this form of development.

Treatment. Niclosamide or praziquantel is the agent of choice in North America. Failure of treatment or reinfection is indicated by the appearance of eggs in the stool about 4 weeks after the last dose.

TREMATODES (FLUKES)

Schistosoma haematobium, S. mansoni, S. japonicum. These are the main species of blood flukes that cause human schistosomiasis; less common species are *S. intercalatum* and *S. mekongi.* The infection affects about 200 million people, and more than 500 million are considered at risk. Geographically, schistosomiasis is widely distributed over the South American continent and certain Caribbean islands (*S. mansoni*), much of the Arabian Peninsula and Africa (*S. mansoni* and *S. haematobium*), and China, the Philippines, and Indonesia (*S. japonicum*). Infected snails act as intermediate hosts for fresh-water transmission of the infection, which continues to spread as the development of agricultural and water resources increases. Schistosomal disease, which is generally correlated with the intensity of infection, primarily involves the liver, spleen, and gastrointestinal tract (*S. mansoni* and *S. japonicum*) or the genitourinary tract (*S. haematobium*).

Treatment. *Praziquantel* is now considered to be the drug of choice for treating all species of schistosomes that infect man. The drug is safe and effective when it is given in single or divided oral doses on the same day. These properties make praziquantel particularly suitable for population-based chemotherapy, although the cost of the drug may limit its use. Although not effective clinically against *S. haematobium* and *S. japonicum,* oxamniquine has proven to be effective for treatment of *S. mansoni* infections, particularly in South America, where the sensitivity of most strains may permit single-dose therapy. However, resistance has been reported, in both the field and the laboratory, and higher doses of the drug are required to treat African than Brazilian strains of *S. mansoni.* Metrifonate has been used with considerable success in the treatment of *S. haematobium* infections, but the drug is not effective against *S. mansoni* and *S. japonicum.* Metrifonate is relatively inexpensive and can be used in conjunction with oxamniquine for treatment of mixed infections with *S. haematobium* and *S. mansoni.*

Paragonimus westermani, P. kellicotti. Called *lung flukes,* a number of *Paragonimus* species are pathogenic for man and carnivores. Found in the Far East and on the African and South American continents, these parasites have two intermediate hosts, snails and crustaceans. Man becomes infected by eating raw or under-cooked crabs or crayfish.

Treatment. Although rather refractory to the drug *in vitro*, preliminary clinical results with *praziquantel* are encouraging. Three doses of 25 mg/kg each are recommended daily for two consecutive days, but an optimal dosage schedule is still to be established.

Clonorchis sinensis, Opisthorchis viverrini, O. felineus, Fasciola hepatica. These parasites are all *liver flukes. Clonorchis sinensis*, the *Chinese liver fluke*, and *Opisthorchis* species inhabit the biliary system of man, where they may produce disease. Snails and fish serve as primary and secondary hosts, respectively, for these parasites. *Fasciola hepatica*, the *large liver fluke*, primarily infects herbivorous ruminants but incidentally infects man. Snails and fresh-water plants, such as watercress, serve as primary and secondary hosts for this parasite, which also infects the biliary system of man.

Treatment. Praziquantel has largely replaced older, rather ineffective drugs for treatment of these infections. *Clonorchis sinensis* and *Opisthorchis viverrini* respond well to the drug at doses of 25 mg/kg given three times during a single day. The drug requires more evaluation in human fascioliasis, for which several days of therapy with the daily regimen given above may be required to cause improvement. Praziquantel is effective against *Dicrocoelium dentriticum* infections in sheep.

Fasciolopsis buski, Heterophyes heterophyes, Metagonimus yokogawai. *Fasciolopsis buski*, the giant intestinal fluke, occurs chiefly in Southeast Asia, whereas the other smaller intestinal flukes occur in various parts of the world. These parasites generally cause clinical symptoms only if infection is massive. As is the case for infections with other trematodes, praziquantel is emerging as the drug of choice for these infections.

Abdallah, A., and Saif, M. The efficacy of N-2′-chloro-4′-nitrophenyl-5-chlorosalicylamide in the treatment of taeniasis. *J. Egypt. Med. Assoc.*, **1961**, *44*, 379–381.

Aubry, M. L.; Cowell, P.; Davey, M. J.; and Shevde, S. Aspects of the pharmacology of a new anthelmintic: pyrantel. *Br. J. Pharmacol.*, **1970**, *38*, 332–344.

Austin, W. C.; Courtney, W.; Danilewicz, J. C.; Morgan, D. H.; Conover, L. H.; Howes, H. L., Jr.; Lynch, J. E.; McFarland, J. W.; Cornwall, R. L.; and Theodorides, V. J. Pyrantel tartrate, a new anthelmintic effective against infections of domestic animals. *Nature*, **1966**, *212*, 1273–1274.

Bassily, S.; Farid, Z.; Higashi, G. I.; and Watten, R. H. Treatment of complicated schistosomiasis mansoni with oxamniquine. *Am. J. Trop. Med. Hyg.*, **1978**, *27*, 1284–1286.

Batzinger, R. P., and Bueding, E. Mutagenic activities *in vitro* and *in vivo* of five antischistosomal compounds. *J. Pharmacol. Exp. Ther.*, **1977**, *200*, 1–9.

Bloom, A. Studies of the mode of action of metrifonate and DDVP in schistosomes—cholinesterase activity and the hepatic shift. *Acta Pharmacol. Toxicol. (Copenh.)*, **1981**, *49*, Suppl. V, 109–113.

Blumer, J. L.; Friedman, A.; Meyer, L. W.; Fairchild, E. H.; Webster, L. T., Jr.; and Speck, W. T. Relative importance of bacterial and mammalian nitroreductases for niridazole mutagenesis. *Cancer Res.*, **1980**, *40*, 4599–4605.

Brown, H. D.; Matzuk, A. R.; Ilves, I. R.; Peterson, L. H.; Harris, S. A.; Sarett, L. H.; Egerton, J. R.; Yakstis, J. J.; Campbell, W. C.; and Cuckler, A. C. Antiparasitic drugs. IV. 2-(4′-thiazolyl)-benzimidazole, a new anthelmintic. *J. Am. Chem. Soc.*, **1961**, *83*, 1764–1765.

Brugmans, J. P.; Thienpont, D. C.; van Wijngaarden, I.; Vanparijs, O. F.; Schuermans, V. L.; and Lauwers, H. L. Mebendazole in enterobiasis. Radiochemical and pilot clinical study in 1278 subjects. *J.A.M.A.*, **1971**, *217*, 313–316.

Bulay, O.; Urman, H.; Clayson, D. B.; and Shubik, P. Carcinogenic effects of niridazole on rodents infected with *Schistosoma mansoni. J. Natl Cancer Inst.*, **1977**, *59*, 1625–1629.

Bumbalo, T. S.; Fugazzoto, D. J.; and Wyczalek, J. V. Treatment of enterobiasis with pyrantel pamoate. *Am. J. Trop. Med. Hyg.*, **1969**, *18*, 50–52.

Chavarria, A. P.; Swartzwelder, J. C.; Villarejos, V. M.; and Zeledon, R. Mebendazole, an effective broad-spectrum anthelmintic. *Am. J. Trop. Med. Hyg.*, **1973**, *22*, 592–595.

Clarke, V. de V.; Blair, D. M.; Weber, M. C.; and Garnett, P. A. Dose finding trials of oxamniquine in Rhodesia. *S. Afr. Med. J.*, **1976**, *50*, 1867–1871.

Coles, G. C.; East, J. M.; and Jenkins, S. N. The mode of action of four anthelmintics. *Experientia*, **1974**, *30*, 1265–1266.

Connor, T.; Stoeckel, M.; and Legator, M. S. Niridazole, a direct acting frameshift mutagen, not affected by microsomal enzyme preparation which can be detected in the host mediated assay. *Mutat. Res.*, **1974**, *26*, 456–457.

Dominguez-Vazquez, A.; Taylor, H. R.; Greene, B. M.; Ruvalcaba-Macias, A. M.; Rivas-Alcala, A. R.; Murphy, R. P.; and Beltran-Hernandez, F. Comparison of flubendazole and diethylcarbamazine in treatment of onchocerciasis. *Lancet*, **1983**, *1*, 137–143.

Doyen, A.; Léonard, J.; Mbendi, S.; and Sonnet, J. Influence des doses thérapeutique du CIBA 32644-Ba sur l'hématopoïèse des patients atteints de bilharziose et d'amibiase. *Acta Trop. (Basel)*, **1967**, *24*, 59–77.

Egerton, J. R. The effect of thiabendazole upon *Ascaris* and *Stephanurus* infections. *J. Parasitol.*, **1961**, *47*, Sect. 2, 37.

Eyre, P. Some pharmacodynamic effects of the nematocides: methyridine, tetramisole and pyrantel. *J. Pharm. Pharmacol.*, **1970**, *22*, 26–36.

Faulkner, J. K., and Smith, K. J. Dealkylation and N-oxidation in the metabolism of 1-diethyl-carbamyl-4-methylpiperazine in the rat. *Xenobiotica*, **1972**, *2*, 59–68.

Fayard, C. Ascaridiose et piperazine. Thesis, Paris, **1949**. (Quoted from *Sem. Hop. Paris*, **1949**, *35*, 1778.)

Feldmeier, H.; Doehring, E.; Daffala, A. A.; Omer, A. H. S.; and Dietrich, M. Efficacy of metrifonate in urinary schistosomiasis: comparison of reduction of *Schistosoma haematobium* and *S. mansoni* eggs. *Am. J. Trop. Med. Hyg.*, **1982**, *31*, 1188–1194.

Foster, R. The preclinical development of oxamniquine. *Rev. Inst. Med. Trop. Sao Paulo*, **1973**, *15*, 1–9.

Gautam, S. C.; Sissors, D. L.; and Webster, L. T., Jr. Further observations on the effects of 1-thiocarbamoyl-2-imidazolidinone in cell-mediated immunity. *Immunopharmacology*, **1982**, *4*, 201–212.

Gönnert, R., and Schraufstätter, E. Experimentelle Untersuchungen mit N-(2'-chlor-4'-nitrophenyl)-5-Chlorsalicylamid, einen neuen Bandwurmmittel. I. Mitterlung: Chemotherapeutische Versuche. *Arzneim. Forsch.*, **1960**, *10*, 881–884.

Goodwin, L. G., and Standen, O. D. Treatment of ascariasis with various salts of piperazine. *Br. Med. J.*, **1958**, *1*, 131–133.

Jewsbury, J. M.; Cooke, M. J.; and Weber, M. C. Field trial of metrifonate in the treatment and prevention of schistosomiasis infection in man. *Ann. Trop. Med. Parasitol.*, **1977**, *71*, 67–83.

Jones, W. Niclosamide as a treatment for *Hymenolepis diminuta* and *Dipylidium caninum* infection in man. *Am. J. Trop. Med. Hyg.*, **1979**, *28*, 300–302.

Katz, N.; Zicker, F.; and Pereira, J. P. Field trials with oxamniquine in a schistosomiasis mansoni–endemic area. *Am. J. Trop. Med. Hyg.*, **1977**, *26*, 234–237.

Kaye, B. Oxamniquine: metabolism, pharmacokinetics and mode of action. *WHO Scientific Working Group on the Biochemistry and Chemotherapy of Schistosomiasis*. WHO, Geneva, **1984**, pp. 1–19.

Kaye, B., and Roberts, D. W. The metabolism of oxamniquine in gut wall. *Xenobiotica*, **1980**, *10*, 97–101.

Kaye, B., and Woolhouse, N. M. The metabolism of oxamniquine, a new schistosomicide. *Ann. Trop. Med. Parasitol.*, **1976**, *70*, 323–328.

Keystone, J. S., and Murdoch, J. K. Mebendazole. *Ann. Intern. Med.*, **1979**, *91*, 582–586.

Kohler, P., and Bachmann, R. The effects of the antiparasitic drugs levamisole, thiabendazole, praziquantel, and chloroquine on mitochondrial electron transport in muscle tissue from *Ascaris suum*. *Mol. Pharmacol.*, **1978**, *14*, 155–158.

Kothari, M. L.; Pardnani, D. S.; and Anand, M. P. Niridazole in dracunculiasis. *Am. J. Trop. Med. Hyg.*, **1968**, *17*, 864–866.

Langham, M. E., and Kramer, T. R. The *in vitro* effect of diethylcarbamazine on the motility and survival of *Onchocerca volvulus* microfilariae. *Tropenmed. Parasitol.*, **1980**, *31*, 59–66.

Mahmoud, A. A. F.; Mandel, M. A.; Warren, K. S.; and Webster, L. T. Niridazole: a potent long-acting suppressant of cellular hypersensitivity. *J. Immunol.*, **1975**, *114*, 279–283.

Miller, M. J.; Krupp, I. M.; Little, M. D.; and Santos, C. Mebendazole. An effective anthelmintic for trichuriasis and enterobiasis. *J.A.M.A.*, **1974**, *230*, 1412–1414.

Nordgren, I.; Bengtsson, E.; Holmstedt, B.; and Pettersson, B. M. Levels of metrifonate and dichlorvos in plasma and erythrocytes during treatment of schistosomiasis with BILARCIL. *Acta Pharmacol. Toxicol.* (*Copenh.*), **1981**, *49*, Suppl. V, 79–86.

Omer, A. H. S. Oxamniquine for treating *Schistosoma mansoni* infection in Sudan. *Br. Med. J.*, **1978**, *2*, 163–165.

Omer, A. H. S., and Teesdale, C. H. Metrifonate trial in the treatment of various presentations of *Schistosoma haematobium* and *S. mansoni* infections in the Sudan. *Ann. Trop. Med. Parasitol.*, **1978**, *72*, 145–150.

Partono, F.; Purnomo, O. S.; Oemijati, S.; and Soewarta, A. The long term effects of repeated diethylcarbamazine administration with special reference to microfilaremia and elephantiasis. *Acta Trop.* (*Basel*), **1981**, *38*, 217–225.

Pax, R.; Bennet, J. L.; and Fetterer, R. A benzodiazepine derivative and praziquantel: effects on musculature of *Schistosoma mansoni* and *Schistosoma japonicum*. *Naunyn Schmiedebergs Arch. Pharmacol.*, **1978**, *304*, 309–315.

Pedro, R. de J.; Amato Neto, V.; Rodrigues, M. S. de M.;

Magalhaes, L. A.; and Lucca, R. S. Treatment of schistosomiasis mansoni with oxamniquine: present state of our observations. *Rev. Inst. Med. Trop. Sao Paulo*, **1977**, *19*, 130–137.

Ree, G. H.; Hall, A. P.; Hutchison, D. B. A.; and Weatherley, B. C. Plasma levels of diethylcarbamazine in man. *Trans. R. Soc. Trop. Med. Hyg.*, **1978**, *71*, 542–543.

Reiner, E. Esterases in schistosomes. Reaction with substrates and inhibitors. *Acta Pharmacol. Toxicol.* (*Copenh.*), **1981**, *49*, Suppl. V, 72–78.

Reiner, E.; Krauthacker, B.; Simeon, V.; and Skrinjaric-Spoljar, M. Mechanism of inhibition in vitro of mammalian acetylcholinesterase and cholinesterase in solutions of O,O-dimethyl-2,2,2-trichloro-1-hydroxyethyl phosphonate (TRICHLORPHON). *Biochem. Pharmacol.*, **1975**, *24*, 717–722.

Reiner, E.; Simeon, V.; and Skrinjaric-Spoljar, M. Hydrolysis of O,O-dimethyl-2,2-dichlorovinyl phosphate (DDVP) by esterases in parasitic helminths, and in vertebrate plasma and erythrocytes. *Comp. Biochem. Physiol.* [C], **1980**, *66C*, 149–152.

Rivas-Alcala, A. R.; Greene, B. M.; Taylor, H. R.; Dominguez-Vazquez, A.; Ruvalcaba-Macias, A. M.; Lugo-Pfeiffer, C.; Mackenzie, C. D.; and Beltran, H. F. Chemotherapy of onchocerciasis: a controlled comparison of mebendazole, levamisole, and diethylcarbamazine. *Lancet*, **1981**, *2*, 485–490.

Rogers, E. W. Excretion of piperazine salts in urine. *Br. Med. J.*, **1958**, *1*, 136–137.

Sargent, R. G.; Savory, A. M.; Mina, A.; and Lee, P. R. A clinical evaluation of mebendazole in the treatment of trichuriasis. *Am. J. Trop. Med. Hyg.*, **1974**, *23*, 375–377.

Scheibel, L. W., and Saz, H. J. The pathway for anaerobic carbohydrate dissimilation in *Hymenolepis diminuta*. *Comp. Biochem. Physiol.*, **1966**, *18*, 151–162.

Scheibel, L. W.; Saz, H. J.; and Bueding, E. The anaerobic incorporation of ^{32}P into adenosine triphosphate by *Hymenolepis diminuta*. *J. Biol. Chem.*, **1968**, *243*, 2229–2235.

Singson, C. N.; Banzon, T. C.; and Cross, J. H. Mebendazole in the treatment of intestinal capillariasis. *Am. J. Trop. Med. Hyg.*, **1975**, *24*, 932–934.

Sotelo, J.; Escobedo, F.; Rodriguez-Carbajal, J.; Torres, B.; and Rubio-Donnadieu, F. Therapy of parenchymal brain cysticercosis with praziquantel. *N. Engl. J. Med.*, **1984**, *310*, 1001–1007.

Thienpont, D.; Vanparijs, O.; Niemegeers, C.; and Marsboom, R. Biological and pharmacological properties of flubendazole. *Arzneim. Forsch.*, **1978**, *28*, 605–612.

Tracy, J. W.; Catto, B. A.; and Webster, L. T., Jr. Metabolism of niridazole by adult *Schistosoma mansoni*: correlation with covalent drug binding to parasite macromolecules. *Mol. Pharmacol.*, **1983**, *24*, 291–299.

Tracy, J. W.; Fairchild, E. H.; Lucas, S. V.; and Webster, L. T., Jr. Isolation, characterization and synthesis of an immunoregulatory metabolite of niridazole: 1-(thiocarbamoyl-2-imidazolidinone). *Mol. Pharmacol.*, **1980**, *18*, 313–319.

Tracy, J. W.; Kazura, J. W.; and Webster, L. T., Jr. Suppression of cell-mediated immune responses in vitro by 1-thiocarbamoyl-2-imidazolidinone. *Immunopharmacology*, **1982**, *4*, 187–200.

Tracy, J. W., and Webster, L. T., Jr. The formation of 1-thiocarbamoyl-2-imidazolidinone from niridazole in mouse intestine. *J. Pharmacol. Exp. Ther.*, **1981**, *217*, 363–368.

Valencia, C. I.; Catto, B. A.; Fairchild, E. M.; Wilson, S. B.; Maramba, N. C.; and Webster, L. T., Jr. The concentration-time course of niridazole and six metabolites in the serum of four Filipinos with *Schistosoma japonicum* infection given niridazole. *J. Pharmacol. Exp. Ther.*, **1984**, *230*, 133–140.

Van Belle, H. Alkaline phosphatase. I. Kinetics and inhibition by levamisole of purified isoenzymes from humans. *Clin. Chem.*, **1976**, *22*, 972–976.

Wagner, E. D., and Chavarria, A. P. *In vivo* effects of a new anthelmintic, mebendazole (R-17,635) on the eggs of *Trichuris trichiura* and hookworm. *Am. J. Trop. Med. Hyg.*, **1974**, *23*, 151–153.

Wahlagren, M., and Frolov, I. Treatment of *Dipetalonema perstans* infections with mebendazole. *Trans. R. Soc. Trop. Med. Hyg.*, **1983**, *77*, 422–423.

Watts, S. D. M.; Rapson, E. B.; Atkins, A. M.; and Lee, D. L. Inhibition of acetylcholinesterase secretion from *Nippostrongylus brasiliensis* by benzimidazole anthelmintics. *Biochem. Pharmacol.*, **1982**, *31*, 3035–3040.

Webster, L. T., Jr.; Tracy, J. W.; Blumer, J. L.; Catto, B. A.; and Sissors, D. L. Relationships of niridazole metabolism to antiparasitic efficacy and host toxicity. In, *Proceedings of IUPHAR 9th International Congress.* Macmillan Press, Ltd., London, **1984**, pp. 363–367.

White, R. H. R., and Scopes, J. W. A single-dose treatment of threadworms in children. *Lancet*, **1960**, *1*, 256–258.

Wolfe, M. S., and Wershing, J. M. Mebendazole. Treatment of trichuriasis and ascariasis in Bahamian children. *J.A.M.A.*, **1974**, *230*, 1408–1411.

Xiao, S.; Catto, B. A.; and Webster, L. T., Jr. Effects of praziquantel on different stages of *Schistosoma mansoni in vitro* and *in vivo*. *J. Infect. Dis.*, **1985**, *151*, 1130–1137.

Monographs and Reviews

Andrews, P.; Thomas, H.; Pohlke, R.; and Seubert, J. Praziquantel. *Med. Res. Rev.*, **1983**, *3*, 147–200.

Barrett-Connor, E. Drugs for treatment of parasitic infection. *Med. Clin. North Am.*, **1982**, *66*, 245–255.

Brown, H. W. Anthelmintics, new and old. *Clin. Pharmacol. Ther.*, **1968**, *10*, 5–21.

Brugmans, J. Levamisole in infectious diseases—a review of the literature. *J. Rheumatol.*, **1978**, *5*, Suppl. 4, 115–121.

Campbell, W. C.; Fisher, M. H.; Stapley, E. O.; Albers-Schönberg, G.; and Jacob, T. A. Invermectin: a potent new antiparasitic agent. *Science*, **1983**, *221*, 823–828.

Chirigos, M. A. (ed.). *Immune Modulation and Control of Neoplasia by Adjuvant Therapy*, Vol. 7. *Progress in Cancer Research and Therapy.* Raven Press, New York, **1978**.

Frohberg, H., and Schencking, M. S. Toxicological profile of praziquantel, a new drug against cestode and schistosome infections, as compared to some other schistosomicides. *Arzneimittelforsch.*, **1981**, *31*, 555–565.

Greene, B. M. Onchocerciasis. In, *Tropical and Geographical Medicine.* (Warren, K. S., and Mahmoud, A. A. F., eds.) McGraw-Hill Book Co., New York, **1984**, pp. 413–422.

Hawking, F. Diethylcarbamazine and new compounds for the treatment of filariasis. *Adv. Pharmacol. Chemother.*, **1979**, *16*, 129–194.

Hewitt, R. I.; White, D. E.; Kushner, S.; Wallace, W. S.; Stuart, M. W.; and Subba Row, Y. Parasitology of piperazines in the treatment of filariasis. *Ann. N.Y. Acad. Sci.*, **1948**, *50*, 128–140.

Janssen, P. A. J. The levamisole story. In, *Progress in Drug Research*, Vol. 20. (Jucker, E., ed.) Birkhäuser Verlag, Basel, **1976**, pp. 347–383.

Janssen, P. A. J., and Van den Bossche, H. Treatment of helminthiasis. *Scand. J. Infect. Dis.*, **1982**, *36*, Suppl., 52–57.

Keeling, J. E. D. The chemotherapy of cestode infections. *Adv. Chemother.*, **1968**, *3*, 109–152.

Marsden, P. D. (ed.). *Clinics in Gastroenterology*, Vol. 7, No. 1. W. B. Saunders Co., Ltd., London, **1978**, pp. 1–243.

Miller, M. J. Use of levamisole in parasitic infections. *Drugs*, **1980**, *19*, 122–130.

Ottesen, E. A. Filariases and tropical eosinophilia. In, *Tropical and Geographical Medicine.* (Warren, K. S., and Mahmoud, A. A. F., eds.) McGraw Hill Book Co., New York, **1984**, pp. 390–412.

Pearson, R. D., and Guerrant, R. L. Praziquantel: a major advance in anthelminthic therapy. *Ann. Intern. Med.*, **1983**, *99*, 195–198.

Renoux, G. The general immunopharmacology of levamisole. *Drugs*, **1980**, *19*, 89–99.

Saz, H. J., and Bueding, E. Relationships between anthelmintic effects and biochemical and physiological mechanisms. *Pharmacol. Rev.*, **1966**, *18*, 871–894.

Schantz, P. M.; Van den Bossche, H.; and Eckert, J. Chemotherapy for larval echinococcosis in animals and humans: report of a workshop. *Z. Parasitenkd.*, **1982**, *67*, 5–26.

Standen, O. D. Chemotherapy of helminthic infections. In, *Experimental Chemotherapy*, Vol. I. (Schnitzer, R. J., and Hawking, F., eds.) Academic Press, Inc., New York, **1963**, pp. 701–892.

Stürchler, D. Chemotherapy of human intestinal helminthiasis: a review, with particular reference to community treatment. *Adv. Pharmacol. Chemother.*, **1982**, *19*, 129–154.

Symoens, J.; DeCree, J.; Van Beuer, W. F. M.; and Janssen, P. A. J. Levamisole. In, *Pharmacological and Biochemical Properties of Drug Substances*, Vol. 2. (Goldberg, M. E., ed.) American Pharmaceutical Association, Academy of Pharmaceutical Sciences, Washington, D. C., **1979**, pp. 408–464.

Symoens, J., and Rosenthal, M. Levamisole in the modulation of the immune response: the current experimental and clinical state. *J. Reticuloendothel. Soc.*, **1977**, *21*, 175–221.

Symoens, J.; Veys, E.; Mielants, M.; and Pinals, R. Adverse reactions to levamisole. *Cancer Treat. Rep.*, **1978**, *62*, 1721–1730.

Symposium. (Various authors.) The pharmacological and chemotherapeutic properties of niridazole and other antischistosomal compounds. *Ann. N.Y. Acad. Sci.*, **1969a**, *160*, 423–946.

Symposium. (Various authors.) Thiabendazole. *Tex. Rep. Biol. Med.*, **1969b**, *27*, 533–708.

Symposium. (Various authors.) Symposium on common parasitic diseases. (Zaman, V., ed.) *Drugs*, **1978**, *15*, Suppl. 1, 1–110.

Symposium. (Various authors.) Biltricide symposium on African schistosomiasis. (Classen, H. G., and Schramm, V., eds.) *Arzneimittelforsch.*, **1981a**, *31*, 535–618.

Symposium. (Various authors.) Metrifonate and dichlorvos: theoretical and practical aspects. *Acta Pharmacol. Toxicol. (Copenh.)*, **1981b**, *49*, Suppl. V, 7–113.

Van den Bossche, H. Peculiar targets in anthelmintic chemotherapy. *Biochem. Pharmacol.*, **1980**, *29*, 1981–1990.

———. A look at the mode of action of some old and new antifilarial compounds. *Ann. Soc. Belg. Med. Trop.*, **1981**, *61*, 287–296.

Van den Bossche, H.; Rochette, F.; and Horig, C. Mebendazole and related anthelmintics. *Adv. Pharmacol. Chemother.*, **1982**, *19*, 67–128.

Van Neuten, J. M. Pharmacological aspects of tetramisole. In, *Comparative Biochemistry of Parasites.* (Van den Bossche, H., ed.) Academic Press, Inc., New York, **1972**, pp. 101–115.

World Health Organization. *Report of the Expert Committee on Filariasis.* Technical Report No. 359, WHO, Geneva, **1967**.

———. *Report of WHO Scientific Group on Intestinal Protozoan and Helminthic Infections.* Technical Report No. 666, WHO, Geneva, **1981**.

45 DRUGS USED IN THE CHEMOTHERAPY OF PROTOZOAL INFECTIONS
Malaria

Leslie T. Webster, Jr.

Malaria remains the world's most important infection in terms of human suffering and death. Even now, there is a desperate need for practical, effective, and safe drugs, insecticides, and vaccines to combat this protozoal affliction. Large-scale attempts to eradicate malaria from most parts of the world (except Africa) were initiated in the 1950s, but they failed due primarily to development of resistance to insecticides and antimalarial drugs. Although over 30 countries were freed of malaria and others had its incidence and prevalence markedly reduced, most tropical areas where the disease is endemic are experiencing a resurgence. Transmission of malaria is rising, multidrug-resistant strains of *Plasmodium falciparum* are spreading, and the degree of resistance to drugs of this most dangerous and prevalent plasmodial species is increasing. Over 200 million people have malaria, and over 1 million deaths per year are associated with malaria in Africa alone. Although the mosquito-borne infection has been virtually eradicated from the United States, immigration from and travel to endemic regions pose an expanding health problem.

The chief agents employed for the chemotherapy of malaria are *chloroquine* and its congeners, *primaquine, quinine*, and inhibitors of dihydrofolate reductase, such as *pyrimethamine. Sulfonamides, sulfones,* and *tetracyclines* are also used in combination with certain of these drugs. *Mefloquine* is a 4-quinolinemethanol derivative that should be released shortly to combat chloroquine-resistant and multidrug-resistant strains of *P. falciparum* under carefully specified conditions. Other compounds that show promise for this purpose are derivatives of *qinghaosu*, a sesquiterpene lactone undergoing clinical evaluation in mainland China, and *halofantrine*, a 9-phenanthrenemetha-

nol derivative being investigated in the United States. The discovery of technics for continuous maintenance of human malarial parasites *in vitro* has been of fundamental importance for the development of chemotherapeutic agents and vaccines (Trager and Jensen, 1976). A related advance has been the establishment of practical methods to assess the susceptibility of human malarial strains to drugs *in vitro* (Rieckmann *et al.*, 1968, 1978; Desjardins *et al.*, 1979a). The opportunity for experimental chemotherapy of human malarias in a nonhuman primate host has been provided by the successful passage of both falciparum and vivax malarias in the owl monkey (*see* World Health Organization, 1973; Schmidt, 1978).

The biology of malarial infection must be appreciated in order to understand the actions and uses of antimalarial drugs. Accordingly, this topic is summarized first.

BIOLOGY OF THE MALARIAL INFECTION

Human malaria is caused by four species of obligate intracellular Protozoa of the genus *Plasmodium*; they reproduce asexually in man, but sexually in female mosquitoes (genus *Anopheles*). Each species has distinguishing morphological features, and the disease caused by each is also distinctive. (1) *Plasmodium falciparum* causes *malignant tertian malaria*, the most dangerous form of human malaria. It can produce a fulminating infection in the nonimmune patient that, if untreated, may lead rapidly to death. Delay in treatment until after demonstration of parasitemia may lead to an irreversible state of shock, and death may ensue even after the peripheral blood is free of parasites. If treated early, the infection usually responds readily to appropriate antimalarial drugs and relapses will not occur. If treatment is inadequate, however, *recrudescence* of infection may result from multiplication of parasites that persist in the blood. (2) *Plasmodium vivax* causes *benign tertian malaria* and produces milder clinical attacks than those of *P. falciparum. P. vivax* infection has a low mortality rate in untreated adults and is characterized by relapses that occur even as long as 2 years after primary infection. (3) *Plasmodium ovale* causes a rare malarial infection with a periodicity and relapses similar to those of *P. vivax*, but it is milder and more readily cured. (4) *Plasmodium malariae* causes *quartan malaria*, an infection that is common in localized areas of the tropics. Clinical attacks may occur years after infection but are much rarer than after infection with *P. vivax*.

Although malaria can be transmitted by transfusion of infected blood, man is naturally infected by *sporozoites* injected by the bite of infected female anopheline mosquitoes. The parasites rapidly leave the circulation and localize in hepatic parenchymal cells, where they multiply and develop into *tissue schizonts*. This asymptomatic *tissue (preerythrocytic or exoerythrocytic) stage* of infection lasts for 5 to 16 days, depending on the species of plasmodium. The tissue schizonts then rupture, each releasing thousands of *merozoites;* these enter the circulation, invade erythrocytes, and initiate the *erythrocytic stage* or *cycle* of infection. In *P. falciparum* and *P. malariae* infections, tissue schizonts burst more or less simultaneously, leaving no forms of the parasite in the liver. But in *P. vivax* and *P. ovale* infections, some tissue parasites remain dormant (*latent forms* or *hypnozoites*) before they proliferate and produce *relapses* of erythrocytic infection months to years later (*see* Krotoski *et al.,* 1982). Once human plasmodia enter the erythrocytic cycle, they cannot invade other tissues; thus, there is no tissue stage of infection for human malarias that are induced by transfusion. In erythrocytes, most parasites undergo asexual development from young *ring forms* to *trophozoites* and finally to mature *schizonts*. Schizont-containing erythrocytes rupture, each releasing 6 to 24 merozoites, and it is this process that produces the febrile clinical attack. The released merozoites then invade more erythrocytes to continue the cycle, which proceeds until death of the host or modulation by drugs or acquired immunity. The periodicity of parasitemia and febrile clinical manifestations in tertian or quartan malaria thus depends on the timing of schizogony of a generation of erythrocytic parasites.

Some erythrocytic parasites differentiate into sexual forms known as *gametocytes*. After blood is ingested by a female mosquito, exflagellation of the male gametocyte is followed by male gametogenesis and fertilization of the female gametocyte in the gut of the insect. The resulting *zygote*, which develops in the gut wall as an *oocyst*, eventually gives rise to the infective *sporozoite*, which invades the salivary gland of the mosquito. The insect then can infect another human host by taking a blood meal.

CLASSIFICATION OF ANTIMALARIAL AGENTS

Antimalarials can be categorized according to the stage of the parasite that they affect.

Tissue Schizontocides Used for Causal Prophylaxis. These agents act on primary tissue forms of plasmodia within the liver that are destined within a month or less to initiate the erythrocytic stage of infection. Invasion of erythrocytes and further transmission of malaria to mosquitoes is thereby prevented. *Pyrimethamine* is extensively used for causal prophylaxis of falciparum malaria. *Primaquine* also has causal prophylactic activity but is not used for this purpose because of its toxicity.

Tissue Schizontocides Used to Prevent Relapse. These compounds act on the latent or hypnozoite forms of *P. vivax* and *P. ovale* in the liver. Thus, these agents used in conjunction with an appropriate blood *schizontocide* can achieve a *radical cure* of *P. vivax* and *P. ovale* infections. *Primaquine* is the prototypical drug to prevent relapse, and *pyrimethamine* also displays some of this type of activity against *P. vivax*.

Schizontocides (Blood Schizontocides) Used for Clinical or Suppressive Cure. These agents act on asexual erythrocytic stages of malarial parasites to interrupt erythrocytic schizogony and terminate clinical attacks (clinical cure). The term *suppressive cure* refers to the complete elimination of malarial parasites from the body by continued suppressive treatment, the effect of which is longer than the life-span of the infection. *Chloroquine, quinine,* and *mefloquine* are typical fast-acting schizontocides. *Pyrimethamine, sulfonamides,* and *sulfones* also have schizontocidal activity, but they act more slowly.

Gametocytocides. An agent of this type acts by destroying sexual erythrocytic forms of plasmodia, thereby preventing transmission of malaria to the mosquito. Primaquine has this type of activity, particularly against *P. falciparum*. Chloroquine and *quinine* show such activity against *P. vivax* and *P. malariae* but lack it against *P. falciparum*.

Sporontocides. These drugs ablate transmission of malaria by preventing or inhibiting formation of malarial oocysts and sporozoites in infected mosquitoes. *Primaquine* and *chloroguanide* are the major antimalarials with this type of action.

Mechanism of Action. Antimalarial agents may also be classified rather grossly into two groups according to their mechanism of action. The first group includes the older agents, that is, quinine, chloroquine, and primaquine, in addition to mefloquine. These compounds can be recognized, even clinically, by the rapidity of their schizontocidal action and the relative difficulty with which resistance to them develops in sensitive strains of *P. falciparum*. Primaquine differs from other drugs in this category, in that it is much less active against erythrocytic stages than tissue stages of malaria parasites. Multiple mechanisms of action probably exist, but these are poorly defined for this group of antimalarial drugs. (*See* discussion of mechanisms of action under Chloroquine.)

Members of the second group of antimalarials are characterized by a schizontocidal effect that is slow in onset and dependent on the stage of multiplication of the parasites. Resistance to their action is achieved readily in experimental models, and resistance in the field is not uncommon. Their mechanism of action is clearly defined. Agents in this group either interfere with the incorporation of para-aminobenzoate into folate, a process that does not occur in mammals, or they bind to and inhibit dihydrofolate reductase: useful agents in this group have a much higher affinity for plasmodial dihydrofolate reductase than they do for the mammalian enzyme. Drugs in the antifolate group include chloroguanide and pyrimethamine and their derivatives (inhibitors of dihydrofolate reductase), as well as sulfonamides and sulfones (inhibitors of folate biosynthesis).

ACQUIRED RESISTANCE TO ANTIMALARIAL DRUGS

The chief obstacle to successful chemotherapy of malaria is the development of resistance to the available drugs. Acquired drug resistance should not be confused with insensitivity or natural refractoriness to antimalarials. The latter obviously exists but is unrelated to previous exposure to the drug.

Of the plasmodial species that infect man, acquired drug resistance poses a serious clinical problem only with *P. falciparum*. However, this species accounts for 85% of the cases and much of the mortality of human malaria. Resistance to chloroquine, first documented in Thailand and Columbia in 1959 to 1960, now affects large regions of South America and of Asia, east of central India. More recently it has spread in milder form to at least seven countries in East Africa. This situation is further complicated by the development of resistance in *P. falciparum* to pyrimethamine and sulfadoxine, a combination of drugs now considered to be the best alternative to chloroquine for chemoprophylaxis of falciparum malaria. Due to the extensive use of these prophylactic antifolate drugs in areas where resistance to chloroquine is prevalent, there is now a considerable overlap in the geographical distribution of resistance to pyrimethamine-sulfadoxine and to chloroquine. Prophylaxis and treatment of infections caused by such multidrug-resistant strains have necessitated a return to older and effective but more toxic schizontocides, such as quinine. Used in combination with tetracycline, even quinine has limited effectiveness because resistance to this agent is emerging in areas of Southeast Asia where the use of antimalarial drugs has been intensive. The history of increasing tolerance of *P. falciparum* to the current armamentarium of antimalarials dramatically illustrates the need for improved chemotherapeutic agents that act by different mechanisms and are not subject to cross-resistance with each other.

The biochemical basis of acquired resistance to antimalarial drugs has yet to be elucidated. Resistant parasites can be selected in the presence of antimalarial agents in laboratory models. As noted in the previous section, this phenomenon occurs more readily with the antifolates than with the agents related to chloroquine and quinine. There is considerable variation in the infectious behavior of malarial parasites from the same species, and field isolates of *P. falciparum* may contain genetically distinct clones of parasites. The advent of sophisticated methodology for culturing human strains of plasmodia, testing individual clones for resistance to drugs and other properties, and characterizing the genomic DNA of malarial parasites should lead to a greater understanding of these problems, with beneficial implications for the chemotherapy of malaria.

CHLOROQUINE AND ITS CONGENERS

History. Chloroquine is one of a large series of *4-aminoquinolines* investigated as part of the extensive cooperative program of antimalarial research in the United States during World War II. The objective was to discover more effective and less toxic suppressive agents than quinacrine, an acridine derivative that has been abandoned for antimalarial chemotherapy because of its toxicity and inability to cure vivax malaria or to act as a causal prophylactic. Although the 4-aminoquinolines had previously been described as potential antimalarials by Russian investigators, serious attention was not paid to this chemical class until the French reported that 3-methyl-7-chloro-4-(4-diethylamino-1-methylbutylamino) quinoline (SN-6911; SONTOCHIN, SONTOQUIN) was well tolerated and had high activity in human malarias. Beginning in 1943, thousands of these compounds were synthesized and tested for activity in avian malaria and for toxicity in mammals; ten of the series were then examined in human volunteers with experimentally induced malarias. Of these, chloroquine proved most promising and was released for field trial. When hostilities ceased, it was discovered that the chemical had been synthesized and studied under the name of RESOCHIN by the Germans as early as 1934.

Chemistry. Chloroquine has the following structural formula:

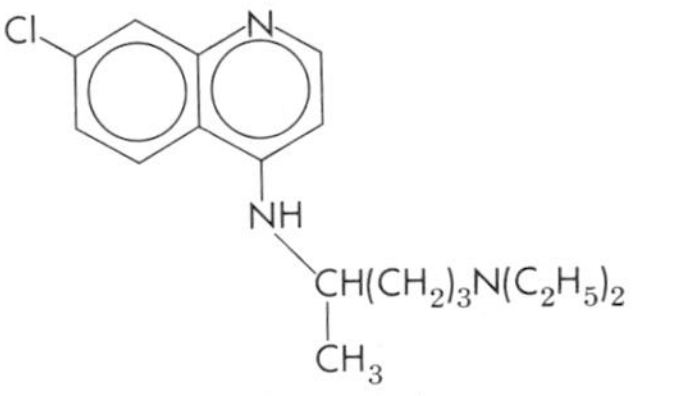

Chloroquine

The diphosphate is a white, bitter powder, soluble in water. Its solutions are stable.

Structure-Activity Relationship. Chloroquine contains the same alkyl side chain as quinacrine (*see* Chapter 46); it differs from the latter in having a quinoline instead of an acridine nucleus and in lacking the methoxy moiety. Chloroquine also bears close resemblance to pamaquine and pentaquine (obsolete 8-aminoquinoline antimalarials); it differs from them in the position of the alkyl side chain and in having a chlorine instead of a methoxy nuclear substituent. The *d*, *l*, and *dl* forms of chloroquine are indistinguishable in potency tests in duck malaria, but the *d* isomer is somewhat less toxic than the *l* isomer in mammals. The 4-aminoquinolines showing the most marked antimalarial activity in both avian and human malarias have a chlorine atom in position 7 of the quinoline. Methyl substitution in position 3 of the quinoline reduces activity, and additional methyl substitution in position 8 completely eliminates activity. The details of the structure-activity relationship of chloroquine

and its congeners are discussed by Berliner and coworkers (1948) and Coatney and colleagues (1953).

Amodiaquine is a congener of chloroquine; its structure is shown below.

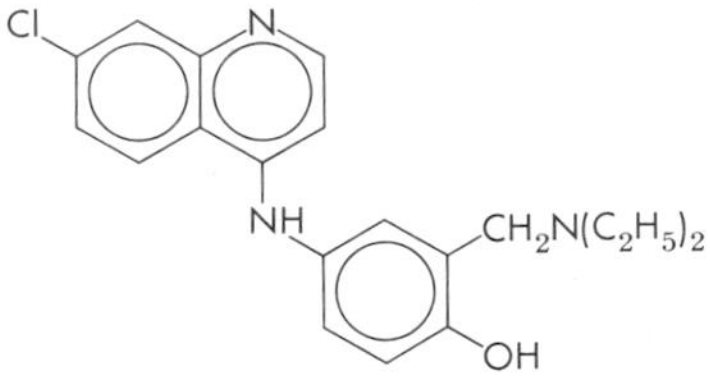

Amodiaquine

This drug is employed much less frequently than chloroquine for the treatment of overt malarial attacks and for suppression. Although it is more active than chloroquine both *in vitro* and *in vivo* against certain strains of *P. falciparum* with decreased sensitivity to chloroquine, amodiaquine is not recommended for routine use in the treatment of such infections. Amodiaquine is not discussed further here because its properties and dosage are largely similar to those of chloroquine. *Hydroxychloroquine,* in which one of the N-ethyl substituents of chloroquine is β-hydroxylated, is considered to be essentially equivalent to the parent molecule. Hydroxychloroquine has been used successfully in place of chloroquine against normally sensitive strains.

Pharmacological Effects. Although chloroquine was developed primarily as an antimalarial agent, it possesses several other pharmacological properties. Its use to treat extraintestinal amebiasis is described in Chapter 46. The anti-inflammatory effects of chloroquine are well known. The drug has been used occasionally in the treatment of *rheumatoid arthritis* and more frequently for *discoid lupus erythematosus;* its efficacy in the latter condition is controversial (*see* Dubois, 1978). Chloroquine has been employed with success to treat *porphyria cutanea tarda, solar urticaria,* and *polymorphous light eruption.* Treatment of these conditions requires much larger doses than are used for malaria, and this mandates proper consideration of the toxicity of this agent. (*See* review by Isaacson *et al.,* 1982.)

Antimalarial Actions. Chloroquine, even in massive doses, exerts no significant activity against the exoerythrocytic tissue stages of plasmodia. The drug is thus not a causal prophylactic agent and does not prevent the establishment of infection. However, it is highly effective against the asexual erythrocytic forms of *P. vivax* and *P. falciparum,* and gametocytes of *P. vivax.* It is superior to quinine in suppressing vivax malaria. In the *acute malarial attack,* chloroquine rapidly controls clinical symptoms and parasitemia; most patients become completely afebrile within 24 to 48 hours after administration of therapeutic doses, and thick smears of peripheral blood are generally negative for parasites by 48 to 72 hours. With the exception of certain strains in Southeast Asia, Central and South America, Africa, and the Indian subcontinent (extending into adjacent land masses), it completely cures falciparum malaria. Chloroquine, like quinine, does not prevent relapses in vivax malaria, but it substantially lengthens the interval between relapses. Chloroquine is well tolerated and is thus easier to administer than quinine. It differs from quinine in that no therapeutic or toxic synergism is manifested when it is given with primaquine.

Mechanism of Antimalarial Action. Although chloroquine causes a number of effects that singly or in combination may relate to its primary mechanism of plasmodicidal action, this process is not yet elucidated.

From early work, it was hypothesized that the drug might exert its effect, at least in part, by an interaction with DNA. Schellenberg and Coatney (1960) found that chloroquine inhibits the incorporation of ^{32}P-labeled phosphate into RNA and DNA by *P. gallinaceum in vitro* and *in vivo,* and by *P. berghei in vitro.* Later it was shown that chloroquine combines strongly with double-stranded DNA. The drug was reported to inhibit DNA polymerase markedly and RNA polymerase less so, in both cases by combining with the DNA primer (Allison *et al.,* 1965; Cohen and Yielding, 1965). Changes in several physical parameters were consistent with an intercalation of chloroquine with guanine-containing double-stranded DNA (Allison *et al.,* 1966). Such intercalation also occurs with primaquine and quinine, but not with mefloquine, an antimalarial structurally related to quinine (*see* Davidson *et al.,* 1977). Failure to demonstrate intercalation in the case of mefloquine, however, does not rule out other types of interactions of these antimalarials with DNA.

Plasmodium-infected erythrocytes exposed to chloroquine rapidly concentrate the drug and also exhibit clumping of malarial pigment that forms as the parasite digests the hemoglobin of the host red cells. The two processes may be related, in that both are energy dependent, saturable, and competitively inhibited by antimalarials such as amodiaquine, quinine, and mefloquine. (For references, *see* Chou *et al.,* 1980.) Recently it has been postulated that aggregates of ferriprotoporphyrin IX, re-

leased during degradation of hemoglobin by parasitized erythrocytes, may serve as a receptor for chloroquine and related antimalarial compounds and thus account for accumulation of the drug (Chou *et al.,* 1980). Either ferriprotoporphyrin IX or complexes of chloroquine with the porphyrin can cause membrane damage with lysis of trypanosomes, erythrocytes, or malarial parasites (Meshnick *et al.,* 1977; Dutta and Fitch, 1983; Fitch, 1983). But whether these agents are actually the physiological mediators of destruction of plasmodia or erythrocytes remains to be established. For example, inhibition of ornithine decarboxylase, the rate-limiting enzyme in polyamine biosynthesis, has recently been proposed as another possible mechanism of action of chloroquine (Konigk and Putfarken, 1983).

Absorption, Fate, and Excretion. Chloroquine is rapidly and almost completely absorbed from the gastrointestinal tract, and less than 10% of the administered dose is found in the stools. About 55% of the drug in the plasma is bound to nondiffusible, unidentified constituents. Excretion of chloroquine is quite slow, but is increased by acidification of the urine. Chloroquine is deposited in the tissues in considerable amounts. In animals, from 200 to 700 times the plasma concentration may be found in the liver, spleen, kidney, lung, and melanin-containing tissues; leukocytes also concentrate the drug. The brain and spinal cord, in contrast, contain only 10 to 30 times the concentration present in plasma.

Chloroquine undergoes appreciable biotransformation. The main metabolite is desethylchloroquine, which accounts for one fourth of the total material appearing in the urine; bisdesethylchloroquine, a carboxylic acid derivative, and other uncharacterized metabolites are found in small amounts. Slightly more than half of the urinary drug products can be accounted for as unchanged chloroquine. Deethylation to the secondary amine results in a substance that is highly active against avian malaria. Metabolic products of chloroquine may thus be partially responsible for antimalarial activity.

Because of the avidity of tissues for the drug, a loading dose is essential if effective plasma concentrations are to be achieved and maintained. When the drug is discontinued after daily dosage for 2 weeks, plasma concentrations and urinary excretion both decrease, with a half-life of 6 to 7 days for the next 4 weeks; subsequently the half-life for urinary excretion increases to about 17 days. Small amounts can be found in the urine for several years. Daily oral dosage of 300 mg of chloroquine base results in a steady-state concentration in plasma of about 125 μg per liter. With a weekly 0.5-g dose, the peak concentration in plasma varies between 150 and 250 μg per liter; just prior to the succeeding dose, the range is between 20 and 40 μg per liter. This compares to therapeutic concentrations of about 30 μg per liter for drug-sensitive *P. falciparum* and 15 μg per liter for *P. vivax*. After single or weekly doses, the half-life of the drug in plasma is about 3 days. Congeners of chloroquine (such as amodiaquine) interfere with its metabolism; with their concurrent use, plasma concentrations of chloroquine are elevated for prolonged periods.

Preparations. *Chloroquine phosphate* (ARALEN PHOSPHATE) is available as tablets containing either 250 or 500 mg of the diphosphate. Approximately 60% of the diphosphate represents the base. Chloroquine hydrochloride is available as an injection (50 mg/ml; equivalent to 40 mg/ml of the base). It is also combined in tablets with primaquine for prophylactic use only.

Hydroxychloroquine sulfate (PLAQUENIL SULFATE) is available in 200-mg tablets, equivalent to 150 mg of the base. For purposes of dosage, 400 mg of hydroxychloroquine sulfate is equivalent to 500 mg of chloroquine phosphate.

Routes of Administration and Dosage. Chloroquine phosphate is given orally in tablet form, either before or after meals. The hydrochloride salt of chloroquine may be employed for parenteral (intramuscular) injection, if necessary.

For the purpose of *suppressive therapy* an oral dose of 500 mg of the phosphate is given to adults on the same day of each week starting 1 week before and continuing for at least 6 weeks after the last exposure in an endemic area. Usual pediatric doses are 5 mg/kg of the base weekly. These regimens may not be sufficient to control infection with certain chloroquine-resistant or multidrug-resistant strains of *P. falciparum*, a topic discussed below.

For the *treatment of the acute attack* of vivax or falciparum malaria, an initial loading dose of 1 g of chloroquine phosphate is administered; this is followed by an additional 500 mg after 6 or 8 hours and a single dose of 500 mg on each of 2 consecutive days, such that a total of 2.5 g is given in 3 days. This dosage is usually sufficient to cure completely most *P. falciparum* infections with chloroquine-sensitive strains and to terminate promptly fever and parasitemia in acute *P. vivax* infections. Freedom from clinical attacks in vivax malaria may then be maintained by suppressive doses of 500 mg weekly.

If parenteral therapy is required for the treatment of coma due to chloroquine-sensitive falciparum malaria, the equivalent of 200 mg of chloroquine base (250 mg of the hydrochloride) can be administered intramuscularly, half the dose in each buttock. This may be repeated at intervals of 6 hours, but the total dose for the first 24 hours should never exceed the equivalent of 800 mg of the base. Parenteral administration should be terminated as soon as the drug can be taken orally.

Dosages administered to infants or children, orally or intramuscularly, should not exceed 10 mg of chloroquine base per kilogram of body weight per day; the usual dose is 5 mg/kg of the base.

Toxicity and Side Effects. The amounts of chloroquine employed for therapy of the acute malarial attack may cause gastrointestinal upset, pruritus, mild and transient headache, and visual disturbances. Prolonged chronic medication for suppressive purposes causes few significant untoward effects, and only rarely must the drug be discontinued because of intolerance. All symptoms readily disappear when the drug is withheld. Chloroquine may cause discoloration of nailbeds and mucous membranes.

Prolonged treatment with chloroquine may cause a lichenoid skin eruption in a few patients; the condition is mild and subsides promptly when the drug is discontinued. Readministration of chloroquine usually does not result in reappearance of the lesion. Large doses given for a year to a group of healthy volunteers occasionally caused some visual symptoms (blurring of vision, diplopia), bleaching of the hair, T wave abnormalities in the ECG, mild skin eruptions, headache, and slight weight loss; the observed toxic effects caused no incapacity and were reversible upon withdrawal of the drug (Alving *et al.*, 1948). These findings emphasize the relative safety of chloroquine in the usual dose range. High daily doses (>250 mg) of chloroquine, used for long-term treatment of diseases other than malaria, can result in irreversible retinopathy. This complication, presumably related to deposition of drug in melanin-rich tissues (Bernstein *et al.*, 1963), can be avoided if the daily dose is 250 mg or less (*see* Dubois, 1978; Olansky, 1982). Rarely, neuropsychiatric disturbances, including unintentional suicide, may be related to overdosage (*see* Good and Shader, 1982). There is no convincing evidence that chloroquine given during pregnancy causes fetal abnormalities.

Precautions and Contraindications. Because of the high concentration that occurs in the liver, chloroquine should be used with caution in the presence of hepatic disease. It should be used cautiously or not at all in the presence of severe gastrointestinal, neurological, or blood disorders. If such disorders occur during the course of therapy, the drug should be discontinued. Concomitant use of gold or phenylbutazone with chloroquine should be avoided because of the tendency of all three agents to produce dermatitis. For patients on long-term, large-dose therapy, ophthalmological examination is recommended before and periodically during treatment (Good and Shader, 1982).

Therapeutic Uses. *Malaria.* Chloroquine has neither prophylactic nor radically curative value in human vivax malarias. However, in well-tolerated doses it is highly effective in terminating acute attacks, and when administered chronically it acts as an effective suppressive agent. When medication is discontinued, relapses may occur but the intervals between their appearance are prolonged. In falciparum malaria, the drug is very effective in controlling acute attacks caused by sensitive strains, and as a rule it completely cures the infection. Chloroquine is superior to quinine in that it is more potent and less toxic and it need be given only once weekly as a suppressive agent. It is the most generally useful of the antimalarial drugs except in those parts of the world where strains of *P. falciparum* occur that are relatively or completely insensitive to the drug.

CHLOROGUANIDE AND CYCLOGUANIL PAMOATE

Known internationally as *proguanil,* chloroguanide is a biguanide derivative that emerged as a product of British antimalarial research during World War II. In mammals, the compound is converted to a triazine metabolite that acts as a *blood schizontocide* by inhibiting plasmodial dihydrofolate reductase. Chloroguanide has been used primarily for long-term prophylaxis and suppression of chloroquine-sensitive strains of *P. falciparum.* The drug is easily administered and causes few side effects. Unfortunately, however, its clinical effectiveness is greatly compromised by the presence or rapid development of drug-resistant strains of *P. falciparum.* Nonetheless, chloroguanide represented an important advance because it opened the field for the development of other antifolates. *Cycloguanil pamoate,* otherwise known as *chloroguanide triazine pamoate,* represented an attempt by Thompson and coworkers (1963) to produce a long-acting preparation of the active triazine metabolite of chloroguanide. This drug must be given intramuscularly. Again, the presence or development of resistance has compromised the clinical efficacy of this preparation. Because chloroguanide and cycloguanil pamoate have been largely replaced by more effective antifolates, their pharmacology is not discussed here further. The reader is referred to *previous editions* of this textbook for more information.

DIAMINOPYRIMIDINES

History. Of the many 2,4-diaminopyrimidines synthesized and tested for antimicrobial activity, two are outstanding. The first, *pyrimethamine,* was developed and used almost solely as an antimalarial agent; the second, *trimethoprim,* was created as an antibacterial agent and found later to have antimalarial properties. Several 2,4-diaminopyrimidines were found to antagonize competitively folic and folinic acids in the growth of *Lactobacillus casei.* The prediction was made that *L. casei* would not be unique in its sensitivity to these substances and that useful chemotherapeutic agents would be developed from this group. Treatment of malaria in experimental animals with diaminopyrimidines bore out prediction; several members of the series had high antimalarial activity. The most active, *pyrimethamine,* was later found to be highly effective against the plasmodia infecting man (*see* Falco *et al.,* 1951; Symposium, 1952), and has since been used widely for prophylaxis and suppression.

Chemistry. *Pyrimethamine* has the following structural formula:

Pyrimethamine

It is a white powder, insoluble in water.

Pharmacological Effects. *Antimalarial Actions and Efficacy.* The antimalarial effects of pyrimethamine are similar to those of chloroguanide. Its potency, however, is considerably greater, undoubtedly owing to the fact that it acts directly and the half-life is much longer than that of the active metabolite of chloroguanide. The major use of pyrimethamine is in prophylaxis, suppression, and combined chemotherapy of chloroquine-resistant strains of falciparum malaria. *Suppressive cure* of some vivax infections may be achieved by continuing prophylactic medication for 10 weeks after leaving a malarious area, and some causal prophylactic activity may occur in vivax infections. The antimalarial effects of both chloroguanide and pyrimethamine have been reviewed by Davey (1963) and Hill (1963).

Mechanisms of Antimalarial Action. In an elegant series of investigations, the 2,4-diaminopyrimidines were shown to act by inhibiting dihydrofolate reductase of plasmodia at concentrations far lower than required to produce comparable inhibition of the mammalian enzymes (Ferone *et al.,* 1969) (*see* Table 45–1). Dihydrofolate re-

Table 45–1.   INHIBITION OF DIHYDROFOLATE REDUCTASES
BY PYRIMETHAMINE AND TRIMETHOPRIM *

| | CONCENTRATION (nM) FOR 50% INHIBITION OF DIHYDROFOLATE REDUCTASES FROM VARIOUS SOURCES | | |
INHIBITOR	*Mammalian* (*rat liver*)	*Bacterial* (*E. coli*)	*Protozoal* (*P. berghei*)
Pyrimethamine	700	2500	~0.5
Trimethoprim	260,000	5	70

* Modified from Ferone, Burchall, and Hitchings, 1969.

ductase catalyzes the reduction of dihydro-folate to tetrahydrofolate, which is in turn required for the biosynthesis of purines, pyrimidines, and certain amino acids (*see* Chapter 57). Inhibition of dihydrofolate reductase by pyrimethamine is manifested in the malarial parasite by failure of nuclear division at the time of schizont formation in erythrocytes and liver.

The concept of inhibiting two steps in an essential metabolic pathway with separate drugs to produce a supra-additive effect explains the synergistic action of the 2,4-diaminopyrimidines with the sulfonamides or sulfones (*see* Hitchings and Burchall, 1965). The two steps involved are the utilization of para-aminobenzoic acid (PABA) in the synthesis of dihydropteroic acid, inhibited by sulfonamides, and the reduction of dihydrofolate to tetrahydrofolate, inhibited by pyrimethamine. About one eighth of the ED50 of pyrimethamine and sulfadiazine administered together was equivalent to the ED50 of either used alone in experimental malarial infections (Rollo, 1955). Hurly (1959) treated African children infected with *P. falciparum* and *P. malariae* with pyrimethamine and sulfadiazine, alone and in combination; clinical cure was obtained with the combination of less than one tenth of the curative dose of pyrimethamine plus less than one fourth of the curative dose of sulfadiazine. Subsequently, trials of several combinations of pyrimethamine and either sulfonamides or dapsone confirmed the augmentative effect both in the suppression and in the treatment of acute falciparum infections (*see* Donno *et al.,* 1969; Lucas *et al.,* 1969).

The value of such combinations lies in preventing or delaying strains of plasmodia from developing resistance to these drugs.

Such strains have arisen readily when small doses of pyrimethamine alone were used for long periods of time. Suitable combinations have shown their value in the treatment and suppression of some multiresistant strains (World Health Organization, 1981). Combinations of trimethoprim, the related diaminopyrimidine, with sulfamethoxazole are of particular value in the treatment of bacterial infections (*see* Chapter 49).

Absorption, Fate, and Excretion. Pyrimethamine is slowly but completely absorbed after oral administration. The compound accumulates mainly in kidneys, lungs, liver, and spleen and is eliminated slowly with a half-life in plasma of about 4 days. Concentrations that are suppressive for drug-sensitive strains remain in the blood for 2 weeks (*see* Brooks *et al.,* 1969; Stickney *et al.,* 1973). Several metabolites of pyrimethamine appear in the urine, but few data are available on either their structure or their antimalarial activity. Pyrimethamine is also excreted in the milk of nursing mothers.

Preparations, Route of Administration, and Dosage. *Pyrimethamine* (DARAPRIM) is marketed in tablets containing 25 mg. However, the drug is nearly always used together with a sulfonamide or a sulfone for antimalarial chemotherapy. For an acute attack, the adult dose of pyrimethamine is 25 mg twice a day for 3 days along with sulfadiazine, 500 mg four times a day for 5 days. *Pyrimethamine* (25 mg) is also available in a fixed-combination tablet with *sulfadoxine* (500 mg) as FANSIDAR. Sulfadoxine is a sulfonamide with a particularly long half-life (7 to 9 days). For prophylaxis and suppressive therapy, one tablet of pyrimethamine-sulfadoxine is taken weekly by adults. The pediatric dose is one eighth to three-quarters of a tablet weekly, depending on the child's weight. The regimen should start 1 week before and continue until 6 weeks after possible exposure. Pyrimethamine (12.5 mg) is also available in combination with *dapsone* (100 mg) as MALOPRIM, which is given weekly for prophylaxis and suppressive therapy.

Toxicity, Precautions, and Contraindications.

At the recommended dosage of 25 mg once weekly, *pyrimethamine* alone causes no significant clinical toxicity except occasional skin rashes and depression of hematopoiesis. Excessive doses do produce a megaloblastic anemia resembling that of folic acid deficiency; this reverses readily on discontinuation of treatment or on administration of folinic acid. The dose of pyrimethamine should not be increased over that recommended for suppression, except when used in combination with other agents for the treatment of strains resistant to multiple drugs. Higher doses of combinations of pyrimethamine and sulfadoxine may produce bone-marrow suppression; aplastic anemia has been reported in a few cases. The weekly dose should be taken regularly to lessen the possibility of selective emergence of resistant strains. In general, the drug should not be used in areas where the plasmodia are predominantly insensitive to the recommended dosage or have become resistant through its misuse. Use of pyrimethamine with either a sulfonamide or dapsone has proven beneficial, however, in areas where multiresistant strains are endemic. Periodic hematological follow-up is recommended under these circumstances, and treatment with folinic acid (10 mg per day) may be helpful.

Therapeutic Uses. *Pyrimethamine* is now used almost exclusively in combination with sulfonamides or sulfones. The drug by itself has little value in the treatment of the acute primary attack of malaria. It is slow in clearing parasitemia, but it prevents development of the fertilized gamete and has some causal prophylactic activity. In combination with a short-acting sulfonamide (*e.g.*, sulfadiazine) or a sulfone, pyrimethamine is useful for the treatment of acute attacks of uncomplicated chloroquine-resistant *P. falciparum* malaria. Quinine should be included in this regimen to assure a prompt schizontocidal effect. A combination of pyrimethamine and a sulfonamide has had considerable use as a prophylactic and suppressive agent and has proven effective against chloroquine-resistant strains of *P. falciparum* if given once weekly. Unfortunately, the increasing prevalence of multidrug-resistant strains of *P. falciparum* is making even this combination less effective. The combina-

tion is not radically curative in vivax malaria, although continuation of suppressive therapy for 10 weeks after leaving a malarious area will provide "suppressive cure" of certain strains.

Pyrimethamine given concurrently with triple sulfonamides is useful in the treatment of toxoplasmosis (*see* Feldman, 1968). Folinic acid should be given concurrently to obviate the hematological toxicity that may occur with continued daily use of pyrimethamine.

MEFLOQUINE

Mefloquine was developed in response to the proliferation of multidrug-resistant strains of *P. falciparum*, particularly in Southeast Asia. Such strains are variously resistant to available schizontocidal drugs and, in general, respond only to quinine or to certain drug combinations. As part of an extensive research program on malaria mounted by the U.S. Army, data collected during the course of World War II (Wiselogle, 1946) were examined to identify compounds with potential activity against these strains. Attention was focused on substances of proven antimalarial activity with some structural resemblance to quinine. These included quinolinemethanols and phenanthrene and pyridine carbinols. Unfortunately interest in these series, which contained many active compounds, had declined because of serious phototoxicity. Phototoxic potential, however, did not always parallel antimalarial activity. Of the many compounds that were then developed and tested for both phototoxicity and antimalarial activity, derivatives of 4-quinoline-methanol showed the most promise, and one of these, *mefloquine*, emerged from eventual clinical trial as a readily tolerated antimalarial drug that is highly active against both the usual and the multidrug-resistant strains of *P. falciparum* (*see* Schmidt *et al.*, 1978; World Health Organization, 1983, 1984). Promising alternatives to mefloquine, including *halofantrine*, have also been identified but require much more extensive clinical evaluation (Canfield, 1980).

Chemistry. Mefloquine has the following structural formula:

Mefloquine

The hydrochloride is a white, odorless, bitter-tasting powder.

Pharmacological Effects. *Antimalarial Actions.* This new antimalarial drug is being developed for the treatment and prevention of chloroquine-resistant strains of falciparum malaria. Such strains not only are resistant to chloroquine but also may show reduced sensitivity to antimalarials of different chemical types. While quinine alone usually controls an acute attack caused by these strains, it not infrequently fails to prevent recurrence. Mefloquine in single, well-tolerated doses has been shown to eliminate fever and parasitemia rapidly in nonimmune volunteers or patients in endemic areas infected with either chloroquine-sensitive or highly chloroquine-resistant strains of *P. falciparum* and to effect a radical cure. It has also been shown to effect suppressive cure against all strains of *P. falciparum* and suppression of *P. vivax*. In *P. vivax* infections, however, malarial attacks recur some time after the end of treatment (Rieckmann *et al.*, 1974; Trenholme *et al.*, 1975; Clyde *et al.*, 1976).

Mechanism of Antimalarial Action. The mechanism of action of mefloquine is unknown. In some respects, mefloquine behaves like quinine, but it does not intercalate with DNA (Davidson *et al.*, 1977). Mefloquine and quinine produce similar morphological changes in early ring stages of *P. falciparum* and *P. vivax* (Schmidt *et al.*, 1978). Mefloquine may affect membranes of malaria parasites (Brown *et al.*, 1979), and, like quinine, it interferes with the clumping of pigment in the parasite produced by chloroquine and related 4-aminoquinolines (Warhurst and Thomas, 1978). Mefloquine also competes for accumulation of chloroquine by infected erythrocytes (Fitch *et al.*, 1979). However, while changes in chloroquine-resistant strains may result in the exclusion of chloroquine, avidity for mefloquine appears to be retained.

Absorption, Fate, and Excretion. Studies in experimental animals have demonstrated that mefloquine is well absorbed after oral administration and is extensively bound to plasma proteins. Peak concentrations in plasma are attained in a few hours and decline slowly over a period of several days. The gastrointestinal system serves as an important compartment for the drug as it undergoes a continuous enterohepatic and enterogastric circulation (Mu *et al.*, 1975). Concentrations in tissues, particularly liver and lungs, are relatively high for extended periods of time. Excretion is mainly in the feces, and only very small amounts of drug appear in the urine. Several metabolites are formed; two have been identified as the 2,8-*bis*-trifluoromethyl-quinoline-4-methanol and a carboxylic acid metabolite. The ratio of the carboxylic acid metabolite to mefloquine in human plasma averages about 5 (World Health Organization, 1983). Subsequent studies in man have confirmed the long sojourn of mefloquine in the body. After a single dose of 1 g, the half-life in blood averages 17 days (Desjardins *et al.*, 1979b).

Preparation, Route of Administration, and Dosage. Mefloquine is an investigational drug that is still undergoing extensive clinical evaluation. In the United States, the compound is supplied in 250-mg tablets by the Walter Reed Army Institute of Research. Administered orally, single doses of 1 to 1.5 g have been effective in curing chloroquine-resistant *P. falciparum* infections in nonimmune patients (Trenholme *et al.*, 1975). Single oral doses of 250 mg weekly, 500 mg every 2 weeks, or 1000 mg every 4 weeks, given to nonimmune volunteers, are completely effective in producing suppressive cure of *P. falciparum* (Smith strain). The strain used for these tests is resistant to 4-aminoquinolines, pyrimethamine, and chloroguanide and has diminished susceptibility to quinine (Clyde *et al.*, 1976). In the same study doses of 250 mg of mefloquine, administered at weekly intervals, suppressed sporozoite-induced *P. vivax* infections. However, malaria developed some time after completing the course of treatment. Persistence of the drug is evident from the observation that exposure to infected mosquitoes 2 weeks after a single oral dose of 1 g did not result in parasitemia.

Toxicity and Side Effects. Mefloquine, given orally in single doses up to 1500 mg or in 500-mg doses each week for 1 year, is well tolerated in man. Side effects such as nausea, vomiting, and dizziness are dose related, self-limiting, and uncommon with single doses of 1 g or less. Rarely, neuropsychiatric disturbances such as disorientation, hallucinations, and depression may occur during the second week after drug administration, but these respond to symptomatic therapy. Studies of mutagenicity, carcinogenicity, and teratogenicity have been negative to date. Very high daily doses of mefloquine given to lactating rats did compromise early postnatal development of the offspring. Because of lack of adequate information, the use of mefloquine in women of childbearing age, infants, and children is not yet recommended.

Therapeutic Use. Mefloquine is indicated only for the treatment and prevention of chloroquine-resistant falciparum malaria. Currently, it is the only agent that, when used alone, is capable of ensuring suppression and cure of infections due to multidrug-resistant strains of *P. falciparum*. The drug should be used *only* for the treatment and prevention of infections with such strains, because its misuse could result in the development of mefloquine-resistant plasmodia. It is possible that it may be used in combination with other drugs (*e.g.*, pyrimethamine and sulfadoxine) to prevent the emergence of mefloquine-resistant *P. falciparum*. The status of mefloquine has been reviewed recently (World Health Organization, 1983, 1984).

PRIMAQUINE

History. In 1891, Ehrlich discovered that methylene blue exhibited weak plasmodicidal activity. Later it was shown that 8-aminoquinoline had weak schizontocidal activity in infected canaries and also that the slight antimalarial potency of methylene blue could be intensified by substitution of a dialkylaminoalkyl group for one of the N-methyl groups of the dye. Because the methoxy group on the quinoline ring, as in quinine, was believed important for antimalarial activity, a large series of quinoline derivatives was synthesized in which both the methoxy and substituted 8-amino groups were present. *Pamaquine* was the first of the 8-aminoquinoline antimalarials to be introduced into medicine (Mühlens, 1926). During the course of the large-scale cooperative antimalarial research program conducted in the United States during World War II, several hundred derivatives of 8-aminoquinoline were explored in an attempt to discover compounds more potent and less toxic than pamaquine itself (*see* Elderfield *et al.,* 1946; Wiselogle, 1946). From this large number, three agents— *pentaquine, isopentaquine,* and *primaquine*—were selected for further study. Of these three, only primaquine, which received extensive field trials with United Nations forces in Korea, is widely used now. *Quinocide,* a substance very similar in structure to primaquine, is employed in some parts of the world.

Chemistry. Primaquine has the following structural formula:

Primaquine

The diphosphate is the commercially available salt; it is soluble in water, and its solutions are stable, although some decomposition may take place on exposure to light and air.

Structure-Activity Relationship. Since a low chemotherapeutic index was a main drawback to the use of pamaquine, the prime value of the newer 8-aminoquinoline derivatives was a reduction in toxicity without concomitant decrease in antimalarial activity. The degree of toxicity is related to the degree of substitution of the terminal amino group. Pamaquine has a tertiary terminal amine, while primaquine has a primary terminal amine. Intermediate between these two lies isopentaquine, isomeric with pamaquine but with a secondary terminal amine. (For a review, *see* Hill, 1963.)

Antimalarial Actions. The great clinical value of primaquine lies in the *radically curative treatment of vivax malarias* and, in unusual situations where chloroquine treatment has proven unsatisfactory, in its use as a supplement to suppression with chloroquine. Primaquine is also highly active against the primary exoerythrocytic forms of *P. falciparum.* Although its causal prophylactic effect is obtained with well-tolerated doses, this activity is of relatively little

practical value. The activity of primaquine against erythrocytic stages of *P. vivax* also has little clinical application; the drug is almost completely ineffective against the asexual blood forms of *P. falciparum,* and it is for this reason that primaquine is almost always used in conjunction with a blood schizontocide. The 8-aminoquinolines exert a marked *gametocytocidal* effect against all four species of plasmodia that infect man, especially *P. falciparum.*

Although resistance of *P. vivax* to primaquine has not yet become a major clinical problem, resistance to 8-aminoquinoline compounds can be developed in experimental animal models, and various strains of *P. vivax* do show different susceptibilities to the action of primaquine in man. Thus, it is of the utmost importance that this drug not be misused and that new drugs of this type be developed (World Health Organization, 1984).

Mechanism of Antimalarial Action. Little is known of the mode of action of 8-aminoquinolines, especially why they are far more active against tissue forms than blood forms of plasmodia. Pentaquine, unlike quinine, chloroquine, and quinacrine, does not inhibit the incorporation of ^{32}P-labeled phosphate into DNA or RNA by *P. gallinaceum* or *P. berghei* (Schellenberg and Coatney, 1960). Nevertheless, binding of 8-aminoquinolines to DNA was demonstrated spectrally (Whichard *et al.,* 1968). There is some evidence that primaquine itself accounts for the antimalarial activity, whereas metabolites of primaquine may be more active than the parent compound in causing hemolysis (*see* World Health Organization, 1984).

Absorption, Fate, and Excretion. After oral administration, the 8-aminoquinoline antimalarial compounds, including primaquine, are promptly absorbed. They are, however, rapidly metabolized, and only a small proportion of the administered dose is excreted as the parent drug. After a single oral dose, the plasma concentration reaches a maximum in about 1 to 2 hours and then falls with an apparent half-life of 3 to 6 hours.

The three oxidative metabolites of primaquine identified to date are 8-(3-carboxyl-1-methyl-propylamino)-6-methoxy-quinoline, 5-hydroxy primaquine, and 5-hydroxy-6-desmethylprimaquine. The carboxyl derivative is the major metabolite found in human plasma (Baker *et al.,* 1982).

These metabolites all have appreciably less antimalarial activity than does primaquine. However, their hemolytic activity, as assessed by formation of methemoglobin *in vitro,* is greater than that of the parent compound (World Health Organization, 1984).

Tarlov and coworkers (1962) outlined a degradation scheme for primaquine modeled after Smith's (1956) proposal for the degradation of pentaquine in monkeys. In this scheme, the 6-methoxy group of primaquine is converted to hydroxy, a second hydroxy group is added in the 5 position, and the resultant compound is converted to a quinonimine by way of the 5,6-quinone derivative of the parent compound. Such a derivative is, or may be, transformed into a resonating compound capable of acting as an oxidation-reduction mediator. Such an agent may accelerate the oxidation of essential substances in sensitive erythrocytes by acting as an electron acceptor and thereby promote hemolysis. This redox behavior could also contribute to antimalarial activity by interfering with parasite electron-transfer pathways or by generating active oxygen species, such as superoxide free radical.

Preparation, Route of Administration, and Dosage. *Primaquine phosphate* is supplied in tablets containing 26.3 mg of the salt, equivalent to 15 mg of base. The dosage is usually expressed in terms of the base.

Primaquine is always given orally. When combined with standard chloroquine therapy, a dose of 15 mg daily of primaquine base for 14 days is effective for the radical cure of infections with primaquine-sensitive strains of *P. vivax.* Patients with intrinsically resistant Chesson or Southwest Pacific strains may require three times the daily dosage of primaquine stated above. The highest-dose regimen has a negligible hemolytic effect upon the erythrocytes of primaquine-sensitive individuals (*see* below). The recommended therapy for patients infected with intrinsically resistant strains of vivax malaria is, therefore, 600 mg of chloroquine base, followed 6 hours later by 300 mg of chloroquine base combined with 45 mg of primaquine base in one dose. Thereafter 300 mg of chloroquine base combined with 45 mg of primaquine base should be given as a single dose on the same day of each week for 7 additional weeks.

Toxicity and Side Effects. In the usual therapeutic doses, primaquine is fairly innocuous when given to Caucasians. Mild-to-moderate abdominal cramps and occasional epigastric distress occur in some individuals given the larger doses, and mild anemia, cyanosis (methemoglobinemia), and leukocytosis have been observed. Higher doses (60 to 240 mg of primaquine

base daily) accentuate the abdominal symptoms and cause methemoglobinemia and cyanosis in most subjects and leukopenia in some. Methemoglobinemia can be severe in individuals with congenital deficiency of nicotinamide adenine dinucleotide (NADH) methemoglobin reductase (Cohen *et al.,* 1968). Hepatic function is unaffected. Abdominal distress can be alleviated by taking the drug at mealtime. Granulocytopenia and agranulocytosis are rare complications of therapy and are usually associated with overdosage. Also rare are hypertension, arrhythmias, and symptoms referable to the central nervous system (CNS).

The toxicity of primaquine in most blacks is as described above; however, there is a fraction of the black population with glucose-6-phosphate dehydrogenase deficiency (about 10% of black males in the United States) who develop anemia due to intravascular hemolysis at daily dose levels of 15 mg (base) and higher. Such primaquine sensitivity of erythrocytes can be more severe in some darker-hued Caucasian ethnic groups, including Sardinians, Sephardic Jews, Greeks, and Iranians, in whom the sensitivity is greater than in blacks.

The incidence of hemolysis (and of the sickle trait) in general follows the same geographical pattern as the distribution of falciparum malaria; erythrocytes that reflect these genetic changes are less subject to malarial infection. A decrease in glucose-6-phosphate dehydrogenase activity has been shown to be characteristic of primaquine-sensitive erythrocytes and appears to represent their major enzymatic deficiency. In normal erythrocytes there are several mechanisms that protect the cells against injury by oxidative drugs such as metabolic derivatives of primaquine. These drugs are capable of accelerating the oxidation of reduced nicotinamide adenine dinucleotide phosphate (NADPH), reduced glutathione, hemoglobin, the free sulfhydryl groups of proteins, and other electron donors. In normal erythrocytes under the stress of oxidant drugs, the rate of NADPH regeneration can be greatly accelerated by increasing the amount of glucose metabolized by means of the pentose phosphate pathway. Sufficient NADPH is therefore readily made available for reduction of oxidized glutathione and (both directly and indirectly) for reduction of methemoglobin. Reduced glutathione also protects the sulfhydryl groups of hemoglobin and vital sulfhydryl-containing enzymes against oxidative destruction, and it is the substrate for glutathione peroxidase, which is the important scavenger of lipid peroxides that may mediate membrane lysis. Primaquine-sensitive erythrocytes are incapable of sufficiently rapid regeneration of NADPH because of their deficiency of glucose-6-phosphate dehydrogenase; consequently, all the NADPH-dependent reductive processes within the cell are compromised (*see* Tarlov *et al.*, 1962; Beutler, 1969). Brewer and colleagues (1960) devised a simple test for detecting such primaquine sensitivity based on the observation that the rate of methemoglobin reduction by erythrocytes from these individuals is markedly slower than normal in the presence of methylene blue. Results from this test correlate very well with the severity of hemolysis. The World Health Organization (1967) and Beutler and Mitchell (1968) have described other simple tests. Since primaquine sensitivity is inherited by a gene carried on the X chromosome, the hemolysis is often of intermediate severity in heterozygous females; because of "variable penetrance," females may be affected less frequently than would be predicted.

Primaquine is the prototype of more than 50 drugs and other substances that are known to be capable of inducing hemolysis. These include antimalarials, sulfonamides, nitrofurans, antipyretics, analgesics, sulfones, vitamin K analogs, fava beans (favism), and certain other vegetables.

The severity of the hemolysis is dependent on the dose of drug used. If the initial dose is not too large, the hemolysis is self-limited even when the same dose of drug is continued. This is because older erythrocytes are most susceptible, and, after their destruction, the remaining younger cells and newly produced reticulocytes are relatively resistant to hemolysis. However, the severity of hemolysis can be enhanced or mitigated by many factors and is often unpredictable. For this reason the administration of primaquine or of any other potentially hemolytic drug should be discontinued immediately if marked darkening of the urine or a sudden decrease in hemoglobin concentration occurs (*see* Kellermeyer *et al.*, 1962).

Precautions and Contraindications. Because of the possibility of hemolytic reactions (*see* above), one should watch for suggestive signs. If a daily dose of more than 30 mg of primaquine base (more than 15 mg daily in possibly sensitive patients such as blacks) is administered, repeated peripheral blood counts and at least gross examination of the urine should be performed during therapy. If the drug is used in schemes for mass administration, supervision is required.

Primaquine is contraindicated in acutely ill patients suffering from systemic disease characterized by a tendency to granulocytopenia, such as very active forms of rheumatoid arthritis and lupus erythematosus. It should not be given to subjects receiving, at the same time, other potentially hemolytic drugs or agents capable of depressing the myeloid elements of the bone marrow.

Therapeutic Uses. Primaquine is used mainly for the *radical cure* of vivax and other relapsing malarias. If it is administered during the long-term latent period of the infection, radical cure can be achieved. Its use during an acute clinical attack will prevent subsequent recrudescences. Primaquine should always be given in conjunction with full doses of a 4-aminoquinoline schizontocide, preferably chloroquine, in order to reduce the possibility of developing drug-resistant strains. In appropriate circumstances it may be used in combination with a 4-aminoquinoline for prophylaxis or for the interruption of transmission, especially of *P. falciparum*.

QUININE AND THE CINCHONA ALKALOIDS

History. Quinine is the chief alkaloid of cinchona, the bark of the cinchona tree indigenous to certain regions of South America. The bark is also called Peruvian, Jesuit's, or Cardinal's bark. It is not clear whether the natives were acquainted with the medicinal properties of cinchona. The first written record of the use of cinchona occurs in a religious book written in 1633 and published in Spain in 1639. The author, an Augustinian monk named Calancha, of Lima, Peru, wrote: "A tree grows which they call 'the fever tree' in the country of Loxa, whose bark, the color of cinnamon, is made into powder amounting to the weight of two small silver coins and given as a beverage, cures the fevers and tertians; it has produced miraculous results in Lima." A variety of colorful and fanciful versions of the discovery of the fever bark exist. A popular and persistent version is that the bark was employed in 1638 to treat Countess Anna del Chinchón, wife of the viceroy to Peru, and that her miraculous cure resulted in the introduction of cinchona into Spain in 1639 for the treatment of ague. There is no evidence that the countess ever used the bark; yet for many years the drug was called *los Polvos de la Condesa*. However, the viceroy did bring a large shipment of cinchona to Spain. By 1640, the drug was being employed for fevers in Europe. Its use was first mentioned in European medical literature in 1643 by a Belgian, Herman van der Heyden.

The term *cinchona* was chosen by Linné (who accidentally misspelled it) for the species of plants yielding the drug. Although this term is probably derived from the name of the countess whose alleged cure led to its wide use, some believe that it comes from a word of Incan origin, *kinia,* which means "bark." The Jesuit fathers were the main importers and distributors of cinchona in Europe, and the name *Jesuit bark* soon became attached to the drug. It was sponsored in Rome chiefly by the eminent philosopher Cardinal de Lugo; hence the drug came to be called *Cardinal's bark*. The conservative medical groups viewed the new antipyretic with disdain because its use did not conform to the teachings of Galen. Others looked upon it with suspicion because the Jesuits used it. For these reasons, the drug was dispensed for many years predominantly by charlatans and in the form of secret remedies. The most fabulous of these quacks was the incomparable Robert Talbor. The first official recognition of cinchona came in 1677, when it was included in an edition of the *London Pharmacopoeia* as "Cortex Peruanus."

For almost 2 centuries the bark was employed for medicine as a powder, extract, or infusion. In 1820, Pelletier and Caventou isolated quinine and cinchonine from cinchona, and the use of the alkaloids as such gained favor rapidly.

Chemistry. While quinine has been synthesized, the procedure is too complex and expensive to provide a practical source of the drug. Quinine and the other alkaloids are, therefore, still obtained entirely from natural sources.

Cinchona contains a mixture of more than 20 alkaloids. The most important of these are two pairs of optical isomers, *quinine* and *quinidine,* and *cinchonidine* and *cinchonine.* Quinine and cinchonidine are levorotatory.

Quinine has the following structural formula:

Quinine

Quinine contains a quinoline group attached through a secondary alcohol linkage to a quinuclidine ring. A methoxy side chain is attached to the quinoline ring and a vinyl to the quinuclidine. *Quinidine* has the same structure as quinine except for the steric configuration of the secondary alcohol group. The many natural alkaloids related to quinine and the semisynthetic chemicals derived from quinine differ mainly in the nature of the substitutions on the side chain. Each alteration in the chemical structure of quinine causes corresponding quantitative but not qualitative changes in the pharmacological actions of the resulting compounds.

Structure-Activity Relationship. The effects of chemical alterations in the quinine molecule on various pharmacological actions have been studied, particularly with regard to antimalarial potency. Since none of the resulting compounds has an antimalarial action superior to that of quinine, the details will not be presented. To summarize, the data indicate that neither the methoxy nor the vinyl radical of the quinine molecule is required for antimalarial activity. In contrast, the secondary alcohol group is absolutely essential, and its reduction in-

creases toxicity and abolishes antiplasmodial potency. Stereoisomerism is a relatively unimportant factor. Thus, quinidine shares the antimalarial activity of quinine.

Further details of the structure-activity relationship in the cinchona alkaloids may be found elsewhere (*see* Oettingen, 1933; Wiselogle, 1946; and others). Historically, this important field has provided the necessary background for the search for more effective and less toxic antimalarials, for example, *mefloquine.*

PHARMACOLOGICAL PROPERTIES

The typical actions of cinchona are largely attributable to its quinine content. The pharmacological properties of quinine are described in abbreviated form below. More complete descriptions and remarks on the properties of related cinchona alkaloids may be found in *earlier editions* of this textbook.

Local Actions. Quinine affects such a large variety of biological systems that it has been called a "general protoplasmic poison"; with some reservations this appraisal is probably correct. It is toxic to many bacteria and other unicellular organisms such as trypanosomes, infusoria, yeast, plasmodia, and spermatozoa. Despite this wide range of activity, quinine does exhibit considerable specificity in its action.

Local Anesthetic Action. Sensory nerves are briefly stimulated and then paralyzed by quinine. Concentrations only slightly higher than those necessary for anesthesia are likely to cause edema, pain, and reactive fibrosis. The anesthesia may last for many hours or days, and in this respect differs sharply from that produced by the conventional local anesthetics.

Irritant Action. Quinine is a marked local irritant. When taken orally, it may cause gastric pain, nausea, and vomiting. Subcutaneous or intramuscular injections of the drug are painful and may cause sterile abscesses. Intravenous administration may result in thrombosis of the injected vein from injury to the intima. Vascular damage is the basis for the occasional use of quinine solutions for sclerosing varicose veins.

Antimalarial Actions and Efficacy. Quinine acts primarily as a schizontocide; it has little effect on sporozoites or preerythrocytic forms of malarial parasites. The alkaloid is also gametocidal for *P. vivax* and *P. malariae* but not for *P. falciparum.* As both a suppressive and therapeutic agent, quinine is more toxic and less effective than chloroquine. However, it is especially valuable for the treatment of severe illness due to chloroquine-resistant and multidrug-resistant strains of *P. falciparum.*

Central Nervous System. Therapeutic doses of quinine have few effects on the CNS other than to cause *analgesia* and *antipyresis.* The discovery that cinchona lowered the fever of malarial patients quickly led to its use in all forms of febrile illnesses. However, quinine is not a potent antipyretic.

Cardiovascular System. The actions of quinine on cardiac muscle are qualitatively similar to those of its isomer, quinidine (*see* Chapter 31). Therapeutic doses of quinine have little, if any, effect on the normal heart or blood pressure in man. When given intravenously, quinine causes a definite and sometimes alarming hypotension, particularly when the injection is made rapidly.

Skeletal Muscle. Quinine and related cinchona alkaloids exert effects on skeletal muscle that have clinical implications. Quinine increases the tension response to a single maximal stimulus delivered to the muscle directly or through the nerve, but it also increases the refractory period of muscle so that the response to tetanic stimulation is diminished. The excitability of the motor end-plate region decreases so that responses to repetitive nerve stimulation and to acetylcholine are reduced. Thus, quinine can antagonize the actions of physostigmine on skeletal muscle as effectively as does curare. Quinine may cause symptomatic relief of *myotonia congenita*. This disease is the pharmacological antithesis of myasthenia gravis, such that drugs effective in one syndrome aggravate the other. Thus, quinine may produce alarming respiratory distress and dysphagia in patients with myasthenia.

Gastrointestinal Tract. The soluble salts of quinine are extremely bitter, and very small amounts of cinchona preparations are occasionally used as *stomachics*. Larger doses may inhibit vagal-mediated gastric secretion. The irritant properties of the cinchona alkaloids cause considerable *gastric distress*. Nausea, vomiting, and diarrhea are prominent when large doses are taken orally. Toxic amounts also produce vomiting by a central action on the medulla. The *musculature* of the intestinal tract is not stimulated by concentrations of the drug reached clinically.

Pancreas. Quinine may lower blood glucose concentrations apparently by stimulating insulin secretion by pancreatic islet cells (Henquin *et al.*, 1975; Herchuelz *et al.*, 1981). Quinine may induce severe hypoglycemia when used parenterally to treat severe falciparum malaria associated with deteriorating consciousness (cerebral malaria) or with pregnancy (White *et al.*, 1983b).

Absorption, Fate, and Excretion. Quinine and its congeners are readily absorbed when given orally. Absorption occurs mainly from the upper small intestine, and is almost complete, even in patients with marked diarrhea. Subcutaneous or intramuscular injection of quinine is contraindicated because of local tissue damage.

Peak plasma concentrations of cinchona alkaloids occur within 1 to 3 hours after a single oral dose. With chronic administration of total daily doses of 1 g of drug, the average plasma quinine concentration approximates 7 μg/ml. After termination of quinine therapy, the plasma concentration falls with a half-time of about 12 hours. A large fraction (approximately 70%) of plasma quinine is bound to proteins. This explains in part why the concentration of the alkaloid in cerebrospinal fluid is only 2 to 5% of that in the plasma. The pharmacokinetic properties of quinine have recently been studied in patients with cerebral and uncomplicated falciparum malaria (White *et al.*, 1982). Quinine readily reaches the tissues of the fetus.

The cinchona alkaloids are extensively metabolized, especially in the liver, so that less than 5% of an administered dose is excreted unaltered in the urine. There is no accumulation of the drugs in the body upon continued administration. The metabolites are excreted in the urine, where many of them have been identified as hydroxy derivatives (Brodie *et al.*, 1951). Renal excretion of quinine is twice as rapid when the urine is acidic as when it is alkaline.

Toxicity. Poisoning by quinine is usually due to clinical overdosage or to hypersensitivity. The fatal oral dose of quinine for adults is approximately 8 g. When quinine is repeatedly given in full doses, a typical cluster of symptoms occurs, termed *cinchonism*. In mild form this consists in ringing in the ears, headache, nausea, and disturbed vision; however, when medication is continued or after large single doses, gastrointestinal, cardiovascular, and dermal manifestations may appear.

Hearing and vision are particularly disturbed. Functional impairment of the eighth nerve results in tinnitus, decreased auditory acuity, and vertigo. Visual signs consist in blurred vision, disturbed color perception, photophobia, diplopia, night blindness, constricted visual fields, scotomata, and mydriasis. It is not known if the visual and auditory effects are directly neural or secondary to vascular changes. Marked spastic constriction of the retinal vessels occurs; the retina is ischemic, the discs are pale, and retinal edema may ensue. In severe cases, optic atrophy results. Degenerative changes in the spiral ganglion cells similar to those noted in the ganglion cells of the retina support the notion that cellular injury from quinine is direct. Perhaps both vascular and neural components of injury are involved.

Gastrointestinal symptoms are also prominent in cinchonism. Nausea, vomiting, abdominal pain, and diarrhea result from the local irritant action of quinine, but the nausea and emesis also have a central basis. The *skin* is often hot and flushed, and sweating is prominent. Rashes frequently appear. Angioedema, especially of the face, is occasionally observed.

CNS symptoms are noted in severer grades of poisoning, particularly headache, fever, vomiting, apprehension, excitement, confusion, delirium, and syncope. *Respiration* is first stimulated and then shallow and depressed. The skin becomes cold and cyanotic as poisoning progresses, the body temperature and the blood pressure fall, weakness is extreme, the pulse is feeble, coma ensues, and death occurs from respiratory arrest. *Death* may result in a few hours or be delayed 1 or 2 days. If the patient recovers, symptoms usually disappear completely except that there may be variable degrees of residual optic and auditory damage in some cases.

At times, *renal damage* may be caused by quinine, and anuria and uremia may ensue. The triad of massive hemolysis, hemoglobinemia, and hemoglobinuria is a rare complication of quinine therapy; it apparently is caused by the drug only in pregnant women or in patients with malaria. Quinine is capable of causing *hypoprothrombinemia;* the simultaneous administration of vitamin K counteracts the prolongation of the prothrombin time. Rarely, quinine may cause symptomatic *purpura* in hypersusceptible individuals, by a thrombocytolytic action. In a few instances, the drug appears to have caused *agranulocytosis. Abortion* may result from quinine overdosage, but this is not necessarily due to an oxytocic action of the drug. The alkaloid may cause *asthma* in hypersensitive individuals. Transient *ventricular tachycardia* may rarely be observed after massive acute overdosage.

When small doses of cinchona alkaloids cause toxic manifestations, the individual is usually hypersensitive to the drug. Cinchonism may appear after a single dose of quinine, but it is usually mild. Cutaneous flushing, pruritus, skin rashes, fever, gastric distress, dyspnea, ringing in the ears, and visual impairment are the usual expressions of hypersensitivity; extreme flushing of the skin accompanied by intense, generalized pruritus is the most common form. Hemoglobinuria and asthma from quinine are rare types of idiosyncrasy.

Contraindications. Quinine must be used with considerable caution, if at all, in patients who manifest idiosyncrasy to it, especially when this takes the form of cutaneous, angioedematous, visual, or auditory symptoms. Quinine should be stopped immediately if evidence of hemolysis appears. The drug should not be employed in patients with tinnitus or optic neuritis. In patients with atrial fibrillation, the administration of quinine requires the same precautions as outlined for quinidine (*see* Chapter 31).

Preparations, Routes of Administration, and Dosages. There are numerous preparations of cinchona alkaloids available, particularly in tropical communities where malaria is endemic and where inexpensive medication is essential. In the United States, the pure alkaloids are employed rather than the galenical preparations.

The most commonly used salt of quinine is the sulfate, which is available in tablets and capsules. The usual oral dose of quinine sulfate is 650 mg three times daily for 10 to 14 days. The drug is given after meals, preferably in capsules, to minimize gastric irritation.

Totaquine contains approximately 75% of the total anhydrous crystallizable cinchona alkaloids, of which 20% is quinine. The drug is cheaper than quinine and available in abundance in parts of the world where quinine is expensive or limited in supply. In proper doses, it is as effective as quinine in malaria inasmuch as it contains cinchona alkaloids with approximately the same order of antimalarial potency as quinine. The usual dosage of totaquine for malaria is 600 mg three times daily after meals.

The *oral route* should be employed for adminis-

tration of quinine whenever possible. Intravenous infusion of the drug is reserved for emergencies, such as fulminant or cerebral malaria; the dihydrochloride salt is employed. An appropriate dosage regimen for adults is 10 mg of base/kg in 250 to 500 ml of 5% glucose in water infused over the first 4 hours, followed by 10 mg/kg given as a 2-hour infusion every 8 hours. An additional dose (10 mg/kg in the first 4-hour infusion) has been advocated (White *et al.,* 1983a).

Therapeutic Uses

Quinine currently has two valid therapeutic applications: the treatment of malaria and the relief of nocturnal leg cramps.

Status as an Antimalarial. The prompt use of intravenous quinine as a rapidly acting schizontocidal drug to treat severe forms of chloroquine-resistant or multidrug-resistant falciparum malaria is mandatory and can be lifesaving in nonimmune patients. The drug should not be used alone, because it is less effective and more toxic than the synthetic antimalarial compounds. It is given concurrently with primaquine to achieve a radical cure of relapsing vivax malaria. Combinations of quinine either with pyrimethamine and a sulfonamide or with tetracycline have been used successfully to effect suppressive cure of patients with multidrug-resistant falciparum malaria (Hall *et al.,* 1975; Reacher *et al.,* 1981).

Nocturnal Leg Cramps. Recumbency leg muscle cramps (night cramps) are usually quickly and effectively relieved by quinine. The dose is 200 to 300 mg before retiring. In some patients, only a brief period of quinine therapy is required to provide long-lasting relief; in a few individuals, even large doses of the drug are ineffective.

ANTIBACTERIAL AGENTS IN ANTIMALARIAL CHEMOTHERAPY

Shortly after their introduction into therapeutics, the sulfonamides were shown to possess antimalarial activity. The sulfones were also shown to be effective; the first trial of dapsone was against *P. falciparum* in 1943. Little attention was paid to the data because of the superiority of other drugs. Current interest stems from their use, usually in combination with pyrimethamine, against resistant strains of falciparum malaria. When antimalarial activity was found in several antibiotics, the tetracyclines and chloramphenicol were tried clinically. Although their action as schizontocides is slow, their activity against drug-resistant malarial parasites is proving useful.

Sulfonamides and Sulfones. Much of the important work on sulfonamides was carried out during the intensive antimalarial program during World War II. This and later work focused attention on sulfadiazine, because of its relatively high activity. It was found, however, to be active only against the asexual blood forms of the human malarial parasites, and to act slowly. The combination of a long-acting sulfonamide, sulfadoxine, and pyrimethamine has been used extensively for the prophylaxis of chloroquine-resistant strains of *P. falciparum*. The utility of this combination is being compromised, however, by the rapid emergence of multidrug-resistant strains. A combination of sulfadiazine and pyrimethamine is preferable for the treatment of *acute attacks* that follow infection with such strains because of the shorter half-life of this sulfonamide. Sulfonamide-pyrimethamine combinations may produce toxic reactions such as hemolysis in patients with glucose-6-phosphate dehydrogenase deficiency or, rarely, exfoliative dermatitis and aplastic anemia. Parallel studies have demonstrated the value of a sulfone, such as dapsone, used in the same way as sulfonamides in combination with pyrimethamine. The danger of producing resistant strains, not only of malarial parasites but also of pathogenic bacteria, by the use of combinations containing sulfonamides or sulfones has been expressed. Neither sulfonamides nor sulfones are as active against *P. vivax* as they are against *P. falciparum*.

Tetracyclines. The use of tetracyclines in the treatment of the acute attack of multiresistant strains of falciparum malaria reflects sadly the sparsity of primary antimalarial drugs effective in such conditions. Their relative slowness of action makes concurrent treatment with quinine mandatory for rapid control of parasitemia. While several tetracyclines appear equivalent, most data have accumulated for tetracycline itself, and this is recommended. Although tetracycline has shown marked activity against primary tissue schizonts of chloroquine-resistant strains of *P. falciparum*, its long-term use as a prophylactic agent cannot be recommended because of the danger of producing antibiotic-resistant pathogenic bacteria (World Health Organization, 1973).

PRINCIPLES OF ANTIMALARIAL PROPHYLAXIS AND CHEMOTHERAPY

The prophylaxis and chemotherapy of the most dangerous forms of human malaria have become more complex and less satisfactory. This is due primarily to the increasing resistance of *P. falciparum* to antimalarial drugs. As of 1984, varying degrees of resistance to chloroquine had been identified in over 30 countries in Asia, South America, and Africa. The incidence of resistance to the combination of pyrimethamine and sulfadoxine is rising in areas of use, and this preparation has already become ineffective for the prophylaxis and treatment of chloroquine-resistant strains of *P. falciparum* malaria in certain parts of southeast Asia. Lack of responsiveness to the usual doses of quinine has even been a problem in these regions. (For review of drug resistance, *see* World Health Organization, 1981, 1984; Symposium, 1982.) Only broad guidelines for the prophylaxis and treatment of malaria are presented here, because specific chemothera-peutic regimens are rapidly changing (World Health Organization, 1984; Wyler, 1985). The Malaria Branch of the Centers for Disease Control is a reliable source of current information about this subject.

With a few important exceptions, the chemotherapy of an acute attack of human malaria is the same for all species of plasmodia; only subsequent treatment is dependent on species. The acute attack requires prompt treatment with a rapidly acting schizontocide; chloroquine is the drug of choice for *P. vivax*, *P. ovale*, *P. malariae*, and chloroquine-sensitive strains of *P. falciparum*. The oral route of administration should be used whenever possible, but chloroquine can be given intramuscularly or even intravenously (except in children, where fatal reactions may occur). For acute attacks with chloroquine-resistant or multidrug resistant strains of *P. falciparum*, the preferred schizontocide is quinine, despite its toxicity. Quinine is given in combination with other effective, but slower acting, blood schizontocides, for example, pyrimethamine-sulfadiazine for chloroquine-resistant strains or tetracycline for multidrug-resistant strains. Quinine is given by the oral route whenever possible, but intravenous preparations can be used when oral medication cannot be taken (White *et al.*, 1982). If intravenous quinine dihydrochloride is not available immediately, quinidine can be substituted (*see* White *et al.*, 1981; Swerdlow *et al.*, 1983). If the diagnosis of chloroquine-resistant falciparum malaria is suspected from a travel history and clinical findings, treatment with quinine should be instituted promptly. It is inadvisable to wait for a definitive diagnosis of *P. falciparum* by hematological findings because the clinical status of the patient may deteriorate rapidly.

Attacks of malaria may recur during or after a course of antimalarial chemotherapy, even in the absence of reinfection. Recurrent attacks of *P. vivax*, *P. ovale*, or *P. malariae* are usually well controlled by another course of chloroquine, combined with primaquine in the case of *P. vivax* and *P. ovale*. Some patients with vivax infection may require more than one course to effect a radical cure. Recrudescence of falciparum malarial attacks or parasitemia after appropriate treatment with chloroquine usually denotes infection with chloroquine-resistant plasmodia (for clinical classification, *see* World Health Organization, 1981). In this situation, treatment with a course of quinine combined with either pyrimethamine-sulfadoxine or tetracycline has provided the best results; the choice of the additional agent depends on the sensitivity to antifolates.

In endemic areas for malaria, chloroquine remains the drug of choice for the prophylaxis and control of infections due to *P. vivax*, *P. ovale*, *P. malariae*, or chloroquine-sensitive strains of *P. falciparum*. Attempts at radical cure of vivax malaria by administration of primaquine should be delayed until the patient leaves an endemic area. In areas where chloroquine-resistant *P. falciparum* is endemic, pyrimethamine-sulfadoxine should be given first to achieve the most effective prophylaxis. However, this regimen may fail to abort attacks with highly resistant or multidrug-resistant strains. If severe, such attacks are best controlled with quinine-tetracycline combination chemotherapy. The introduction of mefloquine given in combination with an antifolate or tetracycline should improve the outcome of prophylaxis and chemotherapy of chloroquine-resistant *P. falciparum.* However, mefloquine has yet to be formulated for parenteral administration.

Prophylaxis and chemotherapy of malaria in children and pregnant women present special problems. With appropriate dosage adjustments, the treatment of children is generally the same as in adults, except that quinine is better tolerated than chloroquine and antifolates should not be prescribed for infants. Malarial infection, particularly with *P. falciparum,* tends to be especially severe in infants and in pregnant women. The latter should be urged to avoid travel to endemic areas, if at all possible. While chloroquine and even quinine may be used during pregnancy, antifolates, tetracyclines and primaquine should be avoided. The exception here is the combination of pyrimethamine and sulfadoxine, which has been used safely for prophylaxis over extended periods.

Allison, J. L.; O'Brien, R. L.; and Hahn, F. E. DNA: reaction with chloroquine. *Science,* **1965,** *149,* 1111–1113.

——. Nature of the deoxyribonucleic acid—chloroquine complex. In, *Antimicrobial Agents and Chemotherapy—1965.* (Sylvester, J. C., ed.) American Society for Microbiology, Ann Arbor, Mich., **1966,** pp. 310–314.

Alving, A. S.; Eichelberger, L.; Craige, B., Jr.; Jones, R., Jr.; Whorton, C. M.; and Pullman, T. N. Studies on the chronic toxicity of chloroquine (SN-7618). *J. Clin. Invest.,* **1948,** *27,* 60–65.

Baker, J. K.; McChesney, J. D.; Hufford, C. D.; and Clark, A. M. High-performance liquid chromatographic analysis of the metabolism of primaquine and the identification of a new mammalian metabolite. *J. Chromatogr.,* **1982,** *230,* 69–77.

Berliner, R. W.; Earle, D. P., Jr.; Taggart, J. V.; Zubrod, C. G.; Welch, W. J.; Conan, N. J.; Bauman, E.; Scudder, S. T.; and Shannon, J. A. Studies on the chemotherapy of the human malarias. VI. The physiological disposition, antimalarial activity, and toxicity of several derivatives of 4-aminoquinoline. *J. Clin. Invest.,* **1948,** *27,* 98–107.

Bernstein, H. N.; Svaifler, N. J.; Rubin, M.; and Mausour, A. M. The ocular deposition of chloroquine. *Invest. Ophthalmol. Visual Sci.,* **1963,** *2,* 384–392.

Beutler, E., and Mitchell, M. Special modifications of the fluorescent screening method for glucose-6-phosphate dehydrogenase deficiency. *Blood,* **1968,** *32,* 816–818.

Brewer, G. J.; Tarlov, A. R.; and Alving, A. S. Methemoglobin reduction test: a new simple, *in vitro* test for identifying primaquine-sensitivity. *Bull. WHO,* **1960,** *22,* 633–640.

Brodie, B. B.; Baer, J. E.; and Craig, L. C. Metabolic products of the cinchona alkaloids in human urine. *J. Biol. Chem.,* **1951,** *188,* 567–581.

Brooks, M. H.; Malloy, J. P.; Bartelloni, P. J.; Sheehy, T. W.; and Barry, K. G. Quinine, pyrimethamine, and sulphorthodimethoxine: clinical response, plasma levels, and urinary excretion during the initial attack of naturally acquired *falciparum* malaria. *Clin. Pharmacol. Ther.,* **1969,** *10,* 85–91.

Brown, R. E.; Stancatto, F. A.; and Wolfe, A. D. The effects of mefloquine on *Escherichia coli. Life Sci.,* **1979,** *25,* 1857–1864.

Chou, A. C.; Chevli, R.; and Fitch, C. D. Ferriprotoporphyrin IX fulfills the criteria for identification as the chloroquine receptor of malaria parasites. *Biochemistry,* **1980,** *19,* 1543–1549.

Clyde, D. F.; McCarthy, V. C.; Miller, R. M.; and Hornick, R. B. Suppressive activity of mefloquine in sporozoite-induced human malaria. *Antimicrob. Agents Chemother.,* **1976,** *9,* 384–386.

Cohen, R. J.; Sachs, J. R.; Wicker, D. J.; and Conrad, M. E. Methemoglobinemia provoked by malarial chemoprophylaxis in Vietnam. *N. Engl. J. Med.,* **1968,** *279,* 1127–1131.

Cohen, S. N., and Yielding, K. L. Inhibition of DNA and RNA polymerase reactions by chloroquine. *Proc. Natl Acad. Sci. U.S.A.,* **1965,** *54,* 521–527.

Davidson, M. W.; Griggs, B. G., Jr.; Boykin, D. W.; and Wilson, W. D. Mefloquine, a clinically useful quinolinemethanol antimalarial which does not significantly bind to DNA. *Nature,* **1975,** *254,* 632–634.

——. Molecular structural effects involved in the interaction of quinolinemethanolamines with DNA. Implications for antimalarial action. *J. Med. Chem.,* **1977,** *20,* 1117–1122.

Desjardins, R. E.; Canfield, C. J.; Haynes, J. D.; and Chulay, J. D. Quantitative assessment of antimalarial activity *in vitro* by a semiautomated microdilution technique. *Antimicrob. Agents Chemother.,* **1979a,** *16,* 710–718.

Desjardins, R. E.; Pamplin, C. L.; von Bredow, J.; Barry, K. G.; and Canfield, C. J. Kinetics of a new antimalarial, mefloquine. *Clin. Pharmacol. Ther.,* **1979b,** *26,* 372–379.

Donno, L.; Sanguineti, V.; Ricciardi, M. L.; and Soldati, M. Antimalarial activity of kelfizina-trimethoprim and kelfizina-pyrimethamine versus chloroquine in field trials in Nigeria. *Am. J. Trop. Med. Hyg.,* **1969,** *18,* 182–187.

Dutta, P., and Fitch, C. D. Diverse membrane-active agents modify the hemolytic response to ferriprotoporphyrin IX. *J. Pharmacol. Exp. Ther.,* **1983,** *225,* 729–734.

Elderfield, R. C., and others. Alkylaminoalkyl derivatives of 8-aminoquinoline. *J. Am. Chem. Soc.,* **1946,** *68,* 1524–1529.

Falco, E. A.; Goodwin, L. G.; Hitchings, G. H.; Rollo, I. M.; and Russell, P. B. 2:4-Diaminopyrimidines—a new series of antimalarials. *Br. J. Pharmacol. Chemother.,* **1951,** *6,* 185–200.

Ferone, R.; Burchall, J. J.; and Hitchings, G. H. *Plasmodium berghei* dihydrofolate reductase: isolation, properties, and inhibition by antifolates. *Mol. Pharmacol.,* **1969,** *5,* 49–59.

Fitch, C. D.; Chan, R. L.; and Chevli, R. Chloroquine resistance in malaria: accessibility of drug receptors to mefloquine. *Antimicrob. Agents Chemother.,* **1979,** *15,* 258–262.

Hall, A. P.; Doberstyn, E. B.; Meltaprakong, V.; and Sonkom, P. Falciparum malaria cured by quinine followed by sulfadoxine-pyrimethamine. *Br. Med. J.,* **1975,** *2,* 15–17.

Henquin, J. C.; Horemans, B.; Nenquin, M.; Verniers, J.; and Lambert, A. E. Quinine-induced modifications of insulin release and glucose metabolism by isolated pancreatic islets. *FEBS Lett.,* **1975,** *57,* 280–284.

Herchuelz, A.; Lebrun, P.; Carpinelli, A.; Thonnart, N.; Sener, A.; and Malaisse, W. J. Regulation of calcium fluxes in rat pancreatic islets; quinine mimics the dual effect of glucose on calcium movements. *Biochem. Biophys. Acta,* **1981,** *640,* 16–30.

Hurly, M. G. D. Potentiation of pyrimethamine by sulphadiazine in human malaria. *Trans. R. Soc. Trop. Med. Hyg.,* **1959,** *53,* 412–413.

Kellermeyer, R. W.; Tarlov, A. R.; Brewer, G. J.; Carson, P. E.; and Alving, A. S. Hemolytic effect of therapeutic drugs: clinical considerations of the primaquine-type hemolysis. *J.A.M.A.*, **1962**, *180*, 388–394.

Konigk, E., and Putfarken, B. Inhibition of ornithine decarboxylase of *in vitro* cultured *Plasmodium falciparum* by chloroquine. *Tropenmed. Parasitol.*, **1983**, *34*, 1–3.

Krotoski, W. A.; Bray, R. S.; Garnham, P. C. C.; Gwadz, R. W.; Killick-Kendrick, R.; Draper, C. C.; Targett, G. A. T.; Krotoski, D. H.; Guy, M. W.; Koontz, L. C.; and Cogswell, F. B. Observations on early and late post-sporozoite tissue stages in primate malaria. II. The hypnozoite of *Plasmodium cynomolgi* bastianelli. *Am. J. Trop. Med. Hyg.*, **1982**, *31*, 211–225.

Lucas, A. O.; Hendrickse, R. G.; Okubadejo, O. A.; Richards, W. H. G.; Neal, R. A.; and Kofie, B. A. K. The suppression of malarial parasitaemia by pyrimethamine in combination with dapsone or sulphormethoxine. *Trans. R. Soc. Trop. Med. Hyg.*, **1969**, *63*, 216–229.

Meshnick, S. R.; Chang, K.-P.; and Cerami, A. Heme lysis of the bloodstream forms of *Trypanosoma brucei*. *Biochem. Pharmacol.*, **1977**, *26*, 1923–1928.

Mu, J. Y.; Israili, Z. H.; and Dayton, P. G. Studies of the disposition and metabolism of mefloquine HCl (WR 142490), a quinolinemethanol antimalarial, in the rat. *Drug Metab. Dispos.*, **1975**, *3*, 198–210.

Mühlens, P. Die Behandlung der naturlichen menschlichen Malaria-Infektion mit Plasmochin. *Naturwissenschaften*, **1926**, *14*, 1162–1166.

Reacher, M.; Campbell, C. C.; Freeman, J.; Doberstyn, E. B.; and Brandling-Bennett, A. D. Drug therapy for *Plasmodium falciparum* malaria resistant to pyrimethamine-sulfadoxine (FANSIDAR). A study of alternate regimens in Eastern Thailand, 1980. *Lancet*, **1981**, *2*, 1066–1069.

Rieckmann, K. H.; Campbell, G. H.; Sax, L. J.; and Mrema, J. E. Drug sensitivity of *Plasmodium falciparum*. An *in vitro* microtechnique. *Lancet*, **1978**, *2*, 22–23.

Rieckmann, K. H.; McNamara, J. V.; Frischer, H.; Stockert, T. A.; Carson, P. E.; and Powell, R. D. Effects of chloroquine, quinine and cycloguanil upon the maturation of asexual erythrocytic forms of two strains of *Plasmodium falciparum in vitro*. *Am. J. Trop. Med. Hyg.*, **1968**, *17*, 661–671.

Rieckmann, K. H.; Trenholme, G. M.; Williams, R. L.; Carson, P. E.; Frischer, H.; and Desjardins, R. E. Prophylactic activity of mefloquine hydrochloride (WR 142490) in drug-resistant malaria. *Bull. WHO*, **1974**, *51*, 375–377.

Rollo, I. M. The mode of action of sulphonamides, PROGUANIL, and pyrimethamine on *Plasmodium gallinaceum*. *Br. J. Pharmacol. Chemother.*, **1955**, *10*, 208–214.

Schellenberg, K. A., and Coatney, G. R. The influence of antimalarial drugs on nucleic acid synthesis in *Plasmodium gallinaceum* and *Plasmodium berghei*. *Biochem. Pharmacol.*, **1960**, *6*, 143–152.

Schmidt, L. H. *Plasmodium falciparum* and *Plasmodium vivax* infections in the owl monkey (*Aotus trivirgatus*). *Am. J. Trop. Med. Hyg.*, **1978**, *27*, 671–737.

Schmidt, L. H.; Crosby, R.; Rasco, J.; and Vaughan, D. Antimalarial activities of various 4-quinolinemethanols with special attention to WR-142,490 (mefloquine). *Antimicrob. Agents Chemother.*, **1978**, *13*, 1011–1030.

Smith, C. C. Metabolism of pentaquine in the rhesus monkey. *J. Pharmacol. Exp. Ther.*, **1956**, *116*, 67–76.

Stickney, D. R.; Simmons, W. S.; De Angelis, R. L.; Rundles, R. W.; and Nichol, C. A. Pharmacokinetics of pyrimethamine (PRM) and 2,4-diamino-5-(3',4'-dichlorophenyl)-6-methyl pyrimidine (DMP) relevant to meningeal leukemia. *Proc. Am. Assoc. Cancer Res.*, **1973**, *14*, 52.

Swerdlow, C. D.; Yu, J. O.; Jacobson, E.; Mann, S.; Winkle, R. A.; Griffin, J. C.; Ross, D. L.; and Mason, J. L. Safety and efficacy of intravenous quinidine. *Am. J. Med.*, **1983**, *75*, 36–42.

Thompson, P. E.; Olszewski, B. J.; Elslager, E. F.; and Worth, D. F. Laboratory studies on 4,6-diamino-1-(p-chlorophenyl)-1,2-dihydro-2,2-dimethyl-s-triazine pamoate (CI-501) as a repository antimalarial drug. *Am. J. Trop. Med. Hyg.*, **1963**, *12*, 481–493.

Trager, W., and Jensen, J. B. Human malaria parasites in continuous culture. *Science*, **1976**, *193*, 673–675.

Trenholme, G. M.; Williams, R. L.; Desjardins, R. E.; Frischer, H.; Carson, P. E.; and Rieckmann, K. H. Mefloquine (WR 142,490) in the treatment of human malaria. *Science*, **1975**, *190*, 792–794.

Warhurst, D. C., and Thomas, S. C. The chemotherapy of rodent malaria. XXXI. The effect of some metabolic inhibitors upon chloroquine-induced pigment clumping (CIPC) in *Plasmodium berghei*. *Ann. Trop. Med. Parasitol.*, **1978**, *72*, 203–211.

Whichard, L. P.; Morris, C. R.; Smith, J. M.; and Holbrook, D. J., Jr. The binding of primaquine, pentaquine, pamaquine, and PLASMOCID to deoxyribonucleic acid. *Mol. Pharmacol.*, **1968**, *4*, 630–639.

White, N. J.; Looareesuwan, S.; Warrell, D. A.; Chongsuphajaisiddhi, T.; Bunnag, D.; and Harinasuta, T. Quinidine in falciparum malaria. *Lancet*, **1981**, *2*, 1069–1071.

White, N. J.; Looareesuwan, S.; Warrell, D. A.; Warrell, M. J.; Bunnag, D.; and Harinasuta, T. Quinine pharmacokinetics and toxicity in cerebral and uncomplicated falciparum malaria. *Am. J. Med.*, **1982**, *73*, 564–572.

White, N. J.; Looareesuwan, S.; Warrell, D. A.; Warrell, M. J.; Chanthavanich, P.; Bunnag, D.; and Harinasuta, T. Quinine loading dose in cerebral malaria. *Am. J. Trop. Med. Hyg.*, **1983a**, *32*, 1–5.

White, N. J.; Warrell, D. A.; Chanthavanich, P.; Looareesuwan, S.; Warrell, M. J.; Krishna, S.; Williamson, D. H.; and Turner, R. C. Severe hypoglycemia and hyperinsulinemia in falciparum malaria. *N. Engl. J. Med.*, **1983b**, *309*, 61–66.

Monographs and Reviews

Albert, A. *Selective Toxicity: The Physico-Chemical Basis of Therapy*, 6th ed. Chapman & Hall, Ltd., London, **1979**.

Beutler, E. Drug-induced hemolytic anemia. *Pharmacol. Rev.*, **1969**, *21*, 73–103.

Bruce-Chwatt, L. J. (ed.). *Chemotherapy of Malaria*, 2nd ed. Monograph Series No. 27. World Health Organization, Geneva, **1981**.

Canfield, C. J. Antimalarial aminoalcohol alternatives to mefloquine. *Acta Trop. (Basel)*, **1980**, *37*, 232–237.

Centers for Disease Control. Prevention of malaria in travelers 1982. *M.M.W.R.*, **1982**, *31*, 15–285.

Clyde, D. F. Clinical problems associated with the use of primaquine as a tissue schizontocidal and gametocytocidal drug. *Bull. WHO*, **1981**, *59*, 391–395.

Coatney, G. R.; Cooper, W. C.; Eddy, N. B.; and Greenberg, J. *Survey of Antimalarial Agents: Chemotherapy of Plasmodium gallinaceum Infections; Toxicity; Correlation of Structure and Action.* Public Health Service Monograph No. 9, U.S. Government Printing Office, Washington, D. C., **1953**.

Davey, D. G. Chemotherapy of malaria. Part 1. Biological basis of testing methods. In, *Experimental Chemotherapy*, Vol. 1. (Schnitzer, R. J., and Hawking, F., eds.) Academic Press, Inc., New York, **1963**, pp. 487–511.

Davidson, D. E.; Ager, A. L.; Brown, J. L.; Chapple, F. E.; Whitmore, R. E.; and Rossan, R. N. New tissue schizontocidal antimalarial drugs. *Bull. WHO*, **1981**, *59*, 463–480.

Dubois, E. L. Antimalarials in the management of discoid and systemic lupus erythematosus. *Semin. Arthritis Rheum.*, **1978**, *8*, 33–51.

Feldman, H. A. Toxoplasmosis. *N. Engl. J. Med.*, **1968**, *279*, 1370–1375, 1431–1437.

Fitch, C. D. Mode of action of antimalarial drugs. In, *Malaria and the Red Cell*. Ciba Foundation Symposium 94. Pitman, London, **1983**, pp. 222–232.

Good, M. I., and Shader, R. I. Lethality and behavioral side effects of chloroquine. *J. Clin. Psychopharmacol.*, **1982**, *2*, 40–47.

Hill, J. Chemotherapy of malaria. Part 2. The antimalarial drugs. In, *Experimental Chemotherapy*, Vol. 1. (Schnitzer, R. J., and Hawking, F., eds.) Academic Press, Inc., New York, **1963**, pp. 513–601.

Hitchings, G. H., and Burchall, J. J. Inhibition of folate biosynthesis and function as a basis for chemotherapy. *Adv. Enzymol.*, **1965**, *27*, 417–468.

Isaacson, D.; Elgart, M.; and Turner, M. L. Antimalarials in dermatology. *Int. J. Dermatol.*, **1982**, *21*, 379–395.

Oettingen, W. F. von. *The Therapeutic Agents of the Quinoline Group*. Chemical Catalog Co., New York, **1933**.

Olansky, A. J. Antimalarials and ophthalmologic safety. *J. Am. Acad. Dermatol.*, **1982**, *6*, 19–23.

Rollo, I. M. Dihydrofolate reductase inhibitors as antimicrobial agents and their potentiation by sulfonamides. *CRC Crit. Rev. Clin. Lab. Sci.*, **1970**, *1*, 565–583.

Sweeney, T. R. The present status of malaria chemotherapy: mefloquine, a novel antimalarial. *Med. Res. Rev.*, **1981**, *1*, 281–301.

Symposium on DARAPRIM. (Various authors.) *Trans. R. Soc. Trop. Med. Hyg.*, **1952**, *46*, 467–508.

Symposium. (Various authors.) The synergy of trimethoprim and sulphonamides. *Postgrad. Med. J.*, **1969**, *45*, Suppl., 3–104.

Symposium. (Various authors.) Malaria. (Cohen, S., ed.) *Br. Med. Bull.*, **1982**, *38*, 115–217.

Tarlov, A. R.; Brewer, G. J.; Carson, P. E.; and Alving, A. S. Primaquine sensitivity. *Arch. Intern. Med.*, **1962**, *109*, 209–234.

Thompson, P. E., and Werbel, L. M. *Antimalarial Agents: Chemistry and Pharmacology*. Academic Press, Inc., New York, **1972**.

Wiselogle, F. Y. (ed.). *A Survey of Antimalarial Drugs, 1941–1945*. J. W. Edwards, Publisher, Inc., Ann Arbor, Mich., **1946**. (Two volumes.)

World Health Organization. *Standardization of Procedures for the Study of Glucose-6-Phosphate Dehydrogenase*. Technical Report No. 366, WHO, Geneva, **1967**.

——. *Chemotherapy of Malaria and Resistance to Antimalarials*. Technical Report No. 529, WHO, Geneva, **1973**.

——. *Chemotherapy of Malaria*, 2nd ed. WHO Monograph Series No. 27, WHO, Geneva, **1981**.

——. Development of mefloquine as an antimalarial drug. *Bull. WHO*, **1983**, *61*, 169–178.

——. *Report of the Steering Committees of the Scientific Working Groups on Malaria*. WHO, Geneva, **1984**.

Wyler, D. J. Malaria-resurgence, resistance, and research. *N. Engl. J. Med.*, **1983**, *308*, 875–878, 934–940.

——. *Plasmodium* species (malaria). In, *Principles and Practice of Infectious Diseases*, 2nd ed. (Mandell, G. L.; Douglas, R. G., Jr.; and Bennett, J. E.; eds.) John Wiley & Sons, Inc., New York, **1985**, pp. 1514–1522.

CHAPTER

46 DRUGS USED IN THE CHEMOTHERAPY OF PROTOZOAL INFECTIONS

[*Continued*]

Amebiasis, Giardiasis, and Trichomoniasis

Leslie T. Webster, Jr.

Three pathogenic protozoal infections are commonly encountered in the United States and other temperate climates, in addition to the tropical world: *amebiasis, giardiasis,* and *trichomoniasis*. These diseases are briefly described here, along with the specific drugs used for their treatment. The reader is referred to the specialized literature and reviews cited at the end of this chapter for more details about the diagnosis and clinical management of these conditions.

Although *amebiasis,* caused by *Entamoeba histolytica,* has a cosmopolitan distribution, it is most severe in subtropical and tropical regions. While endemic amebiasis is relatively rare among the general population of the United States, the infection still has a prevalence of 2 to 4%. It is transmitted by the fecal-oral route and is particularly common under poor hygienic conditions in lower socioeconomic groups, institutionalized individuals, and male homosexuals. Ingested amebic *cysts* from contaminated material change into *trophozoites* that reside in the human colon. There they multiply, encyst, and pass into the environment, thereby completing the cycle. Trophozoites usually exist as commensals in the large intestine; that is, they produce cysts but otherwise cause little harm to the host. However, trophozoites may change into pathogenic forms that invade the tissues. In this case, they produce a variety of local and systemic manifestations, particularly including amebic dysentery and abscesses of the liver and, less frequently, other tissues. The diagnosis of amebiasis and its persistence is made by appropriate examination of rectal scrapings or of the stool. However, the services of a skilled microscopist may be required to distinguish *E. histolytica* from nonpathogenic amebae or white blood cells.

Drugs used to treat amebiasis (amebicides) can be categorized as *luminal, systemic,* or *mixed*. Luminal amebicides, exemplified by *diloxanide furoate* and other *dichloroacetamide derivatives,* are active only against intestinal forms of amebae. These compounds can be used successfully by themselves to treat asymptomatic or mild intestinal forms of amebiasis or, in conjunction with a systemic or mixed amebicide, to eradicate the infection. Systemic amebicides are effective only in invasive forms of amebiasis. These agents have been employed primarily to treat severe amebic dysentery (*dehydroemetine*) or hepatic abscesses (*dehydroemetine* or *chloroquine*), but they are rarely used now unless other drugs fail or cause unacceptable side effects. Mixed amebicides are active against both intestinal and systemic forms of amebiasis. *Metronidazole,* a nitroimidazole derivative, is the prototypical mixed amebicide, and its use has revolutionized the treatment of this protozoal infection. Because it is well absorbed and therefore may fail to reach the large intestine in therapeutic concentrations, this compound is likely to be more effective against systemic than intestinal amebiasis. Antibiotics such as *tetracycline* or the amebicidal aminoglycoside *paromomycin* can be used in conjunction with metronidazole to treat severe forms of intestinal amebiasis. Treatment with metronidazole is often followed by a luminal amebicide to effect a cure.

Giardiasis, caused by the flagellated protozoan *Giardia lamblia,* is the most commonly reported intestinal protozoal infection in developed countries, including the United States. Most infected individuals are asymptomatic. However, these organisms may produce either isolated cases or epidemics of diarrhea; this can be transient or persistent, and it occasionally results in malabsorption, manifested by steatorrhea and weight loss. *Cysts,* in feces or in contaminated food or water, transmit the infection; the organism does not require an intermediate host. Travelers, campers, children and adults living under crowded unhygienic conditions, and male homosexuals are especially at risk. Ingested cysts change into active *trophozoites* that eventually reside and proliferate in the upper small intestine, where they may or may not produce disease. The diagnosis of giardiasis is made by identification of cysts or trophozoites in fecal specimens. Chemotherapy with *quinacrine* or *metronidazole* is usually successful.

Trichomoniasis is caused by the flagellated protozoan *Trichomonas vaginalis.* This organism inhabits the genitourinary tract of the human host, where it can produce vaginitis in women or urethritis in men. Transmission of the infection occurs primarily by sexual contact, and over 200 million people worldwide become affected each year. Only *trophozoite* forms of the parasite have been identified in infected secretions, which are routinely examined for diagnostic purposes. Proper treatment of both partners with either *metronidazole* or related *nitroimidazole compounds* is nearly always successful.

CHLOROQUINE

History. The unique therapeutic value of chloroquine in *extraintestinal amebiasis* in man was first reported by Conan (1948, 1949) and Murgatroyd and Kent (1948). *In-vitro* studies with trophozoites of *E. histolytica* had revealed that chloroquine possesses amebicidal activity greater than that of the halogenated 8-hydroxyquinolines but less than that of emetine. This discovery, combined with the knowledge that chloroquine localizes in the liver in a concentration several hundred times greater than that in the plasma, suggested its use in *hepatic amebiasis.* Clinical trial then revealed that the signs and the symptoms of amebic hepatitis disappeared within a few days after the start of chloroquine therapy and that the disease was adequately controlled and often cured.

Pharmacological Properties. The pharmacology and the toxicology of chloroquine are fully pre-

sented in Chapter 45. Only those features of the drug pertinent to its use in amebiasis are described here.

Chloroquine is now used as a systemic amebicide to treat hepatic amebiasis only when treatment with metronidazole is unsuccessful or contraindicated. The clinical response to chloroquine in patients with hepatic amebiasis is often prompt, and there is no evidence that amebae develop resistance to this agent. The drug is much less effective in amebiasis of the colon, partly because it attains a much lower concentration in the intestinal wall than in the liver and partly because it is almost completely absorbed from the small bowel. Because colonic infection with *E. histolytica* is always the source of extraintestinal amebiasis, a drug effective in intestinal amebiasis is routinely given to all patients receiving chloroquine for hepatic amebiasis; such therapy reduces the relapse rate. Conversely, because of the difficulty of determining whether individuals with colonic amebiasis also have hepatic involvement, it is often wise to administer metronidazole or chloroquine when a luminal amebicide is prescribed.

The conventional course of treatment with chloroquine phosphate for extraintestinal amebiasis in adults is 1 g daily for 2 days, followed by 500 mg daily for 2 to 3 weeks. Because of the low toxicity of the drug, this dose schedule can be increased if necessary. Treatment with chloroquine may be repeated. Extended courses of therapy with chloroquine (10 weeks) have also been recommended (Cohen and Reynolds, 1975).

DILOXANIDE FUROATE

History. *Diloxanide* is a dichloroacetamide derivative that was introduced by Bristow and associates (1956) as a result of the examination of a series of substituted acetanilides for amebicidal activity. Clinical trials showed diloxanide to be effective in cyst-passing patients, but to be relatively ineffective in the treatment of acute intestinal amebiasis. This was attributed to the presence of inadequate concentrations of the drug at the sites of infection. Of the many derivatives of diloxanide prepared in attempts to offset this disadvantage, the furoate ester proved to be appreciably more active than the parent compound in experimentally infected rats (Main *et al.,* 1960). The results of clinical trials showed it to be effective in cases of acute intestinal amebiasis (Shaldon, 1960; Woodruff and Bell, 1960). *Teclozan* and *etofamide* are other dichloroacetamide derivatives that have been used with success as intraluminal amebicides (*see* Neal, 1983).

Chemistry and Preparation. *Diloxanide furoate* (FURAMIDE) has the following structural formula:

Diloxanide Furoate

After oral ingestion the ester is hydrolyzed to diloxanide and furoic acid. In the United States diloxanide furoate is available in 500-mg tablets from the Parasitic Diseases Division, Centers for Disease Control.

Pharmacological Effects. Diloxanide is directly amebicidal when tested *in vitro*. The furoate ester is active at 0.01 to 0.1 μg/ml, and it is thus considerably more potent than emetine. Little is known of its mechanism of action.

Absorption, Fate, and Excretion. In experimental animals, 60 to 90% of an oral dose of diloxanide furoate is excreted in the urine within 48 hours. More than half of this appears within 6 hours. Excretion in the feces accounts for 4 to 9% of the dose. Peak concentrations appear in the blood within 1 hour but fall to a fraction of this within 6 hours. Hence, a major part of an oral dose is rapidly absorbed from the gastrointestinal tract and is rapidly excreted in the urine. The ester is largely hydrolyzed in the lumen or mucosa of the intestine, so that only diloxanide appears in the systemic circulation (Wilmshurst and Cliffe, 1964). The drug appears in the urine largely as the glucuronide.

Route of Administration and Dosage. Diloxanide furoate is given only orally. The recommended dosage is 500 mg, three times daily for 10 days. If necessary, a second course may be given immediately following the first. Children should be given 20 mg/kg per day in three divided doses for 10 days.

Toxicity and Side Effects. Side effects are mild. Flatulence is most commonly reported; vomiting, pruritus, and urticaria occur occasionally (*see* Wolfe, 1973).

Therapeutic Uses. Diloxanide furoate is the drug of choice in the treatment of asymptomatic passers of cysts (administered alone) (Krogstad *et al.*, 1978), or in the treatment of invasive and extraintestinal amebiasis (administered with an appropriate systemic or mixed amebicide). It is ineffective when administered alone in the treatment of extraintestinal amebiasis. There is controversy about its efficacy when used alone in the treatment of acute amebiasis with frank dysentery. While good results have been reported from some areas, other trials have been less successful (*see* Suchak *et al.*, 1962; Wilmot *et al.*, 1962). In trials carried out primarily on asymptomatic subjects passing trophozoites or cysts, or on patients with nondysenteric, symptomatic intestinal amebiasis, treatment with diloxanide furoate resulted in a high percentage of cures (Woodruff and Bell, 1960; Wolfe, 1973). In all cases the drug was well tolerated. The relatively low cost of this compound is also an advantage, particularly in underdeveloped countries.

EMETINE AND DEHYDROEMETINE

Emetine is an alkaloid obtained from ipecac ("Brazil root"); it is also prepared semisynthetically by methylation of cephaëline, another alkaloid in ipecac. The use of this compound as a direct-acting systemic amebicide dates from 1912, when Vedder showed that the drug killed amebae *in vitro*. Since then, emetine has been one of the most widely used agents in the treatment of severe invasive *intestinal amebiasis, amebic hepatitis,* and *amebic abscesses.* Dehydroemetine is a close structural analog of emetine that has similar pharmacological properties, but it is considered to be less toxic. Both drugs are being replaced by mixed amebicides of the *nitroimidazole class,* which are as effective but far safer (*see* below). Thus, emetine and dehydroemetine should not be used unless the nitroimidazoles are ineffective or contraindicated. Disadvantages of these alkaloids are as follows: (1) Both compounds require parenteral administration by subcutaneous or deep intramuscular injection; local reactions ranging from pain to abscess formation are not uncommon. (2) Particularly after prolonged administration, both agents may produce systemic toxic reactions, some of which can be serious or fatal; adverse effects primarily involve the heart and cardiovascular system, the neuromuscular system, the central nervous system, and the gastrointestinal tract. (3) Although their use can occasionally be lifesaving because of direct amebicidal action, neither compound can be used alone for curative purposes. (4) Patients receiving either agent require close medical supervision. (5) Use of either drug is contraindicated in patients who are pregnant or in those who have cardiac, renal, or neuromuscular disease.

Details of the pharmacology and toxicology of emetine and dehydroemetine are presented in *earlier editions* of this textbook (*see also* Yang and Dubick, 1980; Harries, 1982). The dosage for dehydroemetine in adults is 1 to 1.5 mg/kg per day, to a maximal daily dose of 90 mg. This regimen is continued for up to 5 days. The daily pediatric dose is the same, except that one half of it is given every 12 hours. Emetine hydrochloride is available as an injection (65 mg/ml); dehydroemetine is available from the Parasitic Diseases Division, Centers for Disease Control.

8-HYDROXYQUINOLINES

A number of halogenated 8-hydroxyquinolines have been synthesized and utilized clinically as luminal amebicides, particularly to treat asymptomatic passers of cysts. Such direct-acting amebicidal agents have also been used in combination with metronidazole to treat intestinal forms of amebiasis. *Iodoquinol (diiodohydroxyquin)* and *clioquinol (iodochlorhydroxyquin)* are the best known of this class of compounds. They have been widely and all too often indiscriminately employed for the treatment of diarrhea. The use of these drugs, particularly at high doses for long periods, is unfortunately associated with significant risk. The most important toxic reaction, which has been ascribed primarily to clioquinol, is *subacute myelooptic neuropathy* (SMON). This disease is a myelitis-like illness that was first described in epidemic form (thousands of afflicted patients) in Japan; only sporadic cases have been reported elsewhere, but the actual prevalence is unknown. While SMON in

Japan was apparently caused by clioquinol, similar toxic effects have been noted in other countries with other 8-hydroxyquinolines (*see* Oakley, 1973). Administration of iodoquinol in high doses to children with chronic diarrhea, for example, has been associated with optic atrophy and permanent loss of vision. Clioquinol has not been used in Japan since 1970, and severe restrictions were imposed on its sale in other countries, including the United States. Iodoquinol is thought to be safer than clioquinol (probably because the former is less well absorbed after oral administration), and it remains available in the United States. *However, routine use of either compound is not recommended* because members of the less toxic *dichloroacetamide class* of luminal amebicides are available. The dosage of iodoquinol should not exceed 2 g daily for 20 days in adults or 30 to 40 mg/kg per day for 20 days in children. The pharmacology of the 8-hydroxyquinolines is described in greater detail in *previous editions* of this textbook.

METRONIDAZOLE

History. The discovery of *azomycin* (2-nitroimidazole) by Nakamura in 1955 and the demonstration of its trichomonacidal properties by Horie (1956) led to the chemical synthesis and biological testing of many nitroimidazoles. One compound, 1-(β-hydroxyethyl)-2-methyl-5-nitroimidazole, now called *metronidazole*, was found to have particularly high activity *in vitro* and *in vivo* against *T. vaginalis* and *E. histolytica* (Cosar and Julou, 1959; Cosar *et al.*, 1961). Durel and associates (1959, 1960) reported that oral doses of the drug imparted trichomonacidal activity to semen and urine, and they showed that a high cure rate could be obtained in both male and female patients suffering from trichomoniasis. Metronidazole has an extremely broad spectrum of protozoal and antimicrobial activity, which can be used to clinical advantage (*see* below). Other clinically effective 5-nitroimidazoles closely related in structure and activity to metronidazole are currently available in some parts of the world, but not in the United States. These include *tinidazole* (FASIGYN), *nimorazole* (NAXOGIN), and *ornidazole*. *Benznidazole* is another 5-nitroimidazole derivative that is unusual in that it is effective in acute Chagas' infection (*see* Chapter 47).

Chemistry. Metronidazole has the following structural formula:

$$\begin{array}{c}\text{H}-\text{C}-\text{N} \\ \quad\quad \|\quad\quad\diagdown\text{C}-\text{CH}_3 \\ \text{O}_2\text{N}-\text{C}-\text{N} \\ \quad\quad\quad\quad | \\ \quad\quad\quad\quad \text{CH}_2\text{CH}_2\text{OH} \end{array}$$
Metronidazole

It occurs as pale-yellow crystals that are slightly soluble in water and alcohol.

Antiparasitic and Antimicrobial Effects. Metronidazole is directly trichomonacidal. It destroys

99% of the microorganisms in cultures of *T. vaginalis* within 24 hours at a concentration of 2.5 μg/ml. The drug is also exceedingly active against *E. histolytica*. In culture, the morphology of the microorganisms is altered markedly within 6 to 20 hours by concentrations of 1 to 2 μg/ml. Within 24 hours all microorganisms are killed. At a concentration of 0.2 μg/ml, the same effect is seen within 72 hours (Gordeeva, 1965). Trophozoites of *G. lamblia* are probably also directly affected by metronidazole at concentrations of 1 to 50 μg/ml *in vitro* (Jokipii and Jokipii, 1980).

Metronidazole also displays antibacterial activity against all anaerobic cocci and both anaerobic gram-negative bacilli, including *Bacteroides* species, and anaerobic spore-forming gram-positive bacilli. Nonsporulating gram-positive bacilli are often resistant, as are aerobic and facultatively anaerobic bacteria (Chow *et al.*, 1975; Ralph and Kirby, 1975a, 1975b; Sutter and Finegold, in Symposium, 1977; Oldenburg and Speck, 1983).

Metronidazole is clinically effective in *trichomoniasis, amebiasis,* and *giardiasis,* as well as in a variety of infections caused by obligate anaerobic bacteria, including *Bacteroides fragilis*. A related nitroimidazole, *benznidazole,* has shown some promise in the treatment of *American cutaneous leishmaniasis* and *Chagas' disease,* but toxicity may limit its prolonged use (Coura *et al.*, 1978). Other effects of nitroimidazoles include suppression of cellular immunity, mutagenesis, carcinogenesis, and sensitization of hypoxic cells to radiation (*see* Miller, 1980; Voogd, 1981; Brown *et al.*, 1984). Several reviews of the nitroimidazoles are available (Goldman, 1980; Molavi *et al.*, 1982; Oldenburg and Speck, 1983).

The mechanism of action of the nitroimidazoles is reflected in a selective toxicity to anaerobic or microaerophilic microorganisms and for anoxic or hypoxic cells. The nitro group of metronidazole behaves as an electron acceptor for electron-transport proteins such as flavoproteins in mammalian cells and ferredoxins or their equivalent in bacteria. In the former case, a nitro reductase catalyzes the reaction of the flavin radical with the nitro compound; in the latter case, the reduction is catalyzed by iron-sulfur complexes. The source of electrons for the reduction may be a number of endogenous reduced substrates, such as reduced nicotinamide adenine dinucleotide phosphate (NADPH) or sulfide. It is currently thought that chemically reactive reduced forms of the drug produce biochemical lesions that lead to the death of the cell. While earlier work had established that the drug inhibits DNA synthesis in *T. vaginalis* and *Clostridium bifermentans* and causes degradation of existing DNA in the latter microorganism, further studies with mammalian DNA indicate that reduced metronidazole causes a loss of the helical structure of DNA, strand breakage, and an accompanying impairment of its function. Such findings are consistent with the antimicrobial and mutagenic effects of metronidazole and its ability to potentiate the effects of radiation on hypoxic tumor cells (*see* LaRusso *et al.*, 1977; Adams *et al.*, 1980; Edwards, 1980; Edwards *et al.*, 1982).

Absorption, Fate, and Excretion. The pharmacokinetic properties of metronidazole have been summarized by Ralph (1983). The drug is usually well and promptly absorbed after oral administration, reaching concentrations in plasma of about 10 μg/ml in approximately 1 hour after a single 50-mg dose. A linear relationship between dose and plasma concentration pertains for doses between 200 and 2000 mg. Repeated doses every 6 to 8 hours result in some accumulation of the drug. Mean effective concentrations of the compound are 8 μg/ml or less for most susceptible protozoa and bacteria. The bioavailability of metronidazole approaches 100%, its half-life in plasma is about 8 to 10 hours, and its volume of distribution is approximately 1 liter per kilogram. About 10% of the drug is bound to plasma proteins. Metronidazole penetrates well into body tissues and fluids, including vaginal secretions, seminal fluid, saliva, and breast milk. Therapeutic concentrations are also achieved in cerebrospinal fluid (Schwartz and Jeunet, 1976).

Both unchanged metronidazole and several metabolites are excreted in various proportions in the urine of experimental animals and man after oral administration of the parent compound (Ralph, 1983). The liver is the main site of metabolism, and the principal metabolites result from oxidation of side chains and formation of glucuronides. Small quantities of reduced metabolites, including ring-cleavage products, are formed by the gut flora (Koch *et al.*, 1981). The urine of some patients may be reddish-brown due to the presence of unidentified pigments derived from the drug.

Preparations, Routes of Administration, and Dosage. *Metronidazole* (FLAGYL) is available as 250- and 500-mg tablets. The drug is also available in forms for intravenous infusion. *Benzoyl metronidazole*, a tasteless form of metronidazole, is available in some countries as an oral suspension for children.

Many different dosage schedules have been used in the treatment of trichomoniasis in women. However, the currently accepted regimen is one 250-mg tablet, given orally three times daily for 7 days. When repeated courses of the drug are required for stubborn infections, it is recommended that intervals of 4 to 6 weeks elapse between courses. In such cases, leukocyte counts should be carried out before, during, and after each course of treatment. A single oral dose of 2 g of metronidazole has been reported to be effective. Lack of satisfactory response may be due to chronic infection of the cervical glands or of Skene's and Bartholin's glands. Although metronidazole-resistant strains of *T. vaginalis* exist, these are rare and probably only occasionally account for failure of treatment (Müller *et al.*, 1980).

Reinfection by an infected male partner may also cause an unsatisfactory response. If trichomonads are demonstrated in the urogenital tract, the male may be treated by the oral administration of 250 mg, three times daily for 7 days; both partners should be treated over the same 7-day period.

For amebiasis, in all geographical areas and regardless of the virulence of the strains or the form of infection being treated, it is recommended that patients receive 750 mg of metronidazole, three times daily for 5 to 10 days. The daily dose for children is 35 to 50 mg/kg, given in three divided doses for 10 days. Treatment with metronidazole is least effective when the drug is administered to the *asymptomatic* passer of cysts. While metronidazole is still effective, fewer failures result from the use of purely luminal amebicides; the latter are thus preferred alone or in combination with metronidazole. Despite considerable clinical use over the last several years, resistance of *E. histolytica* to metronidazole has not occurred. Indeed, attempts to produce resistance to the drug *in vitro* have been unsuccessful. *Mass treatment* with a large dose of metronidazole once monthly for a few months and then on alternate months has resulted in a marked decrease in the incidence of amebic dysentery in relatively isolated communities with a high degree of endemicity.

While *quinacrine* is the drug of choice in the treatment of giardiasis, its administration is not without unpleasant side effects. Metronidazole is effective in the same dosage as that used for the treatment of trichomoniasis. Others have successfully used a daily dose of 2 g for 3 successive days. Metronidazole is also considered to be an alternative to niridazole for the elimination of the guinea worm in dracunculiasis (Padonu, 1973; Sharma *et al.*, 1979). Recommended dosage is 250 to 500 mg of the drug, given three times daily for 5 to 7 days. Both of these uses are considered to be investigational in the United States.

In 1980, metronidazole was approved by the United States Food and Drug Administration for treatment of serious infections due to susceptible anaerobic bacteria, including *Bacteroides, Clostridium, Fusobacterium, Peptococcus, Peptostreptococcus,* and *Eubacterium*. The drug was also approved for use along with appropriate antimicrobial agents for concomitant infections with aerobic microorganisms. Under these circumstances, metronidazole is usually given intravenously. The recommended intravenous dosage regimen for anaerobic infections includes a loading dose (15 mg/kg), followed 6 hours later by a maintenance dose of 7.5 mg/kg every 6 hours.

Toxicity and Drug Interactions. The toxicity of metronidazole has been reviewed by Roe (1977). Side effects are only rarely sufficiently severe to cause discontinuation of treatment. The most common are referable to the gastrointestinal tract. In particular, nausea, anorexia, diarrhea, epigastric distress, and abdominal cramping may occur. Headache and vomiting are occasionally experienced. A metallic, sharp, and unpleasant taste is not unusual. Furry tongue, glossitis, and stomatitis may occur during therapy and be associated with a sudden intensification of moniliasis. Neurotoxic effects of metronidazole have also been observed. Dizziness, vertigo, and, very rarely, incoordination and ataxia may appear. Numbness or paresthesia of an extremity occurs occasionally, and the drug should be discontinued when this happens. Reversal of serious sensory neuropathies may be slow or incomplete (Coxon and Pallis, 1976). Urticaria, flushing, pruritus, dysuria, cystitis, a sense of pelvic pressure, and dryness of the mouth, vagina, or vulva have been reported. Thrombophlebitis may complicate intravenous use, particularly if the drug solution is not prepared properly. Metronidazole has a well-documented disulfiram-like effect, and a few patients experience abdominal distress, vomiting, flushing, or headache if they drink alcoholic beverages during a course of treatment. Confusional and psychotic states may also occur during concurrent administration of metronidazole and disulfiram.

While related chemicals have caused blood dyscrasias, only a temporary neutropenia, which reverses after therapy, occurs with metronidazole (*see* Lefebvre and Hesseltine, 1965; Goldman, 1980). Metronidazole has been reported to lower concentrations of lipids in plasma (Davis *et al.*, 1983). It also has been suggested that chronic administration of phenobarbital, by increasing the metabolism of metronidazole, may cause failure of treatment for protozoal infections (Gupte, 1983).

Treatment should be discontinued promptly if ataxia, convulsions, or any other symptom of central nervous system (CNS) involvement occurs. Metronidazole is contraindicated in patients with active disease of the CNS or with evidence or a history of blood dyscrasia. The dosage should be reduced in patients with severe hepatic disease.

After prolonged high-dose feeding, metronidazole is carcinogenic in rodents; it is also mutagenic in bacteria. (*See* review by Voogd, 1981.) Furthermore, mutagenic activity associated with metronidazole and several of its metabolites is found in the urine of patients treated with therapeutic doses of the drug (Speck *et al.*, 1976). Two relatively short-term studies of human subjects treated with metronidazole failed to reveal an increased risk of carcinogenesis,

but long-term surveillance is needed (Beard *et al.*, 1979; Goldman, 1980). This evidence should compel the prudent use of the drug. While metronidazole has been given with no apparent adverse effects during all stages of pregnancy (Peterson *et al.*, 1966; Voogd, 1981), its use during the first trimester is not generally recommended.

Therapeutic Uses. The clinical uses of metronidazole have been the subject of several reviews (Goldman, 1980; Molavi *et al.*, 1982; Oldenburg and Speck, 1983). Metronidazole cures genital infections with *T. vaginalis* in both males and females in a high percentage of cases. This efficacy and a probable low incidence of comparatively minor side effects have led to its adoption as the agent of choice. The development of resistance to metronidazole has not proven to be a therapeutic problem. There is also no doubt that persistent reinfection of the female can be prevented if the male partner harboring the parasite is treated concurrently. However, treatment of the male is recommended only if reinfection can be demonstrated to arise from this source.

Metronidazole is an effective amebicide and has become the agent of choice for the treatment of all symptomatic forms of amebiasis. The drug also kills *G. lamblia* and has been shown to be effective in treating giardiasis. Its use in the treatment of dracunculiasis should be considered only as an alternative to niridazole (*see* Chapter 44).

Many studies have indicated that metronidazole may be useful for the treatment of infections with various anaerobic bacteria, particularly *B. fragilis*. The drug is an alternative to clindamycin and chloramphenicol for this purpose. Metronidazole has been employed for the prophylaxis of postsurgical abdominal and pelvic infections and for the treatment of endocarditis caused by *B. fragilis* (*see* Roe, 1977; Symposium, 1977; Galgiani *et al.*, 1978). While information is limited, the drug may also be effective for the treatment of brain abscesses that are not uncommonly caused by such microorganisms.

There is interest in the experimental use of nitroimidazoles to sensitize hypoxic tumor cells to the effects of ionizing radiation. Some success in this endeavor has been achieved *in vitro* and in animals, but metronidazole should not be used clinically for this purpose.

QUINACRINE

Quinacrine is an acridine derivative widely used during World War II as an antimalarial agent. Other drugs with more desirable properties have now replaced quinacrine as an antimalarial and for the treatment of infestations with tapeworms. Currently, the major indication for the administration of quinacrine is for the treatment of *giardiasis* (Wolfe, 1975). For a fuller description of its properties, *earlier editions* of this textbook should be consulted. Quinacrine has the following structural formula:

Quinacrine

Quinacrine is very readily absorbed from the intestinal tract, even in the presence of severe diarrhea. It is widely distributed in the tissues and very slowly liberated. Therefore, the drug accumulates progressively when it is administered chronically. Significant amounts of quinacrine can still be detected in the urine for at least 2 months after therapy is discontinued. The *metabolic fate* of quinacrine in the body is incompletely understood. Whether quinacrine exerts its antiparasitic actions *per se* or after metabolic transformation remains to be determined. However, its ready intercalation into DNA suggests that the parent drug is the active substance, and that its selective toxicity is a function of relative distribution rather than specificity of action (*see* Albert, 1979).

Quinacrine is available as the dihydrochloride, designated *quinacrine hydrochloride (mepacrine hydrochloride;* ATABRINE). It contains approximately 80% quinacrine base and is supplied as tablets containing 100 mg of the dihydrochloride.

In the treatment of *giardiasis,* 100 mg should be given three times daily for 5 to 7 days. A second course of treatment may be given, if necessary, 1 or 2 weeks later. The dosage for children under 8 years of age should be proportionately reduced. The microorganisms disappear from the stools, and symptoms referable to the infection clear rapidly.

Because of its widespread use as an antimalarial drug, the toxic effects of quinacrine are well documented. (*See* review by Findlay, 1951.) The drug frequently causes headache, dizziness, and vomiting. Blood dyscrasias, urticaria, and exfoliative dermatitis may also follow its administration. The skin may acquire a yellow stain from deposition of the drug, and blue or black pigmentation of the nails can occur. Ocular toxicity, similar to that caused by chloroquine, occurs occasionally. The relatively large doses formerly used in the treatment of cestode infection may cause the transitory *toxic psychosis* that is seen in a small proportion of patients receiving lower doses. The duration of the drug-induced psychosis is usually 2 to 4 weeks, and the course is relatively benign. Only symptomatic therapy is indicated.

Great caution should be exercised in administering quinacrine (and other antimalarial compounds) to patients with *psoriasis,* since pronounced exacerbation occurs frequently and exfoliative lesions sometimes develop. Quinacrine is contraindicated in patients receiving antimalarial therapy with primaquine. Concurrent administration of the two drugs results in a markedly elevated concentration of primaquine (or other 8-aminoquinolines) in plasma and greatly enhances its toxicity. Quinacrine should not be given to pregnant women because the drug readily passes the placenta and reaches the fetus.

ANTIBIOTIC AMEBICIDES

A number of antibiotics have been found to be of value in the treatment of intestinal amebiasis, especially *erythromycin, paromomycin,* and some of the *tetracyclines.* Inasmuch as paromomycin is the only one that is directly amebicidal, it is the only one discussed in any detail here. Other antibiotics are not amebicidal directly, but act by interfering with the enteric flora essential for the proliferation of pathogenic amebae. The older tetracyclines—tetracycline itself, chlortetracycline, and oxytetracycline—are the most frequently used, their efficacy probably depending on the relatively large proportion of the administered dose that escapes absorption in the bowel. The better-absorbed agents are much less effective (*see* Chapter 52). If a tetracycline is used, it is recommended that it be administered together with the appropriate drugs for either intestinal or extraintestinal amebic infections.

Paromomycin. This aminoglycoside antibiotic, isolated from cultures of *Streptomyces rimosus,* is amebicidal both *in vitro* and *in vivo.* Many of its properties are similar to those of other antibiotics in this class (*see* Chapter 51). Paromomycin acts directly on amebae but is also antibacterial to normal and pathogenic microorganisms in the gastrointestinal tract. Its structural formula is as follows:

Paromomycin

Paromomycin sulfate (HUMATIN) is supplied in capsules, each containing 250 mg. The recommended dosage is 25 to 35 mg/kg each day, orally in three divided doses at mealtimes, for 5 to 10 days. Higher doses, up to 66 mg/kg, have been used by some investigators. After oral administration, little of the drug is absorbed into the systemic circulation. Side effects are mainly limited to gastrointestinal upset and diarrhea occurring during the course of therapy. Marked renal damage occurs in animals treated parenterally with the drug. A number of clinical trials have been carried out since the introduction of the drug (*see* review by Woolfe, 1965). Experience has shown paromomycin to be effective, but by no means infallible, in the treatment of *intestinal amebiasis;* it is ineffective against extraintestinal forms of the disease. Paromomycin is also effective in the treatment of infections with various tapeworms.

Adams, G. E.; Stratford, I. J.; Wallace, I. G.; Wardman, P.; and Watts, M. E. Toxicity of nitrocompounds towards hypoxic mammalian cells *in vitro*; dependence on reduction potential. *J. Natl Cancer Inst.*, 1980, *64*, 555–560.

Beard, C. M.; Noller, K. L.; O'Fallon, W. M.; Kurland, L. T.; and Dockerty, M. B. Lack of evidence for cancer due to use of metronidazole. *N. Engl. J. Med.*, 1979, *301*, 519–522.

Bristow, N. W.; Oxley, P.; Williams, G. A. H.; and Woolfe, G. ENTAMIDE, a new amoebicide; preliminary note. *Trans. R. Soc. Trop. Med. Hyg.*, 1956, *50*, 182.

Cohen, H. G., and Reynolds, T. B. Comparison of metronidazole and chloroquine for the treatment of amebic liver abscess: a controlled trial. *Gastroenterology*, 1975, *69*, 35–41.

Conan, N. J., Jr. Chloroquine in amebiasis. *Am. J. Trop. Med. Hyg.*, 1948, *28*, 107–110.

———. The treatment of hepatic amebiasis with chloroquine. *Am. J. Med.*, 1949, *6*, 309–320.

Cosar, C.; Ganter, P.; and Julou, L. Etude expérimentale du métronidazole, 8823 R.P., activités trichomonacide et amoebicide. Toxicité et propriétés pharmacologiques générales. *Presse Med.*, 1961, *69*, 1069–1972.

Cosar, C., and Julou, L. Activité de l'(hydroxy-2' ethyl)-1 méthyl-2 nitro-5 imidazole (8,823 R.P.) vis-à-vis des infections expérimentales à *Trichomonas vaginalis*. *Ann. Inst. Pasteur (Paris)*, 1959, *96*, 238–241.

Coura, J. R.; Brindeiro, P. J.; and Ferreira, I. Benznidazole in the treatment of Chagas' disease. In, *Current Chemotherapy*, Vol. 1. *Proceedings of the 10th International Congress of Chemotherapy.* American Society for Microbiology, Washington, D. C., 1978, pp. 161–162.

Coxon, A., and Pallis, C. A. Metronidazole neuropathy. *J. Neurol. Neurosurg. Psychiatry*, 1976, *39*, 403–405.

Davis, J. L.; Schultz, T. A.; and Mosley, C. A. Metronidazole lowers serum lipids. *Ann. Intern. Med.*, 1983, *99*, 43–44.

Durel, P.; Roiron, V.; Siboulet, H.; and Borel, L. J. Trial of an anti-trichomonal derivative of imidazole (8823 R.P.). *C.R. Soc. Fr. Gyn.*, 1959, *29*, 36.

———. Systemic treatment of human trichomoniasis with a derivative of nitroimidazole, 8823 R.P. *Br. J. Vener. Dis.*, 1960, *36*, 21–26.

Edwards, D. I.; Knox, R. J.; and Knight, R. C. Structure-cytotoxicity relationships of nitroimidazoles in an *in vitro* system. *Int. J. Radiat. Oncol. Biol. Phys.*, 1982, *8*, 791–793.

Galgiani, J. N.; Busch, D. F.; Brass, C.; Rumans, L. W.; Mangels, J. I.; and Stevens, D. A. *Bacteroides fragilis* endocarditis, bacteremia and other infections treated with oral or intravenous metronidazole. *Am. J. Med.*, 1978, *65*, 284–289.

Gordeeva, L. M. [A study of the effect of FLAGYL upon *Entamoeba histolytica* in culture.] *Med. Parazitol.* (*Mosk.*), 1965, *34*, 325–329. (In, *Trop. Dis. Bull.*, 1965, *62*, 1115.)

Gupte, S. Phenobarbital and metabolism of metronidazole. *N. Engl. J. Med.*, 1983, *308*, 529.

Horie, H. Anti-*Trichomonas* effect of azomycin. *J. Antibiot.* (*Tokyo*) [A], 1956, *9*, 168.

Jokipii, L., and Jokipii, A. M. M. *In vitro* susceptibility of *Giardia lamblia* trophozoites to metronidazole and tinidazole. *J. Infect. Dis.*, 1980, *141*, 317–325.

Koch, R. L.; Beaulieu, B. B., Jr.; Chrystal, E. J. T.; and Goldman, P. A metronidazole metabolite in urine and its risk. *Science*, 1981, *211*, 398–400.

LaRusso, N. F.; Tomasz, M.; Müller, M.; and Lipman, R. Interaction of metronidazole with nucleic acids *in vitro*. *Mol. Pharmacol.*, 1977, *13*, 872–882.

Lefebvre, I., and Hesseltine, H. C. The peripheral white blood cells and metronidazole. *J.A.M.A.*, 1965, *194*, 15–18.

Main, P. T.; Bristow, N. W.; Oxley, P.; Watkins, T. I.; Williams, G. A. H.; Wilmshurst, E. C.; and Woolfe, G. ENTAMIDE. *Ann. Biochem. Exp. Med.*, 1960, *20*, 441–448.

Müller, M.; Meingassner, J. G.; Miller, W. A.; and Ledger, W. J. Three metronidazole-resistant strains of *Trichomonas vaginalis* from the United States. *Am. J. Obstet. Gynecol.*, 1980, *138*, 808–812.

Murgatroyd, F., and Kent, R. P. Refractory amoebic liver abscess treated by chloroquine. *Trans. R. Soc. Trop. Med. Hyg.*, 1948, *42*, 15–16.

Oakley, G. P., Jr. The neurotoxicity of the halogenated hydroxyquinolines. *J.A.M.A.*, 1973, *225*, 395–397.

Padonu, K. O. A controlled trial of metronidazole in the treatment of dracontiasis in Nigeria. *Am. J. Trop. Med. Hyg.*, 1973, *22*, 42–44.

Peterson, W. F.; Stauch, J. E.; and Ryder, C. D. Metronidazole in pregnancy. *Am. J. Obstet. Gynecol.*, 1966, *94*, 343–349.

Ralph, E. D., and Kirby, W. M. M. Bioassay of metronidazole with either anaerobic or aerobic incubation. *J. Infect. Dis.*, 1975a, *132*, 587–591.

———. Unique bactericidal action of metronidazole against *Bacteroides fragilis* and *Clostridium perfringens*. *Antimicrob. Agents Chemother.*, 1975b, *8*, 409–420.

Schwartz, D. E., and Jeunet, F. Comparative pharmacokinetic studies of ornidazole and metronidazole in man. *Chemotherapy*, 1976, *22*, 19–29.

Shaldon, S. ENTAMIDE FUROATE in the treatment of acute amoebic dysentery. *Trans. R. Soc. Trop. Med. Hyg.*, 1960, *54*, 469–470.

Sharma, V. P.; Rathmore, H. S.; and Sharma, M. M. Efficacy of metronidazole in dracunculiasis. *Am. J. Trop. Med. Hyg.*, 1979, *28*, 658–660.

Speck, W. T.; Stein, A. B.; and Rosenkranz, H. S. Mutagenicity of metronidazole: presence of several active metabolites in human urine. *J. Natl Cancer Inst.*, 1976, *56*, 283–284.

Suchak, N. G.; Satoskar, R. S.; and Sheth, U. K. ENTAMIDE FUROATE in the treatment of intestinal amoebiasis. *Am. J. Trop. Med. Hyg.*, 1962, *11*, 330–332.

Wilmot, A. J.; Powell, S. J.; McLeod, I.; and Elsdon-Dew, R. Some newer amoebicides in acute amoebic dysentery. *Trans. R. Soc. Trop. Med. Hyg.*, 1962, *56*, 85–86.

Wilmshurst, E. C., and Cliffe, E. E. Absorption and distribution of amoebicides. In, *Absorption and Distribution of Drugs.* (Binns, T. B., ed.) E. & S. Livingstone, Ltd., Edinburgh, 1964, pp. 191–198.

Wolfe, M. S. Nondysenteric intestinal amebiasis. Treatment with diloxanide furoate. *J.A.M.A.*, 1973, *224*, 1601–1604.

Woodruff, A. W., and Bell, S. Clinical trials with ENTAMIDE FUROATE and related compounds. I. In a non-tropical environment. *Trans. R. Soc. Trop. Med. Hyg.*, 1960, *54*, 389–395.

Monographs and Reviews

Albert, A. *Selective Toxicity: The Physico-Chemical Basis of Therapy*, 6th ed. Chapman & Hall, Ltd., London, 1979.

Baines, E. J. Metronidazole: its past, present and future. *J. Antimicrob. Chemother.*, 1978, *4*, Suppl. C, 97–111.

Brown, J.; Biaglow, J.; Hall, E.; Kinsella, T.; Phillips, R. C.; Urtasun, R.; Utley, J.; and Yuhas, J. Sensitizers and protectors to radiation and chemotherapeutic drugs. In, *The Interdisciplinary Program for Radiation Oncology Research.* (Wittes, R. E., ed.) *Cancer Treatment Symposia*, Vol. 1. U.S. Government Printing Office, Washington, D. C., 1984, pp. 85–102.

Cavanagh, J. B. Peripheral neuropathy caused by chemical agents. *CRC Crit. Rev. Toxicol.*, 1973, *2*, 365–417.

Chow, A. W.; Patten, V.; and Guze, L. B. Susceptibility of anaerobic bacteria to metronidazole. Relative resistance of non-spore forming gram-positive bacilli. *J. Infect. Dis.*, **1975**, *131*, 182–185.

Edwards, D. I. Mechanisms of selective toxicity of metronidazole and other nitroimidazole drugs. *Br. J. Vener. Dis.*, **1980**, *56*, 285–290.

Findlay, G. M. *Recent Advances in Chemotherapy*, Vol. I. J. & A. Churchill, Ltd., London, **1950**.

————. *Recent Advances in Chemotherapy*, Vol. II. J. & A. Churchill, Ltd., London, **1951**.

Goldman, P. Metronidazole. *N. Engl. J. Med.*, **1980**, *303*, 1212–1218.

Harries, J. Amoebiasis: a review. *J. R. Soc. Med.*, **1982**, *75*, 190–197.

Krogstad, D. J.; Spencer, H. C., Jr.; and Healy, G. R. Amebiasis. *N. Engl. J. Med.*, **1978**, *298*, 262–265.

Miller, J. J. The imidazoles as immunosuppressive agents. *Transplant. Proc.*, **1980**, *12*, 300–303.

Molavi, A.; LeFrock, J. L.; and Prince, R. A. Metronidazole. *Med. Clin. North Am.*, **1982**, *66*, 121–133.

Neal, R. A. Experimental amoebiasis and the development of anti-amoebic compounds. *Parasitology*, **1983**, *86*, 175–191.

Oldenburg, B., and Speck, W. T. Metronidazole. *Pediatr. Clin. North Am.*, **1983**, *30*, 71–75.

Powell, S. J. Therapy of amebiasis. *Bull. N.Y. Acad. Med.*, **1971**, *47*, 469–477.

Ralph, E. D. Clinical pharmacokinetics of metronidazole. *Clin. Pharmacokinet.*, **1983**, *8*, 43–62.

Roe, F. J. C. Metronidazole: review of uses and toxicity. *J. Antimicrob. Chemother.*, **1977**, *3*, 205–212.

Symposium. (Various authors.) *Proceedings of the International Metronidazole Conference*, International Congress Series No. 438. (Finegold, S. M., ed.) Excerpta Medica, Amsterdam, **1977**.

Voogd, C. E. On the mutagenicity of nitroimidazoles. *Mutat. Res.*, **1981**, *86*, 243–277.

Warren, K. S., and Mahmoud, A. A. F. (eds.). *Tropical and Geographic Medicine*. McGraw-Hill Book Co., New York, **1984**.

Wolfe, M. S. Giardiasis. *J.A.M.A.*, **1975**, *233*, 1362–1365.

Woolfe, G. The chemotherapy of amoebiasis. In, *Progress in Drug Research*, Vol. 8. (Jucker, E., ed.) Birkhaüser Verlag, Basel, **1965**, pp. 11–52.

Yang, W. C. T., and Dubick, M. Mechanism of emetine cardiotoxicity. *Pharmacol. Ther.*, **1980**, *10*, 15–26.

47 DRUGS USED IN THE CHEMOTHERAPY OF PROTOZOAL INFECTIONS

[*Continued*]

Leishmaniasis, Trypanosomiasis, and Other Protozoal Infections

Leslie T. Webster, Jr.

In addition to malaria and those pathogenic protozoal infections that are prevalent in the United States, two other major protozoal infections of man cause appreciable morbidity and mortality in tropical countries. *Leishmaniasis* and *trypanosomiasis* in their protean forms can be especially difficult to prevent or cure; effective drugs are either lacking or too toxic. More research is needed to understand the mechanism of action of the older drugs now in use, as well as to identify new biochemical targets in the parasites that can be exploited to chemotherapeutic advantage. The specific compounds used for chemoprophylaxis and therapy of these and some of the less common human protozoal afflictions are presented in alphabetical order. References at the end of the chapter should be consulted for more comprehensive information about this subject.

Leishmaniasis. Human *leishmaniasis* is caused by protozoal species and subspecies of the genus *Leishmania*. The disease occurs on all continents except Australia and probably affects at least 100 million people; the annual incidence is estimated at 12 million cases. Nonhuman mammals are the reservoirs for this infection, which is transmitted to man most often by the bites of infected female phlebotamine sandflies. The parasites are found in two main forms: flagellated *extracellular, free promastigotes,* which live in the gastrointestinal tract and saliva of the insect vector; and *intracellular amastigotes,* located primarily in phagolysosomes of mononuclear tissue phagocytes of the mammalian host (Chang, 1983). The occurrence of localized or systemic disease depends on the species or subspecies of infecting parasite and the host's immunological response to the infected macrophages. In increasing order of systemic involvement and clinical severity, human leishmaniasis can be classified into *cutaneous, mucocutaneous (espundia),*

and *visceral (kala azar)* forms (*see* Wyler and Marsden, 1984). Treatment with *pentavalent antimonials* or second-line drugs, such as *pentamidine* and *amphotericin B,* is unsatisfactory because these agents, even when effective, cause unacceptable levels of toxicity at therapeutic doses. *Allopurinol,* certain *pyrazolopyrimidines,* and *8-aminoquinolines* have shown some promise in experimental leishmaniasis and are being considered for clinical trials (Carson and Chang, 1981; Berman and Webster, 1982; Nelson *et al.,* 1982; Wyler and Marsden, 1984).

Trypanosomiasis. *African trypanosomiasis* is transmitted by tsetse flies of the genus *Glossinia* and is caused by subspecies of the hemoflagellate *Trypanosoma brucei.* The parasite may be detected in the blood and spinal fluid of the human host. Two main types of human trypanosomal disease exist, the *Rhodesian* and the *Gambian. T. brucei rhodesiense* produces a progressive and usually fatal form of disease with early involvement of the central nervous system (CNS), whereas *T. brucei gambiense* causes so-called sleeping sickness, characterized by later involvement of the CNS and a more chronic course. Treatment with standard but toxic agents such as *suramin, pentamidine,* and *melarsoprol* is difficult; it must be of long duration and is often unsuccessful (Apted, 1980). Although *T. brucei* offers several attractive biochemical targets for selective pharmacological intervention, these have yet to be exploited successfully for chemotherapy in man (Clarkson and Brohn, 1976; Berens *et al.,* 1980; Bacchi, 1981; Fairlamb, 1982; Meshnick, 1984).

American trypanosomiasis or *Chagas' disease,* a zoonosis caused by *T. cruzi,* affects more than 10 million people in South America and the Caribbean, where the chronic form of the disease in adults is a major cause of cardiomyopathy, megaesophagus, megacolon, and death. Transmitted by bloodsucking *triatomid bugs,* metacyclic *trypomastigotes* enter host cells and proliferate as intracellular *amastigotes.* These forms then differentiate intracellularly into *trypomastigotes,* which are released into the circulation. Trypomastigotes in the blood stream do not multiply until they invade other cells or are ingested by an insect vector during a blood meal. Chronic disease of the heart and gastrointestinal tract results from destruction of myocardial cells and neurons of the myoenteric plexus. Although nitroheterocyclic drugs such as *nifurtimox* and *benznidazole* can suppress parasitemia and cure or ameliorate the acute stage of Chagas' infection, they have little effect on the chronic phase of the disease (Brener, 1979). *T. cruzi* is especially vulnerable to drugs that form intracellular free radicals. Both nifurtimox and benznidazole have this capability, and other agents with similar potential are being evaluated as antitrypanosomal agents. (*See* review by Docampo and Moreno, 1984.)

Other Protozoal Infections. *Toxoplasmosis,* caused by the intracellular protozoan *Toxoplasma gondii,* is a zoonosis that is a common cause of latent human infection worldwide. Acute infection is particularly threatening to the fetus and the immunocompromised host. The treatment of choice for this infection is pyrimethamine and a sulfonamide (*see* Chapter 49). Examples of less common protozoal infections affecting man are *babesiosis, balantidiasis, pneumocystosis,* and *coccidiosis.* While balantidiasis responds to *tetracyclines* and pneumocystosis to *pentamidine* and *trimethoprim-sulfamethoxazole,* the two other infections are quite refractory to specific chemotherapy.

MELARSOPROL

In 1940, Friedheim described trypanocidal activity of an organic compound of arsenic containing the melamine nucleus. Two compounds made subsequently, the pentavalent melarsen and the trivalent melarsen oxide, were shown to be effective in advanced cases of trypanosomiasis but were considered to be more toxic than tryparsamide, an older pentavalent arsenical. In 1949, Friedheim demonstrated that a dimercaprol derivative of melarsen oxide also could be used effectively and with greater safety in the treatment of such cases; this compound was named *Mel B* and is now known as *melarsoprol.* Of considerable importance was the finding that trypanocidal arsenicals of the melamine type retained their activity against tryparsamide-resistant strains of trypanosomes (VanHoof, 1947).

Chemistry and Preparation. Melarsoprol has the following structural formula:

Melarsoprol

Melarsoprol (Mel B; ARSOBAL) is provided as a 3.6% (w/v) sterile solution in propylene glycol. It is available in the United States only from the Para-

sitic Diseases Division, Centers for Disease Control. The dosage regimens below refer to the 3.6% solution.

Antiprotozoal Effects. Arsenicals react avidly with sulfhydryl groups, including those of proteins, and thereby inactivate a great number and variety of enzymes. As far as is known, the same mechanism by which melarsoprol is lethal to parasites is responsible for its toxicity to host tissues. However, Flynn and Bowman (1969) have demonstrated that arsenical drugs act differently upon the terminal glycolytic enzyme, pyruvate kinase, depending on whether the source of the enzyme is trypanosomal or mammalian. Mammalian tissues oxidize the drug to nontoxic and readily excreted pentavalent compounds more rapidly than does the protozoan. Additionally, melarsoprol may be able to enter the parasite more readily than mammalian tissue cells. So-called arsenic-resistant parasites may resemble host cells in that they have become less permeable to organic arsenicals (*see* Eagle and Doak, 1951).

The pharmacological effects of melarsoprol in man are regarded as toxic effects and are discussed below.

Absorption, Fate, and Excretion. Melarsoprol is usually administered intravenously. A small but therapeutically significant amount of the drug enters into the cerebrospinal fluid and has a lethal effect on trypanosomes infecting the CNS. The substance is excreted quite quickly, and its prophylactic action lasts no more than a few days (*see* Hawking, 1963).

Route of Administration and Dosage. Melarsoprol is administered by slow intravenous injection through a fine needle, and care must be taken to avoid leakage into surrounding tissues, because it is intensely irritating. Patients with advanced meningoencephalitis, or those who are febrile or wasted, should receive preliminary treatment with suramin (two to four doses of 250 to 500 mg on alternate days). Adults in good condition weighing 50 kg or more and whose cerebrospinal fluid contains less than 40 mg of protein per 100 ml should be given up to 3.6 mg/kg daily for 3 or 4 days; this course should be repeated after an interval of 7 days. A third course may be given if required after 10 to 21 days. Lesser doses should be given to children and debilitated patients. Following such regimens, about 80 to 90% of patients are cured. A proportion of those who relapse will be refractory to further treatment with melarsoprol.

Toxicity and Side Effects. Unfortunately, side effects are common during treatment with melarsoprol (*see* Robertson, 1962). A febrile reaction often occurs soon after drug injection, particularly if parasitemia is high. The most serious side effects involve the nervous system. Quite common is a reactive encephalopathy, which usually appears after the first 3- or 4-day course and then subsides; additional treatment does not produce further deterioration. The condition may be fatal, but deaths have become less frequent as experience with this drug has increased. This complication occurs more frequently and is more severe in patients with pronounced cerebrospinal fluid changes. Hemorrhagic encephalopathy during treatment is far less common but is serious and often fatal. Hypersensitivity reactions may occur, particularly during the second or subsequent course of treatment. After recovery, a small dose provokes a lesser reaction, and desensitization may be carried out by starting with a small dose and increasing this slightly, allowing time for recovery, until it is possible to give a final 3- or 4-day course in full dosage. Corticosteroids may be used to control the symptoms during such a procedure. Agranulocytosis is very rare. Occasionally the appearance of numerous casts in the urine or evidence of hepatic disturbance may necessitate modification of treatment. Vomiting and abdominal colic may occur, but their incidence can be reduced by injecting the drug slowly in the supine, fasting patient. The patient should remain in bed and not eat for several hours after the injection is given.

Precautions and Contraindications. Melarsoprol should be given only to patients under hospital supervision so that the dosage regimen may be modified if necessary. It is most important that the initial dosage be based upon clinical assessment of the general condition of the patient, rather than on body weight. Administration of melarsoprol to leprous patients may precipitate erythema nodosum. The use of the drug is contraindicated during epidemics of influenza. Severe hemolytic reactions have been reported in patients with glucose-6-phosphate dehydrogenase deficiency.

Therapeutic Uses. Because of its ability to enter the cerebrospinal fluid, melarsoprol is the drug of choice for treatment of the meningoencephalitic stage of African trypanosomiasis. It is effective in both Gambian and Rhodesian varieties of the disease. Its value is in its quick action against both early and late stages of trypanosomiasis, its effectiveness against tryparsamide-resistant strains of trypanosomes, and its failure to produce ocular toxicity. For these reasons, it has largely superseded tryparsamide. Melarsoprol is also effective in the treatment of the early hemolymphatic stage of the disease; however, because of its toxicity, it is usually reserved for treatment of the late stage. For this reason also, it has no place in prophylaxis.

NIFURTIMOX

Nitrofurans were known to be effective in experimental infections with *T. cruzi,* and numerous congeners have been investigated for their chemotherapeutic usefulness; more recent work has proven promising. One drug, 3-methyl-4(5'-nitro-furfurylidene - amino) - tetrahydro - 4H - 1,4 - thiazine-1,1-dioxide, is quite effective clinically, although more so in acute than in chronic Chagas' infection (Brener, 1979).

Chemistry and Preparation. *Nifurtimox (Bayer 2502;* LAMPIT) has the following structural formula:

Nifurtimox

Nifurtimox is marketed in scored tablets that contain 100 mg of the drug; it is available in the United States only from the Parasitic Diseases Division, Centers for Disease Control.

Antiprotozoal Effects. Nifurtimox is trypanocidal against both the trypomastigote and the amastigote forms of *T. cruzi*. Concentrations of 1 μM have been shown to damage intracellular amastigotes *in vitro* and inhibit their development. Continuous exposure to this concentration of the drug lengthens considerably the intracellular cycle. Trypomastigotes are less sensitive; 10-μM concentrations of nifurtimox inhibit penetration of vertebrate cells by the parasites but do not eliminate this process (*see* Dvorak and Howe, 1977). The trypanocidal action of nifurtimox appears to be related to its ability to form chemically reactive radicals that cause production of toxic, partially reduced products of oxygen, for example, superoxide, hydrogen peroxide, and hydroxyl radicals (*see* Docampo and Moreno, 1984). *T. cruzi* apparently lacks both catalase and glutathione peroxidase, making the parasite extremely vulnerable to hydrogen peroxide. Nifurtimox may also produce damage to mammalian tissues by formation of radicals (Moreno *et al.,* 1980).

Absorption, Fate, and Excretion. Nifurtimox is well absorbed after oral administration. Despite this, only low concentrations of the drug are found in the blood and tissues, and little is present in the urine. High concentrations of several unidentified metabolites are found, however, and it is obvious that biotransformation occurs rapidly. The effect of biotransformation on trypanocidal activity is unknown.

Route of Administration and Dosage. The drug is given orally. *Children* (up to 15 years of age) with *acute* Chagas' disease should receive 25 mg/kg per day in four divided doses for 15 days, followed by 15 mg/kg per day in four divided doses for 75 days. Therapy should be extended to a total of 120 days for *chronic* disease. *Adults* with acute or chronic disease should receive 5 to 7 mg/kg daily for 2 weeks, and this dose is increased by 2 mg/kg per day at intervals of 2 weeks until 15 to 17 mg/kg is given daily by week 10. Treatment with this dose is continued until the patient has taken the drug for a total of 120 days. Gastric upset resulting from drug administration may be alleviated by simultaneous administration of aluminum hydroxide preparations. Weight loss is not uncommon during treatment. If it occurs, dosage should be reduced. The ingestion of alcohol should be avoided during treatment, since the incidence of side effects may increase.

Toxicity and Side Effects. Drug-related side effects are quite common. They range from hypersensitivity reactions, such as dermatitis, icterus, and anaphylaxis, to dose- and age-dependent complications referable to the gastrointestinal tract and both the peripheral and central nervous systems (*see* Wegner and Rohwedder, 1972; Brener, 1979). Peripheral neuropathy and gastrointestinal symptoms are particularly common after prolonged treatment; the latter complication may lead to weight loss and preclude further therapy. Headache, psychic disturbances, and CNS excitation are less frequent. Leukopenia and decreased sperm counts have also been reported. The compound may suppress cell-mediated immune reactions, both *in vivo* and *in vitro* (Lelchuk *et al.*, 1977a, 1977b). Children appear to tolerate nifurtimox better than do adults. Because of the seriousness of the disease and the lack of superior drugs, there are no absolute contraindications to the use of nifurtimox.

Therapeutic Uses. Nifurtimox is employed in the treatment of *trypanosomiasis* caused by *T. cruzi* (Chagas' disease). It is effective in both the acute and, to a lesser extent, the chronic stages of the infection (*see* Brener, 1979). Treatment with nifurtimox has no effect on irreversible organ lesions brought about by the disease process. In the acute stage, drug therapy results in disappearance of parasitemia, amelioration of symptoms, and cure in over 80% of those treated. In the chronic stage, a cure rate of over 90% has been achieved in trials in Argentina, southern Brazil, Chile, and Venezuela. Much poorer results have been obtained in the middle section of Brazil, where the character of the infection is somewhat different. Differences in the susceptibility of various strains of *T. cruzi* to nifurtimox have been described in animal models (*see* Brener, 1979), but whether these account for the variable clinical results is not known.

PENTAMIDINE

The discovery of chemotherapeutic activity in the diamidine group of drugs, of which pentamidine is a member, was quite fortuitous (*see* King *et al.*, 1938; Lourie and Yorke, 1939). Of the compounds of this type, three were found to possess outstanding activity: 4,4′-diamidinostilbene (*stilbamidine*), 4,4′-diamidinophenoxy pentane (*pentamidine*), and 4,4′-diamidinophenoxy propane (*propamidine*). *Pentamidine* is the most valuable because of its stability, low toxicity, and ease of administration. *Hydroxystilbamidine isethionate* (2-hydroxy-4,4′-diamidinostilbene diisethionate) is preferred by some and has proven useful in the treatment of North American blastomycosis (*see* Chapter 54) and visceral leishmaniasis.

Chemistry and Preparation. Pentamidine has the following structural formula:

Pentamidine

Pentamidine isethionate, the preparation that is utilized, is a white powder, soluble in water to the extent of 10%. It is marketed as a dry powder, in vials containing 300 mg of the drug (PENTAM 300). Solutions should be used promptly after preparation and protected from light to avoid formation of hepatotoxic compounds.

Antiprotozoal Effects. The diamidines are toxic to a number of different protozoa, yet show rather marked selectivity of action. For example, the drugs are curative against *T. rhodesiense* and *T. congolense* infections in experimental animals but are ineffective in curing mice infected with *T. cruzi*. They are also capable of curing *Babesia canis* infections in puppies and *Leishmania donovani* infections in hamsters. These experimental results provide the basis for diamidine treatment of human leishmaniasis and trypanosomiasis.

The diamidines are also fungicidal. This can be readily demonstrated *in vitro* against *Blastomyces dermatitidis*, and has led to the successful therapeutic trial of the drugs in systemic blastomycosis. The use of *amphotericin B*, however, has reduced the value of the diamidines in the treatment of this disease. The antibiotic is preferred for initial therapy, but hydroxystilbamidine may prove helpful if an inadequate response is obtained. Although chemotherapy with *trimethoprim-sulfamethoxazole* is preferred, pentamidine may be useful in the treatment of pneumonia caused by *Pneumocystis carinii* (*see* Ivady *et al.*, 1967; Walzer *et al.*, 1974; Hughes *et al.*, 1978; Chapter 49).

Mechanism of Action. The diamidines are concentrated by *T. brucei* via an energy-dependent, high-affinity uptake system, which operates more rapidly in drug-sensitive than in drug-resistant strains (Damper and Patten, 1976a, 1976b). The mechanism of action of the diamidines has not been established. Their trypanocidal activity may emanate from interactions of these positively charged compounds with DNA or nucleotides and their derivatives; another possibility that has been suggested is that these agents interfere with the uptake or function of polyamines (*see* Bacchi, 1981; Meshnick, 1984).

Absorption, Fate, and Excretion. Pentamidine isethionate is fairly well absorbed from parenteral sites of administration. Following a single dose, the drug is detectable in the blood for only a very brief period; it is excreted slowly and unchanged in the urine. In experimental animals, the liver and the kidney are found to store the drug for months (*see* Waalkes *et al.*, 1970). Binding of pentamidine in tissues seems to be the most important factor in its use as a prophylactic agent in trypanosomiasis. However, the drug does not enter the cerebrospinal fluid or the CNS to an appreciable extent.

Therapeutic Uses, Routes of Administration, and Dosage. Pentamidine is best given by intramuscular injection in individual doses of 3 to 4 mg of base per kilogram of body weight, daily or on alternate days. The intravenous route is rarely used now because of severe adverse reactions. In the treatment of *early African trypanosomiasis,* a course of ten injections should be given. The drug is far less effective in *T. rhodesiense* than in *T. gambiense* infections because of the rapidity with which *T. rhodesiense* invades the CNS. Treatment with pentamidine is contraindicated unless infection with *T. rhodesiense* is known to have occurred within the previous 3 or 4 weeks. It is also ineffective in *T. gambiense* infections once the CNS is involved. Pentamidine has been widely used as a *prophylactic* agent in endemic areas. Single intramuscular injections should be given at intervals of not longer than 6 months; various dosages have been used, but all fall within the range of 3 to 5 mg/ kg.

In the treatment of *visceral leishmaniasis* (*L. donovani* leishmaniasis, or *kala azar*), pentamidine has been used successfully in courses of 12 to 15 doses. A second course, given after an interval of 1 to 2 weeks, may be necessary in areas where the infection is known to respond less well to treatment. The drug is particularly useful in cases that have failed to respond to antimonials—for example, in the Sudan, where the disease responds only to high doses of antimonials, and in China, where many patients with kala azar are hypersensitive to antimony. Some success has followed the use of pentamidine in the treatment of *cutaneous (L. tropica) leishmaniasis,* or Oriental sore (*see* Beveridge, 1963). Hydroxystilbamidine is preferred by some practitioners; the choice probably depends upon the local availability of either compound.

Cases of *Pneumocystis carinii pneumonia* should be treated daily with 4 mg/kg intramuscularly, for 12 to 14 days. If treatment is effective, clinical improvement will occur usually 4 to 6 days after the first injection. A high proportion of cures can be expected, depending on supportive therapy and, if possible, elimination of predisposing conditions. The prognosis is less favorable in debilitated patients with altered immunity or neoplastic disease (Walzer *et al.,* 1974). The use of pentamidine has markedly reduced mortality in the epidemic form of infection found in debilitated and premature infants. Alternative treatment, which is preferred, is the administration of trimethoprim-sulfamethoxazole.

Toxicity and Side Effects. Intravenous injection of pentamidine (and other diamidines) is often followed quickly by alarming and sometimes dangerous reactions. These include breathlessness, tachycardia, dizziness or fainting, headache, and vomiting. These reactions are probably connected with the sharp fall in blood pressure that follows too rapid intravenous administration of the drug, and they may be due in part to the release of histamine. Because pentamidine is better tolerated by intramuscular injection, even though sterile abscesses may occur at sites of injection, this route is preferred. Pentamidine has not been observed to give rise to late neuropathies such as have been reported frequently after courses of stilbamidine. Pancreatitis and hypoglycemia and, paradoxically, hyperglycemia have been reported following administration of pentamidine; the hypoglycemia may be life threatening if not recognized (Wang *et al.,* 1970; Sharpe, 1983). Reversible renal dysfunction has been associated with the use of the drug in a small proportion of treated patients (*see* DeVita *et al.,* 1969).

SODIUM STIBOGLUCONATE

The history of the development of leishmanicidal antimonial compounds can be divided into three distinct phases. At first, the use of *antimony potassium tartrate (tartar emetic)* in the treatment of trypanosomiasis was followed by its successful use against cutaneous leishmaniasis and, shortly afterward, in cases of kala azar. Inconvenience in the use of this drug, however, led to the trial of several other trivalent antimonial compounds, notably *antimony sodium tartrate, stibophen,* and *anthiolimine.* These were found to be as effective as and less toxic than tartar emetic. During this period, the successful syntheses of pentavalent antimonial derivatives of phenylstibonic acid were followed by the introduction of a variety of drugs that were as effective as and much less toxic than tartar emetic, thus permitting the use of larger doses and reduction in the period of treatment. Subsequent syntheses reverted to the "tartar-emetic" type of compound in which trivalent antimony was replaced by pentavalent antimony. An early member of this type of compound was *sodium stibogluconate.* This drug is widely used today and, together with *meglumine antimonate* (GLUCANTIME), a compound of the same type that is preferred in French-speaking countries, is the mainstay of the treatment of leishmaniasis by antimony. Full details of the investigations of leishmanicides can be found in the reviews of Findlay (1950) and Beveridge (1963).

Chemistry. Sodium stibogluconate has the following structural formula:

Sodium Stibogluconate

It is a colorless, amorphous powder, readily soluble in water, and contains 30 to 34% pentavalent antimony.

Antiprotozoal Effects. Pentavalent antimony compounds such as sodium stibogluconate have little effect on leptomonads growing in tissue culture. Such a marked contrast between *in-vitro* and *in-vivo* activity of these compounds suggests that reduction of antimony to the trivalent form is necessary for activity. However, the sensitivity of the free flagellated forms could be quite different from that of the morphologically different intracellular stage, which cannot be readily cultured. The mechanism of action of organic antimonials in leishmaniasis is unknown, although antimonials are known to react readily with sulfhydryl groups. Liposome-encapsulated antimonials have been used successfully to treat *L. donovani* infections in hamsters. In this form, the drug is selectively taken up by endocytosis and reaches the phagolysosomes of macrophages where the parasites reside (*see* Steck, 1981b; Chang, 1983).

Absorption, Distribution, and Excretion. The pentavalent antimonials are not bound by erythrocytes and attain much higher concentrations in plasma than do the trivalent compounds. Consequently, they are excreted more rapidly by the kidney. After intramuscular injection, over 80% of an administered dose of the pentavalent antimonial appears in the urine within 6 hours. After intravenous injection, the comparable figure is greater than 95%, indicating that the drug is not metabolized appreciably. About 12% of stibogluconate accumulates in an extravascular compartment, which becomes saturated after 5 days of treatment and from which antimony is slowly released (Rees *et al.*, 1980).

Toxicity. Untoward reactions to pentavalent antimonials are qualitatively similar to those that follow the administration of trivalent compounds, but they are less frequent and usually less severe. In general, sodium stibogluconate is tolerated relatively well. Specific reactions include pain at the injection site after intramuscular administration, muscle pain and stiffness of joints, and gastrointestinal symptoms. Changes in the ECG, which may occur later, include T wave inversion and prolongation of the Q-T interval; these are usually reversible but may precede serious arrhythmias. Abnormalities in renal and hepatic function have been noted, and these parameters should be monitored periodically during therapy. Rarely there is shock and sudden death.

Preparation. *Sodium stibogluconate* (*sodium antimony gluconate;* PENTOSTAM) is available in

sterile, aqueous solution for parenteral administration. Each milliliter contains 330 mg of the drug, equivalent to 100 mg of pentavalent antimony. It is available in the United States only from the Parasitic Diseases Division, Centers for Disease Control.

Routes of Administration, Dosage, and Therapeutic Uses. Sodium stibogluconate may be given either intravenously or by the intramuscular route. In cases of *kala azar,* in which the leishmania are normally sensitive to antimony, the large majority will be cured by a single course of treatment consisting of six daily injections of 6 ml. Against less sensitive strains, three courses, each consisting of ten daily doses of 6 ml intramuscularly and separated by intervals of 10 days, have proven satisfactory. In very debilitated individuals who appear to react unfavorably to the initial injections, it may be advisable to administer the drug on alternate days or at longer intervals. Reduced dosage is indicated in those who have recently received a course of antimony in another form, and in children. Infants and children, however, tolerate rather larger doses in proportion to body weight than do adults. In the treatment of *Oriental sore,* rapid disappearance of parasites has been reported following an infiltration of the solution around the edges of the lesions. The total volume used should not exceed more than 2 ml at any one time. Otherwise, a single course of treatment as outlined above should prove to be effective in nearly all cases. Less is known of the effectiveness of sodium stibogluconate in the treatment of *mucocutaneous leishmaniasis.* Cautious treatment with *amphotericin B* may be successful in this condition (Sampaio *et al.*, 1960).

SURAMIN

Based on the observed trypanocidal activity of the dyestuffs *trypan red, trypan blue,* and *afridol violet,* several years of research in Germany resulted in the introduction of *suramin* into therapy in 1920. Today the drug is used primarily for treatment of *African trypanosomiasis* and for *onchocerciasis* (*see* Chapter 44).

Chemistry and Preparation. *Suramin sodium* (GERMANIN) has the structural formula shown below. It is a white microcrystalline powder, readily soluble in water to yield a neutral solution. Only freshly prepared solutions should be employed. It is marketed in ampuls containing 1.0 g of the drug. Suramin is available in the United States only from

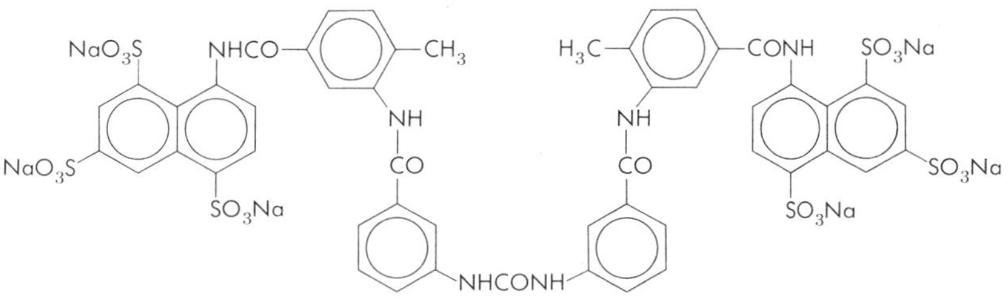

Suramin Sodium

the Parasitic Diseases Division, Centers for Disease Control.

Antiprotozoal Effects. The primary mechanism of action of suramin is not established, particularly because the drug inhibits so many trypanosomal enzymes (*see* Meshnick, 1984). Inhibition of glycerol phosphate oxidase, a parasite enzyme involved in energy metabolism, correlates with the antitrypanosomal activity of several derivatives of suramin (Fairlamb and Bowman, 1977). Furthermore, the energy metabolism of trypanosomes obtained from suramin-treated animals is reduced; the delayed onset of drug activity may be due to slow endocytic uptake by the parasite of a suramin–plasma protein complex (Fairlamb and Bowman, 1980). Williamson and Macadam (1965) have observed changes in suramin-treated trypanosomes characterized by damage to intracellular membranous structures except lysosomes.

Absorption, Fate, and Excretion. Suramin must be administered parenterally. Following its intravenous administration, the concentration in plasma falls fairly rapidly for a few hours, then more slowly for a few days, after which a low concentration is maintained for as long as 3 months. The persistence of suramin in the circulation is due to its firm binding to plasma protein. The large, polar compound apparently does not enter cells readily since none is present in erythrocytes, and tissue concentrations are uniformly lower than those in the plasma. In experimental animals, however, the kidneys have been found to contain considerably more suramin than other organs. This retention in the kidney may account for the fairly frequent occurrence of albuminuria following injection of the drug in man. Suramin does not penetrate into the cerebrospinal fluid in appreciable amounts. Metabolic destruction of the drug appears to be negligible. The protein-bound suramin dissociates slowly to yield effective concentrations of the drug over long periods of time. Thus, suramin has proven valuable in the *prophylaxis* of trypanosomiasis.

Route of Administration and Dosage. Suramin is usually given by slow intravenous injection in 10% aqueous solution. Treatment of active *African trypanosomiasis* should not be started until 24 hours after diagnostic lumbar puncture, and caution is required if the patient has onchocerciasis. The normal single dose for adults is 1 g. It is advisable to employ a small dose of 200 mg initially to test for sensitivity, after which the normal dose is given on days 1, 3, 7, 14, and 21; weekly doses may be given for an additional 5 weeks. Patients in poor condition should be treated cautiously during the first week.

Toxicity and Side Effects. Suramin can cause a variety of untoward reactions. These vary in intensity and frequency with the nutritional status of the patient and can be serious in the debilitated. The most serious immediate reaction consists in nausea, vomiting, shock, and loss of consciousness. Fortunately, the incidence is low (0.1 to 0.3%). Colic and acute urticaria are other immediate reactions. Later reactions, which occur up to 24 hours

after drug administration, are papular eruptions, paresthesia, photophobia, lacrimation, palpebral edema, and hyperesthesia of the palms of the hands and the soles of the feet. Still later reactions consist in albuminuria, hematuria, and cylindruria. Rarely, agranulocytosis or hemolytic anemia may occur.

Precautions and Contraindications. Patients receiving suramin should be followed closely. Therapy should not be continued in patients who show intolerance to initial doses, and the drug should be employed with great caution in individuals with renal insufficiency. A moderate albuminuria is usual during the control of the acute phase, but persisting, heavy albuminuria calls for caution as well as modification of the schedule of treatment. If casts appear, treatment with suramin should be discontinued. The occurrence of palmar-plantar hyperesthesia necessitates caution since it may presage peripheral neuritis.

Therapeutic Uses. Suramin is used to treat *African trypanosomiasis* caused by *T. gambiense* and *T. rhodesiense*. It is of no value in South American trypanosomiasis, caused by *T. cruzi*. When employed alone, the drug is effective only in the early stage of the disease. In later stages of disease with CNS involvement, suramin is commonly used before, or in conjunction with, a course of arsenical therapy because only small amounts of suramin gain access to the cerebrospinal fluid. Suramin is effective in the *prophylaxis* of Rhodesian and Gambian trypanosomiasis. Pentamidine is also useful for this purpose and, indeed, may be a superior agent. Chemoprophylaxis is not recommended for travelers on occasional brief visits to endemic areas since the risk of serious drug toxicity outweighs the risk of acquiring the disease. Suramin is the most effective drug for clearing the adult filariae in *onchocerciasis*. The single dose of 1 g is repeated weekly for 5 or 6 weeks.

Berens, R. L.; Marr, J. J.; and Brun, R. Pyrazolopyrimidine metabolism in African trypanosomes: metabolic similarities to *Trypanosoma cruzi* and *Leishmania* spp. *Mol. Biochem. Parasitol.*, **1980**, *1*, 69–73.

Berman, J. D., and Webster, H. K. *In vitro* effects of mycophenolic acid and allopurinol against *Leishmania tropica* in human macrophages. *Antimicrob. Agents Chemother.*, **1982**, *21*, 887–891.

Carson, D. A., and Chang, K. Phosphorylation and antileishmanial activity of formycin B. *Biochem. Biophys. Res. Commun.*, **1981**, *100*, 1377–1383.

Clarkson, A. B., and Brohn, F. H. Trypanosomiasis: an approach to chemotherapy by inhibition of carbohydrate metabolism. *Science*, **1976**, *194*, 204–206.

DeVita, V. T.; Emmer, M.; Levine, A.; Jacobs, B.; and Berard, C. *Pneumocystis carinii* pneumonia. *N. Engl. J. Med.*, **1969**, *280*, 287–291.

Dvorak, J. A., and Howe, C. L. The effects of LAMPIT (Bayer 2502) on the interaction of *Trypanosoma cruzi* with vertebrate cells *in vitro*. *Am. J. Trop. Med. Hyg.*, **1977**, *26*, 58–63.

Flynn, I. W., and Bowman, I. B. R. Further studies on the mode of action of arsenicals on trypanosome pyruvate kinase. *Trans. R. Soc. Trop. Med. Hyg.*, **1969**, *63*, 121.

Friedheim, E. A. H. L'acide triazine-arsinique dans le traitement de la maladie du sommeil. *Ann. Inst. Pasteur (Paris)*, **1940**, *65*, 108–118.

————. Mel B in the treatment of human trypanosomiasis. *Am. J. Trop. Med.*, **1949**, *29*, 173–180.

Ivady, G.; Paldy, L.; Koltay, M.; Toth, G.; and Kovaks, Z. *Pneumocystis carinii* pneumonia. *Lancet*, **1967**, *1*, 616–617.

King, H.; Lourie, E. M.; and Yorke, W. Studies in chemotherapy. XIX. Further report on new trypanocidal substances. *Ann. Trop. Med. Parasitol.*, **1938**, *32*, 177–192.

Lelchuk, R.; Cardoni, R. L.; and Fuks, A. S. Cell-mediated immunity in Chagas' disease: alterations induced by treatment with a trypanocidal drug (nifurtimox). *Clin. Exp. Immunol.*, **1977a**, *30*, 434–438.

Lelchuk, R.; Cardoni, R. L.; and Lewis, S. Nifurtimox-induced alterations in the cell-mediated immune response to PPD in guinea pigs. *Clin. Exp. Immunol.*, **1977b**, *30*, 469–473.

Lourie, E. M., and Yorke, W. Studies in chemotherapy. XXI. The trypanocidal action of certain aromatic diamidines. *Ann. Trop. Med. Parasitol.*, **1939**, *33*, 289–304.

Moreno, S. N. J.; Palmero, D. J.; de Palmero, K. E.; Docampo, R.; and Stoppani, A. O. M. Stimulation of lipid peroxidation and ultrastructural alterations induced by nifurtimox in mammalian tissues. *Medicina (B. Aires)*, **1980**, *40*, 553–559.

Nelson, D. J.; Lafon, S. W.; Jones, T. E.; Spector, T.; Berens, R. L.; and Marr, J. J. The metabolism of FORMYCIN B in *Leishmania donovani*. *Biochem. Biophys. Res. Commun.*, **1982**, *108*, 349–354.

Sampaio, S. A.; Godoy, J. T.; Paiva, L.; Dillon, N. L.; and Lacas, C. da S. The treatment of American (mucocutaneous) leishmaniasis with amphotericin-B. *Arch. Dermatol.*, **1960**, *82*, 627–635.

VanHoof, L. M. J. J. Observations on trypanosomiasis in Belgian Congo. *Trans. R. Soc. Trop. Med. Hyg.*, **1947**, *40*, 728–761.

Waalkes, T. P.; Denham, C.; and DeVita, V. T. Pentamidine: clinical pharmacological correlations in man and mice. *Clin. Pharmacol. Ther.*, **1970**, *11*, 505–512.

Walzer, P. D.; Perl, D. P.; Krogstad, D. J.; Rawson, P. G.; and Schultz, M. G. *Pneumocystis carinii* pneumonia in the United States. *Ann. Intern. Med.*, **1974**, *80*, 83–93.

Wegner, D. H. G., and Rohwedder, R. W. Experience with nifurtimox in chronic Chagas' infection. Preliminary report. *Arzneimittelforsch.*, **1972**, *22*, 1635–1641.

Williamson, J., and Macadam, R. F. Effect of trypanocidal drugs on the fine structure of *Trypanosoma rhodesiense*. *Trans. R. Soc. Trop. Med. Hyg.*, **1965**, *59*, 367–368.

Monographs and Reviews

Albert, A. *Selective Toxicity: The Physico-Chemical Basis of Therapy*, 6th ed. Chapman & Hall, Ltd., London, **1979**.

Apted, F. I. C. Present status of chemotherapy and chemoprophylaxis of human trypanosomiasis in the eastern hemisphere. *Pharmacol. Ther.*, **1980**, *11*, 391–413.

Bacchi, C. J. Content, synthesis and function of polyamines in trypanosomatids: relationship to chemotherapy. *J. Protozool.*, **1981**, *28*, 20–27.

Beveridge, E. Chemotherapy of leishmaniasis. In, *Experimental Chemotherapy*, Vol. I. (Schnitzer, R. J., and Hawking, F., eds.) Academic Press, Inc., New York, **1963**, pp. 257–287.

Bowman, I. B. R., and Flynn, I. W. Oxidative metabolism of trypanosomes. In, *Biology of the Kinetoplastida*, Vol. 1. (Lumsden, W. H. R., and Evans, D. A., eds.) Academic Press, Inc., New York, **1976**, pp. 435–476.

Brener, Z. Present status of chemotherapy and chemoprophylaxis of human trypanosomiasis in the Western Hemisphere. *Pharmacol. Ther.*, **1979**, *7*, 71–90.

Brown, J.; Biaglow, J.; Hall, E.; Kinsella, T.; Phillips, R. C.; Urtasun, R.; Utley, J.; and Yuhas, J. Sensitizers and protectors to radiation and chemotherapeutic drugs. In, *The Interdisciplinary Program for Radiation Oncology Research*. (Wittes, R. E., ed.) *Cancer Treatment Symposia*, Vol. 1. U.S. Government Printing Office, Washington, D. C., **1984**, pp. 85–102.

Chang, K.-P. Cellular and molecular mechanisms of intracellular symbiosis in leishmaniasis. *Int. Rev. Cytol.*, **1983**, *14*, Suppl., 267–305.

Damper, D., and Patten, C. L. Pentamidine transport and sensitivity in *brucei*-group trypanosomes. *J. Protozool.*, **1976a**, *23*, 349–356.

————. Pentamine transport in *Trypanosoma brucei*—kinetics and specificity. *Biochem. Pharmacol.*, **1976b**, *25*, 271–276.

Docampo, R., and Moreno, S. N. J. Free radical metabolites in the mode of action of chemotherapeutic agents and phagocytic cells on *Trypanosoma cruzi*. *Rev. Infect. Dis.*, **1984**, *6*, 223–238.

Eagle, H., and Doak, G. O. The biological activity of arsenosobenzenes in relation to their structure. *Pharmacol. Rev.*, **1951**, *3*, 107–143.

Fairlamb, A. Biochemistry of trypanosomiasis and rational approaches to chemotherapy. *Trends Biochem. Sci.*, **1982**, *7*, 249–253.

Fairlamb, A. H., and Bowman, I. B. R. *Trypanosoma brucei*: suramin and other trypanocidal compounds: effects on sn-glycerol-3-phosphate oxidase. *Exp. Parasitol.*, **1977**, *43*, 353–361.

————. Uptake of the trypanocidal drug suramin by bloodstream forms of *Trypanosoma brucei* and its effect on respiration and growth rate *in vivo*. *Mol. Biochem. Parasitol.*, **1980**, *1*, 315–333.

Findlay, G. M. *Recent Advances in Chemotherapy*, Vol. I. J. & A. Churchill, Ltd., London, **1950**.

Hawking, F. Chemotherapy of trypanosomiasis. In, *Experimental Chemotherapy*, Vol. I. (Schnitzer, R. J., and Hawking, F., eds.) Academic Press, Inc., New York, **1963**, pp. 129–256.

————. Suramin: with special reference to onchocerciasis. *Adv. Pharmacol. Chemother.*, **1978**, *15*, 289–322.

Hughes, W. T.; Feldman, S.; Chaudhary, S. C.; Ossi, M. J.; Cox, F.; and Sanyal, S. K. Comparison of pentamidine isethionate and trimethoprim-sulfamethoxazole in treatment of *Pneumocystis carinii* pneumonia. *J. Pediatr.*, **1978**, *92*, 285–291.

Meshnick, S. R. The chemotherapy of African trypanosomiasis. In, *Parasitic Diseases*, Vol. 2. (Mansfield, J. M., ed.) Marcel Dekker, Inc., New York, **1984**, pp. 165–199.

Rees, P. H.; Keating, M. I.; Kager, P. A.; and Hockmeyer, W. T. Renal clearance of pentavalent antimony (sodium stibogluconate). *Lancet*, **1980**, *2*, 226–229.

Robertson, D. H. H. Chemotherapy of African trypanosomiasis. *Practitioner*, **1962**, *188*, 80–83.

Sharpe, S. M. Pentamidine and hypoglycemia. *Ann. Intern. Med.*, **1983**, *99*, 128.

Steck, E. A. The chemotherapy of protozoal infections of man. *J. Protozool.*, **1981a**, *28*, 10–16.

————. The chemotherapy of protozoal infections: whither? *Ibid.*, **1981b**, *28*, 30–35.

Wang, J. J.; Freeman, A. I.; Gaeta, J. F.; and Sinks, L. F. Unusual complications of pentamidine in the treatment of *Pneumocystis carinii* pneumonia. *J. Pediatr.*, **1970**, *77*, 311–314.

Warren, K. S., and Mahmoud, A. A. F. (eds.). *Tropical and Geographic Medicine*. McGraw-Hill Book Co., New York, **1984**.

Williamson, J. Chemotherapy and chemoprophylaxis of African trypanosomiasis. *Exp. Parasitol.*, **1962**, *12*, 274–322.

Wyler, D. J., and Marsden, P. D. Leishmaniasis. In, *Tropical and Geographical Medicine*. (Warren, K. S., and Mahmoud, A. A. F., eds.) McGraw-Hill Book Co., New York, **1984**, pp. 270–280.

SECTION
XII

Chemotherapy of Microbial Diseases

CHAPTER

48 ANTIMICROBIAL AGENTS
General Considerations

Merle A. Sande and Gerald L. Mandell

Historical Aspects and Introduction. The concept that substances derived from one living organism may kill another (antibiosis) is almost as old as the science of microbiology. Indeed, the application of antibiotic therapy, without recognition of it as such, is considerably older. The Chinese were aware, over 2500 years ago, of the therapeutic properties of moldy curd of soybean applied to carbuncles, boils, and similar infections and used this material as standard treatment in such disorders. The medical literature has for many centuries contained descriptions of beneficial effects from the application to infections of soil and various plants, most of which probably were sources of antibiotic-forming molds and bacteria.

The first investigators to recognize the clinical potentialities of microorganisms as therapeutic agents were Pasteur and Joubert, who recorded their observations and speculations in 1877. They noted that anthrax bacilli grew rapidly when inoculated into sterile urine but failed to multiply and soon died if one of the "common" bacteria of the air was introduced in the urine at the same time. The same type of experiment in animals produced similar results. They commented on the fact that life destroys life among the lower species even more than among higher animals and plants, and came to the astonishing conclusion that anthrax bacilli could be administered to an animal in large numbers, and it would not sicken, provided that "ordinary" bacteria were given at the same time.

They stated that this observation might hold great promise for therapeutics.

The clinical use of antibiotic agents represents the practical, controlled, and directed application of phenomena that occur naturally and continuously in soil, sewage, water, and other natural habitats of microorganisms. During the latter part of the nineteenth century and the early years of the twentieth century, several antimicrobial substances were demonstrated in bacterial cultures and some were even tested clinically but discarded because they proved to be highly toxic.

The modern era of the chemotherapy of infection started with the clinical use of sulfanilamide in 1936. The "golden age" of antimicrobial therapy began with the production of penicillin in 1941, when this compound was mass-produced and first made available for limited clinical trial. Approximately 30% of all hospitalized patients now receive one or more courses of therapy with antibiotics, and millions of potentially fatal infections have been cured. However, at the same time, these pharmaceutical agents have become among the most misused of those available to the practicing physician. One result of widespread use of antimicrobial agents has been the emergence of antibiotic-resistant pathogens, which in turn has created an ever-increasing need for new drugs. Many of these agents have also contributed significantly to the rising costs of medical care.

The history of antimicrobial agents has thus been dynamic, characterized by the constant emergence of new challenges followed by investigation, discovery, and the production of new drugs. The following pages present both a philosophical and a practical approach to the appropriate use of antimicrobial agents, as well as a discussion of the factors that influence the outcome of treatment with them.

Definition and Characteristics. Antibiotics are chemical substances produced by various species of microorganisms (bacteria, fungi, actinomycetes) that suppress the growth of other microorganisms and may eventually destroy them. The number of antibiotics that has been identified now extends into the hundreds, and nearly 100 have been developed to the stage where they are of value in the therapy of infectious diseases. Antibiotics differ markedly in physical, chemical, and pharmacological properties, antibacterial spectra, and mechanisms of action. Most have been chemically identified, and some have been synthesized. A few are available only as crude or partially purified extracts.

The synthetic chemist has added greatly to our therapeutic armamentarium. Thus, drugs such as isoniazid and ethambutol represent important contributions for the treatment of tuberculosis. While many such antimicrobial agents are not properly termed antibiotics, since they are not produced by living organisms, little distinction should now be made between compounds of natural and synthetic origin. Chemotherapy of viral diseases is currently benefiting from a similar planned approach directed toward purely synthetic drugs as more is learned about mechanisms of viral replication.

Classification and Mechanism of Action. There are several methods used to classify and group antimicrobial agents, and all are hampered by exceptions and overlaps. Historically, the most common classification has been based on chemical structure and proposed mechanism of action, as follows: (1) agents that inhibit synthesis of or activate enzymes that disrupt bacterial cell walls to cause loss of viability and, often, cell lysis; these include the penicillins and cephalosporins, which are structurally similar, and dissimilar agents such as cycloserine, vancomycin, bacitracin, and the imidazole antifungal agents (miconazole, ketoconazole, and clotrimazole); (2) agents that act directly on the cell membrane of the microorganism, affecting permeability and leading to leakage of intracellular compounds; these include the detergents, polymyxin and colistimethate, and the polyene antifungal agents, nystatin and amphotericin B, that bind to cell-wall sterols; (3) agents that affect the function of bacterial ribosomes to cause a reversible inhibition of protein synthesis; these bacteriostatic drugs include chloramphenicol, the tetracyclines, erythromycin, and clindamycin; (4) agents that bind to the 30 S ribosomal subunit and alter protein synthesis, which eventually leads to cell death; these include the aminoglycosides; (5) agents that affect nucleic acid metabolism, such as rifampin, which inhibits DNA-dependent RNA polymerase, and the quinolones (nalidixic acid and congeners) and metronidazole, which inhibit DNA synthesis; (6) the antimetabolites, including trimethoprim and the sulfonamides, which block specific metabolic steps that are essential to microorganisms; (7) nucleic acid analogs, such as vidarabine and acyclovir, which bind to viral enzymes that are essential for DNA synthesis and thus halt viral replication. Additional categories will likely emerge as more complex mechanisms are elucidated; at the present time, the precise mechanism of action of some antimicrobial agents is unknown.

Factors That Determine the Susceptibility and Resistance of Microorganisms to Antimicrobial Agents. When antibiotics are used to treat an infection, a favorable therapeutic outcome is influenced by numerous factors. However, in simple terms, success is dependent on achieving a level of antibacterial activity at the site of infection that is sufficient to inhibit the bacteria in a manner that *tips the balance in favor of the host*. When host defenses are maximally effective, the antibacterial effect required may be minimal, for example, that provided by bacteriostatic agents that slow protein synthesis or prevent microbial cell division.

On the other hand, when host defenses are impaired, complete killing or lysis of the bacteria may be required to achieve a successful outcome. The dose of drug utilized must be sufficient to produce the necessary effect on the microorganisms; however, concentrations of the agent in plasma and tissues must remain below those that are toxic to human cells. If this can be achieved, the microorganism is said to be susceptible to the antibiotic. If the concentration of drug required to inhibit or kill the organism is greater than the concentration that can safely be achieved, the microorganism is considered to be resistant to the antibiotic.

The precise information required to make accurate decisions about concentrations of drugs in various tissues or body fluids is frequently unavailable. Thus, determination of antibiotic sensitivity of microorganisms is at best an inexact science. For example, group-A beta-hemolytic streptococci are exquisitely sensitive to penicillin G and are inhibited and killed by low concentrations (1 ng/ml), yet very high concentrations of penicillin (20 to 100 μg/ml) can be safely achieved in plasma. There is thus a very large margin of "overkill." On the other hand, many gram-negative aerobic bacilli, such as *Pseudomonas aeruginosa,* may require 2 to 4 μg/ml of gentamicin or tobramycin to be inhibited. Such bacilli are considered to be susceptible to these antimicrobials, although peak concentrations in plasma above 6 to 10 μg/ml may result in ototoxicity or nephrotoxicity. Thus, the ratio of toxic to therapeutic concentrations is very low and such agents are difficult to use appropriately. Concentrations of these drugs at certain sites of infection (such as vitreous fluid or cerebrospinal fluid) may be much lower than those in plasma. Thus, the drug may be only marginally effective or ineffective in such cases even though standardized *in-vitro* tests would likely report the microorganism as "sensitive." Conversely, concentrations of drug in urine may be much higher than those in plasma. Microorganisms reported as "resistant" may thus respond to therapy when infection is limited to the urinary tract. Most *in-vitro* sensitivity tests are standardized on the basis of the drug concentrations that can be safely achieved in plasma. They do *not* reflect concentrations that can be attained at sites of infection, nor do they consider any local factors that may affect the activity of the drug. The limitations of such *in-vitro* tests must be understood.

There are multiple factors that determine the relative antimicrobial activity of a drug against a specific microorganism. For an antibiotic to be effective, it must first gain access to the target sites of action on or in the bacterial cell. Microorganisms may resist this passage by several mechanisms (Vaudaux, 1981). Some produce enzymes at or within the cell surface that inactivate the drug. Others possess impermeable cell membranes that prevent influx of the drug. Hydrophilic antibiotics traverse the outer membrane of microbial cells via aqueous channels (pores) comprised of specific proteins (porins). Bacteria deficient in these channels can be resistant to such drugs (Jaffe *et. al.,* 1983). Still others lack the transport systems that are required for entrance of the drug into the bacterial cell (Dickie *et al.,* 1978). Since many antibiotics are organic acids, their penetration may be pH dependent (Bryant, 1984); in addition, permeation may be altered by osmolality or by various cations in the external milieu (Zimilis and Jackson, 1973). The transport mechanisms for certain drugs are energy dependent and are not operative in an anaerobic environment (Verklin and Mandell, 1977).

Once the drug has gained access to the target site, it must exert an effect that is deleterious to the microorganism. If the bacteria are observed to be resistant to an antimicrobial agent, natural or acquired changes in the target sites may afford an explanation.

Acquired Resistance to Antimicrobial Agents. When the antimicrobial activity of a new agent is first tested, a pattern of "sensitivity" and "resistance" is usually defined. Unfortunately, this spectrum of activity can subsequently vary remarkably, since microorganisms have evolved an array of ingenious alterations that allow them to survive in the presence of antibiotics. The phenomenon of drug resistance varies from microorganism to microorganism and from drug to drug. For example, strains of *Staphylococcus aureus* that were resistant to penicillin G appeared shortly after this antibiotic was introduced. The frequency has increased such that up to 80% of both hospital- and community-acquired strains of this bacterium are now insensitive. Emergence of resistance in some other species has occurred more slowly. The gonococcus gradually acquired low-level resistance to penicillin G (*i.e.*, higher doses became necessary for cure) over a period of 20 years, especially in areas where this drug was used excessively. However, since 1974 many gonococcal strains have suddenly emerged that produce penicillinase, an enzyme that inactivates the drug (Washington, 1982). These strains are highly resistant to penicillin G, and infections produced by them are not cured even with high doses of the drug. Likewise, the pneumococcus (*Streptococcus pneumoniae*) has historically been exquisitely sensitive to penicillin G; however, in 1978, strains resistant to this drug emerged in South Africa (Jacobs *et al.*, 1978). Several similar strains have subsequently been isolated in the United States.

The development of resistance to antibiotics may involve a stable genetic change, heritable from generation to generation. Any of the mechanisms that result in alteration of bacterial genetic composition can operate. While *mutation* is frequently the cause, resistance to antimicrobial agents may be acquired through transfer of genetic material from one bacterium to another by *transduction, transformation,* or *conjugation.*

Mutation. Any large population of antibiotic-susceptible bacteria is likely to contain some mutants that are relatively resistant to the drug. Such variants can be isolated when the microorganisms are grown in medium containing the antibiotic, and analysis indicates that these strains have undergone a stable genetic change that may persist in the absence of the drug. There is, however, no evidence that these mutations are actually a result of exposure to the particular drug. Strains of some bacterial species isolated long before certain antibacterial agents were developed have subsequently been found to be naturally highly resistant to these drugs; such was the case with penicillinase-produc-

ing *Staph. aureus.* Such mutations are random events, and the resultant alteration is usually specific for a single drug or class of drugs.

Microorganisms that acquire resistance to a particular antimicrobial agent become important clinically, particularly when the use of an individual drug is widespread. Sensitive strains are suppressed and resistant ones multiply unimpaired; in time, resistant microorganisms predominate. This process is called *selection.*

The acquisition of resistance to antimicrobial agents can follow different temporal patterns. In some instances, a single-step mutation results in a high degree of resistance. For example, when *Escherichia coli* or *Staph. aureus* are exposed to rifampin, highly resistant mutants emerge that contain an altered DNA-dependent RNA polymerase that does not bind the drug (Wehrli, 1983). In other cases the emergence of resistant mutants may be a slow stepwise process, with each step conferring only slight alterations in susceptibility. As mentioned, this has occurred with the gonococcus, where there has been a gradual reduction in accessibility of penicillin G to target sites (penicillin-binding proteins) in the cell envelope of the organism (Sparling *et al.*, 1976).

Mutational changes that confer resistance to a drug may simultaneously alter virulence factors and affect the pathogenicity of the microorganism. For example, some strains of *Staph. aureus* that spontaneously develop resistance to rifampin also produce less catalase and are less virulent in animals (Mandell, 1975). These resistant strains do not persist well in the environment (Sande and Mandell, 1975). Strains of *Neisseria gonorrhoeae* that have acquired stepwise, low-level resistance to penicillin G are less pathogenic and rarely disseminate from the genital sites of primary infection. Such dissemination is more common with their penicillin-sensitive counterparts (Handsfield *et al.*, 1976; Jaffe *et al.*, 1976). Unfortunately, all antibiotic-resistant mutants are *not* less virulent—for example, penicillinase-producing *Staph. aureus.*

Transduction. This process occurs by the intervention of a bacteriophage (a virus that infects bacteria) that can carry bacterial DNA incorporated within its protein coat. If this genetic material includes a gene for drug resistance, a newly infected bacterial cell may become resistant to the agent and capable of passing the trait on to its progeny. Transduction is particularly important in the transfer of antibiotic resistance among strains of *Staph. aureus,* where some phages can carry plasmids (extrachromosomal DNA) that code for penicillinase, while others transfer information for resistance to erythromycin, tetracycline, or chloramphenicol.

Transformation. This method of transferring genetic information involves incorporation of DNA that is free in the environment into bacteria. Although some bacterial cells are capable of excreting transforming DNA during certain phases of growth, the importance of this method of transfer remains unknown.

Conjugation. The passage of genes from cell to cell by direct contact through a sex pilus or bridge is termed conjugation. This is now recognized as an extremely important mechanism for spread of anti-biotic resistance, since DNA that codes for resistance to *multiple* drugs may be so transferred. Conjugation was first recognized in Japan in 1959 after an outbreak of bacillary dysentery caused by *Shigella flexneri* that was resistant to four different classes of antibiotics (Watanabe, 1966). Resistance could be easily transferred to sensitive strains of both *Shigella* and other Enterobacteriaceae. The transferable genetic material consisted of two different DNA sequences. The first sequence codes for the actual resistance and is termed the resistance (R) factor, or the R determinant plasmid. For example, in the case of resistance to aminoglycosides or chloramphenicol, the R factor codes for the synthesis of drug-inactivating enzymes (Davies *et al.*, 1971). The second sequence codes for a sex factor, which is the transfer apparatus (sex pilus) and is termed resistance transfer factor (RTF), or transfer factor plasmid (Datta and Nugent, 1984). Each of these two DNA sequences can be transferred individually, but both must be present for successful transfer of resistance to antibiotics.

Transfer of such information by conjugation occurs predominantly among gram-negative bacilli, and resistance is conferred on a susceptible cell as a single event. Conjugation can take place in the intestinal tract between nonpathogenic and pathogenic microorganisms. While the efficiency of transfer is low *in vitro* and lower *in vivo*, antibiotics can exert a powerful selective pressure to allow emergence of the resistant strain. The proportion of enteric bacteria that carry plasmids for multiple-drug resistance has thus risen slowly in the past 25 years. In some studies, more than 50% of persons have been found to carry multiple-resistant coliform bacilli containing R factors, and such bacteria have been isolated in large numbers from rivers containing untreated sewage. Multiple-resistant Enterobacteriaceae have become a problem worldwide, taxing the physician and creating a constant need for new antibiotics. In several situations where antibiotic usage has been controlled, the rate of emergence of these resistant strains was slowed; in some instances their incidence was actually reduced (Bulger and Sherris, 1968).

The worldwide emergence of *Haemophilus* and gonococci that produce beta-lactamase is a major therapeutic problem. The gene for production of this enzyme is carried on small plasmids. At least some of the gonococcal plasmids are similar in size to the *H. influenzae* gene, and a *Haemophilus* plasmid has been transferred to gonococci by conjugation *in vitro* (Sparling, 1978). Likewise, many gonococcal strains carry a conjugative plasmid that enables sexual transfer to other *Neisseria* and to *E. coli*. It is thus likely that beta-lactamase-producing gonococci initially obtained their plasmid from a *Haemophilus* species and may maintain the potential to transfer it to penicillin-sensitive species such as *N. meningitidis*. Fortunately, some of these genes are unstable, which may explain the reduction in the incidence of these resistant strains in England and their failure to become predominant in the United States.

SELECTION OF AN ANTIMICROBIAL AGENT

Optimal and judicious selection of antimicrobial agents for the therapy of infectious diseases is a complex procedure that requires clinical judgment and detailed knowledge of pharmacological and microbiological factors. Unfortunately, the decision to use antibiotics is frequently made lightly, without regard to the potential infecting microorganism or to the pharmacological features of the drug. *When an antimicrobial agent is indicated, the goal is to choose a drug that is selectively active for the most likely infecting microorganism(s) and that has the least potential to cause toxicity or allergic reactions in the individual being treated (see Table 48–1).*

The first decision a physician must make is whether administration of an antimicrobial agent is indicated. Many physicians reflexly associate fever with treatable infections and prescribe antimicrobial therapy without further evaluation. This practice is irrational and dangerous, since all antibiotics can cause serious toxicity and, as noted above, injudicious use of antimicrobial agents results in the selection of resistant microorganisms. On the other hand, one does not always have the luxury of a definitive identification of a bacterial infection before treatment must be initiated. In the absence of a clear indication, antibiotics may often be used if disease is severe and if it seems likely that withholding therapy will result in failure to manage a potentially life-threatening infection.

Initiation of optimal antibiotic therapy requires the identification of the infecting agent. Since therapy may be required before bacteriological confirmation of identity is available, the physician must make an educated guess, that is, determine the most likely microorganisms responsible for the infection. A number of technics are helpful in this process. Importantly, the clinical picture may suggest the specific microorganism: the therapist must know the microorganisms most likely to cause specific infections in a given host. In addition, simple and rapid laboratory technics are available for the examination of infected tissues. The most valuable and time-tested method for immediate identification of bacteria is the examination of the infected secretion or body fluid with the gram stain. Such tests help to narrow the list of potential pathogens and permit more rational selection of initial antibiotic therapy. However, in some situations, identification of the morphology of the infecting organism may not be adequate to arrive at a specific bacteriological diagnosis, and the selection of a single narrow-spectrum antibiotic may be inappropriate, particularly if the infection is life threatening. Broad antimicrobial coverage is then indicated, pending isolation and identification of the microorganism. *Whenever the clinician is faced with initiating therapy on a presumptive bacteriological diagnosis, cultures of blood and other body fluids should be taken prior to the institution of drug therapy. If the patient has been receiving antibiotics, then beta-lactamase should be added to the culture media or other mechanisms for removal of antibiotics ("antibiotic removal devices") should be employed.*

Testing for Microbial Sensitivity to Antimicrobial Agents. There may be wide variations in the susceptibility of different strains of the same bacterial species to antibiotics. Essential to the choice of drug is information about the pattern of sensitivity of the infecting microorganism. Several tests are now available for determination of bacterial sensitivity to antimicrobial agents.

The most commonly used test of sensitivity to antimicrobial agents is the Kirby-Bauer or disc diffusion technic (Bauer *et al.*, 1966). Although it is simple to perform and relatively inexpensive, it provides only qualitative or semiquantitative information on the susceptibility of a given microorganism to a given antibiotic. The test is performed by applying commercially available filter-paper discs impregnated with specific quantities of the drug onto the surface of agar plates over which a culture of the microorganism has been streaked. After 18 hours of incubation, the size of a clear zone of inhibition around the disc is determined, and this correlates with the activity of the drug against the test strain. Standards for sensitivity vary for each microorganism and, as previously stated, are based on the concentration of drug that can safely be achieved in plasma without producing toxicity. Even though the concentration of the antibiotic in plasma is the standard used for these tests, it may not always reflect the drug concentration at the site of the infection. There are several notable exceptions where the Kirby-Bauer disc diffusion test does not accurately predict therapeutic effectiveness: (1) methicillin-resistant *Staph. aureus*, which may appear to be sensitive to cephalosporins; (2) enterococci, which may appear to be sensitive to cephalosporins and trimethoprim-sulfamethoxazole; and (3) *Shigella* species, which may appear to be sensitive to cephalosporins. These drugs have been proven *not* to be useful in such infections.

Tests that are more reliable, quantitatively, involve serial dilutions of antibiotics in solid agar or broth media containing a culture of the test microorganism. The lowest concentration of the agent that prevents visible growth after 18 to 24 hours of incubation is known as the *minimal inhibitory concentration* (MIC), and the lowest concentration that sterilizes the medium or results in a 99.9% decline in bacterial numbers is known as the *minimal bactericidal concentration* (MBC). The latter test is used only in special instances where very precise knowledge of the ability of a given antimicrobial agent to kill a specific clinical isolate is required, as in the therapy of bacterial endocarditis.

In addition to tests of antimicrobial activity *in vitro*, it would be valuable to have a test to predict efficacy of antimicrobial treatment. One test that has been used for many years is a measure of the bactericidal activity of the patient's serum against the infecting microorganism. This test, first popularized by Schlichter and MacLean (1947), has been used extensively to monitor therapy in patients with bacterial endocarditis and, more recently, in neutropenic patients with disseminated infections (Klastersky and Staquet, 1982). The test simply estimates the dilution of the patient's serum that produces a bactericidal effect. While interpretation is controversial (Coleman *et al.*, 1982) and standardized methods have only recently been established (Stratton *et al.*, 1982), therapists strive to achieve a bactericidal titer in serum of 1:8, taken at the peak of the drug concentration *in vivo*, in patients with endocarditis or neutropenia.

In some increasingly rare instances, antibiotic sensitivity tests need not be carried out, since long experience has indicated that certain microorganisms have remained highly susceptible to specific antibiotics despite years of exposure. For example, group-A beta-hemolytic streptococci have fortunately remained remarkably sensitive to penicillin G; meningococci are always susceptible to penicillin G and to chloramphenicol.

Pharmacokinetic Factors. Although the knowledge that an antibiotic is active *in vitro* against the infecting microorganism is critical, it is not the only factor to be con-

Table 48–1. CURRENT USE OF ANTIMICROBIAL AGENTS IN THE THERAPY OF INFECTIONS

Presentation of choices of specific agents for the treatment of various infections is always provocative of discussion and disagreement because such choices often represent the distillate of personal experiences that may not duplicate those of others. In addition, the current availability of a number of drugs that are approximately equally effective makes an order of choice very difficult, if not impossible. To complicate matters, patterns of sensitivity of a number of microorganisms often vary with the hospital or clinic in which they are isolated; in some instances, this reflects a varying degree of exposure to specific agents. The material presented in this table represents not only the practice of the authors, based on their experience with the management of these infections, but also that of other experts in the United States. These drug selections represent initial therapy only. Each choice must be verified by testing of the etiological isolate for sensitivity to antibiotics. It is important to stress that, as more information accumulates, as recently introduced drugs are used for longer periods, and as entirely new agents are developed, some of the recommendations will require modification not only in the order of choice but even in the specific drugs that are suggested.

DISEASES		DRUG ORDER OF CHOICE		
		1st	2nd[1]	3rd[1]
I. GRAM-POSITIVE COCCI				
Staphylococcus aureus * — Penicillin G sensitive[2]	Abscesses, Bacteremia, Endocarditis, Pneumonia, Meningitis, Osteomyelitis, Cellulitis, Other	Penicillin G	A cephalosporin (G1)[3], Vancomycin	Clindamycin[4]
— Penicillin G resistant		A penicillinase-resistant penicillin	A cephalosporin (G1)[3], Vancomycin	—
— Methicillin resistant		Vancomycin[5]	Trimethoprim-sulfamethoxazole + rifampin[6]	
Streptococcus pyogenes	Pharyngitis, Scarlet fever, Otitis media, sinusitis, Cellulitis, Erysipelas, Pneumonia, Bacteremia, Other systemic infections	Penicillin G, Penicillin V	A cephalosporin (G1)[3,7], Erythromycin	Vancomycin[7]
Streptococcus * (viridans group)	Endocarditis, Bacteremia	Penicillin G ± streptomycin or gentamicin	A cephalosporin (G1)[3]	Vancomycin
Streptococcus agalactiae (group B)	Septicemia	Ampicillin or penicillin G ± an aminoglycoside	A cephalosporin (G1)[3]	Erythromycin
	Meningitis		Cefotaxime	Chloramphenicol[8]

Organism	Infection			
Streptococcus faecalis * (enterococcus)	Endocarditis	Penicillin G + gentamicin or streptomycin	Vancomycin + gentamicin or streptomycin	—
	Urinary tract infection	Ampicillin or penicillin G	Vancomycin	Nitrofurantoin
	Bacteremia			—
Streptococcus bovis	Endocarditis / Urinary tract infection / Bacteremia	Penicillin G ± streptomycin or gentamicin	A cephalosporin (G1) [3] ± streptomycin or gentamicin	Vancomycin
Streptococcus * (anaerobic species)	Bacteremia / Endocarditis / Brain and other abscesses / Sinusitis	Penicillin G [9]	A cephalosporin (G1) [3] Clindamycin [4]	Chloramphenicol [8] Erythromycin [4]
Streptococcus pneumoniae * (pneumococcus)	Pneumonia / Endocarditis / Arthritis / Sinusitis / Otitis	Penicillin G	A cephalosporin (G1) [3] Erythromycin	Chloramphenicol Clindamycin
	Meningitis		Chloramphenicol [8] or cefotaxime	—

* All strains must be examined in vitro for sensitivity to various antimicrobial agents.

[1] Drugs included for second and third choices are (a) indicated in patients hypersensitive to equally or more effective agents, (b) potentially more dangerous than equally active drugs, (c) less likely to produce the desired therapeutic response, or (d) in need, in some cases, of further study in order to allow a valid evaluation of their efficacy.

[2] Minimal inhibitory concentration (MIC) is less than 0.2 μg/ml.

[3] G1 and G3 designate first- and third-generation cephalosporins, respectively. If no generation is specified, certain agents may be preferable to others (see Chapter 50). Therapeutic concentrations of most cephalosporins may not be achieved in the cerebrospinal fluid (exceptions include cefotaxime and moxalactam), and alternative agents should be used to treat infections of the central nervous system (CNS).

[4] Therapeutic concentrations are not achieved in the cerebrospinal fluid, and alternative agents should be used to treat infections of the CNS.

[5] Vancomycin is the only antimicrobial agent proven to be effective for treatment of serious infections due to methicillin-resistant Staph. aureus.

[6] Rifampin is highly active against most strains of Staph. aureus, including some that are resistant to methicillin. Since resistance develops rapidly (one-step mutation) during therapy, a second active drug, such as trimethoprim-sulfamethoxazole, should be used concurrently.

[7] Especially for bacteremia.

[8] Chloramphenicol is effective for infection of the CNS in patients who are allergic to beta-lactam antibiotics.

[9] Large doses of penicillin G may be required.

Table 48–1. CURRENT USE OF ANTIMICROBIAL AGENTS IN THE THERAPY OF INFECTIONS (Continued)

II. GRAM-NEGATIVE COCCI

DISEASES		DRUG ORDER OF CHOICE		
		1st	2nd [1]	3rd [1]
Neisseria gonorrhoeae (gonococcus)				
Genital infections	Penicillin sensitive	Ampicillin or amoxicillin, Penicillin G, A tetracycline	Erythromycin, Spectinomycin	—
	Penicillinase producing	Spectinomycin	Cefoxitin or cefotaxime	Trimethoprim-sulfamethoxazole
Arthritis-dermatitis syndrome		Ampicillin or amoxicillin, Penicillin G	A tetracycline	Erythromycin
Neisseria meningitidis (meningococcus)				
Meningitis Bacteremia		Penicillin G	Cefotaxime or moxalactam	Chloramphenicol [8]
Carrier state		Rifampin	Minocycline	—

III. GRAM-POSITIVE BACILLI

DISEASES	DRUG ORDER OF CHOICE		
	1st	2nd [1]	3rd [1]
Bacillus anthracis *			
"Malignant pustule" Pneumonia	Penicillin G	Erythromycin, A tetracycline	A cephalosporin (G1) [3], Chloramphenicol
Corynebacterium diphtheriae [10]			
Pharyngitis Laryngotracheitis Pneumonia Other local lesions	Penicillin G	Erythromycin	A cephalosporin (G1) [3], Rifampin
Carrier state	Erythromycin	Penicillin G	—
Corynebacterium species, aerobic and anaerobic * (diphtheroids)			
Endocarditis Infected foreign bodies	Penicillin G ± an aminoglycoside, Vancomycin	Rifampin + penicillin G	—
Listeria monocytogenes			
Meningitis Bacteremia Endocarditis	Ampicillin or penicillin G ± an aminoglycoside	Chloramphenicol [8], Erythromycin, A tetracycline	—
Erysipelothrix rhusiopathiae			
Erysipeloid	Penicillin G	Erythromycin, A tetracycline	Chloramphenicol

Organism	Diseases	1st	2nd	3rd [1]
Clostridium perfringens * and other species	Gas gangrene [11]	Penicillin G	Chloramphenicol	A cephalosporin [3] / Clindamycin
Clostridium tetani	Tetanus [11]	Penicillin G [12]	A tetracycline	Erythromycin
IV. GRAM-NEGATIVE BACILLI			DRUG ORDER OF CHOICE	
Escherichia coli *	Urinary tract infection [13]	Ampicillin ± an aminoglycoside / A sulfonamide / Trimethoprim-sulfamethoxazole	A cephalosporin [3] / A tetracycline / An aminoglycoside	Nitrofurantoin
	Other infections / Bacteremia	Ampicillin ± an aminoglycoside	A cephalosporin [3] / An aminoglycoside	Trimethoprim-sulfamethoxazole
Enterobacter aerogenes *	Urinary tract [14] and other infections	Cefamandole, cefuroxime, or another cephalosporin (G3) [3] / An aminoglycoside [15]	An antipseudomonal penicillin [16]	Trimethoprim-sulfamethoxazole
Proteus mirabilis *	Urinary tract [14] and other infections	Ampicillin / An aminoglycoside [15]	A cephalosporin [3]	—
Proteus, other species *	Urinary tract [14] and other infections	An aminoglycoside [15] / A cephalosporin (G3) [3]	An antipseudomonal penicillin [16]	—
Pseudomonas aeruginosa *	Urinary tract infection [14]	An antipseudomonal penicillin [16]	An aminoglycoside [15]	—
	Pneumonia [17] / Bacteremia [17]	An aminoglycoside [15] + an antipseudomonal penicillin [16]	An aminoglycoside [15] + cefoperazone, ceftazidime, or cefsulodin [18]	—

[10] Antibiotics alone do not alter the clinical course of diphtheria, but drugs can eradicate the carrier state.

[11] Adequate debridement is absolutely essential.

[12] Ten to 20 million units of penicillin G daily, with debridement and adsorbed tetanus toxoid.

[13] Sulfonamides, trimethoprim-sulfamethoxazole, and urinary tract antiseptics are useful for acute urinary tract infections, especially cystitis, in the patient without obstructive uropathy or in whom the disease has not become chronic. These agents also prove useful for chronic suppressive therapy in patients with recurrent urinary tract infection. Some clinicians prefer to reserve the antibiotics, such as ampicillin and aminoglycosides, for cases in which there are systemic manifestations—particularly in acute pyelonephritis. In some areas, 20 to 40% of E. coli infections acquired in the community are resistant to ampicillin.

[14] Urinary tract infections caused by microorganisms other than E. coli are less usual and frequently occur in the setting of obstructive uropathy or an indwelling urinary catheter, or following recurrent infections and the use of antibiotics. Therapy must be individualized but is frequently unsuccessful unless the underlying condition is corrected.

[15] Gentamicin, tobramycin, amikacin, or netilmicin only.

[16] Carbenicillin, ticarcillin, piperacillin, mezlocillin, or azlocillin.

[17] While single-drug therapy with an antipseudomonal penicillin or an aminoglycoside is adequate for some infections caused by Pseud. aeruginosa, the combination of the two classes of drug is recommended for therapy of serious infections, especially in the neutropenic patient or in the individual with pneumonia.

[18] Cephalosporins that are most active against Pseud. aeruginosa include cefoperazone, ceftazidime, and cefsulodin, but resistance may develop during therapy.

Table 48-1. CURRENT USE OF ANTIMICROBIAL AGENTS IN THE THERAPY OF INFECTIONS (Continued)

DISEASES	DRUG ORDER OF CHOICE		
	1st [1]	2nd [1]	3rd [1]
IV. GRAM-NEGATIVE BACILLI			
Klebsiella pneumoniae *			
Urinary tract infection [14]	A cephalosporin [5]	An aminoglycoside Mezlocillin or piperacillin	Trimethoprim-sulfamethoxazole
Pneumonia	A cephalosporin [19] + an aminoglycoside	Mezlocillin or piperacillin ± an aminoglycoside	—
Salmonella *			
Typhoid fever Paratyphoid fever Bacteremia	Chloramphenicol Trimethoprim-sulfamethoxazole	Ampicillin [20]	Cefoperazone
Acute gastroenteritis	No therapy or trimethoprim-sulfamethoxazole	—	—
Shigella *			
Acute gastroenteritis	Trimethoprim-sulfamethoxazole	Ampicillin [20]	A tetracycline
Serratia *			
Variety of nosocomial and opportunistic infections	Gentamicin Cefoxitin or another cephalosporin (G3) [3]	Other aminoglycosides Antipseudomonal penicillins [16]	—
Acinetobacter *			
Various nosocomial infections	An aminoglycoside [15]	A cephalosporin (G3) [3]	—
Haemophilus influenzae *			
Otitis media Sinusitis Bronchitis	Amoxicillin or ampicillin [20] Trimethoprim-sulfamethoxazole	Cefaclor	—
Epiglottitis Pneumonia Meningitis	Chloramphenicol Cefotaxime or moxalactam	Cefamandole [21] or cefuroxime [3] Ampicillin [20]	—
Haemophilus ducreyi			
Chancroid	Trimethoprim-sulfamethoxazole	A sulfonamide A tetracycline	Streptomycin
Brucella			
Brucellosis	A tetracycline ± streptomycin [22] or rifampin	Chloramphenicol ± streptomycin [22]	Trimethoprim-sulfamethoxazole
Yersinia pestis			
Plague	Streptomycin ± a tetracycline	A tetracycline	Chloramphenicol

Yersinia enterocolitica	Yersiniosis	No treatment or trimethoprim-sulfamethoxazole [23]	—	—
	Sepsis	An aminoglycoside Chloramphenicol [24]	—	Chloramphenicol
Francisella tularensis	Tularemia	Streptomycin	A tetracycline	—
Pasturella multocida	Wound infection (animal bites) Abscesses Bacteremia Meningitis	Penicillin G	A tetracycline [4] A cephalosporin (G1) [3]	—
Vibrio cholerae	Cholera	A tetracycline	Trimethoprim-sulfamethoxazole	Chloramphenicol
Flavobacterium meningosepticum	Meningitis	Erythromycin + rifampin	—	—
Pseudomonas mallei	Glanders	Streptomycin + a tetracycline	Streptomycin + chloramphenicol	—
Pseudomonas pseudomallei	Melioidosis	A tetracycline ± chloramphenicol	Chloramphenicol	Trimethoprim-sulfamethoxazole
Campylobacter jejuni	Enteritis	No treatment or erythromycin	A tetracycline Clindamycin	—
Campylobacter fetus *	Bacteremia	Chloramphenicol [24] Gentamicin	—	—
Bacteroides species (oral, pharyngeal)	Oral disease Sinusitis Brain abscess Lung abscess	Penicillin G [25] Clindamycin [4]	Metronidazole [25] Cefoxitin or moxalactam	Chloramphenicol [25] Erythromycin A tetracycline
Bacteroides fragilis	Brain abscess Lung abscess Intra-abdominal abscess Empyema Bacteremia Endocarditis	Clindamycin [4] Metronidazole [25,26]	Cefoxitin [4] or moxalactam [25]	Chloramphenicol [25] Piperacillin

19 An increasing number of strains are becoming resistant to the first- and second-generation cephalosporins. Many authorities would use a cephalosporin with an aminoglycoside for treatment of pneumonia.
20 Many strains are now resistant to ampicillin or amoxicillin.
21 Cefamandole should not be used for the therapy of *H. influenzae* meningitis.
22 Such combined therapy is useful in severe infections.

23 Data on treatment are sparse, but therapy with trimethoprim-sulfamethoxazole has been successful in some cases.
24 Most strains are sensitive to aminoglycosides, but chloramphenicol is recommended in CNS infections.
25 Preferred antibiotic for CNS infections.
26 Metronidazole is bactericidal against *B. fragilis* and is thus recommended in endocarditis.

Table 48–1. CURRENT USE OF ANTIMICROBIAL AGENTS IN THE THERAPY OF INFECTIONS (Continued)

	DISEASES	DRUG ORDER OF CHOICE		
		1st	*2nd* [1]	*3rd* [1]
IV. GRAM-NEGATIVE BACILLI				
Fusobacterium nucleatum	Ulcerative pharyngitis Lung abscess, empyema Genital infections Gingivitis	Penicillin G Clindamycin	Cefoxitin Metronidazole	Erythromycin A tetracycline Chloramphenicol
Calymmatobacterium granulomatis	Granuloma inguinale	A tetracycline	Streptomycin	—
Streptobacillus moniliformis	Bacteremia Arthritis Endocarditis Abscesses	Penicillin G	Streptomycin A tetracycline	—
Legionella pneumophila	Legionnaires' disease	Erythromycin ± rifampin	—	

	DISEASES	DRUG ORDER OF CHOICE		
		1st	*2nd* [1]	*3rd* [1]
V. ACID-FAST BACILLI				
Mycobacterium tuberculosis [27]	Pulmonary	Isoniazid + rifampin [28]	Isoniazid + ethambutol [28]	Rifampin + ethambutol
	Miliary, renal, meningeal, and other tuberculous infections	Isoniazid + rifampin Isoniazid + rifampin + streptomycin [29] or ethambutol	—	
Mycobacterium leprae	Leprosy	Dapsone + rifampin	Clofazimine	—

	DISEASES	DRUG ORDER OF CHOICE		
		1st	*2nd* [1]	*3rd* [1]
VI. SPIROCHETES				
Treponema pallidum	Syphilis	Penicillin G	A tetracycline	Erythromycin
Treponema pertenue	Yaws	Penicillin G	A tetracycline	—

| | | DRUG ORDER OF CHOICE | | |
		1st	2nd [1]	3rd [1]
Borrelia recurrentis	Relapsing fever	A tetracycline	Penicillin G	—
Leptospira	Weil's disease Meningitis	Penicillin G	A tetracycline [4,30]	—
Lyme's disease agent	Lyme disease	A tetracycline	Penicillin G	—

| VII. ACTINOMYCETES | DISEASES | DRUG ORDER OF CHOICE | | |
		1st	2nd [1]	3rd [1]
Actinomyces israelii	Cervicofacial, abdominal, thoracic, and other lesions	Penicillin G	A tetracycline	A cephalosporin [3] Chloramphenicol
Nocardia *	Pulmonary lesions Brain abscess Lesions of other organs	A sulfonamide ± ampicillin	A sulfonamide ± minocycline Trimethoprim-sulfa-methoxazole [23]	—

| VIII. MISCELLANEOUS AGENTS | DISEASES | DRUG ORDER OF CHOICE | | |
		1st	2nd [1]	3rd [1]
Ureaplasma urealyticum	Nonspecific urethritis	A tetracycline	Erythromycin	—
Mycoplasma pneumoniae	"Atypical pneumonia"	Erythromycin A tetracycline	—	—
Rickettsia	Typhus fever Murine typhus Brill's disease Rocky Mountain spotted fever Q fever Rickettsialpox	Chloramphenicol A tetracycline	—	—

[27] Second- and third-choice drugs are available for the treatment of disease caused by *M. tuberculosis*; their use, which is complex, is discussed in Chapter 53. The choice of drugs for treatment of infections with atypical mycobacteria is also discussed in Chapter 53.
[28] Use isoniazid, ethambutol, and rifampin when primary resistance is likely.

[29] Recommended by many clinicians for more severe forms of tuberculosis, such as meningitis and the disseminated (miliary) disease. Other physicians use only two of these agents, combining isoniazid and rifampin.
[30] Some physicians favor a tetracycline over penicillin G as the drug of first choice.

Table 48–1. CURRENT USE OF ANTIMICROBIAL AGENTS IN THE THERAPY OF INFECTIONS (Continued)

| VIII. MISCELLANEOUS AGENTS | DISEASES | DRUG ORDER OF CHOICE | | |
		1st	2nd [1]	3rd [1]
Chlamydia psittaci	Psittacosis (ornithosis)	A tetracycline	Chloramphenicol	—
	Lymphogranuloma venereum	A tetracycline	Erythromycin / A sulfonamide	Chloramphenicol
Chlamydia trachomatis	Trachoma	A sulfonamide + a tetracycline [31]	Erythromycin / A tetracycline	Chloramphenicol
	Inclusion conjunctivitis (blennorrhea)	Erythromycin	—	—
	Nonspecific urethritis	A tetracycline	Erythromycin	A sulfonamide
Pneumocystis carinii	Pneumonia in impaired host	Trimethoprim-sulfamethoxazole	Pentamidine	—

| IX. FUNGI | DISEASES | DRUG ORDER OF CHOICE | | |
		1st	2nd [1]	3rd [1]
Candida species	Skin and mucocutaneous lesions	Ketoconazole / Nystatin [32] / Clotrimazole [32]	Amphotericin B	—
	Urinary tract infection	Flucytosine [33] / Amphotericin B [34]	—	—
	Disseminated disease	Amphotericin B	—	—
Coccidioides immitis	Pulmonary/pleural disease	No treatment or ketoconazole	Amphotericin B [35]	—
	Bone/joint or chronic pulmonary infection	Amphotericin B	Ketoconazole	—
	Meningeal disease	Amphotericin B [36]	—	—
Cryptococcus neoformans	Nonmeningeal disease	No treatment or amphotericin B ± flucytosine [37]	—	—
	Meningitis	Amphotericin B ± flucytosine [38]	—	—

Histoplasma capsulatum	Pulmonary disease	No treatment or ketoconazole	—
	Disseminated disease	Amphotericin B [36]	Ketoconazole [4]
Aspergillus	Invasive disease	Amphotericin B [36]	—
Mucor	Invasive disease	Amphotericin B [36]	—
Blastomyces dermatitidis	Blastomycosis (North American)	Amphotericin B	Ketoconazole
Sporothrix schenckii	Sporotrichosis	Iodides	Amphotericin B

	DISEASES	1st	DRUG ORDER OF CHOICE 2nd [1]	3rd [1]
X. VIRUSES				
Herpes simplex virus	Genital disease	Acyclovir [39]	—	—
	Keratoconjunctivitis	Vidarabine [40]	Idoxuridine [32]	—
	Encephalitis	Vidarabine [40]	Acyclovir [40]	—
Influenza virus A	Influenza	Amantadine [41] or rimantadine [41]	—	—

[31] A tetracycline may be given orally alone, or it may be applied locally in the conjunctival sac while a sulfonamide is being administered orally.

[32] Topical application.

[33] A significant percentage of strains may be resistant or may become resistant during therapy.

[34] As a bladder irrigant.

[35] Low-dose treatment for patients disposed to dissemination.

[36] Intrathecal and intravenous treatment with amphotericin B may be necessary.

[37] For progressive disease or when there is evidence of dissemination.

[38] The combination appears to give superior therapeutic results.

[35] Topical application or oral treatment. *See* Chapter 54.

[40] Parenteral.

[41] Effective as prophylaxis for Asian A_2 influenza virus. Some authorities recommend amantadine for treatment of established disease; *see* Chapter 54.

sidered. Successful therapy depends upon achieving antibacterial activity at the site of the infection without significant toxicity to the host. To accomplish this, several pharmacokinetic and host factors must be evaluated.

The location of the infection may, to a large extent, dictate the choice of drug and the route of administration. The minimal drug concentration achieved at the infected site should be at least equal to the MIC for the infecting organism, although in most instances it is advisable to achieve multiples (four to eight times) of this concentration if possible. However, there is evidence to suggest that even subinhibitory concentrations of antibiotics may enhance phagocytosis (Yourtee and Root, 1984) and tip the balance in favor of the host. Scanning electron-microscopic studies of bacteria also demonstrate that effects of drugs on bacteria can be detected at much lower concentrations than those required to inhibit growth in broth (Lorian et al., 1977). Although these observations may explain why some infections are cured even when inhibitory concentrations are not achieved, it should be the aim of antimicrobial therapy to produce antibacterial concentrations of drug at the site of infection during the dosing interval. This can only be achieved if the pharmacokinetic and pharmacodynamic principles presented in Chapters 1 and 2 are understood and employed.

Access of antibiotics to sites of infection depends on multiple factors. If the infection is in the cerebrospinal fluid (CSF), the drug must pass the blood-brain barrier, and many antimicrobial agents that are polar at physiological pH do so poorly. For example, the concentrations of penicillins and cephalosporins in the CSF are usually only 1 to 5% of steady-state concentrations determined simultaneously in plasma (Sande et al., 1978). However, the integrity of the blood-brain barrier is diminished during active bacterial infection; tight junctions in cerebral capillaries open, leading to a marked increase in the penetration of polar drugs. As the infection is eradicated and the inflammatory reaction subsides, penetration reverts toward normal. Since this may occur while viable microorganisms persist in the CSF, drug dosage should not be re-

duced as the patient improves until the CSF is presumed or proven to be sterile.

Penetration of drugs into infected loci almost always depends on passive diffusion. The rate of penetration is thus proportional to the concentration of free drug in the plasma or extracellular fluid. Drugs that are extensively bound to protein thus do not penetrate to the same extent as do congeners that are bound to a lesser extent (Craig and Kunin, 1976).

Controversy exists as to whether the therapeutic effect achieved from constant antibacterial activity at the site of infection is superior to that from high peak concentrations followed by periods of subinhibitory activity. Knowledge of the time required for bacteria to begin to divide after the concentration of drug has dropped below the MIC is required, and this varies from drug to drug and microorganism to microorganism. While some studies in animals suggest that pulse dosing (intermittent administration) of beta-lactam antibiotics and aminoglycosides may be more efficient (equivalent efficacy from less drug) (Täuber et al., 1984), others suggest that constant activity may be superior (Keating et al., 1979; Gerber et al., 1983), even though continuous administration of aminoglycosides causes more toxicity. As a practical matter, it seems reasonable to attempt to achieve antibacterial activity at the site of infection for a major portion of the dosage interval.

Knowledge of the status of the individual patient's mechanisms for elimination of drugs is also essential, especially when excessive plasma or tissue concentrations of the drugs cause serious toxicity. Most antimicrobial agents and their metabolites are eliminated primarily by the kidneys. Specific nomograms are available to facilitate adjustment of dosage of many such agents in patients with renal insufficiency. These are discussed in the chapters dealing with the individual drugs and in Appendix II. One must be particularly careful when using the aminoglycosides, the polymyxins, vancomycin, and flucytosine in patients with impaired renal function, since these drugs are completely eliminated by renal mechanisms and their toxicity appears to correlate with their concentrations in plasma and tissue. Furthermore, a vicious cycle may ensue if care is not exercised, since the toxicity of certain of these drugs is particularly manifested on the kidney. Administration of many tetracyclines is also complicated in patients with impaired renal function; elevated concentrations of these drugs in plasma may worsen uremia because of their catabolic effect.

For drugs that are metabolized or excreted by the liver (erythromycin, chloramphenicol, metronidazole, clindamycin), dosages must be reduced in patients with hepatic failure. Rifampin and isoniazid also have prolonged half-lives in patients with cirrhosis. If there is infection in the biliary tract, hepatic disease or biliary obstruction may reduce the access of drug to the site of the infection. This has been shown to occur with ampicillin, nafcillin, and other drugs that are normally excreted into the bile.

Route of Administration. The discussion of choice of routes of administration that appears in Chapter 1 of course applies to antimicrobial agents. While oral administration is preferred whenever possible, parenteral administration of antibiotics is usually recommended in seriously ill patients in whom predictable concentrations of drug must be achieved. Specific factors that govern the choice of route of administration for individual agents are discussed in the chapters that follow.

Host Factors. Innate host factors, which may appear to be completely unrelated to the infectious disorder being treated, are often the prime determinants not only of the type of drug selected but also of its dose, route of administration, risk and nature of untoward effects, and therapeutic effectiveness.

Host Defense Mechanisms. An important determinant of the therapeutic effectiveness of antimicrobial agents is the functional state of the host's defense mechanisms. Both humoral and cellular immunity are important. Inadequacy of type, quality, and quantity of the immunoglobulins, alteration of the cellular immune system, or either a qualitative or, most important, a quantitative defect in phagocytic cells may result in therapeutic failure despite the use of otherwise-appropriate and effective drugs. Frequently, success-

ful treatment of infection with antimicrobial agents may be achieved by merely halting multiplication of the microorganisms. When the defenses of the host are impaired, this action may be inadequate. In infections where host defenses have been shown to be inefficient, rapidly bactericidal antimicrobial agents have been shown to be essential for cure. Examples include bacterial endocarditis, where phagocytic cells are excluded from the infected site; bacterial meningitis, where phagocytic cells are ineffective due to lack of opsonins; and disseminated gram-negative bacillary infections, especially pseudomonal infections in neutropenic patients, where the total mass of phagocytic cells is reduced.

Local Factors. Cure of an infection with antibiotics depends on an understanding of how local factors at the site of infection affect the antimicrobial activity of the drug. Pus, which consists of phagocytes, cellular debris, fibrin, and protein, binds aminoglycosides and vancomycin, resulting in a reduction in their antimicrobial activity (Bryant, 1984). Large accumulations of hemoglobin in infected hematomas can bind penicillins and tetracyclines and may thus reduce their effectiveness (Craig and Kunin, 1976). The pH in abscess cavities and in other confined infected sites (pleural space, CSF, and urine) is usually low, resulting in a marked loss of antimicrobial activity of aminoglycosides, erythromycin, and clindamycin (Strausbaugh and Sande, 1978). However, some drugs, such as chlortetracycline, nitrofurantoin, and methenamine, are more active in such an acidic environment. The anaerobic conditions found in abscess cavities may also impair activity of the aminoglycosides (Verklin and Mandell, 1977). Penetration of antimicrobial agents into infected areas such as abscess cavities is impaired, since the vascular supply is reduced. Successful therapy of abscesses usually requires drainage.

The presence of a foreign body in an infected site markedly reduces the likelihood of effective antimicrobial therapy. This factor has become increasingly important in the present era of prosthetic cardiac valves, prosthetic joints, pacemakers, vascular prostheses, and various vascular and central nervous system (CNS) shunts. The prosthesis is apparently perceived by the phagocytic cells as foreign. In an attempt to phagocytize and destroy it, degranulation occurs, resulting in the depletion of intracellular bactericidal substances. Thus, these phagocytes are relatively inefficient in killing bacterial pathogens; in fact, microbes may even reside within phagocytes, protected from most antimicrobial agents (Zimmerli *et al.*, 1982). Infections associated with foreign bodies are characterized by frequent relapses and failure, even with long-term, high-dose therapy with antibiotics. Successful therapy usually requires removal of the foreign material. Other infectious agents that reside within phagocytic cells (intracellular parasites) may also be relatively resistant to the action of antimicrobial agents, since many of these drugs penetrate into cells only poorly. This may be a problem in infections with *Salmonella, Brucella, Toxoplasma, Listeria,* and *Mycobacterium,* and, in some instances, even in infections caused by *Staph. aureus.* Rifampin is one drug that is very soluble in lipid, penetrates cells well, and can kill many intraleukocytic microbes.

Another interesting twist that may influence the efficacy of antimicrobial therapy is that these agents have been shown to affect various host immune responses adversely; these include leukocyte chemotaxis, lymphocyte and monocyte transformation, antibody production, phagocytosis, and the microbicidal action of polymorphonuclear leukocytes (Mandell, 1982). While the clinical significance of this immunosuppression is not known, these observations should help discourage the indiscriminate use of antibiotics.

Age. The age of the patient is an important determinant of pharmacokinetic properties of antimicrobial agents (*see* Chapter 1). Mechanisms of elimination, especially renal excretion and hepatic biotransformation, are poorly developed in the newborn; this is particularly true of the premature infant. Failure to make adjustments for such differences can have disastrous consequences (*e.g., see* discussion of the "gray baby syndrome," caused by chloramphenicol, in Chapter 52). Elderly patients may also have significantly reduced rates of creatinine clearance and slower rates of drug metabolism. Also, elderly patients are particularly susceptible to the ototoxic effects of aminoglycosides.

Developmental factors may also determine the *type* of untoward response to a drug. Tetracyclines bind avidly to developing teeth and bones, and their use in young children can result in discoloration or hypoplasia of tooth enamel. Kernicterus may follow the use of sulfonamides in newborn infants because this class of drugs competes effectively with bilirubin for binding sites on plasma albumin. Achlorhydria in young children and in the elderly (or antacid therapy) may alter absorption of orally administered antimicrobial agents (*e.g.,* increased absorption of penicillin G and decreased absorption of ketoconazole).

Genetic Factors. Certain genetic or metabolic abnormalities must be considered when prescribing antibiotics. A number of drugs, including the sulfonamides, nitrofurantoin, and chloramphenicol, may produce acute hemolysis in patients with glucose-6-phosphate dehydrogenase deficiency; more common in black males, the defect is also occasionally found in Caucasians. Patients who acetylate isoniazid rapidly may have suboptimal concentrations of the drug in plasma and an increased risk of hepatotoxicity (Mitchell *et al.,* 1976).

Pregnancy. Pregnancy imposes an increased risk of reaction to some antimicrobial agents for both mother and fetus. For example, hearing loss in the child has been associated with administration of streptomycin to the mother during pregnancy. Tetracyclines can also be particularly toxic to the pregnant female. Pregnant women receiving these drugs may develop fatal acute fatty necrosis of the liver, pancreatitis, and associated renal damage.

Pregnancy also affects the pharmacokinetics of various antibiotics. Plasma concentrations of ampicillin and probably those of other penicillins are lower in pregnant than in nonpregnant females (Philipson, 1977). This phenomenon is likely related to a greater volume of distribution and more rapid clearance of the drug during pregnancy.

The lactating female can pass antimicrobial agents to her nursing child. Both nalidixic acid and sulfonamides in breast milk have been associated with hemolysis in children with glucose-6-phosphate dehydrogenase deficiency. In addition, sulfonamides, even in the small amounts received from breast milk, may predispose the nursing child to kernicterus (Vorherr, 1974).

Drug Allergy. Antibiotics, especially the betalactam derivatives and their degradation products, are notorious for provoking allergic reactions in man. Patients with a history of atopic allergy seem particularly susceptible to the development of these reactions. The sulfonamides, trimethoprim, nitrofurantoin, and erythromycin have particularly been associated with hypersensitivity reactions, especially rash (Arndt and Jick, 1976). Certain viral infections, especially that caused by the Epstein-Barr virus (mononucleosis), dramatically increase the frequency of rash in response to ampicillin and amoxicillin, but this does not imply true allergy to these drugs. When use of a penicillin is contemplated, a history of anaphylaxis (immediate reaction) or hives and laryngeal edema (accelerated reaction) precludes the use of the drug in all but extreme life-threatening situations. Skin testing, particularly of the penicillins, has some value in predicting the life-threatening reactions. However, the controversy over the utility of such tests is only partly resolved (*see* Chapter 50). It should also be noted that antimicrobial agents and other drugs can cause "drug fever," which can be mistaken for a sign of continued infection.

Disorders of the Nervous System. Patients with diseases of the nervous system that predispose to seizures are prone to develop localized or major motor seizures while taking high doses of penicillin G. Neurotoxicity of penicillin and other beta-lactam antibiotics correlates with high concentrations of drug in the CSF and usually occurs in patients with renal insufficiency. Decreased renal function increases concentrations of penicillin in CSF by two mechanisms: reduction of renal elimination of penicillin from plasma, which results in a higher concentration gradient for passive diffusion into CSF; and accumulation of organic acids (in the uremic state), which competitively inhibit the transport mechanism in the choroid plexus that removes penicillin and other organic acids from the CSF. Patients with myasthenia gravis or other neuromuscular problems appear to be particularly susceptible to the neuromuscular blocking effect of the aminoglycosides, polymyxins, and colistin. Patients undergoing general anesthesia who receive a neuromuscular blocking agent are also particularly liable to such antibiotic toxicity.

THERAPY WITH COMBINED ANTIMICROBIAL AGENTS

The simultaneous use of two or more antimicrobial agents has a certain rationale and is recommended in *specifically defined situations* (Table 48–1). However, selection of an appropriate combination requires an understanding of the potential for interaction between the antimicrobial agents. Such interactions may have consequences for *both* the microorganism and the host. Since the various classes of antimicrobial agents exert different actions on the microorganism, one drug has the potential to either *enhance or inhibit* the effect of the second. Similarly, combinations of drugs that might rationally be used to cure infections may have additive or supra-additive toxicities. For example, vancomycin when given alone has minimal nephrotoxicity, as does tobramycin; however, when the drugs are given in combination they cause marked impairment of renal function (Farber and Moellering, 1983).

Methods of Testing Antimicrobial Activity of Drug Combinations. To predict the potential therapeutic efficacy of combinations of antibiotics, methods have been developed to quantitate their effects on bacterial growth *in vitro*. Two distinctly different methods are used. The first employs serial twofold dilutions of antibiotics in broth inoculated with a standard inoculum of the test microorganism in a checkerboard fashion, so that a large number of antibiotic concentrations in different proportions can be tested simultaneously (Figure 48–1). Inhibition of bacterial growth is quantified after 18 hours of incubation. This test determines whether the MIC of one drug is reduced, unchanged, or increased in the presence of another drug. Synergism is defined as inhibition of growth with a combination of drugs when their concentrations are less than or equal to 25% of the MIC of each drug acting alone. This implies that one drug is affecting the microorganism in such a way that it becomes more sensitive to the inhibitory effect of the other. If one half of the inhibitory concentration of each drug is required to produce inhibition, the result is called additive (FIC index = 1), suggesting that the two

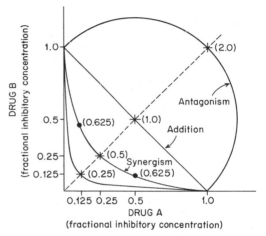

Figure 48–1. *Effect of combinations of two antimicrobial agents to inhibit bacterial growth.*

The effects are expressed as isobols and fractional inhibitory concentration (FIC) indices. The FIC index is equal to the sum of the values of FIC for the individual drugs:

$$\text{FIC index} = \frac{\text{MIC of A with B}}{\text{MIC of A alone}} + \frac{\text{MIC of B with A}}{\text{MIC of B alone}}$$

Points on concave isobols (FIC index < 1) are indicative of synergistic interaction between the two agents, and points on convex isobols (FIC index > 1) represent antagonism. The nature of the interaction is adequately revealed by testing combinations lying along the dotted line (marked +). *See* text for further explanation.

drugs are working independently of each other. If more than one half of the MIC of each drug is necessary to produce the inhibitory effect, the drugs are said to be antagonistic (FIC index >1). When the drugs are tested for a variety of proportionate drug concentrations, such as with the checkerboard technic, an isobologram may be constructed (Figure 48–1). Synergism is shown by a concave curve, the additive effect by a straight line, and antagonism by a convex curve.

The second method for evaluation of drug combinations involves quantitation of their *rate* of bactericidal action. Identical cultures are incubated simultaneously with antibiotics added singly or in combination. If a combination of antibiotics is more rapidly bactericidal than either drug alone, the result is termed *synergism*. Moellering (1985) has recommended that the minimal criterion for synergism should be the observation of a 100-fold additional decrease in the number of microorganisms counted at any one time. If the bactericidal rate of the combination is less than that for either drug alone, *antagonism* is said to occur. If the bactericidal rate is as rapid as that for the more bactericidal drug, the result is called *indifference*. Comparative evaluation of these two distinctly different laboratory technics has, in general, demonstrated a good correlation between the results (Rahal, 1978).

There have been various attempts to predict synergism and antagonism from a knowledge of the action of the two drugs involved. A simple scheme, devised by Jawetz and Gunnison (1952), is still useful. They observed that bacteriostatic antibiotics frequently antagonize the action of a bactericidal drug and that two bactericidal drugs may exhibit synergism. In 1957, Dowling suggested that bactericidal drugs are neither synergistic nor antagonistic to each other, but that additive effects are sometimes observed. Although there are exceptions to this rule, the general principle remains sound. An up-to-date grouping of these bactericidal and bacteriostatic drugs was proposed by Rahal (1978), as follows. Group-1 drugs, which are primarily bactericidal, include the penicillins, cephalosporins, aminoglycosides, and vancomycin. Group-2 agents, which are primarily bacteriostatic, include the tetracyclines, clindamycin, chloramphenicol, and erythromycin. There is frequent antagonism between the drugs of group 1 and those in group 2 because most of the bactericidal agents require active cell division or protein synthesis for expression of their bactericidal activity, and many of the bacteriostatic drugs in group 2 inhibit these processes. However, drugs within group 1 may exhibit synergism by combination of their bactericidal actions. For example, Moellering and colleagues (1971) have demonstrated that the uptake of streptomycin into *Strep. faecalis* is increased markedly following exposure of the organism to penicillin G. It is suggested that the action of penicillin on the cell wall of the bacterium accelerates the uptake of the aminoglycoside, thereby allowing higher concentrations of the latter drug to reach the ribosome. The efficacy of the combination of trimethoprim and sulfamethoxazole is relatively unique, in that synergism results from sequential inhibition of two steps in the pathway of biosynthesis of tetrahydrofolate (*see* Chapter 49).

Indications for the Clinical Use of Combinations of Antimicrobial Agents. Numerous reasons have been given to justify the use of combinations of antimicrobial agents. These will be considered individually.

1. *Treatment of Mixed Bacterial Infections.* Some infections are caused by two or more microorganisms. These include intra-abdominal, hepatic, and brain abscesses and many of the genital tract infections. In such situations it may be necessary to administer different antibiotics with different antimicrobial spectra to obtain the necessary breadth of activity.

Following perforation of a viscus such as the colon, one can expect contamination and, frequently, infection with aerobic Enterobacteriaceae, anaerobic and aerobic gram-positive cocci (streptococci), anaerobic bacilli such as *Bacteroides fragilis*, and anaerobic gram-positive rods such as *Clostridium* species. While a single drug may be ineffective against this mixed infection, a rational combination would be an aminoglycoside for the Enterobacteriaceae, and either clindamycin or metronidazole for the anaerobic microorganisms, including *B. fragilis*. Such combinations may be less necessary if some of the newer, broad-spectrum beta-lactam antibiotics are utilized, although gaps in coverage still exist (Drusano et al., 1982); the efficacy of this therapy awaits clinical confirmation. In most intra-abdominal infections, therapy with antibiotics alone is rarely successful unless there is adequate drainage of pus. The importance of combined therapy has been demonstrated in an animal model of intraperitoneal infection produced by artificial contamination with stool (Joiner et al., 1982). Animals not treated with antimicrobial agents rapidly expired with sepsis due to *E. coli*. Those receiving gentamicin alone were protected from the septic complications of the Enterobacteriaceae, but abscesses containing *B. fragilis* developed in the majority of cases. Treatment with clindamycin alone prevented abscess formation, but animals were again killed by the *E. coli*. When both drugs were used in combination, the majority of animals survived without formation of abscesses. While such studies lend support to the use of combination therapy in mixed microbial infections, not all such infections need to be treated with multiple drugs. For example, cellulitis due to the combination of *Staph. aureus* and group-A streptococci can be treated with a penicillinase-resistant penicillin alone. A drug of this type has antimicrobial activity against both microorganisms. Once results of cultures of aspirated material are known, the minimal number of drugs that will be effective should be used.

2. *Therapy of Severe Infections in Which a Specific Etiology Is Unknown.* Combination chemotherapy is probably most frequently used in the treatment of infections in which the etiological agent has not been or cannot be identified. In these situations, the goal of treatment is to select antibiotic "coverage" for microorganisms that are most likely involved. This selection of antimicrobials must be based on the physician's clinical judgment, which reflects a knowledge of the signs and symptoms of the various infectious diseases and of the microbiology of these diseases and an understanding of the antibiotic spectrum of available drugs. The breadth of the antibiotic blanket that is used is inversely related to one's ability to narrow the list of potential infectious agents.

For example, when a patient has classical signs and symptoms of septic shock with associated upper urinary tract infection, the physician can be relatively certain that the systemic manifestations result from endotoxin released by the gram-negative bacilli disseminated from the kidney. If the patient has not received antibiotics in the immediate past or has not suffered from recurrent urinary tract infections, the agent is most likely *E. coli*. In some geographical locations, ampicillin or amoxicillin would be expected to provide adequate initial coverage. In other areas, resistant strains are common and therapy with an aminoglycoside may be indicated. If the patient had suffered from prior urinary tract infection or had structural abnormalities of the urinary tract, an aminoglycoside plus ampicillin would constitute rational initial coverage. Broadened initial coverage is commonly employed in the severely ill where the penalty for "missing" the microorganism is high. In 24 to 48 hours, the initially obtained cultures of the urine and probably of the blood will likely contain the infecting microorganism, and, once sensitivity tests are available, the coverage can be tailored to treat the infection more specifically.

While the above approach to the severely ill patient can be justified, it is not to be used as a shortcut for a thoughtful analysis of available clinical and laboratory data to facilitate selection of a specific antimicrobial agent. Prolonged administration of broad-spectrum antibiotics may lead to overuse of toxic and expensive drugs. This problem most often arises when the physician fails to obtain adequate cultures *prior* to the initiation of therapy or fails to discontinue the combination chemotherapy *after*

identifying the microorganism and determining sensitivities. There is an understandable reluctance to change antimicrobial agents when a favorable clinical response has occurred. However, the goal of chemotherapy should always be to use the most selectively active drug that produces the fewest adverse effects.

3. *Enhancement of Antibacterial Activity in the Treatment of Specific Infections.* As mentioned above, when two antimicrobial agents are administered together, they may produce a synergistic effect. This may permit a reduction in the dosage of one or both drugs with achievement of a similar therapeutic effect. Alternatively, the combination may produce a more rapid or complete bactericidal effect than could be achieved with either drug alone. There are specific clinical indications for the use of combinations of antimicrobial agents, and they are based on documented proof of efficacy (Sande and Scheld, 1980).

Perhaps the best-documented need for a synergistic combination of antimicrobial agents is in the treatment of enterococcal endocarditis. *In vitro,* a combination of penicillin and streptomycin or gentamicin is bactericidal, while penicillin alone is bacteriostatic against most strains of *Strep. faecalis* (enterococci). Treatment of enterococcal endocarditis with penicillin alone frequently results in relapses, while combination therapy is curative at rates that are comparable to those achieved with endocarditis caused by streptococci that are more sensitive to penicillin (Mandell *et al.*, 1970; Wilson *et al.*, 1984b). This is a clear-cut case where combination therapy produces superior clinical results. Antibiotic therapy of endocarditis caused by strains of penicillin-sensitive *viridans* streptococci may also be improved and the duration of treatment shortened when two drugs are used. Penicillin and streptomycin are synergistic *in vitro* against the vast majority of these strains. In animal models of endocarditis, this combination produces more rapid eradication of bacteria from infected vegetations on heart valves than does penicillin G alone. Wilson and associates (1978) reported a 100% cure rate of patients with this condition who received a short course (2 weeks) of combination chemotherapy; those who advocate treatment with penicillin G alone recommend treatment for 4 weeks (Bisno *et al.*, 1981).

Synergism *in vitro* by a combination of a penicillin and an aminoglycoside has also been demonstrated with *Staph. aureus*. Eradication of the microorganism from infected vegetations was found to be more rapid in an animal model of staphylococcal endocarditis treated with this combination. While these studies demonstrated a more rapid clinical and bacteriological response, there was no change in mortality with the combination (Korzeniowski *et al.*, 1982).

Synergistic antibiotic combinations have been recommended in the therapy of infections with *Pseudomonas* in neutropenic patients. *In vitro*, antipseudomonal penicillins plus an aminoglycoside are synergistic against most strains of *Pseud. aeruginosa.* Studies in animals support the superiority of the combination over either drug alone, and clinical studies suggest improved survival with the combination. Despite the fact that the microorganism is sensitive to gentamicin *in vitro*, administration of gentamicin alone frequently does not cure the infection and may even allow sustained bacteremia. The addition of carbenicillin markedly increases the cure rate, a phenomenon that correlates with a more rapid bactericidal effect *in vitro*. This success may be a reflection of the importance of the use of antibiotics that produce bactericidal effects rapidly when infection occurs in the neutropenic patient (Klastersky and Staquet, 1982).

Sulfonamides combined with trimethoprim are synergistic *in vitro* and are effective against infections caused by microorganisms that may be resistant to sulfonamides alone. A fixed combination of trimethoprim and sulfamethoxazole is available for clinical use and has emerged as an effective treatment of recurrent urinary tract infections, *Pneumocystis carinii* pneumonia, typhoid fever, shigellosis, and certain infections due to ampicillin-resistant *H. influenzae.*

There is considerable interest in the application of a new concept in combination chemotherapy—the use of an inhibitor of beta-lactamase, which has no intrinsic antimicrobial activity, in combination with a beta-lactam antibiotic that is susceptible to beta-lactamase. The prototypical enzyme inhibitor is clavulanic acid; other derivatives are currently being evaluated. This approach may allow successful treatment of infections by microorganisms that produce beta-lactamase. For example, infections caused by beta-lactamase-producing *H. influenzae* may be treatable with ampicillin plus the beta-lactamase inhibitor. Thus, the utility of time-tested antibiotics (*e.g.*, penicillin G and ampicillin) may be restored in infections for which they had become ineffective.

Advances have also been made by combination of synergistic agents in the antimicrobial therapy of fungal infections. The most significant clinical advance to date is in the therapy of cryptococcal meningitis. A combination of flucytosine and amphotericin B has been shown to be synergistic *in vitro* and in animal models of infection. In the therapy of cryptococcal meningitis a combination of flucytosine and a low dose of amphotericin B for 6 weeks was as effective as therapy with a higher dose of amphotericin B for 10 weeks with less renal toxicity (Bennett *et al.*, 1979).

4. *Prevention of the Emergence of Resistant Microorganisms.* The use of combinations of antimicrobial agents was first proposed as a method to prevent the emergence of resistant mutants during therapy. If spontaneous mutation were the predominant means by which microorganisms acquired resistance to antibiotics, combination chemotherapy would, in theory, be an effective means of prevention. For example, if the frequency of mutation for the acquisition of resistance to one drug is 10^{-7} and that for a second drug 10^{-6}, the probability of independent mutation to resistance to both drugs in a single cell is the product of the two frequencies, 10^{-13}. This makes the emergence of such mutant resistant strains statistically unlikely. In practice, however, this method has received extensive use only in the treatment of tuberculosis, where the concomitant use of two or more appropriate agents strikingly reduces the development of drug resistance by the tubercle bacillus.

Disadvantages of Combinations of Antimicrobial Agents. It is important that physicians understand the potential negative results of the use of combinations of antimicrobial agents. The most obvious are the risk of toxicity from two or more agents, the selection of microorganisms that are resistant to antibiotics that may not have been necessary, and increased cost to the patient. In addition, as noted above, antagonism of antibacterial effect may result when bacteriostatic and bactericidal agents are given concurrently. The clinical significance of antibiotic antagonism is not fully understood. Although antagonism of one antibiotic by another has been a frequent observation *in vitro*, well-documented clinical examples are relatively rare. The most notable of these involves the therapy of pneumococcal meningitis.

In 1951, Lepper and Dowling reported that the fatality rate among patients with pneumococcal meningitis who were treated with penicillin alone was 21%, while those patients who received the combination of penicillin and chlortetracycline had a fatality rate of 79%. This study was supported by Mathies and colleagues (1967), who treated children with bacterial meningitis of multiple etiologies with either ampicillin alone or with the combination of ampicillin, chloramphenicol, and streptomycin. The mortality rate among those treated with ampicillin was 4.3%, while those treated with the combination was significantly greater—10.5%.

Antagonism between antibiotics is probably relatively unimportant in *most* infections. If an antagonistic interaction between two antibiotics is to occur, both agents must be active against the infecting microorganism. The addition of a bacteriostatic to a bactericidal drug frequently results in only a bacteriostatic effect. In many infections where host defenses are adequate, this may still be sufficient to tip the balance in favor of the host. Where host defenses are impaired, as in patients with neutropenia, or with special infections, such as endocarditis and meningitis, the bactericidal effect may become more important. Certain studies in experimental animals and in the clinic support this contention. In animals with *Proteus mirabilis* peritonitis, gentamicin alone and a combination of gentamicin and chloramphenicol are equally effective in preventing death. However, if the animals are first irradiated and rendered neutropenic, the antagonistic combination of gentamicin and chloramphenicol is much less effective than gentamicin alone in preventing death (Sande and Overton, 1973). In clinical trials in man, the more rapidly bactericidal combinations of antibiotics have in general been more effective than less rapidly bactericidal or purely bacteriostatic drugs in the therapy of gram-negative infections in neutropenic patients.

THE PROPHYLAXIS OF INFECTION WITH ANTIBIOTICS

A large percentage (from 30 to 50%) of antibiotics administered in the United States are given to *prevent* infection rather than to treat established disease. This practice accounts for some of the most flagrant misuses of these drugs.

Clinical studies have demonstrated that there are some situations in which chemoprophylaxis is highly effective and others in which it is totally without value and may in fact be deleterious. There are still numerous situations where the attempt to use antimicrobial compounds to prevent bacterial infections is controversial. *In general, if a single effective drug is used to prevent infection by a specific microorganism or to eradicate infection immediately or soon after it has become established, then chemoprophylaxis is frequently successful. On the other hand, if the aim of prophylaxis is to prevent colonization or infection by any or all microorganisms present in the environment of a patient, then prophylaxis usually fails.*

Chemoprophylaxis has been employed primarily for three purposes. (1) Prophylaxis may be utilized to protect healthy persons from acquisition of or invasion by specific microorganisms to which they are exposed. Successful examples of this practice include the following: the use of penicillin G to prevent infection by group-A streptococci; prevention of gonorrhea or syphilis after contact; the intermittent use of trimethoprim-sulfamethoxazole to prevent recurrent urinary tract infections usually caused by *E. coli;* the use of rifampin, minocycline, or sulfadiazine to prevent meningococcal disease. (2) Attempts are often made to prevent secondary bacterial infection in patients who are ill with other diseases. Examples of this form of prophylaxis have been efforts to prevent bacterial infection in patients with measles or in those in coma. Likewise, antibiotics are given to prevent infection in patients on respirators. *This form of "total" chemoprophylaxis is usually unsuccessful.* Resistant microorganisms, especially Enterobacteriaceae and fungi, emerge as pathogens and increase in frequency as prophylaxis is prolonged. Although certain centers have reported a decrease in the incidence of bacterial infections in neutropenic patients given trimethoprim-sulfamethoxazole, increased numbers of fungal infections were noted in some series. The normal microbial flora of the host represents an important defense in the prevention of colonization and infection with these pathogens (Sanders and Sanders, 1984). "Shotgun" chemoprophylaxis disrupts this barrier and may be self-defeating. Elaborate technics involving sterile food, life islands, and nonabsorbable antibiotics have shown modest success in decreasing infections in neutropenic patients with hematological malignancies. (3) Chemoprophylaxis *should* be performed to prevent endocarditis in patients with valvular or other structural lesions of the heart who are undergoing dental, surgical, or other procedures that produce a high incidence of bacteremia. Endocarditis results from the bacterial colonization of the cardiac endothelium, particularly that of cardiac valves. The area of colonization is probably a deposit of fibrin and platelets on a damaged valve associated with areas of turbulent blood flow. The prophylactic use of antibiotics is therefore recommended in patients who have cardiac lesions, such as those produced by rheumatic or congenital heart disease that produce turbulence in blood flow. Any procedure that injures a mucous membrane where there are large numbers of bacteria (such as in the oropharyngeal or gastrointestinal tract) will produce transient bacteremia. Streptococci from the mouth, enterococci from the gastrointestinal or genitourinary tract, and staphylococci from the skin have a propensity to produce endocarditis, and chemoprophylaxis directed against these microorganisms is recommended (Medical Letter, 1984). Therapy should not begin until immediately before the procedure, since prolonged administration of antibiotics can lead to colonization by resistant strains. Criteria have been established for the selection of specific drugs and patients who should receive chemoprophylaxis for various procedures (*see* Chapter 50).

Chemoprophylaxis to prevent wound infections after various surgical procedures has created considerable controversy. There are several well-controlled clinical studies that support the use of prophylactic antimicrobial agents in certain surgical procedures. The first such demonstration was by Bernard and Cole (1964), who showed the effectiveness of prophylactic antibiotics in patients undergoing operations involving the stomach, pancreas, and bowel. Wound infection results when a critical number of bacteria are present in the wound at the time of closure. Several factors determine the size of this critical inoculum, and these include the virulence of the bacteria, the presence of devitalized or poorly vascularized tissue, the presence of a foreign body, and the status of the host. Antimicrobial agents directed against the invading microorganisms may reduce the number of viable bacteria below the critical level and thus prevent infection.

Several factors are important to the effective and judicious use of antibiotics in this situation (Sandusky, 1979). First, antimicrobial activity must be present at the wound site at the time of its closure. This has led to the recommendation that the drug be given immediately preoperatively and, perhaps, intraoperatively. Second, the antibiotic must be active against the most likely contaminating microorganisms. This has prompted the wide use of first-generation cephalosporins in this form of chemo-

prophylaxis. Third, there is mounting evidence that the continued use of drugs after the surgical procedure is *unwarranted*. There are no data to suggest that the incidence of wound infections is lower if antimicrobial treatment is continued after the day of surgery (Rowlands *et al.*, 1982). Prolongation of use beyond 24 to 72 hours does, however, lead to the development of a more resistant flora and of wound infections caused by antibiotic-resistant strains. The risk of toxicity and unnecessary expense are, of course, additional disadvantages. In practice, however, this guideline is frequently broken. In a survey of the usage of antibiotics in Pennsylvania, where one third of all antimicrobial agents used were given for chemoprophylaxis, the median duration of such use was 7 days.

Chemoprophylaxis should be used only in selected operative procedures. A number of studies indicate that it can be justified in dirty and contaminated surgical procedures (*e.g.*, resection of the colon), where the incidence of wound infections is high. These include less than 10% of all operations. In clean surgical procedures, which account for approximately 75% of the total, the expected incidence of wound infection is less than 5%, and antibiotics should not be used routinely. Exceptions are rational when the surgical procedure involves insertion of a prosthetic implant. Although clear-cut data are not available to support the use of antibiotics during placement of prosthetic cardiac valves or artificial orthopedic devices, the complications of infection are so drastic that most authorities currently agree with this indication. Of course, the use of systemic antibiotics for chemoprophylaxis during surgical procedures does not reduce the need for clean and skilled surgical technic.

SUPERINFECTIONS CAUSED BY
ANTIMICROBIAL AGENTS

The untoward reactions produced by anti-infective agents include toxic effects and hypersensitivity reactions. These are discussed for individual agents in the chapters that follow. Antibiotics also cause unique reactions that result from alterations in the microbial flora of the host.

All individuals who receive therapeutic doses of these agents undergo alterations in the normal microbial population of the intestinal, upper respiratory, and genitourinary tracts; some develop *superinfection* as a result of such changes. This phenomenon may be defined as the appearance of bacteriological and clinical evidence of a new infection during the chemotherapy of a primary one. It is relatively common and potentially very dangerous because the microorganisms responsible for the new infection are, in many cases, Enterobacteriaceae, *Pseudomonas,* and *Candida* or other fungi; these may be very difficult to eradicate with the presently available anti-infective drugs. Superinfection by these microorganisms is due to removal of the inhibitory influence of the flora that normally inhabits the oropharynx and other body orifices. Many members of the normal flora appear to produce antibacterial substances (bacteriocins), and they also presumably compete for essential nutrients. The more "broad" the effect of an antibiotic on microorganisms, the greater is the alteration in the normal microflora and the greater is the possibility that a single microorganism will become predominant, invade the host, and produce infection. Thus, the incidence of superinfection is lowest with penicillin G, higher with tetracyclines and chloramphenicol, and highest with combinations of broad-spectrum antimicrobials and the expanded-spectrum third-generation cephalosporins. A high incidence of serious superinfections caused by enterococci has been observed in patients receiving moxalactam (Wilson *et al.,* 1984a). It can be expected that further production of agents with increased breadth of antimicrobial activity will lead to more extensive alterations in the normal flora and, thus, more superinfections. The development of agents that kill pathogens selectively while carefully preserving the normal flora would be beneficial. The most specific antimicrobial agent to treat a given infection should be chosen whenever possible. The incidence of superinfection also increases when administration of antibiotics is prolonged.

The fact that harmful effects may follow the therapeutic or the prophylactic use of anti-infective agents must never discourage the physician from their administration in any situation in which they are definitely indicated. It should, however, make the physician very careful in their use when they are required, and very hesitant to employ them in instances in which indications for their application are either entirely lacking or, at most, only suggestive. To do otherwise is to run the risk, at times, of converting a simple, benign, and self-limited disease into one that may be serious or even fatal.

MISUSES OF ANTIBIOTICS

The purpose of this introductory chapter has been to lay the groundwork for the maximally effective utilization of antimicrobial drugs. Unfortunately, in reality, these agents are frequently misused and overused (*see* Symposium, 1978).

Treatment of Untreatable Infections. A common misuse of these agents is in infections that have been proved by experimental and clinical observation to be untreatable. The vast majority of the diseases due to the true viruses will not respond to any of the presently available anti-infective compounds. Thus, the antimicrobial therapy of measles, chickenpox, mumps, and at least 90% of infections of the upper respiratory tract is totally ineffective and, therefore, worse than useless.

Therapy of Fever of Undetermined Origin. Fever of undetermined etiology may be of two types: one that is present for only a few days to a week and another that persists for an extended period. Both of these are frequently treated with antimicrobial agents. Most instances of pyrexia of short duration, in the absence of localizing signs, are probably associated with undefined viral infections, often of the upper respiratory tract, and do not respond to antibiotics. In the bulk of these cases, defervescence takes place spontaneously within a week or less. Studies of prolonged fever have shown that three common infectious causes are tuberculosis, often of the disseminated variety, hidden pyogenic intra-abdominal abscess, and infectious endocarditis. Also, the so-called collagen disorders and various neoplasms, especially lymphoma (often undetectable because it is situated intra-abdominally), are frequently responsible for prolonged and significant degrees of fever. Various types of cancer, metabolic disorders, hepatitis, asymptomatic regional enteritis, atypical rheumatoid arthritis, and a number of other noninfectious disorders may present themselves as cases of fever of unknown etiology (Larson *et al.*, 1982).

It must be stressed that the anti-infective agents are not antipyretics. The most rational approach to the problem of fever of unknown etiology is not one that concentrates on the elevated temperature alone but one that involves a thorough search for its cause. The patient should not be unnecessarily exposed to chemotherapy in the hope, often in vain, that, if one agent is not effective, another one or a combination of drugs will be helpful.

Improper Dosage. Erroneous dosage of antimicrobial agents is of two types: administration of excessive amounts and use of suboptimal quantities. There is little doubt that harm may be produced by overdoses of most antimicrobial agents. The difficulties that may arise from drug overdosage in patients with impairment of drug elimination have already been discussed. It is, however, critical that adequate dosage be given to achieve the desired effects. Drugs such as aminoglycosides are frequently administered in insufficient quantities, probably because of fear of toxicity; the potential for clinical failures is thus increased (Lesar *et al.*, 1982).

Reliance on Chemotherapy with Omission of Surgical Drainage. To rely on anti-infective agents alone to cure some types of infections is to place a demand on them that they cannot always satisfy. The conditions in which this is a problem are usually those with appreciable quantities of purulent exudate or necrotic or avascular infected tissues. Two of many possible examples will be cited. The patient with pneumonia and empyema often fails to be cured by the administration of large doses of an effective drug until drainage of the involved area is established. The patient with renal lithiasis will frequently suffer recurrent episodes of acute pyelonephritis, regardless of the number of times he is treated with antimicrobial agents, until the stones are removed. As a generalization, it may be said that, when an appreciable quantity of pus, or necrotic tissue, or a foreign body is a problem, the most effective treatment is a combination of an antimicrobial agent given in adequate dose plus a properly performed surgical procedure.

Lack of Adequate Bacteriological Information. One half of the courses of antimicrobial therapy administered to hospitalized patients appear to be given in the absence of support from the microbiological laboratory. It is clear that the great bulk of the use of these drugs in hospitals is based on clinical judgment alone. A high proportion of the use is for chemoprophylaxis of questionable value. Bacterial cultures and gram stains of infected material are obtained too infrequently, and the results, when available, are often disregarded in the selection and application of drug therapy. Frequent use of drug combinations is a cover for diagnostic imprecision. The agents selected are more likely to be those of habit rather than for specific indications, and the dosages employed are routine. Antimicrobial drug therapy must be individualized on the basis of the clinical situation, microbiological information, and the pharmacological considerations presented in this chapter and the subsequent chapters of this section. (For discussions of patterns of antibiotic administration by physicians, *see* Symposium, 1978.)

Arndt, K. A., and Jick, H. Rates of cutaneous reactions to drugs. *J.A.M.A.*, **1976**, *235*, 918–922.

Bauer, A. W.; Kirby, W. M. M.; Sherris, J. C.; and Turck, M. Antibiotic susceptibility testing by a standardized single disc method. *Am. J. Clin. Pathol.*, **1966**, *45*, 493–496.

Bennett, J. E., and others. Amphotericin B–flucytosine in cryptococcal meningitis. *N. Engl. J. Med.*, **1979**, *301*, 126–131.

Bernard, H. R., and Cole, W. R. The prophylaxis of surgical infections: the effect of prophylactic antimicrobial drugs on the incidence of infection following potentially contaminated operations. *Surgery*, **1964**, *56*, 151–157.

Bisno, A. L.; Dismukes, W. E.; Durack, D. T.; Kaplan, E. L.; Karchmer, A. W.; Kaye, D.; Sande, M. A.; Sanford, J. P.; and Wilson, W. R. Treatment of infective endocarditis due to *viridans* streptococci. *Circulation*, **1981**, *63*, 730A–733A.

Bryant, R. E. Effect of the suppurative environment on

antibiotic activity. In, *New Dimensions in Antimicrobial Therapy.* (Root, R. K., and Sande, M. A., eds.) Churchill Livingstone, Inc., New York, **1984**, pp. 313–337.

Bulger, R. J., and Sherris, J. C. Decreased incidence of antibiotic resistance among *S. aureus. Ann. Intern. Med.*, **1968**, *69*, 1099–1108.

Coleman, D. L.; Horwitz, R. I.; and Andriole, V. T. Association between serum inhibitory and bactericidal concentrations and therapeutic outcome in bacterial endocarditis. *Am. J. Med.*, **1982**, *73*, 260–267.

Datta, N., and Nugent, M. E. Bacterial variation. In, *Topley and Wilson's Principles of Bacteriology, Virology, and Immunity*, 7th ed., Vol. 1. (Wilson, G. S., and Dick, H. M., eds.) The Williams & Wilkins Co., Baltimore, **1984**, pp. 145–176.

Davies, J.; Brzezinska, M.; and Benveniste, R. R factors: biochemical mechanisms of resistance to aminoglycoside antibiotics. *Ann. N.Y. Acad. Sci.*, **1971**, *182*, 226–233.

Dickie, P.; Bryan, L. E.; and Pichard, M. A. Effect of enzymatic adenylation on dihydrostreptomycin accumulation in *Escherichia coli* carrying an R-factor: model explaining aminoglycoside resistance by inactivating mechanisms. *Antimicrob. Agents Chemother.*, **1978**, *14*, 569–580.

Drusano, G. L.; Warren, J. W.; Saah, A. J.; Caplan, E. S.; Tenney, J. H.; Hansen, S.; Granados, J.; Standiford, H. C.; and Miller, E. H., Jr. A prospective randomized controlled trial of cefoxitin versus clindamycin-aminoglycoside in mixed anaerobic-aerobic infections. *Surg. Gynecol. Obstet.*, **1982**, *154*, 715–720.

Farber, B., and Moellering, R. C., Jr. Retrospective study of the toxicity of preparations of vancomycin from 1974–1981. *Antimicrob. Agents Chemother.*, **1983**, *23*, 138–141.

Gerber, A. U.; Craig, W. A.; Brugger, H.-P.; Feller, C.; Vastola, A. P.; and Brandel, J. Impact of dosing intervals on activity of gentamicin and ticarcillin against *Pseudomonas aeruginosa* in granulocytopenic mice. *J. Infect. Dis.*, **1983**, *147*, 910–917.

Handsfield, H. H.; Wiesner, P. J.; and Holmes, K. K. Therapy of the gonococcal arthritis-dermatitis syndrome. *Ann. Intern. Med.*, **1976**, *84*, 661–667.

Jacobs, M. R.; Koornhof, H. J.; Robins-Browne, R. M.; Stevenson, C. M.; Vermaak, Z. A.; Freiman, I.; Miller, G. B.; Witcomb, M. A.; Isaäcson, M.; Ward, J. I.; and Austrian, R. Emergence of multiply resistant pneumococci. *N. Engl. J. Med.*, **1978**, *299*, 735–740.

Jaffe, A.; Chabbert, Y. A.; and Derlot, E. Selection and characterization of betalactam-resistant *Escherichia coli* K-12 mutants. *Antimicrob. Agents Chemother.*, **1983**, *23*, 622–625.

Jaffe, H. W.; Biddle, J. W.; Thornsberry, C.; Johnson, R. E.; Kaufman, R. E.; Reynolds, G. H.; and Wiesner, P. J. National gonorrhea therapy monitoring study: *in vitro* antibiotic susceptibility and its correlation with treatment results. *N. Engl. J. Med.*, **1976**, *294*, 5–9.

Jawetz, E., and Gunnison, J. B. Studies on antibiotic synergism and antagonism: the scheme of combined antimicrobial activity. *Antibiot. Chemother.*, **1952**, *2*, 243–248.

Joiner, K.; Lowe, B.; Dzink, J.; and Bartlett, J. G. Comparative efficacy of ten antimicrobial agents in experimental infections with *B. fragilis. J. Infect. Dis.*, **1982**, *145*, 561–568.

Keating, M. J.; Bodey, G. P.; Valdivieso, M.; and Rodriguez, V. A randomized comparative trial of three aminoglycosides—comparison of continuous infusions of gentamicin, amikacin, and sisomicin combined with carbenicillin in the treatment of infections in neutropenic patients with malignancies. *Medicine (Baltimore)*, **1979**, *58*, 159–170.

Korzeniowski, O.; Sande, M. A.; and The National Collaborative Endocarditis Study Group. Combination antimicrobial therapy for *Staphylococcus aureus* endocarditis in patients addicted to parenteral drugs and in nonaddicts. *Ann. Intern. Med.*, **1982**, *97*, 496–503.

Larson, E. B.; Featherstone, H. J.; and Petersdorf, R. G. Fever of undetermined origin: diagnosis and follow-up of 105 cases, 1970–1980. *Medicine (Baltimore)*, **1982**, *61*, 269–292.

Lepper, M. H., and Dowling, H. F. Treatment of pneumococcic meningitis with penicillin plus AUREOMYCIN: studies including observations on apparent antagonism between penicillin and AUREOMYCIN. *Arch. Intern. Med.*, **1951**, *88*, 489–494.

Lesar, T. S.; Rotschafer, J. C.; Strand, L. M.; Solem, L. D.; and Zaske, D. E. Gentamicin dosing errors with four commonly used nomograms. *J.A.M.A.*, **1982**, *248*, 1190–1193.

Lorian, V.; Koike, M.; Zak, O.; Zanon, U.; Sabath, L. D.; Grassi, G. G.; and Stille, W. Effects of subinhibitory concentrations of antibiotics on bacteria. In, *Current Chemotherapy: Proceedings of the Tenth International Congress of Chemotherapy*, Vol. I. (Siegenthaler, W., and Lüthy, R., eds.) American Society for Microbiology, Washington, D. C., **1977**, pp. 72–78.

Mandell, G. L. Catalase, superoxide dismutase, and virulence of *Staphylococcus aureus. J. Clin. Invest.*, **1975**, *55*, 561–566.

Mandell, G. L.; Kaye, D.; Levison, M. L.; and Hook, E. W. Enterococcal endocarditis: a review of 38 cases. *Arch. Intern. Med.*, **1970**, *125*, 258–264.

Mandell, L. A. Effects of antimicrobial and antineoplastic drugs on the phagocytic and microbicidal function of the polymorphonuclear leukocyte. *Rev. Infect. Dis.*, **1982**, *4*, 683–697.

Mathies, A. W., Jr.; Leedom, J. M.; Ivler, D.; Wehrle, P. F.; and Portnoy, B. Antibiotic antagonism in bacterial meningitis. *Antimicrob. Agents Chemother.*, **1967**, *7*, 218–224.

Medical Letter. Prevention of bacterial endocarditis. **1984**, *26*, 3–4.

Mitchell, J. R.; Hyman, J. Z.; Ishak, K. G.; Thorgeirsson, U. P.; Timbrell, J. A.; Snodgrass, W. R.; and Nelson, S. D. Isoniazid liver injury: clinical spectrum, pathology, and probable pathogenesis. *Ann. Intern. Med.*, **1976**, *84*, 181–192.

Moellering, R. C., Jr.; Wennersten, C.; and Weinberg, A. N. Studies on antibiotic synergism against enterococci. I. Bacteriologic studies. *J. Lab. Clin. Med.*, **1971**, *77*, 821–828.

Pasteur, L., and Joubert, J. Charbonne et septicemie. *C. R. Acad. Sci. [D] (Paris)*, **1877**, *85*, 101–115.

Philipson, A. Pharmacokinetics of ampicillin during pregnancy. *J. Infect. Dis.*, **1977**, *136*, 370–376.

Rahal, J., Jr. Antibiotic combinations: the clinical relevance of synergy and antagonism. *Medicine (Baltimore)*, **1978**, *57*, 179–195.

Rowlands, B. J.; Clark, R. G.; and Richards, D. G. Single-dose intraoperative antibiotic prophylaxis in emergency abdominal surgery. *Arch. Surg.*, **1982**, *117*, 195–199.

Sande, M. A., and Mandell, G. L. Effect of rifampin on nasal carriage of *Staphylococcus aureus. Antimicrob. Agents Chemother.*, **1975**, *7*, 294–297.

Sande, M. A., and Overton, J. W. *In vivo* antagonism between gentamicin and chloramphenicol in neutropenic mice. *J. Infect. Dis.*, **1973**, *128*, 247–250.

Sande, M. A., and Scheld, W. M. Combination antibiotic therapy of bacterial endocarditis. *Ann. Intern. Med.*, **1980**, *92*, 390–395.

Sande, M. A.; Sherertz, R. J.; Zak, O.; Dacey, R. G.; Bodine, J. A.; and Strausbaugh, L. J. Factors influencing the penetration of antimicrobial agents into the cerebrospinal fluid of experimental animals. *Scand. J. Infect. Dis.*, **1978**, Suppl. 14, 160–163.

Sanders, W. E., Jr., and Sanders, C. C. Modification of normal flora by antibiotics: effects on individuals and the environment. In, *New Dimensions in Antimicrobial Therapy.* (Root, R. K., and Sande, M. A., eds.) Churchill Livingstone, Inc., New York, **1984,** pp. 217–241.

Schlichter, J. G., and MacLean, H. A method of determining the effective therapeutic level in treatment of subacute bacterial endocarditis with penicillin. *Am. Heart J.,* **1947,** *34,* 209–211.

Sparling, F. P. Current problems in sexually transmitted diseases. *Adv. Intern. Med.,* **1978,** *24,* 203–228.

Sparling, F. P.; Guymon, L.; and Biswas, G. Antibiotic resistance in the gonococcus. In, *Microbiology, 1976.* (Schlessinger, D., ed.) American Society for Microbiology, Washington, D. C., **1976,** pp. 494–500.

Stratton, C. W.; Weinstein, M. P.; and Reller, L. B. Correlation of serum bactericidal activity with antimicrobial agent level and minimum bactericidal concentration. *J. Infect. Dis.,* **1982,** *145,* 160–168.

Strausbaugh, L. J., and Sande, M. A. Factors influencing the therapy of experimental *Proteus mirabilis* meningitis in rabbits. *J. Infect. Dis.,* **1978,** *137,* 251–260.

Täuber, M. G.; Zak, O.; Scheld, W. M.; Hengstler, B.; and Sande, M. A. The postantibiotic effect in the therapy of experimental pneumococcal meningitis in rabbits. *J. Infect. Dis.,* **1984,** *149,* 575–583.

Vaudaux, P. Peripheral inactivation of gentamicin. *J. Antimicrob. Chemother.,* **1981,** *8,* Suppl. A, S17–S25.

Verklin, R. M., Jr., and Mandell, G. L. Alteration of effectiveness of antibiotics by anaerobiosis. *J. Lab. Clin. Med.,* **1977,** *89,* 65–71.

Vorherr, H. Drug excretion in breast milk. *Postgrad. Med.,* **1974,** *56,* 97–104.

Washington, A. E. Update on treatment recommendations for gonococcal infections. *Rev. Infect. Dis.,* **1982,** *4,* Suppl., S758–S771.

Watanabe, T. Infectious drug resistance in enteric bacteria. *N. Engl. J. Med.,* **1966,** *275,* 888–894.

Wehrli, W. Rifampin: mechanisms of action and resistance. *Rev. Infect. Dis.,* **1983,** Suppl., S407–S411.

Wilson, W. R.; Geraci, J. E.; Wilkowske, C. J.; and Washington, J. A., II. Short-term intramuscular therapy with procaine penicillin plus streptomycin for infective endocarditis due to *viridans* streptococci. *Circulation,* **1978,** *57,* 1158–1161.

Wilson, W. R., *et al.* Empiric therapy with moxalactam alone in patients with bacteremia. *Mayo Clin. Proc.,* **1984a,** *59,* 318–326.

Wilson, W. R.; Wilkowske, C. J.; Wright, A. J.; Sande, M. A.; and Geraci, J. E. Treatment of streptomycin-susceptible and streptomycin-resistant enterococcal endocarditis. *Ann. Intern. Med.,* **1984b,** *100,* 816–823.

Yourtee, E. L., and Root, R. K. Effect of antibiotics on phagocyte-microbe interactions. In, *New Dimensions in Antimicrobial Therapy.* (Root, R. K., and Sande, M. A., eds.) Churchill Livingstone, Inc., New York, **1984,** pp. 243–275.

Zimilis, V. M., and Jackson, G. G. Activity of aminoglycoside antibiotics against *Pseudomonas aeruginosa:* specificity and site of calcium and magnesium antagonism. *J. Infect. Dis.,* **1973,** *127,* 663–669.

Zimmerli, W.; Waldvogel, F. A.; Vaudaux, P.; and Nydegger, U. E. Pathogenesis of foreign body infection: description and characteristics of an animal model. *J. Infect. Dis.,* **1982,** *146,* 487–497.

Monographs and Reviews

Calderwood, S. B., and Moellering, R. C., Jr. Principles of anti-infective therapy. In, *Internal Medicine.* (Stein, J. H., ed.) Little, Brown & Co., Boston, **1983,** pp. 1139–1152.

Craig, W. A., and Kunin, D. M. Significance of serum protein and tissue binding of antimicrobial agents. *Annu. Rev. Med.,* **1976,** *27,* 287–300.

Ernst, J. D., and Sande, M. A. *In vitro* susceptibility testing and the outcome of treatment of infection. In, *New Dimensions in Antimicrobial Therapy.* (Root, R. K., and Sande, M. A., eds.) Churchill Livingstone, Inc., New York, **1984,** pp. 293–311.

Gleckman, R. A., and Gantz, N. M. (eds.). *Infections in the Elderly.* Little, Brown & Co., Boston, **1983.**

Handbook of Antimicrobial Therapy. Antimicrobial prophylaxis. The Medical Letter, Inc., New Rochelle, N.Y., **1982,** pp. 61–68.

Klastersky, J., and Staquet, M. J. (eds.). *Combination Antibiotic Therapy in the Compromised Host.* Vol. 9, *Monograph Series of the European Organization for Research on Treatment of Cancer.* Raven Press, New York, **1982.**

Lorian, V. *Antibiotics in Laboratory Medicine.* The Williams & Wilkins Co., Baltimore, **1980.**

Moellering, R. C., Jr. Principles of anti-infective therapy. In, *Principles and Practice of Infectious Diseases,* 2nd ed. (Mandell, G. L.; Douglas, R. G., Jr.; and Bennett, J. E.; eds.) John Wiley & Sons, Inc., New York, **1985,** pp. 153–164.

Root, R. K., and Sande, M. A. (eds.). *New Dimensions in Antimicrobial Therapy.* Churchill Livingstone, Inc., New York, **1984.**

Sandusky, W. R. Postoperative infections and antimicrobial prophylaxis for surgical infection. In, *Principles and Practice of Infectious Diseases.* (Mandell, G. L.; Douglas, R. G., Jr.; and Bennett, J. E.; eds.) John Wiley & Sons, Inc., New York, **1979,** pp. 2248–2256.

Sanford, J. P. *Guide to Antimicrobial Therapy 1983.* Sanford, Bethesda, **1983.**

Symposium. (Various authors.) The impact of infections on medical care in the United States. (Kunin, C., and Edelman, R., eds.) *Ann. Intern. Med.,* **1978,** *89,* Suppl., Pt. 2, 737–866.

Symposium. (Various authors.) Reassessment of vancomycin—a potentially useful antibiotic. (Wise, R., and Kory, M., eds.) *Rev. Infect. Dis.,* **1981,** *3,* Suppl., S199–S300.

Symposium. (Various authors.) The use of rifampin in the treatment of nontuberculous infections. (Sande, M. A., ed.) *Rev. Infect. Dis.,* **1983,** *5,* Suppl., S399–S632.

49 ANTIMICROBIAL AGENTS

[*Continued*]

Sulfonamides, Trimethoprim-Sulfamethoxazole, and Agents for Urinary Tract Infections

Gerald L. Mandell and Merle A. Sande

SULFONAMIDES

The sulfonamide drugs were the first effective chemotherapeutic agents to be employed systemically for the prevention and cure of bacterial infections in man. The considerable medical and public health importance of their discovery and their subsequent widespread use were quickly reflected in the sharp decline in morbidity and mortality figures for the treatable infectious diseases. Before penicillin became generally available, the sulfonamides were the mainstay of antibacterial chemotherapy. While the advent of antibiotics has diminished the usefulness of the sulfonamides, they continue to occupy an important, although relatively small, place in the therapeutic armamentarium of the physician. However, the introduction in the mid-1970s of the combination of trimethoprim and sulfamethoxazole has resulted in increased use of sulfonamides for the treatment of specific microbial infections.

The term *sulfonamide* is herein employed as a generic name for derivatives of para-aminobenzenesulfonamide (sulfanilamide). More than 5400 congeneric substances were synthesized and studied in the decade that followed the discovery of sulfanilamide. Yet less than a score of them have attained any therapeutic importance.

History. Investigations at the I. G. Farbenindustrie resulted, in 1932, in a German patent to Klarer and Mietzsch, covering PRONTOSIL and several other azo dyes containing a sulfonamide group. In the same year, Domagk, a research director of the I. G., working with Klarer and Mietzsch, observed that mice with streptococcal and other infections could be protected by PRONTOSIL (Domagk, 1935). To Domagk belongs the credit for the discovery of the chemotherapeutic value of

PRONTOSIL, for which he was awarded the Nobel Prize in Medicine for 1938. In 1933, the first clinical case study was reported by Foerster, who gave PRONTOSIL to a 10-month-old infant with staphylococcal septicemia and obtained a dramatic cure. No great attention was paid elsewhere to these epoch-making advances in chemotherapy until the interest of English investigators was aroused. Colebrook and Kenny (1936) as well as Buttle and coworkers (1936) reported their favorable clinical results with PRONTOSIL and its active metabolite, sulfanilamide, in puerperal sepsis and meningococcal infections. These two reports awakened the medical profession to the new field of antibacterial chemotherapy, and experimental and clinical articles in great profusion soon appeared.

A vast number of derivatives of sulfanilamide were subsequently synthesized; many have been tested for their clinical value in various bacterial, protozoal, and viral diseases. Several achieved important, although temporary, clinical status; relatively few are valuable chemotherapeutic agents today. The major developments have been (1) the introduction of congeners that remain largely unabsorbed in the intestinal tract and hence produce local changes in bacterial flora, (2) the discovery of certain advantages of a combination of sulfonamides (*triple sulfonamides*), (3) the development of sulfonamides with high solubility in urine and hence low renal toxicity, and (4) the establishment of the value of a sulfonamide given in combination with trimethoprim in the therapy of specific infections. One interested in the history of sulfonamides is referred to *earlier editions* of this textbook and the references therein.

Chemistry. The structural formulas of selected sulfonamides are shown in Table 49–1. Most of them are relatively insoluble in water, but their sodium salts are readily soluble. Concentrations of sulfonamides in body fluids are determined by chemical technics rather than by bioassay; the latter technic is used for most antibiotics.

Structure-Activity Relationship. The number of sulfonamides is so vast and the structure-activity data are so complex that only the major features of this subject will be presented. The minimal structural prerequisites for antibacterial action are all embodied in sulfanilamide itself. The $-SO_2NH_2$ group is not essential as such, but the important

Table 49–1.   STRUCTURAL FORMULAS OF SELECTED SULFONAMIDES AND PARA-AMINOBENZOIC ACID *

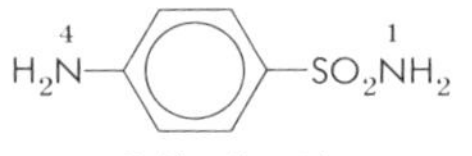

Sulfanilamide

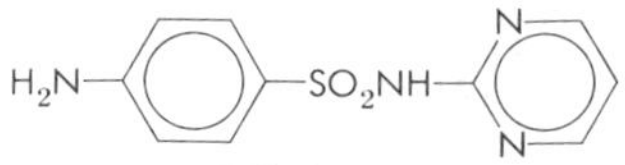

Sulfadiazine

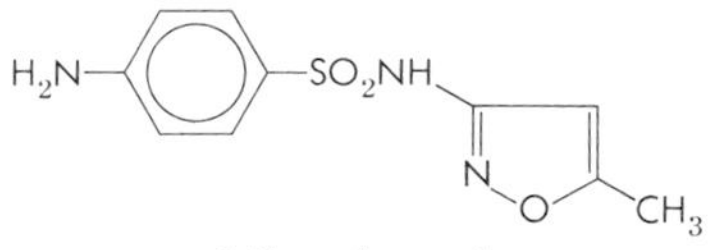

Sulfamethoxazole

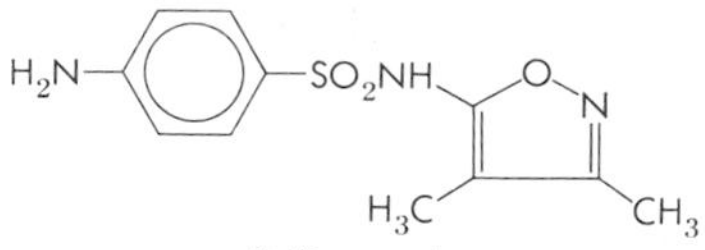

Sulfisoxazole

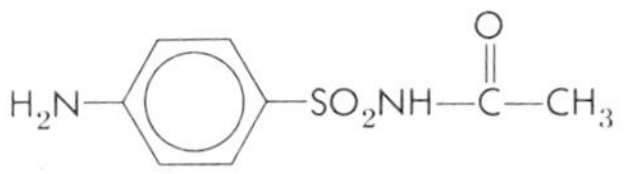

Sulfacetamide

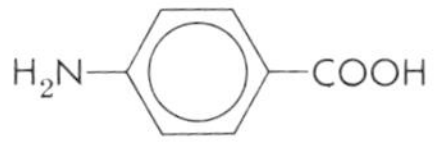

Para-aminobenzoic Acid

* The N of the para-NH_2 group is designated as N^4; that of the amide NH_2, as N^1.

feature is that the sulfur is directly linked to the benzene ring.

The para-NH_2 group (the N of which has been designated as N^4) is essential and can be replaced only by such radicals as can be converted in the tissues to a free amino group. Acylation of the para-NH_2 abolishes *in-vitro* activity; but deacylation may occur *in vivo* with a resulting return of potency, as in the case of the phthalyl derivative of sulfathiazole. Substitutions made in the amide NH_2 group (the N of which has been designated as N^1) have variable effects on antibacterial activity of the molecule. Substitution of heterocyclic aromatic nuclei at N^1 yields highly potent compounds. Bell and Roblin (1942) concluded that the more negative the SO_2 group of an N^1-substituted sulfonamide, the greater is the bacteriostatic activity. They hypothesized that optimal activity had thus been achieved in sulfadiazine. In the main, time has borne out the validity of this prediction. Acetylation at N^1 or its substitution by an amidine group does not interfere with chemotherapeutic activity and may result in compounds with novel properties; for example, the sodium salt of sulfacetamide is nearly neutral in solution, in contrast to the strong alkalinity of sodium salts of other sulfonamides. Substitution in the benzene ring of sulfonamides usually yields inactive compounds.

EFFECTS ON MICROBIAL AGENTS

Sulfonamides have a wide range of antimicrobial activity against both gram-positive and gram-negative microorganisms. With a few exceptions, there is a direct cor-relation between their efficacy *in vitro* and *in vivo*. In general, the sulfonamides exert only a bacteriostatic effect in the body, and cellular and humoral defense mechanisms of the host are essential for the final eradication of the infection.

Antibacterial Spectrum. Among the microorganisms highly susceptible *in vitro* to sulfonamides are *Streptococcus pyogenes*, *Strep. pneumoniae*, some strains of *Bacillus anthracis* and *Corynebacterium diphtheriae*, *Haemophilus influenzae*, *H. ducreyi*, *Brucella*, *Vibrio cholerae*, *Yersinia pestis*, *Nocardia*, *Actinomyces*, *Calymmatobacterium granulomatis*, and *Chlamydia trachomatis*. Minimal inhibitory concentrations range from 0.1 μg/ml for *C. trachomatis* to 4 to 64 μg/ml for *Escherichia coli* (*see* below).

The widespread use of sulfonamides for the treatment of gonorrhea resulted in the appearance of a large number of cases of this disease in which the responsible microorganisms were resistant to these drugs. Therefore, therapy of this infection with the sulfonamides has been replaced completely with the penicillins and other antimicrobial agents. Consequently, there has been a gradual increase in the number of sulfonamide-sensitive gonococci, but this has not reached the point where the use of these compounds is warranted. Although sulfonamides were used successfully for the management of meningococcal infections for many years, a gradual increase in the prevalence of resistant strains became apparent after World War II. By 1963 it was evident that sulfonamide-insensitive strains of *Neisseria meningitidis* were becoming more numerous and producing both the carrier state and disease. The majority of isolates of *N. meningitidis* of serogroups B and C in the United States and group-A isolates from other countries are resistant to sulfadiazine. A similar situation prevails with respect to *Shigella*. By 1965, nearly 60% of *Shigella flexneri* and 90% of *Shig. sonnei* were insensitive to this class of drugs. Most strains of *E. coli* isolated from patients with urinary tract infections (community acquired) that have not previously been treated are susceptible to sulfonamides. *Nocardia asteroides* is highly sensitive.

Mechanism of Action. Sulfonamides are structural analogs and competitive antagonists of para-aminobenzoic acid (PABA), and thus prevent normal bacterial utilization of PABA for the synthesis of folic acid (pteroylglutamic acid, PGA) (*see* Fildes, 1940; Woods, 1940). More specifically, sulfonamides are competitive inhibitors of the bacterial enzyme responsible for the incorporation of PABA into dihydropteroic acid, the immediate precursor of folic acid. Sensitive microorganisms are those that must synthesize their own PGA; bacteria that can utilize preformed PGA are not affected. Bacteriostasis induced by sulfonamides is counteracted by PABA competitively. Sulfonamides do not affect mammalian cells by this mechanism, since they require *preformed* PGA and cannot synthesize it. They are, therefore, comparable to sulfonamide-insensitive bacteria that utilize preformed PGA.

The theory presented above does not explain all the known facts concerning the action of sulfonamides on bacteria. Brown (1962), using cell-free extracts of *E. coli*, found that sulfonamides can also be used as alternative substrates by the enzyme system to form products that are probably analogs of reduced forms of pteroic acid. These analogs could then exert inhibitory effects. The development of knowledge concerning the mode of action of the sulfonamides has been reviewed by Woods (1962).

Synergists and Antagonists of Sulfonamides. One of the most active agents that exerts a synergistic effect when used with a sulfonamide is *trimethoprim* (*see* Bushby and Hitchings, 1968). This compound is a potent and selective competitive inhibitor of microbial dihydrofolate reductase, the enzyme that reduces dihydrofolate to tetrahydrofolate. It is this reduced form of folic acid that is required for one-carbon transfer reactions. The simultaneous administration of a sulfonamide and trimethoprim thus introduces *sequential blocks* in the pathway by which microorganisms synthesize tetrahydrofolate from precursor molecules. The expectation that such a combination would yield synergistic antimicrobial effects has been realized both *in vitro* and *in vivo* (*see* below; Reisberg *et al.*, 1967).

PABA is the most prominent among the sulfonamide antagonists. Certain local anesthetics, such as procaine, that are esters of PABA antagonize these drugs *in vitro* and *in vivo*. PABA may be added to cultures of blood or body fluids in order to block the inhibitory effect of sulfonamides on microbial growth; sensitivity to sulfonamides must be determined in media that are free of PABA. The antibacterial action of these drugs is also inhibited by blood, pus, and tissue breakdown products because the bacterial requirement for folic acid is reduced in media that contain purines and thymidine.

Effects of Sulfonamide Combined with Other Chemotherapeutic Agents. Investigations of the activity of combinations of sulfonamides and antibiotics *in vitro* and in experimental animals suggest an additive effect when sulfonamide is combined with bacteriostatic agents such as the tetracyclines and either an antagonistic or a synergistic effect when bacteria are exposed simultaneously to sulfonamides and a bactericidal antibiotic. The combination of trimethoprim and sulfamethoxazole is discussed below.

Acquired Bacterial Resistance to Sulfonamides. Bacteria initially sensitive to sulfonamides can acquire resistance to the drug both *in vitro* and *in vivo*.

Bacteria resistant to sulfonamide are presumed to originate by random mutation and selection or by transfer of resistance by plasmids (Chapter 48). Such resistance, once it is maximally developed, is usually persistent and irreversible, particularly when produced *in vivo*. Acquired resistance to sulfonamide usually does not imply *cross-resistance* to chemotherapeutic agents of other classes. The *in-vivo* acquisition of resistance has little or no effect either on virulence or on antigenic characteristics of microorganisms.

Mechanism of Resistance. Resistance to sulfonamide is probably the consequence of an altered enzymatic constitution of the bacterial cell; the alteration may be characterized by (1) an alteration in the enzyme that utilizes PABA, (2) an increased capacity to destroy or inactivate the drug, (3) an alternative metabolic pathway for synthesis of an essential metabolite, or (4) an increased production of an essential metabolite or drug antagonist. The latter possibility has received most attention. Woods (1940) was the first to suggest that the resistance of some bacteria to sulfonamide may be based on their ability to synthesize enough PABA to antagonize the drug. Many data support this view. For example, some resistant staphylococci may synthesize 70 times as much PABA as do the susceptible parent strains. Nevertheless, an increased production of PABA is not a constant finding in sulfonamide-resistant bacteria, and resistant mutants may possess enzymes for folate biosynthesis that are less readily inhibited by sulfonamides.

Clinical Aspects and Significance of Resistance to Sulfonamide. Acquired bacterial resistance to sulfonamides plays a significant role in limiting the therapeutic efficacy of these drugs, particularly in infections caused by gonococci, staphylococci, meningococci, streptococci, and shigellae. Sulfonamide-resistant *Strep. pyogenes* emerged during the mass prophylactic use of sulfadiazine in military personnel during World War II. Although one would anticipate that the daily prophylactic use of a sulfonamide in patients who have had rheumatic fever (*see* below) might favor the development of drug-resistant hemolytic streptococci, resistance of clinical importance has not been documented from such medication.

ABSORPTION, FATE AND EXCRETION

Absorption. Except for sulfonamides especially designed for their local effects in the bowel, this class of drugs is rapidly absorbed from the gastrointestinal tract. Approximately 70 to 100% of an oral dose is absorbed, and sulfonamide can be found in the urine within 30 minutes of ingestion. The small intestine is the major site of absorption, but some of the drug is absorbed from the stomach. Absorption from *other sites,* such as the vagina, respiratory tract, or abraded skin, is variable and unreliable, but a sufficient amount may enter the body to cause toxic reactions in susceptible persons or to produce sensitization.

Protein Binding. All sulfonamides are bound in varying degree to plasma proteins, particularly to albumin. The extent to which this occurs is determined by the hydrophobicity of a particular drug and its pK_α; at physiological pH, drugs with a high pK_α exhibit a low degree of protein binding, and *vice versa.* The extent of binding is decreased in patients with severe renal failure, a phenomenon not totally accounted for by low levels of plasma albumin (Andreasen, 1973). In general, a sulfonamide is bound to a somewhat greater extent in the acetylated than in the free form.

Distribution. Sulfonamides are distributed throughout all tissues of the body. The diffusible fraction of sulfadiazine is uniformly distributed throughout the total body water, while sulfisoxazole is largely confined to the extracellular space. The sulfonamides readily enter *pleural, peritoneal, synovial, ocular,* and similar body fluids, and may reach concentrations therein that are 50 to 80% of the simultaneously determined concentration in blood. Since the protein content of such fluids is usually low, the drug is present in the unbound active form.

Cerebrospinal Fluid. After systemic administration of adequate doses, sulfadiazine and sulfisoxazole attain concentrations in cerebrospinal fluid that may be effective in meningeal infections.

At steady state, the concentration ranges between 10 and 80% of that in the blood. Rate and extent of diffusion vary with each drug and depend on many factors, such as the degree of binding by plasma albumin, extent of acetylation, and presence of meningeal inflammation. Inasmuch as the acetylated compounds are more extensively bound by plasma albumin and hence are less available for diffusion, the ratio of free to acetylated drug is higher in the cerebrospinal fluid than in the blood.

Fetus. Sulfonamides readily pass through the placenta and reach the fetal circulation. Equilibration between maternal and fetal blood is usually established within 3 hours after a single oral dose. The concentrations attained in the fetal tissues are sufficient to cause both antibacterial and toxic effects. The concentrations of sulfadiazine in the blood of the fetus are 50 to 90% of those in the maternal blood. The drug appears more slowly in amniotic fluid than in fetal blood.

Metabolism. The sulfonamides undergo metabolic alterations to a varying extent in the tissues, especially in the liver. The major metabolic derivative is the N^4-acetylated sulfonamide. Each sulfonamide is acetylated to a different extent. For example, the percentage of the total plasma sulfonamide that is acetylated ranges between 10 and 40 for sulfadiazine and its methylated derivatives. Acetylation is disadvantageous because the resulting product has no antibacterial activity and yet retains the toxic potentialities of the parent substance. Furthermore, the acetylated forms of some of the older sulfonamides are less soluble and hence contribute to crystalluria and renal complications. Since acetylation is a function of time and hepatic function, the conjugated fraction increases considerably when the sojourn of the drug in the body is prolonged, as in patients with impaired renal function, or decreases when hepatic failure is present. Because of varying degrees of acetylation and other factors, periodic determination of the plasma concentration of free drug is advisable when patients with severe bacterial infections are being treated with large doses of sulfonamide.

Excretion. Sulfonamides are eliminated from the body partly as the unchanged drug and partly as metabolic products. The largest fraction is excreted in the urine, and the half-life of sulfonamides in the body is thus dependent on renal function. Small amounts are eliminated in the feces and in bile, milk, and other secretions.

Renal Elimination. Each sulfonamide, free and acetylated, is handled by the kidney in a characteristic manner. In all cases, glomerular filtration is a major factor. Varying degrees of tubular reabsorption occur for most sulfonamides, although sulfacetamide is not appreciably reabsorbed. Tubular secretion also plays a role in some instances. Marked variations in the rate of renal excretion account for the differences in duration of action of the various sulfonamides, as discussed under the individual drugs. As a generalization, the rate of excretion of sulfonamides increases as their pK_a decreases.

PHARMACOLOGICAL PROPERTIES, PREPARATIONS, AND DOSAGE OF INDIVIDUAL SULFONAMIDES

The sulfonamides may be classified into three groups on the basis of the rapidity with which they are absorbed and excreted: (1) *agents absorbed rapidly and excreted rapidly,* such as sulfisoxazole and sulfadiazine; (2) *agents absorbed very poorly when administered orally* and hence active in the bowel lumen, such as sulfasalazine; and (3) *sulfonamides employed mainly for topical use,* such as sulfacetamide, mafenide, and silver sulfadiazine.

Rapidly Absorbed and Rapidly Eliminated Sulfonamides. *Sulfisoxazole.* Early studies of sulfisoxazole established that it was a rapidly absorbed and rapidly excreted sulfonamide with excellent antibacterial activity (equal to that of sulfadiazine). Since its high solubility eliminates much of the renal toxicity inherent in the use of the older sulfonamides, it has essentially replaced the less soluble agents. Sulfisoxazole should thus be regarded as the prototype of this group.

Sulfisoxazole is extensively bound to plasma proteins, and this explains the fact that the plasma concentration after a given dose is at least twice that for sulfadiazine. Following an oral dose of 2 to 4 g, peak concentrations in plasma of 110 to 250 μg/ml are found in 2 to 4 hours. Both the free and acetylated forms of the drug are much more soluble in urine at pH values encountered clinically than are the respective forms of sulfadiazine. From 28 to 35% of sulfisoxazole in the blood and about 30% in the urine is in the acetylated form. Approximately 95% of a single dose is excreted by the kidney in 24 hours. Concentrations of the drug in urine thus greatly exceed those in blood and may be bac-

tericidal. The cerebrospinal fluid concentration averages about a third of that in the blood.

The recommended daily *oral dose* of sulfisoxazole for children is 150 mg/kg of body weight; one half of this is given initially, followed by one sixth of the daily dose every 4 hours (not to exceed 6 g in 24 hours). The oral dose for adults is 2 to 4 g initially, followed by 1 g every 4 to 6 hours. The *parenteral dose* for adults and children is 100 mg/kg per day, divided into three or four portions. The areas of *clinical usefulness* of sulfisoxazole are discussed below.

Less than 0.1% of patients receiving sulfisoxazole suffer serious *toxic reactions.* The untoward effects produced by this agent are similar to those that follow the administration of other sulfonamides, as discussed below. Because of its relatively high solubility in the urine as compared to sulfadiazine, sulfisoxazole only infrequently produces hematuria or crystalluria (0.2 to 0.3%) and the risk of anuria is very small. Despite this, it is advisable that patients taking this drug ingest an adequate quantity of water. Sulfisoxazole and all sulfonamides that are absorbed must be used with caution in patients with impaired renal function. Like all other sulfonamides, sulfisoxazole may produce hypersensitivity reactions, some of which are potentially lethal. Sulfisoxazole is presently preferred over other sulfonamides by most clinicians, when a rapidly absorbed and rapidly excreted sulfonamide is indicated.

Preparations. *Sulfisoxazole* (GANTRISIN, SK-SOX-AZOLE, others) is available in 500-mg tablets for *oral* use. *Sulfisoxazole diolamine* is available in 4% solution or ointment prepared for *topical* use in the eye; the same salt is marketed for *parenteral injection* (400 mg/ml). Doses are given above. Intravenous administration requires the slow administration of dilute solutions of the drug. *Sulfisoxazole acetyl* is tasteless and hence preferred for *oral* use in children; it is available as a flavored syrup and pediatric suspension (100 mg/ml). The compound is deacetylated by the enzymes in the small intestine, and this results in a relatively slow absorption of the active form of the drug. A flavored emulsion of sulfisoxazole acetyl in vegetable oil (LIPO GANTRISIN) (1 g/5 ml) is a longer-acting preparation. The dose for adults is 4 to 5 g every 12 hours. Sulfisoxazole is also marketed in a fixed-dose combination with phenazopyridine (sulfisoxazole, 500 mg; phenazopyridine, 50 mg; AZO GANTRISIN, others) as a urinary tract antiseptic and analgesic. The urine becomes orange-red soon after ingestion of this mixture because of the presence of phenazopyridine, an orange-red dye. Sulfisoxazole acetyl (600 mg/5 ml) is also marketed in combination with erythromycin ethylsuccinate (200 mg/5 ml) as PEDIAZOLE for use in children with otitis media. The dose is 50 mg/kg per day of the erythromycin component, given in divided doses four times daily.

Sulfamethoxazole. Sulfamethoxazole (GANTANOL) is a close congener of sulfisoxazole, but its rates of enteric absorption and urinary excretion are slower. It is employed for both systemic and urinary tract infections. Precautions must be observed to avoid sulfamethoxazole *crystalluria* because of the high percentage of the acetylated, relatively insoluble form of the drug in the urine. Sulfamethoxazole is available for oral use, as 500-mg and 1-g tablets and as a suspension (100 mg/ml). The *dosage schedule* of sulfamethoxazole for *children* is 50 to 60 mg/kg initially, followed by 25 to 30 mg/kg morning and evening thereafter. The dose for *adults* with mild infections is 2 g, followed by 1 g every 12 hours; for severe disease, the initial dose is 2 g and then 1 g every 8 hours. The half-life of sulfamethoxazole in babies during the first 10 days of life is considerably longer than in adults. It falls rapidly, being about 9 hours at 3 weeks of age and 4 to 5 hours at 1 year. It then increases toward the half-life characteristic for adults, namely, 6 to 12 hours. The clinical uses of sulfamethoxazole are the same as those for sulfisoxazole. It is presently marketed in fixed-dose combinations with phenazopyridine (AZO GANTANOL) as a urinary antiseptic and analgesic, and with trimethoprim (*see* below).

Sulfadiazine. Sulfadiazine given orally is rapidly absorbed from the gastrointestinal tract, and peak blood concentrations are reached within 3 to 6 hours after a single dose. Following an oral dose of 3 g, peak concentrations in plasma are 50 μg/ml. About 55% of the drug is bound to plasma protein at a concentration of 100 μg/ml when plasma protein levels are normal. Therapeutic concentrations are attained in cerebrospinal fluid within 4 hours after a single oral dose of 60 mg/kg.

Sulfadiazine is *excreted* quite readily by the kidney in both the free and the acetylated form, rapidly at first and then more slowly over a period of 2 to 3 days. It can be detected in the urine within 30 minutes after oral ingestion. About 15 to 40% of the excreted sulfadiazine is in the *acetylated* form. This form of the drug is excreted more readily than the free fraction, and the administration of alkali accelerates the renal clearance of both forms by further diminishing their tubular reabsorption.

In *adults* who are being treated with sulfadiazine, the initial dose for oral administration is 2 to 4 g, followed by 2 to 4 g per day in three to six divided doses. *Children* over 2 months of age should receive one half of a calculated daily dose to initiate therapy and then 65 to 150 mg/kg (to a maximum of 6 g) daily in four to six divided doses. Every precaution must be taken to ensure fluid intake adequate to produce a urine output of at least 1200 ml in adults and a corresponding quantity in children. If this cannot be accomplished, sodium bicarbonate may be given to reduce the risk of crystalluria.

Preparations. *Sulfadiazine* is available as tablets that usually contain 500 mg of the drug.

Sulfacytine. Sulfacytine (RENOQUID) is a rapidly excreted sulfonamide for the oral treatment of acute urinary tract infections (Moffat and Wenzel, 1971). The half-life in plasma is shorter than that of sulfisoxazole (4 hours versus 7 hours). Concentrations in blood are lower than those achieved with sulfisoxazole, and this agent should be used only for the treatment of urinary tract infections. A loading dose of 500 mg should be given, followed

by 250 mg four times per day. Sulfacytine is supplied in 250-mg tablets.

Sulfamethizole. Sulfamethizole (THIOSULFIL, others) is a rapidly eliminated sulfonamide; concentrations of the drug in blood are thus low after the administration of conventional doses. It is used for the treatment of urinary tract infections in a dosage of 500 to 1000 mg, given three or four times daily. Sulfamethizole is available in tablets containing 250 or 500 mg.

Sulfonamide Mixtures. A major and frequent toxic reaction to the older sulfonamides was urinary tract injury from precipitation of crystals, usually of acetylated drug, in the renal tubules and ureter. To offset this disadvantage, mixtures of sulfonamides were introduced, since the solubility of one agent is independent of another while antibacterial activity is additive. Because of the availability of newer agents such as sulfisoxazole that are appreciably more soluble than the older sulfonamides, mixtures of these drugs (*e.g., trisulfapyrimidines*) are now little used.

Poorly Absorbed Sulfonamides. *Sulfasalazine* (AZULFIDINE, others) is very poorly absorbed from the gastrointestinal tract. It is used in the therapy of *ulcerative colitis* and regional enteritis, but relapses tend to occur in about one third of patients who experience a satisfactory initial response. Sulfasalazine is preferred to corticosteroids by some gastroenterologists for treatment of patients mildly or moderately ill with ulcerative colitis (Riis *et al.,* 1973). The drug is also being employed as the first approach to treatment of relatively mild cases of *regional enteritis* and *granulomatous colitis* (Singleton, 1977; Summers *et al.,* 1979). Sulfasalazine is broken down in the gut to sulfapyridine, which is absorbed and eventually excreted in the urine, and 5-aminosalicylate, which reaches high levels in the feces (Peppercorn and Goldman, 1973). There is evidence that this latter compound is the effective agent in inflammatory bowel disease (Klotz *et al.,* 1980). Toxic reactions include Heinz-body anemia, acute hemolysis in patients with glucose-6-phosphate dehydrogenase deficiency, and agranulocytosis. Nausea, fever, arthralgias, and rashes occur in up to 20% of patients treated with the drug; desensitization has been effective (Taffet and Das, 1982). The usual daily dose is 1 to 3 g. There is no evidence that the compound alters the intestinal microflora of persons with ulcerative colitis (Gorbach *et al.,* 1967). Sulfasalazine is available in 500-mg tablets and in a suspension (250 mg/5 ml).

Sulfonamides for Topical Use. *Sulfacetamide.* Sulfacetamide is the N^1-acetyl-substituted derivative of sulfanilamide. Its aqueous solubility (1:140) is approximately 90 times that of sulfadiazine. Solutions of the sodium salt of the drug are employed extensively in the management of *ophthalmic infections.* Although topical sulfonamide for most purposes is discouraged because of lack of efficacy and a high risk of sensitization, sulfacetamide has certain advantages. Very high aqueous concentrations are nonirritating to the eye and are effective against susceptible microorganisms. A 30% solution of the sodium salt has a pH of 7.4, whereas the solutions of sodium salts of other sulfonamides are highly alkaline. The drug penetrates into ocular fluids and tissues in high concentration. Sensitivity reactions to sulfacetamide are rare, but the drug should not be used in patients with known hypersensitivity to sulfonamides.

The *usual dose* of sodium sulfacetamide solution applied topically to the eye is 1 or 2 drops of a 10 to 30% solution every 2 hours for severe infections and the same amount three or four times a day for chronic conditions. An ophthalmic ointment may be used instead of the solution, provided there is no wound of the cornea; as a rule, the ointment is reserved for application at bedtime.

Preparations. *Sulfacetamide sodium* (ISOPTO CETAMIDE, SULAMYD SODIUM) is available for topical application to the eye, as an *ophthalmic solution* (10, 15, and 30%) and an *ophthalmic ointment* (10%).

Silver Sulfadiazine (SILVADENE). This drug inhibits the growth *in vitro* of nearly all pathogenic bacteria and fungi, including some species resistant to sulfonamides (Rosenkranz and Rosenkranz, 1972). The compound is used topically to reduce microbial colonization and the incidence of infections of wounds from burns. It should not be used to treat an established infection. Silver is released slowly from the preparation in concentrations that are selectively toxic to the microorganisms (*see* Chapter 41). However, bacteria may develop resistance to silver sulfadiazine (Wenzel *et al.,* 1976). While little silver is absorbed, the plasma concentration of sulfadiazine may approach therapeutic levels if a large surface area is involved. Adverse reactions are infrequent and include burning, rash, and itching (*see* Ballin, 1974). Silver sulfadiazine is considered by most authorities to be the agent of choice for the prevention of infection of burns. It is available as a cream (10 mg/g) to be applied once or twice daily.

Mafenide. This sulfonamide (α-amino-*p*-toluenesulfonamide) is marketed as *mafenide acetate cream* (SULFAMYLON CREAM), which contains 85 mg/g. It is effective, when applied topically, for the prevention of colonization of *burns* by a large variety of gram-negative and gram-positive bacteria. It should not be used in treatment of an established infection. Superinfection with *Candida* may occasionally be a problem. The cream is applied once or twice daily to a thickness of 1 to 2 mm over the burned skin. Cleansing of the wound and removal of debris should be carried out before each application of the drug. Therapy is continued until skin grafting is possible. Mafenide is rapidly absorbed systemically and converted to para-carboxybenzenesulfonamide. Studies of absorption from the burn surface indicate that peak plasma concentrations are reached in 2 to 4 hours (*see* Harrison *et al.,* 1972). Adverse effects include intense pain at sites of application, allergic reactions, and loss of fluid by evaporation from the burn surface, since occlusive dressings are not used. The drug and its primary metabolite inhibit carbonic anhy-

drase. The urine becomes alkaline, and a metabolic acidosis may ensue (White and Asch, 1971). Compensatory tachypnea and hyperventilation with respiratory alkalosis are also observed.

UNTOWARD REACTIONS TO SULFONAMIDES

The untoward effects that follow the administration of sulfonamides are numerous and varied, and may involve nearly every organ system. The overall incidence of reactions is about 5%. (*See* Kutscher *et al.,* 1954; Weinstein *et al.,* 1960.)

Disturbances of the Urinary Tract. The primary factor responsible for the renal damage frequently produced by the older sulfonamides is the formation and deposition of *crystalline aggregates* in the kidneys, calyces, pelves, ureters, or bladder; this leads to the development of irritation and obstruction. Anuria and death may occur in patients in whom no evidence of crystalluria or hematuria can be detected and in whom the lesion found at autopsy is tubular necrosis or necrotizing angiitis.

The risk of crystalluria is minimal with more soluble sulfonamides such as sulfisoxazole. Fluid intake should be such as to ensure a daily urine volume of at least 1200 ml (in adults). Alkalinization of the urine may be desirable if urine volume or pH is unusually low, since the solubility of sulfisoxazole increases greatly with slight elevations of pH.

Disorders of the Hematopoietic System. *Acute Hemolytic Anemia.* The mechanism of the acute hemolytic anemia produced by sulfonamides is not always readily apparent. In some cases, it has been thought to be a sensitization phenomenon. In other instances, the hemolysis is related to an erythrocytic deficiency of glucose-6-phosphate dehydrogenase activity, as discussed on page 1040.

The development of acute hemolytic anemia in the absence of a deficiency of glucose-6-phosphate dehydrogenase may not be dependent on dosage or the concentration of the drug in plasma. Readministration of sulfonamides to individuals who have had an episode of hemolysis provoked by these compounds is accompanied by a 65% incidence of recurrence. Blacks are more susceptible to this reaction than are white-skinned individuals, and children more so than adults. The hemolytic episode occurs abruptly, usually in the first week of therapy. Nausea, fever, vertigo, jaundice, pallor, hepatosplenomegaly, and shock may develop suddenly. There is a marked decrease in erythrocyte and hemoglobin levels, often by 50 to 70% within a few hours, and leukocytosis, reticulocytosis, bilirubinemia, urobilinuria, and hemoglobin casts are common laboratory findings. Acute renal tubular necrosis may follow the hemoglobinuria.

Hemolytic anemia is rare after sulfadiazine (0.05%); its exact incidence following therapy with sulfisoxazole is unknown.

Agranulocytosis. Agranulocytosis occurs in about 0.1% of patients who receive sulfadiazine; it also can follow the use of other sulfonamides. A myelotoxic effect is evident in the bone marrow by a maturation arrest at the myeloblast stage. The granulocytopenia is not related to the dose of drug. While most cases develop after 10 days of medication, the reaction may appear suddenly and without warning, or only after a period of progressive neutropenia. Although return of granulocytes to normal levels may be delayed for weeks or months after sulfonamide is withdrawn, most patients recover spontaneously with supportive care.

Aplastic Anemia. Complete suppression of bone-marrow activity with profound anemia, granulocytopenia, and thrombocytopenia is an extremely rare occurrence with sulfonamide therapy. It probably results from a direct myelotoxic effect, and may be fatal.

Thrombocytopenia. Severe thrombocytopenia rarely arises as a result of therapy with the sulfonamides. Transient, mild decreases in platelet counts are a more common occurrence. The mechanism is unknown.

Eosinophilia. Peripheral eosinophilia may occur as an isolated finding and usually disappears promptly after discontinuation of the sulfonamide. It may also accompany other manifestations of sulfonamide hypersensitivity.

Hypersensitivity Reactions. The incidence of other hypersensitivity reactions to sulfonamides is quite variable. Reactions are seen with greater frequency when long-acting agents are used, and these drugs should thus be avoided.

Vascular lesions, involving various organs including the heart and resembling those present in periarteritis nodosa, may appear rarely in the course of sulfonamide administration. The use of sulfisoxazole has been associated with clinical activation of quiescent systemic lupus erythematosus. A pneumonia characterized by eosinophilic infiltrates may occur.

Among the *skin and mucous membrane manifestations* attributed to sensitization to sulfonamide are morbilliform, scarlatinal, urticarial, erysipeloid, pemphigoid, purpuric, and petechial rashes; and erythema nodosum, erythema multiforme of the Stevens-Johnson type, Behçet's syndrome, exfoliative dermatitis, and photosensitivity. Drug eruptions occur most often after the first week of therapy, but may appear earlier in previously sensitized individuals. Fever, malaise, and pruritus are frequently present simultaneously. The incidence of untoward dermal effects is about 1.5% with sulfadiazine therapy and about 2% with sulfisoxazole.

A syndrome similar to *serum sickness* may appear after several days of sulfonamide therapy. Fever, joint pain, urticarial eruptions, conjunctivitis, bronchospasm, and leukopenia are the outstanding features. In persons previously sensitized to these drugs, immediate reactions of the *anaphylactoid type* are sometimes observed.

Drug fever is a common untoward manifestation of sulfonamide treatment. The incidence approximates 3% with sulfisoxazole. The fever is generally sudden in onset and develops between the seventh and tenth day of sulfonamide administration. It may occur earlier, however, especially if the patient has been previously sensitized to the drug. Headache, chills, malaise, pruritus, and skin rash may accompany the fever. It should be differentiated from the fever that heralds serious toxic reactions to the sulfonamides, such as agranulocytosis and acute hemolytic anemia.

Hepatitis. Focal or diffuse necrosis of the liver due to direct drug toxicity or sensitization occurs in less than 0.1% of patients. Headache, nausea, vomiting, fever, hepatomegaly, jaundice, and laboratory evidence of hepatocellular dysfunction usually appear 3 to 5 days after sulfonamide administration is started, and the syndrome may progress to acute yellow atrophy and death (*see* Dujovne *et al.,* 1967). The development of hepatitis is not influenced by the dose of drug or by the presence of preexisting hepatic disease. Damage to the liver may increase even after drug withdrawal.

Miscellaneous Reactions to the Sulfonamides. Among other untoward effects that may follow the administration of various sulfonamides are *goiter* and *hypothyroidism, arthritis,* and various *neuropsychiatric disturbances.* Coordination and reaction time are not impaired. *Peripheral neuritis* is very rare. *Anorexia, nausea,* and *vomiting* occur in 1 to 2% of persons receiving sulfonamides, and these manifestations are probably central in origin.

The *age* of patients may be an important determinant of the risk of reactions associated with the use of various sulfonamides. The administration of sulfonamides to premature babies may lead to the development of kernicterus due to the displacement of bilirubin from plasma albumin. Sulfonamides should not be given to pregnant women near term.

Drug Interactions. The most important interactions of the sulfonamides involve those with the oral anticoagulants, the sulfonylurea hypoglycemic agents, and the hydantoin anticonvulsants. In each case sulfonamides can potentiate the effects of the other drug by mechanisms that appear to involve primarily inhibition of metabolism and, possibly, displacement from albumin. Dosage adjustment may be necessary when a sulfonamide is given concurrently.

SULFONAMIDE THERAPY

The number of conditions for which the sulfonamides are therapeutically useful and constitute drugs of first choice has been sharply reduced by the development of more effective antimicrobial agents and by the gradual increase in the resistance of a number of bacterial species to this class of drugs. However, the use of sulfonamides has undergone a revival as a result of the introduction of the combination of trimethoprim and sulfamethoxazole (*see* below).

Urinary Tract Infections. The major utility of the sulfonamides in therapeutics is in the treatment of infections of the urinary tract. The vast majority of microorganisms responsible for acute urinary tract infections acquired in the community are *E. coli*, and these are usually sensitive to sulfonamides. Sulfisoxazole (2 g initially followed by 1 g, orally, four times a day for 5 to 10 days) is usually effective. When infections are recurrent, obstruction is present, or bacteremia is suspected, therapy with a sulfonamide alone may not be adequate. In these instances antibiotics may be preferred, and the choice of a specific agent is based on the results of tests of sensitivities of the causative microorganisms. It is important to attempt to distinguish between infections involving the kidney and those that are located in the lower urinary tract. *Acute pyelonephritis* with high fever and other severe constitutional manifestations and the risk of bacteremia and shock is best not treated with a sulfonamide. Most physicians prefer to administer an antibiotic parenterally, selected on the basis of the anticipated antimicrobial sensitivities and later modified, if necessary, by knowledge of the laboratory data. The sulfonamides should be reserved for the management of *acute and chronic cystitis, chronic infections of the upper urinary tract,* and *asymptomatic bacilluria.* Since acute cystitis is most often caused by *E. coli* or *Proteus mirabilis,* the sulfonamides are highly effective.

Recurrent infections of the urinary tract are much more difficult to manage successfully. An integral part of the study of patients with this kind of disease is first to establish whether the chronicity is due to *reinfection* with new microorganisms or whether the same microorganism(s) is persisting, causing *relapse* despite therapy (Turck *et al.,* 1966, 1968). Reinfection occurs most commonly in sexually active females and is related to repeated intraurethral inoculation of perineal bacteria during sexual intercourse. When recurrences are frequent (more than two or three per year), prophylaxis to reduce their number may be employed. Sulfonamides, nitrofurantoin, mandelamine, and trimethoprim-sulfamethoxazole have all been used successfully (Harding and Ronald, 1974; Vosti, 1975), but the last-named preparation is the most effective (*see* below).

Relapse with the same microorganism(s) is often more serious, suggesting a persistent focus of infection in the upper urinary tract that is difficult or impossible to eradicate. This type of infection is often associated with bacteriuria with antibody-coated microorganisms that can be detected by fluorescence microscopy (Thomas *et al.,* 1974). Reasons for this persistence include a functional or mechanical obstruction that interferes with the normal flow of urine or impairment of normal host defenses, as in patients with diabetes mellitus. These patients must be thoroughly evaluated to rule out remediable obstruction. The microorganisms involved include *Escherichia, Enterobacter, Klebsi-*

ella, Proteus, gram-positive cocci (including the enterococcus), and mixtures of microorganisms. Anaerobes are only rarely responsible for urinary tract infections. In some patients the focus of infection may be eradicated by prolonged (6 weeks or more) administration of an antimicrobial agent. However, the cure rate for this type of chronic infection of the urinary tract is relatively low, regardless of the type of antimicrobial therapy employed, and *chronic suppressive therapy or intermittent treatment of symptomatic relapses may eventually be the most reasonable goal.* Chronic suppressive therapy has been shown to decrease the number of symptomatic episodes but has no proven effect on preservation of renal function (Freeman *et al.,* 1975). Agents that have been used include sulfonamides, trimethoprim-sulfamethoxazole, antibiotics, and urinary tract antiseptics.

Bacillary Dysentery (Shigella Diarrhea). Because of the frequency of resistant strains, the sulfonamides are now only infrequently useful in the management of this disease. However, trimethoprim-sulfamethoxazole appears to be effective when given orally. The usual oral dose for adults is 160 mg of trimethoprim plus 800 mg of sulfamethoxazole every 12 hours for 5 days (Nelson *et al.,* 1976; Dupont *et al.,* 1982a).

Meningococcal Infections. Resistance to sulfonamides is now common in the various serological groups of *N. meningitidis.* All forms of disease produced by meningococci should now be treated with large doses of penicillin G or ampicillin; chloramphenicol has been recommended for patients who are allergic to the penicillins. If an epidemic is *proven* to be due to a sulfonamide-sensitive strain of meningococcus, sulfisoxazole or sulfadiazine may be given. In this case, initial sulfonamide therapy is by intravenous administration.

Chemoprophylaxis should be considered for close contacts of patients with meningococcal disease. If the strain of *N. meningitidis* is sensitive to sulfonamides, sulfadiazine (1 g every 12 hours for four doses) should be given. One half of this dose is administered to children 1 to 12 years of age. Penicillin G and several other antibiotics are *not* effective for prophylaxis. Rifampin is now considered the prophylactic agent of choice, since most strains are resistant to sulfonamides. Minocycline is also effective, but its use is not recommended because of a high incidence of vestibular toxicity.

Nocardiosis. Sulfonamides are of value in the treatment of infections due to *Nocardia* species. A number of instances of complete recovery from the disease after adequate treatment with a sulfonamide have been recorded. Sulfisoxazole or sulfadiazine may be given in doses of 6 to 8 g daily. Concentrations of sulfonamide in plasma should be 80 to 160 μg/ml. This schedule is continued for several months after all manifestations have been controlled. The administration of sulfonamide together with an antibiotic has been recommended, especially for advanced cases, and ampicillin, erythromycin, or streptomycin has been suggested for this purpose. The clinical response and the results of sensitivity testing may be helpful in choosing a companion drug. It should be emphasized, however, that there are no clinical data to show that combination therapy is better than therapy with a sulfonamide alone. Trimethoprim-sulfamethoxazole has also been effective, and some authorities consider it to be the drug of choice (*see* below).

Streptococcal Infections. There is presently no indication for the use of sulfonamides in therapy of streptococcal diseases such as pharyngitis, erysipelas, cellulitis, bacteremia, and pneumonia. They are readily managed by administration of penicillin or erythromycin.

Trachoma and Inclusion Conjunctivitis. Systemic therapy with tetracycline (Hoshiwara *et al.,* 1973) or a sulfonamide for 3 weeks appears to be the most effective treatment for *trachoma.* While the topical use of such agents will often suppress signs of infection, it will not eradicate the microorganism. Therapeutic results are best when therapy is initiated early, but even chronic cicatricial cases may respond. The local symptoms may disappear in a few days. Pannus, keratitis, conjunctival granulations, entropion, trichiasis, iritis, and corneal ulcerations improve and may even disappear. Corneal lesions respond more rapidly than do those of the conjunctivae. Blindness may be prevented. Dawson and associates (1968) reported that some of the alleged benefits of chemotherapy in trachoma might be attributable to control of bacterial superinfection.

Many physicians prefer to treat *inclusion conjunctivitis* (inclusion blennorrhea) by the topical application of tetracycline or sulfacetamide ointment (10%), six times a day for 10 days. Administration of tetracycline or erythromycin systemically is also effective.

Lymphogranuloma Venereum and Chancroid. Oral administration of a sulfonamide (1 g of sulfisoxazole four times daily for 21 days) or tetracycline (500 mg four times daily for 21 days) has been successful for the treatment of lymphogranuloma venereum. A similar schedule is recommended for chancroid.

Dermatitis Herpetiformis (Duhring's Disease). Dapsone and sulfonamides have been used for the management of this skin disorder. The preferred sulfonamide appears to be sulfapyridine. Therapy is started with 0.5 g four times a day; this dose may be increased gradually until a total of 4 to 5 g per day is being given, unless intolerance develops. Dermatitis herpetiformis is the only indication for sulfapyridine, an older sulfonamide; it is available in 500-mg tablets for this purpose. Some physicians prefer to use dapsone; the initial dose is 25 to 50 mg per day. If this does not produce suppression of the disease and if there is no evidence of toxicity, the dose is increased by 50 mg per day over a period of several days. Usually a total daily dose of 200 mg is successful.

Toxoplasmosis. Although pyrimethamine is the agent of primary importance in the therapy of infections due to *Toxoplasma gondii,* most clinicians who have had experience with this disease prefer to give full doses of sulfadiazine simultaneously. In patients with severe chorioretinitis, it is advisable to add a corticosteroid to the therapeutic regimen (*see* Remington and Desmonts, 1976).

Use of Sulfonamides for Prophylaxis. The sulfonamides exhibit a degree of effectiveness equal to that of oral penicillin in *preventing streptococcal infections and recurrences of rheumatic fever* among susceptible subjects. Despite the efficacy of sulfonamides for long-term prophylaxis of rheumatic fever, their toxicity and the possibility of infection by drug-resistant streptococci make them less desirable than penicillin for this purpose. They should be used, however, without hesitation in patients who are hypersensitive to penicillin. The recommended dose of sulfisoxazole is 1 g twice daily; for children under 27 kg (60 lb), the dose is halved. If untoward responses occur, they usually do so during the first 8 weeks of therapy; serious reactions after this time are rare. White-cell counts should be carried out once weekly during the first 8 weeks.

TRIMETHOPRIM-SULFA-METHOXAZOLE

The introduction of trimethoprim in combination with sulfamethoxazole constitutes an important advance in the development of clinically effective antimicrobial agents and represents the practical application of a theoretical consideration; that is, if two drugs act on sequential steps in the pathway of an obligate enzymatic reaction in bacteria, the result of their combination will be synergistic (*see* Hitchings, 1961). In much of the world the combination is known as *co-trimoxazole.* (*See* Wormser *et al.,* 1982, for an extensive review.)

Chemistry. Sulfamethoxazole has been discussed on page 1099, and its structural formula is shown in Table 49–1. The history of trimethoprim, a diaminopyrimidine, is discussed in Chapter 45. Its structural formula is as follows:

Trimethoprim

Antibacterial Spectrum. The antibacterial spectrum of trimethoprim is similar to that of sulfamethoxazole, although the former drug is usually 20 to 100 times more potent than the latter. Most gram-negative and gram-positive microorganisms are sensitive to trimethoprim, but resistance can develop when the drug is used alone (Ward *et al.*, 1982). *Pseudomonas aeruginosa, Bacteroides fragilis*, and enterococci are usually resistant. The data presented below refer to the antimicrobial activity of the *combination* of trimethoprim and sulfamethoxazole.

Streptococcus pneumoniae, C. diphtheriae, and *N. meningitidis* are sensitive to trimethoprim-sulfamethoxazole. From 50 to 95% of strains of *Staphylococcus aureus, Staph. epidermidis, Strep. pyogenes*, the *viridans* group of streptococci, *E. coli, Pr. mirabilis, Pr. morganii, Pr. rettgeri, Enterobacter* species, *Salmonella, Shigella, Pseud. pseudomallei, Serratia*, and *Alcaligenes* species are inhibited. Also sensitive are *Klebsiella* species, *Brucella abortus, Pasteurella haemolytica, Yersinia pseudotuberculosis, Y. enterocolitica*, and *Nocardia asteroides*. Methicillin-resistant strains of *Staph. aureus*, although also resistant to trimethoprim or sulfamethoxazole alone, may be susceptible to the combination. A synergistic interaction between the components of the preparation is apparent *even* when microorganisms are resistant to sulfonamide or resistant to sulfonamide and moderately resistant to trimethoprim. However, a *maximal degree* of synergism occurs when microorganisms are sensitive to both components. The activity of trimethoprim-sulfamethoxazole · *in vitro* depends on the medium in which it is determined; for example, low concentrations of thymidine almost completely abolish the antibacterial activity (*see* Symposium, 1969, 1973; Pelton *et al.*, 1977).

Mechanism of Action. The antimicrobial activity of the combination of trimethoprim and sulfamethoxazole results from its actions on two steps of the enzymatic pathway for the synthesis of tetrahydrofolic acid. Sulfonamide inhibits the incorporation of PABA into folic acid, and trimethoprim prevents the reduction of dihydrofolate to tetrahydrofolate. The latter is the form of folate essential for one-carbon transfer reactions, for example, the synthesis of thymidylate from deoxyuridylate. Selective toxicity for microorganisms is achieved in two ways. Mammalian cells utilize preformed folates from the diet and do not synthesize the compound. Furthermore, trimethoprim is a highly *selective* inhibitor of dihydrofolate reductase of lower organisms (*see* Chapter 45). This is vitally important, since this enzymatic function is a crucial one in all species.

The synergistic interaction between sulfonamide and trimethoprim is thus predictable from their respective mechanisms. There is an optimal ratio of the concentrations of the two agents for synergism, and this is equal to the ratio of the minimal inhibitory concentrations of the drugs acting independently. While this ratio varies for different bacteria, the most effective ratio for the greatest number of microorganisms is 20 parts of sulfamethoxazole to

one part of trimethoprim. The combination is thus formulated to achieve a sulfamethoxazole concentration *in vivo* 20 times greater than that of trimethoprim. (*See* articles by Hitchings, Burchall, and Bushby, in Symposium, 1973.) The pharmacokinetic properties of the sulfonamide chosen to be in combination with trimethoprim are thus important, since relative constancy of the concentrations of the two compounds in the body is desired.

Examination of the sensitivity pattern of a typical isolate of *E. coli* illustrates the extent of synergism. The minimal inhibitory concentration for sulfamethoxazole alone is 3 µg/ml, while that for trimethoprim is 0.3 µg/ml. When the combination is tested at a ratio of 20:1, inhibitory concentrations are 1.0 µg/ml and 0.05 µg/ml, respectively. The combination is actually bactericidal for some microorganisms.

Bacterial Resistance. The frequency of development of bacterial resistance to trimethoprim-sulfamethoxazole is lower than it is to either of the agents alone. This is logical, since a microorganism that has acquired resistance to one of the components may still be killed by the other. Trimethoprim-resistant microorganisms may arise by mutation. Resistance in gram-negative bacteria is often associated with the acquisition of a plasmid that codes for an altered dihydrofolate reductase (Burchall *et al.*, 1982). Resistance to trimethoprim in *Staph. aureus* appears to be determined by a chromosomal gene rather than by a plasmid (Nakhla, 1973). The development of resistance to the combination also occurs *in vivo*. While the incidence of resistance of *E. coli* to trimethoprim-sulfamethoxazole increased only from 0.2% to 1.5% over a 5-year period of use (*see* McAllister, 1976), resistance of *Staph. aureus* increased from 0.4% to 12.6% during a similar time span (*see* Chattopadhyay, 1977). Ten to 20% of gram-negative microorganisms were found to be resistant in New York (Wormser *et al.*, 1982).

Absorption, Distribution, and Excretion. The pharmacokinetic profiles of both sulfamethoxazole and trimethoprim are closely but not perfectly matched to achieve a constant ratio of 20:1 in their concentrations in blood and tissues. The ratio in blood is often greater than 20:1, and that in tissues is frequently less (Craig and Kunin, 1973). After a single oral dose of the combined preparation, trimethoprim is absorbed more rapidly than sulfamethoxazole. The concurrent administration of the drugs appears to slow the absorption of sulfamethoxazole. Peak blood concentrations of trimethoprim usually occur by 2 hours in most patients, while peak concentrations of sulfamethoxazole occur by 4 hours after a single oral dose. The half-lives of trimethoprim and sulfamethoxazole are approximately 11 and 10 hours, respectively.

When 800 mg of sulfamethoxazole is given with 160 mg of trimethoprim (the conventional 5:1 ratio), twice daily, the peak concentrations of the drugs in plasma are approximately 40 and 2 μg/ml, the optimal ratio that is sought. Peak concentrations are similar (46 and 3.4 μg/ml) after intravenous infusion of 800 mg of sulfamethoxazole and 160 mg of trimethoprim over a period of 1 hour.

Trimethoprim is rapidly distributed and concentrated in tissues, and about 40% is bound to plasma protein in the presence of sulfamethoxazole. The volume of distribution of trimethoprim is almost nine times that of sulfamethoxazole. The drug enters cerebrospinal fluid and sputum readily. High concentrations of each component of the mixture are also found in bile. About 65% of sulfamethoxazole is bound to plasma protein.

Up to 60% of administered trimethoprim and from 25 to 50% of sulfamethoxazole are excreted in the urine in 24 hours. Two thirds of the sulfonamide is unconjugated. Metabolites of trimethoprim are also excreted. The rates of excretion and the concentrations of both compounds in the urine are significantly reduced in patients with uremia.

(For details of the pharmacology of trimethoprim-sulfamethoxazole and its components, *see* Bushby and Hitchings, 1968; Symposium, 1973.)

Preparations, Routes of Administration, and Dosage. *Sulfamethoxazole and trimethoprim tablets* (BACTRIM, SEPTRA) are available in two sizes: 400 mg of sulfamethoxazole plus 80 mg of trimethoprim, and 800 mg of sulfamethoxazole plus 160 mg trimethoprim. An oral suspension of 200 mg of sulfamethoxazole plus 40 mg of trimethoprim per 5 ml is also available, as is a preparation for intravenous use (400 mg of sulfamethoxazole plus 80 mg of trimethoprim per 5 ml). The usual *adult* dose is 800 mg of sulfamethoxazole plus 160 mg of trimethoprim every 12 hours for 10 to 14 days for management of most infections. Larger quantities have been given in special circumstances in patients with serious or life-threatening disease. Dosage must be reduced in patients with renal insufficiency (*see* Appendix II), and the preparation should not be administered if creatinine clearance is less than 15 ml per minute.

The recommended daily dose for children for treatment of urinary tract infections and otitis media is 8 mg/kg of trimethoprim and 40 mg/kg of sulfamethoxazole, given in two divided doses every 12 hours for 10 days; the same regimen is followed for 5 days to treat shigellosis.

The combination should not be used in infants under 2 months of age, during pregnancy (at term), and during the nursing period.

Trimethoprim is also available as a single-entity preparation (PROLOPRIM, TRIMPEX) in 100- and 200-mg tablets.

Untoward Effects. There is no evidence that trimethoprim-sulfamethoxazole, when given in the recommended doses, induces folate deficiency in normal persons. However, the margin between toxicity for bacteria and that for man may be relatively narrow when the cells of the patient are deficient in folate. In such cases, trimethoprim-sulfamethoxazole may cause or precipitate *megaloblastosis, leukopenia,* or *thrombocytopenia*. In routine use, the combination appears to exert little toxicity. About 75% of the untoward effects involve the *skin*. These are typical of those known to be produced by *sulfonamides*, as already described. However, trimethoprim-sulfamethoxazole has been reported to cause up to three times as many dermatological reactions as does sulfisoxazole when given alone (5.9% versus 1.7%; Arndt and Jick, 1976). *Exfoliative dermatitis, Stevens-Johnson syndrome,* and *toxic epidermal necrolysis* (Lyell's syndrome) are rare, occurring primarily in older individuals. *Nausea* and *vomiting* constitute the bulk of gastrointestinal reactions; *diarrhea* is rare. *Glossitis* and *stomatitis* are relatively common. Mild and transient *jaundice* has been noted and appears to have the histological features of allergic cholestatic hepatitis. Central nervous system reactions consist in *headache, depression,* and *hallucinations,* manifestations known to be produced by sulfonamides. Hematological reactions, in addition to those mentioned above, are various types of *anemia* (including *aplastic, hemolytic,* and *macrocytic*), *coagulation disorders, granulocytopenia, agranulocytosis, purpura, Henoch-Schönlein purpura,* and *sulfhemoglobinemia*. Previous or simultaneous administration of diuretics with trimethoprim-sulfamethoxazole may carry an increased risk of thrombocytopenia, especially in elderly patients with heart failure; death may occur. Permanent impairment of renal function may follow the use of trimethoprim-sulfamethoxazole in patients with renal disease (Kalowski *et al.*, 1973), and a reversible decrease in creatinine clearance has been noted in patients with normal renal function (Symposium, 1973; Shouval *et al.*, 1978).

Patients with acquired immunodeficiency syndrome (AIDS) frequently react adversely when trimethoprim-sulfamethoxazole is administered to treat infection due to *Pneumocystis carinii*. Fever, malaise, rash, and/or pancytopenia were noted in 8 of 18 patients in one series (Jaffe *et al.*, 1983); the incidence was 90% in another (Wharton *et al.*, 1984). Renal allograft recipients may suffer from severe hematological toxicity (Bradley *et al.*, 1980).

Therapeutic Uses. *Urinary Tract Infections.* Treatment of uncomplicated lower urinary tract infections with trimethoprim-sulfamethoxazole is often highly effective, even when the infecting agent is resistant to the sulfonamides alone. A dose of 800 mg of sulfamethoxazole plus 160 mg of trimethoprim every 12 hours for 10 days produces cure in the vast majority of cases. The preparation has been shown to produce a better therapeutic effect than does either of its components given separately when the infecting microorganisms are of the family Enterobacteriaceae. Single-dose therapy (320 mg of trimethoprim plus 1600 mg of sulfamethoxazole) has also been effective for the treatment of acute uncomplicated urinary tract infections (Harbord and Grüneberg, 1981).

The combination appears to have special efficacy in chronic and recurrent infections of the urinary tract (*see* Gleckman, 1975). In females, this may be related to the presence of therapeutic concentrations of trimethoprim in vaginal secretions (Stamey and Condy, 1975). Enterobacteriaceae surrounding the urethral orifice may be eliminated or reduced markedly in number, thus diminishing the chance of an ascending reinfection (*see* Stamey *et al.*, 1977). Trimethoprim is also found in therapeutic concentrations in prostatic secretions and is often effective for the treatment of bacterial prostatitis (Dabhiolwala *et al.*, 1976).

Small doses (200 mg of sulfamethoxazole plus 40 mg of trimethoprim per day, or two to four times these amounts once or twice per week) appear to be effective in reducing the number of recurrent urinary tract infections in females. This correlates with a reduction in the numbers of Enterobacteriaceae inhabiting the vaginal introitus.

It should be remembered that trimethoprim-sulfamethoxazole is a drug combination with toxic potential equal at least to that of the sulfonamide. Furthermore, the cost of a therapeutic course of this combination is considerably more than that of sulfisoxazole alone. Acute, nonrecurrent urinary tract infections need not be treated with the combination; a sulfonamide alone will suffice. Trimethoprim given alone has also been effective for urinary tract infections (Lacey *et al.*, 1980; Iravani *et al.*, 1981). The usual dose for adults is 100 mg every 12 hours for 10 days.

Bacterial Respiratory Tract Infections. Trimethoprim-sulfamethoxazole is effective for *acute exacerbations of chronic bronchitis*. Administration of 1200 mg of sulfamethoxazole plus 240 mg of trimethoprim twice a day appears to be very effective in decreasing fever, purulence and volume of sputum, and sputum bacterial count. The microorganisms involved have been *H. influenzae* and *Strep. pneumoniae* (*see* Carroll *et al.*, 1977; Tandon, 1977). Trimethoprim-sulfamethoxazole should *not* be used to treat streptococcal pharyngitis, since it does not eradicate the microorganism. It is effective for acute otitis media in children and acute maxillary sinusitis in adults caused by susceptible strains of *H. influenzae* and *Strep. pneumoniae* (*see* Cameron *et al.*, 1975; Willner *et al.*, 1978; Hamory *et al.*, 1979). However, bacteremia with resistant pneumococci has been reported (Markman *et al.*, 1982).

Gastrointestinal Infections. The combination has become useful for treatment of shigellosis, since many strains of the causative agent are now resistant to ampicillin (*see* Chang *et al.*, 1977). It is also effective for typhoid fever, but there is some difference of opinion concerning the precise role of trimethoprim-sulfamethoxazole for the management of this disease. The experience of Scragg and Rubidge (1971) suggests that, in children, this drug is not as effective as chloramphenicol. In adults, trimethoprim-sulfamethoxazole appears to be effective when the dose is 800 mg of sulfamethoxazole plus 160 mg of trimethoprim every 12 hours for 15 days. Chloramphenicol remains the drug of choice for typhoid fever in areas where the incidence of strains that are resistant to the drug is low (*see* Ramachandran *et al.*, 1978).

Trimethoprim-sulfamethoxazole appears to be effective in the management of carriers of *S. typhi* and other species of *Salmonella*. One proposed schedule is the administration of 800 mg of sulfamethoxazole plus 160 mg of trimethoprim twice a day for 3 months; however, failures have occurred. It has been suggested that the presence of chronic disease of the gallbladder is associated with a high incidence of failure to clear the carrier state (Brodie *et al.*, 1970). (*See* Symposium, 1969; 1973; Geddes, 1975.) Acute diarrhea due to enteropathogenic *E. coli* can be treated or prevented with either trimethoprim or trimethoprim plus sulfamethoxazole (DuPont *et al.*, 1982a, 1982b).

Infection by Pneumocystis carinii. High-dose therapy (trimethoprim, 15 to 20 mg/kg per day, plus sulfamethoxazole, 75 to 100 mg/kg per day, in three or four divided doses) is effective for this severe infection of impaired hosts. This combination compares favorably to pentamidine for treatment of this disease. However, the incidence of side effects is high for both regimens (Sattler and Remington, 1983; Wharton *et al.*, 1984).

Prophylaxis in Neutropenic Patients. Several studies have demonstrated the effectiveness of low-dose therapy (150 mg/m^2 of trimethoprim and 750 mg/m^2 of sulfamethoxazole) for the prophylaxis of infection by *Pneumocystis carinii* (*see* Hughes *et al.*, 1977). In addition, significant protection against sepsis caused by gram-negative bacteria was noted when 800 mg of sulfamethoxazole plus 160 mg of trimethoprim was given twice daily to severely neutropenic patients (Enno *et al.*, 1978; Gurwith, *et al.*, 1979; Kauffman *et al.*, 1983). The emergence of fungi and resistant bacteria may limit the usefulness of trimethoprim-sulfamethoxazole for prophylaxis (Gualtieri *et al.*, 1983).

Genital Infections. Trimethoprim-sulfamethoxazole is effective in the management of *acute gonococcal urethritis* in both men and women. The special role of trimethoprim-sulfamethoxazole appears to be for oral therapy of oropharyngeal gonorrhea caused by penicillinase-producing strains; the recommended dose is 720 mg of trimethoprim and 3600 mg of sulfamethoxazole daily for 5 days (Centers for Disease Control, 1982). The drug has no effect in preventing incubating *syphilis* or in curing the established disease. *Chancroid* is treated effectively with either erythromycin (500 mg orally four times daily for 10 days) or trimethoprim-sulfamethoxazole (160 mg plus 800 mg orally twice daily for 10 days).

Miscellaneous Infections. *Nocardia* infections have been treated successfully with the combination (Smego *et al.*, 1983), although failures have been reported (Stamm *et al.*, 1983). Trimethoprim-sulfamethoxazole may be effective in the therapy of *brucellosis* even when localized lesions such as arthritis, endocarditis, or epididymo-orchitis are present. Doses have ranged from two tablets (400 mg/80 mg) three times a day for 1 week followed by two tablets a day for 2 weeks to four to eight tablets per day for 2 months. Most patients recover, particularly when the latter dosage schedule is employed; however, relapse has occurred in 4% of cases even with this regimen. Hassan and associates (1971) have suggested that therapy (two to four of the lower-dose tablets per day) be continued for an additional 6 weeks to minimize the risk of relapse.

There is some evidence that *bacterial endocarditis* due to *Pseud. cepacia* may respond favorably, especially when polymyxin is given simultaneously (*see* Moody and Young, 1975).

Intravenous administration of trimethoprim-sulfamethoxazole plus carbenicillin has been used effectively in the treatment of infections in neutropenic patients (Stuart *et al.*, 1980). Trimethoprim-sulfamethoxazole has also been useful in a variety of serious infections in children (Ardati and Dajani, 1979) and adults (Sattler and Remington, 1983). Strains of methicillin-resistant *Staph. aureus* may be susceptible, and the combination with or without rifampin has been effective oral therapy for mild infections. Vancomycin remains the drug of choice for serious infections caused by methicillin-resistant *Staph. aureus*.

AGENTS FOR URINARY TRACT INFECTIONS

The urinary tract antiseptics inhibit the growth of many species of bacteria. They cannot be used to treat systemic infections because effective concentrations are not achieved in plasma with safe doses. However, because they are concentrated in the renal tubules, they can be used to treat infections of the urinary tract. Furthermore, effective antibacterial concentrations reach the renal pelves and the bladder. Treatment with such drugs can be thought of as local therapy in that only in the kidney and bladder, with the rare exceptions mentioned below, are adequate therapeutic levels achieved (*see* Andriole, 1985).

Methenamine. Methenamine is a urinary tract antiseptic that owes its activity to formaldehyde.

Chemistry. Methenamine is hexamethylenetetramine (hexamethyleneamine). It has the following structure:

Methenamine

The compound decomposes in water to generate formaldehyde, according to the following reaction:

$$N_4(CH_2)_6 + 6H_2O + 4H^+ \rightarrow 4NH_4^+ + 6HCHO$$

At pH 7.4 almost no decomposition occurs; however, 6% of the theoretical amount of formaldehyde is yielded at pH 6 and 20% at pH 5. Thus, acidification of the urine promotes the formaldehyde-dependent antibacterial action. The reaction is fairly slow, and 3 hours are required to reach 90% of completion.

Antimicrobial Activity. Nearly all bacteria are sensitive to free formaldehyde at concentrations of about 20 μg/ml. Urea-splitting microorganisms (*e.g.*, *Proteus* species) tend to raise the pH of the urine and thus inhibit the release of formaldehyde. Microorganisms do not develop resistance to formaldehyde.

Pharmacology and Toxicology. Methenamine is absorbed orally, but 10 to 30% decomposes in the gastric juice unless the drug is protected by an enteric coating. Because of the ammonia produced, methenamine is contraindicated in hepatic insufficiency. Methenamine distributes widely into body fluids, but so little decomposes in the blood and tissues that there is no systemic toxicity from ammonia or formaldehyde. Excretion into the urine is nearly quantitative. When the urine pH is 6 and the daily urine volume is 1000 to 1500 ml, a daily dose of 2 g will yield a concentration of 18 to 60 μg/ml of formaldehyde; this is more than the minimal inhibitory concentration for most urinary tract pathogens. Some of the formaldehyde is bound to substances in the urine and in the surrounding tissues, so that daily doses below 0.5 g may not yield much free formaldehyde.

Various poorly metabolized acids can be used to acidify the urine. Low pH alone is bacteriostatic, so that acidification serves a double function. The acids commonly used are mandelic acid, hippuric acid, ascorbic acid, monobasic sodium phosphate, and acid-producing foods such as cranberry juice. Doses of 3 to 6 g or more per day of the acids may be needed to keep the urinary pH at 5.5 or below. Both mandelic and hippuric acids are bacteriostatic *in vitro* in high concentrations, but these levels are not achieved in urine and there is little evidence that they contribute anything more than their effect on the pH (*see* Hamilton-Miller and Brumfitt, 1977).

Gastrointestinal distress frequently is caused by doses greater than 500 mg four times a day, even with enteric-coated tablets. Painful and frequent micturition, albuminuria, hematuria, and rashes may result from doses of 4 to 8 g a day given for longer than 3 to 4 weeks. Once the urine is sterile, a high dose should be reduced. Because systemic methenamine is nontoxic, renal insufficiency does not constitute a contraindication to the use of methenamine alone, but the acids may be detrimental. Methenamine mandelate is contraindicated in renal insufficiency. Crystalluria from the mandelate moiety can occur. Methenamine combines with sulfamethizole (Lipton, 1963) and perhaps other sulfonamides in the urine, which results in mutual antagonism.

Preparations and Dosage. Methenamine is given as tablets in a dose of 0.5 to 2 (usually 1) g, four times a day. *Methenamine mandelate* (MANDELAMINE) is given in an oral suspension or as tablets or granules in the same dose as for methenamine, even though the methenamine equivalence is less. *Methenamine hippurate* (HIPREX, UREX) is usually given in a dose of 1 g, twice a day. The recommended dose of *methenamine and monobasic sodium phosphate,* three tablets (325 mg of each ingredient) four times a day, cannot be considered to yield activity equivalent to the usual doses of the other preparations.

Therapeutic Uses and Status. Methenamine is not a primary drug for the treatment of acute urinary tract infections, but it is of value for chronic suppressive treatment (Freeman *et al.,* 1975). The agent is most useful when the causative organism is *E. coli,* but it can usually suppress the common gram-negative offenders and often *Staph. aureus* and *Staph. epidermidis* as well. *Enterobacter aerogenes* and *Proteus vulgaris* are usually resistant. Urea-splitting bacteria (mostly *Proteus*) make it difficult to control the urine pH. The physician should strive to keep the pH below 5.5. Patient compliance is poor because of the number of tablets required with many products. Methenamine is sometimes employed prophylactically in instrumentation and catheterization of the urinary tract, but studies suggest that it is ineffective for this purpose (Gerstein *et al.,* 1968; Vainrub and Musher, 1977).

The Quinolones. Nalidixic acid and its congeners, the quinolones, are useful agents for the treatment of urinary tract infections. Newer, more potent derivatives may also be effective for certain infections outside the urinary tract. These agents inhibit DNA synthesis during bacterial replication; this effect may result from interference with DNA gyrase activity.

Nalidixic Acid. Nalidixic acid has the following chemical structure:

Nalidixic Acid

Antimicrobial Activity. Nalidixic acid is bactericidal to most of the common gram-negative bacteria that cause urinary tract infections. Brumfitt and Pursell (1971) reported that 99% of strains of *E. coli,* 98% of *Pr. mirabilis* and 75 to 97% of other *Proteus* species, 92% of *Klebsiella-Enterobacter,* and 80% of other coliform bacteria are sensitive to concentrations of 16 μg/ml or less of the drug. *Pseudomonas* species are resistant. It is less active against gram-positive microorganisms. Acquired resistance to the drug occurs during therapy.

Pharmacology and Toxicology. Almost all of orally administered nalidixic acid is absorbed. Plasma concentrations of 20 to 50 μg/ml may be achieved, but the acid is 93 to 97% bound to plasma proteins. In the body some nalidixic acid is converted to an active hydroxynalidixic acid, and both are excreted into the urine. Very high concentrations of nalidixic acid plus its active metabolite are achieved in the urine—100 to 500 μg/ml. Antibacterial activity is not found in prostatic fluid (Stamey *et al.,* 1970). Some nalidixic acid is conjugated in the liver. The plasma half-life is normally about 8 hours, but it may be as long as 21 hours in the presence of renal failure.

Oral nalidixic acid is usually well tolerated, but nausea, vomiting, and abdominal pain may occur. Allergic reactions such as pruritus, urticaria, various rashes, photosensitivity, eosinophilia, and fever occasionally occur, and cholestasis, thrombocytopenia, leukopenia, and hemolytic anemia rarely occur. Liver function tests and blood-cell counts are advisable if treatment lasts longer than 2 weeks. Effects on the central nervous system (CNS), such as headache, drowsiness, malaise, vertigo, visual disturbances, asthenia, and myalgia, are experienced infrequently. In patients with cerebral vascular insufficiency, parkinsonism, or epilepsy, or in normal children given excessive doses, convulsions can occur (*see* Boréus and Sundström, 1967). Pseudotumor cerebri has been described (Rao, 1974).

Therapeutic Uses, Preparations, and Dosage. In the United States, nalidixic acid is approved only for the treatment of urinary tract infections caused by susceptible microorganisms (*see* above). The effectiveness against indole-positive *Proteus* is especially important. Failures in men may be, in part, the result of reinfection from the prostate gland. Whether nalidixic acid can effectively penetrate the renal medulla and be of direct value in the treatment of pyelonephritis is uncertain. Rapid development of bacterial resistance has been reported in a widely varying percentage of cases. Stamey and Bragonje (1976) noted the development of resistance in 7% of patients who were treated with 1 g of the drug four times daily. Others have reported that 25% of patients will harbor resistant microorganisms (Ronald *et al.*, 1966).

Nalidixic acid (NEGGRAM) is available in tablets containing 250, 500, or 1000 mg of the drug and in an oral suspension containing 250 mg/5 ml. The recommended dose for adults is 1 g four times a day for 1 to 2 weeks; thereafter a daily dose of 2 g is suggested. The recommended daily dose for children is 55 mg/kg of body weight, given in four divided doses. The drug should not be used in infants under 3 months of age.

Oxolinic Acid. This drug is very similar to nalidixic acid. Its structural formula is as follows:

Oxolinic Acid

The mechanism of action and spectrum of antimicrobial activity resemble those of nalidixic acid, and cross-resistance between the two agents can be demonstrated. Oxolinic acid is two to four times more potent than nalidixic acid *in vitro*. Adverse reactions are also similar, although oxolinic acid has been associated with a greater incidence of CNS toxicity. Side effects are most frequent in elderly patients, and these include restlessness, insomnia, dizziness, headache, and nausea (*see* Atlas *et al.*, 1969; Ghatikar, 1974). Because of the increased incidence of CNS toxicity compared to nalidixic acid, the latter drug is usually preferred.

Other Quinolones. Cinoxacin is similar in structure to oxolinic acid. Its activity *in vitro* is somewhat better than that of nalidixic acid but less than that of oxolinic acid (Gordon *et al.*, 1976). Peak concentrations in urine are four to eight times higher than those seen with nalidixic acid. Rapid emergence of resistance appears to be less common. Although adverse reactions are similar to those reported with nalidixic acid, they are relatively uncommon (Scavone *et al.*, 1982). *Cinoxacin* (CINOBAC) is available in 250- and 500-mg capsules; the usual dose for adults is 1 g daily in two to four divided portions for 7 to 14 days.

Norfloxacin is a similar, more potent agent with good activity *in vitro* against a large number of gram-negative and gram-positive microorganisms, including *Pseud. aeruginosa, Staph. saprophyticus,* and enterococci (Norrby and Jonsson, 1982).

Ciprofloxacin and *pefloxacin* are two of a group of new quinoline derivatives with even greater activity against gram-negative microorganisms and more activity than norfloxacin against gram-positive cocci (Ito *et al.*, 1980; Muytjens *et al.*, 1983). These agents appear promising not only for use in urinary tract infections but also for serious systemic disease.

Nitrofurantoin. Nitrofurantoin is a synthetic nitrofuran that is used for the prevention and treatment of infections of the urinary tract. Its structural formula is as follows:

Nitrofurantoin

Antimicrobial Activity. Nitrofurantoin inhibits a number of bacterial enzymes, but the basis for its antimicrobial activity and specificity is not known. Bacteria that are susceptible to the drug rarely become resistant during therapy. Nitrofurantoin is active against many strains of *E. coli.* However, most species of *Proteus* and *Pseudomonas* and many of *Enterobacter* and *Klebsiella* are resistant. Nitrofurantoin is bacteriostatic for most susceptible microorganisms at concentrations of 32 μg/ml or less. The antibacterial activity is higher in an acidic urine.

Pharmacology and Toxicity. Nitrofurantoin is rapidly and completely absorbed from the gastrointestinal tract. The macrocrystalline form of the drug is absorbed and excreted more slowly. Antibacterial concentrations are not achieved in plasma following ingestion of recommended doses, because the drug is rapidly eliminated. The plasma half-life is 0.3 to 1 hour; about 40% is excreted unchanged into the urine. The average dose of nitrofurantoin yields a concentration in urine of approximately 200 μg/ml. This amount is soluble at pH values above 5, but the urine should not be alkalinized because this reduces antimicrobial activity. The rate of excretion is linearly related to the creatinine clearance (Sachs *et al.*, 1968), so that in patients with impaired glomerular function the efficacy of the drug may be decreased and the systemic toxicity increased. Nitrofurantoin colors the urine brown.

The most common untoward effects are *nausea, vomiting,* and *diarrhea.* The incidence is less if the drug is administered with milk or other food or is used in a smaller dosage. The macrocrystalline preparation is better tolerated. Various *hypersensitivity reactions* occasionally occur. They may involve the skin, blood, liver, or lungs. They include *chills, fever, leukopenia, granulocytopenia, hemolytic anemia* (when glucose-6-phosphate dehydrogenase deficiency exists in the erythrocyte), *cholestatic jaundice,* and *hepatocellular damage.*

Chronic active hepatitis is an uncommon but serious side effect (Black *et al.,* 1980; Tolman, 1980). *Acute pneumonitis* with fever, chills, cough, dyspnea, chest pain, pulmonary infiltration, and eosinophilia may occur within hours to days of the initiation of therapy (*see* DeMasi, 1967; Strauss and Griffin, 1967); it usually resolves within hours after discontinuation of the drug. More insidious subacute reactions may also be noted, and *interstitial pulmonary fibrosis* can occur in patients on chronic medication. Elderly patients are especially susceptible to the pulmonary toxicity of nitrofurantoin. (*See* Hailey *et al.,* 1969; Holmberg *et al.,* 1980.) Megaloblastic anemia is rare. Various *neurological disorders* are occasionally observed. Headache, vertigo, drowsiness, muscular aches, and nystagmus are readily reversible, but severe *polyneuropathies* with demyelination and degeneration of both sensory and motor nerves have been reported; signs of denervation and muscle atrophy result. Neuropathies are most likely to occur in patients with impaired renal function and in persons on long-continued treatment. However, Lindholm (1967) has detected electromyographic signs of muscle denervation in 62% of nonuremic patients receiving nitrofurantoin chronically. Nitrofurantoin-induced polyneuropathy has been reviewed by Toole and Parrish (1973). Certain adverse reactions may be caused by toxic reactive metabolites (Spielberg and Gordon, 1981).

Nitrofurantoin (FURADANTIN, others) is available in tablets containing 50 or 100 mg of the drug and in an oral suspension containing 25 mg/5 ml. Nitrofurantoin macrocrystals (MACRODANTIN) are available in 25-, 50-, and 100-mg capsules. The oral dose for adults is 50 to 100 mg four times a day, with meals and at bedtime. Alternatively, the daily dose is better expressed as 5 to 7 mg/kg in four divided doses (not to exceed 400 mg). A single 50- to 100-mg dose at bedtime may be sufficient to prevent recurrences (Stamey *et al.,* 1977). The daily dose for children is 5 to 7 mg/kg, but it may be as low as 1 mg/kg for long-term therapy (Lohr *et al.,* 1977). A course of therapy should not exceed 14 days, and repeated courses should be separated by rest periods. Pregnant women at term, individuals with impaired renal function (creatinine clearance less than 40 ml per minute), and children below 1 month of age should not receive nitrofurantoin.

Nitrofurantoin is approved only for the treatment of urinary tract infections caused by microorganisms that are known to be susceptible to the drug. It has been used to prevent recurrent infections and for the prevention of bacteriuria after prostatectomy (Matthew *et al.,* 1978).

Phenazopyridine. *Phenazopyridine hydrochloride* (PYRIDIUM) is *not* a urinary antiseptic. However, it does have an analgesic action on the urinary tract and alleviates symptoms of dysuria, frequency, burning, and urgency. Phenazopyridine is supplied in tablets containing 100 or 200 mg of the drug for oral administration. The usual dose is 200 mg three times daily. The compound is an azo dye, and the urine is colored orange or red; the patient should be so informed. Gastrointestinal upset

is seen in up to 10% of patients; overdosage may result in methemoglobinemia. Phenazopyridine is also marketed in combination with sulfisoxazole (AZO GANTRISIN) and sulfamethoxazole (AZO GANTANOL) (*see* above).

Andreasen, F. Protein binding in plasma from patients with acute renal failure. *Acta Pharmacol. Toxicol. (Kbh.),* **1973,** *32,* 417–429.

Andriole, V. T. Urinary tract agents: nalidixic acid, oxolinic acid, cinoxacin, nitrofurantoin, and methenamine. In, *Principles and Practice of Infectious Diseases,* 2nd ed. (Mandell, G. L.; Douglas, R. G., Jr.; and Bennett, J. E.; eds.) John Wiley & Sons, Inc., New York, **1985,** pp. 244–253.

Ardati, K. O., and Dajani, A. S. Intravenous trimethoprim-sulfamethoxazole in the treatment of serious infections in children. *J. Pediatr.,* **1979,** *95,* 801–806.

Arndt, K. A., and Jick, H. Rates of cutaneous reactions to drugs. *J.A.M.A.,* **1976,** *235,* 918–923.

Atlas, E.; Clark, H.; Silverblatt, F.; and Turck, M. Nalidixic acid and oxolinic acid in the treatment of chronic bacteriuria. *Ann. Intern. Med.,* **1969,** *70,* 713–722.

Ballin, J. C. Evaluation of a new topical agent for burn therapy. Silver sulfadiazine (SILVADENE). *J.A.M.A.,* **1974,** *230,* 1184–1185.

Bell, P. H., and Roblin, R. O., Jr. Studies in chemotherapy. VII. A theory of the relation of structure to activity of sulfanilamide type compounds. *J. Am. Chem. Soc.,* **1942,** *64,* 2905–2917.

Black, M.; Rabin, L.; and Schatz, N. Nitrofurantoin-induced chronic active hepatitis. *Ann. Intern. Med.,* **1980,** *92,* 62–64.

Boréus, L. O., and Sundström, B. Intracranial hypertension in a child during treatment with nalidixic acid. *Br. Med. J.,* **1967,** *2,* 744–745.

Bradley, P. P.; Warden, G. D.; Maxwell, J. G.; and Rothstein, G. Neutropenia and thrombocytopenia in renal allograft recipients treated with trimethoprim-sulfamethoxazole. *Ann. Intern. Med.,* **1980,** *93,* 560–562.

Brodie, J.; MacQueen, I. A.; and Livingstone, D. Effect of trimethoprim-sulfamethoxazole on typhoid and salmonella carriers. *Br. Med. J.,* **1970,** *3,* 318–319.

Brown, G. M. The biosynthesis of folic acid. II. Inhibition by sulfonamides. *J. Biol. Chem.,* **1962,** *237,* 536–540.

Brumfitt, W., and Pursell, R. Observations on bacterial sensitivities to nalidixic acid and critical comments on the 6-centre survey. *Postgrad. Med. J.,* **1971,** *47,* 16–18.

Burchall, J. J.; Elwell, L. P.; and Fling, M. E. Molecular mechanisms of resistance to trimethoprim. *Rev. Infect. Dis.,* **1982,** *4,* 246–254.

Bushby, S. R. M., and Hitchings, G. H. Trimethoprim, a sulphonamide potentiator. *Br. J. Pharmacol. Chemother.,* **1968,** *33,* 72–90.

Buttle, G. A. H.; Gray, W. H.; and Stephenson, D. Protection of mice against streptococcal and other infections by *p*-aminobenzenesulphonamide and related substances. *Lancet,* **1936,** *1,* 1286–1290.

Cameron, G. G.; Pomahac, A. C.; and Johnston, M. T. Comparative efficacy of ampicillin and trimethoprim-sulfamethoxazole in otitis media. *Can. Med. Assoc. J.,* **1975,** *112,* 87S–88S.

Carroll, P. G.; Krejci, S. P.; Mitchell, J.; Puranik, V.; Thomas, R.; and Wilson, B. A comparative study of co-trimoxazole and amoxycillin in the treatment of acute bronchitis in general practice. *Med. J. Aust.,* **1977,** *2,* 286–287.

Centers for Disease Control. Sexually transmitted diseases: treatment guidelines, 1982. *M.M.W.R.,* **1982,** *31,* 35S–62S.

Chang, M. J.; Dunkle, L. M.; Van Reken, D.; Anderson, D.; Wong, M. L.; and Feigin, R. D. Trimethoprim-sulfamethoxazole compared to ampicillin in the treatment of shigellosis. *Pediatrics*, **1977**, *51*, 726–729.

Chattopadhyay, B. Co-trimoxazole resistant *Staphylococcus aureus* in hospital practice. *J. Antimicrob. Chemother.*, **1977**, *3*, 371–374.

Colebrook, L., and Kenny, M. Treatment of human puerperal infections, and of experimental infections in mice, with PRONTOSIL. *Lancet*, **1936**, *1*, 1279–1286.

Craig, A., and Kunin, C. M. Distribution of trimethoprim-sulfamethoxazole in tissues of rhesus monkeys. *J. Infect. Dis.*, **1973**, *128*, Suppl., S575–S579.

Dabhiolwala, N. F.; Bye, A.; and Claridge, M. A study of concentrations of trimethoprim-sulfamethoxazole in the human prostate gland. *Br. J. Urol.*, **1976**, *48*, 77–81.

Dawson, C. R.; Hanna, L.; Wood, T. R.; and Jawetz, E. Double-blind treatment trials in chronic trachoma of American Indian children. In, *Antimicrobial Agents and Chemotherapy—1967*. American Society for Microbiology, Ann Arbor, Mich., **1968**, pp. 137–142.

DeMasi, C. J. Allergic pulmonary infiltrates probably due to nitrofurantoin. *Arch. Intern. Med.*, **1967**, *120*, 631–634.

Domagk, G. Eine neue Klasse von Desinfektionsmitteln. *Dtsch. Med. Wochenschr.*, **1935**, *61*, 829–832.

Dujovne, C. A.; Chan, C. H.; and Zimmerman, H. J. Sulfonamide liver injury: review of the literature and report of a case due to sulfamethoxazole. *N. Engl. J. Med.*, **1967**, *277*, 785–788.

Dupont, H. L.; Evans, D. G.; Rios, N.; Cabada, F. J.; Evans, D. J., Jr.; and Dupont, M. W. Prevention of travelers' diarrhea with trimethoprim-sulfamethoxazole. *Rev. Infect. Dis.*, **1982a**, *4*, 533–539.

Dupont, H. L.; Reves, R. R.; Galindo, E.; Sullivan, P. S.; Wood, L. V.; and Mendiola, J. G. Treatment of travelers' diarrhea with trimethoprim/sulfamethoxazole and with trimethoprim alone. *N. Engl. J. Med.*, **1982b**, *307*, 841–844.

Enno, A.; Catovsky, D.; Darrell, J.; Goldman, J. M.; Hows, J.; and Galton, D. A. G. Co-trimoxazole for prevention of infection in acute leukemia. *Lancet*, **1978**, *1*, 395–398.

Fildes, P. A rational approach to research in chemotherapy. *Lancet*, **1940**, *1*, 955–957.

Freeman, R. B.; Smith, W. M.; and Richardson, J. A. Long-term therapy for chronic bacteriuria in men: U.S. Public Health Service Cooperative Study. *Ann. Intern. Med.*, **1975**, *83*, 133–147.

Geddes, A. M. Trimethoprim-sulfamethoxazole in the treatment of gastrointestinal infections, including enteric fever and typhoid carriers. *Can. Med. Assoc. J.*, **1975**, *112*, 35S–36S.

Gerstein, A. R.; Okun, R.; Gonick, H. C.; Howard, I. W.; Kleeman, C. R.; and Maxwell, M. H. The prolonged use of methenamine hippurate in the treatment of chronic urinary tract infections. *J. Urol.*, **1968**, *100*, 767–771.

Ghatikar, K. N. A multicenter trial of a new synthetic antibacterial in urinary infections. *Curr. Ther. Res.*, **1974**, *16*, 130–136.

Gleckman, R. A. Trimethoprim-sulfamethoxazole vs. ampicillin in chronic urinary tract infections. *J.A.M.A.*, **1975**, *233*, 427–431.

Gorbach, S. L.; Nahas, L.; Plaut, A.; Weinstein, L.; Patterson, J. F.; and Levitan, R. Studies of intestinal microflora. V. Fecal microbial ecology in ulcerative colitis and regional enteritis: relationship to severity of disease and chemotherapy. *Gastroenterology*, **1967**, *54*, 575–587.

Gordon, R. C.; Stevens, L. I.; Edmiston, C. E., Jr.; and Mohan, K. Comparative *in vitro* studies of cinoxacin, nalidixic acid, and oxolinic acid. *Antimicrob. Agents Chemother.*, **1976**, *10*, 918–920.

Gualtieri, R. J.; Donowitz, G. R.; Kaiser, D. L.; Hess, C. E.; and Sande, M. A. Double-blind randomized study of prophylactic trimethoprim/sulfamethoxazole in granulocytopenic patients with hematologic malignancies. *Am. J. Med.*, **1983**, *74*, 934–940.

Gurwith, M. J.; Brunton, J. L.; Lank, B. A.; Harding, G. K. M.; and Ronald, A. R. A prospective controlled investigation of prophylactic trimethoprim-sulfamethoxazole in hospitalized granulocytic patients. *Am. J. Med.*, **1979**, *66*, 248–256.

Hailey, F. J.; Glascock, H. W.; and Hewitt, W. F. Pleuropneumonic reactions to nitrofurantoin. *N. Engl. J. Med.*, **1969**, *281*, 1087–1090.

Hamilton-Miller, J. M., and Brumfitt, W. Methenamine and its salts as urinary tract antiseptics: variables affecting the antibacterial activity of formaldehyde, mandelic acid, and hippuric acid *in vitro*. *Invest. Urol.*, **1977**, *14*, 287–291.

Hamory, B. H.; Sande, M. A.; Sydnor, A.; and Gwaltney, J. M. Etiology and antimicrobial therapy of acute maxillary sinusitis. *J. Infect. Dis.*, **1979**, *139*, 197–202.

Harbord, R. D., and Grüneberg, R. N. Treatment of urinary tract infection with a single dose of amoxycillin, co-trimoxazole or trimethoprim. *Br. Med. J.*, **1981**, *283*, 1301–1302.

Harding, G. K. M., and Ronald, A. R. Controlled study of antimicrobial prophylaxis of recurrent urinary infection in women. *N. Engl. J. Med.*, **1974**, *291*, 597–601.

Harrison, H. N.; Bales, H. W.; and Jacoby, F. J. The absorption into burned skin of SULFAMYLON ACETATE from 5 percent aqueous solution. *J. Trauma*, **1972**, *12*, 994–998.

Hassan, A.; Erian, M. M.; Farid, Z.; Hathout, S. D.; and Sorensen, K. Trimethoprim-sulfamethoxazole in acute brucellosis. *Br. Med. J.*, **1971**, *3*, 159–160.

Hitchings, G. H. A biochemical approach to chemotherapy. *Ann. N.Y. Acad. Sci.*, **1961**, *23*, 700–708.

Holmberg, L.; Boman, G.; Bottiger, L. E.; Eriksson, B. A.; Spross, R.; and Wessling, A. Adverse reactions to nitrofurantoin. *Am. J. Med.*, **1980**, *69*, 733–738.

Hoshiwara, J.; Oster, B.; Hana, L.; Cignett, F.; Colema, V. R.; and Jawetz, E. Doxycycline treatment of chronic trachoma. *J.A.M.A.*, **1973**, *224*, 220–223.

Hughes, W. T.; Kuhn, S.; Chaudhary, S.; Feldman, S.; Verzosa, M.; Aur, J. A. R.; Pratt, C.; and George, S. L. Successful chemoprophylaxis for *Pneumocystis carinii* pneumonitis. *N. Engl. J. Med.*, **1977**, *297*, 1419–1426.

Iravani, A.; Richard, G. A.; and Baer, H. Treatment of uncomplicated urinary tract infection with trimethoprim versus sulfisoxazole with special reference to antibody-coated bacteria and faecal flora. *Antimicrob. Agents Chemother.*, **1981**, *19*, 824–850.

Ito, A.; Hirai, K.; Inoue, M.; Koga, H.; Suzue, S.; Irikura, T.; and Mitsuhaschi, S. *In vitro* antibacterial activity of AM-715, a new nalidixic acid analog. *Antimicrob. Agents Chemother.*, **1980**, *17*, 103–108.

Jaffe, H. S.; Abrams, D. I.; Ammann, A. J.; Lewis, B. J.; and Golden, J. A. Complications of co-trimoxazole in treatment of AIDS-associated *Pneumocystis carinii* pneumonia in homosexual men. *Lancet*, **1983**, *2*, 1109–1111.

Kalowski, S.; Nanra, R. S.; Mathew, T. H.; and Kincaid-Smith, P. Deterioration in renal function in association with co-trimoxazole therapy. *Lancet*, **1973**, *2*, 394–397.

Kauffman, C. A.; Liepman, M. K.; Bergman, A. G.; and Mioduszewski, J. Trimethoprim/sulfamethoxazole prophylaxis in neutropenic patients. *Am. J. Med.*, **1983**, *74*, 599–607.

Klotz, U.; Maier, K.; Fischer, C.; and Heinkel, K. Therapeutic efficacy of sulfasalazine and its metabolites in patients with ulcerative colitis and Crohn's disease. *N. Engl. J. Med.*, **1980**, *303*, 1499–1502.

Kutscher, A. H.; Lane, S. L.; and Segall, R. The clinical

toxicity of antibiotics and sulfonamides: a comparative review of the literature based on 104,672 cases treated systemically. *J. Allergy*, **1954**, *25*, 135–150.

Lacey, R. W.; Lord, V. L.; Gunasekera, H. K.; Leiberman, P. J.; and Luxton, D. E.   Comparison of trimethoprim alone with trimethoprim sulphamethoxazole in the treatment of respiratory and urinary infections with particular reference to selection of trimethoprim resistance. *Lancet*, **1980**, *1*, 1270–1273.

Lindholm, T.   Electromyographic changes after nitrofurantoin (FURADANTIN) therapy in nonuremic patients. *Neurology (Minneap.)*, **1967**, *17*, 1017–1020.

Lipton, J. H.   Incompatibility between sulfamethizole and methenamine mandelate. *N. Engl. J. Med.*, **1963**, *268*, 92–93.

Lohr, J. A.; Nunley, D. H.; Howards, S. S.; and Ford, R. F.   Prevention of recurrent urinary tract infections in girls. *Pediatrics*, **1977**, *59*, 562–565.

McAllister, T. A.   Resistance to co-trimoxazole. *Scand. J. Infect. Dis.*, **1976**, *29*, Suppl. 8, 29–35.

Markman, M.; Mannisi, J.; Dick, J. D.; Filburn, B.; Santos, G. W.; and Rein, S.   Sulfamethoxazole-trimethoprim-resistant pneumococcal sepsis. *J.A.M.A.*, **1982**, *248*, 3011–3012.

Matthew, A. D.; Gonzalez, R.; Jeffords, D.; and Pinto, M. H.   Prevention of bacteriuria after transurethral prostatectomy with nitrofurantoin macrocrystals. *J. Urol.*, **1978**, *120*, 442–443.

Moffat, N. A., and Wenzel, F. J.   The treatment of urinary tract infections with sulfacytine, a new soluble sulfonamide. *Curr. Ther. Res.*, **1971**, *13*, 286–291.

Moody, M. R., and Young, V. M.   *In vitro* susceptibility of *Pseudomonas cepacia* and *Pseudomonas maltophilia* to trimethoprim and trimethoprim-sulfamethoxazole. *Antimicrob. Agents Chemother.*, **1975**, *7*, 836–839.

Muytjens, H. L.; van der Ros–van de Repe, J.; and van Veldhuizen, G.   Comparative activities of ciprofloxacin (Bay o 9867), norfloxacin, pipemidic acid, and nalidixic acid. *Antimicrob. Agents Chemother.*, **1983**, *24*, 302–304.

Nakhla, L. S.   Genetic determinants of trimethoprim resistance in a strain of *Staphylococcus aureus*. *J. Clin. Pathol.*, **1973**, *26*, 712–715.

Nelson, J. D.; Kusmiesz, H.; and Jacobson, L. H.   Comparison of trimethoprim-sulfamethoxazole and ampicillin therapy for shigellosis in ambulatory patients. *J. Pediatr.*, **1976**, *89*, 491–493.

Norrby, S. R., and Jonsson, M.   Antibacterial activity of norfloxacin. *Antimicrob. Agents Chemother.*, **1982**, *23*, 15–18.

Pelton, S. I.; Shurin, P. A.; Klein, J. O.; and Finland, M.   Quantitative inhibition of *Haemophilus influenzae* by trimethoprim-sulfamethoxazole. *Antimicrob. Agents Chemother.*, **1977**, *12*, 649–654.

Peppercorn, M. A., and Goldman, P.   Distribution studies of salicylazosulfapyridine and its metabolites. *Gastroenterology*, **1973**, *64*, 240–245.

Ramachandran, S.; Godfrey, J. J.; and Lionel, N. D. W.   A comparative trial of co-trimoxazole and chloramphenicol in typhoid and paratyphoid fever. *J. Trop. Med. Hyg.*, **1978**, *81*, 36–39.

Rao, K. G.   Pseudotumor cerebri associated with nalidixic acid. *Urology*, **1974**, *4*, 204–207.

Reisberg, B.; Herzog, J.; and Weinstein, L.   *In vitro* antibacterial activity of trimethoprim alone and in combination with sulfonamides. In, *Antimicrobial Agents and Chemotherapy—1966*. American Society for Microbiology, Ann Arbor, Mich., **1967**, pp. 424–427.

Remington, J. S., and Desmonts, G.   Toxoplasmosis. In, *Infectious Diseases of the Fetus and Newborn Infant*. (Remington, J. S., and Klein, J. O., eds.) W. B. Saunders Co., Philadelphia, **1976**, pp. 191–332.

Riis, P.; Anthonisen, P.; Wulff, R.; Folkenborg, O.; Bonnevie, O.; and Binder, V.   The prophylactic effect of salicylazosulphapyridine in ulcerative colitis during long-term treatment. *Scand. J. Gastroenterol.*, **1973**, *8*, 71–74.

Ronald, A. R.; Turck, M.; and Petersdorf, R. G.   A critical evaluation of nalidixic acid in urinary-tract infections. *N. Engl. J. Med.*, **1966**, *275*, 1081–1089.

Rosenkranz, H. S., and Rosenkranz, S.   Silver sulfadiazine: interaction with isolated deoxyribonucleic acid. *Antimicrob. Agents Chemother.*, **1972**, *2*, 373–383.

Sachs, J.; Geer, T.; Noell, P.; and Kunin, C. M.   Effect of renal function on urinary recovery of orally administered nitrofurantoin. *N. Engl. J. Med.*, **1968**, *278*, 1032–1035.

Sattler, F. R., and Remington, J. R.   Intravenous trimethoprim-sulfamethoxazole therapy for *Pneumocystis carinii* pneumonia. *Arch. Intern. Med.*, **1983**, *143*, 1709–1712.

Scavone, J. M.; Gleckman, R. A.; and Fraser, D. G.   Cinoxacin: mechanisms of action, spectrum of activity, pharmacokinetics, adverse reactions and therapeutic indications. *Pharmacotherapy*, **1982**, *2*, 266–271.

Scragg, J. N., and Rubidge, C. J.   Trimethoprim and sulphamethoxazole in typhoid fever in children. *Br. Med. J.*, **1971**, *3*, 738–741.

Shouval, D.; Ligumsky, M.; and Ben-Ishay, D.   Effect of co-trimoxazole on normal creatinine clearance. *Lancet*, **1978**, *2*, 244–245.

Singleton, J. W.   National Cooperative Crohn's Disease Study (NCCDS). Results of drug treatment. *Gastroenterology*, **1977**, *72*, A110/1133.

Smego, R. A.; Moeller, M. B.; and Gallis, H. A.   Trimethoprim-sulfamethoxazole therapy for *Nocardia* infections. *Arch. Intern. Med.*, **1983**, *143*, 711–718.

Spielberg, S. P., and Gordon, G. B.   Nitrofurantoin cytotoxicity. *J. Clin. Invest.*, **1981**, *67*, 37–71.

Stamey, T. A., and Bragonje, J.   Resistance to nalidixic acid. A misconception due to underdosage. *J.A.M.A.*, **1976**, *236*, 1857–1860.

Stamey, T. A., and Condy, M.   The diffusion and concentration of trimethoprim in human vaginal fluid. *J. Infect. Dis.*, **1975**, *131*, 261–266.

Stamey, T. A.; Condy, M.; and Mihara, G.   Prophylactic efficacy of nitrofurantoin macrocrystals and trimethoprim-sulfamethoxazole in urinary infections. Biologic effects on the vaginal and rectal flora. *N. Engl. J. Med.*, **1977**, *296*, 780–783.

Stamey, T. A.; Meares, E. M.; and Winningham, D. G.   Chronic bacterial prostatitis and the diffusion of drugs into prostatic fluid. *J. Urol.*, **1970**, *103*, 187–194.

Stamm, A. M.; McFall, D. W.; and Dismukes, W. E.   Failure of sulfonamides and trimethoprim in the treatment of nocardiosis. *Arch. Intern. Med.*, **1983**, *143*, 383–385.

Strauss, W. G., and Griffin, L. M.   Nitrofurantoin pneumonia. *J.A.M.A.*, **1967**, *199*, 765–766.

Stuart, R. K.; Braine, H. G.; Lietman, P. S.; Saral, R.; and Fuller, D. J.   Carbenicillin-trimethoprim/sulfamethoxazole versus carbenicillin-gentamicin as empiric therapy of infection in granulocytopenic patients. *Am. J. Med.*, **1980**, *68*, 876–885.

Summers, R. W.; Switz, D. M.; Sessions, J. T., Jr.; Becktel, J. M.; Best, W. R.; Kern, F., Jr.; and Singleton, J. W.   National Cooperative Crohn's Disease Study: results of drug treatment. *Gastroenterology*, **1979**, *77*, 847–869.

Taffet, S. L., and Das, K. M.   Desensitization of patients with inflammatory bowel disease to sulfasalazine. *Am. J. Med.*, **1982**, *73*, 520–524.

Tandon, M. K.   A comparative trial of co-trimoxazole and amoxycillin in the treatment of acute exacerbations of chronic bronchitis. *Med. J. Aust.*, **1977**, *2*, 281–284.

Thomas, V.; Shelokov, M.; and Furland, M.   Antibody-coated bacteria in urine and site of urinary tract infections. *N. Engl. J. Med.*, **1974**, *290*, 588–590.

Tolman, K. G. Nitrofurantoin and chronic active hepatitis. *Ann. Intern. Med.*, **1980**, *92*, 119–120.

Toole, J. F., and Parrish, M. L. Nitrofurantoin polyneuropathy. *Neurology (Minneap.)*, **1973**, *23*, 554–559.

Turck, M.; Anderson, K. N.; and Petersdorf, R. G. Relapse and reinfection in chronic bacteriuria. *N. Engl. J. Med.*, **1966**, *275*, 70–73.

Turck, M.; Ronald, A. R.; and Petersdorf, R. G. Relapse and reinfection in chronic bacteriuria. II. The correlation between site of infection and pattern of recurrence in chronic bacteriuria. *N. Engl. J. Med.*, **1968**, *278*, 422–427.

Vainrub, B., and Musher, D. M. Lack of effect of methenamine in suppression of, or prophylaxis against chronic urinary infection. *Antimicrob. Agents Chemother.*, **1977**, *12*, 625–629.

Vosti, K. L. Recurrent urinary tract infection. Prevention by prophylactic antibiotics after sexual intercourse. *J.A.M.A.*, **1975**, *231*, 934–940.

Ward, L. R.; Rowe, B.; and Threlfall, E. J. Incidence of trimethoprim resistance in salmonellae isolated in Britain: a twelve year study. *Lancet*, **1982**, *2*, 705–706.

Wharton, M.; Coleman, D. L.; Fitz, G.; Golden, J.; Wofsy, C.; Luce, J.; and Hopewell, P. Prospective, randomized trial of trimethoprim-sulfamethoxazole versus pentamidine for *Pneumocystis carinii* pneumonia in the acquired immunodeficiency syndrome. *Am. Rev. Respir. Dis.*, **1984**, *129*, A–188.

White, M. G., and Asch, M. J. Acid-base effects of topical mafenide acetate in the burned patient. *N. Engl. J. Med.*, **1971**, *284*, 1281–1286.

Willner, M. M.; Dull, T. A.; and McDonald, H. Comparison of trimethoprim-sulfamethoxazole and ampicillin in the treatment of acute bacterial otitis media in children. In, *Current Chemotherapy: Proceedings of the Tenth International Congress of Chemotherapy*, Vol. I. (Siegenthaler, W., and Lüthy, R., eds.) American Society for Microbiology, Washington, D. C., **1978**, pp. 125–127.

Woods, D. D. Relation of *p*-aminobenzoic acid to mechanism of action of sulphanilamide. *Br. J. Exp. Pathol.*, **1940**, *21*, 74–90.

—————. The biochemical mode of action of the sulphonamide drugs. *J. Gen. Microbiol.*, **1962**, *29*, 687–702.

Monographs and Reviews

Symposium. (Various authors.) The synergy of trimethoprim and sulphonamides. *Postgrad. Med. J.*, **1969**, *45*, Suppl., 3–104.

Symposium. (Various authors.) Trimethoprim-sulfamethoxazole. *J. Infect. Dis.*, **1973**, *128*, Suppl., 425–816.

Weinstein, L.; Madoff, M. A.; and Samet, C. A. The sulfonamides. *N. Engl. J. Med.*, **1960**, *263*, 793–800, 842–849, 900–907.

Wenzel, R. P.; Hunting, K. J.; Ostermary, C. O.; and Sande, M. A. *Providencia stuartii*, a hospital pathogen: potential factors for its emergence and transmission. *Am. J. Epidemiol.*, **1976**, *104*, 170–180.

Wormser, G. P.; Keusch, G. T.; and Rennie, C. H. Cotrimoxazole (trimethoprim-sulfamethoxazole): an updated review of its antibacterial activity and clinical efficacy. *Drugs*, **1982**, *24*, 459–518.

50 ANTIMICROBIAL AGENTS

[*Continued*]

Penicillins, Cephalosporins, and Other Beta-Lactam Antibiotics

Gerald L. Mandell and Merle A. Sande

THE PENICILLINS

Penicillin is one of the most important of the antibiotics. Although numerous other antimicrobial agents have been produced since penicillin became available, it is still a widely used, major antibiotic, and new derivatives of the basic penicillin nucleus are being produced every year. Many of these have unique advantages, such that members of this group of antibiotics are presently the drugs of choice for a large number of infectious diseases.

History. The history of the discovery and the development of penicillin has been recorded by the chief participants. (*See* Fleming, 1946; Florey, 1946, 1949; Abraham, 1949; Chain, 1954.) In 1928, while studying staphylococcus variants in the laboratory at St. Mary's Hospital in London, Alexander Fleming observed that a mold contaminating one of his cultures caused the bacteria in its vicinity to undergo lysis. Broth in which the fungus was grown was markedly inhibitory for many microorganisms. Because the mold belonged to the genus *Penicillium*, Fleming named the antibacterial substance *penicillin*.

A decade later penicillin was developed as a systemic therapeutic agent by the concerted and brilliant researches of a group of investigators at Oxford University headed by Florey, Chain, and Abraham. By May, 1940, the crude material then available was found to produce dramatic therapeutic effects when administered parenterally to mice with experimentally produced streptococcal infections. Despite great obstacles to its laboratory production, enough penicillin was accumulated by 1941 to conduct therapeutic trials in several patients desperately ill with staphylococcal and streptococcal infections refractory to all other therapy. At this stage, the crude amorphous penicillin was only about 10% pure and it required nearly 100 liters of the broth in which the mold had been grown to obtain enough of the antibiotic to treat one patient for 24 hours. Herrell (1945) records that bedpans were actually used by the Oxford group for growing cultures of *P. notatum*. Case 1 in the 1941

report from Oxford was that of a policeman who was suffering from a severe mixed staphylococcal and streptococcal infection. He was treated with penicillin, some of which had been recovered from the urine of other patients who had been given the drug. It is said that an Oxford professor referred to penicillin as a remarkable substance, grown in bedpans and purified by passage through the Oxford Police Force.

A vast research program was soon initiated in the United States. During 1942, 122 million units of penicillin were made available, and the first clinical trials were conducted at Yale University and the Mayo Clinic with dramatic results. By the spring of 1943, 200 patients had been treated with the drug. The results were so impressive that the surgeon general of the United States Army authorized trial of the antibiotic in a military hospital. Soon thereafter, penicillin was adopted throughout the medical services of the United States Armed Forces.

The deep-fermentation procedure for the biosynthesis of penicillin marked a crucial advance in the large-scale production of the antibiotic. From a total production of a few-hundred million units a month in the early days, the quantity manufactured rose to over 200 trillion units (nearly 150 tons) by 1950. The first marketable penicillin cost several dollars per 100,000 units; today, the same dose costs only a few cents.

Chemistry. The basic structure of the penicillins, as shown in Figure 50–1, consists of a thiazolidine ring (*A*) connected to a beta-lactam ring (*B*), to which is attached a side chain (*R*). The penicillin nucleus itself is the chief structural requirement for biological activity; metabolic transformation or chemical alteration of this portion of the molecule causes loss of all significant antibacterial activity. The side chain (*see* Table 50–1, page 1121) determines many of the antibacterial and pharmacological characteristics of a particular type of penicillin. Several natural penicillins can be produced, depending on the chemical composition of the fermentation medium used to culture

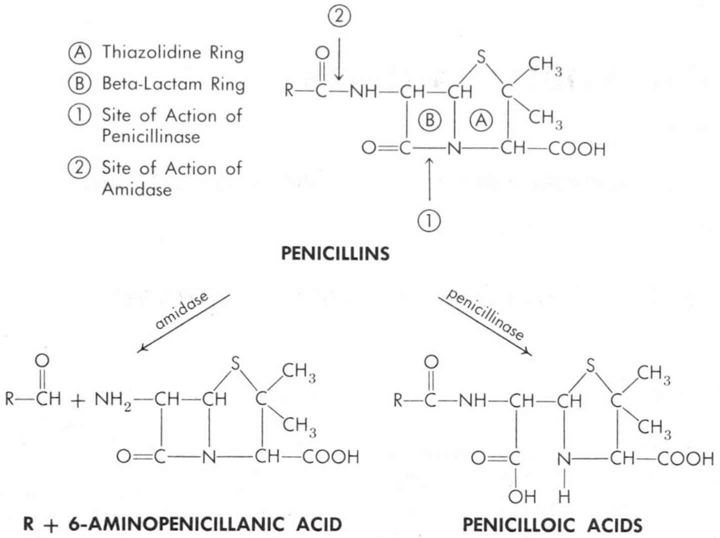

Figure 50–1. *Structure of penicillins and products of their enzymatic hydrolysis.*

Penicillium. Penicillin G (benzylpenicillin) has the greatest antimicrobial activity of these and is the only natural penicillin used clinically.

Semisynthetic Penicillins. The discovery that 6-aminopenicillanic acid could be obtained from cultures of *P. chrysogenum* that were depleted of side chain precursors led to the development of the semisynthetic penicillins. Side chains can be added that alter the susceptibility of the resultant compounds to inactivating enzymes (beta-lactamases) and that change the antibacterial activity and the pharmacological properties of the drug. 6-Aminopenicillanic acid is now produced in large quantities with the aid of an amidase from *P. chrysogenum* (Figure 50–1). This enzyme splits the peptide linkage by which the side chain of penicillin is joined to 6-aminopenicillanic acid.

Unitage of Penicillin. The *international unit of penicillin* is the specific penicillin activity contained in 0.6 μg of the crystalline sodium salt of penicillin G. One milligram of pure penicillin G sodium thus equals 1667 units. Because of the differences in molecular weight, 1.0 mg of pure penicillin G potassium represents 1595 units. The dosage and the antibacterial potency of the semisynthetic penicillins are expressed in terms of weight.

Assay. While various methods are available, microbiological assay is the method of choice for clinical purposes. This technic is widely employed for measurement of penicillin concentrations in blood, urine, and spinal and other body fluids, and for studies on the absorption, fate, and excretion of penicillin.

Mechanism of Action of the Penicillins and Cephalosporins. The beta-lactam antibiotics can kill susceptible bacteria. Although knowledge of the mechanism of this action is incomplete, numerous researchers have supplied information that allows understanding of the basic phenomenon (*see* Neu, 1976, 1983; Yocum *et al.*, 1980).

The cell walls of bacteria are essential for their normal growth and development. Peptidoglycan is a heteropolymeric component of the cell wall that provides rigid mechanical stability by virtue of its highly cross-linked latticework structure. In gram-positive microorganisms, the cell wall is 50 to 100 molecules thick, but it is only 1 or 2 molecules thick in gram-negative bacteria. The peptidoglycan is composed of glycan chains, which are linear strands of alternating pyranoside residues of two amino sugars (N-acetylglucosamine and N-acetylmuramic acid), that are cross-linked by peptide chains. The composition of the peptide cross-links is characteristic of individual microbial species. In *Staphylococcus aureus,* tetrapeptide units are bonded to the acetylmuramic acid residues, and pentaglycine chains bridge between the tetrapeptide moieties on adjacent strands (Figure 50–2).

The biosynthesis of the peptidoglycan involves about 30 bacterial enzymes and may be considered in three stages. The first stage, precursor formation, takes place in the cytoplasm. The product, uridine diphosphate (UDP)–acetylmuramyl-pentapeptide, called a "Park nucleotide" after its discoverer (Park and Stromenger, 1957), accumulates in cells when subsequent synthetic stages are inhibited. The last reaction in this stage is the addition of

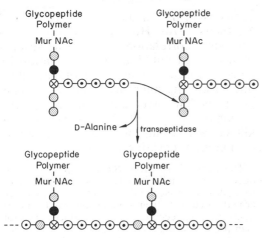

Figure 50–2. *The transpeptidase reaction in* Staphylococcus aureus *that is inhibited by penicillins and cephalosporins.*

See text for details. *Mur NAc* = N-acetyl-muramic acid; ⊘ = L-alanine; ● = D-gluta-mate; ⊗ = L-lysine; ⊖ = D-alanine; ⊙ = glycine.

a dipeptide, D-alanyl-D-alanine. Synthesis of the dipeptide involves prior racemization of L-alanine and condensation catalyzed by D-alanyl-D-alanine synthetase. D-Cycloserine is a structural analog of D-alanine and acts as a competitive inhibitor of both the racemase and the synthetase (*see* Chapter 53).

During reactions of the second stage, UDP-acetylmuramyl-pentapeptide and UDP-acetylglu-cosamine are linked (with the release of the uridine nucleotides) to form a long polymer. The sugar pentapeptide is first attached by a pyrophosphate bridge to a phospholipid in the cell membrane. The second sugar is then added, followed by the addition of five glycine residues as a branch of the heteropentapeptide. The first half of the pentaglycine cross-link is thus formed. The completed unit is then cleaved from the membrane-bound phospholipid, a reaction that is inhibited by vancomycin.

The third and final stage involves the completion of the cross-link. This is accomplished by a *transpeptidation reaction* that occurs outside the cell membrane. The transpeptidase itself is membrane bound. The terminal glycine residue of the pentaglycine bridge is linked to the fourth residue of the pentapeptide (D-alanine), releasing the fifth residue (also D-alanine) (Figure 50–2). It is this last step in peptidoglycan synthesis that is inhibited by the beta-lactam antibiotics. Stereomodels reveal that the conformation of penicillin is very similar to that of D-alanyl-D-alanine (Waxman *et al.,* 1980; Kelley *et al.,* 1982). The transpeptidase is probably acylated by penicillin; that is, penicilloyl enzyme is apparently formed, with cleavage of the —CO—N— bond of the beta-lactam ring.

Various penicillin-binding proteins are associ-ated with the bacterial cell membrane, and beta-lactam antibiotics bind tightly to them. These proteins are probably the transpeptidases and car-boxypeptidases that catalyze some of the terminal reactions in bacterial cell-wall synthesis (Spratt, 1975, 1980). The penicillin-binding proteins vary from one bacterial species to another and in their affinity for different beta-lactam antibiotics.

Beta-lactam antibiotics produce certain charac-teristic morphological effects on bacteria, and these are probably related to the particular penicil-lin-binding proteins that are most affected. These changes are dependent on the antibiotic, its con-centration, and the microbe. Bacteria may form long filamentous forms and fail to divide. Under certain conditions growth may take place at the midportion of a rod with formation of a bulge. Mi-croorganisms may swell and then rupture, with ex-trusion of their contents. In medium that is isos-motic with bacterial cytoplasm, relatively stable cell-wall-deficient bacteria (protoplasts) may be formed. In general, at the lowest effective concen-trations of a beta-lactam antibiotic, cell division is inhibited but elongation continues. As the concen-tration of the antibiotic is increased, growth is in-hibited, bulges may form, and lysis is then ob-served.

Data suggest that *lysis* of bacteria is due to the activity of bacterial enzymes, autolysins, probably including murein hydrolases. These enzymes may function normally in processes related to cell divi-sion. Beta-lactam antibiotics appear to decrease the availability of an inhibitor of murein hydrolase. The uninhibited enzyme can then destroy the struc-tural integrity of the cell. Certain bacterial strains (*e.g.,* strains of *Staph. aureus* and *Streptococcus pneumoniae*) that lack these autolysins have been identified. Beta-lactam antibiotics inhibit the growth of the microorganisms, but lysis does not take place; these bacteria are thus "tolerant" to penicillin (*see* Tomasz and Holtje, 1977; Tomasz, 1979). Patients with staphylococcal endocarditis caused by such microorganisms have been re-ported. Some of these patients may require therapy with agents that have a different mechanism of action, such as vancomycin, rifampin, or an amino-glycoside (*see* Sabath *et al.,* 1977).

Mechanisms of Bacterial Resistance to Penicillins and Cephalosporins. Beta-lac-tam antibiotics cannot kill or even inhibit all bacteria, and various mechanisms of bacte-rial resistance to these agents are operative. The microorganism may be intrinsically resistant because of structural differences in the enzymes that are the targets of these drugs. Furthermore, it is possible for a sen-sitive strain to acquire resistance of this type by mutation. However, in the case of the beta-lactam antibiotics this mechanism for the acquisition of resistance is probably relatively unimportant (*see* Tomasz, 1984).

Other instances of bacterial resistance to the beta-lactam antibiotics are caused by the inability of the agent to penetrate to its site of action (Jaffe *et al.*, 1982; Kobayashi *et al.*, 1982). In gram-positive bacteria the peptidoglycan polymer is very near the cell surface. Only surface macromolecules (capsule) are external to the peptidoglycan. The small beta-lactam antibiotic molecules can easily penetrate to the outer layer of the cytoplasmic membrane and the penicillin-binding proteins, where the final stages of the synthesis of the peptidoglycan take place. The situation is different with gram-negative bacteria. Their surface structure is more complex, and the inner membrane (which is analogous to the cytoplasmic membrane of gram-positive bacteria) is covered by the outer membrane, lipopolysaccharide, and capsule. The outer membrane functions as an impenetrable barrier for certain hydrophilic antibiotics (*see* Richmond, 1978).

Bacteria can destroy beta-lactam antibiotics enzymatically. While amidohydrolases may be present, these enzymes are relatively inactive and do not protect the bacteria. Beta-lactamases or penicillinases, however, are capable of inactivating certain of these antibiotics and may be present in large quantity (*see* Figure 50–1). The different penicillins and cephalosporins vary in their susceptibility to the beta-lactamases that are produced by different bacterial species.

In general, gram-positive bacteria produce a large amount of beta-lactamase that is secreted extracellularly. The information for staphylococcal penicillinase is encoded in a plasmid, and this may be transferred by phage to other bacteria; the enzyme is inducible by substrates. In gram-negative bacteria, beta-lactamases are found in relatively small amounts but are located in the periplasmic space between the inner and outer cell membranes. Since the enzymes of cell-wall synthesis are on the outer surface of the inner membrane, these beta-lactamases are strategically located for maximal protection of the microbe. Beta-lactamases of gram-negative bacteria are encoded either in chromosomes or plasmids, and they may be constitutive or inducible. They may hydrolyze penicillins, cephalosporins, or both (*see* Sykes and Matthew, 1976). However, there is an inconsistent correlation between the susceptibility of an antibiotic to inactivation by beta-lactamase and the ability of that antibiotic to kill the microorganism. For example, penicillins that are hydrolyzed by beta-lactamase (*e.g.*, carbenicillin) are able to kill certain strains of beta-lactamase-producing gram-negative microbes.

The penicillinase from *Bacillus* species is produced commercially (NEUTRAPEN). It can be used to hydrolyze susceptible penicillins to augment growth of cultures from samples obtained from patients who are receiving the drug. Since it is a foreign protein, it must not be used to treat patients who are experiencing an allergic reaction to a penicillin.

Other Factors That Influence the Activity of Beta-Lactam Antibiotics. The density of the bacterial population and the age of an infection influence the activity of beta-lactam antibiotics. The drugs may be several thousand times more potent when tested against small bacterial inocula compared to their activity against a dense culture. Many factors are involved. Among these are the greater number of relatively resistant microorganisms in a large population, the amount of beta-lactamase produced, and the phase of growth of the culture. The clinical significance of this effect of inoculum size is uncertain. The intensity and the duration of penicillin therapy needed to abort or cure experimental infections in animals increase with the duration of the infection. The reason is primarily that the bacteria are no longer multiplying as rapidly as they are in a fresh infection. These antibiotics are most active against bacteria in the logarithmic phase of growth and have little effect on microorganisms in the lag phase, when there is no need to synthesize components of the cell wall.

The presence of proteins and other constituents of pus does not appreciably decrease the ability of beta-lactam antibiotics to kill bacteria. However, bacteria that survive inside viable cells of the host are protected from the action of the beta-lactam antibiotics (*see* Mandell, 1973a). These antibiotics are active when pH or oxygen tension is low.

CLASSIFICATION OF THE PENICILLINS AND SUMMARY OF THEIR PHARMACOLOGICAL PROPERTIES

It is useful to classify the penicillins according to their spectrum of antimicrobial activity (*see* Table 50–1, page 1121; Neu, 1985).

1. Penicillin G and its close congener penicillin V are highly active against gram-positive cocci, but they are readily hydrolyzed by penicillinase. Thus, they are

ineffective against most strains of *Staph. aureus.*

2. The penicillinase-resistant penicillins (methicillin, nafcillin, oxacillin, cloxacillin, dicloxacillin, and floxacillin) have less potent antimicrobial activity against microorganisms that are sensitive to penicillin G, but they are the drugs of choice for infections caused by penicillinase-producing *Staph. aureus.*

3. Ampicillin, amoxicillin, hetacillin, cyclacillin, bacampicillin, and others comprise a group of penicillins whose antimicrobial activity is extended to include such gram-negative microorganisms as *Haemophilus influenzae*, *Escherichia coli*, and *Proteus mirabilis*. All of these drugs and the others listed below that are particularly effective against gram-negative bacteria are readily hydrolyzed by staphylococcal penicillinase.

4. The antimicrobial activity of carbenicillin and its indanyl ester (carbenicillin indanyl), ticarcillin, and azlocillin is extended to include *Pseudomonas*, *Enterobacter*, and *Proteus* species.

5. Other extended-spectrum penicillins include mezlocillin and piperacillin, which have useful antimicrobial activity against *Pseudomonas*, *Klebsiella*, and certain other gram-negative microorganisms. Amdinocillin (also called mecillinam) has poor activity against gram-positive microorganisms but good activity against Enterobacteriaceae. Its use is primarily in combination with other beta-lactam antibiotics, with which it acts synergistically to kill many resistant microorganisms.

While the pharmacological properties of the individual drugs are discussed in detail below, certain generalizations are useful. Following absorption, penicillins are widely distributed throughout the body. Therapeutic concentrations of these agents are readily achieved in tissues and in such secretions as joint fluid, pleural fluid, pericardial fluid, and bile. However, only small amounts of these drugs are found in prostatic secretions, brain tissue, and intraocular fluid, and penicillins do not penetrate living phagocytic cells to a significant extent. Concentrations of penicillins in cerebrospinal fluid (CSF) are variable but are less than 1% of those in plasma when the

meninges are normal. When there is inflammation, concentrations in CSF may rise to be as high as 5% of the plasma value. Penicillins are rapidly eliminated, particularly by glomerular filtration and renal tubular secretion, such that their half-lives in the body are short; values of 30 to 60 minutes are typical. Concentrations of these drugs in urine are thus high.

PENICILLIN G AND PENICILLIN V

Antimicrobial Activity. The antimicrobial spectra of penicillin G (benzylpenicillin) and penicillin V (the phenoxymethyl derivative) are very similar for aerobic gram-positive microorganisms. However, penicillin G is five to ten times more active against gram-negative microorganisms, especially *Neisseria* species, and certain anaerobes.

Penicillin G is highly effective *in vitro* against many, but not all, species of gram-positive and gram-negative cocci. Streptococci, with the exception of enterococci, are very susceptible to the drug, less than 0.01 μg/ml being effective. Whereas most strains of *Staph. aureus* were highly sensitive to similar concentrations of penicillin G when this agent was first employed therapeutically, *most* staphylococci isolated from individuals outside of hospitals are now resistant to penicillin G; in hospitalized patients, the incidence of resistant strains may be as high as 90 to 95%. Many strains of *Staph. epidermidis* are also resistant to penicillin. *Gonococci* are generally sensitive to penicillin G, although continued exposure of this microorganism to the antibiotic has led to a general decrease in sensitivity. Rare strains are highly resistant to penicillin and produce penicillinase. *Meningococci* are quite sensitive to penicillin G. *Pneumococci* of all serological types are, in general, highly susceptible to penicillin G; however, some highly resistant strains have now been described, and hospitals should test their isolates of these bacteria as a means of surveillance.

Although the vast majority of strains of *Corynebacterium diphtheriae* are sensitive to penicillin G, some are highly resistant. This is also true for *Bacillus anthracis*. Most anaerobic microorganisms, including *Clostridium* species, are highly sensitive. *Bacteroides fragilis* is an exception; however, high doses of penicillin (20 million units per day) result in concentrations in blood that inhibit 50 to 80% of strains of this bacterium. *Actinomyces israelii*, *Streptobacillus moniliformis*, *Pasteurella multocida*, and *Listeria monocytogenes* are inhibited by penicillin G. Most species of *Leptospira* are moderately susceptible to the drug. One of the most exquisitely sensitive microorganisms is *Treponema pallidum*. None of the penicillins is effective against *amebae, plasmodia, rickettsiae, fungi,* or *viruses.*

Although many species of *gram-negative bacilli* are resistant to penicillin G, some are affected by moderate-to-high concentrations. The majority of strains of *Pr. mirabilis* are inhibited by 10 μg/ml or less of the drug. Many strains of *E. coli* are also susceptible to high concentrations of penicillin G.

Absorption. *Oral Administration of Penicillin G.* About one third of an orally administered dose of penicillin G is absorbed from the intestinal tract under favorable conditions. Only a small portion is absorbed from the stomach. Gastric juice at pH 2 rapidly destroys the antibiotic. The decrease in gastric acid production with aging, as well as the development of achlorhydria in about 35% of persons over 60 years of age, accounts for better absorption of penicillin G from the gastrointestinal tract of older individuals. Absorption occurs mainly in the duodenum; it is rapid, and maximal concentrations in blood are attained in 30 to 60 minutes. The peak value is approximately 0.5 unit/ml (0.3 μg/ml) after an oral dose of 400,000 units (about 250 mg) in an adult. Two thirds or more of an ingested dose is unabsorbed and passes into the colon, where it is largely inactivated by bacteria; only a small amount is excreted in the feces. The oral dose of penicillin G must be four to five times as large as the intramuscular in order to obtain concentrations in blood of comparable height and duration. The two important points to observe in prescribing penicillin G by mouth are to be certain that the dose is adequate, and that it is taken at least 0.5 hour before a meal and no earlier than 2 to 3 hours after a meal. Ingestion of food interferes with enteric absorption of penicillin, perhaps by adsorption of the antibiotic on food particles. Despite the convenience of oral administration of penicillin G, this route should be used only in those infections in which clinical experience has proven its efficacy.

Oral Administration of Penicillin V. The sole virtue of penicillin V in comparison with penicillin G is that it is more stable in an acidic medium and, therefore, is better absorbed from the gastrointestinal tract. After oral ingestion, the drug escapes destruction in gastric juice, since it is both in-

soluble and stable at a low pH. It goes into solution in the more alkaline medium of the duodenum and is well but incompletely absorbed from the upper portion of the small intestine. On an equivalent oral-dose basis, the compound yields plasma concentrations two to five times greater than those provided by penicillin G. The peak concentration in the blood of an adult after an oral dose of 500 mg is nearly 3 μg/ml. There is some evidence that the drug is better absorbed when ingested after a meal than on an empty stomach. Once absorbed, penicillin V is distributed in the body and excreted by the kidney in the same manner as penicillin G.

Parenteral Administration of Penicillin G. After intramuscular injection, peak concentrations in plasma are reached within 15 to 30 minutes. This value declines rapidly, since the half-life of penicillin G is 30 minutes.

Many means for prolonging the sojourn of the antibiotic in the body and thereby reducing the frequency of injections have been explored. *Probenecid* blocks renal tubular secretion of penicillin, but it is rarely used for this purpose (*see* below and Chapter 38). More commonly, *repository preparations* of penicillin G are employed. The two such compounds currently favored are *penicillin G procaine* and *penicillin G benzathine* (*see* section on preparations). Such agents release penicillin G slowly from the area in which they are injected and produce relatively low but persistent concentrations of antibiotic in the blood.

The injection of 300,000 units of penicillin G procaine produces a peak concentration in plasma of about 1.5 units/ml within 1 to 3 hours; after 24 hours the concentration is reduced to 0.2 unit/ml, and by 48 hours it has fallen to 0.05 unit/ml. A larger dose (600,000 units) yields somewhat higher values that are maintained for as long as 4 to 5 days.

Penicillin G benzathine is very slowly absorbed from intramuscular depots and produces the longest duration of detectable antibiotic of all the available repository penicillins. For example, in adults, a dose of 1.2 million units given intramuscularly produces a concentration in plasma of 0.15 unit/ml on the first, 0.03 unit/ml on the fourteenth, and 0.003 unit/ml on the thirty-second day after injection. The average duration of demonstrable antimicrobial activity in the plasma is about 26 days. Similar pharmacokinetic data are available for newborn

Table 50–1. CHEMICAL STRUCTURES AND MAJOR PROPERTIES OF VARIOUS PENICILLINS

SIDE CHAIN *	NONPROPRIETARY NAME	MAJOR PROPERTIES		
		Absorption after Oral Administration	Resistance to Penicillinase	Useful Antimicrobial Spectrum
(phenyl)—CH_2—	Penicillin G	Variable (poor)	No	*Streptococcus* species, *Neisseria* species, many anaerobes, spirochetes, others
(phenyl)—OCH_2—	Penicillin V	Good	No	
(benzene ring with OCH_3 and OCH_3)	Methicillin	Poor (not given orally)	Yes	
(isoxazolyl ring, R_1, R_2, CH_3, N, O)	Oxacillin ($R_1 = R_2 = H$) Cloxacillin ($R_1 = Cl$; $R_2 = H$) Dicloxacillin ($R_1 = R_2 = Cl$) Floxacillin ($R_1 = Cl$; $R_2 = F$)	Good	Yes	*Staphylococcus aureus*
(naphthalene ring, OC_2H_5)	Nafcillin	Variable	Yes	
R—(phenyl)—CH—NH_2	Ampicillin † ($R = H$) Amoxicillin ($R = OH$)	Good / Excellent	No	*Haemophilus influenzae*, *Proteus mirabilis*, ‡ *Escherichia coli*, ‡ *Neisseria* species
(phenyl)—CH—$COOR$	Carbenicillin ($R = H$) Carbenicillin indanyl ($R = 5$-indanol)	Poor (not given orally) / Good	No	Above plus *Pseudomonas* species, *Enterobacter* species, and *Proteus* (indole positive)
(thiophene ring, S)—CH—$COOH$	Ticarcillin	Poor (not given orally)	No	
(phenyl)—CH—$NHCO$—(imidazolidinone ring, N, O, NH)	Azlocillin	Poor (not given orally)	No	*Pseudomonas* species

* Equivalent to R in Figure 50–1 (page 1116).
† There are various other congeners of ampicillin; *see* the text.
‡ Up to 30% of strains may be resistant to ampicillin.

Table 50-1.   CHEMICAL STRUCTURES AND MAJOR PROPERTIES OF VARIOUS PENICILLINS

SIDE CHAIN *	NONPROPRIETARY NAME	MAJOR PROPERTIES		
		Absorption after Oral Administration	Resistance to Penicillinase	Useful Antimicrobial Spectrum
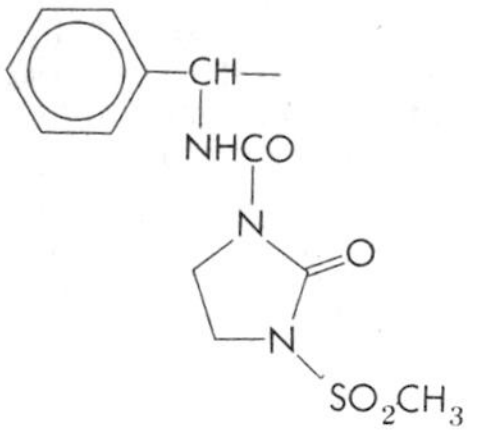	Mezlocillin	Poor (not given orally)	No	*Pseudomonas* species, *Enterobacter* species, many *Klebsiella*
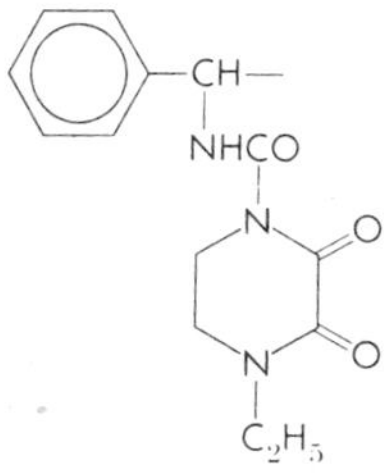	Piperacillin	Poor (not given orally)	No	*Pseudomonas* species, *Enterobacter* species, many *Klebsiella*

infants (Kaplan and McCracken, 1973; Klein *et al.*, 1973).

Absorption from Other Routes. Although suppositories of penicillin G yield detectable concentrations in plasma when inserted in the *rectum* or *vagina,* such therapy is undependable and not advised. The antibiotic is also absorbed from serous surfaces such as the *pleura, pericardium,* and *peritoneum,* and from *joint cavities,* the *subarachnoid space,* and the *respiratory tract.* Penicillin G is not absorbed through the unbroken *skin.*

Intrathecal administration of any of the penicillins is no longer recommended. Penicillin is a potent convulsant when given by this route. Bactericidal concentrations of the drug can be attained in the brain and meninges by the use of other parenteral routes.

Distribution.   Penicillin G is widely distributed throughout the body, but the concentrations in various fluids and tissues differ widely. Its apparent volume of distribution is in about 50% of total body water. More than 90% of the penicillin G in blood is in the plasma and less than 10% is in the erythrocytes; approximately 65% is reversibly bound to plasma albumin. Significant amounts appear in liver, bile, kidney, semen, joint fluid, lymph, and intestine.

While probenecid markedly decreases the tubular secretion of the penicillins, this is not the only factor responsible for the elevated plasma concentrations of the antibiotic that follow its administration. Probenecid produces a significant decrease in the volume of distribution of the penicillins (Gibaldi *et al.*, 1970).

Cerebrospinal Fluid.   Penicillin does not readily enter the cerebrospinal fluid (CSF) when the meninges are normal. A plasma concentration of less than 10 units/ml cannot be depended on to establish therapeutically effective concentrations in the CSF. When the meninges are acutely inflamed, penicillin penetrates into the CSF more easily. Although the concentrations attained vary and are unpredictable, they are usually in the range of 5% of the value in plasma and are often therapeutically effective.

Penicillin and other organic acids are rapidly secreted from the CSF into the blood stream by an active transport process. Probenecid competitively inhibits this transport and thus elevates the concentration of penicillin in CSF (Dacey and Sande, 1974; Spector and Lorenzo, 1974). In uremia, other organic acids accumulate in the CSF and compete with penicillin for secretion; the drug occasionally reaches toxic concentrations in brain and can produce convulsions (Spector and Snodgrass, 1976).

Excretion. Under normal conditions, penicillin G is rapidly eliminated from the body, mainly by the kidney but in small part in the bile and by other channels. The rapid renal excretion of the antibiotic is the reason for the use of measures to prolong its sojourn in the body, such as repository insoluble salts of the drug or the administration of probenecid.

Renal. Approximately 60 to 90% of an intramuscular dose of penicillin G in aqueous solution is eliminated in the urine, largely within the first hour after injection. The half-time for elimination is about 30 minutes in normal adults. Approximately 10% of the drug is eliminated by glomerular filtration and 90% by tubular secretion. Renal clearance approximates the total renal plasma flow. The maximal tubular secretory capacity (Tm) for penicillin in the normal male adult is about 3 million units (1.8 g) per hour.

Clearance values are considerably lower in neonates and infants, because of incomplete development of renal function; as a result, after doses proportionate to surface area, the persistence of penicillin in the blood is several times as long in premature infants as in children and adults. The half-life of the antibiotic in children less than 1 week old is 3 hours; by 14 days of age it is 1.4 hours (McCracken *et al.*, 1973). After renal function is fully established in young children, the rate of renal excretion of penicillin G is considerably more rapid than in adults. For example, following an intramuscular dose of 300,000 units of penicillin G in aqueous solution in a 3- to 4-year-old child, concentrations of the drug in plasma are no longer detectable after 2 to 3 hours. With increasing age and its accompanying decrease in renal tubular excretory function, the rate of elimination of the antibiotic by the kidney is decreased. The renal plasma clearance of penicillin is markedly diminished in the presence of other organic acids that are secreted by the renal tubules.

Approximately 20% of an *oral* dose of penicillin G is excreted in the urine, a reflection of the limited intestinal absorption of the drug; once penicillin has been absorbed, its fate and excretion are the same as for the injected antibiotic.

Anuria increases the half-life of penicillin G from a normal value of 0.5 hour to about 10 hours. When renal function is impaired, 7 to 10% of the antibiotic may be inactivated per hour by the liver. This probably accounts for its failure to accumulate in excessive concentrations in anuric persons given multiple doses. Patients with renal shutdown who require vigorous therapy with penicillin can be treated adequately with 3 million units of aqueous penicillin G followed by additional injections of 1.5 million units every 8 to 12 hours. The dose of the drug must be readjusted during the period of progressive recovery of renal function. If, in addition to renal failure, hepatic insufficiency is also present, the half-life will be prolonged further. It may be necessary to determine the half-life of the drug for the individual patient.

Once penicillin G is released from its repository forms (penicillin G procaine and penicillin G benzathine), it is excreted by the kidney as described above. However, because absorption into the blood from the injection site is continued over a long period, the excretion of active antibiotic in the urine is prolonged. For example, Wright and coworkers (1959) detected penicillin G in the urine of 100% of patients 84 days after an intramuscular injection of 1.2 million units of penicillin G benzathine.

Bile and Other Fluids. Penicillin G is present in human bile, where it is more concentrated and persists longer than in plasma. Biliary excretion of the drug is directly proportional to the adequacy of hepatic function.

A small amount of penicillin G is excreted in human milk and saliva, the concentrations being lower than in plasma. The drug does not appear in detectable quantities in the sweat or tears in man.

Preparations and Dosage. Preparations of penicillin G that are available for parenteral use include aqueous solutions and repository forms that are slowly absorbed from intramuscular depots. In addition, there are many preparations of penicillin G and penicillin V for oral administration. Details of *dosage* of these preparations are presented subsequently, in the discussion of the treatment of specific infections. The use of penicillin G preparations for *inhalational therapy* and for *topical* *application* to skin and mucous membranes is not recommended because they are ineffective and because they produce a high incidence of hypersensitization.

Penicillin G in Aqueous Solution for Parenteral Use. This preparation should be limited to use by the intravenous route. It can be given as an infusion over 20 to 30 minutes or by constant drip. Because of the rapid rate of renal excretion of the drug, intravenous doses should be given at close intervals (usually every 2 to 4 hours) or by constant infusion. The potassium salts are most frequently used. The two penicillin salts for injection are *penicillin G potassium* and *penicillin G sodium*. The preparations are crystalline powders, marketed for parenteral use in sterile dry form in vials containing 200,000 to 20 million units each. It should be remembered that each million units of penicillin G potassium contains about 1.7 mEq of potassium. Because the stability of penicillin G is affected by changes in pH (it is most stable at pH 6 to 7.2), it is physically incompatible with many drugs; other agents should not be mixed with the penicillin solution. Usual doses of intravenous penicillin G for adults are 6 to 20 million units per day in four to six portions or by continuous infusion. Severe infections, such as meningitis, should be treated either by continuous infusion or with doses every 2 to 3 hours. Children should receive 100,000 to 250,000 units/kg per day in four to six portions. Newborns up to 1 week of age should receive 50,000 to 150,000 units/kg per day in two or three portions.

Penicillin G Preparations for Parenteral Use in Repository Form for Prolonged Action. Repository penicillin preparations are designed for deep intramuscular injection, to provide a tissue depot from which the drug is slowly absorbed over a period of 12 hours to several days. The objective is to maintain therapeutic concentrations in plasma with as few injections as possible. *Repository penicillin should never be injected intravenously or subcutaneously or into body cavities.*

Penicillin G procaine suspension (DURACILLIN A.S., WYCILLIN, others) is an aqueous preparation of the crystalline salt that is soluble in water only to the extent of 0.4%. Penicillin G procaine preparations are marketed for intramuscular injection in cartridges and vials, each milliliter usually containing 300,000, 500,000, or 600,000 units of the antibiotic.

Procaine combines with penicillin mole for mole; therefore, a dose of 300,000 units contains approximately 120 mg of procaine. When large doses of penicillin G procaine are given (*e.g.*, 4.8 million units), procaine may reach toxic concentrations in the plasma (*see* Green *et al.*, 1974). If the patient is believed to be hypersensitive to procaine, 0.1 ml of 1% solution of procaine should be injected intradermally; individuals exhibiting a positive local response should not be given penicillin G procaine. A slight anesthetic effect of the procaine accounts in part for the fact that injections of penicillin G procaine are virtually painless.

Penicillin G benzathine suspension (BICILLIN L-A, PERMAPEN) is the aqueous suspension of the salt obtained by the combination of 1 mole of an ammonium base and 2 moles of penicillin G to yield N,N′-dibenzylethylenediamine dipenicillin G. The salt itself is soluble in water only to the extent of 0.02%. It is provided for intramuscular injection in vials containing 300,000 units/ml and in prefilled syringes containing 600,000 units/ml. The long persistence of penicillin in the blood after a suitable intramuscular dose reduces cost, need for repeated injections, and local trauma. The local anesthetic effect of penicillin G benzathine is comparable to that of penicillin G procaine. Penicillin G benzathine should be used only for treatment or prophylaxis of group-A beta-hemolytic streptococcal pharyngitis, treatment of group-A beta-hemolytic streptococcal pyoderma, or treatment of syphilis outside the central nervous system (CNS).

Preparations of Penicillin G and Penicillin V for Oral Use. The oral preparations of penicillin G are *penicillin G potassium tablets, penicillin G potassium powder for oral solution,* and *penicillin G benzathine tablets.* They are marketed as tablets containing from 200,000 to 800,000 units. Various buffer materials are sometimes added; these increase stability of the antibiotic but do not significantly protect against destruction of penicillin G in the acidic gastric contents. Dry salts of penicillin G mixed with flavoring material and various buffers are available for pediatric use.

Penicillin V potassium (PEN-VEE K, V-CILLIN K, others) is supplied for oral use as tablets (125, 250, or 500 mg each) and powders for solution (125 or 250 mg/5 ml). *Penicillin V* is marketed in dosage forms and unitages similar to those for the potassium salt. *Penicillin V benzathine and penicillin V hydrabamine* are additional preparations.

Therapeutic Uses. Penicillin G is the antibiotic of choice for a wide variety of infectious diseases (*see* Table 48–1, page 1072).

Pneumococcal Infections. Penicillin G remains the agent of choice for the management of infections of all types caused by *Strep. pneumoniae.* However, rare strains of pneumococci resistant to usual doses of penicillin G have been encountered in several countries, including the United States (*see* Jacobs *et al.*, 1978), and up to 22% of strains isolated from children are now in the moderately resistant range (minimal inhibitory concentration, 0.5 to 1.0 μg/ml).

Pneumococcal Pneumonia. A variety of dose schedules and types of penicillin have been employed successfully in the treatment of pneumococcal pneumonia. For parenteral therapy, penicillin G or penicillin G procaine are favored, and 300,000 to 600,000 units of procaine penicillin G, given intramuscularly every 12 hours, is adequate therapy for uncomplicated cases. Although oral treatment with 500 mg of penicillin V given every 6 hours has been used with success in this disease, it cannot be recommended for routine initial use. The doses of penicillin G currently used are, in all probability, excessive. Therapy should be continued for 7 to 10 days, including 3 to 5 days after the temperature has returned to normal.

Pneumococcal Empyema. The frequency of this complication of pneumococcal pneumonia has been sharply reduced by penicillin therapy of the primary lung disease. It is not necessary to instill the antibiotic intrapleurally when purulent exudate is present in the pleural space; in such instances, however, the dose of penicillin should be increased to 10 to 20 million units per day, and adequate drainage must be ensured. Patients frequently develop nonpurulent pleural effusions that do not contain pneumococci; these can be treated by drainage, and it is not necessary to increase the dosage of penicillin G.

Pneumococcal Meningitis. Penicillin has reduced the death rate in this disease from nearly 100% to between 8 and 25%. The recommended therapy is 20 to 24 million units of penicillin G daily by constant intravenous drip or divided into boluses given every 2 to 3 hours. The usual duration of therapy is 14 days.

Other Pneumococcal Infections. Penicillin G provides optimal therapy for suppurative *arthritis, osteomyelitis, acute suppurative mastoiditis, endocarditis, peritonitis,* and *pericarditis* due to the pneumococcus. Because of poor penetration of the drug into purulent exudate, the plasma and tissue-fluid concentrations must be high; this is best accomplished by the intravenous administration of large doses of aqueous penicillin G. Doses on the order of 10 to 20 million units per day may be required for cure. Oral and repository penicillins should not be used. The shortest period of treatment for any of these disorders should be 2 weeks. This should be prolonged to at least 4 weeks if there is infection of bone. Infections in the *middle ear* and *paranasal sinuses* caused by the pneumococcus may be treated with 300,000 to 600,000 units of procaine penicillin G intramuscularly every 12 hours or with 250 to 500 mg of oral penicillin V every 6 hours.

Streptococcal Infections. Streptococcal Pharyngitis (Including Scarlet Fever). This is the most common disease produced by *Strep. pyogenes* (group-A beta-hemolytic streptococcus). The preferred oral therapy is with penicillin V, 500 mg every 6 hours for 10 days. Equally good results are produced by the administration of 600,000 units of penicillin G procaine intramuscularly, once daily for 10 days, or by a single injection of 1.2 million units of penicillin G benzathine. Penicillin therapy of streptococcal pharyngitis reduces the risk of subsequent acute rheumatic fever; however, present evidence suggests that the incidence of glomerulonephritis that follows streptococcal infections is not reduced to a significant degree by treatment with penicillin.

Streptococcal Pneumonia, Arthritis, Meningitis, and Endocarditis. While uncommon, when these conditions are caused by *Strep. pyogenes,* they should be treated with daily doses of 10 to 20 million units of penicillin G intravenously for 2 to 4 weeks. Such treatment of endocarditis should be continued for a full 4 weeks.

Streptococcal Otitis Media and Sinusitis. Treatment with an oral preparation, such as 250 to 500 mg of penicillin V every 6 hours for 2 weeks, is usually adequate. Streptococcal mastoiditis is now an uncommon complication of otitis media; it should be treated with high doses of parenteral penicillin G for at least 2 weeks.

Infections Due to Other Streptococci. Group-B (*Strep. agalactiae*) streptococcal infections, including meningitis and bacteremia, are frequent in neonates and should be treated with high doses of penicillin G given parenterally (150,000 to 250,000 units/kg per day).

The *viridans* streptococci are the most common cause of infectious endocarditis. These are nongroupable alpha-hemolytic microorganisms that are usually highly sensitive to penicillin G (minimal inhibitory concentration less than 0.1 μg/ml). Since enterococci may also be beta-hemolytic and certain other alpha-hemolytic strains may be relatively resistant to penicillin, it is important to determine quantitative microbial sensitivities to penicillin G in patients with endocarditis. Patients with penicillin-sensitive *viridans*-group streptococcal endocarditis have been successfully treated with 1.2 million units of procaine penicillin G, given four times daily for 2 weeks, or with daily doses of 6 to 10 million units of intravenous penicillin G for 2 weeks, both regimens in combination with streptomycin, 500 mg intramuscularly twice daily. Some physicians prefer a 4-week course of treatment with penicillin G alone (Bisno *et al.,* 1981).

Enterococcal endocarditis is one of the few diseases that is optimally treated with two antibiotics. The recommended therapy is 20 million units of penicillin G daily, administered intravenously in combination with an aminoglycoside. Some physicians prefer to initiate treatment with streptomycin (500 mg intramuscularly every 12 hours) in combination with penicillin. Others prefer to initiate treatment with gentamicin (1 mg/kg every 8 hours) plus penicillin, since up to 40% of enterococcal strains are highly resistant to streptomycin *in vitro.* If synergism between penicillin and streptomycin is demonstrated (*see* Chapter 48), then therapy with penicillin and streptomycin should be used. Therapy should usually be continued for 6 weeks, but selected patients with a short duration of illness have been treated successfully in 4 weeks (Wilson *et al.,* 1984).

Infections with Anaerobes. Many anaerobic infections are caused by mixtures of microorganisms. The majority are sensitive to penicillin G. An exception is *B. fragilis,* where 20 to 50% of strains may be resistant to high concentrations of this antibiotic. Pulmonary and periodontal infections usually respond well to penicillin G, although a multicenter study indicated that clindamycin is more effective than penicillin for therapy of lung abscess (Levison *et al.,* 1983). Mild-to-moderate infections at these sites may be treated with oral medication (either penicillin G or penicillin V, 400,000 units four times daily). More severe infections should be treated with 10 to 20 million units of penicillin G intravenously. Anaerobic infections involving the gastrointestinal tract and certain pelvic infections may be due in part to *B. fragilis.* The most serious infections should be treated with either clindamycin, chloramphenicol, or metronidazole. Because aerobic gram-negative bacteria may also be involved, an aminoglycoside should be included for the treatment of anaerobic infections originating from the gastrointestinal tract. Brain abscesses also frequently contain several species of anaerobes, and most authorities prefer to treat such disease with high doses of penicillin G (20 million units per day) plus chloramphenicol (2 to 4 g per day, intravenously) or metronidazole (2 to 4 g per day, intravenously).

Staphylococcal Infections. The great majority of staphylococcal infections (80 to 95%) are caused by microorganisms that produce penicillinase. A patient with a staphylococcal infection who requires treatment with an antibiotic should receive one of the penicillinase-resistant penicillins—for example, nafcillin, oxacillin, or methicillin. However, since penicillin G is more active than are the penicillinase-resistant penicillins against the rare staphylococci that do not produce the enzyme, it should be utilized when staphylococcal sensitivity to penicillin G has been demonstrated. Severe infections should be treated with intravenous doses of 10 to 20 million units of penicillin G per day.

Hospitals throughout the world have reported infections due to so-called methicillin-resistant staphylococci. These microorganisms are resistant to penicillin G, all of the penicillinase-resistant penicillins, and the cephalosporins. Isolates may occasionally appear to be sensitive to various cephalosporins *in vitro*, but resistant populations arise during therapy and lead to failure (Chambers *et al.*, 1984). Vancomycin is the drug of choice for infections caused by these bacteria.

Meningococcal Infections. Penicillin G remains the drug of choice for meningococcal disease. Patients should be treated with high doses of penicillin given intravenously, as described for pneumococcal meningitis. It should be remembered that penicillin G does not eliminate the meningococcal carrier state, and its administration is thus ineffective as a prophylactic measure.

Gonococcal Infections. Gonococci have gradually become more resistant to penicillin G, and thus higher doses of the antibiotic are now recommended for treatment of gonococcal infections. In addition, there are rare strains of penicillinase-producing gonococci that are totally resistant to the administration of penicillin G. In spite of this, a penicillin preparation remains the therapy of choice for most gonococcal infections. In view of the nature of the disease and the patient population in which it is most prevalent, it is desirable to complete treatment, if possible, in one visit. Uncomplicated gonococcal urethritis is most common, and, because of safety and acceptability to patients, the oral administration of amoxicillin (3 g) *plus* probenecid (1 g) or ampicillin (3.5 g) plus probenecid is recommended. A total of 4.8 million units of penicillin G procaine injected into two sites combined with oral probenecid (1 g) is equally efficacious. Oral penicillin V or penicillin G is *not* adequate therapy for gonococcal infections, and penicillin G benzathine does not provide adequate therapeutic concentrations. Treatment of contacts of known cases of gonorrhea is the same as is that for gono-

coccal urethritis. Patients with gonococcal pharyngitis respond better to intramuscular procaine penicillin G than to the oral regimens.

Gonococcal arthritis has been treated with a variety of protocols. Some physicians prefer the intravenous administration of 10 million units of penicillin G daily for 3 days, followed by ampicillin or amoxicillin given orally for 5 to 7 additional days. Disseminated gonococcal infections with skin lesions and gonococcemia should be treated similarly. Gonococcal endocarditis is a very rare disease and requires treatment with 10 to 20 million units of penicillin G intravenously daily for at least 3 to 4 weeks. Ophthalmia neonatorum is readily cured by parenteral penicillin G. Some pediatricians prefer aqueous penicillin G for the neonate because of the possibility of adverse reactions to procaine penicillin.

Syphilis. Therapy of syphilis with penicillin G is highly effective. Primary, secondary, and latent syphilis of less than 1 year's duration should be treated with a single intramuscular dose of 2.4 million units of penicillin G benzathine. Patients with latent syphilis of more than 1 year's duration should also be treated with penicillin G benzathine, 2.4 million units weekly for 3 to 4 weeks. Patients with neurosyphilis or cardiovascular syphilis may be treated with a variety of regimens. Since these diseases are potentially lethal and their progression can be halted (but not reversed), intensive therapy with 20 million units of penicillin G daily for 14 days is recommended. This can be followed with benzathine penicillin G (2.4 million units weekly for 3 weeks).

Infants with congenital syphilis discovered at birth or during the postnatal period should be treated for at least 10 days with 50,000 units/kg daily of aqueous penicillin G in two divided doses or 50,000 units/kg of procaine penicillin G in a single daily dose. If the CSF is normal and there is no evidence of neurological involvement, penicillin G benzathine can be given as a single dose (50,000 units/kg).

The vast majority (90% or more) of patients with secondary syphilis develop the Jarisch-Herxheimer reaction. This may also be seen in patients with other forms of syphilis. Several hours after the first injection of penicillin, the patient may develop chills, fever, headache, myalgias, and arthralgias. The syphilitic cutaneous lesions may become more prominent, edematous, and brilliant in color. Manifestations usually persist for a few hours, and the rash begins to fade within 48 hours. It does not recur with the second or subsequent injections of penicillin. This reaction is thought to be due to release of spirochetal antigens, with subsequent host reactions to the products. Therapy should be continued if the Jarisch-Herxheimer reaction occurs.

Actinomycosis. Penicillin G is the agent of choice for the treatment of all forms of actinomycosis. The dose should be 10 to 20 million units of penicillin G intravenously per day for 6 weeks. Some physicians continue therapy for 2 to 3 months with oral penicillin V (500 mg four times daily). Surgical drainage or excision of the lesion may be necessary before cure is accomplished.

Diphtheria. There is no evidence that penicillin or any other antibiotic alters the incidence of complications or the outcome of diphtheria; specific antitoxin is the only effective treatment. However, penicillin G eliminates the carrier state. The parenteral administration of 2 to 3 million units per day, in divided doses for 10 to 12 days, eliminates the diphtheria bacilli from the pharynx and other sites in practically 100% of cases. A single daily injection of penicillin G procaine for the same period produces about the same results. Erythromycin appears to be as effective, and some consider it to be preferable.

Anthrax. Penicillin G is the agent of choice in the treatment of all clinical forms of anthrax. However, strains of *B. anthracis* resistant to this antibiotic have been recovered from human infections. When penicillin G is used, the dose should be 10 to 20 million units per day.

Clostridial Infections. Penicillin G is the agent of choice for *gas gangrene;* the dose is in the range of 10 to 20 million units per day, given parenterally. Adequate debridement of the infected areas is essential. Antimicrobial drugs probably have no effect on the ultimate outcome of *tetanus.* Debridement and administration of human tetanus immune globulin may be indicated. Penicillin is administered, however, to eradicate the vegetative forms of the bacteria that may persist.

Fusospirochetal Infections. Gingivostomatitis, produced by the synergistic action of *Leptotrichia buccalis* and spirochetes that are present in the mouth, is readily treatable with penicillin. For simple "trench mouth," 500 mg of penicillin V given every 6 hours for several days is usually sufficient to clear the disease.

Rat-Bite Fever. The two microorganisms responsible for this infection, *Spirillum minor* in the Orient and *Streptobacillus moniliformis* in America and Europe, are sensitive to penicillin G, the therapeutic agent of choice. Since most cases due to the streptobacillus are complicated by bacteremia and, in many instances, by metastatic infections especially of the synovia and endocardium, the dose should be large; a daily dose of 12 to 15 million units given parenterally, for 3 to 4 weeks, has been recommended.

Listeria Infections. Penicillin G is regarded as the drug of choice in the management of infections due to *List. monocytogenes;* ampicillin is also effective. The recommended dose of penicillin G is 15 to 20 million units parenterally per day, for at least 2 weeks. When endocarditis is the problem, the dose is the same, but the duration of treatment should be no less than 4 weeks.

Pasteurella Infections. The only species of *Pasteurella* highly susceptible to penicillin is *Past. multocida.* Soft-tissue infection, bacteremia, and meningitis are the most common forms of the disease produced by this microorganism in man, and often follow animal bites. Penicillin G, 4 to 6 million units per day parenterally for at least 2 weeks, is effectively curative.

Erysipeloid. The causative agent of this disease, *Erysipelothrix rhusiopathiae,* is sensitive to penicillin. The uncomplicated infection responds well to a single injection of 1.2 million units of penicillin G benzathine. When endocarditis is present, penicillin G, 2 to 20 million units per day, has been found effective; therapy should be continued for 4 to 6 weeks.

Prophylactic Uses of the Penicillins. Demonstration of the effectiveness of penicillin in eradicating microorganisms was quickly, and quite naturally, followed by attempts to prove that it was also effective in preventing infection in susceptible hosts. As a result, the antibiotic has been administered in almost every situation in which a risk of bacterial invasion has been present. As prophylaxis has been investigated under controlled conditions, it has become clear that penicillin is highly effective in some situations, useless and potentially dangerous in others, and of questionable value in still others (*see* Chapter 48).

Streptococcal Infections. The administration of penicillin to individuals exposed to *Strep. pyogenes* affords a predictable and high order of protection. The oral ingestion of 200,000 units of penicillin G or penicillin V twice a day or a single injection of 1.2 million units of penicillin G benzathine has been found effective. Such therapy may promptly and markedly reduce the carrier rate. Some objections have been raised to the routine use of penicillin as prophylaxis in individuals who have had contact with *Strep. pyogenes* on the ground that the risks of reactions to the drug are as great as those associated with the disease. In addition, evidence indicating that the carrier state leads to the development of type-specific immunity has raised serious questions concerning prophylaxis with penicillin, since this tends to suppress or abolish immune responses to *Strep. pyogenes.* This type of prophylaxis finds a rational use in closed populations of young people who are experiencing a high incidence of streptococcal infection. Patients with extensive deep burns are at high risk of developing severe wound infections with *Strep. pyogenes;* several days of "low-dose" prophylaxis appears to be effective in reducing the incidence of this complication.

Recurrences of Rheumatic Fever. The oral administration of 200,000 units of penicillin G or penicillin V every 12 hours produces a striking decrease in the incidence of recurrences of rheumatic fever in susceptible individuals. Because of the difficulties associated with oral treatment, mainly the fact that patients neglect to take the drug, parenteral administration is preferable, especially in children. The intramuscular injection of 1.2 million units of penicillin G benzathine once a month yields excellent results. In cases of hypersensitivity to penicillin, sulfisoxazole or sulfadiazine, 1 g twice a day for adults, is also effective; for children weighing under 27 kg, the dose is halved. Prophylaxis must be continued throughout the year. The duration of such treatment is an unsettled question. It has been suggested that prophylaxis should be continued for life, because instances of acute rheumatic fever have been observed in the fifth and sixth decades. However, the necessity for such prolonged prophylaxis has not been established.

Gonorrhea. Sexual contacts of patients with gonorrhea should receive a course of antibiotics identical to that described for the treatment of gonococcal urethritis.

Syphilis. Prophylaxis for a contact with syphilis consists in the intramuscular administration of 4.8 million units of penicillin G procaine plus 1 g of oral probenecid (this is also effective for gonorrhea) or 2.4 million units of penicillin G benzathine within 24 hours after exposure. A serological test for syphilis should be performed at monthly intervals for at least 4 months thereafter.

Surgical Procedures in Patients with Valvular Heart Disease. About 25% of cases of subacute bacterial endocarditis follow dental extractions. This observation, together with the fact that up to 80% of persons who have teeth removed experience a transient bacteremia, emphasizes the potential importance of chemoprophylaxis for those who have congenital or acquired valvular heart disease of any type and need to undergo dental procedures. Since transient bacterial invasion of the blood stream occurs occasionally after surgical procedures such as tonsillectomy and operations on the genitourinary and intestinal tracts and during childbirth, these too are indications for prophylaxis in patients with valvular heart disease. Bacteremia is not eliminated by the use of penicillin. Whether the incidence of bacterial endocarditis is actually altered by this type of chemoprophylaxis remains to be determined.

Detailed recommendations for both adults and children with valvular heart disease have been formulated by a committee of the American Heart Association and by the Medical Letter (Sande, 1983; Medical Letter, 1984; Durack, 1985).

Penicillin Prophylaxis of No Value. A number of disorders in which penicillin has been used prophylactically have been shown by carefully controlled study to be unaffected by such treatment as far as secondary bacterial invasion is concerned. Among these are numerous viral infections, coma, shock, heart failure, elective and uncontaminated surgical procedures, "clean" wounds, normal obstetrical delivery, catheterization of the urinary tract, and prematurity.

THE PENICILLINASE-RESISTANT PENICILLINS

The penicillins described in this section are not hydrolyzed by staphylococcal penicillinase. Their appropriate use should be restricted to the treatment of infections that are known or suspected to be caused by staphylococci that elaborate the enzyme— the majority of strains of this bacterium that are encountered in the hospital *or* in the general community. These drugs are less active than is penicillin G against other penicillin-sensitive microorganisms, including non-penicillinase-producing staphylococci.

The penicillinase-resistant penicillins remain the agents of choice for most staphylococcal disease despite the increasing incidence of isolates of so-called methicillin-resistant microorganisms. As commonly used, this latter term denotes resistance of these bacteria to all of the penicillinase-resistant penicillins and cephalosporins. Such strains are usually resistant as well to the aminoglycosides, tetracyclines, erythromycin, and clindamycin. Vancomycin is considered to be the drug of choice for such infections, although some physicians use a combination of vancomycin and rifampin. Altered penicillin-binding proteins have been found in some methicillin-resistant strains. From 10 to 40% of strains of *Staph. epidermidis* are also insensitive to the penicillinase-resistant penicillins. As with methicillin-resistant *Staph. aureus,* these strains may appear to be susceptible to cephalosporins on disc sensitivity testing, but there is usually a significant population of microbes that is resistant to cephalosporins and that emerges during such therapy. Vancomycin is also the drug of choice for serious infection caused by methicillin-resistant *Staph. epidermidis.*

Methicillin. This semisynthetic penicillin is prepared from 6-aminopenicillanic acid. Its structural formula is shown in Table 50–1. The drug is highly resistant to cleavage by penicillinase.

Pharmacological Properties. Methicillin is bactericidal for nearly all strains of *Staph. aureus* at concentrations of 1 to 6 μg/ml. Microorganisms that are inhibited only by concentrations in excess of 12.5 μg/ml are considered to be resistant. Penicillinase-producing strains are from 15 to 80 times more susceptible to methicillin than to penicillin G, although methicillin is not as effective as penicillin G against other gram-positive microorganisms. Methicillin is not effective against gram-negative bacteria, some of which may even inactivate it.

Methicillin is not employed by the oral route because it is poorly absorbed and readily destroyed by the acidic gastric contents. When the drug is given intramuscularly, peak concentrations in plasma are reached in about 30 minutes to 1 hour. After the conventional dose of 1 g in adults, plasma concentrations in excess of 10 μg/ml are demonstrable; a 2-g dose provides a peak concentration over 20 μg/ml, and approximately 8 μg/ml is still present after 4 hours. About 40% of the methicillin in plasma is bound to protein. The distribution and excretion of methicillin and penicillin G are essentially identical (*see* above).

Preparations and Routes of Administration. The available preparation is *methicillin sodium for injection* (STAPHCILLIN); it is administered intravenously or intramuscularly. While stable in dry form, the drug is unstable in acidic media and loses potency when dissolved in 0.85% sodium chloride or in dextrose solution at room temperature. This instability, together with the fact that methicillin is excreted rapidly, contraindicates continuous intravenous infusion unless the solutions are buffered to neutrality. The solution should be fresh, and other drugs should not be included, since many are incompatible with methicillin in solution. The usual dose is 4 to 12 g per day for adults and 100 to 200 mg/kg per day for children, given in four or six portions intravenously.

The Isoxazolyl Penicillins: Oxacillin, Cloxacillin, Dicloxacillin, Floxacillin. These four congeneric semisynthetic penicillins are similar pharmacologically and are thus conveniently considered together. Their structural formulas are shown in Table 50–1. All are relatively stable in an acidic medium and are adequately absorbed after oral administration. All are markedly resistant to cleavage by penicillinase. These drugs are not substitutes for penicillin G in the treatment of diseases amenable to it. Furthermore, because of variability in intestinal absorption, oral administration is not a substitute for the parenteral route in the treatment of serious staphylococcal infections that require a penicillin unaffected by penicillinase.

Pharmacological Properties. The isoxazolyl penicillins are potent inhibitors of the growth of most penicillinase-producing staphylococci. This is their valid clinical use. Dicloxacillin is the most active, and most strains of *Staph. aureus* are inhibited by concentrations of 0.05 to 0.8 μg/ml. Comparable values for cloxacillin and oxacillin are 0.1 to 3 μg/ml and 0.4 to 6 μg/ml, respectively. These differences may have little practical significance, however, since dosages are adjusted accordingly. These agents are, in general, less effective against microorganisms susceptible to penicillin G, and they are not useful against gram-negative bacteria.

These agents are rapidly but incompletely (30 to 80%) absorbed from the gastrointestinal tract. Absorption of the drugs is more efficient when they are taken on an empty stomach. Peak concentrations in plasma are attained by 1 hour and approxi-

mate 5 to 10 μg/ml after the ingestion of 1 g of oxacillin. Slightly higher concentrations are achieved after the administration of 1 g of cloxacillin, while the same oral dose of dicloxacillin or floxacillin yields peak plasma concentrations of 15 μg/ml. There is little evidence that these differences are of clinical significance. Since absorption is less than complete, higher plasma concentrations are achieved following intramuscular injection, and larger quantities of the drugs are recoverable in the urine. For example, a 500-mg dose of oxacillin given intramuscularly results in peak concentrations in plasma of approximately 15 μg/ml after 30 to 60 minutes. All these congeners are bound to plasma albumin to a great extent (approximately 90 to 95%); none is removed from the circulation to a significant degree by hemodialysis.

The isoxazolyl penicillins are rapidly excreted by the kidney. Normally, about one half of any of these drugs is excreted in the urine in the first 6 hours after a conventional oral dose. There is also significant hepatic elimination of these agents in the bile. The half-lives for all are between 30 and 60 minutes. Intervals between doses of oxacillin, cloxacillin, and dicloxacillin do not have to be altered for patients with renal failure. The above-noted differences in plasma concentrations produced by the isoxazolyl penicillins are related mainly to differences in rate of urinary excretion and degree of resistance to degradation in the liver.

Preparations and Routes of Administration. *Oxacillin sodium* (BACTOCILL, PROSTAPHLIN) is available for oral use in capsules containing 250 or 500 mg of drug, and as *oxacillin sodium for oral solution* (250 mg/5 ml). The drug is preferably administered 1 or 2 hours before meals, to ensure better absorption. The daily oral dose of oxacillin for adults is 2 to 4 g, divided into four portions; for children, 50 to 100 mg/kg per day is administered similarly. An injectable form of the drug is also available. For adults a total of 2 to 12 g per day, and for children 100 to 300 mg/kg per day, may be given intravenously or intramuscularly, injections being given every 4 to 6 hours.

Cloxacillin sodium (CLOXAPEN, TEGOPEN) is available in capsules (250 and 500 mg) and as a powder for oral solution (125 mg/5 ml). The dose for adults is 250 mg orally every 6 hours for mild-to-moderate infections; for severe infections, it is 500 mg or more every 6 hours. The dose for children is 50 to 100 mg/kg per day, divided into equal quantities and given every 6 hours; for those weighing more than 20 kg, adult doses have been recommended.

Dicloxacillin sodium (DYCILL, DYNAPEN, PATHOCIL, VERACILLIN) is quite stable at acidic pH and at room temperature. The drug is available for oral use in capsules (125, 250, and 500 mg) and as a powder for oral suspension (62.5 mg/5 ml). The dose for adults and for children weighing more than 40 kg is 250 mg or more every 6 hours; for children weighing less than 40 kg, the recommended daily dose is 25 mg/kg, given in four equal portions at intervals of 6 hours. Because there is incomplete information at present, dicloxacillin should not be given to newborn infants.

Floxacillin (*flucloxacillin*) is not currently available in the United States; it closely resembles cloxacillin.

Nafcillin. This semisynthetic penicillin, derived from 6-aminopenicillanic acid, is highly resistant to penicillinase and has proven effective against infections caused by penicillinase-producing strains of *Staph. aureus*. Its structural formula is shown in Table 50–1.

Pharmacological Properties. Nafcillin is slightly more active than oxacillin against penicillin G–resistant *Staph. aureus* (most strains are inhibited by 0.06 to 2 μg/ml). While it is the most active of the penicillinase-resistant penicillins against other microorganisms, it is not as potent as penicillin G.

Nafcillin is inactivated to a variable degree in the acidic medium of the gastric contents. Its absorption after oral administration is irregular, regardless of whether the drug is taken with meals or on an empty stomach. The peak plasma concentration is about 8 μg/ml 60 minutes after a 1-g intramuscular dose. Nafcillin is bound to plasma protein to the extent of about 90%. Peak concentrations of nafcillin in bile are well above those found in plasma. Concentrations of the drug in CSF appear to be adequate for therapy of staphylococcal meningitis.

Preparations and Routes of Administration. Nafcillin sodium (NAFCIL, UNIPEN) is available for oral and parenteral use. Capsules and tablets contain 250 or 500 mg of the drug, and a powder for solution is also marketed for oral use. However, because of its variable absorption from the gastrointestinal tract, the oral route is not recommended. A sterile preparation for injection is supplied in vials. Serious staphylococcal infections should be treated with 6 to 12 g of the drug daily, given in divided doses every 4 hours. Children should receive 100 to 200 mg/kg per day in divided doses given every 4 to 6 hours.

The Aminopenicillins:
Ampicillin, Amoxicillin,
and Their Congeners

These agents have similar antibacterial activity and a spectrum that is broader than the antibiotics heretofore discussed. They are all destroyed by beta-lactamase (from both gram-positive and gram-negative bacteria) and thus are ineffective for most staphylococcal infections.

Antimicrobial Activity. Ampicillin and the related aminopenicillins are bactericidal for both gram-positive and gram-negative bacteria. They are somewhat less active than penicillin G against gram-positive cocci sensitive to the latter agent. The meningococcus, pneumococcus, gonococcus,

and *List. monocytogenes* are sensitive to the drug. *Haemophilus influenzae* and the *viridans* group of streptococci are usually inhibited by very low concentrations of ampicillin. However, strains of type-b *H. influenzae* highly resistant to ampicillin have been recovered from children with meningitis. It is estimated that 5 to 30% of cases of *H. influenzae* meningitis are now caused by ampicillin-resistant strains. Enterococci are about twice as sensitive to ampicillin, on a weight basis, as they are to penicillin G (minimal inhibitory concentration for ampicillin averages 1.5 μg/ml). Although most strains of *E. coli*, *Pr. mirabilis*, *Salmonella*, and *Shigella* were highly susceptible when ampicillin was first used in the early 1960s, an increasing percentage of these species is now resistant. From 30 to 50% of *E. coli*, a significant number of *Pr. mirabilis*, and practically all species of *Enterobacter* are presently insensitive. Resistant strains of *Salmonella* (plasmid mediated) have been recovered with increasing frequency in various parts of the world. Most strains of *Shigella* are now resistant. Most strains of *Pseudomonas*, *Klebsiella*, *Serratia*, *Acinetobacter*, and indole-positive *Proteus* are also resistant to this group of penicillins; these antibiotics are less active against *B. fragilis* than is penicillin G.

Ampicillin. This drug is the prototypical agent of the group. Its structural formula is shown in Table 50–1.

Pharmacological Properties. Ampicillin is stable in acid and is well absorbed after oral administration. An oral dose of 0.5 g produces peak concentrations in plasma of about 3 μg/ml at 2 hours. The drug is detectable in the plasma for about 4 hours after a conventional oral dose. Intake of food prior to ingestion of ampicillin results in less complete absorption. Intramuscular injection of 0.5 or 1 g of sodium ampicillin yields peak plasma concentrations of about 7 or 10 μg/ml, respectively, at 1 hour; these decline exponentially with a half-time approximating 80 minutes. Administration of equal doses of penicillin G and ampicillin results in higher plasma concentrations of the latter agent because of its slower rate of renal elimination.

About one half of an oral dose is cleared by the kidney in the first 6 hours following ingestion. Approximately 80% of an intramuscular or intravenous dose of 500 mg is eliminated in the urine in this time. Severe renal impairment markedly prolongs the persistence of ampicillin in the plasma. Peritoneal dialysis is ineffective in removing the drug from the blood, but hemodialysis removes about 40% of the body store in about 7 hours. Adjustment of the dose of ampicillin is required in the presence of renal dysfunction (*see* Appendix II).

Ampicillin appears in the bile, undergoes enterohepatic circulation, and is excreted in appreciable quantities in the feces. When the common bile duct is obstructed, ampicillin is not detectable in the bile.

Preparations and Routes of Administration. Ampicillin (AMCILL, OMNIPEN, POLYCILLIN, others) is available for oral use in capsules containing 250 or 500 mg; for parenteral use, as the sodium salt; for oral suspension (125 to 500 mg/5 ml); and in pediatric drops (100 mg/ml). The dose varies with the type and the severity of the infection being treated, with renal function, and with age. Newborns (up to 1 week of age) should receive 25 to 50 mg/kg every 12 hours. Infants (1 to 4 weeks of age) should receive 100 to 200 mg/kg per day in three portions, while older children should receive the same daily dose in four portions. For mild-to-moderately severe disease, the oral dose for adults is 2 to 4 g per day, divided and given every 6 hours. For severe infections, it is best to administer the drug parenterally in doses ranging from 6 to 12 g per day. The treatment of meningitis requires the use of large doses, 300 to 400 mg/kg per day parenterally (in equally divided portions given every 4 hours) for children, and 12 g per day for adults. Solutions should be freshly prepared prior to injection.

Amoxicillin. This drug, a penicillinase-susceptible semisynthetic penicillin, is a close chemical and pharmacological relative of ampicillin (*see* Table 50–1). The drug is stable in acid and is designed for oral use. The antimicrobial spectrum of amoxicillin is essentially identical to that of ampicillin, with the important exception that amoxicillin appears to be less effective than ampicillin for shigellosis (Neu, 1979).

Amoxicillin is more rapidly and completely absorbed from the gastrointestinal tract than is ampicillin, which is the major difference between the two. Peak concentrations in plasma are two to two and one-half times greater for amoxicillin than for ampicillin after oral administration of the same dose; they are reached at 2 hours and average about 4 μg/ml when 250 mg is administered. Food does not interfere with absorption. Perhaps because of more complete absorption of this congener, the incidence of diarrhea with amoxicillin is less than that following administration of ampicillin. The incidence of other adverse effects appears to be similar. While the half-life of amoxicillin is similar to that for ampicillin, effective concentrations of orally administered amoxicillin are detectable in the plasma for twice as long as with ampicillin, again because of the more complete absorption. About 20% of amoxicillin is protein bound in plasma, a value similar to that for ampicillin. Approximately 50% of a dose of the antibiotic is excreted in an active form in the urine. Probenecid

delays excretion of the drug. (*See* Gordon *et al.*, 1972; Rolinson, 1973; *see also* Appendix II.)

Preparations and Dosage. Amoxicillin (AMOXIL, LAROTID, others) is available for oral use in tablets and capsules (125 to 500 mg), as a powder for oral suspension (125 or 250 mg/5 ml), and as pediatric drops (50 mg/ml). Usual doses are 0.75 to 1.5 g per day in three divided portions for adults and 20 to 40 mg/kg per day in three portions for children.

Bacampicillin. This agent is the 1-ethoxy-carbonyloxyethyl ester of ampicillin. It is absorbed well after oral administration and is hydrolyzed to ampicillin during absorption from the gastrointestinal tract. Concentrations in blood are about 50% higher than those achieved with amoxicillin, and the drug has been effective when given twice daily. *Bacampicillin hydrochloride* (SPECTROBID) is available in tablets (400 mg; chemically equivalent to 280 mg of ampicillin) and as a powder for oral suspension. The usual dose for adults is 800 to 1600 mg per day divided into two portions (Scheife and Neu, 1982). Children should receive 25 to 50 mg/kg per day.

Hetacillin. This drug is also a chemical modification of ampicillin and is very rapidly hydrolyzed to ampicillin and acetone after administration. It is doubtful that this congener has any advantages to recommend its use in place of ampicillin. *Hetacillin* (VERSAPEN) is available in capsules and a suspension for oral use.

Other Congeners. *Pivampicillin* is the pivaloyloxymethyl ester of ampicillin. It too is active only after conversion to ampicillin *in vivo*. Absorption after oral administration is similar to that for amoxicillin. There is no indication that the use of this drug will offer any advantage. *Talampicillin* is another similar ester of ampicillin. *Epicillin* and *cyclacillin* are aminopenicillins that are also similar to ampicillin and have little or no advantage over the parent compound. None of these drugs, with the exception of cyclacillin (CYCLAPEN-W), is currently available in the United States.

Therapeutic Indications for the Aminopenicillins. *Gonococcal Infections.* Ampicillin and amoxicillin are excellent agents for the treatment of gonococcal urethritis. The uses of these drugs for this and other forms of gonococcal disease are described in more detail above (page 1126).

Upper Respiratory Infections. Ampicillin and amoxicillin are active against *H. influenzae, Strep. pneumoniae,* and *Strep. pyogenes,* which are the major upper respiratory bacterial pathogens. The drugs constitute effective therapy for sinusitis, otitis media, acute exacerbations of chronic bronchitis, and epiglottitis. Ampicillin-resistant *H. influenzae* may be a problem in some areas. Bacterial pharyngitis should be treated with penicillin G or penicillin V, since *Strep. pyogenes* is the major pathogen.

Urinary Tract Infections. Most uncomplicated urinary tract infections are caused by Enterobacteriaceae, and *E. coli* is the most common species. A sulfonamide (*see* Chapter 49) or ampicillin is often considered to be the drug of choice. Enterococcal urinary tract infections are treated effectively with ampicillin alone.

Meningitis. Acute bacterial meningitis in children is most frequently due to *H. influenzae, Strep. pneumoniae,* or *Neisseria meningitidis.* Ampicillin is frequently used for therapy. Since 5 to 30% of strains of *H. influenzae* may be resistant to this antibiotic, it is recommended that chloramphenicol be given concurrently at first until the microorganism is identified and its sensitivities are determined. Alternatives include the use of chloramphenicol alone or a combination of penicillin G and chloramphenicol. Cefuroxime, cefotaxime, ceftizoxime, or the combination of ampicillin and moxalactam have also been effective treatment for meningitis acquired in the community.

Salmonella Infections. Uncomplicated gastroenteritis caused by *Salmonella* should not be treated with antibiotics. Such therapy has little influence on the course of the disease and *prolongs* the period of postconvalescent excretion of the microorganisms. Disease associated with bacteremia, disease with metastatic foci, and the enteric fever syndrome (including typhoid fever) respond favorably to antibiotics. Chloramphenicol is still considered to be the drug of choice, but the administration of high doses of ampicillin (12 g per day for adults) or trimethoprim-sulfamethoxazole is also effective. In some geographical areas (Central America and Southeast Asia) resistance to chloramphenicol is common, and the combination of trimethoprim and sulfamethoxazole has become the agent of choice. The typhoid carrier state has been successfully eliminated in patients without gallbladder disease with ampicillin or trimethoprim-sulfamethoxazole.

Other Infections. The dual administration of ampicillin and an aminoglycoside may be used to treat sepsis caused by gram-negative bacteria acquired in the general community. After sensitivities of infecting microorganisms are known, it is advisable to treat with a beta-lactam antibiotic and to discontinue the aminoglycoside, if possible. Thus, ampicillin may be used alone to treat a variety of serious gram-negative infections once the bacterial sensitivities have been determined.

ANTIPSEUDOMONAL PENICILLINS: THE CARBOXYPENICILLINS AND THE UREIDOPENICILLINS

The carboxypenicillins, carbenicillin and ticarcillin and their close relatives, are active against most isolates of *Pseudomonas aeruginosa* and certain indole-positive *Proteus* species that are resistant to ampicillin and its congeners. They are ineffective against most strains of *Staph. aureus. Bacteroides fragilis* is susceptible to high concentrations of these drugs, but penicillin G

is actually more active on a weight basis (Maki *et al.,* 1978).

Carbenicillin and Carbenicillin Indanyl.

Carbenicillin. This drug is a penicillinase-susceptible derivative of 6-aminopenicillanic acid. Its structural formula is shown in Table 50–1. The major advantage of this agent is that it often cures serious infections caused by *Pseudomonas* species, *Proteus* strains resistant to ampicillin, and certain other gram-negative microorganisms.

Low concentrations of carbenicillin inhibit the growth of *Pr. mirabilis* and many microorganisms sensitive to penicillin G. *Escherichia coli, Enterobacter,* and *Salmonella* are less sensitive. The majority of strains of *Pr. vulgaris* and *Pseud. aeruginosa* are sensitive to 25 μg/ml or less of the drug; 70 to 80% of *Pseudomonas* are inhibited by 100 μg/ml. Penicillin G–resistant staphylococci, *Klebsiella,* and *Serratia* are usually resistant to carbenicillin. Enterococci are suppressed in the range of 50 to 100 μg/ml. Bacterial resistance may appear *in vivo* during treatment with suboptimal doses of carbenicillin.

Carbenicillin is not absorbed from the gastrointestinal tract and, therefore, must be given parenterally. Large doses are often necessary. Intramuscular injection of 1 g produces peak concentrations in plasma of 15 to 20 μg/ml in 0.5 to 2 hours; activity is practically gone at 6 hours. Maximal plasma concentrations are about four times higher after intravenous than after intramuscular administration of the antibiotic. Intravenous infusion at a rate of 1 g per hour results in average plasma concentrations of approximately 150 μg/ml. Intravenous infusion of 4 to 5 g over a 2-hour period every 4 hours will maintain drug concentrations in blood above 100 μg/ml. About 50% of the antibiotic in plasma is protein bound. The distribution of carbenicillin is similar to that of other penicillins. The half-life of carbenicillin in individuals with normal renal function is about 1 hour; it is prolonged to about 2 hours in the presence of hepatic dysfunction. Hemodialysis reduces the concentration of the antibiotic in plasma.

Carbenicillin is excreted primarily by the renal tubules. About 75 to 85% of a dose is recoverable in active form in the urine in 9 hours. Probenecid, by delaying renal excretion of the drug, increases plasma concentrations by about 50%.

Preparations of carbenicillin may cause adverse effects in addition to those that follow use of the other penicillins (*see* below). Congestive heart failure may result from the administration of excessive sodium. Hypokalemia may occur because of obligatory excretion of cation with the large amount of non-reabsorbable anion (carbenicillin) presented to the distal renal tubule. The drug interferes with platelet function, and bleeding may occur because of abnormal aggregation of platelets (*see* Shattil *et al.,* 1980).

Carbenicillin is available for parenteral injection as the disodium salt (GEOPEN, PYOPEN) in sterile vials. The daily dose for adults with serious infections is 30 to 40 g in divided doses given every 4 to 6 hours. Daily doses up to 600 mg/kg have been used to treat children with life-threatening infection. In patients with severe renal failure, the dose should not exceed 2 g every 12 hours; during hemodialysis, the interval between doses may be reduced to 4 to 6 hours. Available preparations of carbenicillin contain approximately 5 mEq of sodium per gram.

Carbenicillin Indanyl. This congener is the indanyl ester of carbenicillin; it is acid stable and is suitable for oral administration. The ester is rapidly converted to carbenicillin *in vivo* by hydrolysis of the ester linkage. The antimicrobial spectrum of the drug is therefore that of carbenicillin. While relatively low concentrations of carbenicillin are achieved in plasma, the active moiety is excreted rapidly in the urine. Thus, the main use of this drug is for the management of urinary tract infections caused by *Proteus* species other than *Pr. mirabilis* and by *Pseud. aeruginosa.*

Carbenicillin indanyl is rapidly absorbed from the small intestine. The peak concentration in plasma, reached about 1 hour after ingestion of 500 mg of the drug, is approximately 5 μg/ml. About 30% of a dose of 500 mg is excreted in the urine in the first 12 hours; an additional 6% is eliminated in the urine over the next 12 hours. Some of the drug is excreted in the bile, and some is detoxified in the liver.

Carbenicillin indanyl sodium (GEOCILLIN) is available in tablets containing 500 mg of the drug (equivalent to 382 mg of carbenicillin). The recommended daily doses are 2 to 4 g, given in four divided portions. The higher end of this range is preferred for treatment of chronic infections or those caused by *Pseudomonas.*

Carbenicillin phenyl sodium (CARFECILLIN) is very similar to carbenicillin indanyl.

Ticarcillin. This semisynthetic penicillin (Table 50–1) is very similar to carbenicillin, but it is two to four times more active against *Pseud. aeruginosa.* Doses are thus usually smaller, and, hopefully, the incidence of toxicity may be decreased. Ticarcillin is now the preferred carboxypenicillin for the treatment of serious infections caused by *Pseudomonas.*

Ticarcillin disodium (TICAR) is available for parenteral injection. Daily doses of the drug are 200 to 300 mg/kg, given in four to six divided portions. Ticarcillin disodium contains about 5 mEq of sodium per gram (*see* Parry and Neu, 1976, 1978).

The Ureidopenicillins. *Azlocillin sodium* (Table 50–1) is a newer penicillin that is about ten times more active than carbenicillin against *Pseudomonas.* It is also more active against streptococci and resembles ampicillin in this regard (Fu and Neu, 1978). The half-life of azlocillin is 60 minutes in normal subjects but is extended to 6 hours when the creatinine clearance is less than 10 ml per minute. Peak concentrations in blood are about 300 μg/ml after the intravenous administration of 4 g; these values are not directly proportional to doses (Bergen, 1983; Neu *et al.,* 1983). Azlocillin (AZLIN) is available as a powder to be dissolved for injection. The preparation contains about 2 mEq of sodium per gram. The usual dose is 8 to 18 g per day, given in divided portions four to six times daily.

Mezlocillin is more active against *Klebsiella* than is carbenicillin; its activity against *Pseudomonas in vitro* is similar to that of ticarcillin. The pharmacokinetic properties of mezlocillin resemble those of azlocillin (*see* McCloskey *et al.,* 1982). Mezlocillin (MEZLIN) is available as a powder to be dissolved for injection and contains about 2 mEq of sodium per gram. The usual dose for adults is 6 to 18 g per day, divided into four to six portions.

Piperacillin is another similar derivative with activity against *Klebsiella* that resembles mezlocillin and activity against *Pseudomonas* similar to that of azlocillin. Pharmacokinetic properties are reminiscent of the other ureidopenicillins (*see* Eliopoulos and Moellering, 1982). The recommended doses are 12 to 24 g per day, given in three to six equal portions. Piperacillin (PIPRACIL) is available as a powder for solubilization and injection and contains about 2 mEq of sodium per gram.

Therapeutic Indications. These penicillins are important agents for the treatment of patients with serious infections caused by gram-negative bacteria. Such patients frequently have impaired immunological defenses, and their infections are often acquired in the hospital. Many authorities feel that a beta-lactam agent, often in combination with an aminoglycoside, should be employed for all such infections. Therefore, these penicillins find their greatest use in treating bacteremias, pneumonias, infections following burns, and urinary tract infections due to microorganisms resistant to penicillin G and ampicillin; the bacteria responsible especially include *Pseud. aeruginosa,* indole-positive strains of *Proteus,* and *Enterobacter* species. Since *Pseudomonas* infections are common in neutropenic patients, therapy for severe bacterial infections in such individuals should include a beta-lactam antibiotic with good activity against these microorganisms. All of these agents are very expensive.

OTHER EXTENDED-SPECTRUM PENICILLINS

Amdinocillin (also known as mecillinam) is a derivative of 6-aminopenicillanic acid with poor activity against gram-positive microorganisms and *Pseudomonas* but with good activity against Enterobacteriaceae. Because of its novel mechanism of action (it appears to bind to different proteins than do other penicillins), it shows significant synergism when utilized concurrently with other beta-lactam antibiotics (Cleeland and Squires, 1983; Symposium, 1983). Amdinocillin is available as COACTIN. It is given intramuscularly or intravenously in doses up to 10 mg/kg every 4 hours for serious infections.

Temocillin is the 6-α-methoxy derivative of ticarcillin. It is resistant to hydrolysis by beta-lactamases produced by gram-negative microorganisms, but it has poor activity against *Pseudomonas* and gram-positive bacteria; activity against Enterobacteriaceae and *H. influenzae* is good. Temocillin is not available in the United States.

UNTOWARD REACTIONS TO PENICILLINS

Hypersensitivity Reactions. Hypersensitivity reactions are by far the most common adverse effects noted with the penicillins, and these agents are probably the most common cause of drug allergy. There is no convincing evidence that any single penicillin differs from the group in its potential for causing true allergic reactions. In approximate order of decreasing frequency, manifestations of allergy to penicillins include maculopapular rash, urticarial rash, fever, bronchospasm, vasculitis, serum sickness, exfoliative dermatitis, Stevens-Johnson syndrome, and anaphylaxis (*see* Levine, 1972). The overall incidence of such reactions to the penicillins varies from 0.7 to 10% in different studies (Idsøe *et al.*, 1968).

Hypersensitivity reactions may occur with any dosage form of penicillin; the presence of allergy to one penicillin exposes the patient to a greater risk of reaction if another is given. On the other hand, the occurrence of an untoward effect does not necessarily imply repetition on subsequent exposures. Hypersensitivity reactions may appear in the absence of previous known exposure to the drug. This may be caused by unrecognized prior exposure to penicillin in the environment (*e.g.*, in foods of animal origin or from the fungus producing penicillin). Although elimination of the antibiotic usually results in rapid clearing of the allergic manifestations, they may persist for 1 or 2 weeks or longer after therapy has been stopped. In some cases, the reaction is mild and disappears even while the use of penicillin is continued. In others, it is of serious import and necessitates immediate cessation of penicillin treatment. In a few instances, it is necessary to interdict the future use of penicillin because of the risk of death, and the patient should be so warned. It must be stressed that fatal episodes of anaphylaxis have followed the ingestion of very small doses of this antibiotic or skin testing with minute quantities of the drug.

Penicillins and breakdown products of penicillins act as haptens after their covalent reaction with proteins. The most important antigenic intermediate of penicillin appears to be the penicilloyl moiety, which is formed when the beta-lactam ring is opened. This is considered to be the *major* (predominant) determinant of penicillin allergy. In addition, *minor* determinants of allergy to penicillins are present. These include the intact molecule itself and penicilloate. These products are formed *in vivo* and can also be found in solutions of penicillin prepared for administration. The terms *major determinant* and *minor determinant* refer to the frequency with which antibodies to these haptens appear to be formed. They do *not* describe the severity of the reaction that may result.

Antipenicillin antibodies are detectable in virtually all patients who have received the drug and in many who have never knowingly been exposed to it (Klaus and Fellner, 1973). Recent treatment with the antibiotic induces an increase in major-determinant-specific antibodies that are skin sensitizing. The incidence of positive skin reactors is three to four times higher in atopic than in nonatopic individuals. Clinical and immunological studies suggest that immediate allergic reactions are mediated by skin-sensitizing or IgE antibodies, usually of minor-determinant specificities. Accelerated and late urticarial reactions are usually mediated by major-determinant-specific, skin-sensitizing antibodies. The recurrent-arthralgia syndrome appears to be related to the presence of skin-sensitizing antibodies of minor-determinant specificities. Some maculopapular and erythematous reactions may be due to toxic antigen-antibody complexes of major-determinant-specific IgM antibodies. Accelerated and late urticarial reactions to penicillin may terminate spontaneously because of the development of blocking antibodies (*see* Levine *et al.*, 1966).

Skin rashes of all types may be caused by allergy to penicillin. Scarlatiniform, morbilliform, urticarial, vesicular, and bullous eruptions may develop. Purpuric lesions are uncommon and are usually the result of a vasculitis; thrombopenic purpura may occur very rarely. Henoch-Schönlein purpura with renal involvement has been a rare complication. *Contact dermatitis* is observed occasionally in pharmacists, nurses, and physicians who prepare penicillin solutions. Fixed-drug reactions have also occurred. More severe reactions involving the skin are exfoliative dermatitis and exudative erythema multiforme of either the erythematopapular or vesiculobullous type; these lesions may be very severe and atypical in distribution and constitute the characteristic Stevens-Johnson syndrome. The incidence of skin rashes appears to be highest following the use of ampicillin, being about 9%; rashes follow the administration of ampicillin in nearly all patients with infectious mononucleosis. When allopurinol and ampicillin are administered concurrently, the incidence of rash also increases. Ampicillin-induced skin eruptions in such patients may represent a ''toxic'' rather than a truly allergic reaction. Positive skin reactions to the major and minor determinants of penicillin sensitization may be absent. The rash may clear even while administration of the drug is continued.

The most serious hypersensitivity reactions produced by the penicillins are *angioedema* and *anaphylaxis*. Angioedema with marked swelling of the lips, tongue, face, and periorbital tissues, frequently accompanied by asthmatic breathing and ''giant hives,'' has been observed after topical, oral, or systemic administration of penicillins of various types.

Acute *anaphylactic* or *anaphylactoid* reactions induced by various preparations of penicillin constitute the most important immediate danger connected with their use. Among all drugs, the penicillins are the most often responsible for this type of untoward effect. Anaphylactoid reactions may occur at any age. Their incidence is thought to be 0.04 to 0.2% in persons treated with penicillins. About 0.001% of patients treated with these agents die from anaphylaxis. It has been estimated that there are at least 300 deaths per year due to this complication of therapy. About 15% of those who succumb have had other types of allergy; 70% have had penicillin previously, and one third of these reacted to it on a prior occasion (Idsøe *et al.*, 1968). Anaphylaxis has most often followed the *injection* of penicillin, although it has also been observed after *oral ingestion* of the drug, and has even resulted from the intradermal instillation of a very small quantity for the purpose of testing for the presence of hypersensitivity. The clinical pictures that develop vary in severity. The most dramatic is sudden, severe hypotension and rapid death. In other instances, bronchoconstriction with severe asthma, or abdominal pain, nausea, and vomiting, or extreme weakness and fall in blood pressure, or diarrhea and purpuric skin eruptions have characterized the anaphylactic episodes.

Serum sickness varies from mild fever, rash, and leukopenia to severe arthralgia or arthritis, purpura, lymphadenopathy, splenomegaly, mental changes, ECG abnormalities suggestive of myocarditis, generalized edema, albuminuria, and hematuria. It is mediated by IgG antibodies. This reaction usually appears after penicillin treatment has been continued for 1 week or more; it may be delayed, however, until 1 or 2 weeks after the drug has been stopped. Serum sickness caused by penicillin may persist for a week or longer.

Vasculitis of the skin or other organs may be related to hypersensitivity to penicillin. The Coombs' reaction frequently becomes positive during prolonged therapy with a penicillin or cephalosporin, but hemolytic anemia is rare. Reversible neutropenia may occur. It is not known if this is truly a hypersensitivity reaction; it has been noted with all of the penicillins and has been seen in up to 30% of patients treated with 8 to 12 g of nafcillin for longer than 21 days. The bone marrow shows an arrest of maturation.

Fever may be the only evidence of a hypersensitivity reaction to the penicillins. It may reach high levels and be maintained, remittent, or intermittent; chills occasionally occur. The febrile reaction usually disappears within 24 to 36 hours after administration of the drug is stopped, but may persist for days.

Eosinophilia is an occasional accompaniment of other allergic reactions to penicillin. At times, it may be the sole abnormality and eosinophils may reach levels of 10 to 20% or more of the total number of circulating white blood cells.

Interstitial nephritis may rarely be produced by the penicillins; methicillin has been implicated most frequently. Hematuria, albuminuria, pyuria, renal-cell and other casts in the urine, elevation of serum creatinine, and even oliguria have been noted. Biopsy shows a mononuclear infiltrate with eosinophilia and tubular damage. IgG is present in the interstitium (*see* Ditlove *et al.*, 1977; Kancir *et al.*, 1978). This reaction is usually reversible.

Management of the Patient Potentially Allergic to Penicillin. Evaluation of the patient's history is the most practical way to avoid the use of penicillin in patients who are at the greatest risk of developing an adverse reaction. The vast majority of patients who give a history of allergy to penicillin should be treated with a different type of antibiotic. In the unusual instance where treatment with a penicillin is essential, skin tests may be of some help (Solley *et al.*, 1982). Lack of a response to *benzylpenicilloyl-polylysine* (PRE-PEN) makes it very unlikely that a patient will develop an immediate or accelerated reaction to penicillin; this preparation is not immunogenic, nor is it likely to provoke severe reactions. Furthermore, only 3% of such patients will develop a delayed reaction (usually rash). Patients with a positive response to benzylpenicilloyl-polylysine are at significant risk of developing a serious reaction, and two thirds of these patients will develop some form of allergic reaction. In order further to reduce the likelihood of an immediate severe reaction, sensitivity to the minor antigenic determinants probably should also be tested. Unfortunately, mixtures of the minor antigenic determinants are not commercially available. A scratch test with a very dilute (5 units/ml) solution of the penicillin to be administered, followed by a test with a more concentrated solution (10,000 units/ml), can be performed; if this is negative, an intradermal test with 0.02 ml of a solution of 100 units/ml should also be done. If these are negative, penicillin may be administered cautiously. Administration of epinephrine is the therapy of choice for an immediate or accelerated reaction to penicillin.

"Desensitization" is occasionally recommended for patients who are allergic to penicillin and who it is felt must receive the drug. This procedure consists of administering gradually increasing doses of penicillin in the hope of avoiding a severe reaction.

This may result in a subclinical anaphylactic discharge and the binding of all IgE before full doses are administered. Penicillin may be given in doses of 1, 5, 10, 100, and 1000 units intradermally in the lower arm with 60-minute intervals between doses. If this is well tolerated, then 10,000 units and 50,000 units may be given subcutaneously. When full doses are reached, penicillin should not be discontinued and then restarted, since immediate reactions may recur. *The patient should be observed constantly during the procedure, an intravenous line must be in place, and epinephrine and equipment and expertise for artificial ventilation must be on hand. It must be emphasized that this procedure may be dangerous and its efficacy is unproven.*

Patients with life-threatening infections (*e.g.*, endocarditis or meningitis) may be continued on penicillin despite the development of a maculopapular rash. The rash often clears as therapy is continued. This is thought to be due to the development of blocking antibodies of the IgG class. The rash may be treated with antihistamines or adrenocorticosteroids, although there is no evidence that this therapy is efficacious. Rarely, such patients develop exfoliative dermatitis with or without vasculitis if therapy with penicillin is continued. Therefore, alternative antimicrobial agents should be used where possible (*see* Green *et al.*, 1977).

Other Adverse Reactions. The penicillins have minimal direct toxicity (*see* Parker, 1975). The actual limit of the dose of penicillin G that can be administered parenterally with safety still remains to be determined. A number of individuals have been treated intravenously with quantities ranging from 40 to 80 million units per day for as long as 4 weeks without untoward effects (Weinstein *et al.*, 1964).

Apparent toxic effects that have been reported include bone-marrow depression, granulocytopenia, and hepatitis. The last-named effect is rare but is most commonly seen following the administration of oxacillin and nafcillin (Onorato and Axelrod, 1978; Kirkwood *et al.*, 1983). The administration of penicillin G, carbenicillin, or ticarcillin has been associated with a potentially significant defect of hemostasis that appears to be due to an impairment of platelet aggregation; this may be caused by interference with the binding of agonists to the platelet surface (Brown *et al.*, 1974; Shattil *et al.*, 1980).

Most common among the *irritative responses* to penicillin are *pain* and *sterile inflammatory reactions* at the sites of intramuscular injections, reactions that are related to concentration. Serum transaminases and lactic dehydrogenase may be elevated as a result of local damage to muscle. Some individuals who receive penicillin intravenously develop *phlebitis* or *thrombophlebitis*. Many persons who take various penicillin preparations by mouth experience nausea, with or without vomiting, and some have mild-to-severe diarrhea. These manifestations are often related to the dose of the drug.

When penicillin is injected accidentally into the sciatic nerve, severe pain occurs and dysfunction in the area of distribution of this nerve develops and persists for weeks. Intrathecal injection of penicillin G may produce *arachnoiditis* or severe and fatal *encephalopathy*. Because of this, intrathecal or intraventricular administration of penicillins should be avoided. The parenteral administration of large doses of penicillin G (greater than 20 million units per day, or less with renal insufficiency) may produce lethargy, confusion, twitching, multifocal myoclonus, or localized or generalized epileptiform seizures. These are most apt to occur in the presence of renal insufficiency, localized CNS lesions, or hyponatremia. When the concentration of penicillin G in CSF exceeds 10 μg/ml, significant dysfunction of the CNS is frequent. The injection of 20 million units of penicillin G potassium, which contains 34 mEq of potassium, may lead to severe or even fatal hyperkalemia in persons with renal dysfunction.

Injection of penicillin G procaine may result in an immediate reaction, characterized by dizziness, tinnitus, headache, hallucinations, and sometimes seizures. This is due to the rapid liberation of toxic concentrations of procaine (Green *et al.*, 1974). It has been reported to occur in 1 of 200 patients receiving 4.8 million units of penicillin G procaine to treat their venereal disease.

Reactions Unrelated to Hypersensitivity or Toxicity. Regardless of the route by which the drug is administered, but most strikingly when it is given by mouth, penicillin changes the composition of the microflora by eliminating sensitive microorganisms. Thus, profound alterations may be observed in the types and numbers of microorganisms present in the intestinal and upper respiratory tracts; the degree of alteration is related directly to the quantity of penicillin administered. Although this occurs in practically all individuals, it is usually of no clinical significance and the normal microflora is reestablished shortly after therapy is stopped. In some persons, however, *superinfection* results from the changes in flora. *Pseudomembranous colitis*, related to overgrowth and production of a toxin by *Clostridium difficile*, has followed oral or, less commonly, parenteral administration of penicillins.

Fever and even vascular collapse and death may follow the use of penicillin in syphilis. This is one manifestation of the Jarisch-Herxheimer reaction. It is thought to be due to hypersensitivity to antigens released during rapid and massive lysis of spirochetes.

THE CEPHALOSPORINS

History and Source. *Cephalosporium acremonium*, the first source of the cephalosporins, was isolated in 1948 by Brotzu from the sea near a sewer outlet off the Sardinian coast. Crude filtrates from cultures of this fungus were found to inhibit the *in-vitro* growth of *Staph. aureus* and to cure staphylococcal infections and typhoid fever in man. Culture fluids in which the Sardinian fungus was cultivated were found to contain three distinct antibiotics, which were named cephalosporin P, N, and C. With the isolation of the active nucleus of cephalosporin C, 7-aminocephalosporanic acid, and with the addition of side chains, it became possible to produce semisynthetic compounds with antibacterial activity very much greater than that of the parent substance. (For a complete historical review and discussion of the biochemistry of the cephalosporins, *see* Abraham, 1962; Flynn, 1972.)

Chemistry. *Cephalosporin C* contains a side chain derived from D-α-aminoadipic acid, which is condensed with a dihydrothiazine beta-lactam ring system (7-aminocephalosporanic acid). Compounds containing 7-aminocephalosporanic acid are relatively stable in dilute acid and highly resistant to penicillinase, regardless of the nature of their side chains and their affinity for the enzyme.

Cephalosporin C can be hydrolyzed by acid to 7-aminocephalosporanic acid. This compound has been subsequently modified by the addition of different side chains to create a whole family of cephalosporin antibiotics. It appears that modifications at position 7 of the beta-lactam ring are associated with alteration in antibacterial activity and that substitutions at position 3 of the dihydrothiazine ring are associated with changes in the metabolism and the pharmacokinetic properties of the drugs (*see* Huber *et al.*, 1972).

The *cephamycins* are similar to the cephalosporins, but have a methoxy group at position 7 of the beta-lactam ring of the 7-aminocephalosporanic acid nucleus. The structural formulas of representative cephalosporins and cephamycins are shown in Table 50–2.

Mechanism of Action. Cephalosporins and cephamycins appear to inhibit bacterial cell-wall synthesis in a manner similar to that of penicillin. This is discussed in detail above (*see* page 1116).

Classification. The explosive growth of the cephalosporins during the past decade has taxed the best of memories and makes a system of classification most desirable. Although cephalosporins may be classified by their chemical structure, clinical pharmacology, resistance to beta-lactamase, or antimicrobial spectrum, the well-accepted system of classification by "generations" is very useful, although admittedly somewhat arbitrary (Table 50–2).

Classification by generations is based on general features of antimicrobial activity (*see* Mandell, 1985). The first-generation cephalosporins, epitomized by cephalothin and cefazolin, have good activity against

Table 50–2. NAMES, STRUCTURAL FORMULAS, DOSAGE, AND DOSAGE FORMS OF SELECTED CEPHALOSPORINS AND RELATED COMPOUNDS

COMPOUND (TRADE NAMES)	R_1	R_2	DOSAGE FORMS, * DOSAGE FOR SEVERE INFECTION, AND HALF-LIVES
First Generation Cephalothin (KEFLIN, SEFFIN)			I: 1 to 2 g every 4 hours $T_{1/2}$ = 0.6 hour
Cephapirin (CEFADYL)			I: 1 to 2 g every 4 hours $T_{1/2}$ = 1.2 hours
Cefazolin (ANCEF, KEFZOL)			I: 1 to 1.5 g every 6 hours $T_{1/2}$ = 1.8 hours
Cephalexin (KEFLEX)		—CH$_3$	C,T,O: 1 g every 6 hours $T_{1/2}$ = 0.9 hour
Cephradine (ANSPOR, VELOSEF)		—CH$_3$	C,O: 1 g every 6 hours I: 2 g every 6 hours $T_{1/2}$ = 0.8 hour
Cefadroxil (DURICEF, ULTRACEF)		—CH$_3$	C,T,O: 1 g every 12 hours $T_{1/2}$ = 1.5 hours
Second Generation Cefamandole (MANDOL)			I: 2 g every 4 hours $T_{1/2}$ = 0.8 hour
Cefoxitin† (MEFOXIN)			I: 2 g every 4 hours or 3 g every 6 hours $T_{1/2}$ = 0.7 hour
Cefaclor (CECLOR)		—Cl	C,O: 1 g every 8 hours $T_{1/2}$ = 0.8 hour
Cefuroxime (ZINACEF)			I: 3 g every 8 hours $T_{1/2}$ = 1.7 hours
Cefonicid (MONOCID)			I: 2 g every 24 hours $T_{1/2}$ = 4.4 hours

Table 50–2. NAMES, STRUCTURAL FORMULAS, DOSAGE, AND DOSAGE FORMS OF SELECTED CEPHALOSPORINS AND RELATED COMPOUNDS (Continued)

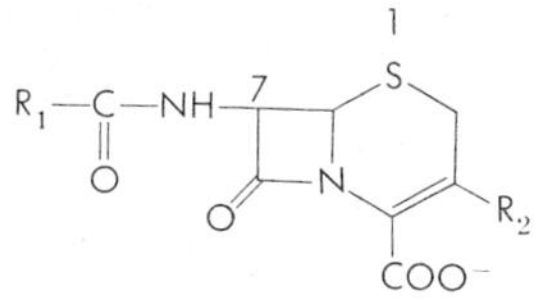

General structure: R_1—C(=O)—NH—7—(β-lactam/dihydrothiazine ring system with S at position 1)—R_2, with COO⁻ at the carboxyl position.

COMPOUND (TRADE NAMES)	R_1	R_2	DOSAGE FORMS,* DOSAGE FOR SEVERE INFECTION, AND HALF-LIVES
Ceforanide (PRECEF)	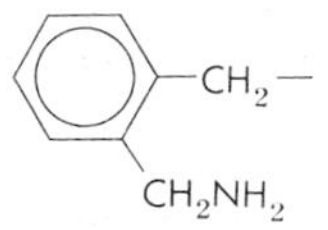 benzyl ring with CH_2— and CH_2NH_2 substituents	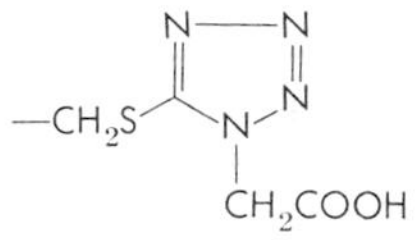 —CH_2S-tetrazole with CH_2COOH	I: 1 g every 12 hours $T_{1/2}$ = 2.6 hours
Third Generation Cefotaxime (CLAFORAN)	aminothiazole H_2N—, ring with C=N—OCH_3	—$CH_2OC(=O)CH_3$	I: 2 g every 4 hours $T_{1/2}$ = 1.1 hours
Moxalactam ‡ (MOXAM)	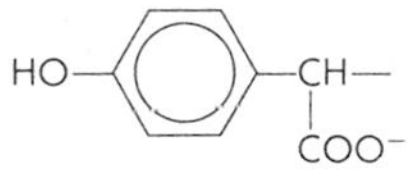 HO—phenyl—CH— with COO⁻	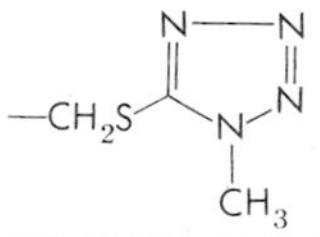 —CH_2S-tetrazole with CH_3	I: 4 g every 8 hours $T_{1/2}$ = 2.1 hours
Ceftizoxime (CEFIZOX)	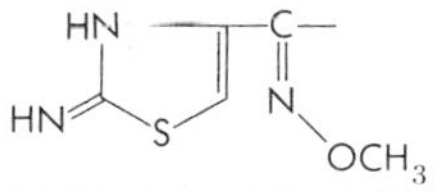 HN, HN—S aminothiazoline ring with C=N—OCH_3	—H	I: 3 to 4 g every 8 hours $T_{1/2}$ = 1.8 hours
Ceftriaxone (ROCEPHIN)	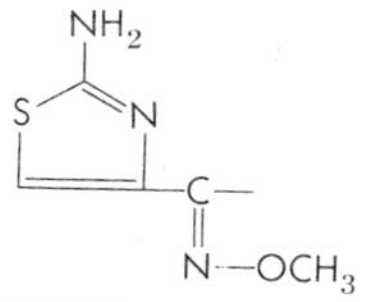 NH_2 aminothiazole S—N ring, C=N—OCH_3	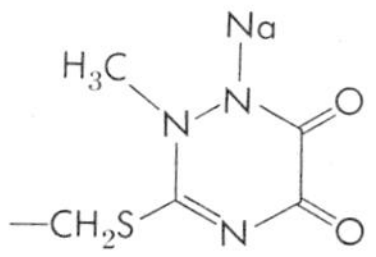 —CH_2S—triazinone ring with H_3C, Na, and two =O	I: 2 g every 12 to 24 hours $T_{1/2}$ = 8 hours
Cefoperazone (CEFOBID)	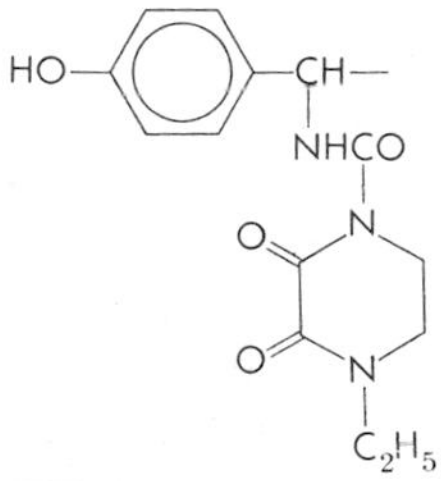 HO—phenyl—CH— with NHCO—piperazinedione (C_2H_5)	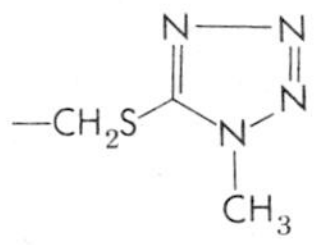 —CH_2S-tetrazole with CH_3	I: 1.5 to 4 g every 6, 8, or 12 hours $T_{1/2}$ = 2.1 hours

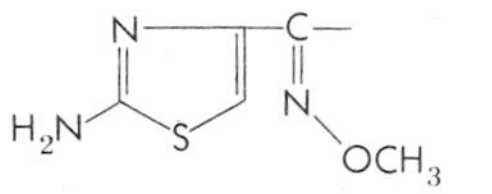

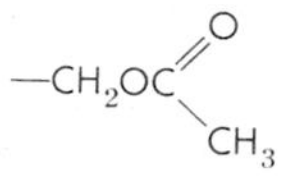

* T = tablet, C = capsule, O = oral suspension, I = injection.
† Cefoxitin, a cephamycin, has a —OCH_3 residue at position 7.
‡ Moxalactam has a —OCH_3 residue at position 7, and oxygen replaces sulfur at position 1.

gram-positive bacteria and relatively modest activity against gram-negative microorganisms. Most gram-positive cocci (with the exception of enterococci, methicillin-resistant *Staph. aureus,* and *Staph. epi-* *dermidis*) are susceptible. Activity against *E. coli, Klebsiella pneumoniae,* and *Pr. mirabilis* is good. The second-generation cephalosporins have somewhat increased activity against gram-negative microorganisms but are much less active than the third-generation agents. Third-generation cephalosporins are generally less active than first-generation agents against gram-positive cocci, but they are much more active against the Enterobacteriaceae, including penicillinase-producing strains. A subset of agents that belong to the third generation is also active against *Pseud. aeruginosa* (Neu, 1982b; Garzone *et al.*, 1983a, 1983b; Schumacher, 1983).

Mechanisms of Bacterial Resistance to the Cephalosporins. Resistance to the cephalosporins may be related to inability of the antibiotic to reach its site of action. Another explanation for resistance could be alterations in the antibiotic-binding proteins, such that interaction does not take place. Bacteria also have the ability to produce enzymes—beta-lactamases (or "cephalosporinases") that can disrupt the beta-lactam ring and render the cephalosporin inactive.

If the antibiotic binds to and inactivates only one enzyme, it is possible that a mutation in the gene coding for that enzyme may lead to resistance. This is probably not a common cause of resistance to the cephalosporins, since most of these agents appear to bind to several different proteins. Bacteria may destroy cephalosporins by hydrolysis of the beta-lactam ring. Many gram-positive microorganisms release relatively large amounts of beta-lactamase into the surrounding medium. Although gram-negative bacteria seem to produce less beta-lactamase, the location of their enzyme in the periplasmic space may make it more effective in destroying cephalosporins as they diffuse to their targets on the inner membrane (Richmond and Sykes, 1973).

The cephalosporins have variable susceptibility to beta-lactamase. Of the first-generation agents, cephaloridine is the most sensitive to beta-lactamases from both gram-positive and gram-negative microorganisms. Cefazolin is more susceptible to hydrolysis by beta-lactamase from *Staph. aureus* than is cephalothin (Farrar and O'Dell, 1978). Cefoxitin, cefuroxime, and the third-generation cephalosporins are the most resistant to hydrolysis by the beta-lactamases produced by gram-negative bacteria (Sykes and Bush, 1983). However, the correlation between antimicrobial activity and resistance to beta-lactamase is not perfect. Some bacterial strains that fail to hydrolyze the antibiotics are nevertheless resistant. Conversely, some bacteria with beta-lactamases that can destroy cephalosporins are susceptible to them (Farrar and Kruse, 1970). Although most of the third-generation cephalosporins are relatively resistant to hydrolysis by bacterial beta-lactamases, there have been reports of the development of resistance to the third-generation agents by *Enterobacter, Serratia,* and *Pseudomonas* species (Sykes and Bush, 1983). Sanders and Sanders (1983) have suggested that the derepression of beta-lactamases in these microorganisms has resulted in the production of enzymes

with a high affinity for the antibiotics, despite the fact that they cannot hydrolyze them. They propose that the third-generation cephalosporins are tightly bound to the beta-lactamases and, thus, are prevented from interacting with their target penicillin-binding proteins.

It is important to remember that none of the cephalosporins has reliable activity against the following microorganisms: penicillin-resistant *Strep. pneumoniae*, methicillin-resistant *Staph. aureus*, methicillin-resistant *Staph. epidermidis, Strep. faecalis, List. monocytogenes, Legionella pneumophila, Legionella micdadei, Clostridium difficile, Pseud. maltophilia, Pseud. putida, Campylobacter jejuni, Acinetobacter* species, and, of course, *Candida albicans.*

General Features of the Cephalosporins. Cephalexin, cephradine, cefaclor, and cefadroxil are absorbed after oral administration and can be given by this route. Cephalothin and cephapirin cause pain when given by intramuscular injection and thus are usually used only intravenously. Most of the other agents can be administered intramuscularly or intravenously.

Cephalosporins are primarily excreted by the kidney; dosage should thus be altered in patients with renal insufficiency. Probenecid slows the tubular secretion of most cephalosporins, but not moxalactam (DeSante *et al.*, 1982). Cefoperazone is an exception, since it is excreted predominantly in the bile. Cephalothin, cephapirin, and cefotaxime are deacetylated *in vivo,* and these metabolites have less antimicrobial activity than the parent compounds. The deacetylated metabolites are also excreted by the kidneys. None of the other cephalosporins appears to undergo appreciable metabolism.

Several cephalosporins penetrate into CSF in sufficient concentration to be useful for the treatment of meningitis. These include cefuroxime, moxalactam, cefotaxime, and ceftizoxime. Cephalosporins also cross the placenta, and they are found in high concentrations in synovial and pericardial fluid. Penetration into the aqueous humor of the eye is relatively good after systemic administration of third-generation agents, but penetration into the vitreous is poor. There is some evidence that concentrations sufficient for therapy of ocular infections due to gram-positive and certain gram-negative microorganisms can be achieved after systemic administration.

Concentrations in bile are usually high, with those achieved after administration of cefoperazone being the highest.

SPECIFIC AGENTS

First-Generation Cephalosporins. *Cephalothin* is not well absorbed orally and is available only for parenteral administration. Because of pain on intramuscular injection, it is usually given intravenously. Peak concentrations in plasma are about 20 μg/ml after an intramuscular dose of 1 g. Cephalothin has a short half-life (30 to 40 minutes) and is metabolized in addition to being excreted. The deacetylated metabolite accounts for 20 to 30% of the excreted drug (Chang and Weinstein, 1963; Klein *et al.*, 1964). Cephalothin does not enter the CSF to a significant extent, and this drug should obviously not be used for the treatment of meningitis. Since cephalothin, among the cephalosporins, is most impervious to attack by staphylococcal beta-lactamase, some authorities consider it to be the cephalosporin of choice in severe staphylococcal infections, such as endocarditis.

Cephapirin is very similar to cephalothin (Renzini *et al.*, 1975).

The antibacterial spectrum of *cefazolin* is similar to that of cephalothin. Although cefazolin is more active against *E. coli* and *Klebsiella* species (Sabath *et al.*, 1973), it is somewhat more sensitive to staphylococcal beta-lactamase than is cephalothin (Regamey *et al.*, 1975; Fong *et al.*, 1976a; Byrant, 1984). Cefazolin is relatively well tolerated after either intramuscular or intravenous administration, and concentrations of the drug in plasma are higher after intramuscular (64 μg/ml after 1 g) or intravenous injection than are concentrations of cephalothin. The half-life is also appreciably longer—1.8 hours (Bergeron *et al.*, 1973). The renal clearance of cefazolin is lower than that of cephalothin; this is presumably related to the fact that cefazolin is excreted by glomerular filtration, whereas cephalothin is also secreted by the kidney tubule. Cefazolin is bound to plasma proteins to a great extent (about 85%). Cefazolin is usually preferred among the first-generation cephalosporins, since it can be administered less frequently because of its longer half-life (Quintiliani and Nightingale, 1978).

Cephalexin is available for oral administration, and it has the same antibacterial spectrum as the other first-generation cephalosporins. However, it is somewhat less active against penicillinase-producing staphylococci. Oral therapy with cephalexin results in peak concentrations in plasma of 16 μg/ml after a dose of 0.5 g; this is adequate for the inhibition of many gram-positive and gram-negative pathogens that are sensitive to cephalothin. The drug is not metabolized, and more than 90% is excreted in the urine (Meyers *et al.*, 1969).

Cephradine is similar in structure to cephalexin, and its activity *in vitro* is almost identical. Cephradine is not metabolized and, after rapid absorption from the gastrointestinal tract, is excreted unchanged in the urine. Cephradine can be administered orally, intramuscularly, or intravenously.

When administered orally, it is difficult to distinguish cephradine from cephalexin; some authorities feel that these two drugs can be used interchangeably. Because cephradine is so well absorbed, the concentrations in plasma are nearly equivalent after oral or intramuscular administration (about 10 to 18 μg/ml after 0.5 g orally or intramuscularly) (Neiss, 1973).

Cefadroxil is the para-hydroxy analog of cephalexin. Concentrations of cefadroxil in plasma and urine are at somewhat higher levels than are those with cephalexin. The drug may be used once or twice a day for the treatment of urinary tract infections. Its activity *in vitro* is similar to that of cephalexin (Hartstein *et al.*, 1977).

Second-Generation Cephalosporins. *Cefamandole* is more active than the first-generation cephalosporins against certain gram-negative microorganisms. This is especially evident for *H. influenzae* (Meyers *et al.*, 1969), *Enterobacter* species, indole-positive *Proteus* species, *E. coli*, and *Klebsiella* species (Meyers and Hirschman, 1978). Heavy inocula of bacteria show decreased susceptibility, and this appears to be related to destruction of the antibiotic by beta-lactamase. Most gram-positive cocci are sensitive to cefamandole. The half-life of the drug is 45 minutes, and it is excreted unchanged in the urine. Concentrations in plasma are 20 to 36 μg/ml after a dose of 1 g given intramuscularly (Fong *et al.*, 1976b; Neu, 1978).

Cefoxitin is a cephamycin produced by *Streptomyces lactamdurans*. It is highly resistant to beta-lactamases produced by gram-negative rods (Kass and Evans, 1979). This antibiotic is more active than cephalothin against certain gram-negative microorganisms, although it is less active than cefamandole against *Enterobacter* species and *H. influenzae*. It is also less active than both cefamandole and the first-generation cephalosporins against gram-positive bacteria. Cefoxitin is more active than other first- or second-generation agents against anaerobes, especially *B. fragilis*. This activity is similar to that of moxalactam and better than that of other third-generation cephalosporins. After an intramuscular dose of 1 g, concentrations in plasma are about 22 μg/ml. The half-life is approximately 40 minutes. Cefoxitin's special role seems to be for treatment of certain anaerobic and mixed aerobic-anaerobic infections, such as pelvic inflammatory disease and lung abscess (Sutter and Finegold, 1975; Bach *et al.*, 1977; Chow and Bednorz, 1978). It is an effective agent for gonorrhea caused by penicillinase-producing *Neisseria* (Greaves *et al.*, 1983).

Cefaclor is used orally. The concentrations in plasma after oral administration are about 50% of those achieved after an equivalent oral dose of cephalexin. However, cefaclor is more active against *H. influenzae*, although some beta-lactamase-producing strains of *H. influenzae* may be resistant (Silver *et al.*, 1977).

Cefuroxime is very similar to cefamandole in structure and antibacterial activity *in vitro* (Smith and LeFrock, 1983), although it is somewhat more resistant to beta-lactamases. The half-life is longer than that of cefamandole (1.7 hours versus 0.8 hour), and the drug can be given every 8 hours. Concentrations in CSF are about 10% of those in plasma, and the drug is effective for meningitis due to *H. influenzae* (including strains resistant to ampicillin), *N. meningitidis,* and *Strep. pneumoniae* (Johansson *et al.,* 1982).

Cefonicid has antimicrobial activity *in vitro* similar to that of cefamandole. The half-life of the drug is about 4 hours, and administration once daily has been effective for certain infections caused by susceptible microorganisms (Gremillion *et al.,* 1983).

Ceforanide is similar in structure and antimicrobial activity to cefamandole; however, it is less active against strains of *H. influenzae* (Barriere and Mills, 1982). Its half-life is about 2.6 hours and it is administered parenterally every 12 hours.

Second-generation cephalosporins that are not available in the United States at the present time include *cefotiam,* which is similar to cefamandole in its antimicrobial activity *in vitro* (Bodey *et al.,* 1981), and *cefmetazole,* which has poor activity against *Enterobacter* but is otherwise similar to cefoxitin.

Third-Generation Cephalosporins. *Cefotaxime* was the first of the third-generation cephalosporins to become available in the United States. The drug is highly resistant to bacterial beta-lactamases and has good activity against many gram-positive and gram-negative aerobic bacteria. However, activity against *B. fragilis* is poor compared to agents such as clindamycin and metronidazole (Neu *et al.,* 1979). Cefotaxime has a half-life in plasma of about 1 hour, and the drug should be administered every 4 to 6 hours for serious infections. The drug is metabolized *in vivo* to desacetylcefotaxime, which is less active against most microorganisms than is the parent compound. Cefotaxime has been utilized effectively for meningitis caused by gram-negative bacteria (Landesman *et al.,* 1981; Cherubin *et al.,* 1982; Mullaney and John, 1983).

Moxalactam has a unique structure (designated oxa-beta-lactam), which is created by the substitution of an oxygen for the sulfur atom in the cephem nucleus (Table 50–2). Moxalactam has the broad antimicrobial activity characteristic of the third-generation cephalosporins (Symposium, 1982). In comparison to cefotaxime, it is less active against gram-positive microorganisms (including streptococci and staphylococci). It is somewhat less active against *H. influenzae* and has very similar activity against most of the Enterobacteriaceae. It is slightly more active against *Pseudomonas* and appreciably more active against *B. fragilis* than cefotaxime. Moxalactam has a half-life in plasma of approximately 2 hours, and the drug is excreted unchanged in the urine (Olson *et al.,* 1981). Clinically significant (and sometimes fatal) bleeding has been described after administration of moxalactam, and it appears that moxalactam can interfere with hemostasis as a result of either hypoprothrombinemia, platelet dysfunction, or, more rarely, immunologically mediated thrombocytopenia (Weitekamp and Aber, 1983). It is recommended that patients who receive moxalactam be given vitamin K pro-

phylactically (10 mg per week). Since platelet dysfunction is dose related, it is suggested that bleeding times be monitored in patients (with normal renal function) who receive more than 4 g of moxalactam per day for more than 3 days.

Ceftizoxime has a spectrum of activity *in vitro* very similar to that of cefotaxime. The half-life is somewhat longer, 1.8 hours, and the drug can thus be administered every 8 hours for serious infections. Ceftizoxime is not metabolized and is excreted in the urine (Neu *et al.,* 1982).

Ceftriaxone has activity *in vitro* very similar to that of ceftizoxime and cefotaxime. A half-life of about 8 hours is the outstanding feature. Administration of the drug twice daily has been effective for patients with meningitis (Del Rio *et al.,* 1983), while dosage once a day has been effective for other infections (Baumgartner and Glauser, 1983). Most of the drug can be recovered from the urine (60%), and about 40% appears to be eliminated by biliary secretion. A single dose of ceftriaxone (125 mg) has been effective in the treatment of gonorrhea, including disease caused by penicillinase-producing microorganisms (Rajan *et al.,* 1982; Handsfield and Murphy, 1983).

Cefotetan is a cephamycin. Its activity *in vitro* against gram-negative bacteria is similar to that of cefotaxime and moxalactam; however, it is less active against *Enterobacter aerogenes* and has no useful activity against *Pseudomonas.* Activity against gram-positive microorganisms is similar to that of moxalactam, but cefotetan is significantly less active against pneumococci. Its activity against anaerobes is similar to that of cefotaxime (Ayers *et al.,* 1982). The half-life is about 3 hours (Phillips *et al.,* 1983).

Cefmenoxime has a spectrum of activity *in vitro* very similar to that of cefotaxime. Its half-life is 1 hour.

Third-Generation Cephalosporins with Good Activity Against Pseudomonas. Cefoperazone is less active than cefotaxime against gram-positive microorganisms and less active than cefotaxime or moxalactam against many species of gram-negative bacteria. However, it is more active than both of these agents against *Pseud. aeruginosa.* Unfortunately, resistant strains may emerge on treatment. Activity against *B. fragilis* is similar to that of cefotaxime. Cefoperazone is slightly less stable to beta-lactamases than are the cefotaxime-like or 7-methoxycephem drugs (Klein and Neu, 1983). Only 25% of a dose of cefoperazone can be recovered from the urine, and most of the drug is eliminated by biliary excretion. The half-life is about 2 hours. Concentrations of cefoperazone in bile are higher than those achieved with any other cephalosporin; concentrations in blood are two to three times higher than those found with cefotaxime. The dose of cefoperazone does not have to be altered in patients with renal insufficiency, but hepatic dysfunction or biliary obstruction affects clearance. Cefoperazone can cause bleeding due to hypoprothrombinemia; this can be reversed by administration of vitamin K. A disulfiram-like reaction has been reported in patients who drink alcohol while taking cefoperazone.

Ceftazidime is about one half as active by weight against gram-positive microorganisms as is cefotaxime. Its activity against the Enterobacteriaceae is very similar, but its major distinguishing feature is good activity against *Pseudomonas*. Ceftazidime has poor activity against *B. fragilis* (Hamilton-Miller and Brumfitt, 1981). Its half-life in plasma is about 1.5 hours, and the drug is not metabolized. Ceftazidime was found to be more active *in vitro* against *Pseudomonas* than was cefsulodin, cefoperazone, or piperacillin (Neu, 1981; Neu and Labthavikul, 1982).

Cefpiramide has good activity against *Pseudomonas* and gram-positive microorganisms (Kato *et al.*, 1982). The half-life is about 4 hours.

Cefsulodin has good activity against *Pseudomonas* and staphylococci but is relatively inactive against most other microorganisms (King *et al.*, 1980).

Adverse Reactions. Hypersensitivity reactions to the cephalosporins are the most common side effects (*see* Petz, 1978), and there is no evidence that any single cephalosporin is more or less likely to cause such sensitization. The reactions appear to be identical to those caused by the penicillins, and this may be related to the shared beta-lactam structure of both groups of antibiotics (Bennett *et al.*, 1983). Immediate reactions such as anaphylaxis, bronchospasm, and urticaria are observed. More commonly, patients develop maculopapular rash, usually after several days of therapy; this may or may not be accompanied by fever and eosinophilia. Fever and lymphadenopathy have been associated with the administration of cephalosporins in the absence of other manifestations of allergic phenomena (*see* Sanders *et al.*, 1974).

Because of the similarity in structure of the penicillins and cephalosporins, patients who are allergic to one class of agents may manifest cross-reactivity when a member of the other class is administered. Immunological studies have demonstrated cross-reactivity in as many as 20% of patients who are allergic to penicillin (*see* Levine, 1973), but clinical reports seem to indicate a lower frequency (5 to 10%) of such reactions. There are no skin tests that can reliably predict whether a patient will manifest an allergic reaction to the cephalosporins.

Patients with a history of a mild or a temporally distant reaction to penicillin appear to be at low risk of developing a rash or other allergic reaction following the administration of a cephalosporin. *However, patients who have had a recent severe, immediate reaction to a penicillin should be given a cephalosporin with great caution, if at all.* A positive Coombs' reaction appears frequently in patients who receive large doses of a cephalosporin. Hemolysis is not usually associated with this phenomenon, although it has been reported. Cephalosporins have produced rare instances of bone-marrow depression, characterized by granulocytopenia (Kammer, 1984).

The cephalosporins have been implicated as potentially nephrotoxic agents, although they are not nearly as toxic to the kidney as are the aminoglycosides or the polymyxins (Barza, 1978). Renal tubular necrosis has followed the administration of cephaloridine in doses greater than 4 g per day; this agent is no longer available in the United States. Other cephalosporins are much less toxic and, in recommended doses, rarely produce significant renal toxicity when used by themselves. High doses of cephalothin have produced acute tubular necrosis in certain instances, and usual doses (8 to 12 g per day) have caused nephrotoxicity in patients with preexisting renal disease (Pasternack and Stephens, 1975). There is good evidence that the concurrent administration of cephalothin and gentamicin or tobramycin causes nephrotoxicity synergistically (Wade *et al.*, 1978). This is especially marked in patients over 60 years of age. Diarrhea can result from the administration of cephalosporins and may be more frequent with cefoperazone, perhaps because of its greater biliary excretion. Intolerance of alcohol (a disulfiram-like reaction) has been noted with cefamandole, moxalactam, and cefoperazone. Serious bleeding related either to hypoprothrombinemia, thrombocytopenia, and/or platelet dysfunction has been reported with several beta-lactam antibiotics (Bank and Kammer, 1983). This appears to be a particular problem with certain patients (elderly, poorly nourished, or those with renal insufficiency) who are receiving moxalactam.

Therapeutic Uses. The cephalosporins are widely used antibiotics. Unfortunately they are often overutilized for conditions where much less expensive antibiotics would provide adequate therapy. Clinical studies have shown them to be effective as both therapeutic and prophylactic agents. In the past it was stated that cephalosporins were not drugs of first choice for any indication. However, they are effective and well tolerated, and indications for their use appear to be changing with the rapid development of new second- and third-generation agents (Neu, 1982a; Brooks and Barriere, 1983). Cephalosporins, either with or without aminoglycosides, have been considered to be the drugs of choice for serious infections caused by *Klebsiella*. Prophylaxis during and after surgery is another area where cephalosporins have found wide use; there are numerous instances where first-generation cephalosporins have been shown to be safe and effective for this purpose. Some of the third-generation cephalosporins are presently the drugs of choice for meningitis caused by gram-negative enteric bacteria because of their antimicrobial activity, good penetration into CSF, and record of clinical successes. Therapeutic trials are in progress to evaluate the role of these agents for meningitis acquired in the community, and it appears that therapy with some second- or third-generation cephalosporins may be equivalent to treatment with a combination of ampicillin and chloramphenicol for meningitis caused by *H. influenzae*.

Cephalosporins are still useful as alternatives to penicillins for a variety of infections in patients who cannot tolerate penicillins. These include streptococcal and staphylococcal infections. Still to be clarified is the role of the third-generation cephalosporins in the treatment of serious infections outside of the CNS caused by gram-negative bacilli. Those relatively uncommon microorganisms that are resistant to other agents are frequently sensitive to third-generation cephalosporins; these drugs should clearly be used in those situations. In other instances, microorganisms may be sensitive to a variety of antibiotics, but third-generation cephalosporins may be the most active *in vitro*. Whether this increased activity *in vitro* will be translated into increased clinical success is unclear, but some infectious disease specialists use the highly active third-generation cephalosporins for selected serious infections caused by gram-negative microorganisms.

Infections with anaerobes are often treated with combinations of antibiotics, since aerobic microorganisms are usually also present. Cefoxitin and several of the third-generation cephalosporins have good activity against anaerobes and are useful alternatives to combination therapy under certain conditions. Infections caused by penicillinase-producing gonococci can be treated effectively with several of the penicillinase-resistant second- or third-generation cephalosporins. The spectrum of activity of some of these agents appears to be excellent for the treatment of pneumonias acquired in the community, *i.e.*, those caused by pneumococci, *H. influenzae* (including strains that produce beta-lactamase), or staphylococci.

Nosocomial infections are frequently caused by microorganisms that are resistant to many of the commonly used agents, such as the first-generation cephalosporins, ampicillin, and some of the aminoglycosides. Third-generation cephalosporins have been useful additions to therapy in these situations. Patients who are severely neutropenic have been treated successfully with either a third-generation cephalosporin plus an aminoglycoside or, for selected patients, a third-generation cephalosporin that is active against *Pseudomonas* (*e.g.*, ceftazidime) without an aminoglycoside. However, resistant strains frequently emerge during therapy of severe infections with *Pseudomonas* when single agents are used.

OTHER BETA-LACTAM ANTIBIOTICS

Agents with a beta-lactam structure that are neither penicillins nor cephalosporins have been developed recently.

Imipenem is derived from a compound produced by *Streptomyces cattleya*. The compound, thienamycin, is unstable, but the N-formimidoyl derivative, imipenem, is stable.

Imipenem, like other beta-lactam antibiotics, binds to penicillin-binding proteins and causes death of susceptible microorganisms. It is very resistant to hydrolysis by most beta-lactamases.

The activity of imipenem is excellent *in vitro* for a wide variety of aerobic and anaerobic microorganisms. Streptococci (including enterococci), staphylococci (including penicillinase-producing strains), and *Listeria* are all susceptible. Although some strains of methicillin-resistant staphylococci are susceptible, many strains are not. Activity against the Enterobacteriaceae is excellent. Most strains of *Pseudomonas* and *Acinetobacter* are inhibited. *Pseud. maltophilia* is resistant. Anaerobes are highly susceptible, including *B. fragilis*. *Clostridium difficile*, the cause of pseudomembranous colitis, is inhibited by concentrations of 6 to 8 μg/ml (Tally *et al.*, 1980; Cullman *et al.*, 1982; Blumenthal *et al.*, 1983).

Imipenem is not absorbed orally. The drug is rapidly hydrolyzed by a dehydropeptidase found in the brush border of the proximal renal tubule (Kropp *et al.*, 1982). Because concentrations of active drug in urine were low, an inhibitor of the dehydropeptidase was synthesized. This compound is called *cilastatin*. A preparation has been developed that contains equal amounts of imipenem and cilastatin (PRIMAXIN). It is not available in the United States.

After the intravenous administration of 500 mg of imipenem (as PRIMAXIN), peak concentrations in plasma are 33 μg/ml. The half-life is 1 hour, and 70% of the active drug is excreted in the urine.

Nausea and vomiting are the most common (1 to 2%) adverse reactions. Although this agent is effective (Eron *et al.*, 1983), its exact place in therapy is unclear. It may be useful for selected severe infections, including those caused by microorganisms resistant to other agents.

Aztreonam (AZACTAM) is a monocyclic beta-lactam compound (a monobactam) isolated from *Chromobacterium violaceum* (Sykes *et al.*, 1981). It interacts with penicillin-binding proteins of susceptible microorganisms and induces the formation of long filamentous bacterial structures. Anaerobic organisms and gram-positive bacteria are resistant. Activity against Enterobacteriaceae is good, as is that against *Pseud. aeruginosa*. The drug is given parenterally and has a half-life of about 2 hours (Scully *et al.*, 1983). The drug is being studied for treatment of serious infections caused by gram-negative bacilli. Its ability to preserve the normal anaerobic and gram-positive flora may prove to be advantageous (Symposium, 1985).

BETA-LACTAMASE INHIBITORS

Certain molecules can bind to beta-lactamases and inactivate them, thus preventing the destruction of beta-lactam antibiotics that are substrates for these enzymes.

Clavulanic acid is produced by *Streptomyces clavuligerus;* its structural formula is as follows:

Clavulanic Acid

It has poor intrinsic antimicrobial activity but is a "suicide" inhibitor of beta-lactamases produced by a wide range of gram-positive and gram-negative microorganisms (Neu and Fu, 1978). Clavulanic acid is well absorbed by mouth and can also be given parenterally. It has been combined with amoxicillin as an oral preparation (AUGMENTIN) and with ticarcillin as a parenteral preparation (TIMENTIN). AUGMENTIN is currently available in the United States as tablets and as powders for oral solution. Amoxicillin plus clavulanic acid appears to be effective *in vitro* and *in vivo* for beta-lactamase-producing strains of staphylococci, *H. influenzae*, gonococci, and *E. coli* (Ball *et al.*, 1980; Yogev *et al.*, 1981). The addition of clavulanic acid to ticarcillin extends its spectrum to some beta-lactamase-producing microorganisms.

Sulbactam is another beta-lactamase inhibitor similar in structure to clavulanic acid. It may be given orally or parenterally along with a beta-lactam antibiotic. Clinical trials are in progress.

Ayers, L. W.; Jones, R. N.; Barry, A. L.; Thornsberry, C.; Fuchs, P. C.; Gavan, T. L.; Gerlach, E. H.; and Sommers, H. M. Cefotetan, a new cephamycin: comparison of *in vitro* antimicrobial activity with other cephems, beta-lactamase stability, and preliminary recommendations for disk diffusion testing. *Antimicrob. Agents Chemother.*, **1982**, *22*, 859–877.

Bach, V. T.; Roy, I.; and Thadepalli, H. Susceptibility of anaerobic bacteria to cefoxitin and related compounds. *Antimicrob. Agents Chemother.*, **1977**, *11*, 912–913.

Ball, A. P.; Geddes, A. M.; Davey, P. G.; Farrell, I. D.; and Brookes, G. R. Clavulanic acid and amoxycillin: a clinical, bacteriological, and pharmacological study. *Lancet*, **1980**, *1*, 620–623.

Barriere, S. L., and Mills, J. Ceforanide: antibacterial activity, pharmacology, and clinical efficacy. *Pharmacotherapy*, **1982**, *2*, 322–327.

Barza, M. The nephrotoxicity of cephalosporins: an overview. *J. Infect. Dis.*, **1978**, *137*, 560–573.

Baumgartner, J., and Glauser, M. P. Single daily dose treatment of severe refractory infections with ceftriaxone. *Arch. Intern. Med.*, **1983**, *143*, 1868–1881.

Bennett, S.; Wise, R.; Weston, D.; and Dent, J. Pharmacokinetics and tissue penetration of ticarcillin combined with clavulanic acid. *Antimicrob. Agents Chemother.*, **1983**, *23*, 831–834.

Bergeron, M. D.; Brusch, J. L.; Barza, M.; and Weinstein, L. Bactericidal activity and pharmacology of cefazolin. *Antimicrob. Agents Chemother.*, **1973**, *4*, 396–401.

Bisno, A. L.; Dismukes, W. E.; Durack, D. T.; Kaplan, E. L.; Karchmer, A. W.; Kaye, D.; Sande, M. A.; Sanford, J. P.; and Wilson, W. R. Treatment of infective endocarditis due to *viridans* streptococci. *Circulation*, **1981**, *63*, 730A–733A.

Blumenthal, R. M.; Raeder, R.; Takemotoa, C. D.; and Freimer, E. H. Occurrence and expression of impemide (N-formimidoyl thienamycin) resistance in clinical isolates of coagulase-negative staphylococci. *Antimicrob. Agents Chemother.*, **1983**, *24*, 61–69.

Bodey, G.; Fainstein, V.; and Hinkle, A. Comparative *in vitro* study of new cephalosporins. *J. Antimicrob. Agents*, **1981**, *20*, 226–230.

Brooks, G. F., and Barriere, S. L. Clinical use of the new beta-lactam antimicrobial drugs. *Ann. Intern. Med.*, **1983**, *98*, 530–535.

Brown, C. H., III; Natelson, E. A.; Bradshaw, M. W.; Williams, T. W., Jr.; and Alfrey, C. P., Jr. The hemostatic defect produced by carbenicillin. *N. Engl. J. Med.*, **1974**, *291*, 265–270.

Bryant, R. E. Effect of the suppurative environment on antibiotic activity. In, *New Dimensions in Antimicrobial Therapy.* (Root, R. K., and Sande, M. A., eds.) Churchill Livingstone, Inc., New York, **1984**, pp. 313–337.

Chain, E. B. The development of bacterial chemotherapy. *Antibiot. Chemother.*, **1954**, *4*, 215–241.

Chambers, H. F.; Hackbarth. C. J.; Drake, T. A.; Rusnak, M. G.; and Sande, M. A. Endocarditis due to methicillin-resistant *Staphylococcus aureus* in rabbits: expression of resistance to beta-lactam antibiotics *in vivo* and *in vitro*. *J. Infect. Dis.*, **1984**, *149*, 894–903.

Chang, T. W., and Weinstein, L. *In vitro* biological activity of cephalothin. *J. Bacteriol.*, **1963**, *85*, 1022–1027.

Chow, A. W., and Bednorz, D. Comparative *in vitro* activity of newer cephalosporins against anaerobic bacteria. *Antimicrob. Agents Chemother.*, **1978**, *14*, 668–671.

Cleeland, R., and Squires, E. Enhanced activity of beta-lactam antibiotics with amdinocillin. *Am. J. Med.*, **1983**, *75*, Suppl., 21–29.

Cullman, W.; Opferkuch, W.; Stieglitz, M.; and Werkmeister, U. A comparison of the antibacterial activities of N-formimidoyl thienamycin (MK0787) with those of other recently developed β-lactam derivatives. *Antimicrob. Agents Chemother.*, **1982**, *22*, 302–307.

Dacey, R. G., and Sande, M. A. Effect of probenecid on cerebrospinal fluid concentrations of penicillin and cephalosporin derivatives. *Antimicrob. Agents Chemother.*, **1974**, *6*, 437–441.

Del Rio, M. A.; Chrane, D.; Shelton, S.; McCracken, G. H.; and Nelson, J. D. Ceftriaxone versus ampicillin and chloramphenicol for treatment of bacterial meningitis in children. *Lancet*, **1983**, *1*, 1241–1244.

DeSante, K. A.; Israel, K. S.; Brier, G. L.; Wolny, J. D.; and Hatcher, B. L. Effect of probenecid on the pharmacokinetics of moxalactam. *Antimicrob. Agents Chemother.*, **1982**, *21*, 58–61.

Ditlove, J.; Weidmann, P.; Bernstein, M.; and Massry, S. G. Methicillin nephritis. *Medicine (Baltimore)*, **1977**, *56*, 483–491.

Eliopoulos, G. M., and Moellering, R. C. Azlocillin, mezlocillin, and piperacillin: new broad-spectrum penicillins. *Ann. Intern. Med.*, **1982**, *97*, 755–760.

Eron, L. J.; Hixon, D. L.; Choong, H. P.; Goldenberg, R. I.; and Poretz, D. M. Imipenem versus moxalactam in the treatment of serious infections. *Antimicrob. Agents Chemother.*, **1983**, *24*, 841–846.

Farrar, W. E., Jr., and Kruse, J. M. Relationship between β-lactamase activity and resistance of *Enterobacter* to cephalothin. *Infect. Immun.*, **1970**, *2*, 610–616.

Farrar, W. E., Jr., and O'Dell, N. M. Comparative betalactamase resistance and antistaphylococcal activities of parenterally and orally administered cephalosporins. *J. Infect. Dis.*, **1978**, *137*, 490–493.

Fong, I. W.; Engelking, E. R.; and Kirby, W. M. M. Relative inactivation by *Staphylococcus aureus* of eight cephalosporin antibiotics. *Antimicrob. Agents Chemother.*, **1976a**, *9*, 939–944.

Fong, I. W.; Ralph, E. D.; Engelking, E. R.; and Kirby, W. M. M. Clinical pharmacology of cefamandole as compared with cephalothin. *Antimicrob. Agents Chemother.*, **1976b**, *9*, 65–69.

Fu, K. P., and Neu, H. C. Azlocillin and mezlocillin—new ureido penicillins. *Antimicrob. Agents Chemother.*, **1978**, *13*, 930–938.

Garzone, P.; Lyon, J.; and Yu, V. L. Third-generation and investigational cephalosporins: I. Structure-activity relationships and pharmacokinetic review. *Drug Intell. Clin. Pharm.*, **1983a**, *17*, 507–515.

———. Third-generation and investigational cephalosporins: II. Microbiologic review and clinical summaries. *Ibid.*, **1983b**, *17*, 615–622.

Gibaldi, M.; Davidson, D.; Plaut, M. E.; and Schwartz, M. A. Modification of penicillin distribution and elimination by probenecid. *Int. Z. Klin. Pharmakol. Ther. Toxikol.*, **1970**, *3*, 182–189.

Gordon, R. C.; Regamey, C.; and Kirby, W. M. M. Comparative clinical pharmacology of amoxicillin and ampicillin administered orally. *Antimicrob. Agents Chemother.*, **1972**, *1*, 504–507.

Greaves, W. L.; Kraus, S. J.; McCormack, W. M.; Biddle, J. W.; Zaidi, A.; Fiumara, N. J.; and Guinan, M. E. Cefoxitin vs penicillin in the treatment of uncomplicated gonorrhea. *Sex. Transm. Dis.*, **1983**, *10*, 53–55.

Green, G. R.; Rosenblum, A. H.; and Sweet, L. C. Evaluation of penicillin hypersensitivity. *J. Allergy Clin. Immunol.*, **1977**, *60*, 339–345.

Green, R. L.; Lewis, J. E.; Kraus, S. J.; and Frederickson, E. L. Elevated plasma procaine concentrations after administration of procaine penicillin G. *N. Engl. J. Med.*, **1974**, *291*, 223–226.

Gremillion, D. H.; Winn, R. E.; and Vandenbout, E. Clinical trial of cefoxicid for treatment of skin infections. *Antimicrob. Agents Chemother.*, **1983**, *23*, 944–946.

Hamilton-Miller, J. M. T., and Brumfitt, W. Activity of ceftazidime (GR20263) against nosocomially important pathogens. *Antimicrob. Agents Chemother.*, **1981**, *19*, 1067–1069.

Handsfield, H. H., and Murphy, V. L. Comparative study of ceftriaxone and spectinomycin for treatment of uncomplicated gonorrhoea in men. *Lancet*, **1983**, *2*, 67–70.

Hartstein, A. I.; Patrick, K. E.; Jones, S. R.; Miller, M. J.; and Bryant, R. E. Comparison of pharmacological and antimicrobial properties of cefadroxil and cephalexin. *Antimicrob. Agents Chemother.*, **1977**, *12*, 93–97.

Huber, F. M.; Chauvette, R. R.; and Jackson, B. G. Preparative methods for 7-aminocephalosporanic acid and 6-aminopenicillanic acid. In, *Cephalosporins and Penicillins.* (Flynn, E. H., ed.) Academic Press, Inc., New York, **1972**, p. 27.

Idsøe, O.; Guthe, T.; Willcox, R. R.; and DeWeck, A. L. Nature and extent of penicillin side-reactions, with particular reference to fatalities from anaphylactic shock. *Bull. WHO*, **1968**, *38*, 159–188.

Jacobs, M. R.; Koornhof, H. J.; Robins-Browne, R. M.; Stevenson, C. M.; Vermaak, Z. A.; Freiman, I.; Miller, G. B.; Witcomb, M. A.; Isaacson, M.; Ward, J. I.; and Austrian, R. Emergence of multiply resistant pneumococci. *N. Engl. J. Med.*, **1978**, *299*, 735–740.

Jaffe, A.; Chabbert, Y. A.; and Semonin, O. Role of porin proteins OmpF and OmpC in the permeation of beta-lactams. *Antimicrob. Agents Chemother.*, **1982**, *22*, 942–948.

Johansson, O., and others. Cefuroxime versus ampicillin and chloramphenicol for the treatment of bacterial meningitis. *Lancet*, **1982**, *1*, 295–298.

Kancir, L. M.; Tuazon, C. U.; Cardella, T. A.; and Sheagren, J. H. Adverse reactions to methicillin and nafcillin during treatment of serious *Staphylococcus aureus* infections. *Arch. Intern. Med.*, **1978**, *138*, 909–911.

Kaplan, J. M., and McCracken, G. H., Jr. Clinical pharmacology of benzathine penicillin G in neonates with regard to its recommended use in congenital syphilis. *J. Pediatr.*, **1973**, *82*, 1069–1072.

Kato, M.; Inoue, M.; and Mitsuhashi, S. Antibacterial activities of SM-1652 compared with those of other broad-spectrum cephalosporins. *Antimicrob. Agents Chemother.*, **1982**, *22*, 721–727.

Kelley, J. A.; Moews, P. C.; Know, J. R.; Frere, J.; and Ghuysen, J. Penicillin target enzyme and the antibiotic binding site. *Science*, **1982**, *218*, 479–481.

King, A.; Shannon, K.; and Phillips, I. *In-vitro* antibacterial activity and susceptibility of cefsulodin, an antipseudomonal cephalosporin, to beta-lactamases. *Antimicrob. Agents Chemother.*, **1980**, *17*, 165–169.

Kirkwood, C. F.; Smith, L. L.; Rustagi, P. K.; and Schentag, J. J. Neutropenia associated with β-lactam antibiotics. *Clin. Pharm.*, **1983**, *2*, 569–578.

Klaus, M. V., and Fellner, M. J. Penicilloyl-specific serum antibodies in man. Analysis in 592 individuals from the newborn to old age. *J. Gerontol.*, **1973**, *28*, 312–316.

Klein, J. O.; Eickhoff, T. C.; Tilles, J. G.; and Finland, M. Cephalothin: activity *in vitro*, absorption and excretion in normal subjects and clinical observations in 40 patients. *Am. J. Med. Sci.*, **1964**, *248*, 640–656.

Klein, J. O., and Neu, H. C. Empiric therapy for bacterial infections: evaluation of cefoperazone. *Rev. Infect. Dis.*, **1983**, *5*, S1–S209.

Klein, J. O.; Schaberg, M. J.; Buntin, M.; and Gezon, H. M. Levels of penicillin in serum of newborn infants after single intramuscular doses of benzathine penicillin G. *J. Pediatr.*, **1973**, *82*, 1065–1068.

Kobayashi, Y.; Takahashi, T.; and Nakae, T. Diffusion

of beta-lactam antibiotics through liposome membranes containing purified porins. *Antimicrob. Agents Chemother.*, **1982**, *22*, 775–780.

Kropp, H.; Sundelof, J. G.; Hajdu, R.; and Kahan, F. M. Metabolism of thienamycin and related carbapenem antibiotics by the renal dipeptidase, dehydropeptidase-I. *Antimicrob. Agents Chemother.*, **1982**, *22*, 62–70.

Landesman, S. H.; Corrado, M. S.; Shah, P. M.; Armengaud, M.; Barza, M.; and Cherubin, M. D. Past and current roles for cephalosporin antibiotics in treatment of meningitis. *Am. J. Med.*, **1981**, *71*, 693–703.

Levine, B. B. Skin rashes with penicillin therapy: current management. *N. Engl. J. Med.*, **1972**, *286*, 42–43.

———. Antigenicity and cross reactivity of penicillins and cephalosporins. *J. Infect. Dis.*, **1973**, *128*, S364–S366.

Levine, B. B.; Redmond, A. P.; Fellner, M. J.; Voss, H. E.; and Levytska, V. Penicillin allergy and the heterogeneous immune responses of man. *J. Clin. Invest.*, **1966**, *45*, 1895–1906.

Levison, M. E.; Mangura, C. T.; Lorber, B.; Abrutyn, E.; Pesanti, E. L.; Levy, R. S.; MacGregor, R. R.; and Schwartz, A. R. Clindamycin compared with penicillin for the treatment of anaerobic lung abscess. *Ann. Intern. Med.*, **1983**, *98*, 466–471.

McCloskey, R. V.; LeFrock, J. L.; Smith, B. R.; and Aronoff, G. R. Microbiology, pharmacology and clinical use of mezlocillin sodium. *Pharmacotherapy*, **1982**, *2*, 300–310.

McCracken, G. H., Jr.; Ginsberg, C.; Chrane, D. F.; Thomas, M. A.; and Horton, L. J. Clinical pharmacology of penicillin in newborn infants. *J. Pediatr.*, **1973**, *82*, 692–698.

Maki, D. G.; Karzynski, T. A.; and Agger, W. A. Carbenicillin for treatment of *Bacteroides fragilis* infections: why not penicillin? *J. Infect. Dis.*, **1978**, *138*, 859–864.

Mandell, G. L. Interaction of intraleukocytic bacteria and antibiotics. *J. Clin. Invest.*, **1973a**, *52*, 1673–1679.

Medical Letter. Prevention of bacterial endocarditis. **1984**, *26*, 3–4.

Meyers, B. R., and Hirschman, S. Z. Antibacterial activity of cefamandole *in vitro*. *J. Infect. Dis.*, **1978**, *137*, 525–531.

Meyers, B. R.; Kaplan, K.; and Weinstein, L. Cephalexin microbiological effects and pharmacologic parameters in man. *Clin. Pharmacol. Ther.*, **1969**, *10*, 810–816.

Mullaney, D. T., and John, J. F. Cefotaxime therapy. *Arch. Intern. Med.*, **1983**, *143*, 1705–1708.

Neiss, E. Cephradine—summary of preclinical studies and clinical pharmacology. *J. Ir. Med. Assoc.*, **1973**, *44*, S1–S12.

Neu, H. C. Mecillinam, a novel penicillanic acid and derivative with unusual activity against gram-negative bacteria. *Antimicrob. Agents Chemother.*, **1976**, *9*, 793–799.

———. Comparison of the pharmacokinetics of cefamandole and other cephalosporin compounds. *J. Infect. Dis.*, **1978**, *137*, S80–S87.

———. Amoxicillin. *Ann. Intern. Med.*, **1979**, *90*, 356–360.

———. In-vitro activity of ceftazidime, a beta-lactamase stable cephalosporin. *J. Antimicrob. Chemother.*, **1981**, *8*, Suppl. B, 131–134.

———. Clinical uses of cephalosporins. *Lancet*, **1982a**, *2*, 252–255.

Neu, H. C.; Aswapokee, N.; Aswapokee, P.; and Fu, K. P. HR756, a new cephalosporin active against gram-positive and gram-negative aerobic and anaerobic bacteria. *Antimicrob. Agents Chemother.*, **1979**, *15*, 273–281.

Neu, H. C., and Fu, K. P. Clavulanic acid, a novel inhibitor of β-lactamases. *Antimicrob. Agents Chemother.*, **1978**, *14*, 650–655.

Neu, H. C., and Labthavikul, P. Antibacterial activity and beta-lactamase stability of ceftazidime, an aminothiazolyl cephalosporin potentially active against *Pseudomonas aeruginosa*. *Antimicrob. Agents Chemother.*, **1982**, *21*, 11–18.

Neu, H. C.; Reeves, D. S.; and Leigh, D. A. (eds.). Azlocillin—an antipseudomonas penicillin. *J. Antimicrob. Chemother.*, **1983**, *11*, Suppl. B, 1–235.

Neu, H. C.; Turck, M.; and Phillips, I. Ceftizoxime, a broad-spectrum beta-lactamase stable cephalosporin. *J. Antimicrob. Chemother.*, **1982**, *10*, Suppl. C, 1–355.

Olson, D. A.; Hoeprich, P. S.; Nolan, S. M.; and Goldstein, E. Successful treatment of gram-negative bacillary meningitis with moxalactam. *Ann. Intern. Med.*, **1981**, *95*, 302–305.

Onorato, I. M., and Axelrod, J. L. Hepatitis from intravenous high-dose oxacillin therapy. Findings in an adult inpatient population. *Ann. Intern. Med.*, **1978**, *89*, 497–500.

Park, J. T., and Strominger, J. L. Mode of action of penicillin. *Science*, **1957**, *125*, 99–101.

Parry, M. F., and Neu, H. C. Ticarcillin for treatment of serious infections with gram-negative bacteria. *J. Infect. Dis.*, **1976**, *134*, S476–S485.

———. A comparative study of ticarcillin plus tobramycin versus carbenicillin plus gentamicin for the treatment of serious infections due to gram-negative bacilli. *Am. J. Med.*, **1978**, *64*, 961–966.

Pasternack, D. P., and Stephens, B. G. Reversible nephrotoxicity associated with cephalothin therapy. *Arch. Intern. Med.*, **1975**, *135*, 599–602.

Petz, L. D. Immunologic cross-reactivity between penicillins and cephalosporins: a review. *J. Infect. Dis.*, **1978**, *137*, S74–S79.

Phillips, I.; Wise, R.; and Leigh, D. A. Cefotetan: a new cephamycin. *J. Antimicrob. Chemother.*, **1983**, *11*, Suppl. A, 1–303.

Quintiliani, R., and Nightingale, C. H. Cefazolin—diagnosis and treatment. *Ann. Intern. Med.*, **1978**, *89*, 650–656.

Rajan, V. S.; Sng, E. H.; Thirumoorthy, T.; and Goh, C. L. Ceftriaxone in the treatment of ordinary and penicillinase-producing strains of *Neisseria gonorrhoeae*. *Br. J. Vener. Dis.*, **1982**, *58*, 314–316.

Regamey, C.; Libke, R. D.; Engelking, E. R.; Clarke, J. T.; and Kirby, W. M. M. Inactivation of cefazolin, cephaloridine, and cephalothin by methicillin-sensitive and methicillin-resistant strains of *Staphylococcus aureus*. *J. Infect. Dis.*, **1975**, *131*, 291–294.

Renzini, G.; Ravagnan, G.; and Oliva, B. *In vitro* and *in vivo* microbiological evaluation of cephapirin, a new antibiotic. *Chemotherapy*, **1975**, *21*, 289–296.

Richmond, M. H. Factors influencing the antibacterial action of β-lactam antibiotics. *J. Antimicrob. Chemother.*, **1978**, *4*, 1–14.

Richmond, M. H., and Sykes, R. B. The β-lactamases of gram-negative bacteria and their possible physiological role. *Adv. Microb. Physiol.*, **1973**, *9*, 31–88.

Rolinson, G. N. Laboratory evaluation of amoxycillin. *Chemotherapy*, **1973**, *18*, Suppl., 1–10.

Sabath, L. D.; Wheeler, N.; Laverdiere, M.; Blazevic, D.; and Wilkinson, B. J. A new type of penicillin resistance. *Lancet*, **1977**, *1*, 443–447.

Sabath, L. D.; Wilcox, C.; Garner, C.; and Finland, M. *In vitro* activity of cefazolin against recent clinical bacterial isolates. *J. Infect. Dis.*, **1973**, *128*, S320–S326.

Sanders, C. C., and Sanders, E. W. Emergence of resistance during therapy with the newer beta-lactam antibiotics: role of inducible beta-lactamases and implications for the future. *Rev. Infect. Dis.*, **1983**, *5*, 639–648.

Sanders, W. E.; Johnson, J. E.; and Taggart, J. G. Adverse reactions to cephalothin and cephapirin. *N. Engl. J. Med.*, **1974**, *290*, 424–429.

Scheife, R. T., and Neu, H. C. Bacampicillin hydrochloride: chemistry, pharmacology, and clinical use. *Pharmacotherapy*, **1982**, *2*, 313–320.

Schumacher, G. E. Pharmacokinetic and microbiologic evaluation of dosage regimens for newer cephalosporins and penicillins. *Clin. Pharm.*, **1983**, *2*, 448–457.

Scully, B. E.; Swabb, E. A.; and Neu, H. C. Pharmacology of aztreonam after intravenous infusion. *Antimicrob. Agents Chemother.*, **1983**, *24*, 18–22.

Shattil, J. S.; Bennett, J. S.; McDonough, M.; and Turnbull, J. Carbenicillin and penicillin G inhibit platelet functions *in vitro* by impairing the interaction of agonists with the platelet surface. *J. Clin. Invest.*, **1980**, *65*, 329–337.

Silver, M. S.; Counts, G. W.; Zeleznik, D.; and Turck, M. Comparison of *in vitro* antibacterial activity of three oral cephalosporins: cefaclor, cephalexin, and cephradine. *Antimicrob. Agents Chemother.*, **1977**, *12*, 591–596.

Smith, B. R., and LeFrock, J. L. Cefuroxime: antimicrobial activity, pharmacology, and clinical efficacy. *Ther. Drug Monit.*, **1983**, *5*, 149–160.

Solley, G. O.; Gleich, G. J.; and Van Dellen, R. G. Penicillin allergy: clinical experience with a battery of skin-test reagents. *J. Allergy Clin. Immunol.*, **1982**, *69*, 238–244.

Spector, R., and Lorenzo, A. V. Inhibition of penicillin transport from the cerebrospinal fluid after intracisternal inoculation of bacteria. *J. Clin. Invest.*, **1974**, *54*, 316–325.

Spector, R., and Snodgrass, S. R. The effect of uremia on penicillin flux between blood and cerebrospinal fluid. *J. Lab. Clin. Med.*, **1976**, *87*, 749–759.

Spratt, B. G. Distinct penicillin binding proteins involved in the division, elongation and shape of *Escherichia coli*, K 12. *Proc. Natl Acad. Sci. U.S.A.*, **1975**, *72*, 2999–3003.

———. Biochemical and genetical approaches to the mechanism of action of penicillin. *Philos. Trans. R. Soc. Lond. [Biol.]*, **1980**, *289*, 273–283.

Sutter, V. L., and Finegold, S. M. Susceptibility of anaerobic bacteria to carbenicillin, cefoxitin, and related drugs. *J. Infect. Dis.*, **1975**, *131*, 417–422.

Sykes, R. B., and Bush, K. Interaction of new cephalosporins with beta-lactamases and beta lactamase-producing gram-negative bacilli. *Rev. Infect. Dis.*, **1983**, *5*, S356–S366.

Sykes, R. B., and Matthew, M. β-lactamases of gram-negative bacteria and their role in resistance to β-lactam antibiotics. *J. Antimicrob. Chemother.*, **1976**, *2*, 115–157.

Sykes, R. B., and others. Monocyclic β-lactam antibiotics produced by bacteria. *Nature*, **1981**, *291*, 489–491.

Tally, F. P.; Jacobus, N. V.; and Gorbach, S. L. *In vitro* activity of N-formimidoyl thienamycin (MK0787). *Antimicrob. Agents Chemother.*, **1980**, *18*, 642–644.

Tomasz, A., and Holtje, J. V. Murein hydrolases and the lytic and killing action of penicillin. In, *Microbiology—1977*. (Schlessinger, D., ed.) American Society for Microbiology, Washington, D. C., **1977**, pp. 209–215.

Wade, J. C.; Smith, C. R.; Petty, B. G.; Lipsky, J. J.; Conrad, G.; Ellner, J.; and Leitman, P. S. Cephalothin plus an aminoglycoside is more nephrotoxic than methicillin plus an aminoglycoside. *Lancet*, **1978**, *2*, 604–606.

Waxman, D. J.; Yocum, R. R.; and Strominger, J. L. Penicillins and cephalosporins are active site-directed acylating agents: evidence in support of the substrate analogue hypothesis. *Philos. Trans. R. Soc. Lond. [Biol.]*, **1980**, *289*, 257–271.

Weinstein, L.; Lerner, P. I.; and Chew, W. H. Clinical and bacteriologic studies of the effect of "massive" doses of penicillin G on infections caused by gram-negative bacilli. *N. Engl. J. Med.*, **1964**, *271*, 525–533.

Weitekamp, M. R., and Aber, R. C. Prolonged bleeding times and bleeding diathesis associated with moxalactam administration. *J.A.M.A.*, **1983**, *249*, 69–71.

Wilson, W. R.; Wilkowske, C. J.; Wright, A. J.; Sande, M. A.; and Geraci, J. E. Treatment of streptomycin-susceptible and streptomycin-resistant enterococcal endocarditis. *Ann. Intern. Med.*, **1984**, *100*, 816–823.

Wright, W. W.; Welch, H. W.; Wilner, J.; and Roberts, E. F. Body fluid concentrations of penicillin following intramuscular injection of single doses of benzathine penicillin G and/or procaine penicillin G. *Antibiotic Med. Clin. Ther.*, **1959**, *6*, 232–241.

Yocum, R. R.; Waxman, D. W.; and Strominger, J. L. The mechanism of action of penicillin. *J. Biol. Chem.*, **1980**, *255*, 3977–3986.

Yogev, R.; Melick, C.; and Kabat, W. J. *In vitro* and *in vivo* synergism between amoxicillin and clavulanic acid against ampicillin-resistant *Haemophilus influenzae* type b. *Antimicrob. Agents Chemother.*, **1981**, *19*, 993–996.

Monographs and Reviews

Abraham, E. P. The action of antibiotics on bacteria. In, *Antibiotics*, Vol. II. (Florey, H. W., *et al.*, authors.) Oxford University Press, New York, **1949**, pp. 1438–1496.

———. The cephalosporins. *Pharmacol. Rev.*, **1962**, *14*, 473–500.

Bank, N. U., and Kammer, R. B. Hematologic complications associated with beta-lactam antibiotics. *Rev. Infect. Dis.*, **1983**, *5*, Suppl. 2, S380–S398.

Bergen, T. Review of the pharmacokinetics and dose dependency of azlocillin in normal subjects and patients with renal insufficiency. *J. Antimicrob. Chemother.*, **1983**, *11*, Suppl. B, 101–114.

Cherubin, C. E.; Neu, H. C.; and Turck, M. Current status of cefotaxime sodium: a new cephalosporin. *Rev. Infect. Dis.*, **1982**, *4*, S281–S488.

Durack, D. T. Prophylaxis of infective endocarditis. In, *Principles and Practice of Infectious Diseases*, 2nd ed. (Mandell, G. L.; Douglas, R. G., Jr.; and Bennett, J. E.; eds.) John Wiley & Sons, Inc., New York, **1985**, pp. 539–544.

Fleming, A. History and development of penicillin. In, *Penicillin: Its Practical Application*. (Fleming, A., ed.) The Blakiston Co., Philadelphia, **1946**, pp. 1–33.

Florey, H. W. The use of micro-organisms for therapeutic purposes. *Yale J. Biol. Med.*, **1946**, *19*, 101–118.

———. Historical introduction. In, *Antibiotics*, Vol. I. (Florey, H. W., *et al.*, authors.) Oxford University Press, New York, **1949**, pp. 1–73.

Flynn, E. H. (ed.). *Cephalosporins and Penicillins: Chemistry and Biology*. Academic Press, Inc., New York, **1972**.

Herrell, W. E. *Penicillin and Other Antibiotic Agents*. W. B. Saunders Co., Philadelphia, **1945**.

Kammer, R. B. Host effects of beta-lactam antibiotics. In, *Contemporary Issues in Infectious Diseases*. Vol. 1, *New Dimensions in Antimicrobial Therapy*. (Root, R. K., and Sande, M. A., eds.) Churchill Livingstone, Inc., New York, **1984**, pp. 101–119.

Kass, E. H., and Evans, D. A. (eds.). Future prospects and past problems in antimicrobial therapy: the role of cefoxitin. *Rev. Infect. Dis.*, **1979**, *1*, 1–244.

Mandell, G. L. Cephaloridine. *Ann. Intern. Med.*, **1973b**, *79*, 561–565.

———. Cephalosporins. In, *Principles and Practice of Infectious Diseases*, 2nd ed. (Mandell, G. L.; Douglas, R. G., Jr.; and Bennett, J. E.; eds.) John Wiley & Sons, Inc., New York, **1985**, pp. 180–187.

Neu, H. C. The *in vitro* activity, human pharmacology, and clinical effectiveness of new beta-lactam antibiotics. *Annu. Rev. Pharmacol. Toxicol.*, **1982b**, *22*, 599–642.

————. Structure-activity relations of new β-lactam compounds and *in vitro* activity against common bacteria. *Rev. Infect. Dis.*, **1983**, *5*, Suppl. 2, S319–S336.

————. Penicillins. *In, Principles and Practice of Infectious Diseases*, 2nd ed. (Mandell, G. L.; Douglas, R. G., Jr.; and Bennett, J. E.; eds.) John Wiley & Sons, Inc., New York, **1985**, pp. 166–180.

Parker, C. W. Drug allergy (third of three parts). *N. Engl. J. Med.*, **1975**, *292*, 957–960.

Sande, M. A. Infectious diseases. In, *Internal Medicine.* (Stein, J. H., ed.) Little, Brown & Co., Boston, **1983**, pp. 1129–1468.

Symposium. (Various authors.) Moxalactam international symposium. (Moellering, R. C., and Young, L. S., eds.) *Rev. Infect. Dis.*, **1982**, *4*, S489–S726.

Symposium. (Various authors.) An international review of amdinocillin: a new beta-lactam antibiotic. *Am. J. Med.*, **1983**, *75*, 1–138.

Symposium. (Various authors.) Aztreonam: a monocyclic beta-lactam antibiotic. *Am. J. Med.*, **1985**, *78*, 1–80.

Tomasz, A. From penicillin-binding proteins to the lysis and death of bacteria: a 1979 view. *Rev. Infect. Dis.*, **1979**, *1*, 434–467.

————. Penicillin binding proteins: their role in beta-lactam action and resistance. In, *Contemporary Issues in Infectious Diseases.* Vol. 1, *New Dimensions in Antimicrobial Therapy.* (Root, R. K., and Sande, M. A., eds.) Churchill Livingstone, Inc., New York, **1984**, pp. 1–16.

CHAPTER

51 ANTIMICROBIAL AGENTS

[*Continued*]

The Aminoglycosides

Merle A. Sande and Gerald L. Mandell

The aminoglycoside antibiotics—gentamicin, tobramycin, amikacin, netilmicin, kanamycin, streptomycin, and neomycin—are discussed in this chapter. As the group name implies, all these drugs contain amino sugars in glycosidic linkage. They are polycations, and their polarity is in part responsible for pharmacokinetic properties shared by all members of the group. For example, none is adequately absorbed after oral administration, inadequate concentrations are found in cerebrospinal fluid (CSF), and all are relatively rapidly excreted by the normal kidney.

The aminoglycosides are used primarily to treat infections caused by gram-negative bacteria; they act to interfere with protein synthesis in susceptible microorganisms. Mutations affecting proteins in the bacterial ribosome, the target for these drugs, can rapidly confer marked resistance to their action. Resistance can also result from the acquisition of a plasmid, and this is associated with the elaboration of drug-metabolizing enzymes. Bacteria that acquire resistance to one aminoglycoside may exhibit resistance to others.

Serious toxicity is a major limitation to the usefulness of the aminoglycosides, and the same spectrum of toxicity is shared by all members of the group. Most notable are ototoxicity, which can involve both the auditory and vestibular functions of the eighth cranial nerve, and nephrotoxicity.

History and Source. The ineffectiveness of penicillin G in the treatment of infections due to gram-negative microorganisms was the primary stimulus for the search for antimicrobial agents effective against such bacteria. The development of streptomycin was the result of a well-planned, scientific search for antibacterial substances. Waksman and coworkers examined a number of soil actinomycetes between 1939 and 1943. In 1943, a strain of *Streptomyces griseus* was isolated that elaborated

a potent antimicrobial substance. The first public announcement of the discovery of this new antibiotic—*streptomycin*—was made by Schatz, Bugie, and Waksman early in 1944, and it was soon shown to inhibit the growth of the tubercle bacillus and a number of gram-positive and gram-negative microorganisms *in vitro* and *in vivo*. In less than 2 years, extensive bacteriological, chemical, and pharmacological investigations of streptomycin had been carried out, and its clinical usefulness was established (*see* Waksman, 1949). However, streptomycin-resistant gram-negative bacilli emerged rapidly and limited its clinical usefulness. Today, it is usually administered in combination with other antimicrobial agents for the treatment of certain types of bacterial endocarditis, tularemia, and plague; it is still used for tuberculosis.

In 1949, Waksman and Lechevalier isolated a soil organism, *Streptomyces fradiae*, which produced a group of antibacterial substances that were labeled "neomycin." One component of this group, *neomycin B*, is still utilized. However, it causes severe renal toxicity and ototoxicity when administered parenterally, and it should be employed only topically and for its local effect on the bowel flora.

Kanamycin, an antibiotic produced by *Streptomyces kanamyceticus*, was first produced and isolated by Umezawa and coworkers at the Japanese National Institutes of Health in 1957. It was shown to be active against a variety of microorganisms and, for several years, was an important antibiotic for the treatment of serious infections with gram-negative bacilli. Because of toxicity and the emergence of resistant microorganisms, kanamycin has largely been replaced by the newer aminoglycosides.

Gentamicin and *netilmicin* are both broad-spectrum antibiotics derived from species of the actinomycete *Micromonospora*. The difference in spelling (-*micin*) compared to that of the other aminoglycoside antibiotics (-*mycin*) reflects this difference in origin. Gentamicin was first studied and described by Weinstein and coworkers in 1963, and isolated, purified, and characterized by Rosselot and colleagues (1964). It has a broader spectrum of activity than kanamycin and is currently used widely for the treatment of severe infections due to gram-negative bacteria. Tobramycin and amikacin were introduced into clinical practice in the 1970s. *Tobramycin* is one of several components of a complex of aminoglycosides (nebramycin) elaborated by *Streptomyces tenebrarius* (Higgins and Kastners, 1967). It is similar in antimicrobial activity and toxicity to gentamicin. In contrast to the other aminoglycosides, *amikacin* and *netilmicin* are semisynthetic products. Amikacin, which is a derivative of kanamycin, was described by Kawaguchi and coworkers (1972); netilmicin, a derivative of sisomicin, is the newest aminoglycoside to be introduced.

Chemistry. The aminoglycosides all consist of two or more amino sugars joined in glycosidic linkage to a hexose nucleus, which is usually in a central position (*see* Figure 51–1). This hexose, or *aminocyclitol,* is either streptidine (found in streptomycin) or 2-deoxystreptamine (characteristic of all other available aminoglycosides). These compounds are thus aminoglycosidic aminocyclitols, although the simpler term *aminoglycoside* is commonly used to describe them.

The aminoglycoside families are distinguished by the amino sugars attached to the aminocyclitol. In the neomycin family, which includes neomycin B, paromomycin (*see* Chapter 46), ribostamycin, and lividomycin (the last two compounds are not used clinically in the United States), there are three amino sugars attached to the central 2-deoxystreptamine, which distinguishes it from the kanamycin

and gentamicin families, which have only two such amino sugars. Neomycin B has the following structural formula:

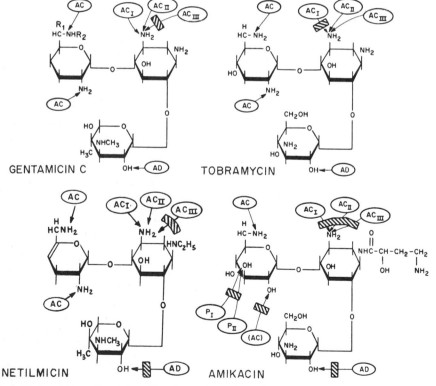

Neomycin B

In the kanamycin family, which includes kanamycins A and B, amikacin, and tobramycin, two amino sugars are linked to a centrally located 2-deoxystreptamine moiety; one of these (in posi-

Figure 51–1. *Sites of activity of various plasmid-mediated enzymes capable of inactivating aminoglycosides.*

The symbol ▨ indicates regions of the molecule that are protected from the designated enzyme (*AC* = acetylase; *AD* = adenylylase; *P* = phosphorylase). In gentamicin C_1, R_1 = R_2 = CH_3; in gentamicin C_2, R_1 = CH_3, R_2 = H; in gentamicin C_{1a}, R_1 = R_2 = H. (Modified from Moellering, 1977. Courtesy of the *Medical Journal of Australia*.)

tion III) is a 3-aminohexose (*see* Figure 51–1 and below for structural formulas). Commercial preparations of kanamycin contain both kanamycins A and B; in the United States the latter must represent less than 5% of the total. The structural formula of kanamycin A is as follows:

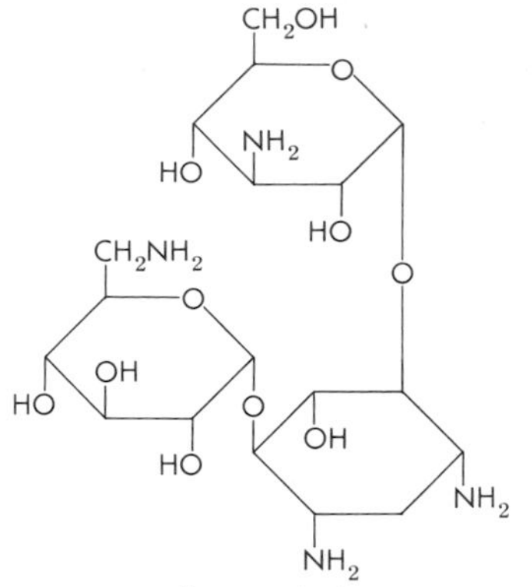

Kanamycin A

Amikacin is a semisynthetic derivative; it is prepared from kanamycin A by acylation of the 1-amino group of the 2-deoxystreptamine moiety with 2-hydroxy-4-aminobutyric acid.

The gentamicin family, which includes gentamicins C_1, C_{1a}, and C_2, sisomicin, and netilmicin (the 1-N-ethyl derivative of sisomicin), has a different 3-amino sugar (garosamine) in position III. Variations in methylation of the amino sugar in position I result in the different components of gentamicin (Figure 51–1). These modifications appear to have little effect on biological activity.

Streptomycin and dihydrostreptomycin (the latter is no longer available because of excessive ototoxicity) differ from the other aminoglycoside antibiotics in that they contain streptidine rather than 2-deoxystreptamine and the aminocyclitol is not in a central position. The structural formula of streptomycin is as follows:

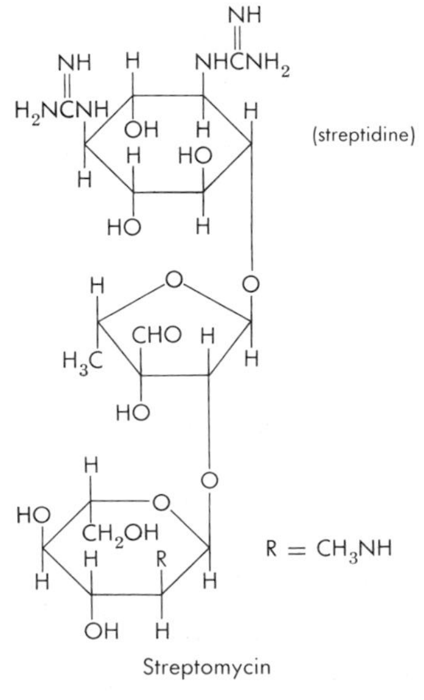

Streptomycin

Mechanism of Action. The aminoglycoside antibiotics are rapidly bactericidal. While much is known about their mechanism of action at the ribosome, where they inhibit protein synthesis and decrease the fidelity of translation of mRNA (Shannon and Phillips, 1982), this does not explain their rapidly lethal effect.

Aminoglycosides diffuse readily through aqueous channels formed by porin proteins in the outer membrane of gram-negative bacteria and thereby enter the periplasmic space (Nakae and Nakae, 1982). Transport of aminoglycosides across the cytoplasmic (inner) membrane is then dependent on electron transport, in part because of a requirement for a membrane potential (interior negative) to drive permeation of these antibiotics (Bryan and Kwan, 1981, 1983; Mates *et al.*, 1983). This phase of transport has been termed energy-dependent phase I, and it can be blocked or inhibited by divalent cations (*e.g.*, Ca^{2+} and Mg^{2+}), hyperosmolarity, a reduction in pH, and anaerobiasis. The last two of these conditions impair the ability of the bacteria to maintain the driving force necessary for transport (membrane potential). Thus, for example, the antimicrobial activity of aminoglycosides is markedly reduced in the anaerobic environment of an abscess, in hyperosmolar acidic urine, and so forth (Bryan and Kwan, 1981). Following transport across the cytoplasmic membrane, the aminoglycosides bind to polysomes and inhibit the synthesis of proteins. This process appears to accelerate the subsequent transport of antibiotic. This phase of aminoglycoside transport, termed energy-dependent phase II (EDP2), is poorly understood; however, it has been suggested that EDP2 is in some way linked with disruption of the structure of the cytoplasmic membrane. This concept is consistent with the observed progression of the leakage of small ions, followed by larger molecules and, eventually, by proteins from the bacterial cell prior to aminoglycoside-induced death. This progressive disruption of the cell envelope may explain the lethal action of aminoglycosides (Bryan, 1984).

The primary intracellular site of action of the aminoglycosides is the 30 S ribosomal subunit, which consists of 21 proteins and a single 16 S molecule of RNA (*see* Mitsuhashi, 1975). Alterations of at least three of these proteins markedly affect the action of streptomycin (Stöffler and Tischendorf, 1975). For example, a single amino acid substitution of asparagine for lysine at position 42 of one ribosomal protein (S_{12}) prevents binding of the drug; the resultant mutant is totally resistant to streptomycin. Another mutant, wherein glutamine is the amino acid at this position, is *dependent* on streptomycin. These microorganisms actually require the presence of the antibiotic for survival. The other aminoglycosides also bind to the 30 S ribosomal subunit; however, they also appear to bind to several sites on the 50 S ribosomal subunit as well (Davies and Courvalin, 1977; Le Goffic *et al.*, 1979).

Aminoglycosides disrupt the normal cycle of ribosomal function by interfering, at least in part, with the first step of protein synthesis that occurs at the ribosome (initiation). Abnormal initiation complexes (or "streptomycin monosomes") accumulate in the cell (Luzzatto *et al.*, 1969). Another effect of the aminoglycosides is their capacity to induce misreading of the genetic code of the mRNA template, and incorrect amino acids are incorporated into the growing polypeptide chains (*see* Tai *et al.*, 1978). The aminoglycosides vary in their capacity to cause misreading, and this property presumably depends on differences in their affinities for specific ribosomal proteins. The mutation to dependence on streptomycin probably results from misreading of the genetic code (*see* Stöffler and Tischendorf, 1975). If there is a mutation at some other site in the bacterial genome that would effectively prevent growth (*e.g.*, an amino acid substitution in a protein essential for normal metabolism), streptomycin-induced misreading of the mutation could result in an acceptable correction of the defect (phenotypic suppression). Bacteria could then resume growth only in the presence of the aminoglycoside. While this is a fascinating phenomenon, it is not of clinical significance.

Microbial Resistance to the Aminoglycosides. Appreciation of the mechanisms of resistance to aminoglycosides is essential to understanding their spectra of antibacterial activity. Bacteria may be resistant to the antimicrobial activity of the aminoglycosides because of failure of permeation of the antibiotic, low affinity of the drug for the bacterial ribosome, or inactivation of the drug by microbial enzymes. The last-named mechanism is by far the most important explanation for the acquired microbial resistance to aminoglycosides that is encountered in clinical practice.

Penetration of drug through the pores in the outer membrane of gram-negative microorganisms into the periplasmic space may be retarded; resistance of this type is unimportant clinically. Once the aminoglycoside does reach the periplasmic space, it may be altered by microbial enzymes that phosphorylate, adenylate, or acetylate specific hydroxyl or amino groups (Figure 51–1). The genetic information for these enzymes is acquired primarily by conjugation and the transfer of DNA as plasmids and resistance transfer factors (*see* Chapter 48). These plasmids have become widespread in nature (especially in hospital environments), and they code for a large number of enzymes (more than 20) that have markedly reduced the antimicrobial spectra of kanamycin and, more recently, gentamicin and tobramycin. Amikacin and, to a lesser extent, netilmicin are less vulnerable to the enzymes that are currently prevalent (Figure 51–1); these drugs may thus have a particularly important role in certain hospital settings. Unfortunately, these plasmids may also spread resistance to other antibiotics simultaneously. The metabolites of the aminoglycosides may compete with the unaltered drug for intracellular transport, but they are incapable of binding effectively to ribosomes and interfering with protein synthesis. In addition, acceleration of drug transport (EDP_2) is not triggered by these altered molecules, and cell death does not occur (Dickie *et al.*, 1978).

Another common form of natural resistance to aminoglycosides is due to failure of permeation of the drug across the cytoplasmic (inner) membrane.

As mentioned above, the transport of aminoglycosides across the cytoplasmic membrane is an oxygen-dependent, active process. Strictly anaerobic bacteria are thus resistant to these drugs, since they lack the necessary transport system. Similarly, facultative bacteria are generally much more resistant when they are grown under anaerobic conditions (Mates *et al.*, 1983). The significance of this so-called permeability barrier as an explanation for resistance to aminoglycosides among aerobic gram-negative bacilli is not known. Natural resistance to amikacin by *Pseudomonas maltophilia* and certain other microorganisms appears to have a similar basis, as does the low-level resistance of some gram-positive cocci, especially enterococci, to aminoglycosides. The addition of antibiotics such as penicillin that alter the structure of the cell wall can markedly increase the entrance of aminoglycosides into these bacteria; this is an excellent example of synergism between antibiotics (*see* Chapter 48).

Resistance that results from alterations in ribosomal structure is less relevant clinically. Single-step mutations in *Escherichia coli* that result in the substitution of a single amino acid in a crucial ribosomal protein may prevent binding of the drug. While such strains are highly resistant to streptomycin (Stöffler and Tischendorf, 1975), they are not widespread in nature. Only 5% of strains of *Pseud. aeruginosa* exhibit such ribosomal resistance to streptomycin. However, from 18 to 40% of strains of enterococci isolated from patients with endocarditis are resistant to high concentrations of streptomycin, and ribosomes from these strains fail to bind streptomycin. For this reason there is no synergistic effect of penicillin and streptomycin against these strains demonstrable *in vitro*. The vast majority of these enterococci are, however, sensitive to a combination of penicillin and gentamicin *in vitro*. Ribosomal resistance to gentamicin is rare among both gram-negative bacilli and gram-positive cocci.

Antibacterial Activity of the Aminoglycosides. The antibacterial activity of gentamicin, tobramycin, kanamycin, netilmicin, and amikacin is primarily directed against aerobic, gram-negative bacilli. As noted above, these antibiotics have little activity against anaerobic microorganisms or facultative bacteria under anaerobic conditions. Their action against most gram-positive bacteria is limited. *Streptococcus pneumoniae* and *Strep. pyogenes* are highly resistant, and, in fact, gentamicin has been added to blood-agar plates to aid in the isolation of these microorganisms from sputum and pharyngeal secretions. Streptomycin and gentamicin are active against enterococci and other streptococci at concentrations that can be achieved clinically only when combined with a penicillin. Such combinations result in a more rapid bactericidal effect than is produced by either drug alone. Both gentamicin and tobramycin are active *in vitro* against more than 95% of strains of *Staphylococcus aureus* and most strains of *Staph. epidermidis*. However, the clinical efficacy of these agents in the treatment of serious staphylococcal infections has not been documented, and they should not be used alone in such situations. Gentamicin-resistant mutant strains of staphylococci emerge rapidly during exposure to the drug.

The aerobic gram-negative bacilli vary in their susceptibility to the major aminoglycosides. Sensitive microorganisms are defined as those inhibited by peak concentrations that can be achieved clinically in plasma but that are not associated with a high incidence of toxicity; this value is 4 to 8 μg/ml for gentamicin, tobramycin, and netilmicin and 8 to 16 μg/ml for amikacin and kanamycin. The mean minimal inhibitory concentration (MIC) and the percentage of clinical isolates considered sensitive are listed in Table 51-1. In general, gentamicin, tobramycin, netilmicin, and amikacin are more active than kanamycin. Tobramycin and gentamicin exhibit similar activity against most gram-negative bacilli, although tobramycin is usually more active against *Pseud. aeruginosa* and against some strains of *Proteus* species. Most gram-negative bacilli (except *Pseud. aeruginosa*) that are resistant to gentamicin because of plasmid-mediated inactivating enzymes will also inactivate tobramycin. However, approximately 50% of *Pseud. aeruginosa* that are resistant to gentamicin remain sensitive to tobramycin (Symposium, 1976b). In some hospitals, the nosocomial flora have undergone considerable alterations in susceptibility to antibiotics during the last 15 years, with a gradual increase in resistance to gentamicin and tobramycin. The relative frequency of these changes varies dramatically—even in different units within a single hospital (Cross *et al.*, 1983). Fortunately, amikacin (Betts *et al.*, 1984) and netilmicin have retained their activity in this setting, a phenomenon attributed to drug resistance to the aminoglycoside-inactivating enzymes. These agents thus have a broad spectrum of activity and are particularly valuable in treating nosocomial infections.

ABSORPTION, DISTRIBUTION, AND ELIMINATION OF THE AMINOGLYCOSIDES

Absorption. The aminoglycosides are highly polar cations; they are thus very poorly absorbed from the intestinal tract. Less than 1% of a dose is absorbed following either oral or rectal administration. The drugs are not inactivated in the intestine, and they are eliminated quantitatively in the feces. Absorption of gentamicin from the gastrointestinal tract may be increased when there is bacillary dysentery (Cox, 1970), but that of neomycin is not altered in the presence of ulcers or inflammatory disease of the bowel (Breen *et al.*, 1972). Repeated oral or rectal administration may, however, result in accumulation to toxic concentrations in patients with renal impairment. Instillation of these drugs into body cavities with serosal surfaces may

result in rapid absorption and unexpected toxicity. Similarly, intoxication may occur when aminoglycosides are applied topically to large wounds, burns, or cutaneous ulcers, particularly if there is renal insufficiency.

All of these antibiotics are absorbed rapidly from intramuscular and subcutaneous sites of injection. Intramuscular injection results in peak concentrations in plasma after 30 to 90 minutes. That peak is similar to the concentration observed 30 minutes after completion of an intravenous infusion of an equal dose over a 30-minute period. In critically ill patients, especially those in shock, absorption of drug may be reduced from intramuscular sites because of poor perfusion.

Distribution. Because of their polar nature, the aminoglycosides are largely excluded from most cells, from the central nervous system (CNS), and from the eye. There is negligible binding of aminoglycosides to plasma albumin; while one half of streptomycin may be so bound, less than 10% of any of the newer aminoglycosides is associated with plasma proteins (Barza and Scheife, 1977). The volume of distribution of these drugs is 25% of lean body weight and approximates the volume of extracellular fluid (Barza *et al.*, 1975).

As would be expected, concentrations of aminoglycosides in secretions and tissues are low. High concentrations are found only in the renal cortex and in the endolymph and perilymph of the inner ear; this presumably contributes to the nephrotoxicity and ototoxicity caused by these drugs. Concentrations in bile approach 30% of those found in plasma as a result of active hepatic secretion, but this represents a very minor excretory route for the aminoglycosides. Penetration into respiratory secretions is likewise poor (Dull *et al.*, 1979; Thys, 1981). Diffusion into pleural and synovial fluid is relatively slow, but concentrations that approximate those in the plasma may be achieved after repeated administration. Inflammation increases the penetration of aminoglycosides into peritoneal and pericardial cavities.

Concentrations of aminoglycosides that can be safely achieved in CSF are very lim-

Table 51–1. ANTIBACTERIAL ACTIVITY OF THE AMINOGLYCOSIDES *

DRUG	PLASMA CONCENTRATION ACHIEVED ($\mu g/ml$)	Staphylococcus aureus †		Escherichia coli		Proteus mirabilis		Pseudomonas aeruginosa		Klebsiella pneumoniae		Enterobacter species		Serratia marcescens	
		MIC	% ‡	MIC	%	MIC	%	MIC	%	MIC	%	MIC	%	MIC	%
Gentamicin	4–8	0.8	88	6.3	87	4.0	97	8.0	87	4.0	97	1.3	90	4.0	95
Tobramycin	4–8	6.3	96	4.0	95	4.0	97	6.3	93	4.0	97	0.8	92	8.0	93
Netilmicin	4–8	0.8	85	1.6	90	4.0	95	20	88	2.0	90	0.8	90	8.0	>90
Amikacin	8–16	2.8	90	4.0	95	4.0	93	16	91	4.0	87	2.7	90	16	95

* Data from Atkinson (1980).
† Mean minimal inhibitory concentration (*see* text).

‡ Percentage of isolated strains considered sensitive to the drug. These values vary among hospitals; most resistant strains are found in hospitals, especially in intensive care units.

ited. In experimental animals and man, concentrations in CSF are less than 10% of those in plasma in the absence of inflammation; this value may approach 20% when there is meningitis (Strausbaugh *et al.,* 1977). The concentrations achieved are therefore *inadequate* for the treatment of gram-negative bacillary meningitis in adults. Intrathecal or intraventricular administration is necessary in such cases (Rahal *et al.,* 1974; Kaiser and McGee, 1975). Therapeutic results of systemic administration alone appear to be better in the treatment of meningitis in neonates (perhaps because of immaturity of the blood-brain barrier), and controlled studies have not shown additional benefit of either intrathecal or intraventricular injection of these drugs (McCracken *et al.,* 1980; McCracken, 1985). Others have suggested that the intraventricular route still merits study (Wright *et al.,* 1981). Similarly, penetration into ocular fluids is so poor that effective therapy of bacterial endophthalmitis requires periocular injections of aminoglycosides (Barza, 1978).

Administration of aminoglycosides to females late in pregnancy may result in accumulation of drug in fetal plasma and amniotic fluid.

Elimination. The aminoglycosides are excreted almost entirely by glomerular filtration, and concentrations in the urine of 50 to 200 μg/ml are achieved. A large fraction of a parenterally administered dose is excreted unchanged during the first 24 hours, with most of this appearing in the first 12 hours. The half-lives of the aminoglycosides in plasma are similar and vary between 2 and 3 hours. Renal clearance is approximately two thirds of the simultaneous creatinine clearance (Barza and Scheife, 1977); this observation suggests some tubular reabsorption of these drugs.

Following the initial doses of an aminoglycoside, disappearance from the plasma exceeds renal excretion by 10 to 20%; however, after 1 to 2 days of therapy, nearly 100% of subsequent doses is recovered in the urine. This lag period probably represents saturation of binding sites in tissues. The rate of disappearance of drug from these sites is considerably longer than from plasma; the half-life for tissue-bound aminoglycoside has been estimated to range from 30 to 700 hours (Schentag and Jusko,

1977). For this reason aminoglycosides can be detected in the urine for 10 to 20 days after dosage is discontinued. All of the administered dose is eventually recovered unchanged in the urine. Aminoglycoside bound to renal tissue appears to exhibit antibacterial activity and protects experimental animals against bacterial infections of the kidney after the drug can no longer be detected in plasma (Bergeron *et al.,* 1982).

The concentration of aminoglycoside in plasma produced by the initial or loading dose is dependent only on the volume of distribution of the drug. Since the elimination of aminoglycosides is almost entirely dependent on the kidney, a linear relationship exists between the concentration of creatinine in plasma and the half-life of all aminoglycosides in patients with moderately compromised renal function. In anephric patients, the half-life varies from 20 to 40 times that determined in normal individuals. *Since the incidence of nephrotoxicity and ototoxicity is related to the concentration to which an aminoglycoside accumulates, it is critical to reduce the maintenance dosage of these drugs in patients with impaired renal function.* This must be done with precision, since the concentration in plasma that is associated with toxicity is not much greater than that required for treatment of many bacterial infections. The size of the individual dose, the interval between doses, or both can be altered. There is no conclusive information on the best approach. A variety of specific recommendations and nomograms may be found in the literature (Hull and Sarubbi, 1976; Barza and Scheife, 1977; Lietman, 1985). The most consistent plasma concentrations are achieved when the loading dose is given in milligrams per kilogram of body weight, and, since aminoglycosides are minimally distributed in fatty tissue, the lean or expected body weight should be used. Methods for calculation of dosage are described in Appendix II.

However, there are obvious difficulties in utilizing any of these approaches for ill patients with rapidly changing renal function (Lesar *et al.,* 1982). In addition, even when known factors are taken into consideration, concentrations of aminoglycosides achieved in plasma after a given dose vary widely between patients (Barza *et al.,* 1975). If extracellular volume is expanded, concentrations will be reduced. For unknown reasons the half-lives of the aminoglycosides are reduced in patients with cystic fibrosis, and the volume of distribution is increased in patients with leukemia (Rosenthal *et al.*, 1977; Spyker *et al.*, 1978). Patients with anemia (hematocrit <25%) have a concentration in plasma that is higher than expected, probably because of a reduction in the number of binding sites on red blood cells (Siber *et al.*, 1975).

Determination of the concentration of drug in plasma is an essential guide to the proper administration of aminoglycosides. Ideally, a plasma concentration at the trough of the fluctuating curve, collected just prior to a dose, and a peak concentration, collected 30 minutes after a dose, should be obtained to ensure adequacy of the antimicrobial activity (peak) and to protect against accumulation of drug (trough). Concentrations should be determined several times per week (more frequently if renal function is changing) and should always be determined within 24 hours after a change in dosage.

Aminoglycosides are removed from the body by either hemodialysis or peritoneal dialysis. Approximately 50% of the administered dose is removed in 12 hours by hemodialysis, and this technic has been used for the treatment of overdosage (Alexander and Gambertoglio, 1985). As a general rule, a dose equal to half of the loading dose administered after each hemodialysis should maintain the plasma concentration in the desired range; however, a number of variables make this a rough approximation at best. Frequent monitoring of drug concentrations in plasma is again crucial.

Peritoneal dialysis is less effective than hemodialysis in removing aminoglycosides. Clearance rates are approximately 5 to 10 ml per minute for the various drugs, but are highly variable (Appel and Neu, 1977). If there is bacterial peritonitis in a patient who requires dialysis, a therapeutic concentration of the aminoglycoside will probably not be achieved in the peritoneal fluid, since the ratio of the concentration in plasma to that in peritoneal fluid may be 10 to 1 (Smithivas *et al.*, 1971). It is thus recommended that antibiotic be added to the dialysate to achieve concentrations equal to those desired in plasma (*i.e.*, 4 µg/ml for gentamicin, tobramycin, and netilmicin; 15 µg/ml for amikacin and kanamycin). This should be preceded by the parenteral administration of a loading dose.

Although excretion of aminoglycosides is similar in adults and children over 6 months of age, half-lives of the drugs may be significantly prolonged in the newborn. Newborn infants who weigh less than 2 kg have half-lives for aminoglycosides of 8 to 11 hours during the first week of life, while those who weigh over 2 kg eliminate these drugs with half-lives of about 5 hours (Yow, 1977). It is thus critically important to monitor concentrations of aminoglycosides during treatment of neonates (Phillips *et al.*, 1982).

Aminoglycosides can be inactivated by various penicillins *in vitro* (Konishi *et al.*, 1983) and in patients with end-stage renal failure (Blair *et al.*, 1982), thus making dosage recommendations even more difficult. Special care must be taken when obtaining serum for determinations of concentra-

tions of these drugs, since inactivation of the aminoglycoside may continue *in vitro* unless the penicillin has been inactivated with beta-lactamase or the specimen has been frozen (Pickering and Gearhart, 1979). Amikacin appears to be the least affected by this interaction. While moxalactam has no effect on the activity of tobramycin *in vitro*, it does appear to increase the clearance of the aminoglycoside (Aronoff *et al.*, 1984).

UNTOWARD EFFECTS OF THE AMINOGLYCOSIDES

All aminoglycosides have the potential to produce reversible and irreversible *vestibular, cochlear,* and *renal* toxicity. These side effects complicate the use of the compounds and make their proper administration difficult. Toxicity may vary between the drugs and, as previously emphasized, can be minimized by careful control of their concentrations in plasma (Appel and Neu, 1977).

Ototoxicity. Both vestibular and auditory dysfunction can follow the administration of any of the aminoglycosides. Studies of both animals and man have documented progressive accumulation of these drugs in the perilymph and endolymph of the inner ear (Huy *et al.*, 1983). Accumulation occurs predominantly when concentrations in plasma are high and diffusion back into the blood stream is slow; the half-lives of the aminoglycosides are five to six times longer in the otic fluids than in plasma. Back diffusion is facilitated when the concentration of drug in plasma reaches a low trough. Thus, ototoxicity is more evident in patients with persistently elevated concentrations of drug in plasma. However, even a single dose of tobramycin can produce slight cochlear dysfunction during periods when the concentration in plasma is at its peak (Wilson and Ramsden, 1977).

Ototoxicity is the result of progressive destruction of vestibular or cochlear sensory cells, which are highly sensitive to damage by aminoglycosides (Brummett and Fox, 1982). Studies in guinea pigs exposed to large doses of gentamicin reveal degeneration of the type-I sensory hair cells in the central part of the crista ampullaris (vestibular organ) and fusion of individual sensory hairs into giant hairs (Wersäll *et al.*, 1973). Similar studies with gentamicin and tobramycin also demonstrate loss of hair cells in the cochlea of the organ of Corti (Theopold, 1977). With increasing dosage and prolonged exposure, damage progresses from the base of the cochlea, where high-frequency sounds are processed, to the apex, necessary for the perception of low frequencies. While these histologic changes correlate with the ability of the cochlea to generate an action potential in response to sound, the biochemical mechanism for ototoxicity is poorly understood. Early changes induced by aminoglycosides may be reversible by calcium. Once sensory cells are lost, however, regeneration does not occur; retrograde degeneration of the auditory nerve follows, resulting in irreversible hearing loss (Lietman, 1985). It has also been suggested that aminoglycosides interfere with the active transport system essential for the maintenance of the ionic balance of the endolymph (Neu and Bendush, 1976); this leads to alteration in the normal concentrations of ions in the labyrinthine fluids, with impairment of electrical activity and nerve conduction. Eventually, the osmotic changes, or perhaps the drugs themselves, damage the hair cells irreversibly.

The degree of permanent dysfunction correlates with the number of destroyed or altered sensory hair cells and is thought to be related to sustained exposure to the drug. Repeated courses of aminoglycosides, each resulting in the loss of more cells, can lead to deafness. Since there appears to be a decrease in the number of cells with age, older patients may be more susceptible to ototoxicity. Drugs such as ethacrynic acid and furosemide potentiate the ototoxic effects of the aminoglycosides in animals (Brummett, 1983); data implicating furosemide are less convincing in man (Moore et al., 1984). Patients with preexisting auditory impairment are also more likely to develop hearing loss following exposure to these agents.

Although all of the aminoglycosides are capable of affecting both cochlear and vestibular function, some preferential toxicity is evident. Streptomycin and gentamicin predominantly produce vestibular effects, whereas amikacin, kanamycin, and neomycin primarily affect auditory function; tobramycin affects both equally. The incidence of ototoxicity is extremely difficult to determine. Data from audiometry suggest that the incidence may be as high as 25% (Moore et al., 1984). The relative incidence appears to be equal for tobramycin, gentamicin, and amikacin. Initial studies in laboratory animals and man suggested that netilmicin is less ototoxic than other aminoglycosides (Brummett and Fox, 1982; Lerner et al., 1983); however, the incidence

of ototoxicity from netilmicin is not low, and 10% of patients developed such complications in one clinical trial of netilmicin (Trestman et al., 1978). A definitive statement on relative ototoxicity awaits further clinical evaluation.

The incidence of vestibular toxicity is particularly high in patients receiving streptomycin; nearly 20% of individuals who received 500 mg twice daily for 4 weeks for enterococcal endocarditis developed clinically detectable, irreversible vestibular damage (Wilson et al., 1984). In addition, up to 75% of patients who received 2 g of streptomycin for more than 60 days showed evidence of nystagmus or postural imbalance.

It is recommended that patients receiving aminoglycosides be carefully monitored for ototoxicity, since the initial symptoms may be reversible; however, deafness may occur several weeks after therapy is discontinued.

Clinical Symptoms of Cochlear Toxicity. A high-pitched tinnitus is often the first symptom of impending difficulty. If the drug is not discontinued, auditory impairment may develop after a few days. The tinnitus may persist for several days to 2 weeks after therapy is stopped. Since perception of sound in the high-frequency range (outside the conversational range) is lost first, the affected individual is not aware of the difficulty, which is not detected unless careful audiometric examination is carried out. If the loss of hearing progresses, the lower sound ranges are affected, and conversation becomes difficult.

Clinical Symptoms of Vestibular Toxicity. Moderately intense headache lasting 1 or 2 days may precede the onset of labyrinthine dysfunction. This is immediately followed by an *acute stage,* in which nausea, vomiting, and equilibratory difficulty develop and persist for 1 to 2 weeks. Vertigo in the upright position, inability to perceive termination of movement ("mental past pointing"), and difficulty in sitting or standing without visual cues are prominent symptoms. Drifting of the eyes at the end of a movement so that focusing and reading are difficult, positive Romberg test, and, rarely, pendular trunk movement and spontaneous nystagmus are outstanding signs. The acute stage ends suddenly and is followed by the appearance of manifestations consistent with *chronic labyrinthitis,* in which, although symptomless while in bed, the patient has difficulty when he attempts to walk or make sudden movements; ataxia is the most prominent feature. The chronic phase persists for approximately 2 months; it is gradually superseded by a *compensatory stage,* in which symptoms are latent and appear only when the eyes are closed.

Adaptation to the impairment of labyrinthine function is accomplished by the use of visual cues and deep proprioceptive sensation for determining movement and position; it is more adequate in the young than in the old, but may not be sufficient to permit the high degree of coordination required in many special trades. Recovery from this phase may require 12 to 18 months, and most patients have some permanent residual damage. Although there is no specific treatment for the vestibular deficiency, early discontinuation of the drug may permit recovery prior to irreversible damage of the hair cells.

Nephrotoxicity. Approximately 8 to 26% of patients who receive an aminoglycoside for more than several days will develop mild renal impairment that is almost always reversible (Smith *et al.,* 1977, 1980). The toxicity is apparently a result of marked accumulation and avid retention of aminoglycoside in the renal cortex by proximal tubular cells (Aronoff *et al.,* 1983; Lietman and Smith, 1983). The initial damage at this site is manifested by the excretion of enzymes of the renal tubular brush border (*e.g.,* alanine aminopeptidase, alkaline phosphatase, and β-D-glucosaminidase) (Patel *et al.,* 1975). After several days there is a defect in renal concentrating ability, mild proteinuria, and the appearance of hyaline and granular casts; the glomerular filtration rate is reduced after several additional days (Schentag *et al.,* 1979). The nonoliguric phase of renal insufficiency has been postulated to be due to the effects that aminoglycosides exert on the distal portion of the nephron. They are thought by some investigators to decrease the sensitivity of the collecting-duct epithelium to endogenous antidiuretic hormone (Appel, 1982). While severe acute tubular necrosis may occur rarely, the most common significant finding is a mild rise in plasma creatinine (0.5 to 2.0 mg/dl); hypokalemia, hypocalcemia, and hypophosphatemia are seen very infrequently. The impairment in renal function is almost always reversible, since the proximal tubular cells have the capacity to regenerate.

Several variables appear to influence nephrotoxicity from aminoglycosides. Toxicity correlates with the total amount of drug administered. Continuous infusion is more nephrotoxic in dogs and rats than is intermittent dosing (Reiner *et al.,* 1978;

Powell *et al.,* 1983), and constant concentrations of drug in plasma above a critical level appear to correlate with toxicity in man (Keating *et al.,* 1979). The nephrotoxic potential varies among individual aminoglycosides. The relative toxicity correlates with the concentration of drug found in the renal cortex in experimental animals; however, clinical studies have not consistently supported this notion. Neomycin, which concentrates to the greatest degree, is highly nephrotoxic in man and should not be administered systemically. Streptomycin does not concentrate in the renal cortex and is the least nephrotoxic. Most of the controversy has concerned the relative toxicities of gentamicin and tobramycin. Gentamicin is concentrated in the kidney to a greater degree than is tobramycin, but several controlled clinical trials have given different estimates of their relative nephrotoxicities (Smith *et al.,* 1977, 1980; Fong *et al.,* 1981; Keys *et al.,* 1981). If differences between these two aminoglycosides do exist in man, they appear to be slight. Similar comparative studies with the new agents (amikacin, sisomicin, netilmicin) have not yet been done. Other drugs, such as amphotericin B, vancomycin, cisplatin, and cyclosporine, may potentiate aminoglycoside-induced nephrotoxicity. Several studies suggest that cephalothin aggravates nephrotoxicity produced by aminoglycosides (Klastersky *et al.,* 1975; Wade *et al.,* 1978). Furosemide enhances the nephrotoxicity of aminoglycosides in rats if concurrent depletion of fluid is not corrected (Mitchell *et al.,* 1977), and it has been suggested that the diuretic-induced loss of potassium might be responsible for this toxicity. Studies in man have not conclusively proven furosemide to aggravate nephrotoxicity (Smith and Lietman, 1983); however, both volume depletion and potassium wasting have been incriminated.

Although advanced age has been suggested as a risk factor for the development of nephrotoxicity from aminoglycosides, data are not convincing. However, in the elderly patient renal function is overestimated from measurement of creatinine concentration in plasma, and overdosing will occur if this value is used as the only guide.

Thus, while aminoglycosides consistently alter the structure and function of renal proximal tubular cells, these effects are usually reversible. The most important result of this toxicity may be reduced excretion of the drug, which in turn will lead to ototoxicity. Meticulous attention to drug clearance and concentrations in plasma is critically important for the effective and safe use of aminoglycosides.

The biochemical events leading to tubular cell damage and glomerular dysfunction are poorly understood, but they may involve perturbations of the structure of cellular membranes. Aminoglycosides inhibit various phospholipases, sphingomyelinases, and ATPases, and they alter the function of mitochondria and ribosomes (Silverblatt, 1982; Queener *et al.*, 1983; Humes *et al.*, 1984). An intriguing observation, which may explain the relationship between tubular damage and the reduction in glomerular filtration rate, is that the aminoglycosides inhibit phosphatidylinositol-specific phospholipase C, a critical enzyme in the synthesis of various prostaglandins. A reduction in the synthesis of these important vasoactive substances may lead to unopposed vasoconstriction by angiotensin II and, thus, a reduction in the rate of glomerular filtration (McNeil *et al.*, 1983). Others have observed morphological changes in glomerular endothelial cells (decreased number of endothelial fenestrations) in animals receiving aminoglycosides (Luft and Evans, 1980) and drug-induced reduction in the glomerular capillary ultrafiltration coefficient (Baylis *et al.*, 1977).

Calcium has been shown to inhibit the uptake and binding of aminoglycosides to the renal brush-border luminal membrane *in vitro*, and supplementary dietary calcium attenuates experimental nephrotoxicity (Bennett *et al.*, 1982; Humes *et al.*, 1984; Quarum *et al.*, 1984). Aminoglycosides are eventually internalized by pinocytosis; morphologically there is clear evidence of accumulation of drug in liposomes. Aminoglycosides are thereby trapped, concentrated (up to 50 times the plasma concentration) (Aronoff *et al.*, 1983), and prepared for extrusion into the urine as multilamellar, phospholipid structures called "myeloid bodies" (Silverblatt, 1982).

Neuromuscular Blockade. The rather unique toxic reaction of acute muscular paralysis and apnea resulting from neuromuscular blockade has been attributed to the various aminoglycosides. A review of 83 reports of prolonged paralysis implicated neomycin as the most frequent cause (Pittinger *et al.*, 1970). In experimental systems the order of decreasing potency is neomycin, kanamycin, amikacin, gentamicin, and tobramycin.

In man, neuromuscular blockade has generally occurred after intrapleural or intraperitoneal instillation of large doses of an aminoglycoside; however, the reaction has followed the intravenous, intramuscular, and even the oral administration of

these agents (Holtzman, 1976). Most episodes have occurred in association with anesthesia or the administration of other neuromuscular blocking agents. Patients with myasthenia gravis are particularly susceptible to this effect. However, others who depend on various degrees of hypoxemia to drive respiration (*e.g.*, patients with chronic obstructive pulmonary disease) should be observed carefully for signs of respiratory depression when an aminoglycoside is used.

Animal studies indicate that the aminoglycosides inhibit prejunctional release of acetylcholine while also reducing postsynaptic sensitivity to the transmitter (Pittinger and Adamson, 1972; Sokoll and Gergis, 1981). Calcium overcomes the effect of the aminoglycoside at the neuromuscular junction, and the intravenous administration of a calcium salt is the preferred treatment of this toxicity (Singh *et al.*, 1978). Inhibitors of cholinesterase (edrophonium, neostigmine) have also been used with varying degrees of success. Since physicians have become aware of this complication, it is now relatively uncommon.

Other Effects on the Nervous System. The administration of streptomycin in particular may produce dysfunction of the *optic nerve*. Scotomas, presenting as enlargement of the blind spot, have been associated with the drug.

Among the less common toxic reactions to streptomycin is *peripheral neuritis*. This may be due either to accidental injection of a nerve during the course of parenteral therapy or to toxicity involving nerves remote from the site of antibiotic administration. Paresthesia, most commonly perioral but also present in other areas of the face or in the hands, occasionally follows the use of the antibiotic and usually appears within 30 to 60 minutes after injection of the drug; it may persist for several hours.

Other Untoward Effects. In general, the aminoglycosides have little allergenic potential; both anaphylaxis and rash are unusual. The rare hypersensitivity reactions, including skin rashes, eosinophilia, fever, blood dyscrasias, angioedema, exfoliative dermatitis, stomatitis, and anaphylactic shock, are discussed in the *sixth and previous editions* of this textbook. Other reactions that have been attributed to these drugs are discussed below.

STREPTOMYCIN

Streptomycin is used today for the treatment of certain unusual infections, generally in combination with other antimicrobial agents. It is also occasionally administered for tuberculosis (*see* Chapter 53).

Preparations, Routes of Administration, and Dosage. *Streptomycin sulfate* is supplied for parenteral injection either as a sterile dry powder or in sterile solutions, which contain 400 or 500 mg/ml.

Streptomycin can be administered by a variety of

routes. *Intermittent, deep intramuscular injection* is the method most often used for parenteral administration. Such intramuscular injection of streptomycin is often painful; hot tender masses may develop at sites of injection. The total daily dose varies from 1 to 2 g (15 to 25 mg/kg); 500 mg to 1 g is injected every 12 hours. In adults, 1 g given intramuscularly produces a peak plasma concentration of 25 to 30 μg/ml. The intramuscular administration of 0.5 g of streptomycin every 8 hours produces *urinary concentrations* ranging from 200 to 1500 μg/ml, depending on renal function and urine volume. Children should receive 20 to 30 mg/kg daily, in two divided doses. Except in tuberculosis and subacute bacterial endocarditis, it is rarely necessary to give streptomycin for more than 7 to 10 days. Dosage schedules for tuberculosis are described in Chapter 53. Streptomycin has also been administered intravenously, intrathecally, and intraperitoneally. There is presently no indication for these methods of administration.

Untoward Effects. Since streptomycin has been available for over 40 years, the extent of its toxicity is more clearly defined than is that of the other aminoglycosides. It is believed that most toxicities are shared by all of the various congeners; detailed description is presented above.

Therapeutic Uses. *Bacterial Endocarditis.* Streptomycin and penicillin produce a synergistic bactericidal effect *in vitro* and in animal models of infection against enterococci, other group-D streptococci, and the various oral streptococci of the *viridans* group. Many authorities administer such antibiotics concurrently for treatment of endocarditis caused by these microorganisms. Penicillin G alone is ineffective in the therapy of enterococcal endocarditis, and either streptomycin (500 mg twice daily) or gentamicin (1 mg/kg three times daily) must also be given to ensure cure. Gentamicin is preferred when the strain shows complete (ribosomal) resistance (MIC greater than 2000 μg/ml) to streptomycin. Both penicillin G and the aminoglycoside are administered for 4 to 6 weeks. Treatment for 4 weeks has been successful in patients who had symptoms for less than 3 months prior to therapy (Wilson *et al.*, 1984). Some authorities recommend gentamicin for all cases of enterococcal endocarditis, since its toxicity is primarily renal and reversible while that of streptomycin is vestibular and irreversible; however, streptomycin has been effective in many patients with enterococcal endocarditis and many other clinicians prefer to use it when microorganisms are susceptible. Tobramycin should not be used because of the resistance of some bacteria (Moellering *et al.*, 1979). Endocarditis caused by penicillin-sensitive streptococci (MIC less than 0.1 μg/ml) has been successfully treated with penicillin G alone for 4 weeks (relapse rate 1 to 2%; Karchmer *et al.*, 1979), penicillin G plus streptomycin (0.5 g twice a day) for 2 weeks (relapse rate 1 to 2%, Wilson *et al.*, 1978), or

penicillin G for 4 weeks combined with streptomycin for the first 2 weeks of therapy (relapse rate 0%; Wolfe and Johnson, 1974). The clinician thus has several options, one of which can be chosen based on the needs of the individual patient. For example, the elderly patient with streptococcal endocarditis due to a penicillin-sensitive strain should probably receive penicillin alone, because of the increased toxicity from streptomycin in this age group. The short, 2-week course of therapy is now recommended for uncomplicated cases (Sande and Scheld, 1980). However, if the infection is on a prosthetic valve, or is caused by a relatively resistant strain (MIC of penicillin greater than 0.2 μg/ml), or is caused by nutritionally deficient (pyridoxal-requiring) streptococci, a longer duration of therapy is prudent (Sande, 1983).

Tularemia. All forms of tularemia benefit dramatically from the administration of streptomycin. The best results are obtained when therapy is instituted early; however, chronicity does not exclude the possibility of complete cure. Most cases respond to the administration of 1 to 2 g of streptomycin per day for 7 to 10 days. The tetracyclines are also highly effective in tularemia and are preferred by some physicians for milder forms of the disease.

Plague. Streptomycin is highly specific and one of the most effective agents for the treatment of all forms of plague. The tetracyclines and chloramphenicol are also beneficial in this disease. When streptomycin is used, a dose of 1 to 4 g per day is given for 7 to 10 days.

Brucellosis. Mild cases of brucellosis respond well to the administration of a tetracycline. Severe cases and especially those due to *Brucella suis* or *Br. melitensis* are best treated with a combination of a tetracycline and streptomycin (1 to 2 g per day), given for 7 to 21 days. Relapses are managed in the same fashion.

GENTAMICIN

Gentamicin is an important agent for the treatment of many serious gram-negative bacillary infections. However, emergence of resistant microorganisms in some hospitals has become a serious problem and may limit the future use of this agent.

Preparations, Routes of Administration, and Dosage. *Gentamicin sulfate* (GARAMYCIN) is available in various forms: vials and prefilled syringes containing 40 mg/ml (or 10 mg/ml for pediatric use), an intrathecal injection (without preservatives) containing 2 mg/ml, an *ointment* and *cream* (0.1%), an *ophthalmic ointment* (0.3%), and *ophthalmic solution* (0.3%). The recommended intramuscular dose for adults is 3 to 5 mg/kg per day, one third being given every 8 hours. Several dosage schedules have been suggested for *infants:* 2 to 2.5 mg/kg every 8 hours has been found to be safe for children up to 2 years of age; 6 mg/kg daily, divided into two equally spaced injections, has been recommended for neonates with severe infections.

While the peak concentration in plasma is approximately 4 μg/ml after the intramuscular administration of 1 mg/kg, careful studies by a number of investigators have emphasized that the recommended doses of gentamicin do not yield reproducible concentrations in plasma and that there is a considerable degree of individual variation. Gentamicin may be present in the plasma in only subinhibitory or undetectable concentrations for several hours after its injection in some patients given the "standard" dose every 8 hours. Periodic determinations of the plasma concentration of the antibiotic are strongly recommended. Although it has not yet been established exactly what plasma concentration is toxic, peak concentrations greater than 10 μg/ml and minimal (predose) values in excess of 2 μg/ml for longer than 10 days have been associated with toxicity.

The presence of any significant degree of renal insufficiency imposes additional difficulty in establishing a regimen of therapy that will yield maximal therapeutic benefit with minimal or no risk of toxic reactions. This problem has been discussed above.

Penicillins and aminoglycosides must never be mixed in the same bottle because the penicillin inactivates the aminoglycoside to a significant degree; similar incompatibilities exist *in vitro* between gentamicin and cephalosporins, amphotericin B, and heparin.

Gentamicin is very slowly absorbed when applied in an *ointment,* but absorption may be more rapid when a *cream* is used topically. When the antibiotic is applied to large areas of denuded body surface, as may be the case in burned patients, plasma concentrations can reach 1 μg/ml, and 2 to 5% of the drug used may appear in the urine.

Untoward Effects. The untoward effects of gentamicin are similar to those of other aminoglycosides. The most important and serious side effect of the use of gentamicin is *irreversible ototoxicity.* This has been discussed in detail above. Gentamicin may produce more *nephrotoxicity* than do the other aminoglycosides that are currently utilized systemically.

Intrathecal or intraventricular administration may cause local inflammation and can result in radiculitis and other complications. Persistent fever and pleocytosis of the CSF have also been attributed to the intrathecal administration of gentamicin.

Therapeutic Uses of Gentamicin and Other Aminoglycosides. Gentamicin, tobramycin, amikacin, and netilmicin can be used interchangeably for the treatment of most of the following infections and will be discussed together. Specific usages will be reviewed under each drug heading. A large variety of infections has been treated successfully

with these aminoglycosides. However, due to their toxicities, prolonged use *must* be restricted to the therapy of life-threatening infections and those for which a less toxic antimicrobial agent is less effective. These antibiotics are frequently used (often in combination with a penicillin or a cephalosporin) for the therapy of proven or suspected serious gram-negative microbial infections, especially those due to *Pseud. aeruginosa, Enterobacter, Klebsiella, Serratia,* and other species resistant to less toxic antibiotics. Among these are urinary tract infections, bacteremia, meningitis, cerebral ventriculitis, infected burns, osteomyelitis, pneumonia, peritonitis, and otitis.

Urinary Tract Infections. Aminoglycosides are not indicated for the treatment of uncomplicated urinary tract infections, although a single intramuscular dose of gentamicin (5 mg/kg) or kanamycin (500 mg) has been effective in curing over 90% of uncomplicated infections of the lower urinary tract (Ronald *et al.,* 1976; Varese *et al.,* 1980). In the extremely ill patient with pyelonephritis, an aminoglycoside alone or in combination with ampicillin offers broad and effective initial coverage. Once the microorganism is isolated and its sensitivities to antibiotics are determined, the aminoglycoside should be discontinued if the infecting microorganism is sensitive to ampicillin or other less toxic antibiotics. The antibacterial activity of aminoglycosides is markedly reduced by low pH (Strausbaugh and Sande, 1978) and hyperosmolarity (Papapetropoulou *et al.,* 1983); however, the very high concentrations achieved in urine in patients with normal renal function are usually sufficient to eradicate sensitive microorganisms. The prolonged release of gentamicin from the renal cortex following discontinuation of therapy has been shown to produce a therapeutic effect for several months in experimental pyelonephritis in rats (Bergeron *et al.,* 1982).

Pneumonia. The frequency of pneumonia caused by various gram-negative bacilli is increasing, especially in hospitalized patients, patients on respirators, and those with impaired defenses (especially granulocytopenia). Selection of an antibiotic depends on the sensitivity of the microorganism. The aminoglycosides are widely used in this setting, but most authorities administer a penicillin or a cephalosporin concurrently, since therapy with an aminoglycoside alone is not very effective. One of the aminoglycosides given concurrently with an antipseudomonal penicillin constitutes effective treatment of pneumonia caused by *Pseud. aeruginosa.* An aminoglycoside plus a cephalosporin, mezlocillin, or piperacillin is used for sensitive strains of *Klebsiella;* an aminoglycoside plus ampicillin is preferred for pneumonia caused by sensitive strains of *E. coli* or *Proteus mirabilis.* All selections should be based initially on the sensitivity patterns at the individual hospital.

Gentamicin- and tobramycin-resistant strains of *Klebsiella, Enterobacter, Serratia, Proteus,* and *Pseudomonas* have emerged in many hospitals. The major reservoirs for these microorganisms are burn units and intensive care units, where these drugs are used extensively. Critically ill patients with tracheostomies and impaired host defenses and those with indwelling intravenous and urinary catheters all appear to acquire resistant bacteria with an increased frequency (*see* Symposium, 1977).

Aminoglycosides are totally ineffective for treatment of pneumonia due to *Strep. pneumoniae,* the most common cause of pneumonia acquired in the community. They should not be considered to be active against any other gram-positive cocci (including *Staph. aureus* or streptococci) or anaerobic bacteria, the microorganisms commonly responsible for suppurative pneumonia or lung abscess. Thus, gentamicin (or other aminoglycosides) should never be used as the sole agent to treat pneumonia acquired in the community or as the initial treatment for pneumonia acquired in the hospital (Kunin, 1977).

Meningitis. Meningitis caused by gram-negative microorganisms presents a grave therapeutic problem. Development of the new third-generation cephalosporins (especially moxalactam and cefotaxime) has reduced the need for treatment with aminoglycosides in most cases, except those caused by resistant isolates (*e.g.,* species of *Pseudomonas* and *Acinetobacter*). If therapy with an aminoglycoside is necessary, it must be administered intrathecally. Rahal and associates (1974) have recommended intramuscular administration of gentamicin in combination with intrathecal injection of 4 to 12 mg every 18 hours for 5 to 10 days. However, even this regimen is associated with a significant number of treatment failures, probably because of coexistent ventriculitis. In such instances, direct administration of gentamicin (or other aminoglycosides) into the cerebral ventricles with an Ommaya reservoir has been suggested. However, in one study children with gram-negative bacillary meningitis failed to show a beneficial effect from such treatment. (For discussion, *see* Kaiser and McGee, 1975; McCracken *et al.,* 1979.) Some authorities recommend the concurrent systemic administration of chloramphenicol because of superior penetration by this drug into the CNS. Unfortunately, chloramphenicol is only bacteriostatic against most gram-negative bacilli, and reports of therapeutic failures have been numerous when this drug is used alone. Chloramphenicol markedly *reduces* the bactericidal activity of the gentamicin *in vitro* and in experimental infections in animals (antibiotic antagonism) (Strausbaugh *et al.,* 1977). Its use in gram-negative bacillary meningitis in man could thus be deleterious; clinical studies of this combination are not available.

Other Infections. Patients who develop peritonitis as a result of peritoneal dialysis may require therapy with an aminoglycoside. Since suboptimal intraperitoneal concentrations of the antibiotic may follow intramuscular administration in patients undergoing dialysis, the procedure should be continued with fluids containing an appropriate concentration of the aminoglycoside (*see* page 1157).

Gentamicin has been given parenterally and applied topically at the same time in the treatment of infected burns; some of the bacteria involved have become resistant to the drug during such therapy.

It has been suggested that this regimen be rigorously restricted to patients with thermal burns that are life endangering, and be used only when other topical agents have failed.

While there are very few indications for the use of aminoglycosides for gram-positive bacterial infections, it may at times be necessary and lifesaving. Methicillin-resistant staphylococci may be sensitive to gentamicin. In cases of enterococcal endocarditis, up to 30% of isolates of enterococci are not killed by penicillin plus streptomycin; these strains are nearly always sensitive to penicillin plus gentamicin (page 1125). However, this is not revealed by testing for sensitivity to a standard dose of gentamicin.

When a patient has granulocytopenia and infection (sepsis) with *Pseud. aeruginosa* is suspected, the administration of an antipseudomonal penicillin in combination with gentamicin, tobramycin, amikacin, or netilmicin is recommended. Treatment of gram-negative bacillary sepsis, especially in neutropenic patients, has been improved by the use of such synergistic combinations (Klastersky *et al.,* 1977; Schimpff, 1977).

TOBRAMYCIN

The antimicrobial activity and pharmacokinetic properties of tobramycin are very similar to those of gentamicin.

Preparations, Routes of Administration, and Dosage. *Tobramycin* (NEBCIN) is available as the sulfate salt for parenteral administration in solutions containing 40 mg/ml. A pediatric injection (10 mg/ml) is also supplied. Tobramycin may be given either intramuscularly or intravenously. Dosages are identical to those for gentamicin. When doses of 1 mg/kg are given intramuscularly every 8 hours, peak concentrations in plasma are typically 5 to 8 μg/ml and minimal concentrations are 1 to 2 μg/ml. Toxicity is most common at peak concentrations of 10 to 12 μg/ml or minimal concentrations that exceed 2 μg/ml for a prolonged period. The latter observation usually suggests impairment of renal function and requires reduction of dosage.

Tobramycin (TOBREX) is also available in ophthalmic ointments and solutions at concentrations of 3 mg/g or 3 mg/ml, respectively.

Untoward Effects. Tobramycin, like other aminoglycosides, causes both nephrotoxicity and ototoxicity, as discussed above. Studies in experimental animals suggest that tobramycin may be less toxic to hair cells in the cochlear and vestibular end organs and cause less renal tubular damage than does gentamicin (Symposium, 1976b, 1978). However, clinical data are less convincing.

Therapeutic Uses. Indications for the use of tobramycin are essentially identical to those for gentamicin. The superior activity of tobramycin against *Pseud. aeruginosa* may make it desirable in the treatment of bacteremia, osteomyelitis, and pneumonia caused by *Pseudomonas* species; it should usually be used concurrently with an anti-pseudomonal penicillin.

In contrast to gentamicin, tobramycin shows poor activity in combination with penicillin against enterococci; a large percentage of strains of *Strep. faecium* is highly resistant (Moellering *et al.*, 1979). Tobramycin is ineffective against mycobacteria, although most other aminoglycosides are active against these microorganisms (Gangadharam *et al.*, 1977).

AMIKACIN

The spectrum of antimicrobial activity of amikacin is the broadest of the group, and, because of its unique resistance to the aminoglycoside-inactivating enzymes, it has a special role in hospitals where gentamicin- and tobramycin-resistant microorganisms are prevalent. Amikacin is similar to kanamycin in dosage and pharmacokinetic properties.

Preparations, Routes of Administration, and Dosage. *Amikacin* (AMIKIN) is available as the sulfate in vials containing either 100, 500, or 1000 mg of the drug. The recommended dose is 15 mg/kg per day, divided into either two or three equal portions. The individual dose or the interval between doses must be altered in patients with renal failure. The drug is rapidly absorbed after intramuscular injection, and peak concentrations in plasma approximate 20 μg/ml after injection of 7.5 mg/kg. An intravenous infusion of the same dose over a 30-minute period produces a peak concentration in plasma of nearly 40 μg/ml at the end of the infusion; this falls to about 20 μg/ml 30 minutes later.

Untoward Effects. Like the other aminoglycosides, amikacin causes both ototoxicity and nephrotoxicity. Auditory deficits are most commonly produced, as discussed above.

Therapeutic Uses. Amikacin or netilmicin has become the preferred agent for initial treatment of serious nosocomial gram-negative bacillary infections in hospitals where resistance to gentamicin and tobramycin has become a significant problem. Some hospitals have restricted their use to avoid emergence of resistant strains, although some suggest that this is not likely (Betts *et al.*, 1984).

Because of its unique resistance to aminoglycoside-inactivating enzymes, amikacin is active against the vast majority of aerobic gram-negative bacilli in both the community and the hospital (Symposium, 1976a, 1977). This includes most strains of *Serratia, Proteus*, and *Pseud. aeruginosa*. It is active against nearly all strains of *Klebsiella, Enterobacter*, and *E. coli* that are resistant to gentamicin and tobramycin. Most resistance to amikacin is found among strains of *Acinetobacter, Providencia*, and *Flavobacter* and strains of *Pseu-*

domonas other than *Pseud. aeruginosa;* these are all unusual pathogens. While amikacin is not active against the majority of gram-positive anaerobic bacteria, it is effective against *Mycobacterium tuberculosis* (99% of strains inhibited by 4 μg/ml) and certain atypical mycobacteria (Gangadharam *et al.*, 1977).

NETILMICIN

Netilmicin, the N-ethyl derivative of sisomicin, is the latest of the aminoglycosides to be marketed. It is similar to gentamicin and tobramycin in its pharmacokinetic properties and dosage. Its antibacterial activity is broad against aerobic gram-negative bacilli; like amikacin, it is not metabolized by the majority of the aminoglycoside-inactivating enzymes, and it may be active against bacteria that are resistant to gentamicin.

Preparations, Routes of Administration, and Dosage. Netilmicin (NETROMYCIN) is available as the sulfate salt in vials containing 100 mg/ml; the pediatric injection contains 25 mg/ml and the neonatal injection contains 10 mg/ml. Netilmicin may be given intravenously or intramuscularly.

Dosages for netilmicin, gentamicin, and tobramycin are identical. Their distribution and elimination are also similar. When given intramuscularly, peak concentrations of netilmicin in plasma approximate 5 μg/ml 30 to 60 minutes after a dose of 2 mg/kg (Humbert *et al.*, 1978). An intravenous infusion of the same dose, given over a 60-minute period, results in a peak plasma concentration of approximately 11 μg/ml (Luft *et al.*, 1978). The half-time for elimination is usually 2.0 to 2.5 hours in adults and increases with renal insufficiency.

Untoward Effects. Netilmicin may also produce ototoxicity and nephrotoxicity. Although studies in animals have suggested that netilmicin may be less toxic (Luft *et al.*, 1976), this remains to be proven in man (Trestman *et al.*, 1978; Bock *et al.*, 1980).

Therapeutic Uses. Netilmicin is a useful antibiotic for the treatment of serious infections due to susceptible Enterobacteriaceae and other aerobic gram-negative bacilli. Developed because of the increasing emergence of bacteria resistant to gentamicin and tobramycin, it has been proven to be effective against certain gentamicin-resistant pathogens (Panwalker *et al.*, 1978).

KANAMYCIN

The use of kanamycin has declined markedly because its spectrum of activity is limited compared to those of other aminoglycosides. It is used orally as an adjunct in the treatment of hepatic coma.

Preparations, Routes of Administration, and Dosage. *Kanamycin sulfate* (KANTREX) is available as injections (250 or 333 mg/ml), a pediatric injection (75 mg/2 ml), and for oral use in capsules containing 500 mg. The daily oral dose of kanamycin for children is 50 mg/kg, divided equally and given at 6-hour intervals; adults may receive up to 8 to 12 g per day by this route. Great care must be exercised when such treatment is carried out in patients with renal insufficiency, and the oral dose must be reduced. The parenteral dose for adults is 15 mg/kg per day (two to three equally divided and spaced doses) with a maximum of 1.5 g per day. The total quantity administered over a period of treatment should not exceed 15 g. For neonates, the intramuscular dose, during the first 3 days of life, is 7.5 mg/kg per day, divided into two to four equal doses; for older infants, it is 5 to 15 mg/kg per day; children may be given up to 15 mg/kg per day.

Untoward Effects. The untoward effects of the oral administration of aminoglycosides are considered under Neomycin, below.

Therapeutic Uses. Kanamycin has been employed to treat tuberculosis in combination with other effective drugs. Since the therapy of this disease is protracted and involves the administration of large total doses of the drug, with the risk of ototoxicity and nephrotoxicity, it should be used only to treat patients who harbor microorganisms that are resistant to the more commonly used agents (*see* Chapter 53).

Prophylactic Uses. Kanamycin can be administered *orally* as adjunct therapy in cases of *hepatic coma*. The rationale for such therapy is described under Neomycin (*see* below). The dose usually employed for these purposes is 6 to 8 g per day; quantities as large as 12 g per day have been given. The effect on intestinal bacteria may not be sustained even when such large doses of kanamycin are administered.

NEOMYCIN

Antibacterial Activity. Neomycin is a broad-spectrum antibiotic. Susceptible microorganisms are usually inhibited by concentrations of 5 to 10 μg/ml or less. Gram-negative species that are highly sensitive are *E. coli, Enterobacter aerogenes, Klebsiella pneumoniae,* and *Pr. vulgaris;* gram-positive microorganisms that are inhibited include *Staph. aureus, Strep. faecalis,* and *M. tuberculosis.* Strains of *Pseud. aeruginosa* are resistant to neomycin.

Preparations, Routes of Administration, and Dosage. *Neomycin sulfate* (MYCIFRADIN, MYCIGUENT, NEOBIOTIC) is available for topical, oral, and parenteral administration. Neomycin sulfate is marketed as 500-mg oral tablets, in a solution (125 mg/5 ml), in *dermatological* and *ophthalmic ointments,* and as a *sterile powder* in vials containing 500 mg for parenteral injection. Ointments or creams contain 5 mg of neomycin sulfate per gram, and should be applied two or three times a day. *Neomycin and polymyxin B sulfates solution for irrigation* (NEOSPORIN G.U. IRRIGANT) contains 40 mg of neomycin and 200,000 units of polymyxin B per milliliter. One milliliter of this preparation is added to 1000 ml of 0.9% sodium chloride solution and is used for continuous irrigation of the urinary bladder through appropriate catheter systems. The goal is to prevent bacteriuria and bacteremia associated with the use of indwelling catheters. The bladder is usually irrigated at the rate of 1000 ml every 24 hours. Neomycin should not be used parenterally. Oral therapy with neomycin sulfate (usually in combination with erythromycin base) either for "preparation" of the bowel for surgery or for the management of hepatic coma requires the ingestion of 4 to 12 g daily, in divided doses.

Neomycin is presently available in many brands of creams, ointments, sprays, and other products both alone and in combination with polymyxin, bacitracin, other antibiotics, and a variety of corticosteroids. There is no evidence that these topical preparations shorten the time required for healing of wounds or that those containing a steroid are more effective.

Absorption and Excretion. Neomycin is poorly absorbed from the gastrointestinal tract and is excreted by the kidney, as are the other aminoglycosides. An *oral* dose of 3 g produces a peak plasma concentration of only 1 to 4 μg/ml; a total daily intake of 10 g for 3 days yields a blood concentration below that associated with systemic toxicity. About 97% of an oral dose of neomycin escapes absorption and is eliminated unchanged in the feces. Although neomycin can be given orally to very young children, in doses as high as 100 mg/kg per day, its use in such patients for longer than 3 weeks should be avoided because of partial absorption from the intestinal tract, especially if it is the site of disease.

Untoward Effects. *Hypersensitivity reactions,* primarily *skin rashes,* occur in 6 to 8% of patients when neomycin is applied topically. Individuals sensitive to this agent may develop cross-reactions when exposed to other aminoglycosides. The most important toxic effects of neomycin are *renal damage* and *nerve deafness.* These are most frequent when relatively large quantities of the antibiotic are used parenterally and are the reason the drug should never be used in this way. Toxicity has even occurred in patients with normal renal function following topical application or irrigation of wounds with 0.5% neomycin solution. Neuromuscular blockade with respiratory paralysis has also occurred after irrigation of wounds or serosal cavities.

The most important *biological effects* resulting from the oral administration of neomycin are *intestinal malabsorption* and *superinfection.* Individuals treated with 4 to 6 g of the drug by mouth per day sometimes develop a *spruelike syndrome* with diarrhea, steatorrhea, and azotorrhea. The outstanding example of drug-induced *malabsorption* is that caused by neomycin. In man, the drug produces a moderate malabsorption syndrome for a variety of substances, including fat, protein, cholesterol, carotene, glucose, lactose, sodium, calcium, cyanocobalamin, and iron. This effect may be produced by as little as 3 g of the drug per day but is more marked with a dose of 12 g per day. Neomycin produces mild morphological changes of intestinal villi; precipitates bile salts within the lumen of the intestine; inhibits intraluminal hydrolysis of long-chain triglycerides, presumably by inhibition of pancreatic lipase activity; increases the fecal bile acid excretion, presumably by decreasing bile acid absorption; and reduces intestinal lactase activity. The antibiotic causes a marked decrease in plasma cholesterol concentrations. This is out of proportion to the moderate malabsorption produced, and small doses of the drug have been used for long periods of time for this purpose. The drug has been shown to produce intestinal crypt-cell necrosis, and, since cholesterol synthesis may occur at these sites, this may account for the effect. *Overgrowth of yeasts* in the intestine may also occur; this is not associated with diarrhea or other symptoms in most cases. The oral administration of even large doses of neomycin usually has no effect on blood levels of prothrombin.

Therapeutic Uses. Neomycin has been widely used for *topical application* in a variety of infections of the skin and mucous membranes caused by microorganisms susceptible to the drug. These include *burns, wounds, ulcers,* and *infected dermatoses.* However, such treatment does not eradicate bacteria from the lesions.

The *oral administration* of neomycin has been employed primarily for *"preparation" of the bowel for surgery* and as an adjunct to the therapy of *hepatic coma.* In a controlled study, concurrent administration of neomycin and erythromycin base to prepare the bowel for surgery was found to reduce the incidence of postoperative wound infections significantly (Clarke *et al.,* 1977).

While the importance of reducing the number of bacteria in the intestine in patients with hepatic coma has not been proven, general clinical experience suggests strongly that this may play an important role in producing a satisfactory outcome in this disease. Blood concentrations of ammonia are reduced during therapy. A daily dose of 4 to 8 g by mouth can be given without difficulty to such patients, provided renal function is normal. Because severe renal insufficiency may develop in the late stages of hepatic failure, treatment with neomycin must be followed with the greatest care and stopped if evidence of ototoxicity or further injury to the kidney appears.

There is presently no indication for the parenteral administration of neomycin. Other equally effective and safer antibiotics have completely replaced it.

Appel, G. B. Aminoglycoside nephrotoxicity: physiologic studies of the sites of nephron damage. In, *The Aminoglycosides: Microbiology, Clinical Use, and Tox-icity.* (Whelton, A., and Neu, H. C., eds.) Marcel Dekker, Inc., New York, **1982,** pp. 269–282.

Appel, G. B., and Neu, H. C. Nephrotoxicity of antimicrobial agents. *N. Engl. J. Med.,* **1977,** *296,* 722–728.

Aronoff, G. R.; Brier, M. E.; Nierste, D. M.; and Sloan, R. S. Interactions of moxalactam and tobramycin in normal volunteers and in patients with impaired renal function. *J. Infect. Dis.,* **1984,** *149,* 9–15.

Aronoff, G. R.; Pottratz, S. T.; Brier, M. E.; Walker, N. E.; Fineberg, N. S.; Glant, M. D.; and Luft, F. C. Aminoglycoside accumulation kinetics in rat renal parenchyma. *Antimicrob. Agents Chemother.,* **1983,** *23,* 74–78.

Atkinson, B. A. Species incidence, trends of susceptibility to antibiotics in the United States, and minimum inhibitory concentration. In, *Antibiotics in Laboratory Medicine.* (Lorian, V., ed.) The Williams & Wilkins Co., Baltimore, **1980,** pp. 607–722.

Barza, M. Factors affecting the intraocular penetration of antibiotics, the influence of route, inflammation, animal species, and tissue pigmentation. *Scand. J. Infect. Dis.,* **1978,** *14,* 151–159.

Barza, M.; Brown, R. B.; Shen, D.; Gibaldi, M.; and Weinstein, L. Predictability of blood levels of gentamicin in man. *J. Infect. Dis.,* **1975,** *132,* 165–174.

Barza, M., and Scheife, R. T. Antimicrobial spectrum, pharmacology, and therapeutic use of antibiotics. *J. Maine Med. Assoc.,* **1977,** *68,* 194–210.

Baylis, C.; Rennke, H. R.; and Brenner, B. M. Mechanisms of the defect in glomerular ultrafiltration associated with gentamicin administration. *Kidney Int.,* **1977,** *12,* 344–353.

Bennett, W. M.; Elliott, W. C.; Houghton, D. C.; Gilbert, D. N.; DeFehr, J.; and McCarron, D. A. Reduction of experimental gentamicin nephrotoxicity in rats by dietary calcium loading. *Antimicrob. Agents Chemother.,* **1982,** *22,* 508–512.

Bergeron, M. G.; Bastille, A.; Lessard, C.; and Gagnon, P. M. Significance of intrarenal concentrations of gentamicin for the outcome of experimental pyelonephritis in rats. *J. Infect. Dis.,* **1982,** *146,* 91–96.

Betts, R. F.; Valenti, W. M.; Chapmen, S. W.; Chonmaitree, T.; Mowrer, G.; Pincus, P.; Messner, M.; and Robertson, R. Five-year surveillance of aminoglycoside usage in a university hospital. *Ann. Intern. Med.,* **1984,** *100,* 219–222.

Blair, D. C.; Duggan, D. O.; and Schroeder, E. T. Inactivation of amikacin and gentamicin by carbenicillin in patients with end-stage renal failure. *Antimicrob. Agents Chemother.,* **1982,** *22,* 376–379.

Bock, B. V.; Edelstein, P. H.; and Meyer, R. D. Prospective comparative study of efficacy and toxicity of netilmicin and amikacin. *Antimicrob. Agents Chemother.,* **1980,** *17,* 217–225.

Breen, K. J.; Bryant, R. E.; Levinson, J. D.; and Schenker, S. Neomycin absorption in man. *Ann. Intern. Med.,* **1972,** *76,* 211–218.

Brummett, R. Animal models of aminoglycoside antibiotic ototoxicity. *Rev. Infect. Dis.,* **1983,** *5,* Suppl. 2, S294–S303.

Brummett, R. E., and Fox, K. E. Studies of aminoglycoside ototoxicity in animal models. In, *The Aminoglycosides: Microbiology, Clinical Use, and Toxicity.* (Whelton, A., and Neu, H. C., eds.) Marcel Dekker, Inc., New York, **1982,** pp. 419–451.

Bryan, L. E., and Kwan, S. Mechanisms of aminoglycoside resistance of anaerobic bacteria and facultative bacteria grown anaerobically. *J. Antimicrob. Chemother.,* **1981,** *8,* Suppl. D, 1–8.

———. Roles of ribosomal binding, membrane potential, and electron transport in bacterial uptake of streptomycin and gentamicin. *Antimicrob. Agents Chemother.,* **1983,** *23,* 835–845.

Clarke, J. S.; Condon, R. E.; Bartlett, J. G.; Gorbach, S. L.; Nichols, R. L.; and Ochi, S. Preoperative oral antibiotics reduce septic complications of colon operations: results of prospective, randomized, double-blind clinical study. *Ann. Surg.*, **1977**, *186*, 251–259.

Cox, C. E. Gentamicin. *Med. Clin. North Am.*, **1970**, *54*, 1305–1315.

Cross, A. S.; Opal, S.; and Kopecko, D. J. Progressive increase in antibiotic resistance of gram-negative bacterial isolates. *Arch. Intern. Med.*, **1983**, *143*, 2075–2080.

Davies, J., and Courvalin, P. Mechanisms of resistance to aminoglycosides. *Am. J. Med.*, **1977**, *62*, 868–872.

Dickie, P.; Bryan, L. E.; and Pichard, M. A. Effect of enzymatic adenylation on dihydrostreptomycin accumulation in *Escherichia coli* carrying an R-factor: model explaining aminoglycoside resistance by inactivating mechanisms. *Antimicrob. Agents Chemother.*, **1978**, *14*, 569–580.

Dull, W. L.; Alexander, M. R.; and Kasik, J. E. Bronchial secretion levels of amikacin. *Antimicrob. Agents Chemother.*, **1979**, *16*, 767–771.

Fong, I. W.; Fenton, R. S.; and Bird, R. Comparative toxicity of gentamicin versus tobramycin: a randomized prospective study. *J. Antimicrob. Chemother.*, **1981**, *7*, 81–88.

Gangadharam, P. R. J.; Candler, E. R.; and Ramakrishna, P. V. *In vitro* anti-mycobacterial activity of some new aminoglycoside antibiotics. *J. Antimicrob. Chemother.*, **1977**, *3*, 285–286.

Hancock, R. F. W. Aminoglycoside uptake and mode of action—with special reference to streptomycin and gentamicin. I. Antagonists and mutants. *J. Antimicrob. Chemother.*, **1981a**, *8*, 249–276.

——. Aminoglycoside uptake and mode of action—with special reference to streptomycin and gentamicin. II. Effects of aminoglycosides on cells. *Ibid.*, **1981b**, *8*, 429–445.

Higgins, C. E., and Kastners, R. E. Nebramycin, a new broad-spectrum antibiotic complex. II. Description of *Streptomyces tenebrarius. Antimicrob. Agents Chemother.*, **1967**, *7*, 324–331.

Holtzman, J. L. Gentamicin neuromuscular blockade. (Letter.) *Ann. Intern. Med.*, **1976**, *84*, 55.

Hull, J. H., and Sarubbi, F. A., Jr. Gentamicin serum concentrations: pharmacokinetic predictions. *Ann. Intern. Med.*, **1976**, *85*, 183–189.

Humbert, G.; Leroy, A.; Fillastre, J. P.; and Oksenhendler, G. Pharmacokinetics of netilmicin in the presence of normal or impaired renal function. *Antimicrob. Agents Chemother.*, **1978**, *14*, 40–44.

Humes, H. D.; Sastrasinh, M.; and Weinberg, J. M. Calcium is a competitive inhibitor of gentamicin–renal membrane binding interactions, and dietary calcium supplementation protects against gentamicin nephrotoxicity. *J. Clin. Invest.*, **1984**, *73*, 134–147.

Huy, P. T. B.; Meulemans, A.; Wassef, M.; Manuel, C.; Sterkers, O.; and Amiel, C. Gentamicin persistence in rat endolymph and perilymph after a two-day constant infusion. *Antimicrob. Agents Chemother.*, **1983**, *23*, 344–346.

Kaiser, A. B., and McGee, Z. A. Aminoglycoside therapy of gram-negative bacillary meningitis. *N. Engl. J. Med.*, **1975**, *293*, 1215–1220.

Karchmer, A. W.; Moellering, R. C.; Maki, D. G.; and Swartz, M. N. Single-antibiotic therapy for streptococcal endocarditis. *J.A.M.A.*, **1979**, *241*, 1801–1806.

Kawaguchi, H.; Naito, T.; Nakagowa, S.; and Fugijawa, K. BBK8, a new semisynthetic aminoglycoside antibiotic. *J. Antibiot.* (*Tokyo*), **1972**, *25*, 695.

Keating, M. J.; Bodey, G. P.; Valdivieso, M.; and Rodriguez, V. A randomized comparative trial of three aminoglycosides—comparison of continuous infusions of gentamicin, amikacin, and sisomicin combined with

carbenicillin in the treatment of infections in neutropenic patients with malignancies. *Medicine* (*Baltimore*), **1979**, *58*, 159–170.

Keys, T. F.; Kurtz, S. B.; Jones, J. D.; and Muller, S. M. Renal toxicity during therapy with gentamicin or tobramycin. *Mayo Clin. Proc.*, **1981**, *56*, 556–559.

Klastersky, J.; Hensgens, C.; and Debusscher, L. Empiric therapy for cancer patients: comparative study of ticarcillin-tobramycin, ticarcillin-cephalothin, and cephalothin-tobramycin. *Antimicrob. Agents Chemother.*, **1975**, *7*, 640–645.

Klastersky, J.; Meunier-Carpentier, F.; and Prevost, J. M. Significance of antimicrobial synergism for the outcome of gram-negative sepsis. *Am. J. Med. Sci.*, **1977**, *273*, 157–167.

Konishi, H.; Goto, M.; Nakamoto, Y.; Yamamoto, I.; and Yamashina, H. Tobramycin inactivation by carbenicillin, ticarcillin, and piperacillin. *Antimicrob. Agents Chemother.*, **1983**, *23*, 653–657.

Kunin, C. M. Blunder drug for pneumonia. (Letter.) *N. Engl. J. Med.*, **1977**, *297*, 113–114.

Le Goffic, F.; Capmau, M. L.; Tangy, F.; and Baillarge, M. Mechanism of action of aminoglycoside antibiotics. Binding studies of tobramycin and its 6'-N-acetyl derivative to the bacterial ribosome and its subunits. *Eur. J. Biochem.*, **1979**, *102*, 73–81.

Lerner, A. M.; Cone, L. A.; Jansen, W.; Reyes, M.; Blair, D. C.; Wright, G. E.; and Lorber, R. R. Randomized controlled trial of the comparative efficacy, auditory toxicity, and nephrotoxicity of tobramycin and netilmicin. *Lancet*, **1983**, *1*, 1123–1126.

Lesar, T. S.; Rotschafer, J. C.; Strand, L. M.; Solem, L. D.; and Zaske, D. E. Gentamicin dosing errors with four commonly used nomograms. *J.A.M.A.*, **1982**, *248*, 1190–1193.

Lietman, P. S., and Smith, C. R. Aminoglycoside nephrotoxicity in humans, *J. Infect. Dis.*, **1983**, *5*, Suppl. 2, S284–S292.

Luft, F. C.; Brannon, D. R.; Stropes, L. L.; Costello, R. J.; Sloan, R. S.; and Maxwell, D. R. Pharmacokinetics of netilmicin in patients with renal impairment and in patients on dialysis. *Antimicrob. Agents Chemother.*, **1978**, *14*, 403–407.

Luft, F. C., and Evans, A. P. Comparative effects of tobramycin and gentamicin on glomerular ultrastructure. *J. Infect. Dis.*, **1980**, *142*, 910–914.

Luft, F. C.; Yum, M. N.; and Kleit, S. Comparative nephrotoxicities of netilmicin and gentamicin in rats. *Antimicrob. Agents Chemother.*, **1976**, *10*, 845–849.

Luzzatto, L.; Apirion, D.; and Schlessinger, D. Polyribosome depletion and blockage of the ribosome cycle by streptomycin in *Escherichia coli. J. Mol. Biol.*, **1969**, *42*, 315–335.

McCracken, G. H., Jr.; Mize, S. G.; and the Neonatal Meningitis Cooperative Study Group. Intraventricular therapy of neonatal meningitis caused by gram-negative enteric bacilli. *Pediatr. Res.*, **1979**, *13*, 464.

McCracken, G. H., Jr.; Mize, S. G.; and Threlkeld, N. Intraventricular gentamicin therapy in gram-negative bacillary meningitis of infancy. *Lancet*, **1980**, *1*, 787–791.

McNeil, J. S.; Jackson, B.; Nelson, L.; and Butkus, D. E. The role of prostaglandins in gentamicin-induced nephrotoxicity in the dog. *Nephron*, **1983**, *33*, 202–207.

Mates, S. M.; Patel, L.; Kaback, H. R.; and Miller, M. H. Membrane potential in anaerobically growing *Staphylococcus aureus* and its relationship to gentamicin uptake. *Antimicrob. Agents Chemother.*, **1983**, *23*, 526–530.

Mitchell, C. J.; Bullocks, S.; and Ross, B. D. Renal handling of gentamicin and other antibiotics by the isolated perfused rat kidney: mechanism of nephrotoxicity. *Antimicrob. Agents Chemother.*, **1977**, *3*, 593–600.

Mitsuhashi, S. (ed.). *Drug Action and Drug Resistance in Bacteria.* Vol. 2, *Aminoglycoside Antibiotics.* University Park Press, Baltimore, **1975.**

Moellering, R. C. Microbiological considerations in the use of tobramycin and related aminoglycosidic aminocyclitol antibiotics. *Med. J. Aust.,* **1977,** *2,* Suppl., 4–8.

Moellering, R. C.; Korzeniowski, O. M.; Sande, M. A.; and Wennersten, C. B. Species-specific resistance to antimicrobial synergism among enterococci. *J. Infect. Dis.,* **1979,** *140,* 203–208.

Moore, R. D.; Smith, C. R.; and Lietman, P. S. Risk factors for the development of auditory toxicity in patients receiving aminoglycosides. *J. Infect. Dis.,* **1984,** *149,* 23–30.

Nakae, R., and Nakae, T. Diffusion of aminoglycoside antibiotics across the outer membrane of *Escherichia coli. Antimicrob. Agents Chemother.,* **1982,** *22,* 554–559.

Neu, H. C., and Bendush, C. L. Ototoxicity of tobramycin: a clinical overview. *J. Infect. Dis.,* **1976,** *134,* S206–S218.

Panwalker, A. P.; Malon, J. B.; Zimelis, V. M.; and Jackson, G. G. Netilmicin: clinical efficacy, tolerance, and toxicity. *Antimicrob. Agents Chemother.,* **1978,** *13,* 170–176.

Papapetropoulou, M.; Papavassiliou, J.; and Legakis, N. J. Effect of the pH and osmolality of urine on the antibacterial activity of gentamicin. *J. Antimicrob. Chemother.,* **1983,** *12,* 571–575.

Patel, V.; Luft, F. C.; Yum, M. N.; Patel, B.; Zeman, W.; and Kleit, S. H. Enzymuria in gentamicin-induced kidney damage. *Antimicrob. Agents Chemother.,* **1975,** *7,* 364–369.

Phillips, J. B.; Satterwhite, C.; Dworsky, M. E.; and Cassady, G. Recommended amikacin doses in newborns often produce excessive serum levels. *Pediatr. Pharmacol. (New York),* **1982,** *2,* 121–125.

Pickering, L. K., and Gearhart, P. Effect of time and concentration upon interaction between gentamicin, tobramycin, netilmicin, or amikacin and carbenicillin or ticarcillin. *Antimicrob. Agents Chemother.,* **1979,** *15,* 592–596.

Pittinger, C., and Adamson, R. Antibiotic blockade of neuromuscular function. *Annu. Rev. Pharmacol.,* **1972,** *12,* 169–184.

Pittinger, C. B.; Eryasa, Y.; and Adamson, R. Antibiotic-induced paralysis. *Anesth. Analg.,* **1970,** *49,* 487–501.

Powell, S. H.; Thompson, W. L.; Luthe, M. A.; Stern, R. C.; Grossniklaus, D. A.; Bloxham, D. D.; Groden, D. L.; Jacobs, M. R.; Discenna, A. O.; Cash, H. A.; and Klinger, J. D. Once-daily versus continuous aminoglycoside dosing: efficacy and toxicity in animal and clinical studies of gentamicin, netilmicin, and tobramycin. *J. Infect. Dis.,* **1983,** *147,* 918–932.

Quarum, M. L.; Houghton, D. C.; Gilbert, D. N.; McCarron, D. A.; and Bennett, W. M. Increasing dietary calcium moderates experimental gentamicin nephrotoxicity. *J. Lab. Clin. Med.,* **1984,** *103,* 104–114.

Queener, S. F.; Luft, F. C.; and Hamel, F. G. Effect of gentamicin treatment on adenylate cyclase and Na$^+$,K$^+$-ATPase activities in renal tissues of rats. *Antimicrob. Agents Chemother.,* **1983,** *24,* 815–818.

Rahal, J. J., Jr.; Hyams, P. S.; Simberkoff, M. S.; and Rubenstein, E. Intrathecal and intramuscular gentamicin for gram-negative meningitis: pharmacologic study of 21 patients. *N. Engl. J. Med.,* **1974,** *290,* 1394–1398.

Reiner, N. E.; Bloxham, D. D.; and Thompson, W. L. Nephrotoxicity of gentamicin and tobramycin given once daily or continuously in dogs. *J. Antimicrob. Chemother.,* **1978,** *4,* Suppl. A, 85–101.

Ronald, A. R.; Boutros, P.; and Mourtada, H. Bacteri-

uria localization and response to single-dose therapy in women. *J.A.M.A.,* **1976,** *235,* 1854–1856.

Rosenthal, A.; Button, L. N.; and Khaw, K. T. Blood volume changes in patients with cystic fibrosis. *Pediatrics,* **1977,** *59,* 588–594.

Rosselot, J. P.; Marquez, J.; Meseck, E.; Murawski, A.; Hamdan, A.; Joyner, C.; Schmidt, R.; Migliore, D.; and Herzog, H. L. Isolation, purification, and characterization of gentamicin. In, *Antimicrobial Agents and Chemotherapy—1963.* (Sylvester, J. C., ed.) American Society for Microbiology, Ann Arbor, Mich., **1964,** pp. 14–16.

Sande, M. A. Infective endocarditis. In, *Internal Medicine.* (Stein, J. H., ed.) Little, Brown & Co., Boston, **1983,** pp. 537–547.

Sande, M. A., and Scheld, M. Antibiotic combinations in infective endocarditis. *Ann. Intern. Med.,* **1980,** *92,* 390–395.

Schatz, A.; Bugie, S.; and Waksman, S. A. Streptomycin, a substance exhibiting antibiotic activity against gram-positive and gram-negative bacteria. *Proc. Soc. Exp. Biol. Med.,* **1944,** *57,* 244–248.

Schentag, J. J.; Gengo, F. M.; Plant, M. E.; Danner, D.; Mangione, A.; and Jusko, W. J. Urinary casts as an indicator of renal tubular damage in patients receiving aminoglycosides. *Antimicrob. Agents Chemother.,* **1979,** *16,* 468–474.

Schentag, J. J., and Jusko, W. J. Renal clearance and tissue accumulation of gentamicin. *Clin. Pharmacol. Ther.,* **1977,** *22,* 364–370.

Schimpff, S. C. Therapy of infection in patients with granulocytopenia. *Med. Clin. North Am.,* **1977,** *61,* 1101–1118.

Siber, G. R.; Echeverria, P.; Smith, A. L.; Paisley, J. W.; and Smith, D. H. Pharmacokinetics of gentamicin in children and adults. *J. Infect. Dis.,* **1975,** *132,* 637–651.

Silverblatt, F. J. Pathogenesis of nephrotoxicity of cephalosporins and aminoglycosides: a review of current concepts. *Rev. Infect. Dis.,* **1982,** *4,* Suppl., S360–S365.

Singh, Y. N.; Harvey, A. L.; and Marshall, I. G. Antibiotic-induced paralysis of the mouse phrenic nerve—hemidiaphragm preparation and reversibility by calcium and by neostigmine. *Anesthesiology,* **1978,** *48,* 418–424.

Smith, C. R.; Baughman, K. L.; Edwards, C. Q.; Rogers, J. F.; and Lietman, P. S. Controlled comparison of amikacin and gentamicin. *N. Engl. J. Med.,* **1977,** *296,* 349–353.

Smith, C. R., and Lietman, P. S. Effect of furosemide on aminoglycoside-induced nephrotoxicity and auditory toxicity in humans. *Antimicrob. Agents Chemother.,* **1983,** *23,* 133–137.

Smith, C. R.; Lipsky, J. J.; Laskin, O. L.; Hellman, D. B.; Mellits, E. D.; Longstreth, J.; and Lietman, P. S. Double-blind comparison of the nephrotoxicity and auditory toxicity of gentamicin and tobramycin. *N. Engl. J. Med.,* **1980,** *302,* 1106–1109.

Smithivas, T.; Hyams, P. J.; Matalon, R.; Simberkoff, M. S.; and Rahal, J. J. The use of gentamicin in peritoneal dialysis. I. Pharmacologic results. *J. Infect. Dis.,* **1971,** *124,* Suppl., S77–S83.

Sokoll, M. D., and Gergis, S. D. Antibiotics and neuromuscular function. *Anesthesiology,* **1981,** *55,* 148–159.

Spyker, D. A.; Sande, M. A.; and Mandell, G. L. Tobramycin pharmacokinetics in patients with cystic fibrosis and leukemia. In, *Eighteenth Interscience Conference on Antimicrobial Agents and Chemotherapy.* American Society for Microbiology, Washington, D. C., **1978,** p. 345.

Stöffler, G., and Tischendorf, G. W. Antibiotic receptor-sites in *E. coli* ribosomes. In, *Drug Receptor Interactions in Antimicrobial Chemotherapy.* Vol. I, *Topics in Infectious Diseases.* (Drews, J., and Hahn, F. E., eds.) Springer-Verlag, New York, **1975.**

Strausbaugh, L. J.; Mandaleris, C. D.; and Sande, M. A. Comparison of four aminoglycoside antibiotics in the therapy of experimental *E. coli* meningitis. *J. Lab. Clin. Med.*, **1977**, *89*, 692–701.

Strausbaugh, L. J., and Sande, M. A. Factors influencing the therapy of experimental *Proteus mirabilis* meningitis. *J. Infect. Dis.*, **1978**, *137*, 251–260.

Tai, P.-C.; Wallace, B. J.; and Davis, B. D. Streptomycin causes misreading of natural messenger by interacting with ribosomes after initiation. *Proc. Natl Acad. Sci. U.S.A.*, **1978**, *75*, 275–279.

Theopold, H. M. Comparative surface studies of ototoxic effects of various aminoglycoside antibiotics on the organ of Corti in the guinea pig. A scanning electron microscopic study. *Acta Otolaryngol.* (*Stockh.*), **1977**, *84*, 57–64.

Thys, J. P. Peak or sustained antibiotic serum levels for optimal tissue penetration. *J. Antimicrob. Chemother.*, **1981**, *8*, Suppl. C, 29–36.

Trestman, I.; Parsons, J.; Santoro, J.; Goodhart, G.; and Kaye, D. Pharmacology and efficacy of netilmicin. *Antimicrob. Agents Chemother.*, **1978**, *13*, 832–836.

Varese, L. A.; Graziolo, F.; Viretto, A.; and Antoniola, P. Single-dose (bolus) therapy with gentamicin in management of urinary tract infection. *Int. J. Pediatr. Nephrol.*, **1980**, *1*, 104–105.

Wade, J. C.; Smith, C. R.; Petty, B. G.; Lipsky, J. J.; Conrad, G.; Ellner, J.; and Lietman, P. S. Cephalothin plus an aminoglycoside is more nephrotoxic than methicillin plus an aminoglycoside. *Lancet*, **1978**, *2*, 604–606.

Wersäll, J.; Bjorkroth, B.; Flock, A.; and Lundquist, P.-G. Experiments on the ototoxic effects of antibiotics. *Adv. Otorhinolaryngol.*, **1973**, *20*, 14–41.

Wilson, P., and Ramsden, R. T. Immediate effects of tobramycin on human cochlea and correlation with serum tobramycin levels. *Br. Med. J.*, **1977**, *1*, 259–261.

Wilson, W. R.; Geraci, J. E.; Wilkowske, C. J.; and Washington, J. A., II. Short-term intramuscular therapy with procaine penicillin plus streptomycin for infective endocarditis due to *viridans* streptococci. *Circulation*, **1978**, *57*, 1158–1161.

Wilson, W. R.; Wilkowske, C. J.; Wright, A. J.; Sande, M. A.; and Geraci, J. E. Treatment of streptomycin-susceptible and streptomycin-resistant enterococcal endocarditis. *Ann. Intern. Med.*, **1984**, *100*, 816–823.

Wolfe, J. C., and Johnson, W. D., Jr. Penicillin-sensitive streptococcal endocarditis. *Ann. Intern. Med.*, **1974**, *81*, 178–181.

Wright, P. F.; Kaiser, A. B.; Bowman, C. M.; McKee, K. T., Jr.; Trujillo, H.; and McGee, Z. A. The pharmacokinetics and efficacy of an aminoglycoside administered into the cerebral ventricles in neonates: implications for further evaluation of this route of therapy for meningitis. *J. Infect. Dis.*, **1981**, *143*, 141–147.

Yow, M. O. An overview of pediatric experience with amikacin. *Am. J. Med.*, **1977**, *62*, 954–958.

Monographs and Reviews

Alexander, D. P., and Gambertoglio, J. G. Drug overdose and pharmacologic considerations in dialysis. In, *Introduction to Dialysis*. (Cogan, M. G., and Garovoy, M. R., eds.) Churchill Livingstone, Inc., New York, **1985**, pp. 261–292.

Atkinson, B. A. Species incidence, trends of susceptibility to antibiotics in the United States, and minimum inhibitory concentration. In, *Antibiotics in Laboratory Medicine*. (Lorian, V., ed.) The Williams & Wilkins Co., Baltimore, **1980**, pp. 607–722.

Barza, M.; Brown, K. B.; Shen, D.; Gibaldi, M.; and Weinstein, L. Predictability of blood levels of gentamicin in man. In, *Clinical Pharmacy and Clinical Pharmacology*. (Gouveia, W. A.; Tognoni, G.; and van der Kleijn, E.; eds.) North-Holland Publications, Amsterdam, **1976**, pp. 207–222.

Bryan, L. E. Mechanisms of action of aminoglycoside antibiotics. In, *Contemporary Issues in Infectious Diseases*. Vol. 1, *New Dimensions in Antimicrobial Therapy*. (Root, R. K., and Sande, M. A., eds.) Churchill Livingstone, Inc., New York, **1984**, pp. 1–8.

Conference on Kanamycin. (Various authors.) Appraisal after eight years of clinical application. *Ann. N.Y. Acad. Sci.*, **1966**, *132*, 773–1090.

Lietman, P. S. Aminoglycosides and spectinomycin: aminocyclitols. In, *Principles and Practice of Infectious Diseases*, 2nd ed. (Mandell, G. L.; Douglas, R. G., Jr.; and Bennett, J. E.; eds.) John Wiley & Sons, Inc., New York, **1985**, pp. 192–206.

McCracken, G. H., Jr. New developments in the management of neonatal meningitis. In, *Contemporary Issues in Infectious Diseases*. Vol. 3, *Bacterial Meningitis*. (Sande, M. A.; Smith, A. L.; and Root, R. K.; eds.) Churchill Livingstone, Inc., New York, **1985**, pp. 159–166.

Shannon, K., and Phillips, I. Mechanisms of resistance to aminoglycosides in clinical isolates. *J. Antimicrob. Chemother.*, **1982**, *9*, 91–102.

Symposium. (Various authors.) Advances in aminoglycoside therapy: amikacin. *J. Infect. Dis.*, **1976a**, *134*, S235–S460.

Symposium. (Various authors.) Tobramycin. *J. Infect. Dis.*, **1976b**, *134*, S1–S234.

Symposium. (Various authors.) Amikacin. *Am. J. Med.*, **1977**, *62*, 863–966.

Symposium. (Various authors.) Tobramycin — comparative toxicity of aminoglycoside antibiotics. *J. Antimicrob. Chemother.*, **1978**, *4*, Suppl. A, 1–101.

Symposium. (Various authors.) *Contemporary Issues in Infectious Diseases*. Vol. 2, *Endocarditis*. (Sande, M. A.; Kaye, D.; and Root, R. K.; eds.) Churchill Livingstone, Inc., New York, **1984**.

Waksman, S. A. (ed.). *Streptomycin, Nature and Practical Applications*. The Williams & Wilkins Co., Baltimore, **1949**.

Tetracyclines, Chloramphenicol, Erythromycin, and Miscellaneous Antibacterial Agents

Merle A. Sande and Gerald L. Mandell

TETRACYCLINES

History. The development of the tetracycline antibiotics was the result of a systematic screening of soil specimens collected from many parts of the world for antibiotic-producing microorganisms. The first of these compounds, *chlortetracycline*, was introduced in 1948. Two years later, *oxytetracycline* became available. Elucidation of the chemical structure of these agents confirmed their similarity and furnished the basis for the production of a third member of this group, *tetracycline*, in 1952. In 1957, a new family of tetracyclines was developed, characterized chemically by the absence of the ring-attached CH₃ group present in the others. One of these, *demethylchlortetracycline*, subsequently given the official name *demeclocycline*, became available for general use in 1959. *Methacycline*, a derivative of oxytetracycline, was introduced in 1961; *doxycycline* became available in 1966; and *minocycline*, in 1972.

Soon after their initial development, the tetracyclines were found to be highly effective against rickettsiae, a number of gram-positive and gram-negative bacteria, and the agents responsible for lymphogranuloma venereum, inclusion conjunctivitis, and psittacosis, and hence became known as "broad-spectrum" antibiotics. With establishment of their *in-vitro* antimicrobial activity, effectiveness in experimental infections, and pharmacological properties, the tetracyclines rapidly became widely used in therapy. (*See* Dowling, 1955; Lepper, 1956.)

Although there are specific and useful differences between the tetracyclines currently available in the United States, they are in the main very much alike. This permits discussion of these drugs as a group.

Source. *Chlortetracycline* and *oxytetracycline* are elaborated by *Streptomyces aureofaciens* and *Streptomyces rimosus*, respectively. The antibiotics are produced in broth by deep-tank fermentation. *Tetracycline* is produced semisynthetically from chlortetracycline; it has also been obtained from a species of *Streptomyces*. *Demeclocycline* is the product of a mutant of the strain of *Streptomyces aureofaciens* from which chlortetracycline was first obtained. *Methacycline, doxycycline,* and *minocycline* are all semisynthetic derivatives.

Chemistry and Stability. The tetracyclines are closely congeneric derivatives of the polycyclic naphthacenecarboxamide. Their structural formulas are shown in Table 52–1.

The crystalline bases are faintly yellow, odorless, slightly bitter compounds. They are only slightly soluble in water at pH 7 (0.25 to 0.5 mg/ml), but they form soluble sodium salts and hydrochlorides. While the bases and the hydrochlorides are quite stable as dry powders, most of these agents lose activity relatively rapidly when in solution.

Effects on Microbial Agents. The tetracyclines possess a wide range of antimicrobial activity against gram-positive and gram-negative bacteria, which overlaps that of many other antimicrobial drugs. They are also effective against some microorganisms that are resistant to agents that exert their effects on the bacterial cell wall,

Table 52–1. STRUCTURAL FORMULAS OF THE TETRACYCLINES

Tetracycline

CONGENER	SUBSTITUENT(S)	POSITION(S)
Chlortetracycline	—Cl	(7)
Oxytetracycline	—OH,—H	(5)
Demeclocycline	—OH,—H; —Cl	(6; 7)
Methacycline	—OH,—H; =CH₂	(5; 6)
Doxycycline	—OH,—H; —CH₃,—H	(5; 6)
Minocycline	—H,—H; —N(CH₃)₂	(6; 7)

such as *rickettsiae, Mycoplasma, Chlamydia* (the agents of *urethritis, lymphogranuloma venereum, psittacosis, inclusion conjunctivitis,* and *trachoma*), some *atypical mycobacteria,* and *amebae.* They have little activity against fungi.

In vitro, these drugs are primarily bacteriostatic. Only multiplying microorganisms are affected. The sensitivity or resistance of a particular microorganism to each of the congeners is similar. However, minocycline is usually the most active, followed by doxycycline. Tetracycline and oxytetracycline are the least active. Strains inhibited by 4 μg/ml or less of a tetracycline are considered sensitive.

Bacteria. In general, gram-positive microorganisms are affected by lower concentrations of tetracycline than are gram-negative species. However, these agents are less useful for infections caused by gram-positive bacteria because of problems of resistance and the availability of superior antimicrobial agents. More than 25 μg/ml of tetracycline or doxycycline is required to inhibit 90% of strains of group-B and group-D streptococci and *Staphylococcus aureus* in current isolates. Corresponding values for *Streptococcus pyogenes* are 6.3 μg/ml and 0.8 μg/ml for tetracycline and doxycycline, respectively. Both drugs are quite active against most strains of pneumococci (minimal inhibitory concentration for 90% of strains [MIC 90] = 0.4 to 0.8 μg/ml). Although as many as 30% of pneumococcal strains have been found to be resistant in some geographical areas, the prevalence of such resistance to tetracyclines is low in most regions (Neu, 1978).

Neisseria gonorrhoeae and many strains of *N. meningitidis* are inhibited by tetracyclines (MIC 90 = 1 to 2 μg/ml).

While the tetracyclines were initially useful for treatment of infections with aerobic gram-negative bacilli, many species are now relatively resistant. However, more than 90% of strains of *Haemophilus influenzae* may still be sensitive to either tetracycline or doxycycline. While all strains of *Pseudomonas aeruginosa* are resistant, 90% of strains of *Pseud. pseudomallei* are sensitive. Nearly 100% of strains of *Campylobacter* are sensitive, but clinical studies demonstrating efficacy have not been reported. Most strains of *Brucella* are also susceptible. Tetracyclines are particularly useful for infections caused by *H. ducreyi, Brucella,* and *Vibrio cholerae.* These drugs also inhibit the growth of *Yersinia pestis, Y. enterocolitica, Francisella tularensis,* and *Pasteurella multocida.* The tetracyclines are active against many anaerobic and facultative microorganisms, and their activity against *Actinomyces* is particularly relevant. Anywhere from 70% to 100% of the various anaerobic species are sensitive to doxycycline, the most active congener of tetracycline. Seventy-five percent of strains of *Bacteroides fragilis* are inhibited by 4 μg/ml of doxycycline, compared to 42% for tetracycline. Nevertheless, tetracyclines are less active against *B. fragilis* than is chloramphenicol, clinda-

mycin, or metronidazole, and these agents have replaced the tetracyclines in the therapy of most anaerobic infections (Standiford, 1985).

Rickettsiae. Like chloramphenicol, all the tetracyclines are highly effective against the rickettsiae responsible for *Rocky Mountain spotted fever, murine typhus, epidemic typhus, scrub typhus, rickettsialpox,* and *Q fever.*

Miscellaneous Microbial Agents. The tetracyclines are active against many spirochetes, including *Borrelia recurrentis, Treponema pallidum,* and *T. pertenue.* The activity of tetracyclines against *Chlamydia* and *Mycoplasma* has become particularly relevant. Strains of *Mycobacterium marinum* are also susceptible.

Effects on Intestinal Flora. Since many of the tetracyclines are incompletely absorbed from the gastrointestinal tract, high concentrations are reached in the intestinal contents. Within 48 hours after daily administration of conventional doses of these agents, the enteric flora is markedly altered. Many aerobic and anaerobic coliform microorganisms and gram-positive spore-forming bacteria are sensitive and may be markedly suppressed during chronic medication before resistant strains reappear. The stools become softer and odorless and acquire a yellow-green color. However, as the fecal coliform count declines, tetracycline-resistant microorganisms, particularly yeasts, enterococci, *Proteus,* and *Pseudomonas,* overgrow and the total fecal microbial count may actually increase. Tetracycline occasionally produces so-called antibiotic-associated colitis. Normal intestinal flora is restored several days after antibiotic medication is withdrawn.

Mechanism of Action. The site of action of tetracyclines is the bacterial ribosome, but at least two processes appear to be required for these antibiotics to gain access to the ribosomes of gram-negative bacteria (Chopra and Howe, 1978). The first is passive diffusion through hydrophilic pores in the outer cell membrane. These structures have been specifically located within protein IA, one of three proteins in the envelope. Minocycline and perhaps doxycycline are more lipophilic than the other congeners and pass directly through the lipid bilayer. The second process involves an energy-dependent active transport system that pumps all tetracyclines through the inner cytoplasmic membrane. Such transport may require a periplasmic protein carrier. Although permeation of these drugs into gram-positive bacteria is less well understood, it too requires an energy-dependent system. Once the tetracyclines gain access to the bacterial cell, they inhibit protein synthesis and, like the aminoglycosides, bind specifically to 30 S ribosomes. They appear to prevent access of aminoacyl tRNA to the acceptor site on the mRNA-ribosome complex. This prevents the addition of amino acids to the growing peptide chain. Only a small portion of the drug is irreversibly bound, and the inhibitory effects of the tetracyclines can be reversed by washing. Therefore, it is probable that the reversibly bound antibiotic is responsible for the antibacterial action. These compounds also impair protein synthesis in mammalian cells at high concentrations; however, the host cells lack the active transport system found in bacteria. Tetracyclines, even in subinhibitory concentrations, have been shown to reduce the ability of *Escherichia coli* to adhere to mammalian epithelial cells *in vitro*. The details of the extensive studies in this field have been reviewed by Pratt (1977).

Resistance to the Tetracyclines. Resistance to the tetracyclines produced *in vitro* appears slowly in a graded, stepwise fashion similar to that observed with penicillin. Microorganisms that have become insensitive to one tetracycline frequently exhibit resistance to the others. Resistance to the tetracyclines in *E. coli* and probably in other bacterial species is mediated by a plasmid and is an inducible trait; that is, the bacteria become resistant only after exposure to the drug. However, the drug itself is not altered. Plasmids that impart resistance contain genetic information for a number of proteins that appear to affect transport of the drug into the cell. In *E. coli*, at least one of these proteins has been located on the inner cytoplasmic membrane, where it may interfere with the energy-dependent accumulation of tetracycline (Chopra and Howe, 1978).

Absorption, Distribution, and Excretion.
Absorption. Most of the tetracyclines are adequately but incompletely absorbed from the gastrointestinal tract. The percentage of an oral dose that is absorbed (when the stomach is empty) is lowest for chlortetracycline (30%); intermediate for oxytetracycline, demeclocycline, and tetracycline (60 to 80%); and high for doxycycline (95%) and minocycline (100%) (Barza and Scheife, 1977). The percentage that is not absorbed rises as the dose increases. Most absorption takes place from the stomach and upper small intestine and is greater in the fasting state; it is much less complete from the lower portions of the intestinal tract. Absorption of these agents is impaired by milk products, aluminum hydroxide gels, sodium bicarbonate, calcium and magnesium salts, and iron preparations. The mechanisms responsible for the decreased absorption appear to be chelation and an increase in gastric pH.

The wide range of plasma concentrations present in different individuals following the oral administration of the various tetracyclines is related in large measure to the irregularity of their absorption from the gastrointestinal tract. These drugs can be divided into three groups based on the dosage and frequency of oral administration required to produce effective plasma concentrations.

Oxytetracycline and *tetracycline* are incompletely absorbed. After a single *oral* dose peak plasma concentrations are attained in 2 to 4 hours. These drugs have half-lives in the range of 6 to 12 hours, and they are frequently administered two to four times daily. The administration of 250 mg every 6 hours produces peak plasma concentrations of approximately 3 μg/ml.

Demeclocycline and *methacycline* are usually administered in lower daily dosage than are the above-mentioned congeners. Their absorption is also incomplete, but their half-lives are about 16 hours and effective plasma concentrations may thus persist for 24 to 48 hours. This is particularly true for demeclocycline. Poor absorption of methacycline may lead to lower plasma concentrations than with recommended doses of tetracycline, despite the difference in half-life. The peak concentration of methacycline is approximately 2 μg/ml after an oral dose of 500 mg.

Doxycycline and *minocycline* should be administered in even lower daily dosage by the oral route, since their half-lives are long (16 to 18 hours) and they are well absorbed. After an oral dose of 200 mg of doxycycline, plasma concentrations of the drug reach a maximum of 3 μg/ml at 2 hours and are maintained above 1 μg/ml for 8 to 12 hours. Plasma concentrations are equivalent when doxycycline is given by the oral or parenteral route. Food does not interfere with the absorption of doxycycline or minocycline.

Distribution. The volume of distribution of many of the tetracyclines is relatively larger than that of the body water. They are bound to plasma proteins in varying degree. The approximate values are as follows: *doxycycline*, 80 to 95%; *demeclocycline*, 65 to 90%; *methacycline*, about 80%; *minocycline*, about 75%; *tetracycline*, about 65%; and *oxytetracycline*, 20 to 40%. However, the values reported in the literature are highly variable (*see* Appendix II).

All the tetracyclines are concentrated in the liver and excreted, by way of the bile, into the intestine, from which they are partially reabsorbed. Biliary concentrations of these agents average at least five to ten times higher than the simultaneous values in plasma. Decreased hepatic function or obstruction of the common bile duct results in reduction in the biliary excretion of these agents and their consequent persistence in the blood. Because of their enterohepatic circulation, the tetracyclines may be present in the blood for a long time after cessation of therapy.

Inflammation of the meninges is not a prerequisite for the passage of tetracyclines into the cerebrospinal fluid (CSF); route and duration of treatment are major determinants. The intravenous injection of a tetracycline results in the gradual appearance of the drug in the spinal fluid over a period of 6 hours. Oral therapy yields very low spinal fluid concentrations.

Penetration of these drugs into most other fluids and tissues is excellent. Concentrations in synovial fluid and the mucosa of the maxillary sinus approach that of plasma. Minocycline reaches a sufficient concentration in tears and saliva to eradicate the meningococcal carrier state; this characteristic is unique to minocycline among the tetracyclines and has been attributed to its greater solubility in lipid. The tetracyclines are stored in the reticuloendothelial cells of the liver, spleen, and bone marrow, and in bone and the dentine and enamel of unerupted teeth (see below). Tetracyclines cross the placenta and enter the fetal circulation and amniotic fluid. Concentrations of tetracycline in umbilical cord plasma reach 60% and in amniotic fluid 20% of those in the circulation of the mother. Relatively high concentrations of these drugs are also found in milk.

Excretion. All the tetracyclines are excreted in the urine and the feces, the primary route for most being the kidney. Since renal clearance of these drugs is by glomerular filtration, their excretion is significantly affected by the state of renal function (see below). Twenty to 60% of an intravenous dose of 0.5 g of *tetracycline* is excreted in the urine during the first 24 hours; from 20 to 55% of an oral dose, regardless of size, is excreted by this route. Ten to 35% of a dose of *oxytetracycline* is excreted in active form in the urine, in which it is detectable within 30 minutes and reaches a peak concentration in about 5 hours after it is administered. The rate of renal clearance of *demeclocycline* is less than half that of tetracycline. About 50% of *methacycline* is excreted in unchanged form in the urine, while about 5% is excreted in the feces over a period of 72 hours.

Minocycline is recoverable from both urine and feces in significantly lower amounts than are the other tetracyclines, and it appears to be metabolized to a considerable extent. Renal clearance of minocycline is low. The drug persists in the body after its administration is stopped; this may be due to retention in fatty tissues. The half-life of minocycline is apparently not prolonged in patients with hepatic failure.

An important distinction should be made in the case of *doxycycline.* It is clear that, with conventional doses, doxycycline is not eliminated via the same pathways as are other tetracyclines, and it does not accumulate significantly in the blood of patients with renal failure. It is thus one of the safest of the tetracyclines for the treatment of extrarenal infections in such individuals. The drug is excreted in the feces, largely as an inactive conjugate or perhaps as a chelate; for this reason it has relatively less impact on the intestinal microflora. The half-life of doxycycline may be shortened from approximately 16 to 7 hours in patients who are receiving chronic treatment with barbiturates or phenytoin.

As mentioned, the intestine is an important avenue of elimination of the tetracyclines. Because these agents are incompletely absorbed from the bowel when given orally or when excreted into the intestine in the bile, they are present, in varying concentrations, in the feces. Elimination from the intestinal tract occurs even when the drugs are given parenterally, as a result of excretion in the bile.

Preparations, Routes of Administration, and Dosage. *Oxytetracycline hydrochloride* (TERRAMYCIN, others), *tetracycline hydrochloride* (ACHROMYCIN, others), *demeclocycline hydrochloride* (DECLOMYCIN), *methacycline hydrochloride* (RONDOMYCIN), *doxycycline hyclate* (VIBRAMYCIN, others), and *minocycline hydrochloride* (MINOCIN) are available in a wide variety of forms for oral, topical, and parenteral administration.

The tetracyclines are usually prescribed for *oral* use, but most may be administered by intravenous injection. Topical administration is best avoided because of the high risk of sensitization, except for use in the eye. *The tetracyclines should never be injected intrathecally and they are rarely given intramuscularly.*

Preparations for Oral Administration. All the tetracyclines listed above are available for oral administration, usually as capsules and occasionally in tablet form, in appropriate dosages ranging from 50 to 500 mg, depending on the preparation. Some of the tetracyclines are also marketed as flavored powders for oral suspension, ophthalmic suspensions and ointments, solutions for injection, and syrups for pediatric use.

The *oral dose* of the tetracyclines varies with the nature and the severity of the disease. For *tetracycline* and *oxytetracycline*, it ranges from 1 to 2 g per day in adults. The recommended dose of *demeclocycline* is somewhat lower, being 150 mg every 6 hours in moderately severe infections and 300 mg every 6 hours when the disease is more serious. The doses for children and infants are calculated on a weight basis. The oral dose of *methacycline* for adults is 150 mg every 6 hours or 300 mg every 12 hours; for children it is 10 mg/kg per day, divided into equal-sized quantities given every 8 hours. The dose of *doxycycline* for adults is 100 mg every 12 hours during the first 24 hours, followed by 100 mg once a day, or twice daily when severe infection is present. Children should receive 4 to 5 mg/kg per day, divided into two equal doses given at a 12-hour interval during the first day, after which a single dose of half this amount is administered; in serious disease, the same quantity is given every 12 hours. The dose of *minocycline* for adults is 200 mg initially, followed by 100 mg every 12 hours; for children it is 4 mg/kg initially, followed by 2 mg/kg every 12 hours.

Because the incidence of gastrointestinal distress and particularly of tetracycline-resistant bacterial enteritis rises as the dose of the antibiotic is increased, the minimal dosage compatible with the desired therapeutic response is recommended. Gastrointestinal distress, nausea, and vomiting can be minimized by administration of the tetracyclines with meals. Milk, antacids containing aluminum or magnesium hydroxide or silicate, and iron interfere with the absorption of the drugs and should not be ingested at the same time as is a tetracycline.

Preparations for Parenteral Administration. Injectable preparations of oxytetracycline, tetracycline, doxycycline, and minocycline are designed for intravenous use, while preparations of tetracycline and oxytetracycline for intramuscular injection are also available. For intravenous use, the concentration of antibiotic should not exceed 5 mg/ml, and the solution should be infused slowly.

Intravenous administration of the tetracyclines can be used in severe illness in which the dose may be large and cause nausea and vomiting if given orally, in patients unable to ingest medication, and when the response to oral therapy is inadequate. However, it should be emphasized that there are currently very few indications for intravenous administration of these drugs, since better alternatives are usually available. The total daily intravenous dose of oxytetracycline or tetracycline for most acute infections is 500 mg to 1 g, usually administered in two equal portions at 12-hour intervals. Up to 2 g per day may be given in severe infections, but this dose may cause difficulty in some patients (*see* below); quantities larger than 2 g per day must not be given parenterally. The recommended daily intravenous dose for children and infants is 10 to 20 mg/kg of body weight. Because of local irritation and poor absorption, *intramuscular administration* of these tetracyclines is generally unsatisfactory and is rarely indicated. The usual intravenous dose of doxycycline is 200 mg in one or two infusions on the first day and 100 to 200 mg on subsequent days. The dose for children who weigh less than 45 kg is 4.4 mg/kg on the first day, and this is then reduced correspondingly.

Preparations for Local Application. Except for local use in the eye, topical use of the tetracyclines is not recommended. Ophthalmic preparations include *chlortetracycline hydrochloride ophthalmic ointment, tetracycline hydrochloride ophthalmic ointment,* and *tetracycline hydrochloride ophthalmic suspension.* One or 2 drops are instilled in the conjunctival sac two to six times daily, or more. The usual concentration of a tetracycline for ophthalmic use is 0.5 to 1%.

UNTOWARD EFFECTS

Toxic Effects. *Gastrointestinal.* The tetracyclines all produce *gastrointestinal irritation* to a varying degree in some but not all individuals; such effects are more common after oral administration of the drugs. Epigastric burning and distress, abdominal discomfort, nausea, and vomiting may occur. The larger the dose, the greater is the likelihood of an irritative reaction. If troublesome, gastric distress can be controlled by administration of the tetracyclines with food (not milk or milk products) or antacids that do not contain aluminum, magnesium, or calcium. Nausea and vomiting often subside as medication continues and can frequently be controlled by temporary reduction in dose or by the use of smaller amounts at frequent intervals. Esophageal ulcers have been reported (Winckler, 1981), as has an association with pancreatitis (Elmore and Rogge, 1981). *Diarrhea* may also result from the irritative effects of the tetracyclines given orally. In such cases, the stools, while frequent and fluid, do not contain blood or leukocytes. *It is imperative that this type of diarrhea be promptly distinguished from that which results from pseudomembranous colitis caused by overgrowth of Clostridium difficile,* a potentially life-threatening complication (*see* below).

Phototoxicity. Demeclocycline, doxycycline, and, to a lesser extent, other derivatives may produce mild-to-severe reactions in the skin of treated individuals exposed to sunlight; this phenomenon is a *phototoxic reaction.* Onycholysis and pigmentation of the nails may develop simultaneously. The incidence of the ''sunburn'' reaction was found to be 40 in 2682 patients treated with demeclocycline (Carey, 1960). Phototoxicity is evident only when the skin is exposed to sunlight containing rays in the range of 270 to 320 nm; these are filtered out by ordinary window glass.

Hepatic Toxicity. Hepatic toxicity due to tetracycline was first observed by Lepper in 1951 in patients receiving large doses of tetracycline orally or intravenously. Microscopic study of the liver reveals fine vacuoles, cytoplasmic changes, and increase in fat (Zimmerman and Lewis, 1984). Oxytetracycline and tetracycline appear to be less hepatotoxic than are the other drugs of this group. Most reactions of this type develop in patients receiving 2 g or more of drug per day parenterally; however, this effect may also occur when large quantities are administered orally. *Pregnant women appear to be particularly susceptible to severe, tetracycline-induced hepatic damage.* Jaundice appears first, and azotemia, acidosis, and irreversible shock may follow. The livers are diffusely infiltrated with fat. Although hepatic fat is increased during pregnancy, the quantity appears to be even greater after exposure to a tetracycline. Disseminated intravascular coagulation has been reported in a pregnant woman who developed hepatorenal failure after being given only two doses of 100 mg each of tetracycline intramuscularly (Pride *et al.*, 1973).

Renal Toxicity. Tetracyclines may aggravate uremia in patients with renal disease by inhibiting protein synthesis, provoking a catabolic effect, and thereby increasing azotemia from metabolism of amino acids (Shils, 1963). Doxycycline has been reported to produce fewer renal side effects than do other tetracyclines; however, a possible association between this drug and the production of renal failure has been suggested (Orr *et al.*, 1978). Kuzucu (1970) has called attention to the possibility of the development of severe renal failure in patients who receive tetracycline after being anesthetized with methoxyflurane; in those who died, the kidneys contained numerous calcium oxalate crystals. Diabetes insipidus has been observed in some patients receiving demeclocycline, and this phenomenon has been exploited for the treatment of chronic, inappropriate secretion of antidiuretic hormone (Forrest *et al.*, 1978; *see* Chapter 37).

A clinical picture characterized by nausea, vomiting, polyuria, polydipsia, proteinuria, acidosis, glycosuria, and gross aminoaciduria—a form of the *Fanconi syndrome*—has been observed in patients ingesting outdated and degraded tetracycline. All manifestations disappear in about a month after cessation of treatment. A facial lesion typical of systemic lupus erythematosus, as well as sensitivity to sunlight, has also been observed following ingestion of outdated and degraded tetracycline.

Effects on Calcified Tissues. Children receiving long- or short-term therapy with a tetracycline may develop *brown discolorations of the teeth.* The larger the dose of drug relative to body weight, the more intense the discoloration of enamel. The duration of therapy appears to be less important than the total quantity of antibiotic administered. The risk of this untoward effect is highest when the tetracycline is given to neonates and babies prior to the first dentition. However, pigmentation of the permanent dentition may develop if the drug is given between the ages of 2 months and 5 years, when these teeth are being calcified. An early characteristic of this defect is a yellow fluorescence of the dental pigment, which has an ultraviolet spectrum with an absorption peak at 270 nm. The *deposition of the drug in the teeth and bones* is probably due to its chelating property and the formation of a tetracycline-calcium orthophosphate complex. As time progresses, the yellow fluorescence is replaced by a nonfluorescent brown color that may represent an oxidation product of the antibiotic, the formation of which is hastened by light. This discoloration is permanent.

Treatment of pregnant patients with tetracyclines may produce discoloration of the teeth in their offspring. The period of greatest danger to the teeth is from midpregnancy to about 4 to 6 months of the postnatal period for the deciduous anterior teeth, and from 6 months to 5 years of age for the permanent anterior teeth, the periods when the crowns of the teeth are being formed. However, children up to 7 years old may be susceptible to this complication of tetracycline therapy.

Tetracyclines are deposited in the *skeleton* of the human fetus and young child. A 40% depression of bone growth, as determined by measurement of fibulas, has been demonstrated in premature infants treated with these agents (Cohlan *et al.*, 1963). This is readily reversible if the period of exposure to the drug is short.

Miscellaneous Effects. The intravenous administration of the tetracyclines is frequently followed by *thrombophlebitis*, especially when a single vein is used for repeated infusion. The highly irritative effects of these agents are emphasized by the severe pain that they produce when injected intramuscularly without a local anesthetic.

Long-term therapy with tetracyclines may produce changes in the peripheral blood. *Leukocytosis, atypical lymphocytes, toxic granulation of granulocytes,* and *thrombopenic purpura* have been observed.

The tetracyclines may cause *increased intracranial pressure* and tense bulging of the fontanels (pseudotumor cerebri) in young infants, even when given in the usual therapeutic doses. Except for the elevated pressure, the spinal fluid is normal. Discontinuation of therapy results in prompt return of the pressure to normal. This complication may occur rarely in older individuals (Walters and Gubbay, 1981).

Patients receiving *minocycline* may experience *vestibular toxicity,* manifested by dizziness, ataxia, nausea, and vomiting. The symptoms occur soon after the initial dose and generally disappear within 24 to 48 hours after drug administration is stopped. The frequency of this side effect is directly related to the dose and has been noted more often in women than in men (Fanning *et al.,* 1977).

Hypersensitivity Reactions. Various skin reactions, including *morbilliform rashes, urticaria, fixed drug eruptions,* and generalized *exfoliative dermatitis,* may follow the use of any of the tetracyclines, but they are rare. Among the more severe allergic responses are *angioedema* and *anaphylaxis;* anaphylactoid reactions can occur even after the oral use of these agents. Other effects that have been attributed to hypersensitivity are *burning of the eyes, cheilosis, atrophic or hypertrophic glossitis, pruritus ani or vulvae, and vaginitis;* these effects often persist for weeks or months after cessation of tetracycline therapy. The exact cause of these reactions is unknown, but they could represent the results of subtle changes in the bacterial flora of the patient. *Fever* of varying degree and *eosinophilia* may occur when these agents are administered. Asthma has also been observed.

It should be emphasized that *cross-sensitization among the various tetracyclines is common.*

Biological Effects Other Than Allergic or Toxic. Like all antimicrobial agents, the tetracyclines administered orally or parenterally may lead to the development of *superinfections* that are usually due to strains of bacteria or yeasts resistant to these agents. Vaginal, oral, pharyngeal, and even systemic infections with yeasts and fungi are observed. The incidence of these infections appears to be much higher with the tetracyclines than with the penicillins.

Among the most important superinfections associated with the administration of the tetracyclines are those that involve the intestinal tract; they may occur with either oral or parenteral therapy. The possibility that drug-induced diarrhea may be due to active infection of the bowel merits serious consideration in every instance.

Pseudomembranous colitis is characterized by severe diarrhea, fever, and stools containing shreds of mucous membrane and a large number of neutrophils. It has been attributed to the overgrowth of toxin-producing bacteria (*Cl. difficile*). The toxin is cytotoxic to mucosal cells and causes shallow ulcerations that can be seen by sigmoidoscopy. Discontinuation of the drug, combined in some instances with the oral administration of vancomycin, is curative.

The oral administration of tetracyclines may result in an increase in the quantity of bilirubin and a decrease in the concentration of urobilinogen in the urine. This may cause diagnostic confusion in instances in which differentiation of obstructive from hepatocellular jaundice is important. Plasma prothrombin may be depressed to low levels by the oral administration of tetracyclines given for even moderate periods; this is probably related to the changes in intestinal flora induced by these drugs.

To decrease the incidence of toxic effects, the following precautions should be observed in the use of the tetracyclines. They should not be given to pregnant patients; they should not be employed for the therapy of the common infections in children under the age of 12 years, and unused supplies of these antibiotics should be discarded.

THERAPEUTIC USES

The tetracyclines have been used extensively both for the treatment of infectious diseases and as an additive to animal feeds to facilitate growth. Both uses have resulted in increasing bacterial resistance to these drugs. Because of this and the development of new antimicrobial agents that are more effective for specific infections and less toxic, the number of indications for the use of tetracyclines has declined. These agents are useful in rickettsial and bacterial diseases, in infections produced by some *Mycoplasma,* and in disorders caused by *Chlamydia.* The status of the tetracyclines for the therapy of various infections is given in Table 48–1 (page 1072).

Rickettsial Infections. The tetracyclines and chloramphenicol are effective and may be lifesaving in rickettsial infections, including Rocky Mountain spotted fever, recrudescent epidemic typhus (Brill's disease), murine typhus, scrub typhus, rickettsialpox, and Q fever. Fever usually subsides in 1 to 3 days, and the rash disappears in 3 to 5 days; striking clinical improvement is often evident within 24 hours after initiation of therapy.

Mycoplasma Infections. *Mycoplasma pneumoniae* is sensitive to the tetracyclines. Treatment of pneumonia with either tetracycline or erythromycin results in a shorter duration of fever, cough, malaise, fatigue, pulmonary rales, and roentgenographic changes in the lungs. Mycoplasma may persist in the sputum following cessation of therapy despite rapid resolution of the active infection.

Chlamydia. *Lymphogranuloma Venereum.* The tetracyclines are currently the treatment of choice in this infection. Tetracycline should be given in oral doses of 500 mg four times a day for at least 2 weeks; longer treatment may be required in more chronic cases. Doxycycline, 100 mg orally twice daily for 2 weeks, may be as effective but has not been extensively studied. Decided reduction in the size of buboes is observed within 4 days, and inclusion and elementary bodies entirely disappear from the lymph nodes within 1 week. Lymphogranulomatous proctitis is promptly improved. Rectal pain, discharge, and bleeding are markedly decreased. When relapses occur, treatment is resumed with full doses and is continued for longer periods.
Psittacosis. The tetracyclines are also of value in proven cases of psittacosis. Drug therapy for 12 to 14 days is usually adequate.
Inclusion Conjunctivitis. This disease responds clinically to topical administration of tetracycline, in ointment or liquid form, four times a day for 3 weeks. However, this treatment does not always eradicate the microorganisms. Systemic therapy with tetracycline or a sulfonamide for 3 weeks is preferred in adults. In infants, erythromycin has been used systemically, but experience is limited (Bowie and Holmes, 1985).
Trachoma. Although the sulfonamides are preferred by some for the treatment of trachoma, the tetracyclines have proven very effective. While topical therapy has been used, oral administration of an antimicrobial agent is now recommended. The most effective regimen has been doxycycline given once daily for 40 days in a dose of 2.5 to 4 mg/kg (Hoshiwara *et al.*, 1973).

Nonspecific Urethritis. Nonspecific urethritis is now known to be caused by *Chlamydia trachomatis.* This microorganism is sensitive to tetracycline; the oral administration of 500 mg every 6 hours for 7 days is recommended. Up to 45% of patients with gonococcal urethritis have been found to have coexistent infection with *C. trachomatis.* A diagnosis of gonorrhea has thus become an indication to treat for *Chlamydia* as well (Washington, 1982).

Sexually Transmitted Diseases. Although penicillin G is still the drug of choice for *gonorrhea,* it cannot be used in some patients because of hypersensitivity. In such cases, the administration of 0.5 g of tetracycline orally every 6 hours for 7 days (or doxycycline, 100 mg orally twice daily for 7 days) is effective for uncomplicated gonococcal infections of the urethra or pharynx. Although tetracycline can be used for anorectal gonorrhea in men, relapse rates of 14 to 17% have been found, compared to 1.6 to 4% after treatment with procaine penicillin G (Washington, 1982). A tetracycline may also be used in disseminated gonococcal infections, except in pregnant women. For *gonococcal salpingitis* (pelvic inflammatory disease), tetracycline should be given for 10 days. *Epididymitis* in males less than 35 years of age is usually caused by the gonococcus or *C. trachomatis* and is effectively treated with tetracycline (*see* above).

Tetracyclines are effective in the therapy of *syphilis* in patients unable to tolerate penicillin. A dose of 500 mg of tetracycline given every 6 hours for 15 days is recommended for early syphilis (less than 1-year duration), but therapy should be continued for 30 days if the disease has been present for longer than 1 year. Tetracyclines are also effective in *chancroid* and *granuloma inguinale,* but their use in these diseases entails the risk of masking a luetic infection that may have been contracted at the same time. If they are employed, the dose and duration of treatment should be the same as those used to treat syphilis.

Endocervical or *rectal infections* caused by *Chlamydia* should be treated with either tetracycline, 500 mg orally four times daily for 7 days, or doxycycline, 100 mg twice daily for 7 days. When disease occurs in pregnant women, erythromycin, 500 mg orally four times daily for 7 days, should be used. When *Chlamydia* is identified (or suspected) as a cause of *acute pelvic inflammatory disease* (*endometritis, salpingitis, parametritis,* and/or *peritonitis*), doxycycline, 100 mg intravenously twice daily, is recommended for at least 4 days or 48 hours after defervescence, followed by oral therapy at the same dosage to complete a 10- to 14-day course. Doxycycline is usually combined with cefoxitin (2 g intravenously four times daily) to cover microorganisms that may be resistant to doxycycline (anaerobes, facultative aerobes, and some strains of penicillinase-producing *N. gonorrhoeae*). *Acute epididymo-orchitis* is often caused by either *C. trachomatis* or *N. gonorrhoeae.* Effective regimens include either tetracycline, 500 mg orally four times daily for at least 10 days, or doxycycline, 100 mg orally twice daily for at least 10 days. Sexual partners of patients with any of the above conditions should also be treated with either tetracycline or doxycycline for 7 days.

Bacillary Infections. *Brucellosis.* Treatment with the tetracyclines produces excellent results in infections caused by *Brucella melitensis, suis,* and *abortus.* Both acute and chronic forms of the disease respond dramatically. Good results are usually obtained in acute brucellosis with full doses of a tetracycline for 3 weeks. Clinical and bacteriological relapses are not the result of the development of resistant strains of *Brucella* and usually respond to a second course of therapy. The tetracyclines given with streptomycin (1 g daily, intramuscularly) also provide prompt results in patients severely ill with acute brucellosis. Whether such therapy results in a lower incidence of relapse than that observed with a tetracycline alone (for 6 weeks) is unsettled.

Tularemia. Although streptomycin is preferable, therapy with the tetracyclines also produces prompt results in tularemia. Both the ulceroglandular and typhoidal types of the disease respond well. Fever, toxemia, and clinical signs and symptoms are all improved; the bacteria rapidly disappear from blood, sputum, and pleural fluid; and complications are usually prevented.

Cholera. In a controlled trial of the effects of oral antibiotics in the management of cholera in children in Pakistan, Lindebaum and associates (1967) found that tetracycline was the most effective of the agents studied in reducing stool volume, intravenous fluid requirement, and the duration of diarrhea and positive stool culture. Only 1% of the children given tetracycline had diarrhea for more than 4 days. Treatment with tetracycline was significantly more effective than intravenous fluid therapy alone, regardless of the severity of the disease. When oral drug therapy was given for only 48 hours, bacteriological relapse developed in 20% of the cases despite a good clinical response. It must be emphasized that antimicrobial agents are not substitutes for fluid and electrolyte replacement in this disease. The effectiveness of tetracycline as a prophylactic agent in families of cholera patients was demonstrated by McCormack and coworkers (1968). They noted that the administration of the drug for 5 days was effective in preventing infection in contacts.

Other Bacillary Infections. Therapy with the tetracyclines is not uniformly effective in infections caused by *Shigella* and *Salmonella,* because of the increase in incidence of resistant strains; consequently, tetracyclines are not the drugs of choice. A similar situation holds for infections of various types caused by *E. coli* and *Enterobacter aerogenes.* Doxycycline has been used successfully to reduce the incidence of traveler's diarrhea, especially that caused by enterotoxin-producing strains of *E. coli* (Sack *et al.,* 1978). Emergence of resistant strains and the potential for an increased incidence of salmonellosis will likely limit the usefulness of this approach.

Coccal Infections. The tetracyclines are no longer indicated for infections caused by *staphylococci* or by *Strep. pyogenes* because of the high frequency of resistant strains. The existence of tetracycline-resistant strains of *Strep. pneumoniae* has also decreased the utility of these drugs in the management of pneumococcal pneumonia. None of the tetracyclines should be used to treat meningococcal infections when other effective drugs are available. Although *minocycline* has been found, when given in a dose of 100 mg every 12 hours for 5 days, to *prevent the development of meningococcal disease* and markedly to *lower the carrier rate,* its use for this purpose is not recommended because of the vestibular disturbances that this drug can cause (*see* above).

Urinary Tract Infections. Although the tetracyclines were initially very valuable in the management of urinary tract infection due to gram-negative bacilli, their usefulness has been appreciably reduced by the increase in the number of drug-resistant microorganisms involved in this kind of infection. As a rule, these drugs are not active against *Proteus* and *Pseud. aeruginosa.* Therapy of urinary tract infections with a tetracycline *should* be undertaken only if the strain isolated from the urine is sensitive. Therapy is usually continued for 7 to 10 days. For severe acute pyelonephritis, tetracyclines should be used only if no other antimicrobial agent is effective. The acute urethral syndrome in women has been effectively treated with doxycycline (100 mg twice daily for 10 days) (Stamm *et al.,* 1981). While doxycycline may be given to patients with high-grade renal dysfunction, the drug concentration in the urine will then not be sufficient for such therapy.

Other Infections. *Actinomycosis,* although most responsive to penicillin G, may be successfully treated with a tetracycline; in severe infections, intravenous therapy for 1 week, followed by oral administration of drug for a month or more, may be required. Minocycline has been suggested for the treatment of *nocardiosis,* but a sulfonamide should be used concurrently. *Yaws* and *relapsing fever* respond favorably to the tetracyclines and penicillin (Salih and Mustafa, 1977). Although either tetracycline or penicillin G is used to treat *leptospirosis,* evidence of efficacy is not convincing with these or any other antimicrobial agent. *Lyme disease,* recognized only recently, is characterized by fever, skin lesions, arthritis, and aseptic meningitis; it is caused by a spirochete (Steere *et al.,* 1980). It responds to either penicillin V or tetracycline (500 mg every 6 hours for 7 days). The tetracyclines have been used to treat atypical mycobacterial diseases, including those caused by *Mycobacterium marinum* (Izumi *et al.,* 1977).

Chronic Obstructive Pulmonary Disease. A large number of studies have suggested that the oral administration of 0.5 g per day of tetracycline or corresponding doses of the congeneric agents is effective in reducing the number of acute pulmonary infections in individuals with chronic lung disease, especially bronchitis or obstructive disorders such as emphysema. In some instances, such prophylaxis has been used only during the winter months; in others, it has been more prolonged. Although many of the reports are enthusiastic about this procedure, universal agreement as to its effectiveness and safety is lacking. The danger of this kind of prophylaxis is superinfection with drug-resistant bacteria and with fungi that may be very difficult or impossible to eradicate; death has occurred as a result of such a complication in a number of patients treated in this manner.

Intestinal Disease. Patients with *Whipple's disease* may respond to tetracycline with a prompt and dramatic cessation of fever, diarrhea, and arthralgia, and with a sustained gain of weight; relapses may disappear promptly on re-treatment. The administration of tetracycline to some patients with *tropical sprue* may be associated with repletion of folate, a favorable hematological response, decrease in diarrhea, improvement in the enzymatic activity and morphology of the superficial epithelium of the jejunal mucosa, gain in weight, and reversal of the abnormal pattern of lipid distribution. Tetracyclines may also be of value in the *blind-loop syndrome*.

Acne. Tetracyclines have been used for the therapy of acne, and good results have been reported by some workers. Benefit has been produced by very small doses. It has been suggested that these drugs may act by decreasing the fatty acid content of sebum. Although it is generally accepted that the tetracyclines or other antibiotics have a beneficial effect in acne, some placebo crossover studies raise doubt concerning the value of this kind of therapy. Use of tetracycline seems to be associated with few side effects when given in doses of 250 mg orally twice a day. Other drugs useful in the treatment of acne are listed in the Index.

CHLORAMPHENICOL

History and Source. *Chloramphenicol* is an antibiotic produced by *Streptomyces venezuelae,* an organism first isolated by Burkholder in 1947 from a soil sample collected in Venezuela. Filtrates of liquid cultures of the organisms were found to possess marked effectiveness against several gram-negative bacteria and also to exhibit antirickettsial activity; a crystalline antibiotic substance was then isolated (Bartz, 1948) and named CHLOROMYCETIN because it contained chlorine and was obtained from an actinomycete. When the structural formula of the crystalline material was determined, the antibiotic was prepared synthetically. Pharmacological studies in animals and man were soon undertaken by Smadel and Jackson. Late in 1947, the small amount of available chloramphenicol was employed in an outbreak of epidemic typhus in Bolivia, with dramatic results. It was then tried with excellent success in cases of scrub typhus on the Malay peninsula. By 1948, chloramphenicol was produced in amounts sufficient for general clinical use, and was then found to be of value in the therapy of a variety of infections. By 1950, however, it became evident that the drug could cause *serious and fatal blood dyscrasias.* The emergence of ampicillin-resistant strains of *H. influenzae* and an awareness of its activity against anaerobic bacteria, especially *B. fragilis,* have accounted for increased use of chloramphenicol in recent years. However, new drugs have emerged that will challenge these indications.

Chemistry. Chloramphenicol has the following structural formula:

Chloramphenicol

The antibiotic is unique among natural compounds in that it contains a nitrobenzene moiety and is a derivative of dichloroacetic acid. The biologically active form is levorotatory. It is only slightly soluble in water (1:400). The antibiotic is extremely stable. Chloramphenicol is inactivated by enzymes present in filtrates of certain bacteria, which reduce the nitro group and hydrolyze the amide linkage; it is also acetylated (*see* below).

Mechanism of Action. Chloramphenicol inhibits protein synthesis in bacteria and, to a lesser extent, in eukaryotic cells. The drug readily penetrates into bacterial cells, probably by a process of facilitated diffusion. Chloramphenicol acts primarily by binding reversibly to the 50 S ribosomal subunit (near the site of action of the macrolide antibiotics and clindamycin, which it inhibits competitively). This prevents the binding of the amino acid–containing end of aminoacyl tRNA to one of its binding sites on the ribosome. It has been suggested that the drug specifically attaches either to the acceptor site (the initial site of binding of aminoacyl tRNA) (*see* Werner *et al.*, 1975) or to the peptidyl (or donor) site, which is the critical binding site for the elongating peptide chain during the translocation step (*see* Hahn and Gund, 1975). Chloramphenicol may act as an analog of a dipeptide and an antagonist of the peptidyl substrate for the enzyme. Peptide bond formation is prevented as long as the drug remains bound to the ribosome.

Chloramphenicol can also inhibit mitochondrial protein synthesis in mammalian cells, perhaps because mitochondrial ribosomes resemble bacterial ribosomes (both are 70 S) more than they do the 80 S cytoplasmic ribosomes of mammalian cells. The peptidyl transferase of bovine mitochondrial ribosomes, but not cytoplasmic ribosomes, is susceptible to the inhibitory action of chloramphenicol. Mammalian erythropoietic cells seem to be particularly sensitive to the drug.

Effects on Microbial Agents. Chloramphenicol possesses a fairly wide spectrum of antimicrobial activity. Strains are considered sensitive if they are inhibited by concentrations of 12.5 μg/ml or less. It is primarily bacteriostatic, although it may be bactericidal to certain species, such as *H. influenzae.* Over 95% of strains of the following gram-negative bacteria are inhibited *in vitro* by 6.3 μg/ml of chloramphenicol: *H. influenzae, N. meningitidis, N. gonorrhoeae, Salmonella typhi, Brucella* species, and *Bordetella pertussis.* Likewise, most anaerobic bacteria, including gram-positive cocci and *Clostridium* species and gram-negative rods including *B. fragilis,* are inhibited by this concentration of the drug. Some aerobic gram-positive cocci, including *Strep. pyogenes, Strep. agalactiae* (group-B streptococci), and *Strep. pneumoniae,* are sensitive to 6.3 μg/ml, while fourfold higher concentrations are required to inhibit over 95% of strains of *Staph. aureus* (Standiford, 1985).

The Enterobacteriaceae have a variable sensitivity to chloramphenicol; while 95% of strains of *E. coli* are inhibited by 12.5 μg/ml, only 75% of *Klebsiella pneumoniae,* 50% of *Enterobacter,* and 33%

of *Serratia marcescens* are inhibited. Ninety percent of strains of *Proteus mirabilis* are inhibited by 12.5 μg/ml. All strains of *Pseud. pseudomallei* are inhibited by this concentration, while *Pseud. aeruginosa* is resistant to even very high concentrations of chloramphenicol. Eighty-four percent of *V. cholerae* are inhibited by 6.3 μg/ml, as are 90% of *Shigella*. Chloramphenicol exerts marked prophylactic and therapeutic effects in experimental infections produced by all rickettsiae. The drug, as a rule, only suppresses rickettsial growth. Chloramphenicol is also effective against *Chlamydia* and *Mycoplasma*.

Resistance to Chloramphenicol. The resistance of gram-positive and gram-negative microorganisms to chloramphenicol *in vivo* is a problem of increasing clinical importance. Resistance of gram-negative bacteria to the drug is usually due to the presence of a specific plasmid acquired by conjugation. The resistance of such strains to chloramphenicol is due to the presence of a specific acetyltransferase, which inactivates the drug by using acetyl coenzyme A as the donor of the acetyl group. At least three types of enzyme have been characterized (Gaffney and Foster, 1978). Acetylated derivatives of chloramphenicol fail to bind to bacterial ribosomes (Piffaretti and Froment, 1978). Several strains of *H. influenzae* that are resistant to chloramphenicol contain resistance factors that can be transferred to *E. coli* and to other strains of *H. influenzae*. These plasmids also invariably code for resistance to tetracyclines and may also code for a beta-lactamase that mediates resistance to ampicillin (Roberts *et al.*, 1980). Plasmid-mediated resistance to chloramphenicol in *S. typhi* emerged as a significant problem during the epidemic of 1972–1973 in Mexico and the United States. However, the prevalence of resistance to chloramphenicol is negligible today, except in some areas of Southeast Asia (Baine *et al.*, 1977). Resistance of staphylococci to this antibiotic has also increased in incidence; it varies from one hospital to another and is as high as 50% or more in some. Shaw and Brodsky (1968) demonstrated that resistant *Staph. aureus* contains an inducible form of chloramphenicol acetyltransferase. While loss of sensitivity to chloramphenicol is usually due to enzymatic degradation of the drug, both decreased permeability of the microorganisms (which has been found in *E. coli* and *Pseudomonas*) and mutation to ribosomal insensitivity have also been described (Sompolinsky and Samra, 1968; Baughman and Fahnestock, 1979).

Absorption, Distribution, Fate, and Excretion. The recent development of more specific assay technics for chloramphenicol has greatly contributed to our knowledge of disposition of the drug. Methods used previously were nonspecific and did not distinguish between the active drug and a variety of inactive metabolites.

Chloramphenicol is available for oral administration in two dosage forms: the active drug itself and the inactive prodrug, chloramphenicol palmitate. Hydrolysis of the ester bond of chloramphenicol palmitate is accomplished rapidly and almost completely by pancreatic lipases in the duodenum under normal physiological conditions (Kauffman *et al.*, 1981). Chloramphenicol is then absorbed from the gastrointestinal tract, and peak concentrations of 10 to 13 μg/ml occur within 2 to 3 hours after the administration of a 1-g dose. The bioavailability is greater for chloramphenicol than for chloramphenicol palmitate, probably due to the incomplete hydrolysis of the latter (Smith and Weber, 1983). Differences in the rate and extent of absorption may be particularly noticeable in patients with gastrointestinal disease or in newborns (Lietman, 1979). The preparation of chloramphenicol for parenteral use is the inactive succinate ester. Absorption after intramuscular injection is highly unpredictable, and this route is not recommended. It is unclear where the hydrolysis of chloramphenicol succinate occurs *in vivo*, but esterases of the liver, kidneys, and lungs may all be involved. After intravenous administration of the succinate ester, peak concentrations of active chloramphenicol are similar to those that follow oral dosage (Yogev *et al.*, 1981). Chloramphenicol succinate itself is also rapidly cleared from plasma by the kidneys. This renal clearance of the prodrug may affect bioavailability, since elimination of up to 20 to 30% of the dose may occur prior to hydrolysis. Poor renal function in the neonate and other states of renal insufficiency result in increased concentrations of chloramphenicol succinate, and thus of chloramphenicol, in plasma (Slaughter *et al.*, 1980b; Mulhall *et al.*, 1983). Decreased esterase activity has been observed in the plasma of neonates and infants. This results in a prolonged period of time to reach peak concentrations of active chloramphenicol (up to 4 hours) and a longer period of time over which renal clearance of chloramphenicol succinate can occur (Kauffman *et al.*, 1981).

Chloramphenicol is well distributed in body fluids and readily reaches therapeutic concentrations in CSF, where values are approximately 60% of those in plasma (range, 45 to 99%) in the presence or absence of meningitis (Friedman *et al.*, 1979). The drug may actually concentrate in brain tissue (Kramer *et al.*, 1969). Chloramphenicol is present in bile, is secreted into milk, and readily traverses the placental barrier. It also penetrates into the aqueous humor after subconjunctival injection.

The major route of elimination of chloramphenicol is hepatic metabolism to the inactive glucuronide. This metabolite, as well as chloramphenicol itself, is excreted in the urine by filtration and secretion. Over a 24-hour period, 75 to 90% of an orally administered dose is so excreted; about 5 to 10% is in the biologically active form. Patients with hepatic cirrhosis have decreased metabolic clearance, and dosage should be adjusted in these individuals. The half-life of chloramphenicol has been correlated with plasma bilirubin concentrations (Koup *et al.*, 1979). Additionally, binding of chloramphenicol to plasma proteins is lower in cirrhotic patients (42%, compared to 53% in normals), as it is in neonates (32%) (Koup *et al.*, 1979; Blouin *et al.*, 1980). The half-life of the active drug (4 hours) is not significantly changed in patients with renal failure compared to those with normal renal function. Full doses of chloramphenicol must still be given to achieve therapeutic concentrations of the active drug in uremia. The extent to which hemodialysis removes chloramphenicol from plasma does not appear to be sufficient to warrant adjustment of dosage (Blouin *et al.*, 1980). However, when patients undergoing dialysis have other complications, such as cirrhosis, the clearance due to dialysis may be important relative to that by other routes. In such cases it may be best to administer the maintenance dose at the end of hemodialysis to minimize this effect (Slaughter *et al.*, 1980a). The variability in the pharmacokinetic parameters of chloramphenicol in neonates, infants, and children necessitates monitoring of drug concentrations in plasma.

Preparations, Routes of Administration, and Dosage. *Chloramphenicol* (CHLOROMYCETIN, MYCHEL) is marketed in capsules containing 250 and 500 mg for oral use. *Chloramphenicol palmitate* is a water-insoluble powder; 1.7 g of this preparation is equivalent to 1 g of chloramphenicol base. *Chlor-*amphenicol palmitate oral suspension* contains an amount of chloramphenicol palmitate equivalent to 150 mg of chloramphenicol base, mixed with suitable dispersing and flavoring agents, in each 5 ml. *Chloramphenicol sodium succinate* is marketed as the dry powder; it is intended for solution for *intravenous use*, and it may not be effective when given by the intramuscular route.

Chloramphenicol may be administered orally or intravenously. Dosage schedules for the therapy of specific infections are presented below. Adjustment in dose must be made when chloramphenicol palmitate is used, as indicated above.

Untoward Effects. Chloramphenicol inhibits the synthesis of enzymes of the inner mitochondrial membrane, probably by inhibition of the ribosomal peptidyl transferase. Other enzymes that are affected are the cytochrome oxidases, ATPase, and ferrochelatase, the final enzyme in heme biosynthesis. Much of the toxicity observed with this drug can be attributed to these effects (Smith and Weber, 1983).

Hypersensitivity Reactions. Although relatively uncommon, *macular* or *vesicular skin rashes* occur as a result of hypersensitization to chloramphenicol. *Fever* may appear simultaneously or be the sole manifestation. Angioedema is a rare complication. *Herxheimer reactions* have been observed shortly after institution of chloramphenicol therapy for syphilis, brucellosis, and typhoid fever.

Hematological Toxicity. The most important adverse effect of chloramphenicol is on the *bone marrow;* of all the drugs that may be responsible for *pancytopenia,* chloramphenicol is the most common cause (Wallerstein *et al.*, 1969). Changes in peripheral blood include *leukopenia, thrombocytopenia,* and *aplasia of the marrow* with *fatal pancytopenia.* These reactions may represent an idiosyncratic reaction to the drug, resulting in inhibition of nucleic acid synthesis in the stem cells. The incidence is not related to dose; however, it seems to occur more commonly in individuals who undergo prolonged therapy and especially in those who are exposed to the drug on more than one occasion. A genetic predisposition is suggested by the occurrence of pancytopenia in identical twins. Although the incidence of the reaction is low, one in approximately 30,000 or more courses of therapy, the fatality rate is high when bone-marrow aplasia is complete, and there is a high incidence of acute leukemia in those who recover.

A compilation of 576 cases of blood dyscrasia due to chloramphenicol indicates that aplastic anemia was the most common type reported, accounting for about 70% of the cases; hypoplastic anemia, agranulocytosis, thrombocytopenia, and bone-marrow inhibition made up the remainder. Among the patients with pancytopenia the outcome was apparently unrelated to the dose of chloramphenicol taken. However, the longer the interval between the last dose of chloramphenicol and the appearance of the first sign of the blood dyscrasia, the greater was the mortality rate; nearly all patients in whom this interval was longer than 2 months died. In most cases the condition for which chloramphenicol had been prescribed did not justify its use (Polak *et al.*, 1972).

Holt (1967) noted the absence of reported instances of aplastic anemia following parenteral administration of chloramphenicol and suggested that absorption of a toxic breakdown product from the gastrointestinal tract might be responsible. Subsequently, four such cases have been described; however, in all instances, the association with parenterally administered chloramphenicol is not clear. In two patients other drugs known to affect the bone marrow were also given (phenylbutazone and glutethimide). The issue thus remains unsettled (Polin and Plaut, 1977), but it seems unlikely that the mode of administration influences the incidence of aplastic anemia (Kucers, 1980). The structural feature of chloramphenicol that is responsible for aplastic anemia is assumed to be the nitro group, which may be metabolized to a toxic intermediate. However, the exact biochemical mechanism has not yet been elucidated (Skolimowski *et al.*, 1983).

The risk of aplastic anemia does not contraindicate the use of chloramphenicol in situations in which it is necessary; however, it emphasizes that the drug should never be employed in diseases readily, safely, and effectively treatable with other antimicrobial agents or in undefined situations.

A second hematological effect of chloramphenicol is a predictable but reversible erythroid suppression of the bone marrow that is probably due to its inhibitory action on mitochondrial protein synthesis. The result is a reduction of uptake of ^{59}Fe by normoblasts and of the incorporation of this isotope into heme (Ward, 1966). The clinical picture is featured initially by reticulocytopenia, which occurs 5 to 7 days after the initiation of therapy, followed by a decrease in hemoglobin, an increase in plasma iron, cytoplasmic vacuolation of early erythroid forms and granulocyte precursors, and normoblastosis with a shift to early erythrocyte forms (Scott *et al.*, 1965). Severe leukopenia and thrombocytopenia may also occur. The incidence and severity of this syndrome are related to dose. It occurs regularly when plasma concentrations are 25 μg/ml or higher and is observed during the use of large doses of chloramphenicol, prolonged treatment, or both. Dose-related suppression of the bone marrow has been reported to progress to fatal aplasia, but this does not occur predictably (Daum *et al.*, 1979).

The administration of chloramphenicol in the *presence of hepatic disease* frequently results in *depression of erythropoiesis;* this is most intense when ascites and jaundice are present (Suhrland and Weisberger, 1963). About one third of patients with renal insufficiency exhibit the same reaction.

Toxic and Irritative Effects. *Nausea, vomiting, unpleasant taste, diarrhea,* and *perineal irritation* may follow the oral administration of chloramphenicol. Among the rare toxic effects produced by this antibiotic are *blurring of vision* and *digital paresthesias.* *Optic neuritis* occurs in 3 to 5% of children with mucoviscidosis who are given chloramphenicol; there is symmetrical loss of ganglion cells from the retina and atrophy of the fibers in the optic nerve (Godel *et al.*, 1980).

Fatal chloramphenicol toxicity may develop in *neonates,* especially premature babies, when they are exposed to excessive doses of the drug. The illness, the *"gray syndrome,"* usually begins 2 to 9 days (average, 4 days) after treatment is started. The manifestations in the first 24 hours are vomiting, refusal to suck, irregular and rapid respiration, abdominal distention, periods of cyanosis, and passage of loose green stools. All the children are severely ill by the end of the first day and, in the next 24 hours, develop flaccidity, an ashen-gray color, a decrease in temperature, and a refractory lactic acidosis. Death occurs in about 40% of the patients, most frequently on the fifth day of life. Those who recover exhibit no sequelae.

Two mechanisms are apparently responsible for this toxic effect in neonates (Craft *et al.*, 1974): (1) *failure of the drug to be conjugated with glucuronic acid,* due to inadequate activity of glucuronyl transferase in the liver, which is characteristic of the first 3 to 4 weeks of life; and (2) *inadequate renal excretion of unconjugated drug* in the newborn. At the time of onset of the clinical syndrome, the chloramphenicol concentrations in plasma usually exceed 100 µg/ml, although they may be as low as 75 µg/ml (Burns *et al.*, 1959). Excessive plasma concentrations of the glucuronide conjugate are also present, despite low rate of formation, because tubular secretion, the pathway of excretion of this compound, is underdeveloped in the neonate. Children 1 month of age or younger should receive chloramphenicol in a daily dose no larger than 25 mg/kg of body weight; after this age, daily quantities up to 50 mg/kg may be given without difficulty. Toxic effects have not been observed in the newborn when as much as 1 g of the antibiotic has been given every 2 hours to women in labor.

Chloramphenicol is removed from the blood to only a very small extent by either peritoneal dialysis or hemodialysis. However, both exchange transfusion and charcoal hemoperfusion have been used to treat overdosage with chloramphenicol in infants (Kessler *et al.*, 1980; Mauer *et al.*, 1980).

Other organ systems that have a high rate of oxygen consumption may also be affected by the action of chloramphenicol on mitochondrial enzyme systems; encephalopathic changes have been observed (Levine *et al.*, 1970), and cardiomyopathy has also been reported (Biancaniello *et al.*, 1981).

Biological Effects Other Than Allergic or Toxic. The effects of chloramphenicol on the normal microflora and the consequences of such alterations are similar to those discussed above for the tetracyclines.

Drug Interactions. Chloramphenicol irreversibly inhibits hepatic microsomal enzymes of the cytochrome P-450 complex (Halpert, 1982), and thus may prolong the half-life of drugs that are metabolized by this system. Such drugs include dicumarol, phenytoin, chlorpropamide, and tolbutamide. Severe toxicity and death have occurred because of failure to recognize such effects. The inhibitory effect of chloramphenicol on hepatic enzymes may protect the liver from the toxic effects of carbon tetrachloride, since metabolism is apparently necessary to convert carbon tetrachloride to toxic products.

Conversely, other drugs may alter the elimination of chloramphenicol. Chronic administration of phenobarbital shortens the half-life of the antibi-

otic, presumably because of enzyme induction, and may result in subtherapeutic concentrations of the drug (Powell *et al.*, 1981).

Therapeutic Uses. *Therapy with chloramphenicol must be limited to those infections for which the benefits of the drug outweigh the risks of the potential toxicities. When other antimicrobial drugs are available that are equally effective but potentially less toxic than chloramphenicol, they should be used* (*see* Kucers, 1980; Feder *et al.*, 1981).

Typhoid Fever. Chloramphenicol is still an important drug for the treatment of typhoid fever and other types of systemic salmonella infections. However, epidemics in some parts of the world have been due to strains of *S. typhi* highly resistant to the drug. Ampicillin and amoxicillin are also effective in the management of such infections, and some authorities now recommend these agents as the treatment of choice for typhoid fever in the United States (DuPont and Pickering, 1980). There appear to be fewer carriers and fewer relapses after ampicillin than after chloramphenicol (Snyder *et al.*, 1976). The occurrence of resistance to the drug makes it necessary to determine the sensitivity of the microorganisms recovered from patients with these diseases. Trimethoprim-sulfamethoxazole has also been used successfully for the treatment of typhoid fever caused by chloramphenicol-resistant *S. typhi* (Gilman *et al.*, 1975).

Within a few hours after chloramphenicol is administered, *S. typhi* disappears from the blood. Stool cultures frequently become negative in a few days. Clinical improvement is often evident within 48 hours, and fever and other signs of the disease commonly abate within 3 to 5 days. The patient usually becomes afebrile before the intestinal lesions heal; as a result, intestinal hemorrhage and perforation may occur at a time when the clinical condition is rapidly improving. The incidence and the duration of the *carrier state* are not altered. The *dose* of chloramphenicol employed in adults with typhoid fever is 1 g every 6 hours for 4 weeks. Although both intravenous and oral routes have been used, the response is more rapid with oral administration. Relapses usually respond satisfactorily to re-treatment; microorganisms isolated during recurrences are usually still sensitive to the antibiotic *in vitro*.

Bacterial Meningitis. Treatment with chloramphenicol produces excellent results in *H. influenzae meningitis* that are equal to or better than those achieved with ampicillin (Jones and Hanson, 1977; Koskinniemi *et al.*, 1978). The total daily dose for children should be 50 to 75 mg/kg of body weight, divided into four equal doses given intravenously every 6 hours for 2 weeks. Such therapy is still recommended for strains of *H. influenzae* that are resistant to ampicillin; furthermore, dual administration of ampicillin and chloramphenicol has been recommended for *initial* treatment of bacterial meningitis in *children* prior to evaluation of the results of cultures. Excellent results have also been obtained with several new cephalosporins, including moxalactam, cefotaxime, ceftriaxone, cefuroxime, and ceftizoxime (Freedman *et al.*, 1983; Bryant, 1984). Although chloramphenicol is bacteriostatic against most microorganisms, it is bactericidal for many meningeal pathogens, such as *H. influenzae* (Rahal and Simberkoff, 1979). There is no evidence of antagonism when it is combined with ampicillin, and, in fact, an additive or synergistic effect may result (Feldman, 1978). Rare strains of *H. influenzae* resistant to chloramphenicol have produced meningitis (Centers for Disease Control, 1984), and sensitivity tests should be obtained on all isolates. Chloramphenicol remains an alternate drug for the therapy of meningitis caused by *N. meningitidis* and *Strep. pneumoniae* in patients who are allergic to penicillin. Several new beta-lactam antibiotics have been shown to be efficacious, and they may replace chloramphenicol for this indication (*see* Bryan, 1984; Chapter 50). Since some strains of *Strep. pneumoniae* may be inhibited but not killed by chloramphenicol, lumbar puncture should be repeated 2 to 3 days after treatment has been initiated to ensure that an adequate response has occurred (Scheld *et al.*, 1979). Higher doses of chloramphenicol (100 mg/kg per day) may be required in some instances.

Anaerobic Infections. Chloramphenicol is quite effective against most anaerobic bacteria; it may be used instead of clindamycin in patients with serious anaerobic infections originating from foci in the bowel or pelvis. Chloramphenicol, together with penicillin, is used for the treatment of brain abscesses. However, many authorities now recommend penicillin plus metronidazole. Most of these infections are caused by anaerobic or mixed aerobic-anaerobic bacteria, including *B. fragilis*. While chloramphenicol and metronidazole both concentrate in brain tissue, clindamycin is largely excluded from the brain and CSF. Chloramphenicol may also be used in conjunction with a penicillin and an aminoglycoside for the treatment of intra-abdominal or pelvic abscesses, which are frequently caused by anaerobic bacteria (especially *B. fragilis*). However, either clindamycin or metronidazole can be substituted for chloramphenicol. Antimicrobial therapy should be accompanied by surgical drainage whenever possible.

Rickettsial Diseases. The tetracyclines are often the preferred agents for the treatment of rickettsial diseases. However, in patients sensitized to these drugs, in those with reduced renal function, in pregnant women, and in certain patients who require parenteral therapy because of severe illness, chloramphenicol is the drug of choice. *Epidemic, murine, scrub,* and *recrudescent typhus* as well as *Rocky Mountain spotted fever* and *Q fever* respond favorably to the antibiotic. The same dose schedule is applicable in all the rickettsial diseases. For adults, 1 g every 6 to 8 hours or 500 mg every 4 hours is recommended. Oral therapy is preferred, whenever possible. The daily dose of chloramphenicol for children with these diseases is 75 mg/kg of body weight, divided into equal portions and given

every 6 to 8 hours; if chloramphenicol palmitate is used, the daily maintenance dose is 100 mg/kg, given at the same intervals. Therapy should be continued until the general condition has improved and fever has been absent for 24 to 48 hours. The duration of illness and the incidence of relapses and complications are greatly reduced.

Brucellosis. Chloramphenicol is not as effective as the tetracyclines in the treatment of brucellosis. In cases in which the use of a tetracycline is contraindicated, 750 mg to 1 g of chloramphenicol orally every 6 hours may produce a beneficial effect in both the acute and chronic forms of the disease. Relapses usually respond to re-treatment.

Urinary Tract Infections. Chloramphenicol, once commonly used for therapy in urinary tract infection, is now rarely indicated. It should be reserved for cases of acute pyelonephritis in which no other effective and safer agent is available.

Miscellaneous Uses. Rarely, chloramphenicol (1 g intravenously every 6 hours) may be useful therapy for infections caused by strains of *K. pneumoniae* resistant to cephalosporins and aminoglycosides. Although chloramphenicol therapy is quite effective in *lymphogranuloma venereum, psittacosis,* and infections caused by *M. pneumoniae* and *Y. pestis,* other antimicrobial agents are preferred.

ERYTHROMYCIN

History and Source. *Erythromycin* is an orally effective antibiotic, discovered in 1952 by McGuire and coworkers in the metabolic products of a strain of *Streptomyces erythreus*, originally obtained from a soil sample collected in the Philippine Archipelago. These investigators also carried out the initial *in-vitro* observations, determined the range of toxicity, and demonstrated the effectiveness of the drug in experimental and naturally occurring infections due to gram-positive cocci.

Chemistry. Erythromycin is one of the macrolide antibiotics, so named because they contain a many-membered lactone ring to which are attached one or more deoxy sugars. It is a white crystalline compound, soluble in water to the extent of 2 mg/ml. The structural formula of erythromycin is as follows:

Erythromycin

Antibacterial Activity. Erythromycin may be either bacteriostatic or bactericidal, depending on the microorganism and the concentration of the drug. The bactericidal activity is greatest against a small number of rapidly dividing microorganisms and increases markedly as the pH of the medium is raised over the range of 5.5 to 8.5. The antibiotic is most effective *in vitro* against gram-positive cocci such as *Strep. pyogenes* and *Strep. pneumoniae*, for which the MIC is from 0.001 to 0.2 μg/ml (Steigbigel, 1985). Resistant strains of these bacteria are rare and are usually isolated from populations of people who have been recently exposed to macrolide antibiotics. For example, only 5% of group-A streptococcal strains isolated in Oklahoma were resistant to erythromycin (Istre *et al.*, 1981), but 60% of such strains were found to be resistant in a single study in Japan (Maruyama *et al.*, 1979). The difference likely reflects the wide use of erythromycin in Japan for respiratory infections. Strains of *Strep. pneumoniae* and *Strep. pyogenes* that have been selected for resistance to erythromycin are often also resistant to clindamycin. Streptococci of the *viridans* group are often inhibited by 0.02 to 3.1 μg/ml. While some staphylococci are sensitive to erythromycin, the range of inhibitory concentrations is great (MIC for *Staph. epidermidis*, 0.2 to 100 μg/ml; for *Staph. aureus*, 0.005 to 100 μg/ml). Erythromycin-resistant strains of *Staph. aureus* are frequently encountered in hospitals, and resistance may emerge during treatment of an individual patient; cross-resistance with other macrolide antibiotics and with clindamycin is common. Many other gram-positive bacilli are also sensitive to erythromycin; values of MIC are from <0.1 to 8 μg/ml for *Cl. perfringens*, from 0.006 to 3.1 μg/ml for *Corynebacterium diphtheriae*, and from 0.1 to 0.3 μg/ml for *Listeria monocytogenes*.

Erythromycin is not active against most aerobic gram-negative bacilli. It has moderate activity *in vitro* against *H. influenzae* (MIC, 0.1 to 6 μg/ml) and *N. meningitidis* (MIC, 0.1 to 1.6 μg/ml), and excellent activity against most strains of *N. gonorrhoeae* (MIC, 0.005 to 0.4 μg/ml). Useful antibacterial activity is also observed against *Past. multocida*, *Borrelia*, *Bord. pertussis*, and less than half of the strains of *B. fragilis* (the MIC ranging from 0.1 to 100 μg/ml). It is quite active against over 90% of strains of *Campylobacter jejuni* (Vanhoof *et al.*, 1980). Erythromycin is effective against *M. pneumoniae* (MIC, 0.001 to 0.02 μg/ml) and the agent of Legionnaires' disease, *Legionella pneumophila* (MIC, <0.5 μg/ml). Most strains of *C. trachomatis* are inhibited by 0.1 to 0.5 μg/ml of erythromycin. It is without effect on viruses, yeasts, and fungi. Some of the atypical mycobacteria are sensitive to erythromycin *in vitro*, where approximately 85% of strains of *Mycobacterium scrofulaceum* and nearly all of *M. kansasii* are sensitive to 0.5 to 2 μg/ml of the drug; the remainder are inhibited by 4 to 16 μg/ml. Nearly all strains of *M. fortuitum* are resistant, while strains of *M. intracellulare* vary in sensitivity (Molavi and Weinstein, 1971).

Mechanism of Action. Erythromycin and other macrolide antibiotics inhibit protein synthesis by binding to 50 S ribosomal subunits of sensitive mi-croorganisms. Erythromycin can interfere with the binding of chloramphenicol, which also acts at this site. Certain resistant microorganisms with mutational changes in components of this subunit of the ribosome fail to bind the drug. The association between erythromycin and the ribosome is reversible and takes place only when the 50 S subunit is free from tRNA molecules bearing nascent peptide chains. The production of small peptides goes on normally in the presence of the antibiotic, but that of highly polymerized homopeptides is suppressed. Gram-positive bacteria accumulate about 100 times more erythromycin than do gram-negative microorganisms. The nonionized form of the drug is considerably more permeable to cells, and this probably explains the increased antimicrobial activity that is observed at alkaline pH (Sabath *et al.*, 1968b; Vogel *et al.*, 1971).

Absorption, Distribution, and Excretion. *Erythromycin base* is adequately absorbed from the upper part of the small intestine; it is inactivated by gastric juice, and the drug is thus administered as an enteric-coated tablet that dissolves in the duodenum. Food in the stomach delays its ultimate absorption. Peak concentrations in plasma are only 0.3 to 0.5 μg/ml 4 hours after oral administration of 250 mg of the base and are 0.3 to 1.9 μg/ml after a single dose of 500 mg. Various esters of erythromycin have been prepared to attempt to improve stability and facilitate absorption. However, concentrations of erythromycin in plasma are little different if the *stearate* is given orally, and its bioavailability is decreased when administered with food. *Erythromycin estolate* is less susceptible to acid than is the parent compound; it is better absorbed than other forms of the drug, and this is not appreciably altered by food. A single, oral 250-mg dose of the estolate produces peak concentrations in plasma of approximately 1.5 μg/ml after 2 hours, and a 500-mg dose produces peak concentrations of 4 μg/ml. At the peak, this includes both the ester and the free base, with the "active" component comprising 20 to 35% of the total. Thus, the actual concentration of erythromycin base in plasma may be similar for the three preparations.

The actual antibacterial activity of the estolate ester of erythromycin is difficult to measure *in vitro*. Only the free base binds to bacterial ribosomes. However, strains of *Staph. aureus* are more susceptible to the estolate ester than to the base if bacteria are exposed for short periods (10 minutes). This suggests that the estolate penetrates into the bacterial cell more rapidly and is hydrolyzed by bacterial enzymes to the active component. Such esterases have been isolated from various species of bacteria.

Erythromycin ethylsuccinate is another ester that is adequately absorbed following oral administration, particularly when the stomach is empty. Peak concentrations in plasma are 1.5 μg/ml (0.5 μg/ml of base) 1 to 2 hours after administration of a 500-mg dose.

High concentrations of erythromycin can be achieved by intravenous administration. Values are approximately 10 μg/ml 1 hour after intravenous administration of 500 to 1000 mg of *erythromycin lactobionate* or *gluceptate*.

Only 2 to 5% of orally administered erythromycin is excreted in active form in the urine and from 12 to 15% after intravenous infusion. When large doses of erythromycin are given by mouth, the feces may contain as much as 0.5 mg/g. The antibiotic is concentrated in the liver and excreted in active form in the bile, which may contain as much as 250 μg/ml when plasma concentrations are very high. Some of the drug may be inactivated by demethylation in the liver. The plasma half-life of erythromycin is approximately 1.6 hours. Although some reports suggest a prolonged half-life in patients with anuria, reduction of dosage is not routinely recommended. The drug is not removed by either peritoneal dialysis or hemodialysis.

Erythromycin diffuses readily into intracellular fluids, and antibacterial activity can be achieved at essentially all sites *except* the brain and CSF. Erythromycin is one of the few antibiotics that penetrates into prostatic fluid; concentrations are approximately 40% of those in plasma. The extent of binding of erythromycin to plasma proteins varies among the different forms of the drug but probably exceeds 70% in all cases. Erythromycin traverses the placental barrier, and concentrations of the drug in fetal plasma are about 5 to 20% of those in the maternal circulation.

Preparations, Routes of Administration, and Dosage. *Erythromycin* (E-MYCIN, ILOTYCIN), *erythromycin stearate* (ETHRIL), *erythromycin estolate* (ILOSONE), and *erythromycin ethylsuccinate* (E.E.S.,

PEDIAMYCIN) are available in a wide variety of preparations for oral administration, including tablets, chewable tablets, capsules, oral suspensions, and drops. *Erythromycin gluceptate* (ILOTYCIN GLUCEPTATE) and *erythromycin lactobionate* (ERYTHROCIN LACTOBIONATE–I.V.) are available for *intravenous* injection in the form of sterile dry powders.

The usual *oral* dose of erythromycin for *adults* ranges from 1 to 2 g per day, in equally divided and spaced amounts, usually given every 6 hours, depending on the nature and severity of the infection. Daily doses of erythromycin as large as 8 g orally, given for 3 months, have been well tolerated. Food should be avoided, if possible, immediately before or after oral administration of erythromycin base; this precaution need not be taken when the estolate is administered. The *oral* dose of erythromycin for *children* is 30 to 50 mg/kg per day, divided into four portions. *Intramuscular injection* of erythromycin is not recommended because of the pain it causes. *Intravenous administration* is used infrequently and is reserved for the therapy of severe infections. The usual dose is 0.5 to 1 g every 6 hours; 1 g of erythromycin gluceptate has been given intravenously every 6 hours for as long as 4 weeks with no difficulty except for thrombophlebitis at the site of injection.

Untoward Effects. Serious untoward effects are only rarely caused by erythromycin. Among the *allergic reactions* observed are *fever, eosinophilia,* and *skin eruptions,* which may occur alone or in combination; each disappears shortly after therapy is stopped. *Cholestatic hepatitis* is the most striking side effect. It is caused primarily by *erythromycin estolate* and only rarely by the ethylsuccinate or the stearate (*see* Ginsburg and Eichenwald, 1976). The illness starts after about 10 to 20 days of treatment and is characterized initially by nausea, vomiting, and abdominal cramps. The pain often mimics that of acute cholecystitis, and unnecessary surgery has been performed. These symptoms are followed shortly thereafter by jaundice, which may be accompanied by fever, leukocytosis, eosinophilia, and elevated activities of transaminases in plasma; the cholecystogram is usually negative. Biopsy of the liver reveals cholestasis, periportal infiltration by neutrophils, lymphocytes, and eosinophils, and, occasionally, necrosis of neighboring parenchymal cells. All manifestations usually disappear within a few days after cessation of drug therapy and rarely are prolonged. The syndrome may represent a hypersensitivity reaction to the estolate ester (*see* Tolman *et al.,* 1974).

Artifactual elevation of glutamic oxalacetic transaminase activity may be reported when serum from patients taking erythromycin estolate is assayed by the colorimetric procedure; the enzymatic assay method is not affected (*see* Sabath *et al.*, 1968a). However, mild elevations of the SGOT were also noted in 16 of 161 pregnant women who received 250 mg of erythromycin estolate orally four times a day for 3 to 6 weeks during the second trimester. In 4 of the 16 pregnant women, transaminase activities had returned to normal by the last day of treatment. Three of 97 patients treated with erythromycin stearate reacted similarly (McCormack *et al.*, 1977).

Oral administration of erythromycin, especially of large doses, is very frequently accompanied by epigastric distress, which may be quite severe. Intramuscular injection of quantities larger than 100 mg produces extremely severe pain that persists for hours. Intravenous infusion of 1-g doses, even when dissolved in a large volume, is predictably followed by thrombophlebitis; this can be minimized by slow rates of infusion.

Transient auditory impairment is a rare complication of treatment with erythromycin that has been observed to follow intravenous administration of large doses of the gluceptate or lactobionate (4 g per day) or oral ingestion of large doses of the estolate (Karmody and Weinstein, 1977). Hypertrophic pyloric stenosis was observed in five infants during administration of erythromycin estolate (Filippo, 1976).

Erythromycin has been reported to potentiate the effects of carbamazepine, corticosteroids, and digoxin, probably by interfering with their metabolism. In addition, high and potentially toxic concentrations of theophylline may result when erythromycin is administered concomitantly (Kozak *et al.*, 1977; May *et al.*, 1982).

Therapeutic Uses. Extensive studies of the clinical application of erythromycin have demonstrated its usefulness in a variety of infections, but it is currently the preferred drug for only a few.

Mycoplasma pneumoniae Infections. Erythromycin (given orally in doses of 500 mg three or four times daily, or, if oral administration is not tolerated, given intravenously) reduces the duration of fever caused by *M. pneumoniae*. In addition, the rate of clearing as noted in the chest x-ray is accelerated (Rasch and Mogabgab, 1965). Tetracycline is just as effective.

Legionnaires' Disease. Erythromycin is currently recommended for the treatment of pneumonia caused by *Legionella pneumophila* or *L. micdadei* (Muder *et al.*, 1983). The antibiotic may be given orally (0.5 to 1 g four times daily) or intravenously (1 to 4 g per day). Clinical evidence and studies in guinea pigs suggest that erythromycin is the most active antimicrobial agent available (*see* Balows and Fraser, 1979).

Chlamydia Infections. Chlamydia infections can be treated effectively with erythromycin. It is specifically recommended as an alternative to tetracycline in patients with uncomplicated urethral, endocervical, rectal, or epididymal infections (500 mg orally every 6 hours for at least 7 days). During pregnancy, erythromycin becomes the drug of choice for chlamydial urogenital infections; it is also preferred for chlamydial pneumonia of infancy (50 mg/kg per day in four divided doses for at least 3 weeks), when tetracyclines are contraindicated because of their effects on tissues that are calcifying (Center for Disease Control, 1982).

Diphtheria. Erythromycin is very effective in eradicating the acute or chronic *diphtheria bacillus carrier state*. Erythromycin estolate (250 mg four times daily for 7 days) was found to be effective in 90% of adults. Most of the failures were due to lack of patient compliance (McClosky *et al.*, 1971). It must be remembered, however, that neither erythromycin nor any other antibiotic alters the course of an acute infection with the diphtheria bacillus or the risk of complications.

Pertussis. If administered early in the course of whooping cough, erythromycin may shorten the duration of illness. The drug has little influence on the disease once the paroxysmal stage is reached, although it may eliminate the microorganisms from the nasopharynx (*see* Bass *et al.*, 1969). Erythromycin can prevent whooping cough in susceptible individuals who are exposed to the disease.

Streptococcal Infections. Pharyngitis, scarlet fever, and *erysipelas* produced by *Strep. pyogenes* respond to erythromycin. The oral administration of 250 to 500 mg every 6 hours or 20 mg/kg per day (of the estolate) or 30 mg/kg per day (for other forms of erythromycin) for 10 days cures these diseases, prevents the appearance of suppurative complications, and suppresses the formation of antistreptococcal antibodies. Treatment with erythromycin appears to produce a rate of cure about equal to that obtained with penicillin G (Shapera *et al.*, 1973). *Pneumococcal pneumonia* responds promptly to oral therapy with 250 to 500 mg of erythromycin every 6 hours. Erythromycin is thus a valuable alternative for the treatment of streptococcal infections in patients who are allergic to penicillin.

Staphylococcal Infections. Erythromycin is an alternative agent for the treatment of relatively minor infections caused by either penicillin-sensitive or penicillin-resistant *Staph. aureus*. However, the emergence of appreciable numbers of strains that are resistant to erythromycin limits the use of the drug. The availability of the penicillinase-resistant penicillins and the cephalosporins has reduced the need to use erythromycin for the treatment of serious staphylococcal disease. The oral administration of 500 mg of erythromycin every 6 hours for 7 to 10 days is effective treatment for staphylococcal infections of the skin or of wounds in patients who are allergic to penicillins and cephalosporins.

Campylobacter Infections. The treatment of gastroenteritis caused by *Campylobacter jejuni* with erythromycin (250 mg orally four times a day) has been shown to hasten the eradication of the microorganism from the stools; however, when therapy is initiated 4 or more days after the onset of symptoms, erythromycin does not alter the clinical course (Blaser and Reller, 1981; Anders *et al.*, 1982). Nevertheless, the drug is recommended in patients with protracted or severe illness.

Tetanus. Erythromycin (500 mg orally every 6 hours for 10 days) may be given to eradicate *Cl. tetani* in patients with tetanus who are allergic to penicillin. The mainstays of therapy are debridement, physiological support, tetanus antitoxin, and drug control of convulsions.

Syphilis. Erythromycin in doses of 2 to 4 g per day for 10 to 15 days has been employed successfully in the treatment of early syphilis in the patient who is allergic to penicillin (Sanford, 1984).

Gonorrhea. Both erythromycin estolate and the base have been used in the therapy of gonococcal urethritis. However, the relapse rate is nearly 25% after the oral administration of 9 g over a 4-day period; this is unacceptably high for routine use. Erythromycin may be useful for disseminated gonococcal disease in the pregnant patient who is allergic to penicillin (since tetracyclines should be avoided during pregnancy). Patients who were treated with 500 mg of erythromycin estolate or stearate, given orally every 6 hours for 5 days, showed rapid clinical and bacteriological responses.

Prophylactic Uses. Although penicillin is the drug of choice for the *prophylaxis of recurrences of rheumatic fever,* another antistreptococcal agent must be used in individuals who are allergic to this antibiotic. The sulfonamides are cheap and effective for this purpose. In some instances, however, it may be preferable to use erythromycin, which is also efficacious.

Erythromycin is recommended as an alternative to penicillin in allergic patients for prevention of bacterial endocarditis following dental or oropharyngeal procedures. The dose is 1 g orally 1.5 to 2 hours before the procedure, followed by 500 mg every 6 hours for eight doses (American Heart Association Committee, 1977) or 1 g given 1 hour before the procedure and a single 500-mg dose given 6 hours later (Medical Letter, 1984).

LINCOMYCIN

Lincomycin is elaborated by an actinomycete, *Streptomyces lincolnensis,* so named because it was isolated from soil collected near Lincoln, Nebraska; it was the first lincosamide antibiotic to be used clinically. *Clindamycin,* the 7-deoxy, 7-chloro derivative of lincomycin, is more active and causes fewer unwanted effects. There are thus few, if any, valid reasons to use lincomycin (LINCOCIN) in the United States. Its properties are discussed in the *fifth edition* of this textbook.

CLINDAMYCIN

Chemistry. *Clindamycin* is a derivative of the amino acid trans-L-4-*n*-propylhygrinic acid, attached to a sulfur-containing derivative of an octose. As mentioned above, it is a congener of lincomycin. The structural formula of clindamycin is as follows:

Clindamycin

Mechanism of Action. Clindamycin and lincomycin bind exclusively to the 50 S subunit of bacterial ribosomes and suppress protein synthesis. Although clindamycin, erythromycin, and chloramphenicol are not structurally related, they all act at this site, and the binding of one of these antibiotics to the ribosome may inhibit the reaction of the other. There are no clinical indications for the concurrent use of these antibiotics. Plasmid-mediated resistance to clindamycin (and erythromycin) has been found in *B. fragilis* (Tally *et al.*, 1979); it may be due to methylation of bacterial RNA found in the 50 S ribosomal subunit (Steigbigel, 1985).

Antibacterial Activity. In general, clindamycin is similar to erythromycin in its activity *in vitro* against pneumococci, *Strep. pyogenes,* and *viridans* streptococci. Almost all such bacterial strains are inhibited by concentrations of 0.04 μg/ml (Steigbigel, 1985), although resistant microorganisms are encountered (Maruyama *et al.*, 1979; Linares *et al.*, 1983). It is also active against many strains of *Staph. aureus,* but not methicillin-resistant strains. Strains that are resistant to clindamycin are often also resistant to erythromycin. In some hospitals, such resistance has been found in 20% of isolates. Resistance to clindamycin has developed during treatment of experimental staphylococcal endocarditis. Clindamycin is inactive against enterococci and *N. meningitidis* in concentrations that can be achieved clinically.

Clindamycin is more active than erythromycin against many anaerobic bacteria, especially *B. fragilis* (MIC, 0.03 to >32 μg/ml), and over 90% of strains are inhibited by 2 μg/ml. A recent survey in the United States found only 6% of strains of *B. fragilis* resistant to clindamycin (MIC more than 4 μg/ml) (Tally *et al.*, 1983). Minimal inhibitory concentrations for other anaerobes are as follows: *B. melaninogenicus,* 0.1 to 1 μg/ml; *Fusobacterium,* <0.5 μg/ml (although most strains of *F. varium* are resistant); *Peptostreptococcus,* <0.1 to 0.5 μg/ml; *Peptococcus,* 1 to 100 μg/ml (with 10% of strains resistant); and *Cl. perfringens,* <0.1 to 8 μg/ml. Ten to 20% of clostridial species, other than *Cl. perfringens,* are resistant (Bartlett, 1982). Strains of *Actinomyces israelii* and *Nocardia asteroides* are sensitive. Essentially all aerobic gramnegative bacilli are resistant, as is *M. pneumoniae.* Strains of *Toxoplasma gondii* have been inhibited by clindamycin in experimental ocular infections (Tabbara *et al.*, 1979). Clindamycin has some activity against strains of *Plasmodium falciparum* and *P. vivax,* but a cure rate of only 50% of patients with malaria was observed in one study (Hall *et al.*, 1975).

Absorption, Fate, and Excretion. Clindamycin is nearly completely absorbed following oral administration, and peak plasma concentrations of 2 to 3 μg/ml are attained within 1 hour after the ingestion of 150 mg. The presence of food in the stomach does not reduce absorption significantly. The half-life of the antibiotic is about 2.7 hours, and modest accumulation of drug is thus expected if it is given at 6-hour intervals.

Clindamycin palmitate, an oral preparation for pediatric use, is an inactive prodrug, but the ester is hydrolyzed rapidly *in vivo*. Its rate and extent of absorption are similar to those of clindamycin. After several oral doses at 6-hour intervals, children attain plasma concentrations of 2 to 4 μg/ml with the administration of 8 to 16 mg/kg.

The phosphate ester of clindamycin, which is given parenterally, is also rapidly hydrolyzed *in vivo* to the active parent compound. Following intramuscular injection, peak concentrations in plasma are not attained until 3 hours in adults and 1 hour in children. The recommended intramuscular dosages provide peak plasma concentrations of approximately 6 μg/ml after a 300-mg dose and 9 μg/ml after a 600-mg dose in adults. Immediately following a 20- to 45-minute infusion of 600 mg, the concentration in plasma is approximately 10 μg/ml.

While clindamycin is widely distributed in many fluids and tissues, including bone, significant concentrations are not attained in CSF, even when the meninges are inflamed. The drug readily crosses the placental barrier. Ninety percent or more of clindamycin is bound to plasma proteins. (*See* Panzer *et al.*, 1972; Philipson *et al.*, 1973.) Clindamycin accumulates in polymorphonuclear leukocytes and alveolar macrophages (Klempner and Styrt, 1981; Prokesch and Hand, 1982); the clinical relevance of this phenomenon is unknown. Clindamycin is also concentrated in abscesses in experimental animals (Joiner *et al.*, 1981).

Only about 10% of administered clindamycin is excreted unaltered in the urine, and small quantities are found in the feces. However, antimicrobial activity persists in feces for 5 or more days after parenteral therapy with clindamycin is stopped; growth of sensitive microorganisms in colonic contents remains suppressed for up to 2 weeks (Kager *et al.*, 1981). Most of the drug is inactivated by metabolism to N-demethylclindamycin and clindamycin sulfoxide, which are excreted in the urine and bile. The half-life of clindamycin may be lengthened in patients with markedly impaired renal function; dosage should be adjusted as necessary based on measurements of the concentration of drug in plasma. Accumulation of drug can also occur in patients with severe hepatic failure unless dosage is adjusted.

The clinical pharmacology of clindamycin is discussed by Balanchandar and colleagues (1973) and Steigbigel (1985).

Preparations, Routes of Administration, and Dosage. *Clindamycin hydrochloride* (CLEOCIN HCL) is supplied for oral administration in capsules containing 75 or 150 mg. *Clindamycin palmitate hydrochloride* (CLEOCIN PEDIATRIC) is a preparation of flavored granules for solution to a concentration of 75 mg/5 ml. *Clindamycin phosphate* (CLEOCIN PHOSPHATE) is for intramuscular or intravenous use.

The *oral* dose of clindamycin for *adults* is 150 to 300 mg every 6 hours; for severe infections, 300 to 450 mg every 6 hours. *Children* should receive 8 to 12 mg/kg per day of the palmitate hydrochloride in three or four divided doses; for severe infections, 13 to 25 mg/kg per day. However, children weighing less than 10 kg should receive ½ teaspoonful of clindamycin palmitate hydrochloride (37.5 mg) three times daily as a minimal dose.

For serious infections due to aerobic gram-positive cocci and the more sensitive anaerobes (not generally including *B. fragilis, Peptococcus,* and

Clostridium species other than *Cl. perfringens*), intravenous or intramuscular administration is recommended in dosages of 600 to 1200 mg per day, divided into two to four equal portions for adults. For more severe infections, particularly those proven or suspected to be caused by *B. fragilis*, *Peptococcus*, or *Clostridium* species other than *Cl. perfringens*, parenteral administration of 1200 to 2700 mg per day of clindamycin is suggested. In life-threatening situations due to aerobes or anaerobes, these doses may be increased. Daily doses as high as 4800 mg have been given intravenously to adults. *Children* should receive 10 to 40 mg/kg per day in three or four divided doses; in severe infections, a minimal daily dose of 300 mg is recommended, regardless of body weight.

Untoward Effects. The reported incidence of *diarrhea* associated with the administration of clindamycin ranges from 2 to 20%; the average appears to be about 8%. A number of patients (variously reported as 0.01 to 10%) have developed *pseudomembranous colitis,* characterized by diarrhea, abdominal pain, fever, and mucus and blood in the stools. Proctoscopic examination reveals white-to-yellow plaques on the mucosa of the colon. *This syndrome may be lethal.* It is caused by a toxin secreted by clindamycin-resistant strains of *Cl. difficile* (Rifkin *et al.,* 1977; Bartlett, 1979; George *et al.,* 1980). This disease, now termed *antibiotic-associated colitis,* can be caused by most antibiotics, but it is particularly common with clindamycin. It is not related to dosage and may occur after either oral or parenteral therapy. Disease may begin during therapy, or it may be delayed for several weeks following discontinuation of the drug. The toxin can be detected in nearly all patients' stool by a cytotoxicity assay. If significant diarrhea or colitis occurs during therapy with clindamycin, the drug should be discontinued immediately; *vancomycin,* given orally in doses of 125 to 500 mg every 6 hours for 7 to 10 days, is effective in reducing the frequency of diarrhea (Tedesco, 1977). Oral metronidazole and bacitracin also appear to be effective (George *et al.,* 1980), and cholestyramine (4 g, given three or four times daily) has proven beneficial. Agents that inhibit peristalsis, such as opioids, may prolong and worsen the condition. While the incidence of this problem is unknown, it is clear that the therapeutic indications for clindamycin should be considered very seriously before it is given.

Skin rashes occur in approximately 10% of patients treated with clindamycin. Other reactions, which are uncommon, include exudative erythema multiforme (Stevens-Johnson syndrome), reversible elevation of SGOT and SGPT, granulocytopenia, thrombocytopenia, and anaphylactic reactions. Local thrombophlebitis may follow intravenous administration of the drug. Clindamycin can inhibit neuromuscular transmission and may potentiate the effect of a neuromuscular blocking agent administered concurrently (Fogdall and Miller, 1974).

Therapeutic Uses. While a number of infections with gram-positive cocci will respond favorably to clindamycin, the high incidence of diarrhea and the occurrence of colitis require limitation of its use to infections in which it is clearly superior to other agents. Clindamycin is particularly valuable for the treatment of infections with anaerobes, especially those due to *B. fragilis* (Bartlett, 1982). It has been used successfully in combination with an aminoglycoside for infections resulting from fecal spillage (intra-abdominal or pelvic abscesses and peritonitis), and this regimen is superior to combinations of an aminoglycoside and penicillin or cephalothin (DiZerega *et al.,* 1979). Other drugs that are effective against anaerobes, such as metronidazole, cefoxitin, chloramphenicol, or ticarcillin, appear to be as efficacious as clindamycin in this setting (Harding *et al.,* 1980; Bartlett, 1982). Clindamycin is not useful for the treatment of brain abscesses, since penetration into the central nervous system (CNS) is poor; either metronidazole or chloramphenicol in combination with penicillin is preferred (Thadepalli *et al.,* 1973).

A recent prospective study demonstrated that parenteral clindamycin (600 mg intravenously every 8 hours) was superior to penicillin (1 million units intravenously every 4 hours) for the treatment of lung abscesses (Levison *et al.,* 1983). Although questions have been raised (Bartlett and Gorbach, 1983), this study may reflect the increasing rate of isolation of penicillin-resistant (beta-lactamase-producing) strains of various species of *Bacteroides* from bronchopulmonary infections. The therapeutic role of clindamycin in the treatment of aspiration pneumonia, postobstructive pneumonia, or lung abscesses has yet to be settled, but it appears to be a reasonable alternative to penicillin. While clindamycin is effective topically or orally (150 mg twice daily) in acne vulgaris (Dhawan and Thadepalli, 1982), less toxic forms of therapy are preferred.

SPECTINOMYCIN

Source and Chemistry. *Spectinomycin* is an antibiotic produced by *Streptomyces spectabilis.* The drug is an aminocyclitol; its structural formula is as follows:

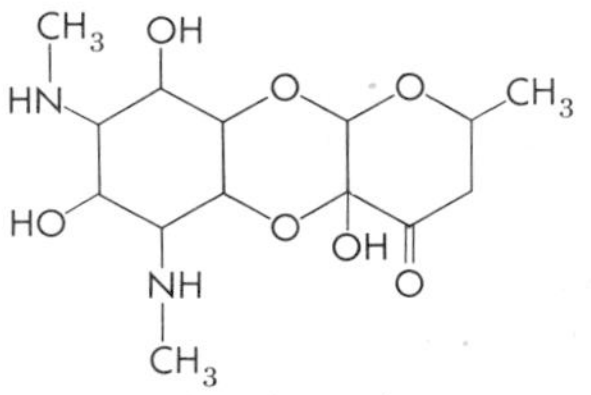

Spectinomycin

Antibacterial Activity and Mechanism. While spectinomycin is active against a number of gram-negative bacterial species, it is inferior to other drugs to which such microorganisms are susceptible (Schoutens *et al.*, 1972). Its only use is in the treatment of gonorrhea, and it inhibits gonococci at concentrations of 7 to 20 µg/ml; these concentrations are achieved in plasma by the administration of recommended doses.

Spectinomycin selectively inhibits protein synthesis in gram-negative bacteria. The antibiotic binds to and acts on the 30 S ribosomal subunit. There are similarities in its action to that of the aminoglycosides; however, spectinomycin is not bactericidal and does not cause misreading of polyribonucleotides. A high degree of bacterial resistance may develop as a result of mutation.

Absorption, Distribution, and Excretion. Spectinomycin is rapidly absorbed after intramuscular injection. A single dose of 2 g produces peak concentrations in plasma of 100 µg/ml at 1 hour; a 4-g injection, 160 µg/ml. Eight hours after injection of 2 or 4 g, the concentrations in plasma are 15 µg/ml or 30 µg/ml, respectively. The drug is not significantly bound to plasma protein, and all of an administered dose is recovered in the urine within 48 hours after injection.

Preparations. *Spectinomycin hydrochloride* (TROBICIN) is supplied as a sterile powder for reconstitution with water containing 0.9% benzyl alcohol. This solution is for intramuscular injection only.

Untoward Effects. Spectinomycin, when given as a single intramuscular injection, produces few significant untoward effects (Duncan *et al.*, 1972). *Urticaria, chills,* and *fever* have been noted after single doses, as have *dizziness, nausea,* and *insomnia.* The injection may be painful. Ototoxicity and nephrotoxicity have not been reported.

Therapeutic Uses. Spectinomycin is primarily recommended for the treatment of uncomplicated gonococcal infections (*i.e., acute genital and rectal gonorrhea*) in patients who are allergic to penicillin or in those who are infected with penicillinase-producing microorganisms. The recommended dose for both men and women is a single deep intramuscular injection of 2 g. The rate of cure for these forms of gonorrhea is about 95%. Spectinomycin is also the preferred drug for patients with such infec-

tions who have not been cured by other treatment regimens. High rates of failure (50%) have followed single-dose treatment with spectinomycin for gonococcal pharyngitis. Multiple doses of spectinomycin (2 g intramuscularly, twice a day for 3 days) are recommended for the treatment of disseminated gonococcal infections (arthritis-dermatitis syndrome) caused by penicillinase-producing strains of *N. gonorrhoeae* (*see* Center for Disease Control, 1979). It must be emphasized that spectinomycin is without effect on incubating or established syphilis, and it is not active against *Chlamydia.*

POLYMYXIN B AND COLISTIN

Because of the extreme nephrotoxicity associated with parenteral administration of these drugs, they are now rarely used except orally for prophylaxis (Enno *et al.*, 1978; Gurwith *et al.*, 1979) or topically for certain gram-negative bacillary infections. Information regarding parenteral administration of these agents can be found in the *fifth edition* of this textbook.

Source and Chemistry. The *polymyxins*, discovered in 1947, are a group of closely related antibiotic substances elaborated by various strains of *Bacillus polymyxa*, an aerobic spore-forming rod found in soil. *Colistin* (polymyxin E) is produced by *Bacillus (Aerobacillus) colistinus*, a microorganism isolated from a soil sample obtained from Fukushima Prefecture, Japan. These drugs, which are cationic detergents, are relatively simple, basic peptides with molecular weights of about 1000. The structural formula for polymyxin B, which is itself a mixture of polymyxins B_1 and B_2, is as follows:

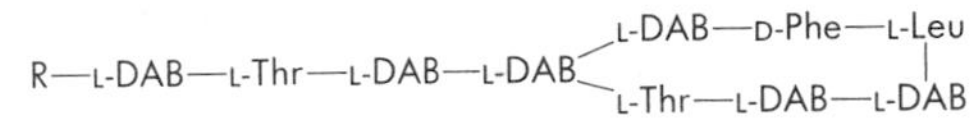

Polymyxin B_1: R = (+)-6-Methyloctanoyl
Polymyxin B_2: R = 6-Methylheptanoyl
DAB = α,γ-Diaminobutyric Acid

Colistin is polymyxin E, and it has a similar structure; it is available for clinical use as colistin sulfate, for oral use, and as colistimethate sodium, a parenteral preparation.

Antibacterial Activity and Mechanism of Action. The antimicrobial activity of polymyxin B and colistin are similar and are restricted to gram-negative bacteria, including *Enterobacter, E. coli, Klebsiella, Salmonella, Pasteurella, Bordetella,* and *Shigella,* which are usually sensitive to concentrations of 0.05 to 2.0 µg/ml. Most strains of *Pseud. aeruginosa* are inhibited by less than 8 µg/ml *in vitro.*

Polymyxins are surface-active agents, containing lipophilic and lipophobic groups separated within the molecule. They interact strongly with phospholipids and penetrate into and disrupt the structure of cell membranes. The permeability of the bacterial membrane changes immediately on contact with the drug. Sensitivity to polymyxin B is apparently related to the phospholipid content of the cell wall-membrane complex (Brown and Wood, 1972). The cell wall of certain resistant bacteria may prevent access of the drug to the cell membrane (*see* Pratt, 1977).

Absorption, Distribution, and Excretion. Neither polymyxin B nor colistin is absorbed when given orally. They are also poorly absorbed from mucous membranes and the surface of large burns.

Preparations, Routes of Administration, and Dosage. *Polymyxin B sulfate* is available for ophthalmic and topical use in combination with a variety of other compounds. While parenteral preparations are still marketed, they are not recommended. *Colistin sulfate* (COLY-MYCIN S) is marketed as a powder to be suspended in distilled water prior to dispensing. It has been administered *orally* to infants and children with diarrhea caused by bacteria susceptible to the drug; the dose is 5 to 15 mg/kg daily, in three divided portions. Colistimethate sodium, a parenteral preparation, is seldom used.

Untoward Effects. Polymyxin B applied to intact or denuded skin or mucous membranes produces no systemic reactions because of almost complete lack of absorption of the antibiotic from these sites. *Hypersensitization* is uncommon when the antibiotic is used in this way. Nausea, vomiting, and diarrhea are produced by large doses (600 mg) taken orally. Adverse effects that follow the parenteral administration of these drugs are discussed in the *fifth edition* of this textbook.

Therapeutic Uses. Infections of the skin, mucous membranes, eye, and ear due to polymyxin B–sensitive microorganisms respond to local application of the antibiotic in solution or ointment. *External otitis*, frequently due to *Pseudomonas*, may be cured by the topical use of the drug. *Pseudomonas aeruginosa* is a common cause of infection of *corneal ulcers;* local application or subconjunctival injection of polymyxin B is often curative.

VANCOMYCIN

History and Source. *Vancomycin* is an antibiotic produced by *Streptomyces orientalis,* an actinomycete isolated from soil samples obtained in Indonesia and India. Purification of the antibiotics was accomplished and its antimicrobial properties were described within a short time after its discovery (McCormick *et al.,* 1956).

Chemistry. Vancomycin is a complex and unusual glycopeptide with a molecular weight of about 1500. Its structural formula was determined only recently by x-ray analysis (Sheldrick *et al.,* 1978). Vancomycin hydrochloride is a white powder, soluble in water to a concentration of over 100 mg/ml.

Antibacterial Activity. Vancomycin is primarily active against gram-positive bacteria. Strains of *Staph. aureus,* including those resistant to methi-

cillin, are inhibited by concentrations of 0.1 to 2 μg/ml. Rare strains of *Staph. aureus* are resistant to concentrations of the antibiotic that can be achieved clinically, but there has been no increase in the incidence of such resistance during the 25 years that the drug has been used. Synergism between vancomycin and gentamicin or tobramycin has been demonstrated *in vitro* against *Staph. aureus,* including methicillin-resistant strains (Watanakunakorn and Tisone, 1982). The minimal inhibitory concentrations of vancomycin for *Staph. epidermidis* range from 0.4 to 1.5 μg/ml; for *Strep. pyogenes,* from 0.15 to 2 μg/ml; for *Strep. pneumoniae,* from 0.1 to 0.3 μg/ml; for the *viridans* streptococci, from 0.3 to 1.5 μg/ml; and for *Strep. faecalis,* from 0.3 to 2.5 μg/ml. Vancomycin is not generally bactericidal for *Strep. faecalis;* however, 40 to 70% of strains are sensitive to a synergistic bactericidal effect when vancomycin and streptomycin are used concurrently (Mandell *et al.,* 1970), and nearly all strains are killed by a combination of vancomycin and gentamicin (Harwick *et al.,* 1973). In experimental endocarditis, vancomycin and streptomycin together are more effective in reducing bacterial counts in cardiac vegetations than is vancomycin alone (Hook *et al.,* 1975). *Corynebacterium* species (diphtheroids) are inhibited by less than 0.04 to 3.1 μg/ml of vancomycin, most species of *Actinomyces* by 5 to 10 μg/ml, and *Clostridium* species by 0.39 to 6 μg/ml. Essentially all species of gram-negative bacilli and mycobacteria are resistant (*see* Cunha and Ristuccia, 1983).

Mechanism of Action. Vancomycin inhibits the synthesis of the cell wall in sensitive bacteria by binding with high affinity to precursors of this structure. The D-alanyl-D-alanine portion of the cell-wall precursor units appears to be a crucial site of attachment (*see* Figure 50–2, page 1117; Nieto and Perkins, 1971a, 1971b). The drug is rapidly bactericidal for dividing microorganisms (Watanakunakorn, 1981).

Absorption, Distribution, and Excretion. Vancomycin is poorly absorbed after oral administration, and large quantities are excreted in the stool. For parenteral therapy, the drug should be administered intravenously. A single intravenous dose of 500 mg in adults produces plasma concentrations of 6 to 10 μg/ml at the end of 1 to 2 hours, 2 to 4 μg/ml after 6 hours, and 1 to 2 μg/ml after 12 hours; the drug has a half-life in the circulation of about 6 hours. Approximately 55% of vancomycin is bound to plasma protein. Vancomycin appears in various body fluids, including the CSF when the meninges are inflamed; bile; and pleural, pericardial, synovial, and ascitic fluids (Fekety, 1982). More than 90% of an injected dose is excreted by glomerular filtration. Dangerously high concentrations may accumulate if renal function is impaired (Cunha *et al.,* 1981; Moellering *et al.,* 1981), and dosage adjustments must be made under these circumstances. The drug is not removed from the plasma by hemodialysis or peritoneal dialysis (Ayus *et al.,* 1979; Magera *et al.,* 1983). Patients with impaired hepatic function also eliminate vancomycin more slowly than normal, and dosage adjustments may be necessary (Brown *et al.*, 1983).

Preparations, Routes of Administration, and Dosage. *Vancomycin hydrochloride* (VANCOCIN HCL) is marketed for *intravenous* use as a sterile powder for solution. The desired dose is preferably diluted and injected intravenously over a 30- to 60-minute period. The dose of vancomycin for adults is 500 mg every 6 hours or 1 g every 12 hours; this will yield an average steady-state concentration of 15 μg/ml (*see* Moellering *et al.*, 1981). The daily dose for children is 44 mg/kg in equally divided and spaced quantities every 6 to 12 hours. The amount administered daily to premature infants and neonates ranges from 6 to 15 mg/kg (Schaad *et al.*, 1981). Because of incompletely developed renal function in this age group, the drug must be used with caution. Alteration of dosage is required for patients with impaired renal function (*see* Appendix II). The drug has been used effectively in functionally anephric patients (who are being dialyzed) by the administration of 1 g (approximately 15 mg/kg) each week. When 1 g is given intravenously to such patients, the peak concentration in plasma is 40 to 50 μg/ml; this falls to a value of 15 μg/ml in 3 to 5 hours. After 7 days, concentrations in plasma are usually still in the therapeutic range (5 to 7 μg/ml). Measurement of the concentration of antibiotic in plasma is recommended.

Vancomycin can be administered *orally* to patients with "antibiotic-associated" colitis (*see* discussion of clindamycin, above) or for the treatment of diarrhea due to other toxin-producing microorganisms that are sensitive to vancomycin. The dose for adults is 500 mg every 6 hours; the total daily dose for children is 44 mg/kg, given in divided doses. *Vancomycin hydrochloride for oral solution* is available for this purpose.

Untoward Effects. Among the *hypersensitivity reactions* produced by vancomycin are *macular skin rashes* and *anaphylaxis*. *Phlebitis* and *pain* at the site of intravenous injection are relatively uncommon. *Chills, rash,* and *fever* may occur, and a *shocklike state* (so-called *red-neck syndrome*) may happen rarely during the course of intravenous infusion (Newfield and Roizen, 1979). The most significant untoward reactions have been *ototoxicity* and *nephrotoxicity*. Auditory impairment, which is frequently although not always permanent, may follow the use of this drug. Ototoxicity is associated with excessively high concentrations of the drug in plasma and is extremely unusual if concentrations are maintained below 30 μg/ml. Ototoxicity may be potentially worsened by simultaneous treatment with aminoglycosides or high-ceiling diuretics such as ethacrynic acid and furosemide. Nephrotoxicity was formerly quite common but has become an unusual side effect when appropriate doses are used, as judged by renal function and determinations of the concentration of the antibiotic in blood. The drug should be avoided when other ototoxic or nephrotoxic drugs are administered concurrently (Farber and Moellering, 1983),

or in patients with impaired renal function if other effective and less toxic antibiotics are available.

Therapeutic Uses. Vancomycin should be employed only to treat serious infections and is particularly useful in the management of infections due to methicillin-resistant staphylococci, including *staphylococcal pneumonia, empyema, endocarditis, osteomyelitis,* and *soft-tissue abscesses* (Sorrell *et al.*, 1982). The drug is also extremely valuable in severe staphylococcal infections in patients who are allergic to penicillins and cephalosporins (Geraci, 1977). Treatment with vancomycin is effective and convenient when there is disseminated staphylococcal infection or localized infection of a shunt in a patient with irreversible renal disease who is being maintained by hemodialysis or peritoneal dialysis (Nolan *et al.*, 1980; Krothapalli *et al.*, 1983). Intraventricular administration of vancomycin (via a shunt or reservoir) has been necessary in a few cases of CNS infections due to susceptible microorganisms that did not respond to intravenous therapy alone (Visconti and Peter, 1979; Sutherland *et al.*, 1981).

Administration of vancomycin is an effective alternative for the treatment of endocarditis caused by *viridans* streptococci in patients who are allergic to penicillin. In combination with an aminoglycoside, it may also be used for endocarditis caused by *Strep. faecalis*. As an oral agent, vancomycin benefits patients with colitis caused by toxin-producing bacteria such as *Cl. difficile* and *Staph. aureus*.

BACITRACIN

History and Source. *Bacitracin* is an antibiotic produced by the Tracy-I strain of *Bacillus subtilis*, isolated in 1943 from the damaged tissue and street dirt debrided from a compound fracture in a young girl named Tracy; hence the name *bacitracin*. The history, properties, and uses of bacitracin have been reviewed by Meleney and Johnson (1949).

Chemistry. The bacitracins are a group of polypeptide antibiotics; multiple components have been demonstrated in the commercial products. The major constituent is *bacitracin A*. Its probable structural formula is as follows:

Bacitracin

A *unit* of the antibiotic is equivalent to 26 μg of the USP standard.

Antibacterial Activity. A variety of gram-positive cocci and bacilli, *Neisseria, H. influenzae,* and *T. pallidum* are sensitive to 0.1 unit or less of bacitracin per milliliter. *Actinomyces* and *Fusobacte-*

rium are inhibited by concentrations of 0.5 to 5 units/ml. Enterobacteriaceae, *Pseudomonas, Candida, Torula,* and *Nocardia* are resistant to the drug. Bacitracin inhibits bacterial cell-wall synthesis.

Absorption, Fate, and Excretion. While bacitracin has been employed parenterally in the past, current use is essentially restricted to topical application. The reader is referred to *earlier editions* of this textbook for descriptions of the pharmacokinetics of this antibiotic.

Preparations, Route of Administration, and Dosage. Only information pertinent to topical application will be presented. *Bacitracin* (BACIGUENT) is available in *ophthalmic* and *dermatological ointments;* the antibiotic is also available in the form of a *powder* for the preparation of topical solutions. The ointments are applied directly to the involved surface one or more times daily. A number of topical preparations of bacitracin to which neomycin or polymyxin or both have been added are available, and some contain the three antibiotics plus hydrocortisone.

Untoward Effects. Serious *nephrotoxicity* results from the parenteral use of this antibiotic. *Hypersensitivity reactions* result from topical application, but this is uncommon.

Therapeutic Uses. *Topical* bacitracin alone or in combination with other antimicrobial agents has no established value in the treatment of *furunculosis, pyoderma, carbuncle, impetigo,* and *superficial and deep abscesses.* For open infections such as *infected eczema* and *infected dermal ulcers,* the local application of the antibiotic may be of some help in eradicating sensitive bacteria. Bacitracin has an advantage over other antibiotics in that topical administration, even in an ointment, rarely produces hypersensitivity. *Suppurative conjunctivitis* and *infected corneal ulcer* respond well to the topical use of bacitracin when they are caused by susceptible bacteria. Oral bacitracin is presently being evaluated for the treatment of antibiotic-associated diarrhea caused by *Cl. difficile.*

American Heart Association Committee. Prevention of bacterial endocarditis. *Circulation,* **1977,** *56,* 139A–143A.

Anders, B. J.; Lauer, B. A.; Paisley, J. W.; and Reller, L. B. Double-blind placebo controlled trial of erythromycin for treatment of *Campylobacter* enteritis. *Lancet,* **1982,** *1,* 131–132.

Ayus, J. C.; Eneas, J. F.; Tong, T. G.; Benowitz, N. L.; Schoenfeld, P. Y.; Hadley, K. L.; Becker, C. E.; and Humphreys, M. H. Peritoneal clearance and total body elimination of vancomycin during chronic intermittent peritoneal dialysis. *Clin. Nephrol.,* **1979,** *11,* 129–132.

Baine, W. B.; Farmer, J. J.; Gangarosa, E. J.; Hermann, G. T.; Thornsberry, C.; and Rice, P. A. Typhoid fever in the United States associated with the 1972–1973 epidemic in Mexico. *J. Infect. Dis.,* **1977,** *135,* 649–653.

Balanchandar, V.; Collipp, P. J.; and Rising, B. J. Intramuscular clindamycin phosphate in children. *Clin. Med.,* **1973,** *80,* 24–30.

Balows, A., and Fraser, D. (eds.). International symposium on Legionnaire's disease. *Ann. Intern. Med.,* **1979,** *90,* 489–707.

Bartlett, J. G. Antibiotic-associated pseudomembranous colitis. *Rev. Infect. Dis.,* **1979,** *1,* 530–539.

————. Anti-anaerobic antibacterial agents. *Lancet,* **1982,** *2,* 478–481.

Bartlett, J. G., and Gorbach, S. L. Penicillin or clindamycin for primary lung abscesses? (Editorial.) *Ann. Intern. Med.,* **1983,** *98,* 546–548.

Bartz, Q. R. Isolation and characterization of CHLOROMYCETIN. *J. Biol. Chem.,* **1948,** *172,* 445–450.

Barza, M., and Scheife, R. T. Antimicrobial spectrum, pharmacology, and therapeutic use of antibiotics. *J. Maine Med. Assoc.,* **1977,** *68,* 194–210.

Bass, J. W.; Klenk, E. L.; Klotheimer, J. B.; Linnemann, C. C.; and Smith, M. H. D. Antimicrobial treatment of pertussis. *J. Pediatr.,* **1969,** *75,* 768–781.

Baughman, G. A., and Fahnestock, S. F. Chloramphenicol resistance mutation in *Escherichia coli* which maps in the major ribosomal protein gene cluster. *J. Bacteriol.,* **1979,** *137,* 1315–1323.

Biancaniello, T.; Meyer, R. A.; and Kaplan, S. Chloramphenicol and cardiotoxicity. *J. Pediatr.,* **1981,** *98,* 828–830.

Blaser, M. J., and Reller, L. B. *Campylobacter* enteritis. *N. Engl. J. Med.,* **1981,** *305,* 1444–1452.

Blouin, R. A.; Erwin, W. G.; Dutro, M. P.; Bustrack, J. A.; and Rowse, K. L. Chloramphenicol hemodialysis clearance. *Ther. Drug Monit.,* **1980,** *2,* 351–354.

Brown, M. R. W., and Wood, S. M. Relation between cation and lipid content of cell walls of *Pseudomonas aeruginosa, Proteus vulgaris* and *Klebsiella aerogenes* and their sensitivity to polymyxin B and other antibacterial agents. *J. Pharm. Pharmacol.,* **1972,** *24,* 215–228.

Brown, N.; Ho, D. H. W.; Fong, K.-L. L.; Bogerd, L.; Maksymiuk, A.; Bolivar, R.; Fainstein, V.; and Bodey, G. P. Effects of hepatic function on vancomycin clinical pharmacology. *Antimicrob. Agents Chemother.,* **1983,** *23,* 603–609.

Bryan, L. E. Mechanisms of action of aminoglycoside antibiotics. In, *Contemporary Issues in Infectious Diseases.* Vol. 1, *New Dimensions in Antimicrobial Therapy.* (Root, R. K., and Sande, M. A., eds.) Churchill Livingstone, Inc., New York, 1984, pp. 17–36.

Burns, L. E.; Hodgman, J. E.; and Cass, A. B. Fatal circulatory collapse in premature infants receiving chloramphenicol. *N. Engl. J. Med.,* **1959,** *261,* 1318–1321.

Carey, B. W. Photodynamic response of a new tetracycline. *J.A.M.A.,* **1960,** *172,* 1196.

Center for Disease Control. Gonorrhea. Recommended treatment schedules, 1979. *Ann. Intern. Med.,* **1979,** *90,* 809–811.

————. Sexually transmitted diseases: treatment guidelines, 1982. *Rev. Infect. Dis.,* **1982,** *4,* Suppl., S729–S746.

Centers for Disease Control. Ampicillin and chloramphenicol resistance in systemic *Haemophilus influenzae* disease. *M.M.W.R.,* **1984,** *33,* 35–37.

Cohlan, S. Q.; Bevelander, G.; and Tiamsic, T. Growth inhibition of prematures receiving tetracycline: clinical and laboratory investigation. *Am. J. Dis. Child.,* **1963,** *105,* 453–461.

Craft, A. W.; Brocklebank, J. T.; Hey, E. N.; and Jackson, R. H. The "grey toddler": chloramphenicol toxicity. *Arch. Dis. Child.,* **1974,** *49,* 235–237.

Cunha, B. A.; Quintiliani, R.; Deglin, J. M.; Izard, M. W.; and Nightingale, C. H. Pharmacokinetics of vancomycin in anuria. *Rev. Infect. Dis.,* **1981,** *3,* Suppl., S269–S272.

Cunha, B. A., and Ristuccia, A. M. Clinical usefulness of vancomycin. *Clin. Pharm.,* **1983,** *2,* 417–424.

Daum, R. S.; Cohen, D. L.; and Smith, A. L. Fatal aplastic anemia following apparent "dose-related" chloramphenicol toxicity. *J. Pediatr.*, **1979**, *94*, 403–405.

Dhawan, V. K., and Thadepalli, H. Clindamycin: a review of fifteen years of experience. *Rev. Infect. Dis.*, **1982**, *4*, 1133–1153.

DiZerega, G.; Yonekura, L.; Roy, S.; Nakamura, R. M.; and Ledger, W. J. A comparison of clindamycin-gentamicin and penicillin-gentamicin in the treatment of postcesarean section endometritis. *Am. J. Obstet. Gynecol.*, **1979**, *134*, 238–242.

Duncan, W. C.; Holder, W. R.; Roberts, D. P.; and Know, J. M. Treatment of gonorrhea with spectinomycin hydrochloride: comparison with standard penicillin schedules. *Antimicrob. Agents Chemother.*, **1972**, *1*, 210–214.

DuPont, H. L., and Pickering, L. K. Salmonellosis. In, *Current Topics in Infectious Disease.* (Greenough, W. B., III, and Merigan, T. C., eds.) Vol. 2, *Infections of the Gastrointestinal Tract: Microbiology, Pathophysiology, and Clinical Features.* Plenum Medical Book Co., New York, **1980**, pp. 83–128.

Elmore, M. F., and Rogge, J. D. Tetracycline induced pancreatitis. *Gastroenterology*, **1981**, *81*, 1134–1136.

Enno, A.; Darrell, J.; Hows, J.; Catovsky, D.; Goldman, J. M.; and Galton, D. A. G. Co-trimoxazole for prevention of infection in acute leukemia. *Lancet*, **1978**, *2*, 395–397.

Fanning, W. L.; Gump, D. W.; and Safferman, R. A. Side effects of minocycline: a double-blind study. *Antimicrob. Agents Chemother.*, **1977**, *11*, 712–717.

Farber, B. F., and Moellering, R. C., Jr. Retrospective study of the toxicity of preparations of vancomycin from 1974 to 1981. *Antimicrob. Agents Chemother.*, **1983**, *23*, 138–141.

Feder, H. M.; Osler, C.; and Maderazo, E. G. Chloramphenicol: a review of its use in clinical practice. *Rev. Infect. Dis.*, **1981**, *3*, 479–491.

Fekety, R. Vancomycin. *Med. Clin. North Am.*, **1982**, *66*, 175–181.

Feldman, W. E. Effect of ampicillin and chloramphenicol against *Haemophilus influenzae.* *Pediatrics*, **1978**, *61*, 406–409.

Filippo, J. A. Infantile hypertrophic pyloric stenosis related to ingestions of erythromycin estolate: a report of five cases. *J. Pediatr. Surg.*, **1976**, *11*, 177–180.

Fogdall, R. P., and Miller, R. D. Prolongation of a pancuronium-induced neuromuscular blockade by clindamycin. *Anesthesiology*, **1974**, *41*, 407–408.

Forrest, J. N.; Cox, M.; Hong, C.; Morrison, G.; Bia, M.; and Singer, I. Superiority of demeclocycline over lithium in the treatment of chronic syndrome of inappropriate secretion of antidiuretic hormone. *N. Engl. J. Med.*, **1978**, *298*, 173–177.

Freedman, J. M.; Hoffman, S. H.; Scheld, W. M.; Lynch, M. A.; da Silva, H. R.; and Sande, M. A. Moxalactam for the treatment of bacterial meningitis in children. *J. Infect. Dis.*, **1983**, *148*, 886–891.

Friedman, C. A.; Lovejoy, F. C.; and Smith, A. L. Chloramphenicol disposition in infants and children. *J. Pediatr.*, **1979**, *95*, 1071–1077.

Gaffney, D. F., and Foster, T. J. Chloramphenicol acetyltransferase determined by R plasmids from gram-negative bacteria. *J. Gen. Microbiol.*, **1978**, *109*, 351–358.

George, W. L.; Rolfe, R. D.; and Finegold, S. M. Treatment and prevention of antimicrobial agent–induced colitis and diarrhea. *Gastroenterology*, **1980**, *79*, 366–372.

Geraci, J. E. Vancomycin. *Mayo Clin. Proc.*, **1977**, *52*, 631–634.

Gilman, R. H.; Terminel, M.; Levine, M. M.; Hernandez-Mendosa, P.; Calderone, E.; Vasquez, V.; Martinez, E.; Snyder, M. J.; and Hornick, R. B. Comparison of trimethoprim-sulfamethoxazole and amoxicillin in therapy of chloramphenicol-resistant and chloramphenicol-sensitive typhoid fever. *J. Infect. Dis.*, **1975**, *132*, 630–636.

Ginsburg, C. M., and Eichenwald, H. F. Erythromycin: a review of its uses in pediatric practice. *J. Pediatr.*, **1976**, *86*, 272A.

Godel, V.; Nemet, P.; and Lazar, M. Chloramphenicol optic neuropathy. *Arch. Ophthalmol.*, **1980**, *98*, 1417–1421.

Gurwith, M. J.; Brunton, J. L.; Lank, B. A.; Harding, G. K. M.; and Ronald, A. R. A prospective controlled investigation of prophylactic trimethoprim/sulfamethoxazole in hospitalized granulocytopenic patients. *Am. J. Med.*, **1979**, *66*, 248–256.

Hahn, F. E., and Gund, P. A structural model of the chloramphenicol receptor site. In, *Drug Receptor Interactions in Antimicrobial Chemotherapy*, Vol. I. (Drews, J., and Hahn, F. E., eds.) Springer-Verlag, New York, **1975**, pp. 245–266.

Hall, A. P.; Doberstyn, E. B.; Nanakorn, A.; and Sonkom, P. Falciparum malaria semiresistant to clindamycin. *Br. Med. J.*, **1975**, *2*, 12–14.

Halpert, J. Further studies of the suicide inactivation of purified rat liver cytochrome P-450 by chloramphenicol. *Mol. Pharmacol.*, **1982**, *21*, 166–172.

Harding, G. K. M.; Buckwold, F. J.; Ronald, A. R.; Marrie, T. J.; Brunton, J. L.; Koss, J. C.; Gurwith, M. J.; and Albritton, W. L. Prospective, randomized comparative study of clindamycin, chloramphenicol, and ticarcillin, each in combination with gentamicin, in therapy for intraabdominal and female genital tract sepsis. *J. Infect. Dis.*, **1980**, *142*, 384–393.

Harwick, H. J.; Kalmanson, G. M.; and Guze, L. B. *In vitro* activity of ampicillin or vancomycin combined with gentamicin or streptomycin against enterococci. *Antimicrob. Agents Chemother.*, **1973**, *4*, 383–387.

Holt, R. The bacterial degradation of chloramphenicol. *Lancet*, **1967**, *1*, 1259–1260.

Hook, E. W., III; Roberts, R. B.; and Sande, M. A. Antimicrobial therapy of experimental enterococcal endocarditis. *Antimicrob. Agents Chemother.*, **1975**, *8*, 564–570.

Hoshiwara, I.; Ostler, B.; Hanna, L.; Cignetti, F.; Coleman, V. R.; and Jawetz, E. Doxycycline treatment of chronic trachoma. *J.A.M.A.*, **1973**, *224*, 220–223.

Istre, G. R.; Welch, D. F.; Marks, M. I.; and Moyer, N. Susceptibility of group A beta-hemolytic *Streptococcus* isolates to penicillin and erythromycin. *Antimicrob. Agents Chemother.*, **1981**, *20*, 244–246.

Izumi, A. K.; Hanke, C. W.; and Higaki, M. *Mycobacterium marinum* infections treated with tetracycline. *Arch. Dermatol.*, **1977**, *113*, 1067–1068.

Joiner, K. A.; Lowe, B. R.; Dzink, J. L.; and Bartlett, J. G. Antibiotic levels in infected and sterile subcutaneous abscesses in mice. *J. Infect. Dis.*, **1981**, *143*, 487–494.

Jones, F. E., and Hanson, D. R. *H. influenzae* meningitis treated with ampicillin or chloramphenicol, and subsequent hearing loss. *Dev. Med. Child Neurol.*, **1977**, *19*, 593–597.

Kager, L.; Liljeqvist, L.; Malmborg, A. S.; and Nord, C. E. Effect of clindamycin prophylaxis on the colonic microflora in patients undergoing colorectal surgery. *Antimicrob. Agents Chemother.*, **1981**, *20*, 736–740.

Karmody, C. S., and Weinstein, L. Reversible sensorineural hearing loss with intravenous erythromycin lactobionate. *Ann. Otol. Rhinol. Laryngol.*, **1977**, *86*, 9–11.

Kauffman, R. E.; Thirumoorthi, M. C.; Buckley, J. A.; Aravind, M. K.; and Dajani, A. S. Relative bioavailability of intravenous chloramphenicol succinate and oral chloramphenicol palmitate in infants and children. *J. Pediatr.*, **1981**, *99*, 963–967.

Kessler, D. L.; Smith, A. L.; and Woodrum, D. E.

Chloramphenicol toxicity in a neonate treated with exchange transfusion. *J. Pediatr.*, **1980**, *96*, 140–141.

Klempner, M. S., and Styrt, B. Clindamycin uptake by human neutrophils. *J. Infect. Dis.*, **1981**, *144*, 472–479.

Koskinniemi, M.; Pettay, O.; Raivio, M.; and Sarna, S. *Haemophilus influenzae* meningitis. A comparison between chloramphenicol and ampicillin therapy with special reference to impaired hearing. *Acta Paediatr. Scand.*, **1978**, *67*, 17–24.

Koup, J. R.; Lau, A. H.; Brodsky, B.; and Slaughter, R. L. Chloramphenicol pharmacokinetics in hospitalized patients. *Antimicrob. Agents Chemother.*, **1979**, *15*, 651–657.

Kozak, P. P.; Cummins, L. H.; and Gilman, S. A. Administration of erythromycin to patients on theophylline. *J. Allergy Clin. Immunol.*, **1977**, *60*, 149–151.

Kramer, P. W.; Griffith, R. S.; and Campbell, R. L. Antibiotic penetration of the brain: a comparative study. *J. Neurosurg.*, **1969**, *31*, 295–302.

Krothapalli, R. K.; Senekjian, H. O.; and Ayus, J. C. Efficacy of intravenous vancomycin in the treatment of gram-positive peritonitis in long-term peritoneal dialysis. *Am. J. Med.*, **1983**, *75*, 345–348.

Kucers, A. Current position of chloramphenicol in chemotherapy. *J. Antimicrob. Chemother.*, **1980**, *6*, 1–9.

Kuzucu, E. Y. Methoxyflurane, tetracycline and renal failure. *J.A.M.A.*, **1970**, *211*, 1162–1164.

Levine, P. H.; Regelson, W.; and Holland, J. F. Chloramphenicol associated encephalopathy. *Clin. Pharmacol. Ther.*, **1970**, *11*, 194–199.

Levison, M. E.; Mangura, C. T.; Lorber, B.; Abrutyn, E.; Pesanti, E. L.; Levy, R. S.; Macgregor, R. R.; and Schwartz, A. R. Clindamycin compared with penicillin for the treatment of anaerobic lung abscesses. *Ann. Intern. Med.*, **1983**, *98*, 466–471.

Lietman, P. S. Chloramphenicol and the neonate—1979 view. *Clin. Pharmacol. Ther.*, **1979**, *6*, 151–162.

Linares, J.; Garau, J.; Dominquez, C.; and Perez, J. L. Antibiotic resistance and serotypes of *Streptococcus pneumoniae* from patients with community-acquired pneumococcal disease. *Antimicrob. Agents Chemother.*, **1983**, *23*, 545–547.

Lindebaum, J.; Greenough, W. B.; and Islam, M. R. Antibiotic therapy of cholera in children. *Bull. WHO*, **1967**, *37*, 529–538.

McClosky, R. V.; Eller, J. J.; Green, M.; Mauney, C. U.; and Richards, S. E. M. The 1970 epidemic of diphtheria in San Antonio. *Ann. Intern. Med.*, **1971**, *75*, 495–503.

McCormack, W. M.; Chowdhury, A. M.; Jahangir, N.; Fariduddin Ahmed, A. B.; and Mosley, W. H. Tetracycline prophylaxis in families of cholera patients. *Bull. WHO*, **1968**, *38*, 787–792.

McCormack, W. M.; Donner, G. H.; Kodgis, L. F.; Alpert, S.; Lower, E. W.; and Kass, E. H. Hepatotoxicity of erythromycin estolate during pregnancy. *Antimicrob. Agents Chemother.*, **1977**, *12*, 630–635.

McCormick, M. H.; Stark, W. M.; Pittenger, G. E.; Pittenger, R. C.; and McGuire, J. M. Vancomycin, a new antibiotic. I. Chemical and biologic properties. In, *Antibiotics Annual, 1955–1956.* Medical Encyclopedia, Inc., New York, **1956**, pp. 606–611.

Magera, B. E.; Arroyo, J. C.; Rosansky, S. J.; and Postic, B. Vancomycin pharmacokinetics in patients with peritonitis on peritoneal dialysis. *Antimicrob. Agents Chemother.*, **1983**, *23*, 710–714.

Mandell, G. L.; Lindsey, E.; and Hook, E. W. Synergism of vancomycin and streptomycin for enterococci. *Am. J. Med. Sci.*, **1970**, *259*, 346–349.

Maruyama, S.; Yoshioka, H.; Fujita, K.; Takimoto, M.; and Satake, Y. Sensitivity of group A streptococci to antibiotics. *Am. J. Dis. Child.*, **1979**, *133*, 1143–1145.

Mauer, S. M.; Chavers, B. M.; and Kjellstrand, C. M. Treatment of an infant with severe chloramphenicol in-

toxication using charcoal-column hemoperfusion. *J. Pediatr.*, **1980**, *96*, 136–139.

May, D. C.; Jarboe, C. H.; Ellenburg, D. T.; Roe, E. J.; and Karibo, J. The effects of erythromycin on theophylline elimination in normal males. *J. Clin. Pharmacol.*, **1982**, *22*, 125–130.

Meleney, F. L., and Johnson, B. A. Bacitracin. *Am. J. Med.*, **1949**, *7*, 794–806.

Moellering, R. C.; Krogstad, D. J.; and Greenblatt, D. J. Vancomycin therapy in patients with impaired renal function: a nomogram for dosage. *Ann. Intern. Med.*, **1981**, *94*, 343–346.

Molavi, A., and Weinstein, L. *In vitro* activity of erythromycin against atypical mycobacteria. *J. Infect. Dis.*, **1971**, *123*, 216–219.

Muder, R. R.; Yu, V. L.; and Zuravleff, J. J. Pneumonia due to the Pittsburgh pneumonia agent: new clinical perspective with a review of the literature. *Medicine (Baltimore)*, **1983**, *62*, 120–128.

Mulhall, A.; de Louvois, J.; and Hurley, R. The pharmacokinetics of chloramphenicol in the neonate and young infant. *J. Antimicrob. Chemother.*, **1983**, *12*, 629–639.

Neu, H. C. A symposium on tetracyclines: a major appraisal. Introduction. *Bull. N.Y. Acad. Med.*, **1978**, *54*, 141–155.

Newfield, P., and Roizen, M. F. Hazards of rapid administration of vancomycin. *Ann. Intern. Med.*, **1979**, *91*, 581.

Nieto, M., and Perkins, H. R. Physicochemical properties of vancomycin and iodovancomycin and their complexes with diacetyl-L-lysyl-D-alanyl-D-alanine. *Biochem. J.*, **1971a**, *123*, 773–787.

———. The specificity of combination between ristocetins and peptides related to bacterial cell wall mucopeptide precursors. *Ibid.*, **1971b**, *124*, 845–852.

Nolan, C. M.; Flanigan, W. J.; Rastogi, S. P.; and Brewer, T. E. Vancomycin penetration into CSF during treatment of patients receiving hemodialysis. *South. Med. J.*, **1980**, *73*, 1333–1334.

Orr, L. H., Jr.; Rudisill, E., Jr.; Brodkin, R.; and Hamilton, R. W. Exacerbation of renal failure associated with doxycycline. *Arch. Intern. Med.*, **1978**, *138*, 793–794.

Panzer, J. D.; Brown, D. C.; Epstein, W. L.; Lipson, R. L.; Mahaffrey, H. W.; and Atkinson, W. H. Clindamycin levels in various body tissues and fluids. *J. Clin. Pharmacol.*, **1972**, *12*, 259–262.

Philipson, A.; Sabath, L. D.; and Charles, D. Transplacental passage of erythromycin and clindamycin. *N. Engl. J. Med.*, **1973**, *288*, 1219–1221.

Piffaretti, J. C., and Froment, Y. Binding of chloramphenicol and its acetylated derivatives to *Escherichia coli* ribosomal subunits. *Chemotherapy*, **1978**, *24*, 24–28.

Polak, B. C. P.; Wesseling, H.; Herxheimer, A.; and Meyler, L. Blood dyscrasias attributed to chloramphenicol. *Acta Med. Scand.*, **1972**, *192*, 409–414.

Polin, H. B., and Plaut, M. E. Chloramphenicol. *N.Y. State J. Med.*, **1977**, *77*, 378.

Powell, D. A.; Nahata, M. C.; Darrell, D. C.; Durrell, D. C.; Glazer, J. P.; and Hilty, M. D. Interactions among chloramphenicol, phenytoin, and phenobarbital in a pediatric patient. *J. Pediatr.*, **1981**, *98*, 1001–1003.

Pratt, W. B. *Chemotherapy of Infection.* Oxford University Press, New York, **1977**, pp. 128–175.

Pride, G. L.; Cleary, R. E.; and Hamburger, R. J. Disseminated intravascular coagulation associated with tetracycline-induced hepatorenal failure during pregnancy. *Am. J. Obstet. Gynecol.*, **1973**, *115*, 585–586.

Prokesch, R. C., and Hand, W. L. Antibiotic entry into human polymorphonuclear leukocytes. *Antimicrob. Agents Chemother.*, **1982**, *21*, 373–380.

Rahal, J. J., Jr., and Simberkoff, M. S. Bactericidal and bacteriostatic action of chloramphenicol against meningeal pathogens. *Antimicrob. Agents Chemother.*, **1979**, *16*, 13–18.

Rasch, J. R., and Mogabgab, W. J. Therapeutic effect of erythromycin on *Mycoplasma pneumoniae* pneumonia. *Antimicrob. Agents Chemother.*, **1965**, *5*, 693–699.

Rifkin, G. D.; Fekety, F. R.; and Silva, J. Antibiotic-induced colitis: implication of a toxin neutralized by *Clostridium sordellii* antitoxin. *Lancet*, **1977**, *2*, 1103–1106.

Roberts, M. D.; Swenson, C. D.; Owens, L. M.; and Smith, A. L. Characterization of chloramphenicol-resistant *Haemophilus influenzae*. *Antimicrob. Agents Chemother.*, **1980**, *18*, 610–615.

Sabath, L. D.; Gerstein, D. A.; and Finland, M. Serum glutamic oxalacetic transaminase: false elevations during administration of erythromycin. *N. Engl. J. Med.*, **1968a**, *279*, 1137–1139.

Sabath, L. D.; Gerstein, D. A.; Loder, P. B.; and Finland, M. Excretion of erythromycin and its enhanced activity in urine against gram-negative bacilli with alkalinization. *J. Lab. Clin. Med.*, **1968b**, *72*, 916–923.

Sack, D. A.; Kaminsky, D. C.; Sack, R. B.; Itotja, J. N.; Arthur, R. R.; Kapikian, A. Z.; Orskov, F.; and Orskov, I. Prophylactic doxycycline for travelers' diarrhea. Results of a prospective double-blind study of Peace Corps volunteers in Kenya. *N. Engl. J. Med.*, **1978**, *298*, 758–763.

Salih, S. Y., and Mustafa, D. Louse-borne relapsing fever: II. Combined penicillin and tetracycline therapy in 160 Sudanese patients. *Trans. R. Soc. Trop. Med. Hyg.*, **1977**, *71*, 49–51.

Schaad, U. B.; Nelson, J. D.; and McCracken, G. H., Jr. Pharmacology and efficacy of vancomycin for staphylococcal infections in children. *Rev. Infect. Dis.*, **1981**, *3*, Suppl., S282–S288.

Scheld, W. M.; Brown, R. S., Jr.; Fletcher, D. D.; and Sande, M. A. Bactericidal versus bacteriostatic antibiotic therapy of experimental pneumococcal meningitis. *Ann. Clin. Res.*, **1979**, *27*, 355a.

Schoutens, E.; Peromet, M.; and Yourassowsky, E. Microbiological and clinical study of spectinomycin in urinary tract infections: reevaluation with hospital strains. *Curr. Ther. Res.*, **1972**, *14*, 349–357.

Scott, J. L.; Finegold, S. M.; Belkin, G. A.; and Lawrence, J. S. A controlled double-blind study of the hematologic toxicity of chloramphenicol. *N. Engl. J. Med.*, **1965**, *272*, 1137–1142.

Shapera, R. M.; Hable, K. A.; and Matsen, J. M. Erythromycin therapy twice daily for streptococcal pharyngitis. Controlled comparison with erythromycin or penicillin phenoxymethyl four times daily or penicillin G benzathine. *J.A.M.A.*, **1973**, *226*, 531–555.

Shaw, W. V., and Brodsky, R. F. Characterization of chloramphenicol acetyltransferase from chloramphenicol-resistant *Staphylococcus aureus*. *J. Bacteriol.*, **1968**, *95*, 28–36.

Sheldrick, G. M.; Jones, P. G.; Kennard, O.; Williams, D. H.; and Smith, G. A. Structure of vancomycin and its complex with acyl-D-alanyl-D-alanine. *Nature*, **1978**, *271*, 223–225.

Shils, M. E. Renal disease and the metabolic effects of tetracycline. *Ann. Intern. Med.*, **1963**, *58*, 389–408.

Skolimowski, I. M.; Knight, R. C.; and Edwards, D. I. Molecular basis of chloramphenicol and thiamphenicol toxicity to DNA *in vitro*. *J. Antimicrob. Chemother.*, **1983**, *12*, 535–542.

Slaughter, R. L.; Cerra, F. B.; and Koup, J. R. Effect of hemodialysis on total body clearance of chloramphenicol. *Am. J. Hosp. Pharm.*, **1980a**, *37*, 1083–1086.

Slaughter, R. L.; Pieper, J. A.; Cerra, F. B.; Brodsky, B.; and Koup, J. R. Chloramphenicol sodium succinate kinetics in critically ill patients. *Clin. Pharmacol. Ther.*, **1980b**, *28*, 69–77.

Smith, A. L., and Weber, A. Pharmacology of chloramphenicol. *Pediatr. Clin. North Am.*, **1983**, *30*, 209–236.

Snyder, M. J.; Gonzalez, O.; Palomino, C.; Music, S. I.; Hornick, R. B.; Perroni, J.; Woodward, W. E.; Gonzalez, C.; DuPont, H. R.; and Woodward, L. E. Comparative efficacy of chloramphenicol, ampicillin, and cotrimoxazole in the treatment of typhoid fever. *Lancet*, **1976**, *2*, 1155–1157.

Sompolinsky, D., and Samra, Z. Mechanism of high-level resistance to chloramphenicol in different *Escherichia coli* variants. *J. Gen. Microbiol.*, **1968**, *50*, 55–66.

Sorrell, T. C.; Packham, D. R.; Shanker, S.; Foldes, M.; and Munro, R. Vancomycin therapy for methicillin-resistant *Staphylococcus aureus*. *Ann. Intern. Med.*, **1982**, *97*, 344–350.

Stamm, W. E.; Running, K.; McKevitt, M.; Counts, G. W.; Turck, M.; and Holmes, K. K. Treatment of the acute urethral syndrome. *N. Engl. J. Med.*, **1981**, *304*, 956–958.

Standiford, H. C. The tetracyclines and chloramphenicol. In, *Principles and Practice of Infectious Diseases*, 2nd ed. (Mandell, G. L.; Douglas, R. G., Jr.; and Bennett, J. E.; eds.) John Wiley & Sons, Inc., New York, **1985**, pp. 206–212.

Steere, A. C.; Malawista, S. E.; Newman, J. H.; Spieler, P. N.; and Bartenhagen, N. H. Antibiotic therapy in Lyme disease. *Ann. Intern. Med.*, **1980**, *93*, 1–8.

Suhrland, L. F., and Weisberger, A. S. Chloramphenicol toxicity in liver and renal disease. *Arch. Intern. Med.*, **1963**, *112*, 747–754.

Sutherland, G. E.; Palitang, E. G.; Marr, J. J.; and Luedke, S. L. Sterilization of Ommaya reservoir by instillation of vancomycin. *Am. J. Med.*, **1981**, *71*, 1068–1070.

Tabbara, K. F.; Dy-Liaco, J.; Nozik, R. A.; O'Connor, G. R.; and Blackman, H. J. Clindamycin in chronic toxoplasmosis. Effect of periocular injections on recoverability of organisms from healed lesions in the rabbit eye. *Arch. Ophthalmol.*, **1979**, *97*, 542–544.

Tally, F. P.; Cuchural, G. J.; Jacobus, N. V.; Gorbach, S. L.; Aldridge, K. E.; Cleary, T. J.; Finegold, S. M.; Hill, G. B.; Iannini, P. B.; McClosky, R. V.; O'Keefe, J. P.; and Pierson, C. L. Susceptibility of the *Bacteroides fragilis* group in the United States in 1981. *Antimicrob. Agents Chemother.*, **1983**, *23*, 536–540.

Tally, F. P.; Snydman, D. R.; Gorbach, S. L.; and Malamy, M. H. Plasmid-mediated transferable resistance to clindamycin and erythromycin in *Bacteroides fragilis*. *J. Infect. Dis.*, **1979**, *139*, 83–88.

Tedesco, F. J. Clindamycin and colitis: a review. *J. Infect. Dis.*, **1977**, *135S*, 95–98.

Thadepalli, H.; Gorbach, S. L.; Broido, P. W.; Norsen, J.; and Nyhus, L. Abdominal trauma, anaerobes, and antibiotics. *Surg. Gynecol. Obstet.*, **1973**, *137*, 270–276.

Tolman, K. G.; Sannella, J. J.; and Freston, J. W. Chemical structure of erythromycin and hepatotoxicity. *Ann. Intern. Med.*, **1974**, *81*, 58–60.

Vanhoof, R.; Gordts, B.; Dierickx, R.; Coignau, H.; and Butzler, J. D. Bacteriostatic and bactericidal activities of 24 antimicrobial agents against *Campylobacter fetus* subs. *jejuni*. *Antimicrob. Agents Chemother.*, **1980**, *18*, 118–121.

Visconti, E. B., and Peter, G. Vancomycin treatment of cerebrospinal fluid shunt infections. *J. Neurosurg.*, **1979**, *51*, 245–246.

Vogel, Z.; Vogel, T.; and Elson, D. The effect of erythromycin on peptide bond formation and the termination reaction. *FEBS Lett.*, **1971**, *15*, 249–253.

Wallerstein, R. O.; Condit, P. K.; Kasper, C. K.; Brown, J. W.; and Morrison, F. R. Statewide study of chloramphenicol therapy and fatal aplastic anemia. *J.A.M.A.*, **1969**, *208*, 2045–2050.

Walters, B. N. J., and Gubbay, S. S. Tetracycline and benign intracranial hypertension: report of five cases. *Br. Med. J.*, **1981**, *282*, 19–20.

Ward, H. P. The effect of chloramphenicol on RNA and heme synthesis in bone marrow cultures. *J. Lab. Clin. Med.*, **1966**, *68*, 400–410.

Washington, A. E. Update on treatment recommendations for gonococcal infections. *Rev. Infect. Dis.*, **1982**, *4*, Suppl., S758–S771.

Watanakunakorn, C. The antibacterial action of vancomycin. *Rev. Infect. Dis.*, **1981**, *3*, Suppl., S210–S215.

Watanakunakorn, C., and Tisone, J. C. Synergism between vancomycin and gentamicin or tobramycin for methicillin-susceptible and methicillin-resistant *Staphylococcus aureus* strains. *Antimicrob. Agents Chemother.*, **1982**, *22*, 903–905.

Werner, R.; Kollak, A.; Nierhaus, D.; Schreiner, G.; and Nierhaus, K. H. Experiments on the binding sites and the action of some antibiotics which inhibit ribosomal functions. In, *Drug Receptor Interactions in Antimicrobial Chemotherapy*, Vol I. (Drews, J., and Hahn, F. E., eds.) Springer-Verlag, New York, **1975**, pp. 217–234.

Winckler, K. Tetracycline ulcers of the oesophagus; endoscopy, histology, and roentgenology in two cases, and review of the literature. *Endoscopy*, **1981**, *13*, 225–228.

Yogev, R.; Kolling, W. M.; and Williams, T. Pharmacokinetic comparison of intravenous and oral chloramphenicol in patients with *Haemophilus influenzae* meningitis. *Pediatrics*, **1981**, *67*, 656–660.

Zimmerman, H. J., and Lewis, J. H. Hepatic toxicity of antimicrobial agents. In, *Contemporary Issues in Infectious Diseases*. Vol. 1, *New Dimensions in Antimicrobial Therapy*. (Root, R. K., and Sande, M. A., eds.) Churchill Livingstone, Inc., New York, **1984**, pp. 153–202.

Monographs and Reviews

Bowie, W., and Holmes, K. K. *Chlamydia* trachomatis (trachoma, inclusion conjunctivitis, lymphogranuloma venereum). In, *Principles and Practice of Infectious Diseases*, 2nd ed. (Mandell, G. L.; Douglas, R. G., Jr.; and Bennett, J. E.; eds.) John Wiley & Sons, Inc., New York, **1985**, pp. 1464–1476.

Bryant, R. E. Effect of the suppurative environment on antibiotic activity. In, *Contemporary Issues in Infectious Diseases*. Vol. 1, *New Dimensions in Antimicrobial Therapy*. (Root, R. K., and Sande, M. A., eds.) Churchill Livingstone, Inc., New York, **1984**, pp. 313–338.

Chopra, I., and Howe, T. G. B. Bacterial resistance to the tetracyclines. *Microbiol. Rev.*, **1978**, *42*, 707–724.

Dowling, H. F. *Tetracycline*. Medical Encyclopedia, Inc., New York, **1955**.

Lepper, M. H. AUREOMYCIN (*Chlortetracycline*). Medical Encyclopedia, Inc., New York, **1956**.

Medical Letter. Prevention of bacterial endocarditis. **1984**, *26*, 3–4.

Pratt, W. B. *Chemotherapy of Infection*. Oxford University Press, New York, **1977**.

Sanford, J. P. *Guide to Antimicrobial Therapy, 1984*. Sanford, Bethesda, **1984**.

Steigbigel, N. H. Erythromycin, lincomycin and clindamycin. In, *Principles and Practice of Infectious Diseases*, 2nd ed. (Mandell, G. L.; Douglas, R. G., Jr.; and Bennett, J. E.; eds.) John Wiley & Sons, Inc., New York, **1985**, pp. 224–232.

53 ANTIMICROBIAL AGENTS

[*Continued*]

Drugs Used in the Chemotherapy of Tuberculosis and Leprosy

Gerald L. Mandell and Merle A. Sande

The pharmacological characteristics and the therapeutic use of each class of compounds employed in the chemotherapy of tuberculosis and leprosy are discussed in this chapter. The treatment of infections in man caused by mycobacteria is still an important and challenging problem. For years, patients with tuberculosis and leprosy were cared for in specialized hospitals. Physicians who treated these patients developed concepts of therapy that at times seemed discordant with those that pertained to the management of other infections. It is now clear that the basic tenets of antimicrobial therapy also apply to these diseases. However, since the microorganisms grow slowly and the diseases are often chronic, there are special therapeutic problems particularly related to patient compliance, drug toxicity, and the development of microbial resistance.

I. Drugs for Tuberculosis

The introduction in the 1960s of two new drugs for the chemotherapy of tuberculosis—ethambutol and rifampin—changed many of the concepts and practices that were prevalent until that time. Drugs used for this disease may be divided into two major categories. "First-line" agents combine the greatest level of efficacy with an acceptable degree of toxicity; these include isoniazid, rifampin, ethambutol, streptomycin, and pyrazinamide. The large majority of patients with tuberculosis can be treated successfully with these drugs. Administration of rifampin in combination with the older but still dominant agent isoniazid may

represent optimal therapy for all forms of disease caused by sensitive strains of *Mycobacterium tuberculosis*. In areas where primary resistance to isoniazid is high, therapy is usually initiated with three drugs—rifampin, isoniazid, and ethambutol (or another "first-line" agent)—until sensitivity tests are completed. If the isolate is sensitive to isoniazid and rifampin, the third drug is discontinued. Occasionally, however, because of microbial resistance or patient-related factors, it may be necessary to resort to a "second-line" drug; this category of agents includes ethionamide, aminosalicylic acid, amikacin, kanamycin, capreomycin, and cycloserine.

ISONIAZID

This agent is still considered to be the primary drug for the chemotherapy of tuberculosis, and all patients with disease caused by isoniazid-sensitive strains of the tubercle bacillus should receive the drug if they can tolerate it.

History. The discovery of isoniazid was somewhat fortuitous. In 1945, Chorine reported that nicotinamide possesses tuberculostatic action. Examination of the compounds related to nicotinamide revealed that many pyridine derivatives possess tuberculostatic activity; among these are congeners of isonicotinic acid. Because the thiosemicarbazones were known to inhibit *M. tuberculosis*, the thiosemicarbazone of isonicotinaldehyde was synthesized and studied. The starting material for this synthesis was the methyl ester of isonicotinic acid, and the first intermediate was isonicotinyl-hydrazide (isoniazid). The interesting history of these chemical studies has been reviewed by Fox (1953).

Chemistry. *Isoniazid* is the hydrazide of isonicotinic acid; the structural formula is as follows:

Isoniazid

The isopropyl derivative of isoniazid, *iproniazid* (1-isonicotinyl-2-isopropylhydrazide), also inhibits the multiplication of the tubercle bacillus. This compound, which is a potent inhibitor of monoamine oxidase, is too toxic for use in man. However, its study led to the use of monoamine oxidase inhibitors for the treatment of depression (*see* Chapter 19).

Antibacterial Activity. Isoniazid is bacteriostatic for "resting" bacilli but is bactericidal for rapidly dividing microorganisms. The minimal tuberculostatic concentration is 0.025 to 0.05 µg/ml. The bacteria undergo one or two divisions before multiplication is arrested.

Among the various atypical mycobacteria, only *M. kansasii* is usually susceptible to isoniazid. However, sensitivity must always be tested *in vitro*, since the inhibitory concentration required may be rather high.

Isoniazid is highly effective for the treatment of experimental tuberculosis in animals and is strikingly superior to streptomycin. Unlike streptomycin, isoniazid penetrates cells with ease and is just as effective against bacilli growing within cells as it is against those growing in culture media.

Bacterial Resistance. When tubercle bacilli are grown *in vitro* in increasing concentrations of isoniazid, mutants are readily selected that are resistant to the drug, even when the drug is present in enormous concentrations. However, cross-resistance between isoniazid and other tuberculostatic drugs does not occur. Present evidence suggests that the mechanism of resistance is related to failure of the drug to penetrate or to be taken up by the microorganisms.

As with the other agents described, treatment with isoniazid also leads to the emergence of resistant strains *in vivo*. The shift from primarily sensitive to mainly insensitive microorganisms occasionally occurs within a few weeks after therapy is started; however, there is considerable variation in the time of appearance of this phenomenon from one case to another. Approximately one in 10^6 tubercle bacilli will be genetically resistant to isoniazid; since tuberculous cavities may contain as many as 10^7 to 10^9 microorganisms, it is not surprising that treatment with isoniazid alone results in the selection of these resistant bacteria. The incidence of primary resistance to isoniazid in the United States appears to be fairly stable at 2 to 5% of isolates of *M. tuberculosis*, but it may be much higher in certain populations, including Asians and Hispanics (Carpenter *et al.*, 1982; Centers for Disease Control, 1983).

Mechanism of Action. While the mechanism of action of isoniazid is unknown, there are several hypotheses. These include effects on lipids, nucleic acid biosynthesis, and glycolysis (Herman and Weber, 1980). Takayama and associates (1975) have suggested a primary action of isoniazid to inhibit the biosynthesis of mycolic acids, important constituents of the mycobacterial cell wall. Low concentrations of the drug may prevent elongation of the very-long-chain fatty acid precursor of the molecule. Since mycolic acids are unique to mycobacteria, this action would explain the high degree of selectivity of the antimicrobial activity of isoniazid. Exposure to isoniazid leads to a loss of acid fastness and a decrease in the quantity of methanol-extractable lipid of the microorganisms. Only isoniazid-sensitive tubercle bacilli take up the drug. This uptake appears to be an active process, although most of the drug within the bacilli is the isonicotinic acid metabolite (Jenne and Beggs, 1973).

Absorption, Distribution, and Excretion. Isoniazid is readily absorbed when administered either orally or parenterally. Aluminum-containing antacids may interfere with absorption (Hurwitz and Schlozman, 1974). Peak plasma concentrations of 3 to 5 µg/ml develop 1 to 2 hours after oral ingestion of usual doses.

Isoniazid diffuses readily into all body fluids and cells. The drug is detectable in significant quantities in pleural and ascitic fluids; concentrations in the cerebrospinal fluid (CSF) are about 20% of those in the plasma. Isoniazid penetrates well into caseous material. The concentration of the agent is initially higher in the plasma and muscle than in the infected tissue, but the latter retains the drug for a long time in quantities well above those required for bacteriostasis.

From 75 to 95% of a dose of isoniazid is excreted in the urine in 24 hours, mostly as metabolites. The main excretory products in man are the result of enzymatic acetylation, acetylisoniazid, and enzymatic hydrolysis, isonicotinic acid. Small quantities of an isonicotinic acid conjugate, probably isonicotinyl glycine, one or more isonicotinyl hydrazones, and traces of N-methylisoniazid are also detectable in the urine.

Human populations show genetic heterogeneity with regard to the rate of acetylation of isoniazid (Evans *et al.*, 1960). There is bimodal distribution of slow and rapid inactivators of the drug due to differences in the activity of an acetyltransferase. The rate of acetylation significantly alters the concentrations of the drug that are achieved in plasma and its half-life in the circulation. The half-life of the drug may be prolonged in the presence of hepatic insufficiency.

The frequency of the rate of acetylation of isoniazid is dependent upon race but is not influenced by sex or age. Fast acetylation is found in Eskimos and Japanese. Slow acetylation is the predominant phenotype in most Scandinavians, Jews, and North African Caucasians. The incidence of slow inactivators among the various racial types in the United States is 50% (La Du, 1972). Since high acetyltransferase activity (fast acetylation) is inherited as an autosomal dominant trait, rapid inactivators of isoniazid are either heterozygous or homozygous. The average concentration of active isoniazid in the circulation of rapid inactivators is about 30 to 50% of that present in persons who acetylate the drug slowly. In the whole population, the half-life of isoniazid varies from less than 1 to more than 3 hours. The mean half-life in rapid acetylators is approximately 70 minutes, while a value of 3 hours is characteristic of slow inactivators. However, it is important to emphasize that there is no conclusive evidence of a difference in therapeutic efficacy or in the incidence of toxicity related to rate of acetylation of isoniazid in patients receiving the drug every day.

The clearance of isoniazid is dependent to only a small degree on the status of renal function, but patients who are slow inactivators of the drug may accumulate toxic concentrations if their renal function is impaired. It has been suggested (Bowersox et al., 1973) that 300 mg per day of the drug can be administered safely to individuals in whom the plasma creatinine concentration is less than 12 mg/dl.

Preparations, Routes of Administration, and Dosage. *Isoniazid* (*isonicotinic acid hydrazide;* NYDRAZID, others) is available in tablets containing 50, 100, and 300 mg; as a syrup containing 10 mg/ml; and as an injection in a concentration of 100 mg/ml. The commonly used total daily dose of the drug is 5 mg/kg, with a maximum of 300 mg; oral and intramuscular doses are identical. Isoniazid is usually given orally in a single daily dose but may be given in two divided doses. While doses of 10 mg/kg with a maximum of 600 mg are occasionally employed in severely ill patients, there is no evidence that this regimen is more effective. Children under 4 years of age should receive 10 mg/kg per day. Isoniazid may be used as intermittent therapy for tuberculosis. After 1 to 4 months of daily therapy, patients may be treated with twice-weekly doses of isoniazid (15 mg/kg, orally) plus twice-weekly doses of either rifampin (10 mg/kg, up to 600 mg per day) for 9 months or streptomycin (25 to 30 mg/kg, intramuscularly) or ethambutol (50 mg/kg, orally) for 18 months.

Pyridoxine (15 to 50 mg per day) should be administered with isoniazid to minimize adverse reactions (*see* below), especially in malnourished patients and those predisposed to neuropathy (*e.g.,* the elderly, pregnant women, diabetics, alcoholics, and uremics) (Snider, 1980).

Untoward Effects. The incidence of adverse reactions to isoniazid was estimated to be 5.4% among more than 2000 patients treated with the drug; the most prominent of these reactions were *rash* (2%), *fever* (1.2%), *jaundice* (0.6%), and *peripheral neuritis* (0.2%) (Pitts, 1977). Hypersensitivity to isoniazid may result in *fever,* various *skin eruptions, hepatitis,* and *morbilliform, maculopapular, purpuric,* and *urticarial rashes. Hematological reactions* may also occur (agranulocytosis, eosinophilia, thrombocytopenia, anemia). *Vasculitis* associated with *antinuclear antibodies* may appear during treatment but disappears when it is stopped (Rothfield *et al.,* 1978). *Arthritic symptoms* (*back pain,* bilateral proximal interphalangeal *joint involvement, arthralgia* of the knees, elbows, and wrists, and the *"shoulder-hand" syndrome*) have been attributed to this agent.

If pyridoxine is not given concurrently, *peripheral neuritis* is the most common reaction to isoniazid and occurs in about 2% of patients receiving 5 mg/kg of the drug daily. Higher doses may result in peripheral neuritis in 10 to 20% of patients. The prophylactic administration of pyridoxine prevents the development not only of peripheral neuritis but also of most other nervous system dysfunction in practically all instances, even when therapy is carried on for as long as 2 years.

Isoniazid may precipitate *convulsions* in patients with seizure disorders and, rarely, in patients with no prior history of seizures. *Optic neuritis* and atrophy have also occurred during therapy with the drug. *Muscle twitching, dizziness, ataxia, paresthesias, stupor,* and *toxic encephalopathy* that may terminate fatally are among other manifestations of the neurotoxicity of isoniazid. A number of *mental abnormalities* may appear during the use of this drug; among these are *euphoria, transient impairment of memory, separation of ideas and reality, loss of self-control,* and *florid psychoses.*

Signs and symptoms of *excessive sedation* or *incoordination* may develop when isoniazid is given to patients with seizure disorders who are simultaneously being treated with phenytoin or other hydantoins. Isoniazid is known to inhibit the parahydroxylation of phenytoin, and toxicity occurs in approximately 27% of patients given both drugs (Miller *et al.*, 1979). Concentrations of phenytoin in plasma should be monitored and adjusted if necessary. The dosage of isoniazid should not be changed.

Although jaundice has been known for some time to be an untoward effect of exposure to isoniazid, it was not until 1970 that it became apparent that *severe hepatic injury* leading to death may occur in some individuals receiving this drug (Garibaldi *et al.*, 1972). Additional studies in adults and children have confirmed this observation; the characteristic pathology is bridging and multilobular necrosis. Continuation of the drug after symptoms of hepatic dysfunction have appeared tends to increase the severity of damage. The mechanisms responsible for this toxicity are unknown, although acetylhydrazine, which is a metabolite of isoniazid, causes hepatic damage in adults (Mitchell *et al.*, 1976). A contributory role of alcoholic hepatitis has been noted (Gronhagen-Riska *et al.*, 1978). Age appears to be the most important factor in determining the risk of hepatotoxicity due to isoniazid. Hepatic damage is rare in patients less than 20 years old; the complication is observed in 0.3% of those 20 to 34 years old, and the incidence increases to 1.2% and 2.3% in individuals 35 to 49 and greater than 50 years of age, respectively (Public Health Service, 1974). A much larger percentage of patients receiving isoniazid (up to 12%) may have elevated plasma transaminase activities (Bailey *et al.*, 1974). Patients receiving isoniazid should be carefully evaluated at monthly intervals for symptoms of hepatitis (anorexia, malaise, fatigue, nausea, and jaundice). Some also prefer to determine serum glutamic-oxalacetic transaminase (SGOT) activities at monthly intervals (Byrd *et al.*, 1979). They feel that an elevation greater than five times normal is cause for discontinuation of the drug. Most hepatitis occurs 4 to 8 weeks after the start of therapy. Isoniazid should be administered with great care to those with preexisting hepatic disease. (*See* Maddrey and Boitnott, 1973.)

Among miscellaneous reactions associated with isoniazid therapy are *dryness of the mouth, epigastric distress, methemoglobinemia, tinnitus,* and *urinary retention*. In those with the predisposition to *pyridoxine-deficiency anemia,* the administration of isoniazid may result in its appearance in full-blown form. Treatment with large doses of the vitamin gradually returns the blood picture to normal in such cases (*see* Goldman and Braman, 1972). A drug-induced syndrome resembling systemic *lupus erythematosus* has been reported (Rothfield *et al.*, 1978). Overdose of isoniazid, as in attempted suicide, may result in coma, seizures, metabolic acidosis, and hyperglycemia.

Therapeutic Status. Isoniazid is still the most important drug for the treatment of all types of tuberculosis. Toxic effects can be minimized by prophylactic therapy with pyridoxine and careful surveillance of the patient. The drug must be used concurrently with another agent for treatment, although it is used alone for prophylaxis.

Details of the use of isoniazid in the chemotherapy of tuberculosis are described below.

RIFAMPIN

The rifamycins are a group of structurally similar, complex macrocyclic antibiotics produced by *Streptomyces mediterranei;* rifampin is a semisynthetic derivative of one of these—rifamycin B.

Chemistry. Rifampin is a zwitterion and is soluble in organic solvents and in water at acidic pH. It has the following structure:

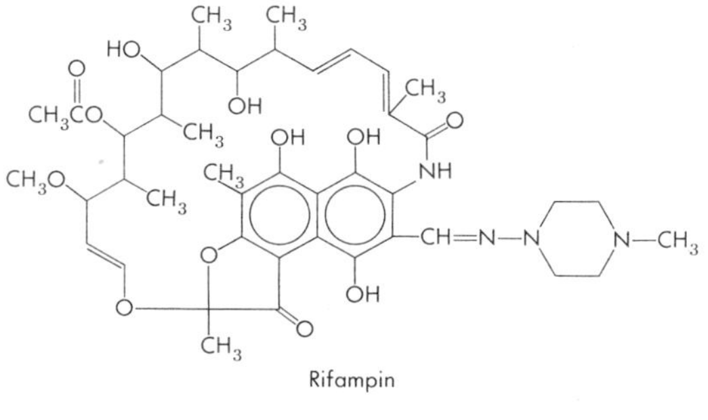

Rifampin

Antibacterial Activity. Rifampin inhibits the growth of most gram-positive bacteria, as well as many gram-negative microorganisms such as *Escherichia coli, Pseudomonas,* indole-positive and -negative *Proteus,* and *Klebsiella* (*see* Atlas and Turck, 1968; Kunin *et al.,* 1969). Rifampin is very active against *Staphylococcus aureus;* bactericidal concentrations range from 3 to 12 ng/ml (Tuazon *et al.,* 1978). The drug is also highly active against *Neisseria meningitidis* and *Haemophilus influenzae;* minimal inhibitory concentrations range from 0.1 to 0.8 μg/ml (Ivler *et al.,* 1970). Rifampin is also very inhibitory to *Legionella* species in cell culture and in animal models (Thornsberry *et al.,* 1983).

Rifampin in concentrations of 0.005 to 0.2 μg/ml inhibits the growth of *M. tuberculosis in vitro.* Among atypical mycobacteria, *M. kansasii* is inhibited by 0.25 to 1 μg/ml. The majority of strains of *M. scrofulaceum* and *M. intracellulare* are suppressed by concentrations of 4 μg/ml, but certain strains may be resistant to 16 μg/ml. *Mycobacterium fortuitum* is highly resistant to the drug (Molavi and Weinstein, 1971). Rifampin increases the *in-vitro* activity of streptomycin and isoniazid, but not that of ethambutol, against *M. tuberculosis* (Hobby and Lenert, 1972).

Bacterial Resistance. Microorganisms, including mycobacteria, may develop resistance to rifampin rapidly *in vitro* as a one-step process, and one of every 10^7 to 10^8 tubercle bacilli is resistant to the drug. This also appears to be the case *in vivo,* and therefore the antibiotic must not be used alone in the chemotherapy of tuberculosis. When rifampin has been used for eradication of the meningococcal carrier state, failures have been due to the appearance of drug-resistant bacteria after treatment for as short a period as 2 days (Devine *et al.,* 1971). Microbial resistance to rifampin is due to an alteration of the target of this drug, DNA-dependent RNA polymerase. Certain rifampin-resistant bacterial mutants have decreased virulence. Tuberculosis caused by rifampin-resistant mycobacteria has been described in patients who had not received prior chemotherapy, but this is very rare.

Mechanism of Action. Rifampin inhibits DNA-dependent RNA polymerase of mycobacteria and other microorganisms, leading to suppression of initiation of chain formation (but not chain elongation) in RNA synthesis. More specifically, the β subunit of this complex enzyme is the site of action of the drug. Nuclear RNA polymerase from a variety of eukaryotic cells does not bind rifampin, and RNA synthesis is correspondingly unaffected. While rifampin can inhibit RNA synthesis in mammalian mitochondria, considerably higher concentrations of the drug are required than for the inhibition of the bacterial enzyme. Rifampin is bactericidal for both intracellular and extracellular microorganisms. (*See* Wehrli, 1983.)

Absorption, Distribution, and Excretion. The oral administration of rifampin produces peak concentrations in plasma in 2 to 4 hours; after ingestion of 600 mg this value is about 7 μg/ml, but there is considerable variability. Aminosalicylic acid may delay the absorption of rifampin, and adequate plasma concentrations may not be reached. If these agents are used concurrently, they should be given separately at an interval of 8 to 12 hours (*see* Radner, 1973).

Following absorption from the gastrointestinal tract, rifampin is rapidly eliminated in the bile, and an enterohepatic circulation ensues. During this time there is progressive deacetylation of the drug, such that nearly all of the antibiotic in the bile is in the deacetylated form after 6 hours. This metabolite retains essentially full antibacterial activity. Intestinal reabsorption is reduced by deacetylation (as well as by food), and metabolism thus facilitates elimination of the drug. The half-life of rifampin varies from 1.5 to 5 hours and is increased in the presence of hepatic dysfunction; it may be *decreased* in patients receiving isoniazid concurrently who are slow inactivators of this drug. There is a progressive shortening of the half-life of rifampin by about 40% during the first 14 days of treatment, due to induction of hepatic microsomal enzymes with acceleration of deacetylation of the drug. Up to 30% of a dose of the drug is excreted in the urine; less than half of this may be unaltered antibiotic. Adjustment of dosage is *not* necessary in patients with impaired renal function.

Rifampin is distributed throughout the body and is present in effective concentrations in many organs and body fluids, including the CSF (Sippel *et al.,* 1974). This is perhaps best exemplified by the fact that the drug may impart an orange-red color to the urine, feces, saliva, sputum, tears, and sweat; patients should be so warned. (For various aspects of rifampin metabolism, *see* Furesz, 1970; Jenne and Beggs, 1973; Radner, 1973.)

Untoward Effects. Rifampin does not cause untoward effects with great frequency. When given in usual doses, less than 4% of patients with tuberculosis develop significant adverse reactions; the most common are *rash* (0.8%), *fever* (0.5%), and *nausea and vomiting* (1.5%) (*see* Grosset and Leventis, 1983). The most notable problem is the development of *jaundice* (Scheuer *et al.*, 1974). Sixteen deaths associated with this reaction have been recorded in 500,000 treated patients. Hepatitis from rifampin rarely occurs in patients with normal hepatic function; likewise, the combination of isoniazid and rifampin appears generally safe in such patients. However, chronic liver disease, alcoholism, and old age appear to increase the incidence of severe hepatic problems when rifampin is given alone or concurrently with isoniazid (Gronhagen-Riska *et al.*, 1978).

Administration of rifampin on an intermittent schedule (less than twice weekly) and/or daily doses of 1200 mg or greater is associated with frequent side effects, and the drug should not be used in this manner. A *flulike syndrome* with fever, chills, and myalgias develops in 20% of patients so treated. The syndrome may also include *eosinophilia, interstitial nephritis, acute tubular necrosis, thrombocytopenia, hemolytic anemia*, and *shock* (Flynn *et al.*, 1974; Girling and Hitze, 1979).

Since rifampin is a potent inducer of hepatic microsomal enzymes (Ohnhaus *et al.*, 1979), its administration results in a decreased half-life for a number of compounds, including prednisone, digitoxin, quinidine, ketoconazole, propranolol, metoprolol, clofibrate, and the sulfonylureas. There is a similar and significant interaction between rifampin and oral anticoagulants of the coumarin type, which leads to a decrease in efficacy of the latter agents. This appears about 5 to 8 days after rifampin administration is started and persists for 5 to 7 days after it is stopped (O'Reilly, 1975; Romankiewicz and Ehrman, 1975). Rifampin also appears to enhance the catabolism of a variety of steroids (Buffington *et al.*, 1976), and for this reason it decreases the effectiveness of oral contraceptives (Skolnick *et al.*, 1976). Methadone metabolism is also increased, and the precipitation of withdrawal syndromes has been reported. Rifampin may reduce biliary excretion of contrast media used for visualization of the gallbladder.

Gastrointestinal disturbances produced by rifampin (*epigastric distress, nausea, vomiting, abdominal cramps, diarrhea*) have occasionally required

discontinuation of the drug. Various symptoms related to the nervous system have also been noted, including *fatigue, drowsiness, headache, dizziness, ataxia, confusion, inability to concentrate, generalized numbness, pain in the extremities*, and *muscular weakness*. Among hypersensitivity reactions are *fever, pruritus, urticaria*, various types of *skin eruptions, eosinophilia*, and *soreness of the mouth and tongue. Hemolysis, hemoglobinuria, hematuria, renal insufficiency*, and *acute renal failure* have been observed rarely; these are also thought to be hypersensitivity reactions. *Thrombocytopenia, transient leukopenia*, and *anemia* have occurred during therapy. Since the potential teratogenicity of rifampin is unknown, it is best to avoid the use of this agent during pregnancy; the drug is known to cross the placenta.

Immunoglobulin light-chain proteinuria (either kappa, lambda, or both) has been noted by Graber and associates (1973) in about 85% of patients with tuberculosis treated with rifampin. None of the patients had symptoms or electrophoretic patterns compatible with myeloma. Renal failure has, however, been associated with light-chain proteinuria (Warrington *et al.*, 1977).

Rifampin suppresses the transformation of antigen-sensitized lymphocytes by the antigen. The administration of rifampin in conventional doses has been noted to suppress T-cell function (Gupta *et al.*, 1975) and cutaneous hypersensitivity to tuberculin (Mukerjee *et al.*, 1973). Rifampin also causes immunosuppression in animal models (Bassi *et al.*, 1973); this may be related to inhibition of protein synthesis by cells involved in the immune process (Buss *et al.*, 1978). However, rifampin does not suppress the antibody response to influenza vaccine (Albert *et al.*, 1978), and there is no evidence that rifampin-induced immunosuppression causes deleterious effects in patients receiving the drug (Farr and Mandell, 1982).

Preparations and Dosage. *Rifampin* (RIFADIN, RIMACTANE) is supplied in capsules containing 150 or 300 mg. The drug is also available as a fixed-dose combination with isoniazid (150 mg of isoniazid, 300 mg of rifampin; RIFAMATE). The dose for therapy of tuberculosis in adults is 600 mg, given once daily, either 1 hour before or 2 hours after a meal. Children should receive 10 mg/kg, with a daily maximum of 600 mg, given in the same way. Doses of 15 mg/kg or higher are associated with increased hepatotoxicity in children (3.2%) (Centers for Disease Control, 1980). Higher doses are reserved for other (short-term) uses. To prevent meningococcal disease (*see* below), adults and children may be treated with 600 mg twice daily or 20 mg/kg for 2 days. For prophylaxis of *H. influenzae* (type-B) meningitis, some authorities recommend a dose of 20 mg/kg daily for 4 days.

Therapeutic Status. Rifampin and isoniazid are the most effective drugs for the treatment of tuberculosis. Rifampin (like isoniazid) should never be used alone for this disease because of the rapidity with which resistance may develop. The combination of isoniazid and rifampin is probably as effective, for sensitive microorganisms, as are programs that utilize three or more agents (*see* British Thoracic and Tuberculosis Association, 1975). Despite the long list of untoward effects from rifampin, their incidence is low and treatment seldom has to be interrupted. The use of rifampin in the chemotherapy of tuberculosis is detailed below.

Rifampin is a drug of choice for chemoprophylaxis of meningococcal disease and meningitis due to *H. influenzae* in household contacts of patients with such infections. The drug also shows promise in the treatment of certain nonmycobacterial diseases (Symposium, 1983). Combined with a beta-lactam antibiotic or vancomycin, rifampin may be useful for therapy of selected cases of staphylococcal endocarditis (on both natural and prosthetic valves) or osteomyelitis, especially those caused by penicillin-"tolerant" staphylococci. Rifampin may be indicated for therapy of infections in patients with inadequate leukocytic bactericidal activity and for eradication of the staphylococcal nasal carrier state in patients with chronic furunculosis (Wheat *et al.*, 1983).

ETHAMBUTOL

Chemistry. Ethambutol is a water-soluble and heat-stable compound. The structural formula is as follows:

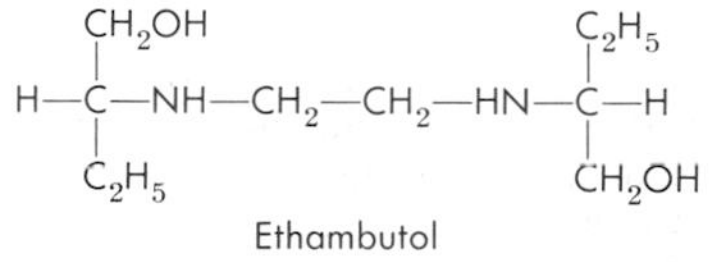

$$H-\underset{\underset{C_2H_5}{|}}{\overset{\overset{CH_2OH}{|}}{C}}-NH-CH_2-CH_2-HN-\underset{\underset{CH_2OH}{|}}{\overset{\overset{C_2H_5}{|}}{C}}-H$$

Ethambutol

Antibacterial Activity. Nearly all strains of *M. tuberculosis* and *M. kansasii* are sensitive to ethambutol. The sensitivities of other atypical organisms are variable (Karlson, 1961). Ethambutol has no effect on other bacteria. It suppresses the growth of most isoniazid- and streptomycin-resistant tubercle bacilli. Resistance to ethambutol develops very slowly and with difficulty *in vitro*.

Mycobacteria take up ethambutol rapidly when the drug is added to cultures that are in the exponential growth phase. However, growth is not significantly inhibited before about 24 hours; the drug is tuberculostatic. The mechanism of action of ethambutol is unknown (*see* Jenne and Beggs, 1973).

The therapeutic activity of ethambutol given orally to animals infected with *M. tuberculosis* is similar to that of isoniazid. When given parenterally, it is superior to streptomycin. Bacterial resistance to the drug develops *in vivo* when it is given in the absence of another effective agent.

Absorption, Distribution, and Excretion. About 75 to 80% of an orally administered dose of ethambutol is absorbed from the gastrointestinal tract. Concentrations in plasma are maximal in man 2 to 4 hours after the drug is taken and are proportional to the dose. A single dose of 15 mg/kg produces a plasma concentration of about 5 μg/ml at 2 to 4 hours. The drug has a half-life of 3 to 4 hours. One to two times as much ethambutol is present in the erythrocytes as in the plasma. Red blood cells thereby may serve as a depot from which the drug slowly enters the plasma.

Within 24 hours, two thirds of an ingested dose of ethambutol is excreted unchanged in the urine; up to 15% is excreted in the form of two metabolites, an aldehyde and a dicarboxylic acid derivative (Place and Thomas, 1963; Peets *et al.*, 1965). Renal clearance of ethambutol is approximately $7 \text{ ml} \cdot \text{min}^{-1} \cdot \text{kg}^{-1}$, and thus it is evident that the drug is excreted by tubular secretion in addition to glomerular filtration.

Preparations, Route of Administration, and Dosage. *Ethambutol hydrochloride* (MYAMBUTOL) is available in tablets containing 100 or 400 mg of the *d* isomer. The usual adult dose is 15 mg/kg, given once a day. Some physicians prefer to institute therapy with a dose of 25 mg/kg per day for the first 60 days and then to reduce the dose to 15 mg/kg per day.

Ethambutol accumulates in patients with impaired renal function, and adjustment of dosage is necessary (*see* Appendix II). Ethambutol is not recommended for children under 13 years of age because of concern about the ability to test their visual acuity reliably (*see* below).

Untoward Effects. Ethambutol produces very few reactions. Daily doses of 15 mg/kg are minimally toxic. Less than 2% of nearly 2000 patients who received 15 mg/kg of ethambutol developed adverse reactions; 0.8% experienced *diminished visual acuity*, 0.5% had a *rash*, and 0.3% developed *drug fever* (Pitts, 1977). Other side effects that have been observed are *pruritus, joint pain, gastrointestinal upset, abdominal pain,* *malaise, headache, dizziness, mental confusion, disorientation,* and possible *hallucination. Numbness* and *tingling of the fingers* due to *peripheral neuritis* are infrequent. *Anaphylaxis* and *leukopenia* are rare.

The most important side effect is *optic neuritis,* resulting in *decrease of visual acuity* and *loss of ability to differentiate red from green.* The incidence of this reaction is proportional to the dose of ethambutol and is observed in 15% of patients receiving 50 mg/kg per day, 5% of patients receiving 25 mg/kg per day, and less than 1% of patients receiving daily doses of 15 mg/kg. The intensity of the visual difficulty is related to the duration of therapy after decrease in visual acuity first becomes apparent, and it may be unilateral or bilateral. *Tests of visual acuity and red-green discrimination prior to the start of therapy and periodically thereafter are thus recommended.* Recovery usually occurs when ethambutol is withdrawn; the time required is a function of the degree of visual impairment (Place and Thomas, 1963).

Therapy with ethambutol results in an increased concentration of urate in the blood in about 50% of patients, due to decreased renal excretion of uric acid. The effect may be detectable as early as 24 hours after a single dose or as late as 90 days after treatment is started. This untoward effect is possibly enhanced by isoniazid and pyridoxine (Postlethwaite *et al.,* 1972).

Therapeutic Status. Ethambutol has been used with notable success in the therapy of tuberculosis of various forms when given concurrently with isoniazid. Because of a lower incidence of toxic side effects and better acceptance by patients, it has essentially replaced aminosalicylic acid (*see* Bobrowitz, 1974).

The use of ethambutol in the chemotherapy of tuberculosis is described below.

STREPTOMYCIN

A discussion of the pharmacology of streptomycin, including its adverse effects and its uses in infections other than tuberculosis, is presented in Chapter 51. Only those features of the drug related to its anti-

bacterial activity and therapeutic effects in the management of diseases caused by mycobacteria are considered here.

History. Streptomycin was the first clinically effective drug to become available for the treatment of tuberculosis, and from 1947 to 1952 it was the only effective agent available to treat the disease. At first, it was given in large doses, but problems related to toxicity and the development of resistant microorganisms seriously limited its usefulness. This led to administration of the antibiotic in smaller quantities, but streptomycin administered alone still proved to be far from the ideal agent for the management of all forms of this disease. However, after the discovery of other tuberculostatic compounds that, given concurrently with the antibiotic, reduced the rate at which microorganisms became drug resistant despite prolonged exposure, streptomycin reached its full potential in the therapy of tuberculosis.

Antibacterial Activity. Streptomycin is bactericidal for the tubercle bacillus *in vitro.* Concentrations as low as 0.4 μg/ml may inhibit growth. The vast majority of strains of *M. tuberculosis* are sensitive to 10 μg/ml. *M. kansasii* is frequently sensitive, but other atypical mycobacteria are only occasionally susceptible.

The activity of streptomycin *in vivo* is essentially suppressive. When the antibiotic is administered to experimental animals prior to inoculation with the tubercle bacillus, the development of disease is not prevented. Infection progresses until the animals' immunological mechanisms respond. The presence of viable microorganisms in nonsloughing abscesses at the sites of injection and in the regional lymph nodes, together with the fact that omission of the drug, after many months of therapy, results in rapid spread of infection, adds support to the concept that the activity of streptomycin *in vivo* is to suppress, not to eradicate, the tubercle bacillus. This may be related to the observation that streptomycin does not readily enter living cells and thus cannot kill intracellular microbes.

Bacterial Resistance. Large populations of all strains of tubercle bacilli include a number of cells that are markedly resistant to the antibiotic because of mutation. However, primary resistance to streptomycin is found in only 2 to 3% of isolates of *M. tuberculosis.*

Selection for resistant tubercle bacilli occurs *in vivo* as it does *in vitro.* In general, the longer therapy is continued, the greater is the incidence of resistance to streptomycin. When streptomycin was used alone, as many as 80% of patients harbored insensitive tubercle bacilli after 4 months of treatment; many of these microorganisms were not inhibited by concentrations of drug as high as 1000 μg/ml.

Preparations, Routes of Administration, and Dosage. The preparations and routes of administration of streptomycin are considered in detail in Chapter 51. The dosage schedules used in the treatment of various forms of tuberculosis are discussed below.

Untoward Effects. Untoward effects of streptomycin are considered in detail in Chapter 51. Of 515 patients with tuberculosis who were treated with this aminoglycoside, 8.2% developed adverse reactions; half of these involved the auditory and vestibular functions of the eighth cranial nerve, and other relatively frequent problems included rash (in 2%) and fever (in 1.4%) (Pitts, 1977).

Therapeutic Status. Since other effective agents have become available, the use of streptomycin for the treatment of pulmonary tuberculosis has been sharply reduced. Many clinicians prefer to give three drugs, of which streptomycin may be one, for the most serious forms of tuberculosis, such as disseminated disease or meningitis.

The use of streptomycin in the chemotherapy of tuberculosis is described below.

PYRAZINAMIDE

Chemistry. Pyrazinamide is the synthetic pyrazine analog of nicotinamide. It has the following structural formula:

Pyrazinamide

Antibacterial Activity. Pyrazinamide exhibits bactericidal activity *in vitro* only at a slightly acidic pH. Tubercle bacilli within monocytes *in vitro* are killed by the drug at a concentration of 12.5 μg/ml. Resistance develops rapidly if pyrazinamide is used alone.

Absorption, Distribution, and Excretion. Pyrazinamide is well absorbed from the gastrointestinal tract, and it is widely distributed throughout the body. The oral administration of 1 g produces plasma concentrations of about 45 μg/ml at 2 hours and 10 μg/ml at 15 hours. The drug is excreted primarily by renal glomerular filtration; urinary concentrations are 50 to 100 μg/ml for several hours after a single dose (Stottmeier *et al.*, 1968). Pyrazinamide is hydrolyzed to pyrazinoic acid and subsequently hydroxylated to 5-hydroxypyrazinoic acid, the major excretory product (Weiner and Tinker, 1972).

Preparation, Route of Administration, and Dosage. *Pyrazinamide* is marketed in tablets containing 500 mg. The daily dosage is 20 to 35 mg/kg orally, given in three or four equally spaced doses.

The maximal quantity to be given is 3 g per day, regardless of weight.

Untoward Effects. Injury to the *liver* is the most common and serious side effect of pyrazinamide. When a dose of 3 g per day (40 to 50 mg/kg) is administered orally, signs and symptoms of hepatic disease appear in about 15% of patients, jaundice supervenes in 2 to 3%, and death due to *hepatic necrosis* results in rare instances (McDermott *et al.*, 1954). Elevations of the plasma glutamic-oxalacetic and glutamic-pyruvate transaminases are the earliest abnormalities produced by the drug. Regimens employed currently (20 to 35 mg/kg per day) are much safer (Girling, 1978; Zierski and Bek, 1980; Pilheu *et al.*, 1981). All patients who are being treated with pyrazinamide should have studies of hepatic function carried out before the drug is administered; these should be repeated at frequent intervals during the entire period of treatment. If evidence of significant hepatic damage becomes apparent, therapy must be stopped. Pyrazinamide should not be given to individuals with any degree of hepatic dysfunction, unless this is absolutely unavoidable.

The drug inhibits excretion of urate, and acute episodes of gout have occurred. Among other untoward effects that have been observed with pyrazinamide are *arthralgias, anorexia, nausea and vomiting, dysuria, malaise,* and *fever*.

Therapeutic Status. Pyrazinamide has become an important component of short-term (6-month) multiple-drug therapy, especially for ambulatory patients in underdeveloped countries where primary resistance is high (Zierski and Bek, 1980; Dutt and Stead, 1982; British Thoracic Association, 1983).

ETHIONAMIDE

Chemistry. Synthesis and study of a variety of congeners of thioisonicotinamide revealed that an alpha-ethyl derivative, ethionamide, is considerably more effective than the parent compound. Ethionamide is a yellow substance, practically insoluble in water, with a faint-to-moderate sulfide odor. It has the following structural formula:

Ethionamide

Antibacterial Activity. The multiplication of human strains of *M. tuberculosis* is suppressed by concentrations of ethionamide ranging from 0.6 to 2.5 μg/ml. Resistance can develop rapidly *in vitro*. Approximately 75% of photochromogenic mycobacteria are inhibited by a concentration of 10 μg/ml or less; the scotochromogens are more resistant. Ethionamide is very effective in the treatment of experimental tuberculosis in animals, although its activity varies greatly with the animal model studied.

Absorption, Distribution, and Excretion. The oral administration of 1 g of ethionamide yields peak concentrations in plasma of about 20 μg/ml in 3 hours; the concentration at 9 hours is 3 μg/ml. The drug has a shorter half-life than does isoniazid. About 50% of patients are unable to tolerate a single dose larger than 500 mg because of gastrointestinal intolerance.

Ethionamide is rapidly and widely distributed; the concentrations in the blood and various organs are approximately equal. Significant concentrations are present in CSF. Ethionamide, like aminosalicylic acid, inhibits the acetylation of isoniazid *in vitro*.

Less than 1% of ethionamide is excreted in active form in the urine. Metabolites detected in the urine include three dihydropyridines: carbamoyl, thiocarbamoyl, and S-oxocarbamoyl (Bieder *et al.*, 1966).

Preparation, Route of Administration, and Dosage. *Ethionamide* (TRECATOR-SC) is administered only by the oral route. Tablets containing 250 mg of the drug are available. The initial dose for adults is 250 mg, given twice a day. This is increased by 125 mg per day every 5 days until 1 g is being given daily; this dose must not be exceeded. The drug is best taken with meals in order to minimize gastric irritation.

Untoward Effects. The most common reactions to ethionamide are *anorexia, nausea,* and *vomiting*. A metallic taste may also be noted. *Severe postural hypotension, mental depression, drowsiness,* and *asthenia* are common. *Convulsions* and *peripheral neuropathy* are rare. Other reactions referable to the nervous system include *olfactory disturbances, blurred vision, diplopia, dizziness, paresthesias, headache, restlessness,* and *tremors. Severe allergic skin rashes, purpura, stomatitis, gynecomastia, impotence, menorrhagia, acne,* and *alopecia* have also been observed. *Hepatitis* has been associated with the use of the drug in about 5% of cases (Simon *et al.*, 1969). The signs and symptoms of hepatotoxicity clear when treatment is stopped. Hepatic function should be assessed at regular intervals in patients receiving ethionamide.

Therapeutic Status. Ethionamide is a secondary agent, to be used concurrently with other drugs only when therapy with primary agents is ineffective or contraindicated. (*See* Schwartz, 1966.)

AMINOSALICYLIC ACID

Chemistry. The structural formula of aminosalicylic acid is as follows:

Aminosalicylic Acid

Antibacterial Activity. Aminosalicylic acid is bacteriostatic. *In vitro,* most strains of *M. tuberculosis* are sensitive to a concentration of 1 μg/ml. The antimicrobial activity of aminosalicylic acid is highly specific, and microorganisms other than *M. tuberculosis* are unaffected. Most atypical mycobacteria are not inhibited by the drug.

Studies of the treatment of experimental infections caused by *M. tuberculosis* indicate that this drug exerts a beneficial effect on the disease. However, the doses of aminosalicylic acid required are relatively large, and the compound must be present continuously. Aminosalicylic acid alone is of little value in the treatment of tuberculosis in man; it is much less effective than either streptomycin, isoniazid, or rifampin.

Bacterial Resistance. Strains of tubercle bacilli insensitive to several hundred times the usual bacteriostatic concentration of aminosalicylic acid can be produced *in vitro*. In general, resistance to aminosalicylic acid is somewhat more difficult to induce *in vitro* than is that to streptomycin.

Resistant strains of tubercle bacilli also emerge in patients treated with aminosalicylic acid, but much more slowly than with streptomycin.

Mechanism of Action. Aminosalicylic acid is a structural analog of para-aminobenzoic acid, and its mechanism of action appears to be very similar to that of the sulfonamides (*see* Chapter 49). Since the sulfonamides are ineffective against *M. tuberculosis* and aminosalicylic acid is inactive against sulfonamide-susceptible bacteria, it is probable that the enzymes responsible for folate biosynthesis in various microorganisms may be quite exacting in their capacity to distinguish various analogs from the true metabolite.

Absorption, Distribution, and Excretion. Aminosalicylic acid is readily absorbed from the gastrointestinal tract. A single oral dose of 4 g of the free acid produces maximal concentrations in plasma of about 75 μg/ml within 1.5 to 2 hours. The sodium salt is absorbed even more rapidly. The drug appears to be distributed throughout the total body water and reaches high concentrations in pleural fluid and caseous tissue. However, values in CSF are low, perhaps because of active outward transport (Spector and Lorenzo, 1973).

The drug has a half-life of about 1 hour, and concentrations in plasma are negligible within 4 to 5 hours after a single conventional dose. Over 80% of the drug is excreted in the urine; more than 50% is in the form of the acetylated compound in man. The largest portion of the remainder is made up of the free acid; small quantities of free and acetylated para-aminosalicyluric and 2,4-dihydroxybenzoic acids are present in the urine. Excretion of aminosalicylic acid is greatly retarded in the presence of renal dysfunction, and the use of the drug is not recommended in such patients. Probenecid decreases the renal excretion of this agent.

Preparation, Routes of Administration, and Dosage. *Aminosalicylate sodium* (TEEBACIN) is available in tablets containing 500 or 1000 mg. Aminosalicylic acid is administered orally in a daily dose of 8 to 12 g. To obtain an equivalent amount of aminosalicylic acid, the dose of the Na^+ salt must be increased 38%. Because it is a gastric irritant, the drug is best administered after meals, the daily intake being divided into three or four equal-sized doses.

Untoward Effects. The incidence of untoward effects associated with the use of aminosalicylic acid is approximately 10 to 30%. Gastrointestinal problems, including anorexia, nausea, epigastric pain, abdominal distress, and diarrhea, are predominant (Pitts, 1977), and patients with peptic ulcer tolerate the drug poorly. Compliance is often poor because of gastrointestinal distress. Hypersensitivity reactions to aminosalicylic acid are seen in 5 to 10% of patients. *High fever* may develop abruptly, with intermittent spiking, or it may appear gradually and be low grade. *Generalized malaise, joint pains,* or *sore throat* may be present at the same time. *Skin eruptions of various types* appear as isolated reactions or accompany the fever. Among the hematological abnormalities that have been observed are *leukopenia, agranulocytosis, eosinophilia, lymphocytosis,* an atypical mononucleosis syndrome, and *thrombocytopenia. Acute hemolytic anemia* may appear in some instances.

Therapeutic Status. Aminosalicylic acid is now a "second-line" agent. Its importance in the management of pulmonary and other forms of tuberculosis has markedly decreased since more active and better tolerated drugs, such as rifampin and ethambutol, have been developed (*see* discussion of chemotherapy of tuberculosis, below).

CYCLOSERINE

Cycloserine is a broad-spectrum antibiotic produced by *Streptomyces orchidaceus.* It was first isolated from a fermentation brew in 1955 and was later synthesized.

Chemistry. Cycloserine is D-4-amino-3-isoxazolidone; the structural formula is as follows:

Cycloserine

The drug is stable in alkaline solution but is rapidly destroyed when exposed to neutral or acidic pH.

Antibacterial Activity and Mechanism of Action. Cycloserine is inhibitory for *M. tuberculosis* in concentrations of 5 to 20 μg/ml *in vitro.* There is no cross-resistance between cycloserine and other tuberculostatic agents. While the antibiotic is effective in experimental infections caused by other microorganisms, studies *in vitro* reveal no suppression of growth in cultures made in conventional media. Hoeprich (1963) determined that this is due to the presence of D-alanine in the commonly used

culture media and that the amino acid blocks the antibacterial activity of cycloserine. The two compounds are structural analogs, and cycloserine inhibits reactions in which D-alanine is involved in bacterial cell-wall synthesis (*see* Chapter 50). The use of media free of D-alanine reveals that the antibiotic inhibits the growth *in vitro* of enterococci, paracolon strains, *E. coli, Staphylococcus aureus, Nocardia* species, and *Chlamydia.*

Absorption, Distribution, and Excretion. When given orally, cycloserine is rapidly absorbed. Peak concentrations in plasma are reached 3 to 4 hours after a single dose and are in the range of 20 to 35 μg/ml in children who receive 20 mg/kg; only small quantities are present after 12 hours. In adults, doses of 750 mg, given at 6-hour intervals, produce plasma concentrations in excess of 50 μg/ml. Multiple doses lead to accumulation of the drug in the circulation after 3 days.

Cycloserine is distributed throughout body fluids and tissues. There is no appreciable blood-brain barrier to the drug, and CSF concentrations in all patients are approximately the same as those in plasma.

About 50% of a parenteral dose of cycloserine is excreted, in unchanged form, in the urine in the first 12 hours; a total of 65% is recoverable in the active form over a period of 72 hours. Approximately 35% of the antibiotic is metabolized. The drug may accumulate to toxic concentrations in patients with renal insufficiency; it may be removed from the circulation by dialysis.

Preparation, Route of Administration, and Dosage. *Cycloserine* (SEROMYCIN) is available in capsules containing 250 mg for oral administration. The usual dose for adults is 250 mg twice a day; this is associated with a small risk of toxic reactions. In more severely ill individuals, 500 mg may be given twice a day for short periods. The dose should be adjusted to yield plasma concentrations no greater than 30 μg/ml in order to minimize toxicity.

Untoward Effects. Reactions to cycloserine most commonly involve the central nervous system (CNS). They tend to appear within the first 2 weeks of therapy and usually disappear when the drug is withdrawn. Among the *central manifestations* are somnolence, headache, tremor, dysarthria, vertigo, confusion, nervousness, irritability, psychotic states with suicidal tendencies, paranoid reactions, catatonic and depressed reactions, twitching, ankle clonus, hyperreflexia, visual disturbances, paresis, and tonic-clonic or absence seizures. Large doses of cycloserine or the ingestion of ethyl alcohol increases the risk of seizures. Cycloserine is contraindicated in individuals with a history of epilepsy and may be dangerous in persons who are depressed or are experiencing severe anxiety.

Therapeutic Status. Cycloserine should be used only when re-treatment is necessary or when microorganisms are resistant to other drugs. When cycloserine is employed to treat tuberculosis, it must be given together with other effective agents.

OTHER DRUGS

The agents grouped in this section are similar in several aspects. They are all "second-line" drugs that are used only for therapy of disease caused by resistant microorganisms or by atypical mycobacteria. They all must be given parenterally, and they have similar pharmacokinetics and toxicity. Since these agents are potentially ototoxic and nephrotoxic, two drugs in this group should not be employed simultaneously, and they should not be used in combination with streptomycin.

Kanamycin, an aminoglycoside that is discussed in Chapter 51, inhibits the growth of *M. tuberculosis in vitro* in a concentration of 10 μg/ml or less. Small groups of patients with tuberculosis have been treated with 1 g of kanamycin daily, and a slight therapeutic effect has been observed; toxic effects have been common.

Amikacin is also an aminoglycoside (*see* Chapter 51). It is extremely active against several mycobacterial species and may become an important drug for treatment of disease caused by atypical mycobacteria (*see* Sanders *et al.*, 1976; Dalovisio and Pankey, 1978).

Capreomycin is an antimycobacterial cyclic peptide elaborated by *Streptomyces capreolus*. It consists of four active components—capreomycins IA, IB, IIA, and IIB—the structures of which have largely been elucidated by Bycroft and associates (1971). The agent used clinically contains primarily IA and IB. The drug is effective both *in vitro* and in experimental tuberculosis (Wilson, 1967). Bacterial resistance to capreomycin develops when it is given alone; such microorganisms show cross-resistance with kanamycin.

Capreomycin must be given intramuscularly. The recommended daily dose is 20 mg/kg or 1 g for 60 to 120 days, followed by 1 g two to three times a week. Capreomycin should be administered together with another effective tuberculostatic agent. It has proven of value in the therapy of "resistant," or treatment-failure, tuberculosis when given with ethambutol or isoniazid (Wilson, 1967; Donomae, 1968). *Capreomycin sulfate* (CAPASTAT SULFATE) is supplied in vials containing 1 g of the drug.

The reactions associated with the use of capreomycin are hearing loss, tinnitus, transient proteinuria, cylindruria, and nitrogen retention. Severe renal failure is rare. Eosinophilia is common. Leukocytosis, leukopenia, rashes, and fever have also been observed. Injections of the drug may be painful.

CHEMOTHERAPY OF TUBERCULOSIS

The availability of effective agents has so altered the treatment of tuberculosis that most patients are now treated in the ambulatory setting. Patients with tuberculosis are admitted to general hospitals. After a period sufficient to establish the diagnosis and to initiate and stabilize therapy, patients may, with uncommon exception, be returned to their homes. Prolonged bed rest is not necessary or even helpful in speeding recovery. The patients must be seen at frequent intervals to follow the course of their disease and treatment. The local health department should be notified of all cases. Contacts should be investigated for the possibility of disease and for the appropriateness of prophylactic therapy with isoniazid.

The vast majority of previously untreated tuberculosis in the United States is caused by microorganisms that are sensitive to isoniazid, rifampin, ethambutol, and streptomycin. To prevent the development of resistance to these agents that frequently occurs *during* the course of therapy of the individual patient, *treatment must include at least two drugs to which the bacteria are sensitive.* Isoniazid should be included in such a regimen if at all possible, and rifampin should be used if isoniazid cannot be given. The combination of isoniazid and rifampin is probably the most effective treatment available. However, in life-threatening disease, large cavitary disease, or renal tuberculosis, three drugs should be used initially to be certain that the mycobacteria are sensitive to at least two of them.

Therapy of Specific Types of Tuberculosis. Optimal therapy for uncomplicated *pulmonary tuberculosis* consists of isoniazid, 5 mg/kg (up to 300 mg per day), plus rifampin, 600 mg once daily. Pyridoxine, 15 to 50 mg per day, should also be included for most adults. The usual regimen for infants and children is isoniazid, 10 to 20 mg/kg per day (300 mg maximum), plus rifampin, 10 mg/kg per day (600 mg maximum). Therapy should be continued for 9 to 12 months (American Thoracic Society, 1980). Another effective regimen for mild or moderately severe pulmonary tuberculosis is isoniazid (300 mg daily) plus ethambutol (15 mg/kg per day) for 18 to 24 months. Six-month programs that include isoniazid, rifampin, streptomycin, and pyrazinamide (the latter two drugs for 2 months) have been effective and may be useful in selected patients. Surgery is rarely indicated (Kucers and Bennett, 1979; Hopewell, 1983; Des Prez and Goodwin, 1985).

Certain patients should receive three drugs initially to ensure that the microorganisms will be susceptible to at least two of the agents. These patients include: (1) those known to have been exposed to drug-resistant microorganisms; (2) Asians and Hispanics, especially if they are recent immigrants; (3) those with miliary tuberculosis or other extrapulmonary disease; (4) those with meningitis; and (5) those with extensive pulmonary disease. The microorganisms should be cultured for determination of their sensitivity to antimicrobial agents, but results will not be available for several weeks. The third agent may be either ethambutol or streptomycin (1 g daily). The dosage of streptomycin is reduced to 1 g twice weekly after 2 months.

Clinical improvement is readily discernible in the vast majority of patients with pulmonary tuberculosis if the treatment is appropriate. Efficacy usually becomes obvious within the first 2 weeks of therapy and is evidenced by a reduction of fever, decrease in cough, gain in weight, and increase in the sense of well-being. There is also progressive roentgenographic improvement. Over 90% of patients who receive optimal treatment will have negative cultures within 3 to 6 months, depending on the severity of the disease. Cultures that remain positive after 6 months frequently yield resistant microorganisms; the value of using an alternative therapeutic program should then be considered.

Disseminated tuberculosis, including tuberculous meningitis and cases with renal, bone, or joint involvement, is treated initially with isoniazid and rifampin plus either ethambutol or streptomycin. While some clinicians increase the dose of isoniazid to 10 mg/kg in these conditions, this is not of proven benefit. When the microorganisms are found to be susceptible to both isoniazid and rifampin, the third drug may be discontinued.

Failure of chemotherapy may be due to (1) irregular or inadequate therapy (resulting in persistent or resistant mycobacteria) due to poor patient compliance during the protracted therapeutic regimen; (2) the use of a single drug, with interruption necessitated by toxicity or hypersensitivity; (3) an inadequate initial regimen; or (4) the primary resistance of the microorganism.

Problems in Chemotherapy. *Bacterial Resistance to Drugs.* One of the more important problems in the chemotherapy of tuberculosis is bacterial resistance. For this reason concurrent administration of two or more drugs should be employed in the treatment of all active tuberculous disease.

A spate of publications has appeared on the incidence of resistance of bacilli isolated from untreated patients. Results depend on the population studied (*e.g.,* patients in Veterans Administration hospitals harbor more resistant microorganisms than do those in the United States as a whole), geographical location, and ethnic and socioeconomic factors. Most observers believe that the frequency of bacterial resistance is presently not rising at a rate such that the effectiveness of programs of concurrent drug therapy is threatened (Centers for Disease Control, 1983). However, *the physician must obtain sensitivity data at the beginning of therapy to assure the selection of a proper combination of drugs.* Disease caused by strains of *M. tuberculosis* that are found to be resistant to the drugs being used should be treated with two or three drugs to which the microorganisms are known to be susceptible.

Where drug resistance is suspected but sensitivities are not yet known (such as in patients who have undergone several courses of treatment), therapy should be instituted with five or six drugs, including two or three that the patient has not received in the past. Such a program might include isoniazid, rifampin, ethambutol, streptomycin, pyrazinamide, and ethionamide. Some physicians include isoniazid in the therapeutic regimen even if microorganisms are resistant because of some evidence that disease with isoniazid-resistant mycobacteria does not "progress" during such therapy. Others prefer to discontinue isoniazid to lessen the possibility of toxicity. Therapy should be continued for at least 24 months.

Nontuberculous (Atypical) Mycobacteria. These microorganisms have been recovered from a variety of lesions in man. Because they are frequently resistant to many of the commonly used agents, they must be examined for sensitivity *in vitro* and drug therapy selected on this basis. In some instances, surgical removal of the infected tissue followed by long-term treatment with effective agents is necessary.

Mycobacterium kansasii causes disease similar to that caused by *M. tuberculosis* but it may be milder. The microorganisms may be resistant to isoniazid. Therapy with isoniazid, rifampin, and ethambutol has been successful (Davidson, 1976; Nicholson, 1976; Pezzia *et al.,* 1981). *Mycobacterium avium-intracellulare* complex (also known as Battey bacillus) can cause a disease with symptoms that resemble chronic bronchitis. Cavities are found in the lung in most patients. The microorganisms are often highly resistant to drugs *in vitro.* Therapy with isoniazid, rifampin, streptomycin, ethambutol, and cycloserine has been successful (*see* Sanders, 1985). Patients with acquired immunodeficiency syndrome are a special problem, since they develop disseminated disease that progresses rapidly. *Ansamycin,* an experimental rifamycin, and *clofazimine* (*see* below) plus other drugs have been used, but results of therapy have been poor (Sanfilippo *et al.,* 1980; Greene *et al.,* 1982). *Mycobacterium marinum* causes skin lesions. A combination of rifampin and ethambutol is probably effective; minocycline (Loria, 1976) or tetracycline is active *in vitro* and is used by some physicians (Izumi *et al.,* 1977). *Mycobacterium scrofulaceum* causes cervical lymphadenitis, especially in children. Surgical excision still seems to be the therapy of choice (Lincoln and Gilberg, 1972). Microbes of the *M. fortuitum* complex (including *M. chelonei*) are usually saprophytes, but they may cause chronic lung disease and infections of skin and soft tissues. The microorganisms are highly resistant to most drugs, but amikacin, cefoxitin, and tetracyclines are active *in vitro* (Sanders *et al.,* 1977; Sanders, 1982).

Chemoprophylaxis of Tuberculosis. Prophylactic therapy can effectively prevent the development of active tuberculosis in certain instances (Des Prez and Goodwin, 1985). There are three categories of patients for whom prophylactic therapy should be considered: those exposed to tuberculosis but who have no evidence of infection; those with infection (positive tuberculin test; more than 10 mm of induration to 5 units of PPD) and no apparent disease; and those with a history of tuberculosis but in whom the disease is presently "inactive" (*see* Public Health Service, 1974; Edwards, 1977; Snider and Farer, 1978).

Household contacts and other close associates of patients with tuberculosis who have negative tuberculin tests should receive isoniazid for at least 3 months after the contact has been broken. This is especially important for children. If the tuberculin skin test becomes positive, therapy should be continued for 12 months.

Persons without apparent disease whose skin test has converted from negative to positive within the preceding 2 years should probably receive isoniazid for 12 months. These patients are considered to be "infected" but not to have clinical disease. Some authorities feel that those with positive skin tests, no matter when they became so, who are under 35 years of age or who are at risk of infection because of such factors as immunosuppressive therapy, leukemia, lymphoma, or silicosis should receive isoniazid for 1 year (Comstock, 1981). Others feel that the benefit of preventive therapy does not clearly outweigh the risk of toxicity (Taylor *et al.*, 1981).

Patients with old "inactive" tuberculosis who have not received adequate chemotherapy in the past should be considered for 1 year of treatment with isoniazid (*see* Comstock, 1983).

Prophylaxis with isoniazid is contraindicated for patients who have hepatic disease or who have had reactions to the drug. There are insufficient data on the advisability of prophylaxis with alternative drugs, such as rifampin. In pregnant women, prophylaxis should usually be delayed until after delivery (Public Health Service, 1974). For prophylaxis, isoniazid is generally given to adults in a daily dose of 300 mg. Children should receive 10 mg/kg to a maximal daily dose of 300 mg.

II. Drugs for Leprosy

Although leprosy is rarely seen in the United States, it is estimated that there are 12 million patients with this disease worldwide (WHO, 1977). Most patients can be managed outside of hospitals because of the development of effective chemotherapy for leprosy.

SULFONES

The sulfones, as a class, are derivatives of 4,4'-diaminodiphenylsulfone (dapsone, DDS), all of which have certain pharmacological properties in common. They are discussed here as a class; only *dapsone* and *sulfoxone* will be considered individually.

History. The sulfones first attracted interest because of their chemical relationship to the sulfonamides. Dapsone was found in 1937 to be 30 times

more active and only 15 times as toxic as sulfanilamide when used in streptococcal infections in mice. In the 1940s sulfones were found to be effective in suppressing experimental infections with the tubercle bacillus and for rat leprosy; this was soon followed by successful clinical trials in human leprosy. The sulfones are presently the most important drugs for the treatment of this disorder.

Chemistry. All the sulfones of clinical value are derivatives of dapsone. Despite the study and development of a large variety of sulfones, this drug remains the agent most useful clinically. The structures of dapsone and sulfoxone sodium are as follows:

$$H_2N-\text{C}_6H_4-\underset{O}{\overset{O}{\text{S}}}-\text{C}_6H_4-NH_2$$

Dapsone

$$NaO_2SCH_2NH-\text{C}_6H_4-\underset{O}{\overset{O}{\text{S}}}-\text{C}_6H_4-NHCH_2SO_2Na$$

Sulfoxone Sodium

Antibacterial Activity. Because *Mycobacterium leprae* does not grow on artificial media, conventional methods cannot be applied to determine its susceptibility to potential therapeutic agents *in vitro*. Crude sensitivities *in vivo* can be determined by injecting microorganisms into the foot pads of mice and treating them with the agents to be tested. After 6 to 8 months the mice are sacrificed, foot pads are homogenized, and microscopic counts are made of acid-fast microorganisms (Shepard *et al.*, 1976). Dapsone is bacteriostatic, but not bactericidal, for *M. leprae*, and the estimated sensitivity to the drug is between 1 and 10 ng/ml for microorganisms recovered from untreated patients (Levy and Peters, 1976). *Mycobacterium leprae* may become resistant to the drug during therapy.

The mechanism of action of the sulfones is probably similar to that of the sulfonamides since both possess approximately the same range of antibacterial activity and both are antagonized by para-aminobenzoic acid.

Dapsone-resistant strains of *M. leprae* are termed "secondary" if they emerge during therapy. This is usually seen in lepromatous (multibacillary) patients treated with a single drug. The incidence is as high as 19% (WHO Study Group, 1982). Partial-to-complete primary resistance (seen in previously untreated patients) has been described in from 2.5 to 40% of patients, depending on geographical location (Centers for Disease Control, 1982).

Untoward Effects. The reactions induced by various sulfones are very similar. The most common untoward effect is *hemolysis* of varying degree. This develops in almost every individual treated with 200 to 300 mg of dapsone per day. Doses of 100 mg or less in normal healthy persons and 50 mg or less in healthy individuals with a glucose-6-phosphate dehydrogenase deficiency do not cause hemolysis (DeGowin, 1967). *Methemoglobinemia* is also common, and Heinz-body formation may occur. While diminished red-cell survival usually occurs during the use of sulfones, and is presumed to be a dose-related effect of their oxidizing activity, *hemolytic anemia* is unusual unless there is a disorder either of the erythrocytes or of the bone marrow (Pengelly, 1963). The hemolysis may be so severe that manifestations of hypoxia become striking.

Anorexia, nausea, and *vomiting* may follow the oral administration of sulfones. Isolated instances of *headache, nervousness, insomnia, blurred vision, paresthesia, reversible peripheral neuropathy* (thought to be due to axonal degeneration), *drug fever, hematuria, pruritus, psychosis,* and a variety of *skin rashes* have been reported (Rapoport and Guss, 1972). An *infectious mononucleosis–like syndrome,* which may be fatal, occurs occasionally (Leiker, 1956). The sulfones may induce an *exacerbation of lepromatous leprosy;* this is thought to be analogous to the Jarisch-Herxheimer reaction. This "sulfone syndrome" may develop 5 to 6 weeks after initiation of treatment in malnourished people. Its manifestations include fever, malaise, exfoliative dermatitis, jaundice with hepatic necrosis, lymphadenopathy, methemoglobinemia, and anemia (DeGowin, 1967).

The sulfones may be given safely for many years in doses adequate for the successful therapy of leprosy if proper precautions are observed. Treatment should be initiated with a small dose and the quantity then increased gradually. Patients must be under consistent and prolonged laboratory and clinical supervision. The reactions induced by the sulfones, especially those related to exacerbation of the leprosy, may be very severe and may require the cessation of treatment as well as the institution of specific measures to reduce the threat to life.

Absorption, Distribution, and Excretion. Dapsone is slowly and nearly completely absorbed from the gastrointestinal tract. The disubstituted sulfones, such as sulfoxone, are incompletely absorbed when administered orally, and large amounts are excreted in the feces. Peak concentrations of dapsone in plasma are reached in 1 to 3 hours after administration, and its half-life of elimination ranges from 10 to 50 hours, with a mean of 28 hours. Twenty-four hours after oral ingestion of 100 mg, plasma concentrations range from 0.4 to 1.2 μg/ml (Shepard *et al.,* 1976), and a dose of 100 mg of dapsone per day produces an average of 2 μg of "free" dapsone per gram of blood or nonhepatic tissue. About 70% of the drug is bound to plasma protein. Concentrations in plasma following conventional doses of sulfoxone sodium are 10 to 15 μg/ml. These values fall relatively rapidly; however, appreciable quantities are still present at 8 hours.

The sulfones are distributed throughout the total body water and are present in all tissues. They tend to be retained in skin and muscle, and especially in liver and kidney; traces of the drug are present in these organs up to 3 weeks after therapy is stopped. The sulfones are retained in the circulation for a long time because of intestinal reabsorption from the bile; periodic interruption of treatment is advisable for this reason. Dapsone is acetylated in the liver, and the degree of acetylation is genetically determined.

The urinary excretion of sulfones varies with the type of drug; about 70 to 80% of a dose of dapsone is so excreted. The drug is present in urine as an acid-labile mono-N-glucuronide and mono-N-sulfamate in addition to an unknown number of unidentified metabolites (Shepard, 1969). Probenecid decreases the urinary excretion of the acid-labile dapsone metabolites significantly and that of free dapsone to a lesser extent (Goodwin and Sparell, 1969).

Preparations, Route of Administration, and Dosage. *Dapsone (DDS)* is available in tablets containing 25 or 100 mg. It is given by the oral route. Several dosage schedules have been recommended (*see* Trautman, 1965; Bullock, 1985). Daily therapy with 50 mg has been successful in adults. If the clinical response is not adequate, the daily dose may be increased to 100 mg. Doses of 100 to 400 mg twice weekly have also been effective. Therapy is usually begun with smaller amounts, and dosage is increased to those recommended by 1 to 2 months. Therapy should be continued for at least 2 years and may be necessary for the lifetime of the patient (*see* below).

Sulfoxone sodium may be substituted for dapsone in patients in whom the latter drug produces sufficient gastric distress to impede effective therapy. It is available for oral administration as enteric-coated tablets containing 165 mg. The recommended daily dose is 330 mg.

The use of sulfones in *malaria* resistant to the usual antimalarial drugs is discussed in Chapter 45.

RIFAMPIN

This antibiotic has been discussed above with regard to its use in tuberculosis. Rifampin is rapidly bactericidal for *M. leprae,* and the minimal inhibitory concentration is less than 1 μg/ml. Infectivity of patients is rapidly reversed by therapy that includes rifampin (Bullock, 1983). Because of the prevalence of resistance to dapsone, a regimen of multiple drugs, including rifampin, is now recommended by the WHO Study Group (1982).

CLOFAZIMINE

Clofazimine is a phenazine dye with the following structural formula:

Clofazimine

Clofazimine may inhibit the template function of DNA by binding to it (Morrison and Marley, 1976). It is weakly bactericidal against *M. leprae*. The drug also exerts an anti-inflammatory effect and prevents the development of erythema nodosum leprosum. Clofazimine is now recommended as a component of multiple-drug therapy for leprosy (*see* below). The compound is also useful for treatment of chronic skin ulcers (Buruli ulcer) produced by *M. ulcerans*, and it has some activity against the *Mycobacterium avium-intracellulare* complex.

Clofazimine is absorbed by the oral route and appears to accumulate in tissues. This makes possible discontinuous therapy with individual doses separated by 4 weeks. Human leprosy from which dapsone-resistant bacilli have been recovered has been treated with clofazimine with good results. However, unlike dapsone-sensitive microorganisms in which killing occurs immediately after dapsone is administered, dapsone-resistant strains do not exhibit appreciable effect until 50 days after therapy with clofazimine has been initiated. The dose of clofazimine is 100 to 300 mg; the optimal interval between doses in man remains to be determined. (*See* Convit *et al.*, 1970; Shepard *et al.*, 1971; Levy *et al.*, 1972.) Patients treated with clofazimine may develop red discoloration of the skin; this may be very distressing to light-skinned individuals (Levy and Randall, 1970). Eosinophilic enteritis has also been described as an adverse reaction to the drug (Mason *et al.*, 1977).

Clofazimine (LAMPRENE) is available only from the National Hansen's Disease Center, Carville, Louisiana 70721.

MISCELLANEOUS AGENTS

Thalidomide seems to be effective for the treatment of *erythema nodosum leprosum* (Iyer *et al.*, 1971). Doses of 100 to 300 mg per day have been effective. The marked teratogenicity of thalidomide limits its use; it is not available in the United States.

Ethionamide has been discussed above as an agent for treatment of tuberculosis. It can be used as a substitute for clofazimine in oral doses of 250 to 375 mg per day.

CHEMOTHERAPY OF LEPROSY

Few physicians, other than specialists in the field, are called upon to treat leprosy. Consultation is available with physicians at the National Hansen's Disease Center, Carville, Louisiana 70721, or at regional centers. Therefore, the following discussion will serve mainly to familiarize the reader with the progress that has been made in the treatment of this chronic bacterial disease that has proven very resistant to chemotherapy.

Five clinical types of leprosy are recognized. At one end of the spectrum is *tuberculoid leprosy*. This form of the disease is characterized by skin macules with clear centers and well-defined margins; these are invariably anesthetic. *Mycobacterium leprae* is rarely found in smears made from quiescent lesions, but may appear during activity. Virchow cells are not demonstrable. Noncaseating foci with giant cells of the Langhans variety are present. The patient's cell-mediated immune responses are normal, and the lepromin test (intradermal injection of a suspension of heat-killed, bacillus-laden tissue) is invariably positive. The disease is characterized by prolonged remissions with periodic reactivation. At the other end of the spectrum is the widely disseminated *lepromatous* form of the disease. These patients have markedly impaired cell-mediated immunity and are frequently anergic; the lepromin test causes no reaction. *Lepromatous disease* is characterized by diffuse or ill-defined localized infiltration of the skin, which becomes thickened, glossy, and corrugated; areas of decreased sensation may appear. *Mycobacterium leprae* is demonstrable in smears, and granulomas containing bacteria-laden histiocytes (Virchow cells) are present. As the disease progresses, large nerve trunks are involved and anesthesia, atrophy of skin and muscle, absorption of small bones, ulceration, and spontaneous amputations may occur. Three intermediate forms of the disease are recognized: borderline tuberculoid disease, borderline lepromatous disease, and borderline disease (Bullock, 1985).

Patients with tuberculoid leprosy may develop "reversal reactions," which are manifestations of delayed hypersensitivity to antigens of *M. leprae*. Cutaneous ulcerations and deficits of peripheral nerve function may occur. Early therapy with corticosteroids or clofazimine is effective.

Reactions in the lepromatous form of the disease (*erythema nodosum leprosum*) are characterized by the appearance of raised, tender, intracutaneous nodules, severe constitutional symptoms, and high fever. This reaction may be triggered by several conditions but is often associated with therapy. It is thought to be an arthus-type reaction related to release of microbial antigens in patients harboring large numbers of bacilli. Treatment with clofazimine or thalidomide is effective.

The outlook for persons with leprosy has been remarkably altered by successful chemotherapy, surgical procedures that help to restore function and repair disfigurement, and a striking change in the attitude of the public toward patients who have this infection. The social stigma based on ignorance and Biblical castigation of individuals with this affliction is gradually being replaced by the attitude that considers leprosy a disease and not a social stigma. Patients with leprosy can be classified as "infectious" or "noninfectious" on the basis of the type, duration, and effects of therapy. Thus, even "infectious" patients need not be hospitalized, provided adequate medical supervision and therapy are maintained, the home environment meets specific conditions, and the local health officer concurs in the disposition of the case.

Therapy, when effective, heals ulcers and mucosal lesions in months. Cutaneous nodules respond more slowly, and it may take years to eradicate bacteria from mucous membranes, skin, and nerves. The degree of residual pigmentation or depigmentation, atrophy, and scarring depends upon the extent of the initial involvement. Severe ocular lesions show little response to the sulfones. If treatment is initiated before ocular disease is evident, it may be prevented. Keratoconjunctivitis and corneal ulceration may be secondary to nerve involvement.

The World Health Organization now recommends therapy with multiple drugs for all patients with leprosy (WHO Study Group, 1982). The reasons for using combinations of agents include reduction in the development of resistance, the need for adequate therapy when primary resistance already exists, and reduction in the duration of therapy. For patients with large populations of bacteria (multibacillary forms), including lepromatous disease, borderline lepromatous disease, and borderline disease, the following regimen is suggested: dapsone, 50 to 100 mg daily, plus clofazimine, 50 mg daily and a 300-mg dose given once monthly under supervision, plus rifampin, 600 mg once a month under supervision. Some prefer to give a daily dose of rifampin (450 to 600 mg) (Jacobson, 1982). All drugs are given orally. The minimal duration of therapy is 2 years, and treatment should continue until acid-fast bacilli are not detected in lesions.

Patients with a small population of bacteria (paucibacillary disease), including those with tuberculoid, borderline tuberculoid, and intermediate disease, should be treated with dapsone, 100 mg daily, plus rifampin, 600 mg once monthly (under supervision), for 6 months. Relapses are treated by repeating the regimen.

Albert, R. K.; Lakshminarayan, S.; and Miller, W. T. Long-term therapy with rifampin and the secondary antibody response to killed influenza vaccine. *Am. Rev. Respir. Dis.*, **1978**, *117*, 605–607.

American Thoracic Society. Guidelines for short-course tuberculosis chemotherapy. *Am. Rev. Respir. Dis.*, **1980**, *121*, 611–614.

Atlas, E., and Turck, M. Laboratory and clinical evaluation of rifampicin. *Am. J. Med. Sci.*, **1968**, *256*, 247–254.

Bailey, W. C.; Weill, H.; DeRouen, T. A.; Ziskind, M. M.; Jackson, H. A.; and Greenberg, H. B. The effect of isoniazid on transaminase levels. *Ann. Intern. Med.*, **1974**, *81*, 200–202.

Bassi, L.; DiBerardino, L.; Arioli, V.; Silvestri, L. G.; and Cherie Ligniere, E. L. Conditions for immunosuppression by rifampicin. *J. Infect. Dis.*, **1973**, *128*, 736–744.

Bieder, A.; Brunel, P.; and Mazeau, L. Identification de trois nouveaux métabolites de l'ethionamide: chromatographie, spectrophotométrie, polarographie. *Ann. Pharm. Fr.*, **1966**, *24*, 493–500.

Bobrowitz, I. D. Ethambutol-isoniazid versus streptomycin-ethambutol-isoniazid in original treatment of cavitary tuberculosis. *Am. Rev. Respir. Dis.*, **1974**, *109*, 548–553.

Bowersox, D. W.; Winterbauer, R. H.; Stewart, G. L.; Orme, B.; and Barron, E. Isoniazid dosage in patients with renal failure. *N. Engl. J. Med.*, **1973**, *289*, 84–87.

British Thoracic and Tuberculosis Association. Short-course chemotherapy in pulmonary tuberculosis. *Lancet*, **1975**, *1*, 119–124.

British Thoracic Association. A controlled trial of six months chemotherapy in pulmonary tuberculosis. Second report: results during the twenty-four months after the end of chemotherapy. *Am. Rev. Respir. Dis.*, **1983**, *126*, 460–462.

Buffington, G. A.; Dominguez, J. H.; Piering, W. F.; Hebert, L. A.; Kouffman, H. M.; and Lemann, J. Interaction of rifampin and glucocorticoids. *J.A.M.A.*, **1976**, *236*, 1958–1960.

Buss, W. C.; Morgan, R.; Guttman, J.; Barela, T.; and Stalter, K. Rifampicin inhibition of protein synthesis in mammalian cells. *Science*, **1978**, *200*, 432–434.

Bycroft, B. W.; Cameron, D.; Croft, L. R.; Hassanali-Walji, A.; Johnson, A. W.; and Webb, T. Total structure of capreomycin 1B, a tuberculostatic peptide antibiotic. *Nature*, **1971**, *231*, 301–302.

Byrd, R. B.; Horn, B. R.; Solomon, D. A.; and Griggs, G. W. Toxic effects of isoniazid in tuberculosis chemoprophylaxis. *J.A.M.A.*, **1979**, *241*, 1239–1241.

Carpenter, J. L.; Covelli, H. D.; Avant, M. E.; McAllister, C. K.; Higbee, J. W.; and Ognibene, A. J. Drug-resistant *Mycobacterium tuberculosis* in Korean isolates. *Am. Rev. Respir. Dis.*, **1982**, *126*, 1092–1095.

Centers for Disease Control. Adverse drug reactions among children treated for tuberculosis. *M.M.W.R.*, **1980**, *29*, 589–591.

———. Increase in prevalence of leprosy caused by dapsone-resistant *Mycobacterium leprae. Ibid.*, **1982**, *30*, 637–638.

———. Primary resistance to antituberculosis drugs. *Ibid.*, **1983**, *32*, 521–523.

Comstock, G. W. Evaluating isoniazid preventive therapy: the need for more data. *Ann. Intern. Med.*, **1981**, *94*, 817–819.

———. New data on preventive treatment with isoniazid. *Ibid.*, **1983**, *98*, 663–665.

Convit, J.; Browne, S. G.; Languillon, J.; Pettit, J. H. S.; Ramanujam, K.; Sagher, F.; Sheskin, J.; deSouza Lima, L.; Tarabini, G.; Tolentino, J. G.; Waters, M. F. R.; Bechelli, L. M.; and Martinez Dominguez, V. Therapy of leprosy. *Bull. WHO*, **1970**, *42*, 667–672.

Dalovisio, J. R., and Pankey, G. A. *In vitro* susceptibility of *Mycobacterium fortuitum* and *Mycobacterium chelonei* to amikacin. *J. Infect. Dis.*, **1978**, *137*, 318–321.

Davidson, P. T. Treatment and long-term follow-up of patients with atypical mycobacterial infections. *Bull. Int. Union Tuberc.*, **1976**, *51*, 257–261.

Devine, L. F.; Johnson, D. P.; Rhode, S. L., III; Hagerman, C. R.; Pierce, W. E.; and Peckinpaugh, R. D. Rifampin—effect of two-day treatment on the meningococcal carrier state and the relationship to the levels of the drug in sera and saliva. *Am. J. Med. Sci.*, **1971**, *26*, 74–83.

Donomae, I. The combined use of capreomycin and ethambutol in re-treatment of pulmonary tuberculosis. *Am. Rev. Respir. Dis.*, **1968**, *98*, 699–702.

Dutt, A. K., and Stead, W. W. Present chemotherapy for tuberculosis. *J. Infect. Dis.*, **1982**, *146*, 698–704.

Edwards, P. Q. Tuberculosis, now and the future: short-term therapy, preventive therapy, and bacillus Calmette-Guerin. *Bull. N.Y. Acad. Med.*, **1977**, *53*, 526–531.

Evans, D. A. P.; Manley, K. A.; and McKusick, V. A. Genetic control of isoniazid metabolism in man. *Br. Med. J.*, **1960**, *2*, 485–491.

Flynn, C. T.; Rainford, D. J.; and Hope, E. Acute renal failure and rifampicin: danger of unsuspected intermittent dosage. *Br. Med. J.*, **1974**, *2*, 482.

Fox, H. H. The chemical attack on tuberculosis. *Trans. N.Y. Acad. Sci.*, **1953**, *15*, 234–242.

Furesz, S. Chemical and biological properties of rifampicin. *Antibiot. Chemother.*, **1970**, *16*, 316–351.

Garibaldi, R. A.; Drusin, R. E.; Ferebee, S. H.; and Gregg, M. B. Isoniazid-associated hepatitis. Report of an outbreak. *Am. Rev. Respir. Dis.*, **1972**, *106*, 357–365.

Girling, D. J. The hepatic toxicity of antituberculous regimens containing isoniazid, rifampicin and pyrazinamide. *Tubercle*, **1978**, *59*, 13–32.

Girling, D. J., and Hitze, H. L. Adverse reactions to rifampicin. *Bull. WHO*, **1979**, *57*, 45–49.

Goodwin, C. S., and Sparell, G. Inhibition of dapsone excretion by probenecid. *Lancet*, **1969**, *2*, 884–885.

Graber, C. D.; Jebaily, J.; Galphin, R. L.; and Doering, E. Light chain proteinuria and humoral immunocompetence in tuberculous patients treated with rifampin. *Am. Rev. Respir. Dis.*, **1973**, *107*, 713–717.

Greene, J. B.; Gurdip, S. S.; Lewin, S.; Levine, J. F.; Masur, H.; Simberkoff, M. S.; Nicholas, P.; Good, R. C.; Zolla-Pazner, S. B.; Pollock, A. A.; Tapper, M. L.; and Holzman, R. S. *Mycobacterium avium-intracellulare:* a cause of disseminated life-threatening infection in homosexuals and drug abusers. *Ann. Intern. Med.*, **1982**, *97*, 539–546.

Gronhagen-Riska, C.; Hellstrom, P. E.; and Froseth, B. Predisposing factors in hepatitis induced by isoniazid-rifampin treatment of tuberculosis. *Am. Rev. Respir. Dis.*, **1978**, *118*, 461–466.

Grosset, J., and Leventis, S. Adverse effects of rifampin. *Rev. Infect. Dis.*, **1983**, *5*, Suppl. 3, S440–S446.

Gupta, S.; Grieco, M. H.; and Siegel, I. Suppression of T-lymphocyte rosettes by rifampin. *Ann. Intern. Med.*, **1975**, *82*, 484–488.

Herman, R. P., and Weber, M. M. Site of action of isoniazid on the electron transport chain and its relationship to nicotinamide adenine dinucleotide regulation in *Mycobacterium phlei*. *Antimicrob. Agents Chemother.*, **1980**, *17*, 450–454.

Hobby, G. L., and Lenert, T. F. Observations on the action of rifampin and ethambutol alone and in combination with other antituberculous drugs. *Am. Rev. Respir. Dis.*, **1972**, *105*, 292–295.

Hoeprich, P. D. Alanine:cycloserine antagonism. II. Significance of phenomenon to therapy with cycloserine. *Arch. Intern. Med.*, **1963**, *112*, 405–414. III. Quantitative aspects and relation to heating of culture media. *J. Lab. Clin. Med.*, **1963**, *62*, 657–662.

Hurwitz, A., and Schlozman, D. L. Effect of antacids on gastrointestinal absorption of isoniazid in rat and man. *Am. Rev. Respir. Dis.*, **1974**, *109*, 41–47.

Ivler, D.; Leedom, J. M.; and Mathies, A. W., Jr. *In vitro* susceptibility of *Neisseria meningitidis* to rifampin. In, *Antimicrobial Agents and Chemotherapy—1969.* (Hobby, G. L., ed.) American Society for Microbiology, Bethesda, **1970**, pp. 473–478.

Iyer, C. G. S.; Languillon, J.; and Ramanujam, K. WHO coordinated short-term double-blind trial with thalidomide in the treatment of acute lepra reactions in male lepromatous patients. *Bull. WHO*, **1971**, *45*, 719–732.

Izumi, A. K.; Hanke, E. W.; and Higaki, M. *M. marinum* infections treated with tetracycline. *Arch. Dermatol.*, **1977**, *113*, 1067–1068.

Jenne, J. W., and Beggs, W. H. Correlation of *in vitro* and *in vivo* kinetics with clinical use of isoniazid, ethambutol and rifampin. *Am. Rev. Respir. Dis.*, **1973**, *107*, 1013–1021.

Karlson, A. G. The *in vitro* activity of ethambutol (dextro-2-2'-[ethylenediimino]-di-l-butanol) against tubercle bacilli and other microorganisms. *Am. Rev. Respir. Dis.*, **1961**, *84*, 905–906.

Kunin, C. M.; Brandt, D.; and Wood, H. Bacteriologic studies of rifampin, a new semisynthetic antibiotic. *J. Infect. Dis.*, **1969**, *119*, 132–137.

La Du, B. N. Isoniazid and pseudocholinesterase polymorphisms. *Fed. Proc.*, **1972**, *31*, 1276–1285.

Leiker, D. L. The mononuclear syndrome in leprosy patients treated with sulfones. *Int. J. Lepr.*, **1956**, *24*, 402–405.

Levy, L., and Peters, J. H. Susceptibility of *Mycobacterium leprae* to dapsone as a determinant of patient response to acedapsone. *Antimicrob. Agents Chemother.*, **1976**, *9*, 102–112.

Levy, L., and Randall, H. P. A study of skin pigmentation by clofazimine. *Int. J. Lepr.*, **1970**, *38*, 404–416.

Levy, L.; Shepard, C. C.; and Fasal, P. Clofazimine therapy of lepromatous leprosy caused by dapsone-resistant *Mycobacterium leprae*. *Am. J. Trop. Med. Hyg.*, **1972**, *21*, 315–321.

Lincoln, E. M., and Gilberg, L. A. Disease in children due to mycobacteria other than *M. tuberculosis*. *Am. Rev. Respir. Dis.*, **1972**, *105*, 683–714.

Loria, P. R. Minocycline hydrochloride treatment for atypical acid-fast infection. *Arch. Dermatol.*, **1976**, *112*, 517–519.

McDermott, W.; Ormond, L.; Muschenheim, C.; Deuschle, K.; McCune, R. M.; and Tompsett, R. Pyrazinamide-isoniazid in tuberculosis. *Am. Rev. Tuberc.*, **1954**, *69*, 319–333.

Maddrey, W. C., and Boitnott, J. K. Isoniazid hepatitis. *Ann. Intern. Med.*, **1973**, *79*, 1–12.

Mandell, G. L. Interaction of intraleukocytic bacteria and antibiotics. *J. Clin. Invest.*, **1973**, *52*, 1673–1679.

Mason, G. H.; Ellis-Pegler, R. B.; and Arthur, J. F. Clofazimine and eosinophilic enteritis. *Lepr. Rev.*, **1977**, *48*, 175–180.

Miller, R. R.; Porter, J.; and Greenblatt, D. J. Clinical importance of the interaction of phenytoin and isoniazid. *Chest*, **1979**, *75*, 356–358.

Mitchell, J. R.; Zimmerman, H. J.; Ishak, K. G.; Thorgeirsson, U. P.; Timbrell, J. A.; Snodgrass, W. R.; and Nelson, S. D. Isoniazid liver injury: clinical spectrum, pathology, and probable pathogenesis. *Ann. Intern. Med.*, **1976**, *84*, 181–192.

Molavi, A., and Weinstein, L. *In vitro* susceptibility of atypical mycobacteria to rifampin. *Appl. Microbiol.*, **1971**, *22*, 23–25.

Morrison, N. E., and Marley, G. M. Clofazimine binding studies with deoxyribonucleic acid. *Int. J. Lepr.*, **1976**, *44*, 475–481.

Mukerjee, P.; Schuldt, S.; and Kasik, J. E. Effect of rifampin on cutaneous hypersensitivity to purified protein derivatives in humans. *Antimicrob. Agents Chemother.*, **1973**, *4*, 607–611.

Nicholson, D. P. Atypical tuberculosis: features and therapy. *Br. J. Dis. Chest*, **1976**, *70*, 217–218.

Ohnhaus, E. E.; Kirchhof, B.; and Peheim, E. Effect of enzyme induction on plasma lipids using antipyrine, phenobarbital, and rifampicin. *Clin. Pharmacol. Ther.*, **1979**, *25*, 591–597.

O'Reilly, R. A. Interaction of chronic daily warfarin therapy and rifampin. *Ann. Intern. Med.*, **1975**, *83*, 506–508.

Peets, E. A.; Sweeney, W. M.; Place, V. A.; and Buyske, D. A. The absorption, excretion and metabolic fate of ethambutol in man. *Am. Rev. Respir. Dis.*, **1965**, *91*, 51–58.

Pengelly, C. D. R. Dapsone-induced hemolysis. *Br. Med. J.*, **1963**, *2*, 662–664.

Pezzia, W.; Raleigh, J. W.; Bailey, M. C.; Toth, E. A.; and Silverblatt, J. Treatment of pulmonary disease due to *Mycobacterium kansasii*: recent experience with rifampin. *Rev. Infect. Dis.*, **1981**, *3*, 1035–1039.

Pilheu, J. A.; De Salvo, M. C.; and Koch, O. Liver alterations in antituberculosis regimens containing pyrazinamide. *Chest*, **1981**, *80*, 720–724.

Pitts, F. W. Tuberculosis: prevention and therapy. In, *Current Concepts of Infectious Diseases.* (Hook, E. W.; Mandell, G. L.; Gwaltney, J. M., Jr.; and Sande, M. A.; eds.) John Wiley & Sons, Inc., New York, **1977**, pp. 181–194.

Place, V. A., and Thomas, J. P. Clinical pharmacology of ethambutol. *Am. Rev. Respir. Dis.*, **1963**, *87*, 901–904.

Postlethwaite, A. E.; Bartel, A. G.; and Kelley, W. N.

Hyperuricemia due to ethambutol. *N. Engl. J. Med.*, **1972**, *286*, 761–762.

Public Health Service, U.S. Department of Health, Education, and Welfare. Isoniazid-associated hepatitis: summary of the report of the Tuberculosis Advisory Committee and special consultants to the Director, Center for Disease Control. *M.M.W.R.*, **1974**, *23*, 97–98.

Radner, D. B. Toxicologic and pharmacologic aspects of rifampin. *Chest*, **1973**, *64*, 213–216.

Rapoport, A. M., and Guss, S. B. Dapsone-induced peripheral neuropathy. *Arch. Neurol.*, **1972**, *27*, 184–186.

Romankiewicz, J. A., and Ehrman, M. Rifampin and warfarin: a drug interaction. *Ann. Intern. Med.*, **1975**, *82*, 224–225.

Rothfield, N. F.; Bierer, W. F.; and Garfield, J. W. Isoniazid induction of antinuclear antibodies. *Ann. Intern. Med.*, **1978**, *88*, 650–652.

Sanders, W. E., Jr. Lung infection caused by rapidly growing mycobacteria. *J. Respir. Dis.*, **1982**, *3*, 30–38.

Sanders, W. E., Jr.; Cacciatore, R.; Valdez, H.; Schneider, N.; and Hartwig, C. Activity of amikacin against mycobacteria *in vitro* and in experimental infections with *M. tuberculosis. Am. Rev. Respir. Dis.*, **1976**, *113*, 59.

Sanders, W. E., Jr.; Hartwig, E. C.; Schneider, N. J.; Cacciatore, R.; and Valdez, H. Susceptibility of organisms in the *Mycobacterium fortuitum* complex to antituberculous and other antimicrobial agents. *Antimicrob. Agents Chemother.*, **1977**, *12*, 295–297.

Sanfilippo, A.; Della Bruna, C.; Marsili, L.; Morvillo, E.; Pasqualucci, C. R.; Schioppacassi, G.; and Ungheri, D. Biological activity of a new class of rifamycins, spiro-piperidyl-rifamycins. *J. Antibiot. (Tokyo)*, **1980**, *33*, 1193–1198.

Scheuer, P. J.; Summerfield, J. A.; Lal, S.; and Sherlock, S. Rifampin hepatitis. *Lancet*, **1974**, *1*, 421–425.

Schwartz, W. S. Comparison of ethionamide with isoniazid in original treatment cases of pulmonary tuberculosis. XIV. A report of the Veterans Administration–Armed Forces Cooperative Study. *Am. Rev. Respir. Dis.*, **1966**, *93*, 685–692.

Shepard, C. C.; Ellard, G. A.; Levy, L.; Opromolla, V.; Pattyn, S. R.; Peters, J. H.; Rees, R. J. W.; and Waters, M. F. R. Experimental chemotherapy of leprosy. *Bull. WHO*, **1976**, *53*, 425–433.

Shepard, C. C.; Walker, L. L.; Van Landingham, R. M.; and Redus, M. A. Discontinuous administration of clofazimine (B663) on *Mycobacterium leprae* infections. *Proc. Soc. Exp. Biol. Med.*, **1971**, *137*, 725–727.

Simon, E.; Veres, E.; and Banki, G. Changes in SGOT activity during treatment with ethionamide. *Scand. J. Respir. Dis.*, **1969**, *50*, 314–322.

Sippel, J. E.; Mikhail, I. A.; Girgis, N. I.; and Youssef, H. H. Rifampin concentrations in cerebrospinal fluid of patients with tuberculous meningitis. *Am. Rev. Respir. Dis.*, **1974**, *109*, 579–580.

Skolnick, J. L.; Stoler, B. S.; Katz, D. B.; and Anderson, W. H. Rifampin, oral contraceptives, and pregnancy. *J.A.M.A.*, **1976**, *236*, 1382.

Snider, D. E., Jr. Pyridoxine supplementation during isoniazid therapy. *Tubercle*, **1980**, *61*, 191–196.

Snider, D. E., and Farer, L. S. Preventive therapy with isoniazid for "inactive" tuberculosis. *Chest*, **1978**, *73*, 4–5.

Spector, R., and Lorenzo, W. V. The active transport of para-aminosalicylic acid from the cerebrospinal fluid. *J. Pharmacol. Exp. Ther.*, **1973**, *185*, 642–648.

Stottmeier, K. D.; Beam, R. E.; and Kubica, G. P. The absorption and excretion of pyrazinamide. I. Preliminary study in laboratory animals and man. *Am. Rev. Respir. Dis.*, **1968**, *98*, 70–74.

Takayama, K.; Schnoes, H. K.; Armstrong, E. L.; and

Boyle, R. W. Site of inhibitory action of isoniazid in the synthesis of mycolic acids in *Mycobacterium tuberculosis. J. Lipid Res.*, **1975**, *16*, 308–317.

Taylor, W. C.; Aronson, M. D.; and Delbanco, T. L. Should young adults with a positive tuberculin test take isoniazid? *Ann. Intern. Med.*, **1981**, *94*, 808–813.

Thornsberry, C.; Hill, B. C.; Swenson, J. M.; and McDougal, L. K. Rifampin: spectrum of antibacterial activity. *Rev. Infect. Dis.*, **1983**, *5*, Suppl. 3, S412–S417.

Trautman, J. R. The management of leprosy and its complications. *N. Engl. J. Med.*, **1965**, *273*, 756–758.

Tuazon, C. U.; Lin, M. Y. C.; and Sheagren, J. N. *In vitro* activity of rifampin alone and in combination with nafcillin and vancomycin against pathogenic strains of *Staphylococcus aureus. Antimicrob. Agents Chemother.*, **1978**, *13*, 759–761.

Warrington, R. J.; Hogg, G. R.; Paraskevas, F.; and Tse, K. S. Insidious rifampin-associated renal failure with light-chain proteinuria. *Arch. Intern. Med.*, **1977**, *137*, 927–930.

Wehrli, W. Rifampin: mechanisms of action and resistance. *Rev. Infect. Dis.*, **1983**, *5*, Suppl. 3, S407–S411.

Weiner, I. M., and Tinker, J. P. Pharmacology of pyrazinamide: metabolic and renal function studies related to the mechanism of drug-induced urate retention. *J. Pharmacol. Exp. Ther.*, **1972**, *180*, 411–434.

Wheat, I. J.; Kohler, R. B.; Luft, F. C.; and White, A. Long-term studies of the effect of rifampin on nasal carriage of coagulase-positive staphylococci. *Rev. Infect. Dis.*, **1983**, *5*, Suppl. 3, S459–S462.

WHO. A study of two twice-weekly and a once-weekly continuation regimens of tuberculosis chemotherapy including a comparison of two durations of treatment. *Tubercle*, **1977**, *58*, 129–136.

WHO Study Group. Chemotherapy of leprosy for control programmes. WHO Technical Report Series No. 675, WHO, Geneva, **1982**, 7–33.

Wilson, T. M. Current therapeutics. CCXL. Capreomycin and ethambutol. *Practitioner*, **1967**, *199*, 817–824.

Zierski, M., and Bek, E. Side effects of drug regimens used in short course chemotherapy for pulmonary tuberculosis. A controlled study. *Tubercle*, **1980**, *61*, 41–49.

Monographs and Reviews

Bullock, W. E. Rifampin in the treatment of leprosy. *Rev. Infect. Dis.*, **1983**, *5*, S606–S613.

———. *Mycobacterium leprae* (leprosy). In, *Principles and Practice of Infectious Diseases*, 2nd ed. (Mandell, G. L.; Douglas, R. G., Jr.; and Bennett, J. E.; eds.) John Wiley & Sons, Inc., New York, **1985**, pp. 1406–1413.

DeGowin, R. L. A review of the therapeutic and hemolytic effects of dapsone. *Arch. Intern. Med.*, **1967**, *120*, 242–248.

Des Prez, R. M., and Goodwin, R. A. *Mycobacterium tuberculosis*. In, *Principles and Practice of Infectious Diseases*, 2nd ed. (Mandell, G. L.; Douglas, R. G., Jr.; and Bennett, J. E.; eds.) John Wiley & Sons, Inc., New York, **1985**, pp. 1383–1406.

Farr, B., and Mandell, G. L. Rifampin. *Med. Clin. North Am.*, **1982**, *66*, 157–168.

Goldman, A. L., and Braman, S. S. Isoniazid: a review with emphasis on adverse effects. *Chest*, **1972**, *62*, 71–77.

Hopewell, P. C. Tuberculosis and nontuberculous mycobacterial diseases. In, *Internal Medicine*. (Stein, J. H., ed.) Little, Brown & Co., Boston, **1983**, pp. 1404–1419.

Jacobson, R. R. The treatment of leprosy (Hansen's disease). *Hosp. Formulary*, **1982**, *17*, 1076–1091.

Kucers, A., and Bennett, N. M.   Drugs mainly for tuberculosis. In, *The Use of Antibiotics*, 3rd ed. Heinemann
Medical Books, London, **1979**, pp. 798–862.

Pitts, F. W.   Tuberculosis: prevention and therapy. In,
Current Concepts of Infectious Diseases. (Hook,
E. W.; Mandell, G. L.; Gwaltney, J. M., Jr.; and Sande,
M. A.; eds.) John Wiley & Sons, Inc., New York, **1977**,
pp. 181–194.

Sanders, W. E., Jr.   Other *Mycobacterium* species. In,

Principles and Practice of Infectious Diseases, 2nd ed.
(Mandell, G. L.; Douglas, R. G., Jr.; and Bennett, J. E.;
eds.) John Wiley & Sons, Inc., New York, **1985**, pp.
1413–1423.

Shepard, C. C.   Chemotherapy of leprosy. *Annu. Rev.
Pharmacol.*, **1969**, *9*, 37–50.

Symposium. (Various authors.)   The use of rifampin in
treatment of nontuberculous infections. *Rev. Infect.
Dis.*, **1983**, *5*, Suppl., S399–S632.

CHAPTER

54 ANTIMICROBIAL AGENTS
[Continued]
Antifungal and Antiviral Agents

Merle A. Sande and Gerald L. Mandell

I. Antifungal Agents

AMPHOTERICIN B

History and Source. *Streptomyces nodosus*, a soil actinomycete, is the source of two antifungal agents, amphotericins A and B. The preparation of an almost pure *amphotericin B* (containing only 1 to 2% amphotericin A) was accomplished by Vandeputte and coworkers (1956); this is the preparation used clinically.

Chemistry. Amphotericin B and nystatin (*see* below) are polyene antibiotics. Such compounds contain a hydrophilic region (which includes a hydroxylated hydrocarbon backbone) and a sequence of four to seven conjugated double bonds, which is lipophilic. Amphotericin B and nystatin also contain an aminodeoxyhexose, mycosamine. The structural formula of amphotericin B is shown below. Amphotericin B is insoluble in water and is somewhat unstable. The antifungal effects of the antibiotic are maximal between pH 6.0 and 7.5 and decrease at low pH.

Antifungal Activity. *Histoplasma capsulatum, Cryptococcus neoformans, Coccidioides immitis, Candida* species including *Candida glabrata, Rhodotorula, Blastomyces dermatitidis, Paracoccidioides brasiliensis*, many strains of *Aspergillus*, and *Sporothrix schenckii* are sensitive to concentrations of amphotericin B ranging from 0.03 to 1.0 μg/ml *in vitro*. The antibiotic is either fungistatic or fungicidal, depending on the concentration of the drug and the sensitivity of the fungus.

The activity of amphotericin *in vitro* can be enhanced when the drug is combined with certain antimicrobial agents (Odds, 1982; Bennett, 1985). Ri-

fampin, which has no antifungal activity when used alone, reduces the concentration of amphotericin B required to inhibit the growth of *Aspergillus, Histoplasma*, or *Candida in vitro*. While similar effects have also been observed in some experimental infections (Arroyo *et al.*, 1977), this has not been a consistent finding (Ernst *et al.*, 1983). Likewise, minocycline enhances the activity of amphotericin B *in vitro* against *Candida* species and *Cryptococcus* (Lew *et al.*, 1978). There are no clinical data to support the use of either combination.

A useful combination for clinical purposes is that of flucytosine and amphotericin B. Flucytosine reduces the concentration of amphotericin B necessary to inhibit growth of *Candida* and *Cryptococcus in vitro* (Medoff *et al.*, 1971a). There is also benefit from their concurrent use *in vivo* in the treatment of experimental infections caused by *Candida* and *Cryptococcus* and in the therapy of cryptococcal meningitis in man (Arroyo *et al.*, 1977; Sande *et al.*, 1977; Bennett *et al.*, 1979; Craven and Graybill, 1984). The mechanism of this synergistic interaction is not completely understood but may involve increased penetration of flucytosine because of damage to the cell membrane caused by amphotericin B. In contrast, concurrent use of ketoconazole and amphotericin B often causes antagonistic effects (Craven and Graybill, 1984; Iwen *et al.*, 1984).

Mechanism of Action. The antifungal activity of amphotericin B is at least in part dependent on its binding to a sterol moiety, primarily ergosterol, present in the membrane of sensitive fungi. By virtue of their interaction with the sterols of cell membranes, polyenes appear to form pores or channels. The result is an increase in the permeability of the membrane, allowing leakage of a variety of small

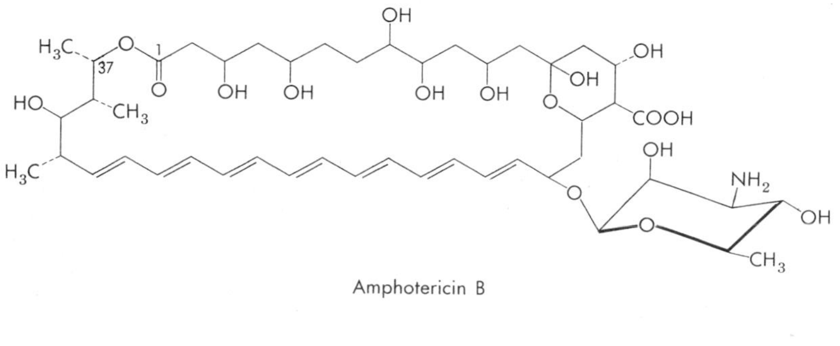

Amphotericin B

molecules (*see* Hamilton-Miller, 1974). However, effects of amphotericin B on the permeability of sterol-free membranes indicate that additional mechanisms may also be involved. Recent data indicate that low concentrations of amphotericin B have paradoxical stimulatory effects on cell proliferation, including that of fungal cells and animal cells in culture. These effects may relate to the fact that the drug has potent humoral and cell-mediated immunostimulant effects in mice. These effects may have clinical relevance, particularly in the immunocompromised host (*see* Medoff *et al.*, 1983).

Fungal Resistance. Strains of *C. albicans* and *Coccid. immitis* serially subcultured in increasing concentrations of amphotericin B become resistant to the drug. Mutants of *C. albicans* that are resistant to the polyene also have an altered colonial morphology, slower rate of growth, and decreased virulence for animals. There are very few instances where *Candida* species have developed resistance *in vitro* (Drutz, 1982).

Absorption, Distribution, and Excretion. Amphotericin B is poorly absorbed from the gastrointestinal tract. The *oral administration* of about 3 g a day produces plasma concentrations of about 0.1 to 0.5 μg/ml. The *intravenous infusion* of 1 to 5 mg of amphotericin B per day initially, followed by the gradual increase of the daily dose to 0.4 to 0.6 mg/kg, yields peak values of approximately 0.5 to 2 μg/ml. The average steady-state concentration of the drug in plasma approaches 0.5 μg/ml (Bindschalder and Bennett, 1969). It is probable that most of the antibiotic is bound to cholesterol-containing membranes in many different tissues. However, details of possible pathways of drug metabolism are unknown. Approximately 95% of the drug circulating in plasma is bound to lipoproteins (Block *et al.*, 1974; Bennett, 1977). Concentrations of amphotericin B in fluids from inflamed pleura, peritoneum, synovium, and aqueous humor are approximately two thirds of trough concentrations in plasma. The drug probably crosses the placenta readily (Bennett, 1985). Little amphotericin B penetrates into cerebrospinal fluid (CSF), vitreous humor, or normal amniotic fluid.

The antifungal agent is excreted very slowly in the urine, and only a small fraction of a given dose is excreted in active form. Biliary excretion may constitute an important route of elimination. When therapy is stopped, the drug can be detected in the urine for at least 7 to 8 weeks. The concentration of amphotericin B in urine roughly parallels that in plasma. There appears to be no significant accumulation of amphotericin B in patients with impaired renal function (Feldman *et al.*, 1973). Hemodialysis does not alter the concentration of amphotericin B in plasma.

The clinical pharmacology of amphotericin B is discussed by Maddux and Barriere (1980) and by Bennett (1985).

Preparations, Routes of Administration, and Dosage. *Amphotericin B* (FUNGIZONE) is available for injection. The sterile, lyophilized powder is marketed in vials containing 50 mg of amphotericin B, plus 41 mg of sodium deoxycholate to effect a colloidal dispersion of the insoluble antibiotic, buffers, and diluent. The contents of the vial should be dissolved, with shaking, in 10 ml of sterile water and then added to 5% dextrose in water to make a final concentration of no more than 0.1 mg/ml. *Solutions of some electrolytes, acidic solutions, or solutions with preservatives should not be used* because they cause precipitation of this antifungal agent (Jurgens *et al.*, 1981). Fresh solutions should be prepared for each infusion. If fever and chills in response to administration of the drug are severe, the addition of 0.7 mg/kg of hydrocortisone may alleviate the symptoms in some patients. Meperidine is also effective (Burks *et al.*, 1980). Intravenous infusion by means of a pediatric scalp-vein needle and the addition of heparin (1000 units per infusion) may decrease the risk of thrombophlebitis. A cream, lotion, and ointment containing 3% amphotericin B are also marketed.

Opinions vary as to the most effective dosage and schedule for administration of amphotericin B. To a certain extent, this is dependent on the type and severity of infection. Most agree that a small test dose (1 mg dissolved in 20 ml of 5% dextrose solution) should first be administered intravenously over 20 to 30 minutes. The temperature, pulse, respiratory rate, and blood pressure should be recorded every 30 minutes for 4 hours. Fever, chills, hypotension, and dyspnea are common. A patient with a severe, rapidly progressing fungal infection, good cardiopulmonary function, and a mild reaction to the test dose can immediately receive 0.3 mg/kg of amphotericin B intravenously dissolved in 500 ml of 5% dextrose in water over a period of 2 to 6 hours (Bennett, 1985). If the patient has a severe reaction to the test dose or cardiopulmonary impairment, a smaller second dose is recommended—for example, 5 to 10 mg. This may then be increased by 5 to 10 mg per day to a final daily dosage of 0.5 mg/kg or, at most, 0.7 mg/kg in patients with normal renal function. While daily maintenance doses of 1 to 1.5 mg/kg have been recommended by some investigators, such regimens often cause renal toxicity and have no documented therapeutic advantage. Others have suggested that smaller daily doses (0.3 to 0.5 mg/kg) can be used effectively for the treatment of most mycoses. They recommend that dosage be adjusted to produce a peak concentration in plasma at least twice that required to inhibit growth of the fungus isolated from the patient (*see* Drutz *et al.*, 1968). Still others have suggested that adjustment of dose on the basis of concentrations in plasma and the sensitivity of the microorganism is of little value, since the technic is difficult and of unproven clinical benefit (Bennett, 1974). Measurement of concentrations of amphotericin B in plasma is probably only of value in situations in which the ability to deliver a given daily dose of amphotericin B is severely restricted. Unusually small doses of the drug given intravenously (10 to 355 mg over 4 to 18 days) have cured some patients with systemic *Candida* infections (Medoff *et al.*, 1971b).

The febrile reactions associated with the administration of amphotericin B usually subside despite consistent use of the drug, and the concurrent use of hydrocortisone can frequently be stopped. Amphotericin B may be administered every other day by doubling the recommended daily dose without sacrifice of therapeutic efficacy (Medical Letter, 1984). The individual dose should not exceed 70 mg in the alternate-day regimen, even if the *daily* dose was greater than 35 mg. There is a greater chance for toxicity and no proof of additional efficacy above this dose. Although this schedule decreases the number of venipunctures and allows more ambulation, there is no reduction in nephrotoxicity and the severity of febrile reactions may increase.

Intrathecal infusion of amphotericin B is necessary in patients with meningitis caused by *Coccidioides*. Up to 0.5 mg of the drug is dissolved in at least 5 ml of spinal fluid and is injected two or three times a week into the lumbar, cisternal, or ventricular CSF. The addition of hydrocortisone (5 to 15 mg) to the injection may reduce side effects, such as fever, headache, and nausea. Use of an artificial reservoir may be necessary for long-term treatment (Posner, 1973); daily doses of up to 0.3 mg infused intraventricularly over a 1-hour period have been used. The incidence of complications with this technic is high (Diamond and Bennett, 1973). Intra-articular doses of 5 to 15 mg have also been administered; this route should be used only when it is deemed necessary to deliver a high dose of the drug to a confined site. The safety of this approach is not established.

Untoward Effects. A large number and variety of untoward effects may be associated with the use of amphotericin B. These include *anaphylaxis, thrombocytopenia, flushing, generalized pain, convulsions, chills, fever, phlebitis, headache, anemia, anorexia,* and *decreased renal function.* About 50% of initial intravenous injections of the drug are associated with chills and about 20% with vomiting; the temperature may rise to as high as 40° C. Fever and chills may develop with every injection in

the same individual, but they usually decrease with sequential injections. There is no clear proof that amphotericin B causes hepatic toxicity (Bennett, 1974), although early reports suggested this association.

Renal function becomes impaired in over 80% of persons given amphotericin B, and this should thus be expected as a result of treatment. The degree of azotemia commonly plateaus at a level that correlates with the daily dose. Renal function usually returns toward normal, even when therapy is continued, but most patients who receive a complete course will be left with some residual reduction in glomerular filtration. The degree of damage is dependent on the total dose of drug. Reduction in dosage is recommended when plasma creatinine increases above 3.5 mg/dl to prevent symptoms of uremia (Bennett, 1985). Adequate hydration remains the most important method of minimizing azotemia. *Mild renal tubular acidosis* and *hypokalemia* are frequent, and supplemental administration of potassium may be required. *Hypomagnesemia* is also observed, but it is not clear if this effect is of renal origin. Pathological changes are seen particularly in the renal tubular cells but also may include thickening and fragmentation of the glomerular basement membrane, hypercellularity, fibrosis and hyalinization of the glomeruli, and nephrocalcinosis (McCurdy *et al.*, 1968; Douglas and Healy, 1969). There may be a synergistic nephrotoxic effect when an aminoglycoside or cyclosporine is used concurrently with amphotericin B (Churchill and Seely, 1977; Kennedy *et al.*, 1983).

Amphotericin B frequently produces normochromic, normocytic *anemia;* the bone marrow reveals a decrease in erythrocyte production; the blood picture usually becomes normal after treatment is stopped. Amphotericin-induced anemia is associated with very low concentrations of erythropoietin (MacGregor *et al.*, 1978). *Leukopenia* and *thrombocytopenia* may occur rarely (Chan *et al.*, 1982).

The *intrathecal injection* of amphotericin B may produce *pain along the distribution of lumbar nerves, headache, paresthesias, nerve palsies* (including *foot-drop*), *chemical meningitis, difficulty in micturition,* and possibly *impairment of vision.* Transient or persistent *parkinsonism* has also been reported (Fischer and Dewald, 1983).

The subconjunctival injection of amphotericin B may produce permanent yellow discoloration of the conjunctiva. When the dose exceeds 5 mg, salmon-colored, raised nodules develop on the conjunctiva; these resolve gradually after treatment is stopped (Bell and Ritchey, 1973).

For a review of the untoward effects of amphotericin B, *see* Maddux and Barriere (1980).

Therapeutic Uses. Amphotericin B is effective in a number of *fungal infections* that, prior to the availability of this drug, were almost invariably fatal. In addition, the empirical use of amphotericin B has become increasingly necessary in severely immunocompromised hosts with fever and unidentified infection (DeGregorio *et al.*, 1982).

The duration of treatment with amphotericin B varies with the nature, severity, and course of the infection, as well as with the development of untoward effects that may necessitate the temporary cessation of therapy or a reduction in dose; recurrences require another full course of drug. Except for treatment of certain infections caused by *Candida*, the period of therapy is usually about 6 to 10 weeks; it may need to be extended to as long as 3 to 4 months in some cases. *All patients requiring amphotericin B must be hospitalized*, at least for the initiation of therapy, and they must be under close observation throughout a course of systemic administration of the drug. Hemograms and urinalyses, as well as determinations of the concentrations of potassium, magnesium, urea nitrogen, and creatinine in plasma, should be made two to three times a week, especially during the period when the dose is being increased. If evidence of significant toxicity appears, the dose may have to be reduced.

NYSTATIN

Source and Chemistry. *Streptomyces noursei* is the source of *nystatin*, and the name of the antibiotic is derived from *New York State*. Nystatin is a polyene antibiotic (Dutcher *et al.*, 1954), and its structure is similar to that of amphotericin B (*see* above). Nystatin is only slightly soluble in water (10 to 20 units per milliliter).

Antifungal Activity. Nystatin is both fungistatic and fungicidal. *Candida, Cryptococcus, Histoplasma,* and *Blastomyces* are sensitive *in vitro* to concentrations ranging from 1.5 to 6.5 μg/ml. It is generally less susceptible to changes in pH than are other antifungal agents. Nystatin is without effect on bacteria, protozoa, or viruses. Since nystatin is too toxic for parenteral use for systemic fungal infections, its predominant use is for the topical treatment of candidiasis.

Mechanism of Action. The mechanism of the antifungal activity of nystatin is similar to that of amphotericin B, described above.

Fungal Resistance. Repeated subculture of *Candida albicans* in increasing concentrations of nystatin results in little development of resistance. However, other species of *Candida* (*C. tropicalis, C. guillermondi, C. krusei,* and *C. stellatoides*) become quite resistant to nystatin and simultaneously

become cross-resistant to amphotericin as well. This resistance is lost when the antibiotic is removed. Resistance does not, as a rule, develop during therapy.

Absorption and Excretion. Absorption of nystatin from the gastrointestinal tract is negligible, and the drug appears in the feces. Persons with renal insufficiency may occasionally develop detectable concentrations of the drug in plasma. Parenteral treatment is not employed.

Preparations, Routes of Administration, and Dosage. Preparations of *nystatin* (MYCOSTATIN, NILSTAT) include *ointments, oral suspensions,* and *oral* and *vaginal tablets. Creams, powders, ointments,* and *suspensions* contain 100,000 units of nystatin per gram or per milliliter; many topical preparations also contain other antibiotics such as neomycin and gramicidin, and triamcinolone acetonide is incorporated in some. Tablets for oral therapy contain 500,000 units; vaginal tablets contain 100,000 units.

The *oral dose for adults* for oral candidiasis is 500,000 to 1 million units, three or four times a day; for *children,* 100,000 to 400,000 units, three to four times per day. Some have prescribed vaginal suppositories *per os,* sucked on like a troche three or four times per day, to produce adequate bathing of the lesions with drug. There is significant controversy over whether these doses (or doses up to 20 million units per day) can really suppress enteric (including esophageal) candidiasis. Doses in excess of 4.5 million units per day have been shown to be required if there is to be any effect at all on enteric colonization by *Candida* species (Drutz, 1982). Topical application is usually made two or three times a day. Vaginal tablets are inserted once or twice daily for 14 days.

Untoward Effects. Untoward effects of nystatin are uncommon. Mild and transitory nausea, vomiting, and diarrhea may occur after oral administration of the drug. A major complaint is the vile taste of nystatin. There is a flavored preparation that can be frozen on a stick ("nystatin popsicle"). Irritation of the skin and mucous membranes does not result from topical application.

Therapeutic Uses. Nystatin is used primarily to treat *Candida* infections of skin, mucous membrane, and intestinal tract. Vaginitis and stomatitis (thrush) caused by this microorganism are usually benefited by topical therapy. Oral, esophageal, and gastric candidiasis are common complications in patients with hematological malignancies, especially those receiving immunosuppressive therapy; such infections may respond to oral nystatin (*see* above). However, if dysphagia is not improved after several days of treatment or if the patient is severely ill, amphotericin B should be administered parenterally. *Vaginal candidiasis* usually responds well to topical application of the drug.

Prophylactic Uses. Nystatin has been administered with the tetracyclines for the purpose of preventing the overgrowth of yeasts and fungi in the bowel of patients predisposed to infections with *Candida*. A controlled study failed to demonstrate a reduction in the incidence of oral candidiasis in patients with acute leukemia who received nystatin orally (Williams *et al.*, 1977).

FLUCYTOSINE

Chemistry. *Flucytosine* is a fluorinated pyrimidine related to fluorouracil and floxuridine. It is 5-fluorocytosine, the formula of which is as follows:

Flucytosine

Antifungal Activity. Flucytosine inhibits the multiplication of *Cryp. neoformans* at concentrations of 0.5 to 4 μg/ml. In some studies, up to 50% of strains of *C. albicans* are resistant (minimal inhibitory concentration [MIC], >100 μg/ml), while susceptible strains of *Candida* are suppressed by concentrations of the drug ranging from 0.4 to 8 μg/ml. Resistance of *C. albicans* is dependent on the serotype and is especially common with serotype A. Strains of *C. glabrata* are inhibited by concentrations of 0.5 to 1 μg/ml. The minimal fungistatic concentrations for *Aspergillus* species range from 0.5 to greater than 100 μg/ml, and the majority of isolates are probably resistant (MIC, >15 μg/ml). Some species of *Cladosporium*, especially *Cladosporium trichoides*, and *Phialophora*, the agents responsible for chromoblastomycosis, are sensitive. The combination of flucytosine and amphotericin B results in synergistic activity *in vitro* against *Cryp. neoformans* and sensitive strains of *C. albicans* and *C. tropicalis*. Flucytosine is without effect on most strains of *Spor. schenckii* and all strains of *B. dermatitidis*, *H. capsulatum*, *Coccid. immitis*, *Rhizopus oryzea*, and *Absidia corymbifer*. Bacteria are generally resistant, although 5-fluorouracil, a metabolite of flucytosine, inhibits a broad range of aerobic bacteria. (*See* Bennett, 1985.)

Fungal Resistance. Resistance to flucytosine is defined as an MIC of greater than 12.5 μg/ml after 48 hours of incubation. Development of resistance to flucytosine *during therapy* has been described in 30% of patients with cryptococcosis (Block *et al.*, 1973), and this has severely restricted its use for the sole treatment of fungal infections. Resistance to flucytosine can also develop during treatment of infections with *C. albicans* (Normark and Schönebeck, 1972). The mechanisms of drug resistance are not completely understood.

Mechanism of Action. Flucytosine is converted in fungal cells to *fluorouracil* by the enzyme cytosine deaminase. Fluorouracil is then metabolized to 5-fluorodeoxyuridylic acid, an inhibitor of thymidylate synthetase (Waldorf and Polak, 1983). Synthesis of 5-fluorouridine triphosphate and RNA that contains this analog may also take place. Mammalian cells do not convert large amounts of flucytosine to fluorouracil. This is crucial for the selective action of this compound. The cytotoxic activity of fluorinated pyrimidines is discussed in detail in Chapter 55.

Absorption, Distribution, and Excretion. Flucytosine is rapidly and well absorbed from the gastrointestinal tract. It is widely distributed in the body, with a volume of distribution approximating the total body water. The drug is minimally bound to plasma proteins. The peak plasma concentration in patients with normal renal function is approximately 70 to 80 μg/ml 1 to 2 hours after a dose of 37.5 mg/kg (Bennett *et al.*, 1979). Approximately 80% of a given dose is excreted in the urine by glomerular filtration in unchanged form; concentrations in the urine range from 200 to 500 μg/ml. The half-life of the drug is 3 to 6 hours in normal individuals. In renal failure, the half-life may be as long as 200 hours. The clearance of flucytosine is approximately equivalent to that of creatinine. Because of the obligate renal excretion of the drug, modification of dosage is necessary in patients with decreased renal function (*see* Appendix II). It is recommended that concentrations of drug in plasma be measured periodically in patients with renal insufficiency. Peak concentrations should range between 50 and 100 μg/ml. Flucytosine is cleared by hemodialysis, and patients undergoing such treatment should receive a single dose of 37.5 mg/kg after dialysis (Bennett, 1985); the drug is also removed by peritoneal dialysis.

Flucytosine is present in CSF at a concentration about 65 to 90% of that simultaneously present in the plasma. The drug also appears to penetrate into the aqueous humor.

Preparations, Route of Administration, and Dosage. *Flucytosine* (ANCOBON) is supplied in capsules containing either 250 or 500 mg for oral administration. There are no parenteral preparations available in the United States. The usual daily dose is 50 to 150 mg/kg, given at 6-hour intervals. This dosage must be altered, as described above, for patients with renal insufficiency.

Untoward Effects. Flucytosine may depress the function of bone marrow and lead to the development of *anemia, leukopenia,* and *thrombocytopenia;* patients are more prone to the appearance of this complication if they have an underlying hematological disorder, are being treated with radiation or drugs that injure the bone marrow, or have a history of treatment with such agents. Other untoward effects, including *nausea, vomiting, diarrhea,* and severe *enterocolitis,* have been noted. In approximately 5% of patients elevation of hepatic enzymes in plasma and *hepatomegaly* have occurred, but these are reversible when therapy is stopped (Steer *et al.,* 1972). All of these complications are more frequent in patients with azotemia, including those who are receiving amphotericin B concurrently, and are markedly increased when concentrations of the drug in plasma exceed 100 μg/ml (Kauffman and Frame, 1977). Some toxicity may be the result of conversion of flucytosine to 5-fluorouracil by the host (Diasio *et al.,* 1978).

Therapeutic Uses. Amphotericin B remains the most effective therapeutic agent for the management of infections due to yeasts and fungi; flucytosine is used predominantly in combination with amphotericin B. It is less toxic than amphotericin B and it can be administered orally. However, except in the treatment of chromoblastomycosis, rapid emergence of flucytosine-resistant strains has restricted its use as a single drug (Mauceri *et al.,* 1974). Flucytosine may be useful for the treatment of infections of the urinary tract with *Candida,* but not if a catheter is in the bladder. The concurrent administration of amphotericin B (0.3 mg/kg per day) and flucytosine (100 to 150 mg/kg per day) has become the treatment of choice for cryptococcal meningitis (*see* page 1228; Utz *et al.,* 1975; Bennett *et al.,* 1979).

GRISEOFULVIN

History and Source. *Griseofulvin* was first isolated from *Penicillium griseofulvum dierckx* by Oxford and coworkers in 1939. Because it was ineffective against bacteria, no further attention was paid to it for some time. In 1946, Brian and associates found a substance in *Penicillium janczewski* that produced shrinking and stunting of fungal hyphae; they named this the *curling factor;* it was later found to be *griseofulvin.* During the next 10 years, the antibiotic was widely employed in the treatment of a variety of fungal diseases in plants and of ringworm of cattle. The search for potential therapeutic compounds for the management of fun-

gal infections of the feet of Scottish miners led Gentles in 1958 to observe that griseofulvin cured experimentally produced mycotic disease of guinea pigs. Soon thereafter, the drug was subjected to clinical trials and became available for general use.

Chemistry. The structural formula of griseofulvin is as follows:

Griseofulvin

The drug is practically insoluble in water. It is remarkably thermostable.

Antifungal Activity. Griseofulvin is fungistatic *in vitro* for various species of the dermatophytes *Microsporum, Epidermophyton,* and *Trichophyton.* The drug has no effect on bacteria or on other fungi, yeasts, *Actinomyces,* or *Nocardia.* Young, actively metabolizing cells may be killed by the drug, but older, more dormant elements are only inhibited.

Fungal Resistance. *Trichophyton, Epidermophyton,* and *Microsporum* can be made resistant to griseofulvin *in vitro,* and such strains remain fully virulent as infectious agents in animals. Isolates from humans receiving the antibiotic appear, with a few exceptions, to retain their sensitivity to the drug when examined *in vitro.* Dermatophytes concentrate griseofulvin by an energy-dependent process, and such uptake is correlated with the sensitivity of the fungi to the antibiotic (*see* El-Nakeeb and Lampen, 1965).

Mechanism of Action. A prominent morphological manifestation of the action of griseofulvin is the production of multinucleate cells as the drug inhibits fungal mitosis (Gull and Trinci, 1973). An explanation for this phenomenon appears to come from studies of the effects of higher concentrations of the antibiotic on mammalian cells. Griseofulvin causes disruption of the mitotic spindle by interacting with polymerized microtubules. While the effects of the drug are thus similar to those of colchicine and the *Vinca* alkaloids, its binding sites on the microtubular protein are distinct. (*See* Malawista *et al.,* 1968; Grisham *et al.,* 1973.)

Absorption, Distribution, and Excretion. The oral administration of griseofulvin produces peak plasma concentrations at about 4 hours, approximately 1 μg/ml when a single dose of 0.5 g is given. These values are quite variable because of the insolubility of griseofulvin. Absorption may be increased if the drug is taken with a fatty meal. Since the rates of dissolution and disaggregation limit the bioavailability of griseofulvin, microsized and ultramicrosized powders are now used in preparations. While the bioavailability of the ultramicrocrystalline preparation is said to be 50% greater than that of the conventional microsized powder, this may not be uniformly correct (Aoyagi *et al.*, 1982). Griseofulvin has a half-life in plasma of about 1 day, and approximately 50% of the oral dose can be detected in the urine within 5 days, mostly in the form of metabolites. The primary metabolite is 6-methylgriseofulvin. Barbiturates decrease the absorption of griseofulvin from the gastrointestinal tract.

The drug is deposited in keratin precursor cells. The antibiotic present in such cells when they differentiate is tightly bound to, and persists in, *keratin* and makes this substance resistant to fungal invasion. For this reason, the new growth of hair or nails is the first to become free of disease. As the fungus-containing keratin is shed, it is replaced by normal tissue. Griseofulvin is detectable in the stratum corneum of the skin within 4 to 8 hours of oral administration. Sweat and transepidermal fluid loss play an important role in the transfer of the drug in the stratum corneum (Shah *et al.*, 1974). Only a very small fraction of a dose of the drug is present in body fluids and tissues.

Preparations, Routes of Administration, and Dosage. *Griseofulvin* microsize (FULVICIN U/F, GRIFULVIN V) is marketed in *capsules* containing 125 or 250 mg and in *tablets* containing 250 or 500 mg; it is also available as an *oral suspension* (125 mg/5 ml). The daily dose recommended for children is 10 mg/kg; for adults, 500 mg to 1 g. Larger doses (1.5 to 2 g per day) may be used for a short time in severe and extensive infections, but the amount should be reduced to 500 mg to 1 g per day when the lesions begin to respond. Best results may be obtained when medication is given at 6-hour intervals. Tablets incorporating an ultramicrosized preparation (FULVICIN P/G, GRIS-PEG) contain 125 to 330 mg of griseofulvin.

Untoward Effects. The incidence of serious reactions associated with the use of griseofulvin is very low. Among the minor effects, the incidence of which may be as high as 15%, is *headache* that is sometimes severe and usually disappears as therapy is continued. Other *nervous system manifestations* include peripheral neuritis, lethargy, mental confusion, impairment of performance of routine tasks, fatigue, syncope, vertigo, blurred vision, transient macular edema, and augmentation of the effects of alcohol. Among the side effects involving the *alimentary tract* are nausea, vomiting, diarrhea, heartburn, flatulence, dry mouth, and angular stomatitis. *Hepatotoxicity* has also been observed. *Hematological effects* include leukopenia, neutropenia, punctate basophilia, and monocytosis; these often disappear despite continuation of therapy. Blood studies should be carried out at least once a week during the first month of treatment or longer. Common *renal effects* include albuminuria and cylindruria, without evidence of renal insufficiency. Reactions involving the *skin* are cold and warm urticaria, photosensitivity, lichen planus, erythema,

erythema multiforme-like rashes, and vesicular and morbilliform eruptions. *Serum-sickness syndromes* and severe *angioedema* develop rarely during treatment with griseofulvin. *Estrogen-like effects* have been observed in children. A moderate but inconsistent increase of *fecal protoporphyrins* has been noted when the drug is used for a long period of time.

Griseofulvin may induce hepatic microsomal enzymes, thus increasing the rate of metabolism of warfarin; adjustment of the dosage of the latter agent may be necessary in at least some patients.

Therapeutic Uses. Mycotic disease of the *skin, hair,* and *nails* due to *Microsporum, Trichophyton,* or *Epidermophyton* responds to griseofulvin therapy. Infections that are readily treatable with this agent include infections of the *hair (tinea capitis)* caused by *M. canis, M. audouinii, T. schoenleinii,* and *T. verrucosum;* "*ringworm*" *of the glabrous skin; tinea cruris* and *tinea corporis* caused by *M. canis, T. rubrum, T. verrucosum,* and *Epidermophyton floccosum;* and *tinea of the hands (T. rubrum, T. mentagrophytes)* and *beard (Trichophyton* species). Griseofulvin is also highly effective in "athlete's foot" or epidermophytosis involving the skin and nails, the vesicular form of which is most commonly due to *T. mentagrophytes,* and the hyperkeratotic type to *T. rubrum.* However, topical therapy is preferred (*see* Chapter 41). *Trichophyton rubrum* and *T. mentagrophytes* infections may require higher-than-conventional doses. Since very high doses of griseofulvin are carcinogenic and teratogenic in laboratory animals, the drug should not be used to treat trivial infections that respond to topical therapy. (For review of griseofulvin therapy, *see* Symposium, 1960; Goldman, 1970.)

HYDROXYSTILBAMIDINE ISETHIONATE

This drug, an aromatic diamidine, is active against fungi and protozoa. Like its congener, *pentamidine* (Chapter 47), it has a suppressive effect on *B. dermatitidis in vitro* and in experimental infections in mice, and has produced favorable results in cutaneous and pulmonary *human North American blastomycosis;* however, the incidence of relapse has been high. The alarming untoward effects that may be produced by the compound are the same as those caused by pentamidine. *Hydroxystilbamidine isethionate* is available in ampuls containing 225 mg of dry, sterile powder. A freshly prepared solution of 225 mg of the drug in 200 ml of 5% dextrose in water or isotonic sodium chloride solution is infused over a period of 2 to 3 hours, every 24 hours; rapid infusion may cause hypotension. The solution must be protected from light. The duration of therapy varies with the location and the severity of the disease. The drug should not be used to treat severe blastomycosis (*see* below), but may be given to selected patients with cutaneous blastomycosis. Anorexia, malaise, and nausea are common untoward responses to hydroxystilbamidine; rash and hepatotoxicity also occur.

IMIDAZOLES

Several substituted imidazole derivatives are currently available for systemic or topical use for the treatment of a variety of fungal infections. The agents that are used topically include *clotrimazole, econazole,* and *miconazole;* they are discussed in Chapter 41. The systemic uses of *ketoconazole* and *miconazole* are described here. Other related agents that are under study include *bifonazole, itraconazole,* and *terconazole.*

Antifungal Activity. Testing *in vitro* has shown these agents to be highly active against a broad spectrum of fungi, including dermatophytes, yeasts, dimorphic fungi, eumycetes, actinomycetes, and some phycomycetes (*see* Heel *et al.,* 1980, 1982; *see also* Chapter 41). However, activity is greatly dependent upon factors such as culture medium, pH, and the size of the inoculum (Minagawa *et al.,* 1983; Van Cutsem, 1983). The data are thus difficult to interpret, and there are no firm indications for performance of sensitivity testing *in vitro* (Bennett, 1985). These imidazole derivatives also inhibit the growth of gram-positive bacteria and certain anaerobes.

Mechanism of Action. The effect of the imidazoles on yeast and other fungi appears to be related to their ability to alter membrane permeability. Ergosterol is the primary cellular sterol of fungi; its synthesis is blocked by these agents. The inhibition of ergosterol synthesis is due in part to the ability of the imidazoles to inhibit the demethylation of lanosterol, a precursor of ergosterol. Both miconazole and ketoconazole have profound effects on the cytochrome P-450 of yeast, which may explain many of the effects of these drugs, including the inhibition of lanosterol demethylase. Ketoconazole inhibits sex steroid biosynthesis, perhaps by a similar mechanism. The imidazole derivatives also interfere with fatty acid synthesis (*see* Drutz, 1982; Borgers *et al.,* 1983).

KETOCONAZOLE

Ketoconazole, administered orally, has broad therapeutic potential for the treatment of a number of superficial and systemic fungal infections. Its structural formula is as follows:

Ketoconazole

Antifungal Activity. Subject to the limitations described above, the MIC of ketoconazole for *Coccid. immitis, Cryp. neoformans, H. capsulatum,* and *B. dermatitidis* ranges from less than 0.125 μg/ml to 0.5 μg/ml. Corresponding values for *Candida* species, *Aspergillus* species, and *Sporothrix* species vary from 6 μg/ml to greater than 100 μg/ml (Hume and Kerkering, 1983).

The concurrent effects of ketoconazole and other antifungal agents have been explored *in vitro* and in animal models of infection. With *Candida,* there is at least an additive effect when the yeast are exposed to both ketoconazole and flucytosine, even with strains that are resistant to usual concentrations of flucytosine (Beggs and Sarosi, 1982). In contrast, exposure of *C. albicans* to ketoconazole causes resistance to the effects of amphotericin B (Sud and Feingold, 1983). Similar conclusions on the utility of such combinations have been reached by study of animal models of cryptococcosis (Craven and Graybill, 1984; Iwen *et al.,* 1984).

Absorption, Distribution, and Elimination. An acidic environment is required for the dissolution of ketoconazole, and drugs that reduce gastric acidity (*e.g.,* H_2-blocking agents and antacids) can reduce the bioavailability of ketoconazole markedly. There are conflicting reports on the effects of meals on absorption of the drug. Peak concentrations of ketoconazole approximate 5 to 9 μg/ml 2 hours after an oral dose of 400 mg (Daneshmend *et al.,* 1984). The distribution of ketoconazole is limited, and its penetration into CSF is minimal (Brass *et al.,* 1982). The drug does, however, appear in milk. More than 90% of the ketoconazole in the circulation is bound to protein.

The rate of elimination of ketoconazole appears to be dose dependent; the elimination half-life is approximately 90 minutes after a 200-mg dose, but it increases to nearly 4 hours when 800 mg is given. Longer half-lives have been reported in other studies (*see* Heel *et al.,* 1982). Very little unchanged drug appears in the urine, and the metabolism takes place in the liver. Ketoconazole may compete with cyclosporine for hepatic metabolism and increase the possibility of nephrotoxicity from the immunosuppressive agent (Dieperink and Moller, 1982; Bennett and Pulliam, 1983). Induction of hepatic microsomal enzymes by rifampin accelerates the metabolic clearance of ketoconazole (Brass *et al.,* 1982). It is advisable to monitor concentrations of ketoconazole in plasma of patients with hepatic failure.

Preparation, Route of Administration, and Dosage. *Ketoconazole* (NIZORAL) is available as 200-mg tablets. The recommended dose is 200 mg, given once daily. In severe infections or when the response is insufficient, 400 mg may be given. For patients with achlorhydria, the drug should be dissolved in 4 ml of 0.2 N HCl. This solution is sipped through a straw to avoid contact with the teeth; the patient should then drink a glass of water.

Untoward Effects. Nausea and vomiting are the most common side effects of ketoconazole, but the incidence may be reduced by administration of the drug with food. Other less common adverse effects include anorexia, headache, epigastric pain, photophobia, paresthesias, gingival bleeding, rash, and thrombocytopenia (Dismukes *et al.*, 1983). Gynecomastia has been reported (Defelice *et al.*, 1981). Studies in animals have shown that ketoconazole inhibits stimulation of testicular synthesis of androgens by chorionic gonadotropin. Ketoconazole also displaces sex steroids from sex hormone–binding globulin (Grosso *et al.*, 1983). Studies in animals and man have shown that ketoconazole significantly blunts the response of cortisol to the administration of ACTH (Pont *et al.*, 1982). Hepatic dysfunction has also been associated with ketoconazole. Mild asymptomatic elevation of transaminase activities in plasma occurs in approximately 5 to 10% of patients. The incidence of symptomatic, potentially serious hepatic toxicity is low and approximates 1 in 15,000 persons. Pathological findings have included acute hepatocellular damage, cholestatic injury, or a mixed process (Janssen and Symoens, 1983; Lewis *et al.*, 1984). This reaction does not appear to be dependent on dose.

Therapeutic Uses. Ketoconazole is particularly useful in the treatment of histoplasmosis involving the lungs, bones and joints, or skin and soft tissues, as well as the progressive disseminated disease (Hawkins *et al.*, 1981; Dismukes *et al.*, 1983). Since ketoconazole penetrates into the CSF poorly, it is not recommended for cryptococcal meningitis; however, the drug has been effective in nonmeningeal cryptococcal disease. Ketoconazole has proven therapeutic efficacy in paracoccidioidomycosis, blastomycosis, certain forms of coccidioidomycosis, some dermatomycoses, and infections caused by *Candida* species (*i.e.*, mucocutaneous candidiasis, vaginitis, and thrush). Ketoconazole has several limitations. It is administered orally, and absorption may be erratic. The response to treatment is typically slow, and this agent is thus less useful in acute, severe fungal infections; it is desirable for

chronic suppressive therapy. It is of limited utility for infections of the urinary tract, since it is metabolized extensively before excretion. Treatment with very high doses of ketoconazole may be useful in the treatment of infections of the central nervous system (CNS), but only when other alternatives are not available. Testing of the susceptibility of isolates *in vitro* is often not useful for predicting the clinical response (Drutz, 1982; Dismukes *et al.*, 1983; Medical Letter, 1984; Bennett, 1985). Ketoconazole should probably not be used in combination with amphotericin B, since antagonism may occur (Iwen *et al.*, 1984).

MICONAZOLE

Miconazole is used primarily as a topical agent (*see* Chapter 41). It is also used parenterally for the treatment of systemic fungal infections (*see* Bennett, 1985). However, because of its toxicity and limited efficacy, indications for such use are few.

Absorption, Distribution, and Excretion. Intravenous administration of 600 mg of miconazole over a period of 15 minutes results in peak concentrations in plasma of 2 to 6 μg/ml in subjects with normal renal function. Higher peak concentrations (up to 33 μg/ml) are achieved in patients with renal insufficiency, due to a decreased initial volume of distribution. The distribution of miconazole over 4 to 8 hours results in concentrations in plasma of 0.1 to 0.6 μg/ml (Lewi *et al.*, 1976; Stevens *et al.*, 1976). Thus, inhibitory concentrations for susceptible fungi (2 to 8 μg/ml) are maintained in plasma for only a few hours. Penetration into CSF is poor, and intrathecal administration of the drug is necessary in meningitis. The elimination half-life of miconazole is about 24 hours, and most of the drug is metabolized. About 90% of miconazole is bound to plasma protein, primarily to albumin.

Preparation, Routes of Administration, and Dosage. *Miconazole for infusion* (MONISTAT I.V.) is available as a solution containing 10 mg/ml. Miconazole is usually administered intravenously every 8 hours, and the total daily dose for adults ranges from 200 to 3600 mg, depending on the infection. Doses of up to 20 to 30 mg, given by various intrathecal routes, have been used to treat coccidioidal meningitis (Sung *et al.*, 1977; Stevens, 1983). Such doses produce concentrations of miconazole in CSF of at least 1 μg/ml for 24 hours (Deresinski *et al.*, 1977).

Untoward Effects. Adverse reactions are frequent after the intravenous administration of miconazole. Those that are attributed to miconazole itself include nausea, vomiting, anemia, thrombocytosis, and hyponatremia. Anaphylactoid reactions, CNS toxicity (euphoria, tremors, confusion, dizziness, hallucinations, blurred vision, and seizures), arthralgia, and weakness have also been reported. Other adverse reactions have been attributed to the vehicle, CREMOPHOR EL, which contains polyethylene glycol, castor oil, and parabens. These reactions include hyperlipidemia, pruritus, formication, thrombocytosis, and cardiorespiratory arrest (Drutz, 1982). The last-named reaction appears to be related to the rate and duration of drug administration, and it is thus recommended that no less than 200 ml of diluent be used and that the infusion be administered over at least 2 hours (Fainstein and Bodey, 1980).

Miconazole appears to inhibit the metabolism of phenytoin and warfarin significantly (Rolan *et al.*, 1983; Stevens, 1983).

Therapeutic Uses. Miconazole given parenterally is not the drug of choice for any fungal infection because of its toxicity. It is useful only in rare and difficult circumstances, such as the critically ill patient with *Pseudoallescheria boydii* infection (Bennett, 1985) or in those who are not able to tolerate amphotericin B. The drug has also been used with limited success in other forms of coccidioidomycosis, paracoccidioidomycosis, and petriellidiosis (Stevens, 1977; Stevens *et al.*, 1978; Lutwick *et al.*, 1979). There are few data to support its use in the treatment of systemic candidiasis and cryptococcosis.

CLOTRIMAZOLE

This antifungal agent is used primarily for topical treatment of vulvovaginal candidiasis or cutaneous infections due to susceptible pathogens (*see* Chapter 41). The 10-mg clotrimazole troche has been used successfully for the treatment of oral candidiasis (Kirkpatrick and Alling, 1978; Yap and Bodey, 1979; Shechtman *et al.*, 1984). Clotrimazole troches have also been shown to be effective prophylaxis for oral candidiasis in certain immunocompromised patients, recipients of renal transplants, and patients with solid tumors (Owens *et al.*, 1984). Clotrimazole troches are well tolerated when used as an oral lozenge.

THERAPY OF SYSTEMIC FUNGAL INFECTIONS

Therapeutic regimens for the treatment of systemic fungal infections have been reviewed by Medoff and Kobayashi (1980), Drutz (1982), and Bennett (1985).

Cryptococcosis. Cryptococcal infection may primarily involve the lungs or the meninges or be widely disseminated. Meningeal or disseminated infections always require therapy, since mortality without treatment is nearly uniform. Some patients with symptomatic cryptococcal pneumonia may also benefit from treatment with amphotericin B. Treatment of cryptococcal meningitis with high doses of amphotericin B (1 mg/kg daily for 6 weeks) results in favorable clinical responses in 75% of patients, but relapse occurs in up to one third of these individuals after treatment is discontinued (Sarosi *et al.*, 1969). In addition, the incidence of toxicity is extremely high. Low doses of amphotericin B (0.4 mg/kg daily for 10 weeks) are equally efficacious and cause less toxicity (Drutz *et al.*, 1968). The concurrent administration of low doses of amphotericin B (0.3 mg/kg per day) plus

flucytosine (150 mg/kg per day) for 6 weeks has been compared with amphotericin B alone (0.4 mg/kg per day) for 10 weeks. Results suggest that the combination is superior, as measured by a more rapid rate of sterilization of the CSF, reduced nephrotoxicity, and the overall rate of cure (Bennett *et al.*, 1979). However, this dose of flucytosine commonly causes bone-marrow toxicity, and it is often necessary to stop administration of the drug. Nonmeningeal cryptococcosis may respond to treatment with ketoconazole, whereas cryptococcal meningitis does not, despite adequate concentrations of the drug in plasma and CSF (Perfect *et al.*, 1982; Dismukes *et al.*, 1983).

Histoplasmosis. *Histoplasma capsulatum* produces a variety of clinical syndromes. Acute pulmonary histoplasmosis is usually self-limited and rarely requires treatment. However, when symptoms are severe or persist beyond 14 days, patients will often respond rapidly to an abbreviated course of amphotericin B (0.4 to 0.7 mg/kg per day for a total dose of 800 to 1000 mg) (Fosson and Wheeler, 1975; Naylor, 1977). For chronic cavitary histoplasmosis, administration of a total of 1.5 to 2 g of amphotericin B over a period of 10 weeks has been successful therapy (Sutliff, 1972; Goodwin and Des Prez, 1978). Progressive disseminated histoplasmosis has a mortality rate of 80 to 90% if untreated and requires intensive treatment with amphotericin B (Smith and Utz, 1972); the usual course is a total of 2 g of amphotericin B given over a period of 10 weeks (Goodwin and Des Prez, 1978). Ketoconazole has also been used successfully in chronic pulmonary and disseminated disease; the drug is given in a dose of 400 to 800 mg per day for 6 to 12 months. Ketoconazole has even been effective after relapse following treatment with amphotericin B (Hawkins *et al.*, 1981; Bennett, 1985).

Coccidioidomycosis. Amphotericin B has been recommended for treatment of disseminated coccidioidomycosis. While primary pulmonary coccidioidomycosis usually does not require treatment, amphotericin B may be of benefit when symptoms are severe. Doses of 1 mg/kg given every other day may be required for prolonged periods. Amphotericin B is less effective in the treatment of coccidioidomycosis than it is for most other fungal infections, even though antifungal activity *in vitro* may be quite similar. This may be due to the ability of each spherule of the microorganism to produce 200 to 500 endospores ("population explosion"), whereas *H. capsulatum* and most other fungi (except *Paracoccidioides brasiliensis*) produce only a single daughter cell each (Drutz, 1983). Treatment of meningitis requires intrathecal administration of 0.5 to 1 mg of amphotericin B three times per week. As mentioned above, direct intraventricular administration with a reservoir may be used, and treatment should probably be continued for at least 3 months after the CSF appears sterile or no longer gives a positive complement-fixation test for antibody to *Coccid. immitis* (Goldstein *et al.*, 1972; Bennett, 1981). Relapsing and resistant cases of coccidioidomycosis have responded to immunotherapy with transfer factor plus amphotericin B (Graybill, 1977).

Ketoconazole (400 to 800 mg per day) appears to have only a suppressive effect on nonmeningeal forms of coccidioidomycosis. With disease involving the skin, the response is favorable; it is less so for arthritis and pneumonia (Dismukes et al., 1983; Stevens et al., 1983; Bennett, 1985). Meningitis has developed during treatment with ketoconazole (Catanzaro et al., 1982); nevertheless, meningitis has responded in a few cases to treatment with high doses of the drug (1200 mg per day).

Blastomycosis and Paracoccidioidomycosis. Both of these diseases respond to treatment with amphotericin B. Recommended doses are similar to those for disseminated histoplasmosis—a total dose of 1.5 g, given over 6 to 10 weeks. Sulfonamides have been used to treat patients with paracoccidioidomycosis (South American blastomycosis), and favorable clinical responses occur, but patients invariably relapse when therapy is discontinued (Abernathy, 1973). Paracoccidioidomycosis responds to ketoconazole (200 to 400 mg per day), and it is now considered the drug of first choice (Bennett, 1985). Hydroxystilbamidine isethionate is effective for cutaneous or localized pulmonary blastomycosis. However, it is less effective than amphotericin B and should not be used in patients with disseminated disease. Ketoconazole (400 to 800 mg per day) may be used as an alternative to amphotericin B for the treatment of nonmeningeal blastomycosis (Drouhet and DuPont, 1983; Medical Letter, 1984).

Sporotrichosis. Amphotericin B in standard doses (total dose of 1.5 to 2 g over 6 to 10 weeks) has been used successfully in the therapy of systemic sporotrichosis, especially when the disease involves bones and joints (Crout et al., 1977). The cutaneous-lymphatic form of sporotrichosis usually responds to the oral administration of iodide (Hernandez, 1979). Sporotrichosis shows only a minimal response to ketoconazole, especially in patients with bone or joint disease (Dismukes et al., 1983).

Candidiasis. Amphotericin B is the preferred drug for the treatment of disseminated candidiasis. Most patients with this disease have suppressed immunological responses, are neutropenic, and some show evidence of fungemia (positive blood cultures for *Candida*). Amphotericin B is effective in eradicating the fungus in some instances; total doses have varied from 100 mg (or less) to 2500 mg (Young et al., 1974). A dose of 40 mg, given every other day, to a total dose of 600 to 1000 mg is probably adequate in many instances. Very low doses of amphotericin B (20 mg daily for 10 days) have been used to treat esophagitis caused by *Candida* (Medoff et al., 1972). The response is usually dramatic, with a reduction in symptoms and disappearance of the plaquelike lesions. Endocarditis produced by *Candida* species that involves natural or prosthetic valves may respond clinically to amphotericin B (with or without concurrent adminis-

tration of flucytosine), but cure almost always requires surgical removal of the infected valve.

Oral, esophageal, and vaginal candidiasis in patients with normal immunological function responds well to ketoconazole (200 to 400 mg per day). While chronic mucocutaneous disease also responds to such therapy, long-term treatment is usually necessary (Peterson et al., 1980; Drouhet and DuPont, 1983; Bennett, 1985). In the treatment and prevention of oral thrush in immunocompromised patients, ketoconazole (600 mg per day) is more effective than nystatin. Concentrations of ketoconazole in saliva fall rapidly, and this may necessitate multiple daily doses for optimal efficacy (Meunier-Carpentier, 1983; Bennett, 1985).

Other Infections. Invasive infections caused by *Aspergillus* species and *Zygomycetes* respond erratically to treatment with amphotericin B (Meyer et al., 1973). Ketoconazole has been effective in the treatment of tinea versicolor, but reinfection remains a problem for this disease (Borelli, 1980). Infections due to dermatophytes ("ringworm") have responded to treatment with ketoconazole, even when griseofulvin has not been effective. However, relapse is common after discontinuation of therapy (Legendre and Steltz, 1980; Bennett, 1985).

II. Antiviral Agents

The development of compounds useful for the prophylaxis and therapy of viral disease has presented more difficult problems than those encountered in the search for drugs effective in disorders produced by other microorganisms. This is so because, in contrast to most other infectious agents, viruses are obligate intracellular parasites that require the active participation of the metabolic processes of the invaded cell. Thus, agents that may inhibit or cause the death of viruses are also very likely to injure the host cells that harbor them. Although the search for substances that might be of use in the management of viral infections has been long and intensive, few agents have been found to have clinical applicability. Indeed, even these have exhibited very narrow activity, limited to one or only a few specific viruses. These drugs are described briefly here. (*See* Hirsch and Swartz, 1980; Hayden and Douglas, 1985.)

ACYCLOVIR

Chemistry and Antiviral Activity. *Acyclovir* is a synthetic purine nucleoside analog, 9-[(2-hydroxyethoxy)methyl]guanine, in which a linear side chain has been substituted for the cyclic sugar of the naturally occurring guanosine molecule. Its structural formula is as follows:

Acyclovir

Acyclovir has antiviral activity that is essentially confined to the herpes viruses; it is particularly active against herpes simplex type I (concentrations of 0.02 to 0.2 μg/ml will reduce viral plaque formation *in vitro* by 50%) and herpes simplex type II (corresponding values are 0.2 to 0.4 μg/ml). Varicella-zoster virus is less sensitive but is inhibited by concentrations that can be achieved clinically (0.8 to 1.2 μg/ml), while Epstein-Barr virus may be inhibited only at concentrations of at least 1.6 μg/ml. Cytomegalovirus is inhibited when concentrations of acyclovir are greater than or equal to 20 μg/ml (Hayden and Douglas, 1985). *In vitro*, acyclovir is more than 100 times more active than vidarabine and 10 times more active then idoxuridine against herpes simplex type I, but it has activity similar to that of vidarabine against varicella-zoster.

Mechanism of Action. There is a 300- to 3000-fold difference in the toxicity of acyclovir for the herpes viruses compared to that for mammalian cells. This degree of specificity is impressive and can be understood on the basis of major differences between certain normal cellular enzymes and their counterparts that are encoded by viral DNA. Thymidine kinase is particularly important in this regard. While mammalian and herpes virus thymidine kinases have similar affinities for thymidine and idoxuridine, there are marked differences in the interactions of acyclovir with the two enzymes (*see* Table 54–1). The affinity of the viral enzymes for acyclovir is 200 times greater than is that of the mammalian enzyme, and phosphorylation of acyclovir by the mammalian enzyme proceeds at a negligible rate. After synthesis of acyclovir monophosphate (acyclo-GMP) in virally infected cells, normal cellular enzymes catalyze the sequential synthesis of acyclo-GDP and acyclo-GTP. The amount of acyclo-GTP formed in herpes virus-infected cells is 40 to 100 times greater than that in uninfected cells. Acyclo-GTP then acts as a significantly more potent inhibitor of the viral DNA polymerase than of the cellular polymerases. In addition, acyclo-GTP is incorporated into viral DNA, where it causes termination of biosynthesis of the viral DNA strand (*see* Elion, in Symposium, 1982; McGuirt and Furman, in Symposium, 1982).

Resistance. Mutant strains of varicella-zoster virus that are resistant to acyclovir have been isolated *in vitro;* they produce altered thymidine kinase and/or DNA polymerase. These strains appear to be less virulent than the wild type (Field and Darby, 1980; Field, 1982), although this is not a constant finding (Darby and Field, 1981). Resistant strains of herpes simplex virus have been found after treatment with intravenous and topical acyclovir (Crumpacker *et al.,* 1982; Sibrack *et al.,* 1982; Corey and Holmes, 1983). They are also found as a small subpopulation in viral isolates from 40% of patients prior to therapy (Parris and Harrington, 1982). The clinical significance of acyclovir-resistant mutants has not been determined, but it is a matter of considerable concern.

Absorption, Elimination, and Excretion. Usual intravenous doses of acyclovir (5 mg/kg) result in peak concentrations in plasma of 10 μg/ml; these values decline to an average value of 0.7 μg/ml at 8 hours. Comparable concentrations are achieved in pediatric patients after intravenous administration of 250 mg/m^2 (de Miranda and Blum, 1983). The elimination half-life of acyclovir is about 2.5 hours in patients with normal renal function; this value is about 3.8 hours in neonates (Hintz *et al.,* in Symposium, 1982). Acyclovir is predominantly eliminated as such by glomerular filtration and tubular secretion, and only about 10% or less of an administered dose is recovered in the urine as an inactive metabolite, 9-carboxymethoxymethylguanine (Whitley *et al.,* in Symposium, 1982). Acyclovir ac-

Table 54–1. SPECIFICITIES OF THYMIDINE KINASES FROM HERPES VIRUS (TYPE I) AND FROM CULTURED MAMMALIAN (VERO) CELLS *

| | THYMIDINE KINASE | | | |
| | Herpes Virus | | Vero Cells | |
SUBSTRATE	K_m (μM)	V_{rel} [†]	K_m (μM)	V_{rel} [†]
Thymidine	0.6	100	1.3	3.4
Idoxuridine	0.5	115	1.2	3.2
Acyclovir	100	36	20,000	<0.00001

* Modified from Elion, in Symposium, 1982.

[†] Relative velocity at 1 mM substrate concentration with rate of Herpes virus enzyme for thymidine = 100.

cumulates in patients with renal failure, and the half-life of the drug in patients with end-stage renal disease is about 20 hours. The extent of binding of acyclovir to plasma proteins is low (about 15%), and the drug is readily removed by hemodialysis (Laskin *et al.* and Kransy *et al.*, in Symposium, 1982; de Miranda and Blum, 1983). Concentrations of acyclovir in CSF are approximately one half of those in plasma (Hayden and Douglas, 1985).

Oral administration of 400 mg of acyclovir results in peak concentrations in plasma of 1.2 μg/ml (after approximately 1.5 hours). The bioavailability of the oral preparation is only approximately 20% (de Miranda and Blum, 1983).

Preparations, Routes of Administration, and Dosage. *Acyclovir sodium* (ZOVIRAX) is available in 200-mg capsules, as an ointment (5%) in a polyethylene glycol base, and as a powder to be reconstituted for intravenous use. For initial therapy of genital herpes, 200 mg of acyclovir is given orally every 4 hours (five times a day) for 10 days. Dosage for chronic suppressive therapy of recurrent disease is 200 mg three to five times daily for up to 6 months. Topical treatment of lesions caused by herpes simplex should be initiated as early as possible by application (with a fresh finger cot) of a 1.25-cm ($\frac{1}{2}$-in.) ribbon of ointment per 25 cm^2 [4 sq in.] of affected surface area. Care should be taken to prevent autoinoculation. The ointment is for cutaneous use only and is not to be used in the eye or the vagina. Transcutaneous absorption of the drug occurs to a minimal degree (plasma concentrations are less than 1 μg/ml). It is not known whether acyclovir is excreted in milk, and caution is thus advised for nursing mothers. Acyclovir should be given slowly by the intravenous route. The usual dose for adults is 5 mg/kg every 8 hours; the infusion is given over a 1-hour period.

Toxicity. The toxicity of topical acyclovir is limited to local irritation and a transient burning when the preparation is applied to genital lesions (Corey and Holmes, 1983); this may be caused by the polyethylene glycol base.

The intravenous preparation appears to be tolerated quite well. Rarely, infusions have been associated with local phlebitis, rash, diaphoresis, nausea, vomiting, and hypotension (Keeney *et al.*, 1983). Intravenous acyclovir may cause transient renal dysfunction (rise in plasma creatinine) in 5 to 25% of patients. This toxic reaction appears to be dependent on dose and is more common when patients are dehydrated,

have renal insufficiency, and/or receive rapid bolus infusions (Bean *et al.*, 1982; Balfour *et al.*, 1983).

In a study conducted on patients who had received bone-marrow transplants, 4% showed evidence of neurotoxicity. Manifestations included lethargy, coma, confusion, hallucinations, tremors, and seizures. While associated temporally with intravenous administration of acyclovir (750 to 3000 mg/m^2 per day), the previous use of intrathecal methotrexate and the simultaneous administration of interferon in these patients make interpretation difficult (Wade and Meyers, 1983). Discontinuation of acyclovir was associated with improvement in all patients.

Little toxicity has been reported to date with the oral administration of acyclovir, with the exception of occasional nausea, amnesia, or headaches (Balfour *et al.*, 1983).

Therapeutic Uses. Acyclovir has proven to be effective in the treatment of herpes simplex virus type-I and type-II infections, including chronic and recurrent mucocutaneous herpes in the immunologically impaired host (Straus *et al.*, 1982), primary and secondary genital herpes, and neonatal herpes (Whitley and the NIAID Study Group, 1983). Acyclovir is currently being tested for encephalitis caused by herpes simplex type I (Whitley and the NIAID Study Group, 1983). The drug is useful in varicella-zoster infections, especially in patients whose cellular immune responses are impaired (Hirsch and Schooley, 1983). Therapeutic uses are discussed in more detail below. (*See also* Hayden and Douglas, 1985.)

IDOXURIDINE

Idoxuridine (HERPLEX, STOXIL) is 5-iodo-2'-deoxyuridine. It is soluble in water (2 mg/ml) and stable at temperatures up to 65° C but sensitive to light. Preparations include an ophthalmic ointment (0.5%) and an ophthalmic solution (0.1%).

Idoxuridine resembles thymidine. It is phosphorylated within cells, and the triphosphate derivative is incorporated into both viral and mammalian DNA. Such DNA is more susceptible to breakage, and altered viral proteins may result from faulty transcription (*see* Pratt, 1977). Thus, the activity of idoxuridine is largely limited to DNA viruses, primarily members of the herpes virus group. The drug is active *in vitro* against vaccinia virus, herpes simplex virus, varicella virus, cytomegalovirus, and others at concentrations of 10 μg/ml or less (Prusoff and Ward, 1976). The development of resistance of viruses to the drug *in vitro* occurs readily and has also been documented in man (Field, 1983).

The primary clinical use of the drug has been in *herpes simplex keratitis*. Maxwell (1963) reported on 1500 cases; he noted a correlation between the type of infection and the response to therapy. Epithelial infections, especially initial attacks in which a dendritic figure is present, respond best. The results are less favorable when the stroma is involved. In recurrent episodes, the acute disease is often controlled. *Herpes simplex* type II does not respond to the drug. When applied topically to the conjunctiva, irritation, pain, pruritus, inflammation or edema of the eyelids, and photophobia may develop. Punctate areas may appear in the cornea; it is difficult to ascertain whether these are related to the disease or to therapy. Topical *vidarabine* is equally effective and probably less irritating and allergenic (Pavan-Langston and Buchanan, 1976).

The *dose* of the 0.1% solution of idoxuridine is 1 drop in the conjunctival sac every hour during the day and every 2 hours during the night until definite improvement is apparent, after which the same quantity is applied every 2 hours during the day and every 4 hours at night. When the 0.5% ointment is used, it is applied every 4 hours during the day and once before bedtime. Therapy is continued for 3 to 5 days after healing is complete, as demonstrated by fluorescein staining.

AMANTADINE

Amantadine (1-adamantanamine) is a synthetic antiviral agent first described in 1964 by Davies and associates. It is a water-soluble, tricyclic amine of unusual structure unrelated to that of any of the other antimicrobial agents. Its structural formula is as follows:

Amantadine

Amantadine inhibits replication of strains of influenza A virus at an early point, probably the stage of uncoating. Attachment of the virus to cells and penetration are not impaired (Skehel *et al.*, 1978). Using a sensitive plaque-reduction assay, most strains of influenza A viruses, including H3N2, Hsw1N1, and H1N1 subtypes, are inhibited by 0.4 µg/ml of amantadine or less. Higher concentrations (25 to 50 µg/ml) are required to inhibit influenza B, rubella, and other viruses (Hayden and Douglas, 1985).

Amantadine is almost completely absorbed from the gastrointestinal tract. Approximately 90% of an orally administered dose is excreted in the urine (50% within 20 hours) in unchanged form; the drug is not metabolized in the body.

A number of studies have demonstrated the effectiveness of this compound in *preventing* infection of tissue cultures and experimental animals by different strains of influenza A viruses. An adequate number of studies have been performed to indicate that amantadine has prophylactic value when administered to humans who have had contact with an active case of influenza A or who have served as experimental subjects for this infection. The drug is valuable in both nosocomial and community settings (*see* Hayden and Douglas, 1985). In double-blind, placebo-controlled studies of amantadine in patients with naturally occurring infections due to influenza A virus, the drug is been found to produce a therapeutic effect even when given within 48 hours after onset of illness (Little *et al.*, 1976, 1978). A decrease in the frequency and quantity of shedding of virus has also been observed (Knight *et al.*, 1970). The development of specific antibody is not suppressed (Nafta *et al.*, 1970).

In the presence of a documented influenza A virus epidemic, amantadine is recommended for unimmunized patients of all ages who have a high risk of development of complications from influenza. Prophylactic administration of amantadine to high-risk patients should be initiated as soon as influenza A activity is documented in the community and continued for the duration of the epidemic (usually 5 to 6 weeks). Since the drug does not impair the immune response to influenza vaccine, patients can be vaccinated at the same time and amantadine discontinued after 2 weeks. The administration of amantadine to patients with established disease is controversial. Some suggest that treatment is worthwhile if it can be instituted within 48 hours of the onset of symptoms. The dosage is 200 mg per day for 5 to 7 days (Hayden and Douglas, 1985).

The discovery that amantadine is also useful in the treatment of parkinsonism was an act of serendipity. This therapeutic application is discussed in Chapter 21. *Rimantadine,* an analog of amantadine, is currently being evaluated for efficacy and toxicity (*see* Van Voris *et al.*, 1981; Hayden *et al.*, 1983).

Amantadine hydrochloride (SYMMETREL) is available in capsules containing 100 mg and as a syrup (50 mg/5 ml). The daily dose for children 1 to 9 years of age is 4.4 to 8.8 mg/kg, but it should not exceed a total of 150 mg per day. For older children and adults, the dose is 200 mg once daily or 100 mg twice daily. Peak concentrations in plasma are 0.3 to 0.6 µg/ml after ingestion of a 200-mg dose. The drug accumulates in patients with impaired renal function. Plasma concentrations of 1 to 5 µg/ml are associated with CNS toxicity, including nervousness, confusion, hallucinations, seizures, and coma. One to 5% of patients with normal renal function who receive amantadine (200 mg once daily) report minor neurological symptoms, including insomnia and difficulty in concentrating (LaMontagne and Galasso, 1979). Symptoms may be reduced by administration of 100 mg twice a day (Monto *et al.*, 1979). Persons with cerebral atherosclerosis, psychiatric disorders, or a history of epilepsy must be observed closely when taking this drug. It should be avoided in pregnant women and nursing mothers. Rimantadine may cause less CNS toxicity, but it seems to create more gastrointestinal disturbances.

VIDARABINE

Vidarabine (adenine arabinoside, ara-A) is an analog of adenosine (arabinose is the 2'-epimer of ribose). Its structural formula is as follows:

Vidarabine

Vidarabine is phosphorylated to the corresponding nucleotides within the cell and acts by inhibiting viral DNA polymerase; mammalian DNA synthesis is inhibited to a lesser extent (Muller *et al.*, 1977). Vidarabine is also metabolized to the less active hypoxanthine arabinoside, which may act synergistically with the parent compound to inhibit the replication of large DNA viruses (Champney *et al.*, 1978). The drug is active *in vitro* against vaccinia virus, herpes simplex virus, cytomegalovirus, and varicella-zoster virus (inhibited by 3 μg/ml or less) (Luby *et al.*, 1975). The drug is not active against other DNA viruses, such as adenoviruses or papovaviruses, nor against RNA viruses.

Preparations and Dosage. The recommended daily dose of vidarabine for treatment of encephalitis caused by herpes simplex virus is 15 mg/kg. Since vidarabine is only slightly soluble in water, large volumes of fluid are needed to dissolve the compound (*e.g.*, 2.5 liters). The drug should be given intravenously at a constant rate over a 12- to 24-hour period daily, for 10 days. Treatment of herpes simplex keratoconjunctivitis is with a 3% ophthalmic ointment, which is administered topically every 3 hours (five times daily).

Vidarabine (VIRA-A) is available for injection in 5-ml vials that contain 200 mg/ml of the monohydrate in a suspension (equivalent to 187 mg of vidarabine). The drug is also supplied as a 3% ophthalmic ointment (VIRA-A OPHTHALMIC).

Adverse Effects. Vidarabine causes relatively few side effects, but these can include nausea, vomiting, diarrhea, rash, weakness, and thrombophlebitis at the site of drug administration. Effects on the CNS, such as hallucinations, psychoses, ataxia, tremor, and dizziness, have been noted with high doses (20 mg/kg per day). The dosage should be reduced in patients with renal insufficiency. There is evidence that vidarabine is mutagenic and carcinogenic. It obviously should not be used to treat trivial infections.

Therapeutic Uses. Vidarabine has proven to be effective in the treatment of herpes simplex encephalitis. Mortality of this serious disease was reduced from 70% in controls to 28% in patients who received 15 mg/kg per day (Whitley *et al.*, 1977). There was also a reduction in neurological sequelae, but patients already in coma at the time of initiation of therapy did not benefit from the drug. Infections with herpes simplex virus in neonates are also effectively treated with vidarabine (Whitley and the NIAID Study Group, 1983).

In herpes zoster infections in immunocompromised patients, vidarabine is effective in reducing the formation of new vesicles; it also accelerates the clearance of virus from vesicles, reduces pain, and decreases the risk of dissemination (Whitley *et al.*, 1976; Whitley *et al.*, 1982b). The drug should not be used to treat unimpaired hosts with uncomplicated herpes zoster, nor is it useful for treatment of recurrent or primary herpes genitalis (Adams *et al.*, 1976).

As previously mentioned, vidarabine given topically is as effective for herpes simplex keratoconjunctivitis as idoxuridine and is less irritating (Pavan-Langston and Buchanan, 1976). *Trifluridine* (*trifluorothymidine;* VIROPTIC), a new halogenated pyrimidine, is currently being used as a 1% ophthalmic solution for topical therapy of ocular infections caused by herpes simplex. It has been effective in patients who have not responded to vidarabine or idoxuridine (Hayden and Douglas, 1985).

HUMAN INTERFERON

Interferons are glycoproteins that have a variety of biological effects; these include the induction of resistance to viral infection and the regulation of other cell functions, including proliferation and immunological responses. Endogenous production and release of interferon occur in response to viral infection, and synthesis of the protein can be induced by double-stranded RNA. There are three major types of human interferons, designated α, β, and γ (Houglum, 1983). Interferons used in clinical trials have been produced by induction of synthesis by human leukocytes, fibroblasts, or lymphoblastoid cells and, more recently, by recombinant DNA technics in bacteria.

In a controlled trial in patients with lymphoma, early treatment of herpes zoster with human, leukocyte-derived interferon prevented distant cutaneous and visceral spread of infection and, in addition, stopped the spread of the infection in the primary dermatome (Merigan *et al.*, 1978). Since interferon has a uniquely broad spectrum of antiviral activity *in vitro*, clinical trials have been undertaken in patients infected with exotic agents such as Ebola-Marburg virus and rabies virus and with the ubiquitous hepatitis B virus (Greenberg *et al.*, 1976). In the last-named infection, interferon has shown promising additive effects when used in combination with vidarabine. Now that large quantities of interferon are available, numerous clinical trials are in progress. Preliminary results from some of these studies suggest that interferon is not as useful in the therapy of viral infections as initially suspected.

THERAPY OF VIRAL INFECTIONS

Herpes Viruses. The infections caused by the herpes simplex viruses are usually divided into those caused by type-I and type-II viruses, although there is overlap between the anatomical sites of infection and the clinical features that distinguish infection by these two agents.

Herpes Simplex Virus I. Mucocutaneous lesions of the face and oropharynx are usually caused by herpes simplex type I. Oral-labial lesions (fever blisters) are not effectively treated with existing antiviral agents. While the morbidity and mortality of encephalitis caused by type-I virus are reduced by antiviral chemotherapy (Whitley *et al.*, 1981), patients with severe neurological dysfunction at the time of initiation of therapy still do very poorly. Intravenous vidarabine (15 mg/kg per day for 10 days) is considered to be the treatment of choice; however, parenteral acyclovir (10 mg/kg every 8 hours for 10 days) may be as effective and less toxic. Results of ongoing comparative studies are pending (Whitley and the NIAID Study Group, 1983).

Herpes simplex type-I infections are usually more severe in patients with impairment of their cellular immune functions; a simple blister of the lip may progress to an invasive oral-pharyngeal necrotizing lesion, esophagitis, pneumonia, or disseminated disease. In such situations, intravenous or oral acyclovir (5 to 10 mg/kg every 8 hours for 5 to 7 days) has been shown to be effective in severe chronic and recurrent mucocutaneous herpes (Straus *et al.*, 1982), and prophylactic oral use of the drug (200 to 400 mg four times a day) can prevent reactivation of infection in patients with bone-marrow transplants (Wade *et al.*, 1984b). However, the use of acyclovir for treatment of mucocutaneous herpes simplex infections in such patients was subsequently associated with more frequent recurrences of infection (Wade *et al.*, 1984a).

Herpes simplex type I also causes keratitis, a serious infection of the eye that can result in blindness. Trifluridine (one drop of a 1% solution every 2 hours), idoxuridine (one drop of a 0.1% solution every 1 to 2 hours), and vidarabine (a 1.25-cm [½-in.] ribbon of 3% ointment five times daily) are all effective when applied topically.

Herpes Simplex Virus II. This type of herpes virus most commonly causes genital disease, but it may also be responsible for meningitis. Primary genital herpes can be treated with acyclovir. Therapy results in more rapid healing, reduction in viral titers, and more rapid disappearance of pain. Topical application (5% ointment, five or six times daily for 10 days) can be utilized for mild-to-moderate disease. Experience with oral therapy (200 mg five times daily for 10 days) is currently limited, but it appears to be preferable. There is a reduction in the formation of new lesions, a decrease in the duration of viral shedding, and a marked abatement of clinical symptoms in both sexes (Bryson *et al.*, 1982; Nilsen *et al.*, 1982). Parenteral treatment is also effective but is reserved for severely ill patients who require hospitalization (Mindel *et al.*, 1982).

Recurrence of genital herpes is not prevented by treatment of the primary disease with acyclovir, and recurrent lesions respond less dramatically than does the primary infection. Topical therapy is completely ineffective; oral acyclovir has some salutary effect on healing and the shedding of virus. Oral administration of acyclovir (200 mg two to five times daily) has also been shown to prevent recurrences of genital herpes, but infections recur at their former frequency when the drug is stopped (Douglas *et al.*, 1984; Straus *et al.*, 1984). There are as yet no data on the treatment of meningitis caused by herpes simplex type II.

Neonatal infections with herpes simplex virus are often severe and are characterized by progressive dissemination and death. Although therapy with vidarabine (15 to 30 mg/kg per day for 10 days) decreases morbidity and mortality, the disseminated infection is still fatal in 60% of patients. Intravenous acyclovir (10 mg/kg every 8 hours for 10 days) also appears to be effective, and comparative trials are ongoing (Whitley and the NIAID Study Group, 1983).

Varicella-Zoster Virus. Shingles, caused by varicella-zoster virus, is usually confined to one dermatome, and routine antiviral therapy is not recommended. Several studies have demonstrated that intravenous or oral acyclovir (15 mg/kg per day) will reduce the duration of viral shedding, decrease erythema and pain, and accelerate healing. However, there is no apparent effect on postherpetic neuralgia. Thus, use of acyclovir for varicella-zoster in the normal host should probably be reserved for patients with severe disease. In patients with impaired cellular immune responses, varicella-zoster infection may be severe, with widespread dissemination to skin and vital organs. Studies have demonstrated that both vidarabine (10 mg/kg per day for 5 days) and acyclovir (10 mg/kg every 8 hours for 7 days or 1500 mg/m^2 per day for 7 days) produce similar local beneficial effects and prevent dissemination to distant cutaneous and visceral sites (Whitley *et al.*, 1982b; Hirsch and Schooley, 1983). Interferon is also effective (Arvin *et al.*, 1982). While the specific utility of vidarabine and acyclovir has yet to be clearly defined, therapy for varicella-zoster infection is recommended in patients with severe deficits in immunological function.

Varicella (chickenpox) is often a severe disease in patients with immunological deficiencies. Both vidarabine (10 mg/kg per day for 5 days) and intravenous acyclovir (for 7 days) cause a reduction in cutaneous lesions and fever; there is also a lower incidence of visceral complications (Prober *et al.*, 1982; Whitley *et al.*, 1982a).

There is currently no effective antiviral therapy for infections caused by the other herpes viruses, Epstein-Barr virus, or cytomegalovirus, although some investigational nucleoside analogs appear promising.

Influenza. Both influenza A and B viruses can produce severe respiratory and systemic diseases. Amantadine, given orally in doses of 200 mg daily, prevents both infection and illness from influenza A. It also results in reduction of fever and respiratory tract symptoms when administered in similar doses up to 48 hours after the onset of symptoms. There is as yet no specific therapy for influenza B or respiratory syncytial virus, although an investigational antiviral agent, *ribavirin*, shortens the course of illness in patients when given as an aerosol.

Rhinoviruses. There is currently no effective treatment for the common cold. However, α-interferon, administered intranasally, has been shown to reduce the symptoms and shedding of virus in experimental infections with rhinovirus (Hayden and Gwaltney, 1984).

Abernathy, R. S. Treatment of systemic mycoses. *Medicine (Baltimore),* **1973,** *52,* 385–394.

Adams, H. G.; Benson, E. A.; Alexander, E. R.; Vontver, L. A.; Remington, M. A.; and Holmes, K. K. Genital herpetic infection in men and women: clinical course and effect of topical application of adenine arabinoside. *J. Infect. Dis.,* **1976,** *133,* Suppl., A151–159.

Aoyagi, N.; Ogata, H.; Kaniwa, N.; Koibuchi, M.; Shibazaki, T.; and Ejima, A. Bioavailability of griseofulvin from tablets in humans and the correlation with its dissolution rate. *J. Pharm. Sci.,* **1982,** *71,* 1165–1169.

Arroyo, J.; Medoff, G.; and Kobayashi, G. S. Therapy of murine aspergillosis with amphotericin B in combination with rifampin or 5-fluorocytosine. *Antimicrob. Agents Chemother.,* **1977,** *11,* 21–25.

Arvin, A. M.; Kushner, J. H.; Feldman, S.; Baehner, R. L.; Hammond, D.; and Merigan, T. C. Human leukocyte interferon for the treatment of varicella in children with cancer. *N. Engl. J. Med.,* **1982,** *306,* 761–765.

Balfour, H. H., Jr., and others; Burroughs Wellcome Collaborative Acyclovir Study Group. Acyclovir halts progression of herpes zoster in immunocompromised patients. *N. Engl. J. Med.,* **1983,** *308,* 1448–1453.

Bean, B.; Braun, C.; and Balfour, H. H., Jr. Acyclovir therapy for acute herpes zoster. *Lancet,* **1982,** *2,* 118–121.

Beggs, W. H., and Sarosi, G. A. Combined activity of ketoconazole and 5-fluorocytosine on potentially pathogenic yeasts. *Antimicrob. Agents Chemother.,* **1982,** *21,* 355–357.

Bell, R. W., and Ritchey, J. P. Medical therapy for *Aspergillus* corneal ulcer. *Arch. Ophthalmol.,* **1973,** *90,* 402–404.

Bennett, J. E. Amphotericin B binding to serum beta lipoprotein. In, *Recent Advances in Medical and Veterinary Mycology.* (Iwata, K., ed.) University of Tokyo Press, Tokyo, **1977,** pp. 107–109.

———. Treatment of cryptococcal, candidal, and coccidioidal meningitis. In, *Current Clinical Topics in Infectious Diseases,* Vol. 2. (Remington, J. S., and Swartz, M. N., eds.) McGraw-Hill Book Co., New York, **1981,** pp. 54–67.

Bennett, J. E., and others. A collaborative study. Amphotericin B–flucytosine in cryptococcal meningitis. *N. Engl. J. Med.,* **1979,** *301,* 126–131.

Bennett, W. M., and Pulliam, J. P. Cyclosporine nephrotoxicity. *Ann. Intern. Med.,* **1983,** *99,* 851–854.

Bindschalder, D. D., and Bennett, J. E. A pharmacologic guide to the clinical use of amphotericin B. *J. Infect. Dis.,* **1969,** *120,* 427–436.

Block, E. R.; Bennett, J. E.; Livoti, L. G.; Klein, W. J.; Brandriss, M. W.; MacGregor, R. R.; and Henderson, L. Flucytosine and amphotericin B: hemodialysis effects on the plasma concentration and clearance. *Ann. Intern. Med.,* **1974,** *80,* 613–617.

Block, E. R.; Jennings, A. E.; and Bennett, J. E. Experimental therapy of cladosporiosis and sporotrichosis with 5-fluorocytosine. *Antimicrob. Agents Chemother.,* **1973,** *3,* 95–99.

Borelli, D. Treatment of pityriasis versicolor with ketoconazole. *Rev. Infect. Dis.,* **1980,** *2,* 592–595.

Borgers, M.; Van den Bossche, H.; and De Brabander, M. The mechanism of action of the new antimycotic ketoconazole. *Am. J. Med.,* **1983,** *74,* 2–8.

Brass, C.; Galgiani, J. N.; Blaschke, T. F.; Defelice, R.; O'Reilly, R. A.; and Stevens, D. A. Disposition of ketoconazole, an oral antifungal, in humans. *Antimicrob. Agents Chemother.,* **1982,** *21,* 151–158.

Bryson, Y. J.; Dillon, M.; Lovett, M.; Acuna, G.; Taylor, S.; Cherry, J. D.; Johnson, B. L.; Weismeier, E.; Growdon, W.; Creagh-Kirk, T.; and Keeney, R. Treatment of first episodes of genital herpes simplex virus infection with oral acyclovir: a randomized double-blind controlled trial in normal subjects. *N. Engl. J. Med.,* **1982,** *308,* 916–921.

Burks, L. C.; Aisner, J.; Fortner, C. L.; and Wiernik, P. H. Meperidine for the treatment of shaking chills and fever. *Arch. Intern. Med.,* **1980,** *140,* 483–484.

Catanzaro, A.; Einstein, H.; Levine, B.; Ross, B.; Schillaci, R.; Fierer, J.; and Friedman, P. J. Ketoconazole for treatment of disseminated coccidioidomycosis. *Ann. Intern. Med.,* **1982,** *96,* 436–440.

Champney, K. J.; Lauter, C. B.; Bailey, E. J.; and Lerner, A. M. Anti-herpesvirus activity in human sera and urines after administration of adenine arabinoside. *J. Clin. Invest.,* **1978,** *62,* 1142–1153.

Chan, C. S. P.; Tuazon, C. U.; and Lessin, L. S. Amphotericin B–induced thrombocytopenia. *Ann. Intern. Med.,* **1982,** *96,* 332–333.

Churchill, D. N., and Seely, J. Nephrotoxicity associated with combined gentamicin-amphotericin B therapy. *Nephron,* **1977,** *19,* 176–181.

Corey, L., and Holmes, K. K. Genital herpes simplex virus infections: current concepts in diagnosis, therapy, and prevention. *Ann. Intern. Med.,* **1983,** *98,* 973–983.

Craven, P. C., and Graybill, J. R. Combination of oral flucytosine and ketoconazole as therapy for experimental cryptococcal meningitis. *J. Infect. Dis.,* **1984,** *149,* 584–590.

Crout, J. E.; Brewer, N. S.; and Tompkins, R. B. Sporotrichosis arthritis. Clinical features in seven patients. *Ann. Intern. Med.,* **1977,** *86,* 294–297.

Crumpacker, C. S.; Schnipper, L. E.; Marlowe, S. I.; Kowalsky, P. N.; Hershey, B. J.; and Levin, M. J. Resistance to antiviral drugs of herpes simplex virus isolated from a patient treated with acyclovir. *N. Engl. J. Med.,* **1982,** *306,* 343–346.

Daneshmend, T. K.; Warnock, D. W.; Ene, M. D.; Johnson, E. M.; Potten, M. R.; Richardson, M. D.; and Williamson, P. J. Influence of food on the pharmacokinetics of ketoconazole. *Antimicrob. Agents Chemother.,* **1984,** *25,* 1–3.

Darby, G., and Field, H. J. Altered substrate specificity of herpes simplex virus thymidine kinase confers acyclovir-resistance. *Nature,* **1981,** *289,* 81–83.

Defelice, R.; Johnson, D. G.; and Galgiani, J. N. Gynecomastia with ketoconazole. *Antimicrob. Agents Chemother.,* **1981,** *19,* 1073–1074.

DeGregorio, M. W.; Lee, W. M. F.; Linker, C. A.; Jacobs, R. A.; and Ries, C. A. Fungal infections in patients with acute leukemia. *Am. J. Med.,* **1982,** *73,* 543–548.

de Miranda, P., and Blum, M. R. Pharmacokinetics of acyclovir after intravenous and oral administration. *J. Antimicrob. Chemother.,* **1983,** *12,* Suppl. B, 29–37.

Deresinski, S. C.; Lilly, R. B.; Levine, H. B.; Galgiani, J. N.; and Stevens, D. A. Treatment of fungal meningitis with miconazole. *Arch. Intern. Med.,* **1977,** *137,* 1180–1185.

Diamond, R. D., and Bennett, J. E. A subcutaneous reservoir for intrathecal therapy for fungal meningitis. *N. Engl. J. Med.*, **1973**, *288*, 186–188.

Diasio, R. B.; Lakings, D. E.; and Bennett, J. E. Evidence for conversion of 5-fluorocytosine to 5-fluorouracil in humans. Possible factor in 5-fluorocytosine clinical toxicity. *Antimicrob. Agents Chemother.*, **1978**, *14*, 903–908.

Dieperink, H., and Moller, J. Ketoconazole and cyclosporin. (Letter.) *Lancet*, **1982**, *27*, 1217.

Dismukes, W. E., and others. Treatment of systemic mycoses with ketoconazole: emphasis on toxicity and clinical response in 52 patients. *Ann. Intern. Med.*, **1983**, *98*, 13–20.

Douglas, J. B., and Healy, J. K. Nephrotoxic effects of amphotericin B, including renal tubular acidosis. *Am. J. Med.*, **1969**, *46*, 154–162.

Douglas, J. M.; Critchlow, C.; Benedetti, J.; Mertz, G. J.; Connor, J. D.; Hintz, M. A.; Fahnlander, A.; Remington, M.; Winter, C.; and Corey, L. A double-blind study of oral acyclovir for suppression of recurrences of genital herpes simplex virus infection. *N. Engl. J. Med.*, **1984**, *310*, 1551–1556.

Drouhet, E., and DuPont, B. Laboratory and clinical assessment of ketoconazole in deep-seated mycoses. *Am. J. Med.*, **1983**, *74*, 30–47.

Drutz, D. J. Newer antifungal agents and their use, including an update on amphotericin B and flucytosine. In, *Current Clinical Topics in Infectious Diseases*, Vol. 3. (Remington, J. S., and Swartz, M. N., eds.) McGraw-Hill Book Co., New York, **1982**, pp. 97–135.

———. Amphotericin B in the treatment of coccidioidomycosis. *Drugs*, **1983**, *26*, 337–346.

Drutz, D. J.; Spickard, A.; Rogers, D. E.; and Koenig, M. G. Treatment of disseminated mycotic infections: a new approach to amphotericin B therapy. *Am. J. Med.*, **1968**, *45*, 405–418.

Dutcher, J. D.; Boyak, G.; and Fox, S. The preparation and properties of crystalline fungicidin (nystatin). In, *Antibiotics Annual, 1953–1954*. Medical Encyclopedia, Inc., New York, **1954**, pp. 191–193.

El-Nakeeb, M. A., and Lampen, J. O. Uptake of griseofulvin by microorganisms and its correlation with sensitivity to griseofulvin. *J. Gen. Microbiol.*, **1965**, *39*, 285–293.

Ernst, J. D.; Rusnak, M.; and Sande, M. A. Combination antifungal chemotherapy for experimental disseminated candidiasis: lack of correlation between *in vitro* and *in vivo* observations with amphotericin B and rifampin. *Rev. Infect. Dis.*, **1983**, *5*, Suppl. 3, S626–S630.

Fainstein, V., and Bodey, G. P. Cardiorespiratory toxicity due to miconazole. *Ann. Intern. Med.*, **1980**, *93*, 432–433.

Feldman, H. A.; Hamilton, J. D.; and Gutman, R. A. Amphotericin therapy in an anephric patient. *Antimicrob. Agents Chemother.*, **1973**, *4*, 402–405.

Field, H. J. Development of clinical resistance to acyclovir in herpes simplex virus–infected mice receiving oral therapy. *Antimicrob. Agents Chemother.*, **1982**, *21*, 744–752.

———. The problem of drug-induced resistance in viruses. In, *Problems of Antiviral Therapy: The Fifth Beecham Colloquium*. (Stuart-Harris, C. H., and Oxford, J. S., eds.) Academic Press, Ltd., London, **1983**, pp. 71–107.

Field, H. J., and Darby, G. Pathogenicity in mice of strains of *Herpes simplex* virus which are resistant to acyclovir *in vitro* and *in vivo*. *Antimicrob. Agents Chemother.*, **1980**, *17*, 209–216.

Fischer, J. F., and Dewald, J. Parkinsonism associated with intraventricular amphotericin B. *J. Antimicrob. Chemother.*, **1983**, *12*, 97–99.

Fosson, A. R., and Wheeler, W. E. Short-term amphotericin B treatment of severe childhood histoplasmosis. *J. Pediatr.*, **1975**, *86*, 32–36.

Goldstein, E.; Winship, M. J.; and Pappagianis, D. Ventricular fluid and the management of coccidioidal meningitis. *Ann. Intern. Med.*, **1972**, *77*, 243–246.

Goodwin, R. A., Jr., and Des Prez, R. M. Histoplasmosis. *Am. Rev. Respir. Dis.*, **1978**, *117*, 929–956.

Graybill, J. R. Clinical course of coccidioidomycosis following transfer factor therapy (for the Coccidioidomycosis Cooperative Treatment Group). In, *Coccidioidomycosis: Current Clinical and Diagnostic Status*. (Libero Ajello, L., ed.) Symposia Specialists, Miami, **1977**, pp. 335–345.

Greenberg, H. B.; Pollard, R. B.; Lutwick, L. I.; Gregory, P. B.; Robinson, W. S.; and Merigan, T. C. Effect of human leukocyte interferon on hepatitis B virus infection in patients with chronic active hepatitis. *N. Engl. J. Med.*, **1976**, *295*, 517–522.

Grisham, L. M.; Wilson, L.; and Bensch, K. Antimitotic action of griseofulvin does not involve disruption of microtubules. *Nature*, **1973**, *244*, 294–296.

Grosso, D. S.; Boyden, T. W.; Pamenter, R. W.; Johnson, D. G.; Stevens, D. A.; and Galgiani, J. N. Ketoconazole inhibition of testicular secretion of testosterone and displacement of steroid hormones from serum transport proteins. *Antimicrob. Agents Chemother.*, **1983**, *23*, 207–212.

Gull, K., and Trinci, A. P. J. Griseofulvin inhibits fungal mitosis. *Nature*, **1973**, *244*, 292–294.

Hamilton-Miller, J. M. T. Fungal sterols and the mode of action of the polyene antibiotics. *Adv. Appl. Microbiol.*, **1974**, *17*, 109–134.

Hawkins, S. S.; Gregory, D. W.; and Alford, R. H. Progressive disseminated histoplasmosis: favorable response to ketoconazole. *Ann. Intern. Med.*, **1981**, *95*, 446–449.

Hayden, F. G., and Gwaltney, J. M., Jr. Intranasal interferon alpha-2 treatment of experimental rhinovirus colds. *J. Infect. Dis.*, **1984**, *150*, 174–180.

Hayden, F. G.; Hoffman, H. E.; and Spyker, D. A. Differences in side effects of amantadine hydrochloride and rimantadine hydrochloride relate to differences in pharmacokinetics. *Antimicrob. Agents Chemother.*, **1983**, *23*, 458–464.

Heel, R. C.; Brogden, R. N.; Carmine, A.; Morley, P. A.; Speight, T. M.; and Avery, G. S. Ketoconazole: a review of its therapeutic efficacy in superficial and systemic fungal infections. *Drugs*, **1982**, *23*, 1–36.

Heel, R. C.; Brogden, R. N.; Pakes, G. E.; Speight, T. M.; and Avery, G. S. Miconazole: a preliminary review of its therapeutic efficacy in systemic fungal infections. *Drugs*, **1980**, *19*, 7–30.

Hernandez, A. D. *Sporothrix schenckii*. In, *Principles and Practice of Infectious Diseases*. (Mandell, G. L.; Douglas, R. G., Jr.; and Bennett, J. E.; eds.) John Wiley & Sons, Inc., New York, **1979**, pp. 2015–2018.

Hirsch, M. S., and Schooley, R. T. Treatment of herpes virus infections. *N. Engl. J. Med.*, **1983**, *309*, 963–970, 1034–1039.

Houglum, J. E. Interferon: mechanism of action and clinical value. *Clin. Pharm.*, **1983**, *2*, 20–28.

Hume, A. L., and Kerkering, T. M. Ketoconazole. *Drug. Intell. Clin. Pharm.*, **1983**, *17*, 169–174.

Iwen, P. C.; Miller, N. G.; and McFadden, H. W., Jr. Treatment of murine pulmonary cryptococcosis with ketoconazole and amphotericin B. *J. Infect. Dis.*, **1984**, *149*, 650.

Janssen, P. A. J., and Symoens, J. E. Hepatic reactions during ketoconazole treatment. *Am. J. Med.*, **1983**, *74*, 80–85.

Jurgens, R. W., Jr.; DeLuca, P. P.; and Papadimitriou, D. Compatibility of amphotericin B with certain large-volume parenterals. *Am. J. Hosp. Pharm.*, **1981**, *38*, 377–378.

Kauffman, C., and Frame, P. T. Bone marrow toxicity associated with 5-fluorocytosine therapy. *Antimicrob. Agents Chemother.*, **1977**, *11*, 244–247.

Keeney, R. E.; Kirk, L. E.; and Bridgen, D. Acyclovir tolerance in humans. *Am. J. Med.*, **1983**, *75*, Suppl., 176–181.

Kennedy, M. S.; Deeg, H. J.; Siegel, M.; Crowley, J. J.; Storb, R.; and Thomas, E. D. Acute renal toxicity with combined use of amphotericin B and cyclosporine after marrow transplantation. *Transplantation*, **1983**, *35*, 211–215.

Kirkpatrick, C. H., and Alling, D. W. Treatment of chronic oral candidiasis with clotrimazole troches. *N. Engl. J. Med.*, **1978**, *299*, 1201–1203.

Knight, V.; Fedson, D.; Baldini, J.; Douglas, R. G.; and Couch, R. B. Amantadine therapy of epidemic influenza A2 (Hong Kong). *Infect. Immun.*, **1970**, *1*, 200–204.

LaMontagne, J. R., and Galasso, G. J. Report of a workshop on clinical studies of the efficacy of amantadine and rimantadine against influenza virus. *J. Infect. Dis.*, **1979**, *138*, 928–931.

Legendre, R., and Steltz, M. A multi-center, double-blind comparison of ketoconazole and griseofulvin in the treatment of infections due to dermatophytes. *Rev. Infect. Dis.*, **1980**, *2*, 586–591.

Lew, M.; Beckett, K. M.; and Levin, M. J. Combined activity of minocycline and amphotericin B *in vitro* against medically important yeasts. *Antimicrob. Agents Chemother.*, **1978**, *14*, 465.

Lewi, P. J.; Boelaert, J.; Daneels, R.; DeMeyere, R.; Van Landuyt, H.; Heykants, J. J. P.; Symoens, J.; and Wynants, J. Pharmacokinetic profile of intravenous miconazole in man; comparison of normal subjects and patients with renal insufficiency. *Eur. J. Clin. Pharmacol.*, **1976**, *10*, 49–54.

Lewis, J. H.; Zimmerman, H. J.; Benson, G. D.; and Ishak, K. G. Hepatic injury associated with ketoconazole therapy. *Gastroenterology*, **1984**, *86*, 503–513.

Little, J. W.; Hall, W. J.; Douglas, R. G., Jr.; Hyde, R. W.; and Speers, D. M. Amantadine effect on peripheral airways abnormalities in influenza. *Ann. Intern. Med.*, **1976**, *85*, 177–182.

Little, J. W.; Hall, W. J.; Douglas, R. G., Jr.; Mudholkar, G. S.; Speers, D. M.; and Patel, K. Attenuation of airway hyperreactivity by amantadine in natural influenza A infection. *Am. Rev. Respir. Dis.*, **1978**, *118*, 295–303.

Luby, J. P.; Jones, S. R.; Johnson, M. T.; and Mikulec, D. Sensitivities of herpes simplex virus types 1 and 2 and varicella-zoster virus to adenine arabinoside. In, *Arabinoside: An Antiviral Agent.* (Pavan-Langston, D., ed.) Raven Press, New York, **1975**, pp. 171–175.

Lutwick, L. I.; Rytel, M. W.; Yañez, J. P.; Galgiani, J. N.; and Stevens, D. A. Deep infections from *Petriellidum boydii* treated with miconazole. *J.A.M.A.*, **1979**, *241*, 272–273.

McCurdy, D. K.; Frederic, M.; and Elkinton, J. R. Renal tubular acidosis due to amphotericin B. *N. Engl. J. Med.*, **1968**, *278*, 124–131.

MacGregor, R. R.; Bennett, J. E.; and Ersley, A. J. Erythropoietin concentration in amphotericin B–induced anemia. *Antimicrob. Agents Chemother.*, **1978**, *14*, 270–273.

Maddux, M. S., and Barriere, S. L. A review of complications of amphotericin B therapy: recommendations for prevention and management. *Drug Intell. Clin. Pharm.*, **1980**, *14*, 177–181.

Malawista, S. E.; Sato, H.; and Bensch, K. G. Vinblastine and griseofulvin reversibly disrupt the living mitotic spindle. *Science*, **1968**, *160*, 770–772.

Mauceri, A. A.; Cullen, F. I.; Vandevelde, A. G.; and Johnson, J. E. Flucytosine in effective oral treatment for chromomycosis. *Arch. Dermatol.*, **1974**, *109*, 873–876.

Maxwell, E. Treatment of herpes keratitis with 5-iodo-2-deoxyuridine (IDU): a clinical evaluation of 1500 cases. *Am. J. Ophthalmol.*, **1963**, *56*, 571–573.

Medical Letter. Drugs for the treatment of systemic fungal infections. **1984**, *26*, 36–38.

Medoff, G.; Comfort, M.; and Kobayashi, G. S. Synergistic action of amphotericin B and 5-fluorocytosine against yeast-like organisms. *Proc. Soc. Exp. Biol. Med.*, **1971a**, *138*, 571–574.

Medoff, G.; Dismukes, W. E.; Meade, R. H., III; and Moses, J. M. A new therapeutic approach to *Candida* infections. *Arch. Intern. Med.*, **1972**, *130*, 241–245.

———. Therapeutic program for *Candida* infection. In, *Antimicrobial Agents and Chemotherapy—1970.* (Hobby, G. L., ed.) American Society for Microbiology, Bethesda, **1971b**, pp. 286–290.

Merigan, T. C.; Rand, K. H.; Pollard, R. B.; Abdallah, P. S.; Jordan, G. W.; and Fried, R. P. Human leukocyte interferon for the treatment of herpes zoster in patients with cancer. *N. Engl. J. Med.*, **1978**, *298*, 981–987.

Meunier-Carpentier, F. Treatment of mycoses in cancer patients. *Am. J. Med.*, **1983**, *74*, 74–79.

Meyer, R. D.; Young, L. S.; Armstrong, D.; and Yu, B. Aspergillosis complicating neoplastic disease. *Am. J. Med.*, **1973**, *54*, 6–15.

Minagawa, H.; Kitaura, K.; and Nakamizo, N. Effects of pH on the activity of ketoconazole against *Candida albicans. Antimicrob. Agents Chemother.*, **1983**, *23*, 105–107.

Mindel, A.; Adler, M. W.; Sutherland, S.; and Fiddian, A. P. Intravenous acyclovir treatment for primary genital herpes. *Lancet*, **1982**, *1*, 697–700.

Monto, A. S.; Gunn, R. A.; Bandy, K. M. G.; and King, C. L. Prevention of Russian influenza by amantadine. *J.A.M.A.*, **1979**, *241*, 1003–1007.

Muller, W. E. G.; Zahn, R. K.; Bittlingmaier, K.; and Falke, D. Inhibition of herpes virus DNA synthesis by 9-D-arabinofuranosyladenine in cellular and cell-free systems. *Ann. N.Y. Acad. Sci.*, **1977**, *284*, 34–48.

Nafta, I.; Turcanu, A. G.; Braun, I.; Companetz, W.; Simionescu, A. B. E.; and Florea, V. Administration of amantadine for the prevention of Hong Kong influenza. *Bull. WHO*, **1970**, *42*, 423–427.

Naylor, B. A. Low-dose amphotericin B therapy for acute pulmonary histoplasmosis. *Chest*, **1977**, *71*, 404–406.

Nilsen, A. E.; Aasen, T.; Halsos, A. M.; Kinge, B. R.; Tiotta, E. A.; Wikström, K.; and Fiddian, A. P. Efficacy of oral acyclovir in the treatment of initial and recurrent genital herpes. *Lancet*, **1982**, *2*, 571–573.

Normark, S., and Schönebeck, J. *In vitro* studies of 5-fluorocytosine resistance in *Candida albicans* and *Torulopsis glabrata. Antimicrob. Agents Chemother.*, **1972**, *2*, 114–121.

Odds, F. C. Interactions among amphotericin B, 5-fluorocytosine, ketoconazole, and miconazole against pathogenic fungi *in vitro. Antimicrob. Agents Chemother.*, **1982**, *22*, 763–770.

Owens, N. J.; Nightingale, C. H.; Schweizer, R. T.; Schauer, P. K.; Dekker, P. T.; and Quintiliani, R. Prophylaxis of oral candidiasis with clotrimazole troches. *Arch. Intern. Med.*, **1984**, *144*, 290–293.

Parris, D. S., and Harrington, J. E. Herpes simplex virus variants resistant to high concentrations of acyclovir exist in clinical isolates. *Antimicrob. Agents Chemother.*, **1982**, *22*, 71–77.

Pavan-Langston, D., and Buchanan, R. A. Vidarabine therapy of simple and IDU- complicated herpetic keratitis. *Trans. Am. Acad. Ophthalmol. Otolaryngol.*, **1976**, *81*, 813–827.

Perfect, J. R.; Durack, D. T.; Hamilton, J. D.; and Galis, H. A. Failure of ketoconazole in cryptococcal meningitis. *J.A.M.A.*, **1982**, *247*, 3349–3351.

Petersen, E. A.; Alling, D. W.; and Kirkpatrick, C. H. Treatment of chronic mucocutaneous candidiasis with ketoconazole. *Ann. Intern. Med.*, **1980**, *93*, 791–795.

Pont, A.; Williams, P. L.; Loose, D. S.; Feldman, D.;

Reitz, R. E.; Bochra, C.; and Stevens, D. A. Ketoconazole blocks adrenal steroid synthesis. *Ann. Intern. Med.*, **1982**, *97*, 370–372.

Posner, J. B. Reservoirs for intraventricular chemotherapy. (Editorial.) *N. Engl. J. Med.*, **1973**, *288*, 212.

Prober, C. G.; Kirk, L. E.; and Keeney, R. E. Acyclovir therapy of chickenpox in immunosuppressed children—a collaborative study. *J. Pediatr.*, **1982**, *101*, 622–625.

Prusoff, W. H., and Ward, D. C. Nucleoside analogs with antiviral activity. *Biochem. Pharmacol.*, **1976**, *25*, 1233–1239.

Rolan, P. E.; Somogyi, A. A.; Drew, M. J. R.; Cobain, W. G.; South, D.; and Bochner, F. Phenytoin intoxication during treatment with parenteral miconazole. *Br. Med. J.*, **1983**, *287*, 1760.

Sande, M. A.; Bowman, C. R.; and Calderone, R. A. Experimental *C. albicans* endocarditis. Characterization of the disease and response to therapy. *Infect. Immun.*, **1977**, *17*, 140–147.

Sarosi, G. A.; Parker, J. D.; Doto, I. L.; and Tosh, F. E. Amphotericin B in cryptococcal meningitis: long-term results of treatment. *Ann. Intern. Med.*, **1969**, *71*, 1079–1087.

Shah, V. P.; Epstein, W. L.; and Riegelman, S. Role of sweat in accumulation of orally administered griseofulvin in skin. *J. Clin. Invest.*, **1974**, *53*, 1673–1678.

Shechtman, L. B.; Funaro, L.; Robin, T.; Bottone, E. J.; and Cuttner, J. Clotrimazole treatment of oral candidiasis in patients with neoplastic disease. *Am. J. Med.*, **1984**, *76*, 1–4.

Sibrack, C. D.; Gutman, L. T.; Wilfert, C. M.; McLaren, C.; St. Clair, M. H.; Keller, P. M.; and Barry, D. W. Pathogenicity of acyclovir-resistant *Herpes simplex* virus type I from an immunodeficient child. *J. Infect. Dis.*, **1982**, *146*, 673–682.

Skehel, J. J.; Hay, A. J.; and Armstrong, J. A. On the mechanism of inhibition of influenza virus replication by amantadine hydrochloride. *J. Gen. Virol.*, **1978**, *38*, 97–110.

Smith, J. W., and Utz, J. P. Progressive disseminated histoplasmosis. A prospective study of 26 patients. *Ann. Intern. Med.*, **1972**, *76*, 557–566.

Steer, P. O.; Marks, M. I.; Klite, P. D.; and Eickhoff, T. C. 5-Fluorocytosine: an oral antifungal compound. A report on clinical and laboratory experience. *Ann. Intern. Med.*, **1972**, *76*, 15–22.

Stevens, D. A. Miconazole in the treatment of systemic fungal infection. *Am. Rev. Respir. Dis.*, **1977**, *116*, 801–806.

———. Miconazole in the treatment of coccidioidomycosis. *Drugs*, **1983**, *26*, 347–354.

Stevens, D. A.; Levine, H. B.; and Deresinski, S. C. Miconazole in coccidioidomycosis. II. Therapeutic and pharmacologic studies in man. *Am. J. Med.*, **1976**, *60*, 191–202.

Stevens, D. A.; Restrepo, M. A.; Cortes, A.; Betancourt, J.; Galgiani, J. N.; and Gomez, I. Paracoccidioidomycosis (South American blastomycosis): treatment with miconazole. *Am. J. Trop. Med. Hyg.*, **1978**, *27*, 801–807.

Stevens, D. A.; Stiller, R. L.; Williams, P. L.; and Sugar, A. M. Experience with ketoconazole in three major manifestations of progressive coccidioidomycosis. *Am. J. Med.*, **1983**, *74*, 58–63.

Straus, S. E.; Smith, H. A.; Brickman, C.; de Miranda, P.; McLaren, C.; and Keeney, R. E. Acyclovir for chronic mucocutaneous herpes simplex virus infection in immunosuppressed patients. *Ann. Intern. Med.*, **1982**, *96*, 270–277.

Straus, S. E.; Takiff, H. E.; Seidlin, M.; Bachrach, S.; Lininger, L.; DiGiovanna, J. J.; Western, K. A.; Smith, H. A.; Lehrman, S. N.; Creagh-Kirk, T.; and Alling, D. W. Suppression of frequently recurring genital herpes. *N. Engl. J. Med.*, **1984**, *310*, 1545–1550.

Sud, I. J., and Feingold, D. S. Effect of ketoconazole on the fungicidal action of amphotericin B in *Candida albicans*. *Antimicrob. Agents Chemother.*, **1983**, *23*, 185–187.

Sung, J. P.; Grendahl, J. G.; and Levine, H. B. Intravenous and intrathecal miconazole therapy for systemic mycoses. *West. J. Med.*, **1977**, *126*, 5–13.

Sutliff, W. D. Histoplasmosis cooperative study. V. Amphotericin B dosage for chronic pulmonary histoplasmosis. *Am. Rev. Respir. Dis.*, **1972**, *105*, 60–67.

Utz, J. P.; Garriques, I. L.; Sande, M. A.; Warner, J. F.; Mandell, G. L.; McGehee, R. F.; Duma, R. J.; and Shadomy, S. Therapy of cryptococcosis with a combination of flucytosine and amphotericin B. *J. Infect. Dis.*, **1975**, *132*, 368–373.

Van Cutsem, J. The antifungal activity of ketoconazole. *Am. J. Med.*, **1983**, *74*, 9–15.

Vandeputte, J.; Wachtel, J. L.; and Stiller, E. T. Amphotericins A and B, antifungal antibiotics produced by a streptomyces. II. The isolation and properties of the crystalline amphotericins. In, *Antibiotics Annual, 1955–1956*. Medical Encyclopedia, Inc., New York, **1956**, pp. 587–591.

Van Voris, L. P.; Betts, R. F.; Hayden, F. G.; Christmas, W. A.; and Douglas, R. G. Successful treatment of naturally occurring influenza A/USSR/77/H1N1. *J.A.M.A.*, **1981**, *245*, 1128–1131.

Wade. J. C.; Day, L. M.; Crowley, J. J.; and Meyers, J. D. Recurrent infection with herpes simplex virus after marrow transplantation: role of the specific immune response and acyclovir treatment. *J. Infect. Dis.*, **1984a**, *149*, 750–756.

Wade, J. C., and Meyers, J. D. Neurologic symptoms associated with parenteral acyclovir treatment after marrow transplantation. *Ann. Intern. Med.*, **1983**, *98*, 921–925.

Wade, J. C.; Newton, B.; Flournoy, N.; and Meyers, J. D. Oral acyclovir for prevention of herpes simplex virus reactivation after marrow transplantation. *Ann. Intern. Med.*, **1984b**, *100*, 823–828.

Waldorf, A. R., and Polak, A. Mechanisms of action of 5-fluorocytosine. *Antimicrob. Agents Chemother.*, **1983**, *23*, 79–85.

Whitley, R. J., and the NIAID Collaborative Antiviral Study Group. Interim summary of mortality in herpes simplex encephalitis and neonatal herpes simplex virus infections: vidarabine versus acyclovir. *J. Antimicrob. Chemother.*, **1983**, *12*, Suppl. B, 105–112.

Whitley, R. J.; Ch'ien, L. T.; Dolin, R.; Galasso, G. J.; Alford, C. A.; and the NIAID Collaborative Antiviral Study Group. Adenine arabinoside therapy of herpes zoster in the immunosuppressed. *N. Engl. J. Med.*, **1976**, *294*, 1193–1199.

Whitley, R. J.; Hilty, M.; Haynes, R.; Bryson, Y.; Connor, J. D.; Soong, S.-J.; Alford, C. A.; and the NIAID Collaborative Antiviral Study Group. Vidarabine therapy of varicella in immunosuppressed patients. *J. Pediatr.*, **1982a**, *101*, 125–131.

Whitley, R. J.; Soong, S.-J.; Dolin, R.; Betts, R.; Linnemann, C., Jr.; Alford, C. A., Jr.; and the NIAID Collaborative Antiviral Study Group. Early vidarabine therapy to control the complications of herpes zoster in immunosuppressed patients. *N. Engl. J. Med.*, **1982b**, *307*, 971–975.

Whitley, R. J.; Soong, S.-J.; Dolin, R.; Galasso, G. J.; Ch'ien, L. T.; Alford, C. A.; and the NIAID Collaborative Antiviral Study Group. Adenine arabinoside therapy of biopsy-proved herpes simplex encephalitis. *N. Engl. J. Med.*, **1977**, *297*, 289–294.

Whitley, R. J.; Soong, S.-J.; Hirsch, M. S.; Karchmer, A. W.; Dolin, R.; Galasso, G.; Dunnick, J. K.; Alford, J. K.; and the NIAID Collaborative Antiviral Study Group. Herpes simplex encephalitis. Vidarabine therapy and diagnostic problems. *N. Engl. J. Med.*, **1981**, *304*, 313–318.

Williams, C. J.; Whitehouse, J. M. A.; Lister, T. A.; and

Wrigley, P. F. M. Oral anticandidal prophylaxis in patients undergoing chemotherapy for acute leukemia. *Med. Pediatr. Oncol.*, **1977**, *3*, 275–280.

Yap, B., and Bodey, G. P. Oropharyngeal candidiasis treated with a troche form of clotrimazole. *Arch. Intern. Med.*, **1979**, *139*, 656–657.

Young, R. C.; Bennett, J. E.; Geelhoed, G. W.; and Levine, A. S. Fungemia with compromised host resistance. *Ann. Intern. Med.*, **1974**, *80*, 605–612.

Monographs and Reviews

Bennett, J. E. Chemotherapy of systemic mycoses. *N. Engl. J. Med.*, **1974**, *290*, 30–32, 320–323.

———. Antifungal agents. In, *Principles and Practice of Infectious Diseases*, 2nd ed. (Mandell, G. L.; Douglas, R. G., Jr.; and Bennett, J. E.; eds.) John Wiley & Sons, Inc., New York, **1985**, pp. 263–270.

Goldman, L. Griseofulvin. *Med. Clin. North Am.*, **1970**, *54*, 1339–1345.

Hayden, F. G., and Douglas, R. G., Jr. Antiviral agents. In, *Principles and Practice of Infectious Diseases*, 2nd ed. (Mandell, G. L.; Douglas, R. G., Jr.; and Bennett, J. E.; eds.) John Wiley & Sons, Inc., New York, **1985**, pp. 270–286.

Hirsch, M. S., and Swartz, M. N. Antiviral agents. *N. Engl. J. Med.*, **1980**, *302*, 903–907, 949–953.

Medoff, G.; Brajtburg, J.; Koragrashi, G.; and Bolard, J. Antifungal agents useful in the therapy of systemic fungal infection. *Annu. Rev. Pharmacol. Toxicol.*, **1983**, *23*, 303–330.

Medoff, G., and Kobayashi, G. S. Strategies in the treatment of systemic fungal infections. *N. Engl. J. Med.*, **1980**, *302*, 145–155.

Pratt, W. B. *Chemotherapy of Infection.* Oxford University Press, New York, **1977**.

Sanford, J. P. *Guide to Antimicrobial Therapy, 1984.* Sanford, Bethesda, **1984**.

Symposium. (Various authors.) Griseofulvin and dermatomycoses. *Arch. Dermatol.*, **1960**, *81*, 650–882.

Symposium. (Various authors.) Symposium on acyclovir. *Am. J. Med.*, **1982**, *73*, Suppl., 1–392.

XIII

Chemotherapy of Neoplastic Diseases

INTRODUCTION

Paul Calabresi and Robert E. Parks, Jr.

Fundamental advances continue in the chemotherapy of neoplastic diseases. The greatest progress in recent years has been not in the discovery of new, useful chemotherapeutic agents but at the conceptual level: the design of more effective regimens for concurrent administration of drugs; the acquisition of knowledge of the mechanisms of action of many antitumor agents, which facilitates the design of new methods to prevent or minimize drug toxicity; the increased use of adjuvant chemotherapy (*e.g.*, the design of chemotherapeutic approaches to destroy micrometastases and prevent the development of secondary neoplasms after removal or destruction of the primary tumor by surgery or irradiation); and increased knowledge about such vital processes as tumor initiation and the dissemination, implantation, and growth of metastases. Of great importance is recognition of the problems imposed by the heterogeneity of tumors, with the realization that individual tumors may contain many subpopulations of neoplastic cells that differ in crucial characteristics, such as karyotype, morphology, immunogenicity, rate of growth, the capacity to metastasize, and, significantly, responsiveness to antineoplastic agents (Calabresi *et al.*, 1979; Calabresi and Dexter, 1982). Information also continues to accumulate in the fields of molecular and cellular biology, resulting in a greater understanding of cellular division and differentiation, tumor immunology, and viral and chemical carcinogenesis. Particularly significant are recent discoveries of the role of oncogenes in carcinogenesis. These genes, introduced into cells by retroviruses, are activated forms of normal cellular proto-oncogenes that have been altered by chromosomal translocation or by point mutations that affect single amino acid residues. Certain of the proteins encoded by viral oncogenes are related to cellular growth factors or their receptors. For example, striking homology has been shown between the protein encoded by the *v-erb-B* oncogene of the avian erythroblastosis virus and the receptor for epidermal growth factor; the protein encoded by the *v-sis* oncogene is homologous with platelet-derived growth factor. It is hoped that these discoveries will provide new targets for therapy.

To appreciate the progress made in the field during the past half century one need only examine *earlier editions* of this textbook. The first edition, published in 1941, does not have a chapter that discusses the chemotherapy of neoplasia. Indeed, the rubric ''cancer'' does not appear in the index. Significantly, in the years between the appearance of the first and second editions, the original authors, Louis S. Goodman and Alfred Gilman, initiated the clinical investigation of the first major antineoplastic agent, nitrogen mustard, a drug that continues to have an important place in therapeutics. By 1965, significant palliative results had been achieved with chemotherapy for a number of human neoplasms, and the first indications had emerged that choriocarcinoma in women could be cured by treatment with methotrexate. Today, we can list a substantial number of neoplastic diseases that need not shorten life if treated with drugs alone or with drugs in combination with other modalities. These include choriocarcinoma in women; acute leukemia, Wilms' tumor, Ewing's sarcoma, rhabdomyosarcoma, and retinoblastoma in children; and Hodgkin's disease, diffuse histiocytic lymphoma, Burkitt's lymphoma, mycosis fungoides, and testicular carcinoma. Despite these impressive advances, there is the sobering realization that many of the most prevalent forms of human cancer still resist effective chemotherapeutic intervention.

The entire population of neoplastic cells must be eradicated in order to obtain these desired results. The concept of "total cell-kill" applies to chemotherapy as it does to other means of treatment; total excision of tumor is necessary for surgical cure, and complete destruction of all cancer cells is required for a cure with radiation therapy. By investigation of a model tumor system, the L1210 leukemia of mice, Skipper and colleagues established a number of important principles that have guided and redirected modern cancer chemotherapy. These may be briefly summarized as follows: (1) A single clonogenic malignant cell can give rise to sufficient progeny to kill the host; to achieve cure it is thus necessary to destroy every such cell. Since the doubling-time of most tumors is relatively constant during logarithmic growth, the life-span of the host is inversely related to the number of malignant cells that are inoculated or that survive therapeutic measures. (2) In contrast to antimicrobial chemotherapy where, in most instances, there are major contributions by the immune mechanisms and other host defenses, these play a negligible role in the therapy of neoplastic disease unless only a small number of malignant cells is present. (3) The cell-kill caused by antineoplastic agents follows first-order kinetics; that is, a constant percentage, rather than a constant number, of cells is killed by a given therapeutic maneuver. This finding has had a profound impact on clinical cancer chemotherapy. For example, a patient with advanced acute lymphocytic leukemia might harbor 10^{12} or about 1 kg of malignant cells. A drug capable of killing 99.99% of these cells would reduce the tumor mass to about 100 mg, and this would be apparent as a complete clinical remission. However, 10^8 malignant cells would remain, any of which could cause a relapse in the disease. The logical outgrowth of these concepts has been the attempt to achieve total cell-kill by the use of several chemotherapeutic agents concurrently or in rational sequences. The resulting prolonged survival of patients with acute lymphocytic leukemia through the use of such multiple-drug regimens has encouraged the application of these principles to the treatment of other neoplasms.

An understanding of cell-cycle kinetics is essential for the proper use of the current generation of antineoplastic agents. Many of the most potent cytotoxic agents act at specific phases of the cell cycle and, therefore, have activity only against cells that are in the process of division. Accordingly, human malignancies that are currently most susceptible to chemotherapeutic measures are those with a large growth fraction, that is, a high percentage of cells in the process of division. Similarly, normal tissues that proliferate rapidly (bone marrow, hair follicles, and intestinal epithelium) are subject to damage by some of these potent antineoplastic drugs, and such toxicity often limits drug utility. On the other hand, slow-growing tumors with a small growth fraction, for example, carcinomas of the colon or lung, are often unresponsive to cytotoxic drugs. Although differences in the duration of the cell cycle occur between cells of various types, all cells display a similar pattern during the division process. This may be characterized as follows: (1) there is a presynthetic phase (G_1); (2) the synthesis of DNA occurs (S); (3) an interval follows the termination of DNA synthesis, the postsynthetic phase (G_2); and (4) mitosis (M) ensues—the G_2 cell, containing a double complement of DNA, divides into two daughter G_1 cells. Each of these may immediately reenter the cell cycle or pass into a nonproliferative stage, referred to as G_0. The cells of certain specialized tissues may differentiate into functional cells that are no longer capable of division. On the other hand, many cells, especially those in slow-growing tumors, may remain in the G_0 state for prolonged periods, only to be recruited into the division cycle again at a much later time. Most antineoplastic agents act specifically on processes such as DNA synthesis, transcription, or the function of the mitotic spindle and, therefore, are regarded as cell-cycle specific. Some agents may act during several or all stages of the cell cycle; while not cell-cycle specific, their cytotoxic effects may still be dependent on proliferation. It is obvious that further understanding of the cell cycle and of the factors that regulate the recruitment of G_0 cells into the cycle should prove of great value in future attempts to develop chemotherapeutic measures for slow-growing tumors.

A great variety of compounds has been investigated in experimental animals, and a few have proven sufficiently useful in the clinical treatment of human neoplasms, at acceptable levels of toxicity, to deserve the designation of chemotherapeutic agents. It should be emphasized that the compounds selected for discussion represent, for the most part, those that are generally available and have withstood the test of time, although a few have been included either because they illustrate special circumstances or because they are representative of newer developments. Not discussed are several biologically active alkylating agents, hormones, antibiotics, and other compounds that are not commonly used in clinical practice, either because their structural variations offer no particular advantage over existing drugs or because additional investigation is deemed to be necessary. It is also important, in this rapidly changing field, continually to reappraise the current status of available agents, with respect not only to new additions but also to appropriate deletions of compounds the clinical importance of which has declined. Information concerning drugs in the latter category may be found in *earlier editions* of this textbook. Other compounds, particularly certain antimetabolites that were originally developed as antineoplastic agents, have now assumed such important roles in the management of nonneoplastic disorders that they belong more properly in other chapters. Indeed, this spin-off in cancer chemotherapy research represents an area of increasing interest and practical importance to medicine in general. Illustrative examples of such stimulating developments include the effectiveness of allopurinol in controlling hyperuricemia and gout, the beneficial effects of fluorouracil and methotrexate in psoriasis, the inhibitory actions of analogs of pyrimidine and purine nucleosides on the proliferation of certain viruses of the DNA type, and the use of various cytotoxic agents for the suppression of immune responses.

The use of cytotoxic drugs to cause immunosuppression has played an essential role in establishing the feasibility of renal transplantation across histocompatibility barriers. Success has improved significantly with transplantation of other organs, including bone marrow, endocrine glands, heart, and liver. The drugs most commonly used to prevent rejection of a homograft are the potent new immunosuppressive agent cyclosporine, the purine antimetabolite azathioprine, the alkylating agent cyclophosphamide, and the adrenocorticosteroid prednisone. Other agents with immunosuppressive properties include methotrexate, cytarabine, thioguanine, dactinomycin, various alkylating agents, and antilymphocyte globulin. They are not as frequently used, however, because of greater toxicity, difficulty of administration, or lesser efficacy. Encouraged by the immunosuppressive activity of these drugs in experimental systems and their effectiveness in renal transplantation, clinical investigators have explored their utility in a number of diseases that are characterized by altered immunological reactivity and manifestations of autoimmunity. These include various collagen-vascular disorders (*e.g.*, systemic lupus erythematosus, necrotizing vasculitis, scleroderma, polymyositis, rheumatoid arthritis, and related entities such as Wegener's granulomatosis), as well as regional enteritis, ulcerative colitis, chronic active hepatitis, glomerulonephritis, the nephrotic syndrome, Goodpasture's syndrome, autoimmune hemolytic anemia, idiopathic thrombocytopenic purpura, pemphigus, and others. (For detailed reviews and references to the original literature, *see* Kaplan and Calabresi, 1973; Sartorelli and Johns, 1975; Cupps and Fauci, 1981; Fauci *et al.*, 1983; Felson and Anderson; 1984.) Although immunosuppressive agents are widely employed and recommended by experienced clinicians for specific clinical situations, such use is not generally approved in the United States and remains largely investigational. Because of the complex and poorly understood etiologies of these conditions, it is not entirely clear whether the beneficial effects of these drugs are exerted through an immunosuppressive, anti-inflammatory, or other mechanism. Recent advances in the understanding of the biochemical properties of lymphocytes, which have stemmed from studies of states of congenital and acquired

Table XIII–1. CHEMOTHERAPEUTIC AGENTS USEFUL IN NEOPLASTIC DISEASE

CLASS	TYPE OF AGENT	NONPROPRIETARY NAMES (OTHER NAMES)	DISEASE *
Alkylating Agents	Nitrogen Mustards	Mechlorethamine (HN₂)	Hodgkin's disease, non-Hodgkin's lymphomas
		Cyclophosphamide	Acute and chronic lymphocytic leukemias, Hodgkin's disease, non-Hodgkin's lymphomas, multiple myeloma, neuroblastoma, breast, ovary, lung, Wilms' tumor, rhabdomyosarcoma
		Melphalan (L-sarcolysin)	Multiple myeloma, breast, ovary
		Uracil mustard	Chronic lymphocytic leukemia, non-Hodgkin's lymphomas, Hodgkin's disease, ovary, primary thrombocytosis
		Chlorambucil	Chronic lymphocytic leukemia, primary macroglobulinemia, non-Hodgkin's lymphomas
	Alkyl Sulfonates	Busulfan	Chronic granulocytic leukemia
	Nitrosoureas	Carmustine (BCNU)	Hodgkin's disease, non-Hodgkin's lymphomas, primary brain tumors, multiple myeloma, malignant melanoma
		Lomustine (CCNU)	Hodgkin's disease, non-Hodgkin's lymphomas, primary brain tumors, small-cell lung
		Semustine (methyl-CCNU)	Primary brain tumors, stomach, colon
		Streptozocin (streptozotocin)	Malignant pancreatic insulinoma, malignant carcinoid
	Triazenes	Dacarbazine (DTIC; dimethyltriazenoimi-dazolecarboxamide)	Malignant melanoma, Hodgkin's disease, soft-tissue sarcomas
Antimetabolites	Folic Acid Analogs	Methotrexate (amethopterin)	Acute lymphocytic leukemia, choriocarcinoma, mycosis fungoides, breast, head and neck, lung, osteogenic sarcoma
	Pyrimidine Analogs	Fluorouracil (5-fluorouracil; 5-FU)	Breast, colon, stomach, pancreas, ovary, head and neck, urinary bladder, premalignant skin lesions (topical)
		Cytarabine (cytosine arabinoside)	Acute granulocytic and acute lymphocytic leukemias
	Purine Analogs	Mercaptopurine (6-mercaptopurine; 6-MP)	Acute lymphocytic, acute granulocytic, and chronic granulocytic leukemias
		Thioguanine (6-thioguanine; TG)	Acute granulocytic, acute lymphocytic, and chronic granulocytic leukemias

* Neoplasms are carcinomas unless otherwise indicated.

CLASS	TYPE OF AGENT	NONPROPRIETARY NAMES (OTHER NAMES)	DISEASE *
Natural Products	Vinca Alkaloids	Vinblastine (VLB)	Hodgkin's disease, non-Hodgkin's lymphomas, breast, testis
		Vincristine	Acute lymphocytic leukemia, neuroblastoma, Wilms' tumor, rhabdomyosarcoma, Hodgkin's disease, non-Hodgkin's lymphomas, small-cell lung
		Vindesine	Lymphomas, blastic crisis of chronic granulocytic leukemia, systemic mastocytosis
	Epipodophyllotoxins	Etoposide Teniposide	Testis, small-cell lung and other lung, breast, Hodgkin's disease, non-Hodgkin's lymphomas, acute granulocytic leukemia, Kaposi's sarcoma
	Antibiotics	Dactinomycin (actinomycin D)	Choriocarcinoma, Wilms' tumor, rhabdomyosarcoma, testis, Kaposi's sarcoma
		Daunorubicin (daunomycin; rubidomycin)	Acute granulocytic and acute lymphocytic leukemias
		Doxorubicin	Soft-tissue, osteogenic, and other sarcomas; Hodgkin's disease, non-Hodgkin's lymphomas, acute leukemias, breast, genitourinary, thyroid, lung, stomach, neuroblastoma
		Bleomycin	Testis, head and neck, skin, esophagus, lung, and genitourinary tract; Hodgkin's disease, non-Hodgkin's lymphomas
		Plicamycin (mithramycin)	Testis, malignant hypercalcemia
		Mitomycin (mitomycin C)	Stomach, cervix, colon, breast, pancreas, bladder, head and neck
	Enzymes	L-Asparaginase	Acute lymphocytic leukemia
Miscellaneous Agents	Platinum Coordination Complexes	Cisplatin (*cis*-DDP)	Testis, ovary, bladder, head and neck, lung, thyroid, cervix, endometrium, neuroblastoma, osteogenic sarcoma
	Substituted Urea	Hydroxyurea	Chronic granulocytic leukemia, polycythemia vera, essential thrombocytosis, malignant melanoma
	Methyl Hydrazine Derivative	Procarbazine (N-methylhydrazine, MIH)	Hodgkin's disease
	Adrenocortical Suppressant	Mitotane (*o,p'*-DDD)	Adrenal cortex
		Aminoglutethimide	Breast

Table XIII–1. CHEMOTHERAPEUTIC AGENTS USEFUL IN NEOPLASTIC DISEASE (Continued)

CLASS	TYPE OF AGENT	NONPROPRIETARY NAMES (OTHER NAMES)	DISEASE *
Hormones and Antagonists	Adrenocorti-costeroids	Prednisone (several other equivalent preparations available; *see* Chapter 63)	Acute and chronic lymphocytic leukemias, non-Hodgkin's lymphomas, Hodgkin's disease, breast
	Progestins	Hydroxyprogesterone caproate Medroxyprogesterone acetate Megestrol acetate	Endometrium, breast
	Estrogens	Diethylstilbestrol Ethinyl estradiol (other preparations available; *see* Chapter 61)	Breast, prostate
	Antiestrogen	Tamoxifen	Breast
	Androgens	Testosterone propionate Fluoxymesterone (other preparations available; *see* Chapter 62)	Breast

* Neoplasms are carcinomas unless otherwise indicated.

immunodeficiency, may offer the promise of devising important new technics to achieve selective immunosuppression. Deficiencies in the enzymes of purine metabolism, adenosine deaminase and purine nucleoside phosphorylase, are associated with specific impairments of the functions of T and B lymphocytes. Potent inhibitors of adenosine deaminase such as pentostatin (deoxycoformycin) can reproduce many features of the combined immunodeficiency state.

While desirable results may be achieved with cytotoxic chemotherapy in diseases that are associated with altered immunological reactivity, as well as in neoplastic disorders, severe untoward complications can result from their administration. There may be increased susceptibility to infections caused by pathogenic bacteria or opportunistic microorganisms. Some immune responses, particularly cellular immunity mediated by T lymphocytes, are also thought to play important roles in the natural resistance of the host against malignant tumors; others, however, including humoral "blocking factors" produced by B lymphocytes, may be deleterious to the host by interfering with the capacity of cytotoxic lymphocytes to react against neoplastic cells. Coupled with the possibility of genetic damage, the chronic use of immunosuppressive agents carries an increased risk of neoplasia, usually of histiocytic or lymphoid origin. Since cytotoxic drugs can suppress or enhance these immune responses selectively, depending upon dosage and schedule of administration, the subtle interactions between these agents and the immunological defenses of the host represent an increasingly important area of investigation.

The emphasis in Chapter 55 is placed upon the drugs themselves. Although this is appropriate in a textbook of pharmacology, it is also essential to point out the importance of the role played by the patient. It is generally agreed that patients in good nutritional state and without severe metabolic disturbances, infections, or other complications are better candidates for significant improvement from antineoplastic therapy than are severely debilitated individuals. Ideally, the patient also should have adequate renal, hepatic, and bone-marrow function, uncompromised by tumor invasion, previous chemotherapy, or radiation (particularly of the spine or pelvis). Nevertheless, even patients with advanced disease have improved dramatically with chemotherapy. Although methods that would enable accurate prediction of the responsiveness of a particular tumor to a given agent are still investigational (Bogden *et al.*, 1981; Griffin *et al.*, 1983; Selby *et al.*, 1983; Fingert *et al.*, 1984), efforts are being made to establish better clinical and laboratory criteria for the rational selection of patients prior to therapy. Despite efforts to anticipate the development of complications, anticancer agents, like many other potent drugs with only moderate selectivity, may cause severe toxicity. In such circumstances, the physician must have at his disposal adequate facilities for vigorous supportive therapy; some of these, including platelet transfusions and the administration of allopurinol to prevent the complications of hyperuricemia, have been widely adopted, while others, including better methods to combat or prevent infections, are the subject of intensive investigation.

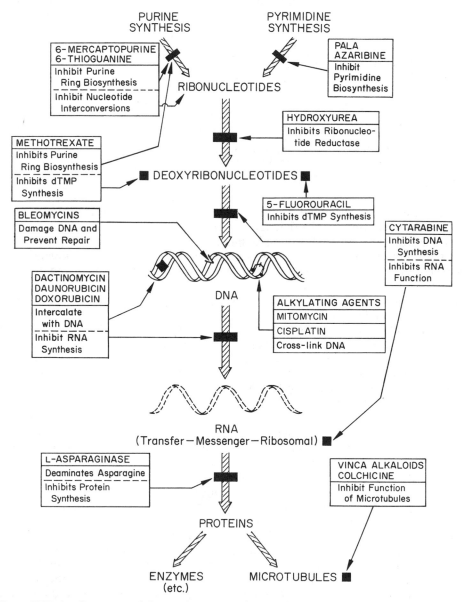

Figure XIII–1. *Summary of the mechanisms and sites of action of chemotherapeutic agents useful in neoplastic disease.*

PALA = N-phosphonoacetyl-L-aspartate.

Drugs currently used in chemotherapy of neoplastic diseases may be divided into several classes, as shown in Table XIII–1. This somewhat arbitrary classification is used in Chapter 55 as a convenient framework for describing the various types of agents; the major clinical indications for the drugs are listed in Table XIII–1 in order to facilitate rapid reference. Dosage regimens, which are often complex, are discussed under the individual drugs.

Mechanistic classification of these agents is increasingly important, particularly as investigators attempt to utilize this information to design "rational" regimens for chemotherapy. A simplified overview of the sites of action of many of the drugs described in Chapter 55 is shown in Figure XIII–1.

CHAPTER

55 ANTIPROLIFERATIVE AGENTS AND DRUGS USED FOR IMMUNOSUPPRESSION

Paul Calabresi and Robert E. Parks, Jr.

I. Alkylating Agents

History. Although synthesized in 1854, the vesicant properties of *sulfur mustard* were not described until 1887. During World War I, medical attention was first focused on the vesicant action of sulfur mustard on the skin, eyes, and respiratory tract. It was appreciated later, however, that serious systemic intoxication also follows exposure. In 1919, Krumbhaar and Krumbhaar made the pertinent observation that the poisoning caused by sulfur mustard is characterized by leukopenia and, in cases that came to autopsy, by aplasia of the bone marrow, dissolution of lymphoid tissue, and ulceration of the gastrointestinal tract.

In the interval between World Wars I and II, extensive studies of the biological and chemical actions of the *nitrogen mustards* were conducted. The marked cytotoxic action on lymphoid tissue prompted Gilman, Goodman, and T. F. Dougherty to study the effect of nitrogen mustards on transplanted lymphosarcoma in mice, and in 1942 clinical studies were initiated. This launched the era of modern cancer chemotherapy (Gilman, 1963).

In their early phases, all these investigations were conducted under secrecy restrictions imposed by the use of classified chemical-warfare agents. At the termination of World War II, however, the nitrogen mustards were declassified and a general review was presented by Gilman and Philips (1946), and shortly thereafter there appeared summaries of clinical research by Goodman and associates (1946), Jacobson and coworkers (1946), and Rhoads (1946). Recent reviews include those by Colvin (1982), Wheeler (1982), Connors (1983), and Ludlum and Tong (1985).

Thousands of variants of the basic chemical structure of the nitrogen mustards have been prepared. However, most attempts at the rational design of "active-site-directed" molecules have failed, and only a few of these agents have proven more useful than the original compound in specific clinical circumstances (*see* below). At the present time five major types of alkylating agents are used in the chemotherapy of neoplastic diseases: (1) the nitrogen mustards, (2) the ethylenimines, (3) the alkyl sulfonates, (4) the nitrosoureas, and (5) the triazenes.

Chemistry. The chemotherapeutic alkylating agents have in common the property of undergoing strongly electrophilic chemical reactions through the formation of carbonium ion intermediates or of transition complexes with the target molecules. These reactions result in the formation of covalent linkages (alkylation) with various nucleophilic substances, including such biologically important moieties as phosphate, amino, sulfhydryl, hydroxyl, carboxyl, and imidazole groups. The cytotoxic and other effects of the alkylating agents are directly related to the alkylation of components of DNA. The 7 nitrogen atom of guanine is particularly susceptible to the formation of a covalent bond with both monofunctional and bifunctional alkylators and may well represent the key target that determines the biological effects of these agents. It must be appreciated, however, that other atoms in the purine and pyrimidine bases of DNA—for example, the 1 or 3 nitrogens of adenine, the 3 nitrogen of cytosine, and the 6 oxygen of guanine—may also be alkylated to a lesser degree, as are the phosphate atoms of the DNA chains and the proteins associated with DNA.

To illustrate the actions of alkylating agents, possible consequences of the reaction of mechlorethamine (nitrogen mustard) with guanine residues in DNA chains are shown in Figure 55–1. First, one 2-chloroethyl side chain undergoes a first-order (S_N1) intramolecular cyclization, with release of a chloride ion and formation of a highly reactive ethylenimonium intermediate. By this reaction the tertiary amine is converted to a quaternary ammonium compound. The ethylenimonium intermediates can react avidly, through formation of a carbonium ion or transition complex intermediate, with a large number of inorganic ions and organic radicals by reactions that resemble a second-order (S_N2) nucleophilic substitution reaction (Price, 1975). Alkylation of the 7 nitrogen of guanine residues in DNA, a highly favored reaction, may exert several

effects of considerable biological importance, as illustrated in Figure 55–1. Normally, guanine residues in DNA exist predominantly as the keto tautomers and readily make Watson-Crick base pairs by hydrogen bonding with cytosine residues. However, when the 7 nitrogen of guanine is alkylated (to become a quaternary ammonium nitrogen), the guanine residue is more acidic and the enol tautomer is favored. Guanine in this form can make base pairs with thymine residues, thus leading to possible miscoding and the ultimate substitution of an adenine-thymine base pair for a guanine-cytosine base pair. Second, alkylation of the 7 nitrogen labilizes the imidazole ring, making possible the opening of the imidazole ring or depurination by excision of guanine residues, either of which can result in serious damage to the DNA molecule

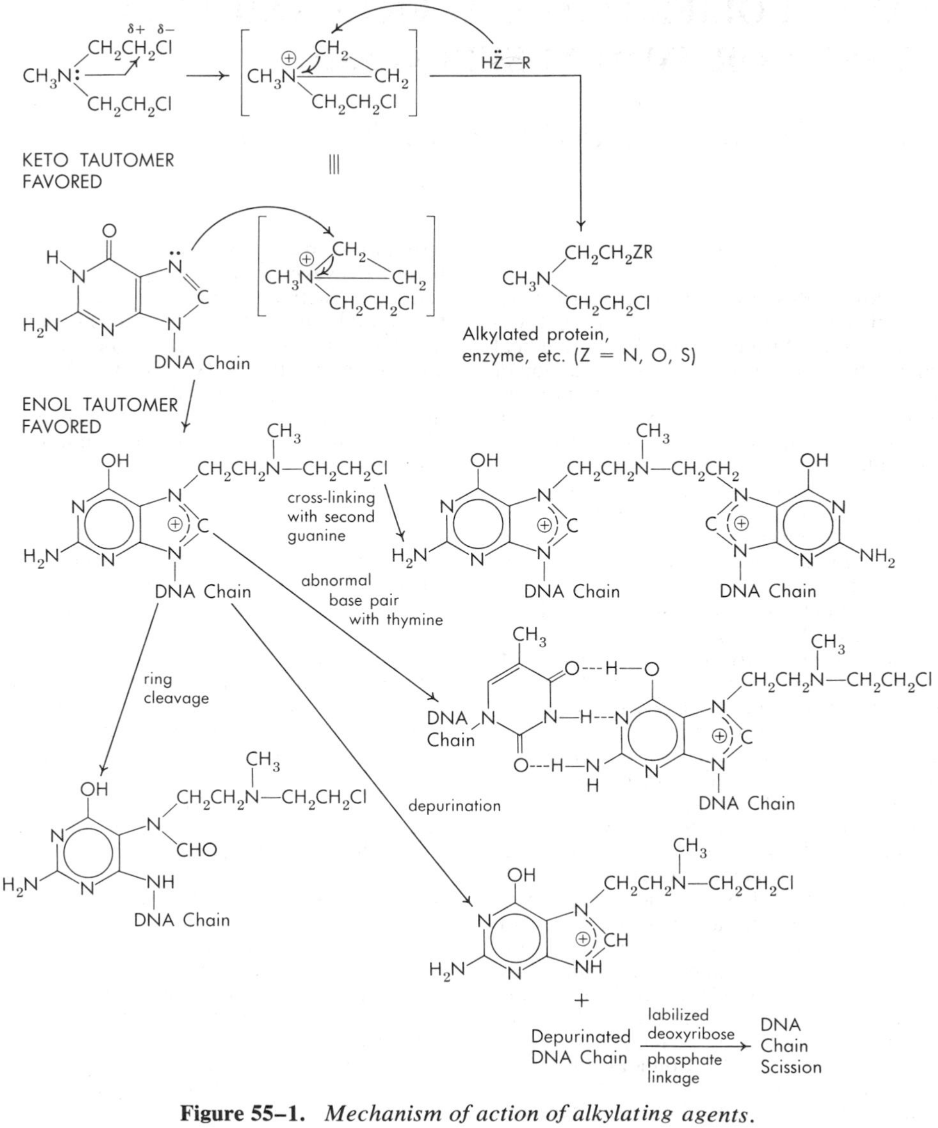

Figure 55–1. *Mechanism of action of alkylating agents.*

(Shapiro, 1968). Third, with bifunctional alkylators, such as nitrogen mustard, the second 2-chloroethyl side chain can undergo a similar cyclization reaction and alkylate a second guanine residue or another nucleophilic moiety, such as an amino group or a sulfhydryl radical of a protein. This can result in the cross-linking of two nucleic acid chains or the linking of a nucleic acid to a protein by very strong covalent bonds, reactions that would cause a major disruption in nucleic acid function. Any of these effects could adequately explain both the mutagenic and the cytotoxic effects of alkylating agents.

In addition to the formation of covalent bonds with purine or pyrimidine residues of DNA, a wide variety of other chemical reactions are possible that can result in a number of other important effects on cellular function and viability.

All nitrogen mustards are chemically unstable but vary greatly in their degree of instability. Therefore, the specific chemical properties of each member of this class of drugs must be considered individually in therapeutic applications. For example, *mechlorethamine* is so hygroscopic and unstable in aqueous form that it is marketed as the dry crystals of the hydrochloride salt. Solutions are prepared immediately prior to injection and, within a few minutes after administration, mechlorethamine reacts almost completely within the body. On the other hand, agents such as *chlorambucil* are sufficiently stable to permit oral administration, and *cyclophosphamide*, which is much less reactive than mechlorethamine, requires biochemical activation by the cytochrome P-450 system of the liver in order to achieve chemotherapeutic effectiveness.

The ethylenimine derivatives react by an S_N2 reaction; however, since the opening of the ethylenimine ring is acid catalyzed, they are more reactive at acidic pH. Busulfan is an atypical alkylating agent with unusual biological properties that differ significantly from substituted nitrogen mustards and ethylenimines (Fox, 1975).

Structure-Activity Relationship. The alkylating agents used in chemotherapy encompass a diverse group of chemicals that have in common the capacity to contribute, under physiological conditions, alkyl groups to biologically vital macromolecules such as DNA. In most instances, physical and chemical parameters, such as lipophilicity, capacity to cross biological membranes, acid dissociation constants, stability in aqueous solution, and so forth, rather than similarity to cellular constituents, have proven crucial to biological activity. With several of the most valuable agents, for example, cyclophosphamide and the nitrosoureas, the active alkylating moieties are generated *in vivo* following complex degradative reactions, some of which are enzymatic. Since many of these physicochemical factors and activation reactions are still unclear, most alkylating agents in use today were discovered by empirical rather than by rational approaches. In most instances where clinically useful agents were uncovered by presumably ''rational'' methods, it was later learned that the original premises were defective, and the biological useful-

ness resulted from factors not considered in the original design.

The nitrogen mustards may be regarded as nitrogen analogs of sulfur mustard. The biological activity of both types of compounds is based upon the presence of the *bis*-(2-chloroethyl) grouping. In sulfur mustard, the two reactive groups are attached to bivalent sulfur; since nitrogen is trivalent, a third substituent must be present on the nitrogen atom. Although a very large number of alkylating agents have been synthesized and evaluated, the methyl derivative, *mechlorethamine,* has received wide clinical use and has been accepted generally as a standard of reference. Various structural modifications have been made in order to achieve greater selectivity and, therefore, less toxicity. *Bis*-(2-chloroethyl) groups have been linked to (1) amino acids (phenylalanine, glycine, DL-alanine); (2) substituted phenyl groups (aminophenyl butyric acid, as in *chlorambucil*); (3) pyrimidine bases (uracil); (4) benzimidazole; (5) antimalarial agents; (6) sugars (mannitol); and (7) several other substances, including a cyclic phosphamide ester. Although none of these modifications has achieved the goal of producing a highly selective and general cytotoxic action for malignant cells, some of the compounds exhibit notable differences in their secondary pharmacological properties and have attracted much clinical, as well as theoretical, interest.

The structural formulas of some of the more commonly used nitrogen mustards are shown in Table 55–1.

There is no definite evidence that the use of special prosthetic groups, such as phenylalanine, a precursor of melanin, conveys unusual selectivity of action on malignant melanoma. The addition of substituted phenyl groups has produced a series of derivatives that retain the ability to react by an S_N1 mechanism; however, the electron-withdrawing capacity of the aromatic ring greatly reduces the rate of carbonium ion formation, and these compounds can therefore reach distant sites in the body before reacting with components of blood and other tissues. Chlorambucil is the most successful example of such aromatic mustards. These molecular modifications of mechlorethamine have not altered its general spectrum of action; however, by reducing the high reactivity characteristic of the parent compound, the derivatives may be administered orally and are more convenient in the treatment of chronic malignancies of the lymphocytic or plasma-cell series, particularly in the presence of extensive infiltration of the bone marrow.

A classical example of the role of the host metabolism in the activation of an alkylating agent is seen with *cyclophosphamide*—now the most widely used agent of this class. The original rationale that guided design of this molecule was twofold. First, if a cyclic phosphamide group replaced the N-methyl of mechlorethamine, the compound might be relatively inert, presumably because the *bis*-(2-chloroethyl) group of the molecule could not ionize until the cyclic phosphamide was cleaved at the phosphorus-nitrogen linkage. Second, it was hoped that neoplastic tissues might possess high phosphatase or phosphamidase activity capable of accomplish-

Table 55–1.   NITROGEN MUSTARDS EMPLOYED IN THERAPY

Mechlorethamine   Cyclophosphamide   Uracil Mustard

Melphalan   Chlorambucil

ing this cleavage, thus resulting in the selective production of an activated nitrogen mustard in the malignant cells. In accord with these predictions, cyclophosphamide displays only weak cytotoxic, mutagenic, or alkylating activity and is relatively stable in aqueous solution. However, when administered to experimental animals or patients bearing susceptible tumors, marked chemotherapeutic effects, as well as mutagenicity and carcinogenicity, are seen. Although a definite role for phosphatases or phosphamidases in the mechanism of action of cyclophosphamide has not yet been demonstrated, it is clearly established that the drug initially undergoes metabolic activation by the cytochrome P-450 mixed-function oxidase system of the liver, with subsequent transport of the activated intermediate to sites of action, as discussed below. Thus, a crucial factor in the structure-activity relationship of cyclophosphamide concerns its capacity to undergo metabolic activation in the liver, rather than to alkylate malignant cells directly. It also appears that the selectivity of cyclophosphamide against certain malignant tissues may result in part from the capacity of normal tissues, such as liver, to protect themselves against cytotoxicity by further degrading the activated intermediates.

Although initially considered as an antimetabolite, the triazene derivative 5-(3,3-dimethyl-1-triazeno)-imidazole-4-carboxamide, usually referred to as *dacarbazine* or DTIC, is now known to function through alkylation. Its structural formula is as follows:

Dacarbazine

This compound bears a striking resemblance to the known metabolite 5-aminoimidazole-4-carboxam-

ide (AIC), which is capable of conversion to inosinic acid by enzymes of purine synthesis. Thus, it was suspected that dacarbazine acts by inhibiting purine metabolism and nucleic acid synthesis. This resemblance to AIC may be fortuitous, since, for chemotherapeutic effectiveness, dacarbazine requires initial activation by the cytochrome P-450 system of the liver through an N-demethylation reaction. In the target cell, there then occurs a spontaneous cleavage liberating AIC and an alkylating moiety, presumably diazomethane (Chabner, 1982d; Oliverio, 1982).

Although the mechanism of action is not yet fully established, it is generally assumed that the *nitrosoureas,* which include compounds such as 1,3-*bis*-(2-chloroethyl)-1-nitrosourea (carmustine, BCNU), 1-(2-chloroethyl)-3-cyclohexyl-1-nitrosourea (lomustine, CCNU), and its methyl derivative (semustine, methyl-CCNU), as well as the antibiotic *streptozocin* (*streptozotocin*), exert their cytotoxicity through the liberation of alkylating and carbamoylating moieties. Their structural formulas are shown in Table 55–2.

The antineoplastic nitrosoureas have in common the capacity to undergo spontaneous, nonenzymatic degradation with the formation of a variety of products. Of these, the methyl carbonium ion (from MNU compounds) and the 2-chloroethyl carbonium ion (from CNU compounds) are strongly electrophilic and can alkylate a variety of substances, including the purine and pyrimidine bases of DNA. Guanine, cytidine, and adenine adducts have been identified; a number of these are derived from the attachment of the haloethyl group to nucleophilic sites on purines or pyrimidines in DNA. Displacement of the halogen atom can then lead to interstrand or intrastrand cross-linking of the DNA. The formation of the cross-links after the initial alkylation reaction is a relatively slow process and can be interrupted by a DNA repair enzyme. As with the nitrogen mustards, it is generally agreed that interstrand cross-linking is associated with the cytotoxicity of nitrosoureas (Colvin, 1982; Hemminki and Ludlum, 1984).

Table 55–2. CLASSIFICATION AND STRUC-TURES OF SOME ANTINEOPLASTIC NITROSOUREAS

METHYLNITROSOUREAS (MNU)

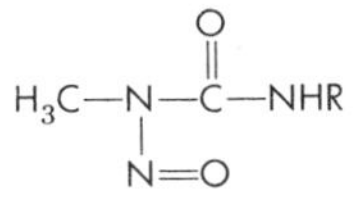

Streptozocin
R = 2-substituted glucose

2-CHLOROETHYLNITROSOUREAS (CNU)

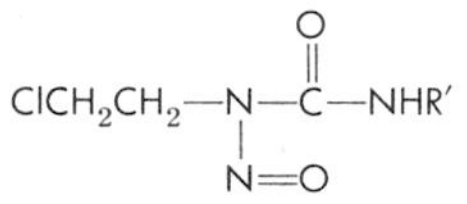

Carmustine (BCNU)
R' = —CH$_2$CH$_2$Cl

Lomustine (CCNU)

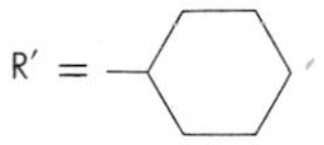

R' =

Semustine (Methyl-CCNU)

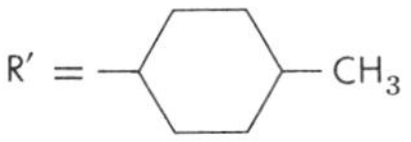

R' =   — CH$_3$

Chlorozotocin
R' = 2-substituted glucose

In addition to the generation of carbonium ions, the spontaneous degradation of nitrosoureas liberates organic isocyanates that are capable of carbamoylating lysine residues of proteins. This reaction can apparently inactivate certain of the DNA repair enzymes, and it has been suggested that high carbamoylating activity might be related to myelosuppression. This has, however, been questioned (*see* Heal *et al.*, 1979). The reactions of the nitrosoureas with macromolecules are shown in Figure 55–2. (For recent reviews of the nitrosoureas, *see* Colvin, 1982; Connors, 1983; Hemminki and Ludlum, 1984; Ludlum and Tong, 1985.)

Since the formation of the ethylenimonium ion constitutes the initial reaction of the nitrogen mustards, it is not surprising that other ethylenimine derivatives or compounds that can produce related structures have antitumor activity. Several agents of this type have been discussed in *earlier editions* of this textbook; these include triethylenemelamine (TEM), triethylenephosphoramide (TEPA), triethylenethiophosphoramide (thiotepa), hexamethylmelamine (HMM), and pentamethylmelamine (PMM). While TEM, TEPA, and thiotepa are cytotoxic, they have no particular clinical advantage over the other alkylating agents. Although there is no evidence that the methylmelamines function as alkylating agents, HMM and PMM are mentioned here because of their chemical similarity to the ethylenimine melamines. The methylmelamines are N-demethylated by hepatic microsomes, with the release of formaldehyde, and there is a relationship between the degree of the demethylation and their activity against murine tumors. HMM requires microsomal activation to display cytotoxicity. The drug appears to have activity against a number of neoplasms that are resistant to

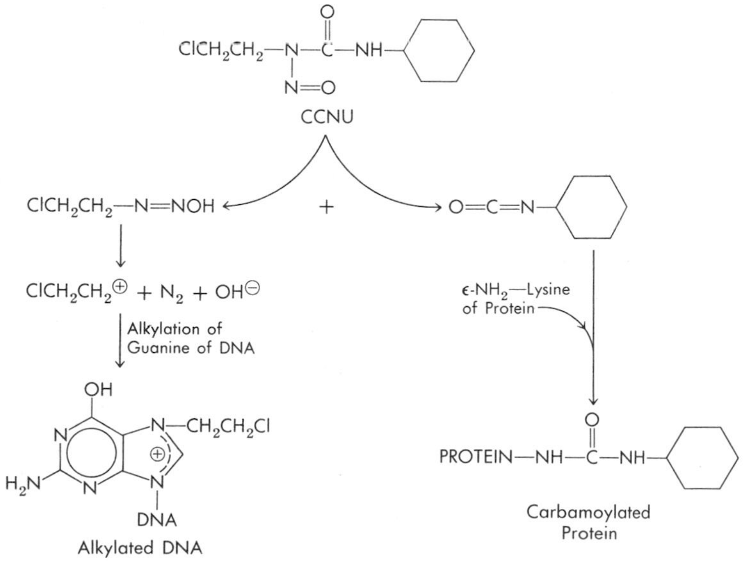

Figure 55–2. *Degradation of lomustine (CCNU) with generation of alkylating and carbamoylating intermediates.*

other alkylating agents. Among these are carcinomas of the ovary, breast, and lung (small cell) and certain lymphomas. Studies are underway to establish the nature of the active metabolite and, hopefully, to identify related compounds with greater therapeutic effectiveness (Rutty and Connors, 1977; Chabner, 1982d).

From a large group of esters of alkanesulfonic acids, synthesized as alkylating agents for chemotherapy of neoplastic disease, several interesting compounds have emerged; one of these, busulfan, is of great value in the treatment of chronic granulocytic leukemia; its structural formula is as follows:

$$H_3C-\underset{\underset{O}{\|}}{\overset{\overset{O}{\|}}{S}}-O-CH_2-CH_2-CH_2-CH_2-O-\underset{\underset{O}{\|}}{\overset{\overset{O}{\|}}{S}}-CH_3$$

Busulfan

Busulfan is a member of a series of symmetrical methanesulfonic acid esters that permit determination of the effects of altering the length of a bridge of methylene groups ($n = 2$ to 10); the compounds of intermediate length ($n = 4$ or 5) possess the highest activities and therapeutic indices. Crosslinked guanine residues have been identified in DNA incubated *in vitro* with busulfan (Tong and Ludlum, 1980).

PHARMACOLOGICAL ACTIONS

The pharmacological actions of the various groups of alkylating agents are considered together in the following discussion. Although there are many similarities, there are, of course, some notable differences. Primary consideration will be given to the cytotoxic actions that follow the administration of a sublethal dose.

Cytotoxic Actions. The most important pharmacological actions of the alkylating agents are those that disturb the fundamental mechanisms concerned with cell growth, mitotic activity, differentiation, and function. The capacity of these drugs to interfere with normal mitosis and cell division in all rapidly proliferating tissues provides the basis for their therapeutic applications and for many of their toxic properties. Whereas certain alkylating agents may have damaging effects on tissues with normally low mitotic indices, for example, liver, kidney, and mature lymphocytes, they are most cytotoxic to rapidly proliferating tissues in which a large proportion of the cells are in division. These compounds may readily alkylate nondividing cells, but

cytotoxicity is seen only if such cells are stimulated to divide. Thus, the process of alkylation itself may be a relatively non-toxic event, as long as the DNA repair enzymes can correct the lesions in DNA prior to the next cellular division.

In contrast to many other antineoplastic agents, the effects of the alkylating drugs, although dependent on proliferation, are not cell-cycle specific, and the drugs may act on cells at any stage of the cycle. However, the toxicity is usually expressed when the cell enters the S phase and progression through the cycle is blocked at the G_2 (premitotic) phase (*see* Wheeler, 1967). While not strictly cell-cycle specific, quantitative differences may be detected when nitrogen mustards are applied to synchronized cells at different phases of the cycle. Cells appear more sensitive in late G_1 or S than in G_2, mitosis, or early G_1. Polynucleotides are more susceptible to alkylation in the unpaired state than in the helical form. During replication of DNA, portions of the molecule are so unpaired.

The cells accumulating behind the block at G_2 may have a double complement of DNA while continuing to synthesize other cellular components, such as protein and RNA. This can result in unbalanced growth, with the formation of enlarged or giant cells that can continue to synthesize DNA, making as much as four or five times the normal complement. Lethal cytotoxic action may occur by so-called interphase death and mitotic death; on the other hand, relatively undifferentiated cells of mammalian germinal tissues may remain nonproliferative during exposure and later undergo nuclear and cytoplasmic hypertrophy, differentiating without further mitosis into more adult cell types. Interphase death is generally regarded as the result of damage to many cellular sites. Nevertheless, this may not be the case; certainly it occurs without any evidence of mitotic activity. For detailed reviews of the cytotoxic and biochemical effects of alkylating agents, *see* Connors (1975) and Colvin, (1982).

Biochemical Actions. The great preponderance of evidence indicates that the primary target of pharmacological doses of alkylating agents is the DNA molecule, as illustrated in Figure 55–1. A crucial distinction that must be emphasized is between the bifunctional agents, in which cytotoxic effects predominate, and the monofunctional agents, which have much greater capacity for mutagenesis and carcinogenesis. This suggests that biochemical events such as the cross-linking of DNA strands, only possible with bifunctional agents, represent a much greater threat to cellular survival than do other effects, such as depurination and chain scission. On the other hand, the latter reactions may cause permanent modifications in DNA structure that are compatible with continued life of the cell and transmissible to subsequent generations; such modifications may result in mutagenesis or carcinogenesis (Colvin, 1982; Ludlum and Tong, 1985).

The remarkable DNA repair systems found in most cells appear to play a key, if not determining, role in the relative resistance of nonproliferating tissues, the selectivity of action against particular cell types, and acquired resistance to alkylating agents. While alkylation of a single strand of DNA may often be repaired with relative ease, inter-strand cross-linkages, such as those produced by the bifunctional alkylating agents, are more difficult to repair and involve more complex mechanisms. Many of the cross-links formed in DNA by these agents at low doses may also be corrected; higher doses cause extensive cross-linkage, and DNA breakdown occurs.

Detailed information is lacking on mechanisms of cellular uptake of alkylating agents. Mechlorethamine appears to enter murine tumor cells by means of an active transport system, the natural substrate of which is choline. Melphalan, an analog of phenylalanine, is taken up by at least two active transport systems that normally react with leucine and other neutral amino acids. The highly lipophilic nitrosoureas, carmustine and lomustine, diffuse into cells passively (Colvin, 1982).

Mechanisms of Resistance to Alkylating Agents. Acquired resistance to alkylating agents is a common event, and the acquisition of resistance to one alkylating agent may impart cross-resistance to other alkylators. While definitive information on the biochemical mechanisms of resistance is lacking, several biochemical mechanisms have been implicated in the development of such resistance by tumor cells. In contrast to the development of resistance to antimetabolites, where single-step mutations can result in almost complete resistance to drug effects, the acquisition of resistance to alkylating agents is usually a slower process, not resulting from single biochemical changes. Resistance of this type may represent the summation of a series of changes, none of which by itself can confer significant resistance. Among the biochemical changes identified in cells resistant to alkylating agents are decreased permeation of the drugs and increased production of nucleophilic substances that can compete with the target DNA for alkylation. The administration of cysteine can considerably reduce the antitumor effects of alkylating agents, and there are several examples of animal tumors with acquired resistance that have greater concentrations of free thiol groups than do the sensitive tumor lines from which they were derived. There has been much speculation about the possibility that increased activity of the DNA repair system may permit cells to acquire resistance to alkylating agents. It has been suggested that cellular resistance to cyclophosphamide may result from increased rates of metabolism of the activated forms of the drug to the inactive keto and carboxy metabolites (*see* Figure 55–3, page 1256). In addition, pleiotropic drug resistance has been documented in experimental and human tumor cell lines; such cells have become resistant to several agents with different chemical structures and mechanisms of action (Connors, 1974; Colvin, 1982; Symposium, 1983a).

Hematological and Immunosuppressive Actions. The hematopoietic system is very susceptible to the effects of alkylating agents. Within 8 hours after administration of a sublethal dose of a nitrogen mustard, cessation of mitosis and disintegration of formed elements may be evident in the marrow and lymphoid tissues. Lymphocytes are more sensitive to the destructive action of the mustards and relatively resistant to the effects of busulfan, an action that is considered responsible for the immunosuppressive effects observed with the former group, particularly cyclophosphamide. Busulfan is more toxic to granulocytes, and suitable combinations of busulfan and chlorambucil, an aromatic mustard, can simulate closely the hematological effects of whole-body x-radiation. The effects of chlorambucil are followed by rapid recovery, except in lymphoid organs, whereas depression of hematopoiesis after busulfan occurs more gradually. In patients treated with mechlorethamine, lymphocytopenia is apparent within 24 hours and becomes more severe for 6 to 8 days; within a few days, granulocytopenia is evident and lasts for 10 days to 3 weeks. Variable depression of platelet and erythrocyte counts may occur during the second or third week after therapy; with ensuing regeneration, hematological recovery is complete at the end of 4 to 6 weeks and rebound hyperplasia may be present from the fifth to the seventh week.

Actions on Reproductive Tissues. In women, amenorrhea of several months' duration sometimes follows a course of therapy with alkylating agents. Impairment of spermatogenesis may be noted in men. Interesting differences and similarities have been found between the effects of these agents and x-rays on the stages of spermatogenesis in rodents. Busulfan mimics most closely the effects of radiation by acting on an early stage of spermatogenesis; this results, after 8 weeks, in a systematic sequential depletion of spermatogonia, spermatocytes, spermatids, and spermatozoa. Triethylenemelamine and the aliphatic mustards affect later stages and produce infertility within 4 weeks. On the other hand, cytotoxic doses of phenylalanine mustard and chlorambucil do not interfere with the fertility of male rats.

Actions on Epithelial Tissues. The intestinal mucosa can be damaged by the parenteral administration of minimal lethal doses of a nitrogen mustard in experimental animals; mitotic arrest, cellular hypertrophy, pyknosis, disintegration, and desquamation of the epithelium are evident. Damage to the hair follicles is much more pronounced with cyclophosphamide than with other mustards and frequently results in alopecia; this effect is usually reversible, even with continued therapy.

Sulfur mustard and the nitrogen mustards are powerful local vesicants. Either direct contact with the compounds or exposure to vapors can lead to serious local reactions. The susceptible tissues are skin, eyes, and respiratory tract. The mustards are not escharotic *per se;* rather, the onset of action is delayed for many hours and the mechanism of tissue injury presumably involves the reaction of their transformation products with essential components of the cell. The vesicant properties of the nitrogen mustards are of concern to the clinician in that local reactions can occur if certain precautions are not observed during the course of administration (*see* below).

Actions on the Nervous System. All nitrogen mustards have effects on the central nervous system (CNS). Nausea and vomiting are prominent side effects, particularly of mechlorethamine, and are presumably the result of CNS stimulation. Convulsions, progressive muscular paralysis, and various cholinomimetic effects have been observed. These effects and a poorly understood "delayed-death" syndrome reported in animals indicate that the cytotoxicity of the alkylating agents extends to cellular functions unrelated to proliferative activity. More detailed descriptions and references appear in the *fourth* and *earlier editions* of this textbook.

NITROGEN MUSTARDS

The chemistry and the pharmacological actions of the alkylating agents as a group, and of the nitrogen mustards, have been presented above. Only the unique pharmacological characteristics of the individual agents are considered below.

MECHLORETHAMINE

Mechlorethamine was the first of the nitrogen mustards to be introduced into clinical medicine and is the most rapidly acting of the drugs in this class. The chemical structure of mechlorethamine has been presented above (*see* Table 55–1).

Absorption and Fate. Severe local reactions of exposed tissues necessitate intrave-

nous injection of mechlorethamine for clinical use. In either water or body fluids, at rates affected markedly by pH, mechlorethamine rapidly undergoes chemical transformation and combines with either water or reactive compounds of cells, so that the drug is no longer present in active form after a few minutes. Indeed, it is possible to protect a given tissue from the effects of the agent by the simple expedient of interrupting the blood supply to the area for a few minutes during and immediately after injection of the drug. Conversely, it is possible, but not always feasible, to localize the action of mechlorethamine or related agents to a large extent in a given tissue by injecting the drug into the arterial blood stream supplying that tissue.

Preparation, Dosage, and Routes of Administration. *Mechlorethamine hydrochloride* (MUSTARGEN) is supplied in vials containing 10 mg of mechlorethamine hydrochloride triturated with 100 mg of sodium chloride. The solution for injection must be freshly prepared before each administration by adding 10 ml of sterile water to the contents of the vial by means of a syringe and needle, with the use of surgical gloves for protection of the hands. The solution should be injected into the tubing of a rapidly flowing intravenous infusion; this not only reduces the possibility of extravasation of the drug but also lowers the concentration of vesicant that comes in contact with the intima of the vein. The exact rate of injection is relatively unimportant, provided it is completed within a few minutes. In patients who have elevated venous pressure in the antebrachial veins because of compression of the great veins by mediastinal tumors, it is advisable to administer the drug through an indwelling catheter inserted into the femoral vein.

A course of therapy with mechlorethamine consists in the injection of a total dose of 0.4 mg/kg of body weight or 10 mg/sq m. Although this total dose may be given in either two or four daily consecutive injections, a single administration is preferable; the therapeutic response is equal, and the patient is spared an additional 2 or 3 days of anorexia, nausea, and vomiting. The recommended total dosage to be given during a single course should be exceeded only by those who are completely familiar with the use of the drug. In the presence of extensive infiltration of bone marrow by neoplastic cells, as is often the case in diffuse lymphoma, it is wise to reduce the dose to 0.3 or even 0.2 mg/kg, at least for the first course of therapy.

A course of mechlorethamine may be repeated only after bone-marrow function has recovered. This is best ascertained by study of the peripheral blood or by evaluation of bone-marrow granulocyte reserve. Usually, at least 6 weeks should elapse between courses of this agent.

Direct intracavitary administration of the drug (0.2 to 0.4 mg/kg) for malignant effusions, particularly of pleural origin, provides valuable palliation.

Therapeutic Uses and Clinical Toxicity. The beneficial results of mechlorethamine in *Hodgkin's disease* and, less predictably, in other *lymphomas* have been extensively confirmed. Although the drug has been effective alone, current practice favors its use in combination with other agents. In generalized Hodgkin's disease (stages III and IV), the so-called MOPP regimen (the combination of mechlorethamine, vincristine [ONCOVIN], procarbazine, and prednisone) is considered the treatment of choice (DeVita *et al.*, 1972).

In patients with generalized *mycosis fungoides,* very dilute solutions (0.02%) of mechlorethamine may be painted on the involved cutaneous areas with marked beneficial results.

In the treatment of leukemias and related myeloproliferative disorders, mechlorethamine has been superseded by other agents. Although palliative results have been observed in carcinomas of the bronchus, ovary, breast, and other solid tumors, alkylating agents of intermediate or slower reactivity are preferable. (*See* Lane, 1977; Colvin, 1982; Calabresi *et al.*, 1985.)

The major toxic manifestations of mechlorethamine include nausea and vomiting, as well as myelosuppression. Leukopenia and thrombocytopenia constitute the major limitation on the amount of drug that can be given in a single course. Rarely, hemorrhagic complications of nitrogen mustard therapy may be due to hyperheparinemia; in such a circumstance, specific therapy with protamine corrects the hemorrhagic diathesis (Chapter 58).

On rare occasions, a maculopapular *skin eruption* may follow therapy with mechlorethamine. The reaction apparently is not one of the hypersensitivity type, does not necessarily recur with subsequent administration of the drug, and does not provide a contraindication to further therapy. *Herpes zoster* is another type of skin lesion frequently associated with nitrogen mustard therapy. A latent viral infection is not uncommonly present in patients with malignant lymphoma, and therapy with either a nitrogen mustard or radiation may be followed by overt manifestations of the viral disease.

Women should be warned that *menstrual irregularities* may be produced by mechlorethamine and, since *fetal abnormalities* have been induced in experimental animals, the drug should not be used if pregnancy exists or is suspected. Breast feeding should be terminated before therapy with mechlorethamine is initiated. After a course of therapy, catamenia may be delayed or several consecutive menstrual periods may be missed. The effect is presumably the result of arrest of maturation of the Graafian follicles, but there appears to be no permanent damage to ovarian function.

Local reactions to extravasation of mechlorethamine into the subcutaneous tissue result in a severe, brawny, tender induration that may persist for a long time. If the local reaction is unusually severe, a slough may result. If it is obvious that extravasation has occurred, the involved area should be promptly infiltrated with an isotonic solution of sodium thiosulfate (⅙ M); an ice compress then should be applied intermittently for 6 to 12 hours. The purpose of the thiosulfate is to provide an ion that reacts avidly with the nitrogen mustard and thereby protects tissue constituents. If thiosulfate solution is not available, prompt injections of isotonic sodium chloride solution may have some value by reducing the local concentration of the vesicant agent.

Thrombophlebitis is a potential complication of therapy with mechlorethamine. It rarely occurs if the drug is injected into the tubing during the course of an intravenous infusion.

CYCLOPHOSPHAMIDE

Efforts to modify the chemical structure of mechlorethamine to achieve greater selectivity for neoplastic tissues led to the development of cyclophosphamide. After studies of the pharmacological activity of cyclophosphamide, clinical investigations by European workers demonstrated its effectiveness in selected malignant neoplasms. (For references to the original literature, *see* Calabresi and Welch, 1962; Symposium, 1967.) The chemical structure of cyclophosphamide and the interesting rationale that led to its synthesis have been presented above (*see* Table 55–1).

Pharmacological and Cytotoxic Actions. None of the severe acute CNS manifestations reported with the typical nitrogen mustards has been noted with cyclophosphamide. Nausea and vomiting, however, may occur. Although the general cytotoxic action of this drug is similar to that of other alkylating agents, some notable differences have been observed. When compared with mechlorethamine, damage to the megakaryocytes and thrombocytopenia are less common. Another unusual manifestation of selectivity consists in more prominent damage to the hair follicles, resulting frequently in alopecia. The drug is not a vesicant, and local irritation does not occur.

Absorption, Fate, and Excretion. Cyclophosphamide is well absorbed orally. As mentioned above, the drug is activated by metabolism in the liver by the mixed-function oxidase system of the smooth endoplasmic reticulum (Brock, 1967); several toxic metabolites have been identified (Colvin, 1982). The current view of the metabolism and fate of cyclophosphamide is presented in Figure 55–3. The hepatic cytochrome P-450 mixed-function oxidase system converts cyclophosphamide to 4-hydroxycyclophosphamide, which is in a steady state with the acyclic tautomer, aldophosphamide. These compounds may be oxidized further by hepatic aldehyde oxidase and perhaps by other enzymes, yielding the metabolites carboxyphosphamide and 4-ketocyclophosphamide, neither of which possesses significant biological activity. It appears that hepatic damage is minimized by these secondary reactions, whereas significant amounts of the activated metabolites, such as aldophosphamide, are transported to the target sites by the circulatory system. It has been proposed that, in cells that are susceptible to cytolysis, the aldophosphamide is cleaved by a β-elimination reaction, generating stoichiometric amounts of phosphoramide mustard and acrolein, both of which are highly cytotoxic. In addition, nor-nitrogen mustard has been identified in the plasma of patients treated with cyclophosphamide. It is not known which of the active metabolites (*e.g.,* phosphoramide mustard, 4-hydroxycyclophosphamide, or nor-nitrogen mustard) plays the key role in the therapeutic and toxic actions of cyclophosphamide. Acrolein may be responsible for the hemorrhagic cystitis seen during therapy with cyclophosphamide. This can be reduced in intensity or prevented by the parenteral administration of N-acetylcysteine or other sulfhydryl compounds; acrolein reacts readily with sulfhydryl groups (Colvin, 1982).

If the cytochrome P-450 system is induced by pretreatment of an animal with phenobarbital or inhibited by administration of proadifen (SK & F 525-A), however, the antitumor activity and therapeutic index of cyclophosphamide are not significantly modified (Sladek, 1972). The explanation proposed for this unexpected finding illustrates several important pharmacological principles. Cy-

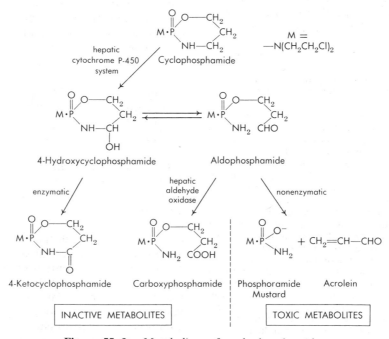

Figure 55–3. *Metabolism of cyclophosphamide.*

clophosphamide, which is biologically relatively inactive, is eliminated from the body very slowly. The activated metabolites (*e.g.*, aldophosphamide) alkylate the target sites in susceptible cells in an "all-or-none" type of reaction or are detoxicated by formation of inactive metabolites that are rapidly excreted by the kidneys. The cytotoxic effects are related to the total amount rather than to the velocity of generation of the activated metabolites. Thus, it seems likely that the biological actions of cyclophosphamide may be affected more drastically by alterations in the rates of detoxication and elimination than by changes in the rate of generation of the activated metabolites.

Urinary and fecal recovery of unchanged cyclophosphamide is minimal after intravenous administration. Maximal concentrations in plasma are achieved 1 hour after oral administration, and a significant amount of unchanged drug is found in the stool when this route is employed. The half-life of cyclophosphamide in plasma is about 7 hours (Bagley *et al.*, 1973). Prior treatment with allopurinol significantly prolongs this value.

Preparations, Dosage, and Routes of Administration. *Cyclophosphamide* (CYTOXAN) is supplied as 25- and 50-mg tablets and as a powder (100 to 2000 mg) in sterile vials. Solutions are prepared by addition of 5 ml of sterile water per 100 mg of drug.

The drug has been administered orally, intravenously, intramuscularly, intrapleurally, and intraperitoneally. A conservative daily dose of 2 to 3 mg/kg, orally or intravenously, has been recommended for patients with more susceptible neoplasms such as lymphomas and leukemias or with compromised bone-marrow function. A higher daily dosage of 4 to 8 mg/kg intravenously for 6 days, followed by an oral maintenance dose of 1 to 5 mg/kg daily, 3 to 5 mg/kg intravenously twice weekly, or 10 to 15 mg/kg intravenously every 7 to 10 days, has been used for the treatment of carcinomas and more resistant neoplasms. Large single doses of 30 mg/kg (750 to 1000 mg/sq m) have been very effective in patients with lymphomas and cause a rapid response approaching that seen with mechlorethamine; in patients without complications or previous therapy, the recommended total initial loading dose is 40 to 50 mg/kg (1500 to 1800 mg/sq m), administered intravenously over a period of 2 to 5 days. Careful evaluation of bone-marrow function is imperative, and prolonged therapy is guided by keeping the total leukocyte count between 2500 and 4000 cells per cubic millimeter of blood or by obtaining the desired response of the tumor.

Therapeutic Uses and Clinical Toxicity. The clinical spectrum of activity for cyclophosphamide is very broad and similar to that of nitrogen mustard. It is an essential component of many effective drug combinations. The drug is effective in Hodgkin's disease and other lymphomas. Complete remissions and presumed cures have been reported in Burkitt's lymphoma and in acute lymphoblastic leukemia of childhood when cyclophosphamide is used concurrently with other agents. It is frequently used in combination with methotrexate and fluorouracil as adjuvant therapy after surgery for carcinoma of the breast when there is involvement of axillary nodes (Bonadonna and Valagussa, 1983).

Notable advantages of this drug are the availability of oral as well as parenteral routes of administration and the possibility of giving fractionated doses over prolonged periods of time. For these reasons it possesses a versatility of action that allows an intermediate range of use, between that of the highly reactive intravenous mechlorethamine and that of oral chlorambucil. Beneficial results have been obtained in multiple myeloma; chronic lymphocytic leukemia; carcinomas of the lung, breast, cervix, and ovary; as well as in neuroblastoma, retinoblastoma, and other neoplasms of childhood. In addition to the combination mentioned above, it is also often used in combination with doxorubicin, vincristine, and prednisone. (*See* Holland and Frei, 1982.)

Because of its potent *immunosuppressive* properties, cyclophosphamide has received considerable attention for the control of organ rejection after transplantation and in nonneoplastic disorders associated with altered immune reactivity, including Wegener's granulomatosis, rheumatoid arthritis, the nephrotic syndrome in children, and autoallergic ocular disease. Appropriate caution is advised when the drug is considered for use in these conditions, not only because of its acute toxic effects but also because of its high potential for inducing sterility, teratogenic effects, mutations, and cancer. The drug should not be used during pregnancy or breast feeding. (*See* Kaplan and Calabresi, 1973; Gershwin *et al.*, 1974; Calabresi, 1979.)

The clinical toxicity of cyclophosphamide differs from that of other nitrogen mustards in that significant degrees of thrombocytopenia are much less common, but there is frequent occurrence of alopecia. Patients should be forewarned of this possible event, which is usually reversible even without interruption of therapy. Nausea and vomiting are common and occur with equal frequency whether the drug is given by the oral or the intravenous route. Mucosal ulcerations, dizziness of short duration, transverse ridging of the nails, increased skin pigmentation, interstitial pulmonary fibrosis, and hepatic toxicity have been reported. Extravasation of the drug into subcutaneous tissues does not produce local reactions, and thrombophlebitis does not complicate intravenous administration. The occurrence of sterile, hemorrhagic cystitis has been reported in 5 to 10% of patients. This has been attributed to chemical irritation produced by reactive metabolites of cyclophosphamide. Its incidence has been reduced by administration of N-acetylcysteine (*see* above). For routine clinical use, ample fluid intake and frequent voiding are recommended. Administration of the drug should be interrupted at the first indication of dysuria or hematuria. The syndrome of inappropriate secretion of antidiuretic hormone (ADH) has been observed in patients receiving cyclophosphamide, usually at doses higher than 50 mg/kg (DeFronzo et al., 1973). It is important to be aware of the possibility of water intoxication, since these patients are usually vigorously hydrated.

MELPHALAN

This phenylalanine derivative of nitrogen mustard is also known as L-sarcolysin. Early clinical studies demonstrated a spectrum of activity similar to that of other alkylating agents.

Chemistry. The chemical structure and the rationale for the synthesis of this amino acid derivative of mechlorethamine have been presented above (see Table 55–1; see also Colvin, 1982; Wheeler, 1982; Vistica, 1983).

Pharmacological and Cytotoxic Actions. The general pharmacological and cytotoxic actions of melphalan are similar to those of other nitrogen mustards. The drug is not a vesicant.

Absorption, Fate, and Excretion. When given orally, melphalan is absorbed in an incomplete and variable manner, and 20 to 50% of the drug is recovered in the stool. The drug has a half-life in plasma of approximately 90 minutes, and 10 to 15% of an administered dose is excreted unchanged in the urine (Tattersall et al., 1978; Alberts et al., 1979b; Colvin, 1982).

Preparation, Dosage, and Route of Administration. Melphalan (ALKERAN) is available in scored, 2-mg tablets. The usual oral dose is 6 mg daily for a period of 2 to 3 weeks, during which time the blood count should be carefully followed. A rest period of up to 4 weeks should then intervene. When the leukocyte and platelet counts are rising, maintenance therapy, ordinarily 2 to 4 mg daily, is begun. It is usually necessary to maintain a significant degree of bone-marrow depression (total leukocyte count in the range of 3000 to 3500 cells per cubic millimeter) in order to achieve optimal results.

Therapeutic Uses and Clinical Toxicity. Although the general spectrum of action of melphalan seems to resemble that of other nitrogen mustards, the advantages of a gradual but continuous administration by the oral route have made the drug useful in the treatment of *multiple myeloma* (Bergsagel, 1972). Beneficial effects have also been reported in malignant melanoma and in carcinoma of the breast and ovary. The clinical toxicity of melphalan is mostly hematological and is similar to that of other alkylating agents. Nausea and vomiting are infrequent. Alopecia does not occur, and changes in renal or hepatic function have not been observed.

URACIL MUSTARD

Uracil mustard was synthesized in an unsuccessful attempt to produce an active-site-directed alkylator by linking the *bis*-(2-chloroethyl) group to the pyrimidine base uracil. Its activity in experimental neoplasms was demonstrated shortly thereafter. No relationship has been demonstrated, however, with the biological functions of uracil.

Chemistry. The structural formula of uracil mustard and its chemical relationship to other alkylating agents are presented above (see Table 55–1). The compound is quite unstable in water.

Pharmacological and Cytotoxic Actions. Uracil mustard may cause nausea and vomiting. The drug is not a vesicant. Cytotoxicity characteristic of the nitrogen mustards has been observed in subacute and chronic toxicity studies of uracil mustard in animals.

Absorption, Fate, and Excretion. Uracil mustard is absorbed quickly but not completely after oral administration in dogs. Concentrations in plasma decline rapidly after either oral (2 mg/kg) or intravenous (1 mg/kg) administration, and no evidence of drug is detected at 2 hours. Less than 1% of the administered dose is recovered unchanged in the urine.

Preparation, Dosage, and Route of Administration. *Uracil mustard* is available in capsules containing 1 mg. Two oral dosage schedules are recommended: (1) 1 to 2 mg daily for 3 weeks, repeated after an interruption of 1 week; and (2) 3 to 5 mg daily for 7 days, then 1 mg daily for 3 weeks.

Therapeutic Uses and Clinical Toxicity. Uracil mustard can be administered orally and, in contrast to cyclophosphamide, does not cause frank alopecia. Its clinical spectrum of action is similar to that of other related alkylating agents. Hematopoietic depression is the major manifestation of toxicity, and uracil mustard has been considered useful for controlling thrombocytosis. Nausea, vomiting, diarrhea, and dermatitis have also been noted.

CHLORAMBUCIL

Initial clinical studies of this aromatic derivative of mechlorethamine demonstrated beneficial results primarily in chronic lymphocytic leukemia, as well as in Hodgkin's disease and related malignant lymphomas. (For references to the early reports, see Calabresi and Welch, 1962.)

Chemistry. The chemical formula of chlorambucil and its relation to the nitrogen mustards are presented above (see Table 55–1).

Pharmacological and Cytotoxic Actions. Although CNS side effects can occur, these have been observed only with large doses. Nausea and vomiting may result from single oral doses of 20 mg or more. Cytotoxic effects on the bone marrow, lymphoid organs, and epithelial tissues are similar to those observed with the nitrogen mustards.

Absorption, Fate, and Excretion. Oral absorption of chlorambucil is adequate and reliable. The drug has a half-life in plasma of approximately 1 hour, and it is almost completely metabolized (Alberts *et al.*, 1979a).

Preparation, Dosage, and Route of Administration. *Chlorambucil* (LEUKERAN) is available in 2-mg tablets for oral administration. The standard initial daily dosage is 0.1 to 0.2 mg/kg, continued for at least 3 to 6 weeks. The total daily dose, usually 4 to 10 mg, is given at one time. With fall in the peripheral total leukocyte count or clinical improvement, the dosage is reduced; maintenance therapy (usually 2 mg daily) is feasible and may be required, depending on the nature of the disease.

Therapeutic Uses and Clinical Toxicity. At the recommended dosages, chlorambucil is the slowest-acting nitrogen mustard in clinical use. It is the treatment of choice in chronic lymphocytic leukemia and in primary (Waldenström's) macroglobulinemia.

In chronic lymphocytic leukemia, chlorambucil may be given orally for long periods of time, achieving its effects gradually and often without toxicity to a precariously compromised bone marrow. Its spectrum of action is similar to that of other alkylating agents, and remissions may be expected in Hodgkin's disease and lymphomas, and sometimes in solid tumors. Clinical improvement comparable to that with melphalan or cyclophosphamide has been observed in some patients with plasma-cell myeloma. Beneficial results have also been reported in disorders with altered immune reactivity, such as vasculitis associated with rheumatoid arthritis and autoimmune hemolytic anemia with cold agglutinins (Livingston and Carter, 1970; Gardner, 1972; Knospe *et al.*, 1974).

Although it is possible to induce marked hypoplasia of the bone marrow with excessive doses of chlorambucil administered over long periods of time, its myelosuppressive action is usually moderate, gradual, and rapidly reversible. Gastrointestinal discomfort, azoospermia, amenorrhea, pulmonary fibrosis, seizures, dermatitis, and hepatotoxicity may be encountered. A marked increase in the incidence of leukemia and other tumors has been noted in a large controlled study of its use for the treatment of polycythemia vera by the National Polycythemia Vera Study Group, as well as in patients with breast cancer receiving long-term adjuvant chemotherapy (Lerner, 1978).

ETHYLENIMINES AND METHYLMELAMINES

TRIETHYLENEMELAMINE (TEM), THIOTEPA (TRIETHYLENETHIOPHOSPHORAMIDE), AND HEXAMETHYLMELAMINE (HMM)

Chemistry. The chemical structures of TEM, thiotepa, and HMM are discussed above in conjunction with the structure-activity relationship of the alkylating agents.

Status. Although still available for clinical use, ethylenimines are now seldom employed as therapeutic agents, having been replaced by selected nitrogen mustards. Their pharmacological properties are described in the *third edition* of this textbook.

Although hexamethylmelamine (HMM) was introduced for clinical trial in the early 1960s, it has recently been shown that the drug has significant activity in small-cell carcinoma of the lung, ovarian cancer, breast carcinoma, and lymphomas, some of which are resistant to alkylating agents. Hexamethylmelamine is available only for investigational purposes in the United States. It is administered orally but is poorly absorbed, and it causes nausea and vomiting, myelosuppression, and neurotoxicity. A more soluble compound, pentamethylmelamine, which is a major metabolite of HMM, has antitumor activity and is under clinical investigation (Chabner, 1982d).

ALKYL SULFONATES

BUSULFAN

During the course of an investigation to determine the antineoplastic properties of a series of alkanesulfonic acid esters, the rather selective action of *busulfan* was detected. This finding led to the use of the drug in patients with chronic granulocytic leukemia. The chemical formula of busulfan is shown on page 1252.

Pharmacological and Cytotoxic Actions. Busulfan is unique in that it exerts virtually no pharmacological action other than myelosuppression. At low doses, selective depression of granulocytopoiesis is evident. Platelets are also affected by relatively small amounts of drug, and erythroid elements may be suppressed as the dosage is raised; eventually, a pancytopenia results. Cytotoxic action does not appear to extend to either the lymphoid tissues or the gastrointestinal epithelium.

Absorption, Fate, and Excretion. Busulfan is well absorbed after oral administration, and it disappears from the blood with a half-time of 2 to 3 hours. Almost all of the drug is excreted in the urine as methanesulfonic acid. The metabolism of busulfan has been reviewed in relation to its mechanism of action by Warwick (1963).

Preparation, Dosage, and Route of Administration. *Busulfan* (MYLERAN) is available in scored, 2-mg tablets. The initial oral dose varies with the total leukocyte count and the severity of the disease; daily doses from 2 to 8 mg are recommended to initiate therapy and are adjusted appropriately to subsequent hematological and clinical responses. It has been reported that reduction of the total leukocyte count to 10,000 or fewer cells per cubic millimeter before discontinuing the drug results in longer remissions. If maintenance doses are required to keep the hematological status under control, 1 to 3 mg may be given daily.

Therapeutic Uses and Clinical Toxicity. The beneficial effects of busulfan in chronic granulocytic leukemia are well established, and remissions may be expected in 85 to 90% of patients after the initial course of therapy.

Reduction in morbidity is readily apparent with symptomatic response, characterized by increased appetite and sense of well-being, which may occur within a few days. Reduction of the leukocyte count is noted during the second or third week, and regression of splenomegaly follows. Beneficial results have been reported in other myeloproliferative disorders, including polycythemia vera and myelofibrosis with myeloid metaplasia. The drug is of no value in acute leukemia or in the "blastic crisis" of chronic granulocytic leukemia.

The major toxic effects of busulfan are related to its myelosuppressive properties, and thrombocytopenia may be a hazard. Occasional instances of nausea, vomiting, diarrhea, impotence, sterility, amenorrhea, and fetal malformation have been reported. The drug may be carcinogenic and leukemogenic (Stott *et al.*, 1977). Hyperuricemia, resulting from extensive purine catabolism accompanying the rapid cellular destruction, and renal damage from precipitation of urates have been noted. To avoid this complication, the concurrent use of *allopurinol* is recommended. A number of unusual complications have been observed in patients receiving busulfan, but their relation to the drug is poorly understood; these include generalized skin pigmentation, cataracts, gynecomastia, cheilosis, glossitis, anhidrosis, and pulmonary and endocardial fibrosis (Calabresi and Welch, 1962; Colvin, 1982).

NITROSOUREAS

The nitrosoureas are important antitumor agents that have demonstrated activity against a wide spectrum of human malignancies; they appear to function chemotherapeutically as bifunctional alkylating agents. Since their introduction by investigators at the Southern Research Institute (Johnston *et al.*, 1963; Schabel, 1973), many nitrosoureas have been synthesized. Certain of these agents, particularly carmustine (BCNU) and lomustine (CCNU), have attracted special interest because of their high lipophilicity and, thus,

their capacity to cross the blood-brain barrier; this enables their use in the treatment of meningeal leukemias and brain tumors. Unfortunately, the nitrosoureas used in the clinic to date, with the exception of streptozocin, cause profound, cumulative myelosuppression that restricts their therapeutic value. In addition, long-term treatment with the nitrosoureas, especially semustine (methyl-CCNU), has resulted in renal failure with lesions that resemble radiation-induced nephritis. As with other alkylating agents, the nitrosoureas are both carcinogenic and mutagenic (Colvin, 1982).

Streptozocin, originally discovered as an antibiotic, is of special interest. This compound has a methylnitrosourea (MNU) moiety attached to the 2 carbon of glucose (*see* Table 55–2). It has special affinity for beta cells of the islets of Langerhans and is employed as a diabetogenic agent in experimental animals. Streptozocin is useful in the treatment of human pancreatic islet-cell carcinoma and malignant carcinoid tumors, as well as other human malignancies (Schein *et al.*, 1973, 1974). Although MNU, the active moiety of streptozocin, is cytotoxic to selected human tumors, it also produces powerful and delayed myelosuppression. Furthermore, MNU is particularly prone to cause carbamoylation of lysine residues of proteins (Figure 55–2). Streptozocin is not myelosuppressive and displays little carbamoylating activity. Thus, the nitrosourea-type moiety has been attached to various carrier molecules, with alterations in crucial properties such as tissue specificity, distribution, and toxicity. Chlorozotocin, an agent in which the 2 carbon of glucose is substituted by the chloronitrosourea group (CNU), was developed and subjected to clinical testing (Green *et al.*, 1982). This compound, unlike streptozocin, is not diabetogenic and, unlike many other nitrosoureas, causes little myelosuppression or carbamoylation. There is reason for optimism that important new nitrosourea-containing derivatives will be prepared (Colvin, 1982; Wheeler, 1982).

CARMUSTINE (BCNU)

This compound was the first of the nitrosourea series to receive extensive clinical evaluation. It is effective against a wide range of experimental tumors.

Pharmacological and Cytotoxic Actions. Carmustine is capable of inhibiting the synthesis of DNA, RNA, and protein in a manner similar but not identical to that of other alkylating agents (Livingston and Carter, 1970). Although bone-marrow suppression is observed, there is an unusually delayed onset of leukopenia and thrombocytopenia that is characteristic of this drug. The nadir of the leukocyte and platelet counts may not be reached until 6 weeks after treatment. Cytotoxic effects on the liver, kidneys, and CNS have been reported (Oliverio, 1973).

Absorption, Fate, and Excretion. Although carmustine is rapidly absorbed by the oral route, it is administered intravenously because tissue uptake and metabolism occur quickly; disappearance from the plasma takes place with a half-life of 90 minutes. Approximately 80% of radioactively labeled drug appears in the urine within 24 hours as degradation products of the parent compound. The pharmacokinetic properties of the drug may be affected by the lipid content of the plasma and the other tissues. Active metabolites may be responsible for the delayed bone-marrow toxicity. Entry of these products into the cerebrospinal fluid (CSF) is rapid, and their concentrations in the CSF of man are 15 to 30% of the concurrent plasma values (Oliverio, 1973, 1976; Levin et al., 1978).

Preparation, Dosage, and Route of Administration. *Carmustine* (BICNU) is a powder at 4° C; it melts to an oily liquid at 27° C and is stable in the anhydrous state. It is available in vials containing 100 mg. The half-life of the drug in 0.9% sodium chloride solution at pH 6 is 24 hours at room temperature. Carmustine is usually administered intravenously at doses of 100 to 200 mg/sq m, given by infusion during a period of 1 to 2 hours, and it is not repeated for 6 weeks. When used in combination with other chemotherapeutic agents, the dose is usually reduced by 25 to 50%.

Therapeutic Uses and Clinical Toxicity. The spectrum of activity of carmustine is similar to that of other alkylating agents, with significant responses observed in Hodgkin's disease and to a lesser extent in other lymphomas and myeloma. Because of its ability to cross the blood-brain barrier, it has been used in meningeal leukemia and in primary and metastatic tumors of the brain, with encouraging results. Beneficial responses have been reported in melanomas, as well as in gastrointestinal, breast, bronchogenic, and renal-cell carcinomas (Young et al., 1971; Carter, 1973; Moertel, 1973; Walker, 1973; Wilson et al., 1976).

The most significant clinical toxicity is the characteristically delayed hematopoietic depression described above. The drug is not a vesicant, but local burning pain has been reported after intravenous administration. Nausea and vomiting occur approximately 2 hours after injection, and flushing of the skin and conjunctiva, CNS toxicity, esophagitis, diarrhea, dyspnea, interstitial pulmonary fibrosis, and renal and hepatic toxicity have been reported (Young et al., 1971; Durant et al., 1979; Wiemann and Calabresi, 1985).

LOMUSTINE (CCNU) AND SEMUSTINE (METHYL-CCNU)

Pharmacological and Cytotoxic Actions. Lomustine and its methylated analog, semustine, were selected for clinical studies because of their lipid solubility and superiority to carmustine in the treatment of certain experimental tumors. The cytotoxic effects of these compounds are similar to those of carmustine, as is their clinical toxicity. Delayed bone-marrow depression, reflected by leukopenia and thrombocytopenia, is characteristic and similar to that caused by carmustine (Moertel, 1973; Wasserman et al., 1975; Wasserman, 1976).

Absorption, Fate, and Excretion. Lomustine and semustine are rapidly absorbed from the gastrointestinal tract and are administered orally. Although lomustine is rapidly and completely metabolized, prolonged plasma half-life of its metabolites, ranging from 16 to 48 hours, has been reported. Approximately 50% of the administered dose is detectable in the urine within 24 hours and 75% within 4 days. Radioactively labeled semustine is not detectable in either plasma or urine. The chloroethyl moiety has a half-life of 36 hours, while the cyclohexyl portion has a biphasic disappearance curve with an early half-life of 24 hours and a slower secondary phase with a half-life of 72 hours. Although neither drug can be detected intact in the CSF, active metabolites appear in significant concentrations within 30 minutes (Oliverio, 1973, 1976; Carter and Slavik, 1974).

Preparations, Dosage, and Route of Administration. *Lomustine* (CEENU) is available in 100-mg, 40-mg, and 10-mg capsules. Semustine is available only for investigational use. The usual oral dose of lomustine is 130 mg/sq m, while the recommended oral dose of semustine is 200 mg/sq m. Both drugs are administered as a single dose, which is not repeated for 6 weeks. When used concurrently with other antineoplastic drugs, the dose is usually reduced by 25 to 50% (Wasserman, 1976).

Therapeutic Uses and Clinical Toxicity. These agents have a wide spectrum of activity. Lomustine appears to be more effective than carmustine in Hodgkin's disease. Beneficial results of therapy with lomustine and particularly semustine, alone and concurrently with other agents, have been reported in patients with malignant gliomas, adenocarcinomas of the gastrointestinal tract, Hodgkin's disease and other lymphomas, carcinoma of the breast, malignant melanoma, hypernephromas, multiple myeloma, and various squamous-cell carcinomas (Symposium, 1973; Carter and Slavik, 1974; Wilson *et al.*, 1976; Moertel, 1978).

The clinical toxicity of both drugs is similar, with the characteristically delayed bone-marrow suppression described above being the dose-limiting effect. Nausea and vomiting are frequently encountered. Nephrotoxicity may occur, particularly when semustine is administered at doses greater than 1500 mg/sq m. The earliest manifestation of this toxic effect may be a decrease in renal size. Both drugs are mutagenic, carcinogenic, and leukemogenic (Green *et al.*, 1982; Calabresi, 1983).

STREPTOZOCIN

This naturally occurring nitrosourea is an antibiotic derived from *Streptomyces acromogenes*. It has been particularly useful in treating functional, malignant pancreatic islet-cell tumors. The drug is capable of inhibiting synthesis of DNA in microorganisms and mammalian cells; it affects all stages of the mammalian cell cycle. Biochemical studies have also revealed potent inhibitory effects on pyridine nucleotides and on key enzymes involved in glyconeogenesis.

Absorption, Fate, and Excretion. Streptozocin is administered parenterally. After intravenous infusions of 200 to 1600 mg/sq m, peak concentrations in the plasma are 30 to 40 μg/ml; the half-life of the drug is approximately 15 minutes. Only 10 to 20% of a dose is recovered in the urine (Schein *et al.*, 1973).

Preparation, Dosage, and Route of Administration. *Streptozocin* (ZANOSAR) is available in 1-g vials as a powder for injection. The intravenous dose is 500 mg/sq m once daily for 5 days; this course is repeated every 6 weeks. Alternatively,

1000 mg/sq m can be given weekly for 2 weeks, and the weekly dose can then be increased to a maximum of 1500 mg/sq m.

Therapeutic Uses and Clinical Toxicity. Streptozocin has been used primarily in patients with metastatic pancreatic islet-cell carcinoma, and beneficial responses are translated into a significant increase in 1-year survival rate and a doubling of median survival time for the responders. It has also been found to be active in Hodgkin's disease, other lymphomas, and occasionally in melanoma and malignant carcinoid tumors (Schein *et al.*, 1974). Broder and Carter (1973) noted nausea and vomiting in almost all of 52 patients treated for islet-cell carcinoma. Renal or hepatic toxicity occurs in approximately two thirds of cases; although usually reversible, renal toxicity may be fatal, and proximal tubular damage is the most important toxic effect. Serial determinations of urinary protein are most valuable in detecting early renal effects. Hematological toxicity, consisting in anemia, leukopenia, or thrombocytopenia, occurs in 20% of patients.

TRIAZENES

DACARBAZINE (DTIC)

Dacarbazine, the chemistry of which is described above, was originally believed to act as an antimetabolite; more recent evidence indicates that it functions as an alkylating agent after metabolic activation in the liver by microsomal enzymes. Dacarbazine appears to inhibit the synthesis of RNA and protein more than that of DNA. It kills cells slowly, and there appears to be no phase of the cell cycle in which sensitivity is increased (Bono, 1976). Minimal immunosuppressive activity has been noted in mice but not clinically (Chabner, 1982d).

Absorption, Fate, and Excretion. Dacarbazine is administered intravenously; after an initial rapid phase of disappearance ($t_{1/2}$ of about 20 minutes), the drug is removed from plasma with a half-time of about 5 hours (Loo *et al.*, 1976). The half-life is prolonged in the presence of hepatic or renal disease. Almost one half of the compound is excreted intact in the urine by tubular secretion. Elevated urinary concentrations of 5-aminoimidazole-4-carboxamide (AIC) are derived from the catabolism of dacarbazine, rather than by inhibition of *de-novo* purine biosynthesis. Concentrations of dacarbazine in CSF are approximately 14% of those in plasma (Chabner, 1982d).

Preparation, Dosage, and Route of Administration. *Dacarbazine* (DTIC-DOME) is available in vials that contain 100 or 200 mg. The recommended regimen is to give 3.5 mg/kg per day, intravenously, for a 10-day period; this is repeated every 28 days. Alternatively, 250 mg/sq m can be given daily for 5 days and repeated every 3 weeks. Extravasation of the drug may cause tissue damage and severe pain.

Therapeutic Uses and Clinical Toxicity. At present, dacarbazine is employed principally for the treatment of malignant melanoma; the overall response rate is about 20%. Beneficial responses have also been reported in patients with Hodgkin's disease, particularly when the drug is used concurrently with doxorubicin, bleomycin, and vinblastine (Santora and Bonadonna, 1979), as well as in various sarcomas when used with doxorubicin (Costanzi, 1976; Gottlieb *et al.*, 1976). Toxicity includes nausea and vomiting in more than 90% of patients; this usually develops 1 to 3 hours after treatment. Myelosuppression, with both leukopenia and thrombocytopenia, is usually mild to moderate. A flulike syndrome, consisting in chills, fever, malaise, and myalgias, may occur during treatment. Hepatotoxicity, alopecia, facial flushing, neurotoxicity, and dermatological reactions have also been reported.

II. Antimetabolites

FOLIC ACID ANALOGS

METHOTREXATE

This class of antimetabolites not only produced the first striking, although temporary, remissions in leukemia (Farber *et al.*, 1948) but also includes the first drug to achieve cures of choriocarcinoma in women (Hertz, 1963). The attainment of a high percentage of permanent remissions in this otherwise-lethal disease provided great impetus to chemotherapeutic investigation. Interest in folate antagonists has increased greatly with the introduction of "rescue" technics that employ leucovorin (folinic acid, citrovorum factor) and/or thymidine to protect normal tissues against lethal damage. These methods permit the use of very high doses of folate analogs such as methotrexate and extend their utility to tumors such as osteogenic sarcoma that do not respond to lower doses.

Methotrexate has also been used with benefit in the therapy of *psoriasis*, a nonneoplastic disease of the skin characterized by abnormally rapid proliferation of epidermal cells (McDonald, 1981). Addi-

tionally, folate antagonists are potent inhibitors of some types of immune reactions and have been employed as *immunosuppressive agents*, for example, in organ transplantation. (For recent reviews, *see* Symposium, 1981b; Chabner, 1982c; Johns and Bertino, 1982; Jackson, 1984.)

Structure-Activity Relationship. Folic acid is an essential dietary factor from which is derived a coenzyme, tetrahydrofolic acid, and a group of structurally related derivatives; these are concerned with the metabolic transfer of one-carbon units. A detailed description of the biological functions and therapeutic applications of folic acid appears in Chapter 57.

Although there are many metabolic loci where folate analogs (antifols) might act, the enzyme dihydrofolate reductase (DHFR) is the primary site of action of most analogs studied to date (*see* Figure 57–1). This enzyme has been purified from a number of species. Important structural differences among the various enzymes have enabled the design of important therapeutic agents for the treatment of bacterial and malarial infections (*see* discussion of trimethoprim, Chapter 49; pyrimethamine, Chapter 45). These inhibitors have much greater activity against the bacterial and protozoal DHFRs than they do against the mammalian enzyme. Such developments have introduced a new level of sophistication into the science of chemotherapy and suggest the possibility of developing new analogs of folate that have unique advantages for the chemotherapy of neoplastic diseases.

Because folic acid and many of its analogs are very polar, they cross the blood-brain barrier poorly and require specific transport mechanisms to enter mammalian cells. Once in the cell, additional glutamyl residues are added to the molecule by the enzyme folylpolyglutamate synthetase. Intracellular methotrexate polyglutamates have been identified in as many as five glutamyl residues. Since these polyglutamates cross cellular membranes poorly, if at all, this serves as a mechanism of entrapment and may account for the prolonged retention of methotrexate in tissues such as liver. Evidence indicates that polyglutamylated folates have substantially greater affinity than the monoglutamate form for enzymes such as thymidylate synthetase. Other findings indicate that distinct differences exist in the folate influx system in certain tumors in comparison with normal tissues (*e.g.*, bone marrow). Novel folate antagonists have been devised to attempt to exploit these differences. The analog 10-deaza,10-ethyl aminopterin is transported into many tumor cells much more

Methotrexate

efficiently than into normal tissues, is poly-glutamylated, and is an excellent inhibitor of DHFR. This promising new compound will be evaluated clinically in the near future (Sirotnak, 1983). In efforts to bypass the obligatory membrane transport system and facilitate penetration of the blood-brain barrier, a number of lipid-soluble folate antagonists have been synthesized; several of these are in the early stages of clinical trial (Johns and Bertino, 1982; Jackson 1984). (For recent reviews, *see* Chabner, 1982c; Goldman *et al.*, 1983; Hitchings, 1983; Jolivet and Chabner, 1983; McGuire *et al.*, 1983; Sirotnak, 1983; Cadman, 1984; Jackson, 1984.)

Mechanism of Action. To understand the mechanism of action of folate analogs such as methotrexate, it is necessary to appreciate the complexities of the metabolism of folate cofactors and their multiplicity of functions; this is discussed in Chapter 57. To function as a cofactor in one-carbon transfer reactions, folate must first be reduced by DHFR to tetrahydrofolate (FH_4). Single-carbon fragments are added enzymatically to FH_4 in various configurations and may then be transferred in specific synthetic reactions. A key metabolic event is catalyzed by thymidylate synthetase and involves the conversion of 2-deoxyuridylate (dUMP) to thymidylate, an essential component of DNA. The methyl group transferred to the uracil moiety of dUMP is donated by N^{5-10}-methylene FH_4. Significantly, this carbon atom is transferred to the pyrimidine ring at the oxidation level of formaldehyde and is reduced to methyl by the pteridine ring of the folate coenzyme; the result is the formation of dihydrofolate (FH_2). Thus, to function again as a cofactor, FH_2 must first be reduced to FH_4 by DHFR. Inhibitors with a high affinity for DHFR prevent the formation of FH_4 and cause major disruptions in cellular metabolism by producing an acute intracellular deficiency of folate coenzymes. The folate coenzymes become trapped as FH_2 polyglutamates, which cannot function metabolically. One-carbon transfer reactions crucial for the *de-novo* synthesis of purine nucleotides and of thymidylate cease, with the subsequent interruption of the synthesis of DNA and RNA (as well as other vital metabolic reactions).

Understanding of these events enables appreciation of the rationale for the use of thymidine and/or leucovorin (N^5-formyl FH_4; folinic acid) in the "rescue" of normal cells from toxicity caused by drugs such as methotrexate. Leucovorin is a fully reduced, metabolically functional folate coenzyme; it enters cells via the specific carrier-mediated transport system and is convertible to other folate cofactors. Thus, it may function directly, without the need for reduction by DHFR in reactions such as those required for purine biosynthesis. On the other hand, thymidine may be converted to thymidylate by thymidine kinase, thus bypassing the reaction catalyzed by thymidylate synthetase and providing the necessary precursor for DNA synthesis.

An important feature of the binding of active folate antagonists with DHFRs is the very low inhibition constants observed (on the order of 1 nM).

Covalent bonds are not involved in the enzyme-inhibitor interactions despite the high affinity of the antagonists for the protein. Substantial progress has been made in defining the chemical basis for the binding of methotrexate to DHFR (*see* Matthews *et al.*, 1978; Chabner, 1982c).

As with most inhibitors of cellular reproduction, a selective effect on neoplastic cells is obtainable to only a partial extent with methotrexate. Folate antagonists kill cells during the S phase of the cell cycle, and evidence indicates that methotrexate is much more effective when the cellular population is in the logarithmic phase of growth, rather than in the plateau phase. Because it is also capable of inhibiting RNA and protein synthesis, however, methotrexate slows the entry of cells into S phase and its cytotoxic action has been referred to as "self-limiting" (Skipper and Schabel, 1982).

Mechanism of Resistance to Antifolates. Although evidence is incomplete, three biochemical mechanisms of acquired resistance to methotrexate have been clearly demonstrated: (1) impaired transport of methotrexate into cells, (2) production of altered forms of DHFR that have decreased affinity for the inhibitor, and (3) increased concentrations of intracellular DHFR. It has been known for years that blood elements with marked increases in the activity of DHFR appear within days after treatment of patients with leukemia with single doses of methotrexate. This may reflect induction of new enzyme synthesis, temporary elimination from the marrow of cells that are susceptible to the drug because of low enzymatic activity, or protection of DHFR against catabolic degradation by intracellular proteases. It is well established that the enzyme, complexed with methotrexate, undergoes conformational changes that render it remarkably resistant to proteolysis.

Of special interest is the phenomenon of gene amplification and its relationship to acquired resistance to methotrexate and, perhaps, other cytotoxic agents. Methotrexate-resistant cell lines have been isolated that have several hundredfold more DHFR than do wild type cells because of comparable increases in the mRNA specific for the enzyme. This is due to the occurrence in these resistant cells of increased numbers of copies of the gene for DHFR. (For further discussion, *see* Schimke *et al.*, 1978; Bertino *et al.*, 1983; Stark and Wahl, 1984.)

Various therapeutic tactics have been recommended to avoid selection of resistant cells. The use of high doses of methotrexate with leucovorin "rescue" may permit the intracellular accumulation of methotrexate in concentrations that inactivate DHFR even when the enzyme is present at markedly elevated levels. Alternation of treatment with methotrexate with other active therapeutic agents that function by different mechanisms is another way to attempt to kill cells that are resistant.

General Toxicity and Cytotoxic Action.
The actions of 4-amino analogs of folate in animals have been studied extensively.

Animals given a minimal lethal dose survive for at least 48 hours and usually die within 3 to 5 days. Anorexia, progressive weight loss, bloody diarrhea, leukopenia, depression, and coma are the outstanding features of fatal intoxication. The major lesions occur in the *intestinal tract* and *bone marrow*. Swelling and cytoplasmic vacuolization of the mucosal cells of the intestinal epithelium are evident within 6 hours. These changes are followed by desquamation of epithelial cells, extrusion of plasma into the lumen of the bowel, and leukocytic infiltration of the submucosa. Terminally, the entire intestinal tract exhibits a severe hemorrhagic desquamating enteritis. Degeneration of bone marrow develops rapidly. Within 24 hours there is evident disturbance in the maturation of erythrocytes. Proliferation of erythroid precursors is inhibited, and significant proportions of primitive erythroid elements have the appearance of megaloblasts. Rapid pathological alteration in myelopoiesis also occurs, and within a few days the bone marrow becomes aplastic. There is diminution in content of lymphoid cells in lymphatic tissue, but there is no evidence of necrosis. The disturbance in hematopoiesis is reflected in the circulating blood by a marked granulocytopenia and reticulocytopenia and a moderate lymphopenia.

Folic acid antagonists seriously interfere with *embryogenesis*. The site of action is on the embryonic mesenchyme. Decidual and placental tissues are unaffected by doses of the drugs that cause fetal death. Young embryos are much more susceptible than are the more developed. The administration of methotrexate during pregnancy obviously is accompanied by great hazards to the fetus.

Absorption, Fate, and Excretion. Methotrexate is readily absorbed from the gastrointestinal tract at doses routinely employed in clinical practice (0.1 mg/kg), but larger doses are incompletely absorbed. The drug is also absorbed from parenteral sites of injection. Peak concentrations in the plasma of 1 to 10 μM are obtained after doses of 25 to 100 mg/sq m, and concentrations of 0.1 to 1 mM are achieved after high-dose infusions of 1.5 g/sq m or more (Chabner, 1982c). A direct relationship exists between dose and plasma concentrations. Following intravenous administration, the drug disappears from plasma in a triphasic fashion (Huffman *et al.*, 1973). The first phase, due to the distribution into body fluids, has a half-time of about 45 minutes. The second phase reflects renal clearance ($t_{1/2}$ of about 2 hours). The final phase has a half-time of approximately 7 hours and begins when the concentration in plasma approximates 0.1 μM. This terminal half-life, if unduly prolonged, may be responsible for major toxic effects of the drug on the marrow and gastrointestinal tract. Distribution of methotrexate into body spaces, such as the pleural or peritoneal cavities, may occur. If such spaces are expanded (*e.g.*, by ascites or pleural effusion), they may act as a site of storage and release of drug with resultant prolonged elevation of plasma concentrations and more severe toxicity.

Approximately 50% of the drug is bound to plasma proteins. Laboratory studies suggest that it may be displaced from plasma albumin by a number of drugs, including sulfonamides, salicylates, tetracycline, chloramphenicol, and phenytoin; caution should be used if these are given concomitantly. Of the drug absorbed, from 40 to 50% of a small dose (2.5 to 15 μg/kg) to about 90% of a larger dose (150 μg/kg) is excreted unchanged in the urine within 48 hours, mostly within the first 8 hours. A small amount of methotrexate is also excreted in the stool, probably through the biliary tract. Metabolism of methotrexate in man does not seem to occur to a significant degree. After high doses, however, metabolites do accumulate; these include a potentially nephrotoxic 7-hydroxylated compound (*see* Chabner, 1982c). The portion of each dose of methotrexate that normally is excreted rapidly gains access to the urine by a combination of glomerular filtration and active tubular secretion. Therefore, the concurrent use of drugs that also undergo tubular secretion, as well as impaired renal function, can influence markedly the response to this drug. Particular caution must be exercised in treating patients with renal insufficiency.

The portion of methotrexate that is retained in human tissues remains for long periods, for example, for weeks in the kidneys and for several months in the liver.

The drug is converted to polyglutamates in hepatocytes, and there is also evidence for enterohepatic recirculation (Chabner *et al.*, 1981).

It is important to emphasize that methotrexate is very poorly transported across the blood-brain barrier; hence, neoplastic cells that have entered the CNS probably are not affected by usual concentrations of drug in the plasma. When high doses of methotrexate are given, followed by leucovorin "rescue" (*see* below), substantial concentrations of methotrexate may be attained in the CNS. The pharmacokinetic properties of methotrexate have been discussed by Goldin (1978); *see also* Appendix II.

Preparations, Dosage, and Routes of Administration. *Methotrexate* (*amethopterin*; FOLEX, MEXATE) is provided in scored, 2.5-mg tablets and also as a dry powder (the sodium salt) in vials containing 20 to 250 mg for preparation of sterile injectable solutions.

Although the standard daily oral dosage of methotrexate ordinarily employed in patients with leukemia has been 2.5 to 5 mg for children and 2.5 to 10 mg for adults, newer therapeutic concepts have emerged involving revised dosage schedules and the use of multiple drugs sequentially and concurrently. Methotrexate induces remission slowly, probably because the cells in advanced leukemia are not in the logarithmic phase of growth. For induction of remission it has been superseded by the more rapid and effective therapy with vincristine plus prednisone, with or without daunorubicin. Methotrexate is of great value in the maintenance of remissions, particularly when administered intermittently at doses of 30 mg/sq m, intramuscularly, twice a week, or by intensive 2-day "pulses" of 175 to 525 mg/sq m at monthly intervals.

The intrathecal administration of methotrexate has been employed, particularly when manifestations of cerebral involvement in either leukemia or choriocarcinoma have appeared, as occurs not infrequently even during systemic remissions. This route of administration achieves high concentrations of methotrexate in the CSF and is effective also in patients whose systemic disease has become resistant to methotrexate, since the leukemic cells in the CNS beyond the blood-brain barrier have survived in a pharmacological sanctuary and retain their original degree of sensitivity to the drug. The recommended intrathecal dose is 0.2 to 0.5 mg/kg, given once or repeated at intervals of 2 to 5 days, depending on the severity of involvement and the response to therapy; another dosage schedule is 12 mg/sq m once weekly for 2 weeks and then monthly. Leucovorin may be administered intramuscularly to counteract the systemic toxicity of methotrexate.

In the treatment of choriocarcinoma with methotrexate, 15 mg/sq m (15 to 30 mg) is administered daily for 5 days orally or parenterally. Courses are repeated at 1- to 2-week intervals, toxicity permitting, and urinary gonadotropin titers are used as a guide for persistence of disease.

Methotrexate has been used in the treatment of severe, disabling *psoriasis* in doses of 2.5 mg orally for 5 days, followed by a rest period of at least 2 days, or 10 to 25 mg intravenously weekly. An initial parenteral test dose of 5 to 10 mg is recommended to detect any possible idiosyncrasy. Complete awareness of the pharmacology and toxic potential of methotrexate is a prerequisite for its use in this nonneoplastic disorder (Weinstein, 1977).

Continuous infusion of relatively large amounts of methotrexate may be employed (from 250 mg to 1 g/sq m, or more, weekly), but only when the technic of leucovorin "rescue" is used. The rationale for the administration of high doses is to achieve an excess of intracellular unbound drug, such that DNA synthesis is inhibited almost completely. Extremely high (0.1 to 1 mM) concentrations of drug must be achieved extracellularly in order to overcome any deficiency of the carrier-mediated transport system. After infusion of methotrexate for 6 hours, leucovorin is injected at a dose of 6 to 15 mg/sq m every 6 hours for 72 hours; the goal is to rescue normal cells and thereby prevent toxicity. The administration of methotrexate in high dosages may be extremely dangerous and should be performed only by experienced chemotherapists who are capable of quantification of the concentrations of methotrexate and leucovorin in plasma. With appropriate precautions, these investigational schedules are surprisingly free of toxicity. It is imperative to maintain the output of a large volume of alkaline urine, since methotrexate precipitates in the renal tubules in acidic urine. In the presence of malignant effusions, delayed clearance may cause severe toxicity. Although the use of methotrexate in high doses with leucovorin "rescue" has been studied clinically for several years with very encouraging results, the optimal timing, dose of leucovorin required, and proof of enhanced therapeutic efficacy remain to be established (*see* Goldin, 1978; Symposium, 1981b; Chabner, 1982c).

Therapeutic Uses and Clinical Toxicity. Methotrexate is a useful drug in the management of *acute lymphoblastic leukemia* in children. However, methotrexate is of very limited value in the types of leukemia seen in adults. It is of established value in *choriocarcinoma* and related trophoblastic tumors of women, with complete and lasting remissions occurring in approximately 75% of women treated sequentially with methotrexate and dactinomycin, and in over 90% when early diagnosis is accompanied by a low concentration of gonadotropin in the urine. A number of these patients are living without evidence of disease more than 25 years after initiation of therapy. In addition, many women with nonmetastatic trophoblastic disease, hydatidiform mole, and chorioadenoma destruens have been treated successfully with methotrexate. Beneficial results have also been reported in patients with mycosis fungoides, Burkitt's and other non-Hodgkin's lymphomas, and carcinomas of the breast, tongue, pharynx, bladder, and testes (in conjunction with chlorambucil and dactinomycin), as well as in occasional patients with other tumors. High-dose methotrexate, with subsequent leucovorin "rescue," can cause substantial tumor regression in at least two tumors highly refractory to most chemotherapeutic agents: carcinoma of the lung and osteogenic sarcoma. (For references, *see* Symposium, 1981b; Chabner, 1982c; Calabresi *et al.*, 1985.) Striking improvement has been observed with the use of methotrexate in the treatment of severe psoriasis. Furthermore, methotrexate is an effective immunosuppressive agent and has been used for prevention of graft-versus-host reactions that result from marrow transplantation, as well as in the management of dermatomyositis, rheumatoid arthritis, Wegener's granulomatosis, and pityriasis rubra pilaris (*see* Weinstein, 1977; Goldin, 1978).

Treatment with methotrexate requires constant surveillance of the patient in order to judge dosage properly and to avoid serious toxic reactions. In persons treated with conventional doses or with concomitant leucovorin, it is frequently possible to avoid severe leukopenia or aplasia of the bone marrow. Thrombocytopenia with bleeding can be treated with platelet transfusions, but it may be difficult to control, particularly in the presence of infection. It is imperative that a skilled medical team and sophisticated facilities, particularly abundant platelet transfusions and measures for preventing and combating infections, be available in order to provide the intensive supportive therapy necessary to control the severe toxic manifestations that may result when intensive dosage schedules are used.

Other untoward reactions also may complicate the use of methotrexate (Wiemann and Calabresi, 1985). Ulcerative stomatitis and diarrhea are frequent side effects and require interruption of the therapeutic regimen; hemorrhagic enteritis and death from intestinal perforation may occur. Additional toxic manifestations include alopecia, dermatitis, interstitial pneumonitis, neurotoxicity, nephrotoxicity, defective oogenesis or spermatogenesis, abortion, teratogenesis, and hepatic dysfunction, usually reversible but sometimes leading to cirrhosis. The long-term complications associated with the use of methotrexate for immunosuppressive therapy are discussed by Schein and Winokur (1975).

PYRIMIDINE ANALOGS

This class of agents encompasses a diverse and interesting group of drugs that have in common the capacity to impede the biosynthesis of pyrimidine nucleotides or to mimic these natural metabolites to such an extent that they interfere with vital cellular activities, such as the synthesis and functioning of nucleic acids. Certain of the drugs in this group are employed in the treatment of a variety of afflictions, including neoplastic diseases, psoriasis, and infections caused by fungi and DNA-containing viruses. When selected members of the group are used together or concurrently with other antimetabolites, synergistic effects have been demonstrated against various experimental tumors, and some of these treatment schedules are being investigated clinically. (*See* reviews by Maley, 1977; Chabner, 1982e.)

General Mechanism of Action. The antineoplastic agents fluorouracil (5-FU) and cytarabine (AraC), the antiviral compound idoxuridine, and the antifungal agent flucytosine (Chapter 54) are the drugs in this group that are established clinically. Other compounds are under clinical investigation, as are potentially synergistic combinations of pyrimidine analogs and other types of inhibitors.

Among the best-characterized agents in this class are the halogenated pyrimidines, a group that includes such compounds as fluorouracil and idoxuridine. If one compares the van der Waals radii of the various substituents (Table 55–3), the dimension of the fluorine atom resembles that of hydrogen, whereas the bromine and iodine atoms are close in size to the methyl group. Idoxuridine has relatively little effect on the biosynthesis of thymidylic acid; like thymidine, however, it is converted enzymatically within cells to phosphorylated derivatives; it is also degraded to the corresponding base, iodouracil, which is converted to uracil and iodide. The phosphorylated forms of idoxuridine inhibit competitively the utilization of the analogous derivatives of thymidine and can lead, in appropriate circumstances, to incorporation of the analog, as iododeoxyuridylic acid, into DNA in place of thymidylic acid. These activities can suppress temporarily the growth of both experimental and human neoplasms; in addition, incorporation of the iodo- or bromo- analogs into DNA renders the latter more susceptible to the injurious effects of radiation.

If the hydrogen on position 5 of the pyrimidine ring is replaced with fluorine, the chemical reactivity of the ring is significantly altered, although the molecule, fluorouracil, behaves as does uracil with several enzymes. Fluorine has an inductive (electron-withdrawing) effect, which is reflected in a much lower pK_a with fluorouracil-containing compounds than with the natural compounds. The ionization that occurs is as follows:

Table 55–3.   STRUCTURAL FORMULAS OF PYRIMIDINE ANALOGS

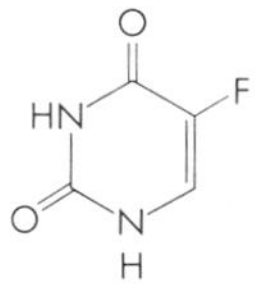

Fluorouracil
(pK$_a$ 8.1)

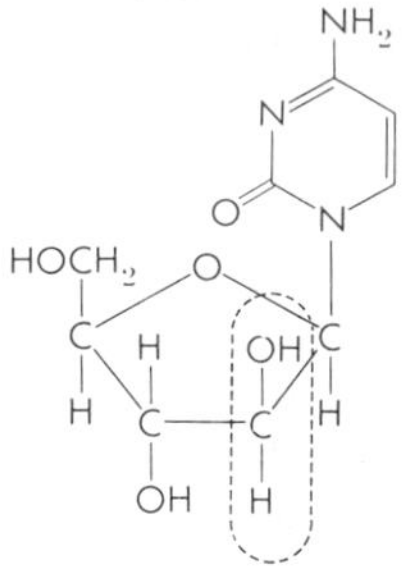

Cytarabine
(Cytosine Arabinoside)
(pK$_a$ 4.5)

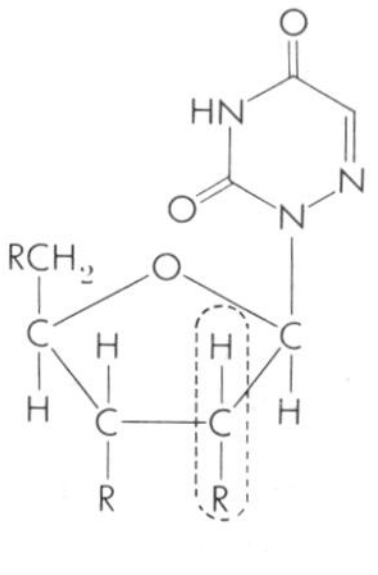

Azauridine: R = —OH

Azaribine: R = —O—C—CH$_3$
(pK$_a$ 6.7)

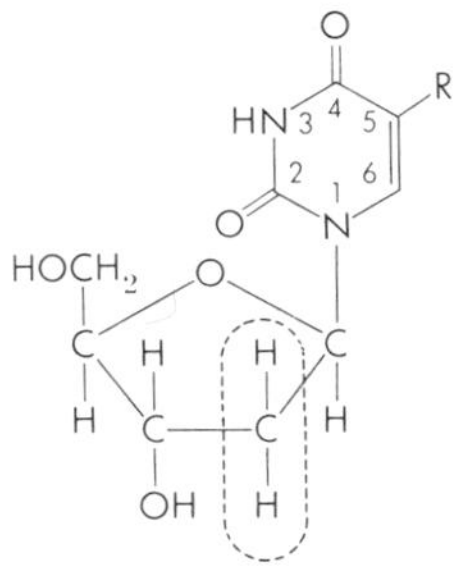

R	van der Waals Radii (Å)	Compound	pK$_a$
H	1.20	Deoxyuridine	9.3
F	1.35	Floxuridine (fluorodeoxyuridine)	7.6
Cl	1.80	Chlorodeoxyuridine	7.9
Br	1.95	Bromodeoxyuridine	7.9
CH$_3$	2.00	Thymidine	9.8
I	2.15	Idoxuridine (iododeoxyuridine)	8.25
CF$_3$	2.44	Trifluoromethyldeoxyuridine	7.35

In addition, the carbon-fluorine bond is stronger than the carbon-hydrogen bond and is less susceptible to enzymatic cleavage. Thus, substitution of a halogen atom of the correct dimensions can produce a molecule that sufficiently resembles a natural pyrimidine to interact with enzymes of pyrimidine metabolism and also to interfere drastically with certain other aspects of pyrimidine action.

Among the various modifications of the sugar moiety attempted, the replacement of the ribose of cytidine with arabinose has yielded a useful chemotherapeutic agent, cytarabine. As may be seen in Table 55–3, the deviation from normal in this case involves the 2′ carbon of the pentose, in which the hydroxyl group is in the opposite configuration from that of the natural ribonucleoside, cytidine. This yields a molecule that sufficiently resembles a deoxynucleoside to be capable of conversion to the nucleotide level, but which blocks the synthesis of DNA (*see* reviews by Chabner, 1982e; Heidelberger, 1982; Kufe and Major, 1982; Pallavicini, 1984).

Several agents are available that inhibit different steps in the synthesis of pyrimidines and that exert synergistic cytotoxicity when used concurrently with a pyrimidine analog such as cytosine arabinoside or 5-fluorouracil. N-phosphonoacetyl-L-aspartate (PALA) is a "transition-state" inhibitor of the enzyme aspartate transcarbamylase, which catalyzes an early step in pyrimidine biosynthesis (Stark and Bartlett, 1983). Two other agents are potent inhibitors of a later step in pyrimidine nucle-

otide synthesis, the coupled enzymatic reactions by which orotate is converted first to the 5′-monophosphate nucleotide (orotidylate) and then decarboxylated to form uridylate. The compounds 6-azauridine and pyrazofuran, after being converted to the corresponding 5′-monophosphate nucleotides, are potent inhibitors of orotidylate decarboxylase. Two other agents, 3-deazauridine and the glutamine antagonist acivicin, block the conversion of uridine triphosphate (UTP) to cytidine triphosphate (CTP). Use of these various agents in combination with cytosine arabinoside has resulted in increased formation of intracellular AraCTP and synergistic cytotoxicity. Recognition that the sugar phosphate, 5-phosphoribosyl-1-pyrophosphate (PRPP), is an essential metabolite for the biosynthesis of both purines and pyrimidines has suggested other synergistic drug combinations. When *de-novo* purine biosynthesis is inhibited by an agent such as methotrexate, the steady-state intracellular concentrations of PRPP rise. This enhances considerably the rate of the lethal synthesis of 5-fluorouridylate from 5-fluorouracil, a reaction that utilizes PRPP. This has led to the clinical trial of timed administrations of methotrexate followed by 5-fluorouracil (Cadman, 1984).

FLUOROURACIL AND FLOXURIDINE (FLUORODEOXYURIDINE)

The chemistry of these analogs is discussed above.

Mechanism of Action. Fluorouracil, as such, is without significant inhibitory activity in mammalian systems, and, in order to inhibit cellular growth, it must first be converted enzymatically to the nucleotide level. Several routes are available for the formation of the 5'-monophosphate nucleotide (F-UMP) in animal cells. Fluorouracil may be converted to fluorouridine by uridine phosphorylase and then to F-UMP by uridine kinase or it may react directly with PRPP, catalyzed by the enzyme orotate phosphoribosyl transferase, to form F-UMP. The latter enzyme is present in higher concentrations in certain tumors than in liver and reacts with orotate as its natural substrate. Many metabolic pathways are available to F-UMP, including incorporation into RNA. A reaction sequence crucial for antineoplastic activity involves reduction of the diphosphate nucleotide by the enzyme ribonucleotide diphosphate reductase to the deoxynucleotide level and the eventual formation of 5-fluoro-2'-deoxyuridine-5'-phosphate (F-dUMP). This complex metabolic pathway for the generation of the actual growth inhibitor, F-dUMP, may be bypassed through use of the deoxyribonucleoside of fluorouracil—floxuridine (fluorodeoxyuridine, FUdR)—which is a substrate for intracellular thymidine kinase. Thus, in a single enzymatic step, the inhibitor of thymidylate synthetase, F-dUMP, can be produced in cells by the use of FUdR. Unfortunately, FUdR is a good substrate for both thymidine and uridine phosphorylases, and it is rapidly degraded to fluorouracil.

There have been notable advances in our understanding of the interaction between F-dUMP and the enzyme thymidylate synthetase, which is an important site of the cytotoxic action of the drug. The folate cofactor, N^{5-10}-methylenetetrahydrofolate, and F-dUMP form a covalently bound ternary complex with the enzyme, which resembles the transition state formed during the normal enzymatic reaction when dUMP is converted to thymidylate. The stable complex inactivates the enzyme. (For details of this mechanism and the nature of the postulated inhibitory ternary complex, see Danenberg and Lockshin, 1981.)

Fluorouracil is incorporated into both RNA and DNA. Incorporation into RNA has been associated with toxicity and has major effects on both the processing and functions of RNA. While the incorporation of FUdR into DNA has been described, its significance is unclear.

Although it has been shown that fluorouracil is much more lethal to logarithmically growing cells than to stationary cells, there is no clearly demonstrated effect at a definite stage of the cell cycle. The phenomenon of "thymineless death" has been invoked to explain the cytotoxic effects of fluorouracil and its derivatives. The blockade of the thymidylate synthetase reaction inhibits DNA synthesis, while cellular production of both RNA and protein continues. An imbalance in growth occurs that is not compatible with cell survival. In accord with this proposal, the administration of thymidine can often reverse the toxicity, presumably through bypass of the block at thymidylate synthetase.

A number of biochemical mechanisms have been identified that are associated with resistance to the cytotoxic effects of fluorouracil or floxuridine. These mechanisms include loss or decreased activity of the enzymes necessary for activation of fluorouracil, decreased pyrimidine monophosphate kinase (which decreases incorporation into RNA), and acquisition of an altered thymidylate synthetase that is not inhibited by F-dUMP. Unfortunately it is not established which (if any) of these mechanisms is associated with inherent or acquired resistance to fluorouracil and its derivatives that is encountered clinically. (For reviews, see Danenberg and Lockshin, 1981; Chabner, 1982e; Heidelberger, 1982; Heidelberger et al., 1983; Valeriote and Santelli, 1984.)

General Toxicity and Cytotoxic Action. The major sites of action of fluorouracil and floxuridine on normal tissues are the bone marrow and the epithelium of the gastrointestinal and oral mucosa. These are described in detail under Therapeutic Uses and Clinical Toxicity (see below).

Absorption, Fate, and Excretion. Fluorouracil and floxuridine are usually administered parenterally, since absorption after ingestion of the drugs is unpredictable and incomplete. Metabolic degradation occurs, particularly in the liver. Floxuridine is converted by thymidine or deoxyuridine phosphorylases into fluorouracil, and the latter is catabolized in much the same way as is uracil. Thus, 5-fluoro-5,6-dihydrouracil is formed, the ring of which is opened to give α-fluoro-β-ureidopropionic acid, which may be degraded further to α-fluoro-β-alanine (Heidelberger, 1975). In man, an important product of the metabolism of fluorouracil is urea.

Rapid intravenous administration of fluorouracil produces plasma concentrations of 0.1 to 1.0 mM; plasma clearance is rapid ($t_{1/2}$ = 10 to 20 minutes). Urinary excretion of intravenously injected fluorouracil-2-^{14}C, given as a single dose, amounts to only 11% in 24 hours; however, during this period, 63% of the radioactivity is expired as carbon dioxide. Given by continuous intravenous infusion for 24 hours, plasma concentrations in the range of 0.5 to 3.0 μM are obtained and the urinary excretion of fluorouracil is only 4%, while the $^{14}CO_2$ excretion rises to 90%. These findings probably account for the lower cytotoxicity of fluorouracil administered by infusion, compared to that seen with single doses. Fluorouracil readily enters the CSF, and concentrations of about 7 μM are reached within 30 minutes after intravenous administration; values are sustained for approximately 3 hours and subside slowly during a period of 9 hours (Fraile *et al .*, 1980; Chabner, 1982e).

Preparations, Dosage, and Routes of Administration. *Fluorouracil (5-FU;* ADRUCIL) is available in sterile ampuls containing 500 mg in 10 ml for intravenous administration. The recommended dose for average-risk patients in good nutritional status with adequate hematopoietic, renal, and hepatic function is 12 mg/kg daily for 4 days, by rapid injection, followed by 6 mg/kg on alternate succeeding days for two to four doses if no toxicity is observed. The maximal daily dose has been established arbitrarily at 800 mg. Treatment should be discontinued at the earliest manifestation of toxicity (usually stomatitis or diarrhea) because the maximal effects of bone-marrow suppression will not be evident until the ninth to fourteenth day. The first course of therapy should be administered either in the hospital or under extremely close supervision in order to establish the tolerance of the individual patient. After a period of 4 weeks from the first injection of the preceding course, a new course of therapy is initiated; the dosage is adjusted on the basis of the previous response and is repeated at monthly intervals. Another type of maintenance schedule is 10 to 15 mg/kg or 500 to 600 mg/sq m, administered weekly as a single rapid injection. It is usually necessary to produce mild-to-moderate toxicity in order to achieve significant antineoplastic effects.

In the selection of patients, the roles of nutritional deficiencies and protein depletion have been stressed, particularly in relation to surgery. Reduced tolerance of the hematopoietic system may be present in elderly patients or as a result of invasion of the bone marrow by either neoplastic cells or myelofibrosis. Patients with compromised bone-marrow function as a result of previous therapy either with alkylating agents or x-ray to the pelvis or vertebrae are particularly sensitive to the myelosuppressive action of these compounds. In patients with extensive liver metastases, catabolism of the drug may be markedly impaired and therapy may be contraindicated; if treatment is instituted, reduced doses must be administered to prevent the hazards of overdosage.

Fluorouracil has been administered by infusion into the hepatic artery with favorable results in patients with metastases to the liver (Ensminger *et al.*, 1978).

Topical fluorouracil as a 1 or 5% cream or a 1 to 5% solution in propylene glycol (EFUDEX, FLUOROPLEX) has been used successfully in dermatology.

Floxuridine (fluorodeoxyuridine; FUDR) is available for injection as a powder, 500 mg in 5-ml containers. It may be administered in schedules identical with those of fluorouracil, except that the individual doses, in milligrams, are twice those

used with the latter agent. Continuous infusion of floxuridine has produced objective responses with $\frac{1}{30}$ to $\frac{1}{60}$ the dose necessary with multiple individual doses, but with similar toxicity. Continuous infusion of fluorinated pyrimidines into the arterial blood supply of localized tumors, particularly in the liver or in the head and neck region, may provide beneficial clinical effects. Intra-arterial infusions, at doses of 0.1 to 0.6 mg/kg per 24 hours, are administered continuously until local toxicity is encountered (Fraile *et al.*, 1980).

Therapeutic Uses and Clinical Toxicity. Clinical use of fluorinated pyrimidines has been concerned primarily with *fluorouracil,* and accumulated experience indicates that the drug can be of palliative value in certain types of carcinoma, particularly of the breast and the gastrointestinal tract; beneficial effects have also been reported in hepatoma, as well as in carcinoma of the ovary, cervix, urinary bladder, prostate, pancreas, and oropharyngeal areas. There is little evidence, however to encourage the expectation that significant overall prolongation of life can be achieved in the majority of patients (Calabresi *et al.*, 1985). Fluorouracil is widely used with very favorable results for the topical treatment of premalignant keratoses of the skin and multiple superficial basal-cell carcinomas. It is also effective in severe recalcitrant psoriasis (Alper *et al.*, 1985).

The clinical manifestations of toxicity caused by fluorouracil and floxuridine are similar and may be difficult to anticipate because of their delayed appearance. The earliest untoward symptoms during a course of therapy are anorexia and nausea; these are followed shortly after by stomatitis and diarrhea, which constitute reliable warning signs that a sufficient dose has been administered. Stomatitis is manifested by formation of a white patchy membrane that ulcerates and becomes necrotic. The occurrence of similar lesions in the stoma of colostomies and at post-mortem examination of the gastrointestinal tract, as well as complaints of dysphagia, retrosternal burning, and proctitis, indicates that enteric injury may occur at any level. The major toxic effects, however, result from the myelosuppressive action of these drugs; clinically, the effects are most frequently manifested as leukopenia, the nadir of which is usually between the ninth and fourteenth day after the first injection of drug. Thrombocytopenia and anemia may complicate the picture. Loss of hair, occasionally progressing to total alopecia, nail changes, dermatitis, and increased pigmentation and atrophy of the skin may be encountered. Neurological manifestations, including an acute cerebellar syndrome, have been reported, and myelopathy has been observed after the intrathecal administration of fluorouracil. Cardiac toxicity may also occur. The low therapeutic indices of these agents emphasize the need for very skillful supervision by physicians familiar with the action of the fluorinated pyrimidines and the possible hazards of chemotherapy.

CYTARABINE (CYTOSINE ARABINOSIDE)

Among the more important antimetabolites is cytarabine (1-β-D-arabinofuranosylcytosine; AraC). Its effectiveness in the treatment of acute leukemia is well established. (For reviews, *see* Chabner, 1982b; Kufe and Major, 1982; Pallavicini, 1984.)

Mechanism of Action. This compound is an analog of 2'-deoxycytidine with the 2'-hydroxyl in a position *trans* to the 3'-hydroxyl of the sugar, as shown in Table 55–3. The 2'-hydroxyl causes steric hindrance to the rotation of the pyrimidine base around the nucleosidic bond. The bases of polyarabinonucleotides cannot stack normally as do the bases of polydcoxynucleotides.

As with most purine and pyrimidine antimetabolites, cytarabine must be "activated" by conversion to the 5'-monophosphate nucleotide, in this case catalyzed by deoxycytidine kinase. The nucleotide analog, AraCMP, can react with appropriate nucleotide kinases to form the diphosphate and triphosphate nucleotides (AraCDP and AraCTP). Accumulation of AraCTP causes potent inhibition of DNA synthesis in many cells. Previously, this was thought to result from competitive inhibition of DNA polymerase by AraCTP. However, studies now indicate that inhibition of DNA synthesis by mammalian cells occurs at AraCTP concentrations $\frac{1}{100}$ or less than those required for inhibition of DNA polymerase, and the incorporation of AraC molecules into alkali-labile internucleotide linkages in DNA has been implicated. There is a significant relationship between inhibition of DNA synthesis and the total amount of AraC incorporated into DNA (Kufe and Major, 1982). Thus, the incorporation of about five molecules of AraC per 10^4 bases in DNA decreases cellular clonogenicity by about 50%. There is also evidence that AraC acts by slowing both chain elongation and the movement of newly replicated DNA through the matrix-bound replication apparatus. In addition, AraC inhibits β-DNA polymerase, an enzyme involved in DNA repair. Of interest, AraCTP can inhibit virally induced reverse transcriptase at low concentrations.

AraC shows relatively high cell-cycle specificity and is most cytotoxic to cells in the S phase; it is thus most active against cells that are actively proliferating. Other important cytokinetic effects have been observed. For example, quiescent tumor cells can be recruited into the cell cycle by AraC. Cells exposed to high concentrations of AraC may be arrested at the G_1-S boundary, but, when released from this block, they traverse the cell cycle at an accelerated rate. This increased rate of transit results from shortening of all phases of the cell cycle.

Another unexplained effect is the induction of terminal differentiation of certain leukemic cell lines exposed to low concentrations of AraC.

Despite a wealth of observation, the precise mechanism of cellular death caused by AraC is not understood. Potentially important is the phenomenon of "unbalanced growth," which results from prolonged suppression of macromolecular syntheses. Thus, inhibition of DNA synthesis by AraC without concomitant inhibition of protein and RNA syntheses can result in marked increases in cellular volume and in cellular death. It is likely that continued inhibition of DNA synthesis for at least one cell cycle is necessary. This mechanism may thus be important when AraC is administered by continuous prolonged infusion. A number of investigations have indicated that the optimal interval between doses of AraC is about 8 to 12 hours. This interval appears to coincide with the time when a large fraction of the cell population is in S phase (Chabner, 1982b; Kufe and Major, 1982; Pallavicini, 1984).

Mechanisms of Resistance to Cytarabine. Both natural and acquired resistance to AraC are seen. A crucial factor is the relative activities of anabolic and catabolic enzymes that influence the conversion of AraC to AraCTP. The rate-limiting enzyme is deoxycytidine kinase, which produces AraCMP. An important degradative enzyme is deoxycytidine deaminase, which deaminates AraC to the relatively nontoxic metabolite, arauridine. This enzyme is found in high activity in many tissues, including some human tumors. A second degradative enzyme, dCMP deaminase, converts AraCMP to the inactive metabolite, AraUMP. Thus, the balance between the anabolic and catabolic enzymes determines the concentrations of AraCTP achieved. Clear relationships have been shown between the synthesis and retention of high concentrations of AraCTP and the duration of complete remission in patients with acute myeloblastic leukemia (Rustum and Priesler, 1979).

Several biochemical mechanisms have been identified in AraC-resistant subpopulations in various murine and human tumor cell lines. Most commonly encountered are alterations in deoxycytidine kinase. Cells may be wholly or partially deficient in this enzyme or may have an enzyme with altered nucleoside binding affinity. Another mechanism of resistance is marked expansion of the dCTP pool due to increased CTP synthetase activity, with or without a deficiency of dCMP deaminase. The increased concentrations of intracellular dCTP presumably can block the actions of AraCTP on DNA synthesis. Other mechanisms include impaired transport of AraC into cells, increased deoxycytidine deaminase activity, and reduced affinity of DNA polymerase for AraCTP.

Tetrahydrouridine, a relatively potent inhibitor of cytidine deaminase, can enhance net synthesis of AraCTP and increase the cytotoxicity of AraC in several cell lines that have high activities of cytidine deaminase. Unfortunately, when the combination of tetrahydrouridine and AraC was subjected to clinical evaluation, marked increases in myelotoxicity were observed, suggesting that the therapeutic index would not be improved. (*See* Chabner, 1982b; Kufe and Major, 1982; Pallavicini, 1984.)

Absorption, Fate, and Excretion. Cytarabine is poorly and unpredictably absorbed after oral administration, with only about 20% of the drug reaching the circulation. Peak concentrations of 2 to 50 μM are measurable in plasma after injection of 30 to 300 mg/sq m intravenously. After intravenous administration the half-time for elimination of cytarabine is about 2.5 hours. Only about 10% of the injected dose is excreted unchanged in the urine within 12 to 24 hours, while 86 to 96% of the radioactivity appears as the inactive, deaminated product, arabinosyl uracil. Higher concentrations of cytarabine are found in CSF after continuous infusion than after rapid intravenous injection. After intrathecal administration of the drug at a dose of 50 mg/sq m, relatively little deamination occurs, even after 7 hours, and peak concentrations of 1 to 2 μM are achieved. The half-life of cytarabine may range from 2 to 11 hours after intrathecal injection (Ho, 1977; Chabner, 1982b; Wiemann and Calabresi, 1985).

Preparation, Routes of Administration, and Dosage. *Cytarabine* (CYTOSAR-U) is marketed as a powder for injection for the treatment of acute leukemias in children and adults. Two dosage schedules are recommended: (1) rapid intravenous injection of 100 to 200 mg/sq m daily for 5 to 7 days; or (2) continuous intravenous infusion of 100 mg/sq m daily for 5 to 7 days. In general, children seem to tolerate higher doses than do adults. *Maintenance* therapy with subcutaneous injections of 1 mg/kg, weekly or every other week, can be used, although the drug appears more effective for the *induction* of remissions in acute leukemia. Intrathecal doses of 30 mg/sq m every 4 days have been used to treat meningeal leukemia.

Therapeutic Uses and Clinical Toxicity. Cytarabine is indicated for induction of remission in acute leukemia in children and adults. When used alone, remission rates of 20 to 40% have been reported. The drug is particularly useful in acute granulocytic leukemia in adults, since chemotherapy is generally disappointing in this disorder. Cytarabine is more effective when used with other agents, particularly thioguanine and daunorubicin; complete remission rates of greater than 50% have been reported. The drug has been studied in patients with a variety of neoplastic diseases. Beneficial effects have been observed in Hodgkin's disease and related lymphomas but very rarely in patients with carcinomas or other tumors. Cytarabine is primarily a potent myelosuppressive agent capable of producing severe leukopenia, thrombocytopenia, and anemia with striking megaloblastic changes. Other toxic manifestations reported include gastrointestinal disturbances and, less frequently, stomatitis, conjunctivitis, hepatic dysfunction, thrombophlebitis at the site of injection, fever, and dermatitis. Seizures and other manifestations of neurotoxicity may occur after intrathecal administration.

AZARIBINE

Azaribine is the triacetyl derivative and prodrug form of azauridine; it was synthesized in order to achieve better absorption following oral administration and to prevent metabolism of azauridine to azauracil by intestinal microorganisms, a factor which contributes to CNS toxicity from azauridine. Azaribine has marked therapeutic activity in psoriasis, mycosis fungoides, and polycythemia vera (McDonald and Calabresi, 1971; Skoda, 1975). Unfortunately, when the drug became available for clinical usage, some patients with psoriasis developed thromboembolic disorders; since evidence indicates an increased incidence of the complication in psoriasis, it is questionable whether this problem should be attributed to the drug or to the disease (McDonald and Calabresi, 1978; Shubin, 1979).

PURINE ANALOGS

Since the pioneering studies of Hitchings and associates, begun in 1942, many analogs of natural purine bases, nucleosides, and nucleotides have been examined in a wide variety of biological and biochemical systems. These extensive investigations have led to the development of several drugs, not only of use in the treatment of malignant diseases (mercaptopurine, thioguanine) but also for immunosuppressive (azathioprine) and antiviral (acyclovir, vidarabine) therapy. The hypoxanthine analog allopurinol, a potent inhibitor of xanthine oxidase, is an important by-product of this effort (*see* Chapter 29). A development of promise has been the discovery of powerful inhibitors of adenosine deaminase, for example, erythrohydroxynonyladenine (EHNA) and pentostatin (2'-deoxycoformycin). In experimental systems these inhibitors of adenosine deaminase have produced marked synergistic effects in combination with various analogs of adenosine, such as vidarabine (arabinosyladenine; AraA); they also show promise as immunosuppressive agents. (*See* reviews by Elion and Hitchings, 1965; Loo and Nelson, 1982; McCormack and Johns, 1982.)

Structure-Activity Relationship. Mercaptopurine and thioguanine, both established clinical agents for the therapy of human leukemias, are analogs of the natural purines hypoxanthine and guanine, in which the keto group on carbon 6 of the purine ring is replaced by a sulfur atom. Substitution in this position by chlorine or selenium also yields antineoplastic compounds. Cytotoxicity is also observed with the β-D-ribonucleoside and β-D-2'-deoxyribonucleoside derivatives. Because these nucleoside analogs are excellent substrates for purine nucleoside phosphorylase, a highly active enzyme in many tissues, the analog nucleosides often serve as prodrugs and liberate the respective hypoxanthine or guanine analogs in tissues. With several important exceptions, analogs of purine bases or nucleosides must undergo enzymatic conversion to the nucleotide level in order to display cytotoxic activity.

Many attempts have been made to modify the structures of such analogs in order to improve their therapeutic indices or tissue selectivity. Azathioprine (Table 55–4) was developed to decrease the rate of inactivation of 6-mercaptopurine by enzymatic S-methylation, nonenzymatic oxidation, or conversion to thiourate by xanthine oxidase. Azathioprine can react with sulfhydryl compounds such as glutathione (apparently nonenzymatically) and thus serves as a prodrug, permitting the slow liberation of mercaptopurine in tissues. Superior immunosuppressive activity is achieved in comparison with mercaptopurine (Elion, 1967).

An important development has been the discovery of potent inhibitors of adenosine deaminase such as pentostatin (2'-deoxycoformycin; K_i = 2.5 pM) and erythro-9-(2-hydroxy-3-nonyl)-adenine (EHNA; K_i = 2 nM). Pentostatin (Table 55–4) may be viewed as an analog of the natural nucleoside 2'-deoxyinosine, in which the six-membered pyrimidine ring is replaced by a seven-membered diazapin ring. This disrupts the natural aromatic and planar purine ring. The keto-enol tautomer of 2'-deoxyinosine is replaced by a secondary alcohol. These structural changes increase the binding of pentostatin to adenosine deaminase by about 10 million-fold compared to that of adenosine. The enzyme-inhibitor complex dissociates with a $t_{1/2}$ of about 25 to 30 hours (Agarwal *et al.*, 1977; Agarwal, 1982). Thus, pentostatin blocks not only the deamination of natural nucleosides but also that of many analogs used in chemotherapy. Genetic deficiency of adenosine deaminase is associated with malfunction of both T and B lymphocytes, with little effect on other normal tissues (Giblett

Table 55–4. STRUCTURAL FORMULAS OF ADENOSINE AND VARIOUS PURINE ANALOGS

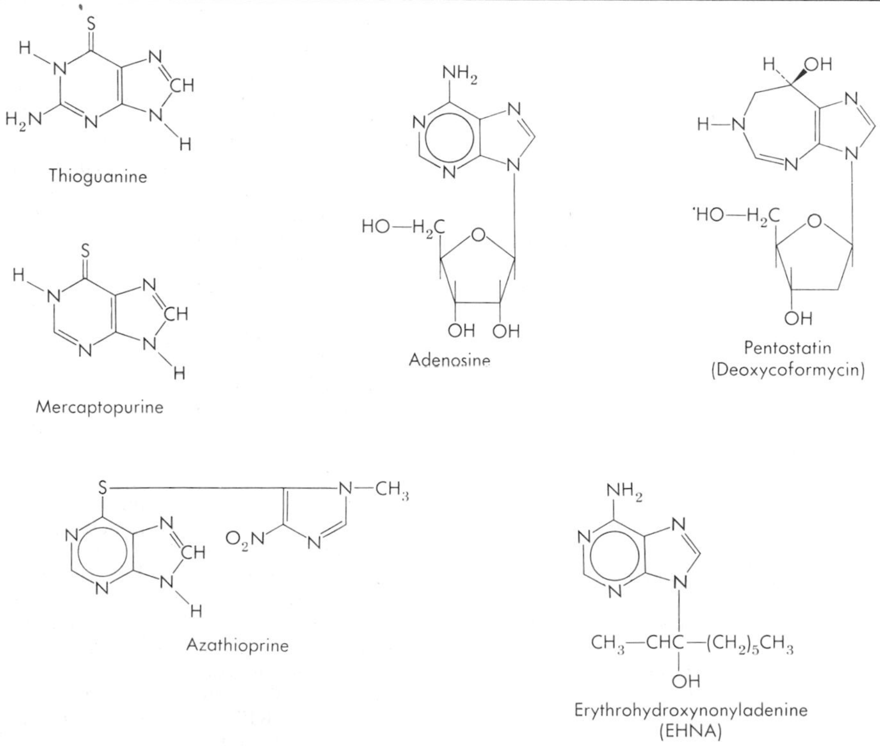

Thioguanine

Mercaptopurine

Adenosine

Pentostatin
(Deoxycoformycin)

Azathioprine

Erythrohydroxynonyladenine
(EHNA)

et al., 1972). Thus, animals treated with pentostatin display marked immunosuppression. Synergistic antineoplastic effects are seen when adenosine analogs, such as vidarabine, are administered concurrently with pentostatin. These synergistic effects are striking in rodent tumor systems, and the concurrent administration of pentostatin and analogs of adenosine is under limited clinical trial in patients with advanced cancer. Treatment with pentostatin alone has induced remissions in T-lymphocyte–related diseases, such as T-cell leukemia and mycosis fungoides. Also reported are antineoplastic effects by low doses of pentostatin in B-lymphocyte–related diseases, such as nodular lymphomas, chronic lymphocytic leukemia, and "hairy-cell" leukemia. Unfortunately, a number of unexplained deaths have occurred in phase-I clinical trials of pentostatin, and further extensive study has thus been restricted. (*See* Symposium, 1984; Tritsch, 1985.)

The glutamine antagonists azaserine (O-diazo-acetyl-L-serine), 6-diazo-5-oxo-L-norleucine (DON), and duazomycin, although not purine analogs, are potent inhibitors of the *de-novo* pathway of purine nucleotide biosynthesis. These glutamine analogs are diazoketones with chemical reactivities resembling those of diazomethane. Recently introduced has been the glutamine analog acivicin, which inhibits important enzymes in the pathways for interconversions of both purine and pyrimidine nucleotides, namely CTP synthetase and guanylate synthetase. Also under preclinical study is tiazofurin, an inhibitor of IMP dehydrogenase and thus of the *de-novo* synthesis of GMP. Although these compounds have only weak cytostatic activity when used alone, they can produce significant potentiation when administered with purine or pyrimidine analogs such as mercaptopurine, thioguanine, or AraC.

Mechanism of Action. Although animal tissues have nucleoside kinases that are capable of converting adenosine or the 2'-deoxyribonucleosides of guanine, hypoxanthine, adenine, and many of their analogs to the corresponding 5'-monophosphates, similar reactions do not occur with inosine, guanosine, or their analogs. The latter compounds must first undergo phosphorolysis by purine nucleoside phosphorylase, which is present in high activity in many human tissues. The liberated bases may then be converted to the corresponding nucleotide by hypoxanthine-guanine phosphoribosyltransferase (HGPRT). Similarly, 2'-deoxyguanosine, 2'-deoxyinosine, and many related analogs may react with purine nucleoside phosphorylase, and the product of this reaction, a purine base or analog, is then converted to the corresponding ribonucleoside 5'-monophosphate.

Although a number of biochemical effects of pentostatin have been observed, it is not yet clear why the loss of adenosine deaminase activity (due to a genetic disorder or the presence of an inhibitor) should cause selective lymphotoxicity. Current hypotheses have focused on the consequences of the intracellular accumulation of 2'-deoxyadenosine and of both the extracellular and intracellular

accumulation of adenosine in various subpopulations of lymphocytes (*see* Symposium, 1983c). For example, in the presence of pentostatin, 2'-deoxyadenosine is a potent inhibitor of the mitogen-induced proliferation of lymphocytes. Possible underlying mechanisms include the accumulation of dATP (and the consequent inhibition of ribonucleotide reductase) and the profound inhibition of S-adenosylhomocysteine hydrolase by 2'-deoxyadenosine. The latter action leads to an accumulation of S-adenosylhomocysteine and inhibition of various methylation reactions, such as protein carboxymethylation. In addition, various lymphocytic functions (such as lymphocyte-mediated cytolysis) are suppressed by the accumulation of adenosine extracellularly (Zimmerman *et al.*, in Symposium, 1983c). These actions appear to involve enhanced synthesis of adenosine 3',5'-monophosphate (cyclic AMP), which results from stimulation of receptors for adenosine. In addition, adenosine can cause an increase in the expression of receptors and antigens in T lymphocytes that are associated with suppressor activity and a decreased expression of antigens associated with T-helper/inducer function (Polmar *et al.*, in Symposium, 1983c).

Both thioguanine and mercaptopurine are excellent substrates for HGPRT and are converted to the ribonucleotides 6-thioguanosine-5'-phosphate (6-thioGMP) and 6-thioinosine-5'-phosphate (T-IMP), respectively. Because T-IMP is a poor substrate for guanylate kinase, the enzyme that converts GMP to GDP, T-IMP accumulates intracellularly. Careful studies have demonstrated, however, that mercaptopurine can be incorporated into cellular DNA in the form of thioguanine, indicating that slow reactions catalyzed by enzymes of guanine metabolism can operate. The accumulation of T-IMP may inhibit several vital metabolic reactions: examples are the conversion of inosinate (IMP) to adenylosuccinate (AMPS) and then to adenosine-5'-phosphate (AMP) and the oxidation of IMP to xanthylate (XMP) by inosinate dehydrogenase. These reactions are crucial steps in the conversion of IMP to adenine and guanine nucleotides. On the other hand, in cells incubated with thioguanine, 6-thioGMP first accumulates; it is a poor, but definite, substrate for guanylate kinase. Thus, there is slow conversion to 6-thioGDP and 6-thioGTP and entry of thioguanine nucleotides into the nucleic acids of the cell. In addition, the concentrations of 6-thioGMP achieved are sufficient to cause progressive and irreversible inhibition of inosinate dehydrogenase, presumably through the formation of disulfide bonds. Furthermore, both 6-thioGMP and T-IMP, as well as a number of other 5'-monophosphate derivatives of purine nucleoside analogs, can cause "pseudofeedback inhibition" of the first committed step in the *de-novo* pathway of purine biosynthesis, the reaction of glutamine and PRPP to form ribosylamine-5-phosphate. This enzyme is a major control point in the biosynthesis of purine nucleotides, and its rate of catalysis is highly responsive to the intracellular concentrations of 5'-mononucleotides (natural, as well as analogs). The synthesis of PRPP is also powerfully inhibited by ADP and ATP or related analogs. In view of the multiplicity of these effects, it can be appreciated that the intracellular accumulation of analogs of various purine nucleotides can produce major metabolic disruptions and, in some instances, may play a key role in cytotoxicity.

Despite extensive investigations, it is still not possible to assess precisely the role of incorporation of thioguanine or mercaptopurine into cellular DNA in the production of either the therapeutic or toxic effects of these drugs. These compounds can cause marked inhibition of the coordinated induction of various enzymes required for DNA synthesis, as well as potentially critical alterations in the synthesis of polyadenylate-containing RNA (Carrico and Sartorelli, 1977).

Other studies indicate that disruption of the synthesis of membrane glycoproteins may be caused by brief exposure to 6-thioguanine. These effects, which are potentially lethal to cellular survival, can occur in model systems at a time before any synthesis of DNA is observed. In view of these diverse biochemical actions, which involve vital systems such as purine biosynthesis, nucleotide interconversions, DNA and RNA synthesis, chromosomal replication, and glycoprotein synthesis, it is not possible to pinpoint a single biochemical event as the cause of thiopurine cytotoxicity. It seems likely that this class of drugs acts by multiple mechanisms (Loo and Nelson, 1982; McCormack and Johns, 1982).

Of many adenosine analogs studied experimentally, *vidarabine* (arabinosyladenine, AraA) has been approved for clinical use in the United States for the treatment of herpetic infections (*see* Chapter 54); its testing as an antineoplastic agent in combination with inhibitors of adenosine deaminase is underway. Vidarabine is converted enzymatically to AraATP. This analog nucleotide can inhibit DNA polymerases by competing with dATP and, in fact, may be incorporated into DNA. In this regard vidarabine resembles the analogous pyrimidine nucleoside antimetabolite cytarabine (AraC). By contrast, vidarabine, when administered alone, is relatively nontoxic and causes minimal immunosuppression. A related compound that has recently been in clinical trial is the analog nucleotide, 2-fluoro-9-β-D-arabinosyladenine-5′-phosphate (2-F-AraAMP), synthesized by Montgomery and Hewson (1969). This analog serves as a prodrug; 2-F-AraA is released by cell membrane–associated 5′-ectonucleotidases. Both 2-F-AraAMP and 2-F-AraA are resistant to enzymatic deamination, which inactivates the parent analog, AraA. Unfortunately, patients who received high intravenous doses of 2-F-AraAMP developed delayed but progressive and fatal CNS toxicity; further clinical study of this agent will likely be curtailed. (For additional discussion and references, *see* Bloch, 1975; Herrmann, 1977; McCormack and Johns, 1982.)

Mechanisms of Resistance to Antipurines. As with other tumor-inhibiting antimetabolites, acquired resistance is a major obstacle to the successful use of antipurines. The most commonly encountered mechanism is deficiency or complete lack of the enzyme HGPRT. In addition, resistance can result from decreases in the affinity of this enzyme for its substrates. Cells that are resistant because of these mechanisms usually show cross-resistance to analogs such as mercaptopurine, thioguanine, and 8-azaguanine.

Another mechanism of resistance identified in cells from leukemic patients is an increase in particulate alkaline phosphatase activity. Other mechanisms include (1) decreased drug transport; (2) increased rates of degradation of the drugs or their intracellular "activated" analogs; (3) alteration in allosteric inhibition of ribosylamine 5-phosphate synthetase; and (4) loss or alterations of the enzymes adenine phosphoribosyltransferase or adenosine kinase (for adenine or adenosine analogs). (For reviews, *see* Brockman, 1974; McCormack and Johns, 1982.)

MERCAPTOPURINE

The introduction of mercaptopurine by Elion and coworkers represents a landmark in the history of antineoplastic and immunosuppressive therapy. Today this antipurine and its derivative, azathioprine, are among the most important and clinically useful drugs of the class. The structure-activity relationship and the mechanism of action and of drug resistance are discussed above. The structural formula of mercaptopurine is presented in Table 55–4.

Absorption, Fate, and Excretion. Absorption of mercaptopurine is incomplete and variable after oral ingestion. About 50% of an oral dose can be accounted for as urinary excretion products in the first 24 hours. After an intravenous dose, the half-life of the drug in plasma is relatively short (about 50 minutes) due to uptake by cells, renal excretion, and rapid metabolic degradation. There are two main pathways for the metabolism of mercaptopurine. The first involves methylation of the sulfhydryl group and subsequent oxidation of the methylated derivatives. The formation of nucleotides of 6-methylmercaptopurine has been shown to occur following administration of mercaptopurine or mercaptopurine ribonucleoside. Substantial amounts of the mono, di, and triphosphate nucleotides of 6-methylmercaptopurine ribonucleoside (6-MMPR) have been identified in the blood and bone marrow of patients treated with mercaptopurine or azathioprine. Desulfuration of thiopurines can occur, and relatively large percentages of the administered sulfur are excreted as inorganic sulfate. The second major pathway for mercaptopurine metabolism involves the enzyme xanthine oxidase, which is present in relatively large amounts in the liver. Mercaptopurine is a good substrate for this enzyme, which oxidizes it to 6-thiouric acid, a noncarcinostatic metabolite.

An attempt to modify the metabolic inactivation of mercaptopurine by xanthine oxidase led to the development of *allopurinol*. This analog of hypoxanthine is a powerful inhibitor of xanthine oxidase, and not only blocks the conversion of mercaptopurine to 6-thiouric acid but also interferes with the production of uric acid from hypoxanthine and xanthine (*see* Chapter 29). Because of its ability to interfere with the enzymatic oxidation of mercaptopurine and related derivatives, allopurinol increases the exposure of cells to the action of these compounds. Although it greatly potentiates the antineoplastic action of mercaptopurine in tumor-bearing mice, allopurinol increases the toxicity as well, and there is no apparent improvement in the therapeutic index (McCormack and Johns, 1982; Zinner and Klastersky, 1985).

Preparation, Dosage, and Route of Administration. *Mercaptopurine* (*6-mercaptopurine;* PURINETHOL) is marketed as scored, 50-mg tablets. The initial average daily oral dose is 2.5 mg/kg. Starting doses usually range from 100 to 200 mg a day; with hematological and clinical improvement, the dose is diminished to an appropriate multiple of 25 mg and, in general, maintenance therapy of 1.2 to 2.5 mg/kg a day is continued. If beneficial effects have not been noted after 4 weeks, the dose may be increased gradually until evidence of toxicity is encountered. The total dose required to produce depression of the bone marrow in patients with nonhematological malignancies is about 45 mg/kg and may range from 18 to 106 mg/kg.

Hyperuricemia with hyperuricosuria may occur during treatment; the accumulation of uric acid presumably reflects the destruction of cells with release of purines that are oxidized by xanthine oxidase, as well as an inhibition of the conversion of inosinic acid to precursors of nucleic acids. This circumstance may be an indication for the use of *allopurinol*. Special caution must be employed if mercaptopurine or its imidazolyl derivative, azathioprine, is used with allopurinol, for reasons presented above. Patients treated simultaneously with both drugs should receive approximately 25% of the usual dose of mercaptopurine (*see* Appendix II).

Therapeutic Uses and Clinical Toxicity. In the early studies with mercaptopurine,

bone-marrow remissions were described in more than 40% of children with *acute leukemia*. In adults with acute leukemia, the results have been much less impressive, but occasional remissions have been obtained. The drug has contributed to the treatment of lymphoblastic leukemia more by maintaining than by inducing remissions. Cross-resistance does not occur between mercaptopurine and other classes of antileukemic agents.

In the treatment of chronic granulocytic leukemia, maintenance therapy with mercaptopurine can be useful. Mercaptopurine has not been of value in chronic lymphocytic leukemia, Hodgkin's disease and related lymphomas, and a wide variety of carcinomas, even at unusually high doses. Although active as an immunosuppressive agent, it has been superseded by its imidazolyl derivative, azathioprine.

The principal toxic effect of mercaptopurine is bone-marrow depression, although, in general, this develops more gradually than with folic acid antagonists; accordingly, thrombocytopenia, granulocytopenia, or anemia may not be encountered for several weeks. When depression of normal bone-marrow elements occurs, cessation of therapy with the drug usually results in prompt recovery. Anorexia, nausea, or vomiting is seen in approximately 25% of adults, but stomatitis and diarrhea are rare; manifestations of gastrointestinal effects are less frequent in children than in adults. The occurrence of jaundice in about one third of adult patients treated with mercaptopurine has been reported; although the pathogenesis of this manifestation is obscure, it usually clears upon discontinuation of therapy. Its appearance has been associated with bile stasis and hepatic necrosis. Dermatological manifestations have been reported. The long-term complications associated with the use of mercaptopurine and its derivative, azathioprine, for immunosuppressive therapy are discussed by Schein and Winokur (1975).

AZATHIOPRINE

Azathioprine, a derivative of 6-mercaptopurine, is used as an immunosuppressive agent. The structural formula is shown in Table 55–4. The rationale that led to its synthesis and its mechanism of action and metabolic degradation have been discussed above.

Azathioprine (IMURAN) is currently approved for use in the United States only as an adjunct for the prevention of rejection in renal transplantation and for the treatment of severe rheumatoid arthritis. All other uses remain investigational. The drug is available in 50-mg tablets and in vials that contain 100 mg of the sodium salt for injection. The initial oral dose of azathioprine varies from 3 to 5 mg/kg daily. For maintenance therapy the dose may be reduced to 1 to 3 mg/kg daily, unless rejection is threatened. Patients with transplanted kidneys or impaired renal function may have reduced clearance of the drug and its metabolites; unless the dose is reduced appropriately, a dangerous cumulative effect may result. Among the conditions for which treatment with azathioprine is being studied are idiopathic thrombocytopenic purpura, autoimmune hemolytic anemias, systemic lupus erythematosus, and other disorders believed to be associated with altered immunological reactivity. The drug has been used alone or concomitantly with corticosteroids and other antiproliferative agents. If allopurinol is administered concurrently, the dose of azathioprine should be reduced to approximately 25%, since inhibition of xanthine oxidase impairs the conversion of azathioprine to 6-thiouric acid and may result in dangerous enhancement of its myelosuppressive effect. Bone-marrow depression, usually leukopenia, is the most common toxic effect of azathioprine. Infection may be a complication of any immunosuppressive regimen. Toxic hepatitis and biliary stasis have been reported. Infrequent complications include stomatitis, dermatitis, fever, alopecia, and gastrointestinal disturbances (McCormack and Johns, 1982).

THIOGUANINE

The synthesis of thioguanine was first described by Elion and Hitchings in 1955. It is of particular value in the treatment of acute granulocytic leukemia when given with cytarabine. The structural formula of thioguanine is shown in Table 55–4, and its mechanism of action is discussed above.

Absorption, Fate, and Excretion. Absorption of thioguanine after oral administration is incomplete and erratic. Peak concentrations in the blood are reached 6 to 8 hours after ingestion, and approximately 40% of the dose is excreted in the urine within 24 hours. When thioguanine is administered to man, the S-methylation product, 2-amino-6-methylthiopurine, rather than free thioguanine appears in the urine. After 8 hours, inorganic sulfate becomes a major urinary metabolite. Lesser amounts of 6-thiouric acid are formed, suggesting that deamination catalyzed by the enzyme guanase does not play a major role in the metabolic inactivation of thioguanine. Accordingly, it may be administered concurrently with allopurinol without reduction in dosage, unlike mercaptopurine and azathioprine.

Preparation, Dosage, and Route of Administration. *Thioguanine* (6-thioguanine, TG) is available in scored, 40-mg tablets. The average daily dose is 2 mg/kg. If there is no clinical improvement or toxicity after 4 weeks, the dosage may be cautiously increased to 3 mg/kg daily.

Therapeutic Uses and Clinical Toxicity. Clinically, the compound has been used in the treatment of acute leukemia and, in conjunction with cytarabine, is one of the most effective agents for induction of remissions in acute granulocytic leukemia; it has not been useful in the treatment of patients with solid tumors. Thioguanine has been used as an immunosuppressive agent, particularly in patients with nephrosis and with collagen-vascular disorders. Toxic manifestations include bone-marrow depression and gastrointestinal effects, although the latter may be less pronounced than with mercaptopurine.

III. Natural Products

VINCA ALKALOIDS

History. The beneficial properties of the periwinkle plant (*Vinca rosea* Linn.), a species of myrtle, have been described in medicinal folklore for many years in various parts of the world. While exploring claims that extracts of the periwinkle might have beneficial effects in diabetes mellitus, Noble and coworkers (1958) observed granulocytopenia and bone-marrow suppression in rats, effects that led to purification of an active alkaloid. Other investigations by Johnson and associates demonstrated activity of certain alkaloidal fractions against an acute lymphocytic neoplasm in mice. Fractionation of these extracts yielded four active dimeric alkaloids: *vinblastine, vincristine, vinleurosine,* and *vinrosidine.* Two of these, vinblastine and vincristine, are important clinical agents. Recently introduced is a semisynthetic derivative, vindesine (desacetylvinblastine carboxamide). (*See* Creasey, 1977; Bender and Chabner, 1982; Johnson, 1982; Bender, 1983.)

Chemistry. The vinca alkaloids are very similar chemically. They are asymmetrical dimeric compounds; the structures of vincristine, vinblastine, and vindesine are as follows:

	Vincristine	Vinblastine	Vindesine
R_1:	—CHO	—CH$_3$	—CH$_3$
R_2:	—OCH$_3$	—OCH$_3$	—NH$_2$
R_3:	—COCH$_3$	—COCH$_3$	—H

No definite information is available regarding metabolic changes that may be necessary for chemical activation or degradative alterations *in vivo.*

Structure-Activity Relationship. Minor differences in structure result in notable differences in toxicity and antitumor spectra among the vinca alkaloids. A number of related dimeric alkaloids are without biological activity. Removal of the acetyl group at C 4 of one portion of vinblastine destroys its antileukemic activity, as does acetylation of the hydroxyl groups. Either hydrogenation of the double bond or reductive formation of carbinols reduces or destroys activity of these compounds.

Mechanism of Action. The vinca alkaloids are cell-cycle–specific agents and, in common with other drugs such as colchicine and podophyllotoxin, block mitosis with metaphase arrest. The biochemical effects of the vinca alkaloids have been explored extensively, and a number of interesting phenomena have been uncovered. It seems likely, however, that most of the biological activities of these drugs can be explained by their ability to bind specifically with the protein tubulin, a key component of cellular microtubules. When cells are incubated with vinblastine, dissolution of the microtubules occurs, and highly regular crystals are formed that contain 1 mole of bound vinblastine per mole of tubulin. Colchicine and podophyllotoxin also can bind specifically with tubulin, but apparently at a site on the protein different from that bound by vinblastine. Through disruption of the microtubules of the mitotic apparatus, cell division is arrested in metaphase. In the absence of an intact mitotic spindle, the chromosomes may disperse throughout the cytoplasm (exploded mitosis) or may occur in unusual groupings, such as balls or stars. The inability to segregate chromosomes correctly during mitosis presumably leads ultimately to cellular death.

In addition to their key role in the formation of mitotic spindles, microtubules have been associated with many other cellular functions. Therefore, it is not surprising that vinca alkaloids may affect these functions as well. Some types of cellular movements, phagocytosis, and certain functions of the CNS appear to involve microtubules, which may explain some of the other effects of vinca alkaloids. (*See* Creasey, 1975.)

Drug Resistance. Despite their structural similarity, a remarkable lack of cross-resistance is seen between the individual vinca alkaloids. Recently, however, attention has been drawn to the phenomenon of pleiotropic drug resistance, in which tumor cells become cross-resistant to a wide range of chemically dissimilar agents. Thus, animal and human tumor cells have been identified that display cross-resistance to vinca alkaloids, the epipodophyllotoxins, anthracyclines, dactinomycin, and colchicine. Chromosomal abnormalities consistent with gene amplification have been observed. Intriguing are reports that calcium channel blockers, such as verapamil, can reverse resistance to vincristine and doxorubicin. (*See* Symposium, 1983a.)

Cytotoxic Actions. Clinical as well as experimental studies have demonstrated that bone-marrow depression, chiefly manifested by leukopenia, is the most important cytotoxic effect on normal cells. In this respect, vincristine is not nearly as potent as vinblastine; with the latter, this is the effect that limits dosage. The relatively low toxicity of vincristine for normal marrow cells makes this agent unusual among antineoplastic drugs, and it is often included in combination chemotherapy with other myelosuppressive agents. Loss of hair, presumably secondary to effects on the epithelial cells of the hair follicles, appears to occur more frequently with vincristine than with vinblastine. No definite explanation is available for the striking differences in the toxicities of these closely related chemical structures.

Neurological Actions. Although neurotoxicity may occasionally be encountered with vinblastine, particularly at high dosage levels, neuromuscular abnormalities are frequently observed with vincristine. Indeed, it is this type of untoward effect that most frequently proves to be the limiting factor during therapy with vincristine. Several types of manifestations have been recognized. In experimental animals, acute toxicity after large doses is characterized by clonic convulsions, muscular weakness, ataxia, tremors, vomiting, and catalepsy. The development of CNS leukemia in patients receiving vincristine and in hematological remission has been interpreted as evidence that the alkaloid penetrates the blood-brain barrier poorly. Although torpor, hallucinations, and coma were observed during exploratory clinical studies with very high doses of vincristine (75 μg/kg weekly), peripheral neuropathy is the most common manifestation of neurotoxicity at usual clinical doses. Numbness and tingling of the extremities, followed by weakness, loss of reflexes, foot-drop, ataxia, muscular cramps, and neuritic pains, have been observed frequently. Clinical neurophysiological studies have demonstrated that asymptomatic depression of the Achilles reflex is the earliest and most consistent sign of vincristine-induced neuropathies. Muscular weakness involving the larynx and the extrinsic muscles of the eye also has been noted. An effect on the autonomic nervous system may be responsible for severe, and even obstructive, constipation that frequently may develop with prolonged administration of vincristine, but it is seen only rarely with vinblastine. Temporary mental depression, occurring on the second or third day after treatment, especially with vinblastine, may be of clinical significance.

Absorption, Fate, and Excretion. Unpredictable absorption has been reported after oral administration of vinblastine, vincristine, or vindesine. At the usual clinical doses the peak concentration of each drug in plasma is approximately 0.4 μM (Bender and Chabner, 1982). Vinblastine and vincristine bind to plasma proteins. They are extensively concentrated in platelets and to a lesser extent by leukocytes and erythrocytes.

After intravenous injection, vinblastine has a multiphasic pattern of clearance from the plasma; after distribution, drug disappears from plasma with half-lives of approximately 1 and 20 hours (Owellen et al., 1977). Vinblastine is metabolized in the liver to the biologically active derivative desacetylvinblastine. Approximately 15% of an administered dose is detected intact in the urine, and about 10% is recovered in the feces after biliary excretion. Vincristine also has a multiphasic pattern of clearance from the plasma; the terminal half-life is about 2.5 hours (Bender et al., 1977). The drug is metabolized in the liver, but no biologically active derivatives have been identified. Greater toxicity is encountered when vincristine is administered to patients with obstructive jaundice. Less is known about the pharmacokinetics of vindesine; its pattern of disappearance from the plasma resembles that of vinblastine. The major route of elimination of the drug is biliary (Bender and Chabner, 1982).

VINBLASTINE

Preparations, Route of Administration, and Dosage. *Vinblastine sulfate* (VELBAN) is supplied in vials containing 10 mg of dry powder for preparation of solutions (10 ml). The drug is given intravenously; special precautions must be taken against subcutaneous extravasation, since this may cause painful irritation and inflammatory changes. The drug should not be injected into an extremity with impaired circulation. After a single dose of 0.1 to 0.15 mg/kg of body weight, hematological responses are observed for 7 to 10 days. If a moderate level of leukopenia (approximately 3000 cells per cubic millimeter) is not attained, the weekly dose may be increased gradually by increments of 0.05 mg/kg of body weight. Beneficial results, however, may occur at lower doses. Once the optimal amount is established, weekly dosage is continued; if the leukocyte count does not return to 4000 cells per cubic millimeter within 10 to 14 days, the treatment schedule is adjusted accordingly.

Therapeutic Uses and Clinical Toxicity. The most important clinical use of vinblastine is with bleomycin and cisplatin (*see* below) in the therapy of metastatic testicular tumors. This regimen is the preferred treatment for these neoplasms, and a substantial number of complete remissions, which are probably cures, have followed its implementation (Williams and Einhorn, 1985). Beneficial responses have been reported in various lymphomas, particularly Hodgkin's disease, where significant improvement may be noted in 50 to 90% of cases. The effectiveness of vinblastine in a high proportion of lymphomas is not diminished when the disease is refractory to alkylating agents. It is also active in Kaposi's sarcoma, neuroblastoma, and Letterer-Siwe disease (histiocytosis X), as well as in carcinoma of the breast and choriocarcinoma in women.

The nadir of the leukopenia that follows the administration of vinblastine usually occurs within 4 to 10 days, after which recovery ensues within 7 to 14 days; with higher dosage, the total leukocyte counts may not return to normal until 3 weeks have elapsed. Other toxic effects of vinblastine include neurological manifestations as described above. Gastrointestinal disturbances, including nausea, vomiting, anorexia, and diarrhea, may be encountered. The syndrome of inappropriate secretion of antidiuretic hormone (ADH) has been reported, and ischemic cardiac toxicity has also been noted. Loss of hair, mucositis of the mouth, and dermatitis may occur infrequently. Extravasation during injection may lead to cellulitis and phlebitis. Local injection of hyaluronidase and application of moderate heat to the area may be of help by dispersing the drug.

VINCRISTINE

Preparations, Route of Administration, and Dosage. *Vincristine sulfate* (ONCOVIN) is available as a solution in vials containing either 1, 2, or 5 mg of drug. Vincristine used together with corticosteroids is presently the treatment of choice to induce remissions in childhood leukemia; the optimal dosages for these drugs appear to be vincristine, intravenously, 2 mg/sq m of body surface, weekly, and prednisone, orally, 40 mg/sq m, daily. In adults, the usual method of administration is to start therapy with intravenous doses of 0.01 mg/kg of body weight. After observation of the patient for 1 week, the dose is raised by weekly increments of 0.01 mg/kg until either the desired response is obtained or toxicity is encountered. Adult patients with carcinomas or lymphomas often will respond to weekly doses of 0.02 to 0.05 mg/kg. When used with other drugs, for example, in the MOPP regimen (*see* below), the recommended dose of vincristine is 1.4 mg/sq m. High doses of vincristine seem to be tolerated better by children with leukemia than by adults, who may experience severe neurological toxicity. Administration of the drug more frequently than every 7 days or at higher doses seems to increase the toxic manifestations without proportional improvement in the response rate. Maintenance therapy with vincristine is not recommended in children with leukemia (*see* below). Precautions should also be used to avoid extravasation during intravenous administration of vincristine. Vincristine (and vinblastine) can be infused into the arterial blood supply of tumors in doses several times larger than those that can be administered intravenously with comparable toxicity, but inadvertent intrathecal administration of vincristine has been lethal (Gaidys *et al.*, 1983; Williams *et al.*, 1983).

Therapeutic Uses and Clinical Toxicity. Vincristine has a spectrum of clinical activity that is similar to that of vinblastine, but there are some notable differences. An important feature is the lack of cross-resistance between these agents, a remarkable finding in view of the very close similarity of their chemical structures. Vincristine is effective in Hodgkin's disease and other lymphomas. While it appears to be somewhat less beneficial than vinblastine when used alone in Hodgkin's disease, when used with mechlorethamine, prednisone, and procarbazine (the so-called MOPP regimen), it is the preferred treatment for the advanced stages (III and IV) of this disease (DeVita and Hellman, 1982). In non-Hodgkin's lymphomas, vincristine is an important agent, particularly when used with cyclophosphamide, bleomycin, doxorubicin, and prednisone. Vincristine is more useful than vinblastine in lymphocytic leukemia. Another area of difference in clinical response to these drugs is acute leukemia, particularly in children; whereas vinblastine is rarely useful in this disease, vincristine is extremely effective.

The rapidity of action of vincristine and its lesser tendency for myelosuppressive action make it a more desirable agent for therapy in the presence of pancytopenia or in conjunction with other myelotoxic agents. It is particularly useful for the *induction* of remission in acute lymphoblastic leukemia in children when given with prednisone. It is the treatment of choice for this purpose and produces complete remissions in approximately 90% of children on the first course of antileukemic therapy (Bloomfield *et al.*, 1985). The approximate rate of second remissions is 70 to 80%. Vincristine and prednisone should be promptly discontinued after remission is induced, since other agents (*e.g.*, methotrexate and mercaptopurine) are more effective for *maintenance*. Vincristine has not prevented the occurrence of leukemia in the CNS. Beneficial responses have been reported in patients with a variety of other neoplasms, particularly Wilms' tumor, neuroblastoma, brain tumors, rhabdomyosarcoma, and carcinomas of the breast, bladder, and the male and female reproductive systems (Calabresi *et al.*, 1985).

The clinical toxicity of vincristine is mostly neurological, as described above. The more severe neurological manifestations may be avoided or reversed by either suspending therapy or reducing the dosage upon occurrence of the earliest symptoms, usually tingling and numbness of the extremities. Severe constipation, sometimes resulting in colicky abdominal pain and obstruction, may be prevented by a prophylactic program of laxatives and hydrophilic agents.

Alopecia occurs in about 20% of patients given vincristine; however, it is always reversible, frequently without cessation of therapy. Although less common than with vinblastine, leukopenia may occur with vincristine, and thrombocytopenia, anemia, polyuria, dysuria, fever, and gastrointestinal symptoms have been reported occasionally. Ischemic cardiac toxicity has been reported. The syndrome of hyponatremia associated with high urinary sodium and inappropriate ADH secretion has been occasionally observed during vincristine therapy. In view of the rapid action of the vinca alkaloids, it is advisable to take appropriate precautions to prevent the complication of hyperuricemia. This can be accomplished by the administration of *allopurinol* (*see* above).

VINDESINE

Preparation, Route of Administration, and Dosage. *Vindesine sulfate* (ELDISINE) is available in 5-mg vials. The drug is given intravenously with precautions to avoid extravasation. Various schedules are being tested, including slow infusion, single weekly injection, and multiple weekly injections. Single weekly doses of 3 to 4 mg/sq m are used in most schedules.

Therapeutic Uses and Clinical Toxicity. The clinical spectrum of activity of vindesine is still being evaluated. The drug appears effective in lymphomas, blastic crises of chronic granulocytic leukemia, and systemic mastocytosis. It is effective in neoplasms that are resistant to vincristine. The major toxic manifestations are moderate leukopenia and mild neurotoxicity.

EPIPODOPHYLLOTOXINS

Podophyllotoxin, extracted from the mandrake plant (or May apple), *Podophyllum peltatum*, was used as a folk remedy by the American Indians and early colonists for its emetic, cathartic, and anthelmintic effects. Two semisynthetic glycosides of the active principle, podophyllotoxin, have been developed that show significant therapeutic activity in several human neoplasms, including small-cell carcinomas of the lung, testicular tumors, Hodgkin's disease, and diffuse histiocytic lymphoma. These derivatives have been referred to as VP-16-213 (etoposide) and VM-26 (teniposide). Although podophyllotoxin binds to tubulin at a site distinct from that for interaction with the vinca alkaloids, etoposide and teniposide have no effect on microtubular structure or function at usual concentrations (Loike and Horwitz, 1976). (For reviews of the epipodophyllotoxins, *see* Bender and Chabner, 1982; Vogelzang *et al.*, 1982; D'Incalci and Garattini, 1983; O'Dwyer *et al.*, 1985.)

Chemistry. The chemical structures of etoposide and teniposide are shown below. They have been selected from many derivatives of podophyllotoxin that have been synthesized during the past 20 years.

Etoposide: **R** = CH$_3$

Teniposide: **R** =

Mechanism of Action. Although the biochemical mechanisms of action are not yet understood, it appears that etoposide and teniposide are similar in their actions and in the spectrum of human tumors affected. Unlike podophyllotoxin, they do not cause mitotic arrest by binding to microtubules. Rather, at low concentrations, they block cells at the S–G$_2$ interface of the cell cycle and, at higher concentrations, cause G$_2$ arrest. Greatest lethality is seen in the S and G$_2$ phases. Single-strand DNA breaks are observed in intact cells but not with purified DNA, suggesting that cellular enzymes are in some way involved. Some evidence indicates that the epipodophyllotoxins stimulate DNA topoisomerase II to cleave DNA (Tewey et al., 1984). It has also been reported that the epipodophyllotoxins, as well as the aglycone, can inhibit nucleoside transport and impair the incorporation of nucleosides into cellular nucleic acids.

ETOPOSIDE

Absorption, Fate, and Excretion. Oral administration of etoposide results in absorption of about 50% of the drug. After intravenous injection, peak plasma concentrations of 30 μg/ml are achieved; there is a biphasic pattern of clearance, with half-lives of about 3 hours and 12 hours. Approximately 45% of an administered dose is excreted in the urine, two thirds as the unchanged drug and one third as metabolites; 15% is recovered in the feces. Concentrations of etoposide in CSF range from 1 to 10% of the simultaneous value in plasma (Bender and Chabner, 1982; Wiemann and Calabresi, 1985).

Preparations, Dosage, and Routes of Administration. Etoposide (VEPESID) is available for intravenous administration. Investigational oral preparations are in the form of a drink ampul or a

hydrophilic soft-gelatin capsule. The recommended intravenous dose is 50 to 100 mg/sq m, daily for 5 days, or 100 mg/sq m, on alternate days, for three doses. When given orally, the dose should be increased two times. Cycles of therapy are usually repeated every 3 to 4 weeks. The drug should be administered slowly during a 30- to 60-minute infusion in order to avoid hypotension and bronchospasm, probably due to the solvents used in the formulation.

Therapeutic Uses and Clinical Toxicity. Clinical use of etoposide has been primarily for testicular tumors that have not responded completely to vinblastine, bleomycin, and cisplatin. Although it is active alone, etoposide is frequently used in combination with cisplatin, bleomycin, and doxorubicin. The drug is active against small-cell and other carcinomas of the lung, Hodgkin's disease and non-Hodgkin's lymphomas, acute nonlymphocytic leukemia, carcinoma of the breast, and Kaposi's sarcoma associated with acquired immunodeficiency syndrome (AIDS). The dose-limiting toxicity of etoposide is leukopenia, with a nadir at 10 to 14 days and recovery by 3 weeks. Thrombocytopenia occurs less often and is usually not severe. Nausea, vomiting, stomatitis, and diarrhea occur in approximately 15% of patients treated intravenously, and in about 55% of patients who receive the drug orally. Alopecia is common but reversible. Fever, phlebitis, dermatitis, allergic reactions including anaphylaxis, and mild hepatic toxicity have been observed. Peripheral neuropathy is usually mild, but more severe if the drug is administered concomitantly with vincristine.

TENIPOSIDE

Teniposide is usually administered intravenously and has a multiphasic pattern of clearance from plasma. After distribution, half-lives of 4 hours and 10 to 40 hours are observed. Approximately 45% of the drug is excreted in the urine but, in contrast to etoposide, as much as 80% is recovered as metabolites. Less than 1% of the drug crosses the blood-brain barrier (Bender and Chabner, 1982; Wiemann and Calabresi, 1985).

Teniposide is available for investigational use. It is administered by intravenous infusion. The clinical spectrum of activity and the toxic manifestations of teniposide have not been fully determined but appear to be similar to those reported with etoposide.

ANTIBIOTICS

DACTINOMYCIN (ACTINOMYCIN D)

History. The first crystalline antibiotic agent to be isolated from a culture broth of a species of Streptomyces was actinomycin A (Waksman and Woodruff, 1940). Many related antibiotics, including actinomycin D, have subsequently been obtained (Waksman Conference on Actinomycins, 1974). Dactinomycin has beneficial effects in the treatment of a number of tumors, particularly certain neoplasms of childhood and choriocarcinoma.

Chemistry and Structure-Activity Relationship. The actinomycins are chromopeptides, and most of them contain the same chromophore, the planar phenoxazone *actinocin,* which is responsible for the yellow-red color of the compounds. The differences among naturally occurring actinomycins are confined to the peptide side chains, and the variations are in the structure, but not in the number or in the configuration of the α carbon, of the constituent amino acids. By varying the amino acid content of the growth medium it is possible to alter the types of actinomycins produced. Changes in the amino acid composition of both polypeptide chains can influence the biological activity of the molecule (Glaubiger and Ramu, 1982; Crooke, 1983). The chemical structure of dactinomycin is as follows:

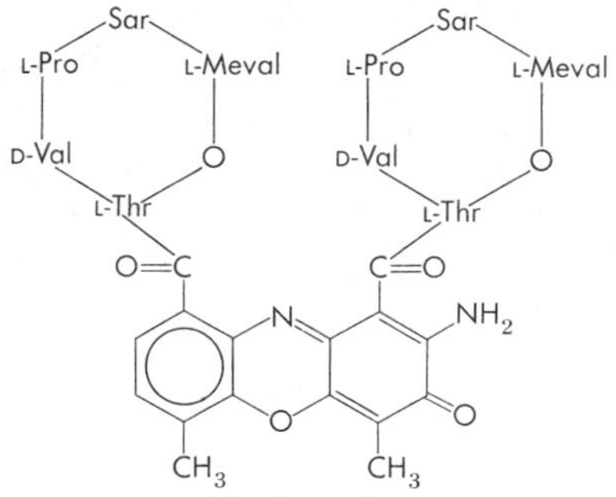

Dactinomycin

$$\left(\begin{array}{l} \text{Sar} = \text{sarcosine} \\ \text{Meval} = \text{N-methylvaline} \end{array} \right)$$

Mechanism of Action. The capacity of actinomycins to bind with double-helical DNA is responsible for their biological activity and cytotoxicity. X-ray studies of a crystalline complex between dactinomycin and deoxyguanosine permitted formulation of a model that appears to explain the binding of the drug to DNA (Sobell, 1973). The planar phenoxazone ring intercalates between adjacent guanine-cytosine base pairs of DNA, where the guanine moieties are on opposite strands of the DNA. The summation of several interactions provides great stability to the dactinomycin-DNA complex, and, as a result of the binding of dactinomycin, the function of RNA polymerase and, thus, the transcription of the DNA molecule are blocked. The DNA-dependent RNA polymerases are much more sensitive to the effects of dactinomycin than are the DNA polymerases. (*See* Waksman Conference on Actinomycins, 1974; Goldberg *et al.,* 1977; Glaubiger and Ramu, 1982.)

Cytotoxic Action. The drug inhibits rapidly proliferating cells of normal and neoplastic origin and, on a molar basis, is among the most potent antitumor agents known. Atrophy of thymus, spleen, and other lymphatic tissues occurs in experi-

mental animals. Detailed studies of the hematological, gastrointestinal, and other toxic effects of dactinomycin in animals have been described. It may produce damage to the hair roots and is capable of marked local inflammatory action. Erythema sometimes progressing to necrosis has been noted in areas of the skin exposed to x-radiation either before, during, or after administration of the drug.

Absorption, Fate, and Excretion. Dactinomycin is much less potent when given orally than when administered by parenteral injection. Very little active drug can be detected in the circulating blood 2 minutes after its intravenous injection. The drug is subsequently released from binding sites in tissues and disappears from plasma with a half-life of 36 hours. Metabolism of the drug is minimal. Dactinomycin does not cross the blood-brain barrier.

Preparation, Dosage, and Route of Administration. *Dactinomycin (actinomycin D;* COSMEGEN) is supplied as a lyophilized powder (0.5 mg in each vial). Solutions should not be exposed to direct sunlight. The usual daily dose is 10 to 15 μg/kg; this is given intravenously for 5 days; if no manifestations of toxicity are encountered, additional courses may be given at intervals of 3 to 4 weeks. Daily injections of 100 to 400 μg have been given to children for 10 to 14 days; in other regimens, 3 to 6 μg/kg, for a total of 125 μg/kg, and weekly maintenance doses of 7.5 μg/kg have been used. Although larger amounts have been given in more prolonged courses, in general the total dose necessary to produce antineoplastic effects has been approximately 2.5 to 5 mg. Although it is safer to administer the drug into the tubing of an intravenous infusion, direct intravenous injections have been given, with the precaution of discarding the needle used to withdraw the drug from the vial in order to avoid subcutaneous reaction.

Therapeutic Uses and Clinical Toxicity. The most important clinical use of dactinomycin is in the treatment of rhabdomyosarcoma and Wilms' tumor in children. In the latter case, remissions that last for several years and increased survival have been reported in patients with advanced disease, including pulmonary metastases (Waksman Conference on Actinomycins, 1974; Pinkel and Howarth, 1985). Antineoplastic activity has been noted in Ewing's tumor, Kaposi's sarcoma, and soft-tissue sarcomas. Its use together with vincristine and cyclophosphamide has been advocated in children with solid tumors. Dactinomycin can be effective in women with methotrexate-resistant choriocarcinoma. It may also be used with chlorambucil and methotrexate for patients with metastatic testicular carcinomas, but this regimen is not preferable to the concurrent use of vinblastine, cisplatin, and bleomycin. It is of limited value in other neoplastic diseases of adults, although a response may sometimes be observed in patients with Hodgkin's disease and related lymphomas. Dactinomycin has also been used to inhibit immunological responses, particularly the rejection of renal transplants.

Toxic manifestations include anorexia, nausea, and vomiting, usually beginning a few hours after administration. Hematopoietic suppression with pancytopenia may occur from 1 to 7 days after completion of therapy. A decrease in the platelet count is often the first manifestation of bone-marrow depression, and pancytopenia may develop rapidly. Proctitis, diarrhea, glossitis, cheilitis, and ulcerations of the oral mucosa are common; dermatological manifestations include alopecia, as well as erythema, desquamation, and increased inflammation and pigmentation in areas previously or concomitantly subjected to x-radiation. Severe injury may occur as a result of local toxic action.

DAUNORUBICIN AND DOXORUBICIN

These anthracycline antibiotics and their derivatives are among the most important of the newer antitumor agents. They are produced by the fungus *Streptomyces peucetius* var. *caesius*. Daunorubicin was isolated independently by DiMarco and by Dubost and their colleagues in 1963. Doxorubicin was identified by Arcamone and coworkers in 1969. Although they differ only slightly in chemical structure, daunorubicin has been used primarily in the acute leukemias, whereas doxorubicin displays activity against a wide range of human neoplasms, including a variety of solid tumors. Unfortunately, the clinical value of both agents is limited by an unusual cardiomyopathy; its occurrence is related to the total dose of the drug, and it is often irreversible. In a search for agents with high antitumor activity but reduced cardiac toxicity, hundreds of anthracycline derivatives and related compounds have been prepared. Several of these have shown promise in the early stages of clinical study, including epirubicin and the synthetic compound mitoxantrone, which is an amino anthracenedione. (For reviews, *see* DiMarco, 1982; Myers, 1982, 1983; Gianni *et al.*, 1983; Myers *et al.*, 1984.)

Chemistry. The anthracycline antibiotics have tetracycline ring structures with an unusual sugar,

daunosamine, attached by glycosidic linkage. Cytotoxic agents of this class all have quinone and hydroquinone moieties on adjacent rings that permit them to function as electron-accepting and -donating agents. Although there are marked differences in the clinical use of daunorubicin and doxorubicin, their chemical structures differ only by a single hydroxyl group on C 14. The chemical structures of daunorubicin and doxorubicin are as follows:

Daunorubicin: R = H
Doxorubicin: R = OH

Mechanism of Action. A number of important biochemical effects have been described for the anthracyclines and anthracenediones, any one or all of which could play a role in the therapeutic and toxic effects of such drugs. These compounds can intercalate with DNA. Many functions of DNA are affected, including DNA and RNA synthesis. Single- and double-strand breaks occur, as does sister chromatid exchange. Thus, the anthracyclines are both mutagenic and carcinogenic. Scission of DNA is perhaps related to the generation of free radicals. The anthracyclines react with microsomal cytochrome P-450 reductase in the presence of reduced nicotinamide adenine dinucleotide phosphate (NADPH) to form semiquinone radical intermediates, which, in turn, can react with oxygen to produce superoxide anion radicals. These can generate both hydrogen peroxide and hydroxyl radicals ($\cdot$OH), which are highly destructive to cells. In addition, intramolecular electron-transfer reactions of the semiquinone intermediates result in the generation of other radicals and, thus, of potent alkylating agents. Furthermore, the anthracyclines can interact with cell membranes and alter their functions; there is evidence that this may play an important role in both the antitumor actions and the cardiac toxicity caused by anthracyclines (Tritton *et al.*, 1978).

As might be expected of compounds that inhibit DNA function, maximal toxicity occurs during the S phase of the cell cycle. At low concentrations of drug, cells will proceed through the S phase and die in G_2.

As discussed above, the phenomenon of pleiotropic drug resistance is observed with the anthracyclines. This appears to result from acceleration of the efflux of anthracyclines and other agents from the cell. A membrane-associated glycoprotein, synthesized in high quantity as a result of gene amplification, has been implicated (Myers, 1982, 1983; Gianni *et al.*, 1983; Myers *et al.*, 1984).

Absorption, Fate, and Excretion. Daunorubicin and doxorubicin are usually administered intravenously, and they are then cleared from the plasma rapidly. The disappearance curve for doxorubicin is multiphasic, with elimination half-lives of 1.5 to 10 hours and 24 to 48 hours. There is rapid uptake of the drugs in the heart, kidneys, lungs, liver, and spleen. They do not appear to cross the blood-brain barrier.

There are notable differences in the metabolism of the two compounds. Daunorubicin is metabolized primarily to daunorubicinol. A significant fraction of doxorubicin is excreted unchanged, and there appear to be multiple metabolites, including, in particular, doxorubicinol. Aglycones result from further metabolism and, after conjugation, they are excreted in the bile. The hepatic clearance of doxorubicin has been estimated to be approximately 60% of hepatic blood flow, and severe clinical toxicity may result if the drug is administered to patients with impaired hepatic function. Renal excretion is modest and occurs mostly during the first 6 hours, resulting in a red discoloration of the urine. Modification of dosage is not required in patients with renal failure but is recommended when severe hepatic dysfunction and hyperbilirubinemia are present (Myers, 1982; Myers *et al.*, 1984; Wiemann and Calabresi, 1985).

Daunorubicin: Preparation, Dosage, and Route of Administration. *Daunorubicin (daunomycin, rubidomycin;* CERUBIDINE) is available as a lyophilized powder in 20-mg vials. The recommended dosage is 30 to 60 mg/sq m daily for 3 days or once weekly. The drug has also been given in doses of 0.8 to 1 mg/kg daily for 3 to 6 days, and other dosage schedules are being investigated. The agent is administered intravenously with appropriate care to prevent extravasation, since severe local vesicant action may result. Patients should be advised that the drug may impart a red color to the urine.

Daunorubicin: Therapeutic Uses and Clinical Toxicity. Daunorubicin is very useful in the treatment of acute lymphocytic and acute granulocytic leukemias. It is the single most active drug in acute nonlymphoblastic leukemia in adults and, given with cytarabine, is the treatment of choice in these conditions. The drug has some activity against solid tumors in children and in lymphomas; its activity against solid tumors in adults appears to be minimal.

The toxic manifestations of daunorubicin include bone-marrow depression, stomatitis, alopecia, gastrointestinal disturbances, and dermatological manifestations. Cardiac toxicity is a peculiar adverse effect observed with this agent. It is characterized by tachycardia, arrhythmias, dyspnea, hypotension, and congestive failure unresponsive to digitalis (*see* below).

Doxorubicin: Preparation, Dosage, and Route of Administration. *Doxorubicin hydrochloride* (ADRIAMYCIN) is supplied as a red-orange lyophilized powder in 10- and 50-mg vials. The recommended dose is 60 to 75 mg/sq m, administered as a single rapid intravenous infusion and repeated after 21 days. Care should be taken to avoid extravasation, since severe local vesicant action and tissue necrosis may result. Patients should be advised that the drug may impart a red color to the urine.

Doxorubicin: Therapeutic Uses and Clinical Toxicity. Doxorubicin is effective in acute leukemias and malignant lymphomas; however, in contrast to daunorubicin, it is also extremely active in a number of solid tumors. Used concurrently with cyclophosphamide, vincristine, bleomycin, and prednisone (BACOP), it is an important ingredient for the successful treatment of non-Hodgkin's lymphomas. In combination with bleomycin, vinblastine, and dacarbazine (ABVD), it is very effective in Hodgkin's disease. Together with cyclophosphamide and cisplatin, it has considerable activity against carcinoma of the ovary. It is a valuable component of various regimens of chemotherapy for carcinoma of the breast and small-cell carcinoma of the lung. The drug is also particularly beneficial in a wide range of sarcomas, including osteogenic, Ewing's, and soft-tissue sarcomas. It is one of the most active single agents for the treatment of metastatic adenocarcinoma of the breast, carcinoma of the bladder, bronchogenic carcinoma, and neuroblastoma. In metastatic thyroid carcinoma, doxorubicin is probably the best available agent. The drug has demonstrated activity in carcinomas of the endometrium, testes, prostate, cervix, and head and neck, and plasma-cell myeloma (DiMarco, 1975; Calabresi *et al.*, 1985).

The toxic manifestations of doxorubicin are similar to those of daunorubicin. Myelosuppression is a major dose-limiting complication, with leukopenia usually reaching a nadir during the second week of therapy and recovering by the fourth week; thrombocytopenia and anemia follow a similar pattern but are usually less pronounced. Stomatitis, gastrointestinal disturbances, and alopecia are common but reversible. Erythematous streaking near the site of infusion ("ADRIAMYCIN flare") is a benign local allergic reaction and should not be confused with extravasation. Facial flushing, conjunctivitis, and lacrimation may occur rarely. The drug may produce severe local toxicity in irradiated tissues (*e.g.*, the skin, heart, lung, esophagus, and gastrointestinal mucosa). Such reactions may occur even when the two therapies are not administered concomitantly.

Cardiomyopathy is a unique characteristic of the anthracycline antibiotics. Two types of cardiomyopathies may occur: (1) An acute form is characterized by abnormal ECG changes, including ST-T wave alterations and arrhythmias. This is brief and rarely a serious problem. Cineangiographic studies have shown an acute, reversible reduction in ejection fraction 24 hours after a single dose. An exaggerated manifestation of acute myocardial damage, the "pericarditis-myocarditis syndrome," may be characterized by severe disturbances in impulse conduction and frank congestive heart failure, often associated with pericardial effusion. (2) Chronic, cumulative dose-related toxicity is manifested by congestive heart failure that is unresponsive to digitalis. The mortality rate is in excess of 50%. Total dosage of doxorubicin as low as 250 mg/sq m can cause myocardial toxicity, as demonstrated by subendocardial biopsies. Nonspecific alterations, including a decrease in the number of myocardial fibrils, mitochondrial changes, and cellular degeneration, are visible by electron microscopy. The most promising noninvasive technic used to detect the early development of drug-induced congestive heart failure is radionuclide cineangiography. Although no completely practical and reliable predictive tests are available, the frequency of serious cardiomyopathy is negligible at total doses below 500 mg/sq m. The risk increases markedly (to >20% of patients) at total doses higher than 550 mg/sq m, and this total dosage should be exceeded only under exceptional circumstances. Cardiac irradiation or administration of cyclophosphamide or another anthracycline or related antibiotic increases the risk of cardiotoxicity. Because doxorubicin is primarily metabolized and excreted by the liver, it is important to reduce the dosage in patients with impaired hepatic function (Minow et al., 1977; Bristow et al., 1978; Myers, 1982; Wiemann and Calabresi, 1985).

BLEOMYCINS

The bleomycins are an important group of antitumor agents discovered by Umezawa and colleagues as fermentation products of *Streptomyces verticillus*. The drug that is currently employed clinically is a mixture of copper-chelating glycopeptides that consists predominantly of two closely related agents, bleomycin A_2 and bleomycin B_2. The various bleomycins differ only in their terminal-amine moiety (*see* below), and the addition of various amines to fermentation broths have made possible the preparation of more than 200 different congeners. Evidence indicates that both the toxic effects and the antitumor spectrum can be modified by such changes.

Bleomycins have attracted great interest because of their activity in a variety of human tumors, including squamous carcinomas of skin, head, neck, and lungs, in addition to lymphomas and testicular tumors. In comparison with many other antineoplastic agents, the bleomycins in current use have minimal myelosuppressive and immunosuppressive activities. They do, however, cause unusual cutaneous and pulmonary toxicity. Since the toxic manifestations of the bleomycins do not overlap significantly with those of most other drugs and since their apparent mechanism of action is also unique (*see* below), the bleomycins have an important place in multidrug chemotherapy. (*See* Umezawa, 1973, 1979, 1982; Chabner, 1982a; Twentyman, 1984.)

Chemistry. The bleomycins are water-soluble, basic glycopeptides that differ from one another in their terminal-amine moieties. The structures of bleomycin A_2 and B_2 are shown on page 1286 (Oppenheimer et al., 1979). The core of the bleomycin molecule is a complex structure containing a pyrimidine chromophore linked to propionamide, a β-aminoalanine amide side chain, and the sugars L-gulose and 3-O-carbamoyl-D-mannose. It also includes a side chain with the amino acids L-histidine and L-threonine, a methylvalerate residue, and a bithiazole carboxylic acid. The terminal amine is coupled through an amide linkage to this carboxylic acid. The bleomycins form equimolar complexes with cupric ions, with ligands involving the β-aminoalanine amide, the pyrimidine ring, the imidazole of L-histidine, and the carbamoyl group of mannose.

Mechanism of Action. While the bleomycins have a number of interesting biochemical properties, it seems most likely that their cytotoxic action relates to their ability to cause chain scission and fragmentation of DNA molecules. Studies *in vitro* indicate that bleomycin causes accumulation of cells in the G_2 phase of the cell cycle, and many of these cells display chromosomal aberrations, including chromatid breaks, gaps, and fragments as well as translocations.

Bleomycin appears to cause scission of DNA by interacting with O_2 and ferrous or cupric ions. Since Cu^{2+} binds to bleomycin more tightly than Fe^{2+}, it is likely that the cytotoxic agent is the copper-bleomycin complex (Lin et al., 1983). In the presence of O_2 and a reducing agent, such as dithiothreitol, the metallobleomycin complex becomes activated and functions mechanistically as a mixed-function oxidase; that is, it resembles the actions of cytochrome P-450 (Ehrenfeld et al., 1985). It has also been shown that metallobleomycin complexes can be activated by reaction with the flavin enzyme, NADPH–cytochrome P-450 reductase. Ble-

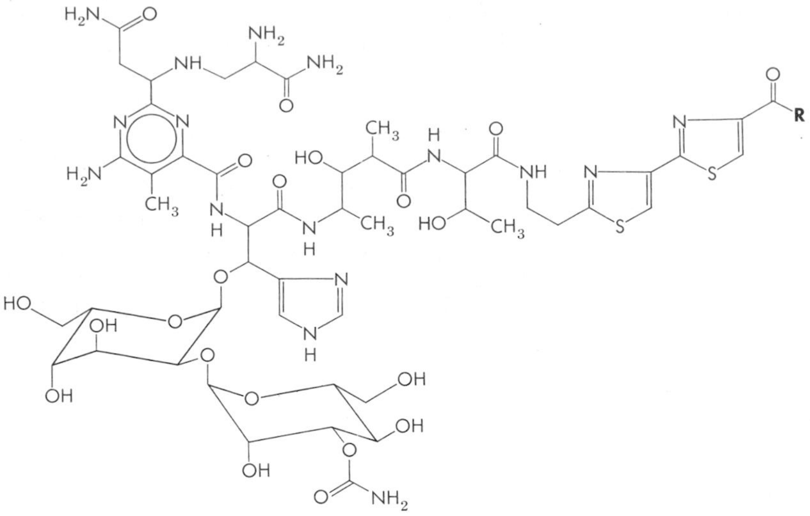

Bleomycinic Acid: **R** = OH

Bleomycin A$_2$: **R** = NHCH$_2$CH$_2$CH$_2$—S$^+$(CH$_3$)(CH$_3$)

Bleomycin B$_2$: **R** = NHCH$_2$CH$_2$CH$_2$CH$_2$NHC(=NH)NH$_2$

omycin binds to DNA through intercalation. It is thought that the metallobleomycin complexes can generate free radicals by transferring electrons to molecular oxygen; the radicals so produced are presumed to be responsible for scission of the DNA chain. (*See* Sausville *et al.*, 1978a, 1978b; Povirk, 1979; Grollman and Takeshita, 1980; Chabner, 1982a.)

Of considerable interest is the apparent mechanism of the selective action of the bleomycins against squamous-cell carcinomas and their toxicity to lung and skin. Most tissues, except lung and skin, have relatively high activities of an enzyme, bleomycin hydrolase, that hydrolyzes the amide group of the β-aminoalanine amide of the bleomycin core and thereby inactivates the molecule. No correlation has been seen, however, between bleomycin hydrolase activity and sensitivity to bleomycin of tumor cells grown *in vitro*. This suggests that mechanisms of resistance other than increased drug degradation are operative (*see* Umezawa, 1979; Lazo *et al.*, 1982; Twentyman, 1984).

Absorption, Fate, and Excretion. Bleomycin is usually administered parenterally, and data on oral absorption are lacking. Relatively high concentrations of the drug are detected in the skin and lungs of experimental animals, the major sites of toxicity. Bleomycin does not cross the blood-brain barrier. In man, bleomycin localizes in various tumors, suggesting a lower level of inactivating enzyme at these sites.

After intravenous administration of a bolus dose of 15 units/sq m, peak concentrations of 1 to 10 mU/ml are achieved in plasma. The half-time for elimination is approximately 3 hours. After continuous intravenous infusion, the clearance of bleomycin is prolonged, with an elimination half-time of approximately 9 hours. The average steady-state concentration of bleomycin in plasma of patients receiving continuous intravenous infusions of 30 units daily for 4 to 5 days is approximately 150 mU/ml, and there is little bound to plasma proteins. Nearly two thirds of the drug is normally excreted in the urine, probably by glomerular filtration. Concentrations in plasma are greatly elevated if usual doses are given to patients with renal impairment. Doses of bleomycin should be reduced in the presence of severe renal failure (*see* Chabner, 1982a; Wiemann and Calabresi, 1985).

Preparation, Dosage, and Routes of Administration. *Bleomycin sulfate* (BLENOXANE) is available as a lyophilized powder in 15-unit vials to be reconstituted with sterile water, saline solution, or 5% dextrose solution. The recommended dose is 10 to 20 units/sq m, weekly or twice weekly, and the drug is most commonly administered intravenously or intramuscularly. It may also be given by subcutaneous or intra-arterial injection. Total courses exceeding 400 units should be given with great caution because of a marked increase in the incidence of pulmonary toxicity; this may occur at lower doses when bleomycin is used concomitantly with other antineoplastic agents.

Therapeutic Uses and Clinical Toxicity. Bleomycin is effective in the treatment of testicular carcinomas. The overall response rate is approximately 30%, and this has increased to 90% when the drug is used with vinblastine. With the addition of cisplatin to this regimen, impressive numbers of complete remissions have been obtained that have lasted for several years (Williams and Einhorn, 1985). Bleomycin is also useful in the palliative treatment of squamous-cell carcinomas of the head, neck, esophagus, skin, and the genitourinary tract, including the cervix, vulva, scrotum, and penis. It is active in Hodgkin's disease and in other lymphomas (*see* Calabresi *et al.*, 1985).

In contrast to most other antineoplastic agents, bleomycin causes minimal bone-marrow toxicity. The most commonly encountered adverse effects are mucocutaneous reactions, including stomatitis and alopecia as well as hyperpigmentation, hyperkeratosis, pruritic erythema, ulceration, and vesiculation of the skin. These changes may begin with swelling and hyperesthesia of the hands or erythematous, ulcerating lesions over the pressure areas of the body. Recrudescence of mucocutaneous complications has been reported when other antineoplastic agents are used within 6 weeks after a course of bleomycin. The most serious adverse reaction to this drug is pulmonary toxicity. Injury to DNA and lipid peroxidation may be the initial lesions (Passero *et al.*, 1983). This poorly characterized manifestation may begin with decreasing pulmonary function, fine rales, cough, and diffuse basilar infiltrates, progressing to severe, and sometimes fatal, pulmonary fibrosis. Approximately 5 to 10% of patients receiving bleomycin develop this severe complication, and about 1% of all individuals treated with the drug have died of pulmonary toxicity. Pulmonary function studies have not been of predictive value. The risk is related to the total dose, with a significant increase in the incidence of pulmonary fibrosis noted at doses higher than 400 units and in patients over 70 years of age or with underlying pulmonary disease. The pulmonary toxicity of bleomycin may be potentiated by the administration of oxygen (Toledo *et al.*, 1982), by combination chemotherapy (Bauer *et al.*, 1983), and by previous radiation to the thorax. The use of corticosteroids has been advocated, but their value in reversing or preventing this complication remains to be established. Other toxic manifestations include hyperpyrexia, headache, nausea, and vomiting, as well as a peculiar, acute fulminant reaction observed in patients with lymphomas. This is characterized by profound hyperpyrexia, hypotension, and sustained cardiorespiratory collapse; it does not appear to be a classical anaphylactic reaction and may possibly be related to release of an endogenous pyrogen. Because this reaction has occurred in approximately 1% of patients with lymphomas and has resulted in deaths, it is recommended that

patients with lymphomas receive a 1-unit test dose of bleomycin, followed by a 24-hour period of observation, before administration of the drug on standard dosage schedules. Unexplained exacerbations of rheumatoid arthritis have also been reported during bleomycin therapy. Raynaud's phenomenon and coronary artery disease have been reported in patients with testicular tumors treated with bleomycin in combination with other chemotherapeutic agents (Chabner, 1982a; Wiemann and Calabresi, 1985).

PLICAMYCIN (MITHRAMYCIN)

This cytotoxic antibiotic was isolated from cultures of *Streptomyces tanashiensis* by Rao and associates in 1962. Although the drug is highly toxic, it has some clinical value in the treatment of advanced embryonal tumors of the testes. Plicamycin appears to have a relatively specific effect on osteoclasts and lowers the plasma calcium concentrations in hypercalcemic patients, including those with various types of cancer and metastatic tumors in bone. The drug has been used experimentally in the treatment of symptomatic Paget's disease, and striking reductions in plasma alkaline phosphatase activity with concomitant relief of bone pain have been observed. For a discussion of the chemistry of plicamycin and related antibiotics, *see* Umezawa (1979). The structural formula of plicamycin is as shown.

Plicamycin

Mechanism of Action. Plicamycin intercalates into DNA in a manner similar to that of dactinomycin, with preferential binding to guanine-cytosine base pairs. In fact, these two drugs compete for the same binding sites on DNA. Inhibition of RNA, DNA, and protein synthesis is observed. However, these effects on macromolecular synthesis occur only at drug concentrations that are higher than those required to block tumor-cell growth. Thus, there is no established correlation between DNA binding and cytotoxicity.

The relatively specific effect of plicamycin on plasma concentrations of calcium suggests that the drug may have a direct action on bone (Robins and Jowsey, 1973). Studies with a tissue culture system of embryonic rat bone showed that the release of calcium caused by the addition of parathyroid hormone can be abolished by simultaneous treatment with low concentrations of plicamycin (Cortes et al., 1972). These effects are thought to be the result of a direct action on osteoclasts (see Glaubiger and Ramu, 1982).

Absorption, Fate, and Excretion. Plicamycin is much less potent when administered orally than when given intravenously. Studies of its clinical pharmacology are lacking, and information on distribution, metabolic fate, and excretion is incomplete.

Preparation, Dosage, and Route of Administration. *Plicamycin (mithramycin;* MITHRACIN) is available as a freeze-dried powder in vials containing 2.5 mg of drug. The recommended dosage for treatment of testicular tumors is 25 to 30 μg/kg daily or on alternate days for eight to ten doses or until toxicity intervenes. The drug is usually diluted in 1 liter of 5% dextrose in water and administered by slow intravenous infusion over a period of 4 to 6 hours. Extravasation can cause local irritation and cellulitis. For the treatment of hypercalcemia or hypercalciuria, 25 μg/kg has been given daily for up to four doses; this is repeated at intervals of 1 week or more.

Therapeutic Uses and Clinical Toxicity. Plicamycin is of limited value in the treatment of neoplastic disease because of its severe toxicity. It has been beneficial in patients with disseminated testicular carcinomas, especially of the embryonal-cell type, but has been largely superseded by other drug regimens, particularly vinblastine, cisplatin, and bleomycin. The drug is useful in treating patients with severe hypercalcemia or hypercalciuria, particularly when associated with advanced or metastatic carcinoma that involves bone or produces parathyroid hormone–like substances. Its effectiveness in severe Paget's disease is encouraging but still considered investigational. Plicamycin is toxic to the bone marrow, liver, and kidneys. It produces a severe hemorrhagic diathesis, which may be the result of impaired synthesis of various clotting factors in addition to thrombocytopenia. Characteristically, this begins with epistaxis and may proceed to generalized hemorrhagic complications and even death. Adverse gastrointestinal, cutaneous, and neurological manifestations are also frequently observed. At the lower total dose recommended above for the treatment of hypercalcemia, toxicity is less severe.

MITOMYCIN

This antibiotic was isolated from *Streptomyces caespitosus* by Wakaki and associates in 1958. Mitomycin contains a urethane and a quinone group in its structure, as well as an aziridine ring, which is essential for antineoplastic activity. Of significance is that it acts through a bioreductive alkylation reaction and may be selectively toxic to hypoxic cells (Crooke and Bradner, 1976; Kennedy et al., 1980; Glaubiger and Ramu, 1982). Its structural formula is as follows:

Mitomycin

Mechanism of Action. After intracellular enzymatic reduction of the quinone and loss of the methoxy group, mitomycin becomes a bifunctional or trifunctional alkylating agent. It inhibits DNA synthesis and cross-links DNA to an extent proportional to its content of guanine and cytosine. In addition, single-strand breakage of DNA is caused by reduced mitomycin; this can be prevented by free radical scavengers. Its action is most prominent during the late G_1 and early S phases of the cell cycle. Mitomycin is teratogenic and carcinogenic in rodents, but its immunosuppressive properties are relatively weak (Crooke and Bradner, 1976; Glaubiger and Ramu, 1982).

Absorption, Fate, and Excretion. Mitomycin is absorbed inconsistently from the gastrointestinal tract, and it is therefore administered intravenously. It disappears rapidly from the blood after injection. Peak concentrations in plasma are 1.5 μg/ml after doses of 20 mg/sq m. Mitomycin is cleared from plasma with a half-time of approximately 35 minutes (Reich, 1979). The drug is widely distributed throughout the body but is not detected in the brain. Inactivation occurs by metabolism, but the products have not been identified. It is metabolized primarily in the liver, and less than 10% of the active drug is excreted in the urine or the bile.

Preparation, Dosage, and Route of Administration. *Mitomycin (mitomycin C;* MUTAMYCIN) is available as deep blue-violet crystals in vials containing 5 or 20 mg. It is soluble in water and is readily reconstituted for administration through a running intravenous infusion. Extravasation may result in severe local injury. The currently recommended dosage is 2 mg/sq m daily for 5 days; this course is repeated after a 2-day interval. The same total dose (20 mg/sq m) may be administered intravenously as a single bolus infusion. The drug may be given again by these schedules after recovery from myelosuppressive toxicity.

Therapeutic Uses and Clinical Toxicity. Mitomycin is useful for the palliative treatment of gastric adenocarcinoma, in conjunction with fluorouracil and doxorubicin. It has produced temporary beneficial effects in carcinomas of the cervix, colon, rectum, pancreas, breast, bladder, head and neck, and lung, and in melanoma. It has also shown activity against lymphomas and leukemia, particularly chronic granulocytic leukemia, but not in myeloma. All responses have been of brief duration and are complicated by severe toxicity. The major toxic effect is myelosuppression, characterized by marked leukopenia and thrombocytopenia; this may be delayed and cumulative. Nausea, vomiting, diarrhea, stomatitis, dermatitis, fever, and malaise have been observed. Interstitial pneumonia and glomerular damage resulting in renal failure are unusual but well-documented complications. Mitomycin may potentiate the cardiotoxicity of doxorubicin when used in conjunction with this drug (Wiemann and Calabresi, 1985).

ENZYMES

L-ASPARAGINASE

History. When L-asparaginase (L-asparagine amidohydrolase) was first introduced into cancer chemotherapy, it was believed that a distinct, qualitative biochemical difference had been detected between normal and certain malignant cells. Although this enzyme has found a limited place in the treatment of acute lymphoblastic leukemia, it is now appreciated that many normal tissues are also sensitive to L-asparaginase. Many toxic effects result from its impairment of the synthesis of secreted proteins, such as insulin, prothrombin and other clotting factors, albumin, and parathyroid hormone (Symposium, 1981a; Liu and Chabner, 1982; Wiemann and Calabresi, 1985).

Mechanism of Action. Most normal tissues synthesize L-asparagine in amounts sufficient for their metabolic needs. Certain neoplastic tissues, however, including acute lymphoblastic leukemic cells in children, require an exogenous source of this amino acid. L-Asparaginase, by catalyzing the hydrolysis of asparagine to aspartic acid and ammonia, deprives these malignant cells of the asparagine available from extracellular fluid, resulting in cellular death. There may be striking synergistic effects when asparaginase is used in combination with other drugs, such as methotrexate or cytarabine. The sequence of drug administration is crucial. For example, synergistic cytotoxicity is seen when methotrexate is administered before asparaginase. When the reverse sequence is used, the toxicity of methotrexate is attenuated. Several patients with refractory acute leukemias have responded favorably to such combinations. (For further discussion, *see* Capizzi and Handschumacher, 1982.)

Absorption, Fate, and Excretion. The enzyme is given parenterally. The rate of clearance from plasma varies considerably with different preparations; the half-life of EC-2 (*see* below) is from 11 to 23 hours (Broome, 1981; Liu and Chabner, 1982).

Preparation, Dosage, and Route of Administration. *Escherichia coli* produces two L-asparaginase isozymes, only one of which (EC-2) has antileukemic activity. The *E. coli* enzyme has been purified to homogeneity and is available for therapeutic use. *Asparaginase* (ELSPAR) is a dry powder in vials containing 10,000 international units (I.U.) per vial. The molecular weight of the enzyme is about 133,000, and it consists of four equivalent subunits (*see* Patterson, 1975). These preparations of *E. coli* L-asparaginase have weak glutaminase activity that may play a role in certain of the biological effects.

L-Asparaginase is administered intravenously or intramuscularly. The suggested dosage for the induction of remission in acute lymphoblastic leukemia is 200 I.U./kg daily for 28 days. Higher daily doses (1000 I.U./kg) for periods not exceeding 10 days have also been proposed as a method of avoiding anaphylaxis, which ordinarily appears only after the tenth day.

Therapeutic Uses and Clinical Toxicity. Unfortunately, L-asparaginase has not fulfilled its early promise of high tumoricidal activity with minimal toxicity in the treatment of human neoplasms. Complete remissions have been observed in acute lymphoblastic leukemia refractory to other antileukemic agents; the duration of these remissions, however, has been disappointingly short. Transient remissions have been observed in other forms of leukemia, and occasional beneficial responses have been reported in a few patients with malignant melanoma and T-cell lymphomas. Objective responses have not been seen with most solid tumors. The role of asparaginase in antineoplastic chemotherapy is currently limited to the treatment of acute lymphoblastic leukemia after standard regimens for induction of remission (*see* Symposium, 1981a).

In contrast to most other antitumor drugs, L-asparaginase has minimal effects on the bone marrow, and it does not damage oral or intestinal mucosa or the hair follicles. On the other hand, severe toxicity has been observed that affects the liver, kidneys, pancreas, CNS, and the clotting mechanism. Biochemical evidence of hepatic dysfunction is present in more than 50% of those treated, and most patients display a substantial elevation of blood ammonia (as great as 700 to 900 μg/dl). Disorders of pancreatic function, including decreased insulin production, are often seen, and approximately 5% of treated adults develop overt pancreatitis; death has resulted from hemorrhagic pancreatitis. CNS dysfunction, ranging from depression to impaired sensorium and coma, has occurred in adults. It is suggested that all or most of these toxic effects result from inhibition of protein synthesis in various tissues of the body. L-Asparaginase has immunosuppressive activity, as seen by inhibition of antibody synthesis, delayed hypersensitivity, lymphocyte transformation, and graft rejection. Thus, both T- and B-lymphocyte functions are affected. Since L-asparaginase is a relatively large, foreign protein, it is antigenic, and hypersensitivity phenomena ranging from mild allergic reactions to anaphylactic shock have been reported in 5 to 20% of treated patients (Wiemann and Calabresi, 1985).

IV. Miscellaneous Agents

CISPLATIN

The platinum coordination complexes are cytotoxic agents that were first identified by Rosenberg and coworkers in 1965. Growth inhibition of *E. coli* was observed when electrical current was delivered between platinum electrodes. The inhibitory effects on bacterial replication were subsequently shown to be due to the formation of inorganic platinum-containing compounds in the presence of ammonium and chloride ions (Rosenberg *et al.*, 1965, 1967). *cis*-Diamminedichloroplatinum (II) (cisplatin) was found to be the most active of these substances in experimental tumor systems and has proven to be of clinical value (Rosenberg *et al.*, 1969; Rosenberg, 1973). Other platinum-containing compounds have subsequently been synthesized and tested; several new agents are currently in clinical trial. Despite pronounced nephrotoxicity and ototoxicity, cisplatin is very useful in combination chemotherapy of metastatic testicular and ovarian carcinoma; encouraging effects have also been reported during treatment of tumors of the bladder and of the head and neck (Rozencweig *et al.*, 1977; Connors, 1982; Zwelling and Kohn, 1982; Roberts, 1983; Hacker *et al.*, 1984; Symposium, 1984).

Chemistry. *cis*-Diamminedichloroplatinum (II) (cisplatin) is an inorganic water-soluble, platinum-containing complex. The *II* indicates the valence of platinum. The structural formula of cisplatin is relatively simple, as follows:

$$\text{Cl}^- \quad \text{Pt}^{2+} \quad \text{NH}_3$$
$$\text{Cl}^- \qquad \qquad \text{NH}_3$$

Cisplatin

The corresponding complex with the ammonia residues in the *trans* configuration lacks antitumor activity.

Mechanism of Action. Cisplatin appears to enter cells by diffusion. The chloride atoms may be displaced directly by reaction with nucleophils such as thiols; hydrolysis of chloride is probably responsible for formation of the activated species of the drug. The platinum complexes can react with DNA, forming both intrastrand and interstrand cross-links. The N(7) of guanine is very reactive, and cross-links between adjacent guanines on the same DNA strand are the most readily demonstrated. It is likely that the geometry of the *cis*, rather than the *trans*, form is more favorable for the formation of both intrastrand and interstrand cross-links. The formation of interstrand cross-links is a relatively slow process and occurs to a much smaller extent. The covalent binding of proteins to DNA has also been demonstrated. At present, there is no conclusive association between a single type of biochemical lesion and cytotoxicity. (*See* Zwelling and Kohn, 1982; Symposium, 1984.)

The specificity of cisplatin with regard to phase of the cell cycle appears to differ among cell types, although the effects on cross-linking are most pronounced during the S phase. Even though cisplatin is mutagenic, teratogenic, and carcinogenic, an increased incidence of second tumors, which has been observed with certain of the alkylating agents, has not yet been reported. Careful observations for a longer period of time are necessary before conclusions can be drawn on this important point.

In addition to its reactivity with DNA, cisplatin can react with other nucleophils, such as thiol groups of proteins. It is speculated that certain of the toxic effects of the drug, such as nephrotoxicity, ototoxicity, and intense emesis, may result from such reactions. This has led to the experimental testing of "rescue" technics that employ molecules with high affinity for heavy metals. One of these, diethyldithiolcarbamate (DDTC), a metabolite of disulfiram, has shown promise. When administered to animals 2 hours after treatment with cisplatin, renal and gastrointestinal toxicity is ameliorated, while the antileukemic effects are not prevented. This compound is under consideration for introduction into the clinic (Zwelling and Kohn, 1982; Borch *et al.*, 1984).

Cisplatin has immunosuppressive activity. Rejection of skin grafts and graft-versus-host responses are suppressed in animals, as is mitogenesis in lymphocytes stimulated by phytohemagglutinin (*see* Connors, 1982; Zwelling and Kohn, 1982; Roberts, 1983; Hacker *et al.*, 1984; Symposium, 1984).

Absorption, Fate, and Excretion. Cisplatin is not effective when administered orally. After rapid intravenous administration, the drug has an initial half-life in plasma of 25 to 50 minutes; concentrations decline subsequently with a half-life of 58 to 73 hours. More than 90% of the platinum in the blood is bound to plasma proteins. High concentrations of cisplatin are found in the kidney, liver, intestines, and testes, but there is poor penetration into the CNS. Only a small portion of the drug is excreted by the kidney during the first 6 hours; after 5 days up to 43% of the administered dose is recovered in the urine. When given by infusion instead of rapid injection, the plasma half-life is shorter and the amount of drug excreted is greater. The extent of biliary or intestinal excretion of cisplatin is unknown (*see* Zwelling and Kohn, 1982; Wiemann and Calabresi, 1985).

Preparation, Dosage, and Route of Administration. *Cisplatin* (PLATINOL) is available as a lyophilized powder in vials that contain 10 or 50 mg of drug. When used alone, the usual intravenous dose is 100 mg/sq m, given once every 4 weeks. Cisplatin is frequently used with other drugs in chemotherapy, and the dosage is reduced in such situations to 50 mg/sq m once every 3 weeks (when given with doxorubicin for ovarian neoplasms) or to 20 mg/sq m daily, for 5 consecutive days, every 3 weeks (when used in combination with bleomycin and vinblastine for testicular tumors). In order to prevent renal toxicity, hydration of the patient is recommended by the infusion of 1 to 2 liters of fluid for 8 to 12 hours prior to treatment. The appropriate amount of cisplatin is then diluted in a solution of dextrose, saline, and mannitol and administered intravenously over a period of 6 to 8 hours. Continued hydration to ensure adequate urinary output is recommended for 24 hours thereafter. Some investigators have advocated the concurrent administration of 40 mg of furosemide. Repeat courses of drug should not be given until all tests of renal and hematopoietic function, as well as auditory acuity, are within acceptable normal limits. Since aluminum reacts with and inactivates cisplatin, it is important not to use needles or other equipment that contain aluminum when preparing or administering the drug.

Therapeutic Uses and Clinical Toxicity. Cisplatin appears to be particularly effective in the treatment of testicular tumors when used alone or, preferably, with bleomycin and vinblastine (Williams and Einhorn, 1985). The drug is also beneficial in carcinoma of the ovary, particularly when used with doxorubicin (Durant and Omura, 1985). Cisplatin may also be useful in the treatment of carcinomas of the bladder, head and neck, and endometrium, as well as for chemotherapy of lymphomas and some neoplasms of childhood (*see* Rozencweig *et al.*, 1977; Sternberg *et al.*, 1977; Randolph *et al.*, 1978; Yagoda *et al.*, 1978; Einhorn and Williams, 1979).

The major toxicity caused by cisplatin is dose-related, cumulative impairment of renal tubular function; this usually occurs during the second week of therapy. When higher doses or repeated courses of the drug are given, irreversible renal damage may occur. Ototoxicity caused by cisplatin is manifested by tinnitus and hearing loss in the high-frequency range (4000 to 8000 Hz). It can be unilateral or bilateral, tends to be more frequent and severe with repeated doses, and may be more pronounced in children. Marked nausea and vomiting occur in almost all patients. Mild-to-moderate myelosuppression may occur with transient leukopenia and thrombocytopenia. Electrolyte disturbances, including hypomagnesemia, hypocalcemia, hypokalemia, and hypophosphatemia, have been encountered. Hypocalcemia and tetany secondary to hypomagnesemia have been observed, and routine measurement of magnesium concentrations in plasma is recommended. Hyperuricemia, peripheral neuropathies, seizures, and cardiac abnormalities have been reported. Anaphylactic-like reactions, characterized by facial edema, bronchoconstriction, tachycardia, and hypotension, may occur within minutes after administration and should be treated by intravenous injection of epinephrine and with corticosteroids or antihistamines (Wiemann and Calabresi, 1985).

HYDROXYUREA

First synthesized in 1869 by Dresler and Stein, hydroxyurea was found to produce leukopenia, anemia, and megaloblastic changes in the bone marrow of rabbits (Rosenthal *et al.*, 1928). It was later shown to have antineoplastic activity against sarcoma 180. Studies of its biological activity and assessments of clinical efficacy have been reviewed (Donehower, 1982). The structural formula of hydroxyurea is as follows:

$$H_2N-\overset{\overset{\displaystyle O}{\|}}{C}-NH-OH$$

Hydroxyurea

Cytotoxic Action. Hydroxyurea is representative of a group of compounds that have as their primary site of action the enzyme ribonucleoside diphosphate reductase. Other members of this class that have shown promise in the laboratory are guanazole and the α-N-heterocyclic carboxaldehyde thiosemicarbazones. A striking correlation has been observed between the relative growth rate of a series of rat hepatomas and the activity of ribonucleoside diphosphate reductase. This enzyme, which catalyzes the reductive conversion of ribonucleotides to deoxyribonucleotides, is a crucial and probably rate-limiting step in the biosynthesis of DNA, and it represents a logical target for the design of chemotherapeutic agents. Nonheme iron is an important component of this enzyme in mammalian tissues, and many of the active inhibitors can chelate or form complexes with iron. These compounds are specific for the S phase of the cell cycle and cause cells to arrest at the G_1–S interface. Since cells are highly sensitive to irradiation in the G_1 phase of the cycle, combinations of hydroxyurea and irradiation cause synergistic toxicity *in vitro* (Agrawal and Sartorelli, 1975; Donehower, 1982).

Two mechanisms of resistance to hydroxyurea have been proposed: the acquisition of ribonucleotide reductases with decreased sensitivity to hydroxyurea and marked increases in ribonucleotide reductase, perhaps due to gene amplification.

Absorption, Fate, and Excretion. In man, hydroxyurea is readily absorbed from the gastrointestinal tract, and peak plasma concentrations of 0.3 to 2.0 μM are reached in 1 to 2 hours; the plasma half-life is about 2 hours. Hydroxyurea readily crosses the blood-brain barrier. Approximately

80% of the drug is recovered in the urine within 12 hours after either oral or intravenous administration (Donehower, 1982).

Preparation, Dosage, and Route of Administration. *Hydroxyurea* (HYDREA) is available for oral use in 500-mg capsules. Two dosage schedules are recommended: (1) intermittent therapy with 80 mg/kg, administered orally as a single dose every third day, and (2) continuous therapy with 20 to 30 mg/kg, administered orally as a single daily dose. Treatment should be continued for a period of 6 weeks in order to determine its effectiveness; if satisfactory antineoplastic results are obtained, therapy can be continued indefinitely, although leukocyte counts at weekly intervals are advisable.

Therapeutic Uses and Clinical Toxicity. At present, the primary role of hydroxyurea in chemotherapy appears to be in the management of selected myeloproliferative disorders, including chronic granulocytic leukemia, polycythemia vera, and essential thrombocytosis. It has also been effective in the hypereosinophilic syndrome (Parrillo *et al.*, 1978) and in achieving rapid reductions of markedly elevated blast cells in the peripheral blood of patients with acute granulocytic leukemia. Hydroxyurea has produced temporary remissions in patients with metastatic malignant melanoma and occasionally in those with other solid tumors, including carcinomas of the head and neck and genitourinary systems. Because of its ability to synchronize neoplastic cells *in vitro* in a radiation-sensitive phase of the cell cycle (G_1), it has been used in combination with radiotherapy in carcinomas of the cervix, head and neck, and lung.

Hematopoietic depression, involving leukopenia, megaloblastic anemia, and occasionally thrombocytopenia, is the major toxic effect; recovery of the bone marrow is usually prompt if the drug is discontinued for a few days. Other adverse reactions include gastrointestinal disturbances and mild dermatological reactions; more rarely, stomatitis, alopecia, and neurological manifestations have been encountered. Inflammation and increased pigmentation may occur in areas previously exposed to radiation.

PROCARBAZINE

A group of antitumor agents, the methylhydrazine derivatives, was discovered among a large number of substituted hydrazines, which had been originally synthesized as potential monoamine oxidase inhibitors. Antineoplastic effects in experimental tumors have been reported with several compounds in this series (Bollag, 1963), including procarbazine, an agent useful clinically in Hodgkin's disease. Comprehensive descriptions of the effects of procarbazine have been published (Oliverio, 1982; Wienkam *et al.*, 1982). The structural formula of procarbazine is as follows:

$$CH_3-NH-NH-CH_2-\langle\bigcirc\rangle-CONH-CH\overset{CH_3}{\underset{CH_3}{\diagdown}}$$

Procarbazine

Cytotoxic Action. Procarbazine itself is inert as a cytotoxic and mutagenic agent, and it must undergo metabolic activation to generate the proximal cytotoxic reactants. The activation pathways are complex and not yet fully understood. The first step involves oxidation of the hydrazine function with formation of the azo analog. This can occur spontaneously in neutral solution by reaction with molecular oxygen and can also occur enzymatically by reaction with the cytochrome P-450 system of the liver. Further oxidations can generate the methylazoxy and benzylazoxy intermediates. It is postulated that the methylazoxy compound can react further to liberate an entity resembling diazomethane, a potent methylating reagent. Free-radical intermediates may also be involved in cytotoxicity. Activated procarbazine can produce chromosomal damage, including chromatid breaks and translocations, that are consistent with its mutagenic and carcinogenic actions. Antimitotic effects have been described in a number of cell types; cells in the G_1 phase of the cell cycle are most susceptible. Inhibition of DNA, RNA, and protein synthesis has been detected both *in vitro* and *in vivo*. Although resistance to procarbazine develops rapidly, there is no clear notion of the mechanism. The highly lipophilic drug enters cells readily by diffusion (*see* Oliverio, 1982; Weinkam, *et al.*, 1982).

Absorption, Fate, and Excretion. Procarbazine is absorbed almost completely from the gastrointestinal tract. After parenteral administration, the drug is readily equilibrated between the plasma and the CSF. It is rapidly metabolized in man, and its half-life in the blood after intravenous injection is approximately 7 minutes. Oxidation of procarbazine produces the corresponding azo compound and hydrogen peroxide. Induction of microsomal enzymes by phenobarbital and other agents enhances the rate of conversion of procarbazine to its active metabolites; the potential for drug interaction thus exists when procarbazine is administered with other agents that are metabolized by microsomal enzymes. From 25 to 70% of an oral or parenteral dose given to man is recovered from the urine during the first 24 hours after administration; less than 5% is excreted as the unchanged compound, and the rest is mostly in the form of a metabolite, N-isopropylterephthalanic acid (Oliverio, 1973; Weinkam *et al.*, 1982).

Preparation, Dosage, and Route of Administration. *Procarbazine hydrochloride* (MATULANE) is marketed in 50-mg capsules. The recommended oral daily dose for adults is 2 to 4 mg/kg for the first week of therapy; then daily doses of 4 to 6 mg/kg are given until maximal response is obtained or toxicity intervenes. Daily maintenance doses of 1 to 2 mg/kg may be used.

Therapeutic Uses and Clinical Toxicity. The greatest therapeutic effectiveness of procarbazine is in Hodgkin's disease, particularly when given with mechlorethamine, vincristine, and prednisone (the MOPP regimen) (DeVita and Hellman, 1982). Of major importance is the apparent lack of cross-resistance with other antineoplastic agents. When used with various other agents, procarbazine has also demonstrated activity against small-cell carcinoma of the lung, non-Hodgkin's lymphomas, myeloma, melanoma, and brain tumors (Oliverio, 1973; Kreis, 1977; Weinkam *et al.*, 1982).

The most common toxic effects include leukopenia, thrombocytopenia, nausea, and vomiting, which occur in 50 to 90% of patients. Myelosuppression may begin during the second week of therapy, and its severity is dose dependent. Other gastrointestinal symptoms as well as neurological and dermatological manifestations have been noted in 5 to 10% of cases; psychic disturbances have also been reported. Because of augmentation of sedative effects, the concomitant use of CNS depressants should be avoided. The ingestion of alcohol by patients receiving procarbazine may cause intense warmth and reddening of the face, as well as other effects resembling the acetaldehyde syndrome produced by disulfiram. Since procarbazine is a weak monoamine oxidase inhibitor, hypertensive reactions may result from its use concurrently with sympathomimetic agents, tricyclic antidepressants, and foods with high tyramine content. Procarbazine is highly carcinogenic, mutagenic, and teratogenic. It is also a potent immunosuppressive agent.

MITOTANE (*o,p'*-DDD)

The principal application of mitotane, a compound chemically similar to the insecticides DDT and DDD, is in the treatment of neoplasms derived from the adrenal cortex. In studies of the toxicology of related insecticides in dogs, it was noted that the adrenal cortex was severely damaged, an effect caused by the presence of the *o,p'* isomer of DDD. Its structural formula is as follows:

Mitotane

Cytotoxic Action. The mechanism of action of mitotane has not been elucidated, but its relatively selective attack upon adrenocortical cells, normal or neoplastic, is well established. Thus, administration of the drug causes a rapid reduction in the levels of adrenocorticosteroids and their metabolites in blood and urine, a response that is useful both in guiding dosage and in following the course of hyperadrenocorticism (Cushing's syndrome) resulting from an adrenal tumor or hyperplasia. Damage to the liver, kidneys, or bone marrow has not been encountered.

Absorption, Fate, and Excretion. Clinical studies indicate that approximately 40% of the drug is absorbed after oral administration. After daily doses of 5 to 15 g, concentrations of 10 to 90 μg/ml of unchanged drug and 30 to 50 μg/ml of a metabolite are present in the blood. After discontinuation of therapy, plasma concentrations of mitotane are still measurable for 6 to 9 weeks. Although the drug is found in all tissues, fat is the primary site of storage. A water-soluble metabolite of mitotane is found in the urine; approximately 25% of an oral or parenteral dose is recovered in this form. About 60% of an oral dose is excreted unchanged in the stool.

Preparation, Dosage, and Route of Administration. *Mitotane* (*o,p'*-DDD; LYSODREN) is supplied in 500-mg scored tablets. Initial daily oral doses of 8 to 10 g are usually given in three or four divided portions, but the maximal tolerated dose may vary from 2 to 16 g per day. Treatment should be continued for at least 3 months; if beneficial effects are observed, therapy is maintained indefinitely. Spironolactone should not be administered concomitantly, since it interferes with the adrenal suppression produced by mitotane (Wortsman and Soler, 1977).

Therapeutic Uses and Clinical Toxicity. Mitotane is indicated in the palliative treatment of inoperable adrenocortical carcinoma. In addition to 138 patients reported by Hutter and Kayhoe (1966), 115 have been studied by Lubitz and associates (1973). Clinical effectiveness has been reported in 34 to 54% of these cases. Apparent cures have been reported in some patients with metastatic disease (Becker and Schumacher, 1975; Ostumi and Roginsky, 1975). Although the administration of mitotane produces anorexia and nausea in approximately 80% of patients, somnolence and lethargy in about 34%, and dermatitis in 15 to 20%, these effects do not contraindicate the use of the drug at lower doses. Since this drug damages the adrenal cortex, administration of adrenocorticosteroids is indicated, particularly in patients with evidence of adrenal insufficiency, shock, or severe trauma (Hogan *et al.*, 1978).

V. Hormones and Related Agents

ADRENOCORTICOSTEROIDS

The pharmacology, major therapeutic uses, and toxic effects of the adrenocorticosteroids are discussed in Chapter 63. Only the applications of the hormones in the treatment of neoplastic disease will be considered here. Because of their lympholytic effects and their ability to suppress mitosis in lymphocytes, the greatest value of these steroids is in the treatment of acute leukemia in children and of malignant lymphoma. They are especially effective in the management of frank hemolytic anemia and the hemorrhagic complications of thrombocytopenia that frequently accompany malignant lymphomas and chronic lymphocytic leukemia.

In acute lymphoblastic or undifferentiated leukemia of childhood, adrenocorticosteroids may produce prompt clinical improvement and objective hematological remissions in 30 to 50% of children. Although these responses frequently are characterized by complete disappearance of all detectable leukemic cells from the peripheral blood and bone marrow, the duration of remission is extremely variable (2 weeks to 9 months) and relapse of the disease invariably occurs; eventually, drug resistance develops. Remissions occur more rapidly with corticosteroids than with antimetabolites, and there is no evidence of cross-resistance to unrelated agents. For these reasons, therapy is often initiated with a steroid and another type of agent, usually vincristine, in order to *induce* remissions. This approach, followed by continuous *maintenance* treatment with various agents, yields more prolonged remissions (*see* section on Methotrexate). Adult leukemia seldom responds to glucocorticoid therapy, but many symptoms of the disease, including the hemorrhagic manifestations of thrombocytopenia, may be controlled effectively, albeit temporarily, without demonstrable changes in platelet counts.

Corticosteroids have been useful in some patients with carcinoma of the breast and other carcinomas; however, palliative effects are of short duration and complications are frequent. Although the overall results in the treatment of carcinoma with these agents are disappointing, the judicious short-term use of corticosteroids may be indicated for specific complications such as hypercalcemia and intracranial metastases.

The adrenocorticosteroids are used in conjunction with x-ray therapy to reduce the occurrence of radiation edema in critical areas such as the superior mediastinum, brain, and spinal cord. These drugs are particularly useful in the symptomatic palliation of patients with severe hematopoietic depression secondary to bone-marrow involvement or previous radiation or chemotherapy. They may produce rapid symptomatic improvement in critically ill patients by temporarily suppressing fever, sweats, and pain, and by restoring, to some degree, appetite, lost weight, strength, and sense of well-being. The symptoms tend to recur after the hormone is withdrawn, which indicates that the effects of the disease, but not necessarily the disease process itself, have been affected. Therefore, the value of this type of therapy is to provide the patient with a relatively asymptomatic period during which the general physical condition may improve sufficiently to permit further definitive therapy.

Several preparations are available and at appropriate dosages exert similar effects (*see* Chapter 63). Prednisone, for example, is usually administered orally in doses as high as 60 to 100 mg, or even higher, for the first few days and gradually reduced to levels of 20 to 40 mg per day. A continuous attempt should be made to lower the dosage required to control the manifestations of the disease.

AMINOGLUTETHIMIDE

Originally developed as an anticonvulsant, aminoglutethimide was subsequently found to inhibit the synthesis of adrenocortical steroids (*see* Chapter 63). Aminoglutethimide inhibits the conversion of cholesterol to pregnenolone, the first step in the synthesis of cortisol. Inhibition of cortisol synthesis, however, results in a compensatory rise in the secretion of ACTH sufficient to overcome the adrenal blockade. Administration of dexamethasone does not prevent the increase in ACTH secretion because aminoglutethimide accelerates the metabolism of dexamethasone. Since the metabolism of hydrocortisone is not affected by aminoglutethimide, this combination produces reliable inhibition of the synthesis of cortisol (Santen *et al.*, 1980). Aminoglutethimide has been used to treat patients with adrenocortical carcinoma and Cushing's syndrome.

Although aminoglutethimide effectively blocks the secretion of cortisol, the production of other adrenal steroids, such as testosterone, dihydrotestosterone, androstenedione, progesterone, and 17-hydroxyprogesterone, is only partially inhibited. In certain tissues, including fat, muscle, and liver, androstenedione is converted by aromatization to estrone and estradiol. In postmenopausal and castrated women, the adrenal gland does not produce estrogens, but it is the most important source of precursors of estrogens. By inhibition of cytochrome P-450–dependent hydroxylation reactions that are necessary for aromatization reactions, aminoglutethimide is a potent inhibitor of the conversion of androgens to estrogens in extra-adrenal tissues. Patients treated with aminoglutethimide and hydrocortisone thus experience a lowering of plasma and urinary concentrations of estradiol that is equivalent to that observed in patients treated by surgical adrenalectomy (Santen *et al.*, 1982).

Therapeutic Uses and Clinical Toxicity. Aminoglutethimide is administered orally at a dose of 250 mg four times a day, together with 40 mg of hydrocortisone in divided doses. The largest dose of hydrocortisone, 20 mg, is given at night.

A major indication for the use of aminoglutethimide is to produce "medical adrenalectomy" in patients with advanced carcinoma of the breast, when the tumor contains estrogen receptors. If women are selected for therapy without regard to the status of estrogen receptors in the tumor, the response rate is 37%; patients whose tumor cells contain estrogen receptors experience a 50% response rate. Skin, soft tissue, and bone lesions respond more frequently than do other sites of metastasis. Such treatment is equal or superior to surgical adrenalectomy or hypophysectomy (Harvey *et al.*, 1979).

Early toxic effects of aminoglutethimide include lethargy, visual blurring, drowsiness, and ataxia. These symptoms usually resolve after 4 to 6 weeks of treatment. A pruritic, maculopapular rash usually appears 10 days after treatment is initiated and resolves after approximately 5 days without withdrawal of the drug. Since the adrenal recovers normal secretory activity and the response to stress 36 hours after aminoglutethimide and hydrocortisone are withdrawn, it is not necessary to taper the administration of these drugs.

PROGESTINS

Progestational agents (*see* Chapter 61) have been found useful in the management of patients with endometrial carcinoma previously treated by surgery and radiotherapy. These compounds were tried initially because of the concept that carcinoma of the endometrium results from the prolonged, unopposed overstimulation by estrogen. This led to the use of progesterone, which would correct this situation because of its physiological effect in producing maturation and secretory activity of the normal endometrium. Apparently a portion of neoplastic cells arising from this tissue is still influenced by normal hormonal controls.

There are several preparations available. Hydroxyprogesterone caproate is usually administered intramuscularly in doses of 500 mg twice weekly; medroxyprogesterone acetate can be administered intramuscularly in doses of 400 mg twice weekly. An alternative oral agent is megestrol acetate (40 to 320 mg daily, in divided doses). Beneficial effects, usually characterized by regression of pulmonary metastases, have been observed in approximately one third of patients. Responses to progestational agents have also been reported in metastatic carcinomas of the breast and prostate, and in hypernephromas.

ESTROGENS AND ANDROGENS

A discussion of the pharmacology of the estrogens and androgens appears in Chapters 61 and 62. Their use in the treatment of certain neoplastic diseases will be discussed here. They are of value in this connection because certain organs that are often the primary site of growth, notably the prostate and the mammary gland, are dependent upon hormones for their growth, function, and morphological integrity. Carcinomas arising from these organs often retain some of the hormonal requirements of their normal counterparts for varying periods of time. By changing the hormonal environment of such tumors it is possible to alter the course of the neoplastic process.

Androgen-Control Therapy of Prostatic Carcinoma. The development of the androgen-control regimen for the treatment of prostatic carcinoma is largely the contribution of Huggins and associates (1941). Although no case of prostatic carcinoma has been cured by androgen-control therapy, life expectancy has been increased and thousands of patients have enjoyed the benefit of its ameliorating effects. Approximately 95% of patients with clinical manifestations of carcinoma of the prostate have nonresectable disease and require androgen-control therapy.

History and Rationale. The relationship between the prostate and testicular function was appreciated early in the nineteenth century, when it was noted that regression of the prostate followed orchiectomy. Huggins observed that, in the dog, shrinkage of the gland and cessation of secretion followed castration and that these effects could be reversed by the administration of androgen. Of even greater significance was the observation that the administration of estrogen could block the effects of the androgen. On the basis of these experimental findings, Huggins and associates (1941) postulated that significant clinical improvement should occur after bilateral orchiectomy in patients with advanced prostatic carcinoma, a theory that proved to be correct. It was also demonstrated that similar results could be obtained by the administration of estrogen (Herbst, 1941). The fundamental mechanism by which the lack of androgen results in regressive changes in normal and neoplastic prostatic cells is unknown. Unfortunately, relapse eventually occurs in patients on androgen-control therapy.

Therapeutic Regimen. Control of prostatic cancer is most effectively obtained by the combined use of orchiectomy and estrogen in patients who, when first treated, are free from metastases. When metastases are already present, orchiectomy seems to be more effective than estrogen therapy, and their combination does not appear to offer any advantage. When either orchiectomy or estrogen alone is employed as a therapeutic measure and the patient relapses, some degree of symptomatic improvement may be obtained by the alternative procedure.

The choice of estrogen is largely determined by cost and convenience. Diethylstilbestrol or a related synthetic compound is usually the preparation of choice. There is no evidence that survival is improved with excessively large doses. An average dose of diethylstilbestrol is 5 mg three times daily. Indeed, many oncologists reduce the daily dose to as little as 1 mg after a few weeks. The dose of other estrogens is in proportion to their potency.

Response to Therapy. Subjective and objective improvements rapidly follow the institution of androgen-control therapy of prostatic carcinoma. From the patient's point of view the most gratifying of these is relief of pain. This is associated with an increase in appetite, weight gain, and a feeling of well-being. Objectively, there are regressions of the primary tumor and soft-tissue metastases, but neoplastic cells do not disappear completely. Elevated plasma acid phosphatase activity usually returns to normal. Alkaline phosphatase activity may first rise and then fall. There is often an associated recovery from anemia. Some patients with prostatic carcinoma show no response to androgen-control therapy. Eventually prostatic tumors become insensitive to the lack of androgen or the presence of estrogen; however, it is now well established that effective palliation is afforded by the therapeutic regimen and that the life expectancy of the treated patient is significantly increased.

Androgen-Control Therapy of Carcinoma of the Male Breast. Carcinoma of the male breast is a rare tumor that is seldom diagnosed sufficiently early to permit definitive surgical intervention. The neoplasm regresses in a high proportion of cases in response to androgen-control therapy. Although this may be achieved by either orchiectomy or the administration of estrogen, it is preferable to initiate treatment with orchiectomy; when evidence of exacerbation appears, estrogen therapy is instituted. Remissions of several years can be achieved with this therapeutic regimen.

Untoward Effects of Androgen-Control Therapy. Androgen-control therapy is one of the safest forms of cancer chemotherapy. The psychic trauma of orchiectomy is not inconsequential, but is often tempered by the age of the patient. After orchiectomy alone, hot flushes are not uncommon; these can be controlled by the administration of estrogen. Estrogens are capable of producing the untoward responses described in detail in Chapter 61. Mild gastrointestinal disturbances may be noted; occasionally, these may be severe enough to require discontinuation of the drug. There may be some expansion of extracellular fluid volume in patients with poor cardiac function. There is also significant mortality from cardiac and cerebrovascular complications. Gynecomastia is frequent and may be a disturbing feature in some patients. In rare instances, carcinoma of the male breast has occurred in patients given estrogen for prolonged periods of time.

Estrogens and Androgens in the Treatment of Mammary Carcinoma. Estrogens and androgens have found application in the treatment of advanced mammary carcinoma. The hormones afford some measure of relief in patients with nonresectable disease in whom the metastatic lesions are too widespread to permit effective radiation.

Therapeutic Regimen. The therapeutic regimen for the use of androgens and estrogens in the treatment of carcinoma of the breast is largely empirical. The first cardinal principle is that hormonal therapy should be reserved for patients for whom surgical treatment or radiotherapy has been fully considered and deemed no longer of value. Once this qualification has been met, androgen therapy may be employed for patients in any age group. Objective remissions are obtained in approximately 20% of patients. Estrogen therapy generally is contraindicated in patients who are not at least 5 years past the menopause, regardless of chronological age. Experience has shown that estrogen may accelerate the neoplastic process in women who are still menstruating. In premenopausal women, oophorectomy is the first recommended procedure to institute hormonal control. On the basis of earlier observations, androgen was said to be preferable for the treatment of bone metastases, whereas estrogen was considered to be the preparation of choice for soft-tissue metastases. Subsequent evidence does not entirely substantiate these findings, however, and it is often the practice to change from one type of hormone to the other in unresponsive patients.

Progress in endocrinology has led to the development of methods that are very useful for the selection of patients for ablative or additive hormonal therapy. Tissues that are responsive to estrogens contain receptors for the hormones that can be detected by ligand-binding technics. Carcinomas that lack specific estrogen-binding capacity rarely respond to hormonal manipulation. The tumors that contain receptors usually do respond and, further-

more, are associated with a better overall prognosis independent of the type of therapy.

Hormonal therapy utilizes doses much larger than those needed for physiological replacement. Androgen therapy with oral agents is preferable; a common regimen is fluoxymesterone, 10 mg orally three times a day. Parenteral androgen therapy may be given as dromostanolone propionate, 100 mg intramuscularly three times weekly.

Compounds with estrogenic activity are numerous. Oral diethylstilbestrol is the most frequently used; it is given initially in doses of 5 mg daily. This dose is gradually increased to a maintenance dose of 5 mg three times daily over a 1- to 2-week period. Ethinyl estradiol is also commonly used, the dosage being gradually increased from 0.5 mg orally once daily to the customary maintenance dose of 3 mg daily, given in three portions. Ethinyl estradiol may be tried if diethylstilbestrol causes intolerable gastrointestinal side effects.

Response to Therapy. The onset of action of the hormones is slow, and it is necessary to continue therapy for 8 to 12 weeks before a decision can be reached as to effectiveness. If a favorable response is obtained, hormonal treatment should be continued until an exacerbation of symptoms occurs. Withdrawal of the hormone at this time may occasionally be followed by another remission. The duration of an induced remission averages about 6 months to 1 year; however, some patients may receive benefit for several years.

Untoward Effects. All the untoward effects that commonly accompany estrogen and androgen therapy have been observed in the use of these agents in the treatment of mammary carcinoma; these effects are described in Chapters 61 and 62. Two toxic manifestations require emphasis. With either hormone, the combined effect of a steroid and osteolytic metastases may result in marked hypercalcemia. The chief dangers are ectopic calcification, particularly in the urinary tract, and the physiological disturbances that may accompany an increase in the concentration of ionized calcium in the extracellular fluid. Patients who show an elevation in plasma calcium should receive a high fluid intake. Severe hypercalcemia, whether spontaneous or drug induced, is a true medical emergency. If an estrogen or androgen is being used, it should be discontinued. Forced hydration, by vein if the patient cannot drink, is mandatory. Further measures may be necessary; these include administration of diuretics, adrenocorticosteroids in large doses, oral or intravenous phosphate supplementation, or the intravenous administration of plicamycin (*see* above; *see also* Chapter 65). When drug-induced hypercalcemia is corrected, further therapy may be cautiously attempted. The incidence of hypercalcemia in patients receiving androgens is approximately 10%; it occurs less frequently with estrogen therapy. Plasma calcium concentrations should be determined routinely in patients receiving hormonal therapy.

Rarely, either estrogen or androgen therapy may cause exacerbation of the neoplastic process; this occurs more frequently as a result of estrogen administration.

ANTIESTROGENS

TAMOXIFEN

About one third of patients with advanced carcinoma of the breast benefit from either endocrine ablation or hormonal therapy. The growth of certain breast cancer cells depends on the presence of estrogens and, in these cases, oophorectomy may suppress tumor growth. A new development has been the introduction of effective and relatively nontoxic antiestrogenic agents that block the peripheral functions of estrogens on target tissues (see Chapter 61). Of various compounds tested, tamoxifen has been approved for clinical use in the United States; it is effective, palliative treatment for certain patients with advanced breast cancer. Tumors that contain estrogen receptors and those whose growth was slowed by prior hormonal therapy tend to respond to tamoxifen; others are often insensitive (see Tormey et al., 1976; Kiang and Kennedy, 1977; Moseson et al., 1978; Jordan, 1982a). The structural formula of tamoxifen is shown in Chapter 61.

Mechanism of Action. Estrogen receptors can be detected in tumor cells of 50% of premenopausal women with breast cancer and 75% of postmenopausal women. Antiestrogens, such as tamoxifen, bind to estrogen receptors in a fashion similar to that of estradiol. The complex of the receptor and the antiestrogen may bind to nuclear chromatin in an atypical manner and for a longer time than the normal hormone-receptor complex. Furthermore, antiestrogens may deplete the cytoplasm of free receptor. Either or both of these effects could severely impair the continued growth of an estrogen-dependent tumor. These observations offer a sound rationale for the use of antiestrogen therapy in combination with various ablative operations—oophorectomy, adrenalectomy, or hypophysectomy. Although any of these procedures may decrease the concentrations of estrogens in tissues, they do not completely eliminate the synthesis of the hormones. For example, after oophorectomy, androgens produced by the adrenals may be converted to estradiol in peripheral tissues. Three antiestrogens have shown useful actions in the treatment of human breast cancer: clomiphene, nafoxidine, and tamoxifen. Of these, tamoxifen is favored because of its relative lack of toxicity (see Legha et al., 1978).

Absorption, Fate, and Excretion. After oral administration, peak concentrations of tamoxifen are found in blood after 4 to 7 hours. The decline in plasma concentration is biphasic; the initial $t_{1/2}$ is 7 to 14 hours, and the terminal $t_{1/2}$ is longer than 7 days. Repeated administration of tamoxifen results in accumulation of the drug, and steady-state concentrations are achieved in 4 weeks. The principal metabolite of tamoxifen in man is N-desmethyltamoxifen. Concentrations of this metabolite in blood are approximately twice those of the parent compound at steady state. Studies in animals indicate that tamoxifen undergoes extensive metabolic conversion by hydroxylation and conjugation. The monohydroxylated derivative has more antiestrogenic activity than does the parent compound or the dihydroxylated metabolite. After enterohepatic circulation, glucuronides and other metabolites are excreted in the stool; excretion in the urine is minimal (Jordan, 1982a).

Preparation, Dosage, and Route of Administration. Tamoxifen citrate (NOLVADEX) is marketed in 10-mg tablets. The recommended dose is 20 to 40 mg daily, administered orally in two divided doses. Objective responses usually occur in 4 to 10 weeks but may be delayed for several months in patients with bone metastases.

Therapeutic Uses and Clinical Toxicity. Tamoxifen is useful in the palliative treatment of advanced carcinoma of the breast in postmenopausal women. Patients who have tumors that contain estrogen receptors are most likely to respond to the drug; those with a recent negative assay for receptor-binding activity are unlikely to benefit. Although a few premenopausal women have responded to this agent, it is more effective in patients who are several years postmenopausal, have metastases to soft tissues rather than to bone, and have derived beneficial effects from previous hormone therapy.

The most frequent adverse reactions include hot flashes, nausea, and vomiting. These may occur in approximately 25% of patients and are rarely severe enough to necessitate discontinuation of therapy. Menstrual irregularities, vaginal bleeding and discharge, pruritus vulvae, and dermatitis have occurred less frequently. The occurrence of pain in tumors, particularly bone metastases, as well as local flare of disease, characterized by increase in size and marked erythema of the lesions, is sometimes associated with good responses. Other infrequent adverse effects include hypercalcemia, peripheral edema, anorexia, depression, pulmonary embolism, light-headedness, headache, mild-to-moderate thrombocytopenia, and leukopenia. Tamoxifen is said to be carcinogenic and teratogenic in animals. (Further information about tamoxifen may be found in the publications of Lerner et al., 1976; Manni et al., 1976; Tormey et al., 1976; Kiang and Kennedy, 1977; Young et al., 1977; Kiang et al., 1978; Legha et al., 1978; Moseson et al., 1978; Furr and Jordan, 1984.)

GONADOTROPIN-RELEASING HORMONE ANALOGS

A recent development of considerable interest is the synthesis of various analogs of gonadotropin-releasing hormone (see Chapter 59). Marked decrease in circulating concentrations of gonadotropins and testosterone can be induced in patients with prostatic carcinoma treated with leuprolide, a peptide analog with high agonist activity. This compound has paradoxical effects on the pituitary; it stimulates initially, but there is subsequent inhibition of secretion of follicle-stimulating hormone

(FSH) and luteinizing hormone (LH). Impressive beneficial effects have been obtained in initial clinical studies, and large-scale clinical trials with leuprolide are in progress. The incidence of side effects, including gynecomastia, edema, thromboembolism, and nausea and vomiting, may be significantly lower in patients treated with leuprolide compared with those receiving therapeutically equivalent doses of diethylstilbestrol (Leuprolide Study Group, 1984; Torti, 1984).

VI. Immunosuppressive Agents

While many agents with immunosuppressive activity are discussed throughout this chapter, cyclosporine is unique in its structure and its mechanism of action. Of great importance, it does not share the relatively general cytotoxic activity of other drugs used for this purpose.

CYCLOSPORINE

Cyclosporine (formerly called cyclosporin A) is a hydrophobic cyclic undecapeptide produced by the fungus *Tolypocladium inflatum*. It is an immunomodulatory substance that acts specifically at an early stage in the activation of T lymphocytes. It displays little myelotoxicity and does not adversely affect the phagocytic cells of the reticuloendothelial system. Thus, in contrast to azathioprine and other cytotoxic agents, cyclosporine makes possible the suppression of T-cell–

mediated cellular immunity without causing major effects on the antibacterial defenses of the body. Its introduction into the clinic in recent years has played a major role in suppression of the immunological reactions that have adversely affected the fields of organ and bone-marrow transplantation in the past. The use of cyclosporine has also been promising in animal models of autoimmune disease, and clinical studies of such therapy have been initiated. (For a comprehensive discussion, *see* Symposium, 1983b.)

Chemistry. Cyclosporine is a complex cyclic peptide. It is comprised of 11 amino acid residues, and it is remarkably hydrophobic. All of the amino acids have the L configuration, except for D-alanine in position 8 and sarcosine (N-methylglycine) in position 3. Seven of the amino acids are N-methylated. The four remaining protonated peptide nitrogen atoms can form hydrogen bonds with carbonyl groups, which contribute substantially to the rigidity of the cyclosporine skeleton. A unique feature of the molecule is the nine-carbon olefin-containing amino acid in position 1. The structure of cyclosporine is shown below.

The total synthesis of cyclosporine has been accomplished, and a number of modified derivatives have been produced. Results to date indicate that the unusual nine-carbon amino acid is intimately involved in the biological actions of the molecule (*see* Wenger, 1983).

Mechanism of Action. Although the precise biochemical events are not yet understood, evidence indicates that cyclosporine blocks an early stage in the activation of

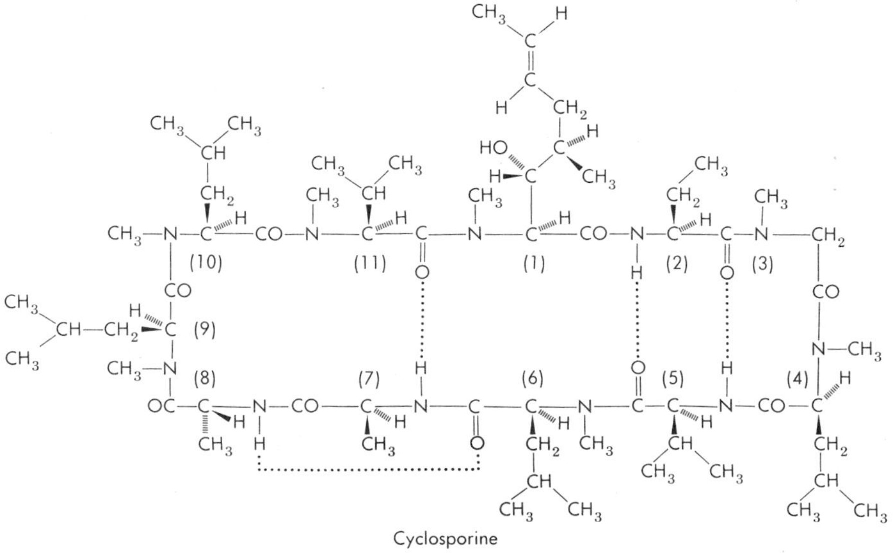

Cyclosporine

cytotoxic T lymphocytes in response to al-loantigens. Several important effects have been observed. Production of the soluble proliferative factor, interleukin II, by acti-vated T-helper cells is blocked; the acquisi-tion of receptors for interleukin II by pre-cursor cytotoxic T cells is inhibited; and the responsiveness of helper/inducer T cells to interleukin I is diminished. Cyclosporine has little effect, however, on the activation and proliferation of suppressor T lympho-cytes or on the responsiveness to interleu-kin II of primed T lymphocytes. Other po-tentially important effects are inhibition of the production of interferon by lympho-cytes and impaired production of macro-phage-specific lymphokines. (For further discussion, *see* Hess *et al.*, 1983; Kahan *et al.*, 1983; Lafferty *et al.*, 1983.)

Specific cytosolic cyclosporine-binding proteins have been discovered in lymphoid tissues. Two closely related proteins have been identified and purified to homogeneity from bovine thymocytes. These basic pro-teins, referred to as cyclophilins, have mo-lecular weights of about 15,000. Cyclo-philins with similar molecular weights but different isoelectric points have been found in cytosolic fractions from murine and human thymus and mature T cells. Cyclophilin has also been identified in non-lymphoid tissues; concentrations are high in brain and kidney, organs that display toxic effects during treatment with cyclo-sporine. It seems likely that cyclophilin plays a crucial role in the activation of T lymphocytes. Its presence in other tissues presumably indicates that it has other important biological functions (Hand-schumacher *et al.*, 1984).

Absorption, Fate, and Excretion. After oral administration, absorption of cyclo-sporine is variable and incomplete, with an absolute bioavailability of approximately 20 to 50%. Peak concentrations in plasma and blood are achieved after approximately 2 to 4 hours; these values are about 1 ng/ml for plasma and 1.4 to 2.7 ng/ml for blood for each milligram of drug administered. About 50% of the drug is found in erythrocytes, 40% in plasma, and 10% in leukocytes. In plasma, approximately 95% is bound to proteins, mostly lipoproteins. Although no major metabolic pathway has been identi-fied, the drug is almost completely metabo-lized, and less than 0.1% of intact com-pound is recovered in the urine. Many metabolites are excreted in the bile. A bi-phasic disappearance curve from blood has been observed, with a terminal half-life of 10 to 27 hours (Kahan *et al.*, 1983; Weil, 1984).

Preparations, Routes of Administration, and Dosage. *Cyclosporine* (SANDIMMUNE) is marketed as an immunosuppressive agent for the prophylaxis and treatment of the rejection of transplanted or-gans. It is provided as an oral solution of 100 mg/ml with 12.5% alcohol and for intravenous administra-tion as a solution of 50 mg/ml, with 33% alcohol and 650 mg of polyoxyethylated castor oil. The usual oral dose is 10 to 15 mg/kg daily, starting a few hours before transplantation and continuing for 1 to 2 weeks; dosage is then reduced gradually to a maintenance level of 5 to 10 mg/kg daily. The drug may be administered intravenously, as a dilute so-lution of 50 mg per 20 to 100 ml of normal saline solution or 5% dextrose in water, by slow infusion over a period of 2 to 6 hours. The intravenous dose is approximately one third the oral dose.

Therapeutic Use and Clinical Toxicity. Cyclo-sporine is a potent immunosuppressive agent and is used for prophylaxis and treatment of organ rejec-tion in allogeneic transplants, usually in conjunc-tion with adrenocorticosteroids. Prolonged sur-vival of allogeneic transplants of the kidney, liver, and heart has been documented in man. There has been more limited, but successful, experience with pancreatic, bone-marrow, and heart-lung trans-plants. The value of cyclosporine in the treatment of autoimmune disease and disorders associated with altered immune reactivity has not been estab-lished and is currently under investigation. There are provocative suggestions that the requirements for insulin in insulin-dependent diabetes can be re-duced substantially by cyclosporine, especially when drug treatment is initiated within 6 weeks of the onset of the disease.

The major toxic manifestations of cyclosporine are renal. Plasma concentrations of creatinine are usually elevated during therapy and require careful monitoring. Hepatotoxicity has been noted, and hepatic function should be assessed carefully. As with other immunosuppressive agents, there may be increased susceptibility to infection and the de-velopment of lymphomas. These lymphomas are associated with reactivation of the Epstein-Barr virus and are frequently similar to Burkitt's lym-phoma (Kahan *et al.*, 1983; Thomson, 1983; Weil, 1984).

Agarwal, R. P. Inhibitors of adenosine deaminase. *Phar-macol. Ther.*, **1982**, *17*, 399–430.

Agarwal, R. P.; Spector, T.; and Parks, R. E., Jr. Tight-binding inhibitors. IV. Inhibition of adenosine deami-nases by various inhibitors. *Biochem. Pharmacol.*, **1977**, *26*, 359–367.

Alberts, D. S.; Chang, S. Y.; Chen, H. S. G.; Larcom, B. J.; and Jones, S. E. Pharmacokinetics and metabolism of chlorambucil in man: a preliminary report. *Cancer Treat. Rev.*, **1979a**, *6*, 9.

Alberts, D. S.; Chang, S. Y.; Chen, H. S. G.; Moon, T. E.; Evans, T. L.; Furner, R. L.; Himmelstein, K.; and Gross, J. F. Kinetics of intravenous melphalan. *Clin. Pharmacol. Ther.*, **1979b**, *26*, 73–80.

Alper, J. C.; Wiemann, M. C.; Rueckl, F. S.; McDonald, C. J.; and Calabresi, P. Rationally designed combination chemotherapy for the treatment of patients with recalcitrant psoriasis. *J. Am. Acad. Dermatol.*, **1985**, *12*.

Bagley, C. M., Jr.; Bostick, F. W.; and DeVita, V. T., Jr. Clinical pharmacology of cyclophosphamide. *Cancer Res.*, **1973**, *33*, 226–233.

Bauer, K. A.; Skarin, A. T.; Balikian, J. P.; Garnick, M. B.; Rosenthal, D. S.; and Canellos, G. P. Pulmonary complications associated with combination chemotherapy programs containing bleomycin. *Am. J. Med.*, **1983**, *74*, 557–663.

Becker, D., and Schumacher, O. P. *o,p'*-DDD therapy in invasive adrenocortical carcinoma. *Ann. Intern. Med.*, **1975**, *82*, 677–679.

Bender, R. A.; Castle, M. C.; Margileth, D. A.; and Oliverio, V. T. The pharmacokinetics of [^{3}H]-vincristine in man. *Clin. Pharmacol. Ther.*, **1977**, *22*, 430–438.

Bertino, J. R.; Carman, M. D.; Weiner, H. L.; Cashmore, A.; Moroson, B. A.; Srimatkandada, S.; Schornagal, J. H.; Medina, W. D.; and Dube, S. K. Gene amplification and altered enzymes as mechanisms for the development of drug resistance. *Cancer Treat. Rep.*, **1983**, *67*, 901–904.

Bloch, A. (ed.). Chemistry, biology, and clinical uses of nucleoside analogs. *Ann. N.Y. Acad. Sci.*, **1975**, *255*, 1–610.

Bogden, A. E.; Cobb, W. R.; Lepage, D. J.; Haskell, P. M.; Gulkin, T. A.; Ward, A.; Kelton, D. E.; and Esber, H. J. Chemotherapy responsiveness of human tumors as first transplant generation xenografts in the normal mouse: six-day subrenal capsule assay. *Cancer*, **1981**, *48*, 10–20.

Bollag, W. The tumor-inhibitory effects of the methylhydrazine derivative Ro 4-6467/1 (NSC-77213). *Cancer Chemother. Rep.*, **1963**, *33*, 1–4.

Bonadonna, G., and Valagussa, P. Chemotherapy of breast cancer: current views and results. *Int. J. Radiat. Oncol. Biol. Phys.*, **1983**, *3*, 279–297.

Bono, V. H., Jr. Studies on the mechanism of action of DTIC (NSC-45388). *Cancer Treat. Rep.*, **1976**, *60*, 141–148.

Bristow, M. R.; Billingham, M. E.; Mason, J. W.; and Daniels, J. R. Clinical spectrum of anthracycline antibiotic cardiotoxicity. *Cancer Treat. Rep.*, **1978**, *62*, 873–879.

Brock, N. Pharmacologic characterization of cyclophosphamide (NSC-26271) and cyclophosphamide metabolites. *Cancer Chemother. Rep.*, **1967**, *51*, 315–325.

Broder, L. E., and Carter, S. K. Pancreatic islet cell carcinoma. II. Results of therapy with streptozotocin in 52 patients. *Ann. Intern. Med.*, **1973**, *79*, 108–118.

Calabresi, P. Principles of oncologic treatment: irradiation, cytotoxic drugs and immunostimulatory procedures. In, *Cecil Textbook of Medicine*, 15th ed. (Beeson, P. B.; McDermott, W.; and Wyngaarden, J. B.; eds.) W. B. Saunders Co., Philadelphia, **1979**, pp. 1922–1941.

————. Leukemia after cytotoxic chemotherapy—a pyrrhic victory? *N. Engl. J. Med.*, **1983**, *309*, 1118–1119.

Calabresi, P.; Dexter, D. L.; and Heppner, G. H. Clinical and pharmacological implications of cancer cell differentiation and heterogeneity. *Biochem. Pharmacol.*, **1979**, *28*, 1933–1941.

Carrico, C. K., and Sartorelli, A. C. Effects of 6-thiogua-

nine on macromolecular events in regenerating rat liver. *Cancer Res.*, **1977**, *37*, 1868–1875.

Cortes, E. P.; Holland, J. F.; Moskowitz, R.; and Depoli, E. Effects of mithramycin on bone resorption *in vitro*. *Cancer Res.*, **1972**, *32*, 74–76.

Costanzi, J. J. Studies in the Southwest Oncology Group. *Cancer Treat. Rep.*, **1976**, *60*, 189–192.

Danenberg, P. V., and Lockshin, A. Fluorinated pyrimidines as tight-binding inhibitors of thymidylate synthetase. *Pharmacol. Ther.*, **1981**, *13*, 69–90.

DeFronzo, R. A.; Braine, H.; and Colvin, O. M. Water intoxication in man after cyclophosphamide therapy. Time course and relation to drug activation. *Ann. Intern. Med.*, **1973**, *78*, 861–869.

Durant, J. R.; Norgard, M. J.; Murad, T. M.; Bartolucci, A. A.; and Langford, K. H. Pulmonary toxicity associated with bischloroethylnitrosourea (BCNU). *Ann. Intern. Med.*, **1979**, *90*, 191–194.

Ehrenfeld, G. M.; Rodrigues, L. O.; Hecht, S. M.; Chang, C.; Basus, U. J.; and Oppenheimer, N. J. Copper (I) bleomycin: a structurally unique complex that mediates oxidative DNA strand scission. *Biochemistry*, **1985**, *24*, 81–92.

Einhorn, L. H., and Williams, S. D. The role of *cis*-platinum in solid tumor therapy. *N. Engl. J. Med.*, **1979**, *300*, 289–291.

Ensminger, W. D.; Rosowsky, A.; Raso, V.; Levin, D. C.; Glode, M.; Come, S.; Steele, G.; and Frei, E., III. A clinical-pharmacological evaluation of hepatic arterial infusions of 5-fluoro-2'-deoxyuridine and 5-fluorouracil. *Cancer Res.*, **1978**, *38*, 3784–3792.

Farber, S.; Diamond, L. K.; Mercer, R. D.; Sylvester, R. F.; and Wolff, V. A. Temporary remissions in acute leukemia in children produced by folic antagonist 4-amethopteroylglutamic acid (aminopterin). *N. Engl. J. Med.*, **1948**, *238*, 787–793.

Fauci, A. S.; Haynes, B. F.; Katz, P.; and Wolff, S. M. Wegener's granulomatosis: prospective clinical and therapeutic experience with 85 patients for 21 years. *Ann. Intern. Med.*, **1983**, *98*, 76–85.

Felson, D. T., and Anderson, J. Evidence for the superiority of immunosuppressive drugs and prednisone alone in lupus nephritis. *N. Engl. J. Med.*, **1984**, *311*, 1528–1533.

Fingert, H. J.; Treiman, A.; and Pardee, A. B. Transplantation of human or rodent tumors into cyclosporine-treated mice: a feasible model for studies of tumor biology and chemotherapy. *Proc. Natl Acad. Sci. U.S.A.*, **1984**, *81*, 7927–7931.

Fraile, R. J.; Baker, L. H.; Buroker, T. R.; Horwitz, J.; and Vaitkevicius, V. K. Pharmacokinetics of 5-fluorouracil administered orally, by rapid intravenous and slow infusion. *Cancer Res.*, **1980**, *40*, 2223–2228.

Furr, B. J. A., and Jordan, V. C. Pharmacology and clinical uses of tamoxifen. *Pharmacol. Ther.*, **1984**, *25*, 127–206.

Gaidys, W. G.; Dickerman, J. D.; Walters, C. L.; and Young, P. C. Intrathecal vincristine. *Cancer*, **1983**, *52*, 799–801.

Gershwin, M. E.; Goetzl, E. J.; and Steinberg, A. D. Cyclophosphamide: use in practice. *Ann. Intern. Med.*, **1974**, *80*, 531–540.

Giblett, E. R.; Anderson, J. E.; Cohen, F.; Pollara, B.; and Meuwissen, H. J. Adenosine-deaminase deficiency in two patients with severely impaired cellular immunity. *Lancet*, **1972**, *2*, 1067–1069.

Gilman, A. The initial clinical trial of nitrogen mustard. *Am. J. Surg.*, **1963**, *105*, 574–578.

Goldin, A. Studies with high-dose methotrexate—historical background. *Cancer Treat. Rep.*, **1978**, *62*, 307–312.

Goodman, L. S.; Wintrobe, M. M.; Dameshek, W.; Goodman, M. J.; Gilman, A.; and McLennan, M. Nitrogen mustard therapy: use of methylbis (B-chlorethyl) amino hydrochloride for Hodgkin's disease, lymphosarcoma, leukemia and certain allied and miscellaneous disorders. *J.A.M.A.*, **1946**, *132*, 126–132.

Gottlieb, J. A., and others. Role of DTIC (NSC-45388) in the chemotherapy of sarcomas. *Cancer Treat. Rep.*, **1976**, *60*, 199–203.

Green, D.; Tew, K. D.; Hisamatsu, T.; and Schein, P. S. Correlation of nitrosourea murine bone marrow toxicity with deoxyribonucleic acid alkylation and chromatin binding sites. *Biochem. Pharmacol.*, **1982**, *31*, 1671–1679.

Griffin, T. W.; Bogden, A. E.; Reich, S. D.; Antonelli, D.; Hunter, R. E.; Ward, A.; Yu, D. T.; Greene, H. L.; and Costanza, M. E. Initial clinical trials of the subrenal capsule assay as a predictor of tumor response to chemotherapy. *Cancer*, **1983**, *52*, 2185–2192.

Handschumacher, R. E.; Harding, M. W.; Drugge, R. J.; Rice, J.; and Speicher, D. W. Cyclophilin: a specific cytosolic binding protein for cyclosporin A. *Science*, **1984**, *226*, 544–547.

Harvey, H. A.; Santen, R. J.; Osterman, J.; Samojlik, E.; White, D. S.; and Lipton, A. A comparative trial of transphenoidal hypophysectomy and estrogen suppression with aminoglutethimide in advanced breast cancer. *Cancer*, **1979**, *43*, 2207–2214.

Heal, J. M.; Fox, P. A.; and Schein, P. S. Effect of carbamoylation on the repair of nitrosourea-induced DNA alkylation damage in L1210 cells. *Cancer Res.*, **1979**, *39*, 82–89.

Heidelberger, C.; Danenberg, P. V.; and Moran, R. C. Fluorinated pyrimidines and their nucleosides. *Adv. Enzymol.*, **1983**, *54*, 57–119.

Hemminki, K., and Ludlum, D. B. Covalent modification of DNA by antineoplastic agents. *J. Natl Cancer Inst.*, **1984**, *73*, 1021–1028.

Herbst, W. P. Effects of estradiol dipropionate and diethyl stilbestrol on malignant prostatic tissue. *Trans. Am. Assoc. Genitourin. Surg.*, **1941**, *34*, 195–202.

Herrmann, C. (ed.). Third conference on antiviral substances. *Ann. N.Y. Acad. Sci.*, **1977**, *284*, 1–197.

Hertz, R. Folic acid antagonists: effects on the cell and the patient. Clinical staff conference at N.I.H. *Ann. Intern. Med.*, **1963**, *59*, 931–956.

Ho, D. H. W. Potential advances in the clinical use of arabinosylcytosine. *Cancer Treat. Rep.*, **1977**, *61*, 717–722.

Hogan, T. F.; Citrin, D. L.; Johnson, B. M.; Nakamura, S.; Davis, T. E.; and Borden, E. C. *o,p'*-DDD (mitotane) therapy of adrenal cortical carcinoma. *Cancer*, **1978**, *42*, 2177–2181.

Huffman, D. H.; Wan, S. H.; Azarnoff, D. L.; and Hoogotraten, B. Pharmacokinetics of methotrexate. *Clin. Pharmacol. Ther.*, **1973**, *14*, 572–579.

Huggins, C.; Stevens, R. E., Jr.; and Hodges, C. V. Studies on prostatic cancer: effects of castration on advanced carcinoma of prostate gland. *Arch. Surg.*, **1941**, *43*, 209–223.

Jackson, R. C. Biological effects of folic acid antagonists with antineoplastic activity. *Pharmacol. Ther.*, **1984**, *25*, 61–82.

Jacobson, L. O.; Spurr, C. L.; Barron, E. S. G.; Smith, T. R.; Lushbaugh, C.; and Dick, G. F. Nitrogen mustard therapy: studies on the effect of methyl-*bis*(betachloroethyl) amine hydrochloride on neoplastic diseases and allied disorders of the hemopoietic system. *J.A.M.A.*, **1946**, *132*, 263–271.

Johnston, T. P.; McCaleb, G. S.; and Montgomery, J. A. The synthesis of antineoplastic agents. XXXII. N-Nitrosoureas. *J. Med. Chem.*, **1963**, *6*, 669–681.

Kaplan, S. R., and Calabresi, P. Drug therapy: immunosuppressive agents. Pt. I. *N. Engl. J. Med.*, **1973**, *289*, 952–954.

Kennedy, K. A.; Rockwell, S.; and Sartorelli, A. C. Preferential activation of mitomycin C to cytotoxic me-

tabolites by hypoxic tumor cells. *Cancer Res.*, **1980**, *40*, 2356–2360.

Kiang, D. T.; Frenning, D. H.; Goldman, A. I.; Ascensao, V. F.; and Kennedy, B. J. Estrogen receptors and responses to chemotherapy and hormonal therapy in advanced breast cancer. *N. Engl. J. Med.*, **1978**, *299*, 1330–1334.

Kiang, D. T., and Kennedy, B. J. Tamoxifen (antiestrogen) therapy in advanced breast cancer. *Ann. Intern. Med.*, **1977**, *87*, 687–690.

Knospe, W. H.; Loeb, V.; and Huguley, C. M. Biweekly chlorambucil treatment of chronic lymphocytic leukemia. *Cancer*, **1974**, *33*, 555–562.

Lazo, J. S.; Boland, C. J.; and Schwartz, P. E. Bleomycin hydrolase activity and cytotoxicity in human tumors. *Cancer Res.*, **1982**, *42*, 4026–4031.

Lerner, H. J. Acute myelogenous leukemia in patients receiving chlorambucil as long-term adjuvant chemotherapy for stage II breast cancer. *Cancer Treat. Rep.*, **1978**, *62*, 1135–1143.

Lerner, H. J.; Band, P. R.; Israel, L.; and Leung, B. S. Phase II study of tamoxifen: report of 74 patients with stage IV breast cancer. *Cancer Treat. Rep.*, **1976**, *60*, 1431–1435.

Leuprolide Study Group. Leuprolide versus diethylstilbestrol for metastatic prostate cancer. *N. Engl. J. Med.*, **1984**, *311*, 1281–1286.

Levin, V. A.; Hoffman, W.; and Weinkam, R. J. Pharmacokinetics of BCNU in man: a preliminary study of 20 patients. *Cancer Treat. Rep.*, **1978**, *62*, 1305–1312.

Lin, P. S.; Kwock, L.; Hefter, K.; and Misslbeck, G. Effects of iron, copper, cobalt, and their chelators on the cytotoxicity of bleomycin. *Cancer Res.*, **1983**, *43*, 1049–1053.

Loike, J. D., and Horwitz, S. B. Effect of VP-16-213 on the intracellular degradation of DNA in HeLa cells. *Biochemistry*, **1976**, *15*, 5443–5448.

Loo, T. L.; Housholder, G. E.; Gerulath, A. H.; Saunders, P. H.; and Farquhar, D. Mechanism of action and pharmacology studies with DTIC (NSC-45388). *Cancer Treat. Rep.*, **1976**, *60*, 149–157.

Lubitz, J. A.; Freeman, L.; and Okun, R. Mitotane use in inoperable adrenal cortical carcinoma. *J.A.M.A.*, **1973**, *223*, 1109–1112.

McDonald, C. J. The uses of systemic chemotherapeutic agents in psoriasis. *Pharmacol. Ther.*, **1981**, *14*, 1–24.

McDonald, C. J., and Calabresi, P. Azaribine for mycosis fungoides. *Arch. Dermatol.*, **1971**, *103*, 158–167.

——. Psoriasis and occlusive vascular disease. *Br. J. Dermatol.*, **1978**, *99*, 469–475.

McGuire, J. J.; Mini, E.; Hsieh, P.; and Bertino, J. R. Folylpolyglutamate synthetase: relation to methotrexate action and as a target for new drug development. In, *Development of Target-Oriented Anticancer Drugs. Progress in Cancer Research and Therapy*, Vol. 28. (Cheng, Y. C.; Goz, B.; and Minkoff, M.; eds.) Raven Press, New York, **1983**, pp. 97–106.

Manni, A.; Trujillo, J.; Marshall, J. S.; and Pearson, O. H. Antiestrogen-induced remissions in stage IV breast cancer. *Cancer Treat. Rep.*, **1976**, *60*, 1445–1450.

Matthews, D. A., and others. Dihydrofolate reductase from *Lactobacillus casei*; x-ray structure of the enzyme-methotrexate-NADPH complex. *J. Biol. Chem.*, **1978**, *253*, 6946–6954.

Minow, R. A.; Benjamin, R. S.; Lee, E. T.; and Gottlieb, J. A. Adriamycin cardiomyopathy-risk factors. *Cancer*, **1977**, *39*, 1397–1402.

Moertel, C. G. Therapy of advanced gastrointestinal cancer with the nitrosoureas. *Cancer Chemother. Rep.*, **1973**, *4*, 27–34.

Montgomery, J. A., and Hewson, K. Nucleosides of 2-fluoroadenosine. *J. Med. Chem.*, **1969**, *12*, 498.

Moseson, D. L.; Sasaki, G. H.; Kraybill, W. G.; Leung, B. S.; Davenport, C. E.; and Fletcher, W. S. The use of antiestrogens tamoxifen and nafoxidine in the treatment of human breast cancer in correlation with estrogen receptor values. *Cancer*, **1978**, *41*, 797–800.

Myers, B. D.; Ross, M. R. C. P.; Newton, L.; Luetscher, J.; and Perlroth, M. Cyclosporine-associated chronic nephropathy. *N. Engl. J. Med.*, **1984**, *311*, 699–705.

Noble, R. L.; Beer, C. T.; and Cutts, J. H. Further biological activities of vincaleukoblastine—an alkaloid isolated from *Vinca rosea* (L.). *Biochem. Pharmacol.*, **1958**, *1*, 347–348.

Oppenheimer, N. J.; Rodrigues, L. O.; and Hecht, S. M. Proton nuclear magnetic resonance study of the structure of bleomycin and the zinc bleomycin complex. *Biochemistry*, **1979**, *18*, 3439–3445.

Ostumi, J. A., and Roginsky, M. S. Metastatic adrenal cortical carcinoma. *Arch. Intern. Med.*, **1975**, *139*, 1257–1258.

Owellen, R. J.; Hartke, C. A.; and Hains, F. O. Pharmacokinetics and metabolism of vinblastine in humans. *Cancer Res.*, **1977**, *37*, 2597–2602.

Parrillo, J. E.; Fauci, A. S.; and Wolff, S. M. Therapy of the hypereosinophilic syndrome. *Ann. Intern. Med.*, **1978**, *89*, 167–172.

Passero, M. A.; Held, J. K.; and Shearer, P. M. Effects of bleomycin, O_2 concentration and H_2O_2 on peroxidation of arachidonic acid. *Am. Rev. Respir. Dis.*, **1983**, *127*, 287.

Povirk, L. F. Catalytic release of deoxyribonucleic bases by oxidation and reduction of an iron bleomycin complex. *Biochemistry*, **1979**, *18*, 3989–3995.

Primack, A. Amelioration of cyclophosphamide-induced cystitis. *J. Natl Cancer Inst.*, **1971**, *47*, 223–227.

Randolph, V. L.; Vallejo, A.; Spiro, R. H.; Shah, J.; Strong, E. W.; Huvos, A. G.; and Wittes, R. E. Combination therapy of advanced head and neck cancer. *Cancer*, **1978**, *41*, 460–467.

Rhoads, C. P. Nitrogen mustards in treatment of neoplastic disease: official statement. *J.A.M.A.*, **1946**, *131*, 656–658.

Rosenberg, B. Platinum coordination complexes in cancer chemotherapy. *Naturwissenschaften*, **1973**, *60*, 399–406.

Rosenberg, B.; VanCamp, L.; Grimley, E. B.; and Thomson, A. J. The inhibition of growth or cell division in *Escherichia coli* by different ionic species of platinum (IV) complexes. *J. Biol. Chem.*, **1967**, *242*, 1347–1352.

Rosenberg, B.; VanCamp, L.; and Krigas, T. Inhibition of cell division in *Escherichia coli* by electrolysis products from a platinum electrode. *Nature*, **1965**, *205*, 698–699.

Rosenberg, B.; VanCamp, L.; Trosko, J. E.; and Mansour, V. H. Platinum compounds: a new class of potent antitumour agents. *Nature*, **1969**, *222*, 385–386.

Rosenthal, F.; Wislicki, L.; and Kollek, L. Über die Beziehungen von schwersten Blutgiften zu Abbauprodukten des Eiweisses. *Klin. Wochenschr.*, **1928**, *7*, 972.

Rosman, M., and Bertino, J. R. Azathioprine. *Ann. Intern. Med.*, **1973**, *79*, 694–700.

Rustum, Y. M., and Priesler, H. D. Correlation between leukemic retention of 1-beta-D-arabinofuranosylcytosine-5′-triphosphate and response to therapy. *Cancer Res.*, **1979**, *39*, 42–49.

Rutty, C. J., and Connors, T. A. *In vitro* studies with hexamethylmelamine. *Biochem. Pharmacol.*, **1977**, *26*, 2385–2391.

Santen, R. J.; Samojlik, E.; and Wells, S. A. Resistance of the ovary to blockade of aromatization with aminoglutethimide. *J. Clin. Endocrinol. Metab.*, **1980**, *51*, 473–477.

Santen, R. J.; Worgul, T. J.; Lipton, A.; Harvey, H. A.; Boucher, A.; Samojlik, E.; and Wells, S. A. Aminoglutethimide as treatment of postmenopausal women with advanced breast carcinoma. *Ann. Intern. Med.*, **1982**, *96*, 94–101.

Santora, A., and Bonadonna, G. Prolonged disease-free survival in MOPP-resistant Hodgkin's disease after treatment with ADRIAMYCIN, bleomycin, vinblastine and dacarbazine (ABVD). *Cancer Chemother. Pharmacol.*, **1979**, *2*, 101–105.

Sausville, E. A.; Peisach, J.; and Horwitz, S. B. Effect of chelating agents and metal ions on the degradation of DNA by bleomycin. *Biochemistry*, **1978a**, *17*, 2740–2745.

Sausville, E. A.; Stein, R. W.; Peisach, J.; and Horwitz, S. B. Properties and products of the degradation of DNA by bleomycin and iron (II). *Biochemistry*, **1978b**, *17*, 2746–2754.

Schein, P.; Kahn, R.; Gorden, P.; Wells, S.; and DeVita, V. T. Streptozotocin for malignant insulinomas and carcinoid tumor. *Arch. Intern. Med.*, **1973**, *132*, 555–561.

Schein, P. S.; O'Connell, M. J.; Blom, J.; Hubbard, S.; Magrath, I. T.; Bergevin, P.; Wiernick, P. H.; Ziegler, J. L.; and DeVita, V. T. Clinical antitumor activity and toxicity of streptozotocin (NCS-86998). *Cancer*, **1974**, *34*, 993–1000.

Schein, P. S., and Winokur, S. H. Immunosuppressive and cytotoxic chemotherapy: long-term complications. *Ann. Intern. Med.*, **1975**, *82*, 84–95.

Selby, P.; Buick, R. N.; and Tannock, I. A critical appraisal of the "human tumor stem-cell assay." *N. Engl. J. Med.*, **1983**, *308*, 129–134.

Shubin, S. TRIAZURE and public drug policies. *Perspect. Biol. Med.*, **1979**, *22*, 185–204.

Sladek, N. E. Therapeutic efficacy of cyclophosphamide as a function of its metabolism. *Cancer Res.*, **1972**, *32*, 535–542.

Stark, G. R., and Bartlett, P. A. Design and use of potent, specific enzyme inhibitors. *Pharmacol. Ther.*, **1983**, *23*, 45–78.

Sternberg, J. J.; Bracken, B.; Handel, P. B.; and Johnson, D. E. Combination chemotherapy (CISCA) for advanced urinary tract carcinoma. *J.A.M.A.*, **1977**, *238*, 2282–2287.

Stott, H.; Fox, W.; Girling, D. J.; Stephans, R. J.; and Galton, D. A. Acute leukemia after busulphan. *Br. Med. J. [Clin. Res.]*, **1977**, *2*, 1513–1517.

Tattersall, M. H. N.; Jarman, M.; Newlands, E. S.; Holyhead, L.; Milstead, R. A. V.; and Weinberg, A. Pharmacokinetics of melphalan following oral or intravenous administration in patients with malignant disease. *Eur. J. Cancer*, **1978**, *14*, 507–513.

Tewey, K. M.; Rowe, T. C.; Yang, L.; Halligan, B. D.; and Liu, L. F. ADRIAMYCIN-induced DNA damage mediated by mammalian DNA topoisomerase II. *Science*, **1984**, *226*, 466–468.

Thomson, A. W. Immunobiology of cyclosporin—a review. *Aust. J. Exp. Biol. Med. Sci.*, **1983**, *61*, 147–172.

Toledo, C. H.; Ross, W. E.; Hood, C. I.; and Block, E. R. Potentiation of bleomycin toxicity by oxygen. *Cancer Treat. Rep.*, **1982**, *66*, 359–362.

Tong, W. P., and Ludlum, D. B. Crosslinking of DNA by busulfan. Formation of diguanyl derivatives. *Biochim. Biophys. Acta*, **1980**, *19*, 643–647.

Tormey, D. C.; Simon, R. M.; Lippman, M. E.; Bull, J. M.; and Myers, C. E. Evaluation of tamoxifen dose in advanced breast cancer: a progress report. *Cancer Treat. Rep.*, **1976**, *60*, 1451–1459.

Torti, F. M. Hormonal therapy for prostate cancer. *N. Engl. J. Med.*, **1984**, *311*, 1313–1314.

Tritsch, G. L. (ed.). Role of adenosine deaminase in disorders of purine metabolism and in immune deficiency. *Ann. N.Y. Acad. Sci.*, **1985**, in press.

Tritton, T. R.; Murphee, S. A.; and Sartorelli, A. C. ADRIAMYCIN: a proposal on the specificity of drug action. *Biochem. Biophys. Res. Commun.*, **1978**, *84*, 802–808.

Twentyman, P. R. Bleomycin—mode of action with particular reference to the cell cycle. *Pharmacol. Ther.*, **1984**, *23*, 417–441.

Valeriote, F., and Santelli, G. 5-Fluorouracil (FUra). *Pharmacol. Ther.*, **1984**, *24*, 107–132.

Vistica, D. T. Cellular pharmacokinetics of the phenylalanine mustards. *Pharmacol. Ther.*, **1983**, *22*, 379–415.

Vogelzang, N. J.; Raghavan, D.; and Kennedy, B. J. VP-16-213 (etoposide): the mandrake root from issykkul. *Am. J. Med.*, **1982**, *72*, 136–144.

Waksman, S. A., and Woodruff, H. B. Bacteriostatic and bactericidal substances produced by a soil actinomyces. *Proc. Soc. Exp. Biol. Med.*, **1940**, *45*, 609–614.

Wasserman, T. H. The nitrosoureas: an outline of clinical schedules and toxic effects. *Cancer Treat. Rep.*, **1976**, *60*, 709–711.

Wasserman, T. H.; Slavik, M.; and Carter, S. H. Clinical comparison of the nitrosoureas. *Cancer*, **1975**, *36*, 1258–1268.

Weinstein, G. D. Methotrexate. *Ann. Intern. Med.*, **1977**, *86*, 199–204.

Williams, M. E.; Walker, A. M.; Bracikowski, J. P.; Garner, L.; Wilson, K. D.; and Carpenter, J. T. Ascending myeloencephalopathy due to intrathecal vincristine sulfate. A fatal chemotherapeutic error. *Cancer*, **1983**, *51*, 2041–2147.

Wilson, C. B.; Gutin, P.; Boldrey, E. B.; Crafts, D.; Levin, V. A.; and Enot, K. J. Single-agent chemotherapy of brain tumors. *Arch. Neurol.*, **1976**, *33*, 739–744.

Wortsman, J., and Soler, N. G. Mitotane-spironolactone antagonism in Cushing's syndrome. *J.A.M.A.*, **1977**, *238*, 2527–2529.

Yagoda, A.; Watson, R. C.; Kemeny, N.; Barzell, W. E.; Grabstald, H.; and Whitmore, W. F., Jr. Diamminedichloride platinum II and cyclophosphamide in the treatment of advanced urothelial cancer. *Cancer*, **1978**, *41*, 2121–2130.

Young, R. C.; DeVita, V. T., Jr.; Serpick, A. A.; and Canellos, G. P. Treatment of advanced Hodgkin's disease with [1,3 *bis*(2-chloroethyl)-1-nitrosourea] BCNU. *N. Engl. J. Med.*, **1971**, *285*, 475–479.

Monographs and Reviews

Agrawal, K. C., and Sartorelli, A. C. α-(N)-heterocyclic carboxaldehyde thiosemicarbazones. In, *Antineoplastic and Immunosuppressive Agents*, Pt. II. (Sartorelli, A. C., and Johns, D. G., eds.) *Handbuch der Experimentellen Pharmakologie*, Vol. 38. Springer-Verlag, Berlin, **1975**, pp. 793–807.

Bender, R. A. Vinca alkaloids. In, *The Cancer Pharmacology Annual.* (Chabner, B. A., and Pinedo, H. M., eds.) Excerpta Medica, Amsterdam, **1983**, pp. 80–87.

Bender, R. A., and Chabner, B. A. Tubulin binding agents. In, *Pharmacologic Principles of Cancer Treatment.* (Chabner, B. A., ed.) W. B. Saunders Co., Philadelphia, **1982**, pp. 256–268.

Bergsagel, D. E. Plasma cell myeloma. An interpretive review. *Cancer*, **1972**, *30*, 1588–1594.

Bloomfield, C. D.; Hurd, D. D.; and Peterson, B. A. Leukemias. In, *Medical Oncology.* (Calabresi, P.; Schein, P. S.; and Rosenberg, S. A.; eds.) Macmillan Publishing Co., New York, **1985**, pp. 523–575.

Borch, R. F.; Bodenner, D. L.; and Katz, J. C. Diethyldithiocarbamate and cis-platinum toxicity. In, *Platinum Coordination Complexes in Cancer Chemotherapy.* (Hacker, M. P.; Douple, E. B.; and Krakoff, I. H.; eds.) Martinus Nijhoff, Boston, **1984**, pp. 154–164.

Brockman, R. W. Resistance to purine analogs. Clinical pharmacology symposium. *Biochem. Pharmacol.*, **1974**, *23*, Suppl. 2, pp. 107–117.

Broome, J. D. L-Asparaginase: discovery and development as a tumor-inhibitory agent. *Cancer Treat. Rep.*, **1981**, *65*, Suppl. 4, 111–114.

Cadman, E. Interaction of methotrexate and 5-fluorouracil. In, *Developments in Cancer Chemotherapy.* (Glazer, R. I., ed.) CRC Press, Inc., Boca Raton, **1984**, pp. 61–90.

Calabresi, P., and Dexter, D. L. Clinical implications of cancer cell heterogeneity. In, *Tumor Cell Heterogeneity: Origins and Implications.* (Owens, A. H., Jr.; Coffey, D. S.; and Baylin, S. B.; eds.) Academic Press, Inc., New York, **1982**, pp. 181–201.

Calabresi, P.; Schein, P. S.; and Rosenberg, S. A. (eds.). *Medical Oncology.* Macmillan Publishing Co., New York, **1985**.

Calabresi, P., and Welch, A. D. Chemotherapy of neoplastic diseases. *Annu. Rev. Med.*, **1962**, *13*, 147–202.

Capizzi, R. L., and Handschumacher, R. E. Asparaginase. In, *Cancer Medicine*, 2nd ed. (Holland, J. F., and Frei, E., III, eds.) Lea & Febiger, Philadelphia, **1982**, pp. 920–932.

Carter, S. K. An overview of the status of the nitrosoureas in other tumors. *Cancer Chemother. Rep.*, **1973**, *4*, 35–45.

Carter, S. K., and Slavik, M. Chemotherapy of cancer. *Annu. Rev. Pharmacol.*, **1974**, *14*, 157–179.

Chabner, B. A. Bleomycin. In, *Pharmacologic Principles of Cancer Treatment.* (Chabner, B. A., ed.) W. B. Saunders Co., Philadelphia, **1982a**, pp. 377–386.

———. Cytosine arabinoside. In, *Pharmacologic Principles of Cancer Treatment.* (Chabner, B. A., ed.) W. B. Saunders Co., Philadelphia, **1982b**, pp. 387–401.

———. Methotrexate. In, *Pharmacologic Principles of Cancer Treatment.* (Chabner, B. A., ed.) W. B. Saunders Co., Philadelphia, **1982c**, pp. 229–255.

———. Nonclassical alkylating agents. In, *Pharmacologic Principles of Cancer Treatment.* (Chabner, B. A., ed.) W. B. Saunders Co., Philadelphia, **1982d**, pp. 340–362.

———. Pyrimidine antagonists. In, *Pharmacologic Principles of Cancer Treatment.* (Chabner, B. A., ed.) W. B. Saunders Co., Philadelphia, **1982e**, pp. 183–212.

Chabner, B. A.; Donehower, R. C.; and Schilsky, R. L. Clinical pharmacology of methotrexate. *Cancer Treat. Rep.*, **1981**, *65*, Suppl. 1, 51–54.

Colvin, M. The alklylating agents. In, *Pharmacologic Principles of Cancer Treatment.* (Chabner, B. A., ed.) W. B. Saunders Co., Philadelphia, **1982**, pp. 276–308.

Connors, T. A. Mechanisms of clinical drug resistance. Clinical pharmacology symposium. *Biochem. Pharmacol.*, **1974**, *23*, Suppl. 2, 89–100.

———. Mechanism of action of 2-chloroethylamine derivatives, sulfur mustards, epoxides, and aziridines. In, *Antineoplastic and Immunosuppressive Agents*, Pt. II. (Sartorelli, A. C., and Johns, D. G., eds.) *Handbuch der Experimentellen Pharmakologie*, Vol. 38. Springer-Verlag, Berlin, **1975**, pp. 18–34.

———. Platinum compounds. In, *Cancer Medicine*, 2nd ed. (Holland, J. F., and Frei, E., III, eds.) Lea & Febiger, Philadelphia, **1982**, pp. 843–849.

———. Alkylating drugs, nitrosoureas and alkytriazenes. In, *The Cancer Pharmacology Annual.* (Chabner, B. A., and Pinedo, H. M., eds.) Excerpta Medica, Amsterdam, **1983**, pp. 29–50.

Creasey, W. A. Vinca alkaloids and colchicine. In, *Antineoplastic and Immunosuppressive Agents*, Pt. II. (Sartorelli, A. C., and Johns, D. G., eds.) *Handbuch der Experimentellen Pharmakologie*, Vol. 38. Springer-Verlag, Berlin, **1975**, pp. 670–694.

———. Plant alkaloids. In, *Cancer 5: A Comprehensive Treatise.* (Becker, F. F., ed.) Plenum Press, New York, **1977**, pp. 379–425.

Crooke, S. T. Antitumor antibiotics II: actinomycin D,

bleomycin, mitomycin C and other antibiotics. In, *The Cancer Pharmacology Annual.* (Chabner, B. A., and Pinedo, H. M., eds.) Excerpta Medica, Amsterdam, **1983**, pp. 69–79.

Crooke, S. T., and Bradner, W. T. Mitomycin C: a review. *Cancer Treat. Rev.*, **1976**, *3*, 121–139.

Cupps, T. R., and Fauci, A. S. The vasculitides. In, *Major Problems in Internal Medicine*, Vol. XXI. (Smith, L. H., Jr., ed.) W. B. Saunders Co., Philadelphia, **1981**.

DeVita, V. T., Jr.; Canellos, G. P.; and Moxley, J. H., III. A decade of combination chemotherapy of advanced Hodgkin's disease. *Cancer*, **1972**, *30*, 1495–1504.

DeVita, V. T., and Hellman, S. Hodgkin's disease and non-Hodgkin's lymphomas. In, *Cancer: Principles and Practice of Oncology.* (DeVita, V. T.; Hellman, S.; and Rosenberg, S. A.; eds.) J. P. Lippincott Co., Philadelphia, **1982**, pp. 1331–1401.

DiMarco, A. Daunomycin and adriamycin. In, *Antineoplastic and Immunosuppressive Agents*, Pt. II. (Sartorelli, A. C., and Johns, D. G., eds.) *Handbuch der Experimentellen Pharmakologie*, Vol. 38. Springer-Verlag, Berlin, **1975**, pp. 593–614.

———. Anthracycline antibiotics. In, *Cancer Medicine*, 2nd ed. (Holland, J. F., and Frei, E., III, eds.) Lea & Febiger, Philadelphia, **1982**, pp. 872–905.

D'Incalci, M., and Garattini, S. Podophyllin derivatives VP-16 and VM-26. In, *The Cancer Pharmacology Annual.* (Chabner, B. A., and Pinedo, H. M., eds.) Excerpta Medica, Amsterdam, **1983**, pp. 87–94.

Donehower, R. C. Hydroxyurea. In, *Pharmacologic Principles of Cancer Treatment.* (Chabner, B. A., ed.) W. B. Saunders Co., Philadelphia, **1982**, pp. 269–275.

Durant, J. R., and Omura, G. A. Gynecologic neoplasms. In, *Medical Oncology.* (Calabresi, P.; Schein, P. S.; and Rosenberg, S. A.; eds.) Macmillan Publishing Co., New York, **1985**, pp. 1004–1044.

Elion, G. B. Biochemistry and pharmacology of purine analogs. *Fed. Proc.*, **1967**, *26*, 898–904.

Elion, G. B., and Hitchings, G. H. Metabolic basis for the actions of analogs of purines and pyrimidines. *Adv. Chemother.*, **1965**, *2*, 91–177.

Fox, B. W. Mechanism of action of methanesulfonates. In, *Antineoplastic and Immunosuppressive Agents*, Pt. II. (Sartorelli, A. C., and Johns, D. G., eds.) *Handbuch der Experimentellen Pharmakologie*, Vol. 38. Springer-Verlag, Berlin, **1975**, pp. 35–46.

Gardner, F. H. Treatment of lymphoproliferative disease. In, *Cancer Chemotherapy II.* (Brodsky, I., and Kahn, S. B. eds.) Grune & Stratton, Inc., New York, **1972**, pp. 361–373.

Gianni, L.; Corden, B. J.; and Myers, C. E. The biochemical basis of anthracycline toxicity and antitumor activity. In, *Reviews in Biochemical Toxicology*, Vol. 5. (Hodgson, E.; Bend, J. R.; and Philpot, R. M.; eds.) Elsevier Science Publishing Co., Inc., New York, **1983**, pp. 1–82.

Gilman, A., and Philips, F. S. The biological actions and therapeutic applications of the β-chlorethylamines and sulfides. *Science*, **1946**, *103*, 409–415.

Glaubiger, D., and Ramu, A. Antitumor antibiotics. In, *Pharmacologic Principles of Cancer Treatment.* (Chabner, B. A., ed.) W. B. Saunders Co., Philadelphia, **1982**, pp. 402–415.

Goldberg, I. H.; Beerman, T. A.; and Poon, R. Antibiotics: nucleic acids as targets in chemotherapy. In, *Cancer 5: A Comprehensive Treatise.* (Becker, F. F., ed.) Plenum Press, New York, **1977**, pp. 427–456.

Goldman, I. D.; Matherly, L. H.; and Fabre, G. Methotrexate, aminopterin and 7-hydroxymethotrexate: recent concepts on the cellular pharmacology of 4-aminoantifolates. In, *Development of Target-Oriented Anticancer Drugs. Progress in Cancer Research and*

Therapy, Vol. 28. (Cheng, Y. C.; Goz, B.; and Minkoff, M.; eds.) Raven Press, New York, **1983**, pp. 19–41.

Grollman, A. P., and Takeshita, M. Interactions of bleomycin with DNA. In, *Advances in Enzyme Regulation.* (Weber, G., ed.) Pergamon Press, Ltd., Oxford, **1980**, pp. 67–83.

Hacker, M. P.; Douple, E. B.; and Krakoff, I. H. (eds.). *Platinum Coordination Complexes in Cancer Chemotherapy.* Martinus Nijhoff, Boston, **1984**.

Hall, E. *Radiobiology for the Radiobiologist*, 2nd ed. Harper & Row, Pub., Hagerstown, Md., **1978**.

Haynie, T. P., III; Johns, M. F.; and Glenn, H. J. Principles of nuclear medicine. In, *Cancer Medicine.* (Holland, J. F., and Frei, E., III, eds.) Lea & Febiger, Philadelphia, **1973**, pp. 567–599.

Heidelberger, C. Fluorinated pyrimidines and their nucleosides. In, *Antineoplastic and Immunosuppressive Agents*, Pt. II. (Sartorelli, A. C., and Johns, D. G., eds.) *Handbuch der Experimentellen Pharmakologie*, Vol. 38. Springer-Verlag, Berlin, **1975**, pp. 193–231.

———. Pyrimidine and pyrimidine nucleoside antimetabolites. In, *Cancer Medicine*, 2nd ed. (Holland, J. F., and Frei, E., III, eds.) Lea & Febiger, Philadelphia, **1982**, pp. 801–823.

Hess, A. D.; Tutschka, P. J.; and Santos, G. W. Effect of cyclosporine on the induction of cytotoxic lymphocytes: role of interleukin-1 and interleukin-2. *Transplant. Proc.*, **1983**, *15*, 2248–2258.

Hitchings, G. H. Rational design of anticancer drugs: here, imminent or illusive. In, *Development of Target-Oriented Anticancer Drugs. Progress in Cancer Research and Therapy*, Vol. 28. (Cheng, Y. C.; Goz, B.; and Minkoff, M.; eds.) Raven Press, New York, **1983**, pp. 227–238.

Holland, J. F., and Frei, E., III (eds.). *Cancer Medicine*, 2nd ed. Lea & Febiger, Philadelphia, **1982**.

Hutter, A. M., Jr., and Kayhoe, D. E. Adrenal cortical carcinoma: clinical features of 138 patients. *Am. J. Med.*, **1966**, *41*, 572–592.

Johns, D. G., and Bertino, J. R. Folate antagonists. In, *Cancer Medicine*, 2nd ed. (Holland, J. F., and Frei, E., III, eds.) Lea & Febiger, Philadelphia, **1982**, pp. 775–789.

Johnson, I. S. Plant alkaloids. In, *Cancer Medicine*, 2nd ed. (Holland, J. F., and Frei, E., III, eds.) Lea & Febiger, Philadelphia, **1982**, pp. 910–919.

Jolivet, J., and Chabner, B. A. Methotrexate polyglutamates in cultured human breast cancer cells. In, *Development of Target-Oriented Anticancer Drugs. Progress in Cancer Research and Therapy*, Vol. 28. (Cheng, Y. C.; Goz, B.; and Minkoff, M.; eds.) Raven Press, New York, **1983**, pp. 89–96.

Jolivet, J.; Curt, G. A.; Clendeninn, N. S.; and Chabner, B. A. Antimetabolites. In, *The Cancer Pharmacology Annual.* (Chabner, B. A., and Pinedo, H. M., eds.) Excerpta Medica, Amsterdam, **1983**, pp. 1–28.

Jordan, V. C. Metabolites of tamoxifen in animals and man: identification, pharmacology, and significance. *Breast Cancer Res. Treat.*, **1982a**, *2*, 123–138.

———. Pharmacology of antiestrogens. In, *Endocrinology of Cancer.* (Rose, D. P., ed.) CRC Press, Inc., Boca Raton, **1982b**, pp. 129–173.

Kahan, B. D.; Van Buren, C. T.; Flechner, S. M.; Payne, W. D.; Boileau, M.; and Kerman, R. H. Cyclosporine immunosuppression mitigates immunologic risk factors in renal allotransplantation. *Transplant. Proc.*, **1983**, *15*, Suppl. 1, 2469–2478.

Kreis, W. Hydrazines and triazenes. In, *Cancer 5: A Comprehensive Treatise.* (Becker, F. F., ed.) Plenum Press, New York, **1977**, pp. 489–519.

Kufe, D. W., and Major, P. P. Studies on the mechanism of action of cytosine arabinoside. *Med. Pediatr. Oncol.*, **1982**, Suppl. 1, 49–67.

Lafferty, K. J.; Borel, J. F.; and Hodgkin, P. Cyclosporine-A (CsA); models for the mechanism of action. *Transplant. Proc.*, **1983**, *15*, Suppl. 1, 2230–2241.

Lane, M. Chemotherapy of cancer. In, *Cancer*, 5th ed. (del Regato, J. A., and Spjut, H. J., eds.) C. V. Mosby Co., St. Louis, **1977**, pp. 105–130.

Legha, S. S.; Davis, H. L.; and Muggia, F. M. Hormonal therapy of breast cancer: new approaches and concepts. *Ann. Intern. Med.*, **1978**, *88*, 69–77.

Liu, Y.-P., and Chabner, B. A. Enzyme therapy: L-Asparaginase. In, *Pharmacologic Principles of Cancer Treatment.* (Chabner, B. A., ed.) W. B. Saunders Co., Philadelphia, **1982**, pp. 435–443.

Livingston, R. B., and Carter, S. K. *Single Agents in Cancer Chemotherapy.* Plenum Press, New York, **1970**.

Loo, T. L., and Nelson, J. A. Purine antimetabolites. In, *Cancer Medicine*, 2nd ed. (Holland, J. F., and Frei, E., III, eds.) Lea & Febiger, Philadelphia, **1982**, pp. 790–800.

Ludlum, D. B., and Tong, W. P. DNA modification by the nitrosoureas: chemical nature and cellular repair. In, *Cancer Chemotherapy*, Vol. II. (Muggia, E. M., and Nishoff, M., eds.) Martinus Nijhoff, Boston, **1985**, pp. 141–154.

McCormack, J. J., and Johns, D. G. Purine antimetabolites. In, *Pharmacologic Principles of Cancer Treatment.* (Chabner, B. A., ed.) W. B. Saunders Co., Philadelphia, **1982**, pp. 213–228.

Maley, F. Pyrimidine antagonists. In, *Cancer 5: A Comprehensive Treatise.* (Becker, F. F., ed.) Plenum Press, New York, **1977**, pp. 327–353.

Moertel, C. G. Current concepts in chemotherapy of gastrointestinal cancer. *N. Engl. J. Med.*, **1978**, *299*, 1049–1052.

Myers, C. E. Anthracyclines. In, *Pharmacologic Principles of Cancer Treatment.* (Chabner, B. A., ed.) W. B. Saunders Co., Philadelphia, **1982**, pp. 416–434.

———. Antitumor antibiotics I: anthracyclines. In, *The Cancer Pharmacology Annual.* (Chabner, B. A., and Pinedo, H. M., eds.) Excerpta Medica, Amsterdam, **1983**, pp. 51–68.

Myers, C. E.; Corden, B.; and Gianni, L. Antitumor antibiotics I: anthracyclines. In, *The Cancer Pharmacology Annual 2.* (Chabner, B. A., and Pinedo, H. M., eds.) Elsevier, Amsterdam, **1984**, pp. 66–79.

O'Dwyer, P. J.; Leyland-Jones, B.; Alonso, M. T.; Marsoni, S.; and Wittes, R. E. Etoposide (VP-16-213). Current status of an active anticancer drug. *N. Engl. J. Med.*, **1985**, *312*, 692–700.

Oliverio, V. T. Toxicology and pharmacology of the nitrosoureas. *Cancer Chemother. Rep.*, **1973**, *4*, Pt. 3, No. 3, 13–20.

———. Pharmacology of the nitrosoureas: an overview. *Cancer Treat. Rep.*, **1976**, 60, 703–707.

———. Derivatives of triazanes and hydrazines. In, *Cancer Medicine*, 2nd ed. (Holland, J. F., and Frei, E., III, eds.) Lea & Febiger, Philadelphia, **1982**, pp. 850–860.

Pallavicini, M. G. Cytosine arabinoside: molecular pharmacokinetic and cytokinetic considerations. *Pharmacol. Ther.*, **1984**, *25*, 207–235.

Paridaens, R. J.; Leclercq, G.; and Heuson, J. C. Steroid hormones, analogs and antagonists. *The Cancer Pharmacology Annual 2.* (Chabner, B. A., and Pinedo, H. M., eds.) Elsevier, Amsterdam, **1984**, pp. 171–192.

Patterson, M. K., Jr. L-Asparaginase: basic aspects. In, *Antineoplastic and Immunosuppressive Agents*, Pt. II. (Sartorelli, A. C., and Johns, D. G., eds.) *Handbuch der Experimentellen Pharmakologie*, Vol. 38. Springer-Verlag, Berlin, **1975**, pp. 695–722.

Pinkel, D., and Howarth, C. B. Pediatric neoplasms. In, *Medical Oncology.* (Calabresi, P.; Schein, P. S.; and Rosenberg, S. A.; eds.) Macmillan Publishing Co., New York, **1985**, pp. 1226–1258.

Price, C. C. Chemistry of alkylation. In, *Antineoplastic and Immunosuppressive Agents*, Pt. II. (Sartorelli, A. C., and Johns, D. G., eds.) *Handbuch der Experimentellen Pharmakologie*, Vol. 38. Springer-Verlag, Berlin, **1975**, pp. 1–5.

Reich, S. D. Clinical pharmacology of mitomycin C. In, *Mitomycin C: Current Status and New Developments.* (Carter, S. K., and Crooke, S. T., eds.) Academic Press, Inc., New York, **1979**.

Roberts, J. Cisplatin. In, *The Cancer Pharmacology Annual.* (Chabner, B. A., and Pinedo, H. M., eds.) Excerpta Medica, Amsterdam, **1983**, pp. 95–117.

Robins, P. R., and Jowsey, J. Effect of mithramycin on normal and abnormal bone turnover. *J. Lab. Clin. Med.*, **1973**, *82*, 576–586.

Rozencweig, M.; Von Hoff, D. D.; Slavik, M.; and Muggia, F. M. *Cis*-diammine dichloroplatinum (II)—a new cancer drug. *Ann. Intern. Med.*, **1977**, *86*, 803–812.

Sartorelli, A. C., and Johns, D. G. (eds.). *Antineoplastic and Immunosuppressive Agents*, Pt. II. *Handbuch der Experimentellen Pharmakologie*, Vol. 38. Springer-Verlag, Berlin, **1975**.

Schabel, F. M., Jr. Historical development and future promise of the nitrosoureas as anticancer agents. *Cancer Chemother. Rep.*, **1973**, *4*, Part 3, No. 3, 3–6.

Schimke, R. T.; Kaufman, R. J.; Alt, F. W.; and Kellems, R. F. Gene amplification and drug resistance in cultured murine cells. *Science*, **1978**, *202*, 1051–1055.

Shapiro, R. Chemistry of guanine and its biologically significant derivatives. *Prog. Nucleic Acid Res. Mol. Biol.*, **1968**, *8*, 73–112.

Sirotnak, F. M. Concepts in new folate analog design. In, *Development of Target-Oriented Anticancer Drugs. Progress in Cancer Research and Therapy*, Vol. 28. (Cheng, Y. C.; Goz, B.; and Minkoff, M.; eds.) Raven Press, New York, **1983**, pp. 77–88.

Skipper, H. T., and Schabel, F. M., Jr. Quantitative and cytokinetic studies in experimental tumor models. In, *Cancer Medicine*, 2nd ed. (Holland, J. F., and Frei, E., III, eds.) Lea & Febiger, Philadelphia, **1982**, pp. 663–684.

Skoda, J. Azapyrimidine nucleosides. In, *Antineoplastic and Immunosuppressive Agents*, Pt. II. (Sartorelli, A. C., and Johns, D. G., eds.) *Handbuch der Experimentellen Pharmakologie*, Vol. 38. Springer-Verlag, Berlin, **1975**, pp. 348–372.

Sobell, H. M. The stereochemistry of actinomycin binding to DNA and its implications in molecular biology. *Prog. Nucleic Acid Res. Mol. Biol.*, **1973**, *13*, 153–190.

Stark, G. R., and Wahl, G. M. Gene amplification. *Annu. Rev. Biochem.*, **1984**, *53*, 447–491.

Symposium. (Various authors.) Cyclophosphamide in pediatric neoplasia. (Oernbach, D. J., ed.) *Cancer Chemother. Rep.*, **1967**, *51*, 315–412.

Symposium. (Various authors.) The nitrosoureas. *Cancer Chemother. Rep.*, **1973**, *4*, Pt. 3, 1–82.

Symposium. (Various authors.) Eighth new drug seminar: L-asparaginase and daunorubicin. *Cancer Treat. Rep.*, **1981a**, *65*, Suppl. 4, 1–130.

Symposium. (Various authors.) Proceedings of the international symposium on methotrexate. *Cancer Treat. Rep.*, **1981b**, *65*, Suppl. 1, 1–189.

Symposium. (Various authors.) Cellular resistance to anticancer drugs. *Cancer Treat. Rep.*, **1983a**, *67*, 855–965.

Symposium. (Various authors.) First international congress on cyclosporine. (Kahan, B. D., ed.) *Transplant. Proc.*, **1983b**, *15*, Suppls. 1 and 2, 2207–3188.

Symposium. (Various authors.) *Regulatory Functions of Adenosine.* (Berne, R. M.; Rall, T. W.; and Rubio, R.; eds.) Martinus Nijhoff, Boston, **1983c**.

Symposium. (Various authors.) Proceedings of the conference on 2′-deoxycoformycin: current status and future directions. *Cancer Treatment Symposia*, Vol. 2,

National Cancer Institute, Washington, D. C., **1984**, pp. 1–104.

Umezawa, H. Studies on bleomycin: chemistry and the biological action. *Biomedicine,* **1973**, *18,* 459–475.

————. Cancer drugs of microbial origin. In, *Methods in Cancer Research, XVI: Cancer Drug Development,* Pt. A. (DeVita, V. T., Jr., and Busch, H., eds.) Academic Press, Inc., New York, **1979**, pp. 43–72.

————. Principles of antitumor therapy. In, *Cancer Medicine,* 2nd ed. (Holland, J. F., and Frei, E., III, eds.) Lea & Febiger, Philadelphia, **1982**, pp. 860–871.

Umezawa, H., and Takita, T. Antitumor antibiotics II: actinomycin D, bleomycin, mitomycin C, neocarzinostatin and other antibiotics. In, *The Cancer Pharmacology Annual 2.* (Chabner, B. A., and Pinedo, H. M., eds.) Elsevier, Amsterdam, **1984**, pp. 80–93.

Waksman Conference on Actinomycins: their potential for cancer chemotherapy. *Cancer Chemother. Rep.,* **1974**, *58,* 1–123.

Walker, M. D. Nitrosoureas in central nervous system tumors. *Cancer Chemother. Rep.,* **1973**, *4,* 21–26.

Warwick, G. P. The mechanism of action of alkylating agents. *Cancer Res.,* **1963**, *23,* 1315–1333.

Weil, C. Cyclosporin A: review of results in organ and bone-marrow transplantation in man. In, *Medicinal Research Reviews,* Vol. 4. John Wiley & Sons, Inc., New York, **1984**, pp. 221–265.

Weinkam, R. J.; Shiba, D. A.; and Chabner, B. A. Nonclassical alkylating agents. In, *Pharmacologic Principles of Cancer Treatment.* (Chabner, B. A., ed.) W. B. Saunders Co., Philadelphia, **1982**, pp. 340–362.

Wenger, R. Synthesis of cyclosporine and analogues: Structure activity relationships of new cyclosporine derivatives. *Transplant. Proc.,* **1983**, *15,* Suppl. 1, 2230–2241.

Wheeler, G. P. Some biochemical effects of alkylating agents. *Fed. Proc.,* **1967**, *26,* 885–892.

————. Alkylating agents. In, *Cancer Medicine,* 2nd ed. (Holland, J. F., and Frei, E., III, eds.) Lea & Febiger, Philadelphia, **1982**, pp. 824–842.

Wiemann, M. C., and Calabresi, P. Pharmacology of antineoplastic agents. In, *Medical Oncology.* (Calabresi, P.; Schein, P. S.; and Rosenberg, S. A.; eds.) Macmillan Publishing Co., New York, **1985**, pp. 292–362.

Williams, S. D., and Einhorn, L. H. Neoplasms of the testis. In, *Medical Oncology.* (Calabresi, P.; Schein, P. S.; and Rosenberg, S. A.; eds.) Macmillan Publishing Co., New York, **1985**, pp. 1077–1088.

Young, R. C.; Lippman, M.; DeVita, V. T., Jr.; Brell, J.; and Tormey, D. Perspectives in the treatment of breast cancer: 1976. *Ann. Intern. Med.,* **1977**, *86,* 784–798.

Zinner, S. H., and Klastersky, J. Infectious considerations in cancer. In, *Medical Oncology.* (Calabresi, P.; Schein, P. S.; and Rosenberg, S. A.; eds.) Macmillan Publishing Co., New York, **1985**, pp. 1327–1357.

Zwelling, L. A., and Kohn, K. W. Platinum complexes. In, *Pharmacologic Principles of Cancer Treatment.* (Chabner, B. A., ed.) W. B. Saunders Co., Philadelphia, **1982**, pp. 309–339.

Drugs Acting on the Blood and the Blood-Forming Organs

A large number of drugs, including many vitamins and minerals, affect the blood and the blood-forming organs, either directly or indirectly. Agents effective in specific anemias include iron, copper, vitamin B_{12}, folic acid, pyridoxine, and riboflavin; these substances are discussed in the following two chapters. In the final chapter of this section, chief attention is devoted to the anticoagulants, heparin and the oral anticoagulants; to thrombolytic agents; and to drugs affecting platelet function.

Many dietary factors are important for normal hematopoiesis, blood coagulation, and the integrity of the vascular wall; some of them are discussed in the section concerning the vitamins. Certain internal secretions can profoundly influence the blood, such as those from the thyroid, the gonads, and the adrenal cortex; these are dealt with in the section devoted to the hormones. A vast array of drugs exert toxic effects on the formed elements of the blood, on hemoglobin, or on the hematopoietic organs. The toxic effects include granulocytopenia, thrombocytopenia, aplastic anemia, hemolytic anemia, and the conversion of hemoglobin into nonfunctional forms. Agents that somewhat selectively depress abnormal proliferation of the cellular elements of the blood are discussed in Chapter 55.

The discovery of liver therapy for pernicious anemia, by Minot and Murphy in 1926, was followed by a marked revival of interest in the field of blood diseases and their therapy. As a result, our knowledge of the mechanisms of blood formation and destruction, the metabolism of iron, the pathological physiology of pernicious and other megaloblastic anemias, and the specificity of hematinic agents is decidedly more complete. The physician now has at his command many reliable procedures for the accurate diagnosis of blood disorders and several drugs for their specific therapy. It is no longer permissible to prescribe these agents without first ascertaining, as nearly as possible, the exact nature of the abnormality. Proper treatment rests upon a clear understanding of the pharmacological properties of the hematopoietic drugs.

The term *nutritional anemias* has been used to indicate the multifactorial nature of anemias that occur in individuals whose diets are inadequate in quantity or quality. Most frequently, deficiencies of iron or protein are responsible; however, in certain geographical areas and in certain individuals with unusual diets, other deficiencies, particularly that of folic acid, are prominent. Each deficiency anemia has its own peculiarities with respect to diet, and more often than not it occurs alone. For the practicing physician, the term *nutritional anemia* now has little value and encourages inappropriate generalization. Possible causes of deficiency need to be considered on an individual basis. All arise from one or more of the following basic causes: inadequate ingestion, absorption, or utilization, or increased requirement, excretion, or metabolic destruction of the nutrient. Knowledge of the food sources and metabolism of nutrients is therefore crucial to determine the causes of such deficiencies; this information is provided in the following two chapters as it relates to iron, folate, vitamin B_{12}, and other nutritional factors that are important for hematopoiesis.

56 DRUGS EFFECTIVE IN IRON-DEFICIENCY AND OTHER HYPOCHROMIC ANEMIAS

Robert S. Hillman and Clement A. Finch

IRON AND IRON SALTS

Iron deficiency is the most common cause of nutritional anemia in man. When severe, it results in a characteristic microcytic, hypochromic anemia secondary to a reduction in the synthesis of hemoglobin. Since more than 80% of the iron present in the body is involved in the support of red-cell production, this is not surprising. However, the impact of iron deficiency is not limited to the erythron (Dallman, 1982). Iron is also an essential component of myoglobin; heme enzymes such as the cytochromes, catalase, and peroxidase; and the metalloflavoprotein enzymes, including xanthine oxidase and the mitochondrial enzyme alpha-glycerophosphate oxidase. Iron deficiency can affect metabolism in muscle independently of the effect of anemia on oxygen delivery. This may well reflect a reduction in the activity of iron-dependent mitochondrial enzymes. Iron deficiency has also been associated with behavioral and learning problems in children and with abnormalities in catecholamine metabolism and, possibly, heat production (Pollit and Leibel, 1982; Martinez-Torres *et al.*, 1984). Awareness of this ubiquitous role of iron has stimulated considerable interest in the early and accurate detection of iron deficiency and also in its prevention.

History. Early in civilization, man learned to mine iron and to forge tools of great strength. This entry into the *iron age* carried with it a belief in the special powers of the metal. Legends and early writings described the many medicinal uses to which this "metal from heaven" could be put (Fairbanks *et al.*, 1971). Iron was used extensively by European physicians through the Middle Ages and the Renaissance, but with little rationale. In the sixteenth century the causative role of iron deficiency in the then-prevalent "green sickness" or chlorosis of adolescent women began to be recognized. It may be that the treatment of this disorder with iron had already enjoyed some vogue in Europe, but Sydenham is properly credited with identifying iron as a specific remedy to take the place of bleedings and purgings. In 1681, he wrote (*see* Latham, 1850): ". . . I comfort the blood and the spirit belonging to it by giving a chalybeate [containing or charged with iron] 30 days running. This is sure to do good. To the worn out or languid blood it gives a spur or fillip, whereby the animal spirits which before lay prostrate and sunken under their own weight are raised and excited. Clear proof of this is found in the effect of steel in chlorosis. The pulse gains strength, the face (no longer pale and deathlike) a fresh ruddy color." In 1713, Lemery and Geoffry provided more direct evidence of the relationship by showing that iron was present in blood (ash) (*see* Christian, 1903). In 1832, the French physician Pierre Blaud wrote that the malady chlorosis ". . . arises from a faulty formation of blood as a result of which the blood is an imperfect fluid or the coloring matter is so defective that it is no longer suitable for stimulating the organism and maintaining the regular exercise of its functions." Blaud recognized that failure in the treatment of chlorosis had been due to the use of too small doses of iron and reported the rapid cure of 30 patients given a mixture of equal parts of ferrous sulfate and potassium carbonate in dosage increasing to as much as 770 mg of elemental iron daily. For many years Blaud's nephew distributed the "veritable pills of Blaud" throughout the world (Neuroth and Lee, 1941). The treatment of anemia with iron followed the principles enunciated by Sydenham and Blaud until the last decade of the nineteenth century and was comparable to modern practice in the amount of iron available for absorption that was prescribed. At that time, however, the teachings of Bunge, Quincke, von Noorden, and others cast doubt on this straightforward approach to the treatment of chlorosis. The dose of iron employed was reduced, and the resulting inefficacy of smaller doses brought discredit on the therapy. It was not until the third and fourth decades of the present century, through the efforts of Faber and Gram, Bloomfield, Heath and associates, and Reimann and coworkers, that the lessons taught by the earlier physicians were relearned (*see* Haden, 1939).

The past half century has brought a clearer understanding of many aspects of iron metabolism in man. In 1937, McCance and Widdowson reported on studies of iron balance that suggested a limited daily absorption and excretion of the element. At the same time, Heilmeyer and Plotner (1937) made quantitative measurements of the concentration of iron in plasma and discussed its function in transport. Laurell in 1947 presented similar information concerning the plasma iron transport protein, which he called *transferrin*. In the early 1940s, Hahn (Hahn *et al.*, 1943) introduced the use of radioactive isotopes of iron as a means to quantitate absorption and demonstrated the capacity of the intestinal mucosa to regulate this function. In the next decade, Huff and associates (1950) initiated isotopic studies of internal iron exchange. In the past 25 years practical clinical measurements of the degree of saturation of transferrin and red-cell protoporphyrin have been developed to a point that permits the accurate detection of iron-deficient erythropoiesis, while quantitation of iron in plasma ferritin and in marrow reveals the status of the body's stores (*see* Bothwell *et al.*, 1979). Even more recently, quantitative methods have been developed for evaluation of the absorption of iron in food, and these have explained the high prevalence of iron deficiency in man as a function of the limited availability of iron in the contemporary diet (Cook and Finch, 1975).

Iron and the Environment. Iron is one of the most abundant elements in the earth's crust; only oxygen, silicon, and aluminum are more common. It exists largely in its trivalent form as ferric oxide or hydroxide or as polymers. In this state, its biological availability is limited unless solubilized by acid or chelates. For example, to meet their needs, bacteria produce high-affinity chelating agents that can extract iron from the surrounding environment (Neilands, 1974). Some plants also have an unique ability to secrete substances that mobilize iron from soils for transport and incorporation into both nonheme and heme-containing enzymes or for storage as phytoferritin. The need for such adaptive mechanisms reflects the poor availability of most environmental iron. In alkaline or high-phosphate soils, plants can, in fact, develop an iron-deficiency disease, chlorosis, manifest by yellowness or blanching of normally green parts. While it might be expected that higher vertebrates would have the greatest problem meeting their requirements because of the high demand for iron to produce hemoglobin, most mammals have little difficulty in acquiring iron. This is probably explained by a more ample iron intake and perhaps also by their greater efficiency in absorbing iron. Man, however, appears to be an exception. While total dietary intake of elemental iron exceeds requirements, the bioavailability of the iron in the diet is limited.

Iron Metabolism in Man. The body store of iron is divided between iron-containing compounds that are essential and those in which excess iron is held in storage. From a quantitative standpoint, *hemoglobin* dominates the essential fraction (Table 56–1). This protein, with a molecular weight of 64,500, contains four atoms of iron per mol-

Table 56–1. THE BODY CONTENT OF IRON

	MALE	FEMALE
	mg/kg of body weight	
Essential iron		
Hemoglobin	31	28
Myoglobin and enzymes	6	5
Storage iron	13	4
Total	50	37

ecule, amounting to 1.1 mg of iron per milliliter of red blood cells. Other forms of essential iron include myoglobin and a variety of heme and nonheme iron-dependent enzymes (Sigel, 1977). *Ferritin* is the protein of iron storage, and it exists as individual molecules or in an aggregated form. Apoferritin has a molecular weight of about 450,000 and is composed of some 24 polypeptide subunits; these form an outer shell within which there is a storage cavity for polynuclear hydrous ferric oxide phosphate (Harrison, 1977). Over 30% of the weight of ferritin may be iron. Aggregated ferritin, referred to as *hemosiderin* and visible by light microscopy, constitutes about one third of normal stores, a fraction that increases as stores enlarge (Wixom *et al.*, 1979). The two predominant sites of iron storage are the reticuloendothelial system and the hepatocytes, although some storage also occurs in muscle (Bothwell *et al.*, 1979).

Internal exchange of iron is accomplished by the plasma protein *transferrin* (Aisen and Brown, 1977). This β_1-glycoprotein has a molecular weight of about 76,000 and two binding sites for ferric iron. Iron is delivered from transferrin to intracellular sites by means of specific receptors in the plasma membrane. The iron-transferrin complex binds to the receptor and is taken up by receptor-mediated endocytosis. Iron subsequently dissociates in a pH-dependent fashion in an acidic, intracellular vesicular compartment, and the receptor returns the ferritin to the cell surface to function again (*see* Brown *et al.*, 1983). The concentration of these receptors for transferrin on a given cell is related to the widely disparate requirement of different tissues for iron. The essential role of transferrin is illustrated by the maldistribution of iron that occurs in congenital atransferrinemia. These patients have iron-deficiency anemia despite excessive concentrations of iron in nonerythroid tissues (Goya *et al.*, 1972).

The flow of iron through the plasma amounts to a total of 30 to 40 mg per day in the adult (about 0.46 mg/kg of body weight) (Finch *et al.*, 1970). The major internal circulation of iron involves the erythron and the reticuloendothelial cell (Figure 56–1). About 80% of the iron in plasma goes to the erythroid marrow to be packaged into new erythrocytes; these normally circulate for about 120 days before being catabolized by the reticuloendothelium. At that time a portion of the iron is immediately returned to the plasma bound to transferrin, while another portion is incorporated into the ferritin stores of the reticuloendothelial cell and is returned to the circulation more gradually. Isotopic studies indicate some degree of iron wastage in this process, wherein defective cells or unused portions of their iron are transferred to the reticuloendothelial cell during maturation, bypassing the circulating blood. In hemolytic anemia the uptake of iron by the erythron may increase five to tenfold, with a corresponding increase in red-cell breakdown. When there

are abnormalities in maturation of red cells, the predominant portion of iron assimilated by the erythroid marrow may be rapidly localized in the reticuloendothelial cell as defective red-cell precursors are broken down; this is termed *ineffective erythropoiesis*. With red-cell aplasia, the rate of turnover of iron in plasma may be reduced by one half or more, with all of the iron now going to the hepatocyte for storage. It should be noted that nonerythroid tissues do not have the ability of erythropoietic cells to increase their number of membrane receptors for transferrin; their capacity to take up iron is thus always limited.

The most remarkable feature of iron metabolism in man is the degree to which the body store is conserved. Only 10% of the total is lost per year from normal men, that is, about 1 mg per day (Green *et al.*, 1968). Two thirds of this iron is excreted from the gastrointestinal tract as extravasated red cells, iron in bile, and iron in exfoliated mucosal cells. The other third is accounted for by small amounts of iron in desquamated skin and in the urine. Physiological losses of iron in the male vary over a relatively narrow range, decreasing to about 0.5 mg in the iron-deficient individual and increasing to as much as 1.5 or possibly 2 mg per day when excessive iron is consumed. Additional losses of iron occur in the female due to menstruation (Hallberg *et al.*, 1966a). While this averages about 0.5 mg per day, 10% of normal menstruating females lose over 2 mg per day. Menstrual losses may be influenced by various types of contraceptive therapy. Loss can be reduced by about one half when estrogen-containing oral contraceptives are used and is increased by intrauterine devices. Pregnancy imposes a requirement for iron of even greater magnitude (Table 56–2). In addition to these physiological losses, there is a great variety of other causes of iron loss. Examples include the donation of blood, the use of anti-inflammatory drugs that cause bleeding from the gastric mucosa, gastrointestinal disease with associated bleeding, and so forth (Fairbanks *et al.*, 1971). Much rarer is the hemosiderinuria that follows intravascular hemolysis, which may result in urinary losses of iron of as much as 20 mg per day; still rarer is pul-

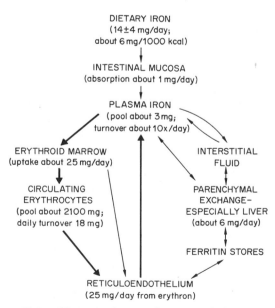

Figure 56–1. *Pathways of iron metabolism in man (excretion omitted).* (*See* text for explanation.)

monary siderosis, wherein iron is deposited in the lungs and becomes unavailable to the rest of the body.

The limited physiological losses of iron point to the primary importance of absorption as the determinant of the body's content of iron. Unfortunately, the biochemical nature of the absorptive process is understood only in general terms (Bothwell *et al.,* 1979). After acidification and partial digestion of food in the stomach, its content of iron is presented to the intestinal mucosa as either inorganic or heme iron. These fractions are taken up by the absorptive cells of the duodenum and upper small intestine, and the iron is either transported directly into the plasma or is stored as mucosal ferritin (Figure 56–2). Absorption is regulated by the relative activity of these two pathways, which is in some manner determined by the internal state of iron metabolism. Recent work suggests that the amount of a specific transferrin-like mucosal protein influences absorption (Huebers *et al.,* 1983). Normal absorption is about 1 mg per day in the adult male and 1.4 mg per day in the adult female. Increased uptake and delivery of iron into the circulation occur when there is iron deficiency, when iron stores are depleted, or when erythropoiesis is increased (Heinrich, 1983). However, there is a ceiling of 3 to 4 mg on the amount of dietary iron that may be absorbed, and this is set not only by the absorptive processes of the intestinal mucosa but also by the amount of available iron in the diet.

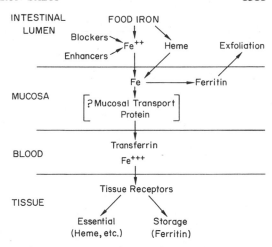

Figure 56–2. *Pathway of iron absorption.* (*See* text for explanation.)

Iron Requirements and the Availability of Dietary Iron. Iron requirements are determined by obligatory physiological losses and the needs imposed by growth. Thus, the adult male has a requirement of only 13 μg/kg per day (about 1 mg), whereas the menstruating female requires about 21 μg/kg per day (about 1.4 mg). In the last two trimesters of pregnancy, requirements increase to about 80 μg/kg per day (5 to 6 mg), and there are similar requirements for the infant due to its rapid growth (Finch, 1976). These requirements (Table 56–3) must be considered in the context of the amount of dietary iron available for absorption.

The dietary content of iron in developed countries is about 6 mg/1000 kcal; this places the average daily iron intake of the adult male between 12 and 20 mg and that of the adult female between 8 and 15 mg. Foods high in iron (greater than 5 mg/100 g) include organ meats such as liver and heart, brewer's yeast, wheat germ, egg yolks, oysters, and certain dried beans and fruits; foods containing intermediate amounts of iron (1 to 5 mg/100 g) include most muscle meats, fish and fowl, most green vegetables, and most cereals; foods low in iron (less than 1 mg/100 g) include milk and milk products and most nongreen vegetables. The general distribution of iron among foods, however, limits the value of manipulation of iron intake by food selection. The content of iron in food is further affected by

Table 56–2. IRON REQUIREMENTS FOR PREGNANCY

	AVERAGE	RANGE
	mg	*mg*
External iron loss	170	150–200
Expansion of red-blood-cell mass	450	200–600
Fetal iron	270	200–370
Iron in placenta and cord	90	30–170
Blood loss at delivery	150	90–310
Total requirement *	980	580–1340
Cost of pregnancy †	680	440–1050

* Blood loss at delivery not included.

† Iron lost to the mother; expansion of red-cell mass not included.

(After Council on Foods and Nutrition, 1968. Courtesy of the *Journal of the American Medical Association.*)

Table 56–3. DAILY IRON INTAKE AND ABSORPTION

SUBJECT	IRON REQUIREMENT (μg/kg)	AVAILABLE IRON IN POOR DIET–GOOD DIET (μg/kg)	SAFETY FACTOR (*Available Iron/ Requirement*)
Infant	67	33–66	0.5–1
Child	22	48–96	2–4
Adolescent (male)	21	30–60	1.5–3
Adolescent (female)	20	30–60	1.5–3
Adult (male)	13	26–52	2–4
Adult (female)	21	18–36	1–2
Mid-to-late pregnancy	80	18–36	0.22–0.45

the manner of its preparation, since iron may be added through contamination with dirt and from cooking in iron pots.

While the iron content of the diet is obviously important, of greater nutritional significance is the bioavailability of iron in food (Hallberg, 1981). Of the two forms of iron that are absorbed, heme iron is by far the more available, and its absorption is independent of the composition of the diet. Its relative absorption is illustrated by the study carried out by Björn-Rasmussen and associates (1974) in which a diet was fed that contained 17.4 mg of iron per day, of which 16.4 mg was nonheme iron and 1 mg was contained in heme; 37% of the heme iron but only 5% of the nonheme iron was absorbed. Thus, heme iron, which constituted only 6% of the dietary iron, represented 30% of that absorbed. Nevertheless, it is the availability of the *nonheme fraction* that deserves the greatest attention, since it represents by far the largest amount of dietary iron and is almost exclusively the form of dietary iron that is ingested by the economically underprivileged. Unfortunately, nonheme iron is usually largely unavailable, and its absorption is profoundly affected by other foods ingested concurrently. In a vegetarian diet, nonheme iron is absorbed very poorly because of the inhibitory action of a variety of components, particularly phosphates (Layrisse and Martinez-Torres, 1971). Two substances are known to facilitate the absorption of nonheme iron—ascorbic acid and meat. Ascorbate forms complexes with and/or reduces ferric to ferrous iron. While meat facilitates the absorption of iron by stimulating production of gastric acid, it is possible that some other effect, not yet identified, is also involved. Either of these substances can

increase availability severalfold. Thus, assessments of available dietary iron should include not only the amount of iron ingested but also an estimate of its availability based on the intake of substances that enhance its absorption (Monsen *et al.*, 1978) (Figure 56–3).

A comparison of iron requirements with available dietary iron is made in Table 56–3. Obviously, pregnancy and infancy represent periods of negative balance. The menstruating woman is also at risk, whereas iron balance in the adult male and nonmenstruating female is reasonably secure. The difference between dietary supply and requirements is reflected in the size of iron stores. These will be low or absent when iron balance is precarious and high when iron balance is favorable. Thus, in the

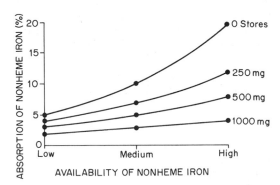

Figure 56–3. *Effect of iron status on the absorption of nonheme iron in food.*

The percentages of iron absorbed from diets of low, medium, and high bioavailability in individuals with iron stores of 0, 250, 500, and 1000 mg are portrayed. (After Monsen, Hallberg, Layrisse, Hegsted, Cook, Mertz, and Finch, 1978. © *American Journal of Clinical Nutrition.* Courtesy of American Society for Clinical Nutrition.)

infant after the third month of life and in the pregnant woman after the first trimester, stores of iron are negligible (Beaton, 1974). Menstruating females have approximately one third the stored iron found in the adult male, indicative of the extent to which the additional average daily loss of about 0.5 mg of iron affects balance (Finch *et al.*, 1977).

Iron Deficiency. Iron deficiency is rampant in human beings, and its victims number in the hundreds of millions (WHO Scientific Group, 1975). The estimate of the prevalence of iron deficiency in the United States and other developed countries depends on the economic status of the population studied and on the methods employed for evaluation. In developing countries as many as 20 to 40% of infants and pregnant women may be affected, while studies in Sweden and the United States suggest that the current prevalence in these countries is 5 to 10% (Hallberg *et al.*, 1979). The difficulty experienced by a substantial proportion of the population in achieving iron balance is recognized by the current practice of fortification of flour with 13 to 16.5 mg of iron per pound, by the use of iron-fortified formulas for infants, and by the prescription of medicinal iron supplements in pregnancy. There have been proposals to increase the current level of fortification of flour in the United States.

Iron-deficiency anemia is due to a dietary intake of iron that is inadequate to meet normal requirements (nutritional iron deficiency), to some condition that produces an increased requirement for iron because of blood loss, or to interference with iron absorption. Most nutritional iron deficiency in the United States is mild. Moderate-to-severe iron deficiency is usually the result of blood loss, either from the gastrointestinal tract or, in the female, from the uterus. *In such patients, no effort should be spared in determining the cause of the bleeding.* Infrequently, impaired absorption of the iron in food results from partial gastrectomy or sprue.

The recognition of iron deficiency rests on an appreciation of the sequence of events that occur with iron depletion. A negative balance first results in a reduction

of iron stores and, eventually, a parallel decrease in red-cell iron and iron-related enzymes (Figure 56–4). In adults, *depleted stores* may be recognized by a plasma ferritin of less than 12 μg per liter and the absence of reticuloendothelial hemosiderin in the marrow aspirate. *Iron-deficient erythropoiesis,* defined as a suboptimal supply of iron to the erythron, is identified by a decreased saturation of transferrin to less than 16% and/or by an increase above normal in red-cell protoporphyrin. *Iron-deficiency anemia* represents that stage where the depletion of essential body iron is associated with a recognizable decrease in the concentration of hemoglobin in blood. However, the physiological variation in the concentration of hemoglobin is so great that only about half of the individuals with iron-deficient erythropoiesis are identified by recognizable anemia (Cook *et al.*, 1976). Critical values in infancy and childhood are different, due to the more restricted supply of iron normally present in plasma at that age (Dallman *et al.*, 1980).

The importance of mild iron deficiency lies more in identifying the underlying cause of the deficiency than in any symptoms related to the deficient state. Because of the frequency of iron deficiency in infancy and in the menstruating or pregnant woman, the need for exhaustive evaluation of such individuals is usually determined by the severity of the anemia. However, in the male and the postmenopausal female, in whom iron balance should be favorable, it becomes important to pursue the search for a site of bleeding whenever iron deficiency is present.

A definite diagnosis of iron deficiency can be more accurately established by laboratory tests than by therapeutic trial, particularly when the deficiency is mild. The presence of *microcytic anemia* is the most commonly recognized indicator of iron deficiency. Other laboratory tests, such as quantitation of *transferrin saturation, red-cell protoporphyrin,* or *plasma ferritin,* are required to distinguish iron deficiency from other causes of microcytosis. Such measurements are particularly useful when circulating red cells are not yet microcytic due to the recent nature of blood loss, but iron supply is nonetheless limiting erythropoie-

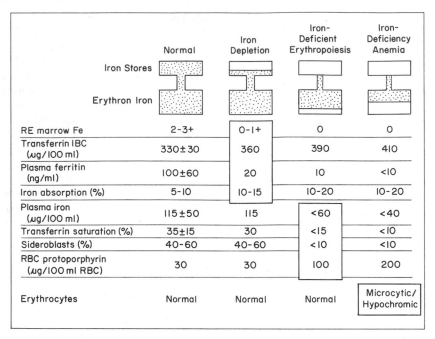

	Normal	Iron Depletion	Iron-Deficient Erythropoiesis	Iron-Deficiency Anemia
RE marrow Fe	2-3+	0-1+	0	0
Transferrin IBC (μg/100 ml)	330±30	360	390	410
Plasma ferritin (ng/ml)	100±60	20	10	<10
Iron absorption (%)	5-10	10-15	10-20	10-20
Plasma iron (μg/100 ml)	115±50	115	<60	<40
Transferrin saturation (%)	35±15	30	<15	<10
Sideroblasts (%)	40-60	40-60	<10	<10
RBC protoporphyrin (μg/100 ml RBC)	30	30	100	200
Erythrocytes	Normal	Normal	Normal	Microcytic/ Hypochromic

Figure 56–4. *Sequential changes (from left to right) in the development of iron deficiency in the adult.*

Rectangles enclose the first appearance of the indicated abnormal test results. IBC = iron-binding capacity. (After Hillman and Finch, 1974, as modified from Bothwell and Finch, 1962. Courtesy of F. A. Davis Co.)

sis. More difficult is the differentiation of true iron deficiency from iron-deficient erythropoiesis due to inflammation (Finch, 1978). In the latter condition, the stores of iron are actually increased, but the release of iron from the reticuloendothelial cell is blocked; the concentration of iron in plasma is decreased, and the supply of iron to the erythroid marrow becomes inadequate. The increased stores of iron in this condition may be demonstrated directly by examination of an aspirate of marrow or may be inferred from determination of an elevated concentration of ferritin in plasma (Lipschitz *et al.*, 1974).

TREATMENT OF IRON DEFICIENCY

General Therapeutic Principles. The response of iron-deficiency anemia to treatment is influenced by several factors, including the cause and severity of the iron-deficient state, the presence of other complicating illness, and the ability of the patient to tolerate and absorb medicinal iron. Effective therapy is followed by an increased rate of production of red cells, and the increase is proportional to the severity of the anemia and the amount of iron made available to the marrow. Some idea of the importance of the relationship of iron delivery to marrow production is found in the studies of Hillman and Henderson (1969). When normal subjects were phlebotomized, erythropoiesis was reduced to less than one third of the normal rate when the concentration of iron in plasma was below 70 μg/dl. In contrast, production increased to more than three times the basal rate when the plasma iron concentration was between 75 and 150 μg/dl. The highest rates of erythropoiesis occurred in subjects with increased destruction of red cells and elevated concentrations of iron in plasma; this situation is observed in patients with ineffective erythropoiesis (*see* above) and/or hemolysis of mature red cells (Hillman and Giblett, 1965).

The level of response of the marrow is also a reflection of the severity of the anemia, and, by inference, the degree of stimulation of marrow precursors by erythropoietin. This assumes, of course, that the marrow can respond normally. An intrinsic disease of the marrow or, more commonly, a complicating illness, such as an inflammatory disorder, can blunt the response to therapy. Continued bleeding will also interfere with the response in terms of hemoglobin, although reticulocytes will increase in number. The ability of the patient to tolerate and absorb medicinal iron is another important factor in determining the rate of response. There are clear limits to the gastrointestinal tolerance for medicinal iron. In addition, the small intestine regulates absorption and prevents the entry of overwhelming amounts of iron into the blood stream. This places a ceiling on how much iron can be provided by oral therapy. In the patient with a moderately severe anemia, maximal doses of oral iron will supply 40 to 60 mg of iron per day to the erythroid marrow, which is sufficient for production of red cells at a rate that is two to three times normal.

The response to iron therapy can be evaluated from the reticulocyte production index and the rate of rise in the level of hemoglobin or the hematocrit. A modest increase in the reticulocyte index may be observed as early as 4 to 7 days after beginning therapy. A measurable increase in the hemoglobin or hematocrit should be evident after 1 week of therapy. If the concentration of hemoglobin before treatment is reduced by more than 3 g/dl, an average increment of hemoglobin of 0.2 g/dl per day is observed with the usual therapeutic doses of iron, administered either orally or parenterally. It should be noted that this is less than the 0.6 g/dl per day (three times basal) that the erythroid marrow can achieve when the supply of iron is optimal. This simply indicates that neither route of administration can provide sufficient iron for maximal erythropoiesis. A decision about the effectiveness of the treatment should not be made for 3 to 4 weeks. An increase of 2 g/dl or more in the concentration of hemoglobin by this time should be considered a positive response to iron, assuming there has been no other change in the patient's clinical status to account for the improvement. It also assumes that the patient has not been transfused during this time.

If the response to oral iron is inadequate, the diagnosis must be reconsidered. A full laboratory evaluation should be carried out, and such factors as the presence of a concurrent inflammatory disease or poor compliance by the patient must be assessed. A source of continued bleeding should obviously be sought. If there is no other explanation, an evaluation of the patient's ability to absorb oral iron should be considered. There is no justification for merely continuing oral iron therapy beyond 3 to 4 weeks if a favorable response has not occurred.

Once a response to oral iron is demonstrated, therapy should be continued until the hemoglobin returns to normal. Treatment may then be extended if it is desirable to establish iron stores. This may require a considerable period of time, since the rate of absorption of iron by the intestine will decrease markedly as iron stores are reconstituted. The prophylactic use of oral iron should be reserved for patients at high risk, including pregnant women, women with excessive menstrual blood loss, and infants. Iron supplements may also be of value for rapidly growing infants who are consuming substandard diets and for adults with a recognized cause of chronic blood loss. Except for infants, where supplementation of formulas is routine, the use of "over-the-counter" mixtures of vitamins and minerals to prevent iron deficiency is to be discouraged. Also to be discouraged are multicomponent preparations, since the availability of their iron for absorption may be reduced.

Therapy with Oral Iron; Preparations, Dosage, and Untoward Effects. Orally administered ferrous sulfate, the least expensive of iron preparations, is the treatment of choice for iron deficiency (Fairbanks *et al.*, 1971; Callender, 1974; Bothwell *et al.*, 1979). Ferrous salts are absorbed about three times as well as ferric salts, and the discrepancy becomes even greater at high dosage (Brise and Hallberg, 1962). Variations in the particular ferrous salt have relatively little effect on bioavailability, and the sulfate, lactate, succinate, glutamate, gluconate, and other ferrous salts are absorbed to approximately the same extent.

Preparations and Dosage. Ferrous sulfate (iron sulfate) is the hydrated salt, $FeSO_4 \cdot 7H_2O$, which contains 20% iron. It is available as tablets, capsules, timed-release preparations, syrups, elixirs, and drops. *Ferrous fumarate* contains 33% iron and is moderately soluble in water, stable, and almost tasteless. It is available in tablets and suspensions. *Ferrous gluconate* and *ferrous lactate* have also been successfully employed in the therapy of iron-deficiency anemia. The gluconate contains 12% iron, and is available in tablets, capsules, and elixirs. The lactate contains 19% iron. Both are tolerated as well as ferrous sulfate. The effective dose of all of these preparations is the same in terms of iron content.

Other iron compounds have utility in fortification of foods. Reduced iron (metallic iron, elemental iron) is considered as effective as ferrous sulfate, provided that the material employed has a small particle size (Elwood, 1968; Cook *et al.*, 1973).

Large-particle *ferrum reductum* and iron phosphate salts have a much lower bioavailability (Cook *et al.,* 1973), and their use for the fortification of foods is undoubtedly responsible for some of the confusion concerning effectiveness. Ferric edetate has been shown to have a suitable bioavailability and to have advantages for maintenance of the normal appearance and taste of food (Viteri *et al.,* 1978).

The amount of iron, rather than the mass of the total salt in iron tablets, is important, since the latter is obviously modified by the mass of the anion and by the degree of hydration of the compound. It is also essential that the coating of the tablet dissolves rapidly in the stomach. Enteric-coated tablets are virtually worthless but are still being marketed. Surprisingly, since iron is usually absorbed in the upper small intestine, certain delayed-release preparations have been reported to be effective and have been said to be even more effective than ferrous sulfate when taken with meals. However, reports of absorption from such preparations vary. Because there are a number of different forms of delayed-release preparations on the market and information on their bioavailability is limited, the effectiveness of most such preparations must be considered questionable.

A variety of substances designed to enhance the absorption of iron have been marketed, including surface-acting agents, carbohydrates, inorganic salts, amino acids, and vitamins. One of the more popular of these is ascorbic acid. When present in an amount of 200 mg or more, ascorbic acid increases the absorption of medicinal iron by at least 30% (Brise and Hallberg, 1962). However, the increased uptake is associated with a significant increase in the incidence of side effects (Hallberg *et al.,* 1966b), and, therefore, the addition of ascorbic acid seems to have little advantage over increasing the amount of iron administered. There is no practical benefit in employing these compounded preparations. It is particularly undesirable to use preparations that contain other compounds with therapeutic actions of their own, such as vitamin B_{12}, folate, or cobalt, since the patient's response to the combination cannot be easily interpreted. Despite the straightforward nature of therapy with iron, it is discouraging to see the frequency with which expensive preparations with worthless additives are prescribed.

The usual therapeutic dose of iron is about 200 mg per day (2 to 3 mg/kg), based on the iron content of the preparation. In selecting the optimal dose for adults, allowance should be made for body size. Children weighing 15 to 30 kg can take half the average adult dose, and smaller children and infants can tolerate relatively larger doses of iron, for example, 5 mg/kg. The dose employed is a practical compromise between the therapeutic action desired and the toxic effects. Prophylaxis and mild nutritional iron deficiency may be managed with modest doses. When the object is the prevention of iron deficiency in pregnant patients, for example, doses of 15 to 30 mg of iron per day, if not taken with meals, are adequate to meet the 3- to 6-mg daily requirement of the last two trimesters. When

the purpose is to treat iron-deficiency anemia, but the circumstances do not demand haste, a total of about 100 mg (35 mg, three times daily) may be used. The average dose for the treatment of iron-deficiency anemia is about 200 mg of iron per day, given in three equal doses of 65 mg.

The responses expected for different dosage regimens of oral iron are given in Table 56–4. However, these effects are modified by the severity of the iron-deficiency anemia and by the time of ingestion of iron relative to meals. Absorption is optimal when the ferrous salt is taken when fasting. As noted previously, food variably reduces the availability of an iron salt, depending on the composition of the diet. Bioavailability of iron ingested with food is probably one half or one third of that seen in the fasting subject (Grebe *et al.,* 1975; Ekenved, 1976). Antacids also reduce the absorption of iron if given concurrently. It is always preferable to administer iron in the fasting state, even if the dose must be reduced because of gastrointestinal side effects. For patients who require maximal therapy to encourage a rapid response or to counteract continued bleeding, as much as 120 mg of iron may be administered four times a day. The timing of the dose is also important. Sustained high rates of red-cell production require an uninterrupted supply of iron. Oral doses should be spaced equally in order to maintain a continuous high concentration of iron in plasma.

The *duration of treatment* is governed by the recovery of hemoglobin and the desire to create iron stores (Norrby, 1974). The former depends on the severity of the anemia. With a daily rate of repair of 0.2 g of hemoglobin per deciliter of whole blood, the red-cell mass is usually reconstituted within 1 to 2 months. Thus, the individual with 5 g of hemoglobin per deciliter may achieve a normal complement of 15 g/dl in about 50 days, whereas the individual with a hemoglobin of 10 g/dl may take only half that time. The creation of stores of iron is a different matter, requiring many months of oral iron administration. The rate of absorption decreases rapidly after recovery from anemia and, after 3 to 4 months of treatment, stores may be increasing at a rate of not much more than 100 mg per month. Much of the strategy of continued therapy depends on the estimated future iron balance of the individual. The person with an inadequate diet may require continued therapy with low doses of iron. The individual whose bleeding has stopped will require no further therapy after the hemoglobin has

Table 56–4.   **AVERAGE RESPONSE TO ORAL IRON**

TOTAL DOSE mg of iron per day	ESTIMATED ABSORPTION		INCREASE IN HEMOGLOBIN g/dl of blood per day
	%	mg	
35	40	14	0.07
105	24	25	0.14
195	18	35	0.19
390	12	45	0.22

returned to normal. For the individual with continued bleeding, chronic therapy is clearly indicated.

Untoward Effects of Oral Preparations of Iron. Contrary to many advertisements, intolerance to oral preparations of iron is primarily a function of the amount of soluble iron in the upper gastrointestinal tract and of psychological factors. Side effects include heartburn, nausea, upper gastric discomfort, constipation, and diarrhea. A good policy, particularly if there has been previous intolerance to iron, is to initiate therapy at a small dosage in order to demonstrate freedom from symptoms at that level and then gradually to increase the dosage to that desired. With a dose of 200 mg of iron per day divided into three equal portions, symptoms occur in approximately 25% of individuals, compared to an incidence of 13% among those receiving placebos; this increases to approximately 40% when the dosage of iron is doubled. Nausea and upper abdominal pain are increasingly common manifestations at high dosage (Sölvell, 1970). Constipation and diarrhea, perhaps related to iron-induced changes in the intestinal bacterial flora, are not more prevalent at higher dosage, nor is heartburn. If an elixir is given, one can place the iron solution on the back of the tongue with a dropper to prevent transient staining of teeth.

Toxicity due to the long-continued administration of iron with the resultant production of iron overload (hemochromatosis) has been the subject of a number of case reports (*see* Bothwell *et al.*, 1979); this is the result of inappropriate therapy. Available evidence suggests that the normal individual is able to control absorption of iron despite high intake, and it is only individuals with underlying disorders that augment the absorption of iron who run the hazard of hemochromatosis.

Iron Poisoning. Large amounts of ferrous salts of iron are toxic but, in adults, fatalities are rare and almost exclusively suicidal. Most deaths occur in childhood and particularly between the ages of 12 and 24 months (Fairbanks *et al.*, 1971; Bothwell *et al.*, 1979). As little as 1 to 2 g of iron may cause death, but 2 to 10 g is usually ingested in fatal cases. The high frequency of iron poisoning obviously relates to its availability in the household, particularly the supply that remains after pregnancy. The colored sugar coating of many of the commercially available tablets gives them the appearance of candy. All such preparations should be kept in child-proof bottles.

Signs and symptoms of severe poisoning may occur within 30 minutes or may be delayed for several hours after ingestion. They are largely those of abdominal pain, diarrhea, or vomiting brown or bloody stomach contents containing pills. Of particular concern are pallor or cyanosis, lassitude, drowsiness, hyperventilation due to acidosis, and cardiovascular collapse. If death does not occur within 6 hours, there may be a transient period of apparent recovery, followed by death in 12 to 24 hours. The corrosive injury to the stomach may result in subsequent pyloric stenosis or gastric scarring. Hemorrhagic gastroenteritis and hepatic damage are prominent findings at autopsy. In the evaluation of the child who is thought to have ingested iron, a color test for iron in the gastric contents and an emergency determination of the concentration of iron in plasma can be performed. If the latter is less than 500 μg/dl, the child is not in immediate danger. However, vomiting should be induced when there is iron in the stomach, and an x-ray should be taken to evaluate the number of pills remaining in the small bowel. Iron in the upper gastrointestinal tract should be precipitated by lavage with sodium bicarbonate or phosphate solution. When the plasma concentration of iron is over 500 μg/dl, deferoxamine should be administered; dosage and routes of administration are detailed in Chapter 69. Shock, dehydration, and acid-base abnormalities should be treated in the conventional manner. Most important is the speed of diagnosis and therapy. With earlier and more effective treatment, the mortality from iron poisoning has been reduced from as high as 45% to about 1% at the present time.

Therapy with Parenteral Iron; Preparations, Dosage, and Untoward Effects. Parenteral administration of iron is the alternative to the use of oral preparations

(Fairbanks *et al.*, 1971; Callender, 1974; Bothwell *et al.*, 1979). The rate of response to such parenteral therapy is similar to that which follows usual oral doses (Pritchard, 1966; Strickland *et al.*, 1977). One of the advantages is that iron stores may be rapidly created, something that would take months to achieve by the oral route. Its most important indication is when disease such as sprue prevents absorption of iron from the gastrointestinal tract or in patients who are receiving parenteral nutrition. Parenteral iron may also be indicated when oral administration is thought to have an adverse effect on inflammatory disease of the bowel and, on rare occasions, when intolerance to oral iron prevents effective therapy. It has also been used in chronic inflammatory states, such as rheumatoid arthritis, where there is a partial block to the absorption of iron. However, the utilization of parenteral iron is probably suboptimal in this situation because of the block in reticuloendothelial iron transport due to inflammation. Other indications have been suggested that do not seem to be soundly based. These include the unsubstantiated beliefs that the response to parenteral iron is faster than that to oral iron, and that patients undergoing dialysis (who absorb oral iron perfectly well) are better managed by the parenteral route. In the occasional patient who presents specific diagnostic problems and who is poorly compliant in taking medication, parenteral iron has been given to ensure the administration of a known amount of iron.

Iron dextran injection (IMFERON) is the parenteral preparation in general use in the United States at the present time. It is a complex of ferric hydroxide with dextrans of 5000 to 7000 daltons in a colloidal solution containing 50 mg/ml of iron. Iron dextran is available in 10-ml vials containing 0.5% phenol for intramuscular use and in 2-ml ampuls for intramuscular or intravenous administration. When given intramuscularly, a variable portion (10 to 50%) may become fixed locally for many months. The remainder enters the blood, mostly through the lymphatic circulation, and elevates the concentration of iron in plasma for days or 1 or 2 weeks due to the presence of the iron-dextran complex. During this time determination of plasma iron does not indicate the amount of iron present in transferrin. The iron dextran must first be phagocytized by reticuloendothelial cells, and the iron is then split from the sugar molecule of the dextran before it becomes available to the body. A portion of the processed iron is rapidly returned to the plasma and made available to the erythroid marrow; however, an even greater portion remains temporarily trapped within the reticuloendothelial cell (Henderson and Hillman, 1969). These iron dextran deposits are very gradually converted into a usable form of iron. While all iron is eventually used (Kernoff *et al.*, 1975), many months are required before this is complete, and, in the interim, iron dextran within the reticuloendothelial cell can confuse the physician who attempts to evaluate the iron status of the patient.

Intramuscular injection of iron dextran has been carried out with an initial dose of 1 or 2 ml, followed by the administration of as much as 10 ml at a time, 5 ml in each buttock. However, local reactions, including long-continued discomfort at the site of injection and local discoloration of the skin, and the concern about malignant change at the site of injection (Weinbren *et al.*, 1978) make the intramuscular route inappropriate except when the intravenous route is inaccessible.

Intravenous administration of iron dextran avoids the deposition of iron in muscle and local reactions at the site of injection. The technic of intravenous administration involves first the injection of 1 or 2 drops of iron dextran over a period of 5 minutes to determine whether any signs or symptoms of anaphylaxis appear. If not, 500 mg of iron may then be injected over a period of 5 to 10 minutes. This dose may be repeated to reach the total amount required. Alternately, the total dose needed to reconstitute red-cell mass and tissue stores may be administered in one infusion over several hours, although this technic is not approved in the United States. Such a dose (in milligrams) may be calculated from the following formula: $0.66 \times$ body weight in kilograms $\times$ (100 − [patient's hemoglobin in g/dl $\times$ 100 ÷ 14.8]). However, such calculations do not take into consideration the delay in the utilization of the material injected or the possibility of continued loss of iron. In practice, more iron needs to be given than might be calculated if an increase in hemoglobin of 0.2 g/dl of whole blood per day is required.

Reactions to intravenous iron include headache, malaise, fever, generalized lymphadenopathy, arthralgias, urticaria, and, in some patients with rheumatoid arthritis, an exacerbation of the disease. Of greatest concern, however, is the rare anaphylactic reaction, which may be fatal in spite of treatment. While only a few such deaths have been reported, it remains a deterrent to the use of iron dextran. Thus, there must be *specific* indications for the parenteral administration of iron.

COPPER

Deficiency of copper is extremely rare in man (Underwood, 1971; Evans, 1973). The amount present in food is more than adequate to provide the needed body complement of slightly over 100 mg. There is no evidence that copper ever needs to be added to a normal diet, either prophylactically or therapeutically. Even in clinical states associated with hypocupremia (sprue, celiac disease, nephrotic syndrome), effects of copper deficiency are usually not demonstrable. However, anemia due to copper deficiency has been described in individuals who have undergone intestinal bypass surgery (Zidar et al., 1977), in those who are receiving parenteral nutrition (Karpel and Peden, 1972; Dunlap et al., 1974), in malnourished infants (Holtzman et al., 1970), and in infants taking copper-deficient diets (Graham and Cordano, 1976). While an inherited disorder affecting the transport of copper in man (Menkes' disease; steely hair syndrome) is associated with reduced activity of several copper-dependent enzymes, this disease is not associated with hematological abnormalities.

Copper deficiency in experimental animals interferes with the absorption of iron and its release from reticuloendothelial cells (Lee et al., 1976). The associated microcytic anemia is related both to a decrease in the availability of iron to the normoblasts and, perhaps even more importantly, to a decreased mitochondrial production of heme. It may be that the specific defect in the latter case is a decrease in the activity of cytochrome oxidase. There are other pathological effects observed in deficient experimental animals that involve the skeletal, cardiovascular, and nervous systems (O'Dell, 1976). In man, the outstanding findings have been leukopenia, particularly granulocytopenia, and anemia. Concentrations of iron in plasma are variable, and the anemia is not always microcytic. When a low plasma copper concentration is determined in the presence of leukopenia and anemia and in a setting conducive to a deficiency of the element, a therapeutic trial with copper is appropriate. Daily doses up to 0.1 mg/kg of copper sulfate have been given by mouth, or up to half this amount may be added to the solution of nutrients for parenteral administration. Copper deficiency usually occurs concurrently with multiple nutritional deficiencies, so that its specific role in the production of anemia is usually difficult to ascertain.

COBALT

The administration of cobalt can produce polycythemia in experimental animals and in the human subject without metabolic disease (Berk et al., 1949). The same effect may be observed in patients with hematological disorders where the underlying proliferative capacity of the marrow is unimpaired (sickle-cell anemia, thalassemia, chronic infection, and renal disease) (Symposium, 1955). In the 1950s cobalt was employed in doses of up to 200 to 300 mg of cobaltous chloride daily, given in divided doses by mouth to patients with various types of anemia. While beneficial effects did not occur in those with aplastic anemia, a response was observed in two patients with pure red-cell aplasia (Voyce, 1963). Cobalt deficiency has not been reported in man.

Cobalt stimulates the production of erythropoietin (Symposium, 1962). It is thought that cobalt acts by inhibition of enzymes involved in oxidative metabolism and that the response is the result of tissue hypoxia. More specifically, cobalt blocks the conversion of pyruvate to acetyl coenzyme A and of α-ketoglutarate to succinate (Webb, 1962). Large amounts of cobaltous chloride depress the production of erythrocytes. Accidental intoxication in children may produce cyanosis, coma, and death. The only disease in which the clinical use of cobalt is still advocated by some is the normochromic, normocytic anemia associated with severe renal failure (Duckham and Lee, 1976). Unwanted effects, including anorexia, nausea and vomiting, and diarrhea, are frequent in these patients, although such effects are said to be reduced by the use of enteric-coated pills in doses below 50 mg per day. In general, the administration of androgens accomplishes the same end and is considered preferable for those with anemia that is associated with renal disease (see Chapter 62).

PYRIDOXINE

The first case of pyridoxine-responsive anemia was described in 1956 by Harris and associates. Subsequent reports suggested that the vitamin might improve hematopoiesis in up to 50% of patients with either hereditary or acquired sideroblastic anemias (Horrigan and Harris, 1968; Harris and Kellermeyer, 1970). Characteristically, these patients show an impairment in hemoglobin synthesis and an accumulation of iron in the perinuclear mitochondria of erythroid precursor cells, so-called ring sideroblasts. Hereditary sideroblastic anemia is an X-linked recessive trait with variable penetrance and expression. Affected males typically show a dual population of normal red cells and microcytic, hypochromic cells in the circulation. In contrast, idiopathic acquired sideroblastic anemia and the sideroblastosis seen in association with a number of drugs, inflammatory states, neoplastic disorders, and preleukemic syndromes show a variable morphological picture. Moreover, erythrokinetic studies demonstrate a spectrum of abnormalities, from a hypoproliferative defect with little tendency to accumulate iron to marked ineffective erythropoiesis with iron overload of the tissues (Solomon and Hillman, 1979a).

Oral therapy with pyridoxine is of proven benefit in correcting the sideroblastic anemias associated with the antituberculosis drugs isoniazid and pyrazinamide, which act as vitamin B_6 antagonists. A daily dose of 50 mg of pyridoxine completely corrects the defect without interfering with treatment, and routine supplementation of pyridoxine is thus recommended (see Chapter 53). In contrast, if pyridoxine is given to counteract the sideroblastic abnormality associated with administration of levodopa, the effectiveness of levodopa in controlling Parkinson's disease is decreased. The sideroblastic abnormalities produced by chloramphenicol and lead are not corrected by pyridoxine therapy.

Patients with idiopathic, acquired sideroblastic anemia are generally older and their nutritional status is marginal. However, a response to pyridoxine cannot be explained simply on the basis of a nutritional deficiency. Those individuals who appear to have a pyridoxine-responsive anemia require therapy with large doses of the vitamin, 50 to 500 mg per day, for prolonged periods. Unfortunately, the early enthusiasm for such treatment with pyridoxine has not been reinforced by more recent studies (Chillar *et al.*, 1976; Solomon and Hillman, 1979a). Moreover, even when a patient responds, the improvement is only partial, since both the ring sideroblasts and the red-cell defect persist and the hematocrit rarely returns to normal. However, in view of the low toxicity of oral pyridoxine, a therapeutic trial with the agent is appropriate.

As shown in studies of normal man, oral pyridoxine in a dose of 100 mg three times daily produces a maximal increase in red-cell pyridoxine kinase and the major pyridoxal phosphate–dependent enzyme, glutamic-aspartic aminotransferase (Solomon and Hillman, 1978). For an adequate therapeutic trial, the drug must be administered for at least 3 months, while monitoring the response by means of the reticulocyte index and the concentration of hemoglobin. It has been suggested that the occasional patient who is refractory to oral pyridoxine will respond to parenteral administration of pyridoxal phosphate (Hines and Love, 1975). However, oral pyridoxine in doses of 200 to 300 mg per day produces intracellular concentrations of pyridoxal phosphate equal to or greater than those generated by therapy with the phosphorylated vitamin (Solomon and Hillman, 1979b). Pyridoxine is further discussed in Chapter 66.

RIBOFLAVIN

A pure red-cell aplasia that responded to the administration of riboflavin was reported in patients with protein depletion and complicating infections (Foy *et al.*, 1961). Lane and associates (1964) induced riboflavin deficiency in man and demonstrated that a hypoproliferative anemia resulted within a month. The spontaneous appearance in man of red-cell aplasia due to riboflavin deficiency is undoubtedly rare, if, in fact, it occurs at all. It has been described in combination with infection and protein deficiency, both of which are capable of producing a hypoproliferative anemia. However, it seems reasonable to include riboflavin in the nutritional management of patients with gross, generalized malnutrition. Riboflavin is further discussed in Chapter 66.

Berk, L.; Burchenal, J. H.; and Castle, W. B. Erythropoietic effect of cobalt in patients with or without anemia. *N. Engl. J. Med.*, **1949**, *240*, 754–761.

Björn-Rasmussen, E.; Hallberg, L.; Isaksson, B.; and Arvidsson, B. Food iron absorption in man. Applications of the two-pool extrinsic tag method to measure haem and non-haem iron absorption from the whole diet. *J. Clin. Invest.*, **1974**, *53*, 247–255.

Blaud, P. Sur les maladies chlorotiques, et sur un mode de traitement, spécifique dans ces affections. *Rev. Med. Fr. Etrang.*, **1832**, *1*, 337–367.

Brise, H., and Hallberg, L. Absorbability of different iron compounds. *Acta Med. Scand.*, **1962**, *171*, Suppl. 376, 23–38. (*See also* related articles by these authors, pp. 7–22 and 51–58.)

Chillar, R. K.; Johnson, C. S.; and Beutler, E. Erythrocyte pyridoxine kinase levels in patients with sideroblastic anemia. *N. Engl. J. Med.*, **1976**, *295*, 881–883.

Christian, H. A. A sketch of the history of the treatment of chlorosis with iron. *Med. Lib. Hist. J.*, **1903**, *1*, 176–180.

Cook, J. D.; Finch, C. A.; and Smith, N. Evaluation of the iron status of a population. *Blood*, **1976**, *48*, 449–455.

Cook, J. D.; Minnich, V.; Moore, C. V.; Rasmussen, A.; Bradley, W. B.; and Finch, C. A. Absorption of fortification iron in bread. *Am. J. Clin. Nutr.*, **1973**, *26*, 861–872.

Dallman, P. R.; Siimes, M. A.; and Stekel, A. Iron deficiency in infancy and childhood. *Am. J. Clin. Nutr.*, **1980**, *33*, 86–118.

Duckham, J. M., and Lee, H. A. The treatment of refractory anaemia of chronic renal failure with cobalt chloride. *Q. J. Med.*, **1976**, *45*, 277–294.

Dunlap, W. M.; James, G. W., III; and Hume, D. M. Anemia and neutropenia caused by copper deficiency. *Ann. Intern. Med.*, **1974**, *80*, 470–476.

Ekenved, G. Iron absorption studies: studies on oral iron preparations using serum iron and different radioiron isotope techniques. *Scand. J. Haematol.*, **1976**, Suppl. 28, 7–97.

Finch, C. A. Iron metabolism. In, *Nutrition Reviews' Present Knowledge in Nutrition*, 4th ed. (Hegsted, D. M., ed.) The Nutrition Foundation, Inc., New York, **1976**, pp. 280–289.

———. Anemia of chronic disease. *Postgrad. Med.*, **1978**, *64*, 107–113.

Finch, C. A.; Cook, J. D.; Labbe, R. F.; and Culala, M. Effect of blood donation on iron stores as evaluated by serum ferritin. *Blood*, **1977**, *50*, 441–447.

Foy, H.; Kondi, A.; and MacDougall, L. Pure red-cell aplasia in marasmus and kwashiorkor treated with riboflavin. *Br. Med. J.*, **1961**, *1*, 937–941.

Goya, N.; Miyazaki, S.; Kodate, S.; and Ushio, B. A family of congenital atransferrinemia. *Blood*, **1972**, *40*, 239–245.

Grebe, C.; Martinez-Torres, C.; and Layrisse, M. Effect of meals and ascorbic acid on the absorption of a therapeutic dose of iron as ferrous and ferric salts. *Curr. Ther. Res.*, **1975**, *17*, 382–397.

Green, R.; Charlton, R. W.; Seftel, H.; Bothwell, T.; Mayet, F.; Adams, B.; Finch, C.; and Layrisse, M. Body iron excretion in man. A collaborative study. *Am. J. Med.*, **1968**, *45*, 336–353.

Haden, R. J. Historical aspects of iron therapy in anemia. *J.A.M.A.*, **1939**, *111*, 1059–1061.

Hahn, P. F.; Bale, W. F.; Ross, J. F.; Balfour, W. M.; and Whipple, G. H. Radioactive iron absorption by the gastrointestinal tract: influence of anemia, anoxia and antecedent feeding; distribution in growing dogs. *J. Exp. Med.*, **1943**, *78*, 169–188.

Hallberg, L.; Hogdahl, A. M.; Nilsson, L.; and Rybo, G. Menstrual blood loss and iron deficiency. *Acta Med. Scand.*, **1966a**, *180*, 639–650.

Hallberg, L.; Ryttinger, L.; and Sölvell, L. Side effects of oral iron therapy. A double blind study of different iron compounds in tablet form. *Acta Med. Scand.*, **1966b**, *181*, Suppl. 459, 3–10.

Henderson, P. A., and Hillman, R. S. Characteristics of iron dextran utilization in man. *Blood*, **1969**, *34*, 357–375.

Hillman, R. S., and Giblett, E. R. Red cell membrane alteration associated with marrow stress. *J. Clin. Invest.*, **1965**, *44*, 1730–1736.

Hillman, R. S., and Henderson, P. A. Control of marrow production by relative iron supply. *J. Clin. Invest.*, **1969**, *48*, 454–460.

Hines, J. D., and Love, D. L. Abnormal vitamin B$_6$

metabolism in sideroblastic anemia: effect of pyridoxal phosphate (PLP) therapy. *Clin. Res.*, **1975**, *23*, 403A.

Holtzman, N. A.; Charache, P.; Cordano, A.; and Graham, G. G. Distribution of serum copper in copper deficiency. *Johns Hopkins Med. J.*, **1970**, *126*, 34–42.

Huebers, H.; Huebers, E.; Csiba, E.; and Finch, C. A. Iron uptake from rat plasma transferrin by rat reticulocytes. *J. Clin. Invest.*, **1978**, *62*, 944–951.

Huebers, H.; Huebers, E.; Csiba, E.; Rummel, W.; and Finch, C. A. The significance of transferrin for intestinal iron absorption. *Blood*, **1983**, *61*, 283–290.

Huff, R. L.; Hennessy, T. G.; Austin, R. E.; Garcia, J. F.; Roberts, B. M.; and Lawrence, J. H. Plasma and red cell iron turnover in normal subjects and in patients having various hematopoietic disorders. *J. Clin. Invest.*, **1950**, *29*, 1041–1052.

Karpel, J. T., and Peden, V. H. Copper deficiency in long-term parenteral nutrition. *J. Pediatr.*, **1972**, *80*, 32–36.

Kernoff, L. M.; Dommisse, J.; and du Toit, E. D. Utilization of iron dextran in recurrent iron deficiency anaemia. *Br. J. Haematol.*, **1975**, *30*, 419–424.

Lane, M.; Alfrey, C. P.; Megel, C. E.; Doherty, M. A.; and Doherty, J. The rapid induction of human riboflavin deficiency with galactoflavin. *J. Clin. Invest.*, **1964**, *43*, 357–373.

Latham, R. G. *The Works of Thomas Sydenham, M.D.*, Vol. 2. C. & J. Adlard, London, **1850**, p. 97.

Lipschitz, D. A.; Cook, J. D.; and Finch, C. A. A clinical evaluation of serum ferritin as an index of iron stores. *N. Engl. J. Med.*, **1974**, *290*, 1213–1216.

McCance, R. A., and Widdowson, E. M. Absorption and excretion of iron. *Lancet*, **1937**, *233*, 680–684.

Monsen, E. R.; Hallberg, L.; Layrisse, M.; Hegsted, D. M.; Cook, J. D.; Mertz, W.; and Finch, C. A. Estimation of available dietary iron. *Am. J. Clin. Nutr.*, **1978**, *31*, 134–141.

Neuroth, M. L., and Lee, C. O. A history of Blaud's pills. *J. Am. Pharm. Assoc., Sci. Ed.*, **1941**, *30*, 60–63.

Norrby, A. Iron absorption studies in iron deficiency. *Scand. J. Haematol.*, **1974**, Suppl. 20, 5–125.

Pritchard, J. A. Hemoglobin regeneration in severe iron deficiency anemia. Response to orally and parenterally administered iron preparations. *J.A.M.A.*, **1966**, *195*, 717–720.

Solomon, L. R., and Hillman, R. S. Vitamin B$_6$ metabolism in human red blood cells. I. Variation in normal subjects. *Enzyme*, **1978**, *23*, 262–273.

——. Vitamin B$_6$ metabolism in idiopathic sideroblastic anaemia and related disorders. *Br. J. Haematol.*, **1979a**, *42*, 239–253.

——. Vitamin B$_6$ metabolism in anaemic and alcoholic man. *Ibid.*, **1979b**, *41*, 343–356.

Sölvell, L. Oral iron therapy—side effects. In, *Iron Deficiency: Pathogenesis, Clinical Aspects, Therapy.* (Hallberg, L.; Harwerth, H.-G.; and Vannotti, A.; eds.) Academic Press, Inc., New York, **1970**, pp. 573–583.

Strickland, I. D.; DeSaintouge, C.; Boulton, F. E.; Francis, B.; Ronbikova, J.; and Waters, J. I. The therapeutic equivalence of oral and intravenous iron in renal dialysis patients. *Clin. Nephrol.*, **1977**, *7*, 55–57.

Viteri, F. E.; Garcia-Ibanez, R.; and Torun, B. Sodium iron NaFeEDTA as an iron fortification compound in Central America. Absorption studies. *Am. J. Clin. Nutr.*, **1978**, *31*, 961–971.

Voyce, M. A. A case of pure red-cell aplasia successfully treated with cobalt. *Br. J. Haematol.*, **1963**, *9*, 412–418.

Weinbren, K.; Salm, R.; and Greenberg, G. Intramuscular injections of iron compounds and oncogenesis in man. *Br. Med. J.*, **1978**, *1*, 683–685.

Zidar, B. L.; Shadduck, R. K.; Zeigler, Z.; and Winkelstein, A. Observations on the anemia and neu-

tropenia of human copper deficiency. *Am. J. Hematol.*, **1977**, *3*, 177–185.

Monographs and Reviews

Aisen, P., and Brown, E. B. The iron-binding function of transferrin in iron metabolism. *Semin. Hematol.*, **1977**, *14*, 31–53.

Beaton, G. H. Epidemiology of iron deficiency. In, *Iron in Biochemistry and Medicine.* (Jacobs, A., and Worwood, M., eds.) Academic Press, Inc., New York, **1974**, pp. 477–528.

Bothwell, T. H.; Charlton, R. W.; Cook, J. D.; and Finch, C. A. *Iron Metabolism in Man.* Blackwell Scientific Publications, Oxford, **1979**.

Bothwell, T. H., and Finch, C. A. *Iron Metabolism.* Little, Brown & Co., Boston, **1962**.

Bottomley, S. S. Porphyrin and iron metabolism in sideroblastic anemia. *Semin. Hematol.*, **1977**, *14*, 169–185.

Brown, M. S.; Anderson, R. G. W.; and Goldstein, J. L. Recycling receptors: the round-trip itinerary of migrant membrane proteins. *Cell*, **1983**, *32*, 663–667.

Callender, S. T. Treatment of iron deficiency. In, *Iron in Biochemistry and Medicine.* (Jacobs, A., and Worwood, M., eds.) Academic Press, Inc., New York, **1974**, pp. 529–542.

Cook, J. D., and Finch, C. A. Iron nutrition. *West. J. Med.*, **1975**, *122*, 474–481.

Council on Foods and Nutrition. Iron deficiency in the United States. *J.A.M.A.*, **1968**, *203*, 119–124.

Dallman, P. R. Manifestations of iron deficiency. *Semin. Hematol.*, **1982**, *19*, 19–20.

Elwood, P. A. Radioactive studies of the absorption by human subjects of various iron preparations from bread. In, *Iron in Flour.* Ministry of Health Reports on Public Health and Medicine, Subject 117. Her Majesty's Stationery Office, London, **1968**, pp. 1–50.

Evans, G. W. Copper homeostasis in the mammalian system. *Physiol. Rev.*, **1973**, *53*, 535.

Fairbanks, V. F.; Fahey, J. L.; and Beutler, E. *Clinical Disorders of Iron Metabolism*, 2nd ed. Grune & Stratton, Inc., New York, **1971**.

Finch, C. A., and Huebers, H. Perspectives in iron metabolism. *N. Engl. J. Med.*, **1982**, *306*, 1520–1528.

Finch, C. A., and others. Ferrokinetics in man. *Medicine (Baltimore)*, **1970**, *40*, 17–53.

Graham, G. G., and Cordano, A. Copper deficiency in human subjects. In, *Trace Elements in Human Health and Disease.* Vol. 1, *Zinc and Copper.* (Prasad, A. S., and Oberleas, D., eds.) Academic Press, Inc., New York, **1976**, pp. 363–372.

Hallberg, L. Bioavailability of dietary iron in man. *Annu. Rev. Nutr.*, **1981**, *1*, 123–147.

Hallberg, L.; Bengtsson, B.; Garby, L.; and others. An analysis of factors leading to a reduction in iron deficiency in Swedish women. *Bull. WHO*, **1979**, *57*, 947–954.

Harris, J. W., and Kellermeyer, R. W. *The Red Cell*, rev. ed. Harvard University Press, Cambridge, Mass., **1970**.

Harrison, P. M. Ferritin: an iron-storage molecule. *Semin. Hematol.*, **1977**, *14*, 55–70.

Heilmeyer, L., and Plotner, K. *Das Serumeisen und die Eisenmangelkrankheit.* Gustav Fischer Verlag, Jena, **1937**.

Heinrich, H. C. Diagnostik Atiologie und Therapie des Eisenmangels unter besonderer Berucksichtigung der 59 Fe retentionsmessung im Gesamtkorperradioaktivitatsdetektor. *Nuklearmedizin*, **1983**, *1*, 137–269.

Hillman, R. S., and Finch, C. A. *Red Cell Manual*, 4th ed. F. A. Davis Co., Philadelphia, **1974**.

Hines, J. D., and Grasso, J. A. The sideroblastic anemias. *Semin. Hematol.*, **1970**, *7*, 86–106.

Horrigan, D. L., and Harris, J. W. Pyridoxine-responsive anemias in man. *Vitam. Horm.,* **1968,** *26,* 549.

Laurell, C. B. Studies on the transportation and metabolism of iron in the body. *Acta Physiol. Scand.,* **1947,** *14,* Suppl. 46, 1–129.

Layrisse, M., and Martinez-Torres, C. Iron absorption from food. *Prog. Hematol.,* **1971,** *6,* 137–160.

Lee, G. R.; Williams, D. M.; and Cartwright, G. E. Role of copper in iron metabolism and heme biosynthesis. In, *Trace Elements in Human Health and Disease.* Vol. 1, *Zinc and Copper.* (Prasad, A. S., and Oberleas, D., eds.) Academic Press, Inc., New York, **1976,** pp. 373–390.

Lynch, R. S., and Morck, T. A. Iron deficiency anemia. In, *Nutrition in Hematology.* Vol. 5, *Contemporary Issues in Clinical Nutrition.* (Lindenbaum, J., ed.) Churchill Livingstone, New York, **1983,** pp. 143–165.

Martinez-Torres, C.; Cobeddu, L.; Dillmann, E.; Brengelmann, G. L.; Leets, I.; Layrisse, M.; Johnson, P. G.; and Finch, C. A. Effect of exposure to low temperature on normal and iron deficient subjects. *Am. J. Physiol.,* **1984,** *246,* R380–R383.

National Research Council, Committee on Medical and Biologic Effects of Environmental Pollutants, Subcommittee on Iron, Division of Medical Sciences, Assembly of Life Sciences. *Iron.* University Park Press, Baltimore, **1979.**

Neilands, J. B. (ed.). *Microbial Iron Metabolism: A Comprehensive Treatise.* Academic Press, Inc., New York, **1974.**

O'Dell, B. L. Biochemistry of copper. *Med. Clin. North Am.,* **1976,** *60,* 687–703.

Pollit, E., and Leibel, R. L. (eds.). *Iron Deficiency: Brain Biochemistry and Behavior.* Raven Press, New York, **1982.**

Sigel, H. *Metal Ions in Biological Systems.* Vol. 7, *Iron in Model and Natural Compounds.* Marcel Dekker, Inc., New York, **1977,** pp. 1–417.

Symposium. (Various authors.) The use of cobalt and cobalt-iron preparations in the therapy of anemia. *Blood,* **1955,** *10,* 852–861.

Symposium. (Various authors.) *Erythropoiesis.* (Jacobson, L. O., and Doyle, M., eds.) Grune & Stratton, Inc., New York, **1962.**

Underwood, E. J. *Trace Elements in Human and Animal Nutrition,* 3rd ed. Academic Press, Inc., New York, **1971.**

Webb, M. The biological action of cobalt and other metals. *Biochim. Biophys. Acta,* **1962,** *65,* 47.

WHO Joint Meeting. Control of nutritional anaemia with special reference to iron deficiency. World Health Organization Technical Report Series No. 580, WHO, Geneva, **1975.**

Wixom, R. L.; Rutkin, L.; and Munro, H. N. Hemosiderin: nature, formation and significance. *Int. Rev. Exp. Pathol.,* **1979,** *22,* 193–225.

CHAPTER

57 VITAMIN B$_{12}$, FOLIC ACID, AND THE TREATMENT OF MEGALOBLASTIC ANEMIAS

Robert S. Hillman

Vitamin B$_{12}$ and folic acid are dietary essentials for man. A deficiency of either vitamin results in defective synthesis of DNA in any cell that attempts chromosomal replication and division. Since tissues with the greatest rate of cell turnover show the most dramatic changes, the hematopoietic system is especially sensitive to deficiencies of these vitamins. Clinically, the earliest sign of deficiency is a megaloblastic anemia, where the derangement in DNA synthesis results in a characteristic morphological abnormality of the precursor cells in the bone marrow. Abnormal macrocytic red blood cells are the product, and the patient becomes severely anemic. Recognition of this pattern of abnormal hematopoiesis, more than 100 years ago, permitted the initial diagnostic classification of such patients as having "pernicious anemia" and the investigations that subsequently led to the discovery of the clinical value of vitamin B$_{12}$ and folic acid. Even today, the characteristic abnormality in morphology is used both for diagnosis and as a therapeutic guide for administration of the vitamins.

History. The discovery of vitamin B$_{12}$ and folic acid is a dramatic story that starts more than 150 years ago and includes two Nobel prize-winning discoveries (*see* Castle, 1961; Kass, 1976). The first descriptions of what must have been megaloblastic anemias are credited to Combe and Addison, who published several case reports between 1824 and 1855. While Combe suggested that the disorder might have some relationship to digestion, it was Austin Flint who, in 1860, first described the severe gastric atrophy and called attention to its possible relationship to the anemia. The name "progressive pernicious anemia" was coined in 1872 by Biermer. This exceptionally colorful term has persisted, for it is still common practice to describe the condition as Addisonian pernicious anemia.

Following the observation by Whipple in 1925 that liver is a source of a potent hematopoietic substance for iron-deficient dogs, Minot and Murphy carried out their Nobel prize-winning experiments that demonstrated the effectiveness of the feeding

of liver in pernicious anemia. Within a few years, Castle defined the need for both an *intrinsic* factor, a substance secreted by the parietal cells of the gastric mucosa, and an *extrinsic factor,* the vitamin-like material provided by crude liver extracts. However, nearly 20 years passed before Rickes and coworkers and Smith and Parker isolated and crystallized vitamin B$_{12}$; Dorothy Hodgkin then determined its crystal structure by x-ray diffraction and subsequently received the Nobel prize for this work.

As attempts were being made to purify extrinsic factor, Wills and her associates described a macrocytic anemia in women in India that responded to a factor present in crude liver extracts but not in the purified fractions known to be effective in pernicious anemia (Wills and Bilimoria, 1932; Wills *et al.,* 1937). This factor, first called Wills' factor and later vitamin M, is now known to be folic acid. The actual term *folic acid* was coined by Mitchell and coworkers in 1941, following its isolation from leafy vegetables (Mitchell *et al.,* 1941).

More recent work has shown that neither vitamin B$_{12}$ nor folic acid as purified from liver or various foodstuffs is the active coenzyme for man. During extraction procedures, active, labile forms are converted to stable congeners of vitamin B$_{12}$ and folic acid, cyanocobalamin and pteroylglutamic acid, respectively. These congeners must then be modified *in vivo* to be effective. While much has been learned of the intracellular metabolic pathways in which these vitamins participate, many questions remain to be answered, especially the relationship of vitamin B$_{12}$ deficiency to the neurological abnormalities that occur with this disorder.

Relationships between Vitamin B$_{12}$ and Folic Acid. The major roles of vitamin B$_{12}$ and folic acid in intracellular metabolism are summarized in Figure 57–1. Intracellular vitamin B$_{12}$ is maintained as two active coenzymes, methylcobalamin and deoxyadenosylcobalamin (Stahlberg, 1967; Linnell *et al.,* 1971). Deoxyadenosylcobalamin is a cofactor for the mitochondrial mutase enzyme that catalyzes the isomerization of L-methylmalonyl CoA to succinyl CoA, an important reaction in both carbohydrate and lipid metabolism (Huennekens, 1968; Weissbach and Taylor, 1968). This reaction

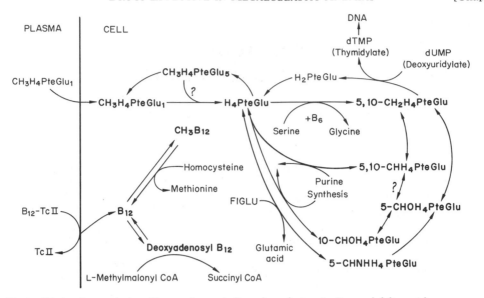

Figure 57–1. *Interrelationships and metabolic roles of vitamin B_{12} and folic acid.*

See text for explanation and Figure 57–5 for structures of the various folate coenzymes. *FIGLU* is formiminoglutamic acid, which arises from the catabolism of histidine.

has no direct relationship to the metabolic pathways that involve folate. In contrast, methylcobalamin supports the methionine synthetase reaction, which is essential for normal metabolism of folate (Weir and Scott, 1983). Methyl groups contributed by methyltetrahydrofolate ($CH_3H_4PteGlu_1$) are used to form methylcobalamin, which then acts as a methyl group donor for the conversion of homocysteine to methionine. This folate-cobalamin interaction is pivotal for normal synthesis of purines and pyrimidines and, therefore, of DNA. The methionine synthetase reaction is largely responsible for the control of the recycling of folate cofactors, the maintenance of intracellular concentrations of folylpolyglutamates, and, through the synthesis of methionine and its product S-adenosylmethionine, the maintenance of a number of methylation reactions.

Since methyltetrahydrofolate is the principal folate congener supplied to cells, the transfer of the methyl group to cobalamin is essential for the adequate supply of tetrahydrofolate ($H_4PteGlu_1$), the substrate for a number of metabolic steps that require folate. Tetrahydrofolate is a precursor for the formation of intracellular folylpolyglutamates; it is also the substrate for the

synthesis of several active coenzymes that are involved in purine and pyrimidine metabolism. Tetrahydrofolate acts as the acceptor of a one-carbon unit in the conversion of serine to glycine, with the resultant formation of 5,10-methylenetetrahydrofolate ($5,10-CH_2H_4PteGlu$). The latter derivative donates the methylene group to deoxyuridylate for the synthesis of thymidylate—an extremely important reaction in DNA synthesis. In the process, the $5,10-CH_2H_4PteGlu$ is converted to dihydrofolate ($H_2PteGlu$). The cycle is then completed by the reduction of the $H_2PteGlu$ to $H_4PteGlu$ by dihydrofolate reductase, the step that is blocked by folate antagonists such as methotrexate (*see* Chapter 55). As shown in Figure 57–1, several other pathways also lead to the synthesis of 5,10-methylenetetrahydrofolate. These pathways are important in the metabolism of formiminoglutamic acid (FIGLU) and both purines and pyrimidines. (*See* reviews by Stokstad and Koch, 1967; Blakely, 1969; Chanarin, 1979; Das and Herbert, 1976; Herbert, 1979; Hoffbrand and Wickremasinghe, 1982; Weir and Scott, 1983.)

In the presence of a deficiency of either vitamin B_{12} or folate, the decreased synthesis of methionine and S-adenosylmethionine interferes with protein biosynthesis, a number of methylation reactions, and the synthesis of polyamines. In addition, the cell responds to the deficiency by redirecting folate metabolic pathways to supply increasing amounts of methyltetrahydrofolate; this tends to preserve essential methylation reactions at the expense of nucleic acid synthesis. With vitamin B$_{12}$ deficiency, methylenetetrahydrofolate reductase activity increases, which directs available intracellular folates into the methyltetrahydrofolate pool (not shown in Figure 57–1). The methyltetrahydrofolate is then trapped by the lack of sufficient B$_{12}$ to accept and transfer methyl groups, and subsequent steps in folate metabolism that require tetrahydrofolate are deprived of substrate. This provides a common basis for the development of a megaloblastic anemia with deficiency of either vitamin B$_{12}$ or folic acid.

The mechanisms responsible for the neurological lesions of vitamin B$_{12}$ deficiency are less well understood (Herbert and Tisman, 1973; Reynolds, 1976; Weir and Scott, 1983). Damage to the myelin sheath is the most obvious lesion in this neuropathy. This led to the early suggestion that the deoxyadenosyl B$_{12}$-dependent methylmalonyl CoA mutase reaction, a step in propionate metabolism, is related to the abnormality. However, recent evidence suggests that the deficiency of methionine synthetase and the block of the conversion of methionine to S-adenosylmethionine is more likely to be responsible (Scott *et al.*, 1981).

Nitrous oxide (N$_2$O) can oxidize the cobalt atom in vitamin B$_{12}$ and can cause megaloblastic changes in the marrow and a neuropathy that resemble those of vitamin B$_{12}$ deficiency (*see* Hoffbrand and Wickremasinghe, 1982). Studies with N$_2$O in experimental animals have demonstrated reduced concentrations of methionine and S-adenosylmethionine; the latter is necessary for methylation reactions, including those required for the synthesis of phospholipids and myelin. Significantly, the neuropathy induced with N$_2$O can be prevented by feeding methionine. A neuropathy similar to that of vitamin B$_{12}$ deficiency has also been reported in dentists who use N$_2$O as an anesthetic (Layzer, 1978).

VITAMIN B$_{12}$

Chemistry. The structural formula of vitamin B$_{12}$ is shown in Figure 57–2 (Smith, 1965; Skeggs, 1967; Pratt, 1972; Herbert, 1979). The three major portions of the molecule are:

1. A planar group or corrin nucleus—a porphyrin-like ring structure with four reduced pyrrole rings (designated A to D) linked to a central cobalt atom and extensively substituted with methyl, acetamide, and propionamide residues.

2. A 5,6-dimethylbenzimidazolyl nucleotide, which links almost at right angles to the corrin nucleus with bonds to the cobalt atom and to the propionate side chain of the D ring.

3. A variable R group—the most important of which is found in the stable compounds cyanocobalamin and hydroxocobalamin and the active coenzymes methylcobalamin and 5-deoxyadenosylcobalamin. While there are a number of other cobalamin derivatives in nature, formed by covalent binding of various ligands to the cobalt atom, these are of no apparent value to man.

The terms *vitamin B$_{12}$* and *cyanocobalamin* are used interchangeably as generic terms for all the cobamides active in man. Preparations of vitamin B$_{12}$ for therapeutic use contain either cyanocobalamin or hydroxocobalamin, since only these derivatives are stable with storage.

Metabolic Functions. The active coenzymes, methylcobalamin and 5-deoxyadenosylcobalamin, are essential for cell growth and replication. Methylcobalamin is required for the formation of methionine and its derivative S-adenosylmethionine from homocysteine. In addition, when concentrations of vitamin B$_{12}$ are inadequate, folate becomes "trapped" as methyltetrahydrofolate to cause a functional deficiency of other vital intracellular forms of folic acid (*see* Figure 57–1 and discussion above). This is the cause of the hematological abnormalities that are observed in vitamin B$_{12}$–deficient patients (Herbert and Zalusky, 1962; Weir and Scott, 1983). 5-Deoxyadenosylcobalamin is required for the isomerization of L-methylmalonyl CoA to succinyl CoA.

Sources in Nature. Man depends on exogenous sources of vitamin B$_{12}$ (Herbert, 1973). In nature, the only original source is certain microorganisms that grow in soil, sewage, water, or the intestinal lumen, and that synthesize the vitamin. Vegetable products are free of vitamin B$_{12}$ unless they are contaminated with such microorganisms, so that animals are dependent on

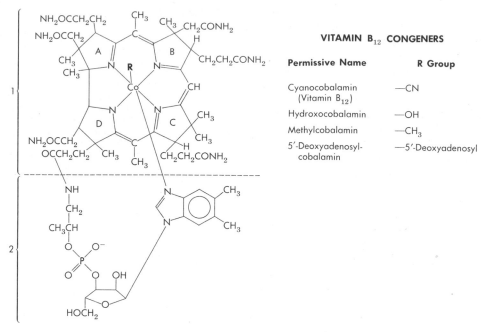

VITAMIN B_{12} CONGENERS	
Permissive Name	R Group
Cyanocobalamin (Vitamin B_{12})	—CN
Hydroxocobalamin	—OH
Methylcobalamin	—CH_3
5'-Deoxyadenosyl-cobalamin	—5'-Deoxyadenosyl

Figure 57–2. *The structure and nomenclature of vitamin B_{12} congeners. (See text for explanation.)*

synthesis in their own alimentary tract or the ingestion of animal products containing vitamin B_{12}. In man, vitamin B_{12} synthesized in the large bowel is unavailable for absorption, and a daily nutritional requirement of 3 to 5 μg must be obtained from animal by-products in the diet. At the same time, strict vegetarians rarely develop vitamin B_{12} deficiency. A certain amount of vitamin B_{12} is available from legumes, which are contaminated with bacteria capable of synthesizing vitamin B_{12}, and vegetarians generally fortify their diets with a wide range of vitamins and minerals.

Absorption, Distribution, Elimination, and Daily Requirements. The development of vitamin B_{12} deficiency during adult life does not usually result from a deficient diet; rather, it reflects some defect in gastrointestinal absorption (*see* Figure 57–3). Classical Addisonian pernicious anemia is caused by a failure of gastric parietal-cell function and production of the glycoprotein *gastric intrinsic factor,* often called the intrinsic factor of Castle in recognition of his major contributions to the field (*see* Castle, 1953). The parietal cells probably fail be-

cause of the presence of cytotoxic autoantibodies (de Aizpurua *et al.,* 1983). Dietary vitamin B_{12}, in the presence of gastric acid and pancreatic proteases, is released from proteins to which it is bound and is then immediately bound to intrinsic factor, a glycoprotein with a molecular weight in the range of 60,000. The vitamin B_{12}–intrinsic factor complex then reaches the ileum, where it interacts with a specific receptor on ileal mucosal cells and is transported to the circulation. Intrinsic factor is required for ileal transport of vitamin B_{12}—both the vitamin in the diet and that which is continuously excreted in the bile (Gräsbeck, 1969; Allen and Mehlman, 1973; Glass, 1974).

Any of a number of intestinal diseases or defects can interfere with the absorption of the intrinsic factor–B_{12} complex. The combination of gastric achlorhydria and decreased secretion of intrinsic factor secondary to gastric atrophy or gastric surgery is a common cause of vitamin B_{12} deficiency in adults. The requirement for pancreatic proteases to release vitamin B_{12} from proteins, such that it can then bind to intrinsic factor, explains the malabsorption of vitamin B_{12} in pancreatic disorders (Allen *et al.,* 1978).

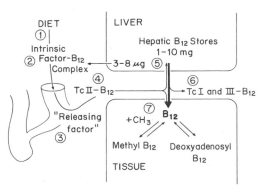

Figure 57–3. *The absorption and distribution of vitamin B$_{12}$.*

Deficiency of vitamin B$_{12}$ can result from a congenital or acquired defect in any one of the following: (*1*) inadequate dietary supply; (*2*) inadequate secretion of intrinsic factor (classical pernicious anemia); (*3*) ileal disease; (*4*) congenital absence of transcobalamin II (Tc II); or (*5*) rapid depletion of hepatic stores by interference with reabsorption of vitamin B$_{12}$ excreted in bile. The utility of measurements of the concentration of vitamin B$_{12}$ in plasma to estimate supply available to tissues can be compromised by liver disease and (*6*) the appearance of abnormal amounts of transcobalamins I and III (Tc I and III) in plasma. Finally, the formation of methylcobalamin requires (*7*) normal transport into cells and an adequate supply of folic acid as CH$_3$H$_4$PteGlu$_1$.

Antibodies to intrinsic factor or to the intrinsic factor–B$_{12}$ complex may also play a role in impaired uptake by ileal cells. Bacterial overgrowth or certain intestinal parasites can prevent an adequate supply of B$_{12}$ from reaching the ileum. Finally, any damage to ileal mucosal cells by disease or surgical procedures can interfere with absorption (Herbert, 1979).

Once absorbed, vitamin B$_{12}$ binds to transcobalamin II, a plasma β-globulin, for transport to tissues (Gräsbeck, 1969; Hall and Finkler, 1971). Two other transcobalamins (I and III) are also present in plasma; their concentrations are related to the rate of turnover of granulocytes. They may represent intracellular storage proteins that are released with cell death (Scott *et al.*, 1974). Vitamin B$_{12}$ bound to transcobalamin II is rapidly cleared from plasma and is preferentially distributed to hepatic parenchymal cells. The liver is thus a storage depot for other tissues. In the normal adult, as much as 90% of the body's stores of vitamin B$_{12}$, from 1 to 10 mg, is in the liver (Chanarin *et al.*, 1966). Vitamin B$_{12}$ is stored as the active coenzyme with a turnover rate of 0.05 to 0.2% per day or 0.5 to 8 μg per day, depending on the size of the body stores (Heyssel *et al.*, 1966; Reizenstein *et al.*, 1966; Adams and Boddy, 1968). The minimal daily requirement of the vitamin is estimated to be as little as 1 μg (Sullivan and Herbert, 1965; FAO/WHO Expert Group, 1970). Recommended dietary allowances are presented in Table XVI–1.

Approximately 3 μg of vitamin B$_{12}$ is secreted into bile each day, and this is normally reabsorbed in the ileum. This enterohepatic cycle is important, since interference with reabsorption by intestinal disease can result in a continuous depletion of hepatic stores of the vitamin. This explains why patients will develop vitamin B$_{12}$ deficiency within 3 to 4 years following major gastric surgery even though a daily requirement of 1 to 2 μg would not be expected to deplete hepatic stores of more than 2 to 3 mg during this period.

The supply of vitamin B$_{12}$ available for tissues is directly related to the size of the hepatic storage pool and the amount of vitamin B$_{12}$ bound to transcobalamin II. Since vitamin B$_{12}$ in liver cannot be easily measured, the concentration of vitamin B$_{12}$ in plasma is the best routine measure of B$_{12}$ deficiency. Normal individuals have plasma concentrations of the vitamin between 200 and 900 pg/ml, while a deficiency state is usually present whenever the value falls below 200 pg/ml. The correlation is excellent except when the concentrations of transcobalamin I and III in the plasma increase as a result, for example, of hepatic disease or a myeloproliferative disorder. Inasmuch as the vitamin B$_{12}$ bound to these transport proteins has a very slow turnover and, therefore, is relatively unavailable to cells, it is possible for there to be a deficiency within tissues at a time when the concentration of vitamin B$_{12}$ in plasma is normal or even high (Retief *et al.*, 1967). A congenital absence of transcobalamin II has been observed in at least two families (Hakami *et al.*, 1971; Hitzig *et al.*, 1974). In the children, megaloblastic anemia was present despite relatively normal concentrations of vitamin B_{12} in plasma. At the same time, the children were quite responsive to doses of parenteral vitamin B_{12} that were sufficient to exceed renal clearance, allow accumulation of the unbound vitamin in plasma, and thereby provide free vitamin B_{12} to cells.

Defects in intracellular metabolism of vitamin B_{12} have been reported in children with methylmalonic aciduria and homocystinuria. Mechanisms involved may include an incapacity of cells to transport vitamin B_{12} or accumulate the vitamin because of a failure to synthesize an intracellular acceptor, a defect in the formation of deoxyadenosylcobalamin, or a congenital lack of methylmalonyl CoA isomerase (Cooper, 1976). Numerous examples of the last-named defect have been reported under the classification of congenital methylmalonic aciduria. In the above-listed situations, large doses of vitamin B_{12} may have a salutary effect.

Vitamin B_{12} Deficiency. Vitamin B_{12} deficiency is recognized clinically by its impact on both the hematopoietic and the nervous systems. The sensitivity of the hematopoietic system relates to its high rate of turnover of cells. There is nothing else unique about the hematopoietic system in this respect, and other tissues with high rates of cell turnover (*e.g.,* mucosa and cervical epithelium) have similar high requirements for the vitamin.

As a result of an inadequate supply of vitamin B_{12}, DNA replication becomes highly abnormal. Once a hematopoietic stem cell is committed to enter a programmed series of cell divisions, the defect in chromosomal replication results in an inability of maturing cells to complete nuclear divisions while cytoplasmic maturation continues at a relatively normal rate. This results in the production of morphologically abnormal cells or death of cells during the maturation phase, a phenomenon referred to as ineffective hematopoiesis (Finch *et al.,* 1956). From the clinical viewpoint, these abnormalities are readily identified by examination of the bone marrow and peripheral blood. Usually, the changes are most marked for the red-cell series. The marrow

shows proliferation of red-cell precursors that is appropriate to the severity of the anemia, but maturation is highly abnormal (megaloblastic erythropoiesis). A majority of the megaloblastic cells die within the marrow, so that the reticulocyte index, the measure of effective red-cell production, is much less than that expected for the level of proliferation in marrow. Finally, those cells that do leave the marrow are highly abnormal, and many cell fragments, poikilocytes, and macrocytes appear in the peripheral blood. The mean red-cell volume increases to values greater than 110 μm^3. When deficiency is marked, all cell lines may be affected, and a pronounced pancytopenia results.

The diagnosis of a vitamin B_{12}–deficiency state can be made by determination of the concentration of vitamin B_{12} in plasma and by tests of gastric function. Measurements of gastric acidity may provide indirect evidence of a defect in parietal-cell function, while the Schilling test can be used to quantitate ileal absorption of vitamin B_{12}. (Isotopically labeled vitamin B_{12} is administered orally, and the radioactivity in urine is quantified.) In addition, the Schilling test performed after the oral administration of intrinsic factor can help to delineate the mechanism of the abnormality of absorption (Schilling, 1953). A less commonly used index of vitamin B_{12} deficiency is the measurement of urinary methylmalonate. While a normal subject excretes only trace amounts of methylmalonate (0 to 3.5 mg per day), the B_{12}-deficient patient will excrete as much as 300 mg in 24 hours (Cox and White, 1962). Finally, the observation of reticulocytosis following a therapeutic trial of vitamin B_{12} confirms the diagnosis.

Vitamin B_{12} deficiency can result in *irreversible* damage to the nervous system. Progressive swelling of myelinated neurons, demyelination, and cell death are seen in the spinal column and cerebral cortex. This causes a wide range of neurological signs and symptoms, including paresthesias of the hands and feet, diminution of sensation of vibration and position with resultant unsteadiness, decreased deep-tendon reflexes, and, in the later stages, loss of memory, confusion, moodiness, and even a loss of central vision. The patient may exhibit delusions, hallucinations, or even an overt psychosis. Since the neurological damage can be dissociated from the changes in the hematopoietic system, especially by the administration of pharmacological doses of folic acid, vitamin B$_{12}$ deficiency must be considered as a possibility in elderly patients with psychosis. However, it is unusual to see patients who are routinely followed by their physicians develop severe neurological complications. The sensitivity of methods for evaluation of the hematopoietic system, the ease of measurement of the concentration of vitamin B$_{12}$ in plasma, and the awareness of the medical profession of the causes of vitamin B$_{12}$ deficiency have made possible an earlier and more accurate diagnosis of B$_{12}$-deficient states, early and adequate therapy, and hence avoidance of neurological complications.

Preparations, Dosage, and Routes of Administration. Vitamin B$_{12}$ is available in pure form for injection or oral administration or in combination with other vitamins and minerals for oral administration. The choice of a preparation must always be made with recognition of the cause of the deficiency. While oral preparations may be used to supplement deficient diets or to prevent vitamin B$_{12}$ deficiency in situations where there is increased utilization, *they are of little value in the treatment of patients with deficiency of intrinsic factor or ileal disease.* Even though small amounts of vitamin B$_{12}$ may be absorbed by simple diffusion, the oral route of administration cannot be relied upon for effective therapy in the patient with a marked deficiency of B$_{12}$ and abnormal hematopoiesis or neurological deficits. Therefore, the preparation of choice for treatment of a vitamin B$_{12}$–deficiency state is cyanocobalamin, and it should be given by intramuscular or deep subcutaneous injection.

Cyanocobalamin injection (REDISOL, RUBRAMIN PC, others) is a clear aqueous solution with a characteristic red color. The aqueous solution is available in concentrations of 30, 100, and 1000 μg/ml. Cyanocobalamin injection is extremely safe when given by the intramuscular or deep subcutaneous route, but it should never be given intravenously. There have been rare reports of transitory exanthema and anaphylaxis following injection. Therefore, if a patient reports a previous sensitivity to injections of vitamin B$_{12}$, an intradermal skin test should be carried out before the full dose is administered.

Cyanocobalamin is administered in doses of 1 to 1000 μg. Tissue uptake, storage, and utilization depend on the availability of transcobalamin II (*see* above). Doses in excess of 100 μg are rapidly cleared from plasma into the urine, and administration of larger amounts of vitamin B$_{12}$ will thus not result in greater retention of the vitamin. Administration of 1000 μg is of value, however, in the performance of the Schilling test. Following oral administration of isotopically labeled vitamin B$_{12}$, the compound that is absorbed can be quantitatively recovered in the urine if 1000 μg of cyanocobalamin is administered intramuscularly. This unlabeled material saturates the transport system and tissue binding sites, so that more than 90% of the labeled and unlabeled vitamin is excreted during the next 24 hours.

A number of multivitamin preparations are marketed either as nutritional supplements or for the treatment of anemia. Many of these contain from 5 to 100 μg of cyanocobalamin without or with intrinsic factor concentrate prepared from the stomachs of hogs or other domestic animals. Purified preparations of intrinsic factor are standardized according to their ability to promote vitamin B$_{12}$ absorption in patients with pernicious anemia. One oral unit of intrinsic factor is defined as that amount of material that will bind and transport 15 μg of cyanocobalamin. Most multivitamin preparations supplemented with intrinsic factor contain 0.5 oral unit per tablet. While the combination of oral vitamin B$_{12}$ and intrinsic factor would appear to be ideal for patients with an intrinsic factor deficiency, *such preparations are not reliable.* Antibodies to human intrinsic factor may effectively counteract absorption of vitamin B$_{12}$. With prolonged therapy, some patients develop refractoriness to oral intrinsic factor, perhaps related to production of an intralumenal antibody against the hog protein (Ramsey and Herbert, 1965). All oral preparations of vitamin B$_{12}$ and intrinsic factor thus carry a warning that patients must be reevaluated at 3-month intervals for recurrence of pernicious anemia.

Hydroxocobalamin given in doses of 100 μg intramuscularly has been reported to have a more sustained effect than cyanocobalamin, a single dose maintaining plasma vitamin B$_{12}$ concentrations in the normal range for up to 3 months. However, a number of patients show reductions of the concentration of B$_{12}$ in plasma within 30 days, similar to that seen after cyanocobalamin. Furthermore, the administration of hydroxocobalamin has resulted in the formation of antibodies to the transcobalamin II–vitamin B$_{12}$ complex (Skouby *et al.*, 1971). *Hydroxocobalamin* (ALPHAREDISOL, others) is thus not recommended.

General Principles of Therapy. Vitamin B$_{12}$ has an undeserved reputation as a health tonic and has been used for a number of diverse disease states. Effective use of the vitamin depends on accurate diagnosis and an understanding of the following general principles of therapy:

1. Vitamin B$_{12}$ should be given prophylactically only when there is a reasonable

indication. Dietary deficiency in the strict vegetarian, the predictable malabsorption of vitamin B_{12} in patients who have had a gastrectomy, and certain diseases of the small intestine constitute such indications. When gastrointestinal function is normal, an oral prophylactic supplement of vitamins and minerals, including vitamin B_{12}, may be indicated. Otherwise, the patient should receive monthly injections of cyanocobalamin.

2. The relative ease of treatment with vitamin B_{12} should not prevent a full investigation of the etiology of the disease. Usually, the initial diagnosis of a deficiency state is made from the characteristic defect in hematopoiesis; a full understanding of the etiology of the disease state involves studies of dietary supply, gastrointestinal absorption, and transport.

3. Therapy should always be as specific as possible. While a large number of multivitamin preparations are available, the use of "shotgun" vitamin therapy in the treatment of vitamin B_{12} deficiency can be dangerous. *With such therapy, there is the danger that sufficient folic acid will be given to result in a hematological recovery; however, this may mask continued vitamin B_{12} deficiency, and neurological damage will develop or progress if already present.*

4. While a classical therapeutic trial with small amounts of vitamin B_{12} can help confirm the diagnosis, the acutely ill, elderly patient may not be able to tolerate the delay in the correction of a severe anemia with resultant tissue hypoxia. Such patients require supplemental blood transfusions and immediate therapy with both folic acid and vitamin B_{12} to guarantee recovery.

5. Long-term therapy with vitamin B_{12} must be evaluated at intervals of 6 to 12 months in patients who are otherwise well. If there is an additional illness or a condition that may increase the requirement for the vitamin (*e.g.*, pregnancy), assessment of treatment should be performed more frequently. The concentration of vitamin B_{12} in plasma should be monitored; peripheral blood counts and parameters of macrocytosis must be evaluated.

Treatment of the Acutely Ill Patient. The therapeutic approach depends on the severity of the patient's illness. The individual with an uncomplicated pernicious anemia, in which the abnormality is restricted to a mild or moderate anemia without leukopenia, thrombocytopenia, or neurological signs or symptoms, will respond quite well to the administration of vitamin B_{12} alone. Moreover, therapy may be delayed until other causes of megaloblastic anemia have been ruled out and sufficient studies of gastrointestinal function have been performed to reveal the underlying etiology of the disease. In this situation, a therapeutic trial with small amounts of parenteral vitamin B_{12} (1 to 10 μg per day) can be extremely valuable in confirming the presence of an uncomplicated vitamin B_{12} deficiency.

In contrast, patients with neurological changes or severe leukopenia or thrombocytopenia associated with infection or bleeding require emergency treatment. The older individual with a severe anemia (hematocrit less than 20%) is likely to have tissue hypoxia, cerebrovascular insufficiency, and congestive heart failure. Effective therapy must not wait for detailed diagnostic tests. Once the megaloblastic erythropoiesis has been confirmed and sufficient blood collected for later measurements of concentrations of vitamin B_{12} and folic acid, the patient should receive intramuscular injections of 100 μg of cyanocobalamin and 1 to 5 mg of folic acid. For the next 1 to 2 weeks the patient should receive daily intramuscular injections of 100 μg of cyanocobalamin, together with a daily oral supplement of 1 to 2 mg of folic acid. Since an effective increase in red-cell mass will not occur for 10 to 20 days, the patient with a markedly depressed hematocrit and tissue hypoxia should also receive a transfusion of 2 to 3 units of packed red cells; if congestive heart failure is present, phlebotomy to remove an equal volume of whole blood can be performed or diuretics can be administered. Disorders of hemostasis secondary to thrombocytopenia should be treated with platelet transfusions (daily or every other day) until the platelet count has increased, and any ongoing infection should be treated aggressively with appropriate antibiotics. However, such patients should not receive chloramphenicol, since this antibiotic can prevent recovery of granulocytes (*see* Chapter 52).

The therapeutic response to vitamin B_{12} is characterized by a number of subjective and objective changes (Figure 57–4). Patients usually report an increased sense of well-being within the first 24 hours after the initiation of therapy. Objectively, memory and orientation can show dramatic improvement, although full recovery of mental function may take months or, in fact, may never occur. In addition, even before there is an obvious hematological response, the patient may report an increase in strength, a better appetite, and an improvement in the soreness of the mouth and tongue.

The first objective hematological change is the disappearance of the megaloblastic morphology of the bone marrow. As the ineffective erythropoiesis is corrected, the concentration of iron in plasma falls dramatically as the metal is used in the formation of hemoglobin. This usually occurs within the

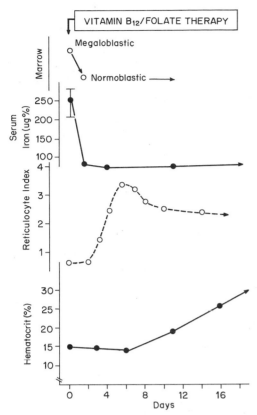

Figure 57–4. *Hematological response to the administration of vitamin B₁₂ or folic acid in patients with deficiency of the administered vitamin.*

Appropriate therapy with vitamin B₁₂ or folic acid results in a predictable series of subjective and objective changes. For the hematopoietic system, these include: an almost immediate reversion of the megaloblastic marrow to normoblastic morphology; a dramatic fall in the plasma iron as efficient erythropoiesis resumes; a rise in the reticulocyte index to values that are three to five times normal in 5 to 7 days; and a gradual increase in the hematocrit beginning in the second week. This pattern of response has been used as the basis for a therapeutic trial. When a small amount of either vitamin B₁₂ (less than 10 μg) or folic acid (less than 100 μg) is administered, the patient will respond only if the appropriate deficiency state is present.

first 48 hours. Full correction of precursor maturation in marrow with production of an increased number of reticulocytes begins on or about the second or third day and reaches a peak 3 to 5 days later. When the anemia is moderate to severe, the maximal reticulocyte index will be between three and five times the normal value, that is, a reticulocyte count of 20 to 40% (Hillman *et al.,* 1968). The

ability of the marrow to sustain a high rate of production of reticulocytes determines the rate of recovery of the hematocrit. Patients with complicating iron deficiency, an infection or other inflammatory state, or renal disease may be unable to maintain a sufficient rate of production to correct their anemia. It is important, therefore, to monitor the reticulocyte index over the first several weeks. If it does not continue at elevated levels for as long as the hematocrit is less than 35%, plasma concentrations of iron and folic acid should again be determined and the patient should be reevaluated for a complicating illness that could inhibit the response of the marrow.

During recovery from a vitamin B₁₂–related thrombocytopenia, the platelet count rises within 10 days to values that exceed normal. This overshoot is a typical response to the correction of an ineffective thrombocytopoietic state. The recovery of the white blood cells is less dramatic. In the absence of infection, the granulocyte count reverts to normal within the first 2 weeks, and large multilobed polymorphonuclear leukocytes gradually disappear from the circulation. Even though the turnover of circulating granulocytes is less than 8 to 12 hours, the continued presence of multilobed polymorphonuclear leukocytes in the peripheral blood reflects continued entry of abnormal cells from the granulocytic pool of the marrow.

Usually, the degree and rate of improvement of neurological signs and symptoms depend on the severity and the duration of the abnormalities. Those that have been present for only a few months disappear quite rapidly. When a defect has been present for months or years, it may require several months for objective improvement, or a full return to normal function may never occur.

The incidence of mortality due to deficiency of vitamin B₁₂ usually correlates with the patient's hematological status. Severe anemia and hypoxia in the elderly patient can overtax the already-compromised cardiovascular and cerebrovascular systems. Heart failure and cardiac arrhythmias are likely causes of death in the severely anemic patient. With marked leukopenia, a complicating infection can also be life threatening.

However, since the hematopoietic abnormalities are completely reversible, the long-term morbidity of vitamin B₁₂ deficiency is restricted to the neurological and gastrointestinal systems. In patients who have had a severe deficiency state with major neurological defects, it is not unusual to see continued difficulties with gait, a loss of position and vibratory sense, and the continued complaint of paresthesias. Chronic problems with gastrointestinal function tend to reflect the etiology of the vitamin B₁₂–deficiency state.

Chronic Therapy with Vitamin B₁₂. Once begun, vitamin B₁₂ therapy must be maintained for life. This fact must be impressed upon the patient and family, and a system should be established to guarantee continued monthly injections of cyanocobalamin. An injection of 100 μg of cyanocobalamin, intramuscularly, every 2 to 4 weeks is sufficient to maintain a normal concentration of vitamin B₁₂ in plasma and an adequate supply for tissues.

Patients with severe neurological symptoms and signs may be treated with larger doses of vitamin B_{12} in the period immediately following the diagnosis. Doses of 100 μg per day or several times per week may be given for several months with the hope of encouraging faster and more complete recovery. Whether recovery is more rapid has not been proven. It is important to monitor vitamin B_{12} concentrations in plasma and to obtain peripheral blood counts at intervals of 3 to 6 months to confirm the adequacy of therapy. Since refractoriness to therapy can develop at any time, evaluation must continue throughout the patient's life.

Other Therapeutic Uses of Vitamin B_{12}. Vitamin B_{12} has been used in the therapy of a number of conditions, including trigeminal neuralgia, multiple sclerosis and other neuropathies, various psychiatric disorders, poor growth or nutrition, and as a "tonic" for patients complaining of tiredness or easy fatigability. There is no evidence for the validity of such therapy in any of these conditions. Maintenance therapy with vitamin B_{12} has been used for the treatment of children with methylmalonic aciduria with some apparent success (Cooper, 1976).

FOLIC ACID

Chemistry and Metabolic Functions. The structural formula of pteroylglutamic acid (PteGlu$_1$) is shown in Figure 57–5. Major portions of the molecule include a pteridine ring linked by a methylene bridge to para-aminobenzoic acid, which is joined by an amide linkage to glutamic acid. While pteroylglutamic acid is the common pharmaceutical form of folic acid, it is neither the principal folate congener in food nor the active coenzyme for intracellular metabolism. Following absorption, PteGlu$_1$ is rapidly reduced at the 5, 6, 7, and 8 positions to tetrahydrofolic acid (H_4PteGlu$_1$), which then acts as an acceptor of a number of one-carbon units. These are attached at either the 5 or the 10 position of the pteridine ring or bridge these atoms to form a new five-membered ring. The most important forms of the coenzyme that are synthesized by these reactions are listed in Figure 57–5. Each plays a specific role in intracellular metabolism, summarized as follows (*see also* previous section on Relationships between Vitamin B_{12} and Folic Acid, as well as Figure 57–1):

1. *Conversion of homocysteine to methionine.* This reaction requires CH_3H_4PteGlu as a methyl donor and utilizes vitamin B_{12} as a cofactor.

2. *Conversion of serine to glycine.* This reaction requires tetrahydrofolate as an acceptor of a methylene group from serine and utilizes pyridoxal phosphate as a cofactor. It results in the formation of 5,10-CH_2H_4PteGlu, an essential coenzyme for the synthesis of thymidylate (dTMP).

3. *Synthesis of thymidylate.* CH_3H_4PteGlu donates a methyl group to deoxyuridylate for the synthesis of thymidylate—a rate-limiting step in DNA synthesis.

4. *Histidine metabolism.* H_4PteGlu also acts as an acceptor of a formimino group in the conversion of formiminoglutamic acid to glutamic acid.

5. *Synthesis of purines.* Two steps in the synthesis of purine nucleotides require the participation of derivatives of folic acid. Glycinamide ribonucleotide is formylated by 5,10-CHH$_4$PteGlu; 5-aminoimidazole-4-carboxamide ribonucleotide is formylated by 10-CHOH$_4$PteGlu. By these reactions carbon atoms at positions 8 and 2, respectively, are incorporated into the growing purine ring.

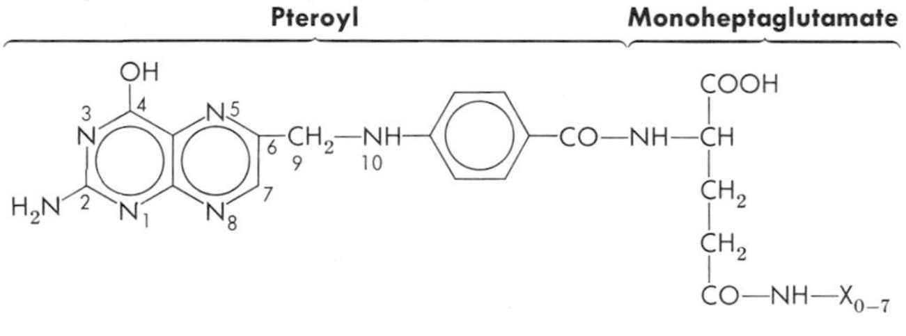

Position	Radical	Congener	
N^5	—CH$_3$	CH$_3$H$_4$PteGlu	Methyltetrahydrofolate
N^5	—CHO	5-CHOH$_4$PteGlu	Folinic acid (Citrovorum Factor)
N^{10}	—CHO	10-CHOH$_4$PteGlu	10-Formyltetrahydrofolate
N$^{5-10}$	—CH—	5,10-CHH$_4$PteGlu	5,10-Methenyltetrahydrofolate
N$^{5-10}$	—CH$_2$—	5,10-CH$_2$H$_4$PteGlu	5,10-Methylenetetrahydrofolate
N^5	—CHNH	CHNHH$_4$PteGlu	Formiminotetrahydrofolate
N^{10}	—CH$_2$OH	CH$_2$OHH$_4$PteGlu	Hydroxymethyltetrahydrofolate

Figure 57–5. *The structures and nomenclature of pteroylglutamic acid (folic acid) and congeners.*

See text for explanation. *X* represents additional residues of glutamate; polyglutamates are storage forms of the vitamin. The subscript that designates the number of residues of glutamate is frequently omitted because this number is variable.

6. *Utilization or generation of formate.* This reversible reaction utilizes $H_4PteGlu$ and 10-$CHOH_4PteGlu$.

Daily Requirements. Virtually all food sources are rich in folates, especially fresh green vegetables, liver, yeast, and some fruits. However, protracted cooking can destroy up to 90% of the folate content of such food (Herbert, 1973). Generally, a standard U.S. diet provides 50 to 500 μg of absorbable folate per day, although individuals with high intakes of fresh vegetables and meats will ingest as much as 2 mg per day. In the normal adult, the minimal daily requirement has been estimated at 50 μg, while the pregnant or lactating female and patients with high rates of cell turnover (as in patients with a hemolytic anemia) may require as much as 100 to 200 μg or more per day. Recommended dietary allowances of folate are presented in Table XVI–1.

Absorption, Distribution, and Elimination. As with vitamin B_{12}, diagnosis and management of deficiencies of folic acid depend on an understanding of the transport pathways and intracellular metabolism of the vitamin (Figure 57–6). Folates present in food are largely in the form of reduced polyglutamates (Tamura and Stokstad, 1973). Absorption requires transport and the action of a pteroyl-γ-glutamyl carboxypeptidase associated with mucosal cell membranes (Rosenberg, 1976). The mucosae of the duodenum and upper part of the jejunum are rich in dihydrofolate reductase and are capable of methylating most, if not all, absorbed, reduced folate. Since most folate is absorbed by the proximal portion of the small intestine, it is not unusual for folate deficiency to occur when there is pathology of the jejunum. Nontropical and tropical sprue are common causes of folate deficiency and megaloblastic anemia (Wellcome Trust Collaborative Study, 1971).

Once absorbed, folate is rapidly transported as $CH_3H_4PteGlu_1$ to tissues. While plasma proteins do bind folate derivatives, they have a greater affinity for nonmethylated analogs. The role of binding to plasma protein in folate homeostasis is not well understood (Rothenberg *et al.*, 1977). An

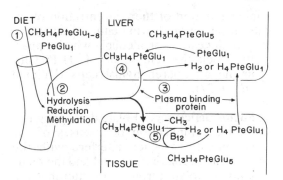

Figure 57–6. *Absorption and distribution of folate derivatives.*

Dietary sources of folate polyglutamates are hydrolyzed to the monoglutamate, reduced, and methylated to $CH_3H_4PteGlu_1$ during gastrointestinal transport. Folate deficiency commonly results from (*1*) inadequate dietary supply and (*2*) small intestinal disease. In patients with uremia, alcoholism, or hepatic disease there may be defects in (*3*) the concentration of folate binding proteins in plasma and (*4*) the flow of $CH_3H_4PteGlu_1$ into bile for reabsorption and transport to tissue (the folate enterohepatic cycle). Finally, vitamin B_{12} deficiency will (*5*) "trap" folate as $CH_3H_4PteGlu$, thereby reducing the availability of $H_4PteGlu_1$ for its essential roles in purine and pyrimidine synthesis.

increase in such binding capacity is detectable during deficiency of folate and in certain disease states, such as uremia, cancer, and alcoholism. Whether this increase interferes with folate transport and tissue supply requires further investigation.

Following uptake into cells, $CH_3H_4PteGlu$ acts as a methyl donor for the formation of methylcobalamin and as a source of $H_4PteGlu$ and other folate congeners, as described above. Folate is stored within cells as polyglutamates (Baugh and Krumdieck, 1969; Hoffbrand *et al.*, 1977).

Supplies of $CH_3H_4PteGlu_1$ are maintained by food and by an enterohepatic cycle of the vitamin. The liver actively reduces and methylates $PteGlu_1$ (and H_2 or $H_4PteGlu_1$) and then transports the $CH_3H_4PteGlu_1$ into bile for reabsorption by the gut and subsequent delivery to tissues (Steinberg *et al.*, 1979). This pathway may provide as much as 200 μg or more of folate each day for recirculation to tissues. The importance of the enterohepatic cycle is suggested by studies in animals that show a rapid reduction of the concentration of folate in plasma following either drainage of bile or ingestion of alcohol, which apparently block the release of $CH_3H_4PteGlu_1$ from hepatic parenchymal cells (Hillman et al., 1977).

Folate Deficiency. Folate deficiency is a common complication of diseases of the small intestine, which interfere with the absorption of folate from food and the recirculation of folate through the enterohepatic cycle. In acute or chronic alcoholism, daily intake of folate in food may be severely restricted, and the enterohepatic cycle of the vitamin may be impaired by the toxic effect of alcohol on hepatic parenchymal cells; this is perhaps the most common cause of folate-deficient megaloblastic erythropoiesis. However, it is also the most amenable to therapy, inasmuch as the reinstitution of a normal diet is sufficient to overcome the effect of alcohol. Disease states characterized by a high rate of cell turnover, such as hemolytic anemias, are often complicated by deficiency of folate (Lindenbaum, 1977). Additionally, drugs that inhibit dihydrofolate reductase (e.g., methotrexate, trimethoprim) or that interfere with the absorption and storage of folate in tissues (e.g., certain anticonvulsants, oral contraceptives) are capable of lowering the concentration of folate in plasma and at times may cause a megaloblastic anemia (Stebbins et al., 1973; Stebbins and Bertino, 1976).

Folate deficiency is recognized by its impact on the hematopoietic system. As with vitamin B_{12}, this reflects the increased requirement of organ systems with high rates of cell turnover. The megaloblastic anemia that results from folate deficiency cannot be distinguished from that caused by a deficiency of vitamin B_{12}. This is to be expected because of the final common pathway of the major intracellular metabolic roles of the two vitamins. At the same time, folate deficiency is rarely if ever associated with neurological abnormalities. Thus, the observation of characteristic abnormalities in vibratory and position sense and in motor and sensory pathways rules against the presence of an isolated deficiency of folic acid.

The appearance of megaloblastic anemia

following deprivation of folate is much more rapid than that caused by the sudden interruption of the absorption of vitamin B_{12} (e.g., gastric surgery). This reflects the fact that stores of folate are quite limited in vivo. In Herbert's classical study of a single normal individual maintained on a diet low in folate for several months, megaloblastic erythropoiesis appeared after approximately 10 to 12 weeks (Herbert, 1962). Subsequent studies have shown that the rate of induction of megaloblastic erythropoiesis varies according to the population studied and the dietary background of the individual (Eichner et al., 1971). A folate deficiency state may appear in 1 to 4 weeks, depending on the individual's dietary habits and stores of the vitamin.

Folate deficiency is best diagnosed from measurements of folate in plasma and in red cells by use of a microbiological assay or a competitive binding technic. The concentration of folate in plasma is extremely sensitive to changes in dietary intake of the vitamin and the influence of inhibitors of folate metabolism or transport, such as alcohol. Normal folate concentrations in plasma range from 4 to 20 ng/ml. A deficiency state may be considered to be present whenever the value is below 4 ng/ml. In the case of the alcoholic, the plasma folate concentration falls rapidly to values indicative of deficiency within 24 to 48 hours of steady ingestion of alcohol, while megaloblastic erythropoiesis becomes apparent after 1 to 2 weeks (Eichner and Hillman, 1971, 1973). At the same time, the plasma folate concentration will quickly revert to normal once such ingestion is stopped, even while the marrow is still megaloblastic. Such rapid fluctuations are but one example of the dynamic state of the concentration of folate in plasma. Thus, while it is an extremely sensitive measure of the supply of the vitamin available for tissues, it must be determined before any therapy is initiated, including the reinstitution of a normal diet. Measurement of folate in red cells or the adequacy of stores in lymphocytes (by use of the deoxyuridine suppression test) may be employed to diagnose a long-standing deficiency of folic acid (Herbert et al., 1973). (In this test, deoxyuridine fails to suppress the synthesis of DNA if normal amounts of folate are present in the cells.) For either test to be positive, a state of deficiency must have existed for a sufficient time to allow the production of a new population of cells with deficient stores of folate.

Preparations. *Folic acid* (FOLVITE) is marketed as oral preparations, alone or in combination with other vitamins or minerals, and as an aqueous solution for injection. Tablets of folic acid contain either 0.1, 0.4, 0.8, or 1 mg of pteroylglutamic acid. *Folic acid injection* is an aqueous solution of the sodium salt of pteroylglutamic acid. *Leucovorin* *calcium injection (folinic acid, 5-CHOH₄PteGlu, citrovorum factor)* is also available for intramuscular injection. The principal indication for the use of folinic acid is to circumvent the action of inhibitors of dihydrofolate reductase, such as methotrexate. It is *not* indicated for use in the treatment of folic acid deficiency. Certainly, leucovorin should never be used for the treatment of pernicious anemia or other megaloblastic anemias secondary to a deficiency of vitamin B_{12}. Just as with folic acid, its use can result in an apparent response of the hematopoietic system, but neurological damage may occur or progress if already present.

Untoward Effects. There have been rare reports of reactions to parenteral injections of both folic acid and leucovorin. If a patient describes such a reaction before the drug is given, caution should be exercised. Oral folic acid is not toxic for man. Even with doses as high as 15 mg per day, there have been no substantiated reports of side effects. Folic acid in large amounts may counteract the antiepileptic effect of phenobarbital, phenytoin, and primidone and increase the frequency of seizures in susceptible children (Reynolds, 1968). While some studies have not supported these contentions, the U.S. Food and Drug Administration has recommended that oral tablets of folic acid be limited to strengths of 1 mg or less.

General Principles of Therapy. The therapeutic use of folic acid is limited to the prevention and treatment of deficiencies of the vitamin. As with vitamin B_{12} therapy, effective use of the vitamin depends on accurate diagnosis and an understanding of the mechanisms that are operative in a specific disease state. The following general principles of therapy should be respected:

1. Prophylactic administration of folic acid should be undertaken only when there is a clear indication. Dietary supplementation is necessary when there is an increased requirement that is not satisfied by normal dietary sources. Pregnancy, with the increased demands of the fetus, or lactation, where as much as 50 μg of folate is lost each day in the breast milk, is an indication for supplementation with folate. The most popular form of supplementation for this situation is a multivitamin preparation that contains 400 to 500 μg of pteroylglutamic acid. Patients with a disease state charac-

terized by high levels of cell turnover (*e.g.,* a hemolytic anemia) should also receive folic acid prophylactically, usually one or two 1-mg tablets of folic acid each day. Finally, any patient who demonstrates folate deficiency because of an undesired effect of a drug (*see* above) may receive supplementation with a preparation of folic acid for oral use.

2. As with vitamin B_{12} deficiency, any patient with folate deficiency and a megaloblastic anemia should be carefully evaluated to determine the underlying etiology of the deficiency state. This should include evaluation of the effects of medications, the amount of alcohol intake, the patient's history of travel, and the function of the gastrointestinal tract.

3. Therapy should always be as specific as possible. Multivitamin preparations should be avoided unless there is good reason to suspect deficiency of several vitamins.

4. The potential complications of mistreating a patient who has vitamin B_{12} deficiency with folic acid must be kept in mind. The administration of large doses of folic acid can result in an apparent improvement of the megaloblastic anemia, inasmuch as PteGlu is converted by dihydrofolate reductase to $H_4PteGlu_1$; this circumvents the methylfolate "trap." Such therapy does not prevent or alleviate the neurological defects of vitamin B_{12} deficiency, and these may become irreversible.

Treatment of the Acutely Ill Patient. As described in detail in the section on vitamin B_{12}, treatment of the patient who is *acutely ill* with megaloblastic anemia should begin with intramuscular injections of both vitamin B_{12} and folic acid. Inasmuch as the patient requires therapy before the exact etiology of the disease has been defined, it is important to avoid the potential problem of a combined deficiency of both vitamin B_{12} and folic acid. When both are present, therapy with only one vitamin will not provide an optimal response. Longstanding nontropical sprue is one example of a disease in which combined deficiency of B_{12} and folate is common. When indicated, both vitamin B_{12} (100 μg) and folic acid (1 to 5 mg) should be administered intramuscularly, immediately, and the patient should then be maintained on daily oral supplements of 1 to 2 mg of folic acid for the next 1 to 2 weeks. Indications and recommendations for further administration of vitamin B_{12} are described above.

Oral administration of folate is generally satisfactory for all patients who are not acutely ill, regardless of the etiology of the deficiency state. Even the patient with tropical or nontropical sprue and a demonstrable defect in absorption of folic acid will respond adequately to such therapy. Abnormalities in the activity of pteroyl-γ-glutamyl carboxypeptidase and the function of mucosal cells will not prevent passive diffusion of sufficient amounts of PteGlu across the mucosal barrier if dosage is adequate, and continued ingestion of alcohol or other drugs will also not prevent an adequate therapeutic response. The effect of most inhibitors of folate transport or dihydrofolate reductase is easily overcome by pharmacological doses of the vitamin. Perhaps the only situation in which this is not true is when there is a severe deficiency of vitamin C. The patient with scurvy may suffer from a megaloblastic anemia despite increased intake of folate and normal or high concentrations of the vitamin in plasma and cells.

An oral dose of 1 mg of folate two or at the most three times a day is generally adequate for adults; children should respond to a daily regimen that contains as little as 1 mg of the vitamin. The therapeutic response may be monitored by study of the hematopoietic system in a fashion identical to that described for vitamin B_{12} (see Figure 57–4). Within 48 hours of the initiation of appropriate therapy, megaloblastic erythropoiesis disappears and, as efficient erythropoiesis begins, the concentration of iron in plasma falls to normal or below-normal values. The reticulocyte count begins to rise on about the second or third day and reaches a peak by the fifth to seventh day; the reticulocyte index reflects the proliferative state of the marrow. Finally, the hematocrit begins to rise during the second week.

It is possible to use this reliable pattern of recovery as the basis for a therapeutic trial. For this purpose, the patient should receive a daily parenteral injection of 50 to 100 μg of folic acid. Administration of doses in excess of 100 μg per day entails the risk of inducing a hematopoietic response in patients who are deficient in vitamin B_{12}, while oral administration of the vitamin may be unreliable because of intestinal malabsorption. A number of other complications may also interfere with the therapeutic trial. The patient with sprue and deficiencies of other vitamins or iron may fail to respond because of these inadequacies. In cases of alcoholism, the presence of hepatic disease, inflammation, or iron deficiency can act to blunt the proliferative response of the marrow and to prevent the correction of the anemia. For these reasons the therapeutic trial has not gained great popularity for the evaluation of the patient with a potential deficiency of folic acid.

Adams, J. F., and Boddy, K. Metabolic equilibrium of tracer and natural vitamin B_{12}—an experimental study. J. Lab. Clin. Med., 1968, 72, 392–396.

Allen, R. H., and Mehlman, C. S. Isolation of gastric vitamin B_{12}–binding proteins using affinity chromatography. I. Purification and properties of human intrinsic factor. J. Biol. Chem., 1973, 248, 3660–3669.

Allen, R. H.; Seetharam, B.; Allen, N. C.; Podell, E. R.; and Alpers, D. H. Correction of cobalamin malabsorption in pancreatic insufficiency with a cobalamin analogue that binds with high affinity to R protein but not to intrinsic factor. J. Clin. Invest., 1978, 61, 1628–1634.

Baugh, C. M., and Krumdieck, C. L. Naturally occurring folates. Ann. N.Y. Acad. Sci., 1969, 186, 7–28.

Chanarin, I.; Hutchinson, M.; MacLean, N.; and Moule, M. Hepatic folate in man. Br. Med. J., 1966, 1, 396–399.

Cox, E. V., and White, A. M. Methylmalonic acid excretion: an index of vitamin B_{12} deficiency. Lancet, 1962, 2, 853–861.

de Aizpurua, H. J.; Cosgrove, L. H.; Ungar, B.; and Tah, B. H. Autoantibodies cytotoxic to gastric parietal cells in serum of patients with pernicious anemia. N. Engl. J. Med., 1983, 309, 625–629.

Eichner, E. R., and Hillman, R. S. The evolution of anemia in alcoholic patients. Am. J. Med., 1971, 50, 218–232.

—————. The effect of alcohol on the serum folate level. J. Clin. Invest., 1973, 52, 584–591.

Eichner, E. R.; Pierce, I.; and Hillman, R. S. Folate balance in dietary induced megaloblastic anemia. N. Engl. J. Med., 1971, 284, 933–938.

FAO/WHO Expert Group. Requirements of ascorbic acid, vitamin D, vitamin B_{12}, folate and iron. WHO Tech. Rep. Ser., 1970, 452, 3–75.

Finch, C. A.; Colman, D. H.; Motulsky, A. G.; Donohue, D. M.; and Reiff, R. H. Erythrokinetics in pernicious anemia. Blood, 1956, 11, 807–820.

Hakami, N.; Nieman, P. E.; Canellos, G. P.; and Lazerson, J. Neonatal megaloblastic anemia due to inherited transcobalamin II deficiency in two siblings. N. Engl. J. Med., 1971, 285, 1163–1170.

Hall, C. A., and Finkler, A. E. Isolation and evaluation of the various B_{12} binding proteins in human plasma. In, Vitamins and Coenzymes. (McCormick, D. B., and Wright, L. D., eds.) Academic Press, Inc., New York, 1971, pp. 108–126.

Herbert, V. Experimental nutritional folate deficiency in man. Trans. Assoc. Am. Physicians, 1962, 75, 307–320.

Herbert, V.; Tisman, G.; Go, L. T.; and Brenner, L. The dU suppression test using ^{125}I-UdR to define biochemical megaloblastosis. Br. J. Haematol., 1973, 24, 713–723.

Herbert, V., and Zalusky, R. Interrelations of vitamin B_{12} and folic acid metabolism: folic acid clearance studies. J. Clin. Invest., 1962, 41, 1263–1276.

Heyssel, R. M.; Bozian, R. C.; Darby, W. J.; and Bell, M. C. Vitamin B_{12} turnover in man: the assimilation of vitamin B_{12} from natural foodstuff by man and estimates of minimal daily dietary requirements. Am. J. Clin. Nutr., 1966, 18, 176–184.

Hillman, R. S.; Adamson, J.; and Burka, E. Characteristics of B_{12} correction of the abnormal erythropoiesis of pernicious anemia. Blood, 1968, 31, 419–432.

Hillman, R. S.; McGuffin, R.; and Campbell, C. Alcohol interference with the folate enterohepatic cycle. Trans. Assoc. Am. Physicians, 1977, 90, 145–156.

Hitzig, W. H.; Dohmann, U.; Pluss, H. J.; and Vischer, D. Hereditary transcobalamin II deficiency: clinical findings in a new family. J. Pediatr., 1974, 85, 622–628.

Hoffbrand, A. V.; Tripp, E.; and Lavoie, A. Folate polyglutamate synthesis and breakdown in cells. In, Folic Acid: Proceedings of a Workshop on Human Folate Requirements, 1975. National Academy of Sciences, Washington, D. C., 1977, pp. 110–121.

Huennekens, F. M. Folate and B_{12} coenzymes. In, Biological Oxidation. (Singer, T. P., ed.) John Wiley & Sons, Inc., New York, 1968, pp. 439–513.

Layzer, R. B. Myeloneuropathy after prolonged exposure to nitrous oxide. Lancet, 1978, 2, 1227–1230.

Lindenbaum, J. Folic acid requirement in situations of

increased need. In, *Folic Acid: Proceedings of a Workshop on Human Folate Requirements, 1975.* National Academy of Sciences, Washington, D. C., **1977**, pp. 256–276.

Linnell, J. C.; Hoffbrand, A. V.; Peters, T. T.; and Matthews, D. M. Chromatographic and bioautographic estimation of plasma cobalamins in various disturbances of vitamin B_{12} metabolism. *Clin. Sci.*, **1971**, *40*, 1–16.

Mitchell, H. K.; Snell, E. E.; and Williams, R. J. The concentration of "folic acid." *J. Am. Chem. Soc.*, **1941**, *63*, 2284.

Ramsey, C., and Herbert, V. Dialysis assay for intrinsic factor and its antibody: demonstration of species specificity of antibodies to human and hog intrinsic factor. *J. Lab. Clin. Med.*, **1965**, *65*, 143–152.

Reizenstein, P.; Ek, G.; and Matthews, C. M. E. Vitamin B_{12} kinetics in man. Implications of total-body-B_{12}-determinations, human requirements and normal and pathological cellular B_{12} uptake. *Phys. Med. Biol.*, **1966**, *11*, 295–306.

Retief, F. P.; Gottlieb, C. W.; and Herbert, V. Delivery of $Co^{57}B_{12}$ to erythrocytes from alpha to beta globulin of normal, B_{12}-deficient, and chronic myeloid leukemia serum. *Blood*, **1967**, *29*, 837–851.

Reynolds, E. H. Mental effects of anticonvulsants and folic acid metabolism. *Brain*, **1968**, *91*, 197–214.

Rothenberg, S. P.; DaCosta, M.; and Fischer, C. Use and significance of folate binders. In, *Folic Acid: Proceedings of a Workshop on Human Folate Requirements, 1975.* National Academy of Sciences, Washington, D. C., **1977**, pp. 82–97.

Schilling, R. F. Intrinsic factor studies. II. The effect of gastric juice on the urinary excretion of radioactivity after the oral administration of radioactive vitamin B_{12}. *J. Lab. Clin. Med.*, **1953**, *42*, 860–866.

Scott, J. M.; Bloomfield, F. J.; Stebbins, R.; and Herbert, V. Studies on derivation of transcobalamin III from granulocytes. *J. Clin. Invest.*, **1974**, *53*, 228–239.

Scott, J. M.; Dinn, J. J.; Wilson, P.; and Weir, D. G. Pathogenesis of subacute combined degeneration: a result of methyl group deficiency. *Lancet*, **1981**, *2*, 334–337.

Skouby, A. P.; Hippe, E.; and Olesen, H. Antibody to transcobalamin II and B_{12} binding capacity in patients treated with hydroxycobalamin. *Blood*, **1971**, *38*, 769–774.

Stahlberg, K. G. Studies on methyl-B_{12} in man. *Scand. J. Haematol.*, **1967**, Suppl. 1, 3–99.

Stebbins, R.; Scott, J.; and Herbert, V. Drug-induced megaloblastic anemias. *Semin. Hematol.*, **1973**, *10*, 235–251.

Steinberg, S.; Campbell, C.; and Hillman, R. S. Kinetics of the normal folate enterohepatic cycle. *J. Clin. Invest.*, **1979**, *64*, 83–89.

Sullivan, L. W., and Herbert, V. Studies on the minimum daily requirement for vitamin B_{12}: hematopoietic responses to 0.1 microgm. of cyanocobalamin or coenzyme B_{12} and comparison of their relative potency. *N. Engl. J. Med.*, **1965**, *272*, 340–346.

Tamura, T., and Stokstad, E. L. R. The availability of food folate in man. *Br. J. Haematol.*, **1973**, *25*, 513–532.

Weissbach, H., and Taylor, R. T. Metabolic role of vitamin B_{12}. *Vitam. Horm.*, **1968**, *26*, 395–412.

Wills, L., and Bilimoria, H. S. Studies in pernicious anaemia of pregnancy: production of macrocytic anaemia in monkeys by deficient feeding. *Indian J. Med. Res.*, **1932**, *20*, 391–402.

Wills, L.; Clutterbuck, P. W.; and Evans, P. D. F. A new factor in the production and cure of macrocytic anaemias and its relation to other haemopoietic principles curative in pernicious anaemia. *Biochem. J.*, **1937**, *31*, 2136–2147.

Monographs and Reviews

Blakely, R. L. *The Biochemistry of Folic Acid and Related Pteridines.* North-Holland Publishing Co., Amsterdam; John Wiley & Sons, Inc., New York, **1969**.

Castle, W. B. Development of knowledge concerning the gastric intrinsic factor and its relation to pernicious anemia. *N. Engl. J. Med.*, **1953**, *249*, 603–614.

————. A century of curiosity about pernicious anemia. *Trans. Am. Clin. Climatol. Assoc.*, **1961**, *73*, 54–80.

Chanarin, I. *The Megaloblastic Anemias*, 2nd ed. Blackwell Scientific Publications, Oxford; F. A. Davis Co., Philadelphia, **1979**.

Cooper, B. A. Megaloblastic anaemia and disorders affecting utilization of vitamin B_{12} and folate in childhood. *Clin. Haematol.*, **1976**, *5*, 631–659.

Das, K. C., and Herbert, V. Vitamin B_{12}–folate interrelations. *Clin. Haematol.*, **1976**, *5*, 697–725.

Glass, G. B. J. *Gastric Intrinsic Factor and Other Vitamin B_{12} Binders: Biochemistry, Physiology, Pathology and Relation to Vitamin B_{12} Metabolism.* George Thieme Verlag, Stuttgart; Intercontinental Medical Book Co., New York, **1974**.

Gräsbeck, R. Intrinsic factor and other vitamin B_{12} transport proteins. *Prog. Hematol.*, **1969**, *6*, 233–260.

Herbert, V. Folic acid and vitamin B_{12}. In, *Modern Nutrition in Health and Disease*, 5th ed. (Goodhart, R. S., and Shils, M. E., eds.) Lea & Febiger, Philadelphia, **1973**, pp. 221–244.

————. Megaloblastic anemias. In, *Cecil-Loeb Textbook of Medicine*, 15th ed. (Beeson, P. B.; McDermott, W.; and Wyngaarden, J. B.; eds.) W. B. Saunders Co., Philadelphia, **1979**, pp. 1719–1729.

Herbert, V., and Tisman, G. Effects of deficiencies of folic acid and vitamin B_{12} on central nervous system function and development. In, *Biology of Brain Dysfunction*, Vol. 1. (Gaull, G., ed.) Plenum Press, New York, **1973**, pp. 373–392.

Hoffbrand, A. V., and Wickremasinghe, R. G. Megaloblastic anemia. In, *Recent Advances in Haematology.* (Hoffbrand, A. V., ed.) Churchill-Livingstone, Ltd., Edinburgh, **1982**, pp. 25–44.

Kass, L. *Pernicious Anemia*, Vol. II. W. B. Saunders Co., Philadelphia, **1976**.

Pratt, J. M. *Inorganic Chemistry of Vitamin B_{12}.* Academic Press, Inc., New York, **1972**.

Reynolds, E. H. Neurological aspects of folate and vitamin B_{12} metabolism. *Clin. Haematol.*, **1976**, *5*, 661–696.

Rosenberg, I. Absorption and malabsorption of folates. *Clin. Haematol.*, **1976**, *5*, 589–618.

Skeggs, H. R. Vitamin B_{12}. In, *The Vitamins: Chemistry, Physiology, Pathology, Methods*, 2nd ed., Vol. VII. (Gyorgy, P., and Pearson, W. N., eds.) Academic Press, Inc., New York, **1967**, pp. 277–301.

Smith, E. L. *Vitamin B_{12}*, 3rd ed. Methuen & Co., London; John Wiley & Sons, Inc., New York, **1965**.

Stebbins, R., and Bertino, J. R. Megaloblastic anemia produced by drugs. *Clin. Haematol.*, **1976**, *5*, 619–630.

Stokstad, E. L. R., and Koch, J. Folic acid metabolism. *Physiol. Rev.*, **1967**, *47*, 83–116.

Weir, D. G., and Scott, J. M. Interrelationships of folates and cobalamins. In, *Nutrition in Hematology.* Vol. 5, *Contemporary Issues in Clinical Nutrition.* (Lindenbaum, J., ed.) Churchill Livingstone, New York, **1983**, pp. 121–142.

Wellcome Trust Collaborative Study. *Tropical Sprue and Megaloblastic Anaemia.* Churchill Livingstone, Ltd., Edinburgh, **1971**.

CHAPTER

58 ANTICOAGULANT, ANTITHROMBOTIC, AND THROMBOLYTIC DRUGS

Robert A. O'Reilly

Interference with hemostasis decreases the morbidity and mortality of thromboembolic disease. This premise provides the basis for therapy with anticoagulant, antithrombotic, and thrombolytic drugs. Unfortunately, studies on animals have contributed little to the clinical application of these drugs, because thrombotic diseases induced by experimental methods seldom simulate the natural diseases of man. Thus, the use of these drugs is empirical and is based on results from clinical trials. Moreover, these therapies are often prophylactic, which can be difficult for physicians to accept. They are too readily aware of therapeutic failures, expressed as further thrombosis or hemorrhage; therapeutic success manifests itself only by the *absence* of thrombosis. Thus, the questionable good, the potential harm, and the many complexities of anticoagulant drugs have earned this therapy a dubious reputation. This pessimism is offset by therapeutic optimism for the drugs that alter platelet function, the antithrombotic drugs, and by the increased usage of thrombolytic agents.

MECHANISMS OF THROMBOGENESIS AND BLOOD COAGULATION

Thrombogenesis. *Hemostasis* is the spontaneous arrest of bleeding from damaged blood vessels. Precapillary vessels contract immediately when cut. Within seconds, thrombocytes or blood platelets are bound to the exposed collagen of the injured vessel by a process called *platelet adhesion*. Platelets also stick to each other, *platelet aggregation*, and, as they lose their individual membranes, a viscous mass is formed (termed *viscous metamorphosis*). This platelet plug can stop bleeding quickly, but it must be reinforced by fibrin for long-term effectiveness. This reinforcement is initiated by the local stimulation of the coagulation process by the exposed collagen of the cut vessel and the released contents and membranes of platelets. Days later, an ingrowth of fibroblasts along a scaffolding of fibrin repairs the vascular rent permanently upon completion of fibrosis.

Thrombogenesis is an altered state of hemostasis. An intravascular thrombus results from a pathological disturbance of hemostasis. The nineteenth century triad of Virchow described thrombogenesis in terms of stasis, hypercoagulability, and change of the vessel wall. This is still the basis for current theories. The *white* or *arterial thrombus* is initiated by the adhesion of circulating platelets to a vessel wall. This initial adhesion and the release of adenosine diphosphate (ADP) from platelets is followed by platelet-platelet interaction or aggregation. The thrombus grows to occlusive proportions in the areas of slower arterial blood flow. When the thrombus finally occludes the blood vessel, hemostasis occurs locally, and a red thrombus forms around the white thrombus. Thus, when occlusion of the artery is total, a mixed white and red thrombus is present. In contrast, a *red* or *venous thrombus* develops in areas of stasis or slow blood flow in veins and resembles a blood clot formed *in vitro*. The bulk of it is a fibrin network enmeshed with red blood cells and platelets. A venous thrombus has a long "tail" that can easily detach and result in embolization of the pulmonary arteries. Thus, arterial thrombi cause serious disease by local ischemia, whereas venous thrombi do so primarily by distant embolization.

A platelet plug formed solely by ADP-stimulated platelet interaction is unstable. After the initial aggregation and viscous metamorphosis of platelets, fibrin becomes an important constituent of a thrombus. Production of thrombin (*see* below) occurs by activation of the reactions of blood coagulation at the site of the platelet mass. This thrombin stimulates further platelet aggregation not only by inducing the release of more ADP from the platelets but also by stimulating the synthesis of prostaglandins—aggregating agents that are more powerful than ADP (*see* Chapter 28). Two classes of prostaglandins with opposite effects on platelet aggregation and thrombogenesis are formed. Thromboxane A_2 (TXA_2) is synthesized by the aggregated platelets and stimulates further aggregation, while prostacyclin (PGI_2) is synthesized by the vessel wall and inhibits thrombosis.

Blood Coagulation. The coagulation of blood entails the formation of fibrin by the interaction of more than a dozen proteins in a cascading series of proteolytic reactions (*see* Figure 58–1). At each step a clotting factor (*e.g.,* XII) undergoes limited proteolysis and itself becomes an active protease (*e.g.,* XIIa) (Table 58–1). This clotting-factor enzyme activates the next clotting factor (XI) until

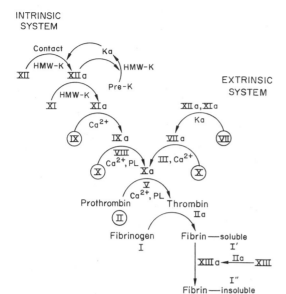

INTRINSIC
SYSTEM

Figure 58–1. *Intrinsic and extrinsic systems of blood coagulation.*

The circled clotting factors are dependent on vitamin K for their activation. Hageman factor (XII) undergoes contact activation and becomes bound to surfaces. This surface-bound factor XII undergoes proteolytic activation by kallikrein (Ka) in the presence of high-molecular-weight kininogen (HMW-K). Factor XIIa constitutes an arm of a feedback loop and activates more Ka from prekallikrein (Pre-K or Fletcher factor), in the presence of HMW-K. Factor XIIa in the presence of HMW-K also activates factor XI. Factor XIa in the presence of Ca^{2+} proteolytically activates factor IX to IXa. Factor VIII, factor IXa, Ca^{2+}, and phospholipid micelles (PL) from blood platelets form a lipoprotein complex with factor X and activate it. Factor V, factor Xa, Ca^{2+}, and PL also form a lipoprotein complex with factor II or prothrombin and activate it to IIa or thrombin. In seconds, thrombin splits two small pairs of peptides off the large fibrinogen (I) molecule, followed by rapid noncovalent aggregation of soluble fibrin monomers (I'). Factor XIII, activated by thrombin to XIIIa, cross-links adjacent fibrin monomers (I') covalently to form the insoluble fibrin clot (I'').

In the extrinsic system, factor VII undergoes proteolytic activation by factors XIIa, XIa, and Ka from the intrinsic system. Factor VIIa, Ca^{2+}, tissue thromboplastin (III), and factor X form a lipoprotein complex that results in activation of factor X. From this step onward the extrinsic system is identical to the intrinsic system. Factor Xa is the principal factor that is inhibited by heparin, following the interaction of heparin with its cofactor, antithrombin III.

ultimately an insoluble fibrin clot is formed. The soluble precursor of fibrin circulates in the blood as fibrinogen (I). Fibrinogen is a substrate for the enzyme thrombin (IIa), a protease that is formed during the coagulation process by activation of a circulating proenzyme, prothrombin (II). Prothrombin is converted to thrombin by activated factor X in the presence of factor V, Ca^{2+}, and phospholipid.

Two separate pathways lead to the formation of activated factor X and the activation of prothrombin. In the *intrinsic system,* all the protein factors necessary for coagulation are present in the circulating blood. In the *extrinsic system,* unidentified lipoproteins called tissue thromboplastin (factor III), which are not present in the circulating blood, activate blood coagulation at the level of factor X (*see* Figure 58–1). In the intrinsic system the prothrombin-activating principle, factor Xa, requires many minutes for formation, whereas the extrinsic system is activated within seconds because the early time-consuming reactions are bypassed. Both pathways must be intact for adequate hemostasis (*see* Ratnoff, 1981; Zwaal and Hemker, 1982).

I. Anticoagulants

HEPARIN

History. In 1916, the medical student McLean, while investigating the nature of ether-soluble procoagulants, made the serendipitous finding of a phospholipid anticoagulant. Soon thereafter, a water-soluble mucopolysaccharide, named *heparin* because of its abundance in liver, was discovered by Howell (1922), in whose laboratory McLean had been working (*see* Jaques, 1978). The use of heparin *in vitro* to prevent the clotting of shed blood led to its use *in vivo* to treat venous thrombosis. Improved purification of the tissue extracts in Canada and in Sweden permitted clinical trials with large

Table 58–1.   BLOOD CLOTTING FACTORS

FACTOR	COMMON SYNONYMS
I	Fibrinogen
I'	Fibrin monomer
I''	Fibrin polymer
II	Prothrombin
III	Tissue thromboplastin
IV	Calcium, Ca^{2+}
V	Labile factor
VII	Proconvertin
VIII	Antihemophilic globulin, AHG
IX	Christmas factor, PTC
X	Stuart factor
XI	Plasma thromboplastin antecedent, PTA
XII	Hageman factor
XIII	Fibrin-stabilizing factor
HMW-K	High-molecular-weight kininogen, Fitzgerald factor
Pre-K	Prekallikrein, Fletcher factor
Ka	Kallikrein
PL	Platelet phospholipid

doses of heparin in 1938. While Best's suggestion in 1948—that endogenous inhibitors that keep blood fluid might be useful clinically—presaged the possibility of therapy with *low doses* of heparin, the efficacy of this procedure was not demonstrated for more than 20 years. Studies *in vitro* by Wessler and Yin in 1970 and clinical trials by Kakkar and colleagues in 1973 led the way for this important improvement in the use of heparin for anticoagulant therapy.

Chemistry and Source. Heparin is a heterogeneous group of straight-chain anionic mucopolysaccharides, called glycosaminoglycans, of molecular weights that average 15,000 daltons (Jaques, 1980). Less than 1% of the native glycosaminoglycans obtained by alkaline hydrolysis from a covalently conjugated protein core is heparin. Commercial heparin consists of polymers of two repeating disaccharide units: D-glucosamine-L-iduronic acid and D-glucosamine-D-glucuronic acid. In the structure that appears below, the upper disaccharide unit is composed of an iduronic acid and a glucosamine residue, while the lower unit contains residues of glucuronic acid and glucosamine. Most samples of heparin contain 8 to 15 sequences of each disaccharide unit, but not necessarily in equal proportions. Heparin is strongly acidic because of its content of covalently linked sulfate and carboxylic acid groups. Sulfamides and sulfate esters are formed at positions 2 and 6, respectively, of glucosamine, and a sulfate ester is also found at the 2-OH group of iduronic acid. Compared with standard heparin, heparin fractions of low molecular weight have a greater inhibitory effect on factor-Xa activity relative to their ability to prolong the partial thromboplastin time. Low-molecular-weight heparin also appears to have less antiplatelet activity (Hoylaerts *et al.*, 1983). However, the translation of these findings into greater efficacy and/or lesser bleeding for any low-molecular-weight fraction of heparin will require clinical trials.

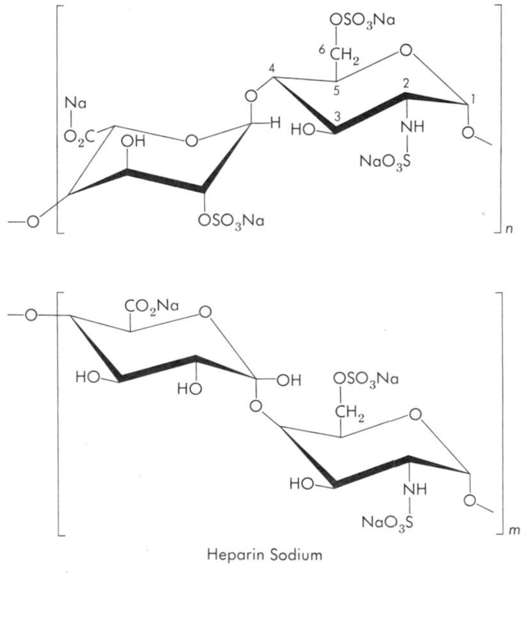

Heparin Sodium

Commercial heparin is prepared from bovine lung and porcine intestinal mucosa, but it can also be obtained from sheep and whales. Although porcine mucosal heparin is more potent in its antifactor-Xa activity and plasma lipolytic activity (*see* below) than is that of bovine lung, all heparins are biologically equivalent. However, the incidence of thrombocytopenia is lower with porcine mucosal heparin (Powers *et al.*, 1979). Since heparin from mammalian-tissue sources is in limited supply, semisynthetic sulfated polymers have been prepared from disaccharides composed of D-glucosamine and D-glucuronic acid. These "heparinoids" have high anticoagulant and lipolytic activities, but their clinical utility has not been tested. New natural heparinoids of low molecular weight may be safer than standard heparin (Henny *et al.*, 1983).

Occurrence and Physiological Function. Heparin occurs intracellularly in mammalian tissues that contain mast cells, but only in a macromolecular form of at least 750,000 daltons. This "big" heparin has only 10 to 20% of the anticoagulant activity of commercial heparin. *Heparan sulfate*, a compound similar to heparin sulfate (in name and chemistry) but with less anticoagulant activity, is a ubiquitous component at the mammalian cell surface (Vernier *et al.*, 1983). When native heparin is released from its bound and inactive state in the metachromatic granules of mast cells, it is ingested and rapidly destroyed by macrophages. Because heparin cannot be detected in the circulating blood and is inactive in its tissue form, its physiological function is still unknown.

PHARMACOLOGICAL PROPERTIES

When injected intravenously, heparin has two major pharmacological effects—impairment of blood coagulation and reduction of the concentration of triglycerides in plasma.

Action on Blood Coagulation and Antithrombin III. The anticoagulant effect of heparin is essentially immediate, and it occurs both *in vitro* and *in vivo*. Heparin acts indirectly by means of a plasma cofactor. The heparin cofactor, or antithrombin III, is an α-globulin and a serine protease inhibitor that neutralizes several activated clotting factors, that is, XIIa, kallikrein (activated Fletcher factor), XIa, IXa, Xa, IIa, and XIIIa. Although antithrombin III was thought to be the only macromolecule able to inactivate thrombin, other plasma proteins are now known to possess this activity. Antithrombin III and the newly described heparin cofactor II form irreversible complexes with thrombin, and, as a result, the proteins are inactivated (Griffith, 1983). Heparin markedly accelerates the velocity, but not the extent, of this reaction. A ternary complex is apparently formed between heparin, antithrombin III, and the clotting factors (Björk and Lindahl, 1982). Low concentrations of heparin increase the activity of antithrombin III, particularly against factor Xa and thrombin; this forms the basis for the administration of *low doses of heparin* as a therapeutic regimen.

Patients who receive intermittent or continuous therapy with heparin have a progressive reduction of antithrombin-III activity to values that approximate one third of normal (Marciniak and Gockerman, 1977). Thus, a heparin-induced reduction of the activity of antithrombin III may paradoxically increase the thrombotic tendency in man. The standard regimens for treatment of thromboembolic diseases may require modification to minimize depletion of antithrombin III during therapy with conventional or high doses of heparin (Kakkar *et al.*, 1980). Estrogen-containing contraceptives also reduce the apparent concentrations of antithrombin III. The thrombotic symptoms that characterize familial deficiency of antithrombin III often are first seen during pregnancy. Because the oral anticoagulants (*see* below) *increase* antithrombin-III activity, they are the treatment of choice for patients with this inherited disorder.

Platelet factor 4 is a cationic, low-molecular-weight protein that is associated with a chondroitin sulfate carrier; this factor is released from aggregated platelets during coagulation, and it binds to and neutralizes heparin. Although its physiological function is unknown, platelet factor 4 may bind heparin locally and thereby facilitate the accumulation of thrombin and clot formation. Since the activity of platelet factor 4 in plasma reflects both the extent of blood clotting and the consumption of platelets, this activity has been measured in many patients with thromboembolic diseases in an effort to detect those at risk from thrombosis.

Lipoprotein Lipase. The effect of injected heparin on plasma lipids, the well-known "clearing" effect of heparin on turbid, lipemic plasma, results from the release into the blood of tissue-bound, lipid-hydrolyzing enzymes. One of these enzymes, lipoprotein lipase, hydrolyzes the triglycerides of chylomicrons and very-low-density lipoproteins bound to capillary endothelial cells into fatty acids and partial glycerides (*see* Chapter 34). These products are then metabolized by extrahepatic tissues. Heparin is thought not to activate these enzymes but to release them from tissues and stabilize them. Lipoprotein lipase activity is high in adipose tissue and skeletal muscle, where the fatty acids released from the catabolism of plasma triglycerides are utilized rapidly.

Miscellaneous Actions. When added to blood, heparin does not alter routine chemical determinations, but it does distort the morphology of red and white blood cells. Heparinized blood is unsuitable for tests that involve complement, isoagglutinins, or erythrocyte fragility, unless the heparin is removed or neutralized *in vitro* by protamine (*see* below), but it may be used for determination of hematocrit, white-blood-cell count, and erythrocyte sedimentation rate. Blood that is sampled from indwelling venous cannulas "flushed" intermittently with heparinized saline solution contains increased concentrations of free fatty acids; these can inhibit the binding to plasma proteins of lipophilic drugs such as propranolol, quinidine, phenytoin, and digoxin and thus interfere with quantification of this parameter.

Heparin has been reported to suppress the secretory rate of aldosterone, increase the concentration of free thyroxine in plasma, inhibit fibrinolytic activators, retard wound healing, depress cell-mediated immunity, suppress graft-versus-host reactions, and accelerate the healing of thermal burns (Jaques, 1982).

Absorption, Fate, and Excretion. Heparin crosses membranes poorly because of its polarity and large molecular size. It is thus not absorbed from gastrointestinal and sublingual sites; fortunately, its passage both across the placenta and into maternal milk is also hindered. The deep subcutaneous or intrafat injection site is used when therapy with low doses of heparin is chosen and for treatment of ambulatory patients. Intramuscular injection of heparin should be avoided because large hematomas can form at the site of injection. Administration of high doses of heparin is accomplished by continuous or intermittent intravenous injection. The anticoagulant activity of heparin disappears from the blood by *apparent* first-order kinetics; nevertheless, the half-life is dependent on the dose. When 100, 400, or 800 units/kg of heparin is injected intravenously, the half-life of the anticoagulant activity is approximately 1, 2.5, and 5 hours, respectively (*see* Appendix II). Surprisingly, steady-state concentrations of heparin may not be reached even after 48 hours of continuous infusion because of dose-dependent kinetics and uptake by the reticuloendothelial system (McAvoy, 1979). Heparin is metabolized in the liver by an enzyme termed *heparinase,* and the inactive metabolic products are excreted in the urine. Heparin itself appears in the urine only after administration of large doses intravenously. In patients with renal failure or hepatic cirrhosis, the half-life of the anticoagulant activity of heparin is significantly longer than in normal subjects. Patients with pulmonary embolism require higher doses of heparin because of more rapid clearance of the drug. Individual variation of both the anticoagulant effect of a given concentration of heparin in plasma and the rate of clearance of the drug have been documented (Whitfield *et al.,* 1982).

Unitage and Preparations. In the absence of a suitable chemical assay, standardization of a sample of heparin is based on comparison *in vitro* with a known standard in a nonspecific assay of anticoagulant activity. The USP unit of heparin is the quantity that will prevent 1.0 ml of citrated sheep plasma from clotting for 1 hour after the addition of 0.2 ml of 1 : 100 $CaCl_2$ solution. *Heparin sodium* derived from lung contains at least 120 USP units/mg, and at least 140 USP units/mg when derived from other tissues. Because the potency (and chain lengths) of different preparations may vary widely, heparin should always be prescribed on a unit basis. The drug is available as *heparin sodium injection* from bovine lung (LIPO-HEPIN/BL) and from porcine intestinal mucosa (LIPO-HEPIN, LIQUAEMIN SODIUM) in sterile water in concentrations of 1000 to 40,000 USP units/ml. *Heparin calcium injection* (CALCIPARINE), widely used in European clinical trials to evaluate low doses of heparin, is reported to cause a significantly lower incidence of local hematoma. It is available in sterile water at a concentration of 25,000 units/ml.

Routes of Administration and Dosage. As mentioned, heparin must be administered parenterally. Blood clotting *in vitro* is fully prevented by a concentration of 1 unit/ml of whole blood. A 10,000-unit bolus of heparin administered intravenously to a 70-kg patient results in an initial plasma concentration of heparin of about 3 units/ml, and anticoagulant activity disappears with a half-life of 1.5 hours. *Intermittent intravenous therapy* is best performed by means of an indwelling, rubber-capped needle (or heparin lock); a dose of 10,000 units initially, followed by doses of 5000 to 10,000 units every 4 to 6 hours, is administered. The size and frequency of the maintenance dose depend on the weight of the patient and especially on the response to previous doses of the anticoagulant. This response should be measured 1 hour before the next dose. For children, the initial dose is 50 to 100 units/kg, the maintenance dose is 50 to 100 units/kg

every 4 hours, adjusted according to the anticoagulant response, and the total daily dose is as much as 500 units/kg of body weight or 20,000 units/m^2 of body surface area.

Administration of *low doses* of heparin preoperatively for primary prophylaxis of deep venous thrombosis is begun 2 hours before surgery with 5000 units of heparin administered *subcutaneously;* this dose is repeated every 8 to 12 hours for 7 days or until the patient is fully ambulatory. However, all patients must be tested before treatment to ensure their hemostatic competence. Bleeding can occur even with low doses of heparin; this particularly includes bleeding and hematomas from the wound postoperatively and hematomas at the injection sites for the heparin. Patients should not receive aspirin, oral anticoagulants, or drugs that inhibit platelet aggregation concurrently; conduction-block anesthesia and neurosurgical procedures are also contraindications. Low doses of heparin are inadequate prophylaxis for any active thrombotic process. They are also inadequate for patients who are at very high risk for venous thromboembolism (*e.g.,* those with major trauma or those having orthopedic operations of the hip or lower extremity or extensive pelvic operations for malignant disease). Low doses of heparin are recommended for patients undergoing major surgery or prolonged hospitalization who are at risk for thromboembolism (*e.g.,* those with congestive heart failure, chronic pulmonary disease, obesity, a history of thromboembolic disease, or chronic venous stasis of the lower extremities) (Nelson *et al.,* 1982). *Ultralow doses* of heparin (1 unit/kg per hour) by continuous intravenous infusion for 3 to 5 days during and after major surgery has been recommended to decrease the incidence of postoperative deep-venous thrombosis and to avoid problems of bleeding, anaphylaxis, impairment of wound healing, and thrombocytopenia. The efficacy of such "ultralow-dose" therapy is comparable to that for "low-dose" treatment (Negus *et al.,* 1980).

Continuous intravenous infusion is initiated with a loading dose of 5000 to 10,000 units of heparin injected directly into the infusion tubing. A constant infusion pump or a mechanical syringe pump controls the flow rate and fluid volume. A solution sufficient for only 6 hours is prepared to avoid accidental overdose. For a 70-kg patient, 6000 units of heparin is added to 100 ml of 5% dextrose or 100 ml of 0.9% saline solution, and this is infused at a rate of 1000 units every hour. The rate of infusion and the amount of heparin added to each 6-hour aliquot are adjusted to keep a measure of blood clotting, the activated partial thromboplastin time, at least twice that of the patient's pretreatment value. Thus, the average-sized patient in 24 hours receives 24,000 units of heparin and 400 ml of fluid and requires four changes of the volume-control unit. The site of heparin-lock needles should be rotated every 2 to 3 days, especially in patients who are neutropenic or otherwise susceptible to infections. *Implantable pumps* for continuous intravenous infusion of heparin have been used successfully for as long as 18 months in patients with recurrent venous thromboembolic disease.

Deep subcutaneous (intrafat) injection of heparin has been used to slow the rate of absorption and thereby prolong the therapeutic concentration in blood. Technics that are helpful to minimize local ecchymoses include use of a very small (#26), 1.25-cm (½-in.) needle; a 1-ml tuberculin syringe; heparin in high concentrations to reduce the injected volume; gentle grasping of a 2.5- to 5-cm (1- to 2-in.) area of iliac or abdominal fat away from the deeper tissues; rotating the sites of injection; cleaning the needle of any heparin solution before injection; positioning the needle perpendicular to the skin surface; clearing the needle with 0.1 ml of air kept at the plunger end of the syringe, which is injected last; and application of firm pressure over the site for 1 to 2 minutes after injection.

Jet-injected subcutaneous administration of low doses of heparin is less painful and faster than needle injection. *Intrapulmonary administration* of aerosolized heparin to human volunteers results in an anticoagulant effect that lasts for days; this technic warrants further study (Jaques, 1982). When heparin is administered *intraperitoneally* during peritoneal dialysis, it often loses its anticoagulant activity locally because of the disappearance of antithrombin-III activity. Heparin may also be inactivated when it is added to the *artificial kidney* because of the influx of calcium, magnesium, and acetate ions from the dialysate.

Side Effects, Toxicity, and Contraindications. Purified commercial preparations of heparin are relatively nontoxic, and side effects from the drug are infrequent. Because heparin is obtained from animal tissue, it should be used cautiously in patients with any history of allergy. A trial dose of 1000 units should precede usual therapeutic doses. Hypersensitivity reactions include chills, fever, urticaria, or anaphylactic shock. Local and systemic allergic reactions to the preservative used in multidose vials have been reported. Heparin intended for use in heart-lung machines is free of preservatives. Increased loss of hair and reversible, transient alopecia have been reported. Osteoporosis and spontaneous fractures occur in patients who have received 15,000 units or more of heparin daily for over 3 months (Megard *et al.,* 1982).

Hemorrhage. The chief complication of therapy with heparin is hemorrhage. Bleeding may be reduced to a minimum by careful control of dosage, careful selection of patients, avoidance of all aspirin-containing medications, and scrupulous respect of the contraindications to the therapy. The anticoagulant effect should be monitored by a test of blood clotting, such as the partial thromboplastin time. Significant gastrointestinal or genitourinary bleeding may be indicative of an underlying occult pathological lesion. Elderly women in particular develop hemorrhagic complications. Increased bleeding in patients with any serious concurrent disease occurs during therapy with heparin.

Thrombocytopenia. Heparin causes transient mild thrombocytopenia in about 25% of patients and severe thrombocytopenia in a few. The mild reaction results from heparin-induced platelet aggregation, while severe thrombocytopenia follows the formation of heparin-dependent antiplatelet antibodies. The latter is characterized by its delayed occurrence (the eighth to twelfth day of treatment), tolerance to the anticoagulant action of heparin, recurrent thromboembolic disease, a platelet count as low as 5000/mm^3, elevated fibrin degradation products in plasma, reduced plasma fibrinogen, adequate megakaryocytes in bone-marrow specimens (consistent with peripheral consumption of platelets), and improvement of thrombocytopenia after discontinuation of the heparin. Most patients with such heparin-induced thrombocytopenia received heparin prepared from bovine lung rather than from porcine intestine (Cipolle *et al.,* 1983). An immunoglobulin G directed against an antigen common to several preparations of heparin has been detected in the plasma of heparinized patients with thrombocytopenia (Trowbridge *et al.,* 1978). It reacts with the heparin-platelet complex to trigger the release reaction of platelets, which results in platelet aggregation and thrombocytopenia. The following considerations apply to all patients given heparin: platelet counts must be monitored frequently; any new thrombus might be the *result* of the heparin therapy; thrombocytopenia sufficient to cause hemorrhage should be considered to be heparin induced; and thromboembolism thought to result from heparin should be treated by discontinuation of heparin and substitution of an agent that inhibits platelet aggregation and/or an oral anticoagulant, if clinically warranted. Severe thrombocytopenia, hemorrhage, and death have occurred even in patients receiving "low-dose" heparin therapy. Low-molecular-weight heparins interact with platelets less readily. Clinical trials are warranted to compare their efficacy and hemorrhagic side effects with those of standard heparins.

Contraindications. Heparin therapy is contraindicated in patients who consume large amounts of ethanol, who are sensitive to the drug, who are actively bleeding, or who have hemophilia, purpura, thrombocytopenia, intracranial hemorrhage, bacterial endocarditis, active tuberculosis, increased capillary permeability, ulcerative lesions of the gastrointestinal tract, severe hypertension, threatened abortion, or visceral carcinoma. Heparin should be withheld during and after surgery of the brain, eye, or spinal cord and should not be administered to patients undergoing lumbar puncture or regional anesthetic block. The drug should be used only when clearly indicated in pregnant women, despite its apparent lack of transfer across the placenta.

Antagonists of Heparin. Mildly excessive anticoagulant effects of heparin are treated by discontinuation of the drug. If the effects are severe and bleeding occurs, administration of a specific antagonist may be indicated. Protamine is available for this purpose.

Protamine Sulfate. The protamines are proteins of low molecular weight that are found in the sperm or mature testes of fish of the family Salmonidae. They are strongly basic because of their high content of arginine. *In vitro,* protamine sulfate combines ionically with heparin to form a stable complex that is devoid of anticoagulant activity. Protamine administered intravenously in the absence of heparin interacts with platelets and with many proteins, including fibrinogen; these interactions may account for its own anticoagulant activity and toxicity. *In vivo,* protamine inhibits the anticoagulant effect of heparin, but the effect of heparin on platelet aggregation may persist; this persistence may be particularly prominent after open-heart surgery (Ellison *et al.,* 1978). The amount of protamine required to antagonize heparin can be estimated; 1 mg of protamine should be administered for every 100 units of heparin

remaining in the patient. Alternatively, the requirement for protamine can be determined directly *in vitro* by titration of the patient's blood with the protein.

Protamine sulfate is available as a solution containing 10 mg/ml and in vials containing 50 or 250 mg of powder. It must be given only by the intravenous route and then slowly (not more than 20 mg/minute, or up to 50 mg in a 10-minute period). Rapid injection may cause dyspnea, flushing, bradycardia, and hypotension, perhaps as a result of the release of histamine. Hypersensitivity reactions have been reported, especially in patients allergic to fish.

Therapeutic Uses. The therapeutic uses of heparin are discussed later in this chapter.

ORAL ANTICOAGULANTS

History. Sweet clover was planted in the Dakota plains and Canada at the turn of the century because it flourished on poor soil and substituted for corn in silage. In 1924, Schofield reported a previously undescribed hemorrhagic disorder in cattle that resulted from the ingestion of spoiled sweet clover silage. After Roderick traced the cause to a toxic reduction of plasma prothrombin, Campbell and Link, in 1939, identified the hemorrhagic agent as bishydroxycoumarin (dicumarol). Many congeners of dicumarol were synthesized in Link's laboratories, the most useful of which, racemic warfarin, was prepared by Ikawa and associates (1944). (*Warfarin* is an acronym for the patent holder, Wisconsin Alumni Research Foundation, plus the cou*marin*-derived suffix.) Initially it was thought to be too toxic for man, but it became the world's most useful rodenticide. In 1951, a man survived an attempted suicide with large and repeated doses of a warfarin-containing rodenticide; this event quickly led to clinical trials that established the safety of its use in humans (Link, 1959). The large multicenter clinical trial of the American Heart Association resulted in a report, in 1954, of seemingly favorable responses of patients with myocardial infarction to dicumarol. This unfortunately led to the overuse of the drug. The oral anticoagulants have since become heuristic models in clinical pharmacology for the study of pharmacokinetics and its correlation with biological effects, genetic control of drug metabolism, and the elucidation of mechanisms of drug interactions.

Chemistry. The structure of the hemorrhagic agent of sweet clover disease was found to be bishydroxycoumarin, a derivative of 4-hydroxycoumarin. Many anticoagulant drugs have been synthesized as derivatives of 4-hydroxycoumarin (Table 58–2) or of the related compound, indan-1,3-dione. A discussion of the indanedione derivatives can be found in the *sixth edition* of this textbook. The essential chemical characteristics of the coumarin derivatives for anticoagulant activity are an

Table 58–2. STRUCTURAL FORMULAS OF THE ORAL ANTICOAGULANTS *

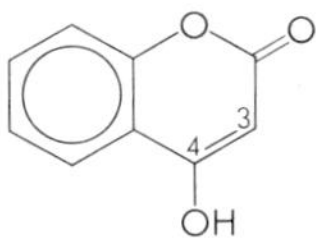

4-Hydroxycoumarin

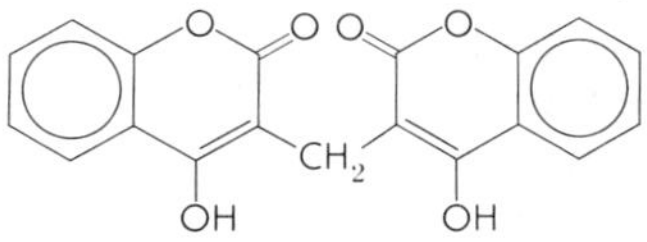

Dicumarol

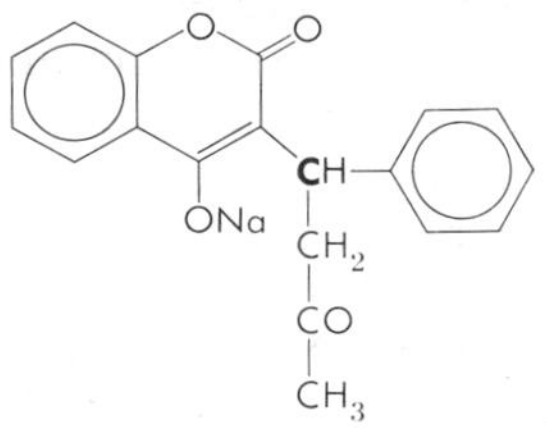

Warfarin Sodium

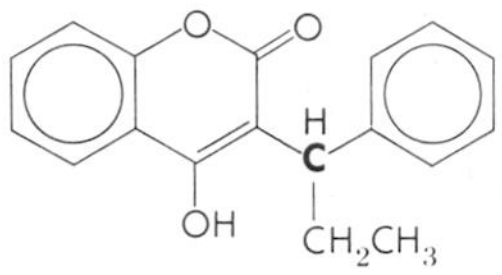

Phenprocoumon

* 4-Hydroxycoumarin is included to indicate the parent molecule from which the oral anticoagulants are derived. Asymmetrical carbon atoms in warfarin and phenprocoumon are indicated in boldface type.

intact 4-hydroxycoumarin residue with a carbon substituent at the 3 position. Phenprocoumon and warfarin both have an asymmetrical carbon atom in the substituent at the 3 position, and the available preparations of the drugs are mixtures of the two optical isomers. The levorotatory or S-(−)-enantiomorphs of warfarin and phenprocoumon are more potent anticoagulants than are the dextrorotatory or R-(+)-enantiomorphs. Some of the drug interactions that have been reported for racemic warfarin are also more prominent with the S-(−)-enantiomorph (O'Reilly, 1976a).

PHARMACOLOGICAL PROPERTIES

The anticoagulant effects of the various oral agents that are available for clinical use differ only quantitatively. However, there are differences in pharmacokinetic properties and toxicity that make racemic warfarin sodium the drug of choice, the prototype, and by far the most widely used oral anticoagulant in the United States.

Effects on Blood Coagulation. The major pharmacological effect of oral anticoagulants is inhibition of blood clotting by interference with the hepatic posttranslational modification of the vitamin K–dependent clotting factors (II, VII, IX, and X). These drugs are often called indirect anticoagulants because they act only *in vivo*, whereas heparin is termed a direct anticoagulant because it acts *in vitro* as well. The therapeutic effect is delayed for 8 to 12 hours

after oral or intravenous administration of racemic warfarin, because it results from an altered balance between the partially inhibited rates of modification and unaltered rates of degradation of the four proteins. The kinetics of the pharmacological effect is thus dependent on the half-lives of these clotting factors in the circulation, which are 6, 24, 40, and 60 hours for factors VII, IX, X, and II, respectively. Larger initial doses of drug (about 0.75 mg/kg of racemic warfarin) hasten the onset of hypoprothrombinemia only to a certain limited extent; beyond this, the rate of onset is independent of the size of the dose. The principal effect of a large loading dose is to prolong the time that the concentration of drug in plasma remains above that required for suppression of modification of clotting factors. The 1- to 3-day delay between the peak concentration of drug in plasma and its maximal hypoprothrombinemic effect is consistent with a kinetic model in which a linear relationship is assumed between the logarithm of the concentration of drug in plasma and the reduction of the *rate of modification* of the vitamin K–dependent clotting factors (Nagashima *et al.*, 1969). The only significant difference that exists in the inherent ability of various oral anticoagulant drugs to produce and maintain hypoprothrombinemia is their half-life (*see* O'Reilly and Aggeler, 1970).

Mechanism of Action. The oral anticoagulants are antagonists of vitamin K (*see* Chapter 67). Their administration to man or other animals leads to the appearance of precursors of the four vitamin K–dependent clotting factors in plasma and liver. These precursor proteins are antigenically active but are biologically inactive in tests of coagulation (Hauschka *et al.*, 1978). The precursor protein to prothrombin can be activated to thrombin nonphysiologically by several snake venoms, demonstrating that the portion of the molecule necessary for this activity is intact. However, the precursor proteins cannot bind divalent cations such as calcium and thus cannot interact with phospholipid-containing membranes, which are their normal sites of activation. The vitamin K–sensitive step in the synthesis of clotting factors is the postribosomal carboxylation of ten or more glutamic acid residues at the amino-terminal end of the precursor protein to form a unique amino acid, γ-carboxyglutamate. These amino acid residues chelate calcium, which is apparently necessary for the binding of the four vitamin K–dependent clotting factors to phospholipid-containing membranes (*see* Symposium, 1980). Both oral anticoagulants and deficiency of vitamin K also reduce the γ-carboxyglutamate content of *osteocalcin,* a protein of bone. This suggests a mechanism for the production of *chondrodysplasia punctata* in infants born of mothers taking oral anticoagulants during the first trimester of pregnancy (Hall *et al.*, 1980).

In hepatic microsomes, the reduction of vitamin K to its hydroquinone form (vitamin KH_2) precedes the bicarbonate-dependent carboxylation of precursor prothrombin, descarboxyprothrombin, to prothrombin (Figure 58–2). This carboxylase activity for the synthesis of prothrombin is linked to an epoxidase activity for vitamin KH_2, which oxidizes the vitamin to vitamin K epoxide (KO). An epoxide reductase, which requires reduced nicotinamide adenine dinucleotide, converts vitamin K epoxide back to vitamin KH_2. This reaction is probably the site of action of warfarin (Whitlon *et al.*, 1978) and the site of genetic resistance to warfarin, which is also characterized by an increased require-

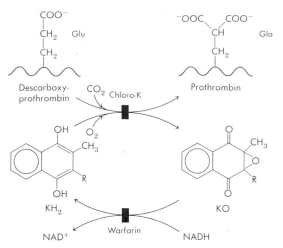

Figure 58–2. *Vitamin K cycle: metabolic interconversions of vitamin K associated with the modification of vitamin K–dependent clotting factors.*

Vitamin K_1 or K_2 is reduced to the hydroquinone form (KH_2). Stepwise oxidation to vitamin K epoxide (*KO*) is coupled to protein carboxylation, wherein descarboxyprothrombin (descarboxy-II) is converted to prothrombin (II) by carboxylation of glutamate residues (*Glu*) to γ-carboxyglutamate (*Gla*). Enzymatic reduction of the epoxide with reduced nicotinamide adenine dinucleotide (*NADH*) as a cofactor regenerates vitamin KH_2. The oxidation of vitamin K is inhibited by the chloro analog of vitamin K (*Chloro-K*), whereas the reduction of vitamin K epoxide is the warfarin-sensitive step (*Warfarin*). The R on the vitamin K molecule represents a 20-carbon phytyl side chain in vitamin K_1 and a 5- to 65-carbon prenyl side chain in vitamin K_2.

ment for vitamin K (O'Reilly, 1971). The vitamin K analog chloro-K_1 (in which the 2-methyl group of vitamin K_1 is replaced by a chloro group) directly inhibits the carboxylase and epoxidase reactions, which are not sensitive to warfarin.

Factors That Affect Activity. Physiological and pathological factors can increase or decrease the response to oral anticoagulant drugs. These factors seldom affect the kinetics of accumulation of the anticoagulant drug, but they do influence its biological effect.

Factors That Increase the Hypoprothrombinemic Response. Inadequate diet, disease of the small bowel, and diseases that hinder the delivery of bile to the small intestine all cause *vitamin K deficiency* and increase the response to oral anticoagulants. Although vitamin K is synthesized by enteric bacteria, antimicrobial agents in general have little effect on anticoagulant therapy unless both dietary and intestinal sources of vitamin K are simultaneously reduced. The effect of the third-generation cephalosporins is more significant (Uotila and Suttie, 1983).

Administration of oral anticoagulants to patients with *hepatic disease* of diverse etiologies results in greater hypoprothrombinemia than when the drugs are given to normal subjects. The effect is ascribable to impaired hepatic synthesis of the clotting factors. Patients in congestive heart failure who are given oral anticoagulants also have an augmented hypoprothrombinemic response; this lessens as myocardial and hepatic functions improve. Variable results have followed the administration of vitamin K to patients with hepatic disease, apparently because many hemostatic abnormalities can occur in such patients, including alterations of platelets and blood vessels and deficiencies of clotting factors I, II, V, VII, IX, X, XI, and XIII. Because of the sporadic unreliability of alcoholic patients, *chronic alcoholism* may be the most common proximate cause of bleeding in subjects taking oral anticoagulants. When compliant subjects receive warfarin, 10 to 20 oz of wine daily at mealtime has no significant effect on the steady-state concentration of prothrombin (O'Reilly, 1979).

Hypermetabolic states, such as fever and hyperthyroidism, increase the responsiveness to oral anticoagulants, whereas myxedematous patients require larger doses of these drugs. The reduced dose requirement for oral anticoagulants in patients with hypermetabolic states results from increased catabolism of the vitamin K–dependent clotting factors. There is also a positive correlation between *patient age* and the degree of response to oral anticoagulants; this effect is independent of body weight, and the pharmacokinetics of warfarin is unaltered (Shepherd *et al.,* 1977).

Factors That Decrease the Hypoprothrombinemic Response. During *pregnancy* a state of decreased responsiveness to oral anticoagulants results from increased activity of factors VII, VIII, IX, and X. However, this affects only the mother, and the fetus is highly susceptible to oral anticoagulants because these drugs cross the placenta freely and the fetus has a limited capacity to synthesize clotting factors. As noted above, heparin does not cross the placenta and its use is thus safer for the fetus, but the many injections required and the hemorrhagic complications for the mother remain as formidable problems. Some patients with the *nephrotic syndrome* have been observed to have a high requirement for warfarin; this may be caused by a shortened half-life of the anticoagulant resulting from proteinuria and the excretion of drug bound to albumin. *Uremia* has little or no effect on the hypoprothrombinemic response of patients receiving warfarin chronically, but it does significantly increase both the fraction of the drug in plasma that is free and the clearance of warfarin from the circulation (Bachmann *et al.,* 1977). *Hereditary resistance* to oral anticoagulants, which has been observed in two human kindreds and in rats in many geographic loci, is an autosomal dominant trait. The metabolism of the drug is normal, but the requirement for vitamin K is markedly increased in both species (O'Reilly, 1971).

Drug Interactions. Chronic treatment with oral anticoagulants is frequently necessary in patients who must also take other drugs for serious disease. Drug interactions with oral anticoagulants are all too common, and the ready occurrence of bleeding renders them indelibly obvious and frequently ominous. Drugs most commonly taken that interact with oral anticoagulants are *barbiturates, salicylates,* and *phenylbutazone*. These and other interactions have been studied extensively because of their importance and because interactions of the oral anticoagulants have come to be regarded as a model for understanding the intricacies of this subject. Interactions of both pharmacokinetic and pharmacodynamic types have been revealed (Serlin and Breckenridge, 1983).

Drugs That Increase the Response to Oral Anticoagulants. It is hazardous to administer any drug containing *acetylsali-*

cylic acid during anticoagulant therapy. Even one 325-mg tablet of aspirin can reduce the release of ADP by platelets and thereby impair their aggregation. Three such tablets will prolong the bleeding time of most normal subjects. The bleeding time is a measure of *primary hemostasis,* wherein platelet "plugs" are formed by collagen-induced aggregation of platelets and thrombin-induced formation of fibrin. When there is impairment of both functions—that is, the formation of fibrin (as in hemophilic patients or during anticoagulant therapy) and the aggregation of platelets (when aspirin is administered)—the hemorrhagic consequences can be catastrophic. Furthermore, large daily doses of aspirin (over 3 g) increase the hypoprothrombinemic response of patients taking oral anticoagulants. *Acetaminophen* and *sodium salicylate* are alternatives to aspirin for analgesia and antipyresis in such patients. These drugs probably do not interact adversely with oral anticoagulants, nor do they affect platelet function. However, there is no good alternative to aspirin for its anti-inflammatory effects in these patients, because other salicylates and even the newer nonsteroidal agents can cause gastrointestinal bleeding and may affect platelet function, even though they do not alter the hypoprothrombinemic response significantly.

Phenylbutazone and *oxyphenbutazone* can cause severe hemorrhage during anticoagulant therapy by impairment of platelet aggregation, induction of peptic ulceration, and augmentation of the hypoprothrombinemia. Phenylbutazone displaces warfarin from albumin and thereby transiently increases the concentration of free warfarin in plasma; chloral hydrate also has this effect. In addition, phenylbutazone interacts stereoselectively with racemic warfarin by inhibiting the metabolism of levowarfarin—the more potent isomer (Lewis *et al.,* 1974). It has little or no effect on the hypoprothrombinemic action of dextrowarfarin (O'Reilly *et al.,* 1980). Other drugs that increase the hypoprothrombinemic effect of warfarin by alteration of its pharmacokinetic parameters include *disulfiram* and *cimetidine,* which inhibit drug metabolism, and *sulfinpyrazone, metronidazole,* and *tri-*

methoprim-sulfamethoxazole, which selectively prolong the half-life of levowarfarin and thus enhance the efficacy of the racemic drug mixture (O'Reilly, 1982a, 1982b, 1984). *Sulfonamides* and other antimicrobial agents have little effect on anticoagulant therapy unless both intestinal and dietary sources of vitamin K are reduced simultaneously.

Clofibrate reduces adhesiveness of platelets and their epinephrine-induced aggregation; it augments the one-stage prothrombin activity; it increases the turnover rate of clotting factors II and X; but it does not affect the steady-state concentration or half-life of racemic warfarin or its enantiomorphs (Bjornsson *et al.,* 1977). Thus, the hemorrhagic complications that occur when therapy with clofibrate and warfarin is concurrent result from an additive hemostatic defect of reduced platelet function and more rapid turnover of the vitamin K–dependent clotting factors. Increased responsiveness to oral anticoagulants occurs with other hypolipidemic drugs, such as *dextrothyroxine,* and also with *anabolic steroids.* The administration of heparin obviously complicates oral anticoagulant therapy because of the combined effect of both drugs on the one-stage prothrombin time. If *heparin* is discontinued and the oral anticoagulant continued at the usual dose (*e.g.,* when a patient leaves the hospital), the prothrombin time may be reduced to the normal range of values of the test.

Drugs That Decrease the Response to Oral Anticoagulants. Induction of hepatic microsomal enzymes by *barbiturates* increases the clearance of oral anticoagulants, which correlates with a decrease in the degree of hypoprothrombinemia. *Glutethimide* has similar effects. Barbiturates have a particularly marked effect on the response to dicumarol because they also interfere with the absorption of this agent. *Benzodiazepines* and *chloral hydrate* have little or no effect during chronic concurrent administration of oral anticoagulants.

Rifampin markedly reduces both the concentrations of drug in the blood and the hypoprothrombinemia produced by oral anticoagulants. *Diuretics* either have no effect or decrease the response to oral anticoagulants. The latter effect may be due to concentration of clotting factors in plasma subsequent to diuresis, as reported for *chlorthalidone* and *spironolactone*. *Cholestyramine* reduces the hypoprothrombinemia and enhances the plasma clearance of oral anticoagulants by increasing the elimination of unchanged drug in the stool. *Antacids* have no effect on the absorption of warfarin or its hypoprothrombinemic effect, although they may impair the absorption of dicumarol. *Vitamin C* in massive doses reduces the hypoprothrombinemic response of some patients on long-term therapy with oral anticoagulants.

Other Concurrent Drug Effects. Case reports of accumulation of *oral hypoglycemic* agents in patients receiving dicumarol have not been substantiated. Intoxication with *phenytoin* may occur with concurrent administration of dicumarol, but not when warfarin is used.

Absorption, Fate, and Excretion. Racemic warfarin sodium is rapidly and completely absorbed, and peak concentrations in plasma are reached within 1 hour after ingestion. The bioavailability of warfarin potassium in man is significantly less than that of warfarin sodium. Food decreases the rate but not the extent of absorption of warfarin.

Racemic warfarin in the circulation is almost totally bound (99%) to plasma albumin during long-term therapy, which largely prevents its diffusion into red blood cells, cerebrospinal fluid, urine, and breast milk. The half-life of racemic warfarin administered by intravenous bolus is 37 hours, and the volume of distribution is that of the albumin space, 11 to 12% of body weight.

In man, the dextrowarfarin enantiomorph is metabolized by side chain reduction to a secondary alcohol, whereas levowarfarin is metabolized by oxidation of the ring, primarily to 7-hydroxywarfarin. These inactive metabolic products are to some extent conjugated with glucuronic acid, undergo an enterohepatic circulation, and are ultimately excreted in the urine and stool.

Preparations, Routes of Administration, and Dosage. *Warfarin sodium* (COUMADIN, PANWARFIN) is available in tablets containing 2, 2.5, 5, 7.5, and 10 mg of drug. Although loading doses of

warfarin have been recommended in the past, most physicians avoid a large loading dose in order to reduce the danger of hemorrhage in sick patients who may be particularly sensitive to the drug. Therapy can be initiated with a daily dose of 10 to 15 mg *without* a loading dose; a daily maintenance dose in the range of 2 to 15 mg is then determined by observation of the one-stage prothrombin activity. Initially, this test is performed daily until the result is stable at about twice the control "prothrombin time" for the laboratory; this represents a prothrombin activity that is 25% of normal (*see* below). The time between tests may then be lengthened gradually to weekly and later to monthly intervals for patients on long-term therapy in whom the results of the test are stable. *Warfarin potassium* (ATHROMBIN-K) is available in tablets containing 5 mg of drug. *Warfarin sodium for injection* is available in vials of 50 mg, but parenteral administration is seldom needed and does not alter the kinetics of response.

Toxic Effects. *Hemorrhage* is the main unwanted effect caused by therapy with oral anticoagulants. *Anticoagulant therapy must always be monitored by determination of one-stage prothrombin times, and the patient must be observed carefully for development of bleeding. Bleeding often occurs even when the prothrombin time is within the expected therapeutic range.* In order of decreasing frequency, complications include ecchymoses, hematuria, uterine bleeding, melena or hematochezia, epistaxis, hematoma, gingival bleeding, hemoptysis, and hematemesis (O'Reilly, 1976b). Particularly *serious bleeding episodes* in patients who are chronically receiving either heparin or oral anticoagulants include compression neuropathy following brachial artery puncture for arteriographic or blood-gas studies, intraperitoneal hemorrhage resulting from rupture of a corpus luteum, retroperitoneal hemorrhage with compression femoral neuropathy, hemopericardium even in the absence of myocardial infarction or pericarditis, intracranial hemorrhage, adrenal hemorrhage, and necrosis of skin and breasts. Identified factors that increase the risk of hemorrhagic complications during long-term therapy include poor supervision of the patient, use of the drug despite medical contraindications, poor control of the drug in relation to laboratory values, administration of large loading doses, administration of therapy that is too intensive for the patient, concomitant administration of interacting drugs, or therapy of the elderly or post-partum patient or those with disorders of the gastrointestinal or genitourinary systems.

The *treatment of hemorrhage* caused by therapy with oral anticoagulants consists in immediate withdrawal of the drug and the oral administration of 10 to 20 mg of vitamin K_1 (*phytonadione*). This regimen will stop minor bleeding and return the prothrombin time to the normal range within 24 hours. Vitamin K_3, or menadione, is *ineffective* as an antidote for hemorrhage from oral anticoagulants. For hemorrhage that is either severe or in a closed body space (*e.g.*, the pericardium or central nervous system), up to 50 mg of vitamin K_1 must be administered intravenously (*see* Chapter 67). If the hemorrhage is not reduced significantly within a few hours, additional vitamin K_1 should be given intravenously and transfusion should be initiated with fresh whole blood, frozen plasma, or plasma concentrates of the vitamin K–dependent clotting factors. After treatment with vitamin K_1, the patient may require higher-than-usual doses of oral anticoagulants when and if such therapy is resumed.

When *elective surgery* is to be performed, the anticoagulant drug may be continued daily, even parenterally, and its hypoprothrombinemic effect partially reversed with one 5-mg tablet of phytonadione the day before surgery or 2.5 mg of phytonadione per day orally for 2 days before surgery. The former method will bring the prothrombin activity from the so-called therapeutic range of 25% of normal to the normal range of 90 to 100% activity; the latter method will bring the value to 50 to 60% of normal activity. The prothrombin activity will return to its previous level of 25% in about 4 days. Alternatively, warfarin may be discontinued and low doses of heparin substituted during the perioperative period for 5 to 7 days, followed by reinstitution of the oral anticoagulant regimen.

Precautions and Contraindications. Long-term anticoagulant therapy of nonhospitalized patients should not be undertaken unless the patient or someone in residence is willing and able to take responsibility for his/her care, has sufficient literacy and vi-

sual acuity to read instructions, and is intelligent enough to understand the serious nature of the therapy and the necessity for close control and supervision (Grand and Collard, 1983). Suitable laboratory facilities must be available and used for accurate control of therapy, and the patient must be consistent in keeping appointments. Oral and parenteral preparations of vitamin K_1 should be readily available, as well as fresh whole blood, frozen plasma, and concentrates of the vitamin K–dependent clotting factors for emergency transfusion.

All of the contraindications listed above for heparin apply to the oral anticoagulants as well. In addition, severe hepatic or renal disease, vitamin K deficiency, chronic alcoholism, and a requirement for intensive salicylate therapy are relative contraindications to the use of oral anticoagulant therapy. Physicians experienced with this therapy give their patients detailed verbal and written instructions about the nature of the therapy. They point out the danger signs of bleeding and symptoms of recurring thromboembolic disease, the times to contact the physician, the danger of relying on memory for the frequency and size of the drug dose, and the value of keeping a calendar or daily diary of the amount of drug actually taken; they instruct the patient to carry on his person a MEDALERT bracelet, "dog tag," or wallet card to alert medical and paramedical personnel in an emergency. They also order a supply of vitamin K_1 tablets for the patient for emergency use.

Therapeutic Uses. The clinical uses of the oral anticoagulant drugs are discussed later in this chapter.

OTHER ORAL ANTICOAGULANTS

Oral anticoagulants other than racemic warfarin are seldom used in the United States because of their less favorable pharmacological properties.

Dicumarol. *Dicumarol* (*bishydroxycoumarin*) is the agent formed in spoiled silage that causes hemorrhagic sweet clover disease in cattle; it is now prepared synthetically. Dicumarol is slowly and incompletely absorbed by man, except when prepared in a micronized form or in propylene glycol. The drug has a half-life in plasma that is dependent on dose. It frequently causes mild gastrointestinal side effects, such as nausea, flatulence, crampy abdominal pain, and diarrhea. The recommended dosage schedule is 200 to 300 mg the first day and 25 to 200 mg on subsequent days, based on the therapeutic response measured by the one-stage prothrombin time. Dicumarol is available in tablets.

Phenprocoumon. *Phenprocoumon* (LIQUAMAR) is used widely in continental Europe as MARCUMAR. Phenprocoumon is a racemic mixture wherein, like warfarin, the levorotatory enantiomorph is a more potent hypoprothrombinemic agent. Its half-life in plasma is long—6 days. Only nausea, diarrhea, and dermatitis have been reported as relatively frequent side effects. Large loading doses are still recommended for the initiation of therapy because of the long half-life: 21 mg the first day, 9 mg the second day, and a maintenance dose of 0.5 to 6 mg according to the one-stage prothrombin activity; it is available in 3-mg tablets.

Indanedione Derivatives. *Anisindione* (MIRADON) remains available commercially in the United States. The toxicity of this agent is greater than that of the coumarin derivatives. Its use is quite limited and is not recommended.

LABORATORY CONTROL OF ANTICOAGULANT MEDICATION

The goal of laboratory evaluation of anticoagulant activity in patients is to reduce the frequency of both bleeding episodes and ineffective treatment. The physician should ask the patient about any previous bleeding history, use laboratory tests before treatment to detect defects of hemostasis, be familiar with regimens for the proper administration of an anticoagulant drug, and monitor the anticoagulant effect of therapy in order to optimize its use.

Heparin. The *partial thromboplastin time* (PTT) has replaced the whole-blood clotting time because it is more reproducible, more sensitive to the effect of the drug, and less costly. Even "low-dose" heparin can prolong the PTT of those who are particularly sensitive, prolong the bleeding time of patients who also are given aspirin, and increase the bleeding of wounds and the size of postoperative hematomas. The PTT should be kept as close as possible to twice the patient's pretreatment baseline time (of 30 to 35 seconds) and should be used to modulate both the continuous and intermittent methods for administration of heparin (Hull and Hirsh, 1983). For the intermittent method, the PTT should be performed daily about 1 hour before a scheduled dose. An unexpected test result in a patient is easily adjusted. A PTT that is too long (over 120 seconds) is readily shortened by omitting a dose, since heparin has a short half-life; a PTT that is too short (less than 50 seconds) is readily pro-

longed by increasing the dose, since the onset of heparin's action is rapid. When "low-dose" heparin therapy is utilized, laboratory tests are generally not necessary to monitor treatment; the dosage and schedule are fixed and hemorrhage rarely occurs.

Heparin and oral anticoagulant drugs often are used together in the acute treatment of thromboembolic disease. The problem in the regulation of such concurrent medication is the *combined effect* of the two drugs on the one-stage prothrombin time. Thus, when heparin is discontinued, the prothrombin time will shorten toward normal because the dosage of the oral agent by itself is insufficient. (Heparin has less effect on the P & P and THROMBOTEST methods of the one-stage test because of the tenfold dilution of the patient's plasma [O'Reilly and Aggeler, 1970].) The impact of an infusion of heparin on the prothrombin time can be ascertained by serial performance of the test: before the heparin infusion, during the infusion before the initiation of treatment with the oral anticoagulant, and during the combined therapy. The effect of heparin on therapy with an oral agent can be minimized by replacing the infusion with intermittent intravenous injections and by determination of the prothrombin time just before the next dose of heparin. The dosage of the oral anticoagulant may need to be increased as the heparin is discontinued.

Oral Anticoagulants. Therapy with oral anticoagulants is best regulated with the original one-stage prothrombin time, by use of a preparation of tissue thromboplastin that has been standardized and a reference plasma from selected patients to form a standard curve (Loeliger and Lewis, 1982). The conversion of the prothrombin time in seconds to percent of normal prothrombin activity partially compensates for variations between different laboratories, but each physician must determine the therapeutic and toxic range for the laboratory he uses. The physician should instruct the patient to use the same laboratory and to notify him when this is not possible. The test is sensitive to the presence of several clotting factors, particularly three of the four that are dependent on vitamin K: II, VII, and X. The prothrombin time should be determined daily when administration of oral anticoagulants is begun and at least once a month in well-controlled patients receiving long-term therapy.

Patients on chronic therapy usually should be maintained at a one-stage prothrombin activity of about 25%, which, expressed in seconds, is about twice the normal baseline of 12 seconds. However, the so-called therapeutic range is based more on the avoidance of bleeding than on the achievement of a proven therapeutic effect. Furthermore, achievement of the therapeutic range during the first few days results primarily from a reduction of the activity of factor VII, which is not involved in intravascular clotting and probably not involved in thrombogenesis (O'Reilly and Aggeler, 1968, 1970). An unexpected laboratory test result is not easily adjusted. A prothrombin time that is too long (over 30 seconds) is not readily shortened by omitting a dose because of the long half-life of oral anticoagulants; a test result that is too short (less than 15 seconds) is not readily lengthened by increasing the daily dose because of the delayed effect of the therapy. A new "plateau" of therapeutic effect is not achieved for 1 to 2 weeks. Wide fluctuations in the patient's prothrombin time are usually the result of poor compliance by the patient or excessive changes of the daily dose of drug by the physician. Often, a graph of the doses of drug and the results of the determinations of prothrombin time may help one to diagnose the difficulty or may reveal a change that can be traced to the administration or discontinuation of an interacting drug.

The concentration of warfarin in plasma should *never* be measured to monitor efficacy; the prothrombin time should be used. Most patients achieve the "therapeutic range" for the prothrombin time (25 ± 5% of normal activity) with a daily dose of 5 to 7.5 mg of warfarin. This dose usually results in a concentration of warfarin in plasma of 2 to 3 μg/ml.

II. Antithrombotic and Thrombolytic Drugs

ANTITHROMBOTIC DRUGS

The antithrombotic drugs suppress platelet function and are used primarily for arterial thrombotic disease, whereas anticoagulant drugs, such as warfarin and heparin, suppress the synthesis or function of clotting factors and are used to control venous thromboembolic disorders. The antithrombotic efficacy of the drugs that prevent platelet aggregation has been inferred from tests of platelet function *in vitro, ex vivo* (platelets obtained from the blood of subjects who have received the drug), and from models in experimental animals. Because platelet plugs form the bulk of arterial thrombi, the best therapeutic strategies may be to utilize agents that interfere with the adherence of platelets to vessel walls and to each other. Nevertheless, the proof of efficacy of any agent will come only from extensive clinical trials, which are still being conducted (*see* Symposium, 1983).

Aspirin. Acetylsalicylic acid inhibits the release of ADP by platelets and their aggregation by acetylating the enzymes of the platelet that synthesize the precursors of prostaglandins and thromboxane A_2 (TXA_2) that stimulate these reactions (*see* Chapters 28 and 29). Although aspirin is cleared from the body within hours, its effects on platelets are irreversible and thus last for the life of the platelet. Doses (0.325 to 1.3 g) used in studies of the antithrombotic effect may prolong the bleeding time for several days after the drug is discontinued (Weiss, 1978). However, aspirin may neither reduce platelet adhesion to subendothelium nor prolong the reduced survival of platelets that is characteristic of thromboembolic disorders. The inhibition of prostacyclin (PGI_2) synthesis in the vessel wall by aspirin may account for these results and reduce its effectiveness as an antithrombotic agent. A large number of studies have been conducted to evaluate the effects of aspirin and other antithrombotic drugs in cardiovascular disease, particularly for the secondary prevention of myocardial infarction and stroke. In general, the results have been disappointing, with either no significant differences or very modest effects (*see* below). However, aspirin does appear to reduce the incidence of myocardial infarction in males with unstable angina. In patients who experience transient cerebral ischemia, aspirin appears to reduce the incidence of such attacks and of stroke; these beneficial effects were also confined to males (*see* Chapter 29).

Sulfinpyrazone. This drug is used for its uricosuric properties (*see* Chapters 29 and 38). It also prolongs the survival of platelets in patients with various thromboembolic disorders. The drug inhibits a number of platelet functions, including the release reaction and adherence to subendothelial cells, and inhibits synthesis of prostaglandins. In large, randomized clinical trials in which 200 mg of sulfinpyrazone was taken four times a day, a reduction in the incidence of sudden death after myocardial infarction was described (ANTURANE Reinfarction Trial Research Group, 1978, 1980); however, the study was subsequently criticized for statistical and methodological reasons (*see* Hampton, 1982). The drug has not been approved by the United States Food and Drug Administration as an antithrombotic agent.

Dipyridamole. This drug is a vasodilator that, in combination with warfarin, inhibits embolization from prosthetic heart valves and, in combination with aspirin, prolongs the survival of platelets in patients with thrombotic diseases. Dipyridamole by itself has little or no clinical effect. It may interfere with platelet function by inhibiting cyclic nucleotide phosphodiesterase activity, thereby increasing the intracellular concentration of adenosine 3',5'-monophosphate (cyclic AMP) and potentiating the effect of PGI_2 (Moncada and Korbut, 1978). A large study of recurrent myocardial infarction called *PARIS* evaluated the use of three regimens. These included daily doses of dipyridamole (225 mg) plus aspirin (1 g), aspirin (1 g), and placebo. No significant differences were found among the three regimens (Buckler and Douglas, 1983). The only current recommended use of dipyridamole is for primary prophylaxis of thromboemboli in patients with prosthetic heart valves; the drug is given in combination with warfarin. Dipyridamole is available in 25-, 50-, and 75-mg tablets (PERSANTINE).

Dextran 70 and Dextran 75. These substances, which are used as plasma expanders, are partially hydrolyzed polymers of glucose that are obtained from the bacterium *Leuconostoc mesenteroides* (*see* Chapter 35). Dextran added to blood *in vitro* has no effect on platelet function; however, the bleeding time, polymerization of fibrin, and platelet function may be impaired *in vivo*. Infusions of dextran increase the colloidal osmotic pressure, which necessitates care in their use in patients with pulmonary edema, congestive heart failure, and decreased renal function. Dextran-induced formation of rouleaux interferes with blood typing, cross matching, and Rh testing, which requires the performance of those tests on blood obtained before dextran infusion. Dextran is contraindicated in patients with significant anemia, severe thrombocytopenia, and reduced concentrations of fibrinogen in plasma. Side effects include occasional urticaria, wheezing, a feeling of tightness in the chest, mild hypotension, and, rarely, severe anaphylaxis. Dextran continues to be studied in randomized double-blind trials for efficacy in the prevention of postoperative thromboembolic disease in surgical patients (*see* Ljungström, 1983). *Dextran 70* (MACRODEX) and *dextran 75* (DEXTRAN 75, GENTRAN 75) are available as a 6% injection with 5% dextrose solution or as a 6% injection with 0.9% sodium chloride solution.

Dazoxiben. This drug, which is an analog of imidazole, selectively inhibits thromboxane synthetase and thereby prevents the formation of TXA_2, a powerful stimulator of platelet aggregation. Dazoxiben markedly inhibits the synthesis of TXA_2 *in vitro*, but does not prevent platelet aggregation unless low doses of aspirin are added to the regimen. The concomitant administration of aspirin appears to inhibit the accumulation of products of the fatty acid cyclooxygenase reaction that occurs during blockade of TXA_2 synthesis; these products can stimulate platelet aggregation (Bertelé et al., 1983). Dazoxiben and other inhibitors of thromboxane synthetase are currently being studied in clinical trials.

Ticlopidine. This drug is a thienopyridine that alters platelet membranes directly, independent of any effect on prostaglandins. It inhibits platelet aggregation and secretion, reduces deposition of platelets and fibrin on artificial surfaces, and prolongs the bleeding time. Ticlopidine has been introduced in Europe, and it is now undergoing clinical trials in the United States. It may be useful in extracorporeal circulation (*see* Symposium, 1983).

Clofibrate. Clofibrate is a hypolipidemic drug that may reduce platelet adhesiveness *in vitro* and increase abnormally short survival of platelets in some patients with coronary artery disease. Previous favorable results with clofibrate in patients with angina pectoris have not been confirmed in a large, randomized clinical trial in patients who had suffered a myocardial infarction (Coronary Drug Project Research Group, 1975). Its use as an antithrombotic agent cannot be recommended. The use of clofibrate in the treatment of hyperlipoproteinemias is discussed in Chapter 34.

THROMBOLYTIC DRUGS

Streptokinase and urokinase are proteins that have demonstrated efficacy for the treatment of acute thromboembolic disease. They promote the dissolution of thrombi by stimulating the activation of endogenous plasminogen to *plasmin* (fibrinolysin), a proteolytic enzyme that hydrolyzes fibrin (*see* Figure 58–3). Because these drugs can profoundly alter hemostasis, they should be used only by physicians who have had extensive experience in the management of thromboembolic disease. Two new approaches may reduce the adverse systemic effects of such therapy. Intra-arterial use of a fibrinolytic drug (*e.g.*,

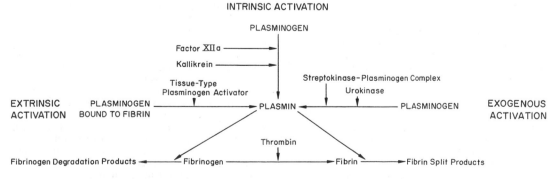

Figure 58–3. *Schematic representation of the pathways for activation of plasminogen and for the lysis of fibrinogen and fibrin.*

intracoronary injection) may reduce systemic bleeding. A second generation of thrombolytic drugs, *tissue-type plasminogen activators,* can induce local fibrinolysis without causing systemic fibrinolysis. Thrombolytic therapy is utilized in patients with extensive pulmonary emboli, in acute coronary thrombosis associated with an evolving transmural myocardial infarction, and in severe iliofemoral thrombophlebitis.

Streptokinase is a protein without known enzymatic activity that is obtained from group-C beta-hemolytic streptococci. It interacts with and activates plasminogen. The complex of streptokinase and plasminogen has protease activity and catalyzes the conversion of plasminogen to plasmin. Following the administration of streptokinase there is a high incidence of bleeding from sites of percutaneous trauma and in wounds, because plasmin lyses fibrin in hemostatic plugs and degrades fibrinogen and factors V and VII. Thus, concurrent use of an anticoagulant or a drug that prevents agglutination of platelets should be avoided when streptokinase (or urokinase) is being given. Fever is common, and allergic reactions and even anaphylaxis result from the formation of antibodies, which may interfere with prolonged or future treatment. Furthermore, naturally occurring antistreptococcal antibodies cross-react with streptokinase and reduce its ability to prolong the thrombin time.

Streptokinase has been used successfully to treat acute pulmonary embolism and deep-vein thrombosis, but randomized, controlled trials are needed to determine whether mortality is lowered. The usual loading dose of streptokinase is 250,000 international units (I.U.), given intravenously over a 30-minute period, followed by 100,000 I.U. per hour, adjusted according to the thrombin time. Therapy is continued for 24 to 72 hours and must be monitored by the thrombin time, which should be prolonged by two to five times the control value. Heparin and oral anticoagulants should be administered after treatment with streptokinase has been completed. Intracoronary administration of streptokinase within the first 6 hours of an acute coronary thrombosis can restore flow in an occluded artery and may reduce mortality (Anderson *et al.,* 1983; Laffel and Braunwald, 1984). Such treatment is based on the experimental finding that reperfusion of an occluded coronary artery in dogs can reduce the size of myocardial infarction if accomplished within a few hours (Jennings and Reimer, 1983). A transmural infarction "in progress" can be converted into a subendocardial infarction. A 20,000-unit bolus of streptokinase followed by 2000 units per minute can be administered until the vessel is patent, and 2000 units per minute can then be given for an additional 30 to 60 minutes. Studies are in progress to evaluate the efficacy of streptokinase when given intravenously rather than into the occluded coronary artery (TIMI Study Group, 1985). Streptokinase has also been used experimentally

with some success in patients with central retinal vein thrombosis (Kwaan *et al.,* 1977). Streptokinase (KABIKINASE, STREPTASE) is available as lyophilized powder for reconstitution in 0.9% saline or 5% dextrose solution.

Urokinase (ABBOKINASE) is a proteolytic enzyme, and its only known natural substrate, plasminogen, is activated by urokinase to the fibrinolytic enzyme plasmin. Urokinase, originally isolated from human urine, is prepared from cultures of human renal cells. A controlled study to evaluate urokinase resulted in the observation of accelerated resolution of pulmonary emboli, but the incidence of bleeding was twofold higher than in heparin-treated patients. Urokinase is contraindicated in children or in patients with any kind of healing wound, recent trauma, visceral or intracranial malignancy, pregnancy, or recent cerebrovascular accident, in addition to *all* of the contraindications listed for heparin and oral anticoagulants. Febrile episodes occasionally occur, but serious allergic reactions are rare. The usual intravenous loading dose of urokinase is 4400 I.U./kg, given over a period of 10 minutes, followed by a continuous infusion of 4400 I.U./kg per hour for 12 hours and then by heparin or oral anticoagulants (Sasahara *et al.,* 1979). It is not necessary to monitor the thrombin time during treatment with urokinase, but it should be evaluated before heparin is given. A course of therapy is very expensive. It should be used when indicated for patients who are allergic to streptokinase. It is available as a lyophilized powder in vials of 5000 or 250,000 I.U. for reconstitution with sterile water; the solution is further diluted with 0.9% saline or 5% dextrose injection just prior to intravenous infusion.

Tissue-type plasminogen activator, an extrinsic activator, preferentially activates plasminogen bound to fibrin, which confines fibrinolysis to a thrombus and avoids systemic activation of plasminogen. Purification of this activator from cultured human melanoma cells and preparation by recombinant DNA technology will facilitate clinical trials with this very promising agent (Pennica *et al.,* 1983; Van de Werf *et al.,* 1984). In preliminary studies, the intravenous administration of tissue-type plasminogen activator to patients with acute myocardial infarction resulted in recanalization of the occluded coronary vessel in about half of the cases (TIMI Study Group, 1985). This value was significantly higher than that achieved with intravenous streptokinase.

Aminocaproic acid (AMICAR) is a specific antidote for an overdose of a fibrinolytic agent. It is also used in patients with hyperfibrinolysis to prevent recurrence of subarachnoid or gastrointestinal hemorrhage, especially when surgery is contraindicated (Graham and Walker, 1982). It is available as an injection, a syrup, and tablets. The usual dose is 5 g initially (orally or intravenously), followed by 1 g per hour until bleeding is under control. The dosage should not exceed 30 g in 24 hours. Rapid intravenous administration should be avoided to prevent hypotension, bradycardia, and other arrhythmias.

III. Therapeutic Uses of Anticoagulant, Antithrombotic, and Thrombolytic Drugs

The anticoagulant model for prevention of thromboembolic disease suggests that slowing the rate of formation of fibrin should have therapeutic efficacy. Because fibrin thrombi occur primarily in the venous system, anticoagulant drugs are used in the prophylaxis of venous thrombosis. Low doses of heparin have been employed for primary prophylaxis in patients who are undergoing elective surgery, to prevent postoperative venous thrombosis. Heparin in conventional doses and oral anticoagulants have been used as secondary prophylaxis to prevent the extension or recurrence of venous thrombi, thrombophlebitis, or pulmonary emboli.

The antithrombotic model for treatment of thromboembolic disease suggests that inhibition of platelet function should have therapeutic efficacy. Because platelet thrombi occur primarily in the arterial system, antithrombotic drugs are used in patients with arterial thrombi in the heart and brain. Several antithrombotic drugs have been and continue to be evaluated as secondary prophylactic agents to prevent recurrence of myocardial infarctions and strokes. While oral anticoagulant drugs have no effect on platelets, they are still utilized in attempts to prevent thrombotic disease in the arterial system, although convincing proof of efficacy is lacking.

The thrombolytic model suggests that activation of the fibrinolytic mechanism by the formation of plasmin will dissolve thrombi that have already formed. Fibrinolytic agents are now available for the treatment of patients with established pulmonary emboli, coronary arterial thrombosis, or proximal venous thrombi, such as occur in iliofemoral thrombosis.

Myocardial Infarction. The acute phase of myocardial infarction was one of the earliest disorders in which therapy with oral anticoagulants was employed. The hope was that anticoagulant therapy would at least reduce the incidence of secondary thromboembolism. While there have been a large number of conflicting studies over several decades, many of the discrepant findings are explained by

failure, at that time, to understand the elements of the randomized, controlled clinical trial (*see* Horwitz and Feinstein, 1981). Despite the lack of convincing data that prove efficacy, oral anticoagulants are widely used in attempts to reduce the risk of recurrent myocardial infarction. Low doses of heparin provide primary prophylaxis against thromboembolism after myocardial infarction, and drugs that prevent aggregation of platelets increase platelet survival and improve the patency of surgically implanted bypass grafts in patients with coronary artery disease. Some large-scale controlled studies on the effects of antiplatelet drugs on mortality after myocardial infarction have been completed and, as mentioned above, have shown little or no effect. Thus, no antithrombotic agent can be recommended unequivocally at this time in the prevention of myocardial reinfarction (Buckler and Douglas, 1983; Bouchier-Hayes, 1983).

Promising strategies for the treatment of acute myocardial infarction and for the prevention of reinfarction come from recent studies on the use of β-adrenergic antagonists (*see* Chapter 9) and thrombolytic agents. Approaches to achieve recanalization by thrombolysis have been discussed in detail by Laffel and Braunwald (1984). In brief, the authors conclude that patients with typical chest pain of less than 4 to 6 hours' duration and with S-T segment elevation that does not respond to sublingual nitroglycerin should be considered for thrombolytic therapy. This is accomplished under arteriographic control by the intracoronary administration of streptokinase (*see* above), which is successful in 75% of the patients. Recanalization is usually achieved in about 30 minutes and is frequently heralded by relief of chest pain, normalization of the S-T segment elevation, *and the onset of ventricular arrhythmias* (although ventricular tachycardia and fibrillation are rare). Intramyocardial hemorrhage may occur, but this does not increase the size of the infarct. However, systemic hemorrhagic complications may be severe; it is hoped that these can be avoided when tissue-type plasminogen activator becomes generally available. After thrombolysis is achieved, patients are treated vigorously with heparin (for 2 to 12 days). Most investigators then recommend administration of oral anticoagulants (*e.g.,* for 3 months); some utilize antiplatelet agents instead of or in addition to anticoagulants. In the absence of contraindications, patients should also receive a β-adrenergic antagonist for at least 1 to 3 years. Patients must also be evaluated for possible percutaneous transluminal angioplasty or coronary bypass surgery. While such a strategy for treatment is both promising and rational, it remains to be proven which components of the approach are the most valuable and how practical it will be on a widespread basis. In particular, it remains to be established that recanalization of a coronary vessel by thrombolysis actually salvages myocardium, improves myocardial performance, and reduces mortality. In view of the costs and the number of variables involved, it will be a formidable task to answer the necessary questions.

Cerebrovascular Disease. Treatment of completed strokes with oral anticoagulants declined because of the high incidence of intracranial bleeding apparently caused by the drugs. In addition, there is little evidence that anticoagulant therapy has any beneficial effect once the deficit is established. Treatment of a stroke-in-progress may be indicated because a hemorrhagic stroke can be ruled out by computerized tomography; heparin is utilized, particularly in the hope of preventing further damage. Surgery is often recommended for a patient with a tightly stenotic lesion who has had a stroke distal to the lesion.

Carotid endarterectomy is the primary treatment for transient ischemic attacks that result from stenosis of a carotid artery. Many investigators suggest that treatment with an oral anticoagulant is useful in this condition if the lesion is inaccessible or if there are other contraindications to surgery. Aspirin has also been investigated widely. While beneficial effects have been documented (see, for example, Canadian Cooperative Study Group, 1978), the magnitude of the effect does not appear to be great. However, in view of the very minimal risk of treatment with aspirin (300 to 600 mg daily), it is widely used for this purpose. (See Kistler et al., 1984.)

The high incidence of deep-vein thrombosis in hemiplegics and quadriplegics has been reduced significantly by the use of low doses of heparin as primary prophylaxis after an acute stroke.

Rheumatic Heart Disease. Thromboembolism occurs in rheumatic heart disease typically as a result of disease of the mitral valve with atrial fibrillation. Primary therapy of these disorders is valvular surgery and conversion of the atrial fibrillation to sinus rhythm; this reduces the thromboembolic risk factor of atrial stasis. When such therapy cannot be used or is not successful in eliminating thromboembolic disease, the administration of oral anticoagulants can reduce the number of embolic episodes. Oral anticoagulants, often in combination with an inhibitor of platelet aggregation like dipyridamole, are also useful in long-term reduction of the incidence of thromboembolism associated with surgical placement of a prosthetic valve, even when the valves are made with the newer, less thrombogenic materials (Chesebro et al., 1983). Some cardiologists advocate the administration of oral anticoagulants for 1 to 2 weeks to patients with atrial fibrillation before attempts are made to convert to sinus rhythm.

Venous Thrombosis and Pulmonary Embolism. *Secondary prophylactic treatment* of these diseases with heparin and the oral anticoagulants is the oldest use of these drugs (Hull and Hirsh, 1983). The recent demonstration of marked antifactor-X activity as a result of heparin-induced antithrombin-III hyperactivity led to the successful application of low doses of heparin for *primary prophylaxis* of deep-vein thrombosis and of pulmonary embolism after surgery. This regimen consists of a

dose of 5000 units of heparin administered subcutaneously, once 2 hours prior to the elective surgery and then every 8 to 12 hours thereafter for at least 7 days. A highly significant reduction in the occurrence of deep-vein thrombosis, with no appreciable increase in the requirement for transfusions or in the incidence of hematoma, has been reported, even for neurosurgical patients (Salzman, 1983). This form of prophylaxis was ineffective, however, in surgical patients who underwent total hip replacement, except when used in combination with *dihydroergotamine mesylate,* a drug that increases venous return from the limbs by constricting capacitance vessels (Kakkar et al., 1979). The many *mechanical means* of preventing venous stasis in the legs include early ambulation, elastic stockings, leg elevation and exercises, intermittent pneumatic compression devices applied to the legs, intermittent galvanic stimulation of the calf muscles, and graduated compression diminishing from the ankle proximally. However, these devices and technics, designed to prevent stasis, have seldom been evaluated by randomized, clinical trials.

The best "treatment" of pulmonary embolus is its prevention by primary prophylaxis of deep-vein thrombosis in the proximal iliofemoral venous system. Such primary prophylaxis with low doses of heparin has been correlated with prevention of deep-vein thrombosis in the distal venous system of the calf in patients at high risk for formation of thrombi, as detected with [^{125}I] fibrinogen. Known *risk factors* include injury; surgery, especially in patients over the age of 40 years; malignancy; congestive heart failure; varicose veins; obesity; pregnancy; the use of oral contraceptives; immobilization from strokes, paraplegia, or heart attacks; and previous venous thromboembolic disease (Colman and Rubin, 1982).

The treatment of pulmonary emboli and deep-vein thrombi is more established by practice than by randomized, control trials. Conventional doses of heparin in the hospital, followed by chronic administration of oral anticoagulants, is the traditional therapy for the prevention of recurrence or extension of these lesions. Dissolution of massive pulmonary emboli by thrombolytic drugs can be lifesaving.

Miscellaneous Uses. Heparin may be of value in selected cases of *disseminated intravascular coagulation* (DIC), a syndrome in which the blood is incoagulable and extensive intravascular fibrin thrombi are present. DIC occurs in patients desperately ill from a variety of serious causes, including obstetrical, infectious, and malignant disorders. The widespread development of thrombi consumes clotting factors, and the resultant bleeding becomes an additional grave problem. Heparin sometimes arrests the intravascular coagulation and thereby allows accumulation of normal amounts of coagulation factors and cessation of bleeding. However, bleeding may sometimes be aggravated by heparin, or DIC may occur during the course of heparin therapy. The administration of protamine may then be necessary. It is difficult to select patients with

DIC who should be treated with heparin and to forecast the outcome (Hamilton *et al.*, 1978).

To avoid thrombus formation in a cannula used for an intravenous infusion, heparin can be added to the solution or can be bound ionically to the surface of the cannula when manufactured. Heparinization of the patient or the extracorporeal device is mandatory for cardiovascular surgery and hemodialysis, to prevent blood coagulation and deposition of thrombotic material in heart-lung machines and dialyzers.

Formation of fibrin is involved in the processes of tumor growth and metastasis. The surfaces of malignant cells commandeer the body's coagulation system, and a "cocoon" of fibrin is built around the cancer, thereby shielding it from antibodies and lymphocytes. Similarly, angiogenesis is induced by the tumor. In a randomized, clinical trial with small-cell carcinoma of the lung, the addition of warfarin to a complex therapeutic regimen resulted in a highly significant prolongation of patient survival (Zacharski *et al.*, 1981).

Anderson, J. L.; Marshall, H. W.; Bray, B. E.; Lutz, J. R.; Frederick, P. R.; Yanowitz, F. G.; Datz, F. L.; Klausner, S. C.; and Hagan, A. D. A randomized trial of intracoronary streptokinase in the treatment of acute myocardial infarction. *N. Engl. J. Med.*, **1983**, *308*, 1312–1318.

Anturane Reinfarction Trial Research Group. Sulfinpyrazone in the prevention of cardiac death after myocardial infarction. *N. Engl. J. Med.*, **1978**, *298*, 289–295.

———. Sulfinpyrazone in the prevention of sudden death after myocardial infarction. *Ibid.*, **1980**, *302*, 250–256.

Bachmann, K.; Shapiro, R.; and Mackiewicz, J. Warfarin elimination and responsiveness in patients with renal dysfunction. *J. Clin. Pharmacol.*, **1977**, *17*, 292–299.

Bertelé, V.; Falanga, A.; Tomasiak, M.; Dejana, E.; Cerletti, C.; and de Gaetano, G. Platelet thromboxane synthetase inhibitors with low doses of aspirin: possible resolution of the "aspirin dilemma." *Science*, **1983**, *220*, 517–519.

Björk, I., and Lindahl, U. Mechanism of the anticoagulant action of heparin. *Mol. Cell. Biochem.*, **1982**, *48*, 161–182.

Bjornsson, T. D.; Meffin, P. J.; and Blaschke, T. F. Interaction of clofibrate with warfarin. I. Effect of clofibrate on the disposition of the optical enantiomorphs of warfarin. *J. Pharmacokinet. Biopharm.*, **1977**, *5*, 495–505.

Bouchier-Hayes, D. Drugs in the treatment of thromboembolic diseases. *Ir. Med. J.*, **1983**, *76*, 101–107, 155–159.

Buckler, P., and Douglas, A. S. Antithrombotic treatment. *Br. Med. J. [Clin. Res.]*, **1983**, *287*, 196–198.

Canadian Cooperative Study Group. A randomized trial of aspirin and sulfinpyrazone in threatened stroke. *N. Engl. J. Med.*, **1978**, *299*, 53–59.

Chesebro, J. H.; Fuster, V.; Elveback, L. R.; McGoon, D. C.; Pluth, J. R.; Puga, F. J.; Wallace, R. B.; Danielson, G. K.; Orszulak, T. A.; Piehler, J. M.; and Schaff, H. V. Trial of combined warfarin plus dipyridamole or aspirin therapy in prosthetic heart valve replacement: danger of aspirin compared with dipyridamole. *Am. J. Cardiol.*, **1983**, *51*, 1537–1541.

Cipolle, R. J.; Rodvold, K. A.; Seifert, R.; Clarens, R.; and Ramirez-Lassepas, M. Heparin-associated thrombocytopenia: a prospective evaluation of 211 patients. *Ther. Drug Monit.*, **1983**, *5*, 205–211.

Coronary Drug Project Research Group. Clofibrate and niacin in coronary heart disease. *J.A.M.A.*, **1975**, *231*, 360–381.

Ellison, N.; Edmunds, L. H., Jr.; and Colman, R. W. Platelet aggregation following heparin and protamine administration. *Anesthesiology*, **1978**, *48*, 65–68.

Graham, D. R., and Walker, R. J. Persistent gastrointestinal bleeding successfully treated with aminocaproic acid. *Postgrad. Med. J.*, **1982**, *58*, 658–661.

Grand, A., and Collard, R. Accidents hemorragiques dus au traitement anticoagulant: 76 observations. *Lyon Med.*, **1983**, *249*, 17–22.

Griffith, M. J. Heparin-catalyzed inhibitor/protease reactions: kinetic evidence for a common mechanism of action of heparin. *Proc. Natl Acad. Sci. U.S.A.*, **1983**, *80*, 5460–5464.

Hall, J. G.; Pauli, R. M.; and Wilson, K. M. Maternal and fetal sequelae of anticoagulation during pregnancy. *Am. J. Med.*, **1980**, *68*, 122–140.

Hampton, J. R. The secondary prevention of heart attacks. *J. Ir. Colleges Physicians Surgeons*, **1982**, *11*, 143–150.

Hauschka, P. V.; Lian, J. B.; and Gallop, P. M. Vitamin K and mineralization. *Trends Biochem. Sci.*, **1978**, *3*, 75–78.

Henny, C. P.; TenCate, J. W.; VanBronswijk, H.; TenCate, H.; Surachno, S.; Wilmink, J. M.; and Ockelford, P. A. Use of a new heparinoid as anticoagulant during acute haemodialysis of patients with bleeding complications. *Lancet*, **1983**, *1*, 890–893.

Howell, W. H. Heparin, an anticoagulant. Preliminary communication. *Am. J. Physiol.*, **1922**, *63*, 434–435.

Hoylaerts, M.; Holmer, E.; DeMol, M.; and Collen, D. Covalent complexes between low molecular weight heparin fragments and antithrombin III—inhibition kinetics and turnover parameters. *Thromb. Haemost.*, **1983**, *49*, 109–115.

Hull, R., and Hirsh, J. Long-term anticoagulant therapy in patients with venous thrombosis. *Arch. Intern. Med.*, **1983**, *143*, 2061–2063.

Ikawa, M.; Stahmann, M. A.; and Link, K. P. Studies on 4-hydroxycoumarins. V. Condensation of alpha, beta-unsaturated ketones with 4-hydroxycoumarin. *J. Am. Chem. Soc.*, **1944**, *66*, 902–906.

Jaques, L. B. Addendum: the discovery of heparin. *Semin. Thromb. Hemostas.*, **1978**, *4*, 350–353.

———. Heparin: a unique misunderstood drug. *Trends Pharmacol. Sci.*, **1982**, *3*, 289–291.

Jennings, R. B., and Reimer, K. A. Factors involved in salvaging myocardium: effect of reperfusion of arterial blood. *Circulation*, **1983**, *68*, Suppl. I, I25–I36.

Kakkar, V. V.; Bentley, P. G.; Scully, M. F.; MacGregor, I. R.; Jones, N. A. G.; and Webb, P. J. Antithrombin III and heparin. *Lancet*, **1980**, *1*, 103–104.

Kakkar, V. V.; Stamatakis, J. D.; Bentley, P. G.; Lawrence, D.; DeHaas, H. A.; and Ward, V. P. Prophylaxis for postoperative deep-vein thrombosis. Synergistic effect of heparin and dihydroergotamine. *J.A.M.A.*, **1979**, *241*, 39–42.

Kwaan, H. C.; Dobbie, J. G.; and Fetkenhour, C. The use of anticoagulants and thrombolytic agents in occlusive retinal vascular disease. In, *Thrombosis and Urokinase*. (Paoletti, R., and Sherry, S., eds.) Academic Press, Inc., New York, 1977, pp. 191–198.

Lewis, R. J.; Trager, W. F.; Chan, K. K.; Breckenridge, A.; Orme, M.; Roland, M.; and Schary, W. Warfarin. Stereochemical aspects of its metabolism and the interaction with phenylbutazone. *J. Clin. Invest.*, **1974**, *53*, 1607–1617.

Ljungström, K.-G. Prophylaxis of postoperative thromboembolism with dextran 70: improvements of efficacy and safety. *Acta Chir. Scand.*, **1983**, *514*, Suppl., 1–39.

Loeliger, E. A., and Lewis, S. M. Progress in laboratory control of oral anticoagulants. *Lancet*, **1982**, *2*, 318–320.

McAvoy, T. J. Pharmacokinetic modeling of heparin and its clinical implications. *J. Pharmacokinet. Biopharm.*, **1979**, *7*, 331–354.

Marciniak, E., and Gockerman, J. P. Heparin-induced decrease in circulating antithrombin-III. *Lancet*, **1977**, *2*, 581–584.

Megard, M.; Cuche, M.; Grapeloux, A.; Bojoly, C.; and Meunier, P. J. Ostéoporose de l'héparinothérapie: Analyse histomorphométrique de la biopsie osseuse. Une observation. *Nouv. Presse Med.*, **1982**, *11*, 261–264.

Moncada, S., and Korbut, R. Dipyridamole and other phosphodiesterase inhibitors act as antithrombotic agents by potentiating endogenous prostacyclin. *Lancet*, **1978**, *1*, 1286–1289.

Nagashima, R.; O'Reilly, R. A.; and Levy, G. Kinetics of pharmacologic effects in man: anticoagulant action of warfarin. *Clin. Pharmacol. Ther.*, **1969**, *10*, 22–35.

Negus, D.; Friedgood, A.; Cox, S. J.; Peel, A. L. G.; and Wells, B. W. Ultra low-dose intravenous heparin in the prevention of postoperative deep-vein thrombosis. *Lancet*, **1980**, *1*, 891–893.

Nelson, P. H.; Moser, K. M.; Stoner, C.; and Moser, K. S. Risk of complications during intravenous heparin therapy. *West. J. Med.*, **1982**, *136*, 189–197.

Olsson, J.-E.; Brechter, C.; Bäcklund, H.; Krook, H.; Muller, R.; Nitelius, E.; Olsson, O.; and Tornberg, A. Anticoagulant vs anti-platelet therapy as prophylactic against cerebral infarction in transient ischemic attacks. *Stroke*, **1980**, *11*, 4–9.

O'Reilly, R. A. Vitamin K in hereditary resistance to oral anticoagulant drugs. *Am. J. Physiol.*, **1971**, *221*, 1327–1330.

———. Stereoselective interaction of warfarin and metronidazole (FLAGYL) in man. *N. Engl. J. Med.*, **1976a**, *295*, 354–357.

———. Lack of effect of mealtime wine on the hypoprothrombinemia of oral anticoagulants. *Am. J. Med. Sci.*, **1979**, *277*, 189–194.

———. Phenylbutazone and sulfinpyrazone interaction with oral anticoagulant phenprocoumon. *Arch. Intern. Med.*, **1982b**, *142*, 1634–1637.

———. Stereoselective interaction of sulfinpyrazone with racemic warfarin and its separated enantiomorphs in man. *Circulation*, **1982a**, *65*, 202–207.

———. Comparative interaction of cimetidine and ranitidine with racemic warfarin in man. *Ibid.*, **1984**, *144*, 989–991.

O'Reilly, R. A., and Aggeler, P. M. Studies on coumarin anticoagulant drugs: initiation of therapy without a loading dose. *Circulation*, **1968**, *38*, 169–177.

O'Reilly, R. A.; Trager, W. F.; Motley, C. H.; and Howald, W. Stereoselective interaction of phenylbutazone with $^{12}C/^{13}C$-warfarin pseudoracemates in man. *J. Clin. Invest.*, **1980**, *65*, 746–753.

Pennica, D.; Holmes, W. E.; Kohr, W. J.; Harkins, R. N.; Vehar, G. A.; Ward, C. A.; Bennett, W. F.; Yelverton, E.; Seeburg, P. H.; Heynekor, H. L.; Goeddel, D. V.; and Collen, D. Cloning and expression of human tissue–type plasminogen activator cDNA in E. coli. *Nature*, **1983**, *301*, 214–221.

Powers, P. J.; Cuthbert, D.; and Hirsh, J. Thrombocytopenia found uncommonly during heparin therapy. *J.A.M.A.*, **1979**, *241*, 2396–2397.

Ratnoff, O. D. The role of haemostatic mechanisms. *Clin. Haematol.*, **1981**, *10*, 261–281.

Salzman, E. W. Progress in preventing venous thromboembolism. (Editorial.) *N. Engl. J. Med.*, **1983**, *309*, 980–982.

Sasahara, A. A.; Ho, D. D.; and Sharma, G. V. R. K. When and how to use fibrinolytic agents. *Drug Ther.*, **1979**, *9*, 111–128.

Serlin, M. J., and Breckenridge, A. M. Drug interactions with warfarin. *Drugs*, **1983**, *25*, 610–620.

Shepherd, A. M. M.; Hewick, D. S.; Moreland, T. A.; and Stevenson, I. H. Age as a determinant of sensitivity to warfarin. *Br. J. Clin. Pharmacol.*, **1977**, *4*, 315–320.

TIMI Study Group. The thrombolysis in myocardial infarction (TIMI) trial. *N. Engl. J. Med.*, **1985**, *312*, 932–936.

Trowbridge, A. A.; Caraveo, J.; Green, J. B., III; Amaral, B.; and Stone, M. J. Heparin-related immune thrombocytopenia: studies of antibody-heparin specificity. *Am. J. Med.*, **1978**, *65*, 277–283.

Uotila, L., and Suttie, J. W. Inhibition of vitamin K–dependent carboxylase *in vitro* by cefamandole and its structural analogs. *J. Infect. Dis.*, **1983**, *148*, 571–578.

Van de Werf, F.; Ludbrook, P. A.; Bergmann, S. R.; Tiefenbrunn, A. J.; Fox, K. A. A.; DeGeest, H.; Verstraete, M.; Collen, D.; and Sobel, B. E. Coronary thrombolysis with tissue-type plasminogen activator in patients with evolving myocardial infarction. *N. Engl. J. Med.*, **1984**, *310*, 609–613.

Vernier, R. L.; Klein, D. J.; Sisson, S. P.; Mahan, J. D.; Oegema, T. R.; and Brown, D. M. Heparan sulfate-rich anionic sites in the human glomerular basement membrane: decreased concentration in congenital nephrotic syndrome. *N. Engl. J. Med.*, **1983**, *309*, 1001–1009.

Whitfield, L. R.; Schentag, J. J.; and Levy, G. Relationship between concentration and anticoagulant effect of heparin in plasma of hospitalized patients: magnitude and predictability of interindividual differences. *Clin. Pharmacol. Ther.*, **1982**, *32*, 503–515.

Whitlon, D. S.; Sadowski, J. A.; and Suttie, J. W. Mechanism of coumarin action: significance of vitamin K epoxide reductase inhibition. *Biochemistry*, **1978**, *17*, 1371–1377.

Zacharski, L. R., and others. Effect of warfarin on survival in small cell carcinoma of the lung: Veterans Administration Study No. 75. *J.A.M.A.*, **1981**, *245*, 831–835.

Monographs and Reviews

Colman, R. W., and Rubin, R. N. Update on pulmonary embolism—modern management. *D.M.*, **1982**, *29*, 4–41.

Hamilton, P. J.; Stalker, A. L.; and Douglas, A. S. Disseminated intravascular coagulation: a review. *J. Clin. Pathol.*, **1978**, *31*, 609–619.

Horwitz, R. I., and Feinstein, A. R. The application of therapeutic-trial principles to improve the design of epidemiologic research: a case-control study suggesting that anticoagulants reduce mortality in patients with myocardial infarction. *J. Chronic Dis.*, **1981**, *34*, 575–583.

Jaques, L. B. Heparins—anionic polyelectrolyte drugs. *Pharmacol. Rev.*, **1980**, *31*, 99–166.

Kistler, J. P.; Ropper, A. H.; and Heros, R. C. Medical progress: therapy of ischemic cerebral vascular disease due to atherothrombosis. *N. Engl. J. Med.*, **1984**, *311*, 27–34, 100–105.

Laffel, G. L., and Braunwald, E. Thrombolytic therapy: a new strategy for the treatment of acute myocardial infarction. *N. Engl. J. Med.*, **1984**, *311*, 710–717, 770–776.

Link, K. P. Discovery of dicumarol and its sequels. *Circulation*, **1959**, *19*, 97–107.

O'Reilly, R. A. Vitamin K and the oral anticoagulant drugs. *Annu. Rev. Med.*, **1976b**, *27*, 245–261.

———. Vitamin K antagonists. In, *Hemostasis and Thrombosis: Basic Principles and Clinical Practice.* (Colman, R. W.; Hirsh, J.; Marder, V. J.; and Salzman, E. W.; eds.) J. B. Lippincott Co., Philadelphia, **1982c**, pp. 955–961.

O'Reilly, R. A., and Aggeler, P. M. Determinants of the response to oral anticoagulant drugs in man. *Pharmacol. Rev.*, **1970**, *22*, 35–96.

Symposium. (Various authors.) *Symposium on Vitamin K Metabolism and Vitamin K–Dependent Proteins.* (Suttie, J. W., ed.) University Park Press, Baltimore, **1980,** pp. 1–592.

Symposium. (Various authors.) Symposium on pharmacokinetic and pharmacodynamic approach to anti-thrombotic therapy. (Buchanan, M. R., and Rosenfeld, J., eds.) *Thromb. Res.,* **1983,** Suppl. 4, 1–190.

Weiss, H. J. Drug therapy. Antiplatelet therapy. *N. Engl. J. Med.,* **1978,** *298,* 1344–1347, 1403–1406.

Zwaal, R. F. A., and Hemker, H. C. Blood cell membranes and haemostasis. *Haemostasis,* **1982,** *11,* 12–39.

Hormones and Hormone Antagonists

INTRODUCTION

Ferid Murad and Robert C. Haynes, Jr.

Preparations that contain the active principles of the endocrine glands may be classified from the pharmacological viewpoint as drugs. Whereas most drugs are considered to be substances foreign to the body, the hormones are natural secretions of the endocrine glands and exert important functional effects upon other tissues. Consequently, there has been a tendency to place hormones in a different category, although there is really no valid reason for doing so; indeed, some endocrine preparations have unobtrusively broken down this arbitrary distinction. For example, epinephrine is much more frequently viewed as a powerful sympathomimetic drug than as a hormone of the adrenal medulla.

Pharmacological studies on the actions of drugs of endocrine origin have contributed greatly to an understanding of the normal functions of the endocrine glands. Conversely, much can be learned about the effects of a hormonally active drug by observing the consequences of a deficiency or an excess of the hormone in question. The diverse actions of cortisol and its congeners, for instance, are strikingly illustrated by the changes from the normal shown by patients suffering from adrenal deficiency on the one hand and by patients with oversecretion on the other.

It has been customary to distinguish between hormones and other active substances of animal origin. By definition, a hormone is a substance secreted by a specific tissue and transported to a distant site, where it exerts its effect upon other specific tissues. One can quibble with the details of this definition in some instances; for example, growth hormone seems to act upon so many tissues that the term *specific* becomes imprecise, and the distance traveled by the hypothalamic releasing hormones is rather short. But there are many active substances derived from tissues or body fluids that may act predominantly at the immediate site of release and thus do not meet the definition of a hormone. The latter compounds are designated as *autacoids* and are discussed in an earlier section (Chapters 26, 27, and 28).

Analogs of the hormones, synthetic compounds resembling the natural products but differing from them in some important respects, have often proven more useful in therapeutics than have the hormones themselves. One aim in endocrinology is the isolation, identification, and synthesis of the active principles of each of the endocrine glands. Sometimes, when these formidable efforts have been successful, the product has been found to be of little use in therapy. It may prove inactive when given by mouth, as are the catecholamines, or it may also be so rapidly degraded that unless injected frequently little effect can be achieved, as in the case of the natural sex hormones. The design of synthetic analogs, compounds altered enough to outwit degradative enzymes but not enough to confuse the receptor sites, is one of the major contributions to endocrine therapy. A striking example was the discovery, 50 years ago, of diethylstilbestrol, a cheap synthetic substance that duplicates the actions of estrogen when given orally. In a number of instances the synthetic analogs, by their more desirable properties, represent striking improvements upon nature. Innovative systems for the regional or targeted delivery of drugs can also influence the therapeutic efficacy of a hormone or analog by allowing control of its site or rate of delivery or its metabolism.

A number of useful drugs can influence the synthesis or secretion of hormones or antagonize their cellular actions. Most endocrine tissues store their hormones or precursors thereof intracellularly, often in granules that contain a prohormone or the biologically active compound itself. Secretion is frequently accomplished by exocytosis of the packaged products, and this process, stimulus-secretion coupling, generally requires calcium ion. Synthesis, storage, and secretion of hormones are regulated at numerous steps. The antithyroid drugs provided the initial example of drugs that inhibit hormone synthesis; they selectively inhibit the synthesis of thyroid hormone, and this action makes them effective in the treatment of hyperthyroidism. Equally specific substances have been developed to block one or another step in the synthesis of the hormones of the adrenal cortex.

Direct inhibition of the action of a hormone upon its receptor sites has been achieved experimentally in several instances and has been put to good use in isolated cases. Inhibition of the action of estrogen accounts for the therapeutic efficacy of clomiphene in reproductive disorders in women. By relieving the inhibitory influence of estrogen upon the pituitary, the substance acts to promote the secretion of gonadotropins.

Usually, when considering the clinical applications of the hormones, one thinks first of their use in replacement therapy—treatment of Addison's disease, myxedema, and so forth, with the appropriate drug. However, if the normal regulatory interactions of an endocrine system are understood, hormones and their antagonists can be exploited for a variety of additional therapeutic and diagnostic purposes. Regulation of the endocrine systems characteristically takes place on a multitude of levels. Many systems are ultimately responsive to neural or neuroendocrine control of either a stimulatory or inhibitory nature or both. A change in the magnitude of such control results in an appropriate alteration of secretion in a dependent target, and this secretion may serve as the immediate regulator of yet another endocrine organ. Any of the intermediate products, but more commonly the final hormonal secretion in such a chain, may "feed back" at any level to regulate the intensity of a controlling signal. Such feedback is predominantly negative; thus, a hormone can inhibit its own synthesis and secretion when its critical concentration is exceeded. Positive feedback systems are, however, occasionally utilized. Blood-borne chemicals, the concentrations of which are subject to hormonal regulation, are also used extensively as feedback regulators in such control systems. This knowledge is useful clinically, and it must be applied in the interpretation of a patient's basal laboratory data and in the performance of a variety of provocative tests of endocrine function. Similarly, therapeutic maneuvers also depend on these regulatory interactions. For example, the activity of the adrenal cortex can be suppressed by an adrenocorticosteroid through inhibition of the secretion of corticotropin; ovulation, if unwanted, can be abolished by ovarian hormones that suppress the secretion of hypophyseal gonadotropins.

The last 25 years have witnessed an explosive increase in knowledge of the mechanisms of hormone action, and this is understood in detail for some endocrine secretions. In a number of cases, hormones interact with specific receptors in cellular plasma membranes that are linked to the enzyme adenylate cyclase, discovered by Sutherland and Rall. This enzyme is stimulated or inhibited by the hormone-receptor complex, and the result is an altered rate of synthesis of adenosine 3′,5′-monophosphate (cyclic AMP) from adenosine triphosphate (ATP) (*see* Figure 2–1, page 38). Cyclic AMP then acts as an intracellular mediator for the hormone, and the system thus functions as a mechanism for transferring and amplifying the information inherent in the extracellular hormone. Cyclic AMP regulates a variety of intracellular processes, and the ultimate effects are dependent on the cell's capacity to respond—its differentiated repertoire. The mechanism of cyclic AMP action involves the activation of protein kinases that phosphorylate cellular constituents and alter the rates at which processes involving these constituents proceed. Cyclic AMP is metabolized to 5′-AMP by specific phosphodiesterases, and inhibitors of these enzymes can sometimes exert hormone-like effects. The hormones discussed in the following chapters that appear to use this mechanism include the trophic hormones of the adenohypophysis, the melanocyte-stimulating hormones, some of the hypothalamic releasing hormones, glucagon, parathyroid hormone, and calcitonin. Many hormones appear to act by altering the uptake, release, and intracellular distribution of calcium ion; calcium, like cyclic AMP, may thus be viewed as an intracellular messenger. There are also situations in which cyclic AMP can influence the distribution and actions of calcium and *vice versa*. These systems are thus frequently interactive. Other molecules are also utilized as intracellular messengers; candidates include guanosine 3′,5′-monophosphate (cyclic GMP), diacylglycerol, and inositol triphosphate (*see* Figure 2–1, page 38).

The steroid hormones utilize a different mechanism of information transfer. They gain access to the intracellular compartment and bind to cytoplasmic receptor proteins. Following this interaction the hormone-receptor complex, without or with some modification, is transported to sites of action within the nucleus. In contrast, thyroid hormones appear to enter the nucleus without interaction with a cytoplasmic receptor. The remaining hormones, which in many ways appear to constitute a group, include growth hormone, somatomedins, prolactin, insulin, and other proteins (not discussed here) such as the various cellular growth factors. Their mechanisms of action remain more obscure; however, in view of their protein nature, it is appealing to envision interaction with the plasma membrane and the subsequent generation of second messengers analogous to cyclic AMP. In some instances altered phosphorylation of proteins is involved.

Finally, mention should be made of methodological advances that have greatly facilitated research and clinical applications in endocrine pharmacology. Foremost, perhaps, is radioimmunoassay, pioneered by Berson and Yalow. Using this sensitive and specific technic, the physician has rapid access to a wealth of analytical information about his patient. Advances in peptide and protein chemistry are also outstanding. The technics for determination of amino acid sequences developed by Edman and for automated peptide synthesis developed by Merrifield are making the clinical use of various peptides a reality. The last several years have also witnessed remarkable advances in molecular biology. Recombinant DNA technology has permitted the incorporation of purified or *synthetic* genes that code for the synthesis of specific human hormones into the bacterial genome. The objective is large-scale microbial synthesis of the human protein. This technic is making a major impact upon the availability of scarce hormones, such as human growth hormone, and should overcome the immunological difficulties that are encountered with the clinical use of animal products such as insulin.

CHAPTER
59 ADENOHYPOPHYSEAL HORMONES AND RELATED SUBSTANCES

Ferid Murad and Robert C. Haynes, Jr.

The hormones of the adenohypophysis regulate many important processes in the body; additionally, they are the mediators of various disturbances in the endocrine system and are themselves sensitive to the aberrations of systemic disease. Their secretion is profoundly influenced by many hormones of the peripheral endocrine glands as well as by stimulatory and inhibitory hormones of hypothalamic origin. Similarly striking effects on their secretion are exerted by many drugs, including natural hormones, hormonal analogs, and inhibitors of hormone synthesis and action.

The interrelationships between the pituitary and the peripheral tissues that it regulates represent elegant examples of feedback regulation. Hormones of the anterior pituitary generally regulate the synthesis and secretion of other hormones and substances in target organs, which, in addition to their other physiological effects, can act on the hypothalamus and/or pituitary to diminish secretion of the adenohypophyseal hormone. These concepts are often utilized to diagnose and treat clinical disorders in endocrinology. Furthermore, these interactions may explain the adverse reactions of many drugs.

Among the vertebrates, ten adenohypophyseal hormones are recognized: growth hormone, prolactin, two gonadotropins, thyrotropin, corticotropin, two melanocyte-stimulating hormones, and two lipotropins. Of these, the first six are demonstrably important in man. However, it would be premature to deny the possibility that there may be others. Since the pituitary gland is rich in polypeptides and small proteins, the isolation of pure compounds can be a formidable undertaking. Generally, proteins destined for secretion are synthesized with an amino-terminal leader sequence in a form that is larger than the secreted product. These larger precursors are referred to as "pro" or "prepro" forms of the hormone. While some of the peptides isolated from the pituitary represent such precursors or proteolytic fragments of the hormones, it would perhaps be surprising if some of them did not have biological properties of physiological importance.

The secretory cells of the anterior pituitary are regulated by peptides and other factors that originate in the hypothalamus and that are delivered via the hypothalamicoadenohypophyseal portal system. Five different cell types in the anterior pituitary function independently to synthesize and release one or more hormones. These are the somatotroph, lactotroph, thyrotroph, gonadotroph, and corticotroph-lipotroph. Conventional staining and immunohistochemical technics have been used to identify these cells in the pituitary.

Elucidation of the amino acid sequences of the recognized hormones of the adenohypophysis has shed light on the amazing diversity of the organ. Three groups of hormones are apparent (Table 59–1). The members of the first group, growth hormone and prolactin, show considerable sequence homology, a fact that accounts, for example, for the lactogenic activity of growth hormone. Amino acid sequences are said to be homologous if the corresponding amino acid residues are either identical or replaced with similar amino acids. It is hypothesized that both proteins evolved from a single, perhaps prolactin-like molecule. The gonadotropins and thyrotropin (TSH) constitute the second group, closely related glycoprotein hormones. These complex proteins are each composed of two different noncovalently linked subunits (α and β). Remarkably, the α subunits of the group are nearly identical, while biological specificity resides in unique β subunits. Thus, hybrid hormones can be formed; for example, the α subunit of luteinizing hormone (LH) can be combined with the β subunit of TSH to yield a molecule with thyroid-stimulating activity. The β subunits of LH and TSH also show significant homology with the α subunits. The remaining group comprises corticotropin (ACTH), the melanocyte-stimulating hormones, and the so-called lipotropins. As part of their sequence, these hormones all share a common heptapeptide (Table 59–1). Detailed understanding of the genes that code for these various proteins will allow additional insights into their evolutionary relationships.

These hormones are not unique to the adenohypophysis, since at least one representative of each group is also produced by the placenta. The placental lactogen is very similar to growth hormone, and chorionic gonadotropin resembles LH. Furthermore, precursors of ACTH and related peptides are found in the placenta, gastrointestinal tract, and brain. Some of these peptides may function as part of peptidergic neural systems.

History. The name *pituitary* comes from the Latin *pituita*, meaning "phlegm." The gland was first thought to be a source of phlegm to moisten the membranes of the nose. In 1887, Minkowski associated the features of acromegaly with a tumor

Table 59–1. PROPERTIES OF THE PROTEIN HORMONES OF THE HUMAN ADENOHYPOPHYSIS AND PLACENTA

HORMONE	MOLECULAR WEIGHT	PEPTIDE CHAINS	AMINO ACID RESIDUES	CARBO-HYDRATE	COMMENTS
Group 1					
Growth hormone (GH)	22,000	1	191	0	Human GH, Prl, and PL have considerably less homology of amino acid sequence, in contrast to the striking degree that is observed in other species
Prolactin (Prl)	23,000	1	198	0	
Placental lactogen (PL)	22,000	1	191	0	
Group 2					
Luteinizing hormone (LH or ICSH)	30,000	2	α-89 β-115	16%	Glycoproteins with nonidentical subunits (α and β); biological specificity is in β subunit
Follicle-stimulating hormone (FSH)	32,000	2	α-89 β-115	18%	The α subunits of LH, FSH, TSH, and CG are nearly identical and interchangeable
Thyrotropin (TSH)	28,000	2	α-89 β-112	13%	FSH-α and FSH-β are similar in amino acid composition
Chorionic gonadotropin (CG)	38,000	2	α-92 β-145	31%	FSH-β and TSH-β share a sequence of 49 amino acid residues, while FSH-β and LH-β share a sequence of 39 residues
					Residues 1 to 115 of CG-β have about 80% homology with the β subunits of LH, FSH, and TSH
					While carbohydrate sequences are incomplete, data suggest heterogeneity, even within each hormone
Group 3					
Corticotropin (ACTH)	4500	1	39	0	This group of peptides is derived from a common precursor, pro-opiomelanocortin
α-Melanocyte-stimulating hormone (α-MSH)	1650	1	13	0	Group shares a common heptapeptide: Met-Glu-His-Phe-Arg-Trp-Gly
β-Melanocyte-stimulating hormone (β-MSH)	2100	1	18	0	ACTH (1-13) = α-MSH
β-Lipotropin (β-LPH)	9500	1	91	0	β-LPH (1-58) = γ-LPH
γ-Lipotropin (γ-LPH)	5800	1	58	0	β-LPH (41-58) = β-MSH β-LPH (61-91) = β-Endorphin β-LPH (61-65) = Met-Enkephalin

of the gland. Although the cause-and-effect relationship was by no means clear at first, by 1900 Hutchinson was able to conclude that ". . . in the pituitary body we appear to have a sort of growth-regulating centre for the entire body, the disturbance of which in early life will produce the phenomena of gigantism, and in later life those of acromegaly."

The induction of growth by the injection of pituitary extract was first accomplished in rats by Evans and Long in 1921; concurrently they noted for the first time the gonadotropic effect. Hypophysectomy as an experimental approach was introduced by Aschner in 1909. However, it was not until 1927 that the true consequences of hypophysectomy in mammals were clarified by Smith's classical experiments in the rat (Smith, 1927, 1930). The failure of growth and the atrophy of the gonads, thyroid, and adrenals that followed hypophy-

sectomy were correctable by hypophyseal implants. This work had been anticipated 10 years earlier by parallel studies on the hypophysectomized tadpole wherein the several functions of the three parts of the pituitary were correctly assigned (*see* Allen, 1917). Smith's work in the rat was quickly followed by the definition of a thyrotropic hormone by Aron and by Loeb and Bassett in 1929, the preparation of an adrenotropic extract by Collip and coworkers in 1933, and the preparation and naming of prolactin by Riddle and associates in the same year. The year 1933 was further notable for the publication by Fevold and coworkers of the separate identity of a follicle-stimulating and a luteinizing hormone.

During the 1950s and 1960s, the development of sophisticated technics of protein purification and analysis greatly facilitated research in this area. Such purification of the hormones provided better products for biological investigation, and the great importance of species specificity came to be recognized. It was most strikingly shown in the case of growth hormone, only the product from the pituitaries of primates being active in monkeys and man (Knobil and Greep, 1959; Raben, 1959). This reopened the field of clinical investigation to the development of effective and new therapeutic applications. Of immense, recent significance in this regard are technics and instruments for automated amino acid sequence analysis and solid-phase peptide synthesis. These capabilities are now making the clinical use of synthetic peptides feasible. The development of recombinant DNA technics during the 1970s and 1980s has ushered in the next era, with the provision of even greater quantities of therapeutic materials and the possibility of their modification.

When it was recognized in the early 1940s that the major vascular supply to the anterior pituitary was made up of blood that had already traversed the capillaries of the median eminence of the hypothalamus, the proper setting for the neurohumoral control of the gland was evident. It is now recognized that hypothalamic cells transmit to the anterior lobe individual factors that regulate the secretion of each of its hormones, and this continues to be an area of intense research activity (see page 1381).

Hypopituitarism. Typically in endocrinology the functions of a gland and its secretions can be surmised from alterations that occur when it is congenitally absent or when the gland is destroyed or removed. A great deal has been learned from the consequences of pituitary deficiency.

Hypopituitarism in the Adult. Post-partum pituitary necrosis, described by Simmonds (1914) and by Sheehan (see Sheehan and Summers, 1949), can amount to complete destruction of the anterior lobe, and the patient may die from adrenal deficiency. If she survives, recovery of strength and well-being is slow and incomplete. The infant cannot be nursed, as there is no milk; the pubic hair, if shaved, does not grow back, and axillary and other body hair later fall out; the menstrual periods do not resume, and the genital tract atrophies. The skin becomes thin, soft, and finely wrinkled, assuming a waxy pallor from the mild anemia and the loss of dermal pigment. Libido is lost. There is reduced thyroid function with sensitivity to cold, lack of sweating, low rate of metabolism, poor accumulation of radioiodine by the thyroid, and increased plasma cholesterol. Various indices of adrenocortical function also show a profound deficit. There is sensitivity to physical stress and to the stress of infection, and there may be frequent episodes of collapse or severe illnesses. Body weight is not grossly altered, but there is a tendency toward plumpness. Sometimes one or more of the clinical features are not present, presumably because destruction of the pituitary is not complete.

Hypopituitarism from local tumors often seems to affect the secretion of some hormones before others. The menstrual cycle may stop several years before the thyroid or adrenals are affected, or failure of growth may be the first manifestation. There may be features of advanced hypopituitarism at a time when the thyroid seems still to be normal. By contrast, the consequences of hypophysectomy in man resemble the complete picture of Sheehan's syndrome.

When hypopituitarism in the adult is treated by replacement with a glucocorticoid, thyroid hormone, and the appropriate sex hormone, complete clinical recovery is apparently achieved. The individual still lacks growth hormone, prolactin, and all other factors that have been detected in the adenohypophysis. However, such patients look like normal people, and they feel well and are capable of normal activities. Gametogenesis is lacking but can be corrected with human gonadotropins. Other deficits are by no means obvious.

Hypopituitary Dwarfism. Failure of the pituitary to develop during embryogenesis is, surprisingly, compatible with almost normal longevity. The most striking feature of the condition is, as the name implies, failure to grow normally. At the age of earliest recognition the child is small, with the deviation from the normal becoming more pronounced with advancing years. The dwarfism affects all parts of the body, and the individual comes to resemble a very small version of a normal child. Although growth is very slow, it does not cease; indeed, because it is not arrested by puberty as it is in the normal case, it continues throughout life.

During the years of childhood, the defect in gonadotropic function cannot be recognized clinically, although it can be detected by sensitive immunoassays of the blood for *gonadotropic hormones*. In the absence of these hormones there is no sexual development in later years. Although there may be no *thyrotropin* or *corticotropin,* there is a small but important amount of activity on the part of the thyroid gland and the adrenal cortex. The dwarfing and retarded osseous development are not as extreme as in cretinism, nor does the hypopituitary dwarf show the mental retardation, the changes of the skin, or the facies of the cretin. However, thyroid function tests indicate hypoactivity, and the thyroid is easily stimulated by thyrotropin. The adrenal cortex is usefully functional also, for quite apart from secretion of aldosterone, which does not require corticotropin, some capacity to make glucocorticoids remains. Addisonian crises are not a feature of the condition, and the subjects withstand the stresses of life and of illness rather well. However, it can be shown that adrenocortical secretions are subnormal. The detection of such thyroid and adrenal deficiency helps to differentiate hypopituitarism from the host of other causes of dwarfism, including the isolated deficiency of secretion of growth hormone by the adenohypophysis.

Hypersecretion of Pituitary Hormones. In acromegaly, the most prominent features are those of excessive action of growth hormone, but it is possible that other hormones are also secreted in excess. One form of Cushing's syndrome is caused by an oversecretion of corticotropin, and in this condition, as in acromegaly, a tumor of the pituitary is often responsible. Increased secretion of prolactin from microadenomata of the pituitary is more common than initially suspected. This disorder in women can result in amenorrhea, galactorrhea, and infertility; in men, it can cause impotence. Precocious sexual development in association with tumors at the base of the brain appears to be due to isolated hypersecretion of the gonadotropins. Pituitary tumors that secrete one or both gonadotropins or thyrotropin are extremely rare. Excessive secretion of the several trophic hormones follows impaired function of the individual target glands, owing to the operation of the normal servomechanism. For example, with ovarian failure of the menopause, concentrations of the gonadotropins are markedly elevated. Similarly, primary disorders of the adrenal or thyroid result in decreased "feedback inhibition" of the pituitary and increases in the rates of secretion of the corresponding trophic hormones.

GROWTH HORMONE

Chemistry. Of all the active principles of the anterior pituitary, growth hormone is easily the most abundant. In the human gland, about 10 to 15% of the dry weight is growth hormone. Current methods of extraction obtain a high percentage of the hormone from the glands in an active form, and it has been used extensively in man.

Growth hormone is a single chain of 191 amino acids. There are two intrachain disulfide bonds, and the complete amino acid sequence of the human hormone is known (Li et al., 1966; Niall et al., 1971). While the bovine and ovine hormones are very similar to the human protein in their general features, there are significant differences in primary structure. These account for their relative inactivity in man.

"Big" and "little" forms of growth hormone have been studied in pituitary extracts and plasma. The larger form is about twice the size of the smaller, which has a molecular weight of 22,000. While both forms are readily detected in radioimmunoassays for the hormone, the smaller form is more active in a radioreceptor assay, which is thought to be a better reflection of biological activity than is the radioimmunoassay. The larger form is converted to the smaller and represents a precursor or progrowth hormone. About 70 to 90% of the immunoreactive growth hormone in plasma in normal individuals and those with acromegaly is the smaller, biologically active species (Gordon et al., 1976).

Recurring regions of amino acid sequence homology within the growth hormone molecule have led to the hypothesis that growth hormone (and the lactogenic hormones) have evolved from smaller ancestors by processes involving the tandem linkage of reduplicated genes (Niall et al., 1971). This concept also suggests the possibility of an "active core" in these hormones. The identification of such an "active core" would be particularly worthwhile, since a relatively small active fragment should prove clinically useful, and synthesis might be practical.

Physiological Actions. The concept of a growth hormone sprang from clinical observations on gigantism and acromegaly and was strengthened by the finding that crude extracts of the pituitary gland of the ox, when injected into dogs and rats, elicited increased growth.

Growth. The stimulus to growth provided by growth hormone administered to the rat affects nearly every organ and tissue of the body, the possible exceptions being the brain and the eye. Organs and tissues of the body respond to growth hormone by a proportional increase in size that is in keeping with the total increase in body weight. The growth of bones is reflected in increased body length; the skin and its appendages grow, and the skeletal muscles enlarge. Growth of the thymus is a sensitive index of the action of growth hormone; like that of the lymph nodes, it can be countered by a direct action of the corticosteroids. Enlargement of the liver and increased cellular proliferation therein follow brief treatment with growth hormone, and accumulation of fat may augment somewhat the increase in weight. There is also slight enlargement of the gonads, adrenals, and thyroid, probably attributable to growth hormone itself rather than to specific trophic hormones that contaminate some preparations.

Studies on the growth effects in other species have not been nearly as detailed as those in the rat; indeed, the animal that has been next best studied is the human being. Such investigation in man represents the first thorough exploration of the effects of growth hormone in the same species from which it was derived. Growth in the human being in response to human growth hormone has been studied largely in dwarfs, and particularly in hypopituitary dwarfs, in whom striking effects, amounting to therapeutic triumphs, have been achieved. The growth is normally proportioned, but there is no sexual maturation, splanchnomegaly, or disproportionate growth of skin or flat bones. No features of gigantism or acromegaly have yet been described. However, in some instances limb growth has exceeded that of the trunk.

Effects on the Metabolism of Nitrogen. Growth connotes increased protoplasm and thus protein, the most abundant nitrogen-containing component of the body. It is thus mandatory that growth be associated with the accumulation of nitrogen in the organism. In several species, and under a variety of conditions, growth hormone has been shown to cause a retention of nitrogen, and this property has come to be equated with its anabolic effect. However, since only 0.3 g of nitrogen need be retained daily to support rapid growth during puberty in man, the positive nitrogen balance caused by growth hormone can be difficult to measure. In fact, when growth hormone is given to human subjects in doses of 5 to 10 mg a day, a total of 3 to 5 g of nitrogen is retained daily—many times the amount needed for a normal rate of growth. Although prolonged balances have not been measured, evidently the effect is evanescent, and the site of storage of this extra nitrogen is unknown.

Along with the retained nitrogen there is, of course, accretion of other constituents of tissue. In the case of calcium, there is a paradoxical increase in the urinary loss of the element that is balanced by an augmented absorption from the intestinal tract.

Animal experiments have shown that treatment with growth hormone increases the transport of amino acids into tissues and accelerates their incorporation into protein. Thus, in man, one of the early effects of growth hormone is a decrease in the concentration of urea in the blood, evidently because of diversion of amino acids into anabolic pathways. A variety of anabolic effects can also be observed with isolated tissues incubated *in vitro,* and in this respect the hormone mimics the action of insulin.

Effects on Metabolism of Carbohydrate and Lipid. Growth hormone has a number of important and complex effects on carbohydrate and lipid metabolism (*see* Frantz, 1976). A large number of hormones, notably growth hormone, insulin, glucocorticoids, catecholamines, and glucagon, play important roles in lipid, carbohydrate, and nitrogen homeostasis. As a first approximation, insulin and growth hormone can be viewed as the major anabolic influences, with the glucocorticoids and catecholamines as their catabolic antagonists. However, the details are not that simple. Each hormone in fact exerts a number of effects at different sites. Although an oversimplification of the facts, it might be said that growth hormone seems to switch over the source of fuel for the body from carbohydrate to fat. Thus, while insulin favors the use of sugar and its conversion to fat, growth hormone has just the opposite effect.

In patients suffering from diabetes mellitus, growth hormone exerts a clear-cut diabetogenic effect that can be offset by a larger dose of insulin. The diabetogenic effects of growth hormone are most apparent when it is administered to hypophysectomized patients with diabetes. For example, patients with severe diabetes who have been hypophysectomized for the palliation of ocular or renal lesions are sometimes exquisitely sensitive to growth hormone. A small fraction of the therapeutic dose for promotion of growth can lead to severe intensification of hyperglycemia and ketosis. However, in the nondiabetic patient with normal pancreatic reserve, the administration of growth hormone has little effect on concentrations of glucose and insulin in plasma.

The prominent metabolic actions of growth hormone resemble those brought about by fasting, and during fasting increased secretion of the hormone may be of central importance in adaptation to lack of food. With fasting there is increasing intolerance to carbohydrate (hunger diabetes), inhibited lipogenesis, mobilization of fat, and ketosis—responses that can be evoked by growth hormone. Circulating growth hormone also increases with exercise, and hypoglycemia is a particularly potent stimulus. In teleological terms it is difficult to understand this response. Growth, in the sense of building of protoplasm, cannot take place without food, and one is led to imagine that, without growth hormone, tissue might be broken down during fasting and used indiscriminately for fuel. Growth hormone might hinder this and thereby enforce the use of fat instead.

Although the effects of fasting mimic some of the actions of growth hormone and may in fact be thus mediated, the analogy by itself cannot be indefinitely extrapolated. On the one hand, growth hormone causes retention of nitrogen, increased assimilation of amino acids by tissue, and growth, whereas starvation has the reverse effects; on the other, growth hormone intensifies those very manifestations of the diabetic state that are ameliorated by fasting. It is difficult to escape the conclusion that the action of growth hormone is closely tied to the action of insulin and that the two hormones work against one another as well as together. When they work together, anabolic effects are dominant. In the fasting state, insulin is inconspicuous but not entirely lacking, and growth hormone then further depresses the use of carbohydrate and promotes the mobilization of fat and mild ketosis; in diabetes, when insulin is lacking or has decreased effectiveness, anabolism is impossible and growth hormone assumes the role of a diabetogenic agent. When growth hormone is lacking, insulin acts unopposed, carbohydrate is burned or converted to fat too quickly, and fasting becomes a major stress because, among other defects, there is difficulty in mobilizing fat for fuel.

Somatomedin (Sulfation Factor). Serum from normal rats increases the incorporation of sulfate into the constituents of cartilage incubated *in vitro*, while serum from hypophysectomized animals is ineffective (Daughaday *et al.*, 1959). However, if growth hormone is injected into the hypophysectomized animals, their sera become endowed with the stimulating property. Added directly to the cartilage or admixed with serum, growth hormone is ineffectual. Normal human serum is also active, that from acromegalic patients more so, and that from patients suffering from hypopituitarism inert. The activity in serum appearing in response to the action of growth hormone was initially referred to as *sulfation factor;* it is now called *somatomedin* because of its diverse actions. The concept has thus emerged that growth hormone acts by means of stimulation of the accumulation of somatomedin, although certain of the effects of the hormone may result from other actions.

It is now apparent that a number of peptides in plasma have somatomedin activity in various biological or protein-binding assays (Daughaday, 1977). These peptides are heat stable and have molecular sizes of 7000 to 8000 daltons. Several somatomedins have now been purified, and they are similar to other growth factors that have been characterized in recent years, such as nonsuppressible insulin-like activity (NSILA-S, also called insulin-like growth factor, or IGF). Indeed, some of these growth factors have been found to be identical, for example, somatomedin-C and IGF-1 (*see* Hintz, 1981). These peptides also have considerable homology with insulin and proinsulin, which explains some of the similarities of their effects and their cross-reactivity in radioreceptor and protein-binding assays (*see* Chapter 64). The number and na-

ture of materials that comprise the somatomedins are unknown. Other growth-promoting factors have been described in plasma that have some of the properties of somatomedins. These include nerve growth factor (NGF), epidermal growth factor (EGF), fibroblast growth factor (FGF), and erythropoietin.

The half-life of growth hormone in the circulation is only about 20 minutes, but its effects are much longer lasting. In the treatment of hypopituitary dwarfism, human growth hormone is effective even when injected at weekly intervals. Several hours after the administration of growth hormone, somatomedins appear in the plasma, where they are bound to several larger proteins; such binding probably accounts for their relatively long half-life of 3 to 4 hours. Experiments in hypophysectomized rats suggest that the liver is the major source of somatomedins. They are synthesized in response to growth hormone, and they are not stored. Somatomedins suppress the secretion of growth hormone in a classical feedback manner. Somatomedins are also produced by kidney, muscle, and perhaps other tissues. In the form of familial dwarfism described by Laron, there is an abundance of circulating growth hormone that is biologically active, but somatomedin activity is lacking and injection of growth hormone fails to stimulate its appearance (Laron, 1982). Concentrations of somatomedins in plasma can be assessed with immunoassays or radioreceptor assays.

Somatomedins from different species can be distinguished immunologically, and there is species specificity in their action in radioreceptor assays; plasma from man and monkeys demonstrates cross-reactivity, but plasma obtained from primates and subprimate species does not. The specificity is thus similar to that for growth hormone. The effects of somatomedins are quite diverse and encompass many of the effects of growth hormone. These include enhanced sulfate incorporation into proteoglycans; increased protein, RNA, and DNA synthesis; and increased amino acid and glucose transport into muscle. In adipose tissue increased glucose oxidation, increased lipid synthesis, and decreased lipolysis are observed. There is evidence that not all of the effects of growth hormone are mediated by somatomedins. For a review of the somatomedins, *see* Phillips and Vassilopoulou-Sellin (1980) and Hintz (1981).

Regulation of the Secretion of Growth Hormone. Growth hormone is synthesized and stored in granules of specific acidophilic cells of the anterior pituitary referred to as *somatotrophs*. These growth hormone–containing cells are probably derived from common stem cells that are also precursors for prolactin-containing cells, or *lactotrophs*.

Detailed information on the secretion of growth hormone has become available since the development of sensitive radioimmunoassays for the protein (*see* Reichlin,

1974; Goldfine, 1978). Such measurements of plasma growth hormone concentration have shown surprisingly large and rapid fluctuations in response to metabolic alterations that are due to changes in the rate of secretion of the hormone from the pituitary. In the resting subject before breakfast, the plasma growth hormone concentration is 1 to 2 ng/ml (range 0 to 3). With continued fasting, the value slowly rises to about 8 ng/ml in 60 hours. After a meal or the drinking of a solution of glucose, the concentration falls rapidly to normal. Hypoglycemia induced by insulin is a particularly potent stimulus, the value rising to 25 to 50 ng/ml in 30 minutes. Hypoglycemia from other causes, as well as interference with the utilization of glucose by 2-deoxyglucose, evokes a similar response. Physical exertion, stress, and emotional excitement are normal stimuli to enhanced secretion of growth hormone. After section of the pituitary stalk, there is no change in the plasma concentration of growth hormone in response to hypoglycemia or to glucose, although the basal concentration of growth hormone is normal. Obesity causes reduction or absence of responses of growth hormone to fasting and other stimuli. Inhibitory influences on secretion of growth hormone are exerted by free fatty acids.

Several provocative tests have been devised to evaluate the capacity of the pituitary to secrete growth hormone. The intravenous infusion of arginine in a dose of 30 g in 30 minutes in adults or 0.5 g/kg in children is safer and just as useful as the induction of hypoglycemia with insulin. Three to 5 hours after a dose of glucose, as used in the glucose tolerance test, there is normally a rise in the concentration of growth hormone in plasma. In this test, excessively obese subjects often do not respond. The administration of levodopa, apomorphine, antagonists of 5-hydroxytryptamine (5-HT), and methylphenidate can also be used to evoke secretion of growth hormone, but there is a relatively high incidence of false-negative responses in these tests.

A consistent finding and probably a most important one is the rise in the concentration of growth hormone in the plasma shortly after the onset of deep sleep. This is not just a reflection of a circadian rhythm; if the subject is kept awake all night or fitfully naps often, the rise does not take place until after he falls fast asleep the next day. In fact, prepubertal children may secrete growth hormone primarily during sleep, while secretion of growth hormone during waking hours becomes more significant in adolescents. Both prepubertal and pubertal boys have higher concentrations of plasma growth hormone than do adult males. Unlike the responses to hypoglycemia and to the other adverse influences mentioned above, this response to sleep makes physiological sense; that is, it fits with one's preconceived notion of how the secretion of growth hormone should be ordered. The old adage to the effect that one grows in his sleep may be right after all.

Normally, secretion of growth hormone is controlled by two hypothalamic factors—growth hormone–releasing factor and growth hormone release-inhibiting hormone (somatostatin) (*see* below)—and it is also inhibited by somatomedins. A variety of drugs can influence the secretion of growth hormone, presumably by altering the secretion or activity of these regulators. For example, large doses of glucocorticoids suppress secretion of growth hormone in normal subjects, and this may contribute to their inhibitory effects on the growth of children. However, steroids may also influence the synthesis or secretion of somatomedin. Dopaminergic agonists acutely increase the secretion of growth hormone in normal subjects, and this is the basis of the levodopa test for growth hormone secretion. In contrast, in some acromegalic patients both levodopa and dopaminergic agonists decrease growth hormone secretion and may be used therapeutically. This area and the role of hypothalamic stimulatory and inhibitory hormones in the regulation of the secretion of growth hormone are discussed below.

Assays. The most commonly used bioassays for growth hormone utilize young hypophysectomized rats. *Gain in weight* during 10 days of daily, subcutaneous injection is roughly proportional to the dose. In the *tibia test,* which is more sensitive, the increase in width of the epiphyseal cartilage is measured microscopically. The substances under test are injected subcutaneously daily for 4 days. Radioimmunoassays for growth hormone are far more sensitive. Radioreceptor assays for growth hormone have also been described (Carr and

Friesen, 1976). This technic is conceptually analogous to that of radioimmunoassay. However, a tissue-binding protein is substituted for the antibody. With this method, sensitivity is usually high, and the technic will detect hormonal derivatives with biological activity that may have lost immunoreactivity.

Therapeutic Uses. Growth hormone (*somatotropin*) is given intramuscularly in doses of 0.05 to 0.1 unit/kg three times weekly. The limited supply of human growth hormone has restricted its therapeutic use almost exclusively to hypopituitary dwarfism. Although improvements in preparative procedures had increased supplies, the distribution of human hormone derived from cadaver pituitaries has recently been halted (*see* below). Fortunately, the human hormone can be produced in bacteria by use of recombinant DNA technology; one such product is currently undergoing clinical evaluation (*see* Seeburg *et al.*, 1978; Martial *et al.*, 1979; Olson *et al.*, 1981).

The first patient to receive prolonged therapy showed the uninterrupted response depicted in Figure 59–1 (Raben, 1962a, 1962b). At age 17, he was 4 ft 2½ in. tall, weighed 68 lb, and exhibited all the features of hypopituitarism. Treatment with thyroid did not promote growth, and cortisone had little clinical effect. Growth hormone was given subcutaneously in a dose of 2 mg three times weekly for the first 14 months, and over the ensuing years the dose was increased by increments to a maximum of 5 mg three times a week. When he had been treated for 3 years, he had grown to a height ot 4 ft 9 in.; although 20 years old, he showed no signs of sexual maturation and, therefore, treatment with androgen was begun. Although he received only 60 mg of testosterone cypionate every 2 weeks, in 4 years there was full development of the penis, growth of axillary and pubic hair, increased body hair, more prominent musculature, and a beginning growth of beard. The bone age, which had advanced slowly with growth hormone, reached 15½ years with androgen therapy. This value is associated with nearly complete closure of the epiphyses of the long bones, implying that growth in height was nearly at an end. As there was an insignificant increase in height during a further 7½ months of treatment, growth hormone was discontinued without stopping the other replacement therapy. He had grown a total of 14 in. in 7 years

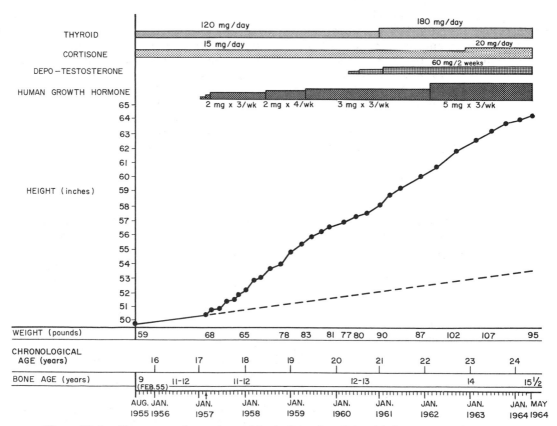

Figure 59–1. *Treatment of a patient with pituitary dwarfism with human growth hormone during replacement therapy with thyroid, cortisone, and testosterone.* (Modified from Raben, 1962b. Courtesy of the *New England Journal of Medicine*.)

and had reached the height of 5 ft 4½ in. at the age of 24.

In the majority of cases pituitary dwarfs respond satisfactorily by an increased rate of growth over many years of treatment. Usually the gain in height declines with succeeding years, and sometimes this is correctable by increasing the dose. Restoration of responsiveness has also been noted after a 3-month interruption of therapy (Rudman *et al.*, 1973).

When there is a poor response or none at all, the diagnosis of hypopituitarism or of isolated deficiency of growth hormone may come into question. While normal children and children with short stature from other causes are less sensitive to growth hormone than are those who are deficient, significant growth responses can be achieved, particularly with larger doses (Van Vliet *et al.*, 1983). Patients with partial deficiency and intermediate concentrations of plasma growth hormone may respond and are candidates for treatment.

To select those cases of short stature that are caused by deficient growth hormone, it is necessary to measure the growth hormone in the plasma and to determine whether there is an appropriate response to a provocative stimulus. Plasma concentrations of somatomedins should also be measured. Requirements for therapy with growth hormone include documentation of the failure to grow and a deficiency of the hormone. Once initiated, therapy should be evaluated for 8 to 12 months for the expected acceleration of growth. An increase in the concentration of somatomedins in plasma after 1 or 2 weeks of therapy may be indicative of subsequent growth response (Rudman *et al.*, 1981). If growth hormone deficiency is the cause and therapy is successful, growth of 5 cm or more in 8 to 12 months can be expected. Evaluation of the growth response to shorter periods of therapy is frequently not possible. Treatment should ideally be continued throughout childhood, and sex hormones, if needed, should be given at the age of puberty to promote normal sexual development (*see* Chapters 61 and 62). The growth response to growth hormone decreases with increasing chronological age or bone age. There is little or no growth response in patients over 20 to 24 years of age. Interestingly, fatter children respond to therapy better than do thinner children (Frasier, 1983).

Treatment with growth hormone has been associated with the development of hypothyroidism. This may be a result of the natural history of hypopituitarism. The development of deficiencies of other pituitary hormones requires therapy. Pain and discomfort from injections of growth hormone are minimal. Subcutaneous injection may lead to local lipoatrophy. Antibodies to human growth hormone are an infrequent cause of resistance; this may be overcome by increasing the dose of growth hormone.

Until the middle of 1985, most of the growth hormone utilized in the United States had been obtained from the National Hormone and Pituitary Program of the National Institutes of Health. *However, distribution of all products derived from human pituitaries was halted after it was determined that at least three individuals who had received human growth hormone in the 1960s and 1970s developed a fatal, degenerative neurological disease* (*Creutzfeldt-Jakob disease*) (Brown *et al.*, 1985; Norman, 1985; Public Health Service, 1985). Since the Creutzfeldt-Jakob virus is difficult to detect, it is uncertain whether contamination of any given preparation with small amounts of virus can either be confirmed or excluded completely. Human growth hormone produced by bacteria as a result of recombinant DNA technology is expected to be available commercially in the future. One such preparation (PROTROPIN) is in clinical trial. Unfortunately, many patients have developed low levels of circulating antibodies to this product (which has one additional amino acid residue), and the utility of this material for long-term treatment is still unknown.

Acromegaly. In acromegaly, the causative hypersecretion of growth hormone is from a pituitary tumor. These tumors can display a spectrum of independence from normal physiological and even pharmacological factors with respect to their secretion. Tumors that secrete growth hormone can be removed surgically or they can be treated with irradiation. While levodopa increases the secretion of growth hormone in normal subjects, it may exert a paradoxical inhibitory effect in some patients with acromegaly. This observation has led to the effective therapeutic use of dopaminergic agonists for the management of acromegaly. Secretion of growth hormone by these tumors can be suppressed successfully with *bromocriptine* (2-bromo-α-ergocryptine) (Wass *et al.*, 1977; Goldfine, 1978). This therapy should be reserved for tumors without suprasellar extension and alterations in visual fields. Oral administration of 10 to 60 mg a day in divided doses is frequently effective. The initial dose of 1.25 to 2.5 mg per day of bromocriptine (PARLODEL) should be increased every few days, if necessary, in order to minimize side effects; these include nausea, vomiting, constipation, and perhaps hypotension. Failure of bromocriptine to lower concentrations of growth hormone in plasma acutely does not necessarily imply that the drug will not be effective during chronic administration. Withdrawal of the drug leads to a resurgence of growth hormone secretion. Increased secretion of prolactin may also occur with acromegaly or other pituitary tumors, due to the removal of inhibitory control from the hypothalamus. Bromocriptine will effectively inhibit prolactin secretion, as discussed below. The dose required for suppression of prolactin is somewhat smaller. Bromocriptine is further discussed in Chapters 21 and 39.

Antagonists of 5-HT such as cyproheptadine and metergoline, as well as α-adrenergic antagonists (*e.g.*, phentolamine), can also inhibit the secretion of growth hormone in acromegaly, but their effects are weaker and inconsistent (Feldman *et al.*, 1976). Somatostatin (growth hormone release-inhibiting hormone) will suppress the secretion of growth hormone, as discussed below. However, somatostatin has not been useful for the treatment of acromegaly because of the need for parenteral administration of the peptide, its short half-life, and its ability to inhibit the secretion of numerous other hormones.

PROLACTIN

Although prolactin was discovered in 1928 and a wealth of information was obtained about its role in a wide variety of species, unequivocal evidence for the existence of the hormone in man was obtained relatively recently. It is now appreciated, however, that prolactin plays an important role in normal human function and in certain pathophysiological states (Thorner, 1977; Frantz, 1978).

Prolactin is widely distributed in the pituitaries of vertebrates. It is synthesized and stored in pituitary lactotrophs, which are probably derived from stem cells similar to those for somatotrophs. Human amniotic fluid has concentrations of prolactin that are considerably higher than those in plasma, and placental tissue can synthesize and secrete the hormone (Golander *et al.,* 1978).

The term *prolactin* was coined for the hormone responsible for the secretion of milk by the crop glands of the pigeon (Riddle *et al.,* 1933). In this bird there is a bilateral outpouching of the esophagus and, prompted by the psychological concomitants of brooding, a glandular structure grows within each pouch so that by the time of hatching a thick secretion (the crop milk), produced as a result of epithelial proliferation and desquamation, becomes available to each parent for regurgitating down the the throats of the young. The response of the bird is a sensitive one; it is sufficient for one partner to see his mate sitting on the eggs for his pituitary to secrete prolactin and provoke the growth of the crop glands. In so naming the hormone, the tenuous analogy between the mammary gland and the crop sac was correctly drawn because it later was clear that prolactin is also of importance in initiating secretion from the breast.

Chemistry. The difficulty in isolating human prolactin is attributable to the facts that growth hormone is very similar in structure, possesses significant lactogenic activity in conventional bioassays for the hormone, and is present in human pituitaries in quantities about 100-fold greater than is prolactin. However, refined bioassay technics permitted verification of the existence of human prolactin (Frantz and Kleinberg, 1970), and the technic of affinity chromatography permitted purification of a primate prolactin and subsequent development of a specific radioimmunoassay (Guyda and Friesen, 1971; Hwang *et al.,* 1971). Progress in the purification, chemistry, and physiology of human prolactin has been rapid since these advances.

Ovine prolactin has been characterized extensively, since the pituitaries of sheep are readily available and constitute a very rich source (Li *et al.,* 1970). The amino acid sequences of human and ovine prolactin are now known to be quite similar (Shome and Parlow, 1977). The general structural features are very similar to those of the growth hormones (Table 59–1), and the proposed evolutionary relationship of these molecules has been discussed above. As with the growth hormones, large (56,000-dalton) and small (23,000-dalton) forms of prolactin have been described (Suh and Frantz, 1974).

Physiological Actions. *Breast.* The mammary gland is a site of immensely complex interactions; a number of hormones and the majority of endocrine organs participate vigorously during pregnancy to prepare the breast for secretion post partum. The hormones of the adrenal cortex, thyroid, and ovaries are all necessary, and their presence is dependent on the trophic hormones of the adenohypophysis. Insulin and perhaps growth hormone exert important anabolic influences. The vital participation of prolactin completes the contribution of the anterior pituitary, with all of its major secretions at work. The role of oxytocin is considered in Chapter 39.

The actions of prolactin on the mammary gland have been studied particularly in explanted rodent tissue. However, investigations of normal and aberrant prolactin secretion assure the existence of comparable functions in the human female. The increasing concentration of prolactin during pregnancy is required for growth and development of the breast in preparation for breast feeding post partum. The high concentrations of estrogens and progestins that are present during pregnancy oppose some of the actions of prolactin. After delivery, the concentrations of the sex steroids decline markedly, and the actions of prolactin become unopposed. In systems *in vitro,* prolactin in the proper hormonal milieu binds to specific receptors and promotes proliferation and subsequent differentiation of mammary ductal and alveolar epithelium. There is a rapid increase in RNA synthesis and induction of the synthesis of milk proteins and of enzymes necessary for lactose synthesis (Topper, 1970; Turkington *et al.,* 1973). At the subcellular level, activation of the development of rough endoplasmic reticulum, Golgi apparatus, and secretory granules is prominent.

These "mammotrophic" actions of prolactin suggest a possible role of prolactin in mammary tumorigenesis (Smithline et al., 1975). Prolonged prolactin administration, the grafting of extra pituitaries, or experimental lesions in the median eminence that cause increased prolactin secretion all result in a high percentage of mammary tumors in susceptible rats and mice. Furthermore, estrogen will not produce tumors in the absence of the pituitary; however, in rats treated with carcinogens, prolactin promotes tumorigenesis in the absence of estrogens or progestins. Moreover, drugs that enhance prolactin secretion (e.g., reserpine, haloperidol—see below) facilitate experimental tumor growth, while those that inhibit secretion (e.g., ergot derivatives) impede growth and reduce the incidence of spontaneous tumors in rodent models. Extrapolation between highly susceptible strains of rodents and man is obviously of questionable value, but these observations may provide additional explanations for the effectiveness of hormonal therapy of breast tumors. They may also relate to some of the conflicting reports of the increased incidence of breast cancer among women who have been treated with reserpine for hypertension (see Frantz, 1978). However, most studies have shown normal concentrations of prolactin in patients with breast tumors, and there is thus no reason to believe that disorders of prolactin metabolism have etiological significance in mammary carcinogenesis in the human female. The hormone may, however, play a permissive role.

Gonads. The effects of prolactin on the ovary are species dependent. While the hormone has in the past also been referred to as *luteotropin,* this description was based on observations on rats and mice. In these species prolactin can prolong the life of the functioning corpus luteum, but it probably does not fulfill the role of a true luteotropic hormone. Notably, prolactin will not stimulate progesterone biosynthesis by corpora lutea in a variety of species, including rats (see Dorfman, 1972). It may, however, function to promote the luteal synthesis of cholesterol, the steroidal precursor. In contrast, luteinizing hormone is uniformly effective in stimulating progesterone synthesis. Surprisingly, evidence suggests that the sharp rise in prolactin secretion seen during proestrus in the rat may be responsible for luteolysis of corpora lutea formed during the previous cycle (Meites et al., 1972).

In human subjects prolactin may inhibit the secretion of gonadotropins or their effects on the gonads (Thorner, 1977). Suckling is a potent stimulus to prolactin secretion for several months post partum. The elevation of prolactin with breast feeding and its inhibitory effects on ovarian function can explain the usual lack of ovulation and infertility during breast feeding. This natural mechanism of contraception becomes ineffective several months post partum as the suckling stimulus to the secretion of prolactin declines. Prolactin-secreting tumors frequently lead to galactorrhea, amenorrhea, anovulatory cycles, and infertility in women, while hyperprolactinemia in men may cause loss of libido and impotence (Thorner, 1977; Frantz, 1978). Paradoxically prolactin may also directly stimulate testicular synthesis of testosterone (Rubin et al., 1976).

Pregnancy. Although concentrations of prolactin increase 20- to 40-fold during human pregnancy, the hormone appears to have no role in maintenance of the pregnancy or the fetus. Normal pregnancies and deliveries have followed inhibition of prolactin secretion with bromocriptine or hypophysectomy (Mehta and Tolis, 1981); however, failure of breast enlargement and lack of post-partum lactation are observed.

Other Effects. Sexual behavior of lower animals and birds is thought to be influenced by gonadotropins and steroids, while parental behavior involving the care, feeding, and protection of offspring may be regulated by prolactin. There is no evidence that similar functions of prolactin occur in man. Although prolactin has effects on salt and water metabolism in lower forms, the consensus is that comparable effects do not occur in man, despite several reports to the contrary; these may be attributable to contaminants in the hormonal preparations used (Baumann and Loriaux, 1976).

Prolactin Secretion. Refined assay technics not only have been instrumental in the identification and purification of human prolactin but also have allowed exploration of physiological, pathological, and pharmacological influences on prolactin secretion (see Friesen, 1973; Thorner, 1977; Frantz, 1978). Concentrations in plasma are high in newborns but decrease to low levels until puberty, when they begin to increase in girls. The normal adult human plasma concentration of prolactin approximates 5 to 10 ng/ml and is somewhat less in males than in females. Prolactin concentrations rise markedly during pregnancy, reaching a maximum at term (values of about 200 ng/ml). After delivery the concentrations of prolactin decline unless the mother breastfeeds. In nursing mothers prolactin secretion is critically controlled by the sucking stimulus or breast manipulation. Prolactin concentration can rise 10- to 100-fold within 30 minutes of stimulation. This response becomes less prominent after several months of breast feeding, and prolactin concentrations decline. Exceptions are noted in some primitive cultures where the response of prolactin to suckling may persist for longer times. In some normal menstruating women, but not in men, breast manipulation may produce small increases in the rate of secretion of prolactin.

Many of the physiological factors that influence the secretion of growth hormone have similar effects on prolactin. These include sleep, stress, hypoglycemia, fluctuations of the concentrations of estrogen, and exercise, which increase the secretion of both hormones. Prolactin shows a circadian rhythm, with peaks during sleep; superimposed on this pattern are minute-to-minute fluctuations due to pulsatile secretion. The half-life of prolactin in plasma is 15 to 20 minutes. A variety of endogenous factors and drugs can alter the secretion of prolactin and are discussed below.

Secretion of prolactin by the pituitary is under predominantly negative control by the hypothalamus, and in this respect it is unique among the pituitary hormones. A prolactin release-inhibiting hormone (PRIH) is secreted by the hypothalamus and is carried by the hypothalamicoadenohypophyseal portal system to the adenohypophysis, where it inhibits prolactin secretion. There is considerable evidence that the release of prolactin is under adrenergic (dopaminergic) control, and PRIH may in fact be dopamine (MacLeod, 1976). Thus, the administration of levodopa in vivo inhibits prolactin secretion, and dopamine is a highly effective inhibitor when instilled into the third ventricle or when applied to the isolated pituitary in vitro. Predictably, the phenothiazine and butyrophenone antipsychotics (e.g., chlorpromazine, haloperidol), which are dopamine antagonists, enhance prolactin secretion, as can metoclopramide, reserpine, and α-methyldopa (see Chapter 19). The antipsychotic agents can cause significant galactorrhea associated with elevated concentrations of prolactin in plasma.

While thyrotropin-releasing hormone (TRH) can stimulate prolactin secretion, the physiological significance of this effect is not known. During suckling the secretions of prolactin and TSH are dissociated. Another factor, designated prolactin-releasing factor (PRF), which is of hypothalamic origin, is thought to play a stimulatory role in the regulation of prolactin secretion, but the nature of this material is not known (Boyd et al., 1976). Estrogens, histamine, and opioids also increase secretion of prolactin, while muscarinic agonists decrease it. The physiological significance, if any, of these effects is unknown (see Mehta and Tolis, 1981).

Hyperprolactinemia. This disorder may be associated with various drugs such as dopaminergic antagonists, infiltrative disorders of the hypothalamus or pituitary that interfere with regulation of prolactin secretion by PRIH, hypothyroidism with accompanying increases in TRH, and the use of oral contraceptives. Prolactin-secreting tumors are another cause, and these may become apparent because of galactorrhea, amenorrhea, and infertility. These tumors can be treated with irradiation, surgical removal, or pharmacological agents. When the tumors are microadenomata that are not associated with suprasellar extension or alterations in vi-

sual fields, pharmacological suppression of prolactin secretion is effective and should be considered. Suppression of galactorrhea by administration of levodopa has been attempted with variable success (Turkington, 1972). Some patients who respond initially become refractory to the drug. More promising clinical results have been achieved with ergot derivatives (Floss et al., 1973). Inhibition of lactation in women suffering from ergotism was observed centuries ago. This phenomenon has gained scientific credence with the discovery that ergot derivatives profoundly inhibit prolactin secretion in vivo and in isolated pituitary preparations in vitro. Since the inhibitory effect in vitro is antagonized by haloperidol, it is likely that ergot alkaloids activate the dopaminergic receptors that inhibit prolactin release. The compound that is most useful is *bromocriptine*, which is available as bromocriptine mesylate in 2.5-mg tablets and 5-mg capsules (PARLODEL). The dosage and side effects of this drug are discussed above with regard to its use in acromegaly. Other ergot derivatives are also effective, but experience with them has been limited (see Parkes, 1977). When bromocriptine is used to suppress prolactin secretion by such functional tumors, the galactorrhea and amenorrhea usually cease within several weeks and pregnancy becomes possible. Pregnancies and offspring have been normal, but it is recommended that bromocriptine be discontinued during pregnancy. Generally galactorrhea, amenorrhea, and infertility will recur in the nonpregnant patient when the drug is stopped. Some prolactin-secreting tumors have decreased in size during administration of bromocriptine; the mechanism of tumor regression is unknown (Mehta and Tolis, 1981). The tumors recur when bromocriptine is discontinued.

Assays. The classical procedure for bioassay of prolactin is based on the original work of Riddle and associates (1933), namely, the increase in weight of the crop sacs of doves and pigeons. Other methods are based on the induction of secretory changes in the suitably prepared mammary glands of guinea pigs and rabbits. As mentioned above, radioimmunoassays have proven invaluable. A radioreceptor assay that utilizes a membrane receptor preparation isolated from rabbit mammary glands is also useful to assess biological activity (Shiu et al., 1973).

Human Placental Lactogen. Preparations from the human placenta contain growth-promoting and lactogenic activity (see Fukushima, 1961); Josimovich and MacLaren (1962) showed that such extracts cross-reacted with antisera to human growth hormone. Purified preparations caused a local response in the crop sac of the pigeon and maintained the function of the corpora lutea of rats but caused little growth in hypophysectomized animals; the active principle was named *placental lactogen*. Friesen (1966) purified the protein to homogeneity and demonstrated that it was strikingly lactogenic in pseudopregnant rabbits.

The chemical similarity of the substance to human growth hormone was shown by Sherwood

(1967), and the complete amino acid sequence has been elucidated by Niall and associates (1971) and Li and coworkers (1973). The resemblance to growth hormone was amply confirmed by these studies, since both hormones contain 191 amino acids that differ in only 32 positions. The greater similarity of amino acid sequence of human placental lactogen and human growth hormone than of human and bovine growth hormones suggests a later evolutionary appearance of the placental lactogen. Because of its resemblance to growth hormone, the unwieldy name *chorionic somatomammotropin* is also in use.

The functions of human placental lactogen have not been clearly defined. It is produced by the syncytiotrophoblasts of the placenta, and concentrations in maternal plasma increase progressively during pregnancy. In addition to promoting growth and development of the mammary gland, it is luteotropic and may stimulate production of steroids by the corpus luteum during pregnancy. The metabolic effects of placental lactogen resemble those of growth hormone, and it is postulated that these effects may be important for fetal nutrition, growth, and development (Chatterjee and Munro, 1977).

GONADOTROPIC HORMONES

The pituitary gland plays an important part in the regulation of gonadal function throughout the vertebrate phylum, but the fullest understanding of the mechanisms involved has been achieved among mammals. The adenohypophysis is physiologically and anatomically so situated that it can mediate neural messages that arise from the environment as well as intercept humoral signals from within. It can regulate such diverse phenomena as the annual growth and regression of the gonads of monestrous mammals in response to the changing length of daylight, the release of ova in the rabbit 10 hours after mating, and the reinitiation of follicular growth when a corpus luteum fails for lack of successful impregnation.

For over 50 years it has been known that two gonadotropins are involved, and it seems a general rule among mammals that follicular growth and development on the one hand and ovulation and the formation of a corpus luteum on the other are separately controlled. These same substances stimulate, respectively, the germinal elements of the testis and the androgen-secreting Leydig cells of the interstitial tissue. In the regulation of the function of the corpus luteum, several adaptations have arisen. In some species luteinizing hormone serves as the luteotropin, in others prolactin plays such a role, while in several species the uterus is somehow involved. During pregnancy the pituitary seems essential in some animals, while in most it is dispensable; luteal function may be autonomous, as in the herbivora, or regulated in part by a placental luteotropin, as in man.

Chemistry. The three gonadotropins considered here (two of pituitary and one of placental origin) are follicle-stimulating hormone (FSH), luteinizing hormone (LH; also called interstitial cell–stimulating hormone, ICSH), and chorionic gonadotropin (CG). The gonadotropins, with thyrotropin (TSH), constitute the glycoprotein group of hormones, and their similarities and general chemical features have been mentioned above (*see* Table 59–1).

FSH, LH, CG, and TSH have been purified and characterized from several sources, including man. These hormones have two nonidentical and noncovalently linked peptide subunits, designated α and β. The α subunits of each hormone are nearly identical; the biological specificity resides in the β subunits (*see* Pierce and Parsons, 1981). A separate gene codes for the synthesis of each subunit. The α subunit of one hormone can be combined with the β subunit of another to yield a hybrid molecule with biological activity of the β-subunit donor. The β subunits also have a great deal of similarity. For example, the β subunit of human chorionic gonadotropin consists of 145 amino acid residues, and residues 1 to 115 are about 80% homologous with the β subunits of LH, FSH, and TSH. The carbohydrate content of each of these glycoproteins is however quite different (Shome and Parlow, 1973, 1974; Lipsett and Ross, 1978). Furthermore, there is some heterogeneity of the carbohydrate residues within each of the hormones.

Secretion and Physiological Actions. Despite an extraordinarily large number of experimental observations of the secretion and actions of gonadotropins, understanding of these areas is far from complete. Most studies have been carried out in species different from that of origin of the hormone, and in some instances impure preparations have been used, which may account for some anomalous responses. Observations on the responses of the normal human gonads to human gonadotropins are still relatively fragmentary.

Secretion. LH and FSH are produced and secreted by the same cell type in the pituitary, gonadotrophs. Secretion of LH and FSH is regulated through feedback inhibition by sex steroids in plasma. As discussed below, a single hypothalamic regulatory factor controls the secretion of both FSH and LH.

In infancy and prepuberty the concentrations of FSH and LH in plasma are measurable, but quite low. At puberty gonadotropin secretion increases about twofold, probably due to diminished feedback inhibition of secretion by sex steroids (*see* Franchimont, 1977). In men, plasma concentrations of FSH and LH are relatively constant while rates of secretion in women are somewhat higher and vary according to the phase of the menstrual cycle. In normal women the daily rate of production of LH is about 500 to 1000 I.U.; this increases about three- to sixfold at ovulation and after menopause. In some gonadal disorders, concentrations of gonadotropins increase due to diminished concentrations of sex steroids and a resultant loss of their feedback inhibition on the pituitary. Gonadotropins are secreted in a pulsatile manner, which accounts for the minute-to-minute oscillations in plasma concentrations. Pituitary tumors may rarely secrete one or both gonadotropins (Friend *et al.*, 1976; Snyder and Sterling, 1976).

Actions on the Ovary. During the follicular phase of the ovarian cycle successive groups of small follicles start to grow, and by the time ovulation is imminent follicles in all stages of development are found. This ovarian response represents the predominant action of FSH, and it is during this phase that estrogen is the main ovarian secretory product (*see* Figure 61–2, page 1416).

Shortly before ovulation is to take place, a series of ovarian changes follow in rapid succession, presumably mediated by a burst of FSH and LH secretion at this time; this is due to a positive feedback effect of estrogen on gonadotropin secretion. The largest follicles expand quickly; those in just the right stage of development to ovulate undergo cytological changes in the granulosa in the direction of luteinization and show intense hyperemia of the theca interna. One area on the surface of the dominant follicle thins and then undergoes dissolution, leaving an aperture through which the viscous follicular fluid oozes, carrying desquamated granulosa cells and the cumulus and its contained ovum with it. Those large follicles not destined to ovulate, perhaps for reasons of improper stage of development, remain avascular and begin to show regressive changes. While ovulation is in progress, widespread atresia involves all the other follicles that shortly before had been flourishing under the influence of FSH, and in certain species the atresic process extends also to the residual corpora lutea of antecedent cycles. It is tempting to attribute the regressive changes in the ovary, which parallel so closely ovulation and luteinization, to an action of LH.

With the earliest stages of preovulatory follicular swelling there is evidence of the first secretion of progesterone. This has been shown in species that require the luteotropic action of prolactin as well as in those that do not. The critical influence is exerted by LH. LH maintains the corpus luteum until the secretion of estrogen and progesterone declines sufficiently to initiate menses, and a new cycle then begins. If pregnancy occurs, chorionic gonadotropin produced by the trophoblastic cells of the placenta maintains the corpus luteum.

Measurements of the gonadotropins in plasma throughout the menstrual cycle show that FSH is elevated during the follicular phase and slowly falls before it rises again at midcycle; it is lowest during the luteal phase. LH shows a striking peak at midcycle, usually on the same day that the FSH is highest (*see* Figure 61–2, page 1416). This surge in the secretion of LH is an immediately preovulatory event (*see* Faiman and Ryan, 1967; Midgley and Jaffe, 1968). Further interactions between the gonadotropins and the sex steroids are discussed in Chapters 61 and 62.

Actions on the Testis. Whereas in the ovary both gonadotropins are involved in the secretion of hormones, LH plays a predominant role in the testis. FSH is primarily a gametogenic hormone in males; it is responsible for the anatomical integrity of the seminiferous tubules and only under its influence are the complex stages of gametogenesis carried through to the production of spermatozoa. In the hypophysectomized animal, the major effect of FSH is stimulation of the seminiferous tubules. As the tubules make up the bulk of the testis, tubular growth is accurately reflected by an increase in testicular weight. Possible effects of FSH on testosterone secretion from the Leydig cells are controversial and are discussed in Chapter 62. LH stimulates the interstitial (Leydig) cells to secrete androgen, but the androgen, in turn, exerts a direct effect upon the tubules so that both components of the testis appear to be stimulated. These effects of LH have led to its alternate designation as interstitial cell–stimulating hormone (ICSH).

Mechanism of Action. LH and FSH bind with specificity to various particulate fractions derived from testis and ovary. Furthermore, both gonadotropins are known to stimulate adenosine $3',5'$-monophosphate (cyclic AMP) synthesis in appropriate gonadal preparations (Marsh *et al.*, 1966; Murad *et al.*, 1969). Cyclic AMP then stimulates conversion of cholesterol to pregnenolone and sex steroid biosynthesis by mechanisms apparently analogous to those operative in the adrenal cortex. The nucleotide also induces luteinization of cultured granulosa cells (Channing and Seymour, 1970) and transplanted ovarian follicles (Ellsworth and Armstrong, 1973).

Chorionic Gonadotropin (CG). Chorionic gonadotropin is a hormone of human pregnancy; it is secreted by the syncytiotrophoblasts of fetal placenta as early as 7 days after ovulation, and it is absorbed into the blood in sufficient quantity to sustain luteal function and forestall the next menstrual period; the secretion of LH remains suppressed because of the rising concentrations of estrogen and progesterone (Lipsett and Ross, 1978).

Chorionic gonadotropin is detectable in the urine by immunoassay several days before the first missed period, and this is the basis of the most commonly used test of pregnancy. The quantity excreted increases rapidly thereafter to a maximum about 6 weeks after ovulation. The urinary content then declines over the next month or so and stabilizes at a lower level for the remainder of pregnancy.

The changes in the corpus luteum in early pregnancy reflect the intense stimulation provided by the LH-like action of chorionic gonadotropin. Furthermore, as noted above, concentrations of placental lactogen increase progressively during pregnancy; it also is luteotropic and may play some role in concert with chorionic gonadotropin to stimulate steroid production by the corpus luteum. With the increasing secretion of estrogen and progesterone by the placenta during the third month, the ovaries and the corpus luteum become unessential to the maintenance of gestation, but the corpus luteum does not undergo a pronounced change at this time. Instead, there is a slow regression that, histologically, is not complete even at the time of delivery. In the presence of the flood of chorionic gonadotropin during pregnancy, the rest of the ovary remains quiescent.

Assays of chorionic gonadotropin and its subunits are also used to diagnose and to evaluate the treatment of trophoblastic tumors (Vaitukaitis *et al.*, 1976). Quantification of the secretion of the hormone by choriocarcinomas and hydatidiform moles can provide an accurate index of tumor regression or recurrence. This ability has contributed to the high rate of successful treatment of these tumors.

The action of chorionic gonadotropin on the testis can hardly be regarded as physiological, for the hormone gains access to the male only *in utero*, when it does cause minimal gonadal stimulation; otherwise the hormone is found in the male only in the rare event of a teratomatous tumor containing chorionic elements. Injected into men, however, chorionic gonadotropin stimulates the interstitial cells of the testis to secrete androgen. Activation of the seminiferous epithelium is minimal and may be mediated entirely by the androgen of Leydig-cell origin.

Chorionic gonadotropin also has some thyrotropic activity, which is thought to be unimportant except in some trophoblastic tumors where the large amounts of hormone can lead to hyperthyroidism (Cave and Dunn, 1976; Morley *et al.*, 1976).

The mechanism of action of chorionic gonadotropin appears to be identical to that of LH.

Absorption, Fate, and Excretion. The gonadotropins of either pituitary or placental origin are effective only if given by injection. The length of survival of the injected and presumably of the endogenously secreted hormones is determined largely by the rate of degradation in the body, because little is excreted in the urine except in the case of chorionic gonadotropin. Studies on the rate of disappearance of endogenous human LH, FSH, and chorionic gonadotropin indicate removal from the plasma with half-lives of 30 minutes, 60 minutes, and 8 hours, respectively. Removal of sialic acid from chorionic gonadotropin greatly decreases its half-life, but this may not be important in its normal metabolism. During the latter part of pregnancy, immunoreactive material appears in the urine in quantities several times greater than the quantity of biologically active hormone, suggesting that there is partial degradation of chorionic gonadotropin before excretion, and this mechanism may be involved in the rapid clearance of the active hormone from the body after delivery of the placenta.

Assays. Bioassay remains a necessary technic for evaluation of functional activity, which often bears no relationship to immunoreactivity. The gonadotropins pose a special problem because many responses to one hormone are modified by the concurrent action of others, and special conditions must be chosen to minimize this influence. References and descriptions of several technics can be found in the *third* and *fourth editions* of this textbook.

For many purposes, particularly the measurement of gonadotropins in blood and urine, radioimmunoassays are more accurate and far simpler than bioassays. References have been cited by Vande Wiele and Dyrenfurth (1973). While some antibodies used in these radioimmunoassays cross-react with the other gonadotropins, specific antibodies against the β chain are available. The use of monoclonal antibodies is expected to circumvent problems of specificity. Radioreceptor assays are also employed.

Preparations and Dosages. For certain purposes, quite crude preparations of gonadotropins from human pituitaries would be suitable, even though they contain both FSH and LH as well as other active principles. While purified human LH and FSH had been available for investigational uses from the National Hormone and Pituitary Program of the National Institutes of Health, distribution of all products derived from human pituitaries was recently discontinued because of possible contamination with Creutzfeldt-Jakob virus (*see* page 1371).

Menotropins for injection (PERGONAL) is a preparation of gonadotropins from the urine of postmenopausal women. While FSH and LH activities are present in equal unitage, chorionic gonadotropin is usually required in conjunction with menotropins to induce ovulation. The recommended initial dose is 75 I.U. of each gonadotropin intramuscularly daily for 9 to 12 days. This is followed by 10,000 I.U. of chorionic gonadotropin. If there is no evidence of ovulation, several treatment cycles may be necessary and the dosage may be increased. In some cases large quantities may be needed.

Chorionic gonadotropin for injection is a preparation derived from the urine of pregnant women, which is sold under various trade names (A.P.L., PREGNYL, others). It is usually given intramuscularly in doses of 500 to 4000 I.U. two or three times weekly for several weeks for the treatment of cryptorchism or hypogonadism in men, and in doses of 5000 to 10,000 I.U. one day following treatment with menotropins to evoke ovulation.

Gonadotropin of pregnant mares' serum has been used clinically to a limited extent for over 4 decades; however, no clear-cut indications have emerged and there are few guidelines to dosage.

Therapeutic Uses. The gonadotropins are used in therapy primarily for the treatment of infertility and cryptorchism.

Infertility. The widest potential usefulness of the gonadotropins is in the induction of ovulation in women who are infertile because of pituitary insufficiency. Extensive clinical experience with menotropins and human chorionic gonadotropin, summarized by Thompson and Hansen (1970), indicated the occurrence of ovulation in 75% of appropriately selected patients treated with the drugs. While ovulation was occasionally seen during administration of menotropins before human chorionic gonadotropin was given, it usually took place about 18 hours after administration of the latter hormone. Pregnancy resulted in approximately 25% of the patients; of these, the abortion rate was 25% and fetal abnormalities occurred in 2%. Twenty percent of pregnancies resulted in multiple births (15% twins and 5% with three or more concepti). Interestingly, in another series the male-to-female sex ratio in single births was 0.88, but only 0.43 for births of twins. The growth and development of children born of mothers receiving gonadotropin treatment have been normal (Hack *et al.*, 1970).

The only complications reported for this therapy have been excessive ovarian enlargement as a result of the maturation of many follicles; this, in turn, may lead to the release of multiple ova and to multiple births. Ovarian hyperstimulation may be seen several days after the administration of chorionic gonadotropin in a few percent of patients. In this condition the enlarged ovaries give rise to pain in the lower abdomen, and, if there is bleeding into the peritoneal cavity, the pain is severe. Under the latter circumstance, hospitalization and observation for ovarian rupture are required. Methods have been devised to avoid these complications (Brown *et al.*, 1969). For example, one can test ovarian responsiveness by measuring the excretion of estrogens in the urine in a preliminary trial and thereby be guided in the dosage appropriate for a therapeutic attempt. If the urinary estrogens exceed 150 μg/24 hours, chorionic gonadotropin should be withheld. Alternatively, several trials may be made with small doses before the larger recommended amounts are used.

It is remarkable how closely the experience with human gonadotropins parallels that following the use of clomiphene (*see* Chapter 61). Further experience will be needed to determine which types of ovarian disorders are best treated with gonadotropin and which with clomiphene; currently clomiphene would seem the better agent in the syndrome of polycystic ovaries whereas gonadotropin would be indicated when the pituitary is primarily at fault.

While the use of human gonadotropin, either from the pituitary gland or from menopausal urine, to promote fertility in the male is a field that has not been extensively explored, men with hypopituitarism have been rendered fertile by this means (Gemzell and Kjessler, 1964; Mancini *et al.*, 1971). As the process of germinal maturation in the tubules requires 10 weeks and the transit of the spermatozoa through the vas deferens several weeks more, investigation of this form of treatment is time consuming. The effectiveness of therapy with gonadotropins when more subtle forms of gametogenic failure are under study is more difficult to evaluate and more extensive experience is required. Often testicular failure appears to be due to an intrinsic fault of the testis itself, and additional gonadotropin would not be expected to be beneficial.

Cryptorchism. Failure of the descent of one testis or both is sometimes noted in childhood; it is most frequent in infancy and is less prevalent with advancing age until it becomes a rare finding in the adult. In the majority of cases, testes undescended in childhood assume their normal position at the time of puberty, a sequence of events that is normal in monkeys. In rare cases, cryptorchism denotes an abnormality of testicular development and in this event descent at puberty does not take place. There is also some indication that testicular development is quite normal if descent is achieved before age seven (Lattimer, 1973). This can often be accomplished by the administration of an androgen or chorionic gonadotropin. Such treatment is more effective when failure of testicular descent is bilateral, in contrast to the unilateral condition. Chorionic gonadotropin is usually used and is customarily given intramuscularly in doses of 500 to 4000 I.U. two or three times weekly for several weeks, but therapy is stopped as soon as the desired result has been achieved. If such treatment is not successful, the undescended testis should be placed in the scrotum surgically or removed, since the incidence of testicular tumors is markedly increased in cryptorchism.

THYROTROPIN (TSH)

The regulatory effects of thyrotropin on the thyroid gland are considered in Chapter 60. The essential chemical features of human thyrotropin are summarized in Table 59–1 (*see also* Pierce, 1971; Burger and Patel, 1977).

Assays. A widely used bioassay is that described by McKenzie (1961). Thyroid stimulation is reflected in increased circulating radioactivity in mice with thyroids prelabeled with radioiodine. Radioimmunoassays for human thyrotropin permit diagnostic studies of the circulating hormone. In primary hypothyroidism, the feedback inhibition of thyroid hormone to regulate the secretion of TSH is reduced or absent, resulting in increased secretion of the trophic hormone. Thus, hypothyroidism with elevated concentrations of TSH in plasma indicates thyroid failure, whereas the occurrence of low concentrations of both thyroid hormone and TSH points to a hypothalamic or pituitary defect. As discussed below and in Chapter 60, the use of thyrotropin-releasing hormone (TRH) is useful to distinguish between the latter two possibilities.

Clinical Application. *Thyrotropin* (THYTROPAR) is not used as a therapeutic agent but to diagnose thyroid disorders. The single clinical application of this bovine preparation is in the evaluation of thyroid function in conjunction with the use of radioiodine. Hypopituitarism can be differentiated from primary myxedema by the stimulation of thyroid accumulation of radioiodine by thyrotropin in the former condition but not in the latter. In the usual procedure, a dose of 10 units is given as a single intramuscular injection followed by a tracer dose of radioiodine 24 hours later. Twenty-four hours after the tracer, the accumulation in hypopituitarism is usually substantially higher than it was before thyrotropin, whereas it usually remains low in spontaneous myxedema. Since thyrotropin concentrations in plasma are elevated in primary myxedema, the availability of radioimmunoassays for thyrotropin has reduced the need for administration of thyrotropin for diagnostic purposes.

OTHER THYROID STIMULATORS

Three other proteins with varying resemblance to pituitary thyrotropin have been described.

Chorionic Thyrotropin. This glycoprotein has a molecular weight of 28,000, of which 3.5% is carbohydrate. It is produced by the human placenta and stimulates the secretion of thyroid hormone much as does TSH. However, the physicochemical and antigenic properties of chorionic thyrotropin are quite different from those of the pituitary hormone. Its significance, if any, is unknown, and its secretion is not influenced by thyrotropin-releasing hormone (TRH) (Hershman, 1972; Chatterjee and Munro, 1977).

Molar Thyrotropin. This material derives its name from its detection in benign and malignant hydatidiform moles, and both *chorionic* and *molar* thyrotropins are thus *trophoblastic* thyrotropins. Molar thyrotropin has also been detected in normal placenta. It appears to have approximately twice the molecular weight of TSH or chorionic thyrotropin (Hershman, 1972). This thyroid stimulator has been responsible for thyrotoxicosis in several patients with hydatidiform mole or choriocarcinoma. In some patients with choriocarcinoma, hyperthyroidism may exist because of marked elevation of the concentration of chorionic gonadotropin, which also possesses some thyrotropic activity (Cave and Dunn, 1976; Morley *et al.,* 1976).

Long-Acting Thyroid Stimulator. In the blood of most patients suffering from Graves' disease (hyperthyroidism) substances have been found that exert a prolonged stimulatory action upon the thyroids of animals. These substances are called *long-acting thyroid stimulators* (LATS) and *long-acting thyroid stimulator-protector* (LATS-P), to distinguish them from thyrotropin. These proteins are immunoglobulins of the IgG class and can bind to antigenic sites on the plasma membrane of thyroid follicular cells (Adams and Kennedy, 1967; McKenzie and Zakarija, 1977). Presumably the binding of these and perhaps other thyroid-stimulating antibodies can mimic the effects of thyrotropin and account for the hyperthyroidism (*see* Kriss, 1970; Volpe, 1978). However the precise role of thyroid-stimulating immunoglobulins in the pathogenesis of Graves' disease remains obscure. Their actions on the thyroid gland are essentially identical to those of thyrotropin, and this may be logical since both TSH and LATS can stimulate the synthesis of cyclic AMP (Yamashita and Field, 1972). The proteins evidently can traverse the placenta and thereby account for hyperthyroidism of the newborn infants of some hyperthyroid mothers.

EXOPHTHALMOS-PRODUCING SUBSTANCE

Injection of pituitary extract into animals can cause protrusion of the eyeballs. The phenomenon, first noted in the duck (Shockaert, 1931), has been studied in the guinea pig and several species of fish. It was thought to be caused by thyrotropin, and this seemed logical at a time when thyrotropin was assumed to be an etiological factor in Graves' disease, which is often associated with exophthalmos. However, it is now known that thyrotropin concentrations are very low in Graves' disease. Furthermore, clinical conditions in which secretion of thyrotropin is elevated are not characterized by such ocular changes. While apparent dissociation of thyroid-stimulating activity and exophthalmos-producing activity was obtained in the past, homogeneous thyrotropin indeed possesses both activities and certain proteolytic fragments of the molecule retain exophthalmos-producing activity after loss of most thyroid-stimulating activity (Kohn and Winand, 1971). It is of course possible that there are other substances that can also cause exophthalmos, and certain reports suggest that exophthalmos is mediated by immunological mechanisms (*see* Volpe, 1978). The etiology of the condition in man is even more obscure than is the etiology of Graves' disease.

CORTICOTROPIN

The essential features of the chemistry of corticotropin (ACTH) are included in Table 59–1, and the structure of the hormone is shown in Figure 63–1. While the discussion of ACTH appears in Chapter 63, the polypeptide precursor of the hormone contains the sequences of several other important peptides, as shown in Figure 59–2; these will be considered here.

LIPOTROPINS

It has long been known that the injection of certain pituitary extracts into animals causes ketosis, lowering of the respiratory quotient, and increased fat in the liver. Subsequent studies have shown increased circulating free fatty acids and a direct lipolytic action on isolated adipose tissue *in vitro,* suggesting that mobilization of depot fat is the primary action concerned. As already noted, this is an important part of the action of growth hormone. While TSH, LH, and ACTH have a similar effect, only the response to TSH is thought to be of possible physiological consequence. However, the pituitary does contain lipolytic factors (lipotropins) that differ from the hormones discussed above. Two such proteins have been purified and analyzed and they are included in Table 59–1 and Figure 59–2.

The presumed initial precursor of the lipotropins, ACTH, and related peptides is termed prepro-ACTH-β-LPH, a protein with a molecular weight of 30,000. After the N-terminal signal peptide is removed, the remainder of the molecule (pro-opiomelanocortin or pro-ACTH-β-LPH) is glycosylated and processed further to give β-LPH; this polypeptide is then finally cleaved to produce many of the peptides shown in Figure 59–2 (*see* Imura and Nakai, 1981).

Despite their designation as β- and γ-lipotropins, these proteins are potent lipolytic agents in certain species, particularly the rabbit. In view of their structural relationship to corticotropin and melanocyte-stimulating hormone, it is likely that these

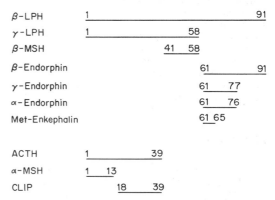

Figure 59–2. *Some structural relationships of certain pituitary peptides.*

CLIP is corticotropin-like intermediate lobe peptide; its functions, if any, are unknown. Other abbreviations are defined in the text. (After Daughaday, 1978. Courtesy of Plenum Medical Book Co.)

materials stimulate lipolysis by a cyclic AMP–dependent mechanism. There is some evidence to favor this hypothesis (Lis *et al.*, 1972). These factors are not lipolytic in the rat, and neither they nor their counterparts from human pituitaries are active in man. The possibility of the presence of additional lipolytic substances in human pituitary remains open. The function of the lipotropins in man may simply be to serve as precursors of the other peptides in Figure 59–2.

ENDORPHINS AND ENKEPHALINS

Oligopeptides have been isolated from extracts of brain and pituitary that possess pharmacological properties similar to those of opioids (Hughes *et al.*, 1975). These morphinomimetic peptides are called *endorphins* and *enkephalins*, and their structural relationship to β-lipotropin is summarized in Figure 59–2. The pentapeptide methionine-enkephalin is identical to the sequence that extends from amino acids 61 through 65 of β-lipotropin (Tyr-Gly-Gly-Phe-Met), while α-endorphin, β-endorphin, and γ-endorphin are identical to amino acids 61 to 76, 61 to 91, and 61 to 77, respectively, in β-lipotropin (Lazarus *et al.*, 1976; Terenius, 1978; Imura and Nakai, 1981). These studies suggest that β-lipotropin may serve as a precursor for some of these morphinomimetic peptides. This topic is also discussed in Chapters 12 and 22.

MELANOCYTE-STIMULATING HORMONE (MSH)

The intermediate lobe of the pituitary is a part of the adenohypophysis, but in most mammals it is separated from the anterior lobe by the hypophyseal cleft and is composed of a sheet of tissue firmly attached to the contiguous surface of the neurohypophysis.

The term *intermedin* was coined by Zondek for the hormone of the intermediate lobe that mediates various pigmentary responses in the lower vertebrates (*see* Zondek and Krohn, 1932). More recently, the term *melanocyte-stimulating hormone* (MSH) has been adopted, a designation that would embrace an action upon the melanocytes of mammalian skin, in keeping with the finding of a darkening of human skin in response to the hormone (Lerner and McGuire, 1964). Three compounds have thus far been isolated from the pituitary extracts and designated α-MSH, β-MSH (Thody, 1977), and γ-MSH.

Chemistry. When strong concentrates of ACTH were first prepared, they were found to be highly active in causing darkening of the skin of frogs. The confusion that arose as a result of this finding was finally resolved when first one component and later two were separated from ACTH. α-MSH and β-MSH are derived from ACTH and β-LPH, respectively, as summarized in Figure 59–2; γ-MSH is derived from the amino-terminal fragment of pro-opiomelanocortin (*see* Krieger *et al.*, 1980). The sequence of 13 amino acids making up the molecule of α-MSH is identical with the first 13 residues of ACTH, and the terminal serine amino group is acetylated. While mammalian α-MSH appears to have a constant amino acid sequence in the species examined, β-MSH is variable between species and is larger than α-MSH. A peptide that is analogous to the β-MSH of other species can be found in the pituitary of man, and its structure is identical to amino acid residues 41 to 58 of the lipotropins. Pure ACTH does have inherent MSH activity, being about 1/40 as active as α-MSH on a molar basis. The bioassays used are based on hormone-induced darkening of the skin of the frog, chameleon, and related species.

Physiological Actions. Melanocyte-stimulating hormones regulate the pigmentation of fish and amphibian skin by causing dispersal of the pigment granules of the melanophores, thus making the cells appear darker. However, the role of MSH in pigmentation in man is debatable. In primary adrenal insufficiency (Addison's disease) and in syndromes characterized by ectopic production of ACTH, increased pigmentation of the skin may be prominent; this is due to the activity of ACTH itself and possibly to lipotropins, rather than to α- or β-MSH. MSH can cause hyperpigmentation when given in large doses (Lerner and McGuire, 1964). While it has been suggested that changes in skin pigmentation during the menstrual cycle and pregnancy may be due to altered secretion of MSH, the hormone has not been detected in human plasma. It is possible that MSH has no function in man and may represent an evolutionary vestige. However, some studies suggest that α-MSH may regulate the secretion of gonadotropins and prolactin (*see* Celis and Volosin, 1982). The MSH-like radioimmunoassayable activity in plasma probably represents β-lipotropin. In lower animals, MSH has natriuretic and lipolytic effects and may increase heart rate, fetal and placental weight, and sebaceous secretions (*see* Thody, 1977). Both MSH and ACTH increase cyclic AMP formation in appropriate tissues (*see* Hadley *et al.*, 1981).

HYPOTHALAMIC CONTROL OF THE ANTERIOR PITUITARY

As a result of the pioneering studies of Harris (1948), it is now well established that the influence of the central nervous system upon adenohypophyseal function is mediated by neurohumoral substances transported to the gland by the hypothalamico-adenohypophyseal-portal system from a capillary network in the region of the median eminence. These substances are referred to as either releasing hormones, releasing factors, or regulatory hormones. Many of these substances have been shown to meet the commonly accepted definition of a hormone and also to influence both the synthesis and release of adenohypophyseal hormones. There is great interest in the identification of hypothalamic regulatory hormones and in their potential use as therapeutic and diagnostic agents. Several reviews are recommended for detailed discussion and references (Guillemin, 1978; Krieger, 1978; Schally, 1978; McCann, 1980).

There is evidence to suggest the existence of at least nine regulatory *activities* in the secretions of the hypothalamus. These activities and the abbreviations used to designate them are listed in Table 59–2. For at least three adenohypophyseal hormones (prolactin, growth hormone, and MSH), there appears to be dual (stimulatory and inhibitory) regulation. ACTH, TSH, LH, and FSH are perhaps subject only to stimulatory control by this mechanism.

The successful isolation and identification of these hormones have required herculean efforts. Tons of hypothalamic starting material containing hundreds of thousands of hypothalami have been required to purify milligram quantities of these substances.

Regulation of Thyrotropin. Thyrotropin-releasing hormone (TRH) was the first to be identified chemically, in 1970. The porcine, ovine, bovine, and human hormones are identical in structure. TRH is a tripeptide with both terminal amino and carboxyl groups blocked: L-pyroglutamyl-L-histidyl-L-proline amide. Pyroglutamate is derived from the cyclization of glutamic acid. Synthetic TRH is available in quantity for clinical diagnostic use. Derivatives of TRH have also been synthesized and studied; 3-methyl-His-TRH is eight to ten times more potent than the naturally occurring hormone. These studies have prompted the search for other analogs that possess even greater activity or that act as antagonists.

An extremely small quantity of TRH is effective at its site of action; picogram amounts are sufficient to release thyrotropin *in vitro*. Human subjects respond to as little as 15 μg administered intravenously, and 400 μg is maximally effective. A dose of 5 mg or more is required orally. In normal man, intravenous TRH provokes a maximal secretion of thyrotropin within 15 to 30 minutes. Plasma concentrations of thyrotropin remain elevated for 2 to 4 hours, although TRH is inactivated rapidly by human plasma and has a half-life *in vivo* of approximately 5 minutes. There is evidence that TRH stimulates the synthesis as well as the secretion of thyrotropin. In addition, prolactin secretion is also enhanced (*see* below). Specific binding of TRH to pituitary membrane receptors has been demonstrated, as has an associated stimulation of cyclic AMP synthesis. It seems likely that the effects of TRH on pituitary thyrotrophs are mediated by cyclic AMP.

The pituitary is the site of negative feedback exerted by the thyroid hormones to inhibit thyrotropin secretion. The action of TRH may be antagonized in part at a molecular site distal to its initial interaction with the plasma membrane, and the number of receptors for TRH on pituitary cells also appears to be reduced (*see* Chapter 60). Sites of thyroid hormone feedback may also exist in the central nervous system. Clinical use is made of TRH in the diagnosis of thyroid disease; with TRH it can be determined whether secondary hypothyroidism is of pituitary or hypothalamic origin, and patients with primary and secondary hypothyroidism can also be distinguished. Patients with hyperthyroidism fail to respond. Testing involves the intravenous administration of TRH (*protirelin*, THYPINONE) in a dose of 200 to 500 μg, followed by serial determinations of thyroid hormones and of plasma thyrotropin by immunoassay (Jackson,

Table 59–2. HYPOTHALAMIC ACTIVITIES THAT CONTROL THE RELEASE OF PITUITARY HORMONES

RELEASING HORMONE OR FACTOR	ABBREVIATION	STRUCTURE
Corticotropin-releasing factor	CRF	Peptide (41 residues)
Thyrotropin-releasing hormone	TRH	Tripeptide
Luteinizing hormone–releasing hormone and follicle-stimulating hormone–releasing hormone (gonadotropin-releasing hormone)	LH-RH/FSH-RH; Gn-RH	Decapeptide
Growth hormone release-inhibiting hormone	GH-RIH; somatostatin; SRIF	Peptides (14 and 28 residues)
Growth hormone–releasing factor	GH-RF; GRF	Peptides (40 and 44 residues)
Prolactin release-inhibiting hormone	PRIH	Probably dopamine
Prolactin-releasing factor	PRF	Unknown
Melanocyte-stimulating hormone release-inhibiting factor	MIF	Tripeptide
Melanocyte-stimulating hormone–releasing factor	MRF	Unknown

1982). Additional discussion of the use of TRH appears in Chapter 60.

Regulation of Gonadotropins. Predictably, this subject is more complex. Convincing evidence indicates that the secretion of luteinizing hormone is regulated by a hypothalamic hormone, LH-RH, and this material has been purified, identified, and synthesized. Porcine and ovine LH-RH is a decapeptide and has the amino acid sequence pyroGlu-His-Trp-Ser-Tyr-Gly-Leu-Arg-Pro-Gly-NH_2. No species specificity for the effect of LH-RH has been demonstrated, suggesting that the decapeptide is similar or identical in a number of species. The major difficulty is that LH-RH stimulates the release of both luteinizing hormone and follicle-stimulating hormone, and it has been proposed that there is but a single gonadotropin-releasing hormone (LH-RH/FSH-RH, also designated Gn-RH).

Synthetic LH-RH is highly active in man. Intravenous administration of 10 to 100 μg causes rapid elevation of plasma gonadotropins; the release of LH is faster than that of FSH. Pulsatile administration results in characteristic and predictable alterations in gonadal function. Ovulation and stimulation of spermatogenesis have been induced in both experimental animals and human subjects. Again, the hormone also stimulates the synthesis of gonadotropin in addition to its release. LH-RH has been used alone or in combination with human menopausal gonadotropin to induce ovulation and promote pregnancy in some amenorrheic women. The use of LH-RH for this purpose may offer an advantage in that superovulation and multiple births have not been observed.

While variations in secretion of luteinizing hormone and follicle-stimulating hormone may be simultaneous, normal divergent patterns of secretion are also well known (*see* Figure 61–2, page 1416). Attempts to explain this in the face of but one gonadotropin-releasing hormone invoke, among other observations, the "feedback" effects of sex hormones, gonadal products such as *inhibin,* and other endogenous regulators on responses to the regulatory decapeptide. While important regulatory effects are thought to occur at neuronal sites in the hypothalamus and elsewhere, direct effects on the pituitary seem probable. Estrogens inhibit the secretion of FSH but have a biphasic effect on the secretion of LH. Inhibin, a peptide with a molecular weight of 15,000 to 30,000 that is derived from the testis or ovary, can feed back and suppress the secretion of both FSH and LH (*see* Franchimont, 1977). Dopamine has been observed to inhibit LH secretion without effect on the secretion of FSH (Leblanc *et al.,* 1976). These interactions are highly complex, and it is impossible at this time to state whether the combined effects of sex hormones, other gonadal products, and one gonadotropin-releasing hormone will supply the necessary controls.

The question of paramount importance involves the existence of a separate FSH-RH. Experimental difficulties with follicle-stimulating hormone itself add to the problem. The fact that LH-RH is also a FSH-RH does not exclude the possibility that an additional regulatory hormone is present.

Synthetic LH-RH (*gonadorelin*) has been approved for diagnostic use, and a commercial preparation (FACTREL) is available. The obvious clinical implications of regulation of gonadotropins have prompted the synthesis and evaluation of hundreds of analogs of LH-RH. LH-RH is rapidly hydrolyzed in plasma and excreted in urine with a half-life of about 4 minutes. No smaller active fragments of LH-RH have been obtained. A variety of amino acid substitutions of the peptide chain have produced analogs with potency increased as much as 10- to 60-fold and a prolonged duration of action. In investigational studies, LH-RH and active analogs have been used successfully to treat cryptorchism and to induce puberty and ovulation in some patients who lack the hormone. Paradoxically, prolonged use of LH-RH and active analogs can suppress secretion of gonadotropins and gonadal steroids, which accounts for their effectiveness in treating precocious puberty and other disorders (Mansfield *et al.,* 1983). Some analogs have been effective after oral, intranasal, or rectal administration (Saito *et al.,* 1977). Prolonged use of high concentrations of LH-RH has caused reversible ovarian and uterine atrophy in animals and has prevented implantation of ova and gestation. In males, high concentrations of LH-RH can inhibit testicular synthesis of testosterone. Some LH-RH analogs also have inhibitory activity and are effective contraceptives (De La Cruz *et al.,* 1976). Other investigational uses have thus included palliative treatment of carcinoma of the breast, prostatic carcinoma, and endometriosis. In these and other experimental studies, significant untoward effects have not been observed. (For additional discussion, *see* Cutler *et al.,* 1985.)

Regulation of Corticotropin. Corticotropin-releasing factor (CRF) was the first to be demonstrated by physiological technics, and these early *in-vitro* studies prompted the purification and characterization of this and other hypothalamic releasing hormones. CRF has now been purified from ovine hypothalami (Spiess *et al.,* 1981). This peptide has 41 amino acid residues and is expected to be similar to the human hormone. Assays of this peptide in plasma and assessment of responses to its administration should assist the clinician in the evaluation of pituitary or adrenal insufficiency. Antidiuretic hormone and fragments thereof also have significant CRF activity, and their effects may be physiologically important. (For additional discussion, *see* Chrousos *et al.,* 1985; Conference, 1985.)

Regulation of Growth Hormone. Growth hormone is subject to regulation by both a GH-RF (or GRF) and a release-inhibiting hormone (GH-RIH). The characterization of GH-RF has been accomplished only recently and indirectly from studies with human tumors (Guillemin *et al.,* 1982; Spiess *et al.,* 1982). Some patients with acromegaly have pancreatic or lung tumors that cause the condition (Frohman and Szabo, 1981). Two peptides with 44 and 40 amino acid residues have been isolated from these tumors, and they stimulate secretion of growth hormone both *in vitro* and *in vivo.* The larger peptide is probably a precursor of the smaller, and both have been found in the human hypothalamus. It is expected that one or both of these peptides will prove to be GH-RF. Interestingly, these peptides have considerable structural homology with glucagon, vasoactive intestinal peptide, and gastric inhibitory peptide. Biological activity of the peptide resides in its first (amino-terminal) 29 residues (Rivier *et al.*, 1982). Although many forms of dwarfism can be treated with growth hormone, variants of the disorder caused by deficiency of GH-RF should respond to this peptide or its analogs.

Brazeau and associates (1973) isolated a tetradecapeptide from the ovine hypothalamus that markedly inhibits the secretion of immunoreactive growth hormone *in vivo* and *in vitro*. The same peptide has also been isolated from porcine hypothalami. Its structure is shown at the bottom of the page. This peptide is thought to represent a GH-RIH, and for simplicity of nomenclature it has been called *somatostatin* (*see* Reichlin, 1983). Somatostatin inhibits secretion of growth hormone that is induced by most stimuli, including arginine, insulin, levodopa, exercise, sleep, and meals (Guillemin and Gerich, 1976). The effect is rapid and immediately reversible when infusion of somatostatin is terminated. Larger peptides with several additional amino acids at the amino terminus have also been isolated and may represent precursors of the tetradecapeptide. A peptide with 28 amino acid residues and similar activity has also been described. With immunohistochemical technics somatostatin has been found in other regions of the brain, and in the spinal cord, D cells of the pancreatic islets, and gastric and duodenal mucosae, as well as in the hypothalamus (Hökfelt *et al.*, 1975).

Somatostatin also inhibits the secretion of TSH, ACTH, insulin, glucagon, gastrin, secretin, pancreozymin or cholecystokinin, pepsin, and renin (Lucke *et al.*, 1975; Fehm *et al.*, 1976; Konturek *et al.*, 1976). In addition, the peptide inhibits the *effects* of pentagastrin and histamine on gastric acid production (Barros D'Sa *et al.*, 1975). Thus, somatostatin can inhibit secretion from a variety of endocrine and exocrine tissues and also the action of some hormones; the full significance of this is unknown. However, somatostatin is known to inhibit the synthesis of cyclic AMP in some types of cells. Current evidence suggests that somatostatin does have local effects in regional tissues where it is stored and released. While these divergent effects are somewhat perplexing, potential clinical applications of somatostatin have been explored. For example, infusion of somatostatin can prevent the development of ketoacidosis in patients with juvenile-type diabetes deprived of insulin for 18 hours; this was attributed to inhibition of glucagon secretion (Gerich *et al.*, 1975). Somatostatin can also decrease the secretion of insulin and gastrin that results from pancreatic tumors (Curnow *et al.*, 1975). However, the short half-life of somatostatin (several minutes) has precluded potential therapeutic uses. Numerous analogs have been prepared that have greater potency (*see* Schally and Meyers, 1982). However, none of the analogs has had an extended duration of action. Some analogs have also shown selective inhibition of the secretion of one hormone with lesser effects on others. Perhaps such studies could provide materials that are useful in the therapy of pituitary disease, diabetes mellitus, acid-pepsin disorders, and syndromes associated with hormone-secreting tumors. Administration of somatostatin to baboons and human subjects has resulted in abnormalities of platelets (Besser *et al.*, 1975; Koerker *et al.*, 1975). Other side effects have included nausea, diarrhea, and abdominal cramps.

Regulation of Prolactin. Several aspects of hypothalamic regulation of prolactin secretion have been discussed above. The inhibitory influence of a prolactin release–inhibiting hormone (PRIH) appears to predominate. Such a material is probably dopamine, and this provides an explanation of the effects of dopaminergic agonists and antagonists on prolactin secretion. While TRH has prolactin-releasing activity, it probably does not serve physiologically as a prolactin-releasing factor (PRF). However, a syndrome characterized by primary hypothyroidism and high circulating prolactin concentration with associated galactorrhea is at least suggestive of a pathological function of TRH in the regulation of prolactin secretion; this syndrome responds to administration of thyroid hormone. Another material in hypothalamic extracts can also stimulate the secretion of prolactin. While this material may be a physiologically important PRF, it has not yet been purified or characterized (Boyd *et al.*, 1976).

Regulation of Melanocyte-Stimulating Hormone. MSH secretion in animals is probably controlled by MSH-releasing factor (MRF), and MSH release-inhibiting factor (MIF), which are thought to originate in the hypothalamus (*see* Thody, 1977). MIF is a tripeptide (L-prolyl-L-leucyl-L-glycine). The structure of MRF is unknown. It has been suggested that both MIF and MRF are derived from oxytocin and represent small fragments of this peptide. Sex steroids and light can increase MSH secretion. The effects of light appear to be mediated through the pineal by means of activation of the biosynthesis of melatonin, which increases the secretion of MSH. Catecholamines can also influence the secretion of MSH. It is interesting to note that administration of MIF to rats prevents tolerance to morphine (Bhargava and Kim, 1982).

Other Peptides. Neurotensin is a tridecapeptide isolated from bovine hypothalami, the structure of which is Glu-Leu-Tyr-Glu-Asn-Lys-Pro-Arg-Arg-Pro-Tyr-Ile-Leu. Immunoreactive material has also been demonstrated in other species, including man. This peptide increases secretion of ACTH, gonadotropins, and glucagon and decreases the secretion

Ala—Gly—Cys—Lys—Asn—Phe—Phe—Trp—Lys—Thr—Phe—Thr—Ser—Cys

of insulin. It can elevate plasma glucose concentrations, lower blood pressure, decrease body temperature, contract smooth muscle in guinea pig ileum, and relax rat duodenum. The effects of neurotensin on insulin, glucagon, and plasma glucose (Carraway *et al.*, 1976) are qualitatively similar but greater than the effects of substance P, an undecapeptide also isolated from hypothalamus (*see* Chapers 12 and 27).

Other peptides that have also been found in the hypothalamus and/or in hypophyseal portal blood include endorphins, vasoactive intestinal peptide, cholecystokinin, and gastrin. The role, if any, of these peptides in regulation of the pituitary is unknown (*see* McCann, 1980).

Regulation of Regulatory Hormones. Although any significant discussion of this important area of neuroendocrinology is beyond the scope of this text, a few points should be made. There is ample evidence to indicate important neural control of regulatory hormone release. Evidence exists for adrenergic, dopaminergic, and tryptaminergic mechanisms that regulate the formation and secretion of various hypothalamic releasing factors. This has been discussed above in regard to the inhibitor of prolactin secretion. Similar evidence implicates adrenergic mechanisms in the secretion of growth hormone, thyrotropin, and gonadotropins. Drugs that alter central adrenergic mechanisms exert significant influences on the secretion of the adenohypophyseal hormones, and these are discussed under the individual agents involved.

Adams, D. D., and Kennedy, T. H. Occurrence in thyrotoxicosis of a gamma globulin which protects LATS from neutralization by an extract of thyroid gland. *J. Clin. Endocrinol. Metab.*, **1967**, *27*, 173–177.

Allen, B. M. Effects of extirpation of the anterior lobe of the hypophysis of *Rana pipiens*. *Biol. Bull. Mar. Biol. Lab., Woods Hole*, **1917**, *32*, 117–130.

Aron, M. Action de la préhypophyse sur la thyroide chez le cobaye. *C. R. Soc. Biol. (Paris)*, **1929**, *102*, 682–684.

Aschner, B. Demonstration von Hunden nach Extirpation der Hypophyse. *Wien. Klin. Wochenschr.*, **1909**, *22*, 1730–1731.

Barros D'Sa, A. A. J.; Bloom, S. R.; and Baron, J. H. Direct inhibition of gastric acid by growth-hormone releasing-inhibiting hormone in dogs. *Lancet*, **1975**, *1*, 886–887.

Baumann, G., and Loriaux, D. L. Failure of endogenous prolactin to alter renal salt and water excretion and adrenal function in man. *J. Clin. Endocrinol. Metab.*, **1976**, *43*, 643–649.

Besser, G. M.; Paxton, A. M.; Johnson, S. A. N.; Hall, R.; Gomez-Pan, A.; Schally, A. V.; Kastin, A. J.; and Coy, D. H. Impairment of platelet function by growth-hormone release-inhibiting hormone. *Lancet*, **1975**, *1*, 1166–1168.

Bhargava, H. N., and Kim, H. S. Structure activity relationship studies with hypothalamic peptide hormones. I. Effect of melanotropin release inhibiting factor and analogs on tolerance to morphine in the rat. *J. Pharmacol. Exp. Ther.*, **1982**, *220*, 394–398.

Boyd, A. E.; Spencer, E.; Jackson, I. M. D.; and Reichlin, S. Prolactin-releasing factor (PRF) in porcine hypothalamic extract distinct from TRH. *Endocrinology*, **1976**, *99*, 861–871.

Brazeau, P.; Vale, W.; Burgus, R.; Ling, N.; Butcher, M.; Rivier, J.; and Guillemin, R. Hypothalamic polypeptide that inhibits the secretion of immunoreactive pituitary growth hormone. *Science*, **1973**, *179*, 77–79.

Brown, P.; Gajdusek, D. C.; Gibbs, C. J., Jr.; and Asher, D. M. "Epidemic" Creutzfeldt-Jakob disease from human growth hormone therapy. *N. Engl. J. Med.*, **1985**, *313*.

Brown, T. B.; Evans, J. H.; Adey, F. D.; Taft, H. P.; and Townsend, L. Factors involved in the induction of fertile ovulation and human gonadotropins. *J. Obstet. Gynaecol. Br. Commonw.*, **1969**, *76*, 289–307.

Carr, D., and Friesen, H. G. Growth hormone and insulin binding to human liver. *J. Clin. Endocrinol. Metab.*, **1976**, *42*, 484–493.

Carraway, R. E.; Demers, L. M.; and Leeman, S. E. Hyperglycemic effect of neurotensin, a hypothalamic peptide. *Endocrinology*, **1976**, *99*, 1452–1462.

Cave, W. T., and Dunn, J. T. Choriocarcinoma with hyperthyroidism: probable identity of the thyrotropin with human chorionic gonadotropin. *Ann. Intern. Med.*, **1976**, *85*, 60–63.

Channing, C. P., and Seymour, J. F. Effects of dibutyryl cyclic-3′,5′-AMP and other agents upon luteinization of porcine granulosa cells in culture. *Endocrinology*, **1970**, *87*, 165–169.

Collip, J. B.; Anderson, E. M.; and Thomson, D. L. The adrenotropic hormone of the anterior pituitary lobe. *Lancet*, **1933**, *2*, 347–348.

Curnow, R. T.; Carey, R. C.; Taylor, A.; Johanson, A.; and Murad, F. Somatostatin inhibition of insulin and gastrin hypersecretion in pancreatic islet cell carcinoma. *N. Engl. J. Med.*, **1975**, *292*, 1385–1386.

Daughaday, W. H.; Salmon, W. D., Jr.; and Alexander, F. Sulfation factor activity of sera from patients with pituitary disorders. *J. Clin. Endocrinol. Metab.*, **1959**, *19*, 743–758.

De La Cruz, A.; Coy, D. H.; and Vilchez-Martinez, J. A. Blockade of ovulation in rats by inhibitory analogs of luteinizing hormone–releasing hormone. *Science*, **1976**, *191*, 195–197.

Ellsworth, L. R., and Armstrong, D. T. Luteinization of transplanted ovarian follicles in the rat induced by dibutyryl cyclic AMP. *Endocrinology*, **1973**, *92*, 840–846.

Evans, H. M., and Long, J. A. The effect of the anterior lobe administered intraperitoneally upon growth, maturity, and oestrous cycles of the rat. *Anat. Rec.*, **1921**, *21*, 62–63.

Faiman, C., and Ryan, R. J. Serum follicle-stimulating hormone and luteinizing hormone concentrations during the menstrual cycle as determined by radioimmunoassays. *J. Clin. Endocrinol. Metab.*, **1967**, *27*, 1711–1716.

Fehm, H. L.; Voigt, K. H.; Lang, R.; Beinert, K. E.; Raptis, S.; and Pfeiffer, E. F. Somatostatin: a potent inhibitor of ACTH—hypersecretion in adrenal insufficiency. *Klin. Wochenschr.*, **1976**, *54*, 173–175.

Feldman, J. M.; Plonk, J. W.; and Bivens, C. H. Inhibitory effect of serotonin antagonists on growth hormone release in acromegalic patients. *Clin. Endocrinol. (Oxf.)*, **1976**, *5*, 71–78.

Fevold, H. L.; Hisaw, F. L.; Hellbaum, A.; and Hertz, A. Sex hormones of the anterior lobe of the hypophysis: further purification of a follicular stimulating factor and the physiological effects in immature rats and rabbits. *Am. J. Physiol.*, **1933**, *104*, 710–723.

Frantz, A. G., and Kleinberg, D. L. Prolactin: evidence that it is separate from growth hormone in human blood. *Science*, **1970**, *170*, 745–747.

Friend, J. N.; Judge, D. M.; Sherman, B. M.; and Santen, R. J. FSH-secreting pituitary adenomas: stimulation and suppression studies in two patients. *J. Clin. Endocrinol. Metab.*, **1976**, *43*, 650–657.

Friesen, H. Lactation induced by human placental lactogen and cortisone acetate in rabbits. *Endocrinology,* **1966,** *79,* 212–215.

———. Human prolactin in clinical endocrinology: the impact of radioimmunoassays. *Metabolism,* **1973,** *22,* 1039–1045.

Fukushima, M. Studies on somatotropic hormone secretion in gynecology and obstetrics. *Tohoku J. Exp. Med.,* **1961,** *74,* 161–174.

Gemzell, C., and Kjessler, B. Treatment of infertility after partial hypophysectomy with human pituitary gonadotropins. *Lancet,* **1964,** *1,* 644.

Gerich, J. E.; Lorenzi, M.; Bier, D. M.; Schneider, V.; Tsalikian, E.; Karam, J. H.; and Forsham, P. H. Prevention of human diabetic ketoacidosis by somatostatin. Evidence for an essential role of glucagon. *N. Engl. J. Med.,* **1975,** *292,* 985–989.

Golander, A.; Hurley, T.; Barrett, J.; Hizi, A.; and Handwergen, S. Prolactin synthesis by human choriondecidual tissue: a possible source of prolactin in the amniotic fluid. *Science,* **1978,** *202,* 311–313.

Gordon, P.; Lesniak, M. A.; Eastman, R.; Hendricks, C. M.; and Roth, J. Evidence for higher portion of "little" growth hormone with increased radioreceptor activity in acromegalic plasma. *J. Clin. Endocrinol. Metab.,* **1976,** *43,* 364–373.

Guillemin, R. P.; Brazeau, P.; Bohlen, P.; Esch, F.; Long, N.; and Wehrenberg, W. B. Growth hormone–releasing factor from a human pancreatic tumor that caused acromegaly. *Science,* **1982,** *21,* 585–587.

Guyda, H. J., and Friesen, H. G. The separation of monkey prolactin from monkey growth hormone by affinity chromatography. *Biochem. Biophys. Res. Commun.,* **1971,** *42,* 1068–1075.

Hack, M.; Brish, M.; Serr, D. M.; Inster, V.; and Lunenfeld, B. Outcome of pregnancies after induced ovulation. Follow-up of pregnancies and children born after gonadotropin therapy. *J.A.M.A.,* **1970,** *211,* 791–797.

Hershman, J. M. Hyperthyroidism induced by trophoblastic thyrotropin. *Mayo Clin. Proc.,* **1972,** *47,* 913–918.

Hökfelt, T.; Efendic, S.; Hellerström, C.; Johansson, O.; Luft, R.; and Arimura, A. Cellular localization of somatostatin in endocrine-like cells and neurons of the rat with special references to the A_1-cells of the pancreatic islets and to the hypothalamus. *Acta Endocrinol. (Kbh.),* **1975,** *80,* Suppl. 200, 5–41.

Hughes, J.; Smith, T. W.; Kosterlitz, H. W.; Fathergill, L. H.; Morgan, B. A.; and Morris, H. R. Identification of two related pentapeptides from the brain with potent opiate agonist activity. *Nature,* **1975,** *258,* 577–579.

Hwang, P.; Guyda, H.; and Friesen, H. A radioimmunoassay for human prolactin. *Proc. Natl Acad. Sci. U.S.A.,* **1971,** *68,* 1902–1906.

Josimovich, J. B., and MacLaren, J. A. Presence in the human placenta and term serum of a highly lactogenic substance immunologically related to pituitary growth hormone. *Endocrinology,* **1962,** *71,* 209–220.

Koerker, D. J.; Harker, L. A.; and Goodner, C. J. Effects of somatostatin on hemostasis in baboons. *N. Engl. J. Med.,* **1975,** *293,* 476–479.

Kohn, L. D., and Winand, R. J. Relationship of thyrotropin to exophthalmos-producing substance. Formation of an exophthalmos-producing substance by pepsin digestion of pituitary glycoproteins containing both thyrotropic and exophthalmogenic activity. *J. Biol. Chem.,* **1971,** *246,* 6570–6575.

Konturek, S. J.; Tasler, J.; Cieszkowski, M.; Coy, D. H.; and Schally, A. V. Effect of growth hormone releaseinhibiting hormone on gastrin secretion, mucosal blood flow and serum gastrin. *Gastroenterology,* **1976,** *70,* 737–741.

Kriss, J. P. The long-acting thyroid stimulator and thyroid disease. *Adv. Intern. Med.,* **1970,** *16,* 135–154.

Laron, Z. Somatomedin, insulin, growth hormone and growth: a review. *Isr. J. Med. Sci.,* **1982,** *18,* 823–829.

Lattimer, J. K. The optimum treatment for undescended testis. *Med. Coll. Va. Q.,* **1973,** *9,* 270–274.

Lazarus, L. H.; Ling, N.; and Guillemin, R. β-Lipotropin as a prohormone for the morphinomimetic peptides endorphins and enkephalins. *Proc. Natl Acad. Sci. U.S.A.,* **1976,** *73,* 2156–2159.

Leblanc, H.; Lachelin, G. C. L.; Abu-Fadil, S.; and Yen, S. S. C. Effects of dopamine infusion on pituitary hormone secretion in humans. *J. Clin. Endocrinol. Metab.,* **1976,** *43,* 668–674.

Lerner, A. B., and McGuire, J. S. Melanocyte-stimulating hormone and adrenocorticotrophic hormone: their relation to pigmentation. *N. Engl. J. Med.,* **1964,** *270,* 539–546.

Li, C. H.; Dixon, J. S.; and Chung, D. Amino acid sequence of human chorionic somatomammotropin. *Arch. Biochem. Biophys.,* **1973,** *155,* 95–110.

Li, C. H.; Dixon, J. S.; Lo, T.-B.; Schmidt, K. D.; and Pankov, Y. A. Studies on pituitary lactogenic hormone. XXX. The primary structure of the sheep hormone. *Arch. Biochem. Biophys.,* **1970,** *141,* 705–737.

Li, C. H.; Liu, W. K.; and Dixon, J. S. Human pituitary growth hormone. XII. The amino acid sequence of the hormone. *J. Am. Chem. Soc.,* **1966,** *88,* 2050–2051.

Lis, M.; Gilardeau, C.; and Chrétien, M. Fat cell adenylate cyclase activation by sheep β-lipotropic hormone. *Proc. Soc. Exp. Biol. Med.,* **1972,** *139,* 680–683.

Loeb, L., and Bassett, R. B. Effect of hormones of anterior pituitary on thyroid gland in the guinea pig. *Proc. Soc. Exp. Biol. Med.,* **1929,** *26,* 860–862.

Lucke, C.; Höffken, B.; and Vonzur Mühlen, A. The effect of somatostatin on TSH levels in patients with primary hypothyroidism. *J. Clin. Endocrinol. Metab.,* **1975,** *41,* 1082–1084.

McKenzie, J. M. Studies on the thyroid activator of hyperthyroidism. *J. Clin. Endocrinol. Metab.,* **1961,** *21,* 635–647.

Mancini, R. E.; Vilar, O.; Donini, P.; and Pérez Lloret, A. Effect of human urinary FSH and LH on the recovery of spermatogenesis in hypophysectomized patients. *J. Clin. Endocrinol. Metab.,* **1971,** *33,* 888–895.

Mansfield, M. J.; Beardworth, D. E.; Loughlin, J. S.; Crawford, J. D.; Bode, H. H.; Rivier, J.; Vale, W.; Kushner, D. C.; Crigler, J. F.; and Crowley, W. F. Long-term treatment of central precocious puberty with a long-acting analogue of luteinizing hormone–releasing hormone. *N. Engl. J. Med.,* **1983,** *309,* 1286–1290.

Marsh, J. M.; Butcher, R. W.; Savard, K.; and Sutherland, E. W. The stimulatory effect of luteinizing hormone on adenosine 3',5'-monophosphate accumulation in corpus luteum slices. *J. Biol. Chem.,* **1966,** *241,* 5436–5440.

Midgley, A. R., and Jaffe, R. B. Regulation of human gonadotropins. IV. Correlation of serum concentrations of follicle stimulating and luteinizing hormones during the menstrual cycle. *J. Clin. Endocrinol. Metab.,* **1968,** *28,* 1699–1703.

Morley, J. E.; Jacobson, R. J.; Melamed, J.; and Hershman, J. M. Choriocarcinoma as a cause of thyrotoxicosis. *Am. J. Med.,* **1976,** *60,* 1036–1040.

Murad, F.; Strauch, B. S.; and Vaughan, M. The effect of gonadotropins on testicular adenyl cyclase. *Biochim. Biophys. Acta,* **1969,** *177,* 591–598.

Niall, H. D.; Hogan, M. L.; Sauer, R.; Rosenblum, I. Y.; and Greenwood, F. C. Sequences of pituitary and placental lactogenic and growth hormones: evolution from a primordial peptide by gene reduplication. *Proc. Natl Acad. Sci. U.S.A.,* **1971,** *68,* 866–869.

Norman, C. News and comment. Virus scare halts hormone research. *Science,* **1985,** *228,* 1176–1177.

Olson, K. C.; Fenno, J.; Lin, N.; Harkins, R. N.; Snider, C.; Kohr, W. H.; Ross, M. J.; Fodge, D.; Prender, G.; and Stebbing, N. Purified human growth hormone from *E. coli* is biologically active. *Nature,* **1981,** *293,* 408–411.

Pierce, J. G. The subunits of pituitary thyrotropin—their relationship to other glycoprotein hormones. *Endocrinology,* **1971,** *89,* 1331–1344.

Public Health Service. Fatal degenerative neurological disease in patients who received pituitary-derived human growth hormone. *MMWR,* **1985,** *34,* 359–366.

Raben, M. S. Growth hormone. 1. Physiologic aspects. *N. Engl. J. Med.,* **1962a,** *266,* 31–35. 2. Clinical use of human growth hormone. *Ibid.,* **1962b,** *266,* 82–86.

Reichlin, S. Regulation of somatotropic hormone secretion. In, *The Pituitary Gland and Its Neuroendocrine Control,* Vol. 4, Pt. 2. Sect. 7, *Endocrinology. Handbook of Physiology.* (Knobil, E., and Sawyer, W. H., eds.) American Physiological Society, Washington, D. C., **1974,** pp. 405–447.

Riddle, O.; Bates, R. W.; and Dykshorn, S. W. The preparation, identification and assay of prolactin—a hormone of the anterior pituitary. *Am. J. Physiol.,* **1933,** *105,* 191–216.

Rivier, J.; Spiess, J.; Thorner, M.; and Vale, W. Characterization of a growth hormone–releasing factor from a human pancreatic islet tumour. *Nature,* **1982,** *300,* 276–278.

Rubin, R. T.; Poland, R. E.; and Tower, B. B. Prolactin-related testosterone secretion in normal adult man. *J. Clin. Endocrinol. Metab.,* **1976,** *42,* 112–116.

Rudman, D.; Kutner, M. H.; Blackston, R. D.; Cushman, R. A.; Bain, R. P.; and Patterson, J. H. Children with normal-variant short stature: treatment with human growth hormone for six months. *N. Engl. J. Med.,* **1981,** *305,* 123–131.

Rudman, D.; Patterson, J. H.; and Gibbas, D. L. Responsiveness of growth hormone–deficient children to human growth hormone. *J. Clin. Invest.,* **1973,** *52,* 1108–1112.

Saito, M.; Kumasaka, T.; Yaoi, Y.; Nishi, N.; Arimura, A.; Coy, D. H.; and Schally, A. V. Stimulation of luteinizing hormone (LH) and follicle stimulating hormone by [D-Leu^6,Des-Gly^{10}-NH$_2$]-LH-releasing hormone ethylamide after subcutaneous, intravaginal and intrarectal administration to women. *Fertil. Steril.,* **1977,** *28,* 240–245.

Seeburg, P. H.; Shine, J.; Martial, J. A.; Ivarie, R. D.; Morris, J. A.; Ullrich, A.; Baxter, J. D.; and Goodman, H. M. Synthesis of growth hormone by bacteria. *Nature,* **1978,** *276,* 795–798.

Sheehan, H. L., and Summers, V. K. The syndrome of hypopituitarism. *Q. J. Med.,* **1949,** *18,* 319–379.

Sherwood, L. M. Similarities in the chemical structure of human placental lactogen and pituitary growth hormone. *Proc. Natl Acad. Sci. U.S.A.,* **1967,** *58,* 2307–2314.

Shiu, R. P. C.; Kelly, P. A.; and Friesen, H. G. Radioreceptor assay for prolactin and other lactogenic hormones. *Science,* **1973,** *180,* 968–971.

Shockaert, J. A. Hyperplasia of thyroid and exophthalmos in treatment with anterior pituitary in young ducks. *Proc. Soc. Exp. Biol. Med.,* **1931,** *29,* 306–308.

Shome, B., and Parlow, A. F. The primary structure of the hormone-specific, beta subunit of human pituitary luteinizing hormone (hLH). *J. Clin. Endocrinol. Metab.,* **1973,** *36,* 618–621.

———. Human follicle stimulating hormone. *Ibid.,* **1974,** *39,* 199–202, 203–205.

———. Human pituitary prolactin (hPrl), the entire amino acid sequence. *Ibid.,* **1977,** *45,* 1112–1115.

Simmonds, M. Über Hypophysisschwund mit tödlichen Ausgang. *Dtch. Med. Wochenschr.,* **1914,** *40,* 322–323.

Smith, P. E. The disabilities caused by hypophysectomy and their repair. *J.A.M.A.,* **1927,** *88,* 158–161.

———. Hypophysectomy and a replacement therapy. *Am. J. Anat.,* **1930,** *45,* 205–256.

Snyder, P. J., and Sterling, F. H. Hypersecretion of LH and FSH by a pituitary adenoma. *J. Clin. Endocrinol. Metab.,* **1976,** *42,* 544–550.

Spiess, J.; Rivier, J.; Rivier, C.; and Vale, W. Primary structure of corticotropin-releasing factor from ovine hypothalamus. *Proc. Natl Acad. Sci. U.S.A.,* **1981,** *10,* 6517–6521.

Spiess, J.; Rivier, J.; Thorner, M.; and Vale, W. Sequence analysis of a growth hormone releasing factor from a human pancreatic islet tumor. *Biochemistry,* **1982,** *24,* 6037–6040.

Suh, H. K., and Frantz, A. G. Size heterogeneity of human prolactin in plasma and pituitary extracts. *J. Clin. Endocrinol. Metab.,* **1974,** *39,* 928–935.

Thompson, C. R., and Hansen, L. M. PERGONAL (menotropins): a summary of clinical experience in the induction of ovulation and pregnancy. *Fertil. Steril.,* **1970,** *21,* 844–853.

Turkington, R. W. Inhibition of prolactin secretion and successful therapy of the Forbes-Albright syndrome with L-dopa. *J. Clin. Endocrinol. Metab.,* **1972,** *34,* 306–311.

Van Vliet, G.; Styne, D. M.; Kaplan, S. L.; and Grumbach, M. M. Growth hormone treatment for short stature. *N. Engl. J. Med.,* **1983,** *309,* 1016–1022.

Wass, J. A. H.; Thorner, M. O.; Morris, D. V.; Rees, L. H.; Stuart, M. A.; Jones, A. E.; and Besser, G. M. Long-term treatment of acromegaly with bromocriptine. *Br. Med. J.,* **1977,** *1,* 875–878.

Yamashita, K., and Field, J. B. Effects of long-acting thyroid stimulator on thyrotropin stimulation of adenyl cyclase activity in thyroid plasma membranes. *J. Clin. Invest.,* **1972,** *51,* 463–472.

Zondek, B., and Krohn, H. Hormon des Zwischenlappens der Hypophyse (Intermedin). *Naturwissenschaften,* **1932,** *8,* 134–136.

Monographs and Reviews

Burger, H. G., and Patel, Y. C. Thyrotropin releasing hormone—TSH. *Clin. Endocrinol. Metab.,* **1977,** *6,* 83–100.

Celis, M. E., and Volosin, M. The physiology of MSH. *Prog. Clin. Biol. Res.,* **1982,** *87,* 113–129.

Chatterjee, M., and Munro, H. N. Structure and biosynthesis of human placental peptide hormones. *Vitam. Horm.,* **1977,** *35,* 149–208.

Chrousos, G. P.; Schuermeyer, T. H.; Doppman, J.; Oldfield, E. H.; Schulte, H. M.; Gold, P. W.; and Loriaux, D. L. Clinical applications of corticotropin-releasing factor. *Ann. Intern. Med.,* **1985,** *102,* 344–358.

Conference. Corticotropin-releasing factor. *Fed. Proc.,* **1985,** *44,* 145–263.

Cutler, G. B.; Hoffman, A. R.; Swerdloff, R. S.; Santen, R. J.; Meldrum, D. R.; and Comite, M. D. Therapeutic applications of luteinizing-hormone-releasing hormone and its analogs. *Ann. Intern. Med.,* **1985,** *102,* 643–657.

Daughaday, W. H. Hormonal regulation of growth by somatomedin and other tissue growth factors. *Clin. Endocrinol. Metab.,* **1977,** *6,* 117–135.

———. Anterior pituitary. In, *The Year in Endocrinology: 1977.* (Ingbar, S. H., ed.) Plenum Medical Book Co., New York, **1978,** pp. 27–71.

Dorfman, R. I. Mechanism of action of gonadotropins and prolactin. In, *Biochemical Actions of Hormones,* Vol. II. (Litwack, G., ed.) Academic Press, Inc., New York, **1972,** pp. 295–316.

Floss, H. G.; Cassady, J. M.; and Robbers, J. E. Influence of ergot alkaloids on pituitary prolactin and prolactin-dependent processes. *J. Pharm. Sci.,* **1973,** *62,* 699–715.

Franchimont, P. Pituitary gonadotropins. *Clin. Endocrinol. Metab.,* **1977,** *6,* 101–116.

Frantz, A. G. Prolactin, growth hormone and human placental lactogen. In, *Peptide Hormones.* (Parsons, J. A., ed.) University Park Press, Baltimore, **1976,** pp. 199–230.

———. Prolactin. *N. Engl. J. Med.,* **1978,** *298,* 201–207.

Frasier, S. D. Human pituitary growth hormone (hGH) therapy in growth hormone deficiency. *Endocr. Rev.*, **1983**, *4*, 155–170.

Frohman, L. A., and Szabo, M. Ectopic production of growth hormone–releasing factor by carcinoid and pancreatic islet tumors associated with acromegaly. *Prog. Clin. Biol. Res.*, **1981**, *74*, 259–271.

Goldfine, I. D. Medical treatment of acromegaly. *Annu. Rev. Med.*, **1978**, *29*, 407–415.

Guillemin, R. Peptides in the brain: the new endocrinology of the neuron. *Science*, **1978**, *202*, 390–401.

Guillemin, R., and Gerich, J. E. Somatostatin: physiological and clinical significance. *Annu. Rev. Med.*, **1976**, *27*, 379–388.

Hadley, M. E.; Heward, C. B.; Hruby, V. J.; Sawyer, T. K.; and Yang, Y. C. S. Biological actions of melanocyte-stimulating hormone. *Ciba Found. Symp.*, **1981**, *81*, 244–262.

Harris, G. W. Neural control of the pituitary gland. *Physiol. Rev.*, **1948**, *28*, 139–179.

Hintz, R. L. The somatomedins. *Adv. Pediatr.*, **1981**, *28*, 293–317.

Imura, H., and Nakai, Y. "Endorphins" in pituitary and other tissues. *Annu. Rev. Physiol.*, **1981**, *43*, 265–278.

Jackson, I. Thyrotropin-releasing hormone. *N. Engl. J. Med.*, **1982**, *306*, 145–155.

Knobil, E., and Greep, R. O. Physiology of growth hormone with particular reference to its action in rhesus monkey and "species specificity" problem. *Recent Prog. Horm. Res.*, **1959**, *15*, 1–69.

Krieger, D. T. Hypothalamus. In, *The Year in Endocrinology: 1977.* (Ingbar, S. H., ed.) Plenum Medical Book Co., New York, **1978**, pp. 1–26.

Krieger, D. T.; Liotta, A. S.; Brownstein, M. J.; and Zimmerman, E. A. ACTH, β-lipotropin, and related peptides in brain, pituitary, and blood. *Recent Prog. Horm. Res.*, **1980**, *36*, 277–344.

Lipsett, M. B., and Ross, G. T. The ovary. In, *The Year in Endocrinology: 1977.* (Ingbar, S. H., ed.) Plenum Medical Book Co., New York, **1978**, pp. 233–254.

McCann, S. M. Control of anterior pituitary hormone release by brain peptides. *Neuroendocrinology*, **1980**, *31*, 355–363.

McKenzie, J. M., and Zakarija, M. LATS in Graves's disease. *Recent Prog. Horm. Res.*, **1977**, *33*, 29–57.

MacLeod, R. M. Regulation of prolactin secretion. In, *Frontiers in Neuroendocrinology*, Vol. 4. (Martini, L., and Ganong, F., eds.) Raven Press, New York, **1976**, pp. 169–194.

Martial, J. A.; Hallewell, R. A.; Baxter, J. D.; and Goodman, H. M. Human growth hormone: complementary

DNA cloning and expression in bacteria. *Science*, **1979**, *205*, 602–606.

Mehta, A. D., and Tolis, G. Prolactin update. *Pathobiol. Annu.*, **1981**, *11*, 337–389.

Meites, J.; Lu, K. H.; Wuttke, W.; Welsch, C. W.; Nagasawa, H.; and Quadri, S. K. Recent studies on functions and control of prolactin secretion in rats. *Recent Prog. Horm. Res.*, **1972**, *28*, 471–516.

Parkes, D. Bromocriptine. *Adv. Drug Res.*, **1977**, *12*, 247–344.

Phillips, L. S., and Vassilopoulou-Sellin, R. Somatomedins. *N. Engl. J. Med.*, **1980**, *302*, 371–379, 438–446.

Pierce, J. G., and Parsons, T. F. Glycoprotein hormones: structure and function. *Annu. Rev. Biochem.*, **1981**, *50*, 465–495.

Raben, M. S. Human growth hormone. *Recent Prog. Horm. Res.*, **1959**, *15*, 71–114.

Reichlin, S. Somatostatin. *N. Engl. J. Med.*, **1983**, *309*, 1495–1501, 1556–1563.

Schally, A. V. Aspects of hypothalamic regulation of the pituitary gland: its implications for the control of reproductive functions. *Science*, **1978**, *202*, 18–28.

Schally, A. V., and Meyers, C. A. Somatostatin, basic and clinical studies. A review. *Mater. Med. Pol.*, **1982**, *12*, 28–32.

Smithline, F.; Sherman, L.; and Kolodny, H. D. Prolactin and breast carcinoma. *N. Engl. J. Med.*, **1975**, *292*, 784–792.

Terenius, L. Endogenous peptides and analgesia. *Annu. Rev. Pharmacol. Toxicol.*, **1978**, *18*, 189–204.

Thody, A. J. The significance of melanocyte-stimulating hormone (MSH) and control of its secretion in the mammal. *Adv. Drug Res.*, **1977**, *11*, 23–74.

Thorner, M. O. Prolactin. *Clin. Endocrinol. Metab.*, **1977**, *6*, 201–222.

Topper, Y. J. Multiple hormone interactions in the development of mammary gland *in vitro*. *Recent Prog. Horm. Res.*, **1970**, *26*, 287–303.

Turkington, R. W.; Majumder, G. C.; Kadohama, N.; MacIndoe, J. H.; and Frantz, W. L. Hormonal regulation of gene expression in mammary cells. *Recent Prog. Horm. Res.*, **1973**, *29*, 417–449.

Vaitukaitis, J. L.; Ross, G. T.; Braunstein, G. D.; and Rayford, P. L. Gonadotropins and their subunits: basic and clinical studies. *Recent Prog. Horm. Res.*, **1976**, *32*, 289–331.

Vande Wiele, R. L., and Dyrenfurth, I. Gonadotropin-steroid interrelationships. *Pharmacol. Rev.*, **1973**, *25*, 189–207.

Volpe, R. The pathogenesis of Graves's disease: an overview. *Clin. Endocrinol. Metab.*, **1978**, *7*, 3–29.

60 THYROID AND ANTITHYROID DRUGS

Robert C. Haynes, Jr., and Ferid Murad

THYROID

The thyroid gland is the source of two fundamentally different types of hormones. *Thyroxine* and *triiodothyronine* are vital for normal growth and development and play an important role in energy metabolism. The other known glandular secretion, *calcitonin,* is considered in Chapter 65.

History. The thyroid gland was first described in 1656 by Wharton. Harington (1935) reviewed the many older and often amusing opinions concerning the function of this gland. Wharton thought, for example, that the viscous fluid within the follicles lubricated the trachea. He also believed that the gland was larger in women to serve a cosmetic function in giving grace to the contour of the neck. Later observers, influenced by the liberal blood supply of the gland, believed that it provided a vascular shunt for the brain. With this function in mind, Rush in 1820 expressed the belief that the larger size of the gland in women was "necessary to guard the female system from the influence of the more numerous causes of irritation and vexation of mind to which they are exposed than the male sex." However, Hofrichter cleverly opposed this theory in the same year by pointing out that, "If it were indeed true that the thyroid contains more blood at some times than at others, this effect would be visible to the naked eye; in this case women would certainly have long ceased to go about with bare necks, for husbands would have learned to recognize the swelling of this gland as a danger signal of threatening trouble from their better halves."

Numerous other theories of thyroid function were advanced, based upon little or no experimental evidence. The belief ultimately became prevalent that the gland served no important physiological role. The thyroid was first recognized as an organ of importance when enlargement was observed to be associated with changes in the eyes and in the heart in the condition we now call hyperthyroidism. It is of interest that this condition, the manifestations of which can on occasion be as striking as any in medicine, escaped description until Parry saw his first case in 1786. Parry's account was not published until 1825 (*see* Parry, 1895) and was followed in 1835 and 1840 by those of Graves and Basedow, whose names became applied to the disorder. It was not until 1874 that Gull first associated atrophy of the gland with the symptoms now known to be characteristic of thyroid deficiency. Hypofunction of the thyroid in adults is still known as *Gull's disease.* The term *myxedema* was applied to the clinical syndrome by Ord (1878) in the belief that the characteristic thickening of the subcutaneous tissues was due to excessive formation of mucus.

Extirpation experiments to elucidate the function of the thyroid were at first misinterpreted because of the simultaneous removal of the parathyroids. However, the pioneer research on the latter organs by Gley (1891) allowed the functional differentiation of these two endocrine glands. It was not until after calcitonin was discovered in 1961 that it was realized that the thyroid itself was also concerned with the regulation of calcium. Murray (1891) was the first to treat a case of hypothyroidism by injecting an extract of the thyroid gland; in the following year, Howitz, Mackenzie, and Fox independently discovered that thyroid tissue was fully effective when given by mouth.

Magnus-Levy (1895) discovered the effect of the thyroid on metabolic rate; he found that Gull's disease was characterized by a low rate of metabolism and that the administration of thyroid to hypothyroid or normal individuals increased oxygen consumption.

Chemistry. The active principles of the thyroid gland are the iodine-containing amino acid derivatives of thyronine—*thyroxine* and *triiodothyronine* (Table 60–1). Thyroxine was first isolated in crystalline form from a hydrolysate of thyroid by Kendall (1915), who found that the crystalline product exerted the same physiological effects as the extract from which it was obtained. It was not until 1926, however, that the structural formula of thyroxine was elucidated by Harington, and in the fol-

Table 60–1.   THE THYROID HORMONES

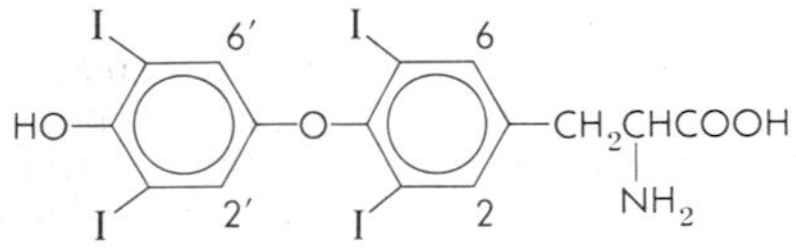

Thyroxine

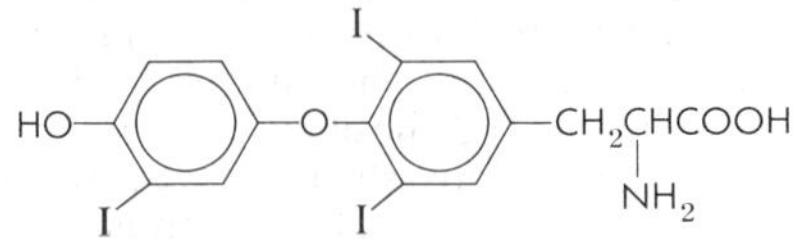

3,5,3'-Triiodothyronine

lowing year Harington and Barger (1927) synthesized the hormone.

Following the isolation and the chemical identification of thyroxine, it was generally believed that all the hormonal activity of thyroid tissue could be accounted for by its content of thyroxine. However, careful studies revealed that crude thyroid preparations possessed greater calorigenic activity than could be accounted for by their thyroxine content. The enigma was resolved with the detection, isolation, and synthesis of triiodothyronine (Gross and Pitt-Rivers, 1952; Roche *et al.*, 1952a, 1952b). Further studies revealed that triiodothyronine is qualitatively similar to thyroxine in its biological action but that it is much more potent on a molar basis (Gross and Pitt-Rivers, 1953a, 1953b).

Structure-Activity Relationship. A great many structural analogs of thyroxine have been synthesized in order to define the structure-activity relationship, to detect antagonists of thyroid hormones, or to find compounds exhibiting one desirable type of activity while not showing unwanted effects. The only significant success has been the partial separation of the cholesterol-lowering action of thyroxine analogs from their calorigenic effect. The D isomer of thyroxine has limited clinical use to lower the concentration of cholesterol in plasma (*see* Chapter 34).

The structural requirements for a significant degree of thyroid hormone activity have been defined (Jorgensen, 1964). The two aromatic rings should be connected by an ether or thioether linkage. However, potent methylene-bridged analogs have been synthesized (Psychoyos *et al.*, 1973). A carboxyl-containing aliphatic side chain in position 1 is important, with L-alanine being the best. Halogen or methyl groups are necessary on positions 3 and 5. Position 4′ should be occupied by a hydroxyl group, an amino group, or a group capable of metabolic conversion to a hydroxyl. For maximal activity, halogen atoms, alkyl, or aromatic substituents are necessary at the 3′ position or at the 3′ and 5′ positions. The 3′-monosubstituted compounds are more active than the 3′,5′-disubstituted molecules. Thus, triiodothyronine is four times more potent than thyroxine, while 3′-isopropyl-3,5-diiodothyronine has seven times the activity.

While the chemical nature of the 3, 5, 3′, and 5′ substituents is important, their effects on the conformation of the molecule are apparently even more so. In thyronine, the two rings are angulated at about 120° at the ether oxygen and are free to rotate on their axes. As depicted schematically in Figure 60-1, when the 3,5 iodines are in place there is some restriction to rotation of the two rings, and they tend to take up positions perpendicular to one another; now positions 2′ and 3′ are no longer equivalent to positions 5′ and 6′. Substituents at the 3′ position can be either distal (on the convex side, as in Figure 60-1) or proximal to the phenylalanine ring, depending on the rotation. Substitution at the more hindered 2′ position probably requires the distal conformation. Much biological evidence indicates that this distal conformation is necessary for activity. Thus, bulky and lipophilic groups in the 3′ position enhance activity, and 2′ substituents

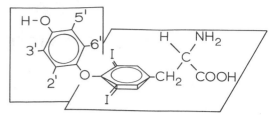

Figure 60-1. *Structural formula of 3,5-diiodothyronine, drawn to show the conformation in which the planes of the aromatic rings are perpendicular to each other.* (After Jorgensen, 1964. Courtesy of The Mayo Association. *See also* Cody and Duax, 1973.)

are tolerated. As mentioned, substitutions in the 5′ position detract from activity. While not potent, even halogen-free derivatives possess some activity if the proper conformation is possible (Pittman *et al.*, 1973). It has been suggested that the iodine atoms of thyroxine are essential for binding to thyroxine-binding globulin in the plasma, as well as for maintenance of the active conformation of the molecule (Cody, 1980).

Synthesis of Thyroid Hormones. The synthesis of the thyroid hormones is unique, complex, and seemingly grossly inefficient. The thyroid hormones are synthesized and stored as amino acid residues of thyroglobulin, a protein constituting the vast majority of the thyroid follicular colloid. The thyroid gland is unique in storing great quantities of potential hormone in this way, and extracellular thyroglobulin can represent a large portion of the mass of the gland. It is a complex glycoprotein made up of two apparently identical subunits of 330,000 molecular weight.

The major steps in the synthesis, storage, release, and interconversion of thyroid hormones are the following: (1) the uptake of iodide ion by the gland, (2) the oxidation of iodide and the iodination of tyrosyl groups of thyroglobulin, (3) the conversion of iodotyrosyl residues to iodothyronyl residues in this protein, (4) the proteolysis of thyroglobulin and the release of thyroxine and triiodothyronine into the blood, and (5) the conversion of thyroxine to triiodothyronine in peripheral tissues. These processes are summarized in Figure 60-2.

1. *Uptake of Iodide.* Iodine ingested in the diet reaches the circulation in the form of iodide. Under normal circumstances the concentration in the blood is very low, 0.2 to 0.4 μg/dl, but the thyroid efficiently and

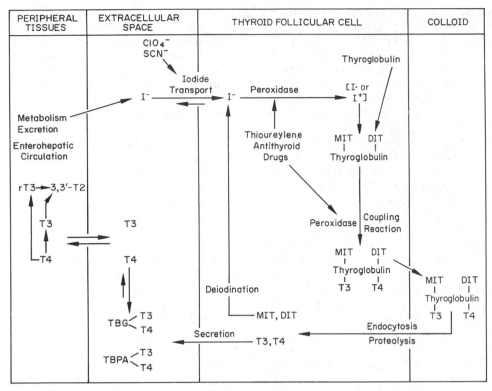

Figure 60–2. *The major pathways of iodine metabolism.*

Abbreviations are as follows: *T3* = triiodothyronine; *T4* = thyroxine; *rT3* = 3,3′,5′-triiodo-thyronine (reverse T₃); *3,3′-T2* = 3,3′-diiodothyronine; *MIT* = monoiodotyrosine; *DIT* = diiodotyrosine; *TBG* = thyroxine-binding globulin; *TBPA* = thyroxine-binding prealbumin.

actively transports the ion. As a result, the ratio of thyroid to plasma iodide concentration is usually between 20 and 50 and can far exceed 100 when the gland is stimulated. The iodide transport mechanism is inhibited by a number of ions such as thiocyanate and perchlorate (*see* below), appears to require concurrent transport of potassium, and is depressed by cardiac glycosides that inhibit the accumulation of potassium by cells (*see* Wolff, 1964).

The transport system is stimulated by thyrotropin (*see* below) and is also controlled by an autoregulatory mechanism. Thus, decreased stores of thyroid iodine enhance iodide uptake, and the administration of iodide can reverse this situation. Some incorporation of iodide into organic form must occur, however, for the inhibitory effect of excess iodide to become apparent (VanderLaan, 1955).

If the further metabolism of iodide is blocked by antithyroid drugs, the iodide-concentrating mechanism can more easily be studied. Thus isolated, the mechanism resembles those found in other bodily structures that concentrate iodide, including the salivary glands, gastric mucosa, midportion of the small intestine, skin, mammary gland, and placenta, all of which maintain a concentration gradient of iodide some 10 to 50 times that of the blood. It has been suggested that the accumulation of iodide by the placenta and the mammary gland may be of importance in providing adequate supplies for the fetus and infant, but no obvious purpose is served by the accumulation of iodide at the other sites. It is evident that the iodide-accumulating system of the thyroid is not unique to the gland and does not account for the specific function of making thyroid hormone.

2. *Oxidation and Iodination.* Consistent with the conditions generally necessary for halogenation of aromatic rings, the iodination of tyrosine residues requires the iodinating species to be in a higher state of oxidation than is the anion. However, the precise nature of the iodinating species is unknown. There is evidence against the participation of I_2 in the reaction; in fact, I_2 inhibits enzymatically catalyzed iodination (Nunez and Pommier, 1982). Possibly the reaction sequence involves the combination of oxidized free radicals of iodine and the tyrosyl acceptor, or the active species may be the iodinium ion (I^+) (DeGroot and Niepomniszcze, 1977). Whatever it may be, the requisite state of oxidation is produced by a peroxidase-catalyzed reaction. The H_2O_2 that serves as a substrate for the peroxidase is presumed to be formed in close proximity to its site of utilization, and the reactions probably involve the oxidation of reduced nicotinamide adenine dinucleotide phosphate (NADPH), although the exact mechanism has not been satisfactorily defined (DeGroot and Niepomniszcze, 1977; Nunez and Pommier, 1982).

Taurog and associates (1970) have purified and characterized a heme-containing peroxidase from thyroid particulate fractions that catalyzes the iodination of tyrosyl residues in protein in the presence of H_2O_2. This enzyme appears to be concentrated in membranes at or near the apical surface of the thyroid cell and to catalyze the iodination of thyroglobulin just prior to its storage in the lumen of the thyroid follicle. The initial products of the reaction are monoiodotyrosyl and diiodotyrosyl residues in thyroglobulin.

3. *Formation of Thyroxine and Triiodothyronine from Iodotyrosines.* The remaining synthetic step is the coupling of two diiodotyrosyl residues to form thyroxine or monoiodotyrosyl and diiodotyrosyl residues to form triiodothyronine. These are also oxidative reactions and appear to be catalyzed by the same peroxidase discussed above (Lamas *et al.*, 1972). The mechanism involves the enzymatic transfer of groups, perhaps as iodotyrosyl free radicals or positively charged ions, within thyroglobulin (DeGroot and Niepomniszcze, 1977). The configuration of the protein is presumed to be important in facilitating this coupling reaction. Iodination of thyroglobulin may be associated with cleavage of peptide bonds; as iodine-poor thyroglobulin is progressively iodinated, the iodine is found increasingly in peptides of 15,000 to 26,000 molecular weight (Dunn *et al.*, 1982, 1983). While many other proteins can serve as substrates for the peroxidase, none is as efficient as thyroglobulin in yielding thyroxine.

The proportions of thyroxine and triiodothyronine formed in the thyroid depend, at least in part, on the relative quantities of monoiodotyrosine and diiodotyrosine available. While a high proportion of monoiodotyrosine seems to favor the formation of triiodothyronine over thyroxine, deficient diiodotyrosine can impair the formation of both thyronines. Thyroxine usually predominates by a factor of severalfold, and about one fourth of the iodine in the thyroid of most species is in the form of thyroxine. When there is a deficiency of iodine in rat thyroid, however, the ratio of thyroxine to triiodothyronine decreases from 4:1 to 1:3 (Greer *et al.*, 1968). Since triiodothyronine is four times as active as thyroxine and contains only three fourths as much iodine, this change could provide little more than a twofold increase in hormonal effect from a given quantity of available iodine.

4. *Secretion of Thyroid Hormone.* Since thyroxine and triiodothyronine are synthesized and stored as parts of the molecule of thyroglobulin, proteolysis is an important part of the secretory process. It is generally believed that thyroglobulin must be completely broken down into its constituent amino acids in order for the hormones to be released. As the molecular weight of thyroglobulin is 660,000 and the protein is made up of about 300 carbohydrate residues and 5500 amino acid residues, only two to five of which are thyroxine (Rall *et al.*, 1964), this is an extravagant process indeed. Evidently evolution has not brought economy to the thyroid or perhaps sufficient intelligence to the scientist to understand the rationale of the process utilized. Thyrotropin appears to enhance the degradation of thyroglobulin by increasing the activity of several thiol endopeptidases of the lysosomes,

the organelles in which the proteolysis is thought to occur (Dunn, A. D., 1984). When thyroglobulin is hydrolyzed, mono-iodotyrosine and diiodotyrosine are liberated also, but they usually do not leave the thyroid. Instead, they are selectively metabolized, and the iodine, liberated in the form of iodide, is reincorporated into protein (Roche *et al.*, 1952c). Normally, all this iodide is reused; however, when hydrolysis is activated intensely by thyrotropin (TSH), some of the iodide reaches the circulation, at times accompanied by trace amounts of the iodotyrosines.

The secretory process is initiated by endocytosis of colloid from the follicular lumen at the apical surface of the cell. This "ingested" thyroglobulin appears as intracellular colloid droplets, which apparently then fuse with lysosomes containing the requisite proteolytic enzymes (Wollman *et al.*, 1964). The liberated hormones presumably exit from the cell at its basal membrane.

5. *Conversion of Thyroxine to Triiodothyronine.* The normal daily production of thyroxine has been estimated to range between 70 and 90 μg, while that of triiodothyronine is between 15 and 30 μg. While triiodothyronine is secreted by the thyroid, the majority (approximately 80%) is synthesized by the metabolism of thyroxine in peripheral tissues. Thus, when thyroxine is given to hypothyroid patients in doses that produce normal concentrations of thyroxine in plasma, the plasma concentration of triiodothyronine also reaches the normal range. This metabolic step has been demonstrated in preparations of a number of different tissues *in vitro;* the liver and kidney are the most active. The enzyme responsible for this reaction (5'-deiodinase) is inhibited by oxidizing agents and by the antithyroid drug propylthiouracil, which appears to form a complex with the enzyme. Methimazole, another antithyroid drug of the thioureylene group, does not inhibit the enzyme and, in fact, antagonizes the inhibition produced by propylthiouracil (Leonard and Rosenberg, 1978). Fasting and a number of acute and chronic illnesses decrease the activity of the 5'-deiodinase, such that the $T_4:T_3$ ratio of the plasma is increased (Braverman and Vagenakis,

1979). The clinical significance of the decreased plasma concentration of triiodothyronine in illness has been discussed by Utiger (1980). The estimation of the total amount of thyroxine eventually converted to triiodothyronine is a difficult one, but it has been calculated to be in the range of 35% (*see* Schimmel and Utiger, 1977).

Transport of Thyroid Hormone in the Blood. Iodine in the circulation is normally present in several forms, with 95% as organic iodine and approximately 5% as iodide. Most of the organic iodine is thyroxine (90 to 95%), while triiodothyronine represents a relatively minor fraction (about 5%). The thyroid hormones are transported in the blood in strong but noncovalent association with certain plasma proteins.

Thyroxine-binding globulin is the major carrier of thyroid hormones. It is an acidic glycoprotein with a molecular weight of approximately 63,000, and it binds one molecule of thyroxine per molecule of protein with a very high association constant (about 10^{10} M^{-1}). Triiodothyronine is bound less avidly. Thyroid hormones are also found associated with *thyroxine-binding prealbumin*. This protein is present in higher concentration than is the thyroxine-binding globulin, but it binds thyroxine and triiodothyronine with association constants near 10^7 M^{-1} and 10^6 M^{-1}, respectively. Despite the fact that the prealbumin has four apparently identical subunits, it has a single high-affinity binding site. Albumin can also serve as a carrier for thyroxine when the more avid carriers are saturated. It is difficult, however, to estimate its quantitative or physiological importance.

Protein binding of thyroid hormones protects them from metabolism and excretion, resulting in their long half-life in the circulation. Only about 0.03% of the total thyroxine in plasma is free (*see* Utiger, 1974). While triiodothyronine is much less firmly bound, the quantity that is free, 0.2 to 0.5%, is still a small percentage of the total. However, the unbound thyroid hormones constitute the fractions available for action, and their concentrations thus assume particular importance.

Certain drugs and a variety of pathological and physiological conditions can alter the binding of thyroid hormones to proteins or the amounts of these proteins. Thus, the total amounts of thyroid hormones in the plasma and the quantities of *free* hormones can vary somewhat independently. For example, pregnancy or the administration of estrogen causes elevation of the concentration of thyroxine-binding globulin. This leads to increased thyroxine binding and could lower the concentration of free hormone. Feedback mechanisms compensate, however, and increased thyroid secretion returns the concentration of free hormone to normal. The result is elevated total and bound thyroxine in plasma and a normal concentration of free thyroxine. Laboratory tests that measure only total thyroxine, therefore, would be subject to misinterpretation. Appropriate tests of thyroid function are discussed below.

Degradation and Excretion. Thyroxine is eliminated slowly from the body; it has a half-life of 6 to 7 days. In hyperthyroidism the half-life is shortened to 3 or 4 days, whereas in myxedema it may be 9 to 10 days. These changes are probably due to altered rates of metabolism of the hormone. In conditions associated with increased binding to the proteins of plasma, as in pregnancy, elimination is retarded; the reverse is observed when there is reduced protein in plasma, as in nephrosis or hepatic cirrhosis, or when binding to protein is inhibited by certain drugs, such as salicylate or dicumarol. Triiodothyronine, which is less avidly bound to protein, has a half-life of 2 days or less.

The liver is the major site of degradation of thyroid hormones; thyroxine and triiodothyronine are conjugated with glucuronic and sulfuric acids through the phenolic hydroxyl group and excreted in the bile. There is an enterohepatic circulation of the thyroid hormones, since they are liberated by hydrolysis in the intestine and reabsorbed. A portion of the conjugated material reaches the colon unchanged, is hydrolyzed there, and is eliminated as the free compounds in the feces. In man, approximately 20 to 40% of thyroxine is eliminated in the stool.

As discussed above, an important route of metabolism of thyroxine is to triiodothyronine. Another compound formed by peripheral metabolism of thyroxine is 3,3',5'-triiodothyronine, often referred to as reverse T3. While the concentration of

this inactive metabolite in plasma varies with diet and disease states, no significant clinical consequences of these changes have been demonstrated (Braverman and Vagenakis, 1979). Triiodothyronine and reverse T3 are deiodinated to 3,3'-diiodothyronine, an inactive metabolite that is a normal constituent of human plasma (Burman, 1978). Additional metabolites in which the diphenyl ether linkage is either intact (Pittman et al., 1972) or cleaved (Wynn and Gibbs, 1962) have been detected both in vitro and in vivo.

Regulation of Thyroid Function. During the last century, it was appreciated that cellular changes occur in the anterior pituitary in association with endemic goiter or following thyroidectomy. The classical experimental observations of Cushing (1912) and the clinical observations of Simmonds (1914) established that ablation or disease of the pituitary causes thyroid hypoplasia. It was eventually determined that the anterior pituitary secretes the specific hormone, thyrotropin (TSH) (Chapter 59).

Although there was evidence that thyroid hormone or lack of it causes cellular changes in the pituitary, the control of secretion of thyrotropin by the negative-feedback action of thyroid hormone was not appreciated fully until its central role in the pathogenesis of goiter was elucidated in the early 1940s. It is now recognized that the rate of secretion of thyrotropin is delicately controlled by thyrotropin-releasing hormone (TRH) and the quantity of thyroid hormone in the circulation. If extra hormone is given, the secretion of thyrotropin is suppressed and the thyroid becomes inactive and regresses, whereas any decrease in the normal rate of secretion of the thyroid evokes an enhanced secretion of thyrotropin and the thyroid is stimulated to increased growth and function. The mechanism of this effect of thyroid hormone on thyrotropin secretion appears, at least in part, to be a reduction in the number of receptors for TRH on pituitary cells (Hinkle and Goh, 1982). The role of TRH is discussed in Chapter 59.

Actions of Thyrotropin on the Thyroid. When thyrotropin is given to experimental animals, the first effect on thyroid hormone metabolism that can be measured is an increased secretion. This can be monitored by detecting the radioactivity in the blood leaving the gland that has been prelabeled with radioactive iodine. Under these circumstances, the response can be seen within minutes. All phases of hormone synthesis and release are eventually stimulated: iodide uptake and organification, hormone synthesis, endocytosis, and proteolysis of colloid. There is increased vascularity of the gland and hypertrophy and hyperplasia of thyroid cells.

A primary action of thyrotropin is to activate thyroid adenylate cyclase and to increase the glandular concentration of adenosine 3',5'-monophosphate (cyclic AMP) (Gilman and Rall, 1968). Cyclic AMP, acting as the intracellular mediator of thyrotropin, appears to be able to reproduce the important actions of the hormone. Thus, iodide uptake and hormone synthesis are stimulated by the cyclic nucleotide, as are endocytosis and secretion of hormone. Protein and nucleic acid synthesis are increased; in fact, cyclic AMP has been shown to be goitrogenic (Pisarev et al., 1970). Several actions of thyrotropin on the intermediary metabolism of thyroid tissue may also be mediated by cyclic AMP, although their immediate importance to hormone metabolism is uncertain. The relationship of cyclic AMP to control of thyroid function has been reviewed by Dumont and associates (1978).

Relation of Iodine to Thyroid Function. Normal thyroid function obviously requires an adequate intake of iodine; without it, normal amounts of hormone cannot be made, thyrotropin is secreted in excess, and the thyroid hypertrophies. The enlarged and stimulated thyroid becomes remarkably efficient in extracting the residual traces of iodide from the the blood. The iodide-concentrating mechanism develops a gradient for the ion that may be ten times the normal, and the vascularity may increase to the point that a bruit is heard over the gland. In this hypertrophied state the thyroid usually succeeds in making sufficient hormone, unless the iodine deficiency is severe.

In some areas of the world *simple* or *nontoxic goiter* is quite prevalent, because iodine is not abundant in most foods. The only rich natural sources commonly eaten are those derived from marine life. Sea fish contain 200 to 1000 μg/kg, shellfish a similar or slightly larger amount, and dried kelp 0.1 to 0.2%, but for those who do not eat marine fish the element can be scarce indeed. To ensure an adequate intake, which is usually taken to be about 100 μg daily,

one would have to eat about 5 kg of vegetables or fruit, or 3 kg of meat or fresh-water fish. Milk and eggs are somewhat better sources, but most potable waters contain a negligible amount. However, unnatural sources of iodine in the environment are becoming prevalent and perhaps of concern. A slice of bread may contain 150 μg of iodate, added as a "conditioner" (London et al., 1965). Other sources are as diverse as food colorings and automobile exhaust.

Iodine has been used empirically for the treatment of goiter for 150 years. However, its modern use was the outgrowth of the extensive studies of Marine, which culminated in the use of iodine to prevent goiter in school children in Akron, Ohio, a region where endemic goiter was prevalent (Marine and Kimball, 1917). The success of these experiments led to the adoption of this form of prophylaxis in many regions of endemic goiter throughout the world.

The most practicable method yet found for providing small supplements of iodine for large segments of the population is the addition of an iodide to table salt, although iodate is now preferred. In some countries, the use of iodine in salt is required by law; in others, including the United States, the use is optional; in some regions of endemic goiter, injection of iodized oil has been used (Thilly et al., 1973); in Japan, supplementation is not needed because kelp is a national delicacy. In the United States, iodized salt provides 100 μg of iodine per gram.

Actions of Thyroid Hormones. The actions of the thyroid hormones are considered under the categories of (1) regulation of growth and development, (2) calorigenic effect, (3) cardiovascular effects, (4) metabolic effects, and (5) inhibition of the secretion of thyrotropin by the pituitary. This last-named action on the pituitary is discussed above.

Growth and Development. It is generally believed that the thyroid hormones exert most if not all of their effects through control of protein synthesis. This is certainly true for the actions of the hormones on the normal growth and development of the organism. Perhaps the most dramatic example is found in the tadpole, which is almost magically transformed into a frog by thyroxine. Not only does the animal grow limbs, lungs, and other terrestrial accouterments, but also the hormone stimulates the synthesis of a host of enzymes and at the same time so influences the tail that it is digested away and used to build new tissue elsewhere.

There is a critically important role of thyroid hormone in the development of the nervous system. Examination of the brain of hypothyroid animals reveals deficient development, particularly of axonal and dendritic networks. Myelinization is severely impaired, and several other deficits in biochemical development are also notable. It has thus been hypothesized that the effect of thyroid hormone is to initiate a series of reactions that lead to differentiation and to terminate the phase of cell proliferation (Hamburgh, 1969). However, the effects of thyroid hormones on protein synthesis and enzymatic activity are certainly not limited to the brain, and a large number of tissues are altered by the administration of thyroid hormone or by its deficiency. The extensive defects in growth and development that are found in cretins provide a vivid reminder of the pervasive effects of thyroid hormones in normal individuals.

Cretinism is usually classified as endemic or sporadic. *Endemic cretinism* is encountered in regions of endemic goiter and is usually due to extreme deficiency of iodine. Goiter may or may not be present. There is a high incidence of nerve deafness in *endemic* but not in *sporadic* cretinism. The latter disease is a consequence of failure of the thyroid to develop normally or the result of a defect in the synthesis of thyroid hormone. Goiter is present if a synthetic defect is at fault.

While detectable at birth, cretinism is often not recognized until 3 to 5 months of age. When untreated, the condition eventually leads to such gross changes as to be unmistakable. The child is dwarfed and the extremities are short, and the child is mentally retarded, inactive, uncomplaining, and listless. The face is puffy and expressionless, and the enlarged tongue may protrude through the thickened lips of the half-opened mouth. The skin may have a yellowish hue and feel doughy, and it is dry and cool to the touch. The heart rate is slow, the body temperature may be low, closure of the fontanels is delayed, and the teeth erupt late. Appetite is poor, feeding is slow and interrupted by choking, constipation is frequent, and there may be an umbilical hernia.

For treatment to be fully effective, the diagnosis must be made long before these obvious changes

have come about. Screening of newborn infants for deficient function of the thyroid is widely established in the United States. Measurements of the concentrations of thyrotropin and thyroxine in umbilical cord blood are performed. The incidence of congenital dysfunction of the thyroid is about one per 6000 births (Fisher, 1977).

It is thus clear that thyroid hormones are important determinants of genetically coded developmental programs. While the precise biochemical mechanisms through which the thyroid controls growth and development are unknown, the thyroid hormones are bound to a limited number of high-affinity sites in the nuclei of many cells. There is no convincing evidence that the hormones bind first to a cytoplasmic receptor, as is thought to be the case with steroid hormones. Both thyroxine and triiodothyronine are bound in nuclei, although thyroxine is bound with lower affinity. Based on the assumption that binding of the hormones represents initiation of their action, it has been calculated that thyroxine accounts for approximately 15% of the total activity of the thyroid hormones. The nuclear binding of thyroid hormones in relation to their actions has been reviewed extensively (Baxter *et al.*, 1979; Oppenheimer, 1981, 1985; Ramsden and Hoffenberg, 1983).

Calorigenic Effect. Thyroid hormones increase the resting or basal metabolic rate of the whole organism, but only certain tissues seem to be affected when their oxygen consumption is measured *in vitro*. Heart, skeletal muscle, liver, and kidney are markedly stimulated by thyroxine, while the adult brain, spleen, and gonads are largely unresponsive. The calorigenic response is important in regulation of temperature in homeotherms, and thyroid secretion is stimulated by exposure to cold. The mechanism of the calorigenic effect of thyroid hormone remains poorly understood, and the field is strewn with discarded hypotheses. For example, it was at one time erroneously believed that thyroid hormones act by uncoupling mitochondrial oxidative phosphorylation. It was also proposed that the increased activity of the Na^+,K^+-ATPase, as assayed in various tissues after treatment with thyroid hormones, indicates that there is enhanced ion pumping that accounts for much of the calorigenic effect. Subsequent studies have shown that the energy required for sodium and potassium transport in liver (Folke and Sestoft, 1977), kidney (Silva *et al.*, 1976), adipose tissue (Fain and Rosenthal, 1971), and skeletal muscle (Biron *et al.*, 1979) is small and contributes little if any to the enhanced oxygen consumption. In a review of the calorigenic effect of thyroid hormones, Sestoft (1980) has suggested that approximately 15% of the increased oxygen consumption is a consequence of an enhanced futile cycle of lipolysis and synthesis of triglycerides in adipose tissue. He has also estimated that stimulation of the heart accounts for 30 to 40% of the increased energy utilized. If these estimates are correct, the explanation for a large fraction of the calorigenic effect remains elusive.

Cardiovascular Effects. Changes in the cardiovascular system are prominent consequences of the action of thyroid hormones. These are most dramatically evident in the cardiac function of hyperthyroid patients (see below). Under the influence of thyroid hormones, the heart beats more rapidly and more forcefully, and cardiac output is thus increased. It would seem reasonable to assume that this represents an adaptation to the load placed on the cardiovascular system by the high rate of metabolism experienced by the body as a whole. To some degree this is certainly true, but a number of observations have indicated that the heart is a direct target of hormone action, rather than merely a passive responder to an increased demand. It has often been stated that the heart is hypersensitive to catecholamines in hyperthyroidism. In support of this it has been observed that the number of myocardial β-adrenergic receptors is increased, and β-adrenergic antagonists are of great value in the treatment of thyrotoxic patients. Furthermore, isolated rat atria exposed to triiodothyronine in vitro develop an enhanced chronotropic response to maximal doses of norepinephrine (Eiden and Ruth, 1981). Nevertheless, several other careful studies have failed to demonstrate an increased sensitivity to β-adrenergic agonists (see Morkin et al., 1983). Decreased muscarinic control of the heart has also been ruled out as a mechanism (Cairoli and Crout, 1967). A biochemical basis for the inotropic effect of thyroid hormone treatment has been proposed: hormone action results in a change in the isozyme pattern of myosin (Hoh et al, 1978), apparently as a result of preferential synthesis of one of the heavy chains of the protein (Flink et al., 1979). This change in isozyme composition enhances the Ca^{2+}-ATPase activity of the myosin, a reaction that may be responsible for generation of force in cardiac muscle (Morkin et al., 1983).

Metabolic Effects. Thyroid hormones appear to stimulate metabolism of cholesterol to bile acids, and hypercholesterolemia is a characteristic feature of hypothyroid states. Some separation of actions has been observed between the effects of thyroxine analogs on cholesterol and on calorigenesis, and D-thyroxine is sometimes used to lower the concentration of cholesterol in plasma (Chapter 34).

Thyroid hormones enhance the lipolytic responses of fat cells to other hormones, for example, catecholamines, and elevated plasma free fatty acid concentrations are seen in hyperthyroidism. In contrast to other lipolytic hormones, thyroid hormones do not directly stimulate the accumulation of cyclic AMP. They may, however, regulate the capacity of other hormones to enhance the accumulation of the cyclic nucleotide by decreasing the activity of a microsomal phosphodiesterase that hydrolyzes cyclic AMP (Nunez and Correze, 1981). There is also evidence that thyroid hormones act to maintain normal coupling of the β-adrenergic receptor to the guanine nucleotide-binding regulatory protein of adenylate cyclase in fat cells (Malbon et al., 1984).

The effects of the thyroid hormones on carbohydrate metabolism are generally consistent with an accelerated utilization of carbohydrate, presumably secondary to increased caloric demand. There is an increased rate of intestinal absorption of glucose that results in higher concentrations of the sugar in plasma during the early phase of an oral glucose tolerance test. In contrast, the increased rate of metabolism of carbohydrate results in a flattened response to intravenous glucose.

In rats, thyroid hormones enhance the hepatic synthesis of glucose under certain conditions. The mechanism and significance of this action are not known (Sestoft, 1980). A recent study demonstrated increased gluconeogenesis in volunteers given triiodothyronine (Sandler et al., 1983).

Thyroid Hyperfunction. Excessive secretion of thyroid hormones may lead to such striking changes that the diagnosis of hyperthyroidism is obvious to the casual observer, or the effects may cause distressing but subtle symptoms that give no clue to their origin. Two major forms of thyroid hyperfunction are recognized. Diffuse toxic goiter (Graves' disease) is characterized by thyrotoxicosis and ophthalmopathy. This disease is now generally considered to be a disorder of the immune response. Antibodies of the IgG type appear to stimulate the thyroid gland by activating receptors for thyrotropin; unknown factors and anti-bodies affect retro-orbital tissue and the eye muscles, leading to the characteristic ophthalmological changes (Volpe, 1978; *see also* Chapter 59). The disease occurs most commonly in young adults. Toxic nodular goiter (Plummer's disease) occurs primarily in older patients and usually arises from long-standing nontoxic goiter; infiltrative ophthalmopathy is uncommon. At times, however, the distinction between these conditions can be difficult.

Most of the signs and symptoms of hyperthyroid-ism stem from the excessive production of heat and from increased motor activity and increased activity of the sympathetic nervous system. The skin is flushed, warm, and moist; the muscles are weak and tremulous; the heart rate is rapid, and the heart beat is forceful; and the arterial pulses are prominent and bounding. The increased expenditure of energy gives rise to increased appetite and, if intake is insufficient, to loss of weight. There may also be insomnia, difficulty in remaining still, anxiety and apprehension, intolerance to heat, and increased frequency of bowel movements. Angina, arrhythmias, and heart failure may be present in older patients. Some individuals may show extensive muscular wasting, suggestive of myopathy. Others have osteoporosis from excessive loss of calcium.

Thyroid Hypofunction. Deficiency of thyroid hormone can be manifested at any age. In the adult, the condition is referred to simply as hypothyroidism or, particularly when severe, as myxedema. If the gland fails to develop or is congenitally incompetent, the deficiency may be noted soon after birth by signs of cretinism (*see* above). Later in childhood, failure of growth and development added to the features of the adult counterpart is recognized as juvenile myxedema.

Myxedema. In its fully developed, classical form, myxedema is associated with degeneration and atrophy of the thyroid gland. The same condition follows surgical removal of the thyroid or its destruction by radioactive iodine. Since it may also occur after Graves' disease, some have speculated that the condition can be the end stage of that disease. Myxedema is sometimes associated with goiter when there is a severe defect in synthesis of thyroid hormone, when the gland is extensively involved in chronic thyroiditis (Hashimoto's disease), or when antithyroid drugs have been given. When the disease is mild, it may be subtle in its presentation. By the time it has become severe, however, all of the signs are overt. The appearance of the patient is pathognomonic. The face is quite

expressionless, puffy, and pallid. The skin is cold and dry, the scalp is scaly, and the hair is coarse, brittle, and sparse. The fingernails are thickened and brittle, the subcutaneous tissue appears to be thickened, and there may be true edema. The voice is husky and low pitched, speech is slow, the hearing is often faulty, and mentality is impaired. The appetite is poor, the gastric juice contains little free hydrochloric acid, gastrointestinal activity is diminished, and abdominal distention and constipation are common. Atony of the urinary bladder suggests that the function of other smooth muscles may also be impaired. The voluntary muscles are weak and flabby, and deep-tendon reflexes are slowed. The heart is often dilated, and cardiac output is diminished. There may also be hydropericardium, hydrothorax, and ascites. Refractory anemia, occasionally hyperchromic and macrocytic in character, is often associated with the disease. Menstrual irregularities are prominent. The patient is prone to be drowsy and to sleep a great deal, and he complains of the cold in winter but not of the heat in summer.

Thyroid Function Tests. The laboratory diagnosis of thyroid disease is complicated by the extremely low quantities of thyroid hormones in plasma; by problems of specificity, particularly when analytical technics are directed at iodine; and by variations in the extent of protein binding of the hormones. The availability of protein-binding assays and radioimmunoassays for the thyroid hormones has greatly improved the laboratory diagnosis of disorders of the thyroid. These specific assays, together with the resin-triiodothyronine-uptake (RT3U) test, which estimates the extent of saturation of thyroid-binding globulin, provide a valuable approach to an accurate diagnosis. Their use permits the estimation of the concentration of free thyroxine in plasma, an excellent index of the activity of the thyroid gland.

As mentioned above, the total concentration of thyroxine in plasma changes with alterations in the concentration of the thyroid-binding globulin, so that, for example, it is high in pregnancy and low in nephrosis even though the patient is euthyroid. From the estimates of the extent of saturation of the thyroid-binding globulin and the measurement of the total concentration of thyroxine in plasma, a free-thyroxine index can be calculated. The measurement of plasma triiodothyronine by radioimmunoassay is also useful for the diagnosis of hyperthyroidism.

The radioimmunoassay of thyrotropin (TSH) is also helpful. Determination of an elevated concentration of this hormone in the plasma can provide confirmation of suspected failure of the thyroid gland. Patients with frank hypothyroidism who have normal or decreased concentrations of TSH in plasma are likely to have hypothyroidism secondary to pituitary or hypothalamic dysfunction. The response of plasma TSH to an injection of thyrotropin-releasing hormone may also be useful in this regard (*see* Chapter 59).

Measurement of the accumulation of radioactive iodine by the thyroid gland as a diagnostic technic is discussed below. The use of laboratory tests in the diagnosis of thyroid disease has been reviewed by Feldman (1977) and Merimee (1978).

Preparations. Thyroid as well as thyroxine and triiodothyronine are official preparations. *Thyroid* is a fine powder made from the thyroids of animals, usually pigs, by defatting and drying with acetone. The USP specifies that the content of iodine be between 0.17 and 0.23%, and, as most thyroid powders are stronger than this, they are diluted by an inert material. Although neither bioassay nor chemical analyses for thyroxine or triiodothyronine are specified, the product is remarkably uniform. *Thyroid tablets* (THYRAR, WESTHROID, others) are made from the compressed powder in numerous sizes from 16 to 325 mg. *Thyroglobulin* (PROLOID) is a purified extract of pig thyroid available in tablets containing from 32 to 200 mg. It conforms to the USP standard for iodine content and is subject to bioassay. Its potency is adjusted to be equivalent to thyroid powder. *Levothyroxine sodium* (SYN-THROID, LEVOTHROID) is the sodium salt of the natural isomer of thyroxine and is dispensed in the form of tablets containing 25 to 300 μg and as a powder for reconstitution for injection. *Liothyronine sodium* (CYTOMEL) is the somewhat uninformative designation for the salt of L-triiodothyronine. It is marketed as tablets containing 5, 25, and 50 μg. Mixtures of the sodium salts of levothyroxine and liothyronine in a ratio of 4:1 by weight are also marketed as *liotrix* (EUTHROID, THYROLAR). Their dubious advantage is replacement therapy with a pure mixture resembling the normal secretion of the gland.

Thyrotropin (THYTROPAR) is a preparation made from bovine pituitaries. It is available in vials containing 10 I.U. of powdered hormone to be reconstituted for injection. This is used only to test the ability of the thyroid to respond to exogenous stimulation. Synthetic *thyrotropin-releasing hormone* (*protirelin;* THYPINONE) is available in ampuls containing 500 μg in 1 ml.

Choice of Preparation. The pure compounds carry the attraction of single, reproducible substances of known and constant composition. However, recent improvements in analytical technics have revealed that the content of thyroxine of some preparations has been less than that stated (Sawin *et al.*, 1984); these discrepancies have presumably been corrected. There is also some evidence that absorption of levothyroxine sodium is variable and incomplete, as much as 30 to 40% being recoverable in the stool (Van Middlesworth, 1960). Depending upon the form in which it is given, the proportion of a single oral dose absorbed may vary from 42 to 74%; this fraction is rapidly absorbed, while the rest traverses the intestine in a bound unabsorbable form. Nevertheless, levothyroxine sodium has been extensively used with satisfaction and is widely held to be superior to thyroid because of better standardization and stability. Variability of absorption also occurs with desiccated thyroid. The two preparations are about the same price.

Liothyronine sodium may occasionally be preferred to levothyroxine sodium when a quicker action is desired. It may be useful, therefore, when hypothyroidism has recently supervened from overtreatment with an antithyroid drug or following treatment with radioiodine or thyroidectomy, and in the rare event of coma due to myxedema. It is perhaps less desirable than the other preparations for prolonged therapy because its briefer action might require more frequent doses for steady response. Other disadvantages include altered normal values for thyroid function tests and high cost.

Comparative Responses to Thyroid Preparations. There is no significant difference in the qualitative response of the patient with myxedema to triiodothyronine, thyroxine, or thyroid. However, there are obvious quantitative differences. Following the subcutaneous administration of a large experimental dose of L-triiodothyronine, a metabolic response can be detected within 4 to 6 hours, at which time the skin becomes detectably warmer and the pulse rate and the temperature increase. With this dose, a metabolic rate of -40% can be raised to normal within 24 hours. The maximal response occurs in 2 days or less, and the effects subside with a half-life of about 8 days. The same single dose of thyroxine exerts much less effect. However, if thyroxine is given in approximately four times the dose of triiodothyronine, a comparable elevation in metabolic rate can be achieved. The peak effect of a single dose is evident in about 9 days, and this declines to half the maximum in 11 to 15 days. In both cases the effects outlast the presence of detectable amounts of hormone; these disappear from the blood with mean half-lives of approximately 2 and 6 days, respectively. Equivalent clinical responses are obtained from the daily administration of approximately 60 mg of thyroid, 60 mg of thyroglobulin, 100 μg of levothyroxine, or 25 μg of liothyronine.

Therapeutic Uses of Thyroid Hormone. The two major indications for the therapeutic use of thyroid hormone are *hypothyroidism* or *myxedema* and *simple goiter*. Inasmuch as they result from thyroid hypofunction, these uses represent true replacement therapy.

Hypothyroidism. It has been said that treatment of adult myxedema is as perfect a form of therapy as any known to medicine. The main objective is to arrive at the proper dose of a suitable thyroid preparation. The dose varies somewhat according to complications, especially those involving the heart. The object of therapy is to restore the patient to normal. However, replacement of thyroid hormone should be done gradually so as not to stress the patient and produce adverse cardiovascular effects. Often the patient may think he is well when the astute observer can see that he is still hypothyroid. The reverse may also be true; the patient can know that he is ill, but the doctor does not recognize the insidious onset of the signs and symptoms of myxedema. Because long-standing hypothyroidism may have undesirable effects, including a predisposition to atherosclerosis, a full replacement dose should be given if possible.

A reasonable therapeutic regimen for adults is to give a daily dose of 50 μg of levothyroxine for 1 to 2 weeks, a daily dose of 100 μg for the next 1 to 2 weeks, then a permanent daily dose of 150 μg, depending on the response of the patient. Although most patients can be managed with a daily dose of 100 to 200 μg, some individuals will require a dose as small as 50 μg while others need as much as 400 μg. Medication should be taken on an empty stomach to minimize irregular absorption. The patient should be carefully observed during the institution of treatment for untoward reactions such as cardiac pain or palpitations. If angina occurs, care should be exercised but therapy should not necessarily be withheld. Cardiac symptoms are the only serious complications of treatment. Arrhythmias have caused death during the initiation of thyroid therapy in myxedema.

In childhood, treatment is the same as in adults, and every attempt should be made to give a fully therapeutic dose without causing symptoms or failure to gain weight normally, in order to ensure normal growth and development. Usually a full adult dose is needed, and the schedule above can be used.

Myxedema Coma. A large number of dosage regimens have been advocated for this emergency, and the following serve as examples. Levothyroxine (200 to 500 μg, intravenously) or liothyronine (10 to 25 μg, intravenously, every 8 to 12 hours, or 100 μg immediately) is preferred initially. Treatment with adrenal steroids is also recommended because of the likelihood of adrenal insufficiency. Further therapy is dictated by the initial clinical response.

Cretinism. Success in the treatment of cretinism depends upon the age at which therapy is started. Unfortunately, many cases do not come to the attention of physicians until the retardation in development has become so obvious as to be alarming to the parents. In such cases, the detrimental effects of the deficiency on mental development will not be completely overcome. If, on the other hand, therapy is started soon after birth, normal physical and mental development may be achieved. Prognosis also depends on the age of onset of the deficiency. If no thyroid develops in the fetus, deficiency probably dates from the fetal age of 3 months, because little hormone is provided from the mother. It is felt, however, that the most critical need for thyroid hormone is the period of central nervous system (CNS) myelination that occurs about the time of birth. Recommended daily doses of levothyroxine are 10 μg/kg for infants under 6 months of age, 8 μg/kg from 6 to 12 months, 6 μg/kg from 1 to 5 years, and 4 μg/kg from 5 to 10 years. Therapy is monitored by determination of the concentrations of thyroxine and TSH and, occasionally, triiodothyronine in the plasma (see Fisher, 1978). Intellectual and physical development are also guides for therapy in this condition, and error, if unavoidable, should be made on the side of higher dosage. Excessive dosage will, however, advance the bone age inappropriately.

Simple Goiter. In simple goiter, or thyroid enlargement without hyperthyroidism, the usual problem is deficient secretion of thyroid hormone, causing an excessive output of thyrotropin. The exceptions are unrecognized cases of subacute thyroiditis and autonomous thyroid tumors. In Hashimoto's thyroiditis, enlargement results from inflammation as well as from increased secretion of thyrotropin. As the cause of the condition is frequently some defect in the production of thyroid hormone, treatment with thyroid can properly be regarded as replacement therapy.

The aim in treatment is to give full replacement doses of thyroid hormone to suppress the secretion of thyrotropin. Usually, this amounts to 100 to 200 μg of levothyroxine daily, but some patients may require 400 μg. The effectiveness of treatment can be judged by the return of the concentration of thyrotropin in plasma to normal values and by the clinical response in the decrease in size of the goiter.

There have been wide differences in the experience of competent observers as to the proportion of cases of goiter that respond to treatment with a decrease in the size of the thyroid. Some have observed that only in a minority of cases is a worthwhile regression achieved. In several large series, however, there has been an appreciable regression in the goiter in about two thirds of the cases and a complete disappearance in half of these. In other series, almost every case showed some response. The degree of response is greatly affected by the duration of the goiter, its cause, and the degree of nodularity. In areas of endemic goiter where deficiency of iodine is the likely cause, thyroid medication has been shown to be prompt and effective unless the goiter had advanced to the stage of nodular degeneration. However, correction of the iodine deficiency is a more direct approach and is advocated for most cases.

Response to treatment of goiter commonly seen in the United States with thyroid hormone may be noticed within a few days; usually, however, it is counted in weeks, and the maximal response may not be seen for many months. Observations on the incidence of relapse when treatment is stopped are insufficient to provide a meaningful figure, but the observation that all do not recur has not been explained.

Nodular Goiter. The transition of diffuse to nodular goiter is much more important than the cosmetic aspect or the infrequent symptoms of compression with difficulty in swallowing. In some instances nodules may secrete hormone and cause hyperthyroidism (toxic nodular goiter); however, they are frequently not functional. Herein lies a controversial area of thyroid therapy, since it is necessary to determine if the nonfunctional nodule is malignant. While some advocate excision or biopsy, many prefer to administer replacement doses of thyroid hormone for several months to determine if the nodule will diminish in size—an unlikely occurrence with nonfunctional malignant nodules. Since there is some evidence that nonfunctional nodules are responsive to thyrotropin, there is logic in such efforts; however, it is more difficult to shrink a nodule than to decrease the size of a diffusely enlarged gland.

Thyrotropin-Dependent Carcinoma. Certain carcinomas of the thyroid gland, particularly those of the papillary type, may remain sensitive to the growth-promoting effects of TSH. If such tumors are not treatable by more definitive technics, the administration of thyroid hormone to suppress the secretion of TSH may cause regression of malignant lesions.

ANTITHYROID DRUGS AND OTHER THYROID INHIBITORS

A large number of compounds are capable of interfering, directly or indirectly, with the synthesis of thyroid hormones. Several are of great clinical value for the temporary or extended control of hyperthyroid states. These will be discussed in detail. Others are primarily of research or toxicological interest and can only be mentioned. The major inhibitors may be classified into four categories: (1) antithyroid drugs, which interfere directly with the synthesis of thyroid hormones; (2) ionic inhibitors, which block the iodide transport mechanism; (3) iodide itself, which in high concentrations suppresses the thyroid; and (4) radioactive iodine, which damages the gland with ionizing radiations. The antithyroid drugs have been reviewed by Cooper (1984).

ANTITHYROID DRUGS

The antithyroid drugs that have clinical utility are thioureylenes; propylthiouracil may be considered as the prototype.

History. Regulatory feedback mechanisms are now well appreciated. Thus, a deficient concentration of circulating thyroid hormone evokes increased secretion of thyrotropin, and the result is thyroid hypertrophy—a goiter. Studies on the mechanism of the development of goiter began with the observation that rabbits fed a diet composed largely of cabbage often developed goiters (Chesney *et al.*, 1928). This result was probably due to the presence of precursors of the thiocyanate ion in cabbage leaves (*see* below). Later, two pure compounds were shown to produce goiter. Sulfaguanidine, used by the Mackenzies and McCollum (1941) to inhibit intestinal flora for nutritional studies, and phenylthiourea, used by Richter and Clisby (1942) for tests on taste, caused goiter in rats. Investigation of the effects of thiourea derivatives revealed that rats became hypothyroid despite hyperplastic changes in their thyroid glands

that were characteristic of intense thyrotropic stimulation. After treatment was begun, no new hormone was made, and the goitrogen had no visible effect upon the thyroid gland following hypophysectomy or the administration of thyroid hormone. This suggested that the goiter was a compensatory change resulting from the induced state of hypothyroidism and that the primary action of the compounds was to inhibit the formation of thyroid hormone (Astwood, 1945). The therapeutic possibilities of such agents in hyperthyroidism were evident and the substances so used became known as *antithyroid drugs*.

Structure-Activity Relationship. The two goitrogens found in the early 1940s proved to be prototypes of two different classes of antithyroid drugs. These two, with one later addition, made up three general categories into which the majority of the agents can be assigned: (1) *thioureylenes* include all the compounds currently used clinically (Table 60–2); (2) *aniline derivatives*, of which the sulfonamides make up the largest number, embrace a few substances that have been found to inhibit the human thyroid; and (3) *polyhydric phenols*, such as resorcinol, which have caused goiter in man when applied to the abraded skin. A few other compounds, mentioned briefly below, do not fit into any of these categories.

Thioureylenes. Thiourea and its simpler aliphatic derivatives and heterocyclic compounds containing a thioureylene group make up the majority of the known antithyroid agents that are also effective in man. Although most of them incorporate the entire thioureylene group, in some a nitrogen atom is replaced by oxygen or sulfur so that only the thioamide group is common to all. Among the heterocyclic compounds, the sulfur derivatives

Table 60–2. ANTITHYROID DRUGS OF THE THIOUREYLENE TYPE

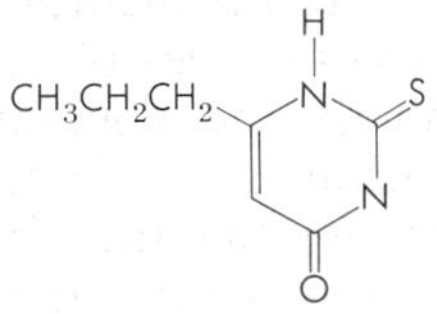

Propylthiouracil

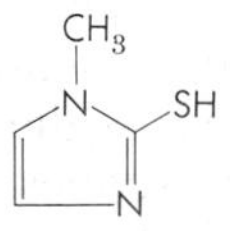

Methimazole

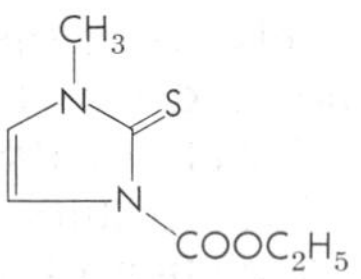

Carbimazole

that are active are representatives of imidazole, oxazole, hydantoin, thiazole, thiadiazole, uracil, and barbituric acid.

Aniline Derivatives. In this group, optimal antithyroid activity in the rat is associated with a para-substituted aminobenzene grouping with or without aliphatic substitution on the amino nitrogen. While sulfathiazole and sulfadiazine possess significant activity, the sulfonamides are not detectably antithyroid in man in doses used clinically. However, aminosalicylic acid, which formerly was given in doses of many grams daily for months, has caused hypothyroidism and goiter.

Polyhydric Phenols. Hypothyroidism and goiter have followed the use of resorcinol in the form of an ointment for the treatment of leg ulcers. Antithyroid activity seems to be associated with meta substitution on the benzene ring with two polar groups.

Individual Compounds of Interest. L-5-Vinly-2-thiooxazolidone (goitrin) is responsible for the goiter that results from consuming turnips or the seeds or green parts of cruciferous plants. These plants are eaten by cows, and the compound is found in cow's milk in areas of endemic goiter in Finland (Arstica *et al.*, 1969); it is about as active as propylthiouracil in man. VanEtten (1969) has reviewed the chemistry of naturally occurring goitrogens.

As the result of industrial exposure, toxicological studies, or clinical trials for various purposes, several other compounds have been noted to possess antithyroid activity. Among compounds used clinically phenylbutazone and thiopental are weakly antithyroid in experimental animals. This is not significant at usual doses in man. However, antithyroid effects in man have been observed from dimercaprol, aminoglutethimide (McLaren and Alexander, 1979), and lithium salts (Schou *et al.*, 1968; Temple *et al.*, 1972).

Mechanism of Action. Antithyroid drugs inhibit the formation of thyroid hormones by interfering with the incorporation of iodine into tyrosyl residues of thyroglobulin; they also inhibit the coupling of these iodotyrosyl residues to form iodothyronines. This implies that they interfere with the oxidation of iodide ion and iodotyrosyl groups. Taurog (1976) proposed that the drugs inhibit the peroxidase enzyme, thereby preventing oxidation of iodide or iodotyrosyl groups to the required active state. Subsequent studies have confirmed that this is, indeed, the mechanism and that the antithyroid drugs bind to and inactivate the peroxidase only when the heme of the enzyme is in the oxidized state (Davidson *et al.*, 1978; Engler *et al.*, 1982). Inhibition of hormone synthesis results, over a period of time, in the depletion of stores of iodinated thyroglobulin as the protein is hydro-

lyzed and the hormones are released into the circulation. Only when the preformed hormone is depleted and the concentrations of circulating thyroid hormones begin to decline do clinical effects become noticeable.

There is some evidence that the coupling reaction may be more sensitive to an antithyroid drug, such as propylthiouracil, than is the iodination reaction (Taurog, 1970). This may explain why patients with hyperthyroidism respond well to doses of the drug that only partially suppress organification.

In addition to blocking hormone synthesis, propylthiouracil also inhibits the peripheral deiodination of thyroxine to triiodothyronine (Geffner *et al.*, 1975; Saberi *et al.*, 1975). Methimazole does not have this effect and, as noted above, can antagonize the inhibition by propylthiouracil. Although the quantitative significance of this inhibition has not been established, it does provide a theoretical rationale for the choice of propylthiouracil over other antithyroid drugs in the treatment of thyroid storm. In this acute situation, a decreased rate of conversion of circulating thyroxine to triiodothyronine would be beneficial.

Absorption, Metabolism, and Excretion. Measurements of the course of organification of radioiodine by the thyroid show that absorption of *effective* amounts of propylthiouracil follows within 20 to 30 minutes after an oral dose. They also show that the duration of action of the compounds used clinically is brief. The effect of a dose of 100 mg of propylthiouracil begins to wane in 2 to 3 hours, and even a 500-mg dose is completely inhibitory for only 6 to 8 hours. As little as 0.5 mg of methimazole similarly stops the organification of radioiodine in the thyroid gland, but a single dose of 10 to 25 mg is needed to extend the inhibition to 24 hours.

Studies with radioactive drugs also reveal rapid absorption of the compounds. The half-life of propylthiouracil in plasma approximates 2 hours, while that for methimazole has been estimated to be between 6 and 13 hours (Marchant *et al.*, 1978). All the useful drugs appear to be concentrated in the thyroid, and methimazole, derived from the metabolism of carbimazole, accumulates after carbimazole is administered (Marchant *et al.*, 1978). Radioactive drugs and metabolites appear largely in the urine.

The antithyroid drugs cross the placenta and can also be found in milk. The use of these drugs during pregnancy is discussed below; women taking these agents should not breast-feed their infants.

Untoward Reactions. The incidence of side effects from propylthiouracil and methimazole as currently used is relatively low. The overall incidence as compiled by VanderLaan and Storrie (1955) from published cases was 3% for propylthiouracil and 7% for methimazole, with 0.44 and 0.12% of cases, respectively, developing the most serious reaction, agranulocytosis. Further observation suggests that there is little, if any, difference in side effects between these two agents, and that an incidence of agranulocytosis of 1 in 500 is a maximal figure. This reaction usually occurs during the first few months of therapy. Since agranulocytosis can develop rapidly, periodic white-cell counts are of little help. Patients should immediately report the development of sore throat or fever, which usually heralds the onset of this reaction. If the drug is discontinued rapidly, recovery is the rule. Mild granulocytopenia, if noted, may be due to thyrotoxicosis or may be the first sign of this dangerous drug reaction. Caution and frequent leukocyte counts are then required.

The most common reaction is a mild, sometimes purpuric, papular rash. It often subsides spontaneously without interrupting treatment but sometimes calls for changing to another drug, since cross-sensitivity is uncommon. Other less frequent complications are pain and stiffness in the joints, paresthesias, headache, nausea, and loss or depigmentation of the hair. Drug fever, hepatitis, and nephritis are very rare.

Preparations and Dosage. The compounds in current use are *propylthiouracil* (6-*n*-propylthiouracil), in the form of 50-mg tablets, and *methimazole* (1-methyl-2-mercaptoimidazole; TAPAZOLE), marketed in 5- and 10-mg tablets. *Methylthiouracil* is not available commercially in the United States at the present time. *Carbimazole* (NEO-MERCAZOLE)

is a carbethoxy derivative of methimazole, which it closely resembles and into which it is converted in the body; it is widely used in Great Britain.

There are no commercial preparations available for parenteral use in the rare event that treatment cannot be given by mouth. For this eventuality and for experimental purposes, the freely water-soluble compound, methimazole, can be dissolved in saline solution and sterilized.

The usual dose of propylthiouracil for the treatment of hyperthyroidism is 75 to 100 mg every 8 hours. In some cases larger doses, up to 1200 mg daily, may be required. Failures of response to treatment with 300 mg daily are sometimes attributable to improper spacing of the doses, since the drug is fully effective for only a few hours. Delayed responses are also sometimes noted when the thyroid is unusually large and when iodine in any form has been given beforehand. When doses larger than 300 mg daily are needed, further subdivision of the time of administration of the daily dose into 4- or 6-hour intervals is perhaps advisable. After the patient is euthyroid, dosage can usually be reduced to one third for maintenance. In mild cases, good control can often be achieved with only one or two daily doses.

The corresponding initial dose of methimazole or carbimazole for the majority of cases is 5 or 10 mg every 8 hours. Because the half-life of methimazole is 6 to 13 hours, this dosage regimen should produce an uninterrupted suppression of the thyroid gland. Methylthiouracil is usually given in a daily dose of 200 mg, divided into two or four equally spaced doses. When a complete response has been achieved, the dose is reduced but the total daily dose is still subdivided. Only when very small amounts are needed is the frequency of dosage reduced to two or even one dose per day.

Therapeutic Uses. The antithyroid drugs are used in the treatment of *hyperthyroidism* in the following three ways: (1) as definitive treatment, to control the disorder in anticipation of a spontaneous remission; (2) in conjunction with radioiodine, to hasten recovery while awaiting the effects of radiation; and (3) to control the disorder in preparation for surgical treatment. There is no uniformity of opinion as to which form of treatment is the most desirable.

Response to Treatment. Hyperthyroidism may be of two kinds, Graves' disease and hyperthyroidism from one or more overfunctioning thyroid nodules; whichever the cause, the hyperthyroidism seems to respond to antithyroid drugs in the same way. After treatment is instituted, there is usually a latent period of a few days to 2 or more weeks before improvement is clearly manifest; however, in a few cases, and particularly when the hyperthyroidism is severe, definite improvement may be seen in 1 or 2 days. In patients with large goiters and particularly if nodular, the response may be slower.

When iodine was commonly used for therapy, it was frequently observed that prior treatment with iodine delayed the response to antithyroid drugs for many weeks. Thus the rate of response is determined by the quantity of stored hormone, the rate of turnover of hormone in the thyroid, and the completeness of the block in synthesis imposed by the dosage given. When large doses are continued, and sometimes with the usual dose, recovery is followed by the development of hypothyroidism. The earliest signs of hypothyroidism call for a reduction in dose; if by chance they have advanced to the point of discomfort, thyroid hormone can be given to hasten recovery. A full dose of 120 to 180 mg daily of thyroid or the equivalent of thyroxine or triiodothyronine for a week will usually suffice. The lower maintenance dose of antithyroid drug discussed above is instituted for continued suppression.

In most cases, treatment with an antithyroid drug requires medical attention only at monthly or bimonthly intervals and adjustment of dosage can be made entirely upon the basis of symptoms and simple clinical signs. If confirmatory tests are desirable, those reflecting the concentration of circulating hormones are the most helpful.

Control of the hyperthyroidism is not associated with further enlargement of the goiter unless hypothyroidism is induced. When this happens, the new enlargement is quickly reversed by giving thyroid hormone. The presumption is, therefore, that thyrotropin is secreted in excessive amounts in response to the hypothyroidism and can be suppressed by thyroid hormone.

Remissions. The antithyroid drugs have been used in many patients to control the hyperthyroidism of Graves' disease until a remission occurs. Solomon and associates (1953) reported that 50% of patients so treated for 1 year remained well without further therapy for long periods, perhaps indefinitely. More recent reports have indicated that a much smaller percentage of patients sustain remissions after such treatment (Wartofsky, 1973; Greer et al., 1977).

Unfortunately, there is no way of predicting before treatment is begun which patients will eventually achieve a lasting remission and which will relapse. It is clear that a favorable outcome is unlikely when the disorder is of long standing, the thyroid is quite large, and various forms of treatment have failed. To complicate the issue further, it is thought that remission and eventual hypothyroidism may represent the natural history of Graves' disease.

During treatment, a fairly certain sign that a remission may have taken place is a reduction in the size of the goiter. The persistence of goiter usually indicates failure, unless the patient becomes hypothyroid. Another favorable indication is continued freedom from all signs of hyperthyroidism when the maintenance dose is small.

The Therapeutic Choice. Because of the low rates of permanent remission of Graves' disease that can be achieved with antithyroid drugs, the majority of patients will eventually require surgery or treatment with radioactive iodine; a 1-year trial of antithyroid agents is not advisable. It may be worthwhile to try prolonged therapy with antithyroid drugs in patients who have minimal enlargement of the thyroid or very mild hyperthyroidism.

Radioiodine or surgery is indicated for definitive therapy in toxic nodular goiter, since spontaneous remissions are not characteristic of this condition.

There is considerable disagreement about the therapy of thyrotoxicosis during *pregnancy.* The antithyroid drugs cross the placenta and can cause fetal hypothyroidism and goiter. Knowledge of thyroid hormone transport to the fetus is poor. There are three choices of therapy; most specialists favor minimal doses of antithyroid drugs. The alternatives are full doses of antithyroid drugs with thyroid hormone supplementation, or surgery. Radioiodine is clearly contraindicated. McLaren and Alexander (1979) have discussed the use of antithyroid drugs in pregnancy and during the neonatal period.

Preoperative Preparation. An important use of antithyroid drugs is in the preparation of the hyperthyroid patient for subtotal thyroidectomy. It is possible to bring virtually 100% of patients to a euthyroid state; as a consequence, the operative mortality for a single-stage thyroidectomy in expert hands is very low. The treatment is continued until the patient is judged to be normal or nearly so, and then iodide is added to the regimen for the 7 to 10 days immediately before the operation. Iodide reduces the vascularity of the gland and makes it less friable, which lessen the difficulties for the surgeon.

Propranolol. This β-adrenergic antagonist does not inhibit the function of the thyroid, but it is useful for the temporary suppression of the signs and symptoms of thyrotoxicosis. As mentioned above, some of the cardiovascular manifestations of hyperthyroidism may be reinforced by the cardiac effects of catecholamines. β-Adrenergic antagonists also reduce the heart rate, tremor, and stare in hyperthyroidism and relieve palpitation, anxiety, and tension. The control of these manifestations is unmistakable and rapid. It is thus valuable in controlling symptoms while awaiting the response to antithyroid drugs or radioiodine, and it is very useful in the rare but potentially lethal complication, thyroid storm (Das and Krieger, 1969). A usual oral dose of propranolol is 20 to 40 mg every 6 hours, but the amount should be adjusted according to the response; the heart rate is a reliable indicator.

IONIC INHIBITORS

The term *ionic inhibitors* serves to designate the substances that interfere with the concentration of iodide ion by the thyroid gland. The effective agents are themselves anions that in some ways resemble iodide ion; they are all monovalent, hydrated anions of a size similar to that of iodide. The most studied example, *thiocyanate*, differs from the others qualitatively; it is not concentrated by the thyroid gland, and in large amounts it inhibits the organification of iodine. Thiocyanate ion is produced following the enzymatic hydrolysis of certain plant glycosides. Thus, the eating of some foods (*e.g.,* cabbage) results in an increased concentration of thiocyanate in the blood and urine. Dietary precursors of thiocyanate may be a contributing factor in endemic goiter in certain parts of the world, particularly when the intake of iodine is very low (Delange and Ermans, 1971).

Wyngaarden and associates (1952) found a number of inorganic ions to be effective in rats; *perchlorate* (ClO_4^-) is ten times as active as thiocyanate and *nitrate* about $\frac{1}{30}$ as active. While perchlorate can be used to control hyperthyroidism, it may cause fatal aplastic anemia and has been abandoned except in very unusual circumstances. Perchlorate can be used to "discharge" inorganic iodide from the thyroid gland in a diagnostic test of organification.

Other ions, selected on the basis of their size, have also been found to be active; fluoborate (BF_4^-) is as effective as perchlorate, whereas fluosulfonate (SO_3F^-) and difluophosphate ($PO_2F_2^-$) are less so (Anbar et al., 1960). Wolff and Maurey (1963) have related the inhibitory properties of a series of anions to their partial molal ionic volumes. A linear relationship was found in the range of 25 to 46 ml per mole, with bromide (Br^-) the smallest and least effective and pertechnetate (TcO_4^-) the largest and most potent. Lithium ion also affects the thyroid and can cause goiter when used therapeutically (*see* Chapter 19).

IODIDE

Iodide is the oldest remedy for disorders of the thyroid gland. Before the antithyroid drugs were used, it was the only substance available for the control of the signs and symptoms of hyperthyroidism. Its use in this way is indeed paradoxical, and the explanation for this paradox is still incomplete.

Response to Iodide in Hyperthyroidism. The response of the patient with hyperthyroidism to iodide is often striking and rapid. The effect is usually discernible within 24 hours, and the basal metabolic rate may fall at a rate comparable to that following thyroidectomy. This provides evidence that the release of hormone into the circulation is quickly interrupted. The maximal effect is attained after 10 to 15 days of continuous therapy when the signs and symptoms of hyperthyroidism may have greatly improved.

The changes in the thyroid gland have been studied in detail; vascularity is reduced, the gland becomes much firmer and even hard to the touch, the cells become smaller, colloid reaccumulates in the follicles, and the quantity of bound iodine increases. The changes are those that would be expected if the excessive stimulus to the gland had somehow been removed or antagonized.

Unfortunately, iodide therapy usually does not completely control the manifestations of hyperthyroidism, and after a variable period of time the beneficial effect disappears. With continued treatment, the hyperthyroidism may return in its initial intensity or may become even more severe than it was at first. It is for this reason that, when iodide was the only agent available for the treatment of hyperthyroidism, it use was usually restricted to preparation of the patient for thyroidectomy.

Mechanism of Action. High concentrations of iodide appear to influence all important aspects of iodine metabolism by the thyroid gland (*see* Ingbar, 1972). The capacity of iodide to limit its own transport has been mentioned above. Acute inhibition of the synthesis of iodotyrosine and iodothyronine by iodide is also well known (the *Wolff-Chaikoff effect*) (Wolff and Chaikoff, 1948). This inhibition is observed only above critical concentrations of iodide, and the intracellular rather than the extracellular concentration of the anion appears to be the major determinant. With time there is "escape" from this inhibition that is associated with an adaptive decrease in iodide transport and a lowered intracellular iodide concentration. The mechanism of the Wolff-Chaikoff effect is not understood. DeGroot and Niepomniszcze (1977) have reviewed the numerous hypotheses that have been proposed as explanations.

The most important clinical effect of high iodide concentration is an inhibition of the release of thyroid hormone. This action is rapid and efficacious in severe thyrotoxicosis. The effect is exerted directly on the thyroid gland, and it can be demonstrated in the euthyroid subject and experimental animals as well as in the hyperthyroid patient.

Iodide antagonizes the ability of both thyrotropin and cyclic AMP to stimulate endocytosis of colloid, proteolysis, and hormone secretion (Pisarev et al., 1971). Several groups of investigators have also reported that iodide attenuates the effect of TSH on the accumulation of cyclic AMP *in vivo* and in isolated tissues (Sherwin and Tong, 1975; Van Sande et al., 1975). Because of the likelihood that cyclic

AMP mediates many, if not all, of the effects of TSH (and presumably the effects of the TSH-imitative immunoglobulins as well), this may help to explain the action of iodide.

Preparations and Dosage. The dosage or form in which iodide is administered bears little relationship to the response achieved in hyperthyroidism, provided not less than the minimal effective amount is given; this dose is 6 mg per day in most, but not all, patients. *Strong iodine solution* (Lugol's solution) is widely used and consists of 5% iodine and 10% potassium iodide. The iodine is reduced to iodide in the intestine before absorption. *Sodium iodide* is available as a 10% solution for intravenous administration. While a dosage of 500 mg of iodide per day is often used, 50 to 150 mg per day seems more reasonable.

Other preparations that contain iodine include several designed for use as antiseptics (*see* Chapter 41) and a large number of compounds that are employed as radiographic contrast media.

Therapeutic Uses. The uses of iodide in the treatment of *hyperthyroidism* are in the immediate preoperative period in preparation for thyroidectomy and in conjunction with antithyroid drugs and propranolol, in the treatment of thyrotoxic crisis. Prior to surgery, iodide is sometimes employed alone, but more frequently it is used after the hyperthyroidism has been controlled by an antithyroid drug. It is then given during the 10 days that immediately antedate the operation. Optimal control of hyperthyroidism is achieved if antithyroid drugs are first given alone. If iodine is also given from the beginning, variable responses are observed; sometimes the effect of iodide predominates, storage of hormone is promoted, and prolonged antithyroid treatment is required before the hyperthyroidism is controlled. These clinical observations may be explained by the ability of iodide to prevent the inactivation of thyroid peroxidase by antithyroid drugs (Davidson *et al.*, 1978).

Iodide salts are also useful *expectorants* when it is desired to liquefy tenacious bronchial secretions, for example, in the later stages of bronchitis, bronchiectasis, and asthma. Potassium iodide is commonly used in a dose of 0.3 g in aqueous solution every 6 hours. Gastrointestinal irritation, anorexia, and vomiting are frequent side effects. The drug should not be administered longer than is actually necessary to "loosen" the cough. However, in some patients with chronic bronchitis or asthma, iodide may be prescribed more or less continuously if it appears to afford relief.

Iodide sometimes aids in the resolution of the granulomatous lesions of tuberculosis, leprosy, syphilis, and various fungal diseases. This does not depend on the effect of iodide on the responsible microorganism. With the advent of more efficacious drugs for the treatment of these diseases, iodide is rarely employed, except in the treatment of sporotrichosis (*see* Seabury and Dascomb, 1964). Another use of iodide is to protect the thyroid after accidental exposure to radioactive isotopes of the element.

Untoward Reactions. Occasional individuals show marked sensitivity to iodide or to organic preparations that contain iodine when they are administered intravenously. The onset of an *acute reaction* may occur immediately or several hours after administration. Angioedema is the outstanding symptom, and swelling of the larynx may lead to suffocation. Multiple cutaneous hemorrhages may be present. Also, manifestations of the serum-sickness type of hypersensitivity, such as fever, arthralgia, lymph node enlargement, and eosinophilia, may appear. Thrombotic thrombocytopenic purpura and fatal periarteritis nodosa attributed to hypersensitivity to iodide have also been described.

The severity of symptoms of *chronic intoxication* with iodide (*iodism*) is related to the dose. The symptoms start with an unpleasant brassy taste and burning in the mouth and throat, as well as soreness of the teeth and gums. Increased salivation is noted. Coryza, sneezing, and irritation of the eyes with swelling of the eyelids are commonly observed. Mild iodism simulates a "head cold." The patient often complains of a severe headache that originates in the frontal sinuses. Irritation of the mucous glands of the respiratory tract causes a productive cough. Excess transudation into the bronchial tree may lead to pulmonary edema. In addition, the parotid and submaxillary glands may become enlarged and tender, and the syndrome may be mistaken for mumps parotitis. There also may be inflammation of the pharynx, larynx, and tonsils. Skin lesions are common, and vary in type and intensity. They usually are mildly acneform and distributed in the seborrheic areas. Rarely, severe and sometimes fatal eruptions (ioderma) may occur after the prolonged use of iodides. The lesions are bizarre, resemble those caused by bromide, and, as a rule, involute quickly when iodide is withdrawn. Symptoms of gastric irritation are common; and diarrhea, which is sometimes bloody, may occur. Fever is occasionally observed, and anorexia and depression may be present. The mechanisms involved in the production of these derangements remain unknown.

Fortunately, the symptoms of iodism disappear spontaneously within a few days after stopping the administration of iodide. The renal excretion of I^- can be increased by procedures that promote Cl^- excretion (*e.g.*, osmotic diuresis, chloruretic diuretics, and salt loading). These procedures may be useful when the symptoms of iodism are severe.

Iodide-Induced Goiter and Myxedema. In a small proportion of individuals given large doses of iodide for long periods, as in the treatment of asthma or chronic bronchitis, goiter and hypothyroidism supervene. The thyroid gland shows hyperplasia and is depleted of stores of iodine. Thyroid hormone corrects the hypothyroidism and causes the goiter to subside, and the same result follows the withdrawal of the iodide.

RADIOACTIVE IODINE

Chemical and Physical Properties. While there are several radioactive isotopes of iodine, greatest use has been made of [131]I. It has a half-life of 8 days, and, therefore, over 99% of its radiant energy is expended within 56 days. Its radioactive emissions include both x-rays and β particles. The short-lived radionuclide of iodine, ^{123}I, emits x-rays with a half-life of only 13 hours. This permits relatively brief exposure to radiation during thyroid scans.

Effects on the Thyroid Gland. The chemical behavior of the radioactive isotopes of iodine is identical to that of the stable isotope, [127]I. [131]I is rapidly and efficiently trapped by the thyroid, incorporated into the iodoamino acids, and deposited in the colloid of the follicles, from which it is slowly liberated. Thus, the destructive beta rays originate within the follicle and act almost exclusively upon the parenchymal cells of the thyroid with little or no damage to surrounding tissue. The x-rays pass through the tissue and can be quantified by external detection. The effects of the radiation depend upon the dosage. When small tracer doses of ^{131}I are administered, thyroid function is not disturbed. However, when large amounts of radioactive iodine gain access to the gland, the characteristic cytotoxic actions of ionizing radiation are observed. Pyknosis and necrosis of the follicular cells are followed by disappearance of colloid and fibrosis of the gland. With properly selected doses of ^{131}I, it is possible to destroy the thyroid gland completely without detectable injury to adjacent tissues. After smaller doses, some of the follicles, usually in the periphery of the gland, retain their function.

Preparations. *Sodium iodide I 131* (IODOTOPE THERAPEUTIC) is available as a solution or in capsules containing ^{131}I suitable for oral administration. Sodium iodide I 131 is essentially carrier free. The information on the label includes the activity at a given hour and date. *Sodium iodide I 123* is available only as an investigational drug.

Therapeutic Uses. Radioactive iodine finds its widest use in the treatment of *hyperthyroidism* and in the *diagnosis of disorders of thyroid function*. Discussion will be limited to the uses of [131]I.

Hyperthyroidism. Radioactive iodine is highly useful in the treatment of hyperthyroidism, and in

many circumstances it is regarded as the therapeutic procedure of choice for this condition.

Dosage and Technic. [131]I is administered orally, either dissolved in half a glass of water or as a capsule. The amount given is so small that it cannot be detected by taste or odor. The effective dose of ^{131}I differs for individual patients. It depends primarily upon the size of the thyroid, the iodine uptake of the gland, and the rate of release of radioactive iodine from the gland subsequent to its deposition in the colloid. To determine these variables insofar as possible, many investigators administer a tracer dose of ^{131}I and calculate the iodine accumulated by the gland and the rate of loss therefrom. The weight of the gland is estimated by palpation. From these data, the dose of isotope necessary to provide from 7000 to 10,000 rads per gram of thyroid tissue is determined. Even when dosage is controlled in this manner, it is difficult to predict the response of an individual to a given amount of the isotope. For these reasons, the optimal dose of ^{131}I, expressed in terms of microcuries taken up per gram of thyroid tissue, varies in different laboratories from 80 to 150 μCi. The usual total dose is 4 to 10 mCi. Lower-dosage ^{131}I therapy (80 μCi/g thyroid) has been advocated to reduce the incidence of subsequent hypothyroidism (Cevallos *et al.*, 1974). While the incidence of hypothyroidism in the early years after such therapy is lower, the ultimate number of patients with late hypothyroidism may go undetected (Glennon *et al.*, 1972).

Course of Disease. The course of Graves' disease in a patient who has received an optimal dose of ^{131}I is characterized by progressive recovery. It is very unusual for any tenderness to be noted in the thyroid region, and most observers have failed to detect any exacerbation of hyperthyroidism from loss of hormone from the damaged gland. Beginning after a variable interval of a few days to a few weeks, the symptoms of hyperthyroidism gradually abate over a period of 2 to 3 months. If therapy has been inadequate, the necessity for further treatment is apparent within 3 months.

Depending to some extent upon the dosage schedule adopted, one half to two thirds of patients are cured by a single dose, one third to one fifth require two doses, and in the remainder three or more doses are needed before the disorder is controlled. Although it is usual to allow only about 3 months to elapse before concluding that an incomplete response calls for another dose, late effects of the radiation make it desirable to wait much longer. But, again, this further delays the recovery.

Propranolol or antithyroid drugs or both can be used to hasten the control of hyperthyroidism while awaiting the full effects of the radioiodine. However, the antithyroid drugs should be withheld for a few days or a week before and after the therapeutic dose of [131]I.

Advantages. The advantages of radioactive iodine in the treatment of Graves' disease are many. No death as a direct result of the use of the isotope has been reported, and only by a gross miscalculation of dose could such an event conceivably occur. In the nonpregnant patient, no tissue other than the thyroid is exposed to sufficient ionizing radiation to be detectably altered. (Nevertheless, the continuing concern about potential effects of radiation on germ cells prompts many specialists to advocate antithyroid drugs or surgery in younger patients who are acceptable operative risks; *see* Dunn, J. T., 1984.) The patient is spared the risks and discomfort of surgery. The incidence of progressive exophthalmos appears to be no different than after surgical treatment. Finally, the cost is low, hospitalization usually is not required, and the patient can indulge in his customary activities during the entire procedure.

Disadvantages. The chief disadvantage of the use of radioactive iodine is the high incidence of delayed hypothyroidism that is induced. Even when elaborate procedures are employed to estimate iodine uptake and gland size, a certain percentage of patients will be overtreated. A distressing feature of this complication is its rising prevalence with the passage of time; the longer the interval after treatment, the higher the incidence. Several analyses of groups of patients treated 10 or more years previously suggest that the eventual rate may exceed 50% (Dunn and Chapman, 1964; Green and Wilson, 1964). However, it now appears that the incidence of hypothyroidism also increases progressively after subtotal thyroidectomy, and such failure of glandular function is suspected to be part of the natural progression of Graves' disease, no matter what the therapy.

Although it is often said that hypothyroidism is not a serious complication because it can so easily be treated with thyroid hormone, its onset may be quite insidious and overlooked for some time. Also, once diagnosed it is difficult to ensure that patients who need the hormone actually take it. Hypothyroidism is obviously a serious complication deserving of painstaking care to make certain that optimal replacement therapy is provided.

Another disadvantage is the long period of time that is sometimes required before the hyperthyroidism is controlled. When a single dose is effective, the response is most satisfactory; however, when multiple doses are needed, it may be many months or a year or more before the patient is well.

Indications. The clearest indication for this form of treatment is hyperthyroidism in older patients and in those with heart disease. Here hyperthyroidism is such a serious disorder that myxedema, as a complication, is of lesser consequence and is correctable. Furthermore, hypothyroidism is not a common sequela following treatment with radioiodine for toxic nodular goiter, the usual cause of hyperthyroidism in the older age group. Radioiodine is also the best form of treatment when hyperthyroidism has persisted or recurred after subtotal thyroidectomy and when prolonged treatment with antithyroid drugs has not led to remission. Other aspects of this problem have been discussed above.

Contraindications. If for no other reason, the risk of hypothyroidism makes radioiodine an unsuitable treatment for hyperthyroidism in childhood. The risk of causing neoplastic changes in the gland has been constantly under consideration since radioiodine was first introduced, and only

small numbers of children have been treated in this way. Indeed, many clinics have declined to treat younger patients for fear of causing cancer and have reserved radioiodine for patients over some arbitrary age, such as 25 to 30 years. Since there is now vast experience with ^{131}I, these age limits are lower than they were in the past. There is no evidence that radioiodine therapy for Graves' disease has caused thyroid or other forms of cancer in adults, although the very large doses that are used to treat cancer may be associated with an increased incidence of leukemia. The use of radioiodine during pregnancy is contraindicated; after the first trimester the fetal thyroid would concentrate the isotope and thus suffer damage, but even during the first trimester radioiodine is best avoided because there may be adverse effects of radiation on fetal tissues.

Hyperthyroidism with Nodular Goiter. It is thought that the risk of inducing hypothyroidism is less in nodular goiter than in Graves' disease, perhaps because of the natural progression of the latter.

Metastatic Thyroid Cancer. Most thyroid carcinomas accumulate very little iodine. However, follicular carcinomas, which comprise 25% of thyroid malignancies, often do so, although they rarely synthesize sufficient hormone to cause thyrotoxicosis. If metastases accumulate iodine, therapy with large doses of ^{131}I may prolong life, particularly in younger patients (Leeper, 1973). In an attempt to stimulate uptake, thyrotropin has been given or secretion of endogenous thyrotropin has been evoked by inducing hypothyroidism by removal or radiation of the thyroid, or by prolonged treatment with antithyroid drugs. The increased uptake thus achieved is usually not large and may be negligible. Moreover, it has been noted by a number of observers that growth of the metastases may be stimulated by these maneuvers, and they have therefore questioned their advisability.

Papillary carcinoma is the most common type of thyroid cancer and may be partially dependent on thyrotropin. Metastatic lesions occasionally regress when thyrotropin secretion is suppressed by administration of thyroid hormone.

Diagnostic Uses. Tracer studies with radioiodine have found wide application in studies of disorders of the thyroid gland. Measurement of the thyroidal accumulation of a tracer dose is helpful in the diagnosis of hyperthyroidism, hypothyroidism, and goiter, and the response of the thyroid to thyrotropin or to suppression by thyroid hormone can be evaluated in this way. Following the administration of a tracer dose, the pattern of localization in the thyroid gland can be depicted by a special scanning apparatus, and this technic is sometimes useful in defining thyroid nodules as functional ("hot") or nonfunctional ("cold") and in finding ectopic thyroid tissue and occasionally metastatic thyroid tumors.

Anbar, M.; Guttmann, S.; and Lewitus, Z. The mode of action of perchlorate ions on the iodine uptake of the thyroid gland. *Int. J. Appl. Radiat. Isot.*, **1960**, *7*, 87–96.

Arstica, A.; Krusius, F.-E.; and Peltola, P. Studies on transfer of thio-oxazolidone-type goitrogens into cow's milk in goiter endemic districts of Finland and in experimental conditions. *Acta Endocrinol. (Kbh.)*, **1969**, *60*, 712–718.

Astwood, E. B. Chemotherapy of hyperthyroidism. *Harvey Lect.*, **1945**, *40*, 195–235.

Biron, R.; Burger, A.; Chinet, A.; Clausen, T.; and Doubois-Ferriere, R. Thyroid hormones and the energetics of active sodium-potassium transport in mammalian skeletal muscle. *J. Physiol. (Lond.)*, **1979**, *297*, 47–60.

Cairoli, V. J., and Crout, J. R. Role of the autonomic nervous system in the resting tachycardia of experimental hyperthyroidism. *J. Pharmacol. Exp. Ther.*, **1967**, *158*, 55–65.

Cevallos, J. L.; Hagen, G. A.; Maloof, F.; and Chapman, E. M. Low-dosage ^{131}I therapy of thyrotoxicosis (diffuse goiters). A five-year follow-up study. *N. Engl. J. Med.*, **1974**, *290*, 141–143.

Chesney, A. M.; Clawson, T. A.; and Webster, B. Endemic goitre in rabbits. I. Incidence and characteristics. *Bull. Johns Hopkins Hosp.*, **1928**, *43*, 261–277.

Cody, V. Role of iodine in thyroid hormones: molecular conformation of a halogen-free hormone analogue. *J. Med. Chem.*, **1980**, *23*, 584–587.

Cody, V., and Duax, W. L. Distal conformation of the thyroid hormone 3,5,3′-triiodo-L-thyronine. *Science*, **1973**, *181*, 757–758.

Cushing, H. *The Pituitary Body and Its Disorders*. J. B. Lippincott Co., Philadelphia, **1912**.

Das, G., and Krieger, M. Treatment of thyrotoxic storm with intravenous administration of propranolol. *Ann. Intern. Med.*, **1969**, *70*, 985–988.

Davidson, B.; Soodak, M.; Neary, J. T.; Strout, H. V.; Kieffer, J. D.; Mover, H.; and Maloof, F. The irreversible inactivation of thyroid peroxidase by methylmercaptoimidazole, thiouracil, and propylthiouracil *in vitro* and its relationship to *in vivo* findings. *Endocrinology*, **1978**, *103*, 871–882.

Delange, F., and Ermans, A. M. Role of a dietary goitrogen in the etiology of endemic goiter on Idjwi Island. *Am. J. Clin. Nutr.*, **1971**, *24*, 1354–1360.

Dunn, A. D. Stimulation of thyroidal thiol endopeptidases by thyrotropin. *Endocrinology*, **1984**, *114*, 375–382.

Dunn, J. T. Choice of therapy in young adults with hyperthyroidism of Graves' disease: a brief, case-directed poll of 54 thyroidologists. *Ann. Intern. Med.*, **1984**, *100*, 891–893.

Dunn, J. T., and Chapman, E. M. Rising incidence of hypothyroidism after radioactive-iodine therapy in thyrotoxicosis. *N. Engl. J. Med.*, **1964**, *271*, 1037–1042.

Dunn, J. T.; Kim, P. S.; and Dunn, A. D. Favored sites for thyroid hormone formation on the peptide chain of human thyroglobulin. *J. Biol. Chem.*, **1982**, *257*, 88–94.

Dunn, J. T.; Kim, P. S.; Dunn, A. D.; Heppner, D. G., Jr.; and Moore, R. C. The role of iodination in the formation of hormone-rich peptides of thyroglobulin. *J. Biol. Chem.*, **1983**, *258*, 9093–9099.

Eiden, L. E., and Ruth, J. A. Acute thyroid hormone increases noradrenergic responsiveness of rat atria *in vitro*. *Eur. J. Pharmacol.*, **1981**, *74*, 91–93.

Engler, H.; Taurog, A.; and Nakashima, T. Mechanism of inactivation of thyroid peroxidase by thioureylene drugs. *Biochem. Pharmacol.*, **1982**, *31*, 3801–3806.

Fain, J. N., and Rosenthal, J. W. Calorigenic action of triiodothyronine on white fat cells: effect of ouabain, oligomycin and catecholamines. *Endocrinology*, **1971**, *89*, 1205–1211.

Fisher, D. A. Screening for congenital hypothyroidism. *Hosp. Pract.*, **1977**, *12*, 73–78.

———. Pediatric aspects. In, *The Thyroid*, 4th ed. (Werner, S. G., and Ingbar, S. H., eds.) Harper & Row, Publisher, Inc., Hagerstown, Md., **1978**, pp. 947–964.

Flink, I. L.; Rader, J. H.; and Morkin, E. Thyroid hormone stimulates synthesis of a cardiac myosin isozyme. Comparison of the two-dimensional electrophoretic patterns of the cyanogen bromide peptides of cardiac myosin heavy chains from euthyroid and thyrotoxic rabbits. *J. Biol. Chem.*, **1979**, *254*, 3105–3110.

Folke, M., and Sestoft, L. Thyroid calorigenesis in isolated perfused liver: minor role of active sodium-potassium transport. *J. Physiol. (Lond.)*, **1977**, *269*, 407–419.

Geffner, D. L.; Azukizawa, M.; and Hershman, J. M. Propylthiouracil blocks extrathyroidal conversion of thyroxine to triiodothyronine and augments thyrotropin secretion in man. *J. Clin. Invest.*, **1975**, *55*, 224–229.

Gilman, A. G., and Rall, T. W. Factors influencing adenosine 3′,5′-phosphate accumulation in bovine thyroid slices. *J. Biol. Chem.*, **1968**, *243*, 5867–5871.

Glennon, J. A.; Gordon, E. S.; and Sawin, C. T. Hypothyroidism after low-dose ^{131}I treatment of hyperthyroidism. *Ann. Intern. Med.*, **1972**, *76*, 721–723.

Gley, E. Sur les effets de l'extirpation du corps thyroide. *C. R. Soc. Biol. (Paris)*, **1891**, *43*, 551–554.

Green, M., and Wilson, G. M. Thyrotoxicosis treated by surgery or iodine-131, with special reference to development of hypothyroidism. *Br. Med. J.*, **1964**, *1*, 1005–1010.

Greer, M. A.; Grimm, Y.; and Studer, H. Qualitative changes in the secretion of thyroid hormones induced by iodine deficiency. *Endocrinology*, **1968**, *83*, 1193–1198.

Greer, M. A.; Kammer, H.; and Bouma, D. J. Short-term antithyroid drug therapy for the thyrotoxicosis of Graves's disease. *N. Engl. J. Med.*, **1977**, *297*, 1973–1976.

Gross, J., and Pitt-Rivers, R. The identification of 3:5:3′-L-triiodothyronine in human plasma. *Lancet*, **1952**, *1*, 439–441.

———. 3:5:3′-Triiodothyronine. 1. Isolation from thyroid gland and synthesis. *Biochem. J.*, **1953a**, *53*, 645–652. 2. Physiological activity. *Ibid.*, **1953b**, *53*, 652–657.

Harington, C. R. Biochemical basis of thyroid function. *Lancet*, **1935**, *1*, 1199–1204, 1261–1266.

Harington, C. R., and Barger, G. Thyroxine. III. Constitution and synthesis of thyroxine. *Biochem. J.*, **1927**, *21*, 169–183.

Hinkle, P. M., and Goh, K. B. C. Regulation of thyrotropin-releasing hormone receptors and responses by L-triiodothyronine in dispersed rat pituitary cell cultures. *Endocrinology*, **1982**, *110*, 1725–1731.

Hoh, J. F. Y.; McGrath, P. A.; and Hale, P. T. Electrophoretic analysis of multiple forms of rat cardiac myosin: effects of hypophysectomy and thyroid replacement, *J. Mol. Cell. Cardiol.*, **1978**, *10*, 1053–1076.

Ingbar, S. H. Autoregulation of the thyroid response to iodide excess and depletion. *Mayo Clin. Proc.*, **1972**, *47*, 814–823.

Jorgensen, E. C. Stereochemistry of thyroxine and analogues. *Mayo Clin. Proc.*, **1964**, *39*, 560–568.

Kendall, E. C. The isolation in crystalline form of the compound containing iodine which occurs in the thyroid: its chemical nature and physiological activity. *Trans. Assoc. Am. Physicians*, **1915**, *30*, 420–449.

Lamas, L.; Dorris, M. L.; and Taurog, A. Evidence for a catalytic role for thyroid peroxidase in the conversion of diiodotyrosine to thyroxine. *Endocrinology*, **1972**, *90*, 1417–1426.

Leeper, R. D. The effect of ^{131}I therapy on survival of patients with metastatic papillary or follicular thyroid carcinoma. *J. Clin. Endocrinol. Metab.*, **1973**, *36*, 1143–1152.

Leonard, J. L., and Rosenberg, I. N. Thyroxine 5′-deiodinase activity of rat kidney: observations on activation by thiols and inhibition by propylthiouracil. *Endocrinology*, **1978**, *103*, 2137–2144.

London, W. T.; Vought, R. L.; and Brown, F. A. Bread— a dietary source of large quantities of iodine. *N. Engl. J. Med.*, **1965**, *273*, 381.

Mackenzie, J. B.; Mackenzie, C. G.; and McCollum, E. V. Effect of sulfanilylguanidine on thyroid of rat. *Science*, **1941**, *94*, 518–519.

Magnus-Levy, A. Über den respiratorischen Gaswechsel unter den Einfluss der Thyroidea sowie unter verschiedenden pathologischen Zustanden. *Berl. Klin. Wochenschr.*, **1895**, *32*, 650–652.

Malbon, C. C.; Graziano, M. P.; and Johnson, G. C. Fat cell β-adrenergic receptor in the hypothyroid rat. *J. Biol. Chem.*, **1984**, *259*, 3254–3260.

Marine, D., and Kimball, O. P. The prevention of simple goiter in man: a survey of the incidence and types of thyroid enlargements in the schoolgirls of Akron, Ohio, from the 5th to the 12th grades, inclusive; the plan of prevention proposed. *J. Lab. Clin. Med.*, **1917**, *3*, 40–48.

Murray, G. R. Note on the treatment of myxedema by hypodermic injection of an extract of the thyroid gland of a sheep. *Br. Med. J.*, **1891**, *2*, 796–797.

Nunez, J., and Correze, C. Interdependent effects of thyroid hormones and cAMP on lipolysis and lipogenesis in the fat cell. *Adv. Cyclic Nucleotide Res.*, **1981**, *14*, 539–554.

Ord, W. M. On myxoedema, a term proposed to be applied to an essential condition in the "cretinoid" affection occasionally observed in middle-aged women. *Med. Chir. Trans. (Lond.)*, **1878**, *61*, 57–78.

Parry, C. H. *Collections from the Unpublished Medical Writings of Dr. C. H. Parry.* Underwood, London, **1895**.

Pisarev, M. A.; DeGroot, L. J.; and Hati, R. KI and imidazole inhibition of TSH and c-AMP induced thyroidal iodine secretion. *Endocrinology*, **1971**, *88*, 1217–1221.

Pisarev, M. A.; DeGroot, L. J.; and Wieber, J. F. Cyclic-AMP production of goiter. *Endocrinology*, **1970**, *87*, 339–342.

Pittman, C. S.; Buck, M. W.; and Chambers, J. B., Jr. Urinary metabolites of ^{14}C-labeled thyroxine in man. *J. Clin. Invest.*, **1972**, *51*, 1759–1766.

Pittman, J. A.; Beschi, R. J.; Block, P., Jr.; and Lindsay, R. H. Thyromimetic activity of 3,5,3',5'-tetramethylthyronine. *Endocrinology*, **1973**, *93*, 201–204.

Psychoyos, S.; Ma, D. S.; Czernik, A. J.; Bowers, H. S.; Atkins, C. D.; Malicki, C. A.; and Cash, W. D. Thyromimetic activity of methylene-bridged thyroid hormone analogs. *Endocrinology*, **1973**, *92*, 243–250.

Richter, C. P., and Clisby, K. H. Toxic effects of bitter-tasting phenylthiocarbamide. *Arch. Pathol.*, **1942**, *33*, 46–57.

Roche, J.; Lissitzky, S.; and Michel, R. Sur la triiodothyronine, produit intermédiare de la transformation de la diiodothyronine en thyroxine. *C. R. Acad. Sci. [D] (Paris)*, **1952a**, *234*, 997–998.

———. Sur la présence de triiodothyronine dans la thyroglobuline. *Ibid.*, **1952b**, *234*, 1228–1230.

Roche, J.; Michel, R.; Michel, O.; and Lissitzky, S. Sur la déshalogénation enzymatique des iodotyrosine par la corps thyroide et sur son rôle physiologique. *Biochim. Biophys. Acta*, **1952c**, *9*, 161–169.

Saberi, M.; Sterling, F. H.; and Utiger, R. D. Reduction in extrathyroidal triiodothyronine production by propylthiouracil in man. *J. Clin. Invest.*, **1975**, *55*, 218–223.

Sandler, M. P.; Robinson, R. P.; Rabin, D.; Lacy, W. W.; and Abumrad, N. N. The effect of thyroid hormones on gluconeogenesis and forearm metabolism in man. *J. Clin. Endocrinol. Metab.*, **1983**, *56*, 479–485.

Sawin, C. T.; Surks, M. I.; London, M.; Chingleput, R.; and Larsen, P. R. Oral thyroxine: variations in biologic

action and tablet content. *Ann. Intern. Med.*, **1984**, *100*, 641–645.

Schou, M.; Amdisen, A.; Jensen, S. E.; and Olsen, T. Occurrence of goitre during lithium treatment. *Br. Med. J.*, **1968**, *3*, 710–713.

Seabury, J. H., and Dascomb, H. E. Results of the treatment of systemic mycoses. *J.A.M.A.*, **1964**, *188*, 509–513.

Sestoft, L. Metabolic aspects of the calorigenic effect of thyroid hormones in mammals. *Clin. Endocrinol. (Oxf.)*, **1980**, *13*, 489–506.

Sherwin, J. R., and Tong, W. Thyroidal autoregulation. Iodide-induced suppression of thyrotropin-stimulated cyclic AMP production and iodinating activity in thyroid cells. *Biochim. Biophys. Acta*, **1975**, *404*, 30–39.

Silva, P.; Torretti, J.; Hayslett, J. P.; and Epstein, F. H. Relation between Na-K-ATPase activity and respiratory rate in the rat kidney. *Am. J. Physiol.*, **1976**, *230*, 1432–1438.

Simmonds, M. Ueber Hypophysisschwund mit todlichem Ausang. *Dtsch. Med. Wochenschr.*, **1914**, *40*, 322–323.

Solomon, D. H.; Beck, J. C.; VanderLaan, W. P.; and Astwood, E. B. Prognosis of hyperthyroidism treated by antithyroid drugs. *J.A.M.A.*, **1953**, *152*, 201–205.

Taurog, A. The mechanism of action of thioureylene antithyroid drugs. *Endocrinology*, **1976**, *98*, 1031–1046.

Taurog, A.; Lothrop, M. L.; and Estabrook, R. W. Improvements in the isolation procedure for thyroid peroxidase: nature of the heme prosthetic group. *Arch. Biochem. Biophys.*, **1970**, *139*, 221–229.

Temple, R.; Berman, M.; Carlson, H. E.; Robbins, J.; and Wolff, J. The use of lithium in Graves' disease. *Mayo Clin. Proc.*, **1972**, *47*, 872–878.

Thilly, C. H.; Delange, F.; Goldstein-Golaire, J.; and Ermans, A. M. Endemic goiter prevention of iodized oil: a reassessment. *J. Clin. Endocrinol. Metab.*, **1973**, *36*, 1196–1204.

VanderLaan, W. P. The biological significance of the iodide-concentrating mechanism of the thyroid gland. *Brookhaven Symp. Biol.*, **1955**, *7*, 30–37.

Van Middlesworth, L. Thyroxine requirement and the excretion of thyroxine metabolites. In, *Clinical Endocrinology I.* (Astwood, E. B., ed.) Grune & Stratton, Inc., New York, **1960**, pp. 103–111.

Van Sande, J.; Grenier, G.; Willems, C.; and Dumont, J. E. Inhibition by iodide of the activation of the thyroid cyclic 3',5'-AMP system. *Endocrinology*, **1975**, *96*, 781–786.

Wartofsky, L. Low remission after therapy for Graves' disease: possible relation of dietary iodine with antithyroid therapy results. *J.A.M.A.*, **1973**, *226*, 1083–1088.

Wolff, J., and Chaikoff, I. L. Plasma inorganic iodide as a homeostatic regulator of thyroid function. *J. Biol. Chem.*, **1948**, *174*, 555–564.

Wolff, J., and Maurey, J. R. Thyroidal iodide transport. IV. The role of ion size. *Biochim. Biophys. Acta*, **1963**, *69*, 58–67.

Wollman, S. H.; Spicer, S. S.; and Burstone, M. S. Localization of esterase and acid phosphatase in granules and colloid droplets in rat thyroid epithelium. *J. Cell Biol.*, **1964**, *21*, 191–201.

Wyngaarden, J. B.; Wright, B. M.; and Ways, P. The effect of certain anions upon the accumulation and retention of iodide by the thyroid gland. *Endocrinology*, **1952**, *50*, 537–549.

Wynn, J., and Gibbs, R. Thyroxine degradation. II. Products of thyroxine degradation by rat liver microsomes. *J. Biol. Chem.*, **1962**, *237*, 3499–3505.

Monographs and Reviews

Baxter, J. D.; Eberhardt, N. L.; Apriletti, J. W.; Johnson, L. K.; Ivarie, R. D.; Schachter, B. S.; Morris, J. A.;

Seeburg, P. H.; Goodman, H. M.; Latham, K. R.; Polansky, J. R.; and Martial, J. A. Thyroid hormone receptors and responses. *Recent Prog. Horm. Res.,* **1979,** *35,* 97–153.

Braverman, L. E., and Vagenakis, A. G. The thyroid. *Clin. Endocrinol. Metab.,* **1979,** *8,* 621–639.

Burman, K. D. Recent developments in thyroid hormone metabolism: interpretation and significance of measurements of reverse T_3, $3,3'T_2$, and thyroglobulin. *Metabolism,* **1978,** *27,* 615–630.

Cooper, D. S. Antithyroid drugs. *N. Engl. J. Med.,* **1984,** *311,* 1353–1362.

DeGroot, L. J., and Niepomniszcze, H. Biosynthesis of thyroid hormone: basic and clinical aspects. *Metabolism,* **1977,** *26,* 665–718.

Dumont, J. E.; Boeynaems, J. M.; Decoster, C.; Erneux, C.; Lamy, F.; Lecocq, R.; Mockel, J.; Unger, J.; and Van Sande, J. Biochemical mechanisms in the control of thyroid function and growth. *Adv. Cyclic Nucleotide Res.,* **1978,** *9,* 723–734.

Feldman, J. M. The practical use of thyroid function tests. *Am. Family Physician,* **1977,** *16,* 159–165.

Hamburgh, M. The role of thyroid and growth hormones in neurogenesis. *Curr. Top. Dev. Biol.,* **1969,** *4,* 109–148.

McLaren, E. H., and Alexander, W. D. Goitrogens. *Clin. Endocrinol. Metab.,* **1979,** *8,* 129–144.

Marchant, B.; Lees, J. F. H.; and Alexander, W. D. Antithyroid drugs. *Pharmacol. Ther. [B],* **1978,** *3,* 305–348.

Merimee, T. J. Thyroid function tests: what they do and do not measure. *Postgrad. Med.,* **1978,** *63,* 113–117.

Morkin, E.; Flink, I. L.; and Goldman, S. Biochemical and physiological effects of thyroid hormones on cardiac performance. *Prog. Cardiovasc. Dis.,* **1983,** *25,* 435–464.

Nunez, J., and Pommier, J. Formation of thyroid hormones. *Vitam. Horm.,* **1982,** *39,* 175–229.

Oppenheimer, J. H. The molecular basis of thyroid hormone action: scattered pieces of a jigsaw puzzle. *Prog. Clin. Biol. Res.,* **1981,** *74,* 45–55.

——. Thyroid hormone action at the nuclear level. *Ann. Intern. Med.,* **1985,** *102,* 374–384.

Rall, J. E.; Robbins, J.; and Lewallen, C. G. The thyroid. In, *The Hormones,* Vol. 5. (Pincus, G.; Thimann, K. V.; and Astwood, E. B.; eds.) Academic Press, Inc., New York, **1964,** pp. 159–439.

Ramsden, D. B., and Hoffenberg, R. The actions of thyroid hormones mediated via the cell nucleus and their clinical significance. *Clin. Endocrinol. Metab.,* **1983,** *12,* 101–115.

Schimmel, M., and Utiger, R. D. Thyroidal and peripheral production of thyroid hormones. *Ann. Intern. Med.,* **1977,** *87,* 760–768.

Taurog, A. Thyroid peroxidase and thyroxine biosynthesis. *Recent Prog. Horm. Res.,* **1970,** *26,* 189–241.

Utiger, R. D. Serum triiodothyronine in man. *Annu. Rev. Med.,* **1974,** *25,* 289–302.

——. Decreased extrathyroidal triiodothyronine production in nonthyroidal illness: benefit or harm? *Am. J. Med.,* **1980,** *69,* 807–810.

VanderLaan, W. P., and Storrie, V. M. A survey of the factors controlling thyroid function, with especial reference to newer views on antithyroid substances. *Pharmacol. Rev.,* **1955,** *7,* 301–334.

VanEtten, C. H. Goitrogens. In, *Toxic Constituents of Plant Foodstuffs.* (Liener, I. E., ed.) Academic Press, Inc., New York, **1969,** pp. 103–142.

Volpe, R. The pathogenesis of Graves' disease: an overview. *Clin. Endocrinol. Metab.,* **1978,** *7,* 3–29.

Wolff, J. Transport of iodide and other anions in the thyroid gland. *Physiol. Rev.,* **1964,** *44,* 45–90.

CHAPTER

61 ESTROGENS AND PROGESTINS

Ferid Murad and Robert C. Haynes, Jr.

The controlled and cyclic formation of estrogens and progesterone is unique to the ovary. These hormones play a vital role in preparing the female reproductive tract for the reception of sperm and implantation of a fertilized ovum. It is of course also well recognized that many features of the female habitus are also influenced by these agents. Current knowledge of the synthesis and action of the ovarian hormones has permitted rational therapeutic intervention in certain diseases. Much more clinical use, however, has been made of agents that can mimic the effects of these hormones and that act as contraceptives.

History. It has long been known that removal of the ovaries results in uterine atrophy and a loss of sexual functions. The hormonal nature of the ovarian control of the female reproductive system was established in 1900 by Knauer when he found that ovarian transplants prevented the symptoms of gonadectomy. This observation was extended by Halban (1900), who showed that, if the glands were transplanted even in immature animals, normal sexual development and function were assured. In 1923, Allen and Doisy devised a simple, quantitative bioassay method for ovarian extracts based upon changes produced in the vaginal smear of the rat. Loewe (1925) first reported a female sex hormone in the blood of various species and, shortly thereafter, Frank and associates (1925) detected an active sex principle in the blood of sows in estrus. Of even greater significance was the discovery by Loewe and Lange (1926) of a female sex hormone in the urine of menstruating women and the observation that the concentration of the hormone in the urine varied with the phase of the menstrual cycle. The excretion of large amounts of estrogen in the urine during pregnancy was also reported (Zondek, 1928). This finding was a boon to the chemists, who soon isolated an active substance in crystalline form (Butenandt, 1929; Doisy *et al.,* 1929, 1930). A few years later its chemical structure was elucidated.

The results of early investigations indicated that the ovary secretes two substances. Beard (1897) had postulated that the corpus luteum serves a necessary function during pregnancy, and supporting evidence was offered by Fraenkel (1903), who showed that destruction of the corpora lutea in pregnant rabbits causes abortion. The contribu-

tions of Corner and Allen (1929) firmly established the hormonal function of the corpus luteum. These investigators showed that the abortion following extirpation of the corpora lutea in pregnant rabbits can be prevented by the injection of luteal extracts.

ESTROGENS

Biosynthesis and Chemistry. The ovary is capable of converting acetate to cholesterol and subsequently to other steroids, as summarized in Figure 61–1. The formation of estrogens by ovarian follicles is regulated by follicle-stimulating hormone (FSH). The effects of this gonadotropin are mediated through the formation and subsequent action of adenosine 3',5'-monophosphate (cyclic AMP). While the actions of this cyclic nucleotide ultimately result in enhanced cleavage of the side chain of cholesterol to yield pregnenolone, the precise mechanism for stimulation of the synthesis of estrogen, as well as other steroids, is unknown. In men, the testis can also produce and secrete small amounts of estradiol and estrone (*see* Chapter 62).

The estrogens are ultimately formed from either androstenedione or testosterone as immediate precursors. The reaction of central importance is the aromatization of ring A. The first step in this reaction involves hydroxylation of C 19, the angular methyl group residing on C 10 of the precursor. Then the newly formed hydroxymethyl group is lost from the nucleus, and ring A is aromatized to yield a phenolic hydroxyl at C 3. In certain pathological conditions, this reaction appears to be defective and the androgenic precursor escapes into the circulation. Some cases of hirsutism and virilism are thought to be caused by this defect.

Of the three main estrogens of human beings, *estradiol-17β* is the most potent and the major secretory product of the ovary; it is readily oxidized to *estrone,* which in turn

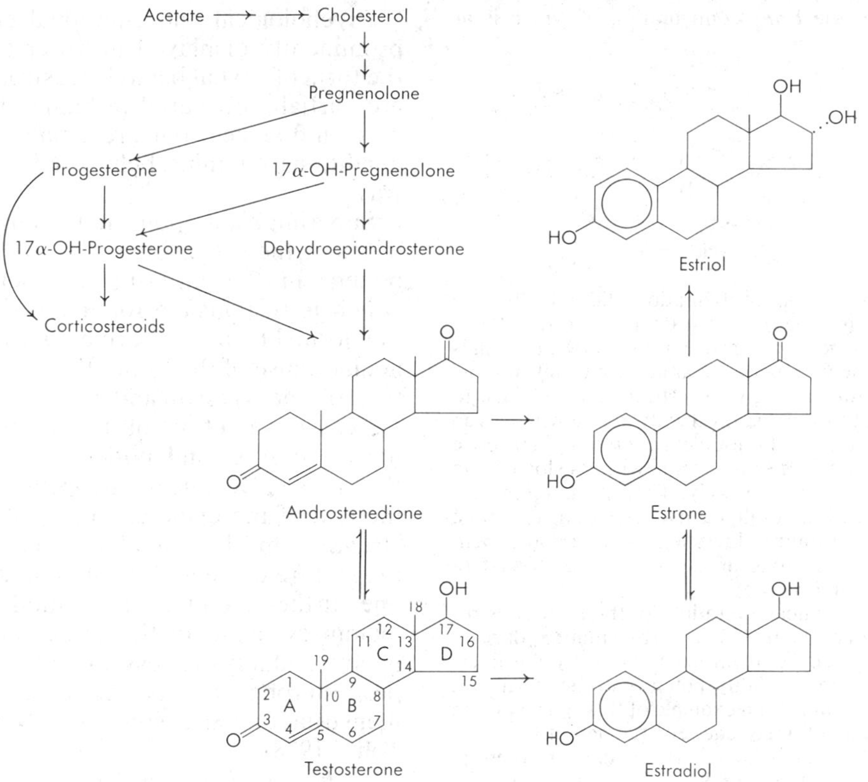

Figure 61–1. *The biosynthetic pathway for the estrogens.* Additional details and structures are shown in Figure 63–3 (page 1465).

can be hydrated to *estriol.* These transformations take place mainly in the liver, where there is free interconversion between estrone and estradiol. All three estrogens are excreted in the urine as glucuronides and sulfates, along with a host of related, minor products in water-soluble complexes. During pregnancy, estrogens are synthesized in large quantities by the placenta by the same enzymatic reactions as occur in the ovary. However, there are complex interactions with the fetus, and the fetal adrenal cortex is required for some synthetic steps that are deficient in the placenta (*see* Kellie, 1971). Human urine of pregnancy is thus an abundant source of natural estrogens. Animals of the genus *Equus,* including the horse, are remarkable estrogen factories. The pregnant mare excretes over 100 mg daily, a record exceeded only by the stallion, who, despite

clear manifestations of virility, excretes into his environment more estrogen than any other living creature.

The formation of estrogens is not limited to the gonads, placenta, and adrenal since peripheral tissues such as liver, fat, skeletal muscle, and hair follicles can form significant quantities of estrogens, particularly estrone, from androstenedione and testosterone (*see* Marcus and Korenman, 1976). This reaction provides a major source of estrogen in males and postmenopausal females, and its contribution to the pool of estrogens is regulated by the availability of the androgenic precursors.

Estrogenic activity is a property shared by a great number of steroidal and nonsteroidal compounds, and many nonsteroidal materials with estrogenic activity have been described in a variety of plants. Among the first nonsteroidal estrogens to be encountered and still the most potent is *diethyl-*

stilbestrol, the *trans* configuration of which is as follows:

Diethylstilbestrol

In this active *trans* configuration, diethylstilbestrol can be seen to be related structurally to the steroidal compounds. Its estrogenic potency in animals varies somewhat with the assay used, but in most tests it is fully as active as estradiol. In contrast to the natural estrogens, it is highly active when given by mouth and the duration of action of a single dose is longer, properties in keeping with its slower rate of degradation in the body. The introduction of a cheap, plentiful, orally active estrogen at a time when the natural products were scarce and expensive was a milestone in the development of effective endocrine therapy.

Certain chemical alterations of the natural estrogens render them effective by mouth, largely through protection from inactivation by the liver. One of the most highly potent estrogens known, *ethinyl estradiol*, is an example of this type wherein the elements of acetylene are attached at C 17. As little as 20 μg daily serves as replacement therapy in the menopause, and 30 to 50 μg may be sufficient to cause withdrawal bleeding. This estrogen and some of its derivatives are widely used and are also incorporated with progesterone-like compounds for regulation of the menstrual cycle and for the control of fertility.

Physiological and Pharmacological Actions. The estrogens are largely responsible for the changes that take place at puberty in girls, and they go a long way toward accounting for the tangible and intangible attributes of femininity. By a direct action, they cause growth and development of the vagina, uterus, and Fallopian tubes. They cause enlargement of the breasts through promotion of ductal growth, stromal development, and the accretion of fat, effects in which pituitary hormones also play a part. They also contribute in a poorly understood manner to molding the body contours, shaping the skeleton, and bringing about changes in the epiphyses of the long bones that condition the puberal spurt in growth and its culmination by fusion of the epiphyses. Growth of axillary and pubic hair and regional pigmentation of the skin of the nipples and areolae and of the genital region are also effects of estrogen.

Psychological and emotional effects, so prominently displayed in lower animals in the form of sexual behavior, estrus, or heat, are partially obscured in human beings by other influences, but presumably estrogen conditions feminine behavior in important ways.

Superimposed upon the feminizing influences of the estrogens is the cyclical component in the intensity of their action, which is responsible for many features of the normal menstrual cycle. During the follicular phase of the cycle, there is proliferation of the vaginal and uterine mucosae, increased secretion of the glands of the uterine cervix, and noticeable fullness of the breasts. Decline in estrogenic activity at the end of the cycle can bring about menstruation and its attendant phenomena. In the mature cycle with ovulation, progesterone further modifies the genital tract and mammary gland in the direction of pregnancy, and it is the cessation of secretion of progesterone that is the determinant of menstruation (Erickson, 1978; Naftolin and Tolis, 1978).

Androgens from the Ovary. A question long of interest is whether the androgens secreted by the normal ovary are physiologically important. Measurements of steroid synthesis by ovarian tissue *in vitro* and fractionation of steroids contained in venous ovarian blood indicate that both testosterone and androstenedione, precursors of estrogens, are normal ovarian secretions. The daily production rates of testosterone and androstenedione in women are about 0.5 and 1.5 mg, respectively (Rosenfield, 1972). Furthermore, studies with rabbit ovary have demonstrated that luteinizing hormone (LH) increases ovarian synthesis and secretion of testosterone (Hilliard *et al.,* 1974).

The complete sexual development that can be brought about by the administration of estrogen alone and the reproduction of all the features of the menstrual cycle (except the ovarian changes) that can be achieved with estrogen and progesterone seem to leave little place for an androgen in the feminine economy. And yet there may be certain features missing when estrogen-progestin therapy replaces ovarian function. The rapid rate of growth at puberty is

hard to explain in view of the limited anabolic and growth-promoting properties of
estrogen. The development of axillary and
pubic hair under the influence of estrogen
alone may not be as complete as it is in the
normal girl, and it may be lacking altogether following therapy with estrogen in
patients with hypopituitarism. When small
doses of androgen are added to the estrogen, growth and distribution of hair on the
body are normal even without the pituitary.
Some aspects of sexual development in
females are thus attributable to adrenal and
ovarian androgens.

Acne, common during puberty in girls, is
closely related to the growth and secretion
of the sebaceous glands. The normal development and function of these structures
cannot be brought about by estrogen or
progesterone, but both can be induced by
the administration of small amounts of androgen. Furthermore, while other treatments are preferred, acne can be effectively
treated and the sebaceous glands caused to
regress by suppressing gonadotropin secretion and ovarian function with estrogen or
with a preparation of an estrogen and a progestin (Briggs, 1976; Kay, 1977).

Although estrogen alone is effective replacement therapy in the menopause, a few
observers believe that a more normal result
is achieved when small amounts of androgen are given as well.

Actions on the Pituitary. The precise
actions of estrogens on the secretory activity of the adenohypophysis have been very
difficult to define. In the normal sexual
cycle of mammals, the structural and the
secretory changes in the ovary are brought
about by the precisely timed and sequential
secretion of gonadotropins from the hypophysis (*see* Franchimont, 1977; Erickson, 1978; Naftolin and Tolis, 1978). The
central mechanisms and events that lead to
the cyclic secretion of gonadotropins and
thereby initiate the onset of puberty and
gonadal development are unknown (Boyer,
1978).

One major difficulty has been the demonstration of a single gonadotropin-releasing
hormone (RH), LH-RH/FSH-RH or Gn-
RH, which increases the pituitary secretion
of both LH and FSH (*see* Chapter 59). The
varying blood concentrations of each go-

nadotropin during the menstrual cycle (Figure 61–2) suggest that another regulatory
hormone might exist to explain the apparent independence of their secretion. However, complex feedback effects of sex steroids and perhaps other gonadal factors on
the pituitary and hypothalamus influence
the secretion and action of Gn-RH, and this
could explain the divergent patterns of release of each gonadotropin. This question is
still open (*see* Schally, 1978).

While generalization is premature, certain interrelations seem definite. As the
ovarian follicle grows under the influence
of FSH, the increasing titer of estrogen that
is produced decreases the release of Gn-RH
and thereby suppresses FSH secretion.
Under the influence of FSH the Graafian
follicle may also secrete *inhibin* or an analogous material that feeds back to decrease
the secretion of FSH (Baker *et al.,* 1975).
Inhibin, a peptide with a molecular weight
of approximately 20,000, was first described in the testis (McCullogh, 1932);
more recently it has been characterized in
cultures of testicular Sertoli cells (Steinberger and Steinberger, 1976) and in ovarian
follicular fluid (DeJong and Sharpe, 1976).
Inhibin suppresses the secretion of FSH
more than it does the secretion of LH.
While estrogens can decrease FSH secretion, they have a biphasic effect on LH.
The rapid swelling of the follicle, culminating in ovulation, is brought about by the
midcycle surge in LH (Figure 61–2), probably due to increased Gn-RH release as well
as to greater estrogen-induced sensitivity of
the pituitary to the regulatory hormone. It
is not known how just one of the many follicles that develop under the influence of
FSH in primates is selected for rupture and
ovulation (Linder *et al.,* 1977; Erickson,
1978).

Progesterone begins to be secreted during the formation of the corpus luteum, and
secretion continues throughout its functional life. The control of the secretion of
the corpus luteum is managed by various
species in quite different ways. In women it
is under the predominant control of LH.

The major mystery is the relatively precise cyclic nature of the pituitary secretion
of gonadotropins and thus ovarian secretion of estrogens and progesterone. In addi-

tion to the more prolonged and larger oscillations in gonadotropins during the menstrual cycle, smaller short-term variations in concentrations of gonadotropins in plasma have been observed in normal women. The significance of the pulsatile secretion that causes these variations is not known.

In contrast, total daily secretion of gonadotropins in men is quite stable, while secretion during the course of the day is variable (Franchimont, 1977). In the male the secretion of both FSH and LH can be inhibited by estrogen and inhibin; as a result, spermatogenesis is arrested, the testicular tubules become atrophic, and the regressive changes in the genital tract show that the secretion of androgen is reduced (*see* Chapter 62).

When the ovaries or testes are removed or cease to function, there is overproduction of FSH and LH, which are excreted in the urine. Measurements of urinary or plasma gonadotropins are valuable clinical

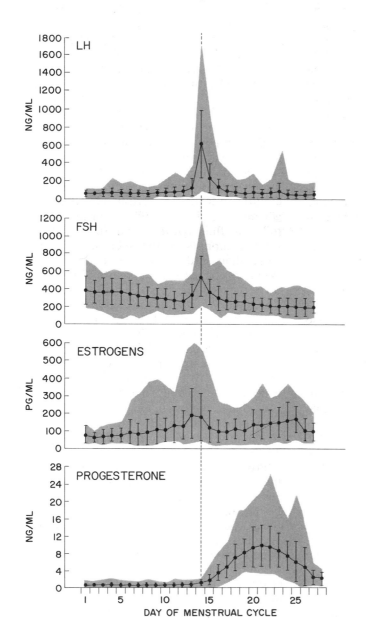

Figure 61–2. *Plasma concentrations of ovarian hormones and gonadotropins in women during normal menstrual cycles.*

Values are the mean ± standard deviation of 40 women. The shaded areas indicate the entire range of observations. Day 1 is the onset of menses. Ovulation on day 14 of the menstrual cycle occurs with the midcycle peak of LH, represented by the dash line. (After Vande Wiele and Dyrenfurth, 1973. Courtesy of *Pharmacological Reviews.* © 1973 The Williams & Wilkins Co., Baltimore.)

tests and can be used to show the effectiveness of replacement doses of estrogen or testosterone, which, in amounts that might be considered physiological, specifically inhibit overproduction.

The regulation of gonadotropin secretion and the actions of FSH and LH are also discussed in Chapter 59.

Estrogens and Menstruation. When the ovaries are not functional or have been removed, menstrual flow can be induced by the administration and subsequent withdrawal of estrogen. Both the size of the dose and the duration of treatment are involved in determining whether bleeding will follow, and, within limits, the two determinants can be varied reciprocally with a similar outcome. Bleeding can be induced by a single large dose or by treatment for several weeks with a much smaller amount. When doses within a certain range are given, menstrual flow (breakthrough bleeding) may ensue even when the treatment is not interrupted. This has been referred to as the "threshold dose."

The action of progesterone upon the estrogen-treated uterus in causing menstruation is quite unrelated to its action in causing the secretory changes seen microscopically. When estrogen is given without interruption, brief treatment with progesterone is followed by menstruation a few days later; as little as 1 mg given in a single dose may be enough, whereas the histological changes in the endometrium require many days to develop.

Menstrual bleeding during continuous treatment with threshold doses of estrogen can be prevented by increasing the dose; however, when a brief treatment with progesterone is introduced, estrogen, even in large doses, will not prevent the ensuing menstruation.

Metabolic Actions. The similarity of the estrogens to the androgens in causing retention of salt and water as well as nitrogen and the elements required for the building of protoplasm is discussed in Chapter 62. Estrogens are weaker anabolic agents than the androgens. Retention of salt and water to the point of causing edema is not a common feature of therapy with estrogen. However, edema may be troublesome when estrogen is given in large doses and particularly if an associated condition predisposes to retention of fluid. While the edema responds well to diuretics, one should discontinue the estrogen if possible. The moderate fluid retention common in the latter half of the menstrual cycle is probably a result of the action of estrogen.

Although estrogens have no effect on fasting plasma glucose concentration, alterations in oral and intravenous glucose tolerance tests may be seen with oral contraceptive agents (Spellacy, 1982; Wynn, 1982); this is discussed below.

Estrogens can cause changes in circulating lipids. They decrease low-density lipoprotein cholesterol and increase that in high-density lipoprotein (Hirvonen *et al.*, 1981; Wahl *et al.*, 1983). These changes may lower the risk of coronary artery disease and contribute to the lower incidence of myocardial infarction in premenopausal women. However, this is by no means clear (*see* below). In addition, the effects of progestins are opposite to those of estrogens (Kalkhoff, 1982; Kay, 1982).

Carcinogenic Action. In several mammalian species, the administration of estrogens is followed by the development of certain tumors. Since the early studies of Lacassagne (1936), it has been known that estrogens can induce tumors of the breast, uterus, testis, bone, kidney, and several other tissues in various animal species. These early studies disseminated a fear of cancer resulting from estrogen use. Until 1971, however, no evidence of a carcinogenic action of estrogens in human subjects had been reported. Since that time there have been many clinical reports of tumors that may be related to estrogens. In the earliest studies (Greenwald *et al.*, 1971; Herbst *et al.*, 1971), an increased incidence of vaginal and cervical adenocarcinoma was noted in female offspring of mothers who had taken diethylstilbestrol or other synthetic estrogens during the first trimester of pregnancy. This has been amply confirmed, and the incidence of clear-cell vaginal and cervical adenocarcinoma in women who were exposed to estrogens *in utero* is estimated to be 0.01 to 0.1% (FDA Drug Bulletin, 1978c). Although most of the affected women have been about 20 to 25 years of age at the time of detection of disease, younger and older individuals have also been affected. Estrogen use during pregnancy can also cause vaginal adenosis (a nonmalignant proliferation of glandular tissue) in female offspring. While males exposed to exogenous estrogens during intrauterine development have an increased incidence of genital abnormalities, tumors have apparently not resulted from such exposure.

Pregnant patients should not be given estrogens, particularly during the first trimester—a time when the fetal reproductive tract is developing and may be influenced by exogenous estrogens.

Data from numerous studies have indicated that the use of estrogen by postmenopausal women is associated with the development of endometrial carcinoma (Smith *et al.*, 1975; Ziel and Finkle, 1975, 1976; Antunes *et al.*, 1979; Jick *et al.*, 1979). The risk is estimated to be increased as much as 5- to 15-fold by estrogen and is related to dose and duration of use. The increased risk declines to normal several years after discontinuation of estrogen. Although epidemiological studies indicate a lower incidence of endometrial carcinoma when low doses of estrogen are administered in a cyclical fashion or when a progestin is also given, adequate prospective studies are not yet available. Also suggested is an apparent association of endometrial carcinoma in premenopausal women with the use of oral contraceptives (Silverberg and Makowski, 1975; Weiss and Sayvetz, 1980). The tumors are usually well differentiated, and the incidence of metastases is low.

Several reports have aroused the suspicion that estrogens or oral contraceptives may increase the incidence of breast tumors (*see* Leis *et al.*, 1976; Kay, 1977). Although numerous factors are associated with an increased risk of breast cancer, some reports have suggested that use of estrogens or oral contraceptives can increase the risk two- to sixfold (Jick *et al.*, 1980; Ross *et al.*, 1980; Lawson *et al.*, 1981). Women who received diethylstilbestrol in pregnancy during the period from 1940 to 1960 were recently found to have a small increase in the incidence of carcinoma of the breast (Greenberg *et al.*, 1984). It should also be noted that many studies have not found an association between use of estrogens and breast cancer.

After a report that the use of oral contraceptives by young women was associated with the occurrence of benign hepatomas (Baum *et al.*, 1973), a number of similar studies have confirmed this relationship. Interestingly, use of estrogens has been associated with a decreased incidence of ovarian tumors.

Mechanism of Action. Considerable progress has been made in the elucidation of the mechanism of action of estrogens (*see* Gorski and Gannon, 1976). Putative receptor proteins for the hormone have been detected in estrogen-responsive tissues (female reproductive tract, breast, pituitary, and hypothalamus). Estrogens are first bound with very high affinity to a cytoplasmic receptor protein. Following modification, the estrogen-protein complex is converted to a species that is translocated to the nucleus, where binding of the estrogen-containing complex to chromatin occurs. As a result of such binding, specific mRNA and certain specific proteins are synthesized. A more general increase in the synthesis of various types of RNA and protein becomes obvious a few hours later, and stimulation of DNA synthesis is an even later event. These effects of estrogens can be blocked by inhibitors of RNA synthesis (dactinomycin) or protein synthesis (cycloheximide). The presence of receptors for estrogen in the tumor cells greatly increases the likelihood of a palliative response to therapy in women with breast cancer (*see* below and Chapter 55).

Absorption, Fate, and Excretion. Estrogens used in therapy are, in general, readily absorbed through the skin, mucous membranes, and gastrointestinal tract. When they are applied for a local action, absorption is often sufficient to cause systemic effects, and in factory workers gynecomastia has followed handling of diethylstilbestrol or other estrogens without gloves, protective garments, and masks. The absorption of most natural estrogens and their derivatives from the gastrointestinal tract is prompt and quite complete. Thus, the limited oral effectiveness of the natural estrogens and their esters is not due to poor absorption but to their metabolism, as discussed below.

The estrogens are practically insoluble in water. When injected dissolved in oil, they are rapidly absorbed and quickly metabolized. The aryl and alkyl esters of estradiol become less and less polar as the size of the substituents increases; correspondingly, the rate of absorption of oily preparations is progressively slowed and the duration of action prolonged. Therapeutic doses of compounds such as estradiol valerate or estradiol cypionate are absorbed over several weeks after a single intramuscular injection.

The estrogens and their esters are handled in the body in much the same way as are the endogenous hormones (*see* Fotherby and James, 1972). Inactivation of estrogen in the body is carried out mainly in the liver. A certain proportion of the estrogen reaching that organ is excreted into the bile, only to be reabsorbed from the intestine. During this enterohepatic circulation, degradation of estrogen occurs through conversion to less active products such as estriol and numerous other estrogens, through oxidation to nonestrogenic substances, and through conjugation with sulfuric and glucuronic acids.

The course of metabolism of *ethinyl estradiol* is different. This compound is active by mouth since its inactivation in the liver and other tissues is very slow. This accounts for the high intrinsic potency of the analog. Similarly the nonsteroidal estrogens are slowly degraded in the body.

The natural estrogens circulate in the blood in association with sex hormone–binding globulin and albumin (Heyns, 1977). A significant proportion of the estrogen is in the form of conjugates, particularly sulfate. These water-soluble conjugates are strong acids and are thus fully ionized in the body fluids; penetration into cells is therefore limited, and excretion by the kidney is favored.

As mentioned above, endogenous estrogens appear in the urine as glucuronides and sulfates of estradiol, estrone, and estriol. Small quantities of a great many other derivatives have also been identified. In the normal menstrual cycle the mean daily excretion of estrogens at the midcycle ovulatory maximum is 25 to 100 μg; the second rise during the luteal phase is more prolonged, but the maximal rates of excretion are somewhat smaller (10 to 80 μg). After the menopause the average excretion of estrogens in normal women totals about 5 to 10 μg daily. As noted above, these estrogens are synthesized from androgenic precursors by nonovarian tissues. The values for normal men average 2 to 25 μg per day, quantities about equal to the urinary estrogens of women during the first week of the menstrual cycle. In young children none is detectable. During the first trimester of pregnancy the placenta becomes the primary source of the urinary estrogens, which continue to increase and reach levels of about 30 mg per day near term. Their serial determination can be used to assess placental and fetal function.

Assays. Most biological assays for estrogen are based upon the original method of Allen and Doisy (vaginal cornification in the spayed rat or mouse) or upon growth of the uterus. The vaginal response is highly specific, and almost by definition a substance giving rise to a cornified vaginal smear is an estrogen. The test is influenced by other factors, however, and it is inhibited by progesterone and androgen; for this reason, tests on compounds of mixed activity may be difficult to interpret. Most tests based upon the increased weight of the uterus are less specific than the vaginal smear.

Local application of substances to the vagina of spayed animals also provides a very sensitive test for estrogen. With the natural estrogens the test is several hundred times more sensitive than tests based on subcutaneous injection, and the method is especially valuable for the assay of biological materials.

Compared to various bioassay methods, competitive protein-binding and radioimmunoassay methods are generally simpler and faster (*see* Vande Wiele and Dyrenfurth, 1973). Since they also usually offer a high degree of sensitivity and specificity, such methods have become routine procedures in many clinical laboratories. However, the immunoassay methods are not useful for studying structure-activity relationship, and it is unlikely that bioassay and sensitive receptor-protein methods will be displaced in research laboratories.

Preparations. Several widely used, orally active nonsteroidal estrogens are available. The most popular have been preparations of *diethylstilbestrol,* available in tablets containing from 0.1 to 5 mg; suppositories containing 0.1 or 0.5 mg are also marketed for vaginal use. *Diethylstilbestrol diphosphate* (STILPHOSTROL) is available as an injection and in 50-mg tablets.

Estradiol is available as 1- and 2-mg tablets of micronized estradiol (ESTRACE) and in the form of various esters. *Estradiol valerate* and *cypionate* are prepared in oil for slow release after intramuscular injection. These preparations contain 1 to 40 mg/ml and are sold under various trade names (*e.g.,* DELESTROGEN). *Polyestradiol phosphate* (ESTRADURIN) is also available for intramuscular use in prostatic carcinoma.

Estrone is the major component of a number of preparations. These include *estrone aqueous sus-*

pension (injections) and *estrogenic substance* (aqueous or oily suspensions; injections). *Estropipate* is crystalline estrone sulfate stabilized with piperazine. It is marketed in tablets containing 0.625 to 5 mg (OGEN). *Conjugated estrogens* (PREMARIN) contain 50 to 65% sodium estrone sulfate and 20 to 35% sodium equilin sulfate. They are available in oral (0.3 to 2.5 mg) and injectable preparations, and as a vaginal cream containing 0.625 mg/g. *Esterified estrogens* (MENEST) contain 75 to 85% sodium estrone sulfate and 6 to 15% sodium equilin sulfate in tablets of 0.3 to 2.5 mg.

Ethinyl estradiol (ESTINYL, FEMINONE) is the most active oral preparation, and the tablets contain 0.02 to 0.5 mg. It is roughly 20 times as potent as diethylstilbestrol. The 3-methyl ether of ethinyl estradiol, *mestranol*, is inactive until it is converted to ethinyl estradiol in the body. Both of these estrogens are widely used in the combination oral contraceptives (*see* below). *Quinestrol* (ESTROVIS) is the 3-cyclopentyl ether of ethinyl estradiol. Since it is stored in fat and released slowly, it can be taken orally once per week in doses of 0.1 to 0.2 mg. It is available in 0.1-mg tablets.

Chlorotrianisene (TACE) is a long-acting oral preparation because of sequestration in adipose tissue and, therefore, is not widely used. It is available in 12-, 25-, and 72-mg capsules and has about one eighth the activity of diethylstilbestrol.

A number of preparations in which estrogen is combined with another agent are also available. Oral contraceptives containing an estrogen and a progestin are discussed later in the chapter. There are no compelling reasons to use formulations of estrogens combined with androgens or antianxiety preparations.

A variety of topical preparations in creams and suppositories are no longer widely used. However, *senile vaginitis* and *kraurosis vulvae* may be effectively treated with such topical preparations. Many of the "over-the-counter" cosmetics and creams that contained estrogens have been removed from the United States market in recent years. While frequent and excessive topical use of estrogens can cause systemic effects, these are minimal when they are used as directed. Intravaginal use of some preparations can lead to significant concentrations of estrogen in blood, since the estrogen is readily absorbed and the initial circulation through the liver is bypassed with this route of administration (Rigg *et al.*, 1978).

Choice of Preparations. Claims have been made that some preparations of estrogen cause fewer side effects than others. However, the prevailing information suggests that all estrogenic materials can cause the same spectrum of side effects. The following parenteral dosages of some estrogens are approximately equivalent: estradiol, 50 μg; ethinyl estradiol, 50 μg; mestranol, 80 μg; diethylstilbestrol, 5 mg; conjugated estrogens, 5 mg. The choice of

preparation is largely determined by cost and convenience to the patient. By all odds oral therapy is the best; the action begins promptly, and treatment can be terminated at will. However, the relative potencies summarized above must be modified to account for diminished efficacy of some agents when given orally; such is the case with estradiol. With substances such as diethylstilbestrol or ethinyl estradiol, which are not quickly inactivated, a single dose each day is usually sufficient. Conjugated natural estrogens are less effective. Parenteral therapy has little to recommend it; frequent injections can be avoided by the use of a long-acting preparation, but then the onset and cessation of action are slow, gradual, and uncertain. The long-acting esters given by injection may be useful for long-continued treatment with large doses in the therapy of patients with cancer. The esters are unsuitable in the management of menstrual disorders or as replacement therapy in menopause when cyclic therapy is desirable; the action slowly declines in a way that is quite unlike the prompt cessation of secretion characteristic of the normal menstrual cycle. Cyclic therapy can be accomplished by interruption of dosage for 1 week per month. As noted below, a progestin may be added to the therapeutic regimen to diminish the incidence of endometrial carcinoma in postmenopausal women. However, the use of progestin may cause other side effects. In premenopausal women the addition of a progestin ensures a more normal menstrual period when estrogen and progestin are terminated together intermittently.

Untoward Responses. The most frequent unpleasant symptom attending the use of estrogen is *nausea*. With large doses there may also be anorexia and even vomiting and mild diarrhea. The nausea is of a peculiar type that seldom interferes with eating and does not cause a loss of weight; it may be noted at various times of the day but, like the "morning sickness" of early pregnancy, it is often troublesome at breakfast time. With continued treatment the symptom usually disappears, and only rarely is it so distressful that treatment must be stopped. Even when very large doses are given, as in the treatment of cancer of the breast, nausea is generally troublesome only for the first 1 or 2 weeks. The symptom can usually be avoided by starting with a small dose and gradually increasing it. Statements that certain preparations are less apt to cause nausea than others may be viewed with skepticism. Other untoward responses are discussed below, under oral contraceptives.

Therapeutic Uses. *Oral Contraception.* A major use of estrogens is in combination with progestins as oral contraceptives; such use is discussed in a separate section later in this chapter.

Menopause. At a variable age, but usually in the late 40s to early 50s, the functions of the ovaries decline. Ovulation is lost first, and anovulatory cycles may continue for 1 or 2 years before menstruation ceases altogether. Irregular menstrual cycles are particularly prevalent at this time due to deficient or poorly cycling estrogen and diminished progesterone soon thereafter. Lack of appreciation of the endocrine basis of the menstrual disturbance usually leads to the conclusion that some mechanical factor, such as fibroid tumors, is at fault.

The decline in the secretion of estrogen by the ovary is a slow and gradual process that continues for some years after menstruation has ceased (see Eskin, 1978). It is a frequent observation that menopausal symptoms are more severe following abrupt removal of estrogen, such as with oophorectomy, than with the natural menopause. Sometimes hot flashes appear for the first time or become more intense if the ovaries are removed after the menopause. The formation of small quantities of estrogens from androgenic precursors by nonovarian tissues may be important in slowing the estrogen withdrawal and the onset of menopausal symptoms in some patients (*see* above).

The decline in ovarian function at the menopause is associated with vasomotor symptoms in about 85% of women. The symptoms are clearly due to deficiency of estrogen. The characteristic hot flashes may alternate with chilly sensations, inappropriate sweating, and paresthesias, including formication. A variety of other symptoms often occur during menopause and include muscle cramps, myalgias, arthralgias, anxiety, overbreathing, palpitation, dizziness, faintness, and syncope. These symptoms may or may not be associated with estrogen deficiency. A few women become chronic invalids and experience years of ill health; some feel genuinely miserable and lack vigor and initiative; many, obviously, tolerate the event quite well. The symptoms lessen and disappear with time. However, about 15 to 25% of menopausal women will seek medical advice or treatment.

Treatment with estrogen is specific and effective. Replacement therapy clearly relieves the hot flashes and other vasomotor symptoms and atrophic vaginitis (*see* Ryan, 1982). The lowest dose needed varies somewhat but can easily be determined by trial. The dose of diethylstilbestrol is about 0.2 to 1 mg once daily by mouth; 0.5 mg is seldom sufficient to cause withdrawal bleeding, 1 mg daily for several weeks sometimes causes bleeding when stopped, and 2 mg often does. Comparable doses of ethinyl estradiol are 0.01 to 0.05 mg; conjugated estrogens may be used in doses of 0.3 to 1.25 mg daily. Therapy with estrogen is best given in a cyclic manner, 3 weeks of treatment followed by 1 week without treatment. If withdrawal bleeding is going to occur, it will begin toward the end of the week of no treatment and the estrogen can be resumed before this induced menstrual period ceases. Menopausal symptoms usually do not return in full intensity during the week without treatment. Occasionally during cyclic therapy with estrogen alone uterine bleeding may continue in an irregular manner after estrogen is resumed. Larger doses of estrogen have been employed to control this bleeding, but the use of a progestin is more uniformly effective. Once a progesterone-withdrawal period has been induced, there may be no further trouble from the use of estrogen alone for many months. While a few physicians prescribe a small dose of androgen along with estrogen, most prefer not to administer any androgen.

Senile or *atrophic vaginitis,* often associated with chronic infection of the atrophic structures, responds well to estrogen. Estrogens are more effective in *preventing* than in reversing atrophic changes of the vagina and the decrease in skin turgor (*see* Eskin, 1978). *Kraurosis vulvae,* a distressingly itchy condition due in part to deficiency in estrogen and in part to scratching and other as-yet-unknown factors, is favorably influenced by estrogen supplemented by local treatment, including the application of adrenocorticosteroids.

Some physicians are disinclined to prescribe estrogens in the menopause; they feel that the symptoms are largely emotional in origin and are better managed by reassurance and with the use of small doses of a sedative. Others prescribe estrogens for periods of months or a few years only. Physicians with these views are undoubtedly concerned about the possible minor and serious side effects of estrogens in light of very little evidence to demonstrate their efficacy in preventing the more serious physical disorders accompanying menopause, such as atherosclerosis. However, indefinite systemic replacement in all menopausal patients, advocated by some, is certainly unwise and unnecessary and may introduce more undesirable effects than the symptomatic improvement warrants. The major indication for replacement therapy is prevention of osteoporosis, as discussed below. Patients receiving estrogens should be examined every 6 to 12 months for possible side effects, and abnormal uterine bleeding should be investigated. Most agree that the risk-to-benefit ratio for estrogen therapy needs to be evaluated for each patient and should be reconsidered periodically; when used, estrogens should be administered in the lowest effective dose for the shortest possible time, and cyclic therapy is preferred.

Pregnancy. In the past, large doses of estrogens have been given during pregnancy in attempts to prevent threatened or habitual abortion or because of abnormalities of urinary estrogen excretion in toxemia of pregnancy. There is little evidence that such uses are of any value. Because of this and the risk of producing vaginal tumors in female offspring and possible teratogenic effects in male offspring (*see* above), *the use of estrogens in pregnancy is not indicated*. The use of progestins in this condition is discussed below.

Dysmenorrhea. Sturgis and Albright (1940) reported the relief of dysmenorrhea by inhibiting ovulation with estrogen. While the mechanisms are not fully understood, such treatment was widely used. Cyclic therapy with an estrogen can often be used successfully month after month if too long an interval is not permitted to elapse between courses. The additional use of an orally active progestin facilitates management. The disorder is probably due to uterine production of prostaglandins; nonsteroidal anti-inflammatory agents are effective and are currently the preferred form of therapy (*see* Chapter 29).

The use of estrogens in the treatment of *endometriosis* is discussed in connection with the therapeutic uses of progestins.

Dysfunctional Uterine Bleeding. This disorder usually occurs at the time of menarche or menopause and results from anovulatory cycles, with continuous secretion of estrogen and endometrial hyperplasia. Insufficient secretion of progesterone results in incomplete sloughing of the proliferative endometrium and excessive bleeding. While estrogen can be used with some success, the cyclic use of a progestin is logically preferred (*see* below).

Failure of Ovarian Development. There are several unusual conditions in which the ovaries do not develop and, in consequence, puberty does not occur. In *ovarian dysgenesis* with dwarfism (Turner's syndrome) diagnosis can often be made before the age of puberty by the associated congenital anomalies and the stature. Therapy with estrogen at the appropriate time replicates the events of puberty, except for the spurt in growth and, of course, the changes in the ovary. The genital structures grow to normal size. The breasts develop, there is growth of axillary and pubic hair, and the body assumes the normal feminine contour. Also, androgens have been used successfully to promote growth (*see* Chapter 62). It is common practice to start with small doses of estrogen, such as 0.2 to 0.5 mg of diethylstilbestrol or 0.02 mg of ethinyl estradiol, and then increase the dose slowly over a year or so before initiating menstrual periods by cyclic treatment with larger doses. It is felt that there may be some merit in thus imitating the normal sequence of events at puberty.

Failure of ovarian development is also a part of the picture of *hypopituitarism* in childhood. Deficiency of the thyroid and the adrenal cortex is easily corrected with replacement therapy, and the failure of sexual development is treated with estrogen as outlined just above. If human growth hormone is used, these girls can achieve a normal adult stature (*see* Chapter 59). Treatment with estrogen at the normal age of puberty can be expected to cause a small acceleration of growth, but the addition of small doses of androgen has a greater growth-promoting effect, as noted in Chapter 62. While estrogens and androgens promote bone growth, they also accelerate epiphyseal fusion, and their premature use can thus result in a shorter ultimate height. Indeed, estrogens have been used in high doses to accelerate epiphyseal closure in tall girls; to be effective, estrogen must be given prior to menarche. This use of estrogen is rarely, if ever, indicated (*see* Wentz, 1977).

Acne. The common form of acne is a feature of puberty in both sexes, and androgens seem to be the essential factor, operating through stimulation of sebaceous glands. Treatment with estrogen is effective in both sexes by suppressing gonadotropins and gonadal androgen secretion, but its usefulness in the male is obviously limited. In young women estrogen is effective therapy in doses designed to suppress the ovary and may be continued with benefit for many months in cyclic fashion. One of the combined oral contraceptive agents is more convenient. It may be given in the same manner as when used to prevent ovulation. However, tretinoin (all-*trans*-retinoic acid) and antibiotics are preferred (*see* Melski and Arndt, 1980); isotretinoin is given orally for severe cystic acne (*see* Chapter 67).

Hirsutism. In most instances, excessive growth of body hair in women cannot be traced to an endocrine cause, but occasionally a mild androgenic influence of ovarian or adrenal origin is suspected. When suppression of the adrenal cortex by the administration of a corticosteroid is ineffectual, suppression of the ovary with an estrogen may be worthwhile. Concentrations of androgens in plasma should be measured and the response to treatment determined. If it is to be tried, suppression of the ovary for about a year with continuous therapy may be needed before it can be ascertained whether the maneuver is successful. Doses of about 2 mg daily of diethylstilbestrol or its equivalent are sufficient. Menstrual periods during this time can be evoked at intervals by cyclic use of an oral progestin, with preference for a progestin that has little androgenic activity.

Prevention of Heart Attacks. In view of the favored position of women in the incidence of fatal myocardial infarction, estrogen therapy has been tried as a prophylactic measure in men. A large-scale study was conducted by the Coronary Drug Project Research Group. The administration of conjugated estrogens daily led to an *increased* incidence of cardiac and thromboembolic complications (Coronary Drug Project Research Group, 1970, 1973). Although the use of estrogen in the form of combination oral contraceptives also increases the incidence of morbidity and mortality from myocardial infarction in premenopausal women (*see* below), the administration of estrogen to postmenopausal women has not been associated with an increased incidence of complications from coronary artery disease (Rosenberg *et al.*, 1976). There is thus no evidence that administration of estrogen delays the progression of atherosclerosis, a previous notion that contributed to their excessive use in postmenopausal women (*see* Weinstein, 1980; Ryan, 1982).

Osteoporosis. Osteoporosis is a disorder of the skeleton associated with the loss of both hydroxyapatite (calcium phosphate complexes) and protein matrix (colloid). The result is thinning and weakening of the bones and an increased incidence of fractures, particularly compression fractures of the vertebrae and fractures of the hip and wrist from minimal trauma. In older patients it is called *senile osteoporosis* and affects both sexes. Coming after menopause it is referred to as *postmenopausal osteoporosis* and occurs in about one third of such women. Unfortunately, substantial bone loss must occur before it can be detected with routine radiographic procedures. Many different methods of treatment have been tried with the aim of increasing bone density and substance. After several months of estrogen replacement in postmenopausal patients, calcium balance becomes positive and bone resorption decreases to normal (Thalassinos *et al.*, 1982). The effects of estrogens in preventing postmenopausal bone loss are dose related. While the equivalent of 15 μg of ethinyl estradiol daily can prevent vasomotor symptoms in menopause, doses of 15 to 25 μg daily are required to prevent bone loss and 25 μg or more per day can result in a net increase in bone density (Horsman *et al.*, 1983). The positive effects of estrogen on calcium balance and bone density are reversed rapidly when treatment is discontinued (Aloia *et al.*, 1985).

The prophylactic effect of estrogen in this condition appears greatest if hormone is given before significant osteoporosis occurs (*see* Gordon, 1978). However, since only 35% of postmenopausal patients develop osteoporosis and because exercise and increased intake of calcium may be equally effective, the routine prophylactic use of estrogen is difficult to justify. In women who have undergone oophorectomy and hysterectomy, such use of an estrogen is more defensible, since one of the possible toxicities, endometrial carcinoma, is no longer an issue. Indeed, the risk-to-benefit ratio is most favorable in this situation (Weinstein, 1980; Richelson *et al.*, 1984). Androgens are less effective than estrogens in the treatment of postmenopausal osteoporosis, but they may be more effective in preventing osteoporosis induced by glucocorticoids (*see* Gordon, 1978). The use of androgens is discussed in Chapter 62, and the use of vitamin D, calcitonin, and fluoride is discussed in Chapter 65.

Breast Cancer. Many carcinomas of the breast are dependent upon the proper hormonal environment for their growth. About 50 to 65% of all breast cancers possess cytosolic estrogen receptors. Alteration of the hormonal environment can be used as a palliative measure in the therapy of metastatic breast cancer. Removal of estrogen by oophorectomy or the administration of antiestrogens (*see* below) or the administration of estrogens themselves can prolong both the quality and duration of life. Favorable responses can be obtained in about 60 to 70% of patients if estrogen or progesterone receptors are present in the tumor, while such re-

sponses are observed in only 10 to 20% if receptors are absent (McGuire, 1975; Kiang *et al.*, 1978; Legha *et al.*, 1978; Clark *et al.*, 1983). This subject is discussed in more detail in Chapter 55.

Prostatic Carcinoma. Since the prostate is a target organ for the actions of androgens, the inhibition of androgen secretion can be used as palliative therapy in patients with metastatic prostatic carcinoma. This can be accomplished by orchiectomy and/or the administration of an estrogen such as diethylstilbestrol. Leuprolide (Gn-RH) appears to be as effective as diethylstilbestrol, and administration of the peptide (1 mg subcutaneously, daily) is associated with fewer side effects (Leuprolide Study Group, 1984). This topic is discussed further in Chapter 55.

Suppression of Post-Partum Lactation. Estrogens, progestins, and androgens have been used to decrease milk production in the post-partum period. However, their use for this purpose has decreased in recent years, since the incidence of painful engorgement is low and this is readily controlled with analgesics.

ANTIESTROGENS

The term *antiestrogen* has been rather broadly applied to several different types of compounds that inhibit or modify the action of estrogen. Progestins and androgens have been described as antiestrogenic; some weak estrogens are antiestrogenic by some criteria, and certain compounds are antiestrogenic when applied locally to the responsive tissue. Two compounds with prominent antiestrogenic activity are currently available for clinical use in the United States—*clomiphene* and *tamoxifen*. The antiestrogens have been reviewed by Jordan (1984).

These highly effective inhibitors of estrogen came from an unexpected direction. The weakly estrogenic compound *chlorotrianisene* (Table 61–1), unlike most estrogens, was noted not to cause enlargement of the pituitary when given to rats in large doses. Estradiol normally causes pronounced enlargement of the pituitary, but when chlorotrianisene was given concurrently the effect was greatly reduced (Segal and Thompson, 1956). The related, nonestrogenic compound *ethamoxytriphetol* was found to be strikingly antiestrogenic. It inhibited endogenous estrogen as well as estrogen given in the form of the natural compounds, diethylstilbestrol, or chlorotrianisene. More extensive human studies have been carried out with the related compounds *clomiphene, tamoxifen,* and *nafoxidine.*

Pharmacological Effects. Initial animal tests with clomiphene showed very slight estrogenic activity and moderate antiestrogenic activity. The striking effect was inhibition of the pituitary's gonadotropic function. Thus, in both sexes the compound was a potent contraceptive. When given to women, however, the most prominent effect was impressive enlargement of the ovaries. Properly applied, the compound has proven to be a most remarkable and useful agent for the treatment of infertility. Greenblatt and coworkers (1962) made extensive and careful studies and found that ovulation could be induced in a high proportion of patients with amenorrhea, the Stein-Leventhal syndrome, and dysfunctional uterine bleeding with anovulatory cycles. Pregnancy followed in a significant number of cases when infertility had been the problem. Excessive enlargement of the ovaries and the formation of ovarian cysts were common features of the treatment when doses of 100 to 200 mg daily were given for 2 or 3 weeks, but with doses of 50 or 75 mg daily this complication was less frequent and the ovaries returned to normal size after treatment had been completed. The substance gave evidence of antiestrogenic effects. Hot flashes were experienced by some patients, vaginal cornification in precocious puberty in young girls was inhibited, and in one case suppression of ovulation with ethinyl estradiol was prevented by clomiphene. There was no clinical evidence of progestational or androgenic effects.

Mechanism of Action. The nonsteroidal compounds in Table 61–1 have some structural similarities to estrogens, which may explain their actions. Clomiphene and related antiestrogens bind to cytoplasmic estrogen receptors, and the modified complex is translocated to the nucleus. Such competition for estrogen binding sites and the resultant diminished amount of estrogen receptor that is available for endogenous hormone explain their antiestrogenic activity (Kato *et al.*, 1968; Legha *et al.*, 1978; Marshall, 1978; Jordan, 1984). Antiestrogens prevent the normal "feedback inhibition" of control of estrogen synthesis in the hypothalamus and pituitary, and this causes an increased secretion of Gn-RH and gonadotropins. The formation of large and cystic ovaries is the result of increased

Table 61–1. STRUCTURAL RELATIONSHIP OF CHLOROTRIANISENE AND THE ANTIESTROGENS

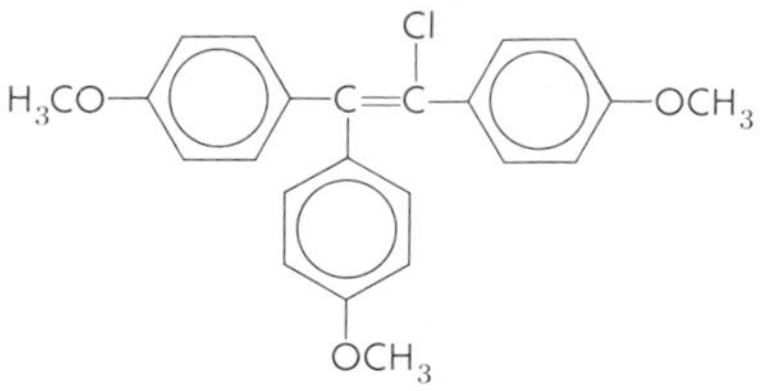

Chlorotrianisene

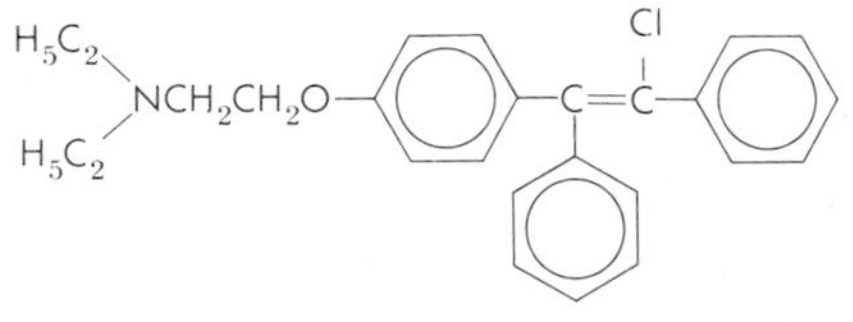

Clomiphene

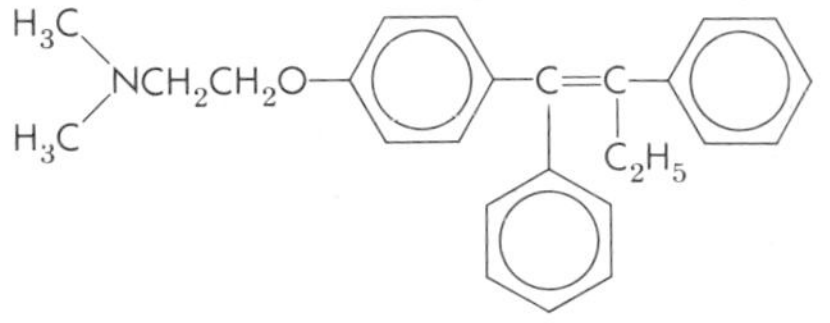

Tamoxifen

concentrations of gonadotropins, leading to ovarian stimulation, ovulation, and sustained function of corpora lutea.

Therapeutic Uses and Preparation. *Clomiphene citrate* (CLOMID, SEROPHENE) has been used clinically for the treatment of infertility in women in doses varying between 25 and 200 mg daily by mouth, for periods of a few days to a few weeks. It is available in 50-mg tablets. In view of the development of enlarged ovaries with higher doses, a dose of 50 mg daily for 5 days is recommended initially. This is started on the fifth day of the menstrual cycle except in patients who have not menstruated recently. In infertility and menstrual disorders, treatment has been repeated at monthly intervals with success. If ovulation and fertility are not achieved, the dose may be increased to 100 mg or even 150 mg per day for 5 days (*see* Marshall, 1978). Ovulation is achieved in most patients whose pituitary and ovaries are capable of stimulated function, and pregnancy occurs in 40 to 50% of such women. The use of clomiphene and gonadotropins in infertility is also discussed in Chapter 59. As with gonadotropins, hyperstimulation of the ovaries with the formation of multiple cysts and a high incidence of multiple births are seen. The incidence of multiple births with clomiphene is about 6 to 8%, compared to an incidence of 15 to 25% when gonadotropins are used to induce ovulation and fertility. About 75% of the multiple births that follow the use of clomiphene are twins. The use of these agents in the palliative treatment of carcinoma of the breast is discussed in Chapter 55.

PROGESTINS

For some years after Corner and Allen had isolated progesterone from the corpora lutea of sows, the small amounts of the hormone available, at first from natural sources and later from synthesis, hampered experimental work and therapeutic application. The hormone had to be given by injection, and the duration of action was brief. With the introduction during the 1950s of new classes of progestational agents with prolonged activity and enhanced oral effectiveness, the structures associated with activity were found to be quite diverse (*see* Rozenbaum, 1982). The number of progestins has proliferated abundantly, and some have had wide clinical use as contraceptive agents.

Chemistry. Some of the progestins have inherent estrogenic or androgenic effects, some show dissociations of effectiveness in various tests, and some have properties that resemble progesterone very closely. The compounds of greatest interest in therapeutics are those that are effective when given by mouth. Some representative progestins are shown in Table 61–2.

The first progestin that was reasonably effective orally was 17α-ethinyltestosterone (*ethisterone*). Derivatives of testosterone lacking the angular methyl group (C 19) attached to C 10, the 19-nortestosterones, were much more effective orally. The parent compound, 19-nortestosterone, is inactive, but a number of 17α-alkyl derivatives are

**Table 61–2. STRUCTURAL RELATIONSHIP OF VARIOUS PROGESTINS
TO PROGESTERONE**

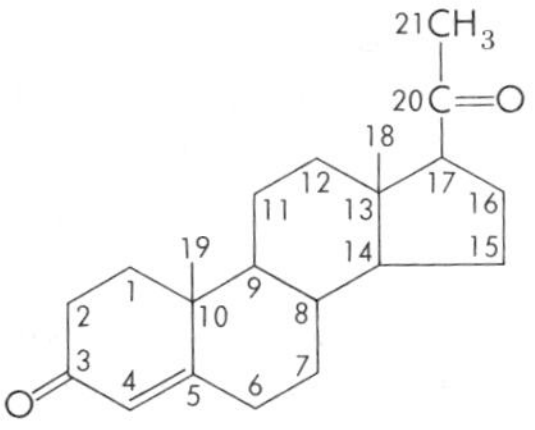

Progesterone

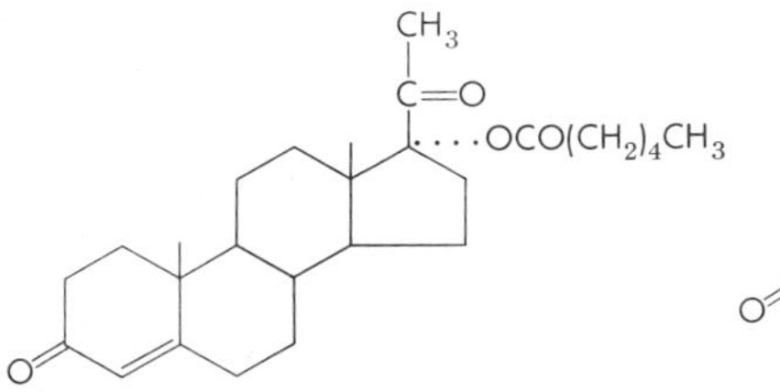

Hydroxyprogesterone Caproate

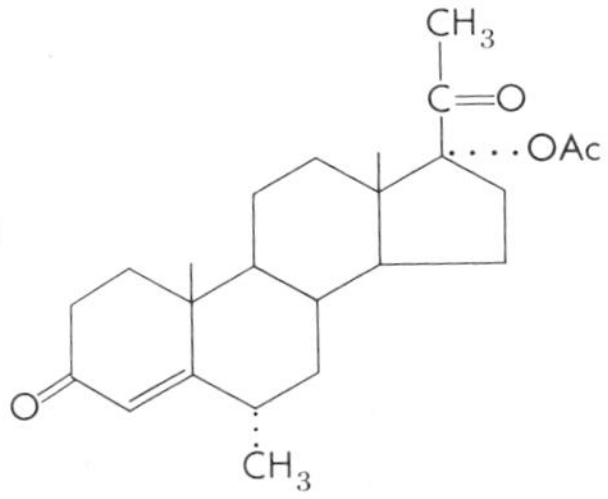

Medroxyprogesterone Acetate

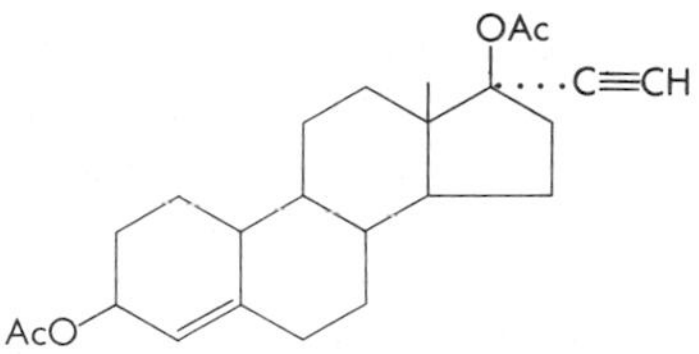

Ethynodiol Diacetate

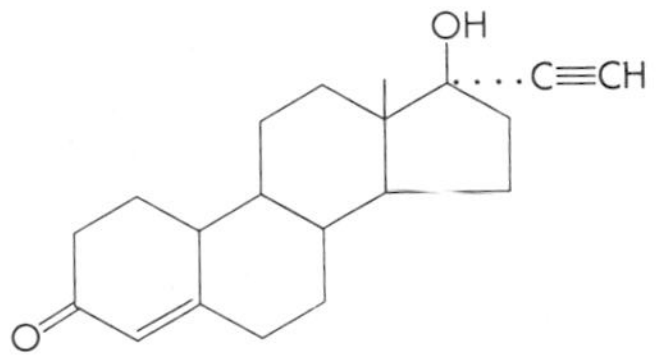

Norethindrone

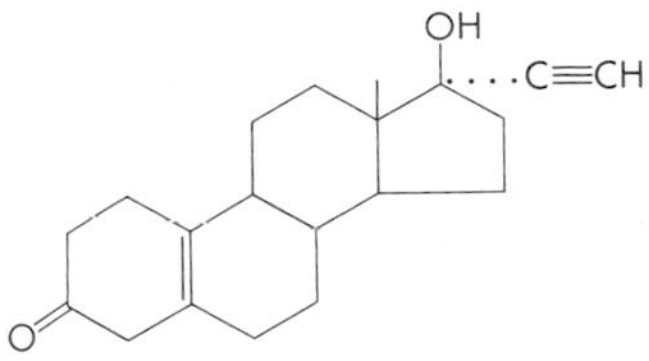

Norethynodrel

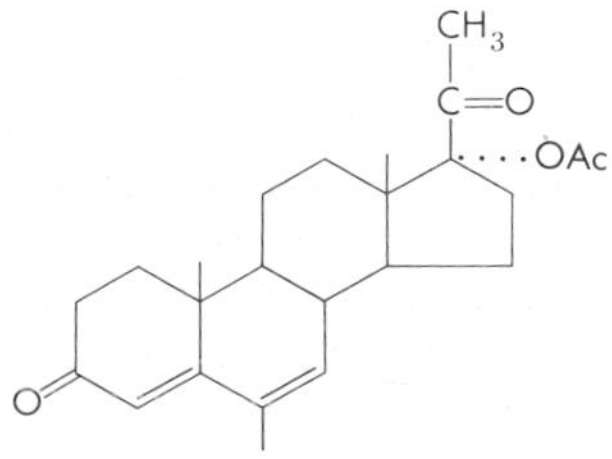

Megestrol Acetate

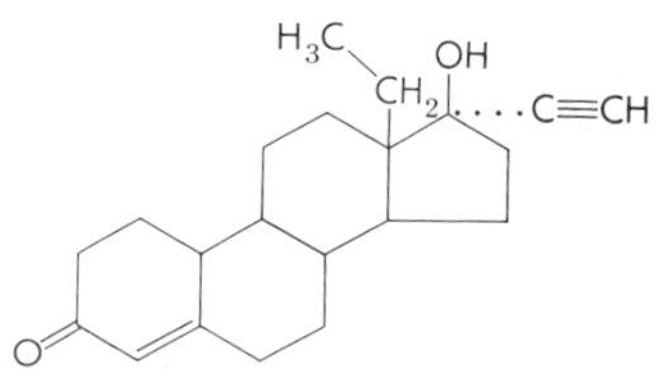

Norgestrel

effective. The 17α-methyl derivative is progestational and androgenic. 17α-Ethyl-19-nortestosterone (*norethandrolone*) is also progestational and androgenic and is used clinically as an anabolic agent. 17α-Ethinyl-19-nortestosterone, or *norethindrone* (*norethisterone*), is a potent oral progestin in man and is only mildly androgenic. Shift of the double bond in norethindrone yields the isomer *norethynodrel*, one of the first compounds to be widely used as a contraceptive. Reduction of the 3-keto group of norethindrone yields a partially reduced derivative of ethinyl estradiol termed *ethynodiol*, the diacetate of which is a particularly potent progestational agent. Removal of the oxygen function at position 3 gives rise to an interesting series of compounds, the *estrenols*, the biological activity of which is critically dependent upon the substituent grouping on C 17. Thus, *ethinylestrenol* is a powerful progestational agent free of androgenic and anabolic effects, *allylestrenol* has progestational and other actions, and *ethylestrenol* (Table 62–3, page 1449) is used as an anabolic agent. The 13-ethyl analog of norethindrone, or 18-homonorethisterone (*norgestrel*), was found to be 100 times as progestational as norethindrone in the Clauberg test, which is based upon the endometrial changes in immature rabbits pretreated with estrogen.

Another series of orally active progestins is typified by the compound *chlormadinone acetate*, which is 6α-chloro-Δ⁶-17α-acetoxy progesterone, a purely progestational agent of high potency previously used in contraceptive formulations. The 6-methyl analog has similar properties and is referred to as *megestrol*.

Additional progestational compounds took origin from a different line of investigation. 17α-Hydroxyprogesterone, first isolated from the adrenal glands in 1940, was virtually inert. On the other hand, the acetic acid ester had appreciable activity and could be taken by mouth, although very large doses were required. When the compound was given by injection in oil, activity was prolonged, a property shared by other esters such as the *valerate* and *caproate*. The caproate has been used extensively as a long-acting progestin, but it is virtually inactive by mouth. Other derivatives of 17α-hydroxyprogesterone were found to be effective orally, and the one most widely studied is the 6-methyl analog, *medroxyprogesterone acetate*. The 16α, 17α-dihydroxy derivative of progesterone in the form of the *acetophenone* is moderately active by mouth but has the property of extremely long action when given parenterally.

Cyproterone acetate is a particularly potent progestin. However, it has had only limited use as a progestin, perhaps because of a greater interest in its use as an antiandrogen (Chapter 62).

Synthesis and Secretion. Progesterone is secreted by the ovary mainly from the corpus luteum during the second half of the menstrual cycle. Secretion actually begins just before ovulation from the follicle that is destined to release an ovum. The formation of progesterone from steroid precursors is summarized in Figure 61–1 and occurs in the ovary, testis, adrenal cortex, and placenta. The stimulatory effect of LH on progesterone synthesis and secretion by the corpus luteum is mediated by an increased synthesis of cyclic AMP.

If the ovum is fertilized, implantation takes place about 7 days later in the human being and almost at once the developing trophoblast secretes its luteotropic hormone, chorionic gonadotropin, into the maternal circulation, and the functional life of the corpus luteum is sustained. Chorionic gonadotropin, detectable in urine several days before the expected time of the next menstrual period, is excreted in progressively increasing amounts for the next 5 weeks or so, and in reduced quantities thereafter throughout pregnancy. During the second or third month of pregnancy the developing placenta begins to secrete estrogen and progesterone in collaboration with the fetal adrenal glands, and thereafter the corpus luteum is not essential to continued gestation. Estrogen and progesterone continue to be secreted in large amounts by the placenta up to the time of delivery.

Measurements of the rate of secretion of progesterone suggest that, from a few milligrams a day secreted during the follicular phase of the cycle, the rate increases to 10 to 20 mg during the luteal phase and to several hundred milligrams during the latter part of pregnancy. Rates of from 1 to 5 mg per day have been measured in men, and are comparable to the values in women during the follicular phase of the cycle.

Physiological and Pharmacological Actions. Progesterone released during the luteal phase of the cycle leads to the development of a secretory endometrium. Abrupt decline in the release of progesterone from the corpus luteum at the end of the cycle is the main determinant of the onset of menstruation. If the duration of the luteal phase is artificially lengthened, either by sustaining luteal function or by treatment with progesterone, decidual changes in the endometrial stroma similar to those seen in early pregnancy can be induced. Under normal circumstances, estrogen antecedes and accompanies progesterone in its action upon the endometrium and is essential to the development of the normal pattern. When the orally active progestins were first tested and given from day 5 of the cycle for 20 days, the endometrial stroma showed intense luteal action while the glands, stimulated at first, actually became atrophic. It turned out that these patterns were caused by progestins with little or no intrinsic estrogenic activity; if estrogen was given as well, the response closely resembled the normal.

The endocervical glands are also influenced by progesterone, and the abundant watery secretion of the estrogen-stimulated structures is changed to a scant viscid material. When the estrogen-stimulated secretion dries on a glass slide, sodium chloride crystallizes to form a dendritic pattern called "ferning." Progestins inhibit this pattern.

The estrogen-induced maturation of the human vaginal epithelium is modified toward the condition of pregnancy by the action of progesterone, a change that can be detected in cytological alterations in the vaginal smear. If the quantity of estrogen concurrently acting is known to be adequate, or if it is assured by giving estrogen, the cytological response to a progestin can be used to evaluate its progestational potency.

Pregnancy. The increasing concentrations of progesterone that are present during the course of pregnancy have been discussed above. While progesterone is very important for the maintenance of pregnancy, in part because it suppresses uterine contractility, other effects may be equally important. For example, progesterone may contribute to a state of "transplantation immunity" and prevent immunological rejection of the fetus (Siiteri *et al.*, 1977). While chorionic gonadotropin was thought to play such a role by inhibiting the functions of T lymphocytes, this action is ascribed to progesterone by some investigators. The effects of progesterone to maintain pregnancy have led to the use of progestins to prevent threatened abortion. However, administration of progestins is of questionable benefit, probably because diminished progesterone is rarely the cause of spontaneous abortion (*see* below).

Mammary Gland. During pregnancy and to a minor degree during the luteal phase of the cycle, progesterone, acting with estrogen, brings about a proliferation of the acini of the mammary gland. Toward the end of pregnancy the acini fill with secretion and the vasculature of the gland is notably increased; however, only after the influences of estrogen and progesterone are withdrawn by the event of parturition does lactation begin. The action of estrogen or estrogen and progesterone, when used post partum for relieving the sensation of engorgement, is probably largely a direct one upon the mammary tissue to inhibit the effects of prolactin and the secretion of milk.

Thermogenic Action. If the body temperature is measured each day throughout the normal menstrual cycle, preferably at the same time before arising each morning, an increase of about 1° F may be noted at midcycle; this correlates with the event of ovulation. The temperature rise persists for the remainder of the cycle until the onset of menstrual flow. The phenomenon is caused by progesterone, as can be shown by giving the hormone to nonovulating women or to men. The minimal detectably effective dose of progesterone is about 5 mg once daily, and a dose of 10 or 20 mg daily is fully effective. These doses also span the range of effectiveness on the changes in the endometrium, cervix, and vagina, as discussed above.

Mechanism of Action. Many studies of the action of progesterone have been performed with the chick oviduct as a model tissue (*see* Chan and O'Malley, 1976). In this tissue progesterone binds to a specific cytosolic receptor with a molecular weight of 225,000 (Schrader *et al.*, 1977). The amount of this receptor protein is increased following pretreatment of animals with estrogen. Following translocation of the progesterone-receptor complex to the nucleus, the synthesis of mRNA for ovalbumin, avidin, and other proteins is markedly stimulated.

Absorption, Fate, and Excretion. Progesterone injected in oily solution is readily absorbed but at a rate that may be too rapid for optimal therapeutic efficiency. In animal tests several doses per day are more effective than the same dose once daily, and less frequent dosage is quite inefficient. Inactivation takes place largely in the liver. Many pregnane derivatives and isomers conjugated with glucuronide or sulfate are found in the urine. One of the major urinary products is the glucuronide of pregnane-3α,20α-diol. The rate of turnover of endogenous progesterone is unusually rapid, the half-life in blood being a few minutes, and doubtless exogenous material is handled in the same way. A small amount of progesterone is stored in body fat, but this is generally regarded as quantitatively unimportant. Although it is quickly disposed of, progesterone given at daily intervals in sufficient dose is thoroughly effective; its actions upon tissue continue after it has disappeared from the plasma. When progesterone is given by mouth, it is much less effective, but a similar proportion is eliminated in the urine as pregnanediol. Absorption from the intestinal tract is prompt, but the compound is rapidly transformed during passage through the liver. Many analogs of progesterone that are less susceptible to hepatic metabolism are more effective than progesterone when given orally. The structures of these agents are shown in Table 61–2.

About 50 to 60% of administered radioactive progesterone appears in the urine and about 10% in feces. Pregnanediol in urine accounts for 12 to 15% of the progesterone metabolized. When progesterone is given for a prolonged period, during the luteal phase of the cycle or during pregnancy, a larger proportion (25 to 30%) appears in the urine as pregnanediol (see Fotherby and James, 1972). Pregnanediol is a notably specific product, and measurements of plasma or urinary pregnanediol provide a valuable index of the secretion and metabolism of progesterone. Approximately 1 mg per day is excreted during the follicular phase of the cycle, after menopause, and by men. During the luteal phase of the cycle 2- to 4-mg amounts are excreted daily, and during pregnancy the values increase to 50 to 70 mg before term.

Assays. Many of the new steroids are not purely estrogenic, progestational, androgenic, or anabolic but show several types of activity. No one bioassay for progesterone-like action adequately characterizes a compound, and each is modified in one way or another by the estrogenic and androgenic potencies of the material being tested; some bioassays are influenced differently from others. A great deal has been learned about the characteristics and limitations of these tests, but none yields an unequivocal estimate of progestational potency of new compounds.

Some bioassay methods are based on changes in the microscopic appearance or carbonic anhydrase activity of the endometrium of animals. Other methods are based upon the maintenance of pregnancy in oophorectomized animals or inhibition of ovulation. The reader is referred to the *fourth edition* of this textbook for a more complete description of bioassay methods used and for references. Various chemical assays for progesterone and pregnanediol are also available. As discussed earlier for estrogens, protein-binding assays and immunoassays are also available, specific, and sensitive (*see* Vande Wiele and Dyrenfurth, 1973).

Preparations. Currently, many orally active and parenteral preparations of progestational agents are available (Table 61–2). Some of these substances in combination with estrogens are used widely as oral contraceptives, which are discussed below.

Progesterone injection (PROGESTAJECT, others) contains 25 to 100 mg of progesterone per milliliter of vegetable oil. Progesterone is peculiar among the commonly used steroids in being locally irritating, and not more than about 100 mg can be given intramuscularly in a single injection. Aqueous suspensions of progesterone are particularly painful and are seldom used. Progesterone is also available in a T-shaped intrauterine contraceptive device that provides continuous delivery of progesterone in the uterine cavity over 1 year. This is marketed under the name of PROGESTASERT and contains 38 mg of progesterone.

Medroxyprogesterone acetate (DEPO-PROVERA) contains 100 or 400 mg/ml in aqueous medium for intramuscular injection, and *medroxyprogesterone acetate tablets* (PROVERA) contain 2.5 or 10 mg each.

Hydroxyprogesterone caproate injection (DELA-LUTIN) is provided as an oily solution of 125 mg/ml (in sesame oil) or 250 mg/ml (in castor oil) for intramuscular injection.

Megestrol acetate (MEGACE, PALLACE) is available in 20- and 40-mg tablets.

Norethindrone (NORLUTIN) and *norethindrone acetate* (NORLUTATE) are available alone in 5-mg tablets and in combination with estrogens as oral contraceptives (*see* below).

A variety of other oral progestin preparations are also combined with estrogens (ethinyl estradiol or mestranol) as oral contraceptives (*see* Table 61–3, page 1432).

It is not possible to give accurate values for the relative clinical effectiveness of the several compounds because careful comparisons are limited in number and different responses have been used in the published studies. In various tests in women, as with different bioassays in animals, the relative potencies of the progestins are not the same. Furthermore, some progestins possess more or less estrogenic and androgenic activities than do others.

Therapeutic Uses. Application of physiological principles in the management of ovarian disorders and contraception has made it possible to use these new agents with notable therapeutic success.

Contraception. This undoubtedly represents the major use of these agents and is discussed later in this chapter.

Dysfunctional Uterine Bleeding. This is a common disorder, characterized by irregular cycles and episodes of prolonged hemorrhage. The condition may arise at any time during menstrual life, but is more frequent in young girls before regular ovulatory cycles are established and again with the approach of menopause. The condition usually results from the continuous action of estrogen, which causes endometrial hyperplasia, combined with an insufficient amount and poor cycling of progesterone. Other causes for uterine bleeding must be excluded before initiating cyclic therapy with progestins.

The immediate goal is to stop the bleeding, and the long-range aim is to regulate the cycle. Both estrogens and androgens have been used effectively, but a progestin is specific. It is best to give an orally active progestin in full doses to stop the bleeding. Five to 10 mg of norethindrone every 4 to 6 hours will usually be effective in 24 hours, and then 5 mg twice daily can be continued for 1 or 2 weeks to give a respite from bleeding. Withdrawal bleeding at the end of treatment will, in effect, be a normal menstrual flow, usually accompanied by cramps; however, it will be self-limited in duration and, if nothing further is done, there will be a free interval of several weeks. Other progestins may also be used, but those without inherent estrogenic activity are more effective if combined with an estrogen such as 1.25 mg of diethylstilbestrol or 0.1 mg of ethinyl estradiol daily. To prevent a recurrence of bleeding, cyclic therapy is called for; an oral progestin, such as norethindrone, in a dose of 5 to 10 mg daily is given for 5 days at monthly intervals, beginning 20 to 25 days after the induced period. Regular menstrual periods can thus be induced for as long as one chooses.

Dysmenorrhea. Relief of dysmenorrhea by inhibiting ovulation is discussed under estrogen. A progestin can be used to advantage either with the estrogen from days 5 to 25 of the cycle or added to the estrogen during the last 5 days. In either case menstruation is prompt, the treatment can be resumed 5 days later, and the cycle can be repeated indefinitely. Such cycles are entirely physiological, lacking only the ovarian components and ovulation. As discussed earlier, nonsteroidal anti-inflammatory agents are the preferred method of therapy.

Premenstrual Tension. This is an ill-defined condition of uncertain etiology. Changes in concentrations of hormones and electrolytes are probably responsible for the irritability, breast tenderness, headache, and weight gain during the luteal phase of the cycle. Progesterone or an oral progestin may offer relief when given during the last week or 10 days of the cycle. Sometimes this is not effective, and the symptoms are sufficiently distressing to warrant inhibition of ovulation with combined progestin-estrogen therapy.

Endometriosis. The severe dysmenorrhea of this condition is not completely understood. In many instances, suppression of ovulation with estrogen is followed by a painless, estrogen-withdrawal period; this suggests that the pain in the two conditions is of similar origin. Treatment of this form of endometriosis thus becomes the treatment of dysmenorrhea. In certain severe cases of endometriosis, the major problem is the development of painful extrauterine masses and infertility. Treatment is aimed at causing regression of the ectopic endometrial growths. Prolonged treatment, designed to prevent menstruation for many months, relieves a major difficulty by preventing bleeding into the endometrial masses or peritoneal cavity. Favorable effects have been achieved even with the continuous use of estrogen alone for this purpose. Better results have been described from the continuous use of oral progestins, and actual regression of the endometrial growths has been observed. Norethindrone acetate may be used in oral doses of 5 mg daily for 2 weeks, after which the dose is increased in increments of 2.5 mg per day every 2 weeks until 15 mg per day is reached. Therapy may be continued for 6 to 9 months. Symptomatic relief can be expected in about 80% of patients and return of fertility in about 50% of patients (Wentz, 1977). Danazol, which is a weak androgen, is also effective for the treatment of endometriosis (*see* Chapter 62).

Threatened and Habitual Abortion. Progestins have been used extensively in attempts to prevent abortion, but there is no evidence that the treatment is effective in the majority of patients. Although the side effects from the administration of progestational agents are usually quite minimal, this does not pertain to the fetus. These agents may cause a variety of fetal anomalies, including virilization and genital deformities of male and female fetuses (Jacobson, 1962; Wentz, 1977; Aarskog, 1979).

There are thought to be a few patients who have an inadequate luteal response to gonadotropins with deficient secretion of progesterone; such women may benefit from treatment with a progestin during the first trimester of pregnancy. To identify such patients, plasma and urinary metabolites of progesterone must be determined to establish that a deficiency exists. The potential risks to the fetus must also be considered.

Suppression of Post-Partum Lactation. While the administration of estrogens and/or progestins is effective in suppressing lactation in the immediate post-partum period as mentioned above, their use for this purpose is decreasing. Significant reduction in milk secretion is seen with concentrations of estrogens and progestins achieved with use of some oral contraceptive preparations.

Endometrial Carcinoma. Progestins may be used as a palliative measure in recurrent or metastatic endometrial carcinoma. When used in this manner, megestrol acetate may be given in oral doses of 40 mg daily for several months as a trial. Alternative therapy is the weekly intramuscular administration of 400 mg of medroxyprogesterone acetate. Improvement can be expected in about one half of the patients treated (*see* Wentz, 1977).

Hypoventilation. Progestins can stimulate respiration and have been used with some success in obese patients with hypoventilation (Pickwickian syndrome). However, other measures, particularly weight reduction and therapy for any pulmonary infection, should be stressed.

ORAL CONTRACEPTIVES

Of drugs requiring a prescription, oral contraceptives are among the most widely used agents. It is estimated that 9 million women in the United States and 55 million worldwide are currently taking these agents. The lives of approximately half of the women in the United States between the ages of 15 and 29 are punctuated daily by the taking of a medicine for a condition from which they do not suffer—a prophylaxis for a contingency that may not materialize.

History. The incredible growth of the world population stands out as one of the fundamental events of our era. The current world population of about 4.5 billion is expected to be 6 billion by the year 2000; most of the growth will be in underdeveloped countries. The Old Testament dictum "Be fruitful, and multiply" (Genesis 9:1) has been religiously followed by readers and nonreaders of the Bible alike. In 1798, Thomas Robert Malthus started a great controversy by opposing the prevailing view of unlimited progress for man by making two postulates and a conclusion. He postulated that "food is necessary to the existence of man," and that sexual attraction between woman and man is necessary and likely to persist, since "towards the extinction of the passion between the sexes, no progress whatever has hitherto been made," barring ". . . individual exceptions." Malthus concluded that "the power of population is infinitely greater than the power in the earth to produce subsistence for man," a "natural inequality" that would someday loom "insurmountable in the way to the perfectibility of society." Malthus' essay sparked great controversy and inquiry into the principle governing the growth of population. In seeking to discover the causes of population increase, T. R. Edmonds in 1832 suggested that "a deterioration in the condition of the English labourers . . . , the destruction of the feeling of self-respect" was such a great distress that "among the great body of the people . . . , sexual intercourse is the only gratification. . . . When they are better fed they will have other enjoyments at command than sexual intercourse, and their numbers . . . will not increase in the same proportion as at present." Today we realize that our sheer numbers have increased so much that they are straining Earth's capacity to supply food, energy, and raw materials. We also know, perhaps better than T. R. Edmonds, where some of the blame for this growth lies. Advances in medicine and public health have led to a significant decline in mortality and an increased life expectancy. Thus, medical science has begun to assume a portion of the responsibility for overpopulation. To this end, drugs in the form of hormones and their analogs have been developed to control human fertility.

As discussed below, oral contraceptives are very effective and are expected to play a major role in control of the world population explosion. The small but definite incidence of serious side effects that results from these agents must be weighed against some of the dire consequences of uncontrolled population growth. Furthermore, in underdeveloped nations the morbidity and mortality of pregnancy and delivery far exceed the incidence of adverse reactions from oral contraceptives. Indeed, in many countries oral contraceptives are available without a physician's prescription.

A comprehensive investigation of the inhibition of ovulation by the use of progestational agents was initiated by Rock, Pincus, and Garcia. The study showed that ovulation could be abolished at will for as long as desired and with great regularity (*see* Rock *et al.,* 1957; Pincus, 1960). The compounds used were derivatives of 19-nortestosterone, given by mouth from day 5 to day 25 of the menstrual cycle (the first day of menses is day 1). Withdrawal bleeding occurred within a few days of completing the course, and treatment was begun again 4 days after the first day of flow. Extensive field studies were started in San Juan, Puerto Rico, in 1955, under the direction of Pincus and associates at the Puerto Rico Family Planning Center. The tablet used was ENOVID, containing 10 mg of the progestin norethynodrel and 0.15 mg of the estrogen mestranol, and it was taken daily on the same schedule. The success of these studies prompted many others, and the results of broad, almost worldwide, experience followed.

Among the first of the orally active steroids to be used in inhibiting ovulation, some had inherent estrogenic activity and some preparations of the progestins were later found to be contaminated with estrogen. In a way this was a happy chance, because it served to show that estrogen enhanced the suppressive effect of the progestin and led to the general use of a mixture of the two. The substance considered to be the most likely estrogenic contaminant of norethynodrel was the 3-methyl ether of ethinyl estradiol, *mestranol,* which was therefore incorporated in ENOVID. As experience has been gained, the doses of progestin and estrogen have been decreased to minimize side effects while maintaining contraceptive efficacy.

Types of Oral Contraceptives.

The most common type of oral contraceptive is the combination preparation, which contains both an estrogen and a progestin. Experience with these preparations shows them to be 99 to 100% effective. This method of reversible contraception is, then, the most effective yet devised. Other modifications of steroidal contraception have also been tried with success. *Sequential* preparations, in which an estrogen is taken for 14 to 16 days and a combination of an estrogen and a progestin is then taken for 5 or 6 days, have been about 98 to 99% successful as oral contraceptives. However, because of reports suggesting an increased incidence of endometrial tumors and a lower efficacy, sequential preparations of this type have been removed from the market. They have been replaced by products that contain relatively low amounts of a progestin and with which the amount of progestin taken is increased during the monthly cycle.

Single-entity preparations are also available. A progestin alone has come to be called the ''minipill,'' while an estrogen alone is a postcoital or ''morning-after-pill.'' The ''minipills'' were introduced in order to eliminate the estrogen, the agent in *combined* preparations that was thought to be responsible for most of the side effects of oral contraceptives. Since the contraceptive efficacy of the ''minipill'' is about 97 to 98%, which is somewhat less than that of the combined preparations, and the menstrual cycles are more irregular, these preparations have been less popular. The intramuscular injection of medroxyprogesterone every few months has been effective but is not approved for use as a contraceptive in the United States because of the development of breast and uterine tumors in animals (FDA Drug Bulletin, 1978b). Diethylstilbestrol is effective as a postcoital contraceptive. Although its *general* use for this purpose is unpleasant and may be dangerous, postcoital contraception with an estrogen can be useful when the desirability of avoiding pregnancy is obvious, as in cases of rape or incest.

Preparations and Dosage. Some of the formulations used as oral contraceptives are listed in Table 61–3. The *combined* preparations contain 0.02 to 0.1 mg of ethinyl estradiol or mestranol and various amounts of a progestin, and are taken for 20 or 21 days. The next course is started 7 days after the last dose or 5 days after the onset of the menstrual flow. It should be noted that ethinyl estradiol is approximately twice as potent as mestranol.

Many contraceptive preparations are dispensed in convenient calendar-like containers that help the user to count the days. Some obviate the need of counting by incorporating seven blank pills in the package to provide 3 weeks of treatment and 1 week off. A pill is taken every day, regardless of when menstruation starts or stops. Iron is included in the ''blank'' pills in some preparations.

The ''minipills'' (MICRONOR and NOR-Q.D., containing 0.35 mg of norethindrone, and OVRETTE, containing 75 μg of norgestrel) are taken daily continually. Since they are less effective and preg-

nancy is possible during their administration, patients should discontinue the ''minipill'' if they have amenorrhea for more than 60 days, and they should be examined for pregnancy. Likewise, if patients have missed one or more pills and have amenorrhea for more than 45 days, they should be similarly evaluated.

Medroxyprogesterone acetate (DEPO-PROVERA) is injected intramuscularly in a dose of 150 mg every 3 months but should be used only if the possibility of permanent infertility is acceptable to the patient. An unpredictable duration of amenorrhea and anovulation can result from such therapy. *Norethindrone (norethisterone) enanthate,* when administered intramuscularly in oil in a dose of 200 mg every 3 months, is also effective for contraception. Although long-acting preparations of a progestin are employed in a number of countries for contraception (*see* Vecchio, 1976), such use remains investigational in the United States.

The postcoital contraceptive diethylstilbestrol is started within 72 hours after sexual intercourse at a dose of 25 mg twice daily for 5 days. To be effective the tablets must be continued for 5 consecutive days in spite of nausea and vomiting, which commonly occur. Since estrogens are not advised in pregnancy because of the possibility of vaginal carcinoma in female offspring (*see* above), abortion should be performed if diethylstilbestrol is not effective.

Effects on Laboratory Tests. A substantial number of laboratory results may be altered by the use of oral contraceptives. These changes are, in general, due to physiological alterations in the patient, rather than to interference with the analysis. Many of the changes are those that occur during pregnancy. A tabulation has appeared in the Medical Letter (1979).

Mechanism of Action. The administration of estrogen and a progestin, as contained in combination preparations, could interfere with fertility in any of several ways. However, it is clear that, as currently used, the mixture inhibits ovulation. The questions then are how is ovulation prevented and what other mechanisms might interfere with impregnation. The effects of ovarian hormones upon the gonadotropic functions of the pituitary are discussed earlier in this chapter; the predominant effect of estrogen is to inhibit the secretion of FSH, while continued action of progesterone serves to inhibit the release of LH. It is clear that ovulation could be prevented either by inhibiting the ovulatory stimulus or by preventing the growth of follicles, and this accords with the experimental observations that follicular growth and ovulation can be prevented by either estrogen or pro-

Table 61–3. COMPOSITION AND DOSES OF SOME ORAL CONTRACEPTIVES

ESTROGEN (mg)	PROGESTIN [1] (mg)	PROGESTATIONAL POTENCY	TRADE NAME
Combinations [2]			
0.02 Ethinyl estradiol	1 Norethindrone acetate	Medium	LOESTRIN 1/20
0.03 Ethinyl estradiol	0.3 Norgestrel	Medium	LO/OVRAL
0.03 Ethinyl estradiol	1.5 Norethindrone acetate	Medium	LOESTRIN 1.5/30
0.03 Ethinyl estradiol	0.15 Levonorgestrel	Medium	NORDETTE
0.035 Ethinyl estradiol	0.4 Norethindrone	Low	OVCON-35
0.035 Ethinyl estradiol	0.5 Norethindrone	Low	BREVICON; MODICON
0.035 Ethinyl estradiol	1 Ethynodiol diacetate	High	DEMULEN 1/35
0.035 Ethinyl estradiol	1 Norethindrone	Low	NORINYL 1+35; ORTHO-NOVUM 1/35
0.05 Mestranol	1 Norethindrone	Low	NORINYL 1+50; ORTHO-NOVUM 1/50
0.05 Ethinyl estradiol	0.5 Norgestrel	High	OVRAL
0.05 Ethinyl estradiol	1 Ethynodiol diacetate	High	DEMULEN
0.05 Ethinyl estradiol	1 Norethindrone	Low	OVCON-50
0.05 Ethinyl estradiol	1 Norethindrone acetate	Medium	NORLESTRIN 1/50
0.05 Ethinyl estradiol	2.5 Norethindrone acetate	Medium	NORLESTRIN 2.5/50
0.075 Mestranol	5 Norethynodrel	Medium	ENOVID 5 MG
0.08 Mestranol	1 Norethindrone	Low	NORINYL 1+80; ORTHO-NOVUM 1/80
0.10 Mestranol	1 Ethynodiol diacetate	High	OVULEN
0.10 Mestranol	2 Norethindrone	Medium	NORINYL 2 MG; ORTHO-NOVUM 2 MG
0.10 Mestranol	2.5 Norethynodrel	Medium	ENOVID-E
Sequential [3]			
0.035 Ethinyl estradiol	0.5 Norethindrone, then 1 Norethindrone	Low	ORTHO-NOVUM 10/11
"Minipills" [4]			
—	0.35 Norethindrone	Low	MICRONOR; NOR-Q.D.
—	0.075 Norgestrel	Low	OVRETTE
Postcoital [5]			
Diethylstilbestrol	—	—	—

[1] Of the progestins used, norethynodrel has no androgenic activity, norgestrel is strongly androgenic, and the other progestins have moderate androgenic activity. The relative progestational potency of each preparation is indicated.

[2] Combination tablets are taken for 20 or 21 days and are omitted for 7 or 8 days. These preparations are listed in order of increasing content of estrogen.

[3] This preparation includes two fixed-dose tablets that both contain the same amount of estrogen; the first is taken for 10 days and the second for 11 days, followed by 7 days of no medication.

[4] "Minipills" are taken daily continually.

[5] Diethylstilbestrol is taken in a dose of 25 mg twice daily for 5 days within 72 hours after sexual intercourse; *see* text for indications.

gesterone given singly. The orally active progestins cannot be equated as a group with progesterone because some are inherently estrogenic, some are androgenic, and some are purely progestational; correspondingly, their ovulation-inhibiting potentialities may be mediated in somewhat different ways.

Measurements of circulating FSH and LH show that estrogen-progestin combinations suppress both hormones. The plasma concentrations of FSH and LH are stable; early follicular FSH and midcycle FSH and LH peaks are not seen (Swerdloff and Odell, 1969; Briggs, 1976).

One might reasonably conclude that the most widely used preparations to date owe their effectiveness in inhibiting ovulation to the estrogenic component and that the progestin serves the major purpose of ensuring that withdrawal bleeding will be prompt, brief, and essentially physiological.

Even if ovulation were not prevented, it is easy to imagine that the contraceptive agents could interfere with impregnation by their direct actions upon the genital tract. It is abundantly clear from animal experiments that the endometrium must be just in the right stage of development under estrogen and progesterone for nidation to take place. It seems unlikely that implantation would be possible in the altered endometrium developed under the influence of most of the suppressants. Similarly, the abundant watery secretion of the cervix at the time of ovulation has always been regarded as essential to the well-being of the sperm and the thick tenacious mucus secreted under the influence of progesterone to be a hostile environment. Little is known of the coordinated contractions of the cervix, uterus, and Fallopian tubes that are presumed to be essential for the transport of spermatozoa to the egg and the precisely timed conveyance of the blastocyst to the uterine lumen, but probably the correct hormonal environment is essential for the execution of these important maneuvers. Although it can easily be imagined that estrogen-progestin mixtures could interfere with impregnation in these ways, there has been no opportunity to find out, because ovulation is almost always prevented when the agents are used in the usual way.

The fear that estrogen may have deleterious effects prompted the use of a *progestin alone* in various ways. Continuous administration of a progestin in sufficient dose abolishes the cycle for as long as it is given and leads to ovarian and endometrial atrophy. Very small doses may alter the structure of the endometrium and the consistency of the cervical mucus without disrupting the cycle or inhibiting ovulation. As currently administered, oral contraceptives that contain only a progestin cause variable suppression of FSH, LH, and ovulation, which may explain their lower degree of efficacy (*see* Briggs, 1976). With continued daily administration, menstruation occurs but the length of the cycle and the duration of bleeding are quite variable, factors that have influenced their popularity.

Long-acting progestins, given by intramuscular injection, are also effective, as noted above. For example, 150 mg of medroxyprogesterone acetate, administered every 3 months starting just after parturition, prevents pregnancy in all; irregular bleeding, troublesome at first, gives way to amenorrhea and an atrophic endometrium in most cases. This form of contraception also utilizes the highly active, purely progestational compounds by incorporating them in pessaries to provide vaginal absorption, in intrauterine devices, or in plastic capsules for subcutaneous application. An intrauterine device containing a reservoir of 38 mg of progesterone is available (*see* above) and releases progesterone continuously into the uterine cavity for 1 year. It is about as effective as other intrauterine devices (97 to 98%), and the side effects are also similar except that the incidence of ectopic pregnancies may be greater (FDA Drug Bulletin, 1978a).

The development of *postcoital* contraceptives is an intriguing subject. A vast number of hormones and other agents are effective in this regard in animals. It has long been known that the use of large doses of estrogen in women is effective in preventing implantation, but such doses are tolerated only in cases of single or very infrequent exposure. There is a rough correlation between the contraceptive potency of these substances and their estrogenic activity.

Large doses of estrogens used as postcoital contraceptives may act by inhibiting fertilization and nidation in several ways. The motility of the oviduct may be altered, the endometrium is changed, and withdrawal from the large doses of estrogens induces bleeding.

Antiprogestational agents could prove to be effective when administered postcoitally or monthly to induce progesterone withdrawal bleeding and abortion. Such drugs are not currently available. The use of prostaglandins to promote abortion is discussed in Chapter 39.

Undesirable Effects. A variety of major and minor side effects have been attributed to the use of oral contraceptives. In some instances the undesirable effects are well documented and their incidence has been determined. Of most concern are cardiovascular side effects and the induction or promotion of tumors. However, a number of possible side effects are not well substantiated. Furthermore, the incidence of some disorders has been lowered by the use of oral contraceptives. An assessment of the risk-to-benefit ratio is essential for each patient in order to provide the most efficacious method of contraception with the least possible risk.

Cardiovascular Disorders. Clinical trials in sizable groups of women had been under way for 5 years or so before side effects of any consequence were described. Instances of *thrombophlebitis,* a rare disorder in healthy young women, then began to be noted, and several reports of *thromboembolism* appeared from England (Inman and Vessey, 1968; Vessey and Doll, 1968). In the latter report it was estimated that the incidence of thrombophlebitis in young women was increased six- to tenfold with oral contraceptives.

These retrospective studies suffered from a statistical dilemma, because what was really studied was the incidence of medication among those with complications versus those without. Retrospective studies are also generally criticized since cause-and-effect relationships cannot be established and because biases are introduced due to the means by which information is obtained.

Because of the British reports, numerous retrospective and prospective studies have since been conducted. The consensus of these reports is that the incidence of thrombophlebitis and thromboembolism is increased, and the incidence of thromboembolism is greater with preparations containing higher doses of estrogens. The Coronary Drug Project Research Group (1973) also found a twofold increase in the incidence of thrombophlebitis and pulmonary embolism in *men* who received conjugated estrogens daily for 4 to 5 years.

The increase in the incidence of thromboembolism is also supported by studies with various clotting factors. Patients taking estrogens or combined oral contraceptives have been found to have accelerated blood clotting and increased blood concentrations of some clotting factors (*see* Stadel, 1981; Meade, 1982a). These effects have not been observed with preparations containing only progestin.

The incidence of cerebral and coronary thrombosis is also increased in "pill" users (Inman *et al.*, 1970). The Collaborative Group for the Study of Stroke in Young Women (1973, 1975) found an increased incidence of thrombotic and hemorrhagic strokes among women taking oral contraceptives. Similarly, in men with prostatic carcinoma the administration of diethylstilbestrol daily was associated with an increased incidence of myocardial infarction and strokes (Veterans Administration, 1967). Users of the "pill" appear to have a two- to fivefold greater incidence of nonfatal and fatal myocardial infarction and a two- to tenfold increase in the frequency of strokes (Mann and Inman, 1975; Mann *et al.*, 1975; Kaplan, 1978; Vessey, 1980). The increased incidence of myocardial infarction is related to the duration of use of oral contraceptives, and the risk may remain elevated after the agent is discontinued (Slone *et al.*, 1981). The increased risk of myocardial infarction with use of oral contraceptives is additive to other risk factors, such as age, smoking, and hypertension; this information has been added to oral contraceptive package inserts.

Most agree that the morbidity and mortality from cardiovascular diseases are increased with the use of *combined* oral contraceptives. The magnitude of the increased mortality is about two- to fourfold and is primarily from ischemic heart disease and cerebrovascular accidents (Royal College of General Practitioners' Oral Contraception Study, 1981; Slone *et al.*, 1981). However, thromboembolism and other cardiovascular disorders also contribute. The increased mortality is most apparent in women over 35 years of age and is greatest in women who smoke or have other risk factors for cardiovascular disorders. Mortality may increase as much as 15- to 18-fold in women over 45 years of age who smoke. Older women with risk factors for cardiovascular disease should be advised to consider other forms of contraception. The cardiovascular disorders that are observed with oral contraceptives may result from alterations in clotting factors, lipoproteins, glucose tolerance, and blood pressure, as discussed below. The use of low-dose preparations reduces the risks but does not eliminate them (*see* Speroff, 1982).

Hypertension has been observed in about 5% of oral contraceptive users (Laragh, 1976; Weinberger, 1982). While the increase in blood pressure is usually gradual, it may be quite severe. Generally the hypertension is reversible within several months of discontinuation of medication. These effects probably result from the retention of sodium and water secondary to increases in circulating concentrations of renin and angiotensin.

While the effects of oral contraceptives on blood pressure, myocardial infarction, and stroke were initially attributed to the estrogen, it has become apparent that many of those untoward effects are related to the amount of progestin in the preparation (*see* Stadel, 1981; Kay, 1982; Meade, 1982b); however, these studies do not discount a significant contribution by the estrogen. The estrogen rather than the progestin appears to contribute to the increased incidence of thromboembolism (Meade, 1982b).

The incidence of thrombophlebitis and other cardiovascular disorders rises during pregnancy and the post-partum period. Furthermore, increased mortality from various causes during pregnancy supports the view that the increased incidence of cardiovascular disorders with oral contraceptives is probably a comparatively minor and acceptable risk, since pregnancy is effectively prevented. Serious complications of pregnancy are perhaps so much more frequent than are those resulting from the use of oral contraceptives that the incidence of difficulties from unwanted pregnancies might be still higher if all couples switched to other methods of contraception, all of which are less effective.

Cancer. Because of the numerous animal studies that demonstrate an increased incidence of several different types of tumors with estrogen, there has also been much concern that similar problems would occur in users of oral contraceptives.

As discussed above, vaginal, uterine, and perhaps breast carcinomas have been caused by the use of estrogens. In addition, a number of cases of benign hepatomas have been associated with the use of oral contraceptives. The primary danger of these benign tumors is rupture and hemorrhage due to their vascularity. The tumors usually regress when oral contraceptives are discontinued. An increased incidence of endometrial carcinoma in premenopausal women receiving oral contraceptives has been observed (Silverberg and Makowski, 1975; Weiss and Sayvetz, 1980; Vessey

et al., 1983). A few studies have suggested an increased incidence of breast tumors, but most have found no association of this disease with the use of oral contraceptives (*see* Leis *et al.*, 1976; Kay, 1977; Pike *et al.*, 1983). The relatively few incriminating reports, despite the vast use of these agents, may reflect the latent period needed for cellular transformation. Additional prospective studies are thus needed to establish whether oral contraceptives are associated with the development of tumors.

Other Effects. The frequent, mild side effects—nausea, occasional vomiting, dizziness, headache, discomfort in the breasts, and gain in weight—are manifestations of early pregnancy and are attributable entirely, or nearly so, to the estrogen in the preparations. These symptoms are more frequent and may be more troublesome than the side effects in menopausal women given estrogen, probably because the contraceptives are not taken for the relief of symptoms. However, most of them are short lived or are noted only in the first cycle or two. Irregular menstrual bleeding, the so-called breakthrough bleeding, is also more frequent at first; it seems to be less troublesome with the preparations containing the larger doses of estrogen. Oral contraceptives can cause intolerance to carbohydrates, with elevations in the concentrations of glucose and insulin in plasma (*see* Spellacy, 1982; Wynn, 1982). The changes tend to be small and are usually reversible. If notable aberrations of this type are seen, oral contraceptives should be discontinued and another form of contraception used. The effects of estrogens and progestins on plasma lipoproteins are mentioned above.

Many other minor disturbances have been attributed to the oral contraceptives (Koide and Ch'iu Lyle, 1975). Some symptoms, including depression of mood, easy fatigue, and lack of initiative, have been attributed to the progestin in the tablets and are less troublesome or even unnoticed with the newer preparations containing smaller amounts. An increase in female-initiated sexual activity that is said to be present at the time of ovulation is suppressed or absent in women using oral contraceptives (Adams *et al.*, 1978).

Various ocular conditions have also been reported, including corneal sensitivity, retinal thrombosis, optic neuritis, diplopia, and others. However, it has not been determined that these are in fact related to oral contraceptives. Skin rashes, photosensitivity, alopecia, and hirsutism seldom occur, but chloasma (brownish macules of the face) may appear with prolonged use of most preparations. Cholestatic jaundice due to the 17-alkyl-substituted steroids in all of the preparations is rare. An increased incidence of gallbladder disease with estrogens has been reported by the Boston Collaborative Drug Surveillance Program (1974). Oral contraceptives increase the concentration of cholesterol in bile, which may provide the biochemical explanation for the increased incidence of cholelithiasis (Bennion *et al.*, 1976). Folate absorption may be decreased, but few patients develop anemia or other signs of deficiency (*see* Briggs, 1976). The resumption of spontaneous menses usually requires about 6 to 10 weeks after oral contraceptives have been discontinued. However, some patients have prolonged periods of anovulation and amenorrhea (sometimes associated with galactorrhea), requiring therapy with clomiphene, gonadotropin, or bromocriptine (*see* Chapter 59). The use of oral contraceptives may in some way provide a setting for the subsequent development of hyperprolactinemia when discontinued. The use of preparations with a low estrogen content may lead to breakthrough bleeding. Preparations with less than 30 to 35 μg of estrogen may also be less efficacious, particularly if the administration of other drugs increases hepatic metabolism of the estrogen. Continuation of intake of oral contraceptives during pregnancy may be associated with congenital limb deformation, masculinization, and cryptorchism in offspring (Janerich *et al.*, 1974; Koide and Ch'iu Lyle, 1975; Heinonen *et al.*, 1977; Rothman and Louik, 1978). Administration of oral contraceptives soon after delivery will decrease lactation and interfere with breast feeding.

In view of these considerations, it seems highly prudent to continue to evaluate each patient and her need for oral contraceptives. The incidence of complications in patients under 30 years of age who do not have risk factors for cardiovascular disease appears to be small. A challenge to the physician is to evaluate the presence of such risk factors in older patients and, if present, to encourage the patient to consider other forms of contraception. Clearly in some patients pregnancy is either very undesirable or contraindicated due to preexisting disease; the additional risks from oral contraceptives seem minor. However, in most patients the decision is more difficult. There are many alternative means of contraception, but none is quite as effective as oral contraceptives. For extensive population control, these agents are extremely useful and a low incidence of complications is to be expected.

If oral contraceptives are prescribed, preparations with low estrogen and progestin content are preferred, and patients require periodic evaluation for side effects. The United States Food and Drug Administration exercises strict control over the labeling of estrogens and oral contraceptives. Contraindications to their use are thromboembolic disorders or a past history of these conditions, markedly impaired hepatic function, known or suspected carcinoma of the breast or other estrogen-dependent neoplasia, and undiagnosed genital bleeding. In addition, various warnings and precautions, as well as the possible adverse reactions outlined above, must be listed. The extent to which these possible adverse reactions should be discussed with the patient at first was left to the discretion of the physician, but now a brief description of the hazards of this form of contraception is included in each package dispensed to the patient.

Aarskog, D. Maternal progestins as a possible cause of hypospadias. *N. Engl. J. Med.*, **1979**, *300*, 75–78.

Adams, D. B.; Gold, A. R.; and Burt, A. D. Rise in female-initiated sexual activity at ovulation and it suppression by oral contraceptives. *N. Engl. J. Med.*, **1978**, *299*, 1145–1150.

Allen, E., and Doisy, E. A. An ovarian hormone: a preliminary report on its localization, extraction, and partial purification, and action in test animals. *J.A.M.A.*, **1923**, *81*, 819–821.

Aloia, J. F.; Cohn, S. H.; Vaswani, A.; Yeh, J. K.; Yuen, K.; and Ellis, K. Risk factors for postmenopausal osteoporosis. *Am. J. Med.*, **1985**, *78*, 95–100.

Antunes, C. M.; Stolley, P. D.; Rosenshein, N. B.; Davies, J. L.; Tonascia, J. A.; Brown, C.; Burnett, L.; Rutledge, A.; Pokempner, M.; and Garcia, R. Endometrial cancer and estrogen use—report of a large case-control study. *N. Engl. J. Med.*, **1979**, *300*, 9–13.

Baum, J. K.; Bookstein, J. J.; Holtz, F.; and Klein, E. W. Possible association between benign hepatomas and oral contraceptives. *Lancet*, **1973**, *2*, 926–929.

Beard, J. *The Span of Gestation and the Cause of Birth.* Gustav Fischer Verlag, Jena, **1897**.

Bennion, L. J.; Ginsberg, R. L.; Garnick, M. B.; and Bennett, P. H. Effects of oral contraceptives on the gallbladder bile of normal women. *N. Engl. J. Med.*, **1976**, *294*, 189–192.

Boston Collaborative Drug Surveillance Program. Surgically confirmed gall bladder disease, venous thromboembolism, and breast tumors in relation to postmenopausal estrogen therapy. *N. Engl. J. Med.*, **1974**, *290*, 15–18.

Butenandt, A. Über "PROGYNON," ein crystallisiertes, weibliches Sexualhormon. *Naturwissenschaften*, **1929**, *17*, 879.

Clark, G. M.; McGuire, W. L.; Hubay, C. A.; Pearson, O. H.; and Marshall, J. S. Progesterone receptors as a prognostic factor in stage II breast cancer. *N. Engl. J. Med.*, **1983**, *309*, 1343–1347.

Collaborative Group for the Study of Stroke in Young Women. Oral contraception and increased risk of cerebral ischemia or thrombosis. *N. Engl. J. Med.*, **1973**, *288*, 871–878.

———. Oral contraceptives and stroke in young women; associated risk factors. *J.A.M.A.*, **1975**, *231*, 718–722.

Corner, G. W., and Allen, W. M. Physiology of the corpus luteum. II. Production of a special uterine reaction (progestational proliferation) by extracts of the corpus luteum. *Am. J. Physiol.*, **1929**, *88*, 326–346.

Coronary Drug Project Research Group. The coronary drug project. Initial findings leading to modifications of its research protocol. *J.A.M.A.*, **1970**, *214*, 1303–1313.

———. The coronary drug project. Findings leading to discontinuation of the 2.5-mg/day estrogen group. *Ibid.*, **1973**, *226*, 652–657.

DeJong, F. H., and Sharpe, R. M. Evidence for inhibin-like activity in bovine follicular fluid. *Nature*, **1976**, *263*, 71–72.

Doisy, E. A.; Veler, C. D.; and Thayer, S. A. Folliculin from the urine of pregnant women. *Am. J. Physiol.*, **1929**, *90*, 329–330.

———. The preparation of the crystalline ovarian hormone from the urine of pregnant women. *J. Biol. Chem.*, **1930**, *86*, 499–509.

FDA Drug Bulletin. PROGESTASERT IUD and ectopic pregnancy. **1978a**, *8*, 10.

———. Approval of DEPO-PROVERA for contraception denied. **1978b**, *8*, 10–11.

———. HEW recommends follow-up on DES patients. **1978c**, *8*, 31.

Fraenkel, L. Die Funktion des Corpus Luteum. *Arch. Gynaekol.*, **1903**, *68*, 483–545.

Frank, R. T.; Frank, M. L.; Gustavson, R. G.; and Weyerts, W. W. Demonstration of the female sex hormone in the circulating blood. I. Preliminary report. *J.A.M.A.*, **1925**, *85*, 510.

Greenberg, E. R.; Barnes, A. B.; Resseguie, L.; Barrett, J. A.; Burnside, S.; Lanza, L. L.; Neff, R. K.; Stevens, M.; Young, R. H.; and Colton, T. Breast cancer in mothers given diethylstilbestrol in pregnancy. *N. Engl. J. Med.*, **1984**, *311*, 1393–1398.

Greenblatt, R. B.; Roy, S.; Mahesh, V. B.; Barfield, W. E.; and Jungck, E. C. Induction of ovulation. *Am. J. Obstet. Gynecol.*, **1962**, *84*, 900–909.

Greenwald, P.; Barlow, J. J.; Nasca, P. C.; and Burnett,

W. S. Vaginal cancer after maternal treatment with synthetic estrogens. *N. Engl. J. Med.*, **1971**, *285*, 390–392.

Halban, J. Ueber den Einfluss der Ovarien auf die Entwicklung des Genitales. *Monatsschr. Geburtshilfe Gynäkol.*, **1900**, *12*, 496–503.

Heinonen, O. P.; Slone, D.; Monson, R. R.; Hook, E. B.; and Shapiro, S. Cardiovascular birth defects and antenatal exposure to female sex hormones. *N. Engl. J. Med.*, **1977**, *296*, 67–70.

Herbst, A. L.; Ulfelder, H.; and Poskanzer, D. C. Adenocarcinoma of the vagina. Association of maternal stilbestrol therapy with tumor appearance in young women. *N. Engl. J. Med.*, **1971**, *284*, 878–881.

Hilliard, J.; Scaramuzzi, R. J.; Pang, C.-N.; Penardi, R.; and Sawyer, C. H. Testosterone secretion by rabbit ovary *in vivo*. *Endocrinology*, **1974**, *94*, 267–271.

Hirvonen, E.; Malkonen, M.; and Manninen, V. Effects of different progestogens on lipoproteins during postmenopausal replacement therapy. *N. Engl. J. Med.*, **1981**, *304*, 560–563.

Horsman, A.; Jones, M.; Francis, R.; and Nordin, C. The effect of estrogen dose on postmenopausal bone loss. *N. Engl. J. Med.*, **1983**, *309*, 1405–1407.

Inman, W. H. W., and Vessey, M. P. Investigation of deaths from pulmonary, coronary and cerebral thrombosis and embolism in women of childbearing age. *Br. Med. J.*, **1968**, *2*, 193–199.

Inman, W. H. W.; Vessey, M. P.; Westerholm, B.; and Engelund, A. Thromboembolic disease and the steroidal content of oral contraceptives. *Br. Med. J.*, **1970**, *2*, 203–209.

Jacobson, B. D. Hazards of norethindrone therapy during pregnancy. *Am. J. Obstet. Gynecol.*, **1962**, *84*, 962–968.

Janerich, D. T.; Piper, J. M.; and Glebatis, D. M. Oral contraceptives and congenital limb-reduction defects. *N. Engl. J. Med.*, **1974**, *291*, 697–700.

Jick, H.; Walker, A. M.; Watkins, R. N.; D'ewart, D. C.; Hunter, J. R.; Danford, A.; Madsen, S.; Dinan, B. J.; and Rothman, K. J. Replacement estrogens and breast cancer. *Am. J. Epidemiol.*, **1980**, *112*, 586–594.

Jick, H.; Watkins, R. N.; Hunter, J. R.; Dinan, B. J.; Madsen, S.; Rothman, K. J.; and Walker, A. M. Replacement estrogens and endometrial cancer. *N. Engl. J. Med.*, **1979**, *300*, 218–222.

Kalkhoff, R. K. Metabolic effects of progesterone. *Am. J. Obstet. Gynecol.*, **1982**, *142*, 735–738.

Kato, J.; Kobayashi, T.; and Villee, C. A. Effect of clomiphene on the uptake of estradiol by the anterior hypothalamus and hypophysis. *Endocrinology*, **1968**, *82*, 1049–1052.

Kay, C. R. Progestogens and arterial disease—evidence from the Royal College of General Practitioners' study. *Am. J. Obstet. Gynecol.*, **1982**, *142*, 762–765.

Kiang, D. T.; Frenning, D. H.; Goldman, A. I.; Ascensao, V. F.; and Kennedy, B. J. Estrogen receptors and responses to chemotherapy and hormonal therapy in advanced breast cancer. *N. Engl. J. Med.*, **1978**, *299*, 1330–1334.

Knauer, E. Die Ovarien-Transplantation. *Arch. Gynaekol.*, **1900**, *60*, 322–376.

Lacassagne, A. Tumeurs malignes appareus au cours d'un traitement hormonal combiné, chez des souris appartenant a'des lignées réfractaires au cancer spontané. *C. R. Soc. Biol. (Paris)*, **1936**, *121*, 607–609.

Lawson, D. H.; Jick, H.; Hunter, J. R.; and Madsen, S. Exogenous estrogens and breast cancer. *Am. J. Epidemiol.*, **1981**, *114*, 710–713.

Leuprolide Study Group. Leuprolide versus diethylstilbestrol for metastatic prostate cancer. *N. Engl. J. Med.*, **1984**, *311*, 1281–1286.

Loewe, S. Nachweis brunsterzeugender Stoffe im

weiblichen Blute. *Klin. Wochenschr.*, **1925**, *4*, 1407–1408.

Loewe, S., and Lange, F. Der Gehalt des Frauenharns an brunsterzeugenden Stoffen in Abhängigkeit von ovariellen Zyklus. *Klin. Wochenschr.*, **1926**, *5*, 1038–1039.

McCullogh, D. R. Dual endocrine activity of the testes. *Science*, **1932**, *76*, 19–20.

Mann, J. I., and Inman, W. H. W. Oral contraceptives and death from myocardial infarction. *Br. Med. J.*, **1975**, *2*, 245–248.

Mann, J. I.; Vessey, M. P.; Thorogood, M.; and Doll, R. Myocardial infarction in young women with special reference to oral contraceptive practice. *Br. Med. J.*, **1975**, *2*, 241–245.

Meade, T. W. Oral contraceptives, clotting factors, and thrombosis. *Am. J. Obstet. Gynecol.*, **1982a**, *142*, 758–761.

———. Effects of progestogens on the cardiovascular system. *Ibid.*, **1982b**, *142*, 776–780.

Medical Letter. Effects of oral contraceptives on laboratory test results. **1979**, *21*, 54–56.

———. Drugs for postmenopausal osteoporosis. **1980**, *22*, 45–46.

Pike, M. C.; Henderson, B. E.; Krailo, M. D.; Duke, A.; and Roy, S. Breast cancer in young women and use of oral contraceptives: possible modifying effect of formulation and age at use. *Lancet*, **1983**, *2*, 926–930.

Pincus, G. Clinical effects of new progestational compounds. In, *Clinical Endocrinology I.* (Astwood, E. B., ed.) Grune & Stratton, Inc., New York, **1960**, pp. 526–531.

Richelson, L. S.; Wahner, H. W.; Melton, L. J., III; and Riggs, B. L. Relative contributions of aging and estrogen deficiency to postmenopausal bone loss. *N. Engl. J. Med.*, **1984**, *311*, 1273–1275.

Rigg, L. A.; Hermann, H.; and Yen, S. S. C. Absorption of estrogens from vaginal creams. *N. Engl. J. Med.*, **1978**, *298*, 195–197.

Rosenberg, L.; Armstrong, B.; and Jick, H. Myocardial infarction and estrogen therapy in postmenopausal women. *N. Engl. J. Med.*, **1976**, *294*, 1256–1259.

Ross, R. K.; Paganini-Hill, A.; Gerkins, V. R.; Mack, T. M.; Pfeffer, R.; Arthur, M.; and Henderson, B. E. A case-control study of menopausal estrogen therapy and breast cancer. *J.A.M.A.*, **1980**, *243*, 1635–1639.

Rothman, K. J., and Louik, C. Oral contraceptives and birth defects. *N. Engl. J. Med.*, **1978**, *299*, 522–524.

Royal College of General Practitioners' Oral Contraception Study. Further analyses of mortality in oral contraceptive users. *Lancet*, **1981**, *1*, 541–546.

Schrader, W. T.; Kuhn, R. W.; and O'Malley, B. W. Progesterone binding components of chick oviduct. Receptor subunit protein purified to apparent homogeneity from laying hen oviducts. *J. Biol. Chem.*, **1977**, *252*, 299–307.

Segal, S. J., and Thompson, C. R. Inhibition of estradiol-induced pituitary hypertrophy in rats. *Proc. Soc. Exp. Biol. Med.*, **1956**, *91*, 623–625.

Siiteri, P. K.; Febres, F.; Clemens, L. E.; Chang, R. J.; Gondos, B.; and Stites, D. Progesterone and maintenance of pregnancy: is progesterone nature's immunosuppressant? *Ann. N.Y. Acad. Sci.*, **1977**, *286*, 384–397.

Silverberg, S. G., and Makowski, E. L. Endometrial carcinoma in young women taking oral contraceptive agents. *Obstet. Gynecol.*, **1975**, *46*, 503–506.

Slone, D.; Shapiro, S.; Kaufman, D. W.; Rosenberg, L.; Miettinen, O. S.; and Stolley, P. D. Risk of myocardial infarction in relation to current and discontinued use of oral contraceptives. *N. Engl. J. Med.*, **1981**, *305*, 420–424.

Smith, D. C.; Prentice, R.; Thompson, D. J.; and Hermann, W. L. Association of exogenous estrogens and endometrial carcinoma. *N. Engl. J. Med.*, **1975**, *293*, 1164–1167.

Spellacy, W. N. Carbohydrate metabolism during treatment with estrogen, progestogen, and low-dose oral contraceptives. *Am. J. Obstet. Gynecol.*, **1982**, *142*, 732–744.

Steinberger, A., and Steinberger, E. Secretion of an FSH-inhibiting factor by cultured Sertoli cells. *Endocrinology*, **1976**, *99*, 918–921.

Sturgis, S. H., and Albright, F. The mechanism of estrin therapy in the relief of dysmenorrhea. *Endocrinology*, **1940**, *26*, 68–72.

Swerdloff, R. S., and Odell, W. D. Serum luteinizing and follicle stimulating hormone levels during sequential and nonsequential contraceptive treatment of eugonadal women. *J. Clin. Endocrinol. Metab.*, **1969**, *29*, 157–163.

Thalassinos, N. C.; Gutteridge, D. H.; Joplin, G. F.; and Fraser, T. R. Calcium balance in osteoporotic patients on long-term oral calcium therapy with and without sex hormones. *Clin. Sci.*, **1982**, *62*, 221–226.

Vessey, M. P. Female hormones and vascular disease—an epidemiologic overview. *Br. J. Fam. Plann.*, **1980**, *6*, Suppl., 1–12.

Vessey, M. P., and Doll, R. Investigation of relation between use of oral contraceptives and thromboembolic disease. *Br. Med. J.*, **1968**, *2*, 199–205.

Vessey, M. P.; Lawless, M.; McPherson, K.; and Yeates, D. Neoplasia of the cervix uteri and contraception: a possible adverse effect of the pill. *Lancet*, **1983**, *2*, 930–934.

Veterans Administration. The Veterans Administration co-operative urological research group: treatment and survival of patients with cancer of the prostate. *Surg. Gynecol. Obstet.*, **1967**, *124*, 1011–1017.

Wahl, P.; Walden, C.; Knopp, R.; Hoover, J.; Wallace, R.; Heiss, G.; and Rifkind, B. Effect of estrogen/progestin potency on lipid/lipoprotein cholesterol. *N. Engl. J. Med.*, **1983**, *308*, 862–867.

Weinberger, M. H. Estrogens and hypertension. *Compr. Ther.*, **1982**, *8*, 71–75.

Weinstein, M. C. Estrogen use in postmenopausal women—costs, risks, and benefits. *N. Engl. J. Med.*, **1980**, *303*, 308–316.

Weiss, N. S., and Sayvetz, T. A. Incidence of endometrial cancer in relation to the use of oral contraceptives. *N. Engl. J. Med.*, **1980**, *302*, 551–554.

Wynn, V. Effect of duration of low-dose oral contraceptive administration on carbohydrate metabolism. *Am. J. Obstet. Gynecol.*, **1982**, *142*, 739–742.

Ziel, H. K., and Finkle, W. D. Increased risk of endometrial carcinoma among users of conjugated estrogens. *N. Engl. J. Med.*, **1975**, *293*, 1167–1170.

———. Association of estrone with the development of endometrial carcinoma. *Am. J. Obstet. Gynecol.*, **1976**, *124*, 735–740.

Zondek, B. Darstellung des weiblichen Sexualhormon aus dem Harn, insbesondere dem Harn von Schwageren. *Klin. Wochenschr.*, **1928**, *7*, 485–486.

Monographs and Reviews

Baker, H. W. G.; Bremner, W. J.; Burger, H. G.; de-Kretser, D. M.; Dulmonis, A.; Eddie, L. W.; Hudson, B.; Keogh, L. J.; Lee, V. W. K.; and Rennie, G. C. Testicular control of FSH secretion. *Recent Prog. Horm. Res.*, **1975**, *32*, 429–444.

Boyer, R. M. Control of the onset of puberty. *Annu. Rev. Med.*, **1978**, *29*, 509–520.

Briggs, M. Biochemical effects of oral contraceptives. *Adv. Steroid Biochem. Pharmacol.*, **1976**, *5*, 66–160.

Chan, L., and O'Malley, B. W. Mechanism of action of sex steroid hormones. *N. Engl. J. Med.*, **1976**, *294*, 1322–1328, 1372–1381, 1430–1437.

Erickson, G. F. Normal ovarian function. *Clin. Obstet. Gynecol.,* **1978,** *21,* 31–52.

Eskin, B. A. Sex hormones and aging. *Adv. Exp. Med. Biol.,* **1978,** *97,* 207–224.

Fotherby, K., and James, F. Metabolism of synthetic steroids. *Adv. Steroid Biochem. Pharmacol.,* **1972,** *3,* 67–165.

Franchimont, P. Pituitary gonadotropins. *Clin. Endocrinol. Metab.,* **1977,** *6,* 101–116.

Gordon, G. S. Drug treatment of osteoporosis. *Annu. Rev. Pharmacol. Toxicol.,* **1978,** *18,* 253–268.

Gorski, J., and Gannon, F. Current models of steroid hormone action: a critique. *Annu. Rev. Physiol.,* **1976,** *38,* 425–450.

Heyns, W. The steroid-binding β-globulin of human plasma. *Adv. Steroid Biochem. Pharmacol.,* **1977,** *6,* 59–79.

Jordan, V. C. Biochemical pharmacology of antiestrogen action. *Pharmacol. Rev.,* **1984,** *36,* 245–276.

Kaplan, N. M. Cardiovascular complications of oral contraceptives. *Annu. Rev. Med.,* **1978,** *29,* 31–40.

Kay, C. R. Oral contraceptives—the clinical perspective. In, *Pharmacology of Steroid Contraceptive Drugs.* (Garattini, S., and Berendes, H. W., eds.) Raven Press, New York, **1977,** pp. 1–24.

Kellie, A. E. The pharmacology of the estrogens. *Annu. Rev. Pharmacol.,* **1971,** *11,* 97–112.

Koide, S. S., and Ch'iu Lyle, K. Unusual signs and symptoms associated with oral contraceptive medication. *J. Reprod. Med.,* **1975,** *15,* 214–224.

Laragh, J. H. Oral contraceptive-induced hypertension—nine years later. *Am. J. Obstet. Gynecol.,* **1976,** *126,* 141–147.

Legha, S. S.; Davis, H. L.; and Muggia, F. M. Hormonal therapy of breast cancer: new approaches and concepts. *Ann. Intern. Med.,* **1978,** *88,* 69–77.

Leis, H. P.; Black, M. M.; and Sall, S. The pill and the breast. *J. Reprod. Med.,* **1976,** *16,* 5–9.

Linder, H. R.; Amsterdam, A.; Solomon, Y.; Tsafriri, A.; Nimrod, A.; Lamprecht, S. A.; Zor, U.; and Koch, Y. Intraovarian factors in ovulation: determinants of follicular response to gonadotropins. *J. Reprod. Fertil.,* **1977,** *51,* 215–235.

McGuire, W. L. Endocrine therapy of breast cancer. *Annu. Rev. Med.,* **1975,** *26,* 353–363.

Marcus, R., and Korenman, S. G. Estrogens and the human male. *Annu. Rev. Med.,* **1976,** *27,* 357–370.

Marshall, J. R. Induction of ovulation. *Clin. Obstet. Gynecol.,* **1978,** *21,* 147–162.

Melski, J. W., and Arndt, K. A. Topical therapy for acne. *N. Engl. J. Med.,* **1980,** *302,* 503–506.

Naftolin, F., and Tolis, G. Neuroendocrine regulation of the menstrual cycle. *Clin. Obstet. Gynecol.,* **1978,** *21,* 17–29.

Rock, J.; Garcia, C. M.; and Pincus, G. Synthetic progestins in the normal human menstrual cycle. *Recent Prog. Horm. Res.,* **1957,** *13,* 323–339.

Rosenfield, R. L. Role of androgens in growth and development of the fetus, child, and adolescent. *Adv. Pediatr.,* **1972,** *19,* 172–213.

Rozenbaum, H. Relationships between chemical structure and biological properties of progestogens. *Am. J. Obstet. Gynecol.,* **1982,** *142,* 719–724.

Ryan, K. J. Postmenopausal estrogen use. *Annu. Rev. Med.,* **1982,** *33,* 171–181.

Schally, A. V. Aspects of hypothalamic regulation of the pituitary gland: its implications for the control of reproductive functions. *Science,* **1978,** *202,* 18–28.

Speroff, L. The formulation of oral contraceptives: does the amount of estrogen make any clinical difference? *Johns Hopkins Med. J.,* **1982,** *150,* 170–176.

Stadel, B. V. Oral contraceptives and cardiovascular disease. *N. Engl. J. Med.,* **1981,** *305,* 612–618, 672–677.

Vande Wiele, R. L., and Dyrenfurth, I. Gonadotropin-steroid interrelationships. *Pharmacol. Rev.,* **1973,** *25,* 189–207.

Vecchio, T. J. Long-acting injectable contraceptives. *Adv. Steroid Biochem. Pharmacol.,* **1976,** *5,* 1–64.

Wentz, A. C. Assessment of estrogen and progestin therapy in gynecology and obstetrics. *Clin. Obstet. Gynecol.,* **1977,** *20,* 461–482.

CHAPTER
62 ANDROGENS

Ferid Murad and Robert C. Haynes, Jr.

Androgens are synthesized in the testis, the ovary, and the adrenal cortex. In the circulation, androgens serve as prohormones for the formation of two classes of steroids: 5α-reduced androgens, which act as the intracellular mediators of most actions of the hormones, and estrogens, which enhance some androgenic effects and block others. Thus, the net effect of the action of endogenous androgens is the sum of the effects of the secreted hormone (testosterone), its 5α-reduced metabolite (dihydrotestosterone), and its estrogenic derivative (estradiol) (*see* Table 62–1). Clear understanding of these interconversions is essential for the rational pharmacological use of these agents.

History. The observation that castration makes the eunuch, properly credited to primitive man, ushered in the dawn of endocrinology. The discovery that the testis is a gland of internal secretion is ascribed to Berthold, who in 1849 showed that the transplantation of gonads into castrated roosters prevented the typical signs of castration. This was the first published experimental evidence for the effect of an endocrine gland (Berthold, 1849). However, it was not this observation but the popular belief that failure of testicular function was the cause of the symptoms of old age in men that stimulated many attempts to isolate an active testicular principle. An example of the wide acceptance of this belief is the experiments of Brown-Séquard (1889), who prepared a testicular extract and administered it to himself. He was convinced that he had gained in vigor and capacity for work from the treatment, but it is now known that his aqueous extract was devoid of any significant quantity of hormone.

Chemistry. The elucidation of the chemistry of the male sex hormones was made possible by the development of methods of assay. The procedure of Koch and coworkers for the determination of

Table 62–1.   METABOLISM OF ANDROGENS

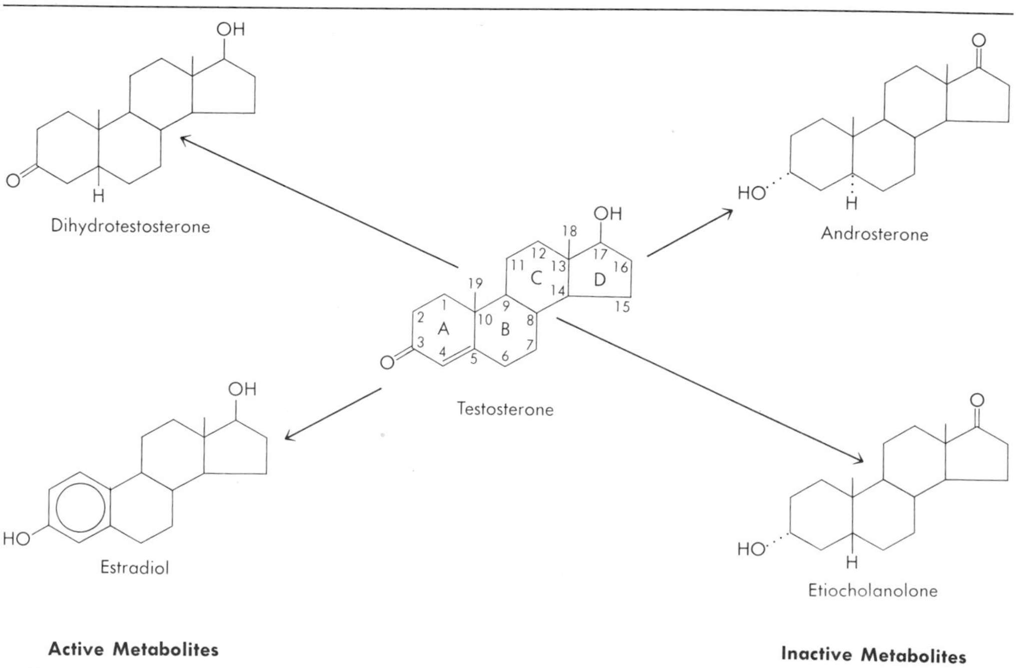

Active Metabolites

Inactive Metabolites

androgenic activity utilizing the growth response of the capon's comb was employed in the first isolation of the urinary principle by Butenandt (1931), who by herculean effort obtained 15 mg of androsterone, a metabolite of testosterone, from 15,000 liters of male urine.

Following the isolation of another androgen from urine (dehydroepiandrosterone—later shown to be of adrenal origin), attention focused on the testes as the source of male sex hormone. Active testicular extracts were prepared as early as 1927 by Loewe, using the mammalian seminal vesicle for assay (*see* Loewe and Voss, 1930). The testicular hormone testosterone was isolated in crystalline form by Laqueur and associates (*see* David *et al.*, 1935); its chemical structure was soon elucidated, and the hormone was then synthesized (Ruzicka and Wettstein, 1935).

Testosterone is the principal androgen secreted by the testis and the main androgenic steroid in the plasma of males. In women, smaller amounts of testosterone are synthesized by the ovary and adrenal. In many target tissues for androgens testosterone is reduced at the 5α position to dihydrotestosterone, which serves as the intracellular mediator of most actions of the hormone. Dihydrotestosterone binds to the cytoplasmic androgen receptor protein about ten times more tightly than does testosterone, and the dihydrotestosterone-receptor complex is more readily transformed to the activated or DNA-binding state than is the testosterone-receptor complex; its greater androgenic potency is thereby explained (*see* below; *see also* Kovacs *et al.*, 1984). A variety of other naturally occurring weak androgens have been described, including the testosterone precursor androstenedione, the adrenal androgen dehydroandrostenedione, and the dihydrotestosterone metabolites 5α-androstane-$3\alpha,17\beta$-diol and androsterone. However, these steroids bind so weakly to the androgen receptor that it is unlikely that they can act directly as androgens at physiological concentrations, and it is now believed that they are androgens only to the extent that they are converted to testosterone and/or dihydrotestosterone *in vivo*. Thus, the prior concept of weak androgens is now one of weak androgen precursors.

The major metabolites of androgens in urine are physiologically inactive (either as free steroids or water-soluble conjugates); these are predominantly etiocholanolone, a 5β-reduced metabolite of testosterone and of other Δ^4,3-keto androgens, and androsterone, a metabolite of dihydrotestosterone (Table 62–1). Testosterone (but not dihydrotestosterone) can also be aromatized to estradiol in a variety of extraglandular tissues, a pathway that accounts for most estrogen synthesis in men and postmenopausal women (Siiteri and MacDonald, 1973). The role, if any, of the approximately 50 μg of estradiol synthesized each day in normal men has never been defined, but either relative or absolute excess of estrogen can cause feminization in men.

Soon after the identification of testosterone as the principal testicular androgen, it became apparent that the hormone cannot be given effectively by mouth or by parenteral injection. Oral administration of testosterone (or dihydrotestosterone) is followed by absorption into the portal blood and prompt degradation by the liver; insignificant amounts of hormone reach the systemic circulation. Parenteral administration is also followed by prompt metabolism. It is thus necessary to modify the androgen molecule to alter its properties or to devise means of administration that circumvent these problems.

The aim of chemical modification has been to retard the rate of catabolism or to enhance the androgenic potency of each molecule. Three general types of modification of testosterone are clinically useful. (1) Esterification of the 17β-hydroxyl group with any of several carboxylic acids decreases the polarity of the molecule, makes it more soluble in the lipid vehicles used for injection, and hence slows release of the injected steroid into the circulation. The longer the carbon chain in the ester, the more lipid soluble the steroid becomes and the more prolonged the action. Such esters are hydrolyzed before the hormone acts, and the effectiveness of drug therapy can thus be monitored by assay of plasma concentrations of testosterone. Most esters must be injected, but two such compounds, methenolone acetate and testosterone undecanoate, have features that make oral administration possible. Testosterone undecanoate is absorbed via the lymphatic circulation rather than the portal system and hence gains direct access to the systemic circulation. The methyl group on the 1 position of methenolone acetate slows hepatic inactivation and hence allows effective concentrations to be achieved in blood. (2) Alkylation at the 17α position (as in methyltestosterone and fluoxymesterone) also allows androgens to be effective orally because the alkylated derivatives are slowly catabolized by the liver. The alkyl group is not removed metabolically, and, hence, the alkylated derivatives mediate the action of the hormone within cells. (3) Other alterations of the ring structure have been made empirically. In some instances the effect is to slow the rate of inactivation; in others the modification enhances the potency; and in still others it alters the pattern of its metabolism. For example, fluoxymesterone is a good androgen but a poor precursor of estrogen, whereas 19-nortestosterone, like dihydrotestosterone, binds more tightly to the androgen receptor.

Synthesis and Secretion of Testosterone. The concentration of testosterone in the plasma of males is relatively high during three periods of life: during the phase of embryonic development in which male phenotypic differentiation takes place, during the neonatal period, and throughout adult sexual life. The concentration starts to rise in male embryos about the eighth week of development and declines prior to birth. It subsequently rises during the neonatal period and then falls to typical prepuberal values within several months after birth. Through poorly understood mechanisms, the pituitary begins to secrete increased amounts of luteinizing hormone (LH) and follicle-stimulating hormone (FSH) at the time of puberty. The increase in the secretion of gonadotropins begins in a cyclic fashion that is synchronized with the sleep cycle. As puberty progresses, however, pulsatile secretion of gonadotropins is observed during both sleep and waking periods (Franchimont 1977; Boyar, 1978). At this stage of development the hypothalamus and pituitary also become less sensitive to feedback inhibition by sex hormones. The initiating event for these phenomena is unknown.

Prior to puberty, concentrations of testosterone in plasma are low (less than 20 ng/dl), although the immature testes are capable of synthesizing androgens if challenged with gonadotropin. In the adult male, plasma testosterone concentrations rise to 300 to 1000 ng/dl, and the rate of production is 2.5 to 11 mg per day (Rosenfield, 1972). Pathways of androgen biosynthesis are shown in Figure 61–1 (page 1413). In plasma, about 98% of testosterone is bound to sex hormone–binding globulin, albumin, and other proteins. About 2% of the steroid is free, and this concentration correlates with the magnitude of androgenic effects (see Dunn et al., 1981).

Androgen-Gonadotropin Relationships. As mentioned, gonadotropins are secreted in a pulsatile manner. In adult men, the concentrations of LH, FSH, and testosterone in plasma fluctuate during the course of the day, while integrated daily values are constant (Naftolin et al., 1973). Similar pulsations in gonadotropins are observed in women, superimposed upon the daily alterations that occur during the menstrual cycle (see Figure 61–2, page 1416).

LH and FSH together are responsible for regulating testicular growth, spermatogenesis, and steroidogenesis. Growth hormone may have a synergistic effect with LH on the testis, while estrogens can decrease the effects of LH on the secretion of testosterone. All of the actions of the gonadotropins are probably mediated through adenosine 3′,5′-monophosphate (cyclic AMP) (Murad et al., 1969; see Eik-Nes, 1971). LH, also called interstitial cell–stimulating hormone

(ICSH), interacts with the interstitial (Leydig) cells of the testes to increase the synthesis of cyclic AMP and subsequently the formation of androgens from acetate and cholesterol. Although cyclic AMP increases the conversion of cholesterol to pregnenolone, the precise mechanism of stimulation of steroidogenesis by cyclic AMP in this and other tissues is unknown. While the major effects of FSH are thought to be on spermatogenesis in the seminiferous tubules and that of LH on testosterone synthesis by Leydig cells, complex interactions exist in the testis. Some studies have indicated that FSH can also enhance testosterone synthesis and can augment the activity of LH (see Bartke et al., 1978; Ewing and Robaire, 1978; Lipsett, 1980). Furthermore, testosterone is required for spermatogenesis and maturation of sperm. With immunohistochemical technics, LH has been localized to Leydig and peritubular cells, and FSH to tubular Sertoli cells (Castro et al., 1972). The Sertoli cells of the seminiferous tubules may also produce small amounts of testosterone in some species (Lacy and Pettit, 1970), and the seminiferous tubules can convert testosterone to dihydrotestosterone. Androgens in the Sertoli cells may act locally and be particularly important for spermatogenesis, whereas the hormone produced by the Leydig cells is released predominantly into the circulation (see Ritzen et al., 1981). Both LH and FSH have growth-promoting effects on the testes. The effects of human chorionic gonadotropin appear to be identical to those of LH in the human testis.

The nature of the mechanism of feedback of the testicular secretions upon the gonadotropic function of the pituitary is a problem of continuing uncertainty. Administration of testosterone to intact animals suppresses the secretion of LH and thereby causes atrophy of interstitial tissue. The administration of testosterone also suppresses the excessive secretion of FSH in eunuchism, but whether testosterone plays a major role in the physiological regulation of FSH secretion is not resolved. Implantation of testosterone in the median eminence of rats inhibits pituitary gonadotropin secretion (see Davidson, 1969) by decreasing the concentration of gonadotropin-releasing hormone (Gn-RH) (Schally, 1978). Likewise, administration of testosterone to hypogonadal men inhibits both the frequency and amplitude of pulses of LH secretion, presumably by inhibition of the release of Gn-RH (Matsumoto and Bremner, 1984).

In normal men, the concentration of estradiol in the spermatic vein exceeds that in peripheral plasma (Kelch *et al.*, 1972; Longcope, 1972); about 15% of the estradiol in the plasma of men is derived from the testes, probably the Leydig cells (*see* Lipsett, 1980). Estrogens are also synthesized from androgens in extraglandular tissue, including the brain (Siiteri and MacDonald, 1973; Marcus and Korenman, 1976). Estrogens formed locally in the brain from administered or endogenous androgen may be responsible in part for the inhibition of gonadotropin secretion that results.

A nonsteroidal substance that inhibits the secretion of FSH is present in testicular extracts and in human seminal plasma (McCullagh, 1932; Keogh *et al.*, 1976; Ramasharma and Sairam, 1982). This material, called *inhibin*, has a molecular weight of approximately 20,000. Inhibin has also been detected in extracts from cultures of Sertoli cells and in ovarian follicular fluid (DeJong and Sharpe, 1976; Steinberger and Steinberger, 1976). Inhibin may act as a feedback regulator of gonadotropin secretion.

Ovarian and Adrenal Androgens. Androgens and androgenic precursors are also normally secreted by the ovary and the adrenal cortex. Androstenedione and dehydroepiandrosterone, which are produced by both the ovary and adrenal, can be converted to testosterone and estrogen in peripheral tissues. The daily rate of production of testosterone in women is about 0.25 mg, and about one half of this is derived from the metabolic conversion of androstenedione to testosterone (*see* Sommerville and Collins, 1970; Rosenfield, 1972; Givens, 1978). The remainder is derived from testosterone produced and secreted by the ovary. Studies with rabbit ovary *in vivo* and *in vitro* have demonstrated that the synthesis and secretion of testosterone are enhanced by the administration of LH (Mills and Savard, 1972; Hilliard *et al.*, 1974).

Alterations in plasma concentrations of testosterone and androstenedione occur during the menstrual cycle. The concentration of testosterone in plasma of women is about 15 to 65 ng/dl. Two peaks of androgen concentration are seen that are qualitatively similar to those of the estrogens at the preovulatory and luteal phases of the cycle (Judd and Yen, 1973). In some ovarian disorders, ovarian secretion of androgens may be increased, resulting in virilization.

In men, production of testosterone by the adrenal cortex is not sufficient to maintain spermatogenesis or secondary sexual features of the adult. In abnormal conditions such as congenital adrenal hyperplasia and adrenal tumors, the adrenal cortex can secrete large quantities of androgens and androgenic precursors.

Physiological and Pharmacological Actions. Androgens serve different functions at different stages of life. During embryonic life, they virilize the urogenital tract of the male embryo, and their action is thus central to the development of the male phenotype. The role of androgens, if any, during the neonatal surge of androgen secretion is not defined but may involve behavioral and functional actions within the central nervous system. At puberty, the hormones act to transform the boy into a man. Minimal androgen secretion from the prepuberal testis and adrenal cortex suppresses secretion of gonadotropins until, at a variable age, secretion of gonadotropins becomes less sensitive to feedback inhibition and the testes start to enlarge (*see* Franchimont, 1977; Boyar, 1978). Shortly thereafter the penis and scrotum begin to grow, and pubic hair appears. Early in puberty penile erections and masturbation become frequent in most individuals. Almost simultaneously the growth-promoting property of androgen causes increase in height and the development of the skeletal musculature, which contributes to a rapid increase in body weight. As the muscles grow there is increased physical vigor. The testes reach adult proportions before all the changes of puberty are completed. As a result of the actions of androgens, the skin becomes thicker and tends to be oily due to a proliferation of sebaceous glands; the latter are prone to plugging and infection, leading to acne in some individuals. Subcutaneous fat is lost, and the veins are prominent under the skin. Axillary hair grows, and hair on the trunk and limbs develops into a pattern typical of the male. Growth of the larynx causes difficulty at first in adjusting the tone of speech and later brings about a permanent deepening of the voice. Growth of beard lags behind the other events of puberty and is the last of the secondary sex characteristics to develop. Concurrently, those whose inheritance so dictates show the first signs of going bald, with recession of the hairline at the temples and thinning of the hair at the crown. At about this time the major spurt in growth comes to an end as the epiphyses of the larger long bones begin to close, and over the next few years only 1 to 2 cm of additional growth is usual.

Androgens may also be responsible in part for the aggressive and sexual behavior of males (*see* Lunde and Hamburg, 1972; Horn, 1977; Wilson, 1982) and, in some species, for organizational effects in the brain during prenatal or early postnatal life (*see* Pardridge *et al.*, 1982). While this is a difficult matter to resolve, the differential behavioral patterns of many male and female animals suggest that sex hormones play an important role. Further, the sexual behavior of female rats is changed to that characteristic of males after treatment with testosterone, either as neonates or as adults (Sachs *et al.*, 1973). Psychopathic behavior in men is not associated with altered patterns of androgen metabolism.

When androgen is given before puberty or to a young eunuchoid man, the events of normal puberty are duplicated, and the time required for complete normal puberty (approximately 2 years) is not significantly shortened. Within 1 or 2 days of the start of treatment erections appear and may be embarrassingly inappropriate and frequent, even to the point of discomfort; with continued treatment at the same dose this response subsides. Increased physical vigor is noted within a few weeks, and a general feeling of well-being prevails. A distinct change in the voice can be noted, and soon thereafter the penis begins to grow and traces of axillary and pubic hair appear. The rapidity of growth is impressive in boys treated at or before the time of normal puberty; the height may increase 10 cm or more during the first year and continue at a somewhat diminished rate for 2 or 3 years. With continued treatment, development follows the course of normal puberty with the growth of a beard as a late expression of therapy.

Failure of Puberty Due to Hypogonadism. The normal actions of androgens are displayed by the consequences of deficiency. If the testes fail to function or are removed in boyhood, there is no puberty. Failure of testicular development may result from the deficiency of gonadotropins or may represent a primary testicular defect. A boy so afflicted continues to grow and becomes abnormally tall; the hands and feet become especially large and the limbs unduly long. The childish appearance and demeanor are in striking contrast to the stature; the larynx does not grow, leaving the voice high pitched. The skeletal musculature is underdeveloped and is made still more inconspicuous by a layer of subcutaneous fat. Accumulation of fat is especially prominent around the shoulders and breasts and over the upper thighs, hips, and abdomen, the whole giving the mistaken impression of femininity. Familial baldness does not appear, the beard is scant or nonexistent, the axillary and pubic hair is sparse, and the body hair is short and fine. The genitalia are those of a child, and there is no sex drive.

Hypogonadism after Puberty. Some of the sex characteristics developed during puberty are self-sustaining, while others must be supported by the continued action of androgen. Hypogonadism in the adult is typified by castration after puberty. The general bodily proportions remain the same, the penis does not shrink, the voice does not change, and the beard and body hair remain unchanged for a long time. Libido is greatly reduced or absent, and erectile potency is usually decreased. The prostate and seminal vesicles are atrophic, and the volume of the semen is small or there is none at all.

Complete failure of the endocrine function of the testis in adult life is not a common event; a partial deficiency is more usual, and it originates from incomplete development at puberty, as in 47,XXY men with the Klinefelter syndrome, or from a disorder during adult life, such as a pituitary tumor or a viral infection of the testis (*see* Odell and Swerdloff, 1978). Testicular function commonly decreases slightly with age; generally this occurs at a slow rate after the sixth or seventh decade. The common decrease in libido in some men after age 40 or 50 usually cannot be attributed to altered testicular function.

Actions on the Testis and Accessory Structures. At about the eighth week of fetal life, testicular androgens begin to be secreted and express their important role in the differentiation and development of the reproductive tract (Jost, 1971). Lack of androgens in the male fetus results in the development of a female external phenotype. The developing testes also produce a peptide hormone (Müllerian inhibiting substance) that causes degeneration of the Müllerian ducts of the fetus (Josso *et al.*, 1975). Subsequently, under the influence of testosterone (or dihydrotestosterone) each of the Wolffian ducts differentiates into the epididymis, vas deferens, and seminal vesicle; fusion of the labioscrotal fold results in the development of the penis (male urethra) and the scrotum, and there is virilization of the urogenital sinus to form the prostate. During the latter part of pregnancy plasma concentrations of androgen in the male fetus begin to decline, and at birth they are essentially undetectable (*see* Rosenfield, 1972).

At puberty and thereafter androgens exert a direct effect upon the testis. Following hypophysectomy in the rat, shrinkage of the testis is slowed by the injection of androgen, and spermatogenesis is maintained for a long time. This effect is also revealed by the biphasic response of the normal animal to androgen; moderate doses produce atrophy of the testis through suppression of gonadotropins, while with larger doses the atrophy is less, possibly because of the direct sustaining effect upon the seminiferous tubules.

Androgens are required for spermatogenesis in the seminiferous tubules and for the maturation of sperm in their passage through the epididymis and vas deferens. These processes are highly ordered and complex, and the nature of the effects of testosterone thereon is unknown. Studies of these events are complicated by the 10 weeks required for completion of spermatogenesis and the several additional weeks needed for passage of sperm through the vas deferens and for maturation of sperm.

In fetal, prepuberal, and puberal life the actions of testosterone result in growth of the clitoris or penis. Androgens are also required for the growth and function of the seminal vesicle and prostate.

Anabolic Effects. The nitrogen-retaining effect of androgen was first demonstrated in castrated dogs injected with androgen-containing extracts from the urine of normal men (Kochakian and Murlin, 1935). Papanicolaou and Falk (1938) showed that the skeletal muscles of male guinea pigs are larger than those of the female and that the difference is abolished by removal of the testes. Injection of testosterone propionate into the female or the castrated male causes pronounced muscular development. The large muscles of the male represent a sex characteristic dependent upon androgen for its expression. In man, the major difference in muscle development between the sexes is in the muscles of the shoulder girdle. The anabolic actions of androgens are mediated by the same receptor protein that mediates the actions of the hormone in other target tissues (*see* below; Saartok *et al.*, 1984). As in the case of other actions of the hormone, the administration of supraphysiological doses of androgen results in no more growth of muscle than is afforded by the normal concentrations of testosterone in the male. Consequently, use of androgens by male athletes in the hope that muscle development may be enhanced has no physiological rationale (*see* Wilson and Griffin, 1980). Furthermore, if these agents are administered during adolescence, premature closure of epiphyses and ultimate short stature are likely.

The anabolic effects of androgen were carefully investigated by Kenyon and associates (*see* Knowlton *et al.*, 1942). The effects are more pronounced in hypogonadal men, in boys before puberty, and in women than in normal men. Indeed, normal men experience only a transient positive nitrogen balance of a slight degree when exogenous androgens are administered. A maximally effective dose of 25 mg of testosterone propionate daily causes an average retention of nitrogen of 63 mg/kg daily in hypogonadal men. There is also retention of potassium, sodium, phosphorus, sulfur, and chloride associated with a gain in weight, which can be accounted for by the water held in association with the retained salts and protein. When the administration of androgen is stopped, sodium, chloride, and water are quickly lost from the body, phosphorus and potassium are lost less rapidly and completely, and the stored nitrogen is retained for weeks. Estradiol benzoate in the large dose of 5 mg daily exerts effects similar to those observed after an equal dose of testosterone propionate (*see* Chapter 61). Progesterone, on the other hand, is mildly catabolic; daily doses of 50 or 100 mg, given intramuscularly, cause a slightly negative balance of nitrogen and a loss of salt in normal men and women.

Effects on Sebaceous Glands. The prevalence of acne at puberty and during treatment with androgens is related to the growth and secretion of the sebaceous glands. Methyltestosterone is active in amounts as small as 5 mg daily, while a dose of 2.5 mg daily of fluoxymesterone has variable effects. However, these effects are not seen in adult males, whose glands are apparently maximally stimulated. When acne results from endogenous androgenic stimulation, estrogens will ameliorate this condition, probably by decreasing the secretion of gonadotropins and androgen (*see* Ebling, 1970; Chapter 61).

Mechanism of Action. At some sites of action, testosterone is not the active form of the hormone. It is converted by a 5α-reductase in target tissues to the more active dihydrotestosterone (*see* Liao and Fang, 1969; Griffin *et al.*, 1982). In one form of male pseudohermaphroditism the target tissues are deficient in the reductase. In this disorder the genotypic male secretes normal amounts of testosterone from the testes, but the hormone is not converted to dihydrotestosterone and male external genitalia fail to develop (Walsh *et al.*, 1974; Griffin and Wilson, 1980; Griffin *et al.*, 1982).

Not all target tissues require the conversion of testosterone to dihydrotestosterone for activity. Virilization of the Wolffian ducts during embryogenesis and regulation of LH production by the hypothalamic-pituitary system are mediated by testosterone itself (*see* Mainwaring, 1977; Givens, 1978; Odell and Swerdloff, 1978).

Testosterone or dihydrotestosterone binds to a cytoplasmic protein receptor, and the hormone-receptor complex acts in the nucleus at specific binding sites on the chromosomes; increased RNA polymerase activity and increased synthesis of specific RNA and protein result. As in other steroid-sensitive cells, the modification of the steroid-receptor complex and the alterations in the synthesis of nucleic acids and protein that occur are complex and incompletely understood (*see* Mainwaring, 1977). In testicular feminization, another type of male pseudohermaphroditism, the genotypic male with normal amounts of testosterone undergoes feminine development because of absence or defective function of the receptor protein for testosterone and dihydrotestosterone (Griffin and Wilson, 1980; Griffin *et al.*, 1982).

Absorption, Metabolism, and Excretion. Testosterone injected as a solution in oil is so quickly absorbed, metabolized, and excreted that the androgenic effect is small. Testosterone given by mouth is readily absorbed but is even less effective, since most of the hormone is metabolized by the liver before reaching the systemic circulation. Alternate means of administration of testosterone have been proposed to circumvent these difficulties. These include implantation of testosterone-filled silastic capsules, oral administration of large amounts of the hormone in particulate form, topical administration in the form of cream, and administration by rectal suppositories or nasal drops. None of the technics appears feasible for effective clinical application.

Testosterone esters are less polar than the free steroid and, when such esters are injected intramuscularly in oil, are absorbed more slowly. For example, testosterone propionate is more active than testosterone, even when each is injected every day. The cypionate and enanthate esters are fully effective when given at 1- or 2-week intervals in proportionately larger doses. Since these esters are hydrolyzed prior to action, the concentrations of testosterone in plasma can be monitored by conventional radioimmunoassay. This greatly facilitates the administration of effective dosages for each patient (Caminos-Torres *et al.*, 1977).

As mentioned earlier, about 98% of testosterone in plasma is bound to protein, mostly to sex hormone–binding globulin (testosterone-estradiol-binding globulin) and albumin (Heyns, 1977; Dunn *et al.*, 1981; Pardridge, 1981). Thus, the concentration of the sex hormone–binding globulin determines the concentration of free testosterone in plasma and thereby its half-life, which is generally 10 to 20 minutes. Testosterone decreases the rate of hepatic synthesis of sex hormone–binding globulin, while estrogens increase its synthesis. For this reason the concentration of the globulin in women is about twice that in men. In disorders characterized by excessive synthesis of androgens, the free concentration of the hormone may be increased disproportionately as a result of diminished synthesis of sex hormone–binding globulin.

Testosterone is inactivated primarily in the liver. Metabolism to androstenedione involves oxidation of the 17-OH group; reduction of ring A of androstenedione leads to formation of androstanedione, with markedly reduced activity. The 3-keto group is reduced to form androsterone; alternatively, androstenedione can be reduced in the 5β position and can undergo 3-keto reduction to form etiocholanolone (Table 62–1). Dihydrotestosterone itself is converted in the liver to androsterone, androstanedione, and androstanediol (*see* Fotherby and James, 1972). Alkylation of androgens at the 17 position markedly retards their hepatic metabolism and permits such analogs to be effective orally. Such alkylated androgens can cause hepatotoxicity (*see* below).

After the administration of radioactive testosterone, about 90% of the radioactivity appears in the urine; 6% appears in the feces after undergoing enterohepatic circulation. Urinary products include androsterone and etiocholanolone. Small amounts of androstanediol and estrogens are also excreted, largely as glucuronide and sulfate conjugates.

Androsterone and etiocholanolone, among many other compounds, are measured as 17-ketosteroids in the usual clinical tests. However, the major fraction of the ketosteroids of urine consists of metabolic products of the adrenal steroids, and only about 30% of urinary 17-ketosteroids are derived from metabolism of testicular hormones. Thus, measurement of the excretion of 17-ketosteroids is an inadequate test for the functional activity of the testis. Low values point to adrenal insufficiency rather than to hypogonadism, and high values almost always are indicative of adrenocortical hyperactivity or tumor. Without the testes, the human male is androgen deficient even though the urinary 17-ketosteroids may be within the normal range. Likewise, in women, measurement of the excretion of 17-ketosteroids is rarely helpful in elucidating whether an excess of androgen originates in the ovary or the adrenal.

The esters of testosterone are hydrolyzed to free testosterone and are subsequently metabolized in the same way as is testosterone itself, but other changes in the molecule (as in methyltestosterone and fluoxymesterone) alter the course of metabolic degradation. Such synthetic androgens are metabolized less rapidly than is testosterone and have longer half-lives. Unaltered compounds, metabolites, and conjugates are excreted in the urine and feces (Fotherby and James, 1972).

Assays. Bioassay is used in the evaluation of androgenic potency of new compounds. The classical assay is based upon the growth of the comb of the capon. Better correlation with clinical effectiveness is given by bioassays in mammals, and the most widely used test depends upon the growth of the seminal vesicles or ventral prostate of the castrated rat.

In clinical medicine, the assay of sex hormone–binding globulin as well as sensitive and specific radioimmunoassays for androgens offer several advantages over bioassay methods (*see* James *et al.*, 1977); the more notable are simplicity, sensitivity, and lower cost. The search for non-androgenic anabolic steroids has made use of assays employing the growth of the kidney or levator ani muscle of castrated animals. Another test for anabolic activity involves examination of nitrogen excretion and the nitrogen-retaining effects of agents given to animals on controlled diets (*see earlier editions* of this textbook for references). Unfortunately, none of these assays is totally satisfactory and able to predict the results obtained in clinical trials, and no pure anabolic steroid without androgenic effects has ever been described. The failure to separate the androgenic and anabolic effects is not surprising, since all known actions of the hormone are mediated by a single receptor protein.

Preparations and Dosage. Some of the preparations of androgens available for clinical use are summarized in Table 62–2.

Androgen therapy is used primarily in androgen-deficient males for the development or maintenance of secondary sex characteristics. When full replacement therapy with androgen is required, the intramuscular preparations are the most effective. Dosage should provide at least 10 mg per day; with testosterone propionate this is met by giving 25 mg three times weekly. With the longer-acting esters, the dose is about 200 mg every 2 weeks. Long-term treatment with these doses ordinarily causes full masculine development, provided they are started sufficiently early in life. When androgen replacement is started late (over the age of 25), the degree of virilization eventually attained is variable, but it may be near normal.

Some preparations of androgens have been introduced primarily for use as anabolic agents, with the expectation that they would be relatively less androgenic than testosterone and its close relatives (Table 62–3). However, none is free of androgenic activity in man.

Various mixtures of androgenic and anabolic steroids with estrogens, vitamins, and other agents are also available. However, the use of these fixed-dose combinations is to be discouraged. In particular, their prolonged use in postmenopausal women and geriatric patients is costly and usually irrational.

Untoward Effects. When used in women, all androgens carry the risk of causing masculinization. Among the earli-

Table 62–2. SOME ANDROGENIC STEROIDS USED IN THERAPY

NONPROPRIETARY NAME AND SOME TRADE NAMES	CHEMICAL STRUCTURE	DOSAGE FORMS AND USUAL DOSAGE FOR ANDROGEN DEFICIENCY *
Testosterone TESTOJECT-50		Aqueous suspension for i.m. use: 10 to 50 mg three times weekly
Testosterone propionate TESTEX	O—COCH₂CH₃	Oily solution for i.m. use: 10 to 25 mg two to three times weekly
Testosterone enanthate DELATESTRYL	O—CO(CH₂)₅CH₃	Oily solution for i.m. use: 50 to 400 mg every 2 to 4 weeks
Testosterone cypionate DEPO-TESTOSTERONE	O—COCH₂CH₂—	Oily solution for i.m. use: 50 to 400 mg every 2 to 4 weeks
Methyltestosterone METANDREN ORETON METHYL		Tablets and capsules: 10 to 40 mg daily Buccal tablets: 5 to 20 mg daily
Fluoxymesterone HALOTESTIN		Tablets: 2 to 10 mg daily
Danazol † DANOCRINE		Capsules: 200 to 800 mg daily

* Dosage schedules for breast carcinoma in females are generally two to three times those for androgen replacement.
† Used predominantly to suppress the pituitary and for the treatment of hereditary angioneurotic edema.

Table 62–3. SOME ANABOLIC STEROIDS USED IN THERAPY

NONPROPRIETARY NAME AND SOME TRADE NAMES	CHEMICAL STRUCTURE	DOSAGE FORMS AND USUAL DOSAGE FOR ANABOLIC EFFECTS
Dromostanolone propionate DROLBAN		Oily solution for i.m. use: 100 mg three times weekly for breast carcinoma
Ethylestrenol MAXIBOLIN		Elixir, tablets: 4 to 8 mg daily
Methandriol		Aqueous and oily solutions for i.m. use: 50 to 100 mg once or twice weekly in oil; 10 to 40 mg daily aqueous
Nandrolone decanoate DECA-DURABOLIN		Oily solution for i.m. use: 50 to 100 mg every 3 to 4 weeks
Nandrolone phenpropionate DURABOLIN		Oily solution for i.m. use: 25 to 50 mg weekly for breast carcinoma
Oxandrolone ANAVAR		Tablets: 5 to 10 mg daily
Oxymetholone ANADROL-50		Tablets: 1 to 5 mg/kg daily for anemia

Table 62–3.   SOME ANABOLIC STEROIDS USED IN THERAPY (Continued)

NONPROPRIETARY NAME AND SOME TRADE NAMES	CHEMICAL STRUCTURE	DOSAGE FORMS AND USUAL DOSAGE FOR ANABOLIC EFFECTS
Stanozolol WINSTROL	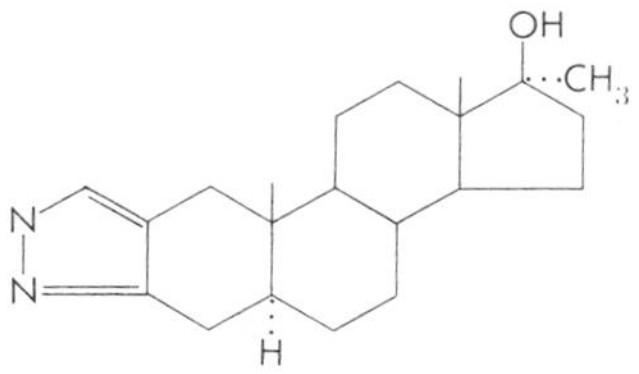	Tablets: 6 mg daily
Testolactone TESLAC	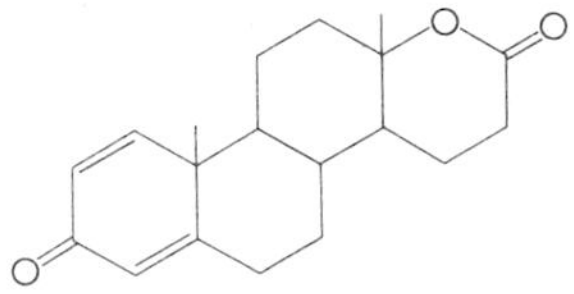	Tablets: 250 mg four times daily for breast carcinoma

est of the undesirable manifestations are acne, the growth of facial hair, and hoarsening or deepening of the voice. Menstrual irregularities will occur if gonadotropin secretion is suppressed. If treatment is discontinued as soon as these are noticed, they slowly subside. With continued treatment, as in the use of androgen in mammary carcinoma, male-pattern baldness, excessive body hair, prominent musculature, and hypertrophy of the clitoris may also develop. With prolonged treatment many of these effects, such as the deepening of the voice, are irreversible. During initial androgen-replacement therapy in hypogonadal males, sustained erections may be seen. This effect subsides with continued therapy at the same or lower doses of androgen.

Serious disturbances of growth and of sexual and osseous development can occur when androgens are given to children. The capacity of androgens to enhance epiphyseal closure in children may persist for as long as several months after discontinuation of the drug. All such agents should be used with great care in children. Androgens should not be used during pregnancy, since they can cause masculinization of the female fetus.

Edema. Retention of water in association with sodium chloride appears to be a consistent effect of the administration of androgen and accounts for most or all of the gain in weight, at least in short-term treat-

ment. In the doses used to treat hypogonadism, retention of fluid usually does not lead to detectable edema, but edema may become troublesome when large doses are given in the treatment of neoplastic diseases. Edema is also problematic in patients with congestive heart failure or renal insufficiency or in patients prone to edema from some other cause, such as cirrhosis of the liver or hypoproteinemia. Salt and water retention from androgens usually responds to the administration of natriuretics.

Jaundice. Methyltestosterone was the first of a number of androgens discovered to cause cholestatic hepatitis, and all androgens with 17α-alkyl substitutions can cause this complication. Disturbance of hepatic function has never been described with the parenteral use of testosterone esters. Jaundice is the prominent clinical feature, and the underlying disturbance is stasis and accumulation of bile in the biliary capillaries of the central portion of the hepatic lobules, without obstruction in the larger ducts (*see* Ishak, 1981). The hepatic cells usually exhibit only minor histological changes and remain viable. If jaundice occurs, it generally develops after 2 to 5 months of therapy. Alterations in various tests of hepatic function occur more commonly than jaundice and include increases in the concentration of bilirubin and the activities of glutamic-oxaloacetic transaminase and alkaline phosphatase in the plasma and reduced elimination of sulfobromophthalein. The severity of the response is dependent on dose and is particularly prominent when large amounts are given, as for palliation in neoplastic diseases. Because of these effects, it has become common practice to use testosterone esters instead of 17α-substituted steroids in virtually all clinical situations (except hereditary angioneurotic edema). In particular, the use of 17α-substituted esters should be avoided in patients with liver disease. Other forms of hepatic disease, such as peliosis hepatitis, have also been associated with use of these agents (*see* Ishak, 1981).

Hepatic Carcinoma. Patients who have received 17α-alkyl substituted androgens for prolonged periods may develop hepatic adenocarcinoma (Bernstein *et al.*, 1971; Johnson *et al.*, 1972; Henderson *et al.*, 1973). Most of the patients described received the derivatives for 1 to 7 years, and the complication may be more common in patients with Fanconi's anemia (*see* Ishak, 1979).

Decreased Spermatogenesis. While androgens are required for spermatogenesis and may maintain spermatogenesis for prolonged periods in animals after hypophysectomy, continued use of androgens in normal men may result in azoospermia due to inhibition of gonadotropin secretion and conversion of androgens to estrogens. For example, administration of 25 mg of testosterone propionate daily for 6 weeks causes a decrease in spermatogenesis. Anabolic steroids may produce the same effect.

Feminizing Side Effects. Paradoxically, feminizing side effects, particularly gynecomastia, can occur in men who receive androgens. The pathogenesis of this phenomenon is poorly understood. As stated above, androgens containing a Δ^4,3-keto configuration can be converted (aromatized) to estrogens in peripheral tissues, and the administration of testosterone esters causes an increase in plasma concentrations of estrogen. The feminizing side effects are particularly severe in children (who have an increased peripheral aromatase activity compared to adults) and in men with liver disease (who have diminished rates of androgen clearance and hence shunt androgen substrate to peripheral sites of aromatization).

Effects on Laboratory Tests. Androgens can decrease the concentration of thyroid-binding globulin in plasma and thereby influence thyroid function tests, increase the excretion of 17-ketosteroids, alter plasma cholesterol, and increase the hematocrit. 17α-Alkyl-substituted steroids cause an increase in the hepatic synthesis and plasma concentrations of a variety of glycoproteins (Barbosa *et al.*, 1971). Alterations in tests of hepatic function are discussed above. Some of these agents also increase the effects of oral anticoagulants; this may require a decrease in the dose of the anticoagulant to prevent bleeding.

Therapeutic Uses. The clearest therapeutic indication for androgens is deficient endocrine function of the testes. In addition, they have been tried in a variety of other situations in the hope that their effects on nongenital tissues would be beneficial. Testosterone esters are the preferred agents in all situations, and the use of alkylated androgens should be restricted to hereditary angioneurotic edema (*see* below) or short-term therapy in patients with serious illnesses.

Hypogonadism. Failure of the testis to secrete androgen usually cannot be recognized in childhood and is first evident when the changes of puberty seem to be delayed. The age of onset of puberty varies widely among individuals, and when there is no evidence of maturation at age 15 to 17, there may be great concern on the part of the patient and his parents. There is a good deal of debate about the use of androgen to hasten the changes of puberty in normal boys with delayed sexual maturation. Most physicians would agree that androgens should be withheld if parental pressures can be overcome.

Patients with delayed puberty should be evaluated for pituitary as well as gonadal function. Hypogonadism may be due to primary testicular failure or to diminished concentrations of gonadotropins. The latter could be due to hypopituitarism, as discussed below, or secondary to low concentrations of the gonadotropin-releasing hormone (Gn-RH). Some patients with the latter disorder have responded to long-term administration of Gn-RH (Hoffman and Crowley, 1982; Skarin *et al.*, 1982; Cutler *et al.*, 1985). The uses of gonadotropins and Gn-RH for secondary hypogonadism are discussed in Chapter 59.

If puberal changes are to be induced with an androgen in the absence of an established diagnosis of hypogonadism, it can be given in courses of 4 to 6 months at a time and stopped for like periods to ascertain whether the testes are enlarging and development is progressing spontaneously. The secretion of gonadotropins must also be reevaluated after discontinuation of androgens.

When there is complete testicular failure and puberty cannot occur, prolonged therapy is required. One of the long-acting esters of testosterone, such as the cypionate or the enanthate, may be given intramuscularly. It is recommended that initial doses of about one half of the eventual maintenance dose be given for 6 months to 1 year; the eventual maintenance dose of the long-acting esters of testosterone is about 200 mg every 2 weeks. Because of the high incidence of effects on hepatic function, 17α-alkyl-substituted androgens should not be used for replacement therapy. Furthermore, the concentration of testosterone in plasma should be titrated to the normal range in all individuals (Caminos-Torres *et al.,* 1977).

When therapy is begun at the time of expected puberty in boys with either primary or secondary hypogonadism, the normal events of puberty proceed in the usual fashion. The normal growth spurt occurs, and penile development, deepening of the voice, and appearance of other secondary sex characteristics are apparent during the first year. Puberty in normal boys extends over several years, and treatment designed to replicate normal development cannot hasten the process greatly. Testosterone exerts its full action only in the presence of a balanced hormonal environment and particularly only in the presence of adequate concentrations of growth hormone. Consequently, prepuberal boys with coexisting deficiency of growth hormone exhibit a diminished response to androgens with regard to both growth and virilization unless growth hormone is given simultaneously.

If therapy is delayed until long after the usual time of puberty, the degree of virilization that can be achieved is variable. Many of these patients undergo a late but relatively complete anatomical and functional male maturation. If hypogonadism is primary and of long duration, suppression of plasma concentrations of LH to the normal range may not occur for many weeks.

In postpuberal testicular failure, even of many years' duration, resumption of normal sexual activity is usual following adequate replacement. The major effect of androgen appears to be on libido; the volume of the ejaculate and other secondary sex characteristics return to normal, and the effects of androgen on hemoglobin, nitrogen retention, and skeletal development are also reproduced. In contrast, administration of testosterone has no effect on libido in men with normal concentrations of the hormone in plasma.

Nitrogen Balance and Muscle Development. Soon after the identification of testosterone as the principal androgen produced by the testis, it was recognized that administration of the hormone to hypogonadal or castrated men has profound effects in addition to those on the male urogenital tract. These effects include reduction in the urinary excretion of nitrogen, sodium, potassium, and chloride and induction of a gain in weight (*see* Wilson and Griffin, 1980). In contrast, in all situations other than hypogonadism, the positive nitrogen balance is short lived (probably lasting no more than 1 to 2 months).

Since androgens have significant effects on muscle mass and on body weight when administered to hypogonadal men, it was assumed, but never proven, that androgens in pharmacological doses could promote growth of muscle above the levels produced by the normal testicular secretion. This assumption was based upon the belief that anabolic and androgenic actions are different, and a concerted effort was made to devise pure "anabolic" steroids that have no androgenic effects. In fact, androgenic and anabolic effects do not result from different actions of the same hormone but represent the same action in different tissues; androgen-responsive muscle contains the same receptor that mediates the action of the hormone in other target tissues. *All anabolic hormones tested to date are also androgenic.* In appropriate doses, all anabolic agents can be used for replacement of androgen. For example, methandrostenolone, which has a greater effect on nitrogen balance per unit weight than does methyltestosterone, is a potent androgen and has been used for replacement therapy in hypogonadal men. Nevertheless, androgens have been tried in a variety of clinical situations other than hypogonadism with the hope that improvement in nitrogen balance and muscle development would outweigh any deleterious side effects.

Catabolic States. Body protein is broken down more rapidly than it is formed following injury or surgery, and excess nitrogen is excreted in the urine as a consequence. During the subsequent recovery phase, nitrogen deficits are replaced. Anabolic steroids can improve the nitrogen balance during the first few days following relatively minor operations in well-nourished subjects, but the diminution in nitrogen loss is minimal and has not been shown to be of significant therapeutic benefit. Likewise, effects of androgens on weight in undernourished, debilitated, or elderly individuals are due predominantly to enhancement of appetite. In appropriately controlled studies, no consistent effects on weight or strength have been documented following treatment with androgen. These negative results are probably the consequence of several factors, including the dependence of anabolic effects on adequate nutrition and health, the paucity of effects of androgens in men with normal concentrations of testosterone, and the temporary nature of any positive nitrogen balance when it does occur. In short, androgens are ineffective in promoting anabolism in acute illness, severe trauma, and protein depletion associated with chronic illness (*see* Wilson and Griffin, 1980). Androgens are also of little value in the management of nitrogen accumulation in chronic renal failure; at best they induce a transient improvement in nitrogen balance that is of doubtful importance. In acute renal failure, androgens cause a decrease in the rate of production of urea and a consequent decrease in the frequency of dialysis required for some patients. Most of these patients do well without androgen therapy.

Athletic Performance. The use of androgens by athletes in the belief that athletic performance will be improved constitutes a remarkably widespread example of drug abuse. Apparently, weight lifters and body builders began to use the drugs first; the abuse of these substances at all levels of athletic competition has become widespread, despite the absence of evidence that the drugs have a positive effect and despite knowledge that the drugs do have significant adverse effects. Three recent reviews have scrutinized more than 25 papers that have addressed the effects of anabolic-androgenic steroids on physical strength and athletic performance in men; the conclusion is that the use of these agents does not cause an increase in muscle bulk, strength, or athletic performance (American College of Sports Medicine, 1977; Wilson and Griffin, 1980; Ryan, 1981). Indeed, in appropriately controlled and designed studies, anabolic steroids do not enhance athletic performance even when phenomenally large doses are used. The commonly observed increase in body weight is due to retention of salt and water. The question of efficacy, interesting though it may be, is independent of the question of the side effects of the drugs. Since most athletes take oral agents rather than testosterone esters by injection, the potential toxic side effects are formidable.

It should be noted that scepticism about the effects of androgens on athletic performance is based solely on their use by men. Although such drugs have a positive effect on nitrogen retention in women and it is presumed that women have used them, no studies of their effects on athletic performance in women have been reported. Such studies are precluded by the inevitable virilizing side effects of the drugs.

Stimulation of Erythropoiesis. The difference in the hematocrit between men and women is the result of a stimulatory effect of testosterone on the formation of erythropoietin. Within 20 days after castration of the male there is a 10% decrease in the mass of red blood cells, a 36% decrease in red-cell diameter, and an increase in osmotic fragility. Occasionally, the anemia may be severe. Administration of androgens to women increases erythropoiesis, and some women develop polycythemia during long-term administration of androgens, as in the treatment of carcinoma of the breast (Shahidi, 1973). In women treated with pharmacological doses of testosterone, the average concentration of hemoglobin increases by 4.3 g/dl and the hematocrit increases by 11 volumes %. The average increase in hemoglobin is about 1 g/dl in normal men given pharmacological doses of testosterone esters. Because of these effects androgens have been used in the treatment of refractory anemias in both men and women (Shahidi, 1973). The capacity to enhance erythropoiesis is shared by all active androgens. In man, some erythropoietin is synthesized by tissues other than the kidney, and the presence of renal tissue is not an absolute requirement for stimulation of erythropoiesis by androgens.

Androgen therapy has been tried extensively in the anemias associated with failure of the bone marrow and/or myelofibrosis and in the anemia of renal failure. Occasional dramatic increases in hemoglobin occur following the administration of androgens to subjects with bone-marrow failure (Azen and Shahidi, 1977). In large numbers of unselected patients treated with androgens approximately half appear to respond, particularly when the bone marrow is hypoplastic or myelofibrotic.

What is uncertain, however, is the frequency with which drug administration and therapeutic response is coincidental (Branda *et al.*, 1977; Camitta *et al.*, 1979). This is a particular problem with regard to acquired anemias, in which spontaneous remission can occur during the course of therapy. Additional randomized prospective studies must be performed before the role of androgens in the routine management of aplastic anemia can be defined. Until such evidence is available, trial with androgens (of limited duration) is probably warranted in selected subjects with aplastic anemia. When an apparent response occurs, it is necessary to stop the drug temporarily to establish a cause-and-effect relationship between the drug and the apparent response.

The role of androgens in treatment of the anemia of renal failure is also uncertain. Androgen-induced increases in concentrations of erythropoietin and hemoglobin are less marked in the anephric state. In addition, the anemia of renal failure may undergo gradual improvement with time following the institution of an adequate dialysis program and correction of other coexisting causes of anemia. Nevertheless, most studies indicate that androgen therapy results in increases in hemoglobin (1 to 5 g/dl) and in red-blood-cell volume (325 to 350 ml), provided that dialysis is adequate and that stores of iron and folate are normal (von Hartizsch *et al.*, 1977). Whether the benefits of such treatment outweigh the potential adverse effects is unclear. When such agents are given to patients with renal failure, it is advisable to discontinue the androgen after 3 months, whether or not a response has occurred, and to resume it in those patients with an initial response only if the hematocrit falls to pretreatment levels.

Hereditary Angioneurotic Edema. In hereditary angioneurotic edema, an autosomal dominant disorder, the plasma contains either a nonfunctional inhibitor of the first component of complement or decreased concentrations of the inhibitor. Thus, there is unopposed activation of the complement cascade, which leads to the generation of factors that enhance the permeability of vessels and cause attacks of angioedema. A variety of 17α-alkylated steroids are efficacious in treating this condition. Such therapy not only increases the activity of the inhibitor in plasma but also restores the concentrations of the components of the complement system that are depleted secondarily. Orally active androgens are effective, and steroids such as danazol that are weak androgens appear to be as or more effective than potent androgens (Medical Letter, 1981). Furthermore, the response of men and women to such oral agents appears to be the same. 17α-Alkylated androgens (but not testosterone or testosterone esters) cause elevations of the concentrations of several plasma glycoproteins that are synthesized in the liver, including several clotting factors and the inhibitor of the first component of complement. The beneficial effect of oral androgens in this disorder is thus likely the result of a side effect of 17α-alkylated steroids on hepatic function rather than of androgen action *per se* (Barbosa *et al.*, 1971; Gralnick and Rick, 1983).

Short Stature. Androgens have been used for the management of growth retardation due to etiologies other than pituitary insufficiency. Their administration prior to epiphyseal closure results in an enhancement of linear growth, and the mean advance of height age is frequently increased more than is skeletal maturation (*see* Wilson and Griffin, 1980). Such therapy, when given for short periods (6 months or less), has no permanent effects on hypothalamic-pituitary or gonadal maturation. This acceleration of growth may be the result of an increase in plasma concentration of growth hormone. Whether such therapy has a beneficial effect on the final adult height is not known. For example, in subjects with 45,X-gonadal dysgenesis, treatment with oral androgens causes a temporary acceleration of growth but has a relatively small effect on mean final height. Furthermore, if given to short children prior to the age of 9 years, such therapy may actually have a deleterious effect on adult height (Bettman *et al.,* 1971). Thus, a role for androgens in the management of any form of short stature other than pituitary dwarfism is not established.

Carcinoma of the Breast. Testosterone propionate has a palliative effect in some women with carcinoma of the breast. The mechanism of this effect is unknown, but the androgen may act as an antiestrogen. The response rates are equivalent to those induced by high doses of estrogen (where an antiestrogenic mechanism may also be operative). No androgen is more efficacious than testosterone, and structural changes in the testosterone molecule that decrease its androgenicity also diminish its effectiveness in breast cancer. Since remission rates are higher with conventional chemotherapy, a significant role for androgens in the management of carcinoma of the breast is not established (*see* Chapter 55).

Other Disorders. Androgen therapy is effective in treatment of the osteoporosis that complicates androgen deficiency; indeed, the histological response to hormonal replacement can be dramatic (Gordon, 1978). A role for androgens in the treatment of osteoporosis unassociated with male hypogonadism has not been established.

Oral androgens cause a modest decrease in total plasma triglyceride and very-low-density lipoprotein triglyceride in occasional subjects with hyperlipidemia. Simultaneous elevation of cholesterol in low-density lipoprotein and reduction of high-density lipoprotein and cholesterol in high-density lipoprotein also result from such therapy. It is not clear if androgen has a net beneficial effect in patients with hyperlipoproteinemias.

ANTIANDROGENS

A search for compounds that might inhibit the synthesis or action of androgen was doubtless prompted by clinical considerations. Treatment of cancer of the prostate was one of the earlier aims; however, the uses of potent antagonists might range from virilization in women to precocious puberty in boys, and from acne to satyriasis in adult men. These compounds might also be valuable as male contraceptives. Recent developments suggest that some of these aspirations can be fulfilled.

Estrogens, in a restricted sense, may be regarded as antiandrogenic. They may have actions of their own upon genital tissues, which differ from those of androgens and in this way seem to antagonize androgen. Their effects on the hypothalamus and pituitary to decrease secretion of gonadotropins can also inhibit testosterone secretion secondarily.

Progesterone comes nearer to being an antiandrogen, albeit a very weak one, and some of the more potent antiandrogens are derivatives of progesterone. Two weak antiandrogens with no known hormonal activity of any other kind are the derivatives dodecahydrophenanthrene (Randall and Selitto, 1958) and A-norprogesterone; the former somewhat resembles progesterone lacking a D ring; the latter is progesterone with one carbon atom missing from ring A (Lerner, 1964). Several other steroids also have weak antiandrogenic activity, although most studies have been confined to animals.

In the search for orally active progestins, steroids with a 1,2-α-methylene substitution were found to be antiandrogenic. Cyproterone acetate is among the most potent. Its structure is as follows:

Cyproterone Acetate

While it is a potent antiandrogen, it also possesses progestational activity and suppresses the secretion of gonadotropins (Neri, 1976; Neumann, 1977, 1982). In androgen-dependent target tissues cyproterone acetate competes with dihydrotestosterone for its receptor site (Brown *et al.,* 1981). Treatment of the pregnant rat with 1 or 10 mg daily led to the remarkable finding that the male fetuses were "feminized," the penis was underdeveloped and resembled a clitoris, the prostate was missing, and the testes were small and undescended. These changes are permanent (Hamada *et al.,* 1963).

In the mature rat, the compound causes atrophy of the seminal vesicles, prostate, levator ani muscle, and other androgen-responsive organs, as well as cellular changes in the pituitary typical of castration with increased gonadotropin secretion (Neumann, 1966). This latter effect is not observed in men (Jackson and Jones, 1972). The testes are unaffected by small or moderate doses, although larger doses can decrease Leydig-cell function and spermatogenesis. In the castrated animal, only about five times as much antagonist as testosterone is needed to reduce the androgenic response by 50%. With large doses of cyproterone acetate the antagonism is almost complete (Neumann *et al.,* 1970).

Laschet and associates (1967) gave doses of cyproterone of 100 to 200 mg daily to men with severe deviations in sexual behavior and noted that male sex drive virtually disappeared in 10 to 14 days. The effect was gone within 2 weeks after discontinuing treatment. This loss of libido precludes its general use as a male contraceptive. Furthermore, its efficacy as a contraceptive in men is inconsistent. Because of its progestational activity and ability to suppress secretion of gonadotropins, it has been used in combination with estrogen as an oral contraceptive in women. Cyproterone acetate has also been tried in the treatment of hirsutism and virilization in women and in acne and baldness in both sexes (*see* Neri, 1976; Neumann, 1977; Dawber, 1982). Side effects other than decreased libido in men include gynecomastia.

Cyproterone has also been used in the therapy of precocious puberty (Kauli *et al.,* 1976). It delays the onset of puberty; decreases breast, testicular, and hair growth; stops menstruation if present; and delays the premature closure of epiphyses. However, in animals, cyproterone acetate can also prevent the anabolic effects of androgens and retard growth. Thus, its efficacy in precocious puberty may be offset by side effects.

Several studies have been encouraging with regard to the use of cyproterone in daily doses of 200 to 300 mg in prostatic carcinoma (*see* Wein and Murphy, 1973). Although cyproterone acetate is the most active antiandrogen so far encountered, closely related analogs are also active. Chlormadinone acetate also has antiandrogenic activity and has been used to treat prostatic carcinoma in doses of 100 mg daily (Nishimura and Shida, 1981). Antiandrogenic drugs are still in the investigational stage and are not yet generally available.

MALE CONTRACEPTIVES

There are many requirements of the ideal contraceptive drug: simplicity, acceptability, reversibility, lack of toxicity, and, of course, efficacy. Although all these criteria have not been attained in the oral contraceptives for women, the agents discussed in Chapter 61 come close. The lack of the development of analogous contraceptives for men reflects many biological and sociological factors. The principal biological factor is that men have fathered children even when sperm counts are lowered 99% (to values of approximately 1 million per milliliter) (*see* Diller and Hembree, 1977; Bialy and Patanelli, 1981; Reyes and Chavarria, 1981).

The highly ordered and precise processes that occur during the genesis and maturation of sperm should allow numerous approaches to their regulation and thus to contraception. A variety of compounds, in addition to the antiandrogens discussed above, can inhibit spermatogenesis. They include antineoplastic agents, cadmium, nitrofuranes, α-chlorhydrin, and dinitropyrrole (*see* Jackson and Jones, 1972; Bremner and DeKretser, 1976; Ewing and Robaire, 1978; Reyes and Chavarria, 1981).

However, the irreversible effects of some and the toxicity of many preclude their clinical use.

Gossypol, a phenolic compound extracted from the cotton plant of the genus *Gossypium,* is effective (about 99.9%) as an oral contraceptive in men. Infertility develops within several months of its use, and fertility is restored within several months of discontinuation of the drug (*see* Lawrence, 1981). Unfortunately, administration of gossypol causes hypokalemia and weakness; diarrhea, edema, dyspnea, neuritis, and paralysis are observed after higher doses are taken. These effects are also seen in cottonseed poisoning.

Gonadal steroids can suppress secretion of FSH and LH, which are required for spermatogenesis and the synthesis of testosterone by the testes (*see* Chapters 59 and 61). While estrogens and progestins are effective contraceptives in males, suppression of testosterone decreases both libido and potency; gynecomastia may also occur. These unacceptable side effects can be overcome by utilizing androgens to inhibit secretion of gonadotropins and spermatogenesis. Although androgens can be used as contraceptives, the treatment is not uniformly effective. The use of androgens alone is thus not encouraging. Estrogens in combination with androgens are also effective (Briggs and Briggs, 1974). Again, however, the side effects of estrogens in men (*e.g.,* gynecomastia and thrombotic disorders) limit the utility of this approach.

Perhaps the most promising regimen to date involves the dual administration of an androgen and progestin (Brenner *et al.,* 1975). Clinical trials in which patients received continuous testosterone and a progestin have resulted in infertility in some men with minimal side effects. The rationale for this combination is to suppress gonadotropin secretion and spermatogenesis with a progestin and to prevent alteration of accessory sexual structures by the simultaneous administration of testosterone (Bremner and DeKretser, 1976; Ewing and Robaire, 1978). Unfortunately, not all subjects develop azoospermia, and sperm counts are suppressed only after several months of treatment. A similar amount of time is required for the recovery of spermatogenesis when the drugs are stopped.

Potent analogs of Gn-RH also have contraceptive actions in men. Paradoxically they can inhibit secretion of gonadotropins after initial stimulation, and these effects are additive to that of testosterone; however, they do not result in uniform azoospermia (Heber and Swerdloff, 1980; Cutler *et al.,* 1985). The use of Gn-RH antagonists with or without androgen may also be effective. All the methods described above for contraception in the male remain investigational.

Azen, E. A., and Shahidi, N. T. Androgen dependency in acquired aplastic anemia. *Am. J. Med.,* **1977,** *63,* 320–324.

Barbosa, J.; Seal, H.; and Doe, R. P. Effects of anabolic steroids on haptoglobin, orosomucoid, plasminogen, fibrinogen, transferrin, ceruloplasmin, α-antitrypsin, β-glucuronidase, and total serum proteins. *J. Clin. Endocrinol.,* **1971,** *33,* 388–398.

Bernstein, M. S.; Hunter, R. L.; and Yachnin, S. Hepatoma and peliosis hepatitis in Fanconi's anemia. *N. Engl. J. Med.*, **1971**, *284*, 1135–1136.

Berthold, A. A. Transplantation der hoden. *Arch. Anat. Physiol. Wiss. Med.*, **1849**, *16*, 42–46.

Bettman, H. K.; Goldman, H. S.; Abramowicz, M.; and Sobel, E. H. Oxandrolone treatment of short stature: effect on predicted mature height. *J. Pediatr.*, **1971**, *79*, 1018–1023.

Bialy, G., and Patanelli, D. J. Potential use of male antifertility agents in developed countries. *Chemotherapy*, **1981**, *27*, 102–106.

Branda, R. F.; Amsden, T. W.; and Jacob, H. S. Randomized study of nandrolone therapy for anemias due to bone marrow failure. *Arch. Intern. Med.*, **1977**, *137*, 65–69.

Brenner, P. F.; Bernstein, G. S.; Roy, S.; Jeckt, E. W.; and Mischell, D. R. Administration of norethandrolone and testosterone as a contraceptive agent for men. *Contraception*, **1975**, *11*, 193–207.

Briggs, M., and Briggs, M. Oral contraceptive for men. *Nature*, **1974**, *252*, 585–586.

Brown, T. R.; Rothwell, S. W.; Sultan, C.; and Migeon, C. J. Inhibition of androgen binding in human foreskin fibroblasts by antiandrogens. *Steroids*, **1981**, *37*, 635–648.

Brown-Séquard, C. E. Des effets produits chez l'homme par des injections souscutanées d'un liquide retiré des testicules frais de cobaye et de chien. *C. R. Soc. Biol. (Paris)*, **1889**, *1*, 420–430.

Butenandt, A. Über die chemische Untersuchung der Sexualhormons. *Z. Angew. Chem.*, **1931**, *44*, 905–908.

Caminos-Torres, R.; Ma, L.; and Snyder, P. J. Testosterone-induced inhibition of the LH and FSH responses to gonadotropin-releasing hormone occurs slowly. *J. Clin. Endocrinol.*, **1977**, *44*, 1142–1153.

Camitta, B. M.; Thomas, E. D.; and Nathan, D. G. A prospective study of androgens and bone marrow transplantation for treatment of severe aplastic anemia. *Blood*, **1979**, *53*, 504–514.

Castro, A. E.; Alonso, A.; and Mancini, R. E. Localization of follicle stimulating and luteinizing hormones in the rat testis using immunohistological tests. *J. Endocrinol.*, **1972**, *52*, 129–136.

David, K.; Dingemanse, E.; Freud, J.; and Laqueur, E. Über krystallinische männliches Hormon aus Hoden (Testosteron), wirksamer als aus Harn oder aus Cholesterin bereitetes Androsteron. *Hoppe Seylers Z. Physiol. Chem.*, **1935**, *233*, 281–282.

Dawber, R. P. R. Alopecia and hirsutism. *Clin. Exp. Dermatol.*, **1982**, *7*, 177–182.

DeJong, F. H., and Sharpe, R. M. Evidence for inhibin-like activity in bovine follicular fluid. *Nature*, **1976**, *263*, 71–72.

Diller, L., and Hembree, W. Male contraception and family planning: a social and historical review. *Fertil. Steril.*, **1977**, *28*, 1271–1279.

Dunn, J. F.; Nisula, B. C.; and Rodbard, D. Transport of steroid hormones: binding of 21 endogenous steroids to both testosterone-binding globulin and corticosteroid-binding globulin in human plasma. *J. Clin. Endocrinol.*, **1981**, *53*, 58–68.

Gralnick, H. R., and Rick, M. E. Danazol increases factor VIII and factor IX in classic hemophilia and Christmas disease. *N. Engl. J. Med.*, **1983**, *308*, 1393–1395.

Hamada, H.; Neumann, F.; and Junkmann, K. Intrauterine antimaskuline Beinflüssung von Rattenfeten durch ein stark Gestagen wirksames Steroid. *Acta Endocrinol. (Kbh.)*, **1963**, *44*, 380–388.

Heber, D., and Swerdloff, R. S. Male contraception: synergism of gonadotropin-releasing hormone analog and testosterone in suppressing gonadotropin. *Science*, **1980**, *209*, 936–938.

Henderson, J. T.; Richmond, J.; and Sumerling, M. D. Androgenic-anabolic steroid therapy and hepatocellular carcinoma. *Lancet*, **1973**, *1*, 934.

Hilliard, J.; Scaramuzzi, R. J.; Pang, C.-N.; Penardi, R.; and Sawyer, C. H. Testosterone secretion by rabbit ovary *in vivo*. *Endocrinology*, **1974**, *94*, 267–271.

Hoffman, A. R., and Crowley, W. F. Induction of puberty in men by long-term pulsatile administration of low-dose gonadotropin-releasing hormone. *N. Engl. J. Med.*, **1982**, *307*, 1237–1241.

Ishak, K. S. Hepatic neoplasms associated with contraceptive and anabolic steroids. *Recent Results Cancer Res.*, **1979**, *66*, 73–128.

Johnson, F. L.; Feagler, J. R.; Lerner, K. G.; Majerus, P. W.; Siegel, M.; Hartmann, J. R.; and Thomas, E. D. Association of androgenic-anabolic steroid therapy with development of hepatocellular carcinoma. *Lancet*, **1972**, *2*, 1273–1276.

Josso, N.; Forest, M. G.; and Picard, J. Y. Müllerian-inhibiting activity of calf fetal testes: relationship to testosterone and protein synthesis. *Biol. Reprod.*, **1975**, *13*, 163–167.

Judd, H. L., and Yen, S. S. C. Serum adrenostenedione and testosterone levels during the menstrual cycle. *J. Clin. Endocrinol. Metab.*, **1973**, *36*, 475–481.

Kauli, R.; Pertzelan, A.; Prager-Lewin, R.; Grünebaum, M.; and Laron, Z. Cyproterone acetate in treatment of precocious puberty. *Arch. Dis. Child.*, **1976**, *51*, 202–208.

Kelch, R. P.; Jenner, M. R.; Weinstein, R.; Kaplan, S. L.; and Grumbach, M. M. Estradiol and testosterone secretion by human, simian, and canine testes in males with hypogonadism and in male pseudohermaphrodites with the feminizing testes syndrome. *J. Clin. Invest.*, **1972**, *51*, 824–830.

Keogh, E. J.; Lee, V. W. K.; Rennie, G. C.; Burger, H. G.; Hudson, B.; and DeKretser, D. M. Selective suppression of FSH by testicular extracts. *Endocrinology*, **1976**, *98*, 997–1004.

Knowlton, K.; Kenyon, A. T.; Sandiford, I.; Lotwin, G.; and Fricker, R. Comparative study of metabolic effects of estradiol benzoate and testosterone propionate in man. *J. Clin. Endocrinol. Metab.*, **1942**, *2*, 671–684.

Kochakian, C. D., and Murlin, J. R. The effect of male hormone on the protein and energy metabolism of castrate dogs. *J. Nutr.*, **1935**, *10*, 437–459.

Kovacs, W. J.; Griffin, J. E.; Weaver, D. D.; Carlson, B. R.; and Wilson, J. D. A mutation that causes lability of the androgen receptor under conditions that normally promote transformation to the DNA-binding state. *J. Clin. Invest.*, **1984**, *73*, 1095–1104.

Lacy, D., and Pettit, A. J. Sites of hormone production in the mammalian testis, and their significance in the control of male fertility. *Br. Med. Bull.*, **1970**, *26*, 87–91.

Laschet, U.; Laschet, L.; Felzner, H.-R.; Glaesel, H.-U.; Mall, G.; and Naab, M. Results in the treatment of hyper- and abnormal sexuality of men with antiandrogens. *Acta Endocrinol. (Kbh.)*, **1967**, *56*, Suppl. 119, 54.

Loewe, S., and Voss, H. E. Der Stand der Erfassung des männlichen Sexualhormons (Androkinins). *Klin. Wochenschr.*, **1930**, *9*, 481–487.

Longcope, C. The metabolism of estrone sulfate in normal males. *J. Clin. Endocrinol. Metab.*, **1972**, *34*, 113–122.

McCullagh, D. R. Dual endocrine activity of the testes. *Science*, **1932**, *76*, 19–20.

Matsumoto, A. M., and Bremner, W. J. Modulation of pulsatile gonadotropin secretion by testosterone in man. *J. Clin. Endocrinol.*, **1984**, *58*, 609–614.

Medical Letter. Danazol and other androgens for hereditary angioedema. **1981**, *23*, 83–84.

Mills, T. M., and Savard, K. *In vitro* steroid synthesis by follicles isolated from the rabbit ovary. *Steroids*, **1972**, *20*, 247–262.

Murad, F.; Strauch, B. S.; and Vaughan, M. The effect of gonadotropins on testicular adenyl cyclase. *Biochim. Biophys. Acta*, **1969**, *177*, 591–598.

Naftolin, F.; Judd, H. L.; and Yen, S. S. C. Pulsatile patterns of gonadotropins and testosterone in man: the effects of clomiphene with and without testosterone. *J. Clin. Endocrinol. Metab.*, **1973**, *36*, 285–288.

Neumann, F. Auftreten von Kastrationszellen im Hypophysenvorderlappen männlicher Ratten nach Behandlung mit einem Antiandrogen. *Acta Endocrinol. (Kbh.)*, **1966**, *53*, 53–60.

Nishimura, R., and Shida, K. Antiandrogenic therapy for the treatment of early stage prostatic cancer. *Prostate*, **1981**, *1*, Suppl., 27–34.

Papanicolaou, G. N., and Falk, E. A. General muscular hypertrophy induced by androgenic hormones. *Science*, **1938**, *87*, 238–239.

Pardridge, W. M.; Gorski, R. A.; Lippe, B. M.; and Green, R. Androgens and sexual behavior. *Ann. Intern. Med.*, **1982**, *96*, 488–501.

Ramasharma, K., and Sairam, M. R. Isolation and characterization of inhibin from human seminal plasma. *Ann. N.Y. Acad. Sci.*, **1982**, *383*, 307–328.

Randall, L. O., and Selitto, J. J. Anti-androgenic activity of a synthetic phenanthrene. *Endocrinology*, **1958**, *62*, 693–695.

Reyes, A., and Chavarria, M. E. Interference with epididymal physiology as possible site of male contraception. *Arch. Androl.*, **1981**, *7*, 159–168.

Ruzicka, L., and Wettstein, A. Synthetische Darstellung des Testishormons, Testosteron (Androsten-3-on-17-ol). *Helv. Chim. Acta*, **1935**, *18*, 1264–1275.

Saartok, T.; Dahlberg, E.; and Gustafsson, J. Relative binding affinity of anabolic-androgenic steroids: comparison of the binding to the androgen receptors in skeletal muscle and in prostate, as well as to sex hormone-binding globulin. *Endocrinology*, **1984**, *114*, 2100–2106.

Sachs, B. D.; Pollak, E. I.; Kreiger, M. S.; and Barfield, R. J. Sexual behavior: normal male patterning in androgenized female rats. *Science*, **1973**, *181*, 770–772.

Shahidi, N. T. Androgens and erythropoiesis. *N. Engl. J. Med.*, **1973**, *289*, 72–80.

Skarin, G.; Nillius, S. J.; Wibell, L.; and Wide, L. Chronic pulsatile low dose GnRH therapy for induction of testosterone production and spermatogenesis in a man with secondary hypogonadotropic hypogonadism. *J. Clin. Endocrinol. Metab.*, **1982**, *55*, 723–726.

Steinberger, A., and Steinberger, E. Secretion of an FSH-inhibiting factor by cultured Sertoli cells. *Endocrinology*, **1976**, *99*, 918–921.

von Hartizsch, B.; Kerr, D. N. S.; and Morley, G. Androgens in the anemia of chronic renal failure. *Nephron*, **1977**, *18*, 13–20.

Walsh, P. C.; Madden, J. D.; Harrod, M. J.; Goldstein, J. L.; MacDonald, P. C.; and Wilson, J. D. Familial incomplete male pseudohermaphroditism. Type 2. Decreased dihydrotestosterone formation in pseudovaginal perineoscrotal hypospadias. *N. Engl. J. Med.*, **1974**, *291*, 944–949.

Wein, A. J., and Murphy, J. J. Experience in the treatment of prostatic carcinoma with cyproterone acetate. *J. Urol.*, **1973**, *109*, 68–70.

Monographs and Reviews

American College of Sports Medicine. Position statement on the use and abuse of anabolic-androgenic steroids in sports. *Med. Sci. Sports*, **1977**, *9*, 11–13.

Bartke, A.; Hafiez, A. A.; Bex, F. J.; and Dalterio, S. Hormonal interactions in regulation of androgen secretion. *Biol. Reprod.*, **1978**, *18*, 44–54.

Boyar, R. M. Control of the onset of puberty. *Annu. Rev. Med.*, **1978**, *29*, 509–520.

Bremner, W. J., and DeKretser, D. M. The prospects for new reversible male contraceptives. *N. Engl. J. Med.*, **1976**, *295*, 1111–1116.

Cutler, G. B.; Hoffman, A. R.; Swerdloff, R. S.; Santen, J.; Meldrum, D. R.; and Comite, F. Therapeutic applications of luteinizing-hormone-releasing hormone and its analogs. *Ann. Intern. Med.*, **1985**, *102*, 643–657.

Davidson, J. M. Feedback control of gonadotropin secretion. In, *Frontiers in Neuroendocrinology*. (Ganong, W. F., and Martini, L., eds.) Oxford University Press, New York, **1969**, pp. 343–388.

Ebling, F. J. Steroids, hormones and sebaceous secretion. *Adv. Steroid Biochem. Pharmacol.*, **1970**, *2*, 1–39.

Eik-Nes, K. B. Production and secretion of testicular steroids. *Recent Prog. Horm. Res.*, **1971**, *27*, 517–535.

Ewing, L. L., and Robaire, B. Endogenous antispermatogenic agents: prospects for male contraception. *Annu. Rev. Pharmacol. Toxicol.*, **1978**, *18*, 167–187.

Fotherby, K., and James, F. Metabolism of synthetic steroids. *Adv. Steroid Biochem. Pharmacol.*, **1972**, *3*, 67–165.

Franchimont, P. Pituitary gonadotropins. *Clin. Endocrinol. Metab.*, **1977**, *6*, 101–116.

Givens, J. R. Normal and abnormal androgen metabolism. *Clin. Obstet. Gynecol.*, **1978**, *21*, 115–123.

Gordon, G. S. Drug treatment of osteoporosis. *Annu. Rev. Pharmacol. Toxicol.*, **1978**, *18*, 253–268.

Griffin, J. E.; Leshin, M.; and Wilson, J. D. Androgen resistance syndromes. *Am. J. Physiol.*, **1982**, *243*, E81–87.

Griffin, J. E., and Wilson, J. D. The syndromes of androgen resistance. *N. Engl. J. Med.*, **1980**, *302*, 198–209.

Heyns, W. The steroid-binding β-globulin of human plasma. *Adv. Steroid Biochem. Pharmacol.*, **1977**, *6*, 59–79.

Horn, H. J. Role of antiandrogens in psychiatry. In, *Androgens and Antiandrogens*. (Martini, L., and Motta, M., eds.) Raven Press, New York, **1977**, pp. 351–355.

Ishak, K. G. Hepatic lesions caused by anabolic and contraceptive steroids. *Semin. Liver Dis.*, **1981**, *2*, 116–128.

Jackson, H., and Jones, A. R. The effects of steroids and their antagonists on spermatogenesis. *Adv. Steroid Biochem. Pharmacol.*, **1972**, *3*, 167–192.

James, V. H. T.; Braunsberg, H.; Rippon, A. E.; Andino, N.; and Parker, V. Measurement of androgens in biological fluids. In, *Androgens and Antiandrogens*. (Martini, L., and Motta, M., eds.) Raven Press, New York, **1977**, pp. 19–35.

Jost, A. Embryonic sexual differentiation. In, *Hermaphroditism, Genital Anomalies and Related Endocrine Disorders*, 2nd ed. (Jones, H. W., and Scott, W. W., eds.) The Williams & Wilkins Co., Baltimore, **1971**, pp. 16–64.

Lawrence, S. U. Gossypol: a potential male contraceptive? *Am. Pharm.*, **1981**, *21*, 57–59.

Lerner, L. J. Hormone antagonists: inhibitors of specific activities of estrogen and androgen. *Recent Prog. Horm. Res.*, **1964**, *20*, 435–476.

Liao, S., and Fang, S. Receptor-proteins for androgens and the mode of action of androgens on gene transcription in ventral prostate. *Vitam. Horm.*, **1969**, *27*, 17–90.

Lipsett, M. B. Physiology and pathology of the Leydig cell. *N. Engl. J. Med.*, **1980**, *303*, 682–688.

Lunde, D. T., and Hamburg, D. A. Techniques for assessing the effects of sex steroids on affect, arousal, and aggression in humans. *Recent Prog. Horm. Res.*, **1972**, *28*, 627–663.

Mainwaring, W. I. P. (ed.). The mechanism of action of androgens. *Monogr. Endocrinol.*, **1977**, *10*, 1–178.

Marcus, R., and Korenman, S. G. Estrogens and the human male. *Annu. Rev. Med.*, **1976**, *27*, 357–370.

Neri, R. O. Antiandrogens. *Adv. Sex Horm. Res.*, **1976**, *2*, 233–262.

Neumann, F. Pharmacology and potential use of cyproterone acetate. *Horm. Metab. Res.*, **1977**, *9*, 1–13.

——. Pharmacology and clinical use of antiandrogens: a short review. *Ir. J. Med. Sci.*, **1982**, *15*, 61–70.

Neumann, F.; Berswordt-Wallrabe, R. von; Elger, W.; Steinbeck, H.; Hahn, J.; and Kramer, M. Aspects of androgen-dependent events as studied by antiandrogens. *Recent Prog. Horm. Res.*, **1970**, *26*, 337–405.

Odell, W. D., and Swerdloff, R. S. Abnormalities of gonadal function in men. *Clin. Endocrinol. (Oxf.)*, **1978**, *8*, 149–180.

Pardridge, W. M. Transport of protein-bound hormones into tissues *in vitro*. *Endocrin. Rev.*, **1981**, *2*, 103–123.

Ritzen, E. M.; Hansson, V.; and French, S. The Sertoli cell. In, *The Testis*. (Burger, H., and DeKretser, D., eds.) Raven Press, New York, **1981**, pp. 171–194.

Ritzen, E. M.; Hansson, V.; and French, S. The Sertoli cell. In, *The Testis*. (Burger, H., and DeKretzer, D., eds.) Raven Press, New York, **1981**, pp. 171–194.

Rosenfield, R. L. Role of androgens in growth and development of the fetus, child, and adolescent. *Adv. Pediatr.*, **1972**, *19*, 172–213.

Ryan, A. J. Anabolic steroids are fool's gold. *Fed. Proc.*, **1981**, *40*, 2682–2688.

Schally, A. V. Aspects of hypothalamic regulation of the pituitary gland: its implications for the control of reproductive processes. *Science*, **1978**, *202*, 18–28.

Siiteri, P. K., and MacDonald, P. C. Role of extraglandular estrogen in human endocrinology. In, *Female Reproductive System*, Vol. 2, Pt. 1. Sect. 7, *Endocrinology. Handbook of Physiology*. (Greep, R. O., and Astwood, E. B., eds.) American Physiological Society, Washington, D. C., **1973**, pp. 615–629.

Sommerville, I. F., and Collins, W. P. Indices of androgen production in women. *Adv. Steroid Biochem. Pharmacol.*, **1970**, *2*, 267–314.

Wilson, J. D. Gonadal hormones and sexual behavior. In, *Clinical Neuroendocrinology*, Vol. II. (Martini, L., and Besser, G. M., eds.) Academic Press, Inc., New York, **1982**, pp. 1–19.

Wilson, J. D., and Griffin, J. E. The use and misuse of androgens. *Metabolism*, **1980**, *29*, 1278–1295.

63 ADRENOCORTICOTROPIC HORMONE; ADRENOCORTICAL STEROIDS AND THEIR SYNTHETIC ANALOGS; INHIBITORS OF ADRENOCORTICAL STEROID BIOSYNTHESIS

Robert C. Haynes, Jr., and Ferid Murad

Adrenocorticotropic hormone (ACTH, corticotropin) and the steroids of the adrenal cortex are considered together in this chapter because the primary physiological and pharmacological effects of ACTH result from the secretion of adrenocortical steroids. Biologically active synthetic analogs of the adrenocorticosteroids are also included, as are substances that alter the pattern of secretion of the adrenal cortex by inhibiting certain biosynthetic reactions. Synthetic steroids and other compounds that inhibit the action of aldosterone on the renal tubule are discussed in Chapter 36.

History. The physiological significance of the adrenals began to be appreciated as a consequence of the description by Addison (1855) of the clinical syndrome resulting from destructive disease of the adrenal glands. His observations interested the physiologist Brown-Séquard (1856), who did the pioneer experiments on the effects of adrenalectomy and concluded that the adrenal glands are essential to life.

By the third decade of this century it was generally recognized that the cortex rather than the medulla is the life-maintaining portion of the gland. Soon the literature was replete with descriptions of the numerous physiological abnormalities exhibited by adrenalectomized animals. The complex nature of adrenocortical deficiency was dramatized in the 1930s by the partisan character of research groups oriented to study either the imbalance of electrolytes or the defects in carbohydrate metabolism present in the deficient state. Renal loss of sodium was convincingly demonstrated to be a characteristic of adrenocortical insufficiency by Harrop and associates (1933) as well as by Loeb and coworkers (1933). Equally convincing was the demonstration of a depletion of carbohydrate stores (Cori and Cori, 1927). Furthermore, hypoglycemia could be corrected by adrenocortical extracts (Britton and Silvette, 1931). Glucose and glycogen, formed under the influence of the adrenal cortex during fasting, appeared to be derived from tissue protein (Long *et al.*, 1940). From these studies there emerged the concepts of two types of adrenocortical hormones. The mineralocorticoids primarily regulate electrolyte homeostasis, and the glucocorticoids are hormones concerned with carbohydrate metabolism. This concept of the dichotomy of "salt" and "sugar" hormones (mineralocorticoids and glucocorticoids) has proven useful and survives at the present time in a modified form.

In 1932, the neurosurgeon Cushing described the syndrome of hypercorticism, which bears his name (Cushing, 1932). The cases Cushing described were those of "pituitary basophilism," recognized subsequently as being a condition characterized by hypersecretion of ACTH. The symptom complex is now known to result from excessive plasma concentrations of adrenocortical hormones, regardless of whether they originate endogenously or as the consequence of therapeutic intervention.

The preparation of adrenocortical extracts with a reasonable degree of activity was first accomplished in 1930 by Swingle and Pfiffner and by Hartman and associates. The existence of biologically active tissue extracts presented a challenge to organic chemists, who by 1942 had isolated, crystallized, and elucidated the structures of 28 steroids from the adrenal cortex (Reichstein and Shoppee, 1943). Five of these compounds—cortisol (hydrocortisone), cortisone, corticosterone, 11-dehydrocorticosterone, and 11-desoxycorticosterone—were demonstrated to be biologically active. Another decade passed before the principal mineralocorticoid was discovered. Deming and Luetscher (1950) found that extracts of urine from patients with edema induced sodium retention and potassium excretion in adrenalectomized rats. The definitive evidence for the source of the active material was provided by Tait and coworkers (1952), who purified the compound with this activity from adrenocortical extracts. The substance was crystallized, the structure was established, and the hormone was eventually named *aldosterone* (Simpson *et al.*, 1954).

Meanwhile, other investigators had turned their attention to the adenohypophysis. The classical studies of Foster and Smith (1926) established the fact that hypophysectomy results in atrophy of the adrenal cortex. By 1933, it had been demonstrated that cell-free extracts of the anterior pituitary had a stimulating effect upon the adrenal cortex of the hypophysectomized animal. Further chemical fractionation of such extracts led to the isolation of a hormone, ACTH, that acted selectively to cause chemical and morphological changes in the adrenal cortex (Li *et al.*, 1943; Sayers *et al.*, 1943; Astwood *et al.*, 1952). The structure of ACTH was established by Bell and coworkers (1956). Within a few years biologically active peptides were synthesized (Hofmann *et al.*, 1961), as was an ACTH of 39 amino acid residues (Schwyzer and Sieber, 1963). The rate of release of ACTH from the adenohypophysis was shown to be determined by the balance of inhibitory effects of the hormones of the adrenal cortex (Ingle *et al.*, 1938) and the excitatory effects of the nervous system. The hypothalamus was established as the "final common path" for the variety of stimuli impinging on the adenohypophysis.

A detailed analysis of the morphology of the adrenal cortex had suggested to Swann (1940) and to Deane and Greep (1946) that the zona glomerulosa of the adrenal cortex functions relatively independently of the pituitary. Following hypophysectomy, the zona glomerulosa thickens, whereas the fasciculata shrinks markedly and the reticularis disappears almost entirely. These morphological observations, together with the fact that the hypophysectomized rat, in contrast to the adrenalectomized animal, can survive without salt therapy, prompted Swann as well as Deane and Greep to assign to the zona glomerulosa the specific function of autonomously elaborating a hormone regulating electrolyte balance. This hormone is now known to be aldosterone. Subsequent experimental studies have shown that the rate of secretion of aldosterone is regulated by a complex system, of which the pituitary is but one element.

In 1949, Hench and coworkers announced the dramatic effects of cortisone and ACTH in the treatment of rheumatoid arthritis. As early as 1929, Hench was impressed by the fact that arthritic patients, when pregnant or jaundiced, experienced a temporary remission; he believed that a metabolite was responsible for the remission. The possibility that the antirheumatic substance might be an adrenocortical hormone was entertained, and as soon as cortisone was available in sufficient quantity it was tested in a case of acute rheumatoid arthritis. Fortunately, an adequate dose was employed and the response was dramatic. Thereafter, the salutary effects of ACTH were also demonstrated. The observations (Hench *et al.*, 1949) immediately evoked

wide interest. Soon, therapeutic applications were extended to other diseases, with results to be presented later in this chapter. The impact upon the medical world can be appreciated from the fact that, in the year following the first published report of the efficacy of cortisone in the treatment of rheumatoid arthritis, the Nobel Prize in Medicine was jointly awarded to Kendall and Reichstein, who were responsible for much of the basic chemical research that led to the synthesis of the steroid, and to Hench, whose contribution has just been described.

In addition to a surge of clinical investigation, the therapeutic success of cortisone stimulated a wave of basic research in the 1950s. In that decade knowledge of the biochemistry of adrenal steroid synthesis and metabolism was brought close to its present level. As noted above, aldosterone was discovered; it was established that ACTH controls the reaction of cholesterol side chain scission (Stone and Hechter, 1954) and acts through the intermediacy of adenosine $3',5'$-monophosphate (cyclic AMP) (Haynes *et al.*, 1959); most synthetic analogs of cortisol used today were introduced, and practical technics for determination of cortisol became available to the clinician.

Effective clinical use of the corticosteroids has become possible because of their isolation, elucidation of structure, and economical synthesis. Manipulation of structure has yielded a variety of synthetic analogs, some of which represent significant therapeutic gains in terms of the ratio of anti-inflammatory potency to effects on electrolyte metabolism. However, hopes for elimination of toxicity have not been fulfilled. For this reason, it cannot be overemphasized that the corticosteroids, in pharmacological doses, are powerful drugs with slow cumulative toxic effects on many tissues, which may not be apparent until made manifest by a catastrophe.

ADRENOCORTICOTROPIC HORMONE

Chemistry. The structure of human ACTH, a peptide of 39 amino acid residues, is shown in Figure 63-1. Loss of one amino acid from the N-terminal end of the molecule by hydrolytic cleavage results in complete loss of biological activity. In contrast, a number of amino acids may be split off the C-terminal end with no effect on potency. A 20–amino acid peptide (sequence 1 through 20, Figure 63-1) retains the activity of the parent hor-

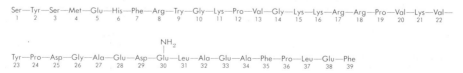

Ser—Tyr—Ser—Met—Glu—His—Phe—Arg—Try—Gly—Lys—Pro—Val—Gly—Lys—Lys—Arg—Arg—Pro—Val—Lys—Val—
1   2   3   4   5   6   7   8   9   10   11   12   13   14   15   16   17   18   19   20   21   22

NH₂
|
Tyr—Pro—Asp—Gly—Ala—Glu—Asp—Glu—Leu—Ala—Glu—Ala—Phe—Pro—Leu—Glu—Phe
23   24   25   26   27   28   29   30   31   32   33   34   35   36   37   38   39

Figure 63–1. *Amino acid sequence of human ACTH.*

Ovine, porcine, and bovine ACTHs differ from human ACTH only at amino acid positions 25, 31, and 33 (Li, 1972).

mone. The structure-activity relationship of ACTH has been reviewed by Otsuka and Inouye (1975). The structural relationships between ACTH, endorphins, lipotropins, and the melanocyte-stimulating hormones are discussed in Chapter 59.

Actions on Adrenal Cortex. ACTH stimulates the human adrenal cortex to secrete cortisol, corticosterone, aldosterone, and a number of weakly androgenic substances. In the absence of the adenohypophysis, the adrenal cortex undergoes atrophy and the rates of secretion of cortisol and corticosterone, which are markedly reduced, do not respond to otherwise-effective stimuli. Although ACTH can stimulate secretion of aldosterone, the rate of secretion is relatively independent of the adenohypophysis, and this explains the nearly normal electrolyte balance in the hypophysectomized animal. The zona glomerulosa is the least affected by atrophic changes that follow hypophysectomy, and it is the glomerulosa that is mainly responsible for the elaboration of aldosterone.

Prolonged administration of large doses of ACTH induces hyperplasia and hypertrophy of the adrenal cortex with continuous high output of cortisol, corticosterone, and androgens.

Mechanism of Action. ACTH acts to stimulate the *synthesis* of adrenocortical hormones; if it facilitates the release of preformed steroids from the adrenal cortex at all, this effect is overshadowed by the greater effect on synthesis. ACTH, as many other hormones, controls its target tissue through the agency of cyclic AMP. Thus, treatment with ACTH causes an increase in concentration of the cyclic nucleotide within adrenocortical cells (Haynes, 1958); cyclic AMP mimics ACTH in stimulating steroidogenesis (Haynes *et al.*, 1959) and in maintaining the weight of the adrenal after hypophysectomy (Ney, 1969). ACTH reacts with a specific hormone receptor in the adrenal-cell plasma membrane, and the result is a stimulation of adenylate cyclase activity and the formation of cyclic AMP.

The principal metabolic site at which steroidogenesis is regulated by the cyclic nucleotide is the oxidative cleavage of the side chain of cholesterol, the reaction that results in the formation of pregnenolone (*see* Figure 63–3, page 1465). This step is rate limiting in the sequence of reactions that leads to the formation of adrenal steroid hormones (Stone and Hechter, 1954). Exposure of adrenocortical cells to ACTH together with aminoglutethimide (to block side chain cleavage; *see* below) leads to increased amounts of cholesterol within the adrenal mitochondria, the locus of the side

chain–cleaving enzyme (Mahaffee *et al.*, 1974). Furthermore, cholesterol bound to cytochrome P-450 is increased by ACTH (Bell and Harding, 1974; Paul *et al.*, 1976). These findings, together with evidence that the availability of cholesterol is the factor that limits the rate of the cleavage reaction in intact mitochondria (Kahnt *et al.*, 1974), suggest that ACTH, via cyclic AMP, stimulates the initial reaction in steroidogenesis from cholesterol by making the substrate available in increased concentration to the enzyme within the mitochondria. ACTH stimulates the formation of free cholesterol in the gland by activating cholesterol esterase, and this activation is apparently accomplished by phosphorylation of the enzyme (Beckett and Boyd, 1975; Pittman and Steinberg, 1977). ACTH also acts to increase the availability of cholesterol by stimulating its uptake from plasma lipoproteins (Gwynne *et al.*, 1976).

The trophic effects of ACTH on the adrenal cortex are little understood beyond the fact that they, like stimulation of steroidogenesis, appear to be mediated by cyclic AMP (Ney, 1969). The regulation of the adrenal cortex by ACTH has been reviewed by Kimura (1981).

Extra-adrenal Effects of ACTH. Large doses of ACTH given to adrenalectomized animals cause a number of metabolic changes, including ketosis, lipolysis, hypoglycemia (early after administration), and resistance to insulin (late after administration). These extra-adrenal effects are of doubtful physiological significance, particularly since large doses are needed to induce them (Engel, 1961). Intravenous administration of ACTH (synthetic or porcine, but not bovine) leads to a transient elevation of the concentration of growth hormone in the plasma of adults but not children (Lee *et al.*, 1973).

Natural and synthetic corticotropins darken the isolated skin of the frog; this is not surprising since the amino acid sequence, 1 through 13, is identical with that of the melanocyte-stimulating hormone, α-MSH. Large doses of highly purified α-MSH and ACTH have been demonstrated to darken the skin of adrenalectomized human subjects. The hyperpigmentation of the skin that occurs in Addison's disease is thought to result from the high concentrations of ACTH that circulate in this condition (Thody, 1977; *see* Chapter 59).

Regulation of the Secretion of ACTH. The fluctuations in the rates of secretion of cortisol, corticosterone, and, to some extent, aldosterone are determined by the fluctuations in the release of ACTH from the adenohypophysis. The adenohypophysis, in turn, is under the influence of the *nervous system* and *negative-feedback control* exerted by *corticosteroids* (*see* Gann *et al.*, 1981).

Nervous System: The Final Common Path. Stimuli that induce release of ACTH travel by neural paths converging on the median eminence of the hypothalamus. The functional link between the median eminence and the adenohypophysis, the final common path, is vascular, not neural. In response to an appropriate stimulus, corticotropin-releasing factor (CRF) is elaborated at neuronal endings in the median eminence and transported in the hypophyseal-portal vessels to the adenohypophysis, where it stimulates the secretion of ACTH. The isolation and synthesis of an ovine CRF were reported by Vale and coworkers (1981). This polypeptide, which contains 41 amino acid residues, increases the concentrations of ACTH and cortisol in plasma when given intravenously to man. It does not change the concentrations of prolactin, growth hormone, thyrotropin, or the gonadotropins (Grossman *et al.*, 1982). Intravenous injection of 100 µg of CRF causes an exaggerated response in patients with Cushing's syndrome due to pituitary hyperfunction. It is thus useful in determining the cause of the disease and helps to rule out ectopic production of ACTH or functional tumors of the adrenal cortex as responsible (Muller *et al.*, 1983). (For additional information, *see* Conference, 1985.)

ACTH is synthesized in basophilic cells of the adenohypophysis and, like many other peptide hormones, it is derived from a larger precursor; the prohormone is a glycoprotein of about 30,000 molecular weight. As indicated in Figure 59–2 (page 1380), the precursor of ACTH includes the sequences of MSH, the lipotropins, and the endorphins. In man, the role of these three groups of active peptides remains conjectural and a subject of active investigation. The complex processing of the prohormone to ACTH, β-lipotropin, and other peptides has been studied extensively (*see* Loh and Loriaux, 1982).

Negative Feedback of the Corticosteroids (Cortisol and Corticosterone). Administration of certain corticosteroids suppresses the secretion of ACTH, reduces the store of ACTH in the adenohypophysis, and induces morphological changes (hyalinization of the basophilic cells) suggestive of functional impairment of the adenohypophysis. The adrenal cortex itself undergoes atrophy. In contrast, adrenalectomized animals and patients with Addison's disease have abnormally high concentrations of ACTH in the blood even under optimal environmental conditions. When a stimulus is applied to an adrenalectomized animal, the concentration of ACTH reaches even higher levels. These observations point out the important inhibitory role of the corticosteroids and clearly demonstrate that ACTH release remains under control of the nervous system in the absence of corticosteroid feedback. Secretion of ACTH at

any instant is determined by the balance of neural excitatory and corticosteroid inhibitory effects.

Mechanism of Feedback by Corticosteroids. Binding of glucocorticoids has been detected in the pituitary, hypothalamus, and other areas of the brain (McEwen, 1979); however, the link between such binding and inhibition of secretion of ACTH has not been established. There is evidence of control at both hypothalamic and hypophyseal sites (*see* Gann *et al.*, 1981). Nakanishi and coworkers (1977) demonstrated that glucocorticoids cause a decrease in the level of mRNA for ACTH in the pituitary, suggesting control may be at least in part at the transcriptional level. It should be noted, however, that glucocorticoids can cause a fall in the plasma concentration of ACTH that is so rapid that other mechanisms may also be utilized (Johnson *et al.*, 1979).

Examples of Effective Stimuli of Secretion. A number of conditions have been demonstrated to stimulate adrenocortical secretion in man. These include the agonal state, severe infections, surgery, parturition, cold, exercise, and emotional stress. Stressful stimuli override the normal negative-feedback control mechanisms, and plasma concentrations of adrenocortical steroids can be elevated within a few minutes of the initiation of an appropriate stimulus.

Diurnal Cycles in Adrenocortical Activity. The rate of secretion of cortisol by the adrenal cortex of a normal human subject under optimal conditions is about 20 mg per day. However, the rate is not steady and exhibits rhythmic fluctuations; concentrations of adrenocortical steroids in plasma are relatively high in the early-morning hours, decline during the day, and reach a minimum about midnight. Plasma concentrations of ACTH are higher at 6 A.M. than at 6 P.M. The diurnal patterns of glucocorticoids and ACTH are not observed in patients with Cushing's disease, and this factor is considered in the diagnosis of the disorder.

Absorption and Fate. ACTH is readily absorbed from parenteral sites, and it is usually administered by intramuscular injection and occasionally by intravenous infusion. The hormone rapidly disappears from the circulation following its intravenous administration; in man, the half-life in plasma is about 15 minutes because of rapid enzymatic hydrolysis.

Bioassay. The USP has adopted the *Third International Standard for Corticotropin* (Bangham *et al.*, 1962) as the reference standard in the United States. Potency is based on an assay in hypophysectomized rats in which depletion of adrenal ascorbic acid is measured after subcutaneous administration of the ACTH. All commercial preparations are now described in these units only.

Preparations, Dosage, and Routes of Administration. *Corticotropin for injection* (ACTH) is available as a lyophilized powder (ACTHAR) for subcutaneous, intramuscular, or intravenous use. The preparation is derived from the pituitaries of mammals used for food. Maximal adrenocortical secretion is obtained in adults with a total dose of 25 USP units infused intravenously for 8 hours.

Repository corticotropin injection (CORTROPHIN GEL, H.P. ACTHAR GEL) is administered either intramuscularly or subcutaneously. It is a highly purified ACTH in gelatin solution. Typical doses are 40 to 80 units, given every 1 to 3 days. *Corticotropin zinc hydroxide suspension* (CORTROPHIN-ZINC) is a preparation of purified corticotropin adsorbed on zinc hydroxide, intended for intramuscular injection. Again, usual doses are 40 to 80 units every 1 to 3 days.

Cosyntropin (CORTROSYN) is a synthetic peptide corresponding to amino acid residues 1 to 24 of human ACTH. This preparation, approved for diagnostic purposes, is given intramuscularly or intravenously in a dose of 0.25 mg (equivalent to 25 units).

Therapeutic and Diagnostic Applications of ACTH. At the present time, the most important use of ACTH is as a *diagnostic agent* in adrenal insufficiency. For this purpose, ACTH is administered and the concentration of cortisol in plasma is determined. A normal increase in plasma cortisol rules out primary adrenocortical failure. If there is no acute response, prolonged or repeated administration of ACTH may be required. In cases of pituitary insufficiency, prolonged treatment can be expected to elicit a rise in plasma cortisol concentration.

Therapeutic uses of ACTH have included the treatment of adrenocortical insufficiency and nonendocrine disorders that are responsive to glucocorticoids. However, therapy with ACTH is less predictable and much less convenient than is that with appropriate steroids. Furthermore, ACTH stimulates secretion of mineralocorticoids and, therefore, may cause acute retention of salt and water. While this generally does not persist with continuing therapy, it is a potentially serious problem in patients who have cardiac insufficiency. ACTH would obviously be of no value in the treatment of primary adrenocortical failure. Furthermore, there is no substantial evidence that therapeutic goals can be attained with ACTH in secondary adrenocortical insufficiency that cannot be attained with appropriate doses of currently available steroids. It must be kept in mind, however, that ACTH and corticosteroids are not pharmacologically equivalent. Treatment with ACTH exposes the tissues to a mixture of glucocorticoids, mineralocorticoids, and androgens, in contrast to the conventional, contemporary practice of administering a single glucocorticoid. It is possible that the steroid mixture resulting from adrenal stimulation by ACTH has effects that differ significantly from those of a single, synthetic glucocorticoid. Thus, Grahame (1969) reported the absence of dermal atrophy in patients treated for prolonged periods of time with ACTH, in contrast to that found with corticosteroid treatment. This has been tentatively attributed to a protective action of androgens against the inhibitory effects of glucocorticoids on fibroblasts (Harvey and Grahame, 1973).

Clinical Toxicity of ACTH. The toxicity of ACTH, aside from rare hypersensitivity reactions, is entirely attributable to the increased rate of secretion of adrenocorticosteroids (*see* below). Hypersensitivity reactions, ranging from mild fever to anaphylaxis and death, have been reported. The synthetic ACTH peptides are thought to be less antigenic than is the parent molecule. Nevertheless, hypersensitivity to them does occur (Forssman and Mulder, 1973). Because it stimulates synthesis and secretion of mineralocorticoids and androgens, ACTH causes more sodium retention, a greater degree of hypokalemic alkalosis, and more acne than do the synthetic congeners of cortisol.

ADRENOCORTICAL STEROIDS

The adrenal cortex synthesizes two classes of steroids: the corticosteroids (glucocorticoids and mineralocorticoids) with 21 carbon atoms and the androgens with 19. A typical corticosteroid, *cortisol,* is shown in Figure 63–2; typical androgens are shown in Figure 63–3.

Adrenocorticosteroid Biosynthesis. Cholesterol is an obligatory intermediate in the biosynthesis of corticosteroids. Although the adrenal cortex synthesizes cholesterol from acetate by processes similar to those in liver, the greater part of the cholesterol (60 to 80%) utilized for corticosteroidogenesis comes from exogenous sources, both at rest and following administration of ACTH. Adrenocortical cells thus have large numbers of receptors that mediate the uptake of low-density lipoprotein, the predominant source of cholesterol (*see* Chapter 34). Cholesterol is enzymatically converted to 21-carbon corticosteroids and 19-carbon weak androgens by a series of steps presented in simplified form in Figure 63–3. Most of the reactions are catalyzed by mixed-function oxidases that contain cytochrome P-450 and require NADPH and molecular oxygen.

In addition to other androgens, the adrenal cortex secretes testosterone; however, about half the plasma testosterone of normal women is derived from androstenedione at an extra-adrenal site.

Adrenocorticosteroids are not stored in the adrenal. The amounts of corticosteroids found in adrenal tissue are insufficient to maintain normal rates of secretion for more than a few minutes in the absence of continuing biosynthesis. For this reason, the rate of biosynthesis is tantamount to the rate of secretion. Table 63–1 shows typical rates of secretion of the physiologically most important corticosteroids in man—cortisol and aldosterone—and also their approximate concentrations in peripheral plasma. The mechanism of control of steroidogenesis by ACTH has been discussed above, and the regulation of aldosterone synthesis by renin and angiotensin is described in Chapter 27.

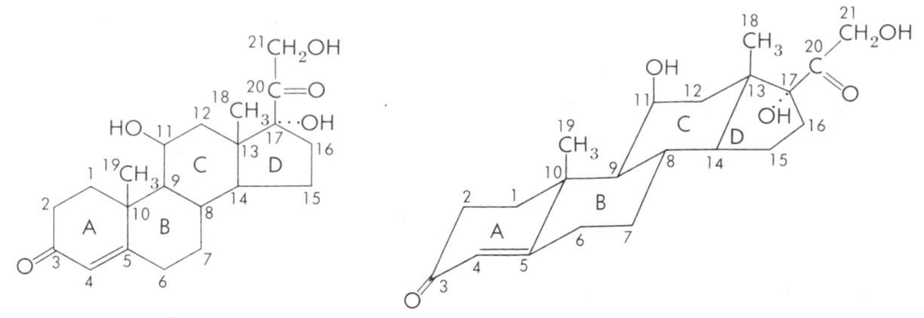

Figure 63–2. *Structure, stereochemistry, and nomenclature of adrenocorticosteroids, as typified by cortisol (hydrocortisone).*

The four rings—A, B, C, and D—are not in a flat plane, as conventionally represented in *I*, but have the approximate configuration shown in *II*. (The planarity of the valence angles about the double bond between C 4 and C 5 prevents the chair form of ring A, as shown, from being an energetically probable conformational state. As a result, ring A is in a half-chair conformation, not easily represented in two dimensions.) Orientation of the groups attached to the steroid ring system is importantly related to biological activity. The methyl groups at C 18 and C 19, the hydroxyl group at C 11, and the two-carbon ketol side chain at C 17 project above the plane of the steroid and are designated β. Their connection to the ring system is shown by full-line bonds. The hydroxy at C 17 projects below the plane and is designated α, and the connection to the ring is shown by a dotted bond. The ketone at C 3 in association with the double bond between C 4 and C 5 in ring A is an important structural feature of the biologically active corticosteroids. Reduction of the ketone at C 3 leads to the formation of two isomers: one, 3β-hydroxy; the other, 3α-hydroxy. Saturation of the 4,5 double bond leads to the formation of two isomers: 5α and 5β. Reduction of the ketone at C 20 creates an asymmetrical carbon at this site, the two possible isomers being designated α and β.

In formal chemical nomenclature, the adrenocortical hormones are described as derivatives of androstane or of pregnane. Double bonds are indicated by the symbol Δ with superscripts to indicate the position of the double bond. In this convention, cortisol is designated 11β,-17α,21-trihydroxy-Δ^4-pregnene-3,20-dione. Dehydroepiandrosterone is designated 3β-hydroxy-Δ^5-androsten-17-one.

PHYSIOLOGICAL FUNCTIONS AND PHARMACOLOGICAL EFFECTS

The effects of the corticosteroids are numerous and widespread. They influence carbohydrate, protein, and lipid metabolism; electrolyte and water balance; and the functions of the cardiovascular system, the kidney, skeletal muscle, the nervous system, and other organs and tissues. Furthermore, the corticosteroids endow the organism with the capacity to resist many types of noxious stimuli and environmental change. The adrenal cortex is the organ, *par excellence*, of homeostasis, being responsible to a large extent for the relative freedom that higher organisms exhibit in a constantly changing environment. In the absence of the adrenal cortex, survival is possible but only under the most rigidly prescribed conditions; for example, food must be available regularly, sodium chloride ingested in relatively large quantities, and environmental temperature maintained within a suitably narrow range.

A given dose of corticosteroid may be *physiological* or *pharmacological*, depending on the environment and the activities of the organism. Under favorable conditions, a small dose of corticosteroid maintains the adrenalectomized animal in a state of well-being. Under adverse conditions a relatively large dose is needed if the animal is to survive. This same large dose given repetitively under optimal conditions induces

Table 63–1. RATES OF SECRETION AND TYPICAL PLASMA CONCENTRATIONS OF THE MAJOR BIOLOGICALLY ACTIVE CORTICOSTEROIDS IN MAN

		CORTISOL	ALDOSTERONE
Rate of secretion under optimal conditions, mg/day		20	0.125
Concentrations in peripheral plasma of man, μg/dl	8 A.M.	16	0.01
	4 P.M.	4	

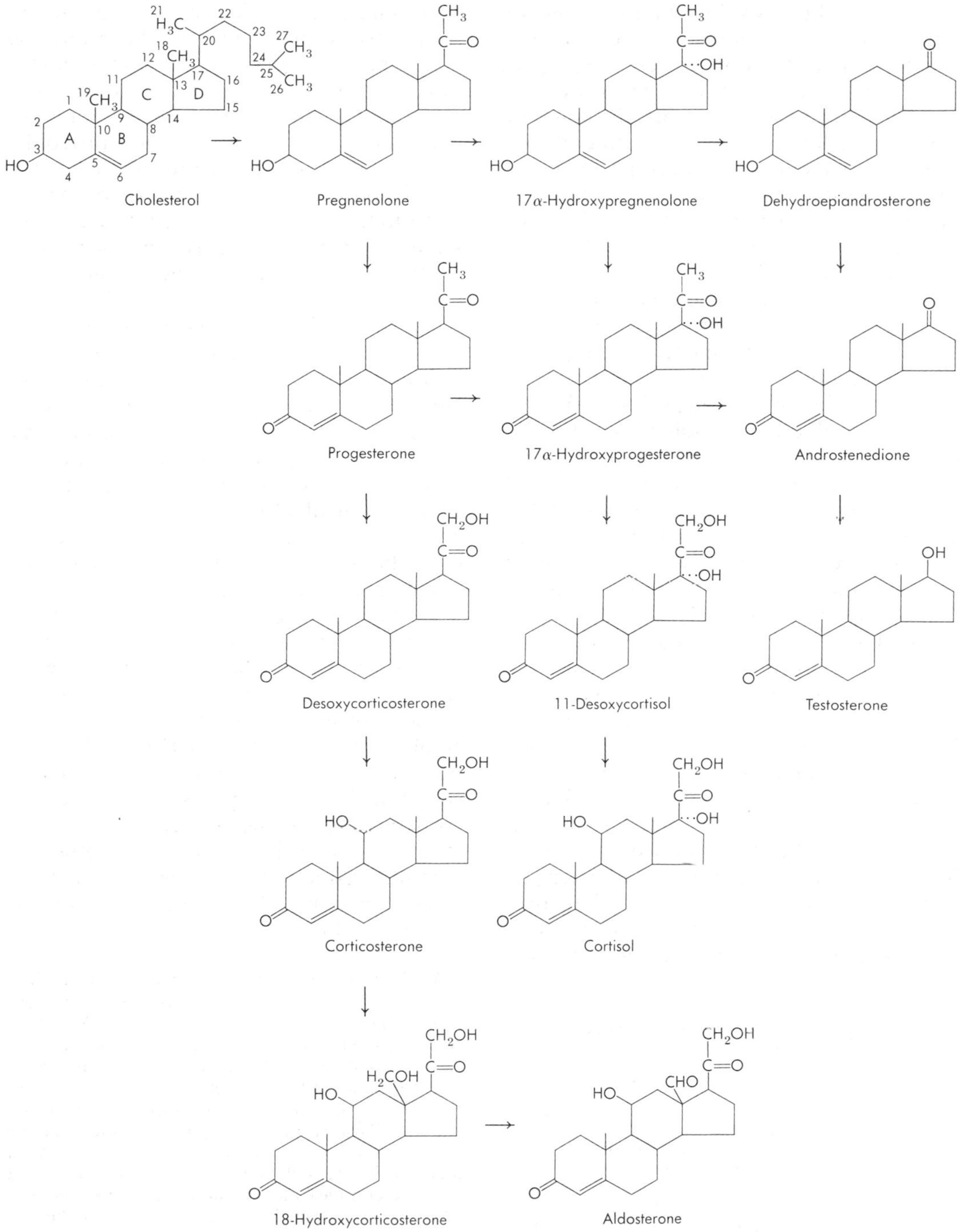

Figure 63–3. *Principal pathways for biosynthesis of adrenocorticosteroids and adrenal androgens.*

hypercorticism, that is, signs of excess of corticosteroid. The fluctuations in the secretory activity of a normal subject are presumed to reflect the varying needs of the organism for corticosteroids.

The actions of corticosteroids are often complexly related to the functions of other hormones. For example, in the absence of lipolytic hormones, cortisol even in large concentrations has virtually no effect on the rate of lipolysis in adipose tissue *in vitro*. Likewise, a sympathomimetic amine has only slight effect on the rate of lipolysis if there is a deficiency of glucocorticoids. However, if a necessary minimal amount of cortisol is added, the lipolytic effect of the sympathomimetic amine becomes evident. The necessary but not sufficient role of corticosteroids acting in concert with other regulatory forces has been termed "permissive" by Ingle (1954).

Certain of the biological actions of the corticosteroids lend themselves to quantitative measurement. Estimates of the potencies of naturally occurring and synthetic corticosteroids in the categories of *sodium retention* (reduction of sodium excretion by the kidney of the adrenalectomized animal), *hepatic deposition of glycogen,* and *anti-inflammatory effect* (inhibition of the action of an agent that induces inflammation) are presented in Table 63–2. It should be noted that such values are not fixed ratios but vary considerably with the conditions of the bioassays used. Potencies of steroids as judged by ability to sustain life in the adrenalectomized animal closely parallel those determined for sodium retention. Potencies based on liver glycogen deposition, anti-inflammatory effect, work capacity of skeletal muscle, and involution of lymphoid tissue closely parallel one another. Dissociations exist between potencies based on sodium retention and on liver glycogen deposition; traditionally the corticosteroids have thus been classified into *mineralocorticoids* and *glucocorticoids,*

according to potencies in the two categories. Desoxycorticosterone, the prototype of the mineralocorticoids, is highly potent in regard to sodium retention but without effect on hepatic glycogen deposition. Cortisol, the prototype of the glucocorticoids, is highly potent in regard to liver glycogen deposition but weak in regard to sodium retention. The naturally occurring corticosteroids cortisol and cortisone as well as synthetic corticosteroids such as prednisolone and triamcinolone are classified as glucocorticoids. However, corticosterone is a steroid that has modest but significant activities in both categories. In contrast, aldosterone is exceedingly potent with respect to sodium retention, with modest potency for liver glycogen deposition. At rates secreted by the adrenal cortex or in doses that exert maximal effects on electrolyte balance, aldosterone has no significant effect on carbohydrate metabolism; it is thus classified as a mineralocorticoid.

In the following descriptions of the physiological functions and the pharmacological effects of the corticosteroids, the terms *mineralocorticoid* and *glucocorticoid* will be employed for convenience. It is to be emphasized that the biological characteristics of the corticosteroids range over a spectrum from that of a strictly mineralocorticoid type at the one end to that of a strictly glucocorticoid type at the other. A comprehensive review of the actions of the glucocorticoids is that edited by Baxter and Rousseau (1979).

Mechanism of Action. Corticosteroids, like other steroid hormones, are thought to act by controlling the rate of synthesis of proteins. As is true with estrogens (Chapter 61), the corticosteroids react with receptor proteins in the cytoplasm of sensitive cells to form a steroid-receptor complex. Such receptors have been identified in many tissues (Ballard *et al.,* 1974). The steroid-receptor complex undergoes a modification, as noted by an increase in the sedimentation constant; following this, the complex moves into the nucleus, where it binds to chromatin. Information carried by the steroid or more likely by the receptor protein directs the genetic apparatus to transcribe RNA. This was established by demonstrations that glucocorticoids, in appropriate tissues, increase the quantity of mRNA that codes for enzymes whose synthesis is stimulated by these hormones (Schutz *et al.,* 1975; Iynedjian and Hanson, 1977). A more precise understanding of the mechanism by which glucocorticoids activate transcription of specific mRNAs

Table 63–2.   RELATIVE POTENCIES OF CORTICOSTEROIDS

	SODIUM RETENTION	LIVER GLYCOGEN DEPOSITION	ANTI-INFLAMMATORY EFFECT
Natural Steroids			
Cortisol	1 *	1	1
Cortisone	0.8 *	0.8	0.8
Corticosterone	15	0.35	0.3
11-Desoxycorticosterone	100	0	0
Aldosterone	3000	0.3	?
Synthetic Steroids			
Prednisolone	<1 *	4	4
Triamcinolone	0	5	5

* Promotes sodium excretion under certain circumstances.

may soon be forthcoming. Glucocorticoids specifically stimulate the rate of viral gene transcription in cultured tumor cells that bear murine mammary tumor virus, and this provides an excellent model system for study of the action of these hormones. The steroid-receptor complex binds *in vitro* to specific sequences of the viral DNA (Payvar *et al.*, 1981). The segments of DNA that are recognized are the long terminal repeat sequences that are known to be sites where transcription is initiated (Govindan *et al.*, 1982).

Steroid hormones thus stimulate transcription and ultimately the synthesis of specific proteins. While this is true for corticosteroids in some tissues, such as the liver, in other tissues, for example, lymphoid cells, the overall effect of the hormones is a catabolic one. This suggests that the steroid-receptor complex may inhibit rather than stimulate transcription in these instances. However, Makman and coworkers (1971) presented evidence suggesting that steroids act in lymphatic cells to stimulate the synthesis of an inhibitory protein, which presumably causes the catabolic effects.

Carbohydrate and Protein Metabolism. The effects of adrenocortical hormones on carbohydrate and protein metabolism are epitomized in the teleological view that these steroids have evolved to protect glucose-dependent cerebral functions by stimulating the formation of glucose, diminishing its peripheral utilization, and promoting its storage as glycogen. Adrenalectomized animals exhibit no marked abnormality in carbohydrate metabolism if food is regularly available. Under such circumstances, normal concentrations of glucose in the plasma are maintained and glycogen is stored in the liver. However, a brief period of starvation rapidly depletes carbohydrate reserves. The concentration of glycogen in the liver, and to a lesser extent that in muscle, decreases and hypoglycemia develops. In light of these facts, it is not surprising that the adrenalectomized animal is hypersensitive to insulin. Patients with Addison's disease have similar abnormalities in carbohydrate metabolism.

Administration of a glucocorticoid such as cortisol corrects the defect in carbohydrate metabolism of the adrenalectomized animal; glycogen stores, particularly in the liver, are increased; concentrations of glucose in plasma remain normal during fasting; sensitivity to insulin returns to normal. Increased excretion of nitrogen accompanies the increased production of glucose, indicating that protein is converted to carbohydrate (Long *et al.*, 1940). Prolonged exposure to large doses of glucocorticoids leads to an exaggeration of these changes in glucose metabolism, so that a diabetic-like state is produced: glucose in the plasma tends to be elevated in the fasting subject, there is increased resistance to insulin, glucose tolerance is decreased, and glucosuria may be present.

The mechanism by which the glucocorticoids inhibit utilization of glucose in peripheral tissues is not understood. Decreased uptake of glucose has been demonstrated in adipose tissue, skin, fibroblasts, and thymocytes as a result of glucocorticoid action.

Glucocorticoids promote gluconeogenesis by both peripheral and hepatic actions. Peripherally these steroids act to mobilize amino acids from a number of tissues. This catabolic action of the glucocorticoids is reflected in the atrophy of lymphatic tissues, reduced mass of muscle, osteoporosis (reduction in protein matrix of bone followed by calcium loss), thinning of the skin, and a negative nitrogen balance. Amino acids funnel into the liver, where they serve as substrates for enzymes involved in the production of glucose and glycogen.

In the liver the glucocorticoids induce *de-novo* synthesis of a number of enzymes involved in gluconeogenesis and amino acid metabolism. For example, the hepatic enzymes phosphoenolpyruvate carboxykinase, fructose-1,6-diphosphatase, and glucose-6-phosphatase, which catalyze reactions of glucose synthesis, are increased in concentration. However, induction of these enzymes requires a matter of hours and cannot account for the earliest effects of the hormones on gluconeogenesis. More rapid effects of glucocorticoids are apparent on hepatic mitochondria, such that they carboxylate pyruvate to form oxaloacetate at an accelerated rate (Adam and Haynes, 1969). This is the first reaction in the synthesis of glucose from pyruvate.

Prolonged, but not acute, treatment with glucocorticoids has been found to elevate the concentration of glucagon in the plasma (Marco *et al.*, 1973; Wise *et al.*, 1973). Inasmuch as glucagon itself stimulates gluconeogenesis, the rise in glucagon should also contribute to the enhanced synthesis of glucose. The deposition of glycogen in the liver found after treatment with glucocorticoids is thought to be the consequence of activation of hepatic glycogen synthase. This activation requires the presence of insulin but is not mediated by a rise in the concentration of insulin (Vanstapel *et al.*, 1982).

Lipid Metabolism. Two effects of corticosteroids on lipid metabolism are firmly established. The first is the dramatic redistribution of body fat that occurs in the hypercorticoid state. The other is the facilitation of the effect of adipokinetic agents in eliciting lipolysis of the triglycerides of adipose tissue. A number of other effects of corticosteroids on lipids have been reported, but in few, if any, instances have they turned out to be direct actions of the corticosteroids themselves.

Administration of large doses of glucocorticoids to human subjects over a long period of time or the hypersecretion of cortisol that occurs in Cushing's syndrome leads to a peculiar alteration in fat distribution. There is a gain of fat in depots in the back of the neck ("buffalo hump"), supraclavicular area, and face ("moon face") and a loss of fat from the extremities. One hypothesis to explain this phenomenon is that of Fain and Czech (1975), who proposed that the adipose tissue that hypertrophies in Cushing's syndrome responds preferentially to the lipogenic and antilipolytic actions of the elevated concentrations of insulin evoked by glucocorticoid-induced hyperglycemia. According to this hypothesis, adipocytes in the extremities, in contrast to those of the trunk, are less sensitive to insulin and more sensitive to the glucocorticoid-facilitated lipolytic effects of other hormones.

The mobilization of fat from peripheral fat depots by epinephrine, norepinephrine, or adipokinetic peptides of the adenohypophysis is markedly blunted in the absence of the adrenal cortex or the adenohypophysis. Cortisol acts in adipose tissue to facilitate the lipolytic response to cyclic AMP, rather than to enhance its accumulation. Hypophysectomy in rats has only a slight effect on the accumulation of cyclic AMP after exposure of adipose tissue to graded doses of epinephrine (Birnbaum and Goodman, 1973); however, hypophysectomy greatly decreases the lipolytic response of adipose tissue to the cyclic nucleotide. Treatment with cortisol restores the normal response to lipolytic hormones and to cyclic AMP (Goodman, 1968). Plasma lipids are not changed consistently in either hypocorticism or hypercorticism.

Electrolyte and Water Balance. Mineralocorticoids act on the distal tubules of the kidney to enhance the reabsorption of sodium ions from the tubular fluid into the plasma; they increase the urinary excretion of both potassium and hydrogen ions. The consequences of these three primary effects in concert with similar actions on cation transport in other tissues appear to account for the entire spectrum of physiological and pharmacological activities that

are characteristic of the mineralocorticoids. Thus, the primary features of *hypercorticism* are positive sodium balance and expansion of the extracellular fluid volume, normal or slight increase in the concentration of sodium in the plasma, hypokalemia, and alkalosis. In contrast, those of the deficient state, *hypocorticism*, are sodium loss, hyponatremia, hyperkalemia, contraction of the extracellular fluid volume, and cellular hydration. A defect of major consequence in adrenocortical insufficiency is the renal loss of sodium. The renal tubules normally reabsorb practically all the sodium filtered at the glomerulus. For example, on an ordinary diet, 99.5% may be reabsorbed to maintain sodium balance. Typically, in a patient with Addison's disease under the same circumstances of dietary intake, maximal reabsorption attainable is 98.5%. Since approximately 24,000 mEq of sodium is filtered per day, the 1% difference between reabsorption in the normal subject and reabsorption in the patient with Addison's disease amounts to a loss of 240 mEq of sodium per day. The gravity of the situation is obvious when one considers that this amount of sodium is normally present in 1.7 liters of extracellular fluid. Proportionately more sodium than water is lost through the kidney and the concentration of extracellular sodium decreases; extracellular fluid becomes hypoosmotic, and water shifts from the extracellular into the intracellular compartment. This shift, together with the renal loss of water, results in a marked reduction in the volume of the extracellular fluid. Cells are hydrated, and the increase in the hematocrit value is due not only to a shrinkage of the plasma volume but also to the swelling of the erythrocytes. Hyperkalemia and the tendency toward acid-base disturbances are a result of impairments in the excretion of potassium and of hydrogen ions. Without administration of mineralocorticoids or sodium chloride solution or both, a rapid downhill course ensues in adrenocortical insufficiency. The shrinkage of extracellular fluid volume, the cellular hydration, and the hypodynamic state of the cardiovascular system combine to cause circulatory collapse, renal failure, and death.

In adrenocortical insufficiency, a basic defect in ion transport occurs in a variety of secretory cells. Not only the kidney but also the salivary glands, the sweat glands, the exocrine pancreas, and the mucosa of the gastrointestinal tract elaborate fluids abnormally high in the concentration of sodium and abnormally low in the concentration of potassium. In the patient with Addison's disease, sweating may contribute significantly to the negative balance of sodium.

Aldosterone is by far the most potent of the naturally occurring corticosteroids with regard to electrolyte balance and plays an important role in the regulation of sodium and potassium balance. Evidence of this is the relatively normal electrolyte balance exhibited by the hypophysectomized animal as a result of continued secretion of aldosterone by the adrenal cortex. The increased rate of secretion of aldosterone that occurs in man when dietary salt is severely limited would appear to be a compensatory adjustment of physiological importance. However, *changes* in the rate of secretion of aldosterone are not the cause of *rapid* changes that may occur in sodium excretion. The latent period of action of the steroid is too long.

The intravenous administration of aldosterone to a normal subject is followed, after a delay of about an hour, by a decrease in the rate of renal sodium ion excretion and an increase in the rate of potassium ion and hydrogen ion excretion. If the administration of relatively large amounts of aldosterone is continued over a period of more than 10 to 14 days, sodium excretion again equals sodium intake. However, potassium ion and hydrogen ion excretion continues at an accelerated rate, resulting in hypokalemic hypochloremic alkalosis. The mechanism of "escape" from acute sodium retention is not understood, but it is not due to suppression of the renin-angiotensin system. The effects of the mineralocorticoids have been reviewed by Mulrow and Forman (1972).

The morphological complexity of the mammalian kidney presents a formidable obstacle to an attack on the question of how aldosterone increases sodium reabsorption. Aldosterone stimulates sodium transport by the toad bladder, and it is understandable that investigators have turned to this structurally simple organ as an experimental system.

Studies with the toad bladder have indicated that aldosterone, like other steroids, probably acts to initiate transcription of RNA that serves as template for the synthesis of a protein or proteins. This hypothetical "aldosterone-induced protein" is thought to facilitate the transport of sodium ions from the lumen of the distal tubules through the tubular cells and into the extracellular fluid. The most widely accepted model to describe the action of aldosterone is the following (Marver, 1980). The sodium ions of the tubular filtrate enter the cells of the distal tubules down a concentration gradient through the cell membrane facing the tubular lumen (apical or mucosal surface). Aldosterone and other mineralocorticoids facilitate this diffusion by increasing the permeability of the apical membrane to sodium ions. Sodium ions therefore enter the cells at an accelerated rate and are pumped out into the extracellular space at the serosal surface by a Na^+,K^+-activated adenosine triphosphatase (Na^+,K^+-ATPase).

The mechanisms of the enhanced excretion of potassium and hydrogen ions are less well understood. For practical purposes one may visualize these ions as being "exchanged" for the additional sodium ions reabsorbed under the influence of the steroids, because the sum of the equivalents of the additional potassium and hydrogen ions excreted is equal to that of the additional sodium ions retained.

The *glucocorticoids* decrease the absorption of calcium from the intestine and increase its renal excretion, thus producing a negative balance of the cation. These effects are considered to be the basis of the favorable therapeutic response to glucocorticoids seen in hypercalcemia (*see* Chapter 65).

Desoxycorticosterone is a natural mineralocorticoid of some historical interest for it was the first corticosteroid to be synthesized and made available for the treatment of Addison's disease. Desoxycorticosterone is practically devoid of glucocorticoid effects. Qualitatively, it is identical to aldosterone in its effects on electrolytes; quantitatively, it is about 3% as potent (*see* Table 63–2). Thus, despite the fact that the concentration of desoxycorticosterone in plasma is approximately the same as that of aldosterone, it apparently is of little physiological significance in the normal individual (Biglieri, 1978).

Cortisol induces sodium retention and potassium excretion, but much less effectively than does aldosterone. Acute treatment with cortisol, unlike that with aldosterone, does not increase net acid secretion (Lemann *et al.*, 1970). In striking contrast to aldosterone, cortisol, under certain circumstances, especially sodium loading, enhances sodium excretion. This may be accounted for by the capacity of cortisol to increase the glomerular filtration rate (GFR). Aldosterone and desoxycorticosterone are ineffective in this regard. Furthermore, cortisol has a significant stimulatory influence on tubular secretory activity.

Impaired water diuresis in response to an administered water load, while not specific for adrenal insufficiency, has been used as a diagnostic criterion. In adrenal insufficiency, GFR is reduced and plasma antidiuretic hormone (ADH) concentration is increased; these factors account for failure to excrete a water load (Ahmed *et al.,* 1967). Administration of cortisol, but not of aldosterone, increases GFR and restores water diuresis (Gill *et al.,* 1962).

Hypercorticism due to administration of large doses of cortisol (or related glucocorticoids) or to excessive secretion of cortisol by the adrenals is sometimes associated with a hypokalemic hypochloremic alkalosis (*see* Chapter 35). However, the changes, particularly the degree of hypokalemia, are moderate in severity and reflect the relatively weak effect of cortisol as compared to aldosterone on electrolyte balance. Muscular weakness associated with glucocorticoid treatment is usually due to a loss of muscle mass rather than of potassium.

Cardiovascular System. The most striking effects of corticosteroids on the cardiovascular system are those that are the consequence of regulation of renal sodium ion excretion. These are seen most vividly in hypocorticism when reduction in blood volume accompanied by increased viscosity can lead to hypotension and cardiovascular collapse. However, the impairment of the cardiovascular system in adrenocortical insufficiency obviously involves additional, poorly understood processes. The corticosteroids exert important actions on the various elements of the circulatory system, including the capillaries, the arterioles, and the myocardium. In the absence of the corticosteroids, there is increased capillary permeability, inadequate vasomotor response of the small vessels, and reduction in cardiac size and output.

An excess of mineralocorticoids occurs in its purest form in *primary aldosteronism,* the result of excessive secretion of this steroid. In this disease the major clinical findings are hypertension and hypokalemia. The hypokalemia is an obvious consequence of the renal effects of aldosterone, but the genesis of the hypertension has not been totally clarified. Development of hypertension requires a prolonged excess of mineralocorticoid and increased sodium intake (Mulrow and Forman, 1972). Hypertension occurs in most cases of Cushing's syndrome but rarely, if at all, as the result of administration of synthetic glucocorticoids lacking mineralocorticoid activity. Steroid-induced hypertension may be the result of prolonged, excessive sodium retention; one hypothesis proposes that this leads to edema within the walls of arterioles, thereby reducing their lumina and increasing peripheral vascular resistance (Tobian, 1960). Another possibility is that salt retention or mineralocorticoids themselves sensitize blood vessels to pressor agents, in particular angiotensin and catecholamines (Brunner *et al.,* 1972; Yard and Kadowitz, 1972). The concentration of renin substrate is elevated in Cushing's syndrome, and this too may play a role (Krakoff *et al.,* 1975). There is also some evidence that ADH plays a role in the pathogenesis of hypertension produced by mineralocorticoids (Share and Crofton, 1982).

Skeletal Muscle. The maintenance of normal function of skeletal muscle requires adequate concentrations of corticosteroids, but excessive amounts of either mineralocorticoids or glucocorticoids lead to abnormalities.

It is well known that one of the outstanding signs of adrenocortical insufficiency is a diminished work capacity of striated muscle. This is manifested in patients with Addison's disease by weakness and fatigue. The most important single factor responsible for this dysfunction appears to be the inadequacy of the circulatory system. Abnormalities in electrolyte balance and carbohydrate metabolism in adrenocortical insufficiency contribute only in small measure to the impairment in skeletal muscle function.

Muscle weakness in primary aldosteronism is in large measure a result of the hypokalemia characteristic of this disease. Glucocorticoids given for prolonged periods in high doses or secreted in abnormal amounts in Cushing's syndrome tend to cause a wasting of skeletal muscle. The mechanism of this is not known. This steroid myopathy is responsible, at least in part, for the weakness and fatigue noted in the syndrome. Steroid-induced myopathy has been reviewed by Mandel (1982).

Central Nervous System. The corticosteroids affect the central nervous system (CNS) in a number of indirect ways; in particular, they maintain normal concentrations of glucose in plasma, an adequate circulation, and the normal balance of electrolytes in the body. The steroids may also have direct effects, but these are as yet poorly defined. An influence of the corticosteroids can be observed on mood, behavior, the EEG, and brain excitability.

Patients with Addison's disease exhibit apathy, depression, and irritability, and some are frankly psychotic. Desoxycorticosterone is ineffective but cortisol is very effective in correcting these abnormalities of psyche and behavior. An array of reactions, varying in degree and kind, is seen in patients to whom glucocorticoids are administered for therapeutic purposes. Most patients respond with elevation in mood, which may be explained in part by the relief of the symptoms of the disease being treated. In some, more definite mood changes occur, characterized by euphoria, insomnia, restlessness, and increased motor activity. A smaller but significant percentage of patients treated with high doses of cortisol become anxious or depressed, and a still smaller percentage exhibit psychotic reactions. There is a high incidence of neuroses and psychoses among patients with Cushing's syndrome. The abnormalities of behavior usually disappear when the corticosteroids are withdrawn or the Cushing's syndrome is effectively treated.

There is usually an increase in the excitability of neural tissue in hypocorticism and a decrease in animals given large doses of desoxycorticosterone; these alterations appear to be related to changes in the concentrations of electrolytes in the brain. In contrast, administration of cortisol increases brain excitability without influencing the concentrations of sodium and potassium in the brain. It is concluded that the influence of desoxycorticosterone on excitability is mediated through its influence on sodium transport, whereas cortisol acts by a different mechanism, presumably mediated by cytoplasmic receptors (McEwen, 1979; Carpenter and Gruen, 1982).

Thresholds for the perception of taste, smell, and sound stimuli are reduced in adrenocortical insufficiency and elevated in hypercorticism. Glucocorticoids restore thresholds to normal, but desoxycorticosterone is without effect (Henkin, 1970).

Formed Elements of Blood. Glucocorticoids tend to increase the hemoglobin and red-cell content of the blood, as evidenced by the frequent occurrence of polycythemia in Cushing's syndrome and a mild, normochromic, normocytic anemia in Addison's disease. The capacity of these steroids to retard erythrophagocytosis may be a factor in the production of polycythemia.

The corticosteroids also affect circulating white cells. Administration of glucocorticoids leads to an increase in the number of polymorphonuclear leukocytes in the blood as the result of an increased rate of entrance into the blood from the marrow and a diminished rate of removal from the circulation (Bishop *et al.*, 1968). In contrast, the lymphocytes, eosinophils, monocytes, and basophils of the blood decrease in number after administration of glucocorticoids. A single dose of cortisol produces a decline of about 70% in circulating lymphocytes and a decline of over 90% in monocytes; this occurs in 4 to 6 hours and lasts for about 24 hours. The decrease in lymphocytes, monocytes, and eosinophils appears to result from redistribution of cells, rather than from their destruction. The cause of the fall in circulating basophils has not been established.

After administration of a glucocorticoid, the thymus-derived lymphocytes (T cells) are decreased proportionately more than those that are derived from the bone marrow (B cells). The profile of cellular responses of the lymphocytes remaining in the blood to various mitogens and antigens is altered when contrasted to that of lymphocytes of untreated subjects. This indicates that subpopulations of lymphocytes are differentially affected by the steroids (*see* Cupps and Fauci, 1982).

Anti-inflammatory Properties. Cortisol and the synthetic analogs of cortisol have the capacity to prevent or suppress the development of the local heat, redness, swelling, and tenderness by which inflammation is recognized. At the microscopic level, they inhibit not only the early phenomena of the inflammatory process (edema, fibrin deposition, capillary dilatation, migration of leukocytes into the inflamed area, and phagocytic activity) but also the later manifestations (capillary proliferation, fibroblast proliferation, deposition of collagen, and, still later, cicatrization).

Although understanding of these effects is unsatisfactory, many observations have been made that have therapeutic relevance and that must be taken into account in explanatory formulations. Perhaps the most important of these for the physician is that corticosteroids inhibit the inflammatory response whether the inciting agent is radiant, mechanical, chemical, infectious, or immunological. In clinical terms, the administration of corticosteroids for their anti-inflammatory effects is palliative therapy; the underlying cause of the disease remains; the inflammatory manifestations are merely suppressed. It is this suppression of inflammation and its consequences that has made the corticosteroids such valuable therapeutic agents—indeed, at times lifesaving. It is also this property that gives them a nearly unique potential for therapeutic disaster. The signs and symptoms of inflammation are expressions of the disease process that are often used by the physician in diagnosis and in evaluating the effectiveness of treatment. These may be missing in patients treated with glucocorticoids. For example, an infection may continue to progress while the patient superficially appears to improve, and a peptic ulcer may perforate without producing clinical signs. This situation has been epitomized in the grimly facetious remark that the corticosteroids, misused, permit a patient to walk all the way to the autopsy room!

Anti-inflammatory effects depend upon the direct local action of the steroids. The most important factor in the anti-inflammatory action of glucocorticoids may be their ability to inhibit the recruitment of neutrophils and monocyte-macrophages into the affected area (Parrillo and Fauci, 1979). Treatment with glucocorticoids decreases the adherence of neutrophils to nylon fibers, and this may reflect a diminished tendency of these cells to adhere to capillary endothelial cells in areas of inflammation (MacGregor, 1977).

In the inflammatory response of delayed sensitivity reactions, lymphocytes previously sensitized to a particular antigen encounter the antigen within a tissue at a site destined to be the location of the inflammatory response. These lymphocytes, activated by the antigen, begin production of a number of soluble factors, *lymphokines*, that control the cellular response. Among the lymphokines is the macrophage migration inhibitory factor (MIF), which causes an accumulation of nonsensitized macrophages in the area by inhibiting their mobility (Bloom and Bennett, 1966). Glucocorticoids do not affect the production of MIF by lymphocytes that have been activated by an appropriate antigen, but the steroids do block the effect of MIF on macrophages; that is, the movement of these cells is no longer impeded, and they do not accumulate locally (Balow and Rosenthal, 1973).

Low concentrations of glucocorticoids inhibit the formation of plasminogen activator by neutrophils (Granelli-Piperano *et al.*, 1977). This enzyme converts plasminogen to plasmin (fibrinolysin), which is thought to facilitate the entrance of leukocytes into areas of inflammation by hydrolysis of fibrin and other proteins. There is also substantial evidence that the glucocorticoids induce the synthesis of a protein that inhibits phospholipase A_2 and thereby diminishes release of arachidonic acid from phospholipids. This decreases formation of prostaglandins, leukotrienes, and related compounds, such as prostaglandin endoperoxides and thromboxane, which may play an important role in chemotaxis and inflammation (Blackwell *et al.*, 1980; Hirata *et al.*, 1980; *see* Chapter 28). As a result of studies on a particular strain of mouse fibroblasts maintained in culture, it was thought that glucocorticoids inhibit the growth of such cells. It is now evident that human fibroblasts are resistant to glucocorticoids; the suppression of late stages of inflammation by inhibition of fibroblast proliferation is probably not a valid model for the anti-inflammatory effects of glucocorticoids (Priestley and Brown, 1980).

Lymphoid Tissue and Immune Responses. Addison was the first to observe the increase in mass of lymphoid tissue that accompanies adrenocortical insufficiency; there is also a lymphocytosis. In contrast, Cushing's syndrome is characterized by lymphocytopenia and decreased mass of lymphoid tissue.

While glucocorticoids cause a rapid lysis of lymphatic tissue in rats and mice, there is no evidence of a comparable effect in man (Claman, 1972). This implies that the changes in lymphoid tissue seen in man in chronic hypercorticosteroid or hypocorticosteroid states must result from changes in rates of cellular formation or destruction that become manifest over a prolonged period of time. As noted above, the acute effects of steroids on circulating lymphocytes are due to sequestration from the blood, rather than to lymphocytolysis. Although glucocorticoids do not produce a sudden, massive lysis of lymphoid tissue in man, cells of acute lymphoblastic leukemia and, in some cases, cells of other lymphatic malignancies are destroyed by glucocorticoids in a manner presumed to be analogous to that which occurs in lymphoid tissue of rodents.

As noted, glucocorticoids and ACTH modify the clinical course of a variety of diseases in which hypersensitivity is believed to play an important role. Although massive doses of methylprednisolone have been shown to cause a modest fall in the concentration of IgG in the plasma of human volunteers, these same subjects produced antibody normally in response to antigenic stimuli (Butler, 1975). On the whole, there is no convincing evidence that the therapeutic use of the corticosteroids has a significant effect on the titer of circulating antibodies, either IgG or IgE, that play a major role in allergic and autoimmune states. Metabolism of complement is likewise probably not significantly affected (Claman, 1975). This is true in spite of the fact that the symptoms of the diseases are often alleviated dramatically by the steroids. It is also now believed that in clinical situations in which the glucocorticoids are used to prevent the consequences of cell-mediated (delayed hypersensitivity) immune reactions, for example, graft rejection, the steroids do not interfere with the development of immune lymphatic cells that are capable of eliciting an inflammatory response upon contact with the sensitizing antigen. Rather, they suppress the inflammatory response, apparently by inhibiting recruitment of leukocytes into the region of contact with the foreign antigen (*see* above; Weston *et al.*, 1973).

Circulating monocytes from individuals who are receiving glucocorticoids display an impaired ability to kill microorganisms, although the process of phagocytosis is not defective (Rinehart et al., 1975).

There are numerous reports of effects of glucocorticoids on lymphatic cells in vitro. Unfortunately, many of these effects are observed at unrealistically high concentrations of steroids, and their significance is unclear. One example of a response that is inhibited by appropriately low concentrations of glucocorticoids in vitro is the proliferation of T cells stimulated by mitogens or mixed leukocyte cultures. This effect is the result of inhibition of the release of interleukin 1 by macrophages. Deficiency of interleukin 1 precludes formation of interleukin 2, the immediate stimulus for proliferation of T cells (Gillis et al., 1979; Smith, 1980).

Growth and Cell Division. Pharmacological doses of glucocorticoids retard or interrupt the growth of children, indicating an adverse effect on the epiphyseal cartilage. Inhibition of growth is a rather widespread effect of the glucocorticoids in tissues of laboratory animals. For example, they inhibit cell division or the synthesis of DNA in thymocytes; normal, developing, and regenerating liver; gastric mucosa; developing brain; developing lung; and human epidermis. Nevertheless, this effect is somewhat selective, and corticosteroids do not characteristically produce the bone-marrow depression or the enteritis that follows exposure to nonspecific antimitotic agents. The mechanism of this effect of the steroids is not known.

ABSORPTION, TRANSPORT, METABOLISM, AND EXCRETION

Absorption. Cortisol and numerous congeners, including synthetic analogs, are effective when given by mouth. Desoxycorticosterone acetate is unusual in that it is ineffective by this route.

Water-soluble esters of cortisol and its synthetic congeners are administered intravenously in order to achieve high concentrations in body fluids rapidly. More prolonged effects are obtained by intramuscular injection of suspensions of cortisol, congeners, and esters. Minor changes in chemical structure may result in large changes in the rate of absorption, time of onset of effect, and duration of action.

Glucocorticoids are absorbed from sites of local application such as synovial spaces, the conjunctival sac, and the skin. The absorption may be sufficient, when administration is chronic or large areas of skin are involved, to cause systemic effects, including adrenocortical suppression.

Transport, Metabolism, and Excretion. In the plasma, 90% or more of the cortisol is reversibly bound to protein under normal circumstances. The binding is accounted for by two proteins. One, corticosteroid-binding globulin, is a glycoprotein; the other is albumin. The globulin has high affinity but low total binding capacity, while albumin has low affinity but relatively large binding capacity. Consequently, at low or normal concentrations of corticosteroids most of the hormone is bound to globulin. When the amount of corticosteroid is increased, concentrations of both free and albumin-bound steroid increase with little change in the concentration of that bound to the globulin. Corticosteroids compete with each other for binding sites on the corticosteroid-binding globulin. Cortisol has high affinity; glucuronide-conjugated steroid metabolites and aldosterone have low affinities.

During pregnancy and during estrogen treatment in both sexes, corticosteroid-binding globulin, total plasma cortisol, and free cortisol increase severalfold. The physiological significance of these facts is not known. The free hormone as opposed to the protein-bound steroid is biologically active, available for hepatic metabolism, and may be excreted by the kidney.

All the biologically active adrenocortical steroids and their synthetic congeners have a double bond in the 4,5 position and a ketone group at C 3. Reduction of the 4,5 double bond can occur at both hepatic and extrahepatic sites and yields an inactive substance. Subsequent reduction of the 3-ketone substituent to a 3-hydroxyl to form tetrahydrocortisol has been demonstrated only in liver. Most of the ring-A–reduced metabolites are enzymatically coupled through the 3-hydroxyl with sulfate or with glucuronic acid to form water-soluble sulfate esters or glucuronides, and they are excreted as such. These conjugation reactions occur principally in liver and to some extent in kidney.

Reversible oxidation of the 11-hydroxyl group has been demonstrated to occur slowly in a variety of extrahepatic tissues and rapidly in liver. Corticosteroids with an 11-ketone substituent require reduction to 11-hydroxyl compounds for their biological activity. Reduction of the 20-ketone group to a 20-hydroxyl configuration yields a substance having little, if any, biological activity. Corticosteroids with a hydroxyl group at C 17 undergo an oxidation that yields 17-ketosteroids and a two-carbon fragment. These 17-ketosteroids are totally lacking in corticosteroid activity but, in a few instances, have weak androgenic properties.

When radioactive-carbon, ring-labeled steroids are injected intravenously in man, most of the radioisotope is recovered in the urine within 72 hours. Neither biliary nor fecal excretion is of any quantitative importance in man. It has been estimated that the liver metabolizes at least 70% of the cortisol secreted.

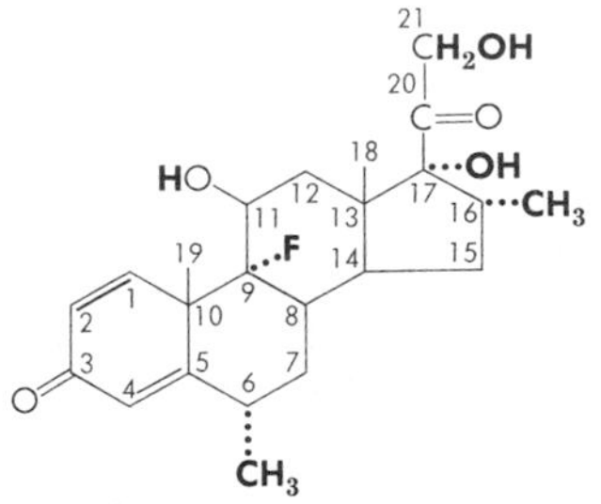

The metabolism of cortisol has been studied more extensively than that of all other corticosteroids, and it is generally assumed that the metabolism of its congeners and synthetic derivatives is qualitatively similar. Cortisol has a plasma half-life of about 1.5 hours. The metabolism of corticosteroids is greatly slowed by introduction of the 1,2 double bond or a fluorine atom into the molecule, and the half-life is correspondingly prolonged.

Clinical laboratories measure urinary cortisol and metabolites with reduced ring A as ''17-hydroxycorticosteroids.'' These compounds and those where the ketone at carbon 20 has been reduced are included in the group referred to as ''17-ketogenic steroids.'' The urinary metabolites that have lost their side chain contribute to the ''17-ketosteroids.''

STRUCTURE-ACTIVITY RELATIONSHIP

Cortisone was the first corticosteroid used for its anti-inflammatory effect. Modifications of structure have led to increases in the ratio of anti-inflammatory to sodium-retaining potency, such that in a number of presently available compounds electrolyte effects are of no serious consequence, even at the highest doses used. However, in all compounds studied to date, effects on inflammation and on carbohydrate and protein metabolism have paralleled one another. It seems very likely that effects on inflammation and metabolism are mediated by the same type of receptor.

Changes in molecular structure may bring about changes in biological potency as a result of alterations in absorption, protein binding, rate of metabolic transformation, rate of excretion, ability to traverse membranes, and intrinsic effectiveness of the molecule at its site of action. In the following paragraphs, modifications of the pregnane nucleus that have been of value in therapeutic agents are described. The molecular sites of alteration are shown in Figure 63–4 in bold lines and letters. Table 63–3 lists the effects of the modifications discussed relative to cortisol. As indicated above, rel-

Figure 63–4. *Structure-activity relationship of adrenocorticosteroids.*

Light lines and letters indicate structural features common to compounds having anti-inflammatory action. Bold lines and letters indicate modifications that enhance or suppress characteristic activities. (After Liddle, 1961. Courtesy of *Clinical Pharmacology and Therapeutics.*)

ative potencies vary to some extent with different conditions of bioassay.

Ring A. The 4,5 double bond and the 3-ketone are both necessary for typical adrenocorticosteroid activity. Introduction of a 1,2 double bond, as in prednisone or prednisolone, enhances the ratio of carbohydrate-regulating potency to sodium-retaining potency by selectively increasing the former. In addition, prednisolone is metabolized more slowly than cortisol.

Ring B. 6α-Substitution has unpredictable effects. In the particular instance of cortisol, 6α-methylation increases anti-inflammatory, nitrogen-wasting, and sodium-retaining effects in man. In contrast, 6α-methylprednisolone has slightly greater anti-inflammatory potency and less electrolyte-regulating potency than prednisolone. Fluorination in the 9α position enhances all biological activities of the corticosteroids, apparently by its electron-withdrawing effect on the 11β-hydroxy group.

Ring C. The presence of an oxygen function at C 11 is indispensable for significant anti-inflammatory and carbohydrate-regulating potency (cortisol versus 11-desoxycortisol) but is not necessary for high sodium-retaining potency, as demonstrated by desoxycorticosterone.

Ring D. 16-Methylation or hydroxylation eliminates the sodium-retaining effect but only slightly modifies potency with respect to effects on metabolism and inflammation.

All presently used anti-inflammatory steroids are 17α-hydroxy compounds. Although some carbohydrate-regulating and anti-inflammatory effects may occur in 17-desoxy compounds (cortisol versus corticosterone), the fullest expression of these activities requires the presence of the 17α-hydroxy substituent.

All natural corticosteroids and most of the active synthetic analogs have a 21-hydroxy group. While some glycogenic and anti-inflammatory activities may occur in its absence, its presence is required for significant sodium-retaining activity.

**Table 63–3. RELATIVE POTENCIES AND EQUIVALENT DOSES
OF CORTICOSTEROIDS**

COMPOUND	RELATIVE ANTI-INFLAMMATORY POTENCY	RELATIVE SODIUM-RETAINING POTENCY	DURATION OF ACTION *	APPROXIMATE EQUIVALENT DOSE † (*mg*)
Cortisol (Hydrocortisone)	1	1	S	20
Tetrahydrocortisol	0	0	—	—
Prednisone (Δ^1-Cortisone)	4	0.8	I	5
Prednisolone (Δ^1-Cortisol)	4	0.8	I	5
6α-Methylprednisolone	5	0.5	I	4
Fludrocortisone (9α-Fluorocortisol)	10	125	S	—
11-Desoxycortisol	0	0	—	—
Cortisone (11-Dehydrocortisol)	0.8	0.8	S	25
Corticosterone	0.35	15	S	—
Triamcinolone (9α-Fluoro-16α-hydroxyprednisolone)	5	0	I	4
Paramethasone (6α-Fluoro-16α-methylprednisolone)	10	0	L	2
Betamethasone (9α-Fluoro-16β-methylprednisolone)	25	0	L	0.75
Dexamethasone (9α-Fluoro-16α-methylprednisolone)	25	0	L	0.75

* S = Short or 8- to 12-hour biological half-life; I = intermediate or 12- to 36-hour biological half-life; L = long or 36- to 72-hour biological half-life (*see* Rose and Saccar, 1978).

† These dose relationships apply only to oral or intravenous administration; relative potencies may differ greatly when injected intramuscularly or into joint spaces.

PREPARATIONS AND ROUTES OF ADMINISTRATION

Organic chemists have synthesized a bewildering number of modified adrenocorticosteroids, many of which share the same properties and differ only with respect to absolute dosage. At the outset it should be reemphasized that, whereas a clear separation has been made between mineralocorticoids and glucocorticoids, there is no member of the latter group that is unique with respect to a separation of therapeutic and toxic effects. A working knowledge of a small number of preparations is sufficient for nearly every clinical purpose.

Corticosteroids are administered orally, parenterally (intravenous, intramuscular, subcutaneous, intrasynovial, and intralesional routes), and topically (dermal ointments, creams, and lotions; ophthalmic ointments and solutions; respiratory aerosols; enemas). Some absorption into the systemic circulation occurs with all forms of topical administration. In the case of most aerosols, absorption is virtually equivalent to that from parenteral or oral administration. Adrenocortical suppression can occur with applications of steroids to the conjunctival sac and to the skin. Absorption from the skin is especially marked when the steroid is applied under plastic film over a large surface area.

Information on available steroid preparations is presented in Table 63–4.

TOXICITY OF ADRENOCORTICAL STEROIDS

Two categories of toxic effects are observed in the therapeutic use of adrenocorticosteroids: those resulting from *withdrawal* and those resulting from *continued use of large doses*. Acute adrenal insufficiency results from too rapid withdrawal of corticosteroids after prolonged therapy. Protocols for discontinuing corticosteroid therapy in patients who have been subjected to suppressive therapy for long periods have been described by Harter and associates (1963) and Byyny (1976). There is a characteristic corticosteroid withdrawal syndrome, consisting in fever, myalgia, arthralgia, and malaise, which may be extremely difficult to distinguish from "reactivation" of rheumatoid arthritis or rheumatic fever (Amatruda *et al.*, 1960). Pseudotumor cerebri with papilledema is a rare reaction that follows reduction or withdrawal of corticosteroid therapy (Levine and Leopold, 1973).

NONPROPRIETARY NAME AND TRADE NAMES	ORAL FORMS	INJECTABLE FORMS	OTHERS [1]
Desoxycorticosterone acetate [2] (DOCA ACETATE, PERCORTEN ACETATE)	—	5 mg/ml (oil) 125 mg (pellets)	—
Desoxycorticosterone pivalate (PERCORTEN PIVALATE)	—	25 mg/ml (susp.)	—
Fludrocortisone acetate [3] (FLORINEF ACETATE)	0.1 mg	—	—
Cortisol [2] (hydrocortisone) (CORTEF, HYDROCORTONE)	5–20 mg	25, 50 mg/ml (susp.)	TA: 0.125–2.5% 100-mg/60-ml enema
Cortisol (hydrocortisone) acetate (CORTEF ACETATE, HYDROCORTONE ACETATE, others)	—	25, 50 mg/ml (susp.)	TA: 0.5–2.5% 15-, 25-mg supposi- tories 10% rectal foam
Cortisol (hydrocortisone) cypionate (CORTEF FLUID)	2 mg/ml (susp.)	—	—
Cortisol (hydrocortisone) sodium phosphate (HYDROCORTONE PHOSPHATE)	—	50 mg/ml	—
Cortisol (hydrocortisone) sodium succinate (A-HYDROCORT, SOLU-CORTEF)	—	100–1000 mg (powder)	—
Beclomethasone dipropionate [4] (BECLOVENT, VANCERIL)	—	—	I: 42 μg per dose
Betamethasone [3] (CELESTONE)	0.6 mg 0.6 mg/5 ml (syrup)	—	—
Betamethasone benzoate (BENISONE, UTICORT)	—	—	TA: 0.025%
Betamethasone dipropionate (DIPROSONE)	—	—	TA: 0.05, 0.1%
Betamethasone sodium phosphate and acetate (CELESTONE SOLUSPAN)	—	6 mg/ml (susp.)	—
Betamethasone valerate (BETA-VAL, VALISONE)	—	—	TA: 0.01, 0.1%
Cortisone acetate [3] (CORTONE ACETATE)	5–25 mg	25, 50 mg/ml (susp.)	—
Dexamethasone [3] (DECADRON, others)	0.25–6.0 mg 0.5 mg/5 ml (elixir) 0.5 mg/0.5 ml (soln.)	—	TA: 0.01, 0.1% O: 0.1%
Dexamethasone acetate (DECADRON-LA, others)	—	2–16 mg/ml (susp.)	—
Dexamethasone sodium phosphate (DECADRON PHOSPHATE, HEXADROL PHOSPHATE, others)	—	4–24 mg/ml	TA: 0.1% O: 0.05, 0.1% I: 100 μg per dose
Methylprednisolone [3] (MEDROL)	2–32 mg	—	—

NONPROPRIETARY NAME AND TRADE NAMES	ORAL FORMS	INJECTABLE FORMS	OTHERS [1]
Methylprednisolone acetate (DEPO-MEDROL, MEDROL ACETATE, others)	—	20–80 mg/ml (susp.)	TA: 0.25, 1% 40-mg/unit enema
Methylprednisolone sodium succinate (A-METHAPRED, SOLU-MEDROL)	—	40–1000 mg (powder)	—
Paramethasone acetate [3] (HALDRONE)	1, 2 mg	—	—
Prednisolone [3] (DELTA-CORTEF, others)	1, 5 mg	—	—
Prednisolone acetate (ECONOPRED, others)	—	25–100 mg/ml (susp.)	O: 0.12–1%
Prednisolone sodium phosphate (HYDELTRASOL, others)	—	20 mg/ml	O: 0.125–1%
Prednisolone tebutate (HYDELTRA-T.B.A.)	—	20 mg/ml (susp.)	—
Prednisone [3] (DELTASONE, others)	1–50 mg 1 mg/ml (syrup)	—	—
Triamcinolone [3] (ARISTOCORT, KENACORT)	1–16 mg	—	—
Triamcinolone acetonide (KENALOG, others)	—	10, 40 mg/ml (susp.)	TA: 0.025–0.5% I: 100 μg per dose
Triamcinolone diacetate (ARISTOCORT, KENACORT DIACETATE, others)	2, 4 mg/5 ml (syrup)	25, 40 mg/ml (susp.)	—
Triamcinolone hexacetonide (ARISTOSPAN)	—	5, 20 mg/ml (susp.)	—
Amcinonide [4] (CYCLOCORT)	—	—	TA: 0.1%
Clocortolone pivalate [4] (CLODERM)	—	—	TA: 0.1%
Desonide [4] (TRIDESILON)	—	—	TA: 0.05%
Desoximetasone [4] (TOPICORT)	—	—	TA: 0.05, 0.25%
Diflorasone diacetate [4] (FLORONE, MAXIFLOR)	—	—	TA: 0.05%
Flumethasone pivalate [4] (LOCORTEN)	—	—	TA: 0.03%
Fluocinolone acetonide [4] (FLUONID, SYNALAR, others)	—	—	TA: 0.01–0.2%
Fluocinonide [4] (LIDEX)	—	—	TA: 0.05%
Fluorometholone [4] (FML LIQUIFILM)	—	—	O: 0.1%

Table 63–4.   **PREPARATIONS OF ADRENOCORTICAL STEROIDS AND THEIR SYNTHETIC ANALOGS** * (Continued)

NONPROPRIETARY NAME AND TRADE NAMES	ORAL FORMS	INJECTABLE FORMS	OTHERS [1]
Flurandrenolide [4] (CORDRAN)	—	—	TA: 0.025, 0.05% 4 μg/sq cm tape
Halcinonide [4] (HALOG)	—	—	TA: 0.025, 0.1%
Medrysone [4] (HMS LIQUIFILM)	—	—	O: 1%

* Preparations above the double line are intended for use as mineralocorticoids.

[1] TA = topical application to skin or mucous membranes in creams, solutions, ointments, gels, lotions, or aerosols. O = ophthalmic solution, suspension, or ointment. I = nasal or oral inhalation.

[2] *See* Figure 63–3 for structure.

[3] *See* Table 63–3 for chemical name.

[4] Beclomethasone, 9α-chloro,16β-methylprednisolone,17,21-dipropionate; amcinonide, 9α-fluoro,16α-hydroxyprednisolone cyclic 16,17-acetal with cyclic pentanone,21-acetate; clocortolone, $\Delta^{1,2}$,6α-fluoro,9α-chloro,16α-methylcorticosterone 21-pivalate; desonide, 16α-hydroxyprednisolone, cyclic 16,17-acetal with acetone; desoximetasone, $\Delta^{1,2}$,9α-fluoro,16α-methylcorticosterone; diflorasone diacetate, 6α,9α-difluoro,16β-methylprednisolone, 17,21-diacetate; flumethasone, 6α,9α-difluoro,16α-methylprednisolone; fluocinolone, 6α,9α-difluoro, 16α-hydroxyprednisolone,16,17-acetal with acetone; fluocinonide, 6α,9α-difluoro,16α-hydroxyprednisolone,16,17-acetal with acetone,21-acetate; fluorometholone, $\Delta^{1,2}$,9α-fluoro,6α-methyl, 11β,17-dihydroxyprogesterone; flurandrenolide, 6α-fluoro,16α-hydroxycortisol,16,17-acetal with acetone; halcinonide, 21-chloro,9α-fluoro,11β,16α, 17-trihydroxypregn-4-ene-3,20-dione,16,17-acetal with acetone; medrysone, 11β-hydroxy,6α-methylprogesterone.

The use of corticosteroids for days or a few weeks does not lead to adrenal insufficiency upon cessation of treatment, but prolonged therapy with corticosteroids may result in suppression of pituitary-adrenal function that can be slow in returning to normal. Graber and coworkers (1965) found that the processes of recovery of normal pituitary and adrenal function required 9 months in some patients. During this recovery period and for an additional 1 to 2 years, the patient may need to be protected during stressful situations, such as surgery or severe infections, by the administration of corticosteroids. Dixon and Christy (1980) have discussed the complex clinical problems that can be provoked by withdrawal from steroid therapy.

In addition to pituitary-adrenal suppression, the principal complications resulting from prolonged therapy with corticosteroids are fluid and electrolyte disturbances; hyperglycemia and glycosuria; increased susceptibility to infections, including tuberculosis; peptic ulcers, which may bleed or perforate; osteoporosis; a characteristic myopathy; behavioral disturbances; posterior subcapsular cataracts; arrest of growth; and Cushing's habitus, consisting in "moon face," "buffalo hump," enlargement of supraclavicular fat pads, "central obesity," striae, ecchymoses, acne, and hirsutism.

Hypokalemic alkalosis and *edema* are infrequently encountered in patients who are treated with synthetic corticosteroid congeners and almost never in patients taking the 16-substituted compounds. *Glycosuria* can usually be managed with diet and/ or insulin, and its occurrence should not be an important factor in the decision to continue corticosteroid therapy or to initiate it in diabetic patients.

Increased susceptibility to infection in patients treated with corticosteroids is not specific for any particular bacterial or fungal pathogen. If infection develops in a patient treated with corticosteroids, the dose may be maintained or increased and the best available treatment for the infection vigorously administered. Corticosteroid therapy may be initiated in patients having known infections of some consequence if effective, specific chemotherapy can be administered concomitantly with the hormones. However, in these circumstances the physician should be confident that the corticosteroid is needed, that the pathogen has been identified, and that chemotherapy will be effective.

Peptic ulceration is an occasional complication of corticosteroid therapy. The high incidence of hemorrhage and perforation in these ulcers and the insidious nature of their development make them severe therapeutic problems. However, there has been disagreement about the incidence of these ulcers, and some studies have concluded that evidence does not support an association between peptic ulcers and treatment with glucocorticoids (Conn and Blitzer, 1976). It is also not known whether there is an interaction between glucocorticoids and nonsteroidal anti-inflammatory drugs, such as aspirin, which, by themselves, can cause ulcers. In a recent survey of the literature, Messer and associates (1983) concluded that steroid therapy approximately doubles the risk of ulcer (see also Spiro, 1983).

Myopathy, characterized by weakness of the proximal musculature of arms and legs and of their associated shoulder and pelvic muscles, is occasionally seen in patients taking large doses of corticosteroids. It may occur soon after treatment is begun and be sufficiently severe to prevent ambulation. It is not specific for synthetic corticosteroid congeners, for it is found in endogenous Cushing's syndrome. It is a serious complication and an indication for withdrawal of therapy. Recovery may be slow and incomplete (see Mandel, 1982).

Behavioral disturbances may take various forms, for example, nervousness, insomnia, changes in mood or psyche, and psychopathies of the manic-depressive or schizophrenic type. Suicidal tendencies are not uncommon. It is no longer believed that previous psychiatric problems predispose to behavioral disturbances during therapy with glucocorticoids. Conversely, the absence of a history of psychiatric illness is no guarantee against the occurrence of psychosis during hormonal therapy.

Posterior subcapsular cataracts have been reported in children receiving corticosteroid therapy. Many patients with rheumatoid arthritis who receive 20 mg of prednisone per day for 4 years develop cataracts (Levine and Leopold, 1973); it is possible that patients with this disease are particularly susceptible to this complication. The problem of corticosteroid-induced cataracts has been reviewed by Lubkin (1977).

Osteoporosis and *vertebral compression fractures* are frequent serious complications of corticosteroid therapy in patients of all ages. Ribs and vertebrae, bones with a high degree of trabecular structure, are generally the most severely affected. Gluco-

corticoids appear to inhibit the activities of osteoblasts directly, and, because of their inhibition of calcium absorption by the intestine, glucocorticoids cause an increased secretion of parathyroid hormone (PTH). PTH stimulates the activity of osteoclasts (Hahn, 1978); thus, there is both decreased formation and increased resorption of bone. As noted above, corticosteroids also increase calcium excretion by the kidney. Osteoporosis is an indication for withdrawal of therapy and should be looked for regularly in radiographs of the spine in patients taking glucocorticoids for longer than a few months. Unfortunately, significant loss of bone must occur before it is apparent from radiography. The possibility of development of osteoporosis should be an important consideration in initiating and managing corticosteroid therapy, especially in postmenopausal women (see Baylink, 1983).

Inhibition or arrest of growth can result from the administration of relatively small doses of glucocorticoids to children. This cannot be overcome with exogenous human growth hormone (Morris et al., 1968). The widespread inhibitory effect of the glucocorticoids on DNA synthesis and cell division discussed above is apparently responsible. Inhibition of growth by glucocorticoids has been reviewed by Loeb (1976).

THERAPEUTIC USES

With the exception of substitution therapy in deficiency states, the use of corticosteroids and their congeners in disease is largely empirical. From the experience accumulated since the introduction of glucocorticoids for clinical use, at least six therapeutic principles may be abstracted, as follows: (1) for any disease, in any patient, the appropriate dose to achieve a given therapeutic effect must be determined by trial and error and must be reevaluated from time to time as the stage and the activity of the disease alter; (2) a *single* dose of corticosteroid, even a large one, is virtually without harmful effects; (3) a few days of corticosteroid therapy, in the absence of specific contraindications, is unlikely to produce harmful results except at the most extreme dosages; (4) as corticosteroid therapy is prolonged over periods of weeks or months, and to the extent that the dose exceeds the equivalent of substitution therapy, the incidence of disabling and potentially lethal effects increases; (5) except in adrenal insufficiency, the administration of corticosteroids is neither etiological nor curative therapy but only palliative by virtue of the anti-inflammatory effects; and (6) abrupt cessation of prolonged, high-dosage corticosteroid therapy is associated with a significant risk of adrenal insufficiency of sufficient severity to be threatening to life.

Translated into the terms of clinical practice, these general principles are equivalent to the following rules. When corticosteroids are to be administered over long periods, the dose must be the smallest one that will achieve a desired effect. This dose must be found by trial and error. Where the goal of therapy is relief of painful or distressing symptoms not associated with an immediately life-threatening disease, for example, rheumatoid arthritis, the initial dose should be small and gradually increased until pain or distress has been reduced to tolerable levels. Complete relief is not sought. At frequent intervals the dose should be gradually reduced until the development of more severe symptoms signals that the minimal acceptable dose has been found. When therapy is directed at an immediately life-threatening state, for example, pemphigus, the initial dose should be a large one, estimated to achieve, almost with certainty, control of the crisis. If some benefit is not observed in a short time, the dose should be doubled or tripled. When potentially lethal disease is controlled by large amounts of corticosteroid, reduction of the dose should be carried out under conditions that permit frequent, accurate observations of the patient. Under these circumstances it is essential to assess constantly the relative dangers of therapy and of the disease being treated.

The apparently innocuous character of a single administration of corticosteroid in amounts within the conventional therapeutic range justifies its use without a definite diagnosis for crises in which there exists some probability that life is threatened by primary adrenal or pituitary insufficiency. If one of these conditions is present, a single intravenous injection of a soluble corticosteroid may prevent immediate death and allow time for diagnostic procedures.

Short courses of systemic corticosteroids in large doses may properly be given for diseases that do not threaten life, in the absence of specific contraindications. The general rule is that long courses of therapy at high dosage should be reserved for life-threatening disease. On occasion, and for definite cause, when the patient is threatened with permanent disability, this rule is justifiably violated.

It is not possible to define the precise dose of glucocorticoids that will produce pituitary and adrenocortical suppression in a given patient, since there is considerable variation. In general, the higher the dose and the more prolonged the therapy, the greater is the likelihood of suppression.

Harter and associates (1963) suggested that some dissociation of therapeutic effects from certain undesirable metabolic effects can be achieved by the administration of a single large dose of corticosteroid every other day, in contrast to the usual daily multiple-dose schedule. A single dose every other day or at even longer intervals is acceptable therapy for some, but not all, patients with a variety of diseases modified by corticosteroid therapy. When this therapeutic regimen is possible, the degree of suppression of the pituitary and adrenal cortex can be minimized. Steroids that are long acting are not suitable for use by this dosage schedule.

Substitution Therapy. Insufficiency of secretion of the adrenal cortex results from structural or functional lesions of the adrenal cortex itself or from structural or functional lesions of the anterior pituitary. In either case, the patient may present with acute, catastrophic adrenal insufficiency (adrenal crisis) or chronic adrenal insufficiency. When the adrenal itself is the site of the lesion, all elements of normal adrenal secretion may be reduced or absent or the deficiency may be selective for one or more components of secretion.

Acute Adrenal Insufficiency. This disease is characterized by gastrointestinal symptoms, dehydration, weakness, lethargy, and hypotension. It is usually associated with disorders of the adrenal, rather than the pituitary, although exceptions occur. It frequently follows abrupt withdrawal of high doses of corticosteroids.

The immediate needs of such patients are water, sodium, chloride, glucose, cortisol, and appropriate therapy for precipitating causes, for example, infection, trauma, or hemorrhage. Inasmuch as these patients have a diminished capacity for a water diuresis and have often undergone some degree of cellular hydration, they are susceptible to water intoxication. The principal intravenous fluid should be isotonic sodium chloride solution. Glucose is required for nutrition and to prevent or treat hypoglycemia, but it should be given intravenously in isotonic sodium chloride solution. The total amount of intravenous fluid administered during the first 24 hours should not, in most instances, exceed 5% of ideal body weight. The patient should be monitored for evidence of rising venous pressure and pulmonary edema, because the functional capacity of the cardiovascular system is reduced by adrenocortical insufficiency. Cortisol (hydrocortisone) sodium succinate or cortisol sodium phosphate must be given in the intravenous fluids at a rate of 100 mg every 8 hours, following an initial intravenous injection of 100 mg. This provides a quantity of cortisol that is equal to the maximal daily rate of secretion in response to stress. In the period of transition from intravenous fluid therapy to normal diet and activity, intramuscular cortisol sodium succinate or sodium phosphate may be used in a dose of 25 mg every 6 or 8 hours.

For the treatment of suspected but unconfirmed acute adrenal insufficiency, 4 mg of dexamethasone sodium phosphate should be substituted for cortisol. In addition, ACTH (5 units per hour) should be given. Concentrations of cortisol and aldosterone in plasma and 17-hydroxycorticosteroids in urine are determined at the outset and at intervals during the course of treatment. A failure to obtain a response to ACTH (stimulation of steroid secretion) is diagnostic of adrenal insufficiency. A lack of response in terms of aldosterone indicates failure of the zona glomerulosa.

Chronic Adrenal Insufficiency. This disease results from adrenal surgery or destructive lesions of the adrenal cortex. It requires the administration of cortisol, 20 to 30 mg per day in divided doses. A common dose schedule is 20 mg on arising and 10 mg in the late afternoon. The circadian pattern of ACTH concentrations should be measured. If it rises above normal, multiple doses of cortisol may be required. Most patients will also require a potent mineralocorticoid. The most convenient drug to use for this purpose is fludrocortisone acetate. The usual adult dose is 0.1 to 0.2 mg daily. Some patients do not need a mineralocorticoid and are adequately treated with cortisone and generous dietary salt. Therapy is guided by the patient's sense of well-being, alertness, appetite, weight, muscular strength, pigmentation, blood pressure, and freedom from orthostatic hypotension.

Congenital Adrenal Hyperplasia. This is a familial disorder in which activity of one of several enzymes required for biosynthesis of corticosteroids is deficient. With diminished or absent production of cortisol, aldosterone, or both, and consequent lack of inhibitory feedback, the adrenal cortex is stimulated to the overproduction of other hormonally active steroids. The clinical presentation, laboratory findings, and treatment depend on which of the six enzyme deficiencies thus far de-

scribed is responsible. Only the syndrome of 21-hydroxylase deficiency will be described here.

In about 90% of the patients with congenital adrenal hyperplasia there is a deficiency of 21-hydroxylase activity. When the deficiency is only partial, the usual case, cortisol is secreted at normal rates as a result of continuous hypersecretion of ACTH, with consequent overproduction of adrenal androgens and their precursors. Aldosterone secretion is approximately normal. Female children undergo virilization, female "pseudohermaphroditism," and male children show precocious development of secondary sex characteristics, "macrogenitosomia." Linear growth is accelerated in childhood, but the height at maturity is reduced by premature closure of the epiphyses.

In about 30% of patients with 21-hydroxylase deficiency, the enzymatic defect is sufficiently severe to compromise increased aldosterone secretion in response to a hypovolemic stimulus. Such patients are unable to conserve sodium normally, in addition to manifesting androgenic effects (Bongiovanni et al., 1967).

All patients with congenital adrenal hyperplasia resulting from a 21-hydroxylase deficiency require substitution therapy with cortisol or a suitable congener, and those with a salt-losing tendency require, in addition, a sodium-retaining steroid. The usual oral dose of cortisol is about 0.6 mg/kg daily in four divided doses, the last one being given as late as possible in order to maintain pituitary suppression overnight. When parenteral substitution therapy is necessary, cortisone acetate may be given intramuscularly every other day. The mineralocorticoid usually given is fludrocortisone acetate, 0.05 to 0.2 mg per day. Therapy is guided by gain in weight and height, by excretion of urinary 17-ketosteroids, and by blood pressure. Sudden spurts of linear growth may indicate inadequate pituitary suppression and excessive androgen secretion, whereas growth failure suggests overtreatment.

A number of rare forms of congenital adrenal hyperplasia are known in which enzyme deficiencies of the adrenal cortex, with similar defects of the gonads, result in clinical and laboratory findings very different from those described above for 21-hydroxylase deficiency. The types described thus far are: "desmolase" deficiency (Camacho et al., 1968), 3β-hydroxysteroid dehydrogenase deficiency (Bongiovanni et al., 1967), 17α-hydroxylase deficiency (Goldsmith et al., 1968), 11β-hydroxylase deficiency (Bongiovanni et al., 1967), and 18-hydroxylase deficiency (David et al., 1968). The clinical and laboratory findings and the treatment in these rare forms are quite different from those in 21-hydroxylase deficiency. The publications cited should be consulted for details.

Adrenal Insufficiency Secondary to Anterior Pituitary Insufficiency. This condition is not usually associated with the dramatic signs and symptoms characteristic of adrenal insufficiency resulting from disease of the adrenal cortex unless there are complicating circumstances, for example, unusual fluid losses, trauma, or starvation. Hypoglycemia is the most frequent cause of symptoms. Quantitation of the electrolytes in plasma often reveals a dilutional hyponatremia. The administration of 20 mg of cortisol on arising and 10 mg in late afternoon is adequate replacement therapy for most patients with anterior pituitary insufficiency. This schedule mimics, to some extent, the normal diurnal cycle of adrenal secretion. Occasional patients require additional doses. When initiating treatment, it is customary to begin cortisol first and to add thyroid replacement therapy after adrenal insufficiency is under some degree of control, on the grounds that the administration of thyroid to a hypopituitary patient may precipitate acute adrenal insufficiency. Additional treatment is necessary during periods of stress. Cortisol, 300 to 400 mg per day, should be given to approximate the normal response to severe stress.

Therapeutic Uses in Nonendocrine Diseases.
Brief outlines of important uses of corticosteroids in diseases other than those involving the pituitary-adrenal complex are set forth below. The disorders discussed are not inclusive, but rather a representative list of the more common diseases for which the glucocorticoids are used.

The dosage of glucocorticoids varies greatly with the condition being treated. In the following discussion approximate doses of a representative corticosteroid congener, usually prednisone, are suggested. It is not meant to imply that prednisone has peculiar merit in general or for any particular disease over the other congeners. For comparison of doses of glucocorticoids, *see* Table 63–3.

Arthritis. In *rheumatoid arthritis,* the criterion for initiating corticosteroid therapy is progressive disease with consequent disability, despite intensive treatment with rest, physical therapy, aspirin-like drugs, gold, and other agents. The decision to embark upon a program of hormone therapy must be made with due consideration for the fact that corticosteroid therapy, once started, may have to be continued for many years or for life, with the attendant risks of serious complications. The initial dose should be small and increased slowly until the desired degree of control is attained. The symptomatic effect of small reductions should be frequently tested in order to maintain the dose as low as possible. Complete relief is not sought. A regimen of rest, physical therapy, and aspirin-like drugs is continued. The usual initial dose is about 10 mg of prednisone (or equivalent) per day in divided doses. Optimal therapy for some patients with painful symptoms confined to one or a few joints may be intra-articular injection of the steroid into the affected joints. Typical doses are 5 to 20 mg of triamcinolone acetonide or the equivalent, depending upon the size of the joint cavity.

In *osteoarthritis,* intra-articular injection of corticosteroids is recommended for treatment of episodic manifestations of acute inflammation: local heat, swelling, and pain. Injections for this purpose should be infrequent because, in both rheumatoid arthritis and osteoarthritis, a significant incidence of painless destruction of the joint, reminiscent of Charcot's arthropathy, may be associated with repeated intra-articular injections of corticosteroids.

Rheumatic Carditis. Corticosteroids are reserved for patients failing to respond to salicylates and as initial therapy for patients severely ill with fever, acute congestive heart failure, arrhythmia, and pericarditis; acute manifestations are more rapidly suppressed by corticosteroids than by salicylates, a possibly lifesaving difference in a moribund patient. A dose of approximately 40 mg of prednisone or equivalent is usually given daily, in divided amounts, although much larger doses may on occasion be required. Reactivation of the disease occurs in a number of instances following withdrawal of steroid therapy. For this reason it has been suggested that salicylates be given concurrently with corticosteroids and be continued through and after the period of withdrawal of hormone therapy.

Renal Diseases. Corticosteroids do not modify the course of acute or chronic glomerulonephritis. However, patients with some forms of the *nephrotic syndrome* attributable to systemic lupus erythematosus or to primary renal disease, except renal amyloidosis, may be benefited by corticosteroid therapy. A typical therapeutic regimen consists in the daily administration, in divided doses, of 60 mg of prednisone or equivalent (2 mg/kg of edema-free body weight in children) for 3 or 4 weeks. If a remission with a diuresis and decreased proteinuria occurs during this period, maintenance treatment is continued for as long as a year. For this, the daily dose of prednisone is given only for the first 3 days of each week (Bacon and Spencer, 1973).

Collagen Diseases. The manifestations of most of the diseases in this group are controlled by glucocorticoids. An exception is *scleroderma,* which is generally considered refractory to these agents. It is important to distinguish between scleroderma and *mixed connective tissue disease syndrome,* which is responsive to steroids (Yount *et al.,* 1973). *Polymyositis, polyarteritis nodosa,* and the granulomatous-polyarteritis group (*Wegener's granulomatosis, temporal-cranial arteritis,* and *polymyalgia rheumatica*) are treated with daily doses of prednisone, approximately 1 mg/kg or equivalent, to induce a remission. The dose is then tapered down to the minimally effective level. Glucocorticoids decrease morbidity in all these diseases and prolong the survival times of patients with polyarteritis nodosa and Wegener's granulomatosis. *In temporal (giant-cell) arteritis, adequate steroid therapy is necessary to prevent the blindness that occurs in about 20% of untreated cases.* Fulminating systemic lupus erythematosus is a life-threatening condition, the manifestations of which should be suppressed by adrenocorticosteroid therapy with doses large enough to produce a prompt effect. Treatment usually consists in a 1-mg/kg daily dose of prednisone or equivalent. Within 48 hours, reduction of fever and improvement in the signs and symptoms of arthritis, pleuritis, or pericarditis should be observed. If not, the dose should be increased in 20-mg increments daily until a favorable response occurs. After the acute episode has been brought under control, corticosteroid therapy should be reduced by small steps, for example, 5 mg of prednisone per week, until signs or symptoms warn against further reductions. Salicylate or related drugs are then introduced and may permit a further reduction of corticosteroid dosage (Robinson, 1962). The treatment of systemic lupus erythematosus with a combination of glucocorticoids and antimetabolites, such as azathioprine, or the alkylating agent cyclophosphamide, is still experimental and not recommended for general use (Deker, 1982).

Allergic Diseases. The manifestations of allergic disease that are of limited duration, such as *hay fever, serum sickness, urticaria, contact dermatitis, drug reactions, bee stings,* and *angioneurotic edema,* can, if necessary, be suppressed by adequate doses of glucocorticoids given as a supplement to the primary therapy. It must be emphasized, however, that the effects of the steroids require some time to develop, and *severe reactions such as anaphylaxis and angioneurotic edema of the glottis require immediate therapy with epinephrine, 0.5 to 1.0 ml of a 1:1000 solution (0.5 to 1.0 mg) subcutaneously.* In life-threatening situations steroids may be given intravenously; dexamethasone sodium phosphate (8 to 12 mg or equivalent) is appropriate. In less severe diseases, such as serum sickness or hay fever, antihistaminic compounds are the drugs of first choice.

Bronchial Asthma. The corticosteroids should *not* be used routinely in the treatment of any asthmatic condition, acute or chronic, that can promptly be brought under moderate control with other measures. In *status asthmaticus,* cortisol sodium succinate (50 to 100 mg) is administered by intravenous infusion over 8 hours. The procedure is repeated daily until the acute attack is under control, following which the patient is given 10 mg of prednisone twice daily for 4 or 5 days. The dose is then reduced in steps and withdrawal planned for about the tenth day after initiation of the prednisone therapy. Under favorable circumstances, the patient can subsequently be managed once again with his prior medication.

In the treatment of *severe chronic bronchial asthma,* or *chronic obstructive pulmonary disease,* uncontrolled by other measures, the administration of a corticosteroid may be considered. The decision must be made with great care since the majority of patients, once started on corticosteroid therapy, remain indefinitely on such therapy. While some patients are effectively managed with inhalation of beclomethasone dipropionate, oral administration of prednisone in daily doses of 5 to 10 mg is required more frequently. Patients who have been taking a glucocorticoid orally must continue this medication in slowly decreasing dosage when inhalation therapy with beclomethasone is begun. Asymptomatic oropharyngeal candidiasis develops in a high percentage of patients using beclomethasone (Webb-Johnson and Andrews, 1977).

Ocular Diseases. Corticosteroids are frequently used to suppress inflammation in the eye, and employed properly they are often responsible for preservation of sight. Levine and Leopold (1973) list 28 disorders of the eye that respond to corticosteroids. They are administered locally for disease of the outer eye and anterior segment. Both natural and synthetic corticosteroids attain therapeutic concentrations in the aqueous humor following instillation into the conjunctival cul-de-sac. For disease of the posterior segment, systemic administration is required.

A typical prescription is 0.1% dexamethasone phosphate solution (ophthalmic), 2 drops in the conjunctival sac every 4 hours while awake, and 0.05% dexamethasone phosphate ointment (ophthalmic) at bedtime. For inflammations of the posterior segment of the eye, usual daily doses are approximately 30 mg of prednisone or equivalent, administered orally in divided doses.

It has been convincingly demonstrated that topical corticosteroid therapy *frequently induces intraocular hypertension* in normal eyes and further increases pressure in eyes with initially elevated pressure. The glaucoma has not always been reversible on cessation of corticosteroid treatment. It has been recommended that intraocular pressure be monitored when corticosteroids are applied to the eye for more than 2 weeks.

The local administration of corticosteroids to patients with bacterial, viral, or fungal conjunctivitis *may mask evidences of progression of the infection until sight is lost.* Corticosteroids are *contraindicated in herpes simplex* (dendritic keratitis) of the eye, because progression of the disease and irreversible clouding of the cornea may occur. Topical steroids should not be used in the treatment of mechanical lacerations and abrasions of the eye. They delay healing and promote the development and spread of infection.

Skin Diseases. The development of corticosteroid preparations suitable for topical administration has revolutionized the therapy of the more common varieties of skin disease. Maibach and Stoughton (1973) have divided 20 dermatological disorders that respond to topical corticosteroids into those that are very responsive and those that require higher concentrations of steroids, occlusion of the drug under a plastic film, or intralesional administration. Attention must be paid to the concentration of steroid used, and there are a large number of preparations of various concentrations available for topical use (Table 63–4). A typical prescription for an eczematous eruption is 1% cortisol ointment applied locally twice daily. Effectiveness is enhanced by application of the cream or ointment under a transparent plastic wrapping. Unfortunately, systemic absorption is also enhanced, occasionally sufficiently to suppress the pituitary-adrenal axis or to produce Cushing's syndrome. Adrenocorticosteroids are administered systemically for severe episodes of acute skin disorders and exacerbations of chronic disorders. The dose is usually 40 mg per day of prednisone or equivalent. Systemically administered corticosteroids may be lifesaving in *pemphigus.* Up to 120 mg of prednisone or equivalent per day may be required to control the disease.

Diseases of the Intestinal Tract. Patients severely ill with untreated *celiac sprue* can often benefit from a course of glucocorticoid therapy given at the same time that management with a gluten-free diet is begun. Prednisolone, 30 mg per day or equivalent, is continued for 3 to 4 weeks. Patients who fail to respond to a gluten-free diet are helped by lower doses of prednisolone (7 to 12 mg per day or equivalent) for an indefinite period (Wall, 1973).

Corticosteroid therapy is indicated in selected patients with *chronic ulcerative colitis.* Mildly ill patients with bowel symptoms but without disabling systemic symptoms usually can and should be managed with rest, diet, sedation, anticholinergic agents, and chemotherapy. However, patients who do not improve should have a trial of methylprednisolone acetate, 40 mg or equivalent, in a nightly retention enema, in an attempt to induce remission. Alternate-day therapy may be effective. Severely ill patients with fever, anorexia, anemia, and malnutrition often improve dramatically when given systemic corticosteroid therapy. Large doses, 60 to 120 mg per day of prednisone, or the equivalent, are recommended. Major complications of ulcerative colitis may occur despite corticosteroid therapy. Signs and symptoms of intestinal perforation and peritonitis may be difficult to detect during corticosteroid treatment (ReMine and McIlrath, 1980).

Cerebral Edema. Corticosteroids are of value in the reduction or prevention of cerebral edema associated with neoplasms, especially those that are metastatic. In spite of widespread use of glucocorticoids for treatment of the cerebral edema due to trauma or cerebrovascular accidents, there is no convincing evidence of their value in these conditions (Nelson and Dick, 1975).

Malignancies. The chemotherapy of *acute lymphocytic leukemia* and *lymphomas* has been greatly improved by the introduction of therapy with multiple agents, and glucocorticoids are used because of their antilymphocytic effects. At the present time these diseases are treated in a complex fashion with rigidly scheduled sequences of combined drug therapy. Prednisone is commonly used in conjunction with an alkylating agent such as cyclophosphamide, an antimetabolite, and a vinca alkaloid (*see* Chapter 55).

Objective tumor regression in *carcinoma of the breast* can be induced by glucocorticoids in about 15% of patients; prednisolone (30 mg per day) has been the usual treatment. The presumed mechanism by which the corticosteroids act in these patients is through adrenocortical suppression, with an accompanying decrease in production of androgens, which are precursors of tumor-stimulating estrogens (Brennan, 1973). A beneficial response should be expected only when the tumor has estrogen and/or progesterone receptors. Other forms of therapy are usually more effective.

Diseases of the Liver. The use of glucocorticoids in the treatment of hepatic diseases has been the subject of controversy. Careful studies have now indicated several diseases of the liver in which therapy with steroids significantly improves survival rates; these are *subacute hepatic necrosis* and *chronic active hepatitis, alcoholic hepatitis,* and *nonalcoholic cirrhosis in females* (Lesesne and Fallon, 1973; Copenhagen Study Group for Liver Diseases, 1974). Only certain patients with chronic active hepatitis should receive steroid therapy. Those who benefit have symptomatic disease, histological evidence of severe disease, and a negative reaction for hepatitis B surface antigen (Berk *et al.,* 1976). Treatment of *subacute hepatic necrosis* and *chronic active hepatitis* includes prednisolone, 60 to 100 mg per day; the dose is tapered as the disease improves. Treatment of *alcoholic hepatitis* with corticosteroids is reserved for patients who are severely ill, with evidence of hepatic encephalopathy. Prednisone (40 mg per day) is given for 1 month, followed by withdrawal over a period of 2 to 4 weeks. *Nonalcoholic cirrhosis in women* should be treated with glucocorticoids if the patient does not have ascites. Daily dosages average 15 to 20 mg of prednisone or equivalent when they are adjusted to the needs of the individual patients. The data indicate that *steroid treatment lowers survival rates when ascites is present.* Treatment of cirrhotic male patients with steroids has not been shown to be beneficial.

Shock. While corticosteroids are often administered to patients in shock, there is no convincing evidence to indicate that such therapy is efficacious.

Miscellaneous Diseases. *Sarcoidosis* is treated with prednisone, approximately 1 mg/kg per day or equivalent, to induce a remission. Maintenance doses, which are often required for long periods of time, may be 10 mg of prednisone per day or less. In this, as in other diseases treated by prolonged steroid therapy, patients with positive tuberculin reactions or other evidence of tuberculosis should receive prophylactic antituberculosis therapy. In *thrombocytopenia,* prednisone, 0.5 mg/kg or equivalent, is used to decrease the bleeding tendency. In severe cases and for initiation of treatment of *idiopathic thrombocytopenia,* daily doses of prednisone, 1 to 1.5 mg/kg, are employed. *Hemolytic anemias* with a positive Coombs' test are treated with prednisone, 1 mg/kg per day or equivalent. If hemolysis is severe, therapy is initiated with 100 mg of cortisol intravenously; as the disease improves, the dose is decreased. Small maintenance doses may be needed for several months if a positive response is obtained. In *organ transplantation,* high doses of prednisone (50 to 100 mg) are given at the time of the transplant surgery, usually in conjunction with immunosuppressive agents. Smaller maintenance doses (10 to 20 mg per day) are continued indefinitely, and the dosage is increased if rejection is threatened. In *aspiration of gastric contents,* prednisone (50 to 100 mg) is given for 2 to 3 days to suppress the inflammatory reaction in the lung and to prevent development of pulmonary abscess. However, corticosteroids are probably effective only if they are administered within several hours of the aspiration.

DIAGNOSTIC APPLICATIONS OF ADRENOCORTICAL STEROIDS

Potent synthetic congeners of cortisol reduce urinary excretion of cortisol metabolites by inhibition of pituitary ACTH release. The dose required is so small, in gravimetric terms, that it contributes only negligibly to the urinary steroids. Liddle (1960) reported that the administration of 0.5 mg of dexamethasone every 6 hours for a total of eight doses results in a marked suppression of excretion of cortisol metabolites in normal persons, but does not suppress urinary steroids in individuals with Cushing's syndrome. This test is useful in distinguishing persons with some nonspecific elevation of steroid excretion, for example, that due to obesity or stress, from patients with Cushing's syndrome. The administration of 2 mg of dexamethasone every 6 hours for a total of eight doses usually causes a suppression of cortisol secretion in patients with pituitary-dependent hypercorticism, but ordinarily has little if any effect on the urinary steroids of patients with adrenal neoplasms or ACTH-producing tumors (Meador *et al.*, 1962). However, "suppressible" tumors have been reported. The results of these tests are likely to be most definite if the urinary steroids are measured daily for 2 days before and for at least 2 days during administration of the suppressing agent. Variations of this procedure (shorter test period and measurement of plasma cortisol rather than urinary metabolites) have been described (Sawin *et al.*, 1968).

INHIBITORS OF THE BIOSYNTHESIS OF ADRENOCORTICAL STEROIDS

Three pharmacological agents have proven most useful as inhibitors of adrenocortical secretion. *Mitotane (o,p'-*DDD), an adrenocorticolytic agent, is discussed in Chapter 55. *Metyrapone* and *aminoglutethimide* are discussed here. The subject has been reviewed by Temple and Liddle (1970).

Metyrapone. Metyrapone reduces cortisol production by inhibition of the 11β-hydroxylation reaction. Metyrapone also inhibits side chain cleavage to some degree (Cheng *et al.*, 1974), but this block is largely overcome when ACTH stimulates the gland. The biosynthetic process is terminated at 11-desoxycortisol (Figure 63–3), a compound that has practically no inhibitory influence on the secretion of ACTH. In the normal person, a compensatory increase in ACTH secretion follows, and the secretion of 11-desoxycortisol, a "17-hydroxycorticoid," is markedly accelerated. Consequently, in normal persons, administration of metyrapone induces increased plasma ACTH and renal excretion of "17-hydroxycorticoids."

Metyrapone is used to test the capacity of the pituitary to respond to a decreased concentration of plasma cortisol. A response that is greater than normal is usually found in patients with Cushing's syndrome of pituitary origin. In most cases of Cushing's syndrome due to ectopic production of ACTH there is no response to the drug. Adminis-

tration of metyrapone to patients with disease of the hypothalamico-pituitary complex who are unable to achieve a compensatory increase in the rate of secretion of ACTH is, of course, not followed by increased renal excretion of 17-hydroxycorticoids.

The ability of the adrenal to respond to ACTH should be demonstrated before metyrapone is employed, for two reasons: (1) administration of metyrapone can be used as a test for normal hypothalamico-pituitary function only if the adrenal glands are capable of responding to ACTH, and (2) the drug may induce acute adrenal insufficiency in patients with reduced adrenal secretory capacity. Metyrapone also inhibits synthesis of aldosterone, which, like cortisol, is an 11β-hydroxylated compound. However, metyrapone does not typically cause a deficiency of mineralocorticoids, with a consequent loss of sodium and retention of potassium, because the inhibition of the 11β-hydroxylation reaction results in an increased production of 11-desoxycorticosterone, a mineralocorticoid.

Metyrapone has been used successfully to treat the hypercortisolism that results from adrenal neoplasms that function autonomously and from ectopic ACTH production by tumors. Its use in treatment of Cushing's syndrome resulting from hypersecretion of ACTH by the pituitary is controversial (Orth, 1978; Gold, 1979). Metyrapone has been used experimentally in patients with Cushing's syndrome during the period of time required for radiation treatment to become effective (Orth, 1978). Long-term treatment with metyrapone can cause hypertension as the result of excessive secretion of desoxycorticosterone.

Metyrapone (METOPIRONE) is 2-methyl-1,2-di-3-pyridyl-1-propanone. The drug is marketed as 250-mg oral tablets. Following two 24-hour control periods, the drug is given orally in the dose of 750 mg every 4 hours for six doses. Maximal urinary excretion of 11-desoxycorticosteroids is observed on the next day.

Aminoglutethimide. This compound, α-ethyl-*p*-aminophenyl-glutarimide, inhibits the conversion of cholesterol to 20α-hydroxycholesterol. This inhibition of the first reaction of steroidogenesis from cholesterol interrupts production of both cortisol and aldosterone.

Aminoglutethimide has been used successfully to decrease the hypersecretion of cortisol in autonomously functioning adrenal tumors and in hypersecretion resulting from ectopic production of ACTH. It has also been used in combination with metyrapone in the treatment of Cushing's syndrome that results from hypersecretion of ACTH by the pituitary (*see* Gold, 1979). Substitution of physiological doses of cortisol may be required to prevent adrenal insufficiency.

Aminoglutethimide (CYTADREN) is marketed as 250-mg oral tablets. The suggested dosage is 250 mg every 6 hours. The dose is increased by 250 mg per day at 1- or 2-week intervals until side effects prohibit further increments or until a daily dose of 2 g is achieved.

Adam, P. A. J., and Haynes, R. C., Jr. Control of hepatic mitochondrial CO_2 fixation by glucagon, epinephrine, and cortisol. *J. Biol. Chem.*, **1969**, *244*, 6444–6450.

Addison, T. *On the Constitutional and Local Effects of Disease of the Suprarenal Capsules.* Samuel Highley, London, **1855**.

Ahmed, A. B. J.; George, B. C.; Gonzalez-Auvert, C.; and Dingman, J. F. Increased plasma arginine vasopressin in clinical adrenocortical insufficiency and its inhibition by glucosteroids. *J. Clin. Invest.*, **1967**, *46*, 111–123.

Amatruda, T. T., Jr.; Hollingsworth, D. R.; D'Esopo, N. D.; Upton, G. V.; and Bondy, P. K. A study of the mechanism of the steroid withdrawal syndrome. *J. Clin. Endocrinol. Metab.*, **1960**, *20*, 339–354.

Astwood, E. B.; Raben, M. S.; and Payne, R. W. Chemistry of corticotrophin. *Recent Prog. Horm. Res.*, **1952**, *7*, 1–57.

Bacon, G. E., and Spencer, M. L. Pediatric uses of steroids. *Med. Clin. North Am.*, **1973**, *57*, 1265–1276.

Ballard, P. L.; Baxter, J. D.; Higgins, S. J.; Rousseau, G. C.; and Tomkins, G. M. General presence of glucocorticoid receptors in mammalian tissues. *Endocrinology*, **1974**, *94*, 998–1002.

Balow, J. E., and Rosenthal, A. S. Glucocorticoid suppression of macrophage migration inhibitory factor. *J. Exp. Med.*, **1973**, *137*, 1031–1039.

Bangham, D. R.; Mussett, M. V.; and Stack-Dunne, M. P. The third international standard for corticotrophin. *Bull. WHO*, **1962**, *27*, 395–408.

Beckett, G. J., and Boyd, G. S. Evidence for the activation of bovine cholesterol ester hydrolase by a phosphorylation involving an adenosine $3':5'$-monophosphate-dependent protein kinase. *Biochem. Soc. Trans.*, **1975**, *3*, 892–894.

Bell, J. J., and Harding, B. W. The acute action of adrenocorticotropic hormone on adrenal steroidogenesis. *Biochim. Biophys. Acta*, **1974**, *348*, 285–298.

Bell, P. H.; Howard, K. S.; Shepherd, R. G.; Finn, B. M.; and Meisenhelder, J. H. Studies with corticotropin. II. Pepsin degradation of β-corticotropin. *J. Am. Chem. Soc.*, **1956**, *78*, 5059–5066.

Berk, P. D.; Jones, E. A.; Plotz, P. H.; Seeff, L. B.; and Wright, E. C. Corticosteroid therapy for chronic active hepatitis. *Ann. Intern. Med.*, **1976**, *85*, 523–525.

Biglieri, E. G. Aldosterone and the renin-angiotensin system. In, *The Year in Endocrinology: 1977.* (Ingbar, S. H., ed.) Plenum Medical Book Co., New York, **1978**, pp. 191–204.

Birnbaum, R. S., and Goodman, H. M. Effects of hypophysectomy on cyclic AMP accumulation and action in adipose tissue. *Fed. Proc.*, **1973**, *32*, 535.

Bishop, C. R.; Athens, J. W.; Boggs, D. R.; Warner, H. R.; Cartwright, G. E.; and Wintrobe, M. M. Leukokinetic studies. XIII. A non-steady-state kinetic evaluation of the mechanism of cortisone-induced granulocytosis. *J. Clin. Invest.*, **1968**, *47*, 249–260.

Blackwell, G. J.; Carnuccio, R.; DiRosa, M.; Flower, R. J.; Parente, L.; and Persico, P. Macrocortin: a polypeptide causing the anti-phospholipase effect of glucocorticoids. *Nature*, **1980**, *287*, 147–149.

Bloom, B. R., and Bennett, B. Mechanism of a reaction *in vitro* associated with delayed hypersensitivity. *Science*, **1966**, *153*, 80–82.

Brennan, M. J. Corticosteroids in the treatment of solid tumors. *Med. Clin. North Am.*, **1973**, *57*, 1225–1239.

Britton, S. W., and Silvette, H. Some effects of corticoadrenal extract and other substances on adrenalectomized animals. *Am. J. Physiol.*, **1931**, *99*, 15–32.

Brown-Séquard, C. E. Recherches expérimentales sur la physiologie et la pathologie des capsules surrenales. *C. R. Acad. Sci.* [*D*] (*Paris*), **1856**, *43*, 422–425.

Brunner, H. R.; Chang, P.; Wallace, R.; Sealey, J. E.; and

Laragh, J. H. Angiotensin II vascular receptors. *J. Clin. Invest.*, **1972**, *51*, 58–67.

Butler, W. T. Corticosteroids and immunoglobulin synthesis. *Transplant. Proc.*, **1975**, *7*, 49–53.

Byyny, R. L. Withdrawal from glucocorticoid therapy. *N. Engl. J. Med.*, **1976**, *295*, 30–32.

Camacho, A. M.; Kowarski, A.; Migeon, C. J.; and Brough, A. J. Congenital adrenal hyperplasia due to a deficiency of one of the enzymes involved in the biosynthesis of pregnenolone. *J. Clin. Endocrinol. Metab.*, **1968**, *28*, 153–161.

Cheng, S. C.; Harding, B. W.; and Carballeira, A. Effects of metyrapone on pregnenolone biosynthesis and on cholesterol–cytochrome P-450 interaction in the adrenal. *Endocrinology*, **1974**, *94*, 1451–1458.

Claman, H. N. Corticosteroids and lymphoid cells. *N. Engl. J. Med.*, **1972**, *287*, 388–397.

———. How corticosteroids work. *J. Allergy Clin. Immunol.*, **1975**, *55*, 145–151.

Conn, H. O., and Blitzer, B. L. Nonassociation of adrenocorticosteroid therapy and peptic ulcer. *N. Engl. J. Med.*, **1976**, *294*, 473–479.

Copenhagen Study Group for Liver Diseases. Sex, ascites, and alcoholism in survival of patients with cirrhosis. Effect of prednisone. *N. Engl. J. Med.*, **1974**, *293*, 271–273.

Cori, C. F., and Cori, G. T. The fate of sugar in the animal body. VII. The carbohydrate metabolism of adrenalectomized rats and mice. *J. Biol. Chem.*, **1927**, *74*, 473–494.

Cushing, H. The basophil adenomas of the pituitary body and their clinical manifestations. *Bull. Johns Hopkins Hosp.*, **1932**, *50*, 137–195.

David, R.; Golon, S.; and Drucker, W. Familial aldosterone deficiency: enzyme defect, diagnosis and clinical course. *Pediatrics*, **1968**, *41*, 403–414.

Deane, H., and Greep, R. O. A morphological and histochemical study of the rat's adrenal cortex after hypophysectomy, with comments on the liver. *Am. J. Anat.*, **1946**, *79*, 117–146.

Deker, J. L. The management of systemic lupus erythematosus. *Arthritis Rheum.*, **1982**, *25*, 891–894.

Deming, Q. B., and Luetscher, J. A., Jr. Bioassay of desoxycorticosterone-like material in urine. *Proc. Soc. Exp. Biol. Med.*, **1950**, *73*, 171–175.

Dixon, R. B., and Christy, N. P. On the various forms of corticosteroid withdrawal syndrome. *Am. J. Med.*, **1980**, *68*, 224–230.

Engel, F. L. Extra-adrenal actions of adrenocorticotropin. *Vitam. Horm.*, **1961**, *19*, 189–227.

Forssman, O., and Mulder, J. Hypersensitivity to different ACTH peptides. *Acta Med. Scand.*, **1973**, *193*, 557–559.

Foster, G. L., and Smith, P. E. Hypophysectomy and replacement therapy in relation to basal metabolism and specific dynamic action in the rat. *J.A.M.A.*, **1926**, *87*, 2151–2153.

Gill, J. R., Jr.; Gann, D. S.; and Bartter, F. C. Restoration of water diuresis in Addisonian patients by expansion of the volume of extracellular fluid. *J. Clin. Invest.*, **1962**, *41*, 1078–1085.

Gillis, S.; Crabtree, G. R.; and Smith, K. A. Glucocorticoid-induced inhibition of T cell growth factor. *J. Immunol.*, **1979**, *123*, 1632–1638.

Goldsmith, O.; Solomon, D. H.; and Horton, E. Hypogonadism and mineralocorticoid excess: the 17-hydroxylase deficiency syndrome. *N. Engl. J. Med.*, **1968**, *277*, 673–677.

Goodman, H. M. Endocrine control of lipolysis. In, *Progress in Endocrinology: Proceedings of the Third International Congress of Endocrinology, Mexico.* (Gual, C., and Ebling, F. J. G., eds.) Excerpta Medica, Amsterdam, **1968**, pp. 115–123.

Govindan, M. V.; Spiess, E.; and Majors, J. Purified glucocorticoid receptor-hormone complex from rat liver cytosol binds specifically to cloned mouse mammary tumor virus long terminal repeats *in vitro*. *Proc. Natl Acad. Sci. U.S.A.*, **1982**, *79*, 5157–5161.

Graber, A. L.; Ney, R. E.; Nicholson, W. E.; Island, D. P.; and Liddle, G. W. Natural history of pituitary-adrenal recovery following long term suppression with corticosteroids. *J. Clin. Endocrinol. Metab.*, **1965**, *25*, 11–16.

Grahame, R. Elasticity of human skin *in vivo*. A study of the physical properties of the skin in rheumatoid arthritis and the effect of corticosteroids. *Ann. Phys. Med.*, **1969**, *10*, 130–136.

Granelli-Piperano, A.; Vassali, J. D.; and Reich, E. Secretion of plasminogen activator by human polymorphonuclear leukocytes. Modulation by glucocorticoids and other effectors. *J. Exp. Med.*, **1977**, *146*, 1693–1706.

Grossman, A.; Perry, L.; Schally, A. V.; Rees, L. H.; Nieuwenhuyzen Kruseman, A. C.; Tomlin, S.; Coy, D. H.; Comaru-Schally, A.-M.; and Besser, G. M. New hypothalamic hormone, corticotropin-releasing factor, specifically stimulates the release of adrenocorticotropic hormone and cortisol in man. *Lancet*, **1982**, *1*, 921–922.

Gwynne, J. T.; Mahaffee, D.; Brewer, H. B.; and Ney, R. L. Adrenal cholesterol uptake from plasma lipoproteins; regulation by corticotropin. *Proc. Natl Acad. Sci. U.S.A.*, **1976**, *73*, 4329–4333.

Harris, G. W. *Neural Control of the Pituitary Gland.* Edward Arnold, London, **1955**.

Harrop, G. A.; Soffer, L. J.; Ellsworth, R.; and Trescher, J. H. Studies on the suprarenal cortex. III. Plasma electrolytes and electrolyte excretion during suprarenal insufficiency in the dog. *J. Exp. Med.*, **1933**, *58*, 17–38.

Harter, J. G.; Reddy, W. J.; and Thorn, G. W. Studies on an intermittent corticosteroid dosage regimen. *N. Engl. J. Med.*, **1963**, *269*, 591–596.

Harvey, W., and Grahame, R. Effect of some adrenal steroid hormones on skin fibroblast replication *in vitro*. *Ann. Rheum. Dis.*, **1973**, *32*, 272.

Haynes, R. C., Jr. The activation of adrenal phosphorylase by the adrenocorticotropic hormone. *J. Biol. Chem.*, **1958**, *233*, 1220–1222.

Haynes, R. C., Jr.; Koritz, S. B.; and Péron, F. G. Influence of adenosine 3',5'-monophosphate on corticoid production by rat adrenal glands. *J. Biol. Chem.*, **1959**, *234*, 1421–1423.

Hench, P. S.; Kendall, E. C.; Slocumb, C. H.; and Polley, H. F. The effect of a hormone of the adrenal cortex (17-hydroxy-11-dehydrocorticosterone; compound E) and of pituitary adrenocorticotropic hormone on rheumatoid arthritis. *Proc. Staff Meet. Mayo Clin.*, **1949**, *24*, 181–197.

Henkin, R. I. The effects of corticosteroids and ACTH on sensory systems. *Prog. Brain Res.*, **1970**, *32*, 270–294.

Hirata, F.; Schiffmann, E.; Venkatasubamanian, K.; Salomon, D.; and Axelrod, J. A phospholipase A_2 inhibitory protein in rabbit neutrophils induced by glucocorticoids. *Proc. Natl Acad. Sci. U.S.A.*, **1980**, *77*, 2533–2536.

Hofmann, K.; Yajima, H.; Yanaihara, N.; Liu, T.; and Lande, S. Studies on polypeptides. XIII. The synthesis of a tricosapeptide possessing essentially the full biological activity of natural ACTH. *J. Am. Chem. Soc.*, **1961**, *83*, 487–489.

Ingle, D. J. Permissive action of hormones. *J. Clin. Endocrinol. Metab.*, **1954**, *14*, 1272–1274.

Ingle, D. J.; Higgins, G. M.; and Kendall, E. C. Atrophy of the adrenal cortex in the rat produced by administration of large amounts of cortin. *Anat. Rec.*, **1938**, *71*, 363–372.

Iynedjian, P. B., and Hanson, R. W. Messenger RNA for renal phosphoenolpyruvate carboxykinase and its regulation by glucocorticoids and by changes in acid base balance. *J. Biol. Chem.*, **1977**, *252*, 8398–8403.

Johnson, L. K.; Baxter, J. D.; and Rousseau, G. G. Mechanisms of glucocorticoid receptor function. In, *Glucocorticoid Hormone Action.* (Baxter, J. D., and Rousseau, G. G., eds.) Springer-Verlag, New York, **1979**, pp. 305–326.

Kahnt, F. W.; Milani, A.; Steffen, H.; and Neher, R. The rate-limiting step of adrenal steroidogenesis and adenosine 3':5'-monophosphate. *Eur. J. Biochem.*, **1974**, *44*, 243–250.

Kimura, T. ACTH stimulation of cholesterol side chain cleavage activity of adrenocortical mitochondria. *Mol. Cell. Biochem.*, **1981**, *36*, 105–122.

Krakoff, L.; Nicolis, G.; and Amsel, B. Pathogenesis of hypertension in Cushing's syndrome. *Am. J. Med.*, **1975**, *58*, 216–220.

Lee, P. A.; Keenan, B. S.; Migeon, C. J.; and Blizzard, R. M. Effect of various ACTH preparations on the secretion of growth hormone in normal subjects and in hypopituitary patients. *J. Clin. Endocrinol. Metab.*, **1973**, *37*, 389–396.

Lemann, J., Jr.; Piering, W. F.; and Lennon, E. J. Studies of the acute effects of aldosterone and cortisol on the interrelationship between renal sodium, calcium, and magnesium excretion in normal man. *Nephron*, **1970**, *7*, 117–130.

Lesesne, H. R., and Fallon, H. J. Treatment of liver disease with corticosteroids. *Med. Clin. North Am.*, **1973**, *57*, 1191–1201.

Levine, S. B., and Leopold, I. H. Advances in ocular corticosteroid therapy. *Med. Clin. North Am.*, **1973**, *57*, 1167–1177.

Li, C. H. Adrenocorticotropin 45. Revised amino acid sequences for sheep and bovine hormones. *Biochem. Biophys. Res. Commun.*, **1972**, *49*, 835–839.

Li, C. H.; Evans, H. M.; and Simpson, M. E. Adrenocorticotropic hormone. *J. Biol. Chem.*, **1943**, *149*, 413–424.

Liddle, G. W. Tests of pituitary-adrenal suppressibility in the diagnosis of Cushing's syndrome. *J. Clin. Endocrinol. Metab.*, **1960**, *20*, 1539–1560.

Loeb, R. F.; Atchley, D. W.; Benedict, E. M.; and Leland, J. Electrolyte balance studies in adrenalectomized dogs with particular reference to the excretion of sodium. *J. Exp. Med.*, **1933**, *57*, 775–792.

Long, C. N. H.; Katzin, B.; and Fry, E. G. Adrenal cortex and carbohydrate metabolism. *Endocrinology*, **1940**, *26*, 309–344.

Lubkin, V. L. Steroid cataract—a review and conclusion. *J. Asthma Res.*, **1977**, *14*, 55–59.

MacGregor, R. R. Granulocyte adherence changes induced by hemodialysis, endotoxin, epinephrine, and glucocorticoids. *Ann. Intern. Med.*, **1977**, *86*, 35–39.

Mahaffee, D.; Reitz, R. C.; and Ney, R. L. The mechanism of action of adrenocorticotropic hormone. The role of mitochondrial cholesterol accumulation in the regulation of steroidogenesis. *J. Biol. Chem.*, **1974**, *249*, 227–233.

Maibach, H. I., and Stoughton, R. B. Topical corticosteroids. *Med. Clin. North Am.*, **1973**, *57*, 1253–1264.

Makman, M. H.; Dvorkin, B.; and White, A. Evidence for induction by cortisol *in vitro* of a protein inhibitor of transport and phosphorylation in rat thymocytes. *Proc. Natl Acad. Sci. U.S.A.*, **1971**, *68*, 1269–1273.

Marco, J.; Calle, C.; Román, D.; Diaz-Ferros, M.; Villanueva, M. L.; and Valverde, I. Hyperglucagonism induced by glucocorticoid treatment in man. *N. Engl. J. Med.*, **1973**, *288*, 128–131.

Meador, C. K.; Liddle, G. W.; Island, D. P.; Nicholson, W. E.; Lucas, C. P.; Nuckton, J. G.; and Luetscher, J. A. Cause of Cushing's syndrome in patients with tumors arising from "nonendocrine" tissue. *J. Clin. Endocrinol. Metab.,* **1962,** *22,* 693–703.

Messer, J.; Reitman, D.; Sacks, H. S.; Smith, H., Jr.; and Chalmers, T. C. Association of adrenocorticosteroid therapy and peptic ulcer disease. *N. Engl. J. Med.,* **1983,** *309,* 21–24.

Morris, H. G.; Jorgensen, J. R.; Elrick, H.; and Goldsmith, R. E. Metabolic effects of human growth hormone in corticosteroid-treated children. *J. Clin. Invest.,* **1968,** *47,* 436–451.

Muller, O. A.; Stalla, G. K.; and v. Werder, K. Corticotropin releasing factor: a new tool for the differential diagnosis of Cushing's syndrome. *J. Clin. Endocrinol. Metab.,* **1983,** *57,* 227–229.

Nakanishi, S.; Kita, T.; Taii, S.; Imura, H.; and Numa, S. Glucocorticoid effect on the level of corticotropin messenger RNA activity in rat pituitary. *Proc. Natl Acad. Sci. U.S.A.,* **1977,** *74,* 3283–3286.

Nelson, S. R., and Dick, A. R. Steroids in the treatment of brain edema. In, *Steroid Therapy.* (Azarnoff, D. L., ed.) W. B. Saunders Co., Philadelphia, **1975,** pp. 313–324.

Ney, R. L. Effects of dibutyryl cyclic AMP on adrenal growth and steroidogenic capacity. *Endocrinology,* **1969,** *84,* 168–170.

Orth, D. N. Metyrapone is useful only as adjunctive therapy in Cushing's disease. *Ann. Intern. Med.,* **1978,** *89,* 128–130.

Otsuka, H., and Inouye, L. K. Structure-activity relationships of adrenocorticotropin. *Pharmacol. Ther.* [*B*], **1975,** *1,* 501–527.

Paul, D. P.; Gallant, S.; Orme-Johnson, N. R.; Orme-Johnson, W. H.; and Brownie, H. C. Temperature dependence of cholesterol binding to cytochrome P-450 of the rat adrenal. Effect of adrenocorticotropic hormone and cycloheximide. *J. Biol. Chem.,* **1976,** *251,* 7120–7126.

Payvar, F.; Wrange, O.; Carlstedt-Duke, J.; Okret, S.; Gustafsson, J.-A.; and Yamamoto, K. Purified glucocorticoid receptors bind selectively *in vitro* to a cloned DNA fragment whose transcription is regulated by glucocorticoids *in vivo. Proc. Natl Acad. Sci. U.S.A.,* **1981,** *78,* 6628–6632.

Pittman, R. C., and Steinberg, D. Activatable cholesterol esterase and triacylglycerol lipase activities of rat adrenal and their relationship. *Biochim. Biophys. Acta,* **1977,** *487,* 431–444.

Priestley, G. C., and Brown, J. C. Effects of corticosteroids on the proliferation of normal and abnormal human connective tissue cells. *Br. J. Dermatol.,* **1980,** *102,* 35–41.

ReMine, S. G., and McIlrath, D. C. Bowel perforation in steroid-treated patients. *Ann. Surg.,* **1980,** *192,* 581–586.

Rinehart, J. J.; Sagone, A. L.; Balcerzak, S. P.; Ackerman, G. A.; and LoBuglio, A. L. Effects of corticosteroid therapy on human monocyte function. *N. Engl. J. Med.,* **1975,** *292,* 236–241.

Robinson, W. D. Management of systemic lupus erythematosus. *Arthritis Rheum.,* **1962,** *5,* 521–528.

Sawin, C. T.; Bray, G. A.; and Idelson, B. A. Overnight suppression test with dexamethasone in Cushing's syndrome. *J. Clin. Endocrinol. Metab.,* **1968,** *28,* 422–424.

Sayers, G.; White, A.; and Long, C. N. H. Preparation and properties of pituitary adrenotropic hormone. *J. Biol. Chem.,* **1943,** *149,* 425–436.

Scherrer, K. Messenger RNA in eukaryotic cells: the life history of duck globin messenger RNA. *Acta Endocrinol. (Kbh.),* **1973,** *180,* Suppl., 95–129.

Schutz, G.; Killewich, L.; Chen, G.; and Feigelson, P. Control of the mRNA for hepatic tryptophan oxygenase during hormonal and substrate induction. *Proc. Natl Acad. Sci. U.S.A.,* **1975,** *72,* 1017–1020.

Schwyzer, R., and Sieber, P. Total synthesis of adrenocorticotropic hormone. *Nature,* **1963,** *199,* 172–174.

Selye, H. General adaptation syndrome and diseases of adaptation. *J. Clin. Endocrinol. Metab.,* **1946,** *6,* 117–230.

Share, L., and Crofton, J. T. Contribution of vasopressin to hypertension. *Hypertension,* **1982,** *4,* Suppl. III, 85–92.

Simpson, S. A.; Tait, J. F.; Wettstein, A.; Neher, R.; Euw, J. V.; Schindler, O.; and Reichstein, T. Konstitution des Aldosterons des neuen Mineralocorticoids. *Experientia,* **1954,** *10,* 132–133.

Smith, K. A. T-cell growth factor. *Immunol. Rev.,* **1980,** *51,* 337–357.

Spiro, H. M. Is the steroid ulcer a myth? *N. Engl. J. Med.,* **1983,** *309,* 45–47.

Stone, D., and Hechter, O. Studies on ACTH action in perfused bovine adrenals: the site of action of ACTH in corticosteroidogenesis. *Arch. Biochem. Biophys.,* **1954,** *51,* 457–469.

Swann, H. G. The pituitary-adrenocortical relationship. *Physiol. Rev.,* **1940,** *20,* 493–521.

Swingle, W. W., and Pfiffner, J. J. Experiments with an active extract of the suprarenal cortex. *Anat. Rec.,* **1930a,** *44,* 225–226.

———. An aqueous extract of the suprarenal cortex which maintains the life of bilaterally adrenalectomized cats. *Science,* **1930b,** *71,* 321–322.

Tait, J. F.; Simpson, S. A.; and Grundy, H. M. The effect of adrenal extract on mineral metabolism. *Lancet,* **1952,** *1,* 122–124.

Thody, A. J. The significance of melanocyte-stimulating hormone (MSH) and the control of its secretion in the mammal. *Adv. Drug Res.,* **1977,** *11,* 23–74.

Tobian, L. Interrelationship of electrolytes, juxtaglomerular cells and hypertension. *Physiol. Rev.,* **1960,** *40,* 280–312.

Vale, W.; Spies, J.; Rivier, C.; and Rivier, J. Characterization of a 41-residue ovine hypothalamic peptide that stimulates secretion of corticotropin and β-endorphin. *Science,* **1981,** *213,* 1394–1397.

Vanstapel, F.; Bollen, M.; deWulf, H.; and Stalmans, W. Induction of hepatic glycogen synthesis by glucocorticoids is not mediated by insulin. *Mol. Cell. Endocrinol.,* **1982,** *27,* 107–114.

Wall, A. J. The use of glucocorticoids in intestinal disease. *Med. Clin. North Am.,* **1973,** *57,* 1241–1252.

Webb-Johnson, D. C., and Andrews, J. L. Bronchodilator therapy. *N. Engl. J. Med.,* **1977,** *297,* 476–482, 758–764.

Weston, W. L.; Mandel, M. J.; Yeckley, J. A.; Krueger, G. G.; and Claman, H. N. Mechanism of cortisol inhibition of adoptive transfer of tuberculin sensitivity. *J. Lab. Clin. Med.,* **1973,** *82,* 366–371.

Wise, J. K.; Hendler, R.; and Felig, P. Influence of glucocorticoids on glucagon secretion and plasma amino acid concentrations in man. *J. Clin. Invest.,* **1973,** *52,* 2774–2782.

Yard, A. C., and Kadowitz, P. J. Studies on the mechanism of hydrocortisone potentiation of vasoconstrictor responses to epinephrine in the anesthetized animal. *Eur. J. Pharmacol.,* **1972,** *20,* 1–9.

Yount, W. J.; Utsinger, P. D.; Puritz, E. M.; and Ortbals, D. W. Corticosteroid therapy of the collagen vascular disorders. *Med. Clin. North Am.,* **1973,** *57,* 1343–1355.

Monographs and Reviews

Baxter, J. D., and Rousseau, G. G. (eds.). *Glucocorticoid Hormone Action.* Springer-Verlag, New York, **1979.**

Baylink, D. J.   Glucocorticoid-induced osteoporosis. *N. Engl. J. Med.*, **1983**, *309*, 306–309.

Bongiovanni, A. M.; Eberlein, W. R.; Goldman, A. S.; and New, M.   Disorders of adrenal steroid biogenesis. *Recent Prog. Horm. Res.*, **1967**, *23*, 375–449.

Carpenter, W. T., and Gruen, P. H.   Cortisol's influence on human mental functioning. *J. Clin. Psychopharmacol.*, **1982**, *2*, 91–101.

Conference. (Various authors.)   Corticotropin-releasing-factor. *Fed. Proc.*, **1985**, *44*, 145–263.

Cupps, T. R., and Fauci, A. S.   Corticosteroid-mediated immunoregulation in man. *Immunol. Rev.*, **1982**, *65*, 133–154.

Fain, J. N., and Czech, M. P.   Glucocorticoid effects on lipid mobilization and adipose tissue metabolism. In, *Adrenal Gland*, Vol. 6. Sect. 7, *Endocrinology. Handbook of Physiology*. (Blashko, H., ed.) American Physiological Society, Washington, D.C., **1975**, pp. 169–189.

Gann, D. S.; Dallman, M. F.; and Engleland, W. C.   Reflex control and modulation of ACTH and corticosteroids. *Int. Rev. Physiol.*, **1981**, *24*, 157–199.

Gold, E. M.   The Cushing's syndromes: changing views of diagnosis and treatment. *Ann. Intern. Med.*, **1979**, *90*, 829–844.

Hahn, T. J.   Corticosteroid-induced osteopenia. *Arch. Intern. Med.*, **1978**, *138*, 882–885.

Liddle, G. W.   Clinical pharmacology of the anti-inflammatory steroids. *Clin. Pharmacol. Ther.*, **1961**, *2*, 615–635.

Loeb, J. N.   Corticosteroids and growth. *N. Engl. J. Med.*, **1976**, *295*, 547–552.

Loh, Y. P., and Loriaux, L. L.   Adrenocorticotropic hormone, β-lipotropin, and endorphin-related peptides in health and disease. *J.A.M.A.*, **1982**, *247*, 1033–1034.

McEwen, B. S.   Influences of adrenocortical hormones on pituitary and brain function. In, *Glucocorticoid Hormone Action*. (Baxter, J. D., and Rousseau, G. G., eds.) Springer-Verlag, New York, **1979**, pp. 467–492.

Mandel, S.   Steroid myopathy. *Postgrad. Med.*, **1982**, *72*, 207–215.

Marver, D.   Aldosterone action in target epithelia. *Vitam. Horm.*, **1980**, *38*, 57–117.

Mulrow, P. J., and Forman, B. H.   The tissue effects of mineralocorticoids. *Am. J. Med.*, **1972**, *53*, 561–572.

Parrillo, J. E., and Fauci, A. S.   Mechanisms of glucocorticoid action on immune processes. *Annu. Rev. Pharmacol. Toxicol.*, **1979**, *19*, 179–201.

Reichstein, T., and Shoppee, C. W.   The hormones of the adrenal cortex. *Vitam. Horm.*, **1943**, *1*, 346–413.

Rose, L. I., and Saccar, C.   Choosing corticosteroid preparations. *Am. Fam. Physician*, **1978**, *17*, 198–204.

Temple, T. E., and Liddle, G. W.   Inhibitors of adrenal steroid biosynthesis. *Annu. Rev. Pharmacol. Toxicol.*, **1970**, *10*, 199–218.

CHAPTER

64 INSULIN AND ORAL HYPOGLYCEMIC DRUGS; GLUCAGON

Joseph Larner

INSULIN

History. Credit for the discovery of insulin is given to Banting and Best, who extracted the active principle from the pancreas and demonstrated its therapeutic effects in diabetic dogs and human subjects in the years 1921 and 1922. However, many investigators had paved the way for the discovery, including E. L. Scott, who in 1911 had extracted an active principle from the pancreas with ethanol and acid. Paulesco also described a pancreatic material that was capable of producing hypoglycemia in animals. Probably of greatest earlier import was the demonstration by von Mering and Minkowski in 1889 that pancreatectomized dogs exhibit a syndrome similar to diabetes mellitus in man, with polyuria, polyphagia, wasting, ketosis, poor wound healing, and infection. They also demonstrated that deprivation of the exocrine function of the pancreas by ligation of the pancreatic duct did not cause diabetes, despite marked atrophy of the gland. The suggestion was made that diabetes occurred in the absence of a factor from the pancreas. Banting approached the problem with two working hypotheses: (1) the islet tissue secreted insulin, and (2) previous difficulties in isolating the active principle had been due in many instances to the proteolytic destruction of insulin by the digestive enzymes of the pancreas during the course of extraction. He devised elegantly simple approaches to circumvent the difficulty. He tied the pancreatic ducts so that the acinar tissue degenerated and left the islet tissue undisturbed, and from the remaining tissue extracted the active principle in relatively high concentration. Later on, normal pancreas was used as a commercial source when it was rediscovered that acidified alcohol not only extracted insulin but also prevented proteolytic destruction.

The first patient to receive the active extracts prepared by Banting and Best was Leonard Thompson, aged 14 (Banting *et al.*, 1922). He appeared at the Toronto General Hospital with a blood glucose of 500 mg/dl, and he was excreting 3 to 5 liters of urine per day. Despite rigid control of diet (450 kcal per day), he continued to excrete large quantities of glucose, and, without insulin, the most likely course was death after a few months. The administration of these extracts induced a reduction in the concentration and excretion of blood glucose. Daily injections were then begun, and there was immediate improvement. The excretion of glucose was reduced from over 100 to as little as 7.5 g per day. Furthermore, ". . . the boy became brighter, looked better and said he felt

stronger." Here was as dramatic an interruption of a fatal metabolic disorder as one will find in the annals of the history of medical science. The early history has been reviewed recently (*see* Bliss, 1983).

Immediately after the discovery of insulin there was justifiable excitement and then unfortunate relaxation, an attitude that the problems of treatment and of etiology of diabetes mellitus had been solved. True, the discovery of insulin was a momentous advance, but as time went by it became apparent that treatment was more than simply injection of insulin, that the etiology was more complex in many instances than mere destruction of islet tissue, and that the explanation of the action of the hormone was an exceedingly complex problem involving the elucidation of the intermediary metabolism not only of carbohydrate but also of protein and fat.

The studies on the etiology of diabetes mellitus took an interesting turn when Houssay reported in 1936 that hypophysectomy ameliorated diabetes in the dog and that extracts of the anterior pituitary exacerbated the condition. Soon thereafter, Young induced permanent diabetes in dogs by prolonged administration of anterior pituitary extract. Long and Lukens provided convincing evidence that the adrenal cortex, as well as the adenohypophysis, exerts effects antagonistic to insulin. A new attitude developed. Diabetes could be caused not only by a deficiency of insulin but also by an excess of certain hormones, for example, growth hormone, glucocorticoids, or glucagon. While hypersecretion of these hormones probably does not occur in the vast majority of diabetic patients, there may be exceptions. Growth hormone has been suggested to play an etiological role in the generation of at least certain forms of the disease (*see* Chapter 59). Furthermore, the concentrations of glucagon in plasma are elevated in many patients with diabetes (Unger and Orci, 1981a, 1981b). The search for the etiology of diabetes mellitus has recently turned from strictly endocrine to immunological, infectious, and genetic factors (*see* below).

Chemistry and Biosynthesis. The chemistry of insulin has progressed from the preparation of active extracts to the preparation of insulin in crystalline form by Abel in 1926, to the establishment of the amino acid sequence of the polypeptide hormone (Sanger, 1960), and, eventually, to the complete synthesis of the molecule (Katsoyannis *et al.*,

1963; Meienhofer *et al.*, 1963). Insulin, with a molecular weight of about 6000, is made up of two chains of amino acids joined together by disulfide linkages (*see* Figure 64–1). Steiner and colleagues and Chance and associates (*see* Steiner, 1977) demonstrated that the β cells of the pancreatic islets synthesize insulin from a single-chain precursor termed *proinsulin* (Figure 64–1). On conversion of human proinsulin to insulin, four basic amino acids and the remaining connector or C-peptide are removed by proteolysis. A thiol-activated protease has been implicated in this reaction (Docherty *et al.*, 1982), as has plasminogen activator (Virji *et al.*, 1980). The resultant insulin molecule has two chains, the A chain with glycine at the amino-terminal residue and the B chain with phenylalanine at the amino terminus. In many commercial preparations of insulin it is possible to detect small amounts of proinsulin and other related molecules resulting from incomplete conversion of the prohormone.

An even larger molecule termed *preproinsulin* has been identified as a precursor of proinsulin. Preproinsulin is extended at the N terminus of the B chain by at least 23 amino acids, many of which are hydrophobic (Chan *et al.*, 1976). It is cleaved to proinsulin in the endoplasmic reticulum, where it is synthesized, and is therefore not a product that accumulates in the β cell.

Insulin is now recognized as one of a family of related peptides, which includes insulin-like growth factors 1 (IGF₁) and 2 (IGF₂), previously termed somatomedins, and nonsuppressible insulin-like activities (NSILAs, *see* below).

Hodgkin and associates (*see* Hodgkin and Mercola, 1972) have determined the three-dimensional structure of insulin by x-ray analysis of single crystals. Insulin can exist as a monomer, a dimer, or a hexamer composed of three such dimers. Two molecules of Zn²⁺ are coordinated in the hexamer, which is presumably the form stored in the granules of the β cell. The biologically active form of the hormone is thought to be the monomer. X-ray analysis has also shown that the two chains are compactly arranged, with the A chain positioned above the central helical portion of the B chain. From each end of this helical region the terminal portions of the B chain extend as arms, and the A chain is enclosed between them.

Many species variations are known, and some are of clinical significance. For example, the major sites of chemical difference among porcine, ovine, equine, and cetacean insulins are in positions 8, 9, and 10 of the A chain. The porcine hormone is most similar to that of man and differs only by the substitution of an alanine residue (for threonine) at the carboxy terminus of the B chain. By the use of porcine insulin as the starting material, human insulin can be synthesized with relative ease (Markussen *et al.*, in Symposium, 1983a). Production of human insulin by cloning of DNA in *Escherichia coli* has also been achieved (Frank and Chance, 1983). This exciting new technology has allowed the production of human insulin on a commercial scale.

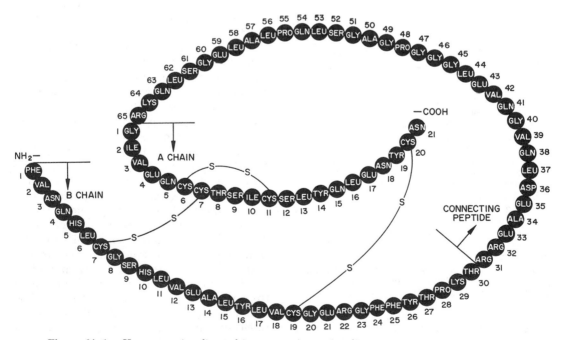

Figure 64–1. *Human proinsulin and its conversion to insulin.*

The amino acid sequence of human proinsulin is shown. By proteolytic cleavage, four basic amino acids (31, 32, 64, 65) and the connecting peptide are removed and proinsulin is converted to insulin. (For details, *see* the text.)

The specific activities of most mammalian insulins are very similar (22 to 27 units/mg). Proinsulin has only slight biological activity, while the separated A and B chains are essentially inactive.

Assay of Insulin in Plasma. In addition to the older *in-vivo* bioassays, which depend on the lowering of blood glucose in rabbits or the production of convulsions in mice, several *in-vitro* methods have attained popularity because of their high degree of sensitivity and their relative simplicity of execution. One method is based on the capacity of insulin to increase the glycogen content or the glucose uptake of the rat diaphragm. Adipose tissue assays are based on the capacity of insulin to stimulate glucose metabolism by the epididymal fat pad of the rat or by suspensions of isolated fat cells. Measured end points are CO_2 production from glucose, incorporation of the ^{14}C of labeled glucose into fat, or glucose uptake from the medium. The sensitivity of the radioimmunoassay for insulin is an order of magnitude greater than the *in-vitro* bioassays and two or more orders of magnitude greater than the *in-vivo* bioassays.

Types of Plasma Insulin. Plasma insulin estimated by bioassay is called *insulin-like activity* (ILA), and plasma insulin estimated by immunoassay is called *immunoreactive insulin* (IRI). IRI and ILA differ both quantitatively and qualitatively. The concentration of plasma IRI of normal persons after an overnight fast is under 20 microunits/ml.

When insulin antibody is added to plasma, a decrease in ILA is observed (suppressible ILA); however, a considerable portion (sometimes over 90%) of the ILA may persist, and this is termed nonsuppressible ILA or NSILA. The amount of suppressible ILA corresponds to the amount of IRI. Thus, estimates of plasma ILA are invariably higher than are those of IRI. NSILA has been intensively studied. Although it is not increased in plasma after the administration of glucose and persists in plasma after pancreatectomy, there is evidence that growth hormone, insulin, thyroxine, and nutritional status regulate its concentration. It behaves like insulin metabolically and, also like insulin, promotes the growth of cells in culture (*see* Zapf *et al.,* 1981). The structures of two components that contribute to NSILA have been defined; these are IGF_1 and IGF_2, mentioned above. Also present is NSILA-P (precipitated in acid-ethanol; molecular weight about 85,000) (Leichter and Poffenbarger, 1978); the structure of this material is not yet known. IGF_1 and IGF_2 interact with two distinct populations of specific cellular receptors to produce several effects that resemble those of insulin. They are normally associated with specific binding proteins in plasma. They are identical with somatomedins (Daughaday, 1982).

Secretion of Insulin: Morphological and Chemical Events. The islet is composed of four recognizable cell types, and each synthesizes a distinct polypeptide: insulin in the β cell, glucagon in the α cell, somatostatin in the D cell, and pancreatic polypeptide in the PP or F cell. Each cell type has a characteristic distribution within the islet (Orci, 1982). The β cells make up about 60% of the islet and form its medulla. The α cells form the outer cortex and constitute about 25%. In the ventral (duodenal) pancreas, α cells are replaced by PP cells. D cells are located between the α and β cells and constitute about 10% of the islet. Specialized connections or tight junctions have been described between cells, through which small molecules pass (Orci, 1982). Paracrine or cell-to-cell control is exerted at a local level (*see* below). Arterioles enter the islets and branch into a glomerular-like capillary mass in the β-cell core. Capillaries then pass through to the rim of the islet and coalesce into collecting venules either in the rim or just outside the islet (Bonner-Weir and Orci, 1982). These studies provide an anatomical basis for the paracrine mechanisms that have been proposed.

Of interest are changes in the morphology of islets that accompany experimental or pathological hypoinsulinemic states. In insulin-dependent diabetes mellitus (IDDM), there is a marked reduction in the volume of β cells (Stefan *et al.,* 1982; Rahier *et al.,* 1983). The mass of α, D, and PP cells appears to be unchanged. In non-insulin-dependent diabetes mellitus (NIDDM), the mass of α cells is increased, without major changes in β, D, or PP cells.

Preproinsulin is synthesized in the membrane-associated polyribosomes of the rough endoplasmic reticulum of the β cells and is converted at this site to proinsulin. Proinsulin is first transferred to the cisternae of the reticulum and then via transitional elements (vesicles) to the Golgi complex, where it is concentrated within immature granules. Here the conversion of proinsulin to insulin begins. Eventually proinsulin- and insulin-containing storage granules bud off from the Golgi apparatus, and the enzymatic conversion of proinsulin to insulin plus C-peptide is completed. The granules may be either stored, destroyed (by lysosomes), or released by exocytosis (*see* Robbins *et al.,* 1984).

Regulation of Insulin Secretion. Gastrointestinal Mechanisms. Insulin release appears to be controlled by the coordinated interplay of the availability of food products, gastrointestinal hormones, and other hormonal and neural stimuli. In the last-named category, both the autonomic nervous system and the central nervous system (CNS) are of major importance.

In keeping with insulin's role to promote the storage of all fuels, it is not surprising that, in addition to glucose, amino acids, fatty acids of all chain lengths, and ketone bodies will call forth its secretion. In man, glucose is most probably the principal stimulus. But in other animals, depending on diet, amino acids or fatty acids may be of primary importance.

It has been known for over 70 years that glucose is more effective in provoking glycosuria when injected intravenously than when administered orally. However, it was recognized only relatively recently that this difference is due to a greater capacity of oral glucose to evoke the secretion of insulin (McIntyre et al., 1964); the same may also be true for other nutrients. This strongly suggests the presence of anticipatory signals (termed *incretins*) from the gastrointestinal tract to the pancreas. Several of the gastrointestinal hormones, including secretin, pancreozymin-cholecystokinin, gastrin, vasoactive intestinal polypeptide (VIP), and gastrointestinal or "gut" glucagon, have been shown to stimulate insulin secretion *in vitro* and *in vivo*. A more recently appreciated polypeptide (43 amino acid residues) termed *gastric inhibitory polypeptide* (GIP) has been purified and its amino acid sequence determined. It is structurally homologous with glucagon, VIP, and secretin and is hypothesized to be the most important β-cell stimulant whose secretion is sensitive to glucose and fat (Brown et al., 1980); however, other polypeptides that contribute to incretin activity may yet be identified. Pancreozymin-cholecystokinin may also play a similar role as a protein- and amino acid–sensitive signal. It is thus clear that the gastrointestinal tract and the pancreas form an enteropancreatic axis responsible not only for digestion and absorption of foods but also for their effective and controlled utilization. (For a review of this rapidly developing field, *see* Jerzy-Glass, 1980.)

Autonomic Mechanisms. The predominant effect of norepinephrine or epinephrine is to inhibit insulin secretion, a response mediated by α-adrenergic receptors. In addition, *selective* activation of β_2-adrenergic receptors results in stimulation of the secretion of insulin. Exercise and pathological states associated with activation of the autonomic nervous system, including hypoxia, hypothermia, surgery, and severe burns, all lead to a suppression of insulin secretion via the α-receptor mechanism. Cholinomimetic drugs and vagal-nerve stimulation enhance insulin release (*see* Porte and Halter, 1981).

The adrenergic and cholinergic systems, which richly innervate the islets, may control the basal rate of secretion of insulin as well as the reaction to stress. Thus, α-receptor blockade raises and muscarinic or β-receptor blockade lowers the basal concentration of insulin in plasma.

The hypothalamus regulates the sympathetic and parasympathetic inputs to the islets. Electrical stimulation of the ventrolateral hypothalamus leads to a rapid increase in insulin secretion, via a vagal pathway. Electrical stimulation of the ventromedial hypothalamus produces a decrease in insulin secretion mediated by the splanchnic nerves. The hypothalamus also controls appetite and integrates feeding behavior, and is thus an important regulator of β-cell secretion (*see* Porte and Halter, 1981; Shimazu and Ishikawa, 1981).

Control by Other Hormones. There is considerable evidence for reciprocal control of secretion of insulin, glucagon, and somatostatin within the pancreatic islet (Unger and Orci, 1981a, 1981b). For example, the secretory activity of α cells is inhibited when insulin secretion from β cells in their vicinity is enhanced (Asplin et al., 1981). Isolated β cells respond to glucose less well than when they are in contact with other islet cells (Pipeleers et al., 1982). The essential features of these relationships are shown in Figure 64–2. Glucagon and related peptides stimulate the secretion of insulin, while insulin inhibits the secretion of glucagon. Somatostatin inhibits the secretion of both insulin and glucagon. Glucagon stimulates somatostatin release, while the effect of insulin on somatostatin is unclear. A variety of other hormones and

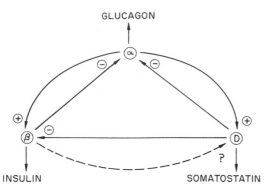

Figure 64–2. *Model of paracrine control of hormone secretion from the islets of Langerhans.*

The effects of insulin, glucagon, and somatostatin on α, β, and D cells are indicated by $\oplus$ or $\ominus$; for details, *see* the text. (Modified from Unger and Orci, 1981a.)

autacoids can also modify the secretory response of the β cell (*see* Porte and Halter, 1981; Robertson, 1983).

Biochemical Mechanisms and Kinetics. While all nutrients stimulate insulin secretion in man, only glucose stimulates both the secretion and biosynthesis of insulin. Indeed, glucose appears to promote the preferential release of newly synthesized insulin irrespective of the secretagogue utilized (Gold *et al.*, 1982); an increased rate of translation of mRNA, rather than stimulation of its synthesis, appears to be involved (*see* Robbins *et al.*, 1984). The importance of glucose is also highlighted by the fact that the effects of all other secretagogues are sensitive to the concentration of glucose. Glucose is thus the primary regulator of the β cell; two models for such regulation have been proposed. In the glucoreceptor model, a specific cell-surface receptor for glucose initiates control, while in the substrate-site model, a signal generated by an intracellular metabolite is utilized. It is now clear that the β cell is relatively permeable to glucose, and the intracellular concentration of the sugar equals that in the extracellular fluid. Thus, the rate of glucose transport far exceeds its rate of phosphorylation. Glucokinase may be the major enzyme responsible for phosphorylation of glucose in β cells, and it may thus be the crucial sensor of the intracellular concentration of free glucose (*see* Ashcroft, 1980). While concentrations of glycolytic intermediates measured in islets after exposure to glucose do not change in a manner sufficient to explain secretion of insulin, there are significant changes in glycolytic flux that can be related to secretion. In general, there is a correlation between the capacity of sugars to undergo glycolysis and their ability to stimulate insulin release. Furthermore, inhibition of glycolysis also inhibits secretion of insulin. Glucose thus appears to serve several

roles; it is hypothesized to act as a secretagogue by means of interaction with a glucoreceptor, and it serves, of course, as an energy source and possibly as the source of another signal within the β cell. Other potential signals that have been suggested include adenosine triphosphate (ATP), glucose-6-phosphate, NADH or NADPH, and phosphoenolpyruvate (Ashcroft, 1980).

The fact that β-adrenergic agonists and glucagon stimulate insulin secretion suggests that adenosine 3',5'-monophosphate (cyclic AMP) has a role in mediating the response. Glucagon and glucose can also increase the concentration of cyclic AMP in islets. The exact role of cyclic AMP is not clear, but it may be related to the requirement for Ca^{2+}. Insulinotropic agents act to evoke sustained secretion of insulin only in the presence of extracellular Ca^{2+}, facilitating its influx and decreasing its efflux.

Of great importance has been the discovery of the biphasic kinetics of the glucose-induced insulin release from the β cell. Both *in vitro* and *in vivo*, there occurs an initial burst of secretion that reaches a peak in minutes and rapidly declines, followed by a second, longer-lasting peak that may duplicate the initial peak value after an hour or longer. The concept of two pools of stored insulin, one more rapidly released than the other, has emerged. The rapidly secreted insulin may be a more important determinant of the rate at which glucose is utilized in the body, and selective hypersecretion or impairment of the early phase of secretion is noted in many "prediabetic" and diabetic patients (*see* below). The first phase of secretion appears to be related to an increased concentration of Ca^{2+} in the cytoplasm as a consequence of decreased Ca^{2+} efflux and release of stored Ca^{2+} within the cell; the second phase is correlated with increased Ca^{2+} influx, together with release of stored Ca^{2+} (Wollheim and Sharp, 1981). Secretion in the second phase may also be related to the assembly of microtubules and/or to the activation of a Ca^{2+}- and calmodulin-stimulated protein kinase (Colca *et al.*, 1983a). A kinetic model that involves feedback control by insulin itself has also been proposed to explain the biphasic pattern of secretion.

Effects of Alloxan, Streptozocin, and Other Toxins. Agents that rather selectively destroy the β cells induce hypoinsulinemic diabetes mellitus. These compounds include alloxan, uric acid, dialuric acid, dehydroascorbic acid, dehydroisoascorbic acid, some quinolones, and streptozocin (streptozotocin). Accidental ingestion of a rodenticide, VACOR (N-3-pyridylmethyl-N'-*p*-nitrophenylurea), has also been shown to destroy β cells and to cause diabetes (Karam *et al.*, 1980). When streptozocin, the N-nitroso derivative of glucosamine produced by *Streptomyces achromogenes,* is injected into rats, degeneration of pancreatic β cells follows. In recent years streptozocin has replaced alloxan as the preferred agent to produce a diabetic state in experimental animals and, in contrast to alloxan, it is useful clinically to treat insulin-secreting tumors (*see* Chapter 55).

Both alloxan and streptozocin may act by breaking DNA strands in β cells. Alloxan appears to do so as a result of generation of free radicals, while streptozocin acts by alkylating the bases of DNA (Uchigata *et al.*, 1983). Alloxan has also been shown to inactivate a Ca^{2+}- and calmodulin-dependent protein kinase, the activity of which is related to insulin secretion (Colca *et al.*, 1983b).

Distribution, Excretion, and Fate. While a fraction of the endogenous or exogenous insulin in plasma may be associated with certain proteins, the bulk appears to circulate in blood and lymph as the free hormone. The volume of distribution of insulin approximates the volume of extracellular fluid. Under fasting conditions, the pancreas secretes 20 μg of insulin per hour into the portal vein; the concentration of insulin in portal blood is 2 to 4 ng/ml (50 to 100 microunits/ml) and that in the peripheral circulation is 500 pg/ml (12 microunits/ml). A small amount of proinsulin is also found in the circulation.

The plasma half-life of insulin injected intravenously is less than 9 minutes in man, and there is no detectable difference between normal and diabetic subjects. However, antibodies to insulin can prolong the half-life. The main sites of destruction are the liver and kidney, and about 50% of the insulin that reaches the liver via the portal vein is destroyed in a single passage, never reaching the general circulation. Insulin is filtered by the renal glomeruli and is reabsorbed by the tubules, which also degrade it. Severe impairment of renal function appears to affect the rate of disappearance of circulating insulin to a greater extent than does hepatic disease, since the liver operates closer to its capacity to destroy the hormone and cannot compensate for such loss of renal catabolic function. Although peripheral tissues such as muscle and fat bind and inactivate insulin, this is of minor quantitative significance.

Proteolytic degradation of insulin in the liver occurs both at the cell surface (Terris and Steiner, 1975) and in lysosomes after internalization of insulin with its receptor (Duckworth *et al.*, 1981). A proteolytic enzyme that degrades insulin has been purified from muscle (*see* Duckworth and Kitabchi, 1981). The enzyme is interesting because its K_m for insulin is within the range of physiological concentrations. An enzyme termed glutathione-insulin transhydrogenase, which utilizes reduced glutathione to reduce the disulfide bridges of insulin and produce separate chains, has also been implicated in the degradation of insulin. A highly purified glutathione-insulin transhydrogenase enzyme without proteolytic activity has been isolated from liver by Varandani and Nafz (1976). Presumably because of the reductive separation of the two chains of insulin, free A chains have been demonstrated in the plasma and urine of normal individuals and diabetic patients.

Insulin and Diabetes Mellitus. Progress has been made in the classification of diabetes mellitus into separate categories. While several schemes have been proposed, only one is described herein: (1) insulin-dependent (previously termed juvenile-onset) diabetes mellitus (IDDM; type 1); (2) non-insulin-dependent (previously termed maturity-onset) diabetes mellitus (NIDDM; type 2); (3) maturity-onset or non-insulin-dependent diabetes in the young—a rare dominantly inherited, mild type of disease; (4) diabetes mellitus or carbohydrate intolerance associated with certain genetic syndromes; (5) secondary diabetes mellitus (drug-induced, pancreatic disease, hormonal, receptor abnormalities, *etc.*); and (6) gestational diabetes mellitus. The first two forms of the disease account for the great majority of cases. Several unusual forms of diabetes not included in the above classification occur in underdeveloped countries. These forms of diabetes are frequently associated with massive pancreatic calculi and concomitant pancreatic destruction. The etiology is unknown, but nutritional and toxic factors have been suggested. The secretion of a structurally abnormal insulin that has reduced biological activity has also been described as a rare cause of diabetes (Shoelson *et al.*, 1983; Haneda *et al.*, 1984).

Insulin-dependent and non-insulin-dependent forms of diabetes mellitus have been recognized clinically for years. Both types of disease have genetic components, and studies of identical twins have indicated a very high degree of concordance for non-insulin-dependent diabetes (*see* Pyke, 1977). There is also a high prevalence of such disease among the offspring of diabetic couples and among first-degree relatives. The genetic mechanism is not completely understood because non-insulin-dependent diabetes probably consists of a group of related diseases and can occur with or without obesity (note the third type above). A polymorphism in the 5' flanking region of the human insulin gene has been suggested to be a possible genetic marker for non-insulin-dependent diabetes

(Rotwein *et al.*, 1983) and for atherosclerosis (Owerbach *et al.*, 1982). Studies of identical twins reveal a lower degree of concordance for insulin-dependent diabetes, suggesting environmental as well as genetic influences. Autoimmune and viral etiologies have been proposed. Antibodies to components of islet cells can be detected in a high proportion of cases if patients are examined early in the onset of the disease, in contrast to non-insulin-dependent disease where they are rarely found. Patients who have antibodies to islet cells tend to have immunoglobulins that react with preparations of adrenal, parathyroid, and thyroid gland as well. There is an association of insulin-dependent diabetes with specific histocompatibility leukocyte antigens (HLA), especially at the B locus (B8 and B15) and at the Dr locus (Dr3 and Dr4) on human chromosome 6. Almost all probands with insulin-dependent diabetes have either Dr3, Dr4, or both (Wolf *et al.*, 1983). This presumably indicates that humoral and cell-mediated immune mechanisms are involved in the etiology of the disease. Direct evidence for a viral etiology in animals (Yoon *et al.*, 1983) and suggestive evidence in man (MacLaren, 1977; Yoon *et al.*, 1979) have also been obtained. Whatever the cause or causes, the final result in insulin-dependent diabetes is a hypoinsulinemic state with an extensive loss of β cells of the islets; there is no such loss of cells in non-insulin-dependent disease.

Numerous studies have demonstrated the absence of insulin in the circulation and in the pancreas in insulin-dependent diabetics. Absence of the C-peptide and proinsulin also indicates failure of the β cell. This form of the disease usually begins with marked hyperglycemia or an episode of ketoacidosis associated with extremely low concentrations of immunoreactive insulin and C-peptide in the plasma. A period of clinical remission follows in some patients, accompanied by improvement in carbohydrate tolerance and a reduction in the requirement for insulin administration. During this time β-cell function returns, as evidenced by restoration of plasma immunoreactive insulin and C-peptide. However, in the fully established disease that follows, the function of the β cell appears to be lost totally (*see* Madsbad, 1983).

Individuals with non-insulin-dependent diabetes have functional β cells, as evidenced by the presence of both immunoreactive insulin and C-peptide in plasma. However, there are abnormalities in the initial secretion of insulin when stimulated by glucose, even in the mildest forms of the disease; these may consist in either increased or decreased secretion. Impaired β-cell function is also revealed by the fact that less insulin is secreted at any given glucose concentration in both diabetic subjects and those with latent disease. The defect may be in the glucose-sensing mechanisms of the β cell (*see* previous section). There is also resistance to insulin in patients in early stages of this form of diabetes. The relative importance of these pathophysiological factors is unclear (*see* DeFronzo and Ferrannini, 1982; Weir, 1982).

The secretory function of α cells of pancreatic islets is also compromised in diabetes mellitus. As mentioned, the mass of α cells is increased in non-insulin-dependent diabetes. Concentrations of immunoreactive glucagon in plasma are elevated in diabetic patients, particularly during ketoacidosis, and the normal suppression of plasma glucagon by hyperglycemia is impaired. Instead, glucagon concentrations may rise paradoxically in response to an oral glucose load, arginine, or a protein meal (Unger and Orci, 1981a, 1981b).

A vitally important and pathognomonic feature of diabetes mellitus is the capillary basement-membrane thickening that occurs early in the course of the disease. This pathological change may be responsible for the major vascular complications of diabetes, including premature atherosclerosis, intercapillary glomerulosclerosis, retinopathy, neuropathy, and ulceration and gangrene of the extremities. Early signs of abnormal vascular permeability are the appearance of immunologically detectable protein in the urine (Viberti *et al.*, in Symposium, 1983b) and increased permeability of retinal vessels to fluorescein (Baudoin *et al.* and Cunha-Vaz, in Symposium, 1983b). (For a recent review, *see* McMillan and Ditzel, in Symposium, 1983b.)

Of considerable interest is the fact that glucose or phosphorylated glucose is able to react covalently with the amino-terminal valine residue of hemoglobin to form a glucosylated protein; the major species that can be quantitated is termed hemoglobin A_1C. Since the rate of formation of hemoglobin A_1C is proportional to the concentration of glucose in blood and the half-life of the derivatized protein is long, its measurement is considered to provide an *integrated index* of the glycemic state and thus an estimate of the long-term effectiveness of the control of the blood glucose concentration. It has been suggested that the nerve lesions and cataracts that are characteristic of diabetes may be caused by the covalent reaction of glucose with endogenous proteins in nerve and crystalline lens, in a manner analogous to the reaction of the hexose with hemoglobin. It has also been hypothesized that the accumulation of sorbitol and resultant osmotic swelling are significant in the etiology of these lesions. Increased concentrations of sorbitol and decreased concentrations of inositol have been observed in sciatic nerve obtained post mortem from diabetic patients (Mayhew *et al.*, 1983). Inhibitors of aldose reductase are therefore being tested for their ability to prevent neuropathy and cataracts (Kikkawa *et al.*, 1983).

It is well established that insulin receptors are altered in diabetes. In general, the number of receptors for the hormone seems to be inversely related to the plasma insulin concentration, perhaps because insulin itself may be able to "down-regulate" the number of its own receptors. In obesity and in non-insulin-dependent diabetes there appears to be a decrease in the number of receptors associated with the hyperinsulinemia. In some rare cases of insulin-resistant diabetes associated with *acanthosis nigricans*, antibodies to the receptors are found, while in other cases the cause of the resistance is thought to be distal to the receptor and in the metabolic machinery of the cell (*see* Roth and Grunfeld, 1981).

Insulin Deficiency: How Insulin Corrects the Metabolic Aberrations of the Diabetic State. Diabetes mellitus due to inadequate insulin secretion by the β cells of the pancreas is characterized by hyperglycemia, hyperlipemia, ketonemia, and azoturia. When deficiency is severe, there may be *diabetic ketoacidosis*. The purpose of the following discussion is to explain these metabolic aberrations in terms of the effects of insulin and glucagon on various tissues and organs. The steps described refer to Figure 64–3.

Hyperglycemia. The hyperglycemia of insulin deficiency and glucagon excess is a consequence of underutilization and overproduction of glucose.

In the absence of insulin there is a marked reduction in the rate of transport of glucose across certain cell membranes. Lundsgaard (1939) first suggested that insulin acted to enhance glucose transport, and Levine and associates (1949) demonstrated that insulin increased the volume of distribution of galactose (which is not metabolized) in the nephrectomized, eviscerated dog. They reasoned that the hormone accelerates transport of certain hexoses, including glucose, across cell membranes (steps Muscle-① [M-①] and Adipocyte-① [A-①], Figure 64–3); the exclusion of glucose from the intracellular compartment by a relatively "impermeable" plasma membrane explained the underutilization of glucose in the diabetic state. However, it could also be explained as an effect on the rate of glucose phosphorylation, the obliga-

tory first step in metabolism. That insulin acts to increase transport of glucose independent of rate of phosphorylation was demonstrated in the isolated rat diaphragm preparation by Park and associates (1955). Normally the concentration of glucose is virtually zero within skeletal muscle cells in the presence or the absence of insulin. Once glucose enters the cell, it is quickly phosphorylated to glucose-6-phosphate (steps Liver-② [L-②], M-②, and A-②, Figure 64–3). Park and coworkers showed that at low temperatures, even though the conversion of glucose to glucose-6-phosphate was slowed, insulin clearly increased the transfer of glucose from the medium into the cells. Likewise, it can be shown that insulin accelerates the transfer of glucose into the fat cell, wherein it is transformed to fat or glycogen or oxidized to CO_2. It is now known that insulin acts to redistribute transport molecules for glucose such that there are more in the plasma membrane and less internally (Karnieli *et al.*, 1981; Kono *et al.*, 1982); this is a novel and interesting mechanism.

Obviously, underutilization of glucose is to an important degree the consequence of a reduced rate of entrance of the sugar into cells. Because of this inability to gain entrance to the metabolic machinery, the oxidation of glucose to CO_2 and its conversion to glycogen and fat are slowed. It is of practical importance to note that exercise increases the rate of transport of glucose into muscle cells, even in the absence of insulin. Vigorous exercise will induce hypoglycemia in the diabetic subject, and the dose and site of insulin injection must be adjusted accordingly. This response may be due to the release of bound insulin from the injection site or from within the muscle itself or its vasculature (Kemmer and Vranic, 1981).

Insulin does not influence the rate of transfer of glucose across all cell membranes. In insulin deficiency, transport of glucose into the hepatic cell (step L-①) is not significantly reduced; this is not a factor of importance in the development of the metabolic aberrations of the hepatic cell. In diabetes, rate of entry of glucose into the brain is unaffected and function of the nervous system remains normal unless a state

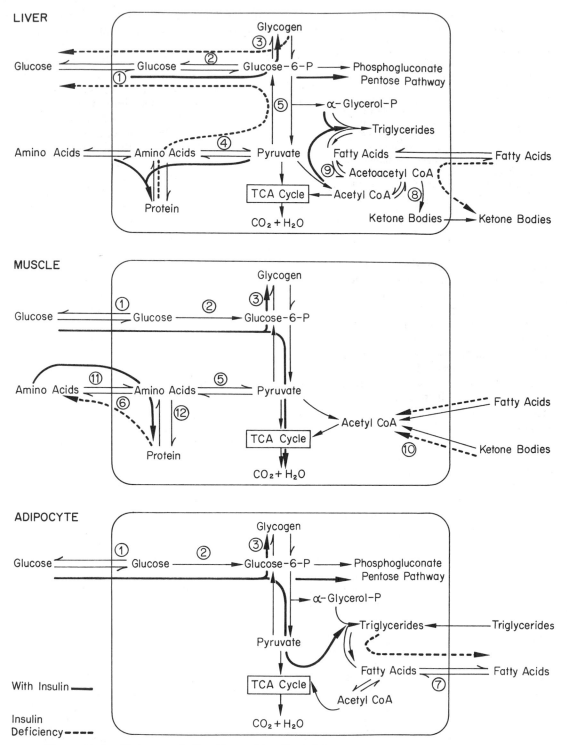

Figure 64–3. *Major metabolic effects of insulin deficiency.*

Thick solid arrows (——▶) show the pathways that are favored in the presence of insulin, while thick broken arrows (····▶) depict those that predominate when the action of the hormone is insufficient. (For explanation, *see* the text.)

of ketoacidosis develops. However, certain nuclei in the hypothalamus are sensitive to insulin (Szabo *et al.*, 1983), and the brain may contain the hormone or a similar molecule as well (Krieger, 1983). Erythrocytes, leukocytes, and cells of the renal medulla take up glucose at a rate designed to meet their needs quite independently of insulin. While a significant reduction in the rate of glucose oxidation characterizes diabetes, the reduction may not be dramatic in quantitative terms.

In the absence of insulin there is a marked reduction in the activity of the enzyme system that catalyzes the conversion of glucose to glycogen. Insulin added to isolated rat diaphragm or injected into the dog increases the activity of the enzyme (glycogen synthase) that is involved in the conversion of glucose to glycogen in skeletal muscle (step M-③), in liver (step L-③), and in the adipocyte (step A-③) (*see* Larner *et al.*, 1982).

In the absence of insulin there is an abnormally high rate of conversion of protein to glucose. In insulin deficiency the quantity of glucose excreted in the urine can far exceed the quantity ingested. One can immediately dismiss fat as a source of the excess glucose, since *net* production of glucose from fat cannot occur. However, proteins and amino acids are converted to glucose at an abnormally high rate when there is a deficiency of insulin and an excess of glucagon. The liver is the site of such conversion (steps L-④ and L-⑤). Protein and amino acids are mobilized from peripheral tissues (*see* the section on azoturia, below). For example, in muscle the branched-chain amino acids are oxidized to pyruvate, which is transaminated to alanine. This amino acid is released into the blood along with large amounts of glutamine. In Figure 64–3, a net loss of amino acid is shown for muscle (step M-⑥); the amino acids so mobilized in insulin deficiency are converted in the liver to glucose (steps L-④ and L-⑤) and to urea.

Hyperlipemia, Ketonemia, and Acidosis. The abnormally high concentration of free fatty acids in the plasma of the diabetic subject is due, in large measure, to their increased mobilization from the peripheral fat depots (step A-⑦). Insulin inhibits the hormone-sensitive lipase concerned with the mobilization of fatty acids, while glucagon, catecholamines, and other hormones enhance lipolysis. The marked hyperlipemia that characterizes the diabetic state may be regarded as a consequence of the uninhibited actions of lipolytic hormones on the fat depots. The antilipolytic and the antigluconeogenic effects of insulin are among the most potent actions of the hormone.

The source of the ketone bodies in the diabetic subject or the fasting normal subject is the liver (step L-⑧). In the absence of insulin, lipolysis, facilitated by various counterregulatory hormones, proceeds unchecked. The liver takes up large quantities of the free fatty acids thus liberated and oxidizes them to acetyl coenzyme A (CoA) (step L- 9). The reduced capacity of the insulin-deficient liver to synthesize fatty acids from acetyl CoA results in the increased diversion of this substrate to ketone bodies (acetone, acetoacetate, and β-hydroxybutyrate; step L-⑧), which appear in the blood in large quantities. Glucagon and perhaps other counterregulatory hormones appear to be necessary for ketone body formation in liver. Some of the ketone bodies are utilized as a source of energy by skeletal muscle, cardiac muscle, and other tissues (step M- ⑩).

The production of large amounts of acetoacetate and β-hydroxybutyrate, which are relatively strong acids, causes the acidosis of severe insulin deficiency. Urinary excretion of these anions is in part responsible for the loss of fixed cation and contributes to the depletion of electrolytes characteristic of diabetic ketoacidosis; the loss of potassium may be particularly severe and averages 5 mEq/kg of body weight in patients with ketoacidosis. Concentrations of potassium in plasma are not usually depressed, however, since intracellular potassium is exchanged for extracellular protons to compensate for the acidosis. Cations are also excreted in combination with phosphate and sulfate, which are lost in the urine in excessive quantities, and as a result of osmotic diuresis due to hyperglycemia.

Azoturia. Insulin deficiency and glucagon excess result in conversion of large amounts of protein to glucose with consequent increased production and excretion of urea and ammonia. Increased excretion of ammonia is a renal homeostatic mechanism stimulated by ketoacidosis. In the absence of insulin there is reduced movement of amino acids into muscle and possibly other cells (step M- ⑪) and reduced incorporation of amino acids into protein (step M- ⑫). Both effects are independent of glucose transport since they can be demonstrated *in vitro* in the absence of glucose in the medium. In insulin deficiency, amino acids do enter the hepatic cell, where they are deaminated and oxidized to yield pyruvate and contribute importantly to the hepatic overproduction of glucose. Hepatic gluconeogenesis from pyruvate and lactate is markedly accelerated by insulin deficiency. Furthermore, the protein catabolic actions of glucagon, adrenocorticosteroids, and thyroid hormones are unopposed in insulin deficiency, thus tilting the protein anabolic-catabolic balance toward catabolism.

Mechanism of Insulin Action.   While certain aspects of the action of insulin are rather well understood, much remains to be done to understand the mechanisms in molecular terms. In general, the actions of the hormone are to stimulate transport of metabolites and ions through cell membranes, biosynthesis of various molecules and macromolecules, and cell growth; this has been termed the pleiotypic response.

The cell-surface receptor for insulin has now been purified to homogeneity, a complementary DNA encoding the protein has been cloned and sequenced, and a model of the receptor is available (Czech and Massague, 1982; Ullrich *et al.*, 1985). The receptor contains two α subunits (molecular weight 125,000) and two β subunits (molecular weight 90,000), joined together by disulfide bonds. Upon addition of insulin and ATP to the receptor *in vitro*, the receptor becomes phosphorylated (apparently autocatalytically) on tyrosine residues of the β subunit. This mechanism is currently of widespread interest. Several products of viral oncogenes are closely related to and were presumably derived from receptors for cellular growth factors (*e.g.*, platelet-derived growth factor, epidermal growth factor); many of these proteins also have tyrosine kinase activity. Hypothetically, these receptors influence intracellular functions by phosphorylation of target proteins. The insulin receptor is also phosphorylated on serine and threonine residues *in vivo*.

Other hypotheses envision the generation of low-molecular-weight second messengers (perhaps peptides) when insulin binds to its receptors. While fractions containing such putative second messengers appear to have activities in broken-cell preparations that are consistent with the hypothesis,

none of these materials has been purified or identified (*see* Larner *et al.*, 1982). This type of mechanism and that involving phosphorylation by the receptor are not mutually exclusive.

The relationship of insulin action to cyclic nucleotide metabolism is of interest. Decreased intracellular concentrations of cyclic AMP (or, perhaps, increased concentrations of cyclic GMP) could explain some of the metabolic effects of insulin. While insulin can cause a lowering of the cyclic AMP concentration in some tissues, this has been observed convincingly only when cyclic AMP synthesis is first stimulated by counterregulatory hormones. Basal concentrations of the cyclic nucleotide are not demonstrably depressed when insulin acts alone. This has been the main argument against a direct relationship between the action of insulin and cyclic AMP. Insulin has been shown to stimulate specific cyclic nucleotide phosphodiesterases (Houslay *et al.*, 1984); it may also inhibit adenylate cyclase modestly.

As described in Chapter 4 (*see* Figure 4–6, page 89), glycogen synthesis and glycogenolysis are controlled by a cascading series of protein phosphorylation reactions. In the presence of cyclic AMP, a protein kinase is activated, and the eventual result is a stimulation of glycogen breakdown and an inhibition of glycogen synthesis. Insulin acts to tip the balance in the other direction—toward glycogen synthesis. The hormone appears to reduce the sensitivity of the protein kinase to cyclic AMP, in effect inhibiting the action of the cyclic nucleotide without the need to lower its concentration (Larner *et al.*, 1982). Glycogen synthase is activated, since a phosphoprotein phosphatase is less opposed and acts to dephosphorylate the enzyme (conversion of the D to the I form); indeed, the phosphatase may also be activated under certain conditions. By analogous mechanisms, the action of insulin results in dephosphorylation of phosphorylase and of a triglyceride lipase; the metabolic sequelae are inhibition of glycogenolysis and lipolysis, respectively.

Pyruvate dehydrogenase, an important mitochondrial enzyme, is also controlled by insulin (and other hormones) by phosphorylation and dephosphorylation reactions (*see* review by Reed *et al.*, 1980). The active form of the enzyme is the dephosphorylated one, and it is increased after insulin treatment by an unknown mechanism. As a result, pyruvate is oxidized or converted to fat and is unavailable for glucose formation. A similar control of acetyl CoA carboxylase by phosphorylation and dephosphorylation has been demonstrated (*see* Cohen, 1982).

In addition to the enhanced synthesis of fat, insulin increases the activity of membrane-bound lipoprotein lipase, which makes fatty acids derived from circulating lipoproteins available to the cell (*see* Steinberg, 1983).

In protein metabolism, insulin promotes amino acid uptake, enhances protein synthesis, and inhibits protein degradation. In general, the effects on protein synthesis have been localized to both transcriptional and translational events. Concentrations of specific mRNAs have been shown to be altered by insulin. For example, mRNAs for hepatic tyrosine aminotransferase and pancreatic amylase increase after administration of insulin; mRNA for hepatic phosphoenolpyruvate carboxykinase decreases. Evidence for translational control of protein synthesis by insulin includes enhancement of polyribosome formation and peptide chain initiation (Perisic and Traugh, 1983; *see also* Rosenfeld and Barrieux, 1979). Insulin may also inhibit intracellular degradation of proteins (Draznin and Trowbridge, 1982).

The capacity of insulin to enhance the transport of glucose into many types of cells is, of course, central to its physiological role. The effect of insulin on the facilitated diffusion of hexoses is to increase the maximal rate of transport; the results are thus consistent with the hypothesis that insulin in some way increases the total number of hexose "transporters" in the plasma membrane. This effect is independent of protein synthesis, and evidence suggests that the mechanism involves the recruitment of transporters from intracellular sites to the surface membrane (*see* Karnieli *et al.*, 1981; Kono *et al.*, 1981; Oka and Czech, 1984).

The action of insulin to promote K^+ uptake into cells, even in the absence of glucose, is classical; a similar effect on Mg^{2+} accumulation has also been demonstrated. Recently it has been shown that stimulation of K^+ uptake by insulin results from a stimulation of the Na^+,K^+-ATPase (Resh *et al.*, 1980). The ability of insulin to control membrane polarization and ion transport, particularly to activate Na^+,K^+-ATPase, has been reviewed by Moore (1983).

Insulin Unitage. Insulin preparations must be bioassayed as described above in order to ascertain their physiological activity. The assay described in the USP is based on the capacity of samples to lower the blood glucose concentration. The potency is expressed in USP units, and the standard of comparison is the USP *Insulin Reference Standard*. The potency of the reference-standard crystals is indicated on the label of each preparation. Newer, more pure preparations of the hormone (*see* below) have potencies of 26 to 30 units/mg.

Preparations. Significant advances and changes have been made in the United States and Europe in the purity and formulation of insulin preparations. These have resulted in the marketing of monospecies insulins (porcine, bovine, and human) of very high purity (*see* Home and Alberti, 1982; Karam and Etzwiler, in Symposium, 1983a). Human insulin is synthesized in *E. Coli* after genetic alteration of the bacteria by recombinant DNA technology.

As a result of a recommendation of the American Diabetes Association's Committee on the Use of Therapeutic Agents, U-40 and U-80 insulins (40 and 80 units/ml) are being eliminated in favor of a single U-100 dosage form for all types of insulin (*see* Committee, 1972). The objective is to reduce the chance of patient error, which is greater with the multiple dosage forms and dually calibrated syringes than with a single dosage form. Concentrated preparations of regular insulin (U-500) are

available for patients who are resistant to the hormone (*see* below).

Prior to 1973, insulin preparations available for therapeutic use contained, as potentially antigenic components, significant amounts of proinsulin and its incompletely converted products as well as other pancreatic hormones. New procedures have been devised to prepare purer preparations of the hormone. Two such preparations are "single-peak" insulin and "single-component" insulin; the latter is designated as "purified." The purity of commercial insulin in the United States is now at least that of "single-peak" insulin (99%). "Purified" insulins contain not more than 10 parts per million of proinsulin, and "purified" porcine insulin is the least immunogenic of the nonhuman insulins available. All new patients should be started on highly purified porcine or human insulin; the choice between the two is not a clear one.

All regular insulin preparations in the United States are now supplied at neutral pH. This has resulted in improved stability of the hormone, and patients need no longer refrigerate the vial of insulin in use. However, excessive heat and sunlight should be avoided. Furthermore, neutral regular insulin can be mixed in any desired proportion with other, modified insulin preparations since all marketed insulin preparations will be at the same pH.

Preparations of insulin are divided into three categories according to promptness, duration, and intensity of action following subcutaneous administration. They are classified as fast-, intermediate-, and long-acting types (*see* Table 64–1). However, it is recognized that a particular insulin preparation can show wide variations of activity in a population of patients and even in a single individual, especially one with labile diabetes. Crystalline insulin is prepared by the precipitation of the hormone in the presence of zinc (as zinc chloride) in a suitable buffer medium. Crystalline insulin when dissolved in water is known as *insulin injection* or regular insulin. Following subcutaneous injection it is rapidly absorbed; action is prompt in onset and relatively short in duration.

By permitting insulin and zinc to react with the basic protein protamine, Hagedorn and associates (1936) prepared a protein complex, *protamine zinc insulin*. When the complex is injected subcutaneously in an aqueous suspension, it dissolves only slowly at the site of deposition, and the insulin is absorbed at a retarded but steady rate.

Isophane insulin suspension is also known as NPH insulin; the *N* denotes a neutral solution (pH 7.2), the *P* refers to the protamine zinc insulin content, the *H* signifies the origin in Hagedorn's laboratory. It is a modified protamine zinc insulin suspension that is crystalline. The concentrations of insulin, protamine, and zinc are so arranged that the preparation has an onset and a duration of action intermediate between those of regular insulin and protamine zinc insulin suspension. Its effects on blood sugar are indistinguishable from those of an extemporaneous mixture of 2 to 3 units of regular insulin and 1 unit of protamine zinc insulin suspension.

Chemical studies revealed that the solubility of

insulin is determined in important measure by its physical state (amorphous, crystalline, size of the crystals) and by the zinc content and the nature of the buffer in which it is suspended. Insulin can thus be prepared in a slowly absorbed, slow-acting form without the use of other proteins, such as protamine, to bind it. Large crystals of insulin with high zinc content, when collected and resuspended in a solution of sodium acetate–sodium chloride (pH 7.2 to 7.5), are slowly absorbed after subcutaneous injection and exert an action of long duration. This preparation is named *extended insulin zinc suspension* (ULTRALENTE insulin). Amorphous insulin precipitated at high pH is almost as rapid in onset and somewhat longer in duration of action than regular insulin. The preparation is named *prompt insulin zinc suspension* (SEMILENTE insulin). The two forms of insulin may be mixed to yield a stable mixture of crystalline (7 parts) and amorphous (3 parts) insulin—*insulin zinc suspension* (LENTE insulin)— that is intermediate in onset and duration of action between SEMILENTE and ULTRALENTE preparations and is similar to NPH insulin.

The properties of the various insulin preparations are presented in Table 64–1. All preparations are usually given by subcutaneous injection. *Only insulin injection can be given by the intravenous or intramuscular route*. The insulins are marketed in 10-ml vials.

Hypoglycemia Associated with Hyperinsulinism. Hypoglycemic reactions may occur in any diabetic subject treated with insulin or with an oral hypoglycemic agent. Reactions are seen frequently in the labile form of the disease, a form characterized by unpredictable spontaneous reductions in insulin requirement. In other instances, precipitating causes are usually responsible, for example, failure to eat, unaccustomed exercise, and inadvertent administration of too large a dose of insulin.

The reaction pattern associated with hypoglycemia has been fully described in connection with insulin shock therapy for schizophrenia (long since outmoded) and in carefully controlled clinical studies in normal and diabetic volunteers. The pattern

Table 64–1. PROPERTIES OF VARIOUS PREPARATIONS OF INSULIN

TYPE	PREPARATION *	APPEARANCE	PROTEIN MODIFIER	APPROX-IMATE TIME OF ONSET † (*hours*)	APPROX-IMATE DURA-TION OF ACTION † (*hours*)	COMPATIBLE MIXED WITH
Fast-Acting	*Insulin Injection* "Insulin made from zinc-insulin crystals" (regular insulin)	Clear solution	None	1	8	All preparations
	Prompt Insulin Zinc Suspension (SEMILENTE insulin)	Cloudy suspension	None	1	14	LENTE preparations
Intermediate-Acting	*Isophane Insulin Suspension* (NPH insulin, isophane insulin)	Cloudy suspension	Protamine	2	24	Insulin injection
	Insulin Zinc Suspension (LENTE insulin)	Cloudy suspension	None	2	24	Insulin injection, SEMILENTE
Long-Acting	*Protamine Zinc Insulin Suspension*	Cloudy suspension	Protamine	4	36	Insulin injection
	Extended Insulin Zinc Suspension (ULTRALENTE insulin)	Cloudy suspension	None	4	36	Insulin injection, SEMILENTE

* Most preparations are available as either porcine or bovine insulin. Human insulin (recombinant DNA origin) is available as regular and isophane insulins and as insulin zinc suspension.

† These figures are representative. The values may be expected to vary over a relatively wide range, depending on the dose and the individual patient. For example, the duration of action of regular insulin is up to 16 hours in some patients.

and the temporal sequence of signs and symptoms are fairly, but by no means absolutely, constant. When the rate of fall in blood glucose is rapid, the early symptoms are those brought on by the compensating secretion of epinephrine; these include sweating, weakness, hunger, tachycardia, and "inner trembling." When the concentration of glucose falls slowly, the symptoms and signs are referable to the brain and include headache, blurred vision, diplopia, mental confusion, incoherent speech, coma, and convulsions. If the fall in blood glucose is rapid, profound, and persistent, all such symptoms may be present. In only a few patients, the onset is heralded by hunger or nausea; bradycardia and mild hypotension may occur in association with the gastrointestinal discomfort.

From a practical point of view, about half of the patients may be expected to call for help; nevertheless, another large fraction will not, presumably because of the confusion attending hypoglycemia or because the reaction may occur during sleep. Fortunately, the patients who have neither signs nor symptoms preceding convulsions and coma are few in number, but they present one of the most difficult problems in the management of diabetes.

The majority of the signs and symptoms of insulin hypoglycemia are the result of functional abnormalities of the CNS, since hypoglycemia deprives the brain of the substrate (glucose) upon which it is almost exclusively dependent for its oxidative metabolism. During insulin coma, oxygen consumption in human brain decreases by nearly half. The reduction in glucose consumption is disproportionately greater, which indicates that the brain is utilizing other substrates. After prolonged fasting in man the brain adapts, and the bulk of the fuel utilized is made up of ketone bodies.

A prolonged period of hypoglycemia causes irreversible damage to the brain, as evidenced in experimental animals by histological changes in the cortex, basal ganglia, and rostral parts of the medulla. There are isolated reports of neurological or mental changes in man following insulin-induced convulsions and coma, including mental retardation, hemiparesis, ataxia,

incontinence, aphasia, choreiform movements, parkinsonism, and epilepsy.

Although the signs and the symptoms of insulin hypoglycemia seem well defined, it is often difficult clinically to distinguish this condition from severe diabetic ketoacidosis (diabetic coma). Unfortunately, many cases of insulin coma have been treated with insulin. The symptoms of hypoglycemia yield almost immediately to the intravenous injection of glucose unless hypoglycemia has been sufficiently prolonged to induce organic changes in the brain. If the patient is not able to take soluble carbohydrate or fruit juice orally and if glucose is not available for intravenous injection, 0.5 to 1 mg of glucagon is given (*see* below). It is important to note that insulin-dependent diabetics who are also receiving β-adrenergic antagonists such as propranolol may have delayed recovery from hypoglycemic episodes; propranolol may also mask many of the signs and symptoms of hypoglycemia. β_1-Adrenergic antagonists are more selective and do not delay recovery from hypoglycemia or mask its signs and symptoms to the same degree as do nonselective antagonists (*see* Chapter 9).

Every diabetic patient taking insulin should carry an identification card or bracelet containing pertinent medical information; in addition, some form of glucose should be carried.

Other Adverse Reactions. Local or systemic allergic reactions are often seen in patients receiving insulin for the first time or when insulin treatment is reinstituted. The local reactions that result from skin sensitivity usually subside spontaneously. Allergic urticaria, angioedema, and anaphylactic reactions occur infrequently and usually can be avoided by changing to insulin obtained from a different species or by utilizing single-component insulin. Rarely, desensitization may be required; insulin-allergy desensitization kits are available (Wentworth *et al.*, 1976).

Patients may experience atrophy of subcutaneous fat at the site of injection (insulin lipoatrophy). Hypertrophy of fat may also occur but is less common. Lipoatrophy is rarely seen with the newer, more highly purified insulins (*see* Home and Alberti, 1982), and injection of these preparations directly into sites of lipoatrophy may facilitate reversal of the process.

Visual disturbances in uncontrolled diabetes that are due to refractive changes are reversed during the early treatment phase. However, since several weeks may be required to stabilize the osmotic equilibrium in the eye, alterations of prescriptions for corrective lenses should be postponed for 3 to 6 weeks. Peripheral edema may occur initially due to retention of sodium, but this disappears with continued administration of insulin.

ORAL HYPOGLYCEMIC AGENTS

History. In 1942, Janbon and coworkers discovered that a sulfonamide (*p*-aminobenzene-sulfonamido-isopropylthiadiazole) induced hypoglycemia. Janbon's colleague, Loubatières, then made the fundamental discovery that the compound exerted no hypoglycemic effect in the completely pancreatectomized animal and suggested that the action was the result of stimulation of the pancreas to secrete insulin. Subsequently, the compound *tolbutamide* was introduced, and it soon became popular for the management of certain diabetic patients. Tolbutamide is a member of the class of oral hypoglycemic agents designated as *sulfonylureas*.

SULFONYLUREAS

Chemistry. A number of sulfonylurea compounds exert hypoglycemic activity. The first-generation agents, *tolbutamide, acetohexamide, tolazamide,* and *chlorpropamide,* have the following structural formulas:

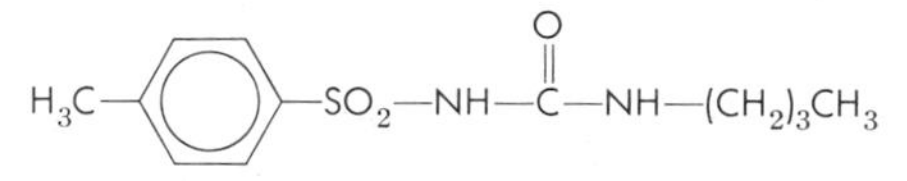

Tolbutamide

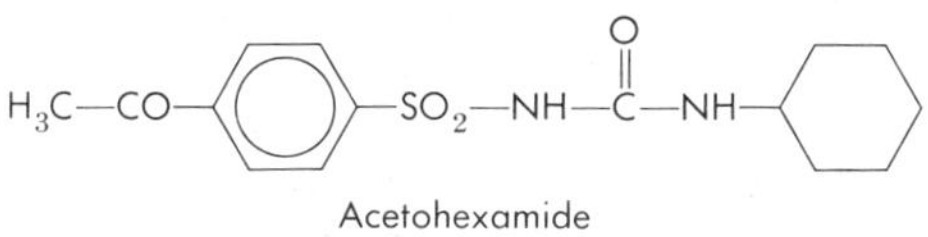

Acetohexamide

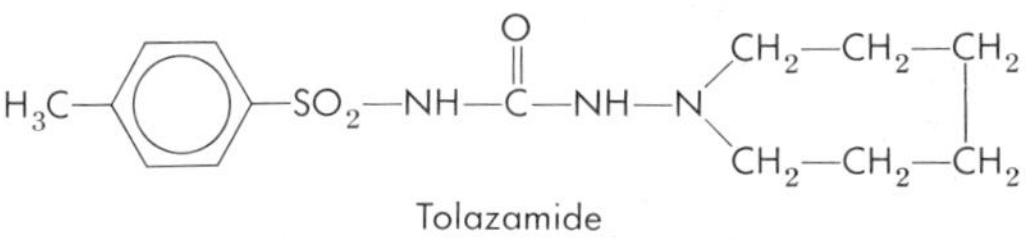

Tolazamide

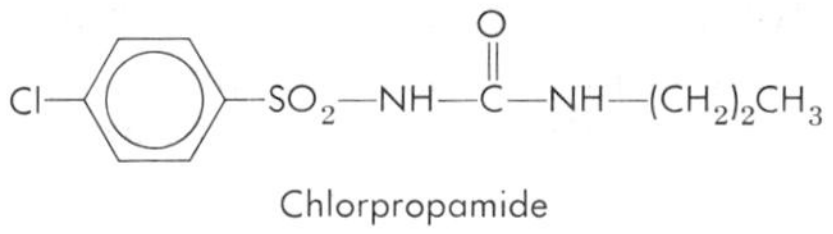

Chlorpropamide

Several members of a large second generation of sulfonylureas are currently in clinical trial. These agents are in general considerably more potent than the first-generation drugs. Two of these, *glyburide* and *glipizide,* have recently been approved for use in the United States. Their structural formulas are as follows:

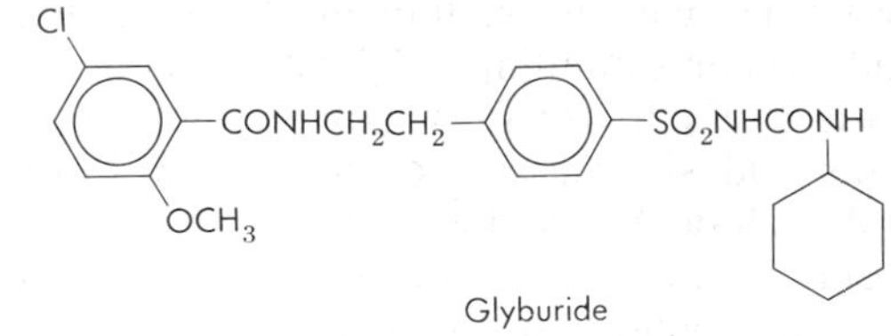

Glyburide

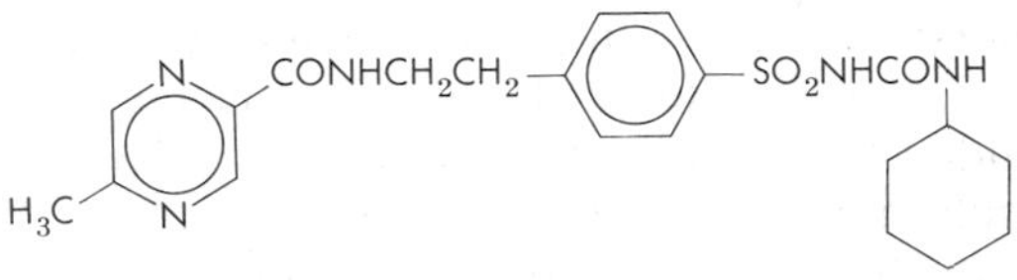

Glipizide

All the effective compounds are arylsulfonylureas with substitutions on the benzene and the urea groups.

Mechanism of Action. The sulfonylureas acutely stimulate the islet tissue to secrete insulin. The evidence, coming as it does from a variety of experimental and clinical studies, unequivocally supports such a conclusion. Administration of sulfonylureas increases the concentration of insulin in the pancreatic vein in cross-circulation experiments. Recipient animals, diabetic or nondiabetic, exhibit hypoglycemia in response to the infusion of pancreatic vein blood from donor animals treated with sulfonylureas but not to the infusion of mesenteric or femoral vein blood from the same animals. Sulfonylureas cause degranulation of the β cells, a phenomenon associated with increased rate of secretion of insulin. Clinical studies demonstrate that the sulfonylureas are ineffective in completely pancreatectomized patients and in insulin-dependent diabetic subjects. On the other hand, they are effective in non-insulin-dependent diabetic patients in whom the pancreas retains the capacity to secrete insulin.

However, an impressive number of studies have now shown that during chronic administration, a significant portion of the hypoglycemic action of the sulfonylureas may be due to extrapancreatic actions. Insulin biosynthesis may actually decrease, and peripheral tissues become more sensitive to a fixed dose of administered hormone, due, possibly, to an increase in the number of insulin receptors (Lebovitz and Feinglos, in *Symposium*, 1983c) or to changes in events subsequent to insulin binding (Lockwood *et al.*, in *Symposium*, 1983d). Extrapancreatic effects of the sulfonylureas have been noted in various organs, including liver, fat, and muscle, and certain of these may potentiate the effects of insulin.

Although the molecular mechanism of action of the sulfonylureas is not understood, pertinent observations have been made. The evoked release of insulin from the pancreas is immediate and is intimately related to the action of glucose, to which the drug may sensitize the β cell (Judzewitsch *et al.*, 1982). Sulfonylureas appear to stimulate Ca^{2+} influx into islet cells (Lebrun *et al.*, 1982). There may be some effect of sulfonylureas on adrenergic control of insulin secretion, since these agents can inhibit the release of catecholamines (Hsu *et al.*, 1975). Sulfonylureas may also increase concentrations of cyclic AMP in pancreatic islets (Jackson and Bressler, 1981a).

In experimental animals and in diabetic patients, conflicting results have been obtained on the effects of sulfonylureas on plasma concentrations of glucagon. Samols and Harrison (1978) have suggested that tolbutamide can enhance glucagon secretion from the α cell, although this may be masked by the effect of the sulfonylurea to stimulate the secretion of insulin. Local actions of insulin within the islet may cause a reduction in the secretion of glucagon; the net effect could be either stimulation or suppression of glucagon secretion.

Duration of Action, Fate, and Excretion. The sulfonylureas are readily absorbed from the gastrointestinal tract. The most important difference among the sulfonylureas, for clinical purposes, is in their duration of action. In increasing order they are tolbutamide; acetohexamide; tolazamide, equal to glipizide and glyburide; and chlorpropamide.

Tolbutamide can be detected in the blood within 30 minutes after oral administration; peak concentrations are reached within 3 to 5 hours. The drug is bound to plasma proteins. Tolbutamide is oxidized in the body to butyl-*p*-carboxyphenylsulfonylurea, which is a major excretory product. The half-life of tolbutamide is about 6 hours. Two or occasionally three doses are required daily.

Acetohexamide is rapidly absorbed, and maximal hypoglycemic activity is observed about 3 hours after ingestion. The total duration of action is 12 to 24 hours. Much of the activity is ascribable to a metabolite, *hydroxyhexamide*, which has a plasma half-life of about 6 hours; the parent compound,

acetohexamide, has a plasma half-life of 1.3 hours. In persons with normal renal and hepatic function, more than 80% is excreted, largely as metabolites, in 24 hours. Two doses are usually required daily.

Tolazamide is slowly absorbed; the onset of hypoglycemic action occurs at 4 to 6 hours and persists at a significant level up to 15 hours after a single dose. Tolazamide is metabolized in the liver to a number of weakly hypoglycemic substances that are largely excreted by the kidney. For most patients controlled by tolazamide, a single daily dose is sufficient; a few patients require administration of the drug twice daily.

Glipizide is absorbed rapidly, and peak concentrations in plasma occur within 1 to 3 hours after an oral dose. Glipizide is 98 to 99% bound to plasma proteins. It is extensively metabolized in the liver, primarily to inactive hydroxylated derivates; these are excreted by the kidney, largely as conjugates. The half-life of glipizide in plasma is approximately 2 to 4 hours, but its hypoglycemic effects may persist for up to 24 hours; some patients can thus be maintained on a single daily dose. The basis of the discrepancy between the half-life of glipizide and its apparent duration of action has not been explained.

Glyburide is absorbed relatively rapidly, and peak concentrations in plasma are detected in 4 hours. As with other sulfonylureas, glyburide is extensively bound to plasma proteins. The drug is excreted as metabolites to an equal extent in the bile and urine. The half-life of glyburide in plasma is about 10 hours, and hypoglycemic effects persist for 24 hours; it is thus usually given once daily. Glyburide is 200 times more potent than tolbutamide.

Chlorpropamide is also rapidly absorbed from the gastrointestinal tract and is bound to plasma proteins. Chlorpropamide is extensively metabolized in the liver, and metabolites are excreted together with unchanged drug (*see* Jackson and Bressler, 1981a). The half-life of a single dose is about 33 hours, but the value can vary considerably depending on urinary pH (*see* Appendix II). Concentrations in blood may not be expected to reach a plateau before 5 to 6 days. Chlorpropamide is administered in a single daily dose.

Toxicity. O'Donovan (1959) analyzed the incidence of side effects to *tolbutamide* in 9168 cases. The total incidence of side effects was 3.2%; the drug was withdrawn in 1.5% of the patients. The reactions have been classified as hematological (0.24%), cutaneous (1.1%), and gastrointestinal (1.4%). Of the 22 subjects exhibiting hematological abnormalities, 19 had a transient leukopenia; in 9 instances, the leukocyte count returned to normal despite continuation of the drug. Paresthesia, tinnitus, and headache may also occur. Tolbutamide can cause a reduction in iodide uptake by the thyroid; hypothyroidism or goiter has not been observed.

The total incidence of untoward reactions is about 6% for *chlorpropamide* (hematological, 0.6; cutaneous, 3; gastrointestinal, 2; and jaundice, 0.4%). The jaundice is of the cholestatic type and is usually transient. Hyponatremia occurs in a small number of patients treated with tolbutamide and chlorpropamide. Inappropriate secretion of antidiuretic hormone has been observed, and chlorpropamide potentiates the renal tubular effects of the hormone.

The frequency and the kinds of toxic reactions produced by *acetohexamide* and *tolazamide* are similar to those encountered with tolbutamide and chlorpropamide. Hematological (leukopenia, agranulocytosis, thrombocytopenia, pancytopenia, and hemolytic anemia), cutaneous (rashes, photosensitivity), gastrointestinal (nausea, vomiting, rarely hemorrhage), and hepatic (increased serum alkaline phosphatase, cholestatic jaundice) reactions have been reported. While experience with *glyburide* and *glipizide* is limited, the incidence of adverse effects observed with their use has been no greater than with the other agents.

Any of the sulfonylureas may cause hypoglycemic reactions, including coma (Seltzer, 1979; *see also* Jackson and Bressler, 1981b). While they are usually not severe, several fatalities have been reported. Hypoglycemic episodes may last for several days so that prolonged or repeated glucose administration is required. Reactions have occurred after one dose, after several days of treatment, or after months of drug administration. Most reactions are observed in patients over 50 years of age, and they are more likely to occur in patients with impaired hepatic or renal function. Overdosage or inadequate or irregular food intake may initiate hypoglycemia. Drugs that may increase the risk of hypoglycemia from sulfonylureas include other hypoglycemic agents, sulfonamides, propranolol, salicylates, clofibrate, phenylbutazone, probenecid, dicumarol, chloramphenicol, monoamine oxidase inhibitors, and alcohol.

Sulfonylureas should not be used in a patient with hepatic or renal insufficiency because of the important role of the liver in their metabolism and of the kidney in the excretion of the drugs and their metabolites. Intolerance to alcohol reminiscent of the disulfiram reaction, with flushing, palpitations, and nausea, occurs occasionally in patients taking sulfonylureas.

These agents are also not recommended for use in pregnancy, but only sparse data have been reported on this point. Teratogenesis in animals has been observed to follow the administration of large doses.

A cooperative clinical trial in 12 university-based clinics (University Group Diabetes Program; UGDP) was established in 1961 to determine if the control of blood glucose concentration helps to prevent or delay vascular disease in non-insulin-dependent diabetic patients. During a period of over 8 years of observation, there were 120 deaths, including 87 from cardiovascular causes; while 10 to 12 cardiovascular deaths occurred in each of the placebo or insulin-treated groups, 26 such deaths (a significantly higher number) were recorded among the patients in each group taking oral hypoglycemic agents. The overall mortality rate was correspondingly higher in this group of diabetic patients. (*See* University Group Diabetes Program, 1982.)

During the decade that followed the appearance of the initial UGDP report, a flood of comments and reports appeared, both critical and supportive of the study. In response to this, at the instigation of the Director of the National Institutes of Health, the Biometric Society appointed a committee to review the UGDP report. The committee concluded that the shortcomings of the study do not invalidate its observations and conclusions. (*See* Chalmers, 1975; Report of the Committee, 1975.) Despite this, debate has continued, fueled more recently by some opportunities to review the original data and patient records. These have revealed deficiencies in patient compliance and selection, among other problems, and have prompted the American Diabetes Association to withdraw its endorsement of the UGDP study. (*See* Feinstein, 1976; Kilo *et al.*, 1979; Kolata, 1979.)

Throughout the controversy, many physicians have maintained an invariant approach to the use of oral hypoglycemic agents, based on cogent arguments. Despite uncertainties about the incidence of serious toxicity caused by these drugs, there *never* has been any proof that their use is beneficial in the prevention of the long-term complications of diabetes. They are capable of controlling mild hyperglycemia and its associated signs and symptoms, but there are more conservative and rational approaches to the management of these problems. Furthermore, if rigorous control of hyperglycemia is proven to be worthwhile for the prevention of long-term complications of diabetes, dietary management and the administration of insulin, as necessary, are more effective. It is thus possible to formulate recommendations for the appropriate therapeutic use of these drugs (*see* below).

Preparations and Dosage. *Tolbutamide* (ORAMIDE, ORINASE) is marketed in the form of 250- and 500-mg tablets. *Acetohexamide* (DYMELOR), is available in 250- and 500-mg tablets. *Tolazamide* (TOLINASE) is supplied in 100-, 250-, and 500-mg tablets. *Chlorpropamide* (DIABINESE) is marketed as 100- and 250-mg tablets. *Glyburide* (DIABETA, MICRONASE) is available in 1.25-, 2.5-, and 5-mg tablets. *Glipizide* (GLUCOTROL) is marketed as 5- and 10-mg tablets.

The usual daily dose of tolbutamide is 1000 mg, while 3000 mg is the maximally effective total dose; corresponding dosages are 500 and 1500 mg for acetohexamide. Tolazamide and chlorpropamide are usually administered in a daily dosage of 250 mg, while 750 to 1000 mg is maximal. The initial daily dose of glyburide is 2.5 to 5 mg, while daily doses of more than 20 mg are not recommended. Therapy with glipizide is usually initiated with 5 mg, given once daily. The maximal recommended daily dose is 40 mg; daily doses of more than 15 mg are usually divided. Treatment with the sulfonylureas must be guided by the individual patient's response, which must be monitored frequently (*see* Lebovitz, in Symposium, 1983c).

Therapeutic Uses. *The sulfonylureas should be used only in patients with diabetes of the non-insulin-dependent type who cannot be treated with diet alone and who are unwilling or unable to take insulin if weight reduction and dietary control fail.* The physician must realize that he is most likely using these agents only to control symptoms associated with hyperglycemia, and that dietary control and exercise with or without insulin is more effective for this purpose. There is no evidence that the oral hypoglycemic agents prevent cardiovascular complications from diabetes, and the best data available, even though controversial, suggest that the incidence of such complications may be increased in patients taking these drugs.

In general, the likelihood of adequate control with an oral hypoglycemic agent is inversely proportional to the dose of insulin required to maintain the patient. When the insulin requirement is in excess of 40 units per day, the chances of success are relatively low. The sulfonylureas are of no value in the insulin-dependent type of diabetes, in which the pancreas has lost all or nearly all of its capacity to secrete insulin. *Such patients require insulin, and attempts to control them with oral therapy are dangerous and doomed to failure.* Deaths from acidosis and dehydration have occurred in patients with unstable ketotic diabetes in whom regulation was attempted with sulfonylureas.

Stimulation of the pancreas of the non-insulin-dependent diabetic can often maintain these subjects under ordinary circumstances. However, when insulin requirements are increased, as in fever, surgical interventions, or trauma, the sulfonylureas are inadequate and the patient must be given insulin.

Weight reduction, dietary therapy, exercise, and education are of the greatest importance in the treatment of diabetes. A vigorous effort must be made by the patient and the physician to reduce the patient's weight to an acceptable level as an integral part of diabetic treatment, irrespective of the drug chosen.

Patients whose diabetes is not controlled by sulfonylureas from the initiation of treatment are said to experience "primary failure." Patients whose diabetes is regulated for a month or more after beginning sulfonylurea treatment, following which inability to maintain control develops, are said to experience "secondary failure." The incidence of this type of failure may be high, regardless of the agent chosen.

TREATMENT OF DIABETES MELLITUS

The Ambulatory Patient. The objectives of therapy are maintenance of health and a symptom-free, productively active life. These are attained by attention to diet, body weight, and activity and, if necessary, by the use of insulin. Inability to use insulin in a given patient with non-insulin-dependent diabetes may necessitate the administration of an oral hypoglycemic agent.

Insulin is required for control of diabetes in most persons in whom the disease has its onset before attainment of adult stature (insulin-dependent diabetes), in most underweight persons in whom it appears after cessation of growth, and in pregnant women whose disorder is not controlled by diet. Insulin will be temporarily required in the treatment of ketoacidosis in the obese patient whose diabetes is otherwise controlled by dietary regulation with or without an oral hypoglycemic agent. Insulin is effective in all forms of diabetes. It is the only effective agent for severe manifestations of diabetes and should be used when these are present or threatened, for example, during surgery or infection or following vascular occlusions, irrespective of previous therapy.

Most patients with onset of diabetes in middle or late life are obese. *A serious effort should be made to regulate their diabetes by diet and weight reduction alone.* In doing so, it is important to avoid confusing weight loss resulting from restricted caloric intake with that resulting from uncontrolled diabetes. Programs of graded physical exercise and education are also important. Weight, glycosuria, and requirement for insulin or oral hypoglycemic agent should diminish.

Insulin therapy can be satisfactorily initiated on an ambulatory basis in an asymptomatic or mildly symptomatic patient with newly discovered diabetes. However, a short period of hospitalization offers superior opportunities for accurate evaluation of the patient, for the rapid attainment of control, and for education of the patient and his family.

A conventional program for treatment of a diabetic patient with insulin is as follows. Urine should be collected from bedtime to breakfast, from breakfast to lunch, from lunch to supper, and from supper to bedtime. A diet calculated for the patient's needs is begun. Many physicians prefer to use regular insulin in multiple daily doses 20 minutes before meals and at bedtime for the first few days. The usual first dose of regular insulin in the nonketotic patient is 10 units. Subsequent doses are determined by the glycosuria, glycemia, and response to preceding doses. After control is achieved, a single dose of modified insulin given before breakfast may be substituted for multiple doses of regular insulin. The total dose of modified insulin is initially equal to 80% of the total daily dose of regular insulin. The basic ingredient of many regimens is an intermediate-acting preparation—isophane insulin suspension or insulin zinc suspension. By adjustment of dose, diet, and exercise, many patients with non-insulin-dependent diabetes can be satisfactorily regulated with a single prebreakfast injection of intermediate-acting insulin. In other patients, persistence of morning glycosuria, despite afternoon and evening aglycosuria, is an indication for addition of a fast-acting insulin (Table 64–1) to the program. In other patients, persistence of nocturnal glycosuria, despite afternoon and evening aglycosuria, is an indication for the addition of long-acting insulin—extended insulin zinc suspension or protamine zinc insulin suspension. A number of patients with severe, labile diabetes must receive supplementary injections of a fast-acting insulin, before meals or before bedtime. An alternative that is often effective is injection of intermediate-acting insulin in two doses, about three fourths of the total requirement before breakfast and the remainder before supper or before retiring.

Two methods for achieving so-called tight control of blood glucose concentrations have been advocated more recently. They rely on determinations of blood glucose concentrations by the patient with a portable reflectance meter. Insulin is given in multiple daily injections or with an open-loop portable pump. In general, multiple daily injections of insulin are with mixtures of intermediate- and short-acting insulin; programmable open-loop portable pumps deliver insulin at a continuous basal rate (about 1 unit per hour), together with boluses on demand at the times of meals (about 1 unit per 100 cal). A nationwide trial is currently underway in several centers to determine the effect of tight control on the progression of vascular complications of diabetes. However, deaths have resulted from the use of pumps, and the seriousness of hypoglycemic episodes has been brought into sharp focus (*see* Polonsky *et al.*, 1982; Unger, 1982). Such programs of tight control are best initiated in a hospital or an outpatient setting where goals of therapy can be set and where patients can be taught to determine blood glucose concentrations and make appropriate adjustments of the dose of insulin. The patient is able to learn to manage the disease in an enlightened fashion and can be motivated to achieve the best results by the fundamental knowledge that he or she is managing the disease. True normalization of blood glucose concentrations and reductions in hemoglobin A_1C concentrations have been achieved in many patients.

Diabetic Ketoacidosis. Diabetic ketoacidosis is a continuum, ranging in severity from slight ketonuria without readily detectable ketonemia (ketosis) to the syndrome of diabetic coma, which is characterized by glycosuria, hypovolemia, ketonuria, ketonemia, metabolic acidosis, and coma, and which may progress to circulatory collapse, anuria, and death. Representative treatment protocols for the more severe form of diabetic ketoacidosis are presented below, but the principles upon which these recommendations are based also govern the treatment of less severe forms of diabetic acidosis.

It is of paramount importance for the patient to be hospitalized and for the physician to remain with the patient until the crisis is past; an accurate running record of all medications, clinical observations, and laboratory tests is essential.

Traditional therapy of diabetic ketoacidosis has involved the administration of large doses of insulin, for example, 2 units/kg initially (divided intravenously and subcutaneously), followed by 1 unit/kg every 2 hours; this regimen is continued until the concentration of glucose in plasma approaches values of approximately 300 mg/dl. Such treatment results in concentrations of insulin in plasma of approximately 1000 microunits/ml, which are presumably far in excess of those usually required to produce a maximal biological response.

Doses of insulin in the range of 2 to 10 units per hour given by continuous intravenous infusion produce concentrations of the hormone in plasma that are nearly maximally effective (50 to 100 microunits/ml). When patients with diabetic ketoacidosis are treated with such doses of insulin, the plasma glucose concentration declines at a rate of approximately 75 to 100 mg/dl each hour and usually reaches values of 200 to 300 mg/dl in 4 to 6 hours. This rate is essentially the same as that achieved with higher doses of the hormone. The advantage of such regimens is that high concentrations of insulin do not persist in the plasma when administration is stopped; complications of hypoglycemia and hypokalemia are thus minimized (*see* Kreisberg, 1978; Burghen *et al.,* 1980).

While most patients with diabetic ketoacidosis respond to low-dose regimens, a few patients are resistant to insulin and require much higher doses. A rare patient may require thousands of units of insulin during the first few hours of treatment. The results of therapy must therefore be monitored carefully, no matter what the regimen, and the dosage of insulin adjusted to the needs of the individual patient.

Appropriate fluid therapy is an essential element in the successful treatment of ketoacidosis and should be started immediately. The first fluid administered to a patient with diabetic coma is usually 0.9% sodium chloride solution, approximately 1 liter for an adult. Subsequently, 0.45% sodium chloride solution is administered. Central venous pressure should be monitored in patients with congestive heart failure, renal insufficiency, or shock. In order to restore the volume of body fluids, most patients with diabetic coma will need to retain an amount of fluid approximating at least 5% of body weight. This should be largely achieved in the first 12 hours of treatment. In the presence of a brisk diuresis resulting from glycosuria, it may be necessary to give intravenous fluids at a rate of 20 ml or more per minute in order to achieve a satisfactory rate of rehydration. Observation of the central venous pressure, the hematocrit, and the cumulative hourly difference between fluid intake and urine volume permits avoidance of overhydration. Reduction in plasma glucose and ketone concentrations signals the need for reduction in the rate of administration of insulin. At this time 0.45% sodium chloride solution containing 5% glucose is administered. Patients who require exceptionally large doses of insulin for control of the critical phase of their acidosis are particularly subject to hypoglycemia for a day or more after the treatment of the critical phase of acidosis, even though insulin may have been completely withdrawn. It is better to tolerate mild glycosuria for 1 or 2 days following treatment of severe acidosis than to risk hypoglycemia.

The administration of alkali is usually not necessary in the treatment of diabetic acidosis (if the blood pH is above 7.1) and may lead to development of alkalosis as insulin corrects the ketoacidosis. However, severe acidosis justifies the adminis-tration of 50 mEq of sodium bicarbonate added to the 0.45% solution of sodium chloride.

Patients with diabetic ketoacidosis usually have a normal or moderately elevated plasma concentration of potassium on admission to the hospital, as a consequence of cellular buffering of metabolic acids. At the same time, there exists an intracellular depletion of potassium that may be of the order of hundreds of milliequivalents in patients with severe or prolonged acidosis (average 5 mEq/kg). During treatment, as the rate of production of ketoacids diminishes, as potassium moves from the extracellular space to the intracellular space under the influence of insulin, and as the patient is rehydrated, hypokalemia may develop, usually beginning after the fourth hour of therapy. When this occurs, there is danger of progressive flaccid paralysis, which may eventually involve muscles of respiration.

Potassium salts usually should not be administered until it is established that the urine flow is at least of the order of 1 ml per minute and that hyperkalemia is absent; otherwise, cardiotoxic concentrations of potassium can readily accumulate in the extracellular fluid. If these conditions are met, potassium chloride should be given. For adults, the administration of 10 mEq of potassium per hour (added to the saline infusion) is a reasonable initial regimen; higher rates of administration may be considered if hypokalemia is severe. The deficit of potassium can, in general, be replaced during the first 24 hours. If the patient is hypokalemic, *cautious* administration of potassium may be necessary despite oliguria.

Deficiency of phosphorus in diabetic ketoacidosis has been known for decades. As a result of such deficiency, there may be lowered concentrations of 2,3-diphosphoglycerate in erythrocytes, with consequent changes in the affinity of hemoglobin for oxygen (*see* Chapter 16). While replacement of phosphate has occasionally been advocated, its efficacy is not known. As with potassium, concentrations of phosphate in plasma may at first be nearly normal despite significant depletion of total stores of the anion. Concentrations in extracellular fluid appear to fall markedly during treatment of ketoacidosis (*see* Kreisberg, 1978). The deficit of phosphorus in ketoacidosis probably averages 1 mmol/kg of body weight. It is often replaced in part by the administration of potassium phosphate rather than potassium chloride. Data are needed to establish the value of this procedure.

After 6 to 8 hours of treatment, most patients are able to tolerate a liquid diet. In patients treated for uncomplicated ketoacidosis, the usual diet can be resumed in 24 hours. Modified insulin should not be given until the patient is eating regularly.

Hyperosmolar Coma. Hyperosmolar coma is a variant form of diabetic ketoacidosis, but it differs in several important respects. Whereas ketoacidosis almost invariably occurs in patients with insulin-dependent diabetes, hyperosmolar coma usually occurs in elderly and obese diabetic patients who often have only mild diabetes and who do not ordinarily require therapy with insulin. The reason for the absence of severe ketosis in hyperosmolar coma is not known with certainty; however, concentrations of insulin in plasma are low to normal in this type of diabetes and may be adequate to inhibit ketogenesis. Typically, infection or other stress causes a worsening of hyperglycemia, followed by glycosuria and osmotic diuresis. In the absence of hyperpnea, vomiting, and other signs of ketoacidosis, the diuresis may be unnoticed and proceed for several days, leading to severe dehydration and decreased renal blood flow. The urinary route for the disposal of glucose is then lost, and the concentration of glucose in plasma increases dramatically, often exceeding 1500 mg/dl; osmolality of the plasma is often greater than 350 mOsm per liter. Coma and death follow quickly unless vigorous treatment is begun. The general principles of treatment are the same as for ketoacidosis. However, it is important to recognize that dehydration is usually much more severe. The fluid deficit may be 8 to 12 liters. Although some patients with hyperosmolar coma appear to be very sensitive to insulin, treatment can be initiated with the same dosages employed for the management of ketoacidosis; concentrations of glucose and potassium in plasma should of course be monitored carefully. The incidence of hyperosmolar coma is probably as great as is that of ketoacidosis. Because of the age of the patient, severity of dehydration, and coincidental illness, the mortality rate is high.

Insulin Resistance. Traditionally, patients requiring more than 200 units of insulin daily were said to be insulin resistant. However, this figure is arbitrary and is undoubtedly too high, and resistance is now defined in terms of a state of relative tissue insensitivity to the action of insulin. A useful point of reference is the daily insulin requirement of pancreatectomized man, frequently as low as 30 units.

Insulin resistance can be acute or chronic. Acute insulin resistance is associated with surgical or other trauma, emotional disturbances, and many infections (especially staphylococcal). It is reasonable to postulate that increased blood concentrations of counterregulatory hormones (including glucagon, epinephrine, and adrenocortical hormones) in response to trauma, anxiety, and infection may be contributory. The treatment of acute insulin resistance is the treatment of the precipitating cause and the administration of large doses of insulin together with needed water and electrolytes.

Chronic insulin resistance is frequently, but not always, associated with large amounts of insulin-binding antibodies in plasma. The incidence of this problem should decline as the more highly purified porcine or human insulins are used more widely. Insulin resistance is a frequent feature of non-insulin-dependent diabetes, and it may be of etiological significance in this disease. Resistance occurs in insulin-dependent diabetes as well. Resistance often appears after resumption of insulin therapy following a period of discontinuance. Identifiable endocrine disturbances (acromegaly, adrenal hypercorticism, and pheochromocytoma) are rarely the cause of chronic insulin resistance and almost never the cause of extreme insulin resistance (daily insulin requirements in excess of 500 units). A rare

and readily recognizable condition associated with chronic insulin resistance is lipoatrophic diabetes, a disorder characterized by absence of normal body fat depots, hyperlipemia and cutaneous xanthomata, hepatomegaly, and cirrhosis, and by insulin-resistant, nonketotic diabetes mellitus (*see* Renold *et al.*, 1978). Other rare forms of chronic insulin resistance are associated with increased degradation of insulin, antibodies to insulin receptors, and postreceptor defects. Patients have also been described who secrete inactive insulins as a result of mutations in the gene for the hormone (Shoelson *et al.*, 1983; Haneda *et al.*, 1984). These are instances of "pseudoresistance," since tissues have been shown to respond normally to the administration of insulin.

In order to supply adequate insulin to those with chronic insulin resistance, it may be convenient to use the preparation containing 500 units/ml. Some patients may be selectively resistant to bovine insulin while remaining sensitive to porcine or human insulin. The insulin requirement may also be reduced if the patient is switched to a highly purified preparation (Home and Alberti, 1982). Chemical alterations have been made to diminish the antigenic properties of porcine insulin. One such modification is dealaninated porcine insulin, where the carboxy-terminal alanine of the B chain is selectively cleaved by enzymatic (carboxypeptidase) action; there is no loss in biological activity. Antibodies to mixed porcine-bovine insulin or to porcine insulin do not react with dealaninated porcine insulin. Sulfated bovine insulin has been used in animal studies and with some success to treat immunologically related insulin resistance (Davidson and DeBra, 1978; Nomura *et al.*, 1983). Sulfonylureas may also reduce the insulin requirement in some insulin-resistant patients.

GLUCAGON

History. Glucagon was discovered by Murlin and coworkers in 1923—2 years after the discovery of insulin. The contrast between the subsequent history of insulin and glucagon, each secreted by adjoining cells in the islets, could hardly be more striking. Because of its immediate therapeutic importance, insulin was well accepted as a hormone and hailed as a major medical advance. Glucagon was of little interest, its discoverers received little recognition, and the hormone was not purified extensively until over 30 years had passed.

Chemistry. Glucagon is a single-chain polypeptide with a molecular weight of nearly 3500. In contrast to insulin, it contains no cysteine and, consequently, no disulfide linkages; the sequence of its 29 amino acids was determined by Bromer and associates in 1956 (*see* Figure 64-4). Of interest is a striking structural analogy between glucagon and the hormone *secretin*, suggesting a common genetic origin. There is also homology with VIP and GIP; glucagon is thus a member of a family of hormones. The structure of human glucagon is identical to porcine and bovine glucagon and probably to

```
                    NH₂
                     |
H—His—Ser—Glu—Gly—Thr—Phe—Thr—Ser—Asp—Tyr—Ser—Lys—Tyr—Leu—Asp—

          NH₂              NH₂              NH₂
           |                |                |
Ser—Arg—Arg—Ala—Glu—Asp—Phe—Val—Glu—Tyr—Leu—Met—Asp—Thr—OH
```

Figure 64–4. *The structure of glucagon.*

the rat and rabbit hormone as well. Glucagon is synthesized *in vivo* as a prohormone with a molecular weight of about 18,000; this is converted to glucagon by a series of proteolytic steps. One of the intermediates is a polypeptide with 69 amino acid residues, termed *glicentin*. Glucagon itself is represented by residues 33 through 61 of glicentin. *Oxyntomodulin* (or enteroglucagon) is represented by residues 33 through 69, while *glicentin-related polypeptide* (GRPP; function unknown) is represented by residues 1 through 31. Glicentin is present in the gut, as well as in the outer rim of pancreatic α cells together with true glucagon (*see* Unger and Orci, 1981a).

Bioassay and Radioimmunoassay of Glucagon in Plasma. A number of bioassays for glucagon have been developed, based on the ability of the hormone to cause hyperglycemia *in vivo* or to stimulate cyclic AMP production, phosphorylase activity, or glucose production *in vitro*. With the advent of radioimmunoassay, this has become the most widely used method to determine the concentration of glucagon. A significant problem has been cross-reaction of antisera with related peptides from the gastrointestinal tract. Since it is now clear that pancreatic and gut glucagons differ chemically and biologically, it is of greatest importance to use specific antisera. The best current methodology yields values for basal plasma pancreatic glucagon concentrations in the range of 50 to 60 pg/ml.

Regulation of Glucagon Secretion. Glucagon secretion, like that of insulin, is controlled by the interplay of gastrointestinal food products and hormones. Glucose is the most potent and important regulator. A rise in plasma glucose concentration leads to an inhibition of glucagon secretion and *vice versa* (*see* Unger and Orci, 1981a, 1981b). As with insulin secretion, glucose given orally is a more effective signal than glucose administered intravenously. A gastrointestinal signal is thus suggested, and, although the evidence is not complete, secretin may play an inhibitory role. Other gut hormones, including gastrin, pancreozymin-cholecystokinin, and gastric inhibitory polypeptide, stimulate the secretion of glucagon. Both insulin and somatostatin inhibit the secretion of glucagon (*see* Figure 64–2). In experimental animals, free fatty acids of various chain lengths and ketones suppress glucagon secretion in a manner analogous to that of glucose; the effects are opposite to those on insulin secretion. A considerable portion of the effects of fuels, particularly glucose, is via their direct effect on the β cells; much of their effect on glucagon secretion is thus indirect.

Of the three primary energy sources, amino acids have a unique effect. Their administration leads to an immediate rise in the concentrations of *both* glucagon and insulin in plasma. It has been argued teleologically that the purpose is to promote gluconeogenesis in the liver. This sugar can then replace that which disappears from the plasma as a result of insulin secretion and action, thus preventing hypoglycemia. If sufficient glucose is administered with amino acids to prevent hypoglycemia, enhanced glucagon secretion is not observed. As in the case of glucose, oral amino acids appear to be more potent secretagogues for glucagon than do those given intravenously. The stimulatory gastrointestinal hormones listed above may again play an important role (*see* Unger and Orci, 1981a).

Glucagon secretion is also controlled by autonomic neural mechanisms; both sympathetic nerve stimulation and sympathomimetic amines, including levodopa, enhance the secretion of the hormone. Conflicting data have accumulated on the effects of acetylcholine, although a number of reports demonstrate an enhanced secretion (*see* Bloom, 1981). Glucagon secretion is also controlled by the CNS (*see* Palmer and Porte, 1981).

Of great importance is the role of relatively or absolutely increased concentrations of glucagon in both insulin-dependent and non-insulin-dependent diabetes. In insulin-dependent diabetes, there is an unrestrained secretion of glucagon due to a lack of suppression of secretion by hyperglycemia. This appears to be corrected by tight control and is thus not considered to be an inherent defect in the α cell (Unger and Orci, 1981b). In non-insulin-dependent diabetes, there is also hyperglucagonemia in the fasting state. It is not clear whether this is a primary defect in the α cell or if it is secondary to β-cell failure and hyperglycemia.

Distribution and Inactivation. Pancreatic glucagon circulating in plasma is the same as that extracted from the organ, although a fraction of the immunoreactive material in plasma is contained in a biologically inactive fraction of higher molecular weight (Von Schenck, 1981). Glucagon is extensively degraded in the liver and kidney, as well as in plasma, and at its tissue receptor sites in plasma membranes (Peterson *et al.*, 1982). Its half-life in plasma is approximately 3 to 6 minutes, which is similar to that of insulin. Enzymatic destruction of glucagon is by proteolysis, and the removal of the amino-terminal histidine leads to loss of biological activity. Cathepsin C inactivates the hormone, as does a proteolytic enzyme purified from rat skeletal muscle that acts on both insulin and glucagon (Duckworth and Kitabchi, 1981).

Physiological and Pharmacological Actions. The hormonal role of glucagon is now well established, and, in general, its actions are antagonistic to those of insulin. Insulin serves as a hormone of fuel storage, while glucagon serves as a hormone of fuel mobilization. Following a meal, β-cell secretion of insulin and suppression of α-cell secretion of glucagon serve to store fuels in liver, muscle, and adipose tissue. Conversely, during starvation, stimulation of glucagon secretion and suppression of insulin secretion direct the breakdown of fuels stored intracellularly to meet the energy needs of the brain and other tissues. A related role for glucagon as the hormone of injury and insult (catabolic illness) has been proposed. For example, impaired glucose tolerance and hyperglycemia noted with infection are associated with increased concentrations of plasma glucagon. Similar increases are seen in patients with myocardial infarctions, burns, and after major trauma (*see* Jaspan, 1981). Here, glucagon acts to stimulate gluconeogenesis and provide the glucose needed under conditions of insult (Jensen *et al.*, 1983).

The known actions of glucagon appear to result from stimulation of the synthesis of cyclic AMP. This is particularly true in liver and adipose tissue, and its metabolic effects at these sites are essentially the same as those of epinephrine (*see* Chapter 4). It is worth noting that studies of the mechanism of the hyperglycemic action of glucagon and epinephrine led to the discovery of cyclic AMP (Rall and Sutherland, 1958). In high concentrations, glucagon has a positive cardiac inotropic effect, also perhaps related to its ability to stimulate the synthesis of the cyclic nucleotide in the heart.

Glucagon is now known to affect motor, vascular, and secretory functions in the gastrointestinal tract. Of significance has been the discovery of the spasmolytic action of the hormone (*see* below). Recent studies have shown that the portion of the glucagon molecule represented by residues 1 to 21, which is not an activator of adenylate cyclase, can relax the guinea pig ileum (Diamant *et al.*, 1981). The mechanism for this effect is unknown. Glucagon is also known to inhibit gastric acid secretion (*see* Christiansen, 1981).

Therapeutic Use and Preparations. Glucagon is useful in the treatment of insulin-induced hypoglycemia when dextrose solution is not available. It may be given intravenously, intramuscularly, or subcutaneously in a dose of 1 mg. When it is given subcutaneously for hypoglycemic coma induced by either insulin or oral hypoglycemic agents, a return to consciousness should be observed within 20 minutes; otherwise, intravenous glucose must be administered as soon as possible. Failure of glucagon to relieve the coma may be due to irreversible brain damage as a consequence of prolonged hypoglycemia or due to marked depletion of glycogen stores in the liver. Nausea and vomiting have been the most frequent adverse effects.

Clinical investigations have been conducted to explore the use of large doses of glucagon in cardiac disorders as an inotropic and chronotropic agent. Unfortunately, it is not very effective. The hormone has also been used experimentally in the diagnosis and treatment of hypoglycemic disorders.

The major use of glucagon is to relax the intestinal tract for radiographic examination (*see* Miller and Chernish, 1981a, 1981b). It is also being used experimentally to treat a number of gastrointestinal disorders associated with spasm, including acute diverticulitis, disorders of the sphincter of Oddi and biliary tract, and impaction of the esophagus. It has not proven useful in intussusception (Franken *et al.*, 1983) or in acute pancreatitis (Debas *et al.*, 1980). Its administration does provide a worthwhile test to distinguish obstructive from hepatocellular jaundice (Berstock *et al.*, 1982).

Glucagon for injection is dispensed as a dry powder of glucagon in 1- or 10-mg vials, packaged with sufficient diluent to make a 1-mg/ml solution.

Miscellaneous Hyperglycemic Agents. *Diazoxide,* a nondiuretic thiazide with antihypertensive activity (*see* Chapter 32), causes hyperglycemia. This effect is usually transitory (maximum of 8 hours) and is apparently due to both decreased insulin secretion and decreased peripheral utilization of glucose (*see* Henquin *et al.*, 1982). Diazoxide appears to exert α-adrenergic-like actions on the islet β cell and it also stimulates the release of endogenous catecholamines. Propranolol may potentiate the action of diazoxide, while α-adrenergic blocking agents and sulfonylureas can overcome its effect. The drug may be used to control hypoglycemia, including that caused by insulin-secreting islet-cell tumors (*see also* Chapter 55). *Diazoxide* (PROGLYCEM) is available in 50-mg capsules and in an oral suspension (50 mg/ml). The usual daily dose for adults and children is 3 to 8 mg/kg, divided into two or three equal portions; for neonates and infants, the usual daily dose is 8 to 15 mg/kg. Other agents that have been utilized experimentally to attempt to ameliorate hypoglycemia include *phenytoin, thiazide diuretics,* and *somatostatin.*

Asplin, C. M.; Paquette, T. L.; and Palmer, J. P. *In vivo* inhibition of glucagon secretion by paracrine β cell activity in man. *J. Clin. Invest.,* **1981,** *68,* 314–318.

Bailly, C.; Imbert-Teboul, M.; Chabardès, D.; Hus-Citharel, A.; Montègut, M.; Clique, A.; and Morel, F. The distal nephron of rat kidney: a target site for glucagon. *Proc. Natl Acad. Sci. U.S.A.*, **1980**, *77*, 3422–3424.

Banting, F. G.; Best, C. H.; Collip, J. B.; Campbell, W. R.; and Fletcher, A. A. Pancreatic extracts in the treatment of diabetes mellitus. *Can. Med. Assoc. J.*, **1922**, *12*, 141–146.

Berstock, D. A.; Wood, J. R.; and Williams, R. The glucagon test in obstructive and hepatocellular jaundice. *Postgrad. Med. J.*, **1982**, *58*, 485–486.

Bonner-Weir, S., and Orci, L. New perspectives on the microvasculature of the islets of Langerhans in the rat. *Diabetes*, **1982**, *31*, 883–889.

Burghen, G. A.; Etteldorf, J. N.; Fisher, J. N.; and Kitabchi, A. E. Comparison of high-dose and low-dose insulin by continuous intravenous infusion in the treatment of diabetic ketoacidosis in children. *Diabetes Care*, **1980**, *3*, 15–20.

Chalmers, T. C. Settling the UGDP controversy. *J.A.M.A.*, **1975**, *231*, 624–625.

Chan, S. J.; Keim, P.; and Steiner, D. F. Cell-free synthesis of rat preproinsulins: characterization and partial amino acid sequence determination. *Proc. Natl Acad. Sci. U.S.A.*, **1976**, *73*, 1964–1968.

Colca, J. R.; Brooks, C. L.; Landt, M.; and McDaniel, M. L. Correlation of Ca^{2+}- and calmodulin-dependent protein kinase activity with secretion of insulin from islets of Langerhans. *Biochem. J.*, **1983a**, *212*, 819–827.

Colca, J. R.; Kotagel, N.; Brooks, C. L.; Lacy, P. E.; Landt, M.; and McDaniel, M. L. Alloxan inhibition of Ca^{2+}- and calmodulin-dependent protein kinase activity in pancreatic islets. *J. Biol. Chem.*, **1983b**, *258*, 7260–7263.

Committee on the Use of Therapeutic Agents of the American Diabetes Association. U100 insulin: a new era in diabetes mellitus therapy. *Diabetes*, **1972**, *21*, 832.

Davidson, J. K., and DeBra, D. W. Immunologic insulin resistance. *Diabetes*, **1978**, *27*, 307–318.

Debas, H. T.; Hancock, R. J.; Soon-Shiong, P.; Smythe, H. A.; and Cassim, M. M. Glucagon therapy in acute pancreatitis: prospective randomized double-blind study. *Can. J. Surg.*, **1980**, *23*, 578–580.

Docherty, K.; Carroll, R. J.; and Steiner, D. F. Conversion of proinsulin to insulin: involvement of a 31,500 molecular weight thiol protease. *Proc. Natl Acad. Sci. U.S.A.*, **1982**, *79*, 4613–4617.

Draznin, B., and Trowbridge, M. Inhibition of intracellular proteolysis by insulin in isolated rat hepatocytes. *J. Biol. Chem.*, **1982**, *257*, 11988–11993.

Duckworth, W. C.; Runyan, K. R.; Wright, R. K.; Halban, P. A.; and Solomon, S. S. Insulin degradation by hepatocytes in primary culture. *Endocrinology*, **1981**, *108*, 1142–1147.

Fabiano de Bruno, L.; Karabatas, L.; Cresto, J. C.; Aparicio, M.; and Basabe, J. C. A comparative study of two insulin secretion inhibitors: somatostatin and diazoxide. *Horm. Metab. Res.*, **1982**, *14*, 351–356.

Feinstein, A. R. Clinical biostatistic 36. The persistent biometric problems of the UGDP study. *Clin. Pharmacol. Ther.*, **1976**, *19*, 472–485.

Franken, E. A.; Smith, W. L.; Chernish, S. M.; Campbell, J. B.; Fletcher, B. D.; and Goldman, H. S. The use of glucagon in hydrostatic reduction of intussusception: a double-blind study of 30 patients. *Radiology*, **1983**, *146*, 687–689.

Gold, G.; Gishizky, M. L.; and Grodsky, G. M. Evidence that glucose "marks" β cells resulting in preferential release of newly synthesized insulin. *Science*, **1982**, *218*, 56–58.

Hagedorn, H. C.; Jensen, B. N.; Krarup, N. B.; and Wodstrup, I. Protamine insulinate. *J.A.M.A.*, **1936**, *106*, 177–180.

Haneda, M., and others. Familial hyperinsulinemia due to a structurally abnormal insulin. *N. Engl. J. Med.*, **1984**, *310*, 1288–1294.

Henquin, J. C.; Charles, S.; Nenquin, M.; Mathot, F.; and Tamagawa, T. Diazoxide and D600 inhibition of insulin release. *Diabetes*, **1982**, *31*, 776–783.

Honey, R. N., and Weir, G. Insulin stimulates somatostatin and inhibits glucagon secretion from the perfused chicken pancreas-duodenum. *Life Sci.*, **1979**, *24*, 1747–1750.

Houslay, M. D.; Wallace, A. V.; Marchmont, R. J.; Martin, B. R.; and Heyworth, C. M. Insulin controls intracellular cyclic AMP concentrations in hepatocytes by activating specific cyclic AMP phosphodiesterases: phosphorylation of the peripheral plasma membrane enzyme. *Adv. Cyclic Nucleotide Protein Phosphorylation Res.*, **1984**, *16*, 159–176.

Hsu, C.-Y.; Brooker, G.; Peach, M. J.; and Westfall, T. C. Inhibition of catecholamine release by tolbutamide and other sulfonylureas. *Science*, **1975**, *187*, 1086–1087.

Jensen, C. B.; Sistare, F. D.; Hamman, H. C.; and Haynes, R. C., Jr. Stimulation of mitochondrial functions by glucagon treatment. *Biochem. J.*, **1983**, *210*, 819–827.

Judzewitsch, R. G.; Pfeifer, M. A.; Best, J. D.; Beard, J. C.; Halter, J. B.; and Porte, D., Jr. Chronic chlorpropamide therapy of non-insulin dependent diabetes augments basal and stimulated insulin secretion by increasing islet sensitivity to glucose. *J. Clin. Endocrinol. Metab.*, **1982**, *55*, 321–328.

Karam, J. H.; Lewitt, P. A.; Young, C. W.; Nowlain, R. E.; Frankel, B. J.; Fujiya, H.; Freedman, Z. R.; and Grodsky, G. M. Insulinopenic diabetes after rodenticide (VACOR) ingestion. *Diabetes*, **1980**, *29*, 971–978.

Karnieli, E.; Zarnowski, M. J.; Hissin, P. J.; Simpson, I. A.; Salans, L. B.; and Cushman, S. W. Insulin-stimulated translocation of glucose transport systems in the isolated rat adipose cell. *J. Biol. Chem.*, **1981**, *256*, 4772–4777.

Katsoyannis, P. G.; Tometsko, A.; and Fukuda, K. Insulin peptides IX: the synthesis of the A-chain of insulin and its combination with natural B-chain to generate insulin activity. *J. Am. Chem. Soc.*, **1963**, *85*, 2863–2865.

Kikkawa, R.; Hatanaka, I.; Yasuda, H.; Kobayashi, N.; Shigeta, Y.; Terashima, H.; Morimura, T.; and Tsuboshima, M. Effect of a new aldose reductase inhibitor, (E)-3-carboxymethyl-5-[(2E)-methyl-3-phenyl-propenylidene]rhodanine (ONO-2235) on peripheral nerve disorders in streptozotocin-diabetic rats. *Diabetologia*, **1983**, *24*, 290–292.

Kilo, C.; Williamson, J. R.; Choi, S. C.; and Miller, J. P. Insulin treatment and diabetic vascular complications. *J.A.M.A.*, **1979**, *241*, 26–27.

Kolata, G. B. Controversy over study of diabetes drugs continues for nearly a decade. *Science*, **1979**, *203*, 986–990.

Kono, T.; Robinson, F. W.; Blevins, T. L.; and Ezaki, O. Evidence that translocation of the glucose transport activity is the major mechanism of insulin action on glucose transport in fat cells. *J. Biol. Chem.*, **1982**, *257*, 10942–10947.

Kono, T.; Suzuki, K.; Dansey, L. E.; Robinson, F. W.; and Blevins, T. L. Energy-dependent and protein synthesis-independent recycling of the insulin-sensitive glucose transport mechanism in fat cells. *J. Biol. Chem.*, **1981**, *256*, 6400–6407.

Lebrun, P.; Malaisse, W. J.; and Herchuelz, A. Modalities of gliclazide-induced Ca^{2+} influx into the pancreatic β-cell. *Diabetes*, **1982**, *31*, 1010–1015.

Leichter, S. B., and Poffenbarger, P. L. The effects of

nonsuppressible insulin-like protein (NSILP) on cyclic nucleotide metabolism in rat liver. *Biochem. Biophys. Res. Commun.*, **1978**, *84*, 403–410.

Levine, R.; Goldstein, M.; Klein, S.; and Huddlestun, B. The action of insulin on the distribution of galactose in eviscerated nephrectomized dogs. *J. Biol. Chem.*, **1949**, *179*, 985–986.

Lundsgaard, E. On mode of action of insulin. *Ups. Läkför. Förh.*, **1939**, *45*, 143–152.

McIntyre, N.; Holdsworth, C. D.; and Turner, D. S. New interpretation of oral glucose tolerance. *Lancet*, **1964**, *2*, 20–21.

Mayhew, J. A.; Gillon, K. R. W.; and Hawthorne, J. N. Free and lipid inositol, sorbitol and sugars in sciatic nerve obtained post-mortem from diabetic patients and control subjects. *Diabetologia*, **1983**, *24*, 13–15.

Meglasson, M. D.; Schinco, M.; and Matschinsky, F. M. Mannose phosphorylation by glucokinase from liver and transplantable insulinoma. *Diabetes*, **1983**, *32*, 1146–1151.

Meienhofer, J.; Schnabel, E.; Brinkoff, O.; Zabel, R.; Sroka, W.; Klostermeyer, H.; Brandenburg, D.; Okuda, T.; and Zahn, H. Synthese der Insulin Ketten und ihre Kombination zu Insulin-aktiven Präparaten. *Z. Naturforsch. [C]*, **1963**, *18b*, 1120.

Nomura, M.; Zinman, B.; Bahoric, A.; Marliss, E. B.; and Albisser, M. Intravenous infusions of sulfated insulin normalize plasma glucose levels in pancreatectomized dogs. *Diabetes*, **1983**, *32*, 788–792.

O'Donovan, C. J. Analysis of long-term experience with tolbutamide (ORINASE) in the management of diabetes. *Curr. Ther. Res.*, **1959**, *1*, 69–87.

Oka, Y., and Czech, M. Photoaffinity labeling of insulin-sensitive hexose transporters in intact rat adipocytes. *J. Biol. Chem.*, **1984**, *259*, 8125–8133.

Owerbach, D.; Billesbolle, P.; Schroll, M.; Johansen, K.; Poulsen, S.; and Nerup, J. Possible association between DNA sequences flanking the insulin gene and atherosclerosis. *Lancet*, **1982**, *2*, 1291–1293.

Park, C. R.; Bornstein, J.; and Post, R. L. Effect of insulin on free glucose content of rat diaphragm *in vitro*. *Am. J. Physiol.*, **1955**, *182*, 12–16.

Perisic, O., and Traugh, J. A. Protease-activated kinase II as the potential mediator of insulin-stimulated phosphorylation of ribosomal protein S6. *J. Biol. Chem.*, **1983**, *258*, 9589–9592.

Peterson, D. R.; Carone, F. A.; Oparil, S.; and Christensen, E. I. Differences between renal tubular processing of glucagon and insulin. *Am. J. Physiol.*, **1982**, *242*, F112–F118.

Pipeleers, D.; Veld, P.; Maes, E.; and Van De Winkel, M. Glucose-induced insulin release depends on functional cooperation between islet cells. *Proc. Natl Acad. Sci. U.S.A.*, **1982**, *79*, 7322–7325.

Polonsky, K.; Bergenstal, R.; Pons, G.; Schneider, M.; Jaspan, J.; and Rubenstein, A. Relation of counterregulatory responses to hypoglycemia in type 1 diabetics. *N. Engl. J. Med.*, **1982**, *307*, 1106–1112.

Rahier, J.; Goebbels, R. M.; and Henquin, J. C. Cellular composition of the human diabetic pancreas. *Diabetologia*, **1983**, *24*, 366–371.

Rall, T. W., and Sutherland, E. W. Formation of a cyclic adenine ribonucleotide by tissue particles. *J. Biol. Chem.*, **1958**, *232*, 1065–1076.

Report of the Committee for the Assessment of Biometric Aspects of Controlled Trials of Hypoglycemic Agents. *J.A.M.A.*, **1975**, *231*, 583–608.

Resh, M. D.; Nemenoff, R. A.; and Guidotti, G. Insulin stimulation of (Na^+, K^+)–adenosine triphosphatase–dependent $^{86}Rb^+$ uptake in rat adipocytes. *J. Biol. Chem.*, **1980**, *255*, 10938–10945.

Robertson, R. P. Hypothesis: PGE, carbohydrate homeostasis and insulin secretion. A suggested resolution of the controversy. *Diabetes*, **1983**, *32*, 231–234.

Rotwein, P. S.; Chirgwin, J.; Province, M.; Knowler, W. C.; Pettitt, D. J.; Cordell, B.; Goodman, H. M.; and Permutt, M. A. Polymorphism in the 5′ flanking region of the human insulin gene: a genetic marker for non-insulin-dependent diabetes. *N. Engl. J. Med.*, **1983**, *308*, 65–71.

Sanger, F. Chemistry of insulin. *Br. Med. Bull.*, **1960**, *16*, 183–188.

Shimazu, T., and Ishikawa, K. Modulation by the hypothalamus of glucagon and insulin secretion in rabbits: studies with electrical and chemical stimulations. *Endocrinology*, **1981**, *108*, 605–611.

Shoelson, S.; Haneda, M.; Blix, P.; Nanjo, A.; Sanke, T.; Inouye, K.; Steiner, D.; Rubenstein, A.; and Tager, H. Three mutant insulins in man. *Nature*, **1983**, *302*, 540–543.

Stefan, Y.; Orci, L.; Malaisse-Lagae, F.; Perrelet, A.; Patel, Y.; and Unger, R. H. Quantitation of endocrine cell content in the pancreas of nondiabetic and diabetic humans. *Diabetes*, **1982**, *31*, 694–700.

Steiner, D. F. Insulin today. *Diabetes*, **1977**, *26*, 322–340.

Sugden, M. C., and Ashcroft, S. J. H. Phosphoenolpyruvate in rat pancreatic islets: a possible intracellular trigger. *Diabetologia*, **1977**, *13*, 481–486.

Szabo, A. J.; Iguchi, A.; Burleson, P. D.; and Szabo, O. Vagotomy or atropine blocks hypoglycemic effect of insulin injected into ventromedial hypothalamic nucleus. *Am. J. Physiol.*, **1983**, *244*, E467–E471.

Terris, S., and Steiner, D. F. Binding and degradation of ^{125}I-insulin by rat hepatocytes. *J. Biol. Chem.*, **1975**, *250*, 8389–8398.

Uchigata, Y.; Yamamoto, H.; Nagai, H.; and Okamoto, H. Effect of poly (ADP-ribose) synthetase inhibitor administration to rats before and after injection of alloxan and streptozotocin on islet proinsulin synthesis. *Diabetes*, **1983**, *32*, 316–318.

Ullrich, A., *et al.* Human insulin receptor and its relationship to the tyrosine kinase family of oncogenes. *Nature*, **1985**, *313*, 756–761.

University Group Diabetes Program. VIII. Evaluation of insulin therapy: final report. *Diabetes*, **1982**, *31*, Suppl. 5, 1–81.

Varandani, P. T., and Nafz, M. A. Insulin degradation XVIII: on the regulation of glutathione-insulin transhydrogenase in the hyperglycemic obese (ob/ob) mouse. *Biochim. Biophys. Acta*, **1976**, *451*, 382–392.

Vassilopoulou-Sellin, R.; Oyedeji, C. O.; and Samaan, N. A. Somatomedin inhibitors in serum and liver of growth hormone–deficient diabetic rats. *Diabetes*, **1983**, *32*, 262–264.

Virji, M. A. G.; Vassalli, J. D.; Estensen, R. D.; and Reich, E. Plasminogen activator of islets of Langerhans: modulation by glucose and correlation with insulin production. *Proc. Natl Acad. Sci. U.S.A.*, **1980**, *77*, 875–879.

Weir, G. C. Non-insulin-dependent diabetes mellitus: interplay between β-cell inadequacy and insulin resistance. (Editorial.) *Am. J. Med.*, **1982**, *73*, 461–464.

Wentworth, S. M.; Galloway, J. A.; Davidson, J. A.; Root, M. A.; Chance, R. E.; and Haunz, E. A. An update of results of the use of "single peak" (SP) and "single component" (SC) insulin in patients with complications of insulin therapy. *Diabetes*, **1976**, *25*, 326.

Westermark, P., and Wilander, E. The influence of amyloid deposits on the islet cell volume in maturity onset diabetes mellitus. *Diabetologia*, **1978**, *15*, 417–421.

Wolf, E.; Spencer, K. M.; and Cudworth, A. G. The genetic susceptibility to type 1 (insulin-dependent) diabetes: analysis of the HLA-DR association. *Diabetologia*, **1983**, *24*, 224–230.

Yoon, J. W.; Austin, M.; Onodera, T.; and Notkins, A. L. Virus-induced diabetes mellitus: isolation of a virus from the pancreas of a child with diabetic keto-acidosis. *N. Engl. J. Med.*, **1979**, *300*, 1173–1179.

Yoon, J.-W.; Melez, K. A.; Smathers, P. A.; Archer, J. A.; and Steinberg, A. D. Virus-induced diabetes in autoimmune New Zealand mice. *Diabetes*, **1983**, *32*, 755–759.

Monographs and Reviews

Ashcroft, S. J. H. Glucoreceptor mechanisms and the control of insulin release and biosynthesis. *Diabetologia*, **1980**, *18*, 5–15.

Bliss, M. *The Discovery of Insulin*. University of Chicago Press, Chicago, **1983**.

Bloom, S. R. Control of glucagon secretion. In, *Glucagon: Physiology, Pathophysiology, and Morphology of the Pancreatic A Cells*. (Unger, R. H., and Orci, L., eds.) Elsevier Publishing Co., New York, **1981**, pp. 99–113.

Brown, J. C.; Frost, J. L.; Kwauk, S.; Otte, S. C.; and McIntosh, C. H. S. Gastric inhibitory polypeptide (GIP): isolation, structure and basic functions. In, *Gastrointestinal Hormones*. (Jerzy-Glass, G. B., ed.) Raven Press, New York, **1980**, pp. 223–232.

Christiansen, J. The possible physiological role of glucagon on gastroesophageal function. In, *Glucagon in Gastroenterology and Hepatology*. (Picazo, J., ed.) MTP Press, Lancaster, England, **1981**, pp. 69–80.

Cohen, P. The role of protein phosphorylation in neural and hormonal control of cellular activity. *Nature*, **1982**, *296*, 613–620.

Czech, M. P., and Massague, J. Subunit structure and dynamics of the insulin receptor. Symposium on cellular dynamics of insulin action. *Fed. Proc.*, **1982**, *41*, 2719–2723.

Daughaday, W. H. Divergence of binding sites, *in vitro* action, and secretory regulation of the somatomedin peptides, IGF-I and IGF-II. *Proc. Soc. Exp. Biol. Med.*, **1982**, *170*, 257–263.

DeFronzo, R. A., and Ferrannini, E. The pathogenesis of non-insulin-dependent diabetes. An update. *Medicine (Baltimore)*, **1982**, *61*, 125–140.

Diamant, B.; Jørgensen, K. D.; and Weis, J. U. Structure-activity relationship for the spasmolytic action of glucagon. In, *Glucagon in Gastroenterology and Hepatology*. (Picazo, J., ed.) MTP Press, Lancaster, England, **1981**, pp. 25–35.

Duckworth, W. C., and Kitabchi, A. E. Insulin metabolism and degradation. *Endocr. Rev.*, **1981**, *2*, 210–233.

Frank, B. H., and Chance, R. E. Two routes for producing human insulin utilizing recombinant DNA technology. *M.M.W.*, **1983**, *125*, 14–20.

Hodgkin, D. C., and Mercola, D. The secondary and tertiary structure of insulin. In, *Endocrine Pancreas*, Vol. 1. Sect. 7, *Endocrinology. Handbook of Physiology*. (Steiner, D. F., and Freinkel, N., eds.) American Physiological Society, Washington, D. C., **1972**, pp. 139–157.

Home, P. D., and Alberti, K. G. M. M. The new insulins. Their characteristics and clinical implications. *Drugs*, **1982**, *24*, 401–413.

Jackson, J. E., and Bressler, R. I. Clinical pharmacology of sulfonylurea hypoglycaemic agents. *Drugs*, **1981a**, *22*, 211–245.

———. II. Clinical pharmacology of sulfonylurea hypoglycaemic agents. *Ibid.*, **1981b**, *22*, 295–320.

Jaspan, J. B. Glucagon: basic pathophysiological considerations. In, *Glucagon in Gastroenterology and Hepatology*. (Picazo, J., ed.) MTP Press, Lancaster, England, **1981**, pp. 1–24.

Jerzy-Glass, G. B. (ed.). *Gastrointestinal Hormones*. Raven Press, New York, **1980**.

Kemmer, F. W., and Vranic, M. The role of glucagon and its relationship to other glucoregulatory hormones in exercise. In, *Glucagon: Physiology, Pathophysiology, and Morphology of the Pancreatic A Cells*. (Unger,

R. H., and Orci, L., eds.) Elsevier Publishing Co., New York, **1981**, pp. 297–331.

Kreisberg, R. A. Diabetic ketoacidosis: new concepts and trends in pathogenesis and treatment. *Ann. Intern. Med.*, **1978**, *88*, 681–695.

Krieger, D. T. Brain peptides: what, where and why? *Science*, **1983**, *222*, 975–985.

Larner, J.; Cheng, K.; Schwartz, C.; Kikuchi, K.; Tamura, S.; Creacy, S.; Dubler, R.; Galasko, G.; Pullin, C.; and Katz, M. Insulin mediators and their control of metabolism through protein phosphorylation. *Recent Prog. Horm. Res.*, **1982**, *38*, 511–552.

MacLaren, N. K. Viral and immunological bases of beta cell failure in insulin-dependent diabetes. *Am. J. Dis. Child.*, **1977**, *131*, 1149–1154.

Madsbad, S. Prevalence of residual β cell function and its metabolic consequences in type 1 (insulin-dependent) diabetes. *Diabetologia*, **1983**, *24*, 141–147.

Miller, R. E., and Chernish, S. M. The response of gastrointestinal tract motility to glucagon. In, *Glucagon in Gastroenterology and Hepatology*. (Picazo, J., ed.) MTP Press, Lancaster, England, **1981a**, pp. 37–53.

———. On the use of glucagon: ancillary effects and other considerations. In, *Glucagon in Gastroenterology and Hepatology*. (Picazo, J., ed.) MTP Press, Lancaster, England, **1981b**, pp. 55–67.

Moore, R. D. Effects of insulin upon ion transport. *Biochim. Biophys. Acta*, **1983**, *737*, 1–49.

Orci, L. Macro- and micro-domains in the endocrine pancreas. *Diabetes*, **1982**, *31*, 538–565.

Palmer, J. P., and Porte, D., Jr. Control of glucagon secretion: the central nervous system. In, *Glucagon: Physiology, Pathophysiology, and Morphology of the Pancreatic A Cells*. (Unger, R. H., and Orci, L., eds.) Elsevier Publishing Co., New York, **1981**, pp. 135–159.

Porte, D., Jr., and Halter, J. B. The endocrine pancreas and diabetes mellitus. In, *Textbook of Endocrinology*, 6th ed. (Williams, R. H., ed.) W. B. Saunders Co., Philadelphia, **1981**, pp. 716–843.

Pyke, D. A. Genetics of diabetes. *Clin. Endocrinol. Metab.*, **1977**, *6*, 285–303.

Reed, L. J.; Pettit, F. H.; Bleile, D. M.; and Wu, T.-L. Structure, function and regulation of mammalian pyruvate dehydrogenase complex. In, *Metabolic Interconversion of Enzymes*. (Holzer, H., ed.) Springer-Verlag, Berlin, **1980**, pp. 124–133.

Renold, A. E.; Mintz, D. H.; Muller, W. A.; and Cahill, G. F., Jr. Diabetes mellitus. In, *Metabolic Basis of Inherited Disease*, 4th ed. (Stanbury, J. B.; Wyngaarden, J. B.; and Fredrickson, D. S.; eds.) McGraw-Hill Book Co., New York, **1978**, pp. 80–110.

Robbins, D. C.; Tager, H. S.; and Rubenstein, A. H. Biologic and clinical importance of proinsulin. *N. Engl. J. Med.*, **1984**, *310*, 1165–1175.

Rosenfeld, M. G., and Barrieux, A. Regulation of protein synthesis by polypeptide hormones and cyclic AMP. *Adv. Cyclic Nucleotide Res.*, **1979**, *11*, 205–264.

Roth, J., and Grunfeld, C. Endocrine systems: mechanisms of disease, target cells, and receptors. In, *Textbook of Endocrinology*, 6th ed. (Williams, R. H., ed.) W. B. Saunders Co., Philadelphia, **1981**, pp. 15–72.

Samols, E., and Harrison, J. Tolbutamide: stimulator and suppressor of glucagon secretion. In, *Glucagon and Its Role in Physiology and Clinical Medicine*. (Foa, P. P.; Bajaj, J. S.; and Foa, N. L.; eds.) Springer-Verlag, Berlin, **1978**, pp. 699–710.

Scott, J., and Poffenbarger, P. L. Tolbutamide pharmacogenetics and the UGDP controversy. *J.A.M.A.*, **1979**, *242*, 45–48.

Seltzer, H. S. Severe drug-induced hypoglycemia: a review. *Compr. Ther.*, **1979**, *5*, 21–29.

Steinberg, D. Lipoproteins and atherosclerosis—a look back and a look ahead. *Arteriosclerosis*, **1983**, *3*, 283–301.

Symposium. (Various authors.) International symposium on human insulin. (Karam, J. H., and Etzwiler, D. D., eds.) *Diabetes Care,* **1983a,** *6,* 1–68.

Symposium. (Various authors.) Proceedings of a conference on diabetic microangiopathy. (McMillan, D. E., and Ditzel, J., eds.) *Diabetes,* **1983b,** *32,* Suppl. 2, 1–104.

Symposium. (Various authors.) New perspectives in noninsulin-dependent diabetes mellitus and the role of glipizide in its treatment. *Am. J. Med.,* **1983c,** *75,* pp. 1–99.

Symposium. (Various authors.) The role of insulin resistance in the pathogenesis and treatment of noninsulin-dependent diabetes mellitus. (Reaven, G. M., ed.) *Am. J. Med.,* **1983d,** *74,* pp. 1–112.

Unger, R. H. Meticulous control of diabetes: benefits, risks and precautions. *Diabetes,* **1982,** *31,* 479–483.

Unger, R. H., and Orci, L. I. Glucagon and the A cell. *N. Engl. J. Med.,* **1981a,** *304,* 1518–1524.

———. II. Glucagon and the A cell. *Ibid.,* **1981b,** *304,* 1575–1580.

Von Schenck, H. Glucagon—biochemistry, physiology and pathophysiology. *Acta Med. Scand.,* **1981,** *209,* 145–148.

Wollheim, C. B., and Sharp, G. W. G. Regulation of insulin release by calcium. *Physiol. Rev.,* **1981,** *61,* 914–973.

Zapf, J.; Froesch, E. R.; and Humbel, R. E. The insulin-like growth factors (IGF) of human serum: chemical and biological characterization and aspects of their possible physiological role. *Curr. Top. Cell. Regul.,* **1981,** *19,* 257–309.

CHAPTER

65 AGENTS AFFECTING CALCIFICATION: CALCIUM, PARATHYROID HORMONE, CALCITONIN, VITAMIN D, AND OTHER COMPOUNDS

Robert C. Haynes, Jr., and Ferid Murad

CALCIUM

Calcium is the fifth most abundant element in the body, and the major portion is in bone. It is present in small quantities in the extracellular fluid and to a minor extent in the structure and cytoplasm of cells of soft tissue. Calcium plays important physiological roles, many of which are not completely understood. It is essential for the functional integrity of nerve and muscle, where it has a major influence on excitability and release of neurotransmitters. It is necessary for muscle contraction, cardiac function, maintenance of the integrity of membranes, and coagulation of the blood.

To carry out these various roles, ionized calcium must be available to the appropriate tissues in the proper concentration. As is the case for other essential constituents of the body, an endocrine control system has evolved that ordinarily keeps the plasma concentration of ionized calcium within narrow limits. This is accomplished in the case of calcium by placing controls at the site of entry of calcium into the system (intestinal absorption) and at a site of exit (the kidney), and by keeping a large store (the skeleton) accessible for deposits or withdrawals depending upon peripheral demand. Intracellular concentrations of ionized calcium are also strictly regulated by control of the exchange of the ion between the cell and its environment and between intracellular compartments. Drugs that affect organ function by blocking channels for calcium ions in the plasma membrane are discussed in Chapter 33.

This chapter will describe the roles of calcium and the three endocrine factors that control its metabolism: parathyroid

hormone (PTH), calcitonin, and vitamin D. The actions of these hormones can be summarized as follows.

PTH is secreted in response to a fall in plasma calcium ion concentration, and the hormone acts to restore calcium to its normal concentration range by accelerating transfer of calcium from the bone compartment, enhancing intestinal absorption of calcium, and increasing reabsorption of calcium by the kidney. In addition, PTH promotes phosphate excretion in the urine. The secretion of calcitonin can be stimulated by a rise in the concentration of calcium ion in plasma; this hormone lowers plasma calcium by decreasing calcium resorption from bone and by increasing the renal excretion of the ion. Vitamin D, now recognized as a hormone, stimulates intestinal absorption of calcium and phosphate and decreases their renal excretion; it also enhances resorption of bone.

Calcium Requirements and Body Stores. The calcium intake varies from 200 to 2500 mg per day, and, in the United States, the predominant source is dairy products. Recommended daily dietary allowances (United States) are presented in Table XVI–1 (page 1546) (*see also* Nordin *et al.*, 1979). The skeleton contains more than 90% of the calcium of the body. The inorganic salts of bone resemble the mineral hydroxyapatite $[Ca_{10} (PO_4)_6 (OH)_2]$. Bone crystals are not pure, however, and contain additional ions in the crystal lattice and in association with the crystals. These include sodium, potassium, magnesium, carbonate, and fluoride (Raisz, 1977). The steady-state content of calcium in the skeleton is a consequence of the net effect of bone resorption and new-bone formation, and the calcium of bone is in a constant exchange with the calcium of the interstitial fluids. The rates of exchange can be modified by drugs, hormones, vitamins, and other factors that influence the level of calcium in the interstitial fluids and also the forms in which the cation is present.

The calcium in plasma is maintained at a fairly constant concentration of about 2.5 mM (5.0 mEq/l; 10 mg/dl). However, this represents the total of three different components: (1) about 40% of the plasma calcium is bound to proteins, primarily albumin; (2) about one tenth is diffusible but complexed with anions (*e.g.*, citrate and phosphate); (3) the remaining fraction represents diffusible ionic calcium. The ionized calcium is the fraction that exerts physiological effects, and symptoms of hypocalcemia occur with its reduction. It is clear that hypocalcemia due to hypoproteinemia and a reduced concentration of protein-bound calcium is not likely to be accompanied by the symptoms and signs of hypocalcemia, unless there is a reduction in the concentration of ionized calcium as well. Hence, the interpretation of the significance of any given value of plasma calcium is impossible without knowledge of the coincident concentration of plasma proteins, and nomograms are available for this purpose. As an approximation, an alteration in plasma albumin of 1 g/dl (from a normal value of 4.0 to 4.4 g/dl) can be expected to change total calcium by 0.8 mg/dl.

Absorption and Excretion. In general, the major portion of intestinal absorption takes place in the more proximal segments of the small bowel; in man, approximately one third of the ingested calcium is absorbed. Intestinal absorption involves the soluble ionized form of calcium and reflects at least two separate steps: (1) calcium uptake at the mucosal pole and (2) efflux at the serosal pole of the intestinal epithelium. Mucosal uptake of calcium is presumably carrier mediated, but the mechanism is not understood (DeLuca and Schnoes, 1983). It is likely that a Ca^{2+}-ATPase is involved at the serosal membrane (Lawson and Davie, 1979).

The factors that clearly augment absorp-

tion of calcium—vitamin D and PTH—are discussed below. It is also generally accepted that a diet low in calcium results in increased fractional absorption of the ion.

Glucocorticoids and other factors depress calcium transport across the small intestine. For example, phytate, oxalate, and probably phosphate in the bowel promote the formation of a complex or insoluble salt of calcium that is not absorbed through the wall of the gut. Disease states such as steatorrhea may result in decreased absorption of calcium. Other diarrheas with chronic gastrointestinal malabsorption may promote increased fecal losses of calcium as well.

Calcium is released into the gastrointestinal tract in saliva, bile, and pancreatic and intestinal secretions. This endogenous calcium and the unabsorbed dietary calcium constitute the sources of the cation excreted in the feces. There is significant loss of calcium in milk during lactation, and also daily losses in sweat.

The *urinary excretion* of calcium is the net result of the quantity filtered and the amount reabsorbed. There is no evidence of renal tubular secretion of calcium. The mechanisms for the renal reabsorption of calcium are unknown, and for unexplained reasons there is, in general, a correlation between the urinary excretion of sodium and calcium. This is true when natriuresis is increased by loading with salt, and it also is noted with diuretics that act at the ascending limb of the loop of Henle and the distal tubule (Davis and Murdaugh, 1970).

In animal studies approximately two thirds of the filtered calcium is reabsorbed in the proximal convolution, 20 to 25% in the loop of Henle, and 10% in the distal convolution (Murayama *et al.*, 1972; Massry and Coburn, 1973).

PTH stimulates the reabsorption of calcium by the kidney apparently by means of an effect on the distal tubule, whereas the active metabolites of vitamin D stimulate proximal tubular reabsorption of calcium (Puschett *et al.*, 1972). Calcitonin inhibits the proximal tubular reabsorption of calcium, thus facilitating excretion of the cation (Paillard *et al.*, 1972).

The influence of renal disease on urinary calcium excretion is variable. In chronic renal failure due primarily to glomerular disease, calcium excretion diminishes as filtration rate falls. However, in those instances where filtration is only minimally depressed and the secretion of hydrogen ions is deficient due to an inability to attain a high concentration gradient for hydrogen ions between tubular cell and lumen (renal tubular acidosis), the excretion of calcium may be enhanced. This hypercalciuria may be diminished by the correction of the systemic acidosis.

PHYSIOLOGICAL AND PHARMACOLOGICAL ACTIONS

The cytoplasmic concentration of ionized calcium is normally maintained at very low values ($\sim$0.1 to 1 μM) by the extrusion of the ion from the cell and by its sequestration within cellular organelles, particularly mitochondria and, in muscle, sarcoplasmic reticulum. The provocative hypothesis has been offered that the need for such transport systems arose in evolution when cells accumulated high concentrations of phosphate for use in energy metabolism (see Kretsinger, 1976). (The solubility product of calcium phosphate is very low.) Given the high gradient of calcium between extracellular and intracellular compartments, use can be made of the ion in mechanisms for transmembrane signaling. Thus, in response to various electrical or chemical stimuli, calcium influx across the plasma membrane or release from internal stores is triggered. This calcium interacts with high-affinity binding sites on specific intracellular proteins (such as troponin or calmodulin) and thereby regulates a number of functional and metabolic processes of the cell.

Local Actions. Certain salts of calcium, notably the chloride, are intensely irritating to tissue and will cause painful sloughing if injected subcutaneously. Therefore, whenever calcium chloride is administered parenterally, it must be given intravenously and every effort should be made to prevent extravasation.

Neuromuscular System. Moderate elevations of the concentration of calcium in the extracellular fluid may have no clinically detectable influences on the neuromuscular apparatus. However, when hypercalcemia becomes extreme, the threshold for excitation of nerve and muscle is increased. This is manifested clinically by muscle weakness, lethargy, and eventually coma. In contrast, modest diminution in the level of ionized calcium may decrease the thresholds of excitation in a striking fashion, leading to positive Chvostek and Trousseau signs and tetanic seizures. The role played by calcium in regulating the excitability of tissues is not completely elucidated. Calcium influx across the plasma membrane is thought to be by means of carrier-mediated facilitated diffusion and by exchange of calcium for sodium, which participates both in excitation and in the maintenance of the steady state. Several calcium channels in cell membranes are regulated by hormones and other ligands as well as by membrane potential. However, in nerve and skeletal muscle, the concentration of cytoplasmic ionic calcium is not controlled by cellular influx and efflux to nearly the same extent that it is by the mitochondria and sarcoplasmic reticulum, which sequester intracellular calcium. Calcium causes relatively small changes in resting membrane potentials but modifies the time-voltage relationships during the action potential in nerve and muscle. In addition, calcium appears to play an important role in the regulation of cell-membrane permeability to sodium and potassium.

Calcium plays additional roles both in coupling excitation with muscle contraction and in the release of neurohumoral transmitters. The action potential in muscle stimulates the release of calcium ions from the sarcoplasmic reticulum, and the divalent cation activates contraction. The binding of calcium to troponin abolishes the inhibitory effect of troponin on the interaction of actin and myosin. Muscle relaxation occurs when ionic sarcoplasmic calcium is pumped back into the sarcoplasmic reticulum, permitting the inhibitory effect of troponin on actin and myosin.

Calcium also plays an important role in stimulus-secretion coupling in most exocrine and endocrine glands. The release of catecholamines from the adrenal medulla, neurotransmitters at synapses, and autacoids from various sites is dependent on calcium ions. Calcium is necessary for exocytosis (Douglas, 1968).

There is an important interrelation between calcium and potassium. A potassium deficiency coincident with hypocalcemia appears to protect against hypocalcemic tetany. Correction of the potassium deficit without attention to the level of calcium may provoke tetany without a change in the concentration of calcium in plasma.

Cardiovascular System. It is probable that the above-described processes relating to nerve and skeletal muscle apply to cardiac muscle as well. In the myocardium, a "slow" inward current occurs during the plateau of the action potential and is dependent on ionic calcium (New and Trautwein, 1972). This "slow" channel allows inward permeation of calcium ions for excitation-contraction coupling. It has long been recognized that there are certain similarities in the effect of calcium and the cardiac glycosides on cardiac muscle (*see* Chapter 30). *Calcium channel blockers* have profound effects on the contractility of cardiac and vascular smooth muscle, and they are also useful in treating cardiac arrhythmias (*see* Chapters 31 and 33).

Miscellaneous Effects. Calcium salts may play a role in maintaining the integrity of mucosal membranes, cell adhesion, and functions of individual cell membranes as well. The use of calcium salts to prevent effusions across capillary endothelial membranes is, however, without demonstrated benefit. Calcium is involved in blood coagulation, but the ion is not used to treat disorders of coagulation. Calcium chloride is an acidifying salt and will promote diuresis; however, ammonium salts are much more effective acidifying agents.

ABNORMALITIES OF CALCIUM METABOLISM

It should be clear from the discussion of some of the factors involved in maintaining calcium homeostasis that there are many ways in which significant alterations in calcium metabolism can occur. Some of these alterations may be accompanied by hypocalcemia and others by hypercalcemia.

Hypocalcemic States. The prominent signs and symptoms of hypocalcemia include tetany and related phenomena such as paresthesias, increased neuromuscular excitability, laryngospasm, muscle cramps, and convulsions (usually tonic-clonic). Some causes of hypocalcemia are discussed below.

Deprivation of calcium and vitamin D may readily promote hypocalcemia. This combination of events is observed in the various malabsorption states and also occurs from inadequate diets. When due to malabsorption, the hypocalcemia is accompanied by a depressed level of phosphorus, total plasma proteins are usually low, and hypomagnesemia is common. During magnesium deficiency, hypocalcemia may be accentuated by diminished secretion and action of PTH (*see* below). Hypocalcemia stimulates the release of PTH, which causes the mobilization of calcium from bone and demineralization. In infants with malabsorption or inadequate calcium intake, the calcium concentration is usually depressed, there is hypophosphatemia, and the resultant bone disease is *rickets* (*see* section on vitamin D).

Hypoparathyroidism may occur spontaneously as a result of a genetic disorder or as a consequence of thyroid or other neck surgery. In these disorders there is distinct hypocalcemia but *hyper*phosphatemia. Although other conditions of hypocalcemia may be associated with opacity of the lens, papilledema, and calcification of the basal ganglia, these occur more commonly with hypoparathyroidism. Other changes include trophic alterations and fungal infections of the skin. Pseudohypoparathyroidism is probably a group of genetic diseases characterized by multiple structural defects and a failure to respond to exogenous PTH (Van Dop and Bourne, 1983). The structural changes are manifested by a round face; short, thick figure; shortening of some of the metacarpal and metatarsal bones; and soft-tissue calcifications. As discussed below, at least one variety of this disease results from a deficiency of calcitriol (1,25-dihydroxycholecalciferol). Another appears to be caused by deficiency of the stimulatory guanine nucleotide–binding regulatory component of adenylate cyclase.

In the period (1 to 4 days) following *removal of a parathyroid adenoma,* hypocalcemia is not unusual, especially if there is bone disease.

Neonatal tetany may result from a temporary hypoparathyroidism that occurs in the newborn of mothers with hyperparathyroidism; indeed, it may be the infant's tetany that provides the clue to the mother's disorder. This is usually transient in the infant and disappears as soon as its own parathyroid glands respond appropriately. Other situations in which neonatal hypocalcemia may supervene include hypernatremia and acute infections.

Hypocalcemia is frequently associated with advanced *renal insufficiency accompanied by hyperphosphatemia.* For reasons that are not clear, many of these patients do not develop tetany unless the severe accompanying acidosis is improved with treatment. High concentrations of phosphate in plasma appear to inhibit the conversion of 25-hydroxycholecalciferol to 1,25-dihydroxycholecalciferol (Haussler and McCain, 1977). Excessive use of potassium phosphate in the treatment of diabetic ketoacidosis can cause hypocalcemia and hypomagnesemia (Winter *et al.*, 1979); potassium chloride is preferred.

Sodium fluoride forms an insoluble salt with calcium and, if ingested in large enough quantities, may induce hypocalcemia and tetany (*see* below).

Hypocalcemia can also occur following massive *transfusions with citrated blood.*

Preparations and Routes of Administration in the Treatment of Hypocalcemia. There are several preparations available if the systemic action of calcium is desired. These differ in calcium content and permissible routes of administration.

Calcium chloride ($CaCl_2 \cdot 2H_2O$) contains 27% calcium and consists of white granules freely soluble in water. It is valuable in the treatment of hypocalcemic tetany. The salt can be given intravenously. *It must never be injected into tissues.* It is somewhat irritating to the gastrointestinal tract. Injections of calcium chloride are accompanied by peripheral vasodilatation and a cutaneous burning sensation. The salt is usually given intravenously in a concentration of 10% (equivalent to 1.36 mEq Ca^{2+}/ml). Injection rate should be slow (not over 1 ml per minute) to prevent a high concentration of calcium from reaching the heart and causing syncope. A moderate fall in blood pressure due to vasodilatation may attend the injection. Since calcium chloride is an acidifying salt, it is usually undesirable in the treatment of the hypocalcemia caused by renal insufficiency.

Calcium gluceptate injection is a 22% solution (18 mg or 0.9 mEq Ca^{2+}/ml). It is administered intravenously in a dose of 5 to 20 ml for the treatment of severe hypocalcemic tetany; the injection may produce a transient tingling sensation. When the intravenous route is not possible, the injection may be given intramuscularly in a dose up to 5 ml, which may produce a mild local reaction.

Calcium gluconate ($[CH_2OH\{CHOH\}_4COO]_2\text{-}Ca \cdot H_2O$) contains 9% calcium. It is available as *calcium gluconate tablets,* containing 500, 650, or 1000 mg of the salt (equivalent to 2.3, 3.0, or 4.5 mEq Ca^{2+}, respectively). It is nonirritating to the gastrointestinal tract. For intravenous injection, *calcium gluconate injection* is administered as a 10% solution (0.45 mEq Ca^{2+}/ml). It is a readily available source of calcium ions, and the intravenous administration of this salt is the treatment of choice for severe hypocalcemic tetany. The intramuscular route should not be employed in children, as abscess formation at the site of injection may result.

Calcium lactate ($[CH_3CHOHCOO]_2Ca \cdot 5H_2O$) contains 13% calcium. Its physical properties are similar to those of the gluconate. Tablets (325 mg or 650 mg) are available for oral administration. In the treatment of tetany, its absorption is apparently enhanced by the simultaneous administration of lactose.

Calcium carbonate is an insoluble, fine, white microcrystalline powder containing 40% calcium; it is available in tablets containing 350 mg to 1.5 g. After ingestion, it is converted to soluble calcium salts in the bowel, and calcium is thereby made available for absorption. Patients with achlorhydria may not solubilize calcium from this preparation. It is also used as an antacid.

Dibasic calcium phosphate, although chiefly used as a gastric antacid, is a valuable source of the calcium ion, especially when it is desired to supply both calcium and phosphorus. It is an insoluble, tasteless white powder that must be given orally.

Calcium levulinate contains 13% calcium. It may be administered orally or parenterally.

Calcium glubionate contains 6.5% calcium and is available as a syrup containing 1.8 g (115 mg of calcium) per 5 ml.

Other calcium preparations are described in connection with gastric antacids.

Therapeutic Uses. Calcium is used in the treatment of deficiency states and as a dietary supplement when intake may be inadequate. Calcium salts are specific in the immediate treatment of *low-calcium tetany* regardless of etiology. In severe manifest tetany, the symptoms are best brought under control by intravenous medication. Five to 20 ml of either 10% calcium gluconate or 22% calcium glucepate solution is injected slowly. For the control of milder symptoms or latent tetany, oral medication suffices. Average doses are *calcium gluconate,* 15 g daily in divided doses; *calcium lactate,* 4 g, plus lactose, 8 g, with each meal; *calcium carbonate* or *calcium phosphate,* 1 to 2 g with meals, as a watery suspension or sprinkled on food.

Hypercalcemic States. Hypercalcemia occurs in a number of diverse clinical conditions and requires differential diagnosis and appropriate corrective measures.

Ingestion of large quantities of a calcium salt is unlikely by itself to cause hypercalcemia except in patients who have hypothyroidism.

Hyperparathyroidism is classically associated with hypercalcemia accompanied by significant hypophosphatemia; the latter is due to the diminished ability of the renal tubules to reabsorb phosphorus, owing to the excessive quantities of PTH. Some patients have renal calculi and peptic ulceration, and a few have mental aberrations with psychotic components. In more advanced stages, characteristic bone lesions are present and the condition can be diagnosed by radiography.

Although very uncommon now, there is the hypercalcemic disorder known as the *milk-alkali syndrome,* caused by the ingestion of large quantities of milk and alkalinizing powders.

Benzothiadiazide diuretics produce a mild hypercalcemia in some individuals.

Vitamin D excess is a cause of hypercalcemia (*see* below).

Sarcoidosis is associated with about a 20% incidence of hypercalcemia. Increased intestinal absorption of calcium is due to an excess production of calcitriol, probably by the sarcoid lesions (Mason *et al.*, 1984). Hypercalcemia peaks during summer months with increased exposure to sunlight.

Neoplasms with or without metastases to the bones may be accompanied by hypercalcemia. Some tumors secrete PTH-like peptides; others appear to secrete an osteoclast-stimulating factor; still others produce prostaglandins that stimulate bone resorption (Odell and Wolfsen, 1978). The hypercalcemia associated with these tumors is usually heralded by lethargy, weakness, nausea, and vomiting and not by renal stones or bone disease.

Occasionally, patients with *hyperthyroidism* have hypercalcemia. This is presumably due to an increased rate of bone resorption.

Disuse atrophy, as may occur when a patient must lie relatively immobile for a long period of time, may lead to hypercalcemia. This is most common after trauma that has involved large areas of the body and when extensive splinting with casts is necessary. Immobilization also often contributes to the hypercalcemia of patients with cancer.

Idiopathic hypercalcemia of infants is an unusual disease of unknown etiology. There are many similarities to intoxication with vitamin D.

Hypercalcemia is uncommonly noted in *adrenocortical deficiency states,* as in Addison's disease or during the period following operation for a hyperfunctioning tumor of the adrenal cortex or removal of bilateral hyperplastic adrenal glands.

Hypercalcemia occurs occasionally following successful *renal transplantation.* This is due to secondary hyperparathyroidism resulting from the previous chronic renal failure.

The *differential diagnosis* of the various causes of hypercalcemia may be difficult. In contrast to former belief, hypophosphatemia is quite common with hypercalcemia of origins other than hyperparathyroidism. Many cases of hypercalcemia are discovered as a result of routine automated analyses of serum samples. The differential diagnosis of hypercalcemia entails the use of many tests, none of which is completely conclusive. Immunoassay of parathyroid hormone in plasma is quite useful, but there are limitations (*see* below). The excretion of adenosine $3',5'$-monophosphate (cyclic AMP) in the urine is increased in hyperparathyroidism, and evaluation of this parameter can facilitate diagnosis. Renal reabsorption of filtered phosphate is diminished in hyperparathyroidism, and this measurement can also be of diagnostic value.

Hypercalcemia of any etiology can have dire consequences. The predominant and most devastating lesion usually occurs in the kidney with reduction of renal function. Pathological changes are prominent in the collecting ducts and distal tubules. Painful bone cysts, osteoporosis, and fractures may also occur if hypercalcemia is due to hyperparathyroidism.

There are occasions when hypercalcemia is in itself a life-threatening situation. The use of agents that augment the excretion of calcium, such as the administration of saline and diuretics, is the treatment of first choice. The employment of steroids to reduce hypercalcemia is of benefit in those situations where the hypercalcemia is a consequence of diseases such as sarcoid. Administration of calcitonin, plicamycin, or phosphate may be necessary and helpful (*see* below). The use of sodium phosphate intravenously, as described by Massry and coworkers (1968), is clearly effective in reducing the concentration of calcium in plasma. However, because of the great danger of precipitating calcium phosphate in soft tissues, oral administration of phosphate is preferred. Intravenous phosphate should be used only in hypophosphatemic patients with severe hypercalcemia who cannot take phosphate orally (Stewart, 1983).

Preparations Used for the Reduction of Hypercalcemia. As indicated above, infusions of saline with or without administration of diuretics such as furosemide are an effective way to promote the excretion of calcium. This constitutes the treatment of choice in most cases.

Prednisone and other steroids with similar characteristics are capable of reducing hypercalcemic concentrations to normal values, particularly when the abnormality is a consequence of sarcoid. Patients with nonmetastatic carcinomas or hyperparathyroidism are less responsive. Frequently, large doses of 30 to 50 mg of prednisone a day may be necessary initially. The response to glucocorticoid therapy is slow, and 1 to 2 weeks may be required before a fall in plasma calcium occurs. A low-calcium intake (virtual elimination of all milk and derivative dairy products) permits the use of the lowest dose of steroid possible to maintain normocalcemia. The complications of the chronic use of steroids must be recalled, and the osteoporosis that results from prolonged administration of glucocorticoids can limit the duration of therapy.

Plicamycin (mithramycin; MITHRACIN) is a cytotoxic antibiotic that can be very useful in decreasing plasma calcium concentration in hypercalcemia (Perlia *et al.,* 1970). This agent probably acts directly on bone and blocks calcium resorption. Reduction in plasma calcium concentration occurs within 24 to 48 hours with relatively low doses of this agent (15 to 25 μg/kg per day for up to 3 to 4 days), and its toxicity is thus less severe (*see* Chapter 55).

Calcitonin (CALCIMAR) may be useful for the treatment of hypercalcemia (*see* below).

Phosphates are given orally four times a day in a total daily dose equivalent to 500 to 1500 mg of phosphorus (Stewart, 1983).

Edetate disodium (EDTA) is a chelating agent that forms soluble complexes with calcium. Chelation occurs in the blood and results in a rapid decrease in the concentration of ionized calcium in plasma before excretion of the complex occurs. Because of potential toxicities this agent is now used only rarely. Among the dangers of such therapy is the possibility that the concentration of calcium may be reduced too quickly and to hypocalcemic levels, thus resulting in tetany, convulsions, severe cardiac arrhythmias, and respiratory arrest.

Indomethacin (INDOCIN) (*see* Chapter 29) has been used to treat hypercalcemia that results from excess production of prostaglandins by tumors. Such treatment is useful only infrequently (Brenner *et al.,* 1982).

PHOSPHATE

In addition to its roles as a dynamic constituent of intermediary and energy metabolism, it is well known that phosphate plays important roles in modifying concentrations of calcium in tissues. Furthermore, the acid-base equilibrium may be modified because phosphate ions are buffers of the intracellular fluid and also play a primary role in the renal excretion of hydrogen ion.

Absorption, Distribution, and Excretion. Phosphate is absorbed from, and to a limited extent secreted into, the gastrointestinal tract. The transport of phosphate from the lumen of the gut is an active, energy-dependent process, and there are factors that appear to modify the degree of its intestinal absorption. The presence of large quantities of calcium or aluminum may lead to the formation of large amounts of insoluble phosphate and may therefore diminish the net absorption of phosphate from the bowel. Vitamin D stimulates phosphate absorption, and this effect precedes the action of the vitamin on transport of calcium (Birge and Miller, 1977). In general, in adults, about two thirds of the ingested phosphate is absorbed from the bowel, and that which is absorbed from the gut is almost entirely excreted into the urine. In growing children, there is a positive balance of phosphate. Concentrations of phosphate in plasma are higher in children than in adults. This "hyperphosphatemia" decreases the affinity of hemoglobin for oxygen and is hypothesized to explain the physiological "anemia" of childhood (Card and Brain, 1973).

Phosphate is present in plasma and extracellular fluid, in cell membranes and intracellular fluid, and in collagen and bone tissue. In the extracellular fluid, phosphate is primarily in inorganic form and only a small component of esterified phosphate is present. Plasma phosphate concentration is inversely related to the rate of renal hydroxylation of 25-hydroxycholecalciferol. A reduction of the plasma phosphate concentration permits the presence of more calcium in the blood and inhibits deposition of new bone salt. An increased concentration of the phosphate anion in plasma facilitates the effect of calcitonin on deposition of calcium in bone (Werner et al., 1972). The concentration of plasma inorganic phosphate may vary with age, and the range has been recorded in great detail by Greenberg and coworkers (1960). The ratio of disodium phosphate and monosodium phosphate in extracellular fluid is 4:1 at a pH of 7.40. The buffer ratio varies, of course, with pH; however, owing to the relatively low concentration, phosphate contributes relatively little to the buffering capacity of extracellular fluid.

The renal excretion of phosphate has been studied quite extensively. More than 90% of the phosphate in plasma is filterable, and the bulk is then actively reabsorbed by the initial segment of the proximal tubule. Phosphate reabsorption takes place to a smaller extent in the pars recta and/or loop of Henle, in the distal convoluted tubule, and possibly in the collecting duct (Kuntziger et al., 1974; Lechene et al., 1978). Expansion of plasma volume causes increased urinary phosphate excretion (Steele, 1970). Phosphate excreted in the urine probably represents the net difference between the amount filtered and that reabsorbed. There is little evidence for tubular secretion of phosphate in the mammalian kidney. Parathyroid hormone increases the urinary excretion of phosphate by blocking reabsorption in all segments proximal to the collecting duct (Lechene et al., 1978). Vitamin D_3 and its metabolites directly stimulate proximal tubular reabsorption of phosphate (Puschett et al., 1972).

Role of Phosphate in the Acidification of the Urine. The interrelations that exist between the rates of excretion of phosphate and titratable acid are referred to in Chapter 35 and in the Introduction to Section VIII. Although the concentration of phosphate is low in the extracellular fluid, the anion is progressively concentrated in the renal tubule and represents the most abundant buffer system in the distal tubule. At this site, the secretion of H^+ by the tubular cell in exchange for Na^+ in the tubular urine converts disodium hydrogen phosphate to sodium dihydrogen phosphate. In this manner, large amounts of acid can be excreted without lowering the pH of the urine to a degree that would block H^+ transport by a high concentration gradient between the tubular cell and luminal fluid.

Actions of the Phosphate Ion. Once phosphate gains access to the body fluids and tissues, it exerts little pharmacological effect. If the ion is introduced into the gastrointestinal tract, the absorbed phosphate is rapidly excreted. If large amounts are given by this route, much of it may escape absorption. This leads to a cathartic action, and, therefore, the phosphate salts are employed as mild laxatives. Inorganic phosphate poisoning following ingestion of laxatives that contain phosphate salts has been reported in adults and children (McConnell, 1971; Levitt *et al.*, 1973). The ingestion of large amounts of sodium dihydrogen phosphate lowers the pH of the urine. If phosphate salts are introduced intravenously in high concentration, they may prove toxic. Toxicity results from reducing the concentration of Ca^{2+} in the circulation and from the precipitation of calcium phosphate in soft tissues.

Phosphate Depletion. There has been a question for some time concerning the possibility of clinical consequences of phosphate depletion. Familial hypophosphatemia is an X-linked dominant trait apparently due to defective intestinal absorption and/or renal reabsorption of inorganic phosphate that results in rickets and dwarfism. In a report by Lichtman and coworkers (1969), a patient with striking hypophosphatemia is described who had a significant depression in the steady-state concentration of erythrocyte adenosine triphosphate (ATP). Certain minimal concentrations of ATP are required for the viability of red cells in the circulation. In addition to reduced ATP, hypophosphatemia causes a marked decrease in concentrations of 2,3-diphosphoglycerate in erythrocytes. Acute hemolytic anemia and impaired oxygenation of tissues can occur in severe hypophosphatemia (Jacob and Amsden, 1971). This raises the possibility that other cellular stores of ATP and other critical organic phosphate compounds may be depleted. These biochemical abnormalities, in turn, could well be responsible for certain features of the clinical syndrome.

In general, the phosphorus present in ordinary foods is an adequate source of the ion. The use of expensive preparations of organic phosphates as "tonics" has no validity.

Pathological Conditions Associated with a Disturbance in Phosphate Metabolism. A defect in phosphate metabolism occurs in a variety of diseases, as briefly mentioned below.

Osteoporosis. This condition is considered to be a primary disorder in the formation of bone matrix. There is no primary defect in phosphate metabolism, and plasma concentrations of phosphorus are within usual limits.

Rickets. The consequences of deficiency of vitamin D with regard to the metabolism of both phosphate and calcium are described below, as are other forms of rickets. *Familial hypophosphatemia* is due to defective absorption and/or excretion of inorganic phosphate and has been mentioned above.

Osteomalacia. The loss of calcium in stools (due to malabsorption) or the loss from body fluids by way of the kidney (essential hypercalciuria or renal tubular acidosis with augmented calcium excretion) promotes a negative balance of calcium. Such loss deprives the body of calcium stores, and the calcium concentration in plasma falls slightly. This, in turn, stimulates the secretion of PTH, which restores the calcium concentration to normal but tends to promote some depression of plasma phosphorus.

Osteitis Fibrosa Cystica. In this disorder, there is a primary increase in the secretion of PTH that is usually accompanied by an increase in plasma calcium, some reduction of plasma phosphorus, and a decreased renal tubular reabsorption of phosphate.

Secondary Hyperparathyroidism. This condition may be seen in patients with chronic renal insufficiency. The sequence of events probably starts with a high plasma concentration of phosphorus and a low value for calcium; this situation stimulates parathyroid secretion. Since the elevated plasma phosphorus is a consequence of renal insufficiency, it persists. The continuing hyperphosphatemia may be modified by the administration of aluminum hydroxide gel, which tends to inhibit the absorption of phosphate from the bowel, owing to the formation of insoluble aluminum phosphates.

Hypoparathyroidism. In this disorder, characterized by deficient parathyroid secretion, there is a rise in plasma phosphorus and a decreased concentration of calcium. This condition can be readily treated with vitamin D with or without calcium supplementation.

Preparations. Only certain of the preparations of *inorganic phosphates* are mentioned here; *calcium phosphates* are described elsewhere.

Phosphate (in the form of sodium and/or potassium salts) is available in tablets, capsules (contents to be diluted with water), and powders for solution. It is also available as *sodium phosphates oral solution,* which is used as a laxative. *Potassium phosphate* and *sodium phosphate injections* are each available in solutions for intravenous administration that contain 3 mmol of phosphate per milliliter.

Therapeutic Uses. The phosphates are of limited therapeutic usefulness. Sodium phosphate has been employed to diminish hypercalcemia. The phosphates have a role in the management of the phosphate-depletion syndrome. Phosphate salts are also effective saline cathartics (*see* Chapter 43).

PARATHYROID HORMONE

History. Although there were many earlier references to the yellow glandular bodies attached to the thyroid, credit for the discovery of the parathyroid gland is usually given to Sandstrom, who in 1880 published an anatomical report that attracted little attention among physiologists. The glands were rediscovered a decade later by Gley, who determined the effects of their extirpation with the thyroid. Vassale and Generali then successfully removed the parathyroids without interfering with the thyroid and noted that tetany, convulsions, and death quickly followed. They thereby demonstrated that this syndrome was specifically due to parathyroid removal. However, the symptoms following parathyroidectomy varied so greatly in different species that the importance of the organs was not appreciated, and controversies continued as to whether they were essential to life. The subsequent discovery of internal and accessory parathyroids accounted for the discrepancies in experimental results and paved the way to the elucidation of the important physiological role played by this endocrine gland.

MacCallum and Voegtlin (1909) first noted the effect of parathyroidectomy on the concentration of plasma calcium. Since Howell and Loeb had previously established the physiological importance of the calcium ion, the relation of low plasma calcium to parathyroprivic symptoms was quickly appreciated and a comprehensive picture of parathyroid function began to form. After various attempts to obtain active extracts of the gland, success was finally attained (Berman, 1924; Collip, 1925; Hanson, 1925). It was readily demonstrated that active extracts could alleviate hypocalcemic tetany in parathyroidectomized animals and raise the concentration of calcium in the plasma of normal animals. For the first time, the relation of certain definite clinical abnormalities to parathyroid hyperfunction was appreciated.

While investigators in the United States, Canada, and England were utilizing the physiological approach to solve the problem of the function of the parathyroid glands, German and Austrian pathologists were associating the skeletal changes of osteitis fibrosa cystica with the presence of parathyroid tumors. In a delightful historical review, Albright (1948) traced the manner in which these two diverse types of investigations finally arrived at the same conclusion.

Chemistry. Human, bovine, and porcine parathyroid hormones are all single polypeptide chains of 84 amino acid residues. Their molecular weights are approximately 9500, and the entire amino acid sequence has been established for each. Biological activity is associated with the N-terminal portion of the peptide; residues 1 to 27 are required. Bovine and porcine PTH differ by only seven amino acid residues, and the amino-terminal segment of the human hormone differs from the equivalent portion of the bovine and porcine molecules by only four and three amino acid residues, respectively. The three differ little in biological activity, but they are immunologically distinguishable; however, they cross-react with a single antibody and this facilitates an immunoassay for PTH, as discussed below. The sequence comprised of the first 34 amino acids of human and bovine PTH has been synthesized and shown to have characteristic biological activity. (*See* Brewer *et al.*, 1974.) The fragment consisting of residues 3 to 34 is an antagonist of PTH *in vitro;* however, to date, studies have failed to reveal antagonism *in vivo* (McGowan, *et al.*, 1983).

Synthesis, Secretion, and Immunoassay. PTH is synthesized initially in a prehormone form. The product of translation that is destined to become PTH is called preproparathyroid hormone, an unfortunate name that grew by accretion in an adaptation to new knowledge of PTH synthesis. This single-chain peptide of 115 amino acids is rapidly converted to proparathyroid hormone by cleavage of a 25 amino-acid peptide fragment from the amino terminus as the peptide is transferred to the intracisternal space of the endoplasmic reticulum. The proparathyroid hormone, which persists somewhat longer than its precursor (15 to 20 minutes, compared to 1 to 2 minutes), moves to the Golgi apparatus and is converted to PTH, again by the cleavage of an N-terminal fragment of six predominantly basic amino acids. The PTH is enclosed within secretory granules, where it remains until released into the circulation. Neither preproparathyroid hormone nor proparathyroid hormone appears in plasma (Habener and Potts, 1978; Cohn and Elting, 1983).

Agents that stimulate adenylate cyclase activity in parathyroid cells increase the secretion of PTH. Among others, these include β-adrenergic agonists and prostaglandins. Calcium probably controls the secretion of PTH by decreasing the cyclic AMP content of parathyroid cells. Synthesis of PTH is not inhibited by calcium, but the extent of proteolytic degradation of the hormone in secretory granules is increased, possibly because more PTH is stored in the presence of elevated concentrations of calcium in plasma (Cohn and Elting, 1983).

Intact PTH has a half-life in plasma of 2 to 5 minutes; removal by the liver and kidney accounts for about 90% of the clearance. Metabolism of PTH results in the production of fragments that circulate in the blood (Hruska *et al.*, 1981). A 6000-dalton fragment from the carboxy terminus is the major circulating peptide that results from PTH metabolism. While this peptide is not active biologically, it does react with antibodies prepared against the intact hormone. The active region of PTH, residues 1 to 27, is, in contrast, poorly reactive immunologically, and fragments from this region tend not to be recognized as PTH by most antibodies. In spite of these problems, management of patients is generally satisfactory with immunoassays that recognize inactive peptides from the carboxy terminus as well as the intact hormone (*see* Broadus and Rasmussen, 1981; Mallette *et al.*, 1982). As noted, measurements of urinary concentrations of cyclic AMP can also provide a useful assessment of parathyroid function.

Physiological Functions. The primary function of PTH is to elicit the adaptive changes that serve to maintain a constant concentration of calcium ion in the extracellular fluid. Processes that are regulated include the absorption of calcium from the gastrointestinal tract, the deposition and mobilization of bone calcium, and the excretion of the ion in urine, feces, sweat, and milk. There is evidence that PTH accomplishes its functions by directly or indirectly influencing all of these mechanisms, but its most prominent effect is to promote the mobilization of calcium from bone.

Regulation of Secretion. The concentration of ionized calcium in the blood (or, perhaps, the concentration of ionized calcium in parathyroid cells) is the primary factor that regulates the secretory activity of the parathyroid gland. When the concentration of ionized calcium is low, the secretion of PTH is increased, and hypertrophy and hyperplasia of the gland result if the hypocalcemia is sustained. If the concentration of ionized calcium is high, the secretion of PTH is decreased, and hypoplasia may result if the hypercalcemia is sustained. *In vitro* studies show that amino acid uptake, nucleic acid and protein synthesis, cytoplasmic growth, and secretion of PTH are stimulated by exposure to low concentrations of calcium and suppressed by exposure to high concentrations. Thus, the calcium ion *per se* appears to regulate growth of the parathyroid gland and its synthesis and secretion of hormone (Roth and Raisz, 1964). Acutely, secretion of PTH can be elicited by hypocalcemia without alteration of the rate of synthesis of PTH (Habener and Potts, 1978; Cohn and Elting, 1983).

Although increased levels of calcium will lower concentrations of cyclic AMP in parathyroid cells, questions remain as to the exact relationship between calcium, the cyclic nucleotide, and regulation of PTH secretion. Brown and colleagues (1978) found that calcium decreases PTH secretion at any given concentration of cyclic AMP, in addition to lowering concentrations of the cyclic nucleotide. The degree of activation of protein kinase, the enzyme through which cyclic AMP is presumed to act, does not appear to change when calcium inhibits PTH secretion severely (Brown and Thatcher, 1982).

Catecholamines may play a role in secretion of PTH. Both epinephrine (Fischer *et al.*, 1973) and dopamine (Brown *et al.*, 1977) can stimulate release of PTH. Calcitriol (*see* below) inhibits secretion of PTH, but whether this is a direct effect of this vitamin D analog or the result of increased calcium in plasma is not certain (Haussler and McCain, 1977).

There appears to be no direct relation between extracellular concentrations of phosphate and the secretion of PTH, except indirectly as changes in phosphate values affect the concentration of calcium. Both hypermagnesemia and hypomagnesemia can inhibit the secretion of PTH (Rude *et al.*, 1976).

Thus, the extracellular concentration of ionized calcium is controlled on a minute-to-minute basis by a feedback system, the afferent limb of which is sensitive to the concentration of calcium and the efferent limb of which releases PTH. The hormone acts on various peripheral tissues to mobilize calcium into the extracellular fluid and thus restores the concentration to normal (Arnaud, 1978).

Effects on Bone. PTH acts on bone to increase the rate of resorption of calcium and phosphate. The site of the resorptive effect appears to be on the stable, older portion of bone mineral and not on the labile fraction.

Resorption of bone is brought about by osteolytic cells—osteoclasts and osteocytes. PTH stimulates the rate of bone resorption by these cells, increases the rate of conversion (differentiation) of mesenchymal cells to osteoclasts, and prolongs the half-life of these latter cells. Twenty minutes after the administration of PTH to some species, activation of osteoclasts is evident by the appearance of ruffled borders on the cells adjacent to bone surfaces (Miller, 1978). With prolonged action of PTH the number of bone-forming osteoblasts is also increased; thus, the rate of bone turnover and remodeling is enhanced. However, individual osteoblasts appear to be less active than normal, and PTH acts to inhibit their synthesis of collagen, a major component of bone matrix.

Biochemical correlates of PTH action have also been studied extensively in bone cultures. PTH causes resorption of cultured bone, and a number of biochemical effects of PTH have been described. A difficulty with this approach is that bone resorption *per se* leads to biochemical changes that may have no relation to specific actions of PTH. PTH stimulates the release of collagenase and other hydrolytic enzymes into the culture medium, stimulates glycolysis, and inhibits the oxidation of citrate—responses that may only reflect the breakdown of bone. Consequently, no satisfactory hypothesis has yet been offered to explain the action of PTH at the biochemical level. Some effects that may be of fundamental importance to the action of PTH include activation of adenylate cyclase with resulting accumulation of cyclic AMP, increased entry of calcium into the cells, change in membrane potential of osteoclasts, and increased incorporation of uridine into osteoclast RNA. How these observations relate to the action of PTH in bone remains to be clarified (*see* Raisz, 1977). There is evidence to support the concept that the ultimate step in PTH-stimulated release of calcium from bone involves calcium-sodium exchange (Krieger and Tashjian, 1980).

Effects on the Kidney. PTH acts on the kidney to increase tubular reabsorption of calcium and to inhibit tubular reabsorption of phosphate. As a result, calcium is retained and its concentration tends to increase in the plasma; phosphate is excreted and the plasma concentration tends to fall.

Calcium. PTH increases tubular calcium reabsorption at a distal site (Agus *et al.*, 1973). Therefore, when the concentration of calcium in plasma is in the normal range, extirpation of the gland decreases tubular reabsorption of calcium and thereby increases calcium excretion in the urine. When the plasma concentration falls significantly (to less than 7 mg/dl), a decrease in calcium excretion occurs because the amount of calcium filtered through the glomeruli is lowered to the point that the cation is almost completely reabsorbed despite the reduced tubular reabsorptive capacity. However, when parathyroidectomized animals are kept on a high-calcium diet and plasma calcium remains higher than 7 mg/dl, the hypercalciuria persists. If PTH is administered to such hypoparathyroid animals or man, tubular reabsorption of calcium is increased and there is initially a decrease in the excretion of calcium. This, along with mobilization of calcium from bone and increased absorption from the gut, results in increased concentration of calcium in plasma. When the value rises above normal, the hypercalciuria so characteristic of hyperparathyroidism ensues.

Phosphate. It is now well established that PTH increases the renal excretion of inorganic phosphate. PTH decreases the reabsorption of phosphate in all or most segments of the nephron proximal to the collecting duct (Lechene *et al.*, 1978).

Cyclic AMP mediates the effects of PTH on the kidney (*see* Brown and Aurbach, 1980). Adenylate cyclase that is stimulated by PTH is located in the renal cortex, and cyclic AMP synthesized in response to the hormone affects tubular transport mechanisms. A portion of the cyclic nucleotide synthesized at this site escapes into the urine, and its assay serves as a measure of parathyroid activity (*see* Chase *et al.*, 1969; *see also* below). Cyclic AMP may inhibit proximal tubular reabsorption of calcium, phosphate, bicarbonate, and sodium. The final effect on calcium excretion is, however, inhibitory, since it stimulates distal calcium reabsorption out of proportion to that of sodium (Agus *et al.*, 1973).

Other Ions. PTH also influences the excretion of other ions, most of which are constituents of bone. Renal excretion of magnesium is reduced by the hormone, and the plasma concentration is elevated; in parathyroidectomized animals, magnesium excretion is usually increased and the plasma concentration is reduced. The hormonal effect on magnesium is probably due, as in the case for calcium, to both increased renal tubular reabsorption of magnesium and its mobilization from the exchangeable compartment of bone (MacIntyre *et al.*, 1963). The excretion of water, amino acids, citrate, potassium, bicarbonate, sodium, chloride, and sulfate is increased, whereas the excretion of hydrogen ion is decreased by PTH. The increased excretion of bicarbonate ion appears to be mainly due to inhibition of proximal tubular reabsorption of this anion; it is antagonized by calcium. Although the effects of PTH on regulation of acid-base metabolism by the kidney are similar to those of acetazolamide, they are independent of the carbonic anhydrase system. The effects of PTH on other ions involve actions on both proximal and distal tubules.

Effects on the Gastrointestinal Tract. PTH acts indirectly to increase intestinal absorption of calcium and phosphate. This effect is now believed to be mediated entirely through the hormone's enhancement of the conversion of calcifediol to calcitriol in the kidney, and the effects of PTH on absorption are the consequence of increased concentrations of calcitriol (*see* section on vitamin D below).

Miscellaneous Effects. PTH decreases the concentration of calcium in milk and saliva. These effects are the opposite from those that would be expected from the concurrent changes in plasma calcium concentration. It appears likely, therefore, that the hormone can conserve calcium in the extracellular fluid not only by its effects on bone, kidney, and gut but also by reducing the rate of calcium transport from extracellular fluid to milk and saliva.

PTH also reduces the calcium concentration in the lens, a fact that explains the prevalence of cataracts in patients with hypoparathyroidism and the increased content of calcium in the lens in hormone-deficient animals.

Hypoparathyroidism. Hypoparathyroidism is only one of the many causes of hypocalcemia and occurs relatively rarely. The deficiency syndrome most commonly follows operative procedures on either the thyroid gland or the parathyroids themselves. Less frequently, disease of the parathyroids is the cause (*idiopathic hypoparathyroidism*). Also uncommon is a genetic disorder in which the target organs do not respond to PTH, despite adequate concentrations of the hormone (*pseudohypoparathyroidism*).

In all varieties of hypoparathyroidism, hypocalcemia and its associated symptoms are encountered clinically. The earliest prodromal symptoms of hypocalcemia are paresthesias in the extremities. Mechanical stimulation of peripheral nerves during physical examination usually produces contraction of the appropriate skeletal muscles. These signs and symptoms may be followed by manifest tetany, consisting in muscle spasms, especially carpopedal spasm and laryngospasm. Eventually, generalized convulsions and other central nervous system (CNS) manifestations occur. It is highly probable that smooth muscle is also affected. For example, hypocalcemia may be followed by spasm of the ciliary muscle, iris, esophagus, intestine, urinary bladder, and bronchi. ECG changes and a marked tachycardia indicate that the heart is involved. Vascular spasm in the fingers and toes is also commonly observed. In *chronic hypoparathyroidism*, ectodermal changes, consisting in loss of hair, grooved and brittle fingernails, defects of the dental enamel, and cataracts are frequently encountered; there is also calcification in the basal ganglia and perhaps other soft tissues. Psychiatric symptoms such as emotional lability, anxiety, depression, and delusions are often present. The EEG may be abnormal.

Hypoparathyroidism is treated primarily with vitamin D (*see* below). Dietary supplementation with calcium may also be necessary.

Hyperparathyroidism. *Primary hyperparathyroidism* results either from hypersecretion of the parathyroid glands (due to hyperplasia, adenoma, or, rarely, carcinoma) or from secretion of PTH-like polypeptides from tumors arising at other sites. In some cases such polypeptides may be distinguished from PTH by immunological technics. Plasma calcium concentrations may be normal with primary hyperparathyroidism, but they are usually elevated and plasma phosphate values are usually decreased. Hyperparathyroidism may also be *secondary* to conditions causing negative calcium balance, such as malabsorption and renal disease; in these cases the concentration of calcium in plasma is low and provides the stimulus for increased secretion of PTH. Hypersecretion of PTH from any cause may lead to a bone disorder known as *osteitis fibrosa generalisata*. However, only one third of cases of hyperparathyroidism exhibit advanced bone changes; another third show minor degrees of decalcification; and the remaining cases present no obvious skeletal abnormalities. However, metabolic studies indicate that resorption of bone is actively occurring in the last-named group; the calcium intake may be sufficient to maintain calcium balance. The symptoms of early decalcification are aching and pain in the bones and joints.

Uncomplicated primary hyperparathyroidism is invariably associated with hypercalciuria and hyperphosphaturia, and is sometimes accompanied by polyuria and polydipsia. The excretion of excessive amounts of calcium and phosphate results in a high incidence of renal calculi, which often cause the presenting symptoms. An equally serious complication is a diffuse nephrocalcinosis, which may progress to a stage of extreme renal insufficiency. It is well to keep in mind that renal insufficiency secondary to nephrocalcinosis or to sequelae of urolithiasis may mask some of the cardinal biochemical features of hyperparathyroidism, namely, hyperphosphaturia, hypercalciuria, and hypophosphatemia.

Hypercalcemia *per se* can be the cause of some of the signs and symptoms of hyperparathyroidism. These include hypotonicity of muscle, with general skeletal muscle weakness and smooth muscle dysfunction leading to constipation, flatulence, anorexia, nausea, and vomiting. Occasionally, cardiac irregularities are observed. A higher-than-normal incidence of peptic ulcers and pancreatitis has been reported in patients with the disease. Neuropsychiatric manifestations also occur in many cases. Advanced cases of osteitis fibrosa generalisata may exhibit anemia and leukopenia.

In addition to laboratory study of calcium and phosphorus, there are certain more specific tests for hyperparathyroidism. The most widely used is the radioimmunoassay of PTH in plasma. However, as discussed above, this test is dependent on the preparation of antibody used. Another method involves determination of the concentration of cyclic AMP in urine, which is elevated by the action of PTH on the kidney (Murad and Pak, 1972; Broadus and Rasmussen, 1981).

Treatment. Surgical resection of the hyperplastic or adenomatous glands is almost always required for the treatment of primary hyperparathyroidism. Surgery can return the patient to a euparathyroid state and prevent continued renal damage and bone dissolution. As discussed earlier, transient hypocalcemia often occurs following surgery, particularly when bone disease is present; this requires brief therapy with calcium. If an excessive amount of parathyroid tissue is removed, permanent hypoparathyroidism may ensue. In this case vitamin D therapy and/or supplementation of the diet with calcium is required. Chronic treatment with oral neutral phosphate, a low-calcium diet, and liberal amounts of fluids is used to lower the plasma calcium concentration in selected patients in whom surgery is contraindicated (Purnell *et al.*, in Symposium, 1974).

Preparations. Parathyroid injection is no longer available commercially for clinical use. *Synthetic parathyroid hormone* (bovine) is available for investigational purposes as the (1-34 amino acid) tetratriacontapeptide.

Absorption, Fate, and Excretion. PTH must be given parenterally. The usual route of administration is subcutaneous or intravenous. The maximal effect is obtained approximately 18 hours after a single subcutaneous injection; the response may last for 36 hours. The peak effect of hormone given intravenously is seen within 1 hour and may last for several hours. Studies in animals with the endogenous hormone assayed by the immunological method demonstrate that its half-life in the body is about 2 to 5 minutes, as noted above. The hormone appears to be transported in the blood, at least in part, in the α-globulin fraction of plasma protein. It is metabolized primarily by the liver to various peptide fragments. Excretion in the urine is minimal (less than 1%).

Clinical Uses. There are currently no valid therapeutic uses of PTH; while it was formerly employed to elevate the concentration of calcium in plasma, this can be accomplished with greater safety by the administration of calcium and/or vitamin D.

PTH has been used for the *diagnosis* of pseudohypoparathyroidism. Since this disease is characterized by target-organ resistance to the hormone, these patients fail to show an increased concentration of calcium in plasma and fail to excrete increased amounts of phosphate and cyclic AMP after the administration of PTH (200 units, intravenously) (*see* Chase *et al.*, 1969).

CALCITONIN

History and Source. A hypocalcemic hormone, the effects of which are generally opposite to those of the parathyroid hormone, was discovered and named *calcitonin* by Copp in 1962 (*see* Copp, 1964). It was demonstrated as a result of perfusion of dogs' parathyroid and thyroid glands with hypercalcemic blood. This caused an immediate transitory hypocalcemic effect in the systemic blood that occurred significantly earlier than does the hypocalcemia observed after total parathyroidectomy. The observations led Copp to conclude that the parathyroid glands secreted calcitonin in response to hypercalcemia and in this way reduced the elevated plasma calcium concentration to normal. Munson and colleagues (Hirsch *et al.*, 1963) noted that parathyroidectomy in rats performed by cauterization caused more severe hypocalcemia than did thyroparathyroidectomy. They thus suspected the existence of a hypocalcemic principle in the thyroid gland. They found that extracts of thyroid produced a hypocalcemic response and named the thyroid factor *thyrocalcitonin*. It is now known that the two factors are the same and that the hormone does originate from the thyroid; however, calcitonin is the name that is generally used.

The parafollicular "C" cells from the thyroid, which are embryologically derived from the ultimobranchial body, are the site of production and secretion of calcitonin. In nonmammalian vertebrates, calcitonin is found only in ultimobranchial bodies, which are separate organs from the thyroid gland. The hormone from both sources, thyroid and ultimobranchial bodies, is the same. In man, calcitonin is present in the thyroid, parathyroid, and thymus, an indication that the "C" cells are widely distributed.

Chemistry and Immunoreactivity. The calcitonins from the thyroid of the pig and a number of other species, including salmon and man, have been isolated, characterized chemically, and totally synthesized. They are all single-chain polypeptides with a molecular weight of 3600, and contain 32 amino acids. A cystine disulfide bridge exists in the 1-7 position at the amino end of the chain; it is essential for biological activity. The carboxyl-terminal amino acid is prolinamide. Calcitonin isolated from human "C"-cell tumors differs from the porcine hormone in 18 of its amino acid residues. The use of synthetic human calcitonin has improved the sensitivity of radioimmunoassays to the point where the hormone can be measured in the blood of normal individuals. There appear to be multiple forms of calcitonin in plasma, including molecules of high molecular weight that may represent polymers of calcitonin, ionically linked aggregates, or calcitonin linked by disulfide bonds to plasma proteins. Antisera vary in their ability to recognize regions of the molecule. These factors make radioimmunoassay of calcitonin a procedure that is not specific for the calcitonin monomer; consequently, values for normal plasma calcitonin concentrations vary from one laboratory to another (*see* Austin and Heath, 1981).

Regulation of Secretion. The secretion and biosynthesis of calcitonin in both animals and man are regulated by the concentration of calcium in plasma. When the calcium concentration is high, the amount of the hormone in plasma increases. When the concentration is low, the amount of the hormone decreases markedly and may be undetectable. Normal basal concentrations of calcitonin in plasma as measured by the radioimmunoassay method are <100 pg/ml in more than 75% of subjects. Calcium infusion increases the basal concentration two- to threefold (Tashjian *et al.*, 1974). The mean concentration of calcitonin in the plasma of women is significantly lower than in men and is less responsive to hypercalcemia (Heath and Sizemore, 1977). The half-life of calcitonin is short (about 10 minutes); hence the hormone most likely is secreted at a fairly continuous rate at normal plasma calcium concentrations. A role of cyclic AMP in the release of calcitonin from "C" cells of the thyroid is indicated by the fact that the dibutyryl derivative of cyclic AMP stimulates its release.

While it is clear that calcitonin secretion can be stimulated by epinephrine, glucagon, gastrin, and cholecystokinin under experimental conditions, the evidence for a physiological role of these hormones is not convincing. It is also not known to what extent normal physiological variations in secretion occur or if calcitonin plays a significant role in calcium homeostasis. High concentrations of calcitonin have been found in plasma, urine, and tumor tissue (50 to 5000 times normal) in patients with medullary carcinoma of the thyroid gland. The tumor cells originate from the parafollicular cells of the thyroid, and this disease represents a true calcitonin-excess syndrome. Measurement of the response of plasma calcitonin to an infusion of calcium gluconate and pentagastrin appears to be a valuable procedure for detection of thyroid medullary carcinoma (Wells *et al.*, 1978). Because one form of this disease is inherited as a dominant trait, relatives of patients should be examined repeatedly (Tashjian *et al.*, 1974).

Mechanism and Actions. There is general agreement from both acute and chronic experiments *in vivo* and culture of bone *in vitro* that the hypocalcemic and hypophosphatemic effects of calcitonin are due predominately to *direct inhibition of bone resorption* by osteoclastic and osteocytic cells. This effect on bone resorption is elicited in parathyroidectomized, nephrectomized, and eviscerated animals. It is not certain if calcitonin stimulates formation of bone by osteoblasts (Austin and Heath, 1981).

Although calcitonin tends to negate the effects of PTH on osteolysis, it does not act as an antiparathyroid hormone. Thus, it does not block the activation of bone-cell adenylate cyclase by PTH and does not inhibit the initial PTH-induced uptake of calcium into bone. The actions of calcitonin are not blocked by inhibitors of RNA and protein synthesis. The hormone produces a decrease in the amount of ruffled border of osteoclasts, indicating their diminished activity in bone resorption (Raisz, 1977). Part of the effect of calcitonin appears to be mediated through increasing the cyclic AMP concentration in bone cells, presumably in cells different from those so activated by PTH (Murad *et al.*, 1970; Brown and Aurbach, 1980).

Calcitonin also antagonizes the inhibitory effects of PTH on pyrophosphatase activity in isolated Ehrlich ascites tumor cells. Pyrophosphate and pyrophosphatase are intimately involved in the processes of bone formation and resorption. Calcitonin decreases glucose utilization and lactate production in bone, effects opposite to those of PTH. As a result of depressed bone resorption, the urinary excretion of calcium, magnesium, and hy-

droxyproline is decreased by calcitonin. Plasma phosphate concentration is also lowered, due mainly to decreased resorption of bone and also to increased urinary phosphate excretion. The direct effects of calcitonin on the kidney are dependent on species. In man, calcitonin increases the excretion of calcium, phosphate, and sodium, effects also mediated in part by cyclic AMP (Murad *et al.*, 1970; Pak, 1971; Paillard *et al.*, 1972). Calcitonin probably does not affect absorption of calcium from the intestinal tract.

Bioassay, Preparations, and Dosage. Bioassay of calcitonin preparations is performed by assessing their ability to lower plasma calcium concentration in the rat. The results are compared with a British Medical Research Council (MRC) Standard and expressed in MRC units. One unit is equivalent to approximately 4 μg of pure porcine calcitonin (*see* Symposium, 1974).

Salmon, porcine, and human calcitonins have been studied experimentally. The hormone from salmon is considerably more potent in man than are the other two, perhaps because it is cleared from the circulation more slowly. Salmon calcitonin is available for clinical use as CALCIMAR, a synthetic preparation supplied in 2-ml vials at 200 MRC units per milliliter. The recommended dosage (administered subcutaneously or intramuscularly) is 4 to 8 units/kg every 6 to 12 hours for hypercalcemia; an initial dose of 100 units per day is used for Paget's disease (*see* below).

Therapeutic Uses. Calcitonin is effective in diminishing hypercalcemia and decreasing concentrations of phosphate in the plasma of patients with hyperparathyroidism, idiopathic hypercalcemia of infancy, vitamin D intoxication, and osteolytic bone metastases. The effect of a single dose lasts for 6 to 10 hours. The decrease in plasma calcium and phosphate is the result of their decreased resorption from bone. Although calcitonin is effective in the initial treatment of hypercalcemia from various causes, other measures are recommended and are generally more practical (*see* section above on hypercalcemia).

Calcitonin is effective in diseases characterized by increased skeletal remodeling (increased bone resorption and bone formation), such as occurs in Paget's disease (Deftos and First, 1981). In this disease, calcitonin given chronically produces symptomatic relief and reduction in alkaline phosphatase activity in plasma, urinary hydroxyproline, and blood flow through the affected area. However, patients may become resistant to therapy after several months. Development of antibodies to porcine or salmon calcitonin does occur with long-term therapy in many patients; this is more common with the porcine preparation and may explain the development of resistance. While optimal dosage has not been established, favorable results were obtained in one study with 100 MRC units of salmon calcitonin given daily or three times a week by subcutaneous injection. The minimal dose for long-term therapy appeared to be 50 MRC units injected three times weekly. Side effects include nausea and swelling and tenderness of the hands; urticaria has also been observed. It is anticipated that human calcitonin will be much less likely to cause resistance and allergic reactions; it is not yet available.

SODIUM ETIDRONATE

This drug is available for the treatment of Paget's disease of bone. It is structurally related to pyrophosphate, which may have a role in bone mineralization, and has the following formula:

$$HO-\underset{\underset{O}{\overset{ONa}{\|}}}{P}-\underset{\underset{CH_3}{\overset{OH}{|}}}{C}-\underset{\underset{O}{\overset{ONa}{\|}}}{P}-OH$$

Sodium Etidronate

This compound (and other diphosphonates), when added to appropriate solutions and suspensions of calcium phosphate, slows the formation and dissolution of crystals of hydroxyapatite. Diphosphonates can protect experimental animals against calcification of soft tissues in vitamin D intoxication (Francis et al., 1969).

The physicochemical action of this drug on the dynamics of crystal formation and dissolution are thought to be responsible for its favorable effects in patients with Paget's disease. In this disease there are foci of increased turnover of bone; these lead to the characteristic alterations of bone structure, which in turn may produce secondary problems, including deafness, spinal cord injuries, high-output cardiac failure, and disabling pain. Sodium etidronate may decrease the elevated plasma alkaline phosphatase activity and the urinary excretion of hydroxyproline that are characteristic of this disease. Most patients experience a decrease in bone pain, but worsening of bone pain has also been reported. There is an increase in the amount of nonmineralized osteoid, especially after treatment with higher doses; this may increase the risk of fractures (Krane, 1982). The drug is effective orally. It is excreted without metabolic alteration by the kidney; dosage must therefore be reduced when there is renal insufficiency (Russell and Fleisch, 1975).

Advantages of this agent over calcitonin include its oral efficacy, lower cost, and lack of antigenicity. In addition, biochemical indices of the rate of bone turnover are more often normalized with etidronate than with calcitonin (Krane, 1982). The relative merits of these two agents or a combination of the two are as yet undetermined.

Etidronate disodium (DIDRONEL) is available in tablets containing 200 or 400 mg. The usual initial dose is 5 mg/kg, given once daily in courses that should be given for no more than 6 months. Such treatment may induce a remission of Paget's disease that can last for years. If symptoms recur, additional courses of therapy may be effective. The drug is also used to reduce heterotopic ossification due to spinal cord injury or that which complicates total hip replacement.

VITAMIN D

Traditionally, vitamin D was assigned a passive role in calcium metabolism in that its presence in adequate concentrations was thought to permit proper absorption of dietary calcium and to allow full expression of the actions of parathyroid hormone. Recent findings indicate a much more active role of vitamin D in the homeostatic mechanisms that control calcium metabolism. It now appears that vitamin D (or its active metabolite) may be considered to be a hormone that plays a major role in the precise control of the concentration of calcium ion in plasma. The following characteristics of vitamin D are consistent with hormonal activity: vitamin D is synthesized in the skin and under ideal conditions probably is not required in the diet; it is transported by the blood to distant sites in the body, where it is activated; its active form then affects target tissues, resulting in increased plasma calcium concentration; and the conversion of vitamin D to its active form is a reaction that is regulated in a negative-feedback system by plasma calcium.

History. Vitamin D is the name applied to two related fat-soluble substances, cholecalciferol and calciferol, that have in common the ability to prevent or cure rickets. Prior to the discovery of vitamin D a high percentage of urban children, especially in the temperate zones, developed rickets. Some thought that the disease was due to lack of fresh air and sunshine; others claimed a dietary factor caused the disease. The work of Mellanby (1919) and Huldschinsky (1919) showed both of these notions to be correct; the addition of cod liver oil to the diet or exposure to sunlight would either prevent or cure the disease. In 1924 it was found that irradiation of animal rations was as efficacious in curing rickets as was irradiation of the animal itself (Hess and Weinstock, 1924; Steenbock and Black, 1924). These observations led to the elucidation of the structures of cholecalciferol and calciferol and eventually to the discovery that these compounds are further metabolized in the body to active compounds. This latter discovery of metabolic activation is primarily attributable to studies conducted in the laboratories of DeLuca in the United States and Kodicek in England (*see* Kodicek, 1974; DeLuca and Schnoes, 1976).

Chemistry and Occurrence. Ultraviolet irradiation of a variety of animal and plant sterols results in their conversion to compounds with vitamin D (antirachitic) activity. Cleavage of the carbon-to-carbon bond between C 9 and C 10 is the essential alteration produced by the photochemical process, but not all sterols that undergo this cleavage possess antirachitic activity. The principal provitamin found in animal tissues is 7-dehydrocholesterol, which is synthesized in the skin. Exposure of the skin to sunlight converts 7-dehydrocholesterol to cholecalciferol (vitamin D_3) (*see* Figure 65–1). Holick and associates have found an intermediate in the photolysis reaction, previtamin D_3, a 6,7-*cis* isomer that accumulates in the skin after exposure to ultraviolet radiation (*see* Holick, 1981). This slowly converts spontaneously to vitamin D_3 and may provide a sustained source of D_3 for some time after exposure to ultraviolet light. The active form of vitamin D is now thought to be *calcitriol* [1,25-(OH)$_2$ cholecalciferol], which is formed by two successive hydroxylations of vitamin D_3.

Ergosterol, which is present in yeasts and fungi, is the provitamin for vitamin D_2 (calciferol). Ergosterol and vitamin D_2 differ from 7-dehydrocholesterol and vitamin D_3, respectively, only by each having a double bond between C 22 and C 23 and a methyl group at C 24. Vitamin D_2 is the active constituent in a number of commercial vitamin preparations as well as in irradiated bread and irradiated

milk. The material historically designated as vitamin D_1 was later shown to be a mixture of antirachitic substances.

In some species the antirachitic potencies of vitamin D_2 and vitamin D_3 differ greatly from each other. In man there is no practical difference between the two, and in the following discussion vitamin D will be used as the collective term for vitamins D_2 and D_3.

METABOLIC ACTIVATION

Dietary vitamin D, or that which is synthesized intrinsically, requires metabolic activation in order to exert its characteristic actions on target tissues. It is now believed that the active form of the vitamin is calcitriol, the product of two successive hydroxylations of D_3. The pathway of activation is shown in Figure 65–1. This subject has been reviewed by DeLuca and Schnoes

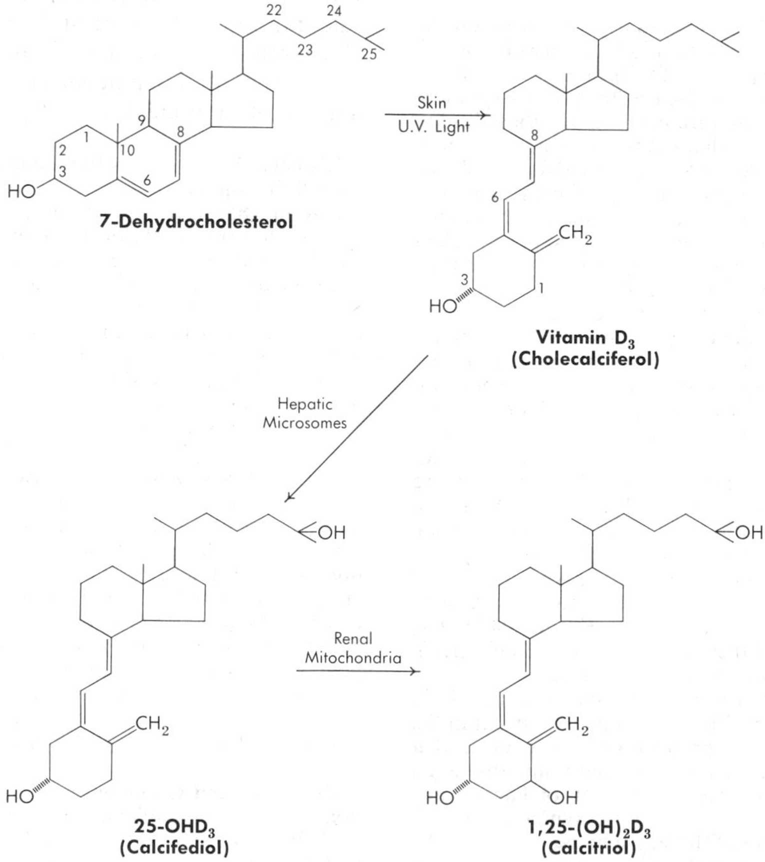

Figure 65–1. *Metabolic activation of vitamin D.* (*See* text for explanation and abbreviations.)

(1976, 1983), Haussler and McCain (1977), and Fraser (1980).

25-Hydroxylation of Vitamin D. In man the initial step in the activation of vitamin D_3 occurs predominantly in the liver, and the product is 25-hydroxycholecalciferol (or calcifediol). The hepatic enzyme system responsible for 25-hydroxylation of vitamin D has not been fully characterized, but it is associated with the microsomal and mito-chondrial fractions of liver homogenates and requires the presence of NADPH and molecular oxygen for the hydroxylation reaction.

1-Hydroxylation of 25-OHD₃. After being produced in the liver, 25-OHD₃ en-ters the blood stream, where it circulates in association with vitamin D–binding globu-lin. Final activation to calcitriol occurs in the kidney. The enzyme system responsible for 1-hydroxylation of 25-OHD₃ is associ-ated with the mitochondria. It too is a mixed-function oxidase and requires mo-lecular oxygen and NADPH as cofactors. Cytochrome P-450, a flavoprotein, and fer-redoxin are components of the enzyme complex.

This enzyme is subject to dietary and endocrine regulations that are of great im-portance for calcium homeostasis. Thus, the activity of the hydroxylase increases in dietary deficiencies of vitamin D, calcium, and phosphate, and it is stimulated by PTH, prolactin, and estrogens. It is suppressed by a high intake of vitamin D. The slowness of the responses to some of these agents and their sensitivity to metabolic inhibitors strongly suggest that the variations in enzy-matic activity represent changes in the quantity of enzyme protein in the kidney. There is also evidence of an acute mecha-nism of control that can change the activity of the hydroxylase within a few minutes. In the case of PTH, this rapid stimulation is probably mediated by cyclic AMP (Larkins *et al.*, 1974; Rost *et al.*, 1981). The model proposed by Haussler and McCain (1977) encompasses the major concepts in this area, but some of these remain controver-sial (*see* Figure 65–2). There is evidence that hypocalcemia can activate the hydrox-

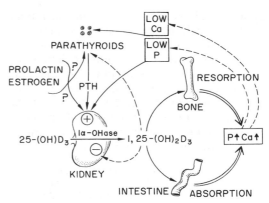

Figure 65–2. *Model for regulation of the bio-synthesis of 1,25-(OH)₂D₃.*

Solid arrows indicate a positive effect; dashed arrows refer to negative feedback (*see* text for explanation). (Modified from Haussler and McCain, 1977. Courtesy of the *New Eng-land Journal of Medicine.*)

ylase directly, in addition to affecting it indirectly by eliciting secretion of PTH (*see* Fraser, 1980). Hypophosphatemia in-creases the activity of the hydroxylase, but it is not known whether this is a direct or indirect effect (Haussler and McCain, 1977; Fraser, 1980; Rosen and Chesney, 1983). Calcitriol exerts negative-feedback control of the enzyme that may be a consequence of a direct action on the renal tissue or by an inhibition of the secretion of PTH. The nature of the regulatory mechanisms of es-trogens and prolactin on the 1α-hydroxylase is not known.

PHYSIOLOGICAL FUNCTIONS,
MECHANISM OF ACTION, AND
PHARMACOLOGICAL PROPERTIES

The physiological role of vitamin D is best characterized as that of a positive reg-ulator in calcium homeostasis. Phosphate metabolism is affected by the vitamin in a parallel manner to that of calcium.

The mechanisms by which vitamin D acts to maintain normal concentrations of cal-cium and phosphate in plasma are to facili-tate their absorption by the small intestine, to enhance their mobilization from bone, and to decrease their excretion by the kid-ney. These processes serve to maintain calcium and phosphate ions at concentrations in plasma that are essential for normal neuromuscular activity, mineralization of bone, and a number of other calcium-dependent functions. A direct role of the vitamin in the mineralization of bone has not been demonstrated; rather, it is thought that normal rates of bone formation occur when calcium and phosphate concentrations in the plasma are adequate.

Intestinal Absorption of Calcium. A defect in intestinal absorption of calcium in vitamin D–deficient rats was demonstrated in the late 1930s (Nicolaysen, 1937). More recently, movement of calcium from the mucosal to the serosal surface of the intestine has been shown to be a process involving a carrier and active transport against an electrochemical gradient (Adams and Norman, 1970). The active-transport mechanism is present in the microvilli of the brush border (luminal side) of the intestinal epithelial cells.

Calcitriol appears to act on the intestine in a manner that is analogous to the way steroid hormones such as estrogens act on target tissues. For example, the cytosol of chicken intestinal cells contains a 3.7 S protein that binds calcitriol specifically and with high affinity. Formation of a complex with this receptor facilitates the transfer of calcitriol to the nuclear chromatin (Brumbaugh and Haussler, 1974). When given *in vivo*, labeled calcitriol can be shown by autoradiographic technics to be located in the nuclei of cells of the intestinal villi and crypts (Zile *et al.*, 1978). Calcitriol stimulates synthesis of RNA and at least two proteins in the intestinal mucosa, alkaline phosphatase and a calcium-binding protein. The latter is absent from vitamin D–deficient animals, and it was proposed that the calcium-binding protein is involved in the transport of calcium. Careful examination of the sequence of events that follow the administration of calcitriol has shown, however, that stimulation of calcium transport is demonstrable 1 hour after calcitriol is given, but synthesis of the calcium-binding protein does not begin for 2 hours (Spencer *et al.*, 1978). Furthermore, cycloheximide blocks calcitriol-stimulated synthesis of intestinal proteins, including alkaline phosphatase and calcium-binding protein, but it does not prevent stimulation of calcium transport (Bikle *et al.*, 1978). Thus, the events that link the binding of calcitriol in the cytoplasm and nucleus of the intestinal cells to the stimulation of calcium and phosphate transport remain obscure.

It has been reported that calcitriol-induced stimulation of intestinal transport of phosphate precedes that of calcium, and it is possible that the primary effect of the vitamin is on phosphate rather than calcium transport (Birge and Miller, 1977). Neither parathyroidectomy nor administration of PTH modifies the response of the intestine to calcitriol (Garabedian *et al.*, 1974).

Mobilization of Bone Salts. Large doses of vitamin D cause decalcification of bone. In 1952,

Carlsson demonstrated that physiological doses of vitamin D promote mobilization of calcium from bone. A requirement for PTH for stimulation of decalcification by vitamin D remains controversial. Calcitriol stimulates resorption of bone in tissue culture in the absence of PTH (Raisz *et al.*, 1972), and dihydrotachysterol, a derivative of vitamin D_2, will promote bone resorption *in vivo* in hypoparathyroid individuals (*see* below). Experimental studies of vitamin D *in vivo*, however, are contradictory with regard to the obligatory role of PTH. It has been reported that administration of calcitriol to thyroparathyroidectomized rats increases bone resorption as in normal animals (Reynolds *et al.*, 1976), whereas Garabedian and associates (1974) concluded that calcitriol has a diminished action on bone after removal of the parathyroids.

The molecular mechanisms responsible for mobilization of bone salts are unclear. Active translocation of calcium across osteocytes (Talmage, 1972) or across a hypothetical bone membrane (Neuman and Ramp, 1971) has been proposed as the mechanism by which plasma calcium is maintained as a supersaturated solution that is not in chemical equilibrium with calcium in bone fluid. In such a scheme, mobilization of calcium from the bone compartment occurs when active transport of calcium from bone fluid to extracellular fluid is enhanced. Thus, vitamin D could promote mobilization of calcium from bone by stimulating active transport of calcium in osteocytes, perhaps by the same mechanisms that stimulate intestinal absorption of calcium. Recent investigations have indicated 1,25-$(OH)_2D_3$ may enhance the differentiation of mononuclear cells into osteoclastic, multinuclear cells (Bar-Shavit *et al.*, 1983). It has been suggested that patients with osteopetrosis, a disease where resorption of bone is deficient, may have a genetic defect that prevents cellular differentiation of osteoclast precursors in response to agents such as calcitriol (Coccia, 1983).

Renal Retention of Calcium and Phosphate. The effects of vitamin D on renal handling of calcium and phosphate have had relatively little study, and their quantitative importance is uncertain. Vitamin D has been shown to increase retention of calcium independently of phosphate. There is evidence that vitamin D enhances the reabsorption of calcium and phosphate by the proximal tubules (Puschett *et al.*, 1972; Costanzo *et al.*, 1974; Harris *et al.*, 1976).

Signs and Symptoms of Deficiency. A deficiency of vitamin D results in inadequate absorption of calcium and phosphate. The consequent decrease in plasma calcium stimulates PTH secretion, which acts to restore plasma calcium at the expense of bone calcium; plasma concentrations of phosphate remain subnormal. In infants and children, this results in a failure to mineralize newly formed osteoid tissue and cartilage matrix, causing the defect in bone growth known as *rickets*. As a consequence of inadequate calcification, the bones of individuals suffering from rickets are unusually soft, and the stress and strain of weight bearing give rise to the characteristic deformities of the disease.

In adults, vitamin D deficiency results in *osteomalacia* or adult rickets, which is most likely to occur during times of increased need for calcium, such as during pregnancy or lactation. The disease is characterized by a generalized decrease in bone density. Unlike osteoporosis, the remaining bone is abnormal in that it contains excessive amounts of uncalcified matrix. Gross deformities of bone occur only in advanced stages of the disease.

Hypervitaminosis. The acute or chronic administration of excessive amounts of vitamin D or enhanced responsiveness to normal amounts of the vitamin leads to a number of clinical syndromes that are the result of deranged calcium metabolism. The physiological or pathological responses to vitamin D are a function of endogenous production of vitamin D, tissue reactivity to the vitamin, and particularly vitamin D intake. Some infants seem to be hyperreactive to relatively small doses of vitamin D. Certain cases of hypervitaminosis D in adults result from the administration of large doses of the vitamin in the attempt to treat conditions that have been wrongly purported to benefit from vitamin D therapy. Other cases are the consequence of excessive doses used in the treatment of hypoparathyroidism. More commonly, toxicity is seen in children as a result of accidental ingestion or excessive administration of the vitamin by parents.

There is wide individual variation in the amount of vitamin D that causes hypervitaminosis. As a rough approximation, it may be stated that the continued ingestion of 50,000 units or more daily by a person with normal parathyroid function and normal sensitivity to vitamin D may result in poisoning. Hypercalcemia is particularly dangerous in patients who are receiving digitalis because the toxic effects of the cardiac glycosides are enhanced (*see* Chapter 30).

Signs and Symptoms. The initial signs and symptoms of vitamin D toxicity are those associated with hypercalcemia and consist in weakness, fatigue, lassitude, headache, nausea, vomiting, and diarrhea. Obtundation and coma may develop. Early impairment of renal function from hypercalcemia is manifest by polyuria, polydipsia, nocturia, decreased urinary concentrating ability, and proteinuria. Some of these effects are due to inhibition of the action of antidiuretic hormone by calcium. With prolonged hypercalcemia there may be deposition of calcium salts in soft tissues, most significantly within the kidney; this results in nephrolithiasis, diffuse nephrocalcinosis, or both. Other sites of calcification may include blood vessels, heart, lungs, and skin. Some individuals exhibit hypertension. The characteristic changes in blood chemistry are elevated concentrations of plasma calcium and nonprotein nitrogen; phosphate concentrations are variable. Mobilization of calcium from bone contributes to the hypercalcemia and is also responsible for the roentgenographic finding of localized or generalized osteoporosis in a significant percentage of cases of hypervitaminosis D.

In children, a single episode of moderately severe hypercalcemia may arrest growth completely for 6 months or more, and the deficit in height may never be fully corrected (Parfitt, 1972).

Vitamin D toxicity may be manifested in the fetus. There is a relationship between excess maternal vitamin D intake or extreme sensitivity to the vitamin and nonfamilial congenital supravalvular aortic stenosis. In infants, this anomaly is often found in association with other stigmata of hypercalcemia. Similar lesions have been produced experimentally in offspring of rabbits treated with large doses of vitamin D during pregnancy (Friedman and Roberts, 1966; Taussig, 1966). Maternal hypercalcemia may also result in suppression of parathyroid function in the newborn, with resultant hypocalcemia, tetany, and seizures.

An occasional sequela resulting from an acute episode of hypercalcemia in patients treated for hypoparathyroidism is a marked increase in response to vitamin D after the disappearance of the hypercalcemia (Leeson and Fourman, 1966).

Treatment of hypervitaminosis D consists in immediate withdrawal of the vitamin, a low-calcium diet, administration of glucocorticoids, and a generous intake of fluid. With this regimen the plasma calcium falls to normal and the calcium in the soft tissue tends to be mobilized. A conspicuous improvement in renal function is often noted with return of the plasma calcium to normal, but this may not occur if renal damage has been severe.

Absorption, Fate, and Excretion. Vitamin D is usually given by mouth, and gastrointestinal absorption is adequate under most conditions. Both vitamin D_2 and vitamin D_3 are absorbed from the small intestine, although vitamin D_3 may be absorbed more completely and more rapidly. The exact portion of the gut that is most effective in vitamin D absorption may be a function of the vehicle in which the vitamin is suspended or dissolved. Most of the vitamin appears first in lymph and primarily in the chylomicron fraction as a lipoprotein complex.

In animals and man, bile is essential for adequate intestinal absorption and deoxycholic acid is the most important constituent of bile in this regard. Thus, hepatic or biliary dysfunction may seriously impair absorption of vitamin D. Likewise, other abnormalities of gastrointestinal function, especially those associated with steatorrhea, may interfere with proper absorption of orally administered vitamin D.

Absorbed vitamin D circulates in the blood in association with vitamin D–binding protein, which is a specific α-globulin. Vitamin D disappears from plasma with a half-life of 19 to 25 hours, but it is stored in the body for prolonged periods (6 months or longer in the rat), apparently in fat deposits throughout the body (Rosenstreich et al., 1971).

As discussed above, the liver is the site of conversion of vitamin D to its 25-hydroxy derivative, which also circulates in association with vitamin D–binding protein. In fact, calcifediol has a higher affinity for the binding protein than does the parent compound. The 25-hydroxy derivative has a biological half-life of 19 days and constitutes the major circulating form of vitamin D. The plasma half-life of calcitriol is estimated to be between 3 and 5 days in man, and 40% of an administered dose is excreted within 10 days (Mawer et al., 1976). Calcitriol is hydroxylated to 1,24,25-$(OH)_3D_3$ by a renal hydroxylase that is induced by calcitriol and suppressed by those factors that stimulate the 25-OHD_3-1α-hydroxylase. This enzyme also hydroxylates calcifediol to form 24,25-$(OH)_2D_2$. Both 24-hydroxylated compounds are less active than calcitriol and presumably represent metabolites destined for excretion. Side chain oxidation of calcitriol also occurs.

The primary route of excretion of vitamin D is in the bile, and only a small percentage of an administered dose is found in the urine.

An important interaction has been demonstrated between vitamin D and phenytoin or phenobarbital. Patients receiving the anticonvulsant agents for a prolonged time have a high incidence of rickets and osteomalacia. Plasma concentrations of calcifediol are decreased in patients receiving these drugs, and it was proposed that phenytoin and phenobarbital accelerate the metabolism of vitamin D to inactive products (Hahn et al., 1972a, 1972b). Furthermore, these drugs protect rats against the toxic effects of high doses of vitamin D (Gascon-Barré and Côte, 1978). However, concentrations of calcitriol in plasma are normal, despite the depression of the concentration of calcifediol, in patients receiving anticonvulsant therapy (Jubiz et al., 1977). A normal concentration of calcitriol in the plasma after such treatment is consistent with the findings of several groups of investigators that anticonvulsant therapy increases target organ resistance to vitamin D and that this is the basis for the interaction. The effects of vitamin D on intestinal absorption of calcium and on bone resorption are diminished by the drugs (see Habener and Mahaffey, 1978). There have been some indications that therapy with glucocorticoids may alter the metabolism of vitamin D. The data relative to this are contradictory, and the issue remains unresolved (Habener and Mahaffey, 1978).

Human Requirements and Unitage. An exhaustive and critical summary of the prophylactic requirements for vitamin D has been compiled by the Committee on Nutrition of the American Academy of Pediatrics (see Committee on Nutrition, 1963). In the more than 60 years that have elapsed since Mellanby demonstrated the efficacy of cod liver oil in the prevention of rickets, the disease has become a clinical rarity in the United States. Although sunlight provides adequate antirachitic prophylaxis in the equatorial belt, in the temperate climates insufficient cutaneous solar radiation may necessitate dietary vitamin D supplementation.

Previously the recommended allowance of vitamin D could be achieved only by the addition of oral vitamin D supplements to a normal diet. Since the advent of the addition of the vitamin to foodstuffs (especially milk, milk products, cereals, and candy), individuals of all ages receive variable and even excessive vitamin D without its special addition to the diet. Thus, the supplemental requirements vary not only with age, pregnancy, and lactation but also with the quality of the diet. Serious toxicity may result from excessive ingestion of the vitamin, and even as little as 1800 USP units per day in infants may lead to inhibition of growth. It is clear, therefore, that any recommendation for vitamin D supplementation must be made only after careful scrutiny of the diet.

In both the premature and the normal infant, a total of 400 units per day of vitamin D ensures full antirachitic prophylaxis and optimal growth. Whether this is obtained by way of the diet, by vitamin D supplementation, or by a combination of both is of no consequence. During adolescence and adulthood this amount is probably also sufficient. There is some evidence that vitamin D requirements are greater than normal during pregnancy and lactation, although a daily intake of 400 units is sufficient in these conditions as well (*see* Table XVI–1, page 1546).

The USP unit is identical with the international unit and is equivalent to the specific biological activity of 0.025 μg of vitamin D_3 (*i.e.*, 1 mg equals 40,000 units).

Bioassay procedures have been used in the past and depend upon evidence of alleviation of the rachitic state. They are still in use for experimental purposes.

Modified Forms of Vitamin D. Two derivatives of vitamin D are of considerable experimental and therapeutic interest.

Dihydrotachysterol (DHT) is an analog of vitamin D that may be regarded as the reduction product of vitamin D_2 (and is sometimes referred to as DHT_2). Although DHT is the compound available for therapeutic use, the corresponding derivative of vitamin D_3 (DHT_3) has been used in experimental studies. Presumably DHT behaves in a manner analogous to that described for DHT_3. DHT is about $1/450$ as active as vitamin D in the usual antirachitic assay, but at high doses it is much more effective than vitamin D in mobilizing calcium from bone (Suda *et al.*, 1970). The latter effect is the basis for the use of DHT to maintain normal concentrations of calcium in plasma in hypoparathyroidism.

Dihydrotachysterol (DHT)

Studies describing the metabolic activation of DHT_3 provide an explanation for the above findings. DHT_3 undergoes 25-hydroxylation to yield 25-hydroxydihydrotachysterol$_3$ ($25-OHDHT_3$), which appears to be the active form of DHT in both intestine and bone. Both DHT_3 and $25-OHDHT_3$ are active in nephrectomized rats, indicating that DHT_3 does not require 1-hydroxylation in the kidney. A comparison of the structures of DHT and $1,25-(OH)_2D_3$ shows that ring A of DHT is rotated so as to place its 3-hydroxyl group in approximately the same geometrical position as the 1-hydroxyl group of $1,25-(OH)_2D_3$. It seems reasonable, therefore, that $25-OHDHT_3$ could interact with receptor sites for $1,25-(OH)_2D_3$ without undergoing 1-hydroxylation in the kidney. Thus, DHT bypasses the renal mechanisms of metabolic control.

1α-*Hydroxycholecalciferol*, $1-OHD_3$, is a synthetic derivative of vitamin D_3 that is hydroxylated in the 1α position. It is readily hydroxylated in the 25 position by the hepatic microsomal system to form $1,25-(OH)_2D_3$ and was therefore introduced as a substitute for this compound. In the chick assays for stimulation of intestinal absorption of calcium and bone mineralization it is essentially equal in activity to calcitriol (Boris, 1977). Because it does not require renal hydroxylation it has been used to treat renal osteodystrophy. This drug is not available in the United States.

Preparations. Many preparations containing vitamin D are marketed. Those containing the vitamin as a single entity are listed below.

Ergocalciferol (*calciferol*) is pure vitamin D_2. *Ergocalciferol capsules* contain 625 μg (25,000 USP units) or 1.25 mg (50,000 USP units) each. *Ergocalciferol oral solution* is a solution of the vitamin in propylene glycol. *Ergocalciferol tablets* contain 1.25 mg (50,000 USP units). An injection (500,000 units/ml) is available for intramuscular administration.

Dihydrotachysterol (HYTAKEROL) is the pure crystalline compound obtained by reduction of vitamin D_2 and is available as tablets (0.125 to 0.4 mg), capsules (0.125 mg), and a solution in oil (0.25 mg/ml). These preparations are all for oral administration.

Calcifediol (25-hydroxycholecalciferol; CALDEROL) is available in capsules containing 20 or 50 μg. The recommended initial dose is 300 to 350 μg per week, administered on a daily or alternate-day schedule.

Calcitriol (*1,25-dihydroxycholecalciferol*; ROCALTROL) is marketed in capsules for oral administration that contain 0.25 or 0.5 μg. Dosage must be individualized but is often effective at 0.5 to 1 μg per day. Dihydrotachysterol, calcifediol, and calcitriol are considerably more expensive than ergocalciferol.

THERAPEUTIC USES

The major therapeutic uses of vitamin D may be divided into three categories: (1) prophylaxis and cure of nutritional rickets, (2) treatment of metabolic rickets and osteomalacia, and (3) treatment of hypoparathyroidism.

Nutritional Rickets. Nutritional rickets results from inadequate exposure to sunlight or a deficiency of vitamin D in the diet. The condition is extremely rare in the United States and other countries where milk and other foods contain added vitamin D. Infants and children receiving adequate amounts of vitamin D–fortified food do not require additional vitamin D; however, breast-fed infants or those fed unfortified formula should receive 400 units of vitamin D daily as a supplement. The usual practice is to administer vitamin A in combination with vitamin D. A number of well-balanced vitamin A and D preparations are available for this purpose. Premature infants are especially susceptible to rickets and may require supplemental vitamin D, since the fetus acquires more than 85% of its calcium stores during the third trimester.

The curative dose of vitamin D for the treatment of *fully developed rickets* is larger than the prophylactic dose. One thousand units daily will produce normal calcium and phosphate concentrations in plasma in approximately 10 days and roentgenographic evidence of healing within about 3 weeks. However, a daily dose of 3000 to 4000 units is often prescribed for more rapid healing; this is of particular importance in severe cases of thoracic rickets when respiration is embarrassed.

There are certain conditions that are known to lead to *poor absorption of vitamin D*. If untreated by vitamin supplementation, a frank deficiency may develop. Therefore, vitamin D may be of definite prophylactic value in such disorders as diarrhea, steatorrhea, biliary obstruction, and any other abnormality in gastrointestinal function in which absorption is appreciably diminished. Parenteral administration may be used in such cases.

Metabolic Rickets and Osteomalacia. This group of diseases, which presents as rickets in infants and children and osteomalacia in adults, is characterized by a failure to respond to physiological doses of vitamin D. Three types of metabolic rickets are discussed below, and the reader is referred to articles by Parfitt (1972), Smith (1972), and Scriver and coworkers (1978) for more complete discussions of other forms of the disease.

Hypophosphatemic vitamin D–resistant rickets is an X-linked inherited disorder of calcium and phosphate metabolism. It is *not* characterized by a defect in vitamin D metabolism, but treatment with large doses of calcitriol in combination with phosphate salts may lead to clinical improvement (Brickman *et al.*, 1973).

Vitamin D–dependent rickets (pseudo-vitamin D deficiency rickets) is an inherited, autosomal recessive disease that appears to be due to an inborn error of vitamin D metabolism involving defective conversion of $25\text{-}OHD_3$ to $1,25\text{-}(OH)_2D_3$ (Fraser *et al.*, 1973). The condition responds to physiological doses of calcitriol (Fraser *et al.*, 1973).

Renal osteodystrophy (renal rickets) is associated with chronic renal failure, and it also is characterized by a decreased ability of the kidney to convert $25\text{-}OHD_3$ to $1,25\text{-}(OH)_2D_3$. The use of calcitriol in this condition can lower the concentrations of PTH and raise the concentration of calcium in plasma and help maintain bone mineralization and growth in children (Berl *et al.*, 1978; Chesney *et al.*, 1978). DHT and $1\text{-}OHD_3$ can also be used effectively, since renal hydroxylation is not required for their activity.

Hypoparathyroidism. Hypoparathyroidism is characterized by hypocalcemia and hyperphosphatemia (*see* above). Dihydrotachysterol has long been used to treat this condition, since it has a more rapid onset of action, a shorter duration of action, and, as noted above, a greater effect on mobilization of bone salts than does vitamin D. Calcitriol is reported to be effective in the management of hypoparathyroidism (Rosen *et al.*, 1977) and at least certain forms of pseudohypoparathyroidism in which an abnormally low concentration of calcitriol is present in plasma (Metz *et al.*, 1977). However, with the exception of the latter rare form of pseudohypoparathyroidism where the hydroxylase is deficient, most hypoparathyroid patients respond to any of the forms of vitamin D. Calcitriol may be the agent of choice for the temporary treatment of hypocalcemia while waiting for a slower-acting form of vitamin D to become effective.

Miscellaneous Uses of Vitamin D. Miscellaneous uses of vitamin D include treatment of the hypophosphatemia seen in the *Fanconi syndrome*. The use of large doses of vitamin D in patients with osteoporosis is of doubtful value and can be dangerous. Furthermore, the indiscriminate use of "over-the-counter" vitamin D preparations for conditions other than the aforementioned is irrational, can be dangerous, and should not be condoned.

FLUORIDE

Fluoride is of interest because of its toxic properties and its effect on dental enamel and bone. Fluoride is widely distributed in nature, and the soils of different regions of the world vary greatly in their fluoride content. Fluoride gains access to plants from the soil as well as from atmospheric sources. The sources of atmospheric fluoride include the burning of soft coal and the manufacturing of superphosphate, aluminum, steel, lead, copper, and nickel. Man obtains fluoride from the ingestion of plants and water. Incidental sources include food additives (*e.g.*, baking powder) that are contaminated with fluoride, and the ingestion of rodenticides and insecticides that contain fluoride compounds.

Absorption, Distribution, and Excretion. Fluorides are absorbed from the gastrointestinal tract, the lungs, and the skin. The gastrointestinal tract is the major site of absorption. The degree of absorption of a fluoride compound is best correlated with its solubility. The relatively soluble compounds, such as sodium fluoride, are almost completely absorbed, whereas relatively insoluble compounds, such as cryolite (Na_3AlF_6) and the fluoride found in bone meal (fluoroapatite), are poorly absorbed. Certain dietary cations (*e.g.*, calcium and iron) retard absorption of fluoride ion by forming low-solubility complexes in the gastrointestinal tract. The second most common route of absorption is by way of the lungs. Pulmonary inhalation of fluoride present in dusts and gases constitutes the major route of industrial exposure. A third, and relatively rare, route of absorption is through the skin.

Fluoride has been detected in all organs and tissues examined; however, there is no evidence that it is concentrated in any tissues except bone, thyroid, aorta, and perhaps kidney. Fluoride is preponderantly deposited in the skeleton and teeth, and the degree of skeletal storage is related to intake and age. This is thought to be a function of the turnover rate of skeletal components, with growing bone showing a greater fluoride deposition than bone in mature animals. Prolonged periods of time are required for mobilization of fluoride from bone. Fluoride is accumulated by the aorta, and concentrations increase with age, probably reflecting the calcification that occurs in this artery.

The major route of fluoride excretion is by way of the kidneys; however, fluoride is also excreted in small amounts by the sweat glands, the lactating breast, and the gastrointestinal tract. Under conditions of excessive sweating, the fraction of total fluoride excretion contributed by sweating can reach nearly one half. About 90% of the fluoride filtered by the glomerulus is reabsorbed by the renal tubules. Whether tubular secretion of fluoride occurs is unknown.

Pharmacological Actions. The pharmacological actions of fluoride, with the possible exception of its effect on bone and teeth, can be classified as toxic. Fluoride is an inhibitor of several enzyme systems and diminishes tissue respiration and anaerobic glycolysis. Fluoride is also a useful anticoagulant *in vitro,* due to its binding of calcium ions. It also inhibits the glycolytic utilization of glucose by erythrocytes, and for this reason is added to specimen tubes that receive blood for glucose determinations.

Fluoride has been used in treating Paget's disease of bone, but more effective therapeutic agents are now available. Fluoride has also been used to treat otosclerosis and osteogenesis imperfecta (Castells, 1973; Daniel et al., 1973). Further studies are required to establish the efficacy of the anion in these disorders. Several clinical studies have reported promising results in the treatment of osteoporosis with sodium fluoride, and two large, double-blind clinical studies are underway to evaluate this therapy (Bikle, 1983). The radioactive nuclide ^{18}F has proven useful in bone imaging and the detection of bone metastases (Jones et al., 1973).

Acute Poisoning. Acute fluoride poisoning is not rare. It usually results from the accidental ingestion of insecticides or rodenticides containing fluoride salts.

Initial symptoms are secondary to the local action of fluoride on the mucosa of the gastrointestinal tract. Salivation, nausea, abdominal pain, vomiting, and diarrhea are frequent. Systemic symptoms are varied and severe. The patient shows signs of increased irritability of the nervous system, including paresthesias, a positive Chvos-

tek sign, hyperactive reflexes, and tonic and clonic convulsions. These signs are related to the calcium-binding effect of fluoride. Hypocalcemia and hypoglycemia are frequent laboratory findings. The signs may be delayed for several hours. Pain in various muscle groups may occur. The blood pressure falls, presumably due to central vasomotor depression as well as direct toxic action on cardiac muscle. The respiratory center is first stimulated and later depressed. Death usually results from either respiratory paralysis or cardiac failure. It is stated that the lethal dose of sodium fluoride for man is about 5 g; however, recovery has been reported in patients ingesting much larger doses, whereas a dose as low as 2 g has been fatal. In children, as little as 0.5 g of sodium fluoride may be fatal. *Treatment* includes the intravenous administration of glucose in saline and gastric lavage with limewater (0.15% calcium hydroxide solution) or other calcium salts to precipitate the fluoride. Calcium gluconate is given intravenously for tetany; urine volume is kept high with parenteral fluid.

Chronic Poisoning. In man, the major manifestations of chronic ingestion of excessive amounts of fluoride are osteosclerosis and mottled enamel. Chronic exposure to excess fluoride causes increased osteoblastic activity. Osteosclerosis is a phenomenon wherein the density and calcification of bone are increased; in the case of fluoride intoxication, it is thought to represent the replacement of hydroxyapatite by the denser fluoroapatite. However, the mechanism of its development remains unknown. The degree of skeletal involvement varies from changes that are barely detectable radiologically to marked thickening of the cortex of long bones, numerous exostoses scattered throughout the skeleton, and calcification of ligaments, tendons, and muscle attachments to bone. In its severest form it is a disabling disease and is designated as *crippling fluorosis.*

Mottled enamel or dental fluorosis is a well-recognized entity that was first described over 50 years ago. The gross changes in very mild mottling consist in small, opaque, paper-white areas scattered irregularly over the tooth surface. In severe cases, discrete or confluent, deep brown- to black-stained pits give the tooth a corroded appearance. Mottled enamel is the result of a partial failure of the enamel-forming cells properly to elaborate and lay down enamel. It is a nonspecific response to a variety of stimuli, one of which is the ingestion of excessive amounts of fluoride.

Since mottled enamel is a developmental injury, the ingestion of fluoride following the eruption of the tooth has no effect. Mottling is one of the first visible signs of an excessive intake of fluoride during childhood. A quantitative relationship between the fluoride concentration of drinking water and mottling has been demonstrated. Continuous use of water containing about 1.0 ppm of fluoride may result in the very mildest form of mottled enamel in 10% of children. The incidence rises to 40 to 50% at about 1.7 ppm; at 2.5 ppm, it is as high as 80%, with 25% classified as moderate or severe; between

4.0 and 6.0 ppm, the incidence approaches 100%, with marked increase in severity.

Some concern has been expressed that fluoridation of public water supplies may result in an increased frequency of cancer or other diseases. Studies carried out by the National Cancer Institute and by the Bureau of Epidemiology of the United States Public Health Service indicate that mortality from cancer and mortality from all causes do not significantly differ between cities with fluoridated and those with nonfluoridated water (Hoover *et al.*, 1976; Erickson, 1978).

Fluoride and Dental Caries. Experiments in controlling the fluoride content of water took an unexpected and significant turn when it was observed that children born at Bauxite, Arkansas, after a new water supply had been obtained, showed a much higher incidence of caries than those who had been exposed to the former fluoride-containing water. This led to extensive studies on the part of the United States Public Health Service to ascertain whether the fluoridation of water could be employed as a practical measure to reduce the incidence of tooth decay. It has now been definitely established on the basis of large-scale studies in a number of communities that the fluoridation of water to a concentration of 1.0 ppm is a safe and practical public health measure that results in substantial reduction in the incidence of caries in permanent teeth.

There are partial benefits for children who begin drinking fluoridated water at any age; however, optimal benefits are obtained at ages before permanent teeth erupt. Topical applications of fluoride solutions by dental personnel appear to be particularly effective on newly erupted teeth and can reduce the incidence of caries by 30 to 40%. The prescription of dietary fluoride supplements should be considered for children whose drinking water contains less than 0.7 ppm of fluoride. Conflicting results have been reported from studies of the effectiveness of fluoride-containing toothpastes.

Adequate incorporation of fluoride into teeth causes the outer layers of enamel to be harder and more resistant to demineralization. The deposition of fluoride ion appears to be an anion-exchange process with hydroxyl or citrate ions. Fluoride occupies the anionic spaces in the enamel apatite crystal surface. The mechanism of prevention of caries exerted by the deposition of minute amounts of fluoride in surface enamel is not completely understood. There is no convincing evidence that fluoride from any source reduces the development of caries after the permanent teeth are completely formed (usually about age 14).

Preparations and Uses. The fluoride salts usually employed in dentifrices are sodium fluoride and stannous fluoride. Sodium fluoride is also available in a variety of preparations for oral and topical use, including tablets, drops, rinses, and gels. Sodium fluoride, sodium fluosilicate (Na_2SiF_6), and cryolite are the salts commonly used for insecticides.

Adams, T. H., and Norman, A. W. Studies on the mechanism of action of calciferol. I. Basic parameters of vitamin D–mediated calcium transport. *J. Biol. Chem.*, **1970**, *245*, 4421–4431.

Agus, Z. S.; Gardner, L. B.; Beck, L. H.; and Goldberg, M. Effects of parathyroid hormone on renal tubular reabsorption of calcium, sodium, and phosphate. *Am. J. Physiol.*, **1973**, *224*, 1143–1148.

Arnaud, C. D. Calcium homeostasis: regulatory elements and their integration. *Fed. Proc.*, **1978**, *37*, 2557–2560.

Bar-Shavit, Z.; Teitelbaum, S. L.; Reitsma, P.; Hall, A.; Pegg, L. E.; and Trial, J. Induction of monocytic differentiation and bone resorption by 1,25-dihydroxyvitamin D_3. *Proc. Natl Acad. Sci. U.S.A.*, **1983**, *80*, 5907–5911.

Berl, T.; Berns, A. S.; Huffer, W. E.; Hammil, K.; Alfrey, A. C.; Arnaud, C. D.; and Schrier, R. W. 1,25 Dihydroxycholecalciferol effects in chronic dialysis. *Ann. Intern. Med.*, **1978**, *88*, 774–780.

Berman, L. A. Crystalline substance from the parathyroid glands that influences the calcium content of the blood. *Proc. Soc. Exp. Biol. Med.*, **1924**, *21*, 465.

Bikle, D. D. Fluoride treatment of osteoporosis: a new look at an old drug. *Ann. Intern. Med.*, **1983**, *98*, 1013–1014.

Bikle, D. D.; Zolock, D. T.; Morrissey, R. L.; and Herman, R. H. Independence of 1,25-dihydroxyvitamin D–mediated calcium transport from *de novo* RNA and protein synthesis. *J. Biol. Chem.*, **1978**, *253*, 484–488.

Birge, S. J., and Miller, R. The role of phosphate in the action of vitamin D on the intestine. *J. Clin. Invest.*, **1977**, *60*, 980–988.

Boris, A. Structure-activity relationships of vitamin D analogues. *Am. J. Med.*, **1977**, *62*, 543–544.

Brenner, D. E.; Harvey, H. A.; Lipton, A.; and Demers, L. A study of prostaglandin E_2, parathormone, and response to indomethacin in patients with hypercalcemia of malignancy. *Cancer*, **1982**, *49*, 556–561.

Brewer, H. B.; Fairwell, T.; Rittel, W.; Littledike, T.; and Arnaud, C. D. Recent studies on the chemistry of human, bovine and porcine parathyroid hormones. *Am. J. Med.*, **1974**, *56*, 759–766.

Brickman, A. S.; Coburn, J. W.; Kurokawa, K.; Bethune, J. E.; Harrison, H. E.; and Norman, A. W. Actions of 1,25-dihydroxycholecalciferol in patients with hypophosphatemic, vitamin-D-resistant rickets. *N. Engl. J. Med.*, **1973**, *289*, 495–498.

Brown, E. M.; Carroll, R. J.; and Aurbach, G. D. Dopaminergic stimulation of cyclic AMP accumulation and parathyroid hormone release from dispersed bovine parathyroid cells. *Proc. Natl Acad. Sci. U.S.A.*, **1977**, *74*, 4210–4213.

Brown, E. M.; Gardner, D. G.; Windeck, R. A.; and Aurbach, G. D. Relationship of intracellular 3′,5′-adenosine monophosphate accumulation to parathyroid hormone release from dispersed bovine parathyroid cells. *Endocrinology*, **1978**, *103*, 2323–2333.

Brown, E. M., and Thatcher, J. G. Adenosine 3′,5′-monophosphate (cAMP)–dependent protein kinase and the regulation of parathyroid hormone release by divalent cations and agents elevating cAMP in dispersed bovine parathyroid cells. *Endocrinology*, **1982**, *110*, 1374–1380.

Brumbaugh, P. F., and Haussler, M. R. 1α,25-Dihydroxycholecalciferol receptors in intestine. II. Temperature-dependent transfer of hormone to chromatin via a specific cytosol receptor. *J. Biol. Chem.*, **1974**, *249*, 1258–1262.

Card, R. T., and Brain, M. C. The "anemia" of childhood: evidence for a physiologic response to hyperphosphatemia. *N. Engl. J. Med.*, **1973**, *288*, 388–392.

Carlsson, A. Tracer experiments on the effect of vitamin D on skeletal metabolism of calcium and phosphorus. *Acta Physiol. Scand.*, **1952**, *26*, 212–222.

Castells, S. New approaches to treatment of osteogenesis imperfecta. *Clin. Orthop.*, **1973**, *93*, 239–249.

Chase, L. R.; Melson, G. L.; and Aurbach, G. D. Pseudohypoparathyroidism: defective excretion of 3′,5′-AMP in response to parathyroid hormone. *J. Clin. Invest.*, **1969**, *48*, 1823–1844.

Chesney, R. W.; Moorthy, A. V.; Eisman, J. A.; Jax, D. K.; Mazess, R. B.; and DeLuca, H. F. Increased growth after long-term oral 1α,25-vitamin D₃ in childhood renal osteodystrophy. *N. Engl. J. Med.*, **1978**, *298*, 238–242.

Coccia, P. F. Cells that resorb bone. *N. Engl. J. Med.*, **1983**, *310*, 456–457.

Cohn, D. V., and Elting, J. Biosynthesis, processing, and secretion of parathormone and secretory protein I. *Recent Prog. Horm. Res.*, **1983**, *39*, 181–209.

Collip, J. B. The extraction of a parathyroid hormone which will prevent or control parathyroid tetany and which regulates the level of blood calcium. *J. Biol. Chem.*, **1925**, *63*, 395–438.

Committee on Nutrition. The prophylactic requirement and toxicity of vitamin D. *Pediatrics*, **1963**, *31*, 512–523.

Costanzo, L. S.; Sheehe, P. R.; and Weiner, I. M. Renal actions of vitamin D in vitamin D deficient rats. *Am. J. Physiol.*, **1974**, *226*, 1490–1495.

Daniel, H. J.; Shambaugh, G. E.; and Fisch, U. Fluoride and clinical otosclerosis. *Arch. Otolaryngol.*, **1973**, *98*, 327–329.

Davis, B. B., and Murdaugh, H. V. Evaluation of interrelationship between calcium and sodium excretion by canine kidney. *Metabolism*, **1970**, *19*, 439–444.

Deftos, L. J., and First, B. P. Calcitonin as a drug. *Ann. Intern. Med.*, **1981**, *95*, 192–197.

Erickson, J. D. Mortality in selected cities with fluoridated and non-fluoridated water supplies. *N. Engl. J. Med.*, **1978**, *298*, 1112–1116.

Fischer, J. A.; Blum, J. W.; and Binswanger, U. Acute parathyroid hormone response to epinephrine *in vivo*. *J. Clin. Invest.*, **1973**, *52*, 2434–2440.

Francis, M. D.; Russell, R. G. G.; and Fleisch, H. Diphosphonates inhibit formation of calcium phosphate crystals *in vitro* and pathological calcification *in vivo*. *Science*, **1969**, *165*, 1264–1266.

Fraser, D.; Kooh, S. W.; Kind, H. P.; Holick, M. F.; Tanaka, Y.; and DeLuca, H. F. Pathogenesis of hereditary vitamin-D-dependent rickets: an inborn error of vitamin D metabolism involving defective conversion of 25-hydroxyvitamin D to 1α,25-dihydroxyvitamin D. *N. Engl. J. Med.*, **1973**, *289*, 817–822.

Friedman, W. R., and Roberts, W. C. Vitamin D and the supravalvular aortic stenosis syndrome. *Circulation*, **1966**, *34*, 77–86.

Garabedian, M.; Tanaka, Y.; Holick, M. F.; and DeLuca, H. F. Response of intestinal calcium transport and bone mobilization to 1,25-dihydroxyvitamin D₃ in thyroparathyroidectomized rats. *Endocrinology*, **1974**, *94*, 1022–1027.

Gascon-Barré, M., and Côte, M. G. Effects of phenobarbital and diphenylhydantoin on acute vitamin D toxicity in the rat. *Toxicol. Appl. Pharmacol.*, **1978**, *43*, 125–135.

Greenberg, B. G.; Winters, R. W.; and Graham, J. B. The normal range of serum inorganic phosphorus and its utility as a discriminant in the diagnosis of congenital hypophosphatemia. *J. Clin. Endocrinol. Metab.*, **1960**, *20*, 364–379.

Hahn, T. J.; Birge, S. J.; Scharp, C. R.; and Avioli, L. V. Phenobarbital-induced alterations in vitamin D metabolism. *J. Clin. Invest.*, **1972a**, *51*, 741–748.

Hahn, T. J.; Hendin, B. A.; Scharp, C. R.; and Haddad, J. G., Jr. Effect of chronic anticonvulsant therapy on serum 25-hydroxycalciferol levels in adults. *N. Engl. J. Med.*, **1972b**, *287*, 900–904.

Hanson, A. M. The hormone of the parathyroid gland. *Proc. Soc. Exp. Biol. Med.*, **1925**, *22*, 560–561.

Harris, C. A.; Sutton, R. A. L.; and Seeley, J. F. Effect of 1,25-(OH)₂-vitamin D₃ on renal electrolyte handling in the vitamin deficient rat: dissociation of calcium and sodium excretion. *Clin. Res.*, **1976**, *24*, 685A.

Heath, H., III, and Sizemore, G. W. Plasma calcitonin in normal man. Differences between men and women. *J. Clin. Invest.*, **1977**, *60*, 1135–1140.

Hess, A. F.; and Weinstock, M. Antirachitic properties imparted to inert fluids and to green vegetables by ultraviolet irradiation. *J. Biol. Chem.*, **1924**, *62*, 301–313.

Hirsch, P. F.; Gauthier, G. F.; and Munson, P. C. Thyroid hypocalcemic principle and recurrent laryngeal nerve injury as factors affecting the response to parathyroidectomy in rats. *Endocrinology*, **1963**, *73*, 244–252.

Holick, M. F. The cutaneous photosynthesis of previtamin D₃: a unique photoendocrine system. *J. Invest. Dermatol.*, **1981**, *76*, 51–58.

Hoover, R. N.; McKay, F. W.; and Fraumeni, J. F., Jr. Fluoridated drinking water and the occurrence of cancer. *J. Natl Cancer Inst.*, **1976**, *57*, 757–768.

Hruska, K. A.; Korkor, A.; Martin, K.; and Slatopolsky, E. Peripheral metabolism of intact parathyroid hormone. *J. Clin. Invest.*, **1981**, *67*, 885–892.

Huldschinsky, K. Heilung von Rachitis durch Kunstliche Hohensonne. *Dtsch. Med. Wochenschr.*, **1919**, *14*, 712–713.

Jacob, H. S., and Amsden, T. Acute hemolytic anemia with rigid red cells in hypophosphatemia. *N. Engl. J. Med.*, **1971**, *285*, 1446–1450.

Jones, A. E.; Ghaed, N.; Dunson, G. L.; and Hosain, F. Clinical evaluation of orally administered fluorine 18 for bone scanning. *Radiology*, **1973**, *107*, 129–131.

Jubiz, W.; Haussler, M. R.; McCain, T. A.; and Tolman, K. G. Plasma 1,25-dihydroxyvitamin D levels in patients receiving anticonvulsant drugs. *J. Clin. Endocrinol. Metab.*, **1977**, *44*, 617–621.

Krane, S. M. Etidronate in the treatment of Paget's disease of bone. *Ann. Intern. Med.*, **1982**, *96*, 619–625.

Krieger, N. S., and Tashjian, A. H., Jr. Parathyroid hormone stimulates bone resorption via a Na-Ca exchange mechanism. *Nature*, **1980**, *287*, 843–845.

Kuntziger, H.; Amiel, C.; Roinel, N.; and Morel, F. Effect of parathyroidectomy and cyclic AMP on renal transport of phosphate, calcium, and magnesium. *Am. J. Physiol.*, **1974**, *227*, 905–911.

Larkins, R. G.; MacAuley, S. J.; Rapaport, A.; Martin, T. J.; Tulloch, B. R.; Byfield, P. G. H.; Matthews, E. W.; and MacIntyre, I. Effects of nucleotides, hormones, ions and 1,25-dihydroxycholecalciferol on 1,25-dihydrocholecalciferol production in isolated chick renal tubules. *Clin. Sci. Mol. Med.*, **1974**, *46*, 569–582.

Lawson, D. E. M., and Davie, M. Aspects of the metabolism and function of vitamin D. *Vitam. Horm.*, **1979**, *37*, 1–67.

Lechene, C.; Colindres, R. E.; and Knox, F. G. Electron probe microanalysis of the renal effect of parathyroid hormone. In, *Endocrinology of Calcium Metabolism.* (Copp, D. H., and Talmage, R. V., eds.) Excerpta Medica, Amsterdam, **1978**, pp. 230–233.

Leeson, P. M., and Fourman, P. Increased sensitivity to vitamin D after vitamin D poisoning. *Lancet*, **1966**, *1*, 1182–1185.

Levitt, M.; Gessert, C.; and Finberg, L. Inorganic phosphate (laxative) poisoning resulting in tetany in an infant. *J. Pediatr.*, **1973**, *82*, 479–481.

Lichtman, M. A.; Miller, D. R.; and Freeman, R. B. Erythrocyte adenosine triphosphate depletion during hypophosphatemia. *N. Engl. J. Med.*, **1969**, *280*, 240–244.

MacCallum, S. G., and Voegtlin, C. On the relation of tetany to the parathyroid glands and to calcium metabolism. *J. Exp. Med.*, **1909**, *11*, 118–151.

McConnell, T. H. Fatal hypocalcemia from phosphate absorption from laxative preparations. *J.A.M.A.*, **1971**, *216*, 147–148.

McGowan, J. A.; Chen, T. C.; Fragola, J.; Puschett, J. B.; and Rosenblatt, M. Parathyroid hormone: effects of the 3-34 fragment *in vivo* and *in vitro*. *Science*, **1983**, *219*, 67–69.

MacIntyre, I.; Boss, S.; and Troughton, V. A. Parathyroid hormone and magnesium homeostasis. *Nature*, **1963**, *198*, 1058–1060.

Mallette, L. E.; Tuma, S. N.; Berger, R. E.; and Kirkland, J. L. Radioimmunoassay for the middle region of human parathyroid hormone using an homologous antiserum with a carboxyterminal fragment of bovine parathyroid hormone as radioligand. *J. Clin. Endocrinol. Metab.*, **1982**, *54*, 1017–1024.

Mason, R. S.; Frankel, T.; Chan, Y.-L.; Lissner, D.; and Posen, S. Vitamin D conversion by sarcoid lymph node homogenate. *Ann. Intern. Med.*, **1984**, *100*, 59–61.

Massry, S. G., and Coburn, J. W. The hormonal and nonhormonal control of renal excretion of calcium and magnesium. *Nephron*, **1973**, *10*, 66–112.

Massry, S. G.; Muella, E.; Silverman, A. G.; and Kleeman, C. R. Inorganic phosphate treatment of hypercalcemia. *Arch. Intern. Med.*, **1968**, *12*, 307–312.

Mawer, E. B.; Backhouse, J.; Davie, M.; Hill, C. F.; and Taylor, C. M. Metabolic fate of administered 1,25-dihydroxycholecalciferol in controls and in patients with hypoparathyroidism. *Lancet*, **1976**, *1*, 1203–1206.

Mellanby, E. An experimental investigation of rickets. *Lancet*, **1919**, *1*, 407–412.

Metz, S. A.; Baylink, D. J.; Hughes, M. R.; Haussler, M. R.; and Robertson, R. P. Selective deficiency of 1,25-dihydroxycholecalciferol. *N. Engl. J. Med.*, **1977**, *297*, 1084–1090.

Miller, S. C. Rapid activation of the medullary bone osteoclast cell surface by parathyroid hormone. *J. Cell Biol.*, **1978**, *76*, 615–618.

Murad, F.; Brewer, H. B.; and Vaughan, M. Effect of thyrocalcitonin on adenosine 3′,5′-cyclic phosphate formation by rat kidney and bone. *Proc. Natl Acad. Sci. U.S.A.*, **1970**, *65*, 446–453.

Murad, F., and Pak, C. Y. C. Urinary excretion of adenosine 3′,5′-monophosphate and guanosine 3′,5′-monophosphate. *N. Engl. J. Med.*, **1972**, *286*, 1382–1387.

Murayama, Y.; Morel, F.; and Le Grimellec, C. Phosphate, calcium and magnesium transfers in proximal tubules and loops of Henle, as measured by single nephron microperfusion experiments in the rat. *Pfluegers Arch.*, **1972**, *333*, 1–16.

Neuman, W. F., and Ramp, W. K. The concept of a bone membrane: some implications. In, *Cellular Mechanisms for Calcium Transfer and Homeostasis.* (Nichols, G., Jr., and Wasserman, R. H., eds.) Academic Press, Inc., New York, **1971**, pp. 197–206.

New, W., and Trautwein, W. Inward membrane currents in mammalian myocardium. *Pfluegers Arch.*, **1972**, *334*, 1–23.

Nicolaysen, R. Studies upon the mode of action of vitamin D. III. The influence of vitamin D on the absorption of calcium and phosphorus in the rat. *Biochem. J.*, **1937**, *31*, 122–129.

Nordin, B. E. C.; Horsman, A.; Marshall, D. H.; Simpson, M.; and Waterhouse, G. M. Calcium requirement and calcium therapy. *Clin. Orthop.*, **1979**, *140*, 216–239.

Odell, W. D., and Wolfsen, A. R. Humoral syndromes associated with cancer. *Annu. Rev. Med.*, **1978**, *29*, 379–406.

Paillard, F.; Ardaillou, R.; Malendin, H.; Fillastre, J. P.; and Prier, S. Renal effects on salmon calcitonin in man. *J. Lab. Clin. Med.*, **1972**, *80*, 200–216.

Parfitt, A. M. Hypophosphatemic vitamin D refractory rickets and osteomalacia. *Orthop. Clin. North Am.*, **1972**, *3*, 653–680.

Perlia, C. P.; Gubisch, N. J.; Wolter, J.; Edelberg, D.; Dederick, M. M.; and Taylor, S. G., III. Mithramycin treatment of hypercalcemia. *Cancer*, **1970**, *25*, 389–394.

Puschett, J. B.; Moranz, J.; and Kurnick, W. S. Evidence for a direct action of cholecalciferol and 25-hydroxycholecalciferol on the renal transport of phosphate, sodium, and calcium. *J. Clin. Invest.*, **1972**, *51*, 373–385.

Raisz, L. G. Bone metabolism and calcium regulation. In, *Metabolic Bone Disease*, Vol. I. (Avioli, L. V., and Krane, S. M., eds.) Academic Press, Inc., New York, **1977**, pp. 1–48.

Raisz, L. G.; Trummel, C. L.; Holick, M. F.; and DeLuca, H. F. 1,25-Dihydroxycholecalciferol: a potent stimulator of bone resorption in tissue culture. *Science*, **1972**, *175*, 768–769.

Reynolds, J. J.; Pavlovitch, H.; and Balsan, S. 1,25-Dihydroxycholecalciferol increases bone resorption in thyroparathyroidectomized rats. *Calcif. Tissue Res.*, **1976**, *21*, 207–212.

Rosen, J. F., and Chesney, R. W. Circulating calcitriol concentrations in health and disease. *J. Pediatr.*, **1983**, *103*, 1–17.

Rosen, J. F.; Fleischman, A. R.; Finberg, L.; Eisman, J.; and DeLuca, H. F. 1,25-Dihydroxycholecalciferol: its use in the long-term management of idiopathic hypoparathyroidism in children. *J. Clin. Endocrinol. Metab.*, **1977**, *45*, 457–468.

Rosenstreich, S. J.; Rich, C.; and Volwiler, W. Deposition in and release of vitamin D_3 from body fat; evidence for a storage site in the rat. *J. Clin. Invest.*, **1971**, *50*, 679–687.

Rost, C. R.; Bikle, D. D.; and Kaplan, R. A. *In vitro* stimulation of 25-hydroxycholecalciferol 1α-hydroxylation by parathyroid hormone in chick kidney slices: evidence for a role for adenosine 3′,5′-monophosphate. *Endocrinology*, **1981**, *108*, 1002–1006.

Roth, S. I., and Raisz, L. G. Effect of calcium concentration on the ultrastructure of rat parathyroid in organ culture. *Lab. Invest.*, **1964**, *13*, 331–345.

Rude, R. K.; Oldham, S. B.; and Singer, F. R. Functional hypoparathyroidism and parathyroid hormone end-organ resistance in human magnesium deficiency. *Clin. Endocrinol. (Oxf.)*, **1976**, *5*, 209–224.

Russell, R. G. G., and Fleisch, H. Pyrophosphate and diphosphonates in skeletal metabolism. *Clin. Orthop.*, **1975**, *108*, 241–263.

Scriver, C. R.; Reade, T. M.; DeLuca, H. F.; and Hamstra, A. J. Serum 1,25-hydroxyvitamin D levels in normal subjects and in patients with hereditary rickets or bone disease. *N. Engl. J. Med.*, **1978**, *299*, 976–979.

Smith, R. The pathophysiology and management of rickets. *Orthop. Clin. North Am.*, **1972**, *3*, 601–621.

Spencer, R.; Charman, M.; Wilson, P. W.; and Lawson, D. E. M. The relationship between vitamin D–stimulated calcium transport and intestinal calcium-binding protein in the chicken. *Biochem. J.*, **1978**, *170*, 93–101.

Steele, T. H. Increased urinary phosphate excretion following volume expansion in normal man. *Metabolism*, **1970**, *19*, 29–39.

Steenbock, H., and Black, A. Fat-soluble vitamins. XVII. The induction of growth-promoting and calcifying properties in a ration by exposure to ultraviolet light. *J. Biol. Chem.*, **1924**, *61*, 405–422.

Suda, T.; Hallick, R. B.; DeLuca, H. F.; and Schnoes, H. K. 25-Hydroxydihydrotachysterol$_3$. Synthesis and biological activity. *Biochemistry*, **1970**, *9*, 1651–1657.

Talmage, R. V. Further studies on the control of calcium homeostasis by parathyroid hormone. In, *Calcium, Parathyroid Hormone, and the Calcitonins.* (Talmage,

R. V., and Munson, P. L., eds.) Excerpta Medica, Amsterdam, **1972**, pp. 422–429.

Tashjian, A. H.; Wolfe, H. J.; and Voelkel, E. F. Human calcitonin. Immunologic assay, cytochemical localization and studies on medullary thyroid carcinoma. *Am. J. Med.*, **1974**, *56*, 840–849.

Taussig, H. B. Possible injury to the cardiovascular system from vitamin D. *Ann. Intern. Med.*, **1966**, *65*, 1195–1200.

Wells, S. A., Jr.; Baylin, S. B.; Linehan, W. M.; Farrell, R. E.; Cox, E. G.; and Cooper, C. W. Provocative agents and the diagnosis of medullary carcinoma of the thyroid gland. *Ann. Surg.*, **1978**, *188*, 139–141.

Werner, J. A.; Gorton, S. J.; and Raisz, L. G. Escape from inhibition of resorption in cultures of fetal bone treated with calcitonin and parathyroid hormone. *Endocrinology*, **1972**, *90*, 752–759.

Winter, R. J.; Harris, C. J.; Phillips, L. S.; and Green, O. C. Diabetic ketoacidosis. Induction of hypocalcemia and hypomagnesemia by phosphate therapy. *Am. J. Med.*, **1979**, *67*, 897–900.

Zile, M.; Bunge, E. C.; Barsness, L.; Yamada, S.; Schnoes, H. K.; and DeLuca, H. F. Localization of 1,25-dihydroxyvitamin D in intestinal nuclei *in vivo*. *Arch. Biochem. Biophys.*, **1978**, *186*, 15–24.

Monographs and Reviews

Albright, F. A page out of the history of hyperparathyroidism. *J. Clin. Endocrinol. Metab.*, **1948**, *8*, 637–657.

Arena, J. M. *Poisoning: Toxicology-Symptoms-Treatments*, 4th ed. Charles C Thomas, Publisher, Springfield, Ill., **1979**.

Austin, L. A., and Heath, H., III. Calcitonin. *N. Engl. J. Med.*, **1981**, *304*, 269–278.

Broadus, A. E., and Rasmussen, H. Clinical evaluation of parathyroid function. *Am. J. Med.*, **1981**, *70*, 475–478.

Brown, E. M., and Aurbach, G. D. Role of cyclic nucleotides in secretory mechanisms and actions of parathyroid hormone and calcitonin. *Vitam. Horm.*, **1980**, *38*, 205–256.

Copp, D. H. Parathyroids, calcitonin, and control of plasma calcium. *Recent Prog. Horm. Res.*, **1964**, *20*, 59–88.

DeLuca, H. F., and Schnoes, H. K. Metabolism and mechanism of action of vitamin D. *Annu. Rev. Biochem.*, **1976**, *45*, 631–666.

———. Vitamin D: recent advances. *Ibid.*, **1983**, *52*, 411–439.

Douglas, W. W. Stimulus-secretion coupling: the concept and clues from chromaffin and other cells. (The First Gaddum Memorial Lecture.) *Br. J. Pharmacol.*, **1968**, *34*, 451–474.

Fraser, D. R. Regulation of the metabolism of vitamin D. *Physiol. Rev.*, **1980**, *60*, 551–613.

Habener, J. F., and Mahaffey, J. E. Osteomalacia and disorders of vitamin D metabolism. *Annu. Rev. Med.*, **1978**, *29*, 327–342.

Habener, J. F., and Potts, J. T. Biosynthesis of parathyroid hormone. *N. Engl. J. Med.*, **1978**, *299*, 580–585, 635–644.

Haussler, M. R., and McCain, T. A. Basic and clinical concepts related to vitamin D metabolism and action. *N. Engl. J. Med.*, **1977**, *297*, 974–983.

Kodicek, E. The story of vitamin D from vitamin to hormone. *Lancet*, **1974**, *1*, 325–329.

Kretsinger, R. H. Evolution and function of calcium-binding proteins. *Int. Rev. Cytol.*, **1976**, *46*, 323–393.

Pak, C. Y. C. Parathyroid hormone and thyrocalcitonin: their mode of action and regulation. *Ann. N.Y. Acad. Sci.*, **1971**, *179*, 450–474.

Stewart, A. F. Therapy of malignancy-associated hypercalcemia: 1983. *Am. J. Med.*, **1983**, *74*, 475–480.

Symposium. (Various authors.) Parathyroid hormone, calcitonin and vitamin D: clinical considerations. (Forscher, B. K., and Arnaud, C. D., eds.) *Am. J. Med.*, **1974**, *56*, 743–870; *57*, 1–62.

Van Dop, C., and Bourne, H. R. Pseudohypoparathyroidism. *Annu. Rev. Med.*, **1983**, *34*, 259–266.

SECTION
XVI
The Vitamins

INTRODUCTION

Robert Marcus and Ann M. Coulston

The diet is the source of some 40 nutrients for man. These are classically divided into energy-yielding dietary components (carbohydrates, fats, and proteins), sources of essential and nonessential amino acids (proteins), essential unsaturated fatty acids (fats), minerals (including trace minerals), and vitamins (water-soluble and fat-soluble organic compounds). In this section, the subject is vitamins.

Centuries ago, physicians described many of the diseases now recognized as vitamin deficiencies, notably night blindness (vitamin A deficiency), beriberi (thiamine deficiency), pellagra (niacin deficiency), scurvy (ascorbic acid deficiency), and rickets (vitamin D deficiency). Long before the era of vitamins, dietary factors were considered to be involved in all these conditions. However, the eventual identification of the active factor in the diet usually required reproduction of the disease in an experimental animal by feeding it a diet similar to that presumed to cause the condition in man, followed by prevention or cure of the disease by addition of certain foods or extracts of foods to the experimental diet. For example, scurvy was identified as a disease in the Middle Ages, and in 1747 Lind showed that citrus fruits could cure scurvy. However, the demonstration in 1907 that a diet of oats and bran causes scurvy in guinea pigs allowed tests for antiscorbutic activity in fractions from citrus fruits; this culminated in the identification of ascorbic acid in 1932. Similarly, beriberi, a form of polyneuritis, has been known for centuries to occur in populations eating polished (refined) rice. In 1897, Eijkman showed that fowl fed polished rice developed a polyneuritis similar to beriberi that could be cured by adding the husks or an extract of the husks back to the polished rice from which they had been derived. This animal model allowed Funk, in 1911, to isolate from the extract an antiberiberi substance, which he believed to be an amine. Being vital for life, he called the substance a *vitamine* and suggested that not only beriberi but also scurvy, pellagra, and possibly rickets were due to the lack of similar organic bases in the diet. The name was shortened to *vitamin* when it was subsequently recognized that dietary factors in this class are not necessarily amines and, indeed, have unrelated structures.

In the meantime, Osborne and Mendel (1911 to 1913) had demonstrated the presence in butter of a factor necessary for the growth of rats. In 1915, McCollum and Davis confirmed its presence in several dietary fats and named it *fat-soluble A,* which they distinguished from *water-soluble B,* another dietary factor necessary for the growth of rats; the latter was subsequently identified as Funk's antiberiberi factor. It soon became apparent that both the fat-soluble and the water-soluble factors (vitamins) consisted of several active components. Fats were shown to contain a factor (vitamin D) that prevented rickets and could be distinguished from the rat growth factor, vitamin A. Subsequent work has identified other fat-soluble factors (vitamins E and K) as essential dietary components. The water-soluble B fraction also proved to contain several components needed by man, namely thiamine, riboflavin, nicotinic acid, pyridoxine, pantothenic acid, biotin, folic acid, and cyanocobalamin (vitamin B_{12}). These were originally grouped together because they could be extracted in high concentration from certain foods, notably liver and yeast, in which the antiberiberi factor B had been identified. When active constituents were separately recognized in factor B, they were assigned the names vitamin B_1, vitamin B_2, and so forth; these have subsequently been replaced by chemical names. The members of the vitamin B complex are quite dissimilar in chemical structure, and they also differ in function. However, their continued classification together is justified by the similarity of their dietary sources and the consequent tendency for deficiency diseases to involve inadequate intakes of more than one member of the group. Finally, the water-soluble, antiscorbutic factor was named vitamin C, or ascorbic acid.

Although the individual vitamins differ widely in structure and function, some general statements do apply. Water-soluble vitamins are stored to only a limited extent, and frequent consumption is necessary to maintain saturation of tissues. Fat-soluble vitamins can be stored to massive degrees, and this property confers upon them a potential for serious toxicity which greatly exceeds that of the water-soluble group. As consumed, many vitamins are not biologically active and require processing *in vivo*. In the case of several water-soluble vitamins, activation includes phosphorylation (thiamine, riboflavin, niacin, pyridoxine) and may also require coupling to purine or pyridine nucleotides (riboflavin, niacin). In their major known actions water-soluble vitamins participate as cofactors for specific enzymes, whereas at least two fat-soluble vitamins, A and D, behave more like hormones and interact with specific intracellular receptors in their target tissues.

Definitions. Vitamins are thus a group of substances of diverse chemical composition. They can be defined as *organic* substances that must be provided in small quantities in the diet for the synthesis, by tissues, of cofactors that are essential for various metabolic reactions. This definition differentiates vitamins from essential trace minerals, which are *inorganic* nutrients needed in small quantities. It also excludes the essential amino acids, which are organic substances needed preformed in the diet in much larger quantities. The Nomenclature Committee of the American Institute of Nutrition recommends that the term *vitamin* be restricted to include only organic substances required for the nutrition of mammals; substances required only by microorganisms and cells in culture should be defined as *growth factors,* in order to prevent scientifically unsound claims for their therapeutic benefit as vitamins for man. When the vitamin occurs in more than one chemical form (*e.g.,* pyridoxine, pyridoxal, pyridoxamine) or as a precursor (*e.g.,* carotene for vitamin A), these analogs are sometimes referred to as *vitamers*.

Vitamin Requirements. *Recommended Dietary Allowances.* In many countries throughout the world, scientific committees periodically assess the evidence about the requirements of the population for individual nutrients. In the United States, the National Academy of Sciences has a Food and Nutrition Board, one of whose functions is to recommend allowances of nutrients that will serve as a goal for good nutrition and will "encourage patterns of food consumption in the United States that will maintain and promote health" (Food and Nutrition Board, 1980). Recommended dietary allowances (RDA) for nutrients to ensure health were first published in 1941 and are periodically revised to incorporate new knowledge by the Dietary Allowances Committee of the Food and Nutrition Board. In 1980, the ninth edition of *Recommended Dietary Allowances* was issued. Its recommendations for males and females of different ages are summarized in Table XVI-1. With the exception of the recommended intakes of energy, these allowances are set at levels sufficiently high to cover the needs of almost all healthy individuals in that age and sex category. This is done because the exact amounts of nutrients needed by each individual in the population are not known, and estimates are made from experiments on a limited number of subjects. If the upper limit of this range is taken as the recommended allowance, it is unlikely that a deficiency will occur in the population. Those with intakes below the recommended allowance will not necessarily develop a deficiency, but the risk of becoming

Table XVI-1. RECOMMENDED DAILY DIETARY ALLOWANCES [a]

	Age	Weight	Height	Energy	Protein	FAT-SOLUBLE VITAMINS			WATER-SOLUBLE VITAMINS							MINERALS					
						Vita-min A	Vita-min D	Vita-min E	Vita-min C	Thia-mine	Ribo-flavin	Nia-cin [e]	Vita-min B$_6$	Fola-cin [f]	Vita-min B$_{12}$	Cal-cium	Phos-phorus	Magne-sium	Iron	Zinc	Io-dine
	(years)	(kg)	(cm)	(kcal)	(g)	(μg R.E.) [b]	(μg) [c]	(mg αT.E.) [d]	(mg)	(mg)	(mg)	(mg)	(mg)	(μg)	(μg)	(mg)	(mg)	(mg)	(mg)	(mg)	(μg)
Infants	0.0–0.5	6	60	kg × 115	kg × 2.2	420	10	3	35	0.3	0.4	6	0.3	30	0.5 [g]	360	240	50	10	3	40
	0.5–1.0	9	71	kg × 105	kg × 2.0	400	10	4	35	0.5	0.6	8	0.6	45	1.5	540	360	70	15	5	50
Children	1–3	13	90	1300	23	400	10	5	45	0.7	0.8	9	0.9	100	2.0	800	800	150	15	10	70
	4–6	20	112	1700	30	500	10	6	45	0.9	1.0	11	1.3	200	2.5	800	800	200	10	10	90
	7–10	28	132	2400	34	700	10	7	45	1.2	1.4	16	1.6	300	3.0	800	800	250	10	10	120
Males	11–14	45	157	2700	45	1000	10	8	50	1.4	1.6	18	1.8	400	3.0	1200	1200	350	18	15	150
	15–18	66	176	2800	56	1000	10	10	60	1.4	1.7	18	2.0	400	3.0	1200	1200	400	18	15	150
	19–22	70	177	2900	56	1000	7.5	10	60	1.5	1.7	19	2.2	400	3.0	800	800	350	10	15	150
	23–50	70	178	2700	56	1000	5	10	60	1.4	1.6	18	2.2	400	3.0	800	800	350	10	15	150
	51+	70	178	2400	56	1000	5	10	60	1.2	1.4	16	2.2	400	3.0	800	800	350	10	15	150
Females	11–14	46	157	2200	46	800	10	8	50	1.1	1.3	15	1.8	400	3.0	1200	1200	300	18	15	150
	15–18	55	163	2100	46	800	10	8	60	1.1	1.3	14	2.0	400	3.0	1200	1200	300	18	15	150
	19–22	55	163	2100	44	800	7.5	8	60	1.1	1.3	14	2.0	400	3.0	800	800	300	18	15	150
	23–50	55	163	2000	44	800	5	8	60	1.0	1.2	13	2.0	400	3.0	800	800	300	18	15	150
	51+	55	163	1800	44	800	5	8	60	1.0	1.2	13	2.0	400	3.0	800	800	300	10 [h]	15	150
Pregnant				+300	+30	+200	+5	+2	+20	+0.4	+0.3	+2	+0.6	+400	+1.0	+400	+400	+150	h	+5	+25
Lactating				+500	+20	+400	+5	+3	+40	+0.5	+0.5	+5	+0.5	+100	+1.0	+400	+400	+150	h	+10	+50

[a] The allowances are intended to provide for individual variations among most normal persons as they live in the United States under usual environmental stresses. Diets should be based on a variety of common foods in order to provide other nutrients for which human requirements have been less well defined.

[b] Retinol equivalents. 1 retinol equivalent = 1 μg of retinol or 6 μg of β-carotene.

[c] As cholecalciferol. 10 μg of cholecalciferol = 400 I.U. of vitamin D.

[d] α-Tocopherol equivalents. 1 mg of d-α-tocopherol = 1 α-T.E.

[e] 1 N.E. (niacin equivalent) is equal to 1 mg of niacin or 60 mg of dietary tryptophan.

[f] The folacin allowances refer to dietary sources as determined by Lactobacillus casei assay after treatment with enzymes ("conjugases") to make polyglutamyl forms of the vitamin available to the test microorganism.

[g] The RDA for vitamin B$_{12}$ in infants is based on the average concentration of the vitamin in human milk. The allowances after weaning are based on energy intake (as recommended by the American Academy of Pediatrics) and consideration of other factors such as intestinal absorption.

[h] The increased requirement during pregnancy cannot be met by the iron content of habitual American diets nor by the existing iron stores of many women; therefore, the use of 30 to 60 mg of supplemental iron is recommended.- Iron needs during lactation are not substantially different from those of non-pregnant women, but continued supplementation of the mother for 2 to 3 months after parturition is advisable in order to replenish stores depleted by pregnancy.

(Modified from Food and Nutrition Board, National Research Council, 1980.)

deficient increases in proportion to the extent to which intake is less than the amount recommended.

It is important to remember that the RDA are subject to periodic reevaluation, and that changes do occur. As subgroups of the population are identified with unique requirements for one or more nutrients (*e.g.*, elderly women), one can anticipate further revisions of the RDA.

A novel feature of the ninth edition of *Recommended Dietary Allowances* is the introduction of *provisional allowances* for some nutrients not previously given RDA. Table XVI–1 lists allowances for only 18 out of the 40 or so known essential nutrients consumed by man. In previous editions of the RDA text a mixed diet was advised in order to include unrecognized nutritional needs and to ensure an adequate intake of essential nutrients for which no allowance could be provided. However, rising consumption of formulated foods, other highly processed foods, and supplements of vitamins and trace elements has increased the risk of imbalances between nutrients, of deficiencies from underconsumption by some members of the population, and of toxicity from overdosage in others. The current RDA text therefore provides allowances for certain additional nutrients in the form of ranges within which adequate intakes are likely to be achieved (Table XVI–2). These provisional allowances include two water-soluble vitamins (pantothenic acid and biotin) and one fat-soluble vitamin (vitamin K), as well as sodium, potassium, chloride, and several trace elements (copper, manganese, fluorine, chromium, selenium, and molybdenum). Although these provisional allowances are presented as recommended ranges of intakes, it is to be emphasized that an intake at one end of the range should not be construed as more desirable than one at the other. Thus, all intakes within the recommended range are considered safe and effective, but consumption of greater or smaller amounts over extended periods of time will increase the risk of marginal toxicity or deficiency, respectively.

There are a number of other constituents in food that have been claimed to be needed by man. As described in the 1980 RDA text, these substances fall into four classes: (1) those known to be essential for some animals but not shown to be needed by man, such as nickel, vanadium, and silicon; (2) substances that act as growth factors only for lower forms of life, such as para-aminobenzoic acid, carnitine, and pimelic acid; (3) substances in foods that are said to be vitamins but whose actions are probably pharmacological or nonexistent, such as rutin, for which claims of antihemorrhagic and other actions have been made but are unsubstantiated; (4) substances for which scientific proof of a nutrient action has not been provided, such as pangamic acid (erroneously designated vitamin B_{15}), laetrile (misnamed vitamin B_{17}), and others promoted in the health-food literature and commercial outlets. Herbert (1979a, 1979b) has written detailed factual reviews of the controversies over laetrile and pangamic acid. The ninth edition of *Recommended Dietary Allowances* (Food and Nutrition Board, 1980) serves as a standard for the intelligent use of vitamin and mineral supplements.

Federal Regulations on Vitamins and Minerals. The United States Food and Drug Administration (FDA), under the authority of the Federal Food, Drug, and Cosmetic Act, regulates the labeling of vitamin and mineral products sold as foods or drugs. (For a review of these regulations, *see* Food and Drug Administration, 1979.) To facilitate the labeling of conventional foods with regard to nutrients, the FDA has designated an official U.S. RDA, which generally represents the highest daily allowance for each nutrient given in the seventh, 1968, edition of *Recommended Dietary Allowances*. Thus, the purchaser can determine what proportion of his daily allowance of each nutrient is provided by a given amount of the food. In addition, the U.S. RDA are used to label the amounts of vitamins and minerals relative to needs in supplements sold to the public. Although the FDA has only limited authority to control the nutrient content of supplements, except those intended for use by children under 12 years of age and by pregnant or lactating women, the label does provide the user with explicit information on content, thus permitting judgment of whether the product purchased contains reasonable amounts, too little, or an excess of each nutrient

Table XVI–2. ESTIMATED SAFE AND ADEQUATE DAILY DIETARY INTAKES OF ADDITIONAL SELECTED VITAMINS AND MINERALS *

	Age (years)	VITAMINS			TRACE ELEMENTS						ELECTROLYTES		
		Vitamin K (μg)	Biotin (μg)	Pantothenic Acid (mg)	Copper (mg)	Manganese (mg)	Fluoride (mg)	Chromium (mg)	Selenium (mg)	Molybdenum (mg)	Sodium (mg)	Potassium (mg)	Chloride (mg)
Infants	0–0.5	12	35	2	0.5–0.7	0.5–0.7	0.1–0.5	0.01–0.04	0.01–0.04	0.03–0.06	115–350	350–925	275–700
	0.5–1	10–20	50	3	0.7–1.0	0.7–1.0	0.2–1.0	0.02–0.06	0.02–0.06	0.04–0.08	250–750	425–1275	400–1200
Children	1–3	15–30	65	3	1.0–1.5	1.0–1.5	0.5–1.5	0.02–0.08	0.02–0.08	0.05–0.1	325–975	550–1650	500–1500
and	4–6	20–40	85	3–4	1.5–2.0	1.5–2.0	1.0–2.5	0.03–0.12	0.03–0.12	0.06–0.15	450–1350	775–2350	700–2100
Adolescents	7–10	30–60	120	4–5	2.0–2.5	2.0–3.0	1.5–2.5	0.05–0.2	0.05–0.2	0.1–0.3	600–1800	1000–3000	925–2775
	11+	50–100	100–200	4–7	2.0–3.0	2.5–5.0	1.5–2.5	0.05–0.2	0.05–0.2	0.15–0.5	900–2700	1525–4575	1400–4200
Adults		70–140	100–200	4–7	2.0–3.0	2.5–5.0	1.5–4.0	0.05–0.2	0.05–0.2	0.15–0.5	1100–3300	1875–5625	1700–5100

* Because there is less information on which to base an allowance, these are not given in the main table of dietary allowances but are provided here in the form of ranges of recommended intakes. Since the toxic levels for many trace elements may be only several times usual intakes, the upper levels for the trace elements given in this table should not be habitually exceeded. (Modified from Food and Nutrition Board, National Research Council, 1980.)

relative to daily allowances. The FDA attempted in 1973 to classify *all* vitamin and mineral preparations in which the dosages exceeded 150% of the U.S. RDA as drugs rather than as special foods, but the regulation was struck by court order. Regulations also developed in 1973 prevented sale to the public of *vitamins A* and *D* in doses exceeding 10,000 international units (I.U.) of the former and 400 I.U. of the latter without a prescription. This was done because of the concern that higher doses of these fat-soluble vitamins can cause toxicity. The regulation was revoked in 1978 because of a court determination that dosages in excess of those amounts could not be *uniquely* classified as drugs by the FDA. Also, an amendment of the Federal Food, Drug, and Cosmetic Act passed by Congress in 1976 limits FDA control of supplements for adult use to cases of demonstrated toxicity but retains the Agency's authority over dietary supplements for children under 12 years and for pregnant or lactating women.

The uses of vitamins and other nutrients to treat disease come under FDA review, either as foods for special dietary use, including food supplements, or as "over-the-counter" or prescription drugs, depending on the purposes for which the product is intended and the claims made for it. Nutrient products designed specifically for special application in medical treatment, such as parenteral solutions for hyperalimentation and so-called medical foods (such as defined formula diets), are evaluated for safety and efficacy, as are "over-the-counter" drugs containing vitamins and minerals. An FDA Over-the-Counter Vitamin, Mineral, and Hematinics Review Panel has recommended appropriate formulations for these preparations (Food and Drug Administration, 1979).

Range of Intakes of Vitamins and Minerals. Many millions of individuals living in the United States regularly ingest quantities of vitamins vastly in excess of the RDA. In 1972, a Study of Health Practices and Opinions (National Analysts, 1972) reinforced previous concern of the FDA that vast numbers of Americans hold some inflated concepts regarding the benefits of taking supplemental vitamins and minerals. Thus, a survey found that more than half the adults interviewed had at one time used vitamin pills. The primary reason for taking vitamin supplements was the erroneous belief that such supplements provide extra energy and made one "feel better," and two thirds of those holding this belief did indeed claim to feel better. This evidence of widespread nutritional self-medication, which is confirmed by other surveys, should be kept in mind when taking a medication history from a patient.

The use of dietary supplements of vitamins is medically advisable in a variety of circumstances where *vitamin deficiencies* are likely to occur. Such situations may arise from inadequate intake, malabsorption, increased tissue needs, or inborn errors of metabolism. In practice, these causes may overlap, as in the case of the alcoholic, who may have an inadequate food intake and also impaired absorption.

Vitamin deficiency due primarily to *inadequate intake* occurs under a variety of circumstances. While gross vitamin deficiencies due to inadequate intakes are still encountered in underdeveloped areas of the world, few florid cases can be seen in the United States; however, a degree of subclinical deficiency of nutrients due to inadequate intake has been documented. Ongoing surveillance of the intake of nutrients has been carried out by the United States Government since 1971. The most recent survey (National Center for Health Statistics, 1983) indicated that mean intake consistently exceeds RDA for several major vitamins (A, thiamine, riboflavin, niacin, ascorbic acid). However, data from this and other surveys (Ten-State Nutrition Survey, 1972) show that individuals living below the poverty level, particularly the elderly and ethnic minorities, may have a substantially greater risk of inadequate intake of some nutrients, especially vitamins A and C. It should be kept in mind that data on intake of nutrients do not take into account such confounding factors as losses of nutrients during food preparation. Furthermore, the data indicate *relative risks* for deficiency, and in no case was a significant incidence of overt vitamin deficiency observed.

Certain individuals are exposed to deficient intakes of vitamins as a result of eccentric diets, such as food faddism, and the avoidance of food because of anorexia. Intakes of vitamins less than those recommended can also occur in subjects on reducing diets and among elderly people who eat little food for economic or social reasons. The consumption of excessive amounts of alcohol can also lead to inadequate intakes of vitamins and other nutrients.

A *disturbance in absorption* of vitamins is also seen in a variety of conditions. Examples are diseases of the liver and biliary tract, prolonged diarrhea from any cause, hyperthyroidism, pernicious anemia, sprue, surgical bypass of the small intestine for the treatment of obesity, and a variety of other disorders of the digestive system. Moreover, since a substantial proportion of vitamin K and biotin is synthesized by the bacteria of the gastrointestinal tract, treatment with antimicrobial agents that alter the intestinal bacterial flora inevitably leads to decreased availability of these vitamins.

Increased tissue requirements for vitamins may cause a nutritional deficiency to develop despite the ingestion of a diet that had previously been adequate. For example, requirements for some vitamins such as pyridoxine may be increased by the use of oral contraceptives and by certain antivitamin drugs (Roe, 1976a, 1976b). Diseases associated with an increased metabolic rate, such as hyperthyroidism and conditions accompanied by fever or tissue wasting, also increase the body's requirements for vitamins.

Finally, an increasing number of cases are recorded in which *genetic abnormalities* lead to an increased need for a vitamin. This is usually due to an abnormality in the structure of an enzyme for which the vitamin provides a cofactor, leading to a decreased affinity of the abnormal enzyme protein for the cofactor (Scriver, 1973).

Role of Vitamins in Therapeutics. Specific diseases caused by vitamin deficiency are relatively rare in the United States, but oral supplements of vitamins are indicated for the conditions that do lead to deficiency. Descriptions of official preparations are given in *The United States Pharmacopeia* (1985) and in the relevant chapters of this textbook. *Decavitamin Tablets and Capsules,* USP, each provide the approximate equivalent of the adult RDA for vitamins A and D, ascorbic acid, thiamine, riboflavin, nicotinamide, pyridoxine, and pantothenate, with somewhat lower levels of folate and vitamin B_{12}. These tablets and capsules contain no minerals.

For patients who cannot consume sufficient regular food for their needs, a number of specially defined formula diets are available. The vitamin content of these is regulated as *medical foods* by the FDA. Some patients require a complete supply of nutrients by the parenteral route. For this purpose, the dosage of water-soluble vitamins may have to be higher because of excessive losses in the urine (Vanamee, 1976; Nicholalds *et al.*, 1977; Moran and Greene, 1979).

In addition to the fact that individual diseases vary in their effects on nutritional requirements, the same disease will make varying demands on nutrients according to its phase and intensity. The need for therapy with vitamins may thus change throughout the course of the illness and, eventually, cure should be associated with cessation of this therapy; this point sometimes escapes the physician, who does not remind the patient to abandon the vitamin supplement.

Food and Drug Administration. Over-the-counter vitamin and mineral drug products for human use. *Federal Register*, **1979**, *44*, No. 53, 16126–16201.

Herbert, V. Laetrile: the cult of cyanide—promoting poison for profit. *Am. J. Clin. Nutr.*, **1979a**, *32*, 1121–1158.

———. Pangamic acid ("vitamin B_{15}"). *Ibid.*, **1979b**, *32*, 1534–1540.

Moran, J. R., and Greene, H. L. The B vitamins and vitamin C in human nutrition. II. "Conditional" B vitamins and vitamin C. *Am. J. Dis. Child.*, **1979**, *133*, 308–314.

National Analysts, Inc. *A Study of Health Practices and Opinions.* National Technical Information Service, Springfield, Va., **1972**, pp. 9–26.

National Center for Health Statistics; Carroll, M. D.; Abraham, S.; and Dress, C. M. Dietary intake source data: United States, 1976–80. *Vital Health Stat.* [*11*],

No. 231. U.S. Government Printing Office, Washington, D.C., **1983**.

Nicholalds, G. E.; Meng, H. C.; and Caldwell, M. D. Vitamin requirements in patients receiving total parenteral nutrition. *Arch. Surg.*, **1977**, *112*, 1061–1064.

Roe, D. A. Antivitamins. In, *Drug Induced Nutritional Deficiencies.* The AVI Publishing Co., Inc., Westport, Conn., **1976a**, pp. 154–185.

———. Nutritional effects of oral contraceptives. *Ibid.*, **1976b**, pp. 222–238.

Scriver, C. R. Vitamin-responsive inborn error of metabolism. *Metabolism*, **1973**, *22*, 1319–1344.

Select Committee on Nutrition and Human Needs, United States Senate. *Dietary Goals for the United States.* U.S. Government Printing Office, Washington, D. C., **1977**.

Ten-State Nutrition Survey, 1968–1970. Center for Disease Control, Department of Health, Education, and Welfare Publication Nos. (HSM) 72-8130-8134. U.S. Government Printing Office, Washington, D. C., **1972**.

The United States Pharmacopeia, 21st rev. The United States Pharmacopeial Convention, Inc. Mack Printing Co., Easton, Pa., **1985**.

Vanamee, P. Parenteral nutrition. In, *Present Knowledge of Nutrition*, 4th ed. (Hegsted, D. M.; Chichester, C. O.; Darby, W. J.; McNutt, K. W.; Stalvey, R. M.; and Stotz, E. H.; eds.) The Nutrition Foundation, Washington, D. C., **1976**, pp. 415–427.

Monographs and Reviews

Food and Nutrition Board, National Research Council. *Recommended Dietary Allowances*, 9th ed. National Academy of Sciences, Washington, D. C., **1980**.

Goodhart, R. S., and Shils, M. E. (eds.). *Modern Nutrition in Health and Disease*, 6th ed. Lea & Febiger, Philadelphia, **1980**.

Hegsted, D. M.; Chichester, C. O.; Darby, W. J.; McNutt, K. W.; Stalvey, R. M.; and Stotz, E. H. (eds.). *Present Knowledge of Nutrition*, 4th ed. The Nutrition Foundation, Washington, D. C., **1976**.

Herbert, V. *Nutrition Cultism, Facts and Fictions*. George F. Stickley Co., Philadelphia, **1980**, pp. 1–234.

Roe, D. A. *Drug Induced Nutritional Deficiencies*. The AVI Publishing Co., Inc., Westport, Conn., **1976**.

Schneider, H. A.; Anderson, C. E.; and Coursin, D. B. (eds.). *Nutritional Support of Medical Practice*. Harper & Row, Pub., Inc., New York, **1983**.

CHAPTER

66 WATER-SOLUBLE VITAMINS

The Vitamin B Complex and Ascorbic Acid

Robert Marcus and Ann M. Coulston

As discussed in the introductory section preceding this chapter, the water-soluble vitamins consist of members of the vitamin B complex and vitamin C (ascorbic acid).

The vitamin B complex comprises a large number of compounds that differ extensively in chemical structure and biological action. The reason for grouping them in a single class was their original isolation from the same sources, notably liver and yeast. Although the classical single-nutrient deficiency diseases were rampant in previous eras, it is far more common in contemporary Western society to see simultaneous deficiency of multiple nutrients.

There are traditionally 11 members of the vitamin B complex, namely, thiamine, riboflavin, nicotinic acid, pyridoxine, pantothenic acid, biotin, folic acid, cyanocobalamin (vitamin B_{12}), choline, inositol, and para-aminobenzoic acid. Folic acid and cyanocobalamin are considered in Chapter 57 because of their special function in hematopoiesis. Para-aminobenzoic acid (PABA) is not a true vitamin for any mammalian species but is a growth factor for certain bacteria, where it is a precursor in the synthesis of folic acid (*see* Chapter 57). The vitamins of the B complex function in intermediary metabolism in many essential reactions; some of these functions are summarized in Figure 66–1, which serves to illustrate their prevalence and importance.

In addition to the vitamin B complex, this chapter also considers ascorbic acid (vitamin C). This water-soluble vitamin is especially concentrated in citrus fruits and is thus obtained mostly from sources differing from those of members of the vitamin B complex. A further series of water-soluble compounds, the flavonoids (*e.g.*, rutin and hesperidin), has been claimed in the past to have vitamin activity beneficial for certain types of hemorrhagic disease. This claim is unsubstantiated. In addition, although the names "vitamin B_{15}" and "B_{17}" have been used in the commercial promotion of pangamic acid and laetrile, respectively, it is emphasized that neither of these products has been shown to be a vitamin or, for that matter, to play any role in human nutrition.

I. The Vitamin B Complex

THIAMINE

History. Thiamine was the first member of the vitamin B complex to be identified. Lack of thiamine produces a form of polyneuritis known as beri-

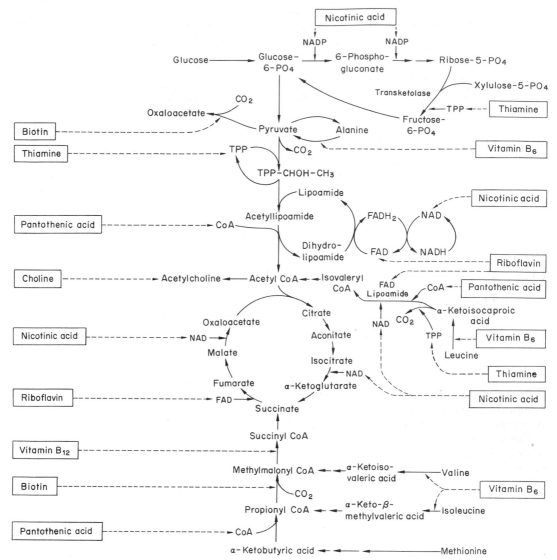

Figure 66–1. *Some major metabolic pathways involving coenzymes formed from water-soluble vitamins.* (Abbreviations are defined in the text.)

beri; this disease became widespread in East Asia in the nineteenth century due to the introduction of steam-powered rice mills, which produced polished rice lacking the vitamin-rich husk. A dietary cause for the disease was first indicated in 1880, when Admiral Takaki greatly reduced the incidence of beriberi in the Japanese Navy by adding fish, meat, barley, and vegetables to the sailors' diet of polished rice. In 1897, Eijkman, a Dutch physician working in Java where beriberi was also common, showed that fowl fed polished rice develop a polyneuritis similar to beriberi and that this could be cured by adding the rice polishings (husks) or an aqueous extract of the polishings back to the diet. He also demonstrated that rice polishings could cure beriberi in humans.

In 1911, Funk isolated a highly concentrated

form of the active factor and recognized that it belonged to a new class of food factors, which he called *vitamines,* later shortened to *vitamins.* The active factor was subsequently named vitamin B_1; in 1926 it was isolated in crystalline form by Jansen and Donath, and in 1936 its structure was determined by Williams. The Council on Pharmacy and Chemistry adopted the name *thiamine* to designate crystalline vitamin B_1, and this is now the official USP name of the vitamin.

Chemistry. Thiamine is an organic molecule containing a pyrimidine and a thiazole nucleus. Thiamine functions in the body in the form of the coenzyme thiamine pyrophosphate (TPP). The structures of thiamine and thiamine pyrophosphate are as follows:

The conversion of thiamine to its coenzyme form is carried out with adenosine triphosphate (ATP) as a pyrophosphate (PP) donor. Antimetabolites to thiamine have been synthesized. The most important of these are neopyrithiamine (pyrithiamine) and oxythiamine.

Pharmacological Actions. Thiamine is practically devoid of pharmacodynamic actions when given in usual therapeutic doses. Even large doses have no effect on the blood glucose concentration despite the physiological role of the vitamin in the intermediary metabolism of carbohydrate. Isolated clinical reports of toxic reactions to the parenteral administration of thiamine probably represent rare instances of hypersensitivity.

Physiological Functions. Thiamine pyrophosphate, the physiologically active form of thiamine, functions in carbohydrate metabolism as a coenzyme in the decarboxylation of α-keto acids such as pyruvate and α-ketoglutarate and in the utilization of pentose in the hexose monophosphate shunt; the latter function involves the thiamine pyrophosphate–dependent enzyme transketolase. Several metabolic changes of clinical importance can be related directly to the biochemical action of thiamine. In thiamine deficiency, the oxidation of α-keto acids is impaired, and an increase in the concentration of pyruvate in the blood has been used as one of the diagnostic signs of the deficiency state. A more specific diagnostic test for thiamine deficiency is based upon measurement of transketolase activity in erythrocytes (Brin, 1968). The requirement for thiamine is related to metabolic rate and is greatest when carbohydrate is the source of energy. This is of practical significance for patients who are maintained by parenteral alimentation and who thereby receive practically all their calories in the form of dextrose. Such patients should be given a *generous* allowance of the vitamin.

In addition to the classical functions of thiamine as a cofactor, it appears that thiamine might serve as a modulator of neuromuscular transmission. Thiamine binds to isolated nicotinic cholinergic receptors, and neurotransmission is impaired by pyrithiamine, a thiamine antagonist (Waldenlind, 1978).

Symptoms of Deficiency. Severe thiamine deficiency leads to the condition known as beriberi. In the East, this is due to consumption of diets of polished rice, which are deficient in the vitamin. In Western countries, thiamine deficiency is most commonly seen in alcoholics. A severe form of acute thiamine deficiency can also occur in infants.

The major symptoms of thiamine deficiency are related to the nervous system (*dry beriberi*) and to the cardiovascular system (*wet beriberi*). Many of the neurological signs and symptoms are characteristic of peripheral neuritis, with sensory disturbances in the extremities, including localized areas of hyperesthesia or anesthesia. Muscle strength is gradually lost and may result in wrist-drop or complete paralysis of a limb. Personality disturbances, depression, lack of initiative, and poor memory may also result from lack of the vitamin.

Cardiovascular symptoms can be prominent and include dyspnea on exertion, palpitation, tachycardia, and other cardiac abnormalities characterized by an abnormal ECG (chiefly low R wave voltage, T wave inversion, and prolongation of the Q-T interval) and cardiac failure of the high-output type. Such failure has been termed *wet beriberi;* there is extensive edema, largely as a result of hypoproteinemia from an inadequate intake of protein together with failing ventricular function.

Symptoms referable to the gastrointestinal tract are also observed in severe cases of deficiency. Loss of appetite occurs early and is followed by constipation.

Human Requirements. Because thiamine is essential for energy metabolism, especially of carbohydrate, requirement for thiamine is commonly related to caloric intake. The minimal thiamine requirement in man approximates 0.3 mg/1000 kcal. To provide a margin of safety, the Dietary Allowances Committee of the National Research Council has designated a Recommended Dietary Allowance (RDA) of 0.5 mg/1000 kcal (*see* Table XVI–1, page 1546). There is evidence that older people utilize thiamine less efficiently and, in consequence, not less than 1 mg daily is recommended for adults of all ages, no matter how low their caloric intake. During pregnancy and lactation, an additional intake of 0.6 mg/1000 kcal is recommended.

Thiamine deficiency may occur in association with an apparently adequate diet, since the vitamin is not stored in the body to a great extent. Thus, an increase in metabolic rate (*e.g.*, hyperthyroidism) or a gastrointestinal disturbance, such as chronic diarrhea, may necessitate an increased intake of thiamine. Thiamine deficiency can also occur from the consumption of large amounts of raw fish containing thiaminase (Murata, 1965) or large quantities of tea, which contains a thiamine antagonist (Vimokesant *et al.*, 1974).

Food Sources. The following foods are particularly rich in thiamine: pork, organ meats, wholegrain and enriched cereals and bread, legumes, and nuts. Thiamine is stable in acidic solution but is destroyed by heat in neutral or alkaline solution.

Absorption, Fate, and Excretion. Absorption of the usual dietary amounts of thiamine from the gastrointestinal tract occurs by sodium-dependent active transport; at higher concentrations, passive diffusion is also significant (Rindi and Ventura, 1972). Absorption is usually limited to a maximal daily amount of 8 to 15 mg, but this can be exceeded by oral administration in divided doses with food.

In adults, approximately 1 mg of thiamine per day is completely degraded by the tissues, and this is roughly the minimal daily requirement. When intake is at this low level, little or no thiamine is excreted in the urine. When intake exceeds the minimal requirement, tissue stores are first saturated. Thereafter, the excess appears quantitatively in the urine as intact thiamine or as pyrimidine, which arises from degradation of the thiamine molecule. As the intake of thiamine is further increased, more of the excess is excreted unchanged, indicating that the capacity of tissues to split thiamine to pyrimidine is limited.

Preparations. Thiamine can be prescribed as the pure vitamin, in mixtures of pure vitamins, or in the form of vitamin-rich concentrates.

Thiamine hydrochloride (vitamin B_1 hydrochloride) occurs as small, white crystals or as a crystalline powder. Tablets can usually be obtained in amounts ranging from 5 to 500 mg each. *Thiamine hydrochloride injection* contains 100 mg/ml. Thiamine is also available as an elixir.

Therapeutic Uses. The only established therapeutic use of thiamine is in the treatment or the prophylaxis of thiamine deficiency. To correct the disorder as rapidly as possible, intravenous doses as large as 100 mg per liter of parenteral fluid are commonly used. Once thiamine deficiency has been corrected, there is no need for parenteral injection or the administration of amounts in excess of daily requirements except in instances when gastrointestinal disturbances preclude the ingestion or absorption of adequate amounts of vitamin.

The syndromes of thiamine deficiency seen clinically can range from beriberi through Wernicke's encephalopathy and Korsakoff's syndrome to alcoholic polyneuropathy. Because normal metabolism of carbohydrate results in consumption of thiamine, it has been observed repeatedly that administration of glucose may precipitate acute symptoms of thiamine deficiency in marginally nourished subjects. This has also been noted during the correction of endogenous hyperglycemia. Thus, in any individual whose thiamine status may be suspect, the vitamin should be given along with dextrose-containing fluids. The clinical findings appear to depend on the amount of deprivation (McLaren, 1978). Encephalopathy and Korsakoff's syndrome result from severe deprivation, whereas beriberi heart disease occurs in less deficient subjects; polyneuritis is observed in milder deprivation. The following discussion describes briefly the varieties of thiamine deficiency and their treatment.

Alcoholic Neuritis. Alcoholism is the most common cause of thiamine deficiency in the United States. Alcoholic neuritis is basically a nutritional deficiency due to an inadequate intake of thiamine. Two factors contribute to such inadequate intake in the chronic alcoholic. Appetite is usually poor. Food consumption drops, and a large portion of the caloric intake is in the form of alcohol. The symptoms of neurological involvement in alcoholics are those of a polyneuritis with motor and sensory defects. Wernicke's syndrome is an additional serious consequence of alcoholism and thiamine deficiency. Certain characteristic signs of this disease, notably ophthalmoplegia, nystagmus, and ataxia, respond rapidly to the administration of thiamine but to no other vitamin. Wernicke's syndrome may be accompanied by an acute global confusional state that may also respond to thiamine. Left untreated, Wernicke's encephalopathy frequently leads to a chronic disorder in which learning and memory are impaired out of proportion to other cognitive functions in the otherwise-alert and responsive patient. This disorder (Korsakoff's psychosis) is characterized by confabulation, and it is less likely to be reversible once established (Victor *et al.*, 1971). It has been problematic that the thiamine stores of some patients with Wernicke's encephalopathy are similar to those in patients without neurological findings. It has recently been shown that patients with Wernicke's encephalopathy have an abnormality in the thiamine-dependent enzyme transketolase, wherein the affinity of the enzyme for the cofactor is reduced. Marginal concentrations of thiamine might thus be sufficient to produce serious neurological damage (Blass and Gibson, 1977).

Chronic alcoholics with polyneuritis and motor or sensory defects should receive 40 mg of oral thiamine daily. The Wernicke-Korsakoff syndrome represents an *acute emergency* that should be treated with daily doses of 100 mg of the vitamin, intravenously.

Infantile Beriberi. Thiamine deficiency also occurs as an acute disease in infancy and may run a rapid and fulminating course. The onset consists in loss of appetite, vomiting, and greenish stools followed by paroxysmal attacks of muscular rigidity. Aphonia due to loss of laryngeal nerve function is a diagnostic feature. Signs of cardiac involvement are also prominent. The pulse becomes weak and rapid, the face is cyanotic, and the neck veins are engorged due to cardiac failure. Death may follow the initial signs within 12 to 24 hours unless vigorous treatment is instituted. Infants with mild forms of this condition respond to oral therapy with 10 mg of thiamine daily. If acute collapse occurs, doses of 25 mg intravenously can be given cautiously, but the prognosis remains poor.

Subacute Necrotizing Encephalomyelopathy. This is a fatal disease of children. Clinical features include difficulties with feeding and swallowing, vomiting, hypotonia, external ophthalmoplegia, peripheral neuropathy, and seizures. Although multiple etiological defects may prove capable of causing the syndrome, many cases appear to be caused by a genetically determined enzyme deficiency that leads to the appearance of a circulating inhibitor of the enzyme that synthesizes thiamine triphosphate from thiamine pyrophosphate in the nervous system (Pincus *et al.*, 1969). Metabolic abnormalities have also been found in liver and muscle from affected infants. A urine test for the presence of the glycoprotein enzyme inhibitor has been described (Pincus *et al.*, 1974). When patients with this syndrome are treated daily with large doses of thiamine, most exhibit marked temporary improvement (Pincus *et al.*, 1973). Other inborn errors of metabolism that are sensitive to the administration of thiamine have also been described (Scriver, 1973).

Cardiovascular Disease. Cardiovascular disease of nutritional origin is observed in chronic alcoholics, pregnant women, persons with gastrointestinal disorders, and those whose diet is deficient for other reasons. When the diagnosis of cardiovascular disease due to thiamine deficiency has been correctly made, the response to the administration of thiamine is striking. One of the pathognomonic features of the syndrome is an increased blood flow due to arteriolar dilatation. Within a few hours after the administration of thiamine, the cardiac output is reduced and the utilization of oxygen begins to return to normal. If edema is present and due to myocardial insufficiency, diuresis results after proper therapy. The rate of improvement is seemingly inversely proportional to the rate of onset and duration of the disease, and individuals suffering from a chronic deficiency may require protracted

treatment. The usual dose of thiamine is 10 to 30 mg three times daily, given parenterally. The dosage can be reduced and the patient maintained on oral medication or by dietary management after signs of the deficiency state have been reversed. It is emphasized that administration of glucose may precipitate heart failure in individuals with marginal thiamine status. All patients potentially in this category should receive thiamine prophylactically; 100 mg is commonly added to the first few liters of intravenous fluid.

Gastrointestinal Disorders. In experimental and clinical beriberi, certain symptoms occur that are referable to the gastrointestinal tract. On this basis, thiamine has been used uncritically as a therapeutic agent for such unrelated conditions as ulcerative colitis, gastrointestinal hypotonia, and chronic diarrhea. Unless the disease being treated is the direct result of a deficiency of thiamine, there is no reason to expect the vitamin to be efficacious.

Neuritis of Pregnancy. Pregnancy increases the thiamine requirement slightly. The neuritis of pregnancy takes the form of multiple peripheral nerve involvement, and the signs and symptoms in well-developed cases resemble those described in patients with beriberi. The problem may occur because of poor intake of thiamine or in patients with hyperemesis gravidarum. Proof that the neuritis is due to thiamine deficiency is gained in those cases in which dramatic clinical improvement follows thiamine therapy. The dose employed is from 5 to 10 mg daily, given parenterally if vomiting is severe.

RIBOFLAVIN

History. At various times from 1879 onward, series of yellow pigmented compounds have been isolated from a variety of sources and designated as flavins, prefixed to indicate the source (*e.g.*, lacto-, ovo-, and hepato-). It was then demonstrated that these various flavins are identical in chemical composition.

In the meantime, water-soluble vitamin B had been separated into a heat-labile antiberiberi factor (B_1) and a heat-stable growth-promoting factor (B_2), and it was eventually appreciated that concentrates of so-called vitamin B_2 had a yellow color, the intensity of which was related to vitamin activity. In 1932, Warburg and Christian described a yellow respiratory enzyme in yeast, and in 1933 the yellow pigment portion of the enzyme was identified as vitamin B_2. All doubt as to the identity of vitamin B_2 and the naturally occurring flavins was removed when lactoflavin was synthesized and the synthetic product was shown to possess full biological activity. The vitamin was designated as *riboflavin* because of the presence of ribose in its structure.

Chemistry. Riboflavin carries out its functions in the body in the form of one or the other of two coenzymes, riboflavin phosphate, commonly called flavin mononucleotide (FMN), and flavin adenine dinucleotide (FAD). The structures of riboflavin, FMN, and FAD are shown below. Riboflavin is converted to FMN and FAD by two enzyme-catalyzed reactions (*see* Wagner-Jauregg, 1972; McCormick, 1975):

$$\text{Riboflavin} + \text{ATP} \longrightarrow \text{FMN} + \text{ADP} \quad (1)$$
$$\text{FMN} + \text{ATP} \longrightarrow \text{FAD} + \text{PP} \quad (2)$$

Pharmacological Actions. No overt pharmacological effects follow the oral or parenteral administration of riboflavin.

Physiological Functions. FMN and FAD, the physiologically active forms of riboflavin, serve a vital role in metabolism as coenzymes for a wide variety of respiratory flavoproteins, some of which contain metals (*e.g.*, xanthine oxidase).

Symptoms of Deficiency. The signs and symptoms of spontaneous or experimentally produced riboflavin deficiency have been reviewed by Rivlin (1970) and by Lane and colleagues (1975). Sore throat and angular stomatitis generally appear first. Later, glossitis, cheilosis (red denuded lips), seborrheic dermatitis of the face, and dermatitis over the trunk and extremities occur, followed by anemia and neuropathy. In some subjects corneal vascularization and cataract formation are prominent.

The anemia that develops in riboflavin deficiency is normochromic and normocytic and is associated with reticulocytopenia; leukocytes and platelets are generally normal. Administration of riboflavin to deficient patients causes reticulocytosis, and the concentration of hemoglobin returns to normal. Anemia in patients with riboflavin deficiency may be related, at least in part, to disturbances in folic acid metabolism.

The problem in the clinical recognition of riboflavin deficiency is that certain features, such as glossitis and dermatitis, are common signs, both in deficiencies of other vitamins and as manifestations of other diseases. Recognition of riboflavin deficiency is also difficult because it rarely occurs in isolation. In nutritional surveys of children in an urban area and of randomly selected hospitalized patients, deficiency of riboflavin was frequently observed, but almost invariably in conjunction with other vitamin deficiencies. Riboflavin deficiency has likewise been observed in association with deficiencies of other vitamins in a large proportion of urban alcoholics of low economic status (Rivlin, 1979). Assessment of riboflavin status is made by correlating dietary history with clinical and laboratory findings. Biochemical tests include evaluation of urinary excretion of the vitamin (excretion of less than 50 μg of riboflavin daily is indicative of deficiency). Although concentrations of flavins in blood are not of diagnostic value, an enzyme activation assay that utilizes glutathione reductase from erythrocytes correlates well with riboflavin status (Prentice and Bates, 1981).

Human Requirements. The Dietary Allowances Committee of the National Research Council recommends a riboflavin intake of 0.6 mg/1000 kcal. This is equivalent to 1.6 mg daily for young adult males and 1.2 mg daily for young adult females. It is recommended that intake for elderly adults should not be less than 1.2 mg daily, even when caloric intake falls below 2000 kcal.

Food Sources. Riboflavin is abundant in milk, cheese, organ meats, eggs, green leafy vegetables, and whole-grain and enriched cereals and bread.

Absorption, Fate, and Excretion. Riboflavin is readily absorbed from the upper gastrointestinal tract by a specific transport mechanism involving phosphorylation of the vitamin to FMN (Jusko and Levy, 1975). Here and in other tissues, riboflavin is converted to FMN by flavokinase, a reaction that is sensitive to thyroid-hormone status and inhibited by chlorpromazine and by tricyclic antidepressants (Rivlin, 1979).

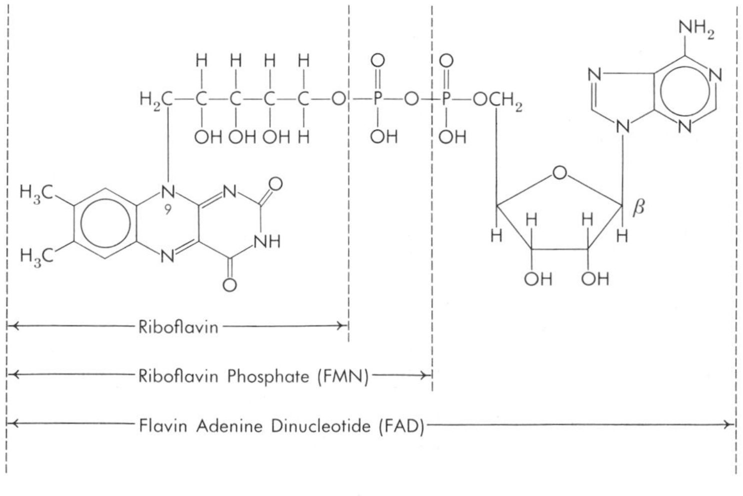

Riboflavin

Riboflavin Phosphate (FMN)

Flavin Adenine Dinucleotide (FAD)

Riboflavin is distributed to all tissues, but concentrations are uniformly low and little is stored. The relationship of riboflavin intake to urinary excretion has been studied extensively (Horwitt *et al.*, 1956). When riboflavin is ingested in amounts that approximate the minimal daily requirement, only about 9% appears in the urine. As the intake of riboflavin is increased above the minimal requirement, a larger proportion is excreted unchanged.

Riboflavin is present in the feces. This probably represents vitamin synthesized by intestinal microorganisms, since, on low intakes of riboflavin, the amount excreted in the feces exceeds that ingested. There is no evidence that riboflavin synthesized by the bacteria in the colon can be absorbed.

Preparations. *Riboflavin (vitamin B$_2$)* is a yellow to orange-yellow crystalline powder with a slight odor. While the vitamin is sparingly soluble in water, it is more so in isotonic sodium chloride solution. When dry, riboflavin is not affected appreciably by light; however, when it is in solution, light induces quite rapid deterioration, especially at alkaline pH. *Riboflavin tablets* are available in amounts ranging from 5 to 100 mg. *Riboflavin injection* contains 50 mg/ml.

Therapeutic Uses. The only established therapeutic application of riboflavin is to treat or prevent disease caused by deficiency. Ariboflavinosis seldom occurs in the United States as a discrete deficiency but may accompany other nutritional disorders. Specific therapy with riboflavin, 5 to 10 mg daily, should thus be given in the context of treating multiple nutritional deficiencies.

NICOTINIC ACID

History. Pellagra (Italian for *pelle agra,* or "rough skin") has been known for centuries in countries where maize is eaten in quantity, notably Italy and North America. In 1914, Funk postulated that the disease was due to a deficiency in the diet, and this was confirmed by the classical work of Goldberger and coworkers of the United States Public Health Service. Goldberger fed deficient diets to dogs and produced the condition known as "black tongue," analogous to human pellagra. In rats, the same diet caused a marked dermatitis that could be cured by dietary measures. The next step was the discovery that black tongue could also be cured by appropriate alterations of diet.

In 1935, Warburg and associates obtained nicotinic acid amide (nicotinamide) from a coenzyme isolated from the red blood cells of the horse. This finding stimulated further studies on the nutritional value of nicotinic acid. Liver extracts were known to be highly effective in curing human pellagra and canine black tongue. Elvehjem and associates prepared concentrates of liver that were highly effective in the treatment of canine black tongue, and, in 1937, they identified the active substance as nicotinamide. Proof was established by the demonstration that synthetic nicotinic acid derivatives were also effective in alleviating the symptoms of black tongue and curing human pellagra. Goldberger and Tanner had previously shown that tryptophan could cure human pellagra; this effect was later determined to be due to the conversion of tryptophan to nicotinic acid. Goldsmith (1958) produced pellagra experimentally in man by feeding a diet deficient in nicotinic acid and tryptophan.

With the recognition of nicotinic acid as the pellagra-preventing vitamin, the compound soon became an official drug. Nicotinic acid is also known as *niacin,* a term introduced to avoid confusion between the vitamin and the alkaloid nicotine. Pellagra is now quite uncommon in the United States, probably as a direct result of supplementation of flour with nicotinic acid since 1939.

Chemistry. Nicotinic acid functions in the body after conversion to either nicotinamide adenine dinucleotide (NAD) or nicotinamide adenine dinucleotide phosphate (NADP). It is to be noted that nicotinic acid occurs in these two nucleotides in the form of its amide, nicotinamide. The structures of nicotinic acid, nicotinamide, NAD, and NADP are shown below, where **R** = H in NAD and **R** = PO$_3$H$_2$ in NADP.

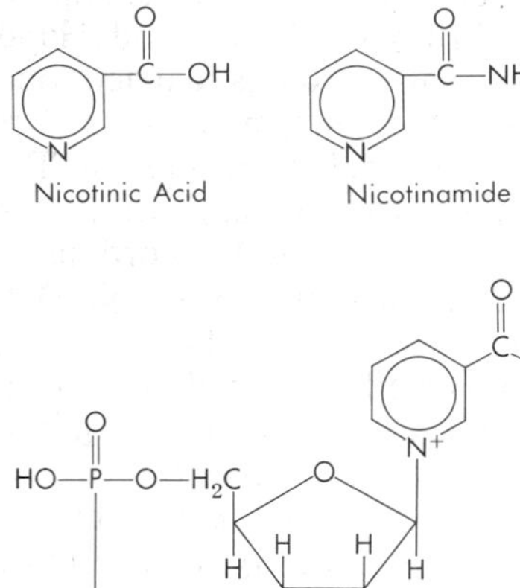

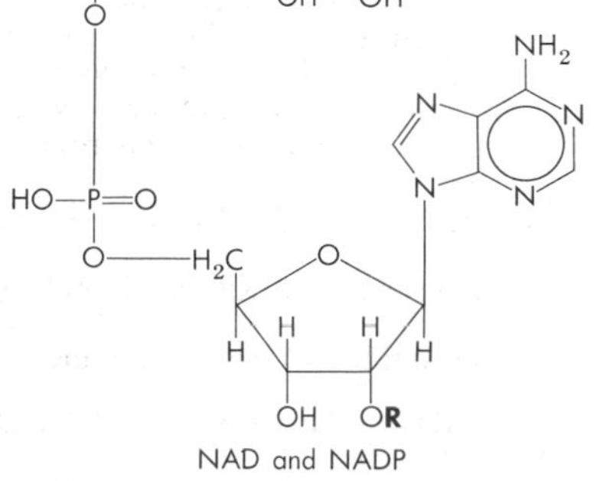

Nicotinic Acid   Nicotinamide

NAD and NADP

Pharmacological Actions. Nicotinic acid and nicotinamide are identical in their function as vitamins. However, they differ markedly as pharmacological agents. The pharmacological effects and toxicity of nicotinic acid in man have been reviewed by Miller and Hayes (1982). These include flushing, pruritus, gastrointestinal distress, hepatotoxicity, and activation of peptic ulcer disease. The compound has been used as a vasodilator and for its effects to lower plasma cholesterol (*see* Chapter 34). Nicotinamide has no such cardiovascular effects.

Physiological Functions. NAD and NADP, the physiologically active forms of nicotinic acid, serve a vital role in metabolism as coenzymes for a wide variety of proteins that catalyze oxidation-reduction reactions essential for tissue respiration. The coenzymes, bound to appropriate dehydrogenases, function as oxidants accepting electrons and hydrogen from substrates and thus becoming reduced. The reduced pyridine nucleotides, in turn, are reoxidized by flavoproteins.

The metabolic pathway by which nicotinic acid is converted into NAD has been elucidated for a variety of tissues, including human erythrocytes (Preiss and Handler, 1958). The conversion is carried out by three consecutive enzyme-catalyzed reactions (*see* 1 to 3 below, where PRPP is 5-phosphoribosyl-1-pyrophosphate). NADP is synthesized from NAD according to reaction 4. The biosynthesis of NAD from tryptophan is more complicated. Tryptophan is converted to quinolinic acid by a series of enzymatic reactions; quinolinic acid is converted to nicotinic acid ribonucleotide (Nishizuka and Hayaishi, 1963), which enters the pathway at reaction 2.

Symptoms of Deficiency. Nicotinic acid is an essential dietary constituent, the lack of which leads to the clinical condition known as pellagra. Pellagra is characterized by signs and symptoms referable especially to the skin, gastrointestinal

tract, and central nervous system (CNS), a triad frequently referred to as dermatitis, diarrhea, and dementia, or the "three Ds." Pellagra now occurs most often in the setting of chronic alcoholism, protein-calorie malnutrition, and deficiencies of multiple vitamins (Spivak and Jackson, 1977). An erythematous eruption resembling sunburn first appears on the back of the hands. Other areas exposed to light (forehead, neck, and feet) are later involved, and eventually the lesions may be more widespread. The cutaneous manifestations are characteristically symmetrical and may darken, desquamate, and scar.

The chief symptoms referable to the digestive tract are stomatitis, enteritis, and diarrhea. The tongue becomes very red and swollen and may ulcerate. There is also excessive salivary secretion, and the salivary glands may be enlarged. Nausea and vomiting are common. Steatorrhea may be present, even in the absence of diarrhea. When present, diarrhea is recurrent and stools may be watery and occasionally bloody.

Symptoms referable to the CNS are headache, dizziness, insomnia, depression, and impairment of memory. In severe cases, delusions, hallucinations, and dementia may appear. Motor and sensory disturbances of the peripheral nerves also occur. The EEG is characterized by excessive theta and delta activity. Common laboratory findings include macrocytic anemia, hypoalbuminemia, and hyperuricemia.

Biochemical assessment of deficiency is attempted by the measurement of urinary excretion of methylated metabolites of nicotinic acid (*e.g.*, N-methylnicotinamide). These tests do not as yet provide unequivocal evidence of deficiency. The measurement of nicotinamide in blood and urine has not been shown to be useful in evaluating niacin status. In most cases, the diagnosis rests on a correlation of clinical findings with the response to supplemental nicotinamide.

Human Requirements. As indicated above, the dietary requirement for this vitamin can be satisfied not only by nicotinic acid but also by nicotinamide and the amino acid tryptophan. Therefore, the nicotinic acid requirement is influenced by the quantity and the quality of dietary protein. Administration of tryptophan to normal human subjects, as well as to patients with pellagra, and analysis of urinary metabolites indicate that an average of 60 mg of dietary tryptophan is equivalent to 1 mg of nicotinic acid. This conversion rate is reduced in women taking oral contraceptives. The minimal requirement of nicotinic acid (including that formed from tryptophan) to prevent pellagra averages 4.4 mg/1000 kcal. The recommended allowance of the Dietary Allowances Committee of the National

$$\text{Nicotinic Acid} + \text{PRPP} \longrightarrow \text{Nicotinic Acid Ribonucleotide} + \text{PP} \qquad (1)$$

$$\text{Nicotinic Acid Ribonucleotide} + \text{ATP} \longrightarrow \text{Desamido-NAD} + \text{PP} \qquad (2)$$

$$\text{Desamido-NAD} + \text{Glutamine} + \text{ATP} \longrightarrow \text{NAD} + \text{Glutamate} + \text{ADP} + \text{P} \quad (3)$$

$$\text{NAD} + \text{ATP} \longrightarrow \text{NADP} + \text{ADP} \qquad (4)$$

Research Council, expressed in nicotinic acid equivalents, is 6.6 mg/1000 kcal (*see* Table XVI–1, page 1546). For people who consume few calories (*e.g.,* the elderly), daily intake should not fall below 13 mg of nicotinic acid or the equivalent.

The relationship between the nicotinic acid requirement and the intake of tryptophan has helped to explain the historical association between the incidence of pellagra and the presence of large amounts of corn in the diet. Corn protein is low in tryptophan, and the nicotinic acid in corn and other cereals is largely unavailable. When cornmeal provides the major portion of dietary protein, pellagra will develop at levels of intake of nicotinic acid that would be adequate if the dietary protein contained more tryptophan. Intake of animal protein is high among Americans; tryptophan thus helps significantly to meet the daily requirement for niacin.

Food Sources. Nicotinic acid is obtained from liver, meat, fish, poultry, whole-grain and enriched bread and cereals, nuts, and legumes. Tryptophan as a precursor is provided by animal protein in particular.

Absorption, Fate, and Excretion. Both nicotinic acid and nicotinamide are readily absorbed from all portions of the intestinal tract, and the vitamin is distributed to all tissues. When therapeutic doses of nicotinic acid or its amide are administered, only small amounts of the unchanged vitamin appear in the urine. When extremely high doses of these vitamins are given, the unchanged vitamin represents the major urinary component. The principal route of metabolism of nicotinic acid and nicotinamide is by the formation of N-methylnicotinamide, which in turn is further metabolized to N-methyl-2-pyridone-5-carboxamide and N-methyl-4-pyridone-3-carboxamide. Nicotinuric acid, the glycine peptide of nicotinic acid, is an additional metabolite.

Preparations. *Niacin* (*nicotinic acid, 3-pyridinecarboxylic acid*) is stable to heat, oxidation, and light. *Niacin tablets* and *capsules* contain from 25 to 500 mg. *Niacin injection* contains 50 or 100 mg/ml.

Niacinamide (*nicotinamide, nicotinic acid amide*) is available in tablets (50 to 500 mg) and as an injection (100 mg/ml).

Therapeutic Uses. Nicotinic acid, nicotinamide, and their derivatives are used for prophylaxis and treatment of pellagra. In the acute exacerbations of the disease, therapy must be intensive. The recommended oral dose is 50 mg, given up to ten times daily. If oral medication is impossible, intravenous injection of 25 mg is given two or more times daily. Pellagra may occur in the course of two metabolic disorders. In Hartnup's disease there is defective intestinal and renal transport of tryptophan (Darby *et al.*, 1976). In some patients with carcinoid tumors large amounts of tryptophan are utilized by the tumor for the synthesis of 5-hydroxytryptophan and 5-hydroxytryptamine (serotonin).

The response to nicotinic acid or its derivatives is dramatic. Within 24 hours, the fiery redness and swelling of the tongue disappear and sialorrhea diminishes. Associated oral infections heal rapidly. Other infections of mucous membranes, notably those involving the pharynx, urethra, vagina, and rectum, also disappear. Nausea, vomiting, and diarrhea may stop within 24 hours, and at the same time the patient is relieved of epigastric distress, abdominal pain, and distention. Appetite also improves. Mental symptoms are quickly relieved, sometimes overnight. Confused patients become mentally clear, and those who are delirious become calm, adjusted to their environment, and remember with insight the events of their psychotic state. So specific are nicotinic acid and its derivatives in this regard that they can be used as diagnostic agents in patients with frank psychoses but with questionable additional evidence of pellagra. Large doses of niacin are recommended, especially when the psychosis is associated with encephalopathy. The dermal lesions blanch and heal, but this occurs more slowly. The vitamin has less effect on cutaneous lesions that are moist, ulcerated, or pigmented. The porphyrinuria associated with pellagra also disappears.

Pellagra may be complicated by thiamine deficiency with associated peripheral neuritis. This complication does not respond to nicotinic acid or its congeners and must be treated with thiamine. Many pellagrins are also benefited by additional therapy with riboflavin and pyridoxine.

The dramatic effect of niacin on the mental status of patients with pellagra led to the advocacy of large doses of the vitamin in the treatment of schizophrenia and other mental disorders. This approach has been reviewed by Lipton and coworkers (1979) and has been found to be without merit.

PYRIDOXINE

History. In 1926, dermatitis was produced in rats by feeding a diet deficient in vitamin B_2. However, in 1936 György distinguished the water-soluble factor whose deficiency was responsible for the dermatitis from vitamin B_2 and named it vitamin B_6. The structure of the vitamin was elucidated in 1939. Several related natural compounds (pyridoxine, pyridoxal, pyridoxamine) have been shown to possess the same biological properties, and therefore all should be called vitamin B_6. However, the

Council on Pharmacy and Chemistry has assigned the name *pyridoxine* to the vitamin.

Chemistry. The structures of the three forms of vitamin B_6—that is, pyridoxine, pyridoxal, and pyridoxamine—are shown below.

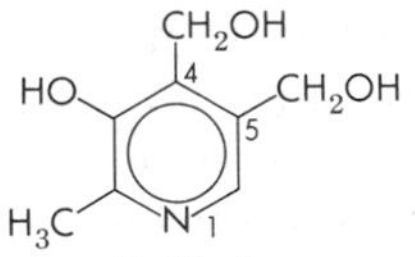

The compounds differ in the nature of the substituent on the carbon atom in position 4 of the pyridine nucleus: pyridoxine is a primary alcohol, pyridoxal is the corresponding aldehyde, and pyridoxamine contains an aminomethyl group in this position. Each of the three forms of the vitamin can be readily utilized by the mammalian organism. The physiologically active forms of vitamin B_6 are pyridoxal phosphate and pyridoxamine phosphate, where the phosphate is esterified with the alcohol at position 5 of the pyridine ring.

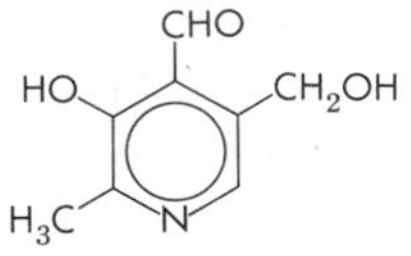

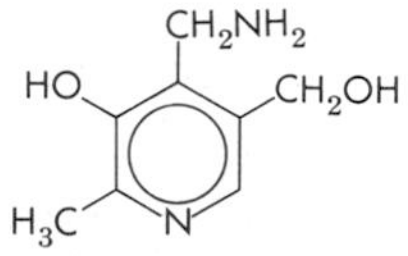

All three forms of vitamin B_6 are converted in the body to pyridoxal phosphate; pyridoxal is converted to pyridoxal phosphate by the enzyme pyridoxal kinase.

Antimetabolites to pyridoxine have been synthesized and are capable of blocking the action of the vitamin and producing signs and symptoms of deficiency. The most active is 4-deoxypyridoxine, in which the substituent on the carbon atom in position 4 is a methyl group. The anti–vitamin B_6 activity of 4-deoxypyridoxine has been attributed to the formation *in vivo* of 4-deoxypyridoxine-5-phosphate, which is a competitive inhibitor of several pyridoxal phosphate–dependent enzymes.

Isonicotinic acid hydrazide (*isoniazid; see* Chapter 53) combines with pyridoxal or pyridoxal phosphate to form hydrazones; as a result, it is a potent inhibitor of pyridoxal kinase. Enzymatic reactions in which pyridoxal phosphate participates as a coenzyme are also inhibited, but only by concentrations about 1000 times as great as that required to inhibit the formation of pyridoxal phosphate. Isoniazid thus appears to exert its anti–vitamin B_6 effect primarily by inhibiting the formation of the coenzyme form of the vitamin.

Pharmacological Actions. Pyridoxine has low toxicity and elicits no outstanding pharmacodynamic actions after either oral or intravenous administration. Extremely large oral doses (in the range of 2 to 6 g/kg) produce convulsions and death in rats and mice (Brin, 1978), but lower doses can be given daily without any obvious effects. In man, oral doses up to 1000 mg daily have not caused adverse reactions (Bauernfeind and Miller, 1978). However, a toxic sensory neuropathy has recently been described in people who consume more than 2000 mg daily on a chronic basis (Schaumberg *et al.*, 1983). Symptoms of dependency have been noted in adults given only 200 mg daily followed by withdrawal (Canham *et al.*, 1964).

Physiological Functions. Pyridoxal phosphate serves an important role in metabolism as a coenzyme for a wide variety of metabolic transformations of amino acids, including decarboxylation, transamination, and racemization, as well as for enzymatic steps in the metabolism of tryptophan, sulfur-containing amino acids, and hydroxyamino acids. In the case of transamination, enzyme-bound pyridoxal phosphate is aminated to pyridoxamine phosphate by the donor amino acid, and the bound pyridoxamine phosphate is then deaminated to pyridoxal phosphate by the acceptor α-keto acid. In the metabolism of tryptophan, vitamin B_6 is involved in a number of enzymatic reactions (Henderson and Hulse, 1978). In vitamin B_6–deficient man and animals a number of metabolites of tryptophan are excreted in abnormally large quantities. The measurement of these metabolites, particularly xanthurenic acid, in urine following tryptophan loading tests has been used to test for vitamin B_6 deficiency. Vitamin B_6 is a cofactor in the conversion of tryptophan to 5-hydroxytryptamine. The conversion of methionine to cysteine is also dependent on the vitamin (Sturman, 1978). In addition to its classical cofactor functions, pyridoxine may be capable of modifying actions of steroid hormones *in vivo* by means of interactions with steroid receptor complexes (DiSorbo *et al.*, 1980; Müller *et al.*, 1980).

Biochemical interactions occur between pyridoxal phosphate and certain drugs and toxins (Bauernfeind and Miller, 1978). Thus, isoniazid increases urinary excretion of vitamin B_6, and prolonged use of penicillamine has caused deficiency of vitamin B_6. The drugs cycloserine and hydralazine are also antagonists of vitamin B_6. Administration of the vitamin reduces the neurological side effects associated with the use of these compounds. Vitamin B_6 enhances the peripheral decarboxylation of levodopa and reduces its effectiveness for the treatment of Parkinson's disease. Vitamin B_6 and multivitamin preparations should thus be avoided in patients receiving levodopa (*see* Chapter 21).

Symptoms of Deficiency. Symptoms referable to pyridoxine deficiency have been produced in all mammalian species that have been studied, including man. It is claimed that the incidence of vitamin B_6 deficiency among alcoholics is 20 to 30% (Li, 1978). Important features of the deficiency observed in more than one species relate to the skin, the nervous system, and erythropoiesis.

Skin. In the rat, a florid dermatitis occurs; this consists in hyperkeratosis and acanthosis of the ears, paws, and snout as well as edema of the corium. In man, seborrhea-like skin lesions about the eyes, nose, and mouth accompanied by glossitis and stomatitis can be produced within a few weeks by feeding a diet poor in vitamin B complex plus daily doses of the vitamin antagonist 4-deoxypyridoxine. The lesions clear rapidly after the administration of pyridoxine but do not respond to other members of the B complex (Mueller and Vilter, 1950).

Nervous System. Rats, pigs, dogs, and man may have convulsive seizures when maintained on a diet deficient in pyridoxine. These seizures can be prevented or cured by the vitamin. In the pig, degenerative changes in peripheral nerves, dorsal root ganglion cells, and posterior columns of the spinal cord have been described. In man, a peripheral neuritis associated with synovial swelling and tenderness, especially of the carpal synovia (*carpal tunnel disease*), has been attributed in some cases to deficiency of pyridoxine; the syndrome is reversible upon treatment with high dosage of the vitamin (Ellis *et al.*, 1979). The general applicability of this approach to patients with carpal tunnel syndrome has not been established.

The electroshock threshold for producing clonic seizures in rats is substantially lowered by pyridoxine deficiency and can be raised to normal by the administration of pyridoxine. The induction of convulsive seizures by pyridoxine deficiency may be the result of a lowered concentration of γ-aminobutyric acid, an inhibitory CNS neurotransmitter, the synthesis of which is carried out by glutamic acid decarboxylase, a pyridoxal phosphate–requiring enzyme (Roberts, 1963). In addition, pyridoxine deficiency leads to decreased concentrations of the neurotransmitters norepinephrine and 5-hydroxytryptamine (Dakshinamurti, 1977).

Erythropoiesis. In the dog, pig, and monkey, pyridoxine deficiency results in microcytic, hypochromic anemia. While dietary deficiency of pyridoxine in man may rarely cause anemia, the usual pyridoxine-responsive anemia of man is apparently not due to inadequate supplies of this vitamin as judged by normal standards. This type of anemia is described in Chapter 56.

Human Requirements. The requirement for pyridoxine increases with the amount of protein in the diet (Linkswiler, 1978). The average adult minimal requirement for pyridoxine is about 1.5 mg per day in individuals ingesting 100 g of protein per day. To provide a reasonable margin of safety and to allow for daily intakes of more than 100 g of protein, a level of 2.2 mg per day is recommended for adult males and 2.0 mg per day for adult females (*see* Table XVI–1, page 1546).

Food Sources. Pyridoxine is supplied by meat, liver, whole-grain breads and cereals, soybeans, and vegetables. There are substantial losses during cooking, and pyridoxine is sensitive to both ultraviolet light and oxidation.

Absorption, Fate, and Excretion. Pyridoxine, pyridoxal, and pyridoxamine are readily absorbed from the gastrointestinal tract. The principal excretory product when any of the three forms of the vitamin is fed to man is 4-pyridoxic acid, formed by the action of hepatic aldehyde oxidase on free pyridoxal. Administration of pyridoxine and pyridoxamine also results in an increased excretion of pyridoxal in man, indicating that both compounds may be first transformed, directly or indirectly, to pyridoxal, which is then oxidized to 4-pyridoxic acid (for review, *see* Brin, 1978).

Preparations. *Pyridoxine hydrochloride* is available in tablets (5 to 500 mg) and as an injection (100 mg/ml).

Therapeutic Uses. Although there is no doubt that pyridoxine is essential in human nutrition, the clinical syndrome of pyridoxine deficiency has not been well defined. Nevertheless, it may be presumed that an individual with a deficiency of other members of the B complex may also have a relative deficiency of pyridoxine. Therefore, pyridoxine therapy may be advantageous in individuals suffering from a deficiency of other members of the B complex. On the basis that pyridoxine is essential in human nutrition, it is incorporated into many multivitamin preparations for prophylactic use. It has already been pointed out that 30% or more of alcoholics have biochemically demonstrable deficiency of vitamin B_6 (Li, 1978).

As indicated above, vitamin B_6 influences the metabolism of certain drugs and *vice versa*. With considerable justification, vitamin B_6 is given prophylactically to patients receiving isoniazid or hydralazine to prevent the development of peripheral neuritis. Biochemical evidence of pyridoxine deficiency has been obtained in a fraction of women taking oral contraceptives containing estrogen (Rose, 1978). As in pregnancy, the administration of estrogen can cause increased urinary excretion of tryptophan metabolites, such as xanthurenic acid, especially following a tryptophan load. There is a reduction in the pyridoxal phosphate concentration in the blood of those who take oral contraceptives, and Rose (1978) considers that 15 to 20% of such women have direct biochemical evidence of vitamin B_6 deficiency. However, the *recommended intakes* of vitamin B_6 appear to be sufficient to meet the requirements of such individuals (Bossé and Donald, 1979; Donald and Bossé, 1979). Several reports have indicated that a subset of women who report symptoms of depression while taking oral contraceptive medication may be deficient in pyridoxine and respond favorably to a daily supplement of 50 mg of the vitamin (Adams *et al.*, 1973).

Pyridoxine-responsive anemia is a well-documented but uncommon condition. The use of the vitamin in this disease is discussed in Chapter 56. Such anemias in patients without apparent pyridoxine deficiency, as well as a seizure disorder in infants that responds to the administration of pyridoxine, and the abnormalities characterized by xanthurenic aciduria, primary cystathioninuria, or homocystinuria appear to constitute a group of genetically determined clinical states of "pyridoxine dependency," manifested by a requirement for large amounts of the vitamin (*see* Mudd, 1971).

PANTOTHENIC ACID

History. Pantothenic acid was first identified by Williams and associates in 1933 as a substance essential for the growth of yeast. Its name, derived from Greek words signifying "from everywhere," is indicative of the wide distribution of the vitamin in nature. The role of pantothenic acid in animal nutrition was first defined in chicks, in which a deficiency disease characterized by skin lesions was known to be cured by fractions prepared from liver extract. Although first thought to be a form of "chick pellagra," it was not cured by nicotinic acid. Shortly thereafter, in 1939, Woolley and co-workers and also Jukes demonstrated that the chick antidermatitis factor was pantothenic acid. This compound also cured graying of the hair of black rats that was produced by feeding certain diets. One must hasten to note, however, that the graying of human hair is not due to a deficiency of pantothenic acid.

Chemistry. Pantothenic acid is an optically active organic acid, and biological activity is characteristic only of the *d* isomer. The vitamin functions in the body following its incorporation into coenzyme A. Their chemical structures are as follows:

Pantothenic Acid

Coenzyme A

The metabolic pathway by which pantothenic acid is converted into coenzyme A involves five consecutive enzyme-catalyzed reactions.

Many analogs of pantothenic acid have been studied in an attempt to find an antimetabolite. Although active antagonists have been synthesized and are of value as research tools, they are not therapeutic agents.

Pharmacological Actions. Pantothenic acid has no outstanding pharmacological actions when it is administered to experimental animals or normal man. The vitamin is essentially nontoxic; as much as 10 g given daily to man produces only minor gastrointestinal disturbance (Miller and Hayes, 1982).

Physiological Functions. Coenzyme A, the physiologically active form of pantothenic acid, serves as a cofactor for a variety of enzyme-catalyzed reactions involving transfer of acetyl (two-carbon) groups; the precursor fragments of various lengths are bound to the sulfhydryl group of coenzyme A. Such reactions are important in the oxidative metabolism of carbohydrates, gluconeogenesis, synthesis and degradation of fatty acids, and the synthesis of sterols, steroid hormones, and porphyrins (Wright, 1976).

Symptoms of Deficiency. Pantothenic acid is essential for the growth of various microorganisms. In animals, deficiency of pantothenic acid is manifested by symptoms of neuromuscular degeneration, adrenocortical insufficiency, and death. By administering a semisynthetic diet low in the vitamin together with a pantothenic acid antagonist, ω-methylpantothenic acid, a syndrome in man is produced that is characterized by fatigue, headache, sleep disturbances, nausea, abdominal cramps, vomiting, and flatulence (Hodges *et al.*, 1959). The subjects complain of paresthesias in the extremities, muscle cramps, and impaired coordination. The eosinopenic response to ACTH is lost and increased sensitivity to insulin develops, but there is no change in the concentration of 17-keto steroids in urine or in the concentration of sodium in blood or urine. Fry and coworkers (1976) have produced the same syndrome by giving human subjects a diet devoid of pantothenic acid for 10 weeks. Pantothenic acid deficiency has not been recognized in man consuming a normal diet, presumably because of the ubiquitous occurrence of the vitamin in ordinary foods.

Human Requirements. Pantothenic acid is a required nutrient, but the magnitude of need is not precisely known. Accordingly, the Committee on Dietary Allowances provides provisional amounts in the form of ranges of intakes (Table XVI–2, page 1548). For adults, the provisional allowance is 4 to 7 mg per day. Intakes for other groups are proportional to caloric consumption. In view of the widespread distribution of pantothenic acid in foods, dietary deficiency is very unlikely.

Food Sources. Pantothenic acid is ubiquitous. It is particularly abundant in organ meats, beef, and egg yolk. However, pantothenic acid is easily destroyed by heat and alkali.

Absorption, Fate, and Excretion. Pantothenic acid is readily absorbed from the gastrointestinal tract. It is present in all tissues, in concentrations ranging from 2 to 45 μg/g. Pantothenic acid apparently is not degraded in the human body since the intake and the excretion of the vitamin are approximately equal. About 70% of the absorbed pantothenic acid is excreted unchanged in the urine.

Preparations. *Calcium pantothenate* is available as tablets containing from 10 to 545 mg.

Therapeutic Uses. No clearly defined uses for pantothenic acid exist, although it is commonly included in multivitamin preparations and in products for enteral and parenteral alimentation.

BIOTIN

History. The discovery of biotin resulted from two different experimental approaches: one, the study of a toxic syndrome, which eventually was proven to be due to a substance *antagonistic* to biotin; the other, a study of the growth requirements of yeast. In 1916, Bateman observed that

rats fed a diet containing raw egg white as the sole source of protein developed a syndrome characterized by neuromuscular disorders, severe dermatitis, and loss of hair (*egg-white injury*). The syndrome could be prevented by cooking the protein or by administering yeast, liver, or extracts of these. In 1936, Kögl and Tönnis isolated a factor in crystalline form from egg yolk that was essential for growth of yeast, which they called *biotin*. It was then demonstrated that biotin and the factor that protected against egg-white toxicity were the same substance (György, 1940). In 1942, duVigneaud established the structural formula of biotin, and shortly thereafter the vitamin was synthesized.

In the meantime, the nature of the antagonist to biotin in egg white received extensive study. The compound is a protein, first isolated by Eakin and associates in 1940 and called *avidin*. Avidin is a glycoprotein that binds biotin with great affinity and thus prevents its absorption.

Chemistry. Biotin is an optically active organic acid, and the active form is the *d* isomer. The vitamin has the following structural formula:

Biotin

Three forms of biotin, apart from free biotin itself, have been found in natural materials. These derivatives are biocytin (ε-biotinyl-L-lysine) and the D and L sulfoxides of biotin. The derived forms of biotin are active in supporting growth of some microorganisms. Their efficacy as substitutes for biotin in human nutrition has not been studied. Biocytin may represent a degradation product of a biotin-protein complex, since, in its role as a coenzyme, the vitamin is covalently linked to an ε-amino group of a lysine residue of the apoenzyme involved.

A number of compounds antagonize the actions of biotin. Among them are biotin sulfone, desthiobiotin, and certain imidazolidone carboxylic acids. The antagonism between avidin and biotin is described above.

Pharmacological Actions. Biotin toxicity has not been reported in man despite administration of large amounts for as long as 6 months (Miller and Hayes, 1982).

Physiological Functions. Biotin is a cofactor for the enzymatic carboxylation of pyruvate, acetyl coenzyme A (CoA), propionyl CoA, and β-methylcrotonyl CoA. As such, it plays an important role in both carbohydrate and fat metabolism. CO_2 fixation occurs in a two-step reaction, the first involving binding of CO_2 to the biotin moiety of the holoenzyme, and the second involving transfer of the biotin-bound CO_2 to an appropriate acceptor (*see* McCormick, 1976).

Symptoms of Deficiency. The ease of producing biotin deficiency varies with the animal species. In a few species, a deficiency state can be produced merely by feeding a synthetic diet deficient in this nutrient. In most, however, presumably owing to synthesis of the vitamin by intestinal bacteria, it is necessary to eliminate bacteria from the intestinal tract, feed raw egg white, or administer antimetabolites of biotin in order to produce the deficiency. The symptoms of deficiency vary with the species and include failure of growth, loss of hair, dermatitis, poor lactation, and loss of muscular control with a spastic gait. Sydenstricker and associates (1942) produced a deficiency syndrome in man by the feeding of egg white that responded to the administration of small doses of biotin. Signs and symptoms included dermatitis, atrophic glossitis, hyperesthesia, muscle pain, lassitude, anorexia, slight anemia, and changes in the ECG. These disappeared on administering biotin. Spontaneous deficiency in man has been observed in some subjects who have consumed raw eggs over long periods (Bonjour, 1977). Inborn errors of biotin-dependent enzymes are known and respond to the administration of massive doses of biotin (Bonjour, 1977).

Symptomatic biotin deficiency has been reported in children and adults who have received chronic parenteral nutrition lacking biotin. The lesions consist of severe exfoliative dermatitis and alopecia, and they are similar to those of zinc deficiency; however, they respond to small doses of biotin. These patients suffered from chronic inflammatory bowel disease, and inadequate synthesis of biotin by gut flora was a probable contributory factor. Few reports have provided biochemical validation of biotin deficiency, but in one case the correction by biotin of an elevated rate of urinary excretion of β-hydroxyisovaleric acid indicates defective function of the biotin-dependent β-methylcrotonyl CoA carboxylase (Gillis *et al.*, 1982).

Human Requirements. The daily requirement of adults for biotin has been assigned a provisional value of 100 to 200 μg by the Committee on Dietary Allowances (Table XVI–2, page 1548). The average American diet provides some 100 to 300 μg of the vitamin. Part of the biotin synthesized by the bacterial flora is also available for absorption.

Food Sources. Organ meats, egg yolk, and peanuts are rich sources of biotin. Biotin is stable to cooking, but less so in alkali.

Absorption, Fate, and Excretion. Ingested biotin is rapidly absorbed from the gastrointestinal tract and appears in the urine predominantly in the form of intact biotin and in lesser amounts as the metabolites *bis*-norbiotin and biotin sulfoxide. Mammals are unable to degrade the ring system of biotin.

Preparations. Although there is no official preparation of biotin, it is available commercially. It is also present in many multivitamin preparations.

Therapeutic Uses. Large doses of biotin (5 to 10 mg daily) are administered to babies with infantile seborrhea and to individuals with genetic alterations of biotin-dependent enzymes. Patients who receive long-term parenteral nutrition should be given vitamin formulations that contain biotin.

CHOLINE

History. In 1932, Best and associates observed that pancreatectomized dogs maintained on insulin developed fatty livers; this could be prevented by inclusion in the diet of crude egg-yolk lecithin or beef pancreas. The substance responsible for this effect was shown to be choline. These studies marked the beginning of an extensive literature on the role of lipotropic substances, especially choline, in animal nutrition. Choline has other important functions in addition to those related to lipid metabolism. For example, it is a precursor of the neurochemical transmitter acetylcholine.

For reasons given below, however, choline should *not* be considered as a vitamin for man.

Chemistry. Choline (trimethylethanolamine) has the following structural formula:

$$H_3C-\overset{\displaystyle CH_3}{\underset{\displaystyle CH_3}{N^+}}-CH_2CH_2OH$$

Choline

Pharmacological Actions. Qualitatively, choline has the same pharmacological actions as does acetylcholine, but it is far less active. The acute toxicity of choline, especially by mouth, is relatively low (about 5 g/kg for rats) in comparison with that of some of its esters and many other quaternary ammonium compounds. The oral LD50 for man is estimated to be of the order of 200 to 400 g. Single oral doses of 10 g produce no obvious pharmacodynamic response.

Physiological Functions. Choline has several roles in the body. It is an important component of phospholipids, affects the mobilization of fat from the liver (lipotropic action), acts as a methyl donor, and is essential for the formation of the neurotransmitter acetylcholine.

Phospholipid Constituent. Choline is a component of the major phospholipid, lecithin, and is also a constituent of plasmalogens, which are abundant in mitochondria, and sphingomyelin, which is found particularly in brain. Choline thus provides an essential structural component of many biological membranes and also of the plasma lipoproteins.

Lipotropic Action. As mentioned, the initial recognition of choline as a significant dietary factor depended on its capacity to reduce the fat content of the liver of diabetic dogs. Substances that stimulate removal of excess fat from the liver are known as lipotropic agents and include choline, inositol, methionine, vitamin B_{12}, and folic acid. Certain of these compounds appear to act by providing methyl groups for the synthesis of choline in the body. Formation of the lipid components of plasma lipoproteins is thus permitted, and this facilitates transport of fat from the liver.

Methyl Donor. Choline can donate methyl groups necessary for the synthesis of other compounds. The first step in transfer is the formation of betaine, which is the immediate donor of the methyl group. Thus, choline can transfer a methyl group to homocysteine to form methionine. The roles of cyanocobalamin and folic acid in the metabolism of one-carbon compounds are discussed in Chapter 57.

Acetylcholine Formation. Acetylcholine is synthesized from choline and acetyl-CoA by choline acetyltransferase and is broken down by acetylcholinesterase (*see* Chapter 4). Choline is transported between the brain and the plasma by a bidirectional system localized in the endothelium of brain capillaries. This system operates by facilitated diffusion, and the amount of choline available to central neurons thus varies as a function of the concentration of choline in the plasma. When rats are given choline chloride, there is a sequential increase in the concentrations of plasma choline, brain choline, and brain acetylcholine. Consumption of lecithin, which contains choline, also causes these changes (Growdon and Wurtman, 1979). These findings are relevant to the treatment of diseases involving reduced capacity to synthesize acetylcholine (*see* below).

Symptoms of Deficiency. The effects of choline deficiency on animals are discussed in two reviews (Griffith and Nye, 1971; Kuksis and Mookerjea, 1978). The deficiency state is really one of available methyl groups, and consequently can only be produced as a result of a combined deficiency of choline and other methyl donors. In animals, the amount of choline needed is affected by growth rate, age, quantity of dietary fat, and quality of dietary protein, as well as by species differences in the capacity to synthesize choline from methyl donors. Some species, such as the guinea pig, have such a low capacity for synthesis that choline is a dietary essential. In such species it is possible to induce choline deficiency with a suitable diet. Not only is there accumulation of fat in the liver, followed by cirrhosis, but hemorrhagic renal lesions and motor incoordination from nerve degeneration have also been observed. Newberne and Chandra (1977) describe damage to the fetus, including atrophy of the thymus, when the pregnant rat is fed a diet with marginal contents of choline, methionine, folate, and vitamin B_{12}. None of these symptoms of deficiency has been identified in man (Kuksis and Mookerjea, 1978).

Human Requirements. The needs of the tissues for choline are met from both exogenous (dietary) and endogenous (metabolic) sources. Biosynthesis of choline occurs by transmethylation of ethanolamine with the methyl group of methionine or by a series of reactions requiring vitamin B_{12} and folate as cofactors (*see* Chapter 57). Thus, an adequate supply of methyl-group donors in the diet is desirable to protect against the hepatic accumulation of lipid. In addition, large amounts of choline appear to have a therapeutic effect on certain diseases of the nervous system, by means of stimulation of the synthesis of acetylcholine. However, none of the functions of choline justifies its classification as a vitamin. It has not been shown to act as a cofactor in any enzymatic reaction, and the doses needed to produce therapeutic effects (several grams) are much greater than those of any vitamin.

Because of the lack of evidence of a choline deficiency syndrome in human subjects, choline cannot be considered an essential dietary constituent for man. In addition, the American diet provides 400 to 900 mg per day of choline as a constituent of lecithin; it is thus difficult to consume a diet that is low in choline. Since human breast milk contains 7 mg choline/100 kcal, the Committee on Nutrition of the American Academy of Pediatrics (1976) recommends the fortification of infant formulas to this level.

Food Sources. Choline is found in egg yolk and in vegetable and animal fat, mostly as lecithin.

Absorption, Fate, and Excretion. Choline is absorbed from the diet as such or as lecithin. The latter is hydrolyzed by the intestinal mucosa to glycerophosphoryl choline, which either passes to the liver to liberate choline or to the peripheral tissues via the intestinal lymphatics. Free choline is not fully absorbed, especially after large doses, and intestinal bacteria metabolize choline to trimethylamine. Since this compound imparts a strong odor of decaying fish to the feces, lecithin is the clearly preferred oral vehicle for the administration of choline.

Preparations. Various preparations of choline are available in tablets containing 250 to 650 mg and as powders. In addition, preparations of lecithin are available, although many of them consist mainly of other phosphatides (Wurtman, 1979).

Therapeutic Uses. The use of choline to treat fatty liver and cirrhosis, usually alcoholic in etiology, has not proven to be consistently effective (Griffith and Nye, 1971). Because of the synthesis of choline from other methyl donors, provision of a well-balanced diet is just as effective in alleviating the symptoms of hepatic damage.

The use of choline in large doses for the treatment of certain disorders of the nervous system has also been advocated (Growdon and Wurtman, 1979). Five such diseases are candidates for treatment with choline (Barbeau, 1978). They include tardive dyskinesia, a disease characterized by choreiform movements that are caused by chronic treatment with some neuroleptic drugs (*see* Growdon, 1978; Chapter 19). Some clinical improvement with choline treatment has also been reported in Huntington's chorea (Growdon, 1978), in which impaired mental function and voluntary muscle contractions are probably associated with reduced acetylcholine synthesis, in Gilles de la Tourette's disease, in Friedreich's ataxia, and in presenile dementia (Barbeau, 1978). Doses of 150 to 300 mg/kg of choline chloride and of 350 mg/kg of lecithin have been administered in these various studies. However, the role of choline as a therapeutic agent for these diseases cannot be considered to be established.

INOSITOL

History. Although inositol was identified more than 100 years ago in the urine of diabetic patients, a role for this substance in animal nutrition was not suspected until 1941, when Gavin and McHenry found that inositol had a lipotropic action in rats. Inositol was subsequently observed to cure alopecia induced in rats and mice by dietary means. A nutritional role for inositol was considerably strengthened when Eagle and colleagues showed in 1957 that this substance is essential for the growth of all human and other animal cells in tissue culture. However, its status as a vitamin for man remains uncertain, for reasons given below.

Chemistry. Inositol (hexahydroxycyclohexane) is an isomer of glucose. There are seven optically inactive and one pair of optically active stereoisomeric forms of inositol possible, of which only one, the optically inactive *myo*-inositol, is nutritionally active. It has the following structural formula:

Myo-Inositol

Pharmacological Actions. Inositol possesses no significant pharmacological actions when given parenterally in doses of 1 to 2 g to human subjects.

Physiological Functions. The physiological role of inositol resembles that of choline in part. Thus, inositol is present in the form of phosphatidylinositol in the phospholipids of cell membranes and plasma lipoproteins. Polyphosphorylated derivatives of inositol (*e.g.*, inositol triphosphate) may be released from such phospholipids in membranes in response to various extracellular signals. Inositol triphosphate appears to play a role as an intracellular second messenger, perhaps by regulation of calcium fluxes (*see* Chapter 2; Berridge, 1984). In addition, inositol has a lipotropic action on fatty livers, and, in the case of the gerbil, will prevent fat accumulation in the intestine (Hegsted *et al.*, 1974). These effects on the transport of fat out of the cells

of the liver and intestine appear to be dependent on the need for inositol in order to complete the fat-carrying lipoprotein molecule in the plasma.

Symptoms of Deficiency. Variable reserves of inositol, its production by gut bacteria, and possibly its synthesis in the cells of the body have made the demonstration of a dietary need for inositol difficult to achieve. However, certain animals can be made deficient; alopecia and fatty infiltration of the liver result. There has been no demonstration of a dietary need by man, but the studies of Eagle and colleagues (1957) showed that 18 human cell lines all needed *myo*-inositol for growth, probably because of its structural role in the formation of cell membranes. In view of the absence of a demonstrable human need for inositol, Eagle and coworkers suggest that it may be synthesized in only a few organs, which then make it available for use by all cells. Experiments with labeled glucose show that the growing rat can synthesize inositol, although this does not exclude a partial dependence on dietary inositol during periods of rapid growth.

Human Requirements. Although there has been no demonstration of a human need for inositol, a high concentration is present in human milk (Committee on Nutrition, Academy of Pediatrics, 1976). As with choline, it may be desirable to add inositol to infant formulas to mimic more closely the content of human milk. The normal daily intake of inositol is about 1 g, mostly from plant sources. Inositol is present in cereals as the hexaphosphate, phytic acid. Inositol in this form is partly available for absorption because of hydrolysis by the enzyme phytase in the intestinal mucosa. Inositol also occurs in vegetable and animal foods in other forms.

Food Sources. Inositol is provided by fruits, plants, and whole-grain cereals as phytic acid.

Absorption, Fate, and Excretion. The consumption of inositol by man is about 1 g per day. The compound is easily absorbed from the gastrointestinal tract. Inositol is readily metabolized to glucose and is about one third as effective as glucose in alleviating starvation ketosis. The concentration of inositol in normal human plasma is about 0.5 mg/dl. Within the tissues, the concentration of inositol is particularly high in heart muscle, brain, and skeletal muscle (1.6, 0.9, and 0.4 g/100 g dry weight, respectively). Urine normally contains only small amounts of inositol, but in diabetic humans and animals the amount is markedly increased, probably because of competition between inositol and glucose for reabsorption by the renal tubule.

Preparations. Inositol is available in tablets containing 250 to 650 mg and as a powder.

Therapeutic Uses. Inositol has been given for the management of diseases associated with disturbances in the transport and metabolism of fat. There is no persuasive evidence that it has therapeutic efficacy. Peripheral nerve from diabetic animals and man contains elevated quantities of free sugars and a decreased level of *myo*-inositol; abnormal incorporation of *myo*-inositol into neural phospholipids has also been demonstrated. The effects of administration of *myo*-inositol on nerve function in human diabetes are unclear. However, improved sensory function has been shown after a few weeks of such treatment (Clements *et al.*, 1979).

II. Ascorbic Acid (Vitamin C)

History. Scurvy, the deficiency disease caused by lack of vitamin C, has been known since the time of the Crusades, especially among northern European populations who subsisted on diets lacking fresh fruits and vegetables over extensive periods of the year (Sharman, 1974). The incidence of scurvy was reduced by the introduction to Europe in the seventeenth century of the potato, an additional source of vitamin C. However, the long sea voyages of exploration in the sixteenth to eighteenth centuries, which were undertaken without a supply of fresh fruits and vegetables, resulted in large numbers of the crew dying from scurvy.

A dietary cause for scurvy had long been suspected. In 1535, Jacques Cartier learned from the Indians of Canada how to cure the scurvy in his crew by making a decoction from spruce leaves, and several subsequent ship captains prevented or cured scurvy by administration of lemon juice. However, a systematic study of the relationship of diet to scurvy had to wait until 1747 when Lind, a physician in the British Royal Navy, carried out a clinical trial on cases of frank scurvy who were given either cider, vitriol, vinegar, sea water, oranges and lemons, or garlic and mustard. Those who received citrus fruits recovered rapidly. The consequent introduction of lemon juice into the British Navy in 1800 resulted in a dramatic reduction in the incidence of scurvy; whereas the Royal Naval Hospital at Portsmouth admitted 1457 cases in 1780, only 2 cases were seen there in 1806. At the present time, frank scurvy is occasionally seen in infants, in older people on restricted diets, and in alcoholics.

The next significant episode in the history of vitamin C was the identification in 1907 of a suitable experimental animal by Holst and Fröhlich, who found that guinea pigs develop scurvy on a diet of oats and bran that is not supplemented with fresh vegetables. It was subsequently shown that most mammals synthesize ascorbic acid; man, the monkey, and the guinea pig are exceptions. The demonstration of scurvy in the guinea pig allowed testing of fractions from citrus fruits for antiscorbutic potency. In 1928, Szent-Györgyi isolated a reducing agent in pure form from cabbage and from adrenal glands; in 1932, Waugh and King identified Szent-Györgyi's compound as the active antiscorbutic factor in lemon juice. The chemical structure of this substance was then soon established in several laboratories, and the trivial chemical name *ascorbic acid* was assigned to designate its function in preventing scurvy. The term *vitamin C* should be used as a generic descriptor for all compounds that exhibit qualitatively the biological activity of ascorbic acid; the latter name should be restricted to that specific substance.

Chemistry. Ascorbic acid is a six-carbon compound structurally related to glucose and other hexoses. It is reversibly oxidized in the body to dehydroascorbic acid. The latter compound possesses full vitamin C activity. The structural formulas of ascorbic acid and dehydroascorbic acid are as follows:

Ascorbic   Dehydroascorbic
Acid   Acid

Ascorbic acid has an optically active carbon atom, and antiscorbutic activity resides almost totally in the L isomer. Another isomer, erythorbic acid (D-isoascorbic acid, D-araboascorbic acid), has very weak antiscorbutic action but has a similar redox potential. Both compounds have therefore been used to prevent nitrosoamine formation from nitrites in cured meats such as bacon. The reason for the lack of a stronger antiscorbutic action of erythorbic acid is probably the incapacity of the tissues to retain it in the quantities that ascorbic acid is stored (Hughes *et al.*, 1971). One consequence of the facile oxidation of ascorbic acid is the readiness with which it can be destroyed by exposure to air, especially in an alkaline medium and if copper is present as a catalyst. Ascorbic acid–2–sulfate is a derivative that is present in tissues and urine; it has no antiscorbutic activity in guinea pigs or monkeys, which may also be correlated with the low capacity of tissues to concentrate this form of ascorbate (Hornig, 1974).

Pharmacological Actions. In the strict sense of the word, vitamin C may be said to possess few pharmacological actions. Administration of the compound in amounts greatly in excess of the physiological requirements causes few demonstrable effects except in the scorbutic individual, whose symptoms are rapidly alleviated. Secondary symptoms accompanying the deficiency disease (scurvy) are likely to be varied and may include anemia, infections, metabolic disturbances, and other symptoms. As a result, an extensive literature has accumulated concerning the effect of vitamin C on practically every function of the body.

Physiological Functions. Ascorbic acid functions in a number of biochemical reactions, mostly involving oxidation. Thus, it is required for or facilitates the conversion of certain proline residues in collagen to hydroxyproline in the course of collagen synthesis (Myllylä *et al.*, 1978), the oxidation of lysine side chains in proteins to provide hydroxytrimethyllysine for carnitine synthesis (Hulse *et al.*, 1978), the synthesis of steroids by the adrenal cortex (Deana *et al.*, 1975), the conversion of folic acid to folinic acid (Stokes *et al.*, 1975), microsomal drug metabolism (Zannoni and Sato, 1975), and tyrosine metabolism. Instead of acting as a cofactor for an enzyme, ascorbic acid has the capacity to protect an enzyme, *p*-hydroxyphenylpyruvic acid oxidase, from inhibition by its substrate. The protection is apparently necessary only after ingestion of large amounts of tyrosine; it does not seem to be required under ordinary dietary conditions. This role of ascorbic acid in tyrosine metabolism is not specific, since various analogs of ascorbic acid and even a dye, 2,6-dichlorophenolindophenol, which has a similar redox potential, can replace the vitamin (La Du and Zannoni, 1961).

At the tissue level, a major function of ascorbic acid is related to the synthesis of collagen, proteoglycans, and other organic constituents of the intercellular matrix in such diverse tissues as tooth, bone, and capillary endothelium (Sebrell and Harris, 1967). Although the effect of ascorbic acid on collagen synthesis has been attributed to its role in the hydroxylation of proline, recent evidence also suggests that there is direct stimulation of collagen peptide synthesis (Murad *et al.*, 1981). Scurvy is associated with a defect in collagen synthesis that is apparent by the failure of wounds to heal, in defects in tooth formation, and in the rupture of capillaries, which leads to numerous petechiae and their coalescence to form ecchymoses. While this last has been attributed to leakage from capillaries because of inadequate adhesion of the endothelial cells, it is also thought that the pericapillary fibrous tissue is defective in

scurvy, leading to inadequate support of the capillary and its rupture under pressure.

Absorption, Distribution, and Excretion. Ascorbic acid is readily absorbed from the intestine, and absorption of dietary ascorbate is nearly (80 to 90%) complete (Kallner *et al.*, 1977). Ascorbic acid is present in the plasma and is ubiquitously distributed in the cells of the body. Concentrations of the vitamin in leukocytes are sometimes taken to represent those in tissue and are less susceptible to depletion than is the plasma. The white blood cells of healthy adults have concentrations of about 27 μg of ascorbic acid per 10^8 cells. It should be noted that the amount of ascorbic acid in leukocytes may be inversely related to their number, and estimates of ascorbic acid status may be falsely low in patients with leukocytosis in whom white-cell ascorbate is measured (Vallance, 1979). Concentrations in plasma also vary with intake. Adequate ingestion is associated with concentrations over 0.5 mg/dl, whereas concentrations of 0.15 mg/dl are seen in individuals with frank scurvy.

When the diet contains essentially no ascorbate, concentrations in plasma fall and, as mentioned, symptoms of scurvy are obvious when a value of 0.15 mg/dl is reached; the total body store of the vitamin at this time approximates 300 mg. When the intake of ascorbate is raised, the concentration in plasma also increases—at first linearly. The daily ingestion of 5 to 10 mg provides a total body store of 600 to 1000 mg of ascorbate. When 60 mg of vitamin C is consumed per day (the recommended dietary allowance for adults), the concentration in plasma reaches about 0.8 mg/dl and the body store is around 1500 mg. If intake is raised beyond 200 mg daily, the body store tends to level off at 2500 mg and the concentration in plasma at 2 mg/dl. However, the renal threshold for ascorbic acid is about 1.5 mg/dl of plasma, and increasing amounts of the ingested ascorbic acid are excreted when the daily intake exceeds 100 mg.

Studies with isotopically labeled L-ascorbic acid have shown that the vitamin is oxidized to CO_2 in rats and guinea pigs, but considerably less conversion can be detected in man. One route of metabolism of L-ascorbate in man involves its conversion to oxalate and eventual excretion in the urine; dehydroascorbate is presumably an intermediate. Ascorbic acid–2–sulfate has also been identified as a metabolite of vitamin C in human urine.

Biosynthesis of Ascorbic Acid. Man and other primates as well as the guinea pig are the only mammals known to be unable to synthesize ascorbic acid; consequently, they require dietary vitamin C for the prevention of scurvy. An explanation for this has come from biochemical studies (*see* Burns, 1959). The rat, a typical species that does not require dietary vitamin C, synthesizes ascorbic acid from glucose through the intermediate formation of D-glucuronic acid, L-gulonic acid, and L-gulonolactone. Man, monkey, and guinea pig lack the hepatic enzyme required to carry out the last reaction, that is, the conversion of L-gulonolactone to L-ascorbic acid.

Symptoms of Deficiency. A deficiency in the intake of vitamin C can lead to scurvy. Cases of scurvy are encountered among elderly people living alone, alcoholics, drug addicts, and others with inadequate diets, including infants.

Experimental scurvy has been produced in man in a number of studies (Crandon *et al.*, 1940; Krebs *et al.*, 1948; Hodges *et al.*, 1969). For example, the surgeon Crandon submitted himself to a diet devoid of vitamin C for 161 days, during which the concentration of ascorbic acid in his plasma fell to negligible values within 41 days, while the concentration in his white blood cells became undetectable after 121 days. Perifollicular hyperkeratosis (an accumulation of epidermal cells around the hair follicles) occurred at 120 days; hemorrhages appeared under his skin (petechiae and ecchymoses) at 161 days, and a wound made into the back failed to heal. In spontaneous cases of scurvy, there is usually loosening of the teeth, gingivitis, and anemia, which may be due to a specific function of ascorbic acid in hemoglobin synthesis. The picture of spontaneous scurvy in clinical practice is often complicated by insufficiencies of other nutrients as well.

Scurvy occurs in infants receiving formula diets prepared at home with inadequate concentrations of ascorbic acid. The infant is irritable and resents being touched because of pain. This is due to hemorrhages under the periosteum of the long bones, and the resulting hematomas are often visible as swellings on the shafts of these bones.

Human Requirements. The daily intake of ascorbic acid must equal the amount that is destroyed by oxidation or excreted. Studies on healthy adult human subjects given [^{14}C] ascorbic acid show an average daily removal rate of 3% of the body store; values of 4% were observed in some subjects (Baker *et al.*, 1971). To maintain a body store of 1500 mg of ascorbic acid or more in an adult man, it would thus be necessary to absorb approximately 60 mg daily. Values for vitamin C requirements of other age groups are based on similar reasoning (Table XVI–1, page 1546).

Under special circumstances, more ascorbic acid appears to be required to achieve normal concentrations in the plasma. Thus, South African miners have been observed to require 200 to 250 mg of vitamin C daily to maintain a plasma concentration of 0.75 mg/dl (Visagie *et al.*, 1975). Concentrations of ascorbate in plasma are lowered by the use of cigarettes (Pelletier, 1977) and of oral contraceptive agents (Rivers, 1975), but the significance of these changes is unclear. Requirements can increase in certain diseases, particularly infectious diseases, and also following surgery (Irvin *et al.*, 1978).

Food Sources. Ascorbic acid is obtained from citrus fruits, tomatoes, strawberries, cabbage greens, and potatoes. Orange and lemon juices are outstanding sources and contain approximately 0.5 mg/ml. Ascorbic acid is readily destroyed by heat, oxidation, and alkali.

Preparations. *Ascorbic acid* is available in a large number of preparations. Tablets contain from 25 to 1500 mg of the vitamin. Solutions for oral use are also available in various concentrations. *Ascorbic acid injection* contains from 50 to 500 mg/ml. *Sodium ascorbate injection* is also available and is preferable to calcium ascorbate, which may cause necrosis at the site of injection. Most multivitamin preparations contain ascorbic acid. The high vitamin content of fruit juices permits their use in therapy in place of pure preparations of the vitamin.

Apart from its role in nutrition, ascorbic acid is commonly used as an antioxidant to protect natural flavor and color of many foods (*e.g.*, processed fruit, vegetables, and dairy products).

Routes of Administration. Vitamin C is usually administered by the oral route; however, in conditions that prevent adequate absorption from the gastrointestinal tract, solutions of the sodium salt may be given by intramuscular or intravenous injection. In addition, ascorbic acid should be given to patients receiving parenteral hyperalimentation. Because of the loss of much of the infused ascorbic acid in the urine, daily doses of 200 mg are needed to maintain normal concentrations in plasma of 1 mg/dl (Nichoalds *et al.*, 1977).

Therapeutic Uses. Vitamin C is used for the treatment of ascorbic acid deficiency, especially frank scurvy, which occurs rather infrequently in infants and in adults.

Human breast milk contains 30 to 55 mg of ascorbic acid per liter, depending on the mother's intake. Consequently, the infant consuming 850 ml of breast milk will receive about 35 mg of ascorbic acid, which has been set as the recommended dietary allowance (Table XVI–1, page 1546). However, during the first week of life, the newborn infant, especially the premature, may have an increased requirement for ascorbic acid to meet the demands of metabolizing large amounts of tyrosine in the diet. To prevent transient accumulation of tyrosine, daily intake of 100 mg of ascorbic acid is recommended. Orange juice may be given to infants to meet such requirements, especially to those who are receiving formulas based on cow's milk. Many commercial formulas are, however, fortified to provide ascorbic acid at these levels. In the rare cases of infantile scurvy, much larger therapeutic doses are used. Adults with scurvy should receive 1 g of ascorbic acid daily. This dose will cause a rapid disappearance of the subcutaneous hemorrhages.

The reducing properties of vitamin C have also been employed to control *idiopathic methemoglobinemia*, although it is less effective than methylene blue. Doses of at least 150 mg of ascorbic acid are needed to be effective in this condition.

In addition to these specific uses of vitamin C, extensive literature has appeared on the application of this vitamin to a wide variety of diseases. Many such claims are associated with megadosage practices, which are stated to prevent or cure viral respiratory infections (Pauling, 1970) and to be beneficial in cancer (Cameron and Pauling, 1978) and other diseases. Creagan and associates (1979) were unable to demonstrate any beneficial effect of high doses of ascorbic acid given to patients with advanced cancer. Anderson (1977) has carried out a series of three carefully designed studies in Canada to test whether vitamin C plays any role in the prevention and treatment of the common cold. No obvious effect on the incidence of headcolds was seen from the administration of ascorbic acid, although there was a slight reduction in the number of days of missed work. Many other studies have yielded negative or inconsistent results (*see* Pitt and Costrini, 1979). Any benefit that might be derived from such use of ascorbic acid seems small when weighed against the expense and the risks of the megadosage treatment. The latter include formation of kidney stones resulting from the excessive excretion of oxalate, rebound scurvy in the offspring of mothers taking high doses (Herbert, 1975), and a similar phenomenon when subjects who are consuming large amounts of vitamin C suddenly stop; a precipitous reduction in ascorbic acid concentration in plasma follows (Anderson, 1977). These rebound phenomena are presumably due to induction of pathways of ascorbic acid metabolism as a result of the preceding high dosage. Excessive doses of ascorbic acid can also enhance the absorption of iron (Cook and Monsen, 1977) and interfere with anticoagulant therapy (Rosenthal, 1971).

Adams, P. W.; Wynn, V.; Rose, D. P.; Seed, M.; Folkard, J.; and Strong, R. Effect of pyridoxine hydrochloride (vitamin B_6) upon depression with oral contraception. *Lancet*, **1973**, *1*, 897–904.

Anderson, T. W. Large scale studies with vitamin C. *Acta Vitaminol. Enzymol. (Milano)*, **1977**, *31*, 43–50.

Baker, E. M.; Hodges, R. E.; Hood, J.; Sauberlich, H. E.; March, S. C.; and Canham, J. E. Metabolism of 14C and 3H-labeled L-ascorbic acid in human scurvy. *Am. J. Clin. Nutr.*, **1971**, *24*, 444–454.

Barbeau, A. Emerging treatments: replacement therapy with choline or lecithin in neurological diseases. *Can. J. Neurol. Sci.*, **1978**, *5*, 157–160.

Bauernfeind, J. C., and Miller, O. N. Vitamin B_6: nutritional and pharmaceutical usage, stability, bioavailability, antagonists, and safety. In, *Human Vitamin B_6 Requirements*. National Academy of Sciences, Washington, D. C., **1978**, pp. 78–110.

Berridge, M. J. Inositol triphosphate and diacylglycerol as second messengers. *Biochem. J.*, **1984**, *220*, 345–360.

Blass, J. P., and Gibson, G. E. Abnormality of a thiamine-requiring enzyme in patients with Wernicke-Korsakoff syndrome. *N. Engl. J. Med.*, **1977**, *297*, 1367–1370.

Bonjour, J. P. Biotin in man's nutrition and therapy—a review. *Int. J. Vitam. Nutr. Res.*, **1977**, *47*, 107–118.

Bossé, T. R., and Donald, E. A. The vitamin B_6 requirement in oral contraceptive users. I. Assessment by pyridoxal level and transferase activity in erythrocytes. *Am. J. Clin. Nutr.*, **1979**, *32*, 1015–1023.

Brin, M. Blood transketolase determination in the diagnosis of thiamine deficiency. *Heart Bull.*, **1968**, *17*, 86–89.

———. Vitamin B_6: chemistry, absorption, metabolism, catabolism and toxicity. In, *Human Vitamin B_6 Requirements*. National Academy of Sciences, Washington, D. C., **1978**, pp. 1–20.

Burns, J. J. Biosynthesis of L-ascorbic acid: basic defect in scurvy. *Am. J. Med.*, **1959**, *26*, 740–748.

Cameron, E., and Pauling, L. Supplemental ascorbate in the supportive treatment of cancer: prolongation of survival times in terminal human cancer. *Proc. Natl Acad. Sci. U.S.A.*, **1976**, *73*, 3685–3689.

Canham, J. E.; Nunes, W. T.; and Eberlin, E. W. Electroencephalographic and central nervous system manifestations of B_6 deficiency and induced B_6 dependency in normal human adults. In, *Proceedings of the Sixth International Congress of Nutrition*. E. & S. Livingstone, Ltd., Edinburgh, **1964**, p. 537.

Clements, R. S.; Vourganti, B.; Kuba, T.; Oh, S. J.; and Darnell, B. Dietary myoinositol intake and peripheral nerve function in diabetic neuropathy. *Metabolism*, **1979**, *28*, Suppl. 1, 477–483.

Committee on Nutrition, Academy of Pediatrics. Commentary on breast-feeding and infant formulas, including proposed standards for formulas. *Pediatrics*, **1976**, *57*, 278–285.

Cook, J. D., and Monsen, E. R. Vitamin C, the common cold and iron absorption. *Am. J. Clin. Nutr.*, **1977**, *30*, 235–241.

Crandon, J. H.; Lund, C. C.; and Dill, D. B. Experimental human scurvy. *N. Engl. J. Med.*, **1940**, *223*, 353–369.

Creagan, E. T.; Moertel, C. C.; O'Fallon, J. R.; Schutt, A. J.; O'Connell, M. J.; Rubin, J.; and Frytak, S. Failure of high-dose vitamin C to benefit patients with advanced cancer. *N. Engl. J. Med.*, **1979**, *301*, 687–690.

Dakshinamurti, K. B vitamins and nervous system function. In, *Nutrition and the Brain*, Vol. 1. (Wurtman, R. J., and Wurtman, J. J., eds.) Raven Press, New York, **1977**, pp. 249–318.

Darby, W. J.; McNutt, K. W.; and Todhunter, E. N. Niacin. In, *Present Knowledge in Nutrition*. (Hegsted, D. M.; Chichester, C. O.; Darby, W. J.; McNutt, K. W.; Stalvey, R. M.; and Stotz, E. H.; eds.) The Nutrition Foundation, Washington, D. C., **1976**, pp. 162–174.

Deana, R.; Bharaj, B. S.; Verjee, Z. H.; and Galzigna, L. Changes relevant to catecholamine metabolism in liver and brain of ascorbic acid deficient guinea pigs. *Int. J. Vitam. Nutr. Res.*, **1975**, *45*, 175–182.

DiSorbo, D. M.; Phelps, D. S.; Ohl, V. S.; and Litwack, G. Pyridoxine deficiency influences the behavior of the glucocorticoid-receptor complex. *J. Biol. Chem.*, **1980**, *255*, 3866–3870.

Donald, E. A., and Bossé, T. R. The vitamin B_6 requirement in oral contraceptive users. II. Assessment by tryptophan metabolites, vitamin B_6, and pyridoxic acid levels in urine. *Am. J. Clin. Nutr.*, **1979**, *32*, 1024–1032.

Eagle, H.; Oyama, V.; Levy, M.; and Freeman, A. Myo-inositol as an essential growth factor for normal and malignant human cells in tissue culture. *J. Biol. Chem.*, **1957**, *229*, 191–205.

Ellis, J.; Folkers, K.; Watanabe, T.; Kaji, M.; Saji, S.; Caldwell, J. W.; Temple, C. A.; and Wood, F. S. Clinical results of a cross-over treatment with pyridoxine and placebo of the carpal tunnel syndrome. *Am. J. Clin. Nutr.*, **1979**, *32*, 2040–2046.

Fry, P. C.; Fox, H. M.; and Tao, H. G. Metabolic response to a pantothenic acid deficient diet in humans. *J. Nutr. Sci. Vitaminol. (Tokyo)*, **1976**, *22*, 339–346.

Gillis, J.; Murphy, F. R.; Boxall, L. B. H.; and Pencharg, P. B. Biotin deficiency in a child on long-term TPN. *J.P.E.N.*, **1982**, *6*, 308–310.

Goldsmith, G. A. Niacin-tryptophan relationship in man and niacin requirement. *Am. J. Clin. Nutr.*, **1958**, *6*, 479–486.

Griffith, W. H., and Nye, J. F. Choline. In, *The Vitamins*, 2nd ed., Vol. III. (Sebrell, W. H., and Harris, R. S., eds.) Academic Press, Inc., New York, **1971**, pp. 3–154.

Growdon, J. H. Effects of choline on tardive dyskinesia and other movement disorders. *Psychopharmacol. Bull.*, **1978**, *14*, 55–56.

Growdon, J. H., and Wurtman, R. J. Dietary influences on the synthesis of neurotransmitters in the brain. *Nutr. Rev.*, **1979**, *37*, 129–136.

György, P. A further note on the identity of vitamin H with biotin. *Science*, **1940**, *92*, 609.

Hegsted, D. M.; Gallagher, A.; and Hanford, H. Inositol requirement of the gerbil. *J. Nutr.*, **1974**, *104*, 588–592.

Henderson, L. M., and Hulse, J. D. Vitamin B_6: relationship in tryptophan metabolism. In, *Human Vitamin B_6 Requirements*. National Academy of Sciences, Washington, D. C., **1978**, pp. 21–36.

Herbert, V. The rationale of massive-dose vitamin therapy. In, *Proceedings, Western Hemisphere Nutrition Congress IV*. Publishing Sciences Group, Inc., Acton, Mass., **1975**, pp. 84–91.

Hodges, R. E.; Baker, E. M.; Hood, J.; Sauberlich, H. E.; and March, S. C. Experimental scurvy in man. *Am. J. Clin. Nutr.*, **1969**, *22*, 535–548.

Hodges, R. E.; Bean, W. B.; Ohlson, M. A.; and Bleiler, R. Human pantothenic acid deficiency produced by omega-methyl pantothenic acid. *J. Clin. Invest.*, **1959**, *38*, 1421–1425.

Hornig, D. Recent advances in vitamin C metabolism. In, *Vitamin C: Recent Aspects of Its Physiological and Technological Importance*. (Birch, G. G., and Parker, K. J., eds.) Applied Science Publishers, Ltd., London, **1974**, pp. 91–103.

Horwitt, M. K.; Harvey, C. C.; Rothwell, W. S.; Cutler, J. L.; and Haffron, D. Tryptophan-niacin relationships in man. *J. Nutr.*, **1956**, *60*, Suppl. 1, 1–43.

Hughes, R. E.; Hurley, R. J.; and Jones, P. R. The retention of ascorbic acid by guinea-pig tissues. *Br. J. Nutr.*, **1971**, *26*, 433–438.

Hulse, J. D.; Ellis, S. R.; and Henderson, L. M. Carnitine biosynthesis. *J. Biol. Chem.*, **1978**, *253*, 1654–1659.

Irvin, T. T.; Chattopadhyay, D. K.; and Smythe, A. Ascorbic acid requirements in postoperative patients. *Surg. Gynecol. Obstet.*, **1978**, *147*, 49–55.

Jusko, W. J., and Levy, G. Absorption, protein binding, and elimination of riboflavin. In, *Riboflavin*. (Rivlin, R. S., ed.) Plenum Press, New York, **1975**, pp. 99–152.

Kallner, A.; Hartman, D.; and Hornig, D. On the absorption of ascorbic acid in man. *Int. J. Vitam. Nutr. Res.*, **1977**, *47*, 383–388.

Krebs, H. A.; Peters, R. A.; Coward, K. H.; Mapson, L. W.; Parsons, L. G.; Platt, B. S.; Spence, J. C.; and O'Brien, J. R. P. Vitamin-C requirement of human adults: experimental study of vitamin-C deprivation in man. *Lancet*, **1948**, *1*, 853–858.

Kuksis, A., and Mookerjea, S. Choline. *Nutr. Rev.*, **1978**, *36*, 201–207.

La Du, B. N., and Zannoni, U. G. The role of ascorbic acid in tyrosine metabolism. *Ann. N.Y. Acad. Sci.*, **1961**, *92*, 175–191.

Lane, M.; Smith, F. E.; and Alfrey, C. P. Experimental dietary and antagonist-induced human riboflavin deficiency. In, *Riboflavin*. (Rivlin, R. S., ed.) Plenum Press, New York, **1975**, pp. 245–277.

Li, T. Factors influencing vitamin B_6 requirement in alcoholism. In, *Human B_6 Requirements*. National Academy of Sciences, Washington, D. C., **1978**, pp. 210–225.

Linkswiler, H. M. Vitamin B_6 requirements of men. In, *Human B_6 Requirements*. National Academy of Sciences, Washington, D. C., **1978**, pp. 279–290.

Lipton, M. A.; Mailman, R. B.; and Nemeroff, C. B. Vitamins, megavitamin therapy, and the nervous system. In, *Nutrition and the Brain*, Vol. 3. (Wurtman, R. J., and Wurtman, J. J., eds.) Raven Press, New York, **1979**, pp. 183–264.

McCormick, D. B. Metabolism of riboflavin. In, *Riboflavin*. (Rivlin, R. S., ed.) Plenum Press, New York, **1975**, pp. 153–198.

———. Biotin. In, *Present Knowledge in Nutrition*. (Hegsted, D. M.; Chichester, C. O.; Darby, W. J.; McNutt, K. W.; Stalvey, R. M.; and Stotz, E. H.; eds.) The Nutrition Foundation, Washington, D. C., **1976**, pp. 217–225.

McLaren, D. Metabolic disorders. In, *Current Therapy*. (Conn, H. F., ed.) W. B. Saunders Co., Philadelphia, **1978**, pp. 409–410.

Miller, D. R., and Hayes, K. C. Vitamin excess and toxicity. In, *Nutritional Toxicology*, Vol. 1. Academic Press, Inc., New York, **1982**, pp. 81–133.

Mudd, S. H. Pyridoxine-responsive genetic disease. *Fed. Proc.*, **1971**, *30*, 970–976.

Mueller, J. F., and Vilter, R. W. Pyridoxine deficiency in human beings induced with desoxypyridoxine. *J. Clin. Invest.*, **1950**, *29*, 193–201.

Müller, R. E.; Traish, A.; and Wotiz, H. J. Effects of pyridoxal 5′-phosphate on uterine estrogen receptor. *J. Biol. Chem.*, **1980**, *255*, 4062–4067.

Murad, S.; Grove, D.; Lindberg, K. A.; Reynolds, G.; Sivarajah, A.; and Pinnell, S. R. Regulation of collagen synthesis by ascorbic acid. *Proc. Natl Acad. Sci. U.S.A.*, **1981**, *78*, 2879–2882.

Murata, K. Thiaminase. In, *Review of Japanese Literature on Beriberi and Thiamine*. (Shimazono, N., and Katsura, E., eds.) Igaku Shoin, Ltd., Tokyo, **1965**, pp. 220–254.

Myllylä, R.; Kuutti-Savolainen, E. R.; and Kivirikko, K. I. The role of ascorbate in the prolyl hydroxylase reaction. *Biochem. Biophys. Res. Commun.*, **1978**, *33*, 441–448.

Newberne, P. M., and Chandra, R. K. *Nutrition, Immunity and Infection: Mechanisms of Interactions*. Plenum Press, New York, **1977**.

Nichoalds, G. E.; Meng, H. C.; and Caldwell, M. D. Vitamin requirements in patients receiving total parenteral nutrition. *Arch. Surg.*, **1977**, *112*, 1061–1064.

Nishizuka, Y., and Hayaishi, O. Studies on the biosynthesis of nicotinamide adenine dinucleotide. I. Enzymic synthesis of niacin ribonucleotides from 3-hydroxyanthranilic acid in mammalian tissues. *J. Biol. Chem.*, **1963**, *238*, 3369–3377.

Pauling, L. Evolution and the need for ascorbic acid. *Proc. Natl Acad. Sci. U.S.A.*, **1970**, *67*, 1643–1648.

Pelletier, O. Vitamin C and tobacco. *Int. J. Vitam. Nutr. Res.*, **1977**, *16*, 147–169.

Pincus, J. H.; Cooper, J. R.; Murphy, J. V.; Rabe, E. F.; Lonsdale, D.; and Dunn, H. G. Thiamine derivatives in subacute necrotizing encephalomyelopathy: a preliminary report. *Pediatrics,* **1973,** *51,* 716–721.

Pincus, H. J.; Cooper, J. R.; Piros, K.; and Turner, V. Specificity of the urine inhibitor test for Leigh's disease. *Neurology (Minneap.),* **1974,** *24,* 885–890.

Pincus, H. J.; Itokawa, Y.; and Cooper, J. R. Enzyme inhibiting factors in subacute necrotizing encephalomyelopathy. *Neurology (Minneap.),* **1969,** *19,* 841–845.

Pitt, H. A., and Costrini, A. M. Vitamin C prophylaxis in marine recruits. *J.A.M.A.,* **1979,** *241,* 908–911.

Preiss, J., and Handler, P. Biosynthesis of diphosphopyridine nucleotide. II. Enzymatic aspects. *J. Biol. Chem.,* **1958,** *233,* 493–500.

Prentice, A. M., and Bates, C. J. A biochemical evaluation of the erythrocyte glutathione reductase test for riboflavin status. *Br. J. Nutr.,* **1981,** *45,* 37–52.

Rindi, G., and Ventura, U. Thiamine intestinal transport. *Physiol. Rev.,* **1972,** *52,* 821–827.

Rivers, J. M. Oral contraceptives and ascorbic acid. *Am. J. Clin. Nutr.,* **1975,** *28,* 550–554.

Rivlin, R. S. Riboflavin metabolism. *N. Engl. J. Med.,* **1970,** *283,* 463–472.

———. Hormones, drugs and riboflavin. *Nutr. Rev.,* **1979,** *37,* 241–246.

Roberts, E. Some thoughts about the γ-aminobutyric acid system in nervous tissue. *Nutr. Rev.,* **1963,** *21,* 161–165.

Rose, D. P. Oral contraceptives and vitamin B_6. In, *Human B_6 Requirements.* National Academy of Sciences, Washington, D. C., **1978,** pp. 193–201.

Rosenthal, G. Interaction of ascorbic acid and warfarin. *J.A.M.A.,* **1971,** *215,* 1671.

Schaumberg, J.; Kaplan, J.; Windebank, A.; Vick, N.; Rasmus, S.; Pleasure, D.; and Brown, M. J. Sensory neuropathy from pyridoxine abuse. A new megavitamin syndrome. *N. Engl. J. Med.,* **1983,** *309,* 445–448.

Scriver, C. R. Vitamin-responsive inborn errors of metabolism. *Metabolism,* **1973,** *22,* 1319–1344.

Sebrell, W. H., and Harris, R. S. (eds.). *The Vitamins: Chemistry, Physiology, Pathology, Methods,* Vol. I. Academic Press, Inc., New York, **1967.**

Sharman, I. M. Vitamin C: historical aspects. In, *Vitamin C: Recent Aspects of Its Physiological and Technological Importance.* (Birch, G. G., and Parker, K. J., eds.) Applied Science Publishers, Ltd., London, **1974,** pp. 1–14.

Spivak, J. L., and Jackson, D. L. Pellagra: an analysis of 18 patients and a review of the literature. *Johns Hopkins Med. J.,* **1977,** *140,* 295–309.

Stokes, P. L.; Melikian, V.; Leeming, R. L.; Portman-Graham, H.; Blair, J. A.; and Cooke, W. T. Folate metabolism in scurvy. *Am. J. Clin. Nutr.,* **1975,** *28,* 126–129.

Sturman, J. A. Vitamin B_6 and the metabolism of sulfur amino acids. In, *Human Vitamin B_6 Requirements.* National Academy of Sciences, Washington, D. C., **1978,** pp. 37–60.

Sydenstricker, V. P.; Singal, S. A.; Briggs, A. P.; DeVaughn, N. M.; and Isbell, H. Observations on the "egg white injury" in man. *J.A.M.A.,* **1942,** *118,* 1199–1200.

Vallance, S. Leucocyte ascorbic acid and the leucocyte count. *Br. J. Nutr.,* **1979,** *41,* 409–411.

Victor, M.; Adams, R. D.; and Collins, G. H. *The Wernicke-Korsakoff Syndrome.* F. A. Davis Co., Philadelphia, **1971,** pp. 1–206.

Vimokesant, S. L.; Nakornchi, S.; Dhanamitta, S.; and Hilker, D. M. Effect of tea consumption on thiamine status in man. *Nutr. Rep. Int.,* **1974,** *9,* 371–374.

Visagie, M. E.; DuPlessis, J. P.; and Laubsher, N. Effect of vitamin C supplementation on black mine-workers. *S. Afr. Med. J.,* **1975,** *49,* 889–892.

Wagner-Jauregg, T. Riboflavin. II. Chemistry. In, *The Vitamins,* 2nd ed., Vol. V. (Sebrell, W. H., and Harris, R. S., eds.) Academic Press, Inc., New York, **1972,** pp. 3–43.

Waldenlind, L. Studies on thiamine and neuromuscular transmission. *Acta Physiol. Scand.,* **1978,** Suppl., *459,* 1–35.

Wright, L. D. Pantothenic acid. In, *Present Knowledge in Nutrition.* (Hegsted, D. M.; Chichester, C. O.; Darby, W. J.; McNutt, K. W.; Stalvey, R. M.; and Stotz, E. H.; eds.) The Nutrition Foundation, Washington, D. C., **1976,** pp. 226–231.

Wurtman, J. J. Sources of choline and lecithin in the diet. In, *Nutrition and the Brain,* Vol. 5. (Barbeau, A.; Growdon, J. H.; and Wurtman, R. J.; eds.) Raven Press, New York, **1979,** pp. 73–81.

Zannoni, V. G., and Sato, P. H. Effects of ascorbic acid on microsomal drug metabolism. *Ann. N.Y. Acad. Sci.,* **1975,** *258,* 119–131.

Monographs and Reviews

American Medical Association Report. *Guidelines for Multivitamin Preparations for Parenteral Use.* Department of Foods and Nutrition, American Medical Association, Chicago, **1975,** pp. 1–27.

Birch, G. G., and Parker, K. J. (eds.). *Vitamin C: Recent Aspects of Its Physiological and Technological Importance.* Applied Science Publishers, Ltd., London, **1974.**

Dodge, P. R.; Prensky, A. L.; and Feigin, R. D. (eds.). *Nutrition and the Developing Nervous System.* C. V. Mosby Co., St. Louis, **1975.**

Food and Nutrition Board, National Research Council. *Recommended Dietary Allowances,* 9th ed. National Academy of Sciences, Washington, D. C., **1980.**

Goldsmith, G. A. Vitamins and avitaminosis. In, *Diseases of Metabolism.* (Duncan, G. G., ed.) W. B. Saunders Co., Philadelphia, **1964,** pp. 567–642.

Goodhart, R. S., and Shils, M. E. (eds.). *Modern Nutrition in Health and Disease,* 6th ed. Lea & Febiger, Philadelphia, **1980.**

Hanck, A., and Ritzel, G. (eds.). Re-evaluation of vitamin C. *Int. J. Vitam. Nutr. Res.,* **1977,** *16,* 1–310.

Hegsted, D. M.; Chichester, C. O.; Darby, W. J.; McNutt, K. W.; Stalvey, R. M.; and Stotz, E. H. (eds.). *Present Knowledge in Nutrition,* 4th ed. The Nutrition Foundation, Washington, D. C., **1976.**

Irwin, M. I., and Hutchins, B. K. A conspectus of research on vitamin C requirements of man. *J. Nutr.,* **1976,** *106,* 823–879.

Lipton, M. A.; Mailman, R. B.; and Nemeroff, C. B. Vitamins, megavitamin therapy, and the nervous system. In, *Nutrition and the Brain,* Vol. 3. (Wurtman, R. J., and Wurtman, J. J., eds.) Raven Press, New York, **1979,** pp. 183–264.

Miller, D. R., and Hayes, K. C. Vitamin excess and toxicity. In, *Nutritional Toxicology,* Vol. 1. Academic Press, Inc., New York, **1982,** pp. 81–133.

Moran, J. R., and Greene, H. L. The B vitamins and vitamin C in human nutrition. I. General considerations and 'obligatory' B vitamins. II. 'Conditional' B vitamins and vitamin C. *Am. J. Dis. Child.,* **1979,** *133,* 192–199, 308–314.

Rechcigl, M. Effect of nutrient deficiencies in man. In, *CRC Handbook Series in Nutrition and Food,* Sect. E. *Nutritional Disorders,* Vol. III. CRC Press, Inc., West Palm Beach, Fla., **1978.**

Scriver, C. R. Vitamin-responsive inborn errors of metabolism. *Metabolism,* **1973,** *22,* 1319–1344.

Sebrell, W. H., and Harris, R. S. (eds.). *The Vitamins,* 2nd ed., Vols. I, II, III, IV, V. Academic Press, Inc., New York, **1971–1974.**

CHAPTER

67 FAT-SOLUBLE VITAMINS
Vitamins A, K, and E

H. George Mandel and Victor H. Cohn

VITAMIN A

History. Night blindness was apparently first described in Egypt around 1500 B.C. Although this disease was not then linked to dietary deficiency, topical treatment with roasted or fried liver was wisely recommended, and Hippocrates later suggested eating beef liver as a cure for the affliction. The relationship to nutritional deficiency was definitively recognized in the last century. Ophthalmia Brasiliana, a disease of the eyes that primarily afflicted poorly nourished slaves, was first described in 1865. In 1887, endemic night blindness was reported to occur among the orthodox Russian Catholics who fasted during the Lenten period. More pertinent was the observation that the nurslings of mothers who fasted were prone to develop spontaneous sloughing of the cornea. Many other reports of nutritional keratomalacia soon followed from all parts of the world, including the United States.

Experimental rather than clinical observations, however, led to the discovery of vitamin A. In 1913, two groups (McCollum and Davis; Osborne and Mendel) independently reported that animals fed on artificial diets with lard as a sole source of fat developed a nutritional deficiency that could be corrected by the addition of a factor contained in butter, egg yolk, and cod liver oil to the diet. An outstanding symptom of this experimental nutritional deficiency was xerophthalmia (dryness and thickening of the conjunctiva). Clinical and experimental vitamin A deficiencies were recognized as related during World War I, when it became apparent that xerophthalmia in human beings was a result of a decrease in the content of butterfat in the diet.

Terminology, Chemistry, and Occurrence. While the term *vitamin A* has been used to denote specific chemical compounds, such as retinol or its esters, it now is used more as a generic descriptor for compounds that exhibit the biological properties of retinol. *Retinoid* refers to the chemical entity retinol or other closely related naturally occurring derivatives. Retinoids also include structurally related synthetic analogs, which need not have retinol-like (vitamin A) activity.

The simple observation of Steenbock (1919) that the vitamin A content of vegetables varies with the degree of pigmentation paved the way for the isolation and discovery of the chemical nature of the vitamin. Subsequently, Euler and associates (1929) and Moore (1929) demonstrated that the purified plant pigment carotene (provitamin A) is a remarkably potent source of vitamin A. β-Carotene, the most active carotenoid found in plants, has the structural formula shown below. In the United States, the average adult receives about half of his daily intake of vitamin A as retinol or retinyl esters and the rest as carotenoids. Major dietary sources of vitamin A are liver, butter, cheese, whole milk, egg yolk, and fish. β-Carotene is present in various yellow or green fruits and vegetables.

Retinol (vitamin A₁), a primary alcohol, is present in esterified form in the tissues of animals and salt-water fish, mainly in the liver. Its structural formula, established by Karrer and associates (1931), is as follows:

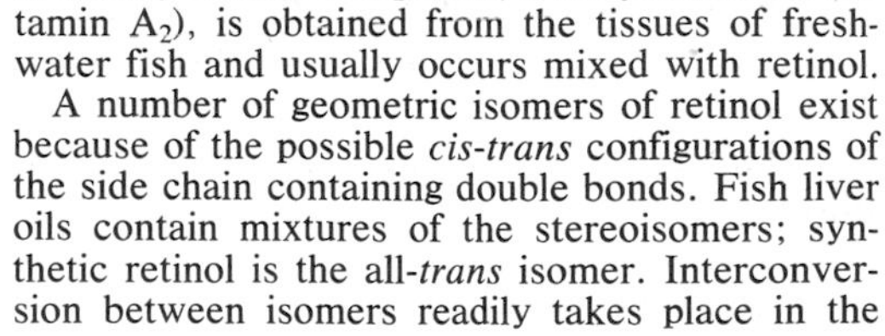

Retinol

A closely related compound, 3-dehydroretinol (vitamin A₂), is obtained from the tissues of freshwater fish and usually occurs mixed with retinol.

A number of geometric isomers of retinol exist because of the possible *cis-trans* configurations of the side chain containing double bonds. Fish liver oils contain mixtures of the stereoisomers; synthetic retinol is the all-*trans* isomer. Interconversion between isomers readily takes place in the

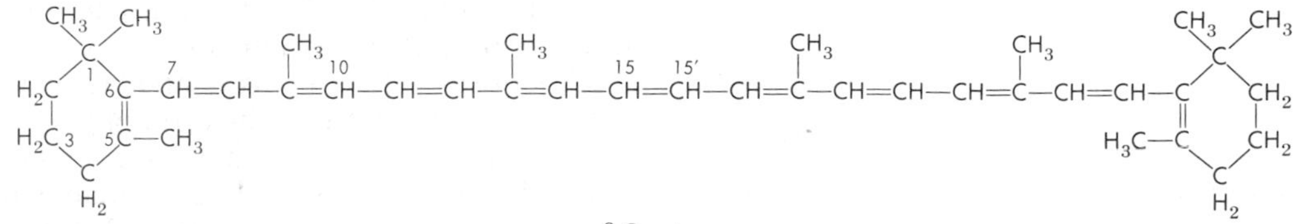

β-Carotene

body. In the visual cycle, the reaction between retinal (vitamin A aldehyde) and opsin to form rhodopsin only occurs with the 11-*cis* isomer.

Certain structural modifications of retinol are possible without destroying its activity. Retinoic acid (vitamin A acid), in which the alcohol group has been oxidized, shares some but not all of the actions of retinol. Retinoic acid is very potent in promoting growth and controlling differentiation and maintenance of epithelial tissue in vitamin A–deficient animals, but it is ineffective in restoring visual or reproductive function in certain species where retinol is effective.

Ethers and esters derived from the alcohol also show activity *in vivo*. The ring structure of retinol (β-ionone), or the more unsaturated ring in 3-dehydroretinol (dehydro-β-ionone), is essential for activity; hydrogenation destroys biological activity. Of all known derivatives, all-*trans*-retinol and its aldehyde, retinal, exhibit the greatest biological potency *in vivo*, although retinoic acid and its derivatives may be 1000-fold more potent in various systems *in vitro* (Newton *et al.*, 1980). Many of these retinoids, however, fail to be transported in plasma via specific binding proteins to target tissues, and they remain inactive *in vivo*.

Physiological Functions and Pharmacological Actions. Vitamin A has a number of important functions in the body. It plays an essential role in the function of the retina. It is necessary for growth and differentiation of epithelial tissue and is required for growth of bone, reproduction, and embryonic development. There is considerable interest in the pharmacological use of retinoids for the prophylaxis and, perhaps, the treatment of malignancies.

The functions of vitamin A are mediated by different forms of the molecule. In vision, the functional vitamin is retinal; retinol is apparently responsible for the actions of the vitamin in reproductive processes, and retinoic acid or a metabolite may be the active form in functions associated with growth, differentiation, and transformation. The major recognized reactions are as follows:

Retinol (transport) ⇌ Retinal → Retinoic Acid

Retinol Esters (tissue storage)   (Visual Pigments)   Inactive Products   Active Metabolite? (growth, tissue maintenance)

light opsin

Retinal and the Visual Cycle. It has long been known that vitamin A deficiency interferes with vision in dim light, a condition known as night blindness (nyctalopia). The fundamental observations of Hecht (1937), Wald and Brown (1965), and Hubbard and colleagues (1965) have contributed greatly to an understanding of this phenomenon (*see* Wald, 1968; Bridges, 1984).

Adaptation to dark is a function of both the rods and the cones. Primary adaptation, accomplished by the cones, is completed in a few minutes. Secondary adaptation is a function of the rods, and is not completed for 30 minutes or longer. The cones act as receptors of high-intensity light and for color vision, whereas the rods are especially sensitive to light of low intensity. The process of adaptation is a chemical one, and consists in the formation of photosensitive pigments in the retina that, upon exposure to light of low intensity, are bleached and undergo chemical reactions that result in the initiation of a receptor potential. After breakdown, the pigment is resynthesized. The photosensitive pigment of the rods of land vertebrates is known as rhodopsin—a combination of the protein, opsin, and a prosthetic group, 11-*cis*-retinal. The known photosensitive pigment of the cones is a combination of retinal with a protein very similar to opsin. Both photosensitive pigments react similarly but to light of different wavelengths.

In the synthesis of rhodopsin, 11-*cis*-retinol is converted to 11-*cis*-retinal in a reversible reaction that requires nicotinamide adenine dinucleotide (NAD) or nicotinamide adenine dinucleotide phosphate (NADP). 11-*Cis*-retinal then combines with the ε-amino group of lysine in opsin to form rhodopsin. Most rhodopsin is located in the membranes of the discs situated in the outer segments of the rods. Photodecomposition begins upon absorption of a photon of light. Although the exact reaction sequence is still disputed, the initial reaction probably involves a conformational change of the protein to form bathorhodopsin, which is followed by the isomerization of 11-*cis*-retinal to the all-*trans* configuration. Rhodopsin is thereby activated.

Rhodopsin interacts with and activates another protein of the retinal rod outer segment, which is termed transducin. Transducin, in sequence, stimulates a guanosine 3′,5′-monophosphate–(cyclic GMP–)specific phosphodiesterase, and the resultant decline in cyclic GMP concentrations is thought to regulate the state of sodium channels in the plasma membrane. An excitatory potential is developed, and action potentials eventually travel to the brain via the optic nerve (*see* O'Brien, 1982; George and Hagins, 1983). Transducin is a guanine nucleotide–binding regulatory protein (G protein) and is homologous to the G proteins that regulate adenylate cyclase activity (Hurley *et al.*, 1984; Harris *et al.*, 1985; Lochrie *et al.*, 1985). The pathway for signal transduction that starts with the receptor for photons (rhodopsin) is thus analogous to that for many hormones and neurotransmitters (*see* Gilman, 1984; Chapter 2).

All-*trans*-retinal can be reconverted to 11-*cis*-retinal directly and recombine with opsin to form rhodopsin. Alternatively, all-*trans*-retinal can be reduced to all-*trans*-retinol, which is first converted to 11-*cis*-retinol and then to rhodopsin in the manner described above. The overall sequence of events in the visual cycle is depicted in Figure 67–1 (*see* Bridges, 1984).

When human beings are fed diets deficient in vitamin A, their ability for dark adaptation is gradually diminished. Rod vision is affected more than cone vision. Upon depletion of retinol from liver and blood (usually at concentrations less than 20 μg of retinol per deciliter of plasma), the concentration of retinol and of rhodopsin in the retina falls. Unless the deficiency is

overcome, opsin, lacking the stabilizing effect of retinal, decays and anatomical deterioration of the rods' outer segments takes place. Irreversible ultrastructural changes leading to blindness then supervene in rats maintained on a vitamin A–deficient diet, a process that takes 10 months.

Following short-term deprivation of vitamin A, dark adaptation can be restored to normal by the addition of retinol to the diet. However, vision does not return to normal for several weeks after adequate amounts of retinol have been supplied. The cause for this delay is unknown.

Vitamin A and Epithelial Structures. The functional and structural integrity of epithelial cells throughout the body is dependent upon an adequate supply of retinol. Retinol plays a major role in the induction and control of epithelial differentiation in mucus-secreting or keratinizing tissues. In the presence of retinol, basal epithelial cells are stimulated to produce mucus. Excessive retinol leads to the production of a thick layer of mucin, the inhibition of keratinization, and the display of goblet cells.

In the absence of retinol, goblet mucous cells disappear and atrophy of epithelium occurs, followed by a proliferation of basal cells at the expense of mucous cells. The new cells, by their continued growth, undermine and replace the original epithelium with a stratified, keratinizing epithelium. The suppression of normal secretions leads to irritation and infection.

Because retinol has the ability to control cell differentiation and proliferation in epithelia, there has been considerable interest in the apparent ability of retinol and related compounds to interfere with carcinogenesis (*see* Moon and Itri, 1984, and related discussions in Sporn *et al.*, 1984). Deficiency of vitamin A appears to enhance susceptibility to carcinogenesis, even in man (Bjelke, 1975); there is marked hyperplasia and enhanced synthesis of DNA by the basal cells of various epithelia and reduced cellular differentiation. The administration of retinol or other retinoids to animals reverses these changes in the epithelium of the respiratory tract, mammary gland, urinary bladder, and skin. Following the studies of Lasnitzki (1955) that demonstrated that treatment with retinoids caused replacement of atypical carcinogen-induced

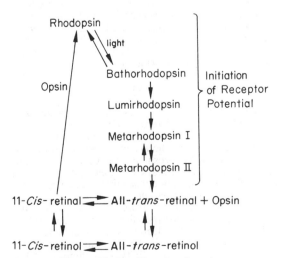

Figure 67–1. *The visual cycle.*

epithelial cells with more normal cells, it was shown that the compounds also prevent the development of epithelial cancer of the tissues mentioned. Thus, the progression of premalignant cells to cells with invasive, malignant characteristics is slowed, delayed, arrested, or even reversed in experimental animals (Hill and Grubbs, 1982). The antitumor effect is seen with chemically and virally induced malignancies, both of epithelial and mesenchymal origin, as well as with transformation induced with radiation or growth factors. Reversal of growth and metastasis of established tumors *in vivo* has been limited, as has prevention of the growth of transplantable neoplasms in animals.

The exact mechanism of the anticarcinogenic effect remains unclear, but obviously it is of enormous interest (Bollag, 1975; Sporn and Roberts, 1983). The effect is observable even if the retinoid is administered many weeks after the exposure to a carcinogen, suggesting interference with the promotion or progression phase of carcinogenesis. Other possible mechanisms that may contribute to the antitumor effect include the induction of differentiation in malignant cells to form morphologically mature normal cells (Strickland and Mahdavi, 1978; Breitman *et al.*, 1980), suppression of the malignant phenotype previously induced by a carcinogen, inhibition of tumor promoter-enhanced carcinogenesis, or an improvement in the host's immune defense mechanisms. A direct cytotoxic action appears unlikely.

Liau and associates (1981) have proposed that retinol, associated with a specific binding protein, reaches the cell nucleus, dissociates from its carrier, binds to chromatin, and modulates gene expression. Nuclear RNA synthesis is diminished in vitamin A–deficient animals, and retinol or retinoic acid stimulates RNA synthesis in this situation. Retinol can regulate the synthesis of specific proteins (*e.g.*, keratin) necessary for the differentiation of epithelial tissues (Fuchs and Green, 1981).

Retinol also appears to have a specific biochemical function in the synthesis of mannose- and galactose-containing glycoproteins and glycolipids. Retinol is converted to retinyl phosphate in epithelial tissues, and this intermediate is in turn metabolized to mannosylretinylphosphate in a reaction that is catalyzed by a microsomal enzyme (Rosso *et al.*, 1975). The glycosylated derivative of retinol mediates the transfer of mannose to specific cell-surface glycoproteins. Thus, the formation of such proteins is sharply curtailed when there is deficiency of vitamin A. Reactions of this type may explain the function of retinol in a number of processes that depend on the integrity of the cell surface.

Signs and Symptoms of Deficiency. Tissue reserves of retinoids in the normal adult are sufficiently large to require long-term dietary deprivation in order to induce deficiency. Vitamin A deficiency occurs more commonly, therefore, in chronic diseases affecting fat absorption, such as biliary tract or pancreatic disease, sprue, colitis, and portal cirrhosis; following partial gastrectomy; or during extreme, chronic dietary inadequacy.

The deficiency is quite widespread in Southeast Asia, the Middle East, Africa, and Central and South America, particularly in children, and is associated with general malnutrition. Vitamin A deficiency and protein malnutrition are the two most serious nutritional deficiency diseases in the world today. Deficiency of vitamin A may be fatal, especially in infants and young children suffering from kwashiorkor or marasmus. It has been estimated that more than one quarter million children in the world go blind every year because of inadequate intake of vitamin A. In the United States, about 15% of the population has concentrations of retinol in plasma or liver below the accepted lower limits of normal (20 μg/dl or 40 μg/g, respectively), indicating a risk of deficiency. Most of these individuals are infants or children, and a disproportionate percentage are Mexican-American or black children.

Signs and symptoms of mild vitamin A deficiency are easily overlooked. Skin lesions, such as follicular hyperkeratosis and infections, are among the earliest signs of deficiency, but the most recognizable manifestation is night blindness, even though its onset occurs only when vitamin A depletion is severe. In general, rapidly proliferating tissues are more sensitive to deficiency of retinol and may revert to an undifferentiated state more readily.

Eye. Keratomalacia, characterized by desiccation, ulceration, and xerosis of the cornea and conjunctiva, is occasionally seen as an acute symptom in the very young who are ingesting severely deficient diets. It is foreshadowed, usually, by night blindness, which appears as the earliest ocular sign of deficiency. Ultimately severe visual impairment and even blindness result.

Bronchorespiratory Tract. Changes in the bronchorespiratory epithelium from mucus secretion to keratinization lead to increased incidence of respiratory infections in the deficiency state. There is also a decrease in elasticity of the lung and other tissues.

Skin. Keratinization and drying of the epidermis occur, and papular eruptions involving the pilosebaceous follicles may be found, especially on the extremities.

Genitourinary System. Urinary calculi are frequent concomitants of vitamin A deficiency. The epithelium of the urinary tract shares in the general pathological changes of all epithelial structures. Epithelial debris may thus provide the nidus around which a calculus is formed. Abnormalities of reproduction include impairment of spermatogenesis, degeneration of testes, abortion, resorption of fetuses, and production of malformed offspring.

Gastrointestinal Tract. The intestinal mucosa shows a reduction in the number of goblet cells but no keratinization. Alterations in intestinal epithelium and metaplasia of pancreatic ductal epithelium are common. They may be responsible for the diarrhea occasionally seen in vitamin A deficiency.

Sweat Glands. These glands may undergo atrophy and keratinizing squamous-cell metaplasia.

Bone. In animals, vitamin A deficiency is associated with faulty modeling of bone (with production of thick, cancellous bone instead of thinner, more compact bone).

Miscellaneous. Often there is an impairment of both taste and smell in vitamin A–deficient individuals, which undoubtedly results from a keratinizing effect. Hearing may also be impaired. Vitamin A deficiency can interfere with erythropoiesis, which may be masked by abnormal losses of fluid. Nerve lesions, increased cerebrospinal fluid pressure, and hydrocephalus have been reported.

Hypervitaminosis A.   An intake of retinoids greatly in excess of requirement results in a toxic syndrome known as hypervitaminosis A. Some 600 cases have been reported in the literature (*see* Kamm *et al.,* 1984). Excess vitamin E appears to protect against hypervitaminosis A.

Most frequently, high intakes in children are the result of overzealous prophylactic vitamin therapy on the part of parents. In adults, toxicity has resulted from extended self-medication, food fads, or the use of high doses of oral retinoids for the therapy of acne or other skin lesions. The daily intake of 3 to 6 mg of retinol for 2 years has led to hypervitaminosis in an adult, although most patients with hypervitaminosis have consumed higher doses for a shorter period (Herbert, 1982). The Food and Nutrition Board of the National Research Council (1980) has warned that the ingestion of more than 7.5 mg of retinol daily is ill advised. Nevertheless, almost 5% of users of vitamin A in the United States exceed that amount.

Early signs and symptoms of *chronic* retinoid intoxication include dry and pruritic skin, skin desquamation, erythematous dermatitis, disturbed hair growth, fissures of the lips, pain and tenderness of bones, hyperostosis, headache, papilledema, anorexia, edema, fatigue, irritability, and hemorrhage. In addition to hepatosplenomegaly, pathological changes in the liver include hypertrophy of fat-storing cells, fibrosis, sclerosis of central veins, and cirrhosis, with resultant portal hypertension and ascites. Intracranial pressure may be increased, and neurological symptoms may mimic those of a brain tumor (pseudotumor cerebri). The activity of alkaline phosphatase in plasma rises because of the increased osteoblastic activity, and a number of cases of hypercalcemia have been reported.

Concentrations of retinol in plasma in excess of 100 μg/dl usually are diagnostic of hypervitaminosis A. Treatment consists in withdrawal of the retinoid. Most signs and symptoms disappear within a week, but the desquamation and hyperostoses remain evident for several months after clinical recovery has occurred.

Acute poisoning in man is known to follow the ingestion of polar bear liver. Signs and symptoms include drowsiness, irritability or irresistible desire to sleep, severe headache due to increased intracranial pressure, dizziness, hepatomegaly, vomiting, papilledema, and, after 24 hours, generalized peeling of the skin. The high content of retinoids in polar bear liver, up to 12 mg of retinol per gram (Russell, 1967), is responsible for the syndrome. The acute consumption of more than 500 mg of retinol in an adult, 100 mg in a young child, or 30 mg in an infant frequently results in toxic effects. As little as 7.5 to 15 mg of retinol daily for 30 days has induced such toxicity in infants (Yaffe and Filer, 1971).

In infants, increased intracranial pressure, a bulging fontanel, and vomiting are seen early, and most symptoms usually disappear within 36 hours after cessation of ingestion of retinol. The toxicity of retinol depends on the age of the patient, the dose, and the duration of administration.

Congenital abnormalities can apparently occur in human infants whose mothers have consumed about 7.5 to 12 mg of retinol daily during the first trimester of pregnancy (Bernhardt and Dorsey, 1974). Obviously, pregnant women should not ingest quantities of retinoids in excess of those recommended. Congenital abnormalities have also been reported in the offspring of hypervitaminotic animals; these include hydrocephalus, encephalocele, urinary tract anomalies, and skeletal deformities.

Human Requirement. Human requirements for vitamin A have been approximated from studies that have attempted to correct experimentally produced deficiency states. The present recommendations of the Food and Nutrition Board of the National Research Council are based upon the amount of retinoid necessary to maintain normal dark adaptation plus an additional factor of safety to cover variations in absorption and utilization of retinol. The recommended daily allowances for the normal male and female adult are 1000 and 800 retinol equivalents per day, respectively (5000 and 4000 units, assuming that 50% of dietary vitamin A is derived from retinol and 50% from β-carotene). For the requirements of infants and children, *see* Table XVI–1 (page 1546) and below.

Absorption, Distribution to Target Cells, Fate, and Excretion. Much of this information has been derived from animal experiments, but it is likely that similar considerations are true for man (*see* Goodman, 1980). More than 90% of the intake of preformed vitamin A is in the form of retinol esters, usually as retinyl palmitate.

Retinol, which is formed by hydrolysis of retinyl esters in the intestine (*see* below), is readily absorbed from the normal gastrointestinal tract. If the amount ingested is not much greater than the requirement, absorption is complete; however, when a large excess is taken, some of the retinol escapes in the feces. Inasmuch as retinol is fat soluble, it is not unexpected to find that its absorption is related to that of lipid and is enhanced by bile; nevertheless, aqueous dispersions of retinol or its ester are absorbed more rapidly than are oily solutions.

In the presence of abnormalities of fat absorption, the absorption of retinol is reduced. In such patients water-miscible preparations should be used. Intestinal absorption of retinol is reduced when diets are low in protein. The absorption of retinol is also disturbed in patients with intestinal infections, cystic fibrosis, and hepatic disease.

Intestinal absorption apparently occurs by a carrier-mediated process and is sensitive to metabolic inhibitors. Retinyl esters are hydrolyzed in the lumen of the intestine by pancreatic enzymes and within the brush border of the intestinal cell before absorption, followed by reesterification, mainly to the palmitate; there may be several cycles of hydrolysis and reesterification. Significant quantities of retinol are also absorbed directly into the circulation.

The long-chain fatty acid ester enters the circulation by transport in the chylomicron fraction of lymph (Goodman *et al.*, 1966), and concentrations of esterified retinol reach a peak in plasma about 4 hours after the administration of retinol. Most of the retinol is stored in the liver, mainly in parenchymal hepatocytes, as the palmitate ester. There are several pools of retinyl esters in the liver, one of which is filled by newly absorbed retinol and which supplies other tissues preferentially; another serves for storage.

The median concentration of retinyl esters in man is about 100 to 300 μg/g of liver, and the normal range of retinol in plasma is 30 to 70 μg/dl. Other tissues, such as kidney, lung, adrenal, and intraperitoneal fat, contain about 1 μg of retinoids per gram, while the retinal pigment epithelium contains ten times this concentration. Administration of low doses of vitamin E markedly increases the tissue storage of retinol. Until hepatic saturation takes place, the administration of retinol leads mainly to its accumulation in the liver rather than in blood.

Prior to entering the circulation from the liver, hepatic retinyl esters are hydrolyzed, and 90 to 95% of the retinol is associated with an α_1-globulin, which has a single binding site for the vitamin. This retinol-binding protein (RBP) is synthesized and secreted by the liver and then circulates in the blood in man complexed with and stabilized by a thyroxine-binding protein. The formation of this complex protects the circulating RBP (and retinol) from metabolism and from glomerular filtration and excretion by the kidney. Normally less than 5% of the total retinoids in the blood is present as the retinyl ester, which is associated with lipoprotein.

When hepatic stores of the vitamin and the RBP carrier system become saturated because of excessive intake of retinol or hepatic damage, up to 65% of the retinoids in plasma may be present as retinyl esters associated with lipoprotein. Similarly, after acute administration of alcohol, retinyl esters accumulate. Since retinol is biologically inert while bound to RBP, these retinyl esters, which are surfactants, may be responsible for much of the toxicity that is observed (Mallia *et al.*, 1975; Smith and Goodman, 1976).

If an individual ingests a diet free of retinol or its precursors, plasma concentrations are maintained over many months at the expense of hepatic reserves. Blood concentrations, therefore, are not an accurate guide to an individual's vitamin A status, but low plasma values of retinol imply that hepatic storage of the vitamin may be exhausted (*see* Underwood, 1984). Signs and symptoms of vitamin A deficiency appear when the plasma concentration falls below 10 to 20 μg/dl or when concentrations of retinoids in liver are less than 5 to 20 μg/g. Hepatic reserves of retinoids decrease with a half-life of about 50 to 100 days; signs of deficiency thus develop only after a prolonged period of inadequate intake. In alcoholic liver disease, hepatic concentrations of retinoids are severely depressed (Leo and Lieber, 1982).

Retinol bound to RBP reaches the cell membrane of the various target organs, and the carrier acts to deliver retinol to specific sites on the cell surface. Retinol then permeates the cell and interacts with another specific protein, the cellular retinol-binding protein (CRBP) (Bashor *et al.*, 1973). This apparent receptor is found in liver, kidney, small intestine, lung, spleen, eye, and testis; by contrast, brain, muscle, thymus, fat, and heart do not contain CRBP (Adachi *et al.*, 1981). The interaction is restricted to retinol and closely related derivatives, and their affinity for CRBP parallels their physiological activity. Retinoic acid does not bind to CRBP but appears to have its own specific receptor (*see* below).

The concentration of RBP in plasma is crucial for the regulation of retinol in plasma and its transport to tissues. In vitamin A deficiency, the synthesis of RBP is maintained, the hepatic content of RBP rises, and its concentration in plasma falls, apparently because the secretion of RBP from the liver is blocked. Once retinol again becomes available, the liver rapidly releases RBP into the plasma for transport of retinol to the tissues. When there is protein deficiency (*e.g.*, caused by malnutrition,

kwashiorkor, or parenchymal liver disease), the concentration of RBP becomes insufficient, and concentrations of retinol in plasma fall despite normal stores in the liver. Replenishment with calories and protein is then required. Deficiency of both RBP and retinol cannot be corrected by the administration of retinol alone.

Other pathological conditions also alter plasma concentrations of retinol and RBP in plasma. Synthesis or release of RBP from the liver is depressed and plasma retinol concentrations are reduced in cystic fibrosis, alcohol-related cirrhosis, and other hepatic diseases. The opposite is true during administration of estrogens or oral contraceptives. In proteinuria, febrile infections, or stress, the concentration of retinol in the blood may be reduced drastically, partially because of increased urinary excretion. In chronic renal disease, RBP catabolism is impaired, and concentrations of the protein and retinol are elevated.

Pregnancy also alters the concentration of retinol in blood. During the first trimester there is a fall in the mean content of retinol in plasma, followed by a slow rise and a return to normal at parturition. It is likely that the increased demands for retinol lead to its withdrawal from the blood at a rate exceeding that of its mobilization from the hepatic reserve. The placental barrier prevents the extensive transfer of retinol or carotenoids. Studies in animals suggest that there is transplacental transport of RBP during early pregnancy; thereafter the fetus begins to synthesize its own RBP. The concentration of retinol in fetal blood is thus less than in maternal blood. Both colostrum and milk offer the newborn an adequate supply of retinol. The concentration of retinol in the milk is maintained at a fixed maximal concentration if the maternal dietary intake of retinol is adequate to permit storage in the liver.

Retinol is in part conjugated to form a β-glucuronide, which undergoes enterohepatic circulation and is oxidized to retinal and retinoic acid. Several other water-soluble metabolites are also excreted in urine and feces. Normally no retinol can be recovered unchanged from human urine.

Retinoic Acid. After oral administration, retinoic acid reaches the circulation by the portal vein and is transported in plasma as a complex with albumin. Unlike retinol, retinoic acid is not stored in the liver but is rapidly excreted. It is metabolized in the liver; there is some isomerization to the 13-*cis* form, and various degradation products are secreted into bile and excreted in urine and feces. Retinoic acid binds to a specific cellular retinoic acid–binding protein (CRABP), which is distinct from CRBP (Ong and Chytil, 1975). The affinity of a series of retinoids for CRABP parallels their growth-promoting ability and their capacity to promote mucous metaplasia of keratinized epithelia in vitamin A–

deficient animals. In adult rats, CRABP is located mainly in thymus, spleen, skin, eye, testis, uterus, and ovary; it is not found in liver, kidney, or lung; however, it is present in human fetal liver, as well as in lung and breast tumor tissue. In the retina CRBP (but not CRABP) is located predominantly in the region of the photoreceptors (Wiggert *et al.*, 1978). This is consistent with the inability of retinoic acid to substitute for retinol in the visual cycle or to be converted to retinal. Following the binding of retinoic acid to CRABP in the cytosol of target tissues, the complex migrates to the nucleus, where it presumably initiates a cascade of specific biochemical events. In many, but not all, biological systems, considerable correlation has been noted between the presence of CRABP or CRBP and the sensitivity of the cell to the antitumor effects of retinoids (Chytil and Ong, 1983).

Carotenoids. Unlike the extensive absorption of retinol, only about one third of β-carotene or other carotenoids is absorbed by man. Absorption depends upon the presence of bile and absorbable fat in the intestinal tract and is greatly decreased by steatorrhea and chronic diarrhea. The ingestion of mineral oil decreases the absorption of carotene, whereas water-soluble dispersing agents enhance absorption. The conversion of carotene to retinol occurs in the wall of the small intestine. Two molecules of retinal are produced by cleavage of the 15,15' double bond. The conversion is influenced by the amount of dietary protein and lipid. Some of the retinal is further oxidized to retinoic acid; only about one half is reduced to retinol, which is then esterified and transported in the lymph, as described above. Carotene is biologically active only following conversion to retinol. Some carotene gains access to the circulation. If very large amounts of carotene are ingested, very high concentrations may be achieved in blood (300 μg/dl), and the hypercarotenemia results in a yellow discoloration of the skin, which is reversible; this can be distinguished from jaundice by the absence of scleral pigmentation. Hypervitaminosis does not develop, however, probably because of a limited conversion to retinol.

Bioassay and Unitage. Most commercial preparations are synthetic retinyl esters. Preparations from animal sources must be biologically assayed to establish their activity. This assay depends upon the ability of retinol to support growth in vitamin-depleted rats of specified age and weight and fed a standard vitamin A–deficient diet over a given period of time. The concentration of suitably purified preparations can be determined by spectrophotometric analysis. One USP vitamin A unit is the spe-

cific biological activity of 0.3 μg of retinol or 0.6 μg of β-carotene. Because of the relatively inefficient dietary utilization of β-carotene compared to retinol, the new nomenclature is in terms of the retinol equivalent, which represents 1 μg of retinol, 6 μg of dietary β-carotene, or 12 μg of other provitamin A carotenoids. One retinol equivalent equals 3.3 USP units of vitamin A activity as supplied by retinol or 10 units of vitamin A activity as supplied by β-carotene (Bieri and McKenna, 1981). The methods for standardizing retinol and carotenoids have been reviewed (Parrish, 1977; Simpson, 1983).

Preparations. There are many types of preparations that contain retinol. These include solutions of pure synthetic retinol and concentrates that contain both retinol and vitamin D in various proportions. In the United States, commercial production of synthetic retinol is about 1000 tons per year. This is approximately equal to the total requirement for the entire world population. Absorption is greatest for aqueous preparations, intermediate for emulsions, and slowest for oil solutions. Whereas oil-soluble preparations may lead to greater hepatic storage of the vitamin, water-miscible preparations usually provide higher concentrations in plasma.

Vitamin A capsules contain 3 to 15 mg of retinol (10,000 to 50,000 USP vitamin A units) per capsule; tablets are also available. A water-miscible preparation (15 mg/ml; 50,000 USP units/ml) can be given intramuscularly for individuals with malabsorption, nausea, vomiting, or severe ocular damage.

Tretinoin (all-trans-retinoic acid; RETIN-A) is available for topical use as a solution (0.05%), a cream (0.05 and 0.1%), and a gel (0.025 and 0.01%). It is an irritant, causes skin peeling, and is used for the treatment of acne and other skin diseases.

Isotretinoin (13-cis-retinoic acid; ACCUTANE) is available for oral use as 10-, 20-, and 40-mg capsules.

Therapeutic Uses. *Vitamin A Deficiency Diseases.* The normal requirement of vitamin A for adults is supplied by an adequate diet. The rational uses of retinol are in the treatment of deficiency of vitamin A and as prophylaxis during periods of increased requirement, such as infancy, pregnancy, and lactation. However, limitation in diet due to economic stress or food fads can give rise to the symptoms of deficiency. Once a vitamin A deficiency has been diagnosed, intensive therapy should be instituted. The patient should then be maintained on a proper diet.

During infancy, pregnancy, or lactation, it is best to supply supplemental retinol rather than to rely solely upon the diet. Infants usually receive retinol in conjunction with vitamin D. A daily intake of 400 to 700 retinol equivalents of vitamin A (400 to 700 μg of retinol) should be provided for infants and growing children. However, ingestion of 6 mg of retinol or more per day for 1 to 2 months by healthy infants or children on good diets is likely to produce signs and symptoms of overdosage. During pregnancy (especially the second and third trimesters) and lactation, the intake of retinoids should be maintained at approximately 1.0 and 1.2 mg of retinol per day, respectively.

Rarely, the absorption, mobilization, or storage of retinol may be adversely affected, and under such circumstances long-continued therapy with retinol may be indicated, as, for example, in an individual with steatorrhea, severe biliary obstruction, cirrhosis of the liver, or following a total gastrectomy. In other disease states where considerable retinol is lost from the body, replacement therapy may be necessary. In various infections in which mucous-cell turnover is accelerated and urinary excretion of retinol is increased, the need for retinol is further enhanced. Individuals already suffering from vitamin A deficiency who develop infections, especially of the respiratory tract, will benefit from the inclusion of adequate amounts of retinoids in the diet. There is no evidence, however, that an excessive intake of retinoids will influence the incidence of infections in an individual whose intake of retinoids is adequate. Although moderate amounts of vitamin A apparently do no harm, hepatotoxicity may be potentiated when such doses are taken by the chronic alcoholic. If vitamin A is prescribed as a dietary supplement, intake of 1.5 mg of retinol represents one and one-half times the recommended daily allowance. Long-term ingestion of much larger amounts may lead to hypervitaminosis.

In kwashiorkor and other severe vitamin A deficiencies in children, a single intramuscular injection of 30 mg of retinol as the water-miscible palmitate has been advocated, followed by intermittent oral treatment with retinoids. The World Health Organization treatment schedule for xerophthalmia in children older than 1 year includes 110 mg of retinyl palmitate orally or 55 mg intramuscularly, plus another 110 mg orally the following day and again prior to discharge (*see* Underwood, 1984). Vitamin E, 40 units, should be coadministered, since it apparently increases the efficacy of retinol. Pregnant women should receive only low doses of retinoids.

Dermatological Diseases. Vitamin A may be helpful in certain diseases of the skin, such as acne, psoriasis, Darier's disease, and ichthyosis. The use of other retinoids in these conditions has largely replaced that of retinol (Symposium, 1982; Peck, 1984).

The topical use of tretinoin for *acne vulgaris* has been advocated, although oral isotretinoin is more efficacious. The retinoids act by increasing epidermal-cell mitosis and cell turnover, resulting in the production of a less cohesive horny cell layer, which is more easily peeled off. The agents thus prevent the formation of comedones, suppress the synthesis of keratin without altering bacterial skin counts, and produce improvement in most patients. The efficacy of topical tretinoin is similar to that of regimens that include methylprednisolone and neomycin, and it may surpass that of benzoyl peroxide. For more severe cases, topical application of tretinoin may be combined with the oral administration of antibiotics or with other topical preparations, but the latter should be used cautiously. Treatment with tretinoin should be continued for

about 3 months. When applied to human skin, about 5% of the compound is recovered in the urine; this is increased when there is acne or psoriasis.

Although many patients tolerate the topical application of tretinoin without undue side effects, erythema and desquamation occur frequently. These adverse effects are not necessary for therapeutic benefit and may be avoided with a less concentrated preparation. The drug sensitizes the skin to sunlight, and may cause severe irritation in patients with eczema. Alterations in hepatic function after tretinoin are minor and reversible. Allergic contact dermatitis and pigmentation changes may require medical attention, as may blistering, crusting, and severe burning or swelling of the skin and irritation of the mucous membranes of the eyes, nose, and mouth. Temporary exacerbation of the acne may occur during the first weeks of treatment, but therapy should be continued. The oral administration of tretinoin is associated with a greater risk of toxicity from hypervitaminosis, but hepatotoxicity is unlikely because this compound, in contrast to retinol, is not stored in the liver.

The oral use of *isotretinoin* is now extensive because of its great effectiveness against severe recalcitrant nodulocystic acne, but it should be reserved for patients who are unresponsive to conventional therapy, including systemic antibiotics. Remission, which may occur within 1 month of treatment, may continue for years after discontinuation of the drug. It is often recommended for inflammatory papulopustular acne with scarring, folliculitis due to gramnegative bacteria, severe acne rosacea, and resistant suppurative hidradenitis. The drug acts by temporarily suppressing the activity of sebaceous glands and sharply diminishing the production of sebum. Growth of *Propionibacterium acnes* on the skin, which is responsible for the inflammation, is also reduced.

The drug is not effective topically. It is rapidly absorbed after oral administration and reaches peak concentrations in plasma in 2 to 3 hours. It has a half-life of 3 to 20 hours, is extensively bound to albumin, and is metabolized and excreted in bile and urine (Brazzell and Colburn, 1982).

Adverse effects are typical of chronic hypervitaminosis A and include major fetal abnormalities and spontaneous abortions, numerous mucocutaneous effects, pseudotumor cerebri, papilledema, corneal opacities, musculoskeletal pain and hyperostosis, abnormalities of liver function, and elevated plasma triglycerides. The drug should be discontinued at least a month before pregnancy is contemplated.

The usual dose of isotretinoin for treatment of acne is 1 mg/kg per day in two doses, preferably with meals, but lower doses may be effective and are less toxic. In patients with severe involvement of the trunk, the dosage may be doubled. The drug is usually given for 15 to 20 weeks, and improvement usually continues after treatment has stopped until clearing of the skin is almost complete. A rest period of at least 8 weeks is recommended in patients (about one third) who need a second course of therapy.

Etretinate has not yet been approved for use in the United States but is available in other countries. This retinoid is employed orally in combination with other drugs for treatment of psoriasis and related disorders of keratinization. Maintenance therapy is required for most psoriatic patients. The incidence and type of toxicities have been reviewed (Ward *et al.,* 1983; Kamm *et al.,* 1984), and they resemble those for isotretinoin. Major toxicities include mucocutaneous effects, alopecia, and the possibility of birth defects. The drug is stored in tissues, and its long half-life (3 months) increases the risk of teratogenicity. Because of the long-term use of this drug in psoriasis, special care is required in the treatment of children to avoid toxicity to bone, premature closure of the epiphyses, and fractures.

Other Uses. The use of retinoids in *rheumatoid arthritis* is currently under investigation because of the ability of retinoids to inhibit production of collagenase. Because of toxicity, routine prophylactic use against *cancer* cannot be recommended. The potential value of retinoids in the prevention of human tumors of the skin, bladder, breast, and other epithelial tissues is, however, currently under investigation.

VITAMIN K

History. Vitamin K is a dietary principle essential for the normal biosynthesis of several factors required for clotting of blood. In 1929, Dam observed that chickens fed on inadequate diets developed a deficiency disease in which the outstanding symptom was spontaneous bleeding, apparently due to a low content of prothrombin in the blood. Subsequently, Dam and coworkers (1935, 1936) found that, although the condition was not cured by any of the known vitamins, it could be rapidly alleviated by feeding an unidentified fat-soluble substance. To this substance Dam gave the name *vitamin K* (*Koagulation* vitamin). Independently, Almquist and Stokstad (1935) described the same hemorrhagic disease in chickens and the method for its prevention.

These investigations were reported at a time when the attention of several groups of workers was centered on the cause of the hemorrhagic tendency in patients with obstructive jaundice and diseases of the liver. For example, Quick and coworkers (1935) observed that the coagulation defect in jaundiced individuals was due to a decrease in the concentration of prothrombin in the blood. In the same year, Hawkins and Whipple reported that animals with biliary fistulas were likely to develop excessive bleeding. Hawkins and Brinkhous (1936) subsequently showed that this was due to a deficiency in prothrombin and that the condition could be relieved by the feeding of bile salts.

The culmination of these experimental studies came with the demonstration of Butt and coworkers (1938) as well as Warner and associates (1938) that combination therapy with vitamin K and bile salts was effective in the treatment of the hemorrhagic diathesis in cases of jaundice. Thus, the relationship between vitamin K, adequate hepatic function, and the physiological mechanisms operating in the normal clotting of blood was established.

Occurrence and Chemistry. The early investigations described above showed that vitamin K is a fat-soluble substance present in hog liver fat and in alfalfa. Subsequently, it has been demonstrated that the vitamin is concentrated in the chloroplasts of plant leaves and in many vegetable oils. The feces of most species of animals contain large amounts of the vitamin, which is synthesized by the bacteria in the intestinal tract (*see* Bentley and Meganathan, 1982).

Vitamin K activity is associated with at least two distinct natural substances, designated as vitamin K_1 and vitamin K_2. Vitamin K_1, or phytonadione (phylloquinone), is 2-methyl-3-phytyl-1,4-naphthoquinone; vitamin K_2 represents a series of compounds (the menaquinones) in which the phytyl side chain of phytonadione has been replaced by a side chain built up of 2 to 13 prenyl units. Phytonadione is found in plants; it is the only natural vitamin K available for therapeutic use. The menaquinones are synthesized, in particular, by gram-positive bacteria.

Phytonadione (Vitamin K_1; Phylloquinone)

Menaquinone (Vitamin K_2) Series

A large number of natural and synthetic quinone derivatives have been tested for their vitamin K activity (*see* review by Isler and Wiss, 1959). Among those that possess activity approaching that of the natural vitamin is 2-methyl-1,4-naphthoquinone, commonly known as menadione or vitamin K_3, which is, depending on the bioassay system used, at least as active on a molar basis as phytonadione.

Menadione

The natural vitamins K and menadione are lipid soluble. It is possible to make active water-soluble derivatives of menadione by forming the sodium bisulfite salt or the tetrasodium salt of the diphosphoric acid ester. These compounds are converted in the body to menadione.

Pharmacological Actions and Physiological Function. In normal animals and man, phytonadione and the menaquinones are virtually devoid of pharmacodynamic activity. In animals and man deficient in vitamin K, the pharmacological action of vitamin K is identical to its normal physiological function, that is, to promote the hepatic biosynthesis of prothrombin (factor II), proconvertin (factor VII), plasma thromboplastin component (PTC, Christmas factor, factor IX), and the Stuart factor (factor X). The role of these factors in blood clotting is discussed in Chapter 58.

The vitamin K–dependent blood clotting factors, in the absence of vitamin K (or in the presence of the coumarin type of anticoagulant), are biologically inactive precursor proteins in the liver. Vitamin K functions as an essential cofactor for a microsomal enzyme system that activates these precursors by the conversion of multiple, peptide-bound residues of glutamic acid in each precursor to γ-carboxyglutamyl residues in the completed protein. The formation of this new amino acid, γ-carboxyglutamic acid, allows the protein to bind calcium ions and in turn to be bound to a phospholipid surface, both of which are necessary in the cascade of events that lead to clot formation (*see* Chapter 58; Nelsestuen, 1978). The exact mechanism of involvement of vitamin K in this carboxylation reaction has not yet been completely elucidated. The active form of vitamin K appears to be the reduced vitamin K hydroquinone, which, in the presence of O_2, CO_2, and the microsomal carboxylase enzyme, is converted to its 2,3-epoxide at the same time γ-carboxylation takes place. The hydroquinone form of vitamin K is regenerated from the 2,3-epoxide by a coumarin-sensitive epoxide reductase (*see* Figure 58–2, page 1346; *see also* Stenflo, 1978; Suttie *et al.*, 1978). γ-Carboxyglutamate has also been found in proteins in bone (osteocalcin), blood (protein S and protein C), kidney, and elsewhere (*see* Galloway *et al.*, 1980). The functions of these newly discovered vitamin K–dependent proteins have yet to be elucidated, but they may share an involvement in calcium metabolism.

Human Requirement. There is no generally accepted figure for the human requirement of vitamin K; it appears to be extremely small. Frick and associates (1967) estimated the daily requirement, in patients made vitamin K deficient by a starvation diet and antibiotic therapy for 3 to 4 weeks, to be a minimum of 0.03 μg/kg of body weight; others place the daily requirement at 0.5 to 1 μg/kg (*see* Suttie, 1978). In the infant, 10 μg/kg of body weight of phytonadione is sufficient to prevent hypoprothrombinemia. Needs are satisfied by the average diet, and, in addition, the vitamin synthesized by intestinal bacteria is also available to the host. Recommendations of the Food and Nutrition Board of the National Research Council, are presented in Table XVI–2 (page 1548).

Symptoms of Deficiency. The chief clinical manifestation of vitamin K deficiency is an increased tendency to bleed. Ecchymoses, epistaxis, hematuria, gastrointestinal bleeding, and postoperative hemorrhage are common; intracranial hemorrhage may occur. Hemoptysis is uncommon. A further discussion of hypoprothrombinemia is presented in the section on oral anticoagulants (Chapter 58). The discovery of a γ-carboxyglutamate-containing protein in bone that is dependent upon vitamin K for its synthesis suggests that the fetal bone abnormalities associated with the administration of oral anticoagulants during the first trimester of pregnancy may be related to a deficiency of the vitamin.

Toxicity. Phytonadione and the menaquinones are nontoxic to animals, even when given in huge amounts. In man, rapid intravenous administration of phytonadione has produced flushing, dyspnea, chest pains, cardiovascular collapse, and rarely death (*see* Barash *et al.*, 1976). Whether these reactions were due to the vitamin itself or to the agents used to disperse and emulsify the preparation is not clear.

The administration of large doses of menadione and its derivatives to animals has resulted in the production of anemia, polycythemia, splenomegaly, renal and hepatic damage, and death. In man, menadione is irritating to the skin and the respiratory tract. Its solutions have vesicant properties. Menadione and its derivatives have been implicated in producing hemolytic anemia, hyperbilirubinemia, and kernicterus in the newborn, especially premature infants (*see* below). Menadione also can induce hemolysis in individuals who are genetically deficient in glucose-6-phosphate dehydrogenase. In patients who have severe hepatic disease, the administration of large doses of menadione or phytonadione may further depress function of the liver (*see* below).

Absorption, Fate, and Excretion. The mechanism of intestinal absorption of compounds with vitamin K activity varies with their solubility. Phytonadione and the menaquinones are adequately absorbed from the gastrointestinal tract only if bile salts are present. Menadione and its water-soluble derivatives, however, are absorbed even in the absence of bile (Shearer *et al.*, 1974). Phytonadione and the menaquinones are absorbed almost entirely by way of the lymph; menadione and its water-soluble derivatives enter the blood stream directly. Phytonadione is absorbed by an energy-dependent, saturable process in proximal portions of the small intestine; menaquinone and menadione are absorbed by diffusion in the distal portions of the small intestine and in the colon. Following intramuscular injection, both natural and synthetic vitamin K preparations are readily absorbed. After absorption, phytonadione is initially concentrated in the liver, but the concentration declines rapidly. Very little vitamin K accumulates in other tissues.

Phytonadione is rapidly metabolized to more polar metabolites that are excreted in the bile and urine. The major urinary metabolites result from shortening of the side chain to five or seven carbon atoms, yielding carboxylic acids that are conjugated with glucuronate prior to excretion. Treatment with a coumarin-type anticoagulant results in a marked increase in the amount of phytonadione-2,3-epoxide in liver and blood. Such treatment also increases the urinary excretion of phytonadione metabolites, primarily degradative products of phytonadione-2,3-epoxide. The biliary metabolites of phytonadione have not been identified (*see* Shearer *et al.*, 1974). Menadione is apparently reduced to the diol (hydroquinone) form and excreted as glucuronide and sulfate conjugates.

Apparently there is little storage of vitamin K in the body. The limited stores of the vitamin present in tissue are slowly destroyed. Under circumstances where lack of bile interferes with absorption of vitamin K, hypoprothrombinemia develops slowly over a period of several weeks.

Assay and Unitage. Drugs with vitamin K activity may be chemically assayed and do not require bioassay. For the determination of the vitamin K content of foods, an assay based upon the ability of the preparation to increase the prothrombin level of deficient chicks is employed.

Preparations. *Phytonadione (vitamin K_1, phylloquinone;* AQUAMEPHYTON, KONAKION, MEPHYTON) is a viscous liquid that is insoluble in water. It is marketed in 5-mg tablets, and in ampuls containing a dispersion of 2 or 10 mg/ml of phytonadione in a solution of buffered polysorbate and propylene glycol (KONAKION) or polyoxyethylated fatty acid derivatives and dextrose (AQUAMEPHYTON). KONAKION is administered only intramuscularly. AQUAMEPHYTON may be given by any parenteral route, although severe reactions including anaphylaxis have followed its intravenous injection; subcutaneous or intramuscular administration is preferred.

Menadione (vitamin K_3) is a bright-yellow crystalline powder that is practically insoluble in water. Menadione is available for oral administration in tablets containing 5 mg. *Menadiol sodium diphosphate* (SYNKAYVITE) is marketed for injection or as 5-mg tablets.

THERAPEUTIC USES

The rational therapeutic use of vitamin K is based on its ability to correct the bleeding tendency or hemorrhage associated with its deficiency. A deficiency of vitamin K and its attendant deficiency of prothrombin and related clotting factors can result from inadequate intake, absorption, or utilization of the vitamin, or as a consequence of the action of a vitamin K antagonist.

Inadequate Intake. After infancy, hypoprothrombinemia arising from a dietary deficiency of vitamin K is extremely rare, because not only is the vitamin present in many foods but also it is synthesized by intestinal bacteria. The combination of an inadequate diet and the prolonged use of drugs that inhibit intestinal bacterial growth may lead, however, to vitamin K deficiency (Frick *et al.*, 1967). Occasionally, the use of a poorly absorbed sulfonamide or a broad-spectrum antibiotic may of itself produce a hypoprothrombinemia that responds readily to small doses of vitamin K and reestablishment of normal bowel flora. The use of such antibiotics in patients who have other causes for hypoprothrombinemia or a deficiency of vitamin K may have profound consequences. Hypoprothrombinemia can occur in patients receiving prolonged intravenous alimentation (Ham, 1971).

Hypoprothrombinemia of the Newborn. Newborn infants have a hypoprothrombinemia due to vitamin K deficiency for a few days after birth, the time required to obtain an adequate dietary intake of the vitamin and to establish a normal intestinal bacterial flora. At birth, the normal infant has only 20 to 40% of the adult plasma concentrations of clotting factors II, VII, IX, and X. These concentrations decline even further during the first 2 or 3 days after birth, before they begin to rise toward the adult values. In premature infants and in infants with hemorrhagic disease of the newborn, these concentrations are depressed even further (*see* Aballi and deLamerens, 1962). Hemorrhagic disease of the newborn has been associated with breast feeding; human milk has low concentrations of vitamin K (*see* Sutherland *et al.*, 1967; Haroon *et al.*, 1982), and, in addition, the intestinal flora of breast-fed infants apparently lacks microorganisms that synthesize the vitamin (Keenan *et al.*, 1971). The recent increase in incidence of hemorrhagic disease of the newborn is believed to be a consequence of increased numbers of births outside of hospital and of breast feeding (*see* O'Connor *et al.*, 1983).

Administration of vitamin K to the normal newborn infant prevents the decline in concentration of the clotting factors on the days following birth; it does not, however, raise these concentrations to the adult level. Premature infants usually display less of a response to the administration of vitamin K. In the infant with hemorrhagic disease of the newborn, the administration of vitamin K raises the concentration of these clotting factors to the level normal for the newborn infant and controls the bleeding tendency within about 6 hours (Wefring, 1962).

Although small doses of menadione and its derivatives are considered safe, moderate doses have produced hemolytic anemia, hyperbilirubinemia, and kernicterus in newborn, especially premature, infants, even when administered to the mother prior to delivery. Menadione is excreted in part as a glucuronide and competes with bilirubin for a detoxication mechanism of limited capacity in the newborn. Moreover, menadione may induce some hemolysis, especially in the newborn infant with a congenital defect in erythrocyte glucose-6-phosphate dehydrogenase or with a low plasma concentration of alpha-tocopherol; this causes a further increase in the concentration of bilirubin.

The routine prophylactic administration of a small dose of phytonadione to the newborn infant is now recommended. Phytonadione is the drug of choice since it appears to be nontoxic. A single dose of 0.5 to 1 mg should be administered parenterally to the infant immediately after delivery. This dose may have to be increased or repeated if the mother has received anticoagulant or anticonvulsant drug therapy, or if the infant develops bleeding tendencies. Alternatively, some clinicians treat mothers who are receiving anticonvulsants with oral vitamin K prior to delivery (20 mg per day for 2 weeks) (*see* Vert and Deblay, 1981).

Infants 1 to 5 months old seem to be quite vulnerable to vitamin K deficiency, especially if they have not received prophylactic administration of the vitamin at birth. Infant formulas that do not contain cows' milk are frequently inadequate in vitamin K. Inadequate intake may be exacerbated by diarrhea, antibiotics that reduce intestinal flora, or any of the malabsorption syndromes (*see* below; *see also* Committee on Nutrition, 1971; Lukens, 1972).

Inadequate Absorption. Hypoprothrombinemia may be associated with either intrahepatic or extrahepatic biliary obstruction, because the lipid-soluble vitamin is poorly absorbed in the absence of bile. A severe defect in the intestinal absorption of fat from other causes can also interfere with absorption of the vitamin.

Biliary Obstruction or Fistula. Bleeding that accompanies obstructive jaundice or biliary fistula responds promptly to the administration of vitamin K. Oral phytonadione administered with bile salts is both safe and effective and should be used in the care of the jaundiced patient, both preoperatively and postoperatively. In the absence of significant hepatocellular disease, the prothrombin activity of the blood rapidly returns to normal. If for some reason oral administration is not feasible, a parenteral preparation should be employed. The usual dose is 10 mg of vitamin K or menadione per day.

The treatment of a patient during hemorrhage is more difficult. Significant hemorrhage will obviously require replacement of blood. In such cases transfusion of fresh blood or reconstituted fresh plasma accomplishes the dual purposes of combating shock and furnishing an immediate supply of prothrombin. Vitamin K should also be given. If biliary obstruction has caused injury to hepatic cells, the response to vitamin K therapy may be poor. Under these circumstances, bleeding associated with hypoprothrombinemia may require continuing administration of fresh blood or reconstituted plasma.

Malabsorption Syndromes. Various disorders that result in inadequate absorption from the intestinal tract may lead to a deficiency of vitamin K and hypoprothrombinemia. These include mucoviscidosis, sprue, regional enteritis and enterocolitis, ulcerative colitis, dysentery, and extensive resection of bowel. Since drugs that greatly reduce the bacterial population of the bowel are frequently used in many of these disorders, the availability of the vitamin may be further reduced. Moreover, dietary restrictions may also limit the availability of the vitamin. For immediate correction of the deficiency, parenteral therapy should be given.

Inadequate Utilization. *Hepatocellular Disease.* Hypoprothrombinemia may accompany or follow hepatocellular disease, for example, toxic or infectious hepatitis, or advanced cirrhosis. Hepatocellular damage may also be secondary to long-lasting obstruction of bile ducts. In these conditions the damaged parenchymal cells may not be able to produce the vitamin K–dependent clotting factors, even if excess vitamin is available. Thus, hypoprothrombinemia under these circumstances is usually not favorably influenced by the administration of vitamin K. However, in some instances an inadequate secretion of bile salts may contribute to the syndrome and some benefit may be obtained from the parenteral administration of 10 mg of phytonadione daily. Paradoxically, the administration of large doses of vitamin K or its analogs in an attempt to correct the hypoprothrombinemia associated with severe hepatitis or cirrhosis may actually result in a further depression of the concentration of prothrombin. The mechanism for this is unknown. The vitamin does not, apparently, further depress hepatic function.

Drug-Induced Hypoprothrombinemia. Anticoagulant drugs such as warfarin and its congeners act as competitive antagonists of vitamin K and interfere with the hepatic biosynthesis of prothrombin and factors VII, IX, and X. The mechanism of this antagonism has been discussed above and in Chapter 58. These proteins then disappear from the blood at rates dependent on their individual turnover rates: factor VII declines first, followed by factor IX, factor X, and prothrombin.

Excessive hypoprothrombinemia or bleeding produced by the administration of oral anticoagulants can be corrected in a period of a few hours by the administration of vitamin K. Phytonadione is much more effective than menadione or its derivatives and should be used to counteract the effects of overdosage or overresponse to these anticoagulants. Mild overdosage may be treated simply by drug withdrawal or reduction of the dose, or by the administration of a single dose of 2.5 to 10 mg of phytonadione. Larger doses of the vitamin may interfere with subsequent oral anticoagulant therapy for several days. If bleeding is severe, the immediate administration of 20 to 40 mg of phytonadione is indicated. Additional doses at 4-hour intervals may be necessary to return the prothrombin time to normal. Transfusion of fresh whole blood, frozen plasma, or concentrates of the vitamin K–dependent clotting factors may also be needed.

If severe hypoprothrombinemia should occur as a result of the administration of large amounts of salicylate, the treatment is the same as that outlined for warfarin-induced hypoprothrombinemia, after withdrawal of the salicylate.

Vitamin K may be of help in combating the bleeding and hypoprothrombinemia following the bite of the tropical American pit viper or other species whose venom destroys or inactivates prothrombin.

VITAMIN E

In animals, the signs of deficiency of vitamin E include structural and functional abnormalities of many organs and organ systems. Attending these morphological alterations are biochemical defects that appear to involve fatty acid metabolism and numerous other enzyme systems. Notable is the fact that many signs and symptoms of vitamin E deficiency in animals superficially resemble disease states in humans; however, there is little unequivocal evidence that vitamin E is of nutritional significance in man.

History. The existence of vitamin E was first demonstrated in 1922 by Evans and Bishop, who found that female rats required a then-unrecognized dietary principle in order to sustain a normal pregnancy. Deficient animals were found to ovulate and conceive normally, but at some time during the period of gestation death and resorption of the fetuses occurred. Lesions in the testes were also described, and for a while vitamin E was referred to as the "antisterility vitamin." Further studies, however, revealed the more widespread effects of deficiency of the vitamin (*see* below).

Chemistry. The vitamin was isolated by Evans and coworkers (1936) from wheat germ oil. Eight naturally occurring tocopherols with vitamin E activity are now known. Alpha-tocopherol (5,7,8-trimethyl tocol) is considered to be the most important tocopherol since it comprises about 90% of the tocopherols in animal tissues and displays the greatest biological activity in most bioassay systems. It was identified chemically by Fernholtz (1938). Optical isomerism affects activity; *d* forms are more active than *l* forms.

Alpha-tocopherol

Alpha-tocopherol bears a striking structural similarity to the 6-chromanol form of coenzyme Q_4, with which it shares biological activity in several systems.

One of the important chemical features of the tocopherols is that they are antioxidants, and this apparently is the basis for most, if not all, of the effects of vitamin E (*see* Machlin, 1980). The tocopherols deteriorate slowly when exposed to air or ultraviolet light.

Pharmacological Actions and Physiological Functions. Aside from relieving symptoms of its deficiency in animals, vitamin E displays no notable pharmacological effects or toxicity. Numerous contradictory findings and claims for the actions and mechanisms of action characterize the literature on vitamin E. In acting as an antioxidant, vitamin E presumably prevents oxidation of essential cellular constituents, such as ubiquinone (coenzyme Q), or prevents the formation of toxic oxidation products, such as the peroxidation products formed from unsaturated fatty acids that have been detected in its absence. Diets high in polyunsaturated fatty acids increase an animal's requirement for vitamin E (*see* Witting, 1972). However, other chemically unrelated substances, such as synthetic antioxidants, selenium, some sulfur-containing amino acids, and the coenzyme Q group, are able to prevent or reverse some of the symptoms of vitamin E deficiency in animal species (*see* Wasserman and Taylor, 1972). In animals, supplemental vitamin E also affords protection against various drugs, metals, and chemicals that can initiate free-radical formation. However, no such protection has been observed in man (*see* Bieri *et al.,* 1983). Some symptoms of vitamin E deficiency in animals are not relieved by other antioxidants, and it is presumed in these cases that the vitamin is acting in a more specific manner (*see* Green, 1972).

There is an apparent relationship between vitamins A and E. The intestinal absorption of vitamin A is enhanced by vitamin E, and hepatic and other cellular concentrations of vitamin A are elevated; this may be related to its protection by the antioxidant properties of vitamin E. In addition, vitamin E seems to protect against various effects of hypervitaminosis A (*see* Underwood, 1984).

Symptoms of Deficiency. Although manifestations of vitamin E deficiency in experimental animals are protean, various effects on the nervous, reproductive, muscular, cardiovascular, and hematopoietic systems are most important because they bear the closest resemblance to the clinical syndromes alleged to be benefited by vitamin E therapy.

Nervous System. In animals, particularly rats, vitamin E deficiency is associated with axonal dystrophy that involves degeneration in the posterior cord and in the gracile and cuneate nuclei. Several recent reports suggest a relationship between vitamin E deficiency and a similar clinical syndrome. Patients with hepatobiliary disease, cystic fibrosis, or other malabsorption syndromes (each of which is associated with decreased absorption or transport of vitamin E) develop similar neurological symptoms, including hyporeflexia, gait disturbances, decreased proprioception, ophthalmoplegia, and retinopathy. Neuropathological lesions, including axonal degeneration of the posterior cord and the gracile nucleus, are comparable to those found in animals deficient in vitamin E. In some studies, treatment of patients with pharmacological doses of vitamin E prevented progression of the neurological abnormalities or caused improvement (*see* Bieri *et al.,* 1983). However, the pathogenesis of these lesions and their relationship to vitamin E are unknown.

Reproductive System. Early evidence indicated that vitamin E is essential for normal reproduction in several mammalian species below the primate level. In the male rat, for example, prolonged deficiency produces irreversible sterility due to degeneration of the germinal epithelium. In the vitamin E–deficient female, pregnancy terminates in about 10 days with fetal death and resorption of the uterine contents. The fundamental mechanism by which vitamin E deficiency interferes with reproduction is apparently related to its antioxidant properties. As mentioned above, the amounts of vitamin E and unsaturated fatty acids in the diet affect reproduction, and antioxidants incorporated into the diet can completely obviate the need for vitamin E for normal growth and reproduction in the rat (*see* Machlin, 1980).

On the basis of such animal studies, vitamin E has been used clinically for the treatment of recurrent abortion and for sterility in both men and women. It has also been used in toxemia of pregnancy, disorders of menstruation, vaginitis, and menopausal symptoms. In spite of early enthusiastic usage of vitamin E, there is no conclusive evidence that the vitamin is beneficial in any of these conditions.

Muscular System. In many species a vitamin E–deficient diet leads to the development of a necrotizing myopathy that resembles muscular dystrophy. In addition to well-defined anatomical lesions, metabolic abnormalities, including creatinuria, increased oxygen uptake of affected muscles, and changes in the activity of numerous enzyme systems, are also seen (Mason, 1973; Machlin, 1980). The anatomical and biochemical changes can be prevented, reversed, or ameliorated with alpha-tocopherol or other lipid-soluble antioxidants. The pathogenesis of the dystrophy is unknown. Tappel and associates (1963) attributed tissue damage to the release of cathepsin, ribonuclease, β-galactosidase, and sulfatase from lysosomes damaged by the action of fatty acid peroxidation products. Even though a similar myopathy accompanies vitamin E deficiency in the monkey, there is no evidence of a vitamin E deficiency or a therapeutic response to the administration of the vitamin in muscular dystrophy in man (Berneske *et al.,* 1960).

Cardiovascular System. The lesions produced in skeletal muscle by a deficiency of vitamin E apparently are also found in cardiac muscle of several species, although involvement of the heart is generally less common and less severe. The cardiac lesions are sometimes associated with ECG alteration, pathological changes, and even heart failure. On this basis, vitamin E has been used in many types of cardiac disorders, including angina and congestive heart failure, and in peripheral vascular disease in man. Carefully controlled clinical studies have failed to demonstrate any benefit from the vitamin (*see* Olsen, 1973).

Hematopoietic System. In several animal species a deficiency of vitamin E is associated with an anemia that has features of both abnormal hematopoiesis and decreased lifetime of erythrocytes. Erythrocytes from such animals have increased susceptibility to hemolysis by oxidizing agents. Indeed, in man this *in-vitro* laboratory test is the only consistent finding associated with low levels of tocopherol in plasma (*see* Leonard and Losowsky, 1967). Presumably, tocopherol protects the lipids in the erythrocyte membrane from peroxidation, which results in membrane destruction and hemolysis. Although the half-life of the human erythrocyte is reduced in individuals with low concentrations of tocopherol in plasma, anemia is not a usual problem. Limited clinical studies in patients with hemolysis due to a genetic deficiency of erythrocytic glucose-6-phosphate dehydrogenase suggest that chronic treatment with large doses of vitamin E may improve survival of erythrocytes and the clinical condition (Corash *et al.,* 1980).

Four clinical situations have been reported to include alpha-tocopherol–responsive anemia (*see* Darby, 1968; Symposium, 1968). (1) A macrocytic, megaloblastic anemia observed in children with severe protein-calorie malnutrition, while unresponsive to treatment with iron, cyanocobalamin, folic acid, or ascorbic acid, was successfully reversed with large doses of alpha-tocopherol acetate. However, subsequent controlled studies have attributed the defective hematopoiesis to deficiency of protein and/or iron rather than to vitamin E (*see* Bieri and Farrell, 1976). (2) Premature infants may develop a hemolytic anemia that is sometimes associated with increased erythrocyte susceptibility to peroxidative hemolysis and low concentrations of tocopherol in plasma. This anemia has been shown to develop only in infants who consume a diet rich in polyunsaturated fatty acids and fortified with iron (Williams *et al.*, 1975). Commercial formulas for premature infants have been modified, such that they now are very low in iron and have an appropriate ratio of vitamin E to fatty acids. It no longer appears to be necessary to administer vitamin E supplements to premature infants on a routine basis (*see* Bieri *et al.*, 1983). (3) Erythrocytes that hemolyze spontaneously *in vitro* constitute one characteristic of the acanthocytosis syndrome. Patients with this rare genetic disease lack plasma β-lipoprotein and, therefore, have little or no circulating alpha-tocopherol. Further, they have impaired intestinal absorption of the vitamin. Parenteral administration of 100 mg of alpha-tocopherol acetate can raise the plasma alpha-tocopherol concentrations and apparently correct the autohemolytic feature of the disease for several weeks. (4) In malabsorption syndromes characterized by steatorrhea (*e.g.*, sprue, mucoviscidosis, chronic pancreatitis), alpha-tocopherol is not absorbed. Here, too, decreased erythrocyte lifetime and increased erythrocyte sensitivity to hydrogen peroxide are coincident with low concentrations of alpha-tocopherol in plasma and are responsive to administration of alpha-tocopherol. Adult man, intentionally deprived of vitamin E over an extended period of time, has similar hematological lesions and responds to alpha-tocopherol (Horwitt *et al.*, 1963).

While the evidence outlined above seems to implicate vitamin E in normal hematopoiesis, other factors must also be considered. Patients with each of the above syndromes have multiple deficiencies. Furthermore, the ability of the coenzymes Q, selenium, other antioxidants, and the sulfur-amino acids to relieve "tocopherol-deficient" syndromes to varying degrees provides further complications for a definitive interpretation. (*See* Bieri and Farrell, 1976; Machlin, 1980.)

Human Requirement. In a long-term controlled study of vitamin E depletion in man, Horwitt and coworkers (*see* Horwitt, 1962) found that vitamin E concentration in plasma declined significantly only after months on a deficient diet. There were no clinical manifestations of the depletion. From these studies, Horwitt estimated that a daily intake of 10 to 30 mg of vitamin E is sufficient to maintain vitamin E concentrations in blood within the normal range. Although some studies have suggested that diets containing large amounts of unsaturated fatty acids increase the daily requirement (Witting,

1972), it should be noted that dietary sources of these fats are also rich in vitamin E (*see* Bieri *et al.*, 1983). Diets containing selenium, sulfur-amino acids, chromenols, or antioxidants decrease the requirement.

The recommendations of the Food and Nutrition Board of the National Research Council include 10 mg of *d*-alpha-tocopherol per day for adult men and 8 mg of *d*-alpha-tocopherol per day for adult women. (*See* Table XVI–1, page 1546.) Human milk (in contrast to cows' milk) has sufficient alpha-tocopherol to meet normal requirements of infants. Tocopherols are present in adequate amounts in the normal adult diet. Indeed, vitamin E deficiency has not been detected as a primary deficiency disease in otherwise-healthy children or adults.

Absorption, Fate, and Excretion. Vitamin E is absorbed from the gastrointestinal tract by a mechanism probably similar to that for the other fat-soluble vitamins; bile is essential (MacMahon and Neale, 1970). When administered as an ester, hydrolysis takes place in the intestine. Vitamin E enters the blood stream by way of the lymph. It appears first in chylomicrons and then is primarily associated with plasma β-lipoproteins. Vitamin E is distributed to all tissues. However, newborn infants have plasma tocopherol concentrations only about one fifth those of their mothers, suggesting poor placental transfer. Tissue stores can provide a source of the vitamin for long periods of time, as evidenced by the long time animals must be kept on a vitamin E–deficient diet before signs of deficiency appear.

Seventy to 80% of an intravenously administered dose of radioactive vitamin E is excreted by the liver over a period of a week; the balance appears as metabolites in the urine. The urinary metabolites are glucuronides of tocopheronic acid and its γ-lactone. Several other metabolites with quinone structures have been found in tissues; dimer and trimer forms of the vitamin are believed to result from reaction with lipid peroxides (*see* Draper and Csallany, 1970).

Plasma concentrations vary widely among normal individuals. Many attempts have been made to correlate the plasma tocopherol values with disease states. In general, tocopherol concentrations in plasma appear to be related more closely to dietary intake and defects in intestinal absorption of fat than to the presence or absence of disease. Low tocopherol values are generally associated, however, with an increased susceptibility of erythrocytes to hemolysis by oxidizing agents (Leonard and Losowsky, 1967).

Assay and Unitage. The vitamin E activity of foods may be determined chemically, or bioassayed for the protection afforded pregnant female rats against death of the fetus. One international unit (I.U.) is equivalent to the activity of 1 mg of *dl*-alpha-tocopheryl acetate. *d*-Alpha-tocopheryl acetate has a potency of 1.36 I.U./mg; *d*-alpha-tocopherol, 1.49 I.U./mg; *d*-alpha-tocopheryl succinate, 1.21 I.U./mg. The activity of 1 mg of *d*-alpha-tocopherol is equal to 1 alpha-tocopherol equivalent.

Preparations. *Vitamin E* is a form of alpha-tocopherol that includes the *d* or the *d* and *l* isomers of alpha-tocopherol, alpha-tocopheryl acetate, or alpha-tocopheryl succinate. Tablets and capsules of many sizes are available (50 to 1000 I.U.), as are injectable forms (200 I.U./ml) and drops (50 I.U./ml).

Therapeutic Uses. The lack of efficacy of vitamin E in treatment of those diseases in man that bear some resemblance to vitamin E deficiency in animals, namely, recurrent abortion, progressive muscular dystrophy, and cardiovascular disease, has been discussed. These are by no means the only disorders in which vitamin E therapy has been studied. The list extends from minor skin ailments to schizophrenia.

The use of vitamin E supplements may be indicated for patients at risk of developing deficiency of the vitamin in order to prevent or ameliorate the consequences of axonal dystrophy (*see* above). Pharmacological doses of vitamin E have been utilized as an antioxidant in premature infants exposed to high concentrations of oxygen; thus, prophylactic use of an oral preparation (100 mg/kg per day) may reduce the incidence and severity of retrolental fibroplasia (*see* Hittner *et al.*, 1981). Only equivocal results have been obtained in the neonatal respiratory-distress syndrome. With the possible exception mentioned above, there is little persuasive evidence that supports a significant therapeutic role for vitamin E in man.

Aballi, A. J., and deLamerens, S. Coagulation changes in the neonatal period and in early infancy. *Pediatr. Clin. North Am.*, **1962**, *9*, 785–815.

Adachi, N.; Smith, J. E.; Sklan, D.; and Goodman, DeW. S. Radioimmunoassay studies of the tissue distribution and subcellular localization of cellular retinol-binding protein in rats. *J. Biol. Chem.*, **1981**, *256*, 9471–9476.

Almquist, H. J., and Stokstad, C. L. R. Hemorrhagic chick disease of dietary origin. *J. Biol. Chem.*, **1935**, *111*, 105–113.

Barash, P.; Kitahata, L. M.; and Mandel, S. Acute cardiovascular collapse after intravenous phytonadione. *Anesth. Analg. Curr. Res.*, **1976**, *55*, 304–306.

Bashor, M. M.; Toft, D. O.; and Chytil, F. *In vitro* binding of retinol to rat-tissue components. *Proc. Natl Acad. Sci. U.S.A.*, **1973**, *70*, 3483–3487.

Berneske, G. M.; Butson, A. R. C.; Gauld, E. N.; and Levy, D. Clinical trial of high dosage vitamin E in human muscular dystrophy. *Can. Med. Assoc. J.*, **1960**, *82*, 418–421.

Bernhardt, I. B., and Dorsey, D. J. Hypervitaminosis A and congenital renal anomalies in a human infant. *Obstet. Gynecol.*, **1974**, *43*, 750–755.

Bieri, J. G., and McKenna, M. C. Expressing dietary values for fat-soluble vitamins: changes in concepts and terminology. *Am. J. Clin. Nutr.*, **1981**, *34*, 289–295.

Bjelke, E. Dietary vitamin A and human lung cancer. *Int. J. Cancer*, **1975**, *15*, 561–565.

Bollag, W. Therapy of epithelial tumors with an aromatic retinoic acid analog. *Chemotherapy*, **1975**, *21*, 236–247.

Brazzell, R. K., and Colburn, W. A. Pharmacokinetics of the retinoids isotretinoin and etretinate. *J. Am. Acad. Dermatol.*, **1982**, *6*, 643–651.

Breitman, T. R.; Selonick, S. E.; and Collin, S. J. Induction of differentiation of the human promyelocytic leukemia cell line (HL60) by retinoic acid. *Proc. Natl Acad. Sci. U.S.A.*, **1980**, *77*, 2936–2940.

Butt, H. R.; Snell, A. M.; and Osterberg, A. E. The use of vitamin K and bile in treatment of hemorrhagic diathesis in cases of jaundice. *Proc. Staff Meet. Mayo Clin.*, **1938**, *13*, 74–80.

Chytil, F., and Ong, D. E. Cellular retinol- and retinoic acid–binding proteins. *Adv. Nutr. Res.*, **1983**, *5*, 13–29.

Committee on Nutrition, American Academy of Pediatrics. Vitamin K supplementation for infants receiving milk substitute infant formulas and for those with fat malabsorption. *Pediatrics*, **1971**, *48*, 483–487.

Corash, L.; Spielberg, S.; Bartsocas, C.; Boxer, L.; Steinherz, R.; Sheetz, M.; Egan, M.; Schlessleman, J.; and Schulman, J. D. Reduced chronic hemolysis during high-dose vitamin E administration in Mediterranean-type glucose-6-phosphate dehydrogenase deficiency. *N. Engl. J. Med.*, **1980**, *303*, 416–420.

Dam, H., and Schønheyder, F. The antihaemorrhagic vitamin of the chick. *Nature*, **1935**, *135*, 652–653.

Dam, H.; Schønheyder, F.; and Tage-Hansen, E. Studies on the mode of action of vitamin K. *Biochem. J.*, **1936**, *30*, 1075–1079.

Draper, H. H., and Csallany, A. S. Metabolism of vitamin E. In, *The Fat Soluble Vitamins*. (DeLuca, H. F., and Suttie, J. W., eds.) University of Wisconsin Press, Madison, **1970**, pp. 347–353.

Euler, B. von; Euler, H. von; and Karrer, P. Zur Biochemie der Carotinoide. *Helv. Chim. Acta*, **1929**, *12*, 278–285.

Evans, H. M., and Bishop, K. S. On the relationship between fertility and nutrition. II. The ovulation rhythm in the rat on inadequate nutritional regimes. *J. Metab. Res.*, **1922**, *1*, 319–356.

Evans, H. M.; Emerson, O. H.; and Emerson, G. A. The isolation from wheat germ oil of an alcohol, α-tocopherol, having properties of vitamin E. *J. Biol. Chem.*, **1936**, *113*, 329–332.

Fernholtz, E. On the constitution of α-tocopherol. *J. Am. Chem. Soc.*, **1938**, *60*, 700–705.

Fisher, K. D.; Carr, C. J.; Huff, J. E.; and Huber, T. E. Dark adaptation and night vision. *Fed. Proc.*, **1970**, *29*, 1605–1638.

Food and Nutrition Board, National Research Council. Fat-soluble vitamins. Vitamin A. In, *Recommended Dietary Allowances*, 9th ed. National Academy of Sciences, Washington, D. C., **1980**, pp. 55–60.

Frick, P. G.; Riedler, G.; and Brögli, H. Dose response and minimal daily requirement for vitamin K in man. *J. Appl. Physiol.*, **1967**, *23*, 387–389.

Fuchs, E., and Green, H. Regulation of terminal differentiation of cultured human keratinocytes by vitamin A. *Cell*, **1981**, *25*, 617–625.

George, J. S., and Hagins, W. A. Control of Ca^{2+} in rod outer segment disks by light and cyclic GMP. *Nature*, **1983**, *303*, 344–348.

Goodman, DeW. S. Vitamin A metabolism. *Fed. Proc.*, **1980**, *39*, 2716–2722.

Goodman, DeW. S.; Blomstrand, R.; Werner, B.; Huang, H. S.; and Shiratori, T. The intestinal absorption and metabolism of vitamin A and β-carotene in man. *J. Clin. Invest.*, **1966**, *45*, 1615–1623.

Green, J. Vitamin E and the biological antioxidant theory. *Ann. N.Y. Acad. Sci.*, **1972**, *203*, 29–44.

Ham, J. M. Hypoprothrombinemia in patients undergoing prolonged intensive care. *Med. J. Aust.*, **1971**, *2*, 716–718.

Haroon, Y.; Shearer, M. J.; Rabin, S.; Bunn, W. G.;

McEnery, G.; and Barkhan, P. The content of phyll-oquinone (vitamin K_1) in human milk, cows' milk, and infant formula foods determined by high-performance liquid chromatography. *J. Nutr.*, **1982**, *112*, 1105–1117.

Harris, B. A.; Robishaw, J. D.; Mumby, S. M.; and Gilman, A. G. Molecular cloning of cDNA for the alpha subunit of the G protein that stimulates adenylate cyclase. *Science*, **1985**, *229*.

Hawkins, W. B., and Brinkhous, K. M. Prothrombin deficiency the cause of bleeding in bile fistula dogs. *J. Exp. Med.*, **1936**, *63*, 795–801.

Hecht, S. Rods, cones, and chemical basis of vision. *Physiol. Rev.*, **1937**, *17*, 239–290.

Herbert, V. Toxicity of 25,000 IU vitamin A supplements in "health" food users. *Am. J. Clin. Nutr.*, **1982**, *36*, 185–186.

Hittner, H. M.; Godio, L. B.; Rudolph, A. J.; Adams, J. M.; Garcia-Prats, J. A.; Friedman, Z.; Kautz, J. A.; and Monaco, W. A. Retrolental fibroplasia: efficacy of vitamin E in a double-blind clinical study of preterm infants. *N. Engl. J. Med.*, **1981**, *305*, 1365–1371.

Horwitt, M. K. Interrelations between vitamin E and polyunsaturated fatty acids in adult men. *Vitam. Horm.*, **1962**, *20*, 541–558.

Horwitt, M. K.; Century, B.; and Zeman, A. A. Erythrocyte survival time and reticulocyte level after tocopherol depletion in man. *Am. J. Clin. Nutr.*, **1963**, *12*, 99–106.

Hubbard, R.; Bownds, D.; and Yoshizawa, T. The chemistry of visual photoreception. *Cold Spring Harbor Symp. Quant. Biol.*, **1965**, *30*, 301–315.

Hurley, J. B.; Simon, M. I.; Teplow, D. B.; Robishaw, J. D.; and Gilman, A. G. Homologies between signal transducing G proteins and *ras* gene products. *Science*, **1984**, *226*, 860–862.

Karrer, P.; Morf, R.; and Schöpp, K. Zur Kenntnis des Vitamins A aus Fischtranen. *Helv. Chim. Acta*, **1931**, *14*, 1431–1436.

Keenan, W. J.; Jewett, T.; and Glueck, H. I. Role of feeding and vitamin K in hypoprothrombinemia of the newborn. *Am. J. Dis. Child.*, **1971**, *121*, 271–277.

Lasnitzki, I. The influence of A hypervitaminosis on the effect of 20-methylcholanthrene on mouse prostate glands grown *in vitro*. *Br. J. Cancer*, **1955**, *9*, 434–441.

Leo, M. A., and Lieber, C. S. Hepatic vitamin A depletion in alcoholic liver injury. *N. Engl. J. Med.*, **1982**, *307*, 597–601.

Leonard, P. J., and Losowsky, M. S. Relationship between plasma vitamin E level and peroxide hemolysis test in human subjects. *Am. J. Clin. Nutr.*, **1967**, *20*, 795–798.

Liau, G.; Ong, D. E.; and Chytil, F. Interaction of the retinol/cellular retinol-binding protein complex with isolated nuclei and nuclear components. *J. Cell Biol.*, **1981**, *91*, 63–68.

Lochrie, M. A.; Hurley, J. B.; and Simon, M. I. Sequence of the alpha subunit of photoreceptor G protein: homologies between transducin, *ras*, and elongation factors. *Science*, **1985**, *228*, 96–99.

Lukens, J. H. Vitamin K and the older infant. *Am. J. Dis. Child.*, **1972**, *124*, 639–640.

McCollum, E. V., and Davis, M. The necessity of certain lipins in the diet during growth. *J. Biol. Chem.*, **1913**, *15*, 167–175.

MacMahon, M. T., and Neale, E. The absorption of α-tocopherol in control subjects and in patients with intestinal malabsorption. *Clin. Sci.*, **1970**, *38*, 197–210.

Mallia, A. K.; Smith, J. E.; and Goodman, D. S. Metabolism of retinol-binding protein and vitamin A during hypervitaminosis in the rat. *J. Lipid Res.*, **1975**, *16*, 180–188.

Moore, T. Relation of carotin to vitamin A. *Lancet*, **1929**, *2*, 380–381.

Nelsestuen, G. L. Interaction of vitamin K–dependent proteins with calcium ions and phospholipid membranes. *Fed. Proc.*, **1978**, *37*, 2621–2625.

Newton, D. L.; Henderson, W. R.; and Sporn, M. B. Structure-activity relationships of retinoids in hamster tracheal organ culture. *Cancer Res.*, **1980**, *40*, 3414–3425.

O'Brien, D. F. The chemistry of vision. *Science*, **1982**, *218*, 961–966.

O'Connor, M. E.; Livingstone, D. S.; Hennah, J.; and Wilkins, D. Vitamin K deficiency and breast-feeding. *Am. J. Dis. Child.*, **1983**, *137*, 601–602.

Olsen, R. E. Vitamin E and its relation to heart disease. *Circulation*, **1973**, *48*, 179–184.

Ong, D. E., and Chytil, F. Retinoic acid binding protein in rat tissue. Partial purification and comparison to rat tissue retinol-binding protein. *J. Biol. Chem.*, **1975**, *250*, 6113–6117.

Osborne, T. B., and Mendel, L. B. The relation of growth to the chemical constituents of the diet. *J. Biol. Chem.*, **1913**, *15*, 311–326.

Quick, A. J.; Stanley-Brown, M.; and Bancroft, F. W. A study of the coagulation defect in hemophilia and in jaundice. *Am. J. Med. Sci.*, **1935**, *190*, 501–511.

Report of the Council on Foods and Nutrition. Deficiencies of the fat-soluble vitamins. *J.A.M.A.*, **1950**, *144*, 34–45.

Rosso, G. C.; DeLuca, L.; Warren, C. D.; and Wolf, G. Enzymatic synthesis of mannosyl retinyl phosphate from retinyl phosphate and guanosine diphosphate mannose. *J. Lipid Res.*, **1975**, *16*, 235–243.

Russell, F. E. Vitamin A content of polar bear liver. *Toxicon*, **1967**, *5*, 61–62.

Simpson, K. L. Relative value of carotenoids as precursors of vitamin A. *Proc. Nutr. Soc.*, **1983**, *42*, 7–17.

Smith, F. R., and Goodman, D. S. Vitamin A transport in human vitamin A toxicity. *N. Engl. J. Med.*, **1976**, *294*, 805–808.

Sporn, M. B., and Roberts, A. B. Role of retinoids in differentiation and carcinogenesis. *Cancer Res.*, **1983**, *43*, 3034–3040.

Steenbock, H. White corn vs. yellow corn, and a probable relation between the fat-soluble vitamin and yellow plant pigments. *Science*, **1919**, *50*, 352–353.

Strickland, S., and Mahdavi, V. The induction of differentiation in teratocarcinoma stem cells by retinoic acid. *Cell*, **1978**, *15*, 393–403.

Sutherland, J. M.; Glueck, H. I.; and Glaser, G. Hemorrhagic disease of the newborn. Breast feeding as a necessary factor in the pathogenesis. *Am. J. Dis. Child.*, **1967**, *113*, 524–533.

Suttie, J. W.; Larson, A. E.; Canfield, L. M.; and Carlisle, T. L. Relationship between vitamin K–dependent carboxylation and vitamin K epoxidation. *Fed. Proc.*, **1978**, *37*, 2605–2614.

Tappel, A. L.; Savant, P. L.; and Shibko, S. Lysosomes: distribution in animals, hydrolytic capacity and other properties. In, *Lysosomes* (a Ciba Foundation symposium). (de Reuck, A. V. S., and Cameron, M. P., eds.) Little, Brown & Co., Boston; J. & A. Churchill, Ltd., London, **1963**.

Vert, P., and Deblay, M. F. Hemorrhagic disorders in infants of epileptic mothers. In, *Epilepsy, Pregnancy and the Child*. (Janz, D.; Bossi, L.; Daum, M.; Helge, H.; Richens, A.; and Schmidt, D.; eds.) Raven Press, New York, **1981**, pp. 387–388.

Wald, G. The molecular basis of visual excitation. *Nature*, **1968**, *219*, 800–807.

Wald, G., and Brown, P. K. Human color vision and color blindness. *Cold Spring Harbor Symp. Quant. Biol.*, **1965**, *30*, 345–361.

Ward, A.; Brogden, R. N.; Heel, R. C.; Speight, T. N.; and Avery, G. S. Etretinate. A review of its pharmacological properties and therapeutic efficacy in psoriasis and other skin disorders. *Drugs*, **1983**, *26*, 9–43.

Warner, E. D.; Brinkhous, K. M.; and Smith, H. P. Bleeding tendency of obstructive jaundice: prothrombin deficiency and dietary factors. *Proc. Soc. Exp. Biol. Med.*, **1938**, *37*, 628–630.

Wefring, K. W. Hemorrhage in the newborn and vitamin K prophylaxis. *J. Pediatr.*, **1962**, *61*, 686–692.

Wiggert, B.; Bergsma, D. R.; Helmsen, R.; and Chader, G. J. Vitamin A receptors. Retinoic acid binding in ocular tissue. *Biochem. J.*, **1978**, *169*, 87–94.

Williams, M. L.; Shott, R. J.; O'Neal, P. L.; and Oski, F. A. Role of dietary iron and fat in vitamin E deficiency anemia of infancy. *N. Engl. J. Med.*, **1975**, *292*, 887–890.

Witting, L. A. The role of polyunsaturated fatty acids in determining vitamin E requirements. *Ann. N.Y. Acad. Sci.*, **1972**, *203*, 192–198.

Yaffe, S. J., and Filer, L. J. The use and abuse of vitamin A. American Academy of Pediatrics, Joint Committee Statement, Committee on Drugs and Nutrition. *Pediatrics*, **1971**, *48*, 655–656.

Monographs and Reviews

Bentley, R., and Meganathan, R. Biosynthesis of vitamin K (menaquinone) in bacteria. *Microbiol. Rev.*, **1982**, *46*, 241–280.

Bieri, J. G.; Corash, L.; and Hubbard, V. S. Medical uses of vitamin E. *N. Engl. J. Med.*, **1983**, *308*, 1063–1071.

Bieri, J. G., and Farrell, P. M. Vitamin E. *Vitam. Horm.*, **1976**, *34*, 31–75.

Bridges, C. D. B. Retinoids in photosensitive systems. In, *The Retinoids*, Vol. II. (Sporn, M. B.; Roberts, A. B.; and Goodman, DeW. S.; eds.) Academic Press, Inc., New York, **1984**, pp. 125–176.

Darby, W. J. Tocopherol-responsive anemias in man. *Vitam. Horm.*, **1968**, *26*, 685–699.

Galloway, P. M.; Lian, J. B.; and Hauschka, P. V. Carboxylated calcium-binding proteins and vitamin K. *N. Engl. J. Med.*, **1980**, *302*, 1460–1466.

Gilman, A. G. G proteins and dual control of adenylate cyclase. *Cell*, **1984**, *36*, 577–579.

Hill, D. L., and Grubbs, C. J. Retinoids as chemopreventive and anticancer agents in intact animals. *Anticancer Res.*, **1982**, *2*, 111–124.

Isler, O., and Wiss, O. Chemistry and biochemistry of the K vitamins. *Vitam. Horm.*, **1959**, *17*, 54–92.

Kamm, J. J.; Ashenfelter, K. O.; and Ehmann, C. W. Preclinical and clinical toxicology of selected retinoids. In, *The Retinoids*, Vol. II. (Sporn, M. B.; Roberts, A. B.; and Goodman, DeW. S.; eds.) Academic Press, Inc., New York, **1984**, pp. 287–326.

Machlin, L. J. (ed.). *Vitamin E: A Comprehensive Treatise*. Marcel Dekker, Inc., New York, **1980**.

Mason, K. E. Effects of nutritional deficiencies on muscle. In, *The Structure and Function of Muscle*, 2nd ed., Vol. 4. (Bourne, G. H., ed.) Academic Press, Inc., New York, **1973**, pp. 155–206.

Moon, R. C., and Itri, L. M. Retinoids and cancer. In, *The Retinoids*, Vol. II. (Sporn, M. B.; Roberts, A. B.; and Goodman, DeW. S.; eds.) Academic Press, Inc., New York, **1984**, pp. 327–371.

Parrish, D. B. Determination of vitamin A in foods—a review. *CRC Crit. Rev. Food Sci. Nutr.*, **1977**, *9*, 375–394.

Peck, G. L. Synthetic retinoids in dermatology. In, *The Retinoids*, Vol. II. (Sporn, M. B.; Roberts, A. B.; and Goodman, DeW. S.; eds.) Academic Press, Inc., New York, **1984**, pp. 391–411.

Shearer, M. J.; McBurney, A.; and Barkhan, P. Studies on the absorption and metabolism of phylloquinone (vitamin K_1) in man. *Vitam. Horm.*, **1974**, *32*, 513–542.

Sporn, M. B.; Roberts, A. B.; and Goodman, DeW. S. (eds.). *The Retinoids*, Vols. I and II. Academic Press, Inc., New York, **1984**.

Stenflo, J. Vitamin K, prothrombin, and gamma-carboxyglutamic acid. *Adv. Enzymol.*, **1978**, *46*, 1–31.

Suttie, J. W. Vitamin K. In, *Handbook of Lipid Research*, Vol. 2. (DeLuca, H. F., ed.) Plenum Press, New York, **1978**, pp. 211–277.

Symposium. (Various authors.) Hematological aspects of vitamin E. *Am. J. Clin. Nutr.*, **1968**, *21*, 1–56.

Symposium. (Various authors.) Oral retinoids—a workshop. (Strauss, J. D.; Windhorst, D. B.; and Weinstein, G. D.; eds.) *J. Am. Acad. Dermatol.*, **1982**, *6*, 573–832.

Underwood, B. A. Vitamin A in animal and human nutrition. In, *The Retinoids*, Vol. I. (Sporn, M. B.; Roberts, A. B.; and Goodman, DeW. S.; eds.) Academic Press, Inc., New York, **1984**, pp. 263–374.

Wasserman, R. H., and Taylor, A. N. Metabolic roles of fat-soluble vitamins D, E, and K. *Annu. Rev. Biochem.*, **1972**, *41*, 179–201.

CHAPTER

68 PRINCIPLES OF TOXICOLOGY

Curtis D. Klaassen

Toxicology is the science of the adverse effects of chemicals on living organisms. The discipline is often divided into several major areas. The *descriptive toxicologist* performs toxicity tests (described below) to obtain information that can be used to evaluate the risk that exposure to a chemical poses to man and the environment. The *mechanistic toxicologist* attempts to determine how chemicals exert deleterious effects on living organisms. Such studies are useful for the development of tests for the prediction of risks, to facilitate the search for safer chemicals, and for rational treatment of the manifestations of toxicity. The *regulatory toxicologist* judges if a drug or other chemical has a low enough risk to be made available for its intended purpose. The Food and Drug Administration (FDA) regulates drugs, medical devices, cosmetics, and food additives in interstate commerce. The Environmental Protection Agency (EPA) is responsible for regulation of pesticides, toxic chemicals, hazardous wastes, and toxic pollutants in water and air. The Occupational Safety and Health Administration (OSHA) determines whether employers are providing working conditions that are safe for employees. The Consumer Products Safety Commission regulates all articles sold for use in the home, school, or recreation, except those products that are regulated by the FDA and the EPA.

Two specialized areas of toxicology are particularly important for medicine. *Foren-sic toxicology,* wherein analytical chemistry and fundamental toxicological principles are hybridized, is concerned with the medicolegal aspects of the use of chemicals that are harmful to animals and man. Forensic toxicologists assist in post-mortem investigations to establish the cause or circumstances of death. *Clinical toxicology* focuses on diseases that are caused by or are uniquely associated with toxic substances. Clinical toxicologists treat patients who are poisoned by drugs and other chemicals and develop new technics for the diagnosis and treatment of such intoxications.

The physician must evaluate the possibility that a patient's signs and symptoms might be caused by toxic chemicals present in the environment or administered as therapeutic agents. Many of the adverse effects of drugs mimic those of disease. Appreciation of the principles of toxicology is necessary for the recognition and management of such problems.

DOSE-EFFECT RELATIONSHIP

Evaluation of the dose-response or the dose-effect relationship is crucially important to toxicologists (*see* Chapter 2). There is both a graded dose-response relationship in an *individual* and a quantal dose-response relationship in the *population.* Graded doses of a drug given to an individual usually result in a greater magnitude of response as the dose is increased. In a quantal dose-effect relationship, the percentage of the population affected increases as the dose is raised; the relationship is quantal in that the effect is specified to be either present or absent in a given individual. This quantal dose-effect phenomenon is extremely important in toxicology and is used to determine the *median lethal dose* (LD50) of drugs and other chemicals.

The LD50 is determined experimentally. The chemical is usually administered to mice or rats (orally or intraperitoneally) at several doses (usually four or five) in the lethal range (*see* Figure 2–6, page 46). To linearize such data, the response (deaths) can be converted to units of *deviation from the mean,* or *probits* (from the contraction of *probability units*). The probit designates the deviation from the median; a probit of 5 corresponds to a 50% response, and, since each probit equals one standard deviation, a probit of 4 equals 16% and a probit of 6 equals 84% (Klaassen, 1985). A plot of percent of population responding, in probit units, against log dose yields a straight line (Figure 68–1). The LD50 is determined by drawing a vertical line from the point where the probit unit = 5 (50% mortality). The slope of the dose-effect is also important. The LD50 for both compounds depicted in Figure 68–1 is the same (10 mg/kg). However, the slopes of the dose-response curves are quite different. At a dose equal to one half of the LD50 (5 mg/kg), less than 5% of the animals exposed to compound B would die, but 30% of the animals given compound A would die.

The quantal or "all-or-none" response is not limited to lethality. Similar dose-effect curves can be constructed for any toxic effect produced by chemicals.

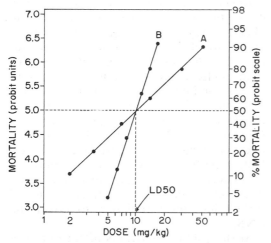

Figure 68–1. *Dose-response relationships.*

The logarithm of the dose is plotted versus the percentage of the population killed by two toxicants in probit units (*see* text).

TOXIC OR SAFE VERSUS RISK OR HAZARD

There obviously are marked differences in the LD50 of various chemicals. Some produce death in doses of a fraction of a microgram (LD50 for botulinus toxin = 10 pg/kg); others may be relatively harmless in doses of several grams or more. While categories of toxicity that are of some practicality have been devised, based on the amount required to produce death, it often is not easy to distinguish between toxic and nontoxic chemicals. Paracelsus (1493–1541) noted . . . "All substances are poisons; there is none which is not a poison. The right dose differentiates a poison and a remedy." *While society wants the toxicologist to categorize all chemicals as either safe or toxic, this is not possible.* The real concern is the *risk* or *hazard* associated with use of the chemical, not whether a chemical is toxic or safe. In the assessment of risk one must also consider the harmful effects of the chemical accrued directly or indirectly through adverse effects on the environment when used in the quantity and in the manner proposed. Depending on the use and disposition of a chemical, a very toxic compound may be less harmful, ultimately, than a relatively nontoxic one.

Assessment of *benefits* to individuals, society, and the environment clearly influences the acceptability of the risks of the use of a chemical. High risks may be acceptable with lifesaving drugs but cannot be tolerated for food additives. The level of acceptable risk depends on a number of factors: (1) the need met by the substance in question, (2) alternatives to the use of the compound, (3) anticipated extent of use by or exposure of the public, (4) economic considerations, (5) effects on the quality of the environment, and (6) conservation of natural resources.

Acute versus Chronic Exposure. Effects of acute exposure to a chemical often differ from those that follow subacute or chronic exposure. Acute exposure occurs when a dose is delivered as a single event. Intravenous and oral doses are usually exposures of short duration, but exposure by inhalation of a volatile substance may be prolonged and repeated, such as throughout an 8-hour work day. Chronic exposure is likely to be to small quantities of a toxic substance over a long period of time, which often results in the slow accumulation of toxic concentrations of the compound in the body. Evaluation of *cumulative* toxic effects is receiving increased attention because of chronic exposure to low concentrations of various natural and synthetic chemical substances in the environment.

SPECTRUM OF UNDESIRED EFFECTS

The spectrum of undesired effects of chemicals may be broad and ill defined. In therapeutics, a drug typically produces numerous effects, but only one is usually sought as the primary goal of treatment; most of the other effects are referred to as *undesirable* or *side effects* of that drug for that therapeutic indication. Mechanistic categorization of such effects is a necessary prelude to their avoidance or, if they occur, to their rational and successful management.

Toxic Reactions. Toxic effects of drugs may be classified as pharmacological, pathological, or genotoxic (alterations of DNA), and their incidence and seriousness are related, at least over some range, to the concentration of the toxic chemical in the body. An example of a pharmacological toxicity is excessive depression of the central nervous system (CNS) by barbiturates; an example of a pathological effect is hepatic injury produced by acetaminophen; and an example of a genotoxic effect is a neoplasm produced by a nitrogen mustard. If the concentration of chemical in the tissues does not exceed a critical level, the effects will usually be reversible. The pharmacological effects usually disappear when the concentration of chemical in the tissues is decreased by excretion from the body. Pathological and genotoxic effects may be repaired. If these effects are severe, death may ensue within a short time; if more subtle damage to DNA is not repaired, cancer may appear in a few months or years in laboratory animals or in a decade or more in man.

Many chemicals are not toxic themselves but are activated by biotransformation into toxic metabolites. The toxic response is then dependent on the balance of the rate at which the toxic metabolite is produced and destroyed.

Phototoxic and Photoallergic Reactions. Many chemicals are activated to toxic metabolites by enzymatic biotransformation. However, some chemicals can be activated in the skin by ultraviolet and/or visible radiation. In photoallergy, radiation absorbed by the drug, such as a sulfonamide, results in its conversion to a product that is a more potent allergen than the parent compound. The clinical manifestations may range from acute urticarial reactions, which develop a few minutes after exposure to sunlight, to eczematous or papular lesions, which appear after 24 hours or more. Phototoxic reactions to drugs, in contrast to photoallergic ones, do not have an immunological component. Drugs, either absorbed locally into the skin or reaching the skin through the systemic circulation, may be the subject of photochemical reactions within the skin; this can lead directly either to chemically induced photosensitivity reactions or to enhancement of the usual effects of sunlight. Tetracyclines, sulfonamides, chlorpromazine, and nalidixic acid are examples of phototoxic chemicals; they are generally innocuous to skin in the absence of exposure to light.

Local versus Systemic Toxicity. Effects of chemicals can be classified by their site of action. Local effects are those that occur at the site of first contact between the biological system and the toxicant. Examples of local effects are ingestion of caustic substances or inhalation of irritant materials. Systemic effects require absorption and distribution of the toxicant; most substances, with the exception of highly reactive chemical species, produce such effects. The two categories are not mutually exclusive. Tetraethyllead, for example, injures skin at the site of contact and is absorbed into the circulation to affect the CNS.

Most systemic toxicants affect one or a few organs predominantly. The target organ of toxicity is not necessarily the site of accumulation of the chemical. For example, lead is concentrated in bone, but its primary toxic action is on soft tissues; DDT is concentrated in adipose tissue but produces no known toxic effects there.

The CNS is most frequently involved in systemic toxicity. Many compounds having prominent effects elsewhere also affect the brain. Next in order of frequency of involvement in systemic toxicity are the circulatory system; the blood and hematopoietic system; visceral organs such as liver, kidney, and lung; and the skin. Muscle and bone are least often affected. With substances that have a predominant local effect, the frequency of tissue reaction depends largely on the portal of entry (skin, gastrointestinal tract, or respiratory tract).

Reversible and Irreversible Toxic Effects. The effects of drugs on man must, whenever possible, be reversible; otherwise the drugs would be prohibitively toxic. If a chemical produces injury to a tissue, the capacity of the tissue to regenerate or recover will largely determine the reversibility of the effect. Injuries to a tissue such as liver, which has a high capacity to regenerate, are usually reversible; injury to the CNS is largely irreversible because the highly differentiated neurons of the brain cannot divide and regenerate.

Delayed Toxicity. Most toxic effects of drugs occur at a predictable (usually short) time after administration. However, such is not always the case. For example, aplastic anemia caused by chloramphenicol may appear weeks after the drug has been discontinued. Carcinogenic effects of chemicals usually have a long latency period, and 20 to 30 years often must pass before tumors are observed. Such delayed effects obviously cannot be assessed during any reasonable period of initial evaluation of a chemical; there is an urgent need for reliably predictive, short-term tests for such toxicity as well as for systematic surveillance of the long-term effects of marketed drugs and other chemicals.

Chemical carcinogenesis is a multistep process. Most carcinogens are themselves unreactive (*procarcinogens* or *proximate carcinogens*) but are converted to *primary* or *ultimate carcinogens* in the body. The cytochrome P-450–dependent monooxygenases of the endoplasmic reticulum often convert the proximate carcinogens to reactive electron-deficient intermediates (electrophils). These reactive intermediates can interact with electron-rich (nucleophilic) centers in DNA to produce a mutation. Such interaction of the ultimate carcinogen with DNA in a cell is thought to be the initial step in chemical carcinogenesis. The DNA may revert to normal if DNA repair mechanisms operate successfully; if not, the transformed cell may grow into a tumor that becomes apparent clinically. A *cocarcinogen* or *promoter* is not a carcinogen by itself, but it potentiates the effects of a carcinogen. Promotion involves facilitation of the growth and development of so-called dormant or latent tumor cells. The time from initiation to the development of a tumor probably depends on the presence of such promoters; for many human tumors the latent period is 15 to 45 years.

Allergic Reactions. *Chemical allergy* is an adverse reaction that results from previous sensitization to a particular chemical or to one that is structurally similar. Such reactions are mediated by the immune systems. The terms *hypersensitivity* and *drug allergy* are often used to describe the allergic state.

For a low-molecular-weight chemical to cause an allergic reaction, it or its metabolic product usually acts as a hapten, combining with an endogenous protein to form an antigenic complex. Such antigens induce the synthesis of antibodies, usually after a latent period of at least 1 or 2 weeks. Subsequent exposure of the organism to the chemical results in an antigen-antibody interaction that provokes the typical manifestations of allergy. Dose-response relationships are usually not apparent for the provocation of allergic reactions.

The allergic responses have been divided into four general categories, based on the mechanism of immunological involvement (Coombs and Gell, 1975). Type-I, or anaphylactic, reactions in man are mediated by IgE antibodies. The Fc portion of IgE can bind to receptors on mast cells and basophils. If the antibody molecule then binds antigen, various mediators (histamine, leukotrienes, prostaglandins) are released, and they cause vasodilatation, edema, and an inflammatory response. The main targets of this type of reaction are the gastrointestinal tract (food allergies), the skin (urticaria and atopic dermatitis), the respiratory system (rhinitis and asthma), and the vasculature (anaphylactic shock). These responses tend to occur quickly after challenge with an antigen to which the individual has been sensitized and are termed *immediate hypersensitivity reactions.*

Type-II, or cytolytic, reactions are mediated by both IgG and IgM antibodies and are usually attributed to their ability to activate complement. The major target tissues are the cells in the circulatory system, and they can be destroyed. Examples of this phenomenon include penicillin-induced hemolytic anemia, methyldopa-induced autoimmune hemolytic anemia, quinidine-induced thrombocytopenic purpura, sulfonamide-induced granulocytopenia, and hydralazine- or procainamide-induced systemic lupus erythematosus. Fortunately, these autoimmune reactions to drugs usually subside within several months after removal of the offending agent.

Type-III, or Arthus, reactions are predominantly mediated by IgG; the mechanism involves the generation of antigen-antibody complexes that subsequently fix complement. The complexes become deposited in the vascular endothelium, where a destructive inflammatory response called serum sickness occurs. This is in contrast to the type-II reaction, in which the inflammatory response is induced by antibodies directed against tissue antigens. The clinical symptoms of serum sickness include urticarial skin eruptions, arthralgia or arthritis, lymphadenopathy, and fever. These reactions usually last for 6 to 12 days and then subside after the offending agent is eliminated. Several drugs, such as sulfonamides, penicillins, certain anticonvulsants, and iodides, can induce serum sickness. Stevens-Johnson syndrome, such as that caused by sulfonamides, is a more severe form of immune vasculitis. Symptoms of this reaction include erythema multiforme, arthritis, nephritis, CNS abnormalities, and myocarditis.

Type-IV, or delayed-hypersensitivity, reactions are mediated by sensitized T-lymphocytes and macrophages. When sensitized cells come in contact with antigen, an inflammatory reaction is generated by the production of lymphokines and the subsequent influx of neutrophils and macrophages. An example of type-IV or delayed hypersensitivity is the contact dermatitis caused by poison ivy.

Idiosyncratic Reactions. *Idiosyncrasy* is defined as a genetically determined abnormal reactivity to a chemical (Goldstein *et al.,* 1974). The observed response is qualitatively similar in all individuals, but it may take the form of extreme sensitivity to low doses or extreme insensitivity to high doses of the agent. For example, many black males (about 10%) develop a serious hemolytic anemia when they receive primaquine. Such individuals have a deficiency of erythrocytic glucose-6-phosphate dehydrogenase (*see* Chapter 45). Genetically determined resistance to the anticoagulant action of warfarin is due to an alteration in the receptor for the drug (*see* Chapter 58).

Interactions between Chemicals. The existence of numerous toxicants requires consideration of their potential interactions (*see also* Chapters 1 to 3 and Appendix III). Concurrent exposures may alter rates of absorption, change the degree of protein binding, or alter the rates of biotransformation or excretion of one or both interacting compounds. The response to combined toxicants may thus be equal to, greater than, or less than the sum of the effects of the individual agents.

Numerous terms describe pharmacological and toxicological interactions. An *additive* effect describes the combined effect of two chemicals that is equal to the sum of the effect of each agent given alone; the additive effect is the most common. A *synergistic* effect is one in which the combined effect of two chemicals is greater than the sum of the effect of each agent given alone. For example, both carbon tetrachloride and ethanol are hepatotoxins, but together they produce much more injury to the liver than expected from the mathematical sum of their individual effects. *Potentiation* is the increased effect of a toxic agent acting simultaneously with a nontoxic one. Isopropanol alone, for example, is not hepatotoxic; however, it greatly increases the hepatotoxicity of carbon tetrachloride. *Antagonism* is the interference of one chemical with the action of another. An antagonistic agent is often desirable as an antidote. *Functional or physiological antagonism* occurs when two chemicals produce opposite effects on the same physiological function. For example, this principle is applied to maintain perfusion of vital organs during certain severe intoxications characterized by marked hypotension and hypoxia, by intravenous administration of dopamine. *Chemical antagonism* or *inactivation* is a reaction between two chemicals to neutralize their effects. For example, dimercaprol (BAL) chelates with various metals to decrease their toxicity. *Dispositional antagonism* is the alteration of the disposition of a substance (its absorption, biotransformation, distribution, or excretion) so that less of the agent reaches the target organ or its persistence there is reduced (*see* below). *Antagonism* at the *receptor* for the chemical entails the blockade of the effect of an agonist with an appropriate antagonist that competes for the same site. For example, the antagonist naloxone is used to treat the respiratory-depressant effects of opioids.

DESCRIPTIVE TOXICITY TESTS IN ANIMALS

Two main principles underlie all descriptive toxicity tests that are performed in animals. First, effects of chemicals produced in laboratory animals, when properly qualified, apply to toxicity in man. When calculated on the basis of dose per unit of body surface, toxic effects in man are usually encountered in the same range of concentrations as are those in experimental animals. On the basis of body weight, man is generally more vulnerable than experimental animals by a factor of about ten. Such information is used to select dosages for clinical trials of candidate therapeutic agents and to attempt to set limits on permissible exposure to environmental toxicants.

The second main principle is that exposure of experimental animals to toxic agents in high doses is a necessary and valid method to discover possible hazards to man. This principle is based on the quantal dose-response concept. As a matter of practicality, the number of animals used in experiments on toxic materials will usually be small compared with the size of human populations potentially at risk. For example, 0.01% incidence of a serious toxic effect (such as cancer) represents 20,000 people in a population of 200 million. Such an incidence is unacceptably high. Yet, detecting an incidence of 0.01% experimentally would likely require a minimum of 30,000 animals. To estimate risk at low dosage, large doses must be given to relatively small groups. The validity of the necessary extrapolation is clearly a crucial question.

Chemicals are first tested for toxicity by determination of the LD50 in two animal species by two routes of administration; one of these is the expected route of exposure. Animals most often used are mice, rats, rabbits, and dogs. In mice and rats the LD50 is usually determined as described above. In larger species the LD50 is approximated by increasing the dose until serious toxic effects are demonstrated. The number of animals that die in a 14-day period after a single dose is tabulated. The animals are also examined for signs of intoxication, lethargy, behavioral modification, and morbidity.

The chemical is next tested for toxicity by subacute exposure, usually for 90 days. The subacute study is most often performed in two species (rat and dog) by the route of intended use or exposure, and at least three doses are employed. A variety of parameters are monitored during this period, and, at the end of the study, organs and tissues are examined by a pathologist.

Long-term or chronic studies are carried out in animals at the same time that clinical trials are undertaken (*see* Chapter 3). The length of exposure depends somewhat on the intended use in man. If the drug would normally be used for short periods under medical supervision, as would an antimicrobial agent, a chronic exposure of animals for 6 months might suffice. If the drug would be used in man for longer periods, a chronic study of 2 years might be required.

Study of chronic exposure is often used to determine the carcinogenic potential of chemicals. These studies are usually performed in rats and mice and cover the average lifetime of the species. Other tests are designed to evaluate teratogenicity, perinatal and postnatal toxicity, and effects on fertility. In addition, drugs are often tested for *mutagenic* potential. The most popular such test currently available, the reverse mutation test developed by Ames and colleagues (Ames *et al.*, 1975), uses a strain of *Salmonella typhimurium* that has a mutant gene for the enzyme phosphoribosyl adenosine triphosphate (ATP) synthetase. This enzyme is required for histidine synthesis, and the bacterial strain is unable to grow in a histidine-deficient medium unless a reverse mutation is induced. Since many chemicals are not mutagenic or carcinogenic unless activated by the endoplasmic reticulum, rat hepatic microsomes are usually added to the medium containing the mutant bacteria and the drug. The Ames test is rapid and sensitive. However, its usefulness for the prediction of the carcinogenic potential of chemicals for man is controversial, and the subject is currently receiving considerable attention.

INCIDENCE OF ACUTE POISONING

The true incidence of poisoning in the United States is not known, but, in 1981, about 50,000 cases were voluntarily reported to the National Clearinghouse for

Poison Control Centers. The number of real or potential poisonings is probably at least tenfold greater than the number reported.

Deaths in the United States due to poisoning number over 4000 per year (Table 68–1). The incidence of poisoning in children (under 5 years of age) has decreased dramatically over the last 2 decades. For example, childhood deaths due to aspirin decreased from 140 in the early 1960s to only 9 in 1979. This favorable trend is probably due to safety packaging of aspirin, prescription drugs, drain cleaners, turpentine, and other household chemicals; improved medical training and care; and increased public awareness of potential poisons. Of the deaths caused by accidental poisoning, about 60% are caused by drugs and the rest by other chemicals.

Marked differences in the incidence of poisoning are seen at different ages. Children under 5 years account for about 60% of the poisoning, but their mortality rate is much less; these cases account for only 2% of the total deaths from poisons. About 50% of accidental poisoning occurs in children 1 to 2 years old, the age at which they actively explore the environment. The agent responsible for poisoning also differs in various age groups. In toddlers, the agents are usually chemicals other than drugs. In 1981, plants were the category most frequently implicated, followed by cleaning agents. As the age of the patient increases, drugs are more frequent causes of poisoning. In people over 15 years of age, about 75% of cases of poisoning are due to drugs.

MAJOR SOURCES OF INFORMATION ON TOXICOLOGY

Pharmacology textbooks are a good source of information on treatment of poisoning by drugs, but they usually say little about other chemicals. Additional information on drugs and other chemicals can be found in various books on poisoning. (*See* Goldfrank, 1982; Haddad and Winchester, 1983; Klaassen *et al.*, 1985.) The most comprehensive book on the subject is *Clinical Management of Poisoning and Drug Overdose,* edited by Haddad and Winchester (1983).

An extremely useful source of information on the treatment of acute poisoning by commercial products is *Clinical Toxicology of Commercial Products* by Gosselin and associates (1984). This book contains seven major sections. One section lists over 17,500 trade names of products that might be ingested accidentally or suicidally. It lists the manufacturer and ingredients of each commercial product and notes components believed responsible for harmful effects. A popular microfiche system for information on toxic substances is POISINDEX (Micromedex, Inc., Denver, Colorado).

There are about 450 poison control centers in the United States, coordinated and served by the Food and Drug Administration's National Clearinghouse for Poison Control Centers, and there are 26 regional poison control centers designated by the American Association of Poison Control

Table 68–1. DEATHS FROM ACCIDENTAL POISONING IN THE UNITED STATES IN 1979 *

TOXICANT	NUMBER OF DEATHS
Analgesics and antipyretics	655
Sedatives and hypnotics	276
Tranquilizers	106
Antidepressants	105
Other psychotropic agents	26
Other drugs acting on nervous system	180
Antibiotics and other antimicrobial agents	41
Cardiovascular drugs	160
Hormones	28
Hematological agents	17
Other drugs	478
Unspecified drugs	472
Subtotal (drugs)	2544
Alcohols	416
Cleaning and polishing agents and paint	14
Petroleum products	74
Pesticides	29
Corrosives and caustics	16
Food and plants	7
Other and unspecified solids and liquids	65
Subtotal (other solids and liquids)	621
Utility gas	170
Carbon monoxide	1116
Nitrogen oxides	8
Freon	30
Other gases	126
Unspecified gases	22
Subtotal (gases)	1472
Total	4637

* Individual poison reports submitted to the National Clearinghouse for Poison Control Centers (Brancato, 1983).

Centers. These centers are a valuable source of information that can be obtained by telephone.

PREVENTION AND TREATMENT OF POISONING

Many acute poisonings could be prevented if physicians provided and parents accepted common-sense instructions about the storage of drugs and other chemicals. These are so widely publicized that they need not be repeated here.

For clinical purposes all toxic agents can be divided into two classes: those for which a specific treatment and antidote exists and those for which there is no specific treatment. For the vast majority of drugs and other chemicals, there is no specific treatment and symptomatic medical care that supports vital functions is the only approach.

Supportive therapy, as in other medical emergencies, is the most important aspect of the treatment of drug poisoning. The adage, "Treat the patient, not the poison," remains the most basic and important principle of clinical toxicology. Maintenance of respiration and circulation takes precedence. Serial measurement and charting of vital signs and important reflexes help to judge progress of intoxication, response to therapy, and the need for additional treatment. This usually requires hospitalization. The classification in Table 68–2 is often used to indicate the severity of CNS intoxication. Treatment with large doses of stimulants and sedatives can often cause more harm than the poison. Chemical antidotes should be used judiciously; heroic measures are seldom necessary.

Treatment of acute poisoning must be prompt. The first goal is to keep the concentration of poison in the crucial tissues as low as possible by preventing absorption and enhancing elimination. The second goal is to combat the pharmacological and toxicological effects at the effector sites.

PREVENTION OF FURTHER ABSORPTION OF POISON

Emesis. Although emesis is indicated after poisoning by oral ingestion of most chemicals, it is contraindicated in certain

Table 68–2. SIGNS AND SYMPTOMS OF CNS INTOXICATION

DEGREE OF SEVERITY	CHARACTERISTICS
	Depressants
0	Asleep, but can be aroused and can answer questions
I	Semicomatose, withdraws from painful stimuli, reflexes intact
II	Comatose, does not withdraw from painful stimuli, no respiratory or circulatory depression, most reflexes intact
III	Comatose, most or all reflexes absent, but without depression of respiration or circulation
IV	Comatose, reflexes absent, respiratory depression with cyanosis or circulatory failure and shock or both
	Stimulants
I	Restlessness, irritability, insomnia, tremor, hyperreflexia, sweating, mydriasis, flushing
II	Confusion, hyperactivity, hypertension, tachypnea, tachycardia, extrasystoles, sweating, mydriasis, flushing, mild hyperpyrexia
III	Delirium, mania, self-injury, marked hypertension, tachycardia, arrhythmias, hyperpyrexia
IV	As in III, plus convulsions, coma, and circulatory collapse

situations. (1) If the patient has ingested a corrosive poison, such as strong acids or alkalis (*e.g.,* drain cleaners), emesis increases the likelihood of gastric perforation and further necrosis of the esophagus. (2) If the patient is comatose or in a state of stupor or delirium, emesis may cause aspiration of the gastric contents. (3) If the patient has ingested a CNS stimulant, further stimulation associated with vomiting may precipitate convulsions. (4) If the patient has ingested a petroleum distillate (*e.g.,* kerosene, gasoline, or petroleum-based liquid furniture polish), regurgitated hydrocarbons can be aspirated readily and cause chemical pneumonitis.

There are marked differences in the capabilities of various petroleum distillates to produce hydrocarbon pneumonia, which is an acute, hemorrhagic necrotizing process. In general, the ability of various hydrocarbons to produce pneumonitis is inversely proportional to the viscosity of the agent: if the viscosity is high, as with oils and greases, the risk is limited; if viscosity is low, as with mineral seal oil found in liquid furniture polishes, the risk of aspiration is high. While induced emesis is contraindicated in most instances of poisoning with petroleum distillates (Ervin, 1983), it should be considered if the solution that is ingested contains potentially dangerous compounds, such as pesticides.

Vomiting can be induced mechanically by stroking the posterior pharynx. However, this technic is not as effective as the administration of ipecac or apomorphine.

Ipecac. The most useful household emetic is syrup of ipecac (not ipecac fluidextract, which is 14 times more potent and may cause fatalities). It is available in 0.5- and 1-fluidounce containers (approximately 15 and 30 ml), which may be purchased without prescription. The drug can be given orally, but it takes 15 to 30 minutes to produce emesis; this compares favorably with the time usually required for adequate gastric lavage. The oral dose is 5 to 10 ml in children less than 1 year of age and 15 ml in older children and adults; this may be repeated after 20 to 30 minutes if vomiting has not occurred. To obtain maximal results, a glass of tepid water should be given after administration of ipecac; emesis may not occur if the stomach is empty.

Ipecac acts as an emetic because of its local irritant effect on the enteric tract (Allport, 1959) and its effect on the chemoreceptor trigger zone (CTZ) in the area postrema of the medulla (Borison and Wang, 1953). Syrup of ipecac may not be effective when antiemetic drugs (such as phenothiazines) have been ingested. Charcoal should not be administered with ipecac, because charcoal can adsorb the ipecac and reduce the emetic effect. Ipecac can produce toxic effects on the heart because of its content of emetine (*see* Chapter 46), but this is usually not a problem with the dose used for emesis (Manno and Manno, 1977). If emesis does not occur, ipecac should be removed by gastric lavage.

Apomorphine. Apomorphine stimulates the CTZ and causes emesis. Its advantage over ipecac is the rapidity of its action, and vomiting usually occurs within 3 to 5 minutes. However, it is not effective orally and must be given parenterally, usually by the subcutaneous route—6 mg for adults and 0.06 mg/kg for children (Goldfrank, 1982). Additionally, the drug is often not readily available. Since apomorphine is a respiratory depressant, it should not be used if the patient has been poisoned by a CNS depressant or if the patient's respiration is slow and labored. Respiratory depression and emesis produced by apomorphine can be reversed by an opioid antagonist such as naloxone, but this usually is not necessary.

Gastric Lavage. Gastric lavage is accomplished by inserting a tube into the stomach and washing the stomach with water, normal saline, or one-half normal saline to remove the unabsorbed poison. The procedure should be performed only if vital functions are adequate or supportive procedures have been implemented, but it should be performed as soon as possible. Lavage may be useful for as long as 6 hours after ingestion of a poison and, if gastric emptying has been delayed, lavage may be useful for as long as 24 hours after ingestion. The contraindications to this procedure are generally the same as for emesis. Unlike emesis, gastric lavage can be used for patients who are hysterical, comatose, or otherwise uncooperative.

The only equipment needed for gastric lavage is a tube and a large syringe. The tube should be as large as possible so that the wash solution, food, and the poison, whether in the form of a capsule, pill, or liquid, will flow freely and lavage can be accomplished quickly. A 36-French tube or larger should be used in adults and a 24-French tube or larger in children. Orogastric lavage is preferred over nasogastric, since a larger tube can be employed. An endotracheal tube with an inflatable cuff should be positioned in the comatose patient before lavage is initiated to prevent aspiration. During gastric lavage the patient should be placed on his left side, due to the anatomical asymmetry of the stomach, with the head hanging over the edge of the examining table and with the face down. If possible, the foot of the table should be elevated. This technic minimizes chances of aspiration (Arena, 1979).

The contents of the stomach should be aspirated with an irrigating syringe and saved for chemical analysis. The stomach may then be washed with saline solution. Saline solution is safer than water in young children because of the risk of water intoxication, manifested by tonic and clonic seizures and coma (Arena, 1975). Only small volumes (120 to 300 ml) of lavage solution should be instilled into the stomach at one time so that the poison is not pushed into the intestine. Lavage should be repeated until the returns are clear, which usually requires 10 to 12 washings and a total of 1.5 to 4 liters of lavage fluid. When the lavage is complete, the stomach may be left empty or an antidote may be instilled through the tube. If no specific antidote is known for the poison, an aqueous suspension of activated charcoal and/or a cathartic is sometimes given.

Chemical Adsorption. Activated charcoal adsorbs drugs and chemicals to the surfaces of the charcoal particles almost irreversibly, thereby preventing absorption and toxicity. The effectiveness of charcoal is dependent on the time since the ingestion and the dose of charcoal; one should attempt to achieve a charcoal:drug ratio of 10:1. Activated charcoal can also interrupt the enterohepatic circulation of drugs and enhance the rate of diffusion of the chemical from the body into the gastrointestinal tract (Levy, 1982).

Activated charcoal is usually prepared as a mixture of about 50 g in a glass of water. The mixture is then administered either orally or via a gastric tube. Since most poisons do not appear to desorb from the charcoal if it is present in excess, the adsorbed poison need not be removed from the gastrointestinal tract. As mentioned, activated charcoal should not be used simultaneously with ipecac.

Activated charcoal must be distinguished from the so-called universal antidote. The universal antidote consists of two parts burned toast (not activated charcoal), one part tannic acid (strong tea), and one part magnesium oxide. In practice, the universal antidote is less effective than activated charcoal alone in detoxifying common drugs (Picchioni *et al.*, 1966). Some of the tannic acid is adsorbed by the charcoal, and less charcoal is thus available for adsorption of the poison (Daly and Cooney, 1978).

As mentioned, the presence of an adsorbent in the intestine may interrupt enterohepatic circulation of a toxicant, thus enhancing its excretion. Activated charcoal is useful to interrupt the enterohepatic circulation of drugs such as tricyclic antidepressants and glutethimide. Poisoning by methylmercury can be treated with a nonabsorbable polythiol resin, which binds mercury excreted into the bile (*see* Chapter 69). Cholestyramine hastens the elimination of cardiac glycosides by a similar mechanism (*see* Chapter 30).

Chemical Inactivation. Antidotes can change the chemical nature of a poison by rendering it less toxic or by preventing its absorption. Formaldehyde poisoning can be treated with ammonia to form hexamethylenetetramine (Goldstein *et al.*, 1974); sodium formaldehyde sulfoxylate can convert mercuric ion to the less soluble metallic mercury (Gosselin *et al.*, 1984); and sodium bicarbonate converts ferrous iron to ferrous carbonate, which is poorly absorbed. However, these technics are seldom used today because valuable time may be lost. Emetics and gastric lavage are rapid and effective.

In the past, neutralization was the usual treatment of poisoning with acids or bases. Vinegar, orange juice, or lemon juice have often been used for the patient who has ingested alkali, and various antacids have often been advocated for treatment of acid burns. The use of neutralizing agents is controversial, since this may produce excessive heat. Carbon dioxide gas produced from bicarbonates used to treat oral poisoning with acids can cause gastric distention and even perforation. The treatment of choice for poisoning with either acids or alkalis is water or milk; neither causes an exothermic chemical reaction (Rumack and Burrington, 1977). Burns on the skin should be treated with copious amounts of water.

Purgation. The rationale for using an osmotic cathartic is to minimize absorption by hastening the passage of the toxicant through the gastrointestinal tract. Few, if any, controlled clinical data are available on the effectiveness of cathartics in the treatment of poisoning. Cathartics are generally considered harmless unless the poison has injured the gastrointestinal tract. Cathartics are indicated after the ingestion of enteric-coated tablets, when the time after ingestion is greater than 1 hour, and for poisoning by volatile hydrocarbons (Rumack and Lovejoy, 1985). Preferred agents are the saline cathartics (sodium sulfate and magnesium sulfate), which act promptly and usually have minimal toxicity.

Inhalation and Dermal Exposure to Poisons. When a poison has been inhaled, the first priority is to remove the patient from the source of exposure. Similarly, the skin should be thoroughly washed with water if it has come in contact with a poison. Even when the poison is a strong acid or base, irrigation with large volumes of water is preferred to neutralization with a base or acid. Contaminated clothing should be removed. Initial treatment of all types of chemical injuries to the eye must be rapid; thorough irrigation of the eye with water for 15 minutes should be performed immediately.

ENHANCED BIOTRANSFORMATION AND EXCRETION OF THE POISON

Biotransformation. Many drugs are metabolized by the cytochrome P-450 system in the endoplasmic reticulum of the liver, and this system can be induced by an array of different compounds (*see* Chapter 1). However, induction of these oxidative enzymes is too slow (days) to be valuable in the treatment of acute poisoning by most chemical agents.

Many chemicals are toxic because they are biotransformed into more toxic chemicals. Thus, inhibition of biotransformation should decrease the toxicity of such drugs. For example, ethanol is used to inhibit the conversion of methanol to its highly toxic metabolite, formic acid, by alcohol dehydrogenase (*see* Chapter 18). Acetaminophen is activated by the cytochrome P-450 system to an electrophilic metabolite that is detoxified by glutathione, a cellular nucleophil. Acetaminophen does not cause hepatotoxicity until concentrations of glutathione are depleted, whereupon the reactive metabolite binds to essential macromolecular constituents of the hepatocyte. The liver can be protected by maintenance of the concentration of glutathione, and this can be accomplished by the administration of N-acetylcysteine (Black, 1980; *see* Chapter 29).

Some drugs are detoxified by conjugation with glucuronic acid or sulfate before elimination from the body, and the availability of the endogenous cosubstrates for conjugation may limit the rate of elimination; such is the case in the detoxication of acetaminophen (Hjelle *et al.*, 1985). When methods become available to replete these compounds, an additional mechanism will be available to treat poisoning. Similarly, detoxication of cyanide by conversion to thiocyanate can be accelerated by the administration of thiosulfate (*see* Chapter 70).

Biliary Excretion. The liver excretes many drugs and other foreign chemicals into bile, but little is known about efficient ways to enhance biliary excretion of xenobiotics for the treatment of acute poisoning. Inducers of microsomal enzyme activity enhance biliary excretion of some xenobiotics, but the effect is slow in onset. Eventually, the procedure may be useful to enhance the elimination of certain compounds with long biological half-lives (Klaassen and Watkins, 1984).

Urinary Excretion. Drugs and poisons are excreted into the urine by glomerular filtration and active tubular secretion (Chapter 1); they can be reabsorbed into the blood if they are in a lipid-soluble form that will penetrate the tubule or if there is an active mechanism for their transport.

There are no methods known to accelerate the active transport of poisons into urine, and enhancement of glomerular filtration is not a practical means to facilitate elimination of toxicants. However, passive reabsorption from the tubular lumen can be altered. Diuretics decrease reabsorption by decreasing the concentration gradient of the drug from the lumen to the tubular cell and by increasing flow through the tubule. Furosemide is used most often, but osmotic diuretics are also employed (Chapter 36). Forced diuresis should be used with caution, especially in patients with renal or cardiac complications. Since nonionized compounds are reabsorbed far more rapidly than ionized, polar molecules, a shift from the nonionized to the ionized species of

the toxicant by alteration of the pH of the tubular fluid may hasten elimination (Chapter 1).

Acidic compounds such as phenobarbital and salicylates are cleared much more rapidly in alkaline than in acidic urine. The effect of increasing urine flow and alkalinization of urine on the clearance of phenobarbital is shown in Figure 68–2. Sodium bicarbonate is used to alkalinize the urine. Renal excretion of basic drugs such as amphetamine can be enhanced by acidification of the urine. This can be accomplished by the administration of ammonium chloride or ascorbic acid. Urinary excretion of an acidic compound is particularly sensitive to changes in urinary pH if its pK_a is within the range of 3.0 to 7.5; for bases the corresponding range is 7.5 to 10.5 (Milne *et al.*, 1958).

Dialysis. Procedures such as peritoneal dialysis or hemodialysis usually have limited use in the treatment of intoxication

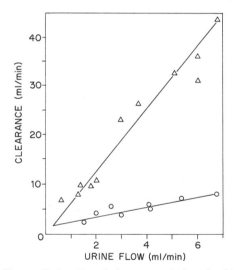

Figure 68–2. *Renal clearance of phenobarbital in the dog as it is related to rate of urine flow.*

The values designated by circles are from experiments in which diuresis was induced by administration of water orally or Na_2SO_4 intravenously and the urinary pH was below 7.0. The values designated by triangles are from experiments in which $NaHCO_3$ was administered intravenously and in which the urinary pH was 7.8 to 8.0. (After Waddell and Butler, 1957. Courtesy of *Journal of Clinical Investigation*.)

with chemicals. However, under certain circumstances, such procedures can be life-saving. The efficiency of dialysis depends on the concentration gradient of the poison between the blood and the dialysis fluid. Thus, if a poison has a large volume of distribution, the plasma will contain too little of the compound for effective dialysis. Extensive binding of the compound to plasma proteins also impairs dialysis greatly. The kinetics of elimination of a toxicant by dialysis is dependent on the rate of dissociation of the compound from binding sites in plasma and tissues, and, for some chemicals, this may be too slow. It is important to keep the concentration of the diffusible form of the poison in the dialysate as low as possible. It may be feasible to add "traps" for the agent in question—for example, albumin for compounds that bind to the protein.

Peritoneal Dialysis. Peritoneal dialysis is performed by the introduction of dialysis fluid into the peritoneal cavity by means of a catheter placed through a small incision in the right section of the mesogastric region. Up to 2000 ml of dialysis fluid can be introduced into the peritoneal cavity of an adult (about 75 to 100 ml/kg is used for infants). The fluid is usually infused over an interval of 5 to 20 minutes, and it is drained about 30 to 90 minutes later. The procedure can be repeated for 48 hours, and the catheter is then removed. Peritoneal dialysis requires a minimum of personnel and can be started as soon as the patient is admitted to the hospital.

Hemodialysis, Hemoperfusion, and Exchange Transfusion. Hemodialysis (extracorporeal dialysis) is being used more frequently in the treatment of acute intoxication. It is usually much more effective than peritoneal dialysis and may be essential in life-threatening intoxications. Passage of blood through a column of charcoal or adsorbent resin (hemoperfusion) is a technic for the extracorporeal removal of a poison (Winchester, 1983). Due to the high adsorptive capacity and affinity of the material in the column, some chemicals that are bound to plasma proteins can be removed. The principal side effect of hemoperfusion is depletion of platelets. Blood-exchange transfusions can be an efficient way to remove poisons that have a small volume of distribution but that are eliminated only slowly by dialysis because, for example, of extensive and avid binding to plasma proteins.

ANTAGONISM OR CHEMICAL INACTIVATION OF AN ABSORBED POISON

Functional and pharmacological antagonism of the effects of absorbed toxicants has been discussed above. If a patient is poisoned with a compound that acts as an agonist at a receptor for which a specific blocking agent is available, administration of the antagonist may be highly effective. Functional antagonism is also a cornerstone of treatment in that support of the patient's vital functions is imperative. However, drugs that stimulate antagonistic physiological mechanisms may be of little clinical value and may even decrease the incidence of survival. It is often difficult to titrate the effect of one drug against another when the two act on opposing systems. An example of such difficulty is the use of CNS stimulants to attempt to reverse respiratory depression. Convulsions are a typical complication of such therapy, and mechanical support of respiration is much preferred. In addition, the duration of action of the poison and the antidote may differ, sometimes leading to poisoning with the antidote.

Specific chemical antagonists of a toxicant are valuable but unfortunately rare. Chelating agents with high selectivity for certain metallic ions provide such examples (*see* Chapter 69). Antibodies offer the potential for the production of specific antidotes for a host of common poisons and for drugs that are frequently abused or misused. A notable example of such success is the use of purified digoxin-specific Fab fragments of antibodies in the treatment of potentially fatal cases of poisoning with digoxin (Smith *et al.*, 1982). The development of human monoclonal antibodies directed against specific toxins has significant potential.

Allport, R. B. Ipecac is not innocuous. *J. Dis. Child.,* **1959,** *98,* 786–787.

Ames, B. N.; McCann, J.; and Yamasaki, E. Methods for detecting carcinogens and mutagens with the *Salmonella*/mammalian microsome mutagenicity test. *Mutat. Res.,* **1975,** *31,* 347–364.

Black, M. Acetaminophen hepatotoxicity. *Gastroenterology,* **1980,** *78,* 382–392.

Brancato, D. J. The FDA's poison control case report category summary: top 10 for calendar years—'79, '80, '81. *Vet. Hum. Toxicol.,* **1983,** *25,* 457–464.

Daly, J. S., and Cooney, D. O. Interference by tannic acid with the effectiveness of activated charcoal in "universal antidote." *Clin. Toxicol.,* **1978,** *12,* 512–522.

Hjelle, J. J.; Hazelton, G. A.; and Klaassen, C. D. Acetaminophen decreases adenosine 3'-phosphate 5'-phosphosulfate and uridine diphosphoglucuronic acid in liver. *Drug Metab. Dispos.,* **1985,** *13,* 35–41.

Levy, G. Gastrointestinal clearance of drugs with activated charcoal. *N. Engl. J. Med.,* **1982,** *307,* 676–677.

Milne, M. D.; Schribner, B. H.; and Crawford, M. A. Non-ionic diffusion and the excretion of weak acids and bases. *Am. J. Med.*, **1958**, *24*, 709–729.

Picchioni, A. L.; Chin, L.; Verhulst, H. L.; and Dieterle, B. Activated charcoal vs "universal antidote" as an antidote for poisons. *Toxicol. Appl. Pharmacol.*, **1966**, *8*, 447–454.

Rumack, B. H., and Burrington, J. P. Caustic ingestions: a rational look at diluents. *Clin. Toxicol.*, **1977**, *11*, 27–34.

Sayid, I. A. Auricular fibrillation after emetine injection. *Lancet*, **1935**, *2*, 556.

Smith, T. W.; Butler, V. P., Jr.; Haber, E.; Fozzard, H.; Marcus, F. I.; Bremner, W. F.; Schulman, I. C.; and Phillips, A. Treatment of life-threatening digitalis intoxication with digoxin-specific Fab antibody fragments. *N. Engl. J. Med.*, **1982**, *307*, 1357–1362.

Waddell, W. J., and Butler, T. C. The distribution and excretion of phenobarbital. *J. Clin. Invest.*, **1957**, *36*, 1217–1226.

Monographs and Reviews

Arena, J. M. *Poisoning: Toxicology, Symptoms, Treatments*, 4th ed. Charles C Thomas, Publisher, Springfield, Ill., **1979**.

———. Poisoning and its treatment. In, *Pediatric Therapy*, 5th ed. (Shirkey, H. C., ed.) C. V. Mosby Co., St. Louis, **1975**, pp. 101–136.

Borison, H. L., and Wang, S. C. Physiology and pharmacology of vomiting. *Pharmacol. Rev.*, **1953**, *5*, 193–230.

Coombs, R. R. A., and Gell, P. G. H. Classification of allergic reactions responsible for clinical hypersensitivity and disease. In, *Clinical Aspects of Immunology*. (Gell, P. G. H.; Coombs, R. R. A.; and Lachmann, P. J.; eds.) Blackwell Scientific Publications, Oxford, **1975**, p. 761.

Ervin, M. E. Petroleum distillates and turpentine. In,

Clinical Management of Poisoning and Drug Overdose. (Haddad, L. M., and Winchester, J. F., eds.) W. B. Saunders Co., Philadelphia, **1983**, pp. 771–779.

Goldfrank, L. R. *Toxicologic Emergencies*. Appleton-Century-Crofts, New York, **1982**.

Goldstein, A.; Aronow, L.; and Kalman, S. M. *Principles of Drug Action: The Basis of Pharmacology*, 2nd ed. John Wiley & Sons, Inc., New York, **1974**.

Gosselin, R. E.; Smith, R. P.; and Hodge, H. C. *Clinical Toxicology of Commercial Products*, 5th ed. The Williams & Wilkins Co., Baltimore, **1984**.

Haddad, L. M., and Winchester, J. F. (eds.). *Clinical Management of Poisoning and Drug Overdose*. W. B. Saunders Co., Philadelphia, **1983**.

Klaassen, C. D. Principles of toxicology. In, *Casarett and Doull's Toxicology: The Basic Science of Poisons*, 3rd ed. (Klaassen, C. D.; Amdur, M.; and Doull, J.; eds.) Macmillan Publishing Co., New York, **1985**.

Klaassen, C. D.; Amdur, M. O.; and Doull, J. (eds.). *Casarett and Doull's Toxicology: The Basic Science of Poisons*, 3rd ed. Macmillan Publishing Co., New York, **1985**.

Klaassen, C. D., and Watkins, J. B., III. Mechanisms of bile formation, hepatic uptake, and biliary excretion. *Pharmacol. Rev.*, **1984**, *36*, 1–67.

Manno, B. R., and Manno, J. E. Toxicology of ipecac: a review. *Clin. Toxicol.*, **1977**, *10*, 221–242.

Rumack, B. H., and Lovejoy, F. H., Jr. Clinical toxicology. In, *Casarett and Doull's Toxicology: The Basic Science of Poisons*, 3rd ed. (Klaassen, C. D.; Amdur, M. O.; and Doull, J.; eds.) Macmillan Publishing Co., New York, **1985**.

Winchester, J. F. Active methods for detoxification: oral sorbents, forced diuresis, hemoperfusion, and hemodialysis. In, *Clinical Management of Poisoning and Drug Overdose*. (Haddad, L. M., and Winchester, J. F., eds.) W. B. Saunders Co., Philadelphia, **1983**, pp. 154–169.

CHAPTER

69 HEAVY METALS AND HEAVY-METAL ANTAGONISTS

Curtis D. Klaassen

Man has always been exposed to heavy metals in the environment. In areas with high concentrations, metallic contamination of food and water probably led to the first poisonings. Metals leached from eating utensils and cookware have also contributed to inadvertent poisonings. The emergence of the industrial age and large-scale mining brought occupational diseases caused by various toxic metals. Metallic constituents of pesticides and therapeutic agents (*e.g.,* antimicrobials) were additional sources of hazardous exposure. The burning of fossil fuels containing heavy metals, the addition of tetraethyllead to gasoline, and the increase in industrial applications of metals have now made environmental pollution the major source of heavy-metal poisoning.

Heavy metals, which, of course, cannot be metabolized, persist in the body and exert their toxic effects by combining with one or more reactive groups (ligands) essential for normal physiological functions. Heavy-metal antagonists (chelating agents) are designed specifically to compete with these groups for the metals, and thereby prevent or reverse toxic effects and enhance the excretion of metals. Heavy metals, particularly those in the transition series, may react with O-, S-, and N-containing ligands, which in the body take the form of —OH, —COO$^-$, —OPO$_3$H$^-$, >C=O, —SH, —S—S—, —NH$_2$, and >NH. The resultant metal complex (or coordination compound) is formed by a coordinate bond—one in which both electrons are contributed by the ligand.

The heavy-metal antagonists discussed in this chapter possess the common property of forming complexes with heavy metals, thereby preventing or reversing the binding of metallic cations to body ligands. These drugs are referred to as *chelating agents.* A

chelate is a complex formed between a metal and a compound that contains two or more potential ligands. The product of such a reaction is a heterocyclic ring. Five- and six-membered chelate rings are the most stable, and a polydentate (multiligand) chelator is typically designed to form such a highly stable complex. Formation of a polydentate chelate results in a far more stable compound than when the metal is combined with only one ligand atom.

The stability of chelates varies with the metal and the ligand atoms. For example, lead and mercury have greater affinities for sulfur and nitrogen than for oxygen ligands; calcium behaves in the opposite manner. These differences in affinity serve as the basis of selectivity of action of a chelating agent in the body.

The effectiveness of a chelating agent for the treatment of poisoning by a heavy metal depends on several factors. These include the relative affinity of the chelator for the heavy metal as compared to essential body metals, the distribution of the chelator in the body compared to the distribution of the metal, and the ability of the chelator to mobilize the metal from the body once chelated.

An ideal chelating agent would have the following properties: high solubility in water, resistance to biotransformation, ability to reach sites of metal storage, ready excretion of the chelate, ability to retain chelating activity at the pH of body fluids, and the property of forming complexes with metals that are less toxic than the free metallic ion. A low affinity for calcium is also desirable, since calcium in plasma is readily available for chelation and a drug might produce hypocalcemia despite high affinity for heavy metals. The most important property is greater affinity for the metal than that possessed by the endogenous ligands.

The large number of available ligands in the body is a formidable barrier to the effectiveness of a chelating agent. Observations *in vitro* on chelator-metal interactions provide only a rough guide to the treatment of heavy-metal poisoning. Empirical observations *in vivo* are necessary to determine the clinical utility of a chelating agent.

LEAD

Lead is virtually ubiquitous in the environment as a result of its natural occurrence and its industrial use. Approximately 10% of the lead mined is used for the production of alkyl lead compounds (*e.g.*, tetraethyllead) to be used as "antiknock" fuel additives (approximately 1 ml per liter of gasoline). The use of lesser amounts of lead in gasoline during the last decade has resulted in a decrease in blood lead concentrations in man (Annest *et al.*, 1983). Overall, human exposure to lead is primarily from food. The average daily intake for an adult in the United States ranges from 0.1 to 2 mg of lead. However, most of the overt toxicity from lead results from environmental and industrial exposure.

Acidic foods and beverages, including tomato juice, fruit juice, cola drinks, cider, and pickles, can dissolve the lead in improperly glazed containers. Food and beverage thus contaminated have caused fatal human lead poisoning. Lead is also a common contaminant of illicitly distilled whisky ("moonshine") made in the United States, since automobile radiators are frequently used as condensers and other components are connected by lead solder. Lead poisoning in children is a fairly common result of their ingestion of paint chips from old buildings. Paints applied to dwellings before World War II, when lead carbonate (white) and lead oxide (red) were common constituents of both interior and exterior house paint, are primarily responsible. In such paint, lead may constitute 5 to 40% of dried solids. Young children are poisoned most often by nibbling lead-painted windowsills and frames. The American Standards Association specified in 1955 that paints for toys, furniture, and the interior of dwellings should not contain more than 1% of lead in the final dried solids of fresh paint (National Academy of Sciences, 1972). Lead poisoning from the use of discarded automobile-battery casings made of wood and vulcanite and used as fuel during times of economic distress has been reported. Sporadic cases of lead poisoning have been traced to miscellaneous sources such as lead toys, lead dust in shooting galleries, soluble lead compounds conveyed in lead pipes, artists'

paint pigments, ashes and fumes of painted wood, jewelers' wastes, home battery manufacture, and lead type.

Occupational exposure to lead has decreased markedly over the last 50 years because of appropriate regulations and programs of medical surveillance. Workers in lead smelters have the highest potential for exposure, since fumes are generated and dust containing lead oxide is deposited in their environment. Workers in storage-battery factories face similar risks.

Absorption, Distribution, and Excretion. The major routes of absorption of lead are from the gastrointestinal tract and the respiratory system. Gastrointestinal absorption of lead varies with age; adults absorb approximately 10% of ingested lead, while children absorb up to 40%. Little is known about lead transport across the gastrointestinal mucosa. It has been speculated that lead and calcium may compete for a common transport mechanism, since there is a reciprocal relationship between the dietary content of calcium and lead absorption. Iron deficiency has also been shown to enhance intestinal absorption of lead. Absorption of inhaled lead varies with the form (vapor versus particle), as well as with concentration. Approximately 90% of inhaled lead particles from ambient air are absorbed (Goyer, 1985).

After absorption, inorganic lead is distributed initially in the soft tissues, particularly the tubular epithelium of the kidney and in the liver. In time, lead is redistributed and deposited in bone, teeth, and hair. About 95% of the body burden of the metal is eventually found in bone. Only small quantities of inorganic lead accumulate in the brain, with most of that in gray matter and the basal ganglia (Task Group, 1973). Nearly all circulating inorganic lead is associated with erythrocytes; only when lead is present in relatively high concentrations does a significant portion remain in the plasma.

The deposition of lead in bone closely resembles that of calcium, but it is deposited as tertiary lead phosphate. Lead in the bone salts does not contribute to toxicity. After a recent exposure, the concentration of lead is often higher in the flat bones than in the long bones (Kehoe, 1961a, 1961b), although, as a general rule, the long bones contain more lead. In the early period of deposition, the concentration of lead is highest in the epiphyseal portion of the long bones. This is especially true in growing bones, where deposits may be detected by x-ray examination as rings of increased density in the ossification centers of the epiphyseal cartilage and as a series of transverse lines in the diaphyses, so-called lead lines. Such findings are of diagnostic significance in children.

Factors that affect the distribution of calcium similarly affect that of lead. Thus, a high intake of phosphate favors skeletal storage of lead and a lower concentration in soft tissues. Conversely, a low phosphate intake mobilizes lead in bone and elevates its content in soft tissues. High intake of calcium in the absence of elevated intake of phosphate has a similar effect, owing to competition with lead for available phosphate. Vitamin D tends to promote the deposition of lead in bone if a sufficient amount of phosphate is available; otherwise, deposition of calcium preempts that of lead. Parathyroid hormone and dihydrotachysterol mobilize lead from the skeleton and augment the concentration of lead in blood and its rate of urinary excretion.

In experimental animals, lead is excreted into the bile, and much more lead is excreted into the feces than into the urine (Klaassen and Shoeman, 1974). In man, urinary excretion is a more important route (Kehoe, 1961a, 1961b), and the concentration of lead in urine is directly proportional to that in plasma (Zielhuis, 1971). However, since most lead in blood is in the erythrocytes, very little is filtered. Lead is also excreted in milk and sweat and is deposited in hair and nails. Placental transfer of lead is also known to occur.

The half-life of lead in blood is 1 to 2 months, and a steady state is thus achieved in about 6 months. After establishment of a steady state early in human life, the daily intake of lead approximates the output, under normal conditions, and concentrations of lead in soft tissues change little. However, the concentration of lead in bone appears to increase (Barry, 1975; Gross *et al.,* 1975), and its half-life in bone has been estimated to be 20 to 30 years. Because the rate of excretion of lead is limited, even a slight increase in daily intake may produce a positive lead balance. The average daily intake of lead is approximately 0.3 mg, while positive lead balance begins at a daily intake of about 0.6 mg. This amount will not ordinarily produce overt toxicity within a lifetime. However, the time to accumulate toxic amounts shortens disproportionately as the amount ingested increases. For example, a daily intake of 2.5 mg of lead requires nearly 4 years for the accumulation of a toxic burden, whereas a daily intake of 3.5 mg requires but a few months, since deposition in bone is too slow to protect the soft tissues during rapid accumulation.

Acute Lead Poisoning. Acute lead poisoning is relatively infrequent and occurs from ingestion of acid-soluble lead compounds or inhalation of lead vapors. Local actions in the mouth produce marked astringency, thirst, and a metallic taste. Nausea, abdominal pain, and vomiting ensue. The vomitus may be milky from the presence of lead chloride. Although the abdominal pain is severe, it is unlike that of chronic poisoning. Stools may be

black from lead sulfide, and there may be diarrhea or constipation. If large amounts of lead are absorbed rapidly, a shock syndrome may develop secondary to massive gastrointestinal loss of fluid. Acute central nervous system (CNS) symptoms include paresthesias, pain, and muscle weakness. An acute hemolytic crisis sometimes occurs and causes severe anemia and hemoglobinuria. The kidneys are damaged, and oliguria and urinary changes are evident. Death may occur in 1 or 2 days. If the patient survives the acute episode, characteristic signs and symptoms of chronic lead poisoning are likely to appear.

Chronic Lead Poisoning. Signs and symptoms of chronic lead poisoning (plumbism) can be divided into six categories: gastrointestinal, neuromuscular, CNS, hematological, renal, and other. They may occur separately or in combination. The neuromuscular and CNS syndromes usually result from intense exposure, while the abdominal syndrome is a more common manifestation of a very slowly and insidiously developing intoxication. In the United States, the CNS syndrome is usually more common among children, while the gastrointestinal syndrome is more prevalent in adults.

Gastrointestinal Effects. Lead affects the smooth muscle of the gut, producing intestinal symptoms that are an important, early sign of exposure to the metal. The abdominal syndrome often begins with vague symptoms, such as anorexia, muscle discomfort, malaise, and headache. Constipation is usually an early sign, especially in adults, but diarrhea occasionally occurs. A persistent metallic taste appears early in the course of the syndrome. As intoxication advances, anorexia and constipation become more marked. Intestinal spasm, which causes severe abdominal pain, or *lead colic,* is the most distressing feature of the advanced abdominal syndrome. The attacks are paroxysmal and generally excruciating. The abdominal muscles become rigid, and tenderness is especially manifested in the region of the umbilicus. In cases where colic is not severe, removal of the patient from the environment in which he was exposed may be sufficient for relief of symptoms. Calcium gluconate administered intravenously is recommended for relief of pain and is usually more effective than morphine.

Neuromuscular Effects. The neuromuscular syndrome, or *lead palsy,* is now rare in the United States. It is a manifestation of advanced subacute poisoning. Muscle weakness and easy fatigue occur long before actual paralysis and may be the only symptoms. Weakness or palsy may not become evident until after extended muscle activity. The muscle groups involved are usually the most active ones (extensors of the forearm, wrist, and fingers and extraocular muscles), and the palsy often occurs only on the dominant side. Wrist-drop and, to a lesser extent, foot-drop with the appropriate history of exposure have been considered almost pathognomonic for lead poisoning. There is usually no sensory involvement. Degenerative changes in the motoneurons and their axons have been described.

CNS Effects. The CNS syndrome has been termed *lead encephalopathy*. It is the most serious manifestation of lead poisoning, and is much more common in children than in adults. The early signs of the syndrome may be clumsiness, vertigo, ataxia, falling, headache, insomnia, restlessness, and irritability. As the encephalopathy develops, the patient may first become excited and confused; delirium with repetitive tonic-clonic convulsions or lethargy and coma follow. Vomiting, a common sign, is usually projectile. Visual disturbances are also present. Although the signs and symptoms are characteristic of increased intracranial pressure, flap craniotomy to relieve intracranial pressure is not beneficial. However, treatment for cerebral edema may become necessary. There may be a proliferative meningitis, intense edema, punctate hemorrhages, gliosis, and areas of focal necrosis. Demyelination has been observed in nonhuman primates. The mortality rate among patients who develop cerebral involvement is about 25%. When chelation therapy is begun after the symptoms of acute encephalopathy appear, approximately 40% of survivors have neurological sequelae, such as mental retardation, EEG abnormalities or frank seizures, cerebral palsy, optic atrophy, or dystonia musculorum deformans (Popoff *et al.*, 1963; Smith *et al.*, 1963; Chisolm and Barltrop, 1979).

Exposure to lead occasionally produces clear-cut, progressive mental deterioration in children. The history of these children indicates normal development during the first 12 to 18 months of life or longer, followed by a steady loss of motor skills and speech. They may have severe hyperkinetic and aggressive behavior disorders and a poorly controlled convulsive disorder. The lack of sensory perception severely impairs learning. Concentrations of lead in blood exceed 60 μg/dl of whole blood, and x-rays may show heavy, multiple bands of increased density in the growing long bones (*see* above). Until recently it was thought that such exposure to lead was largely restricted to children in inner-city slums. However, all children are exposed chronically to low levels of lead in their diets, in the air they breathe, and in the dirt and dust in their play areas. This is reflected in elevated concentrations of lead in blood of many children and may be a cause of subtle CNS toxicity. An increased incidence of hyperkinetic behavior and a statistically significant, although modest, decrease in IQ have been shown in children with blood lead concentrations of 30 to 50 μg/dl (Needleman *et al.*, 1979; Needleman and Devitan, 1982).

Hematological Effects. When the blood lead concentration is near 80 μg/dl or greater, basophilic stippling (the aggregation of ribonucleic acid) occurs in erythrocytes. This is thought to result from the inhibitory effect of lead on the enzyme

pyrimidine-5′-nucleotidase. Basophilic stippling is not, however, pathognomonic of lead poisoning.

A more common hematological result of chronic lead intoxication is a hypochromic microcytic anemia, which is more frequently observed in children. This anemia is morphologically similar to that which results from iron deficiency and is thought to result from two factors: a decreased life-span of the erythrocytes and an inhibition of heme synthesis.

Very low concentrations of lead influence the synthesis of heme. The enzymes necessary for heme synthesis are widely distributed in mammalian tissues, and it is highly probable that each cell synthesizes its own heme for incorporation into such proteins as hemoglobin, myoglobin, cytochromes, and catalases. Lead clearly inhibits heme formation at several points, as shown in Figure 69–1. Inhibition of δ-aminolevulinate (δ-ALA) dehydratase and ferrochelatase, which are sulfhydryl-dependent enzymes, is well documented. Lead poisoning in both man and experimental animals is characterized by accumulation of protoporphyrin IX and nonheme iron in red blood cells, by accumulation of δ-ALA in plasma, and by increased urinary excretion of δ-ALA. There is also increased urinary excretion of coproporphyrin III (the oxidation product of coproporphyrinogen III), but it is not clear whether this is due to inhibition of enzymatic activity or other factors. Increased excretion of porphobilinogen and uroporphyrin has been reported only in severe cases. The pattern of excretion of pyrroles found in lead poisoning differs from that characteristic of symptomatic episodes of acute intermittent porphyria and other hepatocellu-

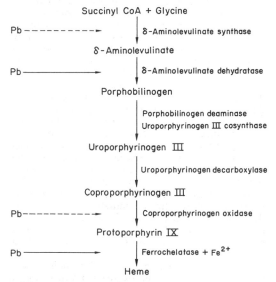

Figure 69–1. *Lead interferes with the biosynthesis of heme at several enzymatic steps.*

Steps that are definitely inhibited by lead are indicated by ——►; steps at which lead is thought to act but evidence is inconclusive are indicated by ‑‑‑►.

lar disorders, as shown in Table 69–1. The increase in δ-ALA synthase activity is due to the reduction of the cellular concentration of heme, which regulates the synthesis of δ-ALA synthase by feedback inhibition.

Measurement of heme precursors provides a sensitive index of recent absorption of inorganic lead salts. δ-ALA dehydratase activity in hemolysates and δ-ALA in urine are sensitive indicators of exposure to lead, and abnormalities of these parameters precede the appearance of symptoms (National Academy of Sciences, 1972). Because they are early signs of abnormal exposure to lead and can be detected by relatively simple laboratory procedures, these measurements are used routinely in diagnosis.

Renal Effects. Although the renal effects of lead are less dramatic than those in the CNS and gastrointestinal tract, nephropathy does occur. Renal toxicity occurs in two forms (Goyer, 1985): a reversible renal tubular disorder (usually seen after acute exposure of children to lead) and an irreversible interstitial nephropathy (more commonly observed in chronic industrial lead exposure). Clinically, a Fanconi-like syndrome is seen with proteinuria, hematuria, and casts in the urine. In some patients, hyperuricemia may be associated with renal insufficiency (Ball and Sorensen, 1969). Histologically, lead nephropathy is revealed by a characteristic nuclear inclusion body, composed of a lead-protein complex (Moore *et al.*, 1973); this appears early and resolves after chelation therapy. Such inclusion bodies have been reported in the urine sediment of workers exposed to lead in an industrial setting (Schumann *et al.*, 1980).

Other Effects. Other signs and symptoms of plumbism are an ashen color of the face and pallor of the lips; retinal stippling; appearance of "premature aging," with stooped posture, poor muscle tone, and emaciation; and a black or grayish so-called lead line along the gingival margin. The lead line, a result of periodontal deposition of lead sulfide, may be removed by good dental hygiene. Similar pigmentation may result from the absorption of mercury, bismuth, silver, thallium, or iron. The carcinogenicity of lead in man is not well established, but it has been suggested (Cooper and Gaffey, 1975), and several case reports of renal adenocarcinoma in lead workers have been published (Baker *et al.*, 1980; Lilis, 1981).

Diagnosis of Lead Poisoning. In the absence of a positive history of abnormal exposure to lead, the diagnosis of lead poisoning is easily missed. Furthermore, the signs and symptoms of lead poisoning are shared by other diseases. For example, the signs of encephalopathy may resemble those of various degenerative conditions. Physical examination does not easily distinguish lead colic from other abdominal disorders, such as peptic ulcer, pancreatitis, or acute intermittent porphyria. Clinical suspicion should be confirmed by determinations of the concentration of lead in blood and protoporphyrin in erythrocytes.

The concentration of lead in blood is one indication of recent absorption of the metal, but measurement of erythrocyte protoporphyrin alone is more cost effective (Berwick and Komaroff, 1982). In normal children and adults, blood lead values range from 10 to 40 μg/dl of whole blood. People with concentrations of 40 to 60 μg/dl exhibit no known functional injury or symptoms; however, they may have a definite decrease in δ-ALA dehydratase activity and a slight increase in urinary excretion of δ-ALA. Patients with a blood lead concentration of 60 to 80 μg/dl have a decrease in δ-ALA dehydratase activity in erythrocytes, an increased urinary excretion of δ-ALA and coproporphyrin, and, usually, nonspecific, mild symptoms of lead poisoning. Erythrocyte protoporphyrin is increased due to the inhibitory effect of lead on ferrochelatase (Figure 69–1). Clear symptoms of lead poisoning are associated with concentrations that exceed 80 μg/dl of whole blood (Kehoe, 1961a, 1961b), and lead encephalopathy is usually apparent when lead concentrations are greater than 120 μg/dl (National Academy of Sciences, 1972). In persons with moderate-to-severe anemia, interpretation of the significance of concentrations of lead in blood is improved by correcting the observed value to approximate that which would be expected if the patient's hematocrit were within the normal range.

Urinary excretion of lead in normal adults is generally less than 80 μg per liter (Kehoe, 1961a, 1961b; Goldwater and Hoover, 1967). Most patients with lead poisoning show concentrations of lead in urine of 150 to 300 μg per liter. However, in persons with chronic lead nephropathy or other forms of renal insufficiency, urinary excretion of lead may be within the normal range.

Because the onset of lead poisoning is usually

Table 69–1. PATTERNS OF INCREASED EXCRETION OF PYRROLES IN URINE OF ACUTELY SYMPTOMATIC PATIENTS *

DISEASE	PYRROLES †			
	ALA	PBG	URO	COPRO
Lead poisoning	+++	o	±	+++
Acute intermittent porphyria	++++	++++	+ to ++++	+ to +++
Acute hepatitis	o	o	o	+ to +++
Acute alcoholism	o	o	±	+ to +++

* Modified from Chisolm, 1967.
† o = normal; + to ++++ = degree of increase; ALA = δ-aminolevulinic acid; PBG = porphobilinogen; URO = uroporphyrin; COPRO = coproporphyrin.

insidious, it is often desirable to estimate the body burden of lead in individuals who are exposed to an environment that is contaminated with the metal. Use of the edetate calcium disodium (CaNa$_2$EDTA) mobilization test helps determine whether there is an increased body burden of lead in those in whom exposure occurred much earlier (Emmerson, 1963). This test is performed by intravenous infusion over 1 hour of 1 g of CaNa$_2$EDTA in 250 ml of a 5% solution of dextrose. All urine is collected for 4 days. The upper limit of excretion of lead by normal adults is 600 μg under these conditions. This test is not used in symptomatic patients or in those whose concentration of lead in blood is greater than 100 μg/dl, because these patients require the proper therapeutic regimen with chelating agents (*see* below).

In summary, the diagnosis of lead poisoning is usually based on the patient's history and clinical presentation and is easily confirmed by laboratory determinations. Other diagnostic information includes characteristic lead lines in the long bones of children, unabsorbed lead seen radiographically in the gastrointestinal tract in a child with recent ingestion, basophilic stippling of erythrocytes associated with anemia, renal dysfunction, and neurological lesions.

Organic Lead Poisoning. Tetraethyllead and tetramethyllead are lipid-soluble compounds and are readily absorbed from the skin, gastrointestinal tract, and lungs. The toxicity of tetraethyllead is believed to be due to its metabolic conversion to triethyllead and inorganic lead.

The major symptoms of intoxication with tetraethyllead are referable to the CNS (Gething, 1975; Seshia *et al.*, 1978). The victim suffers from insomnia, nightmares, anorexia, nausea and vomiting, diarrhea, headache, muscular weakness, and emotional instability. Subjective CNS symptoms such as irritability, restlessness, and anxiety are next evident. At this time there is usually hypothermia, bradycardia, and hypotension. With continued exposure, or in the case of intense acute exposure, CNS manifestations progress to delusions, ataxia, exaggerated muscular movements, and, finally, a maniacal state.

The diagnosis of poisoning by tetraethyllead is established by relating these signs and symptoms to a history of exposure. The urinary excretion of lead may increase markedly, but the concentration of lead in blood remains nearly normal. Anemia is uncommon in organic lead poisoning, and erythrocyte protoporphyrin concentrations are inconsistently elevated (Garrettson, 1983). There is little effect on the metabolism of porphyrins. Basophilic stippling of erythrocytes is uncommon. In the case of severe exposure, death may occur within a few hours or may be delayed for several weeks. If the patient survives the acute phase of organic lead poisoning, recovery is usually complete; however, instances of residual CNS damage have been reported.

Treatment of Lead Poisoning. Initial treatment of the acute phase of lead intoxication involves supportive measures. Prevention of further exposure is important. Seizures are treated with diazepam (Chapter 20); fluid and electrolyte balance must be maintained; cerebral edema is treated with mannitol and dexamethasone. The concentration of lead in blood should be determined prior to initiation of chelation therapy.

Chelation therapy should be instituted in symptomatic patients or in patients with a blood lead concentration in excess of 50 to 60 μg/dl. Three chelators are commonly employed in the treatment of lead intoxication: edetate calcium disodium (CaNa$_2$EDTA), dimercaprol (British antilewisite; BAL), and D-penicillamine. CaNa$_2$EDTA and dimercaprol are usually used in combination, initially, followed by oral penicillamine for long-term treatment.

CaNa$_2$EDTA is employed at a dose of 50 to 75 mg/kg per day in two divided doses, either by deep intramuscular injection or slow intravenous infusion for up to 5 consecutive days. The first dose of CaNa$_2$EDTA should be delayed until 4 hours after the first dose of BAL. An additional course of CaNa$_2$EDTA may be given after an interruption of 2 days. Each course of therapy with CaNa$_2$EDTA should not exceed a total dose of 500 mg/kg. Urine output must be monitored, because the chelator-lead complex is believed to be nephrotoxic. Treatment with CaNa$_2$EDTA can alleviate symptoms quickly. Colic may disappear within 2 hours; paresthesia and tremor cease after 4 or 5 days; coproporphyrinuria, stippled erythrocytes, and gingival lead lines tend to decrease in 4 to 9 days. Urinary elimination of lead is usually greatest during the initial infusion.

Dimercaprol is given intramuscularly at a dose of 4 mg/kg every 4 hours for 48 hours, then every 6 hours for 48 hours, and finally every 6 to 12 hours for an additional 7 days. The combination of dimercaprol and CaNa$_2$EDTA is more effective than is either chelator alone (Chisholm, 1973).

In contrast to CaNa$_2$EDTA and dimercaprol, penicillamine is effective orally and may be included in the regimen at a dose of 250 mg given four times daily for 5 days. During chronic therapy with penicillamine, the dose should not exceed 40 mg/kg per day.

Lead poisoning in children is more dangerous than in adults, primarily because of the greater incidence of encephalopathy. The mortality rate of untreated, severe lead encephalopathy may approach 65%, and neurological sequelae are common in survivors. Hospitalization is recommended for any symptomatic child or any child with a blood lead concentration of 80 μg/dl or greater. Exposure is thereby terminated, and careful monitoring and supportive measures are essential.

Long-term chelation therapy for patients with residual encephalopathy or with blood lead concentrations exceeding 60 μg/dl and with prominent radiographic evidence of lead deposition in bone is most easily accomplished with oral penicillamine (40 mg/kg per day, maximum). One must remember that the oral chelator may promote absorption of lead from the gastrointestinal tract. Avoidance of continued exposure to lead is thus very important.

Treatment of organic lead poisoning is symptomatic. Chelation therapy will promote the excretion of the inorganic lead produced from the metabolism of organic lead, but the increase is not dramatic (Boyd, 1957).

MERCURY

Mercury was an important constituent of drugs for centuries—as an ingredient in many diuretics, antibacterials, antiseptics, skin ointments, and laxatives. More specific and effective modes of therapy have largely replaced the mercurials in recent decades, and drug-induced signs of mercury poisoning have become rare. Mercury poisoning from environmental pollution has, however, become an area of concern. Concentrations of mercury in air, soil, and water have increased because of greater use of fossil fuels, which contain mercury, and the increased use of mercury in industry and agriculture. There have been epidemics of mercury poisoning among wildlife and human populations in many countries. With very few exceptions and for numerous reasons, such outbreaks were misdiagnosed for months or even years. Reasons for these tragic delays included the insidious onset of the affliction, vagueness of early clinical signs, and the medical profession's unfamiliarity with the disease (Gerstner and Huff, 1977).

Chemical Forms and Sources of Mercury. With regard to the toxicity of mercury, three major chemical forms of the metal must be distinguished: mercury vapor (elemental mercury), salts of mercury, and organic mercurials.

Elemental mercury is the most volatile of the inorganic forms of the metal. Human exposure to mercury vapor is mainly occupational and has been known since antiquity. Chronic exposure to mercury in ambient air after inadvertent spills in poorly ventilated rooms, often scientific laboratories, can produce toxic effects.

Salts of mercury exist in two states of oxidation—as monovalent mercurous salts or as divalent mercuric salts. Mercurous chloride or calomel, the best-known mercurous compound, is still used in some skin creams as an antiseptic and was employed as a diuretic and cathartic. Mercuric salts are the most irritating and acutely toxic form of the metal. Mercuric nitrate was a common industrial hazard in the felt-hat industry more than 400 years ago. Occupational exposure produced neurological and behavioral changes depicted by the Mad Hatter in Lewis Carroll's *Alice's Adventures in Wonderland*. Mercuric chloride, once a widely used antiseptic, was also commonly used for suicidal purposes. Mercuric salts are still widely employed in industry, and industrial discharge into rivers has introduced mercury into the environment in many parts of the world. The main industrial uses of inorganic mercury today are in chloralkali production and in electronics. Other uses of the metal include the manufacturing of plastics, fungicides, and germicides and the formulation of amalgams in dentistry.

The organomercurials in use today contain mercury with one covalent bond to a carbon atom. This is a heterogeneous group of compounds, and its members have varying abilities to produce toxic effects. The alkylmercury salts are by far the most dangerous of these compounds; methylmercury is the most common. Alkylmercury salts have been widely used as fungicides and, as such, have produced toxic effects in man. Major incidents of human poisoning from the inadvertent consumption of mercury-treated seed grain have occurred in Iraq, Pakistan, Ghana, and Guatemala. The most catastrophic outbreak occurred in Iraq in 1972. During the fall of 1971, Iraq imported large quantities of seed (wheat and barley) treated with methylmercury and distributed the grain for spring planting. Despite official warnings, the grain was ground into flour and made into bread. As a result, 6530 victims were hospitalized and 500 died (Bakir *et al.*, 1973, 1980).

Minamata disease was also due to methylmercury. Minamata is a small town in Japan, and its major industry is a chemical plant that empties its effluent directly into Minamata Bay. The chemical plant used inorganic mercury as a catalyst, and some of it was methylated before it entered the bay. In addition, microorganisms convert inorganic mercury to methylmercury; the compound is then taken up rapidly by plankton algae and is concentrated in fish via the food chain. Residents of Minamata who consumed fish as a large portion of their diet were the first to be poisoned. Eventually 121 persons were poisoned and 46 died (McAlpine and Shukuro, 1958; Smith and Smith, 1975). In the United States, human poisonings have resulted from ingestion of meat from pigs fed grain treated with an organomercurial fungicide.

Chemistry and Mechanism of Action. Mercury readily forms covalent bonds with sulfur, and it is this property that accounts for most of the biological properties of the metal. When the sulfur is in the form of sulfhydryl groups, divalent mercury replaces the hydrogen atom to form mercaptides, $X—Hg—SR$ and $Hg(SR)_2$, where X is an electronegative radical and R is protein. Organic mercurials form mercaptides of the type $RHg—SR'$. Mercurials even in low concentrations are capable of inactivating sulfhydryl enzymes and thus interfering with cellular metabolism and function. The affinity of mercury for thiols provides the basis for treatment of mercury poisoning by such agents as dimercaprol and penicillamine. Mercury also combines with other ligands of physiological importance, such as phosphoryl, carboxyl, amide, and amine groups.

The various therapeutic and toxic actions of the mercurials are associated with chemical substituents that affect solubility, dissociation, relative affinity for various cellular receptors, distribution, and excretion.

Absorption, Biotransformation, Distribution, and Excretion. *Elemental Mercury.* Elemental mercury is not particularly toxic when ingested because of very low absorption from the gastrointestinal tract due to the formation of droplets and because the metal in this form cannot react with biologically important molecules. However, inhaled mercury vapor is completely absorbed by the lung and is then oxidized to the divalent mercuric cation by catalase in the erythrocytes (Magos *et al.*, 1978). Within a few hours the deposition of inhaled mercury vapor resembles that after ingestion of mercuric salts, with one important difference. Since mercury vapor crosses membranes much more readily than does divalent mercury, a significant amount of the vapor enters the brain before it is oxidized. CNS toxicity is thus more prominent after exposure to mercury vapor than to divalent forms of the metal.

Inorganic Salts of Mercury. The soluble inorganic mercuric salts (Hg^{2+}) gain access to the circulation when taken orally. Gastrointestinal absorption is approximately 10% of that ingested, and a considerable portion of the Hg^{2+} may remain bound to the alimentary mucosa and the intestinal contents. Insoluble inorganic mercurous compounds, such as calomel (Hg_2Cl_2), may undergo some oxidation to soluble compounds that are more readily absorbed. Inorganic mercury has a markedly nonuniform distribution after absorption. The highest concentration of Hg^{2+} is found in the kidneys, where the metal is retained longer than in other tissues. Concentrations of inorganic mercury are similar in whole blood and plasma. Inorganic mercurials do not readily pass the blood-brain barrier or the placenta. The metal is excreted in the urine and feces; studies in laboratory animals indicate that fecal excretion is quantitatively more important (Norseth and Clarkson, 1971; Klaassen, 1976). In general, the body burden of mercury in man has a half-life of about 60 days (Friberg and Vostal, 1972).

Organic Mercurials. Organic mercurials are more completely absorbed from the gastrointestinal tract than are the inorganic salts because they are more lipid soluble and less corrosive to the intestinal mucosa. Over 90% of methylmercury is absorbed from the human gastrointestinal tract. The organic mercurials cross the blood-brain barrier and the placenta and thus produce more neurological and teratogenic effects than do the inorganic salts. Organic mercurials are more uniformly distributed to the various tissues than are the inorganic salts (Klaassen, 1975). A significant portion of the body burden of organic mercurials is in the red blood cells (Swensson and Ulfarsson, 1963). The ratio of the concentration of organomercurial in erythrocytes to that in plasma varies with the compound; for methylmercury, it approximates 20:1 (Kershaw *et al.*, 1980). The carbon-mercury bond of some organic mercurials is cleaved after absorption; with methylmercury the cleavage is

quite slow and the inorganic mercury formed is not thought to play a major role in methylmercury toxicity (Norseth and Clarkson, 1970). Aryl mercurials, like mercurophen, usually contain a labile mercury-carbon bond, and the toxicity of these compounds is similar to that of inorganic mercury. Excretion of methylmercury by man is mainly in the feces; less than 10% of a dose appears in urine. The biological half-life of methylmercury in man is about 65 days (Bakir *et al.*, 1973).

Toxicity. *Elemental Mercury.* Acute exposure to elemental mercury vapor may produce symptoms within several hours; these include weakness, chills, metallic taste, nausea, vomiting, diarrhea, dyspnea, cough, and a feeling of tightness in the chest. Pulmonary toxicity may progress to an interstitial pneumonitis with severe compromise of respiratory function. Recovery, although usually complete, may be complicated by residual interstitial fibrosis.

Chronic exposure to mercury vapor produces a more insidious form of toxicity that is dominated by neurological effects (Friberg and Vostal, 1972). The syndrome is referred to as the *asthenic vegetative syndrome* and consists in neurasthenic symptoms in addition to three or more of the following findings (Goyer, 1985): goiter, increased uptake of radioiodine by the thyroid, tachycardia, labile pulse, gingivitis, dermographia (skin writing), and increased mercury in the urine. With continued exposure, tremor becomes most noticeable and psychological changes consist in depression, irritability, excessive shyness, insomnia, emotional instability, forgetfulness, confusion, and vasomotor disturbances (such as excessive perspiration and uncontrolled blushing, which together are referred to as *erethism*). A common feature of intoxication from mercury vapor is severe salivation and gingivitis. The triad of increased excitability, tremors, and gingivitis has been recognized historically as the major manifestation of exposure to mercury vapor when mercury nitrate was used in the fur, felt, and hat industries. Renal dysfunction has also been reported to result from chronic industrial exposure to mercury vapor.

Inorganic Salts of Mercury. Inorganic, ionic mercury (*e.g.*, mercuric chloride) can produce severe acute toxicity. Precipitation of mucous membrane proteins by mercuric salts results in an ashen-gray appearance of the mucosa of the mouth, pharynx, and intestine and also causes intense pain, which may be accompanied by vomiting. The vomiting is protective, since it removes unabsorbed mercury from the stomach, and should not be inhibited (assuming the patient is awake and alert). The local, corrosive effect of ionic inorganic mercury on the gastrointestinal mucosa results in severe hematochezia with evidence of mucosal sloughing in the stool. Hypovolemic shock and death usually result in the absence of proper treatment. However, these local effects can be overcome readily with prompt corrective treatment. Systemic toxicity may begin within a few hours after exposure to mercury and last for days. A strong metallic taste is followed by stomatitis with gingival irritation, foul breath, and loosening of the teeth. The most serious and, unfortunately, the most frequently encountered systemic effect of inorganic mercury is renal toxicity. Renal tubular necrosis occurs after acute exposure, leading to oliguria or anuria.

Renal injury commonly follows chronic exposure to inorganic mercury; however, glomerular injury predominates. This is the result of both direct effects on the glomerular basement membrane and a later indirect effect mediated by immune complexes (Goyer, 1985).

The symptom complex of acrodynia (pink disease) also commonly follows chronic exposure to inorganic mercury ions. Acrodynia is an erythema of the extremities, chest, and face with photophobia, diaphoresis, anorexia, tachycardia, and either constipation or diarrhea. This symptom complex is seen almost exclusively after ingestion of mercury and is believed to be the result of a hypersensitivity reaction to mercury (Matherson et al., 1980).

Organic Mercurials. Most human toxicological data about organic mercury concern methylmercury and have been collected as the unfortunate result of several large-scale accidental exposures. Symptoms of exposure to methylmercury are mainly neurological in origin and consist in visual disturbance (scotoma and visual-field constriction), ataxia, paresthesias, neurasthenia, hearing loss, dysarthria, mental deterioration, muscle tremor, movement disorders, and, with severe exposure, paralysis and death (Table 69–2). Certain regions of the brain have been found to be particularly sensitive to the toxic effects of methylmercury, namely, the cerebral cortex (especially the visual cortex) and the granular layer of the cerebellum. Effects of methylmercury on the fetus can occur even when the mother is asymptomatic; mental retardation and neuromuscular deficits have been observed.

Diagnosis of Mercury Poisoning. A history of exposure to mercury, either industrial or environmental, is obviously valuable in making the diagnosis of mercury poisoning. Without such a history, clinical suspicions can be confirmed by laboratory analysis. The upper limit of a normal concentration of mercury in blood is generally considered to be 3 to 4 μg/dl. A concentration of mercury in blood in excess of 4 μg/dl should be considered abnormal in adults. Because methylmercury is concentrated in erythrocytes and inorganic mercury is not, the distribution of total mercury between red blood cells and plasma may indicate whether the patient has been poisoned with inorganic or organic mercury. Measurement of total mercury in red blood cells gives a better estimate of the body burden of methylmercury than it does for inorganic mercury. The relationship between concentrations of mercury in blood and the frequency of symptoms that result from exposure to methylmercury is shown in Table 69–2; however, this is only a rough guide. Concentrations of mercury in plasma provide a better index of the body burden of inorganic mercury; however, the relationship between body burden and the concentration of inorganic mercury in plasma is not well documented. The relationship between the concentration of inorganic mercury in blood and toxicity depends on the form of exposure. For example, exposure to vapor results in concentrations in brain about ten times higher than those that follow an equivalent dose of inorganic mercuric salts.

The concentration of mercury in the urine has also been used as a measure of the body burden of the metal. The upper limit for excretion of mercury into urine in the normal population is 25 μg per liter. There is a linear relationship between plasma concentration and urinary excretion of mercury after exposure to vapor; workers in a chloralkali plant exhibited tremors when the concentrations of mercury in urine reached 500 μg per liter (Langolf et al., 1977). In contrast, the excretion of mercury in urine is a poor indicator of the amount of methylmercury in the blood, since it is eliminated mainly in feces (Bakir et al., 1973).

Hair is rich in sulfhydryl groups, and the concentration of mercury in hair is about 300 times that in blood. Furthermore, the most recent growth of hair reflects a fairly current concentration of mercury in blood. Human hair grows about 20 cm a year, and a history of exposure may be obtained by analysis of different segments of hair.

Treatment of Mercury Poisoning. Measurement of the concentration of mercury in blood should be performed as soon as possible after poisoning with any form of the metal.

Table 69–2. FREQUENCY OF SYMPTOMS OF METHYLMERCURY POISONING IN RELATION TO CONCENTRATION OF MERCURY IN BLOOD *

CONCENTRATION OF MERCURY IN BLOOD (μg/ml)	CASES WITH SYMPTOMS (%)					
	Paresthesias	Ataxia	Visual Defects	Dysarthria	Hearing Defects	Death
0.1–0.5	5	0	0	5	0	0
0.5–1.0	42	11	21	5	5	0
1–2	60	47	53	24	5	0
2–3	79	60	56	25	13	0
3–4	82	100	58	75	36	17
4–5	100	100	83	85	66	28

* Based on data in Bakir et al., 1973.

Elemental Mercury Vapor. Therapeutic measures include immediate termination of exposure and close monitoring of pulmonary status. Respiratory support may be necessary acutely. Chelation therapy, as described below for inorganic mercury, should be initiated immediately and continued as indicated by the clinical condition and the concentrations of mercury in blood and urine.

Inorganic Mercury. Prompt attention to fluid and electrolyte balance and hematological status is of critical importance in moderate-to-severe oral exposures. Emesis should be induced if the patient is awake and alert. Alternatively, gastric lavage may be performed to remove mercury from the gastrointestinal tract. Activated charcoal and a magnesium cathartic should then be administered to limit further absorption.

Chelation therapy with dimercaprol (for high-level exposures or symptomatic patients) or penicillamine (for low-level exposures or asymptomatic patients) is routinely used to treat poisoning with either inorganic or elemental mercury. Recommended treatment includes dimercaprol, 5 mg/kg intramuscularly initially, followed by 2.5 mg/kg intramuscularly every 12 hours for 10 days. Penicillamine (250 mg orally every 6 hours) may be used alone or following treatment with dimercaprol. The duration of chelation therapy will vary, and progress can be monitored by following concentrations of mercury in urine and blood.

Hemodialysis may be necessary in the poisoned patient whose renal function declines. Chelators may still be used, because the dimercaprol-mercury complex is removed by dialysis (Giunta *et al.*, 1983).

Organic Mercury. The short-chain organic mercurials, especially methylmercury, are the most difficult forms of mercury to mobilize from the body, presumably due to their poor reactivity with chelating agents. Dimercaprol is *contraindicated* in methylmercury poisoning because it increases brain concentrations of methylmercury in experimental animals. While penicillamine facilitates the removal of methylmercury from the body, its clinical efficacy in the treatment of intoxication with methylmercury is not impressive (Bakir *et al.*, 1976, 1980). The dose of penicillamine normally used in the treatment of poisoning with inorganic mercury (1 g per day) produces only a small reduction in the concentration of methylmercury in blood; larger doses (2 g per day) are needed. During the initial 1 to 3 days of administration of penicillamine the concentration of mercury in the blood increases before it decreases. This is probably due to the mobilization of metal from tissues to blood at a rate more rapid than that at which mercury is excreted into urine and feces.

Methylmercury compounds undergo extensive enterohepatic recirculation in experimental animals (Norseth and Clarkson, 1971). Therefore, introduction of a nonabsorbable mercury-binding substance into the intestinal tract should facilitate their removal from the body. A polythiol resin has been used for this purpose in man and appears to be effective (Bakir *et al.*, 1973). The resin has certain advantages over penicillamine. It does not cause redistribution of mercury in the body with a subsequent increase in the concentration of mercury in blood, and it has fewer adverse effects than do sulfhydryl agents that are absorbed. Clinical experience with various treatments for methylmercury poisoning in Iraq indicates that penicillamine, N-acetyl-D,L-penicillamine, and an oral nonabsorbable thiol resin can all reduce blood concentrations of mercury; however, clinical improvement was not clearly related to reduction of the body burden of methylmercury (Bakir *et al.*, 1980).

Conventional hemodialysis is of little value in the treatment of methylmercury poisoning, because methylmercury concentrates in erythrocytes and little is contained in the plasma. However, it has been shown that L-cysteine can be infused into the arterial blood entering the dialyzer to convert methylmercury into a diffusible form. Both free cysteine and the methylmercury-cysteine complex formed in the blood then diffuse across the membrane into the dialysate. This method has been shown to be effective in man (Al-Abbasi *et al.*, 1978). Recent studies in animals indicate that 2,3-dimercaptosuccinic acid may be more effective than cysteine in this regard (Kostyniak, 1982).

ARSENIC

Arsenic was used more than 2400 years ago in Greece and Rome as a therapeutic agent and poison. The history and folklore of arsenic prompted intensive studies by early pharmacologists. Indeed, the foundations of many modern concepts of chemotherapy derive from Ehrlich's early work with organic arsenicals, and such drugs were once a mainstay of chemotherapy. In current therapeutics, arsenicals are important only in the treatment of certain tropical diseases (*see* Chapter 47). In the United States the impact of arsenic on health is predominantly from industrial and environmental exposures.

Arsenic is found in soil, water, and air as a common environmental toxicant. The element is usually not mined as such but is recovered as a by-product from the smelting of copper, lead, zinc, and other ores. This can result in the release of arsenic into the environment. Mineral-spring waters and the effluent from geothermal power plants leach arsenic from soils and rocks containing high concentrations of the metal (Fowler, 1977). Arsenic has been found in high concentrations in some sources of drinking water. It is also present in coal at variable concentrations and is released into the environment during combustion. Application of pesticides and herbicides containing arsenic has increased its environmental dispersion. Fruits and vegetables sprayed with arsenicals may also be a source of this element, and it is concentrated in many species of fish and shellfish. Arsenicals are sometimes used as feed additives for poultry and other livestock to promote growth. The major source of occupational exposure to arsenic-containing compounds is from the manufacture of arsenical herbicides and pesticides (Landrigan, 1981). The average daily human intake of arsenic is about 300 μg. Almost all of this is ingested with food and water.

Chemical Forms of Arsenic. The arsenic atom exists in the elemental form and in trivalent and pentavalent oxidation states. The toxicity of a given arsenical is related to the rate of its clearance from the body and, therefore, to its degree of accumulation in tissues. In general, toxicity increases in the sequence of organic arsenicals $< As^{5+} < As^{3+} <$ arsine (AsH_3).

The organic arsenicals contain arsenic linked to a carbon atom by a covalent bond, where arsenic exists in the trivalent or pentavalent state. Arsphenamine contains trivalent arsenic; sodium arsanilate contains arsenic in the pentavalent form.

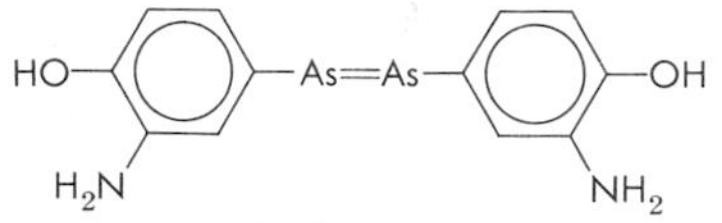

Arsphenamine

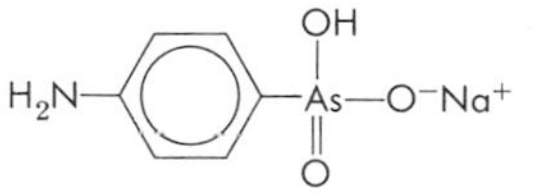

Sodium Arsanilate

The organic arsenicals are usually excreted more rapidly than are the inorganic forms.

The pentavalent oxidation state is found in arsenates (such as lead arsenate, $PbHAsO_4$), which are salts of arsenic acid, H_3AsO_4. The pentavalent arsenicals have very low affinity for thiol groups, in contrast to the trivalent compounds, and are much less toxic. The arsenites, for example, potassium arsenite ($KAsO_2$), and salts of arsenious acid contain trivalent arsenic. Arsine (AsH_3) is a gaseous hydride of trivalent arsenic; it produces toxic effects that are distinct from those of the other arsenic compounds.

Mechanism of Action. Arsenate is a well-known uncoupler of mitochondrial oxidative phosphorylation. The mechanism is thought to be related to competitive substitution of arsenate for inorganic phosphate, with subsequent formation of an unstable arsenate ester that is rapidly hydrolyzed. This process is termed *arsenolysis*.

Trivalent arsenicals, including inorganic arsenite, are regarded primarily as sulfhydryl reagents. As such, trivalent arsenicals inhibit many enzymes by reacting with biological ligands containing available —SH groups. The pyruvate dehydrogenase system is especially sensitive to trivalent arsenicals because of their interaction with two sulfhydryl groups of lipoic acid to form a stable six-membered ring, as shown below.

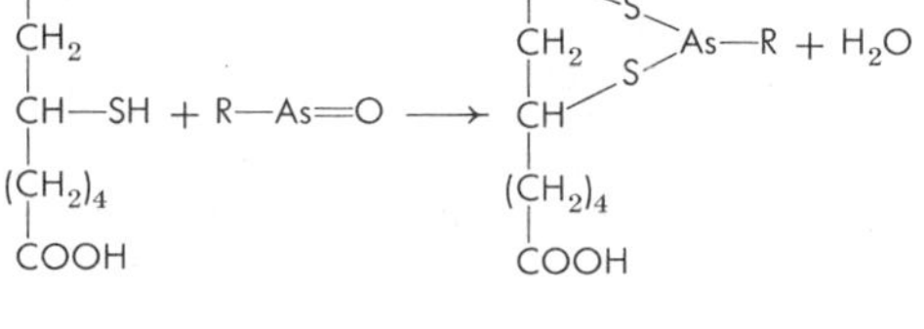

Absorption, Distribution, and Excretion. The absorption of poorly water-soluble arsenicals, such as As_2O_3, greatly depends on the physical state of the compound. Coarsely powdered material is less toxic because it can be eliminated in feces before it dissolves. The arsenite salts are more soluble in water and are better absorbed than the oxide. Experimental evidence has shown a high degree of gastrointestinal absorption of both trivalent and pentavalent forms of arsenic (Tam *et al.*, 1979). Medicinal organic arsenicals vary in their extent of gastrointestinal absorption. Some are well absorbed and are given orally in the treatment of systemic infections; others that are poorly absorbed are used effectively against intraintestinal parasites.

The distribution of arsenic depends upon the duration of administration and the particular arsenical involved. Arsenic is stored mainly in liver, kidney, heart, and lung. Much smaller amounts are found in muscle and neural tissue. Because of the high sulfhydryl content of keratin, high concentrations of arsenic are found in hair and nails. Deposition in hair starts within 2 weeks after administration, and arsenic stays fixed at this site for years. It is also deposited in bone and teeth and is retained there for long periods. Arsenic readily crosses the placental barrier, and fetal damage has been reported in animals and man (Ferm, 1977). Concentrations of arsenic in human umbilical cord blood are equivalent to those in the maternal circulation (Kagey *et al.*, 1977).

Little is known about the biotransformations of arsenicals in man. Some pentavalent arsenicals are partly reduced *in vivo* to the trivalent form. However, the redox equilibria *in vivo* favor the oxidized form, and trivalent arsenic is slowly oxidized in the body to the pentavalent state. The low toxicity and high recovery of pentavalent arsenicals in urine and excreta indicate that very little reduction takes place. It appears that both trivalent and pentavalent forms are methylated in man, because dimethylarsenic acid is a major form of arsenic excreted in urine. Arsenic is eliminated by many routes (feces, urine, sweat, milk, hair, skin, lungs), although most is excreted in urine in man. The half-life for the urinary excretion of arsenic is 3 to 5 days.

Pharmacological and Toxicological Effects of Arsenic. Arsenicals have varied effects on many organ systems. These are summarized below.

Cardiovascular System. Small doses of inorganic arsenic induce mild vasodilatation. This may lead to an occult edema, particularly facial, which has been mistaken for a healthy weight gain and misinterpreted as a "tonic" effect of arsenic. Larger doses evoke capillary dilatation; increased capillary permeability may occur in all capillary beds, but it is most pronounced in the splanchnic area. Transudation of plasma may also occur, and the decrease in intravascular volume may be significant. Myocardial damage and hypotension appear later. ECG abnormalities may persist for months after recovery from acute intoxication.

Gastrointestinal Tract. Small doses of inorganic arsenicals, especially the trivalent compounds, cause mild splanchnic hyperemia. Capillary transudation of plasma, resulting from larger doses, produces vesicles under the gastrointestinal mucosa. These eventually rupture, epithelial fragments slough off, and plasma is discharged into the lumen of the intestine, where it coagulates. Tissue damage and the bulk cathartic action of the increased fluid in the lumen lead to increased peristalsis and characteristic watery diarrhea ("rice-water stools"). Normal proliferation of the epithelium is suppressed, which accentuates the damage. Soon the feces become bloody. Damage to the upper gastrointestinal tract usually results in hematemesis. Stomatitis may also be evident. The onset of gastrointestinal symptoms may be so gradual that the possibility of arsenic poisoning may be overlooked.

Kidneys. The action of arsenic on the renal capillaries, tubules, and glomeruli may cause severe renal damage. Initially, the glomeruli are affected and proteinuria results. Varying degrees of tubular necrosis and degeneration occur later. Oliguria with proteinuria, hematuria, and casts frequently results from exposure to arsenic.

Skin. Acutely, many arsenicals have a vesicant effect on the skin that results in necrosis and sloughing. Chronic ingestion of low doses of inorganic arsenicals causes cutaneous vasodilatation and a "milk and roses" complexion. Prolonged use of arsenic, however, also causes hyperkeratosis, particularly of the palms and soles, and hyperpigmentation over the trunk and extremities. Eventually these actions proceed to atrophy and degeneration, and possibly to cancer. Skin eruptions were common in patients who received inorganic arsenic medication.

Nervous System. Chronic exposure to inorganic but rarely to organic arsenicals may cause peripheral neuritis. In severe cases, the spinal cord may also be involved. After acute ingestion of toxic doses of inorganic arsenic, approximately 5% of the patients have central depression without gastrointestinal symptoms. Neurological symptoms include severe headache, drowsiness, confusion, fever, convulsions, and coma. The most common arsenic-induced neurological lesion is a peripheral neuropathy with a "stocking-glove" distribution of dysesthesia. Muscular weakness also occurs in the extremities, and, with continued exposure, deep-tendon reflexes diminish and muscular atrophy follows. The cerebral lesions are mainly vascular in origin and occur in both the gray and white matter; characteristic multiple, symmetrical foci of hemorrhagic necrosis occur.

Blood. Inorganic arsenicals affect the bone marrow and alter the cellular composition of the blood. Hematological evaluation usually reveals anemia with slight-to-moderate leukopenia; eosinophilia may also be present. Anisocytosis becomes evident with increasing exposure to arsenic. The vascularity of the bone marrow is increased. Some of the chronic hematological effects may result from impaired absorption of folic acid (Van Tongeren *et al.*, 1965). Serious, irreversible blood and bone-marrow disturbances from organic arsenicals are rare. A few cases of agranulocytosis have reportedly been caused by glycobiarsol, an organic arsenical used in the treatment of amebiasis.

Liver. Inorganic arsenicals and a number of now-obsolete organic arsenicals are particularly toxic to the liver and produce fatty infiltration, central necrosis, and cirrhosis; tryparsamide, an antitrypanosomal agent, may induce hepatic damage in therapeutic doses. The damage may be mild or so severe that death may ensue. The injury is generally to the hepatic parenchyma, but in some cases the clinical picture may closely resemble occlusion of the common bile duct, the principle lesions being pericholangiitis and bile thrombi in the finer biliary radicles.

Carcinogenesis and Teratogenesis. Arsenic causes chromosomal breaks in cultured human leukocytes and teratogenic effects in hamsters. There is overwhelming epidemiological evidence that chronic ingestion of arsenic in drinking water or chronic exposure from the use of inorganic arsenicals in sheep-dip or vineyard sprays predisposes to intraepidermal squamous-cell and superficial basal-cell carcinomas of the skin. Evidence has also accumulated that the chronic use of Fowler's solution (potassium arsenite) for psoriasis or other disorders causes skin cancer. Among metal workers, there is a strong correlation between the intensity and duration of exposure to arsenic and lung cancer (Lee and Fraumeni, 1969). More recently, hemangiosarcoma has been found to occur in vineyard workers who are chronically exposed to arsenic (Popper *et al.*, 1978).

Acute Arsenic Poisoning. Federal restrictions on the allowable content of arsenic in food and in the occupational environment not only have improved safety procedures and decreased the number of intoxications but also have decreased the amount of arsenic in use; only the annual production of arsenic-containing herbicides is increasing.

The incidence of accidental, homicidal, and suicidal arsenic poisoning has greatly diminished in recent decades. Arsenic in the form of As_2O_3 used to be a common cause of poisoning because it is readily available, is practically tasteless, and has the appearance of sugar.

Gastrointestinal discomfort is usually experienced within an hour after intake of an arsenical, although it may be delayed as much as 12 hours after oral ingestion if food is in the stomach. Burning lips, constriction of the throat, and difficulty in swallowing may be the first symptoms, followed by excruciating gastric pain, projectile vomiting, and severe diarrhea. Oliguria with proteinuria and hematuria is usually present; eventually anuria may occur. The patient often complains of marked skeletal muscle cramps and severe thirst. As the loss of fluid proceeds, symptoms of shock appear. Hypoxic convulsions may occur terminally, and coma and death ensue. In severe poisoning, death can occur within an hour, but the usual interval is 24 hours. With prompt application of corrective therapy, patients may survive the acute phase of the toxicity only to develop neuropathies and other disorders. In a series of 57 such patients, 37 had peripheral neuropathy and 5 had encephalopathy. The motor system appears to be spared only in the mildest cases; severe crippling is common (Jenkins, 1966).

Chronic Arsenic Poisoning. The most common early signs of chronic arsenic poisoning are muscle weakness and aching, skin pigmentation (especially of the neck, eyelids, nipples, and axillae), hyperkeratosis, and edema. Gastrointestinal involvement is less prominent in chronic exposures. Other signs and symptoms that should arouse suspicion of arsenic poisoning include garlic odor of the breath and perspiration, excessive salivation and sweating, stomatitis, generalized itching, sore throat, coryza, lacrimation, numbness, burning or tingling of the extremities, dermatitis, vitiligo, and alopecia. Poisoning may begin insidiously with symptoms of weakness, languor, anorexia, occasional nausea and vomiting, and diarrhea or constipation. Subsequent symptoms may simulate acute coryza. Dermatitis and keratosis of the palms and soles are common features. Mee's lines are characteristically found in the fingernails (white transverse lines of deposited arsenic that usually appear 6 weeks after exposure). Since the fingernail grows at a rate of 0.1 mm per day, the approximate time of exposure may be determined. Desquamation and scaling of the skin may initiate an exfoliative process involving many epithelial structures of the body. The liver may enlarge, and obstruction of the bile ducts may result in jaundice. Eventually cirrhosis may occur from the hepatotoxic action. Renal dysfunction may also be encountered. As intoxication advances, encephalopathy may develop. Peripheral neuritis results in motor and sensory paralysis of the extremities; usually the legs are more severely affected than the arms, in contrast to lead palsy. The bone marrow is seriously injured by arsenic. With severe exposure, all hematological elements may be affected.

Treatment of Arsenic Poisoning. After acute exposure to arsenic, routine measures are taken to stabilize the patient and prevent further absorption of the poison. In particular, attention is directed to the status of the intravascular volume, since the effects of arsenic on the gastrointestinal tract can result in fatal hypovolemic shock. Hypotension requires fluid replacement and may necessitate pharmacological support of blood pressure with pressor agents such as dopamine.

Chelation therapy should begin with dimercaprol (3 mg/kg intramuscularly every 4 hours) until abdominal symptoms subside and charcoal (if given initially) is passed in the feces. Oral treatment with penicillamine may then be substituted for dimercaprol and continued for 4 days. Penicillamine should be given in four divided doses to a maximum of 1 g per day. If symptoms recur after cessation of chelation therapy, a second course of penicillamine may be instituted.

After chronic exposure to arsenic, treatment with dimercaprol and penicillamine may also be used, but oral penicillamine alone is usually sufficient. The duration of therapy is determined by the clinical condition of the patient, and the decision is aided by periodic determinations of urinary arsenic concentrations. Adverse effects of the chelating agents may limit the usefulness of therapy (see below). Renal dialysis may become necessary with severe arsenic-induced nephropathy; successful removal of arsenic by dialysis has been reported (Vaziri et al., 1980).

Arsine. Arsine gas, generated by electrolytic or metallic reduction of arsenic in nonferrous metal products, is a rare cause of industrial intoxication. Rapid and often fatal hemolysis is a unique characteristic of arsine poisoning and probably results from arsine combining with hemoglobin and then reacting with oxygen to cause hemolysis (Fowler and Weissberg, 1974). A few hours after exposure, headache, anorexia, vomiting, paresthesia, abdominal pain, chills, hemoglobinuria, bilirubinemia, and anuria occur. Jaundice appears after 24 hours. A coppery skin pigmentation is frequently observed and is thought to be due to methemoglobin (Macaulay and Stanley, 1956). Kidneys of persons poisoned by arsine characteristically contain casts of hemoglobin, and there is cloudy swelling and necrosis of the cells of the proximal tubule. If the patient survives the severe hemolysis, death often results from renal failure. Treatment consists of exchange transfusions and forced alkaline diuresis. Dimercaprol has no effect on the hemolysis, and beneficial effects on renal function have not been established; it is thus not recommended.

CADMIUM

Cadmium ranks close to lead and mercury as a metal of current toxicological concern. It occurs in nature in association with zinc and lead, and extraction and processing of these metals thus often lead to environmental contamination with cadmium. The element was discovered in 1817 but was seldom used until its valuable metallurgical properties were discovered approximately 50 years ago. A high resistance to corrosion, valuable electrochemical properties, and other useful chemical properties account for cadmium's wide applications in electroplating and galvanization and its use in plastics, paint pigments (cadmium yellow), and nickel-cadmium batteries. Applications for and production of cadmium will continue to increase. Since less than 5% of the metal is recycled, environmental pollution is an important consideration. Coal and other fossil fuels contain cadmium, and their combustion releases the element into the environment.

Workers in smelters and other metal-processing plants may be exposed to high concentrations of cadmium in the air; however, for most of the population, exposure from contamination of food is most important. Uncontaminated foodstuffs contain less than 0.05 μg of cadmium per gram wet weight, and the average daily intake is about 50 μg. Drinking water normally does not contribute significantly to cadmium intake, but cigarette smoking does. Cigarettes each contain 1 to 2 μg of cadmium, and, with even 10% pulmonary absorption (Elinder et al., 1983), the smoking of one pack of cigarettes per day results in a dose of approximately 1 mg of cadmium per year from smoking alone. Shellfish and animal liver and kidney are among foods that can have concentrations of cadmium higher than 0.05 μg/g, even under normal circumstances. When foods such as rice and wheat are contaminated by cadmium in soil and water, the concentration of the metal may increase considerably (1 μg/g).

In Fuchu, Japan, shortly after World War II, a large number of people complained of rheumatic and myalgic pains; the disease was named *itai-itai* ("ouch-ouch"). It was determined that cadmium had washed into the local rice fields from the effluent from a lead-zinc processing plant.

Absorption, Distribution, and Excretion. Cadmium occurs only in one valency state, 2+, and does not form stabile alkyl compounds or other organometallic compounds of known toxicological significance.

Cadmium is poorly absorbed from the gastrointestinal tract. Studies in laboratory animals indicate the extent of absorption to be only about 1.5% (Klaassen and Kotsonis, 1977; Engstrom and Nordberg, 1979), and limited studies in man indicate a value of about 5% (Rahola *et al.*, 1972). Absorption from the respiratory tract appears to be more complete; cigarette smokers may absorb 10 to 40% of inhaled cadmium (Friberg *et al.*, 1974).

After absorption, cadmium is transported in blood, bound mainly to blood cells and albumin. After distribution, approximately 50% of the total body burden is found in the liver and kidney. These organs also contain metallothionein, a low-molecular-weight protein with high affinity for metals such as cadmium and zinc. One third of the amino acid residues in metallothionein are cysteine (Kägi and Vallee, 1960, 1961). Metallothionein is inducible by exposure to cadmium, and elevated concentrations of this metal-binding protein may be protective by preventing the interaction of cadmium with other functional macromolecules (Goering and Klaassen, 1983, 1984).

The half-life of cadmium in the body is 10 to 30 years. Consequently, with continuous environmental exposure, concentrations of the metal in tissues increase throughout life. The body burden of cadmium in a 50-year-old adult in the United States is about 30 mg (Friberg *et al.*, 1974). Its extremely long biological half-life renders cadmium an environmental poison most prone to accumulation. After a single intravenous injection of cadmium into laboratory animals, the biliary route of excretion is quantitatively more important than the urinary route (Klaassen and Kotsonis, 1977). After multiple exposures the biliary excretion of cadmium is almost abolished because of binding to metallothionein (Klaassen, 1978). Overall, fecal elimination is quantitatively more important than urinary excretion of the metal. Urinary excretion of cadmium becomes significant only after substantial renal toxicity has occurred.

Acute Cadmium Poisoning. Acute poisoning usually results from inhalation of cadmium dusts and fumes (usually cadmium oxide) and from the ingestion of cadmium salts. The early toxic effects are due to local irritation. In the case of oral intake, these include nausea, vomiting, salivation, diarrhea, and abdominal cramps. Acutely, cadmium is more toxic when inhaled. Signs and symptoms, which appear within a few hours, include irritation of the upper respiratory tract, chest pains, nausea, dizziness, and diarrhea. Toxicity may progress to include fatal pulmonary edema or residual emphysema with peribronchial and perivascular fibrosis (Zavon and Meadow, 1970).

Chronic Cadmium Poisoning. The toxic effects of chronic exposure to cadmium differ somewhat with the route of exposure. The kidney is affected following either pulmonary or gastrointestinal exposure; marked effects are observed in the lungs only after exposure by inhalation.

Kidney. When the concentration of cadmium in the kidney reaches a level of 200 μg/g, there is renal injury. It seems probable that binding of the metal by metallothionein protects the organ when concentrations are lower. Proteinuria is due to proximal tubular injury (Lauwerys *et al.*, 1979). The quantitation of β_2-microglobulin in urine appears to be the most sensitive index of cadmium-induced nephrotoxicity (Piscator and Pettersson, 1977). With more severe exposure, glomerular injury occurs, filtration is decreased, and there is aminoaciduria, glycosuria, and proteinuria. The nature of the glomerular injury is unknown but may involve an autoimmune component (Lauwerys *et al.*, 1984).

Lung. The consequence of excessive inhalation of cadmium fumes and dusts is loss of ventilatory capacity, with a corresponding increase in residual lung volume. Dyspnea is the most frequent complaint of patients with cadmium-induced lung disease. The pathogenesis of cadmium-induced emphysema and pulmonary fibrosis is not well understood. However, cadmium specifically inhibits the synthesis of plasma α_1-antitrypsin (Chowdhury and Louria, 1976), and there is an association between severe α_1-antitrypsin deficiency of genetic origin and emphysema in man.

Cardiovascular System. Perhaps the most controversial issue concerning the effects of cadmium on man is the suggestion that the metal plays a significant role in the etiology of hypertension (Schroeder, 1965). The initial study was epidemiological. People dying from hypertension were found to have significantly higher concentrations of cadmium and higher cadmium-to-zinc ratios in their kidneys than people dying of other causes. Others have found similar correlations (Thind and Fischer, 1976; Voors and Shuman, 1977). Cadmium-induced hypertension has been reported in female rats after prolonged exposure to the metal in their drinking water (Kopp *et al.*, 1982), but this effect has not been consistently observed in other laboratories. Hypertension is not prominent in industrial cadmium poisoning. The hypertensive effects of cadmium in man remain unclear.

Bone. One of the hallmarks of *itai-itai* was osteomalacia. However, studies in Sweden and the United Kingdom have failed to corroborate this effect of cadmium poisoning (Friberg, 1950; Kazantzis *et al.*, 1963; Adams *et al.*, 1969). The intake of calcium and fat-soluble vitamins such as vitamin D is much higher in these countries than in Japan. The Japanese victims were mostly multiparous, postmenopausal women. Thus, there may be an interaction between cadmium, nutrition, and bone disease. Body stores of calcium have been found to be decreased in subjects exposed to cadmium occupationally (Scott *et al.,* 1980). This presumed effect of cadmium may be due to interference with renal regulation of calcium and phosphate balance.

Testis. Testicular necrosis, a common characteristic of acute exposure to cadmium in experimental animals, is uncommon with chronic, low-level exposure (Kotsonis and Klaassen, 1978). Cadmium-induced testicular necrosis has not been observed in man.

Treatment of Cadmium Poisoning. Effective therapy for cadmium poisoning has been difficult to achieve. After acute inhalation the patient must be removed from the source, and pulmonary ventilation should be monitored carefully. Respiratory support and steroid therapy may become necessary.

Chelation therapy with $CaNa_2EDTA$ is recommended, although there is no clearly proven benefit. The dosage of $CaNa_2EDTA$ should be 75 mg/kg per day in three to six divided doses for 5 days. After a minimum of 2 days without treatment, a second 5-day course may be given. The total dose of $CaNa_2EDTA$ per 5-day course should not exceed 500 mg/kg. Dimercaprol is *contraindicated* because it increases nephrotoxicity.

Although human data are not available, experimental data in animals have shown that polycarboxylic acid chelators, such as $CaNa_2EDTA$ and calcium disodium diethylenetriaminepentaacetate ($CaNa_2DTPA$), can be effective when administered immediately after exposure to cadmium (Cantilena and Klaassen, 1982a). Unfortunately, there is a rapid decrease in the effectiveness of such chelation therapy with time, due to distribution of the metal to sites that are not reached by the chelators (Waalkes *et al.,* 1983). Therefore, chelation therapy must be instituted as soon as possible after exposure to the metal.

IRON

Although iron is not an environmental poison, accidental intoxication with ferrous salts used to treat iron-deficiency anemias has made iron a frequently encountered source of poisoning in young children. Acute iron poisoning is discussed in Chapter 56.

RADIOACTIVE HEAVY METALS

The widespread production and use of radioactive heavy metals for nuclear generation of electricity, nuclear weapons, laboratory research, manufacturing, and medical diagnosis have generated unique problems in dealing with accidental poisoning by such metals. Since the toxicity of radioactive metals is almost entirely a consequence of ionizing radiation, the therapeutic objective following exposure is not just the chelation of the metals but their removal from the body as rapidly and completely as possible.

Treatment of the acute radiation syndrome is largely symptomatic. Attempts have been made to investigate the effectiveness of organic reducing agents (such as cysteamine), administered to prevent the formation of free radicals. Success has been limited.

Major products of a nuclear accident or the use of nuclear weapons include ^{239}Pu, ^{137}Cs, ^{144}Ce, and ^{90}Sr. Isotopes of Sr and Ra have proven to be extremely difficult to remove from the body with chelating agents. Several factors are involved in the relative resistance of radioactive metals to chelation therapy; these include the affinity of these particular metals for individual chelators and the observation that radiation from strontium and radium in bone destroys nearby capillaries. Blood flow in bone is thereby decreased and the radioisotopes become imprisoned. Many chelating agents have been utilized experimentally, including DTPA, which has been shown to be an effective chelating agent for promoting the excretion of ^{239}Pu (Bair and Thompson, 1974). One gram of DTPA, administered by slow intravenous drip on alternate days, three times per week, has enhanced excretion 50- to 100-fold in animals and in human subjects exposed in accidents. As is commonly seen with heavy-metal poisoning, effectiveness of treatment diminishes very rapidly with an increasing delay between exposure and the initiation of therapy.

HEAVY-METAL ANTAGONISTS

EDETATE CALCIUM DISODIUM

History. *Ethylenediaminetetraacetic acid* (EDTA), its sodium salt (*disodium edetate, Na_2EDTA*), and a number of closely related compounds have been used for many years as industrial and analytical reagents because they chelate many divalent and trivalent metals. The cation used to make a water-soluble salt of EDTA plays an important role in the toxicity of the chelator. Initial studies in animals had shown that Na_2EDTA causes hypocalcemic tetany. However, subsequent studies established the relatively nontoxic nature of the calcium chelate (*edetate calcium disodium, $CaNa_2EDTA$*), and it was soon determined that $CaNa_2EDTA$ could be utilized for treatment of poisoning by metals that have higher affinity for the chelating agent than does Ca^{2+}.

Chemistry and Mechanism of Action. The structure of $CaNa_2EDTA$ is as follows:

Edetate Calcium Disodium

The pharmacological effects of CaNa$_2$-EDTA result from formation of chelates with divalent and trivalent metals in the body. Accessible metal ions (both exogenous and endogenous) with a higher affinity for CaNa$_2$EDTA than calcium will be chelated, mobilized, and usually excreted. Experimental studies in mice have shown that administration of CaNa$_2$EDTA mobilizes several endogenous metals, including Zn, Mn, and Fe (Cantilena and Klaassen, 1982b). The main therapeutic use of CaNa$_2$EDTA is in the treatment of metal intoxications, especially lead intoxication.

The successful use of CaNa$_2$EDTA in the treatment of lead poisoning is due, in part, to the capacity of lead to displace calcium from the chelate. Enhanced mobilization and excretion of lead indicate that the metal is accessible to EDTA. Mercury poisoning, by contrast, does not respond to the drug, despite the fact that mercury displaces calcium from CaNa$_2$EDTA *in vitro*. Mercury is unavailable to the chelate, perhaps because it is too tightly bound by body ligands (—SH) or sequestered in body compartments that are not penetrated by CaNa$_2$EDTA. Due to its ionic character, it is unlikely that CaNa$_2$EDTA penetrates cells significantly and the volume of distribution of CaNa$_2$EDTA is approximately equal to that of extracellular fluid.

Bone provides the primary source of lead that is chelated by CaNa$_2$EDTA (Hammond, 1971). After such chelation, lead is redistributed from soft tissues to the skeleton.

Chelation therapy with CaNa$_2$EDTA has been advocated by some and heralded in the lay press for the treatment of atherosclerosis. The premise is the presence of calcium deposits in atherosclerotic plaques. There is no reasonable rationale for such therapy and, more importantly, no evidence that it is efficacious (Medical Letter, 1981).

Absorption, Distribution, and Excretion. Less than 5% of CaNa$_2$EDTA is absorbed from the gastrointestinal tract. After intravenous administration, CaNa$_2$EDTA disappears from the circulation with a half-life of 20 to 60 minutes. In blood, all of the drug is found in plasma. About 50% is excreted in the urine in 1 hour and over 95% in 24 hours. For this reason, adequate renal function is necessary for successful therapy. Renal clearance of the compound in dogs equals that of inulin, and glomerular filtration accounts entirely for urinary excretion. Altering either the pH or the rate of flow of urine has no effect on the rate of excretion. There is very little metabolic degradation of EDTA. The drug is distributed mainly in the extracellular fluids, but very little gains access to the spinal fluid (5% of the plasma concentration).

Toxicity. Rapid intravenous administration of Na$_2$EDTA causes hypocalcemic tetany. However, a slow infusion (less than 15 mg per minute) administered to a normal individual elicits no symptoms of hypocalcemia because of the ready availability of extracirculatory stores of calcium. In contrast, CaNa$_2$EDTA can be administered intravenously in relatively large quantities with no untoward effects because the change in the concentration of calcium in the plasma and total body is negligible.

The principal toxic effect of CaNa$_2$EDTA is on the kidney. Most notably, the proximal tubule is severely affected with repeated administration. Hydropic vacuolization, loss of the brush border, and, eventually, degeneration of the proximal tubular cells are seen (Catsch and Harmuth-Hoene, 1979). Tubular injury can be produced by large doses of either CaNa$_2$EDTA or Na$_2$EDTA. Changes in distal tubules and glomeruli are less conspicuous. The early renal effects are usually reversible, and urinary abnormalities disappear rapidly upon cessation of treatment.

Renal toxicity may be related to the large amounts of chelated metals that pass through the renal tubule in a relatively short period of time during drug therapy. Some dissociation of chelates may occur because of competition for the metal by physiological ligands or because of pH changes in the cell or the lumen of the tubule (Johnson and Seven, 1960). However, a more likely mechanism of toxicity may be the interaction between the chelator and endogenous metals in proximal tubular cells.

Other less serious side effects have been reported with use of CaNa$_2$EDTA, including malaise, fatigue, and excessive thirst, followed by the sudden appearance of chills and fever. This may, in turn, be followed by severe myalgia, frontal headache, anorexia, occasional nausea and vomiting, and, rarely, increased urinary frequency and urgency. Other possible undesirable effects include sneezing, nasal congestion, and lacrimation; glycosuria; anemia; dermatitis, with lesions strikingly similar to those of vitamin B_6 deficiency; transitory lowering of systolic and diastolic blood pressures; prolonged prothrombin time; and inversion of the T wave of the ECG.

Preparations, Routes of Administration, and Dosage. CaNa$_2$EDTA is available as *edetate calcium disodium* (CALCIUM DISODIUM VERSENATE). For parenteral use, an injection containing 200 mg/ml is employed. Intramuscular administration of CaNa$_2$EDTA results in good absorption, but pain occurs at the injection site. For intravenous use, CaNa$_2$EDTA is diluted in either 5% dextrose or 0.9% saline and is administered slowly by intravenous drip over at least a 1-hour period. A dilute solution is necessary to avoid thrombophlebitis. Regimens for the treatment of intoxications with specific metals are described above. For children, the maximal daily dosage is 75 mg/kg of body weight, divided into two or three doses. To minimize nephrotoxicity, adequate urine production should be established prior to and during treatment with CaNa$_2$EDTA. However, in patients with lead encephalopathy and increased intracranial pressure, excess fluids must be avoided. In such cases, conservative replacement of fluid is advised and either intramuscular or intravenous administration of CaNa$_2$EDTA at a reduced rate is recommended.

Edetate disodium injection is utilized for the emergency treatment of hypercalcemia (*see* Chapter 65).

Therapeutic Uses. The uses of CaNa$_2$EDTA for the treatment of intoxication with various metals are described above under each metal.

DIETHYLENETRIAMINEPENTAACETIC
ACID (DTPA)

DTPA, like EDTA, is a polycarboxylic acid chelator, but it has somewhat greater affinity for most heavy metals (Chaberek and Martell, 1959; Dwyer and Mellor, 1964). Many investigations in animals have shown that the spectrum of clinical effectiveness of DTPA is similar to that of EDTA. Because of its relatively greater affinity for metals, DTPA has been tried in cases of heavy-metal poisoning that do not respond to EDTA, particularly poisoning by radioactive metals. Unfortunately, success has been limited, probably because DTPA also has limited access to intracellular sites of metal storage. Since DTPA rapidly binds calcium, the calcium chelate, CaNa$_2$EDTA is employed. The use of DTPA is investigational.

DIMERCAPROL

History. During World War II, an intensive effort was made to develop an antidote to *lewisite,* a vesicant arsenical war gas. Knowing that arsenicals reacted with SH-containing molecules, Stocken and Thompson, at Oxford University, initiated a systematic study of thiol compounds to find one that would successfully compete with the tissue SH groups for the arsenicals (Stocken and Thompson, 1949). Their investigations indicated that the arsenicals would form a very stable and relatively nontoxic chelate ring with the dithiol compound, dimercaprol (2,3-dimercaptopropanol). When scientists in the United States joined their British colleagues in these studies, they designated dimercaprol as British antilewisite (BAL). Pharmacological investigators revealed that this compound would protect against the toxic effects of other heavy metals as well. At the end of the war, when the results of the work were published, dimercaprol was recognized as effective against poisoning by many heavy metals; such an antidote was a long-sought goal.

Chemistry. Dimercaprol has the following structure:

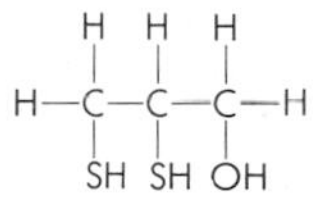

Dimercaprol

It is a clear, colorless, viscous, oily fluid with a pungent, disagreeable odor typical of mercaptans. It is soluble in water (7 g/dl) and is also soluble in vegetable oils, alcohol, and various other organic solvents. Because of its instability in aqueous solutions, peanut oil is the solvent employed in pharmaceutical preparations. Dimercaprol and related thiols are readily oxidized *in vitro* in the presence of a number of catalysts. Presumably, oxidation to a cyclic S—S compound can occur *in vivo.*

Mechanism of Action. The pharmacological actions of dimercaprol are the result of formation of chelation complexes between its sulfhydryl groups and metals. The molecular properties of the dimercaprol-metal chelate have considerable practical significance. With metals such as mercury, gold, and arsenic, the strategy is to attain a stable complex to promote eliminating the metal. Dissociation of the complex and oxidation of dimercaprol can occur *in vivo.* Furthermore, the sulfur-metal bond may be labile in the acidic tubular urine, which may increase delivery of metal to renal tissue and increase toxicity. The dosage regimen is therefore designed to maintain a concentration of dimercaprol in plasma adequate to favor the continuous formation of the more stable 2:1 (BAL:metal) complex and its rapid excretion. However, because of pronounced and dose-related side effects, excessive plasma concentrations must be avoided. The concentration in plasma must therefore be maintained by repeated fractional dosage until the offending metal can be excreted.

Dimercaprol is much more effective when given as soon as possible after exposure to the metal, because it is more effective in preventing inhibition of sulfhydryl enzymes than in reactivating them. This therapeutic principle applies to the use of all chelating agents.

Dimercaprol antagonizes the biological actions of metals that form mercaptides with essential cellular sulfhydryl groups, principally arsenic, gold, and mercury. It is also used in combination with $CaNa_2EDTA$ to treat lead poisoning. Intoxication by selenites, which oxidize sulfhydryl enzymes, is not influenced by dimercaprol.

Absorption, Distribution, and Excretion. Dimercaprol cannot be administered orally; it is given by deep intramuscular injection as a 10% solution in oil. Peak concentrations in blood are attained in 30 to 60 minutes. The half-life is short, and metabolic degradation and excretion are essentially complete within 4 hours. Following injection of dimercaprol into experimental animals, there is a sharp rise in urinary excretion of neutral sulfur, which accounts for approximately 50% of the sulfur administered as dimercaprol. There is no increase in ethereal sulfur. A rise in urinary glucuronic acid suggests that a portion of dimercaprol may be excreted as glucuronide.

Toxicity. In man, the administration of dimercaprol produces a variety of side effects that are usually more alarming than serious; nevertheless, they limit the amount of the dithiol that can be administered. Reactions to dimercaprol occur in approximately 50% of subjects receiving 5 mg/kg intramuscularly. The effects of repeated administration of this dose are not cumulative if an interval of at least 4 hours elapses between injections. One of the most consistent responses to dimercaprol is a rise in systolic and diastolic arterial pressures, accompanied by tachycardia. The rise in pressure is roughly proportional to the dose administered and may be as great as 50 mm

Hg in response to the second of two doses (5 mg/kg) given 2 hours apart. The pressure rises immediately but returns to normal within 2 hours. Other signs and symptoms, many of which tend to parallel the change in blood pressure in time and intensity, are the following, listed in approximate order of frequency: (1) nausea and, in some instances, vomiting; (2) headache; (3) a burning sensation in the lips, mouth, and throat and a feeling of constriction, sometimes pain, in the throat, chest, or hands; (4) conjunctivitis, blepharospasm, lacrimation, rhinorrhea, and salivation; (5) tingling of the hands; (6) a burning sensation in the penis; (7) sweating of the forehead, hands, and other areas; (8) abdominal pain; and (9) occasional appearance of painful sterile abscesses at the injection site. Symptoms are often accompanied by a feeling of anxiety and unrest. Because the dimercaprol-metal complex breaks down easily in an acidic medium, production of an alkaline urine protects the kidney during therapy. Children react as do adults, although approximately 30% may also experience a fever that disappears upon withdrawal of the drug. A transient reduction of the percentage of polymorphonuclear leukocytes may also be observed. Dimercaprol may also cause hemolytic anemia in patients deficient in glucose-6-phosphate dehydrogenase. Dimercaprol is contraindicated in patients with hepatic insufficiency, except when this is a result of arsenic poisoning.

Preparation. *Dimercaprol (2,3-dimercaptopropanol)* is available for injection as a solution in peanut oil. Each milliliter contains 100 mg of dimercaprol. Treatment regimens are described above for the individual metals.

2,3-DIMERCAPTOSUCCINIC ACID

2,3-Dimercaptosuccinic acid has the following structure:

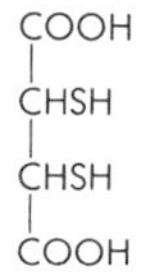

COOH
|
CHSH
|
CHSH
|
COOH

2,3-Dimercaptosuccinic Acid

It is a disulfhydryl compound and is thus similar to dimercaprol. However, it is much less toxic than dimercaprol and is effective orally (Graziano *et al.*, 1978b). While its use is still experimental, 2,3-

dimercaptosuccinic acid is a promising, orally effective, relatively nontoxic chelator for the treatment of not only mercury poisoning (Friedheim and Corvi, 1975) but also poisoning with arsenic (Graziano *et al.*, 1978a) and lead (Friedheim *et al.*, 1976; Graziano *et al.*, 1978b).

PENICILLAMINE

History. Penicillamine was first isolated in 1953 from the urine of patients with liver disease who were receiving penicillin. Discovery of its chelating properties led to its use in patients with Wilson's disease and heavy-metal intoxications (Walshe, 1956; Boulding and Baker, 1957).

Chemistry. Penicillamine is D-β,β-dimethyl-cysteine. Its structure is as follows:

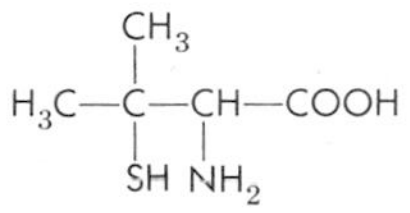

$$H_3C-\overset{\overset{\displaystyle CH_3}{|}}{\underset{\underset{\displaystyle SH}{|}}{C}}-\overset{}{\underset{\underset{\displaystyle NH_2}{|}}{CH}}-COOH$$

Penicillamine

It is prepared by the hydrolytic degradation of penicillin; it has no antibacterial activity. The D isomer is used clinically, although the L isomer also forms chelation complexes. Penicillamine is an effective chelator of copper, mercury, zinc, and lead and promotes the excretion of these metals in the urine.

Absorption, Distribution, and Excretion. Penicillamine is well absorbed from the gastrointestinal tract and, therefore, has a decided advantage over other chelating agents. Peak concentrations in blood are obtained between 1 and 2 hours after administration (Wiesner *et al.*, 1981). It is rapidly excreted in the urine. Unlike cysteine, its nonmethylated parent compound, penicillamine is somewhat resistant to attack by cysteine desulfhydrase or L-amino acid oxidase (Aposhian, 1961). As a result, penicillamine is relatively stable *in vivo*. This probably explains the effectiveness of penicillamine and the lack of effectiveness of cysteine in promoting excretion of metals, although *in vitro* both compounds form stable metal chelates. This explanation is further substantiated by the fact that N-acetylpenicillamine is even more effective than penicillamine in protecting against the toxic effects of mercury (Aposhian and Aposhian, 1959), because the acetylated derivative is more resistant to metabolic degradation than is the parent compound. Hepatic biotransformation is responsible for most of the degradation of penicilla-

mine, and very little is excreted unchanged. Metabolites are found in both urine and feces (Perrett, 1981).

Therapeutic Uses. In addition to its use as a chelating agent for the treatment of copper, mercury, and lead poisoning, penicillamine is used in Wilson's disease (hepatolenticular degeneration due to an excess of copper), cystinuria, and rheumatoid arthritis. The rationale for its use in cystinuria is that penicillamine forms a relatively soluble disulfide compound with cysteine through a disulfide interchange mechanism and thereby decreases the formation of cystine-containing renal stones.

The mechanism of action of penicillamine in rheumatoid arthritis remains uncertain, although suppression of the disease may result from marked reduction in concentrations of IgM rheumatoid factor (Wernick *et al.*, 1983). Uniquely, this decrease is not accompanied by reductions of the concentrations of immunoglobulins in plasma. Other experimental uses of penicillamine include the treatment of primary biliary cirrhosis and scleroderma. The mechanism of action of penicillamine in these diseases may also involve effects on immunoglobulins and immune complexes (Epstein *et al.*, 1979).

Toxicity. Although short-term use of penicillamine as a chelating agent is relatively safe, chronic use in rheumatoid arthritis is associated with marked and varied toxicities. Penicillamine induces several cutaneous lesions, including urticaria, macular or papular reactions, pemphigoid lesions, lupus erythematosus, dermatomyositis, adverse effects on collagen, and other less serious reactions, such as dryness and scaling. Cross-reactivity with penicillin may be responsible for some episodes of urticarial or maculopapular reactions with generalized edema, pruritus, and fever that occur in as many as one third of patients taking penicillamine. For a detailed review of the adverse dermatological effects of penicillamine, *see* Levy and coworkers (1983).

The hematological system may also be affected severely; reactions include leukopenia, aplastic anemia, and agranulocytosis. These may occur at any time during therapy, and they may be fatal. Patients must obviously be monitored carefully.

Renal toxicity induced by penicillamine is usually manifested as reversible proteinuria and hematuria, but it may progress to the nephrotic syndrome with membranous glomerulopathy. More rarely, fatalities have been reported from Goodpasture's syndrome (Hill, 1979).

Toxicity to the pulmonary system is uncommon, but severe dyspnea has been reported from penicillamine-induced bronchoalveolitis. Myasthenia gravis has also been induced by chronic therapy with penicillamine (Gordon and Burnside, 1977). Less serious side effects include nausea, vomiting, diarrhea, dyspepsia, anorexia, and a transient loss of taste for sweet and salt, which is relieved by supplementation of the diet with copper. Contraindications to penicillamine therapy include pregnancy, a previous history of penicillamine-induced agranulocytosis or aplastic anemia, or the presence of renal insufficiency.

Preparations and Dosage. *Penicillamine* is available in capsules containing 125 or 250 mg (CUPRIMINE) or as 250-mg tablets (DEPEN). The drug should be given on an empty stomach to avoid interference by metals in food. For chelation therapy, the usual dose is 500 mg to 1.5 g per day in four divided doses (*see* sections under individual metals). In cystinuria, the urinary excretion of cystine is used to adjust dosage, although 2 g per day in four divided doses is usually employed. Various dosage regimens have been studied for the treatment of rheumatoid arthritis. A single daily dose of 125 to 250 mg is usually used to initiate therapy. Dosage is increased at intervals of 1 to 3 months as necessary. Two or 3 months may be required before improvement is evident. Most patients eventually respond to 500 to 750 mg per day or less. For the treatment of Wilson's disease, four daily doses are taken, and 1 to 2 g per day is usually employed. The urinary excretion of copper should be monitored to determine if the dosage of penicillamine is adequate. During the first 6 months of treatment, sulfurated potash (40 mg) may be given with each dose of penicillamine to minimize absorption of dietary copper.

DEFEROXAMINE

The structure of deferoxamine is shown below. It is isolated as the iron chelate from *Streptomyces pilosus* and is treated chemically to obtain the metal-free ligand. Deferoxamine has the desirable properties of a remarkably high affinity for ferric iron ($K_a = 10^{31}$) coupled with a very low affinity for calcium ($K_a = 10^2$). Studies *in vitro* have shown that it removes iron from hemosiderin and ferritin and, to a lesser extent, from transferrin. Iron in hemoglobin or cytochromes is not removed by deferoxamine. Deferoxamine is poorly absorbed after oral administration, and parenteral administration is required in most cases. Deferoxamine is metabolized principally by plasma enzymes, but the pathways have not yet been defined. The drug is also readily excreted in the urine.

Deferoxamine causes a number of allergic reactions, including pruritus, wheals, rash, and anaphylaxis. Other adverse effects include dysuria, abdominal discomfort, diarrhea, fever, leg cramps, and tachycardia. Occasional cases of cataract formation have been reported. Contraindications to the use of deferoxamine include pregnancy, renal insufficiency, and anuria.

Preparation, Dosage, and Uses. *Deferoxamine mesylate* (DESFERAL MESYLATE) is available in vials containing 500 mg of the drug. In acute iron poisoning the intramuscular route is preferred, unless the patient is in shock. Initially, for adults and children, 1 g is given, followed by 500 mg every 4 hours for two doses. The 500-mg injections may be continued at 4- or 12-hour intervals, depending on the clinical response, but the total amount of drug administered should not exceed 6 g in 24 hours. The intravenous route is required when a patient is in shock. The dosage schedule and limitations are the same as those indicated for the intramuscular route. However, the infusion rate must never exceed 15 mg/kg per hour. As soon as the clinical situation permits, intravenous administration should be discontinued and the drug given intramuscularly. Other aspects of the treatment of acute iron poisoning are discussed in Chapter 56.

For chronic iron intoxication (*e.g.*, thalassemia), an intramuscular dose of 0.5 to 1.0 g per day is recommended, although continuous subcutaneous administration is almost as effective as intravenous administration (Propper *et al.*, 1977). When blood is being transfused to patients with thalassemia, 2.0 g of deferoxamine (per unit of blood) should be given by slow intravenous infusion (rate not to exceed 15 mg/kg per hour) during the transfusion, but not by the same intravenous line. Deferoxamine is

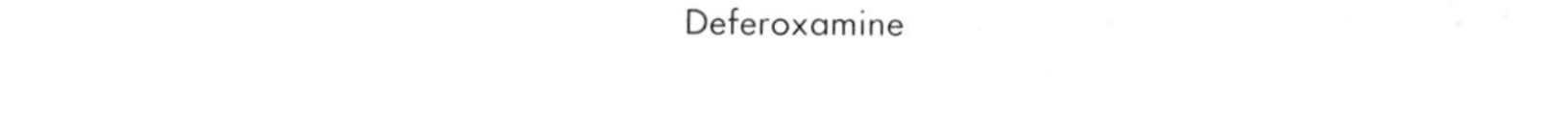

$$H_2N-(CH_2)_5-\underset{\underset{HO}{|}}{N}-\underset{\underset{O}{\|}}{C}-(CH_2)_2-\underset{\underset{O}{\|}}{C}-\underset{\underset{H}{|}}{N}-(CH_2)_5-\underset{\underset{HO}{|}}{N}-\underset{\underset{O}{\|}}{C}-(CH_2)_2-\underset{\underset{O}{\|}}{C}-\underset{\underset{H}{|}}{N}-(CH_2)_5-\underset{\underset{HO}{|}}{N}-\underset{\underset{O}{\|}}{C}-CH_3$$

Deferoxamine

not recommended in primary hemochromatosis; phlebotomy is the treatment of choice.

Adams, R. G.; Harrison, J. F.; and Scott, P. The development of cadmium-induced proteinuria, impaired renal function and osteomalacia in alkaline battery workers. *Q. J. Med.,* **1969,** *38,* 425–443.

Al-Abbasi, A. H.; Kostyniak, P. J.; and Clarkson, T. W. An extracorporeal complexing hemodialysis system for the treatment of methylmercury poisoning. III. Clinical applications. *J. Pharmacol. Exp. Ther.,* **1978,** *207,* 249–254.

Annest, J. L.; Pirkle, J. L.; Makuc, D.; Neese, J. W.; Bayse, D. D.; and Kovar, M. G. Chronological trend in blood lead levels between 1976 and 1980. *N. Engl. J. Med.,* **1983,** *308,* 1373–1377.

Aposhian, H. V. Biochemical and pharmacological properties of the metal-binding agent penicillamine. *Fed. Proc.,* **1961,** *20,* Suppl. 10, 185–188.

Aposhian, H. V., and Aposhian, M. M. N-acetyl-DL-penicillamine, a new oral protective agent against the lethal effects of mercuric chloride. *J. Pharmacol. Exp. Ther.,* **1959,** *126,* 131–135.

Baker, E. L.; Goyer, R. A.; Fowler, B. A.; Khettry, U.; Bernard, O. B.; Adler, S.; White, R.; Babyor, R.; and Feldman, R. G. Occupational lcad exposure, nephropathy and renal cancer. *Am. J. Industr. Med.,* **1980,** *1,* 139–148.

Bakir, F.; Al-Khalidi, A.; Clarkson, T. W.; and Greenwood, R. Clinical observations on treatment of alkylmercury poisoning in hospital patients. *Bull. WHO,* **1976,** *53,* Suppl., 87–92.

Bakir, F.; Damluji, S. F.; Amin-Zaki, L.; Mortadha, M.; Khalidi, A.; Al-Rawi, N. Y.; Tikriti, S.; Dhahir, H. I.; Clarkson, T. W.; Smith, J. C.; and Doherty, R. A. Methylmercury poisoning in Iraq. An interuniversity report. *Science,* **1973,** *181,* 230–241.

Bakir, F.; Rustin, H.; Tikriti, S.; Al-Damluji, S. F.; and Shihristani, H. Clinical and epidemiological aspects of methylmercury poisoning. *Postgrad. Med. J.,* **1980,** *56,* 1–10.

Ball, G. V., and Sorensen, L. B. Pathogenesis of hyperuricemia in saturnine gout. *N. Engl. J. Med.,* **1969,** *280,* 1199–1202.

Barry, P. S. I. A comparison of concentrations of lead in human tissues. *Br. J. Ind. Med.,* **1975,** *32,* 119–139.

Berwick, D. M., and Komaroff, A. L. Cost effectiveness of lead screening. *N. Engl. J. Med.,* **1982,** *306,* 1392–1398.

Boulding, J. E., and Baker, R. A. The treatment of metal poisoning with penicillamine. *Lancet,* **1957,** *2,* 985.

Boyd, P. R. The treatment of tetraethyl lead poisoning. *Lancet,* **1957,** *1,* 181–185.

Cantilena, L. R., and Klaassen, C. D. Decreased effectiveness of chelation therapy for Cd poisoning with time. *Toxicol. Appl. Pharmacol.,* **1982a,** *63,* 173–180.

———. The effect of chelating agents on the excretion of endogenous metals. *Ibid.,* **1982b,** *63,* 344–350.

Chisholm, J. J. Management of increased lead absorption and lead poisoning in children. *N. Engl. J. Med.,* **1973,** *289,* 1016.

Chisolm, J. J., and Barltrop, D. Recognition and management of children with increased lead absorption. *Arch. Dis. Child.,* **1979,** *54,* 249–262.

Chowdhury, P., and Louria, D. B. Influence of cadmium and other trace metals on human α_1-antitrypsin; an *in vitro* study. *Science,* **1976,** *191,* 480–481.

Cooper, W. C., and Gaffey, W. R. Mortality of lead workers. *J. Occup. Med.,* **1975,** *17,* 100–107.

Elinder, C. G.; Kjellstrom, T.; Lind, B.; Linnman, L.; Piscator, M.; and Sundstedt, K. Cadmium exposure from smoking cigarettes. Variations with time and country where purchased. *Environ. Res.,* **1983,** *32,* 220–227.

Emmerson, B. T. Chronic lead neuropathy: the diagnostic use of calcium EDTA and the association with gout. *Aust. Ann. Med.,* **1963,** *12,* 310–324.

Engstrom, B., and Nordberg, G. F. Dose dependence of gastrointestinal absorption and biological half-time of cadmium in mice. *Toxicology,* **1979,** *13,* 215–222.

Epstein, O.; De Villiers, D.; Jain, S.; Potter, B. J.; Thomas, H. C.; and Sherlock, S. Reduction of immune complexes and immunoglobulin induced by D-penicillamine in primary biliary cirrhosis. *N. Engl. J. Med.,* **1979,** *300,* 274–278.

Ferm, V. H. Arsenic as a teratogenic agent. *Environ. Health Perspect.,* **1977,** *19,* 215–217.

Fowler, B. A. Toxicology of environmental arsenic. In, *Advances in Modern Toxicology.* Vol. 2, *Toxicology of Trace Elements.* (Goyer, R. A., and Mehlman, M. A., eds.) Hemisphere Publishing Co., Washington, D. C., 1977, pp. 79–122.

Fowler, B. A., and Weissberg, J. B. Arsine poisoning. *N. Engl. J. Med.,* **1974,** *291,* 1171.

Friberg, L. Health hazards in the manufacture of alkaline accumulators with special reference to chronic cadmium poisoning. *Acta Med. Scand.,* **1950,** *138,* Suppl. 240, 1–24.

Friedheim, E., and Corvi, C. Meso-dimercaptosuccinic acid: a chelating agent for the treatment of mercury poisoning. *J. Pharm. Pharmacol.,* **1975,** *27,* 624–626.

Friedheim, E.; Corvi, C.; and Walker, C. J. Meso-dimercaptosuccinic acid: a chelating agent for the treatment of mercury and lead poisoning. *J. Pharm. Pharmacol.,* **1976,** *28,* 711–712.

Gerstner, H., and Huff, J. Clinical toxicology of mercury. *J. Toxicol. Environ. Health,* **1977,** *2,* 491–526.

Gething, J. Tetramethyl lead absorption: a report of human exposure to a high level of tetramethyl lead. *Br. J. Ind. Med.,* **1975,** *32,* 329–333.

Giunta, F.; DiLandro, D.; and Chiarmda, M. Severe acute poisoning from the ingestion of a permanent wave solution of mercuric chloride. *Hum. Toxicol.,* **1983,** *2,* 243–246.

Goering, P. L., and Klaassen, C. D. Altered subcellular distribution of cadmium following cadmium pretreatment: possible mechanism of tolerance to cadmium-induced lethality. *Toxicol. Appl. Pharmacol.,* **1983,** *70,* 195–203.

———. Tolerance to cadmium-induced hepatotoxicity following cadmium pretreatment. *Ibid.,* **1984,** *74,* 308–313.

Goldwater, L. J., and Hoover, A. W. An international study of "normal" levels of lead in blood and urine. *Arch. Environ. Health,* **1967,** *15,* 60–63.

Gordon, R. A., and Burnside, J. W. Penicillamine induced myasthenia gravis in rheumatoid arthritis. *Ann. Intern. Med.,* **1977,** *87,* 578–579.

Graziano, J. H.; Cuccia, D.; and Friedheim, E. Potential usefulness of 2,3-dimercaptosuccinic acid for the treatment of arsenic poisoning. *J. Pharmacol. Exp. Ther.,* **1978a,** *207,* 1051–1055.

Graziano, J. H.; Leong, J. K.; and Friedheim, E. 2,3-Dimercaptosuccinic acid: a new agent for the treatment of lead poisoning. *Ibid.,* **1978b,** *206,* 696–700.

Gross, J. B.; Pfitzer, E. A.; Yeager, D. W.; and Kehoe, R. A. Lead in human tissues. *Toxicol. Appl. Pharmacol.,* **1975,** *32,* 638–651.

Hammond, P. B. The effects of chelating agents on the tissue distribution and excretion of lead. *Toxicol. Appl. Pharmacol.,* **1971,** *18,* 296–310.

Hill, H. F. H. Penicillamine in rheumatoid arthritis. Adverse effects. *Scand. J. Rheumatol. [Suppl.],* **1979,** *28,* 94–99.

Jenkins, R. B. Inorganic arsenic and the nervous system. *Brain,* **1966,** *89,* 479–498.

Johnson, L. A., and Seven, M. J. Observations on the *in vivo* stability of metal chelates. In, *Metal-Binding in*

Medicine. (Seven, M. J., ed.) J. B. Lippincott Co., Philadelphia, **1960**, pp. 225–229.

Kägi, J., and Vallee, B. Metallothionein: a cadmium- and zinc-containing protein from equine renal cortex. *J. Biol. Chem.,* **1960**, *235,* 3460–3465.

————. Metallothionein: a cadmium- and zinc-containing protein from equine renal cortex. II. Physicochemical properties. *Ibid.,* **1961**, *236,* 2435–2442.

Kazantzis, G.; Flynn, F. V.; Spowage, J.; and Trott, D. G. Renal tubular malfunction and pulmonary emphysema in cadmium pigment workers. *Q. J. Med.,* **1963**, *32,* 165–192.

Kehoe, R. A. The metabolism of lead in man in health and disease. *Arch. Environ. Health,* **1961a**, *2,* 418–422.

————. The metabolism of lead in man in health and disease: The Harben Lectures, 1960. *J. R. Inst. Public Health Hyg.,* **1961b**, *24,* 81–97, 101–120, 129–143.

Kershaw, T. G.; Dhahir, P. H.; and Clarkson, T. W. The relationship between blood levels and dose of methylmercury in man. *Arch. Environ. Health,* **1980**, *35,* 28–36.

Klaassen, C. D. Biliary excretion of mercury compounds. *Toxicol. Appl. Pharmacol.,* **1975**, *33,* 356–365.

————. Effect of metallothionein on the hepatic disposition of metals. *Am. J. Physiol.,* **1978**, *234,* E47–E53.

Klaassen, C. D., and Kotsonis, F. N. Biliary excretion of cadmium in the rat, rabbit and dog. *Toxicol. Appl. Pharmacol.,* **1977**, *41,* 101–112.

Klaassen, C. D., and Shoeman, D. W. Biliary excretion of lead in rats, rabbits, and dogs. *Toxicol. Appl. Pharmacol.,* **1974**, *29,* 447–457.

Kopp, S. G.; Glonek, T.; Perry, H. M.; Erlanger, M.; and Ferry, E. F. Cardiovascular actions of cadmium at environmental exposure levels. *Science,* **1982**, *217,* 837–839.

Kostyniak, P. J. Mobilization and removal of methylmercury in the dog during extracorporeal complexing hemodialysis with 2,3-dimercaptosuccinic acid (DMSA). *J. Pharmacol. Exp. Ther.,* **1982**, *221,* 63–68.

Kotsonis, F. N., and Klaassen, C. D. The relationship of metallothionein to the toxicity of cadmium after prolonged oral administration to rats. *Toxicol. Appl. Pharmacol.,* **1978**, *46,* 39–54.

Landrigan, P. Arsenic—state of the art. *Am. J. Industr. Med.,* **1981**, *2,* 5–14.

Langolf, G. D.; Chaffin, D. B.; Whittle, H. P.; and Henderson, R. Effects of industrial mercury exposure on urinary mercury, EMG and psychomotor functions. In, *Clinical Chemistry and Chemical Toxicology of Metals.* (Brown, S. S., ed.) Elsevier/North Holland Biomedical Press, Amsterdam, **1977**, pp. 213–220.

Lauwerys, R. R.; Bernard, A.; Roels, H. A.; Buchet, J.-P.; and Viau, C. Characterization of cadmium proteinuria in man and rat. *Environ. Health Perspect.,* **1984**, *54,* 147–152.

Lauwerys, R. R.; Roels, H. A.; Buchet, J.-P.; Bernard, A.; and Stanesca, D. Investigations on the lung and kidney function in workers exposed to cadmium. *Environ. Health Perspect.,* **1979**, *28,* 137–146.

Lee, A. M., and Fraumeni, J. F. Arsenic and respiratory cancer in man: an occupational study. *J. Natl Cancer Inst.,* **1969**, *42,* 1045–1052.

Levy, R. S.; Fisher, M.; and Alter, J. N. Penicillamine: review of cutaneous manifestations. *J. Am. Acad. Dermatol.,* **1983**, *8,* 548–558.

Lilis, R. Long-term occupational lead exposure. Chronic nephropathy and renal cancer. A case report. *Am. J. Industr. Med.,* **1981**, *2,* 293–297.

McAlpine, D., and Shukuro, A. Minimata disease. An unusual neurological disorder caused by contaminated fish. *Lancet,* **1958**, *2,* 629–631.

Macaulay, D. G., and Stanley, D. A. Arsine poisoning. *Br. J. Ind. Med.,* **1956**, *13,* 217–221.

Magos, L.; Halbach, S.; and Clarkson, T. W. Role of catalase in the oxidation of mercury vapor. *Biochem. Pharmacol.,* **1978**, *27,* 1373–1377.

Matherson, D. S.; Clarkson, T. W.; and Gelfand, E. W. Mercury toxicity (acradynia) induced by long term injection of gammaglobulin. *J. Pediatr.,* **1980**, *97,* 153–155.

Medical Letter. EDTA chelation therapy for arteriosclerotic heart disease. **1981**, *23,* 51.

Moore, J. F.; Goyer, R. A.; and Wilson, M. H. Lead induced inclusion bodies. Solubility, amino acid content, and relationship to residual acidic nuclear proteins. *Lab. Invest.,* **1973**, *29,* 488–494.

Needleman, H. L., and Leviton, A. Lead associated intellectual defect. *N. Engl. J. Med.,* **1982**, *306,* 367.

Needleman, H. L.; Gunne, C.; Leviton, A.; Reed, R.; Peresie, H.; Maher, C.; and Barrett, P. Defects in psychologic and classroom performance in children with elevated dentine lead levels. *N. Engl. J. Med.,* **1979**, *300,* 689–695.

Norseth, T., and Clarkson, T. W. Studies on the biotransformation of ^{203}Hg-labeled methylmercury chloride in rats. *Arch. Environ. Health,* **1970**, *21,* 717–727.

————. Intestinal transport of ^{203}Hg-labeled methyl mercury chloride. Role of biotransformation in rats. *Ibid.,* **1971**, *22,* 568–577.

Perrett, D. The metabolism and pharmacology of D-penicillamine in man. *J. Rheumatol.* [*Suppl.*], **1981**, *8,* 51–55.

Piscator, M., and Pettersson, B. Plenary lecture. Chronic cadmium poisoning: diagnosis and prevention. In, *Clinical Chemistry and Chemical Toxicology of Metals.* (Brown, S. S., ed.) Elsevier/North Holland Biomedical Press, Amsterdam, **1977**, pp. 143–155.

Popoff, N.; Weinberg, S.; and Feigin, I. Pathologic observations in lead encephalopathy. *Neurology (Minneap.),* **1963**, *13,* 101–112.

Popper, H.; Thomas, L. B.; Telles, N. C.; Falk, H.; and Selikoff, I. J. Development of hepatic angiosarcoma in man induced by vinylchloride, thorotrast, or arsenic. *Am. J. Pathol.,* **1978**, *92,* 349–369.

Propper, R. D.; Cooper, B.; Rufo, R. R.; Nienhuis, A. W.; Anderson, W. F.; Bunn, H. F.; Rosenthal, A.; and Nathan, D. G. Continuous subcutaneous administration of deferoxamine in patients with iron overload. *N. Engl. J. Med.,* **1977**, *297,* 418–423.

Rahola, T.; Aaran, R. K.; and Mietinen, J. K. Half-time studies of mercury and cadmium by whole body counting. International Atomic Energy Agency symposium on the assessment of radioactive organ and body burdens. In, *Assessment of Radioactive Contamination in Man.* The Agency, Vienna, **1972**.

Schroeder, H. A. Cadmium as a factor in hypertension. *J. Chronic Dis.,* **1965**, *18,* 217–228.

Schumann, G. B.; Lerner, S. I.; Weiss, M. A.; Gawronski, L.; and Lohiya, G. K. Inclusion-bearing cells in industrial workers exposed to lead. *Am. J. Clin. Pathol.,* **1980**, *74,* 192–196.

Scott, R.; Haywood, J. K.; Broddy, K.; Williams, E. D.; Harvey, I.; and Paterson, P. J. Whole body calcium deficit in cadmium exposed workers with hypercalciuria. *Urology,* **1980**, *15,* 356–359.

Seshia, S. S.; Rajani, K. R.; Boeckx, R. L.; and Chow, P. N. The neurological manifestations of chronic inhalation of leaded gasoline. *Dev. Med. Child Neurol.,* **1978**, *20,* 323–334.

Smith, H. D.; Boehner, R. L.; Carney, T.; and Majors, W. J. The sequelae of pica with and without lead poisoning. *Am. J. Dis. Child.,* **1963**, *105,* 609–616.

Tam, G. K. H.; Charbenneau, S. M.; Bryce, F.; Pomroy, C.; and Sandi, E. Metabolism of inorganic arsenic (^{74}As) in humans following oral ingestion. *Toxicol. Appl. Pharmacol.,* **1979**, *50,* 319–322.

Thind, G. S., and Fischer, G. Plasma cadmium and zinc in human hypertension. *Clin. Sci. Mol. Med.*, **1976**, *51*, 483–486.

Uldall, P. R.; Khan, H. A.; Ennis, J. E.; McCallum, R. I.; and Grimson, T. A. Renal damage from industrial arsine poisoning. *Br. J. Ind. Med.*, **1970**, *27*, 372–377.

Van Tongeren, J. H. M.; Kunst, A.; Majoor, C. L. H.; and Schilling, P. H. M. Folic acid deficiency in chronic arsenic poisoning. *Lancet*, **1965**, *1*, 784–786.

Vaziri, N. D.; Upham, T.; and Barton, C. H. Hemodialysis clearance of arsenic. *Clin. Toxicol.*, **1980**, *17*, 451–456.

Voors, A. W., and Shuman, M. S. Liver cadmium levels in North Carolina residents who died of heart disease. *Bull. Environ. Contam. Toxicol.*, **1977**, *17*, 692–696.

Waalkes, M. P.; Watkins, J. B.; and Klaassen, C. D. Minimal role of metallothionein in decreased chelator efficacy for cadmium. *Toxicol. Appl. Pharmacol.*, **1983**, *68*, 392–398.

Walshe, J. M. Penicillamine, a new oral therapy for Wilson's disease. *Am. J. Med.*, **1956**, *21*, 487–495.

Wernick, R.; Merryman, P.; Jaffe, I.; and Ziff, M. IgG and IgM rheumatoid factors in rheumatoid arthritis. *Arthritis Rheum.*, **1983**, *26*, 593–598.

Wiesner, R. H.; Dickson, E. R.; Carlson, G. L.; McPhaul, L. W.; and Go, V. L. W. The pharmacokinetics of D-penicillamine in man. *J. Rheumatol.*, **1981**, *8*, 51–55.

Zavon, M. R., and Meadow, C. D. Vascular sequelae to cadmium fume exposure. *Am. Ind. Hyg. Assoc. J.*, **1970**, *31*, 180–182.

Zielhuis, R. L. Interrelationship of biochemical responses to the absorption of inorganic lead. *Arch. Environ. Health*, **1971**, *23*, 299–311.

Monographs and Reviews

Aronaw, R. Mercury. In, *Clinical Management of Poisoning and Drug Overdose*. (Haddad, L. M., and Winchester, J. F., eds.) W. B. Saunders Co., Philadelphia, **1983**, pp. 637–642.

Bair, W. J., and Thompson, R. C. Plutonium: biomedical research. *Science*, **1974**, *183*, 715–722.

Catsch, A., and Harmuth-Hoene, A.-E. Pharmacology and therapeutic applications of agents used in heavy metal poisoning. In, *The Chelation of Heavy Metals.*

(Levine, W. G., ed.) Pergamon Press, New York, **1979**, pp. 116–124.

Chaberek, S., and Martell, A. E. *Organic Sequestering Agents*. John Wiley & Sons, Inc., New York, **1959**.

Chisholm, J. J., Jr. Treatment of lead poisoning. *Mod. Treat.*, **1967**, *4*, 710–727.

Dwyer, F. P., and Mellor, D. P. (eds.). *Chelating Agents and Metal Chelates*. Academic Press, Inc., New York, **1964**.

Friberg, L.; Piscator, M.; Nordberg, G. F.; and Kjellstrom, T. *Cadmium in the Environment*, 2nd ed. CRC Press, Inc., Cleveland, **1974**.

Friberg, L., and Vostal, J. *Mercury in the Environment: An Epidemiological and Toxicological Appraisal*. CRC Press, Inc., Cleveland, **1972**.

Garrettson, L. K. Lead. In, *Clinical Management of Poisoning and Drug Overdose*. (Haddad, L. M., and Winchester, J. F., eds.) W. B. Saunders Co., Philadelphia, **1983**, pp. 649–655.

Goyer, R. A. Toxic effects of metals. In, *Casarett and Doull's Toxicology: The Basic Science of Poisons*, 3rd ed. (Klaassen, C. D.; Amdur, M. O.; and Doull, J.; eds.) Macmillan Publishing Co., New York, **1985**.

Kagey, B. T.; Gumgarner, J. E.; and Creason, J. P. Arsenic levels in maternal-fetal tissue sets. In, *Trace Substances in Environmental Health XI*. (Hemphil, O. D., ed.) University of Missouri Press, Columbia, **1977**, pp. 252–256.

Klaassen, C. D. Biliary excretion of metals. *Drug Metab. Rev.*, **1976**, *5*, 165–196.

National Academy of Sciences. *Lead: Airborne Lead in Perspective*. National Research Council, Washington, D. C., **1972**.

Smith, W. E., and Smith, A. M. *Minamata*. Holt, Rinehart & Winston, New York, **1975**.

Stocken, L. A., and Thompson, R. H. S. Reactions of British antilewisite with arsenic and other metals in living systems. *Physiol. Rev.*, **1949**, *29*, 168–194.

Swensson, A., and Ulfarsson, V. Toxicology of organic mercury compounds used as fungicides. *Occup. Health Rev.*, **1963**, *15*, 5–11.

Task Group on Metal Accumulation. Accumulation of toxic metals with specific reference to their absorption, excretion, and biological half-times. *Environ. Physiol. Biochem.*, **1973**, *3*, 65–107.

70 NONMETALLIC ENVIRONMENTAL TOXICANTS: AIR POLLUTANTS, SOLVENTS AND VAPORS, AND PESTICIDES

Curtis D. Klaassen

Environmental pollution, an undesired spin-off of human activity, was relatively insignificant until urbanization. People dug coal from the ground, used it to heat homes, and thus created an atmosphere of sulfurous smoke above the cities. From the thirteenth century onward, periodic efforts were made to forbid the burning of coal in London, but, on the whole, people have accepted a polluted atmosphere as part of urban life. Power plants burn fossil fuels to generate electricity; steel mills have grown along river banks and lake shores; oil refineries have risen near ports and oil fields; smelters roast and refine metals near great mineral deposits; the automobile is all-prevalent. All these operations pollute the air, water, and soil around them.

When synthetic materials came of age, factories were built to produce them. Little thought was given to the toxicity of chemicals not intended for use in man. Only a few of the three million known chemicals have been tested for toxic effects; many have been indiscriminately disseminated throughout the environment.

AIR POLLUTION

Air pollutants enter the body predominantly through the lungs. Some of these chemicals are absorbed into the blood, whereas the lungs eliminate substances that are not absorbed.

ABSORPTION AND DEPOSITION OF TOXICANTS BY THE LUNGS

The site of deposition of aerosols in the respiratory tract depends on the size of the particle. Particles of 5 μm or larger in diameter are usually deposited in the upper air-

way. Those deposited in the unciliated anterior portion of the nose remain until removed by wiping, blowing, or sneezing. In the posterior portion of the nose, a mucus blanket propelled by cilia carries insoluble particles to the pharynx in minutes. These particles are swallowed and pass to the gastrointestinal tract. Soluble particles dissolved in the mucus may be carried to the pharynx or absorbed through the epithelium into the blood.

Particles of 1 to 5 μm are deposited in the tracheobronchial tree and cleared by the cilia's upward movement of mucus. Although the rate of ciliary movement varies in different parts of the respiratory tract, it is rapid and efficient. Rates of transport are between 0.1 and 1 mm per minute, resulting in half-lives for the particles that range from 30 to 300 minutes. Coughing and sneezing move mucus and particles rapidly toward the glottis. The particles may also be swallowed.

Particles less than 1 μm in diameter remain suspended in the inhaled air and reach the alveolar zone of the lung, where they may be readily absorbed. The surface area is large (50 to 100 sq m); the rate of blood flow is high; and the blood is in close proximity to the alveolar air (10 μm). The factors that govern the rate of absorption of gases are discussed in Chapter 13. Liquid aerosols cross the alveolar cell membranes by passive diffusion in proportion to their lipid solubility. Mechanisms for removal or absorption of particulate matter (usually less than 1 μm in diameter) from the alveolus are less clearly defined and are less efficient than those that remove particles from the tracheobronchial tree. Three processes are apparently operative. The first is physical removal; particles deposited on the fluid layer of the alveoli are believed to be aspirated onto the mucociliary escalator of the tracheobronchial tree. The second is phagocytosis, usually by mononuclear phagocytes or alveolar macrophages. The third is by absorption into the lymphatic system. Particles can remain in lymphatic tissue for long periods of time, and, for this reason, the tissue has been called the dust store of the lungs.

Overall, removal of particulates from the alveolus is relatively inefficient. Only about 20% of such matter is removed during the first day after deposition; that which remains longer than 24 hours is often removed very slowly. The rate of this clearance can be predicted from the solubility of the substance in lung fluids. The least soluble compounds are removed at a slower rate. Such removal is apparently largely due to dissolution and absorption into the blood. Some particles may remain in the alveoli indefinitely if the cells that phagocytize them proliferate and join the reticular network to form an alveolar dust plaque or nodule.

TYPES AND SOURCES OF AIR POLLUTANTS

Five pollutants account for nearly 98% of air pollution. These are carbon monoxide (52%), sulfur oxides (18%), hydrocarbons (12%), particulate matter (10%), and nitrogen oxides (6%) (Amdur, 1985). A distinction is often made between two kinds of pollution. The first is characterized by sulfur dioxide and smoke from incomplete combustion of coal and by conditions of fog and cool temperatures. Because of its chemical nature, it is termed a *reducing type of pollution*. The second is characterized by hydrocarbons, oxides of nitrogen, and photochemical oxidants. It is caused by automobile exhaust and occurs especially in areas such as the Los Angeles basin, where intense sunlight causes photochemical reactions in polluted air masses that are trapped by a meteorological inversion layer. Because of its nature, it is described as an *oxidizing type of pollution* or *photochemical air pollution*.

Five major sources account for 90% of the tons of pollutants that are emitted annually (Amdur, 1985): transportation (particularly automobiles) (60%), industry (18%), electric power generation (13%), space heating (6%), and refuse disposal (3%).

HEALTH EFFECTS OF AIR POLLUTION

Acute episodes of high pollution cause mortality and morbidity. There are three classical examples: 65 people died in the Meuse Valley, Belgium in 1930; 20 people died in Donora, Pennsylvania in 1948; 4000 people died in London in 1952. Each of these incidents occurred during an atmospheric temperature inversion that lasted for 3 to 4 days. During this time the concentration of pollutants surpassed the usual levels for these already heavily polluted areas; since coal was the main fuel, the pollution was the reducing kind. Most of the people who became ill or died were elderly; some had either cardiac or respiratory diseases or both; none could cope with the added stress of breathing heavily polluted air.

Acute effects on health are thus clearly associated with the reducing type of pollution. While there is less evidence to associate photochemical oxidant pollution with such effects on human health, there are significant correlations between levels of oxidants in the air and hospital admissions for allergic disorders, inflammatory disease of the eye, acute upper respiratory infections, influenza, and bronchitis.

TOXICOLOGY OF AIR POLLUTANTS

Sulfur Dioxide. Sulfur dioxide gas is generated primarily by the burning of fossil fuels that contain sulfur. The concentration of sulfur dioxide required to kill laboratory animals is so high that it has little relevance to problems of air pollution. However, daily exposure of rats to 10 ppm of sulfur dioxide for 1 to 2 months thickens the mucus layer in the trachea about fivefold. Although the cilia beat with normal frequency, the thick mucus retards clearance. The abnormal mucus layer is caused by increased numbers of mucus-secreting cells in the main bronchi, where such cells are common, and in the peripheral airways, where they are normally absent (Hirsch *et al.*, 1975).

A basic physiological response to inhalation of sulfur dioxide is a mild degree of bronchial constriction that is dependent on intact parasympathetic innervation. When exposed to 5 ppm of sulfur dioxide for 10 minutes, most human subjects show increased resistance to the flow of air. Asthmatics have an increased sensitivity to sulfur dioxide; bronchoconstriction may occur at concentrations as low as 0.25 ppm (Sheppard *et al.,* 1981).

It appears that an increase in the concentration of atmospheric sulfur oxides, which is generally accompanied by an elevation in the level of particulate matter, significantly affects morbidity and mortality. In heavily polluted cities (London, New York, Cracow), exposure for 24 hours to sulfur dioxide concentrations of 0.11 to 0.15 ppm and total particulate concentrations of 500 to 600 $\mu g/m^3$ results in increased morbidity and mortality, and a temporary decrease in pulmonary function is observed at about 0.1 ppm of sulfur dioxide and 250 $\mu g/m^3$ of particulate matter (Ware *et al.,* 1981).

Sulfuric Acid. A portion of sulfur dioxide in the atmosphere is converted to sulfuric acid, ammonium sulfate, and other sulfates. The conversion to sulfuric acid can be initiated by soot or by trace metals such as vanadium or manganese. Recent evidence indicates that stable sulfite complexes may be formed in the presence of metals such as copper or iron.

Sulfuric acid increases airway resistance in relation to both concentration and particle size (Amdur *et al.,* 1978). Particles of 1 μm (1 mg/m^3) produce a rapid and marked increase in resistance to flow, whereas particles of 7 μm produce only a slight increase because they cannot penetrate beyond the upper respiratory tract. Sulfuric acid produces a greater increase in resistance to flow than does sulfur dioxide after either an acute or chronic exposure.

Particulate Sulfates. Sulfates vary greatly in their effects on respiration, and the sulfate ion *per se* does not alter respiratory function. Zinc ammonium sulfate, a reported constituent of the Donora fog, increases respiratory resistance at a concentration of 0.25 mg/m^3 (Amdur and Corn, 1963); it produces a greater increase in resistance to flow than does sulfur dioxide.

Ozone. The oxidant found in the highest concentrations in polluted atmosphere is ozone (O_3). Several miles above the earth's surface there is sufficient short-wave ultraviolet light to convert O_2 to O_3 by direct absorption. Of the major atmospheric pollutants, nitrogen dioxide is the most efficient in absorbing ultraviolet light. Such absorption leads to a complex series of reactions, which may be simplified as follows:

$$NO_2 \xrightarrow{\text{UV}} NO + O$$
$$O + O_2 \longrightarrow O_3$$
$$O_3 + NO \longrightarrow NO_2 + O_2$$

Since NO_2 is regenerated by the reaction of NO and O_3, the result is cyclical. Simultaneously, oxygen atoms react with hydrocarbons in the atmosphere, especially olefins and substituted aromatics, resulting in oxidized compounds and free radicals that react with NO to produce more NO_2. The re-

sult is accumulation of NO_2 and O_3, while concentrations of NO are depleted.

Ozone is a lung irritant that is capable of causing death from pulmonary edema. Gross pulmonary edema is evident in mice exposed to concentrations above 2 ppm. Ozone causes desquamation of the epithelium throughout the ciliated airways and produces degenerative changes in type-I cells and swelling or rupture of the capillary endothelium in the alveoli (Boatman *et al.,* 1974; Stephens *et al.,* 1974). The type-I cells are later replaced by type-II cells. It is important to note that pulmonary toxicity has been observed in experimental animals after relatively short exposures to concentrations of ozone that occasionally exist for short periods in polluted urban areas.

Long-term exposure to ozone may cause thickening of the terminal respiratory bronchioles. Chronic bronchitis, fibrosis, and emphysematous changes are observed in a variety of species exposed to ozone at concentrations slightly above 1 ppm (Amdur, 1985).

Ozone causes shallow, rapid breathing, a decrease in pulmonary compliance, and subjective symptoms, such as cough, tightness in the chest, and dryness of the throat at 0.25 to 0.75 ppm. Such concentrations of ozone may be present during long, high-altitude flights (Folinsbee, 1983). Ozone also increases the sensitivity of the lung to bronchoconstrictors such as histamine, acetylcholine, and allergens (Lee *et al.,* 1977). It increases the incidence of infection in laboratory animals exposed to an aerosol of infectious microorganisms, which is thought to result from inhibition of clearance mechanisms (Coffin and Blommer, 1967).

The biochemical mechanism of pulmonary injury produced by ozone may be due to the formation of reactive free-radical intermediates (Menzel, 1970). Ozone-induced free radicals may be derived from interaction with sulfhydryl groups, from oxidative decomposition of unsaturated fatty acids, or both. Several lines of evidence indicate that one of the biological actions of ozone is reaction with unsaturated fatty acids. The ozonization of these fatty acids is essentially equivalent to lipid peroxidation. Ozone decreases the concentration of glutathione in the lung (DeLucia *et al.,* 1975). Sulfhydryl compounds and antioxidants (such as ascorbic acid and α-tocopherol) protect against ozone toxicity.

Nitrogen Dioxide. Nitrogen dioxide, like ozone, is a lung irritant that is capable of producing pulmonary edema. This is a risk to farmers, because sufficient amounts of nitrogen dioxide can be liberated from ensilage to produce the symptoms of pulmonary damage known as silo-filler's disease. The LC50 for a 4-hour exposure to nitrogen dioxide is about 90 ppm. As with ozone, nitrogen dioxide damages type-I cells of the alveoli. Chronic exposure of animals to nitrogen dioxide results in emphysematous lesions (Freeman *et al.,* 1972).

Experimental exposure of animals or man to nitrogen dioxide causes measurable alterations in pulmonary function. The pattern of changes resembles that produced by ozone—increased respiratory frequency and decreased compliance. Pulmonary resistance to air flow is minimally altered. The changes in pulmonary function occur when healthy subjects are exposed to 2 to 3 ppm and may happen at far lower concentrations in some asthmatic subjects (Orehek *et al.*, 1976). Short-term or long-term exposure to nitrogen dioxide can increase the susceptibility of experimental animals to respiratory infection (Coffin *et al.*, 1976).

Aldehydes. Aldehydes are formed by oxidation of hydrocarbons by sunlight and by incomplete combustion (automobile exhaust, forest fires); they are released from formaldehyde-containing resins (such as those in plywood, particle board, and urea-formaldehyde foam insulation). The high reactivity of aldehydes results in rather short half-lives of a few hours in the atmosphere. The concentration of aldehydes is 0.0005 to 0.002 ppm in a clean atmosphere, 0.004 to 0.05 ppm in ambient urban air, and up to 0.8 ppm in indoor environments where formaldehyde-emitting materials are found (Committee on Aldehydes, 1981; Woodbury and Zenz, 1983). About 50% of the total aldehyde in polluted air is *formaldehyde* (H_2CO), and about 5% is *acrolein* ($H_2C=CHCHO$). These materials probably contribute to the odor of photochemical smog and the ocular irritation that it causes.

Formaldehyde irritates mucous membranes of the nose, upper respiratory tract, and eyes. Concentrations of 0.5 to 1 ppm are detectable by odor, 2 to 3 ppm produce mild irritation, and 4 to 5 ppm are intolerable to most people. The concentration of formaldehyde may approach 1 ppm in the air of newly built homes, especially mobile homes. A significant correlation was found between the formaldehyde concentration in home air and the incidence of ocular irritation. Other symptoms (*e.g.*, runny nose, sore throat, headache, and cough) are also more frequent in people living in indoor environments with high levels of formaldehyde (Woodbury and Zenz, 1983). The overall pattern of respiratory response to formaldehyde resembles that to sulfur dioxide. Formaldehyde can provoke skin reactions in sensitized subjects, not only by contact but also by inhalation (Maibach, 1983). Inhalation of formaldehyde (6 to 15 ppm) for 2 years induces squamous-cell carcinomas in the nasal cavity of mice and rats (Kerns *et al.*, 1983).

Acrolein is much more irritating than formaldehyde. Acrolein is a major contributor to the irritative quality of cigarette smoke and photochemical smog. The occupational threshold limit value (TLV) for acrolein is 0.1 ppm; 1 ppm causes lacrimation in less than 5 minutes (Committee on Aldehydes, 1981). Acrolein increases airway resistance and tidal volume and decreases respiratory frequency. Aldehydes increase resistance to air flow at concentrations below those that decrease respiratory frequency.

Carbon Monoxide. Carbon monoxide (CO) is a colorless, odorless, tasteless, and nonirritating gas resulting from incomplete combustion of organic matter. CO is the most abundant pollutant in the lower atmosphere, and a large number of accidental and suicidal deaths occur yearly from its inhalation.

The average concentration of CO in the atmosphere is about 0.1 ppm. Natural sources, such as atmospheric oxidation of methane, forest fires, terpine oxidation, and the ocean (where microorganisms produce CO), are responsible for about 90% of the atmospheric CO; human activity produces about 10%.

Inadequate venting of furnaces and automobiles results in many deaths each year. Most victims of fires die from acute CO poisoning rather than from burns. The automobile is the greatest source of CO; concentrations can reach 115 ppm in heavy traffic, 75 ppm in vehicles on expressways, and 23 ppm in residential areas. In underground garages and tunnels, CO levels have been found to exceed 100 ppm for extended periods. The installation of pollution control devices, including catalytic converters in automobile exhaust systems, has reduced CO emissions from about 90 to 3.4 g per mile of automobile travel and should decrease concentrations of CO in urban atmospheres (National Research Council, 1977).

The average concentration of CO in the atmosphere appears to be stabilized by efficient natural means of removal (sinks). The most important sink seems to be the reaction of CO with ambient hydroxyl radicals to form carbon dioxide; the upper atmosphere and the soil also are sinks.

Another source of exposure to CO is smoking. Goldsmith and Landaw (1968) reported a median carboxyhemoglobin (COHb) level of 5.9% in heavy smokers (two packs of cigarettes per day) who inhale.

Reaction of CO with Hemoglobin. According to the classical theory of CO poisoning, toxicity is due to its combination with hemoglobin to form COHb. Hemoglobin in this form cannot carry oxygen, since both gases react with the same group in the hemoglobin molecule. Because the affinity of hemoglobin for CO is approximately 220 times greater than for oxygen, CO is dangerous even at very low concentrations. Since air contains 21% oxygen by volume, exposure to a gas mixture of 0.1% CO (1000 ppm) in air would result in approximately 50% carboxyhemoglobinemia.

The reduction in the oxygen-carrying *capacity* of blood is proportional to the amount of COHb present. However, the amount of oxygen *available* to the tissues is still further reduced by the inhibitory influence of COHb on the dissociation of any oxyhemoglobin (O_2Hb) still available. This can be understood best by comparing an anemic individual having a hemoglobin value of 8.0 g/dl with a person having a hemoglobin value of 16.0 g/dl but with half of it in the form of COHb (*see* Figure 70–1). In each instance the oxygen-carrying *capacity* is the same. The anemic individual may show few, if any, symptoms whereas the person suffering from CO poisoning will be near collapse.

The toxicity of CO is not solely due to the interference of CO with the delivery of O_2 by the blood.

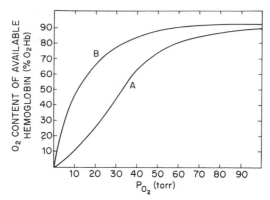

Figure 70–1. *The effect of carboxyhemoglo-bin (COHb) on the dissociation curve of oxy-hemoglobin.*

Curve A represents the normal oxygen dissociation curve, which is unaffected by the presence of anemia (*e.g.*, 8 g hemoglobin/dl blood). Curve B represents the situation when there is 50% COHb and a normal concentration of hemoglobin (16 g hemoglobin/dl blood and half of the binding sites occupied by CO). The oxygen-carrying capacity is the same in both cases; however, when COHb is present, oxygen dissociates from hemoglobin at lower values of P_{O_2}. This effect results from interactions between binding sites for O_2 or CO; there are four such sites per molecule of hemoglobin.

CO also exerts a direct toxic effect by binding to cellular cytochromes, such as those contained in respiratory enzymes and myoglobin (Gutierrez, 1982).

Factors Governing CO Toxicity. Factors that govern the toxicity of CO include the concentration of the gas in the inspired air, the duration of exposure, the respiratory minute volume, the cardiac output, the oxygen demand of the tissues, and the concentration of hemoglobin in the blood. Anemic persons are more susceptible to CO than are individuals with normal amounts of hemoglobin. Increased metabolic rate enhances the severity of symptoms in CO poisoning; this is why children succumb earlier than adults when exposed to a given concentration of the gas.

Change in barometric pressure does not affect the relative affinities of hemoglobin for O_2 and CO. However, at high altitudes and in other situations where oxygen tension is low, the effects of a given concentration of CO will be correspondingly more severe.

Signs and Symptoms of CO Toxicity. The signs and symptoms of CO poisoning are characteristic of hypoxia. They have been correlated with the COHb content of the blood. The relation between symptomatology and COHb concentration is shown in Table 70–1. It should not be inferred that all these symptoms are experienced by any one individual. Although inhalation of a high concentration may produce warning signs (transient weak-

ness and dizziness) before consciousness is lost, there may be no warning at all.

Moderate concentrations of COHb have little effect on vital functions in the human subject at rest. As mentioned previously, the presence of COHb reduces the oxygen-carrying capacity but not the P_{O_2} of arterial blood. As a result, there is no stimulation of respiration by the carotid and aortic chemoreceptor mechanism. Cardiac rate, on the other hand, increases in all subjects when COHb reaches 30%, probably to compensate for peripheral vasodilatation caused by hypoxia.

The clinical findings in patients acutely poisoned by CO are varied. Many patients exhibit symptoms not usually associated with CO poisoning: skin lesions, excessive sweating, hepatic enlargement, bleeding tendency, pyrexia, leukocytosis, albuminuria, and glycosuria.

Pathology of Acute CO Poisoning. The tissues most affected are those most sensitive to oxygen deprivation, such as the brain and the heart, and the lesions are predominantly hemorrhagic. The severe headache following exposure to CO is believed to be caused by cerebral edema and increased intracranial pressure resulting from excessive transudation across hypoxic capillaries. Finck (1966) has cataloged the gross pathological changes observed in 351 fatal cases of accidental CO poisoning. Rapidly fatal cases of CO poisoning are characterized by congestion and hemorrhages in all organs. In less acutely fatal cases, the hypoxic lesions observed are related to the duration of posthypoxic unconsciousness.

Bokonjić (1963) has shown that the maximal period of CO-induced posthypoxic unconsciousness compatible with complete neurological recovery is 21 hours in patients under 48 years of age and 11 hours in older patients. Complete recovery of men-

Table 70–1. CORRELATION BETWEEN % COHb AND SIGNS AND SYMPTOMS OF CO POISONING *

% OF BLOOD SATURATION	SIGNS AND SYMPTOMS
0–10	No symptoms
10–20	Tightness across forehead; possibly slight headache, dilatation of cutaneous blood vessels
20–30	Headache; throbbing in temples
30–40	Severe headache, weakness, dizziness, dimness of vision, nausea and vomiting, collapse
40–50	Same as previous item with greater possibility of collapse or syncope; increased respiration and pulse
50–60	Syncope, increased respiration and pulse; coma with intermittent convulsions; Cheyne-Stokes respiration
60–70	Coma with intermittent convulsions, depressed cardiac function and respiration, possible death
70–80	Weak pulse and slowed respiration; respiratory failure and death

* Modified from Sayers and Davenport, 1930.

tal function was not observed when the CO-induced unconsciousness exceeded 15 hours in the older group or 64 hours in the younger group. Prolonged posthypoxic unconsciousness may damage vital organs severely. Histological studies of the human brain have shown extensive demyelination of the white matter, bilateral necrosis of the globus pallidus, and necrotic lesions of Ammon's horn (Brucher, 1967; Lapresle and Fardeau, 1967). Perhaps the most insidious effect of CO poisoning is the delayed development of neuropsychiatric impairment, which is manifested as inappropriate euphoria and impairment of judgment, abstract thinking, and concentration. The heart is also sensitive to hypoxia and may be permanently damaged by the presence of COHb in the blood. Patients with severe CO poisoning usually exhibit one or more of the following abnormal ECG changes: sinus tachycardia, T wave abnormalities, S-T segment depression, and atrial fibrillation. Evidence of ischemic changes and subendocardial infarction also has been observed. Severe CO poisoning can produce skin lesions varying from areas of erythema and edema to marked blister and bulla formation. Rhabdomyolysis, presumably due to the direct toxic effect of CO on myoglobin, and myoglobinuria with renal failure may also occur.

Diagnosis of Acute CO Poisoning. The presumptive diagnosis of acute CO poisoning is usually facilitated by circumstantial evidence, since the victim is commonly found under circumstances that leave little doubt as to the cause of his condition. COHb is cherry-red in color, and its presence in high concentrations in capillary blood may impart an abnormal red color to the skin, mucous membranes, and fingernails. However, Matthew (1971) has emphasized that the living patient is commonly cyanotic and pale and that "cherry-red cyanosis" is seen only at necropsy. A final diagnosis depends upon the demonstration of COHb in the blood. Therapy is not delayed to perform such a test in a severely poisoned individual, but the demonstration of COHb often has a forensic significance. If a person succumbs in an atmosphere containing CO, a post-mortem blood sample usually contains 60% COHb; however, death sometimes occurs at lower concentrations. If the patient is removed from such an atmosphere while still breathing, the concentration of COHb rapidly declines, and, if respiratory exchange continues to be adequate, the blood is freed of this form of hemoglobin over a course of hours.

Fate and Excretion of CO. COHb is fully dissociable and, once acute exposure is terminated, the CO will be excreted via the lungs. Only a very small amount is oxidized to CO_2.

There is no excretion of CO without active respiration. Furthermore, COHb is extremely stable and is little affected by putrefaction. Therefore, valid measurements of COHb concentrations in the body can be made long after death. Conversely, little or no CO is absorbed post mortem and analysis of the blood in the heart provides an accurate measurement of the concentration of COHb in the blood at death. These factors have great medicolegal importance.

When room air is breathed by a resting subject, the CO content of blood decreases with a half-time of 320 minutes. If 100% oxygen is substituted for air, this value is reduced to 80 minutes; under hyperbaric conditions, the half-time may be less than 25 minutes (Peterson and Stewart, 1970). These facts provide the basic principles for treatment of CO poisoning.

Treatment of CO Poisoning. The first essential is to transfer the patient to fresh air. If respiration has failed, artificial respiration must be instituted immediately. Treatment is then directed toward providing an adequate supply of oxygen to the body cells and hastening elimination of the CO. In severe poisoning, administration of hyperbaric oxygen is the preferred treatment; this not only provides oxygen in solution for the tissues but also hastens the dissociation of COHb. If a hyperbaric chamber is not available, 100% oxygen should be administered with a high rate of flow and a tight-fitting face mask. Oxygen should be given until the level of COHb decreases to at least 10%. Supplementary care includes correction of hypotension and acidosis, as well as monitoring of cardiac function (Tintinalli *et al.*, 1983).

Toxicity of Prolonged and Low-Level Exposure to CO. The cardiovascular system, particularly the heart, is susceptible to adverse effects of low concentrations of COHb. At 6 to 12% COHb there is a shift from aerobic to anaerobic metabolism (Ayres *et al.*, 1970). Experimental and clinical studies have suggested that chronic exposure to CO can facilitate the development of atherosclerosis (Thomsen, 1974). CO also seems to affect human behavior. Performance on tests of vigilance is impaired when there is only 2 to 5% COHb. However, these low levels of COHb probably have no effect on other behaviors, such as driving, reaction time, temporal discriminations, coordination, sensory processes, and complex intellectual tasks (National Research Council, 1977).

The fetus may be extremely susceptible to effects of CO, and the gas readily crosses the placenta. Infants born to women who have survived acute exposure to a high concentration of the gas while pregnant often display neurological sequelae, and there may be gross damage to the brain (Longo, 1977). Persistent low levels of COHb in the fetus of a woman who has smoked during pregnancy may also have effects on the development of the central nervous system (CNS).

Polycythemia develops in the course of chronic exposure to CO. Other compensatory mechanisms are likely, but they have not been demonstrated. Healthy human subjects are exquisitely responsive to any hypoxic stress; they immediately compensate by increasing cardiac output and flow to critical organs. Those with significant cardiovascular disease are more vulnerable to the toxicity of CO because they may be unable to compensate for the hypoxia (*see* Stewart, 1975).

Particulate Material. *Pneumoconiosis* is a category of disease caused by inhalation of dusts. The most common condition of this type is *silicosis*. Next to oxygen, silicon is the most abundant element. Approximately 60% of the rocks in the earth's crust contain silica, and silica dusts are prevalent in many industries, particularly in the mining of gold, iron, and coal; in stonework; and in sandblasting. Particles larger than 10 μm are of little clinical significance, because they seldom reach the alveoli. Particles less than 2 to 3 μm are phagocytized by alveolar macrophages, and these cells are eventually destroyed. Other macrophages proliferate and migrate to sites of reaction, where they may release a soluble substance that stimulates the accumulation of collagen (Heppleston and Styles, 1967). The silicotic nodules that result from such reactions are scattered uniformly throughout both lungs. The disease usually requires 10 to 25 years to develop. As the mass of fibrotic tissue increases, vital capacity decreases and the afflicted individual experiences shortness of breath.

Other pulmonary diseases develop concurrently with silicosis, and their pathogenesis may be facilitated by silica. Long known to enhance susceptibility to tuberculosis, silicosis also increases the risk of infection by other microorganisms.

Asbestosis results from chronic inhalation of asbestos dust. Asbestos is a fibrous substance composed of hydrated silicate minerals. It is widely used in industry because it is nonflammable and flexible, and has high tensile strength, low density, resistance to acids and alkalies, and high electrical resistivity. It is often used for insulation, brake linings, shingles, and draperies.

Asbestosis (a form of pulmonary fibrosis) develops first in areas adjacent to the bronchioles, where there seems to be preferential deposition of longer asbestos fibers. There is also a fibrous pleuritis in which the pleural membrane thickens to encase the lung in a rigid fibrous capsule. Clinical symptoms of asbestosis resemble those of silicosis: dyspnea, tachypnea, and cough. However, tuberculosis is not a prominent complication.

Bronchial cancer associated with inhalation of asbestos occurs some 20 to 30 years after initial exposure. Inhalation of asbestos combined with cigarette smoking significantly increases the incidence of lung cancer over that caused by exposure to either factor alone (Selikoff and Hammond, 1979). *Mesothelioma,* a rapidly fatal malignancy, is also associated with exposure to asbestos fibers. It may appear in the pleura or the peritoneum, usually 25 to 40 years after initial exposure (Selikoff and Hammond, 1979). A high incidence of mesothelioma has been attributed to fibrous tremolite in household stucco and whitewash in Turkey. It thus appears that mesothelioma is not a specific reaction to asbestos, but that any natural or synthetic fibrous material with similar fiber dimensions might be carcinogenic (Elmes, 1980). However, except for chronic inhalation of fibrous matter and the strong suspicion of an increase in risk for persons living adjacent to emissions containing arsenic, there is as yet little convincing evidence that environmental air pollution contributes to the risk of cancer (Kaplan and Morgan, 1981).

Many other occupational pulmonary diseases are caused by chronic inhalation of dusts containing minerals or organic matter. These include coal workers' pneumoconiosis (black lung disease), aluminosis (bauxite lung), baritosis (from barium), beryllium disease, byssinosis (from cotton), and others (*see* Speizer, 1983).

SOLVENTS AND VAPORS

Organic solvents and their vapors are a common part of our environment. Short, incidental exposures to low concentrations of solvent vapors, such as gasoline, lighter fluids, aerosol sprays, and spot removers, may be relatively harmless; however, exposures to paint removers, floor and tile cleaners, and other solvents in home or industry may be dangerous. Because so many industrial workers are exposed to toxic solvents and vapors, considerable effort has gone into determining safe levels of exposure. Threshold limit values (TLV) or maximum allowable concentrations (MAC) have been established for the airborne poisons; a TLV represents the concentration to which most workers may be safely exposed for an 8-hour period.

A variety of anesthetic gases, solvents, and fluorohydrocarbons (used as propellants in aerosol products) cause subjective effects when inhaled and are frequently abused in this way. This dangerous practice, which has caused many deaths, is discussed in Chapter 23.

Aliphatic Hydrocarbons

C_1–C_4 Aliphatic Hydrocarbons. The straight-chain hydrocarbons with four or less carbon atoms are present in natural gas (methane, ethane) and in bottled gas (propane, butane). Methane and ethane produce no general systemic effects. They are "simple asphyxiants"; effects are observed only when their concentration in the air is so high that it decreases the amount of oxygen.

C_5–C_8 Aliphatic Hydrocarbons. The higher-molecular-weight aliphatic hydrocarbons, like most organic solvents, depress the CNS and cause dizziness and incoordination. However, polyneuropathy is the primary toxic reaction to *n*-hexane, a widely used solvent. This was observed first in Japan, where 93 workers engaged in the production of sandals were afflicted by the use of a glue that contained at least 60% *n*-hexane (Iida *et al.*, 1973). 2-Hexanone (methyl *n*-butyl ketone) produces neurological changes similar to those of *n*-hexane. Clinical symptoms include symmetrical sensory dysfunction of the distal portions of the extremities, which progresses to muscle weakness in toes and fingers and loss of deep sensory reflexes. A decrease in nerve conduction velocity precedes the onset of symptoms (Seppäläinen, 1982). The prognosis for recovery is generally good, although the disorder may intensify for months. The cytochrome P-450–mediated biotransformation of *n*-hexane and 2-hexanone to 2,5-hexadione appears to be responsible for the peripheral neuropathy associated with the exposure to these solvents (Couri and Milks, 1982).

Gasoline and Kerosene. Gasoline and kerosene, petroleum distillates prepared by the fractionation of crude petroleum oil, contain aliphatic, aromatic, and a variety of branched and unsaturated hydrocarbons. They are used as illuminating fuels, heating fuels, motor fuels, vehicles for many pesticides, cleaning agents, and paint thinners. Because they are often stored in containers previously used for milk, carbonated drinks, and other beverages, they are a common cause of accidental poisoning in children.

Intoxication by ingestion of gasoline and kerosene resembles that from ethyl alcohol. Signs and symptoms include incoordination, restlessness, excitement, confusion, disorientation, ataxia, delirium, and finally coma, which may last for a few hours or several days. Inhalation of high concentrations of gasoline vapors, as by workmen cleaning storage tanks, can cause immediate death. Gasoline vapors sensitize the myocardium such that small amounts of circulating epinephrine may precipitate ventricular fibrillation; many hydrocarbons have this action. High concentrations of gasoline vapor may also lead to rapid depression of the CNS and death from respiratory failure.

Poisoning from these hydrocarbons results either from inhalation of the vapors or from ingestion of the liquid. Ingestion is more hazardous, because the liquids have a low surface tension and can be easily aspirated into the respiratory tract by vomiting or eructation. Morbidity is attributed to aspiration, whether it occurs at the time of ingestion or during treatment. Pulmonary damage does not result from gastrointestinal absorption of gasoline or kerosene. Chemical pneumonitis, complicated by secondary bacterial pneumonia and pulmonary edema, is the most serious sequel to aspiration. Death caused by hemorrhagic pulmonary edema usually occurs in 16 to 18 hours and seldom later than 24 hours after aspiration.

Examination of tissues from fatal cases reveals heavy, edematous, and hemorrhagic lungs. The alveoli are filled with an exudate that is rich in proteins, cells, and fibrin, often in a pattern resembling that of hyaline membrane disease. Alveolar walls are weakened and may rupture, leading to less frequent sequelae, such as emphysema and pneumothorax. Pulmonary lymph nodes are inflamed, and bronchopneumonia and atelectasis have been noted.

Symptomatic and supportive care is probably the best treatment for intoxication by gasoline or kerosene (Ervin, 1983; Gosselin *et al.*, 1984). Because of the danger of aspiration, emesis or gastric lavage should not be employed unless the risks are justified by the presence of additional toxic substances in the petroleum. Catharsis may be induced with

magnesium or sodium sulfate. Antibiotics and corticosteroids are used if there is a specific indication, such as bacterial pneumonitis or "shock lung." Epinephrine and related substances should be avoided because they may induce cardiac arrhythmias. Treatment should include correction of imbalances of fluid and electrolytes.

HALOGENATED HYDROCARBONS

The excellent solvent properties and low flammability of halogenated hydrocarbons have placed them among the most widely used industrial solvents. Several low-molecular-weight hydrocarbons are found in drinking water. Some of these, such as chloroform, bromodichloromethane, dibromochloromethane, and bromoform, are produced from naturally occurring precursors during chlorination of water; others, such as carbon tetrachloride, dichloromethane, and 1,2-dichloroethane, do not appear to arise from such treatment. Filtration or treatment of water with charcoal prior to chlorination effectively reduces formation of chlorinated hydrocarbons. Because some of these compounds have been shown to be carcinogenic in animals and because correlations have been reported between the chlorination of water and the incidence of cancer of the colon, rectum, and breast, there is a cause for concern about the exposure of a very large percentage of the population to these chemicals in drinking water (*see* Menzer and Nelson, 1985). Since the halogenated hydrocarbons are extremely soluble in lipid, they are readily absorbed after inhalation or ingestion. Like most other organic solvents, halogenated hydrocarbons depress the CNS.

Carbon Tetrachloride. Carbon tetrachloride (CCl_4) has been used for medical purposes and was once commonly employed as a spot remover and carpet cleaner; however, its use has now been abandoned because there are safer alternatives.

Transient exposure to toxic concentrations of CCl_4 vapor results in the following symptoms: irritation of the eyes, nose, and throat; nausea and vomiting; a sense of fullness in the head; dizziness; and headache. If the exposure is soon terminated, symptoms usually disappear within a few hours. Continued exposure or absorption of larger quantities of the chemical may cause stupor, convulsions, coma, or death from CNS depression. Sudden death may occur from ventricular fibrillation or depression of vital medullary centers.

Delayed toxic effects of CCl_4 include nausea, vomiting, abdominal pain, diarrhea, and hematemesis. The most serious delayed toxic effects of CCl_4 result from its hepatotoxic and nephrotoxic actions. Signs and symptoms of hepatic injury may appear after a delay of several hours or 2 to 3 days and may occur in the absence of earlier severe effects on the CNS. Biochemical evidence of hepatic injury often includes greatly elevated activities of transaminases and a variety of other hepatic enzymes in plasma. Alkaline phosphatase activity is, however, only slightly elevated. The chief histological abnormalities include hepatic steatosis and hepatic centrilobular necrosis.

The mechanism of CCl_4-induced hepatic injury has interested many investigators, and the compound has become the reference substance for all hepatotoxic compounds. Injury produced by CCl_4 seems to be mediated by a reactive metabolite—trichloromethyl free radical ($\cdot CCl_3$)—formed by the homolytic cleavage of CCl_4, or by an even more reactive species—trichloromethylperoxy free radical ($Cl_3COO\cdot$)—formed by the reaction of $\cdot CCl_3$ with O_2 (Slater, 1982). This biotransformation is catalyzed by a cytochrome P-450–dependent monooxygenase. Thus, agents such as DDT and phenobarbital, which induce such enzymes, enhance the hepatotoxic effects of CCl_4 strikingly. Conversely, agents that inhibit the drug-metabolizing activity diminish the hepatotoxicity of CCl_4. The toxicity produced by CCl_4 is thought to be due to the reaction of the free radical with the lipids and proteins; however, the relative importance of each in producing injury is controversial. Recknagel and Glende (1973) have proposed that the free radical causes the peroxidation of the polyenoic lipids of the endoplasmic reticulum and the generation of secondary free radicals derived from these lipids—a chain reaction. This destructive lipid peroxidation leads to breakdown of membrane structure and function, and, if a sufficient quantity of CCl_4 has been consumed, damage extends to all cellular membranes (*see* Recknagel and Glende, 1973; Zimmerman, 1978; Plaa, 1985).

Individuals recovering from acute ingestion of ethanol seem more susceptible to the hepatotoxic properties of halogenated hydrocarbons. Other alcohols, such as isopropanol, have an even greater ability to potentiate such effects of CCl_4 (Plaa, 1985). This interaction between isopropanol and CCl_4 was highlighted by an industrial accident in an isopropanol packaging plant, where workers exposed to both agents were adversely affected (Folland *et al.*, 1976).

As hepatic injury develops, signs of renal damage may also be observed and may dominate the clinical picture. Experimental studies in rats indicate that CCl_4 produces an early, reversible lesion of the proximal tubule; initial changes occur in the mitochondria and are followed by cellular swelling, proliferation of the smooth endoplasmic reticulum, and a simultaneous increase in the excretion of sodium salts and water (Striker *et al.*, 1968). Mild poisoning in man may be characterized by a reversible oliguria lasting only a few days. In nonfatal poisoning, recovery of renal function occurs in three phases. In the first, after 1 to 3 days, oliguria stops, but concentrations of creatinine and urea in plasma remain elevated. The second phase starts with a rapid decline in these concentrations. In the third phase, about 1 month after the initial injury, renal blood flow and glomerular filtration begin to improve, and renal function is recovered after 100 to 200 days. In more severe intoxication the oliguria may progress in a week or so to near anuria, with red blood cells and albumin in the scanty urine. Hypertension, acidosis, and terminal uremia develop if renal function is not restored.

Emergency treatment of CCl_4 poisoning should be initiated promptly in any person suspected of having absorbed toxic quantities of the compound. The individual exposed to toxic vapor should be moved to fresh air. If the patient is seen shortly after oral ingestion of CCl_4, the stomach should be emptied immediately, by inducing vomiting if the patient is conscious or by gastric lavage, and a saline laxative should be administered to minimize absorption. If the patient is first seen in the stage of advanced CNS depression, every effort should be made to prevent hypoxia. Oxygen and artificial respiration should be administered if necessary. Under no circumstances should an attempt be made to elevate the blood pressure by the use of sympathomimetic drugs because of the danger of producing serious arrhythmias in the sensitized myocardium.

Treatment of the acute hepatic and renal insufficiency caused by CCl_4 is difficult. Although hepatic insufficiency is a very prominent feature of CCl_4 poisoning, renal failure is the most frequent cause of death. Even though the presenting signs and symptoms may be associated with functional impairment of the liver, renal function should be observed closely and oliguria or anuria anticipated. Fortunately, the basic measures employed in the conservative treatment of acute renal insufficiency—administration of glucose to provide calories and careful maintenance of the volume and composition of the body fluids—apply equally to management of acute hepatic insufficiency.

Other Halogenated Hydrocarbons. Chloroform, dichloromethane (methylene chloride), trichloroethylene, tetrachloroethylene (perchlorethylene), 1,1,1-trichloroethane, and 1,1,2-trichloroethane produce many of the same toxic effects as does CCl_4 (Von Oettingen, 1964). All these compounds produce CNS depression, and some have been used as inhalational anesthetics. They also have the potential to sensitize the heart to arrhythmias produced by catecholamines. The hepatotoxic potential is highest with chloroform and 1,1,2-trichloroethane, and least with trichloroethylene, tetrachloroethylene, 1,1,1-trichloroethane, and dichloromethane; chloroform may be hepatotoxic because it is metabolized to phosgene (Krishna *et al.*, 1978). Chloroform, 1,1,2-trichloroethane, and tetrachloroethylene are also nephrotoxic. Since they produce less organ damage than CCl_4 and chloroform, 1,1,1-trichloroethane, tetrachloroethylene, and trichloroethylene are widely used as dry-cleaning agents and industrial solvents and dichloromethane is employed as a paint stripper. Dichloromethane has an additional toxic effect because it is metabolized to CO by cytochrome P-450 (Kubic and Anders, 1975). Chloroform, trichloroethylene, 1,1,2-trichloroethane, and tetrachloroethane induce hepatic tumors; 1,1-dichloroethane (vinylidene chloride) and 1,2-dichloroethane produce tumors in liver and lung as well as angiosarcomas in mice (Williams and Weisburger, 1985).

Between 1961 and 1980, 330 poisonings and 17 deaths were reported in Great Britain due to inhalation of trichloroethylene, tetrachloroethylene, and

1,1,1-trichloroethane, the three most commonly used solvents in industry (McCarthy and Jones, 1983). Deaths were due to deep narcosis, aspiration of vomitus during anesthesia, or cardiac arrhythmias (Jones and Winter, 1983). Signs of hepatotoxicity were not observed. Exposure to high concentrations of trichloroethylene has been associated with trigeminal neuropathy (Annau, 1981); long-term exposure of workers to halogenated hydrocarbon solvents has resulted in behavioral alterations (Annau, 1981; Lindstrom, 1982).

ALIPHATIC ALCOHOLS

The toxicological properties of ethanol and methanol are discussed in Chapter 18.

Isopropanol. Isopropanol, used for rubbing alcohol, hand lotions, and in deicing and antifreeze preparations, is occasionally the cause of accidental poisoning. Like ethanol and methanol, isopropanol is a CNS depressant, but it does not produce retinal damage or acidosis as does methanol.

In adults, the probable lethal dose of isopropanol is about 250 ml; it is thus more toxic than ethanol. While the signs and symptoms of isopropanol toxicity resemble those of ethanol, there are notable differences. Isopropanol produces a more prominent gastritis, with pain, nausea, vomiting, and hemorrhage. Vomiting with aspiration is a serious threat and dangerous complication. Isopropanol intoxication lasts longer because the compound is oxidized more slowly than ethanol (Gosselin et al., 1984) and because its major metabolite, acetone, is also a CNS depressant. Ketoacidosis and ketones in urine (without glucosuria) support the diagnosis. As with the other alcohols, hemodialysis is a useful procedure for removing isopropanol from the body (King et al., 1970).

GLYCOLS

In addition to their use as heat exchangers, antifreeze formulations, hydraulic fluids, or chemical intermediates, glycols are also employed as solvents for pharmaceuticals, food additives, cosmetics, and lacquers.

Ethylene Glycol. Ethylene glycol ($HOCH_2CH_2OH$) is widely used as antifreeze for automobile radiators, and such products are the usual cause of ethylene glycol poisonings. Like ethanol, ethylene glycol produces CNS depression. Patients who ingest large quantities develop narcosis, which leads to coma and death. In addition to the CNS depression, ethylene glycol produces severe renal injury; most victims experience acute renal failure. Those who die from uremia exhibit marked renal pathology, including destruction of epithelial cells, interstitial edema, focal hemorrhagic necrosis in the cortex, extensive hydropic degeneration, numerous cellular casts, and oxalate crystals in the convoluted tubules (Gosselin et al., 1984).

Initial steps in the oxidation of ethylene glycol to the dialdehyde (glyoxal) and to glyoxylic acid (HCOCOOH) seem to be mediated by alcohol dehydrogenase; decarboxylation of glyoxylic acid yields carbon dioxide and formic acid. Glyoxylic acid is also oxidized to oxalic acid (HOOCCOOH). The glycol probably causes the initial CNS depression; oxalate and the other intermediates seem to be responsible for nephrotoxicity. Formic acid produces the metabolic acidosis of ethylene glycol poisoning, as it does in poisoning with methanol.

The specific treatment of poisoning with ethylene glycol is similar to that for methanol (Gosselin et al., 1984). Metabolic acidosis must be treated with a base such as sodium bicarbonate. Ethanol may be used as a competitive substrate for alcohol dehydrogenase to decrease the rate of formation of metabolites. As with other alcohols, dialysis is effective. Parenteral administration of calcium is recommended for muscle spasms, which may develop because of chelation of calcium by the oxalate formed in the biotransformation of ethylene glycol.

Diethylene Glycol. Diethylene glycol ($HOCH_2CH_2OCH_2CH_2OH$) is used in lacquer, cosmetics, antifreeze, and lubricants, and as a softening agent and plasticizer. Its toxicity was a major problem only when the compound was used in the 1930s as a solvent in a preparation of sulfanilamide (Geiling and Cannon, 1938). In that incident, 105 of 353 people who ingested the sulfanilamide–diethylene glycol preparation died from renal damage. Effects of diethylene glycol resemble those of ethylene glycol, and intoxication should be treated similarly.

Propylene Glycol. The physical properties of propylene glycol ($CH_3CHOHCH_2OH$) are similar to those of ethylene glycol, but it is much less toxic. For this reason propylene glycol is used as a solvent for drugs, cosmetics, lotions, and ointments; in food materials; as a plasticizer; in antifreeze formulations; as a heat exchanger; and in hydraulic fluids. Like ethanol, its primary pharmacological action is to produce CNS depression; however, its elimination is slower and its actions are thus prolonged.

Glycol Ethers. Ethylene glycol monomethyl ether and ethylene glycol monoethyl ether have recently been shown to induce testicular atrophy and infertility in male mice, rats, and rabbits during prolonged inhalation (Miller et al., 1983a; Andrews and Snyder, 1985). In addition, these glycol ethers are teratogenic in rats and rabbits. Both ethylene glycol ethers are metabolized by alcohol dehydrogenase to alkoxyacids. Since methoxyacetic acid also produces testicular toxicity in male rats, it appears that alkoxyacids are responsible for this toxic effect. In contrast, propylene glycol monomethyl ether, which is a poor substrate for alcohol dehydrogenase, does not produce testicular atrophy (Miller et al., 1983b).

AROMATIC HYDROCARBONS

Benzene. Benzene is an excellent solvent. It is widely used for chemical syntheses and is a natural constituent of auto fuels. However, benzene is very toxic.

After acute exposure to a large amount of benzene, by ingestion or by breathing concentrated vapors, the major toxic effect is on the CNS. Symptoms from mild exposure include dizziness, weakness, euphoria, headache, nausea, vomiting, tightness in the chest, and staggering. If exposure is more severe, symptoms progress to blurred vision, tremors, shallow and rapid respiration, ventricular irregularities, paralysis, and unconsciousness.

Chronic exposure to benzene is usually due to inhalation of vapor. Signs and symptoms include effects on the CNS and the gastrointestinal tract (headache, loss of appetite, drowsiness, nervousness, and pallor), but the major manifestation of toxicity is aplastic anemia. Bone-marrow cells in early stages of development are the most sensitive to benzene (Snyder et al., 1977), and arrest of maturation leads to gradual depletion of circulating cells.

A major concern is the relationship between chronic exposure to benzene and leukemia. Epidemiological studies have been conducted on workers in the tire industry (McMichael et al., 1975) and in shoe factories (Aksoy et al., 1974), where benzene is used extensively. Among workers who died from exposure to benzene, death was caused by either leukemia or aplastic anemia, in approximately equal proportions.

The first product of the metabolic oxidation of benzene is postulated to be a highly unstable compound, benzene oxide (Jerina and Daley, 1974). Benzene oxide, formed by introduction of oxygen into the molecule by the cytochrome P-450 system, rearranges to form phenol. The sulfate ester of phenol is the major metabolite in the urine, and the level of exposure of workers to benzene can be estimated by determination of the increase in organic sulfate excreted in the urine. Further hydroxylations of phenol result in the formation of hydroquinone and 1,2,4-benzenetriol. When oxidized, these polyphenols form potentially toxic, covalently binding intermediates that may be responsible for the toxic effects of benzene on the bone marrow (Greenlee et al., 1981).

Toluene. Toluene ($C_6H_5CH_3$) is widely used as a solvent in paints, varnishes, glues, enamels, and lacquers and as a chemical intermediate in the synthesis of organic compounds. Toluene is a CNS depressant, and low concentrations produce fatigue, weakness, and confusion. It is for the CNS effects of solvents such as toluene that "glue sniffers" inhale the vapors of glue. Unlike benzene, toluene produces neither aplastic anemia nor leukemia. However, the solvents in glue are often mixed, and the "glue sniffer" is usually exposed to others beside toluene.

PESTICIDES

Pesticide is a general classification that includes insecticides, rodenticides, fungicides, herbicides, and fumigants. These compounds, manufactured for the sole purpose of destroying some form of life, are classified as pesticides because they are directed against organisms that society deems undesirable. While selective toxicity of pesticides is extremely desirable, all can produce at least some toxicity in man.

Mortality attributed to accidental poisoning by pesticides in the United States has declined during the 1960s and 1970s. Hayes and Vaughn (1977) reported that there were only 52 fatal accidental poisonings with pesticides in 1974, compared to 152 in 1956. During this period the proportion of fatal poisonings in children declined from 61% to 31%. This decline was attributed to increased awareness by poison control centers, pediatricians, and parents of the hazards of pesticides to children.

INSECTICIDES

The use of insecticides in agriculture has grown tremendously since World War II, and there is a great potential for occupational exposure to these chemicals, both in production and in use. However, exposure to insecticides is not limited to occupational incidents; residues often remain on produce, and man is exposed to low levels of the chemicals in food. Numerous incidents of acute poisoning from pesticides have resulted from eating food that was grossly contaminated during storage or shipping. Insecticides used in homes and gardens have caused accidental poisoning in young children.

Organochlorine Insecticides. Organochlorine insecticides include chlorinated ethane derivatives, of which DDT is the best known; cyclodienes, including chlordane, aldrin, dieldrin, heptachlor, and endrin; and other hydrocarbons, including such hexachlorocyclohexanes as lindane, toxaphene, mirex, and chlordecone (KEPONE). From the mid-1940s to the mid-1960s, organochlorine insecticides were widely used in agriculture and in programs for the control of malaria.

DDT. DDT, the most common of the chlorinated ethane derivatives, is also known as *chlorophenothane.*

DDT

Prior to placement of major restrictions on its use in many countries, DDT was the best-known, least-expensive, and probably one of the most effective synthetic insecticides. It was thus widely used after its introduction in the mid-1940s.

DDT has an extremely low solubility in water and very high solubility in fat. It is readily absorbed when dissolved in oils, fats, or lipid solvents but is poorly absorbed as a dry powder or an aqueous suspension. Once absorbed, DDT concentrates in adipose tissue. Storage of DDT in the fat is protective, because it decreases the amount of the chemical at its site of toxic action—the brain. DDT crosses the placenta and its concentration in umbilical cord blood is in the same range as that in the blood of the exposed mother (Saxena *et al.,* 1981).

Since DDT is degraded very slowly in the environment and is stored in the fat of animals, it is a prime candidate for biomagnification; that is, a series of organisms in a food chain accumulate increasingly greater quantities in their fat at each higher trophic level. Ultimately, a species at the top of a food chain is adversely affected. For example, the population of fish-eating birds has declined. The decline is attributed to thinning of the eggshell, a demonstrated result of ingesting DDT and related chlorinated hydrocarbon insecticides.

Due to the ubiquity of DDT, everyone born since the mid-1940s has had a lifetime of exposure to this insecticide and storage of it in fatty tissues. At a constant rate of intake, the concentration of DDT in adipose tissue reaches a steady-state value and remains relatively constant. The concentration of DDT and its metabolites in the fat of man is about 7 ppm (National Academy of Sciences, 1977). The concentration of DDT in the blood of people living downstream from a defunct manufacturing plant was 0.076 ppm, more than five times higher than the average in the United States (Kreiss *et al.,* 1981). When exposure ceases, DDT is eliminated from the body slowly. Elimination has been estimated to be at a rate of approximately 1% of stored DDT excreted per day. Prior to excretion it is slowly dehalogenated and oxidized by cytochrome P-450–dependent monooxygenases; one of the major excretory products is DDA (*bis*[*p*-chlorophenyl] acetic acid) (Peterson and Robison, 1964; Pinto *et al.,* 1965).

DDT has a wide margin of safety and, despite its widespread use and availability, there is no documented, unequivocal report of a fatal human poisoning from DDT. The few human deaths associated with excess exposure to DDT probably resulted from the kerosene solvent rather than the insecticide. The most prominent acute effect of DDT is stimulation of the CNS. In rats, there is a good correlation between concentrations of DDT in brain and signs of toxicity (Dale *et al.,* 1963). Signs and symptoms of poisoning from high doses of DDT in man include paresthesias of the tongue, lips, and face; apprehension; hypersusceptibility to stimuli; irritability; dizziness; tremor; and tonic and clonic convulsions (Murphy, 1985). The mechanism of action of DDT on the CNS is not completely known. The compound is capable of altering the transport of sodium and potassium ions across axonal membranes, resulting in an increased negative afterpotential, prolonged action potentials, repetitive firing after a single stimulus, and spontaneous trains of action potentials. Specifically, DDT seems to inhibit the inactivation of sodium channels and the activation of potassium conductance (Narahashi, 1979, 1983).

In laboratory animals, intravenous administration of DDT causes death by ventricular fibrillation. Apparently, DDT shares with other chlorinated hydrocarbons a tendency to sensitize the myocardium, and, through its action on the CNS and adrenal medulla, it may produce the stimulus necessary for ventricular fibrillation.

Relatively low doses of DDT induce the mixed-function oxidase system of the hepatic endoplasmic reticulum. This has also been demonstrated in exterminators (Kolmodin *et al.,* 1969) and in workers in a DDT factory (Poland *et al.,* 1970). The result is altered metabolism of drugs, xenobiotics, and steroid hormones. It is probably also responsible for the increased frequency of breakage of eggs and the status of the breeding population in the peregrine falcon, sparrow hawk, and golden eagle (*e.g., see* Radcliffe, 1967). Induction of cytochrome P-450 by DDT seems to increase metabolism of estrogens in the birds. This creates an endocrine imbalance that probably affects calcium metabolism, egg laying, and nesting in such a way that total reproductive success and survival of the young may be reduced. To compound the problem, DDT also exerts an estrogenic effect (Kupfer and Bulger, 1982) and inhibits a Ca^{2+}-ATPase that is necessary for the calcification of egg shells (Miller and Kinter, 1976).

Human volunteers have consumed 35 mg of DDT daily, about 1000 times higher than the average human intake, for as long as 25 months without obvious ill effects (Hayes, 1963). However, there is concern that DDT might be carcinogenic following exposure to small amounts of the chemical over a long period. Extensive use of DDT in industrial countries has not been associated with increased hepatic cancer in man. Innes and associates (1969) reported a statistically significant increase in hepatomas in two strains of mice exposed to DDT, and this finding has been confirmed by additional studies sponsored by the International Agency of Research in Cancer (IARC, 1974a). Interpretation of such data is, however, extremely difficult. The long-term effects of pesticides on health is certainly a concern. In a recent survey of the mortality of 3827 licensed pest-control workers, no significant elevation in their standardized mortality ratio was found, but excess deaths were observed from leukemia, particularly myeloid leukemia, and from cancers of the brain and lungs (Blair *et al.,* 1983).

DDT was banned in the United States in 1972 for all but essential public health use and for a few minor uses to protect crops for which there were no effective alternatives. The decision was prompted by the prospect of ecological imbalance from continued use of DDT, the uncertainty of the effect, if any, of continued prolonged exposure and storage of low concentrations of DDT in man, and the development of resistant strains of insects. Several other countries have taken similar actions. As a result, other pesticides have replaced DDT, but many of them are more toxic to man.

Methoxychlor. The structural formula of methoxychlor, a chlorinated ethane derivative, is as follows:

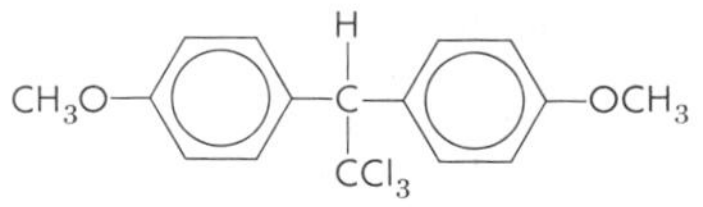

Methoxychlor

The compound is used increasingly as a replacement for DDT. The attractiveness of methoxychlor is that it is much less toxic to mammals than DDT (LD50 in rats is 6000 mg/kg compared to 250 mg/kg for DDT) and does not persist in the body for as long. Methoxychlor is stored in adipose tissue to about 0.2% of the extent of DDT, and its half-life in rats is only about 2 weeks, compared to 6 months for DDT (Murphy, 1985). The shorter half-life is a reflection of more rapid metabolism by O-demethylation (Kapoor *et al.*, 1970); it is then conjugated and excreted in the urine.

Chlorinated Cyclodienes. Structures of the more common chlorinated cyclodienes are shown in Table 70–2. These compounds stimulate the CNS, and many signs and symptoms of poisoning

Table 70–2. CHEMICAL STRUCTURES OF SOME CHLORINATED CYCLODIENES

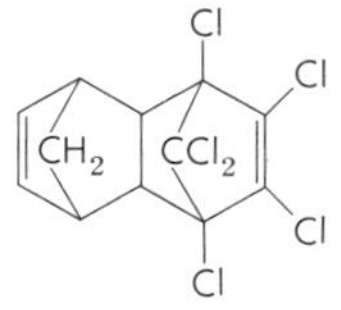

Aldrin

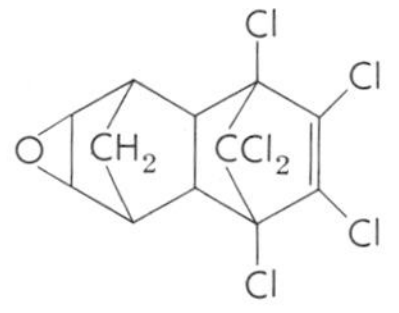

Dieldrin *

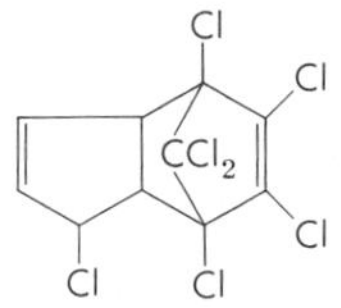

Heptachlor

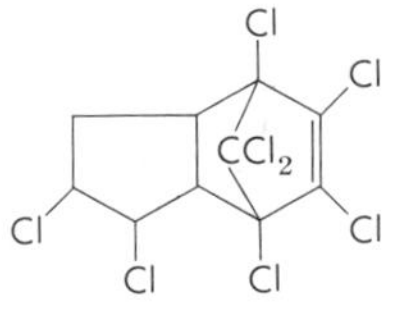

Chlordane

* Endrin is a stereoisomer of dieldrin.

thus resemble those of DDT. Unlike DDT, however, these compounds tend to produce convulsions before other, less serious signs of illness have appeared. Persons poisoned by cyclodiene insecticides have reported headache and nausea, vomiting, dizziness, and mild clonic jerking, but some patients have convulsions without warning symptoms (Hayes, 1963). Electroencephalographic abnormalities are seen in patients without clinical illness, both before and after convulsions. Unlike DDT, cyclodiene insecticides have caused numerous fatalities as a result of acute poisoning.

An important difference between DDT and the chlorinated cyclodienes is that the latter are readily absorbed from intact skin. Cyclodienes may not pose an appreciably greater risk than DDT to the general population exposed to small quantities in food, but manipulation of concentrated solutions of a cyclodiene is more hazardous.

Like DDT, chlorinated cyclodiene insecticides are highly soluble in lipid and are stored in adipose tissue; they induce the mixed-function oxidase system of the liver, are degraded slowly, persist in the environment, and undergo biomagnification through the food chain of animals. This class of insecticides has produced dose-related hepatomas in mice and has the greatest carcinogenic potential among the insecticides (National Academy of Sciences, 1977). For these reasons aldrin and dieldrin were banned in the United States in 1974, and the use of chlordane and heptachlor for agricultural crops was suspended in 1976.

Other Chlorinated Hydrocarbons. This group of insecticides includes lindane, toxaphene, mirex, and chlordecone. These chemicals share many properties with DDT. While they do not modify axonal conduction, they do act on presynaptic nerve terminals in the CNS and enhance the release of neurotransmitters (Shankland, 1982).

Benzene Hexachloride (BHC) and Lindane. Benzene hexachloride (more properly called hexachlorocyclohexane) has the following structural formula:

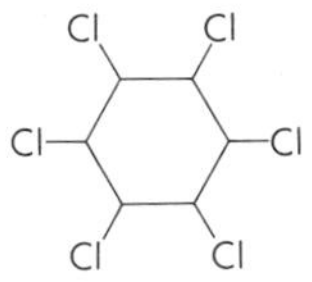

Benzene Hexachloride

It is a mixture of eight isomers, and the γ isomer is referred to as *lindane*. The γ isomer is the most toxic, and virtually all insecticidal activity of BHC resides in lindane. The compound is used clinically as an ectoparasiticide (*see* Chapter 41). Lindane causes signs of poisoning that resemble those produced by DDT: tremors, ataxia, convulsions, and prostration. Violent tonic and clonic convulsions occur in severe cases of acute poisoning. The α and γ isomers are CNS stimulants, but the β and δ isomers are depressants. Lindane induces hepatic microsomal enzymes. Lindane and BHC have been implicated in numerous cases of aplastic anemia (West, 1967); however, a study of 60 cases of aplastic anemia failed to demonstrate an association between the incidence of aplastic anemia and occupational exposure to pesticides (Wang and Grufferman, 1981). A number of the isomers of BHC, including lindane, have been shown to produce hepatomas in rodents (Cueto, 1980).

Biotransformation of the isomers of BHC involves the formation of chlorophenols. Compared to DDT, lindane has a relatively low persistence in the environment.

Toxaphene. For several years this insecticide was ranked first in quantity used in the United States. Toxaphene is a complex mixture of more than 175 C_{10} polychlorinated hydrocarbons, of which only a few are known (*e.g.*, heptachlorobornane) (Turner *et al.*, 1977). Like the other chlorinated hydrocarbon insecticides, the major toxicity of toxaphene is stimulation of the CNS. Toxaphene seems to be metabolized quite readily, and this probably accounts for the low persistence of this preparation in comparison to other chlorinated hydrocarbon insecticides. Toxaphene has been shown to induce hepatic tumors in mice and to produce mutations (Hooper *et al.*, 1979). These observations have resulted in a dramatic reduction in the use of toxaphene.

Mirex and Chlordecone. Mirex and chlordecone (KEPONE) are extremely persistent chlorinated hydrocarbon insecticides, and they are concentrated several thousandfold in the food chain (Waters *et al.*, 1977). Their structural formulas are as follows:

Mirex

Chlordecone

Similar to the other chlorinated hydrocarbon insecticides, mirex and chlordecone produce stimulation of the CNS, hepatic injury, and induction of the cytochrome P-450 system. Inhibition of mitochondrial and synaptosomal ATPases has been suggested to be the basis of neurotoxicity (Desaiah, 1981) and hepatobiliary dysfunction (Mehendale,

1979). Testicular atrophy and reduced sperm production may be due to a direct estrogenic action of chlordecone (Eroschenko, 1981). Mirex and chlordecone are carcinogenic in laboratory animals (Cueto *et al.*, 1976; Waters *et al.*, 1977).

Gross negligence in industrial hygiene resulted in poisoning of 76 of 148 exposed workers engaged in the manufacture of chlordecone in Hopewell, Virginia (Taylor *et al.*, 1978). These workers suffered neurological effects, characterized by tremors, ocular flutter (opsoclonus), hepatomegaly, splenomegaly, rashes, mental changes, and widened gaits. Laboratory tests showed reduced sperm counts and reduced motility of sperm. Contamination of the area surrounding the manufacturing plant resulted in curtailment of fishing and the procurement of shellfish in the James River and threatened portions of the Chesapeake Bay.

Mirex is probably oxidized to chlordecone (Carlson *et al.*, 1976). The main metabolite of chlordecone is chlordecone alcohol, which appears in human bile as glucuronic acid conjugates (Guzelian, 1982). The major route of elimination of chlordecone is in the stool. Cholestyramine (*see* Chapter 34) administered to poisoned patients increases the fecal excretion of chlordecone 3- to 18-fold, shortens its half-life in blood from 140 to 80 days, and enhances the rate of recovery from toxic manifestations (Cohn *et al.*, 1978). Fecal chlordecone originates from both biliary and intestinal excretion (Guzelian, 1982). In man, only 5 to 10% of the chlordecone excreted into bile appears in the stool, which indicates extensive intestinal reabsorption of the chemical (Cohn *et al.*, 1978); bile appears to enhance such reabsorption greatly (Boylan *et al.*, 1979). Thus, cholestyramine may enhance intestinal excretion of chlordecone by binding constituents of bile in the intestinal lumen. Chlordecone has been detected in the milk of women, cows, and rats (Guzelian, 1982). Milk from contaminated cows can be a source of human exposure.

Organophosphorus Insecticides. Organophosphorus insecticides have largely replaced the chlorinated hydrocarbons. The organophosphates do not persist in the environment and have an extremely low carcinogenic potential; however, they have a much higher acute toxicity in man. In fact, parathion is the pesticide most frequently involved in fatal poisoning. The pharmacology and toxicology of these agents are discussed in Chapter 6.

Carbamate Insecticides. The carbamate insecticides resemble the organophosphates in many ways. The most common of these agents is carbaril; since carbaril and related compounds are inhibitors of cholinesterase, they too are discussed in Chapter 6.

Botanical Insecticides. *Pyrethrums* are obtained from flowers of the pyrethrum plant, *Chrysanthemum cincerariaefolium*. The insecticidal activity and toxicity of this group of chemicals reside in a number of structurally similar compounds, and the greatest insecticidal activity resides in *pyrethrin I*. Its structural formula is as follows:

Pyrethrin I

Pyrethrum and synthetic pyrethrin derivatives (pyrethroids) are used in many household insecticides because of their rapid action. Their mechanism of action on neuronal membranes resembles that of DDT (Narahashi, 1983). Pyrethrum is generally rated as the safest insecticide because its primary toxicity is low. The low toxicity of pyrethroids in mammals is due largely to their rapid biotransformation by ester hydrolysis and/or hydroxylation (Aldridge, 1983). The slow biotransformation of pyrethrum in insects is further decreased by its formulation with piperonyl butoxide (which inhibits cytochrome P-450) and thus increases insecticidal efficacy. Unlike mammals, aquatic organisms are extremely sensitive to pyrethroids (Khan, 1983).

The allergenic properties of pyrethrins are marked in comparison with other pesticides. Many cases of contact dermatitis and respiratory allergy have been reported. Persons sensitive to ragweed pollen are particularly prone to such reactions. Preparations containing synthetic pyrethroids are less likely to cause allergic reactions than are the preparations made from pyrethrum powder.

Rotenone is obtained from the roots of plants such as *Derris* and *Lonchocarpus*. It was first used to paralyze fish before being used as an insecticide. Rotenone has the following structural formula:

Rotenone

Human poisoning by rotenone is rare. The compound has been applied directly to treat head lice, scabies, and other ectoparasites. Local effects include conjunctivitis, dermatitis, pharyngitis, and rhinitis. Oral ingestion of rotenone produces gastrointestinal irritation, nausea, and vomiting. Inhalation of the dust is more hazardous; it can cause respiratory stimulation followed by depression and convulsions. Rotenone inhibits the oxidation of NADH to NAD. Consequently, it blocks the oxidation by NAD of substrates such as glutamate, α-ketoglutarate, and pyruvate.

Nicotine is one of the most toxic insecticides (*see* Chapter 10). Poisoning is followed by salivation and vomiting (from ganglionic stimulation), muscular weakness (from stimulation followed by depression at the neuromuscular junction), and, ultimately, clonic convulsions and cessation of respiration (effects on the CNS).

FUMIGANTS

Fumigants are used to control insects, rodents, and soil nematodes. They exert pesticidal action in gaseous form and are used because they will penetrate otherwise-inaccessible areas. Agents used to protect stored foodstuffs include hydrogen cyanide, acrylonitrile (an organic cyanide, $CH_2{=}CHCN$), carbon disulfide, carbon tetrachloride, chloropicrin, ethylene dibromide, ethylene oxide, methyl bromide, and phosphine.

Cyanide. Cyanide (*hydrocyanic acid, prussic acid*) is one of the most rapidly acting poisons. Victims may die within minutes of exposure. Hydrogen cyanide gas is used to fumigate ships and buildings and to sterilize soil. Because of its ability to form complexes with metals, cyanide is used in metallurgy, electroplating, and metal cleaning. In the home, cyanides are present in silver polish, insecticides, rodenticides, and fruit seeds. The major toxicity of *laetrile* is due to its cyanogenic glycoside. Cytochrome P-450–dependent monooxygenases liberate cyanide from organic nitriles (Willhite and Smith, 1981), as do glutathione S-transferases from organic thiocyanates (Ohkawa and Casida, 1971); cyanide is also a metabolite of nitroprusside (Cottrell *et al.*, 1978). Combustion of nitrogen-containing plastics may result in release of HCN. Fire on board airplanes killed 119 passengers in Paris in 1973 and 303 pilgrims in Riyadh, Saudi Arabia in 1980 due to combustion of plastic material that produced HCN (Weger, 1983). Cyanide is also used for executions in so-called gas chambers and was used for more than 900 religious "suicide-murders" in Guyana in 1978.

Cyanide has a very high affinity for iron in the ferric state. When absorbed, it reacts readily with the trivalent iron of cytochrome oxidase in mitochondria; cellular respiration is thus inhibited and cytotoxic hypoxia results. Since utilization of oxygen is blocked, venous blood is oxygenated and is almost as bright red as arterial blood. Respiration is stimulated because chemoreceptive cells respond as they do to decreased oxygen. A transient stage of CNS stimulation with hyperpnea and headache is observed; finally there are hypoxic convulsions and death due to respiratory arrest.

Treatment of cyanide poisoning must be rapid to be effective. Diagnosis may be aided by the characteristic odor of cyanide (oil of bitter almonds). Since toxicity results from binding to the ferric form of cytochrome oxidase, treatment is aimed at prevention or reversal of such binding by providing a large pool of ferric iron to compete for cyanide. An effective mechanism is to administer substances, such as nitrite, that oxidize hemoglobin to methemoglobin. Amyl nitrite is usually administered by inhalation, while a solution of sodium nitrite is prepared for intravenous administration (10 ml of a 3% solution). Methemoglobin competes with cytochrome oxidase for the cyanide ion; the reaction favors methemoglobin because of mass action. Cyanmethemoglobin is formed, and cytochrome oxidase is restored. Alternatively, 4-dimethylaminophenol, which also oxidizes hemoglobin to methemoglobin, can be used in a dose of 3 mg/kg intravenously or intramuscularly (Weger, 1983). Cobalt and carbonyl compounds such as pyruvate also bind cyanide (Way, 1983), and Co_2EDTA has been used successfully in human therapy of cyanide poisoning (Cottrell et al., 1978; Weger, 1983).

The major mechanism for removing cyanide from the body is its enzymatic conversion, by the mitochondrial enzyme rhodanese (transsulfurase), to thiocyanate, which is relatively nontoxic. To accelerate detoxication, thiosulfate is administered intravenously (50 ml of a 25% aqueous solution), and the thiocyanate formed is readily excreted in the urine.

$$Na_2S_2O_3 + CN^- \xrightarrow{\text{Rhodanese}} SCN^- + Na_2SO_3$$

Way and associates (1972) demonstrated that nitrite increases the LD50 of potassium cyanide in mice from 11 mg/kg to 21 mg/kg; administration of thiosulfate increases the value to 35 mg/kg, while with nitrite followed by thiosulfate the LD50 is 52 mg/kg. Chen and Rose (1956) reported that 48 of 49 cases of acute poisoning by cyanide in man were treated successfully with such therapy.

Oxygen alone, even at hyperbaric pressures, has only a slight protective effect in cyanide poisoning; however, it dramatically potentiates the protective effects of thiosulfate or of nitrite and thiosulfate (Sheehy and Way, 1968; Way et al., 1972). The mechanism for this action is not clear, but the intracellular oxygen tension may be high enough to cause nonenzymatic oxidation of reduced cytochromes or oxygen may displace cyanide from cytochrome oxidase by mass action.

If cyanide has been ingested, gastric lavage should follow, not precede, initiation of more specific treatment.

Methyl Bromide. Methyl bromide is used as an insecticidal fumigant and in some fire extinguishers. It is said to have been responsible for more deaths in California in the 1960s among occupationally exposed persons than all the organophosphate insecticides (Hine, 1969). Because methyl bromide is so toxic, chloropicrin (CCl_3NO_2), a powerful stimulator of lacrimation, is added as a warning.

Major signs and symptoms of intoxication with methyl bromide are referable to the CNS. These include malaise, headache, visual disturbances, nausea, and vomiting. Death usually occurs during a convulsion. After severe respiratory exposure, pulmonary edema may prove fatal. The high affinity of methyl bromide for sulfhydryl groups may play a role in its toxic action. Sulfhydryl agents may thus be beneficial as antidotes in poisoning with methyl bromide.

Dibromochloropropane and Ethylene Dibromide. Dibromochloropropane ($ClCH_2CHBrCH_2Br$) and ethylene dibromide (1,2-dibromoethane) are soil fumigants used to control nematodes. In man, they produce moderate depression of the CNS and pulmonary congestion after exposure by inhalation, and they cause acute gastrointestinal distress and pulmonary edema after ingestion. Both agents cause gastric carcinoma in rats and mice (Powers et al., 1975; IARC, 1977). Dibromochloropropane causes sterility and/or abnormally low sperm counts in workmen engaged in its manufacture. Use of both agents is being decreased because of their carcinogenicity and their adverse effects on reproductive function.

Phosphine. Phosphine (PH_3) is a fumigant for grain; it is released gradually, in the presence of atmospheric moisture, from tablets of aluminum phosphide. Phosphine is more toxic than methyl bromide; however, since less is required to fumigate a given volume of grain, it has proven to be safer.

RODENTICIDES

Some rodenticides are quite toxic to man, but the toxicity of others is more selective. In some cases, selectivity is based on a unique aspect of the physiology of rodents; in others, advantage is taken of the habits of these animals. Since rodenticides can be used in baits and placed in inaccessible places, the likelihood of their contaminating the environment is much less than that of insecticides. The toxicological problem posed by rodenticides, therefore, is primarily one of acute accidental or suicidal ingestion.

Warfarin. Warfarin, one of the most frequently used rodenticides, is considered safe because its toxicity depends on repeated ingestion. However, daily intake by man of 1 to 2 mg/kg for 6 days has produced severe illness in an attempted suicide. Warfarin, an oral anticoagulant, is discussed in Chapter 58.

Red Squill. The bulbs of red squill (*Urginea maritima*) have been used for many years as a relatively safe rodenticide. The active principles are scillaren glycosides. These glycosides, like the digitalis glycosides, have cardiotonic actions (*see* Chapter 30). Signs and symptoms associated with ingestion of large doses of red squill include vomiting and abdominal pain, blurred vision, cardiac irregularities, convulsions, and death from ventricular fibrillation. The selective rodenticidal usefulness of squill is due to the inability of rats to vomit (Lisella et al., 1971). Treatment of ingestion in man, if indicated, is the same as for overdosage of digitalis (*see* Chapter 30).

Sodium Fluoroacetate. Sodium fluoroacetate and fluoroacetamide are among the most potent rodenticides. Because they are also highly toxic to other animals, their use is restricted to licensed pest-control operators. Fluoroacetate produces its toxic action by inhibiting the citric acid cycle. The compound is incorporated into fluoroacetyl coenzyme A, which condenses with oxaloacetate to form fluorocitrate. Fluorocitrate inhibits the enzyme aconitase and thereby inhibits conversion of citrate to isocitrate. As might be expected, the heart and CNS are the tissues most critically involved by a general inhibition of oxidative energy metabolism. Thus, the signs and symptoms of fluoroacetate poisoning, in addition to nonspecific signs of nausea and vomiting, include cardiac irregularities, cyanosis, generalized convulsions, and death from ventricular fibrillation or respiratory failure (Brockmann et al., 1955). Provision of large quantities of acetate appears to antagonize fluoroacetate in a competitive manner; monkeys have been successfully protected from fluoroacetate poisoning by the administration of glycerol monoacetate.

Phosphorus. White or yellow elemental phosphorus has poisoned man when it was spread in paste on bread to bait rodents. Shortly after ingestion, phosphorus produces severe gastrointestinal irritation, and, if the dose is sufficient, hemorrhage and cardiovascular failure may prove fatal within 24 hours. The vomitus is luminescent and has a characteristic garlic odor. If the patient survives the initial phase of gastrointestinal injury, secondary systemic poisoning and hepatic necrosis may ensue. Severe acute yellow atrophy of the liver is a delayed sequela that may prove fatal.

Chronic poisoning from phosphorus is characterized by cachexia, anemia, bronchitis, and necrosis of the mandible, the so-called phossy jaw.

Zinc Phosphide. Zinc phosphide reacts with water and HCl in the gastrointestinal tract to produce the gas phosphine (PH_3), which causes severe gastrointestinal irritation. Apparent insensitivity of dogs and cats has been attributed to the emetic qualities of zinc in animals other than rodents. Later phases of toxicity resemble poisoning by yellow elemental phosphorus.

α-Naphthylthiourea. The structural formula of α-naphthylthiourea is as follows:

α-Naphthylthiourea

Its selective rodenticidal properties are due to different susceptibilities of various species. The LD50 in rats is about 3 mg/kg, in dogs 10 mg/kg, in guinea pigs 400 mg/kg, and in monkeys 4 g/kg. The principal toxic effect in susceptible species is massive pulmonary edema and pleural effusion, apparently the result of an action on pulmonary capillaries. Microsomes from rat liver and lung release atomic sulfur from α-naphthylthiourea (Lee et al., 1980). Pulmonary toxicity may result, at least in part, from binding of atomic sulfur to tissue macromolecules. Sulfhydryl blocking agents are effective antidotes for rats in some experimental conditions (Koch and Schwarze, 1956).

Thallium. Thallium sulfate is very hazardous. Since it is not selectively toxic for rodents and many people have been poisoned by thallium, its use is now strictly regulated in many countries. Acute poisoning is accompanied by gastrointestinal irritation, motor paralysis, and death from respiratory failure. Sublethal doses, taken over a period of time, redden the skin and cause alopecia, characteristic signs of thallium poisoning. Pathological changes include perivascular cuffing and degenerative changes in the brain, liver, and kidney. Neurological symptoms are prominent and include tremors, leg pains, paresthesias of hands and feet, and polyneuritis, especially in the legs. Psychoses, delirium, convulsions, and other types of encephalopathy may also be noted. Treatment of thallium intoxication involves the oral administration of ferric ferrocyanide (Prussian blue), hemodialysis, and forced diuresis. Prussian blue binds thallium in the intestine and prevents its absorption. Administration of systemic chelating agents should be avoided, because they may increase uptake of thallium into the brain (Hayes, 1982).

HERBICIDES

The production and use of chemicals for destruction of noxious weeds have increased markedly in the last decade. Herbicides now exceed insecticides in quantities used and values of sales. Although some herbicidal compounds have very low toxicity in mammals, others are highly toxic and have caused human fatalities.

Chlorophenoxy Compounds. The compounds *2,4-dichlorophenoxyacetic acid* (2,4-D) and *2,4,5-trichlorophenoxyacetic acid* (2,4,5-T), as their salts and esters, are probably the most familiar herbicides. Their structural formulas are as follows:

2,4-D   2,4,5-T

They are used to control broad-leaf weeds in fields and to control woody plants along highways and rights-of-way; the compounds act as growth hormones in plants. Animals killed by massive doses of 2,4-D are believed to die of ventricular fibrillation. At lower doses, when death is delayed, there are various signs of neuromuscular involvement, including stiffness of the extremities, ataxia, paralysis, and, eventually, coma. Clinical reports of poisoning from chlorophenoxy herbicides are rare.

These herbicides do not accumulate in animals. They are not extensively metabolized but are actively excreted into the urine (Berndt and Koschier, 1973). Their plasma half-life in man is about 1 day (Gehring *et al.*, 1973).

Chlorophenoxy herbicides have produced contact dermatitis in man, and a rather severe type of dermatitis, chloracne, has been observed in workers involved in the manufacture of 2,4,5-T (Poland *et al.*, 1971). The dermatitis seems due primarily to the action of a contaminant, 2,3,7,8-tetrachlorodibenzo-*p*-dioxin (TCDD), the structure of which is as follows:

TCDD

TCDD is considered to be the most toxic chemical manufactured. It has an LD50 of 0.6 $\mu g/kg$ in guinea pigs. The mechanism of death is not known, but morphological changes in the liver, thymus, and reproductive organs are observed. TCDD shows no toxic effect on cell cultures. Thyroid hormones appear to play a role in TCDD toxicity, since thyroidectomy protects against TCDD-induced lethality in rats (Rozman *et al.*, 1984). TCDD is a potent inducer of aryl hydrocarbon hydroxylase, a microsomal cytochrome P-450–dependent monooxygenase (Poland and Glover, 1974). It is also a very potent teratogen (Neubert *et al.*, 1973) and has been demonstrated to be a carcinogen (Van Miller *et al.*, 1977; Kociba *et al.*, 1978). Hence, there is considerable concern about the contamination of 2,4,5-T with TCDD, and its content is regulated at 0.1 ppm or less in the herbicide.

Accidental human exposures indicate that TCDD has low toxicity for man as compared to that for certain species (*e.g.*, guinea pig) (Holmstedt, 1980). Effects of TCDD poisoning in exposed persons include chloracne, porphyria, hypercholesterolemia, and psychiatric disturbances (Hayes, 1982). Epidemiological studies to support or refute the teratogenicity and carcinogenicity of TCDD in man are still fragmentary and inconclusive.

Dinitrophenols. Several substituted dinitrophenols, alone or as salts of aliphatic amines or alkalies, are used in weed control. Human poisonings by dinitroorthocresol (DNOC) have been reported. The acute toxicity of dinitrophenols is due to the uncoupling of oxidative phosphorylation. The metabolic rate of the poisoned individual can increase markedly, and the body temperature is elevated. Signs and symptoms of acute poisoning in man include nausea, restlessness, flushed skin, sweating, rapid respiration, tachycardia, fever, cyanosis, and, finally, collapse and coma. The illness runs a rapid course; there is death or recovery within 24 to 48 hours. If production of heat exceeds the capacity for its dissipation, fatal hyperthermia

may result. Specific treatment consists in ice baths to reduce fever; oxygen is administered, and fluid and electrolyte imbalances should be corrected.

Bipyridyl Compounds. Paraquat is the most important compound in this class of herbicides from a toxicological viewpoint. The structural formula of paraquat is as follows:

Paraquat

Several hundred cases of accidental or suicidal fatalities from paraquat poisoning have been reported during the last decade. Pathological changes observed at autopsy are indicative of damage to the lungs, liver, and kidneys; myocarditis is sometimes present. The most striking pathological change is a widespread proliferation of fibroblastic cells in the lungs, an effect that is not dependent on the route of administration. Although ingestion of paraquat causes gastrointestinal upset within a few hours, the onset of respiratory symptoms and eventual death by respiratory distress may be delayed for several days.

A biochemical mechanism for paraquat-induced pulmonary injury has been proposed (Bus *et al.*, 1976). Paraquat is believed to undergo a single-electron, cyclic reduction-oxidation, with subsequent formation of superoxide anion radical (O_2^-). Superoxide anion radical is nonenzymatically transformed to singlet oxygen, which attacks polyunsaturated lipids associated with cell membranes to form lipid hydroperoxides. The lipid hydroperoxides are unstable in the presence of trace amounts of transition metal ions and decompose to lipid-free radicals. The chain reaction of lipid peroxidation thus initiated is somewhat similar to that described above for CCl_4.

Due to the serious, delayed pulmonary toxicity produced by paraquat, prompt treatment is important. This involves removal of paraquat from the alimentary tract by gastric lavage and the use of cathartics, prevention of further absorption by oral administration of Fuller's earth, and removal of absorbed paraquat by hemodialysis or hemoperfusion (Cavalli and Fletcher, 1977; Davies *et al.*, 1977).

A recent survey found that 21% of marihuana samples from the Southwestern United States and 3.6% of the samples collected from the entire country were contaminated with paraquat. The source of contamination was an aerial spraying program in Mexico. It is projected that marihuana smokers in the southern region of the United States could be exposed to 0.5 mg or more of paraquat per year by inhalation. However, no clinical case of paraquat poisoning has been recognized among marihuana smokers, although no systematic search for such cases has been undertaken (Landrigan *et al.*, 1983).

Other Herbicides. There are a large number of other herbicides that, for the most part, have relatively low acute toxicities for mammals. These include carbamates (*e.g., propham* and *barban*), substituted ureas (*e.g., monuron* and *diuron*), triazines (*e.g., atrazine* and the related compound *aminotriazole*), aniline derivatives (*e.g., alachlor, propachlor*, and *propanil*), dinitroaniline derivatives (*e.g., triflualin*), and benzoic acid derivatives (*e.g., amiben*).

FUNGICIDES

Fungicides, like other classes of pesticides, comprise a heterogeneous group of chemical compounds. With few exceptions, the fungicides have not been the subject of detailed toxicological research. Although many compounds used to control fungal diseases on plants, seeds, and produce are rather nontoxic acutely, there are some notable exceptions; the mercury-containing fungicides have caused the greatest concern. They have been responsible for many deaths or permanent neurological disabilities resulting from the misdirection of treated seed grains into human and animal food. The toxicities of mercury and its compounds are discussed in Chapter 69.

Dithiocarbamates. Fungicides of this group are commonly used in agriculture. They have a low order of acute toxicity, and values of the oral LD50 in rats range from several hundred milligrams to several grams per kilogram. Except for contact dermatitis induced by dithiocarbamate (Fisher, 1983), there is little evidence of human injury from exposure to these compounds. However, they may have some teratogenic and/or carcinogenic potential (World Health Organization, 1975). Two groups of dithiocarbamates that have been used, the dimethyldithiocarbamates and the ethylenebisdithiocarbamates, have the following general formulas:

Dimethyldithiocarbamates

Ethylenebisdithiocarbamates

The names of the fungicides are derived from the metallic cations. For example, when the cation is zinc or iron, the respective dimethyldithiocarbamate is *ziram* or *ferbam*. With manganese, zinc, or sodium as the cation in the diethyldithiocarbamate series, the respective fungicide is *maneb*, *zineb*, or *nabam*. Some dimethyldithiocarbamates are reported to be teratogenic in animals, and they can form nitrosamines *in vitro* and *in vivo* (IARC, 1974b; World Health Organization, 1975). The ethylenebisdithiocarbamates are also reported to be teratogenic. Furthermore, this group of com-

pounds breaks down to form ethylenethiourea (ETU) *in vivo,* in the environment, and during cooking of foods containing their residues. ETU is carcinogenic, mutagenic, and teratogenic, as well as an antithyroid agent (IARC, 1974b, 1976). Dithiocarbamate fungicides are analogs of disulfiram, and they can produce a disulfiram-like response when ethanol is ingested (*see* Chapter 18).

Hexachlorobenzene. Exposure to hexachlorobenzene results in an increase in hepatic weight, in the quantity of smooth endoplasmic reticulum, and in the activities of cytochrome P-450–dependent monooxygenases (Carlson and Tardiff, 1976). Between 1955 and 1959, more than 300 human poisonings occurred in Turkey as a result of the use of hexachlorobenzene-treated wheat (Schmid, 1960). Some deaths resulted; the major syndrome was cutaneous porphyria with skin lesions, porphyrinuria, and photosensitization. Hexachlorobenzene is eliminated from the body predominantly in the feces as a result of intestinal excretion. This process can be enhanced fivefold in rhesus monkeys by the oral administration of mineral oil (Rozman *et al.*, 1983).

Pentachlorophenol. Pentachlorophenol is used as an insecticide and a herbicide, as well as a fungicide, with major application as a wood preservative. Several cases of human poisoning have been associated with its use. The acute toxic action of pentachlorophenol in man and experimental animals resembles that of the nitrophenolic herbicides—a marked increase in metabolic rate as the result of uncoupling of oxidative phosphorylation. Pentachlorophenol is readily absorbed through the skin. Two cases of fatal poisonings and several nonfatal cases occurred in a hospital nursery; pentachlorophenol had been used as a fungicide in the laundry room and ultimately came in contact with infants through their diapers (Armstrong *et al.*, 1969).

In recent years it has become apparent that many commercial samples of pentachlorophenol are contaminated with polychlorinated dibenzodioxins and dibenzofurans (Buser, 1975). These contaminants are generally less toxic than the tetrachlorodioxin contaminant (TCDD) in 2,4,5-T. Although pentachlorophenol is highly toxic in its own right, some studies suggest that the contaminants may be responsible for some of the untoward effects of the technical-grade product (Johnson *et al.*, 1973; Goldstein *et al.*, 1976). Treatment of intoxication with pentachlorophenol is similar to that for poisoning with dinitrophenols. Fecal excretion of pentachlorophenol can be enhanced by cholestyramine, which interrupts the enterohepatic circulation of the chemical (Rozman *et al.*, 1982).

Aksoy, M.; Erdem, S.; and Dincol, G. Leukemia in shoe-workers exposed to chronic benzene. *Blood,* **1974,** *44,* 837–841.

Amdur, M. O., and Corn, M. The irritant potency of zinc ammonium sulfate of different particle sizes. *Am. Ind. Hyg. Assoc. J.,* **1963,** *24,* 326–333.

Amdur, M. O.; Dubriel, M.; and Creasia, D. A. Respiratory response of guinea pigs to low levels of sulfuric acid. *Environ. Res.*, **1978**, *15*, 418–423.

Armstrong, R. W.; Eichner, E. R.; Klein, D. E.; Barthel, W. F.; Bennett, J. V.; Jonsson, V.; Bruce, H.; and Loveless, L. E.   Pentachlorophenol poisoning in a nursery for newborn infants. II. Epidemiological and toxicologic studies. *J. Pediatr.*, **1969**, *75*, 317–325.

Ayres, S. M.; Giammelli, S., Jr.; and Mueller, H.   Effects of low concentrations of carbon monoxide. Part IV. Myocardial and systemic responses to carboxyhemoglobin. *Ann. N.Y. Acad. Sci.*, **1970**, *174*, 268–293.

Berndt, W. O., and Koschier, F.   *In vitro* uptake of 2,4-dichlorophenoxyacetic acid (2,4,-D) and 2,4,5-trichlorophenoxyacetic acid (2,4,5-T) by renal cortical tissue of rabbits and rats. *Toxicol. Appl. Pharmacol.*, **1973**, *26*, 1114–1117.

Blair, A.; Grauman, D. J.; Lubin, J. H.; and Fraumeni, J. F.   Lung cancer and other causes of death among licensed pesticide applicators. *J. Natl Cancer Inst.*, **1983**, *71*, 31–37.

Boatman, E. S.; Sato, S.; and Frank, R.   Acute effects of ozone on cat lungs. II. Structural. *Am. Rev. Respir. Dis.*, **1974**, *110*, 157–169.

Bokonjić, N.   Stagnant anoxia and carbon monoxide poisoning. *Electroencephalogr. Clin. Neurophysiol.*, **1963**, Suppl. 21, 1–102.

Boylan, J. J.; Cohn, W. J.; Egle, J. L.; Blanke, R. V.; and Guzelian, P. S.   Excretion of chlordecone by the gastrointestinal tract: evidence for a nonbiliary mechanism. *Clin. Pharmacol. Ther.*, **1979**, *25*, 579–585.

Brockmann, J. L.; McDowell, A. V.; and Leeds, W. G.   Fatal poisoning with sodium fluoroacetate. *J.A.M.A.*, **1955**, *159*, 1529–1532.

Brucher, J. M.   Neuropathological problems posed by carbon monoxide poisoning and anoxia. *Prog. Brain Res.*, **1967**, *24*, 75–100.

Bus, J. S.; Cagen, S. Z.; Olgaard, M.; and Gibson, J. E.   A mechanism of paraquat toxicity in mice and rats. *Toxicol. Appl. Pharmacol.*, **1976**, *35*, 501–513.

Buser, H. R.   Analysis of polychlorinated dibenzo-*p*-dioxins and dibenzofurans in chlorinated phenols by mass fragmentography. *J. Chromatogr.*, **1975**, *107*, 295–310.

Carlson, D. A.; Konyhu, K. D.; Wheeler, W. B.; Marshall, G. P.; and Zaylskie, R. G.   Mirex in the environment: its degradation to KEPONE and related compounds. *Science*, **1976**, *94*, 939–941.

Carlson, G. P., and Tardiff, R. G.   Effect of chlorinated benzenes on the metabolism of foreign organic compounds. *Toxicol. Appl. Pharmacol.*, **1976**, *36*, 383–394.

Cavalli, R. D., and Fletcher, K.   An effective treatment for paraquat poisoning. In, *Biochemical Mechanism of Paraquat Toxicity.* (Autor, A. P., ed.) Academic Press, Inc., New York, **1977**, pp. 213–228.

Chen, K. K., and Rose, C. L.   Treatment of acute cyanide poisoning. *J.A.M.A.*, **1956**, *162*, 1154–1156.

Coffin, D. L., and Blommer, E. J.   Acute toxicity of irradiated auto exhaust. Its indication by enhancement of mortality from streptococcal pneumonia. *Arch. Environ. Health*, **1967**, *15*, 36–38.

Coffin, D. L.; Gardiner, D. E.; and Blommer, E. J.   Time-dose response for nitrogen dioxide exposure in an infectivity model system. *Environ. Health Perspect.*, **1976**, *13*, 11–15.

Cohn, W. J.; Boylan, J. J.; Blanke, R. V.; Furiss, M. W.; Howell, J. R.; and Guzelian, P. S.   Treatment of chlordecone (KEPONE) toxicity with cholestyramine. *N. Engl. J. Med.*, **1978**, *298*, 243–248.

Cottrell, J. E.; Casthely, P.; Brodie, J. B.; Pathel, K.; Klein, A.; and Turndorf, H.   Cyanide toxicity with nitroprusside infusions. *N. Engl. J. Med.*, **1978**, *298*, 809–811.

Cueto, C.   Consideration of the possible carcinogenicity of some pesticides. *J. Environ. Sci. Health* [B], **1980**, *15*, 949–975.

Cueto, C.; Page, N.; and Saffiott, V.   *Report of Carcinogenesis, Bioassay of Technical Grade Chlordecone* (KEPONE). National Cancer Institute, Bethesda, **1976**.

Dale, W. E.; Gaines, T. B.; Hayes, W. J., Jr.; and Pearce, G. W.   Poisoning by DDT: relation between clinical signs and concentration in rat brain. *Science*, **1963**, *142*, 1474–1476.

Davies, D. S.; Hawksworth, G. M.; and Bennett, P. N.   Paraquat poisoning. *Proc. Eur. Soc. Toxicol.*, **1977**, *18*, 21–26.

DeLucia, A. J.; Mustaffa, M. G.; Hussain, M. Z.; and Cross, C. E.   Ozone interaction with rodent lung. III. Oxidation of reduced glutathione and formation of mixed disulfides between protein and nonprotein sulfhydryls. *J. Clin. Invest.*, **1975**, *55*, 794–802.

Desaiah, D.   Interaction of chlordecone with biological membranes. *J. Toxicol. Environ. Health*, **1981**, *8*, 719–730.

Elmes, P. C.   Mesotheliomas, minerals and man-made mineral fibres. *Thorax*, **1980**, *35*, 561–563.

Eroschenko, V. P.   Estrogenic activity of the insecticide chlordecone in the reproductive tract of birds and mammals. *J. Toxicol. Environ. Health*, **1981**, *8*, 731–742.

Folland, D. S.; Schaffner, W.; Grinn, H. E.; Crofford, O. B.; and McMurray, D. R.   Carbon tetrachloride toxicity potentiated by isopropyl alcohol. *J.A.M.A.*, **1976**, *236*, 1853–1856.

Freeman, G.; Crane, S. C.; Furiosi, N. J.; Stephens, R. J.; Evans, M. J.; and Moore, W. D.   Covert reduction in ventilatory surface in rats during prolonged exposure to subacute nitrogen dioxide. *Am. Rev. Respir. Dis.*, **1972**, *106*, 563–579.

Gehring, P. J.; Kramer, C. G.; Schwetz, B. A.; Rose, J. Q.; and Rowe, V. K.   The fate of 2,4,5-trichlorophenoxyacetic acid (2,4,5-T) following oral administration to man. *Toxicol. Appl. Pharmacol.*, **1973**, *26*, 352–361.

Geiling, E. M. K., and Cannon, P. R.   Pathologic effects of elixir sulfanilamide (diethylene glycol) poisoning; clinical and experimental correlations: final report. *J.A.M.A.*, **1938**, *111*, 919–926.

Goldsmith, J. R., and Landaw, S. A.   Carbon monoxide and human health. *Science*, **1968**, *162*, 1352–1359.

Goldstein, J. A.; Linder, R. E.; Hickman, P.; and Bergman, H.   Effects of pentachlorophenol on hepatic drug metabolism and porphyria related to contamination with chlorinated dibenzo-*p*-dioxins. *Toxicol. Appl. Pharmacol.*, **1976**, *37*, 145–146.

Greenlee, W. F.; Sun, J. D.; and Bus, J. S.   A proposed mechanism of benzene toxicity. Formation of reactive intermediates from polyphenol metabolites. *Toxicol. Appl. Pharmacol.*, **1981**, *59*, 187–195.

Hayes, W. J., Jr., and Vaughn, W. K.   Mortality from pesticides in the United States in 1973 and 1974. *Toxicol. Appl. Pharmacol.*, **1977**, *42*, 235–252.

Heppleston, A. G., and Styles, J. A.   Activity of a macrophage factor in collagen formation by silica. *Nature*, **1967**, *214*, 521–522.

Hine, C. H.   Methyl bromide poisoning: a review of ten cases. *J. Occup. Med.*, **1969**, *11*, 1–10.

Hirsch, J. A.; Swenson, E. W.; and Wanner, A.   Tracheal mucous transport in beagles after long-term exposure to 1 ppm sulfur dioxide. *Arch. Environ. Health*, **1975**, *30*, 249–253.

Hooper, N. K.; Ames, B. N.; Salek, M. A.; and Casida, J. E.   Toxophane, a complex mixture of polychloroterpenes and a major insecticide, is mutagenic. *Science*, **1979**, *205*, 591–593.

Iida, M.; Yamamoto, H.; and Sobue, I.   Prognosis of *n*-hexane polyneuropathy: follow-up studies on mass outbreak in F district of Mie prefecture. *Igaku No Ayumi*, **1973**, *84*, 199–201.

Innes, J. R. M., and others.   Bioassay of pesticides and industrial chemicals for tumorigenicity in mice: a preliminary note. *J. Natl Cancer Inst.*, **1969**, *42*, 1101–1114.

Jerina, D. M., and Daley, J. R. Arene oxides: a new aspect of drug metabolism. *Science*, **1974**, *185*, 573–582.

Johnson, R. L.; Gehring, P. J.; Kociba, R. J.; and Schwetz, B. A. Chlorinated dibenzodioxins and pentachlorophenol. *Environ. Health Perspect.*, **1973**, *5*, 171–175.

Jones, R. D., and Winter, D. P. Two case reports of deaths on industrial premises attributed to 1,1,1-trichloroethane. *Arch. Environ. Health*, **1983**, *38*, 59–61.

Kapoor, I. P.; Metcalf, R. L.; Nystrom, R. F.; and Sangha, G. H. Comparative metabolism of methoxychlor, methiochlor, and DDT in mouse, insects and in a model ecosystem. *J. Agric. Food Chem.*, **1970**, *18*, 1145–1152.

King, L. H.; Bradley, K. P.; and Shires, D. L. Hemodialysis for isopropyl alcohol poisoning. *J.A.M.A.*, **1970**, *211*, 1855.

Koch, R., and Schwarze, W. Die Hemmung der α-Naphthylthioharnstoffvergiftung durch Cysteamin und seine Derivate. (Zugleich ein Beitrag zur Toxikologie und Strahlenschutzwirkung dieser Sulfhydrylkorper). *Naunyn Schmiedebergs Arch. Exp. Pathol. Pharmakol.*, **1956**, *29*, 428–441.

Kociba, R. J., and others. Result of a 2-year chronic toxicity and oncogenicity study of 2,3,7,8-tetrachlorodibenzo-*p*-dioxin in rats. *Toxicol. Appl. Pharmacol.*, **1978**, *46*, 279–303.

Kolmodin, B.; Azarnoff, D. L.; and Sjoqvist, F. Effect of environmental factors on drug metabolism: decreased plasma half-life of antipyrine in workers exposed to chlorinated hydrocarbon insecticides. *Clin. Pharmacol. Ther.*, **1969**, *10*, 638–642.

Kreiss, K.; Zack, M.; Kimbrough, R. D.; Needham, L. L.; Smreak, A. L.; and Jones, B. T. Cross-study of a community with exceptional exposure to DDT. *J.A.M.A.*, **1981**, *245*, 1926–1930.

Krishna, G.; Pohl, L. R.; and Bhooshan, B. Mechanism of the metabolic activation of chloroform. *Toxicol. Appl. Pharmacol.*, **1978**, *45*, 238.

Kubic, V., and Anders, M. Metabolism of dihalomethanes to carbon monoxide. II. *In vitro* studies. *Drug Metab. Dispos.*, **1975**, *3*, 104–112.

Landrigan, P. J.; Powell, K. E.; James, L. M.; and Taylor, P. R. Paraquat and marijuana: epidemiological risk assessment. *Am. J. Public Health*, **1983**, *73*, 784–788.

Lapresle, J., and Fardeau, M. The central nervous system and carbon monoxide poisoning. II. Anatomical study of brain lesions following intoxication with carbon monoxide (22 cases). *Prog. Brain Res.*, **1967**, *24*, 31–74.

Lee, L. Y.; Bleeker, E.; and Nadel, J. A. Ozone-induced airway hyperirritability in dogs. *Fed. Proc.*, **1977**, *36*, 616.

Lee, P. W.; Arnau, T.; and Neal, R. A. Metabolism of α-naphthylthiourea by rat liver and rat lung microsomes. *Toxicol. Appl. Pharmacol.*, **1980**, *53*, 164–173.

Lindstrom, K. Behavioral effects of long-term exposure to organic solvents. *Acta Neurol. Scand.*, **1982**, *66*, 131–141.

Lisella, F. S.; Long, K. R.; and Scott, H. G. Toxicology of rodenticides and their relation to human health. *J. Environ. Health*, **1971**, *33*, 231–237, 361–365.

Longo, L. D. The biological effects of carbon monoxide on the pregnant woman, fetus, and newborn infant. *Am. J. Obstet. Gynecol.*, **1977**, *129*, 69–103.

McCarthy, T. B., and Jones, R. D. Industrial gassing poisonings due to trichlorethylene, perchlorethylene, and 1,1,1-trichloroethane, 1961–80. *Br. J. Ind. Med.*, **1983**, *40*, 450–455.

McMichael, A.; Spirtas, R.; Kupper, L.; and Gamble, J. Solvent exposure and leukemia among rubber workers: an epidemiological study. *J. Occup. Med.*, **1975**, *17*, 234–239.

Matthew, H. Acute poisoning: some myths and misconceptions. *Br. Med. J.*, **1971**, *1*, 519–522.

Miller, D. S., and Kinter, W. B. Enzymatic basis for DDE-induced eggshell thinning in a sensitive bird. *Nature*, **1976**, *259*, 122–124.

Miller, R. R.; Ayres, J. A.; Young, J. T.; and McKenna, M. J. Ethylene glycol monoethyl ether. 1. Subchronic vapor inhalation study with rats and rabbits. *Fundam. Appl. Toxicol.*, **1983a**, *3*, 49–54.

Miller, R. R.; Hermann, E. A.; Langvandt, P. W.; McKenna, M. J.; and Schwetz, B. A. Comparative metabolism and disposition of ethylene glycol monomethyl ether and propylene glycol monomethyl ether in male rats. *Toxicol. Appl. Pharmacol.*, **1983b**, *67*, 229–237.

National Academy of Sciences. *Drinking Water and Health.* The Academy, Washington, D. C., **1977**, p. 939.

Neubert, D.; Zens, P.; Rothenwallner, A.; and Merker, H. J. A survey of the embryotoxic effects of TCDD in mammalian species. *Environ. Health Perspect.*, **1973**, *5*, 67–79.

Ohkawa, H., and Casida, J. E. Glutathione S-transferases liberate hydrogen cyanide from organic thiocyanates. *Biochem. Pharmacol.*, **1971**, *20*, 1708–1711.

Orehek, J.; Massar, J. P.; Gayrard, P.; Grimaud, C.; and Charpin, J. Effect of short-term, low-level nitrogen dioxide exposure on bronchial sensitivity of asthmatic patients. *J. Clin. Invest.*, **1976**, *57*, 301–307.

Peterson, J. E., and Robison, W. H. Metabolic products of *p,p'*-DDT in the rat. *Toxicol. Appl. Pharmacol.*, **1964**, *6*, 321–327.

Peterson, J. E., and Stewart, R. D. Absorption and elimination of carbon monoxide by inactive young men. *Arch. Environ. Health*, **1970**, *21*, 165–171.

Pinto, J. D.; Camien, M. N.; and Dunn, M. S. Metabolic fate of *p,p'*-DDT. [1,1,1,-trichloro-2,2-*bis*(*p*-chlorophenyl)ethane] in rats. *J. Biol. Chem.*, **1965**, *240*, 2148–2154.

Poland, A. P., and Glover, E. Comparison of 2,3,7,8-tetrachlorodibenzo-*p*-dioxin, a potent inducer of aryl hydrocarbon hydroxylase, with 3-methylcholanthrene. *Mol. Pharmacol.*, **1974**, *10*, 349–359.

Poland, A. P.; Smith, D.; Kuntzman, R.; Jacobson, M.; and Conney, A. H. Effect of extensive occupational exposure to DDT on phenylbutazone and cortisol metabolism in human beings. *Clin. Pharmacol. Ther.*, **1970**, *11*, 724–732.

Poland, A. P.; Smith, D.; Metter, G.; and Possiek, P. A health survey of workers in a 2,4-D and 2,4,5-T plant with special attention to chloracne, porphyria cutanea tarda and psychologic parameters. *Arch. Environ. Health*, **1971**, *22*, 759–768.

Powers, M. B.; Voelker, R. W.; Page, N. P.; Weisburger, E. K.; and Kraybill, H. F. Carcinogenicity of ethylene dibromide (EDB) and 1,2-dibromo-3 chloropropane (DBCP) after oral administration in rats and mice. *Toxicol. Appl. Pharmacol.*, **1975**, *34*, 171–172.

Radcliffe, D. A. Decrease in eggshell weight in certain birds of prey. *Nature*, **1967**, *215*, 208–210.

Rozman, K.; Rozman, T.; and Greim, H. Stimulation of nonbiliary, intestinal excretion of hexachlorobenzene in rhesus monkeys by mineral oil. *Toxicol. Appl. Pharmacol.*, **1983**, *70*, 255–261.

————. Effect of thyroidectomy and thyroxine on 2,3,7,8-tetrachlorodibenzo-*p*-dioxin (TCDD) induced toxicity. *Ibid.*, **1984**, *72*, 372–376.

Rozman, T.; Ballhorn, L.; Rozman, K.; Klaassen, C.; and Greim, H. Effect of cholestyramine on the disposition of pentachlorophenol in rhesus monkeys. *J. Toxicol. Environ. Health*, **1982**, *10*, 277–283.

Saxena, M. C.; Siddiqui, M. K. J.; Bhargava, A. K.; Murti, C. R. K.; and Kutty, D. Placental transfer of pesticides in humans. *Arch. Toxicol.*, **1981**, *48*, 127–134.

Schmid, R. Cutaneous porphyria in Turkey. *N. Engl. J. Med.*, **1960**, *263*, 397–398.

Selikoff, I. J., and Hammond, E. C. Asbestos and smoking. *J.A.M.A.*, **1979**, *242*, 458–459.

Seppäläinen, A. M. Neurophysiological findings among workers exposed to organic solvents. *Acta Neurol. Scand.*, **1982**, *66*, 109–116.

Shankland, D. L. Neurotoxic action of chlorinated hydrocarbon insecticides. *Neurobehav. Toxicol. Teratol.*, **1982**, *4*, 805–811.

Sheehy, M., and Way, J. L. Effect of oxygen on cyanide intoxication. III. Mithridate. *J. Pharmacol. Exp. Ther.*, **1968**, *161*, 163–168.

Sheppard, D. A.; Saisho, A.; Nadel, J. A.; and Boushey, H. A. Exercise increases sulfur dioxide induced bronchoconstriction in asthmatic subjects. *Am. Rev. Respir. Dis.*, **1981**, *123*, 486–491.

Snyder, R.; Lee, E. W.; Kocsis, J. J.; and Witmer, C. M. Bone marrow depressant and leukemogenic actions of benzene. *Life Sci.*, **1977**, *21*, 1709–1722.

Stephens, R. J.; Sloan, M. F.; Evans, M. J.; and Freeman, G. Early response of lung to low levels of ozone. *Am. J. Pathol.*, **1974**, *74*, 31–57.

Striker, G. E.; Smuckler, E. A.; Kohnen, P. W.; and Nagle, R. B. Structural and functional changes in rat kidney during CCl₄ intoxication. *Am. J. Pathol.*, **1968**, *53*, 769–789.

Taylor, J. R.; Selhorst, J. B.; Houff, S. A.; and Martinez, A. J. Chlordecone intoxication in man. 1. Clinical observations. *Neurology (Minneap.)*, **1978**, *28*, 626–635.

Thomsen, H. K. Carbon monoxide–induced atherosclerosis in primates. An electron-microscopic study on the coronary arteries of *Macaca irus* monkeys. *Atherosclerosis*, **1974**, *20*, 233–240.

Turner, W. V.; Engel, J. L.; and Casida, J. E. Toxaphene components and related compounds: preparation and toxicity of some hepta-, octa-, and nonachlorobornanes, hexa-, and heptachlorobornenes and a hexachlorobornadiene. *J. Agric. Food Chem.*, **1977**, *25*, 1394–1401.

Van Miller, J. P.; Lalich, J. J.; and Allen, J. R. Increased incidence of neoplasms in rats exposed to low levels of 2,3,7,8-tetrachlorodibenzo-*o*-dioxin. *Chemosphere*, **1977**, *9*, 537–544.

Wang, H. H., and Grufferman, S. Aplastic anemia and occupational pesticide exposure: a case-control study. *J. Occup. Med.*, **1981**, *23*, 364–366.

Ware, F. H.; Thibodeau, L. A.; Speizer, F. E.; Colome, S.; and Ferris, B. G. Assessment of the health effects of atmospheric sulfur oxides and particulate matter: evidence from observational studies. *Environ. Health Perspect.*, **1981**, *41*, 255–276.

Waters, E. M.; Huff, J. E.; and Gerstner, H. B. Mirex, an overview. *Environ. Res.*, **1977**, *14*, 212–222.

Way, J. L.; End, E.; Sheehy, M. H.; DeMiranda, P.; Feitknecht, O. F.; Bachand, R.; Gibbson, S. L.; and Burrows, G. E. Effects of oxygen on cyanide intoxication. IV. Hyperbaric oxygen. *Toxicol. Appl. Pharmacol.*, **1972**, *22*, 415–421.

West, I. Lindane and hematologic reactions. *Arch. Environ. Health*, **1967**, *15*, 97–101.

Willhite, C. C., and Smith, R. P. The role of cyanide liberation on acute toxicity of aliphatic nitriles. *Toxicol. Appl. Pharmacol.*, **1981**, *59*, 589–602.

Monographs and Reviews

Aldridge, W. N. Toxicology of pyrethroids. In, *Pesticide Chemistry: Human Welfare and the Environment*, Vol. 3. (Miyamoto, J., and Kearney, P. C., eds.) Pergamon Press, Ltd., Oxford, **1983**, pp. 485–490.

Amdur, M. O. Air pollutants. In, *Casarett and Doull's Toxicology: The Basic Science of Poisons*, 3rd ed. (Klaassen, C. D.; Amdur, M. O.; and Doull, J.; eds.) Macmillan Publishing Co., New York, **1985**.

Andrews, L. S., and Snyder, R. Toxic effects of solvents and vapors. In, *Casarett and Doull's Toxicology: The Basic Science of Poisons*, 3rd ed. (Klaassen, C. D.; Amdur, M. O.; and Doull, J.; eds.) Macmillan Publishing Co., New York, **1985**.

Annau, Z. The neurobehavioral toxicity of trichloroethylene. *Neurobehav. Toxicol. Teratol.*, **1981**, *3*, 417–424.

Committee on Aldehydes. *Formaldehyde and Other Aldehydes*. National Academy Press, Washington, D. C., **1981**.

Couri, D., and Milks, M. Toxicity and metabolism of the neurotoxic hexacarbons *n*-hexane, 2-hexanone, and 2,5-hexadione. *Annu. Rev. Pharmacol. Toxicol.*, **1982**, *22*, 145–166.

Ervin, M. E. Petroleum distillates and turpentine. In, *Clinical Management of Poisoning and Drug Overdose*. (Haddad, L. M., and Winchester, J. F., eds.) W. B. Saunders Co., Philadelphia, **1983**, pp. 771–779.

Finck, P. A. Exposure to carbon monoxide: review of the literature and 567 autopsies. *Milit. Med.*, **1966**, *131*, 1513–1539.

Fisher, H. A. Occupational contact dermatitis from pesticides: patch testing procedures. *Cutis*, **1983**, *31*, 483–508.

Folinsbee, L. J. Effects of ozone exposure on lung function in man: a review. *Rev. Environ. Health*, **1983**, *3*, 211–240.

Gosselin, R. E.; Smith, R. P.; and Hodge, H. C. *Clinical Toxicology of Commercial Products*, 5th ed. The Williams & Wilkins Co., Baltimore, **1984**.

Gutierrez, G. Carbon monoxide toxicity. In, *Air Pollution—Physiological Effects*. (McGrath, J. J., and Barnes, C. D., eds.) Academic Press, Inc., New York, **1982**, pp. 127–147.

Guzelian, P. S. Comparative toxicology of chlordecone (KEPONE) in humans and experimental animals. *Annu. Rev. Pharmacol. Toxicol.*, **1982**, *22*, 89–113.

Hayes, W. J., Jr. *Clinical Handbook on Economic Poisons*. Public Health Service Publication No. 476, U.S. Government Printing Office, Washington, D. C., **1963**.

———. *Pesticides Studied in Man*. The Williams & Wilkins Co., Baltimore, **1982**.

Holmstedt, B. Prolegomena to Seveso. *Arch. Toxicol.*, **1980**, *44*, 211–230.

IARC. *Monographs on the Evaluation of the Carcinogenic Risk of Chemicals to Man*. Vol. 5, *Some Organochlorine Pesticides*. International Agency for Research on Cancer, Lyon, France, **1974a**.

———. *Monographs on the Evaluation of the Carcinogenic Risk of Chemicals to Man*. Vol. 7, *Some Antithyroid and Related Substances, Nitrofurans and Industrial Chemicals*. International Agency for Research on Cancer, Lyon, France, **1974b**.

———. *Monographs on the Evaluation of Carcinogenic Risk of Chemicals to Man*. Vol. 12, *Some Carbamates, Thiocarbamates and Carbazides*. International Agency for Research on Cancer, Lyon, France, **1976**.

———. *Monographs on the Evaluation of the Carcinogenic Risk of Chemicals to Man*. Vol. 15, *Some Fumigants, the Herbicides 2,4-D and 2,4,5-T, Chlorinated Dibenzodioxins and Miscellaneous Industrial Chemicals*. International Agency for Research on Cancer, Lyon, France, **1977**.

Kaplan, S. D., and Morgan, R. W. Airborne carcinogens and human cancer. *Rev. Environ. Health*, **1981**, *3*, 329–368.

Kerns, W. D.; Donofrio, D. J.; and Pavkov, K. L. The chronic effects of formaldehyde inhalation in rats and mice: a preliminary report. In, *Formaldehyde Toxicity*. (Gibson, J. E., ed.) Hemisphere Publishing Corp., Washington, D. C., **1983**, pp. 111–131.

Khan, N. Y. An assessment of the hazard of synthetic pyrethroid insecticides to fish and fish habitat. In, *Pesticide Chemistry: Human Welfare and the Environment*,

Vol. 3. (Miyamoto, J., and Kearney, P. C., eds.) Pergamon Press, Ltd., Oxford, **1983**, pp. 115–121.

Kupfer, D., and Bulger, W. H. Estrogenic actions of chlorinated hydrocarbons. In, *Effects of Chronic Exposures to Pesticides on Animal Systems.* (Chambers, J. E., and Yarbrough, J. D., eds.) Raven Press, New York, **1982**, pp. 121–146.

Maibach, H. Formaldehyde: effects on animal and human skin. In, *Formaldehyde Toxicity.* (Gibson, J. E., ed.) Hemisphere Publishing Corp., Washington, D. C., **1983**, pp. 166–174.

Mehendale, H. M. Modification of hepatobiliary function by toxic chemicals. *Fed. Proc., 1979, 38,* 2240–2245.

Menzel, D. B. Toxicity of ozone, oxygen, and radiation. *Annu. Rev. Pharmacol., 1970, 10,* 379–394.

Menzer, R. E., and Nelson, J. O. Water and soil pollutants. In, *Casarett and Doull's Toxicology: The Basic Science of Poisons.* (Klaassen, C. D.; Amdur, M. O.; and Doull, J.; eds.) Macmillan Publishing Co., New York, **1985.**

Murphy, S. D. Toxic effects of pesticides. In, *Casarett and Doull's Toxicology: The Basic Science of Poisons,* 3rd ed. (Klaassen, C. D.; Amdur, M. O.; and Doull, J.; eds.) Macmillan Publishing Co., Inc., New York, **1985.**

Narahashi, T. Nerve membrane ionic channels as the target of insecticides. In, *Neurotoxicology of Insecticides and Pheromones.* (Narahashi, T., ed.) Plenum Press, New York, **1979**, pp. 211–243.

——. Interaction of pyrethroids and DDT-like compounds with the sodium channels in the nerve membrane. In, *Pesticide Chemistry: Human Welfare and the Environment,* Vol. 3. (Miyamoto, J., and Kearney, P. C., eds.) Pergamon Press, Ltd., Oxford, **1983**, pp. 109–114.

National Research Council. Committee on Medical and Biologic Effects of Environmental Pollutants. *Carbon Monoxide.* National Academy of Sciences, Washington, D. C., **1977.**

Plaa, G. L. Toxic responses of the liver. In, *Casarett and Doull's Toxicology: The Basic Science of Poisons,* 3rd ed. (Klaassen, C. D.; Amdur, M. O.; and Doull, J.; eds.) Macmillan Publishing Co., New York, **1985.**

Recknagel, R. O., and Glende, E. H., Jr. Carbon tetrachloride hepatotoxicity: an example of lethal cleavage. *CRC Crit. Rev. Toxicol., 1973, 2,* 263–297.

Sayers, P. R., and Davenport, S. J. *Review of Carbon Monoxide Poisoning.* Public Health Bulletin No. 195,

U.S. Government Printing Office, Washington, D. C., **1930.**

Slater, T. F. Free radicals as reactive intermediates in tissue injury. In, *Biological Reactive Intermediates II: Chemical Mechanisms and Biological Effects.* (Snyder, R.; Parke, D. V.; Kocsis, J. J.; Jollow, D. J.; Gibson, G. G.; and Witmer, C. M.; eds.) Plenum Press, New York, **1982**, pp. 575–589.

Speizer, F. E. Environmental lung diseases. In, *Harrison's Principles of Internal Medicine,* 10th ed. (Petersdorf, R. G.; Adams, R. D.; Braunwald, E.; Isselbacher, K. J.; Martin, J. B.; and Wilson, J.; eds.) McGraw-Hill Book Co., New York, **1983**, pp. 1524–1532.

Stewart, R. D. The effects of carbon monoxide on humans. *Annu. Rev. Pharmacol., 1975, 15,* 409–423.

Tintinalli, J. E.; Rominger, M.; and Kittleson, K. Carbon monoxide. In, *Clinical Management of Poisoning and Drug Overdose.* (Haddad, L. M., and Winchester, J. F., eds.) W. B. Saunders Co., Philadelphia, **1983**, pp. 748–753.

Von Oettingen, W. F. *The Halogenated Hydrocarbons of Industrial and Toxicological Significance.* Elsevier Publishing Co., New York, **1964.**

Way, J. L. Cyanide antagonism. *Fundam. Appl. Toxicol., 1983, 3,* 383–386.

Weger, N. P. Treatment of cyanide poisoning with 4-dimethylaminophenol (DMAP)-experimental and clinical overview. *Fundam. Appl. Toxicol., 1983, 3,* 387–396.

Williams, G. M., and Weisburger, J. H. Chemical carcinogens. In, *Casarett and Doull's Toxicology: The Basic Science of Poisons,* 3rd ed. (Klaassen, C. D.; Amdur, M. O.; and Doull, J.; eds.) Macmillan Publishing Co., New York, **1985.**

Woodbury, M. A., and Zenz, C. Formaldehyde in the home environment: prenatal and infant exposures. In, *Formaldehyde Toxicity.* (Gibson, J. E., ed.) Hemisphere Publishing Corp., Washington, D. C., **1983**, pp. 203–211.

World Health Organization. *1974 Evaluations of Some Pesticide Residue in Food.* World Health Organization Pesticide Residue Series, No. 4, Geneva, Switzerland, **1975**, pp. 261–263.

Zimmerman, H. J. *Hepatotoxicity: The Adverse Effects of Drugs and Other Chemicals on the Liver.* Appleton-Century-Crofts, New York, **1978.**

I   PRINCIPLES OF PRESCRIPTION ORDER WRITING AND PATIENT COMPLIANCE INSTRUCTION

Ewart A. Swinyard

The prescription order is an important therapeutic transaction between the physician and his patient. It brings to focus the diagnostic acumen and therapeutic proficiency of the physician with instructions for palliation or restoration of the patient's health. The most carefully conceived prescription order may become therapeutically useless, however, unless it communicates clearly with the pharmacist and adequately instructs the patient on how to take the prescribed medication.

The importance of clarity in the physician's communication with the pharmacist cannot be overemphasized. Many drugs look alike when they are written or sound alike when spoken. When these like-appearing names are written unclearly, or when like-sounding names are garbled over the telephone, the burden of avoiding misinterpretation falls mainly on the pharmacist who fills the prescription order.

Numerous studies suggest that too many physicians fail to instruct patients adequately on how to take their prescription medication. Reviews of such studies indicate that 25 to 50% of patients in a variety of clinical situations failed to take their prescription medication as directed (Blackwell, 1976; Sackett, 1976). Most errors were related to the prescription order directions; the patient took the medication either in the wrong dose, for the wrong purpose, or at the wrong time. Also, some patients either missed doses or failed to complete the treatment regimen. Data of this kind emphasize the physician's need to understand the basic principles of prescription order writing and how to instruct the patient about his medication.

PRESCRIPTION ORDER WRITING

The practice of writing complex prescription orders containing many active ingredients, adjuvants, correctives, and elegant vehicles has been abandoned in favor of single drugs and mixtures of drugs compounded by pharmaceutical companies. Even when two or more active ingredients are desired for oral administration, they are preferably prescribed separately so that the physician may adjust the dose of each to the individual requirements of the patient. The National Prescription Audit (1983) reveals that 99% of all prescription orders are for precompounded drugs. Only 1% (but still 140 million per year) requires compounding. This is desirable in the great majority of instances, but such simplicity has its drawbacks. Many physicians rely upon fixed-dose combinations rather than adjust the doses of the agents to the particular needs of the patient. For example, the prescription audit referred to above shows that 55 of the 200 most frequently prescribed drugs are combination products.

To be able accurately and speedily to write prescription orders requires practice. The prescription order should be written legibly. It is convenient and the accepted form to have one's name, address, telephone number, office hours, and Drug Enforcement Administration (DEA) registry number printed on the prescription order blank. Because prescription orders are medicolegal documents, they should be written in ink, although this is compulsory only for controlled substances in schedule II. It is also an excellent custom, too infrequently followed, for the doctor to keep an exact or carbon copy for his files. This copy protects him and serves to complete the record of treatment.

Helpful suggestions on prescription order writing may be found in "Prescription Writing and Prescription Labeling," developed by the American Pharmaceutical Association and the American Society of Internal Medicine (1974).

Choice of Drug Name. Most drugs can be prescribed by their official names (*United States Pharmacopeia;* USP), by their nonproprietary names (United States Adopted Names; USAN), or by the manufacturers' proprietary (trade) names. The nonproprietary name is often referred to as the generic name. The latter term, based on strict definition, is properly used to designate a chemical relationship among drugs, such as sulfonamides, barbiturates, and so forth. However, the distinction has been overlooked, and the term *generic* is used almost to the exclusion of *nonproprietary.*

There is much discussion concerning the relative advantages of prescribing by nonproprietary versus proprietary name. Arguments in favor of the use of nonproprietary names are based, for the most part, on the elimination of duplication of drug products and the possibility of an economic benefit to the patient. Arguments against such practice usually include the lack of quality control, variability in the formulation and, consequently, in the biological availability of the drug (*see* Chapter 1), and the fact that many nonproprietary names are difficult to remember and to spell. Arguments on both sides of these questions are being resolved rapidly. Virtually all states have adopted laws that allow the pharmacist to substitute the product of one company for the same formulation from a different manufacturer under specified circumstances. Such laws also speak to mechanisms whereby the clinician can facilitate or prevent such substitution. Clinicians and pharmacists must be familiar with the laws of their own state. The United States Food and Drug Administration (FDA) has prepared a monograph that identifies currently marketed prescription drug products and that contains evaluations of therapeutic equivalence for the multisource approved drug products (Food and Drug Administration, 1983). Use of this volume will minimize the uncertainty associated with prescribing and dispensing nonproprietary drugs. The physician can prevent substitution, however, if he or she writes "dispense as written" on the prescription order, or indicates to the pharmacist in verbal prescription orders that only the product requested is to be dispensed.

Nonproprietary names are now selected by the United States Adopted Name (USAN) Council. The USAN Council is sponsored jointly by the American Medical Association, the United States Pharmacopeial Convention, Inc., and the American Pharmaceutical Association. Provision was made in 1967 for a liaison representative of the United States Food and Drug Administration also to serve on the Council. For details relative to how the USAN Council functions, *see* Jerome and Sagan (1975).

In writing prescription orders it is *best to use the nonproprietary name followed by the name of the manufacturer in parentheses if a specific manufacturer's product has distinct advantages*. This not only eliminates the necessity for memorizing multiple drug names but also assures the physician that the product of a particular manufacturer will be dispensed.

Choice of a System of Weights and Measures. Prescription orders should always be written in the metric system. It is necessary only to designate amounts of drug by numbers and to indicate the metric unit of weight or volume desired. In the prescription order itself, the Arabic number is placed after the official name of the drug and, if several ingredients are prescribed, the decimal points are placed in the same vertical line. Many physicians substitute a vertical line for decimal points, and this "decimal line" may be printed on the prescription order pad. Above this line one may place "g or ml." It should be emphasized, however, that when the decimal line is used all ingredient quantities must be expressed in the basic units of the metric system (g or ml) and this line cannot be used to express decimal fractions of *milligrams*.

Apothecaries' System. Since doses in older publications may appear in units of the apothecaries' system, metric and apothecaries' equivalents are presented in Table A–I–1.

Household Measures. Unfortunately, the drugs prescribed so carefully by the physician in milligrams and milliliters are usually measured by the patient with convenient kitchen utensils. The "drop," which varies in size, presents a special problem. Its size depends on the particular fluid being dropped—its specific gravity, temperature, and viscosity—as well as on the orifice of the dropper and the angle at which the dropper is held. The USP does not sanction the prescribing of doses in drops but provides an official standardized dropper for those who wish to use it. This official dropper, when held vertically, delivers drops of water, each of which weighs between 45 and 55 mg. Although most commercial products provide a calibrated dropper for this type of preparation, all extemporaneous prescription orders for medication to be given in drops should carry the notation "Dispense with calibrated dropper." The size of the household teaspoon also varies considerably. For household purposes, an American Standard Teaspoon has been established by the American National Standards Institute, containing 4.93 ± 0.24 ml. The USP specifies that this teaspoon may be regarded as containing 5 ml. A tablespoon is said to contain 15 ml.

Table A–I–1. METRIC AND APOTHECARIES' EQUIVALENTS

1 milligram	=	$\frac{1}{65}$	grain
1 gram	=	15.43	grains
1 kilogram	=	2.20	pounds
1 milliliter	=	16.23	minims
1 grain	=	0.065	gram
1 ounce	=	31.1	grams
1 minim	=	0.062	ml
1 fluid ounce	=	29.57	ml
1 pint	=	473.2	ml
1 quart	=	946.4	ml

(No. 1)

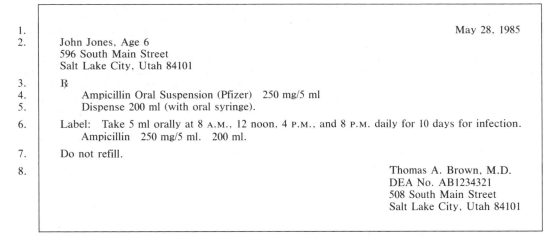

1.		May 28, 1985

1.

2.   John Jones, Age 6
   596 South Main Street
   Salt Lake City, Utah 84101

3.   ℞

4.   Ampicillin Oral Suspension (Pfizer)   250 mg/5 ml

5.   Dispense 200 ml (with oral syringe).

6.   Label: Take 5 ml orally at 8 A.M., 12 noon, 4 P.M., and 8 P.M. daily for 10 days for infection.
      Ampicillin   250 mg/5 ml.   200 ml.

7.   Do not refill.

8.   Thomas A. Brown, M.D.
                              DEA No. AB1234321
                              508 South Main Street
                              Salt Lake City, Utah 84101

Other devices, such as molded plastic cylinders and measuring caps, have been developed for measuring and administering liquid medications. A novel oral syringe may be used to measure and administer drugs to children; these syringes (both glass and plastic) are available in a variety of sizes to assure accurate administration of drugs. Such devices have been strongly recommended by the Committee on Drugs, American Academy of Pediatrics (1975), to replace the usual household utensils. Physicians who find it necessary to prescribe liquid medicines for oral administration should request the pharmacist to supply the appropriate device with the medication in order to assure that the patient can conveniently take the prescribed dose.

Construction of the Prescription Order. Traditionally, a prescription order follows a definite pattern that facilitates its interpretation. This pattern is essentially the same whether the prescription order is for a single drug or a mixture of two or more drugs. Only one prescription should be written on an order blank. The major elements of a model order are illustrated in example No. 1. The numbers at the left call attention to the several parts of a prescription order, which are explained below.

1. *Date.* The date when the prescription order is written is important. Federal law requires that prescription orders for drugs listed in schedules II, III, and IV of the Controlled Substances Act of 1970 be dated; orders for substances in schedules III and IV cannot be filled or refilled more than 6 months after date of issuance.

2. *Name and Address of the Patient.* These are necessary in order to expedite the handling of the prescription order and to avoid possible confusion with medications intended for someone else. The age should also be included. Moreover, the pharmacist should verify the patient's name and age; otherwise it is impossible for him to monitor the prescribed dose. The pharmacist should place the name of the patient on the bottle or container exactly as the doctor has written it. Prescription orders for schedule-II drugs are required to contain the full name and address of the patient.

3. *Superscription.* The superscription consists of the symbol ℞ (not "Rx"), an abbreviation for *recipe*, the Latin for "take thou."

4. *Inscription.* The inscription is the body of the prescription order and contains the name and strength (dose) of the desired drug. Drugs are prescribed in the United States by official English names. Abbreviations should be avoided since their use frequently results in error. When two or more drugs are desired in the same prescription order, the name and amount of each drug are placed together on a separate line directly under the preceding one. Traditionally, the order of ingredients, should there be more than one, is as follows:

Basis. The basis is the principal drug and gives the prescription its chief action.
Adjuvant. As the name suggests, the adjuvant is a drug that aids or increases the action of the principal ingredient.
Corrective. The corrective modifies or corrects undesirable effects of the basis or adjuvant.
Vehicle. The vehicle is the agent used as the solvent in the solution, to increase the bulk, or to dilute the mixture.

In practice, prescription orders seldom contain more than one drug name. However, when three agents are prescribed, the most potent or principal drug is listed first, the other ingredient second, and the vehicle last, as shown below.

5. *Subscription.* The subscription contains the directions to the pharmacist. In prescription orders for a single drug this usually consists in "Dispense 10 tablets," "Dispense 200 ml," "Dispense with oral syringe," and so forth; in the case of prescription orders for two or more drugs it usually consists in either a short sentence such as "Make a solution" or "Mix and place into 10 capsules" or a word such as "Mix."

6. *Signature.* The signature of the prescription order consists in the directions to the patient. The term *signature* does not refer to the physician's name; rather, it is derived from the Latin *signa,* meaning "write," "mark," or "label." Since English is the preferred language, the directions are preceded by the word *Label.* Occasionally, this part of the prescription order is called the *transcription* and the term *signature* is then reserved for the physician's name.

The directions to the patient should always be written in English. The use of Latin abbreviations serves no useful purpose. The directions to the patient contain instructions as to the amount of drug to be taken, the time and frequency of the dose, and other factors such as dilution and route of administration. If a device is involved in the administration of the medication, the physician and/or pharmacist should either demonstrate how it is used or review the instructions with the patient. If the drug is to be used externally only, or to be shaken well before using, or if it is a poison, such facts are included.

Expressions such as "take as directed" and "take as necessary" are *never* satisfactory and should be avoided. Whenever possible, exact times of the day should be specified. If it is therapeutically important to take the medication at specific intervals around the clock or for a specific period of time, this should be stated in the directions to the patient. The physician should be particularly sensitive to the needs of aged, ill, and handicapped patients, as well as those with language difficulties. The directions for these individuals should also be written in greater detail on a separate instruction sheet and left with the patient. To avoid possible error, the first word of the directions to the patient should be employed as a reminder of the correct route of administration. Thus, the directions for a preparation for internal use should start with the word *take;* for an ointment or lotion, the word *apply;* for suppositories, the word *insert;* and for drops to be placed in the conjunctival sac, external auditory canal, or nostril, the word *place.* The directions to the patient should also be employed as a reminder of the intended purpose of the prescription, by including such phrases as "for relief of pain," "for relief of headache," or "to relieve itching." However, directions that would be embarrassing to the patient if placed on the prescription order or label should be given in private.

There are many cogent reasons why the prescription medication and the quantity dispensed should be identified on the label. For example, the rapid identification of a drug and a quick estimate of the amount consumed can help with the initiation of appropriate therapy in the case of adverse drug reactions, or accidental or deliberate overdosage. Therefore, many states require that the name, strength, and quantity of drug dispensed be indicated on the label. When appropriate, the pharmacist should also indicate the expiration date and special storage instructions on the prescription label.

The pharmacist always should be on the alert to detect overdoses of potent drugs in the prescriptions he dispenses. This serves as an added check for the safety of the patient. If it is desirable to administer a drug in a larger amount than is customarily employed, it is best for the prescriber to underline the dose, and to write "correct amount" or "correct dose" and his initials at the side.

7. *Refill Information.* Under the Durham-Humphrey Amendment to the Federal Food, Drug, and Cosmetic Act (*see* page 1658), prescription orders for drugs that bear the caution legend, "Federal law prohibits dispensing without prescription," may not be refilled without the consent of the prescriber. Under the Drug Abuse Control Amendments to the above act (*see* page 1659), prescription orders for schedule-III and schedule-IV drugs cannot be refilled *more than five times* and the prescription order is invalid 6 months from the date of issue. These restrictions are intended to control the overuse and abuse of prescription medications. For these reasons, the physician should indicate his wishes with respect to refills on each original prescription order, irrespective of whether it is for a controlled substance. This may be indicated by instruction to refill a certain number of times or not to refill. Statements such as "Refill prn" and "Refill ad lib" are never appropriate. Such information need not be written on narcotic prescription orders for schedule-II substances, since by law these cannot be refilled.

8. *Prescriber's Signature.* The prescription order is completed by the practitioner writing his signature at the bottom of the blank, with the appropriate professional degree following it. Federal law requires that the physician's address and DEA registry number also appear on every prescription order for controlled drugs and that such an order be signed (last name in full) with ink or indelible pencil.

Classes of Prescription Orders. On the basis of the availability of the prescribed medication, prescription orders may be divided into two classes, *precompounded* and *extemporaneous*. A *precompounded* prescription order is one that calls for a drug or mixture of drugs supplied by the pharmaceutical company by its official or proprietary name and in a form that the pharmacist dispenses without pharmaceutical alteration. An *extemporaneous* prescription order, also called *magistral* or *compounded*, is the type in which the physician selects the drugs, doses, and pharmaceutical form that he desires and the pharmacist prepares the medication. Examples of prescription orders for precompounded and extemporaneous preparations are given below and will serve to illustrate the principles of prescription order writing.

Examples of Prescription Orders for Precompounded Preparations. When writing a prescription order for a precompounded preparation, it is necessary to know the name of the preparation desired, the pharmaceutical form in which it is available (*i.e.,* ointment, tablet, *etc.*), the single dose, the route and the frequency of administration, and the approximate number of days of therapy. Suppose one wishes to renew a prescription order for a 3-month supply of digoxin for an adult with congestive heart failure, who is well stabilized and has been thoroughly instructed regarding compliance. Since digoxin is available under several different trade names, it is good practice to prescribe the drug by its USAN, but to indicate a manufacturer's product that will ensure adequate, dependable bioavailability, as shown below.

(No. 2)

℞

Digoxin Tablets
(Burroughs Wellcome Co.) 0 | 00025

Dispense 100 such tablets.

Label: Take 1 tablet at 9:00 A.M. each morning.
Digoxin, 0.25 mg. 100 tablets.

When the decimal line is used, the unit dose *must* be expressed in grams or decimal fractions thereof. When the decimal line is not used, the unit dose *must be clearly stated.* For example, the above prescription could also be written as follows:

℞

Digoxin Tablets
(Burroughs Wellcome Co.) 0.25 mg

Precompounded prescription orders for orally administered liquid preparations are constructed in a similar manner. It is necessary, however, to know the concentration of the active ingredient(s) in the preparation. Suppose one desires to

prescribe ampicillin suspension (250 mg/5 ml) for a child with otitis media in a dose of 250 mg to be given four times daily. A prescription order providing 7 days of medication may be written as follows:

(No. 3)

℞

Ampicillin suspension, 250 mg/5 ml 150 | 0

Label: Give one teaspoonful every 6 hours for 7 days.

Ampicillin suspension

Do not refill.

Prescription orders for orally administered precompounded remedies, such as solutions, syrups, suspensions, and tinctures, are written as illustrated in the previous example, as are those for preparations that are intended for local application. If special instructions to the pharmacist are necessary, these may be indicated. For example, physicians should remember that the 1970 Poison Prevention Packaging Act was extended in 1974 to require child-resistant containers for *all oral* prescriptions, although several exceptions are permitted (*e.g.,* oral contraceptives). Many patients have difficulty in using the special containers. In such cases the prescriber or patient may request the use of a conventional container.

Examples of Prescription Orders for Extemporaneous Preparations. In writing prescription orders for an extemporaneous preparation for oral administration, it is of course necessary to know the single dose of each ingredient, the number of doses to be taken each day, and the number of days of medication. This knowledge allows the calculation of the total dosage of each ingredient in the prescription. Suppose it is desired to prescribe an antitussive-expectorant mixture to be taken orally every 4 hours. This means that at least four doses will be taken daily. If teaspoonful doses (5 ml) are used and enough medicine is dispensed to last 6 days, approximately 24 doses or a 120-ml total volume will be needed. Calculations are shown below for a mixture of codeine phosphate (antitussive), ammonium chloride (expectorant), and aromatic elixir (vehicle). (*Obviously, these calculations should not appear on the completed prescription order.*)

			Single dose × No. of doses	
Codeine Phosphate	0	24	⟷	10 mg × 24
Ammonium Chloride	7	2	⟷	0.3 g × 24
Aromatic Elixir, to make	120	0	⟷	5.0 ml × 24

Extemporaneous prescription orders for other liquid preparations for oral or local administration are constructed similarly.

The principles of calculation of dosage illustrated above apply also to prescription orders for dry forms of medication to be taken internally. Since pharmacists are not equipped to compound compressed tablets, dry forms of medication are commonly prescribed in capsule form. Whereas it is fairly easy to ingest liquid medicines, it may be difficult to swallow capsules that are too large. Therefore, these are limited to approximately 0.5 g in bulk (for adults) for most medicines. If a larger amount is required for the single dose, then the drug must be divided into 2 or more capsules for each dose. If the ingredients make too small a bulk to be dispensed conveniently in solid form, an inert powder may be added. There are many such powders and excipients (licorice, lactose, *etc.*), and the pharmacist often selects and adds them at his own discretion.

Suppose it is desired to prescribe in capsule form an analgesic mixture containing aspirin, acetaminophen, and amobarbital for a patient with painful myositis. The medicine is to be taken every 4 hours during waking hours (*i.e.,* four doses per day) and enough is to be prescribed to last 5 days. The construction of the prescription order is as follows:

(No. 4)

July 29, 1985

Mary Thomas, Age 54
606 Constitution Avenue, N.W.
Washington, D. C. 20001

℞   Single dose × No. of doses

Aspirin	6|0	⟷	0.3 g	× 20
Acetaminophen	6|0	⟷	0.3 g	× 20
Amobarbital	1|0	⟷	0.05 g	× 20

Mix and divide into 40 capsules.

Label: Take 2 capsules at 8:00 A.M., 12 noon, 4:00 P.M., and 8:00 P.M. for muscle pain. Aspirin, Acetaminophen, and Amobarbital. 40 capsules.

Do not refill.

Prescription orders for medicines to be taken internally may also be written by the *single-dose method*. The pharmacist is then instructed to prepare a given number of doses, and he must carry out the calculations illustrated above. For example, prescription order No. 4, if written by the single-dose method, would appear as follows:

(No. 5)

℞

Aspirin	0|3
Acetaminophen	0|3
Amobarbital	0|05

Make 20 such doses and place in 40 capsules.

Label: *etc.*

The therapeutic efficacy of an ointment is achieved only if the active ingredients are incorporated into the proper ointment base. The ideal ointment base should be compatible with the skin, stable, permanent, smooth and pliable, nonirritating, nonsensitizing, and inert, and should readily release incorporated medication. Four classes of ointment bases are recognized: absorption, emulsion, oleaginous, and water soluble. Unless the physician becomes familiar with the physical properties of the various bases, he should seek the help of a pharmacist in the selection of an appropriate base. The ingredients of an ointment are expressed on a percentage basis. Suppose that it is desired to prescribe an ointment for a fungal infection of the feet, and that benzoic acid (6%) and salicylic acid (3%) are to be incorporated in a base of hydrophilic petrolatum and white petrolatum. If a 60-g amount of ointment is to be dispensed, the order appears as follows:

(No. 6)

℞

Benzoic Acid	3	6
Salicylic Acid	1	8
Hydrophilic Petrolatum		
White Petrolatum, of each an equal amount to make	60	0

Make an ointment.

Label: Apply a thin film to the affected parts night and morning. Benzoic Acid and Salicylic Acid.

When prescribing locally acting drugs, the *percentage form may be used as such* rather than as a basis for calculating absolute amounts of ingredients. The percent employed is always based on weight/weight. Prescription order No. 6 may thus be written as follows:

(No. 7)

℞

Benzoic Acid	6%
Salicylic Acid	3%
Hydrophilic Petrolatum	
White Petrolatum, of each an equal amount to make	60|0

Make an ointment.

Label: *etc.*

A prescription order for a lotion for external use on the skin is similar in construction to that for an ointment in that only the percentages of the ingredients and not absolute doses need be ordered.

Prescription orders for many liquid preparations for local administration, such as ophthalmic solutions, nasal sprays, inhalants, gargles, and douches, are constructed similarly to those cited above. Aqueous solutions prepared for use in the eye are less irritating if they are adjusted to isotonicity with the lacrimal fluid. If it is desired to prescribe an isotonic ophthalmic solution, this fact can be indicated by inserting the phrase, "Sodium Chloride, to make isotonic." Solutions to be used in the nose can also be employed with much greater comfort if made approximately isotonic.

Dosage. Instructions about dosage are an extremely important part of prescription order writing. The number of days for which medication is contemplated, the number of doses per day, and the size of each dose determine the bulk of the prescription. There is *no minimal limit* to the total quantity of prescribed medication, and as little as a single dose may be ordered. On the other hand, a *maximal limit* is indicated for most prescriptions, even when medication is to continue for an indefinite period; this limit is influenced by the stability and cost of the drug and the possible necessity for alteration of the treatment. A major factor that should be a determinant of the quantity of the drug dispensed is the mental state of the patient and the potential toxicity of the drug. If a patient is depressed or potentially suicidal, do not prescribe total quantities of drug that would prove lethal if taken all at one time. If there are no such problems, a convenient rule of thumb is to prescribe only enough medication for 7 to 14 days. *Storage* of unused portions of a prescription and *sharing* of prescriptions with others who were not intended to receive them should be explicitly discussed with any patient who receives an important prescription. Blackwell (1972) reported that 9 of 75 patients used drugs that were prescribed for other individuals.

Size and Form of Medication. The upper limit of the weight of a single capsule or tablet is usually about 0.5 g, for adults. However, this arbitrary limit based on what the patient can comfortably swallow may be exceeded when the drug product is dense. Conversely, even a smaller unit dosage may be indicated for light, bulky medication or for certain patients, especially the very young or old.

Many drugs are commercially available only in a limited variety of dose forms (*e.g.*, only capsules of a single weight). For obvious reasons of convenience and economy, these "standard" forms of medication should be preferred, except under unusual circumstances. Until knowledge of the dosage forms available for the various drugs is acquired through experience, the physician is well advised to rely upon his pharmacist for this information. Other useful sources of information include the sections on preparations in this textbook; *Facts and Comparisons; AMA Drug Evaluations (AMA–DE)*, a publication of the American Medical Association; *Drug Information for the Health Care Provider (USP–DI); Hospital Formulary,* published by the American Society of Hospital Pharmacists; and the *Physicians' Desk Reference (PDR).*

Usual Doses. The physician should consult the above-mentioned references (especially the *USP–DI* or *Facts and Comparisons*) or the package insert for guidance on the recommended *Usual Adult Doses* and *Usual Pediatric Doses.* These represent the doses that should produce the recognized therapeutic effects in adults and children following oral administration unless otherwise specified. The *Usual Dose* is intended to serve only as a guide to the physician, who very frequently must give more or less than what is usual in order to optimize therapy. Some of the above references also give the *Usual Adult Prescribing Limits,* intended primarily to guide the pharmacist with respect to confirmation of prescription orders calling for unusually large dosages.

Vehicles, Flavors, and Coloring Agents. Oral medication should be in the form of tablets and capsules, if at all possible. Children and aged patients, however, usually find the liquid forms of oral medication more acceptable; indeed, if bitter, salty, or other objectionable-tasting drugs could be disguised in a liquid preparation, this would be one of the most useful forms of drug administration for such patients. It is therefore necessary for the physician to know how to prescribe medicines in a form sufficiently palatable so that they will be taken by the patient.

The effective flavoring and coloring of a drug formulation often present formidable problems. Pharmaceutical manufacturers spend considerable sums of money and devote much time and effort to assure that an otherwise-distasteful drug is marketed in an acceptable, elegant form. In such cases, it is probably best to prescribe the drug in a proprietary formulation. Nevertheless, acceptable extemporaneous liquid medications can be obtained by the careful selection of coloring, flavoring, and diluting agents. The physician is well advised to enlist a pharmacist's aid in demonstrating the use of available agents.

Vehicles. The many vehicles available to the physician for flavoring and diluting drugs may conveniently be divided into three groups: elixirs, syrups, and aromatic waters. Elixirs, sweetened hydroalcoholic solutions that contain approximately 25% alcohol, are suitable vehicles for drugs soluble in either water or dilute alcohol. Syrups, concentrated aqueous solutions of sugar, are useful as vehicles for water-soluble drugs. Aromatic waters, saturated aqueous solutions of volatile oils, are used as vehicles for water-soluble substances and salts. Their use is largely governed by flavor, color, and solubility characteristics of the active medicinal agent. Table A–I–2 lists the more commonly employed official vehicles.

Because of its flexibility, iso-alcoholic elixir can be used to advantage in numerous extemporaneous prescription orders. It consists of two formulas, designated as *low-alcoholic elixir* (8 to 10% alcohol) and *high-alcoholic elixir* (73 to 78% alcohol). *Iso-alcoholic elixir* represents a mixture of the two formulas adjusted by the pharmacist to meet the alcoholic requirements of the drugs for which it serves as a vehicle or diluent. For example, if the physician wishes to prescribe an elixir, tincture, or fluidextract in a vehicle in order to increase the volume and thus make the dose more convenient to measure, it is important that the alcoholic strength of the vehicle be approximately the same as that of the preparation to be diluted; otherwise, the active principles may be precipitated. The physician need not remember the particular alcohol concentration required but should merely prescribe the iso-alcoholic elixir. The pharmacist then ascertains how much of the elixirs of low and high alcohol content to mix in order to obtain the same alcohol concentration as the solution of drug that is being prescribed.

Incompatibilities. This term is applied when physical, chemical, or therapeutic problems arise during the compounding, dispensing, or administration of the prescribed medication. A *physical* incompatibility occurs when liquefaction, deliquescence, precipitation, incomplete solution, or other change in physical state takes place. A *chemical* incompatibility occurs when two ingredients in a prescription react chemi-

cally to form new compounds. *Therapeutic* incompatibilities or adverse drug interactions are discussed in Chapter 3 and Appendix III. The avoidance and prevention of physical and chemical incompatibilities are largely the responsibility of the pharmacist and the industrial pharmaceutical research scientist.

Prescription Refills. Prescription drugs were formerly controlled by several federal laws, including the Federal Food, Drug, and Cosmetic Act, the Federal Narcotic–Internal Revenue Regulations (historically known as the Harrison Narcotic Act), and the Federal Marihuana Regulations. On May 1, 1971, the *Comprehensive Drug Abuse Prevention and Control Act* of 1970 became fully effective and, except for the Durham-Humphrey Amendment (Section 503B), repealed all the aforementioned laws controlling prescription drugs.

The Durham-Humphrey Amendment defines certain types of drugs that may be sold by the pharmacist only on the prescription order of a practitioner licensed by law to administer such drugs. These drugs are required to bear the label, *"Caution: Federal law prohibits dispensing without a prescription."* Under the Durham-Humphrey Amendment, a prescription order cannot be refilled unless authorized by the prescriber. The prescriber may indicate the number of times a prescription order may be refilled in the blank space in the statement, "Refill _____ times"; this statement may be printed on the prescription order blank.

The Comprehensive Drug Abuse Prevention and Control Act, commonly referred to as the Controlled Substances Act (*see* below), is designed to control the distribution of all depressant and stimulant drugs (*e.g.*, opioids, barbitu-

Table A–I–2. SELECTED VEHICLES FOR EXTEMPORANEOUS PRESCRIPTIONS

VEHICLE	FLAVOR	COLOR	ACID-BASE PROPERTIES	PERCENT ALCOHOL	USE
Elixirs					
Aromatic	Orange	Colorless	Neutral	21–23	General
Iso-alcoholic	Orange	Colorless	Neutral	8–78	Alcohol-soluble drugs
Syrups					
Acacia	Vanilla	Colorless	Acid	0	Insoluble drugs
Cherry	Cherry	Red	Acid	1–2	Bitter and salty drugs
Cocoa	Chocolate	Brown	Neutral	0	Children
Orange	Orange	Straw	Acid	2–5	Salty drugs
Tolu balsam	Aromatic	Red	Alkaline	3–5	Children
Aromatic Waters					
Orange flower	Orange	Colorless	Neutral	0	General
Peppermint	Peppermint	Colorless	Neutral	0	General

rates, and amphetamines) and other drugs with abuse potential as designated by the Drug Enforcement Administration, Department of Justice. This act requires the pharmacist to keep a record of the receipt and the disposition of all Controlled Substances; such drugs are identified on the label of the *original* container by a symbol, consisting of either the Roman numeral of the schedule within a large letter "C" or the letter "C" followed by the schedule (*e.g.,* C-II). The records must be maintained for a period of at least 2 years and be available for inspection by authorized persons. Prescription orders for Controlled Substances in schedule II must be typewritten, or written in ink or indelible pencil, and signed by the practitioner; such prescription orders *cannot be refilled.* The physician must write a new prescription if administration of the drug is to be continued. Prescription orders for drugs covered by schedule III or IV may be issued either orally or in writing by a practitioner and may be refilled, *if so authorized, not more than five times* and may *not* be filled or refilled *more than 6 months* after date of issue. After five refills or after 6 months, the prescribing practitioner may write or authorize a new prescription order. Drugs in schedule V may be prescribed the same as drugs in schedules III and IV, and, under certain conditions, may be dispensed without a prescription.

Physicians should do all they can to prevent abuses of prescription orders. It is a good practice to write out the number of refills desired during a specific time period on every prescription order; Arabic numerals may easily be altered and, if not indicated, instructions may easily be forged. Furthermore, when an authorization for refill is not given on the prescription order, it cannot be refilled without *personal* authorization by the prescriber.

Controlled Substances Act. Various federal, state, and city laws exist to control the standard of purity of drugs and their manufacture, sale, and dispensing. These laws must be known and observed by the practitioner. The most stringent law takes precedence, whether it be federal, state, or local. The most important laws are embodied in the *Comprehensive Drug Abuse Prevention and Control Act of 1970* (*see* Federal Regulations, April 24, 1971). This act divides opioids and other drugs into five schedules.

Schedule 1. Drugs in this schedule have a high potential for abuse and *no* currently accepted medical use in the United States. Examples of such drugs include heroin, marihuana, peyote, mescaline, psilocybin, tetrahydrocannabinols, LSD, ketobemidone, levomoramide, racemoramide, benzylmorphine, dihydromor-

phine, morphine methylsulfonate, nicocodeine, nicomorphine, methaqualone, and others. Substances listed in this schedule are not for prescription use but may be obtained for research and instructional use or for chemical analysis by application to the Drug Enforcement Administration, Department of Justice (Form 225), supported by a protocol of the proposed use.

Schedule II. Drugs in this schedule have a high potential for abuse with severe liability to cause psychic or physical dependence. Schedule-II controlled substances consist of certain opioid drugs and drugs containing amphetamines or methamphetamines as the single active ingredient or in combination with each other. Examples of substances included in this schedule are opium, morphine, codeine, hydromorphone, methadone, meperidine, cocaine, oxycodone, anileridine, oxymorphone, dextroamphetamine, and methamphetamine. Also included in schedule II are phenmetrazine, methylphenidate, amobarbital, pentobarbital, secobarbital, etorphine hydrochloride, and diphenoxylate.

Schedule III. The drugs in this schedule have a potential for abuse that is less than for those in schedules I and II; their abuse may lead to moderate or low physical dependence or high psychological dependence. This schedule includes compounds containing limited quantities of certain opioid drugs and also certain nonopioid drugs, such as chlorhexadol, glutethimide, methyprylon, sulfondiethylmethane, sulfonmethane, nalorphine, benzphetamine, chlorphentermine, clortermine, phendimetrazine, and certain barbiturates (except those listed in another schedule).

Schedule IV. The drugs in this schedule have a low potential for abuse that leads only to limited physical dependence or psychological dependence relative to drugs in schedule III. In this schedule are barbital, phenobarbital, methylphenobarbital, chloral betaine, chloral hydrate, ethchlorvynol, ethinamate, meprobamate, paraldehyde, methohexital, fenfluramine, diethylpropion, phentermine, the benzodiazepines, mebutamate, and propoxyphene.

Schedule V. The drugs in this schedule have a potential for abuse that is less than those listed in schedule IV and consist of preparations containing moderate quantities of certain opioid drugs, generally for antitussive or antidiarrheal purposes, which may be distributed without a prescription order. Substances in this schedule may be prescribed the same as those in schedules III and IV. In addition, drugs in schedule V may be dispensed without a prescription order provided (1) such distribution is made only by a pharmacist; (2) not more than 240 ml of any schedule-V substance containing opium, nor more than 120 ml or more than 24 solid dosage units of any other controlled substance, is sold to the same consumer in any given 48-hour period without a valid prescription order; (3) the purchaser at retail is at least 18 years of age; (4) the pharmacist obtains suitable identification; (5) a record book is maintained that contains the name and address of the purchaser, name and quantity of Controlled Substance purchased, date of sale, and initials of the pharmacist; and (6) other federal, state, or local law does not require a prescription order.

The label of any Controlled Substance in schedule II, III, or IV, when dispensed to or for a patient pursuant to a prescription order, *must* contain the following warning; *"Caution: Federal law prohibits the transfer of this drug to any person other than the patient for whom it was prescribed."*

In order to prescribe Controlled Substances, a physician must register with the Drug Enforcement Administration, Registration Section, Department of Justice. If a physician has more than one office in which he administers and/or dispenses any of the drugs listed in the five schedules, he then is required to register at each office. The registration must be renewed annually. The number on the certificate of registration must be indicated on all prescription orders for Controlled Substances. The physician must also file an inventory of the Controlled Substances on hand every 2 years; file a revised form if his location is changed; keep a record of controlled substances listed in schedules II through V that he dispenses, if he regularly charges patients either separately or together with professional services for such medication; and *order his supplies of controlled substances listed in schedule II for dispensing or administration on special order forms,* obtainable from the Drug Enforcement Administration, Registration Section, P.O. Box 28083, Central Station, Washington, D. C. 20005.

Both the physician and the pharmacist are legally responsible for the proper prescribing and dispensing of drugs covered by the Controlled Substances Act. There are many technical details in the regulations and, as a result, the physician may innocently violate the law in his professional use of Controlled Substances, especially as related to the use of opioids for patients with incurable diseases or in the management of drug addiction. An outline of the Controlled Substances Act of 1970, entitled *A Manual for the Medical Practitioner,* is especially informative on these problems. Copies may be obtained from the Drug Enforcement Administration at the address indicated in the previous paragraph.

PATIENT COMPLIANCE INSTRUCTION

Most physicians assume that once the diagnosis is made and the prescription order is written the patient will benefit from his diagnostic and therapeutic acumen. Unfortunately, drug treatment of any kind is often compromised by lack of full compliance by the patient. Common errors of compliance to a regimen by a patient may be of omission, purpose (taking medicines for the wrong reasons), dosage, timing or sequence, adding medications not prescribed, or premature termination of drug therapy. In addition, from 3 to 18% of patients fail to have their prescription orders "filled" within 10 days (Boyd *et al.,* 1974). Observations of this kind suggest that attention should be directed to some of the basic principles of instruction of the patient about the importance of compliance.

Factors Associated with Noncompliance. The drug defaulter, like the placebo reactor, is not a readily identifiable individual (Caron and Roth, 1968; Blackwell, 1973). Patients who are unreliable under one treatment regimen may not be under another. Porter (1969), after a detailed study of this problem, concluded that ". . . it has not proved possible to identify an uncooperative type. Every patient is a potential defaulter; compliance can never be assumed." Nevertheless, Gillum and Barsky (1974), based on a critical review of the literature, reported that psychological, environmental, and social factors, characteristics of the drug regimen, and the nature of the physician-patient interaction were most consistently related to noncompliance. Some of these factors are briefly reviewed here in order to indicate some of the steps that the physician can take to improve patient compliance. For a more detailed analysis, the reader is referred to several excellent articles and reviews (Blackwell, 1972, 1976, 1979; Hussar, 1975; Lasagna, 1976; Dunbar and Stunkard, 1979; Leventhal *et al.,* 1984).

The Patient's Illness. After the prescription order has been written, the physician should make sure the patient understands the nature and prognosis of his illness, what he may expect from his medication (both acceptable and unacceptable unwanted effects, as well as signs of efficacy that may help to enforce his compliance). The physician should explain how the medication alters the disease process. Patients frequently discontinue taking a medication such as penicillin for streptococcal pharyngitis because they have not been told the necessity for continuing the drug after the acute symptoms have subsided. Similarly, patients taking antidepressant medication frequently discontinue treatment because the physician failed to mention the untoward effects that might appear or to advise the patient that 10 days or more may elapse before he notices any improvement. Patients with chronic illnesses are prone to lapse in compliance, especially if the treatment is prophylactic or suppressive, the condition is associated with only mild or no symptoms, or the consequences of missing a dose or two are not immediate. In contrast, when relapse is immediate or severe, the patient is much less likely to deviate from the prescribed regimen.

The Patient. Errors and noncompliance occur more frequently at the extremes of age and in patients who live alone. Geriatric patients present problems because of lapses in memory or self-neglect. Poor compliance among children is related to problems of taste and swallowing, although the mother's impression of the severity of the illness has a marked influence on compliance in pediatric patients. The physician must explore the patient's eating, sleeping, and working habits. Otherwise, he might prescribe a drug to be taken three times a day with meals for a patient who either eats only twice a day or sleeps all day and works at night. Educational, economic, ethnic, and personality factors may also influence patient compliance. According to Blackwell (1973), the less educated, poor patient with a risk-prone personality is more likely to be a drug defaulter. In the United States the problem is severe with patients whose primary language is not English, and who may require carefully worded written and oral instructions in that language.

The Physician. Studies by Mazzullo and associates (1974) suggest that physicians who do not explain the reasons for their decisions may be a major determinant of the patient's noncompliance. The physician's relationship with the patient and how clearly he explains the treatment regimen have a powerful impact on compliance. Thus, the physician-patient relationship should be viewed as a process of instruction and motivation for both parties as they enter into a health-related contract. The effectiveness of physician-patient communication is inversely related to the error rate in the taking of drugs. Directions on prescription orders should include all the details necessary for a patient to know how, with what, when, and how long to take the medication.

The Medication Prescribed. Multiple medications, frequent-dose regimens, and the physical features of the medication itself often foster poor compliance. Patients taking three or more medications are less likely to use them as directed. Likewise, the more frequently a medica-

tion is directed to be taken, the less likely it will be taken as prescribed. Hulka and associates (1976) reported that omission rates doubled when the number of medications prescribed was increased from one to four. Likewise, the rates doubled when administration was increased from once daily to four times daily. Considerable confusion may also develop when multiple drugs of similar appearance are prescribed for the same patient, as has been emphasized by Mazzullo (1972) and Mazzullo and Lasagna (1972). They have also stressed the desirability of providing the patient with an identifying name for each medication prescribed, for example, "heart pill" or "water pill," assuming he has been told what each medication is designed to accomplish. The color plates in the *Physicians' Desk Reference* can be used to show patients what their medication will look like.

Patients frequently discontinue medication upon the appearance of minor untoward effects because they have not been told that such reactions are common and not to be feared. Special instruction should be given the patient relative to symptoms that indicate overdosage, such as dizziness from antihypertensive agents. Before this is done, however, the doctor should determine (by taking a nonleading history) whether the patient already has the symptoms that could later be misinterpreted as drug related. Such a misunderstanding could lead to an unjustifiable discontinuation of a very useful drug.

The Treatment Environment. The setting in which the prescribed medication is to be taken has a marked influence on compliance. A series of studies in the same psychiatric hospital revealed that noncompliance increased progressively from 19% in inpatients to 37% in day patients and 48% in outpatients (Hare and Wilcox, 1967). This emphasizes the need to teach the principles of self-medication before the patient leaves the hospital and the added responsibility the physician must assume if he is to achieve satisfactory compliance with patients he sees in clinics and in his private office.

Consequences of Noncompliance. The consequences of noncompliance, although quite apparent, are often not fully appreciated by either the physician or the patient. *Underutilization of the prescribed drug* deprives the patient of the intended therapeutic benefits. This may result in a recurrence or worsening of the illness, emergence of antibiotic-resistant microorganisms, or the prescribing of a larger dose or a more potent agent that could lead to toxicity if compliance is improved. Before a patient is judged to be unresponsive or not optimally controlled with initial therapy, some effort should be made to determine whether the medication is being taken according to instructions. Thus, 75% of patients referred for evaluation of "refractoriness" to phenytoin were found not to be taking the drug as prescribed (Borofsky *et al.*, 1972). The compliance rates of some groups of patients on digoxin, hydrochlorothiazide, and potassium chloride were 92%, 83%, and 60%, respectively (Brook *et al.*, 1971). Hussar (1975) has suggested that the latter illustration indicates that noncompliance is a contributing factor to the frequent cases of hypokalemia and toxicity of cardiac glycosides.

Overutilization of the prescribed drug places the patient at increased risk of adverse reactions. Such problems may develop rather innocently; frequently the patient either forgets a dose and hence doubles the next one or adopts an attitude that if one tablet is good, two must be better. A study of the profile of medications indicates that overutilization of drugs accounts for 65% of problems with compliance (Solomon *et al.*, 1974).

The prevalence of noncompliance has raised questions relative to the effect of this variable on clinical trials of new drugs. Although numerous controls are built into such studies, the difficulties associated with noncompliance must, to some extent, compromise the ability to establish true rates of efficacy and toxicity of any given agent.

The Pharmacist and Patient Compliance. The pharmacist is usually the last professional to be in contact with the ambulatory private patient (or his representative) before medication is started. Pharmacists can effectively cooperate with the physician in education about compliance and can counsel the patient on how to take his medication. Cooperation between physician and pharmacist is in the interest of optimal drug therapy, especially with patients who are likely to make errors in taking drugs. Unfortunately, in certain states such cooperation may be in conflict with laws designed to prevent collusion between pharmacists and physicians.

American Pharmaceutical Association and American Society of Internal Medicine. Prescription writing and prescription labeling. *J. Am. Pharm. Assoc.*, **1974**, *NS 14*, 654.

Blackwell, B. The drug defaulter. *Clin. Pharmacol. Ther.*, **1972**, *13*, 841–848.

——. Patient compliance. *N. Engl. J. Med.*, **1973**, *289*, 249–252.

——. Treatment adherence. *Br. J. Psychiatry*, **1976**, *129*, 513–531.

——. The drug regime and treatment compliance. In,

Compliance in Health Care. (Haynes, R. B.; Taylor, D. W.; and Sackett, D.; eds.) Johns Hopkins University Press, Baltimore, **1979**.

Borofsky, L. G.; Louis, S.; Kutt, H.; and Roginsky, M. Diphenylhydantoin: efficacy, toxicity, and dose-serum level relationships in children. *J. Pediatr.*, **1972**, *81*, 995–1002.

Boyd, J. R.; Covington, T. R.; Stanaszck, W. F.; and Coussons, R. T. Drug defaulting—Part II: Analysis of noncompliance patterns. *Am. J. Hosp. Pharm.*, **1974**, *31*, 485–491.

Brook, R. H.; Appel, F. A.; Avery, C.; Orman, M.; and Stevenson, R. I. Effectiveness of inpatient follow-up care. *N. Engl. J. Med.*, **1971**, *285*, 1509–1514.

Caron, H. S., and Roth, H. P. Patients' cooperation with a medical regimen: difficulties in identifying the noncooperator. *J.A.M.A.*, **1968**, *203*, 922–926.

Committee on Drugs, American Academy of Pediatrics. Inaccuracies in administering liquid medication. *Pediatrics*, **1975**, *56*, 327–328.

Dunbar, J. M., and Stunkard, A. J. Adherence to diet and drug regime. In, *Nutrition, Lipids, and Coronary Heart Disease.* (Levy, R.; Rifkind, B.; Dennis, B.; and Ernest, N.; eds.) Raven Press, New York, **1979**, pp. 391–423.

Food and Drug Administration. *Approved Prescription Drug Products with Therapeutic Equivalence Evaluations*, 4th ed. U.S. Department of Health and Human Services, Washington, D. C., **1983**.

Gillum, R. F., and Barsky, J. Diagnosis and management of patient noncompliance. *J.A.M.A.*, **1974**, *228*, 1563–1567.

Hare, E. H., and Wilcox, D. R. C. Do psychiatric inpatients take their pills? *Br. J. Psychiatry*, **1967**, *113*, 1435–1439.

Hulka, B. S.; Cassel, J. C.; and Kupper, L. L. Disparities between medications prescribed and consumed among chronic disease patients. In, *Patient Compliance.* (Lasagna, L., ed.) Futura Publishing Co., Mount Kisco, N.Y., **1976**, pp. 123–152.

Hussar, D. A. Patient noncompliance. *J. Am. Pharm. Assoc.*, **1975**, *NS 15*, 183–190, 201.

Jerome, J. B., and Sagan, P. The USAN nomenclature system. *J.A.M.A.*, **1975**, *232*, 294–299.

Lasagna, L. (ed.). *Patient Compliance.* Futura Publishing Co., Mount Kisco, N. Y., **1976**.

Leventhal, H.; Zimmerman, R.; and Gutmann, M. Compliance: a topic for behavioral medicine research. In, *Handbook of Behavioral Medicine.* (Gentry, D., ed.) Guilford Press, New York, **1984**.

Mazzullo, J. The nonpharmacologic basis of therapeutics. *Clin. Pharmacol. Ther.*, **1972**, *13*, 157–158.

Mazzullo, J.; Cohn, K.; Lasagna, L.; and Griner, P. Variations in interpretation of prescription instructions. *J.A.M.A.*, **1974**, *227*, 929–931.

Mazzullo, J. M., and Lasagna, L. Take thou . . . but is your patient really taking what you prescribed? *Drug Ther.*, **1972**, *2*, 11–15.

National Prescription Audit: General Information Report, 23rd ed. IMS America, Ltd., Ambler, Pa., **1983**.

Porter, A. M. W. Drug defaulting in general practice. *Br. Med. J.*, **1969**, *1*, 218–222.

Sackett, D. L. The magnitude of compliance and noncompliance. In, *Compliance with Therapeutic Regimens.* (Sackett, D. L., and Haynes, R. B., eds.) Johns Hopkins University Press, Baltimore, **1976**, pp. 9–25.

Solomon, D. K.; Baumgartner, R. P.; Glascock, L. M.; Briscoe, M. E.; and Billups, N. F. Use of medication profiles to detect potential therapeutic problems in ambulatory patients. *Am. J. Hosp. Pharm.*, **1974**, *31*, 348–354.

APPENDIX

II DESIGN AND OPTIMIZATION OF DOSAGE REGIMENS; PHARMACOKINETIC DATA

Leslie Z. Benet and Lewis B. Sheiner

The objective of this appendix is to present pharmacokinetic data in a format that allows the clinician to make rational choices of doses of drugs. Table A–II–1 (pages 1668–1733) contains quantitative information about the absorption, distribution, and elimination of drugs and the effects of disease states on these processes, as well as information concerning the correlation of efficacy and toxicity with measured concentrations of drugs in plasma. The general principles that are used to select the appropriate maintenance dose and dosing interval (and, where appropriate, the loading dose) for the average patient are described in Chapter 1. Discussion of individualization of these variables for a particular patient is presented here.

To utilize the data that are presented, one must understand clearance concepts and their application for the computation of drug-dosage regimens. One must also know average values of clearance for a number of drugs, as well as some measures of the extent and kinetics of drug absorption and distribution. The text that follows defines the eight basic parameters that are listed in the tabular material for each drug, as well as some factors that influence these values in both normal subjects and in patients with particular diseases.

It would obviously be most useful if there was a consensus about the correct value for a given pharmacokinetic parameter, rather than being faced with 10 or 20 separate (and often disparate) estimates of that parameter. Unfortunately, a consensus has been reached for only a very limited number of drugs. In Table A–II–1, single values for each parameter and for its variability (standard deviation) in the population have been selected from the literature, based on the scientific judgment of the authors. Values in the tables are those determined in healthy normal adults, unless otherwise indicated by footnotes. The direction of change for these values in particular disease states is noted next to the average value. Three or four important references are provided for each drug. In most cases, at least one of these references represents a recent review of the clinical pharmacokinetic properties of the drug. Further information can usually be

found in textbooks that detail the effects of disease and altered physiological states on pharmacokinetic parameters (Evans *et al.*, 1980; Gibaldi and Prescott, 1983; Benet *et al.*, 1984).

TABULATED PHARMACOKINETIC PARAMETERS

Each of the eight parameters that are presented in Table A–II–1 has been discussed in detail in Chapter 1. The following discussion focuses on the format in which the values are presented, as well as on factors (physiological or pathological) that influence the parameters.

Availability. The extent of availability of the drug following oral administration is expressed as a percentage of the dose. This value represents the percentage of an oral dose that is available to produce pharmacological actions—the fraction of the oral dose that reaches the left ventricle in an active form. *Fractional availability* (F) is a similar parameter used elsewhere in this appendix; this value varies from 0 to 1. Measures of the *rate* of availability are not provided in Table A–II–1. Since pharmacokinetic concepts are most useful in the design of multiple dosage regimens, the *extent* rather than the rate of availability is more critical to obtain an appropriate concentration of drug in the body (*see* Chapter 1).

It is important to keep in mind that poor patient compliance may be mistaken for decreased bioavailability. A true decrease in bioavailability may result from a poorly formulated dosage form that fails to disintegrate or dissolve in the gastrointestinal fluids, interactions between drugs in the gastrointestinal tract, metabolism of the drug in the gastrointestinal tract, and/or first-pass hepatic metabolism or biliary excretion (*see* Chapter 1). Hepatic disease in particular may cause increased availability either because hepatic metabolic capacity decreases or because of the development of vascular shunts around the liver.

Urinary Excretion of Unchanged Drug. The second parameter in Table A–II–1 is the amount of drug eventually excreted unchanged in the urine, expressed as a percentage of the administered dose. Values represent the percentage expected in a healthy young adult (creatinine clearance greater than 100 ml/min). When possible, the value listed is that determined after bolus intravenous administration of the drug, where availability is assumed to be 100%. If the drug is given orally, this parameter may also reflect loss of drug due to low availability; such values are indicated by a footnote.

Renal disease is the primary factor that causes changes in this parameter. This is especially true when alternate pathways of elimination are available; thus, as renal function decreases, a greater fraction of the dose is available for elimination by other routes. Since renal function decreases as a function of age, the percentage of drug excreted unchanged also usually decreases with age when alternate pathways of elimination are available. For a number of acidic and basic drugs with values of pK_a in the range of the usual pH of urine, changes in the latter will affect the rate or extent of urinary excretion (see Chapter 1).

Binding to Plasma Proteins. The tabulated value is the percentage of drug in the plasma that is bound to plasma proteins at concentrations of the drug that are achieved clinically. In almost all cases the values are from measurements performed in vitro (rather than from measurements of binding to the proteins in plasma that was obtained from patients to whom drug had been administered). When a single mean value is presented, there is no apparent change in this percentage over the range of concentrations normally found in the patient population taking the drug. In cases where saturation of binding is approached at usual plasma concentrations, values are provided at concentrations that correspond to the lower and higher limits of the usual range.

Plasma protein binding is primarily affected by disease states (such as hepatic disease) that alter the concentration of albumin or other proteins in plasma that bind drugs. Some metabolic states and conditions such as uremia also change the affinity of binding for some drugs. Such changes in protein binding as a function of disease can dramatically affect the volume of distribution of a drug.

Clearance. Total systemic clearance of drug from plasma (see equation 3, Chapter 1) is given in Table A–II–1; values are usually reported in units of ml $\cdot$ min^{-1} $\cdot$ kg^{-1}. In some cases, separate values for renal and nonrenal clearance are also provided. For some drugs, particularly those that are predominantly excreted unchanged in the urine, equations are given that relate total or renal clearance to creatinine clearance (also expressed as ml $\cdot$ min^{-1} $\cdot$ kg^{-1}). For those drugs that exhibit saturation kinetics, K_m and V_m are given and represent, respectively, the plasma concentration at which half of the maximal rate of elimination is reached (in units of mass/volume) and the maximal rate of elimination (in units of mass $\cdot$ time^{-1} $\cdot$ kg of body weight^{-1}). The concentration of the drug in plasma (C_p) must, of course, be in the same units as K_m.

As discussed in Chapter 1, intrinsic clearance from blood is the maximal possible clearance by the organ responsible for elimination when blood flow (delivery) of drug is not limiting. Intrinsic clearance is tabulated for a few drugs. Note that intrinsic clearance is defined in terms of the concentration of drug in blood. If one wishes to relate changes in elimination of drug to pathological changes either in the organ itself or to blood flow to the organ, it is necessary to express clearance with respect to concentrations of drug in blood rather than those in plasma. This requires measurement of concentrations in whole blood or knowledge of the distribution of drug between plasma and red blood cells; such information is currently limited. Clearances from plasma are presented in Table A–II–1, since these are most useful to relate dosage of drug to concentrations of drugs in plasma that have been determined previously to be effective or toxic.

Clearance can be determined only when the fractional availability of the drug, F, is known. Therefore, to be accurate, clearances must be determined following intravenous dosage. When such data are not available, the ratio of CL/F is given; values of this kind are indicated by a footnote.

Clearance varies as a function of body size and, therefore, is presented in the table in units of ml $\cdot$ min^{-1} $\cdot$ kg of body weight^{-1}. Although normalization to measures of size other than weight may sometimes be appropriate, weight is so convenient that this offsets any small loss in accuracy, especially when dealing with adults.

Volume of Distribution. The total body volume of distribution at steady state (V_{ss}) is given in Table A–II–1 and is expressed in units of liters/kg.

When estimates of V_{ss} are not available, values for V_{area} are provided (see Chapter 1). These values are obtained by dividing clearance by the terminal rate constant for elimination. V_{area} is a convenient and easily calculated parameter. However, unlike V_{ss}, this volume term varies when the rate constant for drug elimination changes, even though there has been no change in the distribution space. Since the clinician may wish to know whether a particular disease state influences either clearance or the distribution of the drug within the body independently, it is preferable to define volume in terms of V_{ss}, a parameter that is theoretically independent of changes in the rate of elimination.

As is the case for clearance, V_{ss} is usually defined in the table in terms of the concentrations in plasma, rather than in blood. If data were not obtained after intravenous administration of the drug, a footnote will make clear that the parameter determined, V_{ss}/F, contains a measure of availability.

Volume of distribution is primarily a function of body size, and values in the table are given in liters/kg. As mentioned for clearance, normalization to measures of size other than weight may sometimes be appropriate.

Half-life. The time required for one half of the amount of drug in the body to be eliminated is provided. However, drug concentrations in plasma often follow a multiexponential pattern of decline when this value is measured as a function of time. The single number listed in each component of the table corresponds to the rate of elimination that describes the major fraction of total clearance of drug from the body. In many cases this half-life may correspond to the terminal log-linear rate of elimination. For some drugs, however, a more prolonged half-life may be observed at very low plasma concentrations when extremely sensitive assay technics are used. If this component accounts for only 10% of drug clearance, predictions of steady-state concentrations of drug in plasma will be in error by only 10% if this longer half-life is ignored, no matter how large its value. This is true because half-life is a function of both elimination and distribution, as discussed in Chapter 1.

Half-life is usually independent of body size, since it is a function of the ratio of two parameters, clearance and volume of distribution, each of which is proportional to body size.

Effective and Toxic Concentrations. There is no general agreement about the best way to describe the relationship between the concentration of drug in plasma and its effect. Many different kinds of data are presented in the literature, and extraction of a single parameter or even a set of parameters is difficult. Furthermore, there may not be agreement as to which measures are most relevant. Footnotes are common in Table A–II–1 to indicate the meaning and relevance of these values; in many cases reference is made to a chapter in the text for discussion. This is particularly true for antimicrobial agents, since the effective concentration depends on the identity of the microorganism causing infection.

The relationships between the concentration of drug in plasma and the effect of the drug are imperfect, as might be expected (*see* Chapter 2). Little information is available about the variation between individuals of receptor number or affinity or subsequent coupling to a response, or about the effects of disease states on these factors. For many drugs, the form of the relationship between effect and plasma concentration is unknown. Because the concentration of free drug determines the degree of effect, changes in protein binding due to disease may be expected to cause changes in the *total* concentration of drug associated with a desired or an unwanted effect. It is also important to realize that concentration-effect relationships are only meaningful at steady state or during the terminal log-linear phase of the concentration versus time curve, when the ratio of the drug concentration at sites of action to that in the plasma can be expected to remain constant over time. Thus, when attempting to correlate pharmacokinetics with pharmacodynamics, the time of distribution of drug to its site of action must be taken into account (Holford and Sheiner, 1981).

ALTERATIONS OF PARAMETERS IN THE INDIVIDUAL PATIENT

The values in Table A–II–1 represent mean values for populations of normal adults, and it may be necessary to modify them for calculation of dosage regimens for individual patients. The fraction of free drug (α) in a given patient must be known to compute a desired steady-state concentration. The fraction available (F) and clearance must also be estimated to compute a maintenance dose. To calculate the loading dose and to estimate half-life and dosing interval, knowledge of the volume of distribution is needed. The figures in the table and the adjustments apply *only to adults* unless specifically designated otherwise. Although the values may sometimes, with caution, be applied to children in excess of about 30 kg (after proper adjustment for size; *see* below), it is best to consult a textbook of pediatrics or other source for definitive advice.

The segments of the table note the changes in the parameters occasioned by certain disease states. In most cases, a qualitative statement is made, such as "clearance decreased in hepatic disease." A reasonable quantitative translation is to multiply the value of the parameter by 0.5 for each applicable condition that is noted to decrease the parameter and to multiply it by 2 for each condition that is noted to increase the parameter. Such an adjustment can only be approximate; yet, since reliable data are limited, no better approach may be possible. The relevant literature should be consulted for more definitive quantitative information.

Protein Binding. Most acidic drugs that are extensively bound to plasma proteins are bound to albumin. Basic drugs, such as propranolol, are often bound to other plasma proteins (*e.g.,* α_1-acid glycoprotein). The degree of drug binding to proteins will differ in states that cause changes in the concentration of the binding proteins. Unfortunately, only albumin, among binding proteins, is commonly measured. For drugs that are bound to albumin (*alb*), a patient's fraction of free drug (α_{pt}) can be approximated from the following relationship:

$$\alpha_{pt} = 1 \bigg/ \left[\left(\frac{alb_{st}}{alb_{nl}} \right) \left(\frac{1 - \alpha_{nl}}{\alpha_{nl}} \right) + 1 \right] \qquad (1)$$

where alb_{nl} and α_{nl} refer to values of the concentration of albumin in plasma and the fraction of free drug in normal individuals, respectively. Use of this equation assumes that the molar concentration of drug is far less than that of albumin, that only one type of drug binding site is present on albumin, and that there are no cooperative binding interactions. It cannot, therefore, be exact. However, it is a reasonable approximation and, in the absence of actual measurement of the patient's fraction of free drug, can prove quite useful.

Clearance. Clearance must often be adjusted for alterations in renal function. The quantities required for this adjustment are the fraction of normal renal function remaining and the fraction of drug usually excreted unchanged in the urine. The latter quantity appears in the table; the former can be estimated as the ratio of the patient's creatinine clearance to a normal value (120 ml/min per 70 kg). If creatinine clearance has not been measured, it may be estimated from measurements of the concentration of creatinine in serum, using a number of different equations or nomograms. One such is to estimate the fraction of normal renal function present (*rfx*) as the reciprocal of the patient's serum creatinine concentration, minus 0.01 for each year of age over 40. This is a crude estimate, but more accurate ones are seldom justified or necessary, since the whole process of adjustment of clearance is already approximate because of

considerable unpredictable interindividual variation in clearance, which is independent of renal function. The following equation for adjustment of clearance uses the quantities just discussed:

$$rf_{pt} = 1 - fe_{nl}(1 - rfx_{pt}) \qquad (2)$$

where fe_{nl} is the fraction of drug excreted unchanged in normal individuals (*see* table). The renal factor (rf_{pt}) is the value that, when multiplied by normal total clearance, gives the total clearance of the drug adjusted for disturbances of renal function.

Example. Clearance of terbutaline in a patient with depressed renal function (creatinine clearance = 40 ml $\cdot$ min^{-1} $\cdot$ 70 kg^{-1}) may be estimated as follows:

$$\begin{aligned}
rfx_{pt} &= 40 \text{ ml/min} \div 120 \text{ ml/min} = 0.33 \\
fe_{nl} &= 0.57 \ (see \text{ listing for terbutaline}) \\
rf_{pt} &= 1 - 0.57 \ (1 - 0.33) = 0.62 \\
CL_{pt} &= CL_{nl} \cdot rf_{pt} \\
CL_{pt} &= (3.02 \text{ ml} \cdot \text{min}^{-1} \cdot \text{kg}^{-1}) \ (0.62) \\
&= 1.87 \text{ ml} \cdot \text{min}^{-1} \cdot \text{kg}^{-1}
\end{aligned}$$

Adjustment of clearance must also be made for the size of the patient. For convenience, the figures in the table are normalized to weight. However, clearance of drug often varies in proportion to metabolic rate, which is best related to weight to the 0.75 power. To take this into account, the clearance figure in the table can be multiplied by the factor *wf*, instead of by weight:

$$wf = Wt_{nl}(Wt_{pt}/Wt_{nl})^{0.75} \qquad (3)$$

which for weight in kg (where $Wt_{nl} = 70$ kg) becomes:

$$wf = 2.9(Wt_{pt})^{0.75} \qquad (4)$$

Calculation of the weight factor seldom pays for itself by yielding significantly more accurate estimates. It should be done, however, for patients at extremes of size, especially the very obese.

If drug elimination is proportional to the free (rather than the total) concentration of drug in plasma, clearance is then further adjusted by multiplying it by the ratio of the normal free fraction to the free fraction of the patient, calculated as indicated previously.

All the adjustments to clearance should be applied simultaneously. That is, the figure in the table is multiplied by a weight factor (usually weight itself), *and* multiplied by the binding correction, if applicable, *and* multiplied by the renal correction factor, if applicable, *and,* finally, multiplied by the appropriate values of 0.5 and/ or 2 for other factors that are present and qualitatively indicated to modify clearance. Obviously, if a quantitative correction is made for renal function, a qualitative one (multiplication by 0.5) should not also be made for this same factor.

Volume of Distribution. Volume of distribution should be adjusted for the modifying factors indicated in Table A–II–1, as well as for size. The figures in the table are normalized to weight. Unlike clearance, volume of distribution is probably most often proportional to weight itself. Whether or not this is so, however, depends on the actual sites of distribution of drug, and no absolute rule applies.

Whether to adjust volume of distribution for changes in binding to plasma proteins cannot be decided in general, since the decision critically depends on whether the factors that alter binding to plasma proteins also alter binding to tissues. In such cases the qualitative changes in volume of distribution are indicated in the table. Again, each adjustment to volume of distribution should be made independently of any other, and the final estimate should reflect all adjustments simultaneously.

Half-life. Finally, half-life may be estimated from the adjusted estimates of clearance and volume of distribution:

$$t_{1/2} = 0.693 \ V_{pt}/CL_{pt} \qquad (5)$$

Since, historically, half-life has been the parameter most often measured, qualitative changes for this parameter are almost always given in the table.

INDIVIDUALIZATION OF DOSAGE

By using the parameters for the individual patient, calculated as described above, initial dos-ing regimens may be chosen. The maintenance dose may be calculated with equation 16, Chapter 1, and the estimated values for CL and F for the individual patient. The target concentration may need to be adjusted for changes in protein binding in the patient, as described above. The loading dose may be calculated by use of equation 20 in Chapter 1 and the estimated parameters for V_{ss} and F. A particular dosing interval may be chosen; the maximal and minimal steady concentrations can be calculated by using equations 18 and 19 in Chapter 1, and these can be compared with the efficacious and toxic concentrations listed for the drug. As with the target concentration, these values may need to be adjusted for changes in the extent of protein binding. Use of equations 18 and 19 also requires estimates of values for F, V_{ss}, and k ($k = 0.693/t_{1/2}$) for the individual patient.

Note that these adjustments of the pharmacokinetic parameters for an individual patient are suggested for the rational choice of initial dosing regimen. As emphasized in Chapter 1, measurements of drug concentrations in the patient can then be used to adjust the dosage regimen to achieve the desired range of concentrations.

Benet, L. Z.; Massoud, N.; and Gambertoglio, J. G. (eds.). *Pharmacokinetic Basis for Drug Treatment.* Raven Press, New York, **1984.**

Evans, W. E.; Schentag, J. J.; and Jusko, W. J. (eds.). *Applied Pharmacokinetics: Principles of Therapeutic Drug Monitoring.* Applied Therapeutics, Inc., San Francisco, **1980.**

Gibaldi, M., and Prescott, L. (eds.). *Handbook of Clinical Pharmacokinetics.* ADIS Health Science Press, New York, **1983.** (A compilation of review articles that appeared in the journal *Clinical Pharmacokinetics* between 1976 and 1980, with additional references through 1981 added.)

Holford, N. H. G., and Sheiner, L. B. Understanding the dose-effect relationship: clinical application of pharmacokinetic-pharmacodynamic models. *Clin. Pharmacokinet.*, **1981,** *6,* 429–453.

Table A–II–1. PHARMACOKINETIC DATA

AVAILABILITY (ORAL) (%)	URINARY EXCRETION (%)	BOUND IN PLASMA (%)	CLEARANCE ($ml \cdot min^{-1} \cdot kg^{-1}$)	VOL. DIST. (liters/kg)	HALF-LIFE (hours)	EFFECTIVE CONCENTRATIONS	TOXIC CONCENTRATIONS

ACEBUTOLOL [a] (Chapter 9)

AVAILABILITY (ORAL) (%)	URINARY EXCRETION (%)	BOUND IN PLASMA (%)	CLEARANCE ($ml \cdot min^{-1} \cdot kg^{-1}$)	VOL. DIST. (liters/kg)	HALF-LIFE (hours)	EFFECTIVE CONCENTRATIONS	TOXIC CONCENTRATIONS
37 ± 12 [b]	40 ± 11	26 ± 3	6.8 ± 0.8 [c] $\longleftrightarrow$ Urem	1.2 ± 0.3	2.7 ± 0.4 [c] $\longleftrightarrow$ Urem	[a]	—

a An acetylated metabolite, diacetolol, which may have pharmacological activity, is present at steady state at concentrations 2.7 times those of acebutolol.

b Some increase in availability (perhaps to 50%) occurs at higher doses and at steady state.

c Prolonged half-life and decreased clearance of diacetolol in uremia.

ACETAMINOPHEN [a] (Chapter 29)

AVAILABILITY (ORAL) (%)	URINARY EXCRETION (%)	BOUND IN PLASMA (%)	CLEARANCE ($ml \cdot min^{-1} \cdot kg^{-1}$)	VOL. DIST. (liters/kg)	HALF-LIFE (hours)	EFFECTIVE CONCENTRATIONS	TOXIC CONCENTRATIONS
88 ± 15	3 ± 1 $\longleftrightarrow$ Neo, Child	0 at < 60 ng/ml	5.0 ± 1.4 [b] $\downarrow$ Hep [c] $\longleftrightarrow$ Aged $\uparrow$ Obes, HTh	0.95 ± 0.12 [b] $\longleftrightarrow$ Aged, Hep [c], LTh, HTh	2.0 ± 0.4 $\longleftrightarrow$ Urem, Obes $\uparrow$ Neo, Hep [c] $\downarrow$ HTh	$10-20$ μg/ml [d]	>300 μg/ml [e]

a Values reported are for a linear kinetic model for doses less than 2 g; drug exhibits dose-dependent kinetics above this dose.

b Assuming 70-kg weight; reported range, 65–72 kg.

c Acetaminophen-induced hepatic damage.

d Analgesia, antipyresis.

e Hepatic toxicity for these concentrations 4 hours after ingestion; no hepatic toxicity if concentrations < 120 μg/ml 4 hours after ingestion.

N-ACETYLPROCAINAMIDE (Chapter 31)

AVAILABILITY (ORAL) (%)	URINARY EXCRETION (%)	BOUND IN PLASMA (%)	CLEARANCE ($ml \cdot min^{-1} \cdot kg^{-1}$)	VOL. DIST. (liters/kg)	HALF-LIFE (hours)	EFFECTIVE CONCENTRATIONS	TOXIC CONCENTRATIONS
83 ± 12	81 ± 1	10 ± 9	3.1 ± 0.4 $\downarrow$ Urem, Aged, CAD, Obes	1.4 ± 0.2 $\longleftrightarrow$ Urem, Aged, CAD	6.0 ± 0.2 $\uparrow$ Urem, Aged, CAD	21 μg/ml [a] $(12-35$ μg/ml)	—

a 70% reduction in mean frequency of premature ventricular contractions during long-term therapy.

ACETYLSALICYLIC ACID [a] (Chapter 29)

AVAILABILITY (ORAL) (%)	URINARY EXCRETION (%)	BOUND IN PLASMA (%)	CLEARANCE ($ml \cdot min^{-1} \cdot kg^{-1}$)	VOL. DIST. (liters/kg)	HALF-LIFE (hours)	EFFECTIVE CONCENTRATIONS	TOXIC CONCENTRATIONS
68 ± 3	1.4 ± 1.2 $\downarrow$ Urem	49 $\downarrow$ Urem	9.3 ± 1.1	0.15 ± 0.03	0.25 ± 0.03	See Salicylic Acid	See Salicylic Acid

a Values given are for unchanged acetylsalicylic acid. Acetylsalicylic acid is converted to salicylic acid during and after absorption. See salicylic acid for parameters for that compound.

ACYCLOVIR (Chapter 54)

15–30 [a]	75 ± 10	$CL = 3.37\ CL_{cr} + 0.41$ ↓ Neo → Child	0.69 ± 0.19 ↓ Neo → Urem	2.4 ± 0.7 ↑ Urem, Neo → Child	*See* Chapter 54	—

[a] Decreases with increasing dose.

ALFENTANIL (Chapter 14)

—	<1	90	7.6 ± 2.4 ∨ Aged	1.0 ± 0.3 ↔ Aged	1.6 ± 0.2 ↑ Aged	—

ALPRAZOLAM (Chapters 17, 19)

—	20	71 ± 3 ↑ Cirr ↔ Obes, Aged	1.4 ± 0.2 [a] ↓ Obes, Cirr, Aged [b]	1.03 ± 0.14 [a] ↔ Obes, Cirr, Aged	10.6 ± 3.1 ↑ Obes, Cirr, Aged [b]	—

[a] CL/F and V_{area}/F.
[b] In males only.

ALPRENOLOL [a] (Chapter 9)

8.6 ± 5.5 [b]	0.2 ± 0.1	85 ± 3	15 ± 5	3.3 ± 1.2 [c]	2.5 ± 0.6	25 ng/ml [d]	—

[a] Active metabolite, 4-OH alprenolol, present at concentrations of about 75% of those of alprenolol after oral administration.
[b] At a dose of 200 mg. First-pass hepatic metabolism, which is extensive, may be saturable.
[c] V_{area}.
[d] To achieve a 50% decrease in exercise-induced cardioacceleration.

Key: Adult = adults; Aged = aged; Alb = hypoalbuminemia; Arth = arthritis; Atr Fib = atrial fibrillation; AVH = acute viral hepatitis; Burn = burn patients; CAD = coronary artery disease; Celiac = celiac disease; CF = cystic fibrosis; CHF = congestive heart failure; Child = children; Cirr = cirrhosis; COPD = chronic obstructive pulmonary disease; CP = cor pulmonale; CPBS = cardiopulmonary bypass surgery; CRI = chronic respiratory insufficiency; Crohn = Crohn's disease; Cush = Cushing's syndrome; Epilep = epileptic; Fem = female; Hep = Hepatitis; HL = hyperlipoproteinemia; HTh = hyperthyroid; Inflam = inflammation; LTh = hypothyroid; MI = myocardial infarction; Neo = neonate; NS = nephrotic syndrome; Obes = obese; Pneu = pneumonia; Preg = pregnant; Prem = premature; RA = rheumatoid arthritis; Smk = smoking; Tach = ventricular tachycardia; Ulcer = ulcer patients; Urem = uremia

References: *See* end of table.

Table A–II–1. PHARMACOKINETIC DATA (Continued)

AVAILABILITY (ORAL) (%)	URINARY EXCRETION (%)	BOUND IN PLASMA (%)	CLEARANCE ($ml \cdot min^{-1} \cdot kg^{-1}$)	VOL. DIST. (liters/kg)	HALF-LIFE (hours)	EFFECTIVE CONCENTRATIONS	TOXIC CONCENTRATIONS

AMIKACIN (Chapter 51)

| — | 98 | 4 ± 8 [a] | 1.3 ± 0.6 $CL = 0.6\ CL_{cr} + 0.14$ → Obes | 0.27 ± 0.06 ←→ Aged, Child ↓ Obes ↑ Neo | 2.3 ± 0.4 ↑ Urem ←→ Obes ↓ Burn, Child | See Chapter 51 | See Chapter 51 |

[a] At serum concentration of 15 μg/ml.

AMIODARONE [a] (Chapter 31)

| 35 ± 9 | 0 | 96.3 ± 0.6 | 1.9 ± 0.4 [b] | 66 ± 44 | 25 ± 12 days [c] | 0.5–2.5 μg/ml [d] | >2.5 μg/ml [d] |

[a] Significant concentrations of a desethyl metabolite are found (ratio of drug/metabolite ~1); however, the activity of the metabolite has not been determined.
[b] Blood-to-plasma ratio = 0.73 ± 0.06.
[c] Longer half-lives noted in patients (53 ± 24 days); all half-lives may be underestimated because of insufficient sampling.
[d] Suggested upper limit; no definitive data.

AMITRIPTYLINE [a] (Chapter 19)

| 48 ± 11 ←→ Aged | <2 | 94.8 ± 0.8 ←→ Aged ↑ HL | 12.5 ± 2.8 ←→ Aged, Smk | 14 ± 2 ↑ Aged | 16 ± 6 ↑ Aged | 60–220 ng/ml [b] | >1 μg/ml [c] |

[a] Active metabolite is nortriptyline.
[b] Optimal range of amitriptyline plus nortriptyline.
[c] Combined data for toxic effects of tricyclic antidepressants.

AMOXICILLIN (Chapter 50)

| 93 ± 10 | 52 ± 15 | 18 | 5.3 ± 1.3 ↓ Child ↓ Urem | 0.41 ± 0.18 ←→ Urem | 1.0 ± 0.1 ↓ Child ↑ Urem | See Chapter 50 | See Chapter 50 |

AMPHOTERICIN B [a] (Chapter 54)

| — | 3 | >90 | 0.43 ± 0.08 ←→ Urem | 4.0 ± 0.4 | 15 ± 2 days | See Chapter 54 | — |

[a] Based on data from two patients.

AMPICILLIN (Chapter 50)

62 ± 17	82 ± 10	18 ± 2 ↓ Neo	$CL = 1.7\,CL_{cr} + 0.21$ ←→ Cirr, Preg	0.28 ± 0.07 ←→ Urem, Preg ↑ Cirr	1.3 ± 0.2 ↑ Urem, Cirr, Neo ←→ Preg	*See* Chapter 50	*See* Chapter 50

AMRINONE (Chapter 30)

93 ± 12	25 ± 10	35–49	4.3 ± 1.5	1.2 ± 0.3	4.0 ± 1.6 ↑ CHF	—	>2.5 μg/ml [a]

[a] Thrombocytopenia.

ATENOLOL (Chapter 9)

56 ± 30 ←→ Aged, Preg	85	<5 [a]	$CL = 0.77\,CL_{cr} + 0.05$	0.55 ± 0.29 ←→ Urem	6.3 ± 1.8 ←→ Preg. HTh ↑ Urem	1.0 μg/ml [b]	—

[a] Blood-to-plasma ratio = 1.07 ± 0.25.
[b] To achieve a 30% reduction in exercise-induced cardioacceleration.

ATRACURIUM (Chapter 11)

—		—	5.1 ± 0.9	0.15 [a]	0.33 ± 0.04	0.65 μg/ml [b]	1.1 μg/ml [c]

[a] V_{area}.
[b] To achieve 50% depression of twitch tension.
[c] To achieve 90% depression of twitch tension.

Key: Adult = adults; Aged = aged; Alb = hypoalbuminemia; Arth = arthritis; Atr Fib = atrial fibrillation; AVH = acute viral hepatitis; Burn = burn patients; CAD = coronary artery disease; Celiac = celiac disease; CF = cystic fibrosis; CHF = congestive heart failure; Child = children; Cirr = cirrhosis; COPD = chronic obstructive pulmonary disease; CP = cor pulmonale; CPBS = cardiopulmonary bypass surgery; CRI = chronic respiratory insufficiency; Crohn = Crohn's disease; Cush = Cushing's syndrome; Epilep = epileptic; Fem = female; Hep = Hepatitis; HL = hyperlipoproteinemia; HTh = hyperthyroid; Inflam = inflammation; LTh = hypothyroid; MI = myocardial infarction; Neo = neonate; NS = nephrotic syndrome; Obes = obese; Pneu = pneumonia; Prem = premature; RA = rheumatoid arthritis; Smk = smoking; Tach = ventricular tachycardia; Ulcer = ulcer patients; Urem = uremia

References: *See* end of table.

1671

Table A–II–1. PHARMACOKINETIC DATA (Continued)

	AVAILABILITY (ORAL) (%)	URINARY EXCRETION (%)	BOUND IN PLASMA (%)	CLEARANCE $(ml \cdot min^{-1} \cdot kg^{-1})$	VOL. DIST. $(liters/kg)$	HALF-LIFE $(hours)$	EFFECTIVE CONCENTRATIONS	TOXIC CONCENTRATIONS
AZATHIOPRINE [a] (Chapter 55)	60 ± 31 [b]	<2	—	57 ± 31 [c]	0.81 ± 0.65 [c]	0.16 ± 0.07 [c] ←→ Urem	—	—
AZLOCILLIN (Chapter 50)	—	65 ± 9	28 ± 6 ←→ Urem	Dose-dependent [a] → Urem ←→ CF	0.22 ± 0.06 ←→ Urem	1.0 ± 0.2 ↑ Urem, Neo, Prem ←→ CF	See Chapter 50	—
BETAMETHASONE (Chapter 63)	72 [a]	4.8 ± 1.4 ←→ Preg	64 ± 6 [b] ←→ Preg	2.9 ± 0.9 ←→ Preg [c]	1.4 ± 0.3 [d] ←→ Preg	5.6 ± 0.8 ←→ Preg	—	—
BLEOMYCIN (Chapter 55)	—	68 ± 9	—	1.1 ± 0.3	0.27 ± 0.09	3.1 ± 1.7	—	—
BRETYLIUM (Chapter 31)	23 ± 9	77 ± 15	0–8	10.2 ± 1.9 → Urem	5.9 ± 0.8	8.9 ± 1.8 ↑ Urem	—	—

AZATHIOPRINE [a] (Chapter 55)

[a] Values given are for azathioprine. Azathioprine is metabolized to mercaptopurine. *See* mercaptopurine for parameters for that compound.
[b] Determined by the availability of mercaptopurine.
[c] In kidney transplant patients.

AZLOCILLIN (Chapter 50)

[a] For 30-mg/kg dose, $CL = 3.1 \pm 0.7$ ml · min⁻¹ · kg⁻¹; for 80-mg/kg dose, $CL = 2.2 \pm 0.4$ ml · min⁻¹ · kg⁻¹.

BETAMETHASONE (Chapter 63)

[a] Calculated from separate studies of intravenous and oral administration. Predictions based on hepatic first-pass metabolism suggest availability <87%.
[b] Blood-to-plasma ratio = 1.1 ± 0.1.
[c] Increase in CL reported, but values not corrected for body weight of pregnant subjects.
[d] V_{area}.

BLEOMYCIN (Chapter 55)

BRETYLIUM (Chapter 31)

BUSULFAN (Chapter 55)

—	1	—	4.5 ± 0.9 [a]	0.99 ± 0.23 [a]	2.6 ± 0.5	—	—

[a] Oral administration; values are CL/F and V_{area}/F.

CAFFEINE (Chapter 25)

100 ± 13	1.1 ± 0.5	36 ± 7	1.4 ± 0.5 Neo ↑ Smk ↑	0.61 ± 0.02	4.9 ± 1.8 ↑ Neo, Preg ↓ Smk	—	—

CAPTOPRIL (Chapter 27)

65	50	30 ↓ Urem	12.7 ± 3.0	0.70 ± 0.09	1.9 ± 0.5 ↑ Urem	50 ng/ml [a]	—

[a] Complete inhibition of converting enzyme.

CARBAMAZEPINE [a] (Chapter 20)

>70	<1	74 ± 3 ←→ Urem, Hep, Cirr, Epilep, Preg	1.3 ± 0.5 [b,c] ↑ Preg ←→ Child	1.4 ± 0.4 [b] ←→ Child, Neo	15 ± 5 [b,c] ←→ Child, Neo	4–10 μg/ml [a] 6.5 ± 3.0 μg/ml [a,d]	>9 μg/ml [a,e]

[a] A metabolite, the 10,11-epoxide, is equipotent in animal studies; see also data for carbamazepine-10,11-epoxide.

[b] Data from oral, multiple-dose regimen; values are CL/F and V_{area}/F.

[c] Data from multiple-dose regimen. Carbamazepine induces its own metabolism; for a single dose, $CL/F = 0.36 \pm 0.07$ ml · min^{-1} · kg^{-1} and half-life = 36 ± 5 hours.

[d] To achieve control of psychomotor seizures.

[e] Threshold concentration for prominent side effects, such as distinct drowsiness, ataxia, and diplopia.

Key: Adult = adults; Aged = aged; Alb = hypoalbuminemia; Arth = arthritis; Atr Fib = atrial fibrillation; AVH = acute viral hepatitis; Burn = burn patients; CAD = coronary artery disease; Celiac = celiac disease; CF = cystic fibrosis; CHF = congestive heart failure; Child = children; Cirr = cirrhosis; COPD = chronic obstructive pulmonary disease; CP = cor pulmonale; CPBS = cardiopulmonary bypass surgery; CRI = chronic respiratory insufficiency; Crohn = Crohn's disease; Cush = Cushing's syndrome; Epilep = epileptic; Fem = female; Hep = Hepatitis; HL = hyperlipoproteinemia; HTh = hyperthyroid; Inflam = inflammation; LTh = hypothyroid; MI = myocardial infarction; Neo = neonate; NS = nephrotic syndrome; Obes = obese; Pneu = pneumonia; Prem = premature; RA = rheumatoid arthritis; Smk = smoking; Tach = ventricular tachycardia; Ulcer = ulcer patients; Urem = uremia

References: *See* end of table.

Table A–II–1. PHARMACOKINETIC DATA (Continued)

	AVAILABILITY (ORAL) (%)	URINARY EXCRETION (%)	BOUND IN PLASMA (%)	VOL. DIST. (liters/kg)	CLEARANCE ($ml \cdot min^{-1} \cdot kg^{-1}$)	HALF-LIFE (hours)	EFFECTIVE CONCENTRATIONS	TOXIC CONCENTRATIONS
CARBAMAZEPINE-10,11-EPOXIDE [a] (Chapter 20)	90 ± 11 [b]	<1	50	0.74 ± 0.13 [c]	1.4 ± 0.4 [c]	6.1 ± 0.7 [c]	[d]	[d]
CARBENICILLIN (Chapter 50)	—	82 ± 9	50	0.18 [a]	$CL = 0.68\,CL_{cr} + 0.15$	1.0 ± 0.2 ↑ Urem, Hep [b], Prem, Neo	See Chapter 50	See Chapter 50
CARMUSTINE (BCNU) (Chapter 55)	—	—	—	3.3 ± 1.7	56 ± 56	1.5 ± 2.0	—	—
CEFAMANDOLE (Chapter 50)	—	96 ± 3	74 ←→ Urem [a]	0.16 ± 0.05 ←→ Urem	2.8 ± 1.0 ↓ Urem	0.78 ± 0.10 ↑ Urem, Neo, CPBS	See Chapter 50	—
CEFAZOLIN (Chapter 50)	—	80 ± 16	84 ± 1 ↓ Urem	0.12 ± 0.03 [a] ↑ Urem	0.95 ± 0.17 [a] ↓ Urem	1.8 ± 0.4 ↑ Urem	See Chapter 50	—

CARBAMAZEPINE-10,11-EPOXIDE [a] (Chapter 20)

a Active metabolite of carbamazepine.
b Estimated.
c Data from single oral doses (80–200 mg); values are CL/F and V_{area}/F.
d Assumed to be equipotent with carbamazepine. In patients receiving only carbamazepine, ratio of plasma concentrations of epoxide to carbamazepine = 0.12; in patients also receiving phenytoin, primidone, phenobarbital, or valproic acid, ratio ~0.2.

CARBENICILLIN (Chapter 50)

a Assuming 70-kg body weight.
b Half-life is markedly prolonged in oliguric patients with concomitant hepatic dysfunction.

CARMUSTINE (BCNU) (Chapter 55)

CEFAMANDOLE (Chapter 50)

a No difference observed between patients with normal and impaired renal function, but percent bound reported as 32% (range, 17–58%).

CEFAZOLIN (Chapter 50)

a Assuming 70-kg weight.

CEFONICID (Chapter 50)

—	88 ± 6	98	0.32 ± 0.06 ↓ Urem	0.11 ± 0.01 ⟷ Urem	4.4 ± 0.8 ↑ Urem	*See* Chapter 50	—

CEFOPERAZONE (Chapter 50)

—	29 ± 4 ↑ Cirr	89–93 [a]	1.2 ± 0.1 ⟷ Cirr, Urem ↓ Hep	0.09 ± 0.01 [b] ↑ Cirr ⟷ Urem, Hep	2.1 ± 0.3 ↑ Cirr, Hep ⟷ Urem	*See* Chapter 50	—

[a] Nonlinear binding; value decreases from 93% at 25 μg/ml to 89% at 250 μg/ml. [b] V_{area} is about 50% larger than V_{ss} given here.

CEFORANIDE (Chapter 50)

—	84 ± 3	80–82	$CL = 0.26\,CL_{cr} + 0.07$	0.14 ± 0.04 ⟷ Urem	2.6 ± 0.5 ↑ Urem	*See* Chapter 50	—

CEFOTAXIME (Chapter 50)

—	61 ± 8	36	$CL = 1.34\,CL_{cr} + 1.81$	0.24 ± 0.03 ⟷ Urem	1.1 ± 0.2 ↑ Urem ⟷ Hep [a]	*See* Chapter 50	—

[a] Drug-induced hepatic disease; no change in half-life but decrease in fraction of dose converted to desacetyl metabolite.

CEFOXITIN (Chapter 50)

—	78	73	$CL = 3.3\,CL_{cr} + 0.19$	0.31 ± 0.12 ↑ Neo ⟷ Child, Urem	0.65 ± 0.09 ↑ Neo, Urem ↓ Child	*See* Chapter 50	—

Key: Adult = adults; Aged = aged; Alb = hypoalbuminemia; Arth = arthritis; Atr Fib = atrial fibrillation; AVH = acute viral hepatitis; Burn = burn patients; CAD = coronary artery disease; Celiac = celiac disease; CF = cystic fibrosis; CHF = congestive heart failure; Child = children; Cirr = cirrhosis; COPD = chronic obstructive pulmonary disease; CP = cor pulmonale; CPBS = cardiopulmonary bypass surgery; CRI = chronic respiratory insufficiency; Crohn = Crohn's disease; Cush = Cushing's syndrome; Epilep = epileptic; Fem = female; Hep = Hepatitis; HL = hyperlipoproteinemia; HTh = hyperthyroid; Inflam = inflammation; LTh = hypothyroid; MI = myocardial infarction; Neo = neonate; NS = nephrotic syndrome; Obes = obese; Pneu = pneumonia; Preg = pregnant; Prem = premature; RA = rheumatoid arthritis; Smk = smoking; Tach = ventricular tachycardia; Ulcer = ulcer patients; Urem = uremia

References: *See* end of table.

Table A–II–1. PHARMACOKINETIC DATA (Continued)

	AVAILABILITY (ORAL) (%)	URINARY EXCRETION (%)	BOUND IN PLASMA (%)	CLEARANCE $(ml \cdot min^{-1} \cdot kg^{-1})$	VOL. DIST. (liters/kg)	HALF-LIFE (hours)	EFFECTIVE CONCENTRATIONS	TOXIC CONCENTRATIONS
CEFTAZIDIME (Chapter 50)	—	84 ± 4 ⟷ CF	17	$CL = 1.05\ CL_{cr} + 0.12$ ⟷ CF	0.23 ± 0.02 ⟷ Urem, CF	1.6 ± 0.1 ↑ Urem, Prem, Neo ⟷ CF	*See* Chapter 50	—
CEFTIZOXIME (Chapter 50)	—	93 ± 8	28 ± 5 [a]	$CL = 1.1\ CL_{cr} + 0.07$	0.36 ± 0.19 ⟷ Urem	1.8 ± 0.7 ↑ Urem	*See* Chapter 50	—

[a] Values ranging between 28 and 65% have been reported.

	AVAILABILITY (ORAL) (%)	URINARY EXCRETION (%)	BOUND IN PLASMA (%)	CLEARANCE $(ml \cdot min^{-1} \cdot kg^{-1})$	VOL. DIST. (liters/kg)	HALF-LIFE (hours)	EFFECTIVE CONCENTRATIONS	TOXIC CONCENTRATIONS
CEFUROXIME (Chapter 50)	—	96 ± 10	33 ± 6	$CL = 0.94\ CL_{cr} + 0.28$	0.19 ± 0.04 ⟷ Urem, Aged	1.7 ± 0.6 ↑ Urem	*See* Chapter 50	—
CEPHALEXIN (Chapter 50)	90 ± 9	91 ± 18	14 ± 3	4.3 ± 1.1 [a] ↓ Urem	0.26 ± 0.03 [a] ⟷ Urem	0.90 ± 0.18 ↑ Urem	*See* Chapter 50	—

[a] Assuming 70-kg weight.

	AVAILABILITY (ORAL) (%)	URINARY EXCRETION (%)	BOUND IN PLASMA (%)	CLEARANCE $(ml \cdot min^{-1} \cdot kg^{-1})$	VOL. DIST. (liters/kg)	HALF-LIFE (hours)	EFFECTIVE CONCENTRATIONS	TOXIC CONCENTRATIONS
CEPHALOTHIN (Chapter 50)	—	52	71 ± 3	6.7 ± 1.7 [a] ↓ Urem, CPBS	0.26 ± 0.11 [a] ↑ Child	0.57 ± 0.32 ↑ Urem, CPBS	*See* Chapter 50	—

[a] Assuming 70-kg weight; one-compartment model.

CEPHAPIRIN (Chapter 50)

—	48 ± 7	62 ± 4	4.3 ± 1.6 [a] ↓ Urem	0.13 ± 0.05 [a]	1.2 ± 0.3 ↑ Urem	See Chapter 50	—

[a] Assuming 70-kg weight.

CEPHRADINE (Chapter 50)

>90	86 ± 10 [a]	14 ± 3	5.1 ± 1.2 [b] ↓ Urem	0.25 ± 0.01 [b]	0.77 ± 0.30 ↑ Urem	See Chapter 50	—

[a] Oral dose.
[b] Assuming 70-kg weight.

CHLORAMBUCIL (Chapter 55)

—	—	—	0.55 ± 0.38	0.86 ± 0.81	0.95 ± 0.34	—	—

CHLORAMPHENICOL (Chapter 52)

75–90 69 ± 13 [a]	53 ± 5 ↓ Cirr, Prem, Neo ↔ Urem	2.4 ± 0.2 ↓ Cirr, Prem, Neo ↔ Urem	0.94 ± 0.06 ↔ Cirr	4.0 ± 2.0 [b] ↑ Cirr, Prem, Neo ↔ Urem	See Chapter 52	See Chapter 52

[a] After intravenous administration of succinate ester; 27 ± 11% excreted as the ester.
[b] Shorter half-life reported previously due to substantial elimination of the succinate ester. Value given here is for parent drug (i.e., chloramphenicol) only.

Key: Adult = adults; Aged = aged; Alb = hypoalbuminemia; Arth = arthritis; Atr Fib = atrial fibrillation; AVH = acute viral hepatitis; Burn = burn patients; CAD = coronary artery disease; Celiac = celiac disease; CF = cystic fibrosis; CHF = congestive heart failure; Child = children; Cirr = cirrhosis; COPD = chronic obstructive pulmonary disease; CP = cor pulmonale; CPBS = cardiopulmonary bypass surgery; CRI = chronic respiratory insufficiency; Crohn = Crohn's disease; Cush = Cushing's syndrome; Epilep = epileptic; Fem = female; Hep = Hepatitis; HL = hyperlipoproteinemia; HTh = hyperthyroid; Inflam = inflammation; LTh = hypothyroid; MI = myocardial infarction; Neo = neonate; NS = nephrotic syndrome; Obes = obese; Pneu = pneumonia; Preg = pregnant; Prem = premature; RA = rheumatoid arthritis; Smk = smoking; Tach = ventricular tachycardia; Ulcer = ulcer patients; Urem = uremia

References: *See* end of table.

Table A–II–1. PHARMACOKINETIC DATA (Continued)

	AVAILABILITY (ORAL) (%)	URINARY EXCRETION (%)	BOUND IN PLASMA (%)	CLEARANCE ($ml \cdot min^{-1} \cdot kg^{-1}$)	VOL. DIST. (liters/kg)	HALF-LIFE (hours)	EFFECTIVE CONCENTRATIONS	TOXIC CONCENTRATIONS
CHLORDIAZEPOXIDE [a] (Chapters 17, 19)	100	<1	96.5 ± 1.8 ↑ AVH, Cirr ←→ Aged	0.54 ± 0.49 ↓ Aged, AVH, Cirr ↑ Fem ←→ Smk	0.30 ± 0.03 ↑ Aged, Fem, AVH [b], Cirr [b]	10.0 ± 3.4 ↑ Aged, AVH, Cirr	>0.7 µg/ml [c]	—
CHLOROQUINE (Chapter 45)	89 ± 16	55 ± 14	61 ± 9 [a] ←→ RA	10.7 ± 1.7	185 ± 66	8.9 ± 3.1 days	—	0.25 µg/ml [b]
CHLOROTHIAZIDE (Chapter 36)	Dose-dependent [a]	92 ± 5		4.5 ± 1.7 ↓ Urem	0.20 ± 0.08	1.5 ± 0.2 ↑ Urem, CHF [b]	—	—
CHLORPROMAZINE (Chapter 19)	32 ± 19 [a]	<1	95–98 ←→ Urem	8.6 ± 2.9 [b] ↓ Child [c] ←→ Cirr	21 ± 9 [b]	30 ± 7	30–350 ng/ml [d] Children: 40–80 ng/ml	750–1000 ng/ml [e]

CHLORDIAZEPOXIDE

[a] Active metabolites: desmethylchlordiazepoxide, demoxepam, desmethyldiazepam, and oxazepam.

[b] Because of decreased binding to plasma protein; V_{ss} for free drug is unchanged. Other data suggest no change in V_{area} in patients with cirrhosis.

[c] Decrease in anxiety and hostility; reduction in anxiety correlates with steady-state concentrations of metabolites (desmethylchlordiazepoxide and demoxepam) but not with that of chlordiazepoxide.

CHLOROQUINE

[a] Red blood cell–to-plasma ratio = 5.

[b] Diplopia; dizziness.

CHLOROTHIAZIDE

[a] Ranges from 56% for 50-mg dose to 9% for 1-g dose.

[b] May reflect decreased renal function in elderly patients, rather than CHF.

CHLORPROMAZINE

[a] After single dose. Availability may decrease to about 20% with repeated administration.

[b] $CL/F_{intramuscular}$ and $V_{area,\ intramuscular}$.

[c] CL/F_{oral}; there may be induction of metabolism and dose-dependent kinetics.

[d] Values are controversial due to several active and inactive metabolites.

[e] Neurotoxicity (tremors and convulsions).

CHLORPROPAMIDE (Chapter 64)

>90 [a]	20 ± 18 [b]		0.030 ± 0.005 [c,d]	0.097 ± 0.011 [c]	33 ± 6 [e]	—	—

[a] Predicted.
[b] Dependent on urinary pH: acidic urine, 1.4 ± 0.5%, basic urine, 85 ± 11%.
[c] CL/F and V_{area}/F.
[d] Acidic urine, 0.018 ± 0.006 ml · min^{-1} · kg^{-1}; basic urine, 0.086 ± 0.013 ml · min^{-1} · kg^{-1}.
[e] Acidic urine, 69 ± 26 hours; basic urine, 13 ± 3 hours.

CHLORTHALIDONE (Chapter 36)

64 ± 10	65 ± 9 [a] ↓ Aged	75 ± 1 [b]	1.6 ± 0.3 ↓ Aged	3.9 ± 0.8	44 ± 10 [c] ↑ Aged	—	

[a] Value is for 50- and 100-mg doses; renal clearance is decreased at an oral dose of 200 mg, and there is a concomitant decrease in the percentage excreted unchanged.
[b] Blood-to-plasma ratio = 72.5.
[c] Chlorthalidone is sequestered in erythrocytes; the half-life is longer if blood, rather than plasma, is analyzed.

CIMETIDINE (Chapter 26)

62 ± 6 [a]	62 ± 20 ⟷ Cirr	19	7.7 ± 1.8 ↓ Urem, Aged ⟷ Ulcer, Cirr	1.0 ± 0.2 ⟷ Urem, Cirr, Ulcer	1.9 ± 0.3 ↑ Urem ⟷ Ulcer, Cirr	0.78 µg/ml 3.9 µg/ml [b]	—

[a] Oral liquid and tablets are equivalent; value is the same in patients with ulcers.
[b] Concentrations to inhibit gastric acid secretion by 50% and 90%, respectively.

CISPLATIN [a] (Chapter 55)

—	—		17	0.51	0.64	—	

[a] Most studies are of total platinum, rather than the parent compound; values reported here are for cisplatin.

Key: Adult = adults; Aged = aged; Alb = hypoalbuminemia; Arth = arthritis; Atr Fib = atrial fibrillation; AVH = acute viral hepatitis; Burn = burn patients; CAD = coronary artery disease; Celiac = celiac disease; CF = cystic fibrosis; CHF = congestive heart failure; Child = children; Cirr = cirrhosis; COPD = chronic obstructive pulmonary disease; CP = cor pulmonale; CPBS = cardiopulmonary bypass surgery; CRI = chronic respiratory insufficiency; Crohn = Crohn's disease; Cush = Cushing's disease; Epilep = epileptic; Fem = female; Hep = Hepatitis; HL = hyperlipoproteinemia; HTh = hyperthyroid; Inflam = inflammation; LTh = hypothyroid; MI = myocardial infarction; Neo = neonate; NS = nephrotic syndrome; Obes = obese; Pneu = pneumonia; Preg = pregnant; Prem = premature; RA = rheumatoid arthritis; Smk = smoking; Tach = ventricular tachycardia; Ulcer = ulcer patients; Urem = uremia

References: *See* end of table.

Table A–II–1. PHARMACOKINETIC DATA (Continued)

	AVAILABILITY (ORAL) (%)	URINARY EXCRETION (%)	BOUND IN PLASMA (%)	CLEARANCE ($ml \cdot min^{-1} \cdot kg^{-1}$)	VOL. DIST. (liters/kg)	HALF-LIFE (hours)	EFFECTIVE CONCENTRATIONS	TOXIC CONCENTRATIONS
CLINDAMYCIN (Chapter 52)	~87 [a]	9–14 [b]	93.6 ± 0.2	3.5 ± 0.8 ←→ Child	0.66 ± 0.10 [c] ←→ Urem	2.7 ± 0.4 ←→ Child, Urem, Preg ↑ Prem	*See* Chapter 52	—

[a] Clindamycin hydrochloride.
[b] Microbiological assay, which includes active metabolites.
[c] V/F; average value in children, 0.86 liter/kg.

CLOFIBRATE [a] (Chapter 34)	95 ± 10	5.7 ± 2.1 [b]	96.5 ± 0.3 [c] ↓ NS, Cirr, Urem ←→ AVH	0.12 ± 0.01 [b] ↑ NS ↓ Urem ←→ AVH, Cirr	0.11 ± 0.02 [b] ↑ Cirr, Urem	13 ± 3 ↑ Urem	—	—

[a] Clofibrate is the ethyl ester of *p*-chlorophenoxyisobutyric acid (CPIB). All values are for CPIB, since clofibrate is rapidly deesterified upon absorption.
[b] Oral dosage; CL/F and V_{area}/F.
[c] Binding may decrease at high concentrations of CPIB (>200 $\mu g/ml$).

CLONAZEPAM (Chapters 17, 20)	98 ± 31	<1	86 ± 0.5 ↓ Neo	1.55 ± 0.28 [a]	3.2 ± 1.1	23 ± 5	5–70 ng/ml [b]	[c]

[a] CL/F; this value is consistent for a number of studies, but it is higher than the clearance determined in a single study of intravenous administration.
[b] Most patients, including children, whose seizures are controlled by clonazepam have concentrations of the drug in plasma in this range. However, patients who do not respond and those with side effects display similar values.
[c] Occurrence of side effects is apparently not correlated with concentrations of clonazepam or its 7-amino metabolite.

CLONIDINE (Chapters 9, 32)	100	62 ± 11	—	3.1 ± 1.2	2.1 ± 0.4	8.5 ± 2.0 [a]	0.5 ng/ml [b]	1 ng/ml [c]

[a] A longer half-life of about 20 hours is also seen with more sensitive assays.
[b] Reduction in blood pressure.
[c] Sedation, dry mouth.

CLORAZEPATE [a] (Chapters 17, 19, 20)

—	< 1	—	1.8 ± 0.2 [b] ↑ Preg	0.33 ± 0.17 [b] →← Preg	2.0 ± 0.9 ↓ Preg	—

[a] Clorazepate is essentially a prodrug for desmethyldiazepam; *see also* listing for that compound. Values presented here are for clorazepate.

[b] CL/F and V_{area}/F.

CLOXACILLIN (Chapter 50)

43 ± 16 ↑ Urem →← CF	75 ± 14	94.6 ± 0.6 →← CF	2.2 ± 0.5 [a] ↓ Urem ↑ CF	0.094 ± 0.015 [a] ↑ CF, Urem	0.55 ± 0.07 ↑ Urem	*See* Chapter 50

[a] Assuming 70-kg weight.

COCAINE (Chapters 15, 23)

0.5 [a]	—	—	35 ± 9	2.1 ± 1.2	0.71 ± 0.26	—

[a] Intranasal; 100-mg total dose.

CYCLOPHOSPHAMIDE [a] (Chapter 55)

74 ± 22	13	6.5 ± 4.3	1.3 ± 0.5	0.78 ± 0.57	7.5 ± 4.0	—

[a] Cyclophosphamide is activated by hepatic metabolism (*see* Chapter 55); kinetic parameters are for cyclophosphamide itself.

Key: Adult = adults; Aged = aged; Alb = hypoalbuminemia; Arth = arthritis; Atr Fib = atrial fibrillation; AVH = acute viral hepatitis; Burn = burn patients; CAD = coronary artery disease; Celiac = celiac disease; CF = cystic fibrosis; CHF = congestive heart failure; Child = children; Cir = cirrhosis; COPD = chronic obstructive pulmonary disease; CP = cor pulmonale; CPBS = cardiopulmonary bypass surgery; CRI = chronic respiratory insufficiency; Crohn = Crohn's disease; Cush = Cushing's syndrome; Epilep = epileptic; Fem = female; Hep = Hepatitis; HL = hyperlipoproteinemia; HTh = hyperthyroid; Inflam = inflammation; LTh = hypothyroid; MI = myocardial infarction; Neo = neonate; NS = nephrotic syndrome; Obes = obese; Pneu = pneumonia; Preg = pregnant; Prem = premature; RA = rheumatoid arthritis; Smk = smoking; Tach = ventricular tachycardia; Ulcer = ulcer patients; Urem = uremia

References: *See* end of table.

Table A–II–1. PHARMACOKINETIC DATA (Continued)

AVAILABILITY (ORAL) (%)	URINARY EXCRETION (%)	BOUND IN PLASMA (%)	CLEARANCE ($ml \cdot min^{-1} \cdot kg^{-1}$)	VOL. DIST. (liters/kg)	HALF-LIFE (hours)	EFFECTIVE CONCENTRATIONS	TOXIC CONCENTRATIONS

CYCLOSPORINE (Chapter 55)

| 34 ± 11 | <1 | 96 | 9.3 ± 1.0 [a] ←→ Urem [b] | 3.5 ± 2.7 [a] | 16 ± 8 [a] | 100–400 ng/ml [c] | >400 ng/ml [c,d] |

[a] Measurements in blood.
[b] CL in uremia reduced to 6.2 ± 1.4 ml · min⁻¹ · kg⁻¹, but dosage adjustment may not be necessary.
[c] Assay includes some metabolites.
[d] Nephrotoxicity.

CYTARABINE (Chapter 55)

| 20 | 11 ± 8 | 13 | 13 ± 4 | 3.0 ± 1.9 | 2.6 ± 0.6 | — | — |

DAPSONE (Chapter 53)

| [a] | 15 [b] ←→ Urem | 73 ± 1 ←→ Urem | 0.64 ± 0.18 [c] | 1.5 ± 0.5 [c] | 28 ± 3 | — | — |

[a] Slowly and completely absorbed. With low hepatic clearance, availability should be high.
[b] Urine pH = 6–7.
[c] CL/F and V_{area}/F.

DESIPRAMINE (Chapter 19)

| 51 [a] | 3 ± 4 ←→ Urem | 90 ± 1 ←→ Urem | 30 ± 16 [b,c] ↓ Aged | 34 ± 8 [b] | 18 ± 6 ↑ Aged | 40–160 ng/ml | >1 μg/ml [d] |

[a] Estimate assuming erythrocyte:plasma partition of 2.0, hematocrit of 0.45, hepatic blood flow of 1500 ml/min, and complete absorption of the drug.
[b] CL/F and V_{ss}/F. Since F is probably significantly less than 1, actual values may be lower.
[c] Significantly lower in a Chinese population.
[d] Combined data for toxic effects of tricyclic antidepressants.

DESMETHYLDIAZEPAM [a] (Chapters 17, 19, 20)

| 50 [b] | <1 | 97.5 [c] ↓ Urem ←→ Obes, Aged | 0.11 [c] ↑ Smk [d] ↓ Hep, Cirr, Obes [d], Aged [d,e] ←→ Preg [d] | 0.45 [c] ↑ Obes [d], Preg [d] ↓ Hep, Cirr, Aged [d] | 62 ± 16 ↑ Obes, Preg, Aged [e] ↓ Hep, Cirr | — | — |

[a] Desmethyldiazepam is the active species delivered after oral administration of clorazepate and prazepam. It is an active metabolite of diazepam and is itself metabolized to oxazepam.
[b] One subject.
[c] Two subjects; values consistent with reported $CL/F = 0.22$ and $V_{area}/F = 1.05$.
[d] CL/F and V_{area}/F.
[e] In males only.

DEXAMETHASONE (Chapter 63)

78 ± 14 ↔ Smk	2.6 ± 0.6	68 ± 3 ↔ Preg	3.7 ± 0.9 ↑ Preg ↔ Smk	0.82 ± 0.22 ↔ Smk, Preg	3.0 ± 0.8 ↔ Smk, Preg	—

DIAZEPAM [a] (Chapters 17, 19, 20)

100 ± 14	<1	98.7 ± 0.2 ↓ Urem, Cirr, NS, Preg, Neo, Alb [b] ↔ Aged, HTh,	0.38 ± 0.06 ↑ Alb, Epilep [c] Cirr, Hep ↔ Aged, Smk, HTh	1.1 ± 0.3 ↑ Cirr, Aged, Alb ↔ Urem, HTh	43 ± 13 ↑ Aged, Cirr, Hep Epilep [c] ↔ HTh	300–400 ng/ml [d] >600 ng/ml [e]	—

[a] Active metabolites, desmethyldiazepam and oxazepam; *see also* listings for those compounds.
[b] Alcoholics.
[c] Anxiolytic.
[d] Due to administration of other drugs that induce metabolic enzymes.
[e] For control of seizures.

DIAZOXIDE (Chapter 32)

86–96	20–50	94 ± 14 [a] ↓ Urem	0.06 ± 0.02	0.21 ± 0.02	48 ± 12	35 μg/ml [b]	—

[a] Decreased at higher concentrations (*e.g.*, 84% at 250 μg/ml).
[b] 20% reduction in mean arterial pressure.

Key: Adult = adults; Aged = aged; Alb = hypoalbuminemia; Arth = arthritis; Atr Fib = atrial fibrillation; AVH = acute viral hepatitis; Burn = burn patients; CAD = coronary artery disease; Celiac = celiac disease; CF = cystic fibrosis; CHF = congestive heart failure; Child = children; Cirr = cirrhosis; COPD = chronic obstructive pulmonary disease; CP = cor pulmonale; CPBS = cardiopulmonary bypass surgery; CRI = chronic respiratory insufficiency; Crohn = Crohn's disease; Cush = Cushing's syndrome; Epilep = epileptic; Fem = female; Hep = Hepatitis; HL = hyperlipoproteinemia; HTh = hyperthyroid; Inflam = inflammation; LTh = hypothyroid; MI = myocardial infarction; Neo = neonate; NS = nephrotic syndrome; Obes = obese; Pneu = pneumonia; Preg = pregnant; Prem = premature; RA = rheumatoid arthritis; Smk = smoking; Tach = ventricular tachycardia; Ulcer = ulcer patients; Urem = uremia

References: *See* end of table.

Table A–II–1. PHARMACOKINETIC DATA (Continued)

AVAILABILITY (ORAL) (%)	URINARY EXCRETION (%)	BOUND IN PLASMA (%)	CLEARANCE $(ml \cdot min^{-1} \cdot kg^{-1})$	VOL. DIST. $(liters/kg)$	HALF-LIFE $(hours)$	EFFECTIVE CONCENTRATIONS	TOXIC CONCENTRATIONS

DICLOXACILLIN (Chapter 50)

AVAILABILITY (ORAL) (%)	URINARY EXCRETION (%)	BOUND IN PLASMA (%)	CLEARANCE	VOL. DIST.	HALF-LIFE	EFFECTIVE CONC.	TOXIC CONC.
50–85	60 ± 7	95.8 ± 0.2 ↓ Urem ↔ CF	1.6 ± 0.3 [a,b] ↓ Urem ↑ CF [c]	0.086 ± 0.017 [a] ↑ Urem	0.70 ± 0.07 ↑ Urem	See Chapter 50	—

[a] Assuming 70-kg weight.
[b] Possible saturation of renal clearance at doses of 1–2 g.
[c] Concomitant increase in clearance of both drug and creatinine.

DIGITOXIN [a] (Chapter 30)

AVAILABILITY (ORAL) (%)	URINARY EXCRETION (%)	BOUND IN PLASMA (%)	CLEARANCE	VOL. DIST.	HALF-LIFE	EFFECTIVE CONC.	TOXIC CONC.
>90 ↔ Urem, Child	32 ± 15	97 ± 0.5 ↓ NS, Urem ↔ Child	0.055 ± 0.018 ↑ NS, Child ↔ Aged, Urem	0.54 ± 0.14 ↑ Child ↔ Aged, Urem	6.7 ± 1.7 days ↓ NS ↔ Aged, Urem, Child	>10 ng/ml	29, 39, 48 ng/ml [b] ↑

[a] Values for unchanged drug and cardioactive metabolites.
[b] Concentrations causing arrhythmias or other abnormal conduction in 10, 50, and 90% of patients, respectively.

DIGOXIN (Chapter 30)

AVAILABILITY (ORAL) (%)	URINARY EXCRETION (%)	BOUND IN PLASMA (%)	CLEARANCE	VOL. DIST.	HALF-LIFE	EFFECTIVE CONC.	TOXIC CONC.
70 ± 13 [a] ↔ Urem, MI, CHF, LTh, HTh	60 ± 11 ↓ Urem	25 ± 5 ↓ Urem	$CL = (0.88\,CL_{cr} + 0.33) \pm 52\%$ [b,c] ↓ LTh ↑ HTh, Neo, Child	$V = (3.12\,CL_{cr} + 3.84) \pm 30\%$ ↓ LTh ↑ HTh ↔ CHF	39 ± 13 ↓ HTh ↑ Urem, CHF, Aged, LTh ↔ Obes	>0.8 ng/ml [d]	1.7, 2.5, 3.3 ng/ml [e] ↑ Child

[a] Lanoxin tablets; digoxin solutions, elixirs, and capsules may be absorbed more completely.
[b] Equation applies to patients with some degree of heart failure. If heart failure is not present, the coefficient of CL_{cr} must be ml · min^{-1} · kg^{-1}. Units of CL_{cr} is 1.0.
[c] Occasional individuals metabolize digoxin very rapidly to an inactive metabolite, dihydrodigoxin.
[d] Inotropic effect.
[e] Concentrations at which the probability of digoxin-induced arrhythmias are 10, 50, and 90%, respectively.

DILTIAZEM [a] (Chapter 33)

AVAILABILITY (ORAL) (%)	URINARY EXCRETION (%)	BOUND IN PLASMA (%)	CLEARANCE	VOL. DIST.	HALF-LIFE	EFFECTIVE CONC.	TOXIC CONC.
44 ± 10	<4	78 ± 3	11.5 ± 1.8 [b]	5.3 ± 1.7 [c]	3.2 ± 1.3	—	—

[a] Active metabolite, desacetyldiltiazem.
[b] More than a twofold decrease with multiple dosing.
[c] V_{area}.

DIPHENHYDRAMINE (Chapter 26)

51 ± 6	1.9 ± 0.8 ↔ Cirr	78 ± 3 ↓ Cirr	9.8 ± 3.0 [a] ↔ Cirr	6.5 ± 2.6 [a] ↔ Cirr	4.1 ± 0.4 [b] ↑ Cirr	>25 ng/ml [c] >50 ng/ml [d]	>100 ng/ml [e]

[a] Increased CL, decreased V, and no change in half-life in Orientals, presumably due to decreased protein binding.

[b] A longer terminal half-life (9.3 ± 0.7 hours) is observed approximately 8–12 hours after intravenous administration.

[c] Antihistaminic effect.

[d] Sedation.

[e] Marked drowsiness, sleep.

DISOPYRAMIDE (Chapter 31)

83 ± 11 ↔ MI, CHF	55 ± 6 [a]	Dose-dependent [b] Neo ↓ Aged, MI ↑	1.2 ± 0.4 [c] MI, Tach, CHF, Urem	0.59 ± 0.15 [c] Urem ↓ CHF ↔	6.0 ± 1.0 Urem, CHF ↑ MI ↔	>3 µg/ml	—

[a] No effect of urinary pH.

[b] 68% at 0.38 µg/ml and 28% at 3.8 µg/ml.

[c] Unbound clearance, 5.4 ± 2.8 ml · min^{-1} · kg^{-1}; unbound V_{ss}, 1.7 ± 0.8 liters/kg.

DOBUTAMINE (Chapter 8)

—	—	—	59 ± 22 [a]	0.20 ± 0.08 [a]	2.4 ± 0.7 min [a]	—	—

[a] Values for patients with CHF; V, for example, is lower when less edema is present. Values likely represent distribution, rather than elimination.

DOXEPIN [a] (Chapter 19)

27 ± 10 [b]	~0	—	14 ± 3 [c]	20 ± 8 [c,d]	17 ± 6	30–150 ng/ml [e]	—

[a] Active metabolite desmethyldoxepin has a longer half-life (51 ± 17 hours).

[b] Calculated from results of oral administration only, assuming complete absorption, elimination only by the liver, hepatic blood flow of 1500 ml/min, and equal partition between plasma and erythrocytes.

[c] Calculated assuming $F = 0.27$.

[d] V_{area}.

[e] Doxepin + desmethyldoxepin; optimal concentrations have not been defined.

References: *See* end of table.

Table A–II–1. PHARMACOKINETIC DATA (Continued)

	AVAILABILITY (ORAL) (%)	URINARY EXCRETION (%)	BOUND IN PLASMA (%)	CLEARANCE ($ml \cdot min^{-1} \cdot kg^{-1}$)	VOL. DIST. (liters/kg)	HALF-LIFE (hours)	EFFECTIVE CONCENTRATIONS	TOXIC CONCENTRATIONS
DOXORUBICIN (Chapter 55)	—	<15	79–85	17 ± 3	52	36 ± 11 [a]	—	—
DOXYCYCLINE (Chapter 52)	93	41 ± 19 ↓ Urem [a]	88 ± 5 ↓ Urem [a]	0.53 ± 0.18	0.75 ± 0.32	16 ± 6 ←→, ↑ Urem	See Chapter 52	—
EDROPHONIUM (Chapter 6)	—	—	—	9.6 ± 2.7	1.1 ± 0.2	1.8 ± 0.6	<0.15 µg/ml [a]	—
ERYTHROMYCIN (Chapter 52)	35 ± 25 [a] ↓ Preg [b]	12 ± 7	84 ± 3 [c] ←→ Urem	9.1 ± 4.1	0.78 ± 0.44 ↑ Urem	1.6 ± 0.7 ↑ Urem, Cirr	See Chapter 52	—
ETHAMBUTOL (Chapter 53)	77 ± 8	79 ± 3	20–30	8.6 ± 0.8	1.6 ± 0.2	3.1 ± 0.4 ↑ Urem	—	>10 µg/ml [a]

DOXORUBICIN
[a] Prolonged when bilirubin concentration elevated.

DOXYCYCLINE
[a] Changes in plasma protein binding and erythrocyte partitioning yield decrease from 88 ± 5% bound in blood of normals to 71 ± 3% in patients with uremia.

EDROPHONIUM
[a] 80% reversal of 95% blockade due to tubocurarine.

ERYTHROMYCIN
[a] Value for enteric-coated erythromycin base.
[b] Decreased concentrations in pregnancy possibly due to decreased availability (or to increased clearance).
[c] Erythromycin base. Values for the propionate ester range from 90 to 99%.

ETHAMBUTOL
[a] Estimated from kinetics and dosage at which visual toxicity occurs.

ETHANOL (Chapter 18)

100	<3	—	$V_m = 124 \pm 10\ \text{mg} \cdot \text{kg}^{-1} \cdot \text{hr}^{-1}$ [a] $K_m = 82 \pm 29$ mg/l [a]	0.54 ± 0.05 [a]	—	—	1000–1500 mg/l [b]

[a] Ethanol is eliminated by a saturable (Michaelis-Menten) process; the half-life is the fastest possible—that theoretically present at zero concentration.

[b] Legal basis for intoxication in many states of the United States.

ETHOSUXIMIDE (Chapter 20)

—	25 ± 15	0	0.19 ± 0.04 [a,b] ↑ Child	0.72 ± 0.16 [a] ←→ Child	45 ± 8 [a] ↓ Child ←→ Neo	40–100 µg/ml	—

[a] Data from oral, multiple-dose regimen; values are CL/F and V_{area}/F.

[b] CL/F decreases 15% from single dose and may be nonlinear with increasing dose.

FENTANYL (Chapters 14, 22)

—	8	80	13 ± 2	4.0 ± 0.4	3.7 ± 0.4	1 ng/ml [a]	1 ng/ml [b]

[a] Analgesia.

[b] Respiratory depression.

FLUCYTOSINE (Chapter 54)

84 ± 6 ←→ Urem	99 ± 7	4	$CL = CL_{cr}$	0.68 ± 0.04 ←→ Urem	4.2 ± 0.3 ↑ Urem	35–70 µg/ml	>100 µg/ml

FLUNITRAZEPAM [a] (Chapter 17)

~85	<1	77–79	3.5 ± 0.4 [b]	3.3 ± 0.6 [b]	15 ± 5	—	—

[a] Active metabolite, desmethylflunitrazepam.

[b] CL/F and V_{ss}/F.

Key: Adult = adults; Aged = aged; Alb = hypoalbuminemia; Arth = arthritis; Atr Fib = atrial fibrillation; AVH = acute viral hepatitis; Burn = burn patients; CAD = coronary artery disease; Celiac = celiac disease; CF = cystic fibrosis; CHF = congestive heart failure; Child = children; Cirr = cirrhosis; COPD = chronic obstructive pulmonary disease; CP = cor pulmonale; CPBS = cardiopulmonary bypass surgery; CRI = chronic respiratory insufficiency; Crohn = Crohn's disease; Cush = Cushing's syndrome; Epilep = epileptic; Fem = female; Hep = Hepatitis; HL = hyperlipoproteinemia; HTh = hyperthyroid; Inflam = inflammation; LTh = hypothyroid; MI = myocardial infarction; Neo = neonate; NS = nephrotic syndrome; Obes = obese; Pneu = pneumonia; Preg = pregnant; Prem = premature; RA = rheumatoid arthritis; Smk = smoking; Tach = ventricular tachycardia; Ulcer = ulcer patients; Urem = uremia

References: *See* end of table.

Table A–II–1. PHARMACOKINETIC DATA (Continued)

	AVAILABILITY (ORAL) (%)	URINARY EXCRETION (%)	BOUND IN PLASMA (%)	CLEARANCE ($ml \cdot min^{-1} \cdot kg^{-1}$)	VOL. DIST. (liters/kg)	HALF-LIFE (hours)	EFFECTIVE CONCENTRATIONS	TOXIC CONCENTRATIONS
FLUOROURACIL (Chapter 55)	28 [a]	1–4	8–12	16 ± 7	0.25 ± 0.12	11 ± 4 min [b]	—	—
FLURAZEPAM [a] (Chapter 17)	—	<1	96.6	4.5 ± 2.3 [b] ↓ Fem	22 ± 7 [b]	74 ± 24 ↑ Aged [c]	—	
FUROSEMIDE (Chapter 36)	61 ± 17	66 ± 7	98.8 ± 0.2 ↓ Urem, NS, Cirr, Alb ←→ CHF	2.0 ± 0.4 ↓ Urem, CHF, Prem, Neo ←→ Cirr	0.11 ± 0.02 ↑ NS, Neo, Prem, Cirr ←→ Urem, CHF	92 ± 7 min ↑ Urem, CHF, Prem, Neo, Cirr ←→ NS	[a]	25 μg/ml [b]
GENTAMICIN (Chapter 51)	—	>90	<10	$CL = 0.73\ CL_{cr} + 0.06$ ↓ Obes	0.25 ↑ Urem, Aged, CF ←→ Obes ↓	2–3, 53 ± 25 [a] ↑ Urem ←→ Obes ↓ Burn	*See* Chapter 51	*See* Chapter 51

FLUOROURACIL (Chapter 55)

a Higher F with rapid absorption and lower F with slower absorption due to saturable first-pass effect.

b A longer (~20 hour) half-life is seen at very low concentrations of drug.

FLURAZEPAM [a] (Chapter 17)

a Flurazepam is essentially a prodrug for desalkylflurazepam; values presented are for the active metabolite.

b CL/F and V_{area}/F.

c Males.

FUROSEMIDE (Chapter 36)

a Efficacy better correlated with concentration of drug in urine.

b Ototoxicity.

GENTAMICIN (Chapter 51)

a Gentamicin has a very long terminal half-life, which accounts for urinary excretion for up to 3 weeks.

GOLD SODIUM THIOMALATE [a] (Chapter 29)

	60–90	95	7.0 ± 0.6 [b]	0.26 ± 0.05 [b,c]	25 ± 5 days	—	—

[a] Values refer to gold.
[b] Intramuscular dose.
[c] V_{area}.

HALOPERIDOL (Chapter 19)

70 ± 18	Negligible	92 ± 1.4	11.8 ± 2.9	17.8 ± 6.5	17.9 ± 6.4	1 ng/ml [a] ↓ Child	15 ng/ml [a] ↓ Child

[a] For Gilles de la Tourette, 1–3 ng/ml; for psychotic syndromes, 10–15 ng/ml; for mania, 2.5–4.5 ng/ml.

HEPARIN (Chapter 58)

	Negligible	Extensive	1/(0.65 + 0.008D) ± 0.1 [a]	0.058 ± 0.011 [b]	(26 + 0.323D) ± 12 min [a]	See Chapter 58	—

[a] D is dose in I.U./kg. Half-life and clearance are dose dependent, perhaps due to saturable metabolism with end-product inhibition.
[b] V_{area}.

HEXOBARBITAL (Chapter 17)

>90	<1	42–52 ↔ Cirr	3.9 ± 0.7 ↓ Cirr, AVH	1.2 ± 0.3 ↔ Cirr, AVH	3.7 ± 0.9 ↑ Cirr, AVH	—	—

Key: Adult = adults; Aged = aged; Alb = hypoalbuminemia; Arth = arthritis; Atr Fib = atrial fibrillation; AVH = acute viral hepatitis; Burn = burn patients; CAD = coronary artery disease; Celiac = celiac disease; CF = cystic fibrosis; CHF = congestive heart failure; Child = children; Cirr = cirrhosis; COPD = chronic obstructive pulmonary disease; CP = cor pulmonale; CPBS = cardiopulmonary bypass surgery; CRI = chronic respiratory insufficiency; Crohn = Crohn's disease; Cush = Cushing's syndrome; Epilep = epileptic; Fem = female; Hep = Hepatitis; HL = hyperlipoproteinemia; HTh = hyperthyroid; Inflam = inflammation; LTh = hypothyroid; MI = myocardial infarction; Neo = neonate; NS = nephrotic syndrome; Obes = obese; Pneu = pneumonia; Preg = pregnant; Prem = premature; RA = rheumatoid arthritis; Smk = smoking; Tach = ventricular tachycardia; Ulcer = ulcer patients; Urem = uremia

References: *See* end of table.

Table A–II–1. PHARMACOKINETIC DATA (Continued)

AVAILABILITY (ORAL) (%)	URINARY EXCRETION (%)	BOUND IN PLASMA (%)	CLEARANCE ($ml \cdot min^{-1} \cdot kg^{-1}$)	VOL. DIST. (liters/kg)	HALF-LIFE (hours)	EFFECTIVE CONCENTRATIONS	TOXIC CONCENTRATIONS
HYDRALAZINE (Chapter 32)							
16 ± 6 [a,b] 35 ± 4 [c]	1–15	—	56 ± 13 [d,e]	1.5 ± 1.0 [d,e]	0.96 ± 0.28 [d]	100 ng/ml [f]	—

[a] Rapid acetylator.
[b] Availability may increase with large doses that saturate first-pass metabolism.
[c] Slow acetylator.
[d] Same for rapid and slow acetylators after intravenous administration because of other pathways of metabolic alteration.
[e] Blood CL and V_{ss}. Blood-to-plasma concentration ratio = 1.65.
[f] Decrease in mean arterial pressure of 10–20 mm Hg.

AVAILABILITY (ORAL) (%)	URINARY EXCRETION (%)	BOUND IN PLASMA (%)	CLEARANCE ($ml \cdot min^{-1} \cdot kg^{-1}$)	VOL. DIST. (liters/kg)	HALF-LIFE (hours)	EFFECTIVE CONCENTRATIONS	TOXIC CONCENTRATIONS
HYDROCHLOROTHIAZIDE (Chapter 36)							
71 ± 15	>95	64	4.9 ± 1.1 [a] ↓ Urem, CHF [b]	0.83 ± 0.31 [c]	2.5 ± 0.2 ↑ Urem, CHF [b]	—	—

[a] Renal clearance, which should approximate total plasma clearance; calculated assuming 70-kg weight.
[b] Changes may reflect decreased renal function.
[c] Calculated from individual values of renal clearance, terminal half-life, and fraction of drug excreted unchanged; 70-kg weight assumed.

AVAILABILITY (ORAL) (%)	URINARY EXCRETION (%)	BOUND IN PLASMA (%)	CLEARANCE ($ml \cdot min^{-1} \cdot kg^{-1}$)	VOL. DIST. (liters/kg)	HALF-LIFE (hours)	EFFECTIVE CONCENTRATIONS	TOXIC CONCENTRATIONS
IBUPROFEN [a] (Chapter 29)							
>80	<1	>99 [a] ↔ RA, Alb	0.75 ± 0.20 [a,b]	0.15 [c]	2 ± 0.5 [a]	—	—

[a] Nonlinear kinetics observed, probably due to saturable plasma protein binding.
[b] CL/F.
[c] V_{area}/F.

AVAILABILITY (ORAL) (%)	URINARY EXCRETION (%)	BOUND IN PLASMA (%)	CLEARANCE ($ml \cdot min^{-1} \cdot kg^{-1}$)	VOL. DIST. (liters/kg)	HALF-LIFE (hours)	EFFECTIVE CONCENTRATIONS	TOXIC CONCENTRATIONS
IMIPRAMINE [a] (Chapter 19)							
27 ± 8	<2	94.8 ± 0.5 ↑ HI, MI	15 ± 4 ↓ Aged ↑ Smk	23 ± 8 [b]	18 ± 7	100–300 ng/ml [c]	>1 µg/ml [d]

[a] Active metabolite, desipramine.
[b] V_{area}.
[c] Antidepressant effect; combination of imipramine and desipramine.
[d] Concentration of imipramine and desipramine; combined data for toxic effects of tricyclic antidepressants.

INDOMETHACIN [a] (Chapter 29)

98	90 → Alb	15 ± 8	2.0 ± 0.4 [b]	0.26 ± 0.07 [b]	2.4 ± 0.4 [a] → RA, Urem ↑ Neo, Prem	0.3–3 μg/ml	>5 μg/ml

[a] There is significant enterohepatic recycling (~50% after an intravenous dose), which may contribute to low plasma concentrations of the drug for prolonged periods of time.

[b] Assuming 70-kg weight.

ISONIAZID (Chapter 53)

[a]	~0	29 ± 5 [b,c] 7 ± 2 [b,d]	3.7 ± 1.1 [c] 7.4 ± 2.0 [d] → Aged	0.67 ± 0.15 → Aged	1.1 ± 0.1 [d] 3.1 ± 1.1 [c] ↑ AVH, Cirr, Neo, Urem [e] → Aged, Obes, Child	See Chapter 53	—

[a] It is usually stated that isoniazid is completely absorbed; however, good estimates of possible loss due to first-pass metabolism are not available. Absorption is decreased in the presence of food or antacids.

[b] After oral administration; assay includes unchanged drug and its acid-labile hydrazones. Higher percentages have been noted after intravenous administration, suggesting significant first-pass metabolism.

[c] Slow acetylators.

[d] Fast acetylators.

[e] No apparent correlation with degree of renal impairment.

ISOSORBIDE DINITRATE [a] (Chapter 33)

Oral: 22 ± 14 [b] Sublingual: 59 ± 29 [b] Percutaneous: 33 ± 17 [b]	<1	28 ± 12 → Cirr → Smk	45 ± 20 ↓ Cirr → Smk	1.5 ± 0.8	0.8 ± 0.4 → Urem	—	—

[a] Isosorbide dinitrate is metabolized to the 2- and 5-mononitrates. Both metabolites and the parent compound are thought to be active. Values above are for the dinitrate. See also listings for isosorbide mononitrates.

[b] Availability calculations from single doses, since systemic clearance may be decreased after long-term use.

Key: Adult = adults; Aged = aged; Alb = hypoalbuminemia; Arth = arthritis; Atr Fib = atrial fibrillation; AVH = acute viral hepatitis; Burn = burn patients; CAD = coronary artery disease; Celiac = celiac disease; CF = cystic fibrosis; CHF = congestive heart failure; Child = children; Cirr = cirrhosis; COPD = chronic obstructive pulmonary disease; CP = cor pulmonale; CPBS = cardiopulmonary bypass surgery; CRI = chronic respiratory insufficiency; Crohn = Crohn's disease; Cush = Cushing's syndrome; Epilep = epileptic; Fem = female; Hep = Hepatitis; HL = hyperlipoproteinemia; HTh = hyperthyroid; Inflam = inflammation; LTh = hypothyroid; MI = myocardial infarction; Neo = neonate; NS = nephrotic syndrome; Obes = obese; Pneu = pneumonia; Preg = pregnant; Prem = premature; RA = rheumatoid arthritis; Smk = smoking; Tach = ventricular tachycardia; Ulcer = ulcer patients; Urem = uremia

References: *See* end of table.

Table A–II–1. PHARMACOKINETIC DATA (Continued)

	AVAILABILITY (ORAL) (%)	URINARY EXCRETION (%)	BOUND IN PLASMA (%)	CLEARANCE ($ml \cdot min^{-1} \cdot kg^{-1}$)	VOL. DIST. (liters/kg)	HALF-LIFE (hours)	EFFECTIVE CONCENTRATIONS	TOXIC CONCENTRATIONS
ISOSORBIDE-2-MONONITRATE [a] (Chapter 33)	100	—	—	5.8 ± 1.6	0.82 ± 0.34	1.9 ± 0.5 ⟷ CHF, Urem	—	—
ISOSORBIDE-5-MONONITRATE [a] (Chapter 33)	93 ± 13 ⟷ Cirr, Urem	<5	0	1.81 ± 0.26 ⟷ Cirr, Urem	0.79 ± 0.13 ⟷ Cirr	4.4 ± 0.5 ⟷ Cirr, Urem, MI	100 ng/ml	—
KANAMYCIN (Chapter 51)	—	90	0	1.4 ± 0.2 [a] $CL = 0.62\, CL_{cr} + 0.03$	0.26 ± 0.05	2.1 ± 0.2 ↑ Urem, Neo	*See* Chapter 51	*See* Chapter 51
KETAMINE [a] (Chapter 14)	20 ± 7	2.3 ± 0.5	—	19.1 ± 2.5	2.9 ± 0.7	3.6 ± 1.4	100–150 ng/ml [a]	—
KETOPROFEN (Chapter 29)	[a]	<1	98.7 ± 0.2 ⟷ Cirr	1.2 ± 0.3 [b] ↓ Aged ⟷ Cirr	0.11 ± 0.02 [c]	1.5 ± 0.3 ↑ Aged	—	—

ISOSORBIDE-2-MONONITRATE
[a] Active metabolite of isosorbide dinitrate.

ISOSORBIDE-5-MONONITRATE
[a] Active metabolite of isosorbide dinitrate.

KANAMYCIN
[a] Values reported per 1.73 m²; calculated assuming 70-kg weight.

KETAMINE
[a] Norketamine may be an active metabolite.

KETOPROFEN
[a] Completely absorbed; availability likely >90%.
[b] CL/F.
[c] V_{ss}/F.

LABETALOL (Chapter 9)

20 ± 5 ↑ Aged, Cirr	<5	50	22 ± 9 [a] ←→ Urem, Preg, Cirr	10 ± 2	5.2 ± 1.3 [a] ←→ Cirr, Urem, Preg	0.13 μg/ml [b]	—

[a] Shorter half-life and greater clearance values reported by several investigators probably resulting from insufficient length of sampling.

[b] 50% of maximal decrease in blood pressure.

LIDOCAINE (Chapter 31)

35 ± 11 [a] ↑ Neo	2 ± 1 ↑ Neo	70 ± 5 ↓ Neo, ↑ MI, CPBS, Aged, Urem ←→ NS	9.2 ± 2.4 ↓ CHF, Cirr, CPBS [b] ↑ Smk ←→ Urem, AVH [c], Neo, Aged	1.1 ± 0.4 ↓ CHF, CPBS [b] ↑ Cirr, Neo ←→ Urem, Aged	1.8 ± 0.4 ↑ Cirr, MI [d], Neo ←→ Urem, CPBS, CHF [e]	1.5-6 μg/ml	Occasional: 6-10 μg/ml Frequent: >10 μg/ml

[a] Commercial preparations are for parenteral administration.

[b] Decrease (~40%) on day 3 after surgery; return toward normal on day 7.

[c] During acute phase, blood clearance was 13 ± 4 ml · min^{-1} · kg^{-1}, which increased to 20 ± 4 ml · min^{-1} · kg^{-1} after recovery.

[d] Half-life increased when infusion longer than 24 hours, probably related to increased plasma binding.

[e] Short term, no change; long term, marked increase possibly related to increased binding.

LITHIUM (Chapter 19)

100	95 ± 15	0	0.35 ± 0.11 [a] ↑ Urem, Aged Preg	0.79 ± 0.34 [b]	22 ± 8 [c] ↑ Urem, Aged	0.6-1.2 mEq/l	>2.0 mEq/l

[a] Renal clearance of Li$^+$ parallels that of Na$^+$. The ratio of clearances of Li$^+$ and creatinine is about 0.2 ± 0.03.

[b] V_{area}.

[c] A shorter half-life of 5.6 ± 0.5 hours is due to distribution; this influences drug concentrations for at least 12 hours.

Key: Adult = adults; Aged = aged; Alb = hypoalbuminemia; Arth = arthritis; Atr Fib = atrial fibrillation; AVH = acute viral hepatitis; Burn = burn patients; CAD = coronary artery disease; Celiac = celiac disease; CF = cystic fibrosis; CHF = congestive heart failure; Child = children; Cirr = cirrhosis; COPD = chronic obstructive pulmonary disease; CP = cor pulmonale; CPBS = cardiopulmonary bypass surgery; CRI = chronic respiratory insufficiency; Crohn = Crohn's disease; Cush = Cushing's syndrome; Epilep = epileptic; Fem = female; Hep = Hepatitis; HL = hyperlipoproteinemia; HTh = hyperthyroid; Inflam = inflammation; LTh = hypothyroid; MI = myocardial infarction; Neo = neonate; NS = nephrotic syndrome; Obes = obese; Pneu = pneumonia; Prem = premature; Preg = pregnant; RA = rheumatoid arthritis; Smk = smoking; Tach = ventricular tachycardia; Ulcer = ulcer patients; Urem = uremia

References: *See* end of table.

Table A–II–1. PHARMACOKINETIC DATA (Continued)

AVAILABILITY (ORAL) (%)	URINARY EXCRETION (%)	BOUND IN PLASMA (%)	CLEARANCE ($ml \cdot min^{-1} \cdot kg^{-1}$)	VOL. DIST. (liters/kg)	HALF-LIFE (hours)	EFFECTIVE CONCENTRATIONS	TOXIC CONCENTRATIONS

LORAZEPAM (Chapters 17, 19, 20)

93 ± 10	<1	91 ± 2 ↓ Cirr ←→ Aged	1.1 ± 0.4 ←→ Aged, Cirr, AVH	1.3 ± 0.2 [a] ↑ Cirr ←→ Aged	14 ± 5 ↑ Cirr, Neo ←→ Aged, Urem	—	—

[a] V_{area}.

LORCAINIDE [a] (Chapter 31)

Dose-dependent [b]	<2	85 ± 5 ←→ Cirr	17.5 ± 2.8 [c] → Cirr ←→ Aged	6.4 ± 2.4 Aged ←→ Cirr	7.6 ± 2.2 [d] ↑ Cirr	40–200 ng/ml [e]	—

[a] Active metabolite, N-dealkyl lorcainide (norlorcainide).
[b] Saturable first-pass metabolism. F = 1–4% for 100-mg dose; 35–65% for 200-mg dose.
[c] Blood clearance, 23.6 ± 4.2 ml · min⁻¹ · kg⁻¹.
[d] Norlorcainide, half-life = 27 ± 8 hours. Steady-state ratio of norlorcainide to lorcainide = 2.2 ± 0.9.
[e] 80% suppression of premature ventricular contractions.

MELPHALAN (Chapter 55)

71 ± 23	12 ± 7	—	5.2 ± 2.9 → Child	0.62 ± 0.21 ←→ Child	1.4 ± 0.2 [a] ←→ Child	—	—

[a] Approximately equal to half-life of melphalan in vitro in human plasma at 37° C.

MEPERIDINE (Chapter 22)

52 ± 3 ↑ Cirr	1–25 [a]	58 ± 9 [b] ↑ Aged, Urem ←→ Cirr	17 ± 5 → AVH, Cirr ←→ Aged, Preg	4.4 ± 0.9 ↑ Aged ←→ Cirr, Preg	3.2 ± 0.8 [c] ↑ AVH, Cirr, Aged → Preg	0.4–0.7 µg/ml [d]	—

[a] Meperidine is a weak acid ($pK_a = 9.6$) and is excreted to a greater extent in the urine at low urinary pH and to a lesser extent at high pH.
[b] Correlates with the concentration of α_1-acid glycoprotein.
[c] A longer half-life (7 hours) is also observed.
[d] Postoperative analgesia.

MERCAPTOPURINE (Chapter 55)

12 ± 7 [a]	22 ± 12	19	11 ± 4 [b]	0.56 ± 0.38	0.90 ± 0.37	—

[a] Increases to 60% when first-pass metabolism inhibited by allopurinol (100 mg three times daily).

[b] Despite inhibition of intrinsic clearance by allopurinol, hepatic metabolism is limited by blood flow, and clearance is thus little changed by allopurinol.

METHADONE (Chapter 22)

92 ± 21	24 ± 10 [a]	89 ± 1.4	1.4 ± 0.5 [a]	3.8 ± 0.6 [b]	35 ± 12 [b]	—

[a] Inversely correlated with urine pH.

[b] Directly correlated with urine pH.

METHICILLIN (Chapter 50)

—	88 ± 17	39 ± 2	6.1 ± 1.3 ↓↑ Urem CF	0.43 ± 0.10	0.85 ± 0.23 ↑ Urem	*See* Chapter 50

METHOHEXITAL (Chapters 14, 17)

—	<1	—	10.9 ± 3.0	2.2 ± 0.7	3.9 ± 2.1	5 μg/ml

METHOTREXATE (Chapter 55)

65 [a]	85 ± 11	58 ± 7	1.6 ± 0.3 ↓ Urem	0.96 ± 0.20	7.2 ± 2.1 [b]	10 μM (10 μg/ml) [c]

[a] F may be as low as 20% when doses exceed 80 mg/m².

[b] A faster half-life (2 hours) is seen initially.

[c] Bone-marrow toxicity correlated with concentrations greater than 10 μM at 24 hours, greater than 1 μM at 48 hours, or greater than 0.1 μM at 72 hours.

Key: Adult = adults; Aged = aged; Alb = hypoalbuminemia; Arth = arthritis; Atr Fib = atrial fibrillation; AVH = acute viral hepatitis; Burn = burn patients; CAD = coronary artery disease; Celiac = celiac disease; CF = cystic fibrosis; CHF = congestive heart failure; Child = children; Cir = cirrhosis; COPD = chronic obstructive pulmonary disease; CP = cor pulmonale; CPBS = cardiopulmonary bypass surgery; CRI = chronic respiratory insufficiency; Crohn = Crohn's disease; Cush = Cushing's syndrome; Epilep = epileptic; Fem = female; Hep = Hepatitis; HL = hyperlipoproteinemia; Inflam = inflammation; LTh = hypothyroid; MI = myocardial infarction; Neo = neonate; NS = nephrotic syndrome; Obes = obese; Pneu = pneumonia; Preg = pregnant; Prem = premature; RA = rheumatoid arthritis; Smk = smoking; Tach = ventricular tachycardia; Ulcer = ulcer patients; Urem = uremia

References: *See* end of table.

Table A–II–1. PHARMACOKINETIC DATA (Continued)

	AVAILABILITY (ORAL) (%)	URINARY EXCRETION (%)	BOUND IN PLASMA (%)	CLEARANCE ($ml \cdot min^{-1} \cdot kg^{-1}$)	VOL. DIST. (liters/kg)	HALF-LIFE (hours)	EFFECTIVE CONCENTRATIONS	TOXIC CONCENTRATIONS
METHYLDOPA (Chapter 32)	25 ± 16	28 ± 9 ↓ Crohn [a]	1–16 ←→ Crohn	3.1 ± 0.9 ↓ Urem [b]	0.37 ± 0.10	1.8 ± 0.2 ↑ Urem, Neo ←→ Crohn	—	—
METHYLPREDNISOLONE (Chapter 63)	82 ± 13 [a]	4.9 ± 2.3 ←→ NS, RA, CRI	40–60	3.8 ± 0.9 ←→ NS, RA, CRI	0.84 ± 0.18 ←→ NS, RA, CRI	2.5 ± 0.8 ←→ NS, Urem, RA, CRI	—	—
METOPROLOL (Chapter 9)	38 ± 14 ↑ Cirr	10 ± 3	13 [a]	15 ± 3 ↑ HTh ←→ Aged	4.2 ± 0.7	3.2 ± 0.2 ↑ Cirr, Neo ←→ Aged, HTh	25 ng/ml [b]	—
METRONIDAZOLE [a] (Chapter 46)	99 ± 8	<10	10	1.3 ± 0.3 ↓ Cirr, Neo ←→ Preg	1.1 ± 0.4	8.5 ± 2.9 ↑ Neo ←→ Preg, Urem [a]	3–6 μg/ml	—

METHYLDOPA
[a] Interpreted as a decrease in absorption in Crohn's disease.
[b] Clearances of unchanged drug and active metabolites are reduced.

METHYLPREDNISOLONE
[a] May be decreased to 50–60% at high doses.

METOPROLOL
[a] Blood-to-plasma ratio = 1.
[b] To achieve a 10% decrease in resting heart rate.

METRONIDAZOLE
[a] Active hydroxylated metabolite, which accumulates in renal failure.

MEXILETINE (Chapter 31)

87 ± 13	10–15 [a]	63 ± 3 $\longleftrightarrow$ MI	10.3 ± 2.3 [b] $\downarrow$ MI, Urem [c] $\longleftrightarrow$ CHF	9.5 ± 3.4 [b] $\longleftrightarrow$ MI	10.4 ± 2.8 $\uparrow$ MI, CHF, Urem [c]	0.7–2.0 µg/ml	>2.0 µg/ml

[a] Dependent on urinary pH.
[b] Patient population pharmacokinetic data yield $CL = 6.3 \pm 2.7$ ml $\cdot$ min$^{-1} \cdot$ kg^{-1}; $V_{area} =$ 5.3 liters/kg.
[c] Only in patients with $CL_{cr} < 10$ ml/min.

MEZLOCILLIN (Chapter 50)

—	8–22 [a]	16–42	$CL = 1.44\,CL_{cr} + 0.23$ [b] $\rightarrow$ Neo, Prem $\longleftrightarrow$ Urem, Child	Dose-dependent [c] $\rightarrow$ Prem, Neo $\longleftrightarrow$ Urem, Child	1.3 ± 0.4 $\uparrow$ Urem, Prem, Neo $\longleftrightarrow$ Child	—	—

[a] Dose dependent; higher at lower doses.
[b] For 5-g dose, $CL = 2.07\,CL_{cr} + 0.97$.
[c] $V_{ss} = 0.20 \pm 0.06$ for 1-g dose and 0.14 ± 0.05 for 5-g dose.

MINOCYCLINE (Chapter 52)

100	11 ± 2	76	0.30 ± 0.12 $\longleftrightarrow$, $\uparrow$ Urem [a]	0.40 ± 0.12 $\uparrow$ Urem	18 ± 4 $\longleftrightarrow$ Urem	—	—

[a] In patients with reduced CL_{cr}, single-dose infusion studies indicate that clearance is increased, which is consistent with the increased V and unchanged $t_{1/2}$. However, there is no accumulation of drug beyond that seen in normal subjects during repeated administration of minocycline to patients with CL_{cr} between 18 and 45 ml/min.

MINOXIDIL (Chapter 32)

95	12	—	0.15	3.1 ± 0.6	12 ± 3 $\longleftrightarrow$ Urem	—	—

Key: Adult = adults; Aged = aged: Alb = hypoalbuminemia; Arth = arthritis; Atr Fib = atrial fibrillation; AVH = acute viral hepatitis; Burn = burn patients; CAD = coronary artery disease; Celiac = celiac disease; CF = cystic fibrosis; CHF = congestive heart failure; Child = children; Cirr = cirrhosis; COPD = chronic obstructive pulmonary disease; CP = cor pulmonale; CPBS = cardiopulmonary bypass surgery; CRI = chronic respiratory insufficiency; Crohn = Crohn's disease; Cush = Cushing's syndrome; Epilep = epileptic; Fem = female; Hep = Hepatitis; HL = hyperlipoproteinemia; Inflam = inflammation; LTh = hypothyroid; MI = myocardial infarction; Neo = neonate; NS = nephrotic syndrome; Obes = obese; Pneu = pneumonia; Preg = pregnant; Prem = premature; RA = rheumatoid arthritis; Smk = smoking; Tach = ventricular tachycardia; Ulcer = ulcer patients; Urem = uremia

References: *See* end of table.

Table A–II–1. PHARMACOKINETIC DATA (Continued)

	AVAILABILITY (ORAL) (%)	URINARY EXCRETION (%)	BOUND IN PLASMA (%)	CLEARANCE ($ml \cdot min^{-1} \cdot kg^{-1}$)	VOL. DIST. (liters/kg)	HALF-LIFE (hours)	EFFECTIVE CONCENTRATIONS	TOXIC CONCENTRATIONS
MORPHINE (Chapter 22)	20–33	6–10	35 ± 2 ↓ AVH, Cirr, Alb	15 ± 2 ←→ Aged, Cirr	3.3 ± 0.9 ←→ Cirr	3.0 ± 1.2 ←→ Cirr	65 ± 80 ng/ml [a]	—
MOXALACTAM (Chapter 50)	70–100 [a]	76 ± 12	50	$CL = 1.0\,CL_{cr} + 0.071$	0.25 ± 0.08 ←→ Urem, Aged, Neo, Child	2.1 ± 0.7 ↑ Urem, Neo ←→ Child	—	—
NADOLOL (Chapter 9)	34 ± 5	73 ± 4	20 ± 4	2.9 ± 0.6	2.1 ± 1.0 [a]	16 ± 2 ↑ Urem	—	—
NAFCILLIN (Chapter 50)	36 [a]	27 ± 5 ↑ Cirr [b]	89.4 ± 0.2 ↓ Neo	7.5 ± 1.9 ↓ Cirr [c]	0.35 ± 0.09 ↓ Cirr [c]	1.0 ± 0.2 ←→ Cirr [b], Urem	*See* Chapter 50	—
NALOXONE (Chapter 22)	~2 [a]	—	—	25 ↓ Neo	2.0 ↓ Neo	1.2 ↑ Neo	—	—

MORPHINE (Chapter 22)

[a] To achieve surgical analgesia.

MOXALACTAM (Chapter 50)

[a] Intramuscular.

NADOLOL (Chapter 9)

[a] V_{area}.

NAFCILLIN (Chapter 50)

[a] Calculated from mean values of excretion after oral versus intramuscular administration.
[b] Significant increase noted for patients with extrahepatic biliary obstruction.
[c] Significant decrease also noted for patients with extrahepatic biliary obstruction.

NALOXONE (Chapter 22)

[a] Absorption is relatively complete (91%), but most of the drug is subject to hepatic first-pass metabolism.

NAPROXEN (Chapter 29)

99 [a]	99.7 ± 0.1 [b] ↑ Urem, Aged, Cirr	0.13 ± 0.02 [c] → Urem ←→ Aged[d], Cirr[d]	0.16 ± 0.02 [e] ↑ Urem, Cirr ←→ Aged	14 ± 1 ←→ Urem	>50 μg/ml [f]	—

[a] Estimated.
[b] Saturable protein binding yields apparent nonlinear kinetics.
[c] CL/F.
[d] No change in total clearance, but significant (50%) decrease in clearance of unbound drug; it is thus suggested that dosing rate be decreased.
[e] V_{area}/F.
[f] 76% of patients with rheumatoid arthritis responded with trough concentrations in plasma above this value.

NEOSTIGMINE (Chapter 6)

a	—	8.4 ± 2.7 → Urem	0.7 ± 0.3	1.3 ± 0.8 ↑ Urem	—	—

[a] Absorption is presumed to be less than complete, since oral dosage must greatly exceed intravenous to achieve a similar effect.

NETILMICIN (Chapter 51)

80–90 [a]	<10	1.3 ± 0.2 → Urem ←→ CF, Child	0.20 ± 0.02 ←→ Urem	2.3 ± 0.7 / 37 ± 6 [b] ↑ Urem, Neo ↑ CF ←→ Child	See Chapter 51	See Chapter 51

[a] Possibly higher, since drug persists in tissues for a long time.
[b] Netilmicin has a long terminal half-life, which accounts for prolonged urinary excretion.

NICOTINE (Chapters 10, 23)

—	16.7 ± 8.6	4.9 ± 2.8	18.5 ± 5.4	2.6 ± 0.9	2.0 ± 0.7	—

Key: Adult = adults; Aged = aged; Alb = hypoalbuminemia; Arth = arthritis; Atr Fib = atrial fibrillation; AVH = acute viral hepatitis; Burn = burn patients; CAD = coronary artery disease; Celiac = celiac disease; CF = cystic fibrosis; CHF = congestive heart failure; Child = children; Cirr = cirrhosis; COPD = chronic obstructive pulmonary disease; CP = cor pulmonale; CPBS = cardiopulmonary bypass surgery; CRI = chronic respiratory insufficiency; Crohn = Crohn's disease; Cush = Cushing's syndrome; Epilep = epileptic; Fem = female; Hep = Hepatitis; HL = hyperlipoproteinemia; HTh = hyperthyroid; Inflam = inflammation; LTh = hypothyroid; MI = myocardial infarction; Neo = neonate; NS = nephrotic syndrome; Obes = obese; Pneu = pneumonia; Prem = premature; Preg = pregnant; RA = rheumatoid arthritis; Smk = smoking; Tach = ventricular tachycardia; Ulcer = ulcer patients; Urem = uremia

References: *See* end of table.

Table A–II–1. PHARMACOKINETIC DATA (Continued)

AVAILABILITY (ORAL) (%)	URINARY EXCRETION (%)	BOUND IN PLASMA (%)	CLEARANCE ($ml \cdot min^{-1} \cdot kg^{-1}$)	VOL. DIST. (liters/kg)	HALF-LIFE (hours)	EFFECTIVE CONCENTRATIONS	TOXIC CONCENTRATIONS

NIFEDIPINE (Chapter 33)

| 45 ± 28 | ~0 | 98 | 10.3 ± 5.2 | 1.2 ± 0.5 | 3.4 ± 1.2 | — | — |

[a] Sedation and drowsiness.

NITRAZEPAM (Chapters 17, 20)

| 78 ± 16 | <1 | 87 ± 1 ↓ Cirr ←→ Aged | 0.86 ± 0.12 ←→ Aged, Cirr | 1.9 ± 0.3 ↑ Aged ←→ Cirr | 26 ± 3 Aged ←→ Cirr | — | >200 ng/ml [a] |

NITROGLYCERIN [a] (Chapter 33)

| 38 ± 26 [b] | <1 | — | 230 ± 90 [c] | 3.3 ± 1.2 [d] | 2.3 ± 0.6 min | 1.2–11 ng/ml [e] | — |

[a] Active dinitrate metabolites have weak activity compared to nitroglycerin (<10%), but, due to prolonged half-life (~40 min), they may accumulate during administration of sustained-release preparations to yield concentrations in plasma 10–20 times greater than the parent drug.
[b] Sublingual dose rinsed out of the mouth after 8 min. Rinse contained 31 ± 19% of the dose.
[c] Following a prolonged infusion.
[d] V_{area}.
[e] 25% fall in capillary wedge pressure in patients with CHF.

NORTRIPTYLINE (Chapter 19)

| 51 ± 5 | 2 ± 1 | 92 ± 2 ↑ HL | 7.2 ± 1.8 ↓ Aged, Inflam ←→ Smk, Urem | 18 ± 4 [a] | 31 ± 13 ↑ Aged ←→ Urem | 50–140 ng/ml [b] | — |

[a] V_{area}.
[b] At concentrations in plasma above 140 ng/ml, the antidepressant effect appears to be less.

OXACILLIN (Chapter 50)

| 33 | 46 ± 4 | 92.2 ± 0.6 | 6.1 ± 1.7 | 0.33 ± 0.09 [a] ↑ Urem | 0.4–0.7 ↑ Urem | See Chapter 50 | — |

[a] V_{area}.

OXAZEPAM (Chapters 17, 19)

>90 [a]	<1	97.8 ± 2.3 ↑ Urem ↔ Aged, Alb, AVH, Cirr	1.2 ± 0.4 [b] ↑ HTh, Smk, Urem [c] ↔ LTh, Aged, AVH, Cirr	1.0 ± 0.3 [b] ↑ Urem ↔ Aged, AVH, Cirr	7.6 ± 2.2 ↑ Urem, Neo HTh ↔ Aged, AVH, Cirr, LTh, Preg	—	—

[a] Estimated from complete absorption and first-pass hepatic metabolism.
[b] CL/F and V_{area}/F.
[c] CL/F of unbound drug is unchanged in uremia.

PANCURONIUM (Chapter 11)

—	67 ± 18	Small	1.8 ± 0.4 ↓ Aged, Urem	0.26 ± 0.07 ↔ Aged, Urem	2.3 ± 0.4 ↑ Aged, Urem	88 ± 34 ng/ml [a]	—

[a] 50% decrease in twitch tension.

PHENOBARBITAL (Chapters 17, 20)

100 ± 11	24 ± 5 [a] ↔ Cirr, AVH	51 ± 3 ↓ Neo [b] ↔ Preg, Aged	0.062 ± 0.013 ↑ Preg, Child, Neo [b] ↔ Epilep	0.54 ± 0.03 ↑ Epilep [b] ↑ Neo	99 ± 18 ↑ Cirr, Aged Child ↔ Epilep, Neo [b]	10–25 µg/ml [c] 15 µg/ml [d]	>30 µg/ml 65–117 µg/ml [e] 100–134 µg/ml [f]

[a] Increased when urine is alkaline; decreased with decreased urine flow.
[b] Average clearance following daily intravenous dosage: week 1, 0.10; week 4, 0.17. Half-life: week 1, 115 hours; week 4, 67 hours. Insufficient information to determine whether change is due to natural maturation or induction of metabolism by drug.
[c] Tonic-clonic seizures.
[d] Febrile convulsions in children.
[e] Stage III—comatose, reflexes present.
[f] Stage IV—no deep-tendon reflexes.

Key: Adult = adults; Aged = aged; Alb = hypoalbuminemia; Arth = arthritis; Atr Fib = atrial fibrillation; AVH = acute viral hepatitis; Burn = burn patients; CAD = coronary artery disease; Celiac = celiac disease; CF = cystic fibrosis; CHF = congestive heart failure; Child = children; Cirr = cirrhosis; COPD = chronic obstructive pulmonary disease; CP = cor pulmonale; CPBS = cardiopulmonary bypass surgery; CRI = chronic respiratory insufficiency; Crohn = Crohn's disease; Cush = Cushing's syndrome; Epilep = epileptic; Fem = female; Hep = Hepatitis; HL = hyperlipoproteinemia; HTh = hyperthyroid; Inflam = inflammation; LTh = hypothyroid; MI = myocardial infarction; Neo = neonate; NS = nephrotic syndrome; Obes = obese; Pneu = pneumonia; Prem = premature; Preg = pregnant; RA = rheumatoid arthritis; Smk = smoking; Tach = ventricular tachycardia; Ulcer = ulcer patients; Urem = uremia

References: *See end of table.*

Table A–II–1. PHARMACOKINETIC DATA (Continued)

	AVAILABILITY (ORAL) (%)	URINARY EXCRETION (%)	BOUND IN PLASMA (%)	CLEARANCE ($ml \cdot min^{-1} \cdot kg^{-1}$)	VOL. DIST. (liters/kg)	HALF-LIFE (hours)	EFFECTIVE CONCENTRATIONS	TOXIC CONCENTRATIONS
PHENYLBUTAZONE [a] (Chapter 29)	80–100 [b]	~1	96.1 ± 1.1 ↓ Cirr, AVH, Urem, Hep, Aged ↔ Smk	0.023 ± 0.003 [c] ↔ Smk	0.097 ± 0.005 [c] ↑ Urem ↔ Smk	56 ± 8 → Child ↔ Aged, RA, Cirr, Urem	50–150 μg/ml	—
PHENYLETHYLMALONAMIDE [a] (Chapter 20)	91 ± 4	79 ± 5 [b]	Negligible	0.52 ± 0.11 ↓ Urem ↔ Epilep	0.69 ± 0.10 ↔ Epilep	16 ± 3 ↑ Urem, Neo ↔ Epilep	[c]	—
PHENYTOIN (Chapters 20, 31)	98 ± 7	2 ± 8	89 ± 23 → Urem, Hep, Alb, Neo, AVH, Cirr, NS, Preg, Epilep, Burn ↔ Obes	V_m = 7.5 ± 2.0 mg · kg⁻¹ · day⁻¹ → Child; K_m = 5.7 ± 2.9 mg/l [a] ↓ Aged; ↔ Child; ↓ NS, Urem ↑ Prem ↔ AVH, LTh, HTh	0.64 ± 0.04 [c] ↑ Neo, NS, Urem ↔ AVH, LTh, HTh	6–24 [d] ↑ Prem ↑ Urem ↔ AVH, LTh, HTh	>10 μg/ml [e]	>20 μg/ml [f]

PHENYLBUTAZONE footnotes:
a Active metabolites, oxyphenbutazone and γ-hydroxyphenylbutazone.
b Estimate.
c CL/F and V_{area}/F.

PHENYLETHYLMALONAMIDE footnotes:
a One of the two major metabolites of primidone.
b After oral dose.
c Antiepileptic efficacy not established; active in rats.

PHENYTOIN footnotes:
a Significantly decreased in Japanese.
b Comparison of clearances and half-lives with similar doses in normal subjects and patients; nonlinear kinetics not considered.
c V_{area}.
d Apparent half-life is dependent on plasma concentration.
e Suppression of tonic-clonic convulsions.
f Nystagmus; ataxia may not occur until concentrations exceed 30 μg/ml.

PINDOLOL (Chapter 9)

75 ± 9 Urem ↓	54 ± 9	51 ± 3 [a]	8.3 ± 1.8 Urem →	2.3 ± 0.9 Urem ←→	3.6 ± 0.6 Urem ↑	58 ng/ml [b]	—

[a] Blood-to-plasma ratio = 0.69 ± 0.08.

[b] 50% decrease in exercise-induced cardioacceleration.

PIPERACILLIN (Chapter 50)

—	71 ± 14 [a]	2.6 ± 0.7 $CL = 1.36\,CL_{cr} + 1.50$ Child ↑ CF ↓	16, 48 [a]	0.18 ± 0.03 CF ↓ Urem, Child ←→	0.93 ± 0.12 Urem ← Child, CF ↓	—	—

[a] Different studies report 16, 21, and 48%.

PRAZEPAM [a] (Chapters 17, 19)

b	0	140 ± 100 [c]	—	14.4 ± 5.1 [c]	1.3 ± 0.7	—	—

[a] Prazepam is essentially a prodrug for desmethyldiazepam; *see also* listing for that compound. Values above are for prazepam.

[b] Availability of desmethyldiazepam from prazepam is 51 ± 5% of that from clorazepate.

[c] CL/F and V_{area}/F.

PRAZOSIN (Chapter 32)

57 ± 10	95 ± 1 Cirr, Alb ↓ CHF, Urem ←→	3.0 ± 0.3 [a] CHF ↓ Aged ←→	<1	0.60 ± 0.13 [a] Aged ←→	2.9 ± 0.8 CHF ↑ Aged ←→	—	—

[a] Assuming 70-kg weight.

Key: Adult = adults; Aged = aged; Alb = hypoalbuminemia; Arth = arthritis; Atr Fib = atrial fibrillation; AVH = acute viral hepatitis; Burn = burn patients; CAD = coronary artery disease; Celiac = celiac disease; CF = cystic fibrosis; CHF = congestive heart failure; Child = children; Cir = cirrhosis; COPD = chronic obstructive pulmonary disease; CP = cor pulmonale; CPBS = cardiopulmonary bypass surgery; CRI = chronic respiratory insufficiency; Crohn = Crohn's disease; Cush = Cushing's syndrome; Epilep = epileptic; Fem = female; Hep = Hepatitis; HL = hyperlipoproteinemia; HTh = hyperthyroid; Inflam = inflammation; LTh = hypothyroid; MI = myocardial infarction; Neo = neonate; NS = nephrotic syndrome; Obes = obese; Pneu = pneumonia; Preg = pregnant; Prem = premature; RA = rheumatoid arthritis; Smk = smoking; Tach = ventricular tachycardia; Ulcer = ulcer patients; Urem = uremia

References: *See* end of table.

Table A–II–1. PHARMACOKINETIC DATA (Continued)

	AVAILABILITY (ORAL) (%)	URINARY EXCRETION (%)	BOUND IN PLASMA (%)	CLEARANCE ($ml \cdot min^{-1} \cdot kg^{-1}$)	VOL. DIST. (liters/kg)	HALF-LIFE (hours)	EFFECTIVE CONCENTRATIONS	TOXIC CONCENTRATIONS
PREDNISOLONE (Chapter 63)	82 ± 13 → Hep, Cush, Urem, Crohn, Celiac, Smk	15 ± 5 [a]	90–95 (<200 ng/ml) [b] ~70 (>1 µg/ml) ↓ Alb, NS → Hep	8.7 ± 1.6 [c,d] → Hep, Cush, Smk, CRI, NS [c]	1.5 ± 0.2 [c,e] → Hep, Cush, Smk, CRI, NS [c]	2.2 ± 0.5 → Hep, Cush, Smk, Urem, CRI, NS [c]	—	—
PREDNISONE (Chapter 63)	80 ± 11 [a] → Hep, Cush, Urem, Crohn, Celiac, Smk	3 ± 2 [b]	75 ± 2 [c]	3.6 ± 0.8 [d] → Hep	0.97 ± 0.11 [d] → Hep	3.6 ± 0.4 → Smk, Hep	—	—
PRIMIDONE [a] (Chapter 20)	92 ± 18 [b,c]	42 ± 15 [b]	19 [d]	0.94 ± 0.35 [e] ↑ Preg, Urem ↓ → Child	0.59 ± 0.47 [b,e]	8.0 ± 4.8 ↑ Neo, Urem → Child	5–10 µg/ml [f]	>10 µg/ml 70–80 µg/ml [g]

PREDNISOLONE (Chapter 63)

[a] An additional 3 ± 2% is excreted as prednisone.
[b] Extent of binding to plasma proteins is dependent on concentration over range encountered.
[c] Values for unbound drug.
[d] Clearance of unbound drug increases slightly but significantly with increasing dose. Total clearance increases markedly as protein binding is saturated.
[e] Independent of dose. When total drug concentration is measured, V increases due to saturable protein binding.

PREDNISONE (Chapter 63)

[a] Measured relative to equivalent intravenous dose of prednisolone.
[b] An additional 15 ± 5% excreted as prednisolone.
[c] In contrast to prednisolone, no dependence on concentration.
[d] Kinetic values for prednisone are often reported in terms of the values for prednisolone, with which it is interconverted. However, the values above were obtained by measurement of prednisone after the intravenous administration of prednisone.

PRIMIDONE [a] (Chapter 20)

[a] Primidone is metabolized to phenobarbital and phenylethylmalonamide; see also listings for these compounds.
[b] Children.
[c] Based on percentage of dose recovered in urine as primidone and its two primary metabolites.
[d] Based on ratio of drug concentrations in cerebrospinal fluid and plasma. Blood-to-plasma ratio = 0.97 ± 0.12.
[e] Data from oral, multiple-dose regimen; values are CL/F and V_{area}/F.
[f] Concentrations observed in patients with seizures who are improved or controlled by primidone. Concentrations of phenobarbital are considered to be more relevant.
[g] Crystalluria.

PROBENECID (Chapter 38)

| 100 | 1.2 ± 0.2 | 83–95 | Dose-dependent [a] | 0.15 ± 0.02 | Dose-dependent [b] | — | — |

[a] At 0.5-g dose, 0.38 ± 0.17 ml · min^{-1} · kg^{-1}; at 2-g dose, 0.25 ± 0.09 ml · min^{-1} · kg^{-1}.
[b] At 0.5-g dose, 5 ± 3 hours; at 2-g dose, 8 ± 3 hours.

PROCAINAMIDE [a] (Chapter 31)

| 83 ± 16 | 16 ± 5 | $CL = 2.7\, CL_{cr} + 1.7 + 3.2$ (fast)[b] or $+ 1.1$ (slow)[b] | 1.9 ± 0.3 | 3.0 ± 0.6 | 3–14 µg/ml | >14 µg/ml |
| ↓ CHF, COPD, CP, Cirr | | Child, MI ↑, → CHF | ↓ CHF, Obes, Urem, Child | 3.0 ± 0.6, Urem, MI ↑, Child, → Obes | | |

[a] Active metabolite; *see also* data for N-acetylprocainamide.
[b] Clearance depends on acetylation phenotype. Use a mean value of 2.2 if phenotype unknown.

PROPRANOLOL [a] (Chapters 9, 31–33)

| 36 ± 10 | <0.5 | 12 ± 3[c] | 93.3 ± 1.2[b] | 3.9 ± 0.6[c] | 3.9 ± 0.4[c] | 20 ng/ml[d] | — |
| | | ↑ Smk, HTh, Hep; ←→ Aged | ↑ Inflam, Crohn, Preg, Obes; ←→ Urem | ↑ Hep, HTh, Crohn; ←→ Aged | ↑ Hep; ←→ Aged | | |

[a] Active metabolite, 4-hydroxypropranolol.
[b] Drug bound primarily to α_1-acid glycoprotein, which is elevated in a number of inflammatory conditions; blood-to-plasma ratio = 0.74 ± 0.03.
[c] Blood measurements.
[d] To achieve a 50% decrease in exercise-induced cardioacceleration. Antianginal effects are manifest at 15–90 ng/ml. Concentrations up to 1000 ng/ml may be required to control resistant ventricular arrhythmias.

PROTRIPTYLINE (Chapter 19)

| 77–93 [a] | — | 92 ± 0.6[b] | 3.6 ± 0.6[c] | 22 ± 1[d] | 78 ± 11 | 100–200 ng/ml | — |

[a] Estimated from reported values of CL/F, assuming erythrocyte-to-plasma ratio ranges from 0 to 2, complete absorption, hepatic blood flow of 1500 ml/min, and hematocrit of 0.45.
[b] Determined at 24–26° C in heparinized plasma.
[c] CL/F.
[d] V_{area}/F.

Key: Adult = adults; Aged = aged; Alb = hypoalbuminemia; Arth = arthritis; Atr Fib = atrial fibrillation; AVH = acute viral hepatitis; Burn = burn patients; CAD = coronary artery disease; Celiac = celiac disease; CF = cystic fibrosis; CHF = congestive heart failure; Child = children; Cirr = cirrhosis; COPD = chronic obstructive pulmonary disease; CP = cor pulmonale; CPBS = cardiopulmonary bypass surgery; CRI = chronic respiratory insufficiency; Crohn = Crohn's disease; Cush = Cushing's syndrome; Epilep = epileptic; Fem = female; Hep = Hepatitis; HL = hyperlipoproteinemia; HTh = hyperthyroid; Inflam = inflammation; LTh = hypothyroid; MI = myocardial infarction; Neo = neonate; NS = nephrotic syndrome; Obes = obese; Pneu = pneumonia; Preg = pregnant; Prem = premature; RA = rheumatoid arthritis; Smk = smoking; Tach = ventricular tachycardia; Ulcer = ulcer patients; Urem = uremia

References: *See* end of table.

Table A–II–1. PHARMACOKINETIC DATA (Continued)

	AVAILABILITY (ORAL) (%)	URINARY EXCRETION (%)	BOUND IN PLASMA (%)	CLEARANCE (ml · min⁻¹ · kg⁻¹)	VOL. DIST. (liters/kg)	HALF-LIFE (hours)	EFFECTIVE CONCENTRATIONS	TOXIC CONCENTRATIONS
PYRIDOSTIGMINE (Chapter 6)	14 ± 3	80–90	—	8.5 ± 1.7 ↓ Urem	1.1 ± 0.3 ←→ Urem	1.9 ± 0.2 (intravenous) 3.7 ± 1.0 (oral) ↑ Urem	50–100 ng/ml [a]	—

[a] Restoration of neuromuscular transmission in patients with myasthenia gravis.

	AVAILABILITY (ORAL) (%)	URINARY EXCRETION (%)	BOUND IN PLASMA (%)	CLEARANCE (ml · min⁻¹ · kg⁻¹)	VOL. DIST. (liters/kg)	HALF-LIFE (hours)	EFFECTIVE CONCENTRATIONS	TOXIC CONCENTRATIONS
PYRIMETHAMINE (Chapter 45)	[a]	65 [b]	87 ± 1	0.41 ± 0.06 [c]	2.9 ± 0.5 [c]	83 ± 14	—	—

[a] Reported to be well absorbed. Since CL is low, availability is presumably high.
[b] Estimated.
[c] CL/F and V_{area}/F.

	AVAILABILITY (ORAL) (%)	URINARY EXCRETION (%)	BOUND IN PLASMA (%)	CLEARANCE (ml · min⁻¹ · kg⁻¹)	VOL. DIST. (liters/kg)	HALF-LIFE (hours)	EFFECTIVE CONCENTRATIONS	TOXIC CONCENTRATIONS
QUINIDINE (Chapter 31)	Sulfate: 80 ± 15 Gluconate: 71 ± 17	18 ± 5 ←→ CHF	90 ± 3 ↓ Cirr, Hep ←→ Urem, CRI, HL, Aged	4.7 ± 1.8 ↓ CHF, Aged ←→ Cirr	2.7 ± 1.2 ↓ CHF ↑ Cirr ←→ Aged	6.2 ± 1.8 ↑ Aged, Cirr ←→ CHF, Urem	2–6 μg/ml [a]	6, 9, 14 μg/ml [b]

[a] Specific assay methods for quinidine show >75% reduction in frequency of premature ventricular contractions at concentrations of 0.7–5.9 μg/ml, but active metabolites were not measured. Older, less specific assays of both active and inactive metabolites suggested a range of 2–7 μg/ml.

[b] Nonspecific assay; concentrations that cause toxic effects in 10, 30, and 50% of patients, respectively.

	AVAILABILITY (ORAL) (%)	URINARY EXCRETION (%)	BOUND IN PLASMA (%)	CLEARANCE (ml · min⁻¹ · kg⁻¹)	VOL. DIST. (liters/kg)	HALF-LIFE (hours)	EFFECTIVE CONCENTRATIONS	TOXIC CONCENTRATIONS
QUININE (Chapter 45)	—	70	—	1.9 ± 0.5	1.8 ± 0.4	11 ± 2	—	—

RANITIDINE (Chapter 26)

52 ± 11 ↑ Cirr	69 ± 6 → Urem	15 ± 3	10.4 ± 1.1 → Urem, Aged [a]	1.8 ± 0.3 [b] ↔ Cirr	2.1 ± 0.2 ↑ Urem, Aged [a], Cirr	100 ng/ml [c]	—

[a] Related to alterations of renal function.
[b] V_{area}.
[c] IC50 for inhibition of gastric acid secretion.

RIFAMPIN [a] (Chapter 53)

[b]	7 ± 3 ↑ Neo	89 ± 1	3.5 ± 1.6 ↑ Neo, ↑ Urem [c], ↔ Aged	0.97 ± 0.36 ↑ Neo, ↔ Aged	3.5 ± 0.8 [d] ↑ Hep, Cirr, AVH, Urem [c], ↔ Child, Aged	—	—

[a] Active desacetyl metabolite.
[b] Although some studies indicate complete absorption, data are insufficient. Such reports presumably refer to rifampin plus its desacetyl metabolite, since considerable first-pass metabolism would be expected.
[c] Not observed with 300-mg doses, but pronounced differences with 900-mg doses.
[d] Half-life is longer with high single doses and is shorter after repeated administration.

SALICYLIC ACID [a] (Chapter 29)

100	2–30 [b] ↔ Aged, Cirr	Dose-dependent [c] ↓ Urem, Alb, Neo, Preg	0.88 ± 0.16 at 11–16 µg/ml; 0.20 ± 0.01 at 134–157 µg/ml; 0.18 ± 0.02 at 254–312 µg/ml [d] ↑ Neo, ↔ Aged	0.17 ± 0.03 [e] ↔ Cirr	Dose-dependent [f] ↔ Cirr	150–300 µg/ml [g]	>200 µg/ml [h]

[a] Drug displays dose-dependent kinetics.
[b] Dependent on dose and pH of urine.
[c] 95% at 14 µg/ml; 80% at 300 µg/ml; decreases further at higher concentrations.
[d] Note that total clearance does not change over therapeutic range in steady-state studies in normals (urine pH < 6) due to inversely related changes in protein binding and clearance of unbound drug.
[e] At a dose of 1.2 g per day, V increases with increasing dose due to changes in protein binding.
[f] Ranges from 2.4 hours at 300-mg dose to 19 hours and longer when there is intoxication.
[g] Anti-inflammatory effects.
[h] Tinnitus.

Key: Adult = adults; Aged = aged; Alb = hypoalbuminemia; Arth = arthritis; Atr Fib = atrial fibrillation; AVH = acute viral hepatitis; Burn = burn patients; CAD = coronary artery disease; Celiac = celiac disease; CF = cystic fibrosis; CHF = congestive heart failure; Child = children; Cirr = cirrhosis; COPD = chronic obstructive pulmonary disease; CP = cor pulmonale; CPBS = cardiopulmonary bypass surgery; CRI = chronic respiratory insufficiency; Crohn = Crohn's disease; Cush = Cushing's syndrome; Epilep = epileptic; Fem = female; Hep = Hepatitis; HL = hyperlipoproteinemia; HTh = hyperthyroid; Inflam = inflammation; LTh = hypothyroid; MI = myocardial infarction; Neo = neonate; NS = nephrotic syndrome; Obes = obese; Pneu = pneumonia; Preg = pregnant; Prem = premature; RA = rheumatoid arthritis; Smk = smoking; Tach = ventricular tachycardia; Ulcer = ulcer patients; Urem = uremia

References: *See* end of table.

Table A–II–1. PHARMACOKINETIC DATA (Continued)

AVAILABILITY (ORAL) (%)	URINARY EXCRETION (%)	BOUND IN PLASMA (%)	CLEARANCE ($ml \cdot min^{-1} \cdot kg^{-1}$)	VOL. DIST. (liters/kg)	HALF-LIFE (hours)	EFFECTIVE CONCENTRATIONS	TOXIC CONCENTRATIONS
STREPTOMYCIN (Chapter 51)							
—	39 ± 12	48 ± 14	0.39 [a]	0.18 ± 0.11	5.3 ± 2.2 ↑ Urem	—	—

[a] Calculated from average $t_{1/2}$ and V.

SULFADIAZINE (Chapter 49)							
~100	62	54 ± 4 ←→ Aged	0.55 ± 0.17 [a]	0.29 ± 0.04 [a]	7.0 ± 3.9 [a]	—	—

[a] Study included concurrent administration of trimethoprim.

SULFAMETHOXAZOLE (Chapter 49)							
~100	15–30	62 ± 5 ↓ Urem, Alb	0.32 ± 0.04 [a,b] ←→ Urem	0.21 ± 0.02 [a,b] ↑ Urem ←→ Child, CF	10.1 ± 4.6 [b] ↑ Urem ←→ Child ↓ CF	See Chapter 49	—

[a] Assuming 70-kg weight.
[b] Studies included concurrent administration of trimethoprim and variation in urinary pH; these factors had no marked effect on the clearance of sulfamethoxazole.

SULFISOXAZOLE (Chapter 49)							
96 ± 14	49 ± 8 [a]	91.4 ± 1.2 ↓ Urem, Preg, Cirr	0.33 ± 0.01 ↑ Cirr [b]	0.15 ± 0.02 ↑ Cirr [b]	6.6 ± 0.7 ↑ Urem ←→ Cirr	See Chapter 49	See Chapter 49

[a] Dependent on rate of urine formation and pH.
[b] Changes due to differences in protein binding.

TEMAZEPAM (Chapter 17)							
>80	1.5	97.6 ←→ Aged	0.87 ± 0.18 [a] ←→ Aged	1.06 ± 0.31 [a] ←→ Aged	13 ± 3 ←→ Aged	—	—

[a] CL/F and V_{area}/F.

TERBUTALINE (Chapter 8)

15 ± 6 [a]	57 ± 14	25	3.0 ± 0.5 ⟷ Child	1.4 ± 0.4 ⟷ Child	16 ± 3 [b] ⟷ Child	3 ng/ml [c]	—

[a] Decreased when taken with meals.
[b] Significantly shorter half-lives reported in the literature underestimate accumulation.
[c] 50% increase in FEV_1 in asthmatic patients.

TETRACYCLINE (Chapter 52)

77	58 ± 8	65 ± 3	1.67 ± 0.24	1.5 ± 0.08 [a]	10.6 ± 1.5	*See* Chapter 52	—

[a] V_{area}.

THEOPHYLLINE (Chapter 25)

96 ± 8	13 ↑ Neo, Prem	56 ± 4 ↓ Aged, Cirr, Neo	0.65 ± 0.20 [a] ↓ Neo, Prem, Cirr, CHF, CP, Hep, Obes, Pneu ↑ Smk	0.50 ± 0.16 ↓ Obes ↑ Prem, Cirr	9.0 ± 2.1 ↑ Smk ↓ Prem, Neo, Cirr, CHF, Hep, CP	10 µg/ml	20 µg/ml

[a] Nonlinear kinetics due to saturable metabolism, especially in children at steady state. Ratio of % increase in steady-state concentration to % increase in dose was >1.5 in 15% of children changed to a higher dose.

THIOPENTAL (Chapters 14, 17)

—	<1 ↑ Aged, Cirr	85 ± 4 ↓ Aged, Cirr	3.9 ± 1.2 ⟷ Cirr, Aged, Obes; CL_{int} = 28 ± 9 ↓ Cirr	2.3 ± 0.5 ↑ Aged, Obes	9.0 ± 1.6 ↑ Aged, Cirr, Obes	10 µg/ml	—

Key: Adult = adults; Aged = aged; Alb = hypoalbuminemia; Arth = arthritis; Atr Fib = atrial fibrillation; AVH = acute viral hepatitis; Burn = burn patients; CAD = coronary artery disease; Celiac = celiac disease; CF = cystic fibrosis; CHF = congestive heart failure; Child = children; Cirr = cirrhosis; COPD = chronic obstructive pulmonary disease; CP = cor pulmonale; CPBS = cardiopulmonary bypass surgery; CRI = chronic respiratory insufficiency; Crohn = Crohn's disease; Cush = Cushing's syndrome; Epilep = epileptic; Fem = female; Hep = Hepatitis; HL = hyperlipoproteinemia; HTh = hyperthyroid; Inflam = inflammation; LTh = hypothyroid; MI = myocardial infarction; Neo = neonate; NS = nephrotic syndrome; Obes = obese; Pneu = pneumonia; Preg = pregnant; Prem = premature; RA = rheumatoid arthritis; Smk = smoking; Tach = ventricular tachycardia; Ulcer = ulcer patients; Urem = uremia

References: *See* end of table.

Table A–II–1. PHARMACOKINETIC DATA (Continued)

	AVAILABILITY (ORAL) (%)	URINARY EXCRETION (%)	BOUND IN PLASMA (%)	CLEARANCE ($ml \cdot min^{-1} \cdot kg^{-1}$)	VOL. DIST. (liters/kg)	HALF-LIFE (hours)	EFFECTIVE CONCENTRATIONS	TOXIC CONCENTRATIONS
TICARCILLIN (Chapter 50)	—	92 ± 2	65	2.0 ± 0.2 $\downarrow$ Urem	0.21 ± 0.03	1.3 ± 0.1 $\uparrow$ Urem	*See* Chapter 50	—
TIMOLOL (Chapter 9)	50	15	10	7.3 ± 3.3 $\longleftrightarrow$ MI	2.1 ± 0.8 $\longleftrightarrow$ MI	4.1 ± 1.1 $\longleftrightarrow$ MI	15 ng/ml [a]	—

[a] 50% decrease in exercise-induced cardioacceleration.

	AVAILABILITY (ORAL) (%)	URINARY EXCRETION (%)	BOUND IN PLASMA (%)	CLEARANCE ($ml \cdot min^{-1} \cdot kg^{-1}$)	VOL. DIST. (liters/kg)	HALF-LIFE (hours)	EFFECTIVE CONCENTRATIONS	TOXIC CONCENTRATIONS
TOBRAMYCIN (Chapter 51)	—	90 [a]	<10	$CL = 0.66\ CL_{cr}$ $\downarrow$ Obes $\uparrow$ CF	0.26 ± 0.09 $\downarrow$ Obes $\longleftrightarrow$ Urem, Aged, Burn $\uparrow$ CF, Neo	2.2 ± 0.1 100 ± 57 [b] $\uparrow$ Urem, Neo, Prem $\longleftrightarrow$ Obes, CF $\downarrow$ Burn	*See* Chapter 51	*See* Chapter 51

[a] Possibly higher, since drug persists in tissues for long periods of time.
[b] Tobramycin has a very long terminal half-life, which accounts for prolonged urinary excretion.

	AVAILABILITY (ORAL) (%)	URINARY EXCRETION (%)	BOUND IN PLASMA (%)	CLEARANCE ($ml \cdot min^{-1} \cdot kg^{-1}$)	VOL. DIST. (liters/kg)	HALF-LIFE (hours)	EFFECTIVE CONCENTRATIONS	TOXIC CONCENTRATIONS
TOCAINIDE [a] (Chapter 31)	89 ± 5	38 ± 7	10 ± 15	2.6 ± 0.5 $\downarrow$ CHF, Urem $\longleftrightarrow$ MI	3.0 ± 0.2 $\downarrow$ CHF $\longleftrightarrow$ MI, Urem	13.5 ± 2.3 $\uparrow$ Urem $\longleftrightarrow$ MI, CHF	6–15 µg/ml	—

[a] Significant pharmacokinetic differences between R(–) and S(+) enantiomers of this racemic drug.

TOLBUTAMIDE (Chapter 64)

93 ± 10	0	96 ± 1 ↓ AVH, Aged	0.30 ± 0.05 ↑ AVH	0.15 ± 0.03 ←→ AVH	5.9 ± 1.4 ↓ AVH, CRI ←→ Aged, Urem	80–240 μg/ml [a]	—

[a] Decrease in blood glucose concentration of greater than 25%.

TOLMETIN (Chapter 29)

[a]	11 ± 5 [b]	99.4 ± 0.1 ↓ Urem	1.3 ± 0.5 [c] ←→ RA	0.09 ± 0.04 [d] ←→ RA	1.2 ± 0.6 [e]	—	—

[a] Completely absorbed; availability probably >90%.
[b] Oral dosage.
[c] CL/F.
[d] V_{area}/F.
[e] Longer (6–7 hour) terminal half-life also observed; correlates with half-life in synovial fluid.

TRIAMTERENE [a] (Chapter 36)

54 ± 12 [b]	52 ± 10 [b] Cirr [c]	61 ± 2 [d] HL ↓ Urem, Alb, Cirr [e]	63 ± 20 [f] ↓ Cirr, Urem [e]	13.4 ± 4.9 [f]	4.2 ± 0.7 [g] ↑ Urem [e]	—	—

[a] Active metabolite, hydroxytriamterene sulfuric acid ester.
[b] Triamterene plus active metabolite.
[c] Decreased active metabolite; increased parent drug.
[d] For metabolite, percent bound = 90.4 ± 1.3.
[e] Active metabolite.
[f] Since triamterene is predominantly present in plasma as the active metabolite, these values are deceptively high. CL_{renal} = 3.6 ± 0.7 for triamterene and 2.3 ± 0.6 for the metabolite.
[g] Metabolite $t_{1/2}$ = 3.1 ± 1.2 hours.

TRIAZOLAM (Chapter 17)

55 [a]	2	90.1 ± 1.5 ←→ Urem, Alb, Obes, Aged	8.3 ± 1.8 [b] ↓ Obes, Aged	1.1 ± 0.4 [b] ↓ Obes	2.3 ± 0.4 ↑ Obes ←→ Aged	—	—

[a] Estimated.
[b] CL/F and V_{area}/F.

Key: Adult = adults; Aged = aged; Alb = hypoalbuminemia; Arth = arthritis; Atr Fib = atrial fibrillation; AVH = acute viral hepatitis; Burn = burn patients; CAD = coronary artery disease; Celiac = celiac disease; CF = cystic fibrosis; CHF = congestive heart failure; Child = children; Cirr = cirrhosis; COPD = chronic obstructive pulmonary disease; CP = cor pulmonale; CPBS = cardiopulmonary bypass surgery; CRI = chronic respiratory insufficiency; Crohn = Crohn's disease; Cush = Cushing's syndrome; Epilep = epileptic; Fem = female; Hep = Hepatitis; HL = hyperlipoproteinemia; HTh = hyperthyroid; Inflam = inflammation; LTh = hypothyroid; MI = myocardial infarction; Neo = neonate; NS = nephrotic syndrome; Obes = obese; Pneu = pneumonia; Preg = pregnant; Prem = premature; RA = rheumatoid arthritis; Smk = smoking; Tach = ventricular tachycardia; Ulcer = ulcer patients; Urem = uremia

References: *See* end of table.

Table A–II–1. PHARMACOKINETIC DATA (Continued)

	AVAILABILITY (ORAL) (%)	URINARY EXCRETION (%)	BOUND IN PLASMA (%)	CLEARANCE ($ml \cdot min^{-1} \cdot kg^{-1}$)	VOL. DIST. (liters/kg)	HALF-LIFE (hours)	EFFECTIVE CONCENTRATIONS	TOXIC CONCENTRATIONS
TRIMETHOPRIM (Chapter 49)	~100	80–90	35–40 ←→ Urem, Alb	2.2 ± 0.6 [a,b] ↓ Urem	1.8 ± 0.2 [a,b] ←→ Urem, Child, CF	11 ± 1.4 [b] ↑↓ Urem, Child, CF	See Chapter 49	—
TUBOCURARINE (Chapter 11)	—	63 ± 35	50 ± 8 ↑ Burn ←→ Urem, Cirr	2.3 ± 0.7 ↓ Urem	0.30 ± 0.11 ↑ Child	2.0 ± 1.1 [a] ↑ Urem, Child	0.6 ± 0.2 ng/ml [b] ↓ Child	—
VALPROIC ACID (Chapter 20)	100 ± 10	1.8 ± 2.4	93 ± 1 [a] → Urem, Cirr, Preg, Aged, Neo, Burn	0.11 ± 0.02 [b] ↑ Epilep [c], Child [c] ←→ Cirr, Aged	0.13 ± 0.04 [d] ↑ Cirr, Child, Neo ←→ Aged	14 ± 3 [b] ↑ Cirr, Neo Epilep [c], Child [c] ←→ Aged	55–100 µg/ml [e]	—
VANCOMYCIN (Chapter 52)	—	>90	55 ± 3	1.09 ± 0.07 $CL = 0.69\ CL_{cr} + 0.05$ ↓ Urem, Aged ←→ Obes	0.39 ± 0.06 ↓ Obes ←→ Urem	5.6 ± 1.8 ↑ Urem, Obes	See Chapter 52	>80 µg/ml [a]

TRIMETHOPRIM (Chapter 49)

[a] Assuming 70-kg weight.
[b] Studies included concurrent administration of sulfamethoxazole and variation in urinary pH; these factors had no marked effect on the clearance of trimethoprim.

TUBOCURARINE (Chapter 11)

[a] Calculated from two-compartment analysis. Three-compartment analysis suggests a terminal half-life of 3.9 hours.
[b] 50% reduction in twitch tension. Effective concentration is less in the presence of halothane (0.5–0.7% end tidal) and greater in the presence of enflurane (1.3–1.4% end tidal).

VALPROIC ACID (Chapter 20)

[a] Dose dependent; value shown for doses of 250 and 500 mg/day. At 1000 mg/day, % bound = 90 ± 2.
[b] Multiple dosing (500 mg/day). Single-dose value: $0.14 ± 0.04\ ml \cdot min^{-1} \cdot kg^{-1}$; $t_{1/2} = 9.8 ± 2.6$ hours. Total clearance the same at 1000 mg/day, although clearance of free drug increases.
[c] Increased clearance possibly due to enzyme induction due to concomitant administration of other antiepileptic drugs.
[d] V_{area}, dose = 500 mg/day; increases with dose.
[e] For control of seizures.

VANCOMYCIN (Chapter 52)

[a] Ototoxicity.

VERAPAMIL [a] (Chapters 31, 33)

| 19 ± 12
↑ Cirr | 90 ± 2
↑ Cirr
↔ Urem, Atr Fib | 11.8 ± 5.0 [b]
↓ Cirr, Aged
↓ , ↔ Atr Fib | 4.0 ± 0.9
↑ Cirr
↓ , ↔ Atr Fib | 4.8 ± 2.4 [b]
↑ Cirr, Child
↑ , ↔ Atr Fib | 100 ng/ml [c] | — |

[a] Active metabolite, norverapamil, is a vasodilator but has no direct effect on heart rate or P-R interval.
[b] Multiple dosing causes greater than twofold decrease in clearance and prolongation of half-life.
[c] More than 25% reduction in heart rate in atrial fibrillation; more than 10% prolongation of P-R interval; more than 50% increase in duration of exercise in angina patients.

WARFARIN [a] (Chapter 58)

| 100 | 99
↓ Urem
↑ Preg | 0.045 ± 0.024 [b,c]
↔ Aged, AVH | 0.11 ± 0.01 [c]
↔ Aged, AVH | 37 ± 15 [d]
↔ Aged, AVH | 2.2 ± 0.4 μg/ml [e] | — |

[a] Values are for racemic warfarin.
[b] The kinetics of the S(−) and R(+) enantiomers differ; clearance of the R(+) form is about one third that of the S(−) enantiomer.
[c] Conditions leading to decreased binding (e.g., uremia) presumably increase clearance and volume of distribution.
[d] Half-life of the R(+) enantiomer is longer than that of the S(−) form.
[e] The S(−) enantiomer is three to five times more potent than the R(+) form.

Key: Adult = adults; Aged = aged; Alb = hypoalbuminemia; Arth = arthritis; Atr Fib = atrial fibrillation; AVH = acute viral hepatitis; Burn = burn patients; CAD = coronary artery disease; Celiac = celiac disease; CF = cystic fibrosis; CHF = congestive heart failure; Child = children; Cirr = cirrhosis; COPD = chronic obstructive pulmonary disease; CP = cor pulmonale; CPBS = cardiopulmonary bypass surgery; CRI = chronic respiratory insufficiency; Crohn = Crohn's disease; Cush = Cushing's syndrome; Epilep = epileptic; Fem = female; Hep = Hepatitis; HL = hyperlipoproteinemia; HTh = hyperthyroid; Inflam = inflammation; LTh = hypothyroid; MI = myocardial infarction; Neo = neonate; NS = nephrotic syndrome; Obes = obese; Pneu = pneumonia; Preg = pregnant; Prem = premature; RA = rheumatoid arthritis; Smk = smoking; Tach = ventricular tachycardia; Ulcer = ulcer patients; Urem = uremia

References: *See below and pages 1714–1733.*

ACEBUTOLOL

Meffin, P. J.; Winkle, R. A.; Peters, F. A.; and Harrison, D. C. Acebutolol disposition after intravenous administration. *Clin. Pharmacol. Ther.,* **1977,** *22,* 557–567.
———. Dose-dependent acebutolol disposition after oral administration. *Ibid.,* **1978,** *24,* 542–547.
Roux, A.; Flouvat, B.; Chau, N. P.; Letac, B.; and Lucsko, M. Pharmacokinetics of acebutolol after intravenous bolus administration. *Br. J. Clin. Pharmacol.* **1980,** *9,* 215–217.
Smith, R. S.; Warren, D. J.; Renwick, A. G.; and George, C. F. Acebutolol pharmacokinetics in renal failure. *Br. J. Clin. Pharmacol.,* **1983,** *16,* 253–258.

ACETAMINOPHEN

Forrest, J. A. H.; Clements, J. A.; and Prescott, L. F. Clinical pharmacokinetics of paracetamol. *Clin. Pharmacokinet.,* **1982,** *7,* 93–107.
Rawlins, M. D.; Henderson, D. B.; and Hijab, A. R. Pharmacokinetics of paracetamol (acetaminophen) after intravenous and oral administration. *Eur. J. Clin. Pharmacol.,* **1977,** *11,* 283–286.

N-ACETYLPROCAINAMIDE

Atkinson, A. J., Jr.; Lertora, J. J. L.; Kushner, W.; Chao, G. C.; and Nevin, M. J. Efficacy and safety of N-acetylprocainamide in long term treatment of ventricular arrhythmias. *Clin. Pharmacol. Ther.,* **1983,** *33,* 565–576.
Connolly, S. J., and Kates, R. E. Clinical pharmacokinetics of N-acetylprocainamide. *Clin. Pharmacokinet.,* **1982,** *7,* 206–220.

Table A–II–1. PHARMACOKINETIC DATA (Continued)

ACETYLSALICYLIC ACID

Andreasen, F. Protein binding of drugs in plasma from patients with renal failure. *Acta Pharmacol. Toxicol. (Copenh.)*, **1973**, *32*, 417–429.

Roberts, M. S.; Rumble, R. H.; Wanwimolruk. S.; Thomas, D.; and Brooks, P. M. Pharmacokinetics of aspirin and salicylate in elderly subjects and in patients with alcoholic liver disease. *Eur. J. Clin. Pharmacol.*, **1983**, *25*, 253–261.

Rowland, M., and Riegelman, S. Pharmacokinetics of acetylsalicylic acid and salicylic acid after intravenous administration in man. *J. Pharm. Sci.*, **1968**, *57*, 1313–1319.

Rowland, M.; Riegelman, S.; Harris, P. A.; and Sholkoff, S. D. Absorption kinetics of aspirin in man following oral administration of an aqueous solution. *J. Pharm. Sci.*, **1972**, *61*, 379–385.

ACYCLOVIR

Blum, M. R.; Liao, S. H. T.; and de Miranda, P. Overview of acyclovir pharmacokinetic disposition in adults and children. *Am. J. Med.*, **1982**, *73*, Suppl., 186–192.

Laskin, O. L. Clinical pharmacokinetics of acyclovir. *Clin. Pharmacokinet.*, **1983**, *8*, 187–201.

ALFENTANIL

Bovill, J. G.; Sebel, P. S.; Blackburn, C. L.; and Heykants, J. The pharmacokinetics of alfentanil (R39209): a new opioid analgesic. *Anesthesiology*, **1982**, *57*, 439–443.

Camu, F.; Gepts, E.; Rucquoi, M.; and Heykants, J. Pharmacokinetics of alfentanil in man. *Anesth. Analg.*, **1982**, *61*, 657–661.

Helmers, H.; Van Peer, A.; Woestenborghs, R.; Noorduin, H.; and Heykants, J. Alfentanil kinetics in the elderly. *Clin. Pharmacol. Ther.*, **1984**, *36*, 239–243.

Mather, L. E. Clinical pharmacokinetics of fentanyl and its newer derivatives. *Clin. Pharmacokinet.*, **1983**, *8*, 422–446.

ALPRAZOLAM

Abernethy, D. R.; Greenblatt, D. J.; Divoll, M.; Smith, R. B.; and Shader, R. I. The influence of obesity on the pharmacokinetics of oral alprazolam and triazolam. *Clin. Pharmacokinet.*, **1984**, *9*, 177–183.

Greenblatt, D. J.; Divoll, M.; Abernethy, D. R.; Ochs, H. R.; and Shader, R. I. Clinical pharmacokinetics of the newer benzodiazepines. *Clin. Pharmacokinet.*, **1983**, *8*, 233–252.

Juhl, R. P.; Van Thiel, D. H.; Dittert, L. W.; and Smith, R. B. Alprazolam pharmacokinetics in alcoholic liver disease. *J. Clin. Pharmacol.*, **1984**, *24*, 113–119.

Stoehr, G. P.; Kroboth, P. D.; Juhl, R. P.; Wender, D. B.; Phillips, J. P.; and Smith, R. B. Effect of oral contraceptives on triazolam, temazepam, alprazolam, and lorazepam kinetics. *Clin. Pharmacol. Ther.*, **1984**, *36*, 683–690.

ALPRENOLOL

Frisk-Holmberg, M.; Jorfeldt, L.; and Juhlin-Dannfeldt, A. Influence of alprenolol on hemodynamics and metabolic responses to prolonged exercise in subjects with hypertension. *Clin. Pharmacol. Ther.*, **1977**, *21*, 675–684.

Sheiner, L. B.; Benet, L. Z.; and Pagliaro, L. A. A standard approach to compiling clinical pharmacokinetic data. *J. Pharmacokinet. Biopharm.*, **1981**, *9*, 59–127.

AMIKACIN

Bauer, L. A., and Blouin, R. A. Influence of age on amikacin pharmacokinetics in patients without renal disease. Comparison with gentamicin and tobramycin. *Eur. J. Clin. Pharmacol.*, **1983**, *24*, 639–642.

Pechere, J. C., and Dugal, R. Clinical pharmacokinetics of aminoglycoside antibiotics. *Clin. Pharmacokinet.*, **1979**, *4*, 170–199.

Plantier, J.; Forrey, A. W.; O'Neill, M. A.; Blair, A. D.; Christopher, T. G.; and Cutler, R. E. Pharmacokinetics of amikacin in patients with normal or impaired renal function: radioenzymatic acetylation assay. *J. Infect. Dis.*, **1976**, *134*, Suppl., S323–S330.

AMIODARONE

Gillis, A. M., and Kates, R. E. Clinical pharmacokinetics of the newer antiarrhythmic agents. *Clin. Pharmacokinet.*, **1984**, *9*, 375–403.

Holt, D. W.; Tucker, G. T.; Jackson, P. R.; and Storey. G. C. A. Amiodarone pharmacokinetics. *Am. Heart J.*, **1983**, *106*, 840–847.

Latini, R.; Tognoni, G.; and Kates, R. E. Clinical pharmacokinetics of amiodarone. *Clin. Pharmacokinet.*, **1984**, *9*, 136–156.

AMITRIPTYLINE

Braithwaite, R. A.; Crome, P.; and Dawling, S. Amitriptyline overdosage: plasma concentrations and clinical features. *Br. J. Clin. Pharmacol.*, **1979**, *8*, 388P–389P.

Schulz, P.; Turner-Tamiyasu, K.; Smith, G.; Giacomini, K. M.; and Blaschke, T. F. Amitriptyline disposition in young and elderly normal men. *Clin. Pharmacol. Ther.*, **1983**, *33*, 360–366.

Vandel, S.; Vandel, B.; Sandoz, M.; Allers, G.; Bechtel, P.; and Volmat, R. Clinical response and plasma concentration of amitriptyline and its metabolite nortriptyline. *Eur. J. Clin. Pharmacol.*, **1978**, *14*, 185–190.

AMOXICILLIN

Humbert, G.; Spyker, D. A.; Fillastre, J. P.; and Leroy, A. Pharmacokinetics of amoxicillin: dosage nomogram for patients with impaired renal function. *Antimicrob. Agents Chemother.*, **1979**, *15*, 28–33.

Spyker, D. A.; Rugloski, R. J.; Vann, R. L.; and O'Brien, W. M. Pharmacokinetics of amoxicillin: dose dependence after intravenous, oral, and intramuscular administration. *Antimicrob. Agents Chemother.*, **1977**, *11*, 132–139.

Zarowny, D.; Ogilvie, R.; Tamblyn, D.; MacLeod, C.; and Ruedy, J. Pharmacokinetics of amoxicillin. *Clin. Pharmacol. Ther.*, **1974**, *16*, 1045–1051.

AMPHOTERICIN B

Atkinson, A. J., Jr., and Bennett, J. E. Amphotericin B pharmacokinetics in humans. *Antimicrob. Agents Chemother.*, **1978**, *13*, 271–276.

Daneshmend, T. K., and Warnock, D. W. Clinical pharmacokinetics of systemic antifungal drugs. *Clin. Pharmacokinet.*, **1983**, *8*, 17–42.

AMPICILLIN

Ehrnebo, M.; Nilsson, S.-O.; and Boreus, L. O. Pharmacokinetics of ampicillin and its prodrugs, bacampicillin and pivampicillin, in man. *J. Pharmacokinet. Biopharm.*, **1979**, *7*, 429–451.

Jusko, W. J.; Lewis, G. P.; and Schmitt, G. W. Ampicillin and hetacillin pharmacokinetics in normal and anephric subjects. *Clin. Pharmacol. Ther.*, **1972**, *14*, 90–99.

Lewis, G. P., and Jusko, W. J. Pharmacokinetics of ampicillin in cirrhosis. *Clin. Pharmacol. Ther.*, **1975**, *18*, 475–484.

Loo, J. C. K.; Foltz, E. L.; Wallick, H.; and Kwan, K. C. Pharmacokinetics of pivampicillin and ampicillin in man. *Clin. Pharmacol. Ther.*, **1974**, *16*, 35–43.

AMRINONE

Kullberg, M. P.; Freeman, G. B.; Biddlecome, C.; Alousi, A. A.; and Edelson, J. Amrinone metabolism. *Clin. Pharmacol. Ther.*, **1981**, *29*, 394–401.

Park, G. B.; Kershner, R. P.; Angellotti, J.; Williams, R. L.; Benet, L. Z.; and Edelson, J. Oral bioavailability and intravenous pharmacokinetics of amrinone in humans. *J. Pharm. Sci.*, **1983**, *72*, 817–819.

ATENOLOL

Brown, H. C.; Carruthers, G. S.; Johnston, G. D.; Kelly, J. G.; McAinsh, J.; McDevitt, D. G.; and Shanks, R. G. Clinical pharmacologic observations on atenolol, a beta-adrenoreceptor blocker. *Clin. Pharmacol. Ther.*, **1976**, *20*, 524–534.

Fitzgerald, J. D.; Ruffin, R.; Smedstad, K. G.; Roberts, R.; and McAinsh, J. Studies on the pharmacokinetics and pharmacodynamics of atenolol in man. *Eur. J. Clin. Pharmacol.*, **1978**, *13*, 81–89.

Kirch, W., and Görg, K. G. Clinical pharmacokinetics of atenolol—a review. *Eur. J. Drug Metab. Pharmacokinet.*, **1982**, *7*, 81–91.

ATRACURIUM

Weatherley, B. C.; Williams, S. G.; and Neill, E. A. M. Pharmacokinetics, pharmacodynamics and dose-response relationships of atracurium administered I.V. *Br. J. Anaesth.*, **1983**, *55*, 39S–45S.

AZATHIOPRINE

Ding, T. L.; Gambertoglio, J. G.; Amend, W. J. C.; Birnbaum, J.; and Benet, L. Z. Azathioprine (AZA) bioavailability and pharmacokinetics in kidney transplant patients. *Clin. Pharmacol. Ther.*, **1980**, *27*, 250.

Lin, S.-N.; Jessup, K.; Floyd, M.; Wang, T.-P. F.; Van Buren, C. T.; Caprioli, R. M.; and Kahan, B. D. Quantitation of plasma azathioprine and 6-mercaptopurine levels in renal transplant patients. *Transplantation*, **1980**, *29*, 290–294.

AZLOCILLIN

Bergan, T.; Thorsteinsson, S. B.; and Steingrimsson, O. Dose-dependent pharmacokinetics of azlocillin compared to mezlocillin. *Chemotherapy*, **1982**, *28*, 160–170.

Fiegel, P., and Becker, K. Pharmacokinetics of azlocillin in persons with normal and impaired renal functions. *Antimicrob. Agents Chemother.*, **1978**, *14*, 288–291.

Leroy, A.; Humberg, G.; Godin, M.; and Fillastre, J. P. Pharmacokinetics of azlocillin in subjects with normal and impaired renal function. *Antimicrob. Agents Chemother.*, **1980**, *17*, 344–349.

BETAMETHASONE

Loo, J. C. K.; McGilveray, I. J.; Jordan, N.; and Brien, R. Pharmacokinetic evaluation of betamethasone and its water soluble phosphate ester in humans. *Biopharm. Drug Dispos.*, **1981**, *2*, 265–272.

Petersen, M. C.; Collier, C. B.; Ashley, J. J.; McBride, W. G.; and Nation, R. L. Disposition of betamethasone in parturient women after intravenous administration. *Eur. J. Clin. Pharmacol.*, **1983**, *25*, 803–810.

Petersen, M. C.; Nation, R. L.; McBride, W. G.; Ashley, J. J.; and Moore, R. G. Pharmacokinetics of betamethasone in healthy adults after intravenous administration. *Eur. J. Clin. Pharmacol.*, **1983**, *25*, 643–650.

BLEOMYCIN

Crooke, S. T.; Comis, R. L.; Einhorn, L. H.; Strong, J. E.; Broughton, A.; and Prestayko, A. W. Effects of variations in renal function on the clinical pharmacology of bleomycin administered as an iv bolus. *Cancer Treat. Rep.*, **1977**, *61*, 1631–1636.

Kramer, W. G.; Feldman, S.; Broughton, A.; Strong, J. E.; Hall, S. W.; and Holoye, P. Y. The pharmacokinetics of bleomycin in man. *J. Clin. Pharmacol.*, **1978**, *18*, 346–352.

Yee, G. C.; Crom, W. R.; Lee, F. H.; Smyth, R. D.; and Evans, W. E. Bleomycin disposition in children with cancer. *Clin. Pharmacol. Ther.*, **1983**, *33*, 668–673.

BRETYLIUM

Anderson, J. L.; Patterson, E.; Wagner, J. G.; Stewart, J. R.; Behm, H. L.; and Lucchesi, B. R. Oral and intravenous bretylium disposition. *Clin. Pharmacol. Ther.*, **1980**, *28*, 468–478.

Garrett, E. R.; Green, J. R., Jr.; and Bialer, M. Bretylium pharmacokinetics and bioavailabilities in man with various doses and modes of administration. *Biopharm. Drug Dispos.*, **1982**, *3*, 129–164.

Narang, P. K.; Adir, J.; Josselson, J.; Yacobi, A.; and Sadler, J. Pharmacokinetics of bretylium in man after intravenous administration. *J. Pharmacokinet. Biopharm.*, **1980**, *8*, 363–372.

BUSULFAN

Ehrsson, H.; Hassan, M.; Ehrnebo, M.; and Beran. M. Busulfan kinetics. *Clin. Pharmacol. Ther.*, **1983**, *34*, 86–89.

CAFFEINE

Blanchard, J., and Sawers, S. J. A. Comparative pharmacokinetics of caffeine in young and elderly men. *J. Pharmacokinet. Biopharm.*, **1983**, *11*, 109–126.

Bonati, M.; Latini, R.; Galletti, F.; Young, J. F.; Tognoni, G.; and Garattini, S. Caffeine disposition after oral doses. *Clin. Pharmacol. Ther.*, **1982**, *32*, 98–106.

Tang-Liu, D. D.-S.; Williams, R. L.; and Riegelman, S. Disposition of caffeine and its metabolites in man. *J. Pharmacol. Exp. Ther.*, **1983**, *224*, 180–185.

CAPTOPRIL

Cody, R. J.; Schaer, G. L.; Covit. A. B.; Pondolfino, K.; and Williams, G. Captopril kinetics in chronic congestive heart failure. *Clin. Pharmacol. Ther.*, **1982**, *32*, 721–726.

Duchin, K. L.; Singhvi, S. M.; Willard, D. A.; Migdalof, B. H.; and McKinstry, D. N. Captopril kinetics. *Clin. Pharmacol. Ther.*, **1982**, *31*, 452–458.

Singhvi, S. M.; Duchin, K. L.; Willard, D. A.; McKinstry, D. N.; and Migdalof, B. H. Renal handling of captopril: effect of probenecid. *Clin. Pharmacol. Ther.*, **1982**, *32*, 182–189.

CARBAMAZEPINE

Bertilsson, L. Clinical pharmacokinetics of carbamazepine. *Clin. Pharmacokinet.*, **1978**, *3*, 128–143.

Bertilsson, L.; Höjer, B.; Tybring, G.; Osterloh. J.; and Rane. A. Autoinduction of carbamazepine metabolism in children examined by a stable isotope technique. *Clin. Pharmacol. Ther.*, **1980**, *27*, 83–88.

Schneider, H. Carbamazepine: an attempt to correlate serum levels with antiepileptic and side effects. In. *Clinical Pharmacology of Anti-Epileptic Drugs.* (Schneider, H.; Janz, D.; Gardner-Thorpe, C.; Meinardi, H.; and Sherwin, A. L.; eds.) Springer-Verlag, Berlin, **1975**, pp. 151–158.

Westenberg, H. G. M.; van der Kleijn, E.; Oei, T. T.; and de Zeeuw, R. A. Kinetics of carbamazepine and carbamazepine-epoxide determined by use of plasma and saliva. *Clin. Pharmacol. Ther.*, **1978**, *23*, 320–328.

CARBAMAZEPINE-10,11-EPOXIDE

Brodie. M. J.; Forrest, G.; and Rapeport, W. G. Carbamazepine-10,11-epoxide concentrations in epileptics on carbamazepine alone and in combination with other anticonvulsants. *Br. J. Clin. Pharmacol.*, **1983**, *16*, 747–750.

Tomson, T.; Tybring, G.; and Bertilsson. L. Single-dose kinetics and metabolism of carbamazepine-10,11-epoxide. *Clin. Pharmacol. Ther.*, **1983**, *33*, 58–65.

CARBENICILLIN

Hoffman, T. A.; Cestero. R.; and Bullock, W. E. Pharmacodynamics of carbenicillin in hepatic and renal failure. *Ann. Intern. Med.*, **1970**, *73*, 173–178.

Latos, D. L.; Bryan, C. S.; and Stone, W. J. Carbenicillin therapy in patients with normal and impaired renal function. *Clin. Pharmacol. Ther.*, **1975**, *17*, 692–700.

Libke, R. D.; Clarke, J. T.; Ralph, E. D.; Luthy, R. P.; and Kirby, W. M. M. Ticarcillin *vs* carbenicillin: clinical pharmacokinetics. *Clin. Pharmacol. Ther.*, **1975**, *17*, 441–446.

CARMUSTINE (BCNU)

Levin, V. A.; Hoffman, W.; and Weinkam, R. J. Pharmacokinetics of BCNU in man: a preliminary study of 20 patients. *Cancer Treat. Rep.*, **1978**, *62*, 1305–1312.

CEFAMANDOLE

Agbayani, M. M.; Khan. A. J.; Kemawikasit, P.; Rosenfeld, W.; Salazar, D.; Kumar, K.; Glass, L.; and Evans, H. E. Pharmacokinetics and safety of cefamandole in newborn infants. *Antimicrob. Agents Chemother.*, **1979**, *15*, 674–676.

Aziz, N. S.; Gambertoglio, J. G.; Lin, E. T.; Grausz, H.; and Benet, L. Z. Pharmacokinetics of cefamandole using a HPLC assay. *J. Pharmacokinet. Biopharm.*, **1978**, *6*, 153–164.

Neu, H. C., and Srinivasan. S. Pharmacology of cefizoxime compared with that of cefamandole. *Antimicrob. Agents Chemother.*, **1981**, *20*, 366–369.

CEFAZOLIN

Craig, W. A.; Welling. P. G.; Jackson, T. C.; and Kunin, C. M. Pharmacology of cefazolin and other cephalosporins in patients with renal insufficiency. *J. Infect. Dis.*, **1973**, *128*, Suppl., S347–S353.

Nightingale, C. H.; Greene, D. S.; and Quintiliani, R. Pharmacokinetics and clinical use of cephalosporin antibiotics. *J. Pharm. Sci.*, **1975**, *64*, 1899–1927.

Scheld, W. M.; Spyker, D. A.; Donowitz, G. R.; Bolton, W. K.; and Sande, M. A. Moxalactam and cefazolin: comparative pharmacokinetics in normal subjects. *Antimicrob. Agents Chemother.*, **1981**, *19*, 613–619.

CEFONICID

Barriere, S. L.; Hatheway, G. J.; Gambertoglio, J. G.; Lin, E. T.; and Conte, J. E., Jr. Pharmacokinetics of cefonicid, a new broad-spectrum cephalosporin. *Antimicrob. Agents Chemother.*, **1982**, *21*, 935–938.

Dudley, M. N.; Quintiliani, R.; and Nightingale, C. H. Review of cefonicid, a long-acting cephalosporin. *Clin. Pharm.*, **1984**, *3*, 23–32.

CEFOPERAZONE

Barriere, S. L., and Flaherty, J. F. Third-generation cephalosporins: a critical review. *Clin. Pharm.*, **1984**, *3*, 351–373.

Bolton, W. K.; Scheld, W. M.; Spyker, D. A.; and Sande, M. A. Pharmacokinetics of cefoperazone in normal volunteers and subjects with renal insufficiency. *Antimicrob. Agents Chemother.*, **1981**, *19*, 821–825.

Boscia, J. A.; Korzeniowski, O. M.; Snepar, R.; Kobasa, W. D.; Levison, M. E.; and Kaye, D. Cefoperazone pharmacokinetics in normal subjects and patients with cirrhosis. *Antimicrob. Agents Chemother.*, **1983**, *23*, 385–389.

CEFORANIDE

Estey, E. H.; Weaver, S. S.; LeBlanc, B. M.; Brown, N.; Ho, D. H.; and Bodey, G. P. Ceforanide kinetics. *Clin. Pharmacol. Ther.*, **1981**, *30*, 398–403.

Hawkins, S. S.; Alford, R. H.; Stone, W. J.; Smyth, R. D.; and Pfeffer, M. Ceforanide kinetics in renal insufficiency. *Clin. Pharmacol. Ther.*, **1981**, *30*, 468–474.

Pfeffer, M.; Gaver, R. C.; and Van Harken, D. R. Human pharmacokinetics of a new broad-spectrum parenteral cephalosporin antibiotic, ceforanide. *J. Pharm. Sci.*, **1980**, *69*, 398–403.

CEFOTAXIME

Barriere, S. L., and Flaherty, J. F. Third-generation cephalosporins: a critical evaluation. *Clin. Pharm.*, **1984**, *3*, 351–373.

Kampf, D.; Borner, K.; Möller, M.; and Kessel, M. Kinetic interactions between azlocillin, cefotaxime, and cefotaxime metabolites in normal and impaired renal function. *Clin. Pharmacol. Ther.*, **1984**, *35*, 214–220.

Kemmerich, B.; Lode, H.; Belmega, G.; Jendroschek, T.; Borner, K.; and Koeppe, P. Comparative pharmacokinetics of cefoperazone, cefotaxime and moxalactam. *Antimicrob. Agents Chemother.*, **1983**, *23*, 429–434.

Neu, H. C.; Aswapokee, P.; Fu, K. P.; Ho, I.; and Matthijssen, C. Cefotaxime kinetics after intravenous and intramuscular injection of single and multiple doses. *Clin. Pharmacol. Ther.*, **1980**, *27*, 677–685.

CEFOXITIN

Kampf, D.; Schurig, R.; Korsukewitz, I.; and Brückner, O. Cefoxitin pharmacokinetics: relation to three different renal clearance studies in patients with various degrees of renal insufficiency. *Antimicrob. Agents Chemother.*, **1981**, *20*, 741–746.

Regazzi, M. B.; Chirico, G.; Cristiani, D.; Rondini, G.; and Rondanelli, R. Cefoxitin in newborn infants. *Eur. J. Clin. Pharmacol.*, **1983**, *25*, 507–509.

Sonneville, P. F.; Kartodirdjo, R. R.; Skeggs, H.; Till, A. E.; and Martin, C. M. Comparative clinical pharmacokinetics of intravenous cefoxitin and cephalothin. *Eur. J. Clin. Pharmacol.*, **1976**, *9*, 397–403.

CEFTAZIDIME

Barriere, S. L., and Flaherty, J. F. Third-generation cephalosporins: a critical evaluation. *Clin. Pharm.*, **1984**, *3*, 351–373.

Leeder, J. S.; Spino, M.; Isles, A. F.; Tesoro, A. M.; Gold, R.; and MacLeod, S. M. Ceftazidime disposition in acute and stable cystic fibrosis. *Clin. Pharmacol. Ther.*, **1984**, *36*, 355–362.

Leroy, A.; Leguy, F.; Borsa, F.; Spencer, G. R.; Fillastre, J. P.; and Humbert, G. Pharmacokinetics of ceftazidime in normal and uremic subjects. *Antimicrob. Agents Chemother.*, **1984**, *25*, 638–642.

Welage, L. S.; Schultz, R. W.; and Schentag, J. J. Pharmacokinetics of ceftazidime in patients with renal insufficiency. *Antimicrob. Agents Chemother.*, **1984**, *25*, 201–204.

CEFTIZOXIME

Barriere, S. L., and Flaherty, J. F. Third-generation cephalosporins: a critical evaluation. *Clin. Pharm.*, **1984**, *3*, 351–373.

Cutler, R. E.; Blair, A. D.; Burgess, E. D.; and Parks, D. Pharmacokinetics of ceftizoxime. *J. Antimicrob. Chemother.*, **1982**, *10*, Suppl. C, 91–97.

CEFUROXIME

Bundtzen, R. W.; Toothaker, R. D.; Nielson, O. S.; Madsen, P. O.; Welling, P. G.; and Craig, W. A. Pharmacokinetics of cefuroxime in normal and impaired renal function: comparison of high-pressure liquid chromatography and microbiological assays. *Antimicrob. Agents Chemother.*, **1981**, *19*, 443–449.

Foord, R. D. Cefuroxime: human pharmacokinetics. *Antimicrob. Agents Chemother.*, **1976**, *9*, 741–747.

CEPHALEXIN

Finkelstein, E.; Quintiliani, R.; Lee, R.; Bracci, A.; and Nightingale, C. H. Pharmacokinetics of oral cephalosporins: cephradine and cephalexin. *J. Pharm. Sci.*, **1978**, *67*, 1447–1450.

Greene, D. S.; Flanagan, D. E.; Quintiliani, R.; and Nightingale, C. H. Pharmacokinetics of cephalexin: an evaluation of one- and two-compartment model pharmacokinetics. *J. Clin. Pharmacol.*, **1976**, *16*, 257–264.

Table A–II–1. PHARMACOKINETIC DATA (Continued)

Spyker, D. A.; Thomas, B. L.; Sande, M. A.; and Bolton, W. K. Pharmacokinetics of cefaclor and cephalexin: dosage nomograms for impaired renal function. *Antimicrob. Agents Chemother.*, **1978**, *14*, 172–177.

CEPHALOTHIN

Kirby, W. M. M.; DeMaine, J. B.; and Serril, W. S. Pharmacokinetics of the cephalosporins in healthy volunteers and uremic patients. *Postgrad. Med. J.*, **1971**, *47*, Suppl., 41–46.
Nightingale, C. H.; Greene, D. S.; and Quintiliani, R. Pharmacokinetics and clinical use of cephalosporin antibiotics. *J. Pharm. Sci.*, **1975**, *64*, 1899–1927.

CEPHAPIRIN

Bergan, T. Comparative pharmacokinetics of cefazolin, cephalothin, cephacetrile, and cephapirin after intravenous administration. *Chemotherapy*, **1977**, *23*, 389–404.
Cabana, B. E.; Van Harken, D. R.; Hottendorf, G. H.; Doluisio. J. T.; Griffen, W. O., Jr.; Bourne, D. W. A.; and Dittert, L. W. The role of the kidney in the elimination of cephapirin in man. *J. Pharmacokinet. Biopharm.*, **1975**, *3*, 419–438.
Nightingale, C. H.; Greene, D. S.; and Quintiliani, R. Pharmacokinetics and clinical use of cephalosporin antibiotics. *J. Pharm. Sci.*, **1975**, *64*, 1899–1927.

CEPHRADINE

Finkelstein, E.; Quintiliani, R.; Lee, R.; Bracci, A.; and Nightingale, C. H. Pharmacokinetics of oral cephalosporins: cephradine and cephalexin. *J. Pharm. Sci.*, **1978**, *67*, 1447–1450.
Nightingale, C. H.; Greene, D. S.; and Quintiliani, R. Pharmacokinetics and clinical use of cephalosporin antibiotics. *J. Pharm. Sci.*, **1975**, *64*, 1899–1927.
Solomon, A. E.; Briggs, J. D.; McGleachy, R.; and Sleigh, J. D. The administration of cephradine to patients in renal failure. *Br. J. Clin. Pharmacol.*, **1975**, *2*, 443–448.

CHLORAMBUCIL

Ehrsson, H.; Wallin, I.; Nilsson. S.-O.; and Johansson. B. Pharmacokinetics of chlorambucil in man after administration of the free drug and its prednisolone ester (prednimustine, leo 1031). *Eur. J. Clin. Pharmacol.*, **1983**, *24*, 251–253.

CHLORAMPHENICOL

Ambrose, P. J. Clinical pharmacokinetics of chloramphenicol and chloramphenicol succinate. *Clin. Pharmacokinet.*, **1984**, *9*, 222–238.
Nahata, M. C., and Powell, D. A. Bioavailability and clearance of chloramphenicol after intravenous chloramphenicol succinate. *Clin. Pharmacol. Ther.*, **1981**, *30*, 368–372.
Narang, D. P. S.; Datta, D. V.; Nath, N.; and Mathur, V. S. Pharmacokinetic study of chloramphenicol in patients with liver disease. *Eur. J. Clin. Pharmacol.*, **1981**, *20*, 479–483.

CHLORDIAZEPOXIDE

Boxenbaum, H. G.; Greitner, K. A.; Jack, M. L.; Dixon, W. R.; Speigel, H. E.; Symington, J.; Christian, R.; Moore, J. D.; Weissman, L.; and Kaplan, S. A. Pharmacokinetic and biopharmaceutic profile of chlordiazepoxide HCl in healthy subjects: single-dose studies by the intravenous, intramuscular, and oral routes. *J. Pharmacokinet. Biopharm.*, **1977**, *5*, 3–23.
Greenblatt, D. J.; Shader, R. I.; MacLeod, S. M.; and Sellers, E. M. Clinical pharmacokinetics of chlordiazepoxide. *Clin. Pharmacokinet.*, **1978**, *3*, 381–394.
Lin, K.-M., and Friedel, R. O. Relationship of plasma levels of chlordiazepoxide and metabolites to clinical response. *Am. J. Psychiatry*, **1979**, *136*, 18–23.
Sellers, E. M.; Greenblatt, D. J.; Giles, H. G.; Naranjo. C. A.; Kaplan. H.; and MacLeod, S. M. Chlordiazepoxide and oxazepam disposition in cirrhosis. *Clin. Pharmacol. Ther.*, **1979**, *26*, 240–246.

CHLOROQUINE

Gustafson, L. L.; Walker, O.; Alván, G.; Beermann, B.; Estevez, F.; Gleisner, L.; Lindström, B.; and Sjöqvist. F. Disposition of chloroquine in man after single and intravenous oral doses. *Br. J. Clin. Pharmacol.*, **1983**, *15*, 471–479.

CHLOROTHIAZIDE

Gee, W. L.; Lin, E. T.; Brater, D. C.; Gustafson, H. J.; and Benet, L. Z. Chlorothiazide pharmacokinetics following oral and i.v. dosing in man. Presented to Academy of Pharmaceutical Sciences, Anaheim Meeting, April, **1979**, Abstract P-52.
Osman. M. A.; Patel. R. B.; Irwin. D. S.; Craig. W. A.; and Welling. P. G. Bioavailability of chlorothiazide from 50, 100, and 250 mg solution doses. *Biopharm. Drug Dispos.*, **1982**, *3*, 89–94.

CHLORPROMAZINE

Cooper, T. B. Plasma level monitoring of antipsychotic drugs. *Clin. Pharmacokinet.*, **1978**, *3*, 14–38.
Dahl, S. G., and Strandjord, R. E. Pharmacokinetics of chlorpromazine after single and chronic dosage. *Clin. Pharmacol. Ther.*, **1977**, *21*, 437–448.
Rivera-Calimlim, L.; Masrallah. H.; Strass. J.; and Lasagna. L. Clinical response and plasma levels: effect of dose, dosage schedules, and drug interactions on plasma chlorpromazine levels. *Am. J. Psychiatry*, **1976**, *133*, 646–652.

CHLORPROPAMIDE

Balant, L. Clinical pharmacokinetics of sulphonylurea-hypoglycaemic agents. *Clin. Pharmacokinet.*, **1981**, *6*, 215–241.
Monro. A. M., and Welling. P. G. The bioavailability in man of marketed brands of chlorpropamide. *Eur. J. Clin. Pharmacol.*, **1974**, *7*, 47–49.

Neuvonen, P. J., and Kärkkäinen. S. Effects of charcoal, sodium bicarbonate, and ammonium chloride on chlorpropamide kinetics. *Clin. Pharmacol. Ther.*, **1983**, *33*, 386–393.

Taylor. J. A. Pharmacokinetics and biotransformation of chlorpropamide in man. *Clin. Pharmacol. Ther.*, **1972**, *13*, 710–718.

CHLORTHALIDONE

Beermann, B., and Groschinsky-Grind, M. Clinical pharmacokinetics of diuretics. *Clin. Pharmacokinet.*, **1980**, *5*, 221–245.

Colussi, D.; Schoeller, J. P.; Richard, A.; and Sioufi, A. Pharmacokinetics of chlorthalidone in the elderly after single and multiple doses. *Br. J. Clin. Pharmacol.*, **1983**, *16*, 755–756.

Fleuren, H. L. J.; Thien, T. A.; Verwey-van Wissen, C. P. W.; and van Rossum, J. M. Absolute bioavailability of chlorthalidone in man: a cross-over study after intravenous and oral administration. *Eur. J. Clin. Pharmacol.*, **1979**, *15*, 35–50.

CIMETIDINE

Gugler, R.; Fuchs. G.; Dieckmann, M.; and Somogyi, A. A. Cimetidine plasma concentration–response relationships. *Clin. Pharmacol. Ther.*, **1981**, *29*, 744–748.

Schentag, J. J.; Cerra, F. B.; Calleri, G. M.; Leising. M. E.; French, M. A.; and Bernhard. H. Age, disease, and cimetidine disposition in healthy subjects and chronically ill patients. *Clin. Pharmacol. Ther.*, **1981**, *29*, 737–743.

Walkenstein. S. S.; Dubb, J. W.; Randolph, W. C.; Westlake, W. J.; Stote, R. M.; and Intoccia, A. P. Bioavailability of cimetidine in man. *Gastroenterology*, **1978**, *74*, 360–365.

CISPLATIN

Balis, F. M.; Holcenberg, J. S.; and Bleyer, W. A. Clinical pharmacokinetics of commonly used anticancer drugs. *Clin. Pharmacokinet.*, **1983**, *8*, 202–232.

CLINDAMYCIN

DeHaan, R. M.; Metzler, C. M.; Schellenberg, D.; and VandenBosch, W. D. Pharmacokinetic studies of clindamycin phosphate. *J. Clin. Pharmacol.*, **1973**, *13*, 190–209.

DeHaan, R. M.; Metzler, C. M.; Schellenberg, D.; VandenBosch, W. D.; and Masson, E. L. Pharmacokinetic studies of clindamycin hydrochloride in humans. *Int. J. Clin. Pharmacol.*, **1972**, *6*, 105–119.

CLOFIBRATE

Gugler, R.; Kurten, J. W.; Jensen, C. J.; Klehr, U.; and Hartlapp, J. Clofibrate disposition in renal failure and acute and chronic liver disease. *Eur. J. Clin. Pharmacol.*, **1979**, *15*, 341–347.

Hovin, G.; Thebault, J. J.; d'Athis, P.; Tillement, J.-P.; and Beaumont, J.-L. A GLC method for estimation of chlorphenoxyisobutyric acid in plasma. Pharmacokinetics of a single oral dose of clofibrate in man. *Eur. J. Clin. Pharmacol.*, **1975**, *8*, 433–437.

Sheiner, L. B.; Benet, L. Z.; and Pagliaro, L. A. A standard approach to compiling clinical pharmacokinetic data. *J. Pharmacokinet. Biopharm.*, **1981**, *9*, 59–127.

Veenendaal. J. R.; Brooks, P. M.; and Meffin, P. J. Probenecid-clofibrate interaction. *Clin. Pharmacol. Ther.*, **1981**, *29*, 351–358.

CLONAZEPAM

Berlin, A., and Dahlstrom, H. Pharmacokinetics of the anticonvulsant drug clonazepam evaluated from single oral and intravenous doses and by repeated oral administration. *Eur. J. Clin. Pharmacol.*, **1975**, *9*, 155–159.

Khoo, K.-C.; Mendels, J.; Rothbart, M.; Garland, W. A.; Colburn, W. A.; Min. B. H.; Lucek, R.; Carbone, J. J.; Boxenbaum, H. G.; and Kaplan, S. A. Influence of phenytoin and phenobarbital on the disposition of a single oral dose of clonazepam. *Clin. Pharmacol. Ther.*, **1980**, *28*, 368–375.

CLONIDINE

Arndts, D.; Doevendans, J.; Kirsten, R.; and Heintz. B. New aspects of the pharmacokinetics and pharmacodynamics of clonidine in man. *Eur. J. Clin. Pharmacol.*, **1983**, *24*, 21–30.

Davies, D. S.; Wing, L. M. H.; Reid J. L.; Neill, E.; Tippett, P.; and Dollery. C. T. Pharmacokinetics and concentration-effect relationships of intravenous and oral clonidine. *Clin. Pharmacol. Ther.*, **1977**, *21*, 593–601.

Frisk-Holmberg, M.; Edlind, P. O.; and Paalzow, L. Pharmacokinetics of clonidine and its relation to the hypotensive effect in patients. *Br. J. Clin. Pharmacol.*, **1978**, *6*, 227–232.

CLORAZEPATE

Rey, E.; d'Athis, P.; Giraux, P.; de Lauture, D.; Turquais, J. M.; Chavinie, J.; and Olive. G. Pharmacokinetics of clorazepate in pregnant and nonpregnant women. *Eur. J. Clin. Pharmacol.*, **1979**, *15*, 175–180.

CLOXACILLIN

Nauta. E. H., and Mattie, H. Pharmacokinetics of flucloxacillin and cloxacillin in healthy subjects and patients on chronic haemodialysis. *Br. J. Clin. Pharmacol.*, **1975**, *2*, 111–121.

_____. Dicloxacillin and cloxacillin: pharmacokinetics in healthy and hemodialysis subjects. *Clin. Pharmacol. Ther.*, **1976**, *20*, 98–108.

Spino. M.; Chai. R. P.; Isles. A. F.; Thiessen, J. J.; Tesoro, A.; Gold. R.; and MacLeod, S. M. Cloxacillin absorption and disposition in cystic fibrosis. *J. Pediatr.*, **1984**, *105*, 829–835.

COCAINE

Javaid, J. I.; Musa. M. N.; Fischman, M.; Schuster, C. R.; and Davis, J. M. Kinetics of cocaine in humans after intravenous and intranasal administration. *Biopharm. Drug Dispos.*, **1983**, *4*, 9–18.

CYCLOPHOSPHAMIDE

Bramwell, V.; Calvert, R. T.; Edwards, G.; Scarffe, H.; and Crowther, D. The disposition of cyclophosphamide in a group of myeloma patients. *Cancer Chemother. Pharmacol.*, **1979**, *3*, 253–259.

Grochow, L. B., and Colvin, M. Clinical pharmacokinetics of cyclophosphamide. *Clin. Pharmacokinet.*, **1979**, *4*, 380–394.

Juma, F. D.; Rogers, H. J.; and Trounce, J. R. Pharmacokinetics of cyclophosphamide and alkylating activity in man after intravenous and oral administration. *Br. J. Clin. Pharmacol.*, **1979**, *8*, 209–217.

CYCLOSPORINE

Beveridge, T.; Gratwohl, A.; Michot, F.; Niederberger, W.; Nüesch, E.; Nussbaumer, K.; Schaub, P.; and Speck, B. Cyclosporin A: pharmacokinetics after a single dose in man, and serum levels after multiple dosing in recipients of allogenic bone-marrow grafts. *Curr. Ther. Res.*, **1981**, *30*, 5–18.

Follath, F.; Wenk, M.; Vozeh, S.; Thiel, G.; Brunner, F.; Loertscher, R.; Lemaire, M.; Nussbaumer, K.; Niederberger, W.; and Wood, A. Intravenous cyclosporine kinetics in renal failure. *Clin. Pharmacol. Ther.*, **1983**, *34*, 638–643.

Wood, A. J.; Maurer, G.; Niederberger, W.; and Beveridge, T. Cyclosporine: pharmacokinetics, metabolism, and drug interactions. *Transplant. Proc.*, **1983**, *15*, Suppl. 1, 2409–2412.

CYTARABINE

Balis, F. M.; Holcenberg, J. S.; and Bleyer, W. A. Clinical pharmacokinetics of commonly used anticancer drugs. *Clin. Pharmacokinet.*, **1983**, *8*, 202–232.

Harris, A. L.; Potter, C.; Bunch, C.; Boutagy, J.; Harvey, D. J.; and Grahame-Smith, D. G. Pharmacokinetics of cytosine arabinoside in patients with acute myeloid leukaemia. *Br. J. Clin. Pharmacol.*, **1979**, *8*, 219–227.

Wan, S. H.; Huffman, D. H.; Azarnoff, D. L.; Hoogstraten, B.; and Larsen, W. E. Pharmacokinetics of 1-β-arabinofuranosylcytosine in humans. *Cancer Res.*, **1974**, *34*, 392–397.

DAPSONE

Ahmad, R. A., and Rogers, H. J. Pharmacokinetics and protein binding interactions of dapsone and pyrimethamine. *Br. J. Clin. Pharmacol.*, **1980**, *10*, 519–524.

———. Plasma and salivary pharmacokinetics of dapsone estimated by a thin layer chromatographic method. *Eur. J. Clin. Pharmacol.*, **1980**, *17*, 129–133.

DESIPRAMINE

Friedel, R. O.; Veith, R. C.; Bloom, V.; and Bielski, R. J. Desipramine plasma levels and clinical response in depressed outpatients. *Commun. Psychopharmacol.*, **1979**, *3*, 81–87.

Rudorfer, M. V.; Lane, E. A.; Chang, W.-H.; Zhang, M.; and Potter, W. Z. Desipramine pharmacokinetics in Chinese and Caucasian volunteers. *Br. J. Clin. Pharmacol.*, **1984**, *17*, 433–440.

Weiner, D.; Garteiz, D.; Cawein, M.; Dusebout, T.; Wright, G.; and Okerholm, R. Pharmacokinetic linearity of desipramine hydrochloride. *J. Pharm. Sci.*, **1981**, *70*, 1079–1080.

DESMETHYLDIAZEPAM

Abernethy, D. R.; Greenblatt, D. J.; Divoll, M.; and Shader, R. I. Prolongation of drug half-life due to obesity: studies of desmethyldiazepam (clorazepate). *J. Pharm. Sci.*, **1982**, *71*, 942–944.

Klotz, U.; Antonin, K. H.; Brügel, H.; and Bieck, P. R. Disposition of diazepam and its major metabolite desmethyldiazepam in patients with liver disease. *Clin. Pharmacol. Ther.*, **1977**, *21*, 430–436.

Ochs, H. R.; Greenblatt, D. J.; Verburg-Ochs, B.; and Locniskar, A. Comparative single-dose kinetics of oxazolam, prazepam and clorazepate: three precursors of desmethyldiazepam. *J. Clin. Pharmacol.*, **1984**, *24*, 446–451.

Shader, R. I.; Greenblatt, D. J.; Ciraulo, D. A.; Divoll, M.; Harmatz, J. S.; and Georgotas, A. Effect of age and sex on disposition of desmethyldiazepam formed from its precursor clorazepate. *Psychopharmacology*, **1981**, *75*, 193–197.

DEXAMETHASONE

Gustavson, L. E., and Benet, L. Z. Pharmacokinetics of natural and synthetic glucocorticoids. In *Butterworth's International Medical Reviews in Endocrinology*, Vol. 4. *The Adrenal Cortex*. (Anderson, D. C., and Winter, J. S. D., eds.) Butterworth & Co., London, **1985**, pp. 235–281.

Rose, J. Q.; Yurchak, A. M.; Meikle, A. W.; and Jusko, W. J. Effect of smoking on prednisone, prednisolone, and dexamethasone pharmacokinetics. *J. Pharmacokinet. Biopharm.*, **1981**, *9*, 1–14.

Tsuei, S. E.; Moore, R. G.; Ashley, J. J.; and McBride, W. G. Disposition of synthetic glucocorticoids. I. Pharmacokinetics of dexamethasone in healthy adults. *J. Pharmacokinet. Biopharm.*, **1979**, *7*, 249–264.

Tsuei, S. E.; Petersen, M. C.; Ashley, J. J.; McBride, W. G.; and Moore, R. G. Disposition of synthetic glucocorticoids. II. Dexamethasone in parturient women. *Clin. Pharmacol. Ther.*, **1980**, *28*, 88–98.

DIAZEPAM

Greenblatt, D. J.; Allen, M. D.; Harmatz, J. S.; and Shader, R. I. Diazepam disposition determinants. *Clin. Pharmacol. Ther.*, **1980**, *27*, 301–312.

Klotz, U.; Avant, G. R.; Hoyumpa, A.; Schenker, S.; and Wilkinson, G. R. The effects of age and liver disease on the disposition and elimination of diazepam in adult man. *J. Clin. Invest.*, **1975**, *55*, 347–359.

Mandelli, M.; Tognoni, G.; and Garattini, S. Clinical pharmacokinetics of diazepam. *Clin. Pharmacokinet.*, **1978**, *3*, 72–91.

DIAZOXIDE

Ogilvie, R. I.; Nadeau, J. H.; and Sitar, D. S. Diazoxide concentration-response relation in hypertension. *Hypertension.* **1982,** *4,* 167–173.

Pearson, R. M. Pharmacokinetics and response to diazoxide in renal failure. *Clin. Pharmacokinet.,* **1977,** *2,* 198–204.

Pearson, R. M., and Breckenridge, A. M. Renal function, protein binding and pharmacological response to diazoxide. *Br. J. Clin. Pharmacol.,* **1976,** *3,* 169–175.

DICLOXACILLIN

Jusko, W. J.; Mosovich, L. L.; Gerbracht, L. M.; Mattar, M. E.; and Yaffe, S. J. Enhanced renal excretion of dicloxacillin in patients with cystic fibrosis. *Pediatrics,* **1975,** *56,* 1038–1044.

Nauta, E. H., and Mattie, H. Dicloxacillin and cloxacillin: pharmacokinetics in healthy and hemodialysis subjects. *Clin. Pharmacol. Ther.,* **1976,** *20,* 98–108.

Rosenblatt, J. E.; Kind, A. C.; Brodie, J. L.; and Kirby, W. M. M. Mechanisms responsible for the blood level differences of isoxazolyl penicillins. *Arch. Intern. Med.,* **1968,** *121,* 345–348.

DIGITOXIN

Aronson, J. K. Clinical pharmacokinetics of cardiac glycosides in patients with renal dysfunction. *Clin. Pharmacokinet.,* **1983,** *8,* 155–178.

Larsen, A., and Storstein, L. Digitoxin kinetics and renal excretion in children. *Clin. Pharmacol. Ther.,* **1983,** *33,* 717–726.

Sheiner, L. B.; Benet, L. Z.; and Pagliaro, L. A. A standard approach to compiling clinical pharmacokinetic data. *J. Pharmacokinet. Biopharm.,* **1981,** *9,* 59–127.

DIGOXIN

Sheiner, L. B.; Benet, L. Z.; and Pagliaro, L. A. A standard approach to compiling clinical pharmacokinetic data. *J. Pharmacokinet. Biopharm.,* **1981,** *9,* 59–127.

Sheiner, L. B.; Rosenberg, B. G.; and Marathe, V. V. Estimation of population characteristics of pharmacokinetic parameters from routine clinical data. *J. Pharmacokinet. Biopharm.,* **1977,** *5,* 445–479.

DILTIAZEM

Hermann, P.; Roger, S. D.; Remones, G.; Thenot, J. P.; London, D. R.; and Morselli, P. L. Pharmacokinetics of diltiazem after intravenous and oral administration. *Eur. J. Clin. Pharmacol.,* **1983,** *24,* 349–352.

Kölle, E. U.; Ochs, H. R.; and Vollmer, K.-O. Pharmacokinetic model of diltiazem. *Arzneimittelforsch.,* **1983,** *33,* 972–977.

Smith, M. S.; Verghese, C. P.; Shand, D. G.; and Pritchett, E. L. C. Pharmacokinetics and pharmacodynamic effects of diltiazem. *Am. J. Cardiol.,* **1983,** *51,* 1369–1374.

DIPHENHYDRAMINE

Albert, K. S.; Hallmark, M. R.; Sakmar, E.; Weidler, D. J.; and Wagner, J. G. Pharmacokinetics of diphenhydramine in man. *J. Pharmacokinet. Biopharm.,* **1975,** *3,* 159–170.

Carruthers, S. G.; Shoeman, D. W.; Hignite, C. E.; and Azarnoff, D. L. Correlation between plasma diphenhydramine level and sedative and antihistamine effect. *Clin. Pharmacol. Ther.,* **1978,** *23,* 375–382.

Meredith, C. G.; Christian, C. D., Jr.; Johnson, R. F.; Madhavan, S. V.; and Schenker, S. Diphenhydramine disposition in chronic liver disease. *Clin. Pharmacol. Ther.,* **1984,** *35,* 474–479.

Spector, R.; Choudhury, A. K.; Chiang, C.-K.; Goldberg, M. J.; and Ghoneim, M. M. Diphenhydramine in Orientals and Caucasians. *Clin. Pharmacol. Ther.,* **1980,** *28,* 229–234.

DISOPYRAMIDE

Giacomini, K. M.; Swezey, S. E.; Turner-Tamiyasu, K.; and Blaschke, T. F. The effect of saturable binding to plasma proteins on the pharmacokinetic properties of disopyramide. *J. Pharmacokinet. Biopharm.,* **1982,** *10,* 1–14.

Karim, A.; Nissen, C.; and Azarnoff, D. L. Clinical pharmacokinetics of disopyramide. *J. Pharmacokinet. Biopharm.,* **1982,** *10,* 465–494.

Ueda, C. T.; Dzindzio, B. S.; and Vosik, W. M. Serum disopyramide concentrations and suppression of ventricular premature contractions. *Clin. Pharmacol. Ther.,* **1984,** *36,* 326–336.

DOBUTAMINE

Kates, R. E., and Leier, C. V. Dobutamine pharmacokinetics in severe heart failure. *Clin. Pharmacol. Ther.,* **1978,** *24,* 537–541.

DOXEPIN

Biggs, J. T.; Preskorn, S. H.; Ziegler, V. E.; Rosen, S. H.; and Meyer, D. A. Dosage schedule and plasma levels of doxepin and desmethyldoxepin. *J. Clin. Psychiatry,* **1978,** *39,* 740–742.

Ziegler, V. E.; Biggs, J. T.; Wylie, L. T.; Rosen, S. H.; Hawt, D. J.; and Coryell, W. H. Doxepin kinetics. *Clin. Pharmacol. Ther.,* **1978,** *23,* 573–579.

DOXORUBICIN

Balis, F. M.; Holcenberg, J. S.; and Bleyer, W. A. Clinical pharmacokinetics of commonly used anticancer drugs. *Clin. Pharmacokinet.,* **1983,** *8,* 202–232.

Gil, P.; Durand, A.; Iliadis, A.; Cano, J. P.; and Carcassonne, Y. Time dependency of ADRIAMYCIN and adriamycinol kinetics. *Cancer Chemother. Pharmacol.,* **1983,** *10,* 120–124.

DOXYCYCLINE

Fabre, J.; Milek, E.; Kalfopoulos, P.; and Mérier, G. La cinétique des tétracyclines chez l'homme. *Schweiz. Med. Wochenschr.,* **1971,** *101,* 593–598.

Table A–II–1. PHARMACOKINETIC DATA (Continued)

Houin, G.; Brunner, F.; Nebout, T.; Cherfaoui, M.; Lagrue, G.; and Tillement, J. P. The effects of chronic renal insufficiency on the pharmacokinetics of doxycycline in man. *Br. J. Clin. Pharmacol.*, **1983**, *16*, 245–252.

Raghuram, T. C., and Krishnaswamy, K. Pharmacokinetics and plasma steady-state levels of doxycycline in undernutrition. *Br. J. Clin. Pharmacol.*, **1982**, *14*, 785–789.

EDROPHONIUM

Morris, R. B.; Cronnelly, R.; Miller, R. D.; Stanski, D. R.; and Fahey, M. R. Pharmacokinetics of edrophonium and neostigmine when antagonizing *d*-tubocurarine neuromuscular blockade in man. *Anesthesiology*, **1981**, *54*, 399–402.

ERYTHROMYCIN

Hall, K. W.; Nightingale, C. H.; Gibaldi, M.; Nelson, E.; Bates, T. R.; and DiSanto, A. R. Pharmacokinetics of erythromycin in normal and alcoholic liver disease subjects. *J. Clin. Pharmacol.*, **1982**, *22*, 321–325.

Kroboth, P. D.; Brown, A.; Lyon, J. A.; Kroboth, F. J.; and Juhl, R. P. Pharmacokinetics of single-dose erythromycin in normal and alcoholic liver disease subjects. *Antimicrob. Agents Chemother.*, **1982**, *21*, 135–140.

Mather, L. E.; Austin, K. L.; Philpot, C. R.; and McDonald, P. J. Absorption and bioavailability of oral erythromycin. *Br. J. Clin. Pharmacol.*, **1981**, *12*, 131–140.

Welling, P. G., and Craig, W. A. Pharmacokinetics of intravenous erythromycin. *J. Pharm. Sci.*, **1978**, *67*, 1057–1059.

ETHAMBUTOL

Holdiness, M. R. Clinical pharmacokinetics of the antituberculosis drugs. *Clin. Pharmacokinet.*, **1984**, *9*, 511–544.

Lee, C. S.; Brater, D. C.; Gambertoglio, J. G.; and Benet, L. Z. Disposition kinetics of ethambutol. *J. Pharmacokinet. Biopharm.*, **1980**, *8*, 335–346.

Lee, C. S.; Gambertoglio, J. G.; Brater, D. C.; and Benet, L. Z. Kinetics of oral ethambutol in the normal subject. *Clin. Pharmacol. Ther.*, **1977**, *22*, 615–621.

Lee, C. S.; Marbury, T. C.; and Benet, L. Z. Clearance calculations in hemodialysis: application to blood, plasma, dialysate measurements for ethambutol. *J. Pharmacokinet. Biopharm.*, **1980**, *8*, 69–81.

ETHANOL

Rangno, R. E.; Kreeft, J. H.; and Sitar, D. S. Ethanol 'dose-dependent' elimination: Michaelis-Menten vs. classical kinetic analysis. *Br. J. Clin. Pharmacol.*, **1981**, *12*, 667–673.

Vestal, R. E.; McGuire, E. A.; Tobin, J. D.; Andres, R.; Norris, A. H.; and Mezey, E. Aging and ethanol metabolism. *Clin. Pharmacol. Ther.*, **1977**, *19*, 343–354.

Wilkinson, P. K.; Sedman, A. J.; Sakmar, E.; Earhart, R. H.; Weidler, D. J.; and Wagner, J. G. Blood ethanol concentrations during and following constant-rate intravenous infusion of alcohol. *Clin. Pharmacol. Ther.*, **1976**, *19*, 213–223.

Wilkinson, P. K.; Sedman, A. J.; Sakmar, E.; Kay, D. R.; and Wagner, J. G. Pharmacokinetics of ethanol after oral administration in the fasting state. *J. Pharmacokinet. Biopharm.*, **1977**, *5*, 207–224.

ETHOSUXIMIDE

Bauer, L. A.; Harris, C.; Wilensky, A. J.; Raisys, V. A.; and Levy, R. H. Ethosuximide kinetics: possible interaction with valproic acid. *Clin. Pharmacol. Ther.*, **1982**, *31*, 741–745.

FENTANYL

Bentley, J. B.; Borel, J. D.; Nenad, R. E.; and Gillespie, T. J. Age and fentanyl pharmacokinetics. *Anesth. Analg.*, **1982**, *61*, 968–971.

Bower, S., and Hull, C. J. Comparative pharmacokinetics of fentanyl and alfentanil. *Br. J. Anaesth.*, **1982**, *54*, 871–877.

McClain, D. A., and Hug, C. C., Jr. Intravenous fentanyl kinetics. *Clin. Pharmacol. Ther.*, **1980**, *28*, 106–114.

Mather, L. E. Clinical pharmacokinetics of fentanyl and its newer derivatives. *Clin. Pharmacokinet.*, **1983**, *8*, 422–446.

FLUCYTOSINE

Cutler, R. E.; Blair, A. D.; and Kelly, M. R. Flucytosine kinetics in subjects with normal and impaired renal function. *Clin. Pharmacol. Ther.*, **1978**, *24*, 333–342.

Daneshmend, T. K., and Warnock, D. W. Clinical pharmacokinetics of systemic antifungal drugs. *Clin. Pharmacokinet.*, **1983**, *8*, 17–42.

FLUNITRAZEPAM

Boxenbaum, H. G.; Posmanter, H. N.; Macasieb, T.; Geitner, K. A.; Weinfeld, R. E.; Moore, J. D.; Darragh, A.; O'Kelly, D. A.; Weissman, L.; and Kaplan, S. A. Pharmacokinetics of flunitrazepam following single- and multiple-dose oral administration to healthy human subjects. *J. Pharmacokinet. Biopharm.*, **1978**, *6*, 283–293.

FLUOROURACIL

Balis, F. M.; Holcenberg, J. S.; and Bleyer, W. A. Clinical pharmacokinetics of commonly used anticancer drugs. *Clin. Pharmacokinet.*, **1983**, *8*, 202–232.

El Sayed, Y. M., and Sadée, W. The fluoropyrimidines. In, *Pharmacokinetics of Anticancer Agents in Humans.* (Ames, M. M.; Powis, G.; and Kovach, J. S.; eds.) Elsevier, New York, **1983**, pp. 209–227.

Fraile, R. J.; Baker, L. H.; Buroker, T. R.; Horwitz, J.; and Vaitkevicius, V. K. Pharmacokinetics of 5-fluorouracil administered orally, by rapid intravenous and by slow infusion. *Cancer Res.*, **1980**, *40*, 2223–2228.

MacMillan, W. E.; Wolberg, W. H.; and Welling, P. G. Pharmacokinetics of fluorouracil in humans. *Cancer Res.*, **1978**, *38*, 3479–3482.

FLURAZEPAM

Cooper, S. F.; Drolet, D.; and Dugal, R. Comparative bioavailability of two oral formulations of flurazepam in human subjects. *Biopharm. Drug Dispos.*, **1984**, *5*, 127–139.

Greenblatt, D. J.; Divoll, M.; Harmatz, J. S.; MacLaughlin, D. S.; and Shader, R. I. Kinetics and clinical effects of flurazepam in young and elderly noninsomniacs. *Clin. Pharmacol. Ther.*, **1981**, *30*, 475–486.

Kaplan, S. A.; deSilva, J. A. F.; Jack, M. L.; Alexander, K.; Strojny, N.; Weinfeld, R. E.; Puglisi, C. V.; and Weissman, L. Blood level profile in man following chronic oral administration of flurazepam hydrochloride. *J. Pharm. Sci.*, **1973**, *62*, 1932–1935.

FUROSEMIDE

Beermann, B., and Groschinsky-Grind, M. Clinical pharmacokinetics of diuretics. *Clin. Pharmacokinet.*, **1980**, *5*, 221–245.

Benet, L. Z. Pharmacokinetics/pharmacodynamics of furosemide in man: a review. *J. Pharmacokinet. Biopharm.*, **1979**, *7*, 1–27.

Smith, D. E.; Lin, E. T.; and Benet, L. Z. Absorption and disposition of furosemide in healthy volunteers, measured with a metabolite-specific assay. *Drug Metab. Dispos.*, **1980**, *8*, 337–342.

GENTAMICIN

Bauer, L. A., and Blouin, R. A. Gentamicin pharmacokinetics: effect of aging in patients with normal renal function. *J. Am. Geriatr. Soc.*, **1982**, *30*, 309–311.

Schentag, J. J.; Jusko, W. J.; Vance, J. W.; Cumbo, T. J.; Abrutyn, E.; DeLattre, M.; and Gerbracht, L. M. Gentamicin disposition and tissue accumulation on multiple dosing. *J. Pharmacokinet. Biopharm.*, **1977**, *5*, 559–577.

Zaske, D. E.; Cipolle, R. J.; Rotschafer, J. C.; Solem, L. D.; Mosier, N. R.; and Strate, R. G. Gentamicin pharmacokinetics in 1,640 patients: method for control of serum concentrations. *Antimicrob. Agents Chemother.*, **1982**, *21*, 407–411.

GOLD SODIUM THIOMALATE

Massarella, J. W.; Waller, E. S.; Crout, J. E.; and Yakatan, G. J. The pharmacokinetics of intramuscular gold sodium thiomalate in normal volunteers. *Biopharm. Drug Dispos.*, **1984**, *5*, 101–107.

HALOPERIDOL

Holley, F. O.; Magliozzi, J. R.; Stanski, D. R.; Lombrozo, L.; and Hollister, L. E. Haloperidol kinetics after oral and intravenous doses. *Clin. Pharmacol. Ther.*, **1983**, *33*, 477–484.

HEPARIN

Bjornsson, T. D.; Wolfram, K. M.; and Kitchell, B. B. Heparin kinetics determined by three assay methods. *Clin. Pharmacol. Ther.*, **1982**, *31*, 104–113.

Estes, J. W. Clinical pharmacokinetics of heparin. *Clin. Pharmacokinet.*, **1980**, *5*, 204–220.

McAvoy, T. J. Pharmacokinetic modeling of heparin and its clinical implications. *J. Pharmacokinet. Biopharm.*, **1979**, *7*, 331–354.

HEXOBARBITAL

Breimer, D. D.; Honhoff, C.; Zilly, W.; Richter, E.; and van Rossum, J. M. Pharmacokinetics of hexobarbital in man after intravenous infusion. *J. Pharmacokinet. Biopharm.*, **1975**, *3*, 1–11.

Vermeulen, N. P. E.; Rietveld, C. T.; and Breimer, D. D. Disposition of hexobarbitone in healthy man: kinetics of parent drug and metabolites following oral administration. *Br. J. Clin. Pharmacol.*, **1983**, *15*, 459–464.

Zilly, W.; Breimer, D. D.; and Richter, E. Hexobarbital disposition in compensated and decompensated cirrhosis of the liver. *Clin. Pharmacol. Ther.*, **1978**, *23*, 525–534.

HYDRALAZINE

Ludden, T. M.; McNay, J. L., Jr.; Shepherd, A. M. M.; and Lin, M.-S. Clinical pharmacokinetics of hydralazine. *Clin. Pharmacokinet.*, **1982**, *7*, 185–205.

Ludden, T. M.; Shepherd, A. M. M.; McNay, J. L., Jr.; and Lin, M.-S. Effect of intravenous dose on hydralazine kinetics after administration. *Clin. Pharmacol. Ther.*, **1983**, *34*, 148–152.

Shepherd, A. M. M.; Irvine, N. A.; Ludden, T. M.; Lin, M.-S.; and McNay, J. L., Jr. Effect of oral dose size on hydralazine kinetics and vasopressor response. *Clin. Pharmacol. Ther.*, **1984**, *36*, 595–600.

HYDROCHLOROTHIAZIDE

Beermann, B., and Groschinsky-Grind, M. Pharmacokinetics of hydrochlorothiazide in man. *Eur. J. Clin. Pharmacol.*, **1977**, *12*, 297–303.

Beermann, B.; Groschinsky-Grind, M.; and Lindstrom, B. Bioavailability of two hydrochlorothiazide preparations. *Eur. J. Clin. Pharmacol.*, **1977**, *11*, 203–205.

Niemeyer, C.; Hasenfuss, G.; Wais, U.; Knauf, H.; Schäfer-Korting, M.; and Mutschler, E. Pharmacokinetics of hydrochlorothiazide in relation to renal function. *Eur. J. Clin. Pharmacol.*, **1983**, *24*, 661–665.

Williams, R. L.; Davies, R. O.; Berman, R. S.; Holmes, G. I.; Huber, P.; Gee, W. L.; Lin, E. T.; and Benet, L. Z. Hydrochlorothiazide pharmacokinetics and pharmacologic effect: the influence of indomethacin. *J. Clin. Pharmacol.*, **1982**, *22*, 32–41.

Table A–II–1. PHARMACOKINETIC DATA (Continued)

IBUPROFEN

Lockwood, G. F.; Albert, K. S.; Gillespie, W. R.; Bole, G. G.; Harkcom, T. M.; Szpunar, G. J.; and Wagner, J. G. Pharmacokinetics of ibuprofen in man. I. Free and total area/dose relationships. *Clin. Pharmacol. Ther.*, **1983**, *34*, 97–103.

Verbeeck, R. K.; Blackburn, J. L.; and Loewen, G.R. Clinical pharmacokinetics of non-steroidal anti-inflammatory drugs. *Clin. Pharmacokinet.*, **1983**, *8*, 297–331.

IMIPRAMINE

Abernethy, D. R.; Greenblatt, D. J.; and Shader, R. I. Imipramine disposition in users of oral contraceptive steroids. *Clin. Pharmacol. Ther.*, **1984**, *35*, 792–797.

Giardina, E.-G. V.; Louie, M.; Bigger, J. T., Jr.; Brem, R.; and Alchevsky, D. Antiarrhythmic plasma-concentration range of imipramine against ventricular premature depolarizations. *Clin. Pharmacol. Ther.*, **1983**, *34*, 284–289.

Glassman, A. H.; Perel, J. M.; Shostak, M.; Kantor, S. J.; and Fleiss, J. L. Clinical implications of imipramine plasma levels for depressive illness. *Arch. Gen. Psychiatry*, **1977**, *34*, 197–204.

INDOMETHACIN

Alvan, G.; Orme, M.; Bertilsson, L.; Ekstrand, R.; and Palmer, L. Pharmacokinetics of indomethacin. *Clin. Pharmacol. Ther.*, **1975**, *18*, 364–373.

Helleberg, L. Clinical pharmacokinetics of indomethacin. *Clin. Pharmacokinet.*, **1981**, *6*, 245–258.

Kwan, K. C.; Breault, G. O.; Davis, R. L.; Lei, B. W.; Czerwinski, A. W.; Besselaar, G. H.; and Duggan, D. E. Effects of concomitant aspirin administration on the pharmacokinetics of indomethacin in man. *J. Pharmacokinet. Biopharm.*, **1978**, *6*, 451–476.

ISONIAZID

Advenier, C.; Saint-Aubin, A.; Gobert, C.; Houin, G.; Albengres, E.; and Tillement, J. P. Pharmacokinetics of isoniazid in the elderly. *Br. J. Clin. Pharmacol.*, **1980**, *10*, 167–169.

Ellard, G. A., and Gammon, P. T. Pharmacokinetics of isoniazid metabolism in man. *J. Pharmacokinet. Biopharm.*, **1976**, *4*, 83–113.

Holdiness, M. R. Clinical pharmacokinetics of the antituberculosis drugs. *Clin. Pharmacokinet.*, **1984**, *9*, 511–544.

Weber, W. W., and Hein, D. W. Clinical pharmacokinetics of isoniazid. *Clin. Pharmacokinet.*, **1979**, *4*, 401–422.

ISOSORBIDE DINITRATE

Abshagen, U.; Betzien, G.; Endele, R.; Kaufmann, B.; and Neugebauer, G. Pharmacokinetics and metabolism of isosorbide-dinitrate after intravenous and oral administration. *Eur. J. Clin. Pharmacol.*, **1985**, *27*, 637–644.

Bogaert, M. G. Clinical pharmacokinetics of organic nitrates. *Clin. Pharmacokinet.*, **1983**, *8*, 410–421.

Morrison, R. A.; Wiegand, U.-W.; Jähnchen, E.; Höhmann, D.; Bechtold, H.; Meinertz, T.; and Fung, H.-L. Isosorbide dinitrate kinetics and dynamics after intravenous, sublingual, and percutaneous dosing in angina. *Clin. Pharmacol. Ther.*, **1983**, *33*, 747–756.

Platzer, R.; Reutemann, G.; and Galeazzi, R. L. Pharmacokinetics of intravenous isosorbide-dinitrate. *J. Pharmacokinet. Biopharm.*, **1982**, *10*, 575–586.

ISOSORBIDE-2-MONONITRATE

Bogaert, M. G.; Rosseel, M. T.; Boelaert, J.; and Daneels, R. Fate of isosorbide dinitrate and mononitrates in patients with renal failure. *Eur. J. Clin. Pharmacol.*, **1981**, *21*, 73–76.

Straehl, P.; Galeazzi, R. L.; and Soliva, M. Isosorbide 5-mononitrate and isosorbide 2-mononitrate kinetics after intravenous and oral dosing. *Clin. Pharmacol. Ther.*, **1984**, *36*, 485–492.

ISOSORBIDE-5-MONONITRATE

Abshagen, U.; Betzien, G.; Endele, R.; and Kaufmann, B. Pharmacokinetics of intravenous and oral isosorbide-5-mononitrate. *Eur. J. Clin. Pharmacol.*, **1981**, *20*, 269–275.

Major, R. M.; Taylor, T.; Chasseaud, L. F.; Darragh, A.; and Lambe, R. F. Isosorbide 5-mononitrate kinetics. *Clin. Pharmacol. Ther.*, **1984**, *35*, 653–659.

Straehl, P.; Galeazzi, R. L.; and Soliva, M. Isosorbide 5-mononitrate and isosorbide 2-mononitrate kinetics after intravenous and oral dosing. *Clin. Pharmacol. Ther.*, **1984**, *36*, 485–492.

KANAMYCIN

Clarke, J. T.; Libke, R. K.; Regamey, C.; and Kirby, W. M. M. Comparative pharmacokinetics of amikacin and kanamycin. *Clin. Pharmacol. Ther.*, **1974**, *15*, 610–616.

Holdiness, M. R. Clinical pharmacokinetics of the antituberculosis drugs. *Clin. Pharmacokinet.*, **1984**, *9*, 511–544.

Orme, B. M., and Cutler, R. E. The relationship between kanamycin pharmacokinetics: distribution and renal function. *Clin. Pharmacol. Ther.*, **1969**, *10*, 543–550.

KETAMINE

Clements, J. A., and Nimmo, W. S. Pharmacokinetics and analgesic effect of ketamine in man. *Br. J. Anaesth.*, **1981**, *53*, 27–30.

Domino, E. F.; Domino, S. E.; Smith, R. E.; Domino, L. E.; Goulet, J. R.; Domino, K. E.; and Zsigmond, E. K. Ketamine kinetics in unmedicated and diazepam premedicated subjects. *Clin. Pharmacol. Ther.*, **1984**, *36*, 645–653.

Grant, I. S.; Nimmo, W. S.; and Clements, J. A. Pharmacokinetics and analgesic effects of i.m. and oral ketamine. *Br. J. Anaesth.*, **1981**, *53*, 805–809.

Wieber, J.; Gugler, R.; Hengstmann, J. H.; and Dengler, H. J. Pharmacokinetics of ketamine in man. *Anaesthesist*, **1975**, *24*, 260–263.

KETOPROFEN

Upton, R. A.; Williams, R. L.; Guentert, T. W.; Buskin, J. N.; and Riegelman, S. Ketoprofen pharmacokinetics and bioavailability based on an improved sensitive and specific assay. *Eur. J. Clin. Pharmacol.*, **1981**, *20*, 127–133.

Verbeeck, R. K.; Blackburn, J. L.; and Loewen, G. R. Clinical pharmacokinetics of non-steroidal anti-inflammatory drugs. *Clin. Pharmacokinet.*, **1983**, *8*, 297–331.

LABETALOL

Elliott, H. L.; Meredith, P. A.; Sumner, D. J.; and Reid, J. L. Comparison of the clinical pharmacokinetics and concentration-effect relationships for medroxalol and labetalol. *Br. J. Clin. Pharmacol.*, **1984**, *17*, 573–578.

MacCarthy, E. P., and Bloomfield, S. S. Labetalol: a review of its pharmacology, pharmacokinetics, clinical uses and adverse effects. *Pharmacotherapy*, **1983**, *3*, 193–219.

McNeil, J. J., and Louis, W. J. Clinical pharmacokinetics of labetalol. *Clin. Pharmacokinet.*, **1984**, *9*, 157–167.

LIDOCAINE

Follath, F.; Ganzinger, U.; and Schuetz, E. Reliability of antiarrhythmic drug plasma concentration monitoring. *Clin. Pharmacokinet.*, **1983**, *8*, 63–82.

Holley, F. O.; Ponganis, K. V.; and Stanski, D. R. Effects of cardiac surgery with cardiopulmonary bypass on lidocaine disposition. *Clin. Pharmacol. Ther.*, **1984**, *35*, 617–626.

LITHIUM

Groth, V.; Prellwitz, W.; and Jähnchen, E. Estimation of pharmacokinetic parameters of lithium from saliva and urine. *Clin. Pharmacol. Ther.*, **1974**, *16*, 490–498.

Mason, R. W.; McQueen, E. G.; Keary, P. J.; and James, N. McL. Pharmacokinetics of lithium: elimination half-time, renal clearance and apparent volume of distribution in schizophrenia. *Clin. Pharmacokinet.*, **1978**, *3*, 241–246.

Norman, T. R.; Walker, R. G.; and Burrows, G. D. Renal function related changes in lithium kinetics. *Clin. Pharmacokinet.*, **1984**, *9*, 349–353.

LORAZEPAM

Greenblatt, D. J. Clinical pharmacokinetics of oxazepam and lorazepam. *Clin. Pharmacokinet.*, **1981**, *6*, 89–105.

Greenblatt, D. J.; Shader, R. I.; Franke, K.; MacLaughlin, D. S.; Harmatz, J. S.; Allen, M. D.; Werner, A.; and Woo, E. Pharmacokinetics and bioavailability of intravenous, intramuscular, and oral lorazepam in humans. *J. Pharm. Sci.*, **1979**, *68*, 57–63.

Kraus, J. W.; Desmond, P. V.; Marshall, J. P.; Johnson, R. F.; Schenker, S.; and Wilkinson, G. R. Effects of aging and liver disease on disposition of lorazepam. *Clin. Pharmacol. Ther.*, **1978**, *24*, 411–419.

LORCAINIDE

Gillis, A. M., and Kates, R. E. Clinical pharmacokinetics of the newer antiarrhythmic agents. *Clin. Pharmacokinet.*, **1984**, *9*, 375–403.

Kates, R. E.; Keefe, D. L.; and Winkle, R. A. Lorcainide disposition kinetics in arrhythmia patients. *Clin. Pharmacol. Ther.*, **1983**, *33*, 28–34.

Klotz, U.; Müller-Seydlitz, P.; and Heimburg, P. Pharmacokinetics of lorcainide in man: a new antiarrhythmic agent. *Clin. Pharmacokinet.*, **1978**, *3*, 407–418.

MELPHALAN

Alberts, D. S.; Chang, S. Y.; Chen, H.-S. G.; Moon, T. E.; Evans, T. L.; Furner, R. L.; Himmelstein, K.; and Gross, J. F. Kinetics of intravenous melphalan. *Clin. Pharmacol. Ther.*, **1979**, *26*, 73–80.

Bosanquet, A. G., and Gilby, E. D. Pharmacokinetics of oral and intravenous melphalan during routine treatment of multiple myeloma. *Eur. J. Cancer Clin. Oncol.*, **1982**, *18*, 355–362.

Taha, I. A.-K.; Ahmad, R. A.; Rogers, D. W.; Pritchard, J.; and Rogers, H. J. Pharmacokinetics of melphalan in children following high-dose intravenous injection. *Cancer Chemother. Pharmacol.*, **1983**, *10*, 212–216.

MEPERIDINE

Edwards, D. J.; Svensson, C. K.; Visco, J. P.; and Lalka, D. Clinical pharmacokinetics of pethidine: 1982. *Clin. Pharmacokinet.*, **1982**, *7*, 421–433.

McHorse, T. S.; Wilkinson, G. R.; Johnson, R. F.; and Schenker, S. Effect of acute viral hepatitis in man on the disposition and elimination of meperidine. *Gastroenterology*, **1975**, *68*, 775–780.

Verbeeck, R. K.; Branch, R. A.; and Wilkinson, G. R. Meperidine disposition in man: influence of urinary pH and route of administration. *Clin. Pharmacol. Ther.*, **1981**, *30*, 619–628.

MERCAPTOPURINE

Loo, T. L.; Luce, J. K.; Sullivan, M. P.; and Frei, E., III. Clinical pharmacologic observations on 6-mercaptopurine and 6-methylthiopurine ribonucleoside. *Clin. Pharmacol. Ther.*, **1968**, *9*, 180–194.

Zimm, S.; Collins, J. M.; O'Neill, D.; Chabner, B. A.; and Poplack, D. G. Inhibition of first-pass metabolism in cancer chemotherapy: interaction of 6-mercaptopurine and allopurinol. *Clin. Pharmacol. Ther.*, **1983**, *34*, 810–817.

METHADONE

Nilsson, M.-I.; Änggård, E.; Holmstrand, J.; and Gunne, L.-M. Pharmacokinetics of methadone during maintenance treatment: adaptive changes during the induction phase. *Eur. J. Clin. Pharmacol.*, **1982**, *22*, 343–349.

Nilsson, M.-I.; Widerlöv, E.; Meresaar, U.; and Änggård, E. Effect of urinary pH on the disposition of methadone in man. *Eur. J. Clin. Pharmacol.*, **1982**, *22*, 337–342.

Table A–II–1. PHARMACOKINETIC DATA (Continued)

Romach, M. K.; Piafsky, K. M.; Abel, J. G.; Khouw, V.; and Sellers, E. M. Methadone binding to orosomucoid (α₁-acid glycoprotein): determinant of free fraction in plasma. *Clin. Pharmacol. Ther.*, **1981**, *29*, 211–217.

METHICILLIN

Bulger, R. J.; Lindholm, D. D.; Murray, J. S.; and Kirby, W. M. M. Effect of uremia on methicillin and oxacillin blood levels. *J.A.M.A.*, **1964**, *187* 319–322.

Yaffe, S. J.; Gerbracht, L. M.; Mosovich, L. L.; Mattar, M. E.; Danish, M.; and Jusko, W. J. Pharmacokinetics of methicillin in patients with cystic fibrosis. *J. Infect. Dis.*, **1977**, *135*, 828–831.

METHOHEXITAL

Breimer, D. D. Pharmacokinetics of methohexitone following intravenous infusion in humans. *Br. J. Anaesth.*, **1976**, *48*, 643–649.

Hudson, R. J.; Stanski, D. R.; and Burch, P. G. Pharmacokinetics of methohexital and thiopental in surgical patients. *Anesthesiology*, **1983**, *59*, 215–219.

METHOTREXATE

Balis, F. M.; Holcenberg, J. S.; and Bleyer, W. A. Clinical pharmacokinetics of commonly used anticancer drugs. *Clin. Pharmacokinet.*, **1983**, *8,* 202–232.

Edelman, J.; Biggs, D. F.; Jamali, F.; and Russell, A. S. Low-dose methotrexate kinetics in arthritis. *Clin. Pharmacol. Ther.*, **1984**, *35*, 382–386.

Leme, P. R.; Creaven, P. J.; Allen, L. M.; and Berman, M. Kinetic model for the disposition and metabolism of moderate and high-dose methotrexate (NSC-740) in man. *Cancer Chemother. Rep.*, **1974**, *59*, 811–817.

METHYLDOPA

Kwan, K. C.; Foltz, E. L.; Breault, G. O.; Baer, J. E.; and Totaro, J. A. Pharmacokinetics of methyldopa in man. *J. Pharmacol. Exp. Ther.*, **1976**, *198*, 264–276.

Myhre, E.; Brodwall, E. K.; Stenback, Ø.; and Hansen, T. The renal excretion of methyldopa. *Scand. J. Clin. Lab. Invest.*, **1972**, *29*, 201–204.

Myhre, E.; Rugstad, H. E.; and Hansen, T. Clinical pharmacokinetics of methyldopa. *Clin. Pharmacokinet.*, **1982**, *7*, 221–223.

Renwick, A. G.; Higgins, V.; Powers, K.; Smith, C. L.; and George, C. F. The absorption and conjugation of methyldopa in patients with coeliac and Crohn's diseases during treatment. *Br. J. Clin. Pharmacol.*, **1983**, *16*, 77–83.

METHYLPREDNISOLONE

Antal, E. J.; Wright, C. E., III; Gillespie, W. R.; and Albert, K. S. Influence of route of administration on the pharmacokinetics of methylprednisolone. *J. Pharmacokinet. Biopharm.*, **1983**, *11*, 561–576.

Gustavson, L. E., and Benet, L. Z. Pharmacokinetics of natural and synthetic glucocorticoids. In *Butterworth's International Medical Reviews in Endocrinology.* Vol. 4. *The Adrenal Cortex.* (Anderson, D. C., and Winter, J. S. D., eds.) Butterworth & Co., London, **1985**, pp. 235–281.

Narang, P. K.; Wilder, R.; Chatterji, D. C.; Yeager, R. L.; and Gallelli, J. F. Systemic bioavailability and pharmacokinetics of methylprednisolone in patients with rheumatoid arthritis following 'high-dose' pulse administration. *Biopharm. Drug Dispos.*, **1983**, *4*, 233–248.

METOPROLOL

Bengtsson, C.; Johnsson, G.; and Regårdh, C. G. Plasma levels and effects of metoprolol on blood pressure and heart rate in hypertensive patients after an acute dose and between two doses during long-term treatment. *Clin. Pharmacol. Ther.*, **1975**, *17*, 400–408.

Regårdh, C. G. Pharmacokinetic aspects of some β-adrenoceptor blocking drugs. *Acta Med. Scand.*, **1982**, *665*, Suppl., 49–60.

Regårdh, C. G.; Borg, K. O.; Johansson, G.; and Palmer, L. Pharmacokinetic studies on the selective β₁-receptor antagonist metoprolol in man. *J. Pharmacokinet. Biopharm.*, **1974**, *2*, 347–364.

METRONIDAZOLE

Jensen, J. C., and Gugler, R. Single- and multiple-dose metronidazole kinetics. *Clin. Pharmacol. Ther.*, **1983**, *34*, 481–487.

Mattie, H.; Dijkmans, B. A. C.; and van Gulpen, C. The pharmacokinetics of metronidazole and tinidazole in patients with mixed aerobic-anaerobic infections. *Antimicrob. Agents Chemother.*, **1982**, *10*, Suppl. A, 59–64.

Ralph, E. D. Clinical pharmacokinetics of metronidazole. *Clin. Pharmacokinet.*, **1983**, *8*, 43–62.

MEXILETINE

Follath, F.; Ganzinger, U.; and Schuetz, E. Reliability of antiarrhythmic drug plasma concentration monitoring. *Clin. Pharmacokinet.*, **1983**, *8*, 63–82.

Gillis, A. M., and Kates, R. E. Clinical pharmacokinetics of the newer antiarrhythmic agents. *Clin. Pharmacokinet.*, **1984**, *9*, 375–403.

Vozeh, S.; Katz, G.; Steiner, V.; and Follath, F. Population pharmacokinetic parameters in patients treated with oral mexiletine. *Eur. J. Clin. Pharmacol.*, **1982**, *23*, 445–451.

Woosley, R. L.; Wang, T.; Stone, W.; Siddoway, L.; Thompson, K.; Duff, H. J.; Cerskus, I.; and Roden, D. Pharmacology, electrophysiology, and pharmacokinetics of mexiletine. *Am. Heart J.*, **1984**, *107*, 1058–1065.

MEZLOCILLIN

Mangione, A.; Boudinot, F. D.; Schultz, R. M.; and Jusko, W. J. Dose-dependent pharmacokinetics of mezlocillin in relation to renal impairment. *Antimicrob. Agents Chemother.*, **1982**, *21*, 428–435.

Odio, C.; Threlkeld, N.; Thomas, M. L.; and McCraken, G. H., Jr. Pharmacokinetic properties of mezlocillin in newborn infants. *Antimicrob. Agents Chemother.*, **1984**, *25*, 556–559.

MINOCYCLINE

Heaney, D., and Eknoyan, G. Minocycline and doxycycline kinetics in chronic renal failure. *Clin. Pharmacol. Ther.*, **1978**, *24*, 233–239.

Macdonald, H.; Kelly, R. G.; Allen, E. S.; Noble, J. F.; and Kanegis, L. A. Pharmacokinetic studies on minocycline in man. *Clin. Pharmacol. Ther.*, **1973**, *14*, 852–861.

Welling, P. G.; Shaw, W. R.; Uman, S. W.; Tse, F. L. S.; and Craig, W. A. Pharmacokinetics of minocycline in renal failure. *Antimicrob. Agents Chemother.*, **1975**, *8*, 532–537.

MINOXIDIL

Lowenthal, D. T., and Affrime, M. B. Pharmacology and pharmacokinetics of minoxidil. *J. Cardiovasc. Pharmacol.*, **1980**, *2*, Suppl. 2, S93–S106.

MORPHINE

Brunk, S. F., and Delle, M. Morphine metabolism in man. *Clin. Pharmacol. Ther.*, **1974**, *16*, 51–57.

Stanski, D. R.; Greenblatt, D. J.; and Lowenstein, E. Kinetics of intravenous and intramuscular morphine. *Clin. Pharmacol. Ther.*, **1978**, *24*, 52–59.

Stanski, D. R.; Paalzow, L.; and Edlund, P. O. Morphine pharmacokinetics: GLC assay versus radioimmunoassay. *J. Pharm. Sci.*, **1982**, *71*, 314–317.

MOXALACTAM

Barriere, S. L., and Flaherty, J. F. Third-generation cephalosporins: a critical review. *Clin. Pharm.*, **1984**, *3*, 351–373.

Scheld, W. M.; Spyker, D. A.; Donowitz, G. R.; Bolton, W. K.; and Sande, M. A. Moxalactam and cefazolin: comparative pharmacokinetics in normal subjects. *Antimicrob. Agents Chemother.*, **1981**, *19*, 613–619.

Swanson, D. J.; Reitberg, D. P.; Smith, I. L.; Wels, P. B.; and Schentag, J. J. Steady-state moxalactam pharmacokinetics in patients: noncompartmental versus two-compartmental analysis. *J. Pharmacokinet. Biopharm.*, **1983**, *11*, 337–353.

NADOLOL

Dreyfuss, J.; Brannick, L. J.; Vukovich, R. A.; Shaw, J. M.; and Willard, D. A. Metabolic studies in patients with nadolol: oral and intravenous administration. *J. Clin. Pharmacol.*, **1977**, *17*, 300–307.

Dreyfuss, J.; Griffith, D. L.; Singhvi, S. M.; Shaw, J. M.; Ross, J. J.; Vukovich, R. A.; and Willard, D. A. Pharmacokinetics of nadolol, a beta-receptor antagonist: administration of therapeutic single- and multiple-dosage regimens to hypertensive patients. *J. Clin. Pharmacol.*, **1979**, *19*, 712–721.

Frishman, W. Clinical pharmacology of the new beta-adrenergic blocking drugs. Part 9. Nadolol: a new long-acting beta-adrenoceptor blocking drug. *Am. Heart J.*, **1980**, *99*, 124–128.

NAFCILLIN

Marshall, J. P.; Salt, W. B.; Elam, R. O.; Wilkinson, G. R.; and Schenker, S. Disposition of nafcillin in patients with cirrhosis and extrahepatic biliary obstruction. *Gastroenterology*, **1977**, *73*, 1388–1392.

Rudnick, M.; Morrison, G.; Walker, B.; and Singer, I. Renal failure, hemodialysis, and nafcillin kinetics. *Clin. Pharmacol. Ther.*, **1976**, *20*, 413–423.

Waller, E. S.; Sharanevych, M. A.; and Yakatan, G. J. The effect of probenecid on nafcillin disposition. *J. Clin. Pharmacol.*, **1982**, *22*, 482–489.

NALOXONE

Berkowitz, B. A. The relationship of pharmacokinetics to pharmacological activity: morphine, methadone and naloxone. *Clin. Pharmacokinet.*, **1976**, *1*, 219–230.

Fishman, J.; Roffwarg, H.; and Hellman, L. Disposition of naloxone-7,8-^{3}H in normal and narcotic-dependent men. *J. Pharmacol. Exp. Ther.*, **1973**, *187*, 575–580.

Moreland, T. A.; Brice, J. E. H.; Walker, C. H. M.; and Parija, A. C. Naloxone pharmacokinetics in the newborn. *Br. J. Clin. Pharmacol.*, **1980**, *9*, 609–612.

NAPROXEN

Runkel, R. A.; Forchielli, E.; Sevelius, H.; Chaplin, M.; and Segre, E. Nonlinear plasma level response to high doses of naproxen. *Clin. Pharmacol. Ther.*, **1974**, *15*, 261–266.

Upton, R. A.; Williams, R. L.; Kelly, J.; and Jones, R. M. Naproxen pharmacokinetics in the elderly. *Br. J. Clin. Pharmacol.*, **1984**, *18*, 207–214.

Verbeeck, R. K.; Blackburn, J. L.; and Loewen, G. R. Clinical pharmacokinetics of non-steroidal anti-inflammatory drugs. *Clin. Pharmacokinet.*, **1983**, *8*, 297–331.

NEOSTIGMINE

Cronnelly, R.; Stanski, D. R.; Miller, R. D.; Sheiner, L. B.; and Sohn, Y. J. Renal function and the pharmacokinetics of neostigmine in anesthetized man. *Anesthesiology*, **1979**, *51*, 222–226.

Nowell, P. T.; Scott, C. A.; and Wilson, A. Determination of neostigmine and pyridostigmine in the urine of patients with myasthenia gravis. *Br. J. Pharmacol.*, **1962**, *18*, 617–624.

1727

Table A–II–1. PHARMACOKINETIC DATA (Continued)

NETILMICIN

Humbert, G.; Leroy, A.; Fillastre, J. P.; and Oksenhendler, G. Pharmacokinetics of netilmicin in the presence of normal or impaired renal function. *Antimicrob. Agents Chemother.,* **1978,** *14,* 40–44.

Michalsen, H., and Bergan, T. Pharmacokinetics of netilmicin in children with and without cystic fibrosis. *Antimicrob. Agents Chemother.,* **1981,** *19,* 1029–1031.

Welling, P. G.; Baumueller, A.; Lau, C. C.; and Madsen, P. O. Netilmicin pharmacokinetics after single intravenous doses to elderly male patients. *Antimicrob. Agents Chemother.,* **1977,** *12,* 328–334.

NICOTINE

Benowitz, N. L.; Jacob, P., III; Jones, R. T.; and Rosenberg, J. Interindividual variability in the metabolism and cardiovascular effects of nicotine in man. *J. Pharmacol. Exp. Ther.,* **1982,** *221,* 368–372.

NIFEDIPINE

Foster, T. S.; Hamann, S. R.; Richards, V. R.; Bryant, P. J.; Graves, D. A.; and McAllister, R. G., Jr. Nifedipine kinetics and bioavailability after single intravenous and oral doses in normal subjects. *J. Clin. Pharmacol.,* **1983,** *23,* 161–170.

NITRAZEPAM

Jochemsen, R.; Van Beusekom, B. R.; Spoelstra, P.; Janssens, A. R.; and Breimer, D. D. Effects of age and liver cirrhosis on the pharmacokinetics of nitrazepam. *Br. J. Clin. Pharmacol.,* **1983,** *15,* 295–302.

Kangas, L., and Breimer, D. D. Clinical pharmacokinetics of nitrazepam. *Clin. Pharmacokinet.,* **1981,** *6,* 346–366.

Rieder, J. Plasma levels and derived pharmacokinetic characteristics of unchanged nitrazepam in man. *Arzneimittelforsch.,* **1978,** *23,* 212–218.

NITROGLYCERIN

Armstrong, P. W.; Armstrong, J. A.; and Marks, G. S. Pharmacokinetic-hemodynamic studies of intravenous nitroglycerin in congestive cardiac failure. *Circulation,* **1980,** *62,* 160–166.

McNiff, E. F.; Yacobi, A.; Young-Chang, F. M.; Golden, L. H.; Goldfarb, A.; and Fung, H.-L. Nitroglycerin pharmacokinetics after intravenous infusion in normal subjects. *J. Pharm. Sci.,* **1981,** *70,* 1054–1058.

Noonan, P. K., and Benet, L. Z. Incomplete and delayed bioavailability of sublingual nitroglycerin. *Am. J. Cardiol.,* **1985,** *55,* 184–187.

NORTRIPTYLINE

Åsberg, M.; Crönholm, B.; Sjöqvist, F.; and Tuck, D. Relationship between plasma level and therapeutic effect of nortriptyline. *Br. Med. J.* [*Clin. Res.*]. **1971,** *3,* 331–334.

Dawling, S.; Lynn, K.; Rosser, R.; and Braithwaite, R. The pharmacokinetics of nortriptyline in patients with chronic renal failure. *Br. J. Clin. Pharmacol.,* **1981,** *12,* 39–45.

Gram, L. F., and Overø, K. F. First-pass metabolism of nortriptyline in man. *Clin. Pharmacol. Ther.,* **1974,** *18,* 305–314.

OXACILLIN

Dittert, L. W.; Griffen, W. O.; La Piana, J. C.; Shainfeld, F. J.; and Dolusio, J. T. Pharmacokinetic interpretation of penicillin levels in serum and urine after intravenous administration. *Antimicrob. Agents Chemother.,* **1969,** 42–48.

Rosenblatt, J. E.; Kind, A. C.; Brodie, J. L.; and Kirby, W. M. M. Mechanisms responsible for the blood level differences of isoxazolyl penicillins. *Arch. Intern. Med.,* **1968,** *121,* 345–348.

Wirth, K.; Hengstmann, J. H.; Langebartels, F. H.; and Träger, S. Zur Kinetik von Ampicillin. Oxacillin und Carbenicillin nach intravenöser Kurzinfusion beim Menschen. *Arzneimittelforsch.,* **1976,** *26,* 1709–1715.

OXAZEPAM

Abernethy, D. R.; Greenblatt, D. J.; Ochs, H. R.; Weyers, D.; Divoll, M.; Harmatz, J. S.; and Shader, R. I. Lorazepam and oxazepam kinetics in women on low-dose oral contraceptives. *Clin. Pharmacol. Ther.,* **1981,** *33,* 628–632.

Greenblatt, D. J. Clinical pharmacokinetics of oxazepam and lorazepam. *Clin. Pharmacokinet.,* **1981,** *6,* 89–105.

Murray, T. G.; Chiang, S. T.; Koepke, H. H.; and Walker, B. R. Renal disease, age and oxazepam kinetics. *Clin. Pharmacol. Ther.,* **1981,** *30,* 805–809.

PANCURONIUM

Cronnelly, R.; Fisher, D. M.; Miller, R. D.; Gencarelli, P.; Nguyen-Gruenke, L.; and Castagnoli, N., Jr. Pharmacokinetics and pharmacodynamics of vecuronium (org NC45) and pancuronium in anesthetized humans. *Anesthesiology,* **1983,** *58,* 405–408.

Duvaldestin, P.; Saada, J.; Berger, J. L.; D'Hollander, A.; and Desmonts, J. M. Pharmacokinetics, pharmacodynamics and dose-response relationships of pancuronium in control and elderly subjects. *Anesthesiology,* **1982,** *56,* 36–40.

Somogyi, A. A.; Shanks, C. A.; and Triggs, E. J. The effect of renal failure on the disposition and neuromuscular blocking action of pancuronium bromide. *Eur. J. Clin. Pharmacol.,* **1977,** *12,* 23–29.

PHENOBARBITAL

Alvin, J.; McHorse, T.; Hoyumpa, A.; Bush, M. T.; and Schenker, S. The effect of liver disease in man on the disposition of phenobarbital. *J. Pharmacol. Exp. Ther.*, **1975**, *192*, 224–235.

Buchthal, F., and Lennox-Buchthal, M. A. Phenobarbital. Relation of serum concentration to control of seizures. In, *Antiepileptic Drugs.* (Woodbury, D. M.; Penry, J. K.; and Schmidt, R. P.; eds.) Raven Press, New York, **1972**, pp. 335–343.

Wilensky, A. J.; Friel, P. N.; Levy, R. H.; Comfort, C. P.; and Kaluzny, S. P. Kinetics of phenobarbital in normal subjects and epileptic patients. *Eur. J. Clin. Pharmacol.*, **1982**, *23*, 87–92.

PHENYLBUTAZONE

Aarbakke, J. Clinical pharmacokinetics of phenylbutazone. *Clin. Pharmacokinet.*, **1978**, *3*, 369–380.

Krishnaswamy, K.; Ushasri, V.; and Naidu, A. N. The effect of malnutrition on the pharmacokinetics of phenylbutazone. *Clin. Pharmacokinet.*, **1981**, *6*, 152–159.

Verbeeck, R. K.; Blackburn, J. L.; and Loewen, G. R. Clinical pharmacokinetics of non-steroidal anti-inflammatory drugs. *Clin. Pharmacokinet.*, **1983**, *8*, 297–331.

PHENYLETHYLMALONAMIDE

Cottrell, P. R.; Streete, J. M.; Berry, D. J.; Schäfer, H.; Pisani, F.; Perucca, E.; and Richens, A. Pharmacokinetics of phenylethylmalonamide (PEMA) in normal subjects and in patients treated with antiepileptic drugs. *Epilepsia*, **1982**, *23*, 307–313.

Pisani, F., and Richens, A. Pharmacokinetics of phenylethylmalonamide (PEMA) after oral and intravenous administration. *Clin. Pharmacokinet.*, **1983**, *8*, 272–276.

PHENYTOIN

Bauer, L. A., and Blouin, R. A. Age and phenytoin kinetics in adult epileptics. *Clin. Pharmacol. Ther.*, **1982**, *31*, 301–304.

Grasela. T. H.; Sheiner, L. B.; Rambeck, B.; Boenigk. H. E.; Dunlop, A.; Mullen, P. W.; Wadsworth, J.; Richens, A.; Ishizaki, T.; Chiba. K.; Miura. H.; Minagawa, K.; Blain, P. G.; Mucklow. J. C.; Bacon, C. T.; and Rawlins, M. Steady-state pharmacokinetics of phenytoin from routinely collected patient data. *Clin. Pharmacokinet.*, **1983**, *8*, 355–364.

Lund. L. Anticonvulsant effect of diphenylhydantoin relative to plasma levels. *Arch. Neurol.*, **1974**, *31*, 289–294.

Vozeh, S.; Muir, K. T.; Sheiner, L. B.; and Follath, F. Predicting individual phenytoin dosage. *J. Pharmacokinet. Biopharm.*, **1981**, *9*, 131–146.

PINDOLOL

Guerret, M.; Cheymol, G.; Aubry, J. P.; Cheymol, A.; Lavene, D.; and Kiechel, J. R. Estimation of the absolute oral bioavailability of pindolol by two analytical methods. *Eur. J. Clin. Pharmacol.*, **1983**, *25*, 357–359.

Lavene, D.; Weiss, Y. A.; Safar, M. E.; Loria, Y.; Agorus, N.; Georges, D.; and Milliez, P. L. Pharmacokinetics and hepatic extraction ratio of pindolol in hypertensive patients with normal and impaired renal function. *J. Clin. Pharmacol.*, **1979**, *17*, 501–508.

Regårdh, C. G. Pharmacokinetic aspects of some β-adrenoceptor blocking drugs. *Acta Med. Scand.*, **1982**, *665*, Suppl., 49–60.

PIPERACILLIN

Batra, V. K.; Morrison, J. A.; Lasseter, K. C.; and Joy, V. A. Piperacillin kinetics. *Clin. Pharmacol. Ther.*, **1979**, *26*, 41–53.

Lode, H.; Elvers, A.; Koeppe, P.; and Borner, K. Comparative pharmacokinetics of apalcillin and piperacillin. *Antimicrob. Agents Chemother.*, **1984**, *25*, 105–108.

Welling, P. G.; Craig, W. A.; Bundtzen, R. W.; Kwok, F. W.; Gerber, A. U.; and Madsen. P. O. Pharmacokinetics of piperacillin in subjects with various degrees of renal function. *Antimicrob. Agents Chemother.*, **1983**, *23*, 881–887.

PRAZEPAM

Ochs, H. R.; Greenblatt, D. J.; Verburg-Ochs, B.; and Locniskar, A. Comparative single-dose kinetics of oxazolam, prazepam and clorazepate: three precursors of desmethyldiazepam. *J. Clin. Pharmacol.*, **1984**, *24*, 446–451.

Smith. M. T.; Evan. L. E. J.; Eadie. M. J.; and Tyrer, J. H. Pharmacokinetics of prazepam in man. *Eur. J. Clin. Pharmacol.*, **1979**, *16*, 141–147.

PRAZOSIN

Bateman, D. N.; Hobbs, D. C.; Twomey, T. M.; Stevens, E. A.; and Rawlins, M. D. Prazosin, pharmacokinetics and concentration effect. *Eur. J. Clin. Pharmacol.*, **1979**, *16*, 177–181.

Jaillon, P. Clinical pharmacokinetics of prazosin. *Clin. Pharmacokinet.*, **1980**, *5*, 365–376.

PREDNISOLONE

Gustavson, L. E., and Benet, L. Z. Pharmacokinetics of natural and synthetic glucocorticoids. In, *Butterworth's International Medical Reviews in Endocrinology.* Vol. 4. *The Adrenal Cortex.* (Anderson, D. C., and Winter, J. S. D., eds.) Butterworth & Co., London, **1985**, pp. 235–281.

Legler, U. F.; Frey, F. J.; and Benet, L. Z. Prednisolone clearance at steady-state in man. *J. Clin. Endocrinol. Metab.*, **1982**, *55*, 762–767.

Rose, J. Q.; Yurchak, A. M.; and Jusko, W. J. Dose dependent pharmacokinetics of prednisone and prednisolone in man. *J. Pharmacokinet. Biopharm.*, **1981**, *9*, 389–417.

PREDNISONE

Gustavson, L. E., and Benet, L. Z. Pharmacokinetics of natural and synthetic glucocorticoids. In, *Butterworth's International Medical Reviews in Endocrinology.* Vol. 4. *The Adrenal Cor-*

Table A–II–1.   PHARMACOKINETIC DATA (Continued)

tex. (Anderson, D. C., and Winter, J. S. D., eds.) Butterworth & Co., London, **1985**, pp. 235–281.

Schalm, S. W.; Summerskill, W. H. J.; and Go, V. L. W.   Prednisone for chronic active liver disease: pharmacokinetics, including conversion to prednisolone. *Gastroenterology*, **1977**, *72*, 910–913.

PRIMIDONE

Cloyd, J. C.; Miller, K. W.; and Leppik, I. E.   Primidone kinetics: effects of concurrent drugs and duration of therapy. *Clin. Pharmacol. Ther.*, **1981**, *29*, 402–407.

Gallagher, B. B.; Baumel, I. P.; and Mattson, R. H.   Metabolic disposition of primidone and its metabolites in epileptic subjects after single and repeated administration. *Neurology (Minneap.)*, **1972**, *22*, 1186–1192.

Kauffman, R. E.; Habersang, R.; and Lansky, L.   Kinetics of primidone metabolism and excretion in children. *Clin. Pharmacol. Ther.*, **1977**, *22*, 200–205.

Lee, C.-S. C.; Marbury, T. C.; Perchalski, R. T.; and Wilder, B. J.   Pharmacokinetics of primidone elimination by uremic patients. *J. Clin. Pharmacol.*, **1982**, *22*, 301–308.

PROBENECID

Cunningham, R. F.; Israili, Z. H.; and Dayton, P. G.   Clinical pharmacokinetics of probenecid. *Clin. Pharmacokinet.*, **1981**, *6*, 135–151.

PROCAINAMIDE

Benet, L. Z., and Ding, R. W.   Die renale Elimination von Procainamid: Pharmakokinetik bei Niereninsuffizienz. In   *Die Behandlung von Herzrhythmusstörungen bei Nierenkranken.* (Braun, J.; Pilgrim, R.; Gessler, U.; and Seybold, D.; eds.) S. Karger, Basel, **1984**, pp. 96–111.

Follath, F.; Ganzinger, U.; and Schuetz, E.   Reliability of antiarrhythmic drug plasma concentration monitoring. *Clin. Pharmacokinet.*, **1983**, *8*, 63–82.

Karlsson, E.   Clinical pharmacokinetics of procainamide. *Clin. Pharmacokinet.*, **1978**, *3*, 97–107.

PROPRANOLOL

Kornhauser, D. M.; Wood, J. J.; Vestal, R. E.; Wilkinson, G. R.; Branch, R. A.; and Shand, D. G.   Biological determinants of propranolol disposition in man. *Clin. Pharmacol. Ther.*, **1978**, *23*, 165–174.

Regårdh, C. G.   Pharmacokinetic aspects of some β-adrenoceptor blocking drugs. *Acta Med. Scand.*, **1982**, *665*, Suppl., 49–60.

PROTRIPTYLINE

Baldessarini, R. J.   Status of psychotropic drug blood level assays and other biochemical measurements in clinical practice. *Am. J. Psychiatry*, **1979**, *136*, 1177–1180.

Moody, J. P.; Whyte, S. F.; MacDonald, A. J.; and Naylor, G. J.   Pharmacokinetic aspects of protriptyline plasma levels. *Eur. J. Clin. Pharmacol.*, **1977**, *11*, 51–56.

PYRIDOSTIGMINE

Cronnelly, R.; Stanski, D. R.; Miller, R. D.; and Sheiner, L. B.   Pyridostigmine kinetics with and without renal function. *Clin. Pharmacol. Ther.*, **1980**, *28*, 78–81.

Kornfeld, P.; Samuels, A. J.; Wolf, R. L.; and Osserman, K. E.   Metabolism of ^{14}C-labeled pyridostigmine in myasthenia gravis. *Neurology (Minneap.)*, **1970**, *20*, 634–641.

PYRIMETHAMINE

Ahmad, R. A., and Rogers, H. J.   Pharmacokinetics and protein binding interactions of dapsone and pyrimethamine. *Br. J. Clin. Pharmacol.*, **1980**, *10*, 519–524.

Cavallito, J. C.; Nichol, C. A.; Brenckman, W. D., Jr.; DeAngelis, R. L.; Stickney, D. R.; Simmons, W. S.; and Sigel, C. W.   Lipid soluble inhibitors of dihydrofolate reductase. I. Kinetics, tissue distribution, and extent of metabolism of pyrimethamine, metoprurine, and etoprine in the rat, dog and man. *Drug Metab. Dispos.*, **1978**, *6*, 329–337.

QUINIDINE

Follath, F.; Ganzinger, U.; and Schuetz, E.   Reliability of antiarrhythmic drug plasma concentration monitoring. *Clin. Pharmacokinet.*, **1983**, *8*, 63–82.

Ochs, H. R.; Greenblatt, D. J.; and Woo, E.   Clinical pharmacokinetics of quinidine. *Clin. Pharmacokinet.*, **1980**, *5*, 150–168.

Rakhit, A.; Holford, N. H. G.; Guentert, T. W.; Maloney, K.; and Riegelman, S.   Pharmacokinetics of quinidine and three of its metabolites in man. *J. Pharmacokinet. Biopharm.*, **1984**, *12*, 1–21.

QUININE

White, N. J.; Chanthavanich, P.; Krishna, S.; Bunch, C.; and Silamut, K.   Quinine disposition kinetics. *Br. J. Clin. Pharmacol.*, **1983**, *16*, 399–403.

RANITIDINE

Garg, D. C.; Weidler, D. J.; and Eshelman, F. N.   Ranitidine bioavailability and kinetics in normal male subjects. *Clin. Pharmacol. Ther.*, **1983**, *33*, 445–452.

Roberts, C. J. C.   Clinical pharmacokinetics of ranitidine. *Clin. Pharmacokinet.*, **1984**, *9*, 211–221.

Young, C. J.; Daneshmend, T. K.; and Roberts, C. J. C. Effects of cirrhosis and aging on the elimination and bioavailability of ranitidine. *Gut*, **1982**, 23, 819–823.

RIFAMPIN

Acocella, G. Clinical pharmacokinetics of rifampicin. *Clin. Pharmacokinet.*, **1978**, 3, 108–127.

Advenier, C.; Gobert, C.; Houin, G.; Bidet, D.; Richelet, S.; and Tillement, J. P. Pharmacokinetic studies of rifampicin in the elderly. *Ther. Drug Monit.*, **1983**, 5, 61–65.

Holdiness, M. R. Clinical pharmacokinetics of the antituberculosis drugs. *Clin. Pharmacokinet.*, **1984**, 9, 511–544.

Houin, G.; Beucler, A.; Richelet, S.; Brioude, R.; Lafaix, C.; and Tillement, J. P. Pharmacokinetics of rifampicin and desacetylrifampicin in tuberculous patients after different rates of infusion. *Ther. Drug Monit.*, **1983**, 5, 67–72.

SALICYLIC ACID

Furst, D. E.; Tozer, T. N.; and Melmon, K. L. Salicylate clearance, the resultant of protein binding and metabolism. *Clin. Pharmacol. Ther.*, **1979**, 26, 380–389.

Levy, G. Pharmacokinetics of salicylate in man. *Drug Metab. Rev.*, **1979**, 9, 3–19.

Roberts, M. S.; Rumble, R. H.; Wanwimolruk, S.; Thomas, D.; and Brooks, P. M. Pharmacokinetics of aspirin and salicylate in elderly subjects and in patients with alcoholic liver disease. *Eur. J. Clin. Pharmacol.*, **1983**, 25, 253–261.

Verbeeck, R. K.; Blackburn, J. L.; and Loewen, G. R. Clinical pharmacokinetics of non-steroidal anti-inflammatory drugs. *Clin. Pharmacokinet.*, **1983**, 8, 297–331.

STREPTOMYCIN

Holdiness, M. R. Clinical pharmacokinetics of the antituberculosis drugs. *Clin. Pharmacokinet.*, **1984**, 9, 511–544.

Prasad, J. S., and Krishnaswamy, K. Streptomycin pharmacokinetics in malnutrition. *Chemotherapy*, **1978**, 24, 333–337.

SULFADIAZINE

Männistö, P. T.; Mäntylä, R.; Mattila, J.; Nykänen, S.; and Lamminsivu, U. Comparison of the pharmacokinetics of sulphadiazine and sulphamethoxazole after intravenous infusion. *J. Antimicrob. Chemother.*, **1982**, 9, 461–470.

SULFAMETHOXAZOLE

Morgan, D. J., and Raymond, K. Evaluation of slow infusions of co-trimoxazole by using predictive pharmacokinetics. *Antimicrob. Agents Chemother.*, **1980**, 17, 132–137.

Patel, R. B., and Welling, P. G. Clinical pharmacokinetics of co-trimoxazole. *Clin. Pharmacokinet.*, **1980**, 5, 405–423.

Singlas, E.; Colin, J. N.; Rottembourg, J.; Meessen, J. P.; de Martin, A.; Legrain, M.; and Simon, P. Pharmacokinetics of sulfamethoxazole-trimethoprim combination during chronic peritoneal dialysis: effect of peritonitis. *Eur. J. Clin. Pharmacol.*, **1982**, 21, 409–415.

SULFISOXAZOLE

Cello, J. P., and Øie, S. Binding and disposition of sulfisoxazole in alcoholic cirrhosis. *J. Pharmacokinet. Biopharm.*, **1985**, 13, 1–12.

Kaplan, S. A.; Weinfeld, R. E.; Abruzzo, C. W.; and Lewis, M. Pharmacokinetic profile of sulfisoxazole following intravenous, intramuscular, and oral administration to man. *J. Pharm. Sci.*, **1972**, 51, 773–778.

Øie, S.; Gambertoglio, J. G.; and Fleckenstein, L. Comparison of the disposition of total and unbound sulfisoxazole after single and multiple dosing. *J. Pharmacokinet. Biopharm.*, **1982**, 10, 157–172.

TEMAZEPAM

Bittencourt, P.; Richens, A.; Toseland. P. A.; Wicks, J. F. C.; and Latham, A. N. Pharmacokinetics of the hypnotic benzodiazepine temazepam. *Br. J. Clin. Pharmacol.*, **1979**, 8, 37s–38s.

Greenblatt, D. J.; Divoll, M.; Abernethy, D. R.; Ochs, H. R.; and Shader, R. I. Clinical pharmacokinetics of the newer benzodiazepines. *Clin. Pharmacokinet.*, **1983**, 8, 233–252.

Stoehr, G. P.; Kroboth, P. D.; Juhl, R. P.; Wender, D. B.; Phillips, J. P.; and Smith, R. B. Effect of oral contraceptives on triazolam, temazepam, alprazolam, and lorazepam kinetics. *Clin. Pharmacol. Ther.*, **1984**, 36, 683–690.

TERBUTALINE

Nyberg, L., and Wood, C. (eds.). Advances in terbutaline pharmacokinetics. *Eur. J. Respir. Dis.*, **1984**, 65, Suppl. 134, 1–240.

TETRACYCLINE

Doluisio, J. T., and Dittert, L. W. Influence of repetitive dosing of tetracyclines on biologic half-life in serum. *Clin. Pharmacol. Ther.*, **1969**, 10, 690–701.

Jaffe, J. M.; Colaizzi, J. L.; Poust, R. I.; and McDonald, R. H. Effect of altered urinary pH on tetracycline and doxycycline excretion in humans. *J. Pharmacokinet. Biopharm.*, **1973**, 1, 267–282.

Raghuram, T. C., and Krishnaswamy, K. Pharmacokinetics of tetracycline in nutritional oedema. *Chemotherapy*, **1982**, 28, 428–433.

THEOPHYLLINE

Hendeles, L., and Weinberger, M. Theophylline. A "state of the art" review. *Pharmacotherapy*, **1983**, 3, 2–44.

THIOPENTAL

Burch, P. G.; and Stanski, D. R.   The role of metabolism and protein binding in thiopental anesthesia. *Anesthesiology*, **1983**, *58*, 146–152.

Hudson, R. J.; Stanski, D. R.; and Burch, P. G.   Pharmacokinetics of methohexital and thiopental in surgical patients. *Anesthesiology*, **1983**, *59*, 215–219.

Morgan, D. J.; Blackman, G. L.; Paull, J. D.; and Wolf, L. J.   Pharmacokinetics and plasma binding of thiopental. I: Studies in surgical patients. *Anesthesiology*, **1981**, *54*, 468–473.

Pandele, G.; Chaux, F.; Salvadori, C.; Farinotti, M.; and Duvaldestin, P.   Thiopental pharmacokinetics in patients with cirrhosis. *Anesthesiology*, **1983**, *59*, 123–126.

TICARCILLIN

Davies, B. E.; Humphrey, M. J.; Langley, P. F.; Lees, L.; Legg, B.; and Wadds, G. A.   Pharmacokinetics of ticarcillin in man. *Eur. J. Clin. Pharmacol.*, **1982**, *23*, 167–172.

Davies, M.; Morgan, J. R.; and Anand, C.   Administration of ticarcillin to patients with severe renal failure. *Chemotherapy*, **1974**, *20*, 339–341.

Gouyette, A.; Kitzis, M. D.; Guibert, J.; and Acar, J. F.   Pharmacokinetics and bioavailability of intramuscular preparations of ticarcillin. *J. Antimicrob. Chemother.*, **1982**, *10*, 419–425.

Libke, R. D.; Clarke, J. T.; Ralph, E. D.; Luthy, R. P.; and Kirby, W. M. M.   Ticarcillin vs carbenicillin: clinical pharmacokinetics. *Clin. Pharmacol. Ther.*, **1975**, *17*, 441–446.

TIMOLOL

Frishman, W. H.   Atenolol and timolol, two new systemic β-adrenoceptor antagonists. *N. Engl. J. Med.*, **1982**, *306*, 1456–1461.

Regårdh, C. G.   Pharmacokinetic aspects of some β-adrenoceptor blocking drugs. *Acta Med. Scand.*, **1982**, *665*, Suppl., 49–60.

Vedin, J. A.; Kristianson, J. K.; and Wilhelmsson, C.-E.   Pharmacokinetics of intravenous timolol in patients with acute myocardial infarction and in healthy volunteers. *Eur. J. Clin. Pharmacol.*, **1982**, *23*, 43–47.

TOBRAMYCIN

Levy, J.; Smith, A. L.; Koup, J. R.; Williams-Warren, J.; and Ramsey, B.   Disposition of tobramycin in patients with cystic fibrosis: a prospective controlled study. *J. Pediatr.*, **1984**, *105*, 117–124.

Schentag, J. J.; Lasezkay, G.; Cumbo, T. J.; Plaut, M. E.; and Jusko, W. J.   Accumulation pharmacokinetics of tobramycin. *Antimicrob. Agents Chemother.*, **1978**, *13*, 649–656.

Symposium. (Various authors.) Tobramycin: comparative toxicity of aminoglycoside antibiotics. *J. Antimicrob. Chemother.*, **1978**, *4*, Suppl. A, 1–101.

TOCAINIDE

Follath, F.; Ganzinger, U.; and Schuetz, E.   Reliability of antiarrhythmic drug plasma concentration monitoring. *Clin. Pharmacokinet.*, **1983**, *8*, 63–82.

Gillis, A. M.; and Kates, R. E.   Clinical pharmacokinetics of the newer antiarrhythmic agents. *Clin. Pharmacokinet.*, **1984**, *9*, 375–403.

Graffner, C.; Conradson, T.-B.; Hofvendahl, S.; and Ryden, L.   Tocainide kinetics after intravenous and oral administration in healthy subjects and in patients with acute myocardial infarction. *Clin. Pharmacol. Ther.*, **1980**, *27*, 64–71.

Wiegers, U.; Hanrath, P.; Kuck, K. H.; Pottage, A.; Graffner, C.; Augustin, J.; and Runge, M.   Pharmacokinetics of tocainide in patients with renal dysfunction and during haemodialysis. *Eur. J. Clin. Pharmacol.*, **1983**, *24*, 503–507.

TOLBUTAMIDE

Adir, J.; Miller, A. K.; and Vestal, R. F.   Effects of total plasma concentration and age on tolbutamide plasma protein binding. *Clin. Pharmacol. Ther.*, **1982**, *31*, 488–493.

Balant, L.   Clinical pharmacokinetics of sulphonylurea-hypoglycaemic agents. *Clin. Pharmacokinet.*, **1981**, *6*, 215–241.

Nelson, E., and O'Reilly, I.   Kinetics of carboxytolbutamide excretion following tolbutamide and carboxytolbutamide administration. *J. Pharmacol. Exp. Ther.*, **1961**, *132*, 103–109.

Williams, R. L.; Blaschke, T. F.; Meffin, P. J.; Melmon, K. L.; and Rowland, M.   Influence of acute viral hepatitis on disposition and plasma binding of tolbutamide. *Clin. Pharmacol. Ther.*, **1977**, *21*, 301–309.

TOLMETIN

Furst, D. E.; Dromgoole, S. H.; Desiraju, R. K.; and Paulus, H. E.   Clinical pharmacology of tolmetin: comparisons in rheumatoid arthritis patients and normal volunteers. *J. Clin. Pharmacol.*, **1983**, *23*, 329–335.

Verbeeck, R. K.; Blackburn, J. L.; and Loewen, G. R.   Clinical pharmacokinetics of non-steroidal anti-inflammatory drugs. *Clin. Pharmacokinet.*, **1983**, *8*, 297–331.

TRIAMTERENE

Gilfrich, H. J.; Kremer, G.; Möhrke, W.; Mutschler, E.; and Völger, K.-D.   Pharmacokinetics of triamterene after i.v. administration to man: determination of bioavailability. *Eur. J. Clin. Pharmacol.*, **1983**, *25*, 237–241.

Hasegawa, J.; Lin, E. T.; Williams, R. L.; Sörgel, F.; and Benet, L. Z.   Pharmacokinetics of triamterene and its metabolite in man. *J. Pharmacokinet. Biopharm.*, **1982**, *10*, 507–523.

Mutschler, E.; Gilfrich, H. J.; Knauf, H.; Möhrke, W.; and Völger, K.-D.   Pharmakokinetik von Triamteren bei Probanden und Patienten mit Leber-und Nierenfunktionsstörungen. *Klin. Wochenschr.*, **1983**, *61*, 883–891.

TRIAZOLAM

Abernethy, D. R.; Greenblatt, D. J.; Divoll, M.; Smith, R. B.; and Shader, R. I. The influence of obesity on the pharmacokinetics of oral alprazolam and triazolam. *Clin. Pharmacokinet.*, **1984**, *9*, 177–183.

Baktir, G.; Fisch, H. U.; Huguenin, P.; and Bircher, J. Triazolam concentration-effect relationships in healthy subjects. *Clin. Pharmacol. Ther.*, **1983**, *34*, 195–201.

Eberts, F. S., Jr.; Philopoulos, Y.; Reineke, L. M.; and Vliek, R. W. Triazolam disposition. *Clin. Pharmacol. Ther.*, **1981**, *29*, 81–93.

Greenblatt, D. J.; Divoll, M.; Abernethy, D. R.; Ochs, H. R.; and Shader, R. I. Clinical pharmacokinetics of the newer benzodiazepines. *Clin. Pharmacokinet.*, **1983**, *8*, 233–252.

TRIMETHOPRIM

Morgan, D. J., and Raymond, K. Evaluation of slow infusions of co-trimoxazole by using predictive pharmacokinetics. *Antimicrob. Agents Chemother.*, **1980**, *17*, 132–137.

Patel, R. B., and Welling, P. G. Clinical pharmacokinetics of co-trimoxazole. *Clin. Pharmacokinet.* **1980**, *5*, 405–423.

Singlas, E.; Colin, J. N.; Rottembourg, J.; Meessen, J. P.; de Martin, A.; Legrain, M.; and Simon, P. Pharmacokinetics of sulfamethoxazole-trimethoprim combination during chronic peritoneal dialysis: effect of peritonitis. *Eur. J. Clin. Pharmacol.*, **1982**, *21*, 409–415.

TUBOCURARINE

Fisher, D. M.; O'Keeffe, C.; Stanski, D. R.; Cronnelly, R.; Miller, R. D.; and Gregory, G. A. Pharmacokinetics and pharmacodynamics of *d*-tubocurarine in infants, children, and adults. *Anesthesiology*, **1982**, *57*, 203–208.

Meijer, D. K. F.; Weitering, J. G.; Vermeer, G. A.; and Scaf, A. H. J. Comparative pharmacokinetics of *d*-tubocurarine and metocurine in man. *Anesthesiology*, **1979**, *51*, 402–407.

Stanski, D. R.; Ham, J.; Miller, R. D.; and Sheiner, L. B. Pharmacokinetics and pharmacodynamics of *d*-tubocurarine during nitrous oxide–narcotic and halothane anesthesia in man. *Anesthesiology*, **1979**, *51*, 235–241.

VALPROIC ACID

Bauer, L. A.; Davis, R.; Wilensky, A.; Raisys, V.; and Levy, R. H. Diurnal variation in valproic acid clearance. *Clin. Pharmacol. Ther.*, **1984**, *35*, 505–509.

Bowdle, T. A.; Patel, I. H.; Levy, R. H.; and Wilensky, A. J. Valproic acid dosage and plasma protein binding and clearance. *Clin. Pharmacol. Ther.*, **1980**, *28*, 486–492.

Gram, L.; Flachs, H.; Würtz-Jørgensen, A.; Parnas, J.; and Andersen, B. Sodium valproate, serum level and clinical effect in epilepsy: a controlled study. *Epilepsia*, **1979**, *20*, 303–312.

Gugler, R., and von Unruh, G. E. Clinical pharmacokinetics of valproic acid. *Clin. Pharmacokinet.*, **1980**, *5*, 67–83.

VANCOMYCIN

Krogstad, D. J.; Moellering, R. C., Jr.; and Greenblatt, D. J. Single dose kinetics of intravenous vancomycin. *J. Clin. Pharmacol.*, **1980**, *20*, 197–201.

Matzke, G. R.; McGory, R. W.; Halstenson, C. E.; and Keane, W. F. Pharmacokinetics of vancomycin in patients with various degrees of renal function. *Antimicrob. Agents Chemother.*, **1984**, *25*, 433–437.

Rotschafer, J. C.; Crossley, K.; Zaske, D. E.; Mead, K.; Sawchuck, R. J.; and Solem, L. D. Pharmacokinetics of vancomycin: observations in 28 patients and dosage recommendations. *Antimicrob. Agents Chemother.*, **1982**, *22*, 391–394.

VERAPAMIL

Hamann, S. R.; Blouin, R. A.; and McAllister, R. G., Jr. Clinical pharmacokinetics of verapamil. *Clin. Pharmacokinet.*, **1984**, *9*, 26–41.

WARFARIN

Breckenridge, A.; Orme, M.; Wesseling, H.; Lewis, R. J.; and Gibbons, R. Pharmacokinetics and pharmacodynamics of the enantiomers of warfarin in man. *Clin. Pharmacol. Ther.*, **1974**, *15*, 424–430.

O'Reilly, R. A.; Aggeler, P. M.; and Leong, L. S. Studies on the coumarin anticoagulant drugs: the pharmacodynamics of warfarin in man. *J. Clin. Invest.*, **1963**, *42*, 1542–1551.

O'Reilly, R. A.; Welling, P. G.; and Wagner, J. G. Pharmacokinetics of warfarin following intravenous administration in man. *Thromb. Diath. Haemorrh.*, **1971**, *25*, 178–186.

III DRUG INTERACTIONS

Ferid Murad and Alfred G. Gilman

It has become increasingly clear that the effects of many drugs, when given concurrently, are not necessarily predictable on the basis of knowledge of their effects when given alone. Although the earliest observations about drug interactions came from fundamental investigations of the effects of agonists and antagonists on receptors, subsequent knowledge of drug interactions, acquired from experiments on animals, has been used to therapeutic advantage in man. Interactions of multiple types can occur with the same pair of chemicals. When an interaction occurs, the net pharmacological response may result from enhancement of the effects of one or the other drug, the development of totally new effects that are not seen when either drug is used alone, the inhibition of the effect of one drug by another, or no change whatever in the net effect despite the fact that the kinetics and metabolism of one or both of the drugs may be altered substantially.

Estimates of the incidence of drug interactions have ranged from 3 to 5% in patients receiving several medications to 20% or higher in patients taking 10 to 20 drugs. Because the average hospitalized patient is given 6 to 8 drugs, the scope of the problem is significant. Clearly many hospitalizations, illnesses, and deaths result from drug interactions that could often be prevented. In any therapeutic situation, the physician must have expectations of the effects of a drug before it is given and set limits of toxicity beyond which the drug will be discontinued. These requirements are particularly pertinent when multiple drugs are given concurrently.

Knowledge of drug interactions enables a physician to minimize or prevent drug toxicity by adjustment of the dosage or schedule of drug administration or by choice of an alternative agent. The growing use of medications makes it impossible to memorize, catalog, or even recognize all of the significant drug interactions that will confront a physician. However, a physician should find it useful to categorize the multiple mechanisms by which an interaction may occur. The introductory pages of this appendix provide such categorization and thus a framework for the analysis of unanticipated interactions. A list then follows of a large number of drug interactions that are described elsewhere in the textbook. This list is intended to be an index of these interactions and nothing more. It is by no means a complete list of all drug interactions that have been hypothesized or described, or even a complete list of interactions discussed in the textbook. The intention is to focus on those interactions that result in unwanted or adverse effects. Many of the beneficial effects that result from interactions between drugs have become integral factors in the optimal therapy of some diseases, and they are not included in this appendix.

Direct Chemical or Physical Interactions. Two drugs may interact directly, particularly under conditions where their concentrations are high. As a result, the effects of each drug can obviously be modified. For example, heparin is an acidic mucopolysaccharide with anticoagulant activities that can be inhibited or nullified by a basic compound, such as protamine. This electrostatic interaction is used for therapeutic intent to neutralize excessive effects of heparin. Many catecholamines are oxidized when introduced into some intravenous solutions. Other drugs are sensitive to light. It is useful for the physician to have some knowledge of the chemical nature of drugs so that he will use his observational powers in settings where such interactions could occur. Similar examples entail the chelating action of tetracyclines, the adsorbent capacities of resins such as cholestyramine, the ionic properties of the aminoglycoside antibiotics, and others. One must also realize that not all of the physicochemical interactions between drugs will be revealed by the formation of precipitates in bottles used for solutions for intravenous injection. Furthermore, important physicochemical interactions may occur by the adsorption of drugs to the glass or plastic surfaces of such bottles or associated equipment.

Interactions in Gastrointestinal Absorption. Interactions between drugs frequently occur prior to absorption from the intestine. Thus, interaction of a tetracycline with calcium or another metallic cation in the gut prevents absorption of the antibiotic. Drugs that alter gastric or intestinal motility can inhibit or enhance the rate or extent of absorption of a drug administered concurrently. Antacids can decrease the absorption of certain acidic drugs because of the effect of pH on the ionization of the compound. Timing of the administration of two drugs can thus become a crucial determinant of the degree of expression of the drug interaction.

Interactions at the site of absorption can be complex and indirect. For example, antibiotics can alter the gastrointestinal flora, and may thus inhibit the rate of synthesis of vitamin K by intestinal microorganisms. If an oral anticoagulant (vitamin K antagonist) is administered concurrently, the antibiotic will increase its effectiveness. When antibiotics deplete the gut of microorganisms that can conjugate drugs within the intestine, absorption of active drug may increase.

Interactions Due to Protein Binding. Many drugs, particularly those that are acidic, are reversibly bound to plasma proteins, and the extent of competition between drugs for such binding sites depends on the affinity of each for the site and its concentration (*see* Chapter 1). In general, only unbound drug is free to leave the vascular compartment and exert its pharmacological effect. These facts set the stage for an important class of drug interactions, which are most significant for those agents that are extensively bound to plasma proteins at therapeutic concentrations. Tolbutamide and warfarin provide examples of such agents, and their free concentration can be increased significantly in the presence of effective competitors, such as many of the nonsteroidal anti-inflammatory agents. Even a minor percentage change of the extent of binding of drugs that are usually more than 90% bound to plasma proteins may result in a large change in the concentration of the free drug.

Obvious displacement of a bound drug may not occur immediately after initiation of administration of a potential competitor. If the displacing drug has a long half-life and does not reach a plateau concentration for several days after maintenance dosage is started, it may not be present initially in sufficient concentration to cause significant displacement. The pharmacokinetics may be further complicated by enhanced clearance of the displaced drug because of less extensive binding. The intensity of the interaction may thus wane, despite constant dosage. These types of changes may be particularly difficult to recognize, and their kinetics must be understood to avoid undercompensa-

tion, overcompensation, or both at different times.

Interactions at the Receptor Site. Interactions between agonists and antagonists at specific receptor sites are described throughout the text, and many pharmacological agents are obviously valued because of such actions and interactions. What is frequently overlooked, in part because of the convenience of classification, is the lack of specificity of many such drugs. Thus, phenothiazines are effective α-adrenergic antagonists; many antihistamines and tricyclic antidepressants are potent antimuscarinic agents. Such agents have unwanted effects because of their lack of specificity, and these may be most noticeable and troublesome when other drugs are given concurrently and are expected to have their usual efficacy.

Other interactions of an apparent pharmacodynamic nature are poorly understood or are mediated indirectly. Halogenated hydrocarbons, including many general anesthetics, sensitize the myocardium to the arrhythmogenic actions of catecholamines. This effect presumably results from some action on the pathway leading from receptor to effector, but details are unclear. Many signs and symptoms of hypoglycemia are mediated through the adrenergic nervous system and are masked by β-adrenergic blocking agents. Patients taking propranolol may thus fail to note reactions to insulin or oral hypoglycemic agents in time to prevent dangerous consequences, and, furthermore, compensatory mechanisms, such as glycogenolysis, may be blocked by the β-adrenergic antagonist.

Interactions Due to Accelerated Metabolism. Interactions between drugs occur during their metabolism or elimination. Many drugs and a variety of chemicals that are present in the environment, especially insecticides and herbicides, are capable of inducing the synthesis of drug-metabolizing enzymes, particularly those of the hepatic endoplasmic reticulum (*see* Chapter 1). Such induction can enhance the metabolism not only of the inducing agent but also of a variety of drugs administered concurrently and of some endogenous compounds, such as cortisol, bilirubin, and the sex steroids.

Lists of more than 200 agents known to induce their own metabolism and the metabolism of other drugs have been compiled. Much of the data has been obtained from studies of experimental animals and may not be applicable to man. Genetic differences in man also play an important role in determining an individual's response to such enzyme inducers. Despite these variables, which make attempts at prediction imprecise, interactions of this sort are unquestionably important in man. Phenobarbital can dramatically reduce the half-life of quinidine. Rifampin decreases the half-life of estrogens and methadone; the consequences may be an unwanted pregnancy or precipitation of withdrawal from opioids. Enhancement of the rate of metabolism can also result in higher concentrations of active metabolites or of metabolites with unique toxic effects (*see* Chapter 1).

Interactions Due to Inhibition of Metabolism. A number of drug interactions are based on inhibition of metabolism of one drug by another (or by its metabolites). An important example is provided by allopurinol, an inhibitor of xanthine oxidase, which prolongs the half-life and thereby intensifies the effects of 6-mercaptopurine and azathioprine. Profound bone-marrow toxicity will occur if cognizance is not taken of these interactions. The monoamine oxidase inhibitors also provide striking and classical examples of such effects (*see* Chapter 19). Unfortunately, there are few, if any, guidelines to permit predictions of which drugs will inhibit the metabolism of other agents.

Interactions Due to Alteration of Renal Excretion. Urinary pH and the pK_a of a drug influence its renal tubular reabsorption and, thus, the rate of renal excretion. The excretion of an acidic drug such as phenobarbital can be markedly increased by the administration of sodium bicarbonate, while the excretion of a basic drug can be decreased. Some drugs, such as the penicillins, are actively secreted by the renal tubular epithelium. Other agents (*e.g.*, probenecid) can compete for this tubular transport system.

Interactions Due to Alteration of pH or Electrolyte Concentrations. Several drugs, particularly including the diuretics, influence the concentrations of electrolytes and the pH of body fluids. Such changes in pH may produce major alterations in the absorption, distribution, or renal clearance of therapeutic agents, as mentioned above. Interactions of this type may be unwanted, or they may be sought deliberately, particularly to enhance the elimination of a toxicant (*see* Chapters 1 and 68). The same type of effect may alter the activities of a second drug that is given concurrently. A classical example of such is hypokalemia, resulting from the administration of diuretics, which potentiates the activity of digitalis glycosides, often dangerously.

Summary. Although classification of mechanisms of drug interactions should be helpful to the physician, it must be recalled that a single drug may be involved in multiple types of interactions with the same or different drugs. The major task of the physician is to judge whether an interaction has occurred and the magnitude of the change. Many patients see more than one physician for the same purpose. When they do, the physicians do not always know of each other's therapeutic regimens. Likewise, many patients consume drugs that have been prescribed for other diseases or for another patient. In addition, patients may be erratic in their smoking and drinking habits, which can affect a drug's pharmacokinetic or pharmacodynamic properties. There is no easy way to anticipate such problems. There is, therefore, the requirement that an unanticipated turn of events in a patient's course, whether it be accelerated efficacy or the appearance of unusual and untoward events, be considered as a possible consequence of an interaction between drugs.

INDEX